LOTUS MATERIA MEDICA

1,400 Homeopathic and Herbal Remedies

by

Robin Murphy, ND

Third Edition

B. Jain Publishers (P) Ltd.
USA—EUROPE—INDIA

This book is dedicated to
Sant Kirpal Singh Ji, (1894 to 1974)

Acknowledgements

In the past few years of editing the information contained in this book, the author has received inspiration from many people and he would like to thank everyone who has participated in the reprinting of this book. Special thanks are due to the following individuals: Kachina Domenick, Lauren Lupo, Houston Johnson, Alexander Yuan, Ron Surman, Rosko Rosoff, Joan Spiegel, Richard Pitt, Noel Szychowski, Joseph Buttimer, Peter Brodhead, Glenn and Irene Ingram, Greg Cooper, Paula McDonald, John Jezewski, Toraku Yui, Ananda Ruchira, Bryan Murphy, Shelley Murphy, Verna Murphy, Jaylon Carter, Abdul Hayy and Rana Holdijk, Cheyanne West, Kuldeep Jain and Sant Rajinder Singh.

Special thanks go to Kachina Domenick, whose assistance on this edition was invaluable and much appreciated. Also thanks to my Qigong students for helping to keep the author in good health and spirits during this project. The author would like to thank everyone who has purchased books and tapes or attended any Homeopathic or Qigong seminars in 2005 and 2006, your support is greatly appreciated.

LOTUS MATERIA MEDICA
(THIRD EDITION)

First Indian Edition: Sept. 2002
Third Indian Edition: 2010
10th Impression 2020

Published by Kuldeep Jain for
B. JAIN PUBLISHERS (P) LTD.
B. Jain House, D-157, Sector-63,
NOIDA-201307, U.P. (INDIA)
Tel.: +91-120-4933333 • *Email:* info@bjain.com
Website: **www.bjain.com**

Printed in India

ISBN: 978-81-319-0859-4

Publisher's Note

Dr Murphy is one of the most well known teachers of homeopathy. He has extensive teaching and clinical experience including his years spent as the chairman of the Homeopathic Department at the National College of Naturopathic Medicine in Portland.

'Murphy is one of the earliest "seminar" teachers, and is responsible for introducing many people to homeopathy. His teaching style has been described as "laid-back" and he brings a clarity to the inter-relation between philosophy, materia medica and repertory' as quoted by Julian Winston.

We have earlier also published the second edition of this book which has received a tremendous response from the Indian subcontinent. We now hereby present to the profession the third edition of Lotus Materia Medica. This covers 1400 remedies on 2214 pages. It is the most vast and elaborate materia medica ever written in homeopathy. Reading materia medica is always a challenge as remembering so many symptoms from so many books is not an easy task, as one will have to refer to different books for different remedies. This book serves the purpose of giving a comprehensive information on almost all the drugs of homeopathy at one place. The alphabetical schema of the sections in a drug has been followed to keep in line with the repertory style.

This book is one of the very important contributions to the homeopathic literature written by one of the present stalwarts of the field. We hope that the Indian readers will benefit from this publication.

Kuldeep Jain

C.E.O., B. Jain Publisher's (P) Ltd.

PREFACE TO THE THIRD EDITION

Lotus Materia Medica

This is the third edition of the Lotus Materia Medica which was first published in August of 1995. The third editon of the ***Lotus Materia Medica*** was designed to be a complete rewrite and major upgrade of the *second edition*. My attempt has always been to create a modern and easy-to-use materia medica for homeopaths to use in daily practice, while still remaining accessible for use at home and in the classroom.

The changes made in this 3rd edition comprise my attempts to build on that philosophy. *Lotus Materia Medica* contains hundreds of new remedies and thousands of new updates and additions.

The *Lotus Materia Medica, third edition* was updated to be a more clinical, practical and easy-to-use reference guide to the vast homeopathic materia medica. After editing the *second edition*, I continued to add more modern terminology, cross references and corrected any errors that were found. The final step was to systematically survey the homeopathic and herbal literature for reliable additions and updates. The highest priority was to find more clinical information relevant to modern homeopathic, naturopathic and herbal practice.

The writings of Allen, Anshutz, Boericke, Burnett, Clarke, Cooper, Hale, Hahnemann, Hering, Julian, Paracelsus, Phatak and Radamacher formed some of the major resources from which the remedy monographs were compiled, formatted and updated. Each remedy is reviewed as to it's pharmacy, folklore, historical uses, keynotes, generals, provings, case histories and toxicological reports.

Also, traditional herbal lore and information from the ancient medicine was consulted, especially on the use of herbal and spagyric tinctures as therapeutic agents and general tonics.

The result is the *third edition* of *Lotus Materia Medica,* which contains more modern terminology and diseases. Over 200 new remedies, and thousands of new additions and updates, all in a small lightweight book for convenient use. Homeopathic Remedy Guide has been redesigned to better complement the Homeopathic Medical Repertory also written by Robin Murphy, ND.

Similar abbreviations and terminologies were used for both books and the alphabetical schema used in the remedy monographs was designed to relate to the chapters in the Homeopathic Medical Repertory. The *third edition* of *Lotus Materia Medica* has been rewritten over the past few years and the following major changes were made:

Changes to the Third Edition

1. **New Edition** - The Lotus Materia Medica's subtitle has been renamed: *'Lotus Materia Medica: 1,400 Homeopathic and Herbal Remedies'*. This new name was given to represent the 200 new remedies added in the third edition.
2. **New Format** - Lotus Materia Medica has been completely re-formated. The single column plan is replaced with a two column format. This was done to make the book

easier to read and to make more space available for adding new remedies to the book.

3. **New Editing** - Thousands of minor and major corrections have been made in the third edition of this book. Errors in spelling, grammar and formating have been corrected. Also the sentence and paragraph structure was updated and improved.
4. **New Updates** - New cross references with more updated and expanded clinical information added to many remedy monographs.
5. **New Remedies and Updates** - New Remedies added from modern provings. Also additions from Allen, Boericke, Boenninghausen, Burnett, Clarke, Grimmer, Hahnemann, Hering, Julian, Kent, Knerr, Kunzli, Nash, Phatak and many more.

Changes to the Third Edition

6. **Updated Remedy Abbreviations** - The remedy abbreviations of this edition have been updated to match the abreviations in the Homeopathic Medical Repertory.
7. **New Remedy Gradings** - The new remedy gradings for the *Lotus Materia Medica's Repertory* display the strongest remedies in the following manner: <u>**CALC.**</u>, (4 points), bold-capitals and underlined; **CALC.**, (3 points), bold-capitals-type; ***calc.***, (2 points), bold-italics-type; calc., (1 point), plain-small-type.
8. **New Remedies** - Over 200 new remedies were added to this edition. Many new homeopathic provings, herbal remedies, etc. were added in this edition.
9. **New Repertory** - A new clinical repertory has been added to the back of the book.
10. **New Remedy Index** - This expanded list includes the full latin names and common names for many homeopathic and herbal remedies.
11. **New Homeopathic-Herbal Glossary** - A new glossary of Homeopathic, medical and herbal terminology has been added to this edition.
12. **New Homeopathy-Herbal Directory** - Homeopathic and Herbal Resources. A listing of Homeopathic and herbal schools, organizations, pharmacies, bookstores, etc.

Abbreviations: The abbreviations used in this book are:

agg. = aggravated by, worse from or symptoms increased by.

amel. = ameliorated by, better from or symptoms decreased by.

N. O. = Natural order.

The response to previous editions of *Lotus Materia Medica* has been very positive throughout the past 12 years. This demonstrates the need that has existed for many years for a modern materia medica of homeopathic and herbal remedies.

I profoundly thank everyone who has supported this work and I hope this third edition of *Lotus Materia Medica* will be helpful in the study and practice of homeopathic and herbal medicine, worldwide. I welcome any suggestions for corrections and improvements that can be put into any future editions of this work.

Robin Murphy, N.D.
November 9, 2006
Blacksburg, Virginia, U.S.A.

INTRODUCTION

Lotus Materia Medica: 1,400 Homeopathic and Herbal Remedies

The word 'materia medica' originates from the Latin word of 'mater' which means materials and 'medica' which refers to their use in medicine, therefore a materia medica translates as a Book of Medicines. The first Homeopathic Materia Medica was created by Hahnemann which he called the Materia Medica Pura, which translates as the Book of Pure Medicines. Homeopathic remedies were pure because their true medicinal actions were determined via provings not from theories or speculations. These energy medicines were also 'purified' of their earthy matter by the homeopathic method of potentizing substances via dilutions, triturations and succussions.

The Lotus Materia Medica is a book of Natural Medicines, because the homeopathic and herbal remedies have an affect on health and disease by enhancing the vital state of a person. Once the constitutional vitality is increased the healing forces become activated and health can be restored and fortified. This book contains over 1,400 of these Natural Medicines from the homeopathic and herbal materia medicas.

The writings of Allen, Anshutz, Boericke, Burnett, Clarke, Cooper, Hale, Hahnemann, Hering, Julian, Paracelsus, Phatak and Radamacher formed the major resources from which the remedy monographs were compiled, formatted and updated. Each remedy is reviewed as to it's pharmacy, historical uses, keynotes, generals, provings, case histories and toxicological reports. Also, traditional herbal folklore and information from the ancient medicine was consulted, especially on the use of herbal and spagyric tinctures as therapeutic agents and general tonics.

Lotus Materia Medica: Book Outline

1. **Preface** - Acknowledgements and publication information. Updated information about this edtion.
2. **Introduction** - Outline of Remedy Monographs. Homeopathic and Herbal prescribing.
3. **Table of Contents** - Outline of Book. Remedies Lists.
4. **Homeopathic Remedy Guide** - Homeopathic and Herbal Monographs A to Z.
5. **Nature's Repertory** - Clinical Index. Remedy Groups.
6. **Remedy Index** - Common and Latin Names, Synonyms.
7. **Remedy References** - Homeopathic and Herbal References.
8. **Homeopathic-Herbal Glossary** - Homeopathic and Herbal Terminology.
9. **Homeopathic-Herbal Directory** - Homeopathic and Herbal Resources. Homeopathic Schools, Bookstores, Publishers, Pharmacies, Organizations, etc.

Outline of Remedy Monographs

Title - The standard Latin botanical or chemical name, Sub-title - the common name or the remedy's traditional name.

Pharmacy - The remedy's abbreviation is found as it is written in the **Homeopathic Medical Repertory**. The remedy's Latin and common names are given. The abbreviation

N. O., stands for Natural Order or botanical family of the plant. Geographic location. How the remedy is prepared, by tincture or trituration. What parts are used to make the remedy. ***Historical doses:*** This section reviews the doses that have been used of the particular remedy, in a tincture, trituration or potencies. All remedies can be used in potency, but only the non toxic plants should be used for the spagyric and herbal tinctures. Remedies with possible spagyric or herbal uses are marked in the table of contents by underlining the remedy's Latin Name.

Clinical - In the clinical section is an alphabetical list of disorders and conditions that the remedy has helped in the past and present. The disorders in *italic type* are known to have been historically cured by the remedy.

Herbal - This section, shows the herbal remedy's folklore and traditional uses. The medical, herbal or history of the remedy, clinical experiences, herbal signatures, poisonings and case histories are reviewed. This section gives the botanical information of the remedies.

Homeopathic - The homeopathic section gives the remedy's therapeutic and general uses. The remedy's affinities for organs, systems or tissues are covered and the major keynotes, general and particular symptoms, plus the pathological uses of the remedy are given. Information from the homeopathic provings are included.

Mind - This section reviews the mental and emotional symptoms or states. Personality, ego and behavior. Mental functions such as, attention, memory, concentration, reason, thoughts, intellect. Emotions, such as fears, moods, weeping, anxieties, worries, depression, grief, frights, anger, hate, impulses, delusions, delirium, obsessions, gestures. Also, perceptions, self confidence, beliefs, insanity, etc.

Sections - This section of the monograph is an alphabetical schema of anatomical and physiological topics. *Abdomen, Back, Blood, Bones, Brain, Breasts, Causations, Chest, Constitutions, Coughing, Ears, Eyes, Face, Female, Food, Head, Heart, Kidneys, Larynx, Limbs, Liver, Lungs, Male, Mind, Modalities, Mouth, Muscles, Neck, Nerves, Nose, Rectum, Skin, Sleep, Stomach, Stool, Teeth, Temperature, Throat, Tongue, Urine, Vertigo.*

Comments - This section of the book includes historical and modern commentaries, folklore, case histories, remedy reviews, homeopathic provings, etc. Real life experiences and stories from the past are discussed from a practical point of view.

Relations - This part of the remedy monograph gives the various relationships which remedies can have with one another. For example there are antidotal, complementary, remedies which follows each other well and other relationships. ***Compare:*** Here the homeopathic or herbal remedy is compared with other remedies with similar symptoms or therapeutic uses. This section can be used to study similar remedies or to give new ideas for other remedies to consider in complex cases.

References - This section gives the major homeopathic or herbal references for each remedy's outline or commentary that is presented. The name of the author where the original material came from is listed. A list of all sources is found in the back of the book.

Homeopathic Remedies

Homeopathic remedies are energy medicines prescribed on the principle of similarity. Remedies that are in opposition to the immune response are antipathic or allopathic. Sympathy reflects the principle of likes cures likes. There is a sympathetic relationship between the action of the remedy on healthy persons, the provings and the therapeutic action on disease.

Homeopathic remedies contain prana or qi, (vital energy), they are pure prana remedies. When prana is suspended in a fluid or dry medium it can be potentized through a series of dilutions and succusions. The higher the potency means the prana of the remedy has become more pure and more exalted in its healing energy. Therefore these remedies work deeper and last alot longer in their action. Homeopathic remedies have gentle power to restore or to heal. Their function is to neutralize disorders and to arouse the Vix Medicatrix Naturae, (the healing power of nature).

Higher states of vitality and health is a natural consequence of giving the proper homeopathic remedies. The goal in natural therapeutics is to always do the least and also to emphasize hygiene in all chronic disorders. Homeopathic remedies facilitate the self-restoration process. They neutralize the foci of disorder and therefore remove old shocks and traumas to the life principle.

Homeopathic Prescribing Techniques

Acute prescribing - Acute remedies are homeopathic remedies prescribed for acute infections and fevers. Examples: Aconite, Arsenicum album, Baptisia, Belladonna, Bryonia, Chamomilla, Gelsemium, Ferrum phos., Pulsatilla, Pyrogen.

Acute remedies are prescribed in the following manner: (1) Take the acute disease case, consider the keynotes and the major symptoms (2) Diagnose the cause and the type disorder the person has (3) Find a primary rubric or rubrics in the Homeopathic Medical Repertory such as, influenza, pneumonia, etc. (4) Differentiate the major remedies in the primary rubric, (influenza), by reading them in Lotus Materia Medica (5) Choose the most similar remedy (6) Choose the potency, amount and repetition of the dose (7) Follow-up the case and review to determine if the person needs the same remedy and potency, same remedy and different potency, different remedy and potency, etc.

The 30c and 200c are effective potencies for acute and emergency prescribing. When indicated, follow the acute with a deeper acting chronic remedy or a constitutional remedy to help restore health and prevent relapses.

Chronic prescribing - This refers to giving homeopathic remedies for chronic or long term degenerative diseases and weaknesses. Therefore the goals and method of approaching the case is different than in acute or emergency prescribing. Low potencies are very effective for these long term conditions. The homeopathic remedies can be given in a 6c or a LM/1 potency, one to three times a day for weeks or months at a time according to the case. The frequency can be adjusted to once or twice a day if three times a day is two strong for the patient. If after a period of time the 6c or LM/1, stops affecting the vitality, then go up to the next potency in the scale, like 12c or a LM/2 potency. Homeopathic remedies can be also given in a single dose of a high potency remedy which is repeated only after the improvements have relapsed.

Constitutional prescribing - The proper constitutional remedy will enhance and help maintain the general health. Constitutional remedies fortify people through times of stress or help one to recover from infectious or debilitating diseases. When the vitality is weakened, then one's susceptibility is increased to certain diseases. These homeopathic remedies are prescribed for the genetic vitality of the person. Constitutional remedies are often given to children while they are developing and to the weak and elderly. Some important constitutional remedies are: Bar-c., Calc., Calc-p., Sil., Phos., Graph., Sulphur and Lyc.

Emergency prescribing - Homeopathic remedies prescribed for injuries, bites, burns, shocks and traumas in any form. The important things to know are the causative factors and differentials for each emergency condition. Potency is selected as to availability, severity and how much time you have. The 30c and 200c are effective potencies for first aid, emergency and acute dosage. One dose equals a few of the pellets, tablets or two to four drops of liquid remedies. Take one dose of a 30c, 3 times daily for a few days, or as needed or take a dose of 200c, a few times daily for a few days, again repeat as needed. In severe cases, one may need to repeat the remedy more often if needed.

Epidemic prescribing - The epidemic remedies are found by using the frequent appearing symptoms and strong symptoms of the epidemic disease. The epidemic remedy is given in repeated doses for a short period of time, a few days or longer if needed. These conditions are treated as acute diseases with 30c or 200c, or LM potencies. In case of mass epidemics the use of water potencies is essential. Take a few pellets or drops of the remedy and put it into a bottle of water, (4 or 8 oz. size) and shake well. This bottle can be preserved for long periods if 15% to 20% of the bottle is filled with pure alcohol. Also, each medicated remedy solution bottle can be grafted into new bottles by adding a teaspoon of the original to the new bottle and shaking.

Fundamental prescribing - The fundamental remedies give the personality types of the medicine. In some cases, the fundamental will be the same remedy as it is for the pathological layer. In some cases, the constitutional remedy will cover the fundamental and the pathological layers.

Isopathic prescribing - Isopathically using the 'same' substance potentised as a remedy (rather than a 'similar' substance). These remedies are made from discharges, toxins, allergens and nosodes. Isopathic remedies help eliminate toxic chemicals and heavy metals. If there is a strong history that a certain disease, bacteria or virus caused a person's condition then one would consider giving a isopathic remedy.

Miasm prescribing - Miasms are the tendencies and predispositions to certain diseases, like allergies or infectious diseases. If a person has predisposition to get colds and sore throats, then the acute remedy was given and it worked, but the colds and sore throats keep coming back. Here an anti-miasmatic remedy is indicated like Tub., or Bac.

There are five major miasms: Psora, Cancer, Sycosis, Syphilis and the Tuberculosis miasm. Miasms can be dormant or active. Miasms can be acquired by a person during their lifetime or miasms can be inherited from the parents. Miasms should not be treated routinely, but only when they are clearly activated or when one gets stalled in a case and there is a miasm present. Gonorrhea and Cancer are the dominant miasms today.

Acquired miasms are very prevalent, because a lot acute diseases get suppressed by drugs. These suppressed diseases can alter one's susceptibility to the environment and lower their vitality. A family history of certain disease patterns helps to confirm, the presence of an active or dormant miasm. Treat the active miasms when ever they show themselves. Let the dormant miasm alone until they become active.

Pathological prescribing - Pathological remedies are given for their similarity to the disease, as opposed to the fundamental and constitutional remedies which are aimed at the person in general. A pathological state should usually be treated first in many cases because it is the source of much suffering and pain. Pathological states are not limited to physical diseases alone. Also, mental and emotional diseases can form pathological layers and diseases. Examples are depression, mania, personality disorders, senility, violence behavior, insanity, etc. Low potencies in repeated doses are effective for severe pathologies like cancer and for those cases in which the patient is taking allopathic drugs.

Tautopathic prescribing - Tautopathically using the 'same' substance potentised as a remedy (rather than a 'similar' substance). These are the remedies made from allopathic drugs or chemicals. Tautopathics are made from cortisone, morphine, penicillin, histamine, etc. If there is a strong history that a certain drug caused a person's condition then one would consider giving a tautopathic remedy.

Herbal Prescribing Techniques

Herbal Tinctures - The herbal tinctures enhance the vitality and act also as specific tonics for weak organs and the vital systems. Herbal tinctures are plant extracts which stimulate the organs or systems of the body. These tinctures are alcoholic solutions of plant materials. Herbal remedies are often given to children while they are developing or to assist people through times of stress. These remedies also help one recover from infectious or debilitating diseases. When a person's genetic vitality is weakened, then one's susceptibility is increased towards certain diseases.

Herbal Tonics - The word tonic means tone as in musical tones. When the right tone is given it acts as a tonic. If continual vital tones are given then we achieve a sound body and a sound mind. Spagyric or Herbal Remedies give the vital tones that revitalize and restore the weak spirit and the elemental body. These are the vitality remedies that will raise up the health of the whole person. Tonic remedies improve the strength and harmony of the organs and vital systems.

The signs of health emerge from prolonged consumption of the spagyric tinctures in small drop doses. Some of the signs of health are: Wakes refreshed in the morning, clear mind, calm emotions, sense of well-being, strength, flexibility, stamina, adaptable, vitality, clarity and harmony in all the vital systems.

Tonics are given in the following manner: Take the remedy bottle and succuss it 5 times or hit it against a hard book. Then take 5 or more drops of the herbal tincture and put in 1 oz. water, this is stirred or shaken and then consumed. Repeat this three to four times per day, between meals. To adjust the spagyric tonic the person can increase the number of drops taken, from 5 drops go up to 10 drops, etc. If the tonic is too strong the person may reduce the amount of times they take the remedy from 3 times to 1 or 2 times a day or decrease the number of drops.

Spagyric Herbal Tinctures - Spagyria is from two Greek words, 'spao', to draw out, to extract, to divide and 'ageiro' to bind, join, combine, gather. The spagyric art translates as plant alchemy, the art of separating, exalting and recombining medicinal herbs and roots. This word was coined by Paracelsus, a medical alchemist of the 16th century. He also created the phrase: Similia similibus curentur, the famous 'likes cures likes' principle of homeopathy. These preparations are from plant origins. Their therapeutic effect is more tonic and nutritive because they contain the mineral rich plant ashes.

The spagyric herbal tinctures are alcoholic solutions of plant substances. They are prepared by maceration of the plants into pure alcohol and allowing this solution to mature over several weeks. Seven day cycles, usually 14 or 21 days, etc. The work is done at the appropriate planetary day and hour. The mixture is shaken once a week at the right time. After the allotted time has elapsed the mixture is then separated into its liquid and solid components. The plant pulp which most galenic herbalist discard is calcinated, that is, burned to a fine ash. This ash is mineral rich and gives the spagyric a very nutritive and tonic effects. This adds to the remedy an earthy elemental tone to its signature. Thus the spagyric tonics are in a 'stereo mode' while normal herbal remedies are in a 'mono mode'.

Spagyric herbal tinctures are given in the following manner: Take the remedy bottle and strongly shake it 5 times or hit it against a solid object like a book. Then take 5 drops of the spagyric tincture and put in 1 oz. water. This is stirred or shaken and then consumed. Repeat this three to four times per day, between meals. All the spagyric, herbals and homeopathic remedies in low potencies can be given in this same manner. To adjust the spagyric tonic the person can increase the number of drops taken, from 5 drops go up to 10 drops. If the tonic is too strong the person may reduce the amount of times they take the remedy from 3 times to 1 or 2 times a day. There are many levels of spagyric pharmacy and this is a simple method to begin with. The next level is called Spagyric Essences.

LOTUS MATERIA MEDICA

Table of Contents

B

C

D

M

N

O

P

S

R

Similia Similibus Curentur

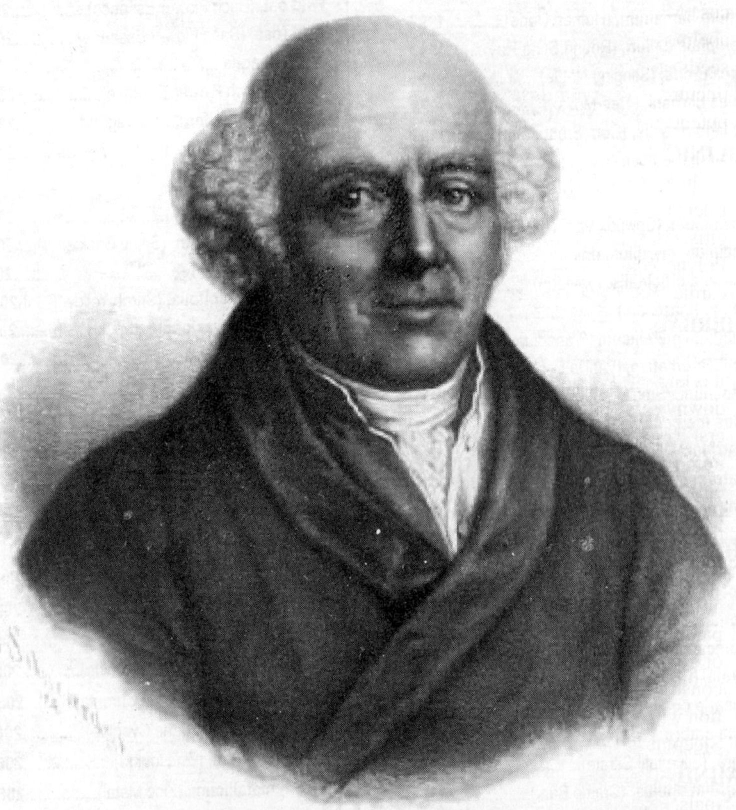

Dr Samuel Hahnemann

born on April 10, 1755, died on July 2, 1843

Founder and Developer

'The Healing Art and Science of Homeopathy'

A

ABELMOSCHUS HIBISCUS

(Musk-seed)

PHARMACY - abel. Abelmoschus hibiscus. Musk-seed. Musk-mallow. Hibiscus abelmoschus. N. O. Malvaceae. The dried seeds are used for making the mother tincture. ***Historical dose:*** Tincture and all potencies.

CLINICAL - Addison's disease. Anemia. Asthma. Delirium. Dysphagia. Dyspnea. Edema. Glaucoma. Headache. Lymphangitis. Migraine. Neuromyelitis. Paralysis. Polyneuritis. Ptyalism. Stomatitis. Tachycardia. Tetany. Trembling.

HERBAL - Abelmoschus is a shrub found in Egypt, the East Indies and Mexico, where it is known as musk-seed. The branches are downy with long leaf stalks and yellow flowers. The fruits appear as capsules containing numerous kidney bean shaped seeds. They emit a pleasant odor like that of musk and their taste is aromatic.

HOMEOPATHIC - Abelmoschus affects the stomach, uterus, mucus membranes and nerves. Trembling and paresis or even paralysis of the limbs with edema. Trembling or paralysis of the lips and jaw. Feeling of constriction in the chest. Excessive salivation with a feeling of dryness in the mouth. Sleepiness, difficulty swallowing.

MIND - Fears at night. Irrational fear of animals. Fear of animals, insects, flies, spiders, scorpions or snakes. Obsession of being attacked by venomous animals. Delirium with hallucinations.

Chest - Sharp pain in the chest.

Ears - Diminished ability to hear, when descending the stairs.

Eyes - Acute and chronic glaucoma. Detachment of the retina. Scotoma with spots before the eyes, impedes the vision. Tearing pain, as if produced by nail.

Face - Face pale, yellow, itching.

Food - Desire for food and cold drinks (Phos.).

Head - Migraine headaches. Heavy feeling in the head, as if it were being clamped in a vice (Crot-c.).

Heart - Feeling of tightness around the precordial region. Rapid beating of the heart with anguish. Tachycardia.

Limbs - Edema of the hands and legs.

Lungs - Asthma. Difficult breathing.

Modalities - Worse at night. Worse from descending the stairs (Calc.).

Mouth - Thick, sticky saliva. Excessive salivation, but feeling of dryness in the mouth. Difficulty with speech. Ptyalism neurotic of pregnancy and mercurial stomatitis. Maxillary trismus.

Stomach - Pain in the pit of the stomach.

Throat - Dysphagia.

RELATIONS - ***Compare:*** (1) Staph., which is also a preventive of mosquito bites. (2) Apis, sharp, stinging and searing pains, partial or general edema, absence of thirst. (3) Ars., anxiety with fear of death. Nocturnal restlessness, worse between 1 a.m. and 3 a.m. Edema of the eyelids, especially the lower lid, thirst for small quantities of iced water.

REFERENCES - Julian.

ABIES CANADENSIS

(Hemlock Spruce)

PHARMACY - abies-c. Abies canadensis. Hemlock Spruce. Canada pitch. Picea alba. Pinus Canadensis. Tsuga canadensis. N. O. Coniferae. Pinaceae. Tincture of fresh bark and young buds. ***Historical dose:*** Tincture and all potencies.

CLINICAL - Aphthous, ulcers. Burns. Chills. Cholera. Colds. Constipation. Croup. Coughs. Diarrhea. Flatulence. Gangrene. Gonorrhea. ***Indigestion.*** Leucorrhea. Liver, disorders. Night-sweat. Prolapsed, anus. Prolapsed, uterus. Rheumatism. Stomach, disorders. Uterine, displacements. Vertigo. Vomiting.

HERBAL - A strong decoction of the bark of this tree is beneficial in leucorrhea, prolapsed uterus, prolapsed anus, diarrhea, etc., administered internally, and used in enema.

It is of service as a local application in gangrene, and in aphthous, and other oral ulcerations.

The essence (oil) of hemlock is diuretic and highly stimulant. As a liniment this oil has been used in croup, rheumatism, and other affections requiring a stimulating local application.

Dr. W. K. Everson states it to be a superior remedy in gastric irritation to allay vomiting in cholera morbus, etc. The dose is 5 or 10 drops in water, every 10 or 20 minutes, until relief is afforded.

It is likewise of value in passive hemorrhages, and is useful topically in scalds and burns. General asthenic state, with feeble digestion, vascular weakness, and pale mucus membranes. Broncho-pulmonary irritation, with profuse secretions. Coughs and colds. Renal torpor. Pyrosis and gastric irritation with vomiting and diarrhea. Never to be used in inflammatory or sthenic conditions.

HOMEOPATHIC - Marked symptoms in mucus membranes and stomach, a catarrhal condition of the stomach is produced. Characteristic cravings and chilly sensations. Useful for women with uterine displacements, probably due to defective nutrition with debility and lack of tone.

The skin is cold and clammy, hands cold, very faint. Respiration and heart action are labored. The right lung and liver feel small and hard. ***Great appetite,*** tendency to overeat. ***Gnawing, hungry, faint feeling*** in epigastrium. Wants to lie down all the time.

MIND - Easily fretful or quiet and careless. Patient wants to lie down all the time on account of nervous weakness and feels faint.

Abdomen - Flatulence disturbs the heart's action. Sick feeling in the bowels. ***Burning and distention*** in abdomen with palpitations. Rumbling in the bowels after eating, with great appetite.

Back - Pain behind the right shoulder blade. Weak feeling in sacral region. Feeling as of cold water between the shoulders.

Eyes - Sensation as of a stye in outer canthus of left eye.

Female - Uterine displacements. Sore feeling at fundus of uterus, relieved by pressure. Prostration, wants to lie down all the time. Sensation as if the uterus is soft and feeble.

Food - Great appetite. ***Tendency to eat far beyond capacity for digestion.*** Craving for meat, pickles, radishes, turnips, and artichokes. Craving for coarse food, such as pickles, radishes, turnips, etc. Canine hunger with torpid liver.

Head - Feels light-headed, tipsy.

Heart - Action of the heart labored. Increased action of the heart with distention of the stomach.

Limbs - Hands cold, shrunken. Lies with the legs drawn up. Very faint, as if top of head were congested. Twitching of the muscles.

Liver - Sensation as if the liver were small and hard, as if bile were deficient.

Lungs - Breathing labored. Sensation as if the right lung were small and hard.

Kidneys - Urinates frequently day and night. Straw colored urine.

Mouth - Dryness of the mouth.

Rectum - Burning in rectum. Constipation.

Sensations - A feeling as if the right lung and liver were small and hard, pain beneath right scapula. The patient lies with the legs drawn up. Shivering as if the blood turned to cold water. Uterus feels soft.

Skin - Clammy and sticky.

Stomach - Catarrhal condition in the stomach, increases the patient's hunger. ***Gnawing, hungry,*** and ***faint feeling*** in the epigastrium. Distention of the stomach and epigastrium, burning.

Temperature - Cold chills, as if blood were ice water (Acon.). Chills run down back. Cold-water feeling between shoulders (Am-m.). Skin clammy and sticky. Night sweat (Chin.).

Vertigo - Tipsy feeling, a swimming of the head, light-headed.

COMMENTS - According to Hale, Abies c. cured a light-headed feeling, attended with a gnawing, hungry and faint feeling at epigastrium. A craving hunger which, if gratified, was followed by distention of the stomach and hard beating of the heart.

RELATIONS - ***Compare:*** (1) Acon. Chin. Am-m.

REFERENCES - Boericke. Clarke. Phatak.

ABIES NIGRA
(Black Spruce)

PHARMACY - abies-n. Abies nigra. Black Spruce. Double Spruce. Picea mariana. Picea nigra. N. O. Coniferae. Pinaceae. North America. Tincture of gum. ***Historical dose:*** Tincture and all potencies.

CLINICAL - Backaches. ***Belching.*** Bone aches. Chills. ***Constipation. Coughs.*** Depression. ***Dyspepsia.*** Fevers. Heartburn. Hemorrhages. Hypochondriasis. Indigestion. Intermittent fever. Malaria. Menses, delayed. Rheumatic pains. ***Stomach, disorders.*** Stomach, pain. ***Tachycardia. Water brash.***

HOMEOPATHIC - Abies-n has been used in many diseases, when they are associated with stomach symptoms. The dyspepsia caused by abuse of tea or tobacco has been cured by it.

Characteristic sensation in the cardiac end of the stomach or in the esophagus, ***"as if a hard body, as a hard-boiled egg had lodged there."*** Where this symptom is present, whether in dyspepsia or lung disease with or without hemoptysis, constipation, Abies-n. will be the most likely remedy. Patients describe this sensation, as if a hard lump is felt in the pit of the stomach or in the lung, which he wants to cough out.

Wakeful at night with hunger. Rheumatic pains and aching in bones. Abies-n in ***dyspeptic troubles of the elderly*** with functional heart symptoms, also after tea or tobacco. Distress in the head with flushed cheeks often accompanies the dyspeptic symptoms of this remedy.

"Pain in the stomach always comes after eating," said Guernsey. ***Constipation.*** Worse after eating. In lung disease when the sensation is as if there was a hard substance to be coughed up. Feeling in the epigastrium as if food were lying there (Puls., Bry.).

MIND - Very low spirited, unable to think or study. Hypochondriasis.

Back - Pain in small of back. Rheumatic pains and aching in bones.

Causations - Useful in indigestion in those who abuse tea drinking, tobacco smoking or tobacco chewing.

Chest - Painful sensation, as if something were lodged in the chest and had to be coughed up. Lungs feel compressed, cannot be fully expanded. Worse from coughing. Water brash succeeds cough. Choking sensation in throat.

Ears - Pain in left external meatus.

Female - Menstruation delayed for three months.

Food - Exceedingly hungry and wakeful at night. ***Great craving for food at noon and night.*** Total loss of appetite in morning.

Head - Hot with flushed cheeks. Low-spirited. Dull during the day, wakeful at night. Unable to think.

Heart - Heavy, slow beating of heart. Sharp, cutting pain in heart. ***Tachycardia*** and bradycardia.

Limbs - Rheumatic pains and aching in the bones.

Lungs - Easily gets out of breath. Difficult breathing, worse lying down.

Modalities - Worse after eating.

Mouth - Offensive breath.

Rectum - Constipation.

Sleep - Sleepy during the day. Wakeful and restless at night with hunger. Very bad dreams.

Stomach - Indigestion. Belchings. ***Pain in stomach always comes on after eating.*** Sensation of a lump that hurts. ***As if a hard-boiled egg*** had lodged in the cardiac end of stomach. Distressing constriction just above the pit of the stomach, as if everything were knotted up.

Temperature - Alternate heat and cold. Chronic intermittent fever with pain in stomach.

Throat - Choking sensation in throat. Sensation of something sticking in esophagus toward its lower end.

COMMENTS - Clarke after giving Abies nigra to one patient, he noted that the coldness around the stomach was removed and general chilliness greatly lessened.

RELATIONS - *Compare:* (1) Lump in stomach, Chin., Bry. Puls. (2) Nux-v. Kali-c. Chin., has the lump under the sternum, but higher up. (3) Also other Conifers - Thuj., Sabina, Cupressus - painful indigestion.

REFERENCES - Boericke. Clarke. Phatak.

ABROMA AUGUSTA RADIX

(Olat Kambal)

PHARMACY - abrom-aug. Abroma augusta radix. Olat kambal. Perennial Indian hemp. Devil's Cotton. Abrome. N. O. Sterculiaceae. Tincture of leaves, roots. ***Historical dose:*** Tincture and all potencies.

CLINICAL - ***Aching, pains.*** Amenorrhea. ***Colicky, pains.*** Constipation. Cough. Debility. ***Dysmenorrhea.*** Dysentery. Edema. Emaciation. Headaches. Hoarseness. Insomnia. ***Itching. Leucorrhea.*** Malaise. ***Menstrual, colic. Menorrhagia. Throbbing, pains.*** Vertigo.

HERBAL - Abroma augusta, indigenous to India, is an evergreen large shrub or a small tree with drooping branches. It grows wild in India's warmer regions, but is also cultivated in gardens for its beautiful deep scarlet flowers. The roots and bark are used as an emmenagogue.

HOMEOPATHIC - The proving, carried out from 1970-1973 by the Central Council for Research in Homoeopathy, consisted of 40 provers and 20 controls. Dr. D. N. Ray, of Calcutta, made a short proving in 1919 and Kishore made one in 1972, all provings are included in the drug picture.

General debility. Feeling of weakness after stool. Tingling and numbness, feeling of warmth and burning. Trembling, lethargy, weakness, uneasiness, drowsiness and heaviness in the whole body.

Body aches particularly in the joints, aggravated by rest, during movement. Malaise, with feverishness, cough. Emaciation and weight loss with general debility. Edema and puffiness in the whole body, first appeared in face and eyes with eruption, aggravated from heat or motion, ameliorated by cold, rest.

MIND - Peevishness. Anxiety. Restless with dislike for everything. ***Quarrelsome.*** Easily excited and easily angered. Contradiction is unbearable. Irritability, moroseness. Indifference, vacantness. Sadness of mind. Feeling of joy. Immoderate laughing from trifles.

Abdomen - Griping pain in the abdomen with dysentery, aggravated in the evening. ***Colicky pains.*** Dislikes a tight band around the abdomen, brings on suffocative attack, with soreness near right hypochondrium. ***Rumbling and ineffectual urging for stool.*** Flatulent distension of upper abdomen with moderate urging before stool. Feeling of warmth in upper abdomen.

Back - Aching, lameness and sharp pains in lumbar region. Bubbling sensation in left lumbar region. ***Sore, bruised pain*** in lumbar region, worse morning on rising, better motion. Aching or tingling in the nape of the neck. Pressure and constriction in the nape of neck.

Chest - Aching pain in the whole chest. Burning in chest. Sharp pain in left infra-clavicular region with catching of breath. Stinging pain in left side of the chest. Aching pain in the left intercostal muscles. Catching pain in the right lower chest with weakness and tiredness, worse movement.

Ears - Pain and soreness with stitching sensation inside the right ear, worse evening, better during the day.

Eyes - Redness of eyes without pain or discharge, ameliorated from cold application. Itching in the right eye with redness, better rubbing the eyes. As if foreign body is lodged in the eyes. ***Heaviness of upper eyelids.*** Watery exudation with redness of left eyeball. Burning in eyeballs with vertigo. Sore pain, aggravated by sunlight, ameliorated by closing the eyes. Aching pain in right eyelid. Agglutination, redness and swelling of eyelids.

Female - Amenorrhea. ***Dysmenorrhea.*** Menses scanty or copious. ***Menstrual colic and heavy bleeding.*** Pain in the lower abdomen, with delayed and scanty menstrual flow. Menses with dark colored clots. ***Leucorrhea with pain in the back and lower abdomen.*** Yellowish, white offensive leucorrhea. Leucorrhea, thin, acrid, whitish discharge. Pain in right ovarian region, better hot applications. Thin, profuse leucorrhea in emaciated young girls.

Food - Voracious appetite. Loss of appetite. Dislike for food with heaviness of abdomen. Increased thirst for cold water with dry mouth. Thirstlessness. Aversion to smoking. Aversion to starchy food. Desire for fish, juicy things. Desire for sweets, Desires coffee and tea. Desires salty foods, sour foods.

Head - Headaches with heaviness and dull aching pains. ***Aching and throbbing pains.*** Burning sensation, better application of cold water. Tingling pain. Heaviness in forehead. Sharp pain in forehead, ameliorated by pressure. Bursting pain. Dullness, dizziness, and heaviness in forehead, ameliorated by bathing. Throbbing pain in temples. ***Heaviness, aching pains.*** Dull pain in vertex, warmth in vertex. Sensation as if being pressed with a blunt object over the supraorbital region.

Heart - Heart, palpitations with undesirable feeling of distress inside the chest, better lying quiet.

Kidneys - Urination followed by weakness and exhaustion. Fishy odor of urine.

Limbs - ***Aching in the limbs*** with weakness. Aching pain in shoulder joints. Tenderness in flexor, pronator group of muscles of forearm. Trembling, burning pain in left hand. Paresis, numbness and tingling in right lower extremely with anxiety, insomnia and restlessness. ***Heaviness of limbs.*** Tiredness in thighs. Aching pain in the knee joints. Lameness and stitching pain. Drawing pain in calf muscles.

Lungs - Shortness of breath with sense of suffocation, with fever, worse during inspiration, lying down on left side. Dry and barking cough. Suffocative cough. Cough with expectoration, whitish or yellowish, salty, mucoid, sticky, thin or thick. Lumpy sputum resembling boiled starch, easily hawked up, worse at night. Must support the chest during cough. Sensation as if the respiratory tract would be torn out.

Male - Lack of sexual desire in males.

Mouth - ***Dryness of tongue and lips.*** Sore pain due to the ulceration of the corners of the mouth. Tenderness and swelling of gums, worse chewing, better cold application. Aching pain with swelling of the gums, worse when eating or from any attempt to move the jaw. Stitching pain in gums on right side.

Nose - ***Sneezing with weakness.*** Burning in the nose with fever and coryza. Profuse coryza, thin, watery, bland discharge with sneezing. Sensation of obstruction of nostrils at night. Thick, yellow, mucopurulent discharge with weakness.

Rectum - Inactivity of rectum. ***Obstinate constipation***. Constipation and headache. Ineffectual desire for stool and rumbling inside abdomen. No desire for stool with pain in abdomen. Hard nodular stool. Weakness after stool. Unfinished sensation after each stool. Constipation with hard, scanty stools. Insufficient, and straining with stools. Stools hard balls like sheep dung.

Skin - ***Intense itching*** all over the body, with pimple-like eruption. ***Dryness and burning sensation of skin,*** worse washing in hot water. Dry small vesicular and papular eruptions (resembling prickly heat) with black discoloration on different parts of the body. Itching without eruptions on the whole body, particularly thighs, during undressing, night, better open air.

Sleep - Insomnia. Sleepiness. Sleep in short naps. Restless tossing in bed with sensation of warmth, ameliorated by hard fanning. ***Sleep disturbed by dreams.*** Vivid dreams about accidents. Dreams ofrobbers and dreadful incidents. Dreams of extreme thirst. Dreams as if somebody is calling him by his name.

Stomach - Eructations, ameliorated by passing flatus. Heaviness in epigastrium with disgust for food and headache. ***Feeling of emptiness.*** Sharp pain in epigastrium. Colicky pain in the epigastrium with fullness of stomach. Nausea while taking food with watery stool, aggravated while eating.

Temperature - Heat all over the body at night with constant chilliness, body aches and sweat, aggravated at night. Temperature ranges between 99° to 100° F. Thirst at night, with fever.

Throat - ***Dryness at night, with great thirst.*** Hoarseness of voice. Soreness with tickling sensation and dry cough. Stinging pain in the left side of throat with headache. Stitching pain on right side of the throat with sore pain. Burning in throat with tickling cough aggravated in the evening.

Tongue - Bitter taste. Stinging pain in tongue, worse at midnight, from warm application. Heaviness and soreness of tongue.

Vertigo - Vertigo and giddiness with headache, worse lying down. Vertigo with nausea.

Vision - ***Blurred vision*** with aching pain in lids, aggravated by sunlight and bright light.

COMMENTS - In the female provers Abroma showed a capacity to relieve menstrual pains and to reduce the tendency to heavy bleeding. None of these provers had a history of leucorrhea but during the proving yellowish white leucorrhoea with offensive odour and pain in the lower abdomen was recorded.

In menstrual disorders it can be compared with Pulsatilla and Viburnum. Pulsatilla patients are generally mild and weep easily, whereas in Abroma the patient is bad-tempered and easily angered.

RELATIONS - ***Compare:*** Puls., Vip., Bry. Mag-p. Ph-ac. Lac-ac. Uran-n. Syzygium.

REFERENCES - Kishore. Ray.

ABROTANUM ARTEMISIA

(Southernwood)

PHARMACY - abrot. Abrotanum artemisia. Southernwood. Lady's Love. Artemisia abrotanum. N. O. Composite. Southern Europe. Tincture of fresh leaves and stems. ***Historical dose:*** Tincture and all potencies.

CLINICAL - Anemia. ***Angioma.*** Arthritis. Ascarides. Brain, congestion. Chlorosis. Contractions. Dyspepsia. Emaciation. Epilepsy. ***Gastralgia.*** Gout. Hydrocele. Indigestion. Influenza. ***Malnutrition. Marasmus.*** Nervousness. Nosebleeds. Otorrhea. Peritonitis. ***Pleurisy.*** Restlessness. ***Rheumatism.*** Sleeplessness. Spinal congestion. Typhoid. Worms.

HOMEOPATHIC - The most prominent symptom of Abrot. is the emaciation in lower limbs. It has also an intense indigestion and morbid appetite. There are burning, gnawing, constricting pains and sometimes vomiting of offensive matters.

Marasmus, especially of lower limbs only, yet with good appetite. Marasmus of children. ***Malnutrition with a failure to thrive***.

The face is wrinkled, pale, old looking, feels cold, blue rings around eyes. Oozing of blood and moisture from navel of newborn. Nosebleed and hydrocele in boys. Chlorosis.

Phagedenic diseases. Contractions of limbs from cramps or following colic. Sudden aching pain in back better by motion. Symptoms are worse at night and in cold air.

A peculiar sensation is as if the stomach were hanging or swimming in water. Weak, sickly feeling, when excited, trembling. Great weakness after influenza (Gels., Kali-p.). A pressing sensation remaining after surgery upon the chest for hydrothorax or empyema (Calen.).

Ill effects of suppressed conditions, especially in gout. Tuberculous peritonitis. Exudative pleurisy and other exudative processes.

Metastasis of states and symptoms. Metastasis of rheumatism from joints to heart, to spine.

Rheumatism from suddenly checked diarrhea, cannot move her head, arms or limbs and suffers much pain, no swelling.

After suppressed gout. Gout, painful and inflamed wrists and ankle joints. Joints stiff with pricking sensation. Painful inflammatory rheumatism before swelling. Aggravation of hemorrhoids, when rheumatism improves.

MIND - Feebleness and dullness of the mind. Easily fatigued by conversation or mental effort. No capacity for thinking, as if all bodily and mental power were gone. Thinks brain is softening. Indolence, aversion to physical exercise. Gloomy, desponding.

Exceedingly peevish. Ill-natured, irritable and violent. Cross, anxious and depressed. Excited, loquacious, feels like shouting. Taciturnity. Feels she would like to do something cruel, no humanity.

Abdomen - Weak, sinking feeling in bowels. Hard lumps are felt in different parts of abdomen. ***Bloated and distended.*** Tuberculosis peritonitis. Blood and moisture oozing from navel of newborn.

Back - Sudden aching pain in the back, worse night, better motion. Pain in lumbar region extending along spermatic cord. Pain in sacrum with hemorrhoids. Back weak with ovarian pain.

Chest - Pain across chest, sharp and severe in region of heart, rheumatism. Pleurisy, when a pressing sensation remains in affected side, which impedes free breathing (Acon., Bry.).

Constitutions - Suited to disorders of newborn children, especially boys. Children with emaciation, especially of legs. Marasmus. Digestive weaknesses in the elderly.

Eyes - Blue rings around dull-looking eyes. Hollow eyed, sunken features.

Face - Dry, cold, wrinkled skin, as if old, with marasmus. ***Angioma of the face***. Acne, comedones with emaciation. Pale, hollow-eyed appearance.

Female - Menses suppressed. Darting pain in left ovary. Back weak with ovarian pain. Twitching in both ovarian regions, seems to extend to back.

Food - Gnawing hunger and whining. Craving for bread boiled in milk. The ***appetite is great, ravenous while emaciating.*** Emaciation progresses with good appetite. ***Marasmus. Loss of appetite.*** Food passes undigested.

Head - Cannot hold the head up on account of weakness of neck. Brain feels tired after conversation or mental effort. Veins distended on forehead. Scalp sore, especially left side, itching.

Heart - Metastasis of rheumatism to heart. Pulse weak and small.

Limbs - Lame and sore all over. Inability to move the limbs, due to rheumatism. Pain in shoulders, arms, ***wrists and ankles***. Joints stiff and lame. Marasmus of lower limbs only. ***Legs are emaciated***. Contraction of limbs from cramps or following colic. Painful contraction of limbs (Am-m.). Chilblains itch, frostbitten limbs. Cold, prickling, numb, fingers and toes. Gout in wrists and ankles.

Lungs - Raw feeling. Impeded respiration. Dry cough following diarrhea. Cold air causes a raw feeling in respiratory tract.

Male - Hydrocele of boys.

Modalities - Better from loose stools. Better motion. Worse in cold air. Worse at night. Worse foggy weather. Worse wet weather. Worse from checked secretions, especially diarrhea.

Mouth - Slimy taste, acidic.

Nose - Nosebleeds. Dryness of nose.

Rectum - Alternating diarrhea with constipation. Food passes undigested. Rheumatism after suddenly checked diarrhea. Destroys worms, especially ascarides (Cina). Protruding hemorrhoids with burning from touch. Hemorrhoids appeared and became worse as rheumatic pains abated. Frequent urging, bloody stools, worse as rheumatic pains abate.

Skin - Flabby and loose skin. Furuncles. Falling out of hair. Skin becomes purplish after suppression of eruptions. Itching chilblains.

Sleep - Restless, frightful dreams.

Stomach - Cutting, gnawing, burning pains, worse at night. ***Gastralgia.*** As if stomach is swimming in cold water. Indigestion with vomiting of large quantities of offensive fluid.

Temperature - High fever, rheumatism. Hectic fever with chilliness, very weakening, and marasmus.

COMMENTS - Characteristic metastasis and marasmus. "Metastasis" is an idea in homeopathy that's not limited to cancer. Metastasis means something disappeared and reappeared. Rheumatic fever followed by sore throat is also known as metastasis. If the throat cleared up but was followed by joint problems, that's a case of metastasis.

Keynote metastasis (Plat.), with a mental state alternating with a physical one. Metastasis in homeopathy is synonymous with "suppression" if there was outside interference. It's perceiving the alternation of states in the person. All the rubrics that say "alternation with..." are metastasis rubrics.

Useful for suppression, can correct the suppression in some cases. Indicated when a disorder has moved from one area and then to another.

Disorders often go to the intestines. Alternation of constipation and diarrhea. Crohn's disease, colitis, and irritable bowel syndrome.

A very powerful children's remedy for malnutrition, malassimilation, failure to thrive, marasmus (Aeth.), colitis and rheumatism. May have a big appetite and still lose weight. Can be emaciated with poor food assimilation (Iod., Cina). Especially useful when failure to thrive is accompanied with muscular weakness.

Loss of muscular strength, of muscle tone. Flaccid. Difficulty holding up head, in older children.

Metastasis of mumps with a large swollen parotid gland, often metastasizes to the testicles or the breasts (Puls., Carb-v.).

Clarke cured with Abrot. indigestion with vomiting of large quantities of offensive fluid (in a middle-aged woman).

RELATIONS - ***Compare:*** (1) Scroph., Bry., Stell. (2) Benz-ac in gout. (3) Iod., Nat-m. in marasmus. (4) Agar, Chin, Led, Nux-v. ***Follows well:*** Acon and Bry in pleurisy.

REFERENCES - Boericke. Clarke. Murphy. Phatak.

ABRUS PRECATORIUS

(Crab's Eye Vine)

PHARMACY - abr. Abrus precatorius. Crab's eye vine. Jequirity. Indian liquorice. N. O. Leguminosae. Papilionoideae. India. Tincture of trituration of the seeds. ***Historical dose:*** Tincture and all potencies.

CLINICAL - Cancer. Conjunctivitis. Epithelioma. Fever. Granular lids. Keratitis. Lupus. Malaise. Ophthalmia. Ulcers. Tumors.

HERBAL - Abrus precatorius is a climbing plant, a native of India, but has been introduced to the Western tropics. It was discovered by the natives of Brazil, who gave it the name Jequirity.

The Treasury of Botany notes that Abrus has small nearly globose seeds, which are of a brilliant scarlet color with a black scar indicating where they were attached to the pods. The seeds are used for necklaces and as a standard of weight under the name of Raté.

Abrus was the plant employed by Professor Nowack to determine weather and telluric forecasts owing to the extreme sensitiveness of its leaves to atmospheric disturbances.

HOMEOPATHIC - Abr. acts chiefly on the eyes, skin and mucus membranes. The general effects are headache, pain in the limbs, fever, and high pulse. Malaise. The roots are used in the same manner as licorice roots.

Eyes - Epithelioma, lupus, ulcers. Granular lids. Purulent conjunctivitis inflammation spreads to face and neck. Granular ophthalmia. Keratitis.

Head - Headache.

Limbs - Pain in limbs.

Skin - Erysipelatous inflammation of skin. Lupus. Indolent ulcers.

Temprature - High temperature and high pulse.

COMMENTS - Shoemaker, of Philadelphia, gave a series of striking cures with the remedy. He showed it to be useful for disorders of the skin showing great cell growth, lupoid conditions, epithelioma and sloughing ulcers.

In a case of ulcerative lupus of both sides of the nose, which was cured by five applications, the first was followed by an enormous amount of inflammation, accompanied by malaise, high fever, which lasted until the crust began to dry.

The preparation he used was made by decorticating two hundred grains of the beans by slightly bruising and crushing them in a mortar, the red hulls were carefully picked from the cotyledons.

The latter were put in a bottle and covered with distilled water. They were macerated for twenty-four hours, then transferred to a mortar and thoroughly triturated to a smooth paste.

Sufficient water was then added to make the whole weight 800 grains. Prepared in this way it was like an emulsion and was applied to the surface to be treated with a large camel hair pencil or mop.

The application of this emulsion to ulcerated surfaces was almost painless, but soon (often within an hour) there was much irritation and inflammation, the edges became red and infiltrated, surrounding tissues edematous and shining.

In the course of from six to twelve hours a desiccated curass-like crust formed which the cracked in twenty-four hours more and the discharge escaped freely. This went on for five or six days, the quantity of discharge diminishing. The crust then separated or was removed by water dressing and disclosed healthy granulations. If any unhealthy granulations were left, the application was repeated.

Shoemaker wrote, "This treatment exercises a destructive action on unhealthy granulated conditions followed by a constructive change. Also promoting under the protective cover of the exudation which it causes, a rapid development if healthy shin and tissue."

But it must be used with caution, for he noted, "It may give rise to erysipelatous inflammation and if used on weak and irritable patients cause great constitutional disturbances."

RELATIONS - ***Compare:*** (1) Jequiritol in cases of trachoma and pannus to engraft a new purulent inflammation. The poisons contained in Jequirity seeds are almost identical in their physiological and toxic properties with the similar principles found in snake venoms.

REFERENCES - Boericke. Clarke.

ABSINTHIUM ARTEMISIA

(Common Wormwood)

PHARMACY - absin. Absinthium artemisia. Common Wormwood. N. O. Compositae. Europe (Not to be confounded with Artemisia vulgaris, which is also called wormwood). Tincture of fresh young leaves and flowers. ***Historical dose:*** Tincture and all potencies.

CLINICAL - Brain, congestion. Chlorosis. Chorea. ***Convulsions.*** Delirium. Dyspepsia. ***Epilepsy. Facial, twitching***. Headaches. Hysteria. Insanity. Insomnia. Impotency. Kleptomania. ***Mushrooms, poisoning.*** Nervousness. Opisthotonos. Otorrhea. Paralysis. Restlessness. Spinal congestion. ***Tremors.*** Typhoid.

HOMEOPATHIC - Absinthium has been proved, but a number of the symptoms were taken from observations made on absinthe drinkers. It causes hyperemia of brain, medulla and spine, more intense when combined with alcohol. Those who take absinthe are liable to hysterical manifestations.

This drug produces a perfect picture of ***epileptiform seizure***. ***Convulsions are preceded by trembling,*** the patient makes grimaces, bites tongue, foams. Marked ***tremors*** of nerves, tongue and heart.

The giddiness and epileptiform attacks are the most important of the symptoms. ***Sudden and severe, giddiness, epileptiform seizures.*** Delirium with hallucinations and loss of consciousness. "A peculiar vertigo on rising with a tendency to fall backward."

Attacks occur in rapid succession.

Useful remedy for nervousness, restlessness, excitement and sleeplessness in children. Cerebral irritation, hysterical and infantile spasms come within range of this remedy.

This remedy has been used for ***mushroom poisonings.*** Opisthotonos. Intoxication. Chorea. Paralysis of inner organs.

MIND - Loss of memory. Forgets what has recently happened after and before convulsion. Wants nothing to do with anybody. Foolish look on face. Hallucinations. Frightful visions. Kleptomania. Insanity. Patient walks about in distress, seeing all sorts of demons. There is exhilaration followed by horrible delirium (Bell.), patient obliged to walk about (Art-v., Cham. and Cina. are better moving about).

Abdomen - Nausea, apparently in region of gallbladder. Bloated around waist and in abdomen, as after ague. Immense accumulation of flatulence in abdomen, wind colic. Liver feels swollen. Pain in spleen, it feels swollen.

Chest - Sensation of weight on chest. Irregular, tumultuous action of heart can be heard in back.

Constitutions - Younger and elderly patients. Chlorosis.

Ears - Discharge from ears after headaches. Otorrhea, especially after hemicrania.

Eyes - Pupils dilated unequally. Injected conjunctiva. Pain in eyes. Itching. Heavy lids.

Face - Foolish look. Rush of blood to the face. ***Spasmodic facial twitching***. Makes grimaces and foams at the mouth in epilepsy. Face blue.

Female - Darting pain in right ovary. Premature menopause. Pains in uterus. Chlorosis. Promotes menses.

Food - Loss of appetite, loathing of food.

Head - Confusion in head. Dull occipital headaches (Gels. Pic-ac.). Wants to lie with the head low. Congestion of the brain and spinal cord.

Heart - Tumultuous action, heartbeats can be heard in back. Tremors of the heart felt toward the back.

Kidneys - Constant desire to urinate. Very strong odor, like horse's urine, deep yellow orange color (Kali-p.).

Limbs - Spasms of the body and limbs. Pain in limbs. Paralytic symptoms. Feet very cold.

Lungs - Cough with liver complaints.

Male - Spermatorrhea with relaxed, enfeebled parts. Impotency.

Mouth - Jaws firmly fixed. Bites his tongue in epilepsy. Tongue trembles, feels as if swollen and too large. Tongue thick, protruding, can scarcely talk. Tongue trembling, feels paralyzed.

Nerves - Falling down, as in epilepsy. Unconsciousness with distortion of the features, followed by spasms of the body and limbs. Bloody foam at mouth and biting of the tongue. Stupidity and the loss of memory afterwards. Opisthotonos, with grinding teeth, followed by stupor. Paralysis of inner organs.

Sleep - Sleeplessness, typhoid with congestion of base of brain. Nervous excitement and sleeplessness in children.

Stomach - Uncomfortable, irritated feeling of stomach. Food lies heavy. Stomach feels cold and oppressed. Nausea, retching, eructation.

Throat - Scalded feeling in the throat. Sensation as if a lump.

Vertigo - Vertigo on rising, with the tendency to fall backward.

COMMENTS - Clarke wrote about a case of epileptic vertigo with signs of constant cerebral and spinal congestion, nausea and tendency to frequent vomiting, persistent tremors, epileptic attacks of hysterical character and opisthotonos. Absinth. first in the tincture and later in 3c, completely cured.

Halbert regarded Absin. as of special service in cases of epilepsy where consciousness is not entirely lost. The characteristic symptoms include a sudden and severe giddiness, epileptiform seizures, delirium with delusions and loss of consciousness. For some time after the attack there is a loss of memory.

RELATIONS - ***Compare:*** (1) Alcohol, Agar., Artemisia, Hydrocy. acid, Cina, Cicuta.

REFERENCES - Boericke. Clarke. Phatak.

ACALYPHA INDICA

(Indian Nettle)

PHARMACY - acal. Acalypha indica. Indian Nettle. Cupameni. Indian acalypha. N. O. Euphorbiacae. East Indies. Tincture of fresh plant. The fresh plant is macerated with two parts by weight of alcohol ***Historical dose:*** Tincture and all potencies.

CLINICAL - Bloody expectorations. Chest, pain. ***Coughs.*** Diarrhea. Emaciation. Flatulence. Hemoptysis. ***Hemorrhages.*** Jaundice. ***Lung, cancer. Tuberculosis.***

HOMEOPATHIC - Acal. is a remedy having a marked action on the alimentary canal and respiratory organs. The herbal tincture of the Acal. is a specific in ***hemorrhage from the lungs***. Hemoptysis. Acal. is indicated in incipient tuberculosis with hard, racking cough, ***bloody expectoration***, arterial hemorrhage, but no febrile disturbance.

All hemorrhages are ***aggravated in the morning***. Very weak in the morning, gains strength during the day. Progressive emaciation, sense of weight in the stomach with sense of burning, flatulence and sputtering diarrhea.

Abdomen - Burning in the intestines. ***Sputtering diarrhea with forcible expulsion of noisy flatus***. Bearing down pains and tenesmus. Rumbling distention and griping pain in abdomen. Rectal hemorrhage, worse in morning.

Chest - Dullness of chest on percussion, constant severe pain in chest.

Constitutions - Tubercular constitution. Hemorrhagic diathesis.

Heart - Pulse soft and compressible.

Lungs - ***Dry, hard coughs, followed by hemoptysis***, worse in morning and at night. ***Expectorates pure blood*** in the morning and dark clotted blood in the evening. Cough most violent at night. ***Lung cancer*** with violent coughs followed by bloody expectoration or ***pure blood***.

Modalities - ***Worse in mornings***. Cough is aggravated at night.

Rectum - Diarrhea. Flatulence and sputtering diarrhea.

Skin - Jaundice. Itching and circumscribed furuncle-like swellings.

Stomach - Burning, sense of a weight in the stomach.

COMMENTS - Dr. Tonnere of Calcutta, India, seems to have been the first to call attention to this plant as a remedy. It first appears in a small work, Additions to the Homeopathic Materia Medica, collected and arranged by Henry Thomas, M. D. and published in London in the year 1858:

Thomas employed a 6x dilution in three cases of tuberculosis. In one case, there was a tuberculous affection of the upper portion of the left lung of two years' standing. Hemoptysis had been going on for three months, the expectoration had been pure blood in the morning, dark lumps of clotted blood in the evening, and the fits of coughing were very violent at night.

In this case, all homeopathic remedies had been tried unsuccessfully, then Thomas accidentally discovered the virtues of the Acalypha Indica, that remedy having been given him by a native for jaundice.

Henry Thomas said, "I prepared the mother tincture upon the homeopathic principle and took 10 drops, which brought on a severe fit of dry cough, followed by spitting of blood. After having noted all the symptoms experienced by myself and finding that they were nearly all similar to those of my patients."

Thomas gave six drops of the 6x dilution in half a tumbler of water. A spoonful was to be taken every half hour, beginning immediately at 9 a.m. At 6 p.m., the blood had stopped. He continued this for eight days and the blood never reappeared. The patient improved and auscultation proved the disease decreased. Thomas was hopeful to effect a cure.

In one case of passive hemorrhage from the lungs, after Arnica was used with little benefit, Acal. benefited and then failed, after which the use of Arnica entirely stopped the hemorrhagic flow.

Grimmer stated that "Lung cancer with a violent cough which followed by bloody expectoration or of pure blood, bright in the morning, dark and clotted in the evening. Dullness of chest on percussion, constant severe pain in chest. Progressive emaciation with a sense of weight in the stomach with burning. Flatulence with a sputtering diarrhea."

RELATIONS - Calc. is an antidote to the Acalypha. ***Compare:*** (1) Mill., Phos., Acet-ac., Kali-n. (2) Also, compare Merl., Manc. and other Euphorbians. (3) Ham., Ip., Acon.

REFERENCES - Anshutz. Boericke. Clarke. Grimmer. Thomas.

ACCUTANE

(Isotretinoin)

PHARMACY - accu. Accutane. Isotretinoin. Allopathic drug for acne. ***Historical dose:*** All potencies.

CLINICAL - ***Acne.*** Allergies. Anemia. ***Birth, defects.*** Bleeding. Bruises. Chest pain. Colitis. Conjunctivitis. Cysts. ***Depression.*** Diarrhea. ***Dry, skin.*** Edema. Emaciation. Eye, disorders. Fatigue. Hair, problems. Headaches. Hematuria. Hepatitis. Herpes. Incoordination. Itching. Joint, pains. Liver, disorders. Nausea. Night blindness. Nosebleeds. Palpitations. Photophobia. Rashes. ***Skin, disorders. Suicidal.*** Sun, sensitivity. Sunburns. Vertigo. Vomiting. Weakness. Wounds.

HOMEOPATHIC - Accutane, a chemical cousin of vitamin A, is prescribed for the treatment of severe, disfiguring cystic acne that has not cleared up in response to other drugs such as antibiotics. It works on the oil glands within the skin, shrinking them and diminishing their output.

Accutane can cause ***severe birth defects***, including ***mental retardation*** and physical malformations. Some people taking Accutane have experienced headaches, nausea, and visual disturbances caused by increased pressure within the skull. Swelling of the optic nerve.

Abnormal hair growth or loss. Allergic reactions. Chest pain. ***Delay in wound healing.*** Dry nose. Fatigue. Flushing. Liver disorders. Pinkeye.

Stomach and intestinal discomfort. Suppression of growth. Swelling due to fluid retention. Weakness. Weight loss.

Abdominal pain. Dizziness. Dry or cracked lips. Facial flushing. Incoordination and clumsiness. Headache, vomiting. Bleeding from the rectum. Severe diarrhea. Inflammatory disease of the bowels.

MIND - Accutane may cause depression or other mental problems. Nervousness. Emotional instability. Depression. Obsessive and compulsive disorders. ***Mental retardation.*** Self mutilation. Aggressive and violent behaviors.

In some cases, it has prompted thoughts of suicide. ***Suicidal depression.*** Some patients taking Accutane have had thoughts about hurting themselves or putting an end to their own lives. Some people tried to end their own lives.

Abdomen - Colitis. Bowel inflammation and pain. Pancreatitis.

Blood - Anemia. Bleeding from, gums, rectum, and nose. Changes in blood sugar or cholesterol levels.

Ears - Hearing problems.

Eyes - Conjunctivitis. Night blindness. Photophobia. Vision problems. Decreased night vision. Decreased tolerance to contact lenses. Swelling of the optic nerve.

Face - Facial flushing.

Female - Menstrual changes.

Head - Headaches.

Heart - Stroke. Irregular heartbeats. Sudden drop in blood pressure (causing unconsciousness).

Kidneys - Blood in urine. Urinary discomfort.

Limbs - Joint pains. Calcification of tissues. Tendon and ligament problems. Peeling palms or soles. Nail disorders.

Liver - Liver disorders. Hepatitis.

Mouth - Dry, mouth. Cracked and bleeding lips. Bleeding gums.

Nose - Dry, nose. Nosebleeds.

Perspiration - Profuse sweating.

Rectum - Bleeding. Diarrhea.

Skin - Dry, fragile skin. Severe cystic acne. Rashes. Skin infections. Sun sensitivity. Sunburn sensitive skin. ***Delay in wound healing.*** Abnormal hair growth. Bruises easily. Herpes. Itching. Changes in skin pigmentation.

Sleep - Drowsiness. Difficulty sleeping.

Stomach - Nausea. Vomiting.

Temperature - Flushing.

Vertigo - Dizziness.

RELATIONS - ***Compare:*** (1) Aur.

REFERENCES - Murphy.

ACETANILIDUM

(Antifebrinum)

PHARMACY - Acetan. Acetanilidum. Antifebrinum. Formed from aniline. Exalgine is a derivative from this Methylacetanilid and has almost identical action. ***Historical dose:*** Trituration and all potencies.

CLINICAL - Albuminuria. Asthma. Collapse. Cyanosis. Edema. Fainting. Palpitations. Thrombosis.

HOMEOPATHIC - Acetan. was used as a sedative and antipyretic for various forms of headache and neuralgia in doses of one to three grains.

Acetan. depresses the heart, respiration, blood pressure and lowers the temperature. Destroys red blood corpuscles, pallor. Cyanosis and collapse. Increased susceptibility to cold. Albuminuria with edema of the feet and ankles.

Several cases of thrombosis of the lower limbs from heart weakness have followed its use. Antifebrinum and Exalgine have produced symptoms of collapse and cyanosis, in some instances fatal, with great rapidity. One patient experienced, after taking Exalgine, a sensation that his head was so large that it seemed to occupy the whole room.

Eyes - Pallor of optic discs, contracted visual field and shrinking retinal vessel, mydriasis.

Head - Enlarged sensation. Fainting. Moral depravity. Given for migraines and in order to reduce fever.

Heart - Weak heart, irregular heartbeat with blue mucus membranes.

Lungs - Difficult respiration, as in a bad attack of asthma. As if the diaphragm ceased working.

RELATIONS - ***Compare:*** (1) Antipyrin., Anilinum, Glon.

REFERENCES - Boericke. Clarke.

ACETICUM ACIDUM

(Acetic acid)

PHARMACY - acet-ac. Aceticum acidum. Acetic acid. Vinegar. Glacial Acetic Acid. Dilutions. ***Historical dose:*** Tincture and all potencies.

CLINICAL - Ascites. ***Anemia. Anesthetics, poisoning.*** Anxiety. Ascarides. Birthmarks. Burns. Corns. Croup. ***Debility.*** Delirium. ***Diabetes.*** Diphtheria. ***Dropsy. Edema. Ebullitions. Emaciation.*** Fevers. Hydrophobia. Nevi. Narcotics, poisoning. Sausage, poisoning. Scalds. Scurvy. Skin, cancer. Stings. Stomach, cancer. Tuberculosis. Varicose, veins. Warts.

HOMEOPATHIC - ***Antidotes the effects of anesthesia*** (Phos.). For dullness or grogginess since anesthesia, with memory problems or chronic fatigue (Phos., Chlf., Nitro-o.).

Keynote waxy pale skin, anemia and severe water brash. The water brash is of a sour regurgitation during pregnancy (Carbo-v., Nat-p.). Intense thirst, burning in throat, nausea, retching and sour rising as met with in cases of cancer and debility. Used in the past as a tonic and to increase digestion.

Profound anemia with some dropsical edema symptoms. Great debility, frequent fainting, dyspnea, weak heart, vomiting, profuse urination and sweat. Hemorrhage from any part. Varicose swellings. ***Emaciation and debility.*** Especially indicated in pale, lean persons with lax, flabby muscles. ***Dropsy of abdomen and legs, anasarca, great thirst, pale, waxen skin.*** Edema, peripheral edema associated with anemia or protein loss through the urine.

Acetic acid has the power to ***liquefy albuminous and fibrinous deposits.*** Dissolves cancer cells.

W. Owens noted that it was useful for epithelial cancer internally and locally. Sycosis with nodules and formations in the joints. Hard chancre, the 1x solution will soften it and cause the formation of pus.

Changes gangrenous ulcers, hospital gangrene, prevents decomposition of animal matter.

There are gnawing, ulcerative pains in stomach, pain and burning in abdomen. Profuse, exhausting diarrhea. ***Ebullitions.*** Diabetes. Scurvy. Putrid and hectic fevers with night sweats.

MIND - Irritable. Very dull and low-spirited. Grieves much, sighs often. Horrible attacks of anxiety with difficult breathing. Borrows trouble, worried about business affairs. Grieves about his sickness and the children. Does not know her own children. Forgets what has recently happened. Confusion of ideas. Alternate stupor and delirium.

Abdomen - Distention of the abdomen, colicky pains. Inflammation of bowels during dentition. Abdomen feels as if sunken in when lying on his back. Frequent watery stools, worse in morning. ***Tympanitic***. Ascites. Hemorrhage from bowels.

Back - Myelitis, with profuse urine, the pain in the back ***relieved only by lying on the abdomen***.

Blood - Hemorrhages from nose, lungs, stomach, bowels, and uterus. Passive hemorrhages. Blood coagulated in veins. Blood vessels contracted. Varicose swellings. Chlorosis, anemia.

Constitutions - Suited to children and old people. For lax, pale, lean anemic persons.

Face - Pale, waxen, emaciated. Expression wild, pupils dilated. Bright red flush on both cheeks. Left cheek red during fever. Sweat on forehead in spots.

Female - Excessive menses. ***Hemorrhages after labor***. Nausea of pregnancy. Metrorrhagia with great thirst after childbirth. Breasts painfully enlarged, distended with milk. Threatening abscess of the breast. Anemia of nursing mothers. Breast milk impoverished, bluish, sour, child droops, lose flesh, gets marasmus.

Food - Greatest burning thirst, with diabetes or dropsy. Insatiable even by taking large quantities. Thirsty with dry lips, which peel off in flakes. No thirst with fever. Cold drinks disagree. Loss of appetite. Disgust for salted things and cold victuals. Bread and butter disagree. Vegetables, except potatoes, disagree.

Head - Blood rushes to head with delirium. Temporal vessels distended. Child does not let its head be touched. Heaviness and dull pains in forehead and vertex. Headache from abuse of tobacco, opium, coffee, or alcohol.

Kidneys - Large quantities of pale urine. Diabetes with great thirst and debility (Ph-ac.).

Limbs - Emaciation. Edema of feet and legs with diarrhea. Varicose swellings.

Lungs - Hoarse, hissing respiration, ***Difficult breathing, cough when inhaling***. Croup. Membranous croup. Irritation of trachea and bronchial tubes. False membrane in throat. Profuse bronchorrhea. Putrid sore throat (gargle). Hurried and laborious breathing. Rattling in chest.

Male - Weakening emissions, semen passes at stool. Prepuce thickened, fissured, can't be retracted and itches fearfully. Sexual passion, but feeble erection.

Mouth - Teeth feel dull, breath foul. Scorbutic ulcers, toothache. Sour taste. Epithelium of mouth quite white. Tongue pale and flabby.

Nose - Nosebleed especially from a fall or blow. Liable to frequent catarrhal attacks.

Rectum - Hemorrhages from bowels. Constipation, with great thirst and excess of pale urine. Chronic diarrhea of emaciated children. Diarrhea with great thirst and swelling of legs and feet. Diarrhea with colic pains. Ascarides.

Skin - Pale, cold, waxen, and edematous. Burning, dry, hot skin or bathed in profuse sweat. Diminished sensibility of the surface of body. Varicose swellings. Scurvy, anasarca. Bruises, sprains. Stings, bites, etc. Tetter-like eruptions. Nevi, warts, corns.

Sleep - Sleepless.

Stomach - Burning water brash and profuse salivation. ***Fermentation*** in stomach. Vomits after every kind of food. Epigastric tenderness. Sour belching and vomiting. ***Violent burning pain in stomach and chest,*** as of an ulcer, followed by coldness of skin and cold sweat on forehead. Stomach feels as if had taken a lot of vinegar. Scirrhus of pylorus. Indurations in stomach. Cancer of stomach.

Temperature - Hectic with drenching night sweats. Red spot on left cheek. No thirst in fever. ***Ebullitions.*** Sweat profuse, cold. Low fever with night sweats. Putrid and typhous fevers.

Throat - False membranes in throat. Hoarse with laryngeal irritation. Children thirsty, but swallow with difficulty. Diphtheria. Hissing respiration, with rattling in the throat.

Vertigo - Vertigo with feebleness and fainting.

COMMENTS - A plump and blooming young woman took a small glass of vinegar daily to reduce size. She soon lost flesh and color. In a month, cough set in with white concocted phlegm, fever. Dyspnea, night sweats, anorexia, dropsy, diarrhea and death. The lungs after death were found stuffed with non-suppurating tubercles.

A German, after working twelve months in a vinegar factory, had to leave from indigestion, dyspnea and ready fatigue.

Equal parts of vinegar and hot water make a refreshing sponge-down for many conditions of fever with or without perspiration. Acetic acid is often given in drop doses: five drops in four ounces of water, take two or three times a day. It was also used in the past as a tonic and to increase digestion. Acet-ac. is useful homeopathically for anemia.

RELATIONS - Acetic acid is antidotal to all anesthetic vapors. Counteracts sausage poisoning. Follows China off. after hemorrhages. ***Compare:*** (1) Am-a. - profuse saccharine urine, patient is bathed in sweat. (2) Benzoin oderiferum - night sweats. (3) Ars., Chin., Dig. (4) Liatris - anasarca in heart and kidney disease, dropsy and chronic diarrhea.

REFERENCES - Boericke. Clarke. Phatak.

ACETONUM

(Acetone)

PHARMACY - aceton. Acetonum. Acetone. It is also called dimethyl ketone, 2-propanone, and beta-ketopropane. Dilutions. ***Historical dose:*** All potencies.

CLINICAL - Birth, defects. Coma. Confusion. Headaches. Menstrual, disorders. Nausea. Unconsciousness. Vertigo. Vomiting.

HOMEOPATHIC - Acetone is used to make plastic, fibers, drugs, and other chemicals, as well as to dissolve other substances. Exposure to moderate to high amounts of acetone can irritate your eyes and respiratory system, causing dizziness. Headaches. Light-headedness. Confusion. Increased pulse rate. Effects on blood. Nausea and vomiting. Shortening of the menstrual cycle in women.

Very high exposure may cause loss of consciousness and coma. Swallowing very high levels of acetone can result in unconsciousness and damage to the skin in your mouth. Skin contact can result in irritation and damage to the skin. Dizzy. Light-headedness. Tobacco smoke, smell of nail polish remover aggravates.

Health effects from long-term exposures are known mostly from animal studies, they include kidney, liver, and nerve damage, increased birth defects, and lowered ability to reproduce (males only). It is not known if these same effects occur in humans.

COMMENTS - Acetone is used to make plastic, fibers, drugs, and other chemicals. It is also used to dissolve other substances.

It occurs naturally in plants, trees, volcanic gases, forest fires, and as a product of the breakdown of body fat. It is present in vehicle exhaust, nail polish, tobacco smoke, and landfill sites. Industrial processes contribute more acetone to the environment than natural processes.

REFERENCES - Murphy.

ACHYRANTHES CALEA

(Herb of Fever)

PHARMACY - achy. Achyranthes calea. Herb of fever. Herba du Tabardilla de Puebla. N. O. Amaranthaceae. Mexico. Tincture of the whole dried plant. ***Historical dose:*** Tincture and all potencies.

CLINICAL - Chickenpox. Encephalitis. Glomerulonephritis. Infectious diseases. Kidney abscess. Measles. Meningitis. Neuritis. Psittacosis. Pyelonephritis. Rubella. Scarlet fever. Septicemia. Typhoid fever.

HERBAL - In herbal medicine, the plant is used as a diaphoretic and a febrifuge. The mother tincture is prepared by using the whole, fresh plant, dried.

HOMEOPATHIC - The homeopathic proving is the work of Dr. De Legarreta, on himself and volunteers. Similar to Aconite in fevers, but of a larger range, also adapted to typhoid states and intermittents. Fever with dry skin. Temperature between 38°C and 40°C. Feeling of heat, which increases when resting.

Muscular pains in the long muscles. Fatigue with need for rest. Sensitive to change in barometric pressure. Face red, swollen as after long exposure to the sun. Muscular rheumatism. Muscular stiffness.

Acute congestive states, feverish with torpor and indifference towards the environment. Congestive, throbbing headache. Dryness and burning of the mucus membranes and of the skin. Acute osteomyelitis in adolescents.

MIND - Desire to be alone in a state of calm, answers in monosyllables. Apathy and indifference towards the environment. Torpor with sudden starting from sleep to return again to a state of torpor. Mental effort tires him and he puts it off until later. Children have nightmares and awake panic-stricken.

Depression. Fear of suffering. Low morale with uneasiness, twinges of conscience, religious preoccupation. Desire to set his conscience right, begs forgiveness and tends to excuse himself for his errors. Suffocates with the intense heat, wants immediate relief. Needs to be well covered despite the feeling of heat of which he complains. Annoyed by light, ameliorated in the dark with the presence of a third, silent person.

Abdomen - Acute epigastric pain from the cold. Acute hemorrhaging pancreatitis. Acute gastritis, colitis, enterocolitis and cholecystitis. Experiences no need for defecation. Feeling of repletion.

Back - Feeling of aching, bruising heaviness of the back and the loins. Feet and hands burning. Acute pain in the back and neck. Cold sweat on the back. Torticollis. Lumbago.

Breasts - Acute mastitis. The breasts are sensitive to the touch.

Chest - Oppression with the need for deep, repeated inhaling. Pain in the pectoral muscles, in the intercostal spaces. Thoracic pain in the pre-sternal and precordial regions.

Ears - Itching, heat and dryness of the auditory canal. The auricle of the ear bright red and tense. Cannot bear noise. Acute congestive otitis media. Acute mastoiditis.

Eyes - Bright, sensitive to light. Feeling of sand in the eyes. Impression of burning in the eyes, watering. Eyes bloodshot, giving a terrifying appearance. Eyelids are hot, heavy, drooping, eyelashes turn upwards. Eyes infected, yellow mucus secretion eased by cold compresses. Painful eyeballs, relieved by pressure of the fingers on the eyeball. Dacryocystitis, blepharitis, conjunctivitis, keratitis and iritis.

Female - Dryness and burning in the vagina. External genital organs relaxed. Menses sometimes relieve the general condition. Valvulitis, bartholinitis, vaginitis, metritis and salpingitis.

Food - Needs to drink to slake thirst. Thirst for cold water, which seems to taste bad. Indifference to food, aversion to solid food.

Head - Severe congestive frontal headache. Beating in the temporal arteries. Strange noises in the head. Headache worse when touched, eased by compression of the head or by placing a heavy pillow on the head.

Heart - Regular yet slow heartbeats, steady with a low, strong and full pulse. Dry pericarditis. Aortitis, syphilitic or atheromatous. Aneurysm of the aorta. Temporal arteritis. Arteritis. Myocarditis. Cardiotonic.

Kidneys - Acute glomerulonephritis. Pyelonephritis. Kidney abscess. Bladder tenesmus, burning in the urethra. Frequent, pressing emission of small quantities of hot, clear urine, which when still, takes on a reddish tint. Urethritis.

Limbs - Acute joint rheumatism. Muscular rheumatism. Acute osteomyelitis in adolescents. Hands and feet also perspire.

Lungs - Breathing is difficult, breaths short, noisy and fast. A light cough, catarrhal and very tiring. Bronchopneumonia. Pneumonia. Pleurisy.

Male - Penis hot and flaccid. Scrotum congested with veins standing out. No sexual desire, aggravated by the cold. Ejaculation rare, erection incomplete. Burning in the urethra after ejaculation. After acute testicular surgery.

Modalities - Better from strong pressure. Better calm, and rest. Worse from movement. Worse cold, damp. Worse on the left, but not exclusively.

Mouth - Hot and dry. Dry, burning tongue. Aphthae, from exposure to the sun or indigestion. Muscular pains in the masseter and zygomatic muscles, which force the mouth to remain open.

Nose - Nose dry, blocked and painful. Black secretion, relief from flowing. Nosebleed on the left side when blowing the nose. Maxillary sinusitis. Frontal sinusitis. Ethmoiditis.

Skin - Skin dry, burning, impression of goose flesh when moving. Burning redness of the skin. Malignant lupus erythematous. Painful dermatitis.

Temperature - Fever after sudden changes of temperature. Temperature level from 38°C to 40°C.

Throat - Dry, burning throat. Needs to swallow often in order to moisten the throat. Prickling in the throat after a cold drink. Hoarseness, difficulty in speaking in cold weather.

COMMENTS - Achyranthes calea is found in Mexico. This herbaceous plant produces a round stem, which, while young is green, but which takes on a bluish-red hue when fully grown. The stem is gnarled and rugged, the leaves oval, spear-shaped and smooth. Small, hermaphrodite flowers with a fruit crowned by a pistil, the pericarp is fine and membranous with reddish dots.

RELATIONS - ***Compare:*** (1) Acon. - Dry, burning skin, but anxious restlessness with a fear of death. (2) Bry - Severe inflammation of the mucus membranes, acute prickling pains aggravated by the slightest movement, ameliorated by pressure. (3) Rhus-t. - Generalized aching. Constant need to change place tongue with red triangle at the tip, painful stiffness of limbs, skin red with vesicular itching eruptions. (4) Pyrog. - Prostration and agitation. Dissociation between pulse and temperature. Cadaverous odor of perspiration and discharges.

REFERENCES - Boericke. Julian.

ACONITINUM

(Aconitine)

PHARMACY - aconin. Aconitinum. Aconitine. Alkaloid of Aconite. Aconitia. N. O. Ranunculacee. An alkaloid obtained from the roots and stems of Aconitum napellus. ***Historical dose:*** All potencies.

CLINICAL - Blindness. Chills. Convulsions. Deaf. Dyspnea. Ears, noises. Esophagus, spasms. Eyes, strained. Hemicrania. Hydrophobia. Liver, disorders. Neuralgia. Paralysis. Spasms. Spleen, enlargement. Tetanus. Tongue, disorders. Trismus. Vomiting.

HOMEOPATHIC - The knowledge of this alkaloid is chiefly derived from cases of poisoning and over-dosing. On local application, first there is a sensation of warmth, then burning with sharp pains and itching. Finally there is numbness and anesthesia.

In one poisoning case, vomiting recurred every two or three minutes and was performed by a sudden jerking action of abdominal muscles, accompanied by a loud shout, probably dependent on a sudden contraction of the diaphragm.

Every attempt to swallow was followed by the spasms, like hydrophobia, but they were not renewed by the sight of water. The slightest touch renewed the spasms.

The numbness, tingling, prickling and heat of the Aconite provings are produced by the alkaloid, but with increased intensity. Tingling sensation. Tinnitus aurium. Heavy feeling as of lead, pains in supra-orbital nerve, ice-cold sensations creep up, hydrophobia symptoms. Aconitine should be helpful in cases of hydrophobia cases, whether of the convulsive or the paralytic kind.

The senses are disordered or lost, including the sight, hearing, and smell.

Symptoms set in with great rapidity and develop with extreme intensity. If recovery occurs it is rapid and complete. There is relaxation of the limbs and every exertion aggravates the symptoms. Worse by mental exertion, by agitation, or touch. Erect position causes nausea.

MIND - Anguish with the fear of death. Intellect perfect, even vivid. Flow of ideas sluggish, long reflection impossible. Power of attention impaired. Feels like one sleeping and dreaming. Forgetfulness and trembling of limbs.

Abdomen - Rumbling in bowels. Sudden contraction of diaphragm. Liver and spleen greatly enlarged.

Ears - Sense of pressure in ears. Roaring in ears. Complete deafness.

Eyes - Strained feeling in eyes. Pupils dilated (both from internal and external use). Complete blindness, accompanying dilatation of pupils, sight returning when pupils contract. Vision hazy with giddiness and nausea. Pupils insensible to light.

Face - Fullness in cheeks and temples gradually changing to painful sense of tension, formication and prickling. Face tense and swollen. Creeping sensation in face and forearms. Peculiar drawing, stretching, pressing sensation in cheeks, upper jaws, forehead.

Head - Fullness in the head with noises in the ears. Head and face ache, often darting pains in face, sometimes accompanied by vomiting. Hemicrania has been cured. Weight about head, unable to hold it up.

Heart - On entering a warm room, pulse is more frequent, then sinks far below normal, small, weak intermittent. Sounds of heart only heard at apex.

Kidneys - Copious diuresis. Difficulty in voiding urine. Dysuria and occasionally retention with hypogastric pain.

Limbs - Weakness, trembling, burning, creeping, tingling, and numbness of limbs.

Liver - Liver and spleen greatly enlarged.

Lungs - Respiration difficult. Oppressive anguish in precordial region. Sighing breathing.

Mouth - Burning on tip of tongue and lips. Burning, constricting, acrid, dry sensation in mouth and fauces. Tongue stiff. Taste disagreeable and disgustingly bitter or completely lost. Taste impaired. Teeth more sensitive when biting. Salivation.

Skin - General formication.

Sleep - Somnolence. Sleep disturbed. Throws himself continually around in bed.

Stomach - Belchings immediately. Severe vomiting, recurring every two or three minutes, from a sudden jerking action of abdominal muscles accompanied by a loud shout. Nausea induced by erect position. Vomiting relieves all symptoms. Warmth most marked in region of stomach.

Temperature - Surface cold, sweating and quite pale. Intense coldness. Head and face became suddenly warm, warmth extended over rest of body, was more intense in region of stomach and was accompanied by sweat.

Throat - Burning anguish in throat. Constriction and burning from mouth to stomach. Every attempt to swallow followed by spasms like hydrophobia but not renewed by sight of water. Difficulty of swallowing and a pain in back of neck and behind jaws in parotid region. Burning in gullet as if a hot coal were there.

Vertigo - Vertigo and confusion with ringing in ears, falls almost immediately. With giddiness, dimness of vision and muscular weakness.

COMMENTS - Found in all species of Aconite except Acon-l. German Aconitine is amorphous, French Aconitine is crystalline and 170 times stronger than the German.

Morson's "English Aconitine" is a secret preparation believed to be made from Acon-f. The alkaloid in Acon-f. differs somewhat from ordinary Aconitine chemically and is called pseudo-Aconitine. The Aconitine of T. H. Smith of Edinburgh is probably identical with Morson's.

Symptoms often proceed from below upwards. "A tingling, prickling sensation, running up leg to spine and head and tingling of fingers." "Ice-cold sensation creeps up from his feet." Fear of death, anguish intense chilliness, feeling of sickness, constricting burning sensation, extending from mouth to stomach. Twitchings and spasms over whole body, especially in face. All symptoms are better by vomiting.

In one poisoning case, the blindness was coincident with sudden dilatation of the pupils and sight partially returned as the pupils contracted. A heavy feeling as of lead all over the body. All parts except head and stomach feel as if filled with lead. Neuralgia of fifth cranial nerve. Creeping on face with feeling of swelling and tension. Pains in supra-orbital nerve were especially prominent.

Postmortem examinations showed the spleen very much enlarged, posterior part of liver dark and almost black. Kidneys hyperemic.

RELATIONS - ***Compare:*** (1) Acon. (2) Hydrophobia, (rabies) symptoms, Bell., Canth., Hyos., Lach., Fagu.

REFERENCES - Boericke. Clarke.

ACONITUM CAMMARUM

PHARMACY - acon-c. Aconitum cammarum. Aconitum neomontanum. Aconitum intermedium. Aconitum stoerckianum. N. O. Ranunculacee. Tincture of fresh root. ***Historical dose:*** All potencies.

CLINICAL - Apathy. Belching. Catalepsy. Eruptions. Headaches. Memory weak. Neuralgias. Paralysis. Pollutions. Salivation. Subsultus tendinum. Tongue, paralysis. Twitching. Vomiting.

HOMEOPATHIC - The main symptoms of Aconitine are reproduced in Acon-c. It has been used for headaches with vertigo and tinnitus. Also cataleptic symptoms, formication of tongue, lips and face. Subsultus tendinum. Twitching.

Aconitum cammarum has formication that begins on the tongue and lips and spreads to the face and finally over the whole body, with this there is distortion of features and dry skin. Headache, worse from bending the body forward. Face pain accompanied by tinnitus aurium and vertigo.

Walking causes weariness and, if continued, causes pains in elbows, knees and hips. Violent belchings, inclination to vomit without vomiting, spasmodic contraction of stomach and abdominal muscles.

Great sensitiveness to light. Erections and pollutions without voluptuous dreams. Small papules and vesicles on lower limbs, filled with serous fluid, very painful. Memory weakened, sense of touch diminished.

MIND - Apathy and indifference. Thought and power of concentration disturbed. Memory weak. Rage. Fear.

Abdomen - Burning in abdomen and sensation of ants crawling around in it.

Face - Black and blue color of face, blue swollen lips. Most remarkable sensation contraction of face.

Heart - The pulse is frequent, afterwards depressed, slow, irregular and intermittent.

Mouth - Paralysis of tongue. Salivation. Fuzzy sensation where the crawling was. Taste and sensation diminished.

Throat - Voice hoarse and rough. Respiration slow, difficult with sensation as if chest and throat constricted.

REFERENCES - Boericke. Clarke.

ACONITUM FEROX

(Himalayan Aconite)

PHARMACY - acon-f. Aconitum ferox. Himalayan Aconite. Indian Aconite. Aconitum heterophyllum. Bisch. Bikh. Ativisha. N. O. Ranunculacee. Himalayas, most poisonous species. Tincture of root. ***Historical dose:*** All potencies.

CLINICAL - Anxiety. Burning pains. Cheyne-Stokes. Chill. Dyspnea. Gastralgia. Neuralgia. Numbness.

HOMEOPATHIC - Aconitum ferox is the most poisonous species known, containing the greatest proportion of Aconitine from the Himalayan Mountains. Rather more violent in its actions than Acon. napellus.

Acon-f. was proved by Dworzack, who also proved Aconitine. The Ferox developed burning pains in greater intensity than the alkaloid, more intense mental activity followed by greater depression. It is more diuretic and less anti-pyretic (fever).

In Aconitum ferox, there was marked suffering. Anxiety and fear of suffocation from paralysis of respiratory muscles, obliged to breathe half-sitting up with head resting on palms of hands. Rapid respiration. Cheyne-Stokes breathing. Cardia dyspnea, neuralgia and acute gout. Dyspnea. Pain in occiput and neck.

MIND - Very active mind, sequence of ideas rapid, talked constantly, remembered easily. Incapable of any mental work, even the simplest addition, comprehension and understanding became confused.

Abdomen - Rumbling in bowels, constant gurgling.

Kidneys - Frequent and very copious evacuations of urine

Limbs - Gait tottering, remarkable weakness in lower limbs, especially right.

Lungs - Dyspnea increased to such a degree that he was obliged to breathe half-sitting up with head resting on palms of hands, constantly feared suffocation from respiratory paralysis.

Modalities - Better cold drinks. Better sitting up. Better warm food. Worse coffee.

Mouth - Tongue almost insensible, feels like a piece of raw leather in month. Tongue covered with a thick yellowish-white fur. Violent burning in mouth (in two minutes), renewed by eating, better by drinking cold water.

Rectum - Two half-watery, dark, not copious stools.

Sleep - Sleeplessness. On waking, violent burning in mouth and throat, warmth in stomach, dull sensation in head.

Stomach - Pressure in stomach with pain. Warmth in stomach. Violent drawing pain in region of stomach and sacral region, soon spreading over the abdomen, worse by pressure on epigastrium. On pressing in stomach, an internal, dull pressing pain.

Temperature - Icy coldness of body, objective and subjective, no amount of wraps and external warmth relieved. Desire to get warm drove him to get out of bed and sit near stove. Tottered to stove, warmth was pleasant, but vertigo, trembling, oppression and nausea ensued and compelled him to return to bed. Fierce heat on forehead, cheek and hands with sensation as if numerous glowing hot wires were stuck into him, better by perspiration.

Throat - Violent burning in pharynx.

COMMENTS - The proving caused a formication that spread over whole body, least noticeable on parts that had been cold. Worse or excited by, change of temperature or motion. It caused a painful unrest so that he could not possibly lie quietly more than a few minutes.

Getting up set up all the train of symptoms, which were better immediately on lying down. Benumbed sensation, as if he had on gloves, on pinching cheeks no pain felt, seemed to walk on woolen carpets.

RELATIONS - ***Compare:*** (1) Curare and Phos. have similar lung paralysis. (2) Achyranthes - Cheyne-Stokes breathing. (3) Eranthis hymnalis, Winter Aconite acts on solar plexus and works upwards causing dyspnea.

REFERENCES - Clarke.

ACONITUM LYCOCTONUM

(Great Yellow Wolfsbane)

PHARMACY - acon-l. Aconitum lycoctonum. Great yellow wolfsbane. Aconitum telyphonum. Badgers bane. N. O. Ranunculacee. Tincture of fresh plant when coming into bloom. The only aconite which does not contain Aconitine. ***Historical dose:*** All potencies.

CLINICAL - Allergies. Constipation. Coughs. Diarrhea. Glands, enlargement. Hodgkin's disease. Liver disorders. Mastitis. Pork, effects. Strangury.

HOMEOPATHIC - The symptoms of Acon. lycoctonum, while resembling those of the other Aconites in some respects, show a marked absence of the cutaneous nerve disorders so prominent in their provings.

Swelling of the cervical, axillary glands and breasts. Clarke has used it with good effect in cases of scrofulous glands and even where Hodgkin's disease has been suspected.

Itching of eyes, nose, anus, and vulva. The skin of the nose is cracked. There is a cough leaving a taste of blood in the mouth. Diarrhea after eating pork.

MIND - Anxiety. Distraction. Dread of work. Instability of ideas. Laughter. Mania. Ferocity.

Abdomen - Right hypochondrium has bruised pain, tearing pain, starting. When breathing both hypochondria feel bruised. Sensation of compression in diaphragm. Anxiety, with beatings in abdomen. Sharp pain after drinking milk.

Back - Swelling of the cervical glands. The neck seems to grow larger. Swelling of the neck on one side only. Pressing pain at the nape of the neck. Shivering in the back. Jerking in the region of the kidneys.

Breasts - Swelling of the breast glands.

Ears - Purulent discharge from ears, redness behind them.

Eyes - Sharp pain in eyes from without inward. Painfulness of lids. Itching in lids. Pressure on lids and difficulty of raising them. Smarting in canthi, dryness at inner canthus.

Face - Face pale, shining. Pain of excoriation around mouth. Pain in facial bones. Tension in facial muscles. Hard pimples of face and lips. Skin of face becomes light brown. Numbness of jaw like incipient paralysis, better by compression and by drinking wine.

Female - Itching at vulva. Fetid menstrual blood. Excoriation of bend of thigh after menses. Leucorrhea, viscid.

Food - Strong relish for dainties, fruits, and cabbage. Increased relish for tobacco in a smoker. Aversion to food in general, especially fatty things and milk, they cause uneasiness. Keen hunger very soon satisfied. Constant thirst even when drinking. Burning thirst. Thirst at night.

Head - Sharp pain in head extending across eyes. Sensation as if a nail were driven into head when moving it. Hammering in temples. Pain like rheumatism in scalp worse by touch.

Kidneys - Desire to urinate with copious emissions. Urging with ineffectual efforts. Hot, turbid urine, depositing a white sediment.

Limbs - On stretching legs, hamstrings feel as if shortened. Jerking in legs. Itching at ankles in evening. Sharp pain at instep when standing. Eruption of hot, red, slightly painful spots on legs and toes. Swelling of axillary glands. Pressure, sharp pains in shoulder joints. Tearing pain in elbow joints. Stiffness in elbows and wrists. Sensation of fullness in hands. Sweat on hands.

Modalities - Worse in afternoon (Lyc.), Better mental exertion. Better after wine. Better during digestion, especially of pork and onions.

Lungs - Difficult respiration. Slight cough with watery expectoration. After a slight chill, leaving a taste of blood in the mouth.

Mouth - Clayey, astringent taste.

Nose - Itching on nose, sensitiveness, lancinations. Compression at root of nose. Skin of nose cracked. Muco-purulent discharge from nose.

Rectum - Constipation, anus feels as if strongly contracted. Diarrhea with violent cutting after eating pork. Whitish stools. After stool, pain in anus as if there was a crack there, shivering. Cramp at anus. Itching at anus. Tenesmus during night.

Sleep - Drowsiness, he sleeps too long. Aberration of hearing during sleep. During sleep, numbness of the parts he lies on.

Stomach - Painful belchings. Belchings are rancid like rotten eggs, acid, with weight on stomach. Hiccough. Inclination to vomit after eating with shivering, vertigo. Vomiting of mucus on getting out of bed, yellowish after drinking with copious urination.

Teeth - Burning pain in upper teeth. Pressing in teeth. Tearing in lower teeth when opening mouth. Gums bluish, ulcerated.

Temperature - Goose bumps. Chilliness of one side only as soon as he is uncovered. In morning external coldness with feeling of heat. Coldness alternating with heat, succeeded by sweat. During fever, pale face, strong appetite, thirst, pain in bowels, restlessness. Sweat continues after fever.

Vertigo - Vertigo with nausea.

RELATIONS - ***Compare:*** (1) Cist, Lap-a., Con., Iod., Spong., Lyc., Carb-an. (2) Puls. in bad effects of pork.

REFERENCES - Boericke. Clarke.

ACONITUM NAPELLUS
(Monkshood)

PHARMACY - acon. Aconitum napellus. Monkshood. Wolfsbane. Common Aconite. Aconitum virosum. N. O. Ranunculacee. Tincture of whole plant with root when beginning to flower. ***Historical dose:*** All potencies.

CLINICAL - Amaurosis. Amenorrhea. Anger. ***Anxiety.*** Asthma. Blindness. Breast-feeding, disorders. Bronchitis. Catalepsy. Catheter, fever. Chickenpox. ***Chills.*** Cholera. Cholera infantum. ***Colds.*** Colic. Conjunctivitis. Convulsions. Cough. ***Croup.*** Cystitis. Dengue fever. Dentition. Diarrhea. Dropsy. Dyspepsia. Dysentery. Dysmenorrhea. Ear, disorders. Enteritis. Erythema. Esophagitis. Eye, disorders. Face, flushing. ***Fears. Fevers. Fright, effects.*** Glossitis. Gonorrhea. Headaches. ***Heart, attack.*** Heart, disorders. Hemorrhages. Hemorrhoid. Hip joint, disease. Hodgkin's disease. ***Influenza.*** Jaundice. Labor, pains. Laryngitis. Lumbago. Lungs disorders. Mania. Mastitis. Measles. Meningitis. Menstruation, disorders. Milk leg. Miscarriage. Mumps. Muscle, pains. Myelitis. Nephritis. ***Nervousness.*** Neuralgias. ***Nightmares.*** Numbness. ***Otitis media. Palpitations. Panic, attacks.*** Paralysis. Peritonitis. Pleurisy, pain. Pneumonia. Puerperal fever. ***Purpura miliaris***. Quinsy. Remittent, fever. Roseola. Scarlatina. ***Shock.*** Sleeplessness. Stiff-neck. Strokes. ***Tachycardia***. Tetanus. Tetany. Throat, disorders. Tingling. Tongue, disorders. Toothache. ***Traumatic, fever.*** Tuberculosis. Urethra, stricture. Urethritis. ***Urine, retention.*** Uterus, prolapsed. Vaccination, effects. Vertigo. Whooping, cough. Yellow fever.

HOMEOPATHIC - Acon. is useful in emergencies and acute diseases. It grows up in the high mountains where there is a lot of wind, storms and activity. Complaints and tension caused by ***exposure to dry, cold weather, winds***, draft of cold air, or checked perspiration. Marked affect on the serous membranes and muscular tissue. Major remedy for inflammation and fevers. A state of ***fear, shock, anxiety***, anguish of mind and body. ***Physical and mental restlessness***.

Acute, sudden and violent illness with high fever. Rapid action, symptoms set in with great intensity, specifically heart attacks, influenza, certain fevers and acute inflammations. Attacks of sudden fear, anxiety and even blindness. Sudden and great sinking of strength. Sudden chills or fever.

Ailments of immune system, especially if caused by suddenly checked sweat or by dry cold air, storms or cold winds. Painful, hot, swollen glands. Neuritis with tingling. ***Influenza and colds.***

Complaints from very ***hot weather***, especially summer diarrhea. Localized blood congestions and inflammations. Tension of arteries, emotional and physical tension. Burning in internal parts. ***Tingling, coldness and numbness***. Does not want to be touched.

Muscular rheumatism with high fever. Joint rheumatism, much fever, restlessness and anxiety. Swellings are red and hot (Bell.), or pale, shifting from one point to another. Shooting, cramps, cracking, loss of power, and drawing pain in joints and tendons.

MIND - ***Mental and emotional shocks.*** Never well since a fright or shock. ***Ailments from fright.*** Fear of death and dying, great anxiety. ***Nightmares, phobias, panic attacks.*** Nightmares after horror stories or movies. Tendency to be startled. Fright followed by panic and shock.

Complaints come suddenly and with great intensity, often with an overwhelming fear of death. ***Great fear, anxiety and restlessness*** accompany every ailment. ***Fears the future***. Panic and anxiety. ***Fear of death.*** Believes that he will soon die, predicts the day. ***Anxiety about heart.***

Forebodings and fears. Panic attacks with restlessness. Agoraphobia. Afraid to go out of the house. Fears a crowds, crossing busy streets. ***Terror stricken.*** Fears of public speaking. Fear of narrow places. ***Fears of going to doctors and dentists***. Anticipation. Fear of the dark. Fear of ghosts.

Oversensitive to pain. Pains are intolerable, drive him crazy. ***Despair from the pains.*** Impatient, beside himself from intensity of pain. Reproaches others for mere trifles.

Inconsolable anxiety. Ailments from anger, from chagrin, child has spells of rage. Desires company. Ideas haunt him, can't get rid of them. Confusion, as after drunkenness. Stupefaction alternating with restlessness.

Delirium and high fever with anxiety, worry, fear and desperation. Nocturnal delirium. Desire for light. ***Restlessness and tossing about.*** Loquacity, speech hurried. Fitful moods, laughing, singing, then sad and fearful. Mania to ridicule.

Music is unbearable, makes her sad (Ambr.). Imagination acute. Clairvoyance. Thinks his thoughts come from the stomach. Thinks that parts of his body are abnormally thick. Feels as if what had just been done was a dream.

Abdomen - ***Colic, forces to bend double, yet no position relieves.*** Wind colic after taking cold. Hot, tense, tympanitic. ***Sensitive to touch.*** Abdominal symptoms better after warm soup. Burning in umbilical region. Hot distended. Incarcerated hernia with bilious vomiting. Burning and cutting pains in intestines. Intestines as if paralyzed, inactive, worse about transverse colon. Loins as if bruised. Burning pain in umbilical region. Umbilical region hard, swollen.

Back - Chilliness and formication down back. Numb, stiff, painful. Numbness in lumbar region. Crawling and tingling, as if bruised. Stiffness in nape of neck. Pain in the back, prevents taking deep inspiration. Bruised pain between shoulders and in sacrum. Burning, shooting pain in spine. Sharp pain between scapulae, on deep breathing. Slightest touch of spine causes spasms. Spinal meningitis after injury or checked sweat.

Bladder - Cystitis. Burning pain in urethra. Hematuria. Urethral chill. Urine suppressed, bloody. Anxiety always on beginning to urinate. Urination painful, difficult, drop by drop. ***Retention with screaming and restlessness*** and handling of genitals. Retention or suppression of urine in newborn due to cold exposure. ***Retention of urine after childbirth.*** Splashing sensation in region of bladder, during urination. Tenesmus and burning at neck of bladder.

Breasts - Mastitis. Milk fever with delirium. Increase of milk in breast. Breasts hot. Milk scanty.

Chest - Constant pressure in left chest. Violent congestion of blood in the chest. Oppression of the chest when moving fast or ascending in heart disease. Blood comes up on hawking. Sharp pain in chest. Lancinating pain through chest. Tingling in chest after coughing. Pressive weight and burning under sternum.

Constitutions - Children. Plethoric persons of a lively character, bilious and nervous constitutions, high color, brown or black hair, are specially suited to Acon. Persons leading a sedentary life, plethora, etc.

Cough - Cough with nervous excitability. ***Hoarse, dry, croupy cough***, loud, labored breathing. Cough better lying on back. Cough from walking in open air. Child grasps at throat every time he coughs. Cough, dry, short, hacking. ***Cough worse at night and after midnight***. Short, barking, ringing or whistling cough, worse every inspiration, at night. Loud, rough, croaking cough, on expiration. Croupy, dry, coarse, suffocating cough. Hemoptysis from mental excitement, wine or exposure to dry, cold air. Cough from tobacco smoke. Cough awakening from sleep. Cough worse after taking cold, drinking cold water.

Ears - ***Otitis media.*** External ear hot, red, painful, swollen (Bell.). ***Earache with pain*** (Bell., Cham.). Tickling and sharp pain in the ears. Tingling and buzzing in the ears. Sensation as if drop of water in left ear. Ringing, humming or roaring noises. ***Sensitive to noises, music is unbearable.*** Left ear deaf, with buzzing in whole head.

Eyes - Red, inflamed. Bloodshot. ***Pain and inflammation after surgery. Injuries to eyes.*** Conjunctivitis. Inflammation from foreign bodies, dust, cinders. Ingrowing eyelashes. Eyes glitter, stare, watery. ***Eyes feels dry and hot***. Shooting pain in eyeballs. Sensation as if sand in eyes. Swelling of the eyes. ***Eyelids swollen, hard and red***. Aversion to light. Can't bear reflection of sun from snow. Profuse watering from ***reflection of snow.*** Profuse lachrymation after exposure to dry, cold winds. Asthenopia from straining eyes. Pupils contracted then dilated.

Face - ***Anxious*** expression. Hippocratic. Face red, hot, flushed, swollen. Pale alternating with red. Burning, lips and tongue, as after eating pepper or smoking. Lips black, dry, peeling off. One cheek red hot other pale and cold (Cham., Ip.). ***Neuralgia, especially on left side with restlessness.*** Tingling, cheeks and numbness. ***Tingling and numbness***. Heavy feeling of the whole face. Sweat on side of face lain on. ***On rising, the red face becomes deathly pale.*** Jaw, pain.

Female - Dysmenorrhea has to bend double, but better in no position. Menses too profuse. Menses with nosebleed. Menses too protracted, late. Frenzy, fury on appearance of menses. Amenorrhea during puberty. ***Suppressed menses from fright, cold***. Ovaritis from sudden checked menstrual flow. Ovaries congested and painful. ***Impending miscarriage from fright or vexation.*** Active uterine hemorrhage. Sharp, shooting pains in uterus. Prolapsed uterus. Labor-pains violent. ***After-pains with fear and restlessness.*** Suppressed lochia. Leucorrhea copious, tenacious, yellowish. Vagina dry, hot, sensitive.

Food - ***Excessive hunger and thirst,*** but eats slowly. Lively sensation of hunger, renewed soon after eating. No appetite, loathing of food, qualmishness. Aversion to tobacco. Better warm soup. Better wine. Anxiety better cold drinks. ***Desires beer, wine.*** Desires brandy, bitter drinks. Worse after iced cold drinks. Milk disagrees. ***Intense thirst***. Thirst for cold water. ***Thirst burning, unquenchable, during all stages of fever.*** Thirst for beer during fever. Thirsty during labor. Everything tastes bitter, except water.

Head - Fullness, pulsating. ***Hot, heavy, bursting sensation***. Burning, undulating sensation. Head excessively hot. ***Congestive headaches.*** Intercranial pressure (Hed.). Burning headache, as if brain were moved by boiling water (Indg.). Violent squeezing or bursting pain in forehead. Pulsation in forehead. Sensation on vertex as if hair were pulled or stood on end. Nocturnal furious delirium. Meningitis. Brain affections of children. Formication of scalp better heat. Scalp sensitive to touch. Scalp sensitive to cold air, strong wind. Sunstroke from sleeping in rays of sun.

Heart - Heart feels swollen. Hypertrophy of heart. ***Heart attacks with anxiety and fear.*** Dreadful oppression and anxiety about heart. Oppression about heart with burning flushes along back. Heart pains into left shoulder, worse sitting erect. ***Tachycardia***. ***Palpitations with anxiety, after fright.*** Palpitations fainting and tingling in fingers, pain down left arm. ***Palpitations during fever.*** Palpitations from motion, on waking. Palpitations from smoking. Arterial tension. Temporal and carotid arteries felt when sitting. ***Pulse fast, full, hard, tense and bounding***. Pulse quicker than heartbeat. Pulse sometimes intermits. Pulse shaking, forcible and tumultuous. Pulse wiry, very irritable.

Kidneys - Anxiety on beginning to urinate. Sharp pains in region of kidneys. Stinging and pressing, in renal region. ***Scanty, red, hot, painful urine***. Kidney region sensitive with shooting pains. Profuse urination with profuse perspiration and diarrhea. Agonizing dysuria. Profuse urination with profuse sweat and diarrhea. Diuresis with headache or profuse sweat. Brown, burning urine, with brick-colored sediment. Urine fiery, scalding hot, red or dark-colored.

Limbs - ***Numbness and tingling***. Numbness of the left arm, tingling in fingers. Shooting pains. Icy coldness and insensibility of hands and feet. Arms feel lame, bruised, heavy, and numb. Arms hang down limp. Red finger tips (Cact. Crot-h., Kalm., Tab.). ***Hot hands and cold feet***. Twitching of fingers and toes. Rheumatic inflammation of joints, worse at night. Red, shining swelling, very sensitive joints. Legs powerless, feel tired during repose. Hip joint and thigh feel lame, especially after lying down. Knees unsteady, disposition of foot to turn (Aesc.). Weak and lax ligaments of all joints. Painless cracking of all joints. ***Bright red hypothenar eminences on both hands***. Sensation as if drops of water trickled down the thigh. Jerking of left or arm. Palms hot. Sharp pains in inflamed joints. Trembling.

Liver - Pressure in the region of the liver, with obstruction of breathing. Burning pain, shooting, stinging and pressure in the liver region, with difficult respiration. Painful sensibility to touch in the region of the liver. Jaundice in newborn children. Jaundice from fright.

Lungs - Asthma after suppression of acute rash. Asthma from active hyperemia of lungs and brain. Hot feeling in lungs. Awaking with danger of suffocation, from tickling in throat. Anxious breathing hard, sits erect. ***Oppressed breathing on least motion***. Agony, sits straight up, can hardly breathe. Deep, slow, sighing. Very sensitive to inspired air. ***Shortness of breath***. Shortness of breath during sleep. Pleurisy. Stitches through chest. ***Croup with fever.*** Sensation as if lungs will not expand. ***Bronchitis. Pneumonia.*** Rusty, thin, frothy, white mucus streaked with bright blood. Sputum absent. Scanty expectoration, falls in round lumps, dark cherry-red, in pneumonia. Blood comes up with hawking. Thin, gelatinous sputum, worse mornings and during day.

Male - Crawling and stinging in glans penis. Orchitis, testicles feel swollen and hard. Bruised pain in testicles, swollen, hard. Stinging and crawling in glans. Scrotum drawn up. Skin of left side of scrotum studded with minute vesicles, with a humid discharge. Frequent erections and emissions. Painful erections. Sexual desire decreased, with relaxed parts, tingling in parts. Fits of lasciviousness. Emissions even after sex.

Modalities - Better in open air. Better from rest. Better warm sweat. Better wine. Better sitting still. ***Worse from fright, shock.*** Worse violent emotions, shock and vexation. ***Worse from being chilled by cold winds. Worse dry weather***. Worse sleeping in the sun. Worse warm room. Worse evening. ***Worse at night***. Worse while sweating, Worse pressure, touch. Worse lying on affected side. Worse getting into bed. Worse noise, music. Worse tobacco smoke. Worse inspiration. Worse light. Worse dentition. Worse during menses.

Mouth - Burning, biting pain in mouth. ***Numb, dry and tingling.*** Lips black, dry, peeling off. Tingling, numbness, burning of lips. Tingling on coughing and swallowing. ***Gums hot and inflamed.*** Everything tastes bitter except water, which has bad taste. Trembling and temporary stammering. Dry burning heat in mouth.

Mouth - Breath cold, in cholera. Breath hot. Orifices of salivary ducts sore, as if corroded. Accumulation of water in mouth. Saliva generally diminished. Saliva frothy, streaked red, sweetish. Trembling and temporary stammering.

Nose - Frequent sneezing. Coryza, much sneezing, throbbing in nostrils. Coryza with headache, roaring in ears, fever, sleeplessness. Hot water runs from nose. ***Pain at root of nose***. Hemorrhage of bright red blood. ***Mucus membrane dry.*** Posterior nares as if dry. ***Nose stopped up, dry or with but scanty watery coryza.*** Numbness with nosebleed. Nosebleed, bright red blood. ***Smell acutely sensitive.***

Perspiration - Bad effects from suppressed sweat. Profuse sweat, wants to uncover. Sweat on uncovered parts or affected parts. ***Sweat on parts lain on.*** Cold or sour sweat. Cold sweat and icy coldness of face. Drenching sweats. Profuse sweat with copious flow of urine and diarrhea.

Rectum - Pain with nightly itching and stitching in anus. ***Cholera.*** Frequent, small stool with tenesmus. Cholera discharges with collapse, anxiety and restlessness. Constipation. Bleeding hemorrhoids (Ham.). Itching and sticking at anus. Sensation as if a warm fluid escaping from the anus. Pain from seatworms.

Skin - Red, hot, swollen, dry, burning. Miliary eruptions. ***Itching relieved by stimulants.*** Itching unchanged by scratching. Rash like measles. ***Purpura miliaris***. Goosebumps. Formication and numbness. Papular erythema. Erythema from sun's rays. ***Dry, hot skin.*** Skin as if ice water on it. Rash of children. Spots like flea-bites.

Sleep - Starting up in sleep. Sleeplessness with restless and tossing about. ***Sleeplessness caused by fear, fright or anxiety.*** Sleeplessness with fear of the future. Nightly ravings. Insomnia of the elderly. ***Children cry and complain, sleepless and restless (Ars., Cham.).*** Spasmodic yawning. Nightmares. ***Anxious dreams.*** Dreams caused by fear, fright or anxiety. Long dreams with anxiety in chest. Vivid dreams of day's occurrences.

Stomach - Pressure in stomach with dyspnea. Burning from stomach to esophagus. Tension in stomach better eructations. Painful hiccough. Nausea and sweating before and after loose stool. Projectile vomiting. Drinks, vomits and declares he will die. Vomiting of clear water, on sitting up. ***Vomiting with fear, heat, profuse sweat and increased urination***. Hematemesis. Vomiting, bilious, mucus and bloody, greenish. Vomiting of lumbrici.

Stools - Bilious diarrhea of infants with colic. Diarrhea from getting wet. Slimy stools alternating with constipation. Clay-colored stools. Involuntary stools, on passing flatus. White stools with red urine. ***Stools of pure blood.*** Slimy, grass green or white stools, worse hot days and cold nights. ***Green stools like chopped herbs***. Frequent, small stool with tenesmus. Dysentery. Watery diarrhea in children on hot days, restless and sleepless.

Teeth - Toothache from cold or dry, cold winds. ***Teeth sensitive to cold.*** Toothache in sound teeth. Throbbing in teeth and head. Grinding of the teeth. ***Gums hot and inflamed.*** Constantly moves lower jaw as if chewing. Sensation as if teeth would fall out. Cold feeling in incisors.

Temperature - Cold stage most marked. Coldness and heat alternate. Evening chilliness soon after going to bed. ***Cold waves pass through him.*** Chills down back. Chill passes through him in waves. Chill or coldness alternating with heat. Chilly if uncovered or touched. Shivering ascends from feet to chest. Dry burning heat in eyelids, nose, mouth, throat, lungs and palms, must uncover. ***High fevers.*** Dry burning heat, red face. Fevers with mental anguish, restlessness. ***Thirst and restlessness***.

Throat - ***Acute inflammation of the throat with high fever.*** Dark redness of throat. Chokes on swallowing, talking. Tingling in the esophagus. ***Burning and stinging pains***. Stinging pain in throat when swallowing. Scraping, tingling sensation of strangling, burning and pricking in the throat. ***Red, dry, constricted***. Numbness and prickling. Sensation of contraction in the throat. Inability to swallow, with hoarseness. ***Hoarseness with pain when talking.*** Hoarseness after speaking or singing. Voice husky, can scarcely speak. Croup with fever. Croaking voice. Laryngitis with fever. Larynx very sensitive. Uvula as if elongated. Tonsillitis. Tonsils dark red. Tonsils swollen and dry.

Tongue - Burning vesicles on tip of tongue. Tongue feels as if swollen. ***Tongue coated white*** (Ant-c.). Tongue coated thick yellow white. Tongue swollen. ***Tongue tip tingles***. Middle of tongue as if dry and numb. Sensation as if cold air passing over tongue. Tongue dry, red on sides, centre thinly coated white. Tongue red and dry.

Vertigo - ***Vertigo, worse on rising*** (Nux-v. Op.), and shaking head. Vertigo on rising from bed. Vertigo on getting up from one's seat. Vertigo on stooping or moving. Sensation of intoxication or dizziness in the head, loss of consciousness. Vertigo with inclination to fail to right side. Vertigo with nausea and vanishing of sight. Vertigo from fright, anger. Vertigo after a shock. Vertigo from heat of sun.

Vision - Dim vision or vision entirely lost. ***Lost vision after fright or shock.*** Optical illusions in dark colors or black. Flickerings make him anxious, fears he might touch people passing by. Total blindness after catching cold. Sparks, with burning and twitching in eyes. Obscuration of vision, when shaking head. Black spots and mist before the eyes.

COMMENTS - Aconite is a tall, upright plant that has dark blue flowers, 4-5 feet tall. Acon. grows in the damp and covered parts of almost every mountainous country in north or middle of Europe, especially in Switzerland, Germany and Sweden. It grows in high altitudes where there is a lot of wind, storms and activity.

It is a very poisonous herb, vinegar in large doses is antidotal to the toxic effects. Aconite in potencies above the 4c is a perfectly safe medicine for any age.

Before Hahnemann's time Aconite had a reputation as a sudorific and in cases of rheumatism, sciatica and tumors, but it was not until Hahnemann proved it that its properties were really understood. Aconite was the remedy by means of which Hahnemann was able to meet most of the conditions, which in his day were treated by bloodletting.

Dr. Hughes has remarked that the condition to which Acon. is homeopathic is one of tension. Emotional and mental tension, as shown in fright or fear and its consequences, anxiety and fear of death, tension of the systemic vessels, as in the effects of a chill.

Asiatic cholera and hemorrhages. Muscular tension, as in tetanus. Tension of involuntary muscles, as in heart spasms. Tension of the semi-involuntary muscular apparatus of respiration, as in asthma.

Hahnemann described it as a tempest, Kent, too. This is the idea of the remedy, it's a storm that has a sudden onset and a sudden dissipation. Keynote sudden onset, a major trigger for this is shocking fright. Violent reactions to fright or weather conditions.

Teste related a remarkable case of an Englishman who had been obliged to take a long sleigh journey in North Russia in midwinter. He suffered thereafter for two years from violent paroxysms of palpitations and acute stitching pains in the heart region, threatening brain strokes.

Aneurysm had been diagnosed by leading physicians in England and on the Continent. Teste localized the affection to neurosis or spasm of the pectoralis major muscle and proved his diagnosis by promptly curing it with Acon.

Chill and fever. Fevers with restlessness and tossing about, often accompanied with anxiety that sometimes leads to fear of death. Acon. can ward off serious results from chill, fright, injury or surgical operation.

It was the feverish restlessness of the Acon. provings that led Hahnemann to infer its similarity to fever states. It is the presence of this restlessness, anxiety, fear and exalted sensibility that are its leading indications in cases of all kinds.

High fevers, sudden surges of body temperature. Inflammatory fevers (Bell. is also inflammatory, Pyrog. and Bapt. are septic). Fevers with wakefulness, anxiety, red and flushed.

"Clean" and functional fevers, no tissue changes, no mucus, no toxic symptoms. Can have thirst with the fever. The skin is dry and hot.

The four keynotes are fear, fright, fast, and fevers. It's a remedy for a lot of fears (Ars.) and any acute problems. Fright followed by speechlessness or shaky trembling speech, shaking of the hands and limbs, dilated pupils, and the patient may be frozen with fear and shaking.

Panic with shaking and trembling. Frail, faint, and anxious. Sudden surges of adrenaline through the body leading to shaking, trembling, fear, panic. Panic attacks with numbness and tingling of fingers or down the arms, in the extremities. Attacks with feeling of anxiety, heart palpitations, fainting. Fear, not that they're going to die (Ars.), but that they're dying right now.

Conditions after fright. Hypersensitivity after a near death situation. Fright leading to shock and panic. Fainting and heart attacks where the main feature is fear.

Fear and apprehension. Dread of crossing streets. Fear of the dark, fear of ghosts. Good for agoraphobia, fear of going outside of the house. They have chronic fears of fatal disasters, fear that something will happen, that they can't go out of the house because they will get into an accident.

The senses are heightened with sensitiveness to pain and a feeling of numbness in parts. Sensation as if bound tightly in the limbs and in other parts (Cact.). Plethora may be classed under increased blood tension. Active, bloody congestions of all kinds, especially those following a chill.

Intolerance to music. Patients may imagine some part of body is deformed, imagine they do all their thinking from the stomach and predict the hour of their death. They sometimes go so far as to predict the day and hour of death (clairvoyance). Extreme sensitiveness to light and sound and all sensations.

Extreme sensitivity to pain (Cham., Coff.). Pains are intolerable, driving to desperation. Tearing, cutting, burning, sharp, stabbing pains, with restlessness, accompanied by numbness, tingling or formication.

Cannot bear the pain, cannot bear to be touched, cannot bear to be covered. Burning pains (Phos.). Feel the blood rushing everywhere. The child or the person screams with pain. Pain causes fright, specifically from heart attack or any acute pain. Frozen from the pain and what that pain means.

Bending double relieves the colic and dysmenorrhea pain (Coloc.). Motion aggravates the pains in muscles, joints and stiffness. There is a great and sudden sinking of strength, fainting on attempting to get up, with anxiety, restlessness, numbness, tingling, formication.

Hemorrhage and shock due to sudden hemorrhaging of bright blood, causing giddiness, faintness, panic (Acon., Bell., Phos.). Active hemorrhages in stout, full-blooded people. Passes almost pure blood in stool. In hemoptysis the blood comes up with great ease by hemming and coughing, bright red in large quantities from cold, dry winds. Bleeding with great fear, anxiety and palpitations.

Toothaches are one-sided with red cheek on same side. Severe toothaches where the teeth are sensitive, painful and the person is in a panic.

Inflammations of the eyes from cold, injury, foreign objects, dust, surgical operations, scrofulous inflammation with enlarged glands. Blindness.

Hirsch of Prague recorded two such cases, one in a man of thirty who went to bed well, having walked home in rough and stormy weather after spending the evening in a hot room. Acon. 3c was given and the following night he perspired freely and in the morning his sight was restored.

Hirsch himself suddenly lost his sight while bathing in hot weather. He took Acon. 3c in water as he had given it to his patient. In two hours he began to perspire and after a six-hours' sleep awoke well.

Every inspiration increases the cough. Tingling sensation in the chest after coughing. Unquenchable thirst, everything tastes bitter except water (Chin.). In croup, the child grasps the throat with every coughing fit. Dry, hacking cough especially from being exposed to a dry, cold wind

Worse exposed to hot weather or cold weather. Coldness, numbness and tingling characterize the paralyzes and neuroses. Facial paralysis from exposure to cold, dry winds. Sunstroke. Diarrhea from heat and sun exposure.

Headaches caused by exposure to the sun, also heat rashes. Headaches are generally better in open air, worse in warm room, toothache and cough worse in open air. Better from uncovering, the bed is intolerable. Worse chill with fever. Sweat on affected or covered parts.

After exposure to cold, croup, severe colds and respiratory problems, bronchitis, infants get pneumonia, and it can go to facial paralysis. Worse cold, dry wind, sudden onset, numbness and tingling of the limbs all keynotes of Aconite. Chills with ailments. Asthma from exposure to cold, dry weather that brings out panic, worse around midnight. Earaches from exposure to cold and wind.

In general for croup, heart attacks, acute bronchitis and colds, and tonsillitis. Sometimes strep throat. First aid for fright. Infantile pneumonia with sudden onset. Childhood diseases with fevers and restlessness, meningitis. Retention of the urine, especially in newborn infants.

Generally aggravated at night, particularly about midnight.

RELATIONS - Aconitum napellus is related in its action to the other Aconites and to Aconitinum, and also to the Ranunculacee, Act-r., Act-sp., Paeon., Podo., Ran-b., Staph. ***Antidoted by:*** Acet-ac., Alcohol, Paris. Acids, wine and coffee, lemonade and acid fruits modify its action. ***Antidotes:*** Cham., Bell., Coff., Spong., Petr., Nux-v., Sep., Sulph. ***Compare:*** (1) Similar to Ars., Bell., Calend., Ferr-p. (2) Cham. and Coffea intense pain and sleeplessness. (3) Agrostis acts like Acon. in fevers and in inflammations, also, Spiranthes. (4) Bapt. or Pyrogen in high fevers with sudden onset. (5) Puls., Lyc., Sec. and Camph. are also better from uncovering. (6) Cham., Hep. and Coff. - intolerance of pain. (7) Chin. - white stool. (8) Gels. - effects of bad news, fright, anger. (9) Nux-v. and Bry. - diarrhea from anger. (10) Bry. - effects of cold, dry winds. (11) Sulph. is the chronic of Acon., it will often complete an action that Acon. begins, and will cure cases in which Acon. is apparently indicated but fails to relieve. ***Complementary to:*** Coff. - in fever, sleeplessness, intolerance of pain. Arn. in bruises, Calend. injury to eye. Sulphur often completes a cure begun with Aconite. ***Follows well:*** Arn., Coff., Sulph., Verat.

REFERENCES - Boericke. Clarke. Murphy.

ACTEA SPICATA

(Baneberry)

PHARMACY - act-sp. Actea spicata. Baneberry. Herb Christopher. Radix christophoriana. N. O. Ranunculacee. Europe and Asia. Tincture of root obtained in autumn. ***Historical dose:*** Tincture and all potencies.

CLINICAL - ***Arthritis.*** Cancer, stomach. Fright, effects. Headaches. Hepatitis. Insomnia. ***Joint, pain.*** Pleurisy. ***Rheumatism.*** Toothache. ***Wrist, pain.***

HOMEOPATHIC - Rheumatism (Cimic.), particularly affecting the small joints and wrists (Caul.). ***Rheumatism of the wrist***, particularly the right wrist and arm. Joints are swollen and pains are worse by touch and movement. Slight fatigue causes swelling of the joints. Violent tearing, drawing and tingling pains. Pains are worse from touch and motion.

Rheumatism like pains in the face. Pains running from decayed tooth to temples. Symptoms are liable to appear from fright and fatigue. Shortness of breath on exposure to cold. Old age. Hypersensitive to cold, weakness. Paralytic weakness of affected part. Pulsations over whole body, especially liver and kidney region. Cardiovascular spasms. Hepatitis. Pleurisy.

MIND - Fearful, starts easily, confused. Fear of death, especially at night in bed. Furious delirium, also during the fever. Effects of exertion of mind, fright, or mental anxiety.

Abdomen - Spasmodic retraction. Sticking pain and distention of hypogastrium. Pain and tenderness in liver region.

Constitutions - Weak, nervous, cold sweat. Rheumatic diathesis. It is especially suited to men (Cimic. to women).

Ears - Twitching pain on sneezing or blowing the nose.

Eyes - Objects seem colored blue. Sharp pains through eyes into head.

Face - Violent pain in upper jaw, running from teeth through malar bones, to temples. Perspiration on face and head. The cheek he lies on sweats. Yellow around mouth. Lips are chapped. Submaxillary glands hurt when chewing.

Female - Menses suppressed by fright or cold.

Food - Hunger with aversion to food. More appetite in morning. Disgust for food. Shuddering after drinking.

Head - Rush of blood to head, excited by drinking coffee. Throbbing in brain. Pain from crown to between eyebrows, heat in forehead, pain in left frontal eminence as if bone were crushed. Itching of scalp alternating with heat. Warm sweat on head. Small pimples on scalp.

Heart - Urging sensation in heart towards abdomen and region of liver with great anxiety at night.

Kidneys - Throbbing in region of kidneys. Urine deposits a white sediment. Kidney stones.

Limbs - Tearing pains in loins. ***Rheumatic pains in small joints, wrist,*** fingers, ankles toes. ***Swelling in joints from slight fatigue. Wrist swollen***, red, worse any motion. Paralytic weakness in the hands. Lame feeling in arms. Pain in knee. Sudden lassitude after talking or eating.

Lungs - Short, irregular breathing at night, while lying. ***Great oppression. Shortness of breath on exposure to fresh air***. Difficult inspiration, stitches in the epigastrium.

Modalities - Worse from change of weather or temperature. Worse cold air. Worse night. Worse touch. Worse slight exertion. Worse fatigue and mental exertion.

Mouth - Increased salivation. Fetid odor.

Nose - Nose red at tip, fluent coryza.

Sleep - Obstinate insomnia, sleeplessness, unable to rest (Coff.).

Stomach - Tearing, darting pains in epigastric region with vomiting. Cramp-like pains in stomach and epigastrium with difficult breathing. Sudden lassitude after eating. Sour vomiting. Cancer of the stomach with tearing, drawing pains.

Temperature - Shuddering after drinking. Shuddering followed by fever during which vomiting supervenes. Belching during the chill.

Throat - Throat sore when speaking, when breathing cold air.

Vertigo - Dizziness, forehead feels empty when stooping. Vertigo with tearing headache, better in open air.

COMMENTS - Rheumatism, arthritis, osteoarthritis. Rheumatoid arthritis, arthritis of the small joints, wrists, fingers and toes (Caul.). Rheumatism, weakness, trembling, spasmodic action of muscles. Epileptic and hysterical convulsions. Sharp pains in various parts. Pains come on suddenly, pains like electric shocks.

Boericke said, "Rheumatic remedy of the small joints and specific for wrist rheumatism." "Worse touch and motion" and "oppression of the chest and shortness of breath."

Grimmer wrote that it had been successfully used in cancer of the stomach. Sour vomiting after drinking with tearing, darting pains in epigastric region. Increased salivation, fetid odor from mouth.

Vertigo, fear of death, especially when in bed at night. Furious delirium, also during fever, mental anxiety. Bad effects from fatigue and fright.

RELATIONS - ***Compare:*** (1) Cimic., Caul., Led. (2) Other Ranunculacee, Arn., Bry. (3) Caul. - Rheumatism of fingers. (4) Lyc., Rhus t., Ruta, Sal-ac., and Stict. - Small joints. ***Complementary:*** Caul., Coloc., Sabin., Stict., Viol-o.

REFERENCES - Boericke. Clarke. Grimmer. Murphy. Phatak.

ADAMAS

(White Diamond)

PHARMACY - adam. Adamas. White Diamond. ***Historical dose:*** All potencies.

CLINICAL - Aphonia. ***Backache.*** Belching. Bladder, disorders. Bone, pains. Brain, tumors. Chilliness. Cold, sores. Constipation. Coughs. Cramps. Diarrhea. Dyspnea. Fever. Fever, blisters. ***Flatulence.*** Hair, loss. ***Headaches.*** Heat. Hemorrhoids. Hyperactive. Insomnia. Itching. Leucorrhea. Moles. Nausea. Nightmares. Nosebleed. Numbness. Palpitations. Photophobia. Pimples. Skin, dryness. Sprained joints. Stiffness. Tingling. Tonsillitis. Varicose, veins. Vertigo. Vomiting.

HOMEOPATHIC - Adamas has associations with the word "Adamantine" meaning unbreakable, impenetrable, impregnable. The Greek word "adamas" means "unyielding, invincible."

Chilliness. Feeling very cold and shivering inside, deep down in bones is freezing cold. Body temperature unusually warm. Sensation of heat all over, all day.

Increased appetite and thirst. Loss of appetite. Craving for coffee, fruit, smoked salmon. Unrefreshing sleep. Frightful dreams. Dryness of skin. Whole body is sensitive, bones aching, skin hurts.

MIND - Irritable and taciturn. Anger towards friends, loved ones. Irritated easily by words and gestures. Does not like to work. Resentful towards others. Does not want to be seen. Aversion to company, talking. ***Desire to be alone.*** Feelings of worthlessness. Loss of self confidence. Critical of others and self. Hard to be pleased.

Mind feels cloudy. Feels separated and detached. Indecision. Does not stick to one decision. Forgetful. Weak memory. Poor concentration. Fumbles in speech with difficulty in getting at certain well-known words. Makes mistakes in speaking. Spelling mistakes. Mixing up words. Mistakes in speech. Slurred speech. Lethargic in morning.

Anxiety about health. Anxiety felt in stomach. Fear of driving car, obsessed with crashing and accidents and death. fear of breast cancer. Despair about their recovery. Delusion they have two pairs of hands, two pairs of arms.

Impatient and intolerant. ***Hurried and impatient.*** Feels rushed, so much to do. Feels overwhelmed. Hyperactive, since beginning of proving. Very excitable as if about to lose control. Sensitive to music. Tearful and oversensitive.

Feels trapped and helpless. Sad and moody. Mood swings. Despair. Lack of joy. Depressed and body feels heavy. Desire for order, everything needs to be in it's place. Fastidious. Feels disorganized. Obsessed with trifles.

Abdomen - Bloated abdomen. Much smelly, nausea-inducing ***flatulence.*** Muscles aches, worse cough, worse movement. Shooting pains in lower abdomen in the evening. Needle like cutting pains. Sharp pain, left hypochondria upwards to left breast and inner left upper arm. Groin hurts when coughs.

Back - Back cold in bed. Chilliness down the back, waist, shoulder blades and spine. Backache, very painful, better heat of bath. Feels better when lying down. Dull aching across back of shoulders, neck with pressure downwards. ***Severe backache*** while walking. Pain aching across lumbar region. Low back pain. Sharp shooting pains.

Bladder - Sharp bladder pain across pubic bone above penis. Very dark, orangey brown urine. ***Diminished urination.*** Urine smells ketonic.

Breasts - Breasts feel enlarged. Fizzy feeling in right breast. Shooting pains through right breast, like needles.

Chest - Spot above left breast. Contracting feeling in chest. As chest if expanded, opened up. Heat rising from chest to face. Pain in base of left ribs corresponding with pain of left vertex. Sharp pain under ribs. Tight chest with cough.

Coughs - Racking, distressing cough. Incessant, exhausting, constant cough. Deep, barking cough. Coughing up bloody mucus, felt cold and clammy. Suffocative cough, difficult to inspire.

Coughs - Cough with chill, shivering and heaviness in limbs, head and eyes. Loose cough with tight chest. Coughing up bloody mucus. Cough with catarrh in nose and throat. Spasmodic cough, better from sips of cold water. Cough, worse deep inspiration, worse morning, aggravated from cold air or drinks. Burning pain with cough. Sharp pain on coughing. Explosive, wet, violent cough. Vomiting from coughing. Wet cough. Cough from anger.

Dreams - Dreams of friends betraying him and felt disappointed. Dream of protection, violence, murder. Dreams of betrayal, conspiracy, lies and deception. Dreams of traveling, water, babies. Dreams of cliffs and chasms.

Ears - Sensation as if ears were filled with water. Buzzing in both ears. Hearing is very sensitive. Hearing impaired.

Eyes - Sticky eyes on waking. eyes watery. Bloodshot. Heat and heavy sensations. Itching, eyes. Photophobia. Twitching. Very tired with gritty eyes. Sensation as if something in the eyes.

Face - Redness of face with burning dry heat. Deep ache in right jaw. Numbness left side of face when in cold air. Dark rings under the eyes. Blemishes on face like spots underneath the skin.

Female - Menses scanty. First day of period very painful. Uterus feels heavy, full aching. Uterus feels as if hanging, suspended in space. Ovarian pain, cramping both sides. Stabbing, knifing pains through abdomen and groin, as if knives were cutting up inside vagina and womb. Severe pulling, as if being dragged down physically by pelvic bone. Pains worse during morning, and when eating. Eruption on right labia with white head. Vagina and labia itching, hot and burning. Voluptuous itch in vagina. Leucorrhea, thick, white, bland vaginal discharge. Heat in vagina with soreness at start of menses. Desire for sex diminished. Aversion to sex.

Food - Aversion to cream, fats, milk. Aversion to white wine. Desires alcohol, cheese, coffee. Desires fruit, dried fruit, sparkling drinks. Desires seafood, fish, smoked salmon. Desires starchy food, potatoes. Desires vegetables, green vegetables. Desires wine, red wine. ***Worse from alcohol.*** Cold drinks aggravates coughs.

Head - ***Headache and hunger.*** Dull and aching pains. Headaches with nausea. Headaches, worse exertion. Hair falling out. Scalp itching and dry. Heat sensation in vertex. Pain over eyebrows. Sharp pains in head. Head feels heavy and congested.

Heart - Heart palpitations. As if heart skips and jumps a beat. Palpitation with anxiety all through day.

Limbs - Cold arms. Chilliness. Hands hot and clammy. Burning pain in ankle. Sensation of heat on soles of feet. Cramp in calves during sleep. Heavy feeling in my arms. Aching pain in wrists and elbows. Sharp pains like pins in hand. Numbness. Sprained joints. Stiffness. Tingling in legs. Varicose veins. Wrists feel weak.

Lungs - Dyspnea. Difficulty breathing in. Burning in lungs on breathing in. Wheeze like a high-pitched whine on breathing. Wheezing and struggling for breath like asthma. Gasping for air on inspiration, during and after coughing fit. Sensitive bronchi.

Male - Penis sore. Low sex drive.

Modalities - Better sunshine. Better fresh air. Worse cloudy days. Worse winter.

Mouth - Dry mouth and throat. Fever blisters. Cold sores. Lips very dry, sore and chafed. Bottom lip cracked in middle, split open. Rawness of palate. Offensive breath better after glass of water. Increased salivation.

Neck - Sore neck, very stiff, aching, better lying down and stretching. Cricking of neck.

Nose - Nosebleed. Catarrh white, stringy, thick and glossy, worse evening. Post-nasal catarrh. Sinuses feel full and congested.

Perspiration - Body odor smells acidic. Perspiration smells garlicky. Hot sweats during day.

Rectum - Urgent desire to pass stool. In the morning has to rush for stool. While going to sleep sudden urging for stool. ***Much flatulence.*** Constipated, dark, round balls. Skin around the anus is raw and sore. Hemorrhoids. Hot itch in anus. Diarrhea, feel weak and drained afterwards. Diarrhea, preceded with gripping cramps. Loose, watery stools. Stool extremely pale. Hard, small stools. Unfinished feeling with bowel movement.

Skin - Dryness of skin. Pale skin. Large, painful cold sores in left corner of upper lip. Moles. Pimples, very sore, red and elevated. Dry, brownish-red eczema-like rash. Itching with redness, especially after a bath. Skin very painful, feels prickling and cold. Itchy pimples on right arm. Bumps and spots on left side of face.

Sleep - Insomnia. Waking frequently. Sleep unrefreshing, awoke tired. Deep yawning. Restless, sleep.

Stomach - Belching. Burning sensation. Cold sensation in stomach. Nausea and distention with headache. Nausea at thought of milk in tea since proving. Feel sick when eating or drinking, worse in morning. Feel nauseous but hungry. Vomiting from coughing. Bruised soreness in epigastric region.

Teeth - Grinding teeth. Teeth feel sharp. Pains in back molar teeth. Bruised sore feeling above right upper canine tooth, worse cold air, pain extends up into the jawbone.

Temperature - Chilliness down the back, waist, shoulder blades and spine. Icy cold body generally. Skin felt icy, freezing. Shaking with cold when sitting still. Chill, unable to keep warm, must go to bed. Cold shivers all over body. Fever, sudden onset. Fever with shaking, heat, sneezing and coughing.

Throat - Sore throat, better eating or drinking hot things. Sensation of needles pricking in throat. Adenoids and tonsils sore from coughing. Tonsils red and inflamed. Aphonia.

Tongue - Burning sensation down the middle of tongue. Tongue feels swollen on the left side. Tongue is coated, white.

Vertigo - Dizzy, worse sitting down, better eating. Sensation on closing the eyes, as if rotating clockwise. Vertigo on closing eyes, floating feeling in head.

COMMENTS - Although extremely hard, diamond is very brittle, being able to tolerate great pressure, yet being sensitive to violent jarring or shock. It will likely to be a remedy that aids recovery from psychological or physical trauma, recent or past.

RELATIONS - ***Compare:*** (1) Plb-i.

REFERENCES - Sankaran. Sherr.

ADELHEID AQUA

(Mineral Springs at Heilbrunn)

PHARMACY - adel. Adelheid aqua. Mineral Springs at Heilbrunn. Adelheidsquelle. Contains among other substances, Iodine, Bromine, Alumina, Natrum, etc. ***Historical dose:*** Tincture and all potencies.

CLINICAL - Diarrhea. Glands, disorders. Goiter. Scrofulous, disorders.

HOMEOPATHIC - This water has been used for hundreds of years for goiter, scrofulous troubles of various kinds, enlarged glands, etc.

MIND - Mental confusion. Reading fatigues them (Nat-m., Ruta). Much trilling and tra-la-ling, which formerly she never did.

Abdomen - Ache in upper abdomen wakes him. Lower abdomen became thick and protruding. Loud rumbling, grumblings and noises in the lower part of the abdomen after every eating or drinking, especially after pears.

Chest - Chest is tired. The whole chest is painfully sensitive, as if inflamed.

Eyes - Eyes feel swollen, as after taking cold, without redness.

Face - Cheeks became full and the face red, was formerly thin and pale.

Food - Increased appetite. Appetite for potatoes and sour fruit. Aversion to meat and roasted articles. Unusual thirst. After drinking water, the appetite increased and then became conversational and lively.

Head - Confusion of head, better in open air.

Limbs - Small, hard indurations in the palm of the hand, very near the last joint of the fourth finger, adherent to the bone. After rising in the morning, cramp in left calf twice disappeared after going around.

Male - Testicles sensitive.

Mouth - Salivation, especially nights.

Neck - Swollen thyroid gland, but not the cervical and inferior maxillary glands.

Nose - Nosebleed and much tossing about the bed at night (Iod.). Nosebleed after beginning to take the waters the second time.

Rectum - Diarrhea, watery, clear brown, then yellow and watery, four or five times a day with much offensive flats, no pains.

Skin - Hard pimples with a red inflamed areola, itching somewhat with a yellow, pustular apex, somewhat moist on scratching it off (like small boils), on neck, chest, fingers and toes (Sil.).

Stomach - Painful flatulent distention in pit of stomach.

RELATIONS - Spirit-nit-dulc., antidotes. Coffee drinking relieved the attacks, especially the rumblings. Nat-c. relieved the diarrhea. ***Compare:*** (1) Iod., Nat-c., Nat-m., Sil.

REFERENCES - Allen.

ADLUMIA FUNGOSA

(Climbing Fumitory)

PHARMACY - adlu. Adlumia fungosa. Climbing fumitory. Fumaria fungosa. N.O. Papaveraceae.

CLINICAL - Bladder, disorders. Chilly. Constipation. Dyspnea. Flatulence. Headache. Impotence. Infertility. Kidney, stones. Nail, disorders. Nausea. Nightmares. Meteorism. Palpitations. Rash. Styes. Vertigo. Weakness.

HERBAL - Fumaria species have long been valued as medicinal herbs for chronic skin rash and kidney stones, in which its success was ascribed to its sweat-inducing capacity, as well as its blood-purifying effect by means of the urinary organs.

French and German physicians prefer it to most other medicines as a purifier of the blood.

Sometimes the dried leaves are smoked in the manner of tobacco, for disorders of the head. The plant was also believed to be useful in infertility.

HOMEOPATHIC - Sense of weakness, must lie down. ***Great weariness towards end of afternoon. must lie down.*** Chilliness, yet better open air. Pain extends to left scapula or to left arm. Meteorismus from smoking. Slow growth of nails.

MIND - Causeless sadness. Sadness and joyless for days. Difficult concentration. Mistakes in writing. Euphoria when weariness subsides.

Abdomen - Flatuence. Distended sensation in abdomen and rumbling. Pressure in hepatic region. Pressing pain in epigastrium after eating, better lying on abdomen. Sensation of weakness in abdomen at 11 p.m.

Chest - Oppression in left side of chest.

Eyes - Styes, lower lid of right eye. Swelling of lower lid of right eye.

Female - Sexual power diminished.

Food - Desires cold milk. Better cold food. Worse beer, fats, sausages. Intolerance to fatty food. Nausea from sausage.

Head - Headache, worse 3 a.m. Headache better fresh evening air, better rainy weather. Headache and nausea and vertigo. Congestion of head and face from flatulence pressing upward. Right-sided headache.

Heart - Palpitations of heart.

Limbs - Pain in finger joints.

Lungs - Dyspnea. Sensation of breathlessness.

Male - Sexual power diminished. Impotence. Too quick ejaculation.

Modalities - Better fresh evening air. Better lying on abdomen. Better pressure. Better coffee. Worse evening. Worse after exposure to heat of sun. Worse 3 a.m. Worse afternoon, 2 p.m. to 5 p.m.

Mouth - Discoloration of tongue. Tongue coated white.

Rectum - Constipation, difficult discharge of soft stool. Ineffectual urging and straining. No stool for days. Frequent urging in afternoon, but passes only yellow mucus. Flatulence and soft stool. Meteorism.

Frequent stools at 4 p.m. to 6 p.m. Hard, knotty stool. Soft, light-colored stool.

Sleep - Disturbed sleep. Wakes at 3 a.m., tosses about and finally falls asleep again. Restless sleep from constipation during daytime. Falling asleep difficult from palpitations of heart. Sleepiness during daytime, worse in afternoon, irresistible desire to lie down. Frequent waking with tormenting thoughts. Nightmares. Frightful dreams, even during short afternoon naps.

Stomach - Pressing pain in stomach after meals. Nausea and pain in epigastrium extending to left scapula. Nausea from smoking. Nausea from beer. Nausea better after eating.

Vertigo - Vertigo on slight exertion. Vertigo with headache and nausea.

REFERENCES - Bayr. Grieve.

ADONIS AESTIVALIS

PHARMACY - adon-ae. Adonis aestivalis. N. O. Ranunculaceae. ***Historical dose:*** All potencies.

CLINICAL - Dyspnea. Heart, disorders. ***Heart, weakness.*** Pulse, rapid.

HOMEOPATHIC - This plant was examined by Italian doctors as to its therapeutic value and Albertoni reported in its favor. His experiments were made on animals and sick and healthy people.

Neither of these species of Adonis has been proved in homeopathy. There were some attempts to prove Adonis vernalis, but the results were very meager. It seems to cause irritation of the bladder, strangury, etc., but all cardiac medicines do that.

In cases of ***insufficiency of heart action***, with feeble, irregular, rapid pulse, diminished arterial pressure, dyspnea and diminished excretion of urine. The administration of the plant in substance produced, in a few days, the return of normal pulse, increase of the pressure of the blood, and disappearance of the respiratory oppression. The quantity of urine increased from eight hundred to three thousand cubic centimeters in a day.

COMMENTS - These good results were not obtained in cases in which the organs susceptible to the influence of Adonis, such as the kidney epithelium, muscular fiber and the nerve apparatus of the heart, had already retrograded to too great an extent.

The dose is 4 to 8 grains a day, given in substance or infusion. The effects manifest themselves about the third day.

REFERENCES - Hale.

ADONIS VERNALIS

(Pheasant's Eye)

PHARMACY - adon. Adonis vernalis. Pheasant's eye. N. O. Ranunculacee. Infusion or tincture of fresh plant, an extract, Adonidin. ***Historical dose:*** Tincture, five to ten drops of the tincture. All potencies.

CLINICAL - Albuminuria. Ascites. Dropsy. ***Dyspnea.*** Fatty, degeneration. ***Heart, disorders.*** Hydrothorax. Myocarditis. Rheumatism. Tinnitus.

HERBAL - Adonis, like Cratageus and Convallaria, is a popular ***herbal heart tonic***. It is used as a heart tonic after rheumatism, influenza or kidney infection. Adonis is not cumulative in action. Compensatory hypertrophy of heart in cardiac stenosis and mitral regurgitation.

Adon. regulates the pulse increases the contracting power of the heart with increased urinary secretion. It is valuable in cardiac dropsy, hydrothorax, ascites and anasarca.

HOMEOPATHIC - Adonis has not been proved, but the indications for its use have been defined from experience. Indications include rapid and feeble action of the heart, dropsy, scanty urine with albumen and casts. Valvular disease and cardiac asthma. There is no record of its uses in the potencies.

Adonis acts predominantly on the heart when it is affected after rheumatism, influenza or nephritis, where the muscles of the heart are in the stage of fatty degeneration. Pains wander from place to place.

Regulates the pulse and increases the power of contractions of heart with more urinary secretions. ***Low vitality with weak heart*** and slow, weak pulse. Most valuable in cardiac dropsy.

Hydrothorax, ascites or anasarca.

MIND - Anxiety about the heart. Apprehension.

Abdomen - Dropsy. Faint feeling in epigastric region with vertigo better out of doors. As if a heavy weight in bowels. Sensation as if intestines would break on bending.

Back - Spine and neck stiff, aching pain with tired feeling. Stiffness of left cervical region and spine.

Ears - Tinnitus.

Eyes - Pupils dilated.

Food - Appetite, easy satiety after a few bites. Gnawing hunger. No thirst.

Head - Feels light headed. Aches across front of head. ***Pain from occiput around temples to eyes***. Scalp feels tight. Pain in occiput, extending to eyes, around temples.

Heart - Weakness of circulatory system and dropsy. Dropsy. Murmurs, valvular disease. Arrhythmia. Heart failure. Mitral and aortic regurgitation. Chronic aortitis. Fatty heart pericarditis. Rheumatic Endocarditis (Kalm.). ***Precordial pain, palpitations and dyspnea***. Marked venous engorgement. Fatty heart. Myocarditis, irregular heart action, constriction and vertigo. Weak, fatty, arrhythmic heart. Precordial pain, palpitations and dyspnea. Trembling and palpitations. Pulse rapid, irregular.

Kidneys - Nephritis. Urging to urinate. Albuminuria, urine scanty, oily pellicle on urine.

Limbs - Aching in nape. Spine stiff and aching. Edema.

Lungs - Cardiac asthma (Queb.). Frequent desire to take a long breath. Feeling of weight on chest. Difficult breathing, worse touching back. Dry tickling, cardiac cough.

Modalities - Better from exertion. Better walking open air. Worse from cold. Worse lying down.

Mouth - Slimy. Tongue dirty, yellow, sore, feels burnt. Sensation as if tongue were scalded.

Skin - Vesicles on the skin.

Sleep - Dozing as soon as eyes are closed. Falling asleep and palpitations. Sleeplessness with rambling thoughts or horrible dreams. Restless with horrible dreams.

Stomach - Heavy weight sensation. Gnawing hunger. Faint feeling in epigastrium. Better out of doors.

Vertigo - Faintness and vertigo, better open air. Vertigo, worse turning or moving head quickly. Vertigo on lying down. Vertigo on rising. Vertigo with palpitations.

COMMENTS - Cash gave great relief to "a water-logged patient of seventy-four" with mitral regurgitation with one-grain doses of Adonidin at eight-hour intervals after the failure of Ars. and Dig. Urinary secretion rose from half a pint to 2 1/2 pints in 24 hours. Breathing was relieved, sleep returned.

RELATIONS - ***Compare:*** (1) Conv., Crat., Dig., Strop.

REFERENCES - Boericke. Clarke. Phatak.

ADOXA MOSCHATELLINA

(Moschatel)

PHARMACY - adox. Adoxa moschatellina. Moschatel. N. O. Caprifliaceae. Adoxaceae. ***Historical dose:*** Tincture and all potencies.

HOMEOPATHIC - This remedy has been used in the past for general prostration. Nervous tremors in some persons. Sleepiness. Vertigo and headaches. Weariness of the eyelids. Dryness of the pharynx and esophagus. Qualmishness in the epigastrium.

RELATIONS - ***Compare:*** (1) Gels. Caust. (2) Dig., Conv., Stroph.

REFERENCES - Allen.

ADRENALINUM

(Adrenal Glands)

PHARMACY - adren. Adrenalinum. Adrenal glands. Extract of adrenal glands. Sarcode. Tincture or trituration. ***Historical dose:*** All potencies.

CLINICAL - ***Addison's disease.*** Adrenalin neuralgias. ***Allergies.*** Angina pectoris. ***Asthma***. Bronzed skin. Debility. Hematuria. Hemorrhages. Hyperemia. Neuralgia. Palpitations. Tachycardia.

HOMEOPATHIC - Adrenaline or Epinephrine, the active principle of the medulla of the suprarenal gland, is employed as a chemical messenger in the regulation of the activities of the body in fact. Its presence is essential to the activity of the sympathetic nerves.

Adrenaline appears to possess a very powerful local action over dilated blood vessels. When injected into the circulation, blood pressure rises, the arteries being contracted. The general muscular system is affected, a slight stimulus producing prolonged contraction.

Adrenalin has been suggested in acute congestion of lungs. ***Asthma***. Addison's diseases and Grave's diseases, Arteriosclerosis, chronic aortitis, angina pectoris, hemophilia, chlorosis, hay fever, serum rashes, acute urticaria, etc.

Adrenalin's chief therapeutic use depends on its ***vaso-constriction*** action, therefore a most powerful and prompt ***astringent and hemostatic*** and invaluable in checking capillary hemorrhages from all parts, where local or direct application is feasible including the nose, ear, mouth, throat, larynx, stomach, rectum, uterus, and bladder.

Clinically effective in ***allergies,*** neuralgia, ***bronzed skin,*** debility, hematuria, palpitations, tachycardia, hyperemia, exceedingly rapid pulse, loss of strength, wasting. May well be needed in cancer patients with adrenal disturbance. Prolonged contraction of the general muscular system. Great loss of strength, rapid emaciation. Rapid pulse and irregular intermitting heartbeats. General marked anemia.

MIND - Despondent and nervous. ***Ailments from overwork and stress.*** Apathy. Lack of interest in anything. No ambition. Disinclination for mental work. Absence of mental stamina and will power. Anxious and restless. Distracted easily. Aversion to mental activity. Cannot concentrate thoughts.

Abdomen - Rumbling in the intestines, borborygmus.

Back - Pain especially on the left side, better by sitting up straight or lying straight.

Ears - Aching in the left ear accompanies the headache, sharp pain in both ears at times. Itching and tickling in right ear, better by boring into ear with finger.

Eyes - Strained feeling as though he wanted to open them wide or press upon them. Pain in the right eye. Pressure on the eyes. Hyperemia of the conjunctiva. Aching in eyeballs, better by pressure and rubbing.

Face - Feels flushed but is not red. Flushes of heat over face and head, flushed throughout evening.

Food - Appetite increased. Ravenous hunger. Less thirst than usual. Thirst at times for large quantities, increased in the evening.

Head - Hot headache in left side, extending to right. Headache, worse by reading and in the morning, with a feeling as though the eyes were strained. Frontal headache with congested nose and eyes. Burning heat in head. Headache extending all over head. Severe pain, better by pressure on the eyes. Headache with nausea and heat in face without redness. Neuralgic headaches. Brain feels swollen as though it were too large for skull. Flushes of heat in the evening over face and head.

Kidneys - Strong odor, hot and scalding, frequent, profuse, pale. Burning before and during urination. Sudden urgent desire to urinate. Amount of urine decreased, solids increased. Crystals of sodium oxalate increased while sodium urate appeared during the proving and was very prominent, no casts.

Limbs - Slight rheumatic pains coming and going down leg. Arms and legs go to sleep easily, numbness and tingling from below upwards. Corns on the toes. Aching in limbs on waking in the morning, aching in the calves. Rheumatic pains in left elbow and little finger on waking. Legs tired and ache, especially in the calves and below the knees. Ankles feel weak and tired. Painful swelling on first finger of right hand, resulting in a felon. Tired aching in arms and legs on waking. Dull pain in arms and legs.

Lungs - Cough from irritation in suprasternal fossa. Expectoration of gelatinous mucus, which is hard to detach. Increase of respiratory movements, soon followed by suffocation and death from paralysis of medulla and pneumogastric.

Male - Sexual desire increased without erections. Erections, lascivious dreams all night causing waking from sleep. Emissions in early morning without any bad effects.

Mouth - Bad taste on waking. Mouth filled with dark brown mucus, which has nasty taste. Tongue coated white, red edge and tip. Tongue clean anteriorly, mouth dry. Tongue coated white at times posteriorly.

Nose - Congested, full feeling in nose. Gelatinous mucus drops from the posterior sinuses, difficult to detach. On going out into the cold air had a copious, watery nasal discharge. Slight stuffiness in the nose with full feeling at the root of the nose.

Rectum - Passage of foul flatus. Stool loose, brown, semi-solid, passed quickly with fetid odor. Sudden spluttering diarrhea, all over in a minute, followed with burning in anus.

Sleep - Great sleepiness and drowsiness. Sleepy in evening and after a good night's sleep. Dullness and sleepiness from 3 p.m. to 6 p.m.

Stomach - Belching after meals. Sensation of nausea as though he would vomit. Pain in stomach passing from right to left, coming and going suddenly. Nausea before meals, though appetite is good after beginning to eat.

Throat - Much hawking to clear throat. Vocal cords inflamed, laryngeal catarrh, profuse secretion from the pharyngeal glands of whitish gelatinous mucus which was difficult to loosen. Right side swollen and sore, red and inflamed, worse by swallowing.

COMMENTS - Leading features include bronzing of the skin, loss of strength, wasting, and exceedingly rapid pulse. It has cured a case of hematuria accompanied by pain in the adrenal region.

Adrenaline has cured a number of cases of Addison's disease and has arrested others. It has been used locally in cases of hyperemia of the conjunctiva, dissipating it almost immediately and thus rendering operations possible.

Dr. P. Jousset reports success in treating, homeopathically, cases of angina and aortitis, sub-acute and chronic, when Adrenalin has been prescribed per os and in infinitesimal dose. The guiding symptom is a sensation of thoracic constriction with anguish. This, with vertigo, nausea and vomiting have been produced by the drug. Abdominal pain. Shock or heart failure during anesthesia.

Adrenaline causes very prompt rise of blood pressure by its action on nerve endings in the vessel wall.

REFERENCES - Allen. Boericke. Clarke. Grimmer. Phatak.

AEGLE FOLIA

PHARMACY - aegle-f. Aegle folia. N. O. Rutaceae. Tincture of the leaves. ***Historical dose:*** Tincture and all potencies.

CLINICAL - Anemia. ***Ascites.*** Asthma. Beriberi. Bites. Bronchitis. Colic. Constipation. Coughs. Diarrhea. ***Dropsy.*** Dysentery. Edema. Fever. Gonorrhea. Headaches. Heart, disorders. Hemorrhages. Hemorrhoids. Impotency. Indigestion. Influenza. Jaundice. Kidney stones. Leprosy. Liver, disorders. Phlegm. Pneumonia. Rabies. Ringworm. Water brash.

HERBAL - In Bengal, the leaves of this plant are kept in the drinking pot of patients suffering from dropsy with the belief that drinking this water will accelerate the cure.

The leaves of the Aegle-f. are used by the Sannyasi (monks and ascetics) of India to suppress sexual desires and excitement (Agn.) as they have found it produces sexual impotency. For seminal weakness and impotency.

HOMEOPATHIC - Dr. Pramada Prasanna Biswas of Padna, Bengal, made a short proving of this drug using a preparation from the leaves.

This remedy destroys phlegm, and is useful for fevers associated with catarrhal symptoms. Generally useful for bowel complaints. Diarrhea and dysentery. Alternating diarrhea and constipation, it acts as a mild stimulant to the intestinal mucus membrane. It can act as a laxative for existing constipation. Intestinal colic.

Dropsy, particularly when due to heart disease. Continued fever associated with dropsy, especially of children. Dropsy in certain parts or throughout entire body. Bruised pains. Diminished appetite. Sensation of heat worse movement, better rest. Weakness.

Leprosy. Bites from venomous animals such as snake, rabid dog and scorpion. Coughs, asthma, gonorrhea. Jaundice, ascites associated with liver disorders. Bleeding piles. Hemorrhages. Anemia. Kidney stones. Diseases of heart and hemicrania.

MIND - Mistakes in spelling. Anxiety with heat and bruised feeling. Lack of concentration while studying.

Abdomen - ***Pain, griping in the lower abdomen, worse after eating.*** Gripping pain in abdomen, worse sitting, better from walking.

Back - Eruptions in scapular regions of back, red, small pimples, painful with thick white pus, itching worse covering, rubbing, better open air. ***Pain, lumbar region.*** Bruised pain, worse sitting, walking.

Chest - Sharp pain, worse during cough.

Eyes - Pain, soreness in the right eye, worse deep inspiration, sunlight, pressure. Sensation, as if sand in the eye. Watery discharge, left eye, better closing eyes. Agglutination of eyelids, worse morning.

Face - Jaw, aching with soreness in throat worse chewing. Jaw, right soreness and tenderness with enlarged cervical lymph nodes on the right side worse chewing, swallowing, better warmth.

Food - Appetite diminished with bad taste in mouth. Appetite diminished during fever. Appetite, increased with increased thirst and sleepiness. Thirst for large quantity of water at short intervals. Desires rice, meat, milk.

Head - ***Heaviness of head.*** Heaviness, better after tea. Heaviness of head with sneezing, malaise, chilliness. Heaviness with soreness in right eye. Heaviness, with throat pain. Heaviness with thirst. ***Pain in frontal region better open air, better pressure.*** Bursting pain, in forehead. Pressing pain in the right frontal region, with profuse sweat all over the body.

Kidneys - Kidney stones. Urine yellow.

Limbs - Bruised pain, shoulders, hips, knee joints with sleepiness worse motion, better pressure. Aching pain in the right hand worse movement of hand, holding anything by hand, better pressure. ***Pain in the knee joints worse motion.*** Eruptions, both hands, pimples like, painful worse touch, pressure, better cold bathing. Eruptions, lower limbs with itching, worse covering, warmth, better open air, undressing.

Lungs - Dyspnea, worse inspiration.

Mouth - Bitter taste in mouth. Salivation, profuse. Taste, bad with diminished appetite. Taste, bitter. Thick yellow coating on the tongue during fever. Tongue flabby with imprints of teeth on edges. Tongue thick, moist and yellow coating.

Nose - Watery discharge bland, white, worse bathing, change in temperature, better hot inhalation. ***Coryza, bland white or watery discharge.*** Sneezing with heaviness of head, malaise, chilliness. Sneezing worse pungent odor. Tickling sensation with thin watery, bland discharge. Thick, bland and yellowish discharge with profuse salivation, disturbed sleep.

Perspiration - Profuse sweat, all over the body, followed by weakness. Profuse, offensive sweat.

Skin - Pimple-like eruptions. Eruptions, papular, dark red, painful. ***Urticaria with itching.*** Urticaria with redness and swelling with restlessness. Itching, worse warmth, covering, better cold bathing, undressing.

Sleep - Sleepiness day and night with uneasiness. Sleepiness with increased appetite and thirst.

Stomach - Nausea, vomiting with weakness. ***Nausea at the sight of food.*** Vomiting of watery fluid containing food particles, sour smelling.

Stools - Semi-solid stool with diminished appetite and bad taste in mouth.

Temperature - ***Fever with weakness, diminished appetite.*** Heat worse at midnight with bursting pain in forehead. ***Fever without chill worse at night.*** Fever with thirst for large quantities of cold water.

Throat - Pain, bruised, amel. hot drinks. Pain, stitching with dry cough worse during deglutition, amel. hot drinks. Soreness, worse swallowing. Soreness with aching in jaw worse chewing.

Vertigo - ***Vertigo worse lying down.*** Vertigo worse physical exertion, better lying down. ***Vertigo worse on walking and standing.*** Vertigo with darkness before eyes.

COMMENTS - An anti-psoric remedy, historically used for skin diseases such as itches and ringworm. An anti-bilious and febrifuge remedy.

Headache due to congestion. Headache between 4 a.m. and 8 p.m. (Lyc.). Heat in the vertex appears in the evening, relieved by eating something. In the afternoon and evening, flushes of heat come out from the eyes and face, and in the ear. All these symptoms disappear after eating.

Irregularity or disorder of the stomach, abdomen is distended and flatus passes with a loud sound, worse in the afternoon. Water brash. Accumulation of wind in the lower abdomen. Constipation with flatus (Lyc.). Indigestion, abdominal colic, piles and constipation (Nux-v.). Chronic gastrointestinal catarrh with flatulent colicky pains. Decreased quantity of urine.

Slight pain in the back and lumbar region that is worse in the afternoon. All pains in the limbs are aggravated after four p.m. Beriberi, with a full, strong and regular pulse (Dig., with irregular or intermittent pulse). Swollen upper eyelids. Anasarca, ascites and edema of all sorts. Full, strong and regular pulse (Bell.).

Chronic fevers associated with hepatic and splenic disorders, with swollen feet, burning in the eye, face, hands, and feet, no appetite, diminished urine, and cough. Continual fever. Fever with swelling in the hands, legs and face. Catarrhal fevers in children. Fever with dropsy and diarrhea. Influenza, with fever and swollen face and eyelids. Bronchitis and pneumonia.

Lt. Col. R. N. Chopra asserted that none of the preparations appear to possess any specific therapeutic properties to cure either amoebic or bacillary dysentery, but its efficacy is certain in chronic cases with the keynote symptoms.

Ghose noted the case of Babu Sarat Chandra Jana, aged 28, who had sudden swellings of his legs and feet on March 2, 1932. His urine was examined, but there was no albumen present. The urine became scanty and high-colored. Pain over the hepatic region. Giddiness of head and heart palpitations.

Ghose prescribed Boerhaavia Diffusa in drop doses to be taken thrice daily. The medicine was continued for six days and the patient got rid of the swelling and other complaints within ten days.

Ghose had a second case, Babu Santiram Roy, aged 28, who had an epidemic dropsy on May 30, 1932. He was treated by several well-known allopaths of Calcutta, but nothing could lessen the swelling. Ghose was called in on June 14.

The patient complained of a terrible headache, principally on the right side. Preexisting liver derangement, at the time it was congested and painful to touch or pressure. Swollen hands, feet and abdomen. Scanty, high-colored urine.

Cough with thick, white mucus expectoration. Throbbing pain in the cardiac region felt off and on. Ghose prescribed Boerhaavia in 2-drop doses thrice daily. He was cured within a month.

Ghose cured more than 30 cases of epidemic dropsy with the help of this new drug.

Aegle marmelos contains almost all the identical therapeutic properties ascribed to Aegle folia.

REFERENCES - Ghose.

AEGLE MARMELOS

(Bel Fruit)

PHARMACY - aegle. Aegle marmelos. Bel fruit. Bael fruit. Bael tree. N. O. Rutaceae. *Historical dose:* Tincture and all potencies.

CLINICAL - ***Allergies.*** Asthma. Backache. Bronchitis. Coccygodynia. Conjunctivitis. Constipation. Coryza. ***Dermatitis.*** Diarrhea. Dyspepsia. Dysentery. Dysmenorrhea. Eczema. Headaches. Hoarseness. Infertility. Intermittent fever. Laryngitis. Lumbago. Migraines. Palpitations. Polyps, nasal. Rheumatism. ***Rhinitis.*** Ringworm. Scabies. Spring catarrh. ***Stomatitis. Styes. Vertigo.***

HERBAL - The aegle marmelos tree is indigenous to India and is found wild all over the Sub-Himalayan forests, in Bengali, in Central and South India, and in Burma. It is also cultivated to a great extent.

Different parts of the bel tree are used in Ayurvedic medicine. The root bark is used in the form of a decoction as a remedy in hypochondriasis, melancholia, intermittent fever and palpitation of the heart.

It constitutes an ingredient in the "Dasamul" or ten roots used by the Ayurvedic physicians. The leaves are made into a poultice and applied to inflamed parts. The fresh juice is bitter and pungent, and when mixed with water is praised as a remedy in catarrh and feverishness.

The fruit, both green and ripe, is used against diarrhea and intestinal conditions. For diarrhea and dysentery the roasted or sun-dried unripe fruit cut in slices is general used. The astringent rind of the ripe fruit is employed in dying and tanning and it is also used medicinally.

Ayurvedic physicians note that the ripe fruit is nutritious, delicious, aromatic, alternative and a laxative. It is given with sugar candy to prevent the growth of piles and to remove habitual constipation.

When taken in excess it often causes flatulence. Syrup of ripe fruits is used in dyspepsia. The root bark is a refrigerant, and is given in fevers and asthma, with palpitations of the heart.

In native practice, a poultice of the leaves is applied to the chest in acute bronchitis.

The decoction of the Aegle leaves is given in asthma, a marmalade of bel fruit is a household remedy for diarrhea and dysentery.

HOMEOPATHIC - A proving of Aegle marmelos was done by the Central Council for Research in Homoeopathy of the Ministry of health and family welfare, Government of India, giving a good array of symptoms. It showed a marked affinity for the gastrointestinal tract, skin and upper respiratory tract though it has also evoked symptoms from head, eyes, genitalia, back and extremities.

A study to clinically confirm the symptoms elicited during provings is in progress and the data obtained so far show its positive application in ***vertigo, styes, rhinitis, stomatitis and dermatitis.*** Nocturnal seminal emission with amorous dreams.

Backache and cramps in calf muscles. Lachrymation and burning in eyes, better closing eyes. Allergic conjunctivitis. Styes, especially when accompanied with stitching pain and sensation of dust particles in eyes with lachrymation (Sulph., Staph.). Aphthae with difficulty in eating.

MIND - Disinclination to talk. Disinclination to work, with sadness. Irritability. Hypochondriasis. Melancholy.

Abdomen - Pain in abdomen around umbilicus. Rumbling in abdomen with diarrhea and increased thirst.

Back - Backache, better lying down worse, turning in bed. Pain in right lumbar region, worse walking, stooping. Pain in coccyx, worse getting up, better walking, lying down.

Chest - Burning sensation in chest. Eruptions, small round patches on chest itching, burning, worse from bathing, sun, and friction of clothes.

Eyes - Redness of eyes, worse from straining. Stitching pain in eyes. Swelling of both upper eyelids. Sensation as if dust particles in right eye, worse touch. Stye in the left lower eyelid. Burning lachrymation with irritability and disinclination to talk. Blurred vision in left eye.

Face - Small eruptions on forehead and cheek. Black, raised eruption on chin.

Female - Dysmenorrhea with pain in the back and legs, worse sitting. Menses dark, blackish.

Food - Thirst increased. Appetite increased, with pain in abdomen.

Head - Bursting pain, better from tea, sleep. Pain as if beaten by hammer, with anger and disinclination to talk, worse after sleep. Hammering pain, left side, worse looking at an object or after sleep, better from closing eyes and in the afternoon.

Limbs - Pain in knee and ankle joints, with sadness and disinclination to work, better pressure, bathing, and sitting, worse walking. Sensation as if legs were being cut. Pain and weakness in left leg, cramping pain worse flexing knee, sitting. Pain in left leg worse walking, feels as if stretched. Pain in calf muscles. Itching on both lower limbs.

Male - Nocturnal seminal emissions.

Mouth - Pain in teeth. Itching over tongue with aching. Aphthae.

Nose - Coryza with sensation of heat in whole body and thirstlessness. Coryza with achiness. Sneezing with itching in nostrils, watery discharge. Thick, white nasal discharge. Burning in right nostril with raw and red surface.

Rectum - Constipation. Loose stool. Profuse, yellowish semi-solid stool. Odorless stool with pain and rumbling in abdomen, increased thirst.

Stomach - Sinking sensation in stomach, not relieved by eating.

Throat - Pain, constricting with difficult speech. Voice heavy and hoarseness, worse from talking. Pain in throat and in the right ear, worse morning, evening. Stitching pain, worse swallowing, drinking and eating.

Vertigo - Vertigo with tendency to fall forward. Vertigo with constipation. Vertigo better lying down. Vertigo worse walking, sitting and standing.

COMMENTS - R. N. Khory, in the Materia Medica of India, noted many traditional uses for Aegle. Aegle marmelos is held sacred by the Hindus, and its leaves are presented to Shiva as an offering by the devotees. It is often planted near the temples. The Hindus consider it an emblem of fertility and a very auspicious plant.

No herbal remedy has been longer and better known or appreciated by the inhabitants of India than the bel fruit. Two kinds of fruit are available in the market: a small, wild variety and a cultivated variety. The full-grown fruit of either variety, when it just begins to ripen, is best for medicinal purposes.

The unripe or half-ripe fruit is regarded as an astringent, digestive, stomachic and is said to be an excellent remedy for diarrhea owing to the presence of tannins or mucilaginous substances. It is said to be particularly useful in chronic diarrhea. It is sometimes used in combination with opium by ayurvedic practitioners.

The fruit is also sliced and a configure made from it, which is commonly used by Hindu physicians in the treatment of diarrheas and dysentery.

The ripe fruit is sweet, aromatic and cooling. When taken fresh, it possesses laxative properties. The dried pulp is pale orange or flesh colored, and when mixed with water, yields a pleasant orange-colored food which has mild astringent properties.

REFERENCES - Ghose.

AEGOPODIUM PODAGRARIA
(Goutweed)

PHARMACY - aego-p. Aegopodium podagraria. Goutweed. Ground elder. Jack-jump-about. Bishopweed. Bishopwort. Herb Gerard. N. O. Umbelliferae. ***Historical dose:*** Tincture and all potencies.

CLINICAL - Constipation. Coryza. Coughs. Diplopia. Flatulence. Gout. Nausea. Rheumatism. Sciatica. Vertigo.

HERBAL - Ground elder was apparently introduced to the British Isles during medieval times, when it was cultivated in monastery gardens for medicinal purposes.

The white rootstock is pungent and aromatic, but the flavor of the leaves is strong and disagreeable. Diuretic and sedative.

Can be employed internally for aches in the joints, gouty and sciatic pains, and externally as a fomentation for inflamed parts.

HOMEOPATHIC - Proved in 1989 by Mattitsch on 11 persons, 5 men and 6 women.

Pain in the entire right side of the body, precisely to the middle line. ***Great tiredness.*** Weariness in morning, desire to remain in bed, must force himself to get going. Weariness in evening and heaviness of eyelids.

Chilly. Disturbed sleep with frequent waking in early morning. Sudden headache, bursting pain. Heat of head and face.

Nausea and pressing, sharp pains in stomach. Nausea at night, worse turning in bed, better lying quietly. Nausea on awaking.

Intolerance to clothing due to abdominal flatulence. Offensive urine, brown like beer. ***Heavy sensation in arms and legs. As if limbs were filled with lead.***

MIND - ***Difficult concentration.*** Absent-minded when driving. ***Mental confusion.*** Mistakes in writing. Does not know whether he has actually experienced things or dreamed them.

Offended easily. Unyielding and resentful. Causeless anger with oneself and family. Dwells on past. Resentful about past. ***Aversion to company.*** Restless feeling in company. Resentful about things that happened in the past. ***Aversion to conversation.***

Gloomy, tearful, but indisposed to talk. Consolation aggravates. Withdraws, shuns people. ***Feels better when alone.*** Discontented with or indifferent to oneself. Reproaches or pities oneself.

Sadness. Gloomy and pessimistic. Feeling of an inner void. Indisposition to talk. Indifference to own mistakes. Fear of getting depressed, wants to escape the daily routine and go on holiday.

Delusion of lying in an open grave, that is being filled in. Floating sensation, as if walking on cotton. Delusion as if head were filled with pudding, or with lead. Wants to be dressed in black. Experiences no anxiety but feels resigned and peaceful.

Back - Drawing pain in scapulae as from having carried heavy loads.

Breasts - Burning pain in nipples, nipples very sensitive to touch.

Cough - Dry, hacking cough.

Eyes - Sensation of dryness, worse draft of air. Burning pain in eyes, and dryness. Twitching of right lower lid. Diplopia, worse thinking about it and excitement, better relaxation.

Female - Burning pain in ovaries at time of ovulation. Sexual desire increased.

Food - Appetite increased. Loss of appetite. Thirst for lukewarm water. Aversion to smell of food. Aversion to smell of onions. Desires chocolate. Desires lukewarm water. Desires salt, sour, sweets. Desires for chocolate. Worse smell and sight of food. Better milk. Better eating. Better milk.

Head - Congestion to head and hot ears. Sensation as if head were filled with cotton. Headaches, better cold applications. Headache and sensation as if walking on cotton. Sudden headache, ceasing suddenly.

Limbs - Heaviness in legs. Tingling legs at night, worse cold, draft of air and lying down, better motion and warmth.

Male - Sexual desire increased.

Modalities - Better eating. Better rest. Better warmth. Better motion. Worse smell and sight of food. Worse cold, cold draughts. Worse cold drinks. ***Worse right side.*** Worse morning on awaking. ***Worse evening.*** Worse pressure. Worse motion.

Mouth - Pappy taste in mouth, in morning. Salivation in morning.

Nose - Sensitive to smell of onions and food in general. Coryza, with clear discharge. Coryza with scanty discharge of white mucus, worse warm room, better cold air. Coryza with sneezing on awaking and in evening.

Rectum - Constipation, stool soft and sticky. Fatty stools.

Skin - Dry skin and desquamating. Itching.

Stomach - Nausea, better diversion, eating and motion. Pressing pain in stomach, better milk. Nausea in morning, worse sight and smell of food. Pressing pain in stomach and nausea, better eating, better rest. Sensation of a stone after drin

Throat - Scraping in throat.

Vertigo - Transitory. Vertigo lying down. Vertigo better sitting.

REFERENCES - Mattitsch.

AESCULUS GLABRA

(Ohio Buckeye)

PHARMACY - aesc-g. Aesculus glabra. Ohio Buckeye. Fetid Buckeye. N. O. Sapindaceae. Hippocastanaceae. States of North America watered by Ohio River. Tincture of the whole ripe fruit without the shell. ***Historical dose:*** Tincture and all potencies.

CLINICAL - Constipation. Cough. Cramp in stomach. ***Hemorrhoids.*** Meningitis. Paralysis. Proctitis. Speech, thick. Vertigo. Wryneck.

HOMEOPATHIC - Aesculus glabra, like the horse chestnut, has a marked action on the rectum. In cattle, it produces wryneck and paresis of hind limbs.

Produces hard, knotty stools, very painful. Very painful, dark purple, external hemorrhoids with constipation, vertigo and portal congestion. Dark purple hemorrhoids with lame back, weakness of sacrum and lower limbs. Proctitis.

Fullness and heaviness of the head without pain, the sight may be dim or lost, eyes fixed and expressionless. The tongue is as if lame, speech thick. Cough produced by sudden irritation of throat. Sensation as of a feather tickling the throat, causing hawking and raising of mucus finally streaked with blood. Impaired vision. Paresis.

MIND - Confusion with vertigo, often followed by stupefaction and coma.

Back - Wryneck. Great lameness and weakness of the back.

Eyes - Eyes fixed and dead, expressionless. Sight dim or lost.

Limbs - Trembling of lower limbs. Lower limbs lame, paralysis. Strong tendency to contraction of legs. Trembling. Spasms and convulsions, followed by lameness.

Lungs - Cough from sudden irritation of throat, sensation as of a feather tickling the throat, causing hawking and raising of mucus finally streaked with blood.

Mouth - Speech thick and tongue as if lame.

Rectum - It has hard, knotty stools, very painful. Dark purple hemorrhoids with lame back and lower limbs. Proctitis.

Stomach - Nausea with loathing of food and vomiting. Distention (in cattle). Full sensation. Cramp-like pain.

Vertigo - Vertigo with staggering, reeling, unconsciousness. Vertigo with full, heavy head, dim sight, thick speech, nausea and vomiting, faintness towards evening.

REFERENCES - Boericke. Clarke.

AESCULUS HIPPOCASTANUM

(Horse Chestnut)

PHARMACY - aesc. Aesculus hippocastanum. Horse chestnut. Hippocastanum vulgaris. N. O. Sapindaceae. Hippocastanaceae. Northern India and North America. Tincture of ripe kernel, trituration of dry kernel. Tincture of fruit with capsule according to Hering is the best. ***Historical dose:*** Tincture and all potencies.

CLINICAL - Anal, problems. Ankylosing, spondylitis. Arthritis. ***Backache***. Constipation. Coughs. ***Glandular, swellings.*** Headaches. ***Hemorrhoids***. Hernia. ***Hip joint, disease.*** Intermittents. Jaundice. Joints, pain. Liver, disorders. Lumbago. Malaise. Palpitations. Prostate, disorders. ***Rheumatism. Sacral-iliac pain.*** Taste, altered. Throat, disorders. Tongue, disorders. Uterine prolapse. ***Varicose, veins. Venous stasis.***

HERBAL - In some districts it is a popular custom to carry a chestnut in the pocket as a preventive for hemorrhoids..

HOMEOPATHIC - The action of this remedy is most marked on the lower bowels, producing engorged ***hemorrhoidal veins*** with the characteristic backache and absence of constipation. ***Hemorrhoids***, with much pain but little bleeding. ***Venous stasis*** in general. ***Varicose veins*** of a purple color.

Many of the symptoms which Aesc. produces are due to a deranged liver or reflex from hemorrhoids. Everything is slowed down, digestion, heart, bowels, etc. Torpor and congestion of the liver and portal system with constipation. ***Fullness in various parts***, dry, swollen mucus membranes.

This remedy has great affinity for the pelvis, hips, the sacro-iliac joint and sacrum problems. ***Sacro-iliac problems*** since an injury or a fall. ***Degenerative hip disease.*** Arthritis of the hip. Aching pains in hips and pelvis. Sore muscles, mornings on waking and on motion.

Glandular swellings. Aesculus produces sensation of ***heat, dryness, stiffness and roughness*** in throat, nose, anus, etc. Throat symptoms with hemorrhoid conditions. Mucus membranes ***dry, swollen, burn and feel raw.***

Joints weak. The back aches and gives out. Backache, lumbo-sacral region aches. ***Walking greatly aggravates all symptoms.*** When walking feet turn under. Soles feels sore, tired and swell. Hands and feet swell and become red after washing, feel full.

MIND - Aesc. patients are despondent, gloomy and irritable. Irritable, unable to fix his attention. ***Depressed and irritable.*** Extremely irritable. Loses temper easily. Feels miserably cross. Gloomy and despondent.

Malaise. Dullness of head and mind, fullness at root of nose. ***Dullness, sluggishness on waking in morning, on waking at night.*** Mistakes in localities. ***Wakes up with confusion of mind***, bewildered, especially the children. Doesn't know where she is nor whence came the objects around her.

Abdomen - It has a marked action on the veins of the lower bowels and pelvic organs causing engorged hemorrhoids. Pain at umbilicus. Jaundice, throbbing in hypogastrium and pelvis. Throbbing in abdomen, especially hypogastrium. The most intense action is on the lower bowel and pelvic organs. Veins of portal system are also engorged producing soreness and fullness of the liver and abdomen.

Back - There is a characteristic backache which unfits the patient for business. ***Backache of sacrum and hips, worse walking or stooping***. Pains are sticking or flying all over, hot like lightning. Lameness in neck, aching between shoulder blades. Back region of ***spine feels weak***, back and legs give out. Pain as if back will break. Has to make repeated efforts at rising, worse walking and stooping. Aching in lumbar and sacral regions with stiffness in the back, almost impossible to walk.

Chest - Feels constricted. Heart's action full and heavy, can feel pulsations all over. Laryngitis, coughs ***depending on liver disorders***, hot feeling in chest, pain around heart in hemorrhoid subjects. Feels constricted, hot feeling in chest.

Constitutions - Bilious temperament. Anal troubles. Menopausal years. Varicose veins. For persons with hemorrhoidal tendencies who suffer with gastric, bilious or catarrhal troubles.

Eyes - Eyeballs feel heavy, dull, hot and sore with lachrymation with ***enlarged blood vessels***.

Female - Constant ***throbbing behind symphysis pubis.*** Leucorrhea with ***lameness of back across the sacro-iliac articulation***, dark, yellow, sticky corroding, worse after menses.

Food - Loss of appetite. Considerable thirst. Nausea from tea.

Head - Headache dull, confused, aching as from a cold. Pressure in forehead with nausea, followed by stitches in right hypochondrium. Pain from occiput to frontal region with bruised sensation of the scalp, worse in the morning. Neuralgic stitches from right to left through forehead, followed by flying pains in epigastrium. Bruised pain in occiput to the frontal region with flushes of heat over occiput, neck and shoulders.

Heart - Pain around heart in hemorrhoid subjects. Audible palpitations, when pulsation extends to limbs.

Kidneys - Frequent, scant, dark, muddy, hot urine. Pain in kidneys, especially left and ureter.

Limbs - ***Degenerative hip disease.*** Arthritis of the hip. Aching pains in hips and pelvis. Bruised pain affecting sacrum and hips. ***Takes repeated efforts at rising from seat, worse walking and stooping.*** Aching and soreness in limbs, in left acromion process with pain shooting down arms, fingertips numb. ***Weak feeling in sacro-iliac joints***, as if legs would gave way. Paralytic heaviness of arms, spine, feet.

Limbs - Hands and feet swell and become red after washing. Spine feels weak.

Liver - Tenderness and fullness in region of liver. Soreness and fullness in liver region, the abdomen is sore to touch. Jaundice with bileless stools. Dull aching in liver and epigastrium.

Male - Discharge of prostatic fluid at every stool and urination. Testes as if sore. Testes itch. Drawing pain in left testes. Dull and heavy shooting pain through penis. Shooting pain in right testes. Seminal emissions with amorous dreams.

Modalities - Hemorrhoids better from bleeding. Better in summer. Better in cool, open air. Better bathing. Better continued exertion. Better kneeling. Worse from winter, cold air, cold seasons. Worse after washing. Worse morning. Worse on waking. Worse afternoon. Worse after eating. Worse after stool, urinating. Worse motion. Worse standing. Worse lying. Worse stooping. ***Worse walking,*** which aggravates all symptoms.

Mouth - Thickly coated tongue, tongue and mouth feel as if scalded. Cannot control the tongue so as to form words rightly. Toothache, lower molar, worse warm drinks, better holding cold water in mouth. Salivation. Taste sweet, bitter, metallic. Teeth as if covered with oil.

Nose - Dry inspired air feels cold, ***nasal passages sensitive*** to it, causes burning, rawness and fluent coryza and sneezing. Pressure at root of nose. Membrane over the turbinate bones distended and boggy. Obstruction of nose due to hepatic disorders. Congestive catarrh.

Rectum - Anus raw, sore. ***Burning in anus with chills up and down the back***. As if a bug crawling from anus. Constipation, hard, dry, knotty, white stools. Pains long after stools. ***Feels full of small sticks***. Much pain after stool with prolapse. ***Hemorrhoids*** with sharp shooting pains up the back. ***Hemorrhoids*** blind and bleeding, purple, painful. Hemorrhoids external, worse standing and walking, worse during menopause. Irritation caused by ascarides and aids their expulsion.

Sleep - Disposition to stretch and yawn. Drowsy, falls asleep easily. ***On awaking, knows not where she is.*** Awakened by burning pain in stomach. Sore and tired in morning on awaking. Sleepless from thoughts continually crowding on mind.

Stomach - Heartburn and gulping up of food after eating. Weight of a stone with gnawing, aching pain, most manifest about three hours after meals. Pressure as from a stone with gnawing, aching pain, about three hours after meals. Desire to vomit with constant distress and burning.

Stool - Large, hard, dry stools. Stools first part hard and black, then white and soft.

Temperature - Chill at 4 p.m. Chilliness up and down back. Evening fever, 7 to 12 p.m., skin hot and dry. Sweat profuse and hot with the fever.

Throat - Hot, ***dry***, raw, stitching pain into ears when swallowing. Swollen glands. Follicular pharyngitis connected with hepatic congestion. ***Veins in pharynx distended*** and tortuous. Throat sensitive to inspired air, feels excoriated and constricted, burns like fire on swallowing in afternoon. Feeling of roughness, dryness, stitching or burning like fire on swallowing. Neuralgic pains in the fauces. Hawking of ropy mucus of sweetish taste.

Vertigo - Vertigo when sitting and walking. Slight vertigo while sitting, worse rising from seat. Vertigo with sensation as if he had to balance the head.

COMMENTS - Disordered liver. Soreness and fullness in the liver region, the abdomen is sore to the touch. Jaundice with bileless stools. Throbbing in abdomen, especially hypogastrium. The most intense action is on the lower bowel and pelvic organs. Malaise, dullness of head and mind, fullness at root of nose. Follicular pharyngitis with dryness, burning, roughness, contraction in throat.

Keynote use for hemorrhoids, blind or bleeding, relieved by bleeding. Large, swollen hemorrhoids, like a bunch of grapes. Feeling of dryness in rectum as if little sticks or splinters were pricking the folds of the mucus membrane with weak feeling in sacroiliac joints, as if legs would gave way.

Constipation, large, hard stools, followed by feeling of prolapse of rectum. Boericke noted fullness in the rectum, pain in the anus as if sticks stuck up the rectum.

General aching in lumbar and sacral regions with stiffness in the back, almost impossible to walk. Tearing pain in the small of the back and hips. Great affinity for the hips, the sacroiliac joint, for sacrum problems.

"Hip joint disease," "dislocates easily." May palliate for hip dysplasia. Degenerative hip disease, arthritis of the hip, bursitis. Deep, sore, aching pains. Characteristic worse from rising from a seat. Paralytic feeling in the hip and sacrum, feels weak, lame, and stiff. Ankylosing spondylitis, rigid back that aches and is sore.

For the back giving out during pregnancy, with a white leucorrhea. Ruptured disks, herniated disks, prolapsed disks, with radiating pains. Sacroiliac and lumbosacral problems with aching down both thighs, the backs of the thighs, and strong aching in the back.

Varicose veins (Ham.). "Venous stasis," the veins in the body are weak, producing hemorrhoids and varicose veins. Veins have lost tone and swell up with blood.

RELATIONS - ***Compare:*** (1) Aesc-g., Aloe, Coll., Merc., Nux-v., Podo., Sulph. (2) Phyt. - throat dry, more often in acute cases. (3) Aloe, Collinsonia. Nux-v. Sulph., Puls. (4) Arg-n. has also pain in sacroiliac joints and sensation as if the bones were loose. (5) Negundium americanum. (6) Kali-bi. - throat, but Aesc. h. has not the stringy mucus. (7) Phyt. - follicular pharyngitis. ***Complementary:*** Carb-v., Lach., Mur-ac. Nux-v. antidotes the hemorrhoidal symptoms. ***Follows well:*** Coll., Nux-v., Sulph.

REFERENCES - Boericke. Clarke. Murphy. Phatak.

AETHER

(Ether)

PHARMACY - aether. Aether. Ether. Etherum. Ethyl oxide. Ethylic ether. Sulfuric ether. ***Historical dose:*** All potencies.

CLINICAL - Bronchitis. Catalepsy. Convulsions. Cough. Delirium tremens. Hiccough. Mania. Meningitis. Nausea. Vomiting.

HOMEOPATHIC - Ether is the well-known anesthetic and the effects are those observed in patients under the action of its vapor, administered for the purpose of operation in habitual ether drinkers and on some who have voluntarily experimented with the drug upon themselves.

Ether is closely allied to alcohol, it possesses very similar intoxicating properties, produces visions, frequently pleasurable, hallucination and in some instances a persistent maniacal condition.

Convulsions, spasms and a cataleptic state. Chilliness. Bronchitis is a common after result of ether anesthesia and Belladonna has been observed to be the best antidote for this.

Macerator reported the cure of a woman of 60, who had been confined to bed for weeks with severe neuralgia of the head, raised welts on the scalp like ridges accompanying the pain. Ether 200c cured quickly.

MIND - Exhilaration, furious excitement, flushed face. Pleasant dreams of rapid flight through the air, gorgeous visions and unearthly music. Frightful dreams, fancied he heard the ringing of his own funeral bell. Low-spirited, fearful of some disease, desponding. Loss of consciousness.

Chest - Extreme coldness of the chest, wants it covered. Tightness, irritation and pain.

Ears - Sounds indistinct, seem far off, yet resound violently in the ears.

Eyes - Eyes suffused, lids closed, conjunctive injected. Pupils dilated. Dim vision as if mist or thin cloud before eyes.

Face - Face flushed.

Head - Meningitis. Temporal arteries enlarged, beat violently. Head drops to one side or is thrown back. Severe neuralgia of head with raised welts on scalp.

Heart - Excitement and invigoration of heart's action. Pulse full and bounding.

Limbs - Paralysis of lower limbs.

Lungs - Violent cough from stinging or heat in bronchia. Expectoration of blood. Breathing is quickened, stertorous. Congestion of lungs and brain.

Mouth - Mouth often open. Salivation, slight frothing at mouth. Pronunciation difficult and indistinct.

Stomach - Hiccough persistent. Nausea. Vomiting.

Vertigo - Dizziness, headache with partial blindness follow ether anesthesia.

REFERENCES - Boericke. Clarke.

AETHIOPS ANTIMONALIS

PHARMACY - aethi-a. Aethiops antimonialis. Hydrargyrum stibiato sulfuratum. Aethi-a. is made by triturating two parts of sulphuret of antimony with one of quicksilver. ***Historical dose:*** All potencies.

CLINICAL - Corneal, ulcers. Otorrhea. Scrofula.

HOMEOPATHIC - Aethiops antimonialis is often more effective than Aethiops mercurialus in scrofulous glandular swellings, eruptions, otorrhea and eye affections, corneal ulcers.

REFERENCES - Boericke.

AETHIOPS MERCURIALIS

(Black Sulphide of Mercury)

PHARMACY - aethi-m. Aethiops mercurialis. Black sulphide of mercury. Aethiops mineralis. Mercurius sulphuratus niger. Hydrargyrum sulfuratum nigrum. Mercurius cum kali sulph. Trituration. Made by triturating two parts of sulfuret of antimony with one of quicksilver. ***Historical dose:*** All potencies.

CLINICAL - Ophthalmia. Otorrhea. Scrofula. Skin disorders. Syphilis.

HOMEOPATHIC - Clarke has confirmed its utility in many aggravated skin disorders. Aethiops Mercurialus has not been proved, but it has been used with success in scrofulous, herpetic, eczematous eruptions and discharges. Favus-like eruptions.

Eruptions from fright. Painful, irritating, scabby eruptions of face. ***Scrofulous disorders.*** Scrofulous ophthalmia and otorrhea offensive. Hereditary syphilis. It seems to combine the powers of its various components.

RELATIONS - ***Compare:*** (1) Calc., Sil., Psor. (2) Aethiops Antimonalis.

REFERENCES - Boericke. Clarke.

AETHUSA CYNAPIUM

(Fool's Parsley)

PHARMACY - aeth. Aethusa cynapium. Fool's parsley. N. O. Umbelliferae. Europe. Tincture of whole flowering plant. ***Historical dose:*** All potencies.

CLINICAL - Attention deficit. Anasarca. Brain, weakness. Cholera infantum. Colic. Coma. ***Convulsions.*** Cough. Delirium. Diarrhea. Dyspepsia. Ear, discharge. Ecchymosis. Emaciation. ***Epilepsy.*** Eye, disorders. Gland disorders. Headaches. Herpes. Hiccoughs. ***Idiocy.*** Infantile, paralysis. Insomnia. ***Malnutrition. Marasmus.*** Mental, retardation. Mental, retardation. ***Milk, allergy. Pyloric, stenosis.*** Stomach disorders. Trismus. ***Vomiting, projectile.***

HOMEOPATHIC - Aethusa cynapium affects the brain and nervous system, connected with gastrointestinal disturbances. Keynote violent action. ***Violent vomiting,*** violent convulsions, violent pains, violent delirium. In epileptiform spasms, the thumbs are clenched, face becomes red, ***eyes turned downwards***, pupils dilate and staring, foams at mouth. There is great weakness of mind or body.

Inability to digest milk (Nat-c.). Diarrhea, with marked ***aggravation from drinking milk*** and poor circulation. ***Improperly fed babies*** (Calc-p.). Patient cannot stand, sit up or hold the head up. Children who lack the power to hold their heads up with no particular ailment, sometimes they can't even stand or bear any weight on their limbs. Want of power to stand up. Sharp pains. Parts feel screwed together.

Weak, nervous and prostrated from overwork. Prostration with somnolence. Profound prostration and stupor and lack of reaction, even speechless. Anguish, crying and expression of uneasiness and discontent. Useful for children's summer complaints and diseases during dentition.

MIND - Mind and body become weak. Brain fatigue from over study. ***Inability to think, to fix the attention***. Awkwardness. Mental, retardation. Attention deficit. Idiotic children. Idiocy may alternate with furor and irritability. Weepy, worse as disease progresses. Stupefaction during vertigo.

Fear before sleep to close eyes lest he should never wake. Examination failure from sense of incapacity. Unable to read after overexertion of mental faculties. ***Restlessness, anxious and crying***. Irritability, especially in open air. Irritability during headache.

Feels different from other people. Reserved people with inwardly strong emotions. Feels unconnected to other people. Loners. Great sadness when alone. Lives in his own sentimental world. ***Loves animals,*** talks to animals, looks after them with unnatural passion.

Delirium, better perspiration. Unconscious, delirious. Fancies herself lost on waking. Hallucinations. Delusions of animals. Delirium, sees cats, dogs and rats. Wants to jump out of bed or out of the window.

Abdomen - Cold internal and external with aching pain in bowels. Colic, exhaustion and drowsiness. Colic, followed by vomiting, vertigo and weakness. Black bluish swelling, coldness of abdomen, subjective and objective with coldness of legs with aching in bowels better warm application. Bubbling sensation around navel.

Back - Small of back as if in vice, aching. Want of power to stand to hold up head. Swelling of glands around neck like string of beads. A feeling as if pain in back could be better by straightening out and bending stiffly backwards.

Chest - Crampy constriction in chest. Stitches in left side of chest.

Constitutions - Suited to infants, teething children and cholera disorders of children and the elderly.

Ears - ***Feel blocked***, better by inserting the fingers and drawing the parts apart. Sense of something hot from ears, as if something hot steaming out. Hissing sound.

Eyes - ***Eyes drawn downward***, squinting, pupils dilated. Brilliant and protruding. Cornea sunken. Objects seem larger or double. Photophobia, chronic. ***Swelling of meibomian glands***. Rolling of eyes on falling asleep.

Face - Sunken, pale, ***puffed***, red-spotted, collapsed. Expression anxious, full of pain. ***Linea nasalis*** marked blue white pallor about the lips. puffed, spotted, red.

Female - Sharp pains in sexual organs. Pimples on external parts, itching on getting warm. Menses watery. Swelling of breasts with sharp pains.

Food - Burning thirst with total loss of appetite. Desires wine, but aggravated from it. ***Intolerance of milk.*** Nibbling appetite. Regurgitation of food long after eating. Digestion affected from brain exhaustion.

Glands - Lymphatic glands swollen like strings of beads.

Head - Head feels confused. Head or brain feels as if bound up or in a vise. ***Occipital pain*** extending down spine, better lying down and by pressure. Head symptoms relieved by expelling flatus (Sang.), and by stool. Cannot raise head. ***Hair feels pulled.*** Squeezing headache with vertigo worse walking and looking upward. Dizzy and drowsy.

Heart - Violent palpitations with vertigo, headache and restlessness. Pulse rapid, hard and small, not rhythmical.

Kidneys - Cutting pain in bladder with frequent urging. Pain in kidneys.

Limbs - Want of power to stand up or hold head up. Weakness of lower limbs. Fingers and thumbs bent inwards or clenched. Numbness of hands and feet. Violent spasms. Sensation as if arms had become much shorter. Heaviness, weakness, contraction of fingers. Excoriation of thighs on walking.

Lungs - Difficult, oppressed, anxious respiration, crampy constriction. Short breath interrupted by hiccough. Suffering renders the patient speechless. Cough causes pain in head.

Male - Right testicle drawn up with pain in kidney.

Modalities - Better in open air. Better from walking in open air. Better by conversation and company. ***Worse from milk***. Worse coffee. Worse wine, drunkenness. Worse frequent over eating. Worse from 3 a.m. to 4 a.m. Worse evenings. Worse warmth. Worse summer. Worse warmth of bed. Worse cold water. Worse over exertion. Heat causes all eruptions to itch intolerably.

Mouth - Dryness. Aphthae in the mouth. Tongue seems too long. Burning and pustules in the throat with difficult swallowing. Speech slow, embarrassed. Speechless. Bitter taste, of onions, cheese, sweetish in morning.

Nose - Nose stopped up with much thick mucus. ***Herpetic eruption*** on tip of nose. Frequent ineffectual desire to sneeze. Alae nasi drawn in.

Rectum - Cholera infantum, child cold, clammy, stupid with staring eyes and dilated pupils. Cholera disorders in old age. ***Undigested, thin, greenish stools***, preceded by colic with tenesmus followed by exhaustion and drowsiness. Yellow, green, slimy diarrhea. Obstinate constipation, feels as if all bowel action is lost.

Skin - Excoriation of thighs when walking. Easy perspiration, ***surface of body covered with clammy sweat. Lymphatic glands swollen. Itching eruption around joints*** better from heat. Skin of hands dry and shrunken. Ecchymosis. Anasarca. Whole body may be blue, black.

Sleep - Disturbed by ***violent startings*** or cold perspiration. Dozing after vomiting or stool. Child is so exhausted, it falls asleep at once. Rolling of the eyes or slight convulsion on falling asleep. ***Limpness and deep sleep after vomiting, with a deathly nausea***.

Stomach - ***Intolerance of milk***, vomiting as soon as swallowed or in large curds. Hungry after vomiting. ***Regurgitation, about an half hour after eating***. Nausea at sight of food. Painful contraction of stomach. ***Violent vomiting*** of a white frothy matter. ***Projectile vomiting.*** Vomiting of frothy matter white as milk or yellow fluid. ***Pyloric stenosis.*** Retching. Vomiting with ***sweat and great weakness***, accompanied by anguish and distress, followed by sleepiness. Stomach feels turned upside down with burning feeling up to the chest. Tearing pains in the stomach extending to esophagus.

Temperature - ***Great heat, no thirst***. Profuse, cold sweat. ***Must be covered during sweat.*** Sweating, on slightest physical effort.

Throat - Sensation of constriction, preventing swallowing. Stinging in the throat. Soft palate red, swollen. Pungent heat in mouth and throat.

Vertigo - Vertigo, with sleepiness, can't raise the head. ***Vertigo with drowsiness with palpitation, head hot after vertigo ceases.***

COMMENTS - Ingesting Aethusa plant matter causes severe projectile vomiting. There is also gripping with diarrhea, vomiting, crying. Guernsey said Aeth. is invaluable for adults who complain of regurgitation of food an hour after it has been taken.

Copious vomiting in adults with a great feeling of distress, can't tell what the distress is about, but it still exists. A peculiar expression of great anxiety and pain. Linea nasalis, a surface of pearly whiteness on upper lip bounded by distinct lines from wings of nose to angles of mouth.

Inability to hold down any food. Severe spasmodic vomiting. Malassimilation. Also for vomiting during pregnancy that's very spasmodic and projectile. Good for projectile vomiting, pyloric stenosis, failure to thrive in children.

Keynote intolerance to milk in any form. Milk allergies in children with vomiting and spasm (Nat-c., has gas, bloating and diarrhea). Vomiting of everything taken, especially milk, which is ejected in yellowish or greenish curds. Great weakness and exhaustion after vomiting, the child is so exhausted they fall asleep at once. Wakes hungry, eats and vomits again. "Hungry after vomiting."

Epilepsy in children with emaciation, malassimilation and failure to thrive. Epileptic spasms (Cup.), the thumbs are clenched, the head is drawn back and the eyes go down. Epilepsy with foaming, pupils fixed and dilated. Prostration and sleepiness after attacks. Convulsions with cold limbs.

Sensation of swelling in the head and face on entering a room, sunken cornea, and eyeballs convulsed and directed downwards. Sensation of swelling in hands after walking. Lancinating pains. Swelling of breast or axillary glands with sharp pains. Prostration, stupid.

Tetanus. Alcoholism, with tremors, shaking, malassimilation and emaciation. Late learning to walk. Backward children with muscle weakness, stumbling, falling, late speech. Poor mental and brain development and coordination.

Characteristic inability to think or fix the attention. Stupor, in some cases alternating with a furor. Hallucinations. Delirium, sees cats and dogs. Wants to jump out of bed or out of the window. Irritability, especially in open air. Somnolence.

Clarke sent single doses of Aeth., at rare intervals with great relief, to a little child in an orphan home who suffered from severe headaches and inability to fix his attention on his lessons. The little boy asked for the remedy himself subsequently on a return of the old symptoms.

Clarke gave it to an undergraduate preparing for an examination with complete success. He had been compelled to give up his studies, but was able to resume them and passed a brilliant examination.

Guernsey said "The mental symptoms peculiar to children and frequently of adults, are, great anguish and crying. As the disease progresses the patient becomes more and more retired in his disposition and more inclined to weep."

RELATIONS - ***Compare:*** (1) Ant-c., Calc., Ars., Cic. (2) Athamantha - confused head, vertigo better lying down, bitter taste and saliva. Hands and feet icy cold. (3) Cic., Con., Oena., Ant-c. and Calc. - vomiting of milk. (4) Ars., Asar., Cupr., Ip., Op. ***Complementary:*** Calc., Sil. ***It antidotes:*** Opium, and is antidoted by vegetable acids. Teste places Aeth. in the Sulphur group with Cic., Con., Aster., Bov., Lob., Merc., Kreos.

REFERENCES - Boericke. Clarke. Phatak.

AGARICINUM

(Agaric Acid)

PHARMACY - Agarin. Agaricinum. Agaric acid. It is obtained from the fungus Boletus laricis (White Agaric) and is a white crystalline powder. Triturations and dilutions. ***Historical dose:*** All potencies.

CLINICAL - Cataracts. ***Chorea.*** Emphysema. Erythema. Heart, weakness. Neuralgias. ***Neuritis.*** Tic douloureux.

HOMEOPATHIC - This remedy is employed in severe cases of ***chorea***. Useful for the sweats of tuberculosis, it should be given before retiring. The dose may be repeated once or twice during the night.

Heart dilation, when complicated with emphysema. Fatty degeneration. Weakened heart action from acute diseases and old age, when attended with profuse perspiration and erythema.

Agaricin should be studied when the symptoms are crossed over the body. ***Chorea.*** There is marked twitching of the eyelids, spasmodic movements from simple involuntary motions and jerks of single muscles to a dancing of the whole body.

Trembling of the limbs, soreness of the spine and redness of the eyes. Involuntary movements cease during sleep, symptoms are worse during a thunderstorm.

Neuritis. The parts are red, hot and swollen. There are burning, itching and cramps of the hands and feet. There is twitching of the muscles of the hands and feet. The sleep is restless and disturbed.

COMMENTS - Royal reported that the 3x of Agarin. given three times daily cured a most violent case of Tic douloureux of the left side of face after Ars., Mag-p. and Bell. had failed. A slight touch would cause the paroxysms to recur.

RELATIONS - ***Compare:*** (1) Agar.

REFERENCES - Blackwood.

AGARICUS BLAZEI MURILL

(Brazil Mushroom)

PHARMACY - agar-b-m. Agaricus blazei murill. Brazil mushroom. Tincture of fresh fungus. Also used as a powder and food. ***Historical dose:*** Tincture and all potencies.

CLINICAL - Allergies. Angina pectoris. Asthma. Athlete's, foot. Atopic, dermatitis. Breast cancer. Bronchitis. ***Cancer.*** Colds. Constipation. Cystitis. Dermatitis. Eczema. Hay fever. Heart, disorders. Hemorrhoids. ***Immune, weakness.*** Infections. Influenza. Insomnia. Kidney, disorders. Leukemia. Lymphoma. Psoriasis. Prostate, enlargement. Raynaud's disease. Rhinitis. Septicemia. Skin, cancer.

HERBAL - An agaricus mushroom found in the highlands of Piedade, Brazil. The inhabitants in Piedade enjoy long and good health with very few degenerative disease. The people there rarely suffer from cancer, heart disease, stroke, diabetes, arthritis, allergies, asthma, eczema, ulcers, etc.

In the 1960s, a Japanese descendant living in Brazil visited Piedade and made the observation that the people there eat a special kind of mushroom which is not found anywhere else. He sent samples of the mushroom to Japan for study and cultivation.

About the same time, two scientists from America also visited Piedade and made a similar observation. They proceeded to analyze the nutritional content of the Brazilian mushroom and published the results in scientific journals in 1965.

Experiments showed that not only the Agaricus mushroom is an effective cancer fighter, but also that it is the best cancer fighter among all the medicinal mushrooms known. The mushrooms fight cancer by enhancing the body's own immune system rather than directly trying to kill off the cancer cells. It is therefore as safe as any food substance can be.

Subsequent studies showed that the Agaricus mushroom has a powerful normalizing effect of all body physiological functions.

That is why that clinically it has been effective against many health problems afflicting mankind.

Blood - Raynaud's disease. Septicemia.

Cancer - Breast cancer. Hodgkin's lymphoma. Leukemia. Lymphatic cancer. Ovarian cancer. Skin cancer.

Heart - Angina pectoris. Heart tonic. High blood pressure, and low blood pressure. Hardening of the arteries.

Kidneys - Kidney infection. Kidney failure.

Lungs - Chronic bronchitis. Hay fever, allergic rhinitis, and asthma.

Rectum - Constipation and hemorrhoids.

Skin - Athlete foot. Eczema. Atopic dermatitis. Psoriasis. Skin cancer.

Sleep - Insomnia.

COMMENTS - Dr. Alexander Yuan of Hong Kong reported on this agaricus mushroom noting its usefulness for blood purification, cold hands and feet, frozen shoulder, hangovers. Neck and shoulder pain and low back pain.

Chronic debility. Collagen disease. German measles. Frequent colds and influenza, lack of energy. Insomnia, weak concentration. Pale, sallow complexion. Hyperactivity and improved athletic performance, among other benefits.

RELATIONS - ***Compare:*** (1) Carc.

REFERENCES - Murphy. Yuan.

AGARICUS CAMPANULATUS

PHARMACY - agar-cpn. - Agaricus campanulatus. Agaricus ovalis. A rare species, found in England on dung. N. O. Fungi. ***Historical dose:*** All potencies.

CLINICAL - Asthenopia. Backaches. Belching. Constipation. Delirium. Diarrhea. Flatulence. Hemorrhoids. Jaundice. Neuralgias. Palpitations. Spasms. Toothache. Trembling. Twitching. Vertigo. Vomiting.

HOMEOPATHIC - Poisonous doses produce violent vomiting and diarrhea with numerous nervous phenomena, tonic contractions of smooth muscle fiber, increased glandular and mucus secretions, and persistent anemia of nerve centers from spasm of arterioles.

Chorea-like spasms. Vertigo and general intolerance of the sun. Heavy weight in occiput. A very irritable and sensitive spine. Asthenopia with flickerings. Twitching of eyes and lids.

Gastro-enteric inflammation, with excessive, inodorous flatulence. Irritable bladder. A host of neuralgic pains everywhere, mostly splinter-like, burning and shooting. Particularly valuable in burning of the skin as from a frostbite, especially on the ears and feet.

Chorea-like twitchings of various fibrillae and even groups of muscles. Tremblings, external and internal. Flesh feels bruised, or as if frostbitten, sensitive to touch and to cold air.

General aggravation from walking in the open air, ameliorated when warm in bed. Pains in the limbs may disappear on motion, and return during rest. Symptoms often appear crosswise, as in right arm and left leg, etc. Shooting, splinter-like pains everywhere.

MIND - Delirium, attempts to escape. Incoherent talking. Aversion to mental work. Confusion and vertigo, aggravated by heat of sun.

Abdomen - Flatulent distention, rumblings, cutting, griping, stitches, and tension.

Back - Stiffness and soreness of nape. Backaches. Bruised and strained feelings. Deep stitches, burning, itching along spine and limbs. Spine sore to the touch and on stooping. Extreme pain and soreness in lower dorsal regions, becoming a pulsating on motion. Severe pains in the spine, boring, stitching, drawing, and soreness, mostly in lower dorsal region. Back pains, aggravated by walking in open air.

Bladder - Irritable bladder. Sharp pains. Burning on urinating. Not profuse urine. Lemon-colored urine, discharge of sticky mucus.

Chest - Numerous pains, tearing, pinching, tensive, stinging, burning. Constriction, oppression, heaviness. Rawness.

Ears - External ear burns and itches, as if it had been frozen. Twitchings of the auricular muscles. Numerous ringing and other noises within the ear.

Eyes - Twitching of lids and eyeballs. Margins of lids red, agglutinating. Vision dim on attempting to use the eyes. Flickering, type wavers, with itching and burning.

Face - Pale. Twitching of the muscles. Pains lancinating, tearing in the cheek.

Female - Violent pressing, tearing pains in back and abdomen with the menses. Pruritus pudendi.

Head - Drawing in bones of forehead, to the root of the nose. Shooting pains, mostly in the sides of the head or in small spots. Feeling of icy coldness on the head.

Heart - Palpitations. Tumultuous action. Irregular, intermittent pulse, ameliorated by coffee.

Limbs - Limbs weary and heavy. Trembling. Twitching. Shooting pains, shifting. Pains often ameliorated by motion.

Male - Sexual desire without erections.

Modalites - Better by motion. Better by coffee. Worse by walking in open air. Worse from heat of the sun.

Mouth - Dryness on salivation. Sweet taste. Toothache, neuralgic, aggravated by open air. Splinter-like pains in the tongue. Splinter-like pains through the jaws. Upper lip chapped, smarting, dry, with burning vesicles. Lips twitch.

Nose - Clear water runs from the nose, without inflammatory symptoms.

Perspiration - Profuse inodorous sweat, often localized to the chest. Oily sweat.

Rectum - Burning. Hemorrhoids.

Respiratory - Convulsive paroxysms of cough, sudden, ends with repeated sneezing. Expectoration of balls of mucus. Difficult respiration as if chest were full. Deep breathing and sighing. Noisy respiration at night.

Skin - Jaundice. Redness, stinging, burning as if frostbitten. Itching. White nodular elevations, with intense itching and burning.

Sleep - General sleepiness, especially after eating.

Stomach - Unnatural hunger, in evenings. Belching, empty. Numerous sensations with spasmodic contractions, irritable spine. Pains, gnawings, boring, cramps, and fullness.

Stool - Emission of much inodorous gas. Watery diarrhea. Constipation.

Temperature - Chilliness on motion, in the air, or on lifting the clothes. Burning heat on different spots, mostly local.

Throat - Constriction of larynx. Sharp pain extends through right eustachian tube to ear. General dryness. Contractions. Feels swollen externally, hands feel tight.

Vertigo - Vertigo, aggravated by heat of sun.

RELATIONS - ***Compare:*** Agar. Agar-cps., Agar-em., Agar-ph., Agar-st., Amanita vernus.

REFERENCES - Allen.

AGARICUS CAMPESTRIS

(Common Mushroom)

PHARMACY - agar-cps. Agaricus campestris. Common mushroom. Psalloita campestris. N. O. Fungi. ***Historical dose:*** All potencies.

CLINICAL - Abdominal pain. Abscesses. Boils. Cold. Colic. Cramps. Delirium. Dyspnea. Fever. Gangrene. Inflammatory, swellings. Nausea. Pulse, weak. Quinsies. Vomiting.

HOMEOPATHIC - Agaricus campestris is the common mushroom. This mushroom, common in the North America and in Europe, is esculent, stem only two to three inches high.

COMMENTS - Poisoning symptoms. Slight delirium. Eyes sunken, with livid circles. Face humid, hippocratic. Tongue red and parched. Skin cold, covered with cold sweat. Greenness of the skin. Formation of abscesses, which discharge a thin, ill-conditioned pus, and pass rapidly into suppuration and gangrene.

Abdomen retracted. Great abdominal pain at intervals. Severe colic. Nausea. Purging and vomiting of liquid matter.

Pulse hard, weak, rapid, irregular. Pulse feeble. Respiration irregular. Severe cramps. Kind of tertian fever. Somnolency.

RELATIONS - ***Compare:*** Agar. Agar-cpn., Agar-em., Agar-ph., Agar-st., Amanita vernus.

REFERENCES - Allen.

AGARICUS EMETICUS

PHARMACY - agar-em. Agaricus emeticus. Russula emetica. N. O. Fungi. A small acrid species, found in woods in Europe. Tincture of fresh fungus. ***Historical dose:*** All potencies.

CLINICAL - Anxiety. Belchings. Cold sweat. Diarrhea. Gastritis. Heartburn. Vertigo. Vomiting. Weakness.

HOMEOPATHIC - The symptoms of Agar-em. resemble those of the other Agarics, but while cold water aggravates the symptoms of Agaricus muscarius it speedily and permanently relieves those of Agar-em. Violent burning pains in the stomach.

There is a sudden and violent ***craving for ice-cold water*** during the worst attacks of anxiety, which gives gradual relief. ***All symptoms better from cold water.*** Violent vomiting with anxious sensation, as if the stomach hung on threads which would be momentarily torn in two with ice-cold sweat of face. Gastritis with cold sweat and a vomiting sensation.

Sudden great weakness. Severe vertigo, one must be carried to bed, is not able to sit or stand. Faintness worse by moving head. ***Faintness worse by smelling vinegar***, which is unbearable.

MIND - Attacks of anxiety. Anxiety in stomach.

Abdomen - Distended abdomen. Constantly increasing pain in abdomen.

Eyes - Lachrymation from odors. Lasting weakness of eyes.

Food - Sudden, violent ***desire for ice-cold water***, during the worst attacks of anxiety, which gives gradual relief. Dislike for wine and meat, relieve by cold water.

Modalities - ***Better from cold water.*** Worse from odors. ***Worse by smelling vinegar.***

Mouth - Nauseous taste in mouth. Sharp burning in mouth.

Nose - Sneezing from smells.

Pulse - Pulse rapid, exceedingly weak.

Stomach - Violent vomiting with anxious sensation, with ice-cold sweat of face. Violent burning pain in stomach. Painful pressure in stomach, followed by frequent belchings, repeated attempts to vomit. Constantly increasing anxiety in stomach. Stomach so sensitive that one could not touch it, nor cough.

Vertigo - Vertigo, so severe that one must be carried to bed is not able to sit or stand.

RELATIONS - ***Compare:*** Agar. Agar-cpn., Agar-cps., Agar-pa., Agar-ph., Agar-st., Amanita vernus.

REFERENCES - Allen. Boericke. Clarke.

AGARICUS MUSCARIUS

(Fly Agaric)

PHARMACY - agar. Agaricus muscarius. Fly agaric. Amanita muscaria. Bug agaric. Champignon fou. N. O. Fungi. Grows in Europe, Asia and America in dry places, especially in dry pine woods. Trituration of the carefully dried-up cap. Tincture of the fresh fungus. ***Historical dose:*** All potencies.

CLINICAL - Acne rosacea. ***Alcoholism.*** Blepharospasm. Brain, softening. Bunion. ***Chilblains.*** Chorea. Coldness. Cough. Cramps. ***Delirium tremens.*** Epilepsy. Fever, enteric. ***Frostbite. Gangrene***. Headaches. Hyperpyrexia. Hypothermia. Itching. Jaundice. Lachrymal, fistula. Lichen. Lumbago. Menses, painful. Meningitis. Myopia. Neuralgias. ***Nosebleeds***. Numbness. Nystagmus. Paralysis. Rheumatism. Sacrum, pains. Sebaceous tumors. Sexual excess, effects. Spinal, Irritation. Spleen, disorders. ***Tics***. Toothaches. Tremors. Tuberculosis. ***Twitching.*** Typhoid fever. Typhus.

HOMEOPATHIC - Agaricus contains several toxic compounds, the best known of which is muscarin. The symptoms of poisoning do not develop at once, usually twelve to fourteen hours elapse before the initial attack. Agaricus acts as an intoxicant to the brain, producing more vertigo and delirium than alcohol, followed by profound sleep with lowered reflexes.

Agaricus is used in many parts of the world for making an intoxicating drink. We find in ***alcoholism*** a sphere for its action and also in all states of delirium, mania and even idiocy. Cerebral excitement, as found in delirium of fevers, alcoholism, etc. The delirium is to make verses and prophesy, also silly merriness and incoherent talk with mania, kisses companions.

Frostbite and chilblains, itching, redness and burning. Bunions. ***Sensations if pierced by needles of ice***. Sensitive to pressure and cold air. ***Violent bearing down pains***. Symptoms appear diagonally as ***right arm and left leg***. Pains are accompanied by sensation of cold, numbness and tingling.

General paralysis. Jerking, ***twitching,*** trembling and itching are strong indications. Epilepsy with great exertion of strength. Chorea, ***twitching ceases during sleep***. Various forms of neuralgia and spasmodic disorders and neurotic skin troubles are pictured in the symptomatology of this remedy.

Agar. is a spleen medicine, causing stitch in the side and it has cured stitch in runners, enabling them to run further. Anemia. Incipient tuberculosis is related to the tubercular diathesis. Offensive breath, belchings and stools. Sweat may be oily, but is not offensive.

MIND - Mental depression, languor, indifference. Disinclination to work, confusion. Indisposed to perform any kind of work especially mental. Cannot do anything new, cannot do routine work, or does the opposite. Slow in learning to walk and talk. Awkward and clumsy.

Morose, self-willed, stubborn. Selfish behavior. ***Alcoholism.*** Dull and dizzy as if drunk. ***Delirium tremens.*** Reveals secrets. Pressure on spine causes involuntary laughter. Aversion to being touched.

Hyperactive, clumsy children without any fear or idea about danger. Fearlessness, recklessness and thoughtlessness. Convulsions after being scolded (Ign.).

Makes many revengeful plans. Confusion of mind on waking in morning, better after eating. Knows no one, throws things.

Hysteria after sexual excesses. Memory active, in evening.

Fears to be left alone lest he injure himself in a frenzy. ***Fear of cancer.*** Preoccupied with death, dying, graveyards. Fear of ghosts. Fear after going to bed. Pities herself.

Delirium of fevers. Delirium characterized by makes verses, singing, shouting and muttering, rhymes and prophesies. ***Increased cheerfulness, courage, loquacity, exalted fancy.*** Hilarious. Embraces and kisses hands.

Delirium with much twitching. ***Fearlessness.*** Sings, talks incoherently, but does not answer. ***Loquacity***, changes rapidly from subject to subject, but does not answer.

Great mental excitement and incoherent talking, immoderate gaiety alternates with melancholy. Perception of relative size of objects is lost. Physical strength is increased, can lift heavy loads. Delirium begins with paroxysm of yawning.

Sings, talks incoherently, changes rapidly from subject to subject, but doesn't answer. ***Full of ecstasy.*** Furious or raging delirium. Screaming, raving, wants to injure himself.

Abdomen - Burning in abdomen. Flatulent distention of abdomen. Sharp pains in ***spleen*** (Cean.), and abdomen. Sharp pain in the splenic region in runners. Colic. Cutting, griping pains in bowels. Rumbling and fermenting in bowels. Profuse, inodorous, hot flatus. Sensation of writhing. Abdomen as if empty, hollow or cold.

Back - Painful weakness and soreness. Shooting, burning pains along spine. ***Pain with sensitiveness of spine to touch***, worse in dorsal region. Aching in back after dinner. Burning pains along the spinal cord. ***Pain as if hot and cold needles stabbed into spine.*** Painfulness along spinal cord when stooping. Painful pulsation in spinal canal. Lumbago, worse in open air. Crick in back and neck. ***Twitching of cervical muscles.*** Spine seems short. Muscles of back feel tight, as if they would break on bending. As if cold air were spreading along back. As if cold water were running down back. ***Spinal irritation, due to sexual excesses.*** Sacrum as if beaten or dislocated. Swelling of cervical glands.

Breasts - Metastases from suppressed milk to the brain, abdominal troubles etc. Nipples, itch and burn, look red during pregnancy.

Causations - Blood poisoning. ***Frostbite***. Mental exertion or excitement, over-exertion. Fright. ***Alcoholism***, sexual excess, subjective symptoms arising after sex.

Chest - Anxiety in chest. Stitches under short ribs, left side. Sharp pain behind sternum most at end of expiration. Sharp pain in right lung while walking. Severe burning in chest. Chest as if too narrow. Chest as if too full of blood. Chest as if sprained, worse deep breathing. Burning. biting pimples on chest.

Constitutions - Light hair, skin and muscles lax. Old people with indolent circulation. Venous weakness. Diarrhea. Alcoholics, especially with headaches. Mushrooms are forbidden by Grauvogl to persons with the ***hydrogenoid constitution.*** The patients are exceedingly sensitive to cold and damp.

Cough - Cough with rattling of mucus, without expectoration. Dry cough after dinner. ***Cough ends in a sneeze***. Spasmodic coughing at night after falling asleep. ***Cough with expectoration of little balls of mucus***. Has to sit up in bed, or cough takes his breath. Has to sit down when cough comes. Violent attacks of coughing that can be suppressed by effort of will, worse eating, pain in head while cough lasts. Convulsive, hacking cough, with anxious sweat.

Ears - Itching in the ears with redness and burning pain, as if they had been frozen. Twitching of the muscles about the ears with noises. Rattling, fluttering in tympanic cavity. Sharp pains in left mastoid process. Excessive secretion of wax. Very acute hearing. Feels worse from hearing people talk. Dull hearing.

Eyes - Eyes as if weak, without having exerted them. Asthenopia from prolonged strain. ***Spasms*** of accommodation. ***Twitching of eyelids and eyeballs*** (Cod.). Oscillating eyeballs. Heat in eyes. Lids heavy, as if stuck together. Eyelids thick, dry, burning red, itch and agglutinate. Inner angles very red. Gum in canthi. Narrowing of space between eyelids. Nystagmus, squint. Swelling of tear gland. Vesicles or ulcers on cornea. Lachrymation from smells or coughing. Sensitive to light, even candlelight. Pupils dilated.

Face - Face, blue and puffed. Grimaces. Idiotic expression. ***Facial twitching***. Muscles feel stiff. Face itches and burns. Lancinating, tearing pain in cheeks, as of splinters. ***Neuralgia, as if cold needles*** ran through nerves or sharp ice touched them. Pricking in chin, as from needles. Herpetic eruptions. Pimples changing to vesicles filled with yellow serum. Burning and smarting on lips. Faceache with toothache. Jaws clenched. Eruption about mouth in growing children given to licking of lips.

Female - Spasmodic dysmenorrhea. Labor-like cramps, must lie down. Menses too profuse, earlier. Menses with titillation in genital organs and desire for sex. Tearing, pressive pain in genitals and back, with itching. ***Severe bearing-down pains, especially after menopause***. Bearing down pains on lifting. Leucorrhea, dark, bloody, excoriating, patient is unable to walk. Leucorrhea, with much itching, with sexual desire. Complaints following childbirth and sex. Itching, with sexual desire. Sexual excitement.

Food - Loss of appetite after sex. Thirsty all the time. Much hunger, but no relish for food. Better from coffee. Better for an hour after eating while he is so exhausted, but great sleepiness remains. ***Alcoholism.*** Craving for alcohol. Worse after tobacco. Worse tea and coffee. Wine causes indisposition to work. Coffee accelerates pulse. Meat causes heartburn. Prunes causes pressure in stomach. Smelling vinegar causes faintness. Smell of vinegar unbearable. Drinking cold water aggravates.

Head - Head in constant motion. ***Headache must move head to and fro.*** Falling backward, as if a weight in occiput. Lateral headache, as if from a nail (Coff., Ign.). Dull headache from prolonged deskwork. Headache, must move the head to and fro. ***Headache with nosebleed.*** Headache with thick mucus discharge. Headache better after stool or urination. Headaches of alcoholics. Aching in vertex. Head drawn towards shoulders. ***Pain in small spots.*** Cold spots on head. ***Icy coldness like icy needles or splinters.*** Sharp, tearing, aching and boring pain in occiput. Neuralgia with icy cold head. Desire to cover head warmly (Sil.). Twitching and stitches, more on left side. Scalp tender, sensitive. Itching nettle-rash on scalp.

Heart - Anxious sensation of pressure in heart. Irritable heart of tea and coffee drinkers, and tobacco smokers. ***Irregular, tumultuous palpations*** after tobacco. Heart region oppressed, as if thorax were narrowed. Oppression on bending body down. Palpitations with redness of face. Palpitations during sex and depressed afterwards in both the sexes. Pulse intermittent and irregular.

Kidneys - Lameness in left kidney, sore to touch. Stitches in urethra. Stitches and burning while urinating. Sudden and violent urging to urinate. Frequent urination. Viscid, glutinous, mucus from urethra. Urine, flows slowly or in drops, has to press for passing urine. Urine, cold, profuse, colorless, clear, lemon colored. As if a cold drop of urine were passing. Urine scanty and dark.

Limbs - Stiff all over. Pain over hips. Rheumatism better motion. Weakness in loins. Uncertain gait. ***Frostbite***. Hands and feet very sensitive to cold. ***Itching of toes and feet as if frozen***. Cramps in hands and feet. Cramp in soles of feet. Joints feel as if dislocated. Pain in shin. Neuralgia in locomotor ataxia. Muscular soreness. Paralysis of lower limbs with spasmodic condition of arms. ***Trembling and twitching.*** Numbness of legs on crossing them. Paralytic pain in left arm followed by palpitations. Tearing painful contractions in the calves. Rheumatism better motion.

Liver - Sharp pains in liver. Cirrhosis. Liver weakness from alcohol.

Lungs - Dyspnea while walking, has to stand still to get breath. Suffocative fits with anxiety and fainting. Labored, oppressed breathing. Difficult, noisy breathing. Frequent deep sighing. Dyspnea with rapid beating of heart. Impeded breathing at night, from closure of nose by thick mucus. Rapid breathing, with heat all over and sweat, most in face. ***Easy expectoration of floculi or balls of mucus.*** Large brown lumps. Mucus, worse mornings.

Male - Burning in urethra during sex, worse ejaculation. Sexual desire increased. After sex, great debility, profuse sweat, burning and itching of the skin, tension and pressure under ribs. Hot seminal discharge. Premature ejaculation. Testes painfully retracted. Old gleet. Complaints after sexual debauches.

Modalities - Better from moving about slowly. Worse from open air. ***Worse cold or freezing air***. Worse cold weather. Worse before a thunderstorm. Worse sun. Worse morning. Worse after eating. ***Worse after sex.*** Worse from touch. ***Worse debauchery, alcohol.*** Worse mental exhaustion. Worse fright. Worse during menses. Worse pressure on dorsal spine.

Mouth - Aphthae on roof of mouth. Herpes on lips. Burning and smarting on lips. Offensive breath. Froth at mouth. Swelling and bleeding gums with pain. Angles of mouth droop from paralysis, saliva runs out. Twitching. Sweet, bitter taste. Taste sweet, sharp and bitter. Increased flow of acrid saliva. Salivation during menses. Thirsty all the time. Indistinct, jerky speech.

Nose - Redness of nose. Nervous nasal disturbances. Hay fever, itching of nasopharynx and ears. ***Itching internally and externally.*** Spasmodic sneezing after coughing, sensitiveness, watery discharge. Inner angles very red. Fetid, dark, bloody discharge. ***Nosebleeds in elderly people***. Frequent sneezing without coryza. Flow of clear water without coryza. Redness. Obstruction on stooping. Sensation of soreness in nose and mouth.

Perspiration - Cold sweat on face, neck, chest. Sweats easily. Sweats on alternate sides. Night sweats. Copious sweat when walking, or from least exertion. Greasy sweat, but not offensive. Sweats from anxious palpitations of heart. Sweats during stool.

Rectum - Crampy colic, with passing wind. Sharp itching in rectum. ***Itching, prickling in rectum and anus, as from worms.*** Biting in rectum after emission of flatus. Flatus hot. Emission of much inodorous gas. Constipation with rumbling in bowels during pregnancy. Hemorrhoids. Writhing in rectum. Burning in anus. Warm feeling in anus. Anus as if completely closed. Dysentery.

Skin - Miliary eruptions with severe itching and burning. ***Burning, itching, redness and swelling, as if frozen***. Pimples, hard like small fleabites. Chilblains. Angioneurotic edema, rosacea. Swollen veins with cold skin. Circumscribed erythematous, papular and pustular and edematous lesions. Itching changing place on scratching. Itching over affected part. Skin pains, when cold. Miliary eruptions with intolerable itching and burning. Slight blow causes ecchymosis.

Sleep - Sleeplessness from rush of ideas. Restless from violent itching and burning. On falling asleep, ***starts, twitches and awakens often.*** Drowsy in daytime. Unpleasant dreams awaking from sleep. ***Paroxysms of yawning***. Frequent yawning before pains or spasms as a concomitant. Yawning followed by involuntary laughter. Vivid dreams. Anxiety as if suffocating in dreams. Nightmares of dead people and graveyards.

Stomach - Empty belchings, tasting of apples. Flatulent distention of stomach. Profuse inodorous belchings. Eructation, empty, tasting of apples or of rotten eggs. Belchings and hiccoughs. Eructations alternating with hiccough. Burning in stomach about three hours after a meal, changing into a dull pressure. ***Gastric disturbance with sharp pains in liver region.*** Nervous disturbances with spasmodic contractions, hiccough. As if a lump in epigastrium. Vomiting, bitter with prostration with stitches in rectum and groin.

Stools - Fetid stools. Pappy stools with cutting in abdomen and passing of wind. Very hard stools, at first hard and knotty, then soft, finally diarrheic. Diarrhea with much fetid, garlicky odor flatus. Diarrhea of children with grass green, bilious stools. Diarrhea, morning after rising.

Teeth - Teeth sensitive to touch, pressure, or while chewing. Teeth as if too long. Tearing pain, pulsating, worse cold air. Shooting pain from right upper teeth up to right side of head. Teeth worse, when abdomen gets better. Toothache at beginning of menses and during. Swelling and bleeding gums, with pain.

Temperature - Chills or sweats easily. Chills with warm face, hands and feet. Very sensitive to cool air. Chilliness in open air, strikes through whole body. Shiverings over body, running from above downward. Goosebumps. Violent attacks of fever in evening. Burning spots.

Throat - Stitches along eustachian tube to ear. Feels contracted. Small solid balls of phlegm thrown up. Dryness of pharynx, swallowing difficult. Scratching in throat, cannot sing a note. Burning, cooling feeling. Pressure as from a foreign body sticking in throat, not better swallowing. Dryness and constriction of pharynx. Induration of tonsils and other glands.

Tongue - Tremulous tongue (Lach.). Tongue coated white. Tongue dry, one side numb with vertigo. Tongue as if dry and contracted, as after an astringent. Splinter like pains in tongue with salivation. Sharp pain, soreness or burning at tip of tongue. Bad taste at root of tongue. Tip of tongue studded with small dirty yellow aphthae.

Vertigo - Vertigo in morning. ***Vertigo from sunlight***. Vertigo from heat of sun. Vertigo with palpitations. Vertigo on walking. Vertigo reeling as if drunk. Vertigo with tendency to fall forward. Vertigo with stupefaction and burning in vertex. Vertigo after menses. Vertigo from yawning.

Vision - ***Double vision*** (Gels.). Dim and flickering vision. Flickering vision while writing. Shortsighted. ***Reading difficult, as type seems to move to swim***. Focal distance changes while reading. Dim vision as from a mist. Vibrating specters. Muscae volitantes, brown. Yellow, brown or black spots before left eye.

COMMENTS - Mushrooms are among the articles of diet forbidden to persons of the hydrogenoid constitution, in which the patients are exceedingly sensitive to cold and damp. Agreeing with this, in the provings of Agaricus is a great sensitiveness to cold air. In skin disorders and brain exhaustions, give the lower potencies. A left-sided remedy.

Talcott considered Agar. the most similar to general paralysis of all the remedies, with exalted notions of grandeur and power, hilarity and excitement followed by depression, confusion, imbecility.

Ludicrous behavior, poor perception. Causes delirium, mania and idiocy. Very talkative and loquacious, and tend to be alcoholics (Lach.). Creative, tendency to poetry, prophesy. Incoherent speech. Silly, may have a confused mind, can't think. States of ecstasy and trance. Wants to kiss and embrace everyone (Hyos.).

Mania with great displays of strength. Confusion in the brain as if semi-intoxicated. Tendency to use alcohol or drugs, spaced out, low energy. Disintegrated personality. Severe mood changes, irritability. May alternate between two states, one of being silly, foolish and manic and the other being depressed, sad and indifferent and the states may alternate.

Worse in the morning and during the daytime. Spacey, awkward. Dull, stupid, poor memory. Can't function during the day, relieved at night. Energy in the evening, they become more fluent, increased intellect. Worse mental exertion in general.

Marked and persistent vertigo with constant impulse to fall backward. Very sleepy after meals. Twitching about eyes and face, redness without heat, puffy and distorted. Visual defects along with twitches, may have blurring vision or twitching in the left eye.

Facial twitches, trigeminal neuralgias, tic douloureux.

Spasmodic twitchings throughout body, followed by tremulousness, finally relaxation and exhaustion. Don't twitch during sleep. Drops things. Hands fly open uncontrollably. Arm may snap or twitch without their knowing it (Nux-v.).

Muscular jerking and twitching, good for chorea. Spinal problems associated with twitching or brain problems associated with a retarded mind. Spasms and twitches due to spinal disease, arthritis or injury to the spine. Twitchings are especially marked in the eyes, eyelids and facial muscles. Blepharospasm and tic convulsif.

Awkward people. Ankylosing spondylitis. Spine is as stiff as a board, as if spine would break (Tub., Rhus-t., Nat-m.). Severe arthritis of the spine. Shooting, burning pains in the spinal cord, as if the whole spine is on fire. Tingling deep in the spine. As if hot or cold needles are being stuck in the spine. For cold spots along the spine or very tender places that cannot be touched.

Numbness of the extremities from some spinal problems. Pain in the sacrum followed by general paralysis symptoms, numbness in the limbs. Burning up and down the spine (Phos.). Back and neck feel dislocated, or for slipped discs with severe pain (Bry., Rhus-t.). Formication of the skin as if bugs are crawling under the skin (Cocain.).

Symptoms in extremities are as if the blood was cut off to the feet or hands, severe numbness, tingling, biting, burning of the extremities, as if they are on fire. Spasms and then burning pain and numbness in their legs, intermittent claudication. Better moving, worse rest. Burning cold, numb, twitching. Awkward walk.

Feet feel so cold as if they are frozen, like blocks of ice. Frostbite. Ailments since frostbite or sensation as if frozen. Poor circulation where the hands and feet turn blue, then burn as if on fire. Chilblains, loss of blood to the extremities. Spasms in the arteries and cuts off the blood. Chilblains, worse heat. Creeping, crawling sensations, formication, itching.

Peripheral vascular disease when the blood vessels in the extremities have deteriorated to the threat of gangrene.

Compromised blood flow. Typhoid states. Epilepsy. Brain disorders and fever with rolling of the head.

Pain as if touched or pierced by needles of ice is very characteristic.

Diagonal symptoms, right side and left forearm (Lac-c.). Electric-like shocks with jerking, spasms and twitching, painful. For bone aches as if they would break.

Peculiar headaches, "throbbing headache with sensation of stiffness of muscles of face. Dull, drawing headache in the morning, extending into root of nose with nosebleed or thick mucus discharge. Pain as from a nail in right side of head." Face feels stiff with the headache.

Chilly remedy, worse cold weather, cold air, drinking cold water. They can also have sun headaches (Nat-m.). Worse from storms. Better in the evening, better warmth and better motion.

Ravenous appetite with bolting of food. Desire for eggs, sweets and salt. Used for sudden, morning diarrhea that smells like sulphur (Aloe, Sulph., Rumx.). For diarrhea in children that is grass green (Cham.).

Worse after sex (Ph-ac., Sil.), may have more pains and twitches. Sexual desire enormous and enthusiastic with relaxed penis and impotence.

Bearing down pains in the pelvis as if everything will come with acrid, vaginal discharge with itching of the vagina. Also for spasmodic chronic hiccups (Nux-v.) and herpes on the lips that burn and smart. The nervous patients requiring Agar. pass little urine (opp. Ign.), though the bladder may be irritable.

Clinical for alcoholism, intoxication, hangovers, DTs, the shakes. Worse alcoholic or for "old drunks", spasms, twitches or convulsions, frothing at the mouth with arching of the back (Nux-v.). Muscle quivers and delirium tremors. Disordered speech in alcoholics. Lost continuity of speech.

Children with retarded development. Late learning to walk and talk. For children who have slow minds or mental retardation. Fainting and twitching of children.

Or twitches and spasms ever since puberty or a shock. Excitement brings on twitches and spasms. Uncoordinated children, they stumble, fall, and drop things. It's hard for them to learn.

Very anxious about their health. Fear of cancer (Ars. Nit-ac., Phos. Kali-ar.). Preoccupation with spookiness, fear of ghosts. Talk and dream about the dead, are obsessed with coffins.

RELATIONS - Agar. stands between Stram. and Lach. ***Antidote:*** Absin., Coff., Camph. ***Compare:*** (1) Agar-cpn., Agar-cps., Agar-em., Agar-pa., Agar-ph., Agar-st., Amanita vernus. (2) Muscarine, Atropia exactly opposes Muscarine, resembles Pilocarpine in action. (3) Tamus - chillblains and freckles. (4) Cimic., Cann-i., Hyos., Tarant-h. (5) Bov., Stict., Act-r., Cann-i., Op., Stram. - alcoholism, chorea. (6) Coff. - ecstasy. (7) Cic. - spasm of eyes. (8) Cod. - spasm of the eyelids. Mygal., Tarent., Verat. - icy-cold feeling in head. (9) Ars. - hot needles, Agar. ice-cold needles.

REFERENCES - Boericke. Clarke. Murphy.

AGARICUS PANTHERINUS

(Spotted Amanita)

PHARMACY - agar-pa. Agaricus pantherinus. Spotted amanita. N. O. Fungi. ***Historical dose:*** All potencies.

CLINICAL - Coma. Convulsion. Delirium. Diarrhea. Fatigue. Mania. Spasms. Trembling. Twitchings. Vertigo.

HOMEOPATHIC - Agaricus pantherinus is a brownish species (not reddish, like Agaricus muscarius), found in woods or pastures in England and in the United States, not considered poisonous.

General ***overpowering sense of fatigue.*** Extreme lassitude and torpor. Problems coordinating muscular movements. Convulsive movements. Loss of power. Monosyllabic answers, with annoyance. Vertigo. Loss of consciousness. Violent general spasms. Violent convulsive twitchings of the muscles of the face and limbs. Restless tossing about.

MIND - Delirium. Maniacal disposition to rave. State of consciousness resembling coma. Loss of memory.

Eyes - Eyes partly open. Conjunctiva injected. Red eyes.

Face - Face congested.

Food - Some loss of appetite.

Head - Great heaviness of the head. Heat in the head.

Limbs - Trembling of the hands.

Lungs - Respiration stertorous and irregular. After a few deep inspirations the respirations became weaker and weaker, until at last they ceased entirely for about a quarter of a minute, then there were again deep inspirations.

Mouth - Lips tremble.

Rectum - Slight diarrhea.

Sleep - Invincible drowsiness. Stupor. During sleep, respiration embarrassed, face congested and of a livid hue, pulse rather slow.

Throat - Difficult swallowing.

RELATIONS - ***Compare:*** Agar. Agar-cpn., Agar-cps., Agar-em., Agar-ph., Agar-st., Amanita vernus.

REFERENCES - Allen.

AGARICUS PHALLOIDES

(Amanita Bulbosa)

PHARMACY - agar-ph. Agaricus phalloides. Amanita bulbosa. Agaricus bulbosa. Amanita phalloides. N. O. Fungi. Europe and North America. Tincture of fresh fungus. ***Historical dose:*** All potencies.

CLINICAL - Chills. Cholera. Chorea. Cold. Collapse. Coma. Cramps. Convulsions. Delirium. Diarrhea. Gastritis. Malaise. Trismus. Urine, suppression. Vomiting.

HOMEOPATHIC - Agaricus phalloides is a small stinking fungus common in Europe and North America. The poison is a toxalbumin, resembling the poison in the rattlesnake and the poison excreted by the cholera and diphtheria germs. It acts on the red blood corpuscles, dissolving them so that blood escapes into the alimentary canal and the whole system is drained.

The amount of this toxic principle is small, even handling specimens and breathing the spores affects some people unpleasantly.

The poison is slow in development, even twelve to twenty hours after taking it the patient feels all right.

Symptoms generally begin with vertigo, followed by violent choleraic symptoms with rapid loss of strength, with death preceded by stupor and spasms on the second or third day. Symptoms observed in poisoning cases give a complete picture: Extreme prostration and chilliness, the sweat is cold, marked hippocratic face, the tongue is cold and there is violent thirst.

Debility, prostration. Malaise. Staggers as if intoxicated and with odd gestures, labors to express his sufferings but cannot articulate a syllable. Violent convulsions. Slight convulsive motions in the legs and arms, which generally extend to the muscles of the trunk and cause irregular distortions of the whole body. Constant restlessness.

Very frequent bilious vomiting. Incessant cramps in stomach. Hard, tense abdomen. Frequent whitish watery stools or bilious, bloody stools.

The urine is suppressed, the voice is hoarse. Pulse small intermittent, hardly perceptible. The limbs are cold and there are violent cramps in legs, feet and calves.

Fatty degeneration of liver, heart and kidneys, hemorrhages in lungs, pleura and skin. Lethargic but mentally clear. Sudden changes from rapid to slow and from slow to rapid breathing. Intense thirst for cold water, dry skin.

Extreme collapse. Cholera, cramps in stomach, cold limbs, urine suppressed. Vomiting and purging. Continuous urging to stool, but no gastric, abdominal or rectal pain.

MIND - Mental excitement for three days after taking them. Delirium with faint indistinct dreams. Very averse to lying down.

Restlessness and impatience lead him to make frequent attempts to walk about, but without any fixed object or design. Complete consciousness until death. Stupor. Coma and rattling respiration before death.

Abdomen - Violent pains in epigastrium, which spread rapidly over the whole abdomen, greatly worse by pressure. Abdomen tense, swollen, painful. Unendurable pain in hypogastrium and lumbar region.

Eyes - Eyes sunken, weak and lusterless. Pupils much dilated.

Face - Deathlike pallor, face sunken, cyanotic. Nose and mouth dry. Anxious countenance, hippocratic. Tetanic closure of jaws with at times grating of the teeth.

Head - Frightful pains in head.

Kidneys - Suppression of urine.

Limbs - Cold limbs. Skin of limbs lost its elasticity. Upper limbs swell and become livid, fingertips livid. Cramps of the legs of the calves of the feet with drawing back of the limbs.

Lungs - Respirations short.

Modalities - Worse from pressure.

Mouth - Teeth and gums black. Cold tongue. Breath cold. Trismus. Speech slow, difficult. Stammering.

Perspiration - Sweat cold.

Pulse - Small and intermittent, hardly perceptible, slow and somewhat irregular, hard and frequent. Pulse full and rapid (later action).

Rectum - Anus inflamed. Frequent, bilious, whitish stools as in Asiatic cholera. Frequent, watery, bloody stools.

Skin - Body covered with livid spots.

Sleep - Somnolence.

Stomach - Violent pain in epigastrium, worse pressure. Violent thirst, nausea, vomiting, then diarrhea. Pains in stomach and hypogastrium followed by anxiety and vomiting. Incessant cramps of stomach. Very frequent mucus and bilious vomiting. Vomiting of an offensive greenish-colored fluid of blood.

Temperature - Marked chilliness. Skin cool, afterwards hot.

Throat - Dry throat. Constant burning sensation in the pharynx after vomiting. Voice hoarse.

Vertigo - Vertigo always on rising up without loss of consciousness.

COMMENTS - General cholera symptoms are developed, as with Agar. muscarius. At times, the development of choleraic symptoms saves the patient. Chilliness predominates.

Prominent convulsions. Mental excitement, which has in some cases lasted for three days. Sometimes there is stupor, at other times consciousness remains until death.

The effects do not come on until ten or twelve hours after taking the drug (Colch.).

RELATIONS - ***Compare:*** Agar. Agar-cpn., Agar-cps., Agar-em., Agar-pa., Agar-st., Amanita vernus.

REFERENCES - Boericke. Clarke.

AGARICUS STERCORANIUS

PHARMACY - agar-st. Agaricus stercoranius. N. O. Fungi. ***Historical dose:*** All potencies.

CLINICAL - Coma. Convulsions. Delirium. Headache. Twitching. Vertigo. Vomiting.

HOMEOPATHIC - Thomas Stevenson M. D., writes in Guy's Hosp. Reports, vol. xix, p. 418: R. M., age thirty-nine years, ate food with Agar-st. in it. In half an hour he complained of nausea, some oppression in his breathing, and of severe pain across the forehead, with giddiness.

His wife then noticed a strangeness in his appearance, and that in attempting to walk he kept his eyes fixed on the ground and guided himself with difficulty. He was, however, quite conscious of everything, and opened a book to see if he could read, but found that he was unable to make out any of the letters.

When outdoors he continued to suffer severely from the pain across the forehead, with giddiness, and in addition experienced a feeling as if something was continually over his head, or as if passing "through an arcade." He staggered much.

About 11 p.m., after more than three hours, Mr. Hicks was called to see him. Hicks found him sitting down in a semi-state of stupor, with pupils dilated and inactive, and the pulse slow and feeble, from 55 to 60. On being roused and made to get up he looked completely bewildered, staggered as if tipsy, and said he could not recognize the things in the room, nor the room itself as that which he usually occupied.

He now become more restless, threw his arms about, and seemed anxious to be continually moving from place to place. He also appeared to be somewhat convulsed, with twitching of the muscles of the face, and complained of pickings in his hands, and of a feeling as if they were swelling. He suddenly became more excited, and rushed wildly out of the house into the street. He was found in a neighbor's house, considerably prostrated after his exertions, and in a very lethargic state.

Twenty grains of Zinc sulphate were now administered, and in a short time vomiting ensued, much dark fluid with numerous pieces of fungi being brought up. For a short time afterwards he expressed himself as feeling better, and was allowed to be taken to the door of the cottage.

Almost immediately afterwards, as if moved by a sudden impulse, he again rushed wildly out, but after going a short distance stopped suddenly, as if bewildered. Emetics were again administered and the stomach pump used, and in the course of a few hours he gradually recovered, though feeling much prostrated.

He said that during the whole time he was quite conscious of what was being done, but that at times he felt drowsy and inclined to sleep. When the convulsive paroxysms came on he felt wild and excited, with an irresistible desire to move about and to run. He had no pain in the stomach or bowels at any time, nor did the feeling of oppression of his breathing continue after the first symptoms.

RELATIONS - ***Compare:*** Agar. Agar-cpn., Agar-cps., Agar-em., Agar-pa., Agar-ph., Amanita vernus.

REFERENCES - Stevenson.

AGATHIS AUSTRALIS

(Kauri Tree)

PHARMACY - agath-a. Agathis australis. Kauri tree. ***Historical dose:*** All potencies.

CLINICAL - Asthma. Backache. Bulimia. Catarrh. Colic. Coryza. Coughs. Diarrhea. Flatulence. Hay fever. Headaches. Heat, flushes. Hysteria. Lachrymation. Lassitude. Leucorrhea. Monomania. Numbness. Photophobia. Salivation. Sneezing. Tooth, decay. Toothache. Twitching.

HOMEOPATHIC - Breathing deep ameliorates. Becomes cold easily. Heat flushes with numbness, waves of heat. Sensation of heat on surface of the body, of energy moving up the body. Heaviness sensation. Lassitude, in the afternoon, walking in open air ameliorates.

Waves of numbness. Usually painful complaints are painless. Prickling sensation. Sluggishness. Worse exposure to the sun. Tingling, trickling sensation, like drops. Twitching. Desires to walk. Wavelike sensation. Pins and needles sensations. Muscular weakness. Weariness in the afternoon.

MIND - Mental power increased. Memory active for past events. Yearning for things long past. Abundant ideas. Restlessness. Irritable. Monomania. Tranquility, serenity, calmness. Spaced-out feeling. Stupefaction with sleepiness. Vague thoughts.

Clearness of mind alternating with dullness, with sleeplessness. Dullness, as if drunk, in the afternoon. As if mind enveloped in a fog. Mental exhaustion, brain fag. Confused memory. Memory loss. Weakness of memory. Forgets what was about to do or say. Memory weakness for everyday things, words. Mistakes about left and right sides, in speaking, writing. Transposes words and uses wrong letters, figures. Studying and reading difficult. Erroneous thoughts. Mental confusion. Confusion as to his identity, sense of duality.

Anxiety for the world. Anxiety in chest and heart region. Cares, full of worries. Desires death. Thoughts of death. Despair of recovery. Discontented with himself. Disgust.

Fear of being alone. Fear of poverty. Forsaken feeling. Feels friendless. Aversion to company. Indifference, apathy. Self-loathing, contempt. Remorse. Helpless feelings. Detached. Discouraged. Insecurity. Hatred. Yearning, longing for things lost.

Moods are changeable. Weeping and tearful mood. Weeping and laughing at same time. Loquacity. Cheerful, exuberant and talkative. Ceaseless, childish, hysterical laughing, excessive. Laughs easily, everything seems ludicrous.

As if intoxicated. Gay delirium, exhilaration. Impulsive. High-spirited. Excitement. Audacity. Childish behavior. Makes strange faces. Curses.

Bulimia. Lascivious, lustful. Tendency to lie. Oversensitive. Sensitive to noise. Sensation of being old. Quarrelsome with her family. Quiet disposition. Resignation. Sadness from a dream. Heaviness, sensation alternating with clearness of mind. Dancing ameliorates mental symptoms.

Abdomen - Sensation of something alive, movements. Bubbling sensation. Painful distension. Flatulence. Fluttering sensation. Gurgling in the evening. Heaviness as from a load. Aching, dull pain. Pain as if clutching with nails. Clawing, cramping, griping pain. Pains extending downward. Sharp pain in the sides, in the evening. Rumbling in daytime, evening, as if diarrhea would come on. Stopped sensation. Twitching and jerking in sides. Colic during diarrhea.

Back - Backache. Aching pains in dorsal region, scapulae, spine, lumbar region, sacrum. Boring pain, extending to right shoulder, in dorsal region, scapulae. Burning pain in dorsal region, right scapulae, between scapulae. Cutting pain as if stabbed. Stabbing pain in vertebrae. Digging pain on right side. Lancinating pain in dorsal region. Pain as if someone is poking. Painful stiffness, in sacral region. Tension in dorsal region, scapulae. Twitching. Back pains extending to arms, elbow, lower limbs, shoulder, thighs, wrist.

Bladder - Constant urging to urinate, with thirst. Long, copious, increased urination, brown, dark brown, brown-yellowish, dark, yellow-dark, straw yellow.

Breasts - Pain in breasts, worse evening, night. Cutting, stitching pain, at night.

Chest - Anxiety in chest and heart region. Constriction, tightness, dryness, oppression. Pains evening in bed, at night. Pain from pressure on chest. Pains on sides, left. Burning pain in the sternum, pressure aggravates. Pressing pain in sternum. Cramping pains, under ribs, sides. Cutting, stitching pain, in ribs, sides, evening and night, extending downward. Sore, bruised pain, particularly ribs. Tearing pain and tension in lower ribs.

Cough - Dry, tickling cough, from irritation in larynx. Persistent cough.

Ears - Coldness as from a draft. Formication. Noises in ears like bell of a clock. Ringing in ears. Boring, lancinating, stitching pains. Stopped sensation, afternoon. Heat on one side, left ear very hot.

Eyes - Filmy. Pain in right eye. Itching in the corners of eyes. Itching canthi, eyelids. Photophobia, during headache. Involuntary desire to close the eyes. Heaviness, pressure sensation. Lachrymation. Burning, cutting, sore, stinging pains. Sensation as from a foreign body.

Face - Sensation of collapse. Pale, flushes easily. Stupid expression. Red face. Sensation of forehead wrinkled. Herpetic eruptions about lips, nose. White pimples. Itching, scratching ameliorates, particularly of cheeks. Aching pain, pressing, pulling sensation.

Female - Menses black, inky, pitch-like. Menses too early, and frequent, every two weeks. Menses too short. Clutching and relaxing sensation of uterus. Offensive leucorrhea, like ammonia, old cheese. Leucorrhea yeast-like, thin, watery, transparent. Vagina pain. Burning pain in ovaries. Cramping, grasping pain in uterus. Drawing pain. Lancinating pain, vagina. Piercing pain in pubic bone. Sore pains. Sore vagina. Sharp pain in labia, uterus, vagina. Sexual desire diminished, wanting or increased, insatiable. Swollen before and during menses.

Food - Appetite increased, with menses. Appetite ravenous, canine hunger. Desires bread, meat, fried food, juicy fruits, chocolate, sweets, cold drink and water, and beer in the morning. Aversion to vegetables. Thirst, at night, on waking. Extreme thirst for large quantities.

Head - Tension headaches. Photophobia during headache. Sensation of a current of air passing through head. Boiling sensation on forehead. Congestion, constriction, tension. Empty, hollow sensation. Headaches in the morning, ceases toward evening.

Limbs - Awkwardness. Coldness at night in bed. Cold hands, knee, leg. Cramps in forearm and hand. Heaviness sensation of thigh. Itching on hands, fingers, thighs, knees, ankles. Sensation of lightness. Lumps in elbows, ankles. Numbness in forearm, wrist, ankle. Pain in right shoulder, forearm, and wrist. Aching pain in upper limbs, elbow, legs, wrist, heat ameliorates. Knee aches in evening. Burning pain in forearm. Drawing, pressing pain in shoulder, extending to nape of neck. Shooting pain in upper limbs, shoulder, elbow, wrist. Sore, bruised pain. Wrist as if sprained. Swelling of ankle. Tingling in the forearm, thigh, knee. Tingling in the foot, extending upwards. Twitching in the knee.

Lungs - Anxious, asthmatic breathing. Periodical dyspnea, dyspnea after vexation. Breathing irregular, slow, stertorous. Difficult breathing, as from dust, in the evening, night, worse mental exertion.

Modalities - Worse exposure to the sun. Worse mental exertion.

Mouth - Itching. Salivation, morning in bed. Herpetic ulcers, on lips, around mouth. Painful, sore, smarting ulcers. Dental caries, decayed, hollow teeth. Toothache, pain in roots. Sensation of lips swelling.

Neck - Itching. Stiffness in neck region. Swelling in nape of neck. Tension in cervical region.

Nose - Hay fever with asthmatic breathing. Hay asthma, with sneezing. Catarrh. Coryza. Sneezing, constant, frequent, paroxysmal. Sneezing in sunshine. One sided nasal discharge, at night. Bloody discharge in the morning.

Nose - Dripping discharge. Gummy discharge. Agglutination of nostrils in the morning. Cracks in nostrils. Dryness inside nose, night, painful. Itching. Nasal obstruction, one sided, in morning and night. Pain in root. Tip of nose swelling, in morning and evening. Tingling inside on blowing the nose. Acute smell.

Perspiration - Profuse. Sweetish odor.

Rectum - Diarrhea in afternoon, evening, night. Itching. Rectal pain with diarrhea. Stinging pain with stool. Stools mushy, soft, thin liquid.

Skin - Herpetic eruptions, itching. Heat sensation. Itching, prickling. Herpetic ulcers. Itching, painful, swollen ulcers.

Sleep - Unrefreshing sleep. Bad sleep, disturbed easily by dreams, thoughts. Frequent waking from dreams. Restless from dreams. Semi-conscious. Sleepiness in forenoon, afternoon. Sleepiness with detached sensation and vagueness.

Stomach - Disordered stomach. Belching, gurgling, nausea. Heaviness after eating. Clawing, prickling pains.

Throat - Choking sensation as if grasped. Dryness of throat, worse morning. Dryness after expectoration. Sensation of a foreign body in esophagus. Esophagitis. Sore pain on swallowing. Sensation of swelling. Thick sensation

Tongue - Sensation as if tongue enlarged. Tip numb, swollen.

Vertigo - Floaty feeling. Tendency to fall forward.

Vision - Acute, clear, bright and lucid vision. Blurred and foggy. Blindness.

REFERENCES - Gray. Norland.

AGAVE AMERICANA

(Century Plant)

PHARMACY - agav-a. Agave americana. Century plant. American aloe. N. O. Amaryllidaceae. Agavaceae. Tincture of fresh-chopped leaves. ***Historical dose:*** Tincture and all potencies.

CLINICAL - Gonorrhea. Hydrophobia. Scurvy. Stomach, pain. Strangury.

HERBAL - The fermented juice of Agave americana is the Mexican intoxicating beverage *"Pulque."* The plant has a local reputation as a remedy for hydrophobia. Indicated in stomach ache and painful erections in gonorrhea.

HOMEOPATHIC - Agav-a. is an unproved remedy. According to Hansen, Agav-a. is indicated in scurvy, stomachache and gonorrhea. Hydrophobia. Scurvy, pale countenance, swollen and bleeding gums. Strangury. The legs covered with dark purple blotches, swollen, painful and hard. Appetite poor, bowels constipated.

MIND - Quarrelsomeness, excitement, fright inability to swallow, great anxiety.

COMMENTS - A striking case is quoted by the Homeopathic Recorder from El Siglo Medico. A boy developed the classical symptoms of hydrophobia four and a half months after being bitten. He showed quarrelsomeness, excitement, fright, inability to swallow, small frequent pulse, and great anxiety.

Finally swallowing was impossible, restraint had to be used to prevent him from biting his nurses in the hospital. As a last resource, a piece of Agave was offered to the boy by the doctor in attendance, cut from a hedge of the plant with which the hospital grounds were fenced.

To the astonishment of all, the boy reached for it and ate it greedily, almost without chewing. By evening a decrease in the violence of the nervous attacks was manifest, though they remained as frequent as before. The improvement was slow but steady.

On the fourth day he took some nourishment, but also continued chewing Agave and swallowing the juice. On the fifth day he recovered consciousness but still demanded Agave. On the eighth day he said he did not want any more as "it tasted too bitter and caused a burning in the mouth." He had no further symptoms of the disease.

RELATIONS - ***Compare:*** (1) Anhalonium, Lyss., Lach.

REFERENCES - Boericke. Clarke.

AGAVE TEQUILANA

PHARMACY - agav-t. Agave tequilana. Agave rigida. N. O. Amaryllidaceae. Agavaceae. Pulque and Tequila are drinks made from the plant. Tincture of whole plant. ***Historical dose:*** Tincture and all potencies.

CLINICAL - ***Alcoholism.*** Anorexia. Cancerous conditions. Chronic invalid syndrome. Drug addictions. Emphysema. Hypopituitarism. Laryngitis. Memory, lost. Migraine. Silicosis. Tubercular conditions.

HERBAL - The agaves belong to the Amaryllidaceae family. Their appearance is reminiscent of aloes. The plant is used in the preparation of a popular drink, "pulque," which is obtained by the fermentation of the plant and a liqueur, "Tequila," obtained by distillation. Roughly 170 varieties of agave are in existence and, for the most part, they originate from Northern and Central America.

HOMEOPATHIC - General fatigue, weakness and muscles pains. Anorexia. Insomnia. Erratic rheumatic pains. Impotence. Ovarian pain. ***Alcoholism*** and alcoholic polyneuritis with mental troubles. Desire for alcoholic drinks. Migraine, notably alcoholic. Hypopituitarism, impotence or amenorrhea with genital and mammary atrophy. Laryngitis and bronchitis. Tuberculosis. Emphysema. Silicosis.

MIND - Sadness and pessimism. Desire for the unattainable. Unsatisfied, unrealistic desires. Alcoholism with mental troubles. Voluble state, excitable. Jokes, asks questions is humorous.

State of nervous irritation, stammers, shouts, becomes violent, even aggressive. Hypomania, a state of exaltation, exaggerated over-activity, followed often by a period of depression. Temporary amnesia following the excited state. Dazed state.

Back - Rheumatic pain in the lumbar region and lower limbs.

Ears - Itching of the auditory canal with the urge to scratch with the first object that comes to hand. Buzzing in both ears. Diminution of auditory acuity. Eczema of the auditory canal. Deafness.

Eyes - Conjunctival congestion and itching of the eyelids. Diplopia and impeded vision, more intense in one eye than the other. Burning sensation in the eyes, resulting in rubbing. Blepharitis. Dacryocystitis. Choroiditis.

Face - Feeling of heat about the face, even though he is pale.

Female - Ovarian inflammation and pain. Acute bilateral pain in the ovaries. Weak, painful menstrual flow. Menstrual stomachache relieved by drinking alcohol. Painful Menstruation.

Food - Total lack of appetite. Desire for alcoholic drinks.

Head - Headache when turning the head from one side to the other. Heaviness and slight headache, eased by pressing the head between the hands.

Limbs - Leg cramps, especially when lying down. Rheumatic pains in different places, aggravated by movement. Short, frequent bouts of arthritis and periarthritis often accompanied by nodules both intradermal and beneath the skin.

Liver - Cirrhosis, alcoholic or atrophic.

Lungs - Dilatation of the bronchi. Cough with sticky, yellow-green sputum. Profusion of glairy secretion, which makes breathing difficult. Forcing the subject to sleep almost upright in bed. Laryngitis with tracheitis.

Male - Intermittent pain in the testicles, as if result of contusion. Incomplete erection, but ejaculation in spite of the flaccidity of the penis. Low sexual desire. Impotence. Epididymitis with orchitis, tubercular or sycotic. Cyst, epididymis.

Modalities - Worse from movement. Worse alcoholic drinks.

Nose - Dryness of the nasal mucus membrane. Formation of sticky nasal scabs which block and are difficult to expel and which make breathing painful. Difficulty in wiping the nose, the scabs come off, causing great pain. Nose blocked at night, alternating from one side to the other. Ozaena. Sinusitis.

Sleep - ***Insomnia*** becomes worse after drinking alcohol. Disturbed dreams, having a bearing on the day's events and of an obsessive nature.

Stomach - Heartburn, hyperacidity of the stomach. Acid dyspepsia. Diffuse hypertrophic cirrhosis from the alcoholic causes. Feeling of emptiness in the stomach, compulsion to eat, but no hunger.

Throat - Dry throat. Difficulty in swallowing as a result of constriction in the neck. Hoarse voice.

Vertigo - Slight vertigo and troubled vision.

COMMENTS - The Homeopathic proving was directed by De Legarreta using 3x, 15 drops three times a day. In his first proving, he used the mother tincture, prepared from the plant itself. In the second proving, the remedy was prepared from Tequila liqueur.

The symptomatological table was the same in both cases. De Legarreta recommends 15 drops of 3x in the morning, fasting as a preventive treatment for alcoholism, causing aversion to alcoholic drinks.

RELATIONS - ***Compare:*** (1) Bryonia - Dryness of the mucus membranes, severe biting pains, better by pressure and rest, aggravated by the slightest movement. (2) Lachesis - Sad, melancholic in the morning, the sleep disturbed, cannot bear any constriction. Extreme loquacity, especially in the evening. Antidote against the bad effects of alcohol. (3) Ran-b. - Antidote against the bad effects of alcohol. Stinging pain in the eyes. Vesicular eruptions which resemble herpes.

REFERENCES - Julian.

AGNUS CASTUS

(Chaste Tree)

PHARMACY - agn. Agnus castus. Chaste tree. Vitex agnus castus. Verbena verticillata. N. O. Verbenacae. Found on the shores of Mediterranean, Provence and Greece. Tincture of ripe berries. ***Historical dose:*** Tincture and all potencies.

CLINICAL - Abuse, sexual. ***Agalactia.*** Anus, excoriation. Ascites. Breast-milk. Chronic fatigue. Debility. Depression. Dislocations. ***Fatigue.*** Gonorrhea. Gouty, joints. Gums, ulcerated. ***Hormonal, disorders. Impotency. Infertility.*** Knees, coldness. Leucorrhea. ***Masturbation.*** Memory, weak. Mouth, ulcers. Neurotic. Photophobia. ***Premature, aging.*** Rheumatism. Spleen, swelling, induration. Sexual, melancholy. ***Sexual, weakness. Sprains***. Strains. Tachycardia. Testicles, disorders. Toothache. ***Weakness.***

HERBAL - The Vitex Agnus Castus of the Alchemists, the *"chaste berry"* from this tree is taken as a herbal tonic for the sexual organs and hormones. Agnus castus is for low sexual vitality with corresponding mental depression and loss of nervous energy.

The Chaste Tree was used in ancient times by both men and women to suppress their sexual desire. It was used by the Greek monks centuries ago to lower their sex drive.

HOMEOPATHIC - Agnus produces its chief effect on ***sexual organs*** of both the sexes. General debility and depression of vital power are marked. ***Impotence and infertility*** in both sexes, but more pronounced in men.

History of repeated gonorrhea or masturbation. ***Impotency and premature old age*** from loss of sexual power. Nervous debility in unmarried persons.

Weakness from masturbation habit. ***Gnawing itching in all parts, especially eyes***. Tachycardia caused by tobacco in neurotic young men. A remedy for sprains and strains.

MIND - Absent-minded, and forgetful. Distraction of mind. Inability to fix attention when reading. ***Bad memory.*** Unable to recollect things has to read a sentence twice before he can comprehend. Forgetful of purchases, goes off and leaves them.

Depression. Nervous depression and mental forebodings. Fear of death. ***Great sadness with a fixed idea of approaching death*** (Acon.). Sad and despairing, repeats that he will soon die. Desires death. Doubts if anything had existence.

Changeable, moods. Indifference to everything, alternating with cheerfulness. Lack of courage. Discouragement alternating with haughtiness. Lethargy alternating with frenzy. Exhilaration alternating with sadness.

Neurotic. Peevish. Inclined to get angry. Premature old age with apathy and melancholy. ***Mental ailments from sexual excesses, masturbation.*** Sexual melancholy. Self-contempt from sexual abuse (Staph.). Aversion to sex. Sexual thrill absent from excessive masturbation. Illusion of smell, herring, musk. Starting during sleep.

Abdomen - Ascites. ***Abdomen distended after meals.*** Incarcerated flatus. Abdomen sensitive to pressure. Rumbling in abdomen during sleep. Violent contracting pain coming suddenly in morning. Spleen swollen, sore. Swelling and induration of spleen, often with soreness, after intermittent fever. Nausea with ***sensation as if intestines were pressed downwards.*** Bowels as if sinking down, wants to support bowels with hands. Flatus smells like urine, remaining long on clothes.

Back - Creaking noise in vertebrae. Pain in sacrum, from flatus. Sharp, deep pain on and near coccyx. Sharp pain near sacrum.

Breasts - Agalactia. ***Breast-milk absent,*** with sadness. Milk scanty or entirely suppressed. Deficient secretion of milk in lying-in women (Calc-p.).

Chest - Sensation of dryness in chest. Hard pressure in the region of the sternum, especially during a deep inspiration. Pressure in xiphoid cartilage. Hard pressure in right axilla and upper arm, worse touch or motion.

Constitutions - It corresponds to lymphatic, sycotic constitutions. Premature old age with apathy and melancholy. Nervous debility in unmarried persons. Impotence and gleet in old offenders.

Cough - Coughs during the evening. Coughs in bed, before going to sleep. Coughs with raising of blood, followed by copious mucus. Coughs in paroxysms. Coughs with palpitations and epistaxis. Coughs when inhaling cold air.

Ears - Roaring in the ears. Hardness of hearing.

Eyes - Gnawing itching in eyes. Corrosive itching over and on eyebrows and lids, and below eyes. Sensation as if one had received a blow on eye. Burning pain when reading in evening. ***Pupils dilated*** (Bell.). Photophobia. Dim vision before menses.

Face - Corrosive itching on the cheeks. Formication in cheeks. Tearing under right lower jaw. Long sharp pain followed by fine pricking itching. Rending, tearing pain under alveoli of right lower jaw. Erysipelas on left cheek, spreading from nose over face and head.

Female - Menses are suppressed with abdominal pains. Bearing down pains. Suppressed menses. Scanty menses. ***Infertility*** with suppressions of menses and no sexual desire (Sep.). Swelling of uterus. Leucorrhea staining yellow, transparent. Relaxation of genitals with leucorrhea. Transparent vaginal discharge passes imperceptibly from the very relaxed genital. Retained placenta. ***Ailments due to masturbation, sexual excesses.*** Sexual thrill absent from excessive masturbation. ***Aversion to sex.***

Food - Appetite lessened. Food makes him feel uneasy and replete. Only the most simple food agrees. Relishes food, but it doesn't agree with him. Warm food and drink cause teeth to ache. Thirst during heat. Thirstlessness, and aversion to all drink.

Head - Headache before menses. Tearing pain with pressure in the temples and forehead, worse during motion. Pain in the temple, as from a blow. Heaviness in the head and pressure, as if the head would fall forward. Pain in the vertex. Tension and chilliness in the scalp, which is warm to the touch. Biting-itching on scalp, worse evenings and when falling asleep.

Heart - Hysterical palpitations with nose-bleed in women. Tachycardia caused by tobacco in neurotic young men. Slow and weak pulse, often imperceptible. Palpitations during cough.

Kidneys - Passes more urine, frequently. Pain in bladder. When urinating, pain in kidneys. Red, turbid urine with burning and pressure in urethra. Gets up twice at night and even once during siesta to urinate.

Limbs - Inflammatory, rheumatic swelling of joints. ***Sprains and strains.*** Gouty nodosities. Hard pressure in right axilla and upper arm, worse from touch and motion. ***Strains from lifting a little too much.*** Swelling of the finger joints, with arthritic, tearing pains. Heaviness of right foot, as from a weight. Joints as if dislocated. Feels bruised all over. Cold hands, cold knees, even in bed. Joints easily twisted. Feet easily turn under when walking on stone pavement. Rheumatic and gouty nodosities on joints.

Liver - Aching in region of liver worse touch.

Lungs - Dyspnea worse evening. Dyspnea on going up stairs. Tough, hanging mucus like a rag in fauces.

Male - Itching of genitals. Testicles, cold, swollen, hard and painful. Penis small, flaccid. ***Drawing pain along spermatic cords.*** Loss of prostatic fluid on straining. Gleety discharge. Yellow discharge from urethra. Aversion to sex. ***Impotence with genitals cold and relaxed.*** Impotence, after frequent attacks of gonorrhea, syphilis. No erections. Penis so relaxed that voluptuous fancies excite no erection. Feeble erections without sexual desire. Impotence, with morning erections only. Spermatorrhea with impotence. ***Ailments due to masturbation, sexual excesses.*** Sexual desire almost lost. ***Sexual desire gone*** (Sel., Con., Sabal.). Scanty emission without ejaculation.

Modalities - Better scratching. Better pressure. Worse from over lifting, sprains. ***Worse from sexual excess***. Worse from seminal losses. Worse from masturbation.

Mouth - Mouth very dry. Saliva viscid and tough, drawing out in strings. Ulcers in the mouth and on the gums. Metallic, coppery, bitter taste. Boils. Tongue coated white.

Nose - Hard ache on dorsum of nose, better pressure. Soreness and pain in left side of nose. Illusion of smell, herring, musk.

Perspiration - Sweats, almost only on the hands, when walking in the open air. Sweats easily. Pungent smell, causes dullness and headache. Sweats followed by vomiting and trembling.

Rectum - Anus excoriated. Deep fissures of the anus, often giving pain when walking. Flatus smells like urine, remaining long on clothes. Sensation as of subcutaneous ulceration near the anus, only while walking. Difficulty of passing soft stools. When pressing at stool, discharge of prostatic fluid. Corrosive itching of the perineum. Sensation as if diarrhea would set in, when standing.

Skin - Corrosive itching on different parts of the body, better by scratching, but soon returns. Itching around the ulcers, in the evening. Yellow tint of skin.

Sleep - Sleeplessness. Awaking often, as if alarmed, starting. Anxious dreams. Amorous dreams.

Stomach - Only the most simple food agrees. Belchings, smell like urine. Pinching pain when sitting bent over. Nausea in pit of stomach after eating. Nausea in pit when standing. Nausea as from eating fat food.

Stools - Stools soft, recede, difficult. Diarrhea of children. Chronic diarrhea of adults.

Teeth - Teeth are painful when touched by warm food or drink. Throbbing, tearing pain in left eyetooth. Small boil near tooth, very painful to touch.

Temperature - Chilliness, internal with trembling, the external skin is warm. Chill alternating with heat. Chilly all over, but only hands feel cold to touch. Much chilliness, with cold hands. Flushes of burning heat, principally in the face, with cold knees in the evening in bed.

Throat - Corrosive itching in pit of throat. Voice as if passing through wool. Voice has no timbre.

Vertigo - Vertigo before menses. Vertigo from loss of vital fluids.

COMMENTS - Great sadness with a fixed idea of approaching death, especially after confinement when milk fails to appear. Deficiency of milk with despair of recovery. Absent-minded. Drowsiness.

Illusion of smell, like herrings or musk. Ulcers in mouth and on gums. Tearing pain in lower jaw. Toothache from hot food or drink. Swelling and induration of spleen. Rumbling of flatus during sleep.

Discharge of prostatic fluid while straining at stool. Suppressed menses with abdominal pain. Leucorrhea staining yellow. Infertility. Pain as if dislocated in joints. Joints easily twisted. Rheumatic and gouty nodosities on joints.

Hahnemann became interested in this remedy when he read that the Chaste tree was used by the Greek monks centuries ago to stop their sex drive. They would take tincture doses and they took so much that their testicles and genitals would atrophy.

In Boericke there are descriptions of shrinking and atrophying, "Testicles, cold, swollen, hard, and painful," "lower sexual vitality," and "corresponding depression."

Useful for people who have over exerted themselves sexually, a promiscuous period, and since have lost sex drive, very apathetic. Emaciated, pale, blue circles around their eyes with dilated pupils. Sexual neurasthenia.

Sexual melancholy, depression about not having a lover, gloom, moroseness. All sexual desire is gone. Impotence. History of repeated gonorrhea or promiscuity. The genitals are cold and relaxed, can get no erection.

History of cures of chronic spermatorrhea, chronic dribbling of semen and prostatic fluid because of the weakness in the whole area. Women's abhorrence or aversion to sexual intercourse and infertility (Nat-m., Ph-ac., Sep.).

RELATIONS - Agnus is the only proved member of the Verbena family, though the Labiate or Mint family are closely allied. Teste groups it with Mur-ac. and Hyos. ***Antidoted by:*** Camphor, Nat-m. - headache, strong solutions of table-salt. ***Compare:*** (1) Sel., Con., Nat-m., Sep., Sabal., Ph-ac., Camph, Lyc. Olnd. (2) Leucorrhea staining yellow, Nux-v., Chel., Carb-an., Kreos. ***Followed well by:*** Ars., Bry., Ign., Lyc., Puls., Sulph., Sel.

REFERENCES - Boericke. Clarke. Murphy.

AGRAPHIS NUTANS

(Bluebell)

PHARMACY - agra. Agraphis nutans. Bluebell. Wild hyacinth. Endymion nutans. Scilla nutans. N. O. Liliaceae. Hyacinthaceae. Tincture of fresh plant and growing shoots. ***Historical dose:*** Tincture and all potencies.

CLINICAL - Adenoids. Catarrh. Chill. Deafness. Diarrhea. ***Glands, enlarged.*** Tonsillitis.

HOMEOPATHIC - Agraphis is one of the remedies introduced by Dr. Cooper. The plant grows in sheltered places, and Dr. Cooper gave "better from shelter" as a leading indication. It partakes of the characters of the lilies and corresponds to catarrhal conditions.

Clarke regarded it as one of the leading remedies in cases of adenoids. Dr. Cooper noted ***"Adenoids with enlarged tonsils, frequently accompanying dentition."*** He cured with it mucus diarrhea following a suppressed cold. Obstruction of the nostrils, especially from adenoids and throat deafness. ***Enlarged tonsils, adenoids, throat deafness.*** The action of it is felt towards the root of the nose. Catarrhal conditions.

Patient is prone to take cold on exposure to cold winds (Acon.). Mutism of childhood unconnected with deafness. Chill from cold winds (Sil.). Mucus diarrhea from cold. Throat and ear troubles with ***tendency to free discharge from mucus membranes***.

Rectum - Mucus diarrhea following a suppressed cold.

Throat - Adenoids with enlarged tonsils. Throat deafness.

RELATIONS - ***Compare:*** (1) Hydr., All-c, Calc-p., Sul-i., Calc-i. (2) All-s., Squil.

REFERENCES - Boericke. Clarke.

AGRIMONY

(Bach Flower Essence)

PHARMACY - agr-b. Agrimony. Agrimonia eupatoria. The flowering stalks are floated in a bowl of water and left in the sun for several hours. The water imbued with healing power is used as medicine. ***Historical dose:*** Take two drops from the stock bottle into a one ounce dropper bottle (add brandy, or some other alcohol, if this bottle will be used for days or weeks). This is the dosage bottle, take a few drops straight into the mouth or as needed in a little water.

HOMEOPATHIC - Agrimony, along with Centaury, Walnut and Holly, belongs to the group of "***Over sensitivity to Influences and Ideas***," as classified by Bach. These four remedies help those who are distressed or overly influenced by disturbing factors, powerful impressions in their environment.

Agrimony has been used as an herbal remedy for liver troubles. Liver disturbances may exist. Craving for stimulants is a frequent indication. Restlessness in mind and body. Anxieties and worries. Internal disquiet, nervousness and hurried. Agrimony will greatly ease pain in a patient who is smiling despite pain and internal torture.

Suppression, over-compliance and denial of emotions.

MIND - Desire to not let others down and burden them with their personal problems. Intend to spread cheer and uplift others. Tendency not to express strong emotions which could bring disharmony or strife to oneself or others. Resentment and antagonism nonetheless build up within and may find release unexpectedly in spiteful remarks or in masked, aggressive behavior. Unsettled and restless mind, prone to be distracted. Inner cares and worries. Anxieties build up, restlessness and a sense of dissatisfaction. Grief or other forms of disappointment. Resentment or guilt which are not being worked through. Unresolved conflicts or trauma. Inner restlessness, a sense of boredom. Often finds some relief in drugs, entertainment, or other forms of diversion. Quarrels distress and bring unhappiness.

REFERENCES - Bach.

AGROSTEMA GITHAGO

(Corn Cockle)

PHARMACY - agro. Agrostema githago. Corn cockle. Lychnis githago. N. O. Caryatides. Caryophyllaceae. Trituration of the seeds, which are poisonous and contain Saponin. Preparations of an active principle Githargin. ***Historical dose:*** All potencies.

CLINICAL - Gastritis. Paralysis. Tenesmus.

HOMEOPATHIC - Knowledge of this plant is derived almost entirely from cases of poisoning in persons who have eaten bread containing the seeds.

Agrostema's active constituent is Saponin. Agrostema causes violent sneezing and sharp burning taste, burning in stomach, which extends to esophagus, neck and breast. Sensations of burning. Vertigo, headache and coma. Impaired locomotion, difficulty remaining erect.

Back - Tearing along spine.

Head - Headache. Sensation of heat and burning rises into vertex from left lower jaw, almost makes her crazy. Vertigo.

Mouth - Dry and hot. Palate has a red margin. Burning on palate in a short time.

Rectum - Constipation with tenesmus. Diarrhea with tenesmus. Burning in bowels and rectum.

Stomach - Nausea and vomiting. Burning from stomach along esophagus to throat and in chest. Knife-like pains in stomach at times.

RELATIONS - ***Compare:*** (1) Lath., Sec.

REFERENCES - Clarke.

AIDS NOSODE

PHARMACY - aids. AIDS nosode. ***Historical dose:*** All potencies.

CLINICAL - AIDS. Bites. Breast, tumors. Chills. Coryza. Cystitis. Emaciation. Fevers. Headaches. Heartburn. Hypertension. ***Memory, weakness. Nosebleeds. Ovaries, pain. Palpitations.*** Sinusitis. ***Toothaches.*** Trembling. Wounds.

HOMEOPATHIC - Sluggishness of the body. Coldness of affected parts, lack of vital heat. Heat sensation. Hypertension. Intoxication, after. Stitching pain. Relaxation of connective tissue. Restlessness. Stiffness. Trembling, quivering, tremulous weakness. Wavelike sensations. Bites and wounds.

Headaches with nausea. ***Ovaries aching pain***, worse evening, on the right. Cystitis. Low or diminished sexual desire. ***Palpitations with anxiety.*** Weakness during menses. Weakness with nausea. Rheumatic pain.

MIND - Awkward. ***Mental dullness. Slowness*** of mind. ***Forgetful, weak memory.*** Prostration of mind. ***Concentration is difficult,*** worse afternoon, studying. Mental confusion. Confusion as to his identity. Mistakes at work, when writing. Awkward. ***Timidity.*** Bashful, want of self-confidence. Pathetic, helpless feelings, self pity. Insecure. Weak character. Introspective.

Anxiety. Fear of authority, death, failure, high places, of infection, of closed places, poverty. ***Aversion to company,*** yet fear of being alone. ***Desire for solitude*** alternating with desire for company. Consolation ameliorates. Discontented.

Irritability alternating with cheerfulness, with discouragement. Irritability from difficult concentration. Offended easily, sensitive to reprimands. Ailments from anger. Anger towards husband. Desire to kill everyone he sees. Least provocation would enrage him. Indifference, apathy, particularly in the afternoon, evening. Indifference to loved ones. ***Want of sensitiveness.*** Hardhearted, inexorable. Suspicious.

Stupefaction, as if intoxicated. Persistent thoughts. Pertinacity. Vanishing of thoughts. Calmness alternating with sadness. Seriousness. ***Wants to be quiet.*** Mildness. Laziness.

Alternating moods. ***Crying***, from many causes. ***Forsaken feeling***. Sensation of isolation. Feels unloved, estranged from loved ones. ***Sympathetic.*** Causeless sadness. ***Dwells on the past***. Exalted love for humanity. Lovesick.

Excitement. Exhilaration. ***Optimistic.*** Extravagance. Desires activity. Playful, frivolous. Mischievous. Shameless. Loquacity. Wants to be naked, because it is natural. Industrious, mania for work. ***Restlessness.*** Hurry, haste.

Automatic conduct. Unconsciousness. Time appears shorter or longer, passes too quickly or too slowly. Everything is strange, as if in a dream. ***Delusions that she has lost her shell and protection. Delusions of floating in air.*** All, barriers between him and others are removed. Beautiful delusions of youth, beauty, love and peace. ***Sees bubbles popping,*** rising to the surface. As if brain was moving, wavering, or as if a heavy lump in the left side of brain.

Abdomen - ***Pain***, distension, heat. Abdomen pain after anger. Cramping, griping pain. Lancinating pain. Sore pain on motion, pressure aggravates. Contraction left side. Lancinating pain in inguinal region. Sore pain, near inguinal region. Pain in the hypogastrium, iliac region. Pain, left side extending to right. Stitching pain, in evening, morning, in left iliac region. Tension in inguinal region. Offensive, yellow discharge from umbilicus. Passing flatus with distension. Cramping, griping pain, before stool.

Back - Boils in dorsal region, scapulae. Pain lumbo-sacral region, in the morning, on stooping. Aching pain, dorsal region, left scapulae. Sore pain. Stitching pain after kneeling. Tension in dorsal region, scapulae.

Bladder - Cystitis. Painful, frequent urging to urinate. Ineffectual urging to urinate. Urging to urinate, night, midnight. Cutting pain when not urinating. Urethral pain after urination. Copious, brown-reddish urine.

Breasts - Breast tumors. Breast pain during cough. Breast cancer, left. Sensitive nodules.

Chest - Constriction on left side. Asthmatic constriction. Fullness of chest. Painful oppression. Cutting pain ribs, left side. Pain as if sternum was punched. Perspiration, axilla, evening.

Dreams - Dreams followed by fear. Amorous dreams, having sex with several people. Dreams of animals, dead, injured, suffering, wild. Dreams of old friends, boyfriend, childhood home. Beautiful, big, ornate, palatial buildings, churches. Buildings are neglected outside but beautiful inside. Being buried alive with explosives. Dreams of infections, AIDS. Dreams about children, babies, looking after or rescuing children. Trapped inside a crystal. Teeth falling out. Being bitten by dogs, snakes or toads. Dreams of people on fire. Hair falling out or turning white. Dreams of jewels, rings, diamonds, knives, magical gifts, music. Dreams of danger, storms, war. Dreams of difficulties on journeys. Horrible dreams, robbers, shooting, police, violence. Dreams of being pursued, rape. Nakedness. Crowds of people. Flying an airplane. Dreams of tunnels, train, foreign country, stairs, banisters

Ears - Aching pain. Fetid, offensive, yellow discharges. Itching external ear. ***Noises in ear. Buzzing***, ringing, night. Soreness ear, meatus, left ear. Pain on yawning, right ear.

Eyes - Discharges, morning, watery, yellow. Aching pain, left. Discoloration, red inner canthi. ***Dryness. Itching***, left eye, inner canthi, eyelids. ***Lachrymation left eye.*** Sore pain with itching, left. Stitching pain about the eyes, left. Eye pain, touch aggravates. Eyes sensitive to touch. Swelling, left inner canthi, on waking.

Face - Acne on lower lip. Red eruptions on cheeks, nose. Herpes about the lips. Red, white pimples. Rash on the chin, warmth aggravates.

Female - Bland, bloody, watery, thin, yellow leucorrhea. Bright red menses, mingled with dark clots. Menses copious, at night. Menses too late, too short. Menses painful on waking. ***Ovaries pain***, worse evening, right. Aching pain in right ovaries. Low or diminished sexual desire.

Food - ***Thirst*** for small quantities and often. Thirst from drinking cold water. Thirstless. Appetite diminished. ***Appetite increased***, evening, night, before midnight, morning on waking. Insatiable appetite. Desires bitter drinks, chocolate, fish, ice cream, milk, peaches, sweets. Aggravated from alcoholic drinks, easily intoxicated. Worse from beer, coffee, bread.

Head - Feeling of cotton wool in head, with slight vertigo. Constriction sensation. Enlarged sensation, head feels inflated. Formication, vertex. Heaviness sensation, smoking aggravates. Perspiration of scalp, forehead. Pulsating, temples, right, vertex, morning on waking. Swollen feeling, vertex.

Headaches - Bursting pain, morning on waking. Cutting pain, above left eyes. Headaches with nausea. Forehead pain extending to occiput, neck, nose or teeth, in morning. Pain behind the eyes. Pain extending to neck region. Pain forenoon, morning on waking. Headaches preceded by disagreeable dreams. Pulsating pain. Stitching pain, forehead over left eye, sides, in morning on waking. Feels well especially before the headache attack.

Heart - Palpitations at night. ***Palpitations with anxiety.***

Kidneys - Cutting pain extending to back.

Larynx - Voice hoarseness.

Limbs - Eruptions, rash, red patches or blotches on leg, calf. Pustules, rash. ***Heat in limbs.*** Heat in right hand, left knee, at night after going to bed. One hand cold the other hot. Coldness, right foot. Perspiration at night and on waking, on feet and hands. Itching, as of insect bites, on legs, toes. Rheumatic pain. Sciatica, particularly on the left side, better from warmth and slow motion. Crushed, cutting, dislocated pain, particularly in joints. Cramping in legs, calves, especially when sitting. Limbs, shoulder is stiff in the morning, tension in the limbs, better from motion. Aching pain in lower joints, sore, bruised pain. Stitching pain in lower limbs after kneeling. Pain extends to groin, inner side of thigh. Pain in wrist when grasping. Stitching pain in toes. Tingling in upper limps, worse left, at night. Heavy sensation in lower limbs. Numbness on feet and hands, in the morning. Lameness of the forearm. Joint pain, particularly hips and knees, worse motion. Trembling in left knee, weakness as if knees would knock together. Relaxed joints.

Lungs - Respiration difficult, after exertion, during palpitations. Wheezing. Tickling cough at night.

Male - ***Sexual desire diminished.*** Erections, wanting, morning. Eruptions, pimples, pustules on the penis. Cutting pain in penis after urination.

Modalities - Better after stool or urination. Better lying. Worse in the afternoon. ***Worse on waking in the morning***. Worse after sleep. Worse during menses.

Mouth - Numbness about mouth. Sore pain, gums. Sore pain, palate. Ulcers, mouth, ulcers. ***Jaw pain,*** left. Sore, bruised lower jaws. Stitching pain, jaws. Convulsions, spasms of jaws.

Neck - Constriction. Eruptions, pustules. Sensitive to slightest touch. Sensation of rope around neck. Cannot bear anything tight around neck and waist, clothing aggravates. Swelling of cervical glands. Pain neck during menses. Perspiration. Prickling sensation. Tension cervical region on waking.

Nose - Bleeding eruptions on nose when touched. ***Coryza,*** from change of temperature. Clear discharge. Crusts, scabs, inside nose. Discharge thick, viscid, tough, in evening. ***Nosebleeds,*** bright red blood, clotted, coagulated. Nosebleeds, left side, morning, in bed, on waking, periodic and profuse. ***Nose itching.*** Obstruction, morning on waking. Burning, smarting pain. Sore pain, worse touch. ***Painful sneezing,*** with nosebleed, from dust. Tingling inside nose.

Rectum - Constipation. Flatus. Frequent, ineffectual urging and straining. Sudden diarrhea, in afternoon, evening. Involuntary stool. Dry or watery stool. Soreness, pain during and after stool. Rectal fissure. Hemorrhage from anus after difficult stool. Itching, in the evening.

Sleep - ***Unrefreshing sleep.*** Anxious, ***restless sleep***, from activity of thoughts. ***Heavy sleep. Sleeps on back,*** with arm over head. Sleeps curled up like a dog, with lower limbs stretched out, or with one leg one stretched out the other drawn up. Waking difficult, too early, too late. Weeping on waking. Prolonged sleep. Sleepy in the afternoon, morning.

Skin - Itching and burning, at night. Insect stings.

Stomach - Fullness, heaviness after eating little, in the morning. Soreness, pain, in the epigastrium, in the morning. Heartburn. Cramping before stool.

Teeth - ***Toothache, worse left,*** in incisors, upper teeth. Aching pain, extending to eyes, forehead, nose, left side. Sensitive teeth, tender to cold water. Sensation of loose teeth.

Throat - ***Dryness***, painful on waking. Disposition to hawk from dryness. ***Sensation of a lump,*** on swallowing. Watery mucus, at night, on waking. Rawness, sore pain. Sore throat, in the morning, worse at night, on the left, better warm drinks. Difficult swallowing. Tickling in throat.

Vertigo - Vertigo accompanied by heaviness in the eye, in head. Sensation of ascending, as if floating, as if intoxicated. Vertigo looking at revolving objects, as if everything were turning in a circle. ***Vertigo on rising,*** while sitting up in bed, lying, walking, after looking into mirror. Vertigo in morning.

Vision - Colors before the eyes, black stripes, blue squares, blue stripes, blue spots, green-yellow, in the morning.

RELATIONS - ***Compare:*** (1) Ars., Carc. Syph. (2) Echi., Nit-ac., (3) Bapt., Bry., Gels., Hyos., Lach.

REFERENCES - Norland.

AILANTHUS GLANDULOSA

(Tree of Heaven)

PHARMACY - ail. Ailanthus glandulosa. Tree of Heaven. Ailanthus altissima. Chinese Sumach. N. O. Simarubacae. Eastern Asia. Cultivated as a shade-tree in North America. Tincture from flowers beginning to open. ***Historical dose:*** All potencies.

CLINICAL - Acne. Chancre. Coryza. Diarrhea. Diphtheria. Dysentery. ***Headaches.*** Meningitis. Mumps. Post-partum fever. Rash. Rheumatic fever. Raynaud's disease. Sepsis. ***Scarlatina.*** Streptococcus, infections. Syphilis. ***Tonsillitis.*** Typhoid fever. Typhus fever.

HOMEOPATHIC - Ailanthus acts upon ***blood*** disorganizing it and producing conditions like low fevers, low types of eruptive diseases and hemorrhagic diathesis. Mucus membranes become hemorrhagic and ulcerative (Lach., Ars.). Rapid prostration. ***Malignant and suppressed scarlatina***. General stupor with sighing. Sepsis. Low types of eruptive diseases, diphtheria. Raynaud's disease.

Lividity, stupor, fetor and malignancy. Thin, acrid discharges. The ***skin appears livid or purplish***, face dark as mahogany. Hot, sordes, throat swollen, purple, livid. Purpled appearance of the skin. Rash coming out in patches. Eruptions which are slow in appearing. Rashes often return annually.

Follicular tonsillitis, streptococcus infection. Hemorrhagic diathesis. Low adynamic forms of disease with extreme prostration torpor, vomiting. Prostration at the outset of a disease. The patient is stupid, dull, delirious, weak. Semi-conscious, delirious, weak pulse, general torpor and prostration. Diarrhea, dysentery and ***great weakness***.

MIND - Confused mind, mental depression. Stupor or stoic indifference, with sighing. Dullness, must read a subject several times or figures over and over again. All the antecedents are forgotten. Constant muttering delirium with sleeplessness and restlessness. Raging delirium with brilliant eyes.

Abdomen - Tenderness over liver region. Burning in the stomach and bowels. Tympanites.

Back - Neck tender, and very much swollen. Constant sharp pains through small of back and hips.

Chest - Stitching and aching in chest. Burning in right lung, contracted feeling in left. Chest feels strapped, or as if air-cells stuck together.

Constitutions - Suited to nervous, sensitive persons. Bilious temperament. Stout and robust. Hemorrhagic diathesis.

Ears - Pain in ear when swallowing. Parotid glands tender and enlarged.

Eyes - Conjunctivitis, smarting, aching, lachrymation, purulent discharge. Suffused and congested, startled look when aroused. Photophobia. Pupils dilated and sluggish.

Face - Mahogany colored, dark and swollen. Chronic speckled spotted face, a kind of acne. Face sallow, jaundiced, blue circles around eyes. Face red and hot, covered with a rash. Purplish face. Lips are swollen, cracked, ulcers near commissures.

Female - Malignant puerperal fever. Vomiting of pregnancy.

Food - No appetite, everything tastes insipid, sight of food makes her worse, disgust for food. Hunger and distressing sense of general emptiness during chill. Thirst for cold drinks, brandy.

Head - ***Frontal headache*** with drowsiness, dizziness and red-hot face, cannot sit up. Faint on rising up or vertigo worse lying. Passive congestion headaches. ***Suffused, dilated eyes***, photophobia. Face dusky. Thin, ***copious, ichorous***, bloody nasal discharge.

Heart - Rapid, small pulse, weak, frequent, and irregular. Dull pain and contracted feeling in region of base of heart and through center of left lung.

Kidneys - Urine scanty, suppressed, passed unconsciously.

Lungs - Breathing hurried, irregular, heavy. Dry, hacking cough. Lungs sore and tired. Deep, exhausting cough, with violent fits until sputum is raised. Sputa is blood-mixed, yellow, bitter, worse morning. Aphonia. Croupy choking.

Male - Sore on prepuce, looking like incipient chancre.

Modalities - Better from hot drinks. Better when lying on right side. Worse from suppressions. Worse raising up or sitting up. Worse walking, motion. Worse sight of food.

Mouth - ***Tongue dry and brown***, parched and cracked. Tongue moist, furred white, tip and edges livid.

Neck - The neck is ***tender and swollen***.

Nose - Nostrils congested. Nose dry, secretion suppressed. Coryza, with rawness in nostrils, sneezing. Loss of smell. Thin copious bloody ichorous nasal discharge. Itching and uneasy feeling around the nose.

Pulse - Rapid, small, weak.

Rectum - Diarrhea, dysentery with great weakness. Thin, watery, offensive stools. Passing of involuntary stools with urine. Tapeworms. Sense of insecurity with stool or urine.

Skin - The skin appears ***livid or purplish***. Miliary, livid rash, returns annually. Large blisters filled with dark serum. ***Irregular, patchy, livid eruptions***, disappearing on pressure. Cold skin. Eruptions in dark, sparse patches, appear slowly, disappear on pressure, but return slowly. Scarlatina maligna. Petechae. Skin mottled. Crawling all over the body.

Sleep - Drowsy, restless. Heavy, disturbed, unrefreshing.

Stomach - Vomits food speedily during the chill, suddenly and violently when sitting up, with stupor. Peculiar feeling of emptiness in stomach.

Teeth - Tearing in teeth. The teeth are ***covered with sordes.***

Temperature - Adynamic fever with weak heart. Cold sweat.

Throat - Diphtheria and tonsillitis. Streptococcus infections. Inflamed, edematous, dusky red. Throat dark and swollen. Tonsils studded with many deep ulcers (worse left), with loose pultaceous discharge. ***Much swelling internal and external***. Dry, rough, scraping, choking feeling. Hoarse, croupy voice. ***Pain in swallowing*** extends to the ears. Dry, foul fauces. Irritation and itching of posterior pharynx.

Vertigo - Dizzy when rising up.

COMMENTS - With the low fever of Ail. there is stupor or indifference with sighing. Constant frontal headache of a neuralgic character. Paroxysmal headache with drowsiness during the day, confused mind, depression.

A feeling of fullness everywhere. A sensation of electric current passing from head into limbs was prominent in the provings. The head is burning hot with piercing pains. The parotid glands are sensitive and enlarged. The attacks are characterized by fullness of head with heat, pains burning, darting in temples and occiput, vertigo and nausea.

The throat is severely affected: thick, edematous, dry, choky feeling. Dry, rough, scrapy, worse morning. Livid, swollen with ulcers oozing a fetid discharge. The symptoms are better lying on right side (bronchial affections). Sitting up causes vomiting, dizziness. Motion causes staggering. Toothache is better walking.

RELATIONS - ***Antidoted by:*** Alcohol, Rhus-t., Nux-v. ***Compare:*** (1) Ptel., Xanthoxylae. (2) Am-c., Arn., Arum-t. (3) Aloe, - dull frontal headache. Bapt., Bry., Gels., Hyos., Lac-c. Lach., Nit-ac., Nux-v., Phyt., Hydr-ac., Rhus-t., Stram., Echi.

REFERENCES - Boericke. Clarke.

ALABASTER

(White Gypsum)

PHARMACY - alab. Alabaster. White gypsum. Hydrous calcium sulphate. ***Historical dose:*** All potencies.

CLINICAL - Backache. Belching. Colds. Colic. Conjunctivitis. Constipation. Cough. Cramps. Eczema. Headache. Hoarseness. Insomnia. Leucorrhea. Moles. Nausea. Sciatica. Sinus, congestion. Sneezing. Tinnitus. Toothache. Vaginitis.

HOMEOPATHIC - Plaster of Paris is so named because of the prevalence of gypsum in the Paris basin where it was originally produced. Plaster of Paris is generally the hemihydrate of Calcium Sulphate - CaSO4-2H2O. Alabaster is a fine-grained, massive, opaque or translucent variety of gypsum. It tends to be white in color but can be streaked or tinted with brown, red, yellow, green, etc.

Chemically, alabaster is hydrous Calcium Sulphate manifesting as a monoclinic crystal structure. Gypsum is formed by the evaporation of bedded deposits that are precipitated mainly from evaporating saline water.

It has been used for centuries for making statues, carvings, ornaments and for decorations. The pyramids near Cairo were originally faced in alabaster, but it is now completely weathered away.

Plaster of Paris (and gypsum plaster) is made by the partial (or complete) dehydration of gypsum by heating or burning. When mixed with water, it gives a plastic paste which can be cast or molded. It eventually sets and hardens due to the chemical recombination of the gypsum with water.

MIND - Rocks violently. Muddled mind. Memory poor. Forgetful. Low self confidence. Indecisive. Feeling very impatient and irritable. Tired physically, bright mentally. Feels depleted. Want to be held, feels vulnerable.

Anxious, fretful, worrying. Anxious on waking. Anxious about future. Anxiety about getting breast cancer. Panic attack, anxious and unable to breath. Fear of death. Fear of life. Fear of the dark. Fear of madness.

Restless, but mind doesn't feel as though it wants to think about anything in particular. Hard to relax, feels vulnerable, stupid. Sensation as if smiling. Tired and restless having to do lots of things. Thinking about travelling.

Depressed and hopeless. Sad, melancholic, blue. Very moody and impatient. Woke feeling very low. Sensation as if, too much to do, feel sorry for myself, teary. Craves some peace and quiet. Don't like crowds.

Discontented. Intolerant, irritable. Ennui. Panicky and weepy. Irritable and angry with people at work. Anger towards former work colleagues. Feels irritable in the morning.

Abdomen - Colic. Griping pain in both sides of lower abdomen. Sudden pains in right abdomen, extending to rectum and extending upwards. Abdominal pain after eating. Achey and bloated feeling. Abdomen bloated and tender. Solar plexus feels heavy. Sharp stabbing pain, left side of abdomen. Nausea and pain abdomen after eating.

Back - Neck very stiff. Neck aching. Back aching down spine with pain shooting from lower back down to both ankles. Stiffness down spine. Desire to twist spine for relief. Tingling base of neck at the back. Skin dry and itchy. Pain in upper back, especially right side. Pain sore, nagging, stitching, tender, compressing. Lower back pain. Coldness middle of back. Backache in middle of back, piercing pain. Backache, worse moving around worse sitting.

Bladder - Bladder discomfort. Burning pain. Not passing urine as often as usual.

Breasts - Breast tenderness, worse before menses. Eruptions on outer side of both breasts. Mastitis. Pain in right breast.

Chests - Sides of chest itch. Chest feels tight. Chest and solar plexus feels heavy. Sore pain.

Cough - Weak cough while eating. Cough from a tickle in the throat. Cough with yellow-brown mucus. Tickling cough. Woke in night with coughing and cramping pain right lower leg.

Ears - Very itchy in ear canal. Popping sound in right ear. Right ear burns and feels warm. Achey and sore. Pain deep in right ear. Shooting sensation below right ear extending to nose and eye. Boring sensation in both ears, better rubbing finger in ear. Left ear, shooting pain, at end of conversation. Sensitive hearing to ticking clock. Tinnitus. Ringing in ears. Sounds more acute on left side. Buzzing noise. Hissing noise.

Eyes - Burning sensation outer corner of right eye. Right eye watering. Heavy and aching pain better closed eyes. Eyes sore, as if tired. Aching pain in left eye. As if, conjunctivitis in right eye. Hard to open eyes, scratchy discomfort and watering. Eyes feel very tired, wants to close them. Woke with watering eyes and blocked nose. Sharp pain in right eye on rubbing it in morning. Woke with eyes discharging and gluey, crusted. Eye irritation and puffiness, worse perfumes.

Face - Upper lip hot and burning. Skin very itchy, especially around right eye and cheek. Numbness of upper lip. Skin on face very sensitive. Cheeks warm, especially right side. Bags under eyes after heavy sleep. Face looked pale. Pins and needles sensations in face. Rash on face and neck, red, sore, itchy. Stinging red rash on forehead and right side face.

Female - Cramping in uterus just before period. Bloating and nausea before menses. Menses profuse with clots. Menses scanty. Leucorrhea with fishy discharge. Thrush symptoms, itching and white discharge. Vaginitis. Vagina red and sore. Vaginal irritation better cold water. Discharge, mucus, cream, pale yellow çolor. Discharge pink again and specks of blood.

Food - No appetite. More thirsty. Craved hot chocolate drink.

Head - Head feels hot. Pressure at back of head in a band running from ear to ear. Headache, back of neck very stiff. Dull ache in occiput extending to temples, worse bending forwards. Temples pounding. Headache all day not better for fresh air or drinking cold water. Head feels full, heavy. Woke with a headache. Pain in head, left side. Headache across forehead and temples. Frontal headache. Light headedness worse moving quickly. Pain in forehead, behind eyes, a nauseating pain. Pain as if brain being squeezed.

Heart - Heart feels as if it's beating faster. Dull, bruised pain in heart.

Limbs - Leg area sensitve. Feels like electric shocks, during menses, running from bottom to ankles. Pain in legs like sciatica, worse bending forward, worse sitting. Sciatica pain worse running. Shooting pains down legs. Hands sensitive to washing. Red blotchy rash on back of hands. Eczema elbows. Twinges of rheumatic pain, left hip. Restless legs. Twitching of legs. Legs feel very tired and heavy. Left knee aches. Pin-prick sensation in right knee. Skin on buttocks dry and flakey, not itchy. Legs felt weak when went upstairs. Tingling in hand. Cramps in limbs. Feet very cold. Legs ache. Aching limbs. Ankles cold.

Lungs - Feels breathless. Wheezy. Yellow, brown expectoration.

Male - Burning pain in the root of the penis and lower urinary tract.

Mouth - Metallic taste. Bitter, taste in mouth.Very dry mouth. Roof of mouth feels a bit greasy. Mouth ulcer in right cheek. Tingling in middle of lower lip. Gums puffy round tooth. Gums bleeding, when brushed teeth. Itchy palate.

Nose - Very itchy inside nose. Colds. Sneezing and runny nose. Nose blocked both sides. Nose tender, feels bashed. Feels broken across bridge of nose. Sensitive to house dust while cleaning. Constant sneezing. Nasal catarrh and sneezing. Lots of mucus in back of throat, nose blocked. More sensitive to smells. Sinus congestion. Tickle on end of nose.

Perspiration - More sweaty than usual, sticky armpits. Less sweaty at night.

Rectum - Rectum feels full, doesn't feel empty even after passing a stool. Windy and loose stools, accompanying right sided (hypochondria) pain. Constipation. Smelly stools. Loose stool, a bit explosive.

Skin - Skin is dry and itchy. Skin feels hot. Red rash, sore, itchy, worse cold weather, better being outside. Stinging red rash on forehead and right side face. Moles, bleeding. Mole with slight prickling, scabbed over. Itchy skin after alcohol, especially legs, worse left.

Sleep - Heavy sleep. Panic attack before going to sleep, fearful not sure of what. Sleeplessness. Restless night. Waking up a lot. Woke with restless legs. Woke very fearful. Woke during the night feeling really depressed and hopeless. Anxious dreams. Dreams of dead people. Nostalgic dreams. Dreams of water. Dreams of work. Lots of different, active dreams. Vivid, intense dreams.

Stomach - Belching. Queasy feeling before breakfast. Rumbling and gurgling. Nausea and pain abdomen after eating. Nauseous and sick feeling. Nauseous at thought of food.

Teeth - Slightly clenching teeth. Pain in left upper molars. Toothache, dull pain. Right upper tooth socket bleeds.

Temperature - Cold and clammy. Feels quite warm. Mild fever. Felt hot.

Throat - Voice hoarse but painless. Voice sounded husky and broken. Laryngitis. Mucus, need to keep clearing throat. Mucus, back of throat. Sore throat. Swollen painful throat, hurts to swallow. Throat sore, both sides, dry and stinging. Woke with painful throat. Dry, burning, raw, difficult to swallow. Feeling something stuck in throat. Throat felt constricted. Mucus running down back of throat. Slight nausea in throat. Tickly feeling at back of throat, extends to left ear, sinuses.

Vertigo - Slight dizziness.

RELATIONS - ***Compare:*** Chemically related remedies would be Calc-sulph. (Calcium Sulphate - $CaSO_4$) and Hepar-sulph. (impure Calcium Sulphide - CaS).

REFERENCES - Wilkinson.

ALBIZIA JULIBRISSIN

(Mimosa Tree)

PHARMACY - alb-j. Albizia julibrissin durazz. Mimosa tree. Silk tree. Powderpuff tree. Silky acacia. Pink siris. N. O. Fabaceae. Asia. Tincture from flowers, leaves and stems. ***Historical dose:*** Tincture and all potencies.

CLINICAL - Abscess. ***Anxiety.*** Boils. Bruises. Cancer, lung. Carbuncles. ***Depression.*** Fractures. ***Grief.*** Heart, disease. Hemorrhoids. ***Insomnia***. Pains. Sarcoma. Sores. Sprains. Stress. Swellings. Worms. Wounds.

HERBAL - The Mimosa tree, Albizia julibrissin, was introduced to the United States in 1745 for use as an ornamental plant because of its unusual, attractive and fragrant pom-like flowers and interesting fern-like foliage. This deciduous tree is attractive to bees, butterflies, and birds.

This is a traditional herb used for depression and irritability. The flower heads are carminative, digestive aid, sedative and tonic.

Mimosa flowers are used internally in the treatment of insomnia, irritability, breathlessness and poor memory. The stem bark is anodyne, anthelmintic, carminative, discutient, diuretic, oxytocic, sedative, stimulant, tonic, vermifuge and vulnerary. It is used internally in the treatment of insomnia, irritability, boils and carbuncles.

Externally, it is applied to injuries and swellings. A gummy extract obtained from the plant is used as a plaster for abscesses, boils, etc., and also as a retentive in fractures and sprains.

The flower of the mimosa invigorates blood, calms the spirit. It's used for acute and chronic depression, insomnia, poor memory, and irritability. Problems due to constrained emotions, especially when accompanied by poor memory, epigastric pain and feelings of tightness and pressure in the chest.

MIND - Depression. ***Anxiety.*** Poor memory. Feelings of grief and loss.

Skin - Abscesses. Boils.

Sleep - Insomnia.

COMMENTS - Called the "tree of collective happiness" by the Chinese, mimosa flowers are specifically used for individuals who are experiencing deep feelings of grief and loss.

Micheal Tierra stated that he has used mimosa or albizia flower and bark extract alone or in formula for large numbers of people who might otherwise be given pharmaceutical anti-depressants.

All experienced complete or significant benefit even after a day's use. He recommend taking one half to one teaspoon, three or four times daily. While its flavor leaves something to be desired, it has shown itself to be completely safe and after experiencing its positive effects, one quickly grows used to the flavor.

REFERENCES - Buttimer. Murphy. Tierra.

ALCHEMILLA ARVENSIS

(Parsley Piert)

PHARMACY - alch-a. Alchemilla arvensis. Parsley piert. Field Lady's Mantle. N. O. Rosaceae. Europe. Tincture from leaves and stems. ***Historical dose:*** Tincture and all potencies.

HERBAL - This is a traditional herb for gravel, kidney stones and urinary infections.

REFERENCES - Potter.

ALCHEMILLA VULGARIS

(Lady's Mantle)

PHARMACY - alch-v. Alchemilla vulgaris. Lady's Mantle. Mary's Cape. Lionsfoot. N. O. Rosaceae. Europe. Tincture from leaves and stems. ***Historical dose:*** Tincture and all potencies.

CLINICAL - Bruises. Cuts. Gastritis. Indigestion. Leucorrhea. Menopause. Menstrual, disorders.

HERBAL - Alchemilla means "Hail to the Alchemists." The leaves of Alchemilla fold in such a way as to catch the morning dewdrops like jewels. In Iceland this plant is sacred to the Virgin, called Mariastakker, which gives quiet sleep if placed under the pillow at night.

HOMEOPATHIC - Alchemilla has been used for healing wounds and for women's problems. It is mildly astringent, diuretic and anti-inflammatory. Helps regulate the menses and eases the menopause. Gastritis and enteritis. Used as a douche for leucorrhea.

REFERENCES - Boericke. Clarke.

ALCOHOLUS

(Ethyl Alcohol)

PHARMACY - alco. Alcoholus. Ethyl alcohol. Aethanolum. Spirits of wine. Remedy made from commercial spirits of wine, by re-distillation. ***Historical dose:*** Tincture and all potencies.

CLINICAL - Alcoholism. Coma. Delirium. Dementia. Double vision. Hallucinations. Imbecility. Insanity. Mania. Stupidity.

HOMEOPATHIC - Amid the pleasures of the cup the soldier no longer complains of the campaign, the sailor forgets the dangers of the storm. The weak one grows strong and the despondent bold. The despairing lover leaves his solitude and forgets the indifference of his mistress. From acute alcohol intoxication all weaknesses are exposed and all secrets divulged without reserve, all hypocrisy ceases. Intoxicated persons beget alcoholics.

General excitement of all the senses. Moral and physical exaltation.

Transition from delirium tremens into permanent mania with hectic fever or dropsy.

A feeling of vague and unaccountable dread. Sadness often constant through the whole disease (delirium tremens). Staggering, uncertain gait. Coma, that changes to paralysis of the brain in persons of an apoplectic habit.

Sexual powers at first increased, then diminished. Impotence, want of sexual power. Irregular menstruation. Abortion in the first months. The children of alcoholics may grow up dull, indolent, stupid and become intemperate. Inclination to obesity. Diminished perspiration.

MIND - Mind disturbed, difficulty fixing the attention. General intellectual enfeeblement. Impaired memory. Absence of the senses and of reason. Restlessness and anxiousness, tries to disguise. Solitude and repose in bed increase the anxiety.

Mania with excessive irritability, excited by slightest causes. Mania with disposition to commit murder or start a fire. Impatience of contradiction. Unreasonable inclination to quarrel. Exhilaration. Increased self-esteem and importance. Feels insulted and abused by one's friends. Melancholy, weeping. Depression. Inclination to commit suicide.

Delirium. Rapid and incoherent talk. Thinks himself pursued. Screaming, singing and immoderate merriment. Feeling unusually strong and rich. Various hallucinations of sight, hearing, smell and sensation.

Abdomen - Sense of pressure in both hypochondria. Swelling of spleen. Recti muscles of abdomen become rigid and prominent. Ascites. Rumbling and growling in intestines. Inflammation of the intestines and stomach. Flatulence. Colic pains. Intestinal hemorrhage.

Back - Veins of neck swollen. Temporal and throat arteries throb, jugular veins turgescent or protruding. Weakness, finally in muscles of back, cannot even sit erect.

Chest - Hydrothorax. Emphysema. Congestion of lungs. Sensation of warmth in chest. Tension of chest. Burning sensation back of the sternum.

Constitutions - A sanguine, choleric temperament, sentimental and passionate. Weak-nerved person shows blunted senses and childish. The phlegmatic temperament remains passive and rather falls from his chair before giving loud evidences of his intoxication.

Ears - Dryness in external meatus. Acute sense on hearing. Hearing blunted, perception of sound lessened. Confusion on sounds. Roaring in ears, especially after spasms or with vertigo. Ringing, buzzing or rushing sound in the ears, frequently accompanied with dull, diffused headache. Illusions of hearing. Imaginary voices and sounds.

Eyes - Eyes injected. Red and excited, watery eyes. Eyes fiery, brilliant, fixed and wild. Rigid, gleaming look. Bright and animated or suffused and soft. Spots in the eye and dimness of vision. Catarrhal inflammation of the eyes. Roughness of the margins of the lids. Contraction of the pupils, drooping lids and coma. Effusion and swelling below the eyes. Conjunctiva more or less jaundiced. Yellow tinge of the sclerotica. Dilated and almost insensible pupils. Vision weak, cannot use eyes, objects flicker and become dim. Cannot read or write. Aversion to light. Black before eyes. Flashes of light before eyes. Muscae volitantes in clouds, before the eyes. Double vision. Visual hallucinations.

Face - Distorted face. Face bloated, without expression, stupid, silly. Redness of the cheeks and nose. Face red and swollen. Tetter in the face. Eruption in the face, bluish-red or white vesicles and pimples.

Food - Mania for alcoholic drinks, pepper and other heating things. Longing for spirituous liquors and, if not speedily gratified, becomes raving or has convulsions. At first no desire to eat, afterwards, ravenous hunger. Loss of appetite. Aversion to food and alcoholic drinks. Thirst before breakfast and through the day, often excessive.

Head - Head dull, clouded and hazy. Effusion of water into the membranes and ventricles of the brain. Softening of the brain. Pressing headache, causing stupidity. Drawing in the head. Dull, diffused headache with a buzzing or rushing sound in the ears. Sensation of fullness at the crown and back of the head or at the temples.

Heart - Valvular insufficiency. Organic difficulties of the heart and the large vessels. Hypertrophy of the left side of the heart. Increased activity of the heart and arteries. Pulsation of the heart and arteries violently increased, hard and full. Increased heat and rapidity of action in the heart. Very excited action, violent throbbing of the heart. Palpitations of the heart. Pulse nearly always accelerated, sometimes small and empty, sometimes full and even rather hard.

Kidneys - Sensitiveness, aching and pain in the region of the kidneys.

Limbs - Sudden startings of the limbs, as from electrical shocks. Trembling of limbs. Increased warmth, then coldness. Creeping sensation (formication) under the skin of the hands and feet. Weakness and relaxation of the muscles of locomotion, first in fingers and hands, especially in thumb and index-finger, extending all over both limbs. Limbs numb, as if paralyzed and extremely sensitive to touch and motion.

Liver - Heat, weight and soreness in the region of the liver. Inflammation of the liver. Cirrhosis.

Lungs - Sensation of heat in the larynx. Catarrhal bronchitis. Accumulation of mucus in the air-passages. Disposition to clear the throat. Hoarseness. Sobbing. Hacking, dry cough. Coughing blood. Accelerated breathing. There was a sense of impediment to respiration. Heavy, labored breathing. Snoring respiration. Asthma. Asphyxia.

Modalities - Worse when lying down. Worse when quiet at night.

Mouth - Grinding the teeth. Tongue fissured from middle to the edges, furred or sometimes denuded of epithelium. Papillae at tip of tongue enlarged and red. Sore and dry condition of the tip of the tongue. Dry, red, glazed tongue. Tongue covered with yellow slime in the middle, the margins clean. Tongue smooth and red with tendency to stick to the teeth or roof of the mouth. Tongue moved with difficulty. Convulsive motions of the tongue with stammering and inarticulate speech. Dry state of the mouth. Offensive smell from the mouth. Froth in mouth. Sour, salty or bitter taste in the mouth in the morning. Bitter taste in the mouth. Illusions of the sense of taste. Stammering speech.

Nose - Redness of the nose and cheeks. Redness of the nose, especially at the tip. Vessels of the skin congested. Swelling and inflammation. Red pimples or tubercles. Lining membrane of the sinuses inflamed and ulcerated. Bleeding of the nose. Illusions of the sense of smell.

Rectum - Hemorrhoids and varicose veins. Bleeding hemorrhoids. Paralysis of anus. Feces compact, knotty, black or light gray. Stool black, bilious, slimy and bloody, thin and clay colored. Diarrhea mucus or mealy. Diarrhea often alternating with constipation. Involuntary excretion of stool and urine.

Skin - Skin smutty or yellowish-gray. Jaundice. Skin soft and flabby. Skin becomes dry and hard. Sense of dryness, heat and evident fullness of swelling of the exposed parts of the skin, as the hands and face with general sensation of heat. Tormenting eruption, exceedingly itching, rough, scaly patches. Eczema and prurigo. Acne rosacea. Skin does not heal readily. Large indolent, blue-looking boils or carbuncles. Varicose ulcers.

Sleep - Irresistible sleep. Deep sleep, frequently accompanied by rattling breath. Lethargic with snoring respiration, intermittent pulsation of the heart. Restless sleep. Starts from his sleep with anxiety and restlessness. Insomnia, the patient tosses from side to side during nearly the whole night, getting only broken snatches of sleep and often with frightful dreams.

Stomach - Belchings, sour or foul. Belchings of water. Eructation like rotten eggs. Nausea and vomiting mucus and water. Vomiting of sour and offensive smelling matters. Hematemesis. Fullness and distention after eating. Burning heat in stomach. Pressure in the stomach. Sense of oppression and weight. Weakness of the stomach. Constriction, uncomfortable tension and pressure in epigastrium.

Temperature - Great inclination to sweat. Sweat easy at first. Sweat profuse, cool, sticky, sour smelling, sometimes warm. Increased perspiration moderates intoxication. Sensation of cold with paleness of the body. Fevers. Evening exacerbations. An agreeable warmth spreads over the body. General sensation of heat with increased action of the heart and dryness of the skin.

Throat - Throat red and feels stiff. Granulations on the posterior wall of the throat, also on the base of the tongue. Engorged appearance of the veins of the fauces. Redness, dryness and heat. Aphthous ulcers in the throat. Gangrenous ulcers. Throat full of tough mucus, difficult to hawk up. Paralysis of pharyngeal muscles. Paralysis of the muscles of swallowing. Sensation as if something lodged in the esophagus. Strong efforts to clear the throat or belch or vomit, bring up blood or bloody mucus. Painful swallowing.

Urine - Frequent need to urinate, finally incontinence. Involuntary excretion of urine and stool. Increased quantity of urine. Lessened secretion of urine. Retention of urine. Urine scanty at first, yellowish or deep red, then more copious with sediment. High-colored urine. Albuminous urine. Urine acid, contains serum and bile. Bloody urine.

Vertigo - Attacks of vertigo with sudden faintness and reeling or falling down, but no twitchings. Violent vertigo, nearly changing to a stroke. He staggers while walking and standing. Momentary attacks of vertigo.

COMMENTS - Frenzy, accompanied by violent convulsions. Drunkenness with various manias. Much inconsiderate, confused talking. Talkativeness, by which confessions are drawn from him. Ashamed of his intoxication. Sweet outpourings of friendship and tender confessions. Shamelessness. Moral degradation. Stubbornness. Quarrelsomeness.

Grudges long since forgotten are renewed. Forgetfulness.

All desires and inclinations become uncontrollable. Indescribable serenity of mind with cheerfulness, which the face expresses. Lively imagination. Rapid flow of thought, but he cannot keep his attention fixed continuously on one subject. Immoderate bursts of laughter. Cheerfulness.

Mental inquietude. Dread arising from actual delusions. Believes he is falling, even when on solid ground. Apprehension of nearby evil. Religious ravings, they address confidential and irreverent discourses to the Deity. Absurd fancies. Confuses one person with another.

Dancing, convulsive gestures, like chorea. Convulsions with a feeling as if something in the head is twisted and turned. Convulsions begin in one extremity, can be confined to one side, head can draw back, teeth clench, eyes distorted. Hysterical paroxysms. Epileptic attacks, generally coming on while standing. Epilepsy returns after every excess in drinking. Convulsive-like epileptic attacks.

The whole body trembles, commonly after exertion. Tottering and shaking. Trembling of the whole body. Twitchings or jerkings in muscles on sitting or lying, not in standing, especially on changing position. Persistent muscular tremor, first developed in the limbs.

Muscular inquietude inability to keep the limbs or the body still without a special effort of attention. Drawings in muscles like electric shocks. Trembling and paralysis as usual consequences of a stroke. General paralysis after delirium tremens. Marked sensory paralysis.

Power of directing and coordinating the muscles lessened. Muscular tone and power greatly lessened. The body loses its mobility and becomes more and more destitute of muscular power. Emaciation, want of strength with continued want of appetite. Prostration of the whole body.

Premature old age, face becomes pale and wrinkled, features relaxed, eyes dim, lips pale, the hands and the rest of the limbs tremble, gait unsteady. Indolence of body and mind. Frequent swoons. Hyperesthesia. This numbness is usually superficial, sensitive to deep pressure, sometimes sensitiveness of the whole body is blunted.

Pain and neuralgic tearings, cuttings. Very marked, continuous buzzing or thrilling, passing from above downwards and through the whole system. Sensitiveness to the fresh air, shudder and frost.

RELATIONS - ***Compare:*** (1) Hyos., Lach., Agar.

REFERENCES - Allen.

ALCOHOLUS SULPHURIS

(Liquor Lampadii)

PHARMACY - alco-s. Alcoholus sulphuris. Liquor lampadii. Carburet of sulphur. ***Historical dose:*** All potencies.

HOMEOPATHIC - Homoeopathic Provings by James W. Metcalf, M. D. It may prove useful in some forms of sick headache, especially when the pain commences in the forehead, and extends to one or the other temples. Scrofulous affections of the eyes and lids. Twitching of the eyes and lids, such as occurs in scrofulous, nervous, and verminous children. Some rheumatic and neuralgic affections of the face.

Chronic rheumatism, prurigo, and impetigo. Chronic pharyngitis. Irritation of the pharynx, with much hawking and spitting. Gagging cough from the irritation of an elongated uvula, especially when these symptoms occur in bilious and dyspeptic subjects.

Chronic irritation of the pharynx and larynx, with constant desire to hawk and spit, with hoarseness and short cough. May prove helpful in the first stage of tubercular disease of the lungs. It may prevent the tendency to irritation and congestion of the upper parts of the lungs which to readily lead to the fresh deposit of tubercles in consumptive patients.

Pyrosis, heartburn, and various dyspeptic and bilious derangements. Flatulence, bilious and flatulent colic, and congestion of the liver. It is one of the few drugs which seem to exert a specific action upon the cecum. Cured a case of chronic diarrhea, appearing every four or six weeks, attended with colic, the evacuations were liquid, frothy, yellowish, sour, and attended with tenesmus.

Abdomen - Great inflation of the abdomen, with rumbling of wind and tearing colic. Colic pains after eating. Slight wind-colic from time to time, with desire to urinate. Colic pains with loose stool and flatulence. Paroxysm of disagreeable pain in the left lobe of the liver. Soft stool, preceded by pain in the left lobe of the liver, and followed by pains in the cecal region.

Chest - Sensation of heat in the chest, congestion in the upper part of the lungs. Oppression, fullness in the chest. Slight stitches and pains about the chest.

Ears - Pain in the ears as if some one were striking upon the tympanum with a dull instrument.

Eyes - Burning and itching of the lids. Pustules on the lids, lasting four days. Dilatation of the pupils, with quickness of the pulse. Abundant secretion of whitish yellow mucus in the eyes. Lachrymation of the eyes. Twitching and trembling of the muscles of the eyes and lids.

Face - Redness and puffiness of the face, heat of the face and hands. Lancinating and tearing pains in the cheeks, extending up to the temples and lasting two months.

Fever - Great internal heat, with coldness of the hands and feet. General heat, headache, quick pulse, cramps in the calves of the legs and toes, without much thirst, and no perspiration.

Head - Pain in the forehead, which draws towards the left temple and remains there for two hours. Pressive frontal headache, lasting almost all day, and accompanied with transient pains in the temple. Drawing and tearing pain, stretching from the forehead to the temples, lasting all day, more severe in the room and during rest, relieved by walking in the open air. Dull pain in the frontal region, with nausea and heaviness of the whole head. Thumping pain in both temples. Violent pressive pain in the right temple, with malaise, desire to vomit, and rumbling of wind in the bowels.

Larynx - Heat and irritation of the larynx, hoarseness and irritation of the larynx, with continual desire to hawk. Cough provoked by a tickling at the bifurcation of the bronchi. Slight dry cough.

Limbs - Pains in and eruption upon the arms and legs.

Mouth - Dryness of the lips and mouth, irritation of the cavity and isthmus of the pharynx, followed by a sensation of contraction in the larynx, with gagging cough and quick breathing. Gum boils. Pasty, disagreeable taste in the mouth, with foul taste of the pharyngeal mucus. Bitter sharp taste in the mouth, or very repulsive acrid taste, or sweetish putrid taste. Great accumulation of saliva, with sweetish taste. Very frequent spitting. Pale red swelling of the uvula and vellum Burning and scraping in the pharynx and esophagus.

Skin - Sharp itching and stinging in different part of the skin, as if from nettles. Itching in various part of the skin, much aggravated by scratching. Bleeding and burning of eruptions when scratched (prurigo). Eruptions of impetigo on the back of the hands, the pustules are seated on the inflamed red base, contain a yellowish cloudy serum, and form thick yellowish scabs.

Sleep - Sleep. Sleeplessness from headache, dryness of the skin and general unpleasant heat, so that he is obliged to rise and bathe himself.

Stomach - Stomach. Very abundant eructation, sour burning, acrid regurgitations (pyrosis) occurring one or two hours after eating. Continual acid regurgitations. Regurgitations of air with nausea, discharge of flatulence upwards and downwards. Burning in the stomach and hepatic region. Heat in the epigastric region, which ascends and occupies the whole chest. Violent heat, ascending from the stomach to the head. Fullness in the stomach, with eructations, yawning, desire to vomit, and dizziness.

Stool - Liquid stools. Slimy, watery diarrhea, with violent pain in epigastrium. Sudden diarrhea, after having dined with good appetite. Violent diarrhea, with tenesmus and sour evacuations.

COMMENTS - Lampadius, in 1796, while distilling a mixture of pyrites and charcoal, procured a clear liquid in the receiver, which he named Alcoholus sulphuris, or the Alcohol of Sulphur. It consists of one equivalent of Carbon and two of Sulphur.

REFERENCES - Jahr. Marcy.

ALETRIS FARINOSA

(Star Grass)

PHARMACY - alet. Aletris farinosa. Star grass. Blazing grass. Colic root. Unicorn root. N. O. Hemodoracae. Melanthiaceae. North America. Tincture of root. ***Historical dose:*** Tincture and all potencies.

CLINICAL - Abortion. Anemia. Colic. Constipation. Convulsions. Debility. Dysmenorrhea. Dysuria. Emaciation. Endometritis. Fainting. ***Fatigue.*** Fever. Hemorrhoids. Hysteric colic. Indigestion. Labor-like, pains. Leucorrhea. Menorrhagia. Miscarriage. Muscle, pain. Pregnancy, vomiting. Infertility. Uterus, pain, prolapse.

HOMEOPATHIC - Star grass is said to be the most bitter of all plants. Aletris farinosa particularly affects the female organs. Produces an anemic, relaxed condition, especially of the female organs. Useful for chlorotic girls and pregnant women.

Many symptoms appear in the uterine sphere including uterine atony. Sensation of weight in uterine region and tendency to prolapse. Hemorrhages. Menorrhagia, black clots, fullness and weight. Menses are profuse and premature with labor-like pains or amenorrhea, debility from loss of fluids, protracted illness. Leucorrhea with debility. Obstinate vomiting of pregnancy. Habitual tendency to miscarriage. Infertility.

Characterized by weariness of body and mind. The patient is ***fatigued and tired all the time***, suffers from prolapse, leucorrhea, rectal distress, etc. Marked anemia. Fainting attacks with vertigo. Sensation of weight in occiput as if it would draw the head back. Parts feel heavy. Lack of appetite, in connection with uterine disorders. Disgust for food, nausea, constipation. The least food distends the stomach. Marked emaciation.

MIND - Mental power and energy weakened. Cannot concentrate mind. Confused feelings. Fainting with vertigo.

Abdomen - Colic settling in lower colon, better passing flatus. Scanty, diarrheic stools. Pain, better bending backwards.

Back - Sensation as if back would break just above waist. Backache with dragging in sacral region, with stringy, colorless leucorrhea.

Constitutions - Suited to chlorotic girls and pregnant women. Weak, emaciated people.

Ears - Feel as if open through from one to the other.

Female - ***Premature and profuse menses with labor-like pains*** (Bell., Cham., Kali-c., Plat.). Menorrhagia profuse, black with clots. Retarded and scanty flow (Senec.). Copious menses followed by copious, watery oozing between periods. Leucorrhea white, stringy, due to weakness and anemia. Uterus seems heavy. ***Prolapse uterus*** with pain in right inguinal region. ***Habitual tendency to miscarriage.*** Muscular pains during pregnancy.

Food - ***Want of appetite*** with weakness.

Head - Weight in occiput, as if it would draw the head backwards. Vertigo with fainting, sleepiness, vomiting or purging.

Kidneys - Involuntary urination on walking fast or sneezing.

Limbs - Chronic rheumatism. Dropsy. Leg (right) feels paralyzed below knee, numb, could not bear weight on it.

Lungs - Cough before menses.

Modalities - Better from passing flatus. Better bending backwards. Worse from loss of fluids.

Mouth - Much frothy saliva.

Rectum - Loads up with feces-paretic condition. Large, hard, difficult stool, with great pain. Fearful pain during passing stools, as if forcing a passage. Constipation, as from rectal atony.

Stomach - Want of appetite, disgust for food. Least food causes distress. Flatulent colic. Nervous dyspepsia. Obstinate vomiting of pregnancy. Nausea better by coffee, by dinner with pressure in forehead.

RELATIONS - ***Compare:*** (1) Chin., Hydr., Sabin., Senec., Sep. Tril. (2) Helon. - False Unicorn, not to be confounded with Alet. (3) Dios. - colic worse bending forward. (4) Caust., Puls., Ferr., - discharge of urine during cough. (5) Alum. - constipation, grasps the seat tightly, despairs of having a stool. During stool terrible pains as if a passage were being forced, Alet.

REFERENCES - Boericke. Clarke.

ALFALFA

(Medicago sativa)

PHARMACY - alf. Alfalfa. Medicago sativa. California clover. Lucerne. N. O. Papilionoideae. ***Historical dose:*** Tincture and all potencies.

CLINICAL - ***Anorexia.*** Appendicitis. ***Appetite, loss.*** Ascites. Breast-feeding. Bulimia. ***Cachexia.*** Cancer. Chemotherapy, effects. Colitis. Diabetes. Diarrhea. Dropsy. ***Emaciation.*** Exhaustion. Fatigue. Flatulence. ***Hypoglycemia.*** Insomnia. ***Malnutrition.*** Marasmus. Neurasthenia. ***Nutritional, disorders.*** Polyuria. Prostate, hypertrophy. Radiation, effects. Rheumatic, diathesis. Syphilis. ***Weakness.*** Weight, loss.

HERBAL - This is a leguminous plant, cultivated from ancient times and highly prized as a pasture and forage plant. Those who have observed its influence when employed as a forage for stock must have been impressed with the favorable results.

All of the provers, except one, noted three things in particular: an increased appetite so they could not wait for their regular meals, an increased amount of urine and urea, and a general sense of well-being. Causes ***mental exhilaration,*** increases energy and stamina.

Alfalfa favorably influences nutrition, evidenced in *"toning up"* the appetite and digestion. Acts as a fat producer, corrects tissue waste. Improves appetite and digestion, mental and physical vigor returns with weight gain.

HOMEOPATHIC - Metabolic regulator. Lack of appetite or aversion to all food. ***Emaciation***. Disorders characterized by malnutrition, including neurasthenia, syphilis, insomnia, or nervous digestion. ***Anorexia*** nervosa. Cancer with emaciation.

Failure to thrive in children. ***Deficient breast-milk***, it increases the quality and quantity of milk in nursing mothers. If a baby has failure to thrive, give Alfalfa to the mother and child, the breast milk improves, the mother gets stronger and the baby gains weight.

Pronounced urinary action. Diabetes insipidus and phosphaturia. Useful to allay the bladder irritability of prostatic hypertrophy. Rheumatic diathesis.

Weakness, enervation, exhaustion, prostration, infirmity. Muscle weakness. Convulsive movements. Desires sweets. Sympathicotonia. Worse in the evening, from 6 to 9 p.m.

A concentrated Alfalfa tincture should exercise an influence similar to that of Avena sativa. An herbal infusion used in three cases produced the same results as the alcoholic preparations.

MIND - Alfalfa induces a mental exhilaration of buoyancy. Cheerfulness. Vivaciousness. A general feeling of well being, feels clear and bright, so that all blues are dissipated. ***Exhilaration.*** Mirth, hilarity, liveliness. Clearness of thoughts.

Morose, sulky, cross, fretful, ill humored, peevish. Sadness, despondency, melancholy. Depression from disappointed love. Hypochondriasis. Aversion to mental work. Bad dreams from emotional causes. Bulimia.

Prostration of mind, mental exhaustion, brain fag. Dull, drowsy, stupid (Gels.), gloomy and irritable, worse during evening. Slowness. Mental dullness, sluggishness. Difficulty thinking and comprehending.

Abdomen - Distension. Flatulence with distention. Pain from passing flatus. Shifting, flatulent pain along colon several hours after meals. Frequent loose, yellow, painful stools with burning flatulence. Colitis. Chronic appendicitis. Inflammation, peritonitis, enteritis. Dropsy, ascites, with scanty urination. Cramping, griping pain. Passing flatus aggravates.

Back - Backache.

Bladder - Bladder irritability. Urging to urinate, morbid desire. Frequent urging to urinate.

Breasts - Breast milk, absent or disappearing.

Constitutions - Anorexic, emaciated, broken down constitutions. Cancer diathesis.

Ears - Stuffed feeling in Eustachian tube (Kali-m.) at night, clear in morning.

Eyes - Aching in and above the eyes.

Face - Flushed.

Female - Increased desire. Menses coming earlier than usual.

Food - Increased thirst. ***Appetite wanting with weight loss.*** Sensation of hunger at all times. Appetite is increased. ***Malnutrition.*** Desire for sweets. Sometimes ravenous appetite. ***Hypoglycemia***, must stop and have something to eat in the middle of the morning. Hungry in forenoon (Sulph.).

Head - Dull, heavy feeling in occiput in and above the eyes, worse toward evening. Violent headache. Pain in the left side of the head. Dull heavy feeling comes on about 2 p.m. and gradually increases until 6 p.m., starts at the occiput and becomes severe.

Kidneys - Kidneys are weak, frequent urging to urinate. Polyuria (Ph-ac.). Increased elimination of urea indican and phosphates. Inactivity. Suppression of urine, anuria.

Male - Enlarged prostate gland. Prostatic hypertrophy.

Rectum - Painless, yellow diarrhea, accompanied with flatus and attended with burning. Stools loose and more frequent than usual. Stools two or three times daily. Pasty, papescent stools.

Sleep - Slept better than usual, especially in early morning, it induces quiet, reposeful and refreshing sleep. Insomnia. Sleeplessness during convalescence.

Stomach - Emptiness, weak feeling, faintness, goneness. Hungry feeling not ameliorated by eating. Nervous indigestion.

Urine - Profuse urine, increased. Scanty. Sediment, increased indican, phosphates. Sugar in urine.

COMMENTS - Dr. Houts gathered the fresh Alfalfa leaves, but obtained good results from the use of dried leaves which still retain a green color. Using these, he made an infusion which he gave to patients suffering from backaches.

He found it especially indicated if they were passing small quantities of water while suffering from rheumatic symptoms or backache with muscular aching, with an excessive quantity of uric acid and urates secreted.

Dr. Fearn of Oakland wrote that its action was very soothing upon the kidneys and urinary apparatus. He believed that it could be prepared for human food to as good, if not better, advantage than for animal food.

Dr. Ben Bradley of Hamlet, Ohio, believed that alfalfa is one of our upcoming remedies. He reported a case where a woman had seven children born apparently strong and well, but when they reached the age of eighteen years they wasted away and died.

When the last girl was taken with the symptoms of which the others had died, Dr. Bradley made a saturated tincture of Alfalfa seed concentrated, fully saturated and gave her ten drops four or five times a day. This is reported to have increased her weight from 99 to 133 pounds. She recovered good health.

Mr. D. aged 41, a chief clerk in the general offices of one of our railroad companies, had complained for several months of losing flesh. His appetite was poor, he did not relish his food. There was present an abnormal thirst, a loss of flesh and polyuria.

The quantity of urine for twenty-four hours was eighty ounces, specific gravity 1008. Nothing abnormal apart from an excess of indican. The prostate was enlarged and sensitive to pressure. He complained of some irritation upon urination.

Five drops of the tincture was prescribed four times a day. After two weeks he sent a message for a supply stating it had greatly benefited him. He called at the end of two months having gained ten pounds, the urine at this time was practically normal in quantity. The appetite was fine and he considered himself in a normal condition.

Mr. G, aged 29, complained of a loss of weight and appetite, excessive thirst, polyuria and mental depression. This syndrome had been gradually developing for the past year.

Physical examination showed a man of medium size, emaciated. Heart action weakened. Prostatic portion of urethra hypersensitive. The urine was greatly increased in quantity and of low specific gravity, free from casts and albumin, phosphates were increased.

Five drops of the tincture before each meal and on retiring gradually relieved the condition so that in three months he considered himself well.

RELATIONS - ***Compare:*** (1) Avena Sat., Hydr., Dipodium punct. (2) Ars., Gels., Kali-p., Ph-ac., Zinc.

REFERENCES - Anshutz. Boericke. Clarke. Murphy

ALLANTOIN

(Glyoxyldiureide)

PHARMACY - allan. Allantoin. Glyoxyldiureide (C4H6N4O3). Allantoin is a white, odorless, crystalline powder (when isolated). ***Historical dose:*** All potencies.

CLINICAL - Acne. Burns. Canker, sores. Diaper rash. Fever blisters. Rashes. Skin. disorders. Stretch, marks. Sunburn. Ulcers. Wounds.

HOMEOPATHIC - Allantoin is a botanical extract of the Comfrey plant and is used for its healing, soothing, and anti-irritating properties. Allantoin helps to heal wounds and skin irritations and stimulate growth of healthy tissue. This extract can be found in anti-acne products, sun care products, and clarifying lotions because of its ability to help heal minor wounds and promote healthy skin.

Abate stretch marks naturally. Promotes wound healing, speeds up cell regeneration, and has a keratolytic (skin-softening) effect. Allantoin has been termed a cell proliferant, an epithelization stimulant, and a chemical debrider.

It is said to clean away necrotic tissue, hastening the growth of new healthy tissue. Since Allantoin stimulates new and healthy tissue growth, healing epithelization may take place.

Allantoin has been also termed a counter irritant that helps alleviate the untoward skin-irritation effects of certain cosmetic ingredients such as soap and detergent surfactants, oils, and acidic or alkaline materials.

It produces its desirable effects by promoting and speeding up the healthy, natural processes of the body. It helps the skin to help itself.

It has long been known to enhance the efficacy and desirability of cosmetic creams and lotions by its action as a skin protectant.

Allantoin has also been incorporated into shampoos, lipsticks, shaving creams, suntan products, bath foams, hair gels, baby powders and various aerosol preparations. Most recently, Allantoin has been used in various dental preparations such as toothpaste and mouthwash.

For the temporary protection of minor cuts, scrapes, burns and sunburn. Helps prevent and temporarily protects chafed, chapped, cracked, or wind-burned skin and lips.

Relieves dryness and softens cold sores and fever blisters. Helps treat and prevent diaper rash. Protects chafed skin. Minor skin irritation associated with diaper rash and helps protect from and seal out wetness.

REFERENCES - Murphy.

ALLIUM CEPA

(Red Onion)

PHARMACY - all-c. Allium cepa. Red onion. N. O. Liliaceae. Alliaceae. Tincture of the onion. Tincture of whole fresh plant gathered from July to August. ***Historical dose:*** Tincture and all potencies.

CLINICAL - ***Allergies.*** Anus, fissure. Ascites. Catarrh. ***Colds. Coryza.*** Coughs. Diarrhea. Earache. Facial paralysis. Feet, easily galled. ***Hay fever.*** Hernia. Influenza. Itching. Laryngitis. ***Neuritis.*** Neuroma. Otitis. Panaritium. Pneumonia. Sinusitis. ***Sneezing. Traumatic, neuritis.*** Whitlow. Whooping cough. Worms. Yellow fever.

HOMEOPATHIC - Allium cepa covers more symptoms of ***common colds and hay fever*** than any other remedy. Anyone who has cut up raw onions for cooking knows the irritation upon the eyes and nose. Onions cause active sneezing and lachrymation. If the homeopathic principle of cure is true, it ought to be a good remedy for coryza, and it is.

All-c. affects the mucus membranes of nose, eyes, larynx and bowels, causing increased secretions. ***Hay fever and coryza*** with ***acrid nasal discharges*** and laryngeal symptoms. Burning of the eyelids, nose, mouth, throat, bladder, skin. Acute colds from ***damp cold weather***. Coughs, colds or headache, worse in warm room, better in open air, worse again on returning to warm room. Eye discharges may be bland.

Cough caused by tickling in larynx, constant inclination to hack in order to relieve it. It has cured violent catarrhal laryngitis, hoarse cough with feeling as if it would split and tear the larynx, causing watering of eyes. Cough from inhaling cold air. Nasal secretion is acrid, secretion from eye is bland.

Traumatic neuritis. Neuralgic pains like a ***fine thread***, following amputations or injuries to nerves. Thread-like pains in the face. Left-side facial paralysis. Wounds do not heal. Singer's coryza. Neuroma. Senile gangrene. Sensation of glowing heat in different parts of the body. Symptoms go from left to right. The feet are aggravated by walking.

The toothache is better by cold air or cold washing. Picking or sucking teeth improves the toothache. Sensation of glowing heat on different parts of the body. Desires raw onions. Strangulated hernia has been known to follow the eating abundantly of cooked onions. A raw onion eaten just before going to bed is a popular remedy for sleeplessness.

MIND - Anxious about their health. Despair of recovery. Fear that pain will become unbearable. Melancholy. Indefinable anxiety. Indolence in morning. Confusion of mind, after coffee, wine.

Abdomen - Rumbling offensive flatus. Pains in left hypogastrium. Colic sitting, moving about. Very offensive flatus. Belching with rumbling and puffing up of the abdomen. Violent cutting pain in the left lower abdomen, with frequent desire to urinate. Pains in liver region. Abdomen distended, rumbling, urging, and finally diarrhea.

Back - Intense pain in nape of neck. Pain under right shoulder blade. Chills run down the back with frequent urination, followed by heat and thirst.

Causations - Damp cold wind, weather causes colds and toothache. Colds of spring, hay fever of August, epidemics of spasmodic cough in autumn. Wet feet. Eating spoiled fish, cucumbers, salads. Injuries. Shooting pains after surgical operations.

Constitutions - Especially adapted to phlegmatic patients. Psoric and allergic constitutions.

Ears - Earache, shooting pain in Eustachian tube. Aching extending to throat. Itching in ears from allergies. Otitis media. Discharge of pus from the ear. Hardness of hearing.

Eyes - Itching, biting, burning in the eyes. Eyes red, sensitive to touch. Flow of tears. Much ***burning*** and smarting lachrymation. ***Sensitive to light***. Eyes suffused and watery, profuse, ***bland lachrymation***, better in open air. Burning in eyelids, worse coughing, wants to rub them. Sensation as if eye were hanging by a string or torn. Near objects seem distant, while yawning. Letters appear smaller. Swelling around the eyes.

Face - Thread-like pains in face. Paralysis of left half of face, also in limbs of same side. Facial neuritis.

Food - Thirst. Canine hunger. Appetite, increased or diminished. Strong craving for raw onions, cannot take any other nourishment.

Head - Dull headache, with coryza. Catarrhal headache, in forehead, ***worse in warm room,*** towards evening. Headache ceases during menses, returns when flow disappears. Aching in forehead, extending to eyes and face, better free running coryza. Electric shock passes through head. Skull bones numb. Pain in occiput and down the neck.

Kidneys - Sensation of weakness in bladder and urethra. Frequent and copious urination. Increased secretion of urine with coryza. Strangury after wet feet. Dribbling of urine in elderly people. Urine red, with much urging and burning in urethra.

Limbs - Joints feel lame. Panaritium. Painful disorders of the fingers about the nails, red streaks running up the arm. Limbs, especially arms feel sore and tired. ***Neuralgia of stump.*** Bad effects from getting feet wet. Ulcers when skin is rubbed off by the shoes especially on the heels. Sore feet from long walking.

Lungs - ***Hacking cough on inhaling cold air.*** Acute bronchitis. ***Oppressed breathing*** from pressure in middle of chest. Constricted feeling in region of epiglottis. Violent catarrhal laryngitis, the hoarse cough seemed to split and tear the larynx. Much sneezing and coughing.

Modalities - Better in open air. Better cold room. Better bathing. Better motion. ***Worse in a warm room***. Worse damp weather. Worse spring. Worse wet feet. Worse afternoon and evening. Worse lying down. Worse singing. Rest aggravates, feels better from motion.

Mouth - Bad odor from the mouth and throat.

Nose - Fluent coryza with headache, cough and hoarseness. ***Hay fever*** (Euphr., Sabad., Psor.). Allergies every August. Spring coryza. ***Nose drips.*** Acrid discharge, when singing. ***Sneezing,*** especially when entering a warm room. Constant sneezing with profuse acrid coryza. Burning and smarting in the nose. Burning pain in edges of nose and lips. ***Profuse watery discharge with sneezing***. Acrid burning discharge. ***Nasal discharge excoriating the nose and upper lip***. Feeling of a lump at root of nose. Coryza, headache, cough and hoarseness. Copious acrid watery discharge from nose, with bland watering of eyes. Polyps. Nosebleed. ***Sinusitis.*** Sensitive to odors of flowers and the skin of peaches. Nose stopped, nasal voice. Common colds becomes laryngitis.

Rectum - Diarrhea after midnight and in the morning. Flatus very offensive. Hemorrhoids, tearing, jerking pains in anus. Stitches in the rectum. Cracks at the anus. Itching at the anus. Worms.

Skin - Redness, nettle rash, measles, scarlatina, when the complaints are characterized by the coryza symptoms. Prickling as from pins. Sensation of glowing heat on different parts of the body. Red streaks running up arm. Felon after childbirth.

Sleep - Yawning in deep sleep or with headache and drowsiness and cramp in stomach. Wakes at 2 a.m. Gaping in deep sleep. Dreams of being near water, of battles, precipices, deep wells, of storms, high waves, Annoying dreams in convalescents.

Stomach - Sour belching. Nausea, coming from stomach up the throat into the fauces. Weak, empty feeling in stomach. Pressure in stomach. Pain in region of pylorus.

Temperature - Fever with rumbling in the abdomen, coryza, and thirst. Flitting heat over whole body, and thirst. Coldness alternates with heat during catarrh. Sweats easily and copiously.

Throat - ***Hoarseness.*** Sensation as of a lump in the throat. ***Tickling in larynx.*** Expectoration of a lumpy mucus through the posterior sinuses. ***Sensation as if larynx is split and torn.*** Pain in throat extending to the ear.

COMMENTS - Coryza with frequent sneezing and profuse acrid discharge, corroding upper lip and nose. Lachrymation, also profuse, but bland (Euphr. is the reverse). The action of All-c. seems to be primarily in the nose (Euphr., in the eyes).

Allium Cepa is irritating discharge with burning and itching, from a cold, flu, allergies and hay fever. The nose, the back of the throat, the palate and the throat are itching and burning.

A keynote is that the upper lip is red and irritated. Frequent sneezing (Ars.), with discharge. Strong symptoms from the nose, profuse sneezing (Nat-m.). Another keynote is itching in the back of the throat that drips into the larynx and causes hoarseness and change of voice. Burning in the larynx and voice box.

Allergic asthma. A hay fever that was suppressed with antihistamines that went into the lungs (Ars., Iod.).

Nash found it particularly useful in children when the profuse coryza or cold extended to the bronchials with much mucus coughing and rattling of mucus.

RELATIONS - ***Antidoted by:*** Arn. - toothache. Cham. - abdominal pains. Roasted coffee will remove onion breath. ***Compare:*** (1) Euphr., Wye., Sabad., Arundo, All-s. (2) Acon., Puls., Gels. (3) Nux-v. - coryza recurring in August. (4) Verat. - colic with despondency. (5) Thuj. - offensive breath and diarrhea after eating onions. (6) Lach. - left to right. (7) Calen., Hyper. - neuritis, amputation pain. ***Complementary:*** Phos., Puls., Sars., Ther., Thuj. ***Incompatible:*** All-s., Aloe, Scilla. ***Followed by:*** Calc. and Sil. in polyps.

REFERENCES - Boericke. Clarke. Nash. Murphy.

ALLIUM SATIVUM

(Garlic)

PHARMACY - all-s. Allium sativum. Garlic. N. O. Liliaceae. Alliaceae. Tincture of fresh bulb. ***Historical dose:*** Tincture and all potencies.

CLINICAL - Alopecia. Asthma, periodical. Bronchiectasis. Bronchitis. Catarrhs. Chest, complaints. Colic. Colitis. Constipation. Coughs. Coxalgia. Dandruff. Deafness. Diabetes. Diarrhea. Dropsy. ***Dyspepsia.*** Fevers. Flatus. Headaches. ***Hemoptysis***. Hemorrhoids. ***High blood pressure.*** Hoarseness. Menstrual. Menorrhagia. Ophthalmia. Prolapsed anus. Retained, placenta. Rheumatism. Ringworm. Salivation. Scurvy. Skin, disorders. Sprains. ***Tuberculosis***. Vertigo. Whitlow. Worms.

HERBAL - Garlic has been used as a condiment from ancient times and also as a remedy against worms and fevers. It has a reputation of lowering the blood pressure.

HOMEOPATHIC - All-s., though closely related to All-c., is incompatible with it and not very like it in action. It produces headache in connection with digestive troubles and menstruation. Heavy headache, can hardly open eyes, better onset of menses, worse after.

Teste cured with it chronic dyspepsia in old, fleshy persons, whose bowels were deranged by the least irregularity of diet. He also greatly relieved cases of diabetes mellitus with it. Periodical asthma, a case of permanent dyspnea, rheumatism of hip, swelling of breasts after weaning.

Characteristic respiratory symptoms include a cough, giving rise to fetid breath (Caps.). Bronchial catarrh with profuse, gelatinous, difficult mucus expectoration. Cough when smoking.

All-s. has vaso-dilatory properties. It acts directly on intestinal mucus membrane increasing peristalsis. Colitis with pathological flora. Adapted to fleshy subjects with dyspepsia and catarrhal disorders. High livers.

Patients who eat a great deal more, ***especially meat***, than they drink. The digestion in disordered by slightest irregularities in diet. Pressure in epigastrium and transverse colon, better by pressure and sitting bent. Pain in hip, psoas and illiac muscles.

Stings and bites. Dropsy after protracted intermittent in marshy districts. The child is drowsy, lifeless, extremely pale, bowels torpid, will not walk and the legs do not grow as rapidly as rest of the body.

Breasts swollen and painful to touch. Profuse menses. During menses there is soreness of vulva and thighs, ***Pulmonary tuberculosis***. ***Hemoptysis***. Cough and expectoration diminishes, temperature becomes normal, weight is gained and sleep becomes regular.

MIND - Anxiety and impatience. Sensitive. Fears he won't recover, that he won't able to bear any medicine. Fear of being poisoned. Fear he will never get well. Impulse to run away. Wants many things, pleased with nothing. Weak memory. Sadness when alone. Weeping during sleep.

Abdomen - Pressure in upper abdomen, better by sitting bent and pressing with both hands. Colic from flatus, twisting and pinchings around navel. Emission of fetid flatus. Everything seemed to drag downward. Weight in hypogastrium, immediately after a meal.

Back - Red spots like ringworm on the back. Itching between shoulders. Tearing, cutting pain in sacrum, in morning. Simple pain in coccyx.

Breasts - Breasts swollen and tender during menses. Swelling of breast after weaning. Dull stitches in right breast. Breasts sensitive to touch. Eruption of red blotches between the breasts and around the nipples.

Causations - Drinking bad water, gluttony, meat eating.

Chest - Darting pain in the chest which prevents sleep. Pain in left chest with dark urine. Chest complaints worse after eating.

Constitutions - Rather a gourmand than a glutton. Suited to persons who are disposed to excesses at the table, have strong constitutions, dark complexions, firm flesh, though occasionally disposed to obesity. Persons who eat a great deal more than they drink. Suited to fleshy people and those used to high living.

Ears - Catarrhal deafness. Hardened earwax and crusts (Thuj.).

Eyes - Catarrhal ophthalmia at night, smarting, burning and lachrymation, agglutination, returns every night when he tries to read. Tarsi sore with irritation.

Face - Spots on face. Lips are dry. Sharp pain on one side of the face.

Female - Eruption in vagina, on breasts and vulva during menses. Menses profuse, too early. Headache and dizziness lessen as the flow becomes established. Soreness of vulva and thighs during menses. Suppurating pimples on vulva. During menses extensive excoriations of skin of internal portions of thighs. Retained placenta.

Food - Voracious appetite. Thirst. Hunger and emptiness in stomach without appetite. Desire for butter. Digestion is disordered by slightest error in diet. Complaints from bad water, gluttony.

Head - Heavy, pulsation in temples. Headaches before menses, ceases during, worse after menses. Heaviness in forehead. Dull pain in occiput in morning, while lying on the back. Headache with mucus in the throat in dyspeptic subjects. Dandruff.

Heart - Leaping beats of the heart. High blood pressure.

Kidneys - Urine increased. Whitish very abundant urine, becoming cloudy from nitric acid. A kind of diabetes. Dark brown with copious sediment.

Limbs - Rheumatism of hip. Tearing pain in hip. Pain in psoas and iliacus muscles, worse crossing legs. Painful contraction in arm. Pain in forearm, seems as if paralyzed. Burning, then moisture in palms. Skin peels off the hands. Tearing pains in fingers extending below the nails. Weakness in lower limbs, painful weariness in the thighs. Pain as from a sprain in ankle joint, in toe joints. Tingling in feet, burning in soles, stiffness in feet.

Lungs - Difficult breathing as if sternum compressed. Periodic asthma. Constant rattling of mucus in bronchials. Cough in the morning after leaving bedroom with mucus expectoration. Coughing when smoking. Sensitive to the cold air. Painful irritation of windpipe when coughing. Cough seeming to come from stomach. Dry cough after eating. Bronchiectasis with fetid expectoration. Great difficulty in expectorating a glutinous mucus. Expectoration of thin, yellowish, purulent-looking blood-streaked mucus of putrid odor.

Modalities - Better from sitting bent. Worse from change of temperature. Worse pressure. Worse drinking bad water. Worse gluttony. Walking aggravates pains in limbs. Every step causes excruciating pain in intestines. Worse in evening and night. Worse in morning on waking.

Mouth - Much sweetish saliva after meals and at night. Tickling sensation in the lower teeth. Swelling of lower gums. Dryness of palate. Hot taste in mouth, from throat, strongly reminding him of garlic.

Nose - Coryza rather dry than fluent, with pressive pain from above the root of the nose. Smarting at junction of ale nasi and face. Blowing blood from the nose in the night.

Rectum - Constipation with constant dull pains in bowels. Expels flatus. Stool first fecal, then watery and hot. Involuntary stools. Diarrhea with cuttings in abdomen and loins. Hemorrhoids. Prolapsed anus. Worms.

Skin - Loose, dry, wilted skin. Skin sensitive. Swelling with itching and burning. Red spots, on hands, on chest, on back. Herpetic itching burning, red or whitish spots on a swollen surface.

Sleep - Drowsiness after a meal. Muscles twitch on falling asleep. Sleep prevented by stitches on chest, weight on stomach, or thirst. Coldness felt in sleep and awakening him frequently. Dreams of water and storms. Anxious dreams, continuing after waking.

Stomach - Burning belchings. Slightest error in diet disturbs the stomach. Sensations of cold and or hot ascending esophagus. Burning in stomach, very sensitive to the least pressure. Weight in stomach which prevents sleep. Pressure inward as from a stone in epigastrium.

Temperature - Chilliness on one side only. Shivering before midday and in evening. During coldness, redness of face. Vomiting during the fever. Sweat in afternoon. Sweat acrid, causing itching, fetid.

Throat - Sticky feeling in throat with dryness, tickling, heat, and raw feeling in larynx. Sensation as of something cold rising in throat. Sensation as of a hot and smarting vapor rising in the throat. Mucus accumulations in the throat in the morning.

Tongue - ***Tongue pale red papillae.*** Sensation of a hair on tongue or throat.

Vertigo - Vertigo while reading. Vertigo on looking steadily at anything for a long time. Short-lasting vertigo, and only on rising from a chair.

COMMENTS - Pain, pressive from within outward (Bry.), stinging or stinging and burning or stinging with paralytic weakness or tearing and crampy. Sometimes they increase gradually to a high point and then decrease gradually (Sulph., Stann.). "Hair" sensation on tongue, worse reading. Copious sweetish saliva. The hip is the seat of many rheumatic pains. Tearing in hip. Pain in psoas and iliac muscles worse least movement, though he can lift the limb with the hands. Aggravation from reading (Cina.).

Vertigo, brought on by looking long and steadily at anything. This is probably, in essence, the same modality as worse by reading. Catarrhal ophthalmia returning every night on trying to read. Coryza, moist, dry, thin, fluent with pressive pains above root of nose. Scurvy gums, sore mouth.

RELATIONS - ***Antidoted by:*** All-c., Lyc. ***Compare:*** (1) Ars., Senega, Kali-n. All-c. (2) Ornithogalum umbellatum - stomach disorders. (3) Bry., Caps., (fetid breath with cough). (4) Coloc. - colic, hip-pain, Ign., Kali-bi. (ropy expectoration, hair on tongue). (5) Rhus-t. and Hyos. (fear of being poisoned), Lyc., Nux-v., Seneg. ***Complementary:*** Ars. ***Incompatible:*** Aloe., All-c., Scilla.

REFERENCES - Boericke. Clarke.

ALLOXANUM

(Meoxalylurea)

PHARMACY - allox. Alloxanum. Meoxalylurea. Allopathic drug. It takes the form of rhomboid crystals soluble in alcohol and insoluble in water. The anhydrous crystals are dark yellow in color, the hydrogenized crystals are colorless. ***Historical dose:*** All potencies.

CLINICAL - Aerophagy. Alcoholism. Aphthae. Arthritis. Bedwetting. Blood, disorders. Cardiac neurosis. Catarrh. Conjunctivitis. ***Diabetes.*** Diarrhea. Dysentery. Dyspepsia. Dysuria. Ecchymosis. Eczema. Glossitis. ***Glycosuria.*** Headaches. ***Hypogycemia.*** Insomnia. Laryngitis. Leucorrhea. Myopia. Narcolepsy. Nausea. Neuralgia. Neurasthenia. Nightmares. Numbness. Osteoporosis. ***Pancreas, disorders.*** Pharyngitis. Pimples. Poly-neuritis. Purpura. Rheumatism. Toothache. Toxemia. ***Toxic diabetes.*** Vaginitis. Varicose veins.

HOMEOPATHIC - Alloxan was discovered accidentally by Dum and his collaborators in 1943. The toxicological action can be seen at the level of the pancreas, the kidneys, the liver, the lungs and in the blood. In animals, diabetes mellitus is provoked or, in other words, alloxanic diabetes. There would be a rapid degeneration if the islet Beta cells responsible for the production of insulin.

The homeopathic proving of Alloxan was undertaken by Templeton on two occasions, in 1949 on six provers, when the potencies 6c and 30c were tried out, and in 1951 on nine provers and seven controls.

Lack of heat and vital reaction. Disturbed sleep with nightmares. General indifference. Need for solitude. Dryness of digestive mucus membranes. ***Diabetes mellitus.*** Excessive thirst and frequent urination. Joint pains in the lumbar, sacral and ileocecal regions. Neuralgia of the tongue. Toothache.

Acrid dyspepsia. Spontaneous ecchymosis and eruption of itching pimples. Sensation of body being dispersed into different parts. Osteoporosis and muscular weakness. Decrease of phosphoremia and increase of phosphates in the blood. Glycosuria without hyperglycemia.

MIND - Great forgetfulness. Forgets places, names, things just done, just heard. Loss of short-term memory. Spelling mistakes. Words don't register. Mistakes in spelling. Dyslexia. Silly mistakes in writing simple words. Silly sort of attitude to serious things.

Alcoholic poly-neuritis with mental troubles. Paranoia. Sadness and tearfulness improved by solitude. Need for solitude and uneasiness about the future. Weeping better when alone.

Indifference towards the surrounding environment. Indifference to conversation. Indifference to loved ones. Indifference to work.

Irritable with people, talking, loud voices. Irritability from noise. Fits of anger. Hurried. Dogmatic. Dictatorial. Impatient, taps foot with impatience. Quarrelsome. Hurried, others move too slow. Wants to dash about, wants to do everything quickly.

Confusion as to his identity, as if head was being lifted off. Delusion, as if head were separated from body (Psor.). People talking seemed miles away. Voices seemed far away. Keeps washing hands.

Abdomen - Abdominal distention with profuse rumbling. ***Toxic diabetes.*** Ileocecal pain, aggravated by bending forwards and by movement. Sensation of a band around abdomen.

Back - Stiffness better stretching. Pain and cervical stiffness, aggravated in bed, ameliorated by stretching. Cramping pain in the shoulder blade, cutting pain, aggravated by drinking. Lumbar rheumatism. Arthritis of the spine, preventing movement. Pain in the lower lumbar region, worse in bed, in kneeling position and by standing, better by hot weather. Pain in lumbar region worse cold weather. Pain in lumbo-sacral region extending down legs.

Bladder - Feeling of fullness in the bladder. Coldness in bladder, worse draft of air. Sensation as if bladder is swollen. Incontinence on hurrying to get up, on sneezing. Bedwetting.

Blood - Reduction in the number of phosphates in the blood plasma, normal presence of glucose in the blood, azotemia. Reduction of sedimentation rate.

Chest - Feeling of a heavy weight on the chest. Heaviness better menses. Stitching pain better menses.

Constitutions - The subjects are often phosphoric and very weak. Subjects nervous, uneasy, anxious.

Ears - Deep, drumming pain inside. Itching of the auditory canal. Eczema of the outer ear.

Eyes - Conjunctivitis. Eyelids red, burning and itching. Eyes painful, especially as a result of light and after reading, ameliorated by closing the lids. Sight dim with patches and bright spots. Myopia. Dim vision and twitching of eyelids, on waking (Cycl.). Sparks like fragments of fire.

Female - Inflammation of the vulva and vagina. Feeling of swelling in the vagina, especially after standing for a long time. White leucorrhea, non-irritating, but increasing with the approach of menses. Sensation as if vagina were swollen, worse standing.

Food - Feeling of hunger, quickly sated. ***Hypogycemia.*** Aversion to salt. Desire for cold drinks, refreshing things. Excessive thirst and feeling of dryness. Worse cold drinks, warm drinks. Better warm drinks.

Head - Feeling of constriction and heat in the head, which is cold to the touch. Heaviness of head on waking with sensation of the hair being pulled. Headache better ascending steps, better closing eyes, worse coughing, worse hot room. Headache from hunger, but eating does not relieve. Headache worse laughing, better talking, better travelling.

Heart - Pain as of a punch in the precordial region. Shooting pain in the heart, worse when walking. Retro-sternal cramping pain. Cardiac neurosis.

Kidneys - Kidney pain on the left side on urination. Dysuria. ***Glycosuria.*** Frothy urine, burning as it passes down the urethra. Frequent urination by day. Waking from urging to urinate, morbid desire. Sudden urging, can't hold urine for long.

Limbs - Cramp in the calves and toes in bed. Aching with shivering in the arms, legs, ameliorated by stretching out, aggravated by the cold and by standing. Chronic joint problems. Chronic rheumatism of the hip. Heaviness and prominent veins in the legs. Varicose veins. Varicose hemorrhage. Itching of leg followed by ecchymoses. Numbness of arms when raising them. Numbness of legs when crossing them.

Liver - Pain in liver on breathing, after eating, better eating, better pressure. Pulsating in liver. Bubbling in region of liver.

Lungs - Breathing difficult after meals.

Modalities - Better from climbing stairs. Better closing eyes. Better eating, but if hungry, there is no improvement. Worse by dust, smells. Worse heat. Worse coughing. Worse laughter. Worse physical or mental exertion. Worse noise. Worse left side. Worse between 4 p.m. and 5 p.m.

Mouth - Breath smells like apples. Salty taste on lips. Sweetish taste on lips. Corners of lips cracked. Dry, chapped lips. Lower jaw painful. Toothache, aggravated by sweet things. Tip of tongue painful. Small, superficial ulcers on the mouth and palate. Bitter, acrid taste, sweet taste on the lips. Mouth dry.

Nose - Acute catarrh of the nasal mucus membrane with streaming, sometimes from the right side, sometimes from the left. Aggravated by dust, smells and heat. Catarrh from dust. Sensation of heat in nose on inspiration. Smell in nose as of musty books.

Rectum - Diarrhea, worse between 6 a.m. and 9 a.m., leaving a burning excoriation in the anus. Feeling of insufficient evacuation. Stools clammy and sticky, blood-streaked. Fullness after stool.

Skin - Dry, cracking eczema. Ecchymosis. Rheumatoid purpura. Purpura without fever, beginning suddenly with large, benign ecchymoses. Hands dry, chapped. Spontaneous bruising of the fingers and legs. Skin dirty, with eruption of itching pimples.

Sleep - Troubled sleep with dreams, nightmares. Sleepwalking, somnambulism. Insomnia until 2 a.m. Sleep disturbed by dreams. Dreams of accidents. Dreams being chased by a horse. Dreams of resurrection. Dreams of death of a friend. Dreams of bandits, robbers. Dreams of rats, toads, frogs in the bed. Dreams of being followed or falling. Dreams killing with a knife. Dreams being imprisoned. Dreams of sermons.

Stomach - Nausea before meals and heavy, aching feeling after. Nausea when travelling.

Throat - Acute and chronic laryngitis and pharyngitis. Dry, painful on the left side with burning, grating pain. Swallowing painful, improved with a hot drink. Throat pain better drinking, better expectoration, worse singing, when talking.

RELATIONS - ***Compare:*** (1) Uranium nit. - Excessive thirst, morbid hunger, emaciation. Polyuria. (2) Ph-ac. - Apathy, indifference towards everything, weakness, headaches, diarrhea, abundant urine, seminal discharge, weakness of vertebral column. (3) Arg-n. - Apprehension. Sadness. Weakness of legs. Feeling of a splinter of wood sticking in the pharynx. Urinary incontinence by day and by night, desire for sweet things to eat.

REFERENCES - Julian.

ALNUS RUBRA

(Red Alder)

PHARMACY - aln. Alnus rubra. Red alder. Alnus serrulata. Alnus glutinosa. Black alder. Tag alder. Common alder of Europe. N. O. Cupuliferae. Betulaceae. Tincture of the bark. Tincture of the young shoots. ***Historical dose:*** Tincture and all potencies.

CLINICAL - Amenorrhea. Glands, enlarged. Gleet. hemorrhage. Herpes. Impetigo. Leucorrhea. Psoriasis. Rheumatism. Scrofula. Syphilis.

HERBAL - The bark-tincture of Aln. is used by herbalists as an "alterative" in scrofulous conditions in chronic skin affections, rheumatism, syphilis, gravel and gleet.

Aln. has some reputation as a remedy for skin affections, glandular enlargements and indigestion from imperfect secretion of gastric juice. It stimulates nutrition and thus acts favorably upon strumous disorders, enlarged glands, etc.

HOMEOPATHIC - Among its indications are leucorrhea with erosions which bleed easily, amenorrhea with burning pains from back to pubis and hematuria. Ulcerated mucus membranes of mouth and throat. Fingers covered by crust caused by pustules, disagreeable odor. Indigestion from imperfect secretion of gastric juice.

Female - Leucorrhea with erosions of cervix, bleeding easily. Amenorrhea with burning pains from back to pubis.

Skin - Chronic herpes. Enlarged submaxillary glands. Eczema, prurigo. Purpura hemorrhagica. Poison oak, used topically.

COMMENTS - The plant grows in swamps and marshes. Not to be confused with certain of the Rhamnacae, which are also popularly called Alders.

Cooper, who used a fresh plant tincture of Alnus glutinosa, noted the "Pain in rectum after stool," and "heaviness in head as after being drunk the night before."

Hale gave, as particularly indicating it, "Eruptions on the skin alternating with diseased conditions of mucus membrane."

REFERENCES - Boericke. Clarke. Cooper.

ALOE SOCOTRINA

(Common Aloes)

PHARMACY - aloe. Aloe socotrina. Common aloes. Aloe ferox. Aloe succotrina. N. O. Liliaceae. Aloaceae. Trituration or solution in spirit of the gum of the leaves. ***Historical dose:*** Trituration, tincture and all potencies.

CLINICAL - Abdomen, plethora. Alopecia. ***Anal, weakness.*** Backache. Bronchitis. Cholera. ***Colic. Colitis.*** Constipation. Coryza. Coughs. ***Diarrhea. Dysentery.*** Earache. Flatuence. Gleet. Gonorrhea. Headaches. ***Hemorrhoids***. Hysteria. ***Incontinence.*** Insomnia. Jaundice. ***Lumbago.*** Nausea. Nosebleed. Onanism. Pimples. ***Proctitis.*** Prostate, disorders. Sacrum, pain. Skin, disorders. Tenesmus. Tuberculosis. Uterus, prolapsed. Varicose veins. Vertigo. Vomiting.

HERBAL - Aloe socotrina is one of the oldest and most famous remedies. It is in worldwide use as a purgative and forms a leading ingredient in a large number of patent medicines for regulating the bowels and menstrual functions.

HOMEOPATHIC - Aloe has the anti-psoric property of throwing out internal complaints to the skin. It causes congestion of various parts, especially abdomen, pelvic organs and head. Especially suitable to lymphatic and hypochondriacal patients. Bad effects from sedentary life or habits. Dissatisfied and angry about himself, alternating with lumbago.

Aloe affects ***abdominal veins,*** causing ***congestion, relaxation in rectum,*** liver, colon and pelvis. The rectal symptoms are usually very strong. Prolapse rectum. Burning in rectum. Heat internally and externally. Pulsation in rectum after eating.

Portal congestion. ***Hemorrhoids like a bunch of grapes***, better cold bathing. Burning and stitching in anus and rectum from hemorrhoids, preventing sleep. Hot stool and flatus.

The child goes around the house, dropping little hard, round, marble-like stools. Diarrhea, after eating oysters in the hot season, or of beer drinkers. A lot of mucus is passed with pain in rectum, after lumpy, watery stools.

Rumbling, gurgling in bowels, sudden urging, ***sense of insecurity*** then hurriedly passes a gushing watery stool. Uncertain whether gas or stool will come. Diarrhea with pain in the rectum after stool. Lienteric stools. ***Anal weakness,*** oozes mucus. Stools escape with flatus or when urinating. Stools, mushy, lumpy, watery, gelatinous, bloody, solid stools passed involuntarily, urging to stools with passing flatus only.

Aloe has a diarrhea that is worse in the early morning (Sulph). Diarrhea worse immediately after eating, worse from walking (Aesc., Thuj.), or standing (Sulph.). Feeling of insecurity of bowels on passing gas or before stool (Phos.).

Periodic headaches which alternate with lumbago. Sensation of fullness in the parts. ***Heavy, dragging,*** as of a load. Drawing, downward sensation. Discharges, gelatinous, post nasal, stools, etc. General weakness and weariness. Heat external and internal.

Aloe has been used successfully in the treatment of tuberculosis by giving the pure juice. Carroll Dunham cured a heavy frontal incapacitating headache in an old man occurring in winter and alternating with a diarrhea which occurred in summer when he was free from headache. Dunham also cured incontinence of urine in an old man with enlarged prostate with the diarrhea.

MIND - Ill humor, especially in cloudy weather or with constipation. Taciturn after eating. Sense of insecurity. Discontented, better evening. ***Dissatisfied and angry about himself.*** Sadness in morning, better evening. Hates people, repels everyone. Thinks that she would die in a week.

Fright at slight noises. Restlessness and fear. Fear of men. Exhaustion alternating with activity. Disinclination to mental labor. Life is a burden. Aversion to labor. Lassitude alternating with great mental activity.

Children, with much emotions, chat and laugh.

Hysteria. Extremely excited during pain. Easily excited, angry, revengeful. Wants to destroy object of wrath, better tea or mild stimulants. Trembling from musical sounds and other noises. Imagines that persons are stepping hard or quickly. Time passes too slowly.

Abdomen - Heaviness in hypogastrium. Colic before and during stool. ***Abdominal pains better from passing burning, offensive flatus.*** Colitis. Dragging down in abdomen. ***Abdomen feels full, heavy, hot, bloated.*** Weak feeling, as if diarrhea would come on. Great accumulation of flatus, pressing downwards, causing distress in lower bowels. ***Sensation as if plug between symphysis pubis and coccyx*** with urging to stool. Twisting, griping pains, must sit bent forward. Soreness in sides. ***Rumbling, gurgling in bowels, sudden urging.*** Pain around navel, worse pressure. Pain from navel to rectum. ***Bloated abdomen, more on left side, or along colon and worse after eating.*** Pulsating pain around navel. Pelvis as if filled with hot water.

Back - Backache. Pain in lumbar region, worse moving. Sharp pain through sacrum, extending to loins. ***Lumbago alternating with a headache and hemorrhoids***. Pain in sacrum, worse while sitting, better moving about. Creeping sensation beginning in sacrum, until it was a creeping in bones over whole body. Heaviness and pressure in sacrum worse sitting, better moving about.

Causations - Sedentary habits, poor diet.

Chest - Congestion to the chest. Breathing impeded by stitches in the left side of the chest. Front of chest feels sore on deep inspiration. Weakness of chest.

Constitutions - Adapted to weary people, the aged and phlegmatic, old beer-drinkers. Suited to old people, to women of relaxed phlegmatic habit, to persons of lymphatic or hypochondriac temperament. Allen said it's adapted to weary people with very broken down constitutions and elderly people. Menopausal years.

Coughs - Cough in winter, with itching. Coughs when she would sit down. Cough when standing, or stand up. Cough after sitting, with lachrymation. Dry, irritative, hacking cough with metallic taste in mouth. Cough with scratching in throat. Cough with sharp pain right side of larynx.

Ears - Cracking when chewing when moving jaw. Sudden explosion and clashing in left ear. Tinkling as of some thin, shivered, metallic globe in head. Sticking in left ear, later in right. Earache during menses. Internal and external heat.

Eyes - Lachrymation. Congestion of eyes. Pressure in orbits. Compelled to make small during pain in forehead. ***Pain deep in orbits***. Flickering before eyes. ***Redness of eyes with yellow vision***. Closes eyes partially from pain in forehead. Pain as if in muscles, worse right side.

Face - Lips dry, cracked, swollen, pustular, sore at corners. Lips markedly red, bleeding. Pain while yawning or chewing. Heat of the face when excited, or during headache. Face pale during cloudy weather. Lips moist, white, scaly.

Female - Menses too early, last too long and too profuse. Menstrual flow increased, dark and clotted. Prolapse uterus. Bearing down in rectum, worse standing and during menses. Uterus feels heavy, cannot walk much on that account. Labor-like pains in loins, extend down legs. Menopausal hemorrhage. Heavy congested uterus with labor-like pains, felt in groins and hips worse standing and during menses. Leucorrhea of bloody mucus, preceded by colic. Dysentery after childbirth.

Food - No appetite. ***Hungry during diarrhea.*** Hungry after stools. Thirst with dryness of mouth, awakens at night. Aversion to meat. Desires juicy things, fruits. ***Desires apples. Desires salty food.*** Beer causes diarrhea. Beer relieves pains in anus. Diarrhea after eating oysters. Diarrhea from vinegar. Vinegar relieves colic. Sour food doesn't agree.

Head - Dull, pressive pain, worse heat. Headache alternates with lumbago. Headache alternates with intestinal and uterine disorders. ***Headaches are above forehead with heaviness in eyes, must partially close them.*** Headache better closing eyes. Headache after stool. Headache with heaviness of eyes and nausea. ***Headaches worse heat, better cold applications.*** Heavy pressure on vertex. Clinking in head as from some thin-slivered glass, extending to ears. Headaches with gastro-intestinal irritation and coldness of lower limbs. Congestion to head, compelling one to sit up. Congestion to head and face during stool. Sensitiveness of scalp in spots. Alopecia with chronic headaches. Dryness of hair.

Heart - Strong beat of heart occasionally. Pulse accelerated. Pulse weak, suppressed after vomiting. Pulse slow in afternoon.

Kidneys - Incontinence in aged, bearing-down sensation and enlarged prostate. Every time on passing urine, feeling as if thin stool would escape with it. Burning pain when urinating. Frequent urging, worse at night or in afternoon. Urging so quick he can scarcely retain urine. Scanty, hot and high colored urine. Urine with much mealy sediment or slimy. Urine copious, pale, after stool. Urine saffron-yellow, becoming cloudy.

Limbs - Lameness in all limbs. ***Drawing pains in joints***. Sensation of weakness in the joints of the hands and feet. Sensation as if joints, bruised or dislocated. Pricking, dull twitching in joints. Paralytic drawing in muscles. Soles are painful when walking on the pavement. Cold hands with warm feet. Heaviness of right arm. Weakness of wrist-joints. Weakness of ankle-joint. Varicose veins.

Liver - Fullness in region of liver, pain under right ribs. Tension in the region of the liver. Uneasiness, heat, pressure, and tension in the region of the liver. Pain in the liver, worse on standing, so that he bends forward. Sharp pains in the liver, when drawing a long breath. Chronic types of jaundice with bilious states, the tongue is coated, breath foul, and a sensation of fullness and heaviness in hepatic region.

Lungs - Difficult respiration with sharp pains from liver to chest. Whistling in throat, as if something had fallen into trachea. Yellow, tenacious mucus. Spits up blood.

Male - Offensive sweat on genitals. Epididymis sensitive, to touch or while walking. Penis shrunk and testicles cold. Scrotum relaxed. Prostate enlarged. Involuntary emissions during siesta. Itching of prepuce. Erections after urinating. Premature ejaculation. Sexual irritability after eating, after waking (in children). Increased sexual desire with erections.

Modalities - Better from cool open air. Better cold applications. Better passing flatus. Better closing eyes. Better taking tea or stimulants. Worse in early morning. Worse evenings. Worse summer. ***Worse heat***. Worse hot damp weather or hot dry weather. Worse after eating or drinking. Worse after dysentery. Worse yawning or chewing. Worse stepping hard. Worse evening. Worse standing or walking.

Mouth - Dry mouth, with increased thirst and greater redness of the lips. Lips dry, peeling off, cracked, bleeding. Metallic, bitter or sour taste. Bitter, nauseous taste. Taste like ink or iron. Yellow spots in mouth. Accumulation of saliva in mouth. Sickening smell from mouth. Increased salivation. Inflamed sore spots in mouth and inside of cheeks. Palate swollen. Concave edges of teeth seem sharp and hurt tongue.

Nose - Coldness of tip. Nosebleed in morning on awakening. Full of crusts. Nosebleed from nose after waking. Coryza with burning and pain in nose. Sneezing causes stitches in umbilical region. Redness of nose in open cold air. Dryness of nose in morning, in bed.

Perspiration - Cold sweat after stool. Sweat smells strong. Offensive sweat on genitals. Sweats at night. Sweats after drinking.

Rectum - ***Every morning, on rising, has a hasty desire for stool***. Must run from bed to toilet. Diarrhea, drives him out of bed. Diarrhea from cold, damp room. ***Diarrhea in hot, damp weather.*** Diarrhea when walking or standing. Diarrhea after chagrin. Hospital diarrhea. Colic and diarrhea. Cholera. ***Rumbling, gurgling in rectum, sudden urging.*** Sensation of weakness and loss of power of anal sphincter. ***Sense of insecurity in rectum***, when passing flatus. Uncertain whether gas or stool will come. ***Urging to stool as soon as he eats, or immediately after eating and drinking.*** Constant bearing down in rectum, bleeding, sore and hot, relieved by cold water. Hemorrhoids protrude like grapes. ***Hemorrhoids bleed often and profusely.*** Hemorrhoids very sore and tender, better cold-water application. Hemorrhoids with soreness and constant bearing down in rectum. Burning and sharp pains in anus and rectum, from hemorrhoids, preventing sleep. ***Burning in anus and rectum.*** Burning, copious flatus. Constipation with heavy pressure in lower part of abdomen. ***Pulsation in rectum*** and sexual irritation. Dysentery, after childbirth. Fistula in anus.

Skin - Itching, especially of legs. Spots which, when scratched, pain and become sensitive. ***Itch appears each year, as winter approaches.*** Golden colored skin. Furuncles with disordered liver. Ointments aggravates burning (Sulph.). Pimples on abdomen. Spots which, when scratched, become sensitive.

Sleep - Drowsy, dozing in morning. Spasmodic jerks when falling asleep. Sleeplessness from itching and burning in anus. Insomnia, cannot get to sleep for a long time, thoughts crowd upon him and keep him awake. Awakened by thirst. Awakened by urgency to urinate. Dreams of soiling himself. Oppressive dreams. Dreams of danger, could not cry out.

Stomach - Bitter, acrid or sour eructations. Tasteless belchings with oppressions in stomach. After eating, flatulence and nausea with a headache. Pain in pit when making false step. Sensations as if vomiting were coming on, from rising of flatulence toward throat. Fullness in stomach, followed by distension. Nausea with headache. Nausea with empty feeling in stomach. Nausea with pain at umbilicus. Vomiting of blood.

Stools - Feces and urine escape together, can't pass one without the other. Child goes around house, dropping little hard round marble-like stools. Stool passes without effort, almost unnoticed. Lumpy, watery stool. ***Jelly-like stools*** with soreness in rectum after stool. ***A lot of mucus with pain in rectum after stool***. Stool escapes with flatus or when urinating. Stools mushy, lumpy, watery, gelatinous. Stools bloody. Stools small, brownish, slimy, half fluid. Stools bright yellow.

Temperature - Chill with coryza, in the cold open air. Chill at stool. Shivering. Cold hands, warm feet. Internal heat. Heat in spots, on scalp or face. Heat flushes with anxiety and restlessness.

Throat - Thick lumps of tough mucus. Varicose condition of veins in pharynx. Dry, scrapy feeling. Hawking of thick lumps of jelly-like mucus. Raw and swollen feeling in throat. Fauces raw, hot, as if burned. Scraping in larynx. Voice husky, hawking.

Tongue - Dry tongue. Yellow ulcers on the tongue. Severe fine stitches in under part of tongue when moving it. Tongue coated yellowish-white. Tongue stiff, dry, red. Inflamed sore spots on tongue.

Vertigo - Vertigo with sense of insecurity. ***Vertigo on moving.*** Vertigo as if everything whirled with her, worse going up stairs or turning quickly. Vertigo with anxiety when moving.

Vision - Flickering vision with heat of face. Flickering vision during headache. Yellow vision. Sees yellow rings moving before eyes, with redness of eyes. Dim vision while writing.

COMMENTS - This is Aloe socotrina, not Aloe vera. Keynote incontinent stool, and an early morning sudden urge to diarrhea or stool. Colitis, irritable bowel, and dysentery.

Uneasiness and pains in the liver region. Fullness, heaviness, heat and inflammation. The whole abdomen is painfully sensitive to touch. Rumbling. Feeling as of a plug wedged in between pelvis and coccyx. Abdominal colic. Burning gas, heaviness in the rectum. Strong relationship to Sulphur.

Sudden and continued desire to go to stool. Tenesmus, weak rectum with forceful stool. Desire for stool after each meal (Ars., Chin., Lyc., Podo., Trom., and Ferr. when it's while still eating).

Rumbling and cramping in abdomen before and during stool. The hard stool falls out without being noticed, urging to stool while passing water, every time on passing water feeling as if stool would pass. A hard stool may be passed involuntarily. "Stool passes unnoticed."

Nash noted the case of a child, constipated from birth, who screamed all the time he as being held to stool, could not pass it even after an enema. Yet when not trying, he passed solid pieces in bed without knowing. Cured with Aloe 200c.

Involuntary soft stool while passing wind. With the diarrhea, flatulency, pinching in abdomen, pain in back and rectum and chilliness. Flatus offensive, burning, copious, much flatus with small stool. Burning in anus with passing of flatus.

Lack of confidence of the sphincter ani (Cimic.). Stools like mush, bright yellow, gray, hot, undigested. Mucus and blood in feces. Profuse with jelly-like lumps. Watery stools, worse standing or walking. Watery stool containing lumps "like frog spawn."

Bilious, yellow fecal, bright yellow diarrhea, great rumblings in bowels and escape of much wind. Worse morning and evening in damp weather, from overheating after cold taken in damp room, after chagrin.

Diarrhea driving one out of bed very early in morning (Sulph). Diarrhea with sense of insecurity (Phos.). Faintness after stool with cold sweat. Griping may (Nux-v.), or may not (Merc.), cease after stool. Heaviness, heat, pressing, burning in rectum. Itching, burning, pulsating as from fissures at anus.

After stool there is a cutting, feeling as if more would come, protruding hemorrhoids. Hemorrhoids that protrude like a bunch of grapes, constant bearing-down in rectum, bleeding, sore, tender, hot, better by cold water.

Periodic headache which alternates with lumbago. Darting pains in left temple worse every step. A peculiar dull, heavy, pressing pain in forehead. Worse all exertion, especially mental. Pressure in vertex and forehead as from a weight. Heaviness in the eyes (All-s.). Compelled to make the eyes small during pain in forehead.

In females, pain in hypogastrium as if menses coming on. Labor-like pains drawing into legs. Menses too early and too profuse. During menstruation there is a headache, better by application of cold water, earache, pain in small of back, and pressing down in rectum. Fullness in pelvis. Leucorrhea of bloody mucus preceded by colic. Pain in small of back, worse sitting or awaking at night, better moving about. Lumbago alternating with headache.

RELATIONS - Aloe is related to All-c., All-s., Agave., Scilla, Colch. ***Antidoted by:*** Sulph., Mustard, Camph. relieves for a while, Lyc., and Nux-v. relieve the earache. ***Compare:*** (1) Sulph. similiar in many symptoms, and is of equal importance with Sulph. in chronic diseases with abdominal plethora. (2) Kali-bi., Lyc., All-s. (3) Ail. - dull, frontal headache. (4) Gamb. - diarrhea. (5) Am-m. - abdominal and diarrheic symptoms. (6) Nux-v. - gastric abdominal and uterine troubles: bad effects of sedentary habits. (7) Aesc. - hemorrhoids. (8) Merc., - dysentery. (9) Podo. - alterations between head symptoms and abdominal symptoms. ***Complementary:*** Sulphur.

REFERENCES - Boericke. Clarke. Murphy. Phatak.

ALOE VERA

(Aloe Barbadenis)

PHARMACY - aloe-v. Aloe vera. Aloe barbadenis. Aloe vulgaris. ***Historical dose:*** Tincture and all potencies. Use the Aloe vera gel externally or internally.

CLINICAL - Acne. ***Burns.*** Colitis. Diabetes. Diarrhea. Poison oak. Radiation, burns. Scars. ***Skin, disorders.*** Stomach, ulcers. Sunburn. Tuberculosis. ***Ulcers.*** Wounds.

HERBAL - Topical applications of the gel from the Aloe vera leaf have been used since ancient times for ***burns and skin problems.*** The gel can also be taken internally for diabetes, stomach ulcers, colitis or as a general tonic. Aloe has been used successfully in the treatment of tuberculosis by giving the pure juice.

RELATIONS - ***Compare:*** Calen.

REFERENCES - Murphy.

ALSTONIA CONSTRICTA

(Bitter Bark)

PHARMACY - alst-c. Alstonia constricta. Bitter bark. Native quinine bark. N. O. Apocynaceae. Australia. Tincture of the bark. ***Historical dose:*** Tincture and all potencies.

CLINICAL - Anemia. Breast-feeding, disorders. Breast-milk, excessive. ***Debility.*** Diarrhea. ***Dysentery.*** Fevers. ***Indigestion.*** Intermittent fever. Leucorrhea. Lienteria. Malaria. Nausea. Palpitations. Pregnancy, vomiting. Rheumatic pains. Ulcers. Uterus, debility. Weakness.

HERBAL - Alstonia constricta is an exceedingly bitter herb. It grows in India and the one from Malabar are probably similar in effects to Alstonia scholaris. It has been used as a ***tonic after exhausting fevers.*** Locally, it has been for ulcers and rheumatic pains.

HOMEOPATHIC - Alstonia was proved by Dr. Cathcart of Australia, who found it produce great debility and prostration or low fever often with diarrhea. Characteristic gone sensation in stomach and sinking in abdomen with debility. Malarial disease with diarrhea, dysentery, anemia, and feeble digestion.

Dr. Dietz gave the following as leading indications: debility from lack of digestive power in the stomach or general assimilative power. Tongue generally has a dirty white coat, especially at base, though it may be clean. Nausea, worse morning, before breakfast or at irregular times, when depending on reflex irritation from pelvic organs.

Food seems to remain in stomach a long time undigested. Diarrhea of undigested food immediately after eating, has to leave table before finishing a meal. This symptom was cured by Alst. c. 1x in a patient who had taken a great deal of iron.

Violent purging and cramps in bowels. Heat and irritation in lower bowels. Camp diarrhea, bloody stool. ***Dysentery***. Diarrhea from bad water and malaria. ***Painless watery stools*** (Phos-ac.). Diarrhea immediately after eating.

Leucorrhea and bearing-down worse by walking. Swollen feeling in right ovarian region. Sharp shooting pain from left side of stomach through to back (spleen).

RELATIONS - ***Compare:*** (1) Similar in action to Alstonia scholaris, the Dita bark of India aand Malabar. (2) Ars., Chin. - similar in diarrhea, chronic dyspepsia and debility. (3) Hydr., Ferr-cit., Chin.

REFERENCES - Boericke. Clarke.

ALSTONIA SCHOLARIS

(Dita Bark)

PHARMACY - alst-s. Alstonia scholaris. Dita bark. Satwan. N. O. Apocynaceae. India. Tincture of the bark. ***Historical dose:*** Tincture and all potencies.

CLINICAL - Anemia. Cramps. Debility. ***Diarrhea.*** Dysentery. ***Indigestion.*** Intermittent fever. Malaria. Ulcers.

HERBAL - Alstonia scholaris is an exceedingly bitter herb. It grows in India and the one from Malabar are probably similar in effects to Alstonia constricta. Ditain the active principle is anti-periodic like quinine, but without unpleasant effects. ***A tonic after exhausting fevers.*** Topically used for ulcers and rheumatic pains.

HOMEOPATHIC - Malarial diseases with diarrhea. Dysentery, anemia, feeble digestion, are the general conditions suggesting this remedy. Characteristics are the gone sensation in stomach and sinking in abdomen, with debility.

Diarrhea immediately after eating. ***Diarrhea from bad water.*** Cramps in bowels with violent purging. Irritation and heat in lower bowels. Camp diarrhea. Bloody stool. Dysentery. Diarrhea from malaria. ***Painless watery stools*** (Ph-ac.).

RELATIONS - ***Compare:*** (1) Similar in action to Alstonia constricta, the bitter bark of native quinine of Australia. (2) Ars., Chin. - similar in diarrhea, chronic dyspepsia and debility. (3) Hydr., Ferr-cit., Chin.

REFERENCES - Boericke. Clarke.

ALUMEN CRUDUM

(Potash Alum)

PHARMACY - alumn. Alumen crudum. Potash alum. Potassic-Aluminic Sulphate. Trituration of the crystallized double sulphate of Aluminium and Kalium. Trituration of the pure crystals. ***Historical dose:*** Trituration and all potencies.

CLINICAL - Alcohol, effects. Alopecia. Anus disorders. Asthma. Backaches. Breast, cancer. Bronchitis. Catarrh. ***Cancer.*** Chilblains. Colic. ***Constipation.*** Coughs. Diabetes. Diarrhea. Dysentery. Eczema. ***Emaciation.*** Epithelioma. Esophagus, stricture. Eye, disorders. Eyes, surgery. ***Fungus.*** Glands, indurated. Gleet. Gonorrhea. ***Hemorrhages.*** Hoarseness. ***Indurations.*** Itching, skin. Lead, colic. Leucorrhea. Locomotor ataxia. ***Nausea.*** Noma. Otorrhea. Palpitations. Paralysis. ***Paralytic, weakness***. Polyps. Scurvy. Skin, rough. Strabismus. Teeth, operations. Throat, disorders. Typhoid. ***Ulcers.*** Uterus, disorders. Uvula. Vaginismus. Vertigo. ***Vomiting. Weakness.***

HOMEOPATHIC - The well-known astringent action of Alum. gives a leading indication for its use in practice. On the other hand, it is equally available for the states of relaxation, which corresponds with its secondary action.

Stools as hard as stones. No desire for stool for days. Aggravated constipation and hemorrhage from bowels during the course of typhoid. ***Cancer of uterus and rectum*** with the most ***obstinate constipation***. Constrictions and contractions of sphincters and various parts.

Tendency to ***induration of glands*** and other tissues. Tongue, rectum, uterus etc., are hardened, ulcers with Indurated base. Indurations following inflammation. Lupus or cancer of nose. Scirrhus of the tongue.

Paralytic weakness of all the muscles of the body with typhoid. Relaxation of muscles.

Prolapsed uterus and rectum, excruciating pains. ***Sensation of dryness and constriction***. Mental paresis, dysphagia especially to liquids.

Sluggish action of muscles, hemorrhages of various kinds, large clots in typhoid, relaxed mucus membranes, relaxed uvula, hoarseness and bronchial affections, diarrhea. Sensitive to cold, exposure to air causes roughness and chaps in the skin. Yellow bland discharges.

Useful after operations on the eyes and teeth. ***Hemorrhages from leech bites, extracting teeth,*** etc. Parenchymatous bleeding from mouth, gums, nose, uterus. Hemorrhages of dark blood. Mucus membrane dry in nose, on tongue in mouth, larynx. ***Emaciation.*** Joints of arms, hands and feet feel bruised.

MIND - Nervous tremors from bad news. Doubting people. Lectophobia. Desires to remain in bed. Fear of falling. Spells of rage, attacks people.

Thinking about disease causes palpitations. ***Anxiety at night.*** Anxiety at night with nausea and headache. Sadness in morning. Weeping in morning.

Abdomen - Colic worse by walking, with fullness and heaviness. Potter's colic, lead colic. Abdomen retracted, better from pressure. Contractive sensation deep in pelvis with complaints of rectum and bladder.

Back - Sensation as if cold water were poured down back, with headache. Backache in evening on both sides of spine, with every deep inhalation. Weakness of spine in evening.

Bladder - Irritable bladder alternating with pain in vertex. Catarrh of bladder, mostly with the aged. Discharge of mucus from urethra. Itching of orifice of urethra.

Breasts - Sore, inflamed nipples. Induration of cervix and breasts (Carb-an., Con.). Breast cancer.

Causations - Bad news. Operations on eyes, on teeth.

Constitutions - Adapted to elderly people, especially bronchial catarrhs. Disease of bladder. Children with profuse bronchial catarrh.

Coughs - Cough in morning before breakfast, better after. ***Dry cough, in evening after lying down.*** Chronic morning cough of elderly people. Cough from tickling in larynx caused by talking.

Ears - Heat in both ears and left side of face at night. Purulent otorrhea. Hears every noise in sleep.

Eyes - ***Wild look with spells of rage.*** Bruised feeling on pressure or by moving eyelids. ***Spots on cornea.*** Prolapse of iris after cataract operation. Right eye squints towards the nose. Varicosities of conjunctiva. Purulent ophthalmia of infants. Itching burning on border of lower lids. Dilated pupils. Diplopia by candlelight. Sees double by candlelight.

Female - Induration of cervix. Left ovary affected. Menses scanty, watery. Hands weak, drops things during menses. Chronic gonorrhea, yellow with little lumps along urethra. Weight and prolapse of uterus. ***Affections of left ovary with troublesome constipation.*** Chronic yellow vaginal discharge. Leucorrhea and emaciation with yellow complexion. Vagina very sensitive, and narrowed by swellings of various size. Vaginismus. Itching. Aphthous patches in vagina (Caul.). ***Bleeding after childbirth.***

Food - Appetite increased, even with fullness in stomach. Loathes food. ***Emaciation.*** Thirst, throat dry and increased appetite with heat in stomach, better by drinking cold water, intense with fever. Mouth dry, but no increase of thirst.

Head - Alopecia. Rush of blood to head. Headache, better drinking cold water. ***Burning pain and weight on vertex,*** better ice-cold cloths pressed on the part. Headache shooting through temples with nausea, better drinking cold water. Jerking pain in left forehead, evening. Pains coming and going, from place to place. Headache in morning on awaking.

Heart - Palpitations worse from thinking of her disease. ***Palpitations from lying down on right side***. Palpitation from mental excitement. Pain from heart to lower part of right leg. ***Dilatation of heart.*** Strong pulsation through whole body.

Kidneys - Frequent and painful urging with painful passing of small quantities of urine. Must urinate every hour or two, night and day. Diabetes mellitus. Urine passed with difficulty. ***Oily iridescent film on urine.*** Urine falls down perpendicularly (Hep.). ***Urine scanty, clear flow, containing lumps of blood.*** Urine sediment slimy, tough or membraneous. Scanty, reddish urine in colic.

Limbs - Bruised pain in joints of arms, hands and feet. ***Weakness of all muscles***, especially arms and legs. Constricted feeling around limbs. Cold hands and feet during pain in stomach. Chilblains.

Lungs - Asthma. Croup and bronchitis. Catarrh of chest. Hemoptysis. Great weakness of chest. Difficult to expel mucus. Copious ropy, expectoration in morning in elderly persons. Ropy sputa. Atonic hemoptysis.

Male - Eczema on the back of penis and scrotum. Erections while at dinner. Frequent emissions. Gonorrhea, gleet. Shooting pain from middle line of belly, as along a thread, down into penis. Cutting pain in left side of penis.

Modalities - Worse from cold, except headache, which is relieved by cold. Worse during sleep. Worse lying on right side. Worse bad news.

Mouth - Mouth dry, without thirst. Dryness of mouth, tongue and throat. ***Taste bitter, sourish, astringent.*** Taste sweetish. Disgusting after-taste. Spreading ulcers in mouth. Noma. Profuse salivation, mercurial in origin or not.

Nose - ***Nasal polyps***, left side with rough skin all over the face and body. Lupus or cancer on nose. Dryness of nostrils and choanae. Nosebleed.

Rectum - ***Constipation of the most aggravated kind,*** as in cancer of uterus and rectum. No desire to stool for days. Violent ineffectual urging to stool. No ability to expel stool. ***Marble-like masses pass, but rectum still feels full.*** Itching after stool. Itching in anus. Long lasting pain and smarting in rectum after stool, also hemorrhoids. Yellow like an infant's. Hemorrhage from bowels. Hematemesis of hard drinkers. Passes large clots.

Sensations - Sensation of dryness. Sensation of constriction, as if a cord or band around limbs in paralytic states.

Skin - Skin roughens and chaps after exposure to cold air. Skin dry. Eczema. Proud flesh, chilblains, indolent ulcers. ***Ulcers with indurated base***. Indolent ulcers. Scorbutic ulcers. Indurations resulting from chronic inflammations. Glands inflame and harden. Furuncles on body, on thighs. ***Fungus granulations.*** Alopecia. Epithelioma. Veins become varicose and bleed.

Sleep - Many complaints come on during sleep, like nightmares. Light sleep, hears every little noise. Can't get to sleep on account of orgasm of blood. Sleeplessness from fever. Disturbed by nightmare, at 4 a.m.

Stomach - Burning heat, better by drinking cold water. Sinking sensation, better by eating. The pain is better by pressing on stomach. Nausea with faintness and weakness. ***Attacks of nausea in morning before breakfast.*** Vomits large quantities of glairy mucus or tough, colorless slime. ***Vomiting of everything he eats.*** Vomits blood. Habitual vomiting in alcoholics.

Teeth - Teeth loose. Teeth and gums scorbutic. Gums swollen, inflamed, spongy. ***Profuse bleeding after extraction of tooth***.

Temperature - Chill during nausea. Coldness followed by headache. Coldness of skin followed by heat and tingling. Coldness during pain in stomach, followed by heat with rush of blood to head, can hardly hold it up. Furious delirium. Fever with intense thirst, nausea, etc. Internal heat throughout body. Heat in forehead. Warmth creeps over abdomen.

Throat - Tendency to throat colds. ***Burning and severe pains.*** Hoarseness worse from talking. Aphonia. ***Enlarged and indurated tonsils*** from frequent colds. Every cold settles in throat. Mucus membrane red and swollen. Throat relaxed. Throat sore and dry when swallowing fluids. ***Uvula inflamed and enlarged.*** Uvula elongated, relaxed. Scraping in throat with cough.

Tickling in throat. Burning pain down the esophagus. Constriction, spasms of esophagus, liquids can scarcely be swallowed.

Tongue - Dryness of tongue. Tongue dry, black. Tongue burning in evening. Tongue sour feeling, stitches worse at tip. Tongue clean, except a slight coating of slime on back part. Scirrhus of tongue.

Vertigo - Vertigo with weakness in the pit of stomach, better opening eyes, turning on right side. Vertigo when lying on his back.

COMMENTS - The Alumn. patient is very sensitive to cold, exposure to air roughens and chaps the skin. Slight scratches bleed. Bleeding after tooth extraction. Catarrhal conditions prevail throughout.

Sensations of dryness and contraction. Contractive sensation in abdomen and pelvis and retraction of abdomen as in lead colic. Paralytic states with the sensation as if bound with a tight band.

Tendency to indurations whenever inflammations occur. Scirrhus indurations, indurated glands. Pains are insupportable. Attacks come and go suddenly, periodically.

Many complaints come on during sleep, like nightmares. Turning on right side improves the vertigo. Lying on right side brings on palpitations. There is sensitiveness to all sorts of weather changes and especially to cold.

W. P. Wesselheft cured bronchitis characterized by scraping from upper sternum to throat with free expectoration of thick, yellow mucus, paroxysmal cough, morning cough with gagging.

Aching in chest and in the lower part of the back in region of lower ribs. Profuse expectoration with a scraping pain, for scraping coughs are usually dry. All-c. had helped the preliminary sneezing and coryza.

RELATIONS - ***Antidoted by:*** Cham. - cramps in abdomen. Nux-v., Ip. - nausea and vomiting. Sulph. ***Antidote to:*** Lead poisoning, calomel and other mercurials, Aloe - vomiting blood. ***Compare:*** (1) Alumina, Alum, Aloe. - rectum. (2) Caps. - long uvula. (3) Ferr. - relaxed abdominal walls, prolapsed uterus. (4) Kali-bi. - stringy discharges. (5) Merc. - prolapsed uterus, vagina, rectum, tenesmus. (6) Merc-c., Mur-ac., Nit-ac., Nux-v., Op., Plat. - lead poisoning. (7) Plb., Rat., Stann., Sulph., Sul-ac., Zinc - eyes.

REFERENCES - Boericke. Clarke. Grimmer.

ALUMINUM ACETICUM

(Aluminum Acetate)

PHARMACY - alum-acet. Aluminum aceticum. Aluminum acetate. Solution. ***Historical dose:*** All potencies.

CLINICAL - Hemorrhage. Skin, infections. Uterus, weak. Wounds.

HOMEOPATHIC - Aluminum acetate arrests hemorrhage from inertia of uterus. Externally, it is used as a lotion for putrid wounds and skin infections.

REFERENCES - Boericke.

ALUMINUM OXYDATA

(Aluminum Oxide)

PHARMACY - alum. Aluminum oxydata. Aluminum oxide. Argilla. Pure clay. Oxide of Alum. Trituration. ***Historical dose:*** Trituration and all potencies.

CLINICAL - Aluminum, poisoning. Alzheimer's Disease. Anus disorders. Boils. ***Brain, weakness.*** Bubo. Catarrh. Chlorosis. ***Colds. Colic. Constipation***. Cough. Cracks. Debility. ***Dehydration.*** Dementia. Disappointment. ***Dryness.*** Dysentery. Dyspepsia. Eczema. ***Emaciated.*** Eyes, disorders. ***Fatigue.*** Fissures. Fistulas. Headaches. Hernia. Lead, poisoning. ***Leucorrhea.*** Locomotor ataxia. ***Memory, loss.*** Muscles, weak. Nails, disorders. Otorrhea. ***Ozaena.*** Paraesthesia. ***Paralysis.*** Pregnancy, disorders. Prostatorrhea. Ptosis. Scrofula. Senility. Strabismus. Taste, disordered. Tetters. Throat, disorders. Trismus. Typhus.

HOMEOPATHIC - Alumina causes ***dryness of skin and mucus membranes***, eyes, throat, rectum etc. Irritability and relaxation. It affects the ***cerebro-spinal axis*** causing disturbances in coordination and tendency to ***paretic muscular states***.

Alumina paralyzes the bowels in the same way as lead poisoning to which it is an antidote. ***Constipation with dry stool.*** Obstinate constipation. Lack of urge. Must strain in order to pass a stool. Small and soft stools are passed with great difficulty. Straining to pass even a soft stool, can only evacuate bowels when standing. Strains as if abdomen and rectum were paralyzed. Painful evacuations with spasms of the colon. Must strain at stool in order to urinate. Urine is slow in passing.

Painter's colic. Pregnant women and children with constipation. ***Constipation from artificial baby foods***. Elderly people with constipation, lack of vital heat or prematurely old with debility. Sluggish functions, heaviness, numbness and staggering. Functions become sluggish, actions are delayed, sensory impressions reach the consciousness slowly.

Alumina produces irritation of mucus membranes with dryness or extreme secretion and paralysis of involuntary muscles, like its relative Alumen. It affects the rectum, the nervous and muscular systems generally.

Degeneration of spinal cord. Paraesthesia. Paralysis of the internal rectus muscle of the eye, causing squint. Also ptosis. Drawing, pains appear in the limbs, a sensation of constriction in several organs. Locomotor ataxia. Boenninghausen cured a case of ataxia with Alum.

Craves dry rice and dry food. ***Worse from starch, especially potatoes,*** salt, wine, vinegar, and spirits. Patient is thin, inactive, wants to lie down, but it increases the fatigue. Exhaustion after talking, after menses. Disposition to colds in the head and belchings in spare, dry, thin subjects. Tendency to induration. Vertigo on closing eyes.

MIND - ***Senility and dementia.*** Absent-minded. ***Memory weak or loss.*** Forgets things, loses their way. Alzheimer's disease. The consciousness of reality and judgment is disturbed. Timid. Makes mistakes in speaking and writing. Inability to think coherently. Slowness in answering questions and vague replies. Cloudiness and drunken feeling alternating with pain in kidneys.

Alternating moods. Always groaning, moaning, worrying, fretting. Sneers at everything. ***Contrary.*** Grumbles. Obstinate. Peevish. ***Hasty, hurried***. A feeling of hurry follows, things do not move fast enough. Hasty, but slow of execution, hence makes mistakes in speaking and writing. Contemptuous laughing. Laughs and talks between paroxysms of spasms.

Depressive mental states. ***Low-spirited.*** Everything is viewed in sad light. Ill effects of disappointments. Ailments from anger. Sad, apprehensive, wants to get away. Mental symptoms mostly come on in the morning on waking. Depressed on awakening. Involuntary weeping.

Great stupor with fear of falling forward. Fears loss of reason (Med., Calc.). ***Anxiety of conscience, as if guilty of a crime.*** Impulses. Fears his own impulses. Desire to kill at the sight of a knife or a gun. Suicidal tendency or impulses when seeing a knife or blood.

Confusion as to personal identity. When he sees or states something, he has the feeling, ***as though another person had said*** or seen it, or as though he was placed in another person and could see only them. Things seem unreal. Time passes slowly. Illusions of being larger, numb, smooth, heavy. Sensation as if he would fall forwards, which he greatly fears.

Abdomen - Abdomen as if hanging down heavily, when walking, worse afternoon. ***Left-sided abdominal complaints.*** Colic whenever the body is exposed to a chill. Cutting pain better warmth. ***Lead colic.*** Colic in morning. ***Painter's colic*** (Plb.). Protrusion and incarceration of inguinal hernia. Pressing in both groins toward sexual organs. Sticking pain from below upward. Sharp pains in region of inguinal ring. Shooting pain in region of spleen. Big-bellied children. Flatulence. Reaching too high strains abdominal muscles.

Back - Backache as if bruised. Pain along spinal cord with paralytic weakness. Gnawing pain. ***Sensation as if hot irons were thrust through lower spine.*** Violent sharp pain in middle of back. Back feels bandaged by a cord.

Back - Shooting in right side of neck. Throbbing in lumbar region during stool. Sudden sharp pain, like a stab in lower part of back, with feeling as if she could not straighten spine. Swelling of glands of left side of neck. Itching in nape and of throat. Cervical muscles drew head back during sleep.

Breasts - Nipples itch, burn, look irritated and inflamed during pregnancy.

Causations - Anger, disappointments. Bodily exertion, lifting.

Chest - Congestion of blood to chest and head, with redness of face. Chest feels constricted, worse sitting bent or stooping. Violent oppressive pain, worse at night. Chilliness in chest. Soreness of chest on talking, on lifting. Chest as if too large.

Constitutions - Psoric persons. Infants, constipation, especially when artificial food is used. Big-bellied children. Suited to persons of sedentary habits who suffer from chronic ailments to constitutions with diminished animal heat. Spare habit, dry, thin subjects. Elderly people, hypochondriacal or suffering from chronic diseases, especially catarrhs. Puberty, chlorosis with longing for indigestible substances. Elderly people with lack of vital heat or premature old age with debility.

Coughs - ***Coughs soon after waking in morning.*** Coughs on talking or singing, in morning. Constant, dry, hacking cough, interrupts breathing. Cough on talking or singing. ***Morning cough***. Coughs with sneezing. Coughs from elongated uvula. Dry hacking cough from tickling in throat or irritability in larynx, worse morning, worse using voice. Coughs at times with dyspnea, vomiting or even involuntary escape of urine. ***Continued dry, hacking cough with vomiting and arrest of breathing.*** Dry cough at night, with dryness of throat. Coughs with much expectoration. Cough causes pain in right temple and vertex.

Ears - Sharp pain in ears, evening or night. Eustachian tube feels piugged (Kali-m.). Heat and redness of one ear. Purulent discharge. Humming, roaring. Crackling noises and buzzing in ears when, chewing or swallowing. Sound as of large bells. Sensation as if something lay before ear. Buzzing as if outside ear.

Eyes - Burning pain on waking with photophobia. Chronic conjunctivitis. Eyes are inflamed, burning, agglutination at night, lachrymation during day. Hot or acrid tears. Eyes feel cold. ***Granular lids or chronic blepharitis.*** Itching in canthi and lids. Photophobia in morning. Ptosis. Strabismus. Eyelids are weak, falling. Upper lids difficult to raise as if powerless. Eyelids thickened, dry, burning, smarting. Double squint, worse teething. Inclination to stare. Eyes better from being bathed. Eyelashes fall out.

Face - Gloomy, pale, or red alternating with pale. ***Old look, dusky, wrinkled.*** Coppery cheeks. Feels as if albuminous substance had dried on it. Sensation as if white of egg or a cobweb on face. Rush of blood to face after eating. Tearing and lancinating in malar bone. Twitching of lower jaw. Involuntary spasmodic twitchings of the lower jaw. Maxillary joints feel tight, while chewing or opening mouth. ***Lips dry, chapped.*** Blood-boils and pimples. Nodules or boils on face and nose. Rubs face all the time.

Female - Menses preceded by headache, colic. Menses too early, short. ***Menses scanty, pale, followed by great exhaustion*** (Carb-an., Cocc.). Girls, dried up and wrinkled, at puberty. It takes a woman all her time to recuperate from one menstrual period to the next. ***Leucorrhea acrid, profuse, transparent, ropy.*** Acrid, corrosive leucorrhea, with burning in genitals. Leucorrhea with burning, runs to feet. Leucorrhea, worse during daytime and after menses. Leucorrhea relieved by washing with cold water. Intolerable bearing down pain. Severe painful swelling in ovaries, very sensitive to touch. Painful throbbing in left side of vagina. Tickling and itching in genitals with strong sexual desire. Sexual desire decreased.

Food - Irregular appetite. No desire to eat. ***No appetite, food has no taste***. Thirst all day. Meat has no taste. ***Aversion to meat*** (Graph., Arn., Puls.). ***Aversion to beer.***

Aversion to potatoes. Abnormal cravings for coarse food, indigestible things. ***Desire for starchy foods.*** Cravings for chalk, charcoal, dry food, clean white rags, tea or coffee grounds. Desires fruits, vegetables, dry rice. Desires cloves, acids. Desire for coffee. ***Worse from potatoes.*** Potatoes causes bitter eructations. Onions causes soreness of throat. Hypoglycemia. Worse when hungry causes trembling and weakness. Worse tobacco smoke.

Head - Headache better by lying quiet in bed. ***Chronic catarrh of head.*** Sharp, burning pain in head with vertigo, worse in morning, but relieved by food. Throbbing headache with constipation. Pressure in forehead as from a tight hat. Vertex painful to touch. Inability to walk except with eyes open. Violent sharp pains in the brain with nausea. Increased pulsation of temporal arteries. Headache, as if one were dragged by the hair. Falling of hair. Scalp itches and is numb. Itching of scalp with dry, white scales. Dry hair.

Heart - Palpitations and shocks at heart. Wakes at 4 a.m. to 5 a.m. with anxiety at heart, better after rising. Palpitations irregular, large and small beats alternate.

Kidneys - Muscles of bladder paretic, ***must strain at stool in order to urinate***. Pain in kidneys with mental confusion, worse dancing. Frequent desire to urinate in old people with slow flow. Difficult starting. Fears he will wet the bed. Retention with dribbling. Smarting while urinating. Feeling of weakness in bladder and genitals.

Limbs - Pain in arms and fingers, as if hot iron penetrated. Arms feel heavy, as if paralyzed, short, go to sleep. Legs feel asleep, ***Especially when sitting with legs crossed.*** Locomotor ataxia. ***Staggers on walking.*** Legs feel numb, especially when sitting cross-legged. ***Heels feel numb*** when stepping. Soles tender, on stepping, feel soft and swollen. Pain in shoulder and upper arm. Gnawing beneath fingernails. ***Brittle nails***. Gnawing under nails. Spinal degeneration and paralysis of lower limbs. Festination. Inability to walk except when eyes are open or in daytime. Totters if eyes were closed. Soles are painful on stepping on them, as if they were too soft and on walking. Cramps when crossing legs. Bones feel squeezed.

Liver - Soreness over liver, on stooping. Tearing pain from liver to hip. Painful sensibility of the liver on stooping, followed sometimes by shooting pains.

Lungs - Arrested breathing by copious, thick, tenacious, saltish mucus. Rattling, asthmatic breathing, worse coughing. Wheezing, with tough mucus in larynx. Sneezing interrupts breathing, worse after waking in the morning. Dyspnea, with spasmodic pains in stomach and hypochondria. Dyspnea when lying on back, better when turning on side. Getting tired from exerting voice aggravates. Hoarse, aphonia, tickling in larynx, wheezing, rattling respiration. Sudden loss of voice on taking cold.

Male - Prostatic discharge. Voluptuous itching or tickling in genitals. Pains in the perineum during sex and while erection continues. Left testicle hard and very painful. Light yellow pus from urethra, causes itching of glans penis. Priapism at night. Sensation of weakness in penis. Increased sexual desire, followed by loss of power. Involuntary emissions when straining at stool.

Modalities - Better evenings. Better open air. Better moderate exertion and temperature. Better damp weather. Better cold. Better washing. Better as day advances. Worse periodically. Worse on alternate days. Worse dry weather. Worse full and new moon. Worse in afternoon. ***Worse from warmth of room or bed.*** Worse from artificial food. Worse potatoes, starch, salt. Worse tobacco smoke. Worse from speaking. Worse when waking. Worse sitting. Worse after menses, sex. Worse lifting, exertion.

Mouth - Dry and sore. Musty bad odor from mouth. Gums sore, bleeding. Tensive pain in articulation of jaw when opening mouth or chewing. Mouth feels dry with increased saliva. Tingling, itching on tongue.

Nose - Disposition to head colds. Nasal catarrh with scanty secretion and obstructed nostrils. Discharge of thick yellow mucus. Pain at root of nose. Sense of smell diminished. Fluent coryza with frequent sneezing. Redness of nose. ***Point of nose cracked, red***. Nostrils sore, worse touch. Nosebleed with pressure in forehead and congestion to eyes. ***Scabs with thick yellow mucus***. Tettery redness. ***Ozaena atrophica sicca***. Membranes distended and boggy. Septum of nose swollen, red, and painful to touch.

Perspiration - ***Inability to perspire.*** Sweats at night, toward morning most profuse in face. Sweats frequently only on right side of face.

Rectum - Inactive rectum and bladder. ***Severe, obstinate constipation.*** Constipation of infants (Coll., Psor., Paraf.) and elderly people. Constipation in women of very sedentary habit. Rectum sore, dry inflamed, bleeding. Itching and burning at anus. Pulsating pain in anus. ***Even a soft stool is passed with difficulty. Great straining.*** Pains from rectum to ankle. Can only pass stool when standing. ***Evacuation preceded by painful urging long before stool and then straining at stool.*** Pressure and sense of excoriation in rectum after a small, hard stool. Hemorrhoids worse evening, better after night's rest. Diarrhea on urinating. Diarrhea, worse on alternate days. Corroding diarrhea during menses. Stools of small balls, hard knots. Stools with bright clots of blood. ***Hard, dry, knotty stools with no desire***. Stool like sheep dung. Stools covered with mucus.

Sensations - Sensation of constriction. Pulsations are felt in various parts and pains go upwards.

Skin - ***Dry, tettery, itching eruptions, worse winter.*** Eczema. Dry, rough, cracked skin. Chapped and dry tettery. Itching, burning, over seat of pain. ***Intolerable itching when getting warm in bed***. Must scratch, until it bleeds. Intolerable itching with constipation. Brittle nails. Brittle skin on fingers. Veins distended. Itching and formication with flatulence, dry stools or diarrhea. Ulcerated surface secretes yellow-brown, badly smelling pus. Slightest injuries of the skin smart and become inflamed. Skin symptoms, worse winter, full and new moon.

Sleep - Sleepy in morning. Frequent waking. Sleeplessness forepart of night. Restless sleep, turns frequently, feels too warm, lies uncovered in unrefreshing slumber. Anxious, restless with confused dreams. Dreams about thieves, ghosts. Dreams of boats foundering. Nightmares. Many dreams before menses, on awaking face hot, headache and palpitation.

Stomach - Belchings, sour and acrid. Heartburn, stomach feels constricted. Chronic eructations for years, worse evening. Heartburn with profuse salivation. Distension of stomach. ***Potatoes disagree***. No desire to eat. ***Can swallow but small morsels at a time***. Feels food, whole length of esophagus. Constriction of esophagus. Pain lasting 3 hours after meals. Nausea, with faintness. Frequent nausea and inclination to vomit. Pain, as from excoriation, in the pit of the stomach. Vomiting with hacking cough. Vomiting of food, mucus or bile.

Teeth - The teeth covered with sordes. Teeth feel long, pain extends to other parts down larynx, neck, shoulders.

Temperature - Chill with great thirst. Chilliness, better open air. Shivering, even when near a fire. Chill at night, in bed, not able to warm oneself. Chill all over during stool. During the day chill, fever during the night. Heat with itching. Fever towards the evening with chilliness. Fever at night with anxiety and sweat.

Throat - Irritable and relaxed throat. Looks parched and glazed. Clergyman's sore throat in thin subjects. ***Dry and sore throat***. Food cannot pass, esophagus contracted. Feels as if splinter or plug were in throat. Thick, tenacious mucus drops from posterior sinuses. ***Great dryness which induces frequent clearing of throat in evening.*** Dry, feels full of sticks or constricted, food cannot pass. Constant inclination to clear the throat. Tightness from pharynx down to stomach as if food could not pass, can swallow but small morsels. Swallowing painful, worse solids. Better from empty swallowing, warm drinks. Elongated uvula from condiments or eating irritating things, talking or singing. Throat sore from eating onions. Uvula hangs down.

Vertigo - Vertigo in elderly people with atheromata or earthy deposits on the cerebral or cardiac arteries. Vertigo with nausea, better after breakfast. Worse talking, on closing or opening eyes, before breakfast. Vertigo with white stars before the eyes. Eyes suddenly went out of focus, one has to wait for normal vision, better wiping eyes.

Vision - Objects look yellow. White stars before eyes, with vertigo. Dim vision obliged to wipe eyes constantly, with sensation as if lids would adhere in corners. Fiery spots. Farsighted. Dim vision as if through mist or as if feathers before eyes. Glittering vision after blowing nose.

COMMENTS - Alum. and Plb. (Lead) antidote each other in homeopathy. They're very similar in their pathologies, but Plb. is more severe and painful. The action of Alum. is slow in developing and the remedy must not be changed quickly. Teste grouped Alum. with Sep. and Cop. He considered it the chronic of Sep. as Sil. is of Puls.

A remedy for the elderly and feeble, especially in senile dementia. Pathological memory loss, confusion over their own identity, slowness of mind. A lot of fears, confusion. Great general fatigue, even after a short walk, but chiefly after speaking. Frequent stretching while sitting. The buttocks go to sleep while sitting. Drags the legs, especially the left one.

Sensations are slow in being transmitted to the centers. Keynote delayed nervous reaction. Spinal diseases, local motor ataxias. Slow onset of nerve degeneration, paralysis of the lower limbs with emaciation, wrinkled face and dry skin. Incoordination of the limbs, loss of control of limbs. Tottering gait.

Several painful symptoms appear after the midday meal and continue until evening, when they disappear or are replaced by others which begin only then.

On the other hand, the pains which appear in the morning or in the evening are abated after eating.

Trembling, convulsive movements of the limbs and head, spasms with tears and laughter alternately. There is exaltation of the whole nervous system. Trembling of the whole body with a desire to lie down.

Catarrh with dryness of mucus membranes, The throat looks parched and glazed. The nose is stopped, feels dry and the point of it is cracked. Alum. has the fish-bone sensation in the throat on swallowing. There is profuse leucorrhea running down to the heels, sometimes excoriating.

Itching eruptions, worse from warmth of bed. Eruptions of all indurations, ulcers. Granular eyelids. Hairs fall out all over body. The skin of the face feels as if covered with dried white of egg or as if a cobweb was on it. Fissures.

Severe dryness of the skin and face where the face is wrinkled, symptoms in children where the children's skin wrinkles, ages and dries out. Alum. in physical doses is a drying agent. The first symptom is that the hair dries and flakes, the skin dries. It affects the fluid balances in the body.

Burning pains in the back are common, especially a sensation as if a hot iron were forced through the lower vertebrae. There are pulsations in various parts. The pains go upward. Upper left, lower right affected (opposite of Lyc.). The symptoms are worse on alternate days, periodically. Keynote as if a hot poker is stuck in the spine.

Another keynote is potatoes and starch disagree, especially affects constipation. Constipation of nursing children from being fed artificial food and bottle-fed babies. Aggravated by hot, dry weather, and the moon phases. Worse heat of the bed, worse after menses. Dryness without eruptions. Desires indigestibles like chalk, sand, dirt (Calc., Tarant.).

RELATIONS - ***Antidote to:*** Lead. ***Antidoted by:*** Bry., Nat-m., Cham., Ip., Camph. ***Compare:*** (1) Bry. Plb. (2) Aluminum chloridum. Pains of loco-motor ataxia. Lower trits in water. (3) Slag Silico, Sulphocalcite of Alumina 3x - anal itching, hemorrhoids, constipation, flatulent distention. (4) Sec., Lath., Aluminum acetate solution. (5) Alumen, Arg-n. (clergyman's sore throat, paralysis), (6) Bar-c. - hypochondriasis of elderly, constipation, Bry., Calc., (7) Con. (old people, squint), (8) Ferr. - chlorosis, relaxed abdomen, disgust for meat, etc. (9) Ferr-i. - profuse transparent leucorrhea. (10) Graph. - chlorosis, skin rough, chapped, itching, nails, blepharitis, etc. (11) Lach. - sad on waking, menopause. (12) Ruta - loss of power of internal recti. (13) Sepia - irritable, tearful, ozaena, scanty menses, puberty, prolapsus uteri, inactive rectum, weakness in urinary organs, etc. (14) Sil., Sulph., Zinc. - inner canthus, granular lids, worse from wine. ***Complementary:*** Bry. Plb. ***Follows well:*** Bry., Lach., Sulph.

REFERENCES - Boericke. Clarke. Murphy.

ALUMINUM PHOSPHORICA

(Aluminum Phosphate)

PHARMACY - alum-p. Aluminum phosphorica. Aluminum phosphate. Solution. ***Historical dose:*** All potencies.

CLINICAL - Asthma. Boils. Bronchitis. ***Constipation.*** Diabetes. Diarrhea. Hair, loss. Headaches. Hemorrhages. Hyperventilation. Ingrowing, toenails. Leucorrhea. Lung, disorders. Mental, prostration. Migraines. Osteoporosis. ***Paralysis.*** Petechia. Rickets. Shocks. Somnambulism. Strokes. Tuberculosis. Vertigo. Vomiting.

HOMEOPATHIC - Burning pains. Feeling of numbness and cobwebs. Constriction. Discharges watery, scanty, acrid. Dryness. Hemorrhages of bright red blood. Cerebral hemorrhage. ***Paralysis, ascending.*** One-sided paralysis from hemiplegia. Shocks.

Weakness and nervousness. Diabetes. Strong desire for the open air which relieves. Sensitive to cold which aggravates. Sensitive to thunderstorms. Bruised, burning, pressing pains, worse morning and night. Electric shocks, worse after sleep. Boils on nates and thighs. Ingrowing toenails. Standing is extremely tiresome. Extreme thirst, except during fever.

MIND - Mental prostration. Confusion of mind. Apathetic. Extreme weariness. Irritable. Suited to mental breakdown after overwork or overstudy. Mental exertion aggravates. Chronic effects of grief. Nervous and anxious. Worse from thinking of their symptoms.

Easily frightened. Fear of being alone. Fear of dark. ***Fear of thunderstorms.*** Fear of twilight. Fear of future, disease. Fear of death of family and friends. Fear of knives, blood. Fear of insanity. Fear of own impulses. Fears comes and goes suddenly.

Ailments from mental work. Anxiety and perspiration. Nervous, restless. Hurried. Discontented. Timid, yielding. Complaining, moaning and groaning. Slow to act and answer. Apathetic and depressed. Mental confusion. Lamenting over imaginary misfortune. Suicidal.

Alternating moods. Excitement alternates with dullness. Abundant ideas, clearness of mind, alternates with deficiency of ideas. Indifference alternates with excitement. Ailments from sexual excesses. Weeping in morning on waking (Alum.). Frequent crying.

Bladder - Ineffectual, fruitless, urging at night. Frequent urination at night.

Chest - Pain after herpes zoster. Palpitations of heart after menses.

Ears - Ears hot and red. Sensation of flapping in ears.

Face - Face sickly, bluish red. Sensation of white of egg dried on it.

Female - Excoriating leucorrhea. Menses too early, short. Menses profuse. Menses pale blood. Tiredness after menses.

Food - Extreme thirst. Aversion to warm food. Aversion to meat, fish, oysters. Aversion to beer, salt. Aversion to cold drinks, cold food. Aversion to milk, potatoes, tobacco. Desires dry food, rice, starch. Desires coffee, spices. Desires fish, salt. Desires fruit, sour foods. Better warm drinks. Worse from potatoes, milk. Worse from artificial food. Worse warm food, warm drinks. Worse cold drinks, cold food. Worse from tobacco. Worse alcohol.

Head - Pain in sides of head. Migraines. Loss of hair. Headache after sleep. Headache, worse warm room. Pain in occiput. Pain in sides. One sided headaches. Pressing pain, worse pressure. Pressing pain in occiput at night (Sulph.). Pressing pain in temples at night.

Limbs - Bone problems. Growing pains. Rickets. Osteoporosis. Tingling fingertips. Weakness of thighs. Weakness of knees.

Lungs - Lung disorders. Hyperventilation. Bronchitis. Asthma. Tuberculosis.

Modalities - Better from open air. Better pressure. Better lying on left side. Better damp weather. Worse from cold. Worse motion. Worse from jar, walking, stepping. Worse from lying. Worse standing. Worse from sexual excess. Worse from mental exertion. Worse from thinking of symptoms. Worse dry weather. Worse 9 a.m. and 9 p.m. Worse winter.

Mouth - Mouth dry. Breath offensive, even putrid.

Nose - Nasal discharge, green. Pain, worse pressure. Lost of smell.

Perspiration - Perspiration little or none.

Rectum - Diarrhea. ***Constipation***, dry, hard stools, no urging or great urging. Stool has to be removed by artificial means. Green stools. Hard, tough and greasy stools (Caust.). Knotty stool.

Skin - Itching eruptions worse warm room (Sep.). Dry, peeling skin. Rough skin with cracks. ***Itching,*** scratching until it bleeds. Petechia. Loss of hair.

Sleep - Sleeping on right side, amel. Short sleep. Somnambulism. Worse on waking. Dreams of death. Dreams of falling. Dreams of robbers.

Stomach - Vomiting worse drinking.

Vertigo - Vertigo in morning, on closing eyes. Vertigo, falling, worse closing eyes. Vertigo tendency to fall forwards.

RELATIONS - ***Compare:*** (1) Alum., Sil., Alum-sil.

REFERENCES - Boericke.

ALUMINUM SILICATA

(Aluminum Silicate)

PHARMACY - alum-sil. Aluminum silicata. Alumina silicate. Kaolin. Chinese clay. Porcelain clay. Bolus alba. Andalusite rock. Alumina 63, Silica 37 parts. Kaolin is disintegrated Fel spar. Trituration. ***Historical dose:*** Trituration and all potencies.

CLINICAL - Brain, disorders. Chest, soreness. Convulsions. Croup. Diphtheria. Lead poisoning. Nose, soreness. Spinal disorders.

HOMEOPATHIC - According to J. Landesmann, Alum-sil. is a remedy for croup and bronchitis. Aegidi was the first to use Alum-sil. in cases of croup. In old-school practice it was used *"as a completely inert powder"* in the same way as fuller's earth and also as a basis for making pills.

Alum-sil. is a deep acting remedy for chronic complaints of brain, spinal cord and nerves. Weakness, especially spinal. Aching and burning in spine. Formication, numbness, pain in all limbs.

Constriction, of orifices. Aching and burning in spine. Formication, numbness and pain in all limbs. Epileptiform convulsions. Coldness during pains. Venous distention.

Croup in the lower portion of the larynx or upper part of the trachea, which may be recognized by the much more laboring and sawing respiration.

Chest - Excessive soreness along trachea and chest. ***Soreness***, cannot stand percussion. Catarrh of chest, pain, raw feeling. Feeling of great weakness in chest. Stitching pains.

Head - Congestion of brain. Constriction of scalp. Pain in head, better heat, perspires. Pain in forehead. Pain in eyes, flickering. Frequent coryza. Swelling and ulceration of nose.

Limbs - Heaviness, jerking, numbness, aching and pains.

Lungs - Spasmodic cough with purulent viscid expectoration. Gray sputa. Capillary bronchitis. Larynx and chest sore. Membranous croup, extends down trachea. Husky voice, metallic, rasping breathing and suffocative cough.

Lungs - Croup dipping down into trachea, heavy, labored, sawing respiration.

Modalities - Better warmth. Better fasting. Better resting in bed. Worse cold air. Worse after eating. Worse standing. Worse towards evening. Worse in the night.

Nose - Itching and burning. ***Yellow discharge. Sore, scabby***, stopped up. Nostrils feel sore, scabs form in nose, scanty and blood-streaked secretion.

Skin - Dryness of skin. Formication along course of nerves, veins feel full and distended. Sore to touch and pressure.

Throat - Membranous covering of left side of throat of right side.

COMMENTS - Landesmann confirmed its efficacy and related a case as an example. After Acon., Hep., Spong., Bor., Phos. and Iod. had failed to relieve, Alum-sil. 6c, four or five globules every half-hour, rapidly removed the laboring, sawing respiration and the child was out of danger.

According to Farrington, a leading indication is internal soreness along trachea and the upper part of the chest, the child will not be touched. The use appears to be from the clinical side entirely. Alum-sil. 30c relieved symptoms of lead poisoning in a case of Clarke's.

RELATIONS - ***Compare:*** (1) Alum., Sil., Kali-bi., Spong., Iod., Hep., Acon. (2) Fuller's Earth.

REFERENCES - Boericke. Clarke.

AMBER

(Fossil Resin)

PHARMACY - succ. Amber. Fossil resin. Succinum purum. Amber oil. (A mineralized fossil resin not to be confused with Ambergris, Ambra). Trituration. Solution of the non-rectified oil prepared by dry distillation of Amber. Solution of Succinic acid. ***Historical dose:*** All potencies. Drop doses of the oil.

CLINICAL - Asthma. Fears. Globus. Hay fever. Hiccough. Hysteria. Leucocythemia splenica. Spleen disorders.

HOMEOPATHIC - The fossil resin known as Amber has been used in folk medicine by many cultures.

Dr. Morris Weiner tested Amber, which he prepared himself from Amber, by dry distillation. The fumes of the crude acid, he said, are inflammable and produce asthma, cough, sneezing, weeping, dropping of watery mucus from nostrils, pain in chest and headache.

On this indication he treated thirty persons suffering from hay fever, and cured them all, saving them the necessity of making an annual exodus. He gave one or two grains of the 3x trituration of Amber diluted in twelve teaspoonfuls of water, a teaspoonful every two hours.

Burnett wrote in Diseases of Spleen, that the Amber non-rectified oil is used as an organ remedy in spleen affections, especially when accompanied by nervous and hysterical phenomena. Burnett noted it for hysterical convulsions in women.

The crude oil is a thick, brown liquid having a strong empyreumatic odor. It is a powerful local irritant and has been used with success as such in lumbago, rheumatism and sciatica.

Amber produces many nervous and hysterical symptoms. Asthma. Fear of trains and closed places. Affections of spleen. Symptoms of collapse, the patient aborted, but recovered.

Heaviness externally. Lassitude. Lie down, desire to. Pulse slow. Trembling externally. Twitching. Weakness, daytime afternoon. Weakness after walking.

MIND - Absorbed mentally. Dullness of mind. Stupefaction. Concentration difficult. Forgetful. Feels constantly as if he had forgotten, something. Memory, weakness. Mistakes in time, confounds the present with past. Disoriented. Abstraction of mind.

Confusion of mind. Confusion as to sexual identity. Confusion, knows not where he is. Confusion of past and present. Confusion, as if in a dream. Speech slow. Expressing oneself difficult.

Mood, alternating. Anger. Offended easily. Averse to being disturbed. Aversion to company, yet fear of being alone. Irritability from conversation. Irritability from noise. Dictatorial. Contemptuous. Hatred of men. Wants to fight. Censorious. Attempts to escape. Suspicious. Fastidious. Sadness after midnight, amel. Desires to attack others.

Loathing, of life. Grief. Unfortunate, feels. Sadness from disappointed love. Lovesick. Sentimental. Homesickness. Forsaken feeling. Helplessness. Estranged feelings. Sensation of being isolated. Despair of life. Weary of life. Suicidal thoughts.

Pities herself. Weeping easily. Weeping from menopause. Weeping during menses, during regrets. Weeping from sickness. Weeping when telling of her. Answers in monosyllable. Aversion to answering. Indisposed to talk others.

Anxiety in daytime, morning. Panic attacks with feelings of electricity. Starting startled. Frightened easily. Fear of conscience. Fear of color black. Fear of everything. Fear of dark. Fear of death. Fear from flying in airplane. Fear in insanity. Fear of narrow places. Fear of trains and closed places. Fear of shadows.

Want of self-confidence. Excitement, excitable. Restlessness. Conviction of death. Desires death, Sensation as if dying. Aversion to the color black. Charmed by orange purple. Contented with himself.

Impressionable. Senses acute. Sensitive to all mental impressions. Sensitive to external impressions. Sensitive to music. Sensitive to noise. Sensitive to reprimands and criticism. Sensitive to reproaches. Sensitive to rudeness.

Desire to frighten others. Gossiping. Haughty. Desire to hide. Reproaches himself. Hysteria. Impatience. Indifference. Sensation as if she could easily injure herself. Intolerance. Introspection. Jesting. Desire for sunlight.

Full of cares. Cautious. Remorse. Childish behavior. Coquettish. Aversion to men. Aversion to conversation. Thinking of complaints aggravates. Aversion to certain persons. Aversion to being touched. Aversion to washing.

Serious. Ardent. Religious affections. Thoughts intrude of the past. Tormented thoughts. Time, appears slower. Clairvoyance. Affectionate. Amorous disposition. Veneration for the sun. Singing. Shuns the foolishness of men.

Delusions, she is beautiful. Delusions, things look beautiful. Delusions, has lost affection of friends. Delusions, impression of division, between himself and others. Delusions, put him into a fury, rage. Delusions sees black objects. Delusions, everything seems unreal.

Delusions, surrounded by enemies. Delusions, as if just waking from a dream. Wrong, everything seems. Coma, unconsciousness. Delusions, she would fall if she did not hold onto something. Delusions, has neglected his duty.

Abdomen - Flatulence. Gurgling. Rumbling. Cramping pain, must bend double. Cramping pain before menses. Hypochondria, dragging, bearing down pain. Eruptions, itching. Trembling.

Back - Itching. Backache, motion amel., stretching amel. Backache, turning head agg. Aching pain in cervical region. Lumbar region sore and bruised. Stiffness. Neck pain, sides. Neck stiffness. Back weakness after walking.

Bladder - Frequent urination at night. Urine burning.

Chest - Pains in chest. Constriction in chest. Pain in sternum during cough. Sore bruised pain in ribs, left side.

Cough - Dry cough. Hard cough. Tight cough. Cough, worse, from smoke, tobacco.

Dreams - Nightmares. Frightful dreams. Dreams of monsters. Amorous dreams. Animal dreams. Awake while dreaming. Dreams of old friends. Dreams of being late. Dreams of being pursued. Dreams of being lost. Dreams of death and decay.

Ears - Sensation of fullness. Heat, flushes. Itching. Pain, behind the ear, touch aggravates. Inside sore. Stopped up. Hearing. Acute.

Eyes - Unable to keep the eyes fixed steadily. Granular. Heaviness sensation. Itching from cats, with lachrymation. Lachrymation, daytime. Lachrymation in cold air. Lachrymation when laughing. Opening the eyelids difficult. Burning pain when looking at the fire. Pressing pain left eye. Stinging pain. Sharp pain, left eye. Photophobia. Pupils, contracted. Desire to rub eyes. Styes. Swollen, lids. Twitching, around eyebrows left. Weak eyes.

Face - Discoloration, red. Expression, old looking. Itching. Numbness. Pain, jaw left pulsating, jaw left. Tension, jaw left. Twitching eyes, below. Twitching corners of mouth. Wrinkled skin.

Female - Menses copious. Menopause, during lying amel. Frequent late menses. Menses painful protracted. Metrorrhagia during menopause. Aphthae, vagina. Heat, flushes during menopause. Sexual desire, increased. Weakness during menses.

Food - Appetite, diminished easy satiety. Appetite, wanting with headache. Desires fruits. Desires sweets.

Head - Headaches. Congestion of head. Constriction, forehead vertex. Formication, vertex. Heat in occiput, temples. Heaviness sensation of forehead. Numbness. Headache, better after eating. Headaches from fasting. Headache above the eyes. Headaches from cold air. Pulsating in temples. Headaches, worse light. Headaches better lying, pressure. Itching.

Limbs - Awkwardness, lower limbs. Coldness. Electrical current sensation. Formication of legs. Heaviness sensation. Itching of shoulder hand, back of legs, feet. Jerking. Numbness. Pain, Wandering, shifting pains in left shoulder, while walking. Aching pain. Cramping pain in shoulder. Sore bruised pains. Stiffness of joints, shoulders, arms, hands. Tension in shoulders. Trembling of limbs. Twitching. Weakness, limbs.

Lungs - Asthma. Asthmatic from contact with cats. Congestion of lungs. Deep desire to breathe. Difficult breathing in daytime, morning. Difficult breathing, lying amel. Difficult breathing, after walking. Chronic bronchitis. Incipient tuberculosis. Whooping cough.

Male - Formication of genitalia. Masturbation, disposition. Aching pain in testes. Sexual desire, increased in morning.

Modalities - Better open air. Desire for open air. Aversion to bathing. Worse air, draft. Worse food, alcohol. Worse fats. Worse spices. Worse sweets. Worse cloudy weather. Mental symptoms, worse before or during menses.

Mouth - Bleeding, gums when cleaning them. Dryness in mouth. Neuralgic pain in gums. Salivation. Taste, acrid.

Nose - Coryza. Nasal congestion. Discharge, copious watery. Dryness. Itching, inside. Own body odor agreeable. Nasal obstruction. Pressing, rawness pain. Sinusitis. Tingling, tip of nose. Sneezing, dropping of watery mucus from nostrils.

Rectum - Diarrhea, daytime. Diarrhea after eating. Painless diarrhea. Brown stools, like chocolate. Light colored stools. Mushy stools. Orange stools. Thin stools. Watery stools.

Skin - Formication. Itching. Sensitive.

Sleep - Disturbed. Sleepiness daytime lying, inclination to lying down. Sleeplessness, midnight, after. Waking night, midnight after, 4 a.m. Anxiety, as from early frequent.

Stomach - Cramping pain, eating amel. Dull pain. Persistent hiccough. Belching. Fullness after eating, ever so little hunger, during. Heartburn after sugar. Indigestion. Fasting, amel. Lying down, amel. Nausea on waking. Nausea on eating. Nausea, daytime, morning. Nausea after eating. Nausea after amel. Violent vomiting.

Teeth - Pain left side. Filled tooth, in a. Upper teeth, right molar. Left molar. Wisdom teeth. Neuralgic pain, left side. Pulsating. Sore.

Temperature - Chilly. Lack of vital heat. Coldness of neck.

Throat - Choking sensation. Burning pain, rawness sore, left side. Globus.

Vertigo - Vertigo in morning on rising. Vertigo on closing, eyes. Vertigo, tendency to fall. Vertigo, as if intoxicated. Vertigo, lying down, necessary. Vertigo, with nausea. Vertigo, on rising from seat.

Vertigo from stooping. Vertigo as if rocking. Vertigo with swaying. Vertigo turning in bed. Vertigo on washing hair.

Vision - Dim vision, alternating with bright. Blurred vision. Bright vision. Flickering vision, around outside range of vision. Foggy vision. Weak vision.

COMMENTS - Amber enters into the composition of "Roche's Embrocation," and "Haarlem Oil," and has a popular reputation as a remedy for whooping cough when rubbed into the spine night and morning. A tablespoonful dose, said Murrell, caused persistent vomiting, diarrhea and symptoms of collapse and the patient aborted.

These observations are of value in relation to Burnett's experience. He added half a scruple of Amber oil to six ounces of Acorn-water. They do not mix chemically, but by shaking each time a dose is taken the required division and potency is attained.

Burnett's keynote is "painful spleen disorders where there are convulsive attacks such as the hysterical and hypochondriacal often have."

Burnett related in his book a most remarkable case of "chronic enlargement of the spleen with hyperesthesia, head pain, Dyspnea orthopnea, convulsions" in a young lady "towards the end of her teens."

After years of treatment, Burnett concluded from Rademacher's account of Amber oil. that it might provide the remedy. Amber oil was given in five-drop doses three times a day. In forty-eight hours the convulsive attacks ceased for good and all the phenomena slowly leucocythemia.

A keynote of Burnett's is "Fear of trains and close places." His dose is five drops of Amber oil three times a day.

RELATIONS - ***Compare:*** (1) Succinic acid. - Hay fever. Paroxysmal sneezing, dropping of watery mucus from nostrils, asthma. Inflammation through respiratory tract, causing asthma, chest pains, etc., itching of eyelids and canthi and nose worse drafts. (2) Ars-i., Arundo, Wye., Sabad, Sinapis.

REFERENCES - Boericke. Clarke. Murphy. Phatak.

AMBRA GRISEA

(Ambergis)

PHARMACY - ambr. Ambra grisea. Ambergris. Morbid secretion of the whale. Trituration and tincture. Most probably a morbid product found in the Sperm Whale or floating in the sea. Not to be confounded with Amber Succinum. ***Historical dose:*** Trituration, Tincture and all potencies.

CLINICAL - Anus, irritation. ***Asthma.*** Bashfulness. Brain, softening. Cardiac asthma. Convulsions. Coughs. Deafness. ***Emaciation.*** Face, pimples. Forgetful. ***Hearing, impaired. Hypertension***. Hysteria. Jaundice. Melancholy. Menstrual, irregularity. Music, intolerance. Nervousness. Nosebleed. Nymphomania. Pruritus vulvae. Puerperal convulsions. Ranula. Reaction defective. Spleen, pain. Tympanites. ***Vertigo***. Weakness.

HOMEOPATHIC - Ambr. produces faintness (Mosch.), nervousness, jerks and twitches. Reflex action is increased. In old age, helpful for asthma and colds.

Ambr. affects the nerves, causing nervousness, twitches and jerks. A great remedy for the elderly people with impairment of all functions. Weakness, coldness and numbness, usually of single parts, fingers, arms, etc. Also for patients ***weakened by age or overwork***, who are anemic and sleepless. ***Emaciation.*** Weakness of upper parts of the body with trembling of lower part.

There is defective reaction in nervous patients. Sensation of icy coldness in abdomen. ***Extreme nervous hypertension***. Patients are worn out, yet over-impressionable. ***Music aggravates symptoms***. External numbness of whole body in the morning and weakness.

Symptoms suddenly change places. One-sided complaints call for it. Numbness and torpor of the whole body especially in the morning. Coldness of the body with twitching. Tearing in muscles and joints often on one side.

Adapted to hysterical subjects or those suffering from spinal irritation with convulsive cough, belching, etc. Coughs are worse when many people are present.

Slight or unusual things aggravates the breathing and the heart, start the menses etc.

MIND - The patient has an embarrassed feelings. ***Bashful state*** is very characteristic. Intensely shy, blushes easily. Cannot do anything in presence of others. Embarrassed in company, ***cannot have others present during urination and stool*** (Nat-m.).

The memory is impaired, slow comprehension. Forgetful. Awkward. Dread of people and desire to be alone. Dwells upon unpleasant things. Melancholy, sits for days weeping. Dreamy. Time passes slowly. Thinking difficult in the morning with old people. Cannot understand what one reads.

Music causes weeping and trembling. Sad. Despair, loathing of life. Fantastic illusions. Bashful, blushes easily. Loss of love of life. Restless, excited, very loquacious. Hearing others talk or talking himself affects him. Aversion to laughter. As if in a dream.

Flitting, flighty talker, modern society girls. Jumping from one subject to another, never waiting to have first question answered. Fixed disagreeable fancies. Imagines diabolic faces, sights.

Abdomen - Flatulence. Incarcerated flatus. Tension and inflation of the abdomen, principally after eating and drinking. Sensation of coldness in the abdomen. Sweat on abdomen and thighs. Pressive pain in the epigastrium. Heaviness in the belly. Cutting pains with diarrhea. Pain in the spleen, as if something were torn off. Flatulent colic in the night.

Back - Pressive, drawing pain in the neck and back. Heaviness in the back, with pain in the belly, as if the intestines were compressed. Shooting pain in the loins. Stiffness in the loins after sitting long.

Causations - Shock due to business failure or due to the deaths, one after another, in the family. Effects of domestic shock, business worry. Loss of near relatives. Imaginations.

Chest - Oppression feit in the chest and between the scapulae. Sensation of rawness in the chest. Itching in the chest and in the thyroid gland. Rheumatic pain, as from a bruise in the chest.

Constitutions - Suited to excitable, nervous children. Young, modern society girls. Nervous persons. Lean persons. Elderly people with a nervous and bilious temperament. ***"Dried-up"*** nervous persons. ***"Thin, scrawny women."*** Hysterical subjects who are weakened by age and overwork to the elderly with impairment of all functions.

Ears - Hardness of hearing with cold sensation in abdomen. Deaf in one, roaring and whistling in the other.

Eyes - Stitching in the eyelids as if a stye were being formed. Eyelids, heavy, cannot open them though awake. Spots float before the eyes after sewing.

Face - Twitching of the facial muscles. Cramps in lips, lips hot. Left cheek red. Flushes of the face, jaundiced color. Embarrassed look. Tetanus, lockjaw in newborn.

Female - The sexual desire is increased. Nymphomania. ***Itching of pudendum with soreness and swelling***. Menses too early and too profuse. Itching in labia. Profuse, bluish leucorrhea, worse at night. ***Discharge of blood between periods, at every little incident***, worse after hard stools, walking a little longer etc. Lying down aggravates uterine symptoms.

Food - Thirstlessness. Want of appetite.

Head - Pressure on front part of head with mental depression. ***Tearing pain in upper half of brain.*** Brain, feels loose, falls to side lain on. Softening of brain. Rush of blood to head, when listening to music. ***Hearing impaired***. Profuse bleeding from teeth. Hair falls out. Confusion in occiput, also sprained feeling in. Headache worse blowing nose.

Heart - ***Palpitation with pressure in chest as if from a lump lodged there or as if the chest were obstructed***. Conscious of the pulse. Palpations in open air with pale face. Anxiety in heart.

Kidneys - Cannot pass urine in presence of others. Pain in bladder and rectum at the same time. Burning in orifice of urethra and anus. ***Feeling in urethra as if a few two drops passed out***. Burning and itching in urethra while urinating. ***Urine turbid, even during emission***, forming a brown sediment. Urinates more than drinks. Urine sour during whooping cough. Burning, smarting, itching in vulva during urination.

Limbs - ***Cramps in hands*** and fingers, worse grasping anything. ***Arms, numbness***. Left leg becomes quite blue during menses. Twitching of limbs with coldness of body during sleep. Cramps in legs and calves. Limbs go to sleep easily. Finger nails brittle. Drops what one is carrying. Coldness of hand (left) with headache. Sore and raw between thighs.

Liver - Aching in small spot in the region of the liver, better pressure. Liver pains, pressive.

Lungs - Asthma of elderly people and of children. Asthma with eructation of gas. ***Asthma when attempting sex.*** Wheezing in the chest. ***Nervous spasmodic cough*** with hoarseness and eructation, on waking in morning. Worse in presence of people. ***Hollow, spasmodic and barking cough,*** coming from deep in chest, then eructation. Tickling in throat, larynx and trachea, chest oppressed, gets out of breath when coughing. Choking when hawking up phlegm. Bluish, white expectoration. Cough worse music, talking, reading aloud, lifting weight. Loss of breath from cough. Cough with emaciation.

Male - Voluptuous excitement of and itching in genitals. Voluptuous itching of scrotum. Parts externally numb, burn internally. Violent erections without voluptuous sensations. Impotence.

Modalities - Better slow motion. Better in open air. Better lying on painful parts. Better cold drinks. Worse music. ***Worse presence of others. Worse from any unusual thing.*** Worse embarrassment, agitation, worry. Worse thinking of problems. Worse in morning. Worse from over lifting. Worse warmth, warm room, warm milk.

Mouth - Profuse bleeding from the gums, offensive breath. Insipid or rancid taste. Sour mouth, worse after milk. Salivation with cough. Small growths under tongue. Ranula.

Nose - Nosebleed, while washing face in the morning, during menses. Stoppage mostly at night, must breathe through the mouth, with chronic coryza.

Rectum - Flatulence, cannot have others present during urination and stool, worse during pregnancy. Constipation during pregnancy and after delivery. Frequent ineffectual urging for stool. Large flow of blood with stools.

Sensations - Sensation of coldness, numbness in spots or of single parts, fingers, arms etc. with twitching. Itching with trembling and flushing. General pulsation.

Skin - Itching and soreness, especially around genitals. Numbness of skin.

Sleep - Retires tired, wakeful as soon as touches the pillow. ***Cannot sleep from worry, must get up***. Anxious dreams. Coldness of body and twitching of limbs during sleep.

Stomach - ***Distention of stomach and abdomen*** after midnight. Sensation of coldness in abdomen. After eating, cough and gasping, and a feeling as if food did not go down into the stomach. Belching with a violent, convulsive cough. Acid belching like heartburn. Heartburn from drinking milk.

Temperature - Frequent flushes of heat at short intervals. Sweat on slightest exertion especially on abdomen and thighs.

Throat - Sensation as if a plug in throat with difficulty swallowing. Sore, raw from exposure to air, worse motion of tongue.

Vertigo - Senile vertigo with weakness in head and stomach. ***Senile dizziness***.

COMMENTS - The pelvic organs are painfully influenced. There is voluptuous itching on the scrotum and some rawness below the thighs in the male. In the female, there is a discharge of blood between the periods at every little accident, as straining at stool or extra work. Severe itching on pudenda. During urination, itching, tickling, burning of vulva and urethra.

Nymphomania with discharge of bluish white mucus. After childbirth, obstinate constipation and tenesmus with bashfulness, cannot make the attempt to stool if any one is present, even the nurse.

There is a tickling, spasmodic cough. Cough excited by speaking. Night cough. Cough followed by copious belching. Itching in chest. The limbs go to sleep easily. Fingernails are brittle. Sweat on slightest exertion. Sleepless from worry, retires tired, wakeful as soon as touches pillows.

RELATIONS - ***Antidoted by:*** Camph., Coff., Nux-v., Puls., Staph. ***Antidote to:*** Staph. - especially the voluptuous itching of scrotum, Nux-v. ***Follows well:*** Moschus frequently follows advantageously. ***Compare:*** (1) Ol-suc. - hiccough. (2) Sumb., Cast., Asaf., Croc., Lil-t. (3) Moschus (faintness, hysteric asthma), (4) Castor., Asaf., Psor. and Valer. (defective reaction), (5) Coca (bashfulness), (6) Kali-br., Nux-v. (increased reflexes), (7) Nux-v. (thin, nervous persons), (8) Ars. - Asthma, Phos. - asthma, nervous excitability, "irritable weakness," slender build, (9) Bov. - flow of blood between the periods. (10) Lach. and Sep. - worse from over lifting. (11) Coff., Chin., Ign., Sulph., Puls., Staph., (12) Sec. - scrawny women. ***Related remedies:*** Bar-c, Ign. Do not confound with Amber succinum.

REFERENCES - Boericke. Clarke.

AMBROSIA ARTEMISIEFOLIA

(Ragweed)

PHARMACY - ambro. Ambrosia artemisiaefolia. Ragweed. Roman wormwood. Hog-weed. N. O. Composite. America. Tincture of fresh flower heads and young shoots. ***Historical dose:*** Trituration, Tincture and all potencies.

CLINICAL - ***Allergies.*** Colds. Coryza. ***Diarrhea.*** Dysentery. ***Hay fever.*** Itching. Lachrymation. Nasal, congestion. ***Nosebleed.*** Sinus, congestion. Whooping cough.

HOMEOPATHIC - Ambrosia is a remedy for lachrymation, ***hay fever*** and intolerable itching of the eyelids (Euphr.). Nosebleeds. Stuffed feeling in nose and head. Some forms of whooping cough. The respiratory tract in its entire length stopped up.

Hay fever with itching, watery eyes. Sneezing to the point of nosebleeds. Hay fever with a tickling cough, can go into asthma. Allergic asthma. ***Severe allergies to ragweed.*** Reactions to allergy shots or drops for ragweed allergy. Also as a preventative, given before ragweed season, if person has a strong history.

Good for children with nondescript stuffy noses and no symptoms or modalities (Acon.). ***Many forms of diarrhea***, especially during summer months, also dysentery. Loose stool (Ars.).

Eyes - Redness. Smart and burn. ***Hay fever with itching, watery eyes.*** Lachrymation. Intolerable itching of eyelids.

Lungs - Respiratory tract is congested. Irritation of trachea and bronchial tubes with asthmatic attacks (Aral., Eucal.). Wheezy cough. Whooping cough.

Nose - Nasal, congestion. ***Allergies.*** Coryza. Watery coryza, sneezing, watery discharge. ***Hay fever.*** Sinus, congestion. ***Nosebleed.*** Stuffed up feeling of nose and head.

Rectum - Loose stool (Ars.). Many forms of diarrhea. Summer diarrhea. Dysentery.

COMMENTS - The fresh leaves and flowers are pounded to a pulp and macerated with two parts by weight of alcohol. In the 1889 Homeopathic Recorder, Dr. C. F. Millspaugh, wrote "Of late years much attention has been called to the species of the genus Ambrosia (the Rag Weeds) as being, through the agency of their pollen, the cause of hay fever."

Dr. E. T. Marsh and another experimenter suffered severely from symptoms of coryza and hay fever while working with the pollen of this plant. Ambrosia should therefore be of service in similar disorders.

RELATIONS - ***Compare:*** (1) In hay fever: All-c., Euphr., Sabad. (2) Wye., Succ-ac., Ars-i., Arund.

REFERENCES - Boericke. Clarke. Murphy.

AMETHYST
(Gemstone)

PHARMACY - ameth. Amethyst. Gemstone. *Historical dose:* Tincture and all potencies.

CLINICAL - Amblyopia. Ataxia. Backaches. Headaches. Insomnia. Migraines. Tinnitus. Trembling.

HOMEOPATHIC - Affects the nervous and endocrine systems, useful in states of nervous tension where the five senses (especially hearing) are overtaxed. Helpful when the hormonal system is affected by excessive adrenalin, creating mood swings and nervous excitation followed by exhaustion.

Profoundly affects sleep patterns, can soothe troubled sleep or induce somnolence in the insomniac. Has been found effective in easing mental disorders where there is too much excitement of the senses.

Nervous tension with an inability to relax. For damaged nerves in the spinal column, especially where the neural pathways are interrupted causing difficulties in relaying sensations or when nerve pains become all consuming, causing the patient to be unable to function normally.

Internal trembling, especially felt in the legs. When exhaustion has set in and nerves no longer respond as efficiently as they should. In low potency, follows well after Mag. Carb. For those who feel the need of stimulants to revive them or to "steady their nerves," bringing them to the point of addictiveness. Addiction rooted in nervous tension and psychic fears. Fear of addiction.

Deeply syphilitic. Nervous diseases such as motor neuron disease, MS and ataxia. Likely to make an improvement on the quality of life in patients suffering these conditions. Arthritic conditions.

MIND - Anxiety and tension. Fear of not being able to achieve all that one sets out to do. Lack of confidence in ability to complete allotted tasks, especially true in those who feel called to a spiritual or caring profession. Sense of thwarted mission where the difficulties seem to be self generated and self perpetuated. Sense of having "done all this before and now I'm getting it wrong again!" Too tired to be able to finish tasks or fulfill role properly due to excessive tension (Oak.).

Negative outlook. Becomes withdrawn and intense when anxious or displeased. Apprehensive of his own position in a general state of difficulty where others are involved. Wonders what will become of him. Tries but finds it difficult not to betray his inner sense of preoccupation and unease. Deeply affected by sad news.

Inexplicable fearfulness, held in the solar plexus. Fears of being overburdened, of becoming too anxious and fixated on one thing to the exclusion of everything else, and of the past and what may come back to influence the present. Deep sense of longing, particularly in connection with places which make one feel spiritually "at home." In cases where one would expect to find despair but instead there is deep pathology.

Difficulty relaxing. Tense and miserable from lack of sleep, nervous tics or tremors from night watching. Indecisive, forgetful, cannot hold many ideas in the mind at the same time so becomes limited to routine functioning. Feels cut off from the real world, floats off into a state of dreaminess. Reluctant to face reality, especially after great tension.

Abdomen - Trembling in the abdomen.

Back - Backaches. Pains in cervical area which extend down the spine, worse emotional turmoil. Tension in the lumbar region with sciatic type pains in either leg. Feels the top half of the spine (or body) is unconnected with the bottom half. Persistent symptoms after manipulative treatment on the spine. Patient enjoys massage and goes for a lot of it but it never holds for long.

Bladder - Tendency to frequent urination. Has to get up at night to pass water, especially worse 3 a.m. to 4 a.m. Cannot drink late at night without having to rise. Must hurry to pass water once the urging is there. Needs to be advised to drink more water as this will ease the tension in the bladder and slow the frequency of urging.

Dreams - Dreams of being held down or held back, of struggling against the odds. Dreams of floating or drifting away but this can be into nothingness, of intoxication.

Ears - Hardness of hearing, but hears soft noise, and things that are not there. Tension in the inner ear. Tinnitus, worse intermittently, after emotional stress.

Eyes - Feels he cannot trust what he sees and needs to look again. Floaters. Amblyopia. Wants to rub the eyes to clear the vision. Sees things that are not there, out of corner of eye, causes anxiety.

Food - ***Desires alcohol and stimulants.*** Either over-interested in food or have no appetite, only eating out of necessity. Forgets to eat. Will drink rather than eat.

Head - Headaches and migraines. Pains felt in the occiput and frontal region, brain feels muzzy. Light-headed with a need to sit down in case they faint. Wants to hold a cool flannel to the forehead or rub the temples gently. Brain feels a bit loose, worse jarring of footsteps. Headaches and backaches.

Limbs - Arthritis. Stiffening of joints with difficulty and pain on moving them in the early morning. Stiffness temporarily better alcohol, sunshine and warmth.

Liver - Sluggish and over-loaded.

Lungs - Easily out of breath, especially rushing around. Chest feels tight and restricted, sense of tension between the front and back ribs as if there is an anterior/posterior compression. Cannot take a full breath, feels as if the top part of the lungs do not expand fully.

Modalities - Better spring and summer. Better sun and warmth. Worse alcohol, except the joints. Worse emotional upsets, contradiction. Worse lifting heavy weights, it aggravates the joints and nervous tension.

Rectum - Constipation with stasis in the lower bowel. Tendency to hemorrhoids, which bleed passively with dark blood.

Sleep - Difficulty getting to sleep either from worry or hormonal imbalances, especially during menopause. Lies in bed feeling tense and stiff. Wakes at 3 a.m. and cannot go back off to sleep. Must get up to urinate and have a drink, usually not water but tea or juice. Restless, tosses and turns. Wakes up unrefreshed. Wakes feeling tense and full of expectations of the worst.

Stomach - Tension in the stomach. Indigestion.

Throat - Sense of drawing or tension pulling downwards internally. Voice becomes higher pitched from tension or from overuse in stressful situations. Difficulty in expressing emotions with the throat center as it tends to close up (Lach.). Recurrent sore throats in tense situations, especially in those requiring cool judgment and quick decisiveness.

COMMENTS - Amethyst can be used as a blood purifier in alcoholics.

REFERENCES - Murphy.

AMMONIACUM GUMMI

(Gum Ammoniac)

PHARMACY - ammc. Ammoniacum gummi. Gum ammoniac. N. O. Umbelliferae. Gum-ammoniac is obtained from Dorema Ammoniacum. Trituration of the gum. ***Historical dose:*** Trituration and all potencies.

CLINICAL - Appendicitis. Asthenopia. Asthma. ***Bronchitis. Eyes, disorders.*** Dyspnea. Glands, disorders. Heart, disorders. Hemorrhages. Hydrocele. Panaritium.

HOMEOPATHIC - The heartbeats too strong, worse lying on left side. Great accumulations of mucus. There are many rheumatic pains in the limbs and loins. Marked sensitiveness to cold, worse in cold weather.

Stitches were prominent in the provings. Stitches in the cecum at 7 p.m., alternating with pains elsewhere. Appendicitis. Diminished secretions from the mucus membranes, then increased. A remedy for the ***elderly and feeble***, especially in chronic bronchitis.

Stars and fiery points before the sight. Sees smoke in circles. Dim sight from a blow on the head, from excessive reading. Sensation of burning and scratching in neck and esophagus. Hydrocele.

Hemorrhages that causes abundant serous discharges. Dropsical complaints.

Gout not developing in usual form of attacks, but disturbing general health. Scrofulous tumors or enlarged joints.

MIND - ***Ill humor***.

Constitutions - Suited to bronchial disorders in old people brought on by cold weather.

Eyes - Dim sight. Stars and fiery points float before eyes. Easily fatigued from reading.

Food - Want of appetite.

Head - Catarrhal headache due to closure of frontal sinuses.

Heart - Heartbeats stronger, extends to pit of stomach.

Lungs - Coarse rattling of chest in elderly people. ***Difficult breathing***. Chronic bronchial catarrh. Large accumulation of pus and feeble expectoration, worse from cold weather. Mucus tough and hard.

Throat - Throat dry, worse inhaling fresh air. Full feeling, burning and scraping sensation. Immediately after eating, sensation as if something stuck in esophagus, causing swallowing.

RELATIONS - ***Antidotes:*** Bry., Arn. ***Compare:*** (1) Senega., Ant-t., Bals-p.

REFERENCES - Boericke. Clarke.

AMMONIUM ACETICUM

(Ammonia Acetate)

PHARMACY - am-acet. Ammonium aceticum. Ammonia acetate. Spiritus Mindereri. Aqueous solution. ***Historical dose:*** All potencies.

CLINICAL - Diabetes. Fever. Sweat.

HOMEOPATHIC - This is a very old medicine in great use in old-school practice for *"fever mixtures."*

Ammonium aceticum has been experimented with by Wibmer, who experienced the following symptoms: "Scraping in throat. Increased warmth in abdomen in the skin, especially of face. Heaviness in the head." ***"Bathed in sweat"*** is a leading indication. It causes profuse flow of urine, said to contain sugar.

REFERENCES - Boericke. Clarke.

AMMONIUM BENZOICUM

(Ammonia Benzoate)

PHARMACY - am-be. Ammonium benzoicum. Ammonia benzoate. Solution in distilled water. ***Historical dose:*** Trituration and all potencies.

CLINICAL - ***Albuminuria.*** Dropsy. Gout. Indigestion. Ranula. Rheumatism.

HOMEOPATHIC - One of the remedies for albuminuria, especially in the gouty. The chief symptoms are that the head feels heavy, dull and stupid. Scanty, smoky urine. Right kidney sensitive to pressure. Gout with fluid in great toe joint or with deposits in the joints.

Back - Pain across sacrum with urgency to stool. Soreness in region of right kidney.

Face - Bloated, swollen eyelids. Swelling under tongue like granula.

Head - Heavy, stupid feeling.

Kidneys - Urine is smoky, scanty. ***Albuminuria.*** Albuminous urine and thick deposits. Urinary incontinence in the aged.

RELATIONS - ***Compare:*** (1) Ter., Benz-ac., Ammonia salts, Caust. (2) In albuminuria - Kalm., Helon, Merc-c., Berb., Canth.

REFERENCES - Boericke. Clarke.

AMMONIUM BROMATUM

(Ammonia Bromide)

PHARMACY - am-br. Ammonium bromatum. Ammonia bromide. Ammonium hydrobromicum. Solution in distilled water. ***Historical dose:*** Trituration and all potencies.

CLINICAL - Ciliary neuralgia. Coryza. Cough. Epilepsy. Kidney, pains. Larynx, catarrh. Nails, biting. ***Obesity.*** Ophthalmia, scrofulous. Ovaries, disorders. Pharyngitis. Pterygium. Whooping cough.

HOMEOPATHIC - This salt has been well proved by A. M. Cushing. Nervous constitutions. Markedly affects the eyes and ovaries. In the morning, the eyes are red and sore with mucus in corners (worse left eye). Dull pain in left ovary, with hard swelling. ***Obesity.***

Indicated in laryngeal and pharyngeal catarrh. Chronic laryngeal catarrh of speakers. Sudden strangling, suffocating, cough. Suffocating sensation before epilepsy. Irritable feeling in fingernails, better by biting it. Constrictive pain in head, chest, legs.

Eyes - Edges of lids red and swollen, also Meibomian glands. Eyeballs feel large. Pain around eyes into head.

Head - Cerebral congestion. Feeling of a band above ears. Sneezing, thick nasal discharge.

Lungs - Sudden, short cough, strangling. Tickling in trachea and bronchial tubes. Wakes at 3 a.m. with cough. Feels suffocated, continuous cough, when lying down at night, sharp pain in lungs. Whooping cough. Dry, spasmodic cough on lying down.

Modalities - Better from warmth and warm drinks. Worse in open air. Worse cold air. Many symptoms occur on waking. Worse 3 a.m.

Throat - Smarting in mouth. Tickling in throat with ***inclination to dry, spasmodic cough, especially at night***. Burning in fauces. White, sticky mucus. Chronic speakers' catarrh.

COMMENTS - The mucus of Am-br. is apt to be stringy. A sudden desire to cough, so sudden it causes strangling. Sudden, short cough when rising in morning from accumulation of mucus in throat. Cough at 3 a.m.

Indicated in epilepsy when the aura begins with a fainting or suffocating sensation at epigastrium, rising up both sides of sternum to throat.

There is an irritable feeling under fingernails, better only by biting them. Must walk about for fear of suffocation.

RELATIONS - ***Compare:*** (1) Hyos., Con., Arg-n., Kali-bi.

REFERENCES - Boericke. Clarke.

AMMONIUM CARBONICUM

(Ammonia Carbonate)

PHARMACY - am-c. Ammonium carbonicum. Ammonia carbonate. Sal volatile. Sesqui carbonate of Ammonia. Solution in distilled water. ***Historical dose:*** Trituration and all potencies.

CLINICAL - Anxiety. Asthma. Bedwetting. Bronchitis. Colic. Cough. Dislocations, pains. Emphysema. Erysipelas. ***Fainting.*** Goiter. Gums, sensitive. ***Heart, weakness. Hemorrhages.*** Hemorrhoids. Hysteria. Lungs, edema. Measles. Military eruptions. ***Nosebleeds***. Nose, disorders. ***Obesity.*** Parotiditis. ***Pneumonia***. Rickets. Scarlatina. Spotted fever. Sprains. Sternum, pain. Toothache. Uremia. Whitlow.

HOMEOPATHIC - Am-c. has a condition of poor oxygenation that underlies a large proportion of its symptoms. This remedy is found in rather stout patients who are always ***tired and weary, catches colds easily***. Those that suffer from cholera-like symptoms before menses. ***Obese patients with a weak heart***, wheezing, feel suffocated.

The venous under-oxygenated condition of the medicine again appears in the excessive sleepiness produced in the daytime. Sleepiness with many conditions. Mucus membranes of the respiratory organs are especially affected.

Tickling cough. Bloody expectoration accompanying the cough. Asthma. Cough from 2 a.m. to 5 a.m. Anguish at heart, palpitation and faintness. Pain as from fatigue (hip joint, legs, thighs). Pains as from dislocation or sprain (wrist, great toe). Pain as of contraction of tendons. Numbness and stiffness of arms and hands. The pains are ulcerative, shooting, digging.

Chilly with great sensitiveness to cold, open air. Worse in wet, stormy weather, from washing, from wet poultice, better by warmth. Right-sided, and a venous medicine. Worse at night, 3 a.m.

Hemorrhagic. Bleeding hemorrhoids, at every menstrual period bleeding from rectum. Nosebleed, especially in the morning, on washing, after a meal. Menses are premature and copious, the blood dark (colic and pains in loins or toothache accompanying). Scorbutic condition, the muscles are soft and flabby, teeth drop out, hemorrhages, hectic. There is the scorbutic condition of bleeding gums.

Old age problems. Uncleanliness in bodily habits. Erythema, then vesication. Finally gangrenous degeneration. Very sensitive to cold air. Great aversion to water, cannot bear to touch it. Too frequent and profuse menses.

Lymphatic and parotid gland swollen and indurated. Hard swelling of parotid and cervical glands. Pains are bruised and sore. There is internal raw burning. Malignancy. Prostration from trifles.

Lies down from debility or soreness of whole body. Malignant scarlatina with somnolence, swollen glands, dark red sore throat, faintly developed eruption. Uremia. ***Heaviness in all the organs***. Swelling of parts, glands, etc. Discharges are hot, acrid, adherent. Prostration from trifles.

MIND - The mental faculties are slow, weak memory, heedlessness, absence of mind. Sadness, disposition to weep. Timidity. Apprehensive. Ill humor. Heedless and unruly. Forgetful, gloomy during ***stormy weather***. Vacant mind. Loss of memory, worse vexation. Talking and hearing others talk affects them greatly.

Sad, weepy, unreasonable. Tendency to make mistakes in speaking, writing and calculating. Depressed with weakness of intellect. Aversion to work. Peevish, fretting, as if crime has been committed. ***Uncleanliness*** (Sulph.). Great aversion to water, cannot bear to touch it.

Timidity of character. Sadness, with disposition to weep. Apprehensions and anguish in the evening. Anxiety with weakness and nightmares. Disgust with life. Ill humor in the morning. Morose. Disobedient and unruly. Excessive gaiety. Heedlessness.

Great absence of mind and weakness of memory. Tendency to make mistake in speaking, in writing, or in calculating. Impairment of the intellectual faculties. In the night there are dreams of specters of death and attacks of anguish.

Abdomen - Flatulent, painful colic. Flatulent hernia. Colic with pain between the scapulae. Pain in the abdomen, with diarrhea. Spasmodic colic with nausea, and accumulation of water in the mouth. Noise and pain in abdomen.

Back - Pains in the lumbar region and pains in the nape of the neck. Painful swelling of the glands of the neck and of the axillary glands. Goiter. Drawing tension in the back and in the loins.

Blood - Hemorrhages are dark and thin. Hemorrhagic diathesis from fluidity of blood and dissolution of red blood corpuscles, tendency to gangrenous ulcerations. Hemorrhages are dark from nose, gums and bowels.

Causations - Ill effects of charcoal fumes. Nosebleed comes on when washing the face.

Chest - Shootings in the chest and in the sides. Feeling of fatigue in the chest. Congestion towards the chest. Heaviness in the chest, as from congestion of blood to the chest. Burning in the chest.

Constitutions - Adapted to overweight patients with weak hearts, wheezing and a suffocated feeling. Suited to scrofulous children, stout and sedentary women. Women who are always having recourse to the smelling-bottle. Most of the carbonates are suited to states of obesity.

Ears - Hardness of hearing. Shocks through ears, eyes and nose, when gnashing teeth. Itching above the ears, spreads over the whole body.

Eyes - Burning of eyes with aversion to light. Eye strain (Nat-m.). Burning and dry. Prolonged use of eyes cause asthenopia with appearance of yellow spots on looking at white objects. Flood of tears. Large black spots float after sewing. Pain in the eyes better afternoon sleep. Sore canthi.

Face - Boils and pustules during menses. Corners of the mouth are sore, cracked and burn. Cracks and burning in lip. Hard swelling of the cheek.

Female - Itching, swelling and burning of pudendum. Copious leucorrhea, burning, acrid, watery. Aversion to the other sex. Irritation of clitoris. Menses too ***frequent, profuse***, early, copious, clotted, black, colicky pains and hard, difficult stool with ***fatigue***, especially of thighs, yawning and chilliness. Cholera-like symptoms with menses. Menses flow more at night, then dyspnea or weakness.

Food - Continual thirst, no appetite, excepting for bread and cold food. Great hunger and appetite, yet a small quantity satiates. Unconquerable appetite for sugar.

Head - Obstinate headache. Headache with nausea. Pulsating forehead, better pressure and in a warm room. Shocks, through head, eyes, ears and nose, on biting. ***Violent headache.*** Full, bursting pain in forehead. Brain seems loose. Hammering, pressure, and beatings in the head. Headache, as if from carbonic acid gas. Soreness of the scalp and of the hair. Itching in the head. Falling off of the hair.

Heart - ***Heart weakness***, collapse, wakes with difficult breathing and palpitations. Audible palpitation with fear, cold sweat, lachrymation inability to speak, loud breathing and trembling hands. Angina pectoris. Circulation becomes sluggish and under-oxygęnation of blood produces ***lividity, weakness*** and drowsiness. Vitality becomes low, lack of reaction.

Kidneys - Frequent desire, involuntary at night. Involuntary urination towards morning. Tenesmus of bladder. Urine, white, bloody, sandy, copious, turbid and fetid.

Limbs - Parts lain on become numb. Tearing in joints relieved by heat of bed inclination to stretch limbs. Hands cold and blue, distended veins. Ganglion. Fingers and hands swell, when arms are hanging down. Whitlow. Panaritium, deep-seated periosteal pain. Right arm heavy and weak. Cramps in calves and soles. Big toe painful and swollen. Felons in the beginning. Heel painful on standing. Tearing in ankle and bones of feet, better when warm in bed. ***Inclination to stretch limbs.*** Tearing pain better by heat of bed. Right foot numb. Aching in bones, better change of weather.

Liver - Pressure, pain as from excoriation and burning in the hepatic region. Piercing shootings in the liver, when seated in the evening.

Lungs - Increasing difficulty in breathing, it wakes him, better cool air. Hoarseness. Chest feels tired. Emphysema. ***Much oppression in breathing***, worse after any effort and ***entering warm room*** or ascending even a few steps. Asthenic ***pneumonia***. Slow labored, stertorous breathing, bubbling sounds. Winter catarrh with slimy sputum and specks of blood. Pulmonary edema. Rattling in chest but gets up little. Cough every morning about three o'clock with dyspnea, palpitation, burning in chest, worse ascending. Cough after influenza. Congestion of lungs. Expectoration of pure blood after cough.

Male - Itching and pain of scrotum and spermatic cords. Persistent erections without desire or violent sexual desire without erection. Seminal emissions, frequent after sex.

Modalities - Better from pressure. Better lying on painful side right side, abdomen, and on stomach. Better in dry weather. Better eating. ***Worse cold, cloudy days. Worse damp cold, wet weather***. Worse open air. Worse evenings. Worse new moon. Worse from applications. Worse washing. Worse 3 a.m. to 4 a.m. Worse during menses. Worse falling asleep. Worse motion. Worse chewing, pressing teeth. Worse bending down.

Mouth - Great dryness of mouth and throat. Vesicles on tongue. Taste sour, metallic. Cracking of jaws on chewing. Tender, bleeding gums. Mouth and throat dry. Vesicles on tongue. Burning, hindering eating and speech. Swelling inside cheek.

Nose - Profuse watery coryza. Discharge of sharp, burning water. ***Stoppage at night with long continued coryza***. Continuous urging to sneeze. ***Cannot breathe through nose. Snuffles*** of children. Inability to blow the nose in children. ***Nosebleeds*** if hands or face are washed after eating or on waking. Ozaena, blows bloody mucus from nose. Tip of nose congested. Boil on tip.

Rectum - Constipation with hard, dry stools. Stools difficult, hard and knotty. ***Bleeding hemorrhoids, worse during menses***. Itching at anus. Protruding hemorrhoids worse after stools or without stools, better lying, cannot walk. Discharge of blood before and after stools. Dark acrid diarrhea.

Skin - Red or mottled skin. Erysipelas in the elderly with brain symptoms. Malignant scarlatina. Violent itching and burning blisters. Scarlet rash. Miliary rash. Faintly developed eruptions from defective vitality. Eczema in the bends of limbs, between legs, about anus and genitals.

Sleep - ***Sleepiness*** during the day. Starts from sleep, strangling. The sooner one goes to bed the better one sleeps.

Stomach - Pain at the pit of stomach with heartburn, nausea, water brash and chilliness. Flatulent dyspepsia. Great appetite, but easy satisfaction.

Teeth - Loose or blunt teeth. Toothache during menses. ***Pressing teeth together sends shocks through head, eyes and ears***.

Temperature - Coldness. Burning heat with thirst.

Throat - Enlarged tonsils and glands of neck. Burning pain all down throat. Tendency to gangrenous ulceration of tonsils. Diphtheria when ***nose is stopped up***, membrane extends to upper lip.

Vertigo - Vertigo, on reading in a sitting posture, in the morning or in the evening, sometimes with nausea.

COMMENTS - Am-c. is for those who lead a sedentary life, have a slow reaction generally and are disposed to frequent use of the smelling-bottle. Am-c. is adapted to stout women who are always tired and weary, take cold easily in winter and suffer from cholera-like symptoms before menses and who lead a sedentary life. Dr. Gallavardin has cured uncleanness in bodily habits with Am-c.

Swelling of glands. Headache worse in morning with nausea. Hammering, pressing, bursting, as if contents would start through forehead. Feeling of looseness of brain, as if it fell from side to side, whichever way the head was moved. Burning in eyes, dryness, black spots, sparks, myopia, cataract, catarrh. Muscular asthenopia from prolonged use of the eyes with appearance of yellow spots on looking at white objects. Pterygium.

Nausea, vomiting, fullness, water brash, worse after eating. Flatulence. Slow, hard evacuations in small pieces. Hemorrhoids during menstrual period.

Miliary eruptions. Dry tetters, excoriations, ulcerations, phagadenic. Restlessness, paralytic weakness. Great prostration with falling temperature. Gout in great toe. Heel painful on standing.

Weak heart, palpitations from the least exertion, state of hypoxia. Heart weakness since congestive heart failure, peripheral edema, hypotension, low blood pressure. Great shortness of breath, fainting spells. Feel weak and have heavy sensations in body. Poor circulation. Flush and faint from odor or emotional upset.

Severe weakness of the lungs since pneumonia (Phos., Kali-c.).

RELATIONS - ***Antidoted by:*** Arn., Camph., Hep., Vegetable acids, Fixed oils. ***Antidotes to:*** Rhus and stings of insects, poisoning from charcoal fumes. ***Compare:*** (1) Ant-t, Carb-v, Glon, Lach, Mur-ac. Rhus-t. (2) Ammonias, Ant-t., Ars. (3) Aur. - crushing weight on sternum, but Aur. has less somnolence and less venous congestion. (4) Lach. - to which Am-c. is inimical. (2) Phos., Puls., Sulph. ***Inimical to:*** Lach. similar in action.

REFERENCES - Boericke. Clarke.

AMMONIUM CAUSTICUM

(Ammonia Hydrate)

PHARMACY - am-caust. Ammonium causticum. Ammonia hydrate. Spirits of Hartshorn. Hydratum ammonia. Solution of the gas in water. ***Historical dose:*** All potencies.

CLINICAL - ***Aphonia.*** Chills. Cyanosis. Esophagitis. ***Exhaustion***. Hemorrhages. ***Fainting***. Nephritis. Rheumatism. Sloughing of tissue. Snakebites. Thirst. Thrombosis. Timidity. Ulcerations. Vomiting.

HOMEOPATHIC - The symptoms of caustic ammonia closely resemble those of the carbonate. The caustic nature of the drug is exemplified in the burning sensations experienced, especially in the throat, gullet and rectum.

Am-caust. is a powerful heart stimulant. In a case of poisoning in a man who took a mouthful of a strong solution of ***"household ammonia"*** by mistake, there was great swelling of mucus membrane of mouth and throat. Stertorous breathing, voice muffled and husky, later, cough with bloodstained expectoration. One night there was headache and delirium and at the same time the urine contained albumen and hyaline casts.

Am-caust. is for ***fainting,*** thrombosis, hemorrhage, snakebites, chloroform narcosis, may be given by inhalation. The edema and ulceration of mucus membranes produced by this powerful drug have been utilized as guiding symptoms for its use, hence in membranous croup with burning in esophagus.

A good remedy in ***aphonia, weak voice low.*** Speech broken. Aphonia with debility or with burning rawness in throat. Great oppression of breathing, the patient gasps for breath.

Excessive exhaustion and muscular debility. Shivering with chills. Rheumatism of shoulders and thighs muscles. hemorrhages occur from mucus surfaces. White patches on tongue and inner side of cheeks. Intense thirst and violent ejection of stomach contents.

MIND - Timidity, great tendency to take fright. Great excitement in evening.

Food - Worse after eating or drinking.

Limbs - Rheumatism of shoulders. Skin hot and dry.

Lungs - Difficult breathing. Accumulation of mucus with incessant coughing. Uvula covered with white mucus.

Nose - Nasal diphtheria with burning excoriating discharge.

Throat - ***Loss of voice. Burning rawness in throat.*** Spasm of the glottis with suffocation, patient gasps for breath. Pain in esophagus on breathing deeply. Scraping and burning in throat and esophagus.

RELATIONS - ***Compare:*** (1) Am-c., Caust.

REFERENCES - Boericke. Clarke.

AMMONIUM IODATUM

(Ammonia Iodide)

PHARMACY - am-i. Ammonium iodatum. Ammonia iodide. ***Historical dose:*** Trituration and all potencies.

HOMEOPATHIC - Ammonium Iodatum is indicated when Iodine has but partially relieved its cases of laryngitis and bronchitis, catarrhal pneumonia, edema of lungs.

Dull headaches, especially in young people. The face is stupid, heavy. Vertigo and Meniere's disease. Laryngitis and bronchitis, catarrhal pneumonia, edema of lungs.

RELATIONS - ***Compare:*** (1) Iodine. (2) Ammonium tartaricum - dry hacking cough after every cold.

REFERENCES - Boericke. Clarke.

AMMONIUM MURIATICUM

(Ammonium Chloride)

PHARMACY - am-m. Ammonium muriaticum. Ammonium chloride. Sal ammoniac. Trituration on aqueous solution. ***Historical dose:*** Trituration and all potencies.

CLINICAL - Anosmia. Bronchitis. Colds. Constipation. Coryza. Cough. Diarrhea. Eyes, inflammation. Fatty tumors. Feet, pains. Glands, enlarged. Hemorrhoids. ***Hoarseness***. Liver, disorders. Melancholy. Menstruation, disorders during. Obesity. Pneumonia. Sciatica. Scurvy. Spleen, pains. Sprains. Stumps, neuralgia. ***Tonsillitis***. Tonsils, swelling. Ulcers.

HOMEOPATHIC - Am-m. is less prominently a right-side medicine than Am-c., Guernsey regarded it as rather left-sided. Both cause paralytic weakness, both are worse in open air. Am-m. has better from warm bath. Am-c. has greater sensibility to cold and to damp weather than the muriate. Both have itching eruptions of all kinds, drowsiness by day with indolence, shivering in the evening.

Am-m. affects ***mucus membranes*** increasing the secretion in the ***lungs*** and gallbladder ducts. Am-c. has fat all over. Fatty tumors. Large buttocks. Obesity. Body fat but the legs are thin.

A state of prostration bordering on a typhoid state is produced by this remedy. Tendency to irregular circulation, blood seems to be in constant turmoil, pulsations.

Many symptoms are accompanied by cough or ***profuse glairy mucus*** discharges with liver trouble. It causes ulceration and ulcerative pains, also dislocation-like pains and tension as if tendons were contracted. ***Boiling sensation.***

Many groups of symptoms are accompanied by cough, ***profuse glairy secretions***.

Am-m. causes ulceration and ulcerative or festering pain. Neuralgic pains in the stumps of amputated limbs. Hemorrhages. Boiling sensation. Tension and tightness, as if the muscles or tendons are too short in groins, hamstrings, lumbar region etc.

MIND -.The mental state is very similar to Am-c. The muriate has perhaps more melancholy and disposition to tears than the other and it has, peculiar to itself, ***"antipathy to certain persons."*** Fear of darkness (Stram.), which is not noted under Am-c. Am-m. covers the consequences of grief. ***Desire to cry, but cannot*** (Nat-m.). Melancholy and apprehensive, as from internal grief. Involuntary, aversion to certain persons (Nat-c.).

Abdomen - Stitches in spleen, while eating or in the morning, with difficult breathing. Pain around navel. Abdominal symptoms appear during pregnancy. Excessive fatty deposit around abdomen. Much flatus. Tense sprained feeling in groins, must walk bent. Groins feel swollen and sore.

Back - Swollen cervical glands. Sore sprain or icy coldness between scapulae, not relieved by warmth. Fatty swelling on nape, extending from ear to ear. Lumbago. Backache, as if in a vise when sitting. Bruise pain in coccyx when sitting.

Causations - Grief.

Chest - Oppression of chest. Pulsation, burning spots in chest.

Constitutions - Adapted to obese and sluggish patients who have respiratory troubles. Adapted to patients who are overweight, puffy and tired with thin limbs, who always feel tired and sore.

Eyes - Mist before eyes in bright light. Optical illusions in incipient cataract, capsular cataract. Flying spots, yellow spots, before the eyes.

Face - Inflammatory face ache. Mouth and lips sore and excoriated. Pale. Lips burning like fire. Lips dry, shriveled cracked, must moisten them with tongue. Burning eruptions, better cold application.

Female - Menses, too early, too free, dark, clotted. ***Menses flow more at night***. Prolapsed uterus. Pain as if sprained in left side of abdomen during pregnancy. Diarrhea, greenish mucus stools and navel pain ***during menses***. Diarrhea, vomiting with menses. Leucorrhea like white of an egg (Alum., Bor., Calc-p.), with pain about the navel. Brown, slimy leucorrhea after ***every urination.***

Food - ***Loss of appetite and thirstlessness***. ***Sometimes extreme thirst***, mostly evenings. Thirsty for lemonade. Want of appetite alternating with canine hunger.

Head - Brain paralysis. Hair falls out with itchiness and dandruff. Feels full, compressed, worse mornings. Heaviness in the forehead, pressive pain towards the root of the nose with a sensation, as if brain were torn.

Kidneys - Profuse and frequent urination. Urging yet a few drops pass, until next stool when it flows freely. Profuse ammoniacal smelling urine.

Limbs - Chronic sprains. Pain as from ulceration in fingertips. ***Shooting and tearing*** in fingertips and toes. Ulcerative pain in heels, fingertips. ***Contraction of hamstring tendons***. Hamstrings as if too short, pain on walking. Sciatica, ***worse left, sitting, better lying***. Neuralgic pain in amputated limbs. Tense sprained feeling in the groins, must walk bent. Offensive sweaty feet. Pain in feet during menses. Large buttocks.

Liver - Chronic congestion of liver. Cough with liver symptoms.

Lungs - ***Hoarseness and burning in larynx***. Dry, hacking, scraping cough, worse lying on back or right side. Stitches in chest. Cough with p rofuse salivation or with liver symptoms. Cough loose in afternoon with profuse expectoration and rattling of mucus.

Lungs - Cannot breathe from coughing. Scanty secretions. Noisy, rattling tenacious mucus in chest. Cough worse lying on back or right side.

Modalities - Better from open air. Better rapid motion. Better walking crooked. Head and chest worse morning. Abdominal symptoms worse afternoons. The skin, limbs and fever worse evenings. Worse walking erect. Worse periodically. Worse night. Worse from 2 a.m. to 4 a.m.

Mouth - Slimy. Burning blisters on tip of tongue.

Nose - Sneezing. ***Loss of smell.*** Free ***acrid, hot watery discharge*** corroding the lip and closing one nostril. ***Obstructed, stuffy feeling,*** constant and unavailing efforts to blow it out. Nose sore to touch, ulcerative pain in nostrils. As of a rough body, obstructing upper sinuses. Sneezing aroused her from sleep with shooting pain in the nape of the neck as far as the shoulders. Coryza in children with bluish discharge. Itching.

Rectum - Burning, smarting in the rectum during and for hours after stools. Itching hemorrhoids, soreness with pustules. Stinging in perineum. Hemorrhoids after suppressed leucorrhea. Scanty, hard, ***crumbly stool*** or covered with glairy mucus, changing color and consistency. Green mucus stools alternate with constipation. Blood from anus or diarrhea during menses.

Skin - Itching on various parts of the body, especially in the evening. Blisters on various parts. Intense burning better cold applications. Bleeding eruptions. Peeling of skin between fingers and wrists. Profuse night sweat. Sweats by every motion.

Sleep - Erotic dreams. Anxious, fearful dreams. Starts out of sleep.

Stomach - Regurgitation of food. Nausea with bitter water brash, worse eating with shuddering. Gnawing burning, stitching in stomach, extending to right axilla and upper arm. Empty sensation in, but no desire to eat anything. Epigastric pain immediately after eating. Cancer of stomach. Stricture of esophagus.

Temperature - Chilly as often as he wakes. ***Chilliness in evenings after lying down*** and on waking, without thirst. ***Prevailing fever.*** Heat in palms and soles. Sub-acute, low fevers due to unhealthy climate.

Throat - ***Tonsillitis***. Throbbing in and swelling of tonsils, can scarcely swallow. Sore spot behind uvula, relieved by eating. Internal and external swelling of throat with ***viscid phlegm***. So tough, it cannot be hawked up. Slimy.

COMMENTS - Am-m. acts specially also on the forehead. The muriate has fullness in head, weight in forehead. Burning in eyes in twilight or in morning with photophobia. Keratitis. Ulceration in corners of mouth.

Sensation in stomach as if fasting, which nevertheless feels full, worse after breakfast. Intermittent pains in both hypochondria. Stitches and burning in liver region. Stitches in spleen, worse sitting. Tension in either groin. Shootings in scapula and ice-cold sensation between scapulae, unrelieved by external wraps.

In the fever, chilliness predominates. Choudhury cured with it a case of intermittent fever characterized by absence of thirst in all stages. Constipation and hemorrhoids with bleeding at stool. Sore, smarting hemorrhoids. Hard stool covered with mucus, mucus secretions generally increased.

Menses too early and too copious (Am-c.), with pains in loins. Vomiting, diarrhea and neuralgic pains in feet during period. Coryza, acrid, watery, scalding hot with cold feeling between shoulders. Loss of smell. Cough and asthmatic symptom worse evening and at night and worse in open air.

Pain as from ulceration at fingertips. Neuralgic pains in stumps of amputated limbs (All-c.). Ulcerative pains in heels (ulcers from friction All-c.). Sciatic pain as if tendons were too short. Worse sitting or walking. Tension in legs on lying. There is improvement when walking crooked, worse on walking erect. Most symptoms are worse at night and from two to four a.m.

RELATIONS - ***Antidotes to:*** Bitter almonds, Coffea, Nux-v., Caust. A hot bath relieves aggravation caused by Am-m. ***Compare:***

(1) Calc., Caust., Seneg. (2) Mag-m, Nat-m., Valer. and Mur-ac. - pains in feet and heels. (3) Rhus-t. - sprains, worse sitting. (4) Seneg. - fat people. (5) Sep., Sulph. - in "aversion to darkness." (6) Calc., Carb-an., Stront., Valer., and Stram.

REFERENCES - Boericke. Clarke.

AMMONIUM PHOSPHORICUM

(Ammonia Phosphate)

PHARMACY - am-p. Ammonium phosphoricum. Ammonia phosphate. Hydro-diammonic phosphate. Solution. ***Historical dose:*** Trituration and all potencies.

CLINICAL - Facial paralysis. Gout. Joints, concretions.

HOMEOPATHIC - Allen said Am-p. has been used with success in some cases of facial paralysis. This salt has been used in cases of chronic gout with nodes of urate of soda on the joints.

For chronic gouty patients, uric acid diathesis. Bronchitis. ***Nodosities of the joints of the fingers*** and backs of the hands. Facial paralysis. Pain in shoulder joint. Tightness around chest. Heaviness of limbs, unsteady tottering gait. Coldness from least draft of air.

Head - Sneezing with excessive running from nose and eyes, ***only in morning***.

Kidneys - Rose-colored sediment.

Lungs - Deep rough cough with greenish expectoration.

REFERENCES - Boericke. Clarke.

AMMONIUM PICRICUM

(Ammonia Picrate)

PHARMACY - am-pic. Ammonium picricum. Ammonia picrate. Picric acid and its combinations are very powerful medicinal substances of the nitric acid group. ***Historical dose:*** Trituration and all potencies, third trituration.

CLINICAL - Bilious headache. Periodical neuralgia. Vertigo. Whooping cough.

HOMEOPATHIC - Am-pic. is intensely bitter and, like Pic-ac. and other picrates, has a strong action on the liver. Hale commended Ammonium picricum in congestion of brain and spinal cord.

Heavy, pressive pains in occiput and mastoid region, on sides of head to temples and eyes. Periodic bilious headache (Sang., Cimic.). Occipital headache (Am-pic.), proceeding down the spine and also a pain traveling the reverse way. Neuralgia. Face darkly flushed. Mind obtuse, disinclined to labor. Malarial fever. Whooping cough.

Head - Periodical neuralgia in ***right side of occiput***, boring extends to ear orbit and jaw. Periodic bilious headaches (Sang.).

Vertigo - Vertigo on rising.

COMMENTS - Hale noted a case he cured with Am-pic. It concerned a middle-aged woman, short, stout, florid, who, every six or eight days, would wake in the morning with violent pain in occipital region, heaviness of head, and vertigo on rising. Pain, worse on getting up, extended over sides of head to temples and eyes. In the afternoon, she had nausea and vomiting of sour bilious matter.

Another case concerned a doctor who had been thrown from his carriage and injured about the back of his head. He seemed more frightened than hurt. In a few days, however, he noticed that on turning in bed or stooping or on any sudden motion he would be seized with a "wild feeling" in the occiput, trembling beating of heart with intermission and great alarm. Am-pic. completely relieved him after other medicines had been given in vain.

Allen noted the indication "Periodical neuralgia in right side of occiput, boring extending to the ear orbit and jaw' vertigo on rising, especially in irregular menstruation."

Clarke gave great relief with Pic-ac. in a case of spinal paresis in which a pain rising up the spine into the head was complained. Clarke thought it was the Pic-ac. element in this ammonia salt that accounts for its action in these cases of Hale's.

REFERENCES - Boericke. Clarke. Hale.

AMMONIUM VALERIANICUM

(Ammonia Valerianate)

PHARMACY - am-val. Ammonium valerianicum. Ammonia valerianate. ***Historical dose:*** Trituration and all potencies.

HOMEOPATHIC - Am-val. is a remedy for nervous, hysterical people suffering with neuralgia headaches and insomnia. Great nervous weakness is always present. Hysteria. Neuralgia headaches and insomnia. Pains in cardiac region. Functional disturbances of the heart, tachycardia.

REFERENCES - Boericke.

AMNIOTIC FLUID

(Amnii liquor)

PHARMACY - amn-l. Amniotic fluid. Amnii liquor. Tincture of the liquid obtained by aseptic puncture. ***Historical dose:*** All potencies.

HOMEOPATHIC - Amniotic fluid is a clear, or limpid, yellowish-white fluid with flocculates. Alkaline or neutral reaction. May contain lanugo, or epidermal cells. May contain pepsin, diatase, fibrinase and anti staphylolysin. Hypotonic. Composition is similar to blood serum, urea 18.25 mg%, uric acid 4.51 mg.%, chlorides 5.93 mg%, creatine 2.33 mg%, CO2, 34.77 vol.%. Source of the organ of secretion is not known. Its role is supportive, and also probably nutritive, it surrounds the embryo.

The provings, published by P. Schmidt in The Journal of the American Institute of Homeopathy, 20:236-248, 1927, consisted of 7 provers and used "one dose of liquor amnii 30c." Schmidt noted that "This remedy seems to act essentially on the head, abdomen and the menstrual periods. It seems to suit better the feminine temperament."

MIND - Increased mental activity. Tends to overwork, industrious. Mania for work. Irritability. Restlessness, nervousness.

Abdomen - Pain in abdomen.

Head - One-sided headaches. Pains in sides of head.

Female - Menstrual disorders.

Sleep - Disturbed sleep. Restless during sleep. Tossing about in the bed.

COMMENTS - Hering related a case of a soldier who, while carrying a wounded comrade, was struck by a spent bullet in the epigastrium. He became pale and weak, "felt the wind knocked out of him" and laid down. A drop of Liquor ammon. in water relieved at once.

REFERENCES - Schmidt.

AMORPHOPHALLUS RIVIERI

(Chinese Umbel)

PHARMACY - amor-r. Amorphophallus rivieri. Chinese umbel. N. O. Spaciflora order and the Araceae family. The tincture is made from the stem, the flower and the root. ***Historical dose:*** Tincture and all potencies.

CLINICAL - Cancer, uterine. Cholera morbus. Dysmenorrhea. Headaches. Infantile, cholera. Leucorrhea. Menopause. Metritis. Metrorrhagia. Typhoid fever.

HERBAL - Amor-r. is an herbaceous plant, growing from 30 to 60 cm high. The starchy rhizome is edible, dried or roasted. This plant flowers only once every seven years, although the cycle may vary in a greenhouse. The whole plant is regarded as medicinal.

HOMEOPATHIC - The proving was the work of Dr. Proceso Sanchez Ortega of Mexico. The provings report weight loss, morbid hunger, bodily swelling and puffiness, and loss of ability to copulate. Repulsive appearance, general puffiness and the stupefied look of enervation.

Feeling of exhaustion, apathy. General discomfort with extreme exhaustion. General uneasiness, extreme weariness. Feels ill, needs to remain in bed. Feverish with intestinal colic. Burning sensation of the orifices and in the throat with numbness of the limbs.

Gastric and intestinal complaints with tiring diarrhea. Female genital complaints with difficult, painful menses and purulent leucorrhea. Burning sensation in the female genitals. Acute or chronic salpingitis.

MIND - Looks bewildered, dazed, exhausted. Total indifference and apathy. Semi-conscious state, does not react. Anxiety and fear.

Abdomen - Intestinal rumbling.

Eyes - Sight weak.

Female - Burning sensation in the vagina and cervix. Painful menstruation with pains in the sacrum and lumbar region, feeling of exhaustion and flow of dark blood. The menses is prolonged, with the blood decomposed, greenish and irritating. Fetid leucorrhea with a greenish, purulent appearance. Irritating leucorrhea with discharge of thick pus. Inflammation of the Bartholin glands. Metritis before menopause, with profuse menstruation and metrorrhagia. Uterine cancer.

Food - Intense thirst. Discomfort during naps, although the food had settled. Cannot bear alcoholic drinks.

Head - Persistent frontal headache, spreading at first to the right temple and then the left. Head pains by day in the morning and afternoon. Periodic head pains, every eight days and throughout the day until bed-time.

Modalities - Better from nourishment. Worse from alcoholic drinks.

Rectum - Normal stools or diarrhea, coffee-colored, preceded by abdominal pains. Diarrhea every two hours with tenesmus, fatigue and weakness.

Stomach - Burning in the stomach, causing great discomfort. Heaviness of the stomach when eating, which disappears after three to four hours. Nausea, especially on waking, ameliorated by nourishment. Nausea at the sight of food. Acidity after introducing food to the stomach.

Vertigo - Slight vertigo, especially while walking and the sensation of walking crookedly.

RELATIONS - ***Compare:*** (1) Ars. - Prostration, violent vomiting after drinking, diarrhea with burning, black stools, excoriation around the anus. Painful menses with black blood and burning, putrid, corrosive leucorrhea. (2) Verat. - Prostration and feeling of coldness, vomiting and diarrhea, painful menses. (3) Camphora - State of collapse, feeling of general cracking, cannot bear to be covered, even though the body may be ice-cold.

REFERENCES - Julian.

AMPELOPSIS QUINQUEFOLIA

(Virginia Creeper)

PHARMACY - ampe-qu. Ampelopsis quinquefolia. Virginia creeper. American Ivy. Vitis quinquefolia. N. O. Vitacae. Tincture of plant. Decoction of chopped inner bark. ***Historical dose:*** Tincture and all potencies.

CLINICAL - Cholera. Dropsy. Hoarseness. Hydrocele. Kidney, dropsies. Vomiting.

HERBAL - S. M. Worthington cured with it kidney dropsies that had resisted other treatment and a case of hydrocele. He found the decoction to be the best preparation.

HOMEOPATHIC - Our knowledge of Ampe-qu. is due to observations on two children poisoned by chewing the leaves. They were quickly seized with violent vomiting and purging with considerable tenesmus, then collapse, sweating and faint pulse, then deep sleep for two hours from which they were aroused by the return of the vomiting and purging. Pupils were dilated for hours after commencement of attack.

Hansen gave as an indication: "Chronic hoarseness in patients who were scrofulous in their youth."

Kidney dropsies, hydrocele and chronic hoarseness in scrofulous patients have been benefited by this drug. Cholera symptoms. Generally worse about 6 p.m. Dilated pupils. Left coastal region sore and sensitive. Elbow joint pains, back sore. Soreness of all limbs. Vomiting, purging with tenesmus. Rumbling in abdomen.

REFERENCES - Allen. Boericke. Clarke.

AMPHETAMINUM SULFURICUM

(Amphetamine)

PHARMACY - amphet. Amphetaminum sulfuricum. Amphetamine. ***Historical dose:*** All potencies.

CLINICAL - ADHD. ***Anorexia.*** Arrhythmia. Constipation. Dermatitis. Diarrhea. Dizziness. Dryness. Dyslexia. Emaciation. Fatigue. Headaches. Heart, disorders. ***Hyperactivity. Insomnia.*** Narcolepsy. Nausea. Nervousness. Palpitations. Tachycardia. Tourette's, syndrome. Vasculitis. Vomiting. Weight, loss.

HOMEOPATHIC - Tourette's syndrome, uncontrolled movements of the head, neck, arms and legs. Trembling. Hyper-reflexia. Vasculitis. General fatigue. Weight loss. Sexual changes of libido. Increased perspiration. Hyperthermia.

MIND - ***Nervousness and restlessness.*** Irritability. Mental depression. Psychosis. Euphoria. False sense of well-being.

Eyes - Blurred vision.

Female - Changes in libido.

Head - Headache.

Heart - Arrhythmia. Tachycardia. Palpitations with chest pain.

Limbs - Uncontrolled movements of the head, neck, arms and legs.

Male - Decreased sexual ability. Changes in libido.

Mouth - Dryness of mouth. Unpleasant taste.

Rectum - Constipation. Diarrhea.

Skin - Dermatitis.

Sleep - Narcolepsy. Insomnia. Drowsiness.

Stomach - Loss of appetite. Nausea. Stomach cramps or pain. Vomiting.

Vertigo - Dizziness. Light-headedness.

REFERENCES - Murphy.

AMPHISBENA VERMICULARIS

(Lizard)

PHARMACY - amph. Amphisbaena vermicularis. Lizard. N. O. Lacertilia. Snake-like lizard without limbs. The jaw containing the poison is removed and triturated. ***Historical dose:*** Trituration, Tincture and all potencies.

CLINICAL - Constipation. Cramps. Debility. Depression. Headache. Hernia. Jaw, pains. Toothache.

HOMEOPATHIC - Mure is the authority for its effects. It is prepared from the jaw as well as the poison of the animal and has symptoms indicating action on bone like that of Silica.

Amph. acts markedly on the jaws, causing swelling and pain, especially in the right jaw, worse by air and dampness. Many kinds of severe headache, pains are frequent. Eruptions of vesicles and pimples. Right-sided action. Generally aggravated from motion.

MIND - Boredom. Depression. Tender sadness, which disposes one to be gentle and meek. Sadness and lassitude in the morning. Impatience.

Abdomen - Protrusion of umbilical hernia. Tearing pain at the navel, all day. Lancination in the navel, as from a stiletto. Suppuration of inguinal hernia. The hernia is painful and air is felt in it.

Back - Violent pain in the whole of the vertebral column, worse when walking, moving the arms or stooping.

Ears - Pain in the meatus, as if air were rushing in.

Eyes - Weariness of the eye in the evening, with pain and pricking when looking at the light. Constriction of the right eye, as if strung together with a cord. Sensation as of a grain of sand in the right eye. Constant twitching at the upper eyelids, especially the left. Pain at the inner canthus of the right eye, as if a stye would form. Shooting pain in the left eye. Lachrymation and constriction of the left eye.

Face - Prickling and heat at the right malar eminence. Painful and large pimple on the left side of upper lip, suppurating. Pains in the right lower jaw and considerable swelling, aggravated by air and dampness. Dull pain in the right lower jawbone.

Head - Horrible headache with sensation as if the feet were in the brain. Weight in the forehead and parietal regions. Repeated beating at the right side of the forehead, as if hailstones fell upon it. Lancination and pain all through the right side of the head. Sweat about the head.

Limbs - Breaking out of little pimples, especially on the forearm. Painful swelling of the arm. Painless drawing up of the legs. Cramp in the left leg, it remains behind in walking, as if paralyzed.

Modalities - Better from evening. Better from itching the eruption. Worse in morning. Worse walking. Worse turning around. Worse itching the eruption. Worse toothache. Worse pains in lower jaw. Worse weariness of the eyes. Worse from sadness or lassitude.

Mouth - The teeth feel elongated and set on edge, especially the right lower molars. Toothache is worse in the afternoon and evening. Chewing is painful, but not the contact of liquids.

Rectum - Constipation.

Skin - Acute acne rosacea. Painful and large pimples on the left side of the upper lip, suppurating. The miliary acne rosacea spreads over the chest, neck and back with itching. Breaking out of little pimples, especially on the forearm. Gradually, a white vesicle forms on pimples. Pimples discharge a clear serum after which the eruption dries up.

Sleep - Wakes at midnight for ten consecutive nights. Disturbed sleep.

Stomach - Chilliness and pains at the epigastrium.

Throat - Swelling of tonsils. Swallowing is difficult, cannot swallow saliva.

Vertigo - Vertigo, as if one would fall towards one side and is then impelled towards the opposite side by a contrary oscillation. Dizziness when turning around.

RELATIONS - ***Compare:*** (1) Hecla lava, Heloderma, Silica.

REFERENCES - Allen. Clarke.

AMYGDALUS AMARA AQUA

(Bitter Almond)

PHARMACY - amyg-am. Amygdalus amara aqua. Bitter almond. Amygdalus communis amara. N. O. Rosacae. An ounce of alcohol is added to a pound of bitter almonds, then six pounds of water are added and distilled down to three pounds. Hydrocyanic acid is formed by the action of water on the amygdaloids. ***Historical dose:*** Tincture and all potencies.

CLINICAL - Asthma, Coma, Diphtheria. Epilepsy. Headache. Syncope. Tetanus. Urticaria.

HOMEOPATHIC - The symptoms of Amyg-am. are not very distinguishable from those of Hydrocyanic acid. Jerking, hesitating, stuttering speech. Dark red palate and fauces. Swallowing impossible. Vomiting of undigested food and bile.

Cough with soreness of chest extending down to stomach. Stitches under left nipple, going deep in, making exhalations more difficult. Convulsive and at intervals very short respiration with fear of suffocation.

Heaviness in forehead (Laur.). Head drawn backward. Congestion of vessels of brain and general effusion on both hemispheres, dura matter gorged. Opisthotonos. Dullness of left half of the head (Hydr-ac., right). Venous system gorged with dark liquid blood. Blood, muscles and bile of a violet color. Snoring. Surface cold, clammy, pale or blue.

Convulsions. Most violent convulsions, which last almost three-quarters of an hour. The convulsions returned after a quarter of an hour, but less violently. General tetanus. Complete opisthotonos.

Excessive languor. General debility from seven bitter almonds. Feeling of weakness, as if the muscular vigor was deficient and he would fall down. Fainting. Syncope. Death in thirty minutes. General malaise. Weight on the eyes and in the limbs.

MIND - Mild delirium. The patient stammers incoherently. Appearance of intoxication. She is so much affected that she can hardly utter a word (after four hours). The feelings were deeply affected, she began to weep. Extreme anxiety. Falls down unconscious.

Loss of consciousness of voice and of motive power. Senseless. Coma with stertorous respiration and involuntary stool, but she revives suddenly and looks wildly her.

Abdomen - Abdomen relaxed, soft, hardly of natural warmth. Pains in abdomen. Colicky pains, which increase, until the abdomen is distended like a balloon.

Chest - The chest heaved spasmodically and its movements were hurried. Oppression of chest. Several transient stitches and pains.

Ears - Ears white and cold. Humming in the ears.

Eyes - Sunken eyes. The eyes are turned upwards. Eyes glassy. Brilliancy of the eyes. Eyes wide open and motionless. Eyes are closed, cold. Spasmodic movements, especially of the eyelids. Upper eyelids convulsed. Eyeballs protruding from their sockets. Eyes open and rolling from side to side. Contracted pupils. Pupils widely dilated and insensible to light. Motionless pupils. Dimness of sight.

Face - Face becomes deadly pale. Face yellowish-gray and moist. Lips bluish, white and cold. Countenance is very flushed. Spasmodic distortion of the features. Frequent convulsive action of muscles of face and neck. Sardonic laughter, joyful countenance, sparkling eyes.

Head - Heaviness and confusion of head and of thought. Head drawn between shoulders. Violent headache. During the forenoon a sense of heaviness in the forehead. Slight pressure in forehead. Sense of weight and oppression on top of head.

Heart - Heartbeats very feebly. Beat of heart feeble, sometimes intermittent.

Kidneys - Scanty and painful urination.

Limbs - Limbs were completely lax and fell lifeless when lifted. Unsteadiness on the limbs. Upper and lower limbs cold. Could not stand on legs. Formication in the legs with staggering gait. Knees flexed on the abdomen. Heaviness of limbs and whole right thigh.

Lungs - Short, painting respiration, suffocative attacks. Breathing stertorous and at long intervals. Breathing slow and gentle. Respiration heavy. Difficult respiration.

Male - Penis shriveled.

Mouth - Tongue dry and coated. Mouth tightly closed. Froth at the mouth. Breath smells of bitter almonds.

Neck - Swelling and undulatory motion in the jugular veins, the carotids beat quickly and fully.

Nose - Nose white and cold.

Pulse - Pulse strong, frequent and wiry. Pulse at first small, frequent and intermittent, then slow and regular. Pulse slow, vibrating, small, flickering. Diminished pulse, scarcely perceptible.

Rectum - Copious, but especially watery evacuations. Stool seldom.

Skin - Skin blue and bluish-red, especially on scrotum, where it was blue and almost greenish-yellow. Wheals over the whole skin. Urticaria with fever.

Sleep - Yawning with irresistible tendency to sleep. Drowsiness. Inclined to sleep the afternoon. Depression in the afternoon and evening. Inclination to sleep soundly and deeply through the night, difficult to rouse. Deep, stertorous sleep.

Stomach - Nausea and vomiting of food. Vomiting of a bitter, viscid substance, bile smelling strongly of prussic acid.

Temperature - General coldness. Surface cold and clammy.

Throat - Increased discharge of mucus from the larynx. Hoarseness caused by scraping in the larynx. Swallowing is impossible. Burning sensation in throat. Excessive burning heat in laryngo-pharyngeal region.

Vertigo - Vertigo, as if gradually passed off by noon. Vertigo in strong air. Vertigo, as if intoxicated, followed by sudden death (from taking many bitter a almonds).

COMMENTS - Farrington noted "Very brilliant appearance of the eyes without corresponding mental expression. Eyes drawn to left side. Burning heat in laryngo-pharyngeal region. Sharp pains through tonsils."

RELATIONS - ***Antidoted by:*** Op. - convulsions., strong coffee, cold water poured over head. ***Compare:*** (1) Laurocerasus, Hydr-ac., Op. - spasms, stertor, slow pulse, stupor. (2) Stram., Tab., Ant-t. (3) Lach., Naja (heart).

REFERENCES - Allen. Clarke.

AMYGDALUS PERSICA

(Peach Tree Bark)

PHARMACY - amyg-p. Amygdalus persica. Peach tree bark. Persica amygdalus. Persica vulgaris. N. O., Rosacea, Amygdalae. Fresh infusion or tincture. ***Historical dose:*** Tincture and all potencies.

CLINICAL - Gastric and intestinal irritation. Hemorrhage. Morning sickness. Nausea. Vomiting.

HERBAL - Outside the old herbalists, the virtues of the bark and leaves of the peach tree have received little attention. The infusion is made by taking of the bark one part and of boiling distilled water ten parts. Infuse in a covered vessel for one hour and strain. The tincture is made by pounding the fresh bark of the twigs to a pulp and macerating in two parts by weight of alcohol.

HOMEOPATHIC - Amygdalus persica is a most valuable remedy in vomiting of various kinds including ***morning sickness***. Constant nausea and vomiting. Irritation of eyes. Ischuria and hematuria. Hemorrhage from the bladder. Gastric irritation of children, no form of food tolerated. Loss of smell and taste. Gastric and intestinal irritation when the tongue is elongated and pointed, tip and edges red.

COMMENTS - Dr. Oliver S. Haines of Philadelphia contributed his experience: "Apropos of the remarks made by Dr. C. C. Edson upon the efficacy of infusion of peach bark in the gastric irritability of children, we might mention the following authentic case:

"For an adult the dose is five drops and in urgent cases repeat every five to ten minutes until the symptoms subside after which give it at intervals of one to four hours as indicated.

"After ten years use I am thoroughly convinced that any physician once giving it a thorough trial will never again be without it. Of course, it is not a specific for all ***"Upheavals of the inner man,"*** but will I think meet more indications than any other known remedy of its class.

"An infant during its second summer, had been much reduced by acute dyspeptic diarrhea. A marked feature of this case was the persistent vomiting of all food. The stomach would tolerate no form of baby food with or without milk. The child's parents had consulted some eminent physicians of our city. The child had been given homeopathic remedies. None of the remedies chosen seemed to produce the desired effect. After a consultation it was deemed best to send the infant to the mountains. The change aggravated its condition.

"While the parents hourly expected their baby would die, it was suggested that they send for an old practitioner living in the mountains near at hand. "This man had a local reputation as a saver of dying babies. His prescription was as follows: Two or three fresh peach leaves were to be put in a cup of boiling water, the infant to receive a *"drink"* of this infusion at frequent intervals.

"The effects of this were remedy as remarkable in this case as in the case narrated by Dr. Edson. Our child soon retained food and eventually recovered. It seems this ancient disciple of Aesculapius had long used peach leaves and regarded them as possessing specific virtues."

Anshutz noted "Dr. C. C. Edson wrote in the Chicago Medical Times. 1890: Some ten years ago I had a little patient whose principal difficulty seemed to be an inability to retain anything whatever upon its stomach. It would vomit up promptly everything I gave it and I had given it everything I had ever heard of and also had eminent council, but it was no go, I was literally at my rope's end.

"At this juncture an elderly lady neighbor, one of "the good old mothers," timidly suggested an infusion of peach bark. I started to find the coveted bark, which I was fortunate enough to procure. I prepared an infusion, gave the little patient a few swallows and presto! the deed was done, the child cured. It fills all the indications of the leaves and many more. It fills the indications of hydrocyanic acid, ipecac or any other anti-emetic.

It will more frequently allay the vomiting of pregnancy than any remedy I have ever tried. And nearly every case of retching or vomiting (except it be reflex) will promptly yield under its use.

"In recent cases I have very rarely had to give the second prescription to relieve morning sickness. I was visiting a doctor in Quincy, while there he told me he was afraid he would have either to make a lady abort of let her die from the fact that he had failed to stop her vomiting. I happened to have a sample of the medicine with me, I gave it to him, he took it to the lady and in a few days he reported her well. I may say like Dr. Edson, it is a standard remedy with me. I have found it very useful in hemorrhage from the bladder.

"Some of my lady patients find it very good in nervous headache. I have used the tincture prepared from the leaves, but it is far inferior to that prepared from the bark of the young shoots. A medical friend was going to see a lady who had morning sickness, he told me he had thought of advising her to use popcorn, I handed him a small bottle of my Amygdalus and told him to take a couple of ears of corn in his pocket and try both. The next time I met him he said my medicine had done the work."

RELATIONS - ***Compare:*** (1) Amygd. - pains through tonsils, throat dark, difficult swallowing, vomiting, cough with sore chest.

REFERENCES - Anshutz. Boericke.

AMYLENUM NITROSUM

(Amyl Nitrite)

PHARMACY - aml-n. Amylenum nitrosum. Amyl nitrite. Iso amylnitrite. Dilution with alcohol. ***Historical dose:*** All potencies.

CLINICAL - Angina pectoris. ***Anxiety***. Blushing. Chorea. ***Circulation.*** Convulsions. Dyspnea. Epilepsy. Exophthalmos. Flushings. Headaches. ***Heart, attack. Heart, disorders. Hiccoughs. Hot, flushes. Hypertension.*** Hysteria. Menopausal, disorders. ***Palpitations.*** Seasickness. Sunstroke. ***Yawning***.

HOMEOPATHIC - The Nitrite of Amyl was introduced into medicine by the old school as a remedy for angina pectoris and was supposed to act by lessening arterial tension. Vasomotor nerves are affected by Aml-n causing dilatation of all arterioles and capillaries, thereby flushing of face, heat and throbbing in the head are produced.

Homeopathic provings have shown that, in some cases at any rate, Aml-n. has a specific action. Also in paroxysms of asthma, chloroform asphyxia inhalation of the Aml-n. will give immediate relief. For this non-homeopathic application, two to five minims (put up in pearls) dropped on a handkerchief and inhaled may be required.

The most striking action of the drug is the ***deep facial flushing*** it causes and the ***pulsation all over the body***. Superficial arterial hyperemia. ***Palpitations*** of the heart and similar conditions are readily cured by it. Amyl-n. is for all conditions where the ***blood vessels are contracted***, as in angina pectoris. Headaches accompanied by cold, pallor, etc. ***Hiccoughs and yawning***. Seasickness. Often relieves temporarily epileptic convulsions. Weak and emaciated.

The flushings and other discomforts at menopausal are helped. ***Hot flashes***. Flushing heats, followed by drenching sweats are marked symptoms. Cerebral vessels dilate. Weak, emaciated, walking with tottering gait inclined to go to one side when walking. Rigid muscles of limbs. Child has convulsions.

Worse since exposure to the sun, heat stroke, vascular headaches, severe palpitations, and the keynote is a sudden rush of blood to the head with palpitations (Glon.).

MIND - Confused feeling after congestion to head. ***Anxiety, as if something bad might happen, must have fresh air.*** Anxiety can't sit still. Shrieking before convulsion. Melancholy. Mental confusion and a dreamlike state. Trancelike state, everything seems unreal. Increasing sense of stupefaction. Unconsciousness, inability to swallow.

Abdomen - Oppression near liver. Crampy colicky pains, rumbling.

Blood - Intense surging of blood to face and head, later veins turgid (Bell.). ***Rapidly dilates arteries and quickens but weakens circulation.*** Venous and arterial blood are of same hue. ***Hypertension.***

Chest - Pain and constriction around the heart. Dyspnea and asthmatic feelings. Great oppression and fullness of chest, spasmodic, suffocative cough. Aching backward along the left floating rib. Feeling as if a weight on sternum. Sensation of swelling of front of chest.

Constitutions - Nervous, sensitive women and men.

Ears - Throbbing in the ears, bursting, burning. Ears hyperemic.

Eyes - Exophthalmic goiter from grief. Protruding, starting eyes, conjunctiva injected. Ciliary neuralgia, eye injected, face or cheek suffused. Objects appear pea-green or yellow. Sight blurred, wavering. Aching eyes in sunlight, trembling and wavering of objects, lachrymation and sneezing.

Face - Easy flushing or blushing of the face, on slightest emotion. Chewing motion of the lower jaw. Smacking of lips as if in act of tasting. Neuralgia of fifth pair of nerves.

Female - Hemorrhages after-pains with facial flushing. ***Menopausal headache and flushes of heat*** with anxiety and palpitations. Neuralgia during menses. Convulsions immediately after delivery.

Food - Loss of appetite.

Head - ***Bursting sensation*** in the head and ears. Throbbing in head. ***Surging of blood to head and face*** with fiery red face. Sensation as if blood would start through skin with heat and redness. Throbbing. Migraine with pallor, worse left side

Heart - Aching pain and constriction around the heart. ***Angina pectoris*** with great anxiety. ***Tumultuous action of the heart.*** Pain and constriction around heart. Fluttering of heart on least excitement. Full, soft pulse. ***Violent beating of the heart and carotids*** with sense of constriction. The heart has an irregular, rumbling sort of sound. Precordial pain extending to right arm.

Kidneys - Increased quantity of urine increased, with sugar in it.

Limbs - ***Constant stretching for hours.*** Veins of hands dilated, pulsations felt in fingertips.

Lungs - Constriction in throat extended to the chest, with dyspnea and asthmatic feeling in larynx and trachea. Asthma. Hastens and deepens the breathing. Suffocation and cough in paroxysms.

Modalities - Better from open air. Better exercise. Better in open air. Better cold water. Worse from menopause. Worse slight causes, emotions. Worse from heat. Worse closed or warm room.

Sleep - Repeated yawning in coma. Yawns profoundly and repeatedly. Stretches almost constantly, it is almost impossible to satisfy the desire. Stretching and yawning with hiccough.

Stomach - Hot, burning sensation in stomach. Hiccough and yawning with stretching. Nausea with dryness of throat. Crampy pains in epigastrium. Fullness and pressure with belching.

Temperature - ***Flushings, followed by sweat at menopause***, sometimes followed by cold and clammy skin with profuse sweat. ***Abnormal sweat after influenza.*** Throbbing throughout whole body.

Throat - Constriction, collar seems too tight. Choking feeling in the throat.

Vertigo - Great confusion of the head, with vertigo and drowsiness.

COMMENTS - The specific heart symptoms of Aml-n. are the sensation of swelling of the chest as if convex, with a feeling as if the lower end of the sternum made a deep depression bent in towards the spine.

Precordial anxiety. Accelerated intensified beating of the heart. Oppression and tumultuous action. Constriction (relieved by Cact.) and aching pain. Strong, full pulse. Eyes protruding, staring. Exophthalmic goiter from grief. Flushing of face. Flushing on least emotion.

Nash has cured "chronic blushing on least excitement mental or physical" with it. Heat, redness, turgidity. Choking feeling, collar feels tight. Tremor and weakness of limbs.

Better open-air exercise, cold water and cold air. Worse in a warm room.

Other prominent symptoms include anxiety as if something might happen, and a desire for fresh air. Throbbing in head. Bursting-out feeling in ears. Smacking of lips as if in act of tasting. Munching movement of lower jaw as if chewing. Constriction of throat and heart from actual fright ran to window for air. Intense fullness in head, sensation of rushing to vertex.

"Impending apoplexy." Threatened apoplexy. Flushing of the face, heat and throbbing, palpitations. Boericke said, "Flushings followed by sweat at menopausal," hot flashes with a red face during menopause (Lach).

Boericke also notes "chloroform asphyxia," antidote for chloroform.

RELATIONS - ***Antidotes:*** Cactus, Stry., Ergot. ***Compare:*** (1) Bell., Glon., Lach.

REFERENCES - Boericke. Clarke. Murphy

ANACARDIUM OCCIDENTALE

(Cashew Nut)

PHARMACY - anac-oc. Anacardium occidentale. Cashew nut. N. O. Anacardiacae. West Indies. Tincture of the black juice between outer and inner shell. ***Historical dose:*** All potencies.

CLINICAL - Allergies. Blisters. Corns. Dysentery. Erysipelas. Hypochondriasis. Imbecility. Itching. Melancholy. Ophthalmia. Paralysis. Rhus poisoning. Ringworm. Smallpox. Warts.

HERBAL - The Anac-oc. nut is kidney-shaped, that of Anac. is heart-shaped. The juice has been used locally as an application for corns, warts, hard excrescences, ringworm and obstinate ulcers.

Anac-oc. has been applied to the face to remove cuticle and produce a fresher and more youthful appearance. If hands are not washed carefully after handling nuts, they cause itching and painful, burning swellings wherever they touch skin.

The effects of the cashew nut are known through instances of poisoning. It acts powerfully on the skin, causing erysipelas, blisters and swelling. It has been used as an antidote to Rhus poisoning. One woman received a swollen face from exposure to fumes when roasting nuts.

HOMEOPATHIC - Anac-oc. causes weakness of memory and mind like Anac. Scirrhus swellings. Hard excrescences. Proud flesh. Tearing pain in left side of head. Burning and itching of ears and face. General paralytic state. Paralysis and imbecility. Tongue painfully swollen.

Erysipelas, vesicular facial eruptions, anesthetic variety of leprosy, warts, corns, ulcers, cracking of the skin on soles of feet. Itching almost intolerable, umbilicated vesicles as in smallpox. The erysipelas spreads from left to right and it cures erysipelas spreading from right to left, Paralysis with imbecility.

MIND - Difficulty with thinking. Did not know his surroundings. Weak memory. Melancholy. Hypochondriasis. Apathy. Loss of will, cannot control voluntary muscles. Paralysis with imbecility.

Ears - Swelling of ears with burning and itching.

Eyes - Scrofulous ophthalmia.

Face - Erysipelas over whole face from applying juice to destroy marks. Swelling of face with itching and burning, next night after handling nuts. Face swollen, features not discernible.

Female - When juice is applied during menses, it causes erysipelas of the face. Uterine complaints and dropsy.

Head - Head falls forward, difficult to keep it up. Tearing headache on left side.

Kidneys - Increased urination.

Limbs - Large blisters filled with a yellow fluid are raised on hands, followed by desquamation. Warts. Corns.

Male - Stimulates sexual desire. Testicles swollen when touched with hands after handling nuts.

Mouth - Drinks run out of mouth. Aphthae. Cannot speak, only mutters unintelligible sounds. Painfully swollen tongue from handling nuts.

Skin - Corroding or dry tetters. Red itching spots like nettle rash (Rhus-t.), spreading from left to right. Used as a vesicant, i causes itching and burning, then gradual reddening and swelling, followed by vesicles which become pustular. These are large and flat at first and gradually become confluent and break, the epidermis peels off, but leaves the surface swollen, hyperemic and suppurating for days. Proud flesh.

RELATIONS - ***Antidoted by:*** Rhus-t., Iodine locally. ***Compare:*** (1) Anac. orien. (2) Similar to Canth., Mez. - as a vesicant. (3) Crot-t., Rhus-rad., Rhus-tox. (4) The tincture of Iodine was found useful as a local application to parts affected.

REFERENCES - Boericke. Clarke.

ANACARDIUM ORIENTALE

(Marking Nut)

PHARMACY - anac. Anacardium orientale. Marking nut. Malacca bean. Semecarpus anacardium. N. O. Anacardiacae. East Indies. Trituration of layer between shell and kernel of heart shaped nut. ***Historical dose:*** All potencies.

CLINICAL - Abuse, effects. Alcoholism. Alzheimer's disease. Amnesia. Anxiety. ***Bipolar. Brain, disorders.*** Brain, weakness. Constipation. Coughs. Debility. ***Delusions. Dementia.*** Dermatitis. Dysmenorrhea. Dyspepsia. Eczema. Elephantiasis. ***Fears.*** Hallucinations. Headache. Hearing, disorders. Heart disorders. Hemorrhoids. ***Humiliation.*** Hypochondriasis. Hypoglycemia. Hysteria. ***Insanity.*** Lichen planus. ***Manic depression. Memory, loss. Mental, disorders.*** Mental, weakness. ***Multiple, personalities.*** Neuralgia. Neurasthenia. Nervous. Palpitations. Paralysis. Pemphigus. ***Phobias. Poison, ivy. Religious, mania.*** Rheumatism. ***Rhus, poisoning.*** Self-abuse. ***Senile, dementia. Schizophrenia.*** Skin, diseases. Smell, illusions. Spinal, disorders. Stiff neck. Strokes. Tendonititis. Urticaria. Vesicular eruptions. Vomiting, pregnancy. Whooping cough. Warts. Writer's cramp.

HERBAL - The nut is heart-shaped, hence its name Anacardium orientale, and perhaps this may be taken as the ***"signature"*** of its courage imparting properties. Found in Asia, native of East Indies and found in mountainous dry forests. Juice in the external rind of nut is used. Excellent ink made from this nut.

Indians after depriving the nut of its external rind and juice roast and eat it with much relish. The juice which is in cells under the rind is of such acridity that it is used by natives to burn off warts, condylomata and other excrescences and keep down excessive granulation in ulcers.

Ancient writers recommended it chiefly in mental diseases - loss of memory, nervous disorders. Abuse of this drug is harmful leading to madness. Poisonous, acrid, vesicant, purgative and narcotic properties prevail in varying degree throughout the order.

Anacardium has many features in common with its botanical relatives, the different species of Rhus, especially in its action on the skin, muscles, and joints, but it has also very distinct features of its own.

HOMEOPATHIC - Anacardium acts on the mind, nerves, muscles and joints. Its skin symptoms are similar to Rhus-t. and it has proved a valuable ***antidote to poison oak and ivy***. Syphilitic patients often suffer with these conditions.

It is used for neurasthenics, such have a type of nervous dyspepsia, relieved by food. Physical and mental lack of power. Special senses are weakened. ***Sensation of a plug*** in various parts-eyes, rectum, bladder, etc., also of a band. Empty feeling in stomach. Intermittent symptoms.

Gnawing hunger, desire to nibble, hypoglycemia. ***Great emptiness in the stomach with weakness and irritability.*** Worse from fasting or missing a meal. ***Better after eating.*** Indigestion, pain is worse when digestion is complete, lasts until the next meal, then better for some time (Nux-v.). ***Eating temporarily relieves all discomfort***. Dypepsia. Constipation.

Headache worse by mental exertion, better by eating. Stiffness of neck, worse beginning to move. The senses are either too weak or too acute and there are sense illusions, a light has a halo, optical illusions in dark colors, illusions of hearing, illusions of smell: burning tinder, pigeon's dung.

Trembling, on slight exertion, worse knees or arms. Emaciation. Paresis of muscles subject to volition. Paralytic condition. Diseases of spinal cord. Heaviness and fullness of the whole body after piano playing. Cramp like pains in muscles. ***Contraction of joints.*** Injured or strained tendons.

MIND - Anacardium has won for itself a reputation for the ***"fear of examinations"*** and allied conditions. ***Mental disorders.*** There is physical and mental lack of power. ***Brain fatigue.*** Aversion to work, wants to lie or sit continually. ***Nervous exhaustion from overstudy***. Special senses are weakened, sight, hearing touch etc. Cowardly. ***Lack of confidence*** in himself or others. Lack of self-esteem.

Absent-minded. Senile dementia. ***Bad memory.*** Impaired memory. Loss of memory from fright or mortification. ***Forgetfulness makes her low-spirited.*** Suddenly forgets names of those around her. Forgets what she has seen. Vanishing of thoughts, deficiency of ideas and loss of subject without knowing it. Alzheimer's disease.

Phobias. Apprehends trouble from everything. Fear of impending misfortune. Anxiety about every trifle. Hypochondriasis. Anxiety when walking, as if pursued. Fear of examinations in students. Fear of the future. Fear of paralysis. Refuses to eat for fear of being poisoned. Fastidious, can't rest when things are not in proper place.

Extremely irritable, passionate and contradictory. Angry and depressed. ***Very easily offended***. Excessive anger at slight offence, breaking out in violent behaviour. Irresistible desire to swear and curse. ***Tendency to use foul, violent language.*** Malicious, seems bent on wickedness. Great propensity to ***curse, swear and blaspheme*** in persons not usually known to curse. Hard hearted, cruel. Unsociable. Absence of all moral restraint.

Profound depression and hypochondriasis, with tendency to use violent language. ***Manic depression.*** Forsaken feeling. Estrangement from individuals and society. Shuns people. ***Victims of verbal, physical and sexual abuse.*** Despairs of getting well. Feeling of helplessness. ***Ailments from humiliation, punishments.*** Mental dullness and gloom after sexual indulgence. There is a tendency to suicide by shooting (Ant-c.).

Schizophrenia (Lach.). Alcoholism. Suspicious and jealous (Hyos., Lach.). ***Religious mania.*** Senseless talk. Internal conflicts. ***Contradictory impulses.*** Conflicted over sexual desire, intense desire or aversion to sex. Sexual perversions. Clairaudient. ***Hears voices,*** of persons far away, spirits or dead people. Hears voices behind her. Hears voices saying he is going to die.

Fixed ideas and delusions of various kinds. There is no reality in anything, all appears as in a dream. Hallucinations. Delusion he is under superhuman control. ***Delusion that a demon and an angel sit on his shoulders telling him offensive or good things.*** Delusion that he is double. Seems to have two wills, one good, one bad. ***Feels as if he had two wills, one commanding him to do what the other forbids.*** Delusion that her husband is not her husband, her child is not hers. Delusion that the mind and body are separated. Sees everybody's face in mirror except his own.

Abdomen - Abdomen full and distended. Colic. ***Pain as if dull plug were pressed into intestines***. Rumbling, pinching and griping, especially with flatulent colic. Pain as if a dull plug were pressed into intestine. Hardness of abdomen.

Back - Lumbago with painful stiffness. Dull pressure in the shoulders, as from a weight. Stiffness at nape of neck, down back and pain worse motion. As of a heavy weight on sides of neck and back. Tearing pain between scapulae.

Causations - ***Abuse, verbal, physical and sexual.*** Checked eruptions. Examinations. Fright. ***Humiliation.***

Chest - Anxiety in region of sternum. Pressure in chest, as from a dull plug. Oppression of chest with internal heat and anxiety, driving him into open air. Rawness and scraping in chest. As if contracted, while walking, during headache. Itching on chest. Violent eczema on chest and throat. Redness of skin, with little vesicles itching intolerably.

Constitutions - Anac. is suited to neurasthenic patients. Suited to manic-depressives. Ill-natured children. Elderly senile people. Frequently indicated in depressed, nervous and paranoid people. Hypochondriacs. Women during pregnancy, gastric and nervous disorders.

Cough - Cough excited by talking in children after fit of temper. Cough after eating with vomiting of food and pain in occiput. Cough then yawns and sleeps. Paroxysms of coughing every three or four hours. Cough more violent every other or every third day. Violent cough with loss of smell and taste.

Ears - Pressing in the ears as from a plug. Otorrhea. Itching in ears. Painful swelling of external ear. Catarrh of eustachian tubes. Hard of hearing. Imagines whispers in the ears. Humming. Roaring.

Eyes - Eyes as if swollen, but without pain. ***Pressing pain like a plug*** on upper orbit. Lachrymation during coryza. Lids so swollen he can hardly see. Great sensitiveness to light. Dim vision as if looking through mist. ***Objects appear too far off.*** Optical illusions in dark colors. Threads and black spots before the eyes. Shortsighted. Pupils first contracted, then dilated.

Face - Redness of face, in mania. Blue rings around eyes. Face pale with sunken eyes. Expressionless, wild, childish. Eczema of face and neck. Violent burning pain. Tetters around mouth. Rough, scaly skin. White, scaly herpes. Twitching of mouth in sleep.

Female - Frequent but scanty menses with spasmodic pain in abdomen. Pressing pain in uterus, with pain in abdomen. Vaginitis. Leucorrhea with itching and excoriation of the parts. Leucorrhea with soreness and itching. Much loss of blood after miscarriage. Melancholy after childbirth. Morning sickness. Nausea during pregnancy better eating.

Food - ***Loss of appetite*** with fever and skin symptoms. Loss of appetite, alternating with violent hunger. Refuses to eat for fear of being poisoned. Food tastes flat and offensive. Bitter taste in mouth after smoking tobacco. Everything tastes like herring-brine. Thirst for milk with sweat all over. ***Thirst during fever.*** Constant thirst, yet drinking takes breath away.

Head - Gastric and nervous headaches. Hot head, with icy-cold hands and feet. ***Headache worse by mental exertion, better by eating.*** Headache from strong smells. ***Pressing pain, as from a plug,*** in forehead, occiput, temples or vertex. Pressing pain worse coughing, deep breathing after mental exertion. ***Headaches, better after a meal.*** Headaches, better falling asleep. Vertex as if constricted. Violent pressure in right or left temple. Throbbing in occiput. Tearing pain during hard labor. Baldness. Itching and little boils on scalp.

Heart - Restless feeling at heart. Double stitch at the heart, passing into lumbar region. Beating in bloodvessels. Palpitations with coryza in the aged. Sharp pains in heart during inspiration, at night. Rheumatic pericarditis with double stitches.

Kidneys - Constant desire to urinate. Frequent urging with but small discharge. Frequent urination at night. Frequent discharge of clear watery urine, deposits, turbid, clay colored sediment.

Limbs - Tired feeling. Paralytic weakness. Knees feel paralyzed or bandaged. Pressure as from a plug in the glutei. Pain in ankle, as if sprained worse stepping. Painful thumping on the middle upper arm (left). Cramps in the calves worse walking or rising from a seat. Cramps from toe to instep from heel up calf. Dry hands. Fingers swollen with vesicular eruption. Writer's cramp. Neuralgia in thumb. Warts on palms and hands.

Lungs - Asthma, hysterical, ends in flow of tears. Breath stops, on coughing or swallowing. Dyspnea in children who have an uncontrollable temper. Attacks of suffocation. Sweetish, flat tasting mucus. Purulent, tenacious mucus. Greyish-yellow mucus. Expectoration only during day.

Male - Sensation of burning in the penis during and after urination. Cutting pain along penis. Prostatic discharge during the stool. Voluptuous itching of scrotum, exciting sexual desire. Seminal emissions without dreams. Enjoyment absent during sex. Sexual excesses and perversions.

Modalities - Symptoms disappear during dinner, but begin anew after two hours. ***Better from eating.*** Better lying on side. Better from rubbing. Better heat, hot bath. Better being in the sun. ***Worse from mental exertion***. Worse emotions, anger, fright, care. ***Worse from abuse and mortification.*** Worse on application of hot water. Worse stepping hard. Worse motion. Worse drafts, open air. Worse cold. Worse hours after eating. Worse rubbing, scratching. Worse from talking. Worse morning. Worse evening to midnight. Worse from checked eruptions. Worse strong smells.

Mouth - Bad breath and taste. Taste lost. Flat offensive taste. Painful vesicles, fetid odor. Tongue feels swollen and stiff, impeding speech and motion with saliva in mouth. Tongue white, and rough like a grater. Ulcers in mouth. Burning around lips as from pepper. Painful vesicles.

Nose - Chronic coryza, with loss of smell and discharge of purulent mucus. Frequent sneezing, followed by coryza and lachrymation. Violent coryza with palpitation especially in the aged. Soreness in nostrils. Red pustule in right nostril on septum. ***Sense of smell perverted***. Smell lost or acute. Illusory smell of burning tinder.

Perspiration - Sweats better while eating. Clammy sweat on palms especially left. Sweats in evening, on head, abdomen and back, even when sitting quiet. Cold sweat with internal heat.

Rectum - ***Rectum seems powerless.*** Bowels inactive. Soft stool passes with difficulty. ***Ineffectual desire. Rectum as if plugged up***. Spasmodic constriction of anal sphincter. ***Itching of anus.*** Painful hemorrhoids. ***Moisture from rectum***. Hemorrhage during stool. Stools of very pale color. Stools mushy, bloody, brown, liver-like. Painless stools.

Sensations - ***Sensation of a plug*** in various parts. Sensation as if a ***dull pressure,*** is repeated from time to time. Sensations of a band or hoop.

Skin - Itching worse scratching. ***Intense itching.*** Eczema with mental irritability. Neurotic eczema. Skin insensible. Dermatitis. Lichen planus. Ulcer on forearm. Urticaria. Promotes expulsion of splinters. ***Eruption like that of poison-oak*** (Xero., Grind., Croto-t.). Weals, exuding a viscid, yellowish fluid. ***Vesicular eruption, swelling***. Yellow vesicles. Blisters discharging a yellowish transparent liquid. White herpetic spots. Smallpox like eruptions. Warts on palms and hands.

Sleep - Spells of sleeplessness lasting for several nights. Sleeplessness from restlessness, itching. Vivid dreams. Anxious dreams. Dreams of fire. Dreams of dead bodies, tombs.

Stomach - Gastric pain, better by eating, but worse again after 2 to 3 hours. ***Empty feeling in stomach***. Spasmodic pain. Hiccough. Weak digestion with fullness and distention. ***Eating relieves dyspepsia***. Rumbling and fermentation. Heartburn after eating soup. Swallows food and drinks hastily. Eructations, nausea, vomiting. Nausea in morning with empty feeling in stomach. Morning sickness. Nausea with retching. Vomiting of food during pregnancy, better eating. Better from vomiting.

Teeth - Toothache on taking something warm in mouth. Tearing pain in lower incisor, worse contact with tongue and in open air. Teeth of lower jaw seem most affected. Bleeding of gums upon slight rubbing. Swelling of gums.

Temperature - Easily chilled, better sunshine. Chills even in a warm room. Chilliness internal with external heat. Chills over back, as if cold water were poured over it, with heat of face. Internal chills with hot breath. Heat from 4 p.m. until evening passing off after supper. Heat of upper body with cold feet. Internal shiverings and hot breath. Heat of left side.

Throat - Apt to choke when eating or drinking. Firm tough mucus in fauces

Suppuration of tonsils. Sensation as if blunt plugs in throat. Sensation of scraping in throat. Sensation of rawness, during cough. Pressure pain or aching near larynx. Voice hoarse and deep. Rattling in trachea when lying on side.

Vertigo - Vertigo worse walking, stooping and rising from stooping. Vertigo objects seem too distant. Vertigo as if turning in a circle. Vertigo with blackness before eyes. Vertigo as if surroundings or self were tottering.

COMMENTS - Characteristic pressing or penetrating pain as from a plug, which may occur in any locality in connection with neuralgias, ear disorders and hemorrhoids.

Alzheimer's disease (Staph., Hyos.), may be accompanied with personality changes. Brain fatigue. Marked loss of memory. Deafness with loss of memory. Fear of exams and failure.

Cough better by eating. Whooping cough with a gasping and drowsiness after the cough. Morning sickness, better by eating, but returns soon after. Symptoms generally better by eating, recur two hours after. Intermittent symptoms.

"The attacks ceased for one or two days and then continued again for a couple of days." Guided by this indication alone, Custis cured a case of sleeplessness in a pregnant woman with Anacardium 200c. "Spells of sleeplessness lasting for several nights."

Disorders of the palms of the hands. There are warts even on the palms. Skin eruptions in general (Rhus-t.).

Bayes' indications are "brain fatigue before examination," "nerve-exhaustion from over-study." "nervous prostration from seminal emissions," or sexual excess. Conflicted over sexual desire, intense desire or aversion to sex.

Paralyzed feeling in knees. Sensation as if knees were bandaged. Sensation of a hoop or band around the body or about any part is a leading symptom. Sensation of a blunt object anywhere.

It has been used with success in diseases of the spinal cord with this sensation and the feeling of a plug in the spine, worse by any motion which causes a pain as if the plug were sticking still further in. Kent noted it for tendonititis.

Paranoid schizophrenia, multiple personalities (Plat.), manic depression (Lach.), symptoms of Lyc. and Nux-v. combined and intensified. Keynote separation of the will, "delusion" that there's an angel on the right shoulder and a devil on the left shoulder.

The moral consciousness becomes polarized. Keynote that they can hear voices telling them to do evil. Moral struggle to fight impulses to hurt people. Rubrics are "lack of moral feeling," "godlessness," not lack of religious feeling, but a feeling that they can't be punished. Impulses so strong they shake and tremble. Misanthropy. Deep, suppressed anger and humiliation. History of hard-tempered and low confidence. Inner antagonism.

Delusions of sight and smell, fears of spirits, demons, paranoia, hallucinations. Hears voices, keynote. Irresistible desire to curse and swear, can be used for Tourette's syndrome (close to Plat., but Plat. talks about sex.).

Religious mania (Verat., Lach.). Feels that he is possessed. Become frightened of their anger, of their own hardness and uncompassionate nature, moral conflicts, turn to religion to restrain themselves. Fear of losing control. Dramatic alteration of moods, deep guilt and torment about their soul and salvation alternating with a mania, maliciousness and impulsiveness.

Clarke cured with it a man who had a smell of burning wood in his nose, remaining after influenza.

RELATIONS - ***Antidotes:*** Grind., Coffea, Jug-c., Rhus-t, Eucalyptus. ***Compare:*** (1) Anac. occidentale, Rhus-t., Cypr., Chel., Xero. (2) Cereus serpentina - swearing. (3) Com., Rhus-t., Rhus-v. (4) Ant-t., Apis, Cori-r., Ferr., Iod., Jug-c., Lyc., Nit-ac., Nux-v., Ph-ac., Plat., Urt-u., Puls., Nat-m., Caust. (5) Thuj. - fixed ideas. ***Related remedies:*** Ign., Lyc, Plat, Rhus-t. Platina follows well. It is an antidote to Rhus-t. if there are gastric symptoms, or symptoms going from right to left.

REFERENCES - Boericke. Clarke. Murphy.

ANAGALLIS ARVENSIS

(Scarlet Pimpernel)

PHARMACY - anag. Anagallis arvensis. Scarlet pimpernel. Weather-glass. Red¨chickweed. N. O. Primulacae. Tincture of whole fresh plant. The fresh plant of the scarlet-flowered variety, gathered before the development of the flowers is pounded to a pulp and subjected to pressure. The expressed juice is mingled with an equal part by weight of alcohol. ***Historical dose:*** Tincture and all potencies.

CLINICAL - Active mind. Amblyopia. Cataract. Constipation. Convulsions. Dropsy. Epilepsy. Gonorrhea. Gout. hemorrhoids. Headache. Hypochondriasis. Hysteria. Itching. Mania. Neuralgia. Nosebleed. Rheumatism. Ringworm. Skin, unhealthy. Snakebites. Syphilis. Tetters. Ulcers. Wounds.

HERBAL - The Greek name of the plant means to laugh out loud. It produces great exhilaration and over activity of mind. Great hilarity. An ancient medicine for hydrophobia and dropsy. It is a vulnerary of some importance.

Like the Primula obconca, Anagallis has a marked action on the skin, characterized by great itching and tingling everywhere. Possesses power of softening flesh and destroying warts. Ill-conditioned ulcers. It favors expulsion of splinters. Anagallis has been used for snakebites and ulcers.

HOMEOPATHIC - Skin itches all over, becomes dry and rough. Tetters. Vesicles in groups. Ulcers and swellings on joints. Bran-like, ring-shaped tetters on face. Eruption on chest. Skin of hands dry, stick and dirty-looking.

Soreness on chest with pain. Pains in joints going from place to place. Rheumatic and gouty pains. Dropsy. Tensive drawing ascending from left shoulder to nape of neck (Eup-per.). Pain and tightness in bend of left knee.

Tickling and itching in left ear. Dull pains in gums accompanied by very hard stools. Sensation on tongue as if something cold were placed on it. Dryness and scraping in throat. Scraping, scratching of larynx and trachea with hoarseness, worse after eating. Syphilis with nosebleed, deranged mind, pain in small of back and itching skin. Tickling prickling along urethra orifice agglutinated. Tearing in spermatic cord.

MIND - Great hilarity, exhilarated feeling. Cannot collect his thoughts while listening on account of jovial feelings. Mind very active. Despondency. Great prostration after mental exertion.

Abdomen - Distended with wind, weak feeling in abdomen.

Causations - Mental work causes great prostration (Pic-ac.).

Constitutions - Psoric, allergic constitutions.

Eyes - Pain in right eyeball, worse from touching lids.

Head - Headache over supra-orbital ridges with rumbling in bowels and belchings, better from coffee. Sick headache. Pain in facial muscles.

Kidneys - More or less irritation in urethra inclining to sex. Burning pain on urinating with agglutination of orifice. Urine passes in several streams, must press before it passes. Urine is dark, straw-colored, urine escapes in divided stream (Thuj.).

Limbs - Rheumatic and gouty pains. Pain in shoulder and arm. Cramp in ball of thumbs and fingers.

Modalities - Better from coffee, relieves headache. Burning in urethra before and during erection, ceases during sex. Worse by touch. Worse after eating.

Mouth - Viscid saliva in mouth, raised by coughing, water in mouth with tearing pains in molars.

Neck - Tensive drawing, ascending from left shoulder to nape of neck, worse from raising and extending arm.

Nose - Nosebleed. Violent sneezing, expelling lumps of yellow phlegm. Running water from nose. Copious secretion of yellow phlegm.

Pelvis - Violent pain in sacrum when lifting a slight load.

Skin - ***Itching,*** dry, bran-like eruption, especially on ***hands and fingers***. Palms especially affected. ***Ulcers*** and swellings on joints. Rough, dry, bran-like tetters in rings. Groups of small vesicles, smarting and itching, oozing a yellowish-brown lymph, which soon turns into a scurf, new vesicles appearing beneath. Promotes expulsion of splinters (Hep.).

Stools - Hemorrhoids. Offensive flatus. Stools soft and pappy, watery diarrhea. Stools hard like stone, knotty.

Teeth - Pain as from cold.

RELATIONS - ***Compare:*** (1) Primula obcon. Anagallis contains Saponin. (2) Similar to Coffea - joyous, excited. (3) Picric acid - prostration after mental exertion. (4) Cyclamen - sneezing. (5) Lith. - cough skin, ringworm. Sep., Tell. (6) Puls. - chilliness, catarrhs.

REFERENCES - Boericke. Clarke.

ANANTHERUM MURICATUM

(Cuscus grass)

PHARMACY - anan. Anantherum muricatum. Cuscus grass. Andropogon muricatus. Andropogon squarrosus. Vetiver. Viti-vayr. N. O. Gramineae. India. Tincture of root. ***Historical dose:*** Tincture and all potencies.

CLINICAL - Abscesses. Aphonia. Boils. Cancer. Chancre-like sores. Colic. Erysipelas. Glandular inflammation. Hair, loss. Herpes. Hydrophobia. Sycosis. Syphilis. Tic convulsive. Tic douloureux. Tumors. Ulcers.

HOMEOPATHIC - A medicinal grass cultivated in the Markarentas Islands, East India. Anantherum has produced a state of drunkenness and intoxication. Farrington noted if for "Erysipelas with much swelling of arms and legs, dark red or bluish eruptions with tendency to suppurate."

Anantherum is a skin remedy of high order. Abscesses, boils. Abscesses, ulcers and fissures on arms and hands. Tumors of breast, ulcerated indurated.

Herpes and ulcers or scabs on scalp. Tumors, wart-like growths on eyebrows. Falling off of eyebrows and beard. Chancre-like ulcers on penis. Eruptions like itch or lichen. Ulcers at labial commissures. Pustules like smallpox on vulva. Syphilis.

Severe neuralgic headache, as if bells moved about in head, as of steel arrows from forehead to nape. Pains in facial bones as if crushed or ulcerated. Convulsive tic. Plugged sensation. Glandular swellings especially of sub-maxillary and cervical glands. Swelling of tonsils, constriction of throat, inability to swallow. Painful swelling of various parts extending to suppuration.

MIND - Sadness and restlessness with fear of death and the future. Sheds tears easily. Dread of society. Seeks solitude and obscurity. Apathetic. Anger with desire to strike and destroy. Quarrelsome, but after being angry he often regrets what he has done. Jealousy. Foolish joy and absurd complacency.

Changes in his mood and turn of thought. Ardent desire to travel. Blunted intellect and loss of memory. Haste in all his actions. Persistent fear of death during all his suffering. Monomania, as for rowing about in a boat, dressing or walking out in a grotesque manner, always frequenting the same places and doing the same things.

Abdomen - Cramps, lancination and digging in the region of the spleen with loss of respiration. Spleen as if ulcerated and hypertrophied. Burning in the whole abdomen, as if he had erysipelas. Inflammation and swelling of the abdomen, very painful. Abdomen inflated, tense and hard, with tympanitic sound on percussion. Colic, cramps and tearing pains in the abdomen, sensation as if there were a red-hot iron in it.

Breasts - Breasts swollen indurated, nipples excoriated. The breasts are atrophied and become soft. Heat and pain in the breasts, as if they had been gashed with a penknife. Inflammation and swelling. Congestions of the breasts as from accumulation of milk. Lancinating, pulsating and pressive pains. Excoriation of the nipples.

Constitutions - Psoric and allergic constitutions.

Ears - Very copious secretion of cerumen. Heat and smarting in the lobes of the ears. Fissures in the lobes of the ears. Noises, murmurs and hissing in the ears.

Eyes - Heat and burning in the eyes. Pressure and painful stitches in the eyes. Photophobia. The eyelids are inverted and as if scarified. Abundant secretion of mucus and considerable lachrymation, especially in the open air. Trembling of the lids.

Eyes - Swelling and ulceration of the lachrymal glands. Weakness of the eyes.

Face - Face yellowish or red, enlarged inflamed and congested. Face pale, transparent and white as wax. Face gray, cold and frozen looking and paralyzed. Face emaciated, bluish, cyanotic, contracted, shrunken with hollow eyes.

Female - Scirrhus-like swelling of cervix. Prolapsed uterus. Sterility, as from atrophy of the ovaries. Swelling of the uterus. Menstruation very painful and copious, the blood generally bright or light-colored. Menstruation retarded, the blood dark, thick, followed by fetid leucorrhea. Suppression of menses. Menstruation frequent and painful. Great itching and burning in the vulva. Whitish and reddish eruptions on the vulva. Leucorrhea watery, clear or milky and of very bad odor. Thick, purulent, yellow or green leucorrhea.

Food - Morbid hunger, wakes up in night to eat, as if he had a tapeworm. Burning, unquenchable thirst. Longing for aromatic drinks.

Head - Pains pierce brain like pointed arrows, worse in afternoon. Herpes, ulcers and tumors on scalp. Wart-like growth on eyebrows. Boils and tumors on tip of nose.

Heart - Burning and sensation of weight in the heart with sadness, anguish and fear of death. Stitches and formication in the heart with great anxiety.

Kidneys - Turbid, thick urine, full of mucus. Bladder cannot hold smallest quantity. Involuntary. Cystitis. ***Constant urging to urinate*** with stitches and crushing pains in the kidneys. Frequent emission of urine, which is turbid or soon becomes so. Sensation of a numbness and obstruction in the kidneys and bladder were always full and swollen.

Liver - Sensation of heat and of congestion of the liver. Cramps in the hepatic region with sensation as if it were full of painful tuberosities.

Male - Excoriations on the prepuce and urethral meatus. Secretion of a thick substance of very strong odor, between the glans and prepuce, which are swollen. Burning, stitching and pinching in the penis. Syphilitic-looking pimples on the penis with intense pains, traversing from one part of another.

Modalities - Coffee at first worse, then better. Wine and coffee aggravates the toothache.

Mouth - Tongue fissured, as if cut on edges, copious salivation. Constant inclination to clench the teeth. Sensation of cold in the teeth with heat in the gums and the whole mouth. Burning in the teeth, gums and lips, as if they were burned. Gum-boils. Very painful pimples on the tongue with itching and burning.

Rectum - Very long-lasting constipation, followed by dry, brown, bulky stools, then diarrhea. Obstinate constipation with fever, heat, thirst, sweat and debility. Stools difficult, large and hard, knotty like sheep-dung, passed with difficulty, even after the use of injections.

Sleep - Restless sleep with cries, starting up, movements of the limbs and anxious dreams. Comatose sleep with disturbing dreams and snoring. Prolonged sleep in the morning with inclination to lie abed late. Sleep with frequent dreams, alternate coldness and heat and burning of the whole body, intense thirst and fright.

Stomach - Obstinate, convulsive hiccough. Burning in the stomach, as if it were on fire. Excessive and almost continual secretion of phlegm. Vomiting of the food and of bile, with hunger even after eating. Vomiting of food and often of blood after meals. Vomiting of acrid, burning matter, followed by bile and blood. Pains in the stomach with cold sweats on the face and back.

Skin - Itching. Offensive foot sweat. Diseased and deformed nails. Herpes. ***Abscesses***, boils and ***ulcers***. Erysipelas. Chancre-like sores.

COMMENTS - Burning and stitches. Thirsty, but cannot drink. Burning heat alternating with icy coldness in gullet, as of something alive in gullet. Involuntary urination when walking and during sleep.

Formication as from ants. Ulcers yellowish, violet, swollen, everted, syphilitic.

Discharges from ulcers are foul, foul breath and belchings. Sexual desire increased by every attempt to satisfy it until driven to onanism and madness.

RELATIONS - ***Compare:*** (1) Staph., Merc., Thuj.

REFERENCES - Boericke. Clarke.

ANDERSONIA ROHITIKA

(Plihaghati)

PHARMACY - ander. Andersonia rohitika. Plihaghati. N. O. Mediaceae. Stem and root bark. ***Historical dose:*** Tincture and all potencies.

CLINICAL - Biliousness. Debility. Fever. Glands, enlarged. Gonorrhea. Heat, flushes. Jaundice. Leucorrhea. Liver, enlarged. Malaria. Nausea. ***Spleen, disorders.*** Spleen, enlarged. Vomiting.

HERBAL - Rohitaka is a large tree and is generally found in many districts of Bengal. It also grows in Assam, Sylhet and Cachar and also in Western India, Burma, Malacca and some other places this plant can be found.

Rohitaka has been named by Ayurvedic physicians as Plihaghati meaning thereby that it does away with all splenic disorders.

The Ayurvedic physicians have found it to be alternative, astringent and tonic. They prize it as an excellent remedy in the enlargement of liver and spleen, in corpulence and enlarged glands and also in general debility. They have also recommended it in gonorrhea.

Chakradatta, Charaka and other ayurvedic authorities have recommended it in the splenic affections, mucus gonorrhea, and leucorrhea. they have also found it efficacious in hepatic affections and derangements as well. They have recommended it for jaundice, dropsical swellings, chronic fevers and some other diseases.

HOMEOPATHIC - Dr. Pramada Prasanna Biswas of Padna, Bengal, personally proved this drug. The following symptoms set in while it was proved:

MIND - Easily angered. Mistakes in spelling take place. Memory become dull and disordered. Cannot fix mind on any subject or matter.

Abdomen - Heat is felt in the lower abdomen. Pains are felt in the right and left hypochondrium. Enlargement of both liver and spleen and burning sensation is felt here.

Eyes - Eyes, burn.

Face - Face, eyes, burn. Flushes of heat come out of the face.

Head - Heat in the head, especially on the vertex. Giddiness of head. Feeling of warmth or heat in the head, specially on the frontal region. Sensation of pain in the temples associated with heat which is relieved by cold breeze or cold application. Burning sensation is felt in the eyes and face.

Limbs - Hands and feet burn. Burning sensation is felt there. The patient feels great relief if body coverings are thrown off.

Modalities - Open air, cold breeze or cold application generally mitigates or relieves all pains, specially burning of the body.

Mouth - Heat comes out of the mouth. Insipid taste in the mouth. In the morning taste becomes bad and bitter.

Stomach - Burning sensation is felt in the stomach with urging for vomiting. Sensation of heat is felt in the stomach and spasmodic colic due to indigestion ensues. Nausea and vomiting. Also an attempt at vomiting. Water comes out of the mouth.

Temperature - There is feverishness with headache with frontal pains. During fever aching pains are felt. Body becomes hot. Face, eyes hands and feet burn.

COMMENTS - It is alternative, astringent, and tonic, given in enlarged gland, as liver and spleen, in corpulence and in general debility. (R. N. Khory, Materia Medica of India. vol. II, p. 118)

R. N. Chopra in his Indigenous Drugs of India, p. 461, says: "It is an aperient used in enlarged glands, liver and spleen diseases and corpulence."

It is a splendid remedy in all disorders of the spleen, either enlarged or painful.

It is also an excellent medicine in all hepatic derangement.

In chronic slow malarial fevers associated with the enlargement of the spleen and liver its action is supreme. It is particularly useful for patients with bilious temperament.

Fever with headache and burning temperature. Fever with headache and burning sensation of eyes, face, hands and feet, they desire to have cold breeze or cold application which ameliorates all burning sensations experienced by them.

There is constipation which is a characteristic symptom of the drug. There is no desire for food. Taste of the mouth is insipid or bitter. The patient feels laziness while getting out of the bed in the morning.

REFERENCES - Ghose.

ANDROCTONOS AMURREUXI

(Scorpion)

PHARMACY - androc. Androctonos amurreuxi hebraeus. Scorpio europaeus. N. O. Scorpionida. Arachnida. A scorpion of West Asia. Tincture of animals. ***Historical dose:*** All potencies.

CLINICAL - Apathy. Backache. Constipated. Fatigue. Headache. Hemorrhoids. Memory, weak. Nausea. Nightmares. Salivation. Strabismus. Tetanus.

HOMEOPATHIC - The scorpion was a major remedy in ancient Egyptian medicine. A proving of scorpion is written in the medical papyruses, which give a vivid description of Isis allowing herself to be stung to determine the effects of the medicine.

A proving on a middle eastern scorpion was conducted by Jeremy Sherr. Most provers were between age 25 to 40 years old. The symptoms are from the provings and effects of the stings.

Pain and swelling of the injured part are first experienced followed by sleepiness, prostration and possibly tetanus. Strabismus has been observed in some cases and the pupils are dilated.

The bitten part is very swollen with violent pains lasting from one to three days. Heat and pain at bitten spot, sleepiness, sneezing, restlessness, later, abundant saliva, meteorism, later, trismus or tetanus. Complete prostration. Always acute pains in and diminished temperature of the part bitten. Scorpion stings are attended with a certain amount of danger, especially for children.

MIND - Forgetful. Absent-minded. Mind dull and foggy, better while moving and walking. Difficulty applying self. Lack of concentration with daydreaming and difficulty in mental exertion. Mind blank when concentrating. Unable to think of more than one thing at a time. Mistakes in writing and spelling. Speech slurred, answered with difficulty. Conversation difficult.

Weariness. Tired and apathetic. Felt detached, very interested in little things. Dreamy and staring. Felt disconnected from the human race, as if everyone were another species. Depressed and destructive. Aversion to things she usually enjoyed. Averse to work.

Very changeable moods, one moment extremely friendly, nice and amiable, then irritable. Incredible upsurge of energy, felt very high, then low, then high again. Great swings of mood, better from eating. Clumsy. Accident-prone. As if drunk, with increased sexual desire. Desire to be out in the country.

Hurried, restless. Impatient watching others. Time seems to go slowly. Irritable, snappy, oversensitive to noise and bright lights, can't bear music. Argumentative, critical. Feels resentful and abused. Great hostility to those around him. Assertive, impatient, aggressive. Angry with her children and family. Terrible uncontrollable temper. Wanted to kill her husband and children.

Panic-stricken. Fear, as if something terrible would happen. Overwhelmed by terror, panic and fear. Terrified of dogs, fearful while driving. Anguish and worry, anxiety for no reason. Anxiety about health. Anxiety for self, friends and the world, with continual sighing.

Despairing, tearful mood, could see no way out. Sadness and confusion. Feels sorry for herself, better crying. Sympathetic, took on other people's problems. Desires company and sympathy. Indisposed to talk and averse to company. Disappointed with people.

Abdomen - Short, sharp, strong, stabbing cramps below ribs. Clinching feeling of panic in abdomen, as if nearly had an accident. Ache in lower abdomen. Pains in intestines feel bruised and sore. Pain in morning, in a horizontal line in intestine, headache alternates with pain in the abdomen. Pain in liver, a deep stitch, worse exertion, movement, walking fast. Pain upper abdomen, above naval in the morning.

Back - Feeling of cold in back while in bed. Sudden and tremendous pain and stiffness. Pain, cramp and stiffness left side neck. Pain between scapulae extending down spine. Numbness and tingling at middle edge of left scapula. Aching and bruised sensation in sacral region. Backache, worse sitting or beginning motion. Pain radiates to sides, pelvis, diaphragm. Feeling of weight in back as if the affected vertebrae were made of lead. Pain in one vertebra. Sharp pain in back, worse breathing deeply.

Breasts - Felt as if breasts were very big. Held breasts, then walked around massaging breasts.

Chest - Anxiety in chest. Pressure, compression on chest. Oppression as if a cushion were inside chest cavity, pressing organ down to spine. Sensation of expansion of chest. Pain in left breast and lymph glands. Itching axilla.

Dreams - Oppressive dreams before waking. Feeling of jealousy. Vague, troublesome dreams, later part of sleep. Dreams are confused, angry, busy, erotic, frightful, violent, guilty. Dreams of a car crash, climbing ladders, bus steps. Dreams of naked women, of being attacked and murdered. Dreams of past events, of events not yet taken place. Dreams of water, of orange and red walls, of toilets and feces. Dreams of people's heads chopped off, that she was weighing them.

Ears - Sharp pain in ears, down canal, as if a sharp pencil was pushed down into the ear. Pressure inside ears. Pain, aching in left ear, extending to the jaw and moving to the back of the right ear. Discomfort, tickling and ringing in left ear. Itch in left meatus of ear. Wave-like sound within and around ears, worse at night. Loud ringing in the ears. Blocked ears, with slight deafness. Hearing dull, as if cotton wool in ears.

Eyes - Pupils dilated. Strabismus. Aversion to sunlight. Eyes water, red and smarting. Eyes sore and hot, feel strained. Eyelids inflamed. Eyes small, puffy, lusterless and tired. Flashes of blue pinpoints on objects when suddenly moving head or bending down. Flashing ripples when closing eyes in bed. Focusing eyes difficult, can focus on distant objects, but close objects are blurred. Eyes sticky, woke with eyes stuck together. Desire to close the eyes. Eyes are heavy, aching and tired.

Face - Cold sores. Face pale and hollow, drained. Face dark purple, rings around the eyes. Top lip cracked, burning at corners. Sore painful patch in right hand corner of lip, as if would crack. Dry and cracked lips. Cracked lips bleeding after cold wind. Trismus. Jaw aches, worse movement of jaw.

Female - Menses early, short. Pain dragging during menses, worse than usual. Pain gathering, as if parts were in an iron grip, lasting one hour. Sharp, griping pain shooting from uterus to bowel. Pain during menstrual period, extending down back of legs. Pain bearing down during menses. Pink-brown vaginal discharge with dull dragging in sacral region. Sticky yellow vaginal discharge. Genital area felt painfully oversensitive. Pressing pain in ovarian region on urinating, better urinating, worse pressure. Extremely passionate, increased desire. Felt amorous in a giggly, sentimental way, as if drunk. Felt sexually aroused all day. Increased sexual desire which is purely physical rising from irritation of genitals.

Food - Appetite increased even after a meal. Eats little but often. Loss of appetite. Extreme thirst. Thirst, but does not drink. Thirst for cold drinks. Aversion to food. Slight aversion to tobacco. Aversion to courgettes, which left an unpleasant taste and nausea. Craves chocolate.

Food - Desires crusty brown bread. Desires hot drinks, milk. Desires raw vegetables, salad. Desires warm milk, which ameliorates.

Head - Headache from the sun. Headache, better for alcohol. After exposure to cold wind, slight neuralgic pain in left occiput, extending to left jaw, worse inclining head forward. Dull pain in occiput and vertex, as of a tight cap. Tightness in occiput and general dullness in head. Sharp pressing pain, in left occiput, worse on listening intently, better when not concentrating. Pain from back of head to over left eye. Pain in left occiput sharp. Throbbing left temple over eye. Headache in temples. Boring pain in right temple. Head feels delicate, worse sudden movement. Throbbing pain in right temple on movement, sensitive to touch. Throbbing, above and behind left temple. Pressure feeling in the head, settling in the left temple.

Head - Headache alternating with nausea. Pain in the head with vomiting and shivering hands. Migraine during menses with very dim vision, vomiting and debility. Dull headache. Head pain poking on outside, worse bending forward. Dull congested feeling, upper left side of head. Itch in forehead. Head pain, vertex and forehead, feels hot. Heat and cold in the head at the same time. Head pain across vertex and sides. Sensation of pressure. Head pain across forehead, like a rope tightening with a feeling of weakness coming and going in waves. Head pain, better lying flat on back with head over the side of the bed, or lying with head raised. Head heavy, better cold, dry air. Crackling and creaking in head, behind ears and above neck, when walking in the cold wind. Numbness sides of head. Pain bridge of nose. Dull sensation between the eyes, better shutting the eyes. Head feels heavy, better shutting eyes. Pressure on the top of head, left side. Pain front and top of head. Sensation as if head rolling, eyes closing, tightness in head and mild heat, especially forehead. Pain, heaviness around head.

Heart - Palpitations on waking. Palpitations on lying down to sleep. Violent heartbeats, audible and visible. Felt heart pounding after urination.

Kidneys - Woke at night with desire to urinate. Frequent urination. Unfinished feeling, slight burning, dribbling after. Increased desire to urinate, more after lying down. Urge to urinate, passed a few drops with cutting pain in bladder and pubic bone. Frequent urination, large quantities. Urging to urinate, sudden, incomplete. Passes drops after urinating, worse bending. Feeling of incontinence. Pink, orange urine. Bruised pain.

Limbs - Beaten sensation in bones and joints, especially large joints. Pains, better stretching, worse movement, worse lying still. Desire to move and stretch during fever. Bruised sensation in limbs. Felt as if he had the "flu." Hands shivering in cold. Hands turn blue in cold. Feet icy cold. Heavy limbs, especially legs. Knees and ankles feel like jelly. Hands shaking. Shaking knees. Felt pins and needles in hands and arms, as of hot water on skin. Thighs burning and itching. Small boils on thighs. Jerking of left arm. Abscess in finger, below nail bed. Purple band under nails on nail bed. Numbness in hands and fingers. Stiff hands and hips. Pains stitching left upper shoulder. Sharp pains joints, worse exertion. Sensation as if had strained tendons. Limbs aching in the morning, thighs sore and heavy. Cramps in calves in bed at nigh. Sharp pain around ankle. Heels painful to stand. Pains in soles, very painful to stand and painful to walk. Awkward, drops things, trips easily.

Lungs - Breathing difficult 9:00 p.m., gradually worse, felt as if chest wouldn't expand properly. Had an urge to take deep breath, but couldn't. No pain, but felt as though muscles weren't working properly. Sensation that air goes to head. Unproductive cough, little mucus. Tickling, dry cough.

Male - Increase in sexual power and desire. Thoughts of women from many years ago, that he had not seen for years. Sexual desire in presence of any woman. Felt as if he would explode with sexuality. Masturbated frequently. Intensely erotic dreams. Intense orgasms.

Mouth - Saliva abundant. Mouth dry, as after alcohol, metallic taste. Mouth wet, yet very thirsty. Strange taste in mouth when outside and breathing through mouth. Ulcer on right inner cheek, white center. Ulcer on the right side of mouth, a hard lump the size of a grain, stinging. Sensitive aching feeling in gums, lower right side at back of mouth. Sides of mouth sore.

Neck - Neck glands feel enlarged. Large, blind, red spot on right side of neck. Pain in neck left side. Sharp pain left side of neck, moving to right side. Tension in neck and shoulders, with ache in lower back, worse sitting.

Nose - Frequent sneezing with nasal obstruction, coryza. Musty, catarrhal smell, as of an old book. Itch in nose, must poke and scratch. Sneezing, with pain in tooth. Coryza fluent. Bloody discharge on blowing nose. Post-nasal catarrh. Discharge clear, running, thick, white, yellow. Discharge alternating sides, worse warm room, better open air. Large red spots on nose.

Perspiration - Profuse perspiration at night, morning. Perspiration on waking. Perspiration, worse in a warm room, from stress. Perspiration does not ameliorate.

Rectum - Anus itching. Pain in anus, feels ill. Vesicles on anus, extremely sensitive, worse touch. Severe pain around anus and rectum, worse after stool, better pressure. Meteorism. Hemorrhoids, painful, hard, swollen, worse walking, worse sitting. Rectum raw, cracks radiating outwards and up crease to lower back. Rectal pain with desire to vomit. Pain shooting upwards, prickling and sticking, prevents sleep. Urging constant and productive for stool. Urging for stool as if diarrhea would come on but it didn't. Gripes and rumbling, with burning sensation in anus. Dry stool, constipated, abdomen bloated. Very constipated, one difficult bowel motion a week. Stool hard, which is unusual. Feeling of diarrhea in bowels and abdomen, as if diarrhea would explode. Diarrhea, brick red, explosive, hot, painful, smell of rank fish. Bowel action greatly reduced from 3 to 4 times to 1 per day. Sensation of parts above rectum in an iron fist, closing in on parts and dragging them down, better gentle motion, bending double, hot bath, worse touch.

Skin - Skin pale, red, sore, itching eruptions, worse 9 p.m., better by midnight. Red, sore, painful itching on soles of feet and palms, around the veins, alternating sides or on both sides.

Sleep - Sleepiness. Tired, could do nothing. Utterly exhausted, could hardly stay awake, could hardly think nor move. Could not remain awake enough to drive the car. Very tired, needed longer than usual afternoon nap. Tired, morning, rises late. Unrefreshed sleep, slept till late. Better after one half hour. Sleepy feeling, reluctant to get out of bed, exhausted. Very tired after evening meal, slept. Tired at night despite rest in day. Slept very deeply. Restless sleep. Great difficulty falling asleep on account of unpleasant pictures crowding in, became fearful. Wide-awake till after midnight, although physically tired. Woke many times at night with sweating, feeling heavy and confused. Awoke early and could not get back to sleep. Woke more relaxed. Slept on back during acute headache and vomiting episode (normally sleeps on side). Slept on abdomen without a pillow on left side of face with right arm curved around head.

Stomach - Anxiety in stomach. Felt absolutely dreadful, violent stomach pains, nausea and dizziness, lasting from 7:00 a.m. to 11:00 a.m., better in the afternoon. Returning at 6:00 p.m. and lasting till 9:00 p.m., then fine. Sickly pain, rising and falling, combined with hunger, better lying down. Pain in the stomach. Slight discomfort in stomach above naval, with sharp pains. Short sharp, strong, stabbing pains and cramps below ribs, coming in spasms all through the day. Sensation as if stomach was screwed up into a ball which moved around. Empty belchings. Nausea and dizziness, worse orange juice, better hot drinks. Nausea after fish, chicken, egg yolk.

Stomach - Nausea beginning in stomach and progressing downwards, better eating. Nausea at thought of food, better after deciding not to eat. Nausea, worse exertion, motion, in a moving car, standing and sitting up, better lying down, hot water bottle. Nausea with lack of appetite and great thirst for warm drinks. Nausea in the afternoon and evening, after eating even small quantities. Nausea from pain in anal cracks. Awoke with nausea and urging to stool. Desire to vomit, but passed bile only. Vomiting and retching. Violent vomiting, an orange-red color which was similar to the color of his diarrhea.

Teeth - Pain in teeth, worse eating, cold food, drinks, or air, better warmth.

Temperature - Chill with shivering and nausea, sensation of heat in forehead, eyes and lips. Chill in evening, felt shivery, especially around upper back, across shoulders and in anus. Influenza, sore throat radiating to ears, dryness in mouth, eyes and throat, tickling in throat, sneezing, nose running, clear phlegm, eyes heavy. Great thirst. Tired, lethargic, desires to lie down. Feels warm. Fever at night, worse uncovering. During the fever, whole body bruised and sore, as if beaten. Unable to get comfortable in bed, had to change position frequently. Fever, very hot, perspires. Fever, hot and cold in turns. Fever, sudden onset. Skin hot to touch.

Throat - Sore throat, in the evening, better by morning, better from beer. Throat feels rough, sore, better hot drinks. Prickling pain from throat to ear, worse empty swallowing and on waking, better warm drinks and hawking. Throat feels blocked, tickling and sore, worse swallowing. Desire to swallow, as if something stuck in the throat which she felt she could move externally. Uncomfortable sensation in throat with desire to swallow. Throat dry, painful on swallowing, worse speaking, with coarseness and cough. After sex, woke with dry throat and a cold. Dry throat with extreme thirst for cold water which ameliorates. Throat dry but thirstless. Throat dry with tickling on left side. Plugs of green catarrh in throat, worse in the evening and morning and better during the day. Thick and yellow catarrh in throat. Catarrh on tonsils, must clear throat. External throat sensitive to closing, which makes head feel hot.

Tongue - Pain in the tongue. Tongue sensation as if hot needles. Root of tongue and soft palate felt sore and enlarged, better for cold water. Tingling and numbness of tongue.

Vertigo - Vertigo, worse first movement, better continued motion.

COMMENTS - Symptoms from the provings included feeling less nervous before an event than usual. Hearing is acute. Menopausal panic attacks, with sweats and palpitations, worse lying in bed, better sitting up or walking around. Desires cold drink, white wine, fruit, especially oranges. Desires fresh air, which ameliorates, or aversion to air. Must get fresh air with hot flushes.

Permanent tiredness and fatigue. Less dryness of skin. Itch after bathing better. Sleeplessness. Woke very gently. Strong smell of coffee. Itching and soreness in vagina after intercourse. Small horny-like growth with spikes on right little toe. Severe pain, worse touch, worse pressure, could not wear shoes. Worse at 9:00 p.m. Palpitations on waking disappeared. Frequent urination.

Stiffness in morning improved. Although usually short sighted and astigmatic, he had short spells of clear vision. Vision is acute, can see for miles. Things she would normally feel guilt about don't bother her.

Felt unusually well all day. Woke more relaxed and calm than for months, slept late (throughout whole proving). Felt more energetic, self assertive and confident. She had lots of energy, worked hard and exercised. She was very bouncy and happy to be busy.

Felt good, happy, satisfied with life, happier and freer in her relationship. Felt expansive and good. Sense of being "centered." Felt euphoric, relaxed, "spaced out." Feeling extremely calm. Her patience surprised her. Extremely alert. Pretended to feel well, although sick.

A feeling of great energy and confidence, a magnetic state, his emotions were more intense than ever before. In his love affair, he surrendered to his feelings for the first time, and his girlfriend commented that this was the most intense relationship she had ever had.

Desired alcohol and drugs, a feeling of wanting to escape. It seemed as though he was a different person, very similar to the way he had been in adolescence, but in a much more powerful manner.

These emotions were so intense he wanted to rip his chest apart to let them out. He lost all control over his emotions, which seemed to come from a deep and distant part of himself, a darker side. He desired to continue the proving for the rest of his life.

Although he experienced acute nausea, headache and dizziness, he felt calm and happy, not upset by his illness, detached. Felt fed up with all activities he normally enjoyed. Felt detached from everything, as in a dream, reactions slowed down a lot. Feeling of separateness, usual sense of urgency gone. Felt detached from her stomach cramps. Felt she should be busy but couldn't.

Felt despondent and directionless in the evening. In the evening, felt as if in a numbness, "thoughts, feelings, buzzing and confusing me. I feel entirely alone, that I am viewing the world through one hole, for it all seems just a picture, and the rest of the world share a different view finder together. I don't want to join theirs though."

Stomach pain ameliorated as headache starts. Headaches and mental state ameliorated with appearance of sexual symptoms.

All colors seemed bright. Nose, discharge yellow-orange. Vomit, orange-red. Diarrhea, brick red. Urine, pink-orange. Stayed awake till early morning, brain racing, enjoyed himself tremendously.

Felt as if he had taken drugs. His friends thought so too. Desired drugs. Warm drinks ameliorate throat. Warm milk ameliorates. Alcohol ameliorates headache. Beer ameliorates throat. Coffee ameliorates. Cold food and drink aggravates pain in teeth. Eating ameliorates lethargy. Eating ameliorates swings of mood. Eating aggravates pain in teeth. Orange juice aggravates.

Hemorrhages on cutting herself, blood dark and clotted quickly. Heaviness feeling all over. Exhaustion, lethargy and fatigue. Exhausted, run down, better for fresh air. Lethargy worse during menses. Lethargy better shutting eyes. No strength, feels sagging all over, limp and weak.

Feet seem to drag. Lassitude in evening, better lying down, better short sleep. Weakness with trembling. Nausea worse for motion. Sitting or first movement aggravate backache.

Walking aggravates vertigo. Walking and movement ameliorate mentally and generally. Gentle motion ameliorates pain in rectum. Constant change of position ameliorates back. Moving car aggravates nausea and vomiting. Riding in car ameliorates. Occupation ameliorates.

Numbness, tingling and nausea throughout body, during fear. During fever the whole body bruised and sore as if beaten, unable to get comfortable in bed, had to change position frequently and slightly, else felt seized up. Restless.

Extreme mental and physical anguish with restlessness, could not be still for a moment. Beaten sensation in bones and joints, especially large joints, better stretching, worse movement and lying still. Pains poking. Pains radiating outwards. Pains sharp.

Right to left, pain in throat. Left to right, pain in knees. Left to right, ears ringing. Alternating sides, red, painful, itching eruptions on soles of feet and palms. Alternating sides, nasal discharge. Felt hot so uncovered, then cold so covered, then hot so uncovered.

Gentle heat over whole body. Sensation of heat. Warm room aggravates. Warm room aggravates nasal discharge. Hot bath ameliorates pain in cracks around anus. Body warm to touch but feels chilly. Cold, feels. Cold dry air ameliorates. Wet, sore throat after getting. Cold wind causes neuralgia in head. Wind aggravates. Desired and relished being in a strong wind. Tremor. Loss of weight.

Coffee, did not antidote. Bruised sensation, cannot get comfortable in bed.

Tiredness, sore throat, thirst, photophobia and headache. Abscess on small toe, pain stinging and burning, worse from heat and touch.

RELATIONS - ***Compare:*** (1) Vesp., Scol., Tarent., Apis. (2) Arn., Bry., Hyper., Led.

REFERENCES - Allen. Clarke. Sherr.

ANDROGRAPHIS PENICULATA

(Kalmegh)

PHARMACY - androg-p. Andrographis peniculata. Kalmegh. N. O. Acanthaceac. The entire fresh plant. ***Historical dose:*** All potencies.

CLINICAL - Abscesses. Boils. Catarrh. Constipation. Cough. Debility. Diarrhea. Dysentery. Dyspepsia. Fever. Flatulence. Headache. Intermittent, fever. Jaundice. Kala-azar. Liver, disorders. Malaria. Vomiting. Worms. Wounds.

HERBAL - Common in India, specially in Bengal. It is an annual plant, 1 to 3 feet high, common in hedgerows throughout the plains of India from Lucknow to Assam. It is also cultivated in gardens in some parts of India.

The shrub is well-known under the name of Kalmegh and forms the principal ingredient of household medicine called alui which is extensively used in Bengali.

The macerated leaves and juice together with certain spices are made into little globules, which are prescribed for infants to relieve griping, irregular stools and loss of appetite.

The roots and leaves have also reputation of being a febrifuge, tonic, alternative and anthelmintic.

In general debility, dysentery and certain forms of dyspepsia associated with gaseous distension of the bowels, the decoction or infusion of the leaves have been used with satisfactory results.

Ayurvedic physicians used it with success singly or as a principal ingredient with other medicines in worms of children, vomiting of children. Infantile liver, enlargement of liver and spleen. Fever with the enlargement of liver and spleen. Fever with constipation. Fever in malaria. Fever in infantile liver. Fever in kala-azar of children, and also in boils, abscesses and septic wounds.

The people of India prize it to be a highly efficacious remedy in all sorts of liver complaints from very early times.

The Ayurvedic physicians of India use it in enlarged liver or any derangement of liver, especially in children with jaundiced skin or without it, in the first stage of cough and cold, in the general debility and in convalescence after a long - continued fever. They also employ it in cutaneous ailments.

In intermittent fevers, the fever comes on daily between 8 and 9. a.m. or between 10 a.m. and 12 noon. During fever there is slight thirst. ***Loose stools, catarrh, cough and pain in the hepatic region*** are the accompanying symptoms. There may be constipation in place of diarrhea.

Burning sensation in eyes, face hands and feet, especially in the palms are keynote symptoms for its administration. During fever the patient is disinclined to move, desire to keep quiet, during fever there is intermingling of chilliness and burning sensation.

Sometimes the patient likes cold applications. Sometimes he dislikes them, in this way contradictory and conflicting symptoms manifest themselves.

It is generally used in an attack of remittent or intermittent fever where there is double accession of the seizure associated with predominance of bilious symptoms and headache. In some cases, headache may be absent.

In show fevers of children with derangement or enlargement of liver, it is very useful. In infantile jaundice where eyes and urine have become yellow, it is used with efficacy. It is excellent remedy in chronic fever associated with the enlargement of liver and spleen along with burning of hands, feet, eyes and face, and headache. Its efficacy is found also in kala-azar of infants. The following are the principal guiding symptoms of Kalmegh:

Sensation of heat and burning in hands and feet, mental depression and despondency, bad taste in the mouth, bitter and putrid taste over the tongue, constipation, scantiness of stools, changeableness of symptoms, heaviness of the whole body for which the patient walks slowly.

The patient wants to wash the hands and the feet with cold water in order to be relieved of the burning sensation felt over the parts, he feels considerable relief from cold, he does not desire to move.

Kalmegh is a domestic medicine for flatulence and diarrhea of children and it is also used for worm symptoms as it is considered to be anthelmintic. It is used in torpidity of liver, neuralgia, dyspepsia, in general debility, in convalescence after fevers and in the fully developed stage of dysentery. In short, Kalmegh is a sovereign remedy for the above mentioned ailments.

HOMEOPATHIC - Dr. Pramada Prasanna Biswas, of Patna and Dr. N. Sinha made provings of this drug. Both the provings are, no doubt, incomplete and fragmentary, bit they cannot be brushed aside with indifference. They lead us to think that it will urn out to be an excellent remedy in our materia medica.

MIND - Despondency. No desire to do any work. No desire to talk. Restlessness. Easily angered.

Abdomen - Heaviness of abdomen. Heat and burning of abdomen.

Chest - Burning in chest.

Eyes. Redness of eyes. Yellowish tinge of eyes.

Fever - Double type of fever is a grand characteristic of this drug fever is associated with slight chilliness, heat remaining all along, heat marked with burning sensation all over the body. Burning sensation is relieved by cold air and application of cold water. Intermittent and remittent fevers and almost specific in the fever which comes on with double accession. Fever comes on after 11 a.m. and again appears at 7 p.m. or 8 p.m.

Head - Giddiness of head. Throbbing pain on the occiput, sometimes very painful. Heaviness of head. Frontal headache. Headache and thirst.

Liver - Enlargement of liver. Liver painful to touch. Pain felt over liver on pressure. Many disorders of liver. Jaundice. Infantile derangement of the liver and its enlargement.

Modalities - Cold water relieves the burning sensation of the body; sweat also relieves these symptoms; all symptoms are worse during fever; there is an intermingling of contradictory symptoms.

Mouth - Bitter taste in the mouth. White coating of the tongue.

Nose. Watery discharge from the nose. Symptoms of catarrh present. Occasional sneezing.

Rectum - Jaundice and constipation manifest themselves. Ineffectual urging of stool. Loose stools, loose bilious stools. Constipation. Frequent urging for stool, but no evacuation takes place. Blackish hard stools. Yellow loose stools of infants. Sometimes constipation, sometimes easy motion. Tendency to costiveness.

Stomach - Occasional eructations.

Throat - Burning in throat. Dryness of throat.

Urine - Urine high-colored. in infantile jaundice. Urine is thick and yellow.

RELATIONS - ***Compare:*** Chin., Chin-ars.

REFERENCES - Ghose.

ANEMOPSIS CALIFORNICA

(Yerba Mansa)

PHARMACY - anemps. Anemopsis californica. Yerba mansa. Household herb. Saururaceae. ***Historical dose:*** Tincture and all potencies.

CLINICAL - ***Catarrh***. Cuts. Bruises. Flatulence. Indigestion. Malaria. Sinusitis. Sprains. Urethritis.

HERBAL - Yerba Mansa is useful in ***cuts, bruises and sprain,*** as a diuretic and in malaria. Recommended in heart disease, as a quieting agent when unduly excited.

HOMEOPATHIC - Anemps. is a mucus membrane medicine. Useful for profuse mucus or serous discharges in nasal and pharyngeal catarrh, diarrhea and urethritis. ***Catarrhal states*** with a full, stuffy sensation in head and throat. Chronic forms of inflammation of the nasal membranes with profuse discharges. Flatulence. Promotes digestion.

RELATIONS - ***Compare:*** (1) Piper-m. Arn.

REFERENCES - Boericke. Clarke.

ANGELICA ATROPURPUREA

(Great Angelica)

PHARMACY - ange. Angelica atropurpurea. Great angelica. Archangelica officinalis. Angelica archangelica. N. O. Umbelliferae. Tincture of the dried root. ***Historical dose:*** Tincture and all potencies.

HERBAL - Angelica in tincture, five drops, three times daily, produces disgust for liquor.

HOMEOPATHIC - Affects the spleen and liver. For atony of different organs. Enlarged spleen (Cean.). Craves alcoholic drinks. Alcoholism. Dyspepsia, nervous headaches, etc. Chronic bronchitis to increase expectoration of mucus.

RELATIONS - ***Compare:*** (1) Quercus gland., Cean.

REFERENCES - Boericke.

ANGELICA SINENSIS

(Dong-Quay)

PHARMACY - ange-s. Angelica sinensis. Dong-Quay. Dies-Umbelliferous. N. O. Umbelliferae. Tincture of the roots. ***Historical dose:*** Tincture and all potencies.

CLINICAL - Acrocyanosis. Amenorrhea. Anaphrodisia. Erysipelas. Leucorrhea. Lumbago. Premenstrual syndrome. Thyroid, problems. Weight, changes.

HOMEOPATHIC - The clinical provings of Ange-s. seem to be rich in promise for the future, especially for female hormonal problems. Affinity for genital organs, especially female, locomotor, and the skin. Easily tired with backache. Tired on waking up.

According to Dr. Nguyen-van-Nghi, a sweet and sharp taste can be observed, along with action on the meridians, particularly the heart, liver and spleen. It tones up the blood and causes it to circulate, moistens the dryness (lungs), regularizes the intestines, and harmonizes the blood and the energy (meridians). Drained feeling with headaches, lumbar aching, chest and abdominal diseases.

Constipation and expulsion of pus. Toning action on the organs. Effective for cases of hematuria and melaena.

Weight changes, regular loss of weight in obese hypothyroid types. Tendency to plumpness. Reduction in libido. Menses scanty with fainting feeling, breast congestion, diarrhea and occasional vomiting. Joint pains, predominantly on the left side, especially in the hip and pelvis. Spontaneous hematomata. Vesicular eruption. Formation of hard nodular patches.

MIND - Difficulty in concentrating. Reading difficult, because he needs to move, to walk about. General restlessness. Lacks courage, while being restless. State of euphoria, which is mixed with a state of indifference. Feels well, calm, a little tired. Feels more dynamic but more nervous.

Abdomen - Pain in the solar plexus with pulsations in the abdominal aorta. Flatulence. Attacks of colitis and prurigo.

Back - Pains in the scapula and left arm, causing him to wake at night. Pain under the left scapula, in the left shoulder. Lumbar pains. Lumbago as after exertion. Spontaneous hematomata in series, stretching all along the vertebral column and waist.

Breasts - Benign breast tumors, cysts on the breasts. Disappearance of a nodule in left-sided mastitis.

Chest - Pain in the middle of the sternum, sometimes spontaneous. Sternum painful, almost impossible to touch it.

Constitutions - Hydrogenoid, neuro-lymphatic type.

Female - Amenorrhea. Long intervals between menses. Premenstrual syndrome. Premenstrual swelling, breast congestion and legs heavy. Menses scanty. Menopausal complaints. Discomfort, feeling sensation during menses with vomiting and frequent stools. Hot flushes and discomfort and night. Profuse leucorrhea, milky, irritating discharge. Intercourse uncomfortable, sometimes painful. Libido very irregular. Pain and congestion in the left ovary.

Food - Loss of appetite, worse after eating sweets, pastries or sugar.

Head - Headache after meals, at the nape of the neck.

Heart - Palpitations, limbs cold, legs heavy.

Kidneys - Urination not very frequent. Urine very dark in color. Has to get up during the night to urinate once or twice.

Limbs - Acrocyanosis of the hands, legs, cheeks, and inside of the arms. Joint pains in the left shoulder and left hip. Strumous edema of the legs, worse in cold weather.

Lungs - Stifled sensation with need for air. Feeling of heat, respiration difficult, need for fresh air. Grasps for breath. Dyspnea with no apparent cause.

Male - Irregular libido with loss of sexual appetite. Sexually indifferent.

Modalities - Better in fresh air, a need for fresh air. Worse from movement. Worse contact. Worse in the late afternoon.

Mouth - Painful swelling of the gum where there is a bridge. Tongue covered with a white or yellow coating at the back and on the edges.

Neck - Cannot bear the collar of his shirt to be fastened.

Pelvis - Pain in the hip and left sacroiliac joint, appearing especially in the late afternoon. Pain in all the joints of the pelvis. Feeling of stretching of the pelvic joints as after giving birth.

Rectum - Diarrhea, worse after eating sweets, pastries, sugar. Diarrhea after any meals. Tendency to periods of constipation, alternating with soft stools, diarrhea.

Skin - Vesicular, itching eruptions, located on the right knee. Itching patches on the left hip, stretching to the waist, back and slightly on the right hip. Hardening below the skin on the left hip. Small hard patches on the outer side of the right forearm. Loss of hair with scaly, scabby formations on the scalp. Erysipelas. Acrocyanosis. Strumous edema. Knotted erythema.

Sleep - Sleep after meals. Sleep not very good, irregular with sensation of heat, persistently disturbed. Sleep lasts only a short while. Agitated dreams, dreams of death, funerals, falling into deep, black pit.

Temperature - Perspiration appears fairly quickly and chill disappears, takes off woolen clothes. Perspires easily. Varying chilliness, at times cold, then with hot flushes.

Throat - Tension in the thyroid region with blocked, stifled sensation.

COMMENTS - "Case (1) Francine D., 28, came for a consultation on 28/10/74, for a hormonal problem. She began menstruation at 17 and since then has always had irregular periods, up to 5 or 6 days late. Menses are weak, scanty with bright red or brown blood and painful. Between menses, yellowish-green leucorrhea.

"She has been receiving allopathic hormone treatment for 5 years after an examination which revealed the right ovary to be large, smooth and white. Feels tired on waking up, tendency to be constipated, dreams a great deal, complains of dorsal pains.

"Anxious, legs heavy. She has scoliosis, small breasts, gastric ptosis, slight acrocyanosis and infiltrated ankles. She says she has not been receiving hormone treatment for several months.

"Prescription of 25 drops of Radix-Angelicae-Sinensis in 3x on waking up. 15 drops of Radix-Angelicae-Sinensis in 7c on going to bed. Condition generally improved, feels better. Stools regular sleep better and fewer dreams, no tiredness on waking, lost a little weight, which pleased her, 52 kilos, arterial tension 14/8.

"As for menses, she had one period on 8th December 1974, but it was still a little painful. Then on 22nd January 1975, normal, copious and, above all, painless. We maintained the original prescription.

"Case (2). D. St., age 24, came on 9th September 1974. Began menses at 9, always had painful, scanty menses with black, clotted blood. Operated on in January 1972 for a right sided hydrosalpinx and menstrual cycle did not improve afterwards. While, milky leucorrhea, feels swollen intercourse painful.

"Prescription Radix-Angelicae-Sinensis, 3x in the morning, 7c in the evening. The menstrual cycle was restored and she had periods on 27th September, 25th October, 20th November, 21st December 1974 and then 22nd January 1975, 18th February and 22nd March 1975. No more leucorrhea, regular, painless intercourse, no more swelling, regular stools.

"Case (3). Myriane F..., 26, came on 13th July 1974 with obesity and rare, irregular menses. Here is a pattern of her periods when taking Radix-Angelicae-Sinensis, 3x and 7c: 18th July, 30th August, 3rd September, 4th October, 14th November, 19th December, 24th January. She was 1.67m tall, weighing 65 kilos at 13/7/74 and 59 kilos at 24/2/75.

"She is now very well. In fact, these three cases are only given as indications. A closer clinical and biological study is necessary in order to demonstrate its value. We must also point out that a greater dosage of 25 to 50 drops, two to three times a day, can be given in cases of benign breast tumors or secondary amenorrhea, especially after cessation of taking the birth control pill."

RELATIONS - ***Compare:*** (1) Aranea Diadema - Hydrogenoid tendency, faintness, menses with pains in the lumbar and sacral regions, periodicity and feeling of increase in size and weight of the upper limbs. (2) Aristolochia Clematitis - Affinity for the female genital organs. Menses scanty, irregular, joint pains, strumous edema. (3) Histamine hydrochlor. - Thyroid type with pain in the left ovary, burning, cramping pains in the scrotum, joints and muscles, burning, itching, red papules on small areas of the skin. (4) Mandragora Radix - Euphoria, alternating with depression, libido disturbed, menses early or late, leucorrhea and lumbar pains, herpes-type vesicles on the face.

REFERENCES - Julian.

ANGOPHORA LANCEOLATA

(Red Gum)

PHARMACY - ango. Angophora lanceolata. Red gum. Eucalyptus rostata. Kino australiense. Metrosideros Costatus. Pterocarpus marsupium. N. O. Myrtacae. Australia. Tincture or trituration of dried sap or gum. ***Historical dose:*** Trituration, Tincture and all potencies.

CLINICAL - Constipation. Debility. Diarrhea. Dysentery.

HERBAL - This herb resembles eucalyptus in appearance. It was proved by F. Kopp, producing bearing-down and constant inclination to stool. Dry, hard evacuations, accompanied with blood, diarrhea. Headache, nausea, flatulent distention and colicky pains.

Pains and tenesmus only better by lying down flat on the face. Obstinate constipation, then nausea, sickness and diarrhea with vertigo and debility.

RELATIONS - ***Antidoted by:*** Ip.

REFERENCES - Clarke.

ANGUSTURA VERA

(Cusparia febrifuga)

PHARMACY - ang. Angustura vera. Cusparia febrifuga. Galipea cusparia. Galipea officinalis. Bonplandia trifoliata. N. O. Rutacae. Bonplandia trifoliata from Angustura, South America. Trituration and tincture of the bark. ***Historical dose:*** Trituration, Tincture and all potencies.

CLINICAL - Anxiety. Belching. Bone, pains. Chills. ***Coffee, addiction. Decay, tissues.*** Diarrhea. Dyspepsia. Headache. Hemorrhoids. Injuries. Intermittent, fevers. ***Knee, pain.*** Myopia. Palpitations. Paralysis. Rheumatism. Spavin in horses. Tetanus. Toothache. Trismus, neonatorum Ulcers. Varicose veins. Vertigo. Whooping cough.

HOMEOPATHIC - The effects of Ang. are closely allied to those of Nux-v., Ruta and Merc. Clarke has verified the power of Ang over long bones in a case of acute periostitis of the tibia in a scrofulous boy. The 5x trituration speedily arrested inflammation after the failure of Merc. Decay of bones, particular if patient has longing for coffee and has a very touchy, sensitive mind.

Principal action is on spinal motor nerves and mucus membranes. ***Over-sensitive and excitable.*** The slightest offense, a mere trifle, irritates (Nux-v.). Timidity and weakness (Sil.). Characteristic ***strong craving for coffee.***

Decay of tissue. Decay with crumbling off of pieces of bone. ***Decay of long bones.*** Ulcers very painful, penetrate to marrow. Tearing in the bones, worse at rest, better cold applications, better extension, worse exertion and pressure. Exostosis of lower jaw. Rheumatic and paralytic complaints with great difficulty in walking. Crackling in all joints. Drawing, tension, stiffness of muscles and joints, bruised, sore feeling as after a blow.

Constricting sensation in varicose veins. Spinal marrow and extensor muscles are principally affected. Paralysis. Tetanus. Drawing of head of right side, later to left. Heat in forehead at night. Near-sighted.

MIND - Greatly excited and extravagant spirits. ***Oversensitive.*** Sudden attacks of anxiety at night. Anxiety while lying in bed. Anxiety as if she never would get awake again. Easily frightened and starts. Pusillanimity. He has not confidence enough in himself to undertake and perform voluntary motions.

Marked ill humor, everything vexes her. Lachrymose and irritable. Great gloom. Disheartened. ***Offended easily.*** Prone to anger, every trifle irritates. Filled with bitterness, will stand no joking, irritation at least offence. Absence of mind, wants now this, then that thing.

Abdomen - Pain from navel into sternum. Loud rumbling in the abdomen. Emission of stinking flatulence.

Back - Itching along back. Twitching and jerking along back. Pain in cervical vertebrae. Drawing in the neck. Cutting pain from point of right scapula to breast, near nipple (Chel.). Pain in spine, at nape of neck and sacrum, worse on pressure. Bends backwards.

Constitutions - Syphilitic constitutions.

Ears - Heat of the ears and both cheeks. Pinching in the external ear. Heat in the lobes. Sensation as if something were before the ear and as if something were inserted in it. Throbbing pain behind the ears, on the side of the neck, as if the carotid were beating.

Eyes - The eyes are red and burn, agglutinated in the morning. Violent burning in the inner half of the eyes. Pressure in both eyes, as if a bright light were irritating them and they became weary. A few stitches over the eyes. Eyes feel as if there was sand in them.

Food - Aversion to solid food, desires nothing but warm drink. Thirst without desire to drink. ***Irresistible desire to drink coffee.*** Aversion to meat, especially pork. Thirst for cold water, could not drink enough during evening. Wants now one thing, now another, which are refused when offered. He cannot get satisfied without having much appetite.

Head - Oversensitive. Headache with heat of face. Acute pain in cheeks. Drawing in facial muscles. Pain in temporal muscles, worse when opening the jaws. Pain in articulation of jaw in masseter muscles, as if fatigued by chewing too much. Cramp-pain on the zygomatic arch.

Limbs - Stiffness and tension of muscles and joints. Pain in limbs on walking. Arms tired and heavy. Decay of long bones. Coldness of fingers. ***Knee pain.*** Cracking in joints.

Lungs - Cough, as if something weighed on his lungs. Frequent short cough, followed by one hiccough. Expectoration of sour, salty water.

Modalities - Toothache is better application of cold fingers. Palpitations, worse sitting bent and better sitting up. Pain in cervical vertebrae worse moving arms. Loose cough is worse 3 p.m. Worse from exertion. Worse stooping. Worse moving or lifting arms. Worse drinking warm milk. Worse cold application. Worse extension. Worse lying on left side.

Mouth - Great dryness of mouth and lips without any thirst. Much saliva flows from the mouth. Bitter taste in the mouth after the usual smoking.

Nose - Sensation of a corrosive soreness deep in the nose.

Rectum - Diarrhea and colic. Tenesmus with soft stool. Chronic diarrhea with debility and loss of flesh. Burning in anus. Frequent urging in the rectum, as if diarrhea would come on immediately.

Rectum - Hemorrhoids remain protruded, even during the night.

Skin - Decay, very painful ulcers which affect the bone.

Sleep - Restlessness at night. Uneasy sleep, wakes without cause and cannot get to sleep again. Vivid dreams, partly disagreeable, partly anxious. Anxious, distressing dreams, causing her to weep much.

Stomach - Belchings of water. Many empty belchings after a meal. Bilious belchings. Belching with cough (Ambr.). Frequent hiccough. Sense of nausea in the stomach. Nausea with water brash. Nausea, especially during a meal. Empty feeling in stomach. Cutting, tearing in the pit increased by moving the trunk after dinner. Cramp like, pinching pain below the pit of the stomach. Atonic dyspepsia.

Temperature - Chills all over with nausea. At 3 p. m., shivering with goose flesh, abating in the open air without thirst, for several days in succession.

Throat - Frequent roughness in the throat, he must hack without being able to expectorate anything. Roughness and dryness in the back part of the palate and fauces without any thirst.

Vertigo - Periodical vertigo. Vertigo in the open air. Vertigo from the occiput when sitting, throbbing in right temple.

COMMENTS - Trismus neonatorum, where much mercury had been given. Drawing in upper right molar tooth better application of cold finger. Thirst, constant desire to drink. Irresistible desire to drink coffee.

Hiccough after cough. Belching with cough (Ambr.). Dry, hacking cough from scratching in throat or irritation behind sternum. Irritation behind sternum through to back. Every evacuation followed by shivering, crawling sensation over face. Tenesmus with soft stool. Hemorrhoids protrude with hard, knotty stool. Seminal emissions. Itching of tip of glans penis (when walking in open air). Violent itching on scrotum.

RELATIONS - ***Antidoted by:*** Coffea, (not Camph.). Bry. - Bellyache after milk, Chel. - sharp, cutting pain from just beneath right scapula to chest. Ang. is like Ruta in its action on bones and as an antidote to Mercury, also like False Angustura. ***Compare:*** (1) Nux-v., Ruta, Merc. (2) Brucea Bark or Angustura falsa. (3) Bell. - worse 3 p.m. (4) All-c., Cham., Coff. - toothache better by cold. (5) Cic., Ign., Nux-v. - tetanus. (6) Merc., Phos., Sil. - decay of jaw. (7) Aesc., Aloe. - hemorrhoids and backache. (8) Hyper. Led. - punctured wounds. (9) Ran-b. - pain in pectoral muscles.

REFERENCES - Allen. Boericke. Clarke.

ANHALONIUM LEWINII

(Peyote)

PHARMACY - anh. Anhalonium lewinii. Peyote. Peyotl. Lophophora williamsii. Mescal buttons. N. O. Cactaceae. Mexico, Rio Grande. Tinctures, extracts or infusions. ***Historical dose:*** Tincture and all potencies.

CLINICAL - ***Audio-visual, hallucinations.*** Brain-fag. Delirium. Delusions. Depersonalization. Depression. Goiter. Headaches. ***Hearing, disorders.*** Hysteria. Insomnia. ***Intoxication.*** Megrim. Mental, weakness. Neuralgia. Paraplegia. Senses, disordered. Ptosis. Pupils, dilated. Schizophrenia. Suicidal, tendencies. ***Vision, disorders.***

HERBAL - The Anhalonium plant from which the mescal buttons are obtained grows in barren and rocky soil in the valley of the Rio Grande. It is used by some Native American tribes in their religious ceremonies. In the ceremonies the constant beating of tom-toms is an essential feature.

HOMEOPATHIC - Anhalonium has been recently tested and a notable proving was made by Dr. Wier Mitchell. It is a cardiac tonic and respiratory stimulant. It weakens the heart and produces insanity.

The chief feature of the drug's action is the production of colorful visions of overpowering brilliancy, associated with moving shapes of fantastic design, the motion being regulated somewhat in time by music.

It makes "each note upon the piano a center of melody which seems to be surrounded by a halo of color pulsating to the rhythm of the music." Hyperesthesia of all the senses. Acute sensitivity to changes of the weather.

Feeling of cold over the body. General increase in muscular tone. Hypersecretion of the thyroid gland. Hysteria. Allergic persons with hypersensitivity. Loss of sex drive (Sep.). Insomnia. Anxiety and neurosis. Melancholy. Chronic hallucinatory state. Schizophrenia. Impression that the self is double. Suicidal tendencies. Basedow's disease (Goiter).

MIND - Anhalonium is a remedy for brain-weakness, ***audio-visual hallucinations*** with colored brilliant visions. It causes a form of ***intoxication*** accompanied by ***wonderful visions, remarkably beautiful and varied kaleidoscopic changes*** and a sensation of increased physical ability. Visions of monsters and various gruesome forms. Delirium.

Loss of contact with the outside world and escape into a fantasy world. Loss of conception of time. Distrust and resentment. Lazy contentment. Gloomy, sad, dull. Irrational, sudden changes of mood. Egocentric introversion. Noises and touch are perceived through colored vision.

Depersonalization, does not know his identity. Diminution of willpower, apathy and slow reactions. Passive state. ***Existential anguish.*** Impression that objects and his whole body are transparent, sees his own internal organs. Memories exalted.

Ears - Exaggerated reverberation of ordinary sounds. Impressions of sound and visions heightened by any marked stimulation of skin.

Eyes - Pupils dilated. Ptosis. Accommodation impaired. Troubled vision, accommodation and perception. ***Visions in all colors***. Fantastic visions of surpassing brilliance, moving in designs. Moving scenes, dances, affected by beating time. Natural objects seem more brilliant, shadows deepened, flickering of lights greatly exaggerated.

Face - Disinclined to make the slightest movement, eyelids droop, they scarcely move the lips and jaws in articulating.

Head - Headaches with disturbed vision. Frontal headache with visual zigzags. Occipital headache, with disturbed vision. Persistent ache and tired feeling in occipital region.

Limbs - Burning sensation of the limbs. A fine tremor in lower limbs.

Lungs - Breathing shallow.

Modalities - Better lying down. ***Worse on closing eyes.*** The nausea and faintness were worse on movement. There is great disinclination to move.

Mouth - Great difficulty in talking, partly from paralysis of the tongue, partly from slowness of thought.

Nerves - Motor incoordination. Extreme muscular depression increased patellar reflex. Paraplegia. Neuralgias, trigeminal of the ophthalmic nerve, the maxillary nerve, frontal nerve and naso-ciliary nerve.

Nose - The air seemed filled with vague perfume. Smell blunted, could not tell whether or not tincture of asafetida was a perfume.

Sleep - Insomnia and hysteria. Drowsiness, followed by consciousness of unusual energy.

Stomach - Nausea, worse on movement, entirely better on lying down.

Vertigo - Faintness. Vertigo, brain tired.

COMMENTS - One prover, Havelock Ellis said "I first cut up the Peyote buttons into small fragments and poured on boiling water twice, a single infusion is inactive." He noted a distinct slowing of the pulse, slight faintness and shallow breathing, but there were none of the terrible heart symptoms of the other Cacti.

Other symptoms are loss of conception of time, occipital headache, tired feeling in head, nausea. Tremor of muscles increased knee-jerk and loss of power of coordination. Extreme muscular depression, don't want to stir, whole body feels relaxed. Lazy contentment. Fine tremor in lower limbs before the visions, unable to walk without assistance, can with difficulty sit up.

RELATIONS - ***Compare:*** (1) Cann-i. - time sense disordered, fantastic visions. (2) Gels. - paralysis of accommodation. (3) Bell., Stram.,

Op., Pic-ac., Pip-m., Coff., Coca. (4) Plat. - objects seem small and distant. (5) Psor. - better lying down. (6) Agave. (7) The intoxication of Anhalonium is similar to that of Cannabis Ind. and Oenanthe.

REFERENCES - Boericke. Clarke.

ANILINUM

(Amidobenzene)

PHARMACY - anil. Anilinum. Amidobenzene. Amidobenzol. A secondary product of coal tar obtained by reduction of nitrobenzene. ***Historical dose:*** Trituration and all potencies.

CLINICAL - Anemia. Anorexia. Cancer. Cholera. Cyanosis. Eczema, rubrum. Tumors.

HOMEOPATHIC - The symptoms of Anil. have been observed on working people poisoned by inhalation of the fumes and on persons who have worn an aniline-dyed article next the skin.

The symptoms are in many respects like those of Arsenicum. There is vomiting, purging, bursting headache, and epileptiform attacks. ***Face has a purple hue***. Marked cyanosis, swelling and irritation of the skin.

Profound anemia with discoloration of the skin, blue lips, anorexia, gastric disturbances. Pain in penis and scrotum with swelling. Cancerous growths. ***Tumors of urinary passages***. Giddiness and pain in head.

COMMENTS - In old-school practice, injections of aniline blue have been used with some success to destroy cancerous, growths, aniline having a marked affinity for cell nuclei, hence its use in staining microscopic specimens.

In Anil. poisoning cases, evacuants, the inhalation of oxygen, and the free use of stimulants, including brandy, ammonia, chloric ether, cold infusions to the head, and mustard plasters on legs and thighs, have been used with success.

RELATIONS - ***Compare:*** (1) Glon., Ars., Pyrog., Phenacetinum. Antifebrinum.

REFERENCES - Boericke. Clarke.

ANISE STELLATUM

(Star Anise)

PHARMACY - anis. Anise stellatum. Star anise. Chinese anise. Illicium stellatum. Illicium verum. N. O. Magnoliacee. Illecebraceae. Tincture of seeds. ***Historical dose:*** Tincture and all potencies.

CLINICAL - Asthma. Catarrh. Colic. Convulsions. Cough. Dyspnea. Hemoptysis. Lungs disorders. Stomach, catarrh. Rheumatism. Thigh, pain. Vomiting.

HERBAL - Illicium is a genus of Magnoliaceous shrubs or low trees with smooth entire leaves, exhaling when bruised a strong odor of aniseed, owing to the volatile oil contained in minute pellucid dots, which may be seen by the aid of a lens. The star anise fruit is used throughout China, Japan and India as a condiment and is chewed in small quantities after a meal to sweeten the breath.

Anis. has a local repute as a stomachic and carminative and should be remembered in the treatment of flatulent conditions. It has been used for the so-called three months colic, especially if it recurs at regular hours, with much rumbling in abdomen. Colic of babies.

HOMEOPATHIC - The Anis. provings were made by Franz and Mure. Both showed the action of the drug on the nose, mouth and stomach. Franz had many symptoms on the face, especially lips, skin and limbs.

Characteristic ***pain in region of third rib***, about an inch or two from the sternum, generally on right side, but occasionally on left. Frequent cough with this pain. Purulent tracheal and gastric catarrh of old alcoholics. Old asthmatics. Vomiting, epileptiform convulsions with biting of tongue.

Abdomen - Three months colic, especially if it recurs at regular hours, bowels disturbed. Violent wind colic. Rumbling in abdomen. Pain in spleen region.

Back - Pain in back and chest. Cramp-like drawing, as from a cold in left side of dorsal vertebra.

Chest - Pain in region of third rib, about one or two inches from sternum, generally on right side, but occasionally left. Pain about junction of third rib with cartilages, hemorrhage, coughs, congestion and enlarged liver.

Ears - Buzzing in ears. Ringing in ears followed by sleep. Itching over left ear, going off when touching the place.

Face - Stinging sensation in upper lip, as if blood would press out, better from touch. Dryness of upper lip, which is drawn closer to teeth. Burning in inner surface of lower lip with sensation as if it had gone to sleep.

Food - All food, except rye bread, tastes too salty or bitter, yet appetite is good. Rye bread tastes good, its odor is refreshing. Satiety after eating but little.

Head - Pains in head, better evenings, worse mornings.

Heart - Palpitations with aphthae and weakness.

Limbs - Jerking and tearing in bend of left elbow and at same time in palm, a feeling as if an artery had been injured by a blow. Pressure back of right hand, between the two middle metacarpal bones, as though something hard lying between them, worse pressing hand against anything hard, not by touch. Left thigh feels as if broken in the middle while sitting, it disappears on standing.

Lungs - Dyspnea in old asthmatics. Feeling of emptiness after coughing. Frequent cough with pain. Spitting blood in small quantities and with pus-like phlegm, pain in right chest. Whitish expectoration. Tough and viscous phlegm with old alcoholics. Dyspnea. Pain near third intercostal cartilage. Cough with pus-like phlegm. Palpitation with aphthae. Hemoptysis.

Modalities - The pain in thigh is worse sitting, better rising. Pains in the head are worse in morning, better in evening.

Mouth - Tongue covered with aphthae, most on edges. Edges of tongue folded like little bags.

Nose - Acute catarrh. Water discharge from nostrils. Warm, smarting sensation in nose, succeeded by sneezing. Sharp stitches in tip of nose, beneath lip. Acute catarrh. Burning and numbness of inner lower lip.

Rectum - Stools bilious, compact and dark-colored.

Skin - Stitches as with pins in left palm, between first and second fingers, better by scratching, but afterwards return with burning. Dull, painful stitches in skin of lower forearm. Crawling, itching stitches in right palm. Itching in front and above left ear, better by touch.

Sleep - Sleepless at nightfall. Disturbed sleep.

Stomach - Nausea in stomach, extends to chest, then ceases. Nausea with gagging and inclination to vomit. Bloating of stomach, acidity.

Temperature - Heat from abdomen to stomach and chest, running over different places and abating during day.

Throat - Touch, viscid phlegm from stomach with old alcoholics.

COMMENTS - A very remarkable symptom of Franz' has been confirmed by Flora A. Waddell. A man suffering from rheumatism of two years' duration came limping into Dr. Waddell's office, asking if she could do anything for his limb. He complained that when he sat down he couldn't rest in that position at all.

Asked why, he replied: "Whenever I sit down my limb feels as if broken off right here," pointing to the middle of his thigh. He said he often got up to straighten himself in order to make sure. He also had some pain in his arm and severe "sore pain" in his back. Anis. 30x cured all the symptoms.

Mure's Anis. symptoms were noted on head, abdomen, chest and back. Tough white expectoration appears to be a characteristic and there is pain in region of third rib, about one or two inches from sternum (junction of rib with its cartilage), generally on right side, but occasionally on the left.

RELATIONS - ***Compare:*** (1) In chest pains, Pix, Menth-pu. (2) Magn-gr. ***Compatible after:*** Acon. and Bry. in hemoptysis.

REFERENCES - Boericke. Clarke.

ANTHEMIS NOBILIS

(Roman Chamomile)

PHARMACY - anth. Anthemis nobilis. Roman chamomile. Chamomilla romana. N. O. Composite. Infusion of flowers or tincture of whole plant when beginning to flower. ***Historical dose:*** Tincture and all potencies.

CLINICAL - Ascarides. ***Colic.*** Coryza. Dyspepsia. Headache. Liver, congestion.

HERBAL - Anth. is the common chamomile used domestically in the form of a tea made of the flowers. It is not to be confounded with Chamomilla Matricaria.

HOMEOPATHIC - Burnett recorded a case in which violent gastric disturbance and headache were caused by the tea, and Berridge proved the tincture. In Burnett's case there was great coldness and chilliness inside abdomen.

Berridge had feelings of coldness generally and sensitiveness to cold air and the touch of cold things, but slight exertion caused heat and perspiration. Gastric disturbances with coldness. Sensitive to cold air and cold things.

Abdomen - ***Colic.*** Griping and ***chilliness inside of abdomen*** and into legs.

Kidneys - Bladder feels distended. Frequent urination.

Liver - Aching in region of liver.

Lungs - Coryza with much lachrymation, sneezing and discharge of clear water from the nose. Symptoms worse indoors. Constriction and rawness of throat. Tickling cough, worse in a warm room.

Male - Pain along spermatic cord, which feels full, as if has varicose veins.

Rectum - Itching of anus with white putty-like stools.

Skin - Itching of the soles, as if from chilblains. Gooseflesh.

RELATIONS - ***Compare:*** (1) Cina. (2) Chin. is "useful after abuse of chamomile tea when hemorrhage from uterus results" (Hering).

REFERENCES - Boericke. Clarke.

ANTHOXANTHUM ODORATUM

(Sweet Vernal Grass)

PHARMACY - antho. Anthoxanthum odoratum. Sweet vernal grass. N. O. Gramineae. Europe and America. Tincture of fresh flowering herb. ***Historical dose:*** Tincture and all potencies.

CLINICAL - Allergies. Coryza. Hay fever.

HERBAL - A popular remedy for hay fever is ***"hay tea,"*** a decoction made of hay itself. Antho. is used both externally and internally, with success on its effects produced by the pollen grains on those subject to hay fever. Seasonal allergies.

RELATIONS - ***Compare:*** (1) All-c., Ars., Naph., Sabad., Psor. (2) Anan., Avena, Arund., Lol. (3) Sac-alb.

REFERENCES - Boericke. Clarke.

ANTHRACINUM

(Anthrax Nosode)

PHARMACY - anthr. Anthracinum. Anthrax nosode. An alcoholic extract of the anthrax poison prepared from the spleens of affected sheep. ***Historical dose:*** All potencies.

CLINICAL - ***Abscesses.*** Acne. Anthrax. Bites. ***Boils. Blisters.*** Bubo. Cancer, pains. ***Carbuncles.*** Cellulitis. Chills. Coma. Delirium. Depression. Ecchymosis. Edema. ***Erysipelas. Gangrene.*** Gangrenous, ulcers. Glands, swollen. ***Fevers.*** Hemophilia. Hemorrhages. Hydrophobia. Injuries. ***Malignant, pustules.*** Parotiditis, gangrene. Phlegmonous, inflammation. ***Prostration.*** Pustules. Quinsy. Septic, fevers. Septicemia. Smallpox. ***Splenic, fever.*** Sycosis, barbae. Ulceration. ***Ulcers.*** Weakness. Whitlow. Wounds. Zymotic fevers.

HOMEOPATHIC - Anthracinum was introduced into homeopathic practice by Lux, a veterinarian, long before the experiments of Pasteur. The potentized anthrax nosode is the best remedy for the disease from which it is obtained, ***"splenic fever"*** in animals and ***"malignant pustule"*** in human beings. Epidemic spleen diseases of domestic animals and in septic inflammation, ***carbuncles and malignant ulcers.***

This nosode is a very valuable remedy in malignant or septic inflammation of connective or cellular tissue. It produces boils or boil-like eruptions, carbuncles, malignant ulcers, abscesses, bubo, where there is purulent focus. For ***boils*** and boil-like eruptions, acne. ***Succession of boils or carbuncles***. Suppurating, burning abscesses, fetid pus. Recurrent abscesses.

Abscess of nasal septum. Quinsy. ***Gangrene***, dissecting wounds. Offensive gangrenous ulcers. Parotiditis. Foul secretions. Ulceration, sloughing and ***intolerable burning***. ***Hard, stony*** swelling in region of right lower jaw and submaxillary gland. Anthrax quinsy. Whitlow and sloughing. Glands painfully swollen. ***Black or blue blisters.*** Foul erysipelas and gangrenous erysipelas, cellulitis.

Septicemia. Hemorrhages are thick, black tar-like from any orifice. Glands swollen, cellular tissue edematous and indurated. ***Terrible burning with great prostration.*** Black and blue blisters. Insect stings. Bad effects from inhaling foul odors.

Induration, cellular tissue, glands, muscles. Lymphangitis. Inflammation after surgery. Injuries, blows, falls and bruises. Injuries to bones, fractures. Compound fracture. Pain in cancerous affections. Burning pain, external. Pyemia. Swelling of glands. Trembling, paroxysmal. Benign tumors. Angioma. Fungus hematodes. Hemangioma. Atheroma. Steatoma.

Disorganization of blood. Congestion of blood. Convulsions, spasms, particularly in alcoholics. Clonic spasms. External dropsy. Weakness, enervation, exhaustion, prostration, infirmity. Weakness during fever. Weakness from perspiration. Wounds. Bites of dogs, poisonous animals. Snakes bites. ***Ailments from inhaling foul odors.*** Poisoning with sewer gas.

In the treatment of carbuncles, remember the prescription of the prophet Isaiah for King Hezekiah's carbuncle i.e., the pulp of a fig placed on a poultice and applied.

MIND - ***Anxiety, with fever.*** Confusion of mind. Disinclined to work, aversion to mental work. Depression, with debility and chill. Silent grief. Irritability, restlessness, nervousness, at night. Sadness, despondency, depression, melancholy.

Delirium and excitement during fever. Oversensitive. ***Presentiment of death***. Thinks she feels death approaching. Hydrophobia. Makes animals howls, bite, run about, become greatly excited, followed by paralytic symptoms. Collapse, unconsciousness, coma.

Abdomen - Distension. Swelling of the abdomen. Colicky pains. Bellyache with chill. Rumbling noises. Abdominal soreness, in epigastrium with vomiting, cold limbs, dull head. Intestinal anthrax. Mesenteric glands enlarged, size of a walnut. Dark red carbuncle in the omentum. Bubo. Burning, smarting pain.

Back - Axillary glands swollen. Eruptions. ***Carbuncles.*** Opisthotonos.

Blood - Septicemia, blood poisoning. Tendency to hemorrhage. Blood does not coagulate, hemophilia. Bleeding from orifices. Bleeding, clots, dark, ropy, tenacious. Rapidly decomposing blood.

Chest - Sensation as if diaphragm were pushed forward. Sensation of anxiety and constriction, in the precordia. Swelling of axillary lymphatic tissue.

Ears - Ringing in ears. Swelling of ears.

Eyes - Dilatation of pupils. Pale yellowish or greenish swelling. Pale redness above the brows along the forehead.

Face - Acne, boils and pustules. Parotiditis gangrenosa, after scarlatina. Abscess, lips. Cancer. Gland under chin painfully swollen. Tearing pain. Earthy discoloration. Red face and nose. Swelling, face glands, lymphatic tissue. ***Erysipelas.*** Indurations. Sycosis barbae.

Food - Appetite wanting. Diminished appetite with fever. Loss of appetite with chills and gastralgia. Aversion to eggs, odor of eggs. ***Excessive thirst, but can hardly swallow.*** Thirst with fever.

Head - Dullness in head as from narcotics. Headache, as if a smoke with a heating pain was passing through the head. Headache with chill. Carbuncles on head, near the ears or temples. Swelling of head. Cerebral hemorrhage. Erysipelas. Swelling of dura mater.

Heart - Heartbeats frequent but weak. Soft, scarcely frequent pulse. Blood does not coagulate.

Jaws - Tearing pain in lower jaws. Lockjaw, trismus. Stiffness in jaws. Stony swelling around lower jaw.

Kidneys - Kidneys swollen with edema. Suppression of urine, anuria. Swelling.

Limbs - Burning pains. Coldness of lower limbs. Cramps. Severe pains in limbs and joints with the fever. Convulsions, spasms. Tetanic spasms of upper limbs. Cracked skin. Arms and hands covered with a crusty eruption, full of cracks. Felon with sloughing, severe torturing pain and great prostration. ***Boils, blisters. and vesicles. Pustules.*** Whitlow. Gangrene from burns or scalds. Gangrenous ulcers. Ulcers with black base on lower limbs. Swelling of limbs.

Liver - Liver engorged. Congestion, liver.

Lungs - Cyanosis. Breathing frequent, laborious and spasmodic.

Male - Erections, troublesome. Erections, continued, priapism.

Mouth - Flabby taste. Dark red, bloody ecchymoses of mouth. Hemorrhage, oozing of blood. Abscess, lips. Pustules, lips. ***Black, lips.*** Erysipelas, lips. Offensive odor from mouth. Mouth could not be opened. Induration of salivary, submaxillary glands. Inflammation of parotid gland. Saliva increased. Cancer of glands, salivary, submandibular. Swelling of salivary, submaxillary glands.

Nerves - Epileptiform convulsions. Paroxysms of trembling. Clonic spasms, trismus or opisthotonos. Tetanic spasms in upper limbs. Debility and depression, with pain in the limbs.

Nose - Eruptions, inside nose, boils, furuncles. Nose swollen and red, fetid smell from it. Bloody mucus membranes of nose. ***Red discoloration of nose extending to cheek.*** Coryza. Discharge, offensive, fetid. Smells putrid odors, imaginary and real. Swelling, nose.

Perspiration - Sweat all over with debility. Night sweats. Cold sweats. Debilitating, exhausting sweats. Sticky, viscid sweats. Perspiration, suppressed.

Rectum - Vomiting followed by a painless, often bloody diarrhea. Diarrhea with fever. Diarrhea painless. Cholera-like collapse. Diarrhea with bellyache. Retarded stool. Stools, white. Mucus, slimy stools. Odor, putrid. Pasty, papescent stools. Sputtering stools.

Skin - Itching with dry skin. Dryness. Ecchymosis. ***Boils, painful.*** Blood boils. ***Carbuncles, burning.*** Edema, ulcers, gangrene, sloughing whitlows. Blackish eruptions. ***Black or blue blisters.*** Crusty oozing eruption. Sloughing ulcers. Smallpox. Bluish spots, with burning. Red spots. Erysipelas. Pustules and vesicles. Gangrene from burns or scalds. Gangrenous ulcers. Ulcers, cancerous. Ulcers with offensive discharges.

Sleep - Sleeplessness because of the pain. Sleepless, restless and irritated at night. Delirium with sleepiness. Sleep short, not refreshing, more like a stupor. Comatose. Unrefreshing sleep.

Spleen - Spleen, complaints of. Enlarged spleen. ***Epidemic spleen diseases of cattle or horses.***

Stomach - Belching with nausea, and inclination to vomit. Nausea and vomiting with chill. Vomiting of bilious and slimy masses. Vomiting followed by diarrhea. Pressure and burning in the region of the stomach. Burning pains. Vomiting of bile, mucus.

Temperature - ***Creeping chills.*** Debility with chills. ***Chills, alternating with heat.*** Great weakness with fever. Fever with diarrhea. Continued fever, typhus fever. Typhoid fever, with rapidly sinking pulse, loss of strength, fainting, delirium. Puerperal fever. Septic fevers. Zymotic fevers.

Throat - Right tonsil painful. Anthrax quinsy. ***Malignant sore throat.*** Swallowing difficult. Bleeding, oozing, tonsils. Sore throat. Tonsillitis. Swelling, edematous.

Tongue - Tongue often furred, with a thick brown coat, dry.

Urine - Pale urine. Profuse, increased urine. Scanty urine. Watery, clear as water.

Vertigo - Dizziness with headaches. Vertigo with loss of consciousness.

COMMENTS - Great restlessness. Debility and depression with pains in limbs and general sense of malaise, followed by disturbance of the intestines. Restlessness. Clonic and tetanic spasms. Exhaustion and collapse. Terrible burning pains.

Malignant boils. Severe boils that are very painful, with a tendency toward gangrene or cancer, or that refuse to heal (Tarant., Sil., Hep., and Bell.). Boils that come in crops all over the body. Keynote severe burning pains (Canth.). Ulcers with terrible burning. Induration of tissues. Hypersensitivity to the least touch, so they can't wear any clothes.

Completely exhausted, think they feel death. Collapse, with difficulty of breathing, loss of consciousness, death. Cyanosis, asphyxia and the most extreme collapse, followed by death in all cases of bleeding. Hemorrhage of dark blood (Croc.), keynote black, stringy hemorrhages.

RELATIONS - ***Antidoted by:*** Camph., Ars., Rhus-t., Sil., Lach., Carb-v., Puls., Kreos., Carb-ac., Sal-ac., Apis. Similar to: Ars., which it often follows. Tarent-c. ***Compare:*** (1) Ars., Tarent-c., Carb-v., Pyrog., Lach., Crot-h., Hippozaen, Echi. ***Follows well:*** Ars. - burning and ulceration, Ph-ac. ***Followed well by:*** Aur-m-n. - periosteal swelling of lower jaw, Sil. - cellulitis.

REFERENCES - Boericke. Clarke. Murphy.

ANTHRAKOKALI

(Anthracite Coal)

PHARMACY - anthro. Anthrakokali. Anthracokali. Anthracite coal of certain kind, dissolved in boiling caustic potash. Trituration. ***Historical dose:*** Trituration and all potencies.

CLINICAL - Decay. Cracks. Diabetes. Diuresis. Ecthyma. Eczema. Gout. Herpes. Impetigo Lichen. Nostrils, cracked. Priapism. Prurigo. Rheumatism. Scabies. Scrofula. Sycosis. Urticaria.

HOMEOPATHIC - Anthracokali has been used in skin affections, scabies, prurigo and chronic herpes. Chronic cracks and ulcerations of nostrils. Papular-like eruptions with a vesicular tendency, especially on scrotum, also on hands, tibia, shoulders and bottoms of the feet.

Eruptions decrease with the full of the moon. Intense thirst and diuresis, diabetes. Chronic rheumatism, gout, decay, scrofulosis. Bilious attacks, vomiting of bile. Tympanic distention of abdomen.

Abdomen - Inflation of the abdomen, as in tympanitis, colic.

Female - Menses beyond the usual period.

Food - Anorexia, nausea and vomiting. Increased appetite. Burning thirst, before sweat. Insatiable thirst. At first no appetite, but soon after it grew sharper.

Kidneys - Increase in the secretion of urine. Abundant flow of pale urine without sediment. Burning in the urethra while passing water, or itching at the orifice. Retention of urine.

Male - Frequent erections.

Mouth - Dryness of the mouth, foul tongue.

Nose - Chronic cracks and ulcerations of nostrils.

Rectum - Black stools, evacuations like pap, with colic and borborygmi, diarrhea, which continues several days.

Skin - Increased activity of the skin, nettle rash. Chronic erysipelas. Purulent pimples, like papules, with considerable itching.

Sleep - Sleeplessness with agitation and excited pulse.

Stomach - Retching, vomiting of bile, and of black mucus. Sensation of heat in the stomach. Cramps of the stomach.

Temperature - Shivering, alternating with heat, followed by gentle perspiration, and quickness of the pulse. Redness and heat of the skin, disappearing on sweating. Perspiration all over the body.

Throat - Dryness of the throat, with internal heat, extending to stomach, swallowing slightly impeded.

RELATIONS - ***Compare:*** (1) Compare the Carbons. (2) Rhus-t., Dulc. (3) Ferr-i. - eczema impetigenoides. (4) Antimonies.

REFERENCES - Boericke. Clarke.

ANTIMONIUM ARSENICOSUM

(Antimony Arsenite)

PHARMACY - ant-ar. Antimonium arsenicosum. Antimony arsenite. Arsenicum stibiatum. Stibium arsenicosum. Trituration. ***Historical dose:*** Trituration and all potencies.

CLINICAL - Asthma. Catarrhal pneumonia. ***Dyspnea***. Edema. ***Emphysema.*** Heart weakness. Influenza. Low, appetite. ***Lung, disorders.*** Myocarditis. Ophthalmia. Pericarditis. Pleurisy. Pneumonia. Sciatica. Tuberculosis.

HOMEOPATHIC - Ant-ar. has a combination of Antimonium Tart. and Arsenicum symptoms. Ant-ar. is said to affect preferably upper left lung. ***Emphysema with excessive dyspnea and cough***, much mucus secretion. Dyspnea, worse on eating and lying down. Sense of weakness.

Catarrhal pneumonia associated with influenza. Mattes said it is equally effective in right-side cases in old pneumonias and catarrhal pneumonias in children in old pleuritic effusions and in pericardial exudations. Loss of appetite. General sick feeling.

The cough is worse by eating and on lying down. Pleurisy especially of left side with ***exudation*** and pericarditis with effusion. Rush of blood to head. Inflammation of the eyes and edema of the face. Wandering pains in sciatic nerves. Myocarditis and cardiac weakness.

COMMENTS - Boericke said "emphysema with excessive dyspnea," difficulty in breathing, cough with a lot of mucus. Catarrhal pneumonia associated with influenza. Other lung disorders, tuberculosis. Worse on eating and lying down, low appetite. Sense of weakness. Pleurisy, especially of left side, with ***exudation*** and pericarditis with effusion.

RELATIONS - ***Compare:*** (1) Other antimony salts. (2) Ars., Aur., Lach., Puls. - wandering pains, Sulph.

REFERENCES - Boericke. Clarke. Murphy.

ANTIMONIUM CRUDUM

(Native Sulphide of Antimony)

PHARMACY - ant-c. Antimonium crudum. Native Sulphide of Antimony. Antimonium sulphuratum nigrum. Stibium sulfuratum nigrum crudum. ***Historical dose:*** Trituration and all potencies.

CLINICAL - Acne. Alcoholism. ***Amenorrhea.*** Anus, irritation. Arthritis. Backache. ***Belching***. ***Blepharitis***. Boils. Bunions. ***Callosities.*** Catarrh. Chills. Chorea. Constipation. Corns. Deafness. Diarrhea. Dyspepsia. Eczema. Emaciation. Feet, sore. Fever. ***Food, allergies.*** Freckles. ***Gastrointestinal, disorders.*** Gout. Grief. Gum rash. Headaches. Heartburn. Heatstroke. Hemorrhoids. Hoarseness. ***Horny, growths.*** Hysteria. ***Indigestion. Leucorrhea.*** Marasmus. ***Nails, fungus.*** Nails, split. nausea. Nettle rash. Nosebleed. Nymphomania. Obesity. Otorrhea. Premenstrual, syndrome. ***Proctitis***. Prolapsed, rectum. Red gum. Remittent, fever. Rheumatism. Skin, disorders. ***Stomach, disorders.*** Suicidal. Sunstroke. Tendons, inflamed. Tongue, coated. Toothache. ***Urticaria***. Vertigo. Voice, low. Vomiting. ***Warts.*** Whooping cough.

HOMEOPATHIC - Ant-c. is pre-eminently a stomach and skin remedy. It corresponding to constitutions with tendency to growths and rough scaling skin with horny patches. These horny patches are very tender, the patient can hardly bear to walk on them. ***Fungus under nails.*** Nails tend to grow in splits. ***Warts.***

Boericke said, ***"thickly coated white tongue are true guiding symptoms."*** Fissures on corner of the mouth that split and crack (Petr.). Lips are dry and cracked, usually at corners. ***Thickly coated tongue, white, milky-white or like whitewash evenly laid.*** The edges may be red and sore. Sore, cracked and crusty nostrils and corners of mouth.

Chronic indigestion. Patient can have a big appetite, ***eats beyond the capacity of his digestion*** or without discrimination, the mental and skin symptoms can be due to this disturbance. Exceedingly weak condition of the body.

Abnormal hunger, not relieved by eating, emptiness of epigastrium and want of animal heat. ***Gastric derangements, with tongue coated thickly white, with different complaints***. Disgust for all foods. Nursing children throw up a little sour milk as soon as they take the breast or bottle, then refuses to nurse again (Aeth. after vomiting the child sleeps and wakes hungry).

Heartburn, gas. Food allergies, especially to sour wines and vinegar. Intolerance to wine. In one case it produced a feeling of intoxication like that of alcohol, so that the patient refused to take any more of it.

Chronic complaints that are traceable to suppression of eruptions or ulcers. Effects of suppressed eruptions. ***Worse by heat*** (Apis, Puls., Cham., Sec., Camph.). ***Worse from cold washing***, cold water and cold food. Cannot bear heat of sun.

An absence of pain, where it would be expected. Rheumatism and gout if parts are inflamed or swollen. Gout with stomach symptoms. Acute gout having left deposits with gastric symptoms. Inveterate chronic gout without fever. Dark hemorrhages. Dropsical swelling of whole body.

Mucus membranes generally affected. Swelling pain and redness of glands. External parts turn black, dry gangrene. Obesity of young people. Tendency to grow fat. Marasmus of children. Emaciation. Glandular obstructions. Scrofula. Fungus articularis. Metastasis of gout and rheumatism causing gastric catarrh. Anasarca.

MIND - ***Excessive irritability and fretfulness***, with a thickly-coated white tongue. Fretful cross and peevish. Adults are sulky, do not wish to speak with anyone. Angry at every little attention. Homesickness. Weeping and impressionable.

Nervous hysterical girls and women, who are overcome by mellow light from stained-glass windows. ***Sentimental mood by moonlight.*** Dreamy, sentimental. Amativeness. ***Ill effects of disappointed love, grief.*** Ecstasy and exalted love. ***Love sick***, with sulkiness. Sulky, doesn't want to speak with anyone. Either ***sentimental or cross and touchy*** during diarrhea and before menses.

The child is cross, but will scream at every little attention (Cham. wants to be carried). ***Child cannot bear to be touched or looked at*** (Nat-m.). Can't bear to be washed or touched. Anger when touched. ***Peevishness, worse touch or consolation.*** Very sentimental, easily moved, more so in the adult. Nymphomania during suppressed menses. Disposition to start, even at slight noises.

Excitability. Anxious reflections in relation to one's present and future. Can be anxious about their fate, health and future. Cross and contradictive, whatever is done fails to give satisfaction. Sleepy and weary. Talks in rhymes or verses, taciturn. So busy with oneself one forgets to urinate or defecate, eats only when asked. Loathing of food, bathing etc.

Great sadness and woeful mood. Sorrowful, irritable humor. Distrustful. Suicidal depression. Inclination to shoot himself, at night he is obliged to get out of bed because he can't free himself of the idea. Loathing, disgust for life. Abject despair, wants to commit suicide by drowning. Mental symptoms are worse from suppressed eruptions (Mez.). Suicidal thoughts drive him out of bed.

Abdomen - Inflation of the abdomen with a sensation of fullness, chiefly after a meal. ***Abdomen very much distended, with much rumbling.*** Colic with loss of appetite, hard stool, red urine. Sensation of emptiness in the abdomen, as after violent diarrhea. Sensation of swelling and of hardness in the inguinal region, on its being pressed. Incarcerated flatus. ***Flatus in the abdomen with rumbling and borborygmi.*** Cutting in bowels with watery diarrhea. Violent cutting pains, sometimes with want of appetite, red urine and hard stools. Pinching pain and sensation as if diarrhea would come on.

Back - Itching and pain of neck and back. Violent pain in small of back when rising, better when walking. Coccyx heavy. Swelling of cervical glands. Spasmodic drawing, in muscles of nape, reaching to scapulae. Backache evening after lying down and in morning.

Back - Backache worse stooping, exerting arms and turning head to left. Spasmodic stitches in right scapula when sitting.

Causations - Ill effects of disappointed love, grief and suppressed eruptions. Hot weather or sun. Getting over-heated. Overeating.

Chest - Stifling oppression and paralytic orthopnea. Shootings in the chest, when drawing breath and at other times. ***Itching of chest*** with oppression. Pain, as of contusion in the pectoralis major, on raising the arm and on pressure. Sharp pain under left breast. Burning pain in the chest with heat. Pains during fever. Oppression and pressive pains, more right side. Sharp pains in chest when exhaling. Burning and sticking pains. Severe itching upon chest continuing all day.

Constitutions - Suited to infants and children with coated, moist, white tongues and to the elderly. Hydrogenoid constitutions. Tendency to grow fat. Constitutions with tendency to rough scaling skin with horny patches. A scrofulous medicine.

Cough - Cough in paroxysms, as if arising from abdomen, first paroxysm always most severe, subsequent ones weaker and weaker, until the last one only resembles a hacking cough. Burning with dry cough and dyspnea. Burning at every cough. ***Cough in hot sun.*** Cough with hot breath. Cough shaking whole body, with involuntary escape of copious urine. ***Cough on coming into warm room.*** Cough from cold air. Cough with burning sensation in chest, itching of chest, oppression. Looking into fire aggravates cough. Cough after rising in morning.

Ears - Redness and swelling, pain in eustachian tube. Ringing and deafness. Moist eruption around ear. Otorrhea. Deafness, as if bandaged or a leaf lying on ear.

Eyes - Dull, sunken, red, itch inflamed, agglutinated. ***Canthi are raw, fissured*** and cracked, red and moist. Itching in canthi. ***Chronic blepharitis***. Pustules on cornea and on the margins of the lids. Looking into the fire causes cough. Inflammation of lachrymal glands and ducts. Chronic sore eyes of children. Photophobia. Dried mucus in corners. Eyes worse glare of snow.

Face - Acne worse near fire. Dry lips. Eczema about mouth. Pimples, pustules and boils on face. Eruption like nettle-rash. Freckles. ***Yellow crusted eruption on cheeks and chin***. Sallow, haggard or sad. Cracks in the corners of the mouth. Corners of lips and nostrils cracked and sore. Burning, stinging on chin, as from a hot spark. Small, sore, honey colored granules on chin. Sharp pain in left cheek when exhaling. Twitching of facial muscles. Heat and itching on cheeks. Submaxillary glands swollen.

Female - Menses too early and profuse. Premenstrual syndrome. Toothache before menses. ***Amenorrhea.*** Menses suppressed from cold bathing. ***Menses suppressed*** with feeling of tenderness of the ovaries, pressure in womb as if something would come out during menses. Painful ovaries in love sick girls. Leucorrhea watery, acrid, lumpy. Nymphomania from checked menses. Excited, genitals itch. Nausea, vomiting with diarrhea, all during pregnancy. Hemorrhoidal affections during pregnancy. Tenderness of ovarian region, with nausea, vomiting and white tongue. Irritable, painful ovaries of hysterical girls who are dreamers, who suffer from unrequited affections. Watery vaginal discharge causes smarting down thighs.

Food - ***Loss of appetite*** with disgust for food. ***Great desire to eat, but gets no strength.*** Appetite does not return after severe illness. Food leaves an aftertaste or causes constant belching. Good appetite with burning at pit of stomach. Diminished appetite in summer owing to heat. Loathing of food with a bitter taste. ***Long-lasting loss of appetite with disgust for all food.*** Hunger early on waking without appetite, eating does not better it. ***Desire for acids, sour pickles.*** Desire for cucumbers, sour, wine, vinegar. Desire for beer with chill. Intense thirst with dryness of lips, more at night. Patient is a gross feeder, a glutton, he eats beyond the capacity of his digestion or without discrimination.

Head - Headaches, worse in vertex, on ascending. ***Headaches from disordered stomach.*** Headache worse candy or acid wines, fruits, fats, ascending stairs. Headache from alcoholic drinks. Suppressed eruptions. Heaviness in forehead with vertigo, nausea and nosebleed. ***Headaches from bathing in cold water***. Headache after stopped coryza. Headache with great loss of hair. Itching of the head with falling of hair. Tendency to take cold about head. Heaviness in forehead with vertigo, nausea and nosebleed. Lentil-sized, flat tubercles here and there on scalp, painful to pressure, crawling sensation around them. Rush of blood to head, followed by nosebleed.

Heart - Violent palpitations. Pulse extremely irregular, now accelerated and again slow. Pulse changing every few beats. Slow pulsation during fine pricking headache.

Kidneys - Urine is turbid and has a foul odor. Cutting in urethra while urinating. Tenesmus of bladder rouses him from sleep at night. Urination is frequent, profuse with burning and backache. Involuntary urination, on coughing. Gritty sediment. Frequent urination with much mucus, intense burning in urethra and backache during emission.

Larynx - Heat in larynx in open air. ***Voice harsh and badly pitched.*** Voice, lacks control, harsh, badly pitched better using it. Aphonia from overheating. Laryngitis. Rough voice from over use. Hoarseness after cold water bath. Great weakness or entire loss of the voice, chiefly on becoming warm. Sensation of a foreign substance in the larynx with inability to expectorate. Violent spasm in the larynx with sensation of excoriation.

Limbs - Lassitude, tremulous fatigue and heaviness of all limbs. Twitching of muscles. Jerks in arms. Limbs weak during headache. ***Arthritic pain in joints of fingers. Horny or split nails. Nails brittle***, grow out of shape. Horny growth under the nails. Skin beneath nails painfully sensitive. Discolored nails. ***Horny warts*** on hands and soles. Weakness and shaking of hands in writing followed by offensive flatulence. Painful stiffness of knee. Pustules on thighs. Inflamed corns. Pain in heels. Painful inflammation of the tendon of elbows with great redness and curvature of the arms. Shiny elbows. ***Callosities on soles.*** Skin on soles is withered on account of foot sweat. ***Feet very tender, covered with large horny places.*** Rheumatic pain, in legs. Numbness of legs during rest and while sitting. Weakness and shaking of hands in writing, followed by offensive flatus. Crippled feet.

Lungs - Deep, sighing, as from fullness of chest, afternoon and after eating. Unequal breathing, during sleep. Oppression coming from stomach. Constriction almost to suffocation. Spells of sighing. Difficult breathing, with raised shoulders. Respiration deep with sighing. Expectoration of large quantities of mucus, exhausts the patient.

Male - Eruption on scrotum and about genitals. Impotence. Atrophy of penis and testicles. Biting, itching of scrotum with eruptions. Excited sexual desire with uneasiness of the whole body. Nightly pollutions with or without voluptuous dreams. Itching of penis, of tip of glans. Erections when getting warm in bed, with sleeplessness.

Modalities - Better in open air. Better moist warmth. Better during rest. Better lying down. Worse in evening. Worse at night. Worse moonlight. Worse water, wet poultices. ***Worse cold bathing, cold water*** (on head). Worse dampness. Worse radiated heat. ***Worse heat from sun***. Worse from acids, vinegar. Worse sweets, wine, pork. ***Worse overeating***, debauches. Worse after getting drunk. Worse rising up. Worse ascending stairs. Worse touch.

Mouth - Aphthae. Dryness of mouth. Gums bleed easily. Taste bitter. Pappy taste. Salivation, taste salty. ***Tongue coated thick white, as if whitewashed.*** Canker sores. Sore feeling and redness on border of tongue. Much slimy mucus. Pimples around the mouth. Rawness of palate, with expectoration of much mucus.

Nose - Fluent or dry coryza. ***Nostrils chapped and covered with crusts.*** Stuffed nose in a heated room. ***Eczema of nostrils, sore, cracked and scurfy***. Nosebleed after headache. Nosebleed, evenings with rush of blood to head. Feeling of coldness on inhalation. Nose painful when breathing.

Perpiration - Hot sweat. Perspires at same hour every other day. Sweats in morning when awaking, causes shrivelling of fingertips. Sweat soon disappears and followed by dry heat. Cold, clammy sweat from motion. Sweats during rheumatic pains. Sweats during headache.

Rectum - Anal itching. Burning, itching and fissures in the anus. Diarrhea alternating with constipation. Acrid diarrhea. Diarrhea in summer. Diarrhea, worse during headache. Diarrhea with much belching. ***Hemorrhoids,*** blind and running with burning and tingling. Mucus hemorrhoids, prickling and burning with continuous mucus discharge from anus, staining yellow. ***Catarrhal proctitis***. Flow of black blood from the anus. ***Abuse of laxatives.*** Constipation in heat of summer, in childbed. Soreness in rectum as if an ulcer has been torn open, during stool. Expansive pressure in the rectum during stool as if an ulcer had been torn open. Burning furunculus in the perineum. Rectal hemorrhage with solid stools, hemorrhoids. Boils on perineum, burning around them.

Skin - Freckles become numerous. ***Eczema with gastric derangements.*** Pimples, vesicles and pustules. imples and vesicles as from stings of insects. Pustules here and there with brown scurf. Eruptions worse heat of stove, etc. Sensitive to cold bathing. Thick, hard, honey-colored scabs. ***Urticaria***. Urticaria, white with red areola, itching fearfully. Itching when warm in bed. Itching of skin, feels sore when scratched. Skin diseases during pregnancy. Measles-like eruptions. Dry skin. Dry gangrene. Scaly, pustular eruption with burning and itching, worse at night. Callosities from slight pressure. Ulcers become fistulous. Deep, spongy ulcers. Smooth warts. ***Warts*** (Thuj., Sabin., Caust.).

Sleep - Great sleepiness during day. Deep unrefreshing sleep, can hardly rise in morning, so tired. Sleepy and weary. ***Drowsiness in elderly people***. Strong inclination to sleep during the day, chiefly in the evening or morning. Waking with fright during the night. Frequent waking from itching here and there. Sleeplessness with shivering over left side. Dreams, anxious, horrible, voluptuous or painful. Dreams full of quarreling. Anxious dreams, as if he were to be hurt. Horrible dreams, about mutilation of men. Coma with delirium.

Stomach - ***Digestion disordered easily***. Heartburn, nausea, vomiting. Burning, spasmodic pains, driving to despair. ***Gastric derangements, with tongue coated thickly white, with different complaints***. After nursing, the child vomits its milk in curds and refuses to nurse afterwards and is very cross. Great desire to eat, but no strength to do it. ***Eructation tasting of the ingesta***. Gastrointestinal complaints from bread and pastry, acids, sour wine, pork, cold bathing, overheating, hot weather. ***Constant belching***. Gouty moves to stomach and intestines. ***Indigestion, chronic.*** Sweetish water brash. ***Bloating after eating***. Sensation of emptiness in stomach. Stomach seems to be always overloaded. Stomach is painful to pressure. Nausea with diarrhea. Loathing nausea, and desire to vomit. Vomiting, worse eating or drinking, without nausea or relief. Nausea ceases, vomiting continues. Vomiting, fearful with convulsions, which nothing can stop. Vomiting of slimy mucus and bile.

Stool - Stools composed entirely of mucus. Hard and loose stools, with nausea. Stools watery, containing undigested food. Diarrhea after acids, sour wine, baths, overeating. ***Diarrhea alternates with constipation***, especially in elderly people. Diarrhea, watery with cutting pains. Urgent inclination to go to stool. Stools composed entirely of mucus, pappy. Constant secretion of yellowish-white mucus by the anus. Difficult evacuation of hard stools, the feces are too large in size. ***Stools of hard lumps mixed with watery discharge***. Diarrhea during summer after nursing.

Teeth - Gums detach from teeth, bleed easily. Grinding of teeth, when sleeping in sitting position. Pains in hollow teeth. Toothache worse touching tooth with tongue, better walking in open air. Teeth so sore it seems one can hardly bear the dental operation. Toothache in hollow teeth, worse night, touching tooth with tongue causes pain as if nerve were torn. Sharp pains in tooth when inspiring air. Toothache before menses.

Temperature - Chill predominating during day. Violent chill, shaking, toward noon, with thirst. Chill over back, feet cold as ice, with sweat on rest of body. Chill at every motion, with cough. Chill after vomiting. Chill before menses. Chilly even in warm room. Disturbances of stomach during apyrexia in intermittent fevers. Intermittent fever with disgust, nausea, vomiting, belchings, coated tongue, diarrhea. Hot sweat. Great heat from little exercise, especially in the sun. Heat and thirst after sweat. Fever at night. Body hot, limbs cold, during cough. Fever with desire to sleep and want of thirst.

Throat - Much thick yellowish mucus from posterior sinuses. Hawking in open air. Great heat in the throat while moving in the open air. Sensation as if a foreign body had lodged with constant desire to swallow.

Vertigo - Confusion of head, as after long labor in the cold. A feeling of intoxication. Vertigo with nausea and nosebleed. Vertigo with nausea and confused feeling, as if drunk, Vertigo during headache. Vertigo from deranged stomach.

COMMENTS - Restlessness and jerking of muscles. Slight noises startle. Nosebleed with vertigo after headache after rush of blood to head. Gastric and remittent fevers and fevers of children with great thirst and the characteristic white tongue. The fever runs higher at night. Tendency to take cold about head.

Scrofulous ophthalmia, canthi especially affected (Graph. the whole margin).

Otorrhea. Moist eruption behind ears (Graph.). Itching of the scalp and hair falling out.

Fungus infections or deformity of the nails, calluses from pressure, corns, painful bunions, painful warts and horny warts (excrescences). Good for warts that grow next to the nail and bleed and irritate. Thickened skin, spots on the nails, nails that split, "crippled nails." Arthritis and deformative arthritis of the fingers and toes.

Constipation and other intestinal disorders. Severe gastric flu with a white tongue. Chronic indigestion. Diarrhea which alternates with constipation, often found in old people, "stomach weak, digestion easily disturbed in old people." Anal fissures (Graph., Sil.). Continuously oozing hemorrhoids, staining linen.

General symptoms are worse heat of sun, sun gives headache, worse bathing or change of weather. Intoxicated easily from wine (Zinc., Chin., Caps.), face flushes after a couple sips. May cough if they look at a fire or will be aggravated by radiant heat. Worse from heat, but great sensitiveness to cold. Suitable to the hydrogenoid constitutions. Tendency toward obesity.

A student, 17, had twenty-three warts on right hand and thirty-four warts on the left hand. Mainly on backs and fingers, but a few on interior surface of fingers. In addition, inflammation of eyelids. Ant-c. 200x cured her of warts in 7 weeks.

Dr. M. Jousset has recorded a severe case of chorea which resisted all the usual remedies and was cured with Ant-c. prescribed on the digestive symptoms, particularly the characteristic white tongue. Ant-c. corresponds in a sense to the swine, as Ars. does to horses and Puls. to sheep.

RELATIONS - ***Antidote to:*** Stings of insects. ***Antidoted by:*** Calc., Hep., Merc. Bry. ***Compare:*** (1) Nat-m., Ant-t., Antimonium Chloridum. (2) Kermes mineral - Stibiat sulph. rub. - Bronchitis. (3) Also Puls, Ip., Sulph. (4) Aethi-a., Am-m., Apis, Bry., Graph., Ran-b., Rhus-t., Vario., Cham., Chin. and Hep., Rhus-t,

Sep. and Spig. (5) Sulph. - Averse to be washed, digestive condition, loaded tongue and worse from warmth in summer complaints. (6) Stram. - averse to be looked at. ***Complementary:*** Squil., Sulph. Follows well: Puls., Ip. Followed by: Puls., Merc., Sulph.

REFERENCES - Boericke. Clarke. Murphy. Phatak.

ANTIMONIUM IODATUM

(Antimony Teriodide)

PHARMACY - ant-i. Antimonium iodatum. Antimony teriodide. Trituration. ***Historical dose:*** Trituration and all potencies.

CLINICAL - Asthma. Bronchitis. Colds. Coughs. Pneumonia. Uterus, hyperplasia.

HOMEOPATHIC - Recommended by Hale in cases of uterine hyperplasia, also in cases of humid asthma, bronchitis and other pulmonary disorders. Inability to raise the sputum, especially in the aged and weak patients. Pneumonia. Stage of resolution of pneumonia slow and delayed.

In sub-acute and chronic colds in chest which have extended downwards from head and into the bronchial tubes in the form of hard, croupy cough with a decided wheeze.

Indicated by frequent spells of coughing with expectoration of frothy, white or thick yellowish mucus. Loss of appetite and strength. Moderate febrile action. Coated tongue. Yellowish discoloration of skin and conjunctive, sweaty. Dull and drowsy.

REFERENCES - Boericke. Clarke.

ANTIMONIUM MURIATICUM

(Antimony Chloride)

PHARMACY - ant-m. Antimonium muriaticum. Antimony chloride. Butter of antimony. Antimonium chloridum. Stibium muriaticum. Triturations. ***Historical dose:*** Trituration and all potencies.

CLINICAL - Abrasions. Cancer. Lip cancer. Nausea. Prostration. Vomiting.

HOMEOPATHIC - Ant-m. is unproved. Poisoning symptoms show a stupor insensibility, collapse and cold, clammy surface. Inactive pupils, sunken, lusterless eyes. Nausea and vomiting, burning pains in throat and stomach, frequent abortive efforts to defecate.

Ant-m. has been used in cases of ***cancer of the lower lip***. Mucus membranes destroyed. The tissues and peritoneum covered with flocculent matter easily scraped off, they are soft and readily torn. Mouth to jejunum becomes black. Abrasions. Great prostration of strength.

MIND - Stupor, but from which he could be aroused by questions. Stupor with cold feet. Insensibility.

RELATIONS - ***Compare:*** (1) Other antimony salts. (2) Acids, Ars., Carb-v. (3) Con. - cancer of lower lip and ineffectual urging to stool.

REFERENCES - Boericke. Clarke. Grimmer.

ANTIMONIUM OXYDATUM

(Antimonious Oxide)

PHARMACY - ant-o. Antimonium oxydatum. Antimonious oxide. Antimony sesquioxide. Fumes from antimony works. Trituration. ***Historical dose:*** All potencies.

CLINICAL - Bloody urine. Cough. Diarrhea. Dyspnea. Headache. Impotence. Intermittent, fever.

HOMEOPATHIC - Great relaxation of the whole organism.

Abdomen - Distended by incarcerated gases.

Back - Sharp pains in the sacro-lumbar region.

Bladder - Pains and urging at neck of bladder, and burning in the urethra during urination. Discharge of a few drops of mucus from the urethra. Gonorrhea-like discharge from the urethra. Urine of a deep orange-yellow color, almost red. Deep-red and bloody urine, causing burning in the urethra, from which exuded a whitish mucus after cessation of the bloody urine.

Chest - Very great constriction of the chest, with stitches. Sharp stitches through the chest, towards the shoulders and back. Violent stitches in chest, with dry cough.

Head - Lightning-like stitches through the head backward, which suddenly disappear, while the headache in the forehead remains. Slight headache increases to an intolerable degree.

Lungs - Cough violent, shattering, dry, with stitches in chest. Cough dry, painful, finally ends in a difficult expectoration of tenacious mucus. Respiration difficult, with mucus and sibilant rales over the chest.

Male - Penis flaccid. Complete impotence, no ejaculation of semen, and even no erections. Atrophy of testicles and penis. Pains in the testicles.

Mouth - Tongue coated white.

Rectum - Diarrhea, with griping pains in abdomen. Stools troublesome, frequent, consisting of food evacuated soon after eating.

Skin - Pustular eruption on lower abdomen, neck, body. Eruption thickest on genitals, in the bends of the limbs, on nates, and especially on thighs and scrotum. Pustular elevations, like pocks, on the scrotum.

Temperature - Very profuse and debilitating sweats during sleep. Very tormenting, pouring sweat, every time after sleeping, followed by great exhaustion. Complaints assume the form of intermittent fever.

REFERENCES - Murphy.

ANTIMONIUM SULPHURATUM AURATUM

(Gold Sulphuret of Antimony)

PHARMACY - ant-s. Antimonium sulphuratum auratum. Gold sulphuret of antimony. Trituration. ***Historical dose:*** Trituration and all potencies.

CLINICAL - Acne. Amaurosis. ***Bronchial**, **catarrh**.* ***Catarrh.*** Constipation. Corneal spots. Diarrhea. Indigestion. Iris, protruding. Itching. Lung, congestion. ***Nasal**, **catarrh**.* ***Nosebleed.*** Pneumonia.

HOMEOPATHIC - In its provings, the most notable effects were produced in the eye and chest. As with the other Antinomies, there is disordered digestion, pasty mouth and taste in morning. ***Chronic nasal and bronchial catarrh***. Increase of tough mucus in larynx and bronchi, respiration difficult. Dry, hard cough with passive congestion of upper lobe of left lung. Nosebleed on washing. Itching on hands and feet.

Burning in head with eye complaints. Amaurosis (commencing). Spots on cornea and hypopion. Acne.

Abdomen - Pressure, tension and fullness in abdomen. Umbilical region sensitive. Violent colic and rumbling around navel.

Eyes - Amaurosis, commencing. Spots on cornea. Iris protruding through cornea.

Face - Pustular acne.

Food - Loss of appetite, almost a loathing of food.

Head - Pressive pains. Burning pain in head, with eye complaints. Reddish swelling behind right ear, leaving a redness and scurfiness.

Kidneys - Urine increased, dark red.

Limbs - Itching on hands and feet. Arms heavy in morning. Boring and tearing pain in arms and hand-joints. Swelling of fingers.

Lungs - Accumulation of tough mucus in bronchi and larynx. Tickling in larynx. ***Increased mucus*** with fullness in bronchials. Respiration difficult, pressure in bronchi with constriction. Dry, hard cough, no expectoration. ***Congestion of upper lobe of left lung.*** Winter coughs, patient is sore all over. Pneumonia, when hepatization occurred and resolution failed to take place. Increased mucus sputum, mixed with blood of a sweetish taste. Passive congestion of upper lobe left lung with hard, dry cough.

Male - Pustular eruption on scrotum with much itching.

Mouth - Metallic taste. Pasty mouth and taste in morning.

Nose - ***Nosebleed on washing the face***. Increased secretion in nose and throat. Loss of smell.

Rectum - Passage of much flatus with sudden urging, followed by a solid stool at first, then bright yellow and pasty stool. Constipation. Feces hard and passed with difficulty.

Skin - Acne, pustular variety. Itching on hands and feet.

Sleep - Deep sleep. Wakes after midnight with dull headache. Wakes with restlessness and sexual desire. Awoke suddenly with heavy, confused head, pressure in stomach, difficult breathing. Sleep dreamy.

Stomach - Pressure and fullness in stomach and abdomen, umbilical region sensitive.

Stool - Passage of much flatus with sudden urging, followed by a stool, solid at first then bright yellow and pasty, afterwards violent colic and rumbling around navel. Constipation, feces hard and passed with difficulty.

Throat - Increased secretion in nose and throat. Rough and scrapy feeling. Metallic styptic taste. Burning or heat in fauces. Mucus from throat becomes offensive to smell. Pressure in throat as if a plug stuck in it. Scratching, rough feeling in throat in morning. Tickling in larynx. Accumulation of tough mucus in larynx and bronchi.

RELATIONS - ***Compare:*** (1) Other Antimonies. (2) Aur. - chest, Ars., Ferr., Merc-sulph., Sulph. (3) Am-c. - nosebleed after washing.

REFERENCES - Boericke. Clarke.

ANTIMONIUM TARTARICUM

(Tartar Emetic)

PHARMACY - ant-t. Antimonium tartaricum. Tartar emetic. Tartrate of Antimony and potash. Trituration and solutions. ***Historical dose:*** Trituration and all potencies.

CLINICAL - Albuminuria. Alcoholism. Aphthae. ***Asphyxia.*** Asthma. Bilharziasis. Bilious disorders. ***Bronchitis.*** Catarrh. Chickenpox. ***Chills.*** Cholera. Cholera morbus. Colic. ***Coughs.*** Croup. Delirium. Delirium, Tremens. Dyspepsia. ***Emphysema.*** Eruptions. Eyes, inflamed. ***Gasping***. Gastric, disorders. Headache. Hematuria. Hydrocephalus. Impetigo. Intermittent fever. Laryngitis. Leucorrhea. Lumbago. ***Lungs, disorders.*** Lungs, paralysis. Muscle pain. Nausea. Parkinson's disease. Plica polonica. ***Pneumonia.*** Psoriasis. ***Pustules.*** Rheumatism. Ringworm. Smallpox. Stiff-neck. Sycosis. Synovitis. Taste, altered. Thirst. Tongue, coated. Tremors. Vomiting. Warts. Weakness. Whooping cough.

HOMEOPATHIC - Tartar emetic of the Alchemists. Ant-t. resembles closely Ant-c. and the other Antimonies in its action, though the modalities differ. Ant-t. was the favorite emetic historically, and consequently it is one of our best remedies in states of nausea. The nausea is as intense as that of Ip., but less persistent and is better by vomiting.

A correspondent related the case of an apprentice who had been employed for a week making up ***"cough-balls"*** and diuretic balls for horses, both containing powdered antimony. He had been cautioned not to inhale the powder, but his employer believes he did. At the end of the week he was seized with an illness due, his employer thinks and no doubt correctly, to the antimony.

Affects the mucus membranes especially of the bronchials and lungs. Ant-t. has many symptoms in common with Ant-c., but also many peculiar to itself. Cyanosis, depression of vital power.

Rattling of mucus with little expectoration. Great accumulation of mucus with coarse rattling, impeded respiration and labored heart action, defective oxygenation in the circulation of blood.

Complaints arising in digestive sphere. Gastric disorders of alcoholics and gouty subjects. ***Cholera morbus.***

Patient becomes ***increasingly weak, sweats, become drowsy and relaxed with lack of reaction.*** Prostrated in mind and body. Sensation of coldness in blood vessels. ***Bilharziasis***. Ant-t. acts indirectly on the parasites by stimulating the oxidizing action of the protective substance. Lumbago. ***Chills and contractures*** with pain in muscles.

Chronic trembling of head and hands, as in Parkinson's disease. Trembling of whole body, great prostration and faintness. Warts on glans penis. Convulsive twitching. Convulsions when eruptions fail to appear. Ant-t. is homeopathic to dysuria, strangury, hematuria, albuminuria, catarrh of bladder and urethra, burning in rectum, bloody mucus stools, etc.

Nursing infants let go the nipple and cry out as if out of breath. Child continuously wishes to be carried erect, unwilling to be looked at or touched. Children have convulsions if attention is thrust upon them. Clings to attendants.

MIND - Great despondency. Fear of being alone. Fretfulness, whining and crying, before the attack of sickness. Bad mood. Frightened, at trifles. Muttering, delirium and stupor. Stupid on awakening.

Melancholic, complains of numerous suffering. Despairs of his recovery. Anxious, despairing. Anxiety during nausea. Peevish, whining and moaning. Child will not be touched without whining. ***Can't bear to be looked at.*** Child clings to those around, calls for help in a hoarse voice, with cough.

Restlessness in children, better being carried about. Dreads being left alone, lest he should be very nervous. Contradiction between mind and will. Pitiful whining before and during attacks. Hopeless and despairing when awake. Clings to attendants.

Apathy or easily annoyed, wants to be let alone. Furious delirium. Talking to himself. Boldness. Desire to bite. Wild gaiety, towards evening. Consciousness wanes on closing eyes.

Abdomen - Burning pain in abdomen. Feels as if full of stones. Painless rumbling. Flatulence, with rumbling in bowels. ***Violent colic with drowsiness.*** Colic, as if bowels would be cut to pieces. Spasmodic cough, much flatus. Sharp, cutting colic before stool. Colic around umbilicus, better after stool. Pressure in abdomen, especially on stooping forward. Pain in the groins and cold creeps before menses.

Back - Lumbago. ***Violent pain in sacro-lumbar region***. Slightest effort to move may cause retching and cold, clammy sweat. Worse lifting. Sensation as if ***a heavy load was hanging on end of coccyx,*** dragging downwards all time. Twitching of muscles, limbs tremulous. Vertebrae seem to rub against each other. Cramp in muscles of neck. Burning in back.

Causations - Effects of anger (cough) or vexation. Ill effects of vaccination when Thuj. fails and Sil. is not indicated.

Chest - ***Rattling of mucus*** in the chest when breathing. Velvety feeling in chest. Burning sensation in chest, which ascends to throat. Paralysis of the lungs. Anxious oppression of the chest, with a sensation of heat, which ascends to the heart. Rheumatic pain in the left side of the chest. Miliary eruption.

Constitutions - Suited to old people and children. Gouty subjects and alcoholics with gastric disorders. Hydrogenoid type constitutions. Torpid and phlegmatic constitutions. Worn-out constitutions.

Coughs - Gasping for air, before every attack of cough. ***Coarse, loose, rattling cough.*** Cough followed by vomiting or sleep worse anger. ***Lungs seems full of mucus yet less and less is raised***. Must sit up to breathe or cough. Coughs and yawns alternately. ***Coughing and gasping***. Cough excited by eating with pain in chest and larynx. Cough and dyspnea better lying on right side (opposite Bad.). Child bends backwards with cough.

Ears - Roaring. Fluttering before left ear, as from a large bird. Warmth of left ear. Tearing pain. Twitching in right ear.

Eyes - Eyes sunken, surrounded by dark circles. Eyes bloodshot. Weak, tired eyes. Eyeballs as if bruised. Dim, swimming eyes. Burning and smarting pain. Tearing pain in eyes. Collection of mucus in margins of lids (in pneumonia). Conjunctivitis with much lachrymation. Pustular eruptions on the conjunctiva. Lachrymation when yawning. Flickering, sparks before the eyes. Eyes staring. One eye closed. Strabismus. Rheumatic ophthalmia.

Face - Anxious, despairing expression. Face pale and sunken. Pale, bluish or twitching with cough. ***Pale face, covered with cold sweat.*** Sickly, sunken. Burning heat of face. Burning pain as from hot coal, on right side of chin. ***Incessant quivering of chin and lower jaw*** (Gels.). Tearing pains. Pustules, leaving ugly blue-red scars.

Female - Menses of watery blood. Menses too early, weak and only for two days. Leucorrhea of watery blood, worse sitting. Severe bearing down pain in vagina.

Female - Chronic metritis with feeling of weight tugging at coccyx. Eruption of pimples on the genital organs. Pustules on external genitals. Itching of pudenda. Puerperal convulsions, better after the child is born.

Food - Appetite diminished. Loss of appetite, anorexia. Disgust for food during pregnancy. Food seems tasteless, tobacco has no taste. Aversion to milk. Aversion to all kind of nourishment. ***Desires apples, fruits and acids,*** which disagree. Desire for cooling things after vomiting. Great disgust for whiskey. Worse sour things and milk. Thirstlessness. ***Thirst for cold water, little and often.*** Difficult swallowing of liquids.

Head - Confusion in head in morning. Numbness of head, with stupefaction and drowsiness. Band-like feeling over forehead. Headache as from a band compressing (Nit-ac.). Hydrocephalus. Trembling of head, while coughing. As of a lump in forehead. Head better in open air, washing with cold water and motion. Head bent back. Headache with vomiting. Wave-like increase and decrease of pain in forehead. Head hot and sweaty. Scalp very sensitive. Child will not be touched without whining.

Heart - Great precordial anxiety with vomiting of mucus and bile. Palpitation with uncomfortable hot feeling. Palpitations with loose stools. Paralytic depression of heart. Weak quick pulse. Sensation of coldness in blood vessels. Sensation as if heart were strained. Rheumatic dilatation of heart. Pulse rapid, weak, trembling. Pulse full and slow, or contracted and hardly perceptible.

Kidneys - Sharp pains in region of kidneys on moving arms. Burning in urethra during and after urinating. Last drops bloody with pain in bladder. Urging increased. Catarrh of bladder and urethra. Stricture. Involuntary emission of urine. Red urine, which forms blood-red filaments after standing. Deep-brown, acrid, turbid urine.

Limbs - Acute articular rheumatism. Rheumatic and bruised pains. Twitching of muscles. Trembling of the hands. Fingertips icy cold or dead, numb, dry and hard. Restless arms. Feet go to sleep on sitting. Dropsy of synovial membranes. Dropsy of the legs and knee joint (left). Calves as if sore. Tension in hamstring when walking. Synovitis. Joints swollen. Jerking up of limbs during sleep with loose stools. Weakness of all limbs. Constant inclination to stretch.

Liver - Liver region sensitive to touch.

Lungs - ***Asphyxia from drowning.*** Asphyxia neonatorum, child breathless and pale when born. Gasping inspirations, expirations long and slow. ***Edema and impending paralysis of lungs***. Unequal breathing, abdominal breathing. ***Suffocative shortness of breath,*** before cough or alternating with cough. Hoarseness. ***Great rattling of mucus, but very little is expectorated***. "Death rattle." Rapid, short, difficult breathing. Feels as if he would ***suffocate***, must sit up. ***Emphysema of the aged.*** Capillary bronchitis, pneumonia, pleuro-pneumonia. Bronchitis. Bronchial tubes overloaded with mucus. ***Severe pneumonia, last stages.*** Gastric or bilious pneumonia. Complete hepatization. ***Expectoration copious, thick, white.*** Velvety feeling in chest. Dyspnea relieved by eructation. As if a leaflet seems to close the trachea. ***Lungs seems full of mucus yet less and less is raised***. Atelectasis. Hydrothorax. Percussion sound tympanitic.

Male - Pain in testicles after checked gonorrhea. Orchitis. Warts on glans penis. Excitation of sexual system. Pustules on genitals and thighs. Syphilis.

Modalities - Better cold open air. Better from sitting erect. Better lying on right side. Better vomiting. Better belching and expectoration. Better motion. ***Worse from warmth.*** Worse warm room. Worse wraps. Worse warm weather. Worse overheating. Worse cold dampness. Worse from anger. Worse lying, sitting down. Worse rising from a seat. Worse motion. Worse morning. Worse sour things and milk.

Mouth - Aphthae around mouth. Itching vesicles on lips. Upper lip drawn up. Lips dry and scurfy, or cracked. ***Spits all the time.*** Copious accumulation of saliva in the mouth. Copious salivation during pregnancy, nausea. Mouth and lips swollen and excoriated. Mouth remains open after yawning. Bitter, flat taste. Mouth so sore, can scarcely swallow, morning after rising.

Nose - Nostrils widely dilated. ***Alae nasi flapping.*** Stoppage of nose alternating with fluent coryza. Violent fluent coryza with frequent sneezing. Ulcerated nostrils. Loss of smell and of taste. Uncontrollable nosebleed with spongy gums. Nosebleed followed by fluent coryza with sneezing. Nose dry and pointed.

Perspiration - ***Copious cold clammy sweat*** with great faintness. Affected parts sweat most profusely. Sticky sweat. Very copious sweat without relief. Sweats with influenza.

Rectum - Sharp pain in rectum. Burning at anus after loose stool. Constipation, alternating with diarrhea. Desire for stool ineffectual though bowels seem full and pressing. Diarrhea and vomiting. Diarrhea in pneumonia, smallpox, and other eruptive diseases, especially if the eruption has been suppressed. Involuntary evacuations. Palpitations during stools. Cholera morbus. Cholera when vomiting is copious and there is coldness, and threadlike or trembling pulse.

Sensations - Sensation of weight or heaviness in many parts, head, occiput, coccyx, limbs. Sensation of coldness in blood vessels.

Skin - Delayed or receding eruptions. Eruption fails to appear and convulsions set in. Vesicular eruptions over whole body. Itching in the skin. Itching pimples, and miliary eruption. Itching around ulcers. ***Pustular eruption***, leaving a bluish-red mark. Rash mixed with small vesicles and pustules. Rash after vaccination. Smallpox. Thick eruptions like pocks. Eruptions like scabies. Barber's itch. Chickenpox. Smallpox. Impetigo. Blue eruptions. Warts.

Sleep - Sleepiness during sweat. Irresistible inclination to sleep with nearly all complaints. ***Great drowsiness with all complaints.*** Drowsiness from warmth. Yawning with many complaints. Electric-like shocks on falling asleep. Cries during sleep with fixed eyes and trembling. Lies on back with left hand passed under head. Trembling during sleep. Heavy, anxious dreams. Dreams, clearly remembered in morning on waking.

Stomach - Great sensitivity of stomach. Throbbing and pressure. Belchings like bad eggs. Eructations empty, acid, bitter, salty. Violent hiccough. Dryness of esophagus. Cramps in stomach. Sinking at stomach. Fullness and heaviness. Nausea produces fear with pressure in precordial region. ***Nausea, retching and vomiting.*** Nausea with deathly faintness and prostration. ***Nausea comes in waves.*** Nausea with weakness and cold sweat. Vomiting forcible, then exhaustion and sleep. ***Frequent vomiting of bitter, sour substances.*** Violent retching. Vomits with great effort. Vomiting better lying on right side.

Stool - Mucus stools, grass green. Bloody feces. Diarrhea in eruptive diseases. Watery, slimy, bloody diarrhea. Diarrhea with vomiting. Diarrhea with flatulence. Diarrhea of alcoholics. Very offensive diarrheic stools. Stools yellowish-brown. Stools thin, bilious. Stools with heat at anus. Stools slimy, like yeast. Stools of cadaverous smell.

Teeth - Violent toothache in morning. Rheumatic pain of intermittent type. Gums bleed. Gums spongy, with nosebleed. Teeth covered with mucus. Dentition with catarrhal hyperemia.

Temperature - Coldness, trembling and chilliness. Cold creeping chills before menses. Chills as if cold water was poured over one. Chills from within outward. Chills with trembling, worse going into open air. Chill alternating with heat, during day. Intense heat. Intermittent fever with fatigue. Burning sensation. Heat coming from heart.

Throat - Aphonia. Voice weak and changed in evening. Hoarseness in morning, worse talking. Rattling of mucus when coughing or breathing. Much mucus in throat with short breathing. Swallowing painful or impossible.

Throat - Roughness in throat with sensation as if a small leaf obstructed trachea on hawking. Throat, mouth and tongue as if tense. Sharp pain in throat. Burning in fauces. Rapid swelling of tonsils and cervical glands. Child grasps at larynx during cough. Larynx painful to touch.

Tongue - Difficult, even painful, to move tongue. Tongue flaccid, dry. Imprints of teeth on border of the tongue. Tongue red, dry in middle, red in streaks. ***Coated, pasty, thick white with red edges.*** Tongue moist, clean, or loaded with a brown coating. Tongue moist and yellow in middle.

Vertigo - Dizziness with cough. Vertigo with dullness and confusion. Vertigo alternates with drowsiness. Vertigo from lifting head from pillow. Fits of vertigo with sparking before the eyes. Vertigo must lie down. Vertigo with dimness of vision and pressing headache. Vertigo with violent chills.

COMMENTS - Hering said that Antimonium Tartaricum was the invention of the Alchemists. Tartar emetic. It has been used as a poison, similar to Arsenic, usually someone would be dead in 12 to 24 hours. It has a very strong affinity for the lungs and stimulating the secretions of the mucus membranes.

Chest disorders with a great accumulation of mucus with coarse rattling and inability to raise it. "Lies with head back." "A child coughs when angry." Heath cured a case of whooping cough in a child who was very fretful before the cough. The mother said that if the child got angry she immediately had a fit of coughing. "Cough at 4 a.m." is another indication.

Last stages of pneumonia, severe rattling in the lungs, and white, thick mucus. Asthma with white, thick mucus, wet asthma (Puls.). Chronic bronchitis in the elderly with a rattling cough and white, thick mucus that's hard to expectorate. Drowning victims, pulmonary edema, Infantile pneumonia.

For children who get colds often and it goes to the chest with a great accumulation of mucus. Sometimes indicated after gas poisonings, if the gas caused irritation to the mucus membranes and mucus comes up (Carb-v., Bry., Ant-t.). For emphysema when caused by an irritant causing loss of lung space (Sil.).

Respiratory distress due to constriction and mucus in the lungs. There is a great accumulation of mucus in the lungs. The sputum is thick and ropy but it is white and more sticky like glue. No expulsive power. Noisy breathing with severe wet cough. Weakness of the bronchioles where they can't expectorate, can be used chronically. The nostrils flare because they can't breathe. Suffocating, choking because of the mucus.

Gastric and bilious complaints. Constant nausea. Nausea felt in chest (Puls.). Nash found Ant-t. the nearest thing to a specific in cholera morbus, the indications being "nausea, vomiting, loose stools, prostration, cold sweat, stupor or drowsiness."

Deathly nausea (Ip., Puls.). Difficulty vomiting, just like expectoration. They strain, a lack of explosive power. Vomits whatever is eaten. Vomits thick, white, ropy mucus, may have blood or slime in it. Also produces ulcers, ulceration of the mucus membranes. Ulcers that bleed and then they vomit blood.

The tongue has a thick, white, pasty coat with red papillae showing through. Intense nausea and vomiting with great effort with perspiration on forehead. Fullness and sensation of stones in abdomen, especially when sitting bent forward. Anxiety felt in the stomach, apprehension in the stomach. Sensations of a weight or heaviness in the abdomen or various parts of the body. The abdomen is distended, severe cramps or cutting pains.

There is heat about heart and warmth rising up from it. Coldness in the blood vessels. Generally cold hands and feet. The face is pale or cyanotic and the breathing stertorous. Severe weakness from lack of oxygen, tired from coughing. Oppression of the chest.

Great drowsiness or sleepiness with cough and congestion in the lungs (Op., more of a stupor). Can palliate or bring them back if it's possible.

Drowning victims and newborns who are not breathing, or for any severe respiratory problems going into respiratory failure (Carb-v.). Coma.

Arthritis in the smaller joints. Sensation of weight or heaviness in many parts, head, occiput, coccyx, limbs. Pulsations in all the blood vessels. Chronic trembling of head of head and hands (as in Parkinson's disease).

"Sycotic" skin. Clarke verified a symptom given in Hering, "warts at the back of the glans penis." Leprosy, chickenpox. smallpox and impetigo, worse after smallpox vaccination. It has been used instead of vaccines for preventive purposes and a prophylactic power has been claimed for it (Vario.). The terrible backache of smallpox is paralleled by the back-pains of Ant-t., which Clarke found to correspond to more cases of lumbago than any other remedy.

Worse by warmth, but not the excessive sensitiveness to heat and sun of Ant-c. and some of the rheumatic symptoms are better by warmth. Cough worse from warm drink, lying in bed, especially becoming warm there. Suffocates in a warm room, want fresh air (Puls.). Greatly aggravated by the sun. Cough is worse anger and worse after eating.

Thirstlessness, lost any desire for fluids (Puls., Ip.). May vomit water if they try to drink it. As if they have enough fluid already (Apis.). Crave apples and acid fruits, but may be aggravated by sour food or wine, causing severe diarrhea. Great aversion to milk or are aggravated by milk. Loathing of food.

Peevishness, whining and crying (Cham.). Restless, apprehension and agitation. Dullness and bewilderment of head as if benumbed. Irritable, don't want to be looked at or talked to or touched. The whole body feels tender. Children may want to be carried and cling to their mother or may scream on being touched, keynote that they do not want to be bothered. Coughing fits at 4 a.m.

The child looks pale, sunken eyes and have dark rings around the eyes and they have periodic cold sweats. The child cries and may jerk during sleep.

Difficulty nursing and breathing at the same time. Better when held upright and hit on back to break up the mucus.

Children are very anxious and timid, especially in the evening, as if they are anticipating the night because it is so bad for them. They lay down and get congestion and coughing fits. They have apprehension about the future, but it's more the upcoming night. Elderly may feel despair of recovery.

Etiology can be cold, damp weather that seems to bring out the mucus.

RELATIONS - ***Antidoted by:*** Asaf., Chin., Cocc., Con. (pustules on genitals), Ip., Laur., Opium in large doses is the best antidote in poisoning, Puls., Sep. ***Antidotes:*** Bar-c., Bry. (dyspepsia), Camph., Caust. (dyspepsia), Puls., Sepia. Ant-t. differs from Merc. in producing a purely local action on the mouth similar to its action on the skin. The action of Merc. on the mouth is indirect. ***Compare:*** (1) Acon. - croup, Aeth. and Ip. - expression of nausea, Am-c. (2) Ars. - asthma, heart symptoms, gastric catarrh, Bry. - pneumonia, worse left, Ant-t. worse right has nostrils dilated. (3) Verat. - colic, vomiting, coldness, craving for acids. Ant-t. has more jerks, drowsiness, urging to urinate, Verat. more cold sweat and fainting. (4) Op. - cough with drowsiness and yawning, Sang. - pneumonia, face livid. (5) Ip. - Ant-t. has more drowsiness and tendency of lungs to collapse. (6) Thuj. - effects of vaccination when Thuj. fails and Sil. is not indicated. Ant-t. develops smallpox pustule, Thuj. dries it up. ***Compatible:*** Phos. in hydrocephalus, worn-out constitutions, laryngitis, pneumonia. ***Follows well:*** Sil. in dyspnea from foreign substances in larynx, Puls. (nausea in chest, gonorrheal suppressions), Ter. (symptoms from damp cellars), Variolinum.

REFERENCES - Boericke. Clarke. Murphy.

ANTIPYRINUM
(Phenazone)

PHARMACY - antip. Antipyrinum. Phenazone. Antipyrine. Phenyl-dimethyl-pyrazolon. A product of coal tar through Toulon. Solution and trituration. ***Historical dose:*** Trituration, tincture and all potencies.

CLINICAL - Bedwetting. Cheyne-stokes, breathing. Dysmenorrhea. Eczema. Edema. Epilepsy. Erythema. German measles. ***Hallucinations. Headache.*** Heart paralysis. ***Itching. Lachrymation***. Menses, suppressed. Mind, deranged. Nausea. Nosebleed. Pemphigus. Scarlatina. Throat, sore. ***Tinnitus***. Toothache. ***Urticaria.*** Vomiting.

HOMEOPATHIC - Antipyrine is known from the poisonous effects it produced in old-school practice. Many fatal cases were recorded and there can be little doubt that its injudicious use determined a fatal issue in many cases that have remained unrecorded.

Antipyrine's action is very like that of Acetan. in producing collapse, but it has more effect on the skin, causing scarlet rash and edema. It is one of the drugs that induce leucocytosis, similar to ergotine, salicylates and tuberculin.

Antipyrine acts especially on the vasomotor centers, causing dilation of the capillaries of the skin and circumscribed patches of hyperemia and swelling. In large doses, it causes profuse perspiration, dizziness, cyanosis, somnolence, albumen and blood in urine. Acute erythema multiform.

MIND - Fear of going insane. ***Hallucinations of sight and hearing.*** Nervous anxiety,

Ears - Pains and buzzing. ***Tinnitus***.

Eyes - Puffiness of lids. Conjunctiva red and edematous with ***lachrymation***. Red spots (Apis).

Face - Edema and puffiness. Red and swollen.

Female - Itching and burning in vagina. Dysmenorrhea. Menses suppressed. Watery leucorrhea.

Head - Throbbing headache. ***Headache under ears with earache. Sensation of constriction***. Flashes of heat.

Heart - Faintness with sensation of stoppage of heart. Throbbing throughout the body. Rapid, weak, irregular pulse.

Kidneys - Diminished. Penis black.

Lungs - Cheyne-Stokes respiration. Aphonia. Oppression and dyspnea.

Mouth - Swelling of lips. tongue Burning of mouth and gums. Ulceration of lips and tongue, vesicles and bullae. Small lump in cheek. Bloody saliva. Toothache along lower jaw.

Nerves - ***General prostration.*** Epileptiform seizures. Contractures. Trembling and cramps. Crawling and numbness.

Nose - Fluent coryza. Nasal mucus membrane swollen. Dull pains in frontal sinus.

Skin - ***Erythema***, eczema, pemphigus. ***Intense itching. urticaria,*** appearing and disappearing suddenly with internal coldness. Angioneurotic edema. Dark blotches on skin of penis, sometimes with edema.

Stomach - Nausea and vomiting, burning and pain.

Throat - Painful when swallowing. Expectoration of fetid pus. Abscess, white false membrane. Sensation of burning.

COMMENTS - A young female patient who took Antipyrine on her own account whenever she thought she might be going to have a headache, developed intense dysmenorrhea (to which she was not subject) with depression.

This was only removed after she had discontinued the drug. Later, she took Phenacetin with result that an eruption of erythema appeared on both cheeks, which peeled after a few days and recurred persistently.

It would seem that the drug is homeopathic to some forms of neuralgia. One patient had Cheyne-Stokes respiration. Erythema appears first on face and arms, last on legs.

Hansen mentioned its use in bedwetting and nosebleed. Better from hot drinks.

RELATIONS - ***Antidoted by:*** Bell. The symptoms are much intensified in persons addicted to coffee in excess. ***Compare:*** (1) Anilinum - skin symptoms. (2) Acon. - numbness, rapidity of attack. (3) Acetan., Ars., Chloral.

REFERENCES - Boericke. Clarke.

APHIS CHENOPODII GLAUCI

(Aphids)

PHARMACY - aphis. Aphis chenopodii glauci. Aphids. Chenopodii glauci aphis. N. O. Insecta. A tincture is made of the aphids grown on the Chenopodium glaucum. ***Historical dose:*** Tincture and all potencies.

CLINICAL - Chills. Colic. Coryza. Cough. Diarrhea. Headache. Rheumatic, pains. Sneezing. Tenesmus. Toothache.

HOMEOPATHIC - The insect partakes of the properties of the plant it lives on, Chenopodium glaucum being a popular colic remedy and allied to the Polygonacae, Rheum and Rumex. Aphis is peculiar in being the only remedy which has toothache better by sweat, though Cham. has general better by sweat.

Coryza with burning and biting on margins of nostrils, especially of septum. Increase of violent toothaches in bed, only relieved from a general warm sweat breaking out.

Cutting in abdomen and rumbling of flatus. Ineffectual urging in bladder and rectum. In the morning urging after rising, several mush-like stools with pinching, burning in anus with urging. Flatus accompanies stool. Thin stools with slime and spots of dark blood.

Abdomen - Rumblings of flatus in the abdomen. Emission of gas. Frequent pinching pains in the abdomen. Cutting and pinching pains with borborygmi. Congestion of blood towards the abdominal viscera.

Back - Pain in the left shoulder blade.

Ears - Tearing pains, sometimes in one ear, and sometimes in the other.

Eyes - Burning heat in the eyelids during several evenings.

Face - Color pale, yellowish, heat in the face, with head confused as by coryza, at night. Dry lips, sometimes especially in the morning.

Food - No appetite for meat and wheat bread, with chilliness. Increased thirst from sensation of dryness in throat. Much thirst in evening, second week.

Head - Head confused in the evening with transient heat in the face. Pressure and tightening in the forehead or occiput, increased by motion. Tearing shooting in the head.

Kidneys - Tearing shooting in the bladder. Irritation in the urethra, compelling frequent urination. Frequent secretion of a frothy urine, deep yellow. Urine red, brownish, frothy, depositing during the night a thick, yellowish sediment. Burning in the urethra, especially at the orifice, while urinating.

Limbs - Rheumatic pains. Bruise-like pain of the limbs. Tearing shootings in the shoulders and the upper part of the arms. Pulling and tearing above the knee in the morning. Weariness in the legs. Coldness of the feet, extending to the knees. Burning lancinations in corns.

Lungs - Expectoration of mucus. Voice frequently rough and smothered, removed by hawking. Frequent irritation in the larynx, which compels coughing. Dry cough, provoked by irritation in the throat.

Male - Voluptuous excitation of the glans penis.

Mouth - Painful vesicles at the end of the tongue. Dryness of the mouth and of the throat. Increase in the secretion of saliva. Scraping sensation in the palate.

Nose - Pain of excoriation in the nostrils. Violent sneezing. Coryza, with burning and smarting at the edges of the nostrils and at the septum. Fluent coryza.

Rectum - Loose evacuations of the consistency of liquid pap. Flatulency before and after a stool. Liquid, mucus-like stools in the morning, with spots of blood. Tearing shooting in the rectum.

Sleep - Sleeplessness at night, without much pain. Lascivious dreams with pollutions.

Teeth - Toothache with tearing shootings. Nocturnal tearing pains in the teeth, with tearing shootings above the face towards morning.

Temperature - Frequent chills on the whole surface of the body, chiefly of the back. Burning in the palms of the hands. Tendency to perspire in the morning. Hot sweat or general perspiration.

Throat - Secretion of frothy mucus in the mouth and throat. Scraping and burning, as from acrid substances. Sensation of dryness and increase of mucus secretion.

RELATIONS - ***Compare:*** (1) Aeth. - stool after rising, pinching, cutting before, urging after. (2) Nat-s. - stool after rising with discharge of wind. (3) Nux-v. - frequent urging in rectum and bladder. (4) Gels. - chills up and down the back.

REFERENCES - Boericke. Clarke.

APIS MELLIFICA

(Honey Bee)

PHARMACY - apis. Apis mellifica. Honey bee. N. O. Insecta. Hymenoptera. Apium virus is honey-bee venom. Tinctures are made of the whole bee and of dilutions of the poison with alcohol. ***Historical dose:*** All potencies.

CLINICAL - Abscess. Albuminuria. ***Allergic, shock. Allergies.*** Amenorrhea. Ankles, swelling. Asthma. ***Bee stings.*** Bladder, disorders. Carbuncle. Chancre. Constipation. Cystitis. Diarrhea. Diphtheria. Dissection, wounds. Dropsy. Dysmenorrhea. ***Edema.*** Erysipelas. Erythema, nodosum. Eyes, disorders. Gangrene. Goiter. Gout. Hands, swelling. Heart, disorders. ***Hives.*** Housemaid's knee. Hydrocephalus. Hydrothorax. Injuries. Intermittent fever. ***Itching.*** Joints, edema. ***Kidney, diseases.*** Laryngitis. Lymphangitis. ***Meningitis.*** Menstruation, disorders. Metrorrhagia. Miscarriage. ***Nephritis.*** Nephrotic, syndrome. ***Nettle rash.*** Otitis. ***Ovaries, cysts***. Ovarian, tumors. Panaritium. Pannus. Peritonitis. Phlebitis. Photophobia. Pleurisy. ***Premenstrual syndrome.*** Prostatitis. Puberty. Punctured, wounds. ***Rashes.*** Rheumatic pains. Scarlatina. Self-abuse. Staphyloma. ***Stinging, pains.*** Strokes. Suppressed eruptions. Surgery, effects. ***Swellings.*** Sycosis. Synovitis. Syphilis. Throat, sore. Thrombosis. Tongue, edema, ulceration. ***Toxemia. Throat, swollen.*** Tumors. Typhus. ***Urticaria.*** Urethritis. Vaccination. Varicose veins. Variola. Wounds.

HOMEOPATHIC - Apis acts on cellular tissue of eyes, face, throat, ovaries, causing edema of skin and mucus membranes. In the ***serous membranes*** of heart, brain, pleura etc. it produces inflammation with effusion. ***Allergic reactions to bee or wasp stings.*** The effects of a bee sting, ***burning, stinging,*** smarting, prickling, sharp pain with ***excessive swelling,*** are the leading symptoms for the selection of this remedy.

The well-known effects of a bee's sting: burning, stinging, sharp pains with excessive swelling, give leading keynotes for its employment in a great variety of conditions. ***Allergic edema of face, eyelids,*** lips, mouth and throat. Burning, stinging itching. Redness and swelling with stinging and burning pain in eyes, eyelids, ears, face, lips tongue, throat, anus, testicles.

The ***stinging pains*** appears in many diseases and conditions, causing the "cry cerebral" in acute hydrocephalus and meningitis. ***Sudden shrill cries*** in hydrocephalus and meningitis. Extreme sensitivity to touch. General ***bruised, sore pains*** is marked of brain, ***abdomen,*** ovaries, bladder. Stinging pains in hemorrhoids. Edema of the throat may be accompanied with stinging pains. Burning symptoms (Ars.), worse by heat.

Apis produces serous inflammation with effusion, membranes of brain, heart and pleuritic effusion. ***Swelling or puffing up of various parts, edema***, red rosy hue, stinging pains, soreness intolerance of heat and from the slightest touch. Afternoon aggravation are some of the general guiding symptoms. The pains are sudden that extort cries.

Acute ***inflammation of kidneys*** and other parenchymatous tissues are characteristic pathological states corresponding to Apis. ***Constricted*** sensations. Sensation of stiffness and as of something torn off in the interior of the body. Prostration even to faintness.

Trembling, jerking and twitching. Symptoms go from right to left. Numbness. Thrombosis. Lymphangitis. Inflammation of kidneys, bladder. Paralysis after diphtheria and other severe diseases.

MIND - ***Great anxious restlessness and fidgety.*** Fussy and fidgety, hard to please. Fear of being poisoned. Dread of apoplexy. ***Constant whining*** in children. Cannot bear to be left alone. ***Restlessness and constantly busy.*** Ailments from hearing bad news ***Weeping***, cannot help crying, all day and night without any cause.

Absent-minded with impaired memory. Cannot concentrate mind on attempting to read and write. Stupor with sudden sharp cries and startings. ***Awkward, drops things readily***. Listless, cannot think clearly. Couldn't bring his thoughts to bear on anything.

Apathy and indifference. Indifference, says nothing ails him. Indifference with dullness of head. Nothing seems to satisfy, all wrong and out of place. Fruitless activity.

Irritable, excitable and sensitive. Fickle and inconsistent behavior. Childish, silly behavior in women after delivery. ***Hysterical girls at puberty.*** Borrows trouble about everything. ***Jealous, fidgety, hard to please.*** Jealous, fright, rage, vexation, grief. Foolishly suspicious. Whining.

Muttering delirium alternating with stupor. Declares she is well, during delirium. Sudden shrill, piercing screams. Mania from sexual irritation. Sexual mania alternating with stupor in women. Premonition of death. Sensation of dying. Lost of consciousness.

Abdomen - Dropsy of abdomen. Burning, pain and tenderness in epigastrium. ***Sore, bruised pain,*** on pressure, when sneezing. ***Extremely tender***. Rumbling in abdomen. Violent cutting pains. Peritonitis. Swelling in right groin. Ulceration of navel in newborn. Inguinal hernia. Sensitivity of ileocecal region.

Back - Back of the neck stiff. Back as if tired and bruised. Rheumatic pain in back. Burning pressing in coccyx worse when sitting down. Back tired and bruised. Scapulae as if lame. Cervical glands swollen. Violent pain in sacrum, could not sit. Dragging pain in lumbar region with ovarian and uterine diseases.

Bladder - Great irritation at neck of bladder with frequent and burning urination. Burning and soreness when urinating. ***Cystitis.*** Dysuria with stinging pains. ***Last drops burn and smart.*** Incontinence of urine worse night, coughing. ***Retention of urine in newborn.*** Stitching in urethra, with bedwetting. ***Suppressed urine.*** Tenesmus during and after urination. Cannot urinate without a stool. Difficult, frequent or slow urination, must press to pass urine, in prostatic affections.

Breasts - Breasts swollen and hard. Child nurses by day, refuses at night. Milk diminished. Stinging burning pains in breasts. Breast tumors. Cancer of breasts. Breast burning, stinging, swelling, hardness and suppuration. Erysipelas of breast.

Causations - Allergens. Grief. Fright. Rage. Vexation. Jealousy, the queen bee is the most jealous thing in nature. Hearing bad news, mental shock. Suppressed eruptions.

Chest - Pains from below ribs going upwards. Burning or soreness below ribs. Hydrothorax. Burning stinging pains throughout entire front of the chest. Hydrothorax after pleurisy. Chest feels as if beaten or bruised.

Constitutions - Psoric and allergic constitutions.

Cough - Severe cough before midnight. Croupy cough with ringing sound. Dry cough with gagging. Cough with soreness of upper part of chest. Very dry cough. Spasmodic cough morning and evening. Dry cough with gagging, worse lying on left side. Cough with tickling behind pit of throat.

Ears - Redness and swelling of both ears. External ear red inflamed, sore. ***Stinging pains.*** Raises the hand to the back of ear with each scream. Scarlatinal otitis. Tension about ears. Violent pain in left ear, when chewing. Shooting, burning pain. Pain in ears, when swallowing. Impaired hearing. Deafness.

Eyes - ***Allergic puffy eyelids***, swollen, red, and edematous like water bags. Burning, stinging and shooting pain in eyes. Conjunctiva is bright red, puffy. ***Lachrymation hot***. Photophobia, yet covering intolerable. Everted lids. ***Sudden piercing pains***. Pain around orbits. ***Serous exudation, edema and sharp pains.*** Keratitis with ***intense chemosis of ocular conjunction***. Cornea opaque. Perforating corneal ulcer. Staphyloma of cornea. ***Suppurative inflammation of eyes***. Cannot look fixedly at any object or cannot read in artificial light. Fistula lachrymalis. Squinting.

Eyes -Myopia. ***Styes***. Asthenopia during eruptive fevers. Ophthalmia.

Face - ***Red, hot, swollen*** with piercing pains. Waxy pale and edematous. Lips bluish, edematous, upper. ***Bee stings.*** Erysipelas with stinging burning edema. Extends from right to left. Expression happy, terror stricken or apathetic. Jaws stiff, with stiffness of tongue. Paralysis of right side with right eye closed. Desire for washing face with cold water. Formication and prickling in face.

Female - Amenorrhea of puberty. ***Premenstrual syndrome with water retention.*** Menses suppressed with mental and head symptoms, especially in young girls. ***Hysterical girls at puberty.*** Menses last a day or appear at intervals of one day. Dysmenorrhea with scanty discharge of slimy blood or with ovarian pains. Dysmenorrhea, with severe ovarian pains. Bearing-down, as if menses were to appear. Great tenderness over abdomen and uterine region. Metritis. Metrorrhagia profuse with heavy abdomen, faintness, stinging pain. Menorrhagia with the miscarriage. Leucorrhea, profuse, acrid, green. Edema of labia, relieved by cold water. ***Ovarian cysts.*** Soreness and stinging pains. Ovaritis, worse in right ovary. ***Ovarian tumors, with stinging pains.*** Ovaries numb or congested with suppressed menses. Pains in ovaries, worse sex. ***Toxemia.*** Miscarriage during early months. Uterine hemorrhage during pregnancy. Dropsy in later parts of pregnancy with puerperal convulsions. Mania in women from sexual excesses or suppressed menses.

Food - ***Thirstless*** with edema, dropsy. ***Craving for milk*** (Rhus-t.). Better from milk. Craving for sour things. Child nurses by day, refuses at night.

Head - Chronic sick headache. Sudden stabbing in head. ***Sharp shrieks.*** Bores head into pillow and screams out. ***Hydrocephalus*** enlargement of head. ***Rolling of the head*** from side to side in hydrocephalus. Boring of the head backward in pillow in ***meningitis.*** Inability to hold the head up in meningitis. ***Stinging pains.*** Numb, tired headache, better pressure. Flow of tears with headache. Fontanelles sunken. Fontanels reopen. ***Brain feels very tired.*** Heat, throbbing, pains, better on pressure and worse on motion. Aching in forehead and temples. Dull, heavy sensation in occiput, as from a blow. Erysipelas of scalp. Painful hair. Musty head sweat. Head feels swollen. Hair falls out, bald spots. Apoplexy.

Heart - Heart troubles with great feeling of suffocation. Heart stitches backward from apex. Violent palpitations, shake the whole body. Palpitations of heart from scanty secretion of urine. Insufficiency of mitral valves. Organic heart disease. Blowing sound with the diastole. Pericarditis. Pulse is hard small intermittent and quick, weak.

Kidneys - Sore or bruised feeling over region of kidneys. Nephritis. ***Acute nephritis, urine scanty or suppressed.*** Hyperemic state of kidneys. Burning and soreness when urinating. Frequent and involuntary urine. Stinging pain and strangury. ***Scanty, high colored urine***. Urine loaded with casts. Urine milky in hydrocephalus. Albuminuria. Urine profuse, more than he drinks. Urine turbid after standing. Coffee ground sediment. Urine clear and colorless during dentition. Urine of greenish hue. Urethra as if scalded.

Limbs - Edematous. Synovitis. Felon in the beginning with burning, stinging throbbing pains. Knee swollen, shiny, sensitive, sore with stinging pain. Feet swollen and stiff. Feel too large. Rheumatic pain in back and limbs. Tired, bruised feeling. Numbness of hands and fingertips. Hives with intolerable itching. Palms hot. Edema of hands. Limbs, immovable, heavy, numb.. Feet numb and stiff. Legs and feet waxy, pale swollen and edematous. Trembling of hands and feet. Nails feel loose. Hemiplegia from severe mental shock. Staggers when eyes are shut.

Lungs - Asthma with hives. Dyspnea from allergic reactions. Breathing hurried and difficult. ***Panting breathing,*** feels every breath would be his last. Air hunger. Edema of larynx. Feels ***as if he could not draw another breath***. Suffocation short, dry cough, supra-sternal. Painful shock in head and chest from every cough. Larynx drawn in. Hoarseness. Expectoration sweetish.

Male - Affections of prostate gland. Dropsy of the scrotum. Hydrocele and cysts. Testicles painful when touched. Frequent and long-lasting erections. Swelling of testicles, worse right. Violent itching and redness of scrotum, sore to touch. Sexual desire increased or diminished. Discharge of prostatic fluid. Gonorrhea, copious secretion of thin, ichorous discharge. Gonorrhea with burning, stinging pain. Large boils on pubes. Swelling of foreskin.

Modalities - ***Better from cool air.*** Better cold applications. Better cool bathing. Better uncovering. Better slight expectoration. Better motion. Better sitting erect. ***Worse from heat in any form.*** Worse hot weather. ***Worse heat of room.*** Worse heat of fire. Worse hot drinks. ***Worse hot bath.*** Worse warm bed. Worse pressure. ***Worse touch,*** even of hair. Worse in late afternoon. Worse after sleeping in closed and heated rooms. Worse right side. Worse pressure. Worse after sleep. Worse lying down. ***Worse from suppressed eruptions.*** Worse at 4 p.m.

Mouth - Scalding in mouth and throat. Bitter taste. Fetid breath. Viscid, tough, frothy saliva. Gums swollen. Lips swollen, especially upper. Membrane of mouth and throat glossy, as if varnished. ***Red, shining and puffy*** like erysipelas. Vesicles. Raw, burning and painful stinging blisters. Dryness of mouth.

Nose - ***Red, swollen*** inflamed nose with sharp pains. Coldness of tip of nose. Boils in nostril, better cold. Nostrils red and burning. Bridge of nose puffy. Coryza, worse warmth. Coryza with feeling of swelling in nose. Thick, white, fetid, mucus discharge, mixed with blood. Copious nosebleed towards morning.

Perspiration - Sweat slight with sleepiness. Perspiration breaks out and dries up frequently. After perspiration, nettle rash, also with shuddering.

Rectum - ***Anus seems open.*** Anus is sore, swollen with profuse hemorrhage. Anus feels raw, remains open. Prolapsed anus. Hemorrhoids with stinging pain after confinement. ***Cholera infantum.*** Cannot urinate without a stool Constipation, feels as if something would break on straining. Feels tight as if to break, on straining at stool. Electric shocks in rectum before urging to stool.

Sensations - The burning is like hot needles. Sensation of constriction. Sensation of stiffness and as of something torn off the interior part of the body.

Skin - ***Bee stings, insect bites.*** Swellings after bites or stings. Nettle rash. Edematous swellings. ***Allergic dermatitis.*** Sudden puffing up of whole body. ***Hives,*** burning, stinging and itching. Rosy red, sensitive, sore skin. ***Stinging pains.*** Scarlatina. Erysipelas with sensitiveness and swelling, rosy hue. ***Urticaria like bee stings, or stings from other insects, with intolerable itching at night.*** Boils. Carbuncles with burning, stinging pain (Ars., Anthr.). Rough eruptions or stinging-like spots on skin. ***Large urticaria.*** Skin dry, hot, alternating with gushes of sweat. Nettle-rash in warm weather, when one can't sweat.

Sleep - Very drowsy. ***Great inclination to sleep*** but cannot from nervous restlessness. Drowsiness during fever. ***Screams and sudden starting during sleep.*** Kicks off covers during sleep. Yawning after coughing. Dreams full of care and toil. Dreams of being busy going from place to place. Travelling dreams. Flying dreams. Unpleasant dreams.

Stomach - Belchings that tasting of ingesta worse drinking water or flow of water. Bitter or acrid belching. Soreness in the pit of stomach when touched. Gastroenteritis. Nausea and vomiting. Neither eats nor drinks for weeks. Vomiting of frothy mucus. Vomiting with diarrhea. Vomiting of food, bile.

Stool - Profuse hemorrhage from anus. Dark, fetid stool, worse after eating. Bloody, painless stools. Stools odorless. Stools, blackish-brown, green or whitish.

Stool - Stools, odorless or offensive involuntary worse motion. Diarrhea, watery yellow orange-yellow or tomato-sauce like stools. Stools, olive-green, slimy.

Teeth - Sudden involuntary biting teeth together. Grinding of the teeth. Gums as if numb. Gums swollen. Gums bleed easily. Swelling and redness of gums and cheek. Sore and stinging pain in teeth. Dentition. Teeth covered with yellow mucus or brown sordes.

Temperature - Chill, anticipating with dyspnea, urticaria, desire to uncover, alternate with heat. Heat of one part coldness of another. ***Thirstless during fever.*** Thirst during chill. ***Burning heat,*** but chilly when moved. ***Afternoon chill with thirst, worse on motion and heat.*** Worse from heat with smothering feeling. Sleeps after the fever paroxysm.

Throat - Tonsillitis with skin eruptions. Tonsils are swollen, fiery red, stinging pain, while swallowing, better cold drinks. Ulcers on tonsils. ***Swollen throat from allergic reaction.*** Constricted, stinging pains. ***Uvula swollen***, sac-like. Sandy, glossy or translucent better cold, swollen inside and outside. Throat purple. Angina. Diphtheria with early prostration, dirty membrane, edema of uvula. Throat sore, swallowing painful worse solids, sour or hot substances. Sensation as if fishbone in throat. Vascular goitre.

Tongue - Tongue as if scalded, red hot, trembling. ***Cancer of the tongue.*** Tongue fiery red, swollen, sore and raw with vesicles. Tongue feels raw. Tongue hangs out or cannot be protruded. Tongue as if wooden. ***Stinging blisters along edge of tongue.*** Dryness of tongue. Tongue red at tip. Tongue coated white. Tongue trembles, catches in teeth. Tongue first covered thickly white, later covered with a brown crust.

Vertigo - Vertigo with sneezing worse lying or closing eyes. Vertigo with nausea and headache. Vertigo as if she would fall. Vertigo with obscuration of sight, nausea and disgust for food.

Vision - Obscured vision, in meningitis cerebrospinalis. Could only observe light coming in at window when turning herself towards it. Whitish grey mist. Weak vision, with feeling of fullness in eyes. Blindness better stool. Myopia. Objects appear too large. Could see better at night than in daytime. Diplopia after meningitis. Whirling. Indistinct vision, as if a skin were drawn over eye.

COMMENTS - Acute remedy for anaphylactic shock from bee stings, jellyfish, nettles, scorpions, from drugs, from allergic reactions especially to strawberries and to certain foods.

In a severe case, their face swells, first the eyes swell, then the face swells, and then the throat swells. It's also for hives, itching, burning, stinging hives from insect bites, from certain foods, severe allergies. Chronic treatment can lesson sensitivity (Vesp., Carb-ac.).

Burns or sunburns with stinging pain, worse heat, or burns with water-filled blisters.

Has been used for eczema, skin cracked and painful, burning, swollen, suppurating, worse water. PMS with acute, severe edema, water retention, irritability, emotional sensitivity. Right sided ovarian cysts, especially if so painful it's about to burst. Appendicitis.

Acute nephritis with stinging pains. Good for urinary retention, cystitis, bladder infections (Canth.). Bladder feels full and urethra is swollen so urine comes out in painful drops. Pelvis feels full. For puncture wounds when the arm swells, vaccinations. Joint pain from arthritis or injury, the joint swells up.

Toxemia in pregnancy, women have protein in the urine and high blood pressure. Inflammation of the body cavity like peritonitis or fluid collecting around the heart, for meningitis, for hydrocephalic children, for painful inflammation of the scrotum. Brain cry, high pitch shrill, due to inflammation and water on the brain. Never well since meningitis (Bell.).

Originally used for edema. Often edema from the immune system or the kidneys, the histamine is released, the tissues swell. Better heat, look for the stinging pains and worse heat in some type of allergic reaction or bite or sting or some kidney failure type of problem.

Apis has great sensitiveness of the surface to touch. General soreness, every hair is painful to contact. Great debility as if he had worked hard is compelled to lie down. Tired and bruised feeling. Great restlessness and fidgetiness (the Ars. restlessness is more from mental anxiety).

Trembling, jerking and twitching. One half of the body twitching, the other lame or paralyzed. Hemiplegia. Apis is more a right-sided medicine, symptoms proceed from right to left (Rhus-t. left to right) and from above downwards.

Stiffness of lower jaw, soon amounting to a sense of complete fixation. This stiffness extended to tongue and throat, rendering speech difficult and unintelligible and causing a condition of extreme discomfort. The stiffness being accompanied by a feeling of constriction, which excited a single, spasmodic, hacking cough at short intervals.

Some difficulty in breathing, especially in inspiration. These symptoms were accompanied by a terrible restlessness.

On a later occasion there was dyspnea, face purple, head thrown back. The same symptoms as above recurred, but the throat was more swollen and the distress extended below the larynx to the upper part of the lung, which soon became very sore and sensitive. An hour after the sting on this occasion a violent cough came on.

It seemed to be excited by the constrictive feeling in the throat, but it reached down to the sore place in the lungs, causing great distress. It was a deep, hard, ringing cough, lasting without intermission for three hours. Traces of the cough and soreness lasted for months.

Apis has slow action and must not be changed too soon. Increased flow of urine shows it is having a favorable effect. The dropsies of Apis are characterized by a waxy hue of skin, whitish or yellowish, transparent swelling of eyelids, bag-like swelling under eyes, surface of body sore, bruised or burning. In cardiac dropsy the feet swell after walking and are intolerably sore and burning.

In chest disorders there is sensation of contraction (Lach.) and inability to lie down. Tension, swelling and stiffness of limbs. This tight sensation is manifested in another symptom: sensation in abdomen as if something tight would break if too much effort was made to void a constipated stool. Aversion to tight things like Lach. Prostration even to faintness. Paralytic weakness. Paralysis after diphtheria and other severe diseases.

Nervous, restless, over-sensitive or hot and drowsy with or without thirst. Worse from touch or pressure (though the head is better by pressure). Apis has a sensitiveness to heat, especially to heated rooms (Puls., Iod., Kali-i., Sec., Sulph.), worse by warmth of bed. Cold water better. Thirstlessness, there's no desire to drink. Can have fever with thirstlessness.

A keynote is the eyes swell from allergic reactions. The person feels hot, the area is swollen. Sensation as though it would burst, skin becomes very sensitive. Dry skin. Wandering pains. Described as a red-hot needle stuck in and moved around. Shrieking out with pain, keynote. The eyes are glassy, the face is hot and puffy. Bobs head back and forth.

Worse bathing, better cold applications. Fears suffocation. Aggravated by heat, congestion and stuffy room (Puls.). Often has a choking feeling because the throat swells up. Dreams of flying from place to place. Induced jealousy. Arching back of neck.

RELATIONS - ***Antidotes:*** to medium doses and poisonings, Nat-m. in all forms, sweet oil, onions, Ammonia, Lach., Ledum. Ip., also powdered Ip. applied locally. ***It antidotes:*** Canth., Iod., Chin., Dig. ***Compare:*** (1) Apium virus - auto-toxemia with pus products. (2) Puls., Zinc., Canth., Lach. (3) Vespa and snake venoms. (4) Apoc., Acet-ac. - dropsy. (5) Acon., Urt-u. Anac. - urticaria. (6) Arn. - bruised, sore conditions. (7) Ars. - typhoid, gangrene, dropsies, scarlatina, urticaria, chills. (8) Bell. - meningitis, sore throat, erysipelas, scarlatina. (9) Brom. - swelling of ovary during menses. (10) Bry. - meningitis rheumatism. (11) Canth. - burns, erysipelas, urinary symptoms. (12) Euphrasia - conjunctiva. (13) Ferr., Graph., Hep., Hyos., Iod. - synovitis. (14) Lach., Lyc., Merc., Nat-a., Nat-m. - chills, urticaria, tension in ovarian region. (15) Rhus-t. - eyes, but Apis has less tendency to suppuration, vesicular erysipelas but darker than Apis and spreading left to right. Apis right to left, typhoid, restlessness, but Apis is more fidgetiness. ***Complementary:*** Nat-m. the chronic of Apis, Arn., Ars., Hell., Merc-cy., Puls. ***Inimical:*** Rhus-t. in eruptive diseases. ***It follows well:*** Bry. when cephalic cry appears. Hell. when torpor sets in, Iod., Hep., Merc., Lyc., Sulph. ***Is followed well by:*** Graph., tetter on ear lobe. Kali-bi., scrofulous ophthalmia. Ars., hydrothorax. Phos. diphtheria. Stram., mania. Lyc., staphyloma, Sulph., hydrothorax, pleurisy, hydrocephalus. Iod., swollen knee.

REFERENCES - Boericke. Clarke. Murphy.

APIUM GRAVEOLENS

(Common Celery)

PHARMACY - ap-g. Apium graveolens. Common Celery. N. O. Umbelliferae. Tincture of seeds. Tincture of sticks. ***Historical dose:*** Tincture and all potencies.

CLINICAL - Fidgets. Headache. Heartburn. Otorrhea. Post-nasal catarrh. Rumination. Toothache. Urine, retention. Urticaria.

HERBAL - Ap-g. contains a soporific active principle.

HOMEOPATHIC - A proving of tincture of celery seeds produced an unpleasant feeling at stomach with belchings tasting of celery. Heartburn. Spitting up of food. Gone feeling at pit of stomach lasting for hours and partially relieved by eating.

Effects of eating the root include the most obstinant retention of urine during the following day and night, which could only be relieved by the catheter. Another person observed an inability to sit still or lie still in bed from feeling of *"fidgets,"* could not keep mind from thinking.

Allen mentioned "Profuse discharge from granulating ulcers intense constriction over sternum with drawing feeling through to back on lying down," as having been cured by it.

Hering cured with Ap-g. an old abscess near the umbilicus.

Obstinate retention of urine, throbbing headaches and heartburn. Swelling of throat, face and hands. Rheumatic pain in muscles of neck, and in sacrum. Growing pains. Hunger for apples. Dysmenorrhea with sharp, short pains, better flexing legs.

Urticaria, which always appearing with shuddering, intense, stinging, itching, with rapid change of location. Pressure in stomach preceding urticaria and relieved when it appears. Toothache in left molars, better by holding cold water in the mouth.

MIND - Depressed, energetic, feeling of fidgets. Cannot keep mind from thinking.

Abdomen - Sore, sharp sticking pain as if stool was coming on. Nausea increases with pains.

Back - Muscles of back of neck painful on motion, sore to pressure. Dull pain in sacrum with slight bellyache. Pain in sacrum more to left side extending to lumbar region. Red, intensely itching blotches on left sacral region.

Chest - Can count heartbeats by hearing and feeling it in chest.

Constitutions - Sycotic constitutions.

Ears - Partial deafness, worse left, painless pulsation. Troublesome otorrhea.

Eyes - Eyeballs feel as if sunken into sockets.

Female - Sharp sticking pains in both ovarian regions, left, better bending over, by lying on left side with ***legs flexed.*** Tender nipples.

Food - Desire for oranges, oatmeal.

Head - Headache, better eating. Eyeballs feel sunken. Itching in eyes. Itching and smarting in inner canthus of left eye.

Kidneys - Obstinate retention of urine, could only be relieved by catheter.

Limbs - Growing pains in right leg during night. Burning on inside of thighs. Raw, excoriated surfaces on inner thighs. Red, itching blotches on foot and ankle.

Lungs - Tickling, dry cough. ***Intense constriction over sternum*** with drawing feeling through to back on lying down. Throat swollen, dyspnea. Tickling in top of windpipe causing dry cough. Wheezing breathing during the night.

Mouth - Sore spot on tip of tongue. Dull, sore pain on upper and lower teeth. Toothache, better by cold water.

Nose - Nostrils stuffed with pain in forehead. Tough, pearl-colored discharge from nostrils. Sudden dropping of mucus into posterior sinuses. Tickling in right nostril with watery discharge and sneezing.

Rectum - Diarrhea, sharp pain in left iliac region going over to right. Urgent, well-formed stools during the day. Before stool, sharp pain from abdomen directly into rectum.

Skin - Itching blotches, burning, creeping sensation. Profuse discharge from granulating ulcers. Urticaria with shuddering.

Sleep - Unrefreshed sleep. Sleepless, wakes from 1 to 3 a.m. Eating does not help sleep. Not fatigued from loss of sleep.

Stomach - Unpleasant feeling at stomach. Belchings tasting of celery. Heartburn. Spitting up of food. Sore feeling at pit of stomach lasting for hours and partially relieved by eating.

Throat - Soft palate and fauces sore, dark red and swollen. Air rushing down posterior sinuses, hurts back of throat.

COMMENTS - In a proving under the direction of W. P. Wesselheft, a remarkable symptom was "A dull ache in sacrum worse when lying down, better when moving about."

Another symptom was "sensation as if both eyes were sunken back into their sockets." Throbbing headaches, worse by slightest motion, better by rest, mostly left-sided.

REFERENCES - Boericke. Clarke.

APOCYNUM ANDROSAEMIFOLIUM

(Spreading Dogbane)

PHARMACY - apoc-a. Apocynum androsaemifolium. Spreading dogbane. N.O. Apocynaceae. Tincture from the root. ***Historical dose:*** Tincture and all potencies.

CLINICAL - Diarrhea. Dropsy. Nausea. Neuralgia of face. Rheumatic pains. Vomiting. Wandering rheumatism. Worms.

HOMEOPATHIC - Acute rheumatism with great stiffness. General rheumatic pains. Flying pains in different parts. Its pains are of a wandering nature with much stiffness and drawing. The pains go from above downward, are worse when breathing and on turning to left side.

Itching of body and face. Profuse sweat of whole body. Swollen sensations. Trembling and prostration. Worms. Everything smells or tastes like honey.

It has been proved in large doses, its most prominent symptoms included "Heaviness with great desire to sleep. Trembling of the body. Prostration and trembling. Swollen sensations of face and body. Swelling of hands and feet, showing its relation to dropsical states like Apoc. can. and Stroph."

Face - Twitching in face. Violent pain in left zygoma.

Female - Profuse menstruation lasting eight days with violent, pressing pain.

Head - Pains and stiffness in back of head and neck.

Kidneys - Profuse flow of clear urine.

Limbs - Violent pains in all the joints. Much pain in knee and right shoulder. Pain in toes and soles. Tingling pain in toes. Cramps in soles. Profuse sweat with violent heat in soles (Sulph.). Swelling of hands and feet.

Mouth - Pains in all teeth of left lower jaw. Delightful taste in the mouth.

Nose - Everything smells like honey.

Stomach - Vomiting and purging, better from copious evacuation.

COMMENTS - Hale cured with it rheumatic gout, "Acute pains in the joints attended with cramps, bilious stools and flying pains in the teeth. The tincture in drop-doses has been known to expel ascarides and other worms." It has been used for expelling kidney stones and gravel.

RELATIONS - ***Compare:*** (1) Bry. Iris., Colch., Benz-ac. (2) Also Apoc., Alst., Stroph.

REFERENCES - Boericke. Clarke.

APOCYNUM CANNABINUM
(Indian Hemp)

PHARMACY - apoc. Apocynum cannabinum. Indian hemp. American hemp. N. O. Apocynaceae. The whole fresh plant, root included, should be used for making the tincture. ***Historical dose:*** Tincture and all potencies.

CLINICAL - ***Alcoholism***. Anasarca. Arrhythmia. ***Ascites.*** Bedwetting. Bright's disease. Catarrh. ***Cirrhosis. Congested heart failure.*** Coryza. Diabetes insipidus. Diarrhea. ***Dropsy, Edema. Heart, disorders. Heart, dropsy***. Hemoptysis. ***Hydrocephalus. Hydrothorax. Hypotension. Kidney, dropsy***. Menorrhagia. Metrorrhagia. ***Mitral, regurgitation.*** Nausea. Neuralgia. Scarlatina. Snuffles. Tobacco heart. ***Tricuspid, regurgitation.*** Typhus. Urinary, difficulties. Vomiting. ***Watery, stools.***

HOMEOPATHIC - Provings were made with fresh plant tinctures or fresh or powdered root tinctures or infusions. Watery infusions with just enough spirit to keep them from fermenting are said to be more efficacious than tinctures.

The clinical effects of Strophanthus and the symptoms produced on patients to whom it has been given in large doses, clearly show the relationship between it and Apocynum. Both produce intense gastric disturbance, extreme depression of the heart's action and both control dropsical effusions and produce diuresis.

Apocynum depresses the heart, kidneys and intestines, relaxing sphincters. ***Hypotensive, low blood pressure.*** Arrhythmia. ***Congested heart failure with ascites.*** Relaxation of sphincters. ***Mitral and tricuspid regurgitation.*** A diminished frequency of the pulse is a prime indication.

Apocynum is a useful remedy for general dropsies with or without organic disease. Increases secretions of mucus and serous membranes and acts on cellular tissue, producing edema and dropsy and on skin causing diaphoresis. Swelling of every part of the body with scanty urine and sweat, feels if he could only sweat he would get well.

Urinary troubles, especially suppression and strangury. An effective remedy for ***dropsies***, ***edema, ascites, anasarca and hydrothorax.*** Dropsy with great thirst, but water causes pain or is vomited after typhus, scarlatina, cirrhosis. Dropsy after hemorrhage, quinine. Dropsy of serous membranes. Acute inflammatory dropsy.

Acute alcoholism. Useful for the digestive complaints of Bright's disease with nausea, vomiting, drowsiness, and difficult breathing.

In acute hydrocephalus, the child lies in stupor with automatic motion of one arm and leg. Paralysis of left side, one eye motionless other rolling. Weakness is marked. Excretions diminished, especially urine and sweat. Rheumatic stiffness.

MIND - ***Acute or chronic alcoholism***. Confusion of mind during fit of pain. Can't think. Bewildered, nervous, low-spirited. Faints when raised from pillow. Restlessness, nervousness at night.

Abdomen - Bloated. ***Ascites,*** often with chronic diarrhea. Distention after a moderate meal. Dropsy after scarlet fever. Dropsy after abuse of quinine.

Chest - Oppression about epigastrium and chest.

Constitutions - Sanguine constitutions.

Eyes - Hot and red, as if sand in them. One eye motionless and other rolling.

Face - Bloated worse lying down, passes off after sitting up. Face pale, covered with cold sweat in diarrhea. Dry, lips, mouth.

Female - Amenorrhea with bloating of abdomen and legs. Metrorrhagia with nausea, fainting, vital depression. Uterine hemorrhage, blood expelled in large clots or sometimes in fluid state. Hemorrhage at menopause. Ovarian tumor. Cough during pregnancy.

Food - Great thirst with hydrothorax. Great thirst, but water disagrees, causing pain or is immediately thrown off. Thirst on walking.

Head - Dull ache. Hydrocephalus with stupor, vision lost, forehead projecting sutures open, stage of exudation.

Heart - Heart's action is depressed. Mitral and tricuspid regurgitation. Rapid and feeble, irregular cardiac action, low arterial tension, pulsating jugulars, genera cyanosis and general dropsy. Pulse, slow, fluttering, irregular or intermittent.

Kidneys - This remedy acts upon ***urinary organs***, producing diuresis and removing the dropsical effusions. ***Kidney dropsy***. Urine is copious, scanty. Bedwetting in old men. Bladder much distended. Turbid, hot urine with thick mucus and burning in urethra after urinating. Little expulsive power. Dribbling. Strangury. Retention of urine with paralysis of lower limbs.

Limbs - Rheumatic condition. Joints stiff, especially on moving in the morning. Constant involuntary motion of one leg and one arm. Fingernails of bluish red color. Aching in both knees. Edema of feet, ankles, and legs.

Lungs - Sighing. Short, dry cough. ***Breathing is short and unsatisfactory***, difficult. Hydrothorax. Hemoptysis. Violent hoarse cough, worse at night. Cough short, dry, loose and rattling.

Male - Prostate gland enlarged. Penis and scrotum swollen, dropsical.

Modalities - Better from warmth. ***Worse from cold weather***. Worse cold drinks. Worse from uncovering. Worse lying. Worse after sleep. Worse on waking in the morning. Diarrhea is worse immediately after eating. Food or water is immediately ejected, though hungry.

Mouth - Dry tongue, immoderate thirst. Tongue coated. Constant spitting, increase of mucus and saliva.

Nose - Long continued sneezing. Snuffles of children (Samb.). Chronic nasal catarrh with tendency to acute stuffiness with dull, sluggish memory. Dull headache. Takes cold easily, nostrils become congested and blocked up easily. Filled with thick yellow mucus in morning, snuffles of infants.

Rectum - Diarrhea with dropsy, yellow, painless, noisy, gushing stools. Feeling as if anus is open and stools run through out. ***Watery stools***, flatulent with soreness in anus, worse after eating.

Perspiration - Sweats when the skin moistens. Clammy sweats. Body covered with large drops of cold sweat.

Skin - Rough, dry. Cannot sweat.

Sleep - Great restlessness and little sleep. Drowsy in afternoon, restless at night. Stupor. Desire to sleep, but inability to do so. Drowsy before and after nausea and vomiting.

Stomach - Nausea with drowsiness. ***Excessive vomiting***. Dull, heavy, sick feeling. Oppression in epigastrium and chest, impeding breathing (Lob.). Sensation of sinking in the pit of stomach after profuse urination, diabetes insipidus. Uremic vomiting.

Vertigo - Dizzy. Piercing pain in right temple followed by vertigo. Vertigo suddenly appearing and disappearing.

COMMENTS - The dropsies of Apocynum are general dropsies with or without organic disease, swelling of every part of the body, cardiac dropsies. It's specific for edema related to a weak heart, ***congestive heart failure. Edema of the heart, pericardium and the limbs.*** The ankles are swollen because of heart problems.

History of heart attack and weak heart ever since (Am-c., Crat.). ***Hypotensive, low blood pressure.*** Ascites, mitral and tricuspid valve regurgitations (Naja). Alcoholism, delirium tremens. Bright's disease, chronic nephritis. Kidney effect is considered secondary to the heart.

Apoc. causes an intense sinking sensation, drowsiness and a bewildered state of mind. Dizziness. hemorrhages. The excretions are diminished, especially urine and sweat.

Hydrocephalus has been cured with it, "Child lying in stupor with constant involuntary motion of one arm and leg." "Paralysis of left side, one eye motionless, one rolling."

Three cases of neuralgia of the right side, groin, hip and, in one case, region of right kidney, have been cured with this remedy. All were violent, extorting cries. In one case the pain set in very suddenly and the slightest jar aggravated.

Hale said the kidneys are the peculiar seat of the operation of the drug and that it is in kidney dropsies that it is especially curative. It has cured diabetes insipidus with "a sense of sinking in the pit of the stomach with great debility."

Hemorrhages, especially menorrhagia and hemorrhages at the change of life have been cured with it. Hale has found it restore the menses when given in cases of dropsy.

Boericke said to use "tincture (ten drops three times daily)." Less effective in potency (like Echi., Equis., and Crat.).

RELATIONS - ***Compare:*** (1) Apoc-a., Alst., Stroph., Acet-ac. (2) Apis, - thirstless in dropsies. (3) Ars., Bell., Bry., Chin., Colch. (4) Dig. - dropsy, slow pulse. (5) Elat., Hell. - hydrocephalus, ascites. (6) Aloe, Ambr. and Trom. - diarrhea. (7) Kali-caust., Lyc., Merc., Merc-sulph. (8) Sulph., Nux-v., Squil., Ign., Curare, Spig., Verat. (9) Strophanthus - extreme cardiac depression with intense gastric disturbance, dropsy. (10) Aralia Hispida.

REFERENCES - Boericke. Clarke. Murphy.

APOMORPHINUM

(Morphine Alkaloid)

PHARMACY - apom. Apomorphinum hydrochloricum. Morphine alkaloid. Apomorphinum muriaticum. Papaveraceae. Alkaloid from decomposition of Morphine by Hydrochloric Acid. Solution. ***Historical dose:*** All potencies.

CLINICAL - Alcoholism. Constipation. Drug, habit. Faintness. Headache. Heartburn. Hysteria. Insomnia. ***Morning sickness. Nausea.*** Opium, habit. Pregnancy, vomiting. ***Seasickness.*** Vertigo. ***Vomiting.*** Water brash.

HOMEOPATHIC - Apomorphine contains the emetic properties of Opium. The chief power of this drug lies in the speedy and effective vomiting that it produces, which becomes a strong guiding symptom to its homeopathic use. It causes very rapid vomiting, most rapid when injected subcutaneously. Vomiting without previous nausea.

Alcoholism with constant nausea, constipation and insomnia. Drowsiness. Faintness. Specific for ***severe morning sickness.*** Keynote is obstinate, severe morning sickness with a lot of saliva and water brash.

The vomiting is preceded by nausea, lassitude and increased secretion of sweat, saliva, mucus and tears. The peculiar vomiting with its suddenness, completeness and the absence of pain or continued nausea. Pneumonia with vomiting.

Back - Pain between shoulder blades.

Eyes - Dilated pupils.

Head - Hot feeling all over body, especially head.

Stomach - ***Nausea and vomiting***. Violent inclination to vomit. Empty retching and headache, heartburn. Reflex vomiting of pregnancy.

Vertigo - Dizziness. ***Seasickness***.

COMMENTS - Apom. has been used with success in cases of sympathetic vomiting and from pressure of a tumor on the brain.

Halbert has given Apom. 3x with success in a desperate case of combined alcoholism and opium addiction. The symptoms were constant nausea, constipation insomnia, delirious headache, extreme emaciation, pronounced hysteria.

Boericke mentions alcoholism, seasickness, and vomiting, nausea, increased salivation and sweat, nausea and vomiting.

RELATIONS - ***Compare:*** (1) Opium, Hyos., Ip., Ant-t., Cer-ox.

REFERENCES - Boericke. Clarke. Murphy.

AQUA MARINA

(Sea Water)

PHARMACY - aq-mar. Aqua marina. Sea water. Isotonic plasma. Marine plasma. Aqua marina is a sea water taken some miles from the coast of Dieppe and some depth below surface, filtered and diluted with twice as much pure fresh water. Dilutions. ***Historical dose:*** Tincture and all potencies.

CLINICAL - Addison's disease. Anxiety. Biliousness. Constipation. Coryza. Eczema. Emaciation. Flatulence. Gastroenteritis. Goiter. Headache. Hypoglycemia. Hyperthyroid. Loeffler's syndrome. Lupus. Lymphadenitis. Nausea. ***Phlegm***. Polyneuritis. ***Seasickness.*** Seaside, effects. Thyroid problems. Tuberculosis. Varicose, ulcers.

HOMEOPATHIC - Aqua marina is a great ***blood purifier and vitalizer.*** Potentized seawater in weakness, lack of reaction, symptoms are worse by the seaside. For the treatment of diseases of skin, kidneys and intestines.

Lymphadenitis. Goiter. Lupus, eczema, varicose ulcers. Scrofulous disorders of children. Gastroenteritis and tuberculosis.

Aq-mar. acts primarily on the blood, as in toxic, scrofulous conditions, enteritis. It helps detoxifies in cancer cases.

Aq-mar. has been principally used in high potencies for the effects of ***residence near the sea***, which causes biliousness, constipation, headache, etc. It has been used in wine glassful doses and also in potencies as a remedy for ***seasickness***. Worse at seaside or on the sea. Subject anxious and in a feverish state with fetid sweating and head pains. Thoracic pains and back pains, cough with watery or mucus sputum tasting of rust.

Neuralgic pains down right temple and forehead. Face ache left side, cold water intolerable. Sensation of a hair or fishbone in throat, tickling and urging to swallow, causing cough, which does not relieve.

Pain on swallowing, extending to ear and temples. Nausea and nauseous sensation in stomach and abdomen. ***"Constant hawking and raising of phlegm tough and white like cotton."***

General and genital weakness, despite arousal of desires. Vesicular rashes. Alcoholic polyneuritis with mental troubles. Addison's disease. Emaciation. Hypoglycemia. Overactive thyroid. Hyper-secretion from the thyroid. Perspiration. Trembling. Fatigue in the morning, feeling feverish at 10 a.m.

MIND - Absent-minded. Slowness of mind. Intellectual concentration difficult. Feels tormented. Agitated. Tormented by lewd thoughts. Fear of madness. Impression of being spied upon. Finds salvation in religion.

Anxiety aggravated by talking. Anxiety in company. Anxiety by iced drinks. Anxiety worse perspiration. Anxiety improved between 2 p.m. and 4 p.m. Delusion of being watched (Ars.). Aversion to bathing.

Abdomen - Flatulence, sensitivity, pain at the sides of the ribs. Spasmodic colitis. Intestinal parasites. Epigastric pain, aggravated at the tip of the xyphoid cartilage. Pains at 11 p.m., worse by pressure and agitation. Pain better exercise (Coloc.).

Back - Vertebral column affected. Pains in the neck, back and thorax, stiff, heavy or prickling pains. Aggravated by hot drinks, heat, pressure contact. Pain at the nape of the neck with stiffness and difficulty in turning the head. Arthritis of the spine. Arthrosis of the spine. Arthritis of the scapula and shoulder.

Chest - Thoracic pain situated at the level of the third intercostal space, right against the sternum. Pain the lowest three intercostal spaces in the morning when rising, worse with pressure. Pain at the tip of the shoulder blade in the evening.

Constitutions - Hypersensitive subjects, tubercular with a congestion of the veins and mucus membranes in the phosphoric or carbo-phosphoric type with an unstable nervous system.

Ears - Stinging pain in right ear in the evening. Transient stitches.

Face - Face ache on left side of upper and lower jaw, extending under lower jaw to right side. The pain was acute like toothache. Cold water was intolerable.

Food - Appetite and thirst increased, especially at 11.30 a.m. after eating. Aversion to fish. Desires salt, farinaceous food. Worse salt, cold drinks. Better salt, ice cold drinks.

Head - Headaches with vertigo, aggravated by pressure, eating, heat, movement, improved after sleep. Localized head pains in the forehead and occipital region and felt when thinking about them. Occipital headaches, vertigo, buzzing in ears, with visual and psychosomatic complaints. Acute, pressure, neuralgic pain above right frontal portion of head (from inhalation by an atomizer). Severe neuralgic pains down right temple and above right frontal protuberance, very acute and vanishing without a trace, appearing after ten or thirty minutes in left side of neck (near edge of trapezius muscle) (immediately from inhalation by an atomizer).

Limbs - Pain in the right arm from the elbow to the fingertips. Pain in the lower limbs, tenderness at the limbs. Offensive smelling perspiration of the hands, feet and axilla. Pain on exerting pressure on muscles. Trembling of the limbs. Involuntary movement of the legs when they are touching the ground.

Liver - Slight hepatic deficiency.

Lungs - Early tuberculosis. Loeffler's syndrome. Morning cough with cold, watery sputum. Rusty, dirty taste at the back of throat. Difficulty expectorating. Expectoration mucus like cotton.

Male - Libido maintained, but sexual impotence. Seminal discharge followed by weakness, sleepiness and the need to stretch out as a result of muscular pains. Impotence. Increased sexual desire without erections.

Modalities - Better from eating. Better rest. Worse from movement. Worse pressure and heat. Worse afternoon and evening. Worse neuralgic pain in anterior portion of head. Pain in right ear, worse evening. Face pain, worse cold water. Aversion to bathing.

Mouth - White, yellowish mucous. Lips dry, especially at night, split in the middle of the lower lip. Breath fetid, spitting of blood and burning in the mouth. Pain on swallowing, ameliorated by gulping, aggravated by cold drinks. Red rash, painful around the chin. Mucus like cotton (Puls.). Pain as from a splinter.

Nose - Coryza with watery flow, blocking the left nostril. Coryza better tea. Feeling of having a cold at the root of the nose only. Thick, fetid mucus, falling into the back of the throat. Aggravated after eating, by respiration and sleep. Burning and heaviness in the eyelids. Spasmodic rhinitis. Purulent rhinitis. Frontal sinusitis. Obstruction first of right nostril, then of left. Sneezing in morning on waking.

Rectum - Heaviness, pain before and during defecation, even when stools soft. Anal burning, heavy bleeding when first going to stool. Stools, hard at first, then soft in great quantities. Evacuation of small worms.

Skin - Itching of the toes, the inner side of the thighs and the bends of the arms and legs. Vesicular rash on the face, cheeks and chin. Fetid sweating of the feet and hands. Acrocyanosis. Eczema of the palms.

Stomach - Epigastric pain, aggravated by pressure and hot applications. Seasickness. Nausea and nauseous sensation in stomach and abdomen with eructation of wind.

Throat - Sore throat after eating. Pain in the right tonsil, improved by pressure and sleep. Throat congested, especially on the left and trickling of mucus. Mucus fetid when swallowing. Sensation as if a small substance were in the throat causing a desire to cough, but not benefited by coughing. Pain on swallowing, extending into ear and temples.

Vertigo - Vertigo with buzzing in ears. Vertigo with visual disturbances and occipital headaches.

COMMENTS - Aqua marina been used for thyroid problems because of the iodine content of seawater. For people aggravated by seawater, headaches, constipation and seasickness. Mentals are slow and apathetic.

Great fatigue in the morning (Mag-m., Nat-m). Neuralgic pains in the face. Great weakness after sex. They have offensive perspiration (Sil.), offensive sweat on hands, feet, and under the arms.

Seeping of fetid mucus, worse when getting up in the morning. Sore throat with sensation of foreign substance in throat. Pain in the right tonsil, aggravated after eating, ameliorated by pressure and during the night.

Acute, paroxysmal, neuralgic pain in right anterior portion of head all the afternoon and evening (from inhalation by atomizer).

RELATIONS - ***Compare:*** (1) Nat-m. (2) Chlorum - but in addition to its chief ingredient, seawater contains in solution every inorganic substance in the world, also Silica marina.

REFERENCES - Boericke. Clarke. Julian.

AQUA PETRA

(Mineral Springs)

PHARMACY - aq-pet. Aqua petra. Rock water. The mineral springs of Chase and Brittingham. ***Historical dose:*** All potencies.

CLINICAL - Asthma. Coughs. Headaches. Photophobia.

HOMEOPATHIC - The Philadelphia Journal of Homeopathy, Vol. II (1853-1854), page 615, published "Provings of Aqua Petra, From the Mineral Springs of Chase and Brittingham," by D.S. Kimball, M.D.

Kimball's symptoms included an afternoon headache, with fever, eyes that burn and smart, especially the edges of the lids, and ears that itch, the right one snaps on chewing. Throat rough and scrapy. Aching in the lumbar region with weakness. Weakness and lassitude. Full and rapid pulse.

Passing of much flatus towards morning. Aching and faint sense extending from the abdomen to the throat. Urine that is pale, watery, scalds and has little odor, with burning in the urethra during and after passing urine.

Asthmatic breathing. Cough around 10 a.m. and 2 p.m. Expectoration white at first, later yellow and tenacious. Difficult, dark yellow expectoration. ***Saffron yellow colored*** expectoration. Frothy, foamy, opaque, thick, with pieces in it. Transparent, viscid, watery expectoration.

REFERENCES - Murphy.

AQUA PURA

PHARMACY - aq-des. Aqua pura. Alchemical water. ***Historical dose:*** Tincture and all potencies.

CLINICAL - Allergies, Arthritis. Brain tumors. Cancer. Chronic fatigue. Immune disorders. Lung diseases. Kidney disorders. Tumors.

HOMEOPATHIC - Aqua Pura has been used for broken down constitutions and hopeless cases. Shortness of breath, exhaustion, multiple allergies. All kinds of cancer. Chronic fatigue. Lung weakness. Kidney failure.

RELATIONS - ***Compare:*** (1) Ars., Cadm-s., Carc., Thuj., Kali-p. Sil.

REFERENCES - Murphy.

AQUILEGIA VULGARIS

(Garden Columbine)

PHARMACY - aqui. Aquilegia vulgaris. Garden columbine. N. O. Ranunculacee. Tincture of fresh wild plant in bloom. ***Historical dose:*** Tincture and all potencies.

CLINICAL - Clavus. Dysmenorrhea. Globus hystericus. Hysteria. Insomnia. ***Sleeplessness***. Vomiting.

HOMEOPATHIC - Hansen gave the following indications for this unproved drug, "Clavus hystericus during menopause with vomiting of green substance, especially in the morning. Globus hystericus."

Nervous trembling of body, sensitive to light and noise. ***Sleeplessness***. Dysmenorrhea of young girls. Menses scanty with dull, painful, nightly increasing pressure in the right lumbar region.

Women at menopause with vomiting of green substance, especially in the morning.

RELATIONS - ***Compare:*** (1) Acon., Cimic. and other Ranunculacee.

REFERENCES - Boericke. Clarke.

ARAGALLUS LAMBERTI

(White Loco Weed)

PHARMACY - arag. Aragallus lamberti. White loco weed. Rattle weed. ***Historical dose:*** Tincture and all potencies.

CLINICAL - Double vision. Locomotor ataxia. Paralysis.

HOMEOPATHIC - Aragallus lamberti acts principally on nervous system, producing a bewildered, confused state. Symptoms of incoordination and paralysis. Tired in the morning. Diplopia. Burning in eyes. Cracking lower lip. Locomotor ataxia.

MIND - Mental confusion and apathy. ***Bewildered***. Difficulty in concentrating mind, absent-minded. Cannot study. Lack of ambition. Great depression, worse in morning or evening. Desires to be alone. Cross, irritable. Restlessness and aimless wandering.

Limbs - Must concentrate his mind on walking. Weakness of limbs. Pain in left sciatic nerve. Cramps of muscles on front of led while walking.

Lungs - Weight on chest in region of ensiform cartilage. Constriction as of a wide band. Soreness of chest under sternum. Oppression.

Throat - Aches. Feels full. Sore with nausea. Pharynx dark, swollen, glazed.

RELATIONS - ***Compare:*** (1) Astragallus and Oxytropis, two varieties of Locoweed, also Bar-c.

REFERENCES - Boericke. Clarke.

ARALIA HISPIDA

(Wild Elder)

PHARMACY - aral-h. Aralia hispida. Wild elder. N. O. Araliaceae. Solution. ***Historical dose:*** Tincture and all potencies.

HERBAL - Aral-h. is a valuable diuretic, useful in dropsy of the cavities, either due to hepatic or kidney disease with constipation. Urinary disorders, especially with dropsy.

REFERENCES - Boericke. Clarke.

ARALIA RACEMOSA

(American Spikenard)

PHARMACY - aral. Aralia racemosa. American Spikenard. N. O. Araliaceae. Grows in rich woodlands throughout North America. Tincture of fresh root. ***Historical dose:*** Tincture and all potencies.

CLINICAL - ***Asthma.*** Coryza. ***Cough.*** Diarrhea. ***Hay fever.*** Hemorrhoids. Leucorrhea. Nausea. Prolapse, anus. ***Sneezing***.

HERBAL - Aralia was used by the old herbalists as a remedy in tuberculosis and coughs, and for leucorrhea and other female complaints when the secretions are acrid or suppressed.

HOMEOPATHIC - The homeopathic uses have been chiefly based on a proving by Dr. S. A. Jones, in whom it developed an attack of asthma. Jones also experienced diarrhea and prolapsed rectum, soft, yellow stools, and an aching pain in the rectum after stool, extending upwards on the left side. Pain in rectum worse lying on side lain on.

Patient is weak, relaxed and exhausted. Biliousness. ***Asthmatic conditions with cough aggravated on lying down***. Acrid mucus secretions. Drenching sweat during sleep. Extreme sensitiveness to drafts.

The characteristic cough, according to Burnett is: "a fit of coughing occurring before midnight, either immediately on lying down or more commonly after a short sleep." Cough occurring at 11 p.m. after a short sleep.

MIND - Fear of lung disease cannot be shaken off.

Female - Menses suppressed. Foul smelling leucorrhea, acrid with pressing-down pain. Lochia suppressed with tympanites.

Liver - Pain from liver to right scapula.

Lungs - Asthmatic condition with coughing, worse lying down. ***Dry cough coming on after first sleep,*** about middle of night. Raw, burning feeling behind the sternum. Asthma on lying down at night with spasmodic cough, worse after first sleep with tickling in throat. Constriction of chest, ***feels as if a foreign body were in throat.*** Obstruction worse in spring. Whistling breathing. Salty expectoration feels warm in mouth. The least current of air causes sneezing with ***copious watery, excoriating nasal discharge of salty acrid taste***.

Mouth - Aphthae. As if foreign body in throat. Nausea in throat.

Modalities - Better from lying with head high. Better sitting up. Worse from drafts. Worse 11 p.m.. Worse after a short nap.

Nose - ***Hay fever. Frequent sneezing***, worse least drafts with copious, watery excoriating nasal discharge.

COMMENTS - Loud wheezing respiratior coming on immediately on lying down a midnight. Loud inspiration, more difficul than expiration. Right lung more affecte than the left.

On turning to left sided, left side seeme affected and right side became quite free As the attack passed off phlegm came mor freely, had a salty taste and felt warm i the mouth.

RELATIONS - ***Compare:*** (1) Gins., Hed. (Calc. - turning on one side, symptoms go that side, relieving opposite side. (3) Rumex - cough at 11 p.m. (4) Chlorum - opposite of Aral. inspiration easy, expiration difficult. (5) Pecten jacobaeus - humid asthma. Quick, labored breathing. Constriction of chest, especially right side. Asthma preceded by coryza and burning in throat and chest. Attack ends with copious expectoration of tough, frothy mucus. Worse at night. (6) Ars-i., Naph., All-c., Rosa, Sabad., Sinapis. ***Complementary:*** Lob.

REFERENCES - Boericke. Clarke.

ARANEA DIADEMA

(Papal Cross Spider)

PHARMACY - aran. Aranea diadema. Papal cross spider. Diadema aranea. Araneus diadematus. N. O. Arachnida. Araneae. Europe. Tincture of the whole animal. ***Historical dose:*** Tincture and all potencies.

CLINICAL - Acroparesthesia. Allergies. Bones disorders. Cancer. Catalepsy. ***Chills.*** Colic. Diarrhea. Dysmenorrhea. Dyspepsia. ***Hemorrhages.*** Headache. Hemoptysis. Intermittent fever. Leucocytosis. ***Lung, cancer.*** Malarial cachexia. Menstruation, irregularities. Neuralgia. Obesity. Polycythemia. Polyuria. Punctured, wounds. Rickets. Scorbutic, disorders. Scurvy. Spleen, disorders. Toothache. Tuberculosis.

HOMEOPATHIC - Grauvogl is our chief authority for the use of Aranea. The spider poisons powerfully affect the nervous system (Tarent., Mygal.). It is one of the leading remedies for the hydrogenoid constitution as described by him and for intermittent fevers and other intermittent disorders.

By hydrogenoid constitution, Grauvogl meant an abnormal sensitiveness to damp and cold and inability to live near fresh water, either rivers or lakes, or in damp, chilly places. This gives the worse from bathing, from the damp weather, localities or habitations, worse drawing in cold air.

Aran. is the remedy for the constitution favorable to malarial poisoning, where every damp day or place favors chilliness. There is ***abnormal susceptibility to dampness and cold***. Patient feels cold to the very bones, cannot get warm enough. Coldness not relieved by anything.

Inability to live near fresh water, rivers, lakes or in damp chilly places (Dulc., Nat-s.).

Characteristic ***periodicity, coldness,*** and great susceptibility to dampness. Feeling of faintness with nausea, vertigo, trembling and cold sweating. Chilliness followed by little or no fever. Chill not better by external warmth, no sweat with fevers. Shivering, cold sweats. Palpitations. Head and feet cold. Face congested and burning. Rush of blood to the head.

Chill and neuralgic attacks at the same hour every day, every other day, week, month or regular period. Attacks are violent and sudden. Loquacious with painful attacks beginning and ending abruptly. Aggravation from mental exertion, amelioration from pressure on head.

Periostitis. Punctured wounds. ***Feeling as if parts were enlarged and heavier***. Wake up at night with hands feeling twice their natural size. Exhaustion, must lie down.

Swelling of the spleen after malaria suppressed by quinine, malarial attacks worse in wet rainy weather, severe attacks of neuralgia after malaria suppressed by quinine. Neurosis. Periodic neuralgia. Parkinson's syndrome. Acroparesthesia at night. Radicular neuritis. Toxic or viral polyneuritis. Facial neuralgia. Obesity with fat and water retention.

Hemorrhage. Violent hemoptysis of bright red blood in debilitated subjects, bathing and damp places aggravate, coldness as if the bones were made of ice. Pains are like electric shocks. Headache relieved by smoking tobacco. Toothache after lying down at night. Creeping as of ants all over the body. Many symptoms occur on the right side.

MIND - Nervous. Great inner unrest, irritability, fear of death. Stays awake late, uneasiness and the need to move about. Confusion of mind, ***better by smoking in open air***. People and objects seem unreal. Speech is perceived as if far away. Alternately, happy and depressed. Despondent, longs for death. Claustrophobia.

Abdomen - Distention of abdomen. Enlarged spleen. Colic returns same hours. Heaviness in lower abdomen, as of a stone. Pain better by rubbing.

Abdomen - Heaviness and sensation of repletion in the intestines with rumbling, repeated at the same hour each day. Shooting pains going from the gallbladder towards the appendix.

Back - Back icy.

Blood - Polycythemia. Leucocytosis.

Chest - Pain in intercostal nerve from nerve endings to spine. Bright red hemorrhage from lungs (Mill., Ferr-p.).

Constitutions - Hydrogenoid constitution, subject to neuralgia as a result of humid cold. Hemorrhagic diathesis.

Ears - Pricking pain in the right ear and Eustachian tube, spreading towards the left ear. Buzzing in the ears.

Eyes - Double vision. Heat and glittering before eyes, before headache. White is perceived as yellow.

Face - Face pale, yellowish color. Pain in right trifacial nerve from periphery inwards. Cheeks feel as if swollen during toothache.

Female - Menstrual blood has a smell of ammonia. ***Menses, too early, too copious***, accompanied by pain in the lumbar and sacral regions, which is aggravated at the end of the period. Lumbar, abdominal neuralgia with vomiting and yawning during menstrual cycle.

Food - Desire for milk and feeling of being soothed greatly. Thirsty.

Head - Head numbed, head pains, ***improved by smoking.*** Daily headaches, improved by fresh air. Feeling of ants on the nape of the neck. Pain in the trigeminal nerve and occipital nerve.

Heart - Palpitations.

Limbs - Stinging pains in all the joints. Arms and legs feel as if asleep. Bone pains in limbs. Pain in ***os calcis,*** better continued motion. ***Sensation of swelling*** and of parts going to sleep. Numbness of parts supplied by ulnar nerve. Arms and legs feel numb. Bones cold, as if made of ice. Ulcer on heel. Limbs feel heavy. Dull, gnawing aching in the bones of the limbs, on the right side. Pain in the right hip and right knee. Arthritis. Arthrosis.

Lungs - Hemoptysis, bright red. Irritated cough with huskiness.

Kidneys - Acute glomerulonephritis. Nephrotic syndrome. Urine strongly yellow in color. Polyuria. Strong smell of ammonia in the urine. Proteinuria. Oxalate, urate and phosphate crystals. Urochrome and guanidine present.

Modalities - Better smoking tobacco. Better in open air. Better movement. Better in the fresh air. Better summer and pressure. ***Worse from cold, damp weather***. Worse cold bathing. Worse late in afternoon. Worse at midnight. ***Exact periodicity.*** Periodic recurrence at the same time of neuralgic pains and cold shivers. Worse from mental strain, especially of head pains.

Mouth - Sudden violent pain in teeth at night immediately after lying down. Feeling of cold toothache (incisors) in the cold air, pains recur at the same time each day. Bitter taste, better smoking.

Nose - Nose red, copper color.

Rectum - Violent attacks of diarrhea, vertigo and faintness. Stools liquid, accompanied by abdominal pains, improved by rubbing the abdomen. Stools glairy or yellow with repulsive odor. Diarrhea, alternating with constipation.

Sensations - ***As if enormous enlargement*** or numbness of parts, worse on waking or he wakes with such a feeling.

Skin - Yellow color of the face. Small fissures and cracks. Small vesicles which burst easily and dry immediately. Formation of abscesses. Slow healing of small wounds.

Sleep - Sleep disturbed, waking often and feeling that the hands and forearms are fat and swollen, as if enlarged. Anxious dreams, painful awakening. Restless and waking, as if hands and forearms were swollen and heavy.

Stomach - Cramps after eating a little, epigastrium painful to pressure. Nausea. Stomach pains, as though it would burst. Noisy eructation, either tasteless or tasting rotten and repulsive.

Temperature - ***Coldness with pain in long bones*** and feeling of stone in abdomen at the same hour daily. ***Chilly day and night***, always worse during rain. No sweat.

Throat - Throat painful, red and swollen. Prickling, burning pains in the throat.

Vertigo - Vertigo, even when in bed. Vertigo with flickering before the eyes.

COMMENTS - Grimmer said ***cancer of lungs*** with hemorrhage, cases based on the tubercular miasm.

Hydrogenoid constitution. Abnormal sensitiveness to damp and cold, inability to live near fresh water, lakes, rivers, etc. or in damp, chilly places (Nat-s., Thuj.). Very sensitive to dampness and rainy weather. Marked periodicity of symptoms, clock-like regularity, annual recurrence of symptoms and conditions.

Vascular and cerebral tension with insomnia, feverish agitation, clouding of consciousness. Neuralgia at regular intervals, especially of the trigeminal region, occipital nerve and of the limbs.

Gastric and intestinal complaints, as well as genital and urinary complaints, mostly cramping pains. The patient thinks his illness is improved by smoking, but the symptoms always recur at the same hour.

Hemorrhages from many parts, from wounds. Punctured wounds. Exhaustion. Pains like electric currents. Great desire to lie down, many symptoms better lying down. Sensation of swelling in many parts, head, face, hands of numbness of coldness as if bones were made of ice.

RELATIONS - ***It antidotes:*** Chin., Quinine, Merc. ***Antidoted by:*** Smoking tobacco. ***Compare:*** (1) Cedron. Mygale, Tela, Theridion, Tarent., Ip., Nux-v. (2) Ars. - intermittents and bone disorders. (3) Lachesis - has greater loquacity and hypersensitivity to light touch, cannot bear the any constriction, better after menses. (4) Cedron - intermittents of hot climates, Aran. of cold climates chiefly. (5) Apis - Very sharp pains, which are worse by heat and partial or generalized edema, occurring suddenly. (6) Form-ac. - Its action is directed towards cutaneous and mucus allergies, for exudative tendencies. Action on neuritis, arthritis or arthrosis. (7) Paris Quad. - Neuralgias and Barre-Liéou's syndrome. (8) Hypericum.

REFERENCES - Clarke. Grimmer. Julian.

ARANEA IXOBOLA

(Cross-spider)

PHARMACY - aran-ix. Aranea ixobola. Cross-spider. America. Tincture of the whole animal. ***Historical dose:*** All potencies.

CLINICAL - Alcoholic polyneuritis. Facial neuralgia. Goiter. Hashimoto's disease. Muscle pain. Neurasthenia. Neuritis. Psychosis. Thyroiditis.

HOMEOPATHIC - Aranea Ixobola is a Cross-spider which lives in Europe, but was imported from America. Pooch examined the venom, which comes from the Chelicerae. The dried venom represents 30% of the original poison.

J. Mezger undertook a homeopathic proving in 1952 at the Robert Bosch Hospital in Stuttgart, at the time when Dr. Otto Leeser was director there. Thirty-two provers, of whom seven were women and all were doctors, participated.

Action was directed to the digestive system, principally the liver and gallbladder. Neurotropic and vascular action, both central and peripheral. Extreme inner disquiet. Euphoria, depression. Overwhelming need to smoke. Hypersensitive senses of smell and hearing. General and localized feeling of coldness.

Shaking, sensation of inner trembling, need to move about. Spasmodic contracture of the unstriped muscles. Arterial congestion, spasms of the digestive passages. Spasms of the striped muscles. Cramps, tremors, and clonic spasms.

Rheumatic pains. Neuritis with abnormality of cerebrospinal fluid. Painful pulsations of the heart and large vessels. Pain in the liver and gallbladder. Thyroid complaints. Spasmodic instability of the nerves, vessels and muscles. Parathyroid deficiency and tetany. Toxic adenoma of the thyroid. Hashimoto's disease, sub-acute thyroiditis with goiter. Spasmodic cardiovascular complaints. Psychotic, digestive and hepatic disorders.

MIND - Absent-minded. Mental exertion aggravates. Answer, answers snappishly. Snappish. Impolite. Hurried. Restlessness, better open air (Arg-n.). Witty talk. Delusions, everything seems unreal. Delusions of being smaller. Time passes too slowly, appears longer.

Euphoric state, as if he had drunk wine. Teasing disposition and the need to speak. Melancholy, weariness of life. Irritable. Must make a great effort not be impolite or rude.

Incapable of mental concentration inattentive, wants to do nothing. Must make an effort to set to work. Need to move about, feels better in the fresh air. Inner disquiet and hastiness, nothing is finished quickly enough for him. Neurosis from anguish. Mania and depression.

Abdomen - Distension of right hypochondrium. Pain better bending backward. Immediately after meals, nausea with feeling of repletion and heaviness in the hepatic region. Pain in gall bladder. Biliary colic. Sharp, shooting pains in the gallbladder.

Back - Stiffness at the nape of the neck, occurring suddenly and spreading towards the trapezius muscles and the shoulders. Acute pain in the lumbar region, requiring him to stop work for several days.

Chest - Angina pectoris.

Constitutions - Tubercular condition in phosphoric, nervous subjects.

Ears - Hypersensitive to noise.

Female - Menses too early by a week, preceded by blood-streaked leucorrhea. Disorders of libido.

Food - Aversion to fats and rich food. Desires cheese, meat. Strong desire for sugary foods, which are easily digested. Desires sweet food, tobacco. Worse alcohol, fats and rich food. Worse wine. Better coffee, tobacco. Worse by fatty foods, especially pork fat, and alcohol.

Head - Hot feeling in the head and vertigo. Deafening or stinging headache, especially right-sided, worse when bending down or after alcohol, better in fresh air or smoking a cigarette. Headache after mental effort. After copious urination, headache disappears.

Heart - Palpitations of heart immediately after lying. Palpitations extending to epigastrium. Strong palpitations and squeezing feeling. Pressure and tingling in the precordial region. Tachycardia and neurosis with strain in those who worry. Aortic deficiency of arterial origin. Pulse is felt in the carotid artery and abdominal aorta, worse when lying down and resting, better, when moving and after drinking coffee. Acceleration of the pulse.

Kidneys - Overpowering need to urinate and increased or reduced volume of urine. Polyuria.

Limbs - Numbness of single parts. Coldness of painful parts. Pain in left leg, sciatica, better motion. Trembling of hands increased. Rheumatic pains in all the joints, especially in the arms, legs and shoulders. Left-sided sciatic pain after standing for a long time, better by moving the legs. Heavy feeling in the arms, especially the right arm and swollen feeling with clumsiness of the right hand. Numb feeling in the forearm and left hand.

Lungs - Persistent, irritating cough and feeling of soreness in the respiratory passages, every breath is painful. Dry feeling in the trachea and intense thirst after cold drinks. Chronic tracheitis. Chronic asthma. Miller's asthma (false croup).

Male - Low libido with cold genital organs. Increased libido with insufficient erection.

Modalities - Better from drinking coffee and smoking cigarettes. Better motion. Better in fresh air. Better walking. Better getting up. Better leaning backwards. Better lying down and stretching out fully. Better after expelling gas and going to stool. Worse from rest. Worse cold. Worse alcohol. Worse in the morning. Worse warm and wet weather.

Mouth - Dry feeling in the mouth and pharynx, sometimes localized on one side only. Bleeding gingivitis, cracking of the lips, aphthae.

Nose - Sharpened, perverted sense of smell. Irritation of the mucus membranes in the nose. Watery discharge. Hypertrophic rhinitis.

Rectum - Sometimes constipation, but more often pale yellow diarrhea with a repulsive odor. Explosive evacuation and immediately the feeling of not quite having emptied the intestines.

Skin - Cracked lips. Chapped fingers. Acne of the scalp, at the hairline. Desquamation of the hands and nose like that following scarlet fever. Seborrhea of the nose. General itching worse when scratched or from pressure. Erythema like fleabites. Varieties of lupus erythematous, simple or exanthematic. Eczema treated by inoculation of impetigo. Psoriasis of the scalp and hair. Rosy pityriasis. Pityriasis characterized by pimples with a hair in the center.

Sleep - Sleep long in coming, followed by a rush of thoughts and inner unrest. Remains awake for several hours during the night. Sleep disturbed by worrying or frightening dreams. Dreams of quarrel with a friend. Dreams of the death of a close relation or husband. Dreams of violence.

Stomach - Vomiting after drinking alcohol. Vomiting, worse wine (Ant-c.).

Temperature - Constant chilliness, despite staying in a warm room, but no sign of catarrh. Feet cold, not gaining heat when moving. Sweating over the whole body, especially after eating soup. Sudden flushes of heat with headaches and sweating on the forehead. Sweating at night, which wakes him.

Throat - Itching of the throat and difficulty swallowing, as if he had an inflammation, ameliorated by hot drinks. Constant need to scratch the throat and occasional grayish-white sputum. Pulsating in throat with palpitations.

Vertigo - Vertigo with a hot feeling. Vertigo with nausea.

COMMENTS - Hypertrophic cirrhosis without jaundice. Viral hepatitis. Atony of the gallbladder. Acute inflammation of the gallbladder. Gallstones. Chronic cholecystitis without the formation of stones. Cirrhosis of the bladder and enlargement of the spleen. Fibrocystic disease of the pancreas. Chronic pancreatitis. Cystic fibrosis of the pancreas.

RELATIONS - *Compare:* (1) Viscum Album. (2) Tarent. - Nervous complaints with restlessness, anxiety, need to run, palpitations and suffocation, sexual excitement. (3) Theridion - Nervous hypersensitive and intolerance of the slightest sound. Left-sided thoracic pain, nausea and vertigo from closing eyes.

REFERENCES - Julian.

ARANEA SCINENCIA

(Gray Spider)

PHARMACY - aran-s. Aranea scinencia. Gray spider. N. O. Arachnida. Araneae. A gray spider found in Kentucky on old walls. Does not spin a web, N. O. Arachnida. Tincture. ***Historical dose:*** All potencies.

CLINICAL - Debility. Eyes disorders. Headache.

HOMEOPATHIC - Aran-s. has been provéd in 1c and 2c dilutions. One remarkable symptom noticed was ***"Constant twitching of under eyelids,"*** which brings this spider into line with the chorea of Mygale.

Eyes inflamed, weak, watery, lids swollen. Rather profuse flow of saliva, sweet taste in mouth. Dull, stupid headache of considerable intensity, especially in upper back part of head, unable to rest for it, could not collect thoughts with it. Felt as if he had been drinking. All symptoms worse in a warm room.

RELATIONS - *Compare:* (1) Spiders generally. (2) Tela, Agar. (3) Carb-v. - worse warm room, also Puls., Apis, Sulph.

REFERENCES - Boericke. Clarke.

ARBUTUS ANDRACHNE

(Strawberry Tree)

PHARMACY - arbu. Arbutus andrachne. Strawberry tree of the Levant. N. O. Ericaceae. Tincture of young shoots. ***Historical dose:*** Tincture and all potencies.

CLINICAL - Arthritis. Eczema. Gout. Lumbago. Rheumatism. Urine, disorders.

HOMEOPATHIC - The strawberry tree sheds its bark annually, which gives the signature of its use in skin cases. Arbu. is one of Dr. Cooper's remedies. He cured several cases of eczema with it and observed that it produced pains in the joints of a gouty or rheumatic character. Noting these symptoms, he was led to give it in certain inveterate cases of arthritis.

For eczema associated with gouty and rheumatic symptoms. Arthritis, especially larger joints. Lumbago. Symptoms shift from skin to joints. One patient who was benefited by the remedy had worse in North-East winds. The larger joints are principally affected and the slightest movement sets up inflammation.

Bladder symptoms. In one case, the patient noticed that it ***"cleared his urine."*** Arbutin has a reputation among the allopaths as a urinary remedy. Arbutus is allied to Uva ursi, which belongs to the Ericaceae.

RELATIONS - ***Compare:*** (1) Arbutin, Led., Bry., Kalm.

REFERENCES - Boericke. Clarke.

ARECA CATECHU

(Betel Nut)

PHARMACY - arec. Areca catechu. Betel-nut. Areca-nut. N. O. Palmae. Palmaceae. Trituration of the nut. Triturations and solutions of the two alkaloids, Arecoline and Tenaline. ***Historical dose:*** Trituration and all potencies.

CLINICAL - Helminthiasis. Myopia. Parasites. Salivation. Tapeworms. ***Worms.***

HERBAL - The betel-nut is in very common use in the East as a masticatory for sweetening the breath and hardening the gums.

The chief medical use of the Areca nut has been in helminthiasis in dogs, but it is not altogether without danger. According to F. Hobday, Tenaline is a much safer and more certain anthelmintic than Arecoline. He advises a dose of one minim of the solution to the pound-weight of the animal, either given pure or with a little water. It is not to be given by injection.

The Hydrobromate of Arecoline has been used to cause contraction of the pupil. It acts more promptly and more energetically than Eserine, but its duration of action is shorter.

Increases the amplitude of pulsations of the heart. It arrests the heart's action in diastole in poisonous doses and in non-toxic doses increases the amplitude of the pulsations without increasing their frequency.

Acts also as a salivatory, according to Ricapet, it surpasses Pilocarpine as such. Serviceable in glaucoma. Useful for ***worms and parasites.*** It promotes the contractibility of the intestines and as a tineafuge it requires no additional laxative. It should be given in pills coated with gelatin or keratin.

REFERENCES - Boericke. Clarke.

ARGEMONE MEXICANA

(Prickly Poppy)

PHARMACY - arge. Argemone mexicana. Prickly poppy. Argemone ochroleuca. N. O. Papaveraceae. ***Historical dose:*** Tincture and all potencies. Fresh juice is applied to ulcers and warts.

CLINICAL - Bright's disease. Colic. Rheumatism.

HOMEOPATHIC - Argemone mexicana has been used for rheumatic disease associated with Bright's disease. Colicky cramp and spasm of bowels. Painful neuro-muscular conditions, preventing sleep. Rheumatism. Left knee stiff and painful. Feet swollen. Weakness.

Female - Menses suppressed. Diminished sexual desire with weakness.

Head - Throbbing headache in eyes and temples. Head hot. Throat very dry, pain on swallowing.

Kidneys - Passes less urine. Changing color.

Modalities - Worse at noon, weakness.

Stomach - Feels sick like vomiting. Griping

in pit of stomach. No appetite. Belching and passing gas.

REFERENCES - Boericke. Clarke.

ARGENTUM CYANATUM

(Silver Cynaide)

PHARMACY - arg-cy. Argentum cyanatum. Silver cyanide. Trituration. ***Historical dose:*** Trituration and all potencies.

CLINICAL - Angina pectoris. Asthma. Cough. Cramps. Esophagus, spasms.

HOMEOPATHIC - As a result of inhaling fumes while silvering with ***"Argentine"*** a woman experienced some severe poisoning symptoms, among the most prominent were in the throat.

Scraping in throat. Sense of constriction and burning. Violent pain in supra-sternal fossa and under the sternum every time she turned to one side. Suffocative attack. Respiration difficult and short.

Constant dry, spasmodic cough, allowing her to articulate but one word at a time. Painful cramps in feet. The face and tongue were very red. Weakness. Painful cramps in feet.

Arg-cy. has been helpful in cases of ***cancer of the tongue and larynx***. Angina pectoris. Asthma, severe spasmodic cough. Cramps. Spasms of the esophagus.

REFERENCES - Boericke. Clarke.

ARGENTUM IODATUM

(Silver Iodide)

PHARMACY - arg-i. Argentum iodatum. Silver iodide. Trituration. ***Historical dose:*** Trituration and all potencies.

CLINICAL - Catarrh. Hoarseness. Paralysis. Syphilis.

HOMEOPATHIC - Hale suggested Arg-i. as a remedy for conditions presenting symptoms of both the silver or the iodine components.

In practice, Hale found Argentum iodatum of great value in disorders of the throat, pharynx, larynx and bronchia in some peculiar mental disorders, glandular affections, catarrhs and disorders of the heart.

REFERENCES - Boericke. Clarke.

ARGENTUM METALLICUM

(Silver Metal)

PHARMACY - arg. Argentum metallicum. Silver metal. Silver leaf. Precipitated silver. Silver, (Ag., At. Wt. 107.66). Trituration. ***Historical dose:*** Trituration and all potencies.

CLINICAL - Anklosing spondylitis. Bedwetting. Blepharitis. Brain-fag. ***Cartilage, disorders.*** Chlorosis. Conjunctivitis. Cough. Diabetes. Emaciation. Encephalomyelitis. ***Epilepsy.*** Epithelial, disorders. ***Exostosis.*** Keratitis. Headache. Heart, disorders. Hip joint, disease. Hysterical, joints. Influenza. Joints disorders. Laryngitis. ***Leucorrhea. Menopausal, hemorrhage***. Osteomyelitis. Osteoporosis. Ovarian, cysts. Ovaries, disorders. ***Rheumatism.*** Uterus, cancer, prolapsed. Tuberculosis. Voice, loss.

HOMEOPATHIC - Luna of the Alchemists. Argentum metallicum corresponds to deep-seated insidious disease. In the mental sphere it affects the intellect more than the disorders.

Headache of businessmen. Left-sided headache as if in brain substance. Headache and dyspepsia induced by mental agitation, nursing the sick, mental exertion. The more deeply seated the troubles are the more likely are they to be painless.

Argentum metallicum affects all the cartilages and hence all joints and bones with tearing and bruised pains, tenderness and weakness, painful, so-called ***"hysterical"*** joint, joint rheumatism without swelling, pain in rib cartilages and especially the left.

Exostosis on skull. Affects nerves causing convulsive and spasmodic effects. ***Epileptic attacks*** followed by delirious rage, jumping about, striking those near.

Argentum metallicum acts upon joints and their components, bones, condyles, cartilages and ligaments. Arg-m. ***thickens the tissue*** especially ***cartilages***. Emaciation, a gradual drying up, desire for fresh air, dyspnea, sensation of expansion and left-sided pains are characteristic. The larynx is also a special center for this drug.

Emaciation. Symptoms appear slowly, but progressing, deeply penetrating. Decay.

Malfunctioning of the pituitary gland, the optic thalamus, the ovaries and testicles. Infectious encephalomyelitis, caused by influenza. Parkinson's disease. Sensation of electric shocks and nervous trembling over the whole body. Sleeping sickness. Twitching, contraction and trembling of limbs, needs to get up and walk about.

Secretions of mucus membranes are ***thick***, gray or tenacious or like boiled starch. Lies down on account of tiredness and weakness. Pains gradually increase, become violent then suddenly cease, worse by touch. Painless twitching or electric-like shocks. Pains are accompanied by polyuria. Cramps in muscles, limbs feel powerless. Bones are painful, tender. Sore rawness.

MIND - Forgetful. Loss of control over mind and body. ***Loss of mental power.*** Total diminution of memory and difficulty in concentrating. ***Mental exertion aggravates.*** Mental agitation causes headache and indigestion.

Neurosis from worry. Worried, feverish, more or less hasty. Hypochondria. Anxiety about health. Fear of apoplexy during palpitations. Nightly fears in children. Restless anxiety which drives him from place to place. Hurried feeling.

Cries for a long time about trifles, weary, sad, pitiful state. Cries from nervous irritation with talkativeness, agitation and mental strain. Talkative or disinclined to talk in society, changes subjects. Hasty, deceitful. Bars out all sympathy for friends.

Loquacity in daytime. Takes on all sorts of whims often does strange and unaccountable things. Constant feeling of being drunk. Increased cheerfulness and disposition to talk the whole time.

Melancholy. Depressive psychosis. Maniacal and depressive state. Pre-senile and senile dementia. ***Delirium after epilepsy.*** Cerebral inhibition, following psychological stress. Delirious rage with jumping about and striking those near, after epileptic attack. Starting as if electric shocks through body during sleep, wakening her. Time passes slowly.

Abdomen - Loud croaking with hunger in abdomen. Painful soreness of abdomen, worse riding in a carriage. Abdominal distention. Noisy rumblings in the bowels like frogs croaking with drawing, cutting pains. Feeling as though a live worm were coming out of the anus.

Back - Severe backache, must walk bent with oppression of chest. Icy cold feeling near sacrum.

Causations - Onanism. Sunstroke.

Chest - Raw, sore feeling when coughing. ***Great weakness in the chest*** (left), stitches in chest impeding breathing, while reading aloud or talking. ***Feeling of raw spot near supra sterna fossa.*** Boil near the last rib, Pain in left lower ribs. Neuralgic pains along the entire border of left lower rib. Aching and shooting pains in the right side of the chest and sternum. Prickling pains in different areas of the chest.

Constitutions - Suited to thin patients with hollow eyes, pale skin, tendency to tubercle, decay, cancer, deep ulcers, imbecility. It is adapted to tall thin irritable people.

Ears - Itching of ear lobes, has to scratch until it bleeds. Shooting pain in the left ear, spreading to the brain. Blocked feeling in the right ear. Sub-acute ear infection. Diminution in auditive acuity. Buzzing in the ears.

Eyes - Itching in eyelids and canthi. Abundant purulent discharge. Lachrymal stricture. Eyelids and tarsi become thick. Eyelids red and thick. Obscurity of vision. Violent itching of the corners of the eyes. Blepharitis with eyes closed. Catarrhal, purulent conjunctivitis. Follicular conjunctivitis. Ulcerated keratitis. Iritis.

Face - Pale, sallow with weakness. Red. Sudden heat with palpitations. Pain in facial bones.

Female - Ovaries feel too large. Pain in left ovary. Ovarian cysts, tumors. Bearing-down pain. Prolapse uterus with pain in left ovary and small of the back, extending in front and downwards. ***Eroded spongy cervix.*** Palliative in scirrhus of uterus. ***Menopausal hemorrhage***. Sore feeling throughout abdomen. Scirrhus of uterus

Leucorrhea, foul, excoriating, bloody water. Palpitations during pregnancy.

Food - Want of thirst, even during hot stage of fever. Desire for wine. Aversion to even the thought of food. Appetite very much increased, hungry after eating a full meal. ***Great hunger. Hungry in morning, giving her nausea.*** Appetite good, at times loss of appetite with aversion to smoking.

Head - Dull paroxysmal neuralgia over left side, gradually increasing and ceasing suddenly. ***Head feels empty, hollow***. Pain between left eye and frontal eminence. ***Exostosis on skull.*** Crawling and emptiness in head. Scalp very tender to touch. Drilling, boring headache.

Heart - Stops, then trembles, then throbs, better inspiration. Palpitations with cardiac unrest, better by lying on left side. ***Palpitations*** during pregnancy, better deep inhalations. Pulse intermittent and very irregular during palpitation.

Kidneys - Frequent urination, polyuria. Diuresis. ***Urine profuse, turbid***, sweet odor. Diabetes, if there is swelling of the ankles. Urine like whey of sweet odor. Chronic urethritis. Frequent need to urinate and profuse emission of urine. Yellowish-green urinary secretions. Chronic cystitis. Hydronephrosis. Pyelonephrosis. Pyelitis. Proteinuria and glycosuria.

Limbs - Rheumatic disorders of joints, especially elbow and knee. Involuntary contractions of fingers, partial paralysis of forearm, writer's cramp. ***Swelling of ankles***. Arms feel powerless. Legs weak and trembling worse descending stairs. Calves feel as if too short on going down stairs. Swelling of ankles (Diabetes). Writer's cramps. Limbs feel numb or stiff. Burning in corns.

Lungs - Easy expectoration of gray, gelatinous or starchy mucus. ***Cough from laughing***. Hectic fever at noon. On reading aloud, must hem and hawk. Alteration in timbre of voice. Fits of coughing with violent expectoration of mucus resembling cooked starch.

Male - Crushed pain in (right) testicles. Clothing increases pain when walking. ***Seminal emissions without sexual excitement*** and erection. Frequent urination with burning. Yellowish green discharge. Frequent emission of sperm at night. Testicular pain, on the left side, as if bruised. Impotence and nightly seminal discharge. Sterility. Loss of libido. Inflammation of the glands and prepuce. Orchitis. Tumors of the testicle. Acute and chronic inflammation of the prostate gland.

Modalities - Better in open air, cough. Better at night when lying down (opposite Hyos.). Better from motion. Better coffee. Better wrapping up. Worse from touch, pressure. Worse toward noon. Worse 3 p.m. to 6 p.m. Worse from using voice, speaking, singing. Worse from mental strain. Worse cold damp. Worse riding in carriage. Worse from lying on back. Worse sitting, stooping. Worse from entering warm room. Worse in the sun.

Mouth - Dry feeling in the mouth, although the tongue is moist. Stomatitis and gingivitis. Bringing up of thick, sticky, grayish, gelatinous mucus in the morning.

Nose - Copious flow of nasal mucus. Exhausting coryza with sneezing. Violent fluent coryza with frequent sneezing, causing exhaustion. Nosebleed with tickling, worse blowing nose. Nostrils blocked with or without sneezing. Boils on the nose. Adenoids. Chronic rhinitis. Nasal polyps. Lupus of the nose.

Perspiration - Sweats only on abdomen and chest. Sweats during and after meals. Sweats after midnight.

Rectum - Vomiting during stool. Stools soft, passed several times during the day.

Skin - Nervous itching, crawling, tickling on various parts. Itching, burning sensation spread unevenly over the surface of the skin without the need to scratch. Tingling sensation, as if an insect were crawling over the skin. Rosy pityriasis. Prurigo. Itching. Senile pruritus.

Sleep - Electric shocks on dropping to sleep. Nausea in dreams. Sleep disturbed by terrifying dreams, which leave him worried on waking. Sleeping sickness.

Stomach - Feeling of hunger and empty stomach in the morning. Burning in stomach, ascending to the chest. Anxiety and pressure in the pit of stomach. Appetite increased or repugnance to all food. Hiccough on smoking. Nausea in dreams.

Temperature - Hectic fever at noon. Feeling of cold and shivers by day and night. Very high temperature between 11 a.m. and 1 p.m.

Throat - ***Hoarseness*** and aphonia, worse using voice. Larynx feels sore and raw. Total loss of voice in professional singers. ***Worse from use of voice.*** Hawking, viscid, ***gray, jelly-like mucus*** and throat sore, on coughing. Chronic pharyngitis. ***Profuse and easy morning expectoration.*** Tension in throat worse yawning. Fauces numb. Abscess on the tonsils.

Vertigo - Attacks of vertigo on looking at running water. Whirling, as if drunk. Vertigo on entering a room after a walk. Worse entering warm room. Vertigo with intoxicated feeling.

COMMENTS - The muscular system is affected with cramps in limbs, calves feel too short going downstairs, stiffness, numbness, electric-like shocks in joints and limbs, painless twitchings. The heart is especially affected, frequent, spasmodic, though painless twitchings in whole heart muscle, worse lying on back, fears having a stroke.

Sensation as if heart stood still, followed by trembling, then irregular violent throbbing. Palpitation, at night during pregnancy. In social interaction, disinclined to talk, discouraged (Reaction from this is a great inclination to talk, mind very clear.) Frontal headache of businessmen. Headache increasing gradually and ceasing suddenly, at acme as if a nerve being torn, usually left side.

Sticky saliva and mucus expectoration, which is easy. Secretion like boiled starch from the mucus membranes, or there may be a thin and at the same time thick yellow or greenish discharge.

Great hunger even after a full meal. Extreme dryness of mouth, tongue sticks to palate. This symptom with the polyuria points to diabetes in which Arg. is particularly indicated if there is swelling of the ankles. Spasmodic bedwetting at night. Effects of onanism: impotence, atrophy of penis, bruised pains in testicles.

Pains in left ovary, feels enormously swollen, prolapse of uterus (scirrhus). Metrorrhagia, large lumps with violent pains, worse by every motion. Arg-m. acts more on the left side than the right, left ovary is affected. "Prolapse uterus with pains in left ovary."

Juvenile disorders of growth in bones. Fracture of the tip of the second metatarsal bone. Fracture of the scaphoid and tarsal bone. Fracture of the anterior tibia. Deforming arthritis of the hip. Vertebral arthritis.

Prominent tenderness. Tearing pressure and pains in the bones. Joint rheumatism without swelling. Parts feel bruised when pressed on. Hoarseness of singers and speakers, worse speaking or singing. Laughing causes cough. Restless sleep, electric shock through body wakens her.

Very specific for the ligaments and cartilage infections, fibrositis, condylitis (Arg-n.). Severe laryngitis is a keynote, clergyman's sore throat.

RELATIONS - Teste classes Arg-m. with Merc. and with Ars. ***Antidotes:*** Merc., Puls., Zinc., Pall. (ovaries, Pall., right, Arg., left). Stann. - cough excited by laughing. ***Antidoted by:*** Merc., Puls. - an occasional dose of Puls. favors action of Arg-n. in ophthalmia. ***Compare:*** (1) Arg-n. - Anxious unrest with great hastiness. Irritation of the mucus membranes with nervous and muscular weakness. Phobias. (2) Alum., Calc, Plat., Puls, Sel., Sep., Stann., Zinc. (3) Med. - Amnesia for recent facts. Hasty and fidgety, burning of the heels. Itching secretions from the skin and mucus membranes, smell of brine. Joint pains improved at the seaside. Ameliorated by resting in 'knee-chest' position. (4) Psor. - Demineralized weak, chilly. Anxious with periodic migraines and offensive eruptions. (5) Ampelopsis - Chronic hoarseness in scrofulous patients. ***Follows well:*** Alum., Plat. ***Followed well by:*** Calc., Puls., Sep.

REFERENCES - Boericke. Clarke. Julian. Murphy.

ARGENTUM MURIATICUM

(Silver Chloride)

PHARMACY - arg-m. Argentum muriaticum. Silver chloride. (AgCl).Trituration. ***Historical dose:*** Trituration and all potencies.

HOMEOPATHIC - Violent urging to pass urine which must be attended to immediately. Drawing in skin on outer side of left thigh and inner condyle of right elbow. Boring in outside of right ankle and side of right foot.

Tearing in left thumb and hand. Pressing pain in forehead, worse stooping, better coughing. Drawing pain in skin of left temple as of contraction. Tearing in right upper jaw and right eyelid, with stitches.

Eyes - Pain on the right lower orbital border. Tearing below the right eye. Violent stitching in the right lids. Violent stitches in the skin of the right lid.

Face - Tearing in the upper jaw. Tearing in the right upper jaw.

Head - After 4 p.m., frontal headache again, especially on stooping. Awoke with pressing in the forehead, which lasted till 4 p.m.; increased on stooping, relieved by coughing; once, in the open air., even nausea appeared with a more violent attack of the headache, which, in general, was not always equally severe in a given time, but sometimes decreased remarkably, then again without cause, became suddenly very violent. Heaviness and pressure in the frontal bone, with heat in the forehead; increased on stooping; more violent at times, and lasting till he went to sleep. 9:30 a.m. tearing in the frontal bone; again at 4 p.m. Drawing in the skin of the left temple, as if it were contracted. Tearing in the left temple. Tearing in the vertex and in the occiput. Tearing on both sides of the occiput.

Limbs - On walking, drawing in the skin on the external side of the left thigh; drawing in the skin above the inner condyle of the left elbow-joint. Tearing in the left shoulder. Drawing in the skin above the inner condyle of the right elbow. On the evening, boring on the sides of the right foot. Boring outside of the right ankle. Pressing deep in the right leg, on sitting, lasting several minutes, and often returning.

Kidneys - Very frequent and violent urging to urinate; much urine. Violent urging to urinate, with dark yellow, and very acrid urine. Remarkably violent urging to urine, which had to obeyed speedily; much clear urine passed; again in an hour, and several times afterwards, until 4 p.m. In the night, very frequent urination; urine as usual in quality and quantity. Frequent and copious urination, but with less urging.

Mouth - Taste slightly metallic, inclining to bitter.

Throat - Convulsive contraction in the pharynx.

REFERENCES - Boericke.

ARGENTUM NITRICUM

(Silver Nitrate)

PHARMACY - arg-n. Argentum nitricum. Silver nitrate. Lunar caustic. Trituration and solution. ***Historical dose:*** Trituration and all potencies.

CLINICAL - Acidity. Addison's disease. Anemia. ***Anticipation. Anxiety, attacks.*** Chancre. Chemosis. Dyspepsia. Epilepsy. Belchings. Erysipelas. Eyes disorders. Flatulence. ***Fears.*** Fright. Gastric ulcer. Gonorrhea. Hands, swelling. Headache. Heartburn. Herpes zoster. Impetigo. ***Incoordination***. Locomotor ataxia. ***Melancholy.*** Neuralgia. ***Ophthalmia, neonatorum. Panic, attacks.*** Paralysis. Prostate, enlargement. Scarlatina. Smallpox. Spinal irritation. Syphilis. Taste, altered. Throat disorders. Tongue ulcerated. ***Trembling***. Warts.

HOMEOPATHIC - It was the use of Argentum nitricum in ancient times in the treatment of epilepsy which led to the production of the lamentable cases of lead-colored pigmentation of the skin called Argyria.

Arg-n. has irresistible ***desire for sugar,*** which at the same time aggravates. Kent related a case illustrating this. A nursing infant had a grass-green diarrhea which failed to yield to Merc., Ars., and Cham. At last Kent discovered that the mother ate a pound of candy a day.

Arg-n. was given and the candy stopped and the child soon got well.

Grimmer used it for Addison's disease, lead-colored pigmentation of the skin. Mental symptoms are important indications for the use of the remedy, nervous fears and restlessness with trembling hands, ***skin cancers***.

In Arg-n. the neurotic effects are very marked, many brain and spinal symptoms presenting themselves which give certain indications for its homeopathic employment. Symptoms of ***incoordination, loss of control*** and want of balance everywhere, mentally and physically, ***trembling*** in affected parts. Emaciation is progressive. Paraplegia. Ascending paralysis. Parts seem ***enlarged*** or bound up. Pains increase and decrease gradually.

The cases of epilepsy calling for this drug are those caused by fright or occurring at the menstrual period. For days or hours before the attack the pupils are dilated and after the attack the patient is very restless and has trembling of the hands.

Impulse to walk very fast (Lil-t.). Suitable to businessmen, students. Very characteristic is the ***great desire for sweets,*** the splinter-like pains and free muco-purulent discharge in inflamed and ulcerated mucus membranes. Sensation as if a part were expanding and other errors of perception are characteristic. Pains increase and decrease gradually.

Muco-purulent discharges and ***splinter like pains.*** Faint and tremulous. Flatulent state and prematurely aged look. Explosive belching, especially in neurotics. Upper abdominal disorders brought on by undue mental exertion. Paraplegia, myelitis and disseminated sclerosis of brain and cord. ***Intolerance of heat***. Sensation of a sudden pinch (Dudgeon). Destroys red blood corpuscles, producing anemia.

MIND - Nervous impulsive and hurried, yet timid and anxious. Panic and anxiety attacks. Dreads ordeals. ***Anticipation, apprehension and fear,*** when ready to go to doctor, dentist, church, etc. Diarrhea from anticipating upcoming events. ***Performance, anxiety.*** Examinations, fear of taking tests. Thinks that all his undertakings will and must fail.

Fears, phobias and anxieties. Fears projecting corners of buildings and high buildings. ***Fear of heights.*** Fearsome. ***Fear of flying in airplanes.*** Fear of impending evil. Fear of crowds. Fear of dark. Claustrophobia. Fear of fainting. Fear of being too late. Fear of failing. ***Fear of having a panic attack.*** Fear of losing self-control.

Peculiar mental impulses. Impulse to jump when crossing a bridge or from a window. ***Impulsive, wants to do things in a hurry*** (Lil-t.). Walks rapidly from anxiety.

Fear of passing a certain point of high buildings. Imagines he cannot pass a certain point (Kali-br.). The sight of high buildings makes him giddy and causes him to stagger, it seems as if houses on both sides of street would approach and crush him.

Tormented by strange ideas and emotions. Irrational, does strange things and comes to strange conclusions, does foolish things. Hidden irrational motives for actions. ***Delusion he is despised.*** Thinks about killing himself.

Obstinate, against whatever was proposed, he had the queerest objection. Errors of perception. ***Time passes slowly*** (Cann-i.). Time seems short, wants to do things in a hurry, must walk fast, etc. Brain fag. Memory weak. Perversion of senses. Indifference while in company. Loss of ambition.

Melancholic, apprehensive of serious disease. Fear of some incurable disease. Forsaken feeling. Sensation of isolation. Desire to talk. Hesitates, falters in speech in gait, etc. Childish talk. Talks about his sufferings. Talks of one subject. Believes that all his undertakings will fail. Weeps, says he is lost beyond hope.

Abdomen - Rumbling, gurgling. ***Flatulence causing distention and bursting of abdomen.*** Loud, explosive belchings discharged upwards and downwards Shivering through bowels, extending up the back. ***Colic with much gas and distention***. Constriction in bowels, as if tightly tied with a band. Sharp ulcerative pain on left side, below short ribs. Cutting pain with loud rumbling. Spasms of diaphragm.

Back - Much pain. Spine sensitive with nocturnal pains (Ox-ac.). Paraplegia. Posterior spinal sclerosis. Pain in the small of the back worse rising from sitting better standing or walking. Throbbing in spine or weak spine. Glands of the neck indurated. ***Weakness in sacro-iliac symphysis as if bones were loose.*** Heaviness in sacrum, as before menses. Glands of neck indurated.

Breasts - Sore nipples from nursing.

Causations - ***Anticipation.*** Apprehension, fear or fright. Eating ices. Mental strain and worry. Masturbation and sexual excesses. Intemperate habits. ***Sugar.*** Tobacco.

Chest - Angina pectoris with nightly aggravation. Intense spasm of chest muscles. Feels as if a bar were around chest. Painful spots in chest. Pain in the chest on putting boots. As if weight of stone in middle of the sternum.

Constitutions - Withered up and dried constitutions, especially when associated with unusual or long continued mental exertion. It corresponds to Grauvogl's carbo-nitrogenoid constitution (Sulph., Cupr.) in higher to the hydrogenoid or sycotic constitution. Hysteric nervous persons, headaches from mental causes characterized by dullness of head. Women with menstrual disturbances. Cachetic state. Scrawny, feeble, dried-up-looking women. Guernsey put it, "withered and dried up by disease. A child looks like a withered old man."

Cough - Cough is worse laughing, stooping, smoking, ascending stairs before menses. ***High notes causes cough.*** Suffocative cough, at noon. Cough when angered.

Ears - Tearing pain in ears. Sharp pain from right to left ear, with congestion to head. Buzzing in ears with vertigo. Ringing with deafness. Whizzing in left ear, with feeling of obstruction and hard hearing. Fullness and ringing.

Eyes - ***Acute conjunctivitis.*** Great swelling of conjunctiva, ***discharge abundant and purulent***. Eyestrain from sewing, worse in warm room. Aching, tired feeling in eyes, better closing or pressing upon them. Useful in restoring power to the weakened ciliary muscles. ***Inner canthi swollen and red***. Photophobia in warm room. Ophthalmia neonatorum. ***Painful purulent ophthalmia***. Chronic ulceration of margin of lids, sore, thick, swollen. Unable to keep eyes fixed steadily. Opacity of cornea. Ulcer in cornea. Pterygium of pink color. Blepharitis, thick crusts on eyelids. Pupils dilated. Chemosis. Eye symptoms worse with abdominal symptoms.

Face - Sunken, old, pale and bluish. Face yellow, dirty looking. Old man's look, tight drawing of skin over bones. Sickly, sunken, grayish of muddy color. Infraorbital neuralgia, left side. Prosopalgia, almost taking away eyesight. Drops of sweat on face.

Female - Pain in stomach and spasmodic contraction in chest before menses. Menses scanty with dyspnea. Menses, irregular too soon too late or last one day only. Menses with headache. Metrorrhagia with nervous weakness at menopause, also of young widows and childless women. Leucorrhea profuse with erosion of cervix, bleeding easily. Leucorrhea mucus, bloody, corroding, yellow and profuse. Prolapsed uterus. Uterine hemorrhage, two weeks after menses, painful disorders of left ovary. Ovaries painful with pains radiating to sacrum and thighs. Itching of skin and flushes of heat during menopause. Disposition to miscarriage. Infertility. Puerperal convulsions. Orgasms at night. Sex painful, followed by bleeding.

Food - Desire for cheese and salt. Loss of appetite. Appetite good, but every kind of food disagrees. ***Hypoglycemia.*** Eating relives nausea but aggravates stomach pain. Better after warm drinks. Better sour things, smoking. Better after alcohol. ***Great craving for sweets***. ***Craves sugar, which disagrees.*** Desires for cheese and salt. Desires ice cream, fat and sweets. Craves plum sauce. Worse from coffee. Worse cold drinks

Head - Excessive congestion to head, with throbbing carotids. Migraine followed by debility. ***Emotional upsets causes appearance of migraine attacks.*** Migraine, head feels much enlarged.

Head - Nervous headache with ***coldness and trembling***. Headaches, worse mental exertion, dancing, better tight bandaging. Head as if in a vise. ***Sensation of expansion***. Brain fatigue with general debility and trembling. Aching in frontal eminence with ***enlarged feeling in corresponding eye***. Boring pain, ***better on tight bandaging and pressure***. Itching of scalp. Hemicrania, bones of head feel as if separated. As if skull bones were separated. Headache ends in vomiting. Headaches of hysterical young women, delicate literary persons. Itching, crawling sensation on the scalp.

Heart - Angina pectoris. Organic heart troubles of business men, students and brain workers. Burning feeling in region of heart. ***Anxiety with palpitations*** and throbbing throughout the whole body. Palpitations with nausea. ***Palpitations, worse lying on right side*** (Alumn.). Palpitations, worse riding in car, better pressing by hand. Unpleasant sensation of fullness about the heart better fresh open air. Sensation as if heart would stop beating, when sitting quietly. Pulse is irregular intermittent.

Kidneys - Violent pain from kidney to bladder, worse touch, motion and deep inspiration. Touching region of kidneys increases pain. Urethra inflamed with pain, burning, itching, pain as from a splinter. Emission of a few drops after having finished. ***Urethritis with pain, increased gonorrhea, priapism, dysuria, bloody urine and fever.*** Early stage of gonorrhea, profuse discharge and terrible cutting pains, bloody urine. Urging to urinate, urine passes less easily and freely. Retention of urine. ***Sugar in urine.*** Divided stream. Urine passes unconsciously, day and night. Yellow bloody urine. Urine is highly colored, dark red with albumin. Urine scanty and dark.

Limbs - Lassitude and weariness of forearm and legs with trembling. Cannot walk with eyes closed. Trembling with general debility. Trembling of hands, cannot write. Numbness of arms. Numbness of fingertips, ring and little fingers. Fingers half clenched, cannot be separated. Paralysis with mental and abdominal symptoms. Weakness, rigidity or twisting in calves. Walks and stands unsteadily, especially when unobserved. Post-diphtheria paralysis (Gels.). Chorea-like convulsions, with the legs drawn up, arms jerked outwards and upwards. Peripheral neuralgias. Edema of legs. Legs feel as if made of wood or padded. Paraplegia after debilitating causes. As if a weight hanging to coccyx.

Lungs - Asthma, worse summer, cold weather or taking cold. Asthmatic attacks from going up stairs or bodily exertion. Suffocative cough, as if from a hair in throat. Dyspnea. ***Craves fresh air.*** Many people in a room seem to take away his breath. Panting, quick, sibilant breathing. Rawness, soreness, high up in trachea worse coughing. Crowded rooms takes away his breath. Desire to take deep breath which aggravates the dyspnea. Craves fresh air. Asthma, worse in summer in cold weather or taking cold.

Male - Chancre like ulcers, on the prepuce. Testes drawn up high. Genitals shrivel. Desire waning. Cutting in urethra with painful erection. Sex painful, urethra as if put on stretch or sensitive at orifice. Impotency. Erection fails when sex is attempted. Cancer-like ulcers. Ulcers on prepuce.

Modalities - Better from open air, fresh air. ***Better cool air, cold, cold bath.*** Better from hard pressure. Better motion. Better belching. Better from bending double, pressure. ***Worse from emotions. Worse anxiety, apprehension. Worse fear or fright***. Worse from suspense. Worse from mental strain and worry. Worse warmth in any form. Worse at night. Worse from cold food, cold drinks. Worse ice cream. ***Worse sugar, sweets.*** Worse after eating. ***Worse left side***. Worse in a room in closed, small places. Worse lying on right side. Worse looking down. Worse from drinking, crowds. Worse from warmth in any form. Worse before and during menses. Worse from riding. Worse thinking intently.

Mouth - Fetor from mouth. Taste coppery like ink. Canker sores. Stringent, sour or bitter-sour taste. Food escapes from mouth during chewing. Cannot talk, spasms of muscles of tongue and throat. Stammers. Tough mucus in mouth. Ptyalism. Lips dry and viscid, without thirst. Lips tremble while speaking. Lips blue.

Nose - Nasal bones painful as if bruised. Nasal discharge like boiled starch. Discharge of whitish pus, with clots of blood. Nosebleed during menopause. Loss of smell. Violent itching. Coryza with chilliness, lachrymation and headache. Violent itching, rubs it. Ulcers in septum.

Perspiration - Sweats in morning or at night. Profuse sweat on the face in beads. Sweat and chilliness as soon as he gets warm in bed.

Rectum - ***Diarrhea from emotions***, worse immediately after eating and drinking. ***Diarrhea from anticipation.*** Diarrhea after any emotion with flatulence. ***Nervous diarrhea after sugar candy***. Diarrhea of children after weaning. ***Fluids go right through him*** after sweets. Constipation, alternates with diarrhea. Hemorrhoidal pain in morning. Itching of anus. Tenia or threadworms.

Skin - Brown, tense and hard. Drawing in skin, as from a spider-web or dried albuminous substance withered and dried up. Irregular blotches. Ulcers, angry, deep with hard edges. Warty granulations. Adherent crusts. Bedsores. Bluish-black eruption. Scarlet fever.

Sleep - Drowsy stupor. Sleepless from fancies before his imagination. Ailments from long, wearisome, fatiguing night watching. Restless sleep, awakes almost every hour, disturbed with many dreams. Horrible dreams of snakes, wakes in fright. Dreams he is hungry. Dreams of sexual gratification.

Stomach - Alcoholic gastritis. ***Belching*** with most gastric ailments. Ineffectual effort at eructation. Gastroenteritis. ***Flatulence, painful swelling of stomach***. Enormous distension. Painful spot over stomach that radiates to all parts of the abdomen. Gnawing ulcerating pain, burning and constriction. Trembling and throbbing in stomach. Enormous distention. Ulcerative pain in left side under ribs. ***Ulceration with radiating pain***. Deathly nausea during headache, not better after vomiting. Nausea, retching, vomiting of glairy mucus. Astringent sour or bitter vomiting. Vomiting with diarrhea and violent colicky pains.

Stool - Stools, shreddy, mucus, turning green like chopped spinach. Watery, noisy, flatulent stools. ***Stools, green like chopped spinach*** with shreddy mucus and enormous distention of abdomen, very offensive.

Teeth - Gums tender and bleed easily. Pain in healthy teeth. Teeth pain worse chewing, cold things, sour things.

Temperature - Chills with nausea. Chilly when uncovered, yet feels smothered if wrapped up. Chilly with many complaints. Chills with cold hands and feet. Constant chilliness up back and over shoulders. Intermittent fever, with hemorrhage from lungs. Fever with no thirst.

Throat - Burning and dryness in fauces and pharynx. ***Much thick mucus*** in throat and mouth causes hawking. Raw, rough and sore. Uvula and fauces dark red. ***Sensation as if a splinter in throat,*** when swallowing, breathing or moving the neck better cool drinks. Dark redness of throat catarrh of smokers with tickling as of hair in throat. ***Strangulated feeling.*** Swallowing difficult. Chronic induration of tonsils. Food lodges in pharynx. Smoker's catarrh with sensation as of a hair in throat. Loss of voice. Chronic laryngitis of singers. Raising the voice causes cough, ***high notes cause cough.*** Chronic hoarseness.

Tongue - Red streak down middle of tongue. Tongue has prominent papilla. Tongue tip is red and painful. Tongue furred with clean edges. Aphthae on edges of the tongue. Tongue coated white.

Vertigo - Vertigo with buzzing in ears and with nervous disorders. Vertigo before epilepsy. ***Vertigo looking down from heights.*** Vertigo with transient blindness. Vertigo worse closing eyes. Vertigo with cerebral congestion.

Vertigo - Vertigo at sight of high buildings.

Vision - Spots before the vision. Blurred vision. Distorted vision. Misty vision. Diplopia, from rush of blood to head. Sight worse by candlelight, than by daylight. Black motes, before right eye. Dim vision on thinking intently, with headache. Grey spots and serpent-like bodies moving before eyes. Vanishing vision must constantly wipe away mucus. Farsighted. Paralysis of accommodation from errors of refraction.

COMMENTS - Among the key symptoms of Arg-n. are great tremor, nervous feeling, and sensation as if being squeezed in a vice. Feeling of constriction in various parts as if a band of iron around chest or waist.

A feeling as if the body or some part of the body was expanding. Migraine with feeling as if head were enormously enlarged, better tightly bound. Defective coordination. Paralysis of motion and sensation, a peculiar numbness accompanied with hyperesthesia. Sensation of a splinter sticking in various parts. Burning sensations.

In allopathic practice the dyspepsia for which it is given is worse before food, when the stomach is empty. The opposite condition is the leading indication in homeopathic practice. Gowers recorded a case in which the use of Arg-n. for stomach trouble caused (like lead), drop-wrist, gout and albuminuria.

E. P. Brewer recorded a proving in which the prover, a young man, took on three consecutive days one grain a day of Arg-n. triturated with sugar of milk. A number of motor and sensory symptoms were elicited, reminding Brewer of locomotor ataxia for which it has been used with success by old-school practitioners.

This use also has led to many cases of argyria. Among the symptoms of this proving were "Mental operations sluggish, continued thought required special effort, but exertion of mind did not aggravate the heaviness and fullness of head. Lower limbs fatigued, as if they would suddenly fail him. Loss of ambition. Building air castles by day: monstrous dreams by night."

Other symptoms were sore throat with white patches, rheumatic pains in (left) wrist and finger joints with external tenderness of bony prominences, pain on rising in right sacroiliac notch. Sore muscles of neck and back. Urticaria spots in various parts.

In poisoning cases complete loss of consciousness insensibility and convulsions have occurred. Some of the notable digestive symptoms are: "Irresistible desire for sugar. Fluids go right through him." Belching accompanies most gastric disorders.

Green stools are remarkable. Green mucus like chopped spinach in flakes. Stool turning green after remaining on diaper. Stool expelled with much spluttering. Stool shreddy, red, green muco-lymph or epithelial substance.

There is a pain in the small of the back, better on standing or walking, but severe when rising from a seat (Sulph., Caust.). Mucus membranes affected, purulent and bloody discharges, membranous diarrhea with agonizing pains. Epithelium affected (cancers). Intestinal catarrh with shreddy membranous discharges is often cured by Arg-n.

Most symptoms are worse night, very nervous at night. Worse at night or in morning on rising (epileptic attacks). Day half more cough, night half more diarrhea. Worse on awaking. At 11 a.m. nervous attacks better by stimulants. Chill down back every day at noon. A large number of symptoms appear on the left side.

Grimmer notes that it's used along with Natrum Mur to antidote the effects of silver nitrate cauterization. For example, of the nose, and sometimes they do the uterus, the cervix, to stop bleeding, any place. Parkinson's paralysis, or disorders after stroke, loss of motor control, especially on left.

Good for multiple sclerosis. Addison's disease, lead-colored pigmentation of the skin. Mental symptoms are important indications for the use of the remedy, nervous fears and restlessness with trembling hands, skin cancers. Severe blood sugar problems, acute or chronic sugar poisoning, hypoglycemia, diabetes.

Consider Arg-n., a left-sided Lycopodium. Voracious, canine desire for sweets. Bingeing on sweets. Can become angry or irritable after sugar. Also craves salt. Another keynote is gas and bloating, then low blood sugar. They can have a splinter-like sensation in the throat.

It's specific for laryngitis. Hoarseness, sore throat. Epilepsy from frights. Diarrhea from anxiety. Headache from over studying, eye strain. Conjunctivitis, looks like raw meat, pus green and yellow in color.

Major phobia remedy. Panic attacks when low blood sugar. They have a lot of fears of fainting, fears of having a fit in public, fears of epilepsy, the general idea is fears of losing control.

Fear of something bad happening, "impending doom." Superstitions, rituals, conspiracy paranoia. "Fear of being poisoned," anxiety over health. Fear of death, may predict their own death (Agn.). In late stages, fear of their own thoughts. Tormenting thoughts and impulses, repeating thoughts.

Over-active mental plane, anticipation leading to worry. For anticipation, stage fright to the point here they get diarrhea (Gels., Acon.). Gastrointestinal symptoms with anxiety. Vertigo due to anxiety.

Concentration problems, brain degeneration, early senility with strong imaginations. Symptoms worse at night. Hasty walk, keynote, they walk so fast that the upper body is leaned forward. Neurological deficiencies and incoordination of walking, staggering gaits.

Keynote craving of sugar, which aggravates. The aggravation of the sugar is as strong as their craving. Sugar causes headaches, anxiety, irritability, and low blood sugar. Severe gas and bloating. Craves salt and strong cheese (Puls, Ign, Rhus-t.). Worse heat, skin may be cool, but they think they are hot (Sec.).

Desires company, open, forward with a lot of vitality. Strong emotional nature. Impulsive, instinctive expression of emotions. Happy, easy-going high sexual power. High sex drive, loss of erection or premature ejaculation due to overexcitement and anticipation.

RELATIONS - ***Antidoted by:*** Am-caust., effects of tobacco. Nat-m., Ars., Milk. ***Antidotes to:*** Puls., Calc., Sep., next in importance, Lyc., Sil., Rhus-t., Phos., Sulph. ***Compare:*** (1) Ars., Merc., Phos., Puls. (2) Arg-cy. - angina pectoris, asthma, spasm of esophagus. (3) Argent, iodat. - throat disorders, hoarseness, gland affected. (4) Argent. phos. - an excellent diuretic in dropsy. (5) Arg-oxyd. - chlorosis with menorrhagia and diarrhea. (6) Arg-m. - acts on cartilages, Arg-n. more on mucus membranes, skin, bone and periosteum and is suited to herpetic patients. (7) to Aur., Cupr., Kali-bi., Lach., Merc., Merc-c., Merc-i., Nat-m., Nit-ac., Thuj. (8) In complaints from pressure of clothes like Calc., Bry., Caust., Lyc., Sars., Stann. (9) In congestive headaches like Glon. and other Nit-ac., Hep., worse by cold, Arg-n. worse in warm room. (10) Puls. is its nearest analog. ***Inimical:*** Coff. (it increases the nervous headache). ***Follows well:*** Bry., Spig. (dyspepsia), Spongia (goiter), Caust. (urethral affections), Verat-a. (flatus). ***Is followed well by:*** Lyc. (flatus).

REFERENCES - Boericke. Clarke.

ARISTOLOCHIA CLEMATITIS

(Common Birthwort)

PHARMACY - arist-cl. Aristolochia clematitis. Common birthwort. Aristolochia infesta. N. O. Aristolochiaceae. Europe, South America, Asia. Tincture of the root. ***Historical dose:*** Trituration and all potencies.

CLINICAL - After-pains. Amenorrhea. Anorexia. Arthritis. Bedwetting. Bronchitis. ***Chills.*** Colic. Cystic mastitis. Cystitis. Depression. Dysmenorrhea. Eczema. Enteritis. Hormonal, imbalances. Insomnia. Laryngitis. Mastitis. Menopause. Metritis. Nephritis. Premenstrual syndrome. Rheumatism. Spasmodic colitis. Sinusitis. Vaginitis. Varicose veins. ***Vertigo.***

HERBAL - Aristolochia Clematitis, of the Aristolochiaceae family, grows in Southern Europe and South America. Its active principle is clematine, which is identical to the Aristolochia or the Serpentarin as well as to non-purified Aristolochic acid. Aristolochic acid causes menorrhagia, tends towards miscarriage, and has a toxic action on the kidneys and liver parenchyma as well as intestinal mucus membranes.

"Aristos" means better, "locheia" means giving birth. Used in popular medicine to induce birth or stimulant the menses. Also as a diuretic, and against rheumatism. In high doses it is an emetic and cathartic. In South America, some Aristolochia are used for blindness.

HOMEOPATHIC - The proving by Mezger made use of the spring rhizome. The experiment was carried out by eighteen provers, of whom thirteen were women. The potencies 5x, 2x, 12x and the mother tincture were used in the proving. The experiment lasted for twelve weeks.

It produced excess of estrogen hormones. Marked affect on the urinary passages, kidneys, venous system, skin. Irregular menses. Premenstrual insomnia with agitation and congestion of the pelvis. Joint pains improved by movement. State of fatigue, or the opposite. ***Worn out with vertigo, chilliness,*** slightly improved by heat. Hunger pangs and need to eat despite feeling nausea. Tendency to plumpness.

MIND - Sensation of solitude. Fear for the future. Rejects company. Psychosomatic complaints tending towards depression, especially in women who are going through the menopause (Sep.). Depression, ameliorated by fresh air and menses. Mental condition aggravated before and after periods, clearly ameliorated during menstrual flow.

Abdomen - Colic. Spasmodic colitis. Enteritis. Abdomen distended, painful, before and during menses.

Breasts - Pain and feeling of hardening of the left breast. Pain in the breast. Cystic mastitis.

Chest - Chest feels hard, like a breastplate.

Constitutions - Hormonal imbalances. Subjects of a nervous constitution, with extreme sensitivity, and who cry easily. Tubercular conditions of the "worn-out" type.

Eyes - Watering aggravated by light, reading. Burning and itching.

Female - Brown discharge, watery flow. Eczema of the vulva. Sensual itching, aggravated before menses, ameliorated during menses, aggravated after menses. Menses absent, late or short, Blood black, with clotting. Varicocele. Dysmenorrhea. Infrequent menses. Amenorrhea. Metritis. After-pains with laryngitis. Vaginitis.

Food - Anorexia, nausea with vertigo and cold sensations.

Head - Diffuse headaches, improved in the fresh air and by cold, damp compresses. Congestive headache (Bell.).

Kidneys - Pain in the kidneys and bladder with a frequent urination. Bedwetting, especially in older women. Incontinence and compelling need to urinate. Pyelitis. Cystitis. Albuminuria with white discharge.

Limbs - Arthritis in women, with menopause. Rheumatism of the knee. Limbs cold, with chilblains, skin discolored or red. Legs heavy before menses. Joint pains improved by movement, aggravated in the sitting position. Fingers and toes swollen before menses. Swollen, distended varicosities before menses. Varicose veins.

Lungs - Bronchitis. Angina, laryngitis with hoarseness. Morning cough, thorax painful on left side.

Modalities - Better during menses. Better from elimination of secretion. Worse from suppression. Worse before and after menses.

Mouth - Mouth painful, with cracked corners of the lips. Teeth painful, aggravated by cold food, ameliorated by hot food.

Nose - Sinusitis. Coryza in the morning, improved by getting up, by fresh air. Watery flow, improved between 8 a.m. and 9 a.m.

Rectum - Rectum prolapsed after eating. Rectal weakness. Mucus diarrhea, hemorrhoid bleeding between stools, which contain mucus.

Skin - Varicose eczema. Acrocyanosis in young girls. Burns, also for external use in compresses of liquid extract at 15%, diluted 1:50 in water.

Stomach - Acrid dyspepsia.

Temperature - ***Chilliness***.

Throat - Throat discolored, yellow, dry. Tonsils inflamed, swallowing painful. Laryngitis.

Vertigo - Vertigo with headache in the morning, worse when learning forwards.

RELATIONS - ***Compare:*** (1) Puls. - close therapeutic relationship, acting on the same type of patient. (2) Calen. - which is also an excellent healing plant. (3) Rhus-t. - also shows amelioration from movement.

REFERENCES - Julian.

ARISTOLOCHIA MILHOMENS

(Brazilian Snake-Root)

PHARMACY - arist-m. Aristolochia milhomens. Brazilian snake-root. Aristolochia cymbifera. Aristolochia glandifera. N. O. Aristolochiacae. Tincture of the flowers. ***Historical dose:*** Tincture and all potencies.

CLINICAL - Achilles tendon. Diabetes. Extravasations. Heart, pain.

HOMEOPATHIC - In a proving by Mure, prominent among the key symptoms were sharp and pricking pains in various parts. Pain at apex of heart stopping breath. Excoriations of lips and gums. Cramp-like pains in left Achilles tendon.

Stitching pains in various parts. Pain in heels, burning in anus and frequent irritation. The whole leg is covered with ***large irregular patches formed by extravasated blood***. Pain in back and limbs. Stiffness of legs. Itching and swelling around the malleoli.

The mouth is pasty in the morning. Anorexia. Flatulence in stomach and abdomen. Colic followed by diarrhea. Burning at anus. Disturbed rest. Disgusting dreams. Head burning hot. Great thirst and bitter mouth, makes water more frequently than usual.

RELATIONS - ***Compare:*** (1) Aristolochia Serpentaria.

REFERENCES - Clarke.

ARISTOLOCHIA SERPENTARIA

(Virginia Snake-Root)

PHARMACY - arist-s. Aristolochia serpentaria. Virginia snake-root. Serpentary. N. O. Aristolochiacae. Trituration of dried roots. ***Historical dose:*** Tincture and all potencies.

CLINICAL - Colic. Diarrhea. Dyspepsia. Flatulence. Poison oak.

HOMEOPATHIC - Aristolochia serpentaria was proved by Jörg's provers and others. Chief effects were noticed in the gastro-enteric organs, nausea, vomiting, abdominal distention, flatulence and urging to stool. Increased, and afterwards lost, appetite. Symptoms of intestinal tract, diarrhea, meteorism. Flatulent dyspepsia. Distention and cutting pains in abdomen.

Irritation of the urinary and genital organs with frequent desire to urinate. Disturbed rest, also heat of the head (Arist-m.). Brain congestion. Symptoms like those of poison oak.

MIND - Peevish mood. Disinclination for work.

Abdomen - Colic in umbilical region. Distention, rumbling, uneasiness, cutting pains, with emission of flatus, belchings which relieve.

Back - Pressive pain in nape of neck.

Head - Sticking in forehead extending to base of brain. Increased warmth of head.

Kidneys - General irritation of urinary and genital organs. Violent desire to urinate with great increase in quantity of urine. Frequent desire but only a little brownish urine passed.

Mouth - Copious salivation with frequent spitting.

Stomach - Increased appetite, yet able to eat little, since the first morsels satisfy. Loss of appetite. Nausea and vomiting, vomiting did not cease until the stomach was entirely emptied. Distended feeling as if too full. Heaviness better by emission of much flatus.

Stool - Distressing itching about anus. Frequent desire with evacuation of more gas than feces. Frequent desire for stool with evacuation of scanty, hard, tenacious feces with much flatulence.

REFERENCES - Clarke.

ARNICA MONTANA

(Leopard's Bane)

PHARMACY - arn. Arnica montana. Leopard's bane. Brusiewort. Fallkraut. Fall herb. N. O. Composite. Tincture of whole fresh plant. Tincture of root. ***Historical dose:*** All potencies. Arnica should not be used externally where there is broken skin. For torn and lacerated wounds, Calendula can be used locally.

CLINICAL - Abscess. ***Aching, pains.*** Back, pains. Baldness. Bedsores. ***Black eye. Blows. Boils.*** Brain disorders. Breath, fetid. Bronchitis. ***Bruises.*** Carbuncle. Chest, disorders. Chorea. ***Concussions. Contusions.*** Corns. Cramp. Diabetes. Diarrhea. Dysentery. ***Ecchymosis.*** Exhaustion. Eyes. disorders. ***Falls. Fatigue.*** Gout. ***Head, injury.*** Hematemesis, ***Hematoma.*** Hematuria. Headaches. Heart, disorders. Impotence. ***Influenza. Injuries.*** Labor, pains. Lumbago. Mastitis. Meningitis. Mental shock. Miscarriage. ***Over-lifting. Over-working***. Paralysis. Pleurodynia. Purpura. Pyemia. Rheumatism. ***Shock.*** Spleen, pain. ***Sore, pains. Sprains.*** Stings. Strains. ***Strokes.*** Suppuration. ***Swellings.*** Taste, disorders. Thirst. ***Trauma. Traumatic, fever.*** Tumors. Typhoid. Voice disorders. Whooping cough. Wounds. Yawning.

HERBAL - Growing on the mountains, Arnica may be said to possess a native affinity to the effects of falls. As its German name, Fallkraut, attests, its value as a vulnerary has been known from remote times. It may be said to be the traumatic par excellence.

Ussher noted that the local use of Arnica produced an extraordinary growth of hair on a limb. This suggested the use of an oil mixed with Arn. 1x in a case of baldness, which was followed with marked success.

Clarke once ran a piece of wire into the tip of one of his fingers, causing paralyzing pain. He applied Arn., 1x at once and the pain was better instantly seeming to be wiped out from the point of injury up the arm.

HOMEOPATHIC - ***Trauma and its effects, recent or remote*** is met by Arnica as by no other single drug and the provings bring out the appropriateness of the remedy in the symptoms it causes. Tumors in many parts, following injury, have been cured by Arnica including scirrhus tumors of the breast. Nervous disorders as chorea after falls.

Trauma in all its forms, and the recent or remote effects injuries are covered by this remedy. It produces conditions upon the system quite similar to those resulting from ***injuries, falls, blows, contusions.*** Compound fractures. Mental or physical shocks.

After ***traumatic injuries***, overuse of any organ, strains. Tinnitus aurium. It affects blood, causing putrid and septic conditions. ***Putrid phenomena***. Septic conditions, prophylactic of pus infection. Strokes with a red, full face. It is especially suited to cases when any injury, however remote, seems to have caused the present trouble. Trauma of grief, remorse or sudden realization of financial loss.

Arnica is disposed to cerebral congestion. Marked effect on the blood. Acts best in plethoric, feebly in debilitated with impoverished blood, cardiac dropsy with dyspnea. A muscular tonic. Thrombosis. Hematocele. ***Influenza with sore bruised muscles***. Limbs and body ache as if beaten, joints as if sprained. ***Bed feels too hard or full of lumps***.

Great prostration, with a tired feeling. Discharges are ***foul***, breath, taste, flatus, stools etc. Tendency to tissue degeneration, low septic conditions. Abscesses that do not mature. Typhoid, septic fevers. Recurring boils. Thrombosis. ***Sore, lame, bruised feeling.*** Rheumatism of muscles and tendons, especially of back and shoulders. Aversion to tobacco. Vaginitis in females and impotence in males from excessive sexual indulgence.

MIND - Arnica is used after severe mental stress or shock. ***Mental or emotional shocks.*** Never well since a trauma, fright or grief. History of severe physical trauma with chronic mental or emotional effects. ***Accident, trauma victims.*** Nervous, can't bear pain, whole body oversensitive.

Fear of being touched or injured. Feels like a wounded animal. ***Fear of the approach of anyone.*** Fear of sickness. Fear of instant death with heart distress. Fear at night. Fear on awakening. Agoraphobia. Fear of open spaces. Fear of crowds, public places.

Violent attacks of anguish, anxiety with angina pectoris (Acon.). Easily frightened, unexpected trifles cause him to start. Hypochondriacal anxiety. Fear remains at night after fright (Op.). A sudden fear that rouses one from sleep at night especially after an accident (Op.).

Head injury or strokes that effect mental functions. Morose, repentant mood. Overworked and exhausted. Indifference to work. ***Depression from injuries to the head (Nat-s.).*** Forgetful, what he reads quickly escapes his mind. Absent-minded. Forgets the word he is about to say. Unconscious. When spoken to answers correctly, but relapses. Coma. Muttering delirium. Delirium tremens.

Morose, delirious. Nervous and mental shock. Sits as if in thought. ***Says there is nothing the matter with him.*** Feels well in serious cases, because of shock. ***Sends the doctor home.*** Wants to be left alone. Prays quietly for her soul. Stupor, with involuntary discharge of feces, typhoid. Stupefaction, loss of sight and hearing, from concussion of brain.

Abdomen - Colic, with retention of urine. Colic, resembling dysentery. Cramps from epigastrium down over the bowels, then foul stools. Tympanitic distension. Distended with offensive flatus. Flatus smelling of rotten eggs. Bruised pain, in sides of abdomen. Sharp pains from side to side. Sharp thrusts through abdomen. Sharp pain in region of spleen, taking away breath. Swashing in abdomen as from water.

Back - ***Backache from muscle strain, overuse.*** Great soreness and pain in back, as if bruised or beaten. ***Back sore and aches, worse overlifting***. Agonizing pain in back and hips before urination. ***Bruises on back from injuries, blows.*** Violent pain, in spine, as after sudden rising up after long stooping. Cervical vertebrae tender. Muscles of neck weak, head falls backwards or any side. Sacrum as if beaten.

Bladder - Retention of urine in bladder from over exertion after labor. Urine retained, with aching and pressing in bladder. ***Bladder affections after mechanical injuries.*** Bladder tenesmus with very painful urination. Tenesmus of bladder with diarrhea. Bladder feels full and sore, the pressure of urine hurts him. Cutting pain in orifice of urethra at end of urination. Infants scream from pain in bladder. Constant dribbling of urine after labor.

Breasts - Sore nipples. Mastitis from injury. Tumors of breast from injury (Bell-p., Con.). Violent after-pains, worse nursing.

Causations - Mechanical injuries. Fright, financial loss, anger. Overuse of any organ. Surgical operations. Insect stings. Splinters.

Chest - Burning or rawness in chest. Sharp pains under false ribs. ***Bruised, aching sensation in chest on walking.*** Sensation as if all ribs were bruised, when coughing. Bones and cartilages of chest are painful, worse motion, breathing or coughing. Heavy sensation lower chest. Sharp pains in chest, taking the breath away, better pressure. Pain in intercostal muscles. Pleurodynia (Ran-b., Bry., Cimic.).

Constitutions - Adapted to sanguine, plethoric persons, disposed to cerebral congestion. Persons easily made train-sick or seasick. It is suited to persons who are sensitive to mechanical injuries and who feel the effects of them long after. Teste noted it for plethoric red-faced persons.

Cough - Cough produced by weeping and lamenting. Dry cough from tickling low down in trachea. Cough causes bloodshot eyes or nosebleed. ***Violent, spasmodic cough with facial herpes***. Cardiac cough, paroxysmal, at night during sleep, worse exercise. ***Whooping cough, child cries before coughing.*** Cough after measles. Cough in sleep without waking.

Ears - Shooting in and around ears. Blood from ears. Suppurating otitis with stupor. Cartilages of ears as if bruised. Bruised pain in external ears. Sensitive to shrill noise. Sensitivity to loud sounds. ***Hearing impaired from injury to the head.*** Dull hearing, after concussion. Hardness of hearing. Deafness after typhus. Noises in ear caused by rush of blood to the head. Humming.

Eyes - Bloodshot. Eyes sunken. ***Black eye from injury.*** Traumatic ulceration with much hemorrhage into anterior chamber. Expedites absorption of clots, in retinal hemorrhage. Bruised iris after cataract operations. Bruised, sore feeling in eyes after close work. ***Eyes feel tired and weary after sightseeing, moving pictures.*** Lachrymation burning. Photophobia. Right eye protrudes, looks larger than left. Must keep eyes open, dizzy on closing them. Photophobia. Pupils contracted, dilated.

Face - Face hot and red, with cold legs. ***Sunken***, very red, pale. Acne sore and painful. Bruised pains. Chilliness during headache. Herpes in face. Ruddy, congested, bluish red in strokes, fevers. Lower jaw hangs down, paralysis. Redness and burning of one cheek. Cheeks puffed, red. Swelling of parotid gland during measles. Throbbing and stinging pain, in swollen cheeks.

Female - Menses, early, hot, profuse. Uterine hemorrhage from mechanical injury after sex. Hemorrhages bright red or mixed with clots. Bloody discharge between menses. Ulcers of uterus with a tendency to bleed. Labia painfully swollen. Prolapsus caused by concussion. Ovarian region feels as if sprained, obliging her to walk bent. Threatened miscarriage from falls etc. Soreness of the whole body during pregnancy. Feeling as if fetus were lying crosswise. ***Cannot bear fetal movements***, cause nausea and vomiting. ***Labor pains, weak or ceasing.*** Bruised parts after labor. Soreness and lameness of parts after delivery. Puerperal fever. Violent after-pains, worse breast-feeding.

Food - Loss of appetite. Loathing very sight of food. Canine hunger. Loss of appetite and sourness of stomach of brandy drinkers, creates a disgust for brandy. Aversion to milk and meat. Aversion to broth, smoking tobacco. Longing for vinegar. Desires sour, alcoholic drinks. Constant desire to drink, but knows not what for, as all drinks are offensive. Thirst with dry mouth.

Head - ***Hematoma. Head injury.*** Headaches from injury to head. Meningitis from injury to head. Periodical attacks of migraine. ***Hot head with a cold body***. Brain feels tired. Burning in brain. Confused, sensitivity of brain with sharp, pinching pains. ***Stroke victims***, with loss of consciousness, involuntary evacuations from bowels and bladder, paralysis. Head as if too large. Headache as from a nail. Headaches from strong emotions. Cold spot on the forehead. Burning or hot spots on vertex. Head throws backwards while walking. Baldness. Recurring boils on scalp. Scalp feels contracted.

Heart - Sudden pain as if heart is squeezed or had got a shock. ***Strain of heart from violent running.*** Weakened heart muscles. Palpitations after any exertion. ***Palpitations after any shock or injury.*** Palpitations shake the whole body. ***Angina pectoris***, with severe pain in elbow of left arm. Sharp pain in heart. Heart pains, left to right. Horror of constant death with cardiac distress at night. Cardiac dropsy with distressing dyspnea. Fatty heart and hypertrophy. Pulse feeble and irregular. Weak fluttering of pulse. Pulse hurried. Pulse quicker than beat of heart.

Kidneys - Cutting pain in kidneys. Piercing pain, as from knives plunged into kidneys, with chilliness and inclination to vomit. Involuntary dribbling with constant urging. Has to wait a long time for urine to pass. Urine has dark brick-red sediment. Bloody urine from mechanical causes. Urine in small quantity, staining napkin yellow-brown. Red urine in liver complaint. Scanty, red urine, very offensive. Brown clear urine which immediately becomes whitish and turbid.

Limbs - Sore and bruised limbs. ***Soreness after overexertion.*** Sprained and dislocated feeling. Lame feeling. ***Great fear of being touched or approached.*** Pain in back and limbs, as if bruised or beaten. ***Limbs ache as if beaten.*** Everything on which he lies seems too hard. ***Bed feels too hard.*** Heaviness in all limbs. Deathly coldness of forearm. ***Joint, muscle pain from injury.*** Cannot walk erect, on account of bruised pain in pelvic region. ***Sore, aching muscles with influenza.*** Gout. Rheumatism begins low down and works up (Led.). Rheumatism, from exposure to dampness, cold. Rheumatism from excessive muscular strain. Cramps in the fingers, writer's cramp. Pain in arms better hanging down. Want of strength in the hands on grasping. Veins of hands distended. Knee joints suddenly bend when standing. Feet numb.

Liver - Sharp pain in region of liver; painful when turning in bed. Pressure in region of liver. Pain from liver through left chest and down left arm.

Lungs - Asthma with inclination to move about. Asthma with sleeplessness before midnight. Asphyxia neonatorum. Dyspnea with hemoptysis. Short, panting breathing. Children lose their breath when angry. Raw, sore feeling in morning. Pneumonia, approaching paralysis. Can't expectorate, but must swallow whatever is loosened by coughing. Bloody expectoration. ***Hemorrhage after mechanical injuries***. Offensive, green, purulent, blood-streaked expectoration. Spitting up of black, thick, viscid blood, or bright red, frothy blood, mixed with mucus and coagula. Pneumothorax from external injuries. ***Pleurisy after mechanical injuries.*** Pleurodynia (Bry., Ran-b., Cimic.).

Male - Genitals bruised and much swollen. Swelling of penis and scrotum, bluish-red. Hot swelling of scrotum after injury. Spermatic cords painfully swollen. Relaxed testicles. Hematocele. Phimosis from friction. Hydrocele caused by a bruise. Violent continued erections often waking. Seminal emission during caress. Impotence from sexual excess or abuse. Erysipelas of scrotum.

Modalities - ***Better from lying down.*** Better lying outstretched. ***Better with head low.*** Better motion. Better clear, cold, stimulating weather. Worse evening and night. ***Worse from injuries. Worse from falls, blows, bruises, shock.*** Worse jarring, noise. Worse after labor, over-exertion, sprains. Worse least touch. Worse motion. Worse rest. Worse alcohol, wine. Worse damp cold. Worse after sleep. Worse coal gas. Worse lying on left side.

Mouth - Soreness of gums after teeth extraction (Sep.). Dry and thirsty. Bitter taste (Coloc.). ***Taste as from bad eggs. Fetid breath***. Taste disgusting, putrid, slimy. Bad taste after operation. Empyema of maxillary sinus. Bright red, puffy fauces. Saliva diminished. Swallowing is prevented by sort of nausea as if food would not go down. Heat in lips. Lips burn, swollen and cracked. Lower lip trembles, while eating.

Nose - Bruised, from above downward. Swelling of nose. Nosebleeds after injury. Nosebleeds after every fit of coughing after washing face, dark fluid blood. ***Nose feels sore, cold***. Violent sneezing from overlifting. Nose feels sore, cold. Post-nasal drip. Catarrh of antrum. Burning pain in typhoid fever. Nosebleeds during typhoid fever. Ulcerated nostrils. Empyema of maxillary sinus.

Perspiration - Sour sweat at night. Sour or offensive sweat, sometimes cold. Several transitory sweats all over at night, with anguish. Worse when sweating. Sweat partial on front of body. Sweat followed by faintness.

Rectum - Flatus smelling of rotten eggs. Sensation of rumbling in rectum, without stools. Obstinate constipation after a blow on epigastrium. ***Straining of tenesmus in diarrhea.*** Dysentery with dysuria, in summer and autumn. Diarrhea at night, with cutting in intestines. Diarrhea of tuberculosis, worse lying on left side. Prolapsed anus, worse after walking for few minutes only better washing the whole body. Cramps in rectum, while standing. Anus as if bruised. Burning along perineum during urination.

Skin - Ecchymosis. ***Bruises from injury.*** Every little injury makes bruises. ***Black and blue spots***. Eruptions after trauma. Red, hot, edematous. Hot, hard, shining swelling, from insect stings. Dusky, mottled. Acne indurata, characterized by ***symmetry in distribution***. Very sore acne. Itching, burning, eruption of small pimples. After scratching, itching begins somewhere else. Tingling and itching which moves from place to place. ***Crops of small boils*** (Ichthy., Sil.). Carbuncles. Bedsores. Petechiae. Erysipelas. Scarlet fever when the eruption doesn't come out. Erythema nodosum. Corns. Varicose ulcers.

Sleep - Unrefreshing sleep. Involuntary stools during sleep. ***Sleepless and restless when overtired.*** Can't fall asleep, fantastical illusions while lying awake. Frequent yawning in evening, without sleepiness. Yawning before chill. Comatose drowsiness, awakens with hot head, drops to sleep as he answers. ***Nightmares.*** Horrors in the night. When dreaming sees black forms of spectres, ghosts, spirits. Dreams of death. Dreams of being buried alive, suffocation. Dreams of mutilated bodies. Anxious and terrible dreams, awakes in terror, then sleepless. Awful dreams, of robbers and murderers.

Stomach - Belchings, tasting of bad eggs after coughing. Eructations of bitter mucus. Oppressive gases pass upward and downward. Stomach distended with wind. Pain in stomach during eating. Pinching, spasmodic griping pain in stomach. Pressure as from a stone. ***Feeling as if stomach were pressing against spine***. As if a lump in stomach. Hiccough. Motion sickness. Nausea with burning and scratching in throat. Retching at night. Fetid vomiting. Vomiting of dark, red coagulated blood. ***Vomiting of blood after injuries.*** Vomiting of food, mixed with blood.

Stools - Dysenteric stools with muscular pains. Brown or white diarrhea. ***Offensive, brown, bloody, putrid involuntary stools.*** Stools look like brown yeast. Must lie down after every stool. Stools are bloody, foamy, purulent, acrid involuntary during sleep. Ribbon-like stools, from enlarged prostrate or retroverted uterus. Stools consisting of bloody, slimy mucus, with urging and violent bellyache. Undigested stools.

Teeth - Swollen jaw after dental work. ***Pains after dental work, injuries.*** Soreness of gums after teeth extraction (Sep.). Gums sore, swollen during dentition. ***Sore and aching after trauma.*** Beating and tingling in gums, during toothache. Throbbing, toothache. Excruciating, cutting, tearing, in teeth.

Temperature - Chilly with heat and redness of one cheek. Coldness of part lain on. Thirst during chill. Must uncover but it chills him. ***Shivering over whole body.*** Shivering, as if dashed with cold water. Internal chills with external heat. Heat and redness of head with coolness of rest of body. Internal heat, feet and hands cold. Head or face alone hot, body cold. Heat flushes, with thirst. ***Influenza fever.*** Intermittent fever. Typhoid fever. Septic and traumatic fevers.

Throat - Acute tonsillitis, swelling of soft palate and uvula. Bright red, puffy fauces. Burning, when swallowing. Stinging in back of throat. Raw, sore feeling. Crackling in trachea, when lying down. ***Hoarseness from overuse of voice.*** Hoarseness, worse exertion, colds or getting wet. Hoarseness early in morning. Voice deep or low, muttering.

Tongue - Tongue dry, almost black. Biting, burning and scraping at root of tongue. Tongue, dry, almost black. Red stripe down centre of tongue. Tongue coated white. Tongue coated yellow. Tongue dry with brown streak down middle.

Vertigo - Chronic vertigo, objects whirl about especially when walking. Vertigo of the elderly. Vertigo with nausea, vomiting and diarrhea. Vertigo worse walking, sitting erect, closing eyes. Vertigo worse head injury. Vertigo during headache. Vertigo on rising and on moving.

Vision - Diplopia from trauma, muscular paralysis, retinal hemorrhage. Diplopia with vertigo, on looking downward. High objects appear to lean forward and ab to fall. Flickering, worse reading or writing, with headache. ***Lost vision, after a violent blow.*** On reading, print seems to dance in a fog and vanish, must rub eyes. Muscae volitantes. Obscured, lost vision, during headache.

COMMENTS - Arnica is allied to wounds and cures hemorrhages of many kinds including strokes, dilatation and rupture of small blood vessels. Vomiting, coughing, purging, accompanied by streaks of blood in vomit. Extravasation of blood into the conjunctiva as in whooping cough. Hemorrhages into the tissues of internal organs or the skin.

An odd symptom of Arnica is "coldness of the nose." A case of facial (left) neuralgia, face swollen, dark red, very painful to touch, was cured with Arnica (radix), the guiding symptom being "cold nose." Patient had bitter taste, was very excitable and worse at night.

Effects of violent cough or sneezing, the child cries before cough comes on (or with the cough) in whooping cough. Chronic bronchitis when patients have bruised, weak aching in the chest or great sensitiveness of the chest on exertion or walking.

Arn. affects the left upper extremity and the right chest. Putrid excretions (Bapt.), putrid breath, fetid sweat. Incessant passing of stool and urine in putrid states.

Nash gave "Stupor with involuntary discharge of feces and urine." "Fears being touched or struck by those coming near him." "Putrid smell from mouth." "Bruised, sore feeling in uterine region, cannot walk erect." "While answering falls into a deep stupor before finishing." "Head alone or face alone, hot, rest of body cool."

"Many small boils, painful, one after another, extremely sore." "Suddenness" is a feature of Arn. pains and action. P. P. Wells related a cure of double pleuro-pneumonia in a child with sudden stabbing pains on both sides of the chest almost preventing breathing. Arnica instantly caused a violent aggravation, the next instant relief was perfect and the child fell asleep breathing naturally.

Keynote sore, bruised feeling. Bluish discoloration, bruising, better cold applications. The bed feels too hard. Fatigue, "fear of being approached," an animal-like fear of guarding a wounded area. Can believe nothing is wrong when severely injured, sign of shock (Op.). Patient may be irritable and want to be left alone. Can have amnesia, or nightmares after injury or loss of confidence since injury. Intermittent fear of death.

A major gout remedy, afraid of joints being touched. Good for flus and mono when there is a sore, achy feeling all over. Also acute muscle fatigue in athletes. Superficial tissue trauma. Boils that feel sore and bruised.

Comas from trauma and injury. Any fever with a sore, bruised feeling. For chronic weak joints after repeated injuries. Shock due to trauma or shock from the injury itself. For grief and financial shock.

Good for overexertion. It's also used for trauma from blows from blunt instruments, sprains. For post-stroke victims, for injuries and hematomas. For heart attacks from overexertion. For internal bleeding. Achiness and weakness from the weight of the baby in pregnant women. For people who have a tendency to bruise easily.

Vertigo, worse head injuries and strokes. Also for severe illness when the patient goes into the stupor stage. Good after dental work. For vomiting of blood after injury to the abdominal region or injury to the uterus.

Sensitive to cold damp weather, and hot sun. Worse from touch. Alcohol will aggravate the condition, but may crave alcohol to relieve pain. Also worse tobacco. Sensation worse after an adjustment to spine (Ruta., Rhus-t.).

RELATIONS - ***Antidotes:*** Camph. Vitex trifolia. ***Compare:*** (1) Acon., Bapt., Bell-p., Ham., Led., Rhus-t., Hyper., Symph., (2) Abrot., Absin., Calen., Cham., Cina, Gnaph. (3) other Composites. (4) Am-c., Crot-t. - swashing in abdomen. (5) Ars., Bapt. - typhoid states, Bapt. "feels ill," Arn. "feels well." Bry., Rhod., Ruta., Sul-ac. ***Complementary:*** Acon., Ip. ***Follows well:*** Acon., Ip., Verat., Apis. ***Followed well by:*** Acon., Ars., Bry., Ip., Rhus-t. ***Antidote to:*** Am-c., Chin., Cic., Ferr., Ign., Ip., Seneg. ***Antidoted by:*** Camph., Ip. (to massive doses),

Coffee (headache), Acon., Ars., Chin., Ign., Ip. (to potencies).

REFERENCES - Boericke. Clarke.

ARSENICUM ALBUM

(White Oxide of Arsenic)

PHARMACY - ars. Arsenicum album. White oxide of arsenic. Arsenic trioxide. Solution and trituration. ***Historical dose:*** Trituration and all potencies.

CLINICAL - Abscess. Acne rosacea. ***Albuminuria. Alcoholism. Allergies.*** Amenorrhea. ***Anemia.*** Angina pectoris. Anorexia. Antrax. ***Anxiety.*** Aphonia. Aphthae. Ascites. ***Asthma.*** Atrophy. Bronchitis. ***Burning, pains.*** ***Cachexia. Cancer.*** Cancrum, oris. Carbuncle. Cecum, disorders. Chills. Cholera asiatica. Colds. ***Colitis. Coryza.*** Coughs. Croup. Cyanosis. Dandruff. Delirium tremens. ***Despair.*** Diabetes. ***Diarrhea.*** Diphtheria. Dropsy. ***Dysentery.*** Dyspepsia. Ears disorders. Eczema. ***Emaciation.*** Endometritis. Enteric fever. ***Epithelioma.*** Erysipelas. Eye, disorders. Face, eruptions. Fainting. Fatigue. ***Fears. Fevers. Food, poisoning.*** Gangrene. Gastric, ulcers. ***Gastritis. Gastroenteritis.*** Glandular, swellings. Gout. Hay asthma. ***Hay fever.*** Headaches. Heart, disorders. ***Hepatitis.*** Herpes zoster. Hodgkin's disease. Hydrothorax. Ichthyosis. ***Influenza. Intermittent fever.*** Jaundice. Kala-azar. Kidney, diseases. Leucorrhea. ***Leukemia.*** Lichen. Lips, epithelioma. Locomotor ataxia. Lung disorders. Lupus. ***Malaria.*** Malignant, pustules. Measles. Menstruation, disorders. Miliary, eruptions. Myelitis. ***Nausea.*** Nettle rash. ***Nephritis. Nervousness.*** Neuralgias. Numbness. Paralysis. Peritonitis. Pityriasis. Plethora. Pleurisy. Pleurodynia. ***Pneumonia.*** Prostration. Psoriasis. Purpura. Remittent, fever. ***Restlessness.*** Rheumatism. Rickets. Ringworm. Scarlatina. Sciatica. Scrofulous, disorders. Sea-bathing. Seasickness. ***Septic, fever.*** Sneezing. Stomach, disorders. Strains. Suppuration. Throat, sore. ***Tobacco habit.*** Tongue, disorders. Traumatic, fever. Typhlitis. Typhus. Ulcers. Uremia. ***Vomiting. Weakness.*** Whooping cough. Worms Wounds. Yellow fever.

HOMEOPATHIC - Grimmer stated that Ars. helped ***cancer, epithelioma***, lupus, pernicious anemia have yielded to the power of this potent medicine. Typhus and pernicious types of malaria present a fair picture of the range and character of the sickness this remedy has cured.

Arsenicum album is a very deep acting remedy, affecting every organ and tissue. Ars. acts on the nerves producing inveterate neuralgias and multiple neuritis better heat. All-prevailing ***anxiety, exhaustion and restlessness*** with nightly aggravation, are most important. Great exhaustion after the slightest exertion.

Burning pains. Burning relieved by heat. Seaside complaints (Nat-m., Aq-mar.). Pains are maddening, ***burning like fire,*** hot needles or wires, better warmth. Acute and chronic burns. Sudden intense effects. ***Sudden great weakness*** from trivial causes. ***Very restless,*** restless even in affected part, even stupor is interrupted by fits of restlessness with anxious moaning.

Fear, fright and worry. ***Dying patients,*** Ars. gives quiet and ease to the last moments of life when given in high potency. ***Cancer pains.*** The prostration seems to be out of proportion to the rest of his illness. Anemia and chlorosis. Low vitality. ***Putrid cadaveric odors. Emaciation.*** Gradual loss of weight.

Asthma, worse after getting colds in midsummer. Asthma, worse around midnight. Unable to lie down, ***fears suffocation.*** Anxious, must sit up, worse from odors, laughing, ascending, turning in bed or receding eruptions, better coffee or sweet water. ***Hay fever.*** Air-passages constricted from allergies. ***Shortness of breath.*** Suffocative catarrh. Whistling, wheezing breathing.

Ars. should be thought of in ailments from alcoholism, Ptomaine poisoning, stings, dissecting wounds, chewing tobacco. ***Food poisoning.*** Ill effects from decayed food or animal matter, odor of discharges is putrid in complaints that return annually Injurious effects of fruits, especially more watery ones.

Discharges of mucus membranes are ***acrid, thin and scanty, coryza,*** saliva sweat etc. Weakness and emaciation is rapid. Degenerative changes. Gradual loss of weight from impaired nutrition. Reduces the refractive index of blood serum (also Chin. and Ferr-p.). ***Malarial cachexia.*** Septic infections and low vitality. Green discharges. Unquenchable thirst. Infantile Kala-azar.

Infections. ***Alcoholism.*** Frequent fainting. Destructive process, carbuncles, gangrene, cancer, malignancy. ***Dropsy, pale, baggy, swellings.*** Restlessness, then becomes drowsy. Eruptions undeveloped or suppressed.

MIND - Clinging, anxious and desperate. Begs for help. ***Extremely nervous and anxious.*** Deep insecurities and fears. Desires company, fears to be left alone. ***Restlessness, changes place continually***. Inclined to complain and whine to those about her. Indecisive. Weeps and whines, but speaks little.

Full of worries about trifles. Anxiety about the future. ***Anxiety about health.*** Anxiety about others. ***Anguish and restlessness.*** Anxiety on waking from frightful dreams. Anxiety during headache. Anxiety, better motion. Anxiety about trifles.

Fear of death, yet tired of living, worse night. Fear of starvation. Fear of financial loss, poverty. ***Fear of diseases.*** Fear of getting cancer. Fear of catching an infection. Fear of germs, viruses. Fear of being poisoned. Fear of being left alone (Phos., Puls.). Fear of violence. Great fear with cold sweats. Fears something may have happened to relatives.

Children are capricious, want to be carried, want to go from father to mother to nurse (Cham.). Lacks courage. Frighten easily. Desires to be carried fast. Desires company, fears to be left alone. Clings to parents.

Obsessive compulsive disorder. ***Fastidious, upset about disorder, dirt, germs.*** Obsessed with order and tidiness. Sensitive to disorder and confusion. Suspicious. Miserly. Selfish and her desires exceeds her needs. Inclined to malice and satire.

Clinging to a doctor, needing reassurance. Exaggerating symptoms to assure attention. ***Domineering and demanding.***

Angry with himself and others. Fault-finding and reproaches others. Irritability alternating with despondency. Irritability and restlessness during headache.

Melancholy. Despair of recovery. ***Despair drives him from place to place.*** Thinks it useless to take medicine. Consolation aggravates. Moaning and groaning, walks about wringing hands. Groans, moans and weeps during menses.

Insanity. Delirium tremens, cursing and raving, vicious. ***Mania, wants to be held.*** Fixed ideas. Tormenting thoughts. Suicidal impulses, mania, determined to commit suicide, he suffers so. Fear of being left alone, lest he do himself bodily harm (Nat-s.). Has no rest anywhere, rolls about on floor and despairs for his life.

Hallucinations of smell and sight. Delusions, body will putrefy. Sees ghosts day and night. Sees vermin, throws away bugs by handfuls. Carphologia. Imagines house full of thieves, jumps and hides. Fears he has murdered somebody. Self-torture, pulls her hair, bites her nails, tears at own body.

Abdomen - Peritonitis. Ascites and anasarca. ***Gastroenteritis.*** Coldness and chilliness in abdomen. Abdomen swollen and painful. Rumbling in bowels. Periodical colic. ***Burning pains.*** Crampy pains in bowels. Cutting pains. ***Violent pains in abdomen with anguish.*** Violent squeezing and constricting, in umbilical region. Intussusception with pain in abdomen. ***Liver and spleen enlarged and painful.*** Spleen is enlarged in malarial fever, kala-azar. Pain as from a wound in abdomen on coughing. Gnawing, burning pains like coals of fire, relieved by heat. Epigastrium sore, tender. Ulcer above navel. Peritonitis. Swelling of inguinal glands.

Back - ***Burning pains in back*** (Ox-ac.). Weakness in lumbar region. Bruised pain in small of back. Cold, chill creeps up back. As if warm air streaming up spine to the head. Drawing in of shoulders. Stiffness of the back ascends from coccyx to nape. Neck stiff, as if bruised or sprained. Sacrum as if broken. Small of back as if broken, with hemorrhoids.

Back - Cervical glands enlarged, felt like a series of hard nodules under skin. Ulceration of sacrum after typhoid.

Bladder - ***Acute cystitis, with violent burning pains.*** Dysuria. Burning in urethra during urination. Burning at commencement of urinating. Bladder as if paralyzed. Atony of bladder in old persons. ***Retention of urine.*** Retention of urine after confinement. Great desire, but passes no urine. Bedwetting, nocturnal.

Blood - Leukemia, especially in children. Blood is disorganized causing pernicious type of anemia and severe septic conditions. Hemorrhages, of black offensive blood.

Breasts - Burning in breasts, better motion. Mastitis.

Causations - Ill effects of food poisoning, eating ices, poor diet, watery fruits tobacco, quinine, sea bathing and traveling, mountain climbing. Care, grief, fright, ptomaine poisoning, financial loss, poverty. dissecting wounds.

Chest - Angina Pectoris. Chest as if raw or excoriated. Chest as if too narrow. Tightness of chest, as if bound with a hoop. ***Tightness of chest, with great anxiety and restlessness.*** Burning or coldness in chest. ***Darting pain through upper third of right lung.*** Sharp pain in chest when coughing. Sharp pain, in sternum. Oppression, worse stormy weather. Yellowish spots on chest.

Constitutions - It is suited to the full plethoric habit. Psoric constitutions. Nervous constitutions.

Coughs - Coughs dependent upon asthma, cyanosis, heart diseases. Cough worse after midnight, worse lying on back. ***Cough with great exhaustion, collapse, anemia, nervous irritability.*** Dry cough alternating with loose. Cough dry at night, better sitting up, worse drinking. Cough dry, as from sulphur fumes. ***Cough after drinking***. Cough excited by smoking. ***Coughing spells preceded by great anxiety and restlessness.*** Cough with bloody sputum. Deep, dry, unceasing cough. Hemoptysis with pain between shoulders, burning heat all over.

Ears - Rash and heat about ears. Skin within, raw and burning. Roaring in ears during a paroxysm of pain. Ringing. Buzzing and singing, during attacks of intermittent and during apyrexia. ***Thin, excoriating, offensive otorrhea.*** Discharges of cadaverous odour, profuse, ichorous. Yellow discharge from right ear, with dryness of nose; hearing not weakened. Difficult hearing, for the human voice only. Unusual sensitiveness to sound. Impaired hearing, with humming in ears. Sensation as if ears were stopped up.

Eyes - Sunken or protruding. ***Burning in eyes with hot, acrid lachrymation***. Edema around eyes. ***Corrosive tears, making cheeks and eyelids sore.*** Agglutination of lids. Eyelids red, ulcerated, scabby, scaly, granulated. Spasms of the eyelids. Stinging pain, when trying to open lids. Corneal ulceration. ***Intense photophobia,*** better external warmth. Sensitive to sunlight. Ciliary neuralgia with fine burning pain. Left-sided infraorbital pain. Blue spots in white of eye. Bluish circle around cornea. Scrofulous ophthalmia. Conjunctiva is injected, yellow. Conjunctiva looks like a piece of raw beef. Falling of eyelashes. Scrofulous ophthalmia. Ophthalmia of children. Pterygium, with dryness of lids. Pupils contracted or dilated.

Face - Expression of agony. Edematous swelling of face. Swollen, pale, yellow, ***cachetic***, sunken (Acet-ac.). Haggard or distorted, hippocratic. Old look in children. Face is covered with cold sweat. ***Tearing, needle-like pains, burning.*** Angry, circumscribed flush of cheeks. ***Burning, stinging pains as from red-hot needles.*** Twitching of facial muscles. Black dots, acne. Pimples and vesicles, with acrid discharge. Pimples and vesicles itching, burning, worse at night, in cold air, better warmth. Swelling of glands of lower jaw, with bruised pain. Cancerous ulcers on face.

Female - Amenorrhea. Scanty pale menses. Menses too profuse and too soon. Dysmenorrhea, better heat. Menses suppressed in weak, tired careworn women. Sharp pain in rectum during menses. ***Menorrhagi***

with black blood. Dark hemorrhages between menses. Thin, whitish, offensive discharge instead of menses. Profuse acrid, yellowish, thick leucorrhea, worse standing, passing flatus. ***Leucorrhea, acrid, burning offensive, thin.*** Pain as from red-hot wires, worse least exertion, causes great fatigue, better in warm room. Burning, throbbing, lancinating in uterine region. Ovaritis. ***Burning in ovarian region.*** Sharp pain in right ovary. Pressive, sharp pain in ovary into the thigh, which feels numb and lame worse motion or bending. Dryness of vagina. Itching of genitals. Promotes expulsion of moles. Increased sexual desire at menses. Cancer of uterus. Polyps on cervix.

Food - Loss of appetite with thirst with nausea. ***Food poisoning with diarrhea.*** Cannot bear the sight, smell or thought of food. Aversion to sweets, butter, fats, meat. Aversion to farinaceous food, beans and peas, gruel. Desire for something refreshing, strengthening, stimulating. Desires acids, sour things, brandy, coffee. Desires milk or warm drinks, tea. Craves fat, even lard or olive oil. Craves lemon, pungent things, acid fruits. Craves rye bread, alcohol, wine, brandy, warm food. ***Worse from of bad meat, bad water, and watery fruits***. Dyspepsia from vinegar, acids, ice cream, ice water, tobacco. Worse from vegetables, melons, fruits. Worse after ice cream, sour beer, alcoholic drinks, cheese, fruits. Worse after salt fish, salt meat. Hives worse shell fish. ***Colic after spoiled sausages.*** Colic after rotten cheese, or moldy cheese. Worse quinine, chewing tobacco. Irritable heart in smokers and tobacco-chewers. ***Intense, thirst.*** Unquenchable thirst. ***Desires warm drinks. Drinks little and often, craves ice-cold water or warm tea.*** Thirst for warm drinks during fever.

Head - Headaches relieved by cold, other symptoms worse. ***Periodical headaches, with burning pains with restlessness***. Hemicrania with icy feeling of scalp and great weakness. Pain over left eye. Throbbing, stupefying, burning pains. Pulsating in forehead, with nausea. Aching in occiput. ***Pain alternates between head or stomach.*** Headache, alternating with colic or liver complaint. Headache with vomiting of bile. Sensitive head in open air. Restless head, it is in constant motion. Walks with head thrown backwards. ***Scalp itches*** intolerably. Circular patches of bare spots, rough, dirty and covered with dry scales, nightly burning and itching. Dandruff. Scalp very sensitive cannot brush hair. Hair becomes gray early. Falling out of hair. Scabs on hairy scalp. Chronic eruptions filled with pus. Tinea.

Heart - ***Angina pectoris,*** sudden tightness above heart. Heart pains into neck and occiput with anxiety, difficult breathing, fainting spells. Cramp in heart. Hydropericardium. ***Palpitations with anguish, worse lying on back.*** Palpitations ascending stairs. Palpitations, pain, dyspnea, faintness. Palpitations with tremulous weakness after stools. ***Palpitations, worse night.*** Beats audible. Visible pulsations. Weak heart, trembles. ***Irritable heart in smokers and tobacco chewers.*** Dilatation. Cyanosis. Fatty degeneration. Right ventricle hypertrophied. Pericarditis after suppressed measles or scarlatina. Valvular disease with intermittent pulse. ***Pulse more rapid in morning*** (Sulph.). Pulse, accelerated, quick and small. Pulse, quick and weak. Pulse, threadlike, small. Pulse, very frequent and irregular, sometimes imperceptible.

Kidneys - ***Albuminuria.*** Nephritis. Bright's disease. Diabetes. Uremia, with vomiting, colic, spells of suffocation. Feeling of weakness in abdomen after urination. Urine black as if mixed with dung. Urine is scanty, burning involuntary. Epithelial cells, cylindrical clots of fibrin and globules of pus and blood. Urine, dark brown. Urine, dark yellow, turbid. Sediment of red sand. Urine, mixed with pus and blood. Urine like thick beer, rotten smell. Glycosuria. Hematuria. Abscesses in kidneys.

Limbs - Weariness of limbs. ***Excessive weakness and exhaustion of limbs obliging him to lie down.*** Trembling of hands of limbs.

Limbs - Twitching, spasms, weakness, heaviness, uneasiness. Limbs heavy. Paraplegia with atrophy. Paralysis with contraction of limbs. Sciatica better walking and hot applications. ***Burning pains.*** Paralysis of lower limbs with atrophy. Drawing pain from elbow to axilla. Tingling in fingers. Fingers cannot be extended. Nails blue, discolored. ***Restless feet.*** Uneasiness in lower limbs, must move feet constantly or walk about. Feet weak, weary and numb, edematous. Wooden feeling in soles. Sore pain in ball of toes, while walking. Toes bend downwards. Cramps in calves. Swelling of feet. Peripheral neuritis. Diabetic gangrene. Ulcers on heel (All-c., Lam.). Ulcers on finger tips with burning pain. Ulcers on soles and toes.

Liver - ***Hepatitis from bad food or poisoning*** (Phos., Nux-v.). Compression pain in the region of the liver. Burning pain in liver, better from warm drinks. ***Liver and spleen enlarged and painful.*** Induration of liver.

Lungs - Air-passages constricted. Allergies. ***Hay fever.*** Asthma when fatigued. ***Asthma from suppressed eruptions.*** Asthma, worse taking cold in mid-summer. Asthma with pale, cold face. ***Asthma about 2 a.m.*** Whistling, wheezing breathing. Wheezing with cough and frothy sputum. ***Asthma, worse around midnight.*** Hysterical asthma from every little excitement. Suffocative catarrh. Unable to lie down, fears suffocation. ***Suffocative attacks during sleep, must sit up.*** Dyspnea, worse from odors, laughing, ascending. ***Shortness of breath.*** Dyspnea, turning in bed or receding eruptions. Dyspnea, better coffee or sweet water. Pleurisy with tendency to syncope. ***Pneumonia from taking cold.*** Pneumonia during a fatiguing journey. Hydrothorax. Pulmonary edema. Emphysema. Gangrene of lungs, with green ichorous sputum. ***Expectoration scanty, frothy.*** Expectoration thick, yellow, green, bitter, salty. Frothy expectoration, looking like beaten white of egg. Very tenacious mucus in lungs. Bloody expectoration. Mucus streaked with blood.

Male - Scrotum edematous. Erysipelatous inflammation of scrotum. Rawness of scrotum, with a bluish look. Testes swollen. Hydrocele. Epididymitis. Syphilitic ulcers with burning, stitching. Painful swelling of genitals, with gangrene. Glans blue, red, swollen and cracked. Glans blue, red, swollen and cracked. Chronic herpes. Serpiginous ulcers on genitals. Emissions during diarrhea stools. Sexual power lost. Increased desire.

Modalities - Better from company. Better heat, warm drinks and food, warm wraps. ***Better hot dry applications***. Better from motion, walking about. Better lying with head elevated. Better sitting erect. Better sweating. Better open air. ***Worse periodically.*** Worse by the seashore. Worse wet weather, cold damp. Worse from cold air. Worse ices, cold drinks or food. Worse right side. Worse lying on affected part. ***Worse exertion. Worse around midnight.*** Worse after midnight. Worse 11 p.m. to 2 a.m. Worse every 14 days, yearly. Worse quinine, alcohol, tobacco. Worse eruptions undeveloped or suppressed.

Mouth - Swollen bleeding gums, painful to touch. ***Ulceration of mouth with dryness and burning heat.*** Bloody saliva. Metallic taste. ***Gulping up burning water***. Bites tumbler while drinking. Dryness of mouth. ***Aphthae in mouth.*** Fetor oris. Bitter taste, water after eating and drinking. Mouth tastes, sour, foul, salty, sweet in morning. Speech rapid, lisping. Eruptions on lips. Sore lips and ulcers in mouth. Lips covered with brown slime. Constant licking of dry, cracked lips. Cancer of lips. Epithelioma of lips. Lips black, livid. Formication on lips.

Nerves - Paralysis. Trembling, jerking, convulsions and chorea twitchings. Epilepsy, suddenly becomes unconscious with convulsions.

Nose - Acne of nose. Allergies. ***Hay fever and coryza,*** worse in open air, better indoors. ***Thin, watery, excoriating*** discharge. Nose feels stopped up with fluent coryza. Coryza with hoarseness and sleeplessness. ***Burning and itching.*** Sneezing with biting watery coryza. ***Sneezing with-***

out relief. Nose colds descend to chest. Dryness of nasal cavity. Cold sores in nose. Knotty swelling of the nose. Scabs in nostrils. Nosebleed after fit of passion or vomiting. Dyspnea felt in nose. Lupus. Offensive smell before nose. Smells of pitch and sulphur alternately. Cannot bear the sight or smell of food.

Perspiration - Cold, clammy sweats. Cold sweats, on face. Sweats with great thirst, dyspnea or exhaustion. Sour, offensive, copious sweats. Sweats on going to sleep, better after a little sleep. Sweats in bed, causes faintness. ***Sweats relieves, rheumatic pains.*** Sweats in morning without relief. Sweat, stains brownish, yellow. Sweat at end of fever. Sweats with aversion to uncover. Weakening sweats, even to fainting.

Rectum - ***Burning pain and pressure*** in rectum and anus. Dysentery, cholera, in children. Cholera with intense agony, prostration and burning thirst. Tenesmus. Ineffectual urging to stool. Fetid flatus. ***Diarrhea from alcoholic abuse or spoiled meat.*** Diarrhea of a cadaverous smell, scenting whole room. ***Diarrhea with coldness of limbs and face, vomiting, prostration.*** Diarrhea copious, smell of rotten eggs. Constipation, with pain in bowels. Acute prolapsed anus. Painful, spasmodic protrusion of rectum. Dark, offensive hemorrhages from bowels. ***Hemorrhoids burn like fire, relieved by heat.*** Itching and eczematous eruptions around anus. Skin excoriated about anus. Anus red and sore.

Skin - Eczema. Oversensitiveness of skin. ***Skin symptoms alternate with asthma or internal disorders.*** Itching, burning, swellings, edema. Intense itching after suppressed eruption. Skin peels off in large scales. Brownish-white spots on skin. Dry, rough, scaly, dirty, shriveled. Skin like parchment. Desquamation. ***Eruptions, papular, dry, rough, scaly, worse cold.*** Spots, blue, black, white. Pimples, vesicles, burning violently. Hives, worse eating shellfish. Urticaria, with burning and restlessness. ***Urticaria with burning and restlessness.*** Miliary eruptions. Petechiae. Malignant pustules. Anthrax. ***Poisoned wounds.*** Scirrhus. Gangrene. Phagedena. Carbuncles. Psoriasis. Skin cancer. Epithelioma. Ulcers, with burning, cutting pain and bloody offensive discharge. Ulcers with high edges, discharging black, coagulated blood. Painful sensitiveness of old ulcers. Sensation of coldness in ulcers.

Sleep - Disturbed, anxious, restless. Sleeps with hands over head. Must have head raised by pillows. Suffocative fits during sleep. ***Sleeplessness from anxiety, nervous exhaustion, restlessness.*** Sleeplessness till 3 a.m. Talks in sleep. Awakened by pains. Shocks on dropping to sleep. Violent starting with twitching, trembling of limbs during sleep. Drowsy. Sleeping sickness. Yawning with stretching of limbs. Dreams of death. Dreams of dead persons. Dreams full of care, sorrow and fear. Dreams of thunderstorms. Dreams of fire, black water, darkness. Dreams of misfortunes and vexations.

Stomach - Anxiety in pit of stomach. ***Sick from of bad meat, water, vegetables, melons and watery fruits***. Dyspepsia from vinegar, acids, ice cream, ice water, tobacco. ***Heartburn***. Belching, gulping up of acid and bitter substances which seem to excoriate the throat. Hiccough, frequent. ***Burning pain.*** Burning as from red-hot coals in stomach. Qualmishness. Gastritis. Burning pain in stomach better by sweet milk. Stomach extremely irritable, seems raw, as if torn. ***Stomach cancer*** (Hydr.). Induration in stomach. Stomach pain from slightest food or drink. ***Food poisoning with nausea, vomiting.*** Nausea with sweetish taste in mouth. Nausea with heat. Vomiting with diarrhea. Nausea, retching and vomiting after eating and drinking. ***Cannot bear the sight or smell of food.*** Vomiting of clear water. Vomiting of blood, bile, green mucus. Vomiting brown-black mucus mixed with blood. ***Ice cold water distresses the stomach and is vomited immediately.*** Vomit, first water, then thick, glairy, or grass-green mucus, lastly blood.

Stool - Involuntary stools and urine. Diarrhea, slimy, green mucus, with tenesmus. Dysentery dark, bloody, very offensive stools. ***Small offensive, dark stools with much prostration.*** Stools, worse at night, after eating and drinking from chilling stomach. Stools, like rice water. Stools, foul, small, involuntary. Stools, acrid, burning, black, mucus, with much prostration. Stools, first dark green feces, afterwards dark green mucus. Stools, like dirty water. Stools, of blood and water. Stools, black, acrid and putrid.

Teeth - Unhealthy, swollen, easily bleeding gums. Gums, painful to touch. Grinding of the teeth in sleep. Neuralgia of teeth. Teeth feel long and very sore. ***Toothache, worse after midnight, better warmth.*** Painless throbbing in roots of teeth. Teeth become loose, sensitive to pressure and cold water. Dentition with nightly restlessness. Gums and teeth covered with brown or black slime.

Temperature - Internal chills with external heat and red cheeks. Sensitive to cold, yet better in open air. Body cold as ice (Verat.). ***Coldness in spots.*** Blue nails and lips during chill. Waves of icy coldness in blood vessels or intense boiling heat. Externally cold with internal burning heat. Chills irregular, shaking, craves hot drinks during chill, dyspnea. ***Fever at night, with anxiety, restlessness.*** High fever, hectic fever. Septic fevers. It is a prophylactic for malaria, yellow fever. Influenza. Delirium, worse after midnight. Great heat about 3 a.m. Typhoid fever. Sordes. Intermittent fever. ***Paroxysms incomplete with exhaustion.*** Great restlessness. ***Complete exhaustion.*** Heat as of hot water in veins or they burn like lines of fire.

Throat - ***Sore throat, better warm drinks.*** Dryness with soreness, scraping and burning. Swollen, edematous, constricted, burning, unable to swallow. ***Burning pain in throat.*** Everything swallowed seems to lodge in esophagus. Nausea in throat. Malignant sore throat. Blueness of external throat from distension of veins. Diphtheria membrane, looks dry and wrinkled. Ulceration with swollen submaxillary glands. Constriction of larynx during cough. Burning in larynx and trachea. Aphonia. Voice weak, trembling, uneven, hoarse. Voice rough, hollow. Spasm of glottis. Sudden catarrh, threatening suffocation at night. Gangrenous croup.

Tongue - Tongue dry, clean and red, stitching. ***Burning pain in tongue.*** Tongue ulcerated bluish white. Edge of tongue red. Tongue takes imprint of the teeth. ***Tongue burning, trembling, stiff.*** Tongue coated, white, yellowish, brown, black. Swelling about the root of the tongue.

Vertigo - Vertigo with a loss of consciousness. Vertigo during coughing fits. Vertigo in asthmatics. Vertigo before epilepsy. Vertigo with confusion. Vertigo with humming in ears. Vertigo of malarial origin. Vertigo during pregnancy. Vertigo when closing eyes, as if he would fall.

Vision - Dim vision during headache. Snow dazzles, with lachrymation. Vision, everything appears green. Sees as through a white gauze. Flickering vision. Horizontal half-sight, only objects in lowest part of field of vision could be seen.

COMMENTS - The Arsenic habit of the Styrian mountaineers has arisen from the discovery of its power of strengthening the muscles both of the limbs and of the breathing apparatus. The arsenic-eaters of the Tyrol can take as much as a few grains of white arsenic or the sulphide, every two days. They maintain that it imparts a sense of invigoration and enables them to carry enormous loads up steep mountains.

According to one account it is resorted to by populations who live on vegetable food almost exclusively. "It strengthens the muscles, helps to digest our coarse bread and potatoes and allows us to breathe freely and easily."

It is difficult to say how far this is a directly ***"tonic"*** effect and how far curative of the dyscrasia generated by the conditions of life. The fine skin and glossy hair of the young women among the arsenic-eating people is remarkable and is comparable to the fine coats of arsenic fed horses.

On the other hand, ***"staring coat"*** in animals and ***"dry, rough, scaly, unhealthy***

looking skin" in human beings are keynote indications for the remedy. In this connection, the effects on the crew of the ship named Zion may be mentioned, which carried arsenic as a portion of its cargo.

This was exposed somewhat to the sun's rays and the crew noticed a peculiar smell. Soon they all began to notice themselves growing stout and on reaching Philadelphia from England they had all gained much, one to the extent of two stones in weight.

Characteristic great fear of death, extreme restlessness, marked weakness, rapid loss of weight, coldness and lack of vital heat, nightly aggravations, especially after midnight, 2 a. m. to 4 a. m., extreme burning pains, marked tendency to ulcerations and destruction of tissues, low types of disease, malignant fevers, such as typhoid.

Restlessness, even the stupor is interrupted by fits of restlessness with anxious moaning. Patients are anxious, full of the fear of death, restlessness compelling them to frequently change their position.

Nervous affections, notably chorea. Jerks and starts on falling asleep. Irritability, desperately angry, almost furious. Despair, hopelessness, unutterable misery. The irritability and sadness of malarial cachexias of the cachexias of quinine, mercury and syphilis.

Low types of disease, typhoid states. Inflammations of great intensity with tendency to destruction of tissue. Burning, sharp pains. Burning is another leading characteristic of Arsenic. The peculiarity of the "burning pains" is that they are better by heat (herein comparing with Caps.).

Ars. affects the entire digestive tract. The lips are so dry and parched and cracked that the patient often licks them to moisten them. The mouth is aphthous, ulcerated or gangrenous. The burning in the throat is better by eating or drinking hot things. On the other hand, cold food and cold drinks, worse stomach irritations, hence Ars. is of signal use for effects of eating ice and drinking ice water.

According to Teste, Ars. is suited to the effects of excess of vegetable diet, melons, strawberries and fruits in general, especially watery fruits. The stomach is so irritable that the least food or drink causes distress or vomiting or stool or both together. Abdominal pains are intense, causing the patient to turn and twist. Hemorrhoids are exceedingly painful as if burning needles plunged in.

States of lowered vitality. The prostration of Ars. is remarkable. With it there is the desire to move or to be moved constantly. The patient is exhausted from the slightest exertion. Exhaustion is not felt while lying still, but as soon as he moves he is surprised to find himself so weak. The prostration seems out of proportion to the rest of his illness. Must lie down. Exhaustion from hill climbing, breathless, sleepless.

Thirst for little and often (Ant-t., Lyc.), wants it very cold and immediately rejects it (Phos. as soon as it becomes warm). Before and after the cough of Arsenic there is an attack of asthma (Phos.).

Acute coryza and hay fever. The fluent coryza is corrosive, reddening the upper lip and has more burning than either Merc. or All-c.

Worse out of doors and better in warmth (compared to All-c.). Predominantly right-sided. The neuralgias affect the right side most. The right lung has acute, sharp, fixed or darting pain in apex and through upper third of right lung. Right lung is more affected than the left, also the right side of the abdomen, hence typhlitis.

Good for controlling dropsical conditions, especially in cases of hydrothorax. It has been called the "liquid trochar," on account of the expeditious way in which it will remove a watery effusion. The patient cannot lie down, must sit up to breathe, anxious, restless, worse about 1 a.m. Puffiness is one of its characteristics and from this to dropsy.

All mucus membranes are irritated. The skin is cold and clammy. Scurfy eruptions. Bran-colored scales on head coming down to forehead.

Epithelioma of the lips and closely corresponds to the cancerous diathesis. Many cures of cancer have been reported under its use, both in crude and in potencies.

When the subjective symptoms of Ars. are present, it will cure in the potencies. When the similarity is more crude, the lower potencies will be required. In cancer cases the Ars. appears to act directly on the cancerous tissue and cancerous elements in the system.

Hemorrhagic, it acts on both blood and blood vessels. Varicose veins burn like fire. Anemia, chlorosis, pyemia. Weakened states resulting from blood loss, as venesection, metrorrhagia, hemoptysis.

Intermittent fevers and chills. Clarke once treated some members of a family who all had attacks of fever of short duration, recurring regularly every six weeks from living in rooms papered with arsenical papers. Its periodicity comes every day, every third or fourth day, every fortnight, every six weeks, every year.

There is pronounced night aggravation, pains with restlessness. Worse near midnight and after midnight, worse 3 a.m. There is worse from cold and damp, better warmth. Ars. loves warmth like Nux-v., Psor., Hep., Sil., Mag-m. and other hydrogenoid remedies. It is differentiated from Sulph., Ant-c., Iod., Apis and Puls. Ars. hugs the fire and likes warm wraps.

Good for food poisoning, pesticide and chemical poisoning, bad water, acute or chronic. The first symptom is diarrhea. Grimmer noted its use for cancer, epithelioma, lupus, and pernicious anemia.

Typhus and pernicious types of malaria present a fair picture of the range and character of the sickness this remedy has cured.

A major asthma remedy. Good for the flu when they despair over their recovery. Good for cancer, pains of cancer, and the reaction to the diagnosis of cancer. Effective for palliative care of dying patient. Minor diabetes remedy. Good for emaciation, periodic fevers and sweating, especially for AIDS patients. Malaria, yellow fever, dysentery.

Burning pains, the chest, the colon, the rectum burn. Better hot drinks and better warmth. Worse 11:00 at night until 2:00 a.m. They get a lot of asthma attacks and anxiety then. They're very chilly in general.

Fastidiousness, concerned with cleanliness and order, particularly the elderly. Fear of death and dying. Agonizing, tormenting fear of dying. Fear of cancer and AIDS. Obsessive, tormenting fears of getting infections. Despair, fear of being incurable. Fear of suffocation, the dark, being alone, poisoned. Worse right side, better heat and warm drinks. Better company. Sips, drinks often. Restless because of anxiety.

Etiology can be from suppressed skin rash. Serious disease, near death experience can make them feel vulnerable. Emotional deprivation, lack of love, shock of abandonment, sense of intense loss. Can be material loss, sense of being in a dangerous situation, poverty, war.

Behavior stems from underlying needs and sense of loss and feeling threatened. Can become stingy and possessive, insecure, hoarders, manipulative, controlling. Instability, concerned with creating stability, safety. Can become self centered, possessive, dependent on others because of this. Much of their concern is about their health, hypochondriacs. Can become paranoid, hostile, leading to depression or anger.

RELATIONS - ***Antidotes of potencies:*** Camph., Chin., Chin-s., Ferr., Graph., Hep., Iod., Ip., Nux-v., Samb., Tab., Verat. Op., Carb-v., Antidotal to lead poison. ***Chemical Antidotes:*** Charcoal, Hydrated Peroxide of Iron, Lime Water. ***Antidotes to poisonous doses:*** milk, albumen, demulcent drinks, followed by emetics of mustard, Sulphate of Zinc or Sulphate of Copper (Tartar emetic is too irritating). Castor oil is the best purgative. ***Antidote to:*** Carb-v., Chin., Ferr., Graph., Hep., Iod., Ip., Lach., Merc., Nux-v., Phos., Samb., Stry., Tab., Verat. ***Compare:*** (1) The restlessness of Ars. differs from that of Mag-c. must get out of bed and walk the floor to relieve pain. The fear of death is not that of Acon., but is an anxiety and a feeling that it is useless to take medicine as they will surely die (more like Agnus). (2) Bry. drinks much seldom, Ars. little and often, Ars. eats much at a time, Bry. often and little. (3) Ars. stibiatum 3x - Chest inflammations of children, restlessness with thirst and prostration, loose mucus cough, oppression, hurried respiration, crepitant rales. (4) Cenchris contortrix, Iod., Phos., Chin., Verat., Carb-v., Kali-p. (5) Epilobium - intractable diarrhea of typhoid. (6) Hoang Nan. (7) Atoxyl. - Sodium arseniate 3x, sleeping sickness, commencing optic atrophy. (8) Sarcolactic acid - influenza with violent vomiting. ***Complementary:*** Carb-v., Phos., Thuja, Secale. All. sat., Phos. ***Follows well:*** Acon., Agar., Arn., Bell., Cham., Chin., Ip., Lach., Verat. ***Followed well by:*** Aran., Nux-v., Iod., Sulph., Rhus-t. follows well in skin affections, especially in cases treated allopathically with large dose of arsenic.

REFERENCES - Boericke. Clarke. Grimmer. Murphy.

ARSENICUM BROMATUM

(Arsenic Bromide)

PHARMACY - ars-br. Arsenicum bromatum. Arsenic bromide. ***Historical dose:*** Trituration, all potencies.

CLINICAL - Acne. Cancer. Constipation. Diabetes mellitus. Herpes. Intermittent fevers. Locomotor ataxia. Neuralgias. Tumors.

HOMEOPATHIC - Ars-br. has proven a great anti-psoric and anti-syphilitic remedy. Hansen said it is useful for "Acne rosacea with violet papules on the nose. Diabetes mellitus."

Herpetic eruptions, syphilitic growths, glandular tumors and indurations. Carcinoma, locomotor ataxia and obstinate intermittent fevers. ***Acne rosacea*** with violet papules on nose, worse in the spring. ***Acne*** in young people.

Great restlessness, wants to be carried continually. Larynx and trachea invaded; the effort to breathe causes profuse sweating. Irregular brownish stripe on center of tongue, more toward base. Great thirst for large quantities.

COMMENTS - Anshutz's best successes were in obstinate cases of syphilis, in the first stages of tabes dorsalis, in the reconvalescence from exhausting acute diseases, in gastric suppurations inactivity of bowels, tardy digestion, constipation.

In those cases where Chin-s. failed in intermittent fevers, he prescribed Ars-br. twice daily, four drops, each time in a full glass of water. Gradually diminishing it to one daily dose and in four weeks.

Even the most obstinate cases yielded to this treatment. The patient felt encouraged by his increasing vigor, the fever-cakes disappear, the bowels moved regularly and appetite left nothing to be desired. Those mean obstinate cases of intermittent fevers often appearing in the form of unbearable neuralgias, yielded more rapidly to it than to the Quinine.

Anshutz noted the case of "S. T., age 46 years old, contracted syphilis some years ago and was relieved of it by mercurial treatment and by Zittman's decoction. About six years ago he felt out of sorts and a papular eruption appeared on forehead, temples and especially at the root of the nose. Though treatment was immediately instituted, still in a few weeks the face of the patient was covered by ugly, foul-smelling crust.

"Cod liver oil was now taken internally and applied externally until the scurfs fell off and the eruption concentrated on three points. For six months that treatment was kept up, but after being omitted for a few weeks, the eruption spread again to its former extent. Every treatment was tried in rotation without the least benefit.

"In the spring 1856 he entered my clinic. In the center of the forehead, at the root of the nose, on both eyebrows on the temples and right cheek there are moist herpetic eruptions covered with crusts, exuding on least pressure an acrid, burning discharge, with easily bleeding.

"Around these eruptions the skin is injected, reddened interspersed with a large network of veins. Cough and expectoration hint to a beginning of tuberculosis, an heirloom in the family. Little appetite, disturbed digestion, tardy defecation and evening fever.

"He is ordered Solutio Ars-br. twice a day, four drops in a glass of water and already after two weeks the eruption begins to dry up, appetite returns and bowels are regular.

"After two months two crusts fall off and the skin under them is soft, shining, somewhat red. About July all eruption had gone and the cough greatly improved."

He continued by noting that "Ars-br. is also a powerful remedy in diabetes mellitus and insipidus, cured cases where the patient had already been reduced from 138 pounds to 98 and where the urine could be condensed, by boiling into syrupy consistency.

"A diabetic patient needs fresh pure air if he wishes to get well, confinement in a room or in the office prevents the action of any treatment, for it needs ozone to reduce the sugar of the blood into carbonic acid and water.

"Let the patient take three drops thrice daily in a glass of water and after a week the insatiable burning thirst will be quenched and these doses must be continued until the quantity of sugar in the urine is reduced, when the remedy might be taken twice a day and continued for a long time."

REFERENCES - Anshutz. Boericke. Clarke.

ARSENICUM HYDROGENISATUM

(Arseniuretted Hydrogen)

PHARMACY - ars-h. Arsenicum hydrogenisatum. Arseniuretted hydrogen. Arsenic hydrogen. Solution in distilled water. ***Historical dose:*** Trituration and all potencies.

CLINICAL - Collapse. ***Hematuria***. Hemorrhages. Hiccough. Menses, suppressed. Prostration. Sneezing. Urine, suppressed. Vertigo. Vomiting. Yellow fever.

HOMEOPATHIC - Ars-h. was used by Drysdale as a substitute for Arsenic in the collapse stage of cholera. The symptoms set in suddenly but developed slowly. In poisoning cases, death often took place in the second week and one person, who recovered, suffered seven weeks.

Though like Ars. in general symptoms, the gas has symptoms of its own. The general action is the same, but more accentuated. A striking case of sudden suppression of menses was cured with Ars-h. after failure of Ars.

Anemia. Anxiety, despair. ***Hematuria*** with general blood disorganization. Hemorrhages from mucus membranes. Urine suppressed, followed by vomiting. The prepuce and glans of penis are covered with pustules and round superficial ulcers.

Collapse. Coldness, prostration. Sudden weakness and nausea. Skin becomes dark brown.

MIND - Mental activity much impaired. Indifference on hearing most important news. Discouraged. Impeded in talking, answers very slowly. Answers abruptly, shortly. Changeable. Starting during sleep. Thinking of water irritates, as if he would have to vomit, nauseates him.

Anxiety, restlessness with great prostration of strength. Anxious feeling before chill. Full of care and fear about complaints when getting awake at night. Fear of death when alone. Excitable, wants to talk constantly. Impatience. Loud complaining about unbearable pains in spine.

Abdomen - Distension of abdomen during chill. Gurgling noise, Incarcerated flatus. Sensation as from a stone lying in abdomen. Glowing heat in abdomen with cold limbs. Violent cutting pain in region of navel, paroxysmal. Colic with vomiting, before midnight. Burning pain through whole alimentary canal. Softening of spleen. Pain in loins during vomiting.

Back - Sensation as if something were sticking below right scapula. Glow in back after chilliness. Backache causing loud lamentations. Tearing pain in neck during chill. Pressure between shoulders. Crawling over shoulders and back. Shuddering over single parts of back. Violent pain in lumbar region. Violent pain in sacrum. Stiffness of neck and between scapulae.

Chest - Constriction of chest, during chill. As if whole thorax were laced tightly, with rapid breathing. Sore, raw, over whole chest. Crawling, as if warm drops running over chest. Glowing sensation in chest after chilly feeling. Pain in middle of sternum, worse walking about. Pressure over whole chest with great anxiety.

Eyes - Eyes sunken, broad, blue circles around. Eyes lustreless. Conjunctiva reddened during chill. Heavinesss of lids, have to be lifted up with fingers. Blue light before right eye when falling asleep. Dim vision.

Face - Expression of extreme anxiety. Painfully distorted features. Face looks old and bears an expression of pain. Face copper-colored, or dark red. Chilly feeling in face, followed by a glow. Yellowish face at beginning of chill. Pain in maxillary joints, when first opening mouth. Heat in face. Face edematous, worse evening. Face greatly changed. Very painful twitching. Lips colorless. Upper lip sore with chill.

Food - Less appetite, eats without relish. Loss of appetite. Violent thirst and a dry tongue. Much thirst. Sensitive to tobacco. Sweet things taste too sweet.

Head - Head dull and benumbed. Pressure in forehead. Heaviness. Pressing, stupefying sensation at night. Headache above forehead. Pressure in right frontal sinus. Pressure above eyebrows with numbness. Violent pressive frontal headache, worse at night. Head worse warmth. Pain in upper and back part of head when coughing. Pain in forehead during chill.

Heart - Knocking, thumping, in heart, deep in chest. Pulse frequent. Pulse quite imperceptible. Pulse intermits when awaking at night, with anxiety and thoughts of death.

Kidneys - Heat and burning over kidney region. Unpleasant sensation of pressure in region of kidneys. Urging to urinate. Urine dark red and a thick clot of pure blood is formed. Pressure in kidneys with desire to urinate. Large quantities of pale urine. Scanty, foaming urine in morning. Inky urine. Urine very dark, orange-colored.

Limbs - Coldness of limbs.

Liver - Liver painful to pressure.

Lungs - Frequent, with pain in perineum. Talking worse. Coming from front upper part of chest. Coughing causes sweating.

Male - Sensation of numbness. Unbearable pain in both groins. Pain in symphysis pubis, sensitive to touch. Pain in left side of penis. Sexual irritation on glans penis. Whole foreskin and glans covered with little blisters containing pus. Small round flat ulcers.

Modalities - Worse dampness. Worse before thunderstorm. Worse from motion.

Mouth - Mouth hot and dry, little thirst. Bitter taste, with great prostration. Contracting. Sensation of numbness, like a cold feeling. Increased salivation. Ammoniacal odour of breath.

Nose - Unpleasant crawling in nose causes sneezing. Nose as if deadened. Nose feels as if dried up. Violent sneezing. Nose cold, must be wrapped up in warm cloths. Tickling up in nose, causes sneezing. Bloody mucus from nose. Nose and lips somewhat excoriated.

Perspiration - Sweats in large drops on face and whole head. General, warm sweat, after midnight. Attacks of night sweat. Sweats on falling asleep.

Rectum - Urging as to diarrhea. Copious passage of wind and looseness. Frequent bilious stools. Constipation with feeling of heaviness and stiffness, like a weight. Stool with vertigo, weakness and crawling. Weak sensation, as if relaxed. Sensation as if diarrhea would fall out, evening. Thumping, knocking, in region of perineum, near anus. Tearing pain in perineum. Tearing pain upward in anterior wall of rectum.

Skin - Dark brown skin all over.

Sleep - Can't get to sleep for a long while, feels as if he had to move about. ***Total sleeplessness.*** So drowsy that he can hardly open his eyes. Sopor between attacks of vomiting. Moaning in sleep. Sleep interrupted by headache. Sleep interrupted by slightest noise. Sleep disturbed by wind colic towards morning. Frequent starting while falling asleep. Very pleasant, poetical dreams. Dreams he was praying. Dreams of people going and arriving.

Stomach - Irritability of stomach. Burning pain. Weary feeling in stomach with pressure in temples. Belching with taste of food eaten. Spasmodic eructations of tasteless gas. Violent cutting pain in stomach. Pressure in epigastric region during chill. Pressure of hand causes dull pain in pit. Hiccough following eructations. Tormenting hiccough. Incessant retching and vomiting.

Stomach - Vomiting with pain in loins. Vomiting liquid, first bilious and afterwards coffee-colored. Vomiting of green, bitter mucus during colic. Vomits large masses.

Temperature - Chills while walking. Chilly and weak while attempting to rise. Glowing heat in abdomen and cold limbs all night. Much heat and burning in different parts of body.

Throat - Burning and constriction in throat, followed by irritability of stomach. Squeaking voice. Whispering voice. Voice has lost its timbre, sounds as if broken, but not hoarse.

Tongue - Tongue enlarged. Tongue deep, irregular ulcer. Tongue nodular swelling. Sensation of numbness in the tongue. Pricking on tip of tongue. Tongue slimy. Tongue yellow. Yellowish furred tongue during chill. Back part of tongue greyish-white.

Vertigo - Swimming sensation in head and whole body. Violent vertigo, on going up stairs. Vertigo, staggers against sides of stairs. Vertigo with general weakness. Vertigo, with nausea and vomiting. Vertigo, with pressure in frontal sinuses.

RELATIONS - ***Antidoted by:*** Am-a. ***Compare:*** (1) Ars. (2) Sinapis - breathing. (3) Nux-v. - fever, drinks containing sulfuretted hydrogen.

REFERENCES - Boericke. Clarke.

ARSENICUM IODATUM

(Arsenic Iodide)

PHARMACY - ars-i. Arsenicum iodatum. Arsenic iodide. Ought to be prepared fresh and protected from light. Trituration. ***Historical dose:*** Trituration and all potencies.

CLINICAL - Abscess. Acne rosacea. AIDS. ***Allergies.*** Amenorrhea. Anemia. Aneurysm. Angina pectoris. Aphonia. Arteriosclerosis. Axillary tumors. ***Breast, tumor.*** Bronchitis. Broncho-pneumonia. ***Bubo. Cachexia.*** Cancer. Catarrh. Coryza. Coughs. ***Debility.*** Diarrhea. Diphtheria. Dropsy. Dysentery. Dyspnea. Eczema. ***Emaciation. Epithelioma.*** Fever. Gastritis. Goiter. ***Hay fever.*** Heartburn. ***Heart, disorders.*** Hectic, fever. Hydrothorax. ***Hyperactive, children. Ichthyosis.*** Influenza. Laryngitis. Leucorrhea. Leukemia. Lichen. Liver, disorders. ***Lung, cancer.*** Lungs, disorders. Measles. Myocardial, degeneration. Nasal, catarrhs. Otitis, media. Otorrhea. Pernicious, anemia. Pharyngitis. Pleuritis. ***Pneumonia.*** Prostration. Psoriasis. Pyemia. Rheumatism. Scrofulous ophthalmia. Syphilis. ***Tuberculosis.*** Ulcers. Vertigo. Vomiting. Weakness.

HOMEOPATHIC - Produces most characteristically ***excoriations of mucus membranes***, like all arsenical preparations. The discharge irritates the membrane from which it flows and over which it flows. The discharge may be fetid, watery and the mucus membrane is red, angry, swollen, itches and burns.

Ars-i., produces marked emaciation, fatty degeneration, debility, night sweats. Tuberculous and anemic conditions are benefited by it. Also hypertrophy and weakening of heart muscle (degeneration).

It will be indicated by a profound prostration, rapid, irritable pulse, recurring fever and sweats, emaciation. Tendency to diarrhea. Hectic fever and debility. Enlargement of the spleen. Bad effects of malaria or quinine. Threatened pyemia (Pyrog., Meth-b).

In Ars-i., we have a remedy most closely allied to manifestations of tuberculosis. In the early stages of tuberculosis, even though there is an afternoon rise in temperature, Ars-i. is very effective.

This remedy is for tuberculosis with hoarse, racking cough and profuse expectoration of a purulent nature and attended with cardiac weakness, emaciation and general debility. Scrofulous glands. Drenching night sweats.

Ars-i. should be thought of when the discharges of mucus membranes are persistently acrid, profuse, thick, gluey, yellow like honey in chronic disorders and thin in acute conditions.

Discharges cause burning on the parts on which they flow. Influenza, ***hay fever***, old nasal catarrhs and catarrh of middle ear. Swelling of tissues within the nose. Hypertrophied condition of eustachian tube and deafness.

Acrid coryza, influenza, hay fever. There is marked burning in the eyes, nasal passages, mouth and pharynx. Thin, acrid, watery discharges from anterior and posterior nares. Watery discharge drops from tip of the nose. Aphonia. Slight hacking cough, dry stopped nostrils.

Has been use in cancerous affections and in all stages of syphilis. ***Cancer of breast*** after ulceration has set in. ***Epithelioma and lung cancers*** based on tubercular disease. Epithelioma of the lip. Axillary tumors. Great emaciation.

Weakness and debility. Heart weakened by chronic lung disorders. Arteriosclerosis. Fatty degeneration of the heart. Myocarditis. Myocardial degeneration. Senile heart. Chronic aortitis. Feeble irregular pulse.

Disorders of the blood and glands are pronounced. Pernicious anemia. In amenorrhea with anemic palpitations and dyspnea. In chronic pneumonia, when abscess is about to form. Pneumonia following influenza. Chronic pneumonia with abscess in lung.

MIND - Excitable. Hurried. Impatience. Anxiety about health. ***Restlessness at night***, driving out of bed. ***Hyperactive children.*** Oversensitive to noise. Oversensitive to sensual impressions. Averse to being spoken to. Unable to study. Study causes headache. Worse from mental exertion. Sudden impulse to kill.

Abdomen - Abdomen hard and distended with flatus, which is constantly discharged. Large quantities of flatus. Bellyache, better after stools. Chronic splenic enlargement. Enlarged mesenteric glands. Painful swelling in right groin on extending leg. Severe cutting pain in abdomen.

Back - Burning heat in lumbar region, as if clothes were on fire. Soreness of back and neck.

Breasts - Lump in breasts, worse touch. ***Cancer of breast*** after ulceration has set in. Nipple retracted. Emaciation of breasts.

Chest - Burning heat in chest. Axillary tumors.

Constitutions - Suited to those with a tendency to allergies, hay fever and asthma. Tubercular constitutions.

Cough - Hacking cough with dry and stopped up nostrils. Cough dry with little difficult expectoration. Frequent, short, suppressed cough. Frequent cough, worse exertion and at night. Cough often loose, with muco-purulent expectoration.

Ears - Otitis media with fetid, corrosive discharge. Hypertrophy of eustachian tube, deafness from. Sharp pain in ears and forehead when riding in a sharp cold wind. Thickening of tympanum, after scarlet fever.

Eyes - Scrofulous ophthalmia. ***Burning, acrid coryza.*** Eyeballs feel heavy. Smarting about eyes. Weakness of eyes, with burning pain. Secretion of meibomian glands.

Face - Sallow complexion. Pinched cadaverous face. Purple, livid hue of skin. Aching in malar bones. Cancer of lips.

Female - Foul, bloody, yellow irritating leucorrhea with swelling of labia.

Food - Intense thirst with desire for cold water which is ejected at once.

Head - Study, mental exertion causes headache. Dull heavy headache, across forehead or occiput. Unpleasant feeling in head, like a bad cold. Stunning pain above eyes and root of nose. Severe pain in forehead. Hyperemia of brain, with cold feeling in scalp. Head covered with an inflammatory scaly eruption.

Heart - Weak heart. Arteriosclerosis. Myocardial degeneration. Senile heart. Fatty degeneration of heart. Chronic aortitis. Pulse rapid, irritable. Pulse rapid, feeble, weak, irregular. Oppression in warm room, with anxiety in region of heart.

Limbs - Cold limbs. Heaviness of limbs with weariness. Pain in humerus, worse from writing. Clothes feel cold better walking. Tired, weary feeling in calves of both legs while kneeling.

Lungs - Asthma. ***General wheezing on first lying down.*** Breathing too rapid, even when at rest, increasing in rapidity on exertion, soon becoming an audible wheezing. Chronic bronchitis. ***Catarrhal pneumonia with muco-purulent expectoration, dyspnea, night sweats.*** Pneumonia that fails to clear up.

Lungs - Broncho-pneumonia after influenza. Rales and crepitation. Pleuritis. ***Short of breath, air hunger.*** Feeble respiration. ***Expectoration, yellow-green, foul.*** Muco-purulent and occasionally stringy mucus. Pulmonary tuberculosis. Tubercular pleurisy.

Modalities - Better from open air. Better after eating. Worse from dry, cold weather. Worse windy, foggy weather. Worse any exertion. Worse in rooms. Worse apples. Worse tobacco smoke. Worse when hungry. Worse lying on the painful side. Worse warm south winds.

Mouth - Breath fetid.

Nose - ***Hay fever***. Swollen nose. Burning, acrid coryza. Coryza with dyspnea. ***Thin, watery, excoriating discharge from anterior and posterior sinuses***. Drips water, which is hot, green, acrid, reddens upper lip. Irritation and tingling of nose constant desire to sneeze (Pollanin.). Aggravation by sneezing. Frequent sneezing, but unsatisfactory. ***Chronic nasal catarrh***, profuse thick, yellow discharge. ***Nasal membrane sore and excoriated.*** Nasal ulcers. Post-nasal catarrh. Colds with hunger. Violent, acute influenza.

Perspiration - Debilitating night-sweats. ***Drenching night-sweats*** with weakness.

Rectum - Continual aching in anus with seeming inability to keep sphincter closed. Diarrhea and dysentery, stools scalding, white. Urging in morning after moving about. Diarrhea not at night. Almost constant copious watery diarrhea.

Sensations - Sensations of heaviness occurs in many parts.

Skin - Dry, scaly, itching. Psoriasis. ***Marked exfoliation of skin in large scales,*** leaving a raw exuding surface beneath. ***Enlarged scrofulous glands.*** Eczema of the beard, watery, oozing, itching, worse washing. ***Ichthyosis.*** Acne is hard, indurated base with pustule at apex. ***Venereal bubo***. Eczema of beard worse washing.

Sleep - Restless sleep. Constant yawning. Sleeplessness from headache.

Stomach - Pain and heartburn. Intense thirst, water is immediately ejected. Pain in stomach, afternoons, with rising of flatus and a greasy fluid. Pain in stomach worse rising after sitting. Pain in epigastrium. Vomiting an hour after food. Distressing nausea and vomiting.

Temperature - Chilly, cannot endure cold. Influenza. Recurrent fever and sweats. Emaciation.

Throat - Hoarseness. Aphonia. Raw burning pains. Burning in pharynx. Thick membrane from fauces to lips. Chronic follicular pharyngitis. Goiter. Diphtheria. Tonsils swollen. Enlargement and inflammation of tonsils and posterior part of uvula during coryza.

Tongue - Tongue slightly furred.

Vertigo - Vertigo with tremulous feeling, especially in the elderly.

COMMENTS - This is a synthetic remedy, its iodine element makes the person hot and adds an affinity for the glands, so it's a warm-blooded glandular remedy. Good for fever with swollen glands. Acute sore throat with burning and swollen glands, worse heat.

In chronic, watery diarrhea in tubercular subjects in cases of emaciation with good appetite. This remedy can be continued for some time. Clinically, it has been found advisable in tuberculosis to begin with about the 4x and gradually go lower to the 2x trituration, 3 times a day.

Also for hay fever and allergies, usually will look like an infection with swollen glands and fever, not an allergy. Psoriasis (Kali-ar). Affinity for the thyroid, hypothyroid conditions. Good for AIDS patients with emaciation, fever, swollen glands.

Eczema of the beard, psoriasis, diarrhea of phthisis. Emaciation with good appetite. Always chilly, feeble respiration. Chronic splenic enlargement after intermittents or quinine.

RELATIONS - ***Antidote:*** Ars., Bry. relieved pain and heartburn. ***Compare:*** (1) All-c., Ars., Sang., Tub., Kali-br. Ant-i. (2) In hay fever Aralia, Naphthalin., Rosa, Sang-n. (3) Bac. in acrid discharges, Nit-ac., Ail., Arum-t., Ars. Ars-m. and Ars. salts. (4) Useful after Sulph in tuberculosis pulmonalis and after Conium is sensitive lump in breast. ***Complementary:*** Kali-i. Phos.

REFERENCES - Boericke. Clarke.

ARSENICUM METALLICUM

(Arsenic Metal)

PHARMACY - ars-met. Arsenicum metallicum. Arsenic metal, (At. Wt. 749) Trituration. ***Historical dose:*** Trituration and all potencies.

CLINICAL - Apathy. Constipation, Coryza. Diarrhea. Eye disorders. Hemorrhoids. Headaches. Itching. Sciatica. Skin, disorders. Syphilis.

HOMEOPATHIC - The symptoms of Ars-met. are very like those of Ars., but not entirely. The following are the most peculiar: symptoms recur every 14 days, coryza every 21 days. Pains extend from one part to another or leave one part and appear in another. Attacks come suddenly and go slowly or vice versa.

General weakness and debility. Thinking of symptoms aggravates. Many symptoms appear on right side. Swollen feeling of parts. Enlarged or swollen feeling of brain, head, eyelids, hands and fingers.

Syphilis wakes up after being many years dormant. Itching in many parts, skin peels off in small scales. Cutting, burning, stinging pains.

MIND - Memory weak for what he has read, has to read everything two or three times before he comprehends it. Thinking of symptoms aggravates. Moody, doesn't wish to see anybody. ***Desire to be alone.***

Depression with exhaustion. Low spirited. Sad with tearful eyes, but can't weep, even during most painful events. Fear of being poisoned.

Annoyed by visions, causing her to cry. Fearful visions of spectres in bright daylight. Sees threatening people after her and screams horribly. Feels as if she has to run away.

Abdomen - Bloated abdomen. Pain in spleen down to groin. Red rash on abdomen. Painful swelling in right groin. Pulsation in navel.

Back - Chilliness in neck, during headache. Numbness and lameness sensation of right lumbar region. Pain in spine between scapulae. Sharp pain behind scapulae. Crawling sensation on back. Feeling as if a furuncle would form. Weakness of neck. Itching in neck during coryza.

Breasts - Itching of breasts. Pain in breast extends to hip and spleen.

Chest - Chilliness extending into chest. Pulsation under sternum. Small blisters filled with blood on left side of chest. Sensation as if a heavy load were lying on chest.

Ears - Numbness below ears.

Eyes - Eyes, red, swollen and watery, burn with coryza. Hot and corroding lachrymation during coryza. Pterygium, with enlarged bloodvessel. Eyes weak. Can't look into bright light. Eyes painful after reading, sewing. Eye pain from walking in wind.

Face - Face bloated, red and hot, during coryza. Red, itching, burning and swollen. Stiffness in lower jaws when biting. Twitching in left lower jaw.

Female - ***Menses too early and too long-lasting.*** Menses too scanty. Heat in uterus and vagina. Burning when touched. Pains in uterus and vagina during menses.

Food - No appetite. Aversion to wine and alcoholic drinks. Great desire for brandy or alcoholic drinks. Worse after brandy.

Head - Writing and thinking aggravates headaches. Headache over eyes, with chilliness. Head feels too large. Left-sided headache up to eyes and into ears. Headaches, worse stooping and lying down. Edematous swelling of forehead. Laughing aggravates. Falling off of hair.

Heart - Pains in region of heart after mental disturbances. Sharp pain in heart. Can lie only on left side in heart disease. ***Pulse accelerated in morning*** (Sulph.).

Limbs - Limbs feel heavy.

Liver - Sore pain in liver goes through to shoulders and spine.

Lungs - Great difficulty in breathing, with sneezing, coryza, lachrymation.

Kidneys - Hot urine in evening. Red, sandy sediment.

Male - Itching on scrotum. Itching on glans. Prepuce swollen. ***Chancres with burning pain.*** Offensive sweat on genitals.

Modalities - Better darkness. Better pinching, sitting erect. Washing helps the itching of anus. Cold bathing helps the itching of face. Worse stooping. Worse light. Worse on waking in morning. Worse lying on left side (heart). Worse thinking of symptoms. Worse right side. Hot bathing aggravates the pain in hip.

Mouth - Dry mouth. Hot breath. Mouth sore and ulcerated. Lips dry and hot. Gums swollen and sore. Gums feel as if scalded, with salivation. Gums painful when touched.

Nose - Coryza with hot face, itching and hoarseness. Coryza, burning hot water runs from nose, excoriating edges of nostrils. Sore nose. Thick, yellow discharge. Violent itching in tip of nose.

Rectum - Diarrhea, burning watery stools with relief of pain. Sore feeling in rectum, better very hot water, not by cold washing. Intense itching at anus, followed by crawling.

Skin - Itching, has to pinch spot. Skin peels off in small scales. Bluish-red eruptions. Rash and red smooth spots. Red spots over whole body. Small furuncles in face.

Sleep - Great drowsiness in morning. Falling asleep on sitting down. Very sleepy, but can't fall asleep. Dreams of danger on the water.

Stomach - Hot eructations as of bile, with throbbing through whole body. Pressure in region of stomach. Empty retching and cutting in belly. Nausea towards morning. Nausea with headache, in morning.

Temperature - Chilliness on occiput, neck and chest.

Throat - Hoarseness during coryza. Sore throat during coryza. Violently inflamed throat, with pain when swallowing, worse right side. Angina with much heat in throat and several little ulcers. Itching of external throat.

Tongue - The tongue coated white and shows imprint of the teeth. Tongue white, slimy, furred.

RELATIONS - ***Antidoted by:*** Bell., Nat-c. ***Compare:*** (1) Iod., Merc., Nat-c. in syphilis, Nux-v. - drowsy after sound sleep. (2) Rhus-t. - pain in back, hips, etc., Sulph. (pulse), Ars. (3) Useful in pterygium after failure of Nux-v. and Spig.

REFERENCES - Boericke. Clarke.

ARSENICUM SULFURATUM FLAVUM

(Arsenious Sulphide)

PHARMACY - ars-s-f. Arsenicum sulphuratum flavum. Arsenious sulphide. Orpiment. Arsenic trisulph. Trituration. ***Historical dose:*** Trituration and all potencies.

CLINICAL - Decay. Children, emaciated. Diarrhea. Gonorrhea. Indigestion. Jaundice. Laryngeal, tuberculosis. Strokes. Walking, late.

HOMEOPATHIC - Orpiment of the Alchemists. The two sulfides of Arsenic orpiment and Realgar have been used in a somewhat general way in cases combining the strong symptoms of both elements. Independent observations and provings have been made with the two salts.

Grimmer called Ars-s-f. an arsenicum that effects the skin and mucus membrane strongly, malignant and regular ulceration, especially of the stomach, which is the seat of severe burning pains with vomiting and diarrhea. There are symptoms of the two components, there is intense torturing anxiety and apprehension with restlessness.

Ars-s-f. has the burning pains and sensations of both Ars. and Sulph., stitching, tearing and rheumatic pains moving from place to place. Lameness, staggering, trembling. Spasms, colic, vomiting and diarrhea. Annoying twitching. General debility. Chafing of skin about genitals and behind ears of children.

Needle pricks from within outwards in chest, also on forehead, right side. Sticking behind the ear. Difficult respiration. Leucoderma and squamous syphilides. Sciatica and pain around the knee.

MIND - Apprehensive. Intense torturing anxiety and apprehension. Obstinate. Touchy, hasty and restless. Discontented. Aversion to being spoken to. Vanishing of thoughts.

Abdomen - Violent griping pain with convulsions. Violent colic. Swelling of abdomen.

Back - Pain in lumbar vertebrae when moving. Back constantly cold.

Food - Loss of appetite. Aversion to fat, rich food and meat. Desires coffee, sweets, warm food and drinks. Extremely thirsty.

Head - Great weakness in head. Stroke. Needle-like stitches in right frontal region. Forehead cold.

Limbs - Sciatica with pain around knee. Knees pain and totter. Feet burn. Feet cold, offensive sweat.

Lungs - Difficult breathing.

Male - Gonorrhea with terrible pains, discharge copious, yellow, constant, burning day and night along entire urethra with restlessness.

Modalities - Better by steam or hot water. Better lying down. Marked periodicity (Ars., Sulph.). Worse every afternoon and evening.

Mouth - Taste bitter. Tongue furred, yellow-white, stiff, swollen. Dry mouth with disgust for all nourishment. Mouth and throat dry. Herpetic ulcers. Teeth pain as if loose, when chewing food.

Nose - Dry nose. Sneezing.

Rectum - Diarrhea with colic, backache and tenesmus. Diarrhea daily 8 a-m. and several times during day, but not at night. Stool like water, green and slimy and terribly offensive.

Skin - Skin itching, dry, cracked, cracks. Skin scaly and blackish. Leucoderma. Eruption on outer side of left wrist, also on inner side.

Sleep - Starting in sleep, also in falling asleep, as if he would fall out of bed. Restless at night, excited, dreams with seminal emissions.

Stomach - Indigestion. Burning and gnawing in stomach with vomiting and diarrhea. Cramp in stomach with fainting, colic, vomiting, diarrhea. Violent, persistent vomiting. Vomiting of offensive bile relieves.

Temperature - Hectic fever without thirst. Chronic intermittent fever, worse every afternoon and evening. Terrible heat at night.

RELATIONS - ***Compare:*** (1) Ars., Sulph. (2) Calc. - children slow in learning to walk. (3) Ars-s-r.

REFERENCES - Boericke. Clarke. Grimmer.

ARSENICUM SULFURATUM RUBRUM

(Arsenic Sulphide)

PHARMACY - ars-s-r. Arsenicum sulphuratum rubrum. Arsenic sulphide. Realgar. Arsenic disulfide. Trituration. ***Historical dose:*** Trituration and all potencies.

CLINICAL - Acne. Diarrhea. Eczema. Furuncles. Gastritis. ***Influenza.*** Neuralgia. Psoriasis. Sciatica.

HOMEOPATHIC - The Realgar of the ancient Alchemists. The Red Sulphide of Arsenic was introduced and proved by Neidhard, but it has been used somewhat empirically on indications borrowed from its two components.

Clarke found Ars-s-r. useful in many cases of influenza and its sequelae, especially sciatica. ***Influenza with intense catarrhal symptoms***, great prostration and high temperature, purulent discharges. Burning pains, as if coals of fire in stomach, worse drinking cold water. External heat. Bone pains.

Chilly even before a hot stove. Restless sleep with very vivid dreams. Psoriasis, acne and sciatica. Itching in various parts. Pellagra. Convulsions. Itching in various parts. Numbness. All symptoms worse at night. Worse on waking (headache).

MIND - Crossness, irritable and acts with more energy. Indisposed for mental or physical exertion after meals.

Abdomen - Dull pain in bowels. Feeling of fullness. Violent colic with terrible vomiting. Large bluish spots.

Back - After rising in morning a heavy pressing pain, extending from tip of coccyx to anus, soreness of coccyx.

Chest - Chest pains. Wakes at 5 a.m. with sharp cutting pain. Commencing between cartilages of 5th and 6th ribs. Extending inwards and upwards deep into chest. Slightest motion aggravates, had to limit respiration as much as possible.

Ears - Sensations of fulness and pressing outward in right ear. Snapping sound in ear corresponding to pulsation of temporal artery. Ear feels hot. Redness and burning of ear. Tingling similar to frost-bite.

Head - Severe continued pain extending deep into brain in right frontal region, also in right ear, worse by stooping and exercise, better cold application, 5 p-m. Waking often with dull pain in forehead over eyes, extending over top of head to crown. Pain commencing at back of head, extending around sides. Neuralgia right side of face, nose, jaw and through temple.

Heart - Occasional sharp pains through base of heart impeding respiration.

Limbs - Rheumatism from right shoulder down arm as if in bone. Pain in right hip with lameness of leg. Severe pain in left tibia. All joints immovable after recovery from the poison.

Mouth - Bitter taste on waking.

Rectum - Pain in anus worse by efforts to stool or urination, bearing-down would cause heavy sickening sensation.

Stomach - Burning in stomach like coals of fire, worse drinking cold water, could not bear least pressure on region of stomach. Sharp cutting pain in left abdominal region after each meal. Weight and gnawing in stomach.

Stool - Diarrhea, yellow, mushy stools in morning early after getting up and in the evening before going to bed, constant tenesmus in anus.

Throat - Hoarseness with accumulation of thick, tenacious mucus in throat. Mucus membranes of mouth and throat inflamed. Right tonsil enlarged. Intolerable itching in throat inducing short, dry, expulsive cough.

COMMENTS - J. Meredith cured with Ars-s-r. mainly, a young girl who suffered from an occipital headache, profuse, repulsive, nauseating nasal catarrh, leucorrhea, pelvic pains, menstrual troubles and general anemic appearance.

T. N. McLaughlin reported much success in skin cases, especially in cases of psoriasis and also of eczema, acne and furuncles. He gave Ars-s-r. in tablets of 2x trituration. He found patients who could not tolerate Ars. could take Ars-s-r. without any unpleasant symptoms and with marked curative effect. There was no gastric or intestinal irritation in any of his cases.

RELATIONS - ***Compare:*** (1) Ars-s-f., Caps.

REFERENCES - Boericke. Clarke. Grimmer.

ARTEMISIA ANNUA

(Sweet Wormwood)

PHARMACY - art-a. Artemisia annua. Sweet wormwood. Sweet Annie. Qing hao. N. O. Compositae. ***Historical dose:*** Tincture and all potencies.

CLINICAL - Fever. Intermittent fever. ***Malaria.*** Parasites. Stomach, problems. Worms.

HERBAL - This herb has been used in China to treat malaria and fevers. Artemisinin is an alkaloid extracted from the plant that is being used as an anti-malarial drug. It reduces fevers and destroys the malaria organism.

Artemisia annua has been used in tinctures, powders and teas. It is of special use in those areas where anti-malarial drugs like quinine are no longer effective.

HOMEOPATHIC - Art-a. has not been proved homeopathically. Clinically it has been used to treat fevers, stomach problems, and parasites.

RELATIONS - ***Compare:*** (1) Ars., Chin., Art-v.

REFERENCES - Boericke. Clarke. Grimmer.

ARTEMISIA VULGARIS

(Mugwort)

PHARMACY - art-v. Artemisia vulgaris. Mugwort. Wormwood. Beifuss. N.O. Compositae. Tincture of fresh root. ***Historical dose:*** Tincture and all potencies. Locally and internally is injurious to eyes.

CLINICAL - Anorexia. Catalepsy. Chorea. Convulsions. Cramps. Dysmenorrhea. Eclampsia. ***Epilepsy.*** Hydrocephalus. Hysteria. Masturbation. Miscarriage. Sleepwalking. Twitching. Worms. Vertigo.

HOMEOPATHIC - Like the other Artemisias, this remedy has a prominent place in convulsive diseases. Some reputation as a remedy for epileptic conditions and convulsive diseases of childhood and girls at puberty. Acts better when given with wine than with water.

Excitable and irritable before attack of epilepsy. ***Epilepsy after fright or grief after a blow on the head*** with menstrual disturbances with teething.

Attack accompanied or followed by profuse offensive sweat, by seminal ejaculations. Profuse sweat, having a peculiar fetid, cadaverous or garlic-like odor is a characteristic of the remedy.

Attacks frequently repeated, then followed by a long interval of rest. ***Petit mal.*** Epilepsy without aura after fright and other violent emotions. Epilepsy after masturbation. Several convulsions close together. Irregular or deficient menstruation with epileptic convulsions.

Violent cramps in abdomen with irregular insufficient menstruation. Nervous chlorosis with very dry skin. Chorea with inability to swallow. Colored light produces dizziness. Worms. Right side convulsed, left paralyzed.

MIND - Complaints from fright. Catalepsy after fright. ***Epilepsy after fright or grief.*** Weak-minded with epileptic fits. ***Excitable before the attack of epilepsy.*** Sudden whining. Stupor after convulsions.

Peevish and inclined to weep. Very much vexed, irritable, depressed. Walks in the street, suddenly stops, stares into space often mumbles a few words, becomes normal and remembers nothing. Kleptomania. Inclination to steal.

Abdomen - Violent cramps in abdomen.

Causations - Blow on head. Fright, grief or bad news. Masturbation.

Constitutions - It has a prominent place in convulsive diseases of childhood and girls at puberty.

Eyes - ***Colored light produces dizziness***. Pain and burning of vision, better rubbing, worse using eyes. Eyes turned up before attack.

Face - Twitching in the face, mouth drawn to left Face looks older.

Female - Irregular or deficient menstruation with epileptic convulsions. Profuse menses. Violent uterine contractions. Spasms during menses. Prolapsed uterus. Nervous chlorosis, with very dry skin. Violent contractions of pregnant uterus, threatened miscarriage. Checked lochia. Eclampsia.

Food - Hunger, but cannot get the food down.

Head - Drawn back by spasmodic twitchings. Head bent backwards and sideways. Congestion of brain. Sharp shooting pains through the head.

Kidneys - Urine increased, yellowish. Obstinate strangury in a child.

Limbs - Over-fatigue or weakness of the feet after long walks or long illness.

Lungs - Rattling breathing with the spasms. Breathing checked, suddenly a deep inspiration ends the attack, catalepsy.

Male - Nightly pollutions. Seminal ejaculations with the spasm.

Mouth - Mouth drawn to left. Chewing motion of gums, grinding teeth. Lower jaw pressed forward. Bites tongue in spasms. Speech unintelligible, can utter but single words, and these only with great exertion.

Perspiration - ***Profuse sweat, smelling like garlic***. Sweats during epileptic attacks. Sweating is a sign of relief. Warm sweat all over, most on occiput.

Rectum - Greenish diarrhea. Passes feces and urine with the spasms. Worms.

Sleep - Sleepwalking. Gets up at night and works, but remembers nothing in the morning (Luna., Kali-p.).

Stomach - Nausea and vomiting. Cramps in stomach.

Teeth - Grinding of teeth, forth at mouth, thumbs drawn into fist, eyes half open, drawn upwards.

Temperature - Chilly, feels unwell with drawing in limbs Coldness of body.

Throat - Swallowing difficult, food escapes from the mouth.

Vertigo - Vertigo caused by colored lights, but not by white light. Epileptic vertigo.

COMMENTS - Convulsions of nursing or teething children. Epileptic spasms, after cooling off, while over-heated from dancing. Epilepsy from menstrual disturbances. Nightly epilepsy with violent trismus injuring teeth. During epileptic attacks violent sweat of offensive odor. Long and deep sleep after a fit. Sleepwalking. Congestion of the brain and spine. Hydrocephalus.

RELATIONS - ***Compare:*** (1) Absin. - nearest relative. (2) Abrot., Cina, Cham., Arn., Mill. (3) Cic. - staring, jerking head, etc. (4) Cina - eyes. (5) Apis, Hell. (6) Bufo - irritable before fit, Caust., Ruta, Sec. (7) Bry. - chewing motion of jaw. ***Compatible:*** Stram., Puls., Aur. ***Follows well after:*** Acon., Bell., Bry., Hell., Cina, Iod.

REFERENCES - Boericke. Clarke.

ARUM DRACONTIUM

(Green Dragon)

PHARMACY - arum-d. Arum dracontium. Green dragon. Arisaema dracontium. N. O. Araceae. North America. Tincture of root before flowering or after the ripening of the seeds. ***Historical dose:*** Tincture and all potencies.

CLINICAL - Asthma. Coughs. Croup. Headaches. Hoarseness. Impotency. Influenza. Itching. Laryngismus stridulus. Pharyngitis. Sore, throat. Urticaria.

HOMEOPATHIC - Arum-d. has the irritating properties of Arums generally. It has been well proved by Dr. C. P. Hart and tested clinically as well.

Asthmatic attacks from cold. Croupy, hoarse cough with sore throat. Laryngismus between 12 a.m. and 2 a.m., attacks every week or ten days. Pharyngitis with sore, raw and tender throat. Swallowing develops and worsens the throat symptoms.

Dryness and smarting. Throat raw and tender. Hawking. Continual disposition to clear throat by hawking and coughing. Hoarseness on awaking in morning, expectorates thick mucus. Expectoration of thick, heavy, yellowish-white pus. Rattling of mucus on full expiration.

Chronic itching. Eruption of pimples or species of lichen, on nose, a patch of urticaria on right arm near elbow. The symptoms move about and from side to side, especially right to left.

MIND - Great languor and depression of spirits, with asthma at night.

Abdomen - Rumbling and much flatus. Pain in bowels from incarcerated flatus.

Cough - Loose cough with dry soreness of throat, worse at night lying down. Cough from laryngeal irritation, worse at night and when lying down. Croupy, hoarse cough with sore throat. Rattling cough in larynx and swelling of air passages, threatening suffocation.

Head - Heavy, shooting pain in ears, aching pain behind right ear.

Heart - Heart beats so violently as to shake walls of chest.

Kidneys - Irresistible desire to pass urine, burns and smarts.

Male - Frequent and copious emissions of urine. Great diminution, mostly an entire absence of sexual desire. Penis flaccid and relaxed. Fine shooting pains in course of left spermatic cord.

Lungs - Asthmatic at night. Asthma from cold. Oppression of breathing. Rattling of mucus. Paroxysms of dyspnea with considerable secretion of mucus in larynx and trachea. Expectoration thick, heavy.

Rectum - Flatus with eructations. Copious, semi-liquid stool with much flatus. Bilious stools with aching in abdomen and burning in rectum.

Skin - Urticaria and other eruptions. Neurotic eruptions.

Throat - Contant disposition to clear throat. Hoarseness, excess of mucus in larynx. Dry, sore, worse swallowing. Raw and tender throat. Laryngismus.

RELATIONS - Arum Italicum. Arum maculatum. ***Compare:*** (1) Calad. in skin affections, Arum-t. (2) Useful after: Colch. and Ant-t. in laryngismus.

REFERENCES - Boericke. Clarke.

ARUM DRACUNCULUS

PHARMACY - arum-dru. Arum dracunculus. Dracunculus vulgaris. N. O. Araceae. Southern Europe. Tincture of root. ***Historical dose:*** Tincture and all potencies.

CLINICAL - Nettle rash. Pricking pains.

HERBAL - Arum-dru. is commonly cultivated in gardens. It has a fetid smell which is apt to cause headache. A styptic metallic taste at back of mouth was observed after pounding the root and tearing up leaves and stems.

HOMEOPATHIC - Pricking, mingled with intolerable itching in fingers, as if hand plunged among nettles. On rubbing the fingers together, a sensation follows, as if a vast number of stings were driven perpendicularly into them.

REFERENCES - Boericke. Clarke.

ARUM ITALICUM

PHARMACY - arum-i. Arum italicum. N. O. Araceae. Southern Europe. Tincture of root. ***Historical dose:*** Tincture and all potencies.

CLINICAL - Brain-fag. Colic. Fever. Headache. Hoarseness. Itching.

HOMEOPATHIC - Dr. Paul Pitet is the authority for this medicine. He used it for brain-fatigue with headache in occipital region.

The chief symptoms observed were headache, chiefly in occiput, worse in damp weather. Dull pain in brain from least intellectual effort. Colic in umbilical region with diarrhea. Smarting and tearing pains in rectum during stool. Burning behind sternum. Burning in fingers, worse by pressure.

Skin covered with miliary vesicles. Prickling and formication as from hundreds of needles on fingertips. The colic is worse by wine, brandy, coffee. Itching is worse 6 p.m. Hoarseness at 9 p.m. Damp weather worse. Unconquerable drowsiness in morning. Copious night sweat, especially on chest, smelling of ivy.

RELATIONS - ***Compare:*** (1) Aeth., Pic-ac. (2) Anac. - brain-fag.

REFERENCES - Boericke. Clarke.

ARUM MACULATUM

(Cuckoo-pint)

PHARMACY - arum-m. Arum maculatum. Cuckoo-pint. Arum vulgare. N. O. Araceae. Tincture of fresh tuber or corn. ***Historical dose:*** Tincture and all potencies.

CLINICAL - Ascarides. Asthma. Catarrh. Coryza. Hoarseness. Nasal, polyps. Prolapsed anus. Scorbutus. Swallowing, constant.

HOMEOPATHIC - Leading symptoms include inflammation and ulceration of mucus membranes. Violent irritation of nose and eyes. Pain left side of nose. Nasal irritation with polyps. Bleeding from mucus membranes and cavities. Violent convulsions. Great physical depression and lassitude. Irrepressible inclination to sleep after meals, the face becoming redder than usual during sleep.

Tongue swollen, pricking, stinging, burning, excoriated. Burning, stinging pains in mouth and lips ***"as with a hundred needles."*** Tickling and burning in throat. Sensation of a swelling in left side above larynx. Hoarseness. From abdomen ascending to chest an oppression over whole chest with hot breath, it then rose into throat. Burning, constricting pain in stomach. Ascaride. Prolapsed anus.

MIND - Anxiety and fear. Hypochondriacal. Melancholy and depressed. Taciturn.

Abdomen - Sensation of emptiness after breakfast in the abdomen, as after vomiting with contraction in the abdomen, as from anxiety and fear. Severe aching between the navel and the hip, especially when standing upright, lying on the side, or drawing a deep inspiration, with great sensitiveness of the part affected to external pressure.

Eyes - Aching in left eye.

Female - Menses profuse.

Head - Migraine. Headache in left temple and forehead. Headache with dyspepsia.

Kidneys - Clear, watery urine, exhaling a smell of burned horn and depositing a cloudy sediment.

Lungs - Phlegm in the respiratory organs. Violent tight cough with a scanty expectoration. Bloody expectoration. After much coughing, expectoration of mucus streaked with yellow.

Mouth - Gums bleed readily. Tongue so swollen he could not swallow.

Nose - Violent irritation of nose and eyes.

Rectum - Diarrhea. Ascarides. Prolapsed anus.

Skin - Redness and erosions of skin. Blisters. Eczema.

Sleep - Redness of face during sleep. Almost uncontrollable sleepiness, an hour after dinner.

Stomach - Pains in stomach on pressing it. Burning, constricting pains. Vomiting of blood.

Throat - Pain in the throat with difficult deglutition, as if from constriction in the esophagus with constant inclination to swallow after drinking, sensation as if something were attached to the epiglottis. Obstinate hoarseness. Pressure in the larynx. Tickling with inclination to cough.

RELATIONS - ***Antidoted by:*** Sweet oil, milk, butter. Gum relieves pungent effect on mouth. ***Compare:*** (1) Arum-t. Arums.

REFERENCES - Boericke.

ARUM TRIPHYLLUM

(Jack-in-the-Pulpit)

PHARMACY - arum-t. Arum triphyllum. Jack-in-the-Pulpit. Arisaema atrorubens. Indian turnip. N. O. Araceae. North and South America. Tincture of fresh tuber or corm. ***Historical dose:*** Tincture and all potencies.

CLINICAL - Allergies. ***Acrid, discharges***. Brain, inflammation. Clergyman's sore throat. Delirium. Diphtheria. Glandular, swellings. ***Hay fever.*** Headache. ***Hoarseness***. Jaw-joint painful. Laryngitis. Mouth, sore. Scarlatina. Tongue, cracked. Typhoid fever. Voice, hoarse.

HERBAL - Arum-t. is the most important of the Arums. Arum maculatum, Italicum, Dracontium, have the same action as the Triphyllum. They all contain an irritant poison, causing inflammation of mucus surfaces and destruction of tissue.

HOMEOPATHIC - Dr. Lippe, who is one of the greatest authorities on this remedy, said it should not be given low or repeated often. ***"Bores head in pillow"*** is an indication when the brain is involved. Kent pointed out that almost all the discharges are acrid and cause irritation of orifices.

The hoarseness is that of public speakers who, after long exertion, get cold (as from a draft) and suddenly are unable to finish (Rhus-t. the hoarseness is at the beginning and passes off by using the voice.).

Well marked irritating properties, excitable and irritable in mind and body. Raw, bloody surfaces appear on lips, on mouth, on nose, etc. Rawness with itching. ***Discharges are acrid***, causing ***painful sore, rawness and burning*** of parts.

Acrid, mucus membranes of mouth, ***throat*** and larynx. ***Irritating to the nose and throat***. Prominently affects the left side. Headache, worse from hot coffee, from too hot clothing.

Children lose their appetite, do not want to play, lose flesh, have headaches. ***Picks the nose and lips*** until they bleed. Corners of mouth sore, cracked and bleeding also, ***"picking ends of fingers"*** and ***"boring nose"*** Especially side of nose. Tongue cracked and bleeding. Urine scanty or suppressed. Bores head into the pillow. Jerking shooting pain.

Patient passes into unconsciousness and slides down in bed. This with its scarlet rash suggested its appropriateness in cases of scarlatina of malignant type in which it has met with great success. An indication of its curative action in scarlatina is the urine becoming more abundant and watery.

MIND - Restlessness, tossing about in bed. Nervous, bites nails until fingers bleed. Restlessness or irritability. Excessively cross and stubborn. Great delirium. Delirium, bores in nose, picks at one spot or at dry lips.

Forgetful. Absence of mind, giddy.

Abdomen - Sensation of emptiness after breakfast. Severe aching between the navel and the hip, with great sensitiveness of the part affected to external pressure. Contraction in the abdomen, as from anxiety and fear.

Back - Stiff-neck, with intolerable pressing headache. Pain in region of atlas vertebra, extending to right side. Sore, moist places on coccyx.

Chest - Raw feeling in chest. Lungs sore.

Eyes - Quivering of upper left eyelid. Heavy, sleepy. Aversion to light. Quivering of left upper lid. Catarrh of lachrymal sac, bores into side of nose.

Face - Face feels chapped, as if from cold wind, feels hot. Lips dry, swollen, cracked, corners of mouth sore, bleeding, cracked, picks them. Face swollen. Swelling of submaxillary glands.

Female - Cutting pain in either ovary. Menstrual blood darker. Menses checked for two months, returned.

Food - Loss of appetite.

Head - Bores head into pillow. Child puts hand on back of head and cries during headache. Headache from too warm clothing, from becoming hot and hot coffee. Violent headache, pressing on right or both sides, worse from hot coffee, better after dinner, and after breakfast. Head burning hot. Tinea capitis.

Kidneys - Very scanty secretion of urine. Uremia. Frequent discharge of abundant pale urine. Clear, watery urine and smelling like burnt horn, and depositing a cloudy sediment.

Lungs - Accumulation of mucus in trachea. Cough hurts the throat and annoys the patient. Voice, hoarse, squeaky or breaks. Hay asthma.

Male - Tearing pain in right testicle, sometimes extending to abdomen, comes and goes suddenly. Smarting at end of penis.

Modalities - Worse from over use of voice. ***Worse talking, singing.*** Worse from cold winds. ***Worse northwest wind***. Worse cold wet. Worse heat. Worse lying down.

Mouth - ***Raw feeling at roof and palate***. Lips chapped and burning. Lips dry, swollen, cracked corners of the mouth sore. ***Corners of mouth sore and cracked***. Picking lips until they bleed. Mouth painfully raw, sore inflamed. Aphthae. Saliva profuse, acrid, corroding.

Nose - Soreness of nostrils. ***Constant picking at nose until it bleeds*** or picking at lips, fingers, until it is sore, especially children. Nasal obstruction with fetid discharge, sneezing worse at night. Large scabs high up on right side of nose. ***Hay fever*** with pain over root of nose. Coryza, discharge blood-streaked, watery. ***Acrid, excoriating discharge,*** producing raw sores. Nose completely stopped with fluent, acrid discharge, ***must breathe through mouth***.

Rectum - Diarrhea, typhoid-like. Stools like corn meal. Stool dark brown, watery, thin, acrid. Thin feces escape from anus, and keep the parts raw and burning.

Skin - Dry heat of skin. Scarlet rash, ***raw, bloody surfaces*** anywhere. Itching of fingers and toes. Eruptions leave a brilliant red stain. Pemphigus. Impetigo contagiosa. Erythema of scarlet rash, skin peels afterwards. Itching of scarlet eruption.

Sleep - Sleeplessness from soreness of mouth or itching of skin. Starting during sleep.

Stomach - Sensation of emptiness, as after vomiting, with contraction.

Throat - Clergyman's sore throat. ***Hoarseness***. Laryngitis. Expectoration of much mucus. Voice uncertain, uncontrollable. Worse talking, singing. ***Constricted and swollen, burns, raw.*** Constant hawking. Raw, sore, painful on clearing or coughing, yet grasps and wants to scratch it. Swelling of glands on throat and neck.

Tongue - Tongue sore, red papillae elevated. Tongue red, sore, whole mouth raw. Tongue cracked and bleeding. Strawberry tongue.

Vertigo - Vertigo and fullness. Vertigo with absence of mind. Light-headed, sleepy.

COMMENTS - One of the first indications for this remedy is the appearance of raw, bloody surfaces, which may be on the lips, buccal cavity, nose, back of ear, etc. Burning in many parts, ear, lips, tongue, palate, throat, anus, lungs, upper arms.

Child has headache, puts hand on back of head and cries. A raw spot appears on the lip, corners of mouth, or on the nose. Emitting one drop of blood, urine scanty, this raw spot may occur on the hand when the child bores and digs at it. Dull headache, upper part feels cold, as if open and without covering.

Keynote irresistible desire to pick the nose (Cina), from inflammation of the nerve endings in the nose. Hay fever or coryza that leaves ulcers and sores on the upper lip. For hoarseness and laryngitis, "speaker's sore throat." Raw feeling in the palate and throat, burning.

RELATIONS - ***Antidoted by:*** Buttermilk, Lac-ac., Acet-ac., Puls. ***Compare:*** (1) Am-c., All-c. (2) The other Arums and Calad. (3) Ail. - scarlatina, depressing, stupid, drowsy sleep. (4) Cina - boring nose. (5) Am-c. - acrid discharge from nose in scarlatina, but right parotid more decidedly affected in Am-c., drowsiness is very marked. (6) Am-m. (scarlatina), Arg-n. (scarlatina, painful red blotches left side of tongue). (7) Ars., Canth., Caps. (8) Castor. - nasal discharge watery and acrid but with violent tearing pain at root of nose. (9) Caust., All-c., Crocus - elevated papillae, but tongue white. (10) Hep., Hydr-ac., Iod., Kali-i., Lach., Lyc., Merc., Mez., Mur-ac., Nit-ac., Phyt., Sang., Sil., Sulph. (11) Useful after: Hep., Nit-ac., Caust., Seneg. ***Complementary:*** Nit-ac. ***Incompatible:*** Calad.

REFERENCES - Boericke. Clarke.

ARUNDO MAURITANICA

(Reed)

PHARMACY - arund. Arundo mauritanica. Reed. Italian grass. Arundo donax. N. O. Gramineae. Mediterranean. Tincture of the root sprouts. ***Historical dose:*** Tincture and all potencies.

CLINICAL - ***Allergies.*** Catarrh. Coryza. Coughs. Dentition. Diarrhea. Dyspnea. Ear, discharge. Edema. ***Hay fever.*** Hair, loss. ***Itching.*** Nasal, discharges. Ophthalmia. Pustules. Scrofulous, ophthalmia. ***Sneezing.*** Stomach, pain. Urine, deposits. Vertigo.

HOMEOPATHIC - Arundo is a reedy grass and the tincture is made from the root-shoots. It has not been tested much clinically, but its chief sphere has been proved to be in catarrhal conditions. Chagon is the authority for the pathogenesis.

Hay fever, beginning with ***burning and itching of palate and conjunctiva.*** Catarrhal states. Constant watery diarrhea of nursing or teething children. Urine deposits much red sand. Mouth excoriated. Thirst. Coryza and snuffing. Pain in liver. Purulent discharge from the ear.

MIND - Dullness of mind. Indifference to painful sensations. Absence of ideas. Anxiety better open air. Anxiety from coughing. Anxiety from accumulation of mucus in bronchi. Lascivious fancies. Laughs easily, a stupid hilarity.

Abdomen - Movement as from something alive in abdomen. Flatulence, pain at pubic region. Pain in liver. Pricking in spleen. Acute pain at umbilicus.

Back - Acute pain under left scapula. Jerking in neck, crawling on left side of it.

Breasts - Excessive secretion of milk causes pain in left breast. Burning and pain in nipples.

Chest - Pricking in chest.

Ears - Burning and itching in auditory canals. Eczema behind ears. Purulent discharge from ears. Sound of little bells in ears.

Eyes - Ophthalmia in children. Blepharitis. Pricking, itching, burning in conjunctiva. Undulating luminous openings appear wherever he looks. Fluttering luminous objects. Cannot look up.

Face - Erysipelas on right cheek. Pricking in point of chin.

Female - Early, profuse, long-lasting menses, dark, clotted blood. Sexual desire with vaginal itching. Violent desire for sex or aversion to it. Pains start from left side of jaw, extending to shoulders and loins and finally settling on pubis, burning like fire.

Food - Want of appetite. Constant thirst, after waking in morning. Thirst during fever. Food tastes insipid. Water has a bad taste. Craving for acids.

Head - Itching, falling off of hair. Hair falls off entirely in children. Roots of hairs painful. Pustules. Pain in occiput, extends to right ciliary region. Deep seated pain in sides of head. Painful undulation in frontal region. Scurf.

Heart - Pricking in arteries. Abnormal movements of heart. Oppression of heart.

Kidneys - Burning on urinating. After urinating, weight, burning, and itching in urethra. Red sediment (Lyc.), red sand in urine.

Limbs - Itching, burning. Edema of hands and feet. Pain in limbs as if tightly bandaged. Burning and swelling of soles. Copious and offensive sweat of feet.

Lungs - Accumulation of mucus in bronchi causes anxiety. Catarrhal cough. Dyspnea, cough, bluish expectoration. Sputa at first bluish, then white, and alternates. After expectorating, bruised feeling in pit of throat. After cough, burning in the epigastrium, with the larynx obstructed.

Male - Pain in spermatic cord after sex. Sexual desire, lascivious ideas, frequent erections. Difficult breathing after sex.

Mouth - Bleeding of gums. Ulcers and exfoliations in the commissures. Fissures in tongue. Pain in sublingual glands. Salivation. Burning and itching of palate.

Nose - Hay fever begins with burning and ***itching of palate*** and conjunctiva. ***Annoying itching in the nostrils and roof of the mouth*** (Wye.). Coryza, loss of smell (Nat-m.). ***Sneezing, itching of nostrils***.

Perspiration - Tendency to sweat. Motion causes profuse sweat.

Rectum - Burning at anus. Constant diarrhea of nursing or teething children (Cham., Calc-p.). Greenish stools. Stools at first hard, soon become loose. Stools followed by burning at anus. Pricking at anus. Hemorrhoids and prolapsed rectum.

Skin - Eczema, itching and crawling, especially of chest, upper limbs. Fissures in fingers and heels.

Stomach - Coldness in stomach. Longing for acids. Wants to belch but cannot. Burning in esophagus.

Throat - Globus hystericus. Pit of throat as if bruised after expectoration. Burning and pain on swallowing. Obstruction prevents swallowing.

Vertigo - Vertigo on getting out of bed.

COMMENTS - Hay fever remedy, keynote itching in the nostrils. Loss of smell (Puls., Sabad.). Itching of the upper palate, raw and sore, try to scratch palate with their tongue (Wye.).

Burning itching in auditory canals, coincides with pain in sublingual glands. The inflammation of ears begins with shooting pains in concha, extends to external meatus, finally with itching and discharge of blood. Hay fever. Pain at root of nose.

Coryza with snuffling. In the beginning, water runs from nose, later, green mucus and thick, white, slimy masses, with sneezing, pieces of indurated greenish mucus.

RELATIONS - ***Compare:*** (1) Anthroxantum. (2) Anan., Lolium. (3) All-c., Sil., Sulph., Calc., Lyc., Sabad., Psor.

REFERENCES - Boericke. Clarke. Murphy.

ASAFOETIDA

(Gum of the Stinkasand)

PHARMACY - asaf. Asafoetida. Gum of the Stinkasand. Ferula asafoetida. Narthex Asafoetida. Scorodosma foetida. N. O. Umbelliferae. Tincture of the gum resin, obtained by incision from the living root. ***Historical dose:*** Tincture and all potencies.

CLINICAL - Asthma. Belching. ***Bone, diseases.*** Breast-feeding. Chorea. ***Decay, bones. Diarrhea.*** Dyspepsia Fainting, easily. ***Flatulence. Globus, hystericus***. Headaches. Heart, disorders. ***Hypersensitiveness. Hysteria.*** Iritis. Mercury, poisoning. Neuralgias. Obesity. Orbital, neuralgia. Ozaena. Syphilis. Tympanitis. Ulcers. Whitlow.

HERBAL - The fetid smell of Asafoetida may be regarded as one of its *"herbal signatures."*

HOMEOPATHIC - Fetid discharge from the nose, bones affected. ***Offensive discharges.*** Watery stools of most disgusting odor, profuse and greenish, fetid flatus. Belchings smelling like garlic. Flatulent hysteria. Characteristic sensitiveness to touch.

Flatulence and spasmodic contractions of stomach and esophagus with ***reverse peristalsis***, everything comes up, nothing goes down. Excessive abdominal distention and sensation as if everything in the abdomen would burst through the mouth. After belching of wind, strong rancid taste in mouth. Sinking sensation at epigastrium, worse 11 a.m. Hysteria from suddenly suppressed discharges.

Deficient milk with over sensitiveness after confinement. Decay of bones, especially in the syphilitic organism, with ***extreme sensitiveness*** and terrible throbbing, nightly pains. Glands all over the body are hot and throb. Pain, as if a nail or plug driven in.

MIND - Dissatisfied with oneself. Irritable, complains of her troubles. ***Irritability during menses, alternating with indifference.*** Changing moods, fits of joy with burst of laughter. Fickle, cannot persevere in anything. Wants now one thing, then another.

Great excitability and sensitiveness, yet with complete indifference to everything. Ill-humor. Apprehensive. Fear arising from abdomen. Fear from stomach. Apprehension of dying. Fears paralysis or softening of brain.

Hysterical and hypochondriacal. ***Magnifies her symptoms.*** Craves sympathy. ***Hysteria from suddenly suppressed discharges.*** Hysteria with much trouble about throat or esophagus, clutches throat. Walks hither and thither.

Oversensitiveness, mental and physical. Faints from emotional excitement or disturbance. Faintness from noise or from being in crowded streets. Fainting during pain. Faints when he thinks that he has taken medicine. Faints almost without cause in a closed room.

Abdomen - Great distention. Flatulence, sudden, pushing upwards. Flatuent colic with abdominal pulsations. ***Hysterical flatulence.*** Bowels seem knotted. Flatus passing upwards, none downwards. Heat in spleen and abdomen.

Bones - Periosteum painful, swollen, enlarged. Decay of bones and deep ulcerations. Ulcers affecting bones, thin, ichorous pus. Fits of hard, violent throbbing. Pains are pressive, sharp, stitching, extending outwards, associated with numbness. Pains change place and are better by touch. Aching, boring in bones. Darting pain and decay in bones.

Breasts - Breasts turgid with milk, when not pregnant. ***Deficient milk with oversensitiveness.*** Galactagogue, in sensitive, hysterical women.

Causations - Ill effects of checked skin eruptions or suppressed discharges. Neuralgia of stump after operations. Nervous disorders from suppressed skin eruptions. Most pains are accompanied by numbness in the affected parts.

Chest - ***Spasmodic tightness***, as if lungs could not be fully expanded. Palpitation more like a tremor.

Constitutions - Suited to nervous and hysterical people, phlegmatic, scrofulous and syphilitic who have taken much Mercury. Though the patient is of full habit and stout aspect yet he is intolerably nervous and ***oversensitive***. Clumsy children. Obesity.

Ears - Offensive otorrhea with boring pains in mastoid bone. Mastoid disease with pain in temporal region with ***pushing out sensation***. Offensive, purulent discharge. Hardness of hearing.

Eyes - Orbital neuralgia, better pressure and from rest. Iritis and intra-ocular inflammations with boring, throbbing pains at night. Stitches under left frontal eminences. Boring pains in and around eyes. Syphilitic iritis. Superficial corneal ulcer with digging pains, worse at night. Eyelids stick to balls. Numbness about eyes, ulceration of cornea. Syphilitic iritis.

Face - Puffy, purple as if heated. Small tubercles in the cheek. Swelling of the lower lip. Numbness of bones.

Female - Menses too early too scanty last for a short time. ***Irritability during menses, alternating with indifference***

Bearing down in the genital especially while riding in a carriage. Labor-like pains in uterine region, with cutting and bearing down. Leucorrhea, profuse, greenish, thin offensive. Swelling and inflammation of genitals. Excited sexual desire. Uterine ulcer, sensitive and painful. Miscarriages.

Food - Ravenous hunger. Disgust for all food. Aversion to beer. Beer tastes slimy. Desire for strong, cooling food. Desire for wine. Fat food causes indigestion. Heat in face after eating. Diarrhea after eating. Want of thirst. Fever without thirst.

Head - Headaches in occipital region, better stool. Irritable, complains of her troubles, sensitive. ***Pressive pain from within outward.*** Boring pain above eyebrows.

Heart - Palpitations more like a tremor. Heart seems full, distended. Reflex heart symptoms of nervous origin.

Kidneys - Urine brown and of pungent odor. Spasms in bladder during and after urination.

Limbs - Pain and tenderness in tibia intolerable, worse night. Cannot work on account of backache. Cold swelling around ankles. Convulsive tremors better by holding.

Lungs - Asthmatic attacks at least once in a day, worse bodily exertion, sex, satisfying meals. Spasms of the glottis, alternating with contraction of finger and toes.

Male - Needle like stitches in penis. Fainting after seminal emissions.

Modalities - Many symptoms appear while sitting and are better in open air. Touch relieves pain in head, on touch pains cease or change place. Scratching relieves itching. Worse at night. Worse left side. Worse during rest. Worse warm applications, warm wraps. ***Worse after suppressions.*** Worse mercury. Worse noise. Worse sitting. Worse after eating or drinking.

Mouth - Greasy, rancid taste. Constant chewing with frothy saliva from mouth, chorea.

Nose - Offensive discharge from the nose. Syphilitic ozaena with very offensive purulent discharge. ***Decay of nasal bones*** (Aur.). Tension over nasal bones with numbness.

Perspiration - Cold, moist skin. Cold sweat on limbs. Sweats during vertigo. Sweats with drowsiness.

Rectum - Distended, griping with hunger. Obstinate constipation. Pain in perineum, as if something dull pressed out. ***Diarrhea, extremely offensive with meteorism*** and regurgitation of food. Diarrhea, stools dark, watery with disgusting odor. Only mucus is passed.

Skin - Suppressed skin symptoms produce nervous disorders. Itching, better scratching, ulcers painful on edges. Eruptions of vesicles. Bluish ulcers with highly sensitive edges. Itching better scratching. Old scars turn purple and ulcerate. Foul burrowing pus.

Stomach - Explosive belchings smelling like garlic and rancid in taste. Violent gastralgia, cutting and burning in stomach and region of diaphragm. Great difficulty in bringing up flatus. ***Flatulence and regurgitation of liquids.*** Sensation of emptiness and weakness with distention and beating in the stomach and abdomen. Forcible eructation of gas. Gurgling and rolling of flatus, which escapes afterwards with loud and difficult eructation. ***Pulsation in the pit of stomach,*** perceptible to the hand or even visible.

Temperature - Chills runs over body. Chills with coldness and dryness of skin. Chills every day between 3 p.m. and 4 p.m. Coldness and trembling. Chill alternating with heat. Chills during faintness. Heat of face after dinner. Fever with anxiety and sleepiness. Fever without thirst. Heat in toes. Heat of face, with cold hands and feet, and chills of back.

Throat - Sensation as if peristaltic motion were reversed and esophagus were driven from stomach to throat. Sensation as if a ball rises in throat. ***Globus hystericus***. Everything presses towards throat. Spasms of gullet and stomach.

Vertigo - Vertigo with violent pressing in head. Vertigo with vanishing of sight. Vertigo with sweat on forehead and limbs.

COMMENTS - Asafoetida has hiccough-like contractions of diaphragm. Griping pain below navel while standing. Heat in spleen and abdomen. Stitches in right hypochondrium towards the diaphragm.

Affects the left side generally, left side of abdomen, left hypochondrium, left side of neck and nape, left arm, left leg. Hysterical restlessness and anxiety. Eyes inflamed, dry sensation, better in open air.

Characteristic bruised, sore and sensitive bones of the orbits. Iritis after abuse of mercury (Merc. has less sensitiveness). Decay of bones, bone diseases. Multiple nodes on the roof of mouth, discolored, bone deeply involved.

Periosteal disorders ending in ulcers which are so sensitive that no dressing is tolerated. Pressing pains in various parts, especially pressure from within outwards, worse in room, better in open air.

Used for foul flatulence where it is a social, cultural problem. Lingering odor. Regurgitation and bad-smelling and bad-tasting burps. Belchings, the taste stays in their mouth for hours or even days. Used in tincture for giardia and parasites with the symptom of foul smelling flatus.

RELATIONS - ***Antidotes:*** China, Merc. ***Antidoted by:*** Puls., Caust., Camph., Chin., Merc., Valer. ***Compare:*** (1) Aur, Chin, Lach, Merc, Sumb, Valer. (2) Compare family relations: Am-c., Cic., Con. (3) ***Similar to:*** Arg-n. - better open air, Aur. - bone diseases, iritis, Castor., Chin., Caust., Crot-t. (whooping cough), Hep. - sensitiveness round ulcers, faints from pains, (4) .Mosch., Mang. and Kali-i. (5) nodes: Mang., bluish, Kali-i., pink, pain unbearable. Asaf. the nodes are multiple and discolored. (6) Ign., Merc., Phos., Puls., Thuj., Valer. ***Complementary:*** Caust. Puls.

REFERENCES - Boericke. Clarke.

ASARUM CANADENSE

(Wild Ginger)

PHARMACY - asar-c. Asarum canadense. Wild ginger. N. O. Aristolochiaceae. Tincture of the rhizome. ***Historical dose:*** Tincture and all potencies.

HOMEOPATHIC - Colds followed by amenorrhea or gastro-enteritis. Suppressed colds. Headache from suppressed nasal catarrh. Watery, irritating discharge from the nose. Frequent and profuse menses. Miscarriage in the early months. Relieves excessive pain in labor.

REFERENCES - Boericke. Hale.

ASARUM EUROPAEUM

(European Snake-root)

PHARMACY - asar. Asarum europaeum. European Snake-root. Asarum officinale. Asarabacca. Hazelwort. Wild Nard. Wild Nath. N. O. Aristolochiacae. Mountainous woods in Europe. Tinctures of root and whole fresh plant. ***Historical dose:*** Tincture and all potencies.

CLINICAL - Alcoholism. Anus, prolapsed. Asthenopia. Catarrhs. Cough. Deafness. Diarrhea. Dysmenorrhea. Eyes, affections, operations. Faintness. Fidgets. Headache. ***Hypersensitive.*** Hysteria. Leucorrhea. Levitation, sensation. Prolapsed rectum. Typhus. Vertigo. Vomiting.

HOMEOPATHIC - Before Hahnemann's time, Asarum was little known except as an emetic. Hahnemann's proving brought to light some unique characteristics, including that cold air and cold washing ameliorates many of the symptoms.

With a single dose of Asar. 200c, Clarke cured a case of sub-acute inflammation of eyes and lids which had lasted some months after an attack of influenza, the symptoms were better in open air and by washing in cold water.

Deschere reported a case of dysmenorrhea in a nervous, fidgety woman of twenty-seven, who had intense backache during first two days, so severe that the she could not move. It often rose to the dorsal region, when it would take away her breath. Cured with Asar. 50c, one dose every evening.

Hypersensitiveness of nerves. Scratching on silk or linen, rattle of paper is unbearable, even the idea that someone might scratch with fingertip or nail produces a disagreeable thrill, through him. Nervous affections, loss of vital energy with ***excessive nerve sensitivity. Always feels cold.*** Cold shivers from any emotion. Sensation of lightness of the limbs.

Pains and spasmodic muscular actions. Useful for the darting pains remaining after operations on the eyes. Nervous deafness and asthenopia. Tension and contractive sensations. Pressure, tension and contractive sensation are also leading features, patient thinks that his whole body or single parts were being pressed together. Mucus discharges are glairy. For alcoholics.

MIND - Inability to think. Deficiency of ideas better vomiting. Thoughts vanish with drawing pressure in forehead. Thoughts vanish as when falling asleep. Vacant feeling on attempting to concentrate mind. No desire to do anything, from stupid feeling in head.

Nervous irritability and exaltation. ***Sensibility increased, even from mere imagination.*** Feeling of lightness as if floating, when walking in the open air. Delusion he is hovering in air like a spirit. ***Thinks she is gliding through the air*** when she walks.

Oversensitive to slightest noise. Cold shivers from any emotion is also a marked symptom. Ill-humor. Sadness, with weeping. ***Nerves on edge.*** Great merriness alternating with occasional momentary quiet or gloominess. Aversion to sex, kissing and embracing. Wrings hands. Very sensitive to violence.

Abdomen - Oppression around navel, three or four times after each meal, lasting one hour. Pain in region of descending colon, with discharge of stringy mucus.

Back - Paralytic pain in muscles of nape of neck. Weakness with staggering.

Chest - Sharp pressure in region of last ribs as with the back of a knife. Pain around both lungs as if they were constricted by a wire. Frequent stitches in both lungs during inspiration.

Constitutions - Nervous constitutions. It is suitable to people of sedentary habits who shrink from cold or always feel cold. Literary, sedentary people who are sick and chilly.

Ears - Painfully sensitive hearing. Sensation as if plugged up with coryza. Sensation as if skin were stretched over external ear (right). Catarrh with deafness. Heat of external ear. Noises.

Eyes - Watering and burning of the eyes. Feel stiff, burn, feel cold. Better in cold air or water, worse sunlight and wind. Asthenopia. Darting pains in the eye after operations.

Face - Warm feeling in face better cold washing. Burning, stinging, on cheeks. Cutting pain with cramp at joint of lower jaw. Dryness of inner side of lower lip.

Female - Menses too early, long lasting, black. Violent pain in small of back. Tenacious, yellow leucorrhea. Violent pain in small of back at the appearance of menses, scarcely permitting her to breathe, worse motion. Threatened miscarriage from excessive sensibility of nerves.

Food - Want of appetite, even nauseated by food. ***Craving for alcohol.*** Smoking tobacco tastes bitter.

Head - Compressive headache. Tension of whole scalp, cannot bear combing, hair painful (Chin.). Coryza with sneezing.

Limbs - Lightness of all the limbs. Gurgling sensation in patella. Weakness with staggering.

Lungs - Nervous, hacking cough. Short respiration. Asthmatic breathing, worse odors and cold. Both lungs as if constricted by wire. Stitches in larynx better cough.

Modalities - Better from cold bathing of face. Better washing. Better in damp and wet weather. Better on wetting affected parts. Worse in cold dry weather. ***Worse from penetrating noise.*** Worse emotions. Worse retching.

Mouth - Accumulation of cold watery saliva in the mouth with nausea. Tobacco tastes bitter when smoking. Clean tongue. Disgusting taste.

Nose - Coryza with sneezing. Sharp aching pain above root of nose. Bloody mucus from nose. Dry coryza, left nostril stopped up. Tickling in nose, causing a sneeze, and discharge of clear fluid. Violent sneezing.

Perspiration - Sweat is sour, easily excited. Sweats easily, especially on upper body. Sour sweat in axillae. Sweats after lying down in evening.

Rectum - ***Strings*** of odorless, yellow mucus pass from bowels. Diarrhea of tough mucus. ***Undigested food in stools***. Stools worse after eating or drinking. Gelatinous or shreddy mucus in stool. Mucus colitis. Prolapsed rectum.

Sleep - Great drowsiness by day. Short breath by night. Frequent yawning, great drowsiness. Nightly vexatious dreams, about humiliations. Restless sleep.

Stomach - Flatulence, belching and vomiting. Horrible feeling at epigastrium on waking in the morning, alcoholics. Nausea, worse after eating. Accumulation of cold, watery saliva. Violent empty retching. Violent vomiting with diarrhea and violent colic.

Temperature - Chilliness, single parts get icy cold. Cold feeling not better by covering or heat of room.

Vertigo - Great faintness. Elderly people with weak constitutions, who get dizzy easily. Lightness as if floating. ***Sensation that she is gliding through the air,*** when she walks.

COMMENTS - Sensation as though whole body or single parts were being pressed together. Pain as from contraction in forehead, temples and behind ear with watering and burning of the eyes, worse afternoon, better when sitting and by washing. Pressure, tension and contractive sensations. Plugged sensation.

Sensation of skin stretched over right external ear. Deafness. Eyes inflamed, bleary, staring. Weak sight, worse bright light. When reading, sensation as if eyes would be pressed asunder. Accumulation of cold watery saliva in mouth. Hunger in early morning. Constant nausea. Vomiting with diarrhea and violent colic. Stool of jelly-like mucus.

Menstrual colic. Headache before and after menses. Violent pain in small of back which scarcely permits her to breathe, at beginning of menses. Heat, especially of face and in palms of hands. When retching, all symptoms worse except dullness of the head, which is better.

Vertigo as if floating, or can't feel the ground, particularly in the elderly (Calc.). Can get faint or lose sensations in their legs. Sensitive to odors and noises. Can crave alcohol. Also a geriatric remedy for weak constitutions, easily dizzy (Ambr., Con.).

RELATIONS - ***Antidotes:*** Camph., vinegar and vegetables acids. ***Compare:*** (1) Acon., Arg-n, Castor, Ther. (2) Aloe. - stringy stools, Camph. - cholerine, Cupr., Hep., Ip. - cholerine, Merc. - stringy stools. (3) Nux-v., Phos., Podo., Puls. and Sul-ac. - stringy stools, Sep., Stram., Tab. and Verat. - cholerine. Asaf. - over-sensitiveness. (4) Sticta, Calc., Cann-i., Gels., Thuj., Ol-j. - levitation. Mosch., Tarent., Meph., Zinc. - fidgety feet. (5) Ip., especially in diarrhea, Sil., Nux-v., China. ***Complementary:*** Caust, Puls, Sil. ***Followed well by:*** Bism.

REFERENCES - Boericke. Clarke.

ASBESTOS

(Silicate Mineral Fiber)

PHARMACY - asbes. Asbestos. Silicate mineral fiber. Asbestos is a term applied to some mineral silicates present in a fiber form. There are many members of the family: common among these are blue asbestos (crocidolite) white (chrysotile) and brown or grey asbestos (amosite). Other forms of asbestos include anthophyllite, and tremolite, which are present in some commercial talcs. Trituration. ***Historical dose:*** All potencies.

CLINICAL - Asbestosis. Anemia. Ascites. Bronchitis. Cancer. ***Dyspnea.*** Emphysema. Fibrosis. Hoarseness. Lung, cancer. ***Mesothelioma.*** Nausea. Pleural, effusion. Pneumonia.

HOMEOPATHIC - Asbestos is a mineral fiber that was commonly used in a variety of building construction materials for insulation and as fire retardant. The most dangerous asbestos fibers are too small to be visible.

Once they are inhaled, the asbestos fibers can remain and accumulate in the lungs. Breathing high levels of the fibers can lead to an increased risk of lung cancer, mesothelioma (a cancer of the chest and abdominal linings), and asbestosis (irreversible lung scarring that can be fatal). Symptoms of these diseases do not show up until many years after exposure.

The most common symptoms of asbestos exposure are shortness of breath, coughing, and chest pain. ***A dry crackling sound in the lungs while inhaling.*** Pains in the lower back or sides of the chest. Persistent coughs, loss of appetite, weight loss, and recurrent bronchitis or pneumonia.

Less common symptoms may include fever or night sweats. Ascites or fluid buildup in the abdomen, weight loss, nausea, difficulty with bowel movements, anemia, and foot swelling.

Abdomen - Ascites. Peritoneal cancer.

Back - Pains in lower back.

Chest - Pains in sides of chest.

Lungs - Breathing difficulties. Cancer. Shortness of breath, which increases over time. Increased sputum. Chronic and persistent coughs. Coughing up blood. Scarring of lungs and pleura. Pleural effusion.

Food - Loss of appetite. Weight loss and fatigue. Nausea.

Throat - Hoarseness.

COMMENTS - Asbestos has been known and used for as long as 4,500 years. Many centuries ago, Finnish peasants mixed it in pottery and sealed cracks in their log huts with it. The ancient Romans wove asbestos fibers into fabrics to make towels, nets and even head coverings for women.

In the early 1900's, doctors in Europe knew that asbestos workers were dying from respiratory ailments. In 1924, Dr. W. E. Cooke reported in the British Medical Journal cases of pulmonary fibrosis (asbestosis) in workers employed in the asbestos industry.

RELATIONS - ***Compare:*** (1) Sil. (2) Cob., Rado.

REFERENCES - Murphy.

ASCLEPIAS CORNUTI

(Milkweed)

PHARMACY - asc-c. Asclepias cornuti. Milkweed. Silkweed. Asclepias syriaca. N. O. Asclepiadacae. North America. Tincture of root. ***Historical dose:*** Tincture and all potencies.

CLINICAL - Allergies. Bronchitis. Catarrhal fever. Diaphoresis. Dropsy. Dysmenorrhea. Hay fever. ***Headaches.*** Indigestion. Influenza. Menses, scanty. Miscarriage. ***Neuralgia.*** Pleurisy. Rheumatism. Uremia. Uterine pains.

HOMEOPATHIC - Asclepias cornuti is a remedy for dropsy, hepatic, kidney or after scarlet fever. It causes diaphoresis and augments the urinary secretion. Dropsy after heart disease. Uremia. Intermittent, pressing-down uterine pains.

Acts especially on the nervous system and urinary organs. Nervous headache, as if a sharp instrument were thrust through from one temple to the other with vomiting, followed by sweating or profuse urination. Belching of food with its proper taste.

Influenza, catarrhal fever, bronchitis, hay fever. Headache from checked sweat or retention of effete matters. Uterine pains are intermittent, pressing with threatened miscarriage. Coldness of surface after vomiting. Diaphoresis, profuse sweat. Acute rheumatism confined to large joints with much pain and swelling.

Abdomen - Flatuent colic. Rumbling in abdomen, as if diarrhea would set in. Pain and soreness in abdomen, with or without distension. Stitching and aching pains, in left side of abdomen.

Back - Cutting and aching about lowest dorsal vertebra.

Female - Intermittent, bearing-down, labor-like pains, pressing from sacrum to hypogastrium. Scanty flow. Suppression of menses.

Food - Increased appetite, vomiting and headache with constipation. Great appetite even a few hours after a meal.

Head - Constriction across forehead. ***Feels as if a sharp instrument were thrust through from temple to temple.***

Head - Nervous headache after suppressed perspiration, followed by ***increased urine with increase of specific gravity***. Headache from retention of effete matters in system.

Heart - Action of heart lessened, pulse slow. Feeble pulse after vomiting.

Kidneys - Ardor urinae. Increased flow of urine. Pale-colored urine with light specific gravity. Increase of solid matters in urine.

Lungs - Increase of the bronchial secretions. Burning and tickling in fauces. Pain in left side of chest on deep inspiration (pleurisy).

Male - Tickling sensation at the end of the penis.

Perspiration - Diaphoresis, profuse sweat.

Rectum - Diarrhea with nausea and vomiting with excoriation of the anus. Copious stools of soft, fluid consistence, yellowish in color and attended with some griping pain. Constipation, pain in right side, lower limbs, loss of appetite.

Sleep - Drowsy, sleepiness, hard sleep during the night.

Stomach - Excessive nausea with violent headache, violent vomiting and retching. Severe and long-continued vomiting. Sensation of rawness in the stomach and pain.

Temperature - Coldness of the surface of the skin and feeble pulse.

Throat - Burning and tickling in the fauces with nausea and headache.

Tongue - Tongue covered with a white fur.

Vertigo - Vertigo, dullness and stupidity. Vertigo with headache.

RELATIONS - ***Compare:*** (1) Cimic., Bry., Colch., Asc-t. (2) Asclepias Vincetoxicum.

REFERENCES - Boericke. Clarke.

ASCLEPIAS INCARNATA
(Swamp Milkweed)

PHARMACY - asc-i. Asclepias incarnata. Swamp milkweed. N. O. Asclepiadaceae. North America. Tincture of the rhizome. ***Historical dose:*** Tincture and all potencies.

CLINICAL - Amenorrhea. Asthma. Catarrh. Diarrhea. Dropsy. Dysentery. Dyspnea. Leucorrhea. Rheumatism. Syphilis. Worms.

HERBAL - Asclepias Incarnata is diuretic, stomachic, anthelmintic, and in very large doses, emetic. When it is used anthelmintic, the powder of the root has been employed, in doses of ten to twenty grains per day.

As a diuretic in dropsy this herb is of considerable value. It strengthens the heart. Often relieves the heart distress caused by infiltration of the tissues, especially the difficult breathing.

HOMEOPATHIC - Catarrhal discharges. Dropsy with dyspnea. Catarrhal inflammation of the respiratory organs. Dysentery and diarrhea. Leucorrhea. Rheumatism from cold. Dropsies.

COMMENTS - Dr. Tully, of New Haven, has found it useful in catarrh, asthma, syphilis, rheumatism, and worms. Dr. Fowler, of New York, speaks in the most unequivocal terms of its virtues in amenorrhea. Dr. A. C. Jones, of Philadelphia, has given it in several cases of suppressed menstruation, without benefit. Dr. Hale, of Michigan, thinks it is the Asclepias syriaca which is so useful in amenorrhea, and not the Asclepias incarnata.

REFERENCES - Boericke.

ASCLEPIAS TUBEROSA

(Pleurisy Root)

PHARMACY - asc-t. Asclepias tuberosa. Pleurisy root. Butterfly-weed. N. O. Asclepiadacae. North America. Tincture of fresh root. ***Historical dose:*** Tincture and all potencies.

CLINICAL - Alopecia. Asthma. Bilious fever. ***Bronchitis.*** Catarrh. Chancre. Colic. Coughs. Diarrhea. Dyspnea. ***Dysentery.*** Flatulence. Headaches. Heart disorders. ***Influenza.*** Marsh, fever. Ophthalmia. Pericarditis. ***Pleurisy.*** Pleurodynia. ***Pleuro-pneumonia***. ***Pneumonia***. Rheumatism. Scrofula. Syphilis.

HERBAL - Asc-t. is said to be diaphoretic and expectorant, without being stimulant. In large doses, it is often a cathartic. It is thought, by the herbal doctors, to act prominently on the cutaneous system, stimulating the capillary circulation, promoting diaphoresis.

HOMEOPATHIC - Asclepias tuberosa has been used for ***bronchitis and pleurisy***. Marked action on the chest muscles, which has been verified. Also effective in autumn dysentery with painful diarrhea, griping and tenesmus.

Increases the secretions of skin, serous and mucus membranes. Catarrhal states from cold and damp weather. ***Bronchitis and pleurisy***. Pains in lungs better bending forward. Stitches in left side shooting over to right and up to left shoulder. Profuse perspiration in ***pneumonia*** and ***pleuro-pneumonia***.

A general eliminative remedy, acting specially on the sweat glands. ***Influenza*** with pleuritic pains. Cutting pain behind sternum intercostal spaces near sternum tender to pressure. ***Catarrhal complaints from cold and damp weather.*** Bilious marsh fever on rice plantations. High fever with hot sweat.

Sick headache with flatulence in stomach and bowels. Dyspepsia. Sensitive to tobacco. Unfit for business because of pain in bowels and frequent stools. Irritation of larynx with huskiness, grip with pleuritic pain. Diarrhea or rheumatic conditions. Muscular and joint rheumatism with stitching pains, dark red urine and hot, perspiring skin.

MIND - Dullness of mind with difficult thinking. Languid and dull all day both in body and mind. Memory weak. Mood changes, without any cause. Cheerful mood. Excessive dejection. Fretful and peevish.

Abdomen - Flatulence after meals. Colic pains from flatulence. Colic on going upstairs. Rumbling in the bowels with uneasiness, or sharp, cutting pains and soreness. Burning borborygmi. Dull pain in bowels on pressure. Emission of fetid flatulence.

Back - Stiff-neck on waking. Sharp pains in back and between the shoulders. Pains shooting from left chest into left shoulder. Sharp pain in loins near sacrum, lumbago.

Breasts - Sharp pains shooting from left nipple downward, with stiffness of left side of neck. Pain beneath left nipple with palpitations.

Chest - Warm feeling in chest. ***Pleurisy.*** Pleurodynia. Acute pleuritic pain in right side, with dry, hacking cough, and scanty mucus expectoration. Chest pains better bending forward, worse lying, breathing. Pains worse 4 a.m. and 4 p.m. Spaces between ribs close to sternum tender. Pain in lower chest, diaphragm.

Constitutions - Hydrogenoid type, which corresponds to catarrhal complaints, worse from cold and damp weather.

Eyes - Eyes look dull, fatigued, and heavy, as after a long illness. Ophthalmia, with itching and pain in eyes. Feeling of sand in the eyes. Vision disturbed, large spots before the eyes.

Face - Hippocratic face after violent diarrhea. Yellow complexion. Vesicles on lips. Itching of lips.

Female - Profuse menses. Menorrhagia with violent bearing down pain.

Food - Loss of appetite, especially in morning. Insatiable hunger. Sensitive to tobacco.

Head - Headache better after footbath. Headache in the morning on rising. Headache pressing deeply on the base of the skull. Pain in the forehead from coughing. Alopecia.

Heart - Pericardial effusion. Constrictive pain in the heart. Tenderness to pressure over heart. Sharp pains, like pricking of a needle in region of heart. Pulse slightly accelerated.

Kidneys - Sharp pain in urethra, excoriation of glans penis in several places with bloody and purulent secretion. Urine very red, looks as if blood were in it.

Limbs - Rheumatic pain in all the joints. Rheumatic pains that affect the body diagonally, or left upper and right lower or the opposite. Pains near wrists. Joints give sensations as if adhesions being broken up on bending. Itching of thighs and buttocks but no eruption. Pain in right hip. Corns painful.

Lungs - Short of breath and weak on walking. ***Bronchitis and pleurisy***. Dry cough, throat constricted, causes pain in head and abdomen.

Lungs - ***Breathing painful***, at base of left lung. Humid asthma, worse after eating, worse after smoking a little. Oppression and difficulty of breathing, in paroxysms, like asthma. Catarrh with frontal headache and sticky yellow discharge.

Male - Flabbiness, perspiration, and insipid smell of genitals. Excoriation of glans penis in several places with a bloody discharge, better by bathing with urine. Chancre. Weakness, erection without desire.

Modalities - Worse in morning. Worse on rising. Worse by motion. Worse by coughing. Worse from tobacco. Worse from motion. Worse deep breathing. Worse lying down. Worse rising up. Worse coughing.

Mouth - Breath smells like pepper. Tough yellow coating on tongue. Taste, putrid of blood. Teeth yellow-coated. Bleeding of the gums. Tongue covered with a tough yellow coating.

Nose - Sticky yellow nasal discharge, Snuffles of children. Fluent coryza with much sneezing. Blowing of blood from left nostril. Itching of the nose. Snuffles of children.

Rectum - Autumnal dysentery. Tenesmus. ***Catarrhal dysentery with rheumatic pains***. Diarrhea is a worse in winter. Stools with a feeling as stream of fire passing through abdomen. Soft and fetid stool. Early morning diarrhea. Winter diarrhea. Stools like white of eggs, yellow, green, clammy, enveloped in froth, like moss. Stools smell like rotten eggs or burn like fire. Constipation after diarrhea.

Skin - Vesicles, pimples, and pustules all over the body, especially on arms, legs, and face, itching.

Sleep - Drowsy. Uneasy, restless sleep. Troublesome dreams.

Stomach - Fullness, pressure, weight. Belchings. Nausea, and efforts to vomit, in the morning when rising. Stomach pains, burning, disagreeable weight. In evening, violent stomach pain after supper. Cramps.

Temperature - Chill towards noon, with cold feet though room is warm. Feverish afternoon. High fever with hot sweat. Rheumatic, catarrhal, bilious marsh fevers of rice plantations.

Throat - Slight constriction of throat, and pricking in larynx.

Vertigo - Feeling of drunkenness with weakness of sight after smoking a very little. Swimming of the head with dullness behind forehead.

COMMENTS - Sharp, stitching, pricking pains, worse by motion. Sensitive to tobacco. Pain in forehead and abdomen from coughing. Griping and sharp peritoneal pains, worse by pressure. Excessive weakness, walking seems impossible.

Dyspnea. Hard cough, dry or hoarse, croupy with tight breathing and constriction of larynx and acute pleuritic pains. Warm feeling in chest. Pain like pricking of a needle in region of heart. Contracting pain in heart. Sharp pains, starting from left nipple downward with stiffness of left side of neck.

Increased secretions of skin, serous and mucus membranes. Catarrhal states from cold and damp weather. ***Bronchitis and pleurisy*** (often will follow Bry. in pleurisy cases), coughing and pain in the chest and pain on breathing. Pains in lungs, better bending forward.

Stitches in left side shooting over to right and up to left shoulder. Profuse perspiration in ***pleuro-pneumonia***.

RELATIONS - ***Compare:*** (1) Ant-t. (2) Asclepias Incarnata. Periploca greca - Cardiac tonic, acts on circulation and respiratory center, accelerating the respiration in a ratio disproportionate to pulse. (3) Agar., diagonal pains. (4) Bry., Verat. Relieved pains with stool at night. (5) Dulc. - worse cold and damp.

REFERENCES - Boericke. Clarke.

ASCLEPIAS VINCETOXICUM

(Swallow-wort)

PHARMACY - asc-v. Asclepias vincetoxicum. Swallow-wort. Vince. N. O. Asclepiadaceae. ***Historical dose:*** All potencies.

CLINICAL - Dropsy. Diabetes.

HOMEOPATHIC - Asclepias vincetoxicum is a gastro-intestinal irritant. Producing vomiting and purgation. Asc-v. is useful in dropsy, diabetes, great thirst, and profuse urination.

REFERENCES - Boericke.

ASIMINA TRILOBA

(American Papaw)

PHARMACY - asim. Asimina triloba. American papaw. Anona triloba. Paw Paw. Custard Apple. N. O. Anonaceae. Tincture of ripe and unripe fruit, green leaves, bark and root. ***Historical dose:*** Tincture and all potencies.

CLINICAL - Acne. Aphthae. Carbuncle. Cramp. Diarrhea. Fever. Glands, enlarged. ***Hoarseness.*** Scarlatina. Throat, sore. Vomiting.

HOMEOPATHIC - The Anonaceae, to which Asimina belongs, are allied to the Magnolia family. From eating the unripe fruit, five children developed high fever, sore throat and a scarlet eruption with diarrhea, one of them eventually having a carbuncle.

Asimina produces a series of symptoms much like scarlet fever, sore throat, fever, vomiting, scarlet eruption. Tonsils and submaxillary glands enlarged with diarrhea. Fauces are red and swollen. Face swollen.

In provings, the mouth, throat and stomach are irritated. Drinks much, desire for ice cold things and worse after eating. ***Hoarseness talks with difficulty.*** Languid, drowsy irritable.

Acne. Itching in evening on undressing. Thick, yellow nasal discharge in morning. Hard, flaky, dark grey and often offensive nasal discharge. Cramps in chest.

RELATIONS - ***Compare:*** (1) Caps., Bell., Ill. (Colic).

REFERENCES - Clarke.

ASPARAGUS OFFICINALIS

(Garden Asparagus)

PHARMACY - aspar. Asparagus officinalis. Garden asparagus. N. O. Liliaceae. Tincture of young sprouts. ***Historical dose:*** Tincture and all potencies.

CLINICAL - Coryza. Coughs. ***Cystitis.*** Diabetes. Dropsy. Gravel. Heart disorders. Hydrothorax. ***Kidney, disorders.*** Kidney, stones. Migraine. Nasal catarrh. ***Palpitations. Polyuria.*** Pulse, weak. Rheumatic, pains. Urinary disorders.

HERBAL - Asparagus has a marked and immediate action on the urinary secretion. Like other liliaceous plants it acts on the kidneys, heart and dropsical effusions.

HOMEOPATHIC - Cystitis. Frequent urination with fine stinging in the meatus, followed by stitches out of the urethra. After urinating, burning in urethra with sensation as if some were still passing. Increased urine, beer-brown without sediment. Urine is strong smelling, odor peculiar, deposits greasy sediment on sides of vessel, gravel.

Severe coryza and nasal catarrh with profuse secretion of thin, whitish fluid from left nostril, afterwards right. Frequent violent sneezing. Copious discharge of tenacious mucus from the throat, not easily loosened, but brought up by hawking or paroxysms of cough.

Weakness and cardiac depression with dropsy. Rheumatic pains, especially about left shoulder and heart. Fullness in chest, hydrothorax. Visible violent palpitations, while sitting, with anxious restlessness increased by motion or ascending with oppression of chest.

Pulse weak, slow, irregular. Pain at left acromion process, under clavicle and down left arm. Constant desire to be carried about in the arms.

MIND - Constant anxiety and apprehension. Anxiety with palpitations of the heart and ill humor. Calmness of the mind. Fretful and peevish. Disturbed by trifles.

Abdomen - Sensation of fullness in the abdomen, pinching in the umbilical region, at night with painful sensibility to the touch. Inflation of the abdomen, frequent emission of wind.

Back - Pain near the shoulders on touching the part, rheumatic pain between the shoulders. Sensation, as if something passed through kidneys and penetrated to the abdominal vertebrae, on the patient sitting down. Shootings pains, especially below the left shoulder blade. Pains in the region of the false vertebrae.

Chest - Oppression of the chest, especially when writing. Dyspnea brought on by motion, on going upstairs. Pressure on the chest. Emptiness within, with weight on the chest. Severe shooting pain across the right side when sitting down. Hydrothorax.

Eyes - Darting and tingling in the eyes, sight more piercing.

Face - Paleness of the face. Increase of heat in the face, cheeks burning.

Female - Menses continue a day beyond the usual time.

Food - Thirst increased. Feeble appetite. Fullness and oppression after eating and drinking. Vomiting of food taken evening before. Palpitations after eating.

Head - Aching in forehead and root of nose. Morning migraine headaches with scotoma. Aching pain in the temples, aggravated by pressure, weight in the forehead.

Heart - Irregular beating of the heart, rapid, redoubled. Heartbeat almost imperceptible. ***Palpitations with oppression of chest***. Palpitations, which are visible and audible even during very gentle movements with agitation and anxiety. Palpitations from motion and on ascending the stairs, worse when seated. Shooting pains in the region of the heart after a meal. Pulse slightly accelerated, feeble, intermits, weak.

Kidneys - ***Frequent urination with fine stitches in orifice of urethra***, burning of peculiar odor. Kidney stones. ***Cystitis*** with pus, mucus and tenesmus. Urgent inclination to urinate. Frequent and scanty emission of urine, preceded by a sensation as if a foreign body were in the urethra. Diminished secretion of urine, burning in the urethra.

Limbs - Rheumatic pain in back, especially near shoulder and limbs. Pain at acromion process of left scapula under clavicle and down arm with feeble pulse. Pain, as of dislocation in the right hip joint, which causes lameness. Shootings in the knees, at night afterwards under the left patella, on being seated. Bruise-like pains. Severe drawing pains in the calf of the right leg, in the morning, on waking and on extending the limb, cramps in both calves.

Lungs - Great oppression in breathing. Frequent sneezing, hawking with irresistible inclination to cough, but without any power to detach mucus, paroxysms of coughing, which compel the patient to rise from his seat, abating after breakfast, violent cough, attended by oppression of the chest and copious expectoration of mucus. Violent cough inducing retching.

Male - Excitation of sexual appetite, dartings in the glans penis.

Mouth - Taste insipid, sweetish (as of copper), softness of the saliva, as if it were mixed with blood.

Nose - Coryza with profuse, thin fluid.

Rectum - Bilious diarrhea with pain as of excoriation in the anus, colic and dragging in the groins.

Stomach - Belchings, flatulency in the stomach, nausea in the morning, on waking. Vomiting of food, mixed with bile and slimy matter afterwards diarrhea of bile and of fecal matter.

Throat - Throat feels rough with hawking copious, tenacious mucus from throat. Abundant secretion of mucus in the throat, a constant rattling of mucus in the chest with roughness in the throat.

Urine - Urine loaded with phosphates and the urate of ammonia in kidney dropsy. Gravel passes in small quantities with the urine. Straw colored urine, scanty, soon becomes turbid with little white specks. White flaky sediment, the urine deposits a fatty sediment on the sides of the vessel. Urine brown or clear with a fetid smell, a peculiar smell from the urine.

Vertigo - Vertigo in forehead, head confused, as during an attack of vertigo, dizziness in the forehead, followed by aching in the temples.

COMMENTS - Aspar. is a prostate and kidney remedy. The old homeopaths used to give it in tincture for the tendency to form kidney stones or history of kidney stones. Sediment in the urine, urine is gritty and painful. Boericke noted it for cystitis and lithiasis, the predisposition to kidney stones. Diabetes. Dropsy. Heart disorders. Urinary disorders.

RELATIONS - ***Antidote:*** Acon., Apis. ***Antidoted by:*** Acon. (prostration, feeble pulse, pain in shoulder), Apis. ***Antidote to:*** Coffea. ***Compare:*** (1) Conv., Sars., Arn., Aur-m., Cann-i., Dig., Spig. (2) Althea - Marshmallow, contains asparagin, irritable bladder, throat and bronchin. (3) Physalis Alkekengi. Dig., Sars., Spig.

REFERENCES - Boericke. Clarke.

ASPARTAME

(Aspartyl-phenylalanine)

PHARMACY - aspart. Aspartame. Aspartyl-phenylalanine-1-methyl ester. Artificial sweetener. ***Historical dose:*** All potencies.

CLINICAL - Abdominal Pain. Allergies. Arthritis. Attention deficit disorder. Asthma. Brain, cancer. Blood sugar problems. Cancer. Chronic fatigue. Convulsions. Depression. Diabetes. Diarrhea. Edema. Epilepsy. Headaches. Hives. Hyperglycemia. Hypertension. ***Hypoglycemia.*** Insomnia. Itching. Lupus. Memory weakness. Migraines. Multiple sclerosis. Nausea. Rashes. Vertigo. Vomiting.

HOMEOPATHIC - Aspartame is an artificial sweetener and neurotoxin. It chemically breakdowns into very toxic by-products including formaldehyde, formic acid, and methanol. The homeopathic indications are based on Aspartame's many toxic side effects and provings.

Epilepsy. Seizures and convulsions. Autoimmune diseases. Increased susceptibility to infections. Weak immune system. Allergic reactions. Lupus. Pains appear suddenly. Pain in spots. Stabbing pains. Sharp pains.

Hypertension. Blood sugar problems. Hypoglycemia and hyperglycemia. Weariness, worse in evening.

MIND - Mental confusion with headache. Confusion while talking. Poor concentration. Poor memory. Difficulty thinking. Anxiety attacks. Phobias. Depression. Marked personality changes.

Mental prostration. Desires activity. Delusion that he has been poisoned. Mental dullness with headache. Exhilaration. Forgetful during headache. Grief.

Industrious. Indifference during headache. Indifference to important things. Indifference to usual intellectual occupation. Indifference to irritating, disagreeable things.

Irritability, alternating with indifference. Irritability to her family. Irritability, headache amel. Laughing. Loquacious.

Memory weakness for what he is about to do. Memory weakness of memory for what he is about to say. Memory weakness for proper names. Mistakes in speaking, using wrong words. Mistakes in work. Mistakes in time, days of the week.

Prostration of mind - headache, during. Reproaching himself. Senses acute. Time appears longer, passes too slowy. Tranquillity while performing tasks. Untidy. Weakness of will.

Abdomen - Hypogastrium pain. Sharp pains in abdomen. Painful spot beneath navel.

Back - Burning pains in lumbar. Heat in lumbar region on waking from sleep, radiating to body. Aching pain in cervical region. Neck stiffness, creaking as if bones need oiling.

Bladder - Urging to urinate.

Breasts - Sharp pain in left breast.

Chest - Constricted sensation. Oppression of chest. Sore pains. Sharp pains on breathing. Sharp pains between the ribs.

Ears - Heat in ears. Itching in meatus. Hearing loss. Tinnitus.

Eyes - Glassy, appearance. Bloodshot eves. Sensation of a hair in eye. Itching of inner canthi. Eyes staring. Acute vision. Foggy vision. Vision loss.

Face - Dryness of face. Corners of mouth cracked. Eruptions around the mouth. Heat in spots. Bone pains. Stinging pain. Pain in cheeks.

Female - Menses delayed. Menses protracted. Sharp pains in uterus.

Food - Lack of appetite. Appetite increased in morning. Errors in diet aggravates. Aversion to sweets. Desires for sweets.

Head - Heaviness sensation. Bursting pain, better after eating. Cutting pain in forehead. Pains in forehead extending to eyes. Headache worse from light. Headaches are left sided.

Heart - Rapid heartbeat. Palpitations.

Limbs - Heaviness in upper limbs while writing. Tremors. Numbness and tingling of limbs. Sharp pain in lower limbs, motion amel. Sharp pain in knees. Ankle weakness while walking. Knee suddenly gives way while walking (Ruta).

Lungs - Asthmatic reactions. Difficult breathing while eating. Desire to breathe deeply. Difficult breathing after exertion. Chronic cough. Dry cough.

Modalities - Better open air.

Mouth - Saliva frothy, offensive, thick. Salivation profuse. Taste, acute. Burning pain in tongue. Tongue yellow. Ulcer of gums.

Nose - Smell, acute.

Rectum - Constipation. Insufficient urging to stool. Diarrhea. Hard stools. Long, narrow stools. Offensive smelling stools.

Skin - Itching in scars. Hives. Itching. Rashes.

Sleep - Insomnia. Sleepiness. Dreams of dead children.

Stomach - Nausea and vomiting. Diarrhea. Stomach distension. Emptiness in stomach after breakfast. Eructations. Heartburn. Retching with cough.

Temperature - Lack of vital heat. Sensation of heat.

Throat - Dryness of throat. Sensation as if a foreign body in throat.

Vertigo - Vertigo when turning head or moving quickly. Vertigo while walking.

RELATIONS - ***Compare:*** (1) Ars., Carc., Phos. (2) Formaldehyde. Formic acid. Methanol.

REFERENCES - Bocock. Murphy.

ASPEN

(Bach Flower Essence)

PHARMACY - asp-b. Aspen. Populus tremula. Small twigs with leaf buds and clusters of flowers, which are the catkins, are boiled for half an hour. Both the male catkins, which are gray with tinges of red anthers or yellow pollen, and the smaller, gray female catkins are selected. The water is subsequently strained and used as medicine. ***Historical dose:*** Take two drops from the stock bottle into a one ounce dropper bottle (add brandy or another alcohol if this bottle will be used for days or weeks). This is the dosage bottle, take a few drops straight into the mouth or as needed in a little water or juice.

HOMEOPATHIC - The remedy Aspen belongs to the group of ***"For Those who have Fear,"*** as determined by Bach. The other fear remedies are Rock Rose, Mimulus, Cherry Plum and Red Chestnut.

Aspen can greatly benefit those unable to fall asleep due to their fears of letting go. Sleeping disorders and insomnia due to nightmares of an eerie, haunting kind.

Foreboding and anxious disquiet in mind and body. In panic disorders, when no apparent reason can be given for the attacks (Cher-p-b, Rock Rose). Anxiety attacks marked by the typical, vague fears with shaking and trembling. Anxiety about death Mental and emotional withdrawal. Dejected or haunted in appearance.

MIND - In the Aspen state, the mind is overly receptive and too easily impressed. Primordial fears and feelings of doom. Delusions, superstitions, omens, fateful encounters, prophesies and ghost stories.

Some people develop personal rituals to establish a sense of protection.

Forebodings are vague and may be solely imaginary. Intuitive, spiritual or psychic paths of personal development may lead people into the Aspen state. Aspen is indicated in states of fearful delusions and paranoia when fears are based on imaginary content with haunting features.

REFERENCES - Bach.

ASTACUS FLUVIATILIS

(Crawfish)

PHARMACY - astac. Astacus fluviatilis. Crawfish. Cancer astacus. Cancer fluviatilis. River crab. N. O. Crustacea. Europe. Tincture from whole animal. ***Historical dose:*** Tincture and all potencies.

CLINICAL - Biliousness. Colic. Cough. Diarrhea. Fever. Swelling of cervical glands. Intermittent fever. Jaundice. Liver complaints. Nettle rash. Neuralgia. Shivering. Stomach, disorders. Toothache. Tumors.

HOMEOPATHIC - The well-known effects of shellfish, as well as of other fish, in producing nettle rash is exemplified in Astacus more than all other varieties. The lacquer workers of the East have discovered that the river-crab is the best antidote to the effects of Rhus-t., which they employ in their craft.

The liver is markedly affected and a great characteristic is "nettle-rash with liver complaint." Pain and tenderness of the liver, jaundice, stools of pipe-clay color. Jaundice in children. Skin symptoms. ***Urticaria,*** with liver complaints. Itching of various parts. Stinging pains are felt in various parts. Nervous crawls over body.

Crusta lactea with enlarged lymphatic glands. Enlarged glands of the neck in children and the elderly. Tumors. Gout from drinking alcohol. Inward chilliness and sensitiveness to air, worse uncovering. Violent fever with headache, glowing red face inward chilliness.

MIND - Melancholic mood. Apprehensiveness with anxiety in chest. Slight delirium during nettle-rash.

Abdomen - Constricts and may completely close both the duodenum and especially the opening of the gall duct into the duodenum.

Liver - Cramps in liver region. Liver inflamed, worse pressure.

Lungs - Cough, better when walking, but returns as soon as he sits down.

Modalities - Worse from air, uncovering.

Skin - Itching in various parts. Nettle rash over whole body. Crusta lactea with enlarged lymphatic glands. Erysipelas and ***liver infection with nettle rash***. Jaundice.

Temperature - Violent fever with headache, red glowing face. Inward chilliness, very sensitive to air, worse uncovering, violent fever with headache.

RELATIONS - ***Antidoted by:*** Acon. ***Compare:*** (1) Calc., Rhus-t. Apis, Homarus, Chloral, Nat-m. (2) Bombyx - Caterpillar, Itching of whole body, urticaria.

REFERENCES - Boericke. Clarke.

ASTERIAS RUBENS

(Red Starfish)

PHARMACY - aster. Asterias rubens. Red starfish. N. O. Radiata, Echinodermata. Tincture of fish. ***Historical dose:*** All potencies.

CLINICAL - Acne. Axillary, tumor. ***Breast, cancer.*** Cancer. Chorea. Colic. Constipation. Convulsions. Epilepsy. ***Gland, disorders.*** Headaches. Heart, disorders. Hemorrhoids. Herpes zoster. Hysteria. ***Insomnia.*** Neuralgia. Psoriasis. Salivation. Scabies. Strokes. Sycosis. Tetters. Tongue, paralysis, swelling. Ulcers. Uterus, disorders. Vertigo.

HOMEOPATHIC - The starfish was used by Hippocrates in uterine diseases. This shows its pathogenic relationship to Sep. and Murx. It is also an ancient remedy for epilepsy and stroke.

Aster. has been successful in curing ***breast cancers with nightly sharp pains.*** Drawn back feeling in eyes. Nipples feel drawn in. ***Breast cancer.*** Increased sexual desire, sexual excitement.

Powerfully affects the brain and the head, causing severe congestion with red face, strokes.

This remedy produces disturbances of the circulation with pulsations and congestion in head, womb, chest. Sexual desire increased, sexual excitement. A pushing-out sensation in womb, impeding walking (Sep.).

Petroz used Asterias rubens successfully in old skin affections, old ulcers and in cancers. He found that it only acted on the latter when on the left side. H. C. Allen mentions it as a remedy for acne having small puncta with black tips and small red bases.

Nervous disorders include neuralgia, chorea, hysteria and epilepsy. Epilepsy is preceded by twitching over whole body. Chorea, quiet only when the hands are in the pockets. Left-sided symptoms. Symptoms are worse at night, by motion and in cold, damp weather. Tears ameliorate the mental state.

MIND - Easily excited by any emotion. Weeps from least emotion. Sense of impending misfortune. Fears bad news. Fear of apoplexy at night, with feeling as if head would burst. Fear of fainting with sensation of fullness in chest.

Melancholy alternating with cerebral excitement. Cannot bear contradiction. Indifference. Unwilling to think or work. Clearness of mind when headache disappears.

Irritability, necessity of quarrelling with somebody. Irritability before convulsion. Impatience in house. Sadness, desire to weep.

Anxiety during sleep after menses. Feeling of extreme anxiety from noon to 3 p.m. Nervous agitation with erotic thoughts and sexual desire.

Insanity during menopause. Delusion he is under control of strangers. Hallucinations of hearing voices, away from, among strangers. Loss of consciousness in epilepsy.

Abdomen - Shocks of dull pain in the right side of abdomen and near umbilicus. Incarcerated wind. Violent colic, with shuddering, alternating with flushes of heat in the face. Alternate swelling and sinking of the abdomen during the twenty-four hours. Sensation of pressure on lower abdominal organs. Tearing, drawing pain in abdominal walls.

Back - Scrofulous ulcer left neck. Pulling, drawing in the back and sacrum.

Breasts - ***Breast cancer even in ulcerative stage.*** Neuralgia of left breast and arm (Brom.). ***Acute, lancinating, or smarting pains*** in breast tumor, entirely depriving her of rest at night. Nodes and induration of breast gland. Dull aching, neuralgic pain in breast region (Con.). ***Nipples retracted.*** Breasts swell and painful, worse left. ***Left breast feels as if pulled inward***. Pain from breasts extends over inner arm to end of little finger. Slight eruption between breasts. ***Axillary glands swollen hard and knotted.*** Rash or furfuraceous eruption between breasts.

Chest - Enlarged axillary glands, worse at night and in damp weather. ***Axillary glands swollen hard and knotted.*** Ulceration with sharp pains, piercing to scapulae. Pain under sternum and in muscles of precordial region. Full feeling in chest with fear of fainting. Violent itching spot upon chest. Itching in right axilla. Pain under sternum. Lancinating pain.

Constitutions - A remedy for the sycotic diathesis, flabby with ***red face***. Flabby lymphatic constitution.

Ears - Lightning-like stitches in the meatus auditorius. Violent reports in the ears. Noise in the ears as from waves. Noise of rushing water. Dullness of hearing in the right ear.

Eyes - Drawn backwards. Winking of eyelids. Heat and redness in the eyes, weary look. Difficulty of bearing the light. Eyes are drawn backwards. Edges of eyelids reddened. Photophobia. Light fatigues eyes. Twitching of lids.

Face - Red, flushed face. Redness of face, precursor of apoplexy. Acne. Pimples on side of nose, chin and mouth. ***Disposition to pimples at adolescence.*** Pimples, black tips with small red bases. Neuralgia. Livid discoloration of face, during epileptic attack with falling.

Female - Jerking or distress in uterus. Colic and other sufferings cease with appearance of flow. As if something were passing out of uterus. As if something protruded behind uterus. Pushing sensation in uterus. Twitching of uterus. Vagina moist with feeling of ease. Violent and constant sexual desire, not better by sex, with nervous agitation with disposition to weep. Sexual desire increased, worse mornings in bed.

Food - Loss of appetite. Uncertain appetite. Dullness of taste. Aversion to meat. Desires cold drinks. Desires highly seasoned food, strong cheese. Desires liquors, tea. Great desire for cold drinks. Worse from coffee.

Head - Face red, with throbbing carotids. Rushes of blood to head with throbbing. ***Sensation as if head would burst, precursor to stroke.*** Sensation as if head would split. Shocks in brain, throbbing. ***Heat in head, as if surrounded by hot air.*** Bones of skull and scalp sore. Pain in occiput, right side. Emptiness in the head. Severe pressure in forehead. Boring pain, above left eye. Burning pains in head. Soreness of whole scalp during severe headache.

Heart - Palpitations, pulse hard and frequent. Strong and frequent beating of the heart, jerking palpitations. As if heart had ceased to beat, with dull, prolonged heartbeats. Anxiety at the heart. Violent beating in right carotid artery. ***Pulse hard, full, frequent.***

Kidneys - Heat in the urethra while the urinating. Frequent urination with copious, clear urine. Thick, viscid urine. Urine profuse. Urine thick and slimy.

Limbs - Gait unsteady muscles refuse to obey the will. Numbness of hand and fingers of left side. Numbness of hands, with coldness of the arm. Lassitude and great weakness of the lower limbs. Pain in the left hip. Pain in the joints of the foot. Feeling in all limbs as if beaten, most in arms, when walking in open air. Restlessness in limbs worse covered or in warm room.

Lungs - Short breath with pain in chest when inhaling. Cough with expectoration, morning in bed. Easy hawking of greyish-black mucus during forenoon.

Male - Sexual desire increased, erotic thoughts. Frequent erections during sleep or in the morning.

Modalities - Better appearance of menses. Worse from coffee. Worse at night. Worse cold damp weather. Worse left side. Worse from heat, motion. Worse during menses. Worse from contradiction. Malaise is worse heat.

Mouth - Acute and pressing stitches in the upper teeth. Swelling of the tongue. Pulling pains in the tongue. Heaviness of speech. Profuse flow of saliva. Dry, hard, exceedingly painful pimples on lower lip. Loss of taste. Shooting pain in tongue. Difficulty to move tongue, aversion to speak. Talking difficult with profuse salivation.

Nerves - Gait unsteady, muscles refuse to obey the will. Epilepsy, preceded by twitching over whole body.

Nose - Nosebleed, sneezing and coryza in the morning on waking. Sneezing and coryza in morning on awaking. Pimples on sides of nose and chin.

Rectum - Severe constipation. Ineffectual urging. Obstinate constipation. Stool like olives. Stool hard, round balls. Diarrhea preceded by colic. Diarrhea, watery brown stools gushing out with force. Heat in the rectum. Bleeding hemorrhoids.

Sleep - Sleeplessnes from nightly, pains. ***Insomnia.*** Disposition to sleep after reading a moment. Late falling asleep and late getting up. Agitated sleep, tossing about. Sleep quiet but not refreshing. Many dreams. Dreams about persons and events. Dreams, images vivid and lifelike. Dreams, sees and hears people as if she was awake.

Skin - Acne with black tipped puncta, small red base. Dry, harsh skin, earthy appearance. Destitute of pliability and elasticity. Itching spots. Psoriasis and herpes zoster worse left arm and chest. Eruption on thighs and insteps of small itching vesicles which tear easily and form superficial ulcers. Ulcers with sensitive edges, fetid discharge. Scabies. Tetters.

Stomach - Frequent belchings. Dull or constrictive pain at the precordial region.

Frequent forcible eructations in morning. Nausea. Distress in pit, with great debility.

Temperature - Shivering with sleepiness, followed by hot skin and restless night. Fever followed by coldness. Violent heat, in head, then over whole body. Increased general heat. Heat alternating with cold.

Throat - Dryness and heat in throat. Sore throat with constriction in morning on awaking. Pressing irritation of the throat. Dull pain apparently all along the esophagus.

Throat - Rough sensation in larynx causes cough.

Vertigo - Vertigo, transient, when walking. Vertigo with insensibility of lower limbs. Sudden attacks, like shocks in head. Vertigo, precursor of apoplexy.

COMMENTS - Asterias powerfully affects the mind and head, producing symptoms strongly suggesting a stroke.

The face is red and there is strong congestion to the head, which is hot and feels as if surrounded by hot air. Certain forms of cerebral congestion with obstinate constipation. Electric shocks in the head. Nightly sharp pains in the breasts have led to its successful use in cases of breast cancer.

Teste noted that the malaise is worse by heat. Great desire for cold drinks. Coffee worsens all the symptoms and excites them anew several days after they have disappeared.

Breast cancer in the upper-left quadrant, which is the most frequent place to get breast cancer. Cancer of the left breast that has metastasized to the axillary glands of the armpit. Tumors of the nipple.

Characteristic severe lancinating pains which are worse at night. Sharp, darting pains. Bearing down pains. May complain of a sensation of the breast being drawn inward. Sharp pains that extend to the scapula. Severe, dull, aching pains in the breast. Pains can be related to hormones, can be worse premenstrually. Substernal pains.

Cancer pains, inflamed and swollen glands (Con.). Axillary glands are swollen, indurated and knotted. Knotted in the left side of the neck. Pain extends down the left arm. Swollen breast, can have ulcerations.

The affected breast may develop a red spot that suppurates premenstrually. At times it will become inflamed and discharge with an offensive odor coming out.

For stroke patients, or threatened stroke or epilepsy (Bell., Glon.). They get a red, congested face and are excitable, apprehensive with fears.

Weeping ameliorates the mental state. Worse at night, cold, and motion. Desire cold drinks. Aggravated by coffee. They are very excitable, weepy, and fear something bad will happen, fear of getting bad news or misfortune (common symptoms of cancer patients).

RELATIONS - ***Antidotes:*** Plb., Zinc. ***Antidoted by:*** Plum., Zinc. ***Compare:*** (1) Carc., Con., Carb-an., Ars., Cund., Murex, Sep., Astac., Homarus, Eryth., Crot., Grat., Gamb., Jatr., Thuj., Bell., Lil-t. ***Follows well:*** Bell., Carb-an., Con., Sil., Sulph., Calc. ***Incompatible:*** Coffee, Nux-v. (Ip. relieved after Nux-v. aggravated.) Teste includes Aster. in the Sulphur group of anti-psorics.

REFERENCES - Boericke. Clarke. Murphy.

ASTRAGALUS EXCAPUS

PHARMACY - astra-e. Astragalus excapus. N. O. Papilionoideae. Tincture of the fresh plant with flowers and seeds. ***Historical dose:*** Trituration, tincture and all potencies.

CLINICAL - Migraine. Neuritis. Syphilis. Tabes.

HERBAL - Astra-e. is a leguminous plant which grows in the Canton of Valais. It is a small, herbaceous plant with a short stem and downy leaves. When mature, it has an oval fruit.

HOMEOPATHIC - There is no homeopathic symptomatology for this remedy. The symptoms which follow are from O. A. Julian's toxicology and clinical experimentation.

Alternation of mental and pulmonary complaints. Dyspnea and respiratory spasm. Falls easily and has tension disorders of the organs. Giddiness. Pressing pains in the temples, in the maxillary sinuses. Shooting pains above the right eyebrow. Painful sensation of fullness in the left temporal and maxillary regions.

General paralysis. Cerebral softening. Paretic weakness of the lower limbs. Incoordination of movements, walking difficult of an ataxic type. Paretic walk and pressing temple and maxillary pains. Neuritis of syphilitic type. Tertiary syphilis.

MIND - Unstable moods, excites quickly and loses his dash and assurances easily. Mental confusion in nervous subjects. Psychological state, sees as through a fog. Bewilderment, worse in the morning.

Chest - Weakness of the chest.

Constitutions - Psoric and allergic constitutions. Tubercular types. Nervous, uneasy types with depressive or obsessive tendencies.

Food - Anorexia. Emaciation.

Limbs - Sensation of formication on the right foot from the heel towards the toes. Icy coldness in the left calf. Tumors on the maxillary bones and jaw. Juvenile dystrophy and the bones. Multiple myelomata of the bones. Raynaud's syndrome. Arteritis.

Lungs - Difficulty in breathing, choking sensation, groping for breath. Asthma. Emphysema. Slow, difficult respiration and small or thick plugs of sputum. Rhonchi and bronchial wheezing.

Nose - Permanent head cold with watery, abundant flow, sometimes burning and excoriating. Sinusitis.

Stomach - Burning all along the esophagus. Empty feeling in the stomach with failing and debility. Crises of gastric tabes. Hiatus hernia.

RELATIONS - ***Compare:*** (1) Arg-m. - Paretic type with cramps, chronic laryngitis and pharyngitis. (2) Ars-i. - Chronic coryza inflammation of lymphatic glands and bronchitis, weakness and rapid emaciation. (3) Tuberculinum - Gradual emaciation, headache as though restricted by a headband, nasal and pharyngeal congestion, cough with thick, yellow sputum, sweating. (4) Syphilium - Obsessions, loss of memory, nightly aggravation, especially of the pains in the bones, coughing.

REFERENCES - Julian.

ASTRAGALUS MENZIESII

PHARMACY - astra-me. Astragalus menziesii. N. O. Leguminose. Papilionoideae. Tincture of leaves. ***Historical dose:*** Tincture and all potencies.

CLINICAL - Emptiness, sensation. Facial bones, painful. Headache.

HOMEOPATHIC - After eating some of the green leaves of Astra-me., J. Selfridge experienced burning in his pharynx esophagus, and stomach. Fullness in right temple and right upper jaw, slight nausea with shivering and chilliness, dizziness and fullness of the head.

Astra-me. has weakness and sense of emptiness in stomach, eating relieved empty sensation, but not the weakness. Pressive pains in both temples, slight pain in left maxilla and aching in right maxilla with pressure in both bones.

REFERENCES - Boericke.

ASTRAGALUS MOLLISSIMUS

(Purple Loco-Weed)

PHARMACY - astra-mo. Astragalus mollissimus. Purple loco-weed. Woolly loco-weed. Loco-weed. Papilionoideae. ***Historical dose:*** Tincture and all potencies.

CLINICAL - Mania. Vision, weakness.

HOMEOPATHIC - Purple Loco-Weed causes irregularities in gait, paralytic disorders. Loss of muscular coordination.

Affects animals like the effects of alcohol, tobacco, and morphine in man. After acquiring a taste for the plant, the animals refuse every other kind of food. In the first stage, a period of hallucination or mania with defective eyesight during which the animal performs all sorts of antics.

Second stage brings emaciation, sunken eyeballs, lusterless hair and feeble movements. After a few months, the victim dies from starvation.

Head - Fullness in right temple and upper jaw. Pain over left eyebrow. Dizzy. Pressive pain in temples.

Face - Painful facial bones. Pain and pressure in maxillae.

Limbs - Purring sensation in right foot, outer side from heel to toe. Icy coldness of left calf.

Stomach - Weakness and emptiness. Burning in esophagus and stomach.

RELATIONS - ***Compare:*** (1) Aragallus Lamberti - White Loco-Weed, Rattleweed, Bar-c., Oxytropis.

REFERENCES - Boericke.

ATHAMANTHA CRETENSIS

PHARMACY - atha. Athamanta cretensis. Athamanta oreoselinum. Peucedanum oreoselinum. Grundheil." N. O. Umbelliferae. Tincture of fresh plant. ***Historical dose:*** Tincture and all potencies.

CLINICAL - Head, confused. Headache. Indigestion. Vertigo.

HOMEOPATHIC - Athamanta was proved by Franz and has produced some peculiar symptoms. There is a dull, befogged condition of brain, recalling Aethusa. A stupefaction and confusion rises like a vapor from the lower part of occiput, on motion and walking. Vertigo, better lying. Sleep heavy and profound, prolonged in the morning to later period than usual.

Pressure and numbness of head and upper teeth. Pressure on one eyeball from below upward. Bitter taste and bitter mucus in air passages. Icy coldness of feet and hands.

RELATIONS - ***Compare:*** (1) Umbelliferae, especially Aethusa.

REFERENCES - Boericke.

ATISTA INDICA

(Ban Nimbu)

PHARMACY - atista. Atista indica. Ban Nimbu. Glycosmis pentaphylla. Correa root. ***Historical dose:*** Tincture and all potencies.

CLINICAL - Biliousness. Chill. Chlorosis. Colic. Cough. Dysentery. Fever. Jaundice. Rheumatism. Snake, bite. Spasms. Tonsilitis. Worms.

HERBAL - Description: A small evergreen, glabrous, fragrant shrub. Flowers small white, fragrant in erect terminal or lateral pubescent. Fruit a berry, white pink or blue.

In the opinion of Ayurvedic physicians it causes rheumatism and is a useful medicine in bilious complaints, cough, worms, jaundice, fever and chlorosis. Lt. Col. R. N. Chopra in his Indigenous Drugs of India, has written that its "Root is used in snake-bite".

HOMEOPATHIC - Proving was done in March, 1997, by Dr. Kati Kumar Bhattacharjee, homeopath.

An excellent remedy in breaking and stopping fevers which appear on alternate days or on every third day with or without malarial infection.

MIND - Memory weak. Vigorless, indifferent mood.

Abdomen - Flatulence, colicky pain, griping pain round the navel. Unbearable pain in the umbilicus making the patient senseless. Biliary colic.

Face - Spasms of facial muscles.

Food - Canine hunger, aversions to liquid food and strong desire for lime juice.

Head - Gnawing pain in the temple generally on one side.

Limbs - Weakness in the muscles of the legs, legs' go to sleep' they seem to give way at every step; cramping while getting straight.

Male - Sexual desire almost nil. Erections at night without any lascivious talk prior to it.

Mouth - Dryness, unbearable thirst during hot stage.

Rectum - All sorts of worm complaints. All types of dysentery with colic felt at navel.

Sleep - Transient, unrefreshing sleep.

Throat - Tonsils swollen, pain and inflammation persist for a few weeks after the fever is over.

Temperature - Chill without thirst. Heat with intense thirst. Every alternate day, third day fever. Fever at 5 a.m.

REFERENCES - Desai.

ATRAX ROBUSTUS

(Sidney Funnelweb Spider)

PHARMACY - atra-r. Atrax robustus. Sidney Funnelweb Spider. Australia. Arachnida. ***Historical dose:*** Tincture and all potencies.

CLINICAL - Earaches. Exophthalmic goiter. Glaucoma. Headaches. Insomnia. Mental exhaustion. Neuralgias. Tubercular states. Worms.

HOMEOPATHIC - Atra-r. is a venomous spider, a spinner mygale from Australia. Its bite produces a serious toxic syndrome, atraxism, which is characterized by a phase of excitement followed by a period of stupor and sleepiness with hypothermia. Death comes after a phase of intense agitation with salivary and lachrymal secretions.

Sankaran undertook the proving in 1969, at the suggestion of D. W. Everitt of London. There were four provers, of whom one acted as control. The potency used was 30c, at the rate of one daily dose for a month.

Gets up in the morning with a feeling of fatigue which then gradually disappears. Feeling of general exhaustion. Sensation of protrusion of the throat and eyes. Asthenia of the body. Drawing pain in the ears. Weakness of the lower limbs, predominantly on the left.

MIND - Mental exhaustion in the evening. Incapable of doing the least physical or intellectual exercise.

Abdomen - Pain around the umbilical region, starting in the morning. Pain worse after breakfast, from leaning backwards, walking, standing, improving with pressure, lying on the stomach or leaning forwards.

Ears - Drawing sensation in the outer ear as if pulled by a string. Impression of tugging behind the ears, passing from left to right.

Eyes - Eyelids stuck together in the morning. Pain below the left orbit when lying down. Heavy, yellowish-white secretion during the night. Eyeballs painful with feeling of protrusion, especially on the left side.

Face - Neuralgia of the face and under the orbits.

Kidneys - Urine slightly irritating. Frequent urination at night. Feeling in the bladder of not being empty after urination. Last drop hot and irritating.

Limbs - Sudden sensation of weakness in the limbs, especially the legs. Need to lie down and condition improved by continual pressure. Joint pains in the knees.

Lungs - Cough with thick, greenish sputum which comes up easily.

Modalities - Better from pressure, lying on the stomach. Worse from walking. Worse standing still. Worse leaning backwards.

Nose - Nasal discharge of thick, yellowish liquid, sometimes black and sticky.

Sleep - Insomnia until 1 a.m.

Throat - Feeling of obstruction in the throat, worse when lying on the back. Throat red, dry, painful, especially on the left side and when swallowing. Dryness of the throat not improved by drinking water, worse from drinking cold drinks. Feeling of protrusion of the thyroid cartilage.

Vertigo - Feeling of vertigo, lasting only a short while in the evening, around 7 p.m.

RELATIONS - ***Compare:*** (1) Aranea Diadema - Exhaustion with strong desire to go to bed. Icy cold feeling in the bones. Drilling pains in the heels. (2) Spigelia - Pains in the eyeballs, as if the eyes were too big for the sockets. Neuralgic pain starting at the back of the head, spreading to the frontal region and ending above the eye, especially the left side.

REFERENCES - Julian.

ATROPINUM PURUM

(Atropine)

PHARMACY - atro. Atropinum purum aut sulphuricum. Atropine. N. O. Solanaceae. Atropine is an alkaloid of Belladonna. The effects of the Sulphate of Atropine, the preparation most in use, are included. Solution. ***Historical dose:*** Trituration and all potencies.

CLINICAL - Bedwetting. Blepharospasm. Convulsions. Epilepsy. Eyes, disorders. Gastric ulcer. Locomotor ataxia. Mania. Neuralgias. Pancreatitis. Peritonitis. Spinal irritation.

Stammering. Tetanus. Vision, disorders. Torticollis.

HOMEOPATHIC - Atropine, as the most active principle in Belladonna, produces most of the characteristic effects of that drug, but at the same time the two are not identical. Atropine has shown an affinity for the pancreas, which relates it to Iod., Kali-i. and Iris. It can produce a hypersensitivity of the sensory nerves.

Numerous eye symptoms. All kinds of illusions of vision. Motes seen over everything. All kinds of illusions of sight. Everything appears large (Plat. opposite). On reading, words run together, double vision, all objects seem to be elongated.

Clarke once cured with Atro. a woman who had an appearance of shadows passing over whatever she looked at.

Difficulty of speech. Frequent stuttering, especially at difficult to pronounce words. Indistinct articulation, rapid and chattering.

Great dryness of throat, almost impossible to swallow. Chronic stomach disorders with great pain and vomiting of all food. Peritonitis. Hypochlorhydria, heartburn. Eustachian tube and tympanic congestion. Affinity for the pancreas. Hyperacidity of stomach. Paroxysm of gastric pain, ovarian neuralgia.

Mind - Sad and morose, prefering solitude and a dark room to society of friends. Fear of her condition being observed. Meddlesome. Mistakes in localities, in time. Rambling speech. Speech embarrassed, loud, slow, unintelligible in sleep. Wandering thoughts. Mirthful.

Frightful delirium. Delusions, sees frightful images. Delusions sees people in room at bedside. Delusions familiar things seem strange. Answers to imaginary questions. Refuses obstinately to swallow anything or to answer questions in any way than by a grunt.

Back - Constant burning in back. Large portion of spine so sensitive that she cried out on pressure. Painful affections from spinal irritation.

Chest - Burning under sternum.

Ears - Morbid sensitiveness to sounds and objects.

Eyes - Sharp neuralgic pains in and about eyes. Neuralgic pain. Eyelids heavy and difficult to keep open. ***Corneal ulcers*** with spasmodic winking. Irritability of eye. Conjunctivitis with lachrymation. Dim vision with dilated pupils. Vertical diplopia, apparent object below real one.

Face - Deep red distorted face. Deathly pallor.

Female - Severe cutting or drawing pains, in left ovary, extorting screams, must bend double. Left ovary swollen and tender during menses. Puerperal convulsions.

Food - Appetite often considerable, sometimes absent. Thirst after vomiting.

Head - Periodical headache, coming on suddenly, increasing rapidly, until intensely severe. Dull pain in temples. Sticking pain in back of skull and over eyes, worse every motion, stepping. Severe headache beginning in occiput, passing over right side, locating over eyes. Headache with flushing of face and head. Headache with rush of blood to head. Sensation as if head were screwed up. Headache of epileptics. Headache with great weakness.

Kidneys - Congestive states of kidneys. ***Chronic albuminuria.*** Involuntary urination, but scanty discharge of urine.

Limbs - Throwing about limbs. Spasms worse when disturbed. Gouty affection of right wrist, with stiffness. Clenching of thumbs. Involuntary movements of hands towards head. Locomotor ataxia. Edema of legs.

Mouth - Pappy taste. Dryness of mouth and throat. Unability to speak from dryness of mouth, tongue nearly adherent to roof of mouth. Dryness of mouth after two hours suddenly gave way to a viscid, acrid secretion, very highly offensive odor.

Rectum - Diarrhea with constipation. During stool, felt badly weak, terribly nervous, with general sweat.

Sleep - Drowsiness with tendency to quiet dreams and delirium. Somnolence with nervous startings. Prolonged yawning Restless sleep, sleeps only towards morning. Sleep much disturbed by gastric pains. Starting as if frightened on falling asleep.

Stomach - Constant burning under stomach. Constant retching and empty eructations, immediately after eating. Nausea with pressure at stomach. Vomiting of food. Fluttering in stomach. Vomiting seldom with nausea. Vomiting at times extremely violent. Stomach very sensitive to pressure.

Teeth - Grinding of teeth.

Throat - Burning from coughing. Dark red, husky hue. Difficult swallowing from great dryness. Voice husky. Dryness of larynx causes dry cough and difficult swallowing.

Tongue - Tongue seems partially paralyzed, speech indistinct, rapid and chattering. Tongue hard, parched and cracked. Tongue coated white.

Vertigo - Vertigo on rising in morning. Vertigo on turning head suddenly.

RELATIONS - ***It antidotes:*** Muscarine and Op. It is ***Antidoted by:*** Op. and Phys. ***Compare:*** Like Bell., it is a right-side medicine.

REFERENCES - Boericke. Clarke.

AURUM ARSENICUM

(Gold Arsenate)

PHARMACY - aur-ar. Aurum arsenicum. Gold arsenate. Trituration. ***Historical dose:*** Trituration and all potencies.

CLINICAL - Anemia. Anxiety. Aortitis. ***Cancer.*** Chlorosis. Depression. Headaches. Lupus. Syphilis. Tuberculosis.

HOMEOPATHIC - Aur-ar. was first used by Chrestien in cases of tuberculosis. Later it has been used by others in syphilis, especially chronic syphilitic headaches, chlorosis, anemia, ***cancer,*** chlorosis, lupus.

The first effect of the Aur-ar. is to cause rapid increase of appetite. The peristaltic contractions of stomach and intestines are excited and absorption accelerated. Blood, glands and bones are centers frequently involved.

MIND - The depression of Aurum metallicum and the anxiety of Arsenic are often present in cases needing this remedy. Weary of life, wants to jump out of window. Averse to being spoken to. Always in a hurry and excited. Impatient and restless. Neglects his family and children. Fault-finding and critical.

Constitutions - Cancer based on the tuberculosis miasm or syphilitic constitution.

Eyes - Pupils contracted.

Face - Face hot with suffering expression.

Food - Increase of appetite. Aversion to food and meat. Desire for alcoholic stimulants. Desire cold drinks and milk.

Head - Chronic syphilitic headaches.

Lungs - Dyspnea, desire for open air. Tuberculosis.

Modalities - Better heat, warm bed. Better summer. Worse open air. Worse cold, wet weather. Worse mental and physical exertion.

Mouth - Breath offensive and putrid. Grinding of teeth at night.

Stomach - Bitter eructations.

REFERENCES - Clarke. Grimmer.

AURUM BROMATUM

(Gold Bromide)

PHARMACY - aur-br. Aurum bromatum. Gold bromide. Trituration. This is an unproved salt of gold. ***Historical dose:*** Trituration and all potencies.

CLINICAL - Epilepsy. Headaches. Heart, disorders. Migraine. Neurasthenia. Night terrors. Sleepwalking.

HOMEOPATHIC - Aurum bromatum was recommended by Dr. E. M. Hale as being superior to other preparations of gold, especially in certain nervous disorders of an epileptiform character, such as migraine, night terrors, sleepwalking.

Valvular diseases of the heart and hypertrophy, attacks of faintness with coldness and feeble pulse alternating with attacks of congestion and red face with palpitations. In headaches with neurasthenia, megrim, night terrors, valvular diseases.

COMMENTS - Hale writes: "In the physiological hypertrophies of young persons at puberty, of pregnant women, and at the climacteric period, I prefer the bromide of gold in the 6x trituration.

It will prevent the pathological hypertrophy which often threatens."

"Besides the class of disorders enumerated, this preparation of gold is very useful in reflex mental affections from uterine or ovarian irritation. I do not consider the suicidal despondency a necessary symptom. It is often indicated in just the opposite state when there is exalted sensitiveness, great mental exhilaration and unnatural gaiety."

REFERENCES - Clarke. Hale.

AURUM IODATUM

(Gold Iodide)

PHARMACY - aur-i. Aurum iodatum. Gold iodide. ***Historical dose:*** Trituration and all potencies.

CLINICAL - Arteriosclerosis. Larynx spasm. Leucorrhea. Lupus. Myomata uterus. Osteitis. Ovarian, cysts. Ozaena. Palpitations. Pericarditis. Senile paresis. Syphilis. Thyroid, enlarged. Valvular, diseases.

HOMEOPATHIC - Aur-i. is another unproved gold salt brought forward by Hale and used by him with success in cases of chronic pericarditis, valvular diseases, arteriosclerosis, ozaena, lupus, osteitis, ovarian cysts, and myomata uterus. Senile paresis.

Obstruction of nose, thick, yellow, purulent, offensive discharge. Nostrils ulcerated. Strong desire for and feels better in open air. Constriction of chest. Tumultuous palpitations. Thyroid enlarged, right side, pulse rapid, eyes protrude. Ravenous appetite. Extreme thirst. Constipation. Aching in testes. Induration of uterus and ovaries. Leucorrhea with thick, yellow discharge.

MIND - Excited. Restlessness. Sensitive to noise. Aversion to company.

REFERENCES - Clarke. Hale.

AURUM METALLICUM

(Gold Metal)

PHARMACY - aur. Aurum metallicum. Gold metal. Aurum foliatum. Foliatum colloidale. Gold, (Au, At. Wt. 1968). Trituration. ***Historical dose:*** Trituration, Tincture and all potencies.

CLINICAL - ***Alcoholism.*** Amenorrhea. Angina pectoris. Anthropophobia. ***Arteriosclerosis***. Ascites. Asthma. Bone, disorders. Breath, offensive. Colic. ***Depression.*** Double, vision. Dropsy. Dyspnea. Ears, disorders. Erysipelas. Exostosis. Eye, disorders. Fatigue. Flatus. Fevers. Glaucoma. Gonorrhea. ***Grief.*** Headaches. ***Heart, disease.*** Hemorrhages. Hemorrhoids. Hemiopia. Hepatitis. ***Hopelessness.*** Hydrocele. ***Hypertension. Infertility.*** Inguinal, hernia. ***Insomnia.*** Jaundice. Leucorrhea. Lipoma. Locomotor ataxia. Melanosis. Mercurial poisoning. Miscarriages. Nasopharyngeal catarrh. Night terrors. Obesity. ***Orchitis. Otorrhea***. Ozaena. Palpitations. Paralysis. ***Photophobia***. Pining, boys. Pustules. Scrofula. Smell, disordered. ***Suicidal, depression. Syphilis.*** Testicles, affections. Tongue, nodules. Tuberculosis. Tumors. Uterus, disorders. Vaginismus. Vertigo. Vision, disordered. Warts. Weakness.

HOMEOPATHIC - Sol of the Alchemists. This use of gold as an anti-venereal and anti-scrofulous remedy is very ancient, but has been forgotten until rediscovered by homeopathy.

Gold profoundly affects the entire organism, exercising a solvent action on the tissues, producing ulcerations and the disappearances of new growths. It is one of the best antidotes to mercurial over-dosing and especially in cases of syphilis. Scrofula and bone decay. Produces rushes of blood and hemorrhages. ***"Worse from sunset to sunrise***."

Ulcers which attack the bones. Warts, scrofulous, syphilitic, mercurial. Exostosis, decay, nightly bone pains, especially cranial, nasal and palatine. Glands swollen in scrofulous subjects. Palpitations and congestions. Frequently indicated in secondary syphilis and for the effects of mercury.

Ascites often in conjunction with heart disorders. Ozaena. Sexual hypersensitivity. ***Arteriosclerosis***. High blood pressure. Nightly paroxysms of pain behind sternum. Sclerosis of liver, arterial system, brain.

Shelton has recorded effects on girls working with gold leaf, including the occurrence of a "thick leucorrheal discharge, not offensive, white or yellowish, occasionally profuse invariably worse by walking."

MIND - Mental states of great depression. No remedy produces more ***acute mental depression*** than Aurum met. There is a condition of ***melancholy, hopelessness and profound depression.*** Acute depression. Future looks dark. Hopelessness with heart disease. Want of self-confidence and thinks others have none which makes her unhappy.

Complaints after grief, fright, anger, disappointed love, contradiction, reserved displeasure. Ailments from unusual responsibilities. Duty-bound. Workaholic, industrious, always busy and working, never finished. ***Grief and depression.*** Financial loss. ***Hopelessness.*** Aggravation from strong emotions. ***Forsaken feeling.*** Sadness when alone. Homesickness.

Despondent and great desire to commit suicide. Profound despondency, with increased blood pressure. Loss of love of life. ***Disgust of life and thoughts of suicide.*** Despair from pain, wants to jump out of window. ***Talks of committing suicide***. Every opportunity is sought for self-destruction. ***Tendency to suicide and longing for death.***

Mental derangements. Weak memory. Melancholy, imagines he is unfit for this world, never can succeed. She does everything wrong. Thinks had neglected something, her friends, her duty. Pining boys, low spirited, lifeless, weak memory. Self-reproach, self-criticism. Feeling of self-condemnation and utter worthlessness.

Peevish and vehement at least contradiction. ateful and quarrelsome. Dictatorial. Grumbling. ***Boredom***. Indisposed to talk. Vexed mood. Enraged by least contradiction. ***Oversensitive to contradiction,*** resulting in explosive fits of anger and violence. Anger at absent persons. Hatred of persons who had offended. Trembling when he can't satisfy his anger.

Changing moods. Brooding melancholy, alternating with irritability and moroseness. Excitement and confusion. Hysteria, laughs and cries alternately. Weeping when meeting people. Weeping, because he imagines he has lost the affection of his friends.

Anthrophobia. Great fear of death. Fears the least noise. Fear of persons intruding. Frightened easily on falling asleep.

Oversensitive to pain, to smell, taste, hearing and touch. ***Hypersensitive to noise***, causes excitement, confusion. Excitement about absent persons during pain. Loquacity. Constant rapid questioning without waiting for reply. Rapid questioning without waiting for a reply. Speaks continually in questions. Cannot do things fast enough.

Delirium with exaltation of strength. Religious mania, imagines herself irretrievably lost. Violent hysteria, with desperate actions, thrashes oneself about. ***Weeping, praying and self-reproaching.*** Delusion has neglected his duty and deserves reproach. Imagines to see obstacles in his way everywhere. Wrings the hands.

Abdomen - Ascites with heart disorders. Colic, with sensation of great uneasiness and inclination to evacuate. Incarcerated flatus. Abdomen inflated. Grumbling and rumbling. Right hypochondrium hot and painful. Swelling and suppuration of inguinal glands. Inguinal hernia of children. Tendency of hernia to protrude. Swelling and suppuration of the inguinal glands. Frequent gas, very fetid wind.

Back - Stinging pains in small of back. As if lower spine bulged backwards. Lumbar muscles painfully stiff, thigh cannot be raised. Swollen cervical glands like knotted cord. Tension in neck as if muscles too short, even at rest, worse stooping. Pains, drawing and acute, in the back and sometimes so violent as to prevent any motion of the limbs.

Bones - Destruction of bones like secondary syphilis. Pain in bones of head, lumps under scalp, exostosis with nightly pains in bones. Decay of nasal, palatine and mastoid bones. Soreness of affected bones, better in open air, worse at night.

Causations - Ill effects of grief, fright, anger, disappointed love, contradiction, reserved displeasure. Prolonged anxiety, unusual responsibility. Loss of property.

Chest - Aching in left side of the chest. Crushing weight under sternum, worse ascending. Stitches in the sternum. Constrictive oppression of the chest. Pain, as if there were a plug placed under the ribs. Much congestion in the chest. Oppression of chest with faceache. Inflammatory swelling of axillary glands.

Constitutions - Suited to sanguine people with black hair and dark eyes, olive-brown complexion. Syphilitic and mercurial patients. When syphilis is implanted on the scrofulous constitution.

Constitutions - It is adapted to nervous, hysterical women, girls at puberty. Also light-haired scrofulous persons. Pining boys and old age. Old people with heart disease. Persons who are low-spirited, lifeless, weak memory, yet sensitive to pain, which drives them to despair.

Cough - Cough from want of breath at night. Cough with tough yellow sputum on awaking in morning. Dry, nervous spasmodic cough, peculiar to women from sunset to sunrise. Cough from want of breath, at night.

Ears - Congestion to ears. Burning, prickling, itching. Decay of the mastoid process. ***Obstinate fetid ottorrhea*** after scarlatina. Flow of fetid pus from the ears. External meatus bathed in pus. Labyrinthine disease due to syphilis. Menière's disease. Nerve deafness with embarrassed speech. Oversensitive to noise, but better music. Hardness of hearing with embarrassed speech. Humming, buzzing and rushing in the ears. Roaring in the ears.

Eyes - Orbits feel sore. Feels tense. Violent pains in bones around eye (Asaf.). Intestinal keratitis. ***Vascular cornea***. Pains from without inward. ***Sticking pains inward***. Trachoma with pannus. Glaucoma. ***Extreme photophobia***. Constant lachrymation. Styes. Eyes better moonlight and after active muscular exercise.

Face - Anxious expression. Inflammation of the bones of the face. Congested, bluish-red. Face puffed, and shining as if from sweat. Tearing in zygoma. Mastoid and other facial bones inflamed. Red eruption, which peels off, on the forehead and on the nose. Painful swelling of the submaxillary glands. Parotids swollen, painful to touch. Swelling of the cheeks.

Female - Amenorrhea with great sadness. Delayed menarche. Menses too late, and scanty or absent. Before menses, swelling of axillary glands. Uterine troubles worse reaching high with arms. Uterus enlarged and prolapsed. Induration and ulceration of the womb from repeated miscarriages. ***Uterine disorders with depression.*** Prolapsus uterus with heaviness in abdomen. Prolapsus uterus, with backache, worse during menses. Vaginismus. Great sensitiveness of vagina. Burning-smarting of vulva. Labia majora red, swollen. Leucorrhea profuse and corroding. Leucorrhea yellow, thick white, not offensive. Leucorrhea, worse walking. ***Infertility***, also of those women who are mentally depressed on account of their barrenness. Depression during pregnancy. Despair from labor pains. Labor pains make her desperate. Suppressed breast-milk.

Food - Loathing of food. Bulimia. Loss of appetite in pining boys. Appetite and thirst increased with qualmishness. Excessive hunger and thirst. Aversion to meat. Craves nothing but sour things. Desire for milk and coffee. Desire for alcohol, wine. Desire bread, delicacies such as pastries. Water tastes foul. Worse after drinking. Worse after wine.

Head - Rush of blood to head. ***Violent pain in head, worse during the night***, outward pressure, causing confusion. Roaring in head. Vertigo. Tearing through brain to forehead. Pain in bones extending to face. Congestion to head. Head hot, full. Headache of students with precordial anxiety and flushes of heat to the head. As if air passed over the brain. Exostosis with boring pain. Lumps under scalp. Baldness from syphilis. Boils on scalp.

Heart - Angina Pectoris. Oppression at the heart. ***High blood pressure.*** Carotids and temporal arteries throb visibly. Valvular lesions of arteriosclerosis. Heart feels loose on walking. Palpitations compels him to stop. Violent palpitation, at puberty. ***Sensation as if heart stopped beating*** for two or three seconds, immediately followed by tumultuous rebound with sinking at the epigastrium. ***Palpitations with rush of blood to chest.*** Heart bruised, sore worse suppressed foot sweat. Aortic disease. Fatty degeneration of heart. Hypertrophy. Endocarditis. Carotids and temporal arteries throb visibly. ***Pulse rapid, feeble, irregular***. Pulse small but accelerated.

Kidneys - Nephritis with cardiac and hepatic diseases. Painful retention of urine with urgent inclination to urinate. Pressure on the bladder. Constant urging. Urine turbid, like buttermilk. Urine scanty, greenish-brown. Urine with thick mucus-like sediment. Frequent emission of watery urine. Hematuria. Urine increased, pale.

Limbs - Holds the left arm during attack of palpitations. Nightly leg pains. All the blood seems to rush from head to lower limbs. Dropsy of lower limbs. Orgasm, as if blood were boiling in all veins. Paralytic, tearing pains in joints. Knees weak. Pains in both the knees as if tightly bandaged. Paralytic feeling in legs. Nails turn blue. Trembling feet. Hot bruised soles, at night. Cold foul foot sweat.

Liver - Liver region hot and painful. Hepatitis. Liver with heart symptoms. Jaundice of pregnancy.

Lungs - Asthma, from congestion to chest. Cardiac asthma with weak pulse, mental depression and great debility. Asthma worse open air. Suffocative attacks, with spasmodic constriction of chest. Dyspnea worse laughing, at night. Always takes a deep breath and cannot get enough air. Frequent, deep breathing, stitches in sternum. Accumulation of mucus in the trachea, which is expectorated with difficulty. Tough yellow mucus, on awaking in morning.

Male - ***Pain and swelling of testicles***. Chronic induration of testicles. ***Atrophy of testicles in boys***. Undeveloped testes. Itching of scrotum. Hydrocele of children. ***Orchitis.*** Chronic induration of testicles. Epididymitis. Sarcocele. Flow of prostatic fluid, with flaccidity of the penis. Bubo. Chancre. Condylomata around corona glandis. Violent erections. Sexual desire greatly increased. Nocturnal erections and pollutions. Ulcers on scrotum.

Modalities - Better from cool, open air. Better cold bathing. Better becoming warm. Better music. Better walking. Better moonlight. Worse from emotions, depressing affections. Worse mental exertion. Worse in cold weather. Worse when getting cold. ***Worse cloudy weather, winter.*** Worse at night. ***Worse sunset to sunrise.*** Worse mercury, alcohol, iodide.

Mouth - Aphthae on mouth. Copious saliva. Saliva sweetish. Fetid smell of the mouth, like rotten cheese. Foul breath in girls at puberty. Taste putrid or bitter. Metallic taste. Milky or sweetish taste, foul even to water. Ulceration of gums. Ulcers on palate. Inside of mouth blistered. Gums swollen, dark red, bleeding.

Nose - Nose red and swollen. Inflammation of nose. Decay with fetid discharge, purulent, bloody. Red, knobby tip of nose. Ozaena. Snubbed. ***Ulcerated, painful***, swollen, obstructed. Boring pains in nose, worse at night. ***Horrible odor*** from nose and mouth. Putrid smell from nose. Fetid discharge, purulent, bloody. Complaints from strong odors. Sensitive smell (Carb-ac.).

Perspiration - Cold sweat and damp all over. Sweat about genitals. Copious general perspiration. Early morning sweats, mostly about genitals. Profuse sweat in endocarditis.

Rectum - Fetid flatus. Constipation, stool very large in size, or very hard and knotty. Constipation better during menses. Copious stool. Offensive stool during pregnancy. Stools offensive, painful, greyish, ashy. Diarrhea alternating with constipation. Nightly diarrhea with burning in the rectum. Hemorrhoids with rectal catarrh. Hemorrhoids bleed during stool. Prolapse of rectum during menses. Warts around the anus.

Skin - Acne. Large red pimples. Lipoma.

Violent itching. Indurations under the skin, like wheals. Pustules in the face and on the neck and chest. Formication, here and there, over the body. Transient but intense itching of the abdomen, hips, knees, arms and wrists. Fine papular eruption on face. Deep ulcers. Warts.

Sleep - Weary, but cannot rest or sleep. Sleeplessness after midnight. ***Chronic insomnia with depression.*** Nocturnal mumbling in the form of questions. Sobs aloud in sleep. ***Moaning and crying out in sleep.*** Sobs aloud in sleep. Disturbed by sexual excitement. Drowsiness after meals. ***Awakened by bone pains with despair.*** Unrefreshing sleep.

Sleep - Fatigue and weakness in the morning on waking. Vivid, frightful dreams. Frightful dreams. Restless sleep, with anxious dreams. Dreams of thieves. Dreams of dead, death and corpses. Dreams towards morning.

Stomach - Swelling of epigastrium. Burning at stomach and hot belchings. Burning, drawing, and cutting pain, pressure. Pain in the stomach, as if from hunger. Uneasiness in the epigastrium. Stinging pain when touching stomach. Nausea from mental labor. Sour eructations.

Teeth - Decay of teeth. Toothache, with heat and congestion in the head. Looseness of the teeth. Sensation as if too long. Ulcers in the gums, with swelling of the cheeks. Toothache worse at night, worse drawing cold air into mouth. Gums swollen, dark red, bleeding.

Temperature - Painfully sensitive to cold, shivering in bed. Febrile chills over the whole body, while in bed in the evening. Coldness of the entire body, with bluish color of the nails, nauseous taste, with inclination to vomit. Heat of the face, with cold in the hands and feet.

Throat - Voice nasal. Stitches when swallowing, pain in glands. Decay of the palate. Drinks come through nose. Stinging in throat when swallowing. Tonsils swollen and ulcerated. Red and swollen tonsils.

Tongue - Aphthae on tongue. Tongue swollen, with scirrhus-like hardness. Flabby taste with clean tongue. Tongue trembling and dry. Tongue leathery, hard. Tongue dry and coated. Tongue coated at back. Ulcers on tongue. Warts on tongue.

Vertigo - Stupefaction during vertigo. Vertigo when stooping. Vertigo as if turning in a circle, better on rising. Vertigo as if drunk when walking in open air, feels as if he would fall to left, must lie down.

Vision - Double vision. ***Hemiopia, upper half of objects invisible.*** Hemiopia from straining eyes. Yellow crescent bodies floating obliquely upward. Sees fiery objects. Sees fog or smoke before eyes. Everything looks blue. Black spots, flames, sparks before the eyes. Irregular pupils. Optical illusions in bright colors.

COMMENTS - Boring pains and burning stitches predominate. The head is giddy, full, hot. Rush of blood to the head. Vertigo as if turning in a circle when stooping, goes away on rising. As if drunk when walking in the open air. Sensation as if a current of air were rushing through the head if not kept warm. Bones of skull painful, especially lying down.

Vertical half-sight. Fiery sparks. Decay of mastoid process of bones of nose. Ozaena. In the abdominal region there is swelling of liver, jaundice (Merc.). Hernia inguinal or umbilical and in children. Onanism.

The sexual organs are markedly affected. Induration of testes. Undeveloped testicles in puny boys. Swelling or neuralgia of testicle. Uterus prolapsed and indurated, the weight of it causes prolapses. The chloride of gold and sodium acts more powerfully in these conditions.

Suffocative attacks with oppression of chest. Anxious palpitations from congestion to the chest. Palpitation with anguish and tremulous fearfulness. Pain in heart region extending down left arm to fingers. Boring pains in bones, worse at night.

Hysterical spasms with laughing and crying alternately. Hypersensitive to all pains. Great ebullitions with congestion to the head and chest and palpitation of the heart.

Frightful dreams, sobs aloud when asleep. Chilliness predominates, shivering in open air, coldness of hands and feet, sometimes lasting all night. Heat, only in the face.

Perspiration in the morning hours, mostly on and around the genitals. Paralytic drawing in the limbs in the morning when awaking and on getting cold.

Severe heart disease, arteriosclerosis, cerebral arteriosclerosis, high blood pressure, with depression. Sensation of the heart not beating or getting heart pains or that it is beating too fast. Fear of heart disease.

Also for arthritis or for the ill effects of gold shots. Tennis elbow. Sinus infections, breaking down in nasal septum. Late stage syphilis. Chronic, severe, unrelenting insomnia that no medication can help. Hair falls out.

Suicidal depression or severe depression with no hope of recovery. Giving Aurum is giving a ray of hope back, that the actual remedy is like potentized light, because in their life there's no light or hope.

May have history of attempted suicide from financial loss, from the loss of money and property, loss of love. Manic depression. Suicidal tendencies from pain. Kent describes losing the will to live as the deepest illness one can have

Religious mania with deep guilt (Nat-m.). Depression after death of a loved one. Over investment, possessiveness followed by loss. Over responsible, strong sense of duty and loyalty.

Keynote insomnia, drives a person crazy, particularly in the elderly. Geriatric remedy for people who feel they've lost their purpose or value in life, but act stoic. "Hippocratic countenance," as if their face was chiseled out of stone. Flat tone to voice, can have lack of emotion but with a happy façade.

Pathologically independent and can have difficulty expressing themselves. Resigned to depression. Introverted. Kent gave the etiologies as prolonged anxiety, grief, and unusual responsibilities that were heaped on someone and they failed. Financial loss, abuse of mercury as a medicine, or a history of suppressed syphilis.

Craves sunshine, finds dull, cloudy days unbearable. Depressed, dejected, tired of life, discontented.

Depression worse at night. Deep self-condemnation, guilt complex, easily frightened, feels worthless. Restless, hurried, fidgety.

Quarrelsome, may have wild outbursts of rage followed by remorse, worse contradiction. Sensitive to pain and cold. Chilly, likes to be wrapped up but may still like fresh air. Worse from sunset to sunrise. May have a history of syphilis, especially if there is bone pain. Worse grief or emotional stress.

RELATIONS - ***Antidoted by:*** Bell., Chin., Cocc., Coff., Cupr., Merc., Puls., Spig., Sol-n. ***Antidote to:*** Merc., Spig., Chronic effects of alcohol, Kali-i. ***Compare:*** (1) Aur-ars. (2) Aur-mur-kali. - in uterine induration and hemorrhage. (3) Aur-sulph. (4) Also, Asaf. - in decay of bones of ears and nose. (5) Syphilis, Kali-i., Hep., Merc., Mez., Nit-ac., Phos., Syph. (5) Bell., Caps. - Caries of mastoid, corpulency. (6) Calc. - night terrors, leuco-phlegmatic. (7) Dig., Ferr., Glon. - hyperemia of lung from heart. (8) Kali-br. - anguish at heart and desire to move about. (9) Lach., Lyc., Merc., Nit-ac., (10) Nux-v., - hernia, prolapsed uterus. (11) Tarent. - Heart as if turned around.

REFERENCES - Boericke. Clarke. Murphy.

AURUM MURIATICUM

(Gold Chloride)

PHARMACY - aur-m. Aurum muriaticum. Gold chloride. ***Historical dose:*** Trituration, Tincture and all potencies.

CLINICAL - Albuminuria. Amaurosis. Angina pectoris. Anus, fistula. Asthma. Brachial neuritis. Bubo. ***Cancer.*** Decay. Condylomata. Dropsy. Eczema. Fistula. Gland, disorders. Gonorrhea. Hair, loss. Heart, disorders. Hemorrhage. Hemorrhoids Indurations. Infertility. Leucorrhea. Liver, disorders. Morvan's disease. Multiple sclerosis. Ophthalmia. Ozaena. Periostitis. Pudenda, over-sensitiveness. Spinal, sclerosis. Spleen, enlarged. Syphilis. Tuberculosis. Uterus, tumors, Uterus, hemorrhage. Vaginitis. Voice, hoarse. ***Warts.***

HOMEOPATHIC - Gold salts, like mercury salts, dissolve organic tissues, they stimulate the heart more, but act on fluid tissues less powerfully than mercury. This salt has been proved.

The symptoms are mostly identical with those of the metal, but some are peculiar or more pronounced in the one than in the other. The Muriatic element is seen in the heart symptoms, violent palpitations, sore aching, heaviness and sensation of rigidity in heart, hyperemia from heart disease.

Aurum muriaticum is a sycotic remedy, causing suppressed discharges to reappear. Marked catarrhal and glandular disorders. Burning, yellow, acrid leucorrhea. Heart symptoms, glandular affection. Warts appear on various parts on tongue, genitals. Sclerotic and exudative degeneration of the nervous system.

Indescribable weariness in whole body. Sclerotic and exudative degenerations of nervous system. Hypertrophy of all the fingers. Drawing pains in various parts, especially the limbs.

Multiple sclerosis, pains and tremors, it will often help in sclerotic and exudative degenerations. Valuable in menopausal hemorrhages from the womb. Diseases of frontal sinus. Stitching pain in left side of forehead. Weariness, aversion to all work. Drawing feeling in stomach.

MIND - Great depression of mind. ***Suicidal disposition***, with frequent weeping. Tired of life. Everything is disagreeable, dreary, even nature around. Sadness, as when homesick. Sad, as if a great misfortune impended. Aversion to weeping. Ailments after mortification. Laziness, aversion to all work. Desires company. Irritable without cause.

Great restlessness, changes his position every moment. Restlessness, nervousness better open air. Great anxiety with palpitations. Full of whims and notions. Delusion that he has every disease. If left alone thinks of nothing but of one's ailments and becomes more out of humor. Anger when thinking of his ailments. Starting from sleep, on waking as if suffocated.

Abdomen - Distension of abdomen. Redness, heat, itching and biting at umbilicus. Spleen enlarged. Abdomen sensitive to touch. Swollen abdomen. Ascites. Stiffness in region of groins. Swelling of inguinal glands.

Back - Tension in dorsal vertebrae. Dull drawing pain in neck while sitting. Burning, pricking, cutting pains and stiffness in back. Very severe backache.

Causations - Ill effects of chagrin, fright, vexation.

Chest - Anxious contraction of chest. Pressure under sternum. Pleuritic pains left side of chest, changing place.

Constitutions - In this remedy the sycotic miasm unites with the syphilitic and psoric miasms to produce constitutions that are feeble and prone to degenerative diseases. Suited to the lymphatic, scrofulous constitutions.

Cough - Short, dry cough, in paroxysms. Frequent hard cough, with white sputa mingled with threads of blood. Frequent, loud sounding cough. Loose, with thick yellow sputum.

Ears - Burning and itching behind ears worse night. Tinkling sound in ears followed by deafness, as if interior of ears were large and empty. Buzzing in left ear and sensitivity. Ringing and roaring in ears. Music relieves. Redness of ears. Scurf behind ears.

Eyes - Sudden blindness after childbirth. Neuralgic pains in left eye. Scrofulous phlyctenular ophthalmia. Chronic inflammation of margins of lids. Fistula lachrymalis. Burning, pricking, itching and tickling in eyes and lids. Red sclerotics. Burning heat and prickling. Lachrymation. Difficulty in keeping eyes shut. Lids agglutinated in morning. Chronic inflammation of edges of eyelids.

Face - Acne rosacea. Red face. Pale face with red spots. Hair falling out of eyebrows and head. Exostosis of right cheekbone. Induration of lips. Burning like pepper on lips. Cancerous ulcers on lips. Painful swelling of maxillary glands.

Female - Amenorrhea. ***Suppressed menses.*** Menses too early and profuse, blood acrid, excoriating. ***Painful induration of os uteri.*** Metritis. ***Gonorrheal discharge with swelling of both groins.*** Hemorrhage from the uterus at menopausal. Constant discharges from vulva. Burning stitching of vulva. Heat and itching in vagina. Leucorrhea, light yellow, especially mornings. ***Vaginitis.*** Leucorrhea and red pustules on labia before menses. Leucorrhea acrid, excoriating thighs with itching of genitals. Gonorrheal discharge with swellings in each groin.

Food - Slow digestion. Appetite increased or lost. Thirst. Disgust for sweetened coffee. Coffee, tea, wine aggravates.

Head - Head hot, limbs cool. Cold sensation on vertex. Dullness in head. Drawing pain in forehead. Constant burning in whole head. Burning in forehead. Throbbing pains in left temple. Tearing pain in bones of skull. Head feels insensible. Pressure on brain, along sagittal suture. Congestion increasing to delirium. Tickling itching on forehead. Falling out of hair, eyebrows and beard.

Heart - ***Angina pectoris.*** Sharp pains above the heart. Palpitations with anxiety, worse emotions. Palpitation when thinking about his diseases. Heartbeats increased, too strong. Rheumatic endocarditis. Irregular heartbeats with severe constriction of chest.

Kidneys - Burning on urinating. Urine feels as if too hot. Incontinence of urine. Tenesmus of bladder. Kidney pain with pale, clear urine. Burning, tickling and heat in urethra. Scanty urine. Turbid urine with brick-red sediment.

Limbs - Morvan's disease, hypertrophy of fingers. Swelling of the wrists with tension on reversing the hand and lancinations in grasping an object, tearing pains in middle finger after meals. Legs swollen and very tender along inside of tibia. Exostosis. Periostitis after typhoid.

Liver - Induration of liver with dropsy.

Lungs - Loud cough with thick yellow expectoration. Asthma worse at night. Impeded breathing, from pressure on chest. Difficult breathing, from stagnation of blood. Suffocation at night.

Male - Diminished virility. Increased desire. Exhausting erections. Violent itching of glans penis wakes him at night. Drawing along spermatic cord. Painful drawing in left testis extends towards inguinal ring, recurring by paroxysms. Chancres. Condylomata. ***Syphilitic gonorrhea.*** Excrescences from glans up to sacrum. Warts on prepuce.

Modalities - Better from cold washing, weather. Better gentle motion. Worse from ascending stairs. Worse from warmth, throws off bed-covers.

Mouth - Dryness of mouth. Increased saliva, frequent desire to swallow. Metallic taste. Mouth filled with aphthae. Flat, bad taste. Taste entirely lost. Burning itching and biting in mouth.

Nose - Offensive, watery discharge, irritating upper lip. Pressing pain in nose. Ozaena scrofulosa. Tingling, burning and itching in nose. Redness and inflammation with itching. Red swelling with ulcerated nostrils. Dry yellow crusts. Sensation of stoppage. Deep crack in alae nasi. Sudden running of pus from nose. Blowing of blood from nose. Snuffles. Nostrils stuffed up with hard crusts.

Perspiration - Copious sweats, offensive smell. Copious sweats, cold. Promotes sweat in smallpox.

Rectum - Obstinate constipation. Hemorrhoids, bleeding during stool. Condylomata at anus. Excoriation at anus and between thighs. Fistula. Diarrhea after eating. Diarrhea, worse night after eating with pain in bowels. Frequent fluid stools. Stools, greyish-white, yellow, watery.

Sleep - Yawning after eating. Sleepy by day, even at work. Comatose sleep. Sleeplessness from excitement. Sleeplessness from palpitations. Frequent starting. Dreams with sadness. Tormenting dreams.

Stomach - Gastritis. Putrid eructations and nausea. Hot feeling in stomach. Cramps. Burning, cutting, stitching in stomach, cramps. Nausea, distension. Fullness of stomach, after eating. Nausea, worse fasting, better after breakfast. Painful drawing in pit worse eating, drinking. Vomiting of a green fluid.

Temperature - Violent chill and fever. Hectic fever, with dropsy, after scarlatina.

Teeth - Looseness of teeth. Front teeth sensitive. Dental fistula. Toothache with thrilling pains. Great tenderness of gums with salivation. Gums inflamed or white, bluish.

Throat - Scraping and pricking in throat. Hoarseness, speaking difficult. Dyspnea, sensation in larynx as if closed. Laryngeal disorders in syphilis and mercurio-syphilis. Frequent desire to swallow, feeling of a plug in throat. Suppurating ulcer on tonsil.

Tongue - Redness, dryness and excoriation of tongue. Cancer of the tongue. Tongue hard as leather, hardly movable. Indurated tongue, warts, cancer, ulcers. Induration after glossitis. Yellow coated tongue. Warts on tongue.

Vertigo - Vertigo as if walking in air.

Vision - Slow accommodation for near or far objects. Sudden blindness in childbed. Sudden blindness after scarlatina. Pupils don't react to light. Letters disappear in evening when reading at candlelight. Paper seems white, as if not printed upon.

COMMENTS - Grimmer said that the patient needing this medicine is sensitive to heat and relieved in wet weather, he is as restless as Arsenicum and as depressed as Aurum. ***Cancerous warts*** on the tongue and genitals have been cured with this medicine.

Aur-m. is particularly valuable in hemorrhages from the womb at menopausal and after, which are frequently of sycotic origin. Violent chill and fever. Hectic fever. Sensitive to heat and relieved in wet weather, restless (Ars.).

Depressed (Aur.), with suicidal conflict. Will discuss and plan suicide, but fear of it. Both "desires death" and "loathing of life." Boericke noted this conflict, similar to Nat-s., but with Nat-s. they are constantly trying to restrain themselves. For Aur-m., the plans content them, a wonderful secret that they can rely on.

Catarrhal and glandular disorders are marked. Warts appear in various parts, on the tongue, on the genitals. Digestion is slow. Diarrhea after eating.

A sycotic remedy, causing suppressed discharges to reappear.

Halbert gave Aur-m. 2x with much success in cases of sclerotic and exudative degeneration of the nervous system. He narrated a case of disseminated sclerosis, the result of a fall, one of exudative localized meningitis and one of Morvan's disease greatly improved under its use.

This patient, a male cook, had hypertrophy of all the fingers. In some of them this had progressed until the painless whitlows appeared.

Analgesia and anesthesia were present and some atrophy of the muscles of the hand and arm. Brachial neuritis appeared to be the causative factor in the case. Remarkable improvement occurred under Aur-m. 2x.

RELATIONS - ***Antidoted by:*** Bell., Cann-i., Merc. Sulphur springs are incompatible. ***Compare:*** (1) Acon., Am-c., Arg-m., Arg-n., Ars., Aurum met. Bell., Cann-i., Ferr., Glon., Hecla., Lyc., Merc., Nit-ac., Phos., Plat., Sil., Sulph.

REFERENCES - Boericke. Clarke. Grimmer. Murphy.

AURUM MURIATICUM KALINATUM

(Potassium Chloroaurate)

PHARMACY - aur-m-k. Aurum muriaticum kalinatum. Potassium chloroaurate. Double Chloride of Potassium and Gold. ***Historical dose:*** Trituration and all potencies.

CLINICAL - Uterus, hemorrhage induration.

HOMEOPATHIC - An unproved gold salt, recommended by Dr. Burford and others as the best preparation of gold in cases of uterine induration and hemorrhage.

RELATIONS - ***Compare:*** (1) Aur-m-n., Hydrin-m.

REFERENCES - Clarke.

AURUM MUR. NATRONATUM

(Sodium Chloroaurate)

PHARMACY - aur-m-n. Aurum muriaticum natronatum. Sodium chloroaurate. Double Chloride of Gold and Sodium. ***Historical dose:*** Trituration and all potencies.

CLINICAL - Amaurosis. Amenorrhea. Arteriosclerosis. Ascites. Bright's disease. Bubo. Cancer. Cervicitis. Chancres. Cirrhosis. Dyspepsia. Erysipelas. ***Gastroenteritis.*** ***Fibroids.*** Hemorrhoids. Hair, loss. Headaches Hectic fever. Hypertension. ***Indurations*** Infertility. ***Jaundice.*** Leucorrhea. Miscarriage. Nephritis. Ovarian, tumors. Prolapsed uterus. Psoriasis, syphilitica. Rhinoscleroma

Scrofula. Sycosis. Syphilis. Syphilitic, ataxia. Tongue, disorders. Tuberculosis. ***Tumors.*** Ulcers. ***Uterus, indurations. Uterus, tumors.*** Warts.

HOMEOPATHIC - This double salt of natrum and chloride of gold shows more of the syphilitic miasm present, carcinoma on a syphilitic base. Burnett stated that Aur-m-n. has more power over ***uterine tumors*** than any other remedy.

Anshutz wrote, "Never have I observed gold so startling in its action as in the following case: The patient is a type of the scrofulous habit, reddish hair, pasty complexion, thick nose, coarse features.

"About thirty years of age. He has had the misfortune of being infected by syphilis and the still greater ill-luck of being treated by mercury and iodine to excess. All these circumstances conjoined helped to produce a complication of morbid conditions which would put medical art to a severe test."

A case of rhinoscleroma was reported cured by Aur-m-n. in 5x by Kranz-Busch. Old cases of rheumatism or gouty pains. Scrofula. Burnett considered it to have more power over uterine tumors than any other gold preparation. Aur-m-n. has been proved, but it has been chiefly used on general Aurum indications.

Aur-m-n. has ***induration*** of one part, softening of another. This remedy has a pronounced effect on the female organs. ***Fibroids of uterus***. Enormous induration of an ovary. Cancer of breast and uterus. Cancerous warts on tongue. Corrosive leucorrhea, pustules on genitals.

Arteriosclerosis. High blood pressure due to disturbed functions of the nervous system. Warts on tongue. White stools with jaundice. Swelling of testicle. Bright's disease. Old cases of rheumatism and gouty pains. Hepatic cirrhosis. Interstitial nephritis.

Affections of the bones and glands. Boring pains are very marked in the pathogenesis of this salt, over left eye, skull, chest, tibia and bones generally. Periosteal swelling on lower jaw. Psoriasis syphilitica. Chancres, ulcers, warts. Bubo. Syphilitic ataxia.

MIND - Depression and anger. Ailments from anger. Hysteria. Mental activities are disordered. Feeling of unrest and impatience. Reproaches, himself. Yielding. Anxiety of consciousness. Remorse. Ailments after reproaches.

Ailments from grief. Fear of failure and rejection. Cautiousness. Fear of undertaking anything new. Fear of strangers. Compulsive disorders. Sarcastic. Self pity. Tendency to daydream.

Abdomen - Coldness in abdomen. Dropsy. ***Gastroenteritis.*** Pressure in the right hypochondrium. Dropsy without fever but threatening suffocation.

Back - Cracking in cervical vertebrae on bending head. Burning and drawing, tension and pressure in muscles to left of nape extending to shoulder, worse bending head to right, at times unbearable during rest. Pustular eruption on back.

Causations - Vexation (jaundice).

Constitutions - Suited to Carbo-nitrogenoid and mercurio-syphilitic constitutions.

Eyes - Amaurosis. Ophthalmia, scrofulous, cancerous, at the same time, nose scurfy.

Face - Ulcers in cavities of upper jaw. Pallor of face. Ulcer in right corner of mouth.

Female - ***Indurated cervix.*** Chronic metritis and prolapsed uterus. Uterus fills up whole pelvis. Leucorrhea with spasmodic contraction of vagina. Leucorrhea, corroding the parts. Ovaries indurated. Ovarian dropsy. Enlargement of ovary. Sub-involution. Ossified uterus. ***Fibroids of uterus. Uterus, tumors.*** Scirrhus cancer of uterus. Carcinoma of breast and uterus. Pustules on genitals. Miscarriage from uterine indurations. Ulceration of neck of womb and vagina. Ulcers with induration of uterus.

Fever - Remarkable coldness of back. Remarkable heat in skin. Sweats only on right side, left (affected) side of head remains dry. Excessive perspiration.

Food - No appetite in jaundice.

Head - Hair falls out. Every morning pressure over eyes, pains in forehead, dullness in head, lasting until afternoon, better in evening, nasal discharge bloody, fetid, ichorus. Continual humming in head with beating of carotids. Violent headache, in left side of head, mostly over eye.

Heart - Palpitations of young girls. Irregular heartbeats with anxiety and short breath, while sleeping. Severe violent beats of the heart with sensation of pressure while standing.

Kidneys - Dark urine in jaundice. Turbid urine.

Limbs - ***Rheumatism or gouty pains.*** Burning in skin of right axilla. Pressure in right deltoid. Boring and pressing pains in arms and elbow-joints. Boring pain in bones. Painful stitching in fingertips. Boring pains in thighs, knees, tibia (first right then left). Boring in both sides right Achilles tendon when sitting. Stitches in tips of toes in bunion.

Liver - Hepatic cirrhosis. Pressure in liver region. Jaundice after vexation.

Male - Ulcers on foreskin, warts around them. Ulcers on glans eating deeply. Chancre on internal surface of prepuce. Bubo in fold of groin.

Modalities - Worse in cold, wet weather. Worse from October to spring (headache). Worse by rest.

Mouth - Redness and swelling of palate behind upper incisors. Salivation. Bitter taste. Fetid odor from mouth.

Neck - Burning pain in skin of nape. Heat in nape rising into head and cheeks.

Nose - ***Ulcers, caries.*** Ozaena. Nose swollen, hard, shining (scrofulous), if he takes cold, erysipelas sets in. Destruction of nasal bones. Scurfy, oozing tetter on nose.

Perspiration - Sweats only on right side. ***Excessive sweats***. Suppressed sweats.

Rectum - Clay-like feces. Hemorrhoid which protrudes and is painful. Stools hard. Feces like whitish clay.

Skin - Intolerable itching all over body, sores followed by an eruption of little lumps, several covered with dark-looking scabs. Jaundice. Deep-spreading syphilitic ulcers on skin.

Teeth - Teeth get loose, look dirty, gums recede.

Throat - Swelling and inflammation of fauces. Small blisters on fauces.

Tongue - Burning, stitches and induration. Burning on tip of tongue. Tongue coated white in jaundice. Warts on tongue.

COMMENTS - Hale considered this the most active of all the preparations of gold. In toxic doses it causes ***"violent gastroenteritis"*** accompanied by cramps, convulsive trembling insomnia, priapism and insensibility.

In pathogenetic doses it causes epigastric pain, nausea, loss of appetite and constipation. The constipation is like that of Hydr., being accompanied with catarrh.

Hale used it with success in nervous dyspepsia with a tendency to diarrhea after eating in gastric and duodenal catarrh with or without jaundice.

He stated that the primary effect of the salt is to cause congestion, irritation of the uterus and ovaries, sub-acute metritis, ovaritis, profuse and premature menses, habitual abortion, nymphomania, ulceration of uterus, cervicitis. For these, the potencies are suitable.

The secondary effects are "Atonic amenorrhea, scanty and delaying menses, deficient sexual desire, infertility from ovarian torpor, ovarian dropsy," for these, Hale recommended the lowest triturations.

He suggested its use in puerperal mania with sexual excitement, ovaritis, gastro-intestinal irritation and suicidal impulses. Also in corresponding states in men.

Aur-m-n. is a specific for asymptomatic ovarian tumors and asymptomatic fibroids.

RELATIONS - ***Compare:*** (1) Arg-n., Ars., Bad., Bry., Crot., Con. (2) Graph., Hep., Iod., Kali-bi., Kali-i. (3) Lyc., Merc., Nit-ac., Phos., Sulph., Thuj.

REFERENCES - Boericke. Clarke. Grimmer. Murphy.

AURUM SULPHURATUM

(Gold Sulphide)

PHARMACY - aur-s. Aurum sulphuratum. Gold sulphide. Auric sulphide. ***Historical dose:*** Trituration and all potencies.

CLINICAL - Bedwetting. Goiter. Head, nodding. Impotence. Jaundice. Breasts disorders. Nightmare. Nose, swelling. Parkinson's disease. Pruritus vulvae. Staggering.

HOMEOPATHIC - This valuable gold preparation has been used with success in Aurum met. cases with some Sulphur indications.

Aur-s. has been proved and the most striking symptoms include constant nodding of head. Lancinations in occiput. Redness and swelling of nose, crusts, dry coryza, great sensitiveness to least contact.

Sensitiveness to touch was observed in other parts. Inclined to vomit after eating. Bedwetting. Impotence. Lancinations in penis. Heaviness in genitals. Heat, lancinations and itching of vulva.

Swelling of the breasts, painful to touch. Cracked nipples, sharp pain in point of nipples. Thick yellowish leucorrhea, especially in morning. Staggering gait. Weariness. Frightful dreams.

Indurations, ulcerations around nose, lips and genitals with intense itching of skin. Parkinson's disease, constant nodding of the head. Affections of the breasts, swelling pain, cracked nipples with sharp pains.

MIND - Desire for solitude. Disgust for life.

Breasts - Swelling of breasts, painful to touch. Cracks on nipples.

Eyes - Redness of eyelids. Morning agglutination. Stye near outer canthus. Photophobia.

Face - Cracked lips.

Female - Thick, yellowish leucorrhea, especially in the morning. Irregular menstruation. Sensitiveness of uterus to touch.

Head - Constant nodding of head. Continual rush of blood to had. Lancinations in occiput. Itching of scalp, worse night. Burning and smarting of scalp. Falling out of hair.

Heart - Palpitation when ascending a height.

Kidneys - Nocturnal bedwetting. Thick, yellow, red and sandy urine.

Lungs - Nightly paroxysms of loud cough. Hard cough with scanty expectoration of pure blood. Suffocating attacks at night.

Male - Frequent erections with desire for embrace, but ceasing immediately. Impotence.

Mouth - Redness, swelling and bleeding of gums. Aphthae.

Nose - Redness and swelling of nose. Crusts on nose. Sensitiveness to least contact.

Sleep - Troublesome frightful dreams of thieves of assassins.

Stomach - Great thirst. Watery belchings tasting of ingesta. Frequent hiccough. Very slow digestion.

Throat - Swelling of thyroid.

REFERENCES - Clarke. Grimmer.

AVENA SATIVA

(Oatstraw)

PHARMACY - aven. Avena sativa. Oatstraw. Common Oat. N. O. Gramineae. Tincture of fresh plant in flower. The fresh green plant, gathered in August is pounded to a pulp and macerated with two parts by weight of alcohol. ***Historical dose:*** Tincture and all potencies.

CLINICAL - ***Addictions.*** Alcoholism. Amenorrhea. Brain, fatigue. Cholera. Chorea. Coffee. ***Colds. Coryza.*** Debility. Delirium, tremens. ***Drug, abuse.*** Dysmenorrhea. Endocarditis. Epilepsy. Headaches. ***Heroin.*** Impotency. ***Insomnia.*** Influenza. Masturbation. Nervous, disorders. ***Neurasthenia. Opium, morphine, addiction.*** Palpitations. Sexual, weakness. ***Sleeplessness.*** Spermatorrhea. Tobacco. Tuberculosis. ***Weakness.***

HERBAL - Aven. improves the nutrition of brain and nervous system. One of the best tonics for debility after exhausting diseases. Valuable in enabling a patient to overcome the morphine or heroin habit.

Aven. has been used in substantial doses of 5 to 15 drops of the tincture in a large number of cases of nerve weakness. The only symptom that has been observed to be caused by it is a pain at the base of the brain from 20-drop doses.

For acute coryza, take 20 drop doses in hot water hourly for a few doses.

HOMEOPATHIC - Selective action on brain and nervous system, favorably influencing their nutritive function. Leading indications are nervous exhaustion, sexual debility, and general weakness. ***Sleeplessness with nervous exhaustion and weakness.*** Chronic insomnia. Delirium tremens.

Drug addictions. Bad effects of ***morphine or heroin addiction.*** Addicted to cocaine, marijuana, nervines, tranquilizers or sedatives. Alcoholism. ***Insomnia due to drugs or alcohol.*** Post-diphtheria paralysis. Rheumatism of heart.

Colds and coryza. Nervous palpitations. It is useful in nervous exhaustion, sexual debility, debility after exhausting diseases. Weakness of the mind when due to masturbation or sexual irregularities.

Nervous states of the female and male sexual systems. Nervous tremors of the aged. Parkinson's disease, chorea and epilepsy.

MIND - Prostration of mind, mental exhaustion, brain fag, with sleeplessness. Symptoms from mental or physical overwork. ***Mental exertion aggravates.*** Dullness, sluggishness. Difficulty of thinking and comprehending. Inability to keep mind on any one subject.

Nervous exhaustion in brain workers, or from worry and anxiety. ***Difficult concentration from masturbation.*** Brain fatigue with sleeplessness. ***Morphine or heroin addiction.*** Alcoholism, dipsomania to help withdrawal. Hypochondriasis.

Constitutions - Nervous constitution.

Female - Amenorrhea. Dysmenorrhea with weak circulation.

Head - Nervous headache at menstrual period with burning at top of head. Occipital headache with phosphatic urine. Aching deep in brain. Vertex headache during menses.

Heart - Inflammation of heart, carditis. Endocarditis. Rheumatic heart. Palpitations.

Limbs - Numbness, as if paralyzed. Weakness, twitching, trembling of hands. Strength of hand diminished. Numbness, insensibility. Paralytic weakness. Rheumatic pains.

Male - ***Disposition to masturbation.*** Troublesome erections, wanting. ***Seminal emissions*** aggravates. Seminal emissions without erection. Spermatorrhea. Impotency after sexual excesses. Diminished sexual desire.

Nose - ***Coryza.*** Acute colds. Watery discharge. Rhinitis.

Rectum - Cholera. Diarrhea.

Sleep - ***Chronic insomnia***, worse during convalescence. ***Sleeplessness*** after worry, mental exertion, ***after influenza***, from weakness. Insomnia, aggravated by exhaustion, alcohol. Sleeplessness in alcoholics, with delirium tremens.

Urine - Sediment, phosphates increased.

COMMENTS - Aven. is pre-eminently an anti-neurotic, quieting the nervous system to a remarkable degree. Its special sphere of action seems to be upon the male sexual organs, regulating the functional irregularities of these parts perhaps as much as any remedy can.

Aven. is indicated in the sleeplessness of the weak and elderly. Also for children who are nervous and weak. It is a most useful remedy in all cases of nervous exhaustion, general debility, nervous palpitation of the heart insomnia inability to keep the mind fixed upon any one subject. More especially when any or all of these troubles is apparently due to nocturnal emissions, masturbation, or sexual over activity.

This is a specific remedy for drug addiction, mainly heroin and morphine, but also tobacco, cocaine, marijuana and valium. Boericke noted it for alcohol addiction.

It is one of the most valuable means for overcoming morphine addiction. In most cases in which the habit has not used more than four grains daily the opiate may be abruptly discontinued and even substituted without any serious results.

If a larger quantity than this amount has been taken for some time, it is better to gradually reduce the daily dose of morphine in the usual manner, simply prescribing the Avena in addition. The latter should be given in the same dose, as a rule, regardless of the amount of morphine taken.

In other words, it is not necessary to increase the Avena as the opiate is withdrawn. When the quantity of morphine has not exceeded four grains daily it should be stopped at once, as stated above and Avena given in its stead in fifteen-drop doses, four times a day in wine glassful of hot water.

By this method the disagreeable after-effects will be much less than though the dose of morphine is gradually reduced and the patient will find life quite bearable, as a rule, at the end of a week.

Avena sativa should always be given in appreciable doses of the tincture. Fifteen drops three or four times a day, well diluted, will usually meet the case. It may be given in doses of from five to sixty drops in rare instances.

It should, however, never be given in larger quantities than twenty minims unless the patient is thoroughly accustomed to the remedy and has found the usual dose insufficient.

Otherwise, there is danger of getting the physiological effect of the drug, which is pain at the base of the brain. When this symptom makes its appearance the medicine should be discontinued for a day or two and then given in reduced doses.

There seems to be no danger whatever of forming the habit of taking this remedy, as it can be suddenly abandoned at any time without evil consequences, even when given in large quantities. In one case it was prescribed in sixty drop doses, night and morning, for one year and then abruptly stopped. Nothing was substituted, without bad effects.

Whenever a quick action is desired and in all cases where Avena is given to overcome the morphine habit, it should be prepared in hot water. It is also a good plan to prescribe it in this fashion wherever indigestion complicates the case.

Anshutz employed this drug in his private practice for a number of years with the most gratifying results. He has very rarely found it to fail when indicated and on account of his high opinion of the remedy he has taken great pleasure in thus bringing it prominently to the attention of the medical profession.

RELATIONS - ***Compare:*** (1) Alfalfa - general tonic similar to Avena sativa. Alfalfa, also for scanty and suppressed urine. (2) Passiflora, Valerian.

REFERENCES - Anshutz. Boericke. Clarke. Murphy.

AZADIRACHTA INDICA

(Neem Bark)

PHARMACY - aza. Azadirachta indica. Neem bark. Margosa bark. Nim. Melia azadirachta indica. Antelaea azadirachta. N. O. Meliacae, Tribe, Meliee. India and Burma. Tincture of the bark. The fresh bark is pounded to a pulp and macerated in two parts by weight of alcohol. ***Historical dose:*** Tincture and all potencies.

CLINICAL - Acroparesthesia. Amnesia. Boils. Constipation. Depression. Diarrhea. Eczema. Gonorrhea. Hypochondria. ***Intermittent, fever.*** Leprosy. Leucorrhea. ***Malaria.*** Miscarriages. Quinine, effects. Rheumatism, acute. Senile dementia. Spleen, congested. Typhoid fever. Vomiting. Worms.

HERBAL - Azadirachta Indica is a large tree. The leaves, bark, wood, roots, fruits and every part of this tree, are ***intensely bitter.*** The vast range of its action is chiefly due to azaserine, margocine and catechin, the three active principles found in this tree.

This is an Indian remedy from very ancient times. The bark, known as Margosa bark, is the best-known medicinal portion. The tincture for the provings were made from the bark by Dr. P. C. Majumdar of Calcutta, India.

Majumdar contributed a synopsis of Aza. According to Ayurveda, the different parts of this tree possess different medicinal properties. Sanskrit authors agree that Azadirachta Indica bark, though very disagreeable in taste, is generally used with success.

The Neem tree is used for treatment of bacterial, viral, fungal infections and for the ***treatment and prevention of malaria***. Its action on fevers is well-known in India, the native physicians use Neem as the principal substance in their febrifuge medicines. It is especially useful in cases previously maltreated with quinine.

In Kenya the tincture of Neem in the 2x dilution has been used as a treatment for three weeks to neutralize the malaria organism from the body. A decoction of fresh leaves is used as a favorite wash to cure old ulcers of long standing.

It removes within a short time the sloughs and promotes the healing. The fruit is purgative, demulcent and is used in some forms of skin disorders.

A kind of oil is produced from the seed of ripe fruits and this oil is said to cure leprosy, eczema and some other obstinate skin diseases. Neem is also praised by some of the allopathic physicians for its tonic, anti-septic, astringent and anti-periodic properties.

HOMEOPATHIC - Aza. has been used in cases of lassitude, thirst, cough, fever. Loss of appetite, helminthiasis, boils, bilious derangements. Catarrh, vomiting, skin diseases, hiccough, gonorrhea. Its leaves are used in some forms of ophthalmic diseases, parasites, worms and disorders brought on by deranged bile or from the use of poisonous things.

Aza. is used in a variety of complaints, especially of the eyes, digestive derangements and skin disorders. An afternoon fever and rheumatic pains in various parts are caused by this remedy. Pain in sternum and ribs in back and shoulders and limbs.

Giddy on rising, headaches, scalp sensitive, eyes burn, pain in right eyeball. Heat, pricking and aching in hands. Loss of memory. Thirsty for large quantities of water at long intervals. Tendency to miscarriage. Copious leucorrhea.

MIND - Mind, weak and dull, full of anxiety inactive. No desire to go out or walk out. Depressed. Mistakes in writing and spelling words. Senile dementia. Hypochondriasis. Amnesia. Loss of memory. Forgetful.

Abdomen - Great uneasiness in the abdomen, with flatulent rumbling in the bowels, twisting pain in the epigastric region, no tenderness in the abdomen, clutching pain in the umbilical region, obliging to bend forwards, which affords some relief. Abdomen a little distended, passing of offensive flatus. Painful tension in the hypochondria region.

Back - Itching of the body, especially the back, worse in the open air and in the afternoon. Pain and aching at the nape of the neck.

Chest - Pain in sternum and ribs. Aching in the lower part of the right chest below the nipple. Stitches in the chest. Crampy pains in the lower part of chest. Transitory stitches in the chest, especially in the right side. Cramping pains at the base of the lungs.

Constitutions - Nervous or rheumatic constitutions.

Ears - Buzzing in the ears. A peculiar cracking sound is heard in the ear like tickling with a feather, which is increased on opening the mouth.

Eyes - Burning, dull and heavy. Pain in the eye, from slightest pressure. Red, sunken, congested, with slight coryza. Sense of pressure in the right eye.

Face - Flushing and heat in the face. Pale. Alternating heat and pallor of the face.

Female - Copious leucorrhea. Metritis of the cervix. Metrorrhagia. Recurring miscarriages.

Fever - Fever commences with very slight chill or without chill at 4:30 p.m. and abates at 7:30 p.m. Afternoon fever. Glowing heat and burning, especially in the face, eyes, palms of the hands and soles of the feet, in open air.

Food - Thirsty for large quantities of water at long intervals. Keen appetite. Desires cold drinks and sweets.

Head - Right-sided headache with throbbing of the temporal artery and pain in the right eyeball, worse in the open air. Scalp and hair painful and sensitive to the touch.

Heart - Pulse rapid and strong, or rapid and weak. Pulse is quick and hard, feeble.

Kidneys - Urine purple in color. Urine scanty and high colored and scalding, urine white, clear and copious, urine of strong odor.

Limbs - Numbness of the limbs, as if the limbs are paralyzed. Rheumatic pains in the lower limbs. Gnawing in the legs. Strength of the hand diminished. Burning of the hands and soles of the feet. Numbness of the hands only, especially the right hand.

Lungs - Sighing, breathing at intervals. Hot breath, rapid respiration. Short dry cough in the afternoon. Violent cough with thick, white, jelly-like sputum, which is difficult to expel. Cough after bathing. Cough with grayish expectoration, thick sputa. Cough with tasteless white sputa.

Male - Great excitement of sexual organs. Sexual desire a little diminished.

Modalities - Worse in the open air. Worse in the afternoon.

Mouth - No thirst, but mouth is clammy, water has relish, good taste. Mouth is bitter. A painful burning sensation, as if scalded, is felt on the sides and surface of the tongue, papillae seem to be enlarged and prominent. Putrid taste in the mouth. Saliva coming out which tastes salty. Slight difficulty in deglutition, especially water and meat.

Neck - Pain and debility in the nape of the neck.

Nose - Running of watery fluid from the nose.

Perspiration - Copious sweat, especially on the forehead, neck and upper part of the body. Sweating commences on the forehead, gradually extending towards the trunk, no sweat in lower part of the body.

Rectum - Diarrhea, no satisfaction after stool. Feeling after stool, that the rectum is not empty. Constipation with ball-like stools which are hard and small, alternating with diarrhea. Insufficient, constipated, stools hard, small and knotty, stools hard. Copious, soft, semi-solid stools.

Skin - Itching of various parts of the body without the appearance of any eruption. Sudamina on the back.

Sleep - Insomnia and agitation in bed. Wakes frequently. Dreams of fights and quarrels in the second half of the night. Sleeplessness and tossing in the bed, dreamy and interrupted sleep at night.

Stomach - No thirst, appetite very acute and keen. Very great thirst for large quantity of cold water, at long intervals. Heartburn and water brash. Uneasy sensation in the thorax.

Throat - Bitter taste in the throat. Slight hoarseness. Left-sided sore throat.

Vertigo - Sensation of drunkenness, especially on lifting the head and around 10 a.m.

COMMENTS - The most peculiar feature of the proving is the fever, which commences with a very slight chill or none at all, at about 3 p.m. to 4:30 p.m. and abates around 7:30 p.m.

Glowing heat and burning, especially in face, eyes, palms of hands and soles of feet in open air.

Sweat copious, commencing on forehead, gradually extending towards trunk, no sweat on lower part of body.

RELATIONS - ***Compare:*** (1) Cedron, Chin., Ars., Nat-m. (2) Guarea. (3) Ars. - Prostration, anxiety, restlessness. Cadaverous odor of secretions. Aggravation from 1 a.m. to 3 a.m. (4) Chin. - General weakness from loss of liquid. Thirst for large quantities of water. Hemorrhaging from the mucus membranes. Sensitive scalp. (5) Sulph. - Quarrelsome with grandiose ideas. Burning pains, weakness in the morning. Need for fresh air and fear of water. Morbid alternations. (6) Med.- Forgets names and recent events. Restlessness, precipitation, desire for drinks. Irritating leucorrhea. Breasts cold. Heels sensitive. Sleeps in knee-chest position.

REFERENCES - Anshutz. Boericke. Clarke.

B

BACILLINUM

(Tuberculosis Nosode)

PHARMACY - bac. Bacillinum. Tuberculosis nosode. A nosode prepared from human tuberculous sputum. Nosodes. ***Historical dose:*** All potencies.

CLINICAL - Addison's disease. Alopecia. ***Asthma. Bronchitis. Colds. Coughs. Dyspnea.*** Eczema. Growth, defective. Headache. Hydrocephalus. Idiocy. ***Infections.*** Insanity. Joints, disorders. ***Lung, disorders.*** Meningitis. Melancholy. Night-sweats. ***Phlegm.*** Pityriasis. Pyorrhea. Quinsy. ***Ringworm***. Scrofulous, glands. Teeth, defective. Tabes, mesenterica. ***Throat, sore. Tonsillitis. Tuberculosis***.

HOMEOPATHIC - Bacillinum is a nosode of tuberculosis named and first described by Dr. Burnett, for whom it was prepared from tuberculosis sputum by Dr. Heath. As this preparation has been experimented with separately, its symptoms are given apart from the other nosodes of tuberculosis. Useful as an intercurrent remedy.

Bacillinum has been used for the treatment of tuberculosis, generally causing the sputum to decrease and less become less purulent. Tubercular meningitis. It has a ***disposition to catch colds and sore throats.*** Respiratory and lung weakness. ***Chronic reoccurring sore throats and coughs.*** Glands of the neck are enlarged and tender. Night-sweats.

Bacillinum is indicated for the weak lungs of elderly people and for children with chronic catarrhal conditions and attacks of suffocation at night with difficult cough. Suffocative catarrh. ***The patient expectorates very little***. Chronic catarrhal conditions of the lungs when bronchial mucus and dyspnea are present. Tubercular meningitis. Ringworm.

Dr. Burnett has shown that ringworm of the scalp and pityriasis versicolor on the body are indications of tubercular diathesis and they respond to this remedy. He cured a case of insanity and ringworm.

Tuberculosis patients are better in dry sunny climates in mountains areas and in the pine forests. Sunlight helps to prevent tuberculosis, also there has been many cures of tuberculosis via sunbathing and the milk diet, which these patients crave.

Dr. Cartier has found it particularly useful in cases where there was excessive muco-purulent bronchial secretion threatening to occlude the lungs. It should be compared with Bacillinum testium, Tuber. Bovinum, Tuber. Aviaire and Tuber. Koch.

MIND - Taciturn, sulky, snappish, and irritable. Does not want to be disturbed. Fretful ailing, whines and complains. Great weakness. Morose. Depressed and melancholic, even to insanity. Tendency to be frightened, fear of dogs.

Abdomen - Abdominal pains, enlarged glands in groin. Tabes mesenterica, grinds teeth, indurated and swollen glands. Spleen region bulging out. Inguinal glands indurated and visible, excessive sweats, chronic diarrhea.

Back - Glands of neck enlarged and tender. Sensation of damp clothes on spine. Very sharp pain in left scapula, worse lying down in bed at night, better by warmth.

Chest - Sharp pain in precordial region arresting breathing.

Constitutions - Tubercular constitutions. For cases stemming from a tubercular inheritance with extreme soreness of affected parts, patients of rheumatic tendencies with syphilitic taints in the bloodstream, general muscular soreness.

Ears - Otitis after sore throats.

Eyes - Eczema of the eyelids.

Face - Indolent, pimple on left cheek, breaking out from time to time and persisting for many weeks.

Food - Poor appetite.

Head - Severe headache, deep in, recurring from time to time, worse shaking head. Terrible pain in the head as if he had a tight hoop of iron around it. Meningitis. Ringworm. Alopecia areata.

Kidneys - Increased quantity of urine, pale with white sediment. Rises several times in the night to urinate.

Limbs - Trembling of hands. Hands blue. Pain in left knee while walking. Tubercular inflammation of knee.

Lungs - Weak lungs. ***Humid asthma.*** Colds with sore throats. Hacking cough. Hard cough, shaking patient. Coughing, more during sleep, but it did not waken him. ***Catarrhal dyspnea.*** Muco-purulent expectoration of bronchitis. Congestion of the lung. Tuberculosis. ***Bubbling rales and muco-purulent expectoration***. Coughing, that wakes him in night, easy expectoration. Expectoration of non-viscid easily detached, thick phlegm from air passages.

Modalities - Worse night and early morning. Worse from cold air.

Nose - Nasal congestion. Coryza.

Perspiration - Night-sweats.

Rectum - Sudden diarrhea before breakfast, with nausea. Obstinate constipation with offensive flatus. Severe hemorrhages from bowels. Stitching pain through hemorrhoids. Passes much ill-smelling flatus.

Skin - ***Ringworm***. Pityriasis. Eczema. Glands enlarged and tender.

Sleep - Absolute sleeplessness. Talks in sleep. Drowsy during day, restless at night. Many dreams.

Stomach - Windy dyspepsia, with pinching pains under ribs of right side in breast line.

Teeth - Pyorrhea. Aching in teeth, especially lower incisors, very sensitive to air. Grinds teeth in sleep. Imperfectly developed teeth. Favors falling off of tartar of teeth.

Temperature - Flush of heat, some perspiration, severe headache. Fever, with emaciation, abdominal pains and discomfort. Restless at night, glands of both groins enlarged and indurated, cries out in sleep, strawberry tongue.

Throat - Tickling in fauces, compelling cough. Pricking in larynx with sudden cough.

COMMENTS - In the provings, a constant symptom was a severe headache, deep in, worse by motion. Also a slight cough with easy expectoration of phlegm. Tends to do better in chronic cases of tuberculosis, as compared to acute cases.

There are leading indications for it when present in combination with other disorders. An inter-current course of Bacillinum will often make a wonderful change in patients who have a personal or family history of chest disorders. Bacillinum is an acute miasm remedy for Phosphorus and Calcarea constitutions in particular.

Grimmer used it for cases stemming from a tubercular inheritance with extreme soreness of affected parts, patients of rheumatic tendencies with syphilitic taints in the bloodstream, general muscular soreness.

Dr. Young recorded the cure of several cases of cretinism. A case of insanity with pityriasis yielded rapidly to the remedy. Pityriasis has been cured by it when all attempts to kill the body lice by chemicals were useless. Clarke has found an eczematous condition of the margins of the eyelids a strong indication for it.

Bacillinum is made from tuberculosis bacilli, and Tuberculinum is from bovine tuberculosis. Tuberculinum is a deeper and more chronic remedy. Bacillinum tends to be more for acutes, but there's a lot of overlap. If a Bacillinum case keeps relapsing, follow with Tuberculinum. Miasmatic remedy, history of tuberculosis in family.

Good for children or adults with a tendency to get colds and sore throats frequently, particularly if they react well to acute remedies, but keep coming back. For children who get a cold at every change in the weather. Often swollen glands in the throat. Weight on the chest (Phos.). Mucus in the lungs, bronchitis. Good for the elderly with a tendency to colds and bronchitis. Lingering colds. The majority of the symptoms are gone, but a lingering cough or sore throat. Nondescript coughs.

Ringworm (Sep., Thuj., Tell.), and the tendency to ringworm. Diarrhea, especially with a cold, sore throat (Ars.).

RELATIONS - ***Compare:*** (1) Phos., Dros., Mercury. Its effects seem to be identical to that of Koch's Tuberculinum. Both are useful in the tubercular diathesis before tuberculosis has developed. In the early stages of tubercular disease of glands, joints, skin and bones. (2)

Psor. (3) Bac-t. (4) Ant-t., Iod., Lach., Ars-i., Myosotis. ***Complementary:*** Kali-c., Calc-p., Lach., goes with this remedy very well. ***Follows well:*** Levico, 5-10 drops, follows as an intercurrent where much debility is present (Burnett).

REFERENCES - Boericke. Clarke. Mur-

BACILLIUM TESTIUM

PHARMACY - bac-ts. Bacillinum testium. Nosode prepared from human tuberculous testicle. ***Historical dose:*** All potencies.

CLINICAL - Bedwetting. Inguinal glands, disease. Leucorrhea. Lipomas. Mesenteric glands, disease. Pneumonia. Testicles, tubercles. Tuberculosis. Tumors.

HOMEOPATHIC - This preparation has been used by Burnett; it has a more direct relation to the lower half of the body than the pulmonary Bac., but it is not an exclusive distinction.

Tuberculosis. Pneumonia. Inguinal glands and mesenteric glands are affected. Eruptions in inguinal region. Abscesses with suppurations. Benign tumors or lipomas. Bedwetting with a weak bladder. Frequent urination. Excoriating leucorrhea, smells like fish brine. Testicles have tubercles. ***Picking in the nose*** with fingers.

Abdomen - Cracks on surface of abdomen and groin. Eruptions in inguinal region. Pain in gallbladder.

Back - Soreness and pain in coccyx. Fatty tumors on neck.

Constitutions - Tubercular constitutions.

Chest - Pneumonia. Perspiration of axilla. Tumors, lipoma.

Female - Itching, acrid discharges. Leucorrhea is excoriating, greenish offensive like fish brine. Menses are painful, dysmenorrhea.

Food - Appetite wanting, worse mornings. Aversion to bread, eggs, tea, tomatoes. Desires chocolate, fried fish, sweets. Nausea and vomiting.

Head - Forehead pain.

Kidneys - Urination, frequent. Carbuncle, vascular bleeding, tumor of urethra.

Limbs - Eruption in the bends of joints. Eczema. Felon, panaritium. Flat, pointed warts on hands. Rheumatic pains in thighs and knees.

Lungs - Asthmatic breathing. Morning cough.

Modalities - Worse at the seaside. Worse during the summer months.

Mouth - Odor offensive. ***Cracked***, middle of lower lips (Nat-m.).

Nose - ***Picking*** the nose. ***Boring*** in nose with fingers. ***Catarrh***.

Rectum - Diarrhea. Itching.

RELATIONS - ***Compare:*** (1) Bac., Cina, Tub.

REFERENCES - Boericke. Clarke.

BACILLUS SEVEN

(Bacillus Asiaticus)

PHARMACY - ba-sv. Bacillus seven. Bacillus asiaticus. Bacillus cloacae. Bacillus freundi. ***Historical dose:*** All potencies.

CLINICAL - Asthma. Arthritis. Backache. Bronchitis. Cardiac arrest. Constipation. Deafness. Exhaustion. ***Fatigue. Fibrositis.*** Flatulence. Hemorrhoids. Mental fatigue. Menorrhagia. Metrorrhagia. Myocardial, weakness. Osteo-arthritis. Osteoporosis. Quinsy. ***Rheumatoid, arthritis. Rheumatism***. Senility. Tonsillitis.

HOMEOPATHIC - This remedy is so named as it was the seventh non-lactose fermenting type of bacillus observed in the laboratory. As it did not confirm to any of the previously known groups, it was given the number "Seven."

Extreme mental and physical fatigue. Its site of action is the neuro-muscular junction. Unfit for mental exertion, leading to extreme physical exhaustion. Asthma, catarrh, sticky mucous. Low blood pressure and myocardial weakness.

Flatulence, fullness after food. Feeble urinary flow, loss of sexual function, premature senility. Rheumatic nodules. Backache, cannot stand long. Faints easily. Sensitive to cold. All the symptoms can be related to general lack of nerve and muscle tone.

MIND - The outstanding symptom is mental fatigue, a feeling of unfitness for any mental effort, which produces a sense of extreme physical exhaustion. ***Tense and tired.*** Th thought of doing anything is sufficient to exhaust him.

Abdomen - Flatulence. A sense of fullness after food, flatulence and distention of the stomach. Flabby abdomen. Pain in liver region.

Back - Backache, cannot stand long without feeling of faintness. ***Fibrous rheumatism of neck and back.*** abdominal muscles, shoulders and arms. Spinal osteo-arthritis.

Chest - Some pain.

Constitutions - More suitable for the elderly and the debauch.

Ears - Catarrhal deafness.

Eyes - Thrombosis central retinal vein. Eyes closed, lasted one week.

Face - Dark, pale, puffy. Angio-neurotic edema.

Female - Pain in vulvae, no leucorrhea. Menorrhagia and metrorrhagia.

Food - Averse to fat.

Head - Dull headaches.

Heart - Myocardial weakness. Sudden cardiac arrest. Slow pulse rate, often with lowered blood pressure.

Kidneys - Feeble urinary flow.

Limbs - Poor muscle tone. Joints swollen and painful. ***Fibrositis.*** Fibrous rheumatism thighs. Limbs stiff. ***Osteo-arthritis*** of the ***knees.*** Left hip fixed, arthritis. Rheumatoid arthritis, knees and ankles. Stabbing pain in hip. Pain shoots up and down leg. Cramps in leg at night. Pes planus. Feet painful. Gout in left toe. Wrists and ankles immobile. ***Rheumatism of the wrists.*** Ganglion right hand. Fingers swell. Blood vessels burst in fingers.

Lungs - Asthma. Bronchitis. Bronchial catarrh, tough sticky mucus, difficult to raise. Worse at 2 a.m. (Kali-c.).

Male - Loss of sexual function. Premature senility.

Modalities - Sensitive to cold to drafts and cold, damp air. Backache, better heat and rest. Worse damp and cold. Worse on commencing to move.

Neck - Stiff neck "cracks like a nut." ***Fibrositis of neck and shoulders.***

Nose - Nasal catarrh.

Perspiration - Excessive perspiration.

Rectum - Constipation. Hemorrhoids.

Skin - Cracks in knuckles, fingertips, palms. Circinate eruption hands, palms, hot, nippy and scaly. Paronychia fingers.

Sleep - Light sleeper. Wakes 2 or 3 a.m. Takes hours to fall off to sleep.

Stomach - Belching.

Throat - Tonsillitis. Quinsy.

Vertigo - Tendency to syncope after sudden exertion. Faintness on standing long and after sudden exertion.

COMMENTS - Rheumatoid arthritis shoulders, elbow, wrists. Relaxed fibrous tissue with tendency to the formation of "rheumatic nodules".

RELATIONS - This bacillus has a closer relationship to the two halogens, *Bromine* and *Iodine* often in combination with Potassium. ***Compare:*** (1) Bromine, Iodine and particularly the Kali salts, especially Kali-c. (2) Among remedies related to this nosode are many iodides. (3) Calc-f.

REFERENCES - Paterson.

BACILLUS TEN

PHARMACY - ba-tn. Bacillus ten. This is so named as it was the tenth non-lactose fermenting type of bacillus observed in the laboratory. ***Historical dose:*** All potencies.

CLINICAL - Allergy. ***Asthma.*** Anorexia. Cough. Dermatitis. Headache. ***Itching. Leucorrhea.*** Nasal catarrh. Paronychia. Pruritus, ani. ***Pruritis, vulvae.*** Rheumatism. ***Ringworm.*** Vomiting. ***Warts.***

HOMEOPATHIC - Allergy to drugs given for asthma.

MIND - Anxious. Overactive mind. Irritable and depressed.

Abdomen - Pain in gallbladder.

Back - Pain in left iliac fossa and right iliac fossa.

Chest - Panniculitis, chest wall. Lipoma, lower ribs

Food - Anorexia. Averse to egg, bread, tomato, tea and to breakfast. Aggravated by eggs and fat. ***Craves sweets, chocolates, fried fish.***

Female - ***Pruritis vulvae. Leucorrhea,*** fishy odor, greenish, corrosive. Groin skin is raw, dry and cracked. Urethral caruncle.

Head - Headache in forehead, left eye.

Kidneys - Frequent urination.

Limbs - Tenderness coccyx. Rheumatism of thigh. Rheumatoid arthritis left knee. Paronychia.

Lungs - ***Asthma***. Cough, worse in the morning, sputum difficult.

Mouth - Spongy gums. Offensive breath.

Neck - Fatty cyst.

Nose - Nasal catarrh.

Rectum - Bowel motion first thing in the morning. Sluggish bowel motion. Pruritus ani.

Skin - ***Warts on hands***, numerous flat or pointed (after working with pickled hams). Dermatitis of skin flexures. ***Ringworm.*** Perspiration in axilla.

Stomach - Nausea, vomiting.

REFERENCES - Paterson.

BACOPA MONNIERI

(Brahmi)

PHARMACY - baco. Bacopa monnieri. Brahmi. Water Hyssop. Thyme-leafed gratiola. Moneywort. Herpestris monnieria. Moniera euneifolia. Lysimachia monnieri. N. O. Plantaginaceae. Historical dose: Tincture and all potencies.

CLINICAL - Anemia. Ascites. Biliousness. Blood, disorders. Diarrhea. Epilepsy. Fevers. Indigestion. Leprosy. Leucoderma. ***Memory, disorders.*** Scabies. Spleen. Syphilis. Tumors. Ulcers.

HERBAL - Bacopa monnieri is a perennial, creeping herb whose habitat includes wetlands and muddy shores. It commonly grows in marshy areas throughout India.

Bacopa monnieri is an herb used in India for memory, epilepsy, and as a mild sedative. It has been used for centuries to treat epilepsy, improve memory capacity, increase concentration, and reduce stress-induced anxiety.

Traditionally, it was used as a ***brain tonic*** to enhance memory development, learning, and concentration, and to provide relief to patients with anxiety or epileptic disorders.

Patients taking Bacopa say that they can better handle difficult mental tasks and stress. It improves the memory. Increased learning abilites. Protects the brain from the effects of aging. Alleviate anxiety. Mental and brain fatigue. Attention-deficit disorders.

The plant has also been used in India and Pakistan as a cardiac tonic. Digestive aid. Improves respiratory function in cases of broncho-constriction.

According to Unani medicine, it is bitter, aphrodisiac, good in scabies, leucoderma, syphilis etc. It is a blood purifier and useful in diarrhea and fevers.

Bacopa is bitter, pungent, heating, emetic, laxative and useful in bad ulcers. Also used to treat anemia, ascites, enlargement of spleen, biliousness, indigestion, inflammations, leprosy, tumors, etc.

COMMENTS - In India, this herb has also been used traditionally to consecrate new born babies in the belief that it will stimulate the intelligence. Studies suggest bacopa may improve intellectual activity in children.

Recent research has focused primarily on Bacopa's cognitive-enhancing effects, specifically memory, learning, and concentration, and results support the traditional Ayurvedic herbal claims.

Also, research on anxiety, epilepsy, bronchitis and asthma, irritable bowel syndrome, and gastric ulcers also supports the traditional uses of Bacopa.

RELATIONS - Compare: Ginko, Kali-p. Gotu kola.

REFERENCES - Murphy.

BADIAGA

(Freshwater Sponge)

PHARMACY - bad. Badiaga. Freshwater sponge. Spongilla fluviatilis. Trituration of the dried sponge gathered in autumn. ***Historical dose:*** Trituration and all potencies.

CLINICAL - Basedow's disease. ***Breast, cancer.*** Bruises. Buboes. Catarrh. Chilblains. Cracks. ***Coryza.*** Coughing. ***Dandruff***. Edema. Eyes, pains. Glands disorders. Hay fever. Headache. Hemorrhoids. Heart disorders. Indurations. Influenza. Metrorrhagia. Ophthalmia. Neuralgia. Palpitations. Paresis. Rheumatism

Roseola. Scrofula. ***Soreness.*** Syphilitic, buboes. Syphilis. Tibia, pain. Thyroid, disorders. Tonsillitis. Whooping cough.

HOMEOPATHIC - Badiaga is the Russian name for the river sponge, which is a popular Russian remedy. Among the peculiar symptoms and indications are headache with aching in backs of eyeballs, 2 p.m. to 7 p.m., worse motion. Severe headache in vertex better night, returning severely after breakfast. Headache with inflamed eyes. Pains in eyeballs extending to head.

General soreness of muscles and tissues, feeling as if beaten, worse motion and friction of clothes with sensitiveness to cold. Soreness of anterior muscles of legs, toes bend while walking as if extensors were paralyzed. Left cheek and malar bone sore to touch. Sharp pains in stomach, liver, below scapulae, urethra, chest.

Swollen glands. General paresis. Influenza. Basedow's disease. Syphilis, bubo, roseola. Buboes. Infantile syphilis. Chronic rheumatism, worse by cold, especially in cold air. Chancres suppressed by cauterizations. Breast cancer.

Cough, causes sneezing, profuse coryza, coming from nostril with a gush. Occasional severe fit of coughing ejecting viscid mucus, flying out of mouth. Cough caused by tickling in larynx as if a particle of sugar was dissolving in throat, better in warm room. Pleuritic stitches in chest, neck and back.

Tremulous palpitations, worse lying right side. Palpitations after pleasurable emotions. Edema. It has lessened a hard, cellular swelling of both legs. Sharp stinging in back of right heel, worse least pressure.

MIND - Mind generally clear, active in spite of headache. Palpitations after pleasurable emotions. Desire for mental work.

Abdomen - Sharp pain with a bounding movement in region of liver. Indurated inguinal glands. Syphilitic buboes.

Back - Stitches in nape of neck, scapula. Pain in small of back, hips and lower limbs. Very stiff neck. ***Muscles and skin sore,*** as if beaten.

Breasts - Indurations. ***Breast cancer*** (Aster., Carc., Con., Carb-an., Plum-i.).

Ears - Slight sounds are very accentuated.

Eyes - Eyeballs tender, aching in eyeballs. ***Twitching of left upper lid***. Intermittent sore pain in eyeball, coming on at 3 p.m. Neuralgia of eyeballs extending to temple.

Face - Blue color under the eyes.

Female - Metrorrhagia, worse at night with feeling of enlargement of head (Arg-n.).

Food - Much thirst.

Head - Headache, better at night after sleep. Dull, dizzy feeling in head. Sensation of enlargement and fullness. Pain in forehead and temple, ***extending to eyeballs***, worse in afternoon. Headache with inflammation of eyes. ***Dandruff***. Scalp sore, tetter-like.

Heart - Tremulous palpitations. Heartbeats are felt from chest to neck, worse lying on right side. Indescribable bad feeling about the heart with soreness and pain, flying stitches all over.

Lungs - Cough, worse in afternoon, better in warm room. Cough excited by sweets, candies etc. The ***mucus flies out of mouth and nostrils***. Whooping cough with thick yellow expectoration, flies out. Hay fever with asthmatic breathing.

Male - Syphilis of infants. Chancres. Buboes.

Modalities - Better by heat, warm room. Worse from cold air. Worse stormy weather. Worse afternoon. Worse pressure and touch.

Mouth - Hot. Breath hot.

Nose - ***Coryza***, sneezing, watery discharge with asthmatic breathing and suffocative cough.

Skin - Sore to touch. ***Freckles.*** Cracks. Raised and discolored scars.

Stomach - Sharp pain in pit of stomach, extending to vertebra and scapula.

Throat - Tonsils inflamed, swollen, worse swallowing solids.

COMMENTS - J. A. Biegler cured a case in which a woman had, off and on for months, a severe pain in her right eyeball, which extended to her forehead over the eye, then to her temple, always worse in the afternoon. Scalp sore, dry, itching, scurf, tetters.

RELATIONS - *Compare:* (1) Merc. similar but opposite generals. (2) Hydr., Phyt., Con. (3) Seneg. - cough caused by sneezing, opposite of Bad. (4) Grind. - respiration ceases on falling asleep. (5) Spong. - cough with much sneezing. Kali-c. - phlegm flies from mouth. (6) Calc-s. - indurations, Carb-an. - indurations, buboes. (7) Cist. - scrofula. (8) Clem., Hep., Iod., Kali-i., Lach., Merc., Merc-i., Nit-ac., Sil., Sulph. ***Complementary:*** Iod., Merc., Sulph. ***Followed well by:*** Lach.

REFERENCES - Boericke. Clarke.

BALSAMUM PERUVIANUM

(Balsam of Peru)

PHARMACY - bals-p. Balsamum peruvianum. Balsam of Peru. Myroxylon Pereire. Myroxylon peruvianum. Peruvianum, balsamum. N. O. Leguminose. Caesalpinioideae. Tincture of the balsam that flows from the stems. ***Historical dose:*** Tincture and all potencies.

CLINICAL - Bronchitis. Catarrh. Cracks. Diarrhea. ***Hectic, fevers.*** Nosebleed. Scabies. Tuberculosis. Ulcers. Vomiting.

HOMEOPATHIC - Peruvian Balsam has been proved by Lembke. It has been chiefly used empirically in catarrhal tuberculosis or bronchial catarrh with copious purulent expectoration. Sputa thick, creamy, yellowish white, loud rales, night sweats, hectic.

Bals-p. is useful in bronchial catarrh with copious, purulent expectoration. ***Debility and hectic fever***. Cracks of nipples and fingers.

Chest - Cough, mucus and purulent expectoration. Tuberculosis of mucus type, vomit in lungs. Loud rales in chest (Kali-s., Ant-t.).

Kidneys - Scanty urine, with much mucus sediment. Urination more frequent and copious. Catarrh of bladder (Chim.). Sticking and cutting in urethra.

Limbs - Oppressive pain in right wrist. Severe pain in left tibia. Boring in right tibia.

Lungs - Bronchitis and tuberculosis with ***muco-purulent, thick, creamy expectoration***. Tuberculosis of mucus type, vomit in lungs. Very loose cough, mucus and purulent expectoration.

Nose - Profuse, thick discharge. Chronic, fetid, nasal catarrh. Bleeding from right nostril. Ozaena with ulceration. Eczema with ulceration.

Perspiration - Night-sweats.

Stomach - Vomiting of food and mucus. Catarrh of stomach.

Stool - Mucus diarrhea. Copious liquid stool, painless. Passage of blood with normal stool.

Temperature - Hectic fever and night-sweats with irritating, short cough and scanty expectoration.

Throat - Scraping in larynx in forenoon, dry cough. Continued scraping of fauces.

COMMENTS - Hale used it with success in "chronic, purulent, fetid anterior or posterior nasal catarrh with or without ulceration." He said that a cerate of the Balsam is the best application next to Glycerol of Aloes for indolent ulcers, cracked nipples, cracks in fingers and palmar surfaces of hands or fissured and chapped lips.

Bals-p. is used locally as a stimulant to raw surfaces in indolent ulcers, scabies, cracked nipples. Promotes granulation, removes the fetid odor. A one percent solution in alcohol or ether may be used with the atomizer in respiratory disorders.

Internally, it is used as an expectorant in chronic bronchitis. Used externally for killing scabies. All parts affected are gently rubbed with it at night and a bath taken in the morning. A single application is sufficient.

RELATIONS - *Compare:* (1) Balsamum Tolutanum. (2) Oleum Caryophyllum - oil of cloves in profuse expectoration, 3 to 5 minims in milk or capsules.

REFERENCES - Boericke. Clarke.

BALSAMUM TOLUIFERUM

PHARMACY - bals-t. Balsamum toluiferum. Balsamum tolutanum. Balsam of Myroxylon toluifera. N. O. Caesalpinioideae. ***Historical dose:*** Tincture and all potencies.

HOMEOPATHIC - Chronic bronchitis with profuse expectoration.

RELATIONS - ***Compare:*** (1) Ant-t., Balsam of Peru, Bac.

REFERENCES - Boericke.

BAMBUSA ARUNDINACEA

(Bamboo)

PHARMACY - bamb-a. Bambusa arundinacea. Bamboo. N. O. Gramineae. ***Historical dose:*** All potencies.

CLINICAL - Acne. Ankylosing spondylitis. ***Arthritis.*** Backache. Belching. Colds. Constipation. Cystitis. ***Depression.*** Diarrhea. Dyspepsia. Gingivitis. Headaches. Heartburn. Indigestion. Influenza. Insomnia. Joint, pains. ***Leucorrhea.*** Motion sickness. Nausea. Neck, pain. Neuralgic, pains. Nightmares. ***Post-partum, depression. Rheumatism.*** Ringworm. Sciatica. Spinal, injuries. ***Stiffness.*** Tendonitis. Torticollis. Tuberculosis. Vertigo. ***Vomiting.***

HERBAL - In folk medicine, the leaves have been used to treat blood diseases and inflammation. The hardened material inside bamboo has been used for tuberculosis, asthma and leprosy. The shoots are said to be an appetite stimulant and digestion aid.

The root has been used for ringworm. The juice from the flowers has been used for earache and deafness. Some modern studies confirm its anti-inflammatory and anti-tumor effects and its action on the uterus.

HOMEOPATHIC - ***Arthritis and rheumatism.*** Back pain and sciatica. Spinal injuries. Tension and ***stiffness of joints, worse from damp,*** cold weather. Clumsiness and awkwardness. Radiating pains. Wandering and wave-like pains. Numbness and tingling. ***Post-partum depression*** (Sep.). Generally chilly, better from warmth and worse cold and damp.

MIND - Everything seems uncertain. Emotionally sensitive, vulnerable. Yielding disposition. Sadness with weeping. Crying over trivial things. Conscientious about trifles. Capricious. Restless, tosses about in bed. Startled as from a fright.

Cannot handle things anymore, overwhelmed by stress. Mental exhaustion, brain fag. Anxiety, felt in chest. Anxiety during vertigo. Anxiety of conscious. Bites nails. Anxiety about the future, finances. Worries about money. Depression with a strong fear of poverty.

Overpowering panic attacks. Fear of losing self-control, of misfortune, of failure. Fear during pregnancy. Fear of impending disease. ***Fear of something wrong in her head***. Fear of brain tumor, epileptic convulsions. ***Fear of lumps in breast***. Fear of something wrong in head, Fear of being observed. Fear of saying something wrong. Fear of vertigo. Hypochondriasis.

Moods changeable, variable. Jealous. Brooding. Domineering, Morose, sulky, cross, fretful, ill-humor, peevish. Anger from noises. Cursing, swearing. Quarrelsome, scolding. Averse to being disturbed. ***Irritable towards husband, children***, better in the evening. Irritable, when spoken to. Easily offended. Sensitive to reprimands, criticism.

Post-partum depression. Depression with a feeling that they would never get well again. General feeling of betrayal and desertion. ***Forsaken feeling.*** New mother feels stressed, drained, overwhelmed, and trapped.

Feelings of helplessness. Pities herself. Feels inferior, poor self confidence. Timidity about appearing in public. Discontented, dissatisfied with himself, everything. ***Desire for change.*** Ennui, boredom. ***Feels cut off from life.*** Indifference, apathy to everything. Sadness alternating with indifference. Depression before menses, in morning on waking, ***afternoon, worse 4 pm.*** Desire for solitude.

Mental dullness, sluggishness. Difficulty thinking and comprehending. Concentration difficult while driving, studying, reading, writing.

Confusion of mind in morning, as if in a dream. Mistakes about time. ***Confounds the days of the week.*** Mistakes in writing, omitting letters. Absent-mindedness. Memory weakness, from mental exertion. Forgetful.

Delusions, imagines that she is alone in the world. ***Blames her partner for her bad mood***. Imagines he is deceived, deserted, forsaken. Delusions everything will fail. Imagines he has ruined his health. ***Delusions, that left and right side are not the same.***

Delusions that body parts are distorted. Foolish behavior. Attempts to escape.

Abdomen - Gas and bloating. Obstructed flatulence. Rumbling noises. Bilious complaints. Tenderness in the gallbladder region.

Back - Backaches. Spinal injuries. Ankylosing spondylitis. Burning along the spine. Stiffness and tension. Cramping, aching and dragging pains. A knotted feeling in the back. Heat waves, flushes. Numbness and tingling. Sacroiliac pains. Coccyx pain, after injuries. stiffness. Stiffness, shoulders. Neuralgic and rheumatic pains, shoulders.

Bladder - Cystitis, from taking cold. Dragging pains. ***Pain comes in waves.***

Causations - Ailments from anger, vexation, suppressed anger, anticipation, foreboding, excitement, wounded pride, honor.

Chest - Sensation of a lump near sternum.

Ears - Hissing noises in ear. Stopped sensation. Pulsation during headache.

Eyes - Blinking. Itching, swelling of eyelids.

Face - Acne. Painful pimples. Numbness. Pain in facial bones.

Female - Dysmenorrhea. Profuse menses. Suppressed menses. ***Offensive leucorrhea. Post-partum depression,*** accompanied by a stiff neck, back pain or sciatica (Cimic.). Prolonged lochia. Menstrual problems after childbirth. Excoriation of cervix. Tearing pain in ovaries.

Fever - Influenza (Rhus-t.).

Food - Strong aversion to fat and to beer. Desires wine, cheese spicy foods. Desires stimulants, like coffee. Worse from fats, beer and wine.

Head - Headaches are worse from physical exertion, cold wind, and bending the head forward. Pressing pain.

Heart - Stitching, burning pain and stiffness. Dragging sensation in heart region.

Limbs - Rheumatic pains. ***Stiffness, worse from damp,*** cold weather. Sciatica, as if painful electric currents running down the sciatic nerve to the hollow of the knee. Sharp, stitching pains. Numbness and tingling. Twitching of limbs. Radiating pains. Wandering and wave-like pains. Icy cold hands and feet. Weakness and heaviness. Swelling of the ankles.

Limbs - Weak ankles. Burning in the soles of the feet. Icy cold feet. Weakness of the hand, difficulty in writing. Contractions and spasms.

Liver - Pressing pain.

Male - Atrophy, shriveled genitals. Troublesome erections. Priapism.

Modalities - Pains are better from rest, heat, hot drinks. Worse in the morning on waking, Worse from cold and damp.

Mouth - Profuse salivation. Gingivitis.

Neck - ***Stiffness, worse from damp,*** cold weather. Tension in neck. Very difficult to turn the neck. Torticollis.

Nose - Colds. Nasal congestion. Dryness and numb. Sensitive to odors.

Perspiration - Profuse night-sweats. ***Odor of sweat, like fresh coffee***. Offensive, sweetish sweats. Sticky, viscid sweats.

Rectum - Anal, itching. Constipation, with soft stool. Diarrhea, like gushing water. Greasy and fatty stools. Involuntary stool.

Skin - Excoriation. Itching during sleep. Painful scars. ***Sensitive to hot water***. Stings, from insects.

Sleep - Insomnia. Sleeplessness, from an overactive mind. Constantly turning ideas over in the mind. Wakes 3:30 a.m. to 4:30 a.m. Confused dreams. Nightmares Dreams of accidents, misfortune, disease deaths. Dreams of animals, water. Dreams children, old friends. Dreams of teeth falling out. Amorous dreams.

Stomach - Belching. Heartburn, worse from excitement, beer. Indigestion. Dyspepsia Empty, weak, hungry feeling. Nausea from odors. Nausea with headaches. Motion sickness. Lump sensation. ***Vomiting after nuts.*** Vomiting, evening.

Teeth - Toothaches, pain worse from sweets.

Temperature - Alternating fever and chills. Chilliness, worse at night. Shaking, shivering with chills.

Throat - Sore throat. Tonsillitis. Tonsils, suppuration. Coldness sensation. Redness. Lump, plug sensation. Mucus, tenacious, difficult to hawk up. Difficult swallowing. Hoarseness. Roughness sensation. Ulcerative pain.

Tongue - Burning, raw pains. As if tongue was burnt. Formication. Tingling and prickling sensations. Metallic, offensive, sour, putrid taste.

Urine - Dark color, frothy, foamy urine. Profuse, increases amounts urine. Scanty urine. Strong, putrid odor, like rotten eggs, sulphur.

Vertigo - Vertigo with staggering. As if intoxicated. Worse from looking downward. Motion sickness.

Vision - Double vision. Foggy, dim vision. Blurred vision with lachrymation.

COMMENTS - Bernd Schuster related several cases of his experiences with Bamb-a. The first concerned Karen, a 29-year-old mother, who could not look after her 12-week-old baby because of severe headaches. The baby was delivered by caesarian and her headaches started shortly afterwards.

Initially, the pain was felt only when she shook her head or cleaned her teeth, but by the time the baby was three weeks old she could only lie down. She could not bear the sound of her child crying. Pain was better if she lay down or supported her head. There was a feeling of heaviness or enlargement of her head. Menstruated immediately after childbirth.

Irritable. She said she wished her little boy would get lost. Then she laughed and said she didn't mean it and then cried and said, I feel guilty enough about not looking after him properly. After being given Bamb-a., her head and neck pain did not return and her mood improved markedly

The second case concerned Lisa, a 35-year-old new mother, who reported "The stress of the birth completely changed me. It was difficult. I am nervous and a wreck. Breastfeeding makes me feel weaker while nursing I have a terrible feeling. My mood is the same as when my mother died. I always weep when I am nursing. I feel empty, miserable, depressed, drained of all my energy."

She was completely stressed and almost felt persecuted by her crying baby. She lay in bed all day. She was afraid to be solely responsible for the child. "I imagined the relationship with the child to be closer, but I need someone to help me I need more support."

After being given Bamb-a., Lisa was more at ease with her baby; the weakness, emptiness and depression have gone and she had more energy. She found it easier to tell friends how she really felt and to accept help.

The third case concerned Judy, a 38-year-old mother of two, who suffered from headaches, backaches, sciatica and a feeling of stiffness in the morning, all of which were worse for three days before her period. She had been diagnosed with postnatal depression in the past. She described it as "feeling down."

"My children are not babies any more, but still everything to do with them depends very much on me. My husband is never there. My parents have now moved here and they are always wanting something. And I have to do a lot of jobs physically which women don't usually do. They all come to me when they want something but no one ever asks if they can help me. It bothers me for the future if I get ill, no one will be there for me."

She has had other homeopathic remedies and chiropractic, which both worked well, but it was not until she was given Bamb-a. that her mood improved profoundly, she changed the dynamics in her relationships and her pain and stiffness disappeared.

RELATIONS - ***Compare:*** (1) Sep., Puls., Placenta. (2) Rhus-t., Dulc., Cimic., Eup-per.

REFERENCES - Schuster.

BANISTERIOPSIS CAAPI

(Ayahuasca)

PHARMACY - bani-c. Banisteriopsis caapi. Ayahuasca. Spirit Vine. Yagé. Psychotria viridis. N. O. Malpighiaceae. South America. Amazon. ***Historical dose:*** All potencies.

CLINICAL - AIDS. Allergies. Asthma. Autism. Cancer. Chronic, fatigue. Clairvoyance. Delusions. ***Digestive, problems.*** Drug, abuse. Emphysema. ***Hallucinations.*** Insomnia. Kyphosis. Malnutrition. Nausea. Numbness. Parkinson's, disease. Scoliosis. Sexual, abuse. Vomiting. Worms.

HERBAL - Ayahuasca, commonly called *yagé*, or *yajé* in Colombia. *Ayahuasca* in Ecuador and Peru. Inca "vine of the dead, vine of the souls," *aya* means in Quechua "spirit," "ancestor," "dead person," while *huasca* means "vine," "rope," and *caapi* in Brazil. Ayahuasca brew is prepared from segments of a species of the vine *Banisteriopsis,* a genus belonging to the *Malpighiaceae.*

HOMEOPATHIC - Tiredness, exhaustion, debility. Unable to move from tiredness. Shakiness and disorientation. Unable to recover one's energy with rest. Feelings of detachment, poor memory and vagueness with the exhaustion. Rushes of energy which are associated with raised heartbeat and that cause some anxiety. Heightened sensitivity of all senses, mostly vision and hearing.

Muscular soreness and weakness from tiredness. Limbs go to sleep, pins and needles sensations. Tightness, tingling, aching, and drawing in the spine. Numbness and general malaise. Anesthesia. Muscle wastage. Tissue necrosis. Easy dislocation of joints. Crumbling of bone tissue.

Digestive tract malfunction. Poor assimilation and metabolism. Imbalance of bowel flora causing psychological symptoms such as depression. Pains can be sharp, sudden on appearance and quick to go, tend to be worse night. Autism. Ailments from injuries, worse spine or the head. AIDS. Cancer. Chronic fatigue. Parkinson's disease. Strong history of drug abuse. Multiple allergy syndrome.

MIND - Confusion of mind. Cannot think straight. Difficult concentration, comprehension. Dullness, sluggishness. Mistakes about time. Memory weakness. Forgetfulness. Thoughts intrude and crowd around each other. Tormenting, persisting thoughts. Amorous thoughts.

Clear-sighted, increased precision of mind. Sensitive to all external impressions. Senses are acute. Oversensitive to light, noise, shrill sounds, sad stories. ***Charmed by colors, especially red.*** Easily startled.

Moods are changeable, variable, swings between extremes of rage and well being. Impulsive. Restless, nervous. Impatient, hurried, everybody moves too slow.

Stressed mentally and emotionally. Full of worries, forebodings. Insecure. Anxious, desperate. Anxiety from palpitations, on waking. Anxiety about salvation. Overpowering panic attacks. Prolonged anguish and fear which has heightened every sense.

Irritability from any disturbance, when questioned. Fastidious. Obstinate, headstrong. Rage, fury. Impulse to kill. ***Anger during meetings***. Jealousy associated with sexual excitement. Suspicious, mistrustful.

Weeping, causeless. Pessimistic. Dwells on past disagreeable events. Homesick, nostalgic. Sadness, depression, crying difficult. Ailments from grief, sorrow. ***Grief of the deepest kind.*** Forsaken feeling. Worse from consolation, company. Aversion to company. Indifference, apathy towards friends. Despair of life. Unmitigated misery. Suicidal thoughts. Loquacity alternating with sadness. Loss of self-control.

Feelings of being disconnected, worse fatigue, stress, anxiety or fear. Inability to feel connected to the mother. Desire for sympathy. Inability to remember childhood. Loss of purpose. Sense of uselessness and frustration at not being able to find one's path. Sense of having been derailed. Work fatigue easily. Sympathetic, compassionate.

Fear that something bad will happen. Fear of insanity, of losing self-control. ***Fear of crossing a bridge***, of falling. Fear of ghosts, evil. Fear of impending death, feels as if soul were escaping from body. Fear of terrible dreams.

Disoriented. Sense of unreality. Feels as if intoxicated, drugged. Blissful. Cheerfulness. Euphoria. Tranquility, serenity, calmness. Thoughtless. Out-of-body states. Feeling of lightness. Fearlessness. No conception of time. Incorrect judge of sizes.

Trance. Clairvoyant and clairaudient. Telepathic phenomena. Psychic abilities that may be illusory. Hears voices or receives psychic messages. False messages. Pride about psychic abilities, may be deluding themselves.

Delusions, visions and hallucinations on closing eyes. ***Floating in air***, that he is a bird, of flying, that he has no weight.

Delusions that body parts are immaterial, that the head is separated from body, that the mind and body are separated.

Religious delusions, that he lost his salvation, of gods, goddesses, angels, devils, ghosts, spirits. Frightful images, phantoms. ***Delusions of dangerous animals, crocodiles, tigers.*** Delusions of leopards, reptiles, snakes. Delusions of seeing monsters.

Visions of suffering, cruelty, torture, of being at war. Delusions of danger, of being surrounded by the enemy, of being watched, that another person is in the room. Delusions of events long past. Delusions that death is approaching, ***about the death of others.***

Abdomen - Flatuence. Malabsorption and malnutrition from defective gut.

Back - Injuries to the spine and coccyx. Tension in the neck. Scoliosis and kyphosis.

Dreams - Exhausting, frightful or joyful dreams. Unremembered dreams. ***Dreams of animals***, reptiles. ***Dreams of crossing bridges***, flying, ***musical instruments***, music, food. Amorous, lewd, lascivious, sexual dreams. Dreams of previous events, old friends, people not seen for years. Dreams of anger of cruelty, enemies, death, dying, war, being taken prisoner, strife, being wounded.

Ears - Hears acutely. Hears as if from a distance.

Eyes - Acute vision or blurred. Sees images superimposed on whatever is being looked at. Doubts what is seen, has to look again.

Female - Total loss of libido after use of hallucinatory drugs. Heightened libido, which can lead to excessive masturbation. Excessive libido in those who enjoy it as if it were only a spiritual experience. Sex with detached feelings. Sexual abuse followed by a crippled sex-life. Difficult, prolonged or late periods.

Food - ***Craves alcohol, stimulants*** such as coffee and tea. No appetite, would prefer to do without food.

Head - Sensation of being stuffed up with cotton wool. Heat in the vertex or cold as ice.

Heart - Congenital heart disease. Real or phantom pains. Raised heart rate. Palpitations.

Kidneys - Weak kidneys. Frequent urinary infections or pains in the kidneys.

Limbs - Muscle wasting. Poor extension and abduction of limbs due to inelasticity of tendons and ligaments. ***Poor circulation***, coldness and numbness of extremities. Possible remedy for gangrenous states.

Lungs - Restricted breathing from emotional disturbances. Emphysema. Asthma, chronic constricted airways.

Male - Prostate trouble relating to impotency. Total loss of libido after use of hallucinatory drugs. Heightened libido, which can lead to excessive masturbation. Excessive libido as if it were a spiritual experience. Sexual abuse followed by a crippled sex-life.

Perspiration - Offensive, strong, sweetish odor.

Rectum - Constipation, ineffectual urging and straining.

Sleep - ***Sleeps as if dead***. Full of dreams. Many and varied dreams. Dreams seem more real than life. Desire to go back into the dream to continue it. Insomnia, from drug abuse or from over-use of sleeping pills.

Stomach - Sensitive stomach, reacts to many foods. Nausea and vomiting after stimulant food and drink. Feels relieved from vomiting. Nausea and vomiting with anxiety and dread.

COMMENTS - Ayahuasca has been noted to produce lethargy, immobility, a desire to close the eyes and a sense of withdrawal from the environment. Visions or dreams, most commonly of snakes which portend either good or evil: they appear either with an open mouth that threatens to swallow, or in motion. Results are different among non-native users.

Extreme spiritual fear, often followed by giddiness, nervousness, nausea and sometimes vomiting accompanied by profuse sweating.

Flashes of light, which can be followed by a bluish haze on closing the eyes.

General lassitude and a heightened awareness and appreciation of colors. Deep and dream filled sleep. On waking there is a common urgency to pass diarrhea. The net result of the whole experience is one of peace of mind and a physical purging.

Sleep-like trance, in which the person would want to keep the eyes closed, but in which there would be a sense of alertness with greatly increased intensity of awareness and insight into metaphysics or into personal problems of the moment.

Users described various themes, including the separation of soul and body separate, often with a sense of flight, sometimes at high speed. Visions of jungle animals. Mystical visions of angels, Christ or the Devil. Clairvoyance, vision of a future event. Visual experience of an event from the past that in some way illuminates the present.

RELATIONS - ***Compare:*** Anac., Ahal. Op.

REFERENCES - Murphy. Wansbrough.

BAPTISIA CONFUSA ACETICA

(Australian Baptisia)

PHARMACY - bapt-c. Baptisia confusa acetica. Australian baptisia. N. O. Leguminosae. Papilionoideae. Acetum of stem and leaves. ***Historical dose:*** Tincture and all potencies.

CLINICAL - Dyspnea. Headaches. Oppression. Spleen pain. Typhoid. Vision, weak.

HOMEOPATHIC - Pain in the right jaw and oppression in left hypochondrium, producing dyspnea and a necessity to assume an erect position.

COMMENTS - J. Meredith noted his experience with this shrub. He showed symptoms including congestion of the forepart of head. Weak vision. Hectic flush after tea. Right molar felt too long, worse by pressure intermittent, right jaw (later both jaws) stiff and painful at joint. Sciatica left side. Appetite increased, more energy for mental work. Improved sleep.

He was also relieved of a distressing symptom, that has troubled him for many months, and for which the ordinary Bapt. tincture in any preparation had failed to relieve. He described it as "a really distressing left hypochondrium oppression, fullness and actual dyspnea, impelling me to assume an erect position."

This oppression would continue half the night. The distress was located either in the spleen or splenic curve of the colon. It was uninfluenced by eating. Bapt-c. seemed to relieve the symptom very rapidly, causing something to move to the left and downwards, after which he went to sleep.

A case simulating typhoid was rapidly relieved by the remedy, showing its relation to Bapt. tinct.

REFERENCES - Boericke. Clarke.

BAPTISIA TINCTORIA

(Wild Indigo)

PHARMACY - bapt. Baptisia tinctoria. Wild indigo. N. O. Leguminosae. N. O. Papilionoideae. North America. Tincture of fresh root and its bark. ***Historical dose:*** Tincture and all potencies.

CLINICAL - Appendicitis. Biliousness. ***Blood, poisoning.*** Brain, softening. Cancer. ***Delirium.*** Delusions. ***Diarrhea.*** Diphtheria. Dysentery. ***Epidemic, influenza***. Enteric fever. Esophagus, stricture. Eye disorders. ***Fevers.*** Gallbladder, disorders. ***Gastric, fever.*** Headaches, bilious. Hectic, fever. ***High, fever***. Hysteria. ***Infections. Influenza. Intestinal toxemia.*** Mumps. Miscarriage, threatened. ***Plague. Prostration***. ***Putrid, discharges.*** Relapsing, fever. ***Septic, fever. Septicemia***. ***Sewer gas, poisoning.*** Shivering. Stomatitis. Strokes. Tabes mesenterica. Tinea capitis. Tongue, ulcerated. ***Toxemia.*** Tuberculosis. ***Typhoid fever. Typhus.*** Vaccinations. Variola. Worms.

HOMEOPATHIC - Baptisia, the wild indigo of America, has its reputation as a remedy for ***typhoid fever.*** In low potency it increases the resistant power of the body against typhoid.

In one case, that of an old man, food could be swallowed and retained some days, but not on others. He had always liked very hot food. The esophagus was red and granular. Bapt. 12c cured.

Hale considered it specific in threatened miscarriage from mental depression, shock of bad news, watching, fasting or low septic fevers. Patients in these conditions often complain of ***"dreadful sinking at the stomach,"*** fetid breath and other symptoms of Baptisia.

Many cases of tuberculosis are relieved by this remedy when the symptoms and type of fever correspond. It has cured hysteria with prostration, numbness and fear of paralysis, wanting to die, rubbing hands continually, restlessness.

Baptisia tinctoria has the ill effects of anti-typhoid serum vaccinations. It affects the blood, causing septic conditions, like low fevers and malaria poisoning. The symptoms of this remedy are of an asthenic type, simulating low fevers, ***septicemia conditions*** of the blood, malarial poisoning and extreme prostration.

Restlessness, does not sleep quietly, wants to be on the move. ***Indescribable sick feeling all over***. Tired, bruised, sick feeling in all parts of the body. Great languor, wants to lie down. Weak and tremulous, as if recovering from a severe illness. Prostration with disposition of fluids to decompose. ***Great muscular soreness and putrid states are present***. All the secretions are offensive, breath, stool, urine, sweat, etc.

It has proved specific in a large number of cases is ***epidemic influenza***. Besotted look, bleary eyes, aching head, sore throat, pains and soreness all over the body and profound prostration.

Chronic intestinal toxemia of children with fetid stools and belchings. ***Foul odor*** of the body, breath of excretions, stools, sweat, urine etc. Brown, sordes, stools, menses.

Discharges, stools, hemorrhages etc. are dark in color, fetid. Dark spots appear upon the body. Mucus membranes that become dark. Ulceration of the mucus membranes, especially of the mouth, with tendency to putrescence.

Feeling of ***soreness, heaviness and aching of muscles***. ***Prostration is rapid,*** bed feels too hard on account of soreness of muscles, yet he feels too weak to move.

Lifeless body but restless mind. Restless, always rubs the hands, hysterical. Insensitive to pain. Parts feel numb or too large. Bed sores. Intermittent pulse, especially in the elderly. Numbness, prickling and paralytic feeling over the whole body, especially left side.

MIND - Dull and confused mind. Inability to think. Mind wanders as soon as eyes are closed. ***Confusion, as if intoxicated.*** Ideas confused. Aversion- to mental and bodily exertion. Hopeless of recovery and certain of death. Melancholia with stupor. Indifference, doesn't care to do anything. Aversion to hear conversation about sickness or injuries. Falls asleep while answering or does not complete his sentence.

Delirium, wandering, muttering. Wild, wandering feeling. Bewildered. Sense of duality. Illusion of divided personality. ***Thinks he is broken or double and tosses about the bed trying to get pieces together.*** Imagines his limbs are talking to each other. Sensation as if some person touched him gently while dozing. ***Parts feel separated.*** Worse when thinking of pains in various parts of body.

Abdomen - Distended and rumbling. Fullness and distention of the abdomen. Severe colic in umbilical and hypogastric region. ***Intestinal toxemia.*** Soreness of abdomen in region of liver. Right side markedly affected. Right, iliac region sensitive. Pain in region of spleen. Abdominal muscles sore on pressure. Sharp, rheumatic pains in groins, worse from walking. Glands of left groin swollen, painful on walking.

Back - Back and hips very stiff, ache severely, worse walking. Symptoms radiate from small of back. Back sore and bruised. Feels as if lying on board. Neck tired, cannot hold it easy in any position. Dull pain in sacrum. Pain in sacrum around hips and legs. Bedsores. Stiffness and lameness of neck muscles, worse on moving head. Rheumatic pains in muscles of back, followed by burning.

Breasts - Dull stitches in left nipple.

Chest - Constriction and oppression of the chest. Weakness of chest. Sharp pains in center of sternum. Weight and oppression in precordial region, with a feeling of unsatisfied breathing, afternoon.

Ears - Ears feel hot and burn, yet cold to touch. Soreness in right ear, running down neck. Roaring in ear, with mental confusion. Dull hearing. Early deafness in typhoid conditions. Delirium with almost complete deafness.

Eyes - Blood vessels congested, eyes look red, inflamed. Eyes feel swollen. ***Eyelids heavy.*** Half closed. Cannot bear light. Feeling as if eyes would be pressed into head. Eyeballs feel sore with great confusion of sight. Visually, everything appears to move. Severe pains in eyes on reading, compelling to stop. Partial paralysis of lids. Photophobia, eyes burn, but don't water. Chronic ophthalmia.

Face - Anxious, frightened look. Dusky, stupid. ***Besotted look***. Dark red. Heat and redness of face. Sweats on face and forehead. Face and whole head feel numb. Pain at root of nose. Burning, prickling of left side of face and head. Cheeks burn. Muscles of jaw rigid. Cracked, bleeding lips. Pain in left parotid gland. Lower jaw drops.

Female - Menses too early and too profuse. Threatened miscarriage from mental depression, shock, night-watching, low fevers. Lochia acrid, fetid. Puerperal fever. Stomatitis of nursing mothers.

Food - No appetite. Constant desire for water. Great thirst. Loss of appetite. Averse to nourishment and stimulants. Child can drink nothing but milk. All symptoms worse from beer (Kali-bi.).

Head - Congestive headache. ***Headache, as if intoxicated.*** Dull, bruised feeling in occiput. ***Headache, fever and delirium.*** Frontal headache, with pressure at root of nose. ***Headache, with stupor and confusion.*** Excitement of brain, with delirium at night. Feels too large. ***Heavy, numb feeling in head***. Brain feels sore. As if a blow or heavy pain on occiput. Vertex feels as if would fly off. Brain feels sore. Skin of forehead feels tight, seems drawn to back of head.

Heart - Heartbeats seem to fill the chest. Feeling of greatly increased frequency of heart's pulsations, seem to fill chest. Audible palpitations. Pulse first accelerated, then slow and faint.

Kidneys - Sharp pain in region of right kidney. Shooting pain in left kidney. Burning when urinating. Increased secretion of urine at night. Urine is scanty, dark red, alkaline and fetid. Light-green urine. Uremia.

Limbs - ***Muscles ache, sore and bruised pains***. Feels as if lying on a board, changes position often. ***Bed feels too hard***, worse in region of sacrum. Great weakness, especially in lower limbs. Stiffness and pain, aching and drawing in arms and legs. Wandering pains in all the limbs with dizziness. Bedsores.

Liver - Soreness over region of gallbladder with diarrhea. Pain in liver, from right lateral ligament to gallbladder, can scarcely walk. Constant pain in stomach and liver, worse walking, hot sensation, heavy aching in liver. Pain in liver region on going upstairs.

Lungs - Asthmatic oppression of chest, with frequent yawning. Bronchial asthma. Craves air. Afraid to go to sleep on account of ***sense of suffocation*** and nightmares. Snoring. Awakes with great difficulty of breathing. ***Lungs feel tight and compressed.*** Breathing difficult from weakness of chest, worse on waking, better standing. Cough from tickling in throat.

Male - Dull pain in right groin and testicle. Orchitis. Pressing pain in testes as if squeezed.

Modalities - Better drinking liquids. Better open air. Better motion. Worse from open air, cold wind. Worse autumn. Worse hot weather, humid heat. Worse fog. Worse indoors. Worse from pressure. Worse on waking, walking. Worse mental exertion. Worse swallowing solids. Worse during sleep.

Mouth - Mouth and tongue very dry in fevers. Filthy taste with flow of saliva. Flat, bitter taste. Foul or bitter nauseous taste. ***Putrid, offensive breath.*** Breath fetid. ***Can swallow liquids only***, least solid food gags. Lower jaw drops. Sore mouth of nursing child. Thick speech. Soft palate swollen. Putrid ulcers with salivation. Saliva viscid. Ulcers in the mouth. Sordes on lips. Dark red, tumid mouth and throat.

Nose - Dull pain at root of nose. Nosebleed of dark blood. Sensation of fullness, edema. Sneezing and feeling as after a severe cold. Thick mucus from nose. Right nostril stopped up. Illusion of smell of burnt feathers.

Perspiration - Fetid sweat. Beginning of typhus when the nervous symptoms predominate, causes sweat to break out and relieve. Typhus with sweat on forehead and face.

Rectum - ***Intestinal toxemia*** of children with fetid stools and belchings. Constipation with fullness of abdomen. ***Offensive diarrhea day and night.*** Diarrhea sudden, horribly foul, mushy, painless, dark or bloody stools. Aphthous diarrhea. Very fetid exhausting diarrhea. Dysentery of the elderly people with pain in limbs, small of back and rigors. Painless dysentery with fever. Stricture from hemorrhoids. ***Stools very offensive, thin, dark, bloody***. Stool like sheep dung, dry and crumbling. Stool papescent, with large quantities of mucus.

Sensations - As if bruised or beaten all over the body. Bed feels too hard, makes him feel sore and bruised. Feels as if lying on a board, changes position.

Skin - Livid spots all over body and limbs. Burning and heat in skin (Ars.), worse in face. Eruption like measles or urticaria. Confluent smallpox, tardy eruption. Foul, gangrenous, eating syphilitic sores. Putrid ulcers with stupor, low delirium and prostration.

Sleep - Fears going to sleep on account of nightmare and sense of suffocation. ***Drowsy, stupid and languid, slides down in bed.*** Drowsiness, can only keep awake by great effort. Falls asleep when answering a question. Lies curled up like a dog on one side. ***Sleepless and restlessness.*** Sleeplessness with wandering of mind. Weary, as if he had not slept enough. Cannot get herself together, feels scattered about bed. Troubled with dreams, but inability to remember them. Nightmares and frightful dreams.

Stomach - Gastric fever. Can swallow only liquids. Cramp in stomach, evening. ***Constriction at cardiac orifice.*** Cardiac orifice contracted convulsively. Ulcerative inflammation of stomach and bowels. ***Dreadful sinking feeling in the stomach.*** Pain in epigastric region. Feeling of hard substance (Abies-n.). Nausea with eructations, followed by painful vomiting. Easy vomiting. Sudden attacks of vomiting and diarrhea, with fever. Vomiting due to spasm of esophagus.

Teeth - Sordes on the teeth and lips. Teeth and gums sore, ulcerated. Gums oozing of large quantities of blood on pressure with finger.

Temperature - Chill with rheumatic pains and soreness all over body. Chilly with soreness of body. ***High fever, sudden onset.*** Sweat relieves. ***Gastric influenza.*** Typhoid and cerebral forms of fever. Shipboard fever. Heat all over with occasional chills. ***Septic fevers***. The whole surface hot and dry with occasional chills, mostly up and down the back. ***Typhoid fever.*** Flashes of heat, feeling as if sweat would break out. Uncomfortable burning all over surface, especially face.

Throat - Aphonia. Larynx sore to touch, painful swallowing or speaking. ***Septic sore throat.*** Fauces red, dark, putrid ulcers. ***Painless sore throat and offensive discharge.*** Numb inside but sensitive outside. Mucus rattles in throat. ***Can swallow liquids only***, ***least solid food***

gags. Spasms of gullet. ***Constriction*** at cardiac orifice of esophagus. Constrictive feeling in throat causing frequent efforts at swallowing. Dark redness of tonsils and soft palate. Tonsils and soft palate dark red and swollen. Sharp pain in right tonsil. Ragged ulcers in the throat.

Tongue - Burning at root of tongue. ***Tongue feels burned***. Tongue feels thick. Brown down the center, cracked, sore, ulcerated. Tongue is dry, glistening edges. Yellow-brown coating in center, edges dark-red and shining. Tongue cracked, bleeds, heavily coated. Numb, pricking sensation in tongue. Root of tongue feels numb.

Vertigo - Confused, swimming feeling in head. Vertigo, with paralysis of eyelids. Vertigo, with severe nausea. Vertigo with a weak feeling, especially of lower limbs and knees. Vertigo as if intoxicated, worse walking. Vertigo, pressure at root of nose.

COMMENTS - Stupor, falls asleep while being spoken to, confused as if drunk. Cannot keep his mind together, a wild wandering feeling. This scattered feeling is further exemplified by the illusion that the body is double, limbs separated and conversing with each other. Can't sleep because body seems scattered about and cannot collect pieces. Indifferent and apathetic.

There is a dull, heavy sensation in the head with drowsiness and heavy eyelids. The head feels large with a numb feeling of head and face. Bruised headache, as if soreness in brain, bruised feeling in occiput, heavy feeling at base of brain with drawing in of cervical muscles. Frontal headache with pressure at root of nose. The neck is tired, cannot hold head easy in any position. The jaw drops, prostration.

The eyes cannot bear light, burn, are weak, painful on reading. Weight on eyes, eyeballs sore, feels lame on moving eyes. Blear-eyed. Lids partially paralyzed. An illusion of smell "as of burnt feathers" has been caused and cured by it. Pain in left parotid gland.

Flat, bitter taste. Tongue swollen, feels numb, speech difficult. Whitish yellow coating and feels burnt or scalded. Dry, parched, brown center, cracked and ulcerated. Canker sores in mouth. Ropy saliva. Sore mouth in nursing children. Thirsty. Sore throat with abscessed tonsils and pus (Merc.). Painlessness is a feature in the sore throat, putrid, painless, dark ulcers.

Esophagus feels constricted down to stomach, can only swallow liquids, cases of convulsive contraction of esophagus and cardiac orifice with regurgitation of food have been cured by it. Nausea, retching and vomiting. For food poisoning from bad water.

Gastric flus with nausea, loss of appetite and diarrhea (Nux-v., Ars.). Sinking, gone feeling.

Pain in liver and gallbladder. Pain in spleen, in right iliac region, in groin, swollen glands. Soreness of abdominal muscles in right iliac region. Fetid, exhausting diarrhea, dysentery in autumn or hot weather. Bleeding from the colon, dark, offensive blood. Worms.

The urine is high-colored, scanty, alkaline, and fetid. Orchitis, squeezed pain in testes.

Lumbar backache. Feels as if lying on a board, bed feels hard. Pain in sacrum. Weakness of lower limbs. Much prickling and numbness in left foot. Numbness and soreness. Excessive drowsiness. Bedsores with offensive discharge (Hyper., Led.). Offensive, putrid discharges, like something is decomposing. The sweat is putrid, cadaver-like odor.

Threatened miscarriage (Pyrog., Caul.), from overexertion, excitement, emotional stress, morning sickness, or lifting.

Sudden onset septic fevers. Overall feeling of toxicity. Drugged look, "besotted appearance," "dusky appearance." Septic infection from blood poisoning from an infected wound, or after childbirth or surgery. Good for toxic flu.

On a spectrum, Gelsemium is the mild toxic flu, then Baptisia, then Pyrogen for the most toxic. The first keynote is a bad taste in the mouth, foul mucus in the back of the throat.

Used in the past as the primary remedy for typhoid, contemporary interest for AIDS, as they share many symptoms. Possible remedy for toxic fever with an AIDS case, with diarrhea, emaciation, and chronic recurring fever.

RELATIONS - ***Compare:*** (1) Echinacea angustifolia is perhaps its nearest analog. (2) Gels., Arn., Ars., Pyrog., Bry. or Ars. may be needed to complete the favorable reaction. (3) Ailanthus differs, being more painful. Bapt. more painless. (4) Rhus-t., Mur-ac., Hyos., Kali-m., Lach., Mur-ac. and Nit-ac.. ***Follows well:*** Ars. ***Followed well by:*** Ter., Nit-ac. Ham., in typhoid Nux-v., Op., Rhus-t. Sil. has like Bapt., ability to swallow only liquids like milk, but unlike Bapt., Sil. has aversion to milk.

REFERENCES - Boericke. Clarke. Murphy. Phatak.

BAROSMA CRENULATUM

(Buchu)

PHARMACY - baros. Barosma crenulatum. Buchu. Barosma betulina. Barosma sanatifolia. N. O. Rutacae, genus, Diosmee. South Africa. Tincture of dried leaves. ***Historical dose:*** Tincture and all potencies.

CLINICAL - Bladder disorders. Calculus. Catarrh. Gravel. Leucorrhea. Prostate, disorders.

HERBAL - The leaves of several species of Barosma contain in vitae a volatile oil, having a warm camphor-like taste and an odor something like mint.

HOMEOPATHIC - Buchu has a markedly specific effect on mucus membranes and especially on the genito-urinary system, closely resembling that of Sabal, Populus, Copaiva and Thuja. There are no provings of the remedy and the only uses made of it have been with the tincture.

Muco-purulent discharges. Hale gave as indications chronic disorders of genito-urinary organs with muco-purulent discharges, abundance of epithelium mixed with pus and mucus corpuscles.

Irritable bladder with catarrh or gravel with spasmodic stricture. Prostatic disorders. Vaginal leucorrhea. Undue secretions from mucus follicles of urethra, seminal vesicles or prostate produced by excessive sex or masturbation.

RELATIONS - ***Compare:*** (1) Cop., Thuj., Pop., Chim. (2) Diosm.

REFERENCES - Boericke. Clarke.

BARYTA ACETICA

(Barium Acetate)

PHARMACY - bar-acet. Baryta acetica. Barium acetate. Trituration. ***Historical dose:*** Trituration and all potencies, second and third trituration.

CLINICAL - Forgetful. ***Paralysis***. Rheumatic pain.

HOMEOPATHIC - Hering and Hahnemann combined the two, Baryta acetica and Baryta carbonate. Hering said there is hardly any difference between the two and certainly none in the symptoms cured. Bar-a. produces paralysis beginning at the limbs and spreading upward (Con.). Pruritus of aged.

MIND - Absent-minded. Forgetful. Foggy mind. Childish and stupid. Lack of self confidence. Wavering long between opposite decisions. Weak mind.

Back - Lumbago. Fine stitches in neck. Suppurating pimples. Spinal disease with tinea capitis.

Eyes - Immovable pupils.

Face - Feeling of cobweb in face. Cadaverous pallor. Pale face. Drawn features, eyebrows rather drooping. Dark redness of cheeks. Mouth drawn to one side.

Head - Tinea capitis. Very disagreeable formication and pricking under skin of head and face.

Heart - Dull, deep sounds of heart. Pulse very small and frequent.

Kidneys - Frequent urination. When appetite improved and thirst lessened, urinary secretions became very considerable. Clear and abundant urine. Incontinence of urine and feces.

Limbs - Crawling pain with burning stitches. ***Paralysis of limbs***. Rheumatic pain in muscles and joints. Drawing pain down whole left leg.

Liver - Sensation as of a ball in liver. Region of liver as if swollen and cold.

Rectum - Involuntary stools. Rumbling in bowels. Diarrhea. Semi-liquid stool followed by constipation.

Lungs - Breathing gradually more and more embarrassed. Imperfect and very frequent respiration. Respiratory sound almost inaudible. Inability to cough, to expectorate. Inability to articulate words.

Skin - Skin cool and rather moist. Skin covered with profuse sweat.

Sleep - Wants to sleep all the time. Restless sleep. Moaning and muttering during sleep.

Stomach - Retching. Nausea followed by sudden and very copious vomiting of bile. Severe attacks of very copious vomiting. Vomiting almost regularly every hour for twenty-four hours.

Tongue - Cold tongue, somewhat black.

RELATIONS - ***Compare:*** (1) Bar-c., Bar-m.

REFERENCES - Boericke.

BARYTA CARBONICA

(Barium Carbonate)

PHARMACY - bar-c. Baryta carbonica. Barium carbonate. Bar-c. with which are included symptoms of Baryta acetica. Trituration of carbonate. ***Historical dose:*** Trituration and all potencies.

CLINICAL - Amenorrhea. ***Aneurysm.*** Arteriosclerosis. Asthma. Atheroma. Atrophy. Baldness. Brain disorders. Bronchitis. ***Down's, syndrome.*** Dwarfish, children. Colds. Cysts. Dyspepsia. Emaciation. Esophagus, spasms. ***Fatty tumors. Foot sweats. Glandular, swellings.*** Hemorrhoids. Heart, disorders. High blood pressure. Impotency. Leucorrhea. ***Lipomas.*** Marasmus. Memory, defective. ***Mental, retardation.*** Ophthalmia. Palpitations. Paralysis. Parotiditis. Photophobia. ***Prostate, enlarged.*** Quinsy. Sarcoma. ***Senile, dementia. Strokes.*** Throat, sore. ***Tonsillitis. Tonsils, enlarged.*** Tumors. Warts. Vertigo. Waterbrash. Wens.

HOMEOPATHIC - Bar-c. is especially indicated in infancy and old age. Dwarfish children and childish old people. Elderly people who are overweight. It has cured a case of fetid foot sweat with spells of despondency, seeking solitude, sobbing and crying.

Bar-c. has cured tumors of several kinds. Induration in the breasts. Sarcoma in neck with burning. Fatty tumors, especially about the neck. Swelling and induration of glands.

Has cured baldness in young people, tinea, wens. The scalp is very sensitive to touch. Enlarged glands in occiput and neck. It has proved curative in the habitual colic of children who do not thrive, enlarged mesenteric glands. Hungry, but refuses food, painful swallowing.

It's a cardio-vascular poison acting on the muscular coats of heart and vessels. Arterial fibrosis. Blood vessels soften and degenerate, become distended and aneurysms, ruptures and apoplexies result.

Affects glandular structures and useful in general degenerative changes, especially in coats of arteries and senility. Many cases of ***aneurysm*** have been cured with Bar-c. It corresponds to the atheromatous condition.

For those liable to ***take cold easily***, sore throat from cold, glandular disorders. There is a tendency to ***enlargement of the glands*** with indurations especially tonsils, cervical and ***prostate***. Takes cold easily and then ***always have swollen tonsils***. Catarrh of posterior sinuses with frequent nosebleeds.

This remedy brings aid to scrofulous children, if they are backward mentally and physically. Dull, and apathetic. ***Down's syndrome, delayed development.*** Marasmus. Dwarfish, they do not grow and develop. Scrofulous ophthalmia with a swollen abdomen. Persons subject to quinsy, which is prone to suppurate, gums bleed easily.

Diseases of old men when degenerative changes begin in cardiac and cerebral vascular. Old men who have ***enlarged prostate*** or indurated testes. Offensive foot sweats. Very sensitive to cold. Very weak and weary, must sit or lie down or lean on something. Averse to meeting strangers.

Often useful in the dyspepsia of the young who have masturbated and who suffer from seminal emissions together with cardiac irritability and palpitations. Cysts. Sarcoma with burning. Vascular softening and dilation, aneurysm, ruptures, strokes. ***Lipomas, fatty tumors.*** Emaciation of persons who were well nourished. Prostration, weariness, constant inclination to lie down, sit or lean on something. Upper half of the body feels stiff and numb. Too tired even to eat. Paralytic effects.

MIND - Increasing mental weakness. Beclouded mind. Difficult concentration. ***Irresolution.*** Confusion. Idiocy. ***Senile dementia. Slow mental grasp***. Loss of memory tries to recollect past events. Forgets her errand or word in her mouth. ***Slow, inept and backward.*** Thinking of ailments worse. Mental dullness. Irresolute. Lost confidence in himself. Mental functions loss after a stroke.

Bashful. Timid. ***Cowardly.*** Shy of strangers. Aversion to strangers, shuns, avoids strangers and unfamiliar faces. Dread of strangers. Mistrustful. Hides behind the furniture and keeps the hands over the face, peeping through the fingers. Easily frightened and afraid of strangers. Childish and thoughtless behavior, worse since a stroke.

Idiocy. Whining mood. ***Silly***, absurd. ***Mental retardation.*** Children cannot remember to learn. Slow in learning to talk. ***Difficult concentration in children.*** Talking mania during menses in young girls. Child does not want to play but sits in the corner doing nothing. Excessively busy, without any aim.

Anxiety about future. Anxiety about domestic affairs. Censorious, critical. Conscientious about trifles. Grief over trifles. Suspicious that people are talking about her. Imagines being criticised and laughed at. Thinks one is being laughed at and made fun of. ***Homesickness.*** Oversensitiveness of all senses. Heedless. Loquacity during menses. Sadness about trifles. Exaltation of fancies at night.

Abdomen - Habitual colic of children who do not thrive and though apparently hungry refuse food. ***Children with large abdomen.*** Hard and tense, tender, distended with emaciation of body. Colicky pains. Pain in abdomen swallowing food. Colic with hunger, but food is refused. As if intestines fell from one side to other on turning in bed. Mesenteric glands hard and swollen.

Back - Burning in back. ***Glands swollen*** in nape and occiput. Weakness of spine. Pulsation in back after emotions. Bruised pain between scapulae. ***Indurated cervical glands, like knotted cords.*** Stiffness in sacrum. Throbbing in back after emotions. Fatty tumors upon the neck. Chronic torticollis. Itching on lumbar region. Cramp in neck.

Causations - Ill effects of checked foot sweat. Vaccinations.

Chest - Sharp pain in chest, worse inspiration. Pains in the chest, mitigated partly by belching and by external heat. Sensation of soreness in the chest. Fullness and pressive heaviness, especially when ascending. Chest as if sore when coughing. Pain in axillary glands, which are swollen. Chest sensitive to pressure. Itching and burning stinging in moist, pustular eruption on chest.

Constitutions - Marked influence on the ***growth*** especially of children and old people, who become childish. In children the growth is retarded, they become dwarfish mentally and physically. Children are late coming into maturity to take on their responsibilities and do their work. It is a remedy for early senility and when degenerative changes in old men begin in heart, brain and vascular system.

Cough - Dry suffocative cough in old people, full of mucus but lacking strength to expectorate. ***Cough after getting feet wet, or least exposure to cold air.*** Cough is worse every change of weather (Seneg.). Cough worse in the presence of strangers, eating warm food. Chronic cough, in scrofulous children, with swollen glands and enlarged tonsils.

Ears - Hardness of hearing. ***Crackling noise,*** worse swallowing, walking. ***Glands around ears painful and swollen***. Itching in ears. Eruptions on lobes of ears. Eruption on and behind ears. Suppuration of middle ear. Reverberation on blowing nose. Roaring in right ear. Buzzing and jingling.

Eyes - Burning and pressure in eyes after exerting vision. Feeling of sand in eyes. Redness of conjunctiva, with swollen lids. Itching in eyes. Photophobia. Pressure deep in eyes, better looking downward. Light dazzles and hurts eyes. Opaque cornea. Agglutination of lids. Eyelids are granular, thickened. Pupils dilate and contract quickly. Cataracts (Calc-p., Phos., Sil.).

Face - Expression stupid and vacant, always whining. Tension as from a cobweb (Alum.). Sensation as if white of egg had dried on face. Parotitis after scarlatina. Face deep red with purple lips and great congestion of the blood. Prosopalgia. Eruption on the face. Lips dry and cracked. Swelling of upper lip, with burning pain. Lips pendulous. Acute pain in the joint on closing the jaws. Swelling of the submaxillary glands, with induration.

Female - Amenorrhea. Menses scanty, last only one day. Before menses, pain in stomach and lumbar back. Menses of long duration. Tearing pain in vulva. Leucorrhea, immediately before menses. Genitals feel numb. Atrophy of ovaries and breasts.

Food - Loss of appetite, though food has natural taste. Food has a sour taste. Hungry, but refuses food. Sudden disgust while eating. Aversion to sweet things, fruits especially plums. Desire for sweets. Worse after warm food. Better from cold diet. Weakness of digestion. Thirst during chill.

Head - Head sensitive to cold, disposed to catch cold when washing head. Brain feels loose, better cold air. Heavy pressure over eyes. Stitching pain when standing in sun. Pulsation in temples. Crawling over scalp, as from ants, in spots. Wens on scalp. Dry eruptions or moist crusts on the scalp. Tension as if skin were too tight. Hair falls out. Baldness of vertex. Premature baldness, even in very young men.

Heart - Arteriosclerosis. High blood pressure. ***Aneurysm.*** Cardiac symptoms after suppressed foot sweat or after masturbation. Heart feels bruised, sore. Palpitations and distress in region of heart. Palpitations when lying on left side, when thinking of it. Palpitation felt in head. Violent, long-lasting palpitations. Pulse full and hard. Pulse, slow, small.

Kidneys - Burning in urethra on urinating. Every time patient urinates, his hemorrhoids come down. Urging to urinate, cannot retain the urine. Renewed straining after urination, with dribbling of urine. Frequent urination. Passes much urine at night. Urine is dark brown, scanty.

Limbs - Pain in axillary glands. Pain in deltoid on raising arms. Limbs feel numb. Numbness from knees to scrotum, better when sitting. Fingers numb. Pain in joints, burning pains in lower limbs. Trembling of feet and hands while writing. Cold, foul foot sweat. Pain in the knees, while kneeling. Cold, clammy feet (Calc.). ***Fetid foot sweats***. Toes and soles sore, soles painful when walking. Soles feel hot or bruised at night during sleep.

Lungs - Asthma of old people, worse wet, warm air. Chronic bronchitis. Oppressed, breathing with anguish. Paralytic aphonia. Larynx feels as if smoke were inhaled. Lungs feel full of smoke. Paralysis of lungs in elderly people.

Male - ***Enlarged prostate gland.*** Flabby genitals. Genitals feel numb. Indurated testicles. Small retracted testicles. Impotency. Premature emissions. Diminished desire. Erections when riding. Erections only in morning before rising. Falling asleep during sex. Painful nodes in breast in old fat men. Moisture and soreness between scrotum and thighs. Sweats about scrotum.

Modalities - Better walking in open air. Better cold food. Better warm wraps, warm atmosphere. Better when alone, standing. Worse while thinking of symptoms. Worse company. ***Worse mental exertion, emotions.*** Worse raising arms. Worse sitting. Worse lying on painful side. Worse left side. Worse from cold air, cold damp, Worse cold exposure to feet and head. Worse washing. Worse odors. Worse warm food and after eating. ***Worse supressed foot sweat.*** Headache is worse from heat of sun or being near a warm stove.

Mouth - Mouth feels numb. Sour, bitter taste. Whole mouth filled with vesicles, especially inside the cheek. Saliva runs out, while asleep. Dribbling of saliva at dawn. Fetor oris, unnoticed by himself. Awakes with dry mouth. Sudden accumulation of water in mouth.Much tough mucus in mouth.

Nose - Dry, sneezing, worse blowing it. ***Coryza with swelling of upper lip and nose.*** Coryza worse mornings. Tip and edges of nose are painful. Sensation of smoke in nose. Discharge of thick, yellow mucus. Frequent nosebleeds. Nosebleeds before menses. Scabs around wings of nose. Smell sensitive.

Perspiration - Sweats on single parts, one hand, one foot, Sweats on one side of body, face. ***Fetid foot sweats***. Stinking sweat of feet. ***Worse supressed foot sweat.*** Debilitating at night.

Rectum - Burning in anus and rectum during stool. Crawling in rectum. Ascarides. Hemorrhoids protrude while urinating. Shooting pain in hemorrhoids. Constipation with hard, knotty stools. Diarrhea with lumbar ache. Diarrhea, with bloody mucus. Anus sore and moist. Oozing at anus. Anus as if excoriated.

Skin - Acne. ***Lipomas***. Cysts. Whitlows. Intolerable itching and tingling over the whole body at night. Sensation like the pricks of burning needles, itching and crawling sensations. Burning sarcoma. Excoriation and oozing in several parts of the skin. Injuries in the skin heal with difficulty. Swelling and induration of the glands. Warts.

Sleep - Sleepy and can't sleep. Sleepiness in the daytime. Sleepiness and weariness on slightest exertion. Talking in sleep, awakens frequently, feels too hot. Twitching during sleep. Sleep, agitated. Frequent waking and anxious dreams. Almost constant dreaming, causes anxiety at night.

Stomach - Sensitivity of stomach. ***Spasms of esophagus*** as soon as food enters esophagus, causes gagging and choking (Merc-c., Graph.). Pain and weight immediately after a meal with epigastric tenderness (Kali-c.). Pain while fasting and after eating. Sore spot in stomach. Weak digestion of old people with possible malignancy, better cold food. Dyspepsia of young masturbators or with seminal emissions. Long-lasting nausea. Morning sickness and vomiting. Vomiting fluid, water and chalk, followed by prostration. Waterbrash, hiccough and eructation, which relieves pressure as of a stone.

Teeth - Rapid decay of teeth. Gums bleed and retract. Gums hurt when touched. Toothache with swelling of gums. Toothache, worse before menses. Involuntary chattering of teeth. Fistula dentalis. Abscesses at roots.

Temperature - Strong disposition to chilliness. Chilliness relieved by external heat. Flushes of heat, more at night.

Throat - Submaxillary glands and tonsils swollen. ***Takes cold easily with stitches and smarting pain.*** Tonsils inflamed with swollen veins. ***Suppurating tonsils from every cold.*** Enlarged tonsils. ***Quinsy.*** Smarting pain when swallowing, worse empty swallowing. Feeling of a plug in pharynx. ***Tendency to tonsillitis.*** Can swallow liquids only. Sudden waterbrash. Sore throat with salivation. Throat troubles from over use of voice. Stinging pain in tonsils, pharynx or larynx. Submaxillary gland swollen. Much burning in throat. Chronic torticollis.

Tongue - Tongue, weak, hard, cannot speak. Paralysis of tongue. Smarting, burning, in tip of tongue. Burning soreness or vesicles on tip or under the tongue. Tongue as if swollen, with dryness, early in morning. Tip of tongue cracked and sore. As if blisters were on side of tongue.

Vertigo - Vertigo with confusion, in morning. Vertigo when standing in the sun, sharp pain extending through head. Vertigo of elderly people. Vertigo with nausea, worse stooping. Vertigo when lifting arms up.

Vision - Amblyopia. Gauze before eyes. Fiery sparks before eyes in dark. Sparks before eyes in dark. Diplopia. Weakness of sight caused by old age. Flying webs and black spots. Optical illusions, generally in bright colors. Sees everything as in a fog when closing eyes and pressing balls. Sees a cloud before left eye. Weak vision, worse during day, evening. Weak vision in candlelight

COMMENTS - A paralytic condition runs throughout the pathogenesis. There is paralysis of mind and body. Mistrust, lack of self-confidence, aversion to strangers. The child does not want to play.

Deficient memory. Children cannot remember and learn. Sensation as if the brain is loose.

Vertigo with nausea from stooping, or when lifting arms up in old people. Pressure and sticking in brain at vertex, on waking.

Rough, dry and herpetic eruptions on the face. Dark redness. Tension of whole face as if egg white had dried on it, as if a cobweb (Bar-acet.), over face, temples and scalp. Painful swelling of parotid and of submaxillary glands. The sense of smell is very acute, may have an illusion of the smell of pine smoke. Nosebleed before menses. The tongue is paralyzed. Salivation, saliva runs out during sleep.

The digestion is weak after eating. Pressing in the stomach, pain in hard, swollen abdomen. Stomach feels sore while eating, it feels as if the food had to force its way through some raw place.

The anus is sore and humid. Hemorrhoids protrude with urination as well as stool. Constipation with hard, knotty stools, hemorrhoids, burning and soreness. The paralytic condition appears in the sexual organs. Soreness and moistening between scrotum and thighs. Impotence. Enlarged prostate.

Paralytic condition of the respiratory organs. Feeling in the larynx as if inspiring smoke or pitch. Hoarseness and loss of voice from cough, mucus in larynx and trachea. Suffocating catarrh and paralysis of lungs in old people. Sensation as if lungs are full of smoke.

There is a spasmodic cough, like whooping cough, from roughness and tickling in the throat and the pit of stomach. Cough is worse evening until midnight. Worse after getting feet cold, exercise, lying left side, cold air, thinking of it.

Palpitations with soreness of heart, worse lying on left side, worse thinking of it. Violent, long-lasting palpitation felt in head. Palpitations worse on exertion. Slightest exertion makes him feel tired and sleepy. Aneurysm and atheroma.

Marked pulsation in the back. Stiffness and tension in small of back in the evening, especially while sitting, allowing one to neither rise nor bend backwards. Painfulness of arms and swelling of axillary glands. Cold feet. Fetid perspiration of feet. Corns with burning and stinging. Burning and drawing pains are frequent in lower limbs. Tearing in limbs with chilliness. Tension and shortening of muscles

Intolerable irritation all over like prickings and tingling, waking him at night. Itching, sore and humid skins. Warts. General soreness and sensitiveness. Small wounds ulcerate and get very sore. Offensive sweat of one side (mostly the left). Cold, clammy feet (Calc.). Chilliness predominates. Left side much affected. After eating, so weak cannot raise his hands. Too weak to masticate.

Down's syndrome, delayed development. Slow learning, slow speech, slow walking and coordination, delayed dentition. Difficulty making connections between words and objects, communication problems. Weak long-term memory, forgetfulness, poor attention span. Simian fold, a straight line across the palms.

Retarded development of growth, or of a specific organ. Stimulates the growth hormone (Pituin. 6x) if child is still growing. Also for pituitary tumors. Growth could be stopped by trauma, vaccination, or shock. Delayed development of the genitalia, especially the ovaries and the testicles. Undescended testicles (Aur., Clem.).

Very shy, gentle, and docile. They have very poor self-confidence. Inability to make decisions. The Bar-c constitution has floppy hands and feet, and giggling, spacey eyes. Simple mindedness. Symptoms of autism, dreamy. Never leave childish state, dependent.

Dumbfounded look on their face, clumsy, dull. Can have night terrors (Calc.).

Post-apoplectic in the elderly, when they revert to a childhood-like states. They become very shy and sensitive and can't make decisions. Also from epilepsy or head injury. Elderly have poor memory and indecision, some of the symptoms of Alzheimer's. Premature senility. Can have high blood pressure, swollen glands. Hormonal problems which age them quickly. Both the elderly and children need a specific routine, structure, to be happy.

Children can have recurring tonsillitis (Bar-m.). Tendencies to colds, with swollen glands. A lot of adenoid problems. Can have skin problems. Chilly. Can get emaciation easily, especially after infections. Lymphatic problems with a history of glandular problems. They have an enlarged abdomen (Sil., Calc., Sanic.). Offensive foot sweats (Sil., Nit-ac., Graph., Calc.).

Clarke cured an advanced case of thoracic aneurysm with the 3x. A case has been recorded in which Bar-c. removed from an old man a pain that came suddenly in the hollow of the knee and ran down the back of the leg like a thin stream of hot fluid or molten metal running down under the skin.

RELATIONS - Antidote for poisonous doses: Epsom salts. ***Antidoted by:*** Ant-t., Bell., Camph., Dulc., Merc., Zinc. ***Compare:*** (1) Dig., Rad-br., Arag., Oxyt., Astrag. Alum. (2) Ant-t. - paralysis of lungs. (3) Bell., Calc. - scrofulosis, coryza, etc. Calc-i. - large tonsils, Caust. - paralysis, Cham., Chin. (4) Con. - old people, Dulc. - catching cold, Fl-ac. - old people, Iod. - glands, Lach., Lyc. (tonsils). (5) Mag-c., Merc. - colds, glands, diarrhea, Nat-c., Phos., Puls., Sep. (tinea), (6) Sil. - glands, fetid foot sweat, but Bar-c. lacks the head-sweat of Sil. and Sil. has self-will instead of the weak-mindedness of Bar-c. (7) Sulph., Tell. ***Compatible:*** after Scilla, Ars. Before and after Sulph. ***Complementary:*** Dulc., Silica, Psor. ***Incompatible:*** Calc.

REFERENCES - Boericke. Clarke. Murphy.

BARYTA IODATA

(Barium Iodide)

PHARMACY - bar-i. Baryta iodata. Baric iodide. Trituration. ***Historical dose:*** Trituration and all potencies.

CLINICAL - Breast, cancer. Cancer. Glands, enlargement. ***Indurated, glands. Leucocytosis.*** Ophthalmia. ***Quinsy.*** Tumors.

HOMEOPATHIC - Bar-i. has been used empirically, especially in cases of glandular enlargement and new growths. The indications are suggested by its two elements. This remedy is used clinically for enlarged and ***indurated glands*** especially the tonsils and breasts.

Bar-i. has been used in breast cancer, breast tumors, ***breast cancer after trauma*** (Arn., Bell-p., Calen., Con.). Tumors and cancers following blows or other injuries (Con.), cuts, punctured wounds, or abrasions.

Acts on the lymphatic system, ***increased leucocytosis. Quinsy.*** Strumous ophthalmia with tumefaction of cervical glands and stunted growth.

Modalities - Better from cold open air. Worse from walking.

COMMENTS - Grimmer noted that Bar-i. has been used for ***breast cancer,*** breast tumors and enlarged glands. ***Breast cancers after trauma***. Tumors and cancers following blows or other injuries, cuts punctured wounds, abrasions. Indications are from the provings of the two remedies making up the compound.

RELATIONS - ***Compare:*** (1) Acon. lycotonum - swelling of cervical, axillary and breast glands. (2) Lapis, Con. Merc., Iod., Carb-an.

REFERENCES - Boericke. Grimmer.

BARYTA MURIATICA

(Barium Chloride)

PHARMACY - bar-m. Baryta muriatica. Barium chloride. ***Historical dose:*** Trituration and all potencies.

CLINICAL - ***Aneurysm.*** Anus, abscess. ***Arteriosclerosis.*** Asthma. ***Bronchial, disorders***. Convulsions. Deafness. Dyspepsia. Fistula. ***Glandular, swellings.*** Gleet. Gonorrhea. Headache. Hypertension. Idiocy. Influenza. Leucorrhea. Mania. Mumps. Multiple sclerosis. Nymphomania. Otorrhea. ***Pancreas, induration***. Pancreatitis. Paralysis. Paresis. Quinsy. Scrofula. Infertility. Testicles, disorders. Tinea capitis. Tinnitus. ***Tonsillitis.*** Tumors. Vertigo.

HOMEOPATHIC - The symptoms of Bar-m. are like those of the other Barium salts, but it has a distinct character of its own. Convulsions are more marked in the muriate. Many cases of aneurysm have been benefited by Bar-m. Both elements have a strong action on the heart and arteries. It has cured whizzing and buzzing in ears, noises on chewing and swallowing.

In one poisoning case, that of a girl, the instant she swallowed the solution she exclaimed that she was on fire; vomitings, convulsions, pain in the head and complete deafness supervened and death in an hour.

Bar-m. causes vascular degeneration, causing hypertension when high systolic pressure with a comparatively low diastolic is present with cerebral and cardiac symptoms. Arteriosclerosis (Aur., Sec.), and cerebral disorders due to this condition. Increased tension of pulse. Vertigo, due to cerebral anemia and noises in ears.

Acts on the lower digestive tract, especially rectum, on muscles and joints, giving stiffness and weakness as from walking too much. Indurated and ***narrowing of the cardiac orifice with pain***, immediately after eating, and epigastric tenderness.

Multiple sclerosis of brain and cord. ***Voluntary muscular power gone but perfectly sensible***. Paresis after influenza and diphtheria. ***Icy coldness of body with paralysis.*** Convulsions. Convulsive attacks occur periodically with starting and excessive tossing about. Electric shocks with convulsions.

General feeling of lassitude in the morning, especially weakness of the legs with muscular stiffness. Great weakness, wants to lie down. Enlargement of the glands and induration tonsils, pancreas. Chronic hypertrophy of the tonsils.

Nymphomania and satyriasis. In every form of mania when the sexual desire is increased. Children who go around with their mouth open and who talk through the nose. Child lies on the abdomen all the time to shun the light. Stupid appearing, hard of hearing. Headaches, but without acute crisis, occurring in old people, heaviness rather than pain.

MIND - Answers confusedly as if thinking of something else. Anxiety in evening. Irresolution. Sense of oppressive anxiety. Sadness in morning. Dejection and dread of men. Suspicious. Talking in sleep. Sexual mania in every form when sexual desire is increased.

Dullness of mind. Stupid appearance. Idiocy. Startles easily. Children are inattentive when studying, sit in corners and give confused answers. Indisposition to play in children.

Abdomen - Distressing throbbing in abdomen (Sel.). ***Induration of pancreas***. Abdominal aneurysm. Inguinal glands swollen.

Back - Enlargement and induration of cervical glands. Pains in the back. Eruption at the nape of the neck.

Chest - Catarrh with heat. Heat in the upper part of the chest. Oppression.

Constitutions - Useful in old age and childhood, when mental and physical dwarfishness is present (Bar-c.). Acts on parotid glands and pancreas. Suited to scrofulous children. Attacks of tonsillitis occurring in spring and autumn.

Ears - Earache, better sipping cold water. Offensive otorrhea. Inflates middle ear on blowing nose. Hard of hearing. Noises on chewing and swallowing or sneezing. Whizzing and buzzing.

Eyes - Eyes fixed and immovable. Pupils

dilated and insensible, with fixed look. Blennorrheal of the eyes, of the ears, and of the nose. Shuns light, child lies all the time on its face.

Face - Pulling pains in the muscles of the face. Painful nodosity at the point of the nose with slight pricking. Parotids swollen.

Female - Induration of ovaries. Tumor or atrophy of ovaries. Infertility. Menses too early. Pains as from a bruise, in the pelvis. Leucorrhea. Nymphomania.

Food - Loss of appetite. Thirst.

Head - Headache with vomiting. Heaviness of head in elderly people. Very purulent eruptions on the scalp. Scabby eruptions on the head and neck.

Heart - Throbbing of the heart accelerated. Palpitation of the heart. Irregular heart-beats, pulse scarcely perceptible.

Kidneys - ***Great increase in uric acid***, diminution of chlorides. Frequent, involuntary, and painful urine. Very offensive urine, yellowish, with whitish sediment.

Limbs - Toes cramp up, better drawing up the limbs. Fatigue of legs as from long walk with stiffness of joints.

Lungs - Weak voice. Dry cough. Great accumulation and rattling of mucus with difficult expectoration. ***Facilitates expectoration***. Senile asthma. ***Bronchial disorders of elderly people*** with cardiac dilation. Chronic cough of scrofulous children.

Male - Frequent emission of semen. Swelling of the testes. Buboes after suppressed gonorrhea.

Mouth - Swelling of the salivary glands and palate. Tongue loaded. Tongue and mouth dry. Fetor of the mouth, as if from mercury. Putrid taste in the mouth, also of food.

Nose - Coryza. Sneezing in sleep without waking.

Perspiration - Increased perspiration. Cold sweat.

Rectum - Spasmodic pain in rectum. Feces slimy, jelly-like with blood. Stools white, hard as stones. Easy evacuation. Chronic, painless diarrhea or diarrhea with violent colic.

Skin - Burning and pricking in excoriated places. Small, itchy eruptions on the head, nape of the neck, abdomen, and thighs. Glands are inflamed and ulcerated. Hemorrhage.

Stomach - Burning pain in the stomach. Sensation of heat, ascending from the stomach to the chest and head. ***Gone feeling at epigastrium***. Retching and vomiting. Vomiting in the morning, with anxiety. Vomiting of a small quantity of water, with nausea.

Temperature - General dry heat, night and day. Redness and heat of the face. Pulse frequent and full. Tertian fever.

Throat - Suppuration of tonsils after every cold. Swallowing difficult. Tonsillitis. ***Tonsils enlarged and infected***. Uvula elongated. Paresis of pharynx and Eustachian tubes with sneezing and noises. Throat feels too wide open. Varicose veins of throat.

Vertigo - Vertigo due to cerebral anemia and noises in the ears. Vertigo, swimming before the eyes, things turnaround. Head confused and heavy.

COMMENTS - Periodical attacks of convulsions with excessive excitement of the limbs. Idiocy. Mania with increase of sexual desire, "in every form of mania as soon as the sexual desire is increased." Offensive otorrhea. Parotid glands hard and swollen, especially right. Earache is better by sipping cold water. Deafness.

Great salivation and odor from mouth as from mercurialization. Swelling of salivary glands. Disposition to tonsillitis. Great indigestion. A hardness below the stomach to left, from which paroxysms of dyspnea come. Induration of pancreas. Distressing throbbing in abdomen with abdominal aneurysm.

RELATIONS - ***Compare:*** (1) In sclerotic degenerations, especially of spinal cord, liver and heart. Plb. met. and Plb-i. (2) Aur-m. (3) Con. - indurations of abdominal glands. (4) Iod., Kali-i. and Iris (pancreas), Sel. (pulsations in abdomen). (5) Useful after Ars. in extravasations of blood. (6) The vomiting is antidoted by Absinthe.

REFERENCES - Boericke. Clarke.

BARYTA SULPHURICA

(Barium Sulphide)

PHARMACY - bar-s. Baryta sulphurica. Barium sulphide. ***Historical dose:*** All potencies.

CLINICAL - Arteriosclerosis. Cancer. Dementia. Emaciation. Glands, swelling. Growth, disorders. Headaches. Hemorrhoids. Leucorrhea. Tonsilitis. Varicose veins. Weakness.

HOMEOPATHIC - Arteriosclerosis. Pressing pains. Weakness. Emaciation. Dwarf growth. Swelling of glands. Cancer of the glands. Tonsils swollen and inflamed. Pain in heart, radiating to throat. Varicose veins.

MIND - Dementia. Idiocy. Retarded development. Very anxious, especially during fever. Suspicious. Timidity, bashful. Anxiety. Fear of people. Cowardice. Anthropophobia. Always in a hurry. Loss of willpower. Marked irritability.

Ears - Roaring in ears. Hearing impaired.

Eyes - Eyes worse light. Vision dim on exertion of eyes.

Female - Leucorrhea copious, smarting.

Food - Cannot bear hunger. Craving for salt, sour, pickles. Desires sweets and chocolate.

Head - Itching of scalp. Headaches. Pain in sides of head. Throbbing in the occiput or in whole head.

Limbs - Corns sore, sting, burning, painful. Small warts, stinging pain.

Modalities - Desire for and better open air. Better walking in open air. Worse morning. Worse forenoon, night. Worse hearty meals. Worse bathing. Worse before and during menses. Worse lying on left side.

Nose - Nose dry, internally.

Rectum - External hemorrhoids. Constant moisture at anus.

Sleep - Restlessness sleep.

Stomach - Pressing in stomach after eating.

REFERENCES - Murphy.

B.C.G.

(Myobacterium Tuberculosis Vaccine)

PHARMACY - bcg. B.C.G. Myobacterium tuberculosis vaccine. Tuberculosis bovine vaccine. Nosodes. Vaccinations. ***Historical dose:*** All potencies.

CLINICAL - Abscess. Adenitis. Anorexia. Asthma. Blepharitis. Bronchitis. Catarrh. Chilliness. ***Colds.*** Conjunctivitis. Cystitis. Dysthyroidism. Dysuria. Eczema. Emaciation. Eosinophilia. Erythema, nodosum. ***Fatigue. Gland, disorders.*** Granulomas. Hematuria. Hypersensitive. Hyperthyroid. Hypochondriasis. Hypotension. Ichthyosis. Incontinence. ***Insomnia.*** Keratitis. Leukocytosis. ***Lung, disorders.*** Lupus, vulgaris. Lymphadenitis. ***Lymphogranulomatosis.*** Malaise. Melancholy. Nausea. Nocturia. Osteomyelitis. Peritonitis. Pleuritis. Pleurodynia. Pneumonia. Pulmonary, granulomas. Sore, throat. Tonsillitis. ***Tuberculosis***. Tumors, benign. Urticaria. Vaccinations. Vertigo. Vomiting. Weakness.

HOMEOPATHIC - BCG, or Bacille Calmette-Guérin, is a vaccine for tuberculosis. BCG is used in many countries with a high prevalence of TB to prevent childhood tuberculous meningitis and miliary disease. However, BCG is not generally recommended for use in some countries because of the low risk of infection with Mycobacterium tuberculosis, the variable effectiveness of the vaccine against adult pulmonary TB, and the vaccine's potential interference with tuberculin skin test reactivity.

Leukocytosis. Eosinophilia. Lymphadenitis. ***Lymphogranulomatosis.*** Inflammation of glands, adenitis. ***Tuberculosis of glands.*** Dysthyroidism with tendency to hyperthyroidism. Benign tumors. Hypotension.

Malaise. Emaciation. Lack of vital heat. Weakness and exhaustion. Tendency to take colds. Intoxication. Tobacco, aversion to smoking his accustomed cigar. Ill effects after vaccinations.

MIND - Mental excitability. ***Exaggerated cares and worries.*** Sensitive, oversensitive. Restlessness and nervousness. Prostration of mind, mental exhaustion, brain fag. Dull ness, sluggishness, difficulty of thinking and comprehending. Memory weakness. Loss of memory.

Easily irritated, angered, depressed. Any noise annoys him. Hypochondriasis. Anxiety, vertigo, feeling that death is imminent. Presentiment of death. Depressive psychoneurosis. Sadness, despondency. Melancholy.

Abdomen - Abdominal pain. Peritonitis, enteritis. Colitis. Cramping, griping pain. Stitching, sticking, pains.

Back - Backache.

Bladder - Cystitis. Dysuria. Hematuria. Paralysis of the bladder. Incontinence. Nocturia.

Chest - Pleurodynia. Chest pains. Oppression of the chest, sternum.

Constitution - Constitutional emaciation, especially in tubercular types. Phosphoric or carbo-phosphoric types. Hypersensitive, nervous, uneasy, restless.

Coughs - Dry cough. Exhausting cough. Hacking cough. Hoarse cough. Whooping cough.

Ears - Stitching pains, worse left.

Eyes - Catarrh. Blepharitis. Conjunctivitis. Interstitial keratitis. Swelling, eczema on the eyelids.

Face - Discoloration pale. Dry lips. ***Pain in left cheekbones, worse chewing.***

Female - Diminished sexual desire.

Food - Anorexia. Wanting appetite. Appetite increased, hunger in general.

Head - Brain feels dull. Headache in school children, students, and over-worked intellectuals. Headaches with disturbed sleep. Sensitive scalp. Heaviness sensation.

Heart - Oppression of heart. Palpitations.

Limbs - Joint pains, worse in small joints. ***Cramps in toes***, lower limbs.

Liver - Stitching, sticking pains, worse lying down.

Lungs - Asthma in children. Bronchitis. Pneumonia. Pleuritis. Pulmonary granulomas. Pulmonary infections.

Male - Diminished sexual desire.

Modalities - Better from cold application. Better lying down. Better after eating. Worse from physical or mental exertion. Worse evening. Worse 6 p.m. to 9 p.m. Worse 9 p.m. to 5 a.m.

Mouth - Cracks in corners of mouth. Bitter, pasty taste.

Neck - Inflammation of lymphatic tissue. ***Neck pain, better motion.*** Pain in cervical region on turning head to right.

Nose - Icy coldness. Dryness inside. Sneezing. Prolonged, chronic coryza. Chronic rhinitis. Nasal obstruction, better open air, worse in a room. Polyps.

Rectum - Constipation. Rectal, anal fissures.

Skin - Dry skin, with fissures. Scaly skin, ichthyosis. Abscess with recurrent discharge. Granulomas. Lupus vulgaris. Histiocytoma. Hidradenoma. Urticaria. Erythema nodosum. Erythema multiforme. Red papules.

Sleep - Sleeplessness after midnight. ***Insomnia in school children.*** Sleep disturbed by dreams. Restless sleep.

Stomach - Slow digestion. Stomach distension. Nausea, worse in the morning, on and after rising, better after eating. Retching, gagging with distention. Vomiting.

Temperature - Chills. Fever. Flu-like symptoms.

Throat - Sore throat. Tonsillitis. ***Pain in tonsils on swallowing, worse right.*** Scraping.

Tongue - Coated, discolored yellow, white tongue. Bitter, pasty taste.

Vertigo - Vertigo, feeling that death is imminent. Dizziness.

COMMENTS - Made from a stock of Myobacterium tuberculosis of the bovine variety. The vaccinating mother-stock suspension of the homeopathic attenuations is made from a film of this bacillus, cultivated on a background of Santon fluid.

A Hahnemannian Proving was conducted by O. A. Julian in 1960-61 on six provers, using the 5c, 7c, and 9c (1977). Symptoms included extreme fatigue, persistent asthenia, and a heavy head, with diffuse pain in the occipital region. Head dull, face pale. Dry skin, with fissures.

Dry, tiring cough. Pleurodynia. Frequent head colds, eyes red, earache. Glandular infections. Extreme chilliness. Chilly, cannot bear noise, headaches, with disturbed sleep.

Rare fever, lasting only a short time.

Anorexia, persistent nausea. Tubercular conditions in thin types, always tired, and with chronic constipation. Asthenic, thin, hypersensitive, constipated type. Aversion to cigarettes.

Julian noted "in clinical practice, B.C.G. is shown to be a polycrest, and has a definite value in all para-tubercular and psychosomatic cases. It is worthy of replacing the nosode Marmoreck."

RELATIONS - ***Compare:*** Tub., Bac., Phos.

REFERENCES - Julian. Murphy.

BEECH

(Bach Flower Essence)

PHARMACY - beech-b. Beech. Fagus sylvatica. The remedy is prepared by the boiling method. Small twigs and male and female flowers, they are found on the same tree, are boiled for half an hour. The boiled water is strained and used as medicine. ***Historical dose:*** Take two drops from the stock bottle into a one ounce dropper bottle, (add brandy or alcohol, if this bottle will be used for days or weeks). This is the dosage bottle, take a few drops straight into the mouth or as needed in a little water or juice.

HOMEOPATHIC - Together with the remedies Rock Water, Vine, Vervain and Chicory, this remedy belongs to Bach's group of ***Over-care for Others' Welfare.*** These five remedies deal with attitudes of control and over-care towards others.

People in need of Beech may appear haughty and rigid in body posture, in some cases, frequently raised eyebrows can be observed. Faultfinding, criticism and intolerance are predominant traits. The attitude may also be less condescending, more nagging and dissatisfied.

In the treatment of persecutory delusions or paranoid personality disorders, Beech lessens the tendency to overly criticize others and fit them into a specific image with threatening features (Holly-b., Will-b.).

MIND - Bach described the indications for the remedy, "The mind is narrowed in perception, tolerance and judgment, although one believes oneself to have the right attitude and capacity for assessment. This results in self-deception. The ego raises itself above others with the self-appointed right to assume critical judgment on another's expression of life. It is a state of arrogance, an attempt to impress upon others one's own standards of assessment considered special or perfect.

"Judging others creates superiority and those criticized are held low, condescended against. Oftentimes, one actually does not want them to measure up to one's own perfect style, so that one may continue to consider oneself special. The mind does not want others to move up in standard and it gives more personal satisfaction to keep them in their place.

"There is often an underlying sadness, a personal loss of a more perfect reality that is mourned. To have personal perfect standards and finding reality wanting implies a loss, a sense of being let down. In many cases, if grief was not allowed to be fully worked through there may develop a Beech state. The event or person is criticized or rejected, instead of mourned."

REFERENCES - Bach.

BELLADONNA

(Deadly Nightshade)

PHARMACY - bell. Belladonna. Deadly Nightshade. Atropa belladonna. N. O. Solanaceae. Europe. Greece, Italy, Britain. Tincture of whole plant when beginning to flower. ***Historical dose:*** All potencies.

CLINICAL - Abscess, Acne. Airsickness. Amaurosis. Bladder weakness. ***Boils.*** Brain disorders. Bronchial glands, disease. Carbuncle. Colic. Constipation. Convulsions. Cough. Croup. ***Delirium. Delusions.*** Diarrhea. ***Diplopia***. Dysentery. ***Ear, disorders. Epilepsy.*** Erysipelas. ***Eye, disorders. Exophthalmic, goiter. Fevers.*** Glandular, swellings. Goiter. Gout. ***Hallucinations***. Hemorrhoids. ***Headaches.*** Heart, disorders. ***High, fevers.*** Hydrocephalus. ***Hydrophobia.*** Hyperemia. ***Infections.*** Influenza. Intestinal fever. Kidney disorders. Lung, disorders. ***Mania. Mastitis***. Measles. ***Meningitis.*** Menses. Mumps. ***Otitis media.*** Neuralgia. Nymphomania. Paralysis.

Peritonitis. Phlegmasia alba dolens. ***Photophobia***. Pleurisy. Pneumonia. Pregnancy, disorders. Puerperal mania. ***Rabies.*** Rheumatism. ***Rheumatic, fever.*** Roseola. ***Scarlet fever.*** Sleep, disorders. Strangury. Strokes. ***Throbbing, pains. Throat, sore.*** Tongue disorders. ***Tonsillitis.*** Tuberculosis. Ulcers. Uterine disorders. ***Vaccinations.*** Vertigo. Whooping cough. Worm fever.

HOMEOPATHIC - Bell. acts upon brain and nerve centers, producing twitching, convulsions and pain. Produces an active congestion, furious excitement, perverted special senses. ***Glands swollen, tender, red.*** Marked action on the vascular system, skin and glands.

Hot, red face, semi-stupor, every little while starting or jumping in sleep as if it might go into convulsions. Excited mental state, hyperesthesia of all senses, delirium, restless sleep. ***Spasms, shocks, jerks and twitching. Constrictions*** occur in parts of the body like throat, vagina etc. or in whole body.

Fullness, congestion especially to head, and ***swelling***. ***Pains are throbbing, sharp, cutting, shooting*** or clawing of maddening severity, coming and going in repeated attacks. ***Severe neuralgic pain,*** that come and go suddenly (Oxyt.).

Violent attacks and sudden of onset. Complaints come suddenly. ***Hot, red skin, flushed face, dilated pupils, throbbing carotids.*** Marked ***burning heat, bright redness and dryness***. Red streaks. Hot body, part, etc. Discharges are hot and scanty. Hot hemorrhages.

Convulsive movements. Epileptic attacks are followed by nausea and vomiting. Spasms are followed by prolonged unconsciousness. Throws the body forwards and backwards, chorea. Convulsions commence in the arm.

Scarlet fever, also as a prophylactic. ***Exophthalmic goiter*** with extreme thyroid toxemia. ***Sensitive to light, noise, jarring.*** Dry mouth and throat with aversion to water. No thirst. ***Hydrophobia.***

Right sided symptoms. Good for children (Cham.).

MIND - ***Acuteness of all senses***. Overactive mind. Changeable moods. Quarrelsome. Constant moaning. Disinclined to talk. Memory impaired. Forgets in a moment what he was about to do. Mental confusion, worse motion. Mind disordered so that speech didn't correspond to thought. Mistrustful. Hides things.

Anxious and confused. Fears she is about to die. ***Fear of imaginary animals.*** Fright, with weeping. Starts in fright at approach of others. ***Fear of dogs.*** Anxiety during menses. Anxiety during sleep.

Stupefaction with congestion to head and dilated pupils. Hypochondriac depression. Consolation aggravates. Sadness, with indifference. Suicidal disposition while walking in open air. Weary of life, with desire to drown herself. Rather desires death than fears it. Weeping and screaming, worse consolation. Loss of consciousness.

Wildly delirious. Delirium, furious, rages, bites, strikes. Rage, doesn't know his relatives. Delirium wants to escape or hide himself. Delirium, better after sleep. ***Rage during headache.*** Restlessness during headache. Delirium with quick movements. Delirium with springing out of bed.

Violent delirium with livid face, injected and protruding eyes, dilated pupils, strong pulsation in carotids. full, hard, frequent pulse and inability to swallow. ***Imagines himself dreaming when awake.*** Carphologia, picking at bedclothes as if looking for something lost, with confused muttering. Hands constantly in motion, tries to catch things in air.

Desire to escape or hide himself. ***Mania***, rages, bites, strikes. ***Very restless.*** Spits on faces of other people. Tendency to dance, laugh, sing, whistle. Plays antics. Excitable, easily weeps. Disposed to tear things to pieces. ***Hydrophobia.*** Abhorrence of liquids. Liquid poured out makes her furious.

Delirium, sees frightful images. Fear of imaginary things, wants to run away from them. ***Delusions, hallucinations, sees monsters, hideous faces.*** Imagines he sees ghosts, hideous faces and various insects. ***Horrible visions in the dark.***

Visions of fire. Sees black animals, dogs, wolves, etc. ***Sees faces on closing eyes.*** Praying. Rage leading to violent deeds. Insanity with increased strength.

Abdomen - Flatulent colic. Distended, hot abdomen. ***Extreme sensitiveness to touch***, bedclothes, etc. (Lach.). ***Cramps and colic***, as if a hand has clutched some parts. ***Colic pains, comes quickly and goes quickly.*** Bearing down in abdomen as if all the viscera would protrude through genitals. ***Tender, swollen abdomen.*** Transverse colon distends and protrudes during abdominal colic. ***Colic from gall-stones.*** Cutting pain in epigastrium, better bending backwards. Cutting pain across, stitches in left side of abdomen, when coughing, sneezing or touching it. Clawing pain around the navel. Incarcerated hernia. Itching on abdomen. Pain in splenic region, worse sneezing, coughing, touch.

Back - Back feels broken. As if lumbar region would break. Pressure on dorsal region, most painful. Lumbago with pain in hips and thighs. Curvature of lumbar vertebrae. Hyperemia of spine, with difficulty in walking. Pain in sacrum. ***Swelling of glands of neck***. Sour smelling sweat only on neck. Stiff neck and shoulder (right). Pain in nape, as if it would break.

Bladder - Cystitis. ***Retention of urine*** with paralysis of bladder. Postpartum retention of urine. Sensation of motion in bladder as of a worm. Bladder region is sensitive. Dull pressing pain in bladder during night. Shooting pain in bladder when moving. Incontinence, continuous dripping.

Breasts - Breasts feel heavy, hard and red. ***Mastitis with throbbing, redness***. Red streaks radiate from nipple. Tumors of breast, pain worse lying down. Discharge of milk from women not pregnant. Erysipelatous inflammation of breasts, worse from weaning.

Causations - Ill effects of hair cutting, head getting wet. Sausages. Sunstroke. Walking in the wind or a draft.

Chest - Burning pain in right chest. Pressive pains in chest. Sharp pain in chest when coughing. Constriction across chest, as if pressed inwards from both sides. Heat in sternum. Corroding, gnawing, beneath cartilages of last ribs, right side. Swelling of axillary glands. Eruption of scarlatina begins on throat and chest.

Constitutions - Suited to plethoric persons with red face and to conditions where there is local plethora, inflammatory states with pain, throbbing, shiny redness as in acute gout. Suited to the bilious, lymphatic temperament. Light hair and complexion, blue eyes. It grows in dry limestone soils and is the acute correlative of Calc. Its influence is felt more in intelligent and plethoric persons who are jovial and entertaining when well, but violent when sick, therefore a great children's remedy.

Cough - Barking cough, whooping cough with pain in stomach before attack, with expectoration of blood. ***Tickling, short, dry cough, worse at night.*** Cough, worse fine dust in air, yawning. Cough with pain in left hip. Stitches in chest when coughing. Child cries before cough. Cough with stiffening of body. Tickling, short, dry, worse night. Dry, barking cough, sometimes spasmodic, caused by scraping or pain in larynx. Violent cough in sleep, with grinding of teeth.

Ears - ***Otitis media.*** Otorrhoea. Hematoma auris. Inflammatory swelling of ears. ***Hot, sensitive and painful ears.*** Bulging and red eardrums. ***Child cries out in sleep***, throbbing and beating pain deep in ear, synchronous with heartbeat. Tearing pain in middle and external ear. ***Pain causes delirium.*** Earache worse least noise. Pa rotid gland swollen. Acute conditions o eustachian tube. Noises in ears. Humming roaring, ringing noises. Hearing ver acute. Intolerance of noises. Autophony hearing one's voice in the ear. Impaire hearing from taking cold. Deafness, as a skin were drawn over ears.

Eyes - ***Pupils dilated***. Throbbing deep eyes on lying down. Eyes feel swolle and protruding, ***Staring, brilliant, co junctiva red, dry***. Burning, shooting pa in eyes. ***Photophobia,*** worse artifici light. ***Conjunctivitis, with great infla mation.*** Sensation as if eyes were h closed. Eyelids swollen, congested, f sore. Squinting, spasms of lids. Everted lids. Fundus congested. Exophthalmus. Lachrymation like brine. Ciliary neuralgia appearing and disappearing suddenly, with photophobia and congestion. Sudden ophthalmia. Eyeballs in constant motion. Mydriasis, resulting from nervous headache. Inflammation of optic nerve and retina. Strabismus. Yellow sclera. Ulcers or spots on cornea. Thickening of cornea.

Face - Becomes pale and red alternately. ***Red, hot, swollen and shining face.*** Face mottled, bluish red. Swelling of upper lip. Facial neuralgia with twitching muscles and flushed face. Spasmodic distortion of mouth (risus sardonicus). Convulsive motions of muscles of face. Lower jaw, as if drawn backwards. Cutting, tearing pain, worse right side. Parotid glands swollen. Pustules on face. Sweats only in face.

Female - Amenorrhea, with congestion to head. ***Menses bright red, too early, too profuse.*** Menses gushing. ***Menses and lochia very offensive and hot***. Ovarian pain with appearance of menses. Flow of blood between periods. Dragging around loins. ***Painful menstrual cramps with bright red flow.*** Cutting pain from hip to hip. Badly smelling hemorrhages. Hot gushes of blood. Metritis. ***Violent bearing down towards genitals***, as if everything would fall out, better standing and sitting erect, worse lying down. Spasmodic contractions of uterus. Ovaritis. Leucorrhea, white mucus with colic. Bearing down pain with leucorrhea. Dryness and heat of vagina. Rigidity of the cs. Labor pains come and go suddenly or ceasing. Diminished lochia. Afterpains, confinement. Retained placenta. Hemorrhage after confinement or after miscarriage. Menopause with sudden hot flushes.

Food - Loss of appetite. Distaste for acids, coffee, beer. Aversion to meat and milk. ***Desire for lemonade or lemons*** (which agree). Desire sour food, vegetables, sweets. Craving for undigestible things. Craving for snuff. Beer causes internal heat. Desire for lemonade during headache. Headache from abuse of coffee. Shortness of breath after drinking coffee. Bread tastes sour. Wine aggravates dyspnea. ***Great thirst for cold water***. Dread of drinking, abhorrence of liquids. Drinks in sips. Thirst for water changed into thirst for beer.

Head - Rush of blood to head, pulsation of cerebral arteries, throbbing in brain. ***Congestive headaches with a red face.*** Meningitis. Sunstroke. Vascular headaches. ***Throbbing, hammering headache,*** worse temples, motion. Headache better letting hair down, laying the hand on head, bending head backwards. Much throbbing and heat. ***Pain, fullness, especially in forehead***, occiput and temples. Headache from suppressed catarrhal flow. Sensitive to least contact. Sudden outcries. ***Headache, worse light, noise, jar, lying down and in afternoon***, better by pressure and sitting in a semi-erect posture. Headache worse on right side and when lying down. ***Headache worse from having hair cut.*** Hydrocephalus with boring of head in the pillows, head drawn backward and rolls from side to side. ***Head sensitive to drafts and cold or washing hair.*** Feeling in the brain like swashing of water, rises and falls in waves. Cold sensation in head at the middle of the forehead. Sinusitis, maxillary or frontal. Pulls her hair. Hair splits, is dry and comes out. Hematoma.

Heart - Heart seemed too large. ***Throbbing in carotid and temporal arteries.*** Throbbing all through body. Bubbling at the region of the heart. Violent palpitations, reverberating in head with labored breathing. Palpitations from least exertion. Gurgling at heart, when going up stairs. Pressure in cardiac region, arresting breath and causing anxiety. Dichrotism. Rapid but weakened pulse. Pulse full, hard, tense. Pulse slow, thready, irregular.

Kidneys - Stinging, burning pain from region of kidneys to bladder. Acute urinary infections. Involuntary urination, on lying down or when standing or at night, when sleepy during day. ***Frequent and profuse urination***. Hematuria where no pathological condition can be found. Spasmodic, crampy pains along ureter, during passage of kidney stones. Urine scanty with tenesmus. ***Urine dark and turbid.*** Urine loaded with phosphates. Fiery red urine. Urine deep red, with white sediment. Urine turbid like yeast, with reddish sediment. Urine copious, pale and watery.

Limbs - Joints swollen, red, shining with radiating red streaks. Jerks, spasms, or trembling in limbs. ***Cramping pains of limbs.*** Spasms. Heaviness and paralytic feeling in limbs. Shifting rheumatic pains. Shooting pains along limbs. Phlegmasia alba dolens. ***Cold limbs.*** Lies or sits with feet crossed, cannot uncross them. Weakness and tottering gait. Involuntary limping. Violent convulsions, distortions of all muscles.

Liver - Acute pain in liver region, extending to shoulder and neck, worse lying on it. ***Gallstone colic.*** Jaundice with stones in gall bladder.

Lungs - Asthma in hot, damp weather. Asthmatic attacks with sensation of dust in lungs. Difficult, short, quick respiration. Respiration oppressed, unequal. Cheyne-Stokes respiration (Cocain., Op.). ***Moaning at every breath.*** Oppressed, quick, unequal breaths. Heavy and stertorous breathing. Dyspnea after rising in morning, better open air. Bloody mucus, in morning, with bloody taste in mouth.

Male - Testicles hard, drawn up, inflamed. Weakness and relaxation of genitals. Nocturnal emissions with relaxation of penis. Nocturnal sweat of genitals. Flow of prostatic fluid. Prostatitis. Hypertrophy of prostate. Soft, painless tumor on glans. Drawing pain in spermatic cord during urination. Increased sexual desire, with great inclination to masturbation. Diminished desire.

Modalities - Better from light covering. Better wrapped up well in a warm room. Better bending backward, semi-erect. Better rest in bed. Better standing. Better from leaning head against something. Better bending or turning the affected part. Worse from heat of sun. Worse if heated. ***Worse drafts on head.*** Worse getting hair cut. Worse washing head. Worse after taking cold. Worse from light, noise. Worse jarring. ***Worse checked sweat.*** Worse touch. Worse company. Worse pressure. Worse motion. Worse from hanging down affected part. Worse afternoon. Worse lying down. Worse looking at shining objects. Worse running water. Worse morning, afternoon. Worse 3 p.m., 11 p.m. Worse after midnight. Worse night.

Mouth - Dry and hot. Mouth feels scalded. Hot breath. Taste salty, sour, bitter, pappy, offensive. Chewing or sucking motions of the mouth. Scraping in mouth and throat. Mouth as if constricted. Soft palate bright red and swollen. Thick whitish mucus in mouth and throat, with constant inclination to hawk and swallow. Lockjaw. Stammering speech. Hemorrhage from mouth and nose. Salivation worse lying down. Increased flow of saliva.

Nose - Drying in nose, fauces, larynx and trachea. Red and swollen. Tip of nose, shining red and burning. Tingling in tip of nose. ***Nosebleeds with red face.*** Coryza, mucus mixed with blood. Fluent coryza from one nostril only. Frequent sneezing with tickling in nostrils. Imaginary odors. Offensive smell in nose as from herring brine or sour beer. Odor of tobacco intolerable. Nostrils and corners of lips ulcerated.

Perspiration - Hot sweat. Sweats on covered parts. Perspiration, dry only on head. All over, dry only on head. Perspiration of chest at night, during menses. Cold sweat on limbs.

Rectum - Stinging pain in rectum. Spasmodic stricture. Straining and urging to stool, with scanty evacuations. Hemorrhoids with back pain as if breaking. Hemorrhoids more sensitive with backache. Violent itching with constrictive sensation in anus. Prolapsed anus (Ign., Podo.). Shuddering during stool. Mucus membrane of anus seems swollen and pressed out. Diarrhea with bearing down pain in uterus. Diarrhea worse motion (Rheum and Crot-t.). Escape of faeces when passing flatus.

Skin - Skin hot, moist alternating with dry. ***Dry and hot skin.*** Skin imparts a burning sensation to the examining hand. Swollen, sensitive, scarlet, smooth skin

Intense dermatitis. ***Bright, red,*** glossy. Redness of whole body, with quick pulse. Erythema, pustules on face. Erythema, very sensitive. ***Alternate redness and paleness of the skin***. Indurations following inflammations. Acne rosacea. ***Scarlet fever.*** Intense erysipelatous fever, with inflamed swellings, passing even into gangrene. Urticaria during profuse menses. Eruptions resembling measles. ***Boils***, returning every spring. Red scaly eruptions. Suppurative wounds.

Sleep - Sleep prevented by fever, anxiety. Sleeplessness with drowsiness. Kept awake by pulsation of blood vessels. Moans and tosses about in sleep. ***Jerks during sleep.*** Kicks in sleep. Restless, crying out, gritting of teeth. Screams out in sleep. ***Staring when closing the eyes during sleep***. Sleeps with hands under the head (Ars., Plat.). Heavy sleep with hot skin. Restless, crying out, grinding of teeth. Kept awake by pulsation of bloodvessels. Screams out in sleep. ***Sees frightful visions on closing eyes,*** dreams of quarrels, fire, robbers, assassins. Frequent yawning. Waking at night full of fear. Woken constantly by fearful dreams and twitching. Frightful dreams. Dreams of quarrels. Dreams of fire, robbers, assassins. ***Dreams of falling.*** Vivid dreams, but can't remember them. Dreams of swimming.

Stomach - Burning pain in stomach. Pain in stomach extending to shoulder and throat worse pressure. Constriction, pain runs to spine. ***Cramps in stomach.*** Spasms of stomach. Spasmodic pain in epigastrium. Painless throbbing and beating at pit. Violent hiccoughs. Spasmodic hiccough with sweat and convulsions. Esophagus is dry, feels contracted. Nausea and vomiting. Empty retching. Uncontrollable vomiting. Vomits everything with paleness and weakness. Vomiting of mucus. Vomiting of bile and mucus. Vomiting of undigested food. Hematemesis with ringing in ears, red cheeks.

Stool - Dysenteric stool in lumps like chalk. Retarded stools. Involuntary stools. Stools are thin, green, dysenteric or contain chalky lumps. Stools thin, green mucus. Stool sometimes bloody. Diarrhea of green mucus and blood after a haircut. Stools clay-colored, chalky white. Stools with granular, slimy mucus, smell sour.

Teeth - Throbbing pain in teeth. Pain becomes intolerable. Toothache, better biting. Toothache with red, hot face and throbbing in head. Teeth feel on edge. Teeth feel elongated. Toothache with earache. Gums as if ulcerated. ***Grinding of teeth***. Heat and redness of gums during dentition. Painful swelling of gums. Gumboils. Bleeding of gums.

Temperature - Chill alternating with heat. Chill without thirst. Feet icy cold. Shuddering during stool. Shivering chills running down back. ***Burning, pungent, steaming, heat***. Distended blood vessels. Skin hot, but moist and dry alternately. ***High fever without thirst. Hot head with cold limbs.*** Burning, pungent, steaming heat with internal coldness. ***Delirium and fever.*** Internal heat, with anxiety and restlessness. Fever with redness and puffiness of face.

Throat - ***Dry, red, hot throat.*** Dry throat, as if glazed, angry-looking congestion (Gins.). Throat feels constricted. ***Redness, worse on right side***. Tonsils enlarged. Spasms in throat. ***Tonsillitis worse right side.*** Chokes easily, things go down wrong way. Swallowing difficult, worse liquids. ***Sore, bright red throat with fever.*** Muscles of swallowing very sensitive. Must take a drink to swallow solid food. When swallowing, bends head forward and lifts up knees. Sensation of a lump. ***Larynx feels sore, very painful***. Larynx feels as if a foreign body were in it with cough. ***Laryngitis.*** Painless hoarseness, voice loss. ***High piping voice. Spasms in throat.*** Urging to swallow with choking. Scraping sensation. Hypertrophy of mucus membrane. Clutches at throat during epilepsy. Aversion to tight collars.

Tongue - Tongue is red, hot, swollen and painful. ***Strawberry tongue.*** Edges of tongue red. Red streak in middle of tongue, wider at tip. Tongue hangs out of the mouth in children. Forepart of the tongue cold and dry. ***Tongue hot, dry, red, cracked.*** Tongue white centre with red edges. Tongue difficult to move, scalded feeling. Papillae of tongue of deep red color. Tongue covered with white clammy fur. Trembling of tongue when protruded.

Vertigo - Vertigo with falling to left side or backwards. Vertigo, worse stooping and rising from stooping. Vertigo with vanishing of sight and flickering before eyes. Vertigo with rush of blood to head, roaring in ears, dim vision, etc. Vertigo on motion, on turning over in bed.

Vision - Diminished vision from doing fine work. Lost vision after severe congestive headache. Attacks of blindness, then yellow vision. Clouded vision before menses. ***Diplopia***. Triplopia. Squinting, spasms of eyelids. Moonlight blindness. Lines appear crooked when reading. Objects appear upside down. Objects appear double, and seem to revolve and run backwards. Sees red flashes before vision. Flickering, sparks. Bright sparks. Farsightedness. Amblyopia.

COMMENTS - Cases of Belladonna poisoning have frequently been mistaken for cases of scarlatina. Can control and act as a prophylactic for cases presenting a smooth, even, red surface. When such an epidemic is about, those who may be exposed to infection may obtain almost certain immunity by taking Belladonna two or three times a day.

A striking picture of Bell. is sometimes seen in cases of worm-fever. Lutze reported a case of a pale, feeble child, aged 3, who awoke, or at least sat up, at night in bed screaming, could not be pacified. Wet the bed at night, passed worms now and then. Cheeks and ear-tips were brilliant scarlet, other parts of the face, especially around the mouth, were white as snow.

Eyes brilliant, staring, pupils dilated. Skin dry and hot like fire. On being spoken to, flew into a violent rage. Cina 200c ameliorated. Bell. 100,000c cured permanently.

Corresponds to the symptoms of *"air-sickness"* in aviators. Can be given as a preventive. Has cured a very severe headache in a nervous man that occurred whenever he was exposed to tobacco smoke.

An enormous number of the symptoms of Bell. are developed in and from the head and sensorium. The pains of Bell. run downwards, away from the head (Sil. and Gels. have a pain running up the back). Characteristic heat, redness and burning.

All the symptoms come and go quickly. Predominantly a right-side medicine. Worse lying down. May want something bitter or sour with their fever. They like lemons and are thirsty in general for cold water. Generally aggravated at 3 p.m. and 9 p.m.

Great general sensitiveness and also sensitiveness of the special senses. Sensitive to light, to slightest noise, to motion or jar as when someone touches the bed. Photophobia. Mania, rage, disposition to bite, scratch and tear things. Fantastic illusions when closing eyes. Dull and sleepy, half asleep and half awake. Delirium with fevers, especially with kidney infections. Hallucinations.

Chilly. Sensitive to changes from warm to cold, to drought of air, to damp weather, to chilling from having the head uncovered or having the hair cut. Better from being wrapped up warmly in a room.

Remarkable quickness of sensation or of motion, the eyes snap and move quickly. The pains come and go suddenly no matter how long they may last. Pains are throbbing, burning and stabbing, "stabbing from one temple to the other." Throbbing pains anywhere in the body.

Head pains, headache. Headache with flushed face and brilliant eyes, dilated pupils. Feeling in brain like swashing of water. Throbbing, pulsating headache with beating arteries and violent palpitation of the heart. Congestion of blood to the head. Migraine headaches, vascular headaches, where all the blood rushes to the head. Palpitations, feels as if head would burst. Headache from sudden exposure to cold air or the sun (Acon.). Sun headache.

Blood congestion. The blood rushes to one part of the body and becomes hot and throbbing. Congestion, inflammation, throbbing blood vessels. Hemorrhaging, nosebleeds, uterine bleeding. The blood may feel hot.

Vertigo, mostly at night on turning over in bed or when getting up in the morning, also when walking and on every change of position. Starting, twitching or jumping in sleep. "Sleepy, but cannot sleep." Moaning in sleep.

Marked spasms and twitchings. Neuralgias and cramps. Convulsions. Epilepsy. Spasms from congestion or heat. Meningitis with sudden onset, high fever, dilated glassy eyes, rolling their head back.

The face is purple, red and hot, or yellow. Redness and pallor alternate. Skin is "uniform, smooth, shining, scarlet redness, so hot that it imparts a burning sensation to the hand of one who feels it. Sweat on covered parts only." Burning rashes, smooth and shiny. Scarlet fever.

Acute sinusitis, especially with nasal discharge that dries up (Kali-bi.) and throbbing. Bronchitis. Strep throat, ear infections. Earaches that come on fast with a high fever. Photophobic with earache.

Tonsillitis, throat and tonsils are red (Ars.). The mouth is exceedingly dry without thirst. Stinging in esophagus, worse swallowing or talking. Esophagus feels contracted. Affinity for sore throats, especially for children. May have swollen glands, high fever.

Vision disorders. Child has glassy eyes. Eye injuries (Acon., Calen.) with inflammation, pain and photophobia. Pupils are dilated and the eye gets red and hot. Very sensitive to light. Sparks before eyes.

Cough short, dry, tickling (Rumx. and Phos.). Whooping cough with crying or pains before the attack, flushed face, nosebleed and bloody expectoration.

Paralysis of lungs and heart (vagus nerve). Violent palpitation of heart. Stitches in chest. Swellings of breast with bright red streaks radiating from center of inflammation. Rheumatism worse by motion. Sweat on covered parts only.

"Tenderness of abdomen, worse by least jar. Pressing downward as if contents of abdomen would issue through vulva, worse mornings often associated with pain in back as if it would break."

Lumpy stool, like chalk. Spasmodic contraction of anus, obstinate constipation. Involuntary stool and urine. Bladder infections with congestion. Cramps and spasms on trying to urinate. Bleeding hemorrhoids, back pains as if breaking. Sensation of a hand clutching intestines. Stitches in spleen. Appendicitis, acute pancreatitis, gallstone colic.

The menstrual flow is hot, light color or bad smell. Ovarian cysts, especially on the right. Bearing down symptoms, stabbing pains (Sep.). Pelvic inflammatory disease with severe cramps and high fever.

Can be used prophylactically or to treat rabies, or bad reaction to rabies shot (Lyss., Hydrophoninum). Appropriate in hydrophobia.

The almost absolute deafness in cases is noteworthy in connection with Dr. Cooper's cure of a very chronic case of deafness with single drop doses of Bell.

RELATIONS - Calc. is often required after Bell. Antidotes to Belladonna: Camph, Coff., Op., Acon. ***Compare:*** (1) Glon., Hyos., Stram. (2) Sanguisorba officinalis - Profuse, long-lasting menses, especially in nervous patients with congestive symptoms to head and limbs. Passive hemorrhages at menopausal. Chronic metritis. Hemorrhage from lungs. Varicose veins and ulcers. (3) Mandragora - A narcotic of the ancients. Restless excitability and bodily weakness. Desire for sleep. Anti-periodic properties like Chin. and Aranea. Useful in epilepsy and hydrophobia, also Cetonia. (4) Hyos. - less fever, more agitation, Stram. - more sensorial excitement, frenzy. (5) Hoitzia - A Mexican drug, similar in action to Bell. It useful in fever, scarlatinal eruption, measles, urticaria, etc. High fever with eruptive fevers. Dry mouth and throat, red face injected eyes, delirium. ***Complementary:*** Bor., Hep., Merc., Nat-m. Calc. Especially in semi-chronic and constitutional diseases. ***Incompatible:*** Acet-ac.

REFERENCES - Boericke. Clarke. Murphy.

BELLIS PERENNIS

(English Daisy)

PHARMACY - bell-p. Bellis perennis. English daisy. N. O. Composite Tincture of whole fresh flowering plant. ***Historical dose:*** Tincture and all potencies.

CLINICAL - Acne. ***Aching, pains.*** Arteriosclerosis. Artery diseases. ***Boils. Blows.*** Brain, softening. ***Breast, tumors. Bruises.*** Cancer. Carpal tunnel syndrome. Conjunctivitis. Debility. Ecchymosis. Exudations. ***Falls. Fatigue.*** Giddiness. Gout. Headaches. Hematoma. Hemorrhages. Hemoptysis. Herpes. Indigestion. ***Injuries.*** Joint, pains. ***Lameness.*** Masturbation. Miscarriages. Menopause. Muscle, pains. Mydriasis. Neuragias. Neuritis. Organ, injury. ***Over-work.*** Pregnancy, complaints. Psoriasis. Railway spine. Repetitive strain. ***Rheumatism.*** Sleeplessness. Spleen, disorders. ***Sprains. Sore, pains.*** Stasis. Stomatitis. ***Strains. Strokes. Swelling. Tendonitis. Trauma. Tumors.*** Uterus, fatigued. Uterus prolapsed. Varicose, veins. ***Venous, stasis.***

HERBAL - The old name of *"Wound-wort" or "Bruise-wort,"* shows one of the main spheres of the action of Bellis and allies it in action with its fellow composites, Arnica and Calendula. The daisy is a flower that is repeatedly trodden upon and always comes up smiling afterwards. Being the *"day's eye"* may be the sign of its propensities for waking too early.

Burnett said "It is a princely remedy for old laborers, especially gardeners." Overworked old laborers and workmen, head sufferings of elderly working gardeners, commercial travelers, railway spine. Burnett generally gave it in the mother tincture.

HOMEOPATHIC - Dr. Burnett is the chief authority for its homeopathic uses. "It acts very much like Arnica, even to the production of erysipelas." He has cured with its aid several cases of tumors originating in a blow. ***"Stasis" and "fatigue"*** are the principal notes of the action. Exudations and swellings of many kinds. Fagged womb. Varicose veins. The giddiness of elderly people (cerebral stasis).

Bell-p. acts upon the muscular fibers of the blood vessels. Lameness of joints, as if sprained. Debility of limbs after gout. Venous congestion due to mechanical causes. Arteriosclerosis. Vascular cerebral sclerosis. ***Venous stasis***, swelling, ***varicose veins.*** Hemorrhages.

Injuries to the deeper tissues. Septic wounds to the internal organs, after major surgical work (Calen.). ***Sprains and bruises*** (Arn.). Near and remote ***effects of blows,*** falls, accidents.

Soreness, swelling due to injuries. Injuries to the nerves with intense soreness, better by cold bathing. Feeling of bruising of the whole body, especially the back. ***Tumors or cysts from injury.*** Exhaustion with need to move, which eases the pain. Muscular and joint pains. Pain in the right deltoid muscle.

Rheumatic symptoms. Pains are hard, aching, squeezing or throbbing. Unbearable pain that drives to distraction, worse heat better cold. Patients feel tired and exhausted, desire to lie down. Trigeminal neuralgia. Development of chronic conditions that may become cancerous.

Trauma of the pelvic organs from kicks, blows and surgery. ***Sore, bruised feeling in the pelvic region***, worse since childbirth. It removes the ill effects of excess of masturbation.

Externally in nevi. Acne. ***Boils all over.*** Acrid pus, destroying hair. Belchings.

MIND - Impulse to move. Ideas slow, difficult. Very excitable, makes himself noticed by those around him. Insomnia between 3 a.m. and 5 a.m. Dreams of anger.

Abdomen - Abdominal muscles lame. ***Soreness of abdominal walls.*** Soreness of abdomen in pregnancy. Fullness about the spleen. Sharp pain in spleen. Spleen sore, enlarged. Bloated, rumbling in bowels. ***Injuries, blows to abdominal organs.*** Post-operative pain and ecchymosis. Sharp pain in the right iliac cavity. Polyps of the buccal and intestinal mucus membranes. Pain in the appendix. Chronic appendicitis.

Back - Sore, aching pains. Backache from overlifting and strain. ***Sprains with great soreness.*** Backache or strain during pregnancy. Lumbago form physical labor. Falls on coccyx. ***Railway spine***. Itching on back and flexor surface of thighs.

Breasts - Breasts and uterus engorged. ***Breast tumor or cancer after injury.***

Causations - Ill effects of ***cold drinks***, exposure to wet or getting chilled when overheated. Affections due to cold wind. Blows, falls, injury, accidents, surgical operations. ***Childbirth.*** Overexertion, overwork.

Chest - Angina pectoris.

Constitutions - Suited to old gardeners, farmers, laborers and commercial travelers. Carbo-fluorica types with tendency to visceral ptosis, laxity of the ligaments and hemorrhages.

Eyes - Eye injury or strain. Catarrhal conjunctivitis. Conjunctivitis with excoriation and irritating discharge.

Female - Painful menses. Injury to female organs. Uterus prolapsed. Prolapse of the bladder and vagina. Uterus tumors. Pelvic cramping pain, spreading to the back. ***Uterus feels sore, as if squeezed.*** Tendency to hemorrhage. Viscous, irritating leucorrhea. ***Injuries, blows to pelvic organs.*** Feeling of downward pressure in the uterus. ***Soreness of uterus.*** Metrorrhagia. Metritis. Cervicitis. ***Varicose veins with pregnancy.*** Uterine strain, soreness from prolonged standing or pregnancy. ***Inability to walk during pregnancy.*** Sore, aching pains after childbirth.

Food - Insatiable hunger. Desire for exotic food. Effects of cold or iced drinks when heated.

Head - Headache from occiput to top of vertex. Forehead feels contracted. ***Bruised soreness***. Shooting pain. Head heavy on waking with feeling of blood in the head. Attack of migraine with pain in the eyes and watery nasal secretion. Drawing pains in the head and around the trigeminal region. Headache better by holding the head tightly. Itching around scalp and over back, worse from hot bath and bed.

Heart - Enlargement of heart. Rhythmic anomalies. Irregular pulse. Extra systole. Palpitations. Spasms and precordial pain, spreading to the right shoulder. Coronary thrombosis. Angina pectoris. Non-inflammatory lesion of the myocardium. Cardiac neurosis.

Limbs - ***Injuries, blows, strains to limbs.*** Muscular and joint rheumatism. ***Sprains with great soreness.*** Joints sore, muscular soreness. Hematoma. Tendonitis. ***Bruised, aching, sore pains from injury or strain.*** Post-traumatic and rheumatic myalgic pains. ***Rheumatism*** in old laborers. ***Swellings from injuries.*** Pain down anterior of thigh. Wrist feels contracted as from elastic band around joint. Carpal tunnel syndrome. Repetitive strain. ***Hip pains, worse exertion.*** Itching on back and flexor surfaces of thighs. ***Varicose veins with bruised sore feeling.***

Liver - Tingling in the hepatic region. Chronic inflammation of the gallbladder.

Lungs - Acute bronchitis. Hemoptysis. Pulmonary atelectasis.

Modalities - Better from continued motion. Better pressure. Better cold applications. Better heat and food. ***Worse from injuries, blows, sprains.*** Worse exertion, lifting. Worse surgical operations. ***Worse left side***. Worse immobility. ***Worse touch***. Worse hot bath. Worse warmth of bed. ***Worse becoming chilled when hot.*** Worse before storms. Worse cold wind. ***Worse cold baths, cold drinks.***

Mouth - Stomatitis. Angina. Pain in the tongue and mucus membranes of the mouth. Small ulcerations and cracks and chapping of the lips. Lip herpes. Burning sensation on the tip of the tongue and edges of the tongue are red. Improved by drinking cold water. Toothache improved by heat. Impression that the teeth are too long. Dental neuralgia.

Nose - Watery, irritating secretion. Loss of sense of smell. Nosebleeds. Sinusitis. Rhinitis.

Rectum - Diarrhea and large amounts of gas. Yellow, painless diarrhea, foul odor, worse at night.

Skin - Ecchymosis, swelling, very sensitive to touch. ***Bruises and swellings.*** Venous congestion due to mechanical causes. Hematoma. Acne. Herpes. Red papules and blisters. ***Boils with itching and burning sensation.*** Skin dry, cracked. Itching, aggravated by heat in bed and in a hot bath, improved by the cold. Exudations and swellings. Anthrax. Seeping eczema. Nevus.

Sleep - Sleeplessness due to sore, aching pains. Wakes early in morning and cannot get to sleep again. Dreams of anger.

Stomach - Indigestion or stomach ache. Acrid dyspepsia. Aerophagy. Heavy feeling, vomiting, acrid belching. Cannot bear the weight of clothing on the stomach. Worse cold drinks. Worse when overheated, touch. Pain improved by eating and by pressure. Vomiting, or regurgitation.

Temperature - Fever with shivering.

Throat - Pain on swallowing, feeling of itching in the throat. Huskiness. Feeling of rawness of the mucus membranes, heavy cough. When coughing, feels a sharp pain the thorax. Acute and chronic laryngitis.

Vertigo - Vertigo in elderly persons with cerebral stasis. Headaches with vertigo, improved by fresh air and by leaning over.

COMMENTS - Marked action on the female sexual organs, especially on engorged uterus and breasts. It relieves troubles of pregnancy including the inability to walk, varicose veins, weakness of bladder, constipation, hemorrhoids, prolapses. Given after childbirth, it will relieve pain and bleeding, help the sore, bruised tenderness of uterine area.

Bearing down pains, sense of weight or a ball in the uterus of rectum, weak bladder or uterus since childbirth (Sep.). Mechanical symptoms, the "heavy, tired womb." For toning the uterus after many births. For profuse bleeding or weakness in the uterus since pregnancy, miscarriage or abortion, with muscle soreness and bruised feeling. Sensation of being kicked, deep soreness (Arn.).

Near and remote effects of blows, falls, accidents (trauma). Tumors or cysts from trauma. For sports injuries with chronic aches and pains, or arthritis in the joints from overexertion and bending. Tennis elbow, sprains. Aches and pains in the elderly and laborers are worse with weather changes.

Stasis and stagnation. Loss of tone after injury or trauma, especially to soft tissue. Sleeplessness from overwork. Fatigue from masturbation. Tired feeling with desire to lie down. Can cause sleeplessness. Waking at 3 a.m. "Waking up too early in the morning and cannot get to sleep again."

Stitches in spleen. For severe injury to spleen, sore and enlarged, knife-like pain, area becomes congested and bluish. It has produced acne, boils, rheumatic pains, giddiness. Headache from occiput to front, contracted feeling in front brain. A pain in inner side of right arm as if a boil were developing.

Ill-effects of sudden, wet chill to heated stomach or body surface (Rhus-t.). Keynote "effects of cold or iced drinks when heated," dyspepsia, amenorrhea, skin disorders, rheumatism from this cause. Pre-eminently left-side medicine.

Burnett had a case of a tumor in the abdomen after injury to a rib. It became inoperable, he gave Bellis tincture, and seventeen days later the tumor was gone. He also gave it as a remedy for debility following acute attacks of gout, classing it with Vanadium of which it is a complement in degenerative states, as brain softening and atheroma of arteries.

Bell-p. has been observed to cause dilatation of the pupil when used locally.

RELATIONS - ***Compare:*** (1) Compare with Arn. - aggravation from the slightest touch and from movement. (2) Calen., Hyper., Con. Ars., Ham., Staph. (3) In effects of brain fag Pic-ac. Vanad. - degenerative states. (4) Ign - Unstable, nervous, weeping easily. (5) Sepia - Affects of childbirth. After pains.

REFERENCES - Boericke. Clarke. Julian Murphy.

BENZOICUM ACIDUM

(Benzoic Acid)

PHARMACY - benz-ac. Benzoicum acidum. Benzoic acid. It is obtained by sublimation from Gum benzoin or from several aromatic hydrocarbons. Tincture or trituration. ***Historical dose:*** Trituration, tincture and all potencies.

CLINICAL - Asthma. ***Bedwetting.*** Bladder, disorders. Bunions. Cracks. Diarrhea. Eye, tumors. Ganglion. Gonorrhea. ***Gout.*** Joints, disorders. ***Kidney, disorders.*** Knee, pain. Rheumatism. Sycosis. Throat, sore. Tongue, sore. Tonsils, enlarged. Ulcers. ***Uric, acid. Urine, offensive.*** Wens.

HOMEOPATHIC - The leading keynote is the occurrence, as a concomitant of any morbid condition, of ***strong smelling urine***, generally also dark. It produces and cures symptoms of a ***uric acid diathesis*** with highly colored and very offensive urine and ***gouty symptoms***. Patient gives out a very strong urine-like odor. Symptoms fluctuate according to the fluctuation of urine. Urination profuse and scanty alternately.

Gouty and asthmatic. Painful gouty nodes. Kidney insufficiency. Joints crack when moving. Hygroma, bunions. Meniere's disease. Marked action on the metabolism.

Pains suddenly change their locality but are mostly felt in the region of the heart or they alternate with urinary symptoms. Pains alternate with heart symptoms. Chilly, symptoms are worse in open air, by uncovering, better by heat. Symptoms appear left side first, then right. Child wants to be nursed in the arms, will not be laid down.

MIND - Activity of mind while at work, followed by anxiety. Fear following hurry. Anxiety while sitting. Anxiety while sweating. Omits words in writing. Child cross, wants to be nursed in arms, will not be laid down.

Depression. Prone to dwell on unpleasant things in the past. Shudders if he sees anyone deformed. Delusion hears confused voices, worse swallowing or walking in open air.

Abdomen - Cutting about navel, better stool.

Back - Pressure on spinal column. Coldness in sacrum. Dull pain in region of kidneys, worse wine. Trembling in lumbar region.

Chest - Chest very tender. Cannot tolerate pressure of clothes on chest. Pain in region of heart.

Constitutions - Gouty constitutions.

Ears - Noise, as of confused voices in ears, worse swallowing or walking in open air.

Face - Copper-colored spots. Red with little blisters. Circumscribed redness of cheeks.

Female - Prolapse of uterus with foul urine.

Head - Headaches when urine becomes scanty. Throbbing in temporal arteries, causes puffing around ears. Noises when swallowing. Ulceration of tongue. Swelling behind ears (Caps.). Cold sweat on the forehead. Pricking, puckered constriction of mouth, bluish and bleeding gums. Wens.

Heart - Pains change places, but are most constant about the heart. Awakes after midnight with violent pulsation or burning at heart.

Kidneys - ***Urine is hot, dark brown, strong foul odor*** of horse urine, ammoniacal. Excess of uric acid. Cystitis. ***Kidney insufficiency.*** Kidney gravel, stones. Dribbling of urine. Retention of urine in infants. ***Bedwetting***, the sheets are stained brown. ***Offensive urine of old men***. Bladder catarrh from suppressed gonorrhea.

Limbs - Gouty deposits. Joints crack on motion. Rheumatic gout, nodes very painful. Tearing with stitches. Cracking, pain and swelling in knees. ***Pain in Achilles tendon*** at the os calcis with pain in heart, when stepping on foot. Ganglion, swelling of the wrist. Bunion of great toe. Tearing pain in great toe.

Liver - Stitching in liver region.

Lungs - Hoarse in morning. Asthma with rheumatic complaints. Asthmatic cough, worse night, lying on right side. Hard, dry cough, followed by expectoration of green mucus.

Modalities - Better from heat. Better profuse urination. Worse from open air, Worse cold. Worse changing weather. Worse by uncovering. Motion aggravates most symptoms, but headache is worse at rest and toothache is worse lying down.

Mouth - Involuntary biting of lower lip, while eating. Tongue, spongy on surface with deep cracks and spreading ulcers. Mouth and throat symptoms are better eating. Toothache worse lying down.

Nose - Itching of septum. Pain in nasal bones. Seems to smell cabbage, dust or something stinking.

Perspiration - Profuse sweat without relief. Night sweats. Sweat with aromatic odor.

Rectum - Frothy ***offensive, liquid***, light-colored like soapsuds, bowel movements mostly windy. Stitches and ***constricted*** feeling. Puckering constriction of rectum. Itching and watery elevations around anus. Copious grayish stools like soap suds of a pungent urine-like odor, very foul, white.

Skin - Red spots. Itching with agreeable sensation on being scratched, but leaving a burning.

Stomach - Sweat while eating, pressure in stomach, sensation of a lump. Vomiting of salty or bitter substance.

Temperature - Hands, feet, back, knees cold, as from a cold wind. Chilliness, cold sweat. Internal heat on awakening.

Throat - Sensation as of a lump, swelling and constriction better eating.

Vertigo - Vertigo inclination to fall sideways.

COMMENTS - Ganglion of wrist and bunion of great toe have been frequently cured with Benz-ac. In these cases, an ointment of the 3x is a useful external adjunct. Asthma has been cured by it, especially in rheumatic persons. "Most of the symptoms appear on the left side, but may subsequently come on the right." Inclination to dwell on unpleasant subjects and shuddering on seeing anyone deformed.

Inflammation of bronchi and lungs with great tenderness of chest, cough worse night, lying on right side.

Long-continued, dry cough after suppressed gonorrhea. Sensation of lump (as of food) in pit of throat of swelling and constriction. Throat symptoms are better by eating. Tongue is spongy on the surface with deep cracks and spreading ulcers.

Watery, light, very offensive stools (in children), stools like soapsuds with usually strong-smelling urine. Shivering before stool. Bedwetting at night, urine dark, strong-smelling, heavy, hot, smelling like horse's urine.

Gout (Colch.), kidney infections, with strong-smelling and offensive urine (Nit-ac.). Joints are red and swollen, sensitive to the touch, gout can migrate. Tearing and stitches in great toe, especially right (gout). Swelling and pain of right knee. Gouty concretions. Kidney stones or gravel in the urine, or for the tendency to form gravel. Uric acid diathesis (Colch., or Urt-u. in tincture).

RELATIONS - ***Antidoted by:*** Copaiva. ***Compare:*** (1) Nit-ac. - urine smelling like horse's. (2) Calc., Am-c. benz., Sabina, Tropeleum, Garden Nasturtium, (fetid urine). (3) Cop., Ferr., Zinc., Tropeolum. (4) Useful in gout after Colch. after abuse of Copaiva. (5) In suppression of gonorrhea in bedwetting after failure of Nitrum. ***Incompatible:*** Wine, which aggravates pains in kidneys, drawing in knees, etc. Useful after Colch. fails in gout after Copaiva in gonorrhea.

REFERENCES - Boericke. Clarke. Murphy.

BENZOINUM ODERIFERUM

(Spicebush)

PHARMACY - benzo. Benzoinum oderiferum. Spicebush. Fever-bush. Lindera benzoin. Laurus benzoin. Benzoe. N. O. Lauracae. Tincture of twigs. ***Historical dose:*** Tincture and all potencies.

CLINICAL - Fever. Hair, oily. Hip, pain. Vertigo.

HOMEOPATHIC - The symptoms of Benzo. as shown in a short proving, somewhat resemble those of Laur. Sense of touch fine, quic and pleasant. The hair is oily. Feverish.

Empty sensation at the stomach and lower part of bowels. Wakes from sleep with a sick feeling in stomach and bowels, tired feeling, turns often in bed at night.

MIND - Unpleasant, fearful feeling.

Head - Hair oily.

Limbs - Hips feel crushed. Pains in knees. Feet and legs cold up to knees, remained cold in bed.

Modalities - Worse after sleep. Worse on lying down. Head swims with sinking sensation, which makes lying down in bed unpleasant.

Stool - Soft stool, with pain before stool in lower bowel.

Urine - Urine more frequent, small quantity, dark color, had to rise twice in night to urinate.

Vertigo - Head swims with sinking sensation, worse lying down.

RELATIONS - ***Compare:*** (1) Laur. (2) Lach. - worse after sleep.

REFERENCES - Clarke.

BENZOLUM

(Benzol)

PHARMACY - benz. Benzolum. Benzol. Benzinum. Benzene. Coal naphtha. Benzoline. A product of distillation from coal tar. Tincture with alcohol. ***Historical dose:*** Tincture and all potencies.

CLINICAL - Coma. Dysentery. Fever. Headache. Insomnia. ***Myeloid, leukemia.*** Photophobia. Sweat. Typhoid fever. Vision disorders.

HOMEOPATHIC - Our knowledge of this medicine is derived from observations on a worker in a rubber factory, who for weeks had his hands and arms daily bathed in benzine and drank water impregnated with it.

Benz. affects the blood. In the provers it resulted in a ***decrease of the red and increase of white cells***. It may to be of use in acute myeloid leukemia. Patients are tired and nervous. Pain travels from below upwards. Striking eye symptoms. Sense of falling through bed and floor. Hallucinations, epileptiform attacks, coma and anesthesia.

MIND - Hallucination as of a great white hand appeared to him in darkness.

Eyes - Illusion of vision with wide-open eyes. Twitching of lids. Photophobia, objects blurred. Aching in eyes and lids. Marked dilation of pupils. Failure to react to light, particularly daylight.

Head - Sense of falling through bed and floor. Dizzy. Tired and nervous. Pains from below upward. Pressing feeling in head. Frontal headache to root of nose. Right-sided headache.

Limbs - Heavy limbs and cold legs, exaggerated knee-jerk. Pains from below upward.

Male - Swelling of right testicle. Severe pain in testicles. Itching of scrotum. Profuse urination.

Modalities - Worse at night, right side.

Nose - Profuse fluent coryza, especially in afternoon. Violent sneezing.

Skin - Eruption like measles. Perspiration on side not lain upon. Itching all over back.

COMMENTS - Benz. caused a profound disturbance of mind and body, weeping at trifles, irritability, pain darting upwards in occiput. Could not turn eyes upward without severe aching and throbbing.

A sort of clairvoyant state in which a great white hand appeared to him in the darkness, coming outspread towards his face, causing him in terror to scream for the watcher. A sense of falling through the bed and floor. Insomnia and visual illusions. Pains travel from below upward (headache, pain in anus), chills.

RELATIONS - ***Compare:*** (1) T. N. T. (2) Benzin. - Petroleum ether, not as pure a compound as Benzene, (Benzol). It is the same, but with a mixture of various hydrocarbons. Oxyhemoglobinemia. It seems to exercise a special influence on the nervous system and the blood. Physical weakness, cramps, exaggeration of knee jerks, nausea, vomiting, dizziness, Heaviness and coldness of limbs. Tremor of eyelids and tongue. (3) Benzin. dinitricum.

REFERENCES - Boericke. Clarke

BENZOLUM DINITRICUM

PHARMACY - benz-d. Benzolum dinitricum. Di-Nitrobenzol. A crystalline substance obtained from the further action of Nitric Acid on Nitrobenzol at higher temperatures. Solution in alcohol. ***Historical dose:*** Tincture and all potencies.

CLINICAL - Amblyopia. Anemia. ***Color-blindness.*** Impotence. Peripheral, neuritis. Retinitis. ***Scotoma***. Spastic paralysis, Urine, black.

HOMEOPATHIC - Benz-d. is used in the manufacture of the higher explosives. The effects on workers were recorded by Simeon Snell in the British Medical Journal of March 3, 1894. The symptoms observed strongly resemble those of Benz-n.

The most obvious results of poisoning by skin absorption are changes in the red blood corpuscles and liver degeneration. Anemia with a murmur in the pulmonary artery. Headaches, giddiness, staggering, with numbness and paralytic sensations. Impotence in men. Distaste for tobacco. Dyspnea was marked in all, accounting partly for the inability to smoke.

Amblyopia, color-blindness, retinitis, ***"a small central scotoma for red and green."*** Field of vision contracted. The retinal veins were found much engorged, probably part of the general venous engorgement and cyanosis. The blood is altered and turned black, and the urine is black without containing blood.

MIND - Delirious, complaining of great pain in head. Raving behavior and unconscious from 5 p.m. to 10 p.m., the doctor gave him up, but he recovered.

Eyes - Blindness. ***Color-blindness, central scotoma for red and green***. Disc pale, grayish, edges defined, retinal vessels full, especially the veins. Retinal hyperesthesia. Veins much larger than the arteries. Conjunctive jaundiced.

Face - Face pale, lips blue. Face bluish, asphyxiated look.

Head - Giddiness, compelling to sit down. Reels as if drunk, even fell off a stool when sitting, stumbled getting into a train. Could not walk many yards without falling. Occipital headache, unable to work on account of headache. Frontal headache with delirium. Color of hair altered from golden to a sort of red.

Heart - Engorgement of venous system. Bruit in pulmonary artery. Pulse very frequent (115), small and compressible. Anemia. Blood black.

Kidneys - Urine dark like ink.

Limbs - Want of sensation in arms and legs, prickly feeling. Legs numbs to knees and arms to elbows. Stiffness about hands and feet, especially the fingers. Hands and feet cold, feet numb and sore. Fingertips feel cold to the touch, though she herself is not aware of it.

Lungs - Breath very short, rendering smoking very difficult. Short breath with giddiness. Asphyxia.

Male - Sexual desire lost, power diminished (restored when taking liquid strychnine after leaving off the work).

Stomach - Intolerance of alcohol, ***"it made him fell so bad."*** Occasional nausea and vomiting.

RELATIONS - ***Antidoted by:*** Strychnine. ***Compare:*** (1) Benz., Benz-n., Hydr-ac., Ars.

REFERENCES - Clarke.

BENZOLUM NITRICUM

(Nitro-benzene)

PHARMACY - benz-n. Benzolum nitricum. Nitro-benzene. Essence of Morbane. Artificial Oil of Bitter Almonds. Prepared by heating Benzol with Nitric Acid, the oily fluid formed is washed and rectified, it is miscible with alcohol and has an odor of bitter almonds. Solution in alcohol. ***Historical dose:*** Tincture and all potencies.

CLINICAL - Amaurosis. Convulsions. Cyanosis. Diuresis. ***Epilepsy.*** Nystagmus. Respiration, slow. Strabismus. Tetanus. Trismus.

HOMEOPATHIC - Nitro-benzene is a very poisonous substance and our knowledge of its action is due to numerous cases of poisoning that have occurred. Slows the respiration until death occurs.

Rolling of eyeballs in their vertical axis, pupils dilated. Nystagmus. Blue lips, tongue, skin, face, conjunctive and fingernails.

Flapping of nasal alae. Burning taste in mouth. Burning in throat and stomach. Sweat on forehead and face. Whole body covered with profuse cold sweat. Secretions smell strongly of bitter almonds. Nausea, vomiting of food eaten. Pains in abdomen. Involuntary evacuations.

Paralysis of all limbs. Faintness, sinking, convulsions, twitchings, stupor. Head drawn backward and to the left side in spasms. Punctiform ecchymoses. Dark, black blood, that coagulates with difficulty. Venous blood, hyperemia of the brain and general venous engorgement. Respiration very slow, difficult, sighing. Cold skin, pulse small, weak, breathing slow and irregular, unconsciousness, symptoms of apoplectic coma.

MIND - Loquacity, following drowsiness, soon passing into stupor. Extreme mental excitement, soon became unconscious with inarticulate, confused speech.

Ears - Violent roaring in ears and sounds.

Eyes - Eyes staring. Rolling of the eyeballs in their vertical axis. Constant turning of the eyeballs, inward and outward in a slow, regular motion with the visual axes perfectly parallel. Constant slow movement of eyeballs from left to right under closed lids. Nystagmus. Great injection of conjunctiva of bulbs. Eyeballs seemed enlarged. Strabismus. Pupils dilated, insensible to light. Distorted vision and flashes of strange light and colors.

Head - Head drawn backwards and to the left in spasms.

Kidneys - Diuresis, urine brownish red, odor of bitter almonds. Urine and feces passed involuntarily.

Limbs - Paralysis of all limbs. Twitchings in hands and feet. Arms spasmodically flexed, sometimes extended afterwards relaxed.

Lungs - Dyspnea. Snoring. Sighing, frequently interrupted. Breathing, slow, difficult.

Mouth - Tongue white and swollen, thick and soft. Burning taste, followed by numbness and tingling of tongue and lips. Tenacious saliva. Stammering speech.

Neck - Stiff-neck, trismus and twitchings in masseter muscles.

Pulse - Pulse rapid, weak, irregular, scarcely perceptible. Pulse full and slow.

Rectum - Involuntary evacuation.

Skin - Skin cold and livid, bluish-gray. Punctiform ecchymosis. Bruised spots, bluish-black, beneath scalp and on gluteal muscles.

RELATIONS - ***Compare:*** (1) Benzin., Amyg. am., Camph. Hydr-ac.

REFERENCES - Boericke. Clarke.

BERBERIS AQUIFOLIUM

(Oregon Grape)

PHARMACY - berb-a. Berberis aquifolium. Oregon grape. Mahonia. Mountain grape. N. O. Berberidacae. The fresh root and stem is pounded to a pulp and macerated in two parts by weight of alcohol. Fluid extract or tincture of root. ***Historical dose:*** Tincture and all potencies.

CLINICAL - Biliousness. Bladder, stones. Blisters. Bronchitis. Eczema. Face, roughness. Headache. Herpes. Kidney, stones. Leucorrhea. Nausea. ***Pimples***. Pityriasis. Psoriasis. Pustules. ***Scald, head.*** Spleen disorders. Stomatitis. Syphilis. Typhoid. Voice disorders.

HERBAL - Berberis aquifolium belongs to the Mahonia group of the Barberry family. It has been used by eclectics in chronic syphilis, chronic skin diseases in scrofulous cachexia and for removing pimples from the faces of girls.

A tea made of the leaves of Berb-a. Mahonia has a local reputation in the *mountain typhoid* of the Rockies and the provings of Berb-a. show febrile symptoms and a marked action on the spleen. It has a reputation for making *"a new man of an old one."*

Hale reported a case of very advanced secondary syphilis cured with it and some characteristic cases of psoriasis. In all these conditions Berb-a. tincture has been given in 5 to 10 drops doses.

HOMEOPATHIC - Keynotes include an intense, pulsating headache in the forehead. Nausea, vomiting. Pains in the bladder. Rheumatic pains in the joints of the hands and in the lumbar and sacral regions, worse at night.

Pruritus and psoriasis-type eruptions. The skin becomes dry, rough, scaly, pimply. Clears the complexion. Eruptions on scalp extending to face and neck. Acne. Psoriasis. Dry eczema.

For chronic catarrhal affections, secondary syphilis. Hepatic torpor, lassitude and other evidences of incomplete metabolism. Stimulates all glands and improves nutrition. Heavy feeling in the stomach, liver and bladder. Pains in the region of the bladder. Rapid peristalsis.

MIND - Unhappiness and depression, sometimes coming on suddenly. Hysterical crying at frequent intervals. Nervous, restless. Disinclined to move or do anything, dullness, stupidity.

Abdomen - Uneasy feeling without desire for stool. Pain in the hypogastrium. Biliousness and waxy, jaundiced hue. Intense burning in spleen and feeling as if pounded. Distressing soreness in spleen.

Back - Pain in the dorsal vertebrae. Pain in the sacrum.

Breasts - Breast tumor with pain.

Chest - Oppression and weakness of upper part of chest. Burning heat in lower left lung.

Constitutions - Psoric and the sycotic constitution. Biliary types and allergic reactions. Types with a predominance of allergies with chronic mesenchymal poisoning.

Eyes - Feeling that the eye is falling from the socket. Conjunctiva injected. Sensation of film before eyes. Eyes look hollow and weak, as if tired, burning feeling and aching as from strain.

Face - Acne. Blotches and pimples. Clears the complexion. Waxy, yellowish white skin. Flashes of heat to cheeks. Pinched expression.

Female - Slight burning in vagina, bearing-down pains and aching as if menses about to come on.

Food - Anorexia, aversion to food. Hunger, even soon after eating, without desire for food. Sudden nausea after eating.

Head - Sensation of a band just above ears. Bilious headache. ***Scald head.*** Scaly eczema. Cramping pains located in the forehead, spreading towards the occiput. Sensation that the hair is stiff. Pulsating vascular pains.

Kidneys - Stitching, crampy pains, thick mucus and bright-red, mealy sediment. Frequent need to urinate in small quantities. Pain in the region of the kidneys, worse when seated, with frequent need to urinate and burning pain in the bladder. Urine increased or decreased in quantity.

Limbs - Rheumatic pain in the joints of the hands and fingers with slight swelling of the joints between the phalanges. Sense of numbness and feeling as if there was no strength of will to lift the part. Pain severe as after a heavy blow. Peculiar prickling as from electricity on back of hand and outside forearm. Rheumatic tensions and stiffness of legs.

Lungs - Bilious colds, expectoration yellow and then greenish. Dry, irritating cough. Scanty, tenacious, blood-streaked expectoration.

Male - Drawing and pressure in testicles.

Modalities - Better from cold water. Worse in the evening and at night. Aggravation from rest at night, but also from prolonged movement.

Mouth - Fetid breath. Blisters on the edge of the tongue. Tongue thickly coated, yellowish-brown, pasty white, feels blistered. Bilious taste after eating. Soreness in lower teeth and salivary glands.

Nose - Stuffy feeling, with discharge of greenish-yellow mucus. Itching within nose with desire to sneeze.

Rectum - Large, dark stools. Hot, bilious diarrhea. After loose stools, light-colored, constipated stools. Stools too large, expelled with difficulty.

Skin - Acne. ***Pimples with a dry, rough, scaly skin.*** Dry eczema. ***Eruption on scalp extending to face and neck.*** Psoriasis. Glandular induration. Pruritus, at first in localized places, then spreading over the whole surface of the skin. Appearance of rashes, blisters, pustules, papules, urticaria. Amelioration from washing in cold water.

Sleep - Drowsy in daytime.

Stomach - Heartburn. Burning in stomach. Nausea and severe straining to vomit. Nausea and hunger after eating.

Temperature - Diurnal rise of temperature and pulse. Flashes of heat and burning of palms. Flashes of heat to cheeks.

Throat - Dry throat. Throat choked with mucus. Voice rough and somewhat hoarse. Voice seemed cut off, as if a damper had closed. Lack of timbre in voice.

Vertigo - Dizzy sensation, worse sleeping or moving.

COMMENTS - J. D. W. C. in the Recorder, 1896, detailed his personal experiences with does of 10 to 15 drops a day. On the third day he felt nausea and dull-headed. Later, there was straining to vomit without vomiting. Then came a peculiar headache, strong compression, as if a band of iron two inches wide passed entirely around head just above ears. It kept growing tighter and tighter.

Strong black coffee relieved this after a time, but left him tremulous in nerves and unsteady in gait. Even after that, a single drop of Berb-a. on the tongue was sufficient to avert an attack of biliousness when threatening, and saved him much trouble of the kind to which he had formerly been liable.

Clarke verified its usefulness in secondary syphilis.

RELATIONS - ***Compare:*** (1) Sulph. - Principal remedy for allergy with burning pains, need for cool air, but aggravation from washing or bathing. Pain in the lumbar and sacral regions with stiffness. Dry, scaly, itching rashes. (2) Psor. - This is a principal nosode remedy for allergic conditions. Chilliness, itching, sometimes fetid eruptions. Subject aggravated by the cold, but the eruption is aggravated by the heat in bed. Occipital and frontal migraine improved by eating. (3) Ars. - Burning pains improved by heat. Nightly aggravation between 1 a.m. and 3 a.m. Scaly, burning, itching rashes, improved by hot, damp compresses. (4) Carb-ac., Euonym., Berb., Hydr.

REFERENCES - Anshutz. Boericke. Clarke. Julian.

BERBERIS VULGARIS

(Barberry)

PHARMACY - berb. Berberis vulgaris. Barberry. N. O. Berberidacae. Britain. Tincture of the bark of the root. ***Historical dose:*** Tincture and all potencies.

CLINICAL - Aphthae. Arthritis. Bilious attack. ***Bladder, disorders.*** Chills. Colic. Coryza. Cystitis. Diarrhea. Duodenum, catarrh. ***Dysmenorrhea.*** Dysuria. ***Eczema.*** Fevers. Fistula. ***Gallstone, colic. Gallstones.*** Gravel. Heartburn. Hematuria. Hemorrhoids. Herpes. ***Itching.*** Jaundice. Joint, disorders. ***Kidney, colic. Kidney, disorders. Kidney, stones.*** Knee, pain. Leucorrhea. Liver, disorders. Lumbago. Menstrual complaints. ***Nausea. Nephritis. Neuralgias.*** Ophthalmia. Oxaluria. Polyps. Prostate, enlarged. Rheumatism. Sacrum, pain. Side pain. Spermatic cords, neuralgia. Spleen, disorders. Tonsillitis. Tumors. ***Urinary, disorders.*** Vaginismus. Venous, stasis. Vertigo .

HERBAL - The usual preparations of Berberis vulgaris are made from the root bark. Affections of liver and kidneys are strongly marked, but Berb. is a medicine of wide range.

HOMEOPATHIC - Berb. is often useful in arthritic and hepatic disorders with urinary, hemorrhoidal or menstrual complaints. Venous stasis occurs in the pelvic region, causing hemorrhoids. It acts upon the urinary organs, when there is tendency to the formation of kidney stones.

Berb. causes ***inflammation of the kidneys*** with hematuria. Marked pain in the region of the kidneys, hence its use in kidney and bladder troubles. ***Severe pains from kidney stones***. Gallstones and bladder catarrh. Sharp or tearing, ***bubbling pains in region of kidneys,*** worse stooping and rising again, sitting or lying, better standing.

Violent sticking pains in bladder, extending from kidneys into urethra with urging to urinate. The emission of urine is frequently accompanied by pains in thighs and loins. During urination burning in urethra or bladder, pressure in bladder, cutting, burning or stitches in urethra.

Dragging or sharp pains in spermatic cord, extending into testes.

Affects the liver markedly, promotes the flow of bile. Useful for fleshy persons with good livers, but with little endurance. ***Gallstone colic,*** followed by jaundice. Sticking pain in region of liver and gall-bladder shooting up to left shoulder, worse by pressure.

Pains rapidly change their locality and character. ***Pains are radiating from one point***, shooting outward or all over, sticking, burning, smarting, soreness. Pains may be felt all over body, emanating from small of back. Spinal irritation. Cold feeling in prepuce, glans, testes and scrotum.

Movement aggravates complaints (Bry.). Sharp pains are frequent and a ***bubbling sensation***. Bubbling and sharp pains are characteristic. A bubbling feeling as if water were coming up through the skin. Tearing, burning pains or bubbling sensation in joints.

Rapid changes of symptoms. Thirst alternates with thirstless, hunger and loss of appetite. Chills and fever. Coldness of body with hot face, commencing 11 a.m., burning heat in afternoon, worse during night.

MIND - The mental condition of Berb. is one of indifference, apathy. Aversion to the darkness. Melancholy, inclination to weep. Fretful humor with weariness of life.

Patient is mentally and physically tired, not inclined to do anything. Mental work requiring close thinking is very difficult, the least interruption breaks the chain of thought. Vanishing of thoughts when interrupted. Objects seem twice as large as natural.

Apathetic. Indifference and pensiveness, with disinclination to speak. Anxiety before sleep in evening. Anxiety while sitting, standing or moving. Sees terrifying apparitions in twilight, especially children. Desires death during menses.

Abdomen - Burning in or under skin of abdomen. Rumbling in bowels. Colic pains from gallbladder to abdomen, worse pressure. Torn loose feeling in the epigastrium. Sharp pains in front of kidneys extending to liver, spleen, stomach, groins. Cramplike contraction in splenic region. Sticking deep in ileum. Pressure and tension in groins, as if a hernia would develop. Sharp pain in region of umbilicus. Severe pain in inguinal region. Varicose veins near right inguinal ring.

Back - Back as if beaten, disabled or stiff. ***Bubbling sensation*** in back. Tearing, sticking with stiffness, which making rising difficult. Numbness, bruised sensation. Lumbago (Ant-t., Rhus-t.). Post-operative pain in lumbar region. Soreness with sharp pains, with frequent urination. Stitches in the spine. Constant pulsating, sharp pains in sacrum. Sharp pains in neck and back, worse respiration. Pustules. Pimples on scapulae. Inflammation of the glands of the neck.

Bladder - Cystitis. Burning pains in bladder region. Dysuria, frequent urination. Urethra burns when not urinating. ***Pain in the thighs and loins on urinating.*** Cutting and burning in urethra during and after urinating. Sensation as if some urine remained after urinating. Crampy, contractive, or aching pains in bladder, when bladder is full or empty. Burning in urethra during menopause. Constant urging, with pain in neck of bladder, mostly burning and scanty discharge.

Breasts - Pressure in breasts, especially at nipple. Sensation as if breasts were swollen, after menses. Pressure behind left nipple.

Chest - Oppression of the chest, especially at night, with violent flowing of the coryza. Painful shootings in the left side of the chest. Sensation of excoriation in the chest. ***Tearing, sharp pains in chest and region of heart.*** Stinging, pulsating, pressing or tensive pains in muscles of chest. Pimples on chest and scapulae. Itching, smarting and burning in axillae. Itching returns after scratching, with smarting stitches or burning.

Constitutions - Acts well in fleshy persons with good livers, but with little endurance. Prematurely old and worn out men and women. Old gouty constitutions. Suited to bilious diathesis. Cases where kidney or bladder symptoms are prominent.

Ears - Itching with small pustules on the outer parts of the ears. Heat alternating with coldness of external ear. Sensation of coldness or bubbling in ears. Stopped up feeling with pressure. ***Beating or fluttering noise in ear.*** Nodes on auricle. Throbbing and roaring. Acute and shooting pains in the interior of the ear and in other parts. Sharp pains in the ear. Small tumor, size of hazelnut, under and behind ear, enlarged gland.

Eyes - Conjunctivitis, with inflamed lachrymal caruncle. Dryness of eyes with burning and redness of conjunctiva. Aching and sensation of burning in the eyes. Eyes sunken with dark-bluish circles around. Burning and dryness in the eyes, which are dull. As if sand between the lids and eyes. Eyes feel cold as from a cool wind with lachrymation on closing the eyes. Shootings in the eyes. Itching in the canthi, eyebrows, and eyelids. Ophthalmia. Painful eyes on reading by candlelight. Sensitive to the sunlight. Shuns light.

Face - Face hot and red. Sunken cheeks and eyes with bluish circles. Dirty gray, pale, sickly. Bilious. Greenish face, with blue rings and pink eyes. Sensation as if cold drops were spurted into the face when going into the open air. Dryness of the lips. Sensation of tingling on the lips. Burning in lips. Suppurating acne.

Female - Menses, consisting of gray mucus or brown blood. ***Menses, with pain in kidneys and chilliness, pain down thighs.*** Scanty menses, of black drops of filthy slime. Menses, watery blood or brown. Gray mucus replaces menses. Dysmenorrhea with blood looking like gray serum. ***Dysmenorrhea, with pains radiating in every direction.*** Leucorrhea, grayish mucus with painful urinary symptoms. Acrid leucorrhea, very prostrating. Neuralgia of ovaries and vagina. Pain changes sides. Vagina sensitive. Vaginismus. Vulva itching and burning. Pinching constriction in mons veneris, contraction and tenderness of vagina. Burning and soreness in vagina. Urinary symptoms with menses and leucorrhea. Cutting pain during sex. Enjoyment absent during sex. Prostration after sex. Desire diminished. Suppressed sexual desire with long delayed orgasm.

Food - Appetite either increased or decreased. Excessive appetite, almost like bulimia. Very slow digestion. Acid, bitter taste, especially after a meal. Want of appetite, with bitter, bilious taste. Food appears insipid. Alcoholic drinks aggravates. Thirst and dryness of the mouth.

Head - Dullness of head, as from coryza. Confusion and heaviness of the head. Frontal headache. Cold sensation in right temple. Cold temples. Chilliness in back and occiput. Heat in head from exertion. Skin of head and face as if numb. ***Headache, worse by movement, better in open air.*** Headache with hepatic or rheumatic arthritic complaints. ***Headache with affections of urinary organs.*** Darting and shooting pains in the head after changing the locality. Sensation as if the head were becoming larger. ***Sensation of a tight cap pressing upon the whole scalp***. Tearing pain in auricle and gouty concretions. Pustules in the tissues of the head and in the face.

Heart - Squeezing with shooting pains in the region of the heart. Frequent palpitations. Sharp pains about the heart. Very painful contracting, shooting pain in region of heart. Pulse becomes very slow. Pulse slow and weak. Pulse full, hard and rapid.

Kidneys - ***Radiating, shooting pains*** from kidneys into bladder. ***Kidney colic from kidney stones.*** Pain from kidney, extending along ureter or to liver, stomach, spleen, arresting breathing. ***Bubbling sensation*** in region of kidneys. ***Kidney stones.*** Burning, soreness in kidney region. Stinging, burning, gnawing, on small spot near kidneys, worse hard pressure. ***Sensitiveness in region of kidneys*** so great that any jarring motion, riding in a wagon, jumping from it, was intolerable. Clear discharge from meatus before urinating. ***Urine with thick mucus and bright-red.*** Urine turbid, yellow. Urine red, mealy, sandy or slimy sediment. ***Passes small calculi.*** Urine smells like coffee. Urine blood-red.

Limbs - ***Bruised feeling in limbs.*** Rheumatic paralytic pain in shoulders, arms, hands and fingers, legs and feet. Swelling of joints. ***Neuralgia under fingernails*** with swelling of the finger joints. Sensation of cold on outside of thighs. Heels pain, as if ulcerated. Sharp pains between metatarsal bones as from a nail when standing. Pain in balls of feet on stepping. Intense weariness and lameness of legs after walking a short distance.

Liver - ***Liver troubles with sticking pains in region of gall bladder.*** Shooting, aching pains in the hepatic region, increased by pressure. Pressure in the liver. ***Gallstones***. Sharp pain in region of gallbladder, worse pressure, extending to stomach. ***Gallstone attack with severe pains.*** Violent stabbing, in region of liver, taking breath, must bend over. Catarrh of the gallbladder with constipation and yellow complexion.

Lungs - Increased deep breathing, with dry cough. Shortness of breath when going up stairs. Obstruction of breath when raising arms. ***Gallbladder or kidney colic arresting breathing.*** Short, dry cough with sharp pains in chest. Expectoration of a quantity of thick, yellow, jelly-like mucus.

Male - Genitals cold and sweaty. ***Neuralgia of spermatic cord and testicles.*** Constricting pain in testicles. Testicles drawn up. Smarting, burning, stitching in testicles in prepuce and scrotum. Itching on scrotum. Pain changes sides. Prostate gland enlarged, with pressure in perineum. Prepuce and glans cold and numb. Penis hard and contracted, bends upwards. Suppressed sexual desire. Straining during and after ejaculation of semen.

Modalities - Better after urination. Better open air. Worse from motion. Worse jarring. Worse stepping hard. Worse rising from sitting, Worse fatigue. Worse urinating. Worse twilight. ***Worse standing***, it brings on, or increases, urinary complaints. Worse deep pressure.

Mouth - Aphthae. Burning and acrid taste in the mouth. Bitter taste. Offensive metallic odor from mouth. Sticky, viscid, foamy, saliva like cotton (Nux-m.). White, sticky tongue, viscid saliva resembling soapsuds. Diminished saliva. Ugly bluish-red spots in mouth. Gums dirty gray. Small white nodes in the gums. Teeth feel as if too long or too large.

Nose - Dryness in the nose. Crawling and itching in nostrils. Pricking pain in tip of nose. Coryza with the yellowish serum discharge, afterwards of purulent. Obstinate catarrh of left nostril. Catarrh whitish, yellowish, or greenish mucus, especially in the morning. Titillating irritation to sneeze. Drops of blood from left nostril.

Perspiration - Everything excites sweat.

Rectum - Constant urging to stool. Diarrhea painless, clay-colored. Burning and smarting in anus and perineum. Bearing down pain in anus and in sacrum. ***Changing stools.*** Scanty, thin-formed stool, hard or soft. Hard stools, like sheep dung, with burning in the anus. Stools are dirty gray, smarting tough, watery with jaundice. Tearing pain around anus. Fistula in anus, itching with chest complaints. Copious hemorrhage from anus after increased exercise. Hemorrhoids. Herpes around anus.

Skin - ***Itching, burning and smarting, worse scratching***, better cold applications. Small pustules over whole body. ***Eczema of anus and hands***. Eruptions leave a brown stain. ***Circumscribed pigmentation*** following eczematous inflammation. Red marbled spots changing into brown spots. Boils, hastens suppuration and prevents return. Flat warts.

Sleep - Sleepiness during the day. Restless sleep, disturbed by burning itching of the skin or by anxious dreams. Frequent waking, and fatigue, as from want of sleep. Sleep greatly prolonged. Unrefreshing sleep. Difficult awaking in morning, followed by headache, exhaustion, and want of recollection. Anxious dreams.

Stomach - Bitter eructations. Heartburn. Eructations, without bad taste or smell. Bilious risings. Frequent eructations alternating with yawning. ***Nausea before breakfast, better after***. Pains from stomach to back, or the reverse. Shiverings in the epigastrium. Burning, shooting pains in the stomach. Sticking or whirling pain in gastric region.

Teeth - Teeth as if too long or too large. Pain as if gums were torn, or teeth pulled out. Scraping, gnawing pains. Tearing pain in left upper molar. Piercing pain in hollow tooth of lower jaw. Sharp pains. Gums dirty grey. Small white nodes in gums. Dingy red edges of gums. Gums bleed easily. Sore gums during dentition.

Temperature - Chilly. Cold sensation in various parts, as if spattered with cold water. Cold single parts. Chills as if in bones, with warmth of skin. Chills before dinner, with ice-cold feet. Chills in region of kidneys. Warmth in lower part of back, hips and thighs. Heat in the hands and head in the afternoon, continuing for several days. Typhoid and putrid fevers.

Throat - Inflammation of the tonsils and pharynx, with swelling and fiery redness. Hoarseness with soreness. Sensation of plug in the side of the throat with dryness. Scratching and burning as from sand in throat. Tonsillitis. Pain in tonsils, when speaking or swallowing. Polyps of larynx.

Tongue - Tongue feels scalded. Vesicles on tongue. Painful pimple on tip. Tongue smarts when touched. Slimy furred tongue.

Vertigo - Vertigo, with sensation of fainting and great weakness. Vertigo on stooping and on making use of the arms. Feeling of intoxication and giddiness.

Vision - Dim vision, all objects looking dark, as if through a veil, or running together. Dim vision with itching around eyes and in face, preceded by incipient catarrh, succeeded by itching on legs.

COMMENTS - There is great weakness like fainting after a walk, with perspiration and heat on the upper part of the body, cold, pale, sunken face and oppression of breathing. Great relaxation with disinclination to do anything. Great sleepiness during day and after dinner. Vertigo and heaviness.

Heat of head after dinner or in afternoon. Puffy feeling in head, as if it were becoming larger. Scalp tense. The face is pale with a dingy gray tinge, sunken cheeks. Deep-set eyes, surrounded with bluish and black-gray border. Mouth dry and sticky, painful white blisters on tip of tongue.

Darting and shooting pains often changing their localities, worse movement, better open air. Changeable pains. Dry mucus membranes. Discharges or skin is dirty gray. Cold feeling in the bones, eyes, ears etc. Numbness insensible to extreme heat and cold. Metatarsus and metacarpus feel sprained. Neuralgia under fingernails.

Lumbago, pains extend from back, around body, down leg, with red sediment in urine. Many old troubles in the back. Sufferings worse by fatigue. Aching in small of back, worse sitting or lying in the morning on awakening.

Chest affected after operations, hemorrhoids, fistula, etc. The pit of the stomach is puffed up. Gnawing pain in right hypochondrium, shooting up to left scapula. Pains shoot down from tenth rib to navel. Burning in either inguinal region (especially right).

Constipation, stool like sheep-dung. Diarrhea. Hemorrhoids with itching or burning, particularly after stool, which is frequently hard and covered with blood. Anal fistula with painful pressure in perineum, extending deep into pelvis (left side).

Nephritis, acute kidney infections, kidney pain from passing a stone, kidney colic from polyhephritis. Numbness, stiffness and lameness in kidney region. Great sense of weakness in kidney region, after exertion. Kidneys are worse walking, especially down stairs, worse jar, bubbling sensation.

Bladder infections with achy kidneys, burning on urination, worse motion (Bry.). Cramping pain while urinating with urinary infection. Profuse amount of urine alternating with little urine.

Frequent urging to urinate. Urine is dark yellow and red, becoming turbid, copious, mucus sediment or transparent, jelly-like or reddish, bran-like sediment. Urine slimy when passed, depositing copious foamy yellowish sediment. Greenish urine depositing mucus.

A liver remedy and gallstone colic with the same pain as passing a stone from the gallbladder, sharp pain that radiates.

Gallstone colic with jaundice. Absence of pleasurable sensation during sex, in women. Uterine symptoms and leucorrhea associated with painful urinary symptoms. Dysmenorrhea, pains radiating in all directions down thighs, etc. Vagina intensely painful, reddened. Violent pain in back with menses, which are too scanty.

Guernsey admirably summed up Berb. "Affects particularly the lumbar region, kidneys, uterus. The patient is sometimes unable to tell the exact locality, but the pain is somewhere in the back and shoots up the back or into the spermatic cord or testes, bladder, buttocks or legs.

"The pain may shoot up or down or both ways. Pains may be felt all over the body, emanating from the back, the pains are of a sticking, pricking, sharp or jerking character, flying about now here and there. There is often a bubbling sensation in the region of the kidneys."

On the indication "tumors and sessile growths," Ozanam cured a case of polyps of the vocal cords, red with a sessile base. Thuja had failed. Berb. 200c was given at first with good effect, the potency being gradually reduced with increasingly good effect until the growth disappeared entirely under the 1x.

B. Simmons verified a symptom of Berb. A gentleman of 52 complained of rheumatic pains in his legs and loss of walking power. After he had walked a short distance, he was compelled to stop from a feeling of intense weariness, heaviness, lameness and stiffness of the legs, which felt sore as if bruised. A single dose affected a complete cure, improvement commencing on the fourth day.

Stuart Close recorded the cure with Berb. 200c of a woman who had cutting, burning pains in the balls of the feet on stepping. On standing with most of the weight on the heels, she had no pain. On rising in morning, there was a sensation in soles as if stepping on needles.

RELATIONS - ***Antidotes:*** Camphor, Bell. ***Antidoted by:*** Camph., Bell. ***Antidote to:*** Acon. ***Compare:*** (1) Ipomea, Aloe, Lyc., Ox-ac., Nux-v., Sars. Xanthorrhea arborea. Xanthorrhiza apifolia. (2) Aloe., Ant-t., Ars. (3) Calc-p. - fistula in ano, chest symptoms, especially after surgical operation. (4) Canth., Carb-v., Cham., Chin., Lyc., Nat-m., Nit-ac., Nux-v., Puls. Rheum. (5) In burning and pricking pains in anus. Lyc., Thuj. (6) In duodenal catarrh: Chin., Lyc., Hydr., Podo., Ric., Merc. (6) In aversion to darkness: Stram., Am-m., Calc., Carb-an., Stroph., Valer. (6) In pains in feet on stepping: Cycl. (7) Podo., Caul., Berb-a. ***Complementary:*** Mag-m. Follows well: Bry., Kali-bi., Rhus-t, Sulph.

REFERENCES - Boericke. Clarke. Murphy.

BERYLLIUM METALLICUM

PHARMACY - beryl. Beryllium metallicum. Glucinium metallicum. ***Historical dose:*** Trituration and all potencies.

CLINICAL - Allergic conditions. Cancerous conditions. Chronic fatigue. Dermatitis. Eczema. Emphysema. Erythema nosodum. Gingivitis. Kidney stones. Lichen planus. Lipomas. Myocarditis. Sarcoidosis. Stomatitis. Tubercular conditions. Tumors.

HOMEOPATHIC - Beryllium, a light metal closely resembling Aluminium, was isolated in 1828 by Bussy, thirty-one years after Vauquelin's discovery of the oxide which he named glucinium, because of the sweet taste of its salts. Beryl exists in America, especially in Columbia; Madagascar; Russia and France.

The homeopathic symptomatology was undertaken by Templeton in 1951-52 on seven provers, using the 3x, 6x, 7x, 12x, and 30c. Some symptoms can be attributed to the fluorine if it is a question of impure beryllium containing beryllium fluoride.

The usefulness of the remedy should be noted for kidney stones with hyper-production. It is especially a remedy for respiratory deficiency with audible heartbeat.

Slight fever with gradual weight loss. Gradual emaciation and sub-febrile state. Anorexia. Faintness with weakness of the legs. Asthenia. Sleepiness, desire to eat, general weakness, rapid pulse.

Throbbing headache and pain going from the left to right mastoid.

Dyspnea, dry cough, painful with blood-stained sputum, difficult to expectorate. Dorsal and lumbar pains, as if produced by needles. Disorders of the bones of the limbs. The skin is weeping, burning with an itching eruption. Acrid, abrasive coryza. Tendency to skin tumors.

Abdomen - Diaphragmatic hernia. Chronic pancreatitis. Fibrocystic disease of the pancreas.

Back - Lumbar osteoarthritis. Pain in the back, aggravated by bending head forwards and lying down. Stitching pain and cold feeling in the dorsal and lumbar region.

Blood - Hyperchromic anemia. Increase of leucocytes. Elevation of calcium. Elevation of total protein. Elevation of the sedimentation rate. Albumin-Globulin ratio inverted.

Chest - Angina pectoris. Burning pain behind the sternum.

Eyes - Conjunctivitis with photophobia. Catarrhal conjunctivitis. Follicular conjunctivitis.

Face - Facial neuralgia.

Food - Capricious appetite. Anorexia, followed by keen appetite, which improves the condition. Aggravation from the sight or smell of food from riding in a bus. Aversion to sweets.

Head - Beating or bursting headache, improved by fresh air, lying on the painful side and aggravated by the least movement. Occipital pain extending to the mastoid. Pain from one mastoid to the other, from left to right.

Heart - Rhythmic anomaly. Rheumatic myocarditis. Sclerous myocarditis. Cardiac palpitations and feeling of thoracic constriction.

Kidneys - Porphyrins increased in urine.

Limbs - Rheumatism. Pain in the arms as if bruised. Buttocks cold. Clubbed fingers. Blue discoloration of the hands. Sarcoidosis of the bones. Deposits around the inter-phalangeal joints.

Liver - Liver weakness and deficiency. Acute inflammation of the gallbladder and bile ducts. Chronic cholecystitis with or without stones.

Lungs - Respiration painful, aggravated by movement. Deep, dry, painful cough, aggravated by bending backwards, from smoke, better in a very warm room. Sputum streaked with blood. Cyanosis, cough accelerating the respiratory rhythm. Spasmodic cough with pain behind the sternum. Appearance similar to tuberculosis or sarcoidosis. Pulmonary sarcoidosis. Pulmonary tuberculosis, early stage. Emphysema. Tracheitis and bronchitis. Capillary bronchitis. Dilation of the bronchi. Pneumoconiosis.

Modalities - Better from the cold and fresh air. Worse from physical exercise. Worse heat. Worse movement.

Mouth - Lips dry, cracking. Small ulcerations on lips and tip of tongue. Ulcers of the mouth and tongue. Glazed appearance of the palate. Stomatitis, gingivitis. Lichen planus of the mouth.

Nose - Acute and chronic rhinitis. Seasonal rhinitis, hay fever. Acrid, excoriating coryza, improved in the open air, aggravated in a warm room. Bruised pain inside the nose.

Rectum - Painful, explosive stool, worse by breathing in.

Skin - Nodules and papules, itching and burning. Development of granulomata and papillomata. Hypodermic sarcoids. Lichen planus. Eczema. Dermatitis. Erythema nosodum. Tumors, syphilitic, tubercular or parasitic. Cysts and lipomas.

Stomach - Capricious appetite, nausea at the sight or smell of food and from traveling in a bus.

Temperature - Feverish, goose flesh, shivering, aggravated by the slightest movements.

Throat - Shiny, painful, burning, pain going from left to right mastoid. Constant need to swallow. Stridulous laryngitis. Chronic non-specific laryngitis. Tubercular laryngitis. Polyps and papilloma of the larynx.

COMMENTS - The extraction of the metal is made from the iron ore, beryl, which is ground and roasted, usually with sodium fluoro-silicate. The double fluoride of Be and Na thus obtained is transformed into beryllium oxyfluoride. The metal is isolated by electrolysis in the presence of barium.

Oxidized beryllium can also be treated with sulfuric acid and transformed into Be sulphate from which glucinium is extracted, the latter can be used directly in the manufacture of alloys or to pure Be after treatment by ammonium fluoride.

Workers are exposed at different stages of preparation to the inhalation of fine particles of dust and noxious fumes, formed particularly by fluoride derivatives as well as derivatives of glucinium.

Beryllium is used in, among other things, the manufacture of light bulbs, radio and TV sets' incandescent casings, glass making and ceramics and synthetic precious stones.

Accidental poisoning can occur during the crushing process or the thermal treatment necessary to produce the powders. Chronic berylliosis is essentially caused by its insoluble compounds, especially beryllium, zinc manganese silicate.

These compounds are dangerous because of their fumes and particularly the dust particles, even at a rate lower than half a milligram per cubic meter.

The finer dust particles, are particularly noxious. These form veritable aerosols, which spread over a distance (which explains cases near factories) and which impregnate worker's clothes easily (this explains cases in the family, resulting from brushing the clothes).

The element causes proliferation in the mesenchyme, which ends in the formation of alveolar granuloma. This in turn causes difficulty in the diffusion of oxygen through the alveolar walls with subsequent anoxaemia.

The fixation is above all made in the ethmoid bones and is permanent. It is of the same nature and rapidity in the liver and kidneys, but less prolonged. Elimination is brought about through the urine, at first rapid and profuse, then slow and sparse.

In a subject who died from berylliosis, Martland showed spectrographically that beryllium was present, especially in the kidneys and skeleton.

RELATIONS - ***Compare:*** (1) Bry. - Aggravated by movement with a dry, painful cough. (2) Lach. - Failing from cardiac weakness, suffocation, dry, rending cough.

REFERENCES - Julian.

BETA VULGARIS

(Beet-root)

PHARMACY - beta. Beta vulgaris. Beet-root. Sugar beet. N. O. Chenopodiaceae. Tincture of the juice. ***Historical dose:*** Trituration and all potencies.

CLINICAL - Catarrhal. Tuberculosis.

HOMEOPATHIC - The salt of Betainum hydrochloricum obtained from the beet root itself seems to be the best adapted to tuberculosis patients. Children with tuberculosis yield very quickly to the action of the remedy. Influences chronic catarrhal states and tuberculosis.

REFERENCES - Clarke.

BISMUTHUM SUBNITRICUM

(Magistrate of Bismuth)

PHARMACY - bism. Bismuthum subnitricum. Magistrate of Bismuth. Bismuthum oxidum. Precipitated Sub-Nitrate of Bismuth. The oxidum of Hahnemann and Kent. Trituration. ***Historical dose:*** Trituration and all potencies.

CLINICAL - Abdominal surgery, vomiting after. Anemia. Angina pectoris. ***Cancer.*** Cholera. Colds. Coughs. Cystitis. Delirium tremens. Diaphragm, inflamed. Flatulence. Gangrene. Gastralgia. Gastritis. Headaches. ***Hemorrhages. Nausea.*** Nosebleeds. Phlegmasia alba dolens. ***Stomach, cancer. Stomach, cancer. Stomach, disorders.*** Stomatitis. Toothache. ***Ulcers. Vomiting.***

HOMEOPATHIC - Bismuth, including the sub-nitrate, was used by alchemists to prepare the *"Magistrate of Bismuth."* According to Teste, Bism. corresponds to slow digestion with fetid belchings. It is hardly ever indicated where belchings are not odorous or sour.

Bism. exerts its chief action on stomach and alimentary canal, causing irritation and catarrhal inflammation of the digestive tract.

Gastric disorders with ***vomiting, purging and prostration.*** The surface of the patient is generally warm. In summer complaints of children there is cadaverous smell of flatus or stool. Desires company, child holds on to its mother's hand.

Gastralgia, not associated with catarrh (Nux-v.). Stomach pain is accompanied by habitual constipation without vomiting or with vomiting of insipid, ropy mucus. The stools are preceded by crampy, pinching pains in the stomach.

Cancer of the stomach, nausea after every meal relieved by cold drinks. ***Water is vomited as soon as it reaches the stomach***, violent belching with a putrid smell. Violent retching and vomiting of bile and brownish fluid with extreme pain. Burning, griping, sharp with dull pain in back or spasmodic vomiting.

Oppressive anxiety, with a small pulse, vertigo and prostration. Hemorrhage of dark blood. Prostration. Pains are tearing, pinching, burning, and screwing. Sensation of heaviness in internal parts. Ailments after abdominal surgery.

MIND - Apathetic. Fickle minded, begins this, then that, holds but a short time to any one thing. ***Anguish, never long in one place or position.*** Restlessness.

Discontented and dissatisfied. Complains about his condition. Irritability in daytime, better evening. Fear of being alone on waking. Solitude is unbearable. ***Desire for company.*** Children hold on to mother's hand.

Abdomen - Flatulence. ***Distended abdomen.*** Abdomen bloated in ridges. Rumbling along colon. Pinching pain in lower abdomen with rumbling.

Back - Boring and burning pains. Tensive pressure on right side of neck near cervical vertebrae. Pain in left side of back, as after stooping too long. Pressure in spine better bending backward.

Chest - Angina pectoris, pain around heart, left arm to fingers. Burning and piercing in the chest and back. Flushes of heat in chest and head. Aching in right half of chest, near sternum. Pressure and squeezing across the chest. Hot, burning, constriction of the chest.

Ears - Pressure and drawing pains in left external meatus.

Eyes - Aching of the eyeballs. Thickened mucus in both canthi. Secretion of mucus in the corner of the eyes. Stupor, with mist before the eyes. Foggy, dim vision, during vertigo.

Face - Earthy, blue around the eyes. Aching pain in cheekbones, better running about and holding cold water in mouth. Face pale and cold. Face pain alternating with gastric pain.

Female - Menstrual blood dark, pitchy.

Food - Intolerable thirst. ***Craves cold drinks***, which are vomited.

Head - ***Headache alternates with stomach pain.*** Neuralgic pain, as if torn by pincers involves face and teeth, worse eating, better cold. Cutting or pressure above right orbit extending to occiput. ***Headache extending to the root of nose.*** Pressure in occiput, worse motion with heaviness. Headaches return in winter. Cutting pain in brain.

Heart - Angina pectoris, pain around heart, left arm to fingers. Violent heartbeat.

Kidneys - Urine, frequent, watery, copious and pale. Emission of urine entirely suppressed.

Limbs - Cramps in hands and feet. Tearing in wrist. Paralytic weakness, especially in right arm. Tearing in fingertips under nails (Berb.). Itching erosion near tibia and back of feet near joints. Dry palms and soles. Limbs cold. Blue color of forearm and thigh.

Lungs - Dyspnea, from burning, constriction in chest. Cough, day and night with copious expectoration. Pinching in middle of diaphragm, extending transversely through chest. Dark, bloody or blood-streaked.

Male - Aching pains in the testes. Gonorrhea. Nocturnal pollutions without dreams. Pressing, aching in the (right) testicle. Seminal emissions with lascivious dreams.

Modalities - Better from cold drinks. Better cold applications. Better bending backwards. Worse motion. Worse from eating, over eating. Worse when alone.

Worse summer, winter.

Mouth - Metallic, sweetish, sour taste on back part of tongue. Taste bitter. Inflammation of mouth, with whitish excoriations and fissures. ***Gums swollen***. Profuse salivation, teeth loose. Constant secretion of a brownish, thick saliva. Tongue coated white, swollen. Black, gangrenous looking wedges on dorsum and sides of tongue.

Nose - Nosebleeds, with dark blood. Heaviness at the root of the nose.

Perspiration - Surface covered with warm sweat.

Rectum - Painless discharge of blood from rectum. Cholera infantum, when the body remains warm. ***Cholera morbus and summer complaint, when vomiting predominates.*** Watery diarrhea with a putrid smell. Painless diarrhea with great thirst and frequent urination and vomiting. Stools papescent, foul, watery, smell cadaverous. Prostration after stool.

Skin - Burning, smarting in the skin. Ulcers, gangrenous black, bluish. Dry gangrene, parchment-like.

Sleep - Frequent waking, as if in a fright. Sleepy in morning, a few hours after eating. Restless on account of voluptuous dreams, with or without emissions. Drowsy while working. Starts in sleep, thinks that he is falling, awakes in a fright. Unrefreshing sleep. Lascivious, vivid dreams, sometimes without, frequently with seminal emissions.

Stomach - Eructation after drinking. ***Burning, feeling of a load***. Will eat for several days, then vomit. Bilious vomiting after eating. ***Slow digestion with fetid belchings***. Pain from stomach through to spine. ***Gastritis, better from cold drinks***, but vomiting when stomach becomes full. Stomach pains, better bending backwards. Pressure as from a load in one spot, alternating with burning, crampy pain and heartburn. Atrophy of stomach. Stomach hangs down, hard lumps are felt below navel. Nausea after eating or nursing. Nausea and pressure in stomach after eating, during headache. ***Stomach cancer,*** vomiting brownish water. Vomits with convulsive gagging and pain. ***Water is vomited as soon as it reaches the stomach***. Vomits all fluids. Vomiting with vertigo and prostration. Bilious vomiting, after eating. ***Vomiting and purging***, with great prostration, flatulence, white tongue and cadaverous stools.

Teeth - ***Gums swollen***, with pain like excoriation. Pressive, pains. Toothache, better from cold water in the mouth, worse when it becomes warm (Coff.).

Temperature - Chill with deathly coldness of whole body. Chilliness intermittent, periodical. Coldness of the whole body, externally. Great heat. Flushes of heat, especially on head and chest. Intermittent fever, small pulse.

Throat - Inflammation of the throat. Burning pain in the throat, sometimes insupportable. Difficult swallowing of fluids, which return through nose. Sore throat, awaking at night and paining very much, with short cough and retching. Ulceration of uvula with burning and tearing.

Vertigo - Giddiness in the morning. Vertigo from violent exercise. Vertigo as if the brain were turning in a circle. Violent vertigo with pressing pain in forehead.

COMMENTS - Grimmer wrote that it's good for stomach cancer, nausea after every meal relieved by cold drinks, water is vomited as soon as it reaches the stomach. Great affinity for disorders of the right upper limb or forehead. The patient is restless, moving about, anxiety. Desires company (Phos.).

Violent risings of a putrid smell with violent retching and vomiting of bile and brownish fluid with extreme pain. Pressing heaviness with stomach pains. Headache alternating with gastralgia.

The pains are chiefly piercing, tearing, burning, cramping and screwing. There are tearing pressing pains in the bones of the hands and feet, spasmodic disorders of the muscles of face and limbs.

Sensation of heaviness in inner parts. Oppressive anxiety, small pulse, vertigo and prostration. Hemorrhage, with dark, pitchy blood. Anemia, with an itch-like eruption. Corrosive itching on side of tibia. Gangrene and gangrenous ulcers, bluish or dried, parchment-like.

Craves cold drinks, which ameliorate symptoms, but aggravates after it warms up. Cold drinks and cold bathing improve the headache and toothache. Summer complaints. Headache returning in winter. Motion relieves most symptoms, but aggravates some headaches. Pressure in spine is better bending backward.

O. W. Smith verified "Pain in stomach, better bending backward and eructation, tasting of food eaten twenty-four hours before."

Teste cured with the oxide a wearing, nightly cough in a hysteric woman and a case of sub-acute cystitis with irregular paroxysms of crampy pains in the bladder, also a case of phlegmasia alba dolens (left). Petroz cured another such case.

RELATIONS - ***Antidotes:*** Nux, Caps., Calc. Bismuth is ***Antidoted by:*** Calc., Caps., Coff., Nux-v. Is isomorphic with: Ant-c., Ars., Phos. Useful after: Euonymus (headache). ***Compare:*** (1) Phos. - vomiting, Bism. vomits immediately, Phos. vomits water as soon as it becomes warm in stomach. (2) Ant-c. - vomiting, white tongue, gastritis. (3) Ars. - anxiety, gastritis, cancer, gangrene, vomiting. (4) Bell. - gastralgia, cancer, flatus in ridges. (5) Bry. - toothache, gastritis. (6) Calc., Caps., Chin., Ign., Kali-c., Kreos. (7) Lach. - sore throat, sleep, ulcers. (8) Lyc., Merc. (9) Nux-v. - gastralgia, urging to stool. (10) Plb. - abdomen in ridges, gastralgia, better bending backward, heart disease. (11) Puls., Rhus-t. - better by motion. (12) Sep., Sil., Staph.

REFERENCES - Boericke. Clarke.

BIXA ORELLANA

PHARMACY - Bixa orellana. ***Historical dose:*** Tincture and all potencies.

CLINICAL - Eczema. Elephantiasis. Leprosy.

HERBAL - Bixa is a South American herb that's related to the Chaulmoogra plant, recommended for leprosy, eczema and elephantiasis.

REFERENCES - Boericke.

BLATTA AMERICANA

(American Cockroach)

PHARMACY - blatta-a. Blatta americana. American Cockroach. Periplaneta americana. Kakerlac insignis. N. O. Orthoptera. Trituration of insect with milk sugar. ***Historical dose:*** Trituration and all potencies.

CLINICAL - Asthma. Dropsy. Jaundice.

HOMEOPATHIC - Mure, who proved Blatta-a., noted that it developed symptoms of jaundice, yellow sclerotics and complexion. Ascites. Various forms of dropsy. Extreme weariness. General prostration and weariness on going upstairs.

Blatta-a. has been used as a remedy for dropsy and has a popular reputation in jaundice. Pain shifting from back to shoulder blade. Acute pain in chest with want of breath (Blatta.). Heat in urethra when urinating (Canth.).

RELATIONS - ***Compare:*** (1) Blatta.

REFERENCES - Boericke. Clarke.

BLATTA ORIENTALIS

(Indian Cockroach)

PHARMACY - blatta. Blatta orientalis. Indian Cockroach. Periplaneta orientalis. N. O. Orthoptera. Trituration of whole insect with milk sugar. ***Historical dose:*** Trituration and all potencies.

CLINICAL - ***Asthma. Bronchitis.*** Colds. ***Coughs. Dyspnea.*** Emaciation. Obesity. Lockjaw. ***Lung, disorders.*** Lung, weakness. ***Mucus. Pneumonia. Suffocation.*** Tuberculosis. Unconsciousness.

HOMEOPATHIC - Blatta orientalis was found accidentally to relieve asthma in a patient who took tea in which a cockroach had been infused. More effective in low potencies for acute attacks, the higher potencies being given in the more chronic stages.

Asthma, especially when associated with bronchitis (after Ars., when it is insufficient). Acts best in stout and corpulent patients. Much pus-like yellow mucus. ***Threatened suffocation threatened by great accumulation of mucus.***

Asthmatic fits at night, coughs during the day with slight expectoration and hurried breathing.

Bronchitis and tuberculosis, with shortness of breath. ***Cough with dyspnea*** in bronchitis and tuberculosis. Chronic bronchitis. Colds that bring on bronchitis with fever, may develop into asthma. Emaciation.

MIND - Anxiety about health.

Chest - Chronic inflammation of bronchial tubes.

Constitutions - Obesity, suited to corpulent people. Malarial cases and cases worse in rainy weather. Asthmatic constitutions.

Limbs - Weakness in hollow of knee.

Lungs - Severe chronic asthma. Shortness of breath. Difficult breathing, better from expectoration. ***Suffocation from great accumulation of mucus.*** Purulent tough, viscid, yellow mucus. ***Cough with dyspnea***. Pneumonia. Bronchitis and tuberculosis. Spasmodic cough at short intervals with slight expectoration.

Modalities - Worse from dust. Worse during the rain. Worse winter

COMMENTS - Asthma with a lot of mucus and rattling, yellow brown phlegm (Nat-s.). Bronchitis with yellow mucus, difficulty breathing. Keynote worse dust (Sil.), sensitivity to dust (Poth.), especially in dry climates. Great oppression of the chest, "as if a weight or a heaviness on the chest," with asthma. "Feeble lungs," totally inability to expectorate the thick, yellow mucus (Hydr.).

Easier breathing with head bend forward or supporting head with elbows while sitting. Must sit up in bed. Loud, coarse wheezing, like a saw through pinewood. Spasmodic, debilitating coughs. Great fear of suffocation and dying. Lack of ambition to live, great weariness in this remedy.

Clammy, cold sweat. General swelling of the body. Tends to stooped shoulders, barrel-chest. Bronchial spasms. Locked jaws. Unconsciousness.

Used in tuberculosis epidemics, especially the last stages. Characteristic lung weakness, the doctor would have to put their ear next to the person's mouth to hear the case (Stann.). Aggravated at 9:00 p.m. (Cham., Bell.).

Dr. Ray recorded a case, one of the first for this remedy, in which a man had a 25-year history of severe asthma cured with Blatta. He was emaciated, had nightly attacks, troublesome cough and very frothy mucus. Worse lying down. Stooped shoulders and a stiff neck. Despaired, feeble, could not expectorate, speechless, so weak he could not talk (Stann.).

Anshutz recorded 4 cases concerning the use of Blatta. The first, "A young man, aged thirty-four, had been suffering from asthma for some years. He was invariably worse during the rains and the winter and chronic bronchitis was almost a constant accompaniment. He tried allopathic and lots of patent drugs with only temporary amelioration of the trouble. At last in November, 1888, he came to my office.

"On examination of his chest I found there was a chronic bronchitis. He said that slight difficulty of breathing with hacking cough used to trouble him every night, besides a cold would be followed by a severe attack of asthma, so its periodicity of recurrence was irregular. I treated him with Ipecac, Arsenicum alb., etc. The first-named medicine did him the most good, but he never got entirely well.

"In July, 1889 I put him under tincture Blatta orientalis 3x, drop doses, three or four times daily. Under its use he began to improve steadily and had only two or three attacks of asthmatic fits since he used this drug, which were promptly relieved by the same drug in 1x potency.

"Euphrasia off. was prescribed for his cold whenever he had it. He is free from all trouble for the last year and a half. His general condition is so much changed that there is no apprehension of the recurrence of his former illness."

The second case, "A shoemaker, aged forty-two, robust constitution, has been suffering with asthma for three or four years. He came to my office on the 6th of November, 1890. He had been getting asthmatic fits almost every night since October last. During the day a troublesome cough comes with slight expectoration and hurried breathing made him unable to attend his business.

"Tincture Blatta orientalis 1x, one drop doses, six times daily, was given. The very first day he perceived the good effect of the medicine and continued the same for a month, when he got well and discontinued the medicine. He has been keeping well ever since."

Anshutz's third case concerned "A gentleman, the keeper of a common shop, aged forty-four, belonging to a village, had been suffering from asthma for the last eight years and had always been under treatment of native kabiraj (medical men). In June, he came to the city and I was called to see him on the 14th of June to treat him for his asthma. The day previous he had an attack, for which he took no medicine. Each of his attacks usually lasted four or five days.

"I gave him Blatta orientalis 1x trituration., one grain every two hours and left him six such powders to be taken during the day. He took them and felt better the next day. He stayed here two or three days more and when well he wanted to proceed home, which was some couple of hundred miles.

"He took with him two drachm phials of Blatta orientalis, one of 1x and the other of 3x trituration. He continued the 3x, one grain doses, two or three times daily, for a month and discontinued afterward. He had no more asthmatic fits.

"In January last, 1891, I had a letter from him, thanking me for his recovery and asking for some of the same medicine for a friend of his, who had been suffering from asthma. The friend of his who used the same drug, Blatta orientalis, was equally benefited."

The fourth case, "Mrs. Datta, a thin lady, aged thirty-eight, mother of several children, had been exposed to cold, which brought on an attack of bronchitis with fever. This in the course of a fortnight, developed into a regular fit of asthma.

"She was all this time treated by an old school physician, but when the husband of the lady saw that she was daily getting worse and a new disease crept in, he made up his mind to change the treatment, I was called to see her in the morning of the 8th of June, 1890.

"She became very much emaciated, could not take any food, had fever with acute bronchitis, hurried respiration, difficulty of breathing, this she was complaining of bitterly, owing to which she could not lie down in bed, but had to sit up day and night. There was a prolonged fit of spasmodic cough at short intervals with slight expectoration, but these coughing fits would make her almost breathless.

"This was the first time I prescribed Blatta orientalis 1x in a case of asthma with fever and acute bronchitis. It answered my purpose well. She had only ten powders during the day and passed a comparatively better night.

"Next morning when I saw her she was better except the coughing fits, which were continuing as before. The same medicine was repeated. On the 10th of June she had no asthmatic trouble at night, but there was not much improvement in her cough, Ant-t. and Bry. were needed to complete the cure."

RELATIONS - ***Compare:*** (1) Ars., Hydr. (2) Puls., Sil., Kali-s.

REFERENCES - Anshutz. Boericke. Clarke. Murphy.

BOLDO FRAGRANS

PHARMACY - bold. Boldo fragrans. Boldus peumus. Peumus boldo. Ruizia fragrans. Nyctaginaceae. Tincture of the leaves. ***Historical dose:*** Tincture and all potencies.

CLINICAL - Abscess. Asthma. Bladder, atony. Bronchitis. Catarrh. Cholecystitis. Constipation. Gallstones. ***Liver, disorders.*** Lung, disorders. Malaria. Pulmonary, edema.

HOMEOPATHIC - Bold. has been used for cholecystitis and biliary calculus. Atonic states of stomach and intestinal canal. Bitter taste in mouth. No appetite. Constipation. Hypochondriasis. Exhaustion.

Burning weight in region of liver and stomach. Liver disorders following malaria. Abscess of liver. Congestion of liver. Burning weight in liver and stomach. Painful hepatic diseases. Asthma, bronchitis, catarrh and edema of lungs.

REFERENCES - Boericke. Clarke.

BOLETUS LARICIS
(White Agaric)

PHARMACY - bol. Boletus laricis. White agaric. Boletus purgans. Agaricus laricis. Larch agaric. Polyporus officinale. N. O. Fungi. Trituration. Tincture of the dried mushroom. ***Historical dose:*** Trituration and all potencies.

CLINICAL - Chills. Diarrhea. Dysentery. Faintness. Fever. Gallbladder, disorders. Headaches. Intermittent fever. Liver disorders.

HOMEOPATHIC - Burt proved the crude substance and the third trituration. The gastroenteric irritation common to the fungus was very well marked. Motion will aggravate the headache. Disposition to yawn and stretch when chilly. Great restlessness after midnight. Faintness after stool. Aching distress in all joints.

MIND - Very gloomy and despondent. Irritated at the least trifle. Absent-minded.

Abdomen - Aching in liver and umbilicus. Severe cutting pains in abdomen every few minutes. Dull, aching distress in umbilicus and loud rumbling in bowels all night. Severe, aching pain just below stomach, causing great faintness.

Back - Chilliness along spine with frequent hot flashes of fever. Dull, aching distress in back and legs.

Eyes - Agglutination of eyelids morning with dull, aching pains in eyeballs.

Face - Hot and flushed with severe frontal headache. Hands hot and dry.

Head - Head feeling very light and hollow with deep frontal headache and great faintness.

Liver - Heavy dragging pains in liver, more in right lobe. Dull, burning distress, drawing, aching in right lobe of liver with frontal headache. Sharp cutting pains in right lobe of liver and whole dorsal region on full inspiration. Sharp cutting pains near gallbladder. Burning distress in region of gallbladder all afternoon with sharp pains in stomach and heavy aching in liver.

Mouth - Teeth and gums very sore.

Perspiration - ***Profuse perspiration at night*** with hectic chills and fever. Sweat is light and without relief. Night-sweat in tuberculosis.

Rectum - Thin, yellow pasty stool, mixed with something looking like oil in large and small drops. Black, lumpy, dry stools mixed with bile, blood and mucus, with high fever. Lienteric. Straining after stool.

Skin - Hot and dry, especially in palms. Itching more between scapulae and on forearms.

Stomach - Constant nausea and vomiting. Feeling in fauces as if would vomit. Great faintness at epigastrium. Severe cutting pains in stomach.

Temperature - Quotidian intermittent fever. Chilliness along spine with frequent, hot flashes. Yawns and stretches when chilly. Severe aching in shoulders and joints and small of back. Waking at midnight in a profuse perspiration.

Tongue - White coat, thick yellow coat showing marks of teeth. Taste is flat, coppery, unnatural of all food, lost.

COMMENTS - Anshutz noted two cases. The first consisted of a case of fever. "Intermittent fever: Type Quotidian Duplex. In a large lymphatic woman, weight about 180 lbs., aged thirty-nine. November 4th. For the last five weeks has had the ague. At first it was simple quotidian. Took quinine, which broke it for four days, when it returned took quinine in massive doses, which checked it for one week.

"It returned two weeks since in the form of a double quotidian. The chill comes on every day at 10 a.m. and 5 p.m. The chill lasts from one to two hours each time, hands and feet get icy cold, chills run up and down the spine with severe pains in the head, back and limbs, followed by high fever for three hours and then profuse sweat.

"Tongue furred whitish yellow with large fissures in the tongue, flat, bitter taste, has had no appetite for five weeks, craves cold water all the time, bowels rather costive, has nausea during every chill, but no vomiting, very weak, can only sit up about one hour in the morning.

Great depression, cried during the whole examination, face very much jaundiced.

"Treatment: Ars. 2c, every two hours, for three days. It produced constant nausea and lessened the chills, but aggravated the fever. I then determined to try the Boletus 1c, two grains every two hours. Took two doses when the chills came on, she then ceased to take the medicine until 5 p.m.

Took three doses and then fell asleep. 8th. She says she is feeling a little Better continued treatment, 10 a.m., commenced to have a severe diarrhea, an effect of the medicine, discontinued the powders until 5 p.m.

"The fever did not come on until 3 p.m., had no chill, fever lasted three hours, perspired profusely all night, slept well for the first time in a number of weeks. 9th. Feeling much better. Fever came on at 4 p.m., had no chill, fever lasted four hours, nausea all the evening, sweat all night. 10th. Feeling quiet well. Had no more fever, but had night sweats for a week after. Convalescence was very slow, she had no more fever it was three weeks before she felt perfectly well.

"This case demonstrated the fact to us that the Boletus is superior to our greatest remedial agents in the case of intermittent fevers. I believe if I had not been acquainted with the therapeutic properties of the Boletus I would have been compelled to treat this lady every few weeks for two or three months with our usual remedies."

His second case, "Intermittent fever: Type quotidian. November first, Mrs. B., aged fifty-six. Temperament nervous. Three weeks since had an abscess in left ear, which made her quite sick for a week.

"Since then has had fever every afternoon and night. Feels chilly whenever she moves. Walking produces nausea. Does not perspire any. Tongue coated white. Loss of appetite, bowels loose. Very restless at night, cannot sleep any, getting very weak, keeps to her bed most of the time. Gave Boletus laricis. She had the fever but one day after."

RELATIONS - ***Compare:*** (1) Boletus luridus. Boletus satanus. Cocc. (head hollow). (2) Agaricin, active constituent of Polyporus officinale - tubercular and other enervating night-sweats 1-4 to 1-2 grains doses, also in chorea in dilatation of heart with pulmonary emphysema, fatty degeneration, profuse perspiration and erythema.

REFERENCES - Anshutz. Clarke.

BOLETUS LURIDUS

PHARMACY - bol-lu. Boletus luridus. Boletus nigrescens. N. O. Fungi. Trituration. ***Historical dose:*** Trituration and all potencies.

CLINICAL - Delirium. Meteorism. Pain. Subsultus tendinum. Urticaria tuberosa.

HOMEOPATHIC - Poisoning effects show delirium, sunken features, cold sweat, and a violet color of nose and lips. Intense thirst with a loss of stool, subsultus tendinum, urticaria tuberosa, and violent pain in the epigastrium.

REFERENCES - Boericke. Clarke.

BOLETUS SATANUS

PHARMACY - bol-s. Boletus satanas. N. O. Fungi. Trituration. ***Historical dose:*** Trituration and all potencies.

CLINICAL - Cramps. Debility. Diarrhea. Dysentery. Faintness. Vomiting. Weakness.

HOMEOPATHIC - There are two fragmentary provings of this fungus and observations on six persons poisoned. It produces gastro-intestinal disturbances very similar to its two relatives.

Dysentery, vomiting, great debility. Faintness while vomiting. Cold sweat over whole body. Cold limbs, spasm of limbs and face. Sudden sensation through all his limbs as if he would be attacked with a stroke. Violent and extremely painful cramps in the muscles of the limbs and face.

MIND - Fear and restlessness.

Abdomen - Obstinate tension of abdomen. Sunken and frightfully painful abdomen.

Eyes - Sparks before eyes, alternating with obscure vision.

Mouth - Troublesome dryness in mouth and throat.

Rectum - A profuse diarrhea of blood and of the mucus lining of the intestines. Watery evacuations.

Stomach - Unquenchable thirst. Sudden desire to vomit, no nausea between attacks. Vomited twenty times in three hours. Frightful pain in stomach.

Throat - Violent burning and scraping in throat.

REFERENCES - Boericke. Clarke.

BOMBYX PROCESSIONEA

(Procession Moth)

PHARMACY - bomb-pr. Bombyx processionea. Procession Moth. Thaumetopoea processionnea. N. O. Lepidoptera. Tincture of caterpillars. ***Historical dose:*** Trituration and all potencies.

CLINICAL - Delirium. Fever. Itching. Tubercles. Urticaria.

HOMEOPATHIC - Contact with the caterpillars or the emanations from a nest of them causes intense irritation. Large, hard tubercles with a red areola formed, so thick as to leave hardly any space between. Sometimes they are formed in a linear manner, most marked near joints. .

In one case, that of a boy who shook a large number of the caterpillars from a tree onto his naked breast, it caused an itching so severe that the boy had to run home for assistance, then fever, somnolence, delirium and finally death ensued.

Burning heat of skin. Sensation as if a foreign body were under the skin. Itching of whole body. Itching, in evenings, not relieved by anything. In one victim it caused frequent waking at night and dreams that his arms were being cauterized and arrows thrust into the muscles.

RELATIONS - ***Compare:*** (1) Apis, Astac. fl., Rhus-t.

REFERENCES - Boericke. Clarke.

BORAX VENETA

(Sodium Biborate)

PHARMACY - bor. Borax veneta. Sodium biborate. Natrum biboracicum. Trituration and solution. ***Historical dose:*** Trituration and all potencies.

CLINICAL - Albuminuria. ***Aphthae. Aphthous, ulcers***. Chilblains. Colic. Collapse. Corns. Coryza. Cystitis. Dentition. Diarrhea. ***Dysmenorrhea***. Ear, discharge. Emaciation. Entropion. Erysipelas. Eyes, disorders. Finger, joints. Finger, ulcers. ***Galactorrhea.*** Headache. Hematuria. ***Herpes, simplex.*** Herpes zoster. Infertility. Leucorrhea. Marasmus. Menstruation, painful. Nephritis. Nipples, sore. Nose, disorders. Pleurisy. Pleurodynia. Plica, polonica. ***Psoriasis***. Screaming. ***Seasickness.*** Sore, throat. Taste, disordered. ***Thrush***. Trichinosis. ***Ulcers.*** Urine, offensive. Vertigo.

HOMEOPATHIC - The nervous symptoms are very characteristic and have frequently been verified, especially in the therapeutics of children. Useful in epilepsy. ***Sensitiveness to sudden noises***, as a distant shot, which causes violent starting. Gastro-intestinal irritation. Eructation, when painful parts are pressed.

Dread of downward motion in nearly all complaints. Symptoms are worse going down stairs. ***Seasickness*** when the downward motion is felt most: "Every time the ship goes down, everything in me comes up." Child screams when nurse puts it into cot or when she rocks it.

Aphthous mouth ulcers of the mucus membranes. ***Thrush. Herpes of the mouth.*** Salivation, nausea, vomiting. Aphthae, mouth of child feels hot to mother's nipple, child lets go nipple and cries with pain and vexation, or else refuses breast altogether.

Painful nursing, pain after nursing, empty feeling in breasts, they ache because they are empty, keynote better by pressure. Mother's milk is thick and tastes badly. Poorly nourished, soft and flabby, children. General emaciation. Marasmus.

Skin and mucus membranes shriveled. Child screams before urinating from inflammation of mucus membrane. Colic, diarrhea, collapse, albuminuria, casts and bladder spasms. Diarrhea with pain or soft yellow stools accompanying aphthae. Hematuria.

Discharges are thick, hot, biting. Clear, copious, albuminous, unnaturally hot leucorrhea. Favors easy conception. Infants cyanotic from birth.

Heat in single parts, mouth, vagina, palms etc. Sticking or drawing pains internal intercostal, soles etc. Skin eruptions. Parts which are usually red turn white. Sensation of cobweb, on hands, face. Restlessness in afternoon. Delirium, visual changes.

MIND - Great anxiety and sleepiness. ***Dread of downward motion, causes anxiety.*** Afraid of falling. Excessively nervous, easily frightened. ***Fear of thunder.*** Fear of being infected by some contagious disease. ***Fear of falling.***

Sensitive to sudden noises. Startles from hearing bad news or from excitement. ***Easily frightened and startled with least noise.*** Frightened easily at sneezing. Starting at hawking, at sneezing. Oversensitive to noise during labor. Violent fright from sound of a gun, even at a distance.

Fretful, ill-humored, indolent and discontented. Irritability. Fault finding. Changes from one business to another from one room to another. Confusion, better after stool. Disposition to be angry, with ill humor and passion. Becomes vehement and swears. Does not wish to do anything. Dread of labor.

Fidgety, fickle. Irritable before stool, cheerful and happy after. Babies cry and scream, when nursing or before passing stool or urine. Children awake, suddenly, scream, hold the sides of cradle without any apparent cause. All the mental symptoms are better at 11 p.m. Laughing alternating with weeping.

Abdomen - Colic with tendency to diarrhea after smoking tobacco. Accumulation of flatus in the abdomen, and frequent escape of wind. After every meal inflation of the abdomen with diarrhea and colic. Belly soft, flabby, sunken. Distention after eating, vomiting. Pain as if diarrhea would set in. Pulling from spleen to chest. Catch in groin on coughing. Stitching pains in the groins before or during menses.

Back - Pain in back, inability to stoop. Sharp and drawing pains between the shoulder blades. Furunculus in the armpit. Itching and crawling, aching or burning in the sacrum, when seated or stooping.

Breasts - ***Galactorrhea***, flow of milk, which curdles speedily (Calc., Con., Bell.). ***When nursing, pain in opposite breast***. Empty feeling in breasts after child nurses with stitches better compressing. Mother's milk is thick and tastes badly. Aphthae so tender they prevent child nursing.

Chest - Pain in chest, better lying on back, washing with cold water, or pressure. ***Sharp pains in chest*** with inspiration and cough. Pleurodynia, worse upper part of right chest. Sticking pain in chest (intercostal), worse coughing, inspiration, yawning or any physical exertion. Sneezing with violent shootings in right side of the chest.

Constitutions - Suited to the period of dentition, to persons with light hair, lax skin and muscles, wrinkled skin, consequences of getting cold in cold and wet weather, riding, or eating fruit.

Ears - Inflammation and swelling of the ears. Shootings in the ears, with pain as of excoriation. ***Very sensitive to slightest noise***, not so much disturbed by louder ones. Buzzing and murmuring in the ears. As if ear opened and closed.

Eyes - Itching in the eyes. Redness about eyes. Pressure on the eyes. ***Eyelashes turn inward.*** Entropion. Gummy, crusty, sticky eyelids. Granular eyelids. Eyelids inflamed, lids cut against eyeball. Visions of bright waves. Sparkling before the eyes when writing. Sensitivity to candlelight.

Face - Erysipelas in face. Pale, earthy with suffering expression. Swollen with pimples on nose and lips. Puffy face, bluish in infants. Cobweb sensation. As of a bug crawling over lip. Anxious during downward motion.

Female - Labor pains with frequent belchings. Leucorrhea, like egg whites, with sensation as if warm water was flowing. ***Menses too soon, profuse,*** with gripping, nausea and pain in stomach extending into the small of back. ***Membranous dysmenorrhea***. Itching of vulva and eczema. Sensation of distention in clitoris with sticking. Indifference to sex. Infertility. Easy conception.

Food - Appetite moderate, especially at supper. Loss of taste. Thirst in the morning. Desire for acid drinks, sour things.

Head - Headache, with shootings in the ears. Headache with nausea and trembling of the whole body. Fullness in the head, and pressure above the eyes. Hot head in babies. Hair tangled, cannot be separated, as in plica polonica (Vinc.).

Heart - Violent palpitations. Feels as if on right side and being squeezed. Infants cyanotic from birth.

Kidneys - Nephritis. Cystitis. Urgent inclination to urinate. Frequent emission of urine even in the night. Ineffectual urge to urinate. Hot acrid, smarting urine of pungent smell. Child afraid to urinate, screams before urinating (Sars.). Small red particles on diaper.

Limbs - Want of strength, especially in joints. Limbs tremble at 10 a.m. As if warm water running down thighs. Weakness in calves. ***Sharp pains in sole***. Pain in heel. Burning pain in great toe, inflammation of balls of toes. Eczema of toes and fingers with loss of nails. Feeling as of cobwebs on hands. Palms hot. Itching on back of finger joints and hands. Throbbing pain in tip of thumb.

Lungs - Shortness of breath, worse ascending stairs, stitches on speaking. Arrest of breathing when lying, is obliged to jump and catch breath, which causes pain in right side. Dry, hectic cough, caused by a tickling and scraping in the throat. Hacking and violent cough. Expectoration, blood streaked or moldy taste and smell.

Male - Indifference to sex, low sexual desire. Erections, with painful tension, on waking in the morning. Gonorrhea. Chancres studding prepuce. Sticking, sore pain, worse when touched.

Modalities - Better at 11 p.m., evening, cold weather, pressure. ***Worse from downward or upward motion***, rocking, being dangled up and down. Worse from cold, wet. Worse least uncovering. Worse warm weather. Worse fruit. Worse smoking. Worse after menses.

Mouth - Mouth hot and tender. ***Aphthous ulcers*** in the mouth and on the tongue, which bleed easily. Aphthous after taking sour or salty food. ***Oral thrush.*** White fungus-like growth. Dry cracked or puffy indented tongue. Bitter taste in the mouth on eating or on swallowing the saliva (Bry., Puls., Cupr.). Palate, hard and wrinkled, as if burnt, pains when chewing, while nursing in children.

Nose - Itching in the nose with tingling. Acrid coryza. Nostrils ulcerated. Dry scabs in the nose. Sneezing. Stoppage of nostrils alternately with lachrymation. Red nose of young women (Nat-c.). Red and shining swelling with throbbing and tensive sensation. Tip swollen and ulcerated. Blood follows on blowing the nose. Accumulation of thick and greenish mucus in the nose.

Perspiration - Perspiration during the morning sleep.

Rectum - Burning in rectum during stool. Pain as if diarrhea would result. Stools, turning green or persistently green like boiled starch. Mucus diarrhea, then weakness. ***Loose, pasty, offensive stools in children***. Stools slender. Diarrhea offensive, preceded by colic, mucus stools with aphthous sore mouth.

Skin - Unhealthy skin, slight injuries suppurate. Wilted, wrinkled skin. ***Skin, dry,*** festers easily, won't heal. ***Psoriasis***. Eruptions on fingers and hands, itching and stinging eczema. Whitish pimples with areola. Ulcerations on feet from rubbing of shoe or boots. Herpes (Nat-m., Rhus-t.). Erysipelatous inflammation with swelling and tension. Chilblains relieved in open air.

Sleep - Anxious cries of children during sleep with convulsive movements of the hands. Child cries out in sleep, as if frightened (Bell.). Voluptuous dreams, dreams of sex. Cannot sleep on account of heat, especially in head. Starts from deep as if to fall. Sleepiness during the day and sleeplessness at night.

Stomach - Fullness and pressure in the stomach after having eaten fruit, pears and apples. Gastralgia, reflex from uterine troubles. Belchings, on pressing painful part. Nausea, when thinking hard with trembling of body and weakness of knees. Vomiting of sour mucus after drinking. Pain in the region of stomach after heavy lifting. Stitching, extending to small of back. Sweat on stomach.

Teeth - Toothache, worse wet weather, better by smoking. Shooting pains in decayed teeth. Pressive tingling in the teeth, immediately after supper or breakfast. Ulcers in the gums with swelling of the cheek. Bleeding gums. Painful gumboil.

Temperature - Flushes of heat. Shivering, shuddering or cold with trembling. Chilliness especially during sleep. Thirst before or during the cold, or else after the sweat. Heat in the evening in bed, with shivering on being the least uncovered.

Throat - Dryness in the throat. Hoarseness in the throat with drawing shootings on coughing and sneezing. Tenacious mucus in the throat with difficult expectoration.

Vertigo - Fits of vertigo with fainting. Vertigo, with fullness in the head. Vertigo, worse from ascending stairs or any elevation.

COMMENTS - A piece of borax, the size of a pea, dissolved in the mouth, acts magically in restoring the voice in cases of sudden hoarseness brought on by cold and frequently for an hour or so, it renders the voice silvery and clear. It has even cured *"shot-shyness"* in sporting dogs.

Herpetic eruptions, pleuritic symptoms (upper right chest) and cough with expectoration of a mushy, moldy odor. Parts usually red turn white. White fungus-like growths. Stitching pains predominate. Starts with pain. Cobweb sensations. Restlessness with ebullitions, especially after talking with nausea.

Sore muco-cutaneous surfaces. Ingrown eyelashes. Otorrhea and inflammation of auricle, "starts with the pains." Nostrils ulcerated, soreness, pain and swelling of tip of nose. For oral thrush, oral candida. Aphthous ulcers, round and white, like canker sores. Thrush in AIDS cases, with or without aphthous ulcers.

Dysmenorrhea with excessive pain during flow. Leucorrhea preceding and following menses, albuminous, acrid (Graph.).

For infected or cracked nipples while nursing. For babies with sores from nursing (Nat-m., and Sul-ac.), hot and burning. Diaper rash, ulcers and sores around the rectum, candida rashes of the anus. Diarrhea, offensive stools, excoriating. Child screams out in sleep, wakes frightened and clinging.

Laughter alternating with weeping. Idles through the afternoon, does not really get to work, changes from one business to another from one room to another. Fretful, ill humored, indolent and discontented before easy stool in the afternoon, after it, lively, contented and cheerful. Excessively nervous, a slight noise arouses. Patients tend to pale, earthy, fleshy and flabby.

RELATIONS - ***Antidoted by:*** Cham., Coffea. ***Compare:*** (1) Calc., Bry., Nux-v., Bry., Lyc., Merc., Puls., Rhus-t, All-c., Sil., Sanicula, Sulph., Sulphuric acid. (2) Ars., Bell., Graph., Ign., Kali-bi., Phos. (3) Am-c. and Mag-m. - right nostril stopped. (4) Calc. - inclination to breathe deeply. (5) Kali-bi. - tough mucus. (6) Aur. and Puls. - laughter alternately with weeping. (7) Sars., Lyc. (8) Benz-ac. - strong urine, crying before urination, but these three have gravel: with Borax it is from inflammation of mucus membrane. (9) Arum-t. - sore mouth, Graph. - trichiasis. (10) Bell. - hot leucorrhea. (11) Sep. - small ulcers about joints. (12) Bar-c. - cobweb-sensation. (13) Nat-s. - cheerful after stool. ***Incompatible:*** Acet-ac., Vinegar, Wine.

REFERENCES - Boericke. Clarke.

BORIC ACIDUM

(Boric Acid)

PHARMACY - bor-ac. Boricum acidum. Boric acid. Solution of crystals in alcohol. ***Historical dose:*** Trituration and all potencies.

CLINICAL - Antiseptic. Colds. ***Conjunctivitis.*** Dermatitis. ***Diabetes.*** Dermatitis. Edema. Erythema. Eyes, disorders. Headache. Impetigo. Edema. Menopausal, flushings. Kidney colic. Vomiting. Whitlow. Wounds.

HOMEOPATHIC - Bor-ac. has been largely used as an antiseptic dressing for wounds, as a lotion for the eyes and whitlow, and as a wash in catarrh of the bladder. Arrests fermentation and putrefaction. It is much less irritating than Carbolic acid, but it has also produced skin eruptions.

Bor-ac. affects the skin causing an extensive exfoliative dermatitis.

Pain along ureters with frequent urination. Edema around the eyes. ***Diabetes.*** Tongue dry, red and cracked. ***Coldness*** (Helo.). Cold saliva. Vagina cold as if packed with ice. Useful in menopausal flushing.

Eyes - ***Conjunctivitis.*** Edema of tissues around eyes.

Female - Menopausal flushings (Lach., Amyl-n.). Vaginal coldness, as if packed with ice.

Kidneys - Frequent urination with burning and tenesmus.

Modalities - Better from walking in open air.

Skin - Exfoliating dermatitis. Multiform erythema of trunk and upper limbs.

COMMENTS - Poisonings and provings with Bor-ac. have caused headache, vertigo, noises in the ears, prostration, cold saliva, vomiting of tough, greenish stuff, uncontrollable vomiting, hiccough, pasty stool, pain in region of ureters or increased urine and increased call to urinate, albuminuria, and an erythematous eruption on face, body and thighs followed by pearly vesicles on face and neck.

Three cases of poisoning have been reported from packing the vagina with the dry acid, kept in by tampons until liquefaction took place. Symptoms included formication of hands and feet, later of face.

Sad spirits, great nervous depression. Burning skin, became swollen and charred and all motions were painful.

One case went into collapse, temperature subnormal, sighing and weeping by turns. Prominent coldness, vagina felt "cold as if packed with ice."

In the 3x potency, Cooper found it give great relief in menopausal flushings.

One woman took 30 grains of boric acid per day for a month, when there appeared a multiform erythema of trunk extending to upper limbs, at the same time there appeared a painful swelling of upper lids with conjunctivitis and photophobia.

Finally the edema was so intense as to close the eyes and give the appearance of sclerosed tissue. The symptoms began to abate when the Bor-ac. was discontinued and disappeared in a week.

RELATIONS - ***Compare:*** (1) Bor., Carb-ac. (2) Kali-bi. - tough mucus.

REFERENCES - Boericke.

BORON METALLICUM

PHARMACY - bor-met. Boron metallicum. Boron metal. ***Historical dose:*** Trituration and all potencies.

CLINICAL - Anemia. Aphthae. Arthritis. Bronchitis. Conjunctivitis. Constipation. Cystitis. Diarrhea. Ear, infections. Eczema. Epilepsy. Gastritis. Herpes. Joint pains. Leucorrhea. Mastitis. Motion sickness. Nausea. Osteoporosis. Parkinson's disease. Sterility. Vertigo. Vomiting.

HOMEOPATHIC - Retarded development, late walking, late talking, late being toilet trained. Growth disorders. Hair tangled. Nails drop off. Anemia.

Dizziness with feeling of falling backwards or sliding down, as if in a lift. Parkinson's disease. Epilepsy. Watery, sometimes green discharges.

MIND - Mentally confused. Slow mind. Disoriented. Lack of concentration. Forgetful. Dementia. Confusion of identity. Sympathetic. Obsessive behavior. Psychosis caused by stress. Delirium.

Nervous, and restless. Timid, unsure of themselves. Indecisive. Low self confidence. Fear of failing. Doubts oneself. Easily discouraged. Desire support from others. Listless and apathetic. Gloomy disposition. Suicidal.

Startled easily from sudden noises. Vague fears. Fear of the unknown. Fear of diseases, infections, germs. Fear of death. Fear of going down stairs. Delusions voices that tell them who they are and what they should do.

Bladder - Cystitis. Inflammations of bladder. Bladder spasms.

Breasts - Mastitis. Inflammation of breasts, pain on the opposite side from the one the baby is suckling from. Late birth, child prefers the right breast.

Chest - Sharp pains in chest.

Ears - Ear infections. Sensitive to noises.

Eyes - Conjunctivitis. Inverted eyelids.

Face - Face pale, tip of nose red.

Female - Menses frequent, profuse, with stomach and back pains. Sterility. Clitoris painful and swollen, eczema. Leucorrhea white, sticky and stringy. Leucorrhea like egg-white. Sexually immature. Low estrogen levels.

Food - Aversion to lettuce, fruit, meat, vegetables. Desires apples, pears, potatoes, sweet, cheese, bread. Worse from fruit, pears, bananas, wine, coffee, sour, salt, coffee. Worse fats.

Kidneys - Crying before urination. Urine contains blood and protein.

Limbs - Osteoporosis. Joint pains. Pain at tip of thumb, soles and ball of feet.

Lungs - Bronchitis. Hard cough. Sharp pains in lungs. Lungs feel as if pressed in.

Male - Atrophy of testes. Sexually immature. Low testosterone levels.

Modalities - Better after stools and urination. Better crying. Worse loud noises. Worse 8 am. Worse downward motion. Worse going down stairs, Worse elevators. Worse chlorine. Worse cold weather. Worse damp weather. Worse thunder.

Mouth - Infections in mouth, aphthae, thrush. Herpes on lips. Salivation aggravates. Taste and smell of fungus. Fissured tongue, red and bleeding. Fungus taste.

Rectum - Constipation. Diarrhea. Stools soft with mucus.

Skin - Cobweb sensation on skin. Eczema around mouth, on cheeks, fingers and toes.

Sleep - Sleeps a long time. Talking during sleep.

Stomach - Gastritis. Inflammations of the stomach. Stomach acidity. Nausea on exertion. Vomiting. Motion sickness.

Vertigo - Dizziness with feeling of falling backwards or sliding down, as if in a lift.

REFERENCES - Scholten.

BOTHROPS LANCEOLATUS

(Yellow Viper)

PHARMACY - both-l. Bothrops lanceolatus. Yellow viper. Lachesis lanceolatus. Vipera jaune. Fer-de-lance. N. O. Crotalide. Martinique Island. Solution of the poison in glycerin. Potencies in rectified spirit. ***Historical dose:*** All potencies.

CLINICAL - Abscesses. Amaurosis. Anthrax. Aphasia. Blindness. ***Blood, clots.*** Bones, necrosis. Day-blindness. Edema. Emaciation. Erysipelas. Gangrene. Hematemesis. Hemiplegia. ***Hemorrhages.*** Lockjaw. Lungs, congestion. Lymphangitis. Nervous, trembling. Paralysis. ***Phlebitis.*** Pulmonary, congestion. Septic, fever. Septicemia. Snake, bites. Thrombosis. Trembling. Tongue, paralysis. Wounds.

HOMEOPATHIC - The venom of the yellow viper is a coagulant, therefore it is expected to be useful in thrombosis and thrombotic disorders.

After being bitten in the little finger of one hand, paralysis began in the fingertips of the other hand and extended over the whole of that side. Intolerable pain in right great toe (patient bitten in left thumb). Marked diagonal course of symptoms.

Ozanam noted some peculiar symptoms, including amaurosis. Day blindness, can scarcely see her way after sunrise. Deep gangrene, dissecting, bones laid bare and necrotic.

Hemorrhages from every orifice of the body. Black spots. Blindness from hemorrhage into retina. Pulmonary congestion, oppressed breathing and bloody expectoration, more or less profuse. Hemorrhages from the wounds.

Great lassitude and sluggishness. Nervous trembling. Syncope. Sudden or rapid debility and emaciation. Slight shivering, followed by profuse sweat. Aphasia, inability to articulate, without any tongue problems. Hemiplegia, with aphasia. Paralysis of one arm or one leg only.

MIND - Persistent hypochondriasis. ***Mental symptoms after having a stroke.*** Behaves as if he had a stroke. Aphasia, inability to articulate. Forgetful of words while speaking. Mistakes, using wrong words. Stupefaction, as if intoxicated. Anguish. Stupor, syncope. Unconsciousness, coma.

Abdomen - Tympanitis.

Back - Opisthotonos.

Blood - Septicemia. ***Hemorrhages from every orifice of the body.*** Blood being fluid and black. Lymphangitis. Dissecting gangrene. ***Blood clots.*** Thrombosis.

Constitutions - Broken-down and hemorrhagic constitutions, septic states.

Eyes - Conjunctival hemorrhage. Blindness from hemorrhage into retina. Day-blindness. Amaurosis without any notable pupillary dilatation.

Face - Swollen and puffy. Besotted expression. Swollen, injected, cyanotic. Lockjaw.

Head - Hemicrania, stupor, vertigo. Migraine headaches. One-sided headaches.

Heart - Heart pains. Precordial pains, syncope. Frequent, tight pulse.

Kidneys - Hematuria.

Limbs - Abscess, leg. Edema. Heaviness, lower limbs. Paralysis of the right leg. Paralysis of the right arm. Muscular tissues are filled with black blood. Numbness. ***Phlebitis.*** Consecutive necrosis. Suppuration, leg. Varicose veins. ***Leg is badly infected after surgery for varicose veins.*** Swollen veins. Gangrene, toes, legs. Gangrenous ulcers.

Lungs - Bloody expectoration, pneumonia. Pulmonary congestion, oppressed breathing and bloody expectoration, more or less profuse. Spitting of blood.

Modalities - Worse on right side.

Mouth - Trismus. Aphasia, inability to articulate words, while the tongue retains all its functions.

Nerves - Hemiplegia. Nervous, trembling.

Perspiration - Clammy sweats. Profuse sweats. Chills with abundant sweats. Abundant cold sweats at the beginning and end of the malady.

Rectum - Tympanitis and bloody stools.

Skin - Formication and itching. Burning pains. Skin bluish, as from deep and extensive contusion. Skin yellow, as in yellow fever. Blackish skin. Swollen, livid skin, cold with hemorrhagic infiltration. Anthrax. Gangrene. Lymphatics swollen. Malignant erysipelas. Septic wounds and ulcers. Scars, bleeding and break open. Wounds heal slowly.

Sleep - Tendency to sleep, somnolence; coma, deeper and deeper until death.

Stomach - Intense hematemesis. Epigastric distress. Nausea and vomiting. Black vomiting. Gastric mucosa is red and dotted.

Temperature - Septic fever. Coldness. General heat. Chills with abundant sweats.

Throat - Red, dry, constricted, swallowing difficult, cannot pass liquids.

COMMENTS - The main idea of Bothrops is thrombosis and phlebitis. Tendency to form blood clots (Lach.).

Eizayaga used this remedy for clots in the legs, specifically for clots that form in the veins in the legs, and then go somewhere else. Also for "milk leg," phlebitis in nursing women.

RELATIONS - ***Compare:*** (1) Other snake poisons, notably Lachesis. (2) Bell. has night-blindness. (3) Toxicophis. Trachinus.

REFERENCES - Boericke. Clarke. Murphy.

BOTULINUM

PHARMACY - botul. Botulinum. Bacillus botulinum. Toxin of Bacillus botulinum. Nosodes. ***Historical dose:*** Trituration and all potencies.

CLINICAL - Albuminuria. Aphonia. Bulbar paresis. Coma. Constipation. Convulsions. Diphtheria. Diplopia. Dizziness. Dysphagia. Dyspnea. Eye, disorders. Food, poisoning. Hydrophobia. Muscular, weakness. Mydriasis. Paralysis. Ptosis. Vision, disorders. Strabismus. Vomiting.

HOMEOPATHIC - Botulism is classified under the heading of meat poisoning. Meat infected by it has no putrid odor, though a characteristic rancid smell is described. Fish, as well as any sort of preserved meat, may form a suitable medium for its growth.

The symptoms of poisoning set in 24 to 36 hours after taking the infected material. Vomiting is usually the first symptom, but the gastro-intestinal tract is little affected in patients attacked by the bacillus botulinus and its toxin.

There is generally constipation rather than diarrhea. Following the first vomiting a train of nerve symptoms develope. Eye symptoms, ptosis, double vision, blurred vision, mydriasis, strabismus, paralysis of accommodation.

Botulism poisoning produced a clinical picture of bulbar paresis. Repeated suffocative attacks have been often observed and after large doses convulsions. General muscular weakness, successive dryness and hypersecretion of the buccal and pharyngeal mucus membranes.

Aphonia, and retention of urine. Difficulty in swallowing and breathing, choking sensation. Weakness and uncertainty in walking, ***blind staggers,*** dizziness. Thickening of speech. Cramping pain in stomach. ***Mask-like expression of face***, due to weakness of facial muscles. Severe constipation.

COMMENTS - The therapeutic applications spring from the recorded symptoms. The drug is to be thought of in hydrophobia, bulbar paralysis and allied affections, diphtheritic paralyses, and the dyspnea attacks and coma of diabetes.

Paroxysmal dyspneas occurring in various diseases, in so far as they are central in origin, should be aided by Botulinum , and it is interesting to note that it is precisely repeated attacks of dyspnea that Dr. Schepens has found himself able to cure with the drug.

His first recorded case is that of a lady of 70, with arteriosclerosis, slight albuminuria, and a small pleural effusion, who suffered from nocturnal dyspnea attacks of an alarming kind. Phos., Ars., Lach., Spong., and Hyos. all did little or nothing. After fifteen days Botul. 30c was given, one dose.

Short aggravation followed by amelioration ensued. The dose was repeated in two days' time, and the same phenomena occurred, but the improvement was more marked. In another two days another dose, and no more, was required. Nine days from the first dose the effusion had disappeared, and albuminuria and attacks of dyspnea followed suit.

The second patient was a man of over 50. An erysipelatous eruption of the right leg disappeared under Apis, Iod., and Kali-i., but when the patient returned to work he was at once attacked by paroxysms of dyspnea, preventing him from lying down and causing great distress. Traces of albumen were found in the urine. Rhus-t. and Lach. did little.

Botul. 50c, two doses within an interval of two days, caused amelioration, after two days more, Botul. 30c, one dose. The next day the albumen had disappeared. One more dose after four days was all that was required, and the patient returned to work restored fully to health.

RELATIONS - ***Compare:*** Bell., Bry., Rhus-t., Sulph., Agar., Hydr-ac., Lach., Ant-t. Ars., Phos., and Tab.

REFERENCES - Boericke. Wheeler.

BOVISTA LYCOPERDON

(Puff-Ball)

PHARMACY - bov. Bovista lycoperdon. Puff ball. Bovista gigantea. Warted puff-ball. Lycoperdon bovista. N. O. Fungi. Trituration. Tincture of the spores of the mushroom. ***Historical dose:*** Trituration and all potencies.

CLINICAL - Absent minded. ***Acne.*** Asphyxia. Boils. Chills. Coccyx, itching. ***Colic.*** Constipation. Corns. Cough. Cysts. Diabetes mellitus. ***Diarrhea.*** Ear, eczema. Eczema. Fever. Flatulence. Ganglion. Gleet. ***Headache. Hemorrhages.*** Heart, disorders. Herpes. Hiccough. Jaundice. Joints, disorders. Leucorrhea. Menstruation, disordered. Metrorrhagia. Morning sickness. Nausea. Neuritis. Nosebleed. Ovarian, cysts. Ovaries, disorders. Palpitations. Pellagra. Rheumatic, disorders. Scurvy. ***Stammering.*** Tetters. Tongue, ulcers. Tumors. ***Urticaria.*** Vertigo. Vomiting. Warts. Whitlow. Wounds.

HOMEOPATHIC - Clarke stated "This globular fungus, which, according to report is eaten in Italy before it is ripe, becomes filled, while ripening with a black dust that breaks the husk which contains it with a slight noise."

Corresponding to this signature, "bloated, puffy condition of body surface," and a sense of "enlargement," leading features of the Bov. pathogenesis include flatulent distention and noisy passage of flatus. Guernsey added "We may always think of Bov. when we see a very 'tettery' person, one who has tetters here and there, all over the body. These tetters may be either moist or dry."

The puffball exerts its influence on the ***circulation,*** causing relaxation of the capillary system, thereby producing ***hemorrhagic diathesis.*** There is a general puffiness, bloated condition of body surface, which produces easy indentations with a blunt instrument (scissors etc.). Eczema-like eruption. Herpes. Marked languor and lassitude.

Laxity, especially felt in joints, which seem loose. Great weakness of the joints (has cured where Rhus-t. seemed indicated and failed). Nervous joints. Enlarged or swollen feeling in head, heart, etc.

Stage of numbness and tingling in multiple neuritis. Asphyxia due to charcoal fumes. Effects of over-exertion and application of tar locally.

MIND - Awkward in speech and action, drops things. ***Everything falls from hands***. Absent-minded. Weak memory. Inattentive. Slowness of understanding and comprehension. Dullness, with restlessness.

Alternating moods. Laughs and cries alternately. Sensitive, takes offense at everything. Ill-humor, aversion to all things. Quarrelsome. Wants to fight. Fear of insanity on waking from a dream. Irritable, takes everything amiss.

Confusion on waking. Confusion while standing. Confusion when stooping. ***Enlarged sensation*** (Arg-n.). Stares vacantly into space. Sad when alone. Cheerful in company. Mental symptoms from sexual excesses.

Abdomen - Bloatedness of abdomen. Cannot bear tight clothing around the waist. Flatulence or rumbling with constipation. Pain around umbilicus. Abdominal colic, with bright red urine. Flatulent colic. ***Colic relieved by eating*** and bending double. Offensive flatus. Sharp pain through perineum towards rectum and genitals. Coldness sensation moving about in abdomen. Ulceration in bowels.

Back - Pain in the back with heaviness after stooping. ***Tip of coccyx itches intolerably.*** Pain and stiffness of back after stooping. Stiffness of neck in morning. Shooting pains between the shoulders are better from bending, straightening up. Sharp pains in neck.

Causations - Antidotes effects of charcoal fumes.

Chest - Oppression of chest, as from constriction, with desire to loosen clothes. Sharp pains in various parts of chest. ***Sweat in axilla, onion smell***. Burning in outer chest.

Constitutions - Hemorrhagic diathesis. Adapted to old maids with palpitation and stammering children.

Ears - Boil in right ear with pain, worse swallowing. Discharge of fetid pus. Indistinct hearing, misunderstands muc that is spoken.

Eyes - Eyes look weak and dim. Inflammation of eyelids, with nightly agglutination. Pressure in orbits. Vertical half-sight. Objects seem to be nearer than they really are. Stares at one point. Loss of vision from paralysis of optic nerve.

Face - Frequent violent alternations of color. ***Acne***, worse in summer, due to use of cosmetics. Cheeks and lips swollen. Crusts about corners of mouth. Twitching of muscles, before asthma. Pale swelling of cheek after toothache.

Female - Burning pain in genitals. Menses too early. ***Menses too profuse, worse at night***. Menses every two weeks, much dark and clotted blood. Soreness of pubes during menses. ***Traces of menses between menstruation***. Leucorrhea a few days before or a few days after menses. Leucorrhea like white of egg, when walking. ***Leucorrhoea acrid, thick, tough, greenish***, leaving green spots on linen worse while walking after menses. Metrorrhagia. ***Cannot bear tight clothing around waist*** (Lach.). Ovarian cysts. Voluptuous sensation.

Food - Excessive hunger, even after meals. No appetite for cooked food, desire for bread only. Desire for brandy, wine, milk. Hot food relieves. Worse spirituous liquors, wine, cold food. Confusion from spirituous liquors, after wine. Thirst for cold drinks. Thirst during chill and heat.

Head - Dull, bruised pain in brain. Confusion on waking. Staggering, confusion and numbness in head after sex. ***Tension headaches***, worse early morning, open air, lying. Stupefying headache in forehead and vertex. ***Sensation as if head were enlarging***, especially of occiput. As if wedge is pressed in occiput. Scalp itches, worse warmth, sensitive, must scratch until sore. Falling out of hair. Scalp tender to touch.

Heart - Heart feels enormously large. Palpitations as if heart working in water. Palpitations with tremor of hands, worse bathing, excitement. Palpitations worse after eating. Palpitations with restlessness, nausea and headache. Palpitations during menses. Visible palpitations of the heart.

Kidneys - Frequent desire to urinate, even immediately after urination. Diabetes mellitus. Stinging, itching, burning in urethra. Bright red urine. Urine bright yellow. Urine with slowly forming cloud, turbid. Urine like loam water. Urine with violet sediment.

Limbs - Great weakness of all joints, clumsiness with her hands, drops things from hands. Weariness of hands and feet. Moist eczema on back of hand. Weak hands. Heavy, painful legs. Itching of feet and legs. ***Tip of coccyx itches intolerably***. Edematous swelling of (right) foot even years after a sprain. Edema of joints after fracture.

Lungs - Asthma preceded by twitching of facial muscles. Shortness of breath on moving the arms. Viscid expectoration. Spasmodic laughing and crying with asthma. Dry cough, caused by tickling in throat and chest. Cough after coming into room from cold air. Loose cough in evening, dry in morning.

Male - Increased sexual desire. Reeling and confusion in head after sex.

Modalities - Better from bending double. Better eating, hot food. ***Worse before and during menses.*** Worse hot weather, getting warm. Worse full moon. Worse from cold food, coffee, and wine. Worse at night. Worse after eating. Worse when blowing nose. ***Easily intoxicated, worse wine.***

Mouth - Putrid taste. Stammering when reading with inability to pronounce several words rapidly. ***Stammering*** (Stram., Merc.). Mouth dry, as if sand were in it. Numbness. Increased saliva. Offensive odor from mouth. Gums bleed easily on sucking them. Bleeding after tooth extraction. Lips chapped, cracked, crusty. Pale swelling of upper lip. Scurf and crusts about nostrils and corners of mouth. Corners of mouth sore.

Nose - Nose stopped up, cannot breathe, worse lying down. Scurf and crusts about nostrils and corners of mouth. ***Discharge from nose, stringy,*** tough. Watery coryza with dizziness. Bleeding of nose and gums. Nosebleed with menstrual irregularity, or from trauma. Bleeding early in the morning (during sleep), a few drops escape on sneezing.

Perspiration - ***Sweat in axilla, onion smell***. Sweats in morning, most profuse on chest.

Rectum - Offensive flatus. Flatulence or rumbling with constipation. Constipation. Fruitless urging to stool. ***Sharp pains through perineum towards rectum and genitals.*** First portion of stool is hard, latter part thin and watery. ***Diarrhea worse before and during menses.*** Chronic diarrhea of elderly people, worse at night and early morning. Diarrhea, better after breakfast. Itching in rectum, as from worms.

Skin - Eczema, red, burns, itches, disturbs sleep. ***Eczema, moist formation of thick crusts.*** Jaundice of newborns. Pellagra. Itching on getting warm. Itching eruptions, oozing, forming thick crusts or scabs with pus beneath. ***Urticaria on excitement*** with rheumatic lameness, palpitations and diarrhea (Dulc.). Urticaria covering whole body with diarrhea or metrorrhagia. Urticaria on waking in the morning, worse from bathing. Pimples cover the entire body. Scurvy. Herpetic eruptions. Shooting pain in corns and warts. Blunt instruments leave deep impression on the skin. Tetter, moist or dry, red, scabby eruptions.

Sleep - Spasmodic yawning before asthma, morning sweat in bed. Night Great drowsiness in afternoon and early evening and after eating. rest disturbed by burning and itching of nettle-rash. Restless sleep with many anxious, frightful dreams.

Stomach - Empty eructations. Intolerant of tight clothing around waist. Hiccough before and after dinner. Sensation as if a lump of ice in stomach. Pressure and fulness in pit. Nausea better breakfast. Nausea with chilliness, whole forenoon. Morning sickness, vomits only water. Vomits watery fluid.

Temperature - Chills with pain. Chills after going to bed at night. Chill predominating, even near a warm stove. Chills all night. Shivering in evening, spreading from back. Shuddering alternating with flying heat. Fever with thirst, anxiety and restlessness. Fever heat during sleep.

Throat - Burning pain in throat. Sharp pain in throat before asthma. Sore throat with scratching and burning in esophagus. Scratching sensation in larynx with viscid mucus. Rawness in larynx, mornings, with catarrhal speech. Hoarseness in morning, with scraping in throat.

Tongue - Soreness or ulcers on edges of tongue. Burning in tip of tongue early in morning on waking. Cutting pain in tongue, before asthma. Numbness of posterior portion of tongue early in morning on waking. Tongue feels almost like wood.

Vertigo - Vertigo with feeling of stupidity in head on rising. Vertigo and confusion of head after sex. Vertigo, falls over, momentarily unconscious in morning. Sudden attacks of vertigo while standing.

COMMENTS - Relaxation of entire capillary system. The heart feels enormously large. Hemorrhagic diathesis. Hemorrhage from menstrual irregularities, from trauma. Hemorrhage between the periods. Menstrual flow occurring only or chiefly at night. Ovarian cysts.

Puffy condition of the body, surface instruments (e.g., scissors) indent the fingers in an unusual degree. Sweat of axilla, smells like onions. Early morning sweat, worse on chest. Many symptoms are worse in early morning, including the diarrhea. Sensitive to touch, cannot bear clothing. Sensitive to drafts, chilliness predominates.

Warts and corns with shooting pains. Ebullitions with great thirst. "Itching at top of coccyx." The corners of the mouth are broken out. Numb, pithy feeling in mouth There is stuttering and stammering speech. Awkwardness, misapplies words in speaking and writing.

Colic, causing the patient to bend double (Coloc.), better by eating, sometimes accompanied by voiding of red urine.

M. L. Sircar recorded a striking cure of such a case with Bov. 3x, the pain being griping-twisting intermittent, starting be low umbilicus and diffusing itself towards epigastrium, some constipation, urine scanty and reddish. Nothing gave relief except eating.

Teste observed psoric eruptions appear on the hands and feet of a patient to whom he gave Bov. for a headache. He cured with it "red, crusty eruptions on thighs and bends of knees of eighteen years' duration." It disappeared for weeks, reappearing in hot weather and at the full moon.

W. S. Gee recorded a case concerning a widow, 55. She had an eruption, which she thought to be erysipelas, on her right foot. Some years before, she had an eruption on her left foot, which discharged much water and was "cured" by the use of a salve. A few months later, the left knee became affected and the limb was amputated above the joint.

The current eruption was fiery red, covered with yellowish-brown scales, thick as an old-fashioned wafer. There were also rheumatic pains in the leg. After Rhus-t. had been given without benefit, she was cured with Bov. 4c.

Dr. Gee elicited additional symptoms including "Occasional spells of short breathing, especially from working with the hands. Frequent desire to urinate, even immediately after urinating. Sleep disturbed by burning and itching and also by anxious, frightful dreams, headache when waking from sleep."

Lilienthal noted "moist vesicular eruptions with formation of thick crusts"; Bov. was given with steady improvement and eventual cure.

A case of cyst in the broad ligament was cured. It was accompanied by metrorrhagia, flow at night or early morning, easily provoked from slight over-exertion during menses. Could bear nothing tight around body. Menses were preceded and followed by diarrhea. Acrid, corrosive leucorrhea, flowing at night only, follows menses.

RELATIONS - ***It antidotes:*** Effects of Tar applied locally. ***Compare:*** (1) Calc., Cic., Rhus-t., Sep., Phos., Puls., Staph., Sulph., Verat., Bell., Bry., Carb-v., Caust., Kali-c., Lyc., Merc., Nat-m., Sil., Spig., Stront., Valer. Aur., Puls., Lyc. (2) Stram. - laughter alternately with weeping. (3) Ars., Lyc., Sulph. - sinking immediately after eating. (4) Bufo - sensation as if heart in water. (5) Zinc. - worse from wine. (6) Coloc. - colic better bending double. (7) Am-c. - poisoning by charcoal fumes. (8) Stram. - stammering. (9) Ambra - hemorrhage between periods. (10) Sec., Ust. ***Followed well by:*** Alum., Calc., Rhus-t., Sep. Teste puts Bov. in his Sulphur group. ***Antidoted by:*** Camph. Bov. antidotes coal tar applications. Suffocation from gas. After Rhus-t. in chronic urticaria.

REFERENCES - Boericke. Clarke.

BRACHYGLOTTIS REPENS

(Puka Puka)

PHARMACY - brach. Brachyglottis repens. Puka puka. N. O. Eupatoriacae. New Zealand. Compositae. Tincture of green leaves and flowers. ***Historical dose:*** Tincture and all potencies.

CLINICAL - Albuminuria. Back, pain. ***Bright's disease.*** Cystitis. Dysmenorrhea. Nephritis. Writer's cramp.

HERBAL - The Maoris use the leaves to apply to old sores and ulcers. Horses eating young shrubs lose all power over their hind legs and spine.

HOMEOPATHIC - Brachyglottis was proved by C. L. Fischer. A large number of symptoms were produced in all regions of the body, but few have been tested clinically.

Kidney and bladder symptoms predominate. ***Bright's disease.*** Produces symptoms of albuminuria. Urgency in passing urine, pain in neck of bladder. Pain in bladder after urinating. Pain in urethra and stinging in penis. A large quantity of pale-colored urine voided of low specific gravity and containing albumen.

Causes lassitude, weakness, and flesh loss. ***Fluttering sensation*** (Calad.). Throbbing pains. Pains in back and limbs. Oppression of chest. Writer's cramp. Chilliness predominates. Itching in ears and nostrils.

Dysmenorrhea with fluttering in abdomen, right ovary has been cured with it.

Abdomen - Isolated throbbing in left groin. Fluttering sensation in abdomen. Feeling as if something rolling about.

Back - First dorsal vertebra sore to touch. Cutting under left shoulder. Aching in lumbar region. Isolated throbbing in right side of back. Feeling as if whole back would contract backward and muscles of neck were affected.

Bladder - Cystitis. Sense of swashing in bladder. Pressure in neck of bladder, urging to urinate. Soreness in urethra, feeling as if urine could not be retained.

Chest - Pains flying about chest and precordial region. Throbbing in sternum.

Ears - Tingling, itching, pricking in ears. Throbbing about right ear, from ear to eyes, and throat to neck.

Eyes - Soreness around eyes, as if bruised. Dim sight during pressure in forehead.

Face - Twitching in left side of face (evening). Soreness right zygomatic process. Flushed face. Face ache left side, submaxillary glands affected.

Female - Fluttering in region of ovary. Dysmenorrhea with fluttering in abdomen and right ovary.

Head - Cold sensation and tightness about scalp. Throbbing in left temple. Headache over left or right eye. Headache and faceache become very severe and prevent sleep during night.

Kidneys - Bright's disease. Nephritis. Urine contains mucous, cells, albumen and casts. Passing urine preceded by pains in bowels. Urine abundant, contains mucus and albumen.

Limbs - Great weakness in limbs, weariness and prostration. Cramp in fingers, thumb and wrist when writing, soreness extending along flexor carpi ulnaris.

Lungs - Oppression of breathing, better by sighing.

Male - Throbbing in penis and desire to pass urine, pressure in bladder.

Mouth - Pain, numbness, pricking, soreness of tongue. Heat in mouth. Toothache right side.

Nose - Nostrils, sore, itching. Irritation in nose.

Rectum - Ineffectual urging for stool. Diarrheic stools in evening. Tendency to diarrhea. Constipation. Evacuation of dry feces with sore, constrictive pain in anus. Feces like balls and knotty. Dry stool, like balls, evacuated with sore, constrictive pain in anus, evening.

Sleep - Great sleepiness during day with constant yawning. Restless and sleepless nights. Talking in sleep. Sleeplessness after waking. Confused dreams. Full of dreams.

Stomach - Nausea in stomach. Fluttering. Soreness in evening. Throbbing in stomach, right side.

Temerature - Chilliness and shivering. Coldness of hands and feet. Nervous chills.

Throat - Soreness, rawness, scraping in throat, worse by swallowing.

Vertigo - Vertigo with flushed face. Vertigo with pain in forehead.

RELATIONS - ***Compare:*** (1) Helon., Merc-c., Plb. (2) Apis - soreness, stinging in urethra, Arn. - bruised, sore feeling. (3) Bov. albuminuria, Helonias, Merc-c. - albuminuria, urging to urinate and defecate. (4) Nux-v. - urging to urinate and defecate. (5) Op. - constipation, Plb. - feces like balls, painful urination, albuminuria. (6) Eupatoriacae.

REFERENCES - Boericke. Clarke.

BRANDY

(Spirit of Wine)

PHARMACY - bran. Brandy. Spirit of wine. Aqua vitae. Tincture. ***Historical dose:*** Tincture and all potencies.

CLINICAL - Burns. Colds. Indigestion. Insomnia. Shock. Toothaches. Wounds.

HOMEOPATHIC - Brandy is distilled wine - wine with most of the water removed - which changes the taste and makes the alcohol content higher.

"Brandy" is derived from brandywijn, a word of Dutch origin for "burnt". Created in a still to leave the water and remove the alcoholic vapor which condenses back into liquid form as it cools. In other languages too, it is the burning that is the essential feature.

Concentrated spirits of wine were used in ancient Greece and Rome, both as an antiseptic and as a primitive anesthetic.

From the 12th to the 14th centuries alchemists in Europe began experimenting with the distillation of many items, but medicines were still mostly given as infusions or decoctions of single herbs. Arabic writings and universities in Spain began to influence Christian schools of medicine in Italy and France.

Two contemporary 13th century Spanish alchemists, Arnold de Villanova and Raymond Lully, introduced wine spirits, which they called aqua vitae (water of life), as a solvent into European medicine.

This later became known as brandy, shortened from the Dutch term for "burnt wine." In the 14th century during the Black Death brandy began to be used as a medicine by itself. It was thought of as a polycrest, a remedy of many virtues.

Brandy is a stimulant, tonic and has restorative powers. Teaspoon doses of brandy were given to patients with low fevers, typhus. Sleep aid, helps prevent and treat colds. Warms the body and improves the circulation.

RELATIONS - ***Compare:*** (1) Alco., Vitis.

REFERENCES - Murphy.

BRASSICA NAPUS

(Rape Seed)

PHARMACY - brass. Brassica napus. Rape seed. Cole seed. Wild corn. Wild kale. N. O. Cruciferae. Tincture of whole fresh plant.

Historical dose: Tincture and all potencies.

CLINICAL - Amenorrhea. Arthritis. Bulimia. Carpal tunnel. Contractures, joints. Cough. Cramps. Dropsy. Dysphagia. Edema. Gangrene. Insomnia. Jaundice. Liver, enlargement. Myalgia. Nails, shedding. Numbness. Pes, equinnus. Raynauds disease. Scleroderma. Scurvy. Ulcers. Wasting, muscles. Weakness.

HOMEOPATHIC - Our knowledge of the toxic effects of Brassica napus is derived from the experience of the Irish famine during which people ate it freely.

Brass. has all the symptoms of impoverished blood, such as growth of downy, colorless hair. Dropsical swellings, scorbutic mouth, voracious appetite.

Tympanitic abdomen. Skin blotches like burns. Dropping off of nails and gangrene. Weariness, strength loss. Wasting, extreme weight loss. Jaundice.

MIND - Irritability. Anxiety. Depression. Distress. Memory disorders

Abdomen - Enlargement of liver. Tympanitic abdomen. Enlargement of spleen. Liver disease.

Back - Pitting edema.

Chest - Pulmonary edema. Chest wall restricted from motion. Pain. Pulmonary hypertension.

Cough - Non-productive cough.

Eyes - Sicea syndrome, reduced or no lachrymation with consequent dryness and inflammation of conjunctiva.

Face - Edema. Scleroderma. Swollen to an enormous extent, the distended state of eyelids and upper lip producing great deformity. Burn-like blotches on nose and forehead (also hands and feet), varying from discoloration to ulceration.

Female - Transient amenorrhea.

Food - Appetite increased, sometimes voracious.

Head - Alopecia. Very distressing frontal headache and tension.

Kidneys - Urine deficient and irritating.

Limbs - Chronic pain. Hands and feet dry and shrunken, with blotches of a deep red, like burns, on backs of hands and dorsa of feet, the fingers and toes being frequently cold and livid, ulceration, loss of nails. Myalgia. Contractures, joints. Claw-hand. Hands, feet. Genu-flexum. Pes Equinnus. Raynauds disease. Cramps, muscles. Wasting, muscles. Arthritis. Arthralgia. Loss of reflex. Weakness. Numbness. Carpal Tunnel Syndrome. Tenderness.

Lungs - Pneumonia. Dyspnea, worse exertion. Respiratory failure.

Mouth - Mucus membrane of mouth and throat inflamed, ulcerated in parts, gums spongy.

Rectum - Bowels torpid.

Skin - Sallow and muddy-looking, covered with downy hair. Edema. Pitting edema. Tenderness. Itching. Blotches, deep red, like burns, on backs of hands, feet, nose and forehead, varying from simple discoloration to most troublesome ulceration. Destruction of cuticle and dropping off of nails. Gangrene. Skin rash. Maculopapular rash. Jaundice. Scleroderma. Hyperaesthesia. Hypoaesthesia. Atrophy. Hyperpigmentation.

Sleep - Sleep disturbances. Insomnia.

Throat - Dysphagia. Mucus membrane of mouth and throat inflamed, ulcerated in parts, gums spongy.

Vision - Xeropthalmia.

COMMENTS - Allen gives this account of Brass. poisoning: They all exhibited indications of deteriorated health, the hue of the skin being uniformly sallow and muddy-looking, totally different from the brown discoloration caused by exposure to the sun, the surface was always covered with that colorless downy hair, so characteristic of what the country people here call "impoverished blood."

An edematous state prevailed generally of the whole body, but a always of the face and lower extremities, the former sometimes being swollen to an enormous extent, the distended state of the eyelids and upper lip especially producing remarkable deformity

The abdomen was tympanitic. The bowels torpid. The mucous membrane of the mouth and pharynx was inflamed, and in some parts ulcerated, and the gums spongy. The appetite was usually greater than natural in some cases voracious. The urinary secretion was deficient and irritating, and that of the skin suspended.

Very distressing frontal headache and tension was also complained of, but the most curious symptom, next to the edematous appearance of the patient, was the state of the hands and feet, which were dry and shrunken, with blotches of a deep red, resembling burns, on the backs of the hands and dorsum of the feet, the fingers and toes being frequently cold and livid.

Similar blotches existed on the nose and forehead, and these varied in their consequence from simple discoloration to ulceration of a most troublesome description, terminating in loss of the cuticle, and dropping off of the nails, with a marked disposition in the aggravated cases to gangrene.

RELATIONS - ***Compare:*** (1) Raph., Armoracea, Sinapis, Sec.

REFERENCES - Allen. Clarke. Murphy. Sherr.

BROMIUM

(Bromine)

PHARMACY - brom. Bromium. Bromine. (Br, At. Wt. 799). Halogens. Must be prepared fresh, as it is predisposed to rapid deterioration. Solution in distilled water. ***Historical dose:*** Tincture and all potencies.

CLINICAL - Aphthae. ***Asthma.*** Breast, cancer. Bronchitis. Cancer. Coughs. Croup. ***Diphtheria.*** Dysmenorrhea. Emaciation. Emphysema. Encysted, tumors. Fainting. Feet, pain. Fistula, lachrymalis. ***Glands, enlargement.*** Goiter. Heart, diseases. Headache. Laryngismus. Migraine. ***Mumps***. Nosebleeds. Palpitations. Parotid gland. Parotid, induration. Respiration, disorders. Scrofula. Seaside, effects. Strokes. Testicles, induration. Throat, sore. Tonsils, enlarged. Tonsils, inflamed. Trachea, irritation. Tuberculosis. Tumors, breast. Ulcers. Uterus, air in. Vagina, air in. Vertigo. Vomiting.

HOMEOPATHIC - Bromine forms a leading constituent in the mineral waters of Kreutzach and Wood hall. Bromine is useful in scrofulous children with enlarged glands, which are swollen and indurated, but seldom suppurate. Like the other Halogens, Bromine is a strong antiscorbutic.

Marked effects on the respiratory tract, especially larynx and trachea. Constriction and membranous formation occur in larynx, spreading upwards. A sense of suffocation. Cough, worse entering warm room. Nosebleed, accompanies many problems especially those pertaining to chest and respiratory tract.

Excoriating discharges. Profuse sweats and great weakness. Weak and easily overheated, then sweaty and sensitive to drafts. Fainting. Tremulous all over. Tendency to spasmodic attacks. Emaciation. Headache worse from drinking milk or from stooping.

Boring pains in bones. Cancer. Breast cancer. Enlarged and indurated glands. ***Glands which become hard, but seldom suppurate. Left-sided mumps***. Complaints from being over-heated. Complaints are worse at seaside, sailors coming ashore suffer from asthma, which is relieved when they go to sea again.

MIND - Much anxiety of the mind. Fears a stroke. Fear of ghosts. Quarrelsome. ***Very bad humor.*** Takes no interest in the household duties. ***Loss of ideas.*** Forgetfulness. Aversion to any kind of work, even reading.

Sad. Indifferent. Low spirited, inconsolable. Does not feel normal, but cannot tell why. Sits alone in her room without doing anything. Looks constantly in one direction without saying anything.

Desires to be carried. Crying and lamentations, with hoarse voice. Cheerful mood, desire for mental labor. Visions when in the dark. Expects to see something jump around the floor. Delusion that strange persons are looking over patient's shoulder and that she would see someone on turning.

Abdomen - Tympanitic abdomen, bloated. Enlargement and induration of spleen. Passage of much wind.

Back - Neck stiff. Goiter. ***Glands of neck much swollen.*** Encysted tumors on sides of the neck. Aching at inner border left scapula. Boring in spinous processes of different vertebrae. Glands of neck enlarged. Cystic tumors on both sides of neck.

Breasts - Tumors in breasts with sharp pains, worse left. Sharp pains from breast to axilla. Sharp, shooting pains in left breast, worse pressure. Suppression of menses in scirrhus breasts. Hard, uneven tumor in right breast.

Chest - Violent cramping of chest. Chest pains run upward. ***Cold sensation when inspiring.***

Constitutions - Suited to scrofulous children with enlarged glands. Blue-eyed, fair people, especially children with thin, pale, delicate skins and very light hair and eyebrows to scrofulous constitutions. Blondes.

Ears - Hard swelling of the parotid gland, warm to touch after eruptive fevers. Noise in ears.

Eyes - Lachrymation with swelling of tear glands. Pupils dilated. Protruding eyes. Flashes before eyes. Darting through the left eye.

Face - Ashy gray. Pale, red, alternating. Swelling and hardness of parotid gland, feeling warm to the touch. Suppuration of left parotid, swelling remaining hard and unyielding. Sensation of cobweb. Seems drawn to a point at nose.

Female - Menses, bright red blood. Menses flow passive with much exhaustion. Dysmenorrhea. Depressed before menses. Queer ill feeling a few days before menses. Menses too early, too profuse, with membranous shreds. Violent contractive spasms before or during menses. Chronic ovaritis. Dull, constant pain, in left ovary. Swelling of ovaries. Itching in vagina. Flatus from vagina, noisy. Vagina as if sore. Suppression of menses in scirrhus breasts. Prolapsed uterus, with mental derangement.

Food - Desire for acids, which aggravate and cause diarrhea. Water tastes salty.

Head - Head congested, fears a stroke. Headache worse drinking milk, stooping. Headache in sun, passes off in shade. Headaches, deep in the vertex with palpitations. Megrim of left side, worse stooping, especially after drinking milk. Headache, worse heat of sun and from rapid motion. Sharp pain through eyes.

Heart - Hypertrophy from gymnastics with palpitations. Cutting pain running upwards, with heart disease. Violent palpitation worse lying on left side. Nervous palpitations with nausea with headache.

Kidneys - Constant desire to urinate with tickling sensation in tip of urethra. Dribbling of urine with burning, after urinating. Urine scanty and dark. Urine turbid, deposits a whitish sediment adhering to vessel. Urine leaves a red coating on vessel. Urine contains large flakes of white mucus. High colored urine with eczema.

Limbs - Icy cold forearms or hands. Boring pain in one or both tibiae. Left arm, lame in cardiac affections.

Lungs - Whooping cough. ***Dry cough with hoarseness and burning pain behind sternum.*** Suffocative fits, choked, croupy or wheezing cough, with palpitations. ***Spasmodic cough with rattling of mucus*** in the larynx, suffocative. Thick white expectoration. Spasms of glottis. Croup after febrile symptoms have subsided. Fibrinous bronchitis. Bronchial tubes feel filled with smoke. Wants to take a deep breath, but it excites cough. Lungs feel coated with down. Every inspiration provokes cough. Colds start in larynx, go upward and downward. Deep hoarseness if heated. Difficult and painful breathing. Larynx is cold. ***Laryngeal diphtheria***, membrane begins in larynx and spreads upward. Dyspnea with great swelling. ***Asthma, difficulty in getting air into lung*** (Chlor. in expelling air). Asthma of sailors going ashore. Better at sea.

Male - Swelling and induration of testes, worse slight jar. Sharp pain in glans and sides of penis. ***Swelling of left testicle, with sore pain, or sensation of coldness.*** Increased sexual desire. Nightly emissions.

Modalities - Better from any motion. Better exercise. Better riding on horseback. Better at sea. Better from nosebleed, shaving. ***Worse from warmth. Worse damp warm.*** Worse Worse overheating. Worse from evening, until midnight. Worse when sitting. Worse in warm room. Worse heat of sun. Worse chilled when hot. Worse cold and damp weather and cold air. Worse water or diet. Worse from sea bathing. Worse dust. Worse draft. Worse lying on left side.

Mouth - Dry, parched. Aphthae with affection of eyes. Water tastes salty.

Nose - ***Tickling, smarting, as from cobwebs***. Fan-like motion of ale (Lyc.). Nosebleed, relieving the chest. Stoppage of right nostril. Long continued, obstinate coryza. Acrid, burning coryza, with violent sneezing and soreness of the nose. Pressure at root of nose.

Perspiration - Sweats from least exertion or exercise. Sweats on palms. Viscous sweat, with cool skin.

Rectum - Painful hemorrhoids with black stool. Hemorrhoids, bleed, intensely painful, worse application of cold or warm water. Diarrhea after eating oysters and sour things.

Skin - Acne, pimples and pustules. Boils on arms and face. ***Glands stony, hard, especially on lower jaw*** and throat. Hard goiter (Spong.). Gangrene.

Sleep - Great drowsiness when reading. Continued yawning in respiratory troubles, with drowsiness. Full of dreams and anguish, jerking and starting during sleep, full of fantasy and illusions, difficult to go to sleep at night, cannot sleep enough in morning, trembling and weak on awaking.

Stomach - Sharp burning from tongue to stomach. Pressure like from a stone. Stomach pain, better eating. Sour things disagree. Vomiting like coffee grounds, bloody mucus. Aversion to customary tobacco smoking.

Temperature - Chills with yawning and stretching, repeated every other day, as a chilliness, and cold feet. Chills on alternate days, with cold feet. Internal burning heat, as if between skin and flesh.

Throat - Tonsils, swollen, deep red, with network of dilated blood vessels. Pain, worse swallowing fluids than solids. Feels raw, evening with hoarseness. Tickling in trachea during inspiration. Hoarseness coming on from being overheated. Even a small goiter oppresses. Stony hard, swollen glands. Diphtheria.

Vertigo - Dizzy when crossing a stream of water. Vertigo worse on bridge. Vertigo at the sight of running water. Vertigo with nosebleed. Vertigo with a tendency to fall backward.

COMMENTS - Migraine, chiefly on left side, worse from stooping, especially after drinking milk. Sensation deep in the brain as if vertigo would come on. Vertigo with a tendency to fall backward, worse at the sight of running water or if he put his foot on a bridge, worse in damp weather. Vertigo with nosebleed.

The glands (thyroid, testes, maxillary, parotid) are swollen and indurated. Tuberculosis, especially of right lung. Hypertrophy of the heart and palpitations. Pain in heart going up to axilla. Exertion causes oppression at heart.

Soreness and crusts inside nose. Nosebleed accompanies many affections, especially of chest. There is a peculiar headache with coryza. Loud emissions of air from the vagina.

Particularly affects the internal head, left side. Predominantly a left-side medicine. Better at the seaside (opposite Nat-m.), but worse in sailors when coming ashore.

Guernsey noted that cases of diphtheria begin in the larynx and run up. In croup with all the croupy sound, there is a loose rattling in the larynx with the breathing and coughing, but no choking in the cough, as there is in Hepar sulph.

RELATIONS - ***Antidotes:*** Am-c., Camph. Salt inhibits the action of Brom. ***Antidoted by:*** Camph., Am. c., Mag-c., Op. Useful after: Iod., Phos., Spong. ***Compare:*** (1) Iod. - but Iod. has worse morning, dark hair and eyes. (2) Chlorum, Lach., Spong., Fl-ac., Hep., Apis, Arg-n., Chin., Con., Coff., Cina., Cupr., Lyc., Merc., Phos. (3) Rhus-t. - cardiac hypertrophy, also Spong., Arn. from over-exertion. (4) Sep., Sulph., Ant-t. (5) Puls. - blondes. Fear of ghosts or visions, also, Acon., Ars., Carb-v., Phos., Sulph. (6) Con., Aster., Hydrobromic acid. ***Compatible:*** Arg-n. - generally after Brom. Kali-c. - emphysema.

EFERENCES - Boericke. Clarke. Murphy. Phatak.

BRUCEA ANTIDYSENTERICA

(Angustura Spuria)

PHARMACY - bruc. Brucea antidysenterica. Angustura spuria. Angustura falsa. Nux vomica cortex. N. O. Loganiacae. Bark of Nux vomica or angustura falsa. Tincture or trituration. ***Historical dose:*** Trituration and all potencies.

CLINICAL - Abdomen, throbbing. Belches. Borborygmi. Headaches. Hypochondriasis. Pain. Tetanus.

HOMEOPATHIC - Although the Brucea symptoms are similar to the pathogenesis of Nux-v., the bark has been experimented with independently. The homeopathic preparation of Nux-v. is prepared from the seed. Brucea contains strychnine, and the symptoms are included in the pathogenesis of Stry. and Nux-v..

Paralyzed lower limbs, worse least touch, ***cries for fear of being touched.*** Tetanic spasms with undisturbed consciousness, worse from noise or liquids. Painful jerking of legs, cramp-like pain in knees, rigid and lame limbs of paralytics.

Disposition to stretch the limbs and to yawn. Great weariness when walking. In the evening, nervous excitement, trembling and tottering when walking. Painful sensation of fatigue in the limbs. Pinching in several parts of the limbs. In the evening, stiffness in the joints and acute drawing pains in the limbs with shootings in the head in the ears and in the chest. "Headache with extreme drowsiness, disappearing in evening."

"Sensation of throbbing in pit of stomach and in entire abdomen." For the pain in the passing of kidney stones or gallstones.

MIND - Irritability, augmented in the evening. Dejection, with want of sleep. Taciturnity and hypochondriasis. Gloomy, melancholy humor with indolence and lassitude. Sad and gloomy on waking in the morning.

Abdomen - Throbbing felt in the abdomen. Painful pinching in the abdomen. Squeezing, as from claws in the abdomen, followed by frequent, small, slimy evacuations. Borborygmi in the abdomen. The pains in the abdomen cease after the first evacuation. Shootings in the umbilicus after the evacuations. Loose evacuations, followed by fainting, which enforces lying down.

Back - Sensation of squeezing in the back.

Chest - On breathing, sensation of great weight on the whole chest. Oppression of the chest with chilly disposition and great sensibility in the open air. In the morning, pain as from a bruise on the outside of the chest, with tight pains on breathing deeply. Pains like excoriation in the interior of the chest, especially in bed at night, which are most violent when lying on the side.

Eyes - Dull and swollen eyes. Eyes red in the corners, in the evening. Eyes red and burning in the morning. Itching in the eyelids. Painful sensation in the eyes, as from sand, rendering it necessary to rub them.

Face - Mealy, itching tetters on the face, followed by peeling off of the skin. Paleness in the face. Slight convulsive, rapid movements in the lips.

Fever - Sweats on walking, with shiverings, which appear chiefly during rest. Chilly disposition and aversion to the open air. Shivering and excessive coldness.

Food - Weak appetite, food at dinner and breakfast appears insipid. After a meal, violent beating of the heart, aggravation of headache, fermentation in the intestines and inclination to evacuate.

Head - Headache, aggravated by sitting, as well as after eating. Shootings in the head, aggravated by walking, especially in the sun. Heaviness and confusion in the head with sleepiness, disappearing in the evening. Digging, crawling in the top of the head. Headache in the evening after having walked a while in the sunshine. Headaches behind the eyebrows, which seem to be swollen.

Limbs - Pains, as of fatigue, in the thighs and loins. Cramp-like pain in the back of the hand. Miliary eruption, red, raised and itching on the back of the hand and on the body. In the evening, sensation of paralysis in the thigh. Weariness in the knees. Curvature of the joint of the foot, so that one walks almost on the anklebone. Sensation of burning in corns.

Mouth - Acute pains in the teeth and gums, especially on drinking cold water. Accumulation of saliva in the mouth, forcing one to spit continually. Dryness and burning pain in the gullet, as if from rancid fat.

Rectum - Evacuations too soft, in too small quantity, and of too light a color. Strong disposition to loose evacuations with colic and flatulency. Loose evacuations in the morning and in the evening. Itching in the anus in the evening.

Sleep - Sleepiness during the entire day, especially when seated, in the morning, early in the evening, and particularly in the afternoon. Sleepiness alternately with want of appetite. Sleep full of dreams, with ebullition of the blood. Sleep troubled with confused or frightful dreams.

Stomach - Clammy taste. Empty belches. Sensation in the stomach, as if nothing had been eaten for a long time. Sensation of burning, heat in the pit of the stomach. Sensation of throbbing in the pit of the stomach and in the entire abdomen. Pressure in the stomach, immediately after eating or drinking. In the evening, attack of nausea with cramp-like pains in the abdomen, vomiting of food and loose evacuations with great prostration.

Vertigo - Vertigo, which occasions falling in the evening.

COMMENTS - Under the name of Brucea antidysenterica, a quantity of Nux-v. bark got upon the drug market and was at first supposed to be Angustura bark. Many poisonings ensued before the mistake was discovered and the bark received the name Angustura falsa in contradistinction to the true Angustura.

RELATIONS - ***Compare:*** (1) The following also have drowsiness with headache: Gins., Hera., Nux-m., Nat-s., Sulph. (2) Gels. - difficult to keep the eyes open.

REFERENCES - Clarke.

BRUCELLA MELITENSIS

(Brucella Nosode)

PHARMACY - brucel. Brucella melitensis. Brucella nosode. ***Historical dose:*** All potencies.

CLINICAL - Anorexia. Backaches. Brucellosis. Chills. Cirrhosis. Coma. Constipation. Depression. Emaciation. Epilepsy. Faintness. Fatigue. Fever. Glands, swollen. Headaches. Hemochromatosis. Insomnia. Intermittent, fever. Joint, pains. Muscle, pain. Perspiration, excessive. Undulant, fever. Vertigo. Weakness. Weight, loss.

HOMEOPATHIC - Brucellosis, also known as undulant fever or Mediterranean fever, is caused by the bacterium Brucella. Undulant fever derives its name from the undulating, or up-and-down, temperature.

Brucella bacteria infect cattle, goats, camels, dogs, and pigs. Transmission of the disease to humans occurs by contact with infected meat, the placenta of infected animals, or ingestion of unpasteurized milk or cheese. The illness may be chronic and persist for years.

Acute brucellosis may begin with mild flu-like symptoms with fever, chills, sweating, muscle aches, joint aches and malaise. Fever spikes occur every afternoon to levels around 104° Fahrenheit.

Common symptoms include fever and chills, excessive sweating, weakness, weight loss and fatigue. Loss of appetite. Anorexia, emaciation. Febrile state with profuse sweat, at night, from the least effort. Headache. Insomnia. Vertigo. Faintness.

Muscular and joint pains, especially of the lower limbs. Back pain. Joint and muscle pain. Swollen glands and lymph nodes. Vesicular eruptions. Abdominal pain. Enlarged liver. Constipation, dry and hard stools.

Weariness in the morning with strong desire to sleep. Pricking pains everywhere. Wandering diffuse pains particularly in lumbar region, in thighs, hips, better by motion. Alternation of symptoms, for example the joint pains disappear and cough appears. Periodical complaints, worse in winter, spring, summer, every 2 to 4 weeks.

MIND - Changes mood and behavior. Emotional instability. Irritability and nervousness. Apathy and indifference. Depression. Coma.

Abdomen - Abdominal pain.

Back - Feeling of coldness with shivers in the back. Back pain. Pains in lumbar region, better by motion.

Glands - Swollen glands and lymph nodes.

Limbs - Muscular and joint pains, especially of the lower limbs.

Liver - Cirrhosis. Enlarged liver.

Modalities - Better by occupation. Better in company. Better motion. Better heat, particularly of the sun. Worse from prolonged exercise. Worse when rising from sitting. Worse when motionless. Worse after alcohol, eating. Worse from changes of temperature or weather. Worse warm room. Worse hot summer. Worse damp, wet. Worse storms. Worse in morning. Worse from sea, wind.

Perspiration - Excessive sweating.

Rectum - Constipation, dry and hard stools.

Skin - Blotches and rashes. Vesicular eruptions.

Temperature - Fever and chills. Chills with shivers. Fever, with profuse sweat, depression.

Vertigo - Vertigo with loss of sight and feeling of coldness.

COMMENTS - Roger Schmidt recorded two cases, published in Annales Hom. Fr., No. 2. 1959. The first case concerned M. W. R., a butcher who was 43 years old. He called on Schmidt on the 18th October, 1948, for a fever of 103.4 F in the evening which he's had for three days. Profuse sweat on the upper part of the body, preceded by shivering, which jerks him from head to foot. Restless during the fever, hungry, and has the desire to drink cold water.

While telling Schmidt his history, he noted having been treated for acute brucellosis in 1935, and that half of the workers of the same firm were affected. At that time, M. W. R. stopped his work for a year. The fever, he said caused his hair to fall out, but it, fortunately, grew back.

In 1940 and 1941, he had two new attacks that were treated by serum. In 1949, he relapsed again, complicated with anemia, and was treated by penicillin and vaccines. He told Schmidt that since that time he has always felt weak.

Gels. 6c ameliorated the fever in 24 hours. The temperature did not rise above 99.5° F. One week later, the patient had diarrhea with profuse sweats, rapidly ameliorated by Chin. 6c.

During the next month, he gained 8 pounds and was feeling better. Schmidt's intention was to complete the cure by the nosode, but he did not get the chance because, in order to resume his work, M. W. R. was forced to see the doctors who treated him before.

Schmidt's second case concerned Mrs. H. B. of San Diego, married, age 69. She came to see Schmidt in September 1950, complaining of some gastric troubles, which she had for several months. She was also suffering from gas, vomiting, regurgitations, and a stubborn constipation.

She was constantly depressed and weak, nervous, restless and had shiverings. She felt sudden weakness, had vertigo by the least movement. While she was young she suffered from a perforated appendix. Physical examination was negative, except for a distended abdomen.

After her return to San Diego she asked Schmidt to prescribe by mail. Ars., Sulph., Nux-v., Carb-v., Kali-p., and Carbo-s. all did her some good, but the variety of remedies showed that the case was jumbled when it was difficult to get a simillium.

Finally in July, 1951, Schmidt had the idea that this may be a case of Brucel. The sudden attack of fever and sweats, weight loss (seven pounds), and the persistence of some symptoms indicated the diagnosis.

Schmidt gave her Brucel. 10m. Without any delay, the patient informed Schmidt that this was the first remedy that gave her almost instantaneous result. She soon took up weight, but after six weeks she complained anew of serious vertigo and the stubborn constipation. She was given Brucel. 30c, and for 3 months her condition was satisfactory.

On December 6th, 1951, her fever returned with profuse sweat and abdominal pains. Schmidt gave her Brucel. 10m, which caused a moderate aggravation but clearly ameliorated during the next two weeks, with a maximum temperature of 100° F during the day, which ended in a long period of amelioration lasting for 3 years.

RELATIONS - ***Compare:*** (1) Nat-m. - Emaciation with anemia, cachexia. depression, headaches, constipation, sensitiveness to cold, desire for salt, mapped tongue. (2) Gels. - General weakness with tremblings; headache with heaviness; weakness of limbs, slow pulse. (3) Ferr-p - Febrile states with full, rapid and soft pulse, thirst and sweats that does not ameliorate.

REFERENCES - Julian. Murphy.

BRUCINUM

(Brucine)

PHARMACY - brucin. Brucinum. Brucine. An alkaloid obtained from the bark and seeds of Strychnos nux vomica. N. O. Loganiacae. Tincture or trituration. ***Historical dose:*** All potencies.

CLINICAL - Headaches. Paralysis.

HOMEOPATHIC - Lepelletier noted that Brucin. caused sudden jerking, especially of the lower limbs, spreading generally, but not accompanied by trismus or tetanus, and not extending to the esophagus and pharynx as with Strychnia. Twitching in the paralyzed as well as healthy muscles. A fever of short duration ends the attacks, after which deep sleep comes on.

RELATIONS - ***Compare:*** (1) Stry., Nux-v., Brucea antidys.

REFERENCES - Clarke.

BRYONIA ALBA

(Wild Hops)

PHARMACY - bry. Bryonia alba. Wild hops. Bryonia dioica. White Bryony. N. O. Cucurbitaceae. Tincture of root procured before flowering. ***Historical dose:*** Tincture and all potencies.

CLINICAL - Alcoholism. Amenorrhea. Anger, effects. Angina pectoris. Ankle, injuries. ***Appendicitis.*** Aphthae. ***Arthritis.*** Asthma. ***Backache. Bilious attack.*** Bones, broken. Brain disorders. Breast-feeding, disorders. Breast inflamed. Bronchitis. Cancer. Chills. Chlorosis. Constipation. Coryza. ***Coughs.*** Dehydration. Dentition. Diaphragm, rheumatism. Diarrhea. Dropsy. Dyspepsia. Eczema. Edema. Enteric fever. Gastroenteritis. Glaucoma. Hemorrhages. Hands, swollen. ***Headaches.*** Heart, pain. Hernias. Hiccoughs. Hydrocele. Hydrocephalus. ***Influenza. Injuries.*** Intermittent fevers. Jaundice. ***Joints, pain.*** Knee, injuries. Liver, disorders. Lumbago. ***Lymphangitis.*** Mastitis. Measles. Meningitis. Menstruation, vicarious. ***Migraine.*** Milk fever. Muscle pain. Nephritis. Nosebleeds. Ovaritis. Peritonitis. Phlegmasia alba dolens. ***Pleurodynia. Pleurisy. Pneumonia.*** Pregnancy. Puerperal fever. Pyuria. Relapsing fever. Remittent fever. ***Rheumatism.*** Scarlatina. Sciatica. Spina bifida. Stiff-neck. Strokes. Suppressed, eruptions. Tongue, coated. Toothache. Trachea, pain. Tuberculosis. Vertigo. Waterbrash. Whooping cough. Yellow fever.

HERBAL - The common Bryony of England is the Bryonia dioica, which has been substituted for the Bryonia alba and has probably identical properties, but the alba alone has been proved, and consequently this should always be dispensed. Bryonia dioica is a popular remedy for "black-eye" as a local application.

HOMEOPATHIC - Bry. is one of the polycrest remedies of the homeopathic Materia Medica. Less rapid in its action than Acon., but it goes deeper in its effects and often takes up the work where Acon. leaves off. It not only disorders the circulation, but alters the blood itself. Vicarious bleeding. Corresponds to fevers of almost all kinds, especially rheumatic, typhoid, bilious and remitting.

Affects on all serous membranes and the viscera they contain, causing inflammation and exudation. ***Mucus membranes are all dry***. Discharges are scanty and adherent. Dryness everywhere, of mouth, throat etc. ***Dry hacking painful coughs*** in pleurisy, pneumonia. ***Streaks of red in lymphangitis.*** Dry, parched lips and mouth. ***Excessive thirst,*** bitter taste in the mouth.

Rheumatic pains and swellings, dropsical effusions into synovial and serous membranes. Aching in joints and muscles. ***Injury of the joints*** (when Arn. fails). Every spot in the body is painful to pressure. ***Pains are bursting***, stitching or heavy sore, going backwards, ***tearing, worse by motion, better rest***. Stitching pains in the chest. Muscles become hard after neuralgia.

Pressure headaches. Severe headaches. ***Bursting, splitting headaches***. Vertigo from raising the head. Physical weakness, on slightest exertion. Dropsical swellings gradually increase as the day progresses and disappear during the night. Sensitive epigastrium and feeling of a stone in the stomach. Stools large, dry, hard.

Complaints develop slowly but forcibly. ***Aggravation from motion, movement*** of all kinds. Avoids even the movement of the eyes, raising head from pillow causes faintness, nausea and vomiting. ***Better from pressure,*** from lying on painful side. Right-sided effects. Tendency to great ***irritability*** and bad temper.

Children dislike to be carried or raised. Persons who over-eat or eat excessively of meat, and have strong constitutions.

MIND - Effects of anger, fright, chagrin or pain. ***Exceedingly irritable***, everything puts him out of humor. Very morose, ill-humored. Ugly in behavior. Easily angered, with biliousness, headache, dyspepsia. Quarrelsome. Worse from arguments, which will give them a headache and pain.

Capricious, hard to please and satisfy. Desire for things that are rejected when offered (Cham., Calc-p.). Desire for things that can't be had. Weeping mood, with headache and other complaints. Hasty disposition.

Easily startled, during headache. Restlessness, wants change.

Determined. Taciturn. Aversion to being disturbed. Intolerance of contradiction. Contradiction causes anger. Irritability during menses. ***Wants to be let alone.*** Aversion to company. Desire to be independent, difficulty asking for help. Aversion to being touched.

Fright, fear and vexation. Apprehension and dread for future. ***Talks of business.*** Worried about money and the future. ***Fearful of poverty.*** Fear of thunderstorm. Insecure. Despair of being cured with fear of death. Worry about their health. Despair of recovery. Anxiety better open air.

Mental state, better from cool temperature, wants windows open. Oversensitiveness of senses to external impressions. ***Child dislikes to be carried or to be touched.*** Dullness of mind. Weakness of mind, so that his ideas disappear. Delirium, wants to go home, thinking he is not there.

Abdomen - Distension of abdomen with colic after eating. Abdomen very sore to touch, with constipation. Appendicitis. Peritonitis. Gastroenteritis. Abdominal wall very tender. Griping, pinching colic. ***Burning, sharp pain, worse from pressure, coughing, breathing***. Movements, loud rumbling or a gurgling and soreness and dragging downward. Pain from movement of flatus. Epigastrium, tender, throbbing. Groin sore before menses.

Back - Complaints from over lifting, concussion. Backache from over lifting. ***Severe painful back injuries, worse any motion.*** Scapular numbness or pain going to epigastrium or from left scapula to heart. ***Slipped disks with sharp pains.*** Lumbago, worse stooping. ***Sharp pains and stiffness in lumbar region***. Pain in the small of back worse walking or turning. Sharp pain in lumbar region during cough. Backache from sudden changes of weather. ***Vertebrae out of place causing much pain and immobility.*** Joints and muscles of lumbar region stiff and tender, preventing motion and stooping, worse standing or sitting, better lying. Brachial neuragia.

Back - ***Painful stiffness of neck, worse motion.*** Drawing and stiffness in muscles of right side of neck. Cervical glands sore to touch. Spina bifida.

Breasts - Pain in breasts at menstrual period. Mastitis, stony hard breasts. ***Breasts hot and painful, hard***. Abscess of breasts. Milk fever. Swollen breasts.

Causations - Ill effects of anger, fright, chagrin. Complaints from taking cold drinks in hot weather. Alcohol. Gluttony. Suppressed eruptions and discharges. Constipation. Broken bones, joint injury, wounds. Cold winds.

Chest - Angina pectoris. Holds chest or presses the sternum when coughing. ***Sharp pains in chest, worse motion, deep breathing and coughing.*** Sticking pain, in chest, better pressure or lying upon painful side. Sticking pain in sternum when pressing upon it. Heaviness beneath the sternum extending towards the right shoulder. Internal heat in chest. Sharp pains in cardiac region. Sharp pain from left to right side of chest, during inspiration. Rheumatism of muscles of chest. Ribs sore, as if beaten.

Constitutions - Suited to a robust, firm fiber and dark complexion with tendency to leanness and irritability. Gastro-bilious-rheumatic constitutions. Choleric, bilious tendency with firm fleshy fiber. Adapted to nervous, dry, slender people.

Cough - ***Dry, hacking cough*** from irritation in upper trachea. ***Cough, dry, hard, very painful,*** at night as if from stomach. Cough with sneezing. ***Coming into warm room excites cough*** (Nat-c.). Cough with feeling as if head and chest would fly to pieces. ***Very painful coughs must hold the chest.*** Nausea excites cough, and coughing often excites vomiting. Coughs with gagging, without nausea. ***Cough with sharp pains in sides of chest.*** Cough compels patient to spring up in bed involuntary and immediately. Whooping cough. Coughs, worse motion, talking and laughing. Painful coughs with bronchitis, pleurisy, pneumonia.

Ears - As if stopped-up. Otorrhea following inflammation. Boil in front of ear.

Vicarious bleeding from ears. Intolerance of noise. Aural vertigo. Roaring, buzzing, ringing, humming in ears. Chirping, as from locusts. Humming in left ear, resembling pouring of water over a dam.

Eyes - Eyeballs sore. Burning in eyes, inflammation, worse warmth. Pains behind the eyeballs. Glaucoma. Pressing, crushing, aching pains. Aching and pulsation in left orbit. Lachrymation during day, especially in the sun. Lids swollen and puffed. Sore to touch. ***Sore when moving eyes.*** Sharp pain like a needle going through eye. Itching and burning of margins of lids. Sensation as if sand in eyes. Gout shifting to eyes. Aversion to light, especially sunlight.

Face - Dark red, hot, bloated. Yellowish paleness. Heat of face with redness and thirst. Redness of face after getting angry. Face bluish-red, during difficult respiration. Lips, dry, as if burnt, parched, cracked, wants to moisten them. Picking of lips. Burning of lower lip in old smokers. Chewing motions in brain disorders of children. Twitching in corners of mouth. Small nodules and induration. Tetters in face.

Female - Menstrual irregularities with gastric symptoms. Menses, dark, foul. Menses too early, too profuse, worse from motion, with tearing pains in legs. ***Menses suppressed with vicarious discharge or splitting headache***. Frequent bleeding of nose at appearance of menses. Ovaritis. ***Inter-menstrual pain with a great abdominal and pelvic soreness*** (Ham.). Pain in right ovary as if torn, extending to thigh (Lil-t., Croc.). Sharp pains in ovaries on taking a deep inspiration, very sensitive to touch.

Food - Craves what he cannot relish. Loathing for food. Canine hunger after nausea. Irritability after eating. Aversion to greasy food. Aversion to milk, but when he takes it he relishes it. ***Great desire for coffee, wine and acid drinks.*** Desire for meat, oysters, sweets. Desire for warm drink, and better by it. Worse bread. Cabbage causes diarrhea. ***Sauerkraut, cabbage, potatoes and other vegetables, disagree.*** Worse warm drinks, which are vomited. Gastric derangement after old sausages, old cheese, cabbage, sauerkraut, fruit, turnips, salads, milk, etc. Drinks hastily and eagerly. ***Thirst, for large quantity of cold water,*** also for warm drinks, which ameliorate.

Head - Gastric, rheumatic, congestive, bilious headaches. ***Migraine headaches, worse on any motion***, even that of the eyeballs, better from closing eyes. Pressure in head, as if brain were too full, worse sitting. ***Bursting, splitting headache***, as if everything would be pressed out. Bursting pain, with dry, parched lips. ***As if hit by a hammer from within, worse from motion, stooping, opening eyes.*** Pain over left eye, pressive, going to occiput, then spreading over whole body. ***Severe sharp pains in head, worse motion.*** Headache in occiput. Headache from ironing. Headache when constipated. Frontal headache, frontal sinuses involved. Bones drawing in towards zygoma. Vertex as if bruised. Headaches better from tying up head. Mental exertion aggravates head pains. Rheumatic pains, in cold, damp, wet seasons. Scalp very sensitive, can't bear even a soft brush, every hair pains. Dandruff, rough and uneven. ***Hair very greasy***. Cold sweat on head.

Heart - Angina pectoris. ***Sharp pain in cardiac region, worse motion.*** Sharp pain, cramp in region of heart, worse walking, motion or slightest exertion. Heart beats violently and rapidly. Palpitations with dyspnea. Fluttering and palpitations on going up stairs. Burning in veins. Endocarditis. Pulse frequent at night, slower during day. Pulse tense and hard. ***Pulse full and quick.*** Intermittent pulse with strong orgasm of blood.

Kidneys - Pain in region of kidneys. Involuntary urination during exertion. Involuntary discharge of urine from cough. Burning and cutting pain before urination. Burning in urethra, when not urinating. Urination frequent, but scanty. Obliged to rise at night to urinate. Urine, red, brown, like beer, scanty, hot. Urine whitish, turbid.

Limbs - Joints with sharp and tearing pains, worse on least movement. ***Sprained, injured and painful joints, worse motion.*** Severe pain from broken bones. ***Joints red, swollen, hot.*** Swelling of elbow. Painful stiffness of limbs. ***Pains in joints and limbs better warmth.*** Every spot is painful on pressure. Constant motion of left arm and leg with sighing (Hell.). Sciatica, better lying quietly and on painful side. Knees stiff and painful. ***Ankle or knee injury, swollen, painful and worse motion.*** Knees totter and bend under him when walking. Hot swelling of feet. Pins and needles in soles, preventing walking. Ulcers on fingers and toes. Weariness and heaviness in all limbs.

Liver - Liver heavy, swollen, sore, tensive, better lying on it. Jaundice. Symptoms of inflammation of liver. Burning and sharp pain in hepatic region.

Lungs - Bronchitis. Asthma. Paroxysms of asthma, at night. ***Pleurisy with sharp pains, worse motion.*** Difficult, quick respiration, worse every movement, caused by sharp pains in chest. Croup and pleuro-pneumonia. ***Dyspnea, must sit up, worse after eating or drinking, with sharp pain in chest.*** Dyspnea painful, so that he could not talk. Sighing and sobbing. Dyspnea with rapid breathing. Wants to take deep breath, but cannot or it excites cough. ***Pneumonia with painful cough.*** Rusty, tenacious sputum. Brick colored, blood-streaked sputum. Sputum like lumps of jelly. Tough mucus in trachea, loosened only with much hawking. Yellowish mucus. Dry, friction sound.

Male - Sharp pains in right testicle and spermatic cord. Sharp pains in testicles when sitting. Red, itching eruption on glans penis. Increased sexual desire.

Modalities - ***Better from lying on painful side. Better from pressure.*** Better bandaging. ***Better rest, being quiet.*** Better drawing knees up. Better sitting up, descending. ***Better from cold things.*** Better cold food or drink. ***Better cool open air.*** Better cloudy, damp days. Better heat to inflamed part. Better exhaling.

Modalities - ***Worse from least motion.*** Worse lying on the painless side. ***Worse raising up, stooping. Worse coughing, deep breathing. Worse exertion, touch.*** Worse from dry cold or heat. ***Worse becoming hot. Worse in room.*** Worse hot weather. Worse drinking while hot. Worse from eating, vegetables, acids. ***Worse from anger, vexation.*** Worse calomel. Worse suppressions. Worse taking cold. Worse 3 a.m. to 4 a.m. Worse evening, 9 p.m. Worse in the early morning. Worse summer.

Mouth - ***Dryness of mouth, tongue and throat with excessive thirst.*** Offensive smell from mouth, with hawking of offensive, tough mucus. ***Taste bitter,*** cannot swallow food, better cold drinks. Soapy, frothy saliva. Burning in lower lip in old smokers. ***Lips parched, dry, cracked.*** Sore mouth in infants, child does not want to take hold of breast, but after mouth becomes moist it nurses well.

Nose - Fluent coryza, watery or greenish. Headache following checked coryza. Descending colds. Dry nasal catarrh. Coryza with shooting and aching in the forehead. ***Vicarious nosebleeds,*** when menses should appear. Nosebleeds in pregnancy. Nosebleeds in the morning relieving the headache. Swelling of tip of nose, feels as if it would ulcerate when touched. Inflamed and ulcerated nostrils. Boils. Sneezing between coughs. Loss of smell.

Perspiration - Sweat, sour or oily after slight exertion. Easy, profuse perspiration. Profuse sweat at night and in morning. Suppressed sweat, during confinement and ill-effects therefrom. Oily sweat. Sweats in short spells and on single parts. Perspiration relieves.

Rectum - Burning in anus with stools. Burning in rectum during evacuation of stool and urine. As if a plug in anus. ***Constipation.*** Hard stool passed with great exertion, with confusion of head. Constipation on going to sea. Constipation of nursing babies and lying-in women. Constipation during pregnancy. Diarrhea after castor oil. Diarrhea alternating with constipation. Diarrhea after suppression of exanthemata. Aching hemorrhoids. Passage of offensive flatus. Prolapse of rectum during stool.

Skin - Dry skin. Skin, yellow, pale swollen, dropsical. Slow development or sudden receding of rash in eruptive fevers. ***Undeveloped measles.*** Burning, itching eruptions. Itching, better scratching, worse walking rapidly. Erysipelas. Seborrhea. Nettle-rash. Red elevated rash, like eruptions, over whole body. Rash, better getting warm in bed. Hard nodes in various parts of body. Cold feeling in putrid ulcers.

Sleep - Drowsy, starting when falling asleep. Sleepiness during and after stool. Frequent yawning the whole day. Somnambulism. Restless sleep before midnight. Sleeplessness on account of heat and thirst. Sleeplessness from crowding of thoughts. ***Sleeps on back.*** Kicks covers off. Talks irrationally when he first wakes out of sleep. Dreams of hard work. Dreams about household affairs, business of the day. Anxious dreams and screaming out. Dreams of dispute and vexation.

Stomach - Dyspeptic ailments during summer heat. Burning pain in stomach. Tasteless eructations. ***Stomach sensitive to touch.*** Throbbing in pit. ***Pressure in stomach after eating, as of a stone***. Soreness in stomach when coughing. Shooting pain, with belching. Sharp pain in stomach on motion, arresting breathing. Numbness in stomach. Constant nausea with constipation. ***Nausea and faintness when rising up.*** Nausea lying on right side. ***Nausea and vomiting from slightest motion.*** Bitter vomiting of bile and water, immediately after eating. Vomiting of blood. Vomits solid food only. Vomiting of bitter, musty or putrid liquid, which leaves a similar taste in mouth. Worse warm drinks, which are vomited.

Stools - ***Stools, large dry, very hard.*** Stools, as if burnt. Stools, brown, thick, bloody. Stools, loose, painless, undigested. Stools, ***worse in morning,*** worse from ***moving***, worse after being heated from cold drinks, worse every spell of hot weather. Involuntary stool during sleep. Yellow, mushy stools. Lumps of tough mucus after stools. Gushing diarrhea, worse in the morning, on rising, eating cabbage. Stools offensive, bilious, acrid, smelling like old cheese.

Teeth - Gums pain as if sore and raw, with painful loose teeth. Aching of gums with teething children (Dol.). Toothache when coughing. Toothache, better cold water, worse brushing teeth. Jerking pain when smoking or chewing tobacco. Toothache about 3 a.m. Teeth feel too long. Toothache, as if an exposed nerve in a hollow tooth was in pain from cold air.

Temperature - Chilliness predominates. Chill with external coldness, dry cough, stitches. Chill with hot head and red face, worse warm room. Chill after anger. Coldness and rigors during stool. Dry burning heat, with worsening of all symptoms. Blood seems hot. Fever with desire to uncover. Rheumatic fever and typhoid fever marked by gastro-hepatic complications. Painful continued fevers.

Throat - Hoarseness, worse in open air. Dryness, sticking on swallowing, scraped and constricted (Bell.). Hawks brown lumps with effort. Dryness and rawness of throat worse in warm room. Back of throat seems swollen. Aphthous patches, recurring. ***Sharp pain when swallowing.*** Pressive pain in right tonsil. Pain, pressure and soreness in trachea, pain worse talking and smoking. Soreness in larynx and trachea. Tough mucus in larynx and trachea, loosened only after much hawking, worse coming into warm room. Voice nasal or raised.

Tongue - Dryness of tongue. Dry, white, filthy tongue. Aphthae on tip of tongue. Tongue coated yellowish, dark brown. Tongue coated heavily white in gastric derangement. Tongue coated along centre, red at base. Trembling of tongue. Tongue thinly coated yellow, with longitudinal fissure. White tongue with red edges.

Vertigo - Aural vertigo (Aur., Nat-sal., Sil., Chin.). Vertigo, nausea, confusion. ***Vertigo, dizzy or faint on rising up.*** Vertigo felt in occiput. Vertigo, as though all objects are whirling. ***Vertigo worse on least motion.*** Vertigo, as if sinking deep down in the bed, better cold. Vertigo, as if brain were turning around. Vertigo on turning head or on stooping.

Vision - Dim vision. Every object appears covered with rainbow colors, followed by photophobia. Letters run together when reading. Bluish haze.

COMMENTS - Primary distinguishing symptoms are a slow onset of a disease, dryness of the mouth and skin and a thirst for cold drinks. Any complaint is worse motion, patient will immobilize affected area, frozen with pain.

Intermitting fever, chill mixed with heat. During chill, head hot, cheeks deep red, decided thirst, generally for large quantities at long intervals, sweat worse by least motion, sour or oily. Fever with a stupid, drowsy condition or mild delirium in which the patient has the delusion that he is somewhere else and "wants to go home." Chilliness predominates.

Dry, burning heat as if blood burning in veins. Sweat profuse at night and morning, sour or oily.

Headache or neuralgia in (left) side of head and face, better from hard pressure and cold applications, worse moving. Dull headache, frontal or bursting, splitting. Headache is worse by any motion or by the concussion of cough, and it goes from the front to back of head. The headache of alcoholics, of over-feeding or constipation. Nausea and faintness when rising up, better when lying still.

Migraines with splitting, sharp pain, throbbing nausea and vomiting. They want to go into a dark room and be left alone. Sensation of hammers hitting their head (Nat-m.). Better hard pressure, can be worse light touch. Worse motion, light, sound, any stimulation. Headache with bursting pain, as if their head will explode. Eye movement can cause severe pain, occipital pain is sharp. With sinus headache, sinuses become dry.

Dry mucus membranes, especially those of the mouth and stomach, deficient secretion. Serous membranes are inflamed, the seat of sharp, stitching pains, worse from motion, later on there is exudation.

Muscles are inflamed and sore. Flu with soreness and aching in the joints, pain, worse motion.

The respiratory organs and heart are profoundly affected. Lungs are dry, good for dry, hacking cough that goes into the chest in pneumonia and bronchitis. Respiration becomes worse with deep breathing, try to breath as little as possible. Cough, worse morning. "Frequent desire to take a long breath, must expand the lungs" Want open, fresh air, felt better in cold air.

Hemorrhages. Nosebleeds, especially in the night, 3 to 4 a.m., which is characteristic. This may or may not be preceded by a sense of fullness in the head. Nosebleeds consequent on suppression of the menses is characteristic.

Mouth very dry, tongue coated white down the middle, the edges may be quite clean, later it becomes yellow with bitter taste. Lips are dry and cracked.

Toothache, better by pressing head into pillow, by cold applications. Tendency to chew lips, pick nose or cracked lips, or grind teeth. Brain disorders with a constant motion of the mouth as if chewing. Dirty wash-leather, foul tongue, congested eyes, bitter nausea.

Food lies at the epigastrium like a stone, better bringing up wind. The digestion is worse in summer. Symptoms worse after a meal. A coarse feeder. Bry. is a gourmand (Nux-v., an epicure). There is intolerance of vegetable food. Everything tastes bitter. Gastric derangement "absolutely requires water as a dissolvent." Thirst for large quantities. Burning thirst, for cold drinks, worse from beer. Dehydration in the GI, causing constipation, and joint, causing arthritis.

"Belchings of tasteless gas." Sour stomach. Constipation, atony of the bowels. Stool large, dry, hard, brown or black, as if burnt or charred, crumbling (Plat. has sticky, tenacious stool, sticks to rectum). Stools smell of old cheese. Can have no desire to stool. Diarrhea worse in the morning.

The liver is tender and inflamed. The kidneys also are inflamed, the urine being dark red without deposit (from excess of coloring matter). Appendicitis with nausea, vomiting, fever and rebound tenderness (Bell.). Mastitis, hard, tender. Left ovarian pain, better lying on painful side.

Dropsical swellings, swellings of the legs, sensitive to touch. "Joints red, swollen, stiff with stitching pain from slightest motion." Synovial swellings. Symptoms are worse with stiffness.

Ankle injuries, the slightest movement causes severe pain. Trauma injuries. Low back problems, slipped disks. Whiplash where the neck is frozen with pain and they don't want to be touched, will immobilize neck as movement causes great pain.

Fixation due to pain worse from motion. Worse with any effort, they move only because there is pain. Will cling to support. Lying on the painful part keeps the part at rest. There is also an intense headache, dull throbbing or sharp stabbing pains, sharp pain in or over eyes. Head greasy, scalp tender, eyeballs tender. All their symptoms become worse at 9 p.m. and 3 a.m.

Irritable. Constantly finding dissatisfaction. Hasty speech. Dreams of the occupations of the day. The child kicks the covers off. Often of a dark complexion and hair, choleric, bilious tendency with firm fleshy fiber, tendency to great irritability and bad temper.

Clarke cured a case of congenital hydrocele with Bry.

Van den Berghe found Bry. singularly curative in chlorosis, with diarrhea and constipation. Diarrhea occurs in the morning "as soon as he moves" from cold drinks in warm weather, on every spell of hot weather.

Teste took Bryonia as the type of a group which includes All-s., Lyc., Dig., Nux-v., Coloc. and Ign. All these act with much more power on carnivorous than on herbivorous animals. They are thus appropriate to persons who over-eat or eat excessively of meat and have strong constitutions, "persons accustomed to rich living with rich blood, firm resisting flesh." Teste regarded the digestive canal, and more particularly the stomach, as the principal seat of the action of Bry.

A case of facial eczema was cured with it in an infant five months old, presenting the additional symptoms of constipation, peevish, fretful, thirsty, face and lips are cracked and sore. The child scratched continually. The mother had a similar eruption for some years and it disappeared suddenly at the sixth month of her pregnancy.

RELATIONS - ***Antidotes:*** Acon., Cham., Nux-v.. Bryonia is ***Antidoted by:*** Acon., Alum., Camph., Cham., Chel., Clem., Ign., Mur-ac., Nux-v., Puls., Rhus-t., Seneg. Teste found by accident, Ferr-m. the best antidote in his experience. ***It antidotes:*** Alum., Chlorum, Chin., Frag., Merc., Rhus-t. ***Compare:*** (1) Asc-t., Kali-m., Ptelia. (2) The Cucurbitaceae - all have belching with unaltered taste of food. (3) Acon. - pallor on rising up. Acon. has more restlessness and tossing about is full of fears, Bry. must keep still. (4) Amm., Ant-c. (nausea, vomiting and diarrhea, aversion to milk), Arn. (hemorrhages, wounds, soreness all over, also Bapt.), Ars. (unlike Bry. drinks often and little and eats seldom but much), Asc-t. (pleurisy). (5) Bell. (delirium, hasty speech, hasty drinking. Bell. has headache worse lying down, Bry. must lie down, Bell. has worse lying on painful side, Bry. better lying on painful side. (6) Bell. has *"chewing motion of jaws"* but without the dry, cracked lips of Bry.). (7) Calc. like Bry., Chin. and Bell., has *"as soon as he closes his eyes sees all sorts of objects"*, Carb-v. (miliaria), Caust., Cham., Ign., Ip. (miliaria). (8) Kali-c., chest affections, sharp pains in right hypochondrium shooting up into chest, sharp pain coming from lower lobe right lung, but Kali-c. has not necessarily worse by motion. (9) Kreos., Lach., Lyc., Merc., Nat-s. (morning diarrhea), (10) Nat-m.. - headache in morning, oily, sour sweat on face, Bry. on head generally, cracked lips, Bry. and Nat-m. go well together and are often complementary. ***Complementary:*** Alum., Rhus-t. Alum. is the *"chronic"* of Bry. and Kali-c. and Nat-m., hold a similar but less pronounced relation to it. ***Complementary:*** Upas when Bryonia fails. Rhus-t., Alumina.

REFERENCES - Boericke. Clarke. Murphy. Phatak.

BUFO RANA

(Toad Poison)

PHARMACY - bufo. Bufo rana. Toad poison. Bufo satytiensis. Bufo vulgaris. N. O. Bufonide, Batrachide. Europe, Asia, Japan. Solution of the poison expressed from the cutaneous glands on the back. ***Historical dose:*** Tincture and all potencies.

CLINICAL - Brain, softening. Brain, tumors. ***Breast, cancer.*** Buboes. Cancer. Carbuncles. Convulsions. Decay. Dropsy. Chorea. Convulsions. ***Dropsy. Epilepsy.*** Gout. Heart disorders. Imbecility. ***Impotency.*** Intermittent fever. Leucorrhea. Lumbago. ***Lymphangitis***. Malignant pustules. ***Masturbation, effects.*** Meningitis. Nosebleed. ***Panaritium***. Paralysis. Parkinson's disease. Pemphigus. Phlegmasia alba dolens. Plague. Sciatica. Self-abuse. ***Septic, lymphangitis***. Skin disorders. ***Spasms***. Stammering. Suppuration. Whitlow.

HOMEOPATHIC - Mure proved the common variety, Bufo rana and the Brazilian toad, Bufo Satytiensis. Shakespeare was correct in speaking of the toad as having *"sweltered venom."*

The poison is excreted by glands in the skin of the back. *"Quintessence of toads"* figured largely in the therapy of Salmon's Doron Medicon (1583), where it is commended as a *"Specific in the Dropsy."* Homeopathic provings and poisonings have shown that this reputation is founded on fact.

The chief laurels of Bufo have been won in the treatment of epilepsy. Bojanus cured many cases, and no medicine has served better in the treatment of this disease.

Few people who have witnessed a characteristic epileptic seizure can have failed to notice the curiously toad-like aspect assumed by the subject.

The epileptic seizure and the status epileptic give the clearest correspondence to the Bufo range of action. Epilepsy is often found among the effects of self-abuse in the young.

Remarkable action on nervous system and sexual organs.

Epileptic symptoms. Epileptic seizures occur during night, connected with sexual sphere. Variety of symptoms occur before epileptic spasms. Seizures at the time of menses in women when sexual desire is excited in young men due to onanism or during sex. Falls down unconscious with a blood-curdling scream.

Bufo is indicated in epilepsy when the attacks occur during sleep at night. The patient may or may not be awakened by the attack, if not, when he does awaken he will have violent headache. Epileptic symptoms worse warm room.

Symptoms of Parkinson's disease. Convulsions from suppurative conditions. Fetid discharges and exhalations. Injuries to fingers, pain runs in streaks up the arms. ***Septic lymphangitis,*** due to injuries, when pain runs up in streaks. Striking rheumatic symptoms. As if a peg in joint.

Marked periodicity, quartan fever. Dropsy. Paralysis. Carbuncle. Buboes. Causes low grades of inflammatory action, fetid exhalations and discharges. Cancer. Severe late cancer conditions. Clarke has removed the fetor in hopeless cases of cancer with this remedy.

Affects circulation, causing heat flushings, burning in different parts. Anesthetic spots on skin. Marked uterine symptoms. ***Spasms in children after nursing***, angry or frightened mother. Causes a desire for intoxicating drink and produces impotence. Extremely sensitive to light and noise, the latter is intolerable.

MIND - Confusion and loss of memory, bordering on imbecility. Prematurely senile. Great weakness of memory, idiotic. The mind remains childish, only the body grows. Of use in feeble-minded children. ***Feeble-minded.*** Idiocy, silly, tittering. Talks nonsense, then angry if not understood.

Anxious about health. Fears animals, strangers. Fear of mirrors in room. Biting nails. Nervousness and trembling worse open air. Music is unbearable. Lamenting alternating with crying. Easily laughs or cries. Cries much with epilepsy. Easily startled.

Sad, restless. Sadness on waking. Dullness better evening. Walks the floor and wrings the hands. Ill-humour after menses. Irritability in morning on waking. Irritability at night after retiring. Irritability after menses.

Delirium or apathy, with hot head. Stupor and inability to speak. Deceitfulness. Rage while alone. Propensity to bite. Howling, impatient, nervous, imbecility. Longs for solitude, yet dreads being alone.

Anger before convulsions. Stupefaction between convulsions. ***Unconsciousness after convulsions.***

Moral depravity. Derangements of the sexual sphere. Depravities due to bad inheritance. ***Desire for solitude to practice masturbation.*** It arouses lowest passions, patient is not only low minded but develops low type of disease also.

Abdomen - Colicky pain after drinking milk, and after smoking. ***Violent colic with convulsive movements of jaws and limbs.*** Sensation as if cold balls running through bowels. ***Buboes in groins.*** Convulsive movements in abdomen after spasms. Spasms end by convulsive movements in abdomen. Epileptic attacks originate in abdomen.

Back - Jerks in nape of neck, epileptic attacks. Lumbago, worse rising up or least motion. Swelling of bone, size of a fist. Decay of dorsal vertebrae. Stiff neck after sleep.

Breasts - Mastitis. Bloody oozing from nipples. Bloody milk. ***Breasts cancer.*** Induration in breast glands. Violent pain in breasts, worse at night. Palliative in cancer of breasts. Offensive bloody discharge from breast.

Chest - Sensation as if chest and heart were constricted. Burning like fire in chest. Rapid motion of diaphragm.

Constitutions - Feeble-minded children. Prematurely senile.

Cough - Suffocative. [11] From any emotion. From burning or stitches in larynx. At night, provoked towards 3 or 4 AM by tickling in larynx, which he feels only at this hour. In consequence of cold feet. Violent, with vomiting. Dry, with sharp pain or burning in chest.

Ears - Music is intolerable (Ambr.). Every little noise distresses. Purulent otorrhea, ulceration and bleeding of external ears. Heartbeats reverberate in ears, in meningitis. Pains worse cold washing. Swelling of ears and parotids.

Eyes - Eyes red, injected. Itching, swollen, painful. Eyes sunken during epileptic attack. Burning, itching and ulceration of lids. Left eyelid paralyzed. Little blisters form on eye. Right eye open, left nearly closed. Eyeballs rolled upward and to left before attack. Strabismus. Aversion to the sight of brilliant objects. Pupils dilated.

Face - Face greyish. Burning and redness of swollen face. Lips black. Face bloated and distorted, mouth and eyes convulsed. Bathed in sweat during spasms. Sweat runs down face. Momentary hot flushes of face. Phlegmonous erysipelas, which leaves face deformed. Cold water causes pricking of face.

Female - Menses too early, too copious. ***Epilepsy with menses.*** Menses with headache. Menstrual pains run into legs. After menses, ill-humored. Offensive, bloody discharge, clots. Watery leucorrhea. Offensive purulent leucorrhea. Burning and swelling in ovaries and uterus. Burning heat and sharp pain in ovaries. Hydatids in ovaries. ***Ulceration of cervix,*** with burning pains. Tumors and polyps of the womb. Milk-leg. Veins swollen. Cord like swelling from groin to knee, milk leg. Sexual excitement with epileptic attacks. Cancer of uterus. Veins swollen. Swelling and great sensitiveness of ovarian region.

Food - Desire for sweet drinks. Desire for sugar-water. Longing for brandy, delights in getting drunk. Aversion to food and drink.

Head - Face bathed in sweat. Congestive headaches with flushed face. Pillow hurts occiput. Pressure like two iron hands holding temples. Headaches after breakfast. One-sided headaches, worse by light and noise. Numbness of brain before epileptic attack. ***Headache with epilepsy.*** Head at first drawn to one side, then backwards before an attack. Lancinating pain in occiput, inclining head to fall backward, in meningitis. Violent orgasm in head. Profuse sweat on head. Hair falls out. Sensation as if hot vapor rose to top of head.

Heart - Feels too large. Heaviness about heart. Rapid heart action in exophthalmos. Palpitations with headache during menses. Constriction about heart. Palpitations after eating. Palpitations with nausea. Palpitations on awaking. Heart seems to float in water or air. Sticking pain about apex of heart. Palpitations and oppression from walking fast. Paralysis of heart. Pulse more rapid and threadlike as epileptic attacks multiplied.

Kidneys - Burning pain in kidneys, with oppressed breathing and faintness. Involuntary urination. ***Hematuria in childbed.*** Frequent discharge of pale urine. Suppression of urine. Urine brown, offensive.

Limbs - Trembling of limbs. Limbs become stiff, numb. Cramps in limbs worse cold air. Bruised pains, trembling, cramps, arthritic swellings. Arms go to sleep easily. Swelling of hands and arms, burning pains. ***Lymphangitis*, *red streaks under skin.*** Staggering gait. Feeling as if a peg were driven in joint. ***Panaritium***, swelling blue-black around nail, pain in streaks up arm. Sciatica. Contusive pains in arms, legs and loins, during motion. Arthritic pains, worse after sleep. Swelling of bones. Epileptic attacks preceded by restless movements of limbs and body.

Liver - Enlargement of liver. Pulsating, pain in liver like an abscess, with vomiting of bile.

Lungs - Burning like fire in lungs. Suffocative cough. Asthma. Difficult breathing from compression of larynx, trachea and heaviness of chest, must sit up or bend forward. Anxious, difficult, gets shorter and shorter, during fever. Dyspnea, pants like a dog. Mucus or bloody expectoration, or pure blood, raised most in morning and evening, with sensation of cold in chest.

Male - ***Buboes***. Disposition to fondle organ (Hyos., Zinc.). ***Disposition to masturbation.*** Effects of onanism. Involuntary emissions. ***Impotence***, ejaculation too quick. Spasms during sex.

Male - Semen is discharged too quickly, without pleasurable sensation, sometimes with cramps or painful heaviness in limbs.

Modalities - Better from cold bathing. Better putting feet in hot water. Better cool air. Better bleeding. Worse from warm room. Worse sexual excitement. Worse from masturbation. Worse least motion and injuries. Worse on waking. Worse with a full moon.

Mouth - Burning in mouth, as from acid, worse cold water. Bloody saliva. ***Constant licking of lips.*** Fetid odor from mouth. Stuttering and stammering, angry when not understood. Falling out of teeth. Convulsions after extracting teeth. Mouth wide open before epileptic attack. Ejection of frothy, bloody saliva from mouth during epileptic attack.

Nose - Nosebleed with flushed faced and pain in forehead. Better after nosebleed. Nosebleed almost producing faintness. Sneezing in evening, when going to bed. Coryza, pimples on upper lip. Discharge of greenish-yellow, putrid mucus, worse evening. Mucus descends into posterior nares. Ulcerated, burning nostrils. Loss of smell.

Perspiration - Profuse sweat, oily, on head and face. Profuse sweat with weakness. Sweats during spasms. Sweats during sleep, towards morning. Cold sweat. Copious, clammy sweat, on hands and arms. Sweats during epilepsy.

Rectum - ***Dysentery with delirium, headache and sleeplessness.*** Bowels torpid. Ascarides. Hemorrhoids, discharging bright red blood. Stools white. Difficult, hard stool, with cold body and hot head.

Skin - Itching and burning. ***Lymphangitis*, *red streaks under skin.*** Patches of skin lose sensation. ***Pustules, suppuration from every slight injury.*** Pustules, tetters and eruption of small nodules. Pemphigus. Yellow bullae, yellowish, corrosive fluid oozes out. Blisters on hands occurring annually. Blisters on palms and soles Large yellow blisters. ***Epidemic, infectious carbuncles.*** Carbuncles. Goose bumps. Ulcers with burning pain. Anthrax

Chilblains. Yellowness of skin.

Sleep - Irresistible sleepiness after eating. Drowsy, but can't sleep, from agitation, constantly turning in bed. Sleepiness after smoking in forenoon. Comatose after spasms. Sleepy after meals. Sleepiness after having been in open air. Constant yawning, can't keep lids open. Starting in sleep, awakens as if frightened. All symptoms worse on waking.

Stomach - Burning pain in stomach. Weak, faint feeling in stomach. Eructations, as from rotten eggs. Nausea and vomiting from nervous excitement. Vomiting after drinking. Yellow fluid in vomit. Vomiting of blood and bile.

Temperature - Coldness and shivering, with moist skin, nervousness and trembling, worse going into open air. Fever with apathy or delirium, and cold feet. Burning heat in various parts. Limbs burning hot during fever.

Throat - Convulsive and constrictive motion in throat, with sensation like a stone there. Dryness in throat, impeding swallowing, in morning. Difficult swallowing, can hardly swallow saliva. Burning, excoriation in larynx. Bleeding fissures, causes quick, jerking cough.

Tongue - Tongue is cracked, bluish black. ***Lapping of or playing with tongue.*** Paralysis of tongue, lapping motion before the attacks. Bites tongue. Dry tongue.

Vertigo - Vertigo, as if house was turned upside down. Vertigo with heaviness of head. Vertigo, as if floating or swimming in water or air. Dizzy, drunken feeling after dinner.

Vision - Dim vision, with itching in eyes. Can't bear sight of brilliant objects. Objects appear crooked. Objects appear as if seen through a veil.

COMMENTS - Bufo provokes the tendency to the practice, or even causes impotence. The Indian women of Brazil are aware of this last property and administer the venom to their husbands in food or drink when they wish to free themselves from their marital attentions.

L. Guthrie told a story of an Italian peasant, apparently dying of dropsy, whose wife, weary of the interminable length of his illness, thought to hasten his end by putting a toad into his wine. The man was completely cured.

According to Lippe, Bufo is especially indicated in epilepsy when the attacks occur during sleep at night. The patient may or may not be awakened by the attack, if not, when he does awaken he will have a violent headache.

Epileptic symptoms are worse in warm room, but there is also great sensitiveness to cold air and wind. Epilepsy that's worse with a full moon. For epilepsy in children with delayed development (Bar-c.). Keynote masturbation in children or with epilepsy.

Lymphangitis. Swollen glands, buboes, particularly in groin and armpits. May go systemic, pus and suppuration. Infection leading to swollen glands and fever (Carb-an.). ***"Low state,"*** decomposition, breakdown in tissues with pus and septic states. Difficult to heal. Cancers with deterioration (Kreos.) in the late stages.

Greasy skin, foul discharges and odors. Carbuncles, boils, large water-filled vesicles (bullae). Marked periodicity, quartan fevers. Hemorrhages. Boericke noted a ***"desire for solitude"*** in order to masturbate.

Guernsey commended it in panaritium where the pain runs in streaks, all the way up the arm. Also when the fingers have been injured and look black, with pains running in streaks up the arm.

E. E. Case reported a cure with Bufo cinereus of "nosebleed daily for several weeks with flushed face, heat and pain in forehead better by the bleeding, there was also easy, perspiration in general, apt to be offensive, especially on the feet."

RELATIONS - ***Antidoted by:*** Lach., Seneg. ***Compare:*** (1) Bar-c., Aster., Salamand. (Epilepsy and softening of brain). (2) Cubeb. in convulsions from low grades of suppuration. (3) Ars., Canth., Lach. and Tarent. in epilepsy aura starting in solar plexus. (4) Art-v., Calc., Nux-v., Sil., (5) aura starting in arm, Lach., Sulph. (6) in chorea, patient cannot walk, must run or jump, Kali-br., Nat-m., as if heart in water, Bov., (7) in masturbation, impotence, etc., Hyos., Merc., Sulph., (8) in malignant pustule, Anthrax., Ant. c., Lach. (9) in bullae, panaritium, etc., Hep., Lach., Ph-ac., Sil., Dios. (10) Head drawn to either side, Camph. ***Complementary:*** Salamandra. Helo., Amphisbena is complementary in epilepsy and brain-softening (Hering).

REFERENCES - Boericke. Clarke. Murphy.

BUNIAS ORIENTALIS

PHARMACY - buni-o. Bunias orientalis. N.O. Cruciferae. Tincture of the seeds. ***Historical dose:*** Tincture and all potencies.

CLINICAL - Adenitis. Allergies. Amaurosis. Arthritis. Asthma. Brachial neuralgia. Cancer. Coccydynia. Congenital malformations. Dyspnea. Eczema. Emaciation. Fever. Headaches. Hoarseness. Hodgkin's disease. Intermittent fever. Leucorrhea. Menorrhagia. Metrorrhagia. Nausea. Neuralgia. Neuritis. Proteinuria. Scars. Syphilitic, adenitis. Tubercular, adenitis. Vertigo.

HERBAL - Bunias is a biennial plant, measuring up to 120 cm. It flowers in May and June, and grows near lucerne fields and along the roads all over Europe.

Prinzing used the seeds of the Norwegian stock of the plant in homeopathic potencies. His attention was drawn towards this plant after learning that a doctor in the North was using Bunias to treat cancerous subjects with interesting results.

HOMEOPATHIC - The homeopathic clinical proving involved one hundred and three patients during a period of two years, and a series of forty patients observed for ten years. The remedy as found to be suitable for tubercular and sycotic types with arthritic neurotic tendencies, for women with syphilitic afflictions, and especially for cancerous subjects.

Allergic, psoric or syphilitic conditions, pre-cancerous conditions. Hodgkin's disease. Intermittent attacks of fever, beginning with a fit of shivering at around 11 p.m. chattering teeth, heat and ending in the morning.

Brachial neuralgia. Pains go around in circles, quickly change place, burning, stinging or cramping. Diffuse nerve pains, behind the mastoid process, the top of the radius top of the fibula the end of the 12th rib. Neuralgia of the left sciatic nerve.

The sudden appearance and disappearance of all symptoms. Rapid emaciation of no apparent reason, (pre-cancerous condition). Tiredness, weakness, loss of vitality. Every difficult previously overcome with ease is now arduous and faced with gritting of the teeth. Need to lie down after a few hours work. Cannot stay awake in the evening.

Sensory complaints decreased vision and hearing. Feeling of stabbing the chest. Sensation that the head is increased in size of swelling in the upper part of the body in the hand. Feeling of coldness in the head, stomach, fingers and back. Sensation of lightness and of hovering in the air, then of falling violently into a bottomless pit.

Itching eruption followed by adenitis. Subacute infections of rheumatic or of the female genital organs. Neuritis and neuralgia.

Irregular menses, nauseating leucorrhea. Abnormal pregnancy. Children weak puny, premature, syphilitic types. Babies born with congenital malformations.

Profuse bleeding after birth with large placenta. Scars. Bloodstained lochia continuing for three to four months. Vulvar varicosity during pregnancy. Metrorrhagia during menopause.

MIND - Neurotic condition with anguish and unrest. Irrational anxiety, can lead to suicide. Depressive psychosis in the pre-cancerous subject. Psychological exhaustion. Depressed. Depressive psychosis, which can end in suicide.

Abdomen - Copies flatulence during the day.

Constitutions - Psoric and allergic constitutions. Cancerous, syphilitic conditions.

Ears - Tinnitus-like bells ringing, or water boiling.

Eyes - Visual complaints. Sees clouds or black circles before the eye. Temporary amaurosis.

Female - Menses painful, irregular, abundant or scanty flow with purplish blood and clotting. Infrequent menses. Headaches and dyspnea before menses. Vulvar congestion with red-brown coloring. Vulvar eczema. Irritating leucorrhea, yellow or brownish, foul-smelling, nauseating. Menorrhagia in young girls. Pre-menopausal menorrhagia. Metrorrhagia through premature placenta or hematoma behind the placenta. Abnormal pregnancy.

Kidneys - Urine irritating of a strong odor, albuminous or streaked with blood. Proteinuria. Indol in urine. Bacteria in urine.

Limbs - Bouts of rheumatoid arthritis with swollen joints. Localized edema, coming and disappearing suddenly, on the back of the hand, collarbones and axillae. Coccydynia.

Lungs - Sharp, sudden hoarseness. Dyspnea. Asthma, appearing suddenly at the age of 40. Wheezy respiration, dyspnea, sensation of restriction in the chest, pain on the left side of the sternum.

Modalities - Better from walking. Better changing position. Better open air. Worse at night. Worse on the side of the body compressed for a long time. Worse on left side. Worse from over-exertion. Worse from heavy, fatty foods.

Rectum - Stools suddenly turn to diarrhea in attacks lasting 2-3 days, then reverting to normal. Attacks of constipation with hard stools, difficult with nausea. Tendency to sudden appearance of hemorrhoids.

Skin - Eruption of red spots or vesicles, red-brick or pale purple in color, located on the nose, cheeks, palms, forearms, thighs, legs. Vesicles on the tip of the tongue, the periphery of the mouth and around the anus. Itching eruption, aggravated by scratching. Pruritus premonitory to malignant adenitis.

Sleep - Sleep light, disturbed, frequently woken. Tosses and turns constantly from one side to the other to fall asleep exhausted when the morning comes.

Temperature - Fever every 21 days in short attacks, coming between 11 p.m. and 12 p.m. with shivering, thoracic pains on the left side, weakness and vomiting. Two to four hours after the shivering comes sweating, which soothes.

Vertigo - Vertigo with a feeling of uncertainty, coming suddenly, lasting only a short while in the early morning.

RELATIONS - ***Compare:*** (1) Bapt. - Considerable nervous depression, face red, bewildered, extreme agitation, putrid-smelling breath, fetid diarrhea, lived marks on the body and limbs. (2) Syph. - Pains in the bones, at night, appearing and disappearing slowly. Breath fetid and painless constipation or diarrhea in the morning. Profuse, acrid, yellowish leucorrhea. (3) Syph. - Changing moods, difficulty in assembling thoughts, loss of memory, especially for proper nouns. (4) Ars. - Rapid prostration, anxiety, agitation, cadaverous odor of the secretions, aggravation at night between 1 a.m. and 3 a.m. (5) Sec. - Post-partum hemorrhage. Hemorrhage of black blood in exhausted women.

REFERENCES - Julian.

BUTHUS AUSTRALIS

(Scorpion Venom)

PHARMACY - buth-aust. Buthus australis. Scorpion venom. Buthus prionuris. Androctonos funestus. Buthus occitanus. Algerian scorpion. Common yellow scorpion. N. O. Arachnida. Tincture is prepared from the scorpion venom. ***Historical dose:*** Tincture and all potencies.

CLINICAL - Chills. Fever. Headaches. Hypotension. Prostration. Salivation.

HOMEOPATHIC - Buthus Australis is a scorpion belonging to the arthropod order of the arachnid class.

The scorpions are insects distinguished by the division of their bodies into three sections: the head and thorax, the pre-abdomen (seven segments) of the same form as the head and thorax, and the post-abdomen (six segments), mistakenly called the tail, which is very mobile and ends with a venomous, curved sting.

The chelicerae have three joints, the last sections forming the pincers. The leg-jaws are very long and end in fat pincers. These animals are viviparous, carnivorous, feed on insects and spiders, which they catch with their pincers and have a defense organ.

Azam first carried out a proving on himself by taking one drop of pure venom orally. A second proving was undertaken by Azam and carried out with the help of eight provers (three women and five men), using the 6x potency for thirty days. Only four provers continued to the end of the thirty days.

Symptoms included an inhibition of will power and reduced activity. Head heavy, frontal headache. Vertigo on walking. Excessive salivation. Attacks of fever with shivering. Limbs are cold with burning pain in the skin. Upset by climatic changes with mental depression and shivering.

Anguish, thoracic constriction. Sensation of a piece of wood nailed between the heart and lungs. Hypotension in infectious conditions. Infectious conditions with fever, shivering, prostration, aggravated at night. Respiratory difficulty during pulmonary or cardiac illnesses.

MIND - Intellectual work arduous or trying. Alternating moods, at times loquacious, at times taciturn, sometimes prostrate, sometimes restless. Irresistible need to speak. Anguish. Indecision and worry. Weepy. Fear of the future, especially after 7 p.m. Sensation of being in a dream.

Abdomen - Pain and chill.

Back - Cervical muscular pains and stiffness of the nape of the neck.

Eyes - Red, weeping with photophobia. Eyeballs sunken. Strabismus.

Head - Throbbing headaches, wandering, very intense.

Heart - Feeling of heat in heart of a piece of wood nailed between heart and lungs.

Limbs - Trembling of the limbs. Hands cold, especially during shivering. Walking painful, and the legs seem to want to move backwards instead of forwards.

Lungs - Difficult respiration, palpitations.

Male - Erection not achieved.

Modalities - Better from eating, rest. Worse from effort, intellectual work. Worse in the late afternoon. Worse when shivering. Periodicity is worse yearly.

Mouth - Profuse salivation. Difficult swallowing.

Nose - Sneezing.

Rectum - Diarrhea.

Skin - Red spots. Formication. Itching. Cold sweating, especially at night. Sensation of coldness, like icy needles pricking the skin.

Sleep - Strong feeling of fatigue, sleepiness and insensitivity.

Throat - Constriction in the throat.

Vertigo - Vertigo on walking.

RELATIONS - ***Compare:*** (1) Lach. - Aggravated by lying down. Spontaneous hematoma. (2) Merc. - Excessive salivation and tongue has a yellowish coating, which retains the imprint of the teeth. (3) Apis - Sensation of being pierced by red hot needles, but with a predominance coldness at the limbs and sensation of icy needles. (4) Verat. - Sensation of icy coldness. (5) Sil. - Throbbing headache, weeping, sneezing, difficulty in swallowing, chilliness, shivering and sweating, but without the feeling of a piece of wood nailed between the heart and lungs.

REFERENCES - Julian.

BUTYRICUM ACIDUM

(Butyric Acid)

PHARMACY - but-ac. Butyricum acidum. Butyric acid. A volatile acid obtained chiefly from butter, being found there in the form of an ester, a triglyceride, and as such constitutes the chief fat of butter and milk. ***Historical dose:*** Tincture and all potencies.

CLINICAL - Ankylosing spondylitis. Anorexia. Belching. Cervicitis. Cramps. Dysidrosis. Dysuria. Edema. Flatulence. ***Foot sweat.*** Gingivitis. Headache. Leucorrhea. Onychomycosis. Palpitations.

HOMEOPATHIC - Butyric acid occurs in the animal organism under a variety of conditions. It constitutes the chief fat of butter and milk. Butyric acid set free by fermentation causes a rancid taste and the odor of contaminated butter.

When milk sours, milk sugar is converted into lactic acid by the lactic ferment of various bacteria. The lactic acid is then acted upon by butyric acid ferment contained in the air.

It may be present in the gastric contents under abnormal conditions, with a markedly diminished hydrochloric acid secretion. In excessive fermentation in the enteric tract, butyric acid may be formed in significant amounts.

Abdominal flatulence. Tremendous formation of gas in the whole belly, much belching of gas, a great deal of gas is passed at the call to stool, which in many cases fails to come.

Marked straining at stool. Stools are small like lumps. Intermittent belly cramps which are below the umbilicus. Pain in the ileocecal region. Complete loss of appetite. Fetid leucorrhea. Offensive sweating of the soles of feet.

MIND - Anxiety and fear. Worries over trifles. Constant fear and nervousness. Impulsive thoughts of suicide, brooding.

Abdomen - Gastric and abdominal flatulence. Cramp in abdomen below umbilicus. Bowels irregular. Atony of the liver and stomach. Epigastric and peri-umbilical pains, awaking at about 2 a.m. Pain in the ileocecal region with feeling of cramp, relieved by expulsion of gas.

Back - Tired feeling and dull pain in small of back, worse walking. Pain in ankles and up back of leg. Pain low down in back and limbs. Ankylosing spondylitis. Morbus coxae senilis.

Female - Foul-smelling leucorrhea, like horses urine. Purulent cervicitis. Dysuria.

Food - Anorexia. Poor appetite.

Head - Headache makes him apprehensive about trifles, worse going upstairs or rapid motion. Dull, hazy ache of head.

Heart - Palpitations, aggravated by eating, with a feeling of abdominal plethora.

Kidneys - Urgent and pressing need to urinate, especially for women. Urine malodorous, smelling like asparagus. Amorphous urate deposits.

Limbs - Dull aching of lumbar and sacral regions, worse standing, spreading towards the hip. Dull aching of arms, legs and calves. Cold feet, with abundant, fetid perspiration. Edema of the feet during menses.

Modalities - ***Worse at night.*** Worse fast walking. Worse going upstairs. ***Worse during menses.***

Mouth - Fetid odor in the mouth. Profuse salivation. Gingivitis. Gums tinged with blood. Gingival secretions, which are offensive smelling and more profuse during menses. Painful gums, worse during menses.

Perspiration - Perspiration on slight exertion. ***Profuse, offensive foot sweat.***

Rectum - Sudden nocturnal cramps with an urgent need to go to stool. ***Offensive smelling stools***, chestnut or light yellow in color. Feeling of heaviness in rectum with pain in the anus. Stool accompanied by pain and straining.

Skin - The fingernails crumble away. Sudamina. Dysidrosis of the palms and soles. Onychomycosis.

Sleep - Sleep disturbed, owing to digestive complaints. Pronounced sleeplessness, dreams of serious nature while asleep.

Stomach - Much gas in stomach and bowels. Cramps in pit of stomach, worse at night. Stomach feels heavy and overloaded.

COMMENTS - The following provings were conducted at the Hahnemann Hospital of Philadelphia, upon students at that institution. The students took the 3c potency of the remedy every two hours; in all, the proving was carried on for approximately seven weeks.

The remedy induces a peculiar effect on the superficial part of the body. Pronounced and awfully malodorous foot sweat.

Students at the Hahnemann College often had to constantly change their socks, a thing quite foreign to the provers under normal conditions.

Crumbling away of the fingernails. Aggravated backache.

All the symptoms are decidedly worse at night. Pronounced sleeplessness.

RELATIONS - ***Compare:*** (1) Bapt. - Putrid smelling breath. Fetid diarrhea and putrid stools. Mental confusion, illusion that the body is double. (2) Verat. - Prostration intense delirium, feeling of chill running over the whole body and cold sweating on forehead, hands and feet. Abdominal colic with copious diarrhea, followed by extreme weakness. (3) Nux-m. - Dryness of the mucus membranes, thirst, gastric and abdominal distention. Constipation with difficulty in expelling stools. Amenorrhea with leucorrhea.

REFERENCES - Anshutz.

BUXUS SEMPERVIRENS

(Box Tree)

PHARMACY - bux. Buxus sempervirens. Box tree. N. O. Euphorbiacae. Tincture of the young leaves and twigs. ***Historical dose:*** All potencies.

CLINICAL - Abdomen, pains. Coldness. Convulsions. Diarrhea. Dizziness. Faintings. Nausea. Rheumatic pain. Sleepiness.

HOMEOPATHIC - Faintings. Strong forcing pains, like those of labor, in the lower part of the abdomen, which varied greatly in intensity, and lasted from twenty or thirty seconds to a minute or longer.

Pretty frequent desire to urinate, but no increase in amount of urine emitted. Slight increase in frequency of pulse. Slight degree of nausea on one or two occasions.

Senseless and unconscious, with ice-cold hands and feet, half-closed eyes, dilated pupils, respiration very slow, almost imperceptible, action of the heart intermitting, scarcely perceptible, anus relaxed, wide open, limbs relaxed. He fell to the ground unconscious, with loud cries and convulsions.

MIND - Mental and physical prostration. Emotional. At times, painful weeping, with grinding of the teeth. Sadness. Wakes in bad humor. She seemed to have some consciousness, as was shown by the look of her eye when her name was called aloud.

Abdomen - Labor like pains in lower abdomen.

Ears - Noise in the ears, extending to the occiput, like letting off steam.

Eyes - Dimness of sight. Optical illusions.

Food - Appetite when beginning breakfast, but it suddenly ceases after taking a little milk.

Head - Giddiness of the head. Weight in the head, especially the top of the forehead, at 4 p.m.

Kidneys - Sudden pain, with lancination, in the urethra, above the fossa navicularis, for two minutes.

Limbs - Rheumatic pain in the right thigh. Trembling of the knees and of all the limbs with violent emotion, when hearing others talk about the disease he is afraid of having. Weakness of the knees when going upstairs. Swelling of the ankles, less at night.

Mouth - Clammy mouth, with bad breath. Bitter mouth.

Perspiration - Profuse sweat during sleep, ceasing on waking. Very fetid sweat under the axilla and on the scrotum.

Rectum - Tenesmus and pressure in the sphincter ani, with pricking, but ineffectual urging to stool. Diarrhea in the morning. Unusually easy stools. Watery, greenish, fetid stools. Copious, light colored, watery, fetid stools.

Sleep - Sleepiness. Drowsiness in daytime. Falls asleep late. Distressing dreams, about wanting to save an asphyxiated child, whose parents will not let him treat it. Dreams about a conflagration, with small flames.

Stomach - Violent vomiting and purging. Heaviness in the stomach all night, relieved by applying the hands. Borborygmi. Vague and transient, but very acute, pains in the stomach.

Temperature - Coldness and shrinking. The whole head, especially the nape of the neck, is cold. Face and limbs cold. Icy coldness under the shoulder-blades, in bed, even when well covered up. Coldness even to the marrow of the bone.

Vertigo - Dizziness. Faintings.

RELATIONS - ***Compare:*** Gels., Chin.

REFERENCES - Desai.

C

CACAO
(Cocoa)

PHARMACY - cac. Cacao. Cocoa. Theobroma cacao. N. O. Sterculiaceae. Tribe, Buettnerieae. Trituration of the seeds. ***Historical dose:*** Trituration and all potencies.

CLINICAL - Aneurism. Angina pectoris. Apoplexy. ***Atheroma***. Asthma. Bladder, paralysis. Brain, congestion. Bronchitis. Diaphragm, rheumatism. Dropsy. Exophthalmic goitre. Fistula. Hematuria. Hemoptysis. Hemorrhage. Headaches. Heart, affections. Heart, hypertrophy. Intermittent fever. Lungs, hemorrhage. Melancholy. Menstruation, painful. Malaria. Neuralgia. Otitis. Ovaries, inflammation. Ovaritis. Pneumonia. Prostate, affections. Rheumatism. Sunstroke. Traumatic fever. Vaginismus.

HERBAL - Theobroma is Greek for "Food of the Gods". Mayan Indian legend has it that the cocoa tree was a gift from the gods. The Mayas believed the drink made from the cocoa seeds would nourish them after death. The Aztecs believed cocoa would relieve their fatigue and stimulate their mental and psychic abilities.

The Spanish invaders were surprised to find that the cocoa beans were valued more than any other substance, even more than gold. The Aztecs used a chocolate drink as a base in many of their medicinal formulas. The Aztec nobility used the chocolate drink favored with vanilla and spices as a pleasurable drink.

HOMEOPATHIC - The main ingredients of chocolate are caffeine, phenylethylamine, theobromine and theophylline. Feeding with waste Chocolate led to fatal poisoning in calves. The animals showed excitement, stared about in all directions, walked with exaggerated strides and had convulsions. One calf died, possibly from heart failure.

Allen noted, "In explaining the nutritive value of Cacao, we must take into account the presence in this substance of a special alkaloid, theobromin, whose physiological effects are identical with those of caffeine and thein.

"Which, retarding the organic waste in the same way as the active principles of coffee and tea, place Cacao high up among the preservative substances or those that check tissue-waste."

"By placing ourselves under the influence of a decoction highly charged with aromatic principles and made from powdered Cacao well roasted, we ascertained that this beverage produces an excitement of the nervous system similar to that caused by a strong infusion of black coffee.

"Since these effects are insignificant if a decoction of the raw bean is employed. It is natural to attribute them to the aromatic essences that are developed in the Cacao by the process of roasting. A still wider difference is observed when we compare the effects on the circulation respectively produced by a decoction of powdered Cacao roasted and one of the same substance in a crude state.

"The former case indicated an excitement of the circulation, as shown by an accelerated pulse, with an increased fullness and diminished arterial pressure.

"When, on the other hand, an infusion of the raw bean is made use of, the action of the theobromin predominates and an entirely different character of pulse is the result, as may be placed beyond doubt by examining the results, obtained from a single individual."

Causation - Damp. Disappointed love. Sun.

Sensations - ***Finger were enlarged on waking.*** Grain of sand under skin. ***Worm under skin which ran away when touched.***

COMMENTS - Allen stated "In order to ascertain the effect of the active ingredients, contained in Cacao, (aromatic essences and theobromin) upon the nervous system. It was necessary to separate those ingredients, as far as possible from the fatty substances (cacao butter) of which the beans are so largely composed. With this view, we prepared a decoction of powdered Cacao in boiling water and conducted our experiments with this liquid.

RELATIONS - ***Compare:*** (1) Chocolate, Coffea, Thea.

REFERENCES - Allen. Desai.

CACTUS GRANDIFLORUS

(Night-blooming Cereus)

PHARMACY - cact. Cactus grandiflorus. Night-blooming Cereus. Cereus grandiflorus. Cactus selenicereus. N. O. Cactaceae. Mexico. West Indies. Tincture of youngest, tender stems and flowers collected in summer. ***Historical dose:*** Tincture and all potencies.

CLINICAL - Aneurysm. ***Angina pectoris.*** Atheroma. Asthma. Bladder, paralysis. Brain, congestion. Bronchitis. Colic. Diaphragmitis. Dropsy. ***Dysmenorrhea***. Ear, inflammation. Exophthalmic, goiter. Fevers. Fistulas. Goiter. Hematuria. ***Hemorrhages.*** Headache. ***Heart, attack. Heart, disorders.*** Indigestion. Intermittent, fevers. Lungs, hemorrhage. Melancholy. Menstruation, painful. Malaria. Neuralgias. Otitis media. Ovaritis. Pneumonia. Prostate, disorders. Rheumatism. ***Spasmodic, pains***. Stroke. Sunstroke. Traumatic fever. Vaginismus.

HERBAL - Given as a ***heart tonic,*** it will benefit a large number of cases of weakened and painful heart. Atheromatous arteries and weak heart. General weakness and prostration. Irregular circulation, causing violent congestion or localized pulsations. Congestion in the esophagus, bladder, etc. Used as an herbal tonic for heart patients with a history of constricting pains.

HOMEOPATHIC - Cactus affects the entire organism powerfully, but its internal operation is on the heart and circulation. In congestive violence it rivals Acon., which is one of its antidotes. The pains are unendurable, they extort screams. Sadness, apprehension, fear of death and a tendency to be easily frightened characterize the mental state, as they do many conditions of heart disease.

Constriction, periodicity and spasmodic pains. ***"As if an iron band*** had prevented its normal movements," or ***"heart as if compressed***, and as violently struggled to burst its bonds." Whole body feels ***as if caged, each wire being twisted tighter***. It affects the circular muscles, thereby producing ***constricting pains in the heart***, throat, chest, bladder, rectum, vagina, and neck.

"Fluttering and palpitation of heart, worse when walking or lying on left side." Pain and numbness in left arm accompanying heart disease. "Heart disease with swelling of left hand only." "Numbness of left arm."

Hemorrhagic remedy, favors formation of clots speedily. Hemorrhages (nose, lungs, rectum, stomach). Bloody congestions, which are in a way a counterpart of the constrictive sensations.

"Periodical attacks of suffocation with fainting, cold sweat on face and loss of pulse." Pulseless, panting and prostration. Low blood pressure from weakness of heart. Congestions, irregular distribution of blood.

Sharp pains in diaphragm and girdle pain around its attachment, with indigestion. Hot gushing into chest. Toxic goiter with cardiac symptoms. Dropsical disorders.

Weakness and coldness of limbs. Twitching of muscles and sensation of constriction produced by touching the affected part. "Rheumatism of all joints, beginning in upper limbs." The pains are very sharp, causing the patient to cry out. "Heavy pain in vertex like a weight."

Great periodicity, neuralgic pains occur periodically. Chill at same hour every day, 11 a.m. or 11 p.m. Many symptoms are worse at night. Menses cease at night.

MIND - Melancholic, taciturn, sad, ill-humored. Sadness and melancholy. Cries, knows not why, worse from consolation. Scream with pain. Love of solitude. Weeping, withou knowing why, worse consolation.

Fear that something bad will happen. Easil frightened. Fear of death. Fear of heart dis ease. Screams with pain. Anxiety on wakin Irresistible inclination to weep. Believes th his disease is incurable. Fears some organi lesion of heart which will cause sudde death. Easily frightened on waking.

Wishes to be alone and not to speak anyone. Slowness, always behind han Impulse to do strange things. Irritabili worse consolation. Sadness during menses. Sensitive to music, noise. Talk of others aggravates. Weeping before menses. Difficulty in expressing ideas when writing.

Delirium at night, ceases on awaking, but returning in sleep. Feels she is dying and thinks she will not live till morning, but has no fear of death. Unwilling to answer. Easily frightened, often awakes in a fright. Felt much alarmed on waking, but could not tell cause of alarm.

Abdomen - Colic with loose stool. Intense burning in abdomen. Sharp pain, shooting through diaphragm and up into chest. As if a cord was tied tighter and tighter around attachment of diaphragm, taking his breath away. Pain and bearing-down in lower abdomen.

Back - Exophthalmic goiter. Cold in back and icy cold hands. Rheumatism of the shoulder. Pain under left shoulder blade with palpitations. Lumbar muscles tender on pressure and stiff, especially on first moving after repose.

Breasts - Inflammation of breasts. Mastitis. Breast tumor.

Causations - Ill effects of sun, dampness, disappointment in love, or grief.

Chest - ***Constriction***, acute pains and stitches in chest. ***Constriction as if bound, hindering respiration***. Oppressed breathing as from a weight on chest. Angina pectoris with suffocation, cold sweat and an iron-band feeling. Palpitation, pain shooting down left arm. Diaphragmitis with great difficulty of breathing. Continuous rattling of mucus in chest.

Constitutions - Sanguine constitutions.

Ears - Pulsation in ears. Hearing diminished by the buzzing in the ears. Singing, ringing in ears.

Eyes - Bloodshot eyes. Exophthalmic goiter. Dimness of sight, cannot see at a distance, objects seem obscured.

Face - Face, red bloated, emaciated. Pale. ***Right-sided facial pain***, constricting pains, returns at same hour daily (Cedr.).

Female - Constriction of vagina preventing sex, vaginismus. Constriction in uterine region and ovaries. Pulsation in ovarian region. ***Dysmenorrhea***, pulsating pain in uterus and ovaries. Vaginismus. Menses early, dark, pitch-like (Cocc., Mag-c.), cease on lying down, with heart symptoms. Menses lumpy, black, too soon. Painful menses, extorting loud cries. Menstrual disorders with heart symptoms.

Food - Appetite good, digestion weak. Complete loss of appetite, stomach rejects everything. Aversion to meat, of which he was fond.

Head - Headache if misses a meal (Ars., Lach., Lyc.). ***Sensation as of a weight on vertex***. Right-sided pulsating pain. Headache worse by seeing opera, noise, light. Periodic pains, compressive and pulsating. ***Congestive headaches***, threatening a stroke. Blood vessels to the head distended. Feels as if head were compressed in a vice.

Heart - ***Feels clutched and released alternately by an iron band*** or feels it expand and contract, seems to turn over. ***Constriction,*** very acute pains and stitches in heart. Pain in apex, shooting down left arm. ***Palpitations,*** worse lying on left side, at the approach of menses, during the day, while walking, from disappointed love. Palpitations with vertigo, dyspnea, flatulence. Pulsations increase on holding the breath. ***Endocarditis with mitral insufficiency together with violent and rapid action***. Murmurs, excessive pulse rate, increased precordial dullness, enlarged ventricle. Pulse feeble, irregular, quick without strength. Low blood pressure. Heart disease with edema of left hand. As if heart would fly to pieces on holding the breath. Hypertrophy. ***Aneurysm of large arteries and heart.*** Heart weakness and arteriosclerosis. Tobacco heart.

Kidneys - Constriction of neck of bladder, causing retention of urine. Urine suppressed in fevers. Hemorrhage from bladder. Clots of blood in urethra. Irritation in urethra. Constant urination. Hematuria, urination prevented by clots in vagina in females. Urine passes by drops, with much burning. Profuse urine of a straw color. Urine has deposits of red sand.

Limbs - Rheumatic pains, in shoulders, upper and lower arms, in hips down to feet, worse in rest and in motion, and in all positions. Left arm numb. Pain in left arm down to fingers. Fingers tingle. Icy cold hands. Edema of left hand in heart disease and of feet, extending to knees. Hands soft, feet enlarged. Restless legs.

Liver - Engorgement of liver due to heart disease.

Lungs - Difficulty breathing. Oppression of breathing, going up stairs. Periodical attacks of suffocation with fainting, sweat on face and loss of pulse. Inflammation of diaphragm with difficulty in breathing. Chronic bronchitis with rattling of mucus. Hemoptysis with convulsive, spasmodic cough. Cough from heart disorders. Catarrhal cough with much viscid expectoration. Cyanotic infants.

Male - Prostatic affections, weight in anus.

Modalities - Better from open air. Better pressure on vertex. Worse from lying down on left side, on occiput. Worse exertion. Worse walking, and going upstairs. Worse from 11 a.m. or 11 p.m. Worse night. Worse noise, light. Worse heat, sun's rays, and damp. Worse from fasting. Worse after eating, as a weight in stomach.

Mouth - Loss of taste for food, with nausea. Tongue purple, thick, brown sordes on teeth. Prickling on point of tongue. Very offensive breath. Dryness of tongue, as if burnt.

Nose - Profuse nosebleed, but soon ceases. Fluent coryza.

Pulse - Pulse, irritable intermittent, feeble. Irregular and intermittent action after forceps delivery.

Rectum - Constipation, hard and black stool. Diarrhea, watery, mucous, bilious. Hemorrhoids, swollen and painful. Sensation of great weight in anus. Itching in the anus. Pricking as from a pin in anus, better slight friction. Fistula in anus with violent palpitations of heart. Hemorrhages from bowels in malarial fevers and with heart symptoms.

Skin - Dry, scaly herpes on the outside of the elbow and on the right internal malleolus.

Sleep - Sleeplessness, on account of strong pulsations in different places. ***Frightful dreams***, lascivious, of falling. Awakes in fright.

Stomach - After eating, weight and distress in stomach. Gastro-enteritis. ***Constriction***, burning pulsation or heaviness in stomach. Vomiting of blood. Pulsation in celiac artery behind the stomach. Nausea in the morning, lasting all day. Acrid, sour fluid in stomach, which rises in throat and mouth.

Temperature - Coldness predominates, cold sweat with great anguish. Chilly, not worse by covering. Persistent ***subnormal*** temperature. Fever every day at same hour. Coldness in back and icy cold hands. Intermittent paroxysms about midday (11 a.m.), incomplete in their stages, accompanied by hemorrhages.

Throat - Suffocative constriction at throat with full, ***throbbing carotids in angina pectoris***. Constriction of esophagus, must drink to swallow. Needs much liquid to get food down. Feeling of warmth about throat and chest. Scraping sensation at soft palate.

Vertigo - Vertigo, worse deep breathing or exertion. Vertigo from blood congestions to head.

COMMENTS - Snader considered Cact. especially indicated where the heart is weak and the arteries atheromatous. This was confirmed by a correspondent of the Hom. World (July, 1898), who, finding his temporal arteries swollen and hard to the touch took several doses of Cact. 1x with the result that in a few days they became normal. Snader used the lower potencies in this condition.

A case of angina pectoris was cured by the 30c with a sensation as though a swarm of hornets were going from pectoral region to heart.

Choudhury reported a case cured, the characteristics included "Chill severe, 11 a.m., thirst, headache, body hot, no separate heat."

Heat with thirst and short breath. At times there is entire absence of sweat.

Keynote constricting pain. The chest feels tight, and keeps getting tighter as their breath goes away. Feels like a hand has reached into the chest and grabbed the heart and is squeezing (Spig., as if a hot burning knife is being stabbed into the heart and pulled out repeatedly, with a pain shooting down the arm).

Heart attack (Lat-m.). Tendency to a heart attack with high blood pressure, chest pain, shortness of breath, with constriction. After a heart attack, with shortness of breath and tightness in the chest.

Tendency to get out of breath and get tightness in the chest (acute or chronic). In some cases, even the throat goes tight. Heart symptoms tend to the left side. Heart pathologies, regurgitation and failure of the valves, tightness and shortness of the breath, suffocated feeling, heart murmurs, palpitation, high or low blood pressure.

Neuralgia around the ribs and heart, feels as if the rib cage or the heart is wrapped with wire and someone is twisting the end of the wire and tightening the wires around the heart. Oppression of the chest (Phos.).

Constriction anywhere in the body. Constriction in the ovaries. Uterine cramps where the uterus feels constricted as if a band is wrapped around it, or as if a hand is grabbing the uterus, squeezing and letting go repeatedly.

Facial neuralgias where the face feels squeezed in together and painful, more often right (Spig., more often left). They constantly look in the mirror to see if they can actually see their face being constricted. Headaches with constricting pain, as if there's a band being tightened. Sunstroke. Many fears (Ars.), fear of death and dying.

Used as an herbal tonic for heart patients with a history of constricting pains. Used in a 30c or 200c for a person with an active heart attack. Low potencies can help to strengthen the heart.

ELATIONS - ***Antidoted by:*** Acon., Camph., Chin., Eup-per. ***Compare:*** (1) Dig., Spig., Conv., Kalm., Naja, Magn-gr. (2) Cer-b., Cer-s., Opun-v. (3) Coc-c. (4) In mental symptoms - Dig., Lach. (5) In congestions to head - Bell., Glon. (6) In pain and pressure in head - Arn., Carb-v., Cor-r., Iod., Nux-v., Op., Spig. (7) Weight in vertex - Aloe., Alum. (8) In heart affections - Acon., Cimic., Amyl-n., Arn., Bell., Bov., Crot-h., Dig., Eup-per., Kalm., Lach., Lil-t., Naja, Puls., Spig., Zinc. (as if a cap over heart). (9) Constrictions of chest - Zinc., Kali-chl., Cadm-s., Alum., Bell., Bov., Arn., Kali-n., Lach. (10) Constrictions - Stram., Murx., (uterus), Kali-c., (vagina) . (11) In menses ceasing at night - Caust. (12) In leucorrhea - Am-m. (13) In intermittents - Ars., Bry., Calc., Eup-per., Nat-m., Rhus-t, Sulph. (14) In dropsies - Dig., Kalm. ***Compatible:*** (1) Dig. - Tumultuous action of heart, slow, irregular pulse, scanty urine, dropsy. (2) Eup-per., Lach., Nux-v., Sulph. - Pleurisy. ***Follows well:*** Acon., Arn., Ars., Bell., Bry., Cham., Gels., Ip., Kali-br. - diaphragmitis. Lach., Nux-v., Rhus-t.

REFERENCES - Boericke. Clarke. Murphy.

CADMIUM BROMATUM

(Cadmium Bromide)

PHARMACY - cadm-br. Cadmium bromatum. Cadmium bromide. Trituration or solution. ***Historical dose:*** Trituration and all potencies.

CLINICAL - Cancer. Diarrhea. Heartburn. Indigestion. Strokes. Throat pain. Tumors. Vomiting.

HOMEOPATHIC - Cadm-br. should be compared to Cadm-s. Three persons experimented with Cadm-br., it produced a burning sensation in mouth, gullet and stomach. Goose flesh. Diarrhea.

Clinically Cadm-br. has been used for apoplexy, threatening stroke and predisposition for strokes. Cerebral hemorrhage. Pulse, imperceptible. Throat pain. Sore throat, pain worse after swallowing.

Stomach pain after lifting. Burning pain in stomach. Burning pain as from an ulcer. Vomiting of blood. Bloody vomit. Sudden vomiting. Cancer of the bowels. Tumors.

COMMENTS - Allen stated: "I found both ladies vomiting severely and complaining of extreme pain and burning sensation in the stomach.

"Mrs. R. who also purging freely, though her daughter was not. The vomiting and purging lasted fully five hours and during a part of the time the pulse was imperceptible in either patient. After this period the symptoms ameliorated and they both fell asleep.

"For several days they were both confined to their beds and were obliged to be extremely careful as to what they took into their stomachs. Mrs. R. has since suffered with some cerebral symptoms which betoken a tendency to strokes. A severe burning sensation in the mouth, esophagus and stomach, which lasted perhaps and hour."

REFERENCES - Allen. Clarke.

CADMIUM FLOURATA
(Cadmium Flouride)

PHARMACY - cadm-f. Cadmium flourata. Cadmium flouride. Cadmium fluoricum. ***Historical dose:*** Trituration and all potencies.

CLINICAL - Adenoma. Bowel, cancer. Cancer. Prostate, cancer. Rectal, cancer. Tumors.

HOMEOPATHIC - Grimmer wrote: "Cadmium fluorata is a remedy that helped one case very much, a late case of cancer of the prostate. There was no question about the diagnosis, which was made by an eminent pathologist in Chicago. The patient was at the point of death.

"I sent my assistant out to see him and get a blood sample. Every test showed the presence of cancer. I never saw this patient, so I didn't report the case, but the doctor informed me there was a big pulsating mass. He could feel it through the patient's rectum and said it was undoubtedly cancer, very far advanced. He didn't think the man would live more than a few days. Nevertheless, we gave him cadmium flour.

"This man lived for a year and part of the time the function of the bladder was restored. He gave up his catheter for quite a while and subsequently used it only occasionally. He left us because he was dissatisfied with his progress. He was an old man and had been put in much more comfort. I lost track of him after a year, but at the end of that year he was better in every way."

REFERENCES - Grimmer. Murphy.

CADMIUM IODATUM
(Cadmium Iodine)

PHARMACY - cadm-i. Cadmium iodatum. Cadmium iodine. ***Historical dose:*** Trituration and all potencies.

CLINICAL - Anal, itching. Bowel cancer. Cachexia. ***Cancer.*** Constipation. Gland, cancer. ***Gland, disorders.*** Goiter. Emaciation. Ileus. Necrosis. Pancreatic cancer. Palpitations. Pruritis ani. Radiation, poisoning. Rectal, prolapse. Spleen, cancer. Thyroid, cancer. ***Thyroid, disorders.*** Tumors. Ulcerative colitis. Ulcers. Uterine, cancer.

HOMEOPATHIC - Grimmer said this remedy is a powerful anti-syphilitic as well as anti-psoric and anti-sycotic. All the Cadmiums cover the three miasms of Hahnemann.

A great remedy for the ***glands***. the cervical glands of the neck, the tonsils, the thyroid, the mammary glands. The entire lymphatic system, the testicles, and the ovaries.

Cancer of the glands with emaciation. Thyroid, cancer. Bowel cancer. Pancreatic cancer. Spleen, cancer. Tumors of glands.

The liver, the spleen, and the pancreas are sooner or later involved under the influence of this remedy. Constipation. Frequent desire to stool, tenesmus. Abdomen bloated. Anal itching with constipation. Itching of anus and rectum felt during the day only.

Characteristic hatred, hates everybody and everything. Atheistic and hateful with a high degree of self-pity.

Aggravated from extreme heat, as well as from extreme cold. As a rule, the patient becomes less chilled than when under the influence of other Cadmiums due to the iodine component of the remedy.

COMMENTS - Grimmer had a patient with some of the above symptoms, together with an ulceration of the transverse colon, which cleared up, under Cadm-i. He lost his hatred became quite human and kind, and gained greatly in weight.

REFERENCES - Grimmer.

CADMIUM METALLICUM

(Cadmium Metal)

PHARMACY - cadm-met. Cadmium metallicum. Cadmium metal (At. Wt. 48). ***Historical dose:*** Trituration and all potencies.

CLINICAL - Aluminum, poisoning. Anemia. Bacillary, dysentery. Backache. Blood, poisoning. ***Cancers. Chemotherapy, effects.*** Chlorosis. Colic. Colitis. Constipation. Coughs. Depression. Diaphragmatic, hernia. Diarrhea. Dyspepsia. Dysentery. Emaciation. Enterocolitis. ***Fatigue, chronic.*** Headaches. Hemorrhoids. Indigestion. ***Influenza.*** Liver, weakness. Lupus, erythematous. Migraines. Nausea. Pharyngitis. ***Radiation, poisoning.*** Tuberculosis. Vomiting.

HOMEOPATHIC - Cadmium met. comes between zinc and mercury with an atomic weight of 48. The toxicology indicates vomiting, loss of appetite, emaciation. Sneezing and coughing with profuse secretion from the respiratory and ocular mucus membranes.

Cadmium met. and other chemical combinations of cadmium have proved curative in many cases of stomach and intestinal cancer.

Many of these cases were caused were caused by irritative actions of alumina toxin resulting from aluminum cooking utensils. The water supply of many cities and towns has been treated with aluminum fluoride, exposing the public to a potent carcinogenic agent that has the potential to activate the disease in all those with inherited tendencies to it.

Cadm-met. and Cadm-o. are the most effective antidotes against the alumina toxins.

The blood changes, anemia and the gastrointestinal tracts are especially affected by the alumina poison. When absorbed by the lungs and intestines, cadmium causes lesions on the pulmonary and digestive epithelium.

Fatigue, with lassitude like influenza, dull aching all over. State of indifference, desire to be alone, improved by appearance of a skin eruption. Anemia. Nausea and vomiting.

Diarrhea with soft stools and the sensation of a foreign body in the rectum. Sneezing, coughing, muco-purulent sputum. Sneezing with influenza and tickling at the back of the throat. Influenza-type rhino-pharyngitis.

MIND - Hypersensitive. Nervous and restlessness. Irritable. Impulsive irritability, on the verge of insanity in its violence, alternating with deep depression.

Depressive psychosis with fear of cancer (Carc.). Loathing of life. Despair. Hopeless and apathetic, all joy is gone. Averse to people. Averse to certain kinds of music. Averse to noise.

Concentration difficult. Mental exertion aggravates. Mistakes, saying and doing the wrong things. Makes simple mistakes. Weak memory. Indifference, does not want to see anyone. Apathy after influenza. Indifference to work.

Abdomen - Diaphragmatic hernia. Colitis and enterocolitis. Bacillary dysentery. Abdominal distention with pain in the region of the umbilicus and epigastrium, better by eating, bending double.

Back - Backache, pain in the scapula.

Blood - Acquired hemolytic jaundice. Anemia. Anemia and chlorosis in young girls. Infantile hereditary anemia.

Breasts - Breasts feel enlarged and sore.

Causations - Aluminum or radiation poisoning.

Chest - Constrictive pain behind the sternum, especially when coughing.

Constitutions - Pre-cancerous. Chronic infection of the reticuloendothelial system. State of psychosomatic, ***post-influenza exhaustion.***

Ears - Buzzing and painfully sensitive. Old ear discharge with pain.

Eyes - Sensitive to light. Eyelids painfully sensitive and burning, worse when reading and in a hot room.

Food - Insatiable hunger, with nausea aggravated by jarring. Loss of appetite.

Head - Extreme, neuralgic headaches with maddening pressing pains throughout the head, extending to eyes and ears. Occipital headaches with vertigo, buzzing in ears, visual and psychosomatic complaints. Headaches, the pains come and go suddenly. Headaches accompanied by nausea. Headache worse by shaking the head, movement. Headache worse reading, sustained intellectual activity, and in the morning on waking. Headaches, better by cold compresses, holding the head, and eating.

Heart - Intense squeezing pain in the region of the heart, with a sense of weakness.

Kidneys - Frequent urination.

Limbs - Numbness of the feet and hands when sitting. Paraesthesia at the limbs. Weakness. Heaviness of the limbs. Trembling of the feet and hands. Feet burning, formication.

Lungs - Difficult respiration, especially with the slightest movement. Cough with muco-purulent, sometimes blood-streaked sputum. Acute bronchial and pulmonary diseases.

Modalities - Better from eating. Better pressure. Better bending double. Better cold application, and with the appearance of an eruption. Worse in the morning. Worse from waking. Worse left side. Worse movement. Worse mental effort.

Mouth - Teeth yellow. Mouth dry, lips itching.

Nose - Sneezing.

Rectum - Constipation with hemorrhoids, aggravated by passing stool. Soft diarrhea with sensation of a foreign body in the rectum. Diarrhea of black, musty stools with intestinal pains. Constipation with clay-colored stools.

Skin - Sensation of heat or burning in small areas of the skin. Localized itching. Erythema, dry eruption, papules, vesicles. General fatigue, diminishes with the appearance of eruption on the skin. Lupus erythematous. Tuberculosis with papules, nodules, vesicles and purpura. Sclerous lichen (isolated or grouped papules, sclerodermic in appearance). Chronic pustular dermatitis, spreading away from the center.

Sleep - Dreams of sickness, causing worry after waking. Dreams of running without reaching anywhere.

Stomach - Acrid dyspepsia. Indigestion. Odors and other unpleasant stimuli induce nausea, even thinking of them.

Temperature - Goose bumps. Shivering without fever. Cold even when near a fire. Glandular fever. Mononucleosis.

Throat - Throat dry in the morning, improved by eating.

Vertigo - Vertigo while looking at moving pictures. Vertigo with a sensation of something taking the breath away. Objects recede and return.

COMMENTS - The first proving was carried out by Burdach in 1827 with a half grain, and later by Petroz. The proving was undertaken again at the instigation of the International League of Homeopathy in 1947 and a report was created by Gutman in 1951. The proving was made on thirty-eight provers, using the 2c, 3c, 6x, 12x and 30c potencies.

In another connection, MacFarland made a proving on four female provers using the Skinner potencies, 10m and 50m. Templeton experimented on nine provers with 2c, Pahud on sixteen provers with 2c, 3c, 6x, 12x and 30x.

Violent vomiting attack with headache, alternating of heat and coldness. Some pressing pains in the liver and spleen. Vomiting of bile and acid. More frequent urination, discoloring the toilet bowl brownish or a deep lemon color, very difficult to wash from the bowl.

Hemorrhage of the bladder and rectum was cured many times by Dr. Grimmer, especially when dark-colored blood with small clots was present. Bright red hemorrhages have also been observed.

Grimmer had a case: "Severe neuralgic pains in the face with plugged sinus, followed by facial paralysis, after large doses of quinine and aspirin, cured with one dose of Cadm-met. 10,000c."

RELATIONS - ***Compare:*** (1) Cadm-s. (2) Bry - Also aggravated by movement, constipated intensely thirsty. (3) Ars. - Agitation with anxiety, burning ameliorated by heat.

REFERENCES - Grimmer. Julian. Murphy.

CADMIUM OXIDATUM

(Cadmium Oxidate)

PHARMACY - cadm-o. Cadmium oxidatum. Cadmium oxidate. Trituration. ***Historical dose:*** Trituration and all potencies.

CLINICAL - Aluminum, poisonings. Arthritis. Asthma. Cancer. Chills. Dyspnea. Emaciation. Fever. Influenza. Neuritis.

HOMEOPATHIC - Cadm-o. is the most active of the cadmiums and has a wide range of action in chronic and intractable conditions of cancer. Useful for degenerative diseases of heart and kidneys and many forms of arthritic and nerve inflammations.

Indispensable and unequalled as an antidote to the alumina toxins which stem from the use of aluminum cooking utensils, as well as from the toxins resulting from water softeners in which aluminum chloride is used.

Those who use the water treated with aluminum chloride for cooking and drinking purposes are sure to suffer from the ill effects of aluminum poisoning, and when so affected will not respond to curative remedies until this toxin is antidoted and eradicated completely from the system. This poison acts like one of the basic miasms of Hahnemann as the patient will not get well until it is entirely removed.

COMMENTS - Grimmer noted a case in which the patient suffered from chronic asthma, despite having excellent homeopathic treatment over a long period of time with only short acting palliation of the asthmatic attacks, which gradually became more intense and wearing.

The patient was greatly reduced in weight and strength with an ever-increasing dyspnea, which made him very depressed with despair of recovery. Then it was discovered that he was poisoned with chronic aluminum from using aluminum cooking ware for a long time.

A dose of Cadm-o. 30c, and later a 200c, brought quick relief which was superseded by an attack of what appeared to be the symptoms of a viral influenza.

In this condition a perfect picture of Hep. was presented. Chill, fever and copious sweat, must be covered in all stages, no relief from sweat. Hep. 30c brought complete relief of the asthma for several weeks without a break and the patient rapidly regained weight and strength.

REFERENCES - Grimmer. Murphy.

CADMIUM SULPHURATUM

(Cadmium Sulphide)

PHARMACY - cadm-s. Cadmium sulphuratum. Cadmium sulphide. Trituration. ***Historical dose:*** Trituration and all potencies.

CLINICAL - Aluminum, poisoning. Anorexia. Aphthae. Asthma. ***Blood poisoning.*** Boils. ***Cancers. Chemotherapy, effects***. Chilblains. Chilliness. Chloasma. Cholera. Colon, cancer. Coma. Drug, overdose. Emaciation. Erysipelas. ***Facial paralysis***. Hair, loss. Herpes. Insomnia. Lead, poisoning. Liver, damage. ***Nausea. Opacity, cornea. Ozaena.*** Poisonings. ***Polyps. Prostration. Radiation, effects. Stomach, cancer***. Stomach, disorders. Strokes. Toxic, exposure. Tympanites. Ulcers. Vaccinations. Vertigo. ***Vomiting.*** Weakness. ***Yellow fever.***

HOMEOPATHIC - The major use of Cadm-s. has been as an antidote to the severe side effects of toxic cancer therapy, especially, chemotherapy and radiation treatments, which can cause weakness, emaciation, nausea, vomiting, liver damage, hair loss, anorexia and which speeds up the time of death.

Cadm-s. chief action centers on the stomach and respiration. Important gastric symptoms. Symptoms corresponding to very low forms of disease. Useful for the last stage of diseases which runs deathward. A notable anti-psoric.

Side effects of ***chemotherapy and radiation treatments. Stomach cancer*** with persistent nausea and vomiting. Cholera and ***yellow fever***, when there is ***emaciation, vomiting and extreme prostration***.

Burning and cutting pain in the stomach. Intense nausea, retching, gagging, vomiting, bringing up tough mucus. Extreme exhaustion and prostration with vomiting. Black vomit. The least thing touching the lips will excite vomiting. Pitchy taste, food tastes like salt. Acts well in alcoholics.

Facial paralysis from the cold winds. ***Chilliness and coldness*** even when near the fire. Patient must keep quiet. Lies with the head low and the hands under it. Restlessness.

Skin blue, yellow, scaly, cracking, damp, suppurating herpes, and chilblains. Formication between the skin and deep tissue. Itching of skin, at night in bed, when touched when cold, better scratching, which causes a voluptuous feeling.

Cutting pains in the joints. Starting of the limbs. Numbness of parts, nose, head etc. Paralyzed parts painful or crawling in. Weakness remaining after epileptic attacks of one arm and one leg. Weakness of affected parts with goose bumps.

MIND - Dullness of mind, unconscious. Horror of solitude and work. Apprehension at the approach of anybody. Excessive irritability. Anxiety, before stool. Effects of anxiety or fits of passion. Restlessness worse sunlight.

Fear of others approaching him. Smiling in sleep. Moaning during sleep. Nervousness during headache. Anxiety. Vexation. Fits of passion aggravates symptoms in general. Unconsciousness between attacks of cough.

Abdomen - Sore, tender, tympanitic. Pain in abdomen with vomiting. Coldness. Stretching in the sides. Compressed feeling, pressure, bruised pain. Pulsation. Lancinations in the left hypochondria. Griping in the lower bowels.

Back - Pain in muscles of neck. Back pain as from the efforts to vomit.

Breasts - Inflamed nipples. Erysipelas of the breasts.

Causations - Chemotherapy, radiation poisoning. Vaccinations. Lead or other toxic poisoning. Grief.

Chest - Chest contracted with asthma. Drawing. Feeling of dilatation or contraction. Feeling as if the lungs adhered to the chest. Swelling of the external chest. Weakness of the chest. Rheumatic pain. Painful blows. Tingling in the chest. Beating near the heart. Chest symptoms, worse squatting.

Constitutions - Cancer miasm and toxic constitution. Broken down constitution from cancer, chemotherapy or radiation treatments.

Ears - Pressure behind the ears. Lacerating pain. Lancinating pain in ears. Abnormal hearing, alternating with abnormal vision. Sounds echo in the head. Clucking noises in the ears.

Eyes - Hollow eyes. ***Opacity of cornea*** from injuries or inflammation. Blue circle around eyes. Lachrymation, hot tears. Blenorrhea. One pupil dilated the other contracted. Swelling of conjunctiva. Scrofulous inflammation of eyes. Idiopathic chronic conjunctivitis. Night blindness. Cannot read small type.

Face - Gloomy countenance. Vexed look. Grayish complexion. Drawing pain in face. ***Facial paralysis,*** left side, worse cold air, cannot close the eyes, difficult talking and swallowing, distortion of the mouth. Crawling sensation in the face. Trembling of lower jaw. Spasmodic motion of the upper lip. Swelling of the lips. Yellow spots on the cheeks and nose.

Food - Thirst, with heat in bed at night. Craves little drinks of cold water that are vomited at once. Nausea and vomiting after eating.

Head - Inflammation of the brain. Strokes. Heat in head. Lancinations, hammering, digging pains. Drawing pains in head. Tingling in head. Heat in head. Pulsation in the temples. Pain in the vertex. Congestion to head, with pains cutting like knives. Rolling of head, with open eyes, in cholera infantum. Inflammation of brain. Apoplexy. Herpes on temples.

Heart - Palpitation with constriction of chest.

Kidneys - Rawness and soreness in urethra. Urine mixed with pus and blood. Griping in the region of the kidneys.

Limbs - Rheumatism. Boring and digging. Suppuration of the axillary glands. Stretching of the arms. Swelling of the arm-bones. Tension in the forearm. Gnawing in the hands. Tearing pain in the metacarpal joints. Jerking of the fingers.

Lancinations in the joints and in the toes. Numbness of the thighs. Trembling in the knee. Pressure in the knee. Tearing pain in the legs. Cramp of the calf. Pain, as if sprained. Heaviness of the feet. Chilblains.

Liver - Region of liver sore.

Lungs - Suffocation on dropping to sleep. Cough with loss of consciousness. Cough with agitation, red face, pain in the stomach or vomiting of bile. Interrupted breathing during sleep On waking, want of air.

Modalities - Better eating and rest. Worse from raising up. Worse least motion. Worse carrying burdens. Worse ascending stairs. Worse walking. Worse swallowing. Worse after sleep. Worse in morning. Worse from stimulants. Worse after intoxication. Worse from vexation. Worse in sunshine. Worse open air. Worse cold, cold air. Worse itching of skin when cold.

Mouth - Difficult swallowing. Salty, pitchy taste. Salivation. Aphthae on the lips. Stringy and offensive exudation on mucus membrane. ***Tongue, dirty brown or black.*** The symptoms of the mouth are aggravated during deglutition. Salty belching.

Nose - Tightness at the root of the nose. Obstruction of the nose by swelling. Numbness of the nose. ***Ozaena.*** Nose-bleed. ***Polyps***, boils. Caries of the nose. Lacerating pain in the nose. Nostrils ulcerated. Decay of nasal bones. Ulcerative, cancerous smell.

Rectum - Clots of blood from bowels. Bloody, black and offensive stools, gelatinous, yellowish green, semi-fluid with urinary suppression.

Skin - Blue, yellow, sallow, scaly, cracking. Chloasma, yellowish stains on nose and cheeks, worse exposure to sun and wind. Itching when touched and during cold, ameliorated by scratching, which excites a voluptuous feeling. Chilblains. Goose bumps after drinking, with hot hands, heartburn.

Sleep - Sleeps with open eyes. Somnolence with broken dreams. Moaning and smiling during sleep. Nightmares. While asleep, the feet are agitated by shocks. Stops breathing on going to sleep, wakes up suffocating. Fears to go to sleep again. Protracted sleeplessness (Carc., Cocc.). Sleepiness in the forenoon. Drowsiness when sitting.

Stomach - Intense nausea with pain and cold. Burning and cutting pain with retching and gagging. Violent ***nausea***, retching. ***Black vomit***, like coffee grounds. Vomiting of mucus, green slime, blood, with great prostration and tenderness over the stomach. Least thing touching lips will excite nausea and vomiting. Stomach symptoms worse carrying burden, better quiet. Stomach cancer, with persistent vomiting.

Temperature - ***Icy coldness*** (Camph., Verat., Helo.), Goose bumps after drinking or with hot hands. Coldness, even when near the fire, with heat in the hands. Coldness after sleeping and after walking. Fever, before midnight. ***Yellow fever*** (Crot-h., Carb-v.). Sweat in the axilla and the palms.

Throat - Chilliness and aching. Sore throat, constant tickling, gagging and nausea, worse from deep breathing. Dysphagia. Esophagus is constricted (Bapt.).

Vertigo - Faintness on rising. Vertigo, room and bed seem to spin around.

COMMENTS - Cadmium sulphuratum is found in nature in intimate association with Zinc, which it resembles in action, but it acts more powerfully. Cadm-s. is a cross between Bry. and Ars. It has the desire to keep quiet of Bry. with the exhaustion and stomach irritability of Ars.

A major cancer remedy. Affinity for cancers of the GI tract, cancers of the esophagus, the stomach, the liver, and the colon (Cadm-met. for bone cancers, Cadm-i. for glandular cancers). Nausea and vomiting in cancer cases. For the ill effects of radiation and chemotherapy. Extreme prostration and fatigue after chemotherapy or radiation, emaciation, sunken features, cachexia.

Nausea, intensified by motion. Vomiting of acid or yellow substances. Black vomit, occurs in severe zymotic diseases. Vomit like coffee grounds. Vomiting during pregnancy, when other remedies fail. Pernicious forms of vomiting, of black blood from chronic ulcers or cancer of the stomach. Nausea and vomiting with cold perspiration bathing the face and cutting pains in the abdomen.

Ulceration of the stomach in alcoholics (Ars.). Beer aggravates the gastric complaints. Salivation, with bitter burning in the mouth and throat, fetid breath, ulcers with dryness, and burning constriction of the throat.

Characteristic coldness, all complaints are made worse from becoming cold, or from cold changes in the weather. Icy coldness even when near a fire. Goose bumps, with hot hands, or after drinking. Sweat in axilla. Effect of a drought or cold air in checking sweat.

Weakness and tiredness, accompanied by a cachectic state that stimulates the cachexia of advanced cancer cases or pernicious anemia. Increased irritability. Horror of solitude and of work.

Ozaena and polyps. Cutting, sharp pains, sense of constriction. Opacity of the cornea, loss of vision. Protracted sleeplessness, insomnia. Sleeps with eyes open, stops breathing on going to sleep. Awakens suffocating after sleep.

RELATIONS - ***Followed well by:*** Carc., Bell. - rolling of head with open eyes in cholera infantum, Carb-v., Lob. inf. In cancer - Hydr., Ars. In yellow fever - Nit-ac. In nausea of pregnancy - Alet. ***Compare:*** (1) Cadm-ox., Cadm-br. - pain and burning in stomach and vomiting. (2) Cadm-i. - Itching of anus and rectum felt during the day only, constipation, frequent desire, tenesmus, abdomen bloated. (3) Zinc., Ars., Carb-v., Verat. (3) Zinc. but in Zinc. the action is primarily on brain in Cadm. primarily on stomach. (4) in constriction across chest with palpitations, Kali-chl. (5) weakness, nausea, vomit and burning, Ars. (6) black vomit, disorders of alcoholism, Ars., Lach. in nausea and retching, Asar., Bry., Crot-t., Cupr., Nux-v., Podo., Ant-t. in deathly nausea, Ip., Tab., greenish gelatinous vomit.

REFERENCES - Boericke. Clarke. Grimmer. Murphy.

CAESALPINIA BONDUCELLA

(Nata)

PHARMACY - caesal. Caesalpinia bonducella. Nata. Fever nut. Bondue nut. N. O. Leguminosae. ***Historical dose:*** Tincture and all potencies.

CLINICAL - Asthma. Hemorrhage. Leprosy. Tuberculosis.

HERBAL - Nata is a well-known wild shrub of India. It grows near the sea-coast in all hot countries, the extensive distribution being due probably to the transport of the seeds by oceanic currents. It is pregnant with climbing prickly points and the shrub is commonly found all over Bengali, Bombay and practically the whole of southern India. The plant has been known for a long time to the Hindu and Mohammedan physicians to contain excellent medicinal properties.

The seeds are considered in India and Persia to be "very hot and dry" and they are found to be very useful in dispersing swellings, arresting hemorrhage and warding off infectious maladies. The seeds, roasted and powdered, are employed for hydrocele internally and externally. They are also used internally in curing leprosy.

The powdered seeds mixed with black pepper are found to be febrifuge and antiperiodic and are used in chronic fevers. The fixed oil expressed from the seeds is emollient and is employed as an embrocation for the purpose of removing freckles from the face, also as a cosmetic and used also to arrest discharges from the ear. A decoction of the roasted seeds is employed against consumption and asthma.

HOMEOPATHIC - Extreme weakness is felt after the remission of fever, so much so that the patient is averse even to have any talk. There is no inclination to do any work. Always likes to sleep. Lies quit with closed eyes. No desire to leave bed.

After the remission of fever the patient feels extreme weakness, is disinclined to do any work. There is no desire to talk even The patient likes to lie down quietly in bed with closed eyes.

The fever appears between 8 a.m. and 10 a.m. or between 2 p.m. and 4 p.m. In the afternoon fever there is no thirst, but in the morning fever there is thirst in hot stage.

The above symptoms are generally observed in intermittent fevers, but in remittent fevers of malarial origin it is also used with benefit.

MIND - Mental depression. Lack of enthusiasm.

Abdomen - there is gurgling in the lower abdomen, sometimes liquid, slimy stools are passed by the patient.

Back - Drawing pains are felt in the back after cold bath.

Eyes - Before the appearance of fever and during its invasion terrible pains are felt in the eyes as if they are burnt; they are relieved by the application of cold water; eyes are sunken and bloodless.

Fever - It is very irregular in appearance. It may come on any time; fever appears with chilliness and shivering one day and again on another day it appears in the afternoon with slight chilliness. The character of fever is changeable. It's is generally felt with chilliness and shivering. Thirst is generally felt in the stage of heat; the stage of sweat lasts for a short time only, sweat breaks out over face, chest, neck, shoulder. the fever does not last more than 6 hours.

Food - Desire to take boiled rice and other hard substance and meat. Aversion to take any liquid food. No desire to take bath.

Head - During fever terrible pains are felt over both the temples of head, relieved by wrapping them up or by pressure.

Liver - The lower lobe is enlarged; before fever sometimes uneasiness in the hepatic region is felt or sometimes slight pain is felt there.

Mouth - During hot stage of the fever thirst is felt; thirst for cold water; face is flushed during fever.

Nose - Hot breath; during fever frequent and hurried respiration takes place.

Skin - Dry, dirty, blackish coloured. Small eruptions like mosquito bite appear on the skin, which disappear generally.

Spleen - Enlargement and hardness of spleen exist and it is painful to touch.

Stool - Hard, saffron colored stools. Stools are sometimes liquid and yellow coloured.

Tongue - Slight white coating on the tongue appears; bloodless white tongue; tongue is moist, but there is thirst.

REFERENCES - Ghose.

CAFFEINE

(Coffee Alkaloid)

PHARMACY - caffe. Caffeine. Alkaloid of Coffee arabica. Coffine. Trituration of the alkaloid and also of the Citrate of caffeine. ***Historical dose:*** Trituration and all potencies.

CLINICAL - Anxiety. Brachialgia. ***Diuresis***. Dizziness. ***Headaches. Insomnia. Nervousness.*** Neuralgias. ***Polyuria.*** Pulmonary edema. Restlessness. Trembling.

HOMEOPATHIC - A crystalline alkaloid, it is a direct heart stimulant and diuretic. One of the best stimulants of the vaso-motor centers. Dropsy depending on cardiac insufficiency. Cardiac insufficiency in pneumonia and other infectious diseases. Myocardial degeneration.

Caffeine raises the blood pressure, increases pulse rate and stimulates the heart muscle, hence a support in extreme feebleness or threatened failure. Stimulates the respiratory center, nerve centers and ***increases diuresis***. Acute pulmonary edema. Brachialgia and other neuralgias characterized by ***nightly aggravations***.

COMMENTS - A proving has been made with this alkaloid, but has brought out no symptoms not included in the pathogenesis of Coff. Marked pulsation of the arteries on the head and temples. Sparks before eyes, roaring in the ears. Vomiting with relief of all symptoms.

The Citrate of caffeine, which is used in allopathic practice, has occasioned dangerous poisonous symptoms in a number of cases. The most characteristic include restlessness and dizziness, inability to keep erect. Palpitations. Violent precordial anxiety. Very rapid pulse.

Abdominal pulsation. Violent trembling of all the limbs. Grating of the teeth. Features expressive of great anxiety. Constriction of the neck and throat, recurring periodically every fifteen minutes.

RELATIONS - ***Compare:*** (1) Acon., Cham., Coffea, Nux-v, Cypr. (2) Caffeine and plants containing it, as Cacao, Kola, Thea, etc.

REFERENCES - Boericke. Clarke.

CAINCA RACEMOSA

(Brazilian Chiococca)

PHARMACY - cahin. Cainca racemosa. Brazilian chiococca. Chiococca densifolia. Chiococca racemosa. N. O. Rubiacae. Brazil. Tincture of dried root bark. ***Historical dose:*** Tincture and all potencies.

CLINICAL - Albuminuria. Ascites. Bright's disease. Cough. Dropsy. Dyspnea. ***Fatigue.*** Kidney, pain. Nephritis. Ophthalmia. Polyuria. Spleen, pain. Traveling, effects. Weakness.

HOMEOPATHIC - Cainca is related botanically to Chin., Ip., and Coff. Clinically, it is very like Apoc. Marked urinary symptoms. It has been given with success in dropsies, especially when associated with dry skin.

General fatigue and weakness. It removes fatigue from riding on horseback too long. Much weakness after dinner, so as to make him lie down. Abdomen sensitive to the touch. Albuminuria with dyspnea on lying down at night. Ascites and anasarca with dry skin. Polyuria while traveling. Slight uneasiness.

MIND - Feeling of anxiety with increased warmth of the lower abdomen.

Abdomen - Stitches in and through the spleen. Warmth about the umbilicus. Fullness, inflation and uncomfortable feeling in the abdomen. After eating, perceptible pulsation of abdominal aorta during rest. Gurgling and rumbling in the abdomen and bowels. Slight colic with borborygmus. Cutting pains in abdomen before evacuation of the bowels. Pain under the umbilicus with desire to go to stool.

Back - Pain in region of kidneys, better lying bent backward.

Chest - Constriction and pressure on chest. Peculiar shooting and beating pain over the trunk. Dartings in the right side of thorax. Piercing pain in the middle part of the right side of the chest. Pricking pain in the lower third of the right side of the chest, with feeling of weight.

Ears - Intolerable hissing in the ears. Roaring and buzzing, as if from a swarm of insects in the air.

Eyes - Burning in the eyes. Increased sensibility of the eyes. Photophobia. Edema of left upper or right lower eyelid. Pressure in the eyeballs from above downwards and from below upwards. Sensation as if the eyeballs were pressed upwards, with troubled vision for five minutes, returning after half an hour.

Face - Heat of the face.

Food - Appetite good in the evening. Absence of appetite. Less appetite than usual for dinner. Thirst.

Head - Very violent headache. Severe headache, particularly in the occiput, forbidding reading and every intellectual exertion. Heaviness of the head. Heaviness, pressure and uneasiness of front of head. Piercing pain in right temple. Pressure in the sinciput. Darting pains in right half of sinciput. Feeling of weight and pressure in occiput.

Kidneys - Constant desire to urinate. Polyuria while traveling. Urine fiery. Burning pain in urethra, especially glandular portion.

Limbs - Pricking pain in left hand. Stretching of lower limbs. Heaviness of the lower limbs. Feeling of lassitude in soles of feet. Constant pressure in the lower third of the under part of right foot. Acute pricking under nail of great toe.

Lungs - Tickling cough with tough, greenish-gray expectoration, waking him at 3 a.m.

Male - Drawing in of testicles and spermatic cord. Pain worse during passage of pungent-smelling urine. Horridly excited sexual impulses. Fearful, lascivious dreams with erections, restlessness awakened by an emission.

Modalities - Better in evening. Better rest. Better after diarrhea. Worse from motion. Worse ascending stairs. Worse from waking. Worse in the morning. Worse siesta. Worse from 4 p.m. to 6 p.m.

Mouth - Offensive smelling breath. Considerable salivation, or saliva no longer seemed to be secreted. Perverted taste, the whole mouth bitter. Mucous, insipid taste. Drug tasted like apple-wine, first sweetish, then bitter and burning. In the evening, tearing pains in the teeth of the upper jaw.

Nose - Violent catarrh of thin mucus, excoriating the nose, especially in the daytime.

Rectum - Frequent calls to stool with escape of nothing but air. Burning at the anus. Tickling in the anus, obliging him to scratch frequently.

Sleep - Yawning with stretching of limbs. Sleepiness in morning. Desire to sleep. Sleepless during the whole night. Restless sleep, with lascivious dreams. Somnolence.

Stomach - Dryness of the throat, trembling of the hands. Belchings, as after small doses of tartar emetic. Much tasteless belching. Nausea and vomiting. Violent vomiting from three spoonfuls. Vomiting and slight shivering, for half an hour. Feeling of cold in the epigastric region.

Temperature - Heightened temperature of the body. Warmth all over. Moist skin, sweating even when at rest. Perspiring more easily than usual, particularly in the evening.

Throat - Voice hoarse and hollow. Ulcers in the throat to the Eustachian tube. Distressing dryness in throat. Obliged to hawk often from irritation of the throat. Burning and grating pain in throat. Scraping in throat, forcing him to cough. Rawness of throat, with taste like that of pepper. Dry, burning heat in the pharynx, at first with sensation as if from pepper. Feeling of itchiness and scraping. Dysphagia. Cold feeling down the esophagus.

Tongue - Tongue coated with mucus. Tongue exceedingly dry with a white and very dark coating. Tongue furred white.

Vertigo - Symptoms of giddiness and sickness. Giddiness, with vomiting, or on going up stairs.

RELATIONS - ***Antidoted by:*** Colch., Rhus-t. (gastralgia), Verat. Cainca follows well: Ars. ***Compare:*** (1) Apocynum, Ars., Bry. (2) Similar to Coffea in relieving effects of fatigue, also Arn.

REFERENCES - Boericke. Clarke.

CAJUPUTUM OLEUM

(Cajuput Oil)

PHARMACY - caj. Cajuputum oleum. Cajuput Oil. Oleum cajuputi. Oleum wittnebianum. Melaleuca leucadendron. White Tea Tree. Weeping Paperbark. N. O. Myrtaceae. Solution of the oil in rectified Spirit. ***Historical dose:*** Tincture and all potencies.

CLINICAL - Cholera. Colic. Coughing. Deafness. Diarrhea. Dropsy. Dyspnea. Epilepsy. Eruptions. Esophagus, stricture. ***Flatulence.*** Gout. Headaches. Heartburn. Hiccoughs. Hysteria. Menstruation, disorders. Paralysis. Rheumatism. Tongue, disorders. Toothaches. Urinary, disorders. Vertigo.

HERBAL - Cajuput oil distilled in water from the leaves of Melaleuca leucadendron. Cajuput Oil acts like Cloves Oil, it has a reputation as a local application in rheumatism and also in cases of dysmenorrhea. Cajuput has cured obstinate hiccoughs from the slightest provocation, talking, laughing, eating or any motion. Symptoms appear and then disappear suddenly, come at 5 a.m., disappear on eating. Many symptoms are worse at night. Smoking causes desire to vomit.

HOMEOPATHIC - The homeopathic proving of Caj. showed a characteristic ***sensation of enlargement.*** A feeling of being too large all over, as if head as large as half a bushel. Feeling as though could not get himself together (Bapt.), could not get his clothes for a time, though they were quite near.

Nervous symptoms, some reflected from the female sexual organs. Persistent choking sensation of hysteria, nervous dyspnea, nervous distention of the bowels. Earache and face ache, the lobe of the ear is red, alae nasal turn red, nose appears swollen.

Neuralgic affections, not inflammatory.

Flatulence and disorders of the tongue. Gout. Nervous dyspnea. Copious perspiration. A measles-like eruption with intense itching. Sensations as if poisoned. As if the arms were tied to the body, heavy, useless. Numb feeling all over.

MIND - Feeling as if he did not want any one to speak. Feel sad and downhearted, as if could cry. Want to walk in a slow and very dignified manner and prefer to walk alone. Can't think of anything, ideas come slow. Can't bear to do any work or study. Feels stupefied and completely intoxicated all the afternoon.

Abdomen - ***Flatulent colic***, tympanites (Tereb.). Nervous distention of the bowels. Griping pain in the bowels on riding. Spasmodic cholera.

Chest - Sharp, steady pain. Soreness. Pain across the chest, in the right lung.

Ears - The lobes of the ears are red and the upper portion remains natural.

Face - Sensation of burning in the face. Yellow appearance, feels puffy, rough to the touch. Can't hurt the skin of the face by pinching it. Pain through the left malar bone. Stiff, dry feeling in the jaws, with neuralgic pains in the malar bones and severe headache all over the head, on waking at 5 a.m. Prosopalgia with the severe headache.

Food - No appetite or thirst. Good appetite, can eat anything, but feels unnatural when eating, the eating seems to be performed mechanically

Head - Feels much enlarged. As if he could not get himself together (Bapt.).

Kidneys - Urine smells badly, like cat's urine. Urine diminished in quantity and has a milky, light-colored appearance.

Limbs - Joints feel enlarged with some pain. Sensation in the arms as if they were tied to the body. Arms feel tired and heavy. Weakness and aching pain in both knees.

Lungs - Severe coughing and strangulation. Coughing almost makes one vomit.

Male - Erections with great desire for an embrace. Erections all night, in the morning, without the least sexual desire. Penis shriveled and shrunk. Loss of sexual desire (Sep.).

Modalities - Better in open air. Better from pressure. Better lying down. Worse at night. Worse about 5 a.m. Worse from bending forward. Worse riding. Worse itching, and scratching.

Mouth - ***Spasmodic stricture of esophagus***. Persistent sensation of choking. Constricted sensation on swallowing solid food. Much water in the mouth, wants to spit a great deal. Profuse flow of saliva. Constant inclination to spit and hawk up large quantities of tough white mucus, can feel drawn through the sinuses. Cool and not unpleasant sensation in the mouth and pharynx. Taste in the mouth of lye. Salty taste after intense thirst. Acrid taste in the pharynx and esophagus for a few minutes. Speech thick and slow.

Nose - Nose is most prominent.

Rectum - Diarrhea, watery, yellowish. Diarrhea by day, and worse by night, bowels moved often.

Skin - An eruption as thick as measles, all over the arms and body. Intense itching, aggravated by scratching.

Sleep - Tired and sleepy. Amorous dreams without emissions. In dreams, felt disposed to swear and act rowdy.

Stomach - ***Hiccough***, on slightest provocation.

Temperature - Feels cold, cold sweat all over the body. Profuse and weakening sweat.

Throat - Burning in the throat down to the stomach. Burning in the lower part of the pharynx. Burning in the esophagus, as if there was lye in it. Can hardly swallow. Esophagus feels sore. Voice hoarse, as if taken cold .

Tongue - Tongue moist, looks white and rough, like a calf's tongue, feels as if it were scalded and as if the skin would peel off. ***Tongue feels swollen***, fills whole mouth.

COMMENTS - The provers of Caj. experienced a "Feeling as if I did not want any one to speak to me" (after twenty-four hours). Did not want to be spoken to, particularly from men. Felt better in the society of ladies, "can laugh and make free with the women (am naturally bashful)," (after two hours).

"Feel sad and down-hearted, as if I could cry (after two hours). I do not want any one to speak to me, nevertheless

I like to be where I can see persons and hear their talk. Can't bear to look inside the books I usually study, can think of a thousand things in a minute (one hour after first dose, second day).

"Want to walk in a slow and very dignified manner and prefer to walk alone (one hour second dose, second day). Can't think of anything, ideas come slow, can't bear to do any work or study (one hour after second dose, second day). Can't think of study (eight day). Felt stupefied and completely intoxicated all the afternoon (after second dose, fifth day)."

RELATIONS - ***Compare:*** (1) Bov. - swollen sensations. Plantago - earache toothache. Colch. - gout and rheumatism. (2) Acon. and Bell. - effects of checked sweat. (3) Bapt., Nux-m., Asaf., Ign., Eucal.. (4) Eugenia caryophyllacea (cloves), Eugenia jambos and the Brazil-nut tree belong to the same order.

REFERENCES - Boericke. Clarke.

CALADIUM SEGUINUM

(American Arum)

PHARMACY - calad. Caladium seguinum. American arum. Arum seguinum. Dumb cane. Dieffenbachia seguine. N. O. Araceae. South America. Tincture of whole fresh plant. ***Historical dose:*** Tincture and all potencies.

CLINICAL - ***Asthma.*** Dropsical, swellings. Gonorrhea. Impotence. Masturbation. Mosquito, bites. Nymphomania. ***Itching. Pruritus, vulvae.*** Spermatorrhea. Threadworms. ***Tobacco, habit. Tobacco, poisoning.*** Typhoid. Typhus. Worms.

HOMEOPATHIC - Like the other Arums, Caladium has an intensely irritating effect on the mucus membranes and skin and produces many burning sensations. Caladium seems to lessen the ***craving for tobacco.*** Mosquito bites that itch and burn intensely.

Marked action on the genital organs and itching of this region. ***Itching of the vagina. Pruritus vulvae*** in females, which may sometimes be due to thread worms finding their way into vagina inducing masturbation and sometimes nymphomania.

Lascivious thoughts in men, but impotent. Masturbation and its results. Nocturnal emissions occurring either without dreams or with non-sexual dreams. ***Spermatorrhea.*** The glans penis is flabby from masturbation. Prepuce, if drawn back, remains so from loss of contractility.

Dryness of parts, which are usually moist. Coldness of single parts and inclination to lie down, with aggravation on lying on left side. Great desire to lie down and aversion to motion, but if he makes the effort he is strong enough.

Asthma, alternating with itching rash. Asthmatic complaints. Catarrhal asthma, mucus not readily raised, but giving relief when it comes up. Tobacco heart.

Fever with drowsiness. Sweet odor of sweat. Attacks like fainting after writing and thinking, when lying down or when rising. Unable to walk with closed eyes. ***Dread from motion.*** Slightest noise startles from sleep.

MIND - Refuses to take medicine. Very careful about health. Fear of catching disease. Afraid of his own shadow. Forgetfulness. Foolish boldness. Nervous excitation. Restless, cannot control himself after smoking. Nervous and craves tobacco.

Abdomen - Sensation as of a long worm writhing in transverse colon.

Causations - Gonorrhea. Masturbation. Tobacco habit, poisoning.

Constitutions - Suited to persons of lax, phlegmatic temperament.

Ears - Sensitive to noise. Slightest noise starts from sleep.

Eyes - Eyes are closed, even while walking in open air.

Face - Sensation as of a cobweb or crawling.

Female - ***Itching of vulva and vagina*** (Ambr., Kreos.). Itching from pinworms or with pregnancy. Voluptuousness. Itching leading to masturbation, with burning. Cramp pains in uterus at night. Sexual weakness or neurasthenia.

Food - Eats without hunger and drinks without thirst. Thirstless for days. ***Craving for tobacco.***

Head - Headaches and mental states of smokers. Very forgetful, does not know about the occurrence of things. Confused headache with pain in shoulder, pressure in eyes and forehead, extremely sensitive to noise, throbbing in ear. Numbness in side of head.

Heart - ***Tobacco heart.*** Heart weakness.

Kidneys - Urine offensive, scanty.

Limbs - Weak, cannot get out of bed. Hands numb. Cannot walk or stand with closed eyes.

Lungs - Catarrhal asthma, mucus not readily raised, but better expectoratión. Hard cough with asthma. Impeded breathing. Sighing respiration. Larynx seems constricted. Fear of going to sleep. Lung cancer.

Male - Erections when half-asleep, cease when fully awake. ***Impotency***, relaxation of penis during excitement. Impotency after gonorrhea, with mental depression. ***Spermatorrhea***. No emission and no orgasm during embrace. Atonic pollution. Prepuce retracted after sex. ***Pruritus***. Organs seem larger, puffed, relaxed, flaccid, sweaty. Genitals cold (Agn.). Thick skin of scrotum. Glans very red, like a rag.

Modalities - Better after sweat. Better after sleeping in the daytime, short nap. Better cold air. Worse from sudden noises. Worse sexual excess. Worse tobacco smoking. Worse motion. Worse falling asleep. Worse lying on left side. Worse warmth. Aversion to cold water, but bathing with cold water improves itching.

Mouth - Food eaten seems too dry, must drink to swallow. Milk tastes sour. Red, dry stripe down center of tongue, widening towards tip. Saliva like egg white.

Nose - Discharge of bloody mucus on blowing nose.

Skin - Itching rash alternates with asthma. ***Burning sensation***. Erysipelatous inflammation. Sweet sweat that attracts flies. Insect bites burn and itch intensely. Feels rough and dry. Burning in spots, must touch the part, but cannot scratch them.

Sleep - Groans and moans anxiously, loudly in sleep. Vivid dreams.

Stomach - Belchings. ***Stomach feels full of dry food*** with asthma. ***Fluttering sensation.*** Burning in the stomach, worse deep breathing, taking tea or chocolate. Gnawing in orifice of stomach, which prevents deep breathing and belchings. Acrid vomiting. Thirstless, tolerates only warm drinks.

Temperature - Cold single parts, feet. Sweat of sweetish odor, attracting flies. Low fevers. Falls asleep during fever, wakes up when it stops.

Vertigo - Vertigo, as if rocked, worse closing eyes and lying down.

COMMENTS - Tobacco heart, tobacco craving, tobacco addiction. Some results for lessening addiction, but often difficult case management. Caladium will lessen the cravings and help with the withdrawal (Lob., Nicot., Fumeris Tabacum). Treatment can cause nausea when smoking, or the patient can develop an allergy to tobacco smoke.

Asthma and emphysema from cigarette smoking. Lung cancer with a history of cigarette smoking. Constriction of the peripheral blood vessels causes coldness of the limbs, weakness of the heart, blood pressure problems. Motion sickness.

H. N. Martin gave a picture: "Caladium is similar to Lycopodium, the patient wants to lie down always. Better from sweat, opposite of Merc., and better after short sleep, opposite of Lach. Perspiration attracts flies. Genitals relaxed and perspire. Patient afraid to go to sleep and doesn't know why. Itching of vulva with burning."

RELATIONS - ***Compare:*** (1) Caps., Phos., Caust., Sel., Lyc. (2) Ikshugandha - sexual weakness, emissions, prostatic enlargement. ***Incompatible:*** Arum triph. ***Complementary:*** Nit-ac.

REFERENCES - Boericke. Clarke. Murphy. Phatak.

CALCAREA ACETICA

(Calcium Acetate)

PHARMACY - calc-acet. Calcarea acetica. Calcium acetate. Tincture. ***Historical dose:*** Trituration and all potencies.

CLINICAL - Anus, itching. Bronchitis. Cancer, pains. ***Coughs.*** Dysmenorrhea. Dyspnea. Headaches. Migraine. Vertigo.

HOMEOPATHIC - Calcarea acetica was one the first of the lime preparations proved by Hahnemann. The symptoms of Calc-acet. are generally identical with those of Calc., both are prepared from oyster shells and are included in the pathogenesis of that medicine.

Calc-acet. has had brilliant clinical results in inflammations of mucus membranes characterized by ***membranous exudation***, otherwise its action and application is like the carbonate.

Cancer pains. Stupefying, pressive pains in the forehead with compression of the whole head. Dulling of the senses while reading, obliged to stop reading.

MIND - Anxieties and worries. Confusion of the mind.

Chest - Constrictive, anxious sensation in chest.

Eyes - ***Senses obscure while reading.***

Female - Membranous dysmenorrhea (Bor.).

Head - ***Migraine*** with great coldness in head and sour taste. Frontal headache, stupefying, pressing pain. Head feels compressed.

Lungs - Violent spasmodic cough. Rattling expiration. ***Loose cough with expectoration of large pieces*** like casts of bronchial tubes. Difficult breathing, better bending shoulders backward.

Rectum - Severe itching of the anus. Profuse, painless, not exhausting diarrhea.

Stomach - Sour, offensive belchings.

Vertigo - Vertigo when walking in the open air.

COMMENTS - Allen's Handbook mentions that Calc-acet. cured some cases of membranous dysmenorrhea and also cases of violent spasmodic cough ending in the expulsion of casts of bronchial tubes (Calc.). It has been used in the excruciating pains of open cancer (Calc-ox.).

Clotar Muller cured many cases of megrim with Calc-acet. The indications he relied on were "Sour taste in mouth, sour belchings, sensation of coldness in the head and of emptiness. Head pain one-sided, affecting the right eye, which was red, causing lachrymation."

RELATIONS - ***Compare:*** (1) Calc., Brom., Bor. (2) also Calc-oxal. in excruciating pains of open cancer.

REFERENCES - Boericke. Clarke.

CALCAREA ARSENICOSA

(Calcium Arsenite)

PHARMACY - calc-ar. Calcarea arsenicosa. Calcium arsenite. Tricalcic arsenite of lime. Diarsenite. Trituration. ***Historical dose:*** Trituration and all.

CLINICAL - Acidity. ***Albuminuria. Alcoholism.*** Anemia. Anger. Ascarides. Asthma. Belching. ***Cancer. Chilliness.*** Cholera. Cirrhosis. Colic. Constipation. Delusions. Diarrhea. Dropsy. Embolus. ***Epilepsy.*** Gastric, ulcer. Headaches. ***Heart, disease.*** Heartburn. Indigestion. Intermittent fever. Kidneys, disorders. Leucorrhea. Liver, disorders. Malaria. ***Nephritis.*** Obesity. ***Palpitations. Pancreas, cancer. Pancreas, disorders.*** Proteinuria. Spleen, disorders. Stroke. Tuberculosis. Tumors. Typhoid. Vertigo.

HOMEOPATHIC - Calcarea Arsenicosa was prepared and proved by Hering in the 4c dilution in 1848. According to P. C. Majumdar, it is the most efficient remedy in the infantile enlarged liver and spleen of India. In albuminuria cases, there is great sensitiveness of the kidney region. Cholera with impeded respiration from heart embolism.

Epilepsy with rush of blood to the head before attack, aura felt in region of heart, flying sensation. Epilepsy with heart disease. Flying sensation or swimming sensation, as if feet did not touch the ground.

Affections of spleen and mesenteric glands. ***Nephritis*** with great sensitiveness in kidney region. Dyspnea with feeble heart.

Hemoglobin and red corpuscles are low. Chronic malaria.

Fleshy women at menopause with ***slightest emotion causing palpitations***. Children with enlarged liver and spleen. Complaints of alcoholics after abstaining (Carbn-s.). ***Chilliness***.

MIND - Great mental depression. Depression and anger. ***Anxiety about future.*** Desire for company. Confusion of mind. ***Dullness of mind***, unable to digest any subject. Unable to attend any business on account of headache. ***Restlessness after midnight, 3 a.m.*** Delirium in evening in the dark.

Delusions and illusions. Wonderful visions passing before eyes, often an indescribable feeling of health, "as if in heaven." It seems to be a great many different things but lasts only a second, it passes like lightning, but is infinitely much.

Abdomen - Colic with looseness of bowels. Very painful shooting, cutting pains across abdomen going from right to left. ***Pancreatic diseases,*** with albuminuria. Relieves burning pain in cancer. ***Burning pain in cancer of pancreas.*** Sensation as if diarrhea would appear, soon after colicky pain around navel with pressure downward. Sensation as if a hernia would be forced out. Swollen inguinal glands with tearing pain in legs.

Back - Pain and stiffness near nape of neck. Stiffness of neck with headache, on waking in morning. Violent backache, throbbing, drives out of bed. ***Violent pain between shoulders and sacrum.*** Frequent shooting pain in lumbar region. Backache during pregnancy. Backache extends to lower limbs.

Chest - Burning heat in chest. Chest feels as if beaten. Sneezing with jerking, shooting pain near left side of sternum, region of 4th and 5th ribs. Dull pressure on chest with roughness of throat.

Constitutions - Suited to lymphatic, scrofulous and tuberculosis constitutions. Overweight women, approaching menopause. Obese persons. Complaints of alcoholics after leaving off alcohol.

Eyes - Blue rings around eyes. Violent pain in right eye and above it. Letters seem to run together.

Face - Face swollen, especially about eyes with albuminuria. ***Pale face and blue rings under eyes with palpitations.*** Tearing pain in upper and lower jaw. Face hot during palpitations.

Female - Amenorrhea. ***Scanty menses.*** Bearing down pain and uterine prolapse. Bearing down pain during pregnancy. Prolapsed vagina during pregnancy. Albuminuria during pregnancy. Offensive, bloody leucorrhea. Cancer of uterus. Burning pain in uterus and vagina.

Food - No appetite, can only enjoy soup. Thirst for cold water. ***Desire for soup. Desire for wine or other spirituous drinks.*** Worse after slightest error in diet. ***Worse eating which often causes eructations and vomiting.*** Worse after drinking wine. Worse after sweet potatoes.

Head - Headache causes feeling of lameness in whole body. ***Congestion to head before epileptic attack.*** Dull, stupefying pain. Rush of blood to the head with vertigo. Weekly headaches. ***Headaches better lying on painful side.*** Headache, goes to side not lain upon. Headache with palpitations, increase and decrease together. Headache worse after slightest error in diet. Benumbing headache, mostly around ears. Sharp pain in forehead. Burning pain in head, first left then right side. Swelling of temples. Head hot, in albuminuria.

Heart - Attacks of pains in heart, and fear of suffocating. Constriction of heart like a rush of blood to left chest, with palpitations and urging to stool. ***Constriction of heart before an epileptic attack.*** Constriction and pain in region of heart, suffocating feeling. Palpitations and heart pains before epileptic attack. ***Palpitations with oppression of chest, disturbing sleep.*** Palpitations, oppression, throbbing and pain in back extending to arms. ***Pains in region of heart and fearful palpitations.*** Beat of heart very strong in albuminuria. Pulse intermittent, every fourth beat regularly.

Kidneys - Burning pain with scanty urine. Nephritis. ***Albuminuria and dropsy.*** Passes urine every hour. ***Kidney region***

sensitive to pressure. Soreness in region of kidneys from drinking wine, with scanty, burning, albuminous urine. Urine containing very much protein.

Limbs - ***Edema of lower limbs with albuminuria.*** Inflammation of veins of lower limbs. Weariness and lameness of lower limbs. ***Pains in upper limbs before epileptic attack.*** Pain in left hand and arm before epileptic fit. Cold hands and fainting after pain in spermatic cords. Heat of hands before palpitations. ***Back of hands edematous with albuminuria.*** Feet feel as if heavy. Neuralgic pain in left knee. Tearing pain in legs, with swelling in groin.

Liver - Enlarged liver and spleen in chronic malaria in children.

Lungs - ***Dyspnea and feeble heart.*** Burning heat in lungs. Feeling as if he would suffocate with palpitations. Asthma. Every night an attack of difficult breathing. Shaking cough of whole chest, caused by a tickling in upper part of throat. Copious hawking of tough white phlegm.

Male - After drinking wine, pain in groins and in spermatic cords.

Modalities - Better rest. Better open air. Better mental exertion but worse after. Worse from slight exertion. Worse errors in diet. Worse cold air. Worse menopause. It is a chilly medicine, the symptoms being worse in cold weather, worse when out of doors.

Mouth - Copious saliva. ***Salivation with tasteless belching.*** Garlicky taste in mouth when swallowing. Flat unpleasant taste, sometimes metallic, sometimes alkaline. Sour taste. ***Itching on upper lip.*** Lips dry with albuminuria. Burning on tip of tongue. ***Tongue dry with albuminuria.*** Pains in decayed molars, extending to ears, recurring weekly.

Nose - Sneezing with fluent coryza in morning. Running catarrh at 3 a.m. with restlessness, sweat and sleeplessness. Catarrh in head before breakfast with spitting of mucus, which falls down from choanae. No phlegm through nose, only from choanae. Crusts in choanae.

Perspiration - Sweats at night, worse after 3 a.m.

Rectum - Burning during stool. Urging to stool with palpitations and oppression of chest. Diarrhea after midnight. Diarrhea, worse sweet potatoes or yams. Infantile diarrhea. Loose stools and colic. Loose stools during pregnancy. Stool with ascarides. Stool with itching at anus from evening until midnight. Stool tardy, but not hard. Hard and difficult stool for months.

Sleep - Drowsy and weary, with sensation of fullness under short ribs. Desire to sleep in middle of day, with heavy legs. Very restless sleep at night, disturbed by headache and palpitations. Turns from one side to another. Rolls about all night, sleeps and wakes, with asthma. After 3 a.m., sleepless, restless and perspiring. Dreams of people he had not seen for years.

Stomach - Anxiety in stomach. Acidity of stomach. Burning heat in stomach. Belching with saliva and beating of heart. Pressing pain as if to belch, ending with a sudden beat of heart. Food seems to lie in stomach without digesting. Sensation as if stomach was expanded, during fever. Digging pain in pit. Nausea when sitting down. Waterbrash with sour taste.

Temperature - Marked malaria. Chilly. Chills crawl over back towards arm and chest. Fever in afternoon, with sensation as if abdomen was puffed up. Fever with much thirst for cold water and loss of appetite in evening. Heat in chest during palpitations.

Throat - Sore throat with sour taste in mouth. Dryness in pit of throat with roughness of voice. Scratchy sensation in throat. Sensation as if a scab was in upper part of throat. Burning in esophagus as from pepper. Burning in throat after belching, with garlicky taste when swallowing. Pressing pain in throat with sour taste and waterbrash. ***Loses voice and afterwards consciousness, before an epileptic attack.*** Drawing as with a thread from larynx backwards.

Vertigo - Vertigo before epilepsy. Vertigo when moving head. Violent rush of blood to head with vertigo. Flying sensation or swimming sensation, as if feet didn't touch ground.

COMMENTS - Calc-ar. is a synthetic remedy that combines a Calcarea person with Arsenicum mentals and burning pains.

Great affinity for the pancreas. Pancreatitis and pancreatic cancer (Hydr., Con., Phos.). Burning in the solar plexus. Liver and spleen somewhat enlarged. Nephritis. Alcoholism.

Vertigo when moving the head. Flying or swimming sensation, as if feet did not touch the ground. Sudden, fleeting visions. Rush of blood to head before an epileptic attack. Epilepsy with heart disease.

Headaches move from front of head to back, worse mornings, going out of doors. Worse on aspect opposite to the one lain on, whether front or back or either side. Weight on vertex, later on occiput.

Well-marked fever symptoms, intermittent, remittent. Hectic fever and masked malaria. Marked chilliness, originates inwardly with a sensation as if skin and adjoining parts were hot. Chilly cramps over back towards arms and chest. Night sweat after 3 a.m.

RELATIONS - ***Antidoted by:*** Carb-v. (palpitations), Glon. (headache), Puls. - headache, tearing pains in the face. ***Compare:*** (1) Lith. - mental symptoms, palpitations. (2) Graph. - obesity. (3) Glon., Puls., Sep. (4) Sulph. - headache. (5) Ars. - alcohol drinking., Nux-v. - desire for wine. (6) Kali-i., Phos. - gastric ulcer. (7) Ars., Ip. - asthma. (8) Carb-v., Dig., Glon. and Lith-c. - heart. ***Compatible:*** Con., Glon., Op., Puls. Acts well in: Cases which have been heavily dosed with Quinine.

REFERENCES - Boericke. Clarke. Murphy.

CALCAREA BROMATA

(Calcium Bromide)

PHARMACY - calc-br. Calcarea bromata. Calcium bromide. ***Historical dose:*** Trituration and all potencies.

CLINICAL - Brain, congestion. Diarrhea. Fretfulness. Insomnia. Irritability. Sleeplessness. Vomiting.

HOMEOPATHIC - Calc-br. is an unproved remedy, recommended by Hale for a variety of children's complaints. Suited to children who are of lax tissue, lymphatic, nervous and irritable.

Calc-br. is for children that are nervous and irritable with gastric and cerebral irritation. ***Tendency to brain diseases***. Insomnia and cerebral congestion. Vomiting and diarrhea. Fretfulness. It removes inflammatory products from uterus.

Constitutions - Both Bromine and Calcarea are suited to fair-haired and fat children, the combination appears to intensify the effect.

RELATIONS - ***Compare:*** (1) Bell., Aeth., Calc., Carc., Brom., Kali-br.

REFERENCES - Clarke.

CALCAREA CARBONICA

(Calcium Carbonate)

PHARMACY - calc. Calcarea carbonica. Calcium carbonate. Calcarea ostrearum. Conchae praeparatae. Impure carbonate of lime. Including symptoms of Calcarea acetica and Calcarea ostrearum. A trituration of the middle layer of oyster shells. Trituration. ***Historical dose:*** Trituration and all potencies.

CLINICAL - Abdomen, large. ***Abscesses***. Acidity. Alcohol, effects. Anemia. Ankles. weak. ***Arthritis.*** Beard, sycosis. Birthmarks. ***Bone, diseases.*** Breast-feeding, defective. Breasts, swollen. Decay, bones. Cataract. Chilblains. Colds. Coryza. Coughs. Coxalgia. Cracks. ***Cramps.*** Croup. Crusta lactea. Debility. Delirium tremens. ***Dentition. Diabetes.*** Diarrhea. Dropsy. Dyspepsia. Ear, disorders. ***Epilepsy.*** Epulis. Eye, disorders. Fever, intermittent. Fistula. Gallstones. Glandular swellings. Gleet.

Goiter. Gonorrhea. Gout. Headaches. Hernia. Herpes. Hydrocephalus. Hysteria. Impotence. Insomnia. ***Joints disorders.*** Kidney, colic. Leucocythemia. Leucorrhea. Lupus. ***Malnutrition.*** Melancholy. Menstrual, disorders. Milk-fever. Miscarriages. Muscles, pain. Neuralgias. ***Nightmares. Obesity.*** Osteomyelitis. ***Osteoporosis.*** Paralysis. Parotiditis. Peritonitis. Perspiration. Plethora. ***Polyps.*** Prosopalgia. Psoriasis. Ranula. ***Rheumatism. Rickets.*** Ringworm. Stones. Teeth, decayed. Toothaches. Tuberculosis. Tumors. Typhoid. Urticaria. Uterus, disorders. Varicose, veins. Vertigo. ***Walking, late***. Warts. Whitlow. ***Worms.***

HOMEOPATHIC - Calcarea carb. is the chief remedy of Calcium compounds. This ***constitutional remedy*** is one of the polycrest remedies and ranks with Sulph. and Lyc. at the head of the ***anti-psorics***. It is essential to a correct appreciation of the Homeopathic Materia Medica that these three medicines should be thoroughly known, as these are, in a sense, the standards around which the rest are grouped.

All three have a very wide range and deep action. They have many symptoms in common, but Calc. is somewhat sharply distinguished form Sulphur in that it is a chilly remedy, the patient seeking warmth, while the Sulph. patient is worse by heat and better by cold.

Cold, clammy feet, ***"as if there wet damp stockings on,"*** (Sulph. has hot, sweaty feet). The ***"sinking sensation"*** common to all three is most marked with Sulph. at 11 a.m., with Lyc. at 4 p.m., and with Calc. at any time.

Calc. is closely allied to Bell., Nux-v., Puls. and Rhus-t. in its action. Like many of the other carbonates, Calc. corresponds to persons of soft tissue with tendency to be fat. Hydrogenoid and sycotic constitution Sensitive to cold and damp, and early morning aggravation. Warts and polyps.

The chief action of Calc. is centered in the vegetative sphere, the keynote being impaired nutrition, the glands, skin and bone, being instrumental in the changes wrought. It alters the blood, causing anemia.

The calcium metabolism is active during childhood and becomes defective after middle age. Improper assimilation of calcium gives rise to defective nutrition of glands, bones and skin. Calc. is a definite stimulant to the periosteum.

Calc. patients are generally fat, fair, flabby, perspiring, cold, damp and sour. Great sensitiveness to cold weather, patients are ***susceptible to cold***. Cold, moist air chills through and through, takes cold easily especially in chest. Chilliness is aggravated from contact with water.

Out of breath easily. ***Sweating is easy,*** partial, on head, chest during sleep. Muscles and skin become fat or flabby, patient grows heavier, but not strong. Great weakness on ascending stairs, on walking, from talking (chest feels weak), or excitement. ***A jaded state, mental or physical, due to overwork.*** In epilepsy the aura spreads up from solar plexus, or as of a mouse running up the arm or down epigastrium to uterus or limbs.

Tendency to strain the muscles and joints easily. Parts lain on become numb. Cramps in muscles which draw limbs. Muscular atrophy. ***Abscesses in deep muscles. Polyps and exostoses***. Polyps, nasal, uterine etc. cysts. Osteomyelitis. Osteoporosis.

Malnutrition. Improper nutrition and indigestion. ***Glandular swelling*** below the jaw and in the neck. Pituitary and thyroid dysfunction. ***Discharges are profuse often sour,*** stools, sweat, odor of the body, saliva etc.

Tendency to the formation of gallstones and kidney stones. Early stage of tuberculosis of lungs with tickling cough, fleeting chest pains, nausea, acidity and dislike for fats. Varicose veins, burning in veins. Raised blood clotting factors (Stront.).

Diarrhea, tremors after burns. Generally feels better when constipated. The diarrhea is generally worse in afternoon. Painless hoarseness, worse in morning.

Swelling and pain in the breasts before the menstrual flow begins (Con.). Menses are scanty or absent with chilliness and cold, clammy feet. Suppression of menses in women after working in water. Bearing-down pains.

Fibroids and cysts. Ovarian or uterine pains, right side, extending down thighs, worse on reading or writing (left side, Lil-t.).

Children crave eggs, eat dirt and other indigestible things. Prone to diarrhea. Emaciated children with a big head and belly. ***Slow in teething,*** walk late. ***Complaints of teething children,*** convulsions, sour diarrhea.

Children do not put their feet down on the ground. Dull, lethargic children, do not want to play. Nightmares, ***dreams of monsters***.

MIND - Rumination and worry. ***Overworked and exhausted.*** Sits and thinks about little affairs that amount to nothing. ***Worries about all their responsibilities and duties. Apprehensive***, worse towards evening. Anxiety with palpitations. Desire to weep, to go home. Suspicious. Cautious. Low-spirited. Apathetic. Depressed. Melancholic or doubting moods. Hopeless of ever getting well.

Forgetful, confused, misplaces words and expresses himself wrongly. Averse to work or exertion. Inability to apply himself. Learns poorly. Easily frightened or offended. Fears of being observed. Fears of misery, ***misfortune***, disaster, contagious disease, insanity. Fear excited by reports of cruelties. ***Fears loss of reason***.

Children are self willed, obstinate. Child is afraid of everything it sees. ***Nightmares and poor sleep.*** Imagines someone in their room. ***Fear of monsters.*** Irritable, cries about trifles, borrows trouble. Visions of fire, murder, rats and mice in delirium. Feels as if she would run up and down, and scream. Sits and breaks sticks etc. all day long.

Abdomen - Increase of fat in abdomen. ***Large and hard*** abdomen. Sensitive to slightest pressure, cannot bear tight clothing around the waist. ***Distention*** with hardness, better slightest pressure. Cutting pain in swollen abdomen. Colic with coldness of thighs after stopped coryza or with cold feeling in abdomen. Incarcerated flatulence. Peritonitis when pain better by cold application. Twisting or cramps about umbilical region. Umbilical hernia. The navel is sore, excrescences like proud flesh in infants. ***Inguinal and mesenteric glands swollen*** and painful.

Back - Pain as if sprained, can scarcely rise, from over lifting. Cannot sit upright in the chair from weakness of back. Neck pains, worse lifting. Neck stiff and rigid. Pain between shoulder blades, impeding breathing. Rheumatism in lumbar region, weakness in small of back. Vertebrae, feel loose, painful on pressure. Curvature of dorsal vertebrae.

Breasts - Breast tender and swollen, before menses. Hot, swelling breasts. Severe stitches in breasts, when nursing. Milk too abundant, disagreeable to child. Deficient breast-feeding with distended breasts in lymphatic women. Nipples, cracked, ulcerated, very tender.

Bones - Faulty development of bones. ***Open fontanelles.*** Curvatures, bone growths, rickets. Osteoporosis. Growing pains (Calc-p.).

Causations - Ill effects of overwork, worry, fright. Poor nutrition, alcohol. Aging. Loss of vital fluids. Suppressed sweat, eruptions, or menses. Strains, over lifting. Affections of stonecutters.

Chest - Sharp pains in chest, going backwards. ***Chest very sensitive to touch, percussion or pressure.*** Weak feeling in chest, cannot even speak.

Constitutions - Anti-psoric constitutional remedy. Persons of scrofulous type, who take cold easily, with increased mucus secretions, children who grow fat, are large-bellied with large head, pale skin, chalky look. Fat, flabby children rather bloated than solid, pale but flushing easily. ***Leuco-phlegmatic temperament***, disorders caused by working in water.

Ears - Throbbing, cracking in ears, stitches pulsating pain as if something would press out. Scrofulous inflammation with ***muco-purulent otorrhea and enlarged glands***. Purulent offensive discharge and enlarged glands. Eruption on and behind ear (Graph., Petr.). Polyps which bleed easily. Aching, when blowing the nose and coughing. Perversions of hearing. Illusory noises, on swallowing, chewing. Cracking noises in ear. Deafness from working in water or quinine. Sensitive to cold about ears and neck.

Eyes - Lachrymation in open air and early in morning. Lachrymal ducts closed from exposure to cold. Itching of lids, swollen, scurfy. Suppurating fistula. ***Spots and ulcers on cornea***. Cataract. ***Dilatation of pupils.*** Sensitive to light. Cannot read in gas light, feels as if she squinted. Dimness of vision, as if looking through a mist, by constant reading, writing etc. Far-sighted. Sees visions on closing eyes, besides field of vision. Easy fatigue of eyes. Ophthalmia in newborn after taking cold.

Face - Pale, puffy, pasty, with deep-seated eyes, surrounded by dark rings. Old, wrinkled. Swelling of upper lip in the morning with cracks and bleeding. Submaxillary glands swollen. Crusta lactea, itching, burning after washing. Goiter. Itching eruptions on chin. Itching of pimples in whiskers. Pain from right mental foramen along lower jaw to ear. Chewing and swallowing in sleep in children.

Female - Before menses, headache, colic, chilliness and leucorrhea. Cutting pains in uterus during menstruation. ***Menses too early, too profuse, too long,*** with vertigo toothache and ***cold, damp feet***. Menses late in fat, flabby girls with palpitation, dyspnea and headache. Absence of menses in plethoric women from fright. Infertility with copious menses. Mental excitement brings on dysmenorrhea or causes menses to rectum. Burning and itching before and after menstruation. Thick, milky, gushing or yellow leucorrhea, worse during urination with itching and burning. Uterine polyps. Uterus easily displaced. Sex followed by sweat and prostration. Itching and burning in genitals. Much sweat about genitals. Increased sexual desire, easy conception. Clumsy, awkward and tired during pregnancy. Cramps in toes or soles during pregnancy.

Food - ***Poor diet and nutrition.*** Loss of appetite, but when he begins to eat, he relishes it. ***Loss of appetite when overworked***. Repugnance to hot food. Ravenous hunger. ***Cravings for eggs,*** ice-creams, salt and sweets. ***Craving for indigestible things,*** dirt, chalk, coal, pencils. Aversion to meat, milk, boiled things, ***fat.*** Worse after eating, smoked meats, milk, or when fasting. Thirst for ***cold drinks***.

Head - Head hot with pale face, with mental exertion. ***Icy coldness*** in and on the head, especially right side. Cold spots on head. ***Vertex icy cold.*** Burning in vertex after grief. Sense of weight on top of head. Headache with cold hands and feet. Headache from over lifting, from mental exertion, with nausea. Chronic hydrocephalus. ***Big head with large hard abdomen.*** Open fontanelles, head enlarged. ***Much perspiration, wets the pillow***. Sweat with palpitations. Itching of the scalp. Scratches head on waking. Falling of hair.

Heart - Weakness. Palpitation at night, after eating. Palpitations with a feeling of coldness, with restless oppression of chest, after suppressed eruption.

Kidneys - ***Kidney colic.*** Irritable bladder. Bedwetting, incontinence when walking. Urine, dark, brown, bloody, sour, foul or of strong odor. White urinary sediment with milky urine. Polyps.

Limbs - Trembling, weakness. Creeping on the limbs like a mouse. Tearing in muscles. Clumsy, awkward, easily falls. Joints as if sprained. Old sprains. Tired from short walk. Rheumatoid pains, as after exposure to wet. Arthritic deformans, nodosities. Arms, weak, lame. Hands numb, when grasping. Want of mobility of fingers. Sweat of hands. Chapped hands. Cold, clammy hands, knees. Swelling of joints, especially knee. ***Cramps in calves*** when stretching out leg at night. Feet turn inward, while walking. ***Soles of feet raw***, burning. ***Cold, damp feet,*** feel as if damp stockings were worn. Sour foot-sweat. Feet feel cold and dead at night. ***Weakness of ankles*** in children. Children are late in learning to walk.

Liver - Liver region painful when stooping. ***Gallstone colic***.

Lungs - ***Painless hoarseness***, worse in the morning. ***Short of breath.*** Emphysema. Habitual cough. Tickling cough as from dust or feather in throat. Cough, worse inspiration, playing on piano, eating.

Suffocating spells, tightness, burning and soreness in chest, ***worse climbing upstairs*** or slightest ascent, must sit down. Ulcers or abscesses in the lungs. Expectoration only during the day, thick, yellow, sour mucus. Purulent, loose, sweet, expectoration. Bloody expectoration with sour sensation in chest. Scanty, salty expectoration. Longing for fresh air (Puls.).

Male - Increased sexual desire with retarded erections. ***Frequent emissions***. Burning with seminal emission. Seminal discharge premature. Sex followed by profound weakness, vertigo, irritability, lameness of back and knees, headache and sweat. Itching and burning in genitals. Impotence from sexual abuse or from overindulgence. Hydrocele of children.

Modalities - Better from dry climate and weather. Better inspiring fresh air. Better uncovers during fever. Better after breakfast. Better from lying on painful side, on back. Better sneezing, rubbing, scratching. Better wiping or soothing with hands. ***Worse from bathing. Worse working in water***, cooling off. Worse walking in open, ***cold, raw air.*** Worse wet weather, change of weather. Worse from exertion, mental or physical. ***Worse ascending.*** Worse standing. Worse lifting, or stooping. ***Worse from pressure of clothes***. Worse letting limbs hang down. Worse eyestrain. Worse light. Worse looking fixedly at any object. Worse looking upward. Worse turning the head. ***Worse from dentition. Worse milk.*** Worse worry. Worse puberty, menopause. Worse at full moon or new moon. Worse at solstice. Worse after midnight. Worse in early morning, on waking.

Mouth - Bleeding of gums. Persistent ***sour taste***. Mouth fills with sour water. Offensive smell. Ranula under the tongue. Epulis, soft, painless. Tongue dry at night, does not like to talk. Burning pain at tip of tongue, worse anything warm taken into stomach.

Nose - Nosebleed, in children inclined to be fat. Nostrils, ***dry, sore, ulcerated.*** Polyps with loss of smell. Swelling at root of nose. Offensive odor in nose, offensive yellow discharge. Coryza with polyuria. Sneezes, frequently without a cold. ***Takes cold at every change of weather.*** Catarrhal symptoms with hunger, coryza alternates with colic. Senile catarrh. Swelling of the nose and upper lip in children.

Rectum - Feels best when constipated. Stool large and hard, whitish, watery, sour. Diarrhea of fetid, undigested food with ravenous appetite, particularly in children. Diarrhea, chronic after burns. Persistent tenesmus after dysentery. Prolapse of anus and burning, stinging hemorrhoids. Hemorrhoids, painful when walking better sitting. Crawling and constriction in rectum. ***Worms,*** tapeworms, ***pinworms,*** roundworms.

Sensations - Pain as if the parts would burst, were pressed or pushed asunder. ***As if cold, damp stockings were on the feet.*** Creeping on the limbs like a mouse. Pain as if sprained in outer parts. Sensation of dust in inner parts as the eye, bronchial tubes. Pricking, darting, jerking, trembling, itching better by scratching.

Skin - Cold, like a snake, flaccid, unhealthy. Visible quivering of skin from head to foot, followed by giddiness. Psoriasis. Glands swollen. Unhealthy, ulcerating, flaccid. Small wounds do not heal readily. Nettle rash, better in cold air. Warts on face and hands. Milk white spots. ***Petechial eruptions***. Recurring blood boils. Boils. Chilblains.

Sleep - Drowsy in early part of evening. Frequent waking at night. Insomnia due to worry. ***Same disagreeable ideas arouses from light sleep.*** Night terrors (Kali-p.). Starts at every noise, fears that she will go crazy. ***Nightmares*** in children, scream after midnight and cannot be pacified. Dreams of the dead, ***of monsters.***

Stomach - Heartburn and loud belching. ***Frequent sour belchings, sour vomiting*** of curdled milk. Cramps in stomach, worse pressure, cold water. Swelling over pit of stomach like a saucer turned bottom up. Pain in epigastric region to touch. Hyperchlorhydria (Phos.). Aggravation while eating. Drinking water, if ever so little, causes nausea, but not if iced. Sensation as if rising something to head.

Stools - Chalky, gray or green, watery stools. Stools at first hard, then pasty, then liquid. Stools, worse eating and drinking. Undigested stools.

Teeth - Difficult and delayed dentition. Toothache, worse cold air or hot things.

Temperature - Chill with thirst. ***Chill at 2 p.m., begins internally in stomach region***. Coldness, icy in different parts of the body, of affected part. Internal heat with external coldness and sweat. ***Fever with sweat***. Hectic fever. Sweat cold, partial. ***Night sweats, especially on head***, neck and chest. Heat, at night during menses. ***Sweat over head in children, so that pillow becomes wet.*** Pulse full and frequent.

Throat - ***Swelling of the tonsils*** and submaxillary glands, with stitches on swallowing. Difficult swallowing. Hawks salty mucous. Small ulcers spreading up to palate. Uvula, swollen, edematous. Goiter. Parotid fistula.

Vertigo - Vertigo on ascending (especially running) and when turning head, worse looking upward. Vertigo with many conditions, worse scratching head, after epilepsy. Tendency to fall to left, to either side, backward.

COMMENTS - Calcium carbonate is the foundation of the structure of our body. One of the dominant constitutions today, it has a profound influence, particularly on growing children.

There's a strong complementary relationship between Calc. and Bell. Calc. has a tendency to go toward Bell. acutes, especially tonsillitis and fevers. It's also closely related to Puls. Calc acutes can become Puls. cases, particularly in children. Adults have a tendency to become Rhus-t., especially the elderly. Calc. can deal with residue from many of these complaints.

Helpful for teething problems, bone problems, spinal problems, and flabby muscles. Children with slow development, a tendency to be sluggish. Tendency to sore throats, swollen glands, and earaches.

Colic. Constipation in babies (Alum.). When constipated, the child cries, moans, does a lot of body movements, and then they pass a large stool. Babies sweat on the back of their head, and they smell sour. Their stool and sweat smell sour, their pillow smells sour.

Insomnia in babies. Nightmares, especially about monsters. Fears, particularly vulnerable and susceptible to watching frightening movies or news (Phos.).

Apprehensive state of mind. Fear of losing reason, that people will notice her mental confusion. Fears she has some fatal disease, especially heart disease. Great desire for order and structure, fear of losing control. Great sense of responsibility, happy when working.

Shuddering and dread as evening draws near. Sees visions on closing eyes (useful in delirium tremens). Cries out, twitches, grasps at flocks, restless and anxious though unconscious (nervous and typhoid fever), beside herself with anguish, on the borders of acute mania. Evil foreboding, talks of mice, rats, murders. Forgetful.

Abnormally sleepy or sleepless. Wakes at 3 a.m. and cannot get to sleep again, tosses about. Horrible phantasms. The child wakes in the night screaming and cannot be pacified, in the morning remembers nothing of it. Chews and swallows in sleep. Frightful dreams of sickness, death and smell of corpses. Insomnia, especially in the elderly. Aversion to darkness.

Slow in movements (Sulph., quick and active). Exhaustion on exertion or excitement, though he may feel well before. Exhaustion in the morning. Cramp in legs at 3 a.m. Tendency toward arthritis. Disposition to strain a part by lifting heavy things.

Scrofulous diseases of bones, spinal curvature, rickets. Swellings. Sciatica, after working in water. Rheumatic and gouty conditions from wetting. Joints crack and crepitate as if dry. Inclination to stretch and put the shoulders back, but straightening aggravates the rheumatism.

Neuralgias and paralyzes. Twitching. Internal trembling sensation on awaking. Fainting, coming on in the street with sensation of something rising from stomach to head. Talking causes a feeling of weakness that compels him to desist.

Epilepsy has an aura spreading up from the solar plexus in which case the convulsion comes on immediately. It may be like a mouse running on the arm, or it may run down from epigastrium into uterus or limbs. Epilepsy from fright, suppressed eruptions and discharges, sexual excesses. Characteristic rush of blood to head, a sensation of something rising up from epigastrium to head.

Sensations of heat and burning. Heat in and on the vertex. Head sweats profusely, wetting the pillow. Sweat chiefly on occiput and forehead (Sil. sweats all over). Better uncovered during the heats (Lyc., opp. of Sil.). Hot breath with heat in mouth.

Sweats relieve. Bloody sweats. Sweats may be sour or odorless. Sour body smell. Burning in soles of feet at night, burning in back of hands. Sour or odorless foot sweat. Soft, cold and moist hands, a boneless hand, inclined to chap.

All the symptoms are made worse by taking cold. Great sensitiveness to cold, damp air. Dread of open air. Cannot bear sun. The slightest change of weather aggravates. Dread of bathing and water. When a cold wind strikes the body it immediately runs to the teeth, causing them to ache.

Rough, scaly skin, inclined to chap. Cracks. Chilblains from wetting. Eruptions, behind right ear. Pricking corns, polyps, cysts, in the leuco-phlegmatic constitutions.

Scrofulous glands. Enlarged and hard lymphatic glands. Swelling of cervical and bronchial glands. Hypothyroidism (Sep.).

Related to the pre-tubercular stage of tuberculosis, especially suited to disorders of the right apex. Stitching in chest and sides of chest when moving and when lying on affected side. Cough when going into a cold room, from chilliness. Tickling cough, sensation of feather in throat. Rattling in the chest, miller's and stone-cutter's tuberculosis, old suppurating cavities.

Sinking sensation. Icy coldness in abdomen. Malnutrition. Ravenous hunger and feeling of emptiness immediately after a meal and in the early morning. Headache from hunger.

Nausea after drinking water, even ever so little, but not if iced. Nausea when fasting.

Craving for eggs, starchy grains, sweets. Craving for indigestible things like chalk, coal, etc. Children with pica. Milk disagrees, sour vomiting of large curds. Inability to swallow solids. Chronic disease of left tonsil, feeling of lump in left side of throat, pain from left tonsil to ear. Semi-lateral swelling of tongue. Ranula.

Sour belchings. Sour diarrhea. Crawling in rectum as from worms. Burning in rectum. Weight in lower rectum. Ardor urine, offensive urine. Stools hard and pasty, like chalk or clay, offensive, undigested. Flatulence or gurgling in right hypochondrium.

Impotence, penis cold and relaxed. Good for weight gain after pregnancy and menopause. Milk leg, better by elevating the limb, worse hanging it down.

Sensation as if in a dream. Sensation of levitation. Vertigo, especially in the elderly.

Dr. Van den Neucker cured a baker of paralysis of both arms with Calc. and also a case of paralysis with many symptoms of locomotor ataxia in a lymphatic blonde girl of nineteen.

Cooper cured psoriasis of the palms with it.

Guernsey said "this remedy is particularly adapted to the real leuco-phlegmatic constitution. Where we find a large head, large features, pale skin with a chalky look and (in infants) open fontanelles, we may think strongly of Calc."

According to Guernsey, Calc. is in general a right-side remedy, particularly the right external head, right eye, right face, right abdominal ring, sexual organs on the right side, right back, right upper limbs. Left side neck and nape of neck, left chest, left lower limbs.

Alexander Villers cured with Calc. 200c a case combining many of the features of the remedy. The patient, a woman, age 20, was very despondent through long-continued depressing circumstances, became very nervous.

She was companion to an exceedingly deaf lady, whose voice was high-pitched.

This, with the strain on her voice to make herself heard, caused headache through her temples, better from rapid motion of head.

Outdoor exercise was accompanied by hard pressure on chest, which only belchings seemed to relieve. Constipated bowels. Menses every fortnight with backache and great prostration. Under the remedy, repeated at rare intervals, the menses came on monthly, headache and pressure on the chest disappeared.

RELATIONS - ***Antidoted by:*** Camph., Ip., Nit-ac., Nit-s-d., Nux-v., Sulph. ***Antidote to:*** Bism., Chin., Chin-s., Dig., Mez. (headache), Nit-ac., Phos. ***Compare:*** (1) Calc-o-t., Calc-ar., Calc-p., and other Calcareas., Lyc., Sulph. - differs in being worse by heat, hot feet. (2) Sil., Calc-f., Calc-p., Calc-br. (3) Lime-water and Calc-caust. (4) Calc-calcin. - calcinated oyster-shell a remedy for warts. (5) Calcarea ovorum - Toasted egg-shells., Calc. lactic. (6) Calc. lacto-phosph. (7) Calc-mur. (8) Arn. (strains, etc.), Ars. (swollen mesenteric glands). (9) In ardor. urine Sep., burning and cutting, Canth., cutting. (10) loss of fluids Chin., Sulph. (11) Leucorrhea, acrid or bland - Graph., Sulph. (12) Acid stomach - Chin., Lyc., Sulph., Puls., Rob. (13) Waking at 3 a.m. - Bellis, Nux-v., Kali-c., Ars., Sep. (14) swelling and painfulness of breasts before menses - Kali-c., Lac-c., Con. (15) Dread of losing senses - Lyc., Med., Nux-v., Sulph. (16) Ravenous hunger - Ars., Calc., Cina., Iod., Sil., Staph. (17) Rhus-t. is a very close analogue of Calc., Bell., Dulc., Nux-v., Puls., and Rhus may be regarded as the acute satellites of Calc. ***Complementary:*** Bell., Rhus-t., Lyc., Sil. Calc. is useful after Sulph. where the pupils remain dilated. When Puls. failed in school girls. ***Incompatible:*** Bry. ***Follows well:*** Cham., Chin., Con., Cupr., Nit-ac., Nux-v., Puls., Sulph. (especially if the pupils dilate). ***Followed well by:*** Lyc., Nux-v., Phos., Plat., Sil.

REFERENCES - Boericke. Clarke. Murphy. Phatak.

CALCAREA CAUSTICA

(Lime-water)

PHARMACY - calc-caust. Calcarea caustica. Lime-water. Aqua calcis. Quicklime is slaked in distilled water. Afterwards alcohol is added and the clear liquid decanted. ***Historical dose:*** Tincture and all potencies.

CLINICAL - Back, pains. Coccyx, pain. Corns. Heel, pain. Hoarseness. Jaw, disorders. Malar bones, pain. Neuralgia. Paralysis. Rheumatism. Spleen, disorders. Stiff-neck. Tapeworm. Toothaches.

HOMEOPATHIC - Lime-water has an ancient repute in allaying inflammation of many kinds. Extensively proved, it rapidly dispelled all inflammatory action in cases of appendicitis and removed all suffering in an aggravated case of hemorrhoids.

Marked difficult thinking. Confusion in the head. Vertigo, as if room turning in a circle. Sticking, tearing, throbbing pains in various parts. Pain in right eye as if a foreign body were in it. Burning and tearing in eyes. Tearing in right cheekbone and in right articulation of jaw.

Mucus in throat, burning, sensation as if a bone were sticking in it. Burning in stomach. Tapeworm passes. Hoarseness with pain in throat, rawness in trachea and cough. Stitches in chest. Stiffness and tearing in all regions of back and in coccyx. Tearing in either shoulder down arms. Tearing in left Achilles tendon, left heel. Sticking in corns.

Worse from working in water, "pains in hands and feet after a foot-bath." Worse from hanging down limb. Toothache every night, 2 a.m. Fuzzy sensation in the teeth and other parts.

MIND - Very difficult thought. Weary and peevish on waking, as if he had been intoxicated.

Abdomen - Sticking in both hypochondria, especially severe in left. Pain in left side of region of spleen, as if a ball were turning on its axis. Constrictive pain in abdomen, griping, stitches. Violent stitches in small intestines when bending forward.

Back - Violent pains in scapulae, extending into small of back when sitting, worse on inspiration. Tearing between the shoulders. Tearing in both scapulae, between shoulders, then through neck and occiput as far as forehead. Sensation in both shoulder blades as if they were fuzzy and had gone to sleep (8 p.m.). Pain in small of back, on waking better by moving about. Pressive, drawing pains, sticking, tearing in small of back. Tearing in coccyx.

Chest - Sternum feels oppressed, pressive sticking under, stitches across. Stitches in left chest.

Eyes - Burning in eyes, in evening by candlelight. Pain in right eye as if foreign body under upper lid in eye, on rising in morning.

Face - Tearing in right cheekbone. Violent pain, swelling, stiffness of right joint of jaw. Lips unusually red.

Female - Menses eight days too early.

Head - Confusion of the head, especially left side. Throbbing in frontal sinus, better by contracting skin of forehead.

Limbs - Trembling in limbs, could not continue work, better by eating a piece of bread. Rheumatic pain alternating in all the joints. Wandering pains. Tearing in shoulders, arms and axilla. Paralyzed condition of right hand. Stitches and tearing in left wrist. Severe tension in lower limbs. Stitches in hip joints. Tearing in knees in right side of right tibia down to toes in left Achilles tendon in left heel. Sticking in a corn. Pains in hands and feet after a foot bath.

Lungs - Feeling of rawness in trachea, cough. Cough with stitches in chest, expectoration of mucus and blood.

Mouth - Mouth offensive, palate feels as if mucus was upon it, but none is expectorated.

Neck - Tearing in nape. Stiffness of neck of back of neck of all neck muscles.

Rectum - Three thin stools before breakfast and one immediately after. Thin, pasty stool with much mucus. Painful stool, as if a nail were scratching in anus. Passed many pieces of tapeworm. Hemorrhoids. Sticking, tearing motions in rectum extending towards anus. Crawling in rectum and anus.

Skin - Rash-like eruption on forehead. Biting, itching vesicles, on neck and back extending later to occiput and behind ears.

Sleep - Restless, many dreams, nightmare.

Stomach - Severe hunger three hours after eating. Nausea followed by vomiting of some fluid.

Teeth - Severe toothache every night, 2 a.m., as if tooth was fuzzy and too large with tensive pain in left ear as if something was sticking in it. Teeth feel too large, fuzzy.

Temperature - A violent chill with chattering teeth 7 to 7. 30 p.m.

Throat - Mucus in throat, difficult to raise, almost causing vomiting. Hawking of granular, glutinous material like cooked rice. Burning in fauces and esophagus caused by water. Sensation as of a bone sticking in pharynx.

Throat - Stitches in larynx, left half. Hoarseness with pain in throat.

Vertigo - Vertigo, as if room turning in a circle, thinks she will fall from chair.

RELATIONS - ***Compare:*** (1) Besides the Calcareas, Rhus-t. - pain in joint of jaw. (2) Mez. and Mag-c. - pain in malar bones. (3) Valer. - pain in heel. (4) Pic-ac. and Sep., (loins). (5) Hep. and Nit-ac. - bone sensation in throat.

REFERENCES - Clarke.

CALCAREA CHLORINATA

(Chlorinated Lime)

PHARMACY - calc-chln. Calcarea chlorinata. Chlorinated lime. Hypochlorate of lime with Calcium chloride and a varying amount of Hydrate of Lime. ***Historical dose:*** Trituration and all potencies.

CLINICAL - Boils. Carbuncles.

HOMEOPATHIC - This preparation has only been used as a local application, for boils and carbuncles, chiefly in the preparation of the Liquor Calcis Chlorate of the British Pharmacopeia.

REFERENCES - Clarke.

CALCAREA FLUORATA

(Calcium Fluoride)

PHARMACY - calc-f. Calcarea fluorata. Calcium fluoride. Calcarea fluorica. Fluorspar. Flouride of Lime. Trituration. ***Historical dose:*** Trituration and all potencies.

CLINICAL - Adenoids. Aneurysm. Blood, tumors. ***Bone, disorders. Bone, deformities. Bone, spurs.*** Breast, indurations. Burns. Cancer. ***Cataract.*** Catarrh. Childbirth. Cold, sores. Corneal, opacities. Cough. ***Croup***. Dental, problems. ***Exostosis.*** Flatulence. ***Glands, enlarged.*** Goiter. Hemoptysis. Herpes. Hodgkin's, disease. Hydrocele. ***Induration***. Joints, cracking. ***Keratitis.*** Liver, disorders. ***Lumbago.*** Nodes. Ozaena. Periosteitis. Post-nasal, catarrh. Rickets. Sarcoma. ***Scoliosis.*** Spavin (horses). Strains. Syphilis. Teeth, deformed. Toothache. ***Tumors.*** Ulcers. ***Varicose, veins***.

HOMEOPATHIC - Calc-f. is Schüssler's *"bone salt."* It is found in the surface of bones, the enamel of teeth, in elastic tissues, and in the cells of the epidermis. A powerful tissue remedy for hard, stony glands, varicose veins and malnutrition of bones.

Calc-f. has cured lumbago after the failure of Rhus-t. Lumbago from strains, worse after rest, better after moving a little and from warmth. Tendon and joint disorders, especially weakness after injury (Ruta.). Joints give way easily. Tendons have nodules and growths after injury or overuse.

Disperses ***bony growths***. Bone spurs and tumors. Ulcerations of the bone, fistula. Periosteitis of lower jaw, ribs etc. Deficient enamel of teeth (Sil.). Nails hypertrophied. General stiffness. Weakness in the morning. Feeling of fatigue all day. Numbness in different parts.

Tendency to adhesions after operations (Calen.). ***Indurations of stony hardness,*** tonsils, tumors, neck after injury, margins of ulcers. Hard knots in breast. ***Induration threatening suppuration***. Grass green discharges. Stinking pus.

Arteriosclerosis, threatened stroke. Veins dilate and become varicose, inflamed. Tuberculosis. ***Glands enlarge and become stony hard.*** Goiter. X-ray, radiation burns. ***Cataract***. Congenital hereditary syphilis manifesting itself in ulceration of mouth and throat, decay and necrosis with boring pains and heat in parts.

MIND - Depression, anxiety, indecision. Groundless fear of financial loss, fear of poverty.

Abdomen - Flatulence, during pregnancy. Sharp pain in hepatic region. Dull weight and discomfort in right hypochondrium.

Back - Scoliosis. ***Chronic lumbago*** from strain, better motion and warmth. Lumbago, worse on beginning to move and ameliorated on continued motion. Tired aching, as from a long ride, with restlessness. Pain in lower part of back with burning. Bone tumors. Exostoses.

Blood - Vascular tumors with dilated blood vessels. ***Varicose or enlarged veins***.

Bones - ***Bony growths,*** bone spurs. Bone deformities. Osteo-sarcoma. Exostosis after injury.

Breasts - Hard knots in breasts. Hard glands in the female breast. Breast nodes, tumors.

Constitutions - Sluggish temperament. Congenital syphilis manifesting itself in ulceration of mouth and throat.

Ears - ***Chronic suppuration of middle ear***. Chronic otorrhea (Sil.). Calcareous deposits on eardrum, sclerosis of temporal bone with deafness, ringing and roaring.

Eyes - ***Cataract.*** Cornea opaque in spots. ***Keratitis.*** Flickering and sparks before the eyes, conjunctivitis. ***Subcutaneous palpebral cysts.*** Aching in eyes, better closing and pressure.

Face - Hard swelling on jawbone. Hard swelling on the cheek with pain or toothache. Small, hard, cold sores on lips.

Female - Excessive menses. Prolapsed uterus. Bearing-down, dragging pains in uterus and thighs. Flatulence in pregnant women. After-pains from feeble contractions.

Head - Cracking noise in head, disturbing sleep. Cephalhematoma of newborn infants (Sil.). Blood tumors of newborn infants. Hard excrescences on the scalp.

Ulcers on the scalp with callous, hard edges.

Heart - Arteriosclerosis. Aneurysm. Valvular disease. Fibroid deposits about the endocardium. When the tuberculosis toxins attack the heart and blood vessels.

Limbs - Cracking in the joints. ***Easy joint dislocations.*** Exostoses. ***Bone spurs***. Synovial swellings. ***Swellings and indurated enlargements,*** having their seat in the tissue and ligaments, tendons of joints. Bursitis. Chronic synovitis of knee joint. Recurrent fibroids in the hollow of the knee. Hip joint disease. Cold wrists and ankles. Ganglia or encysted tumors at the back of the wrist. Gouty enlargements of the joints of the fingers. ***Enlargement of femur in infants.*** Rickets.

Lungs - Difficulty in breathing, as if epiglottis is nearly closed. Hoarseness after laughing or reading aloud. ***Croup***. Spasmodic cough. Cough with expectoration of tiny lumps of yellow mucus with tickling sensation and irritation on lying down.

Male - Induration of testes. Hydrocele. Syphilis, chancre.

Modalities - Better by rubbing. Better continued motion. Better warm applications. Better heat, and warm drinks. Worse from beginning of motion. Worse during rest. Worse sprains. Worse cold, wet. Worse changes of weather. Worse from damp weather, but better from fomentations.

Mouth - Periosteitis of lower jaw.

Neck - Goiter. Indurated cervical glands of stony hardness.

Nose - Cold in the head, stuffy cold, dry coryza. Copious, offensive, thick, greenish, lumpy, yellow nasal catarrh. Ozaena. Atrophic rhinitis, especially if crusts are prominent.

Rectum - Itching of anus, as from pinworms. Fissure of the anus and intensely sore crack near the lower end of the bowel. Fistula. Bleeding hemorrhoids with pain in sacrum. Internal or blind hemorrhoids frequently with pain in back, generally far down on the sacrum and constipation. Much wind in lower bowels, worse with pregnancy. Diarrhea in gouty subjects. Stools, gushing, watery of fetid odor.

Skin - Cracked, dry, hard, alabaster white. Scar tissue, adhesions after operations. ***Indurations are stony hard.*** Suppurations with callous, hard edges. Indolent, fistulous ulcers, secreting thick, yellow pus. Hard, elevated edges of ulcer, surrounding skin is purple and swollen. Fissures or cracks in the palms of the hands or hard skin. Whitlow. Warty growths. Birthmarks.

Sleep - Vivid dreams with sense of impending danger and weeping. Jumps out of bed in a dream. Unrefreshing sleep.

Stomach - Weakness and daintiness of appetite. ***Acute indigestion from fatigue*** and brain-fag. Flatulence. Hiccoughs (Caj., Sul-ac.), when one hawks of mucus. Nausea and distress after eating in young children who are overtaxed by studies. Vomiting of infants of undigested food.

Teeth - ***Deficient enamel of teeth*** (Sil.). Gum-boils with hard swelling on the jaw. Looseness of the teeth in their sockets, with or without pain. Toothache with pain if any food touches the tooth.

Throat - Tonsils rough and irritated, forming plugs of mucus. Hypertrophy of Luschka's tonsil. Follicular sore throat. Pain and burning in throat, better by warm drinks, worse cold drinks. Relaxed uvula, tickling referred to larynx.

Tongue - Cracked appearance of the tongue, with or without pain. Induration of the tongue, hardening after inflammation.

COMMENTS - Bone deformities and bone tumors, bony growths, bone spurs. Tendency for the vertebrae to slip, curvatures of the spine. Bone cancer, cysts, spinal weakness, joint weaknesses. Bone and ligament disturbances. Tendency toward weak ligaments. Diseases where the ligaments are very weak, where the hands, arms, or feet don't function. Marfan's disease.

Calcium deposits in tissues. Tendonitis with calcification, calcified pituitary glands, calcifications in eardrums. Deposits in arthritic joints, fingers deformed with calcium deposits. Dental and enamel problems. Senile cataract. Spots on cornea.

Glandular problems, indurated tonsils and adenoids. Cephalhematoma (Sil.). Ozaena. Herpes, hard and small on lips. Prickly, burning, suffocating sensation in throat. Hemoptysis, causing contraction of the blood vessels. Bleeding hemorrhoids.

Local pains and symptoms can be ameliorated with heat and warm application, but hot weather aggravates. Generally warm-blooded. Worse change of weather with arthritis, stiffness that's better motion (Rhus-t.). Vivid dreams of death. Fear of poverty, indecisiveness.

A giant-celled sarcoma of upper maxilla causing the deformity known as "frog-face" was very greatly relieved by Calc-f. in a short space of time after Silica failed to make much impression.

Dr. Seine had several cases where the child's teeth were turning yellow and the enamel was falling off. Using the Calc-f. cell salt, he had the child's parents rub it into the teeth, and the enamel grew back.

One prover, Dr. Sarah N. Smith, had among other symptoms a peculiar and constant one in the head: a sort of creaking, straining and drawing like the noise of a cornstalk fiddle, greatly interfering with sleep.

Dr. Sarah Hogan gave Calc-f. with complete success in a case of flatulency in a pregnant woman.

The patient passed through the labor quite easily, whereas the previous labor had been very difficult. In many other cases Dr. Hogan found the remedy facilitate labor. She found flatulency a marked indication for the remedy independent of pregnancy.

G. P. Hale with the 3x, removed induration after typhlitis, also encysted tumor of eyelids. He regarded induration threatening suppuration as a marked indication. Induration in the epigastric region after a kick from a horse was cured, also indurated glands of stony hardness.

W. P. Wesselheft cured two cases of syphilitic periosteal swelling, one on the right radius, one on the left ulna, one sensitive, one not, one patient was male, dark, the other was blonde, female. Each case received a dose of Calc-f. 100,00c.

RELATIONS - ***Compare:*** (1) Con., Lap-a., Bar-m., Hecla, Rhus-t. (2) Calc. sulph-stibiata - acts as an hemostatic and absorptive in uterine myoma. (3) Mangifera indica - varicose veins. (4) Calc-p. - ozaena, suppuration of bones. (5) Nat-m. - cold sores. (6) Sil. - Swellings on skulls of infants, suppuration of bones, Ph-ac. (7) Cacodylate of Soda - tumors.

REFERENCES - Boericke. Clarke. Murphy.

CALCAREA HYPOPHOSPHOROSA

(Calcium Hypophosphite)

PHARMACY - calc-hp. Calcarea hypophosphorosa. Calcium hypophosphite. Hypophosphite of lime. Trituration and solution. ***Historical dose:*** Trituration and all potencies.

CLINICAL - Angina pectoris. Arteries, disorders. Asthma. Congestion. Debility. Dyspnea. Emaciation. Headache. Paralysis. Sweating. Tuberculosis.

HOMEOPATHIC - This salt was proved by A. R. Barrett and a friend, who each took one grain of 2x trituration. Calc-hp. is to be preferred when it seems necessary to furnish the organism with liberal doses of phosphorus in consequence of continued abscesses having reduced the vitality.

Indicated in those persons who become pale, weak with violent drenching sweat, rapidly emaciate with extreme debility, on account of vital losses or continued abscesses. Emaciation of children. Loss of appetite, rapid debility, night sweats.

Great fullness and oppression around heart, fullness throughout thorax and head, veins of upper parts and upper limbs stand out like whipcords. Dyspnea, must have air. Tuberculosis, diarrhea and cough, acute pains in chest. Mesenteric tuberculosis. Bleeding from lungs, angina pectoris, asthma, affection of arteries. Veins stand out like whipcords.

Dull, heavy pressure from top of head between frontal and occipital bones, pain generally increased with increasing depression. Pallor of skin. Habitually ***cold limbs***. Acne with pustules. Profuse sweat all over. Complete loss of muscular power with loss of desire to move.

MIND - Excitable nervous and sleepless. Talks rapidly and easily angered.

Abdomen - Sore throbbing in spleen. Mesenteric tuberculosis.

Chest - Veins stand out like whip-cord.

Ears - Frying or sizzling in ears.

Heart - Angina pectoris.

Limbs - Habitually cold limbs.

Lungs - Acute pain in chest. Tuberculosis cough. Bleeding from the lungs. Asthma. Bronchitis.

Modalities - Worse from vital losses. Worse cold wind.

Rectum - Diarrhea of tuberculosis.

Skin - Exhausting night sweat (Merc.). Acne with pustules all over the body.

Sleep - Starts in sleep.

Stomach - Ravenous hunger, worse two hours after meals better when stomach is full. Loss of appetite.

COMMENTS - Has cured attacks of pain occurring two hours after meals, relieved by a cup of milk or light food.

With the first trituration, Nash cured a boy of eight who had several abscesses in and around the knee joint. The tibia was ulcerated and the ragged edge of the bone protruded through the surface. There was emaciation, loss of appetite and he was as pale as a corpse. The appetite returned at once in great force.

RELATIONS - ***Compare:*** (1) Calc-p., Calc-i., Glon., Bar-c. (2) Kali-c. - excessive sweating, weakness, pallor, Cact. - heart and arteries.

REFERENCES - Boericke. Clarke.

CALCAREA IODATA

(Calcium Iodide)

PHARMACY - calc-i. Calcarea iodata. Calcium iodide. Iodide of lime. ***Historical dose:*** Trituration and all potencies.

CLINICAL - Adenoids. ***Breast, tumors.*** Cancer. Catarrh. ***Croup***. Cysts. Flatulence. Glandular, swellings. Goiter. Headaches. Osteomalacia. ***Pneumonia***. Polyps. Scrofulous, disorders. Thyroid, disorders. ***Thyroid, tumors. Tonsils, enlarged.*** Tuberculosis. ***Ulcers.*** Uterine, fibroids. ***Varicose veins***.

HOMEOPATHIC - Calcarea iodata has a short proving, it has been used on the indications suggested by its two components in the diseases named. It is similar to Bar-i. in its action on enlarged glands.

Indicated for ***enlarged tonsils*** honeycombed with little crypts. Induration of glands. ***Thyroid tumors and cysts***. Thyroid gland enlargements about time of puberty. For the treatment of scrofulous disorders.

Weariness of the whole body. Secretions inclined to be profuse and yellow. ***Croup***. Adenoids. Uterine fibroids. Polyps of nose and ear. Indolent ulcers accompanying varicose veins. Headache while riding against a cold wind. Profuse sweat.

MIND - Indifference and indolence.

Abdomen - Rumbling in the bowels with discharge of wind. Constant evacuation of large quantities of wind downward. Slight pain in the abdomen.

Breasts - Indurated growth in breasts, movable, painful on pressure and on movement on arm.

Constitutions - Flabby children subject to colds.

Ears - Numbness and ringing in the ears.

Eyes - Pain over the eyes.

Head - Headache while riding against cold wind. Light-headed. Catarrh, worse at root of nose, sneezing, very little sensation. Constant, severe and dull headache, forehead and temples, worse stooping. Sharp, piercing pain in right temple. Falling out of hair.

Limbs - Dull, heavy lameness in the external portion of the right arm, with numbness of the hands and fingers. Tired feeling in the lower limbs, especially in the calves of the legs. Pain across the anterior surface of the upper third of both thighs, as if he had been beaten.

Lungs - Chronic cough. ***Pneumonia***. Pain in chest, difficulty breathing after syphilis and mercury. ***Croup.*** Hectic fever with green, purulent expectoration.

Mouth - Dry, furred feeling on lips and tongue. Mouth and gums burn like fire. Bitter taste in the mouth, but not disagreeable like myrrh. Astringent taste in mouth, like alum. Taste at first sweetish, afterwards slightly astringent and metallic.

Neck - Stiffness of the back of the neck.

Skin - ***Indolent ulcers, with varicose veins***. Easy perspiration. Copper-colored and papular eruption. Tinea, favus, crusta lactea. Swelling of the glands. Skin is cracked.

Stomach - Inclined to belch wind. Slight hiccough. Slight nausea.

Throat - Enlarged tonsils filled with little crypts. Thyroid enlargement about the time of puberty. Adenoids.

Vertigo - Light-headed. ***Sensation as if the head wasn't there.*** Giddy headache.

COMMENTARY - The main use for this is tonsil and thyroid problems. Thyroid cysts (Thuj.), goiters, and thyroid tumors, especially since a treatment of radioactive iodine. Hyperthyroidism. Large tonsils and adenoids. Thyroids enlarge at puberty. Indurated glands. Generally warm-blooded.

Kent named Calc-i. and Calc-sil. as the remedies for delusions of seeing dead people or dreaming of dead people.

C. L. Nicholls cured a number of cases of breast tumors with the 3x, nodular tumors, movable, tender to touch, painful on moving arm.

RELATIONS - ***Compare:*** (1) Agraphis - adenoids with enlarged tonsils. (2) Sulph-i. follows both Agraphis and Calc-i. (3) Acon-l. - swelling of glands, Hodgkin's disease. (4) also Calc-f., Sil., Merc., Iod. (5) Calc., Bar-c., Calc-p., Carb-v.

REFERENCES - Boericke. Clarke. Murphy.

CALCAREA MURIATICA

(Calcium Chloride)

PHARMACY - calc-m. Calcarea muriatica. Calcium chloride. Chloride of lime. Rademacher's Liquor is 1 part to 2 of distilled water of which take 15 drops in half a cup of water, five times daily. ***Historical dose:*** Tincture and all potencies.

CLINICAL - Abscess. Belchings. Boils. Convulsions. Diarrhea. Eczema. Edema. Faintness. Gastritis. Glandular, swellings. Impetigo. Iritis. Nausea. Paralysis. Pleurisy. ***Ringworm.*** Scrofula. ***Vomiting.***

HOMEOPATHIC - In scrofulous cases, Calc-m. promotes the action of mercury. Under its use, glandular swellings and indurations soften and disappear, hence its use in swollen glands and boils.

Calc-m. in the form of the liquor (1 part of 2 of distilled water), was one of Rademacher's *"Stomach Remedies"* and was used with great success by him in cases of obstinate vomiting. He gave 15 drops of the liquor in half a cup of water five times a day.

Rademacher's indications were vomiting of all food and drink, vomiting when no food had been taken, jaundice, and pain in the left hypochondrium. He also found it indicated in gastric pain, bloating and belchings.

Faintness, anxiety and weakness. Trembling and giddiness. Respiration quick and snoring. Increased secretion of mucus, perspiration and urine. Nausea and vomiting. ***Vomiting of all food and drink with gastric pain.*** Diarrhea. Tender precordium.

Accelerated pulse. Cold sweats, convulsions, paralysis. Glandular swellings. Angio-neurotic edema. Pleurisy with effusion. Boils. Eczema. Eczema in infants. ***Ringworm of the scalp.*** Impetigo.

COMMENTS - C. W. recorded a remarkable instance of the action of this remedy. A scrofulous and rheumatic woman had suffered from abscess of cornea, followed by rheumatic iritis and a dense opacity was left. An old-school practitioner had treated her with mercury during two years in a vain endeavor to "touch her mouth."

C. W. put one grain of Calc-m. in an 8-oz. bottle and directed the patient to take a tablespoonful three times a day. The medicine had not been taken ten minutes before she felt it at her fingers' ends. The mercurial action was evoked and she was in bed a fortnight, terribly salivated. The condition of the eye was unchanged.

RELATIONS - ***Compare:*** (1) Calc-i., Calc-chln., Nat-h.

REFERENCES - Boericke. Clarke.

CALCAREA OVI TESTAE

(Egg-shell)

PHARMACY - calc-o-t. Calcarea ovi testae. Egg-shell. Ovi testa. Testa praeparata. Trituration of the shell, not including the lining membranes. ***Historical dose:*** Trituration and all potencies.

CLINICAL - ***Backache***. Leucorrhea. Warts.

HOMEOPATHIC - Calc-o-t. has the general properties of Calc., but it has been little used clinically. This preparation of Calcium has been used in preference to others in cases of simple bland leucorrhea and warts.

Backache, as if broken in two. Leucorrhea. ***Backache with leucorrhea.*** Tired feeling. Effective in controlling suffering from cancer. Warts.

COMMENTS - Water in which eggs have been boiled is popularly supposed to have the property of causing warts if brought in contact with the hands. This suggests Calc-o-t. as possibly the best Calcarea preparation to prescribe in cases of warts.

REFERENCES - Boericke. Clarke.

CALCAREA PHOSPHORICA

(Calcium Phosphate)

PHARMACY - calc-p. Calcarea phosphorica. Calcium phosphate. Phosphate of lime. Tricalcic phosphate. A mixture of the basic and other phosphates of lime, made by dropping dilute phosphoric acid into lime water. Trituration. ***Historical dose:*** Trituration and all potencies.

CLINICAL - ***Adenoid, growths***. Anemia. Ankles, weak. Back, weakness. Bedwetting. ***Bones, disorders. Bones, fractures.*** Brain-fag. Bright's disease. ***Broken bones.*** Cholera infantum. Chorea. ***Colds. Colic.*** Cretinism. Debility. ***Dentition, slow.*** Diabetes. Dyspepsia. Emissions. Epilepsy. Face, boils. Fistula. ***Fractures.*** Gleet. Gonorrhea. ***Growing, pains.*** Headaches. Hernia. Hydrocele. Joints disorders. Leucorrhea. Lumbago. ***Malnutrition.*** Nymphomania. ***Osteomyelitis. Osteoporosis.*** Polyps. Rheumatism. ***Rickets.*** Sexual, mania. Spermatorrhea. Spina bifida. Stiff-neck. Strabismus. Testicles, swollen. Throat, sore. ***Tobacco habit.*** Tonsils, enlarged. Toothache. ***Tuberculosis.*** Uterus prolapsed.

HOMEOPATHIC - Calc-p., while resembling Calc., has a very distinct individuality. It has been proved and tested clinically and, having been adopted by Schüssler as his leading *"anti-psoric,"* a number of valuable indications have been added by him and his followers.

Generally emaciated (Calc. is generally fat). Dirty-white or brownish (Calc. is chalky-white). Large abdomen (Calc.), but flabby. Craves the salt of smoked meats, and ***"fat bacon."***

Stools are green and slimy, or hot and watery, with fetid flatus (Calc.), sometimes green, generally watery, white and mixed with curds. Open fontanelles, especially the posterior (Calc., the anterior only). The skull is thin and soft, almost cracks like paper when pressed upon.

Affects the ***nutrition of bones*** and glands. The ***bones become soft, thin and brittle. Osteoporosis. Osteomyelitis.*** Spinal curvatures (Calc-f., Sil.). Promotes ossification of bones in the ***non-union of fractures*** (Symph.). It has a special affinity where bones form sutures or symphysis. Bone diseases.

Arthritis. Rheumatism. Shifting pains. A slight draft causes rheumatic pains, every cold causes pains in joints and sutures. Sensation of ***crawling and numbness.*** Trembling or trembling hands with pain or other complaints. Coldness or soreness in spots, vertex, eyeballs, tip of nose, fingers etc.

Predisposition to glandular and bone diseases. Glands are swollen. ***Enlargement of tonsils,*** acute and chronic. Addison's disease. Tendency to perspiration and glandular enlargement (Calc.). Discharges are albuminous. Shortness of breath. Tuberculosis. Diabetes when the lungs are affected. Symptoms are worse from any change of weather.

Malassimilation. Poor nutrition. ***Rickets. Growing pains. Slow development of teeth.*** Slow walking, neck too thin and weak to support head. Indicated in anemic children who are peevish, flabby, have cold limbs and feeble digestion. Anemia after acute diseases and chronic wasting diseases. Chlorosis.

Dyspepsia, pain better for a short time by raising wind. When fasting, the pain goes to the spine. ***Child suffers from colic after every feeding.*** Feeling as if one ought to raise wind and could not. Dyspepsia with indescribable distress in region of stomach, only temporarily better by eating.

MIND - Mental anxiety. Effects of mental strain (Nat-m., Kali-p.). ***Moaning and irritable, hard to please.*** Complaints are worse when thinking of them. Prostration of mind from talking. Mistakes in repeating words. Writes wrong words, or same words twice. Lack of memory. Weak memory, inability to exert mentally. Forgetful after grief and vexation (Ign., Ph-ac).

Great depression. ***Ailments after bad news.*** Unpleasant news brings him beside himself. ***Ailments from grief, disappointed love.*** Vexation and disappointment after grief. Homesickness. Sentimental. Indignation at unpleasant dreams. ***Involuntary sighing.*** Shuns society and seeks solitude, desires to be quiet and alone. Suspicious. Jealousy. ***Discontentment.*** Sadness in girls before puberty. Weeping worse consolation.

Fear of hearing bad news. Anxiety during palpitations. Fear of thunder storms. Anxiety for others. Adverse to company. Over reactive, can be irritable and upset easily. Discontent, peevish, restless, bored easily.

Changeable moods. ***Temper tantrums.*** Sensitive and offended easily. Children are peevish and fretful. ***Obstinate and hard to please.*** Slow comprehension. ***Mental dullness in children.*** Difficulty in performing intellectual operations. Cretinism. Idiocy of children. Slow learning to talk.

Dullness and obtuse. ***Irritability worse consolation.*** Irritability during dentition. Irritability during headache.

Dissatisfaction. Restlessness. ***Constant desire to go from place to place*** (Tub.). Boredom. Always wants to go somewhere. ***Desire to travel.*** Wants to be at home and when at home wants to go out, goes from place to place. Censorious, fault-finding. Nymphomania before menses. Confusion on waking in morning.

Abdomen - Colic, soreness and burning around navel. ***Colic,*** at every attempt to eat, by taking ice cream, cold water or fruits. ***Child suffers from colic after every feeding.*** Cutting, pinching, sharp pains, followed by diarrhea. Flatulent colic. Bellyache better passing wind, after stool or after leucorrhea. Griping pain and rumbling in bowels before menses. Burning pain in abdomen. ***Sunken and flabby***. Aching soreness and pain around navel, better passing fetid flatus. Oozing of bloody fluid from navel of infants. Festering navel. Empty, sinking sensation around navel, or in whole abdomen. Motion in abdomen, as of something alive. Abdominal wall as if numb. Abdominal wall quivering or aching. Warm feeling in groins. Pressure and soreness in left side. Weak, sinking feeling in abdomen, with leucorrhea.

Back - Backache, worse stormy weather. Backache with uterine pains. ***Backache with menses.*** Throbbing or jerking, below scapula. ***Curvature of the spine to the left.*** Violent pain, worse least effort, screams with pain. Lumbar vertebrae bend to the left. Rheumatic pain from draft of air with stiffness and dullness of head. Sacrum numb and lame. Soreness in sacro-iliac sympysis, as if broken (Aesc.). Spina bifida. Pott's disease. Drawing pain in back and limbs, with yawning, stretching, bending backward. Aching, pressure, tearing, soreness and shooting pains in coccyx. Violent stitch at a small spot between left ilium and sacrum, from slightest motion.

Bladder - Painful sensation in neck of bladder, like that when having the stream suddenly stopped. Pain in bladder, worse when empty. Sore aching pain in bladder, worse after urination. Pressing pain, most on right side of bladder. Shooting pain in mouth of bladder. Violent pain, in bladder and prostate with weak stream of urine. Cutting and burning, in urethra, after urinating in males. Pressing down, before urination. Drawing in bladder, extends upward, while urinating. Pressing and cutting pains after urinating, in females.

Breasts - Infant wants to nurse all the time and vomits easily. Breasts sore to touch. ***Child refuses breast, milk tastes sour or salty.*** Milk acid, watery, thin, neutral. Nipples aching, sore. Breasts feel as if larger, as during last half of pregnancy. Weakness after prolonged nursing. Tumors in breasts (left), in men, painful on pressure. Tumors in breasts, painful sensation on pressure. Breasts, sore, feel large. Sexual desire increased during breast-feeding.

Bones - Weak bones, slow to heal. ***Osteoporosis.*** Brittle bones. Demineralization of bones. ***Slow ossification, non-union of bones. Rickets.*** It has an affinity where bones form sutures or symphysis, pain, burning along sutures. ***Broken bones.*** Bone injuries. ***Delayed healing of broken bones.*** Pains in joints and bones. ***Growing pains.*** Delayed growth of bones. Osgood-Schlatter disease. Osteogenesis imperfecta. Paget's disease. Osteomyelitis, acute or chronic (Calc.).

Causations - Ill effects of over-growth. Broken bones, lifting, operations for fistula. Over study. Grief, disappointed love, bad news. Sexual excess or irregularities. Getting wet. Poor diet.

Chest - Chest sore. Pain through lower left lung. Pain in chest from drafts. Sore pain in sternum. Sharp pain, through sternum. Aching pain in chest with soreness to touch. Sharp pain, right side, coming and going. Sharp pain, takes breath away, worse breathing deep. Clavicle sore. Pressing ache in chest. Shooting pain, in left chest. Pains where cartilages and ribs meet. Ulcer over sternum or clavicle. Hard, bluish lumps in axilla.

Constitutions - Patients, especially children, are delicate, tall, thin or scrawny with dirty brownish skin. Suited to scrofulous, gouty constitutions. Anemic children who are peevish, flabby, have cold limbs and weak digestion, they start convulsively when lying on back better lying on side. They lose breath when they are lifted.

Cough - Suffocative cough, better lying down. Cough during dentition. Cough worse sitting up, better lying down. Whooping cough, obstinate cases. Dry, short cough, with soreness and hoarseness. Cough with yellow expectoration, more in morning. Cough with fever, dryness and thirst. Cough from 6 a.m. to 6 p.m. Chronic, of consumptives, who suffer with cold limbs.

Ears - Defective hearing. Sudden swelling of external ear. Coldness of tips of ears, nose and chin. ***Cold feeling in ears***, followed by throbbing, heat and hard hearing. Noises in ears after stools. Tearing, in ears when the weather changes to cold. Aching, pressing, tearing or rending in and around ears, most behind, or below. Burning, on a small spot over right ear, highly sensitive to slightest touch. All bones around ears ache and hurt. Sudden swelling of external ear. Singing or other noises in ears. Inner and outer ear swollen, red, sore, itching, hot. Excoriating discharge from ears. Burning itching of outer ear in warm room. Pimples on ears.

Eyes - Cool feeling behind the eyes. Conjunctivitis during dentition. Eyes red, capillary vessels visible in streaks from corners to cornea. Sensation as if something in eyes, worse thinking of it. Diffused opacity in cornea following abscess. Eyes pain, as if beaten. Hot feeling in lids. Squinting. Cannot use the eyes in gas-light. Sweat of brows and lids. Lachrymation, worse when yawning. Light, candlelight or gaslight, hurts the eyes. Misty vision Letters change into little black points or small round grey spots. Shimmering glittering, fiery circles. Veil over eyes.

Face - Pale, yellowish, earthy, full of pimples. Acne in anemic girls at puberty (Calc-pic). Coppery face, full of pimples. Cold sweat on face. Upper lip swollen painful, hard and burning. Pains in face in upper jaw bone. Pains in face, with every spell of cold weather. Neuralgia at night in cold air, sensitive to pressure worse exertion, better heat. Aching, sore in region of parotid gland. In process zygomaticus. Heat in face, in evening Heat in with chill or other complaints.

Female - Girls slow in maturing. Effects of taking cold during first menses. Menses, early, scanty. Menses, every two weeks, excessive, bright. Late menses, when blood is dark, sometimes first bright then dark. Menses during lactation, with sexual excitement. Dysmenorrhea. ***Menses with violent backache.*** Eruption, worse during menses. ***Leucorrhea like egg white***, worse morning. Burning leucorrhea, albuminous from one term to another, follows pain in abdomen. Prolapsed uterus in debilitated women, worse while passing urine or stool with menses with rheumatic pains. Uterine spasms. Uterine polyps. Uterus, heavy, weak or aching. Uterine displacement with rheumatic pains. Crawling, voluptuous in genitals. Sexual desire increased before menses. Clitoris erect after urination, with sexual desire. Voluptuous feeling as if parts, with increased sexual desire. Nymphomania with aching, pressing or weakness in uterine region (Plat.). Pressure upward over mons veneris. Pressing, drawing and sore feeling as if menses should appear. Abnormal cravings during pregnancy. Weariness in all limbs during pregnancy.

Food - Great hunger with thirst. Much thirst, with dry mouth and tongue. ***Craving for bacon, ham, salted or smoked meats.*** Craving for raw, salty, piquant food. Desire for tobacco smoking, which helps the headache. Craving for salami, sweets. Abnormal cravings during pregnancy. Colic from ice cream, cold water or fruits. Irritability after coffee. Nausea from smoking, after coffee. Confusion after coffee. Wheat bread tastes bitter. Juicy fruit or cider causes diarrhea. Drinking cold water causes cutting in abdomen.

Head - Delayed closure or reopening of fontanelles. Skull soft and thin, cracking like paper, worse at occiput. ***Headache of school children*** near puberty, with diarrhea. Headache, ***worse near the region of sutures.*** Headache, ***worse from change of weather***. Depression on occipital bone. Cannot hold the head up, it wobbles. Burning, worse near sutures. Headache in occiput, down spine better cool bathing or sneezing. Headache with abdominal flatulence. Sensation as if brain was pressed against skull. As of ice in occiput. Head hot, with smarting of roots of hair. Cold or sore vertex. Hydrocephalus. Can't hold head up, it wobbles. Throbbing in forehead during menses. Congestion of blood to head during menses. Headache with diarrhea. Perspiration on scalp during sleep. Impetigo on scalp. Bald spots on head.

Heart - Dropsy from heart disease. Palpitations with trembling weakness in calf. Sharp cutting, shooting, pains in region of heart, interrupts breathing. Palpitations with anxiety, followed by trembling weakness, particularly of calves. Feels beating of pulse, not frequent but quick, while sitting, feels it in nape and left chest.

Kidneys - Urine increased with sensation of weakness. Pain in region of kidneys, worse blowing nose or lifting. Urine increased, with sensation of weakness. Frequent urging to urinate. Dark urine, warmer than usual and of a penetrating odor. Diaper reddish-yellow. Increase of urine, with flocculent sediment.

Limbs - Aching in all limbs, with weariness. ***Broken bones. Delayed healing of broken bones.*** Pains in joints and bones. Pains flying about in all parts of rump and limbs, after getting wet in the rain. ***Growing pains.*** Gouty fingers and toes becoming painful in cold weather. Weary limbs when going upstairs. Rheumatism in cold season. Rheumatism after every cold. Stiffness and pain with ***cold, numb feeling***, worse any change of weather. Crawling and coldness. Cold limbs with digestive troubles. Fingers sore. Pain, burning along edges of nails. As of a splinter under the nails. Trembling of arms and hands with many complaints. Hard bluish lumps in axilla. Buttocks, back and limbs asleep. Weakness of the hips. Hip joint disease. Fistulous ulcers on ankle joint.

Lungs - Breathing more frequent, short and difficult. Child loses breath on being lifted up. Suffocating attacks in children after nursing worse after crying. Suffocative cough, better lying down. ***Involuntary***

sighing. Rattling of mucus in lungs. Must scrape mucus from larynx before one can sing or talk. Tuberculosis with cavities with night sweats, yellow expectoration. ***Tuberculosis with emaciation.*** Obstinate whooping cough.

Male - Stitching pain in perineum extending to penis. Erections while riding in carriage without desire. Shooting pain in root of penis and bladder. Chronic gonorrhea, in anemic subjects. Gonorrhea, gleety discharge, sharp pain in urethra and prostate. Swelling of testicles. Scrotum sore, oozing a fluid. Itching of scrotum with sweating, soreness and pimples. Sexual desire increased with some, with others decreased. Weak feeling in sexual organs after stools.

Modalities - ***Better in summer***. Better warm, dry atmosphere. Better lying down, rest. Better lying on abdomen during restless night. Worse from exposure to damp, cold weather. Worse changes of weather. Worse drafts, cold. Worse melting snow. ***Worse from dentition. Worse puberty. Worse mental exertion.*** Worse when thinking of symptoms. Worse loss of fluids. Worse from motion. Worse lifting. Worse pressure. Worse ascending. Worse fruits, cider. Worse mornings, evenings. Worse artificial light. Worse getting wet in rain.

Mouth - Sore spot inside of right cheek. ***Adenoid growths***. Disgusting taste, worse in morning. Bitter taste in morning, with headache. Bitter taste particularly of wheat bread. Flabby sweetish taste. Bitter taste at begining of menses. Tongue swollen, numb, stiff, with pimples on it. Tip of tongue sore, burning, little blisters on it. Tongue coated white at root, most in morning. Dryness of mouth and tongue, into choanae, with or without thirst.

Neck - Neck painful from drafts. Rheumatic pains in neck from slight draft of air, with stiffness and dullness of head. Neck weak, thin, head bobs about. Neck too slender to support head. Weak, thin neck, head bobs about. Cramplike, in neck, first one side, then the other. Aching in sides of neck, up to ear, worse pressure, and when turning neck.

Nose - ***Tip of nose is icy cold***. Tip of nose itching. Polyps, large, pedunculated. Fluent coryza, forenoon. Coryza with salivation. Coryza, fluent in cool room, stopped in warm air and out-doors. Biting stinging pain in front corner of left nostril, later right nostril. Sneezing and lachrymation. Sneezing and soreness on edges of alae. Nose swollen, with sore nostrils or ulcers. Nosebleeds in afternoon.

Perspiration - Sticky sickly sweat worse head and throat, at night. Perspires on various parts at night, waking out of sleep. Copious sweat at night, on single parts. Sweats towards and in morning.

Rectum - Abscess and boils near or about anus, discharge blood and pus. Itching in anus, worse evening. Bleeding after hard stool. Offensive flatus. Tendency to diarrhea from juicy fruits. Diarrhea during dentition with much flatus. Diarrhea from vexation. Diarrhea, containing white points or flakes/ Diarrhea like pus, scanty with much flatulence. Disposition to intestinal worms in anemic or weakly patients. Stitches in rectum toward anus. Shooting pain in anus. Fistula in anus, alternating with chest symptoms. Fistula of anus, in persons who have pains in joints with every spell of cold, stormy weather. Fissure of anus in tall, slim children. Hemorrhoids, oozing watery fluid all the time. Hemorrhoids, painful, external, send one to bed, itch, burn, discharge a yellow pus. Sore feeling in anus when getting up in morning. Daily watery, very hot stools. Copious soft stool in morning. Soft stool, passed with difficulty. Stools, green, slimy, ***hot***, sputtering, undigested with ***fetid flatus***.

Skin - Dry skin, moist on hands. Dark, brown, yellow. Itching and burning, as from nettles. Itching, biting, most on places years before affected. Pimples in region of joints. Fistulous or scrofulous ulcers, slow to heal. Cholesteatoma. Tetters on lower legs, peeling off, scaling. Furuncles from ulcers. Ulceration from mustard poultice. Scars from amputation ulcerate.

Sleep - ***Children cry and moan in sleep.*** Constant stretching and yawning. Sleepiness during day, before menses. Yawning, with irresistible drowsiness all day. Cannot get awake in early morning. Disturbed sleep, worse before midnight. Drowsiness gloomy mood, inability to think, headache, singing in ears, sweat in face, prostration of limbs. Nightmares. Vivid dreams of late events or last readings. Dreams of travelling. Dreams of fire.

Stomach - ***Weak digestion***, every bite hurts the stomach. Chronic stomach or abdominal pains of schoolchildren. Heartburn. Burning in pit after belching. Burning at stomach and rising of water into mouth. Infant persistently vomits breast milk or other milk. Infant wants to nurse all the time and vomits easily. Stomach feels expanded. ***Much flatulence***, temporarily relieved by sour belchings. Faint feeling in stomach, with too early menses. Nausea on attempting to scrape larynx. Nausea, rising from pit when moving, better rest. Nausea followed by headache and lassitude. Retching from hawking up mucus. Vomiting, while hawking mucus with trembling hands.

Teeth - ***Delayed dentition.*** Teeth develop slowly. Retarded dentition, with emaciation. Convulsions without fever during dentition. Teeth sensitive to chewing. Hollow teeth sensitive to cold air. Teeth, soft. ***Teeth decay easily*** (Calc-f.). In eye and stomach teeth. Shooting pain in molars. Tearing, boring pain, at night, worse warm and cold things. Toothache worse warm and cold things.

Temperature - Easily chilled. Chilly with pains. Chills up the back, but heat down the back. Fever with dentition. Dry fever, in evening, hot breath, noticeable beating of heart, mouth and tongue without thirst, yawning, stretching.

Throat - Sore aching in throat, feels hollow. Sore throat with tickling cough in evening, worse after going to bed. It hurts to swallow saliva, not food. Burning in pit of throat. Pain and burning from other parts towards throat. Burning in larynx following burning at back of tongue. ***Tonsillitis. Swollen tonsils***, cannot open mouth without pain. ***Chronic enlargement of tonsils*** in scrofulous subjects. ***Adenoid growths.*** Throat feels hollow. Sensation of weakness in throat. Dryness in throat at night. Sore throat with fluent coryza. Hawking up phlegm late in evening, at night and in morning, with gagging. Hoarseness and cough, day and night. Must scrape mucus from larynx before one can sing or talk. Catarrhs in scrofulous or gouty constitutions.

Vertigo - Vertigo in windy weather. Vertigo and loss of memory during dinner. Vertigo, worse constipation. Staggering when rising from a seat. Vertigo on motion. When walking in open air. Vertigo of old people. Dizziness when getting up, or rising from sitting. Vertigo with dull headache, nausea, complaints of eyes, neck, aching limbs. Vertigo during menses.

COMMENTS - Affects the parathyroid glands, which affect calcium metabolism. Paget's disease, Osgood-Schlatter disease, osteoporosis, osteomyelitis, acute or chronic (Calc.). Brittle bones.

In a case of osteogenesis imperfecta, Calc-p. lessened the frequency of broken bones and helped to strengthen the bones. Helps to heal broken bones (Symph., Calc-f. if the broken bone begins to decay). For both remedies, make sure that the bones are correctly set before giving the remedy.

For problems associated with bony structures, calcium deficiency related to bone, bone marrow problems and anemia. Defective bone growth, bones thin and brittle. Brittled matrix. Lack of structure and cohesiveness, curvatures (Calc., Sil.).

Flat feet and feet that are turning in too much (Calc.). Growing pains. Slow bone growth, fontanelles not closing properly. Scoliosis, weak tender feet. Stiffness on the neck and knees. Teething delayed and painful.

Children with a lot of glandular problems, adenoid and tonsils problems. Stunted growth. Enlargement of tonsils, acute and chronic. Tumor of the parathyroid gland, hyperparathyroidism.

Useful in cases of fistula and when fistula has been operated on with the symptoms appearing elsewhere. Fistula alternating with chest symptoms.

Shortness of breath. Involuntary sighing. Contraction of chest and difficult breathing, evening until 10 p.m., better lying down, worse getting up. Constant stretching and yawning. Crying out in sleep. Cannot get awake in morning.

Keynote moaning. Moaning in fevers. Children that are peevish and have chronic discontent. Hyperactive, hard to please, irritable, emaciated, and scrawny. Sunken features and blue circles around the eyes.

There is a weak, sinking sensation in the hypogastrium and a sinking, empty feeling in the epigastrium. Poor assimilation problems, may have poor nutrition. Rickets, thin and weak. Flabby stomach (Bar-c.. is hard). Aggravation from fruits, resulting in diarrhea.

Prolapsed uterus, worse during stool or urination. Aching in uterus, cutting through to sacrum. Cream-like leucorrhea. Burning in vagina with pain on both sides of the bladder and uterus, burning like fire up into chest. Flushes of heat and faintness, sweats easily. Profuse sweats (less than Sep.). Menses are profuse and the patient is weak and tubercular.

Nymphomania, all organs in erection with irresistible desire, particularly before menses. Voluptuous feeling, as if all the parts were filled with blood, pulses in all the parts with increased desire after urination.

Grauvogl considered it the most important remedy in chronic hydrocephalus and he gave it as a prenatal remedy during pregnancy to women who had previously borne hydrocephalic children.

Chills, run upward. Hering states: "The chills run up the back, terrible muscular jerks in body, which almost throw him out of his chair." Cold sensation in the limbs as if cold water poured over them, creeping numbness pains and coldness, electric-like shooting pains. Very sensitive to draft. Worse from cold, wet weather. Every exposure increases the rheumatic pains and uterine distress.

Etiologies include a large stress resulting in a decrease of vital energy, like grief, separation, death. They may get sick after not enough sleep (Cocc.). Slow to learn, due to structural problem (Bar-c., neurological). Headaches worse from studying and concentration.

RELATIONS - ***Compare:*** (1) Calc., Sil., Phos., Calc. hypophos. (2) Cheiranthus - effects of cutting wisdom teeth. (3) Conchiolin. - Mother of pearl - has a wide range of action in bone affections, especially when the growing ends are affected. Osteitis. (4) Cham., Ign. Psor., Sulph. ***Complementary:*** Ruta., Hepar.

REFERENCES - Boericke. Clarke. Murphy.

CALCAREA PICRICA

(Calcium Picrate)

PHARMACY - calc-pic. Calcarea picrica. Calcium picrate. Picrate of calcium. ***Historical dose:*** Trituration and all potencies.

CLINICAL - ***Boils.*** Ear, boils. Fatigue. Phlyctenules. Prostration. Skin, disorders. Styes.

HOMEOPATHIC - Houghton noted that the extreme prostration of Picric acid is relieved by this salt also. Picric acid and all its salts are curative in states of intense prostration and fatigue. Indicated by clinical experience for peri-follicular inflammation.

Recurring or chronic ***boils***, particularly when located on parts thinly covered with muscle tissue, as on shinbones, coccyx, or the auditory canal. Minute and excessively painful boils in meatus. Dry, scurfy accumulation and exfoliation of epithelial scales. Styes, phlyctenules.

REFERENCES - Clarke.

CALCAREA SILICATA

(Calcium Silicate)

PHARMACY - calc-sil. Calcarea silicata. Calcium silicate. Trituration. ***Historical dose:*** Trituration and all potencies.

CLINICAL - Anal fistula. Atrophy. Cataracts. ***Chilliness. Cold.*** Cornea, ulcers. Diabetes. Dropsy. ***Emaciation.*** Epithelioma. Flatulence Goiter. Hydrocele. Leucorrhea. Lupus. Polyps Scrofula. Ulcers. Uterus, prolapsed. ***Weak.***

HOMEOPATHIC - This preparation of Calcarea silicata has been used by Ussher in the 1x and 6x potencies in cases of atrophy of children. He found it succeeded where Sil. failed in these cases and in corneal disorders. It causes absorption of corneal exudations. Indicated by ulcers with punched-out edges.

Kent said it cured cataracts, polyps, goiter, epithelioma and lupus. Diabetes mellitus. Hydrocele. Useful in restraining malignant ulceration in the breasts.

Calc-sil. is a deep, long acting medicine for complaints which come on slowly and reach their final development after long periods. ***Weak, emaciated, cold and chilly,*** worse from being overheated, generally sensitive. Atrophy of children.

Aversion to the open air. ***Lack of vital heat.*** Very sensitive to the ***cold.*** Extreme sensitiveness to drafts. Catching colds constantly. Thick greenish-yellow expectoration. Abscesses, catarrhal discharges, ulcers, are marked with thick, greenish-yellow pus.

MIND - Absent-minded. Inability to concentrate. Confusion of mind in the morning. Irritable, irresolute. Lacks self-confidence. Discontent and despair. Weary. ***Fearful.*** Anxiety about health. Fear of brain lesion. Discouraged about her disease, thinks it an incurable disease. Excitable and easily angered, worse after anger. Consolation irritates.

She sits long in one place and looks into space and does not answer when spoken to. Passive delirium, talks and acts like one insane. Talks to people who have long been dead. Mutters foolish things.

Abdomen - Slow digestion, slow action of bowels and liver. Dropsy of the abdomen, enlarged liver. Distention of the abdomen after eating. Flatulence with much rumbling and fullness.

Back - Back feels cold and there is a sensation of coldness in back of neck and sacrum. Hard aching in the back, when rising from a seat. The spine is sore to touch. Stiff neck.

Breasts - Useful in restraining malignant ulceration in the breasts. Excoriation of the nipples. Suppressed or absent milk.

Chest - Pain in chest walls. Constriction of chest. Eruption on chest. Pain in chest during cough, on inspiration, deep breathing.

Constitutions - Hydrogenoid constitution. Constitutional condition in patients suffering from epilepsy, making the fits lighter and farther apart.

Ears - Offensive, purulent, thick and greenish yellow discharge. Itching deep in ears. Noises in ears, cracking in ears when chewing. Increased wax in ears.

Eyes - Corneal exudation. Eyelids are agglutinated with pus. Cataracts. Itching of the eyes. Lachrymation in open air. Paralysis of the optic nerve. Photophobia.

Face - Very pale, an earthy color. Lips bluish, dry and cracked. Red face during headache, circumscribed red cheeks. Eruptions of the face, acne, boils, comedones, eczema, herpes, pimples.

Female - Menstrual flow absent or suppressed, painful and irregular. Flow between periods. Leucorrhea, painful and irregular menses. Uterus is heavy, prolapsed. Ulceration of labia, vagina.

Food - Great thirst. Aversion to food, especially to meat and milk. Some desire for sour things, milk. Many complaints worse from cold food and cold drinks.

Head - Coldness of the head, especially of occiput and vertex. Congestion of the head at night. Constriction of the forehead. Eruptions on the scalp, crusts, eczema, pustules. Perspiration of the whole scalp.

Kidneys - Sudden ineffectual urging. Frequent urination during the night. Involuntary urination during sleep.

Limbs - The muscles, tendons and joints are weak and easily strained. Stiffness of all the limbs, joints. Heaviness of all the limbs. Gouty nodosities. Cramps in hands, lower limbs, calves, feet, soles, toes. Boils on the upper limbs. Cracked hands and fingers. Nails have ceased to grow.

Lungs - Difficult respiration. Breathing fast, asthmatic. Chronic irritation of air passages. Coughs with coldness, weakness, emaciation, worse from cold air. Coughs in tubercular subjects. Copious expectoration, greenish-yellow, bloody.

Male - Enlarged and tender prostate gland. Emission of prostatic fluid when straining to pass stool. Erection at night without thought or dreams. Eruptions on the prepuce. Hydrocele and induration of testes. Foul sweat on genitals.

Modalities - Worse from change of weather. Worse from warm to cold. Worse cold air. Worse becoming cold. Worse after becoming cold, and cold, wet weather. Great aggravation from being overheated. Worse after sex, Worse exertion. Worse motion.

Mouth - Mouth covered with aphthae. Very dry, but at times copious mucus. Offensive, even putrid odor from the mouth. Bad taste, alkaline, bitter in the morning, metallic, putrid, sour. White coated tongue. Tongue is very sore. Difficult speech. Swollen gums and tongue. Bleeding gums.

Nose - Head colds, catarrh of nose and posterior sinus, discharge thick, yellow, hard crusts. Extreme dryness inside. of nose. Nosebleed, bright red blood, on blowing nose. Polyps.

Rectum - Extreme constipation with inactivity of the rectum. Difficult stool, paralyzed feeling in rectum. Constriction of anus. Stricture of the rectum. Fistula in anus. Painless diarrhea. Dysentery with bloody, scanty stools.

Skin - Cold and blue, very sensitive. Cracked skin. Dry, burning skin and inability to perspire. Burning of the skin after scratching. Pimples, comedones, wens. Eczema and herpes. Psoric eruptions. Pimples, pustules, and red rashes. Warts painful, hard. Liver spots.

Sleep - Restless sleep. Easily startled during sleep. Shrieks during sleep. Confused, amorous, frightful, fantastic dreams. ***Dreams of the dead***, of death, murder, disease, fire, anger.

Stomach - Anxiety in the stomach. Sinking sensation at pit. Sensation of coldness, especially when empty. Flatulence and distention after eating. Heartburn. Hiccough. Vomiting and belchings. Vomiting bile, black blood, food, mucus and watery substances.

Teeth - Loose teeth, feel too long. Decay of the teeth. Pain in the teeth at night. Very sore when chewing.

Temperature - ***Cold all the time, lack of vital heat.*** Cold sweat mostly on the limbs. Hectic fevers. When perspiring, a slight draft or cold air will suppress the sweat and he becomes lame and the symptoms in general are worse. Marked periodicity in many symptoms.

Throat - Inflammation of the throat, pharynx and tonsils with dryness and redness. Constant effort to clear the throat. Lump in the throat. Splinter-like pain on swallowing.

Vertigo - Vertigo, in morning, on rising, after rising, in evening, while lying, looking upwards, from mental exertion. Vertigo with a tendency to fall backward during headache.

COMMENTS - The silicate of lime is a very deep-acting remedy. It acts profoundly upon the skin, mucus membranes, bones and glands. Marked emaciation, especially in children who have inherited tuberculosis.

Great weakness, especially in the morning on waking, after least exertion, from mental exertion, or walking in open air. Great nervous weakness. Weakness, night sweats and seminal emission. The least exertion prostrates and increases many symptoms. Stiffness in body, back and limbs when cold, after exertion and after sweating. Wet weather brings out all his sufferings.

Hemorrhage from throat, nose, larynx and chest. Swelling from dropsy and inflammation, swelling of affected parts, of glands with hardness. Mucus secretions increased and greenish-yellow.

RELATIONS - ***Compare:*** (1) Ars,, Tub., Bar-c Iod. (2) Fl-ac., Lap-a.

REFERENCES - Boericke. Clarke. Kent.

CALCAREA SULPHURICA

(Calcium Sulphate)

PHARMACY - calc-s. Calcarea sulphurica. Calcium sulphate. Plaster of Paris. Gypsum. Trituration. ***Historical dose:*** Trituration and all potencies.

CLINICAL - ***Abscesses.*** Anus, abscess. ***Boils.*** Buboes. Burns. Carbuncles. Chilblains. Concussion. Conjunctivitis. Cornea, ulceration. Cough. Crusta, lactea. Cysts. Deafness. Dropsy. Dysentery. Eczema. Fistula. Gland, swellings. Gonorrhea. Headaches. Hemorrhages. Injuries. Lupus, vulgaris. ***Pimples.*** Pneumonia. Polyps. ***Pustules.*** Scarlatina. ***Skin, disorders.*** Spermatorrhea. Syphilis. Tonsillitis. Tumors. Ulcers.

HOMEOPATHIC - Calc-s., which is an impure sulphide of calcium, has a wide sphere and deep action in suppurative processes. Calc-s. is closely related to Hep. It is Dr. Schüssler's connective tissue remedy, and most of the indications for its use are derived from his clinical experience.

Calc-s. affects glands, mucus membranes, bones and skin. ***Mucus discharges are yellow, thick and lumpy.*** Abscess formation. Recurrent or running ***abscesses.***

Tendency to suppuration. Suppurative processes come after pus finds a vent. Pus is thick, yellow, lumpy, bloody. Burns and scalds after suppuration starts in. Malignant growth after ulceration has set in. Torpid glandular swellings.

Tendency to form pus easily. Every cut or scratch will suppurate, create pus. Boils with a lot of pus, boils all over the body (Calc-pic.). Tendency to get boils. Severe acnes with yellow pus coming out and leaving pock marks.

Eczema and torpid glandular swellings. Cystic tumors. Fibroids. Ulcers, malignant, corneal, deep. Fistula. Cutting pains. Poor reaction. Infants with bloody coryza, diarrhea or eczema. Lupus vulgaris.

MIND - Confusion from mental exertion. Forgetful after eating. Loses memory and power of thought suddenly, after lunch. Sits and meditates over imaginary misfortune. ***Changeable moods.*** Liveliness and good spirits change to grief and melancholy, afternoon and evening. Sad in morning, but mirthful in evening. Inclination to weep during perspiration.

Hurried feeling. ***Anxiety in evening.*** Anxiety in bed, at night, better open air. ***Timidity.*** Fear of birds. Sometimes a desire to walk, to attend to something, as soon as she sets out to do it the desire is gone.

Easily angered, followed by weakness. Jealousy. Despises those who do not agree with him. ***Irritability in evening.*** Lamenting because he feels he is not appreciated. Grumbles that others do not understand him.

Abdomen - Colic with rumbling. Colic with diarrhea. Coldness and distension of abdomen after eating. Pain in right side of pelvis, followed by weakness, nausea and pain in stomach. Sensations in lower part of abdomen as if skin was too tight, with pain. Pains in liver region, in right side of pelvis, followed by weakness, nausea and pain in stomach. Buboes, to prevent suppuration.

Back - Curvature of lumbar spine, difficult to sit up. Pains across back of neck. Pains in lower part of back. Chronic pain in os coccygis was greatly aggravated.

Chest - Pain in sternum, becoming so much worse that she was obliged to double up. Pains across chest. Pains in chest with headache. Abscess in axilla.

Constitutions - Psoric and allergic constitutions.

Ears - Deafness with discharge of matter from the middle ear, sometimes mixed with blood. Chronic otorrhea. Otorrhea after scarlet fever, pus thick, bloody and offensive. Otorrhea with sore and enlarged parotids. Flow of dark wax from right ear. Otitis after a slap on ear. Pimple on top of right ear. Pimples around ear.

Eyes - Inflammation of eyes, evening and night. Conjunctivitis with discharge of thick, yellow matter. Conjunctiva yellow. Eyes red like raw beef. Red, itching tarsi. ***Inflammation of the eyes with discharge of thick, yellow matter.*** Sensation as if eyes were sunken, during menses, during headache. Cornea smoky. Deep ulcers on cornea. Ophthalmia neonatorum.

Severe inflammation in canthi. Smarting pain in inner canthi. Injury to eye from a splinter with pus formation. Twitching of eye muscles. Sees only one-half of an object. Diplopia. Occasional blindness, with twitching of eyelids.

Face - Exceedingly pale, sickly appearance. Flushes with heat. ***Pimples and pustules on the face***. Many tender pimples under beard discharge blood or oily transparent matter. Herpes. Boils. Darting pain in right side of face. Soreness of right parotid gland, better walking in open air. Swollen hard pimple on left cheek.

Female - Menses late, long-lasting, with headache, twitching, and great weakness. Vagintis. Thick, white leucorrhea. Itching high up in vagina. Mastitis, when pus begins to form or to prevent suppuration. Twitching during menses. Cutting pain in right ovary.

Food - Excessive appetite and thirst. No appetite for meat. Craves stimulants to overcome the weakness. Desires for both sour and salt. Desires sweets, acid fruit, green fruit. Desires tea, claret, green sour vegetables and fruit. Diarrhea after maple sugar.

Head - Chronic and periodic headache, worse looking up. Severe frontal headache, worse after dinner. Ache across forehead and in vertex. Headache from concussion. Tearing pain around whole head, with nausea. Pulsating headache from becoming cold, better cold air. Painful pimples on scalp leave a yellow scab. Hard tender swellings in scalp in edge of hair, bleeding when scratched. Boil over left eye. Scald head of children, with purulent, yellow discharge or crusts.

Heart - Pains from anterior of heart down extending to lower part of thigh.

Kidneys - Pyelitis. Chronic nephritis. Pain in kidneys. Severe pain, followed by pus in urine, which weakens one rapidly. Catarrh of bladder. Copious, yellow pus in urine. Red urine with hectic fever.

Limbs - Pains in joints. Chilblains, when suppurating. Swelling of phalanges of fingers. Burning in soles with hectic fever. ***Burning, itching of soles of feet***. Inflammation and swelling of little finger. Whitlow when suppuration begins. ***Weakness of legs.*** Weariness in knees after walking. Lameness in inner part of left knee when in bath. Pains in lower limbs worse stretching limb. Sciatica. Stitches in knee. Inflammation of hip-joint. Suppurative stage of hip disease. Painful stiffness of legs. Legs tender to touch. Feet slightly swollen and tender.

Liver - Pain in region of liver.

Lungs - Asthma with hectic fever. Difficult breathing, worse evening and night. Difficult breathing, worse ascending, cough and lying, better cool air. Short-breathed, constipated and cachectic. Pneumonia, late stage. ***Empyema, pus forming in lungs or pleural cavities.*** Rattling of mucus in lungs. Choking croup. Cough with purulent and bloody sputum and hectic fever. Chronic cough with tuberculosis. Purulent, bloody expectoration. Catarrh with thick, lumpy, white-yellow or pus-like secretions.

Male - Gonorrhea in suppurative stage. Chronic syphilis. Spermatorrhea with impotence.

Modalities - Better from open air. Better bathing. Better eating. Better local heat. Better uncovering. Worse from drafts. Worse cold, wet. Worse touch. Worse heat of the room. Worse standing. Worse walking fast.

Mouth - Inside of lips sore. ***Gumboils.*** Gums bleed while brushing teeth. Soreness, left side of roof as if burned, while eating. Sour, soapy, acrid taste. Taste bitter. Sour, soapy, acrid taste. Blister-like sores on right lower lip, ulcerate, ooze bloody matter. On outer lower lip a raw sore, forming a scab. Cracked lips. ***Swollen cheek with toothache, if suppuration threatens.*** Pains in right upper jaw, with swollen and tender gums about a decayed molar. Toothache, molar sensitive to cold air, water. Toothache with swollen cheek. Toothache after dark and in sleep. Toothache first worse cold water, soon better.

Nose - Influenza and sneezing, better open air. Cold in the head with thick, ***yellowish purulent secretion***, frequently tinged with blood. Bloodstreaked mucus from left nostril after a bath. One-sided discharge from nose. ***Yellowish discharge from posterior sinuses.*** Sneezing, better open air. Bloody coryza in infants. Excoriating watery coryza in open air, better in-doors and after washing with cold water. Coryza on right side after a bath, better outdoors. Edges of nostrils sore. Quivering on root of nose. During day right nostril discharges watery mucus, left dry, at night vice versa. Scanty phlegm, mostly from posterior nares, morning and evening. Posterior nares closed, watery coryza from anterior.

Perspiration - Foul, cold foot sweat. Easy sweating, worse coughing. Profuse sweats with hectic fever.

Rectum - Constipation with hectic fever. Constipation with difficult breathing. Diarrhea of children with discharge of pus or bloody pus. Diarrhea with pain in abdomen and from change of weather. Diarrhea after maple sugar and from change of weather. Purulent diarrhea mixed with blood. ***Painful abscesses about the anus.*** Anal fistula. Pus-like, slimy discharge from the bowels. Stools, coated white. Moisture about anus causes itching and smarting.

Skin - ***Unhealthy skin.*** Cuts, wounds, discharging pus, do not heal readily. ***Boils and abscesses.*** Skin affections with yellowish brownish or greenish scabs. ***Skin suppurates easily.*** Many little pimples under the hair, bleeding when scratched. Dry eczema in children. ***Acne with pus filled pimples.*** Eczema, eruption has yellowish scales, and there are many pimples and points of suppuration. Skin cracked in winter, especially the hands after washing. Scarlet rash. Scarlatina with excessive swelling of soft palate. ***Yellow, purulent crusts or discharge.*** Purulent exudation in or upon the skin. Yellowish scabs. Many little pimples under the hair, bleeding when scratched. Dry eczema, worse in infants.

Sleep - Starts from sleep, as if wanting air. Sleepy during day, wakeful at night. Before going to bed, pain in head. Internal lassitude after siesta. Dreamed she had a convulsion from fright, awoke screaming and much exhausted.

Stomach - Indigestion on least provocation. Pains in stomach and burnings. Nausea during vertigo. Nausea during headache. Nausea during pain in pelvis. Sensations of weakness in stomach.

Temperature - Chills beginning in feet. Hectic fever, caused by formation of pus. Averse to covers when cold. Dry heat at night. Easy sweating, worse coughing. Hectic fever with cough and burning in soles.

Throat - Last stage of ulcerated sore throat with discharge of yellow matter. Tonsillitis. Suppurating stage of tonsillitis, when abscess is discharging. Discharge of pus is anticipated. Pharynx red and sore, tonsils affected.

Tongue - Slightly puckered sensation at base of tongue. Tongue seamed with a deep red line. Glossitis, when suppuration begins. Tongue flabby, resembling a layer of dried clay. Yellow coating at base.

Vertigo - Vertigo better open air but worse walking fast. Vertigo while walking. Dizzy in head and weakness. Vertigo with deathly nausea.

COMMENTARY - Calc-s. is a synthetic remedy, useful for a Sulph. and Calc. states. Similar to Hep., which is calcium sulphide (this is calcium sulphate), it's useful for following Hep., or dealing with residue.

Better in open air, better walking in it, desire for it (Hep. cannot bear the slightest exposure). Worse from change of weather (Hep.). Calc-s. has not the excessive sensitiveness to touch found in Hep.

Nash cured a case of suppurating kidney with it. Hansen recommended it in dry eczema in children. Has cured cystic tumors, fibroids and polyps.

RELATIONS - ***Compare:*** (1) Calen., Hep., Kali-m. (2) Nat-s. - post-scarlatinal dropsy. (3) Sil. - hard or suppurating glands, ulcers of cornea tonsillitis, mastitis, frostbite. ***Follows well:*** Kali-m., Nat-s., Sil..

REFERENCES - Boericke. Clarke. Murphy.

CALCULUS RENALIS

(Kidney Stones)

PHARMACY - calcul-r. Calculus renalis. Kidney stones. Calculi urinae. Lapidus renalis. Calcarea renalis. Renal calculi. (Urate of lime, or phosphate of lime, kidney stones) Trituration. ***Historical dose:*** Trituration and all potencies.

CLINICAL - Arthritis. Arthritis, nodosities. Bladder, stones. Gout. Gravel. Joints, nodosities. ***Kidney, pain. Kidney stones.*** Rheumatism. Rigg's disease. Teeth, tartar. Uric acid, stones. Urinary gravel. Vomiting.

HOMEOPATHIC - Bredenoll considered the kidney stones, tartar on the teeth and arthritic nodosities very similar morbid products. Calcul-r. is reported to be peculiarly beneficial in Rigg's disease of the teeth. Arthritic nodosities. It is called for in gouty conditions : in . renal calculi and nodosities of fingers.

Lessens the tendency to the accumulation of tartar on teeth, gravel and kidney stones. Useful where teeth acquire abundant tartar with inflamed gums. ***Horrible anguish and pain from kidney stones.*** Frequent desire to urinate. Urinary gravel. Urine is turbid and bloody. Vomiting of mucus, bile ingesta.

Joints - Arthritis nodosities. Stiffness. Rheumatism.

Kidneys - Severe pain in region of kidneys. ***Kidney colic.*** Violent lancinating, sore or pinching pains. ***Kidney stones.*** Uric acid stones.

Teeth - Tartar on teeth. Rigg's disease.

COMMENTS - The Hom. Recorder of Aug., 1895, reprinted a paper by Dr. Bredenoll of Erwitte in which he gave his experience with this remedy in his own case of intense kidney colic with the passage of uric acid stones.

One of these stones was triturated in the proportion of 5 parts to 95 of milk sugar. Of this, he took 1/2 grain doses for a considerable time, resulting in the formation of stones ceasing. The tartar which had formed on his teeth dropped off, and a nodosity of stony hardness disappeared from the extensor tendon of the right middle finger.

Dr. Bredenoll writes: "In November, 1837, I was suddenly attacked with vomiting, accompanied with violent lancinating, sore or pinching pains in the region of the left kidney. The horrible anguish and pain which I experienced extorted from me involuntary screams, I was writhing like a worm in the dust.

"A calculus had descended into the ureter and had become incarcerated in it. Repeated doses of Nux-v relieved the incarceration and I distinctly felt that the calculus was descending towards the bladder. After twenty-four hours of horrible suffering the vomiting ceased. The pain became duller and was felt in the region where the ureter dips into and becomes interwoven with the tissue of the bladder.

"It continued for three days and then disappeared all of a sudden (the stone had not got into the bladder). Thirty-six hours afterwards the calculus entered the bulb of the urethra. I felt a frequent desire to urinate, the urine was turbid and bloody, until at last a calculus of four grains made its appearance in the urine.

"After this I frequently passed gravel and stones, at times with slight, at times violent pains, sometimes accompanied with vomiting, I kept the larger stones with a view of using them hereafter as a curative agent.

"Professor Nasser of Bonn, where my son studied medicine at the time, has analyzed the stones and has found them to be urate of lime. He advised me to take Merc-d. and the Sulphate of soda for some time, it is scarcely necessary for me to say that I did not follow his advice.

"On the 15th of February, 1839, I felt the precursory symptoms of a new attack which really did break out in all its fury on the 16th and continued on the 17th and 18th I now took 5 grains of my kidney stones to be triturated in my presence with 95 grains of sugar of milk, according to the fashion of Hahnemann and took 1/2 grain in th evening of the 17th, another 1/2 grain i the morning of the 18th.

"On this day I passed very turbid urine wit a considerable quantity of gravel, howeve in the region where the ureter dips into th bladder, I experienced an uncomfortab sensation, but was well otherwise.

"On the 19th I was obliged to visit a patient at the distance of two miles, on my journey I felt that the calculus was descending into the bladder, the urine which I emitted shortly afterwards was very turbid and bloody.

"That same evening after returning home, I left the stone in the bulb of the urethra and on the morning of the 20th it came off during stool, but unfortunately got lost among the excrement.

"To judge from my feeling it must have been larger than any of the preceding stones and also rougher, for its passage through the urethra was very painful and followed by an oozing out of blood.

"The uncomfortable feeling in the region of the left kidney never disappeared completely, it became especially painful when pressing upon that place, when riding on horseback or in a carriage, when taking exercise or turning the body.

"It seems to me that the whole pelvis of the kidneys must have been full of gravel and stones. I now took 1/2 grain at intervals of eight days, the result was that I passed gravel and small stones at every urination.

"On the 30th of November my condition got worse and I continued to take 1/2 grain of Calcul-r., at longer or shorter intervals, until October 18th, 1840. After this period I ceased to pass any gravel and I felt entirely well. On the kidneys must have been full of gravel and stones. I now took 1/2 grain of Calcul-r., another dose on June 3rd.

"On June 17th precursors of another attack, on the 18th vomiting accompanied by all the frightful circumstances which I have detailed above, the vomiting of mucus, bile ingesta, continued at short intervals until the 26th, my tongue was coated with yellow mucus and my appetite had completely disappeared.

"Bry., Nux-v. and Puls. relieved the gastric symptom, on the 26th in the afternoon, I passed a calculus of the size of a pea. I now resumed the use of Calcul-r. in 1/2 grain doses, at irregular intervals.

"On the 23rd of October I passed a stone of the size of a pea without vomiting, there were no other precursory symptoms except the uncomfortable feeling in the region of the kidneys a few days previous. I have felt well ever since and free from all complaint, although I continue the occasional use of 1/2 grain of Calcul-r., lest I should have a relapse.

"Every time I took a dose of Calcul-r. I found that the so-called tartar on the teeth became detached a few days afterwards. A short while ago a nodosity, hard as a stone, which had appeared on the extensor tendon of the right middle finger, about nine months ago and which threatened to increase more and more, disappeared."

RELATIONS - ***Compare:*** Berb., Ox-ac.

REFERENCES - Anshutz.

CALEA ZACATECHCHICHI

(Dream Herb)

PHARMACY - calea. Calea zacatechchichi. Dream herb. Bitter grass. Leaf of God. N. O. Compositae. ***Historical dose:*** Tincture and all potencies.

CLINICAL - Dreams. Dysentery. Fever. Gastrointestinal, disorders. Nausea. Nightmares. Vertigo. Vomiting.

HERBAL - Calea zacatechichi is a medium sized shrub that has reportedly been used by the Chantal indians of Mexico as a hallucinogen. Its dried leaves are used before sleep to increase dreaming. Its effects are not well documented.

HOMEOPATHIC - Calea actions during wakefulness were tested in five subjects after several inhalations and the administration of an infusion.

With high doses, effects included: sensations of well-being and light-headedness, difficulty in bringing events to mind, somnolence, and an intensification of visual imagery, but only with the eyes closed.

Symptoms include lack of physical stamina. Nausea and vomiting. Severe leg cramping. Swelling of the limbs with rash on the feet, between toes. Swelling in the hands, with redness on the fingers. Severe bitter taste in mouth. Drowsiness, mild vertigo.

Euphoria. Mental clarity. It alters the perception of time so that it appears that time is passing more slowly. Makes one feel more 'in control' of things. Vivid dreams. More lucid in dreams. Dreams seem more realistic.

RELATIONS - Compare: Salv-d. Anh.

REFERENCES - Buttimer. Murphy.

CALENDULA OFFICINALIS

(Pot Marigold)

PHARMACY - calen. Calendula officinalis. Pot Marigold. N. O. Composite. Tincture of leaves and flowers. Calendula Succus is made from the fresh plant juice. ***Historical dose:*** Tincture and all potencies. Locally, use tincture for all wounds, one of the greatest healing agents. Also as an injection in leucorrhea internally.

CLINICAL - ***Abrasions.*** Abscess. Balanitis. Breast, infection. Bubo. ***Burns.*** Carbuncles. Chilblains. Cornea, injuries. ***Cuts.*** Deafness. Erysipelas. Eyes, injuries. Fever. Fistula. Glandular, swellings. Gunshot, wounds. ***Injuries.*** Jaundice. ***Knife, wounds. Lacerated, tissue.*** Muscle, tears. Nails, inflamed. Nipples, sore. Perineum, tears. ***Puncture, wounds.*** Septic, wounds. Sunburn. Suppuration. ***Surgery, effects.*** Tetanus. ***Ulcers.*** Uterus, inflammation. Uterus, cancer, discharge. Varicose, ulcers. Whitlow. ***Wounds.***

HERBAL - Calen. belongs to the same family as those other great vulneraries: Arn. and Bell-p. The ***great herbal anti-septic***, it restores the vitality of an wounded part, making it impregnable against the forces of putrefaction. Indicated in lacerated and suppurative wounds.

Unlike Arnica, it has no irritating property capable of producing erysipelas, it is therefore suitable to all cases of injury where the skin is broken. Calendula is all the dressing needed for any open wound or severe laceration. It takes away the local pain and suffering.

Hot lotions are generally preferable to cold, as they conserve the vitality of the injured parts. Hot compresses in pneumonia. Hot fomentations, when intermittently applied, are far better than poultices as applications to forming abscesses. If they do not abort the process, they favor the maturation and ultimate healing.

Kent noted that Calen. tincture cannot be ignored in injuries, in cuts with laceration, surface or open injuries. Diluted Calendula used locally will keep the wound odorless, will reduce the amount of pus and favor granulation in the very best possible manner. Thus it assists the surgeon in healing up surface wounds.

A correspondent of the Hom. World, 1891, "C. W.," mentions that a friend of his who chewed for a few minutes a Calen. leaf noticed that it entirely removed for some days the difficulty of passing water such as is commonly met with in old men.

The application of a sponge saturated with a hot solution of calendula after delivery gives the greatest comfort to the patient.

HOMEOPATHIC - Calen. has not been largely proved, but very definite fever symptoms have been elicited. Fever and chills. Goose bumps. Cases of jaundice have been treated with it successfully.

Calen. acts on muscles, spine, liver and skin. ***A most remarkable healing agent, applied locally or given internally in potency.*** Exhaustion from loss of blood and excessive pain.

Calen. is used for open, torn, cut, lacerated, ragged or suppurating wounds. Wounds raw and inflamed. Wounds painful as if beaten. Pain is excessive and out of all proportion to injury. The parts around the wound become red, with stinging in the wound during the febrile heat. Flesh wounds.

Rapid healing of wounds. ***Wounds, cuts, abrasions, lacerations, broken skin surface.*** Promotes healthy granulations and rapid healing by first intention. Prevents scar tissue formation. Arrests bleeding from wounds, especially to scalp, mouth.

Both prevents and heals infection, pus formation. ***Antiseptic for sores, abscesses, infection at the site of a wounds.*** Pain appears or is worse after bandage is put on. Muscle injuries.

Give Calen. before and after surgery. Exhaustion from blood loss or pain. ***Pains after cuts or surgery***. Ruptures of muscles.

tendon. Fractures or compound fracture. Head injury or concussion. ***Stab wounds.*** Penetrating wounds into joints. Soft tissue injuries.

Useful for open wounds, parts that will not heal, ulcers, etc. It is useful in preventing excessive suppuration and putridity, both keep septic germs from sores and wounds (Sul-ac). Prevents pyemia. Prevents gangrene.

Calen. has the power to produce local exudation and helps to make the acrid discharge healthy and free. ***Burns, scalds, sunburns.*** Caesarean operation. Constitutional tendency to erysipelas.

General pallor and insensibility. Nearly all symptoms appear with a chill. Deafness. Catarrhal conditions. Hemostatic after tooth extraction. Neuroma. ***Great disposition to take cold, especially in damp weather***. Sensitive to damp or open air. Cold hands. Paralysis after a stroke. Cancer, intercurrent remedy.

Valuable in healing or reproducing bone. Sensation as if he would faint, with movements in stomach and abdomen. Feels best when walking about, or when lying perfectly still. Moving causes pain, even after the wound is dressed, rheumatism worse motion.

MIND - Great irritability. Easily frightened. Fretful, sleepy, dreamy. Extremely nervous. Starts with fright. Dread of something bad happening. Bulimia. Anxious, morose and solicitous during the chill.

Abdomen - ***Epigastric distention***. Stretching and dragging in groin. Sticking in the left side of the abdomen. Movements in abdomen causes faint feeling. Griping and anxiety in abdomen during stool. Constant soreness of abdomen and tenderness in left iliac region. Enteritis from foreign body. Dull, coarse stitches in middle of right side of abdomen, on moving. Boring, digging, deep in region of navel, when walking.

Back - Bruised pain at angle of right scapula. Tearing with pressure between the scapulae. ***Pains after back surgery.*** Pain under the right scapula. Rheumatic drawing in the right side of neck. Pressive drawing pain, between scapula.

Causations - Burns. Cuts, punctures, stabs. Wounds. Surgery.

Chest - Pressure on last rib, left side. Drawing pressure in left side of chest, also in sternum. Stitches in right side of chest. Nausea felt in chest. Ribs ache as if pressed together. Pressure and oppression in left side of chest, in evening, when lying in bed. Stitches in right side of chest. Axillary glands sore to touch. Axillae very hot.

Constitutions - Constitutional tendency to erysipelas.

Ears - ***Ruptured eardrum.*** Deafness, worse in ***damp*** surroundings, with eczematous conditions. Hears best on a train and distant sounds. Hearing acute.

Eyes - Eyewash for irritations, abrasions, infections, conjunctivitis. Eye inflammation after trauma. ***Scratched cornea.*** Injuries to the eyes which tend to suppuration. ***Eye pains after surgery***. Blenorrhea of lachrymal sac, yellow vision. ***Lacerated and incised wounds of eyes.*** Eyes black and blue from extravasated blood. ***Foreign objects*** in the eye. Traumatic conjunctivitis, keratitis and iritis. White of eye inflamed, with pressive headache, in forehead, temples. Pupils dilated. Dryness and biting in margin of lid, as from smoke. Lid very much swollen. Wounds of eyelids and brows badly treated with plasters and where suppuration takes place.

Face - Face puffy, much swollen under eyes. Eruption of small vesicles in left corner of lips and on right side of mouth. Lips as if swollen. Burning and stinging. Submaxillary glands swollen and about to suppurate, painful on touch. Drawing, tensive pains, in gland behind left ramus of lower jaw, on moving head.

Female - Menses suppressed with cough. Menorrhagia. Chronic cervicitis. ***Warts on cervix***. Os lower than natural. Profuse offensive watery discharge after forceps delivery. ***Vaginal tears after childbirth***. Hypertrophy of uterus. ***Lacerated vagina from childbirth, sex, surgery, wounds.*** Sensation of weight and fullness in pelvis. Stretching and dragging pain in pelvis. Pain on sudden movements. Uterine pain after taking cold. Cancer of womb with bleeding. Ruptures of cervix and perineum during childbirth. Excoriated and cracked nipples.

Food - Hunger immediately after nursing. Hiccough when smoking. Bulimia. Diminished appetite for dinner, though he relishes food when he eats. Drinks much at night with fever. Aversion to drinks. Crawls on back from cold drinks.

Head - Pains after mechanical injuries. Concussion of brain. ***Lacerated scalp wounds***. Hemorrhages in scalp wounds. Compound fractures of skull. Dull, pressive sensation in occiput. Dull headache, as after a debauch. Fungus of cranium. Tearing pains. Sensation of a weight on brain. Submaxillary glands swollen, painful to touch. Pain in right side of neck. Pain and heat in forehead after eating.

Limbs - Drawing, pressive pains in wrists and ankles during rest. Wounds about joints. Pains after surgical operations, to prevent caries or necrosis. ***Torn tendons and muscles.*** Cold hands and feet. The axillary glands are painful to the touch. ***Varicose swellings and ulcers.*** Foot crushed, erysipelas and gangrene. Pressure and drawing tension in the hand. Tearing, burning in the calf. Spasmodic drawing of the foot, when sitting.

Lungs - Cough with green expectoration, hoarseness, with distention of inguinal ring. Great efforts made to inflate lower lobes of lungs, which were only successful when sitting up. Breathing easier after fever abates.

Kidneys - Frequent urination, with emission of pale, clear, hot, and even burning urine. Tearing in the urethra during the chilliness. Has to urinate often at night. Urine suppressed. Urine colorless as water. Urine is very hot and burning. Urine suppressed, passes less than half her usual quantity of urine.

Male - Excoriation of prepuce after sex.

Modalities - Better from walking about. Better lying perfectly still. Better warmth. Worse in damp. ***Worse heavy, cloudy weather.*** Worse during chill. Worse evening.

Mouth - Bitter phlegm in mouth. Bleeding gums. ***Bleeding after tooth extraction.*** Pains after gum surgery.

Nose - Coryza in one nostril, with much green discharge.

Rectum - Stools curdy. Frequent almost entirely mucus stools. Stool in morning, preceded by griping and anxiety in abdomen, with chi!!. Diarrhea with vomiting of food, with heartburn. Constipation. Perineal abscess. To close the wound after operation. Ruptures of perineum.

Skin - Topical treatment of fissures, varicose ulcers, bedsores, gangrene. Stinging and cutting pains. Skin feels warm to touch. Jaundice. ***Yellow skin***. Goose bumps. Slough, proud flesh and raised edges. ***Burns and scalds.*** Erysipelas (use topically). ***Promotes favorable scar tissue with least amount of suppuration.*** Ulcers, irritable and inflamed. Sloughing of tissues from wounds, ulcers. Varicose ulcers, painful, as if beaten. ***Excessive secretion of pus from ulcers or wounds.*** Wounds, ulcers with surrounding parts red.

Sleep - Restless at night, can rest in no position. Wakes continually. Must urinate frequently and drinks very much. Feels as if he would fall from a height, when falling asleep.

Stomach - Hunger immediately after nursing. ***Heartburn.*** Nausea in chest. Vomiting. Sinking sensation. Hiccough, when smoking. Sinking feeling. Movements in stomach causes faint feeling. Vomiting with pain in uterine region, after taking cold. Induration in stomach and uterus.

Temperature - Shivering and shaking chill from drinking. Violent chill after trauma. Feels shivery and has a kind of gooseflesh, while skin seems warm to touch. ***Coldness, a great sensitiveness to open air***. Shuddering in back. Heat in evening. After dinner, heat in face, hands and feet.

Throat - Scalds, burns of throat. ***Injuries to air passages, in form of cuts or lacerations.*** Foreign bodies in air passages. Bitter phlegm in throat. Painful swelling of submaxillary gland, worse on moving head. Pressure in throat when swallowing. Wounds of esophagus, to prevent esophagitis. Foreign bodies in esophagus having produced laceration. Voice stronger and deeper as soon as fever heat abates, in evening.

COMMENTS - Calendula, largely diluted with water, is highly esteemed by many physicians as a dressing for lacerated wounds, ulcers, and burns. Burns are dressed by applying muslin cloth saturated with dilute calendula night and morning. The cloth should be kept constantly saturated with the agent. It is also used an injection in vaginal and uterine leucorrhoea.

Useful for surgeries, given before and after. Hemorrhage, cuts that keep bleeding and won't heal. Sharp stinging, cutting feelings, redness and rawness. Very good for preventing septic wounds (Pyrog., once septic situations have set in). Torn or wounded muscles. Bedsores.

Hansen noted it for open wounds, very sore and painful, difficult granulation, tendency to inflammation and suppuration. Useful for burns when applied topically (Canth., Urt-u.). Good as local application in phlegmonous erysipelas.

For severe nerve pain (Coff., Phos. is numb and tingling). Nerve injury (when Hyper. fails). Excessive pain out of proportion to the injury (Coff.). Pain under right scapula, or bruised feeling under the right scapula.

Can be used as an eyewash for bloodshot eyes from dust or irritation (Euphr.). Injuries to the eyes from foreign objects and irritants. Tendency to catch colds. Carious root toothache. An excellent hemostatic in tooth extractions and for gum surgery.

Very acute hearing. Hypersensitive hearing (Coff.). Deafness from inflammation. Boericke noted it as being specific for ruptured or torn eardrums (Thiosin. is for eardrum adhesions and ossification of the bones, Kali-m., if deafness is caused by blocked Eustachian tubes).

Ulcers, heartburn, bleeding ulcers. Bleeding hemorrhoids, internally is best. Diuretic (urine feels hot like Bell.).

Nodosities in breast. Helpful for episiotomies, the stinging, cutting pains. Hemorrhage after childbirth. Bad ulcers of os uteri. Offensive leucorrhea. Ludlam recommended it in chronic endocervicitis and scrofulous ulcerations with much purulent leucorrhea. Useful topically after childbirth.

Jahr, who was in Paris during the Coup d'Etat of 1849, treated a number of cases of gunshot wounds with comminuted bones and saved several limbs by means of Calen. It prevented suppuration and pyemia. In some cases of carbuncle it acts with great promptitude, subduing pain and fever. In obstetric practice it is invaluable.

Calen. as been used in Germany in tincture on cancer areas. It helped to stop the spread of cancer and helped to reabsorb it.

Almost all the symptoms appear during the chilly stage of the fever, he feels most comfortable when walking about or else when lying perfectly still.

Cooper said that calen. is worse in cloudy weather. Drinking causes a shaking chill or creeping crawls, even during heat. Very sensitive to cold air. Restless, can't get comfortable in bed. Fear of some overwhelming calamity.

C. R. Crosby gave it internally in the 3x potency, as well as externally. He had excellent results from its use as a hot compress (an ounce to the pint) in pneumonia and other inflammations.

C. W., himself a pharmacist, noticed the following effect on himself when making the fresh-plant tincture: "There was such a feeling as if some overwhelming calamity was hovering over me as to be almost unbearable.

"Three years ago, just after making the tincture, my old enemy the gout nipped me in the middle of the spine and in three days spoiled all my powers of walking and then the dreadful feeling became very much exaggerated." His experience led him to conclude that Calen. has an action on the spinal cord.

RELATIONS - ***Antidote:*** Chel., Rheum. ***Antidoted by:*** Arn. ***Compare:*** (1) Staph., Arn., Ars., Bry., Calc-s., Carb-an., Carb-v., Ham., Hep., Hyper., Led., Nit-ac., Phos., Rhus-t., Ruta, Sal-ac., Sul-ac., Symph. (2) in deafness: Ferr-pic., Kali-i., Calc., Mag-ac, Graph. ***Compatible:*** Arn., Ars., Bry., Nit-ac., Phos., Rhus-t. ***Complementary:*** Hep. Calendula contains much nitrogen and phosphoric acid. ***Followed well by:*** Arn., Hep. ***Incompatible:*** Camph. ***Follows well:*** Ars. i.

REFERENCES - Boericke. Clarke. Kent. Murphy.

CALOTROPIS GIGANTEA

(Madar Bark)

PHARMACY - calo. Calotropis gigantea. Madar bark. N. O. Asclepiadacae. East India. The root-bark is called Mudar, Mirdar, Yercum. Tincture or trituration of bark of root. Tincture of the milky juice or gum. ***Historical dose:*** Tincture and all potencies.

CLINICAL - ***Anemia***. Dysentery. Feet, pains. Fevers. Hand, pains. Leprosy, tubercular. Lupus. ***Obesity. Syphilis.*** Tuberculosis.

HERBAL - The expressed juice, root and bark have been extensively used in the East for their emetic, sudorific, alterative and purgative qualities. The fresh juice is considered a valuable remedy in skin disorders.

HOMEOPATHIC - Calotropis has been used with marked success in the treatment of ***syphilis*** (following Mercury), elephantiasis, leprosy and acute dysentery. Pneumonic tuberculosis. Tuberculosis. Increases the circulation of the skin. Has a powerful effect as a sudorific.

In the secondary symptoms of syphilis, where Mercury has been used but cannot be pushed safely any farther, it rapidly recruits the constitution, heals the ulcers and blotches from the skin and perfects the cure. ***Primary anemia of syphilis. Heat in stomach*** is a guiding symptom. ***Obesity***, while flesh decreases, muscles become harder and firmer.

A short proving brought out a weak, tired feeling, coldness, dizziness, pain and confusion in head, nausea and vomiting of bile.

Frequent urination, pain, soreness and redness of thigh, pain in both legs, swelling of knees, and stiffness and inability to walk. Pains in hands and feet, first left then right, worse movement or putting weight on them.

COMMENTS - Dr. Gramm of Philadelphia used the tincture with great success in cases of syphilis when Mercury can no longer be given, in the anemia of syphilis, secondary syphilis. A sense of warmth in the scrobiculus cordis is a leading indication for the remedy.

In one case of severe and advanced syphilis with enormous thickening of the ends of all the nails, Calo. effected a cure. The remedy was given in one- to five-drop doses of the tincture or in pellets saturated with equal parts of the tincture and 95 percent alcohol.

RELATIONS - Coffee caused vomiting when before there was only nausea, but antidoted many effects. Camph. also antidoted. ***Compare:*** (1) Merc., Kali-i., Berb-a., Sars. (2) Asc-c., Asc-t. (3) Ip. - emetic. (4) Berb-a. - syphilis.

REFERENCES - Boericke. Clarke.

CALTHA PALUSTRIS

(Cowslip)

PHARMACY - calth. Caltha palustris. Cowslip. Marsh marigold. N. O. Ranunculacee. Tincture of fresh shoots and flowers. ***Historical dose:*** Tincture and all potencies.

CLINICAL - Cancer. Itching. Pemphigus. Uterine cancer.

HOMEOPATHIC - This is an unproved remedy, but it has irritant properties like the other Ranunculacee. Hansen gave as indications: "Pemphigus, bullae are surrounded by a ring, much itching. On the third day they are transformed into crusts."

Cooper used it with excellent effect in a case of uterine cancer, giving single doses of the tincture at long intervals.

REFERENCES - Boericke. Clarke. Hansen.

CAMPHORA

(Camphor)

PHARMACY - camph. Camphora. Camphor. Laurus camphora. N. O. Lauracae. A gum obtained from Laurus camphora. Solution in rectified spirit. ***Historical dose:*** Tincture and all potencies, tincture in drop doses, repeated frequently or smelling of Spirits of Camphor.

CLINICAL - Angina, pectoris. Anxiety. Asphyxia, neonatorum. Bedsores. ***Chills. Cholera. Colds.*** Colic. ***Collapse.*** Congestion. Convulsions. Coughs. Cramps. Delirium. ***Diarrhea.*** Epilepsy. Eruptions. Erysipelas. ***Fevers.*** Gonorrhea. Heart, disorders. Hematuria. High, fever. ***Influenza.*** Measles. Memory, loss. Nausea. Priapism. Rheumatism. Sexual, mania. Shiverings. Sleeplessness. Snakebites. Spasms. Strangury. Taste, disordered. Tetanus. Tobacco, habit. Twitching. Urethra, stricture. Urine, suppression. Vomiting.

HOMEOPATHIC - Marked coldness, cramps and convulsions with mental anguish. Affects the digestive tract and cerebro-spinal nerves, urinary organs and nose. For colds and chills. Scrofulous, weakly, irritable children are especially affected.

Shock. ***State of collapse***. Sudden collapse from over-powering influences acting on nervous centers. Sunstroke with ebbing vitality, fainting spells, cold sweat and icy cold body.

First stages of a cold with chilliness and sneezing. Very sensitive to cold and to touch. Great sensitiveness to cold and cold air, which worse pains, takes cold easily. ***Icy coldness*** of the whole body, sudden sinking of strength, pulse small and weak. Low blood pressure after operations, if temperature is subnormal.

Patient will not be covered, notwithstanding the icy coldness of the body, or wants them off and then on alternately with internal burning heat and anxiousness. Limbs cold with cramps.

Camph. has a direct relationship to muscles and fascia. Local rheumatic disorders in cold climates. Awkwardness. Trembling and extreme restlessness. ***Pain better while thinking of it.*** Cracking of joints. Distention of veins.

Convulsions with blue lips, froth at mouth and lock-jaw. Epileptiform convulsions. After effects of measles. ***Violent convulsions*** with wandering and hysterical excitement. Tetanic spasms.

Camph. achieved classical fame in ***cholera epidemics***. In some epidemics, Camph. given early has cured a majority of the cases treated, whether it was given as drop doses of the tincture or in the 30c.

In the collapse of cholera it corresponds rather to the initial chill before either vomiting or diarrhea. The tongue is cold. If he can speak, the voice is either high pitched or husky. Coldness (Verat.), with marked nausea and vomiting, upper lip drawn up.

Acts on the genito-urinary sphere (similar to and antidotes Canth.). Strangury and priapism.

MIND - Afraid of his own thoughts, wants to be diverted from thoughts of himself. Fears to be left alone. Does not like any one near him. Memory lost. Most pains are felt during a half-conscious condition and disappear when thinking of them. Worse from inattention.

Insensibility, vanishing of all senses or anxiety. Awkwardness. Nothing satisfies. Delirium. Mania, religious, puerperal. Wants to jump out of bed or window. Excited, talks constantly, scolds in indecent language.

Feeling that she is going to die, relieved, when she finds herself alive. Attacks of anguish at night. State of frenzy, hysterical, scratches, spits, bites, tears her clothes. Screams and calls for help. Closes her eyes and answers no questions.

Abdomen - Cramps in the abdomen. Cutting colic at night. Bellyache as if diarrhea would follow. Drawing pain, as from a bruise. Sensation of fullness in the abdomen. Cold or of burning heat in the epigastrium and in the abdomen.

Back - Tension and stiffness of the neck. Drawing stitches between shoulder blades. Pressure in small of back. Sensation as if cool air was blowing on back.

Causations - Ill effects of shock from injury, operations, sunstroke, snakebites. Vexation.

Chest - A cold feeling in chest followed by cold breath. Dry feeling at bifurcation of trachea. Cramps in the chest. Shootings in the chest.

Ears - Heat and redness of the ears, especially in the lobes. Abscess in the meatus with deep redness and pressive shooting pain.

Eyes - Fixed, staring, turned upwards or outwards, pupils dilated. Sensation as if all objects were too bright and glittering. Objects appear too bright or move to one side with a jerk. Eyes protrude with mania. Eyes deeply sunken.

Face - Pale, haggard, ***anxious***, distorted, ***bluish***, cold. Cold sweat. Pale and red by turns. Distorted. Grimaces. Upper lip retracted. Lockjaw. Froth or foam at the mouth.

Female - Menses too profuse, or absent. Sexual desire increased. Hot flushes with coldness of abdomen and limbs, at menopause. Labor-like pains. Weakness of sexual system.

Food - Bitter taste of food, especially of meat. Dislike and repugnance to tobacco smoke. Excessive thirst.

Head - Influenza, headache with catarrhal symptoms, sneezing, etc. Cold sweat. Head sore. Feels knotted up. Beating pain in cerebellum. ***Occipital throbbing, synchronous with the pulse,*** better standing, when deprived of sexual intercourse. ***Fleeting stitches in temporal region and orbits***. Head is drawn to one side (in spasms). Pains run from head to fingertips.

Heart - Anxiety at heart. Spasmodic stitches in region of heart. Precordial distress. Palpitations, after eating. Pulse, weak, not perceptible, frequent, small.

Kidneys - Burning and ***strangury*** with tenesmus of the neck of the bladder. Retention with full bladder. Hematuria.

Limbs - Rheumatic pain between the shoulders. Difficult motion. Numbness, tingling and ***coldness***. Cramps in calves. Cracking in joints. Feet cold, pains as if sprained. Icy cold feet, ache as if sprained. Fingers stiff, open, distorted. Thumbs drawn backwards.

Lungs - Asphyxia neonatorum. Asthma, worse from bodily exertion. ***Breath cold***. Breathing anxious, oppressed, sighing, quiet, deep and slow, snoring. Cutting, cold feeling deep in windpipe, causes a slight cough. Hoarse, squeaking voice. Suspended respiration. Violent attacks of dry cough. Suffocative dyspnea.

Male - Sexual excitement. Chordee. ***Priapism***, during dreams Nightly emissions. Satyriasis. Impotence.

Modalities - Better from free discharges, sweat. Better warmth. Better thinking of it. Better drinking cold water. Worse motion. Worse contact. Worse mental exertion, shock. Worse night. Worse when half asleep. Worse from cold air, drafts. ***Worse suppressions***.

Mouth - Breath fetid in the morning. Cold breath. Foam at the mouth. Abundant accumulation of a viscid and slimy saliva. Tongue cold, flabby, trembling, bluish. Speech, broken, feeble, hoarse. Boiling hot tea seems cold.

Nose - ***Cold and pinched***. Inhaled air seems cold. ***Persistent nosebleed with*** goose bumps. Stopped up, sneezing. Fluent coryza on sudden change of weather. Coryza in old age.

Rectum - Black stools, involuntary. Rice water stools. ***Asiatic cholera*** with cramps in calves, coldness of body, anguish, great weakness, ***collapse,*** tongue and mouth cold.

Skin - Dryness of the skin. Skin, bluish and cold, with coldness of the body. ***Old looking***, pale, blue, livid. Cannot bear to be covered (Sec.). Erysipelas. Sequelae of measles. Skin sensitive, even to the slightest touch.

Sleep - Comatose sleep. ***Insomnia*** with cold limbs. Trembling and extreme restlessness.

Stomach - Pressive pain in pit of stomach. ***Coldness***, followed by burning. Burning in stomach, in abdomen. Little vomiting or purging with dry collapse. Vomiting of bile or blood. Sour, bilious vomiting in the morning. Strong pressure in the epigastrium.

Teeth - Toothache, as if from swelling of the sub-maxillary glands. Toothache better beer. Sensation of lengthening of the teeth. Acute shocks in the roots of the incisors. Painful looseness of the teeth.

Temperature - Pulse small, weak, slow. Cold perspiration. ***Icy coldness of the whole body***. Shaking chill with cold skin, wants covers during the hot stage only. ***Congestive chill. Tongue cold***, flabby, trembling. Sudden inflammatory fevers with rapid alternation of heat and cold, followed by rapid prostration. Heat or sweat, better covers. Sweats when covered, body becomes cold when uncovered. Chilly, below scapula, before colds.

Throat - Soreness in the throat on swallowing. Dry, scraping sensation of the palate. Burning heat in the throat. Constriction of larynx, feeling as if throat tied.

Vertigo - Vertigo, with a tendency to unconsciousness, feeling as if he would die.

COMMENTS - Camphor has a special place in homeopathy because it's the major antidote of the remedies along with coffee. Camph. corrects spoiled cases and antidotes most of the medicines, especially from the vegetable kingdom.

Useful as a heart stimulant for emergency use. Give drop doses on sugar as often as every five minutes.

Hahnemann gave it as a remedy for cholera along with Cupr. and Verat. (Cupr. has spasms and cramps, Verat. has voracious thirst), and used it prophylactically. Useful for dehydration. Rice-water stools. Collapse and coldness (Carb-v.).

Internal heat and external coldness. Great coldness of surface with sudden and complete prostration of the vital forces. Feeling as if a cold wind were blowing over body. For all kinds of sudden internal pains arising from chill or other causes.

Tetanic spasms, with drawing up the corners of the mouth, showing the teeth (like Nux-v. and Phyt.), and coldness. Spasmodic movement of head, head drawn to right side, rest of body relaxed, unconscious.

Spasmodic drawing of head laterally or backwards with deathly coldness.

Erysipelas spreading to central membranes. Eruptions. Soft parts drawn in. Skin painfully sensitive.

Salzer said the cases calling for it are those in which "arterial spasm," with difficult breathing (spasm of pulmonary arteries), coldness and lividity are the leading features.

In the form of the ordinary Camph. pilules, Clarke found it an excellent remedy for sleeplessness. In this, as in its effect on colds, it resembles Acon.

RELATIONS - ***Antidotes:*** Opium, Nit-s-d., Phos. Camph. has very important antidotal relations. Camphor antidotes or modifies the action of nearly every vegetable medicine-tobacco, opium, worm medicines, etc. It is ***Antidoted by:*** Op., Nit-s-d., Dulc. and Phos. It antidotes: Am-c., Canth., Carb-v., Cupr., Lyc., Squil., Nat-m., so-called worm-medicines tobacco, bitter almonds and other fruits containing prussic acid. Also the secondary disorders remaining after poisoning with acids, salts, metals, poisonous mushrooms, etc. ***Compare:*** (1) Cupr., Ars., Verat., Aloe. (2) Carb-v. - coldness from undeveloped exanthema, collapse, nosebleed, dark, persistent, low hemorrhages generally. (3) Canth., Dulc. (4) Sec. - skin cold with desire to uncover. (5) Lyc. - head drawn to one side, Lyc. to left, Plb. and Stram. to right, Bufo to either. (6) Op. - narcotism, heart disorders. (7) Phos. - anguish and burning in cholera. (8) Nit-s-d., Squil., Verat. (9) Teste puts Camph. in his Belladonna group with Agar., Lach., Cedr., Stram., Tab. and others. ***Complementary:*** Canth. ***Incompatible:*** Kali-n. Nitrum. Tea, coffee and lemonade, as a rule, do not interfere, but sometimes coffee worse.

REFERENCES - Boericke. Clarke. Murphy.

CAMPHORA BROMATA

(Camphor Monobromide)

PHARMACY - camph-br. Camphora bromata. Camphor monobromide. Monobromata. A compound in which one atom of hydrogen of the camphor has been replaced by one of bromine. Trituration. ***Historical dose:*** Trituration and all potencies.

CLINICAL - Cholera infantum. Chordee. Convulsions. Delirium tremens. Eczema. Gastric, catarrh. Hysteria. Impotence. Influenza. Irritation, skin. Nervous, excitability. Neuralgia. Parkinson's disease. Sleep, disorders. Spermatorrhea.

HOMEOPATHIC - Dr. Cooper found Camph-br. of wide utility in all cases where nervous excitability is present. He has given it chiefly in single doses of 3x trituration. Hale noted it for hysteria, weeping and laughter alternately.

Nervous excitability. Headache in women and young girls due toe to mental excitement and excessive study. Delirium tremens. Parkinson's disease. Cholera infantum and infantile convulsions.

Chordee. Neuralgia of testes and prostate. Impotence. Spermatorrhea. Nightly emissions. Painful erections. Suppression of breast milk. Intensifies the action of Quinine and renders it more permanent.

MIND - Sense of direction is lost. Directions appear reversed, i.e., north seems south and east seems west. ***Nervous excitability***. Mental excitement and excessive study. Hysteria, weeping and laughing alternately. Trance-like state.

COMMENTS - In a case reported by Dr. E. M. Beard, a young man suffered from gastric catarrh in paroxysms which were induced by the sight of physical deformity, the touch of a cold, clammy hand and the mention of odors, the actual presence of which did not affect him.

Complete relief was afforded by 3 gram doses of Camph-br. every 3 or 4 hours.

The drug, however, set up some singular symptoms including: directions appeared to be reversed, north seemed south and east seemed west, innumerable black flies seemed to be flitting over the field of vision, he was sleepless and when he did sleep it was restless and vexed with ghastly dreams.

The reversal of directions lasted many days and the strain on the faculty of attention was so torturing that he became prostrate in mind and body.

REFERENCES - Boericke. Clarke.

CANCHALAGUA

(Centaury)

PHARMACY - canch. Canchalagua. Centaury. Erythraea chironioides. Erythraea chilensis. Centaurium chironioides. Venusta centaury. N. O. Gentianacae. Chile, Peru. Tincture of whole plant when in flower. Must be made from the fresh plant. ***Historical dose:*** Tincture and all potencies.

CLINICAL - Chills. Constipation. Influenza. Intermittents. Nausea. Sleeplessness.

HERBAL - Canch. has been used extensively as a fever remedy and bitter tonic (Gent-b.), anti-malarial and anti-septic.

HOMEOPATHIC - Dr. Richter proved Canch., experiencing symptoms including a congested feeling in the heard, scalp tight, felt as if drawn together by India rubber. Stitches, pain, buzzing and roaring in ears.

Indicated in severe intermittents of hot countries, and influenza. General sore, bruised feeling, nausea and retching. The skin becomes wrinkled like a washer woman's.

Sensation of drops falling from and upon different spots. Constipation, hard, knotty stools. Chills repeatedly down back worse in bed, at night. Sleeplessness. After the proving, a cold wind could be borne better than before.

Head - Congested. Scalp feels tight, head feels as if bound, burning in eyes, buzzing in ears.

Skin - Wrinkled like a washerwoman's. Scalp feels tight, as if drawn together by India-rubber.

Temperature - Chill all over, worse in bed at night. Sensitive to cold, trade-winds. General sore and bruised feeling, nausea and retching.

RELATIONS - ***Compare:*** (1) The Gentians, Chin., Ip.

REFERENCES - Boericke. Clarke.

CANDIDA ALBICANS
(Thrush Fungus)

PHARMACY - cand-a. Candida albicans. Thrush fungus. Monilia albicans. N. O. Fungi, Ascomycetes, Endomycetidae, Saccharomycetaceae. ***Historical dose:*** All potencies.

CLINICAL - Candidiasis. ***Flatulence.*** Indigestion. Leucorrhea. ***Thrush.*** Vaginitis.

Abdomen - Rumbling and gas in the abdomen. Flatulence. Bloated abdomen. Loud rumbling in abdomen while lying.

Female - Leucorrhea. Vaginitis.

Mouth - ***Thrush.***

RELATIONS - ***Compare:*** Cand-p., Carbo-v, Chin., Lyc., Sul-ac.

REFERENCES - Murphy.

CANDIDA PARAPSILOSIS
(Thrush Fungus)

PHARMACY - cand-p. Candida parapsilosis. N. O. Fungi, Ascomycetes, Endomycetidae, Saccharomycetaceae. ***Historical dose:*** All potencies.

CLINICAL - Candidiasis. ***Flatulence.*** Headache. Indigestion. Itching. Leucorrhea. ***Thrush.*** Vaginitis. Vertigo.

HOMEOPATHIC - Candida parapsilosis is a common yeast-like organism that has been implicated in human infection. It has been recovered from respiratory secretions, urine, gastric washings, blood, vagina, oropharynx, skin, transtracheal aspiration, stool, pleural fluid, ear, and nails.

It is implicated in the following human infections: Endopthalmitis, endocarditis, vaginitis, mycotic keratitis, external otomycosis, paronychia, and fungemia. In the vagina, it is found less frequently than Candida albicans and Torulopsis glabrata and is only rarely associated with vulvovaginal candidiasis as it is a less adherent organism.

The people most infected with Candida are those with natural defences depressed by excessive use of antibiotics and steroids or by certain diseases or operative procedures. Oral candidiasis is called thrush.

MIND - Very tired and scatter-brained. Total 'loss of mind': seeing red lights and thinking they were green. Spacey and poor concentration. Unusually irritable. Explosive anger at minor incidents - as though their rights were being infringed upon. Mind races and words come out in wrong order or mispronounced.

Abdomen - Bloating, fullness, cramping of abdomen. Bloating with flatulence.

Female - Egg-white leucorrhea. Dripping discharge.

Food - Increased appetite. Great thirst. Desires salt, garlic, pickles.

Head - Wakes with a headache. Banging sensation. Frontal constriction. Light-headed feeling. Itching of scalp, dry, flaking, reddening spot along hairline. Eczema-like patches on hairline. Red, scaly and itching.

Heart - Sensation of arrhythmias with light-headed feeling. Prominent, quick heartbeat which reverberates through the chest.

Modalities - Better open air. Worse direct sunlight.

Nose - Stuffiness of nose.

Skin - Eczema-like patches. Red, scaly and itching.

Stomach - Bloating, fullness, cramping of stomach.

Vertigo - Vertigo and hot flushes.

RELATIONS - ***Compare:*** Cand-a., Carbo-v, Chin., Lyc., Sul-ac.

REFERENCES - Brown. Lange. Murphy.

CANNABIS INDICA

(Indian Marijuana)

PHARMACY - cann-i. Cannabis indica. Indian marijuana. Hashish. Bhang. Ganja. N. O. Cannabinacae. East India. Tincture of young leaves and twigs. ***Historical dose:*** Tincture and all potencies.

CLINICAL - ***Absent-minded.*** Anxiety. ***Backache.*** Catalepsy. Chordee. Clairvoyance Delirium, tremens. Delusions. Diabetes. Dysmenorrhea. Epilepsy. Flatulence. Fears. Gonorrhea. Headache. Infertility. Insomnia. Intoxication. Kidney, disorders. Mania. ***Memory, weak.*** Menorrhagia. Miscarriage. Nervousness. Paralysis. Paranoia. Prostatitis. Satyriasis. Stammering. Uremia. ***Urinary, disorders.***

HERBAL - The use of Cann-i. in the East as an intoxicant gives the leading note of its sphere of action. Cannabis sativa and Cannabis indica are botanically identical, the difference in their properties is solely due to the difference of soil and climate in which they are grown.

HOMEOPATHIC - Cann-i. produces a ***state of exaltation*** with sublime visions, delusions and hallucinations in great variety. ***Time seems too long***, space illimitable. Paranoid. Apprehensive of approaching death. Fixed ideas. Fear of becoming insane or losing control. Horror of darkness.

Great desire to lie down in the daytime. Thoroughly exhausted after a short walk. Felt so weak that he could scarcely speak and soon fell into a deep sleep.

Soothing influence in many nervous disorders like epilepsy, mania, dementia and irritable reflexes. Catalepsy. Delirium tremens, trembling. Hallucinations. Tendency to become furious. Nausea, unquenchable thirst. Feels weak and all gone to nothing. Diabetes. Exophthalmic goiter.

MIND - Remarkable hallucinations and imaginations. ***Exaggeration of the duration of time and extent of space.*** Misperceptions of time and space. ***Time seems too long, seconds seem ages. A few miles an immense distance***. Heat and cold sensations of the body. Loss of identity. Clairvoyance. Imagines himself in a room of which the walls gradually close in upon him. Double consciousness, subconscious or ***dual nature state***.

Absent-minded. Poor short-term memory. Poor concentration and foggy mind. ***Sudden loss of memory.*** Inability to fix his thoughts on one subject. ***Forgets what he intends to write or speak.*** Sudden loss of speech, begins a sentence but cannot finish it. Lazy but restless. Chronic insomnia due to over activity of the mind.

Drug-induced spaciness, pathologically happy state. Full of fun, mischief and laughs. ***Uncontrollable laughter***. Extremely happy and contented, nothing troubles.

Emotional excitement, rapid change of moods. ***Exaltation of spirits*** with excessive loquacity. Stammering and stuttering. Constantly theorizing. Fixed ideas. Ideas crowd upon each other. Lost in thoughts.

Great agitation, anxiety and nervousness. Mania, must constantly move. Panic attacks, paranoia. Anguish, better in the open air. Constant fear of becoming insane. Horror of darkness. Fear of approaching death. Depression, constant fear of becoming insane.

Abdomen - Throbbing here and there. Rumbling in bowels at night. Flatulence, on rising in morning, with headache. The abdomen feels swollen, better by belching. Sensation of extreme tension in abdominal vessels feel distended to bursting. Sensation as if something alive in abdomen (Thuj.).

Back - Backache, worse during menses, which occur every two weeks and are scanty. Warmth in spine extending to head. Torticollis, chin drawn to the sternum. ***Pain across shoulders and spine, must stoop, cannot walk erect***.

Breasts - Stitches extending from both nipples through chest.

Chest - Oppression of chest with deep, labored breathing. Feels suffocated, has to be fanned.

Ears - Aching, throbbing and fullness in both ears. Extreme sensitiveness to noise, very acute hearing. Noise like boiling water, buzzing and ringing. Periodical singing in the ears during a dreamy spell, ceasing when he came to himself.

Eyes - Eyes bright and shiny. Injection of vessels of conjunctiva of both eyes. Glaucoma. Jerking in corner of the eye and eyelids. Fixed gaze. Weak vision. Twinkling, trembling and glimmering before the eyes. Letters run together when reading. Sees objects outside of visual field. Visual clairvoyance.

Face - Dejected, careworn, wearied, exhausted appearance. Drowsy, stupid look. Skin of face, especially of forehead and chin, feels as if drawn tight.

Female - Menses with violent uterine colic with dysuria. ***Menses profuse***, dark, painful, without clots. Backache during menses. Spasmodic uterine pains returning like labor pains, great agitation and sleeplessness. Sexual desire increased in infertile women or with dysmenorrhea. Infertility (Bor., Sep.). Threatened miscarriage in eighth month, burning on urination with purulent discharge.

Food - Increased appetite. Ravenous hunger. ***Craves sweets. Very thirsty for cold drinks.***

Head - Violent headaches and hallucinations. Vertex seems to open and shut, worse noise. Head seems separated from the body. Feels ***as if top of head were opening and shutting.*** Shocks through brain (Aloe., Coca.). ***Involuntary shaking of head***. Uremic headache. Headache with flatulence. Migraine attack preceded by unusual excitement with loquacity. Pain in the whole right side of the head. Throbbing and weight at occiput. Heavy pressure on the brain, forcing him to stoop. Dull, heavy, throbbing pain with sensation as from a blow, on back of head and neck.

Heart - Palpitations, awaking from sleep. Piercing pain with great oppression. ***Pulse very slow*** (Dig., Kalm., Apoc.). Pressing pain in the heart with dyspnea the whole night. Sensation as if drops were falling from the heart. Stitches in the heart, accompanied by great oppression, the latter relieved by deep breathing.

Kidneys - Dull pain in region of right kidney. Pain in the kidneys when laughing. Burning, aching or sharp stitches in the kidneys. Urging to urinate, but cannot pass a drop. Must wait some time before the urine flows, strain. The urine ***dribbles*** out after the stream ceases. Must force out the last few drops with the hand. Profuse, colorless urine, can have mucus. A white glairy mucus may be squeezed from the urethra. ***Burning and scalding or stinging pain*** in the urethra before, during, and after urination.

Limbs - Weariness in limbs and stiffness and aching in knees, almost paralysis. Thrilling through arms and hands, and from knees down. ***Entire paralysis of the lower limbs.*** Pain in soles and calves, sharp pains in knees and ankles, ***very exhausted after a short walk.*** Paralysis of the right arm. Coldness of right hand with stiffness and numbness of right thumb. On attempting to walk, intensely violent pain as if treading on spikes, which penetrated the soles and ran upward through the limbs. Shooting pains in the joints of the toes of the left foot, worse in great toe, aching and stitching pain in ball of left great toe.

Lungs - Humid asthma. Chest oppressed with deep, labored breathing. Rough cough with scraping immediately under the sternum. Great effort to take a deep inspiration.

Male - ***Sexual desire increased***. Satyriasis, priapism. Prolonged thrill. Erections not caused by amorous thoughts. Violent painful erections. ***Backache*** after sexual intercourse. Oozing of white, glairy mucus from glans. Chordee. Sensation of swelling in perineum or near anus, as if sitting on a ball. Penis relaxed and shrunken. Itching in the glans penis. Sharp pricking like needles in urethra, so severe as to send a thrill to cheeks and hands. Gonorrhea without pain with a very profuse yellowish-white discharge. Feeling as if discharge in urethra.

Modalities - Better from walking about outdoors. Better fresh air. Better cold water. Better rest. Worse from coffee, liquor and tobacco. Worse lying on right side. Worse mornings.

Mouth - ***Gritting and grinding of teeth while sleeping***. Tongue is white, thick, frothy and sticky saliva. ***Dryness of the mouth and lips.*** Lips feel as if glued together. Every article of food is extremely palatable. Stammering and stuttering speech.

Rectum - Sensation in anus as if sitting on a ball. Painless, yellow diarrhea.

Sleep - Sleepy but cannot sleep. Chronic insomnia. Excessive sleepiness, sound sleep with melancholy dreams. Jerking of the limbs while sleeping, causing him to awake. Talks during sleeps. Gritting teeth during sleep. Catalepsy. Nightmares every night as soon as he falls asleep. Dreams are prophetic, of dead bodies, danger and perils to be encountered. Erotic dreams with erection and profuse seminal emission.

Stomach - Pain in the cardiac orifice, relieved by pressure. Suffocative feeling while eating. Distention. Pyloric spasm.

Temperature - Loss of vital heat. General chilliness. Coldness of the face, nose and hands after dinner. Profuse sticky sweat, standing out in drops on his forehead.

Throat - Throat is parched, accompanied by intense thirst for cold water.

Vertigo - Chronic vertigo, as of floating off the ground. Worse on rising with stunning pain in back part of head. Sensation as if the room were falling in pieces about her.

COMMENTS - Cann-i. inhibits the higher faculties and stimulates the imagination to a remarkable degree. A major remedy for drug flashbacks, fears, phobias or panic attacks since a drug overdose. DTs. Clairvoyance and clairaudience.

A condition of intense exaltation in which all perceptions and conceptions, all sensations and emotions are exaggerated to the utmost degree. Hypersensitivity of all the senses. Extreme sensitivity to noise, can hear a whisper in adjoining room and is irritated from it. Startles easily. Fear of loss of control.

Sensation of levitation. Sensation as if in a dream. Vertigo on rising with stunning pain in back part of head. Cann-i. removed a vertigo in which the patient felt as if the house were falling in ruins about her.

Starting, talking, nightmares, during sleep. Grinds teeth while asleep. Wants to sleep but cannot (Gels.). Palpitations, awakens from sleep. Stitches in heart with oppression, better deep breathing.

Dryness of the mouth. Stammering and stuttering. Thirst for cold water, worse warm, stuffy rooms. Craves sweets. Useful when treating hypoglycemia related to smoking marijuana.

Affects the urinary and generative organs. History of kidney problems, cystitis, or gonorrhea. Constant dull pain in region of right kidney. Pains in kidneys when laughing. Sensation in anus as if sitting on a ball, as if anus and part of urethra were filled by a hard, round body.

Frequent urination with burning pain in evening. Urging and straining, but cannot pass a drop. Burning, scalding or stinging in urethra before during and after urination. Dribbling of urine (Thuj., Sabal., Sep.). Urine loaded with slimy mucus after exposure to damp and cold.

Backache worse during menses, which occur every two weeks and are scanty. Very profuse, painful, dark menstruation, but without clots. Tendency to get vaginitis.

Catalepsy. Tingling of paralyzed parts. Paralysis of lower limbs and right arm. Muscle cramps and weak knees.

Headache with flatulence, lasts until flatus can be passed up or down, throbbing of occiput. Scalp sore feeling, crawling on vertex, sensation as though skin tightly stretched over bones of face. Weight at occiput from which pains start up sides of head to temples and vertex. Warmth of spine extending to head.

Sensation as of brain boiling over and lifting cranial arch like a lid, opening and shutting sensation. Shocks through brain on regaining consciousness. Guided by this symptom, Clarke removed a "noise like a crash or explosion during sleep."

Nash related the case of a woman suffering from cardiac dropsy, who, when relieved of the latter, suddenly lost the power of speech. In answer to a question she could begin a sentence, but could not finish it as she could not remember what she wished to say. She was very impatient about it, would cry, but could not finish the sentence, though she could signify assent if any one did finish it for her. Cann-i. cured rapidly.

In one case of overdose the observer experienced a modification of this: absolute forgetfulness of the thought, speech or acts of the previous moment, startled by hearing the echo of the last words of a sentence he has just spoken. Having suggested a walk to a companion and meeting him at the street door, wondered why they were there. Afterwards, he could remember everything.

RELATIONS - ***Compare:*** (1) Cann-s., Bell., Hyos., Stram., Lach., Agar. (2) Anhalon. - time sense disordered, time periods enormously overestimated, thus, minutes seem hours. (3) Cann-s. - in extreme sensitiveness to noise. (4) Nit-ac. - to jarring and rumbling of wagon in street. (5) Coff. - to all sounds, Borax - slightest noise, fall of door latch, rumpling of paper, rustling of silk. (6) Asar. - to scratching of linen or silk or even the thought of it. (7) Levitation - Asar., Calc., Cocc., Ph-ac., Sil., Stict., Sulph., Thuj. (8) As if in a dream - Ambr., Anac., Calc., Con., Cupr., Med., Rheum., Stram., Valer., Verat., Zinc. (9) Horror of darkness - Am-m., Bar-c., Calc., Carb-an., Phos., Stram., Stroph., Valer. (10) Noise like a crash or explosion in head - Aloe.

REFERENCES - Boericke. Clarke. Murphy.

CANNABIS SATIVA

(Marijuana)

PHARMACY - cann-s. Cannabis sativa. Marijuana. Hemp. European hemp. American hemp. N. O. Cannabinacae. Tincture of male and female flowering tops. ***Historical dose:*** Tincture and all potencies.

CLINICAL - Ascites. Asthma. Cataract. Choking. ***Cystitis.*** Fatigue. Forgetful. Glaucoma. ***Gonorrhea.*** Headache. Hysteria. Infertility. ***Impotence.*** Leucorrhea. Memory, weak. Miscarriages. Nausea. Nephritis. Nosebleeds. ***Opacity, cornea***. Ophthalmia. Palpitations. Paralysis. Phimosis. Pleurisy. Pneumonia. Post-partum hemorrhage. ***Polyuria.*** Priapism. ***Sexual, disorders. Stammering.*** Tetanus. Trachea, mucus. Urethral discharges, caruncle. Vaginitis. Vomiting.

HERBAL - Cann-s. and Cann-i. are similar, the difference in their properties is solely due to the difference of soil and climate in which they are grown. Cann-s. has less pronounced mental symptoms and head symptoms and the eye and genito-urinary symptoms are more so than Cann-i.

HOMEOPATHIC - Cann-s. seems to affect especially the ***urinary and sexual organs. Acute and chronic gonorrhea,*** especially when the patient walks with the legs apart. ***Sexual excitement*** in both the sexes. Threatened miscarriage from too frequent sexual intercourse or complicated with gonorrhea. Vaginitis.

Characteristic sensations as of dropping water. Choking in swallowing, things go down the wrong way. Great fatigue from having spoken or written. Feels exhausted after a short walk. Feet feel heavy on going upstairs.

Acute drawing and contractive, pressive pains with sensation of paralysis. Drawing pains in regions of kidneys extending into inguinal glands with anxious sensation of nausea at epigastrium.

Tetanus, chiefly in the upper limbs and in the trunk. Paralysis with tingling of the affected part. Unendurable fine stitching over whole body, as from a thousand needle points, at night, when sweating from warm covering, better uncovering.

MIND - Confusion of thought and speech. ***Stuttering and stammering***. Embarrassed speech, at one time words are wanting, at another the voice fails. ***Very forgetful cannot finish the sentence.*** Vanishing of thoughts, want of words. Wavering speech, hasty, incoherent. Speech stops with anxiety and agony on account of pain in the back. Many errors in writing.

Ideas seem to stand still, he stares in front of him is absorbed in higher thoughts, but in unconscious of them. ***Time seems too long.*** Thinks everything is unreal, ***as if in a dream***. Voices including her own, seem to come from a distance, her own voice seems strange, as if it were somebody else speaking. Clairvoyance.

Loquacity. Laughs immoderately, at mere trifles. Laughs and weeps. Ecstatic, heavenly. Fixed ideas. Mania, sometimes happy, sometimes serious or furious. Sadness and indifference. Irresolution and uncertainty. Moaning and crying. Disposition to be easily frightened or irritated. Fear of going to bed.

Abdomen - Pain as from a bruise in the intestines. Hard and painful swelling of the liver region. Cramp-like pains in the epigastrium. Sensation of soreness. Shuddering sensation, as if cold water were running through abdomen. Painful jerks. Shaking of the intestines, as if they were detached, when the arms are moved. Shocks and pressure towards the outside in the regions of the groins. Pulsation of abdomen from within outward.

Back - Pains in the back, which impede speech and suspend respiration. Shooting pains between the shoulder blades. Pressure towards the outside in the sacral region and coccyx.

Chest - Weight on chest, rattling wheezing breathing. Shootings in the bottom of the chest, especially on breathing, speaking or during movement.

Ears - Throbbing and pressure in the ears, that disappears when one is stooping and reappearing when raising the head again. Hears voices, bells, music. Buzzing in the ears and sensation as if a skin were before them.

Eyes - Glaucoma. Pressure from back of eyes, forward. Eyeballs ache. Cataract from nervous disturbances, abuse of alcohol and tobacco, patient feels deeply approaching blindness. Gonorrheal ophthalmia. ***Opacity of cornea***. Scrofulous eye troubles (Sulph., Calc.). Cramp-like pulling in the eyes. Misty sight. Weakness and confusion of sight, on viewing objects either distant or near. Appearance of a circle of whitish flames before the eyes.

Face - Paleness of the face. Heat of the face and redness of the cheeks. Tingling, itching and smarting in the face, as if from salt. Twitching of the muscles of the face.

Female - ***Acute gonorrhea***. Threatened abortion, complicated with gonorrhea or on account of frequent sexual intercourse. ***Leucorrhea.*** Infantile leucorrhea. Amenorrhea, also with constipation. Profuse menstruation. Miscarriage with convulsions. Great sexual excitement with infertility.

Food - ***Desires sweets and cold drinks.*** Every article of food is extremely palatable. Aversion to meat, of which she was fond.

Head - Headache, as if there were a stone pressing upon it. Sensation of a heavy weight on the vertex. Pressure and tension on the temples. Pressure on root of nose. Congestion in the head, throbbings in the brain, cheeks red and hot with pulsation. Sensation at the scalp, as if something were creeping on it and as if drops of cold water were falling on the head.

Heart - Great anxiety of heart. Painful tension in the heart with palpitations of the heart and anxiety. Beatings of the heart, which are felt lower than their ordinary place. Pulse weak, slow and scarcely perceptible. Pericarditis. Inflammation of the heart. Sensation as if drops were falling from the heart.

Kidneys - Inflamed sensation with soreness to touch. ***Acute gonorrhea***, urethra sensitive, walks with the legs apart. Kidney colic and pains. Pain in kidney, while laughing. Painful urging. Must strain to urinate, has to wait for some time before the urine flows, dribbles after flow ceases. ***Scanty burning urine passed drop by drop***. Urination in split stream. ***Burning while urinating, extending to bladder.*** Urine scalding with spasmodic closure of sphincter. Stitches, zigzag pain along urethra. Urethral caruncle (Eucal.), phimosis. Stoppage of urethra by mucus and pus. Discharge of yellow, watery mucus from the urethra (gonorrhea). Urine, turbid white or reddish and as if mixed with blood and pus. Incontinence of urine. Ejection of a kidney stone on urinating. Retained urine with constipation.

Limbs - Pain in the limbs, worse deep breathing. Pain, as from a bruise in the shoulder and forearm during movement. Entire paralysis of lower limbs. Cramps in the thighs, the calves of the legs and the hams. Weakness, staggering and pains of the knees. Displacement of the patella on going up the stairs. Pulsation and stretching pain in the feet and in the joints of the foot, as after a long walk. Spasmodic contraction of the Achilles tendon with violent pains. Cramps in the hands and the fingers. Sudden paralytic weakness of the hand with trembling on laying hold of an object and inability to hold it firmly.

Lungs - Suffocative attacks. Humid asthma. Difficulty in breathing and palpitations, ***then must stand up.*** As if there were a weight on the chest, with wheezing and rattling in the bronchials. Difficulty of respiration with uneasiness in the throat, worse lying down. Rattling breathing. Inflammation of the lungs, with greenish vomiting and delirium. Cough with green viscid, bloody, expectoration. Cough, violent and dry.

Male - ***Sexual desire increased.*** Priapism. Strong sexual desire or aversion to sex. Erections without amorous thoughts. Erections with tensive pains. ***Acute gonorrhea***. Itching and inflammatory swelling of the prepuce, glans and penis with deep redness and phimosis. The penis feels sore and burnt when walking, walks with legs apart. Cold genitals. Dragging, aching in the testes and tension in the spermatic cord, when standing upright. Swelling of the prostate gland.

Modalities - Better from fresh air. Better cold water. Better rest. ***Worse from urinating.*** Worse after a meal. Worse coffee, liquor or tobacco. ***Worse darkness***. Worse at night. Worse after midnight. Worse open air, and heat. Worse from exercise, exertion. Worse talking. Worse walking. Worse going upstairs. Worse touch. Worse lying down.

Mouth - Grinding of teeth in sleep. ***Dryness of the mouth*** with viscid saliva and absence of thirst. Saliva, white, thick, frothy. Eruption on the border of the lips.

Nose - Swelling of the nose with copper-like redness. Stupefying pressure on the root of the nose. Heat and dryness of the nose. Nosebleed, preceded by a sensation of burning in the nose.

Rectum - Diarrhea, accompanied by cramp-like pains in the abdomen. Pressure in the rectum towards the outside. Sensation as of cold water running from the anus. Constipation and hard feces.

Sensations - As if hot water were poured over him. ***As if drops of cold water were falling on the head, from anus, or from heart.*** As if pinched with pincers in back. Pressure as with a sharp point in coccyx.

Skin - At night, pricking and sensation of burning over the whole skin, as if from boiling water.

Sleep - Sleepy, but cannot sleep. Frightful or erotic dreams. Dreams of the dead. Sensation of greater fatigue on waking in the morning, then when going to bed in the evening. Sleepy during the day.

Stomach - Empty risings. Regurgitation of acrid substances of a bitter sourness. Attack of violent cramps in the stomach. Nausea with inclination for food. Vomiting with sensation of strangulation from the epigastrium to the throat. Vomiting of green bile. Pain in the stomach, on being touched, as if it were ulcerated, better by eating. Aching, pinchings and cuttings in the epigastrium and in the upper part of the stomach.

Temperature - Typhoid fevers, where strangury exists. Shuddering, shivering with thirst. Uneasiness and external cold. Coldness of the body with heat in the face. Heat only in the face. Burning heat over the whole body at night.

Throat - Cannot control voice. Loss of voice. Accumulation of tenacious mucus in the larynx with scraping and difficulty of breathing.

Vertigo - Vertigo, sensation of dropping water on head. Attacks of vertigo on walking or when standing for some time to such an extent as to cause falling. Sensation as if intoxicated.

COMMENTS - In Cann-i., the drug state is often the etiology, but Cann-s stands on its own. Closely related to Med. And Thuj., will often follow Med. Boericke said that lemon juice antidotes Cann-s.

Strong affinity for the genital area and infections. High sex drive (Med.). Acute gonorrhea remedy, with spaciness and a history of drug use. Yellow-green discharges.

Urethral symptoms with burning and smarting (Canth. has more tenesmus). Mucus in urine, burning on urination. The bladder feels full. Non-specific urethritis. Pain in right kidney. Cramps of any kind. The urethra is very sensitive to touch and pressure, the patient cannot bear the legs close together. Urethral caruncle. Phimosis.

Dry mouth, craves sweets, thirst for cold water. Hypoglycemia. Sensitive to stimulants. Limbs feel weak and heavy. Glaucoma. Cataract and opacities of the cornea, gonorrhea of the eyes. Eyeballs aches, pressure in back of the eyes.

Sudden changes from agitation to restless to calm. Distortion in perception, spacey, bad memory. Better with fresh, open air and cold water on their face.

RELATIONS - ***Antidotes:*** Camph., Lemon juice. Antidotes of large doses: lemon juice, Strychnia, Camph., Merc. ***Compare:*** (1) Cann-i., Thuj. Med., Canth., Petros. (2) Sars. - worse going up stairs. (3) In phimosis - Merc., Sulph., Nit-ac., Sep., Thuj. Rhus-t., Sabin. (4) as if something alive in abdomen - Croc., Thuj. (5) Apis, Cop., Cimic., Kali-n. (6) Hedysarum - gonorrhea and inflammation of penis. ***Compatible:*** Bell., Hyos., Lyc., Nux-v., Op., Puls., Rhus-t., Verat.

REFERENCES - Boericke. Clarke. Murphy.

CANTHARIS VESICATORIA

(Spanish Fly)

PHARMACY - canth. Cantharis vesicatoria. Spanish Fly. Lytta vesicator. Meloe vesicatorius. N. O. Insecta, Coleoptera. Tincture or trituration of whole insect. ***Historical dose:*** Trituration, tincture and all potencies.

CLINICAL - ***Bladder, infections.*** Blisters. ***Burns***. Chordee. ***Cystitis.*** Diphtheria. Dysentery. Eczema. Emissions. ***Erysipelas.*** Eyes inflammation. Gastritis. Gonorrhea. Herpes zoster. ***Hydrophobia. Kidneys, disorders.*** Mania. Neuralgia. Nymphomania. Ovaries, disorders. Peritonitis. Pleurisy. Pregnancy, disorders. Retained, placenta. Satyriasis. Scarlatina. ***Sexual, mania.*** Spermatorrhea. Strangury. ***Sunburn.*** Thirst. Throat, sore. Tongue inflammation. Urine, abnormal. Vesicles.

HOMEOPATHIC - Commonly known as Spanish fly, Canth. belongs to the animal kingdom and finds its most prominent sphere of action in exciting the animal passions. There is anger in a very acute degree amounting to paroxysms of rage and a corresponding condition of the bodily tissues.

Rapid and intense action. Characteristic ***irritation***. Hypersensitiveness of all parts. ***Burns and scalds***. ***Vesication***. Erysipelas, blisters. Burning, stitches, shooting pains and exudation are the indications. ***Pains are cutting, smarting or burning, biting*** or as if raw, causing mental excitement. ***Raw, burning pains.***

Inflammations are violently acute or rapidly destructive in the mucus and serous membranes. Violent inflammation of the whole gastro-intestinal canal, especially lower bowel. Puerperal convulsions. Inflammations are often associated with bladder irritation.

In any condition when the urine is scanty, cutting and burning. Intolerable, ***constant urging to urinate***. ***Dysuria*** with any other complaints. Painful urination, as a concomitant in any diseased condition. Acute nephritis.

Gastric, hepatic and abdominal complaints, ***aggravated by drinking coffee*** Gastric derangements of pregnancy.

Inflamed ***sexual organs***, causing frenzied delirium. Amorous frenzy, unbounded sexual desire. Sexual weakness and excitability. ***Sexual excitement during pains.*** Expels dead fetus, placenta, promotes fecundity.

Discharges are bloody, acrid, watery, tenacious. ***Hemorrhages.*** Serous effusions. Sudden attacks of weakness that takes the voice away. Hemiplegia of (right) side with aphasia. Convulsions with dysuria and hydrophobic symptoms. Moles.

MIND - Great restlessness, obliging him to move constantly. ***Anxious restlessness***, ending in rage. Paroxysms of rage with crying, barking, biting and worse by bright objects, by touching the larynx, drinking cold water. Despondent and low-spirited, says she must die. Weeping aggravates.

Furious delirium. Delirium, with dread. Acute mania after erysipelas. Wildness. Excessive sexual desire, not better by sex. ***Acute mania***, generally of a sexual type, amorous frenzy, fiery sexual desire. Sings lewd songs. Striking at imaginary objects about him.

Fear of mirrors in room. Constantly attempts to do something but accomplishes nothing. Insolent, contradictory mood. Disposition to contradict. Irritable, dissatisfied with every one and everything. Whining and complaining, with anxious restlessness, worse motion, better lying quiet.

Exceedingly sensitive to all impressions. Uneasiness day and night, with hot head. Strange ideas crowd on him against his will. Prattles about genitals, urine, feces. Delusion bed were raised. Insanity with increased strength. ***Sudden loss of consciousness*** with red face.

Abdomen - Pain in loins with incessant desire to urinate. Violent burning pain through the whole intestinal tract, with painful sensitiveness to touch.

Back - Emprosthotonos and opisthotonos. Pain in loins with frequent desire to urinate.

Bladder - ***Acute severe cystitis. Constant desire to urinate.*** Urging to urinate from smallest quantity of urine in bladder. ***Intolerable tenesmus.*** Burning, cutting pains before, during and after urination. Severe burning pains in bladder. ***Intense burning pain in urethra***, worse motion, better lying on back. ***Violent burning, cutting pains*** in neck of bladder. Atony of bladder from long retention of urine. Griping in bladder. Heaviness in bladder, feels sore on slightest motion. ***Terrible pains from being catheterized.*** Bladder pains, worse drinking, even small quantities of water. Burning pains when urinating and when not. Must double herself and scream from fearful cutting pains in urethra.

Breasts - Breasts painful, with dysuria.

Chest - Chest pains better belchings. Burning pains in chest. Stitches in chest, at sternum (Bry., Kali-c., Squil.). Pleurisy, as soon as effusion has taken place.

Ears - Sensation as if wind were coming from ear or hot air. Bones about ear painful (Caps.).

Eyes - Objects look yellow. Yellow vision (Sant.). ***Fiery, sparkling, staring look***. Burning in eyes.

Face - Pale and wretched, death-like appearance. Expression of extreme suffering, terror or despair. Hot and red. Jaws tightly closed, acute mania. Itching vesicles on face, burning when touched. Erysipelas of face with burning, biting heat with urinary symptoms.

Female - Retained placenta (Sep.), with painful urination. Expels dead fetuses, membranes, etc. ***Nymphomania*** (Plat.). Pruritus with strong sexual desire, at menopause. Leucorrhea with sexual excitement, causing severe itching and masturbation. Puerperal metritis with inflammation of bladder. Menses too early and too profuse, black. Swelling of vulva with irritation. Constant discharge from uterus, worse false step. Cutting burning in ovaries, ovaritis. Sharp, tearing pain in os coccyx.

Food - Disgust for everything, drink, food, tobacco. Thirst unquenchable. Burning thirst, but aversion to all fluids. Aversion to water. ***Aggravation from drinking coffee***, drinking the smallest quantity increases pain in bladder and is vomited.

Head - Burning in brain. Sensation as if boiling water in brain. Head heavy, aches from bathing or washing. Hair falls when combing.

Heart - Palpitation, pulse feeble, irregular, tendency to syncope. Pericarditis with effusion.

Kidneys - ***Acute nephritis.*** Nephritis with bloody urine. Diabetes insipidus. Bright's disease. Kidney colic. Kidney region very sensitive. Kidney pains and urging to urinate, steadily increasing in severity. Dropsy. ***Urine, burning, scalding with cutting pains and intolerable urging.*** Strangury. Violent paroxysms of cutting and burning in whole renal region, with painful urging to urinate. ***Urine is passed drop by drop, dribbling.*** Bloody urine. Membranous scales looking like bran in water. Urine jelly-like, shreddy. Paroxysmal cutting and burning, in both kidneys, the region very sensitive to slightest touch.

Limbs - Knees totter when ascending steps. Ulcerative pain in soles, cannot step. Tearing in limbs.

Lungs - Voice low, weak feeling. Tenacious mucus in air passages. Pleurisy with ***exudation***. Dyspnea, palpitation, frequent, dry cough. ***Tendency to syncope.*** Short, hacking cough, blood-streaked, ***tenacious*** mucus.

Male - Painful swelling of genitals. Priapism. Pulls at penis. Sexual desire increased not better by sex. Bloody semen. Pollutions. Burning in urethra after sex. ***Strong desire***, painful erection. Pain in glans. Gonorrhea with priapism.

Modalities - Better from rubbing. Better warm applications. Better warmth. Better rest. Worse during or after urination. Worse drinking cold water or coffee. Worse sound of water. Worse bright objects. Worse touch, especially the larynx.

Mouth - Tongue covered with vesicles, deeply furred, edges red. Swollen tremulous tongue, edges raw. ***Burning in mouth, pharynx and throat.*** Vesicles in mouth. Grinding of the teeth with lockjaw. Saliva disgustingly sweet.

Rectum - Dysentery, mucus stools like ***scrapings of intestines***. ***Shreddy burning stools with*** tenesmus of rectum and bladder, with shuddering after stools. Bloody with ***burning***, ***tenesmus and shuddering after stool.*** Dysentery or diarrhea with dysuria. Constipation with retention of urine. Desire for stool while urinating. Cutting in rectum partially better by flatus, entirely by stools.

Skin - ***Burns and scalds*** with rawness and smarting, relieved by cold applications, followed by undue inflammation. Severe sunburns. Eruptions burn when touched. Dermatitis with bleb formation. Eruption with mealy scales. ***Vesicular eruptions,*** turning black with burning and itching. ***Erysipelas***, vesicular type with great restlessness. Secondary eczema about scrotum and genitals, following excessive perspiration. Tendency to gangrene. Burning in soles of feet at night.

Stomach - Burning sensation of esophagus and stomach (Carb.). Very sensitive, ***violent burning.*** Vomiting of blood-streaked membrane. Violent retching and vomiting. Sensitiveness over stomach, slightest pressure produces convulsions.

Temperature - Chilly, as if cold water poured over him during stool. Cold hands and feet, cold sweat. Urinous sweat, on genitals. Soles burn.

Throat - Burnt after taking hot food. As if on fire. Burning in mouth, pharynx and throat. Scalding feeling. ***Great difficulty when swallowing liquids.*** Painfully constricted, aphthous ulceration. Full of blisters. Very ***tenacious mucus*** (Kali-bi.). Violent spasms reproduced by touching larynx.

Vertigo - Vertigo, worse in open air.

COMMENTS - In Canth., the pains are burning and sharp, sharp along the course of a nerve. Tyler wrote that it was "Another vehement drug of storm and stress, tamed by Hahnemann."

Burns and blisters. Severe pain from burns. The part may be treated with a lotion containing a few drops or pills of the Canth. 30c or 200c to the ounce of water, a dilution given internally.

An ointment made with the 3x is a good application for herpes zoster.

Useful for bladder infections (Staph.), with a constant, severe, painful urging, cutting in the urethra (Sars.). Hematuria, blood in the urine, with a severe bladder infection. Pus in the urine. Can pass only a few drops like molten lead. Strangury. Cutting, burning pains from the kidney down to urethra. Irritation of all grades. Worse from a catheter.

The pains are burning and sharp, sharp along the course of a nerve. Neuralgia of head and face from taking cold with loud screams and jerking of muscles. The slightest touch or approach aggravates the mental symptoms. Violent spasms reproduced by touching larynx.

It acts on the brain, producing inflammation of the tissues. Irritation on the skin and serous membranes. Pleurisy with effusion. Diphtheria, inflammation of throat, severe burning, constriction, thirst with aversion to drinking.

The face is generally pale or yellowish with an expression of deep-seated suffering. Erysipelas commencing in nose. The eyes are bright, pupils widely dilated. Conjunctivitis where the eye has burning pains, clawing at the eye (Euphr.).

Pain in abdomen, colic-like, doubling the patient up, cutting, burning, lancinating. Dysenteric stools with tenesmus. Violent dysentery, painful dysentery, with burning on passing the stool with blood and mucus. Extreme superficial sensitiveness in hypogastrium (especially when the bladder is full), attended with unbearable tenesmus of bladder. Inflamed stomach. The sexual appetite is aroused to the point of mania.

H. N. Guernsey observed that Canth. is almost always the remedy for whatever other sufferings there may be, when there is as well frequent urination with burning, cutting pain or if cutting burning pain attends the flow, even when urination is not very frequent.

Guernsey noted that "Canth. expels moles, dead fetus, placenta, promotes fecundity." He also pointed out that Canth. should be studied in treating disorders of the air-passages when the mucus is tenacious.

Guernsey gave as the special indications in rabies and hydrophobia as "moaning and violent cries interspersed with barking." Glassy eyes, dilated pupil, flushed face, and the person is in a violent frenzy. Worse from dazzling objects and by water, completing the hydrophobia picture.

Nash recorded a case in which this observation led him to make a cure. Kali-bi. had completely failed to relieve a woman who had long suffered from bronchitis. The mucus was profuse, tenacious and ropy. One day the patient mentioned that she had great cutting and burning on urinating, which she was obliged to do very frequently. Canth. made a rapid cure.

Canth. has cured a case of malarial cachexia in which the symptoms were always worse when the urine was scanty.

RELATIONS - ***Antidotes:*** Acon., Puls. Camph. antidotes the strangury and retention of urine of Canth., Apis the cystitis, Kali-n. the kidney symptoms. For its throat symptoms it is nearest to Capsicum. Canth. is ***Antidote to:*** Camph., Vinegar, Alcohol. ***Compare:*** (1) Apis, Staph., Ars., Merc-c., Bell. (2) Cann-s. - more burning and smarting, Canth. more tenesmus. (3) Petros. - sudden urging, Caps, Puls. - retained placenta, Ars. - delayed urination after childbirth. (4) Erections, those of Canth. prevent urination, those of Thuj do not. (5) Merc. - semen mixed with blood, Sars. (urine burns like fire, shreddy particles and blood in it), Arum, Arn., Rhus-t., Ran-s. (6) Teste classes Canth. with Senega and Ph-ac. in his Conium group. (7) Cantharidin - Glomerular nephritis. (8) Vesicaria - urinary and kidney remedy. Smarting, burning sensation along urethra and in bladder with frequent desire to void urine often with strangury. Cystitis irritable bladder. (9) Fuschina - Nephritis with albuminuria. Redness of ears, mouth, swollen gums, deep, red urine, red, profuse diarrhea with severe abdominal pains. (10) Androsace lactea - urinary troubles, diuretic, dropsy. ***Compatible with:*** Bell., Merc., Phos., Puls., Sep. ***Complementary:*** Camph. ***Incompatible:*** Coffea.

REFERENCES - Boericke. Clarke. Murphy.

CAPSICUM ANNUUM

(Cayenne Pepper)

PHARMACY - caps. Capsicum annuum. Cayenne pepper. N. O. Solanaceae. South America. West Indies. Tincture of the dried pods. ***Historical dose:*** Tincture and all potencies.

CLINICAL - Amaurosis. Asthma. Brain, irritation. Delirium tremens. Cough. ***Delirium tremens***. Diarrhea. Diphtheria. Dysentery. Ear disorders. Esophagus, stricture. Colic. Gland, disorders. Hemorrhoid. Headache. Heartburn. Hernia. ***Homesickness.*** Intermittents. Lungs, disorders. ***Mastoiditis.*** Measles. Mouth, ulcers. Neuralgia. Nose, disorders. Obesity. Paralysis. Pleuro-pneumonia. Pregnancy, disorders. Rectum, diseases. Rheumatic gout. Rheumatism. Sciatica. Scrofula. Seasickness. ***Stomatitis.*** Throat, sore. Tongue, paralysis. Trachea, tickling. Urine, disorders. Whooping cough. Yellow fever.

HERBAL - Capsicum should be studied in connection with the other great members of the Solanum family, Bell., Stram., Hyos., Dulc., Solan. carolin., Solan. nig., Solan. tub. (Potato) and Lycoper. (Tomato).

HOMEOPATHIC - The well-known burning effects of red pepper is a leading indication for its use. ***Burning pains,*** wherever they occur, demand that Caps. should have consideration, if there are no other determining symptoms in favor of another remedy. Burning, worse from cold water.

Pains are ***burning, smarting,*** pungent or strangling, threadlike, worse by cold water. Burning and pungent pains, worse by application of cold water. Burning, pungent sensation in face worse by slightest draft of cold air. Burning pains and general chilliness.

Burning in throat. Burning blisters in roof of mouth (diphtheria or gangrene). Constriction of throat, spasmodic closure. Throat pain when not swallowing. Burning in rectum, tenesmus. Burning in bladder. Burning on urination.

Fever. Redness of the skin, scarlet eruption (Bell.). Mucus membranes become dark, red, spongy or ooze bloody mucus. Mucus membranes have a sensation of ***constriction***.

Disorders of bones. Pains in bones of face. Inflammation of petrous bone. ***Mastoiditis.*** Marked tendency to suppuration in every inflammatory process. Deep abscesses. Discharges are very foul.

Violent pains in various places, now here now there. Muscle pain, aching and jerking of muscles. Neuralgias. ***Sensation of soreness*** and constriction. Sensation as if cayenne pepper were sprinkled on parts. Sensation as if parts go to sleep. Shuddering during pain or drinking.

Lack of reaction, particularly in persons of lax tissue. Sluggish circulation. Hemorrhages. Bodily irritability. Parts pinched remain in raised position for a long time.

Extreme sensitiveness to cold and damp (Dulc.), aggravates most symptoms. Shuns open air, dreads uncovering, dreads air, especially a draft. Better from heat. Patients who cannot get to sleep without a hot bottle at their back. Spirits become lower as body becomes cooler. Symptoms generally appear on left side. A general ***uncleanliness of body.***

Thirsty, but drinking causes shuddering. Absence of thirst during heat. Prostration and feeble digestion of alcoholics. Abstainers from accustomed alcohol.

MIND - Capricious and changeable mood. If she wants a certain thing, she will oppose, if proposed by someone else. ***Homesickness with red cheeks and sleeplessness with hot feeling in fauces.*** Homesickness with sleeplessness and disposition to suicide. ***Sentimental, nostalgic moods.***

Peevish, irritable, angry, easily offended ***Irritability during chill.*** Confusion during chill. Peppery disposition. Always on the lookout for insults. Obstinacy. Refractory especially children. Wants to be left alone Red cheeks after emotions, fever.

Alternating states, laughs and weeps b turns is now jocose and sings, but become angry from slightest cause. Clumsy. Awk ward, runs into everything. ***Delirium tremen*** Alcoholism. Dreads any kind of exercise

Anxiety and fear, as though he was goin to die. Fearfulness. Fear of slightest dra

Fear of being censured. Frightened easily on waking. Awakens with fright, screams, and remains full of fear. Sensitive to noise.

Abdomen - Flatulent colic. Colic about umbilicus with mucus stools. Violent pulsations of arteries in abdomen.

Back - Lumbar pain after stools. Pain in sacrum with hemorrhoids and dysentery. Pain in the back while drinking water. Sensation as if cold water dropping down back.

Causations - Homesickness.

Chest - ***Constriction*** of chest, arrests breathing.

Constitutions - Suited to those of lax tissues, weak, lazy indolent, fat, red, clumsy, awkward and of unclean habits. Such persons are opposed to physical exertion, averse to go outside of their routine and get homesick easily. Old people who have exhausted their vitality, especially by mental work and poor living. Persons react poorly and are afraid of cold. Abstainers from accustomed alcohol.

Ears - ***Swelling and pain behind ears. inflammation of mastoid. Mastoiditis.*** Otorrhea and mastoid disease before suppuration. ***Tenderness over the petrous bone***, extremely sore and tender to touch (Onos.). Hot ears. Burning and stinging in ears. Otalgia, then deafness. Tympanum perforated. Sub-acute inflammation of Eustachian tube with great pain. Ear affections during pregnancy.

Eyes - Objects appear black. Eyes prominent, with burning and lachrymation during cough.

Face - ***Red, but cold,*** or pale and red alternately. Pain in fine line coursing along the nerve. Lips, swollen, cracked, burning.

Female - Menopausal disturbances with burning of tip of tongue. Pushing or sticking sensation in ovarian (left) region with disorders of menses. Uterine hemorrhage near the menopause, with nausea. Sticking sensation in left ovarian region.

Food - Craves stimulating, pungent things, wants a bracer. ***Much thirst, but drinking causes shuddering.*** Desire for coffee, but it nauseates. Vegetables cause flatulence.

Head - Bursting headache, worse coughing, better heat, movement, lying with head high. Hot face. Red cheeks. Face red, though cold (Asaf.).

Kidneys - Strangury, frequent, almost ineffectual urging. ***Burning in orifice.*** Comes first in drops, then in spurts, neck of bladder spasmodically contracted. Thick, white creamy discharge from urethra, with gonorrhea. Drinking excites urination and stool. Meatus everted.

Limbs - Joints crack, stiff, painful on beginning to move, pain as if paralyzed. Sciatica, worse bending backwards and coughing. Leg (left) atrophied with violent pain. Staggers when walking. Pain from hips to feet, worse coughing. Tensive pain in the knee.

Lungs - Pain at apex of heart or in rib region, worse touch. Dry, hacking cough, expelling an offensive breath from lungs. Dyspnea. Explosive cough. Feels as if chest and head would fly to pieces. Ribs seem dislocated. ***Pain in distant parts on coughing***, bladder, legs, ears, etc. Wants to take deep breath, thinking that it would relieve all her symptoms. Too weak to cough out expectoration. Asthma with redness of face, worse ascending. Hoarseness in singers and preachers. Threatening gangrene of lung.

Male - ***Coldness of the scrotum,*** with impotency, with softening and dwindling. Atrophy, softening of testes with loss of sensibility, spermatic cord shriveled. Prepuce swollen. Cramps in testes after emission. Trembling of the whole body during amorous caresses. Gonorrhea with chordee, excessive burning, pain in prostate.

Modalities - Better from continued motion. Better heat. Better while eating. ***Worse from slight draft,*** even warm. ***Worse cold air.*** Worse cold water. Worse uncovering. Worse dampness. Worse bathing. Worse touch. Worse from empty swallowing. Worse drinking. After eating, the throat or excited urination is worse, in alcoholics. Rest aggravates some forms of headache and improves others. Motion causes headache as if skull would split, as if bruised, asthma, chilliness, stiff joints to crack. Ascending causes asthma.

Mouth - ***Stomatitis. Tongue greenish at base.*** Burning in tip of tongue. Vesicles or flat painful aphthae. Gums, hot, spongy, retracted. Saliva increased. Taste, foul like putrid water, sour to food. ***Fetid odor from mouth***. Herpes of lips (apply one drop of the mother tincture.).

Nose - ***Red but cold,*** tip very hot. Nosebleed in the morning in bed.

Rectum - Dysentery. Mucus diarrhea. ***Bloody mucus with burning and tenesmus***, drawing pain in back after stool. Small, hot, burning stools. ***Thirsty after stool with shivering***, worse drinking. Stinging pain during stool. Burning, ***bleeding from hemorrhoids*** with soreness of anus.

Skin - Burning. Bloated, flabby.

Sleep - Sleeplessness from emotions, homesickness or cough. Sleepy after meals. Yawning by day. As if falling from a height during sleep.

Stomach - Much flatulence, especially in debilitated subjects. Vomiting, sinking at pit of stomach. Water brash. Acid dyspepsia, burning or trembling in stomach or icy coldness or as if cold water.

Temperature - Coldness with ill-humor. Chilly with the pains. Thirst before chill. ***Shivering after drinking***. Chill begins in back with violent thirst, but shivers from every drink with excruciating backache. Chill alternating with heat, mounting to head, then sweat. Coldness of affected part. Sweats easily. Cold sweat on thighs. Fevers after emotions with homesickness. Must have something hot to back.

Throat - Burning, smarting in throat. ***Hot feeling in fauces.*** Constriction of throat with urging to swallow. Inflamed uvula and palate, swollen, elongated and relaxed, feeling as if it were pressing on something hard. ***Pain and dryness in throat*** extending to the ears. ***Sore throat of smokers and drinkers.*** Paralytic dysphagia. Hot, pungent air comes up from the throat, tasting foul when coughing. Pains when coughing.

COMMENTS - A case of poisoning in a worker in a capsicum-plaster factory brought out a severe chill with shaking and it ended in an intense coryza.

Mastoiditis. Glossitis. Cystitis. Dysentery (Canth.). Bloody mucus. Hemorrhage, helps stop blood flow. Ulcers and burning. Herpes, where there is a smarting, burning sensation on the sores. Characteristic cough with fetid breath or bad taste. Cough causing splitting pain in head. Chill at 10:30 a.m., beginning between shoulders and running down back.

Homesickness (Calc-p., Ign., Nat-m.). Weight loss, insomnia, loss of appetite, depression. "Pining." A lot of sighing, respiration..

Clarke cured completely with a few doses of Caps., an Australian girl of florid complexion, who had come to London to study and who was quite incapacitated by homesickness.

Delirium. Successful in delirium tremens, mostly in drachm doses of the tincture, given in milk or tincture of orange peel. Equal parts of tincture of Caps. and glycerin make a liniment for external use in many cases of chronic rheumatism and neuralgia.

Caps. 30c brought speedy relief in a case of tympanites following laparotomy, the concomitant symptoms included cold nose and limbs and cyanosis.

RELATIONS - ***Antidoted by:*** Calad., Camph., Cina, Chin., Sul-ac. or vapor of burning sulphur. It antidotes: Effects of Alcohol, Coffee, Opium or Quinine. ***Compare:*** (1) Arn., Bell., Bry. - headache from cough, Canth. - burning pains, throat symptoms, dysentery, urinary symptoms. (2) Psor. - lack of reaction, despair of recovery, Caps. in persons of lax tissue. (3) Lach - thirst before chill, continues into chill, drinking Worse also Elaps. (4) Nat-m., Carb-v. and Meny. (5) intermittents, Nat-m. is the *"chronic"* of Caps. (6) Carb-an. and Nit-ac. - inflammation behind ears, Aur. and Nit-ac. preferable in abscess, Sil. in chronic suppuration. (7) Ph-ac. - homesickness, Caps. has red face. (8) Ars., Alum., Carb-v., Lyc. have burning pains better by heat. (9) Merc., Nit-ac., Sulph. have passage of blood from bowels. (10) Crot-t. after drinking urging to stool. (11) Hell. - colic with spasm of bladder. (12) Plat. - burning, pungent pain in face, worse slightest drought of air, warm or cold. (13) Puls., Lyc., Bell. (14) Centaurea - surging of blood, homesickness intermittent fever. ***Compatible:*** Bell., Lyc., Puls., Sil.

REFERENCES - Boericke. Clarke. Murphy.

CARBO ANIMALIS

(Animal Charcoal)

PHARMACY - carb-an. Carbo animalis. Animal charcoal. Made from charred ox-hide. Contains Calc-p. Trituration. ***Historical dose:*** Trituration and all potencies.

CLINICAL - Acne, rosacea. Aneurysm. ***Asphyxiation.*** Appetite, disordered. Belchings. ***Breast, cancer.*** Breast-feeding. ***Bronchitis***. Bubo. ***Cancer.*** Cataract. Constipation. Coccyx, pain. Cough. Empyema. Face, eruption. Gangrene. ***Glandular, indurations.*** Hemorrhoids. Headaches. Homesickness. ***Hookworm.*** Hypertrophy. Legs, pain. Leucorrhea. Lumbago. Nose, disorders. Otorrhea. Pancreas, indurated. Perspiration, altered. Pleurisy. ***Pneumonia***. Polyps. ***Scrofula.*** Strabismus. Syphilis. Tongue disorders. Trachea, disorders. ***Ulceration.*** Uterus, cancer. Vision, disorders.

HOMEOPATHIC - Carb-an., or animal charcoal, is made from charred ox hide, it contains Calc-p. in small quantity. The Carbon group all have putrid discharges and exhalations. All act on the skin, causing interrigo and excoriations and Carb-tcl. is said to cause fatty liver (Phos., Kreos., Chlf.).

Carb-an. is often indicated in the ***last stage of cancer, pneumonia, bronchitis, tuberculosis.*** Breast cancer with burning, drawing pains through breast. Right chest is most affected. Uterine cancer, burning pains down thigh. ***Tendency to malignancy.***

Glands enlarge slowly and painfully, burning. Glandular enlargements with catarrhal states, flatulency and asphyxiation. Painful swelling, lancinating, cutting and burning (Con., Merc-i-f.). ***Glands are indurated,*** veins distended, skin blue. Glands are stony hard. Neglected buboes.

Marked tendency to induration of glands and tissues. Indurations after inflammations. ***Ulceration and decomposition***. Hemorrhages. Gangrene. Offensive secretions. Discharges are acrid and foul. Slow, hard, painful processes. Sensations of looseness, crawling as of bugs.

Stitch remaining after pleurisy (Bry.). Venous stasis, blue skin. Local ***congestions without heat***. Copper-colored eruptions. Constitutional syphilis. Gummae.

Paralysis of muscles of feet and hands. Patients are susceptible to colds and easy sprains. Easily strained from lifting. ***Hookworm*** disease (Thymol.).

Especially adapted to scrofulous and venous constitutions. Suited to weak, broken-down constitutions and to the infirmities of old age or those prematurely aged. After debilitating disease with feeble circulation and lowered vitality. Weakness of nursing women, they weep while eating, unable to walk even across the room.

MIND - Alternations of mood and overexcitability, alternating with fretful sadness. Sadness in morning. ***Aversion to company.*** Desire to be alone, sad and reflective. ***Avoids conversation***. Weeps during meals. Whining.

Cheerfulness alternating with sadness. Homesickness, longing for the past. Homesickness in morning. Forsaken feeling in morning. Anger about former vexations, about past events.

Easily frightened. Fear of the dark, worse on closing eyes. Anxiety at night with orgasm of blood. Fear of suffocation on closing eyes. Frightful images before sleep. Starting on falling asleep.

Stupefaction, with vertigo, has to close eyes, when rising after stool. Confusion better epistaxis. Confusion in morning, did not know whether he had been asleep or awake. Difficulty in expressing ideas when writing. Hastiness. Irritability in morning, with heavy and dull head.

Abdomen - Great distention after a operation. As of a hard body in groin (left) worse sitting, better pressure and passing flatus. Feeling of coldness rising into the throat. Induration of pancreas. Neglected bubo.

Back - Coccyx feels bruised, burns when touched, worse sitting or lying. Coldness and aching in lumbar region with cough.

Breasts - Weakness of nursing women. Darting in breast, ***painful indurations*** in breast, especially right, while nursing, arresting breathing. Hard painful nodes in breast. ***Last stages of breast cancer***.

Causations - Ill effects of eating spoiled fish or decayed vegetables. They are over affected by small vital losses. Sprains.

Constitutions - Constitutional syphilis. Suited to old persons, greatly debilitated, especially when there is venous plethora and blueness of skin. Persons whose vitality becomes low on account of some serious or deep seated diseased condition or loss of fluids.

Ears - Parotid gland swollen. Otorrhea with swelling of mastoid. Sharp pain. Hearing confused, ***cannot tell direction of sound.*** Ringing in ears, when blowing the nose.

Eyes - Pains down through (right) eyeball. Sensation as if something lay above eyes, so that she could not look up. As if eyeball were loose in the socket. Objects seem to be far off. Dimness of vision when reading, better rubbing eyes. Senile cataract.

Face - Bluish cheeks and lips. Copper colored eruptions. Acne, large number of pimples.

Female - Menses too early, frequent, long lasting, dark, clotted, putrid, ***followed by great exhaustion.*** So weak can hardly speak (Cocc.). Flow only in the morning (Bor., Sep.). Leucorrhea, watery, burning, biting. Worse walking or standing, stains linen yellow. Nausea of pregnancy, worse at night. Offensive lochia (Kreos., Rhus-t., Sec.), thin, long lasting, with numb limbs. Right ovary seems a heavy ball. Burning in vagina and labia. Indurated os with burning. Uterine hemorrhage with disorders of glands. ***Cancer of uterus,*** burning pain down thighs, pelvic bones pain on sitting.

Head - Rush of blood with confusion. Headache, As if skull had been split or blown to pieces, must press it with both hands, better eating. Brain feels loose, worse motion and coughing. Throbbing headache after menses. Sensation as if something lay above eyes so that she could not look up.

Heart - Palpitations when hearing singing in church or in public places. Coldness in precordial region with goose bumps.

Limbs - Axillary glands, swollen, indurated. ***Night sweat*** fetid and profuse. Wrist pain. Hands numb with chest disorders. Joints weak, easy dislocation. Ankles turn easily. Pain in hip joints at night. Pain in coccyx, burns when touched. Straining and over-lifting produces a great debility. Easy discoloration.

Lungs - Nervous dyspnea. Suffocation on closing eyes. Pleurisy, typhoid character, with remaining stitch. Ulceration of lungs with feeling of coldness in lungs. Cough with discharge of greenish pus. Sputum, dark, brown tough, syrup-like.

Male - Syphilis. Bubo.

Modalities - Better in warm room. Better from laying hand on affected part. Worse from slight causes. Worse losses of vital fluids. Worse after or during menses. Worse from sprains. Worse lifting. Worse touch. Worse taking cold. Worse dry, cold air. Worse after shaving. Worse while eating. Cough is worse lying on right side. Throbbing headache worse in open air. Weakness worse during menses.

Mouth - Salty or sour water runs from the mouth. Knotty indurations in the tongue. Bites cheeks while eating. Teeth loose, worse chewing and least cold. Toothache better eating salty things.

Nose - Hard, red, swollen, hot with itching pimples and desquamation. Brown stripe across the nose. Nose swollen, tip bluish, small tumor on it. Fluent coryza with loss of smell with yawning and sneezing.

Rectum - Anus sore. Moisture, oozing from anus and on perineum.

Skin - Unsightly scars from eruptions. Spongy ulcers, copper-colored eruption. Acne rosacea. Chilblains, worse in evening in bed and from cold. Warts on hands and face of elderly people, with bluish color of limbs. Burning, rawness and fissures, moisture. Bubo.

Sleep - Full of vivid fancies, Talks, groans, sheds tears in sleep. Talking and weeping in sleep.

Stomach - All food distresses the stomach. Repugnance to fat food. Eating tires patient. Weak, empty feeling in stomach. Burning and griping. ***Weak digestion, flatulence***. Heartburn. Retching, vomiting, hiccough with stomach cancer. Sensation of coldness around the stomach better rubbing and pressure. Nausea from smoking, which causes aversion to tobacco. Nausea, worse at night, of pregnancy. Faint gone feeling in stomach not better by eating in nursing women. Ptomaine poisoning.

Temperature - Hot flushes. Sweat, foul, exhausting, at night, staining yellow.

Throat - Raw feeling like heartburn, better eating.

Vertigo - Vertigo after shaving, better reeling. Vertigo followed by nosebleed.

COMMENTS - Carb-an. is animal charcoal (Carb-v. is plant ash) and has similar affects as Bufo. Swollen glands with suppuration. Glands become indurated, have bluish color. Often used in the last stages of cancer with decomposition of tissue and sloughing off of tissue. Swollen inguinal glands that suppurate. Inflamed axillary glands. Buboes.

Affections from loss of animal fluids, especially nursing women. Weakness of nursing women, can hardly walk across the room. "Gone" feeling from loss of fluids. Too weak to eat. Weeps when eating.

Aversion to dark. Aversion to cold (Carb-v. to heat). Sensations of coldness, particularly in chest, about stomach. Coldness of the stomach, better pressure from hand.

Nausea at night. Hunger in early morning. Emptiness, not better by eating (Carb-v. better eating). Constipation where patient thinks bowels will be moved but only wind passes.

Discharges are ichorous, but the discharge from hemorrhoids is odorless. Secretions stain yellow, particularly sweat and leucorrhea.

Ichorous otorrhea and swelling of the periosteum over the mastoid bone. Hearing is confused, cannot tell the direction from which sounds come. Carb-an. 3x trituration has been used for ear polyps.

Hoarse, suffocating cough producing a shaking of the brain as if it were loose. Expectoration is greenish, purulent offensive (Carb-v. yellow, more fetid). Tip of nose red or blue. Disagreeable smoothness of the teeth.

Smothering feeling on closing eyes. Feeling of looseness of eyes in sockets, on motion or coughing. Far-sighted (Carb-v. is near-sighted). Objects seem farther apart and brighter.

Neuralgia of the bone. Injured coccyx, with a dragging, bruised pain, burning when touched. Gnawing pains in tibia (during the night), such as usually followed cold feet. Lumbago when walking, standing and lying, feels as if the back were broken.

A. W. K. Choudhury reports a case of cough of two years' duration in an unhealthy boy of twelve, cured by Carb-an. The symptoms were: "Cough evening and morning or after lying down, especially at night, thick or frothy whitish or yellowish sputa, sweetish when thick, worse lying on right side, worse from exposure to air to which he is very sensitive. Great tendency to catch cold."

RELATIONS - ***Antidoted by:*** Ars., Camph., Nux-v. Vinegar. ***Antidote to:*** Effects of Quinine. ***Compare:*** (1) Thymol., Badiaga, Sep., Sulph., Plb. iod. (2) Calc-p. - nearest analog, Carb-an. contains Calc-p. (3) in indurations, suppurations etc., Bad., Brom. (4) loss of fluids, Chin. (5) Graph., nostrils adhere to septum. (6) Phos., gone feeling, loss of fluids induration of cervix, pressure on back, groins and thighs during menses. (6) Cocc. has similar weakness and prostration as Carb-an. (7) Puls., Sil. (8) in vertigo with nosebleed, Sulph. (9) aversion to darkness, Am-m., Bar-c. Calc., Stroph., Stram. (10) hunger in early morning, Ant-c., Asar., Calc., Sabad. (11) swelling behind ear, Caps., Aur. (12) burning pains, Caps. (13) weakness of nursing women, Olnd. ***Complementary:*** Calc-p.

REFERENCES - Boericke. Clarke. Murphy.

CARBO VEGETABILIS

(Vegetable Charcoal)

PHARMACY - carb-v. Carbo vegetabilis. Vegetable charcoal. Carbo ligni. Contains impure carbon. Trituration. ***Historical dose:*** Trituration and all potencies.

CLINICAL - Acidity, Acne. ***Air hunger.*** Anemia. Angina Pectoris. Aortitis. Aphonia. ***Asphyxiation.*** Asthenopia. ***Asthma. Belching. Body, cold.*** Breast, erysipelas. ***Blood, loss. Breathing, labored.*** Bronchitis. Burns. Carbuncle. Catarrh. Chilblains. ***Chills. Cholera. Coldness.*** Colds. ***Collapse. Coma.*** Constipation. Cough. Deafness. Debility. ***Dehydration.*** Diarrhea. ***Digestion, weak.*** Distention. Dysentery. Dyspepsia. Emphysema. Erysipelas. ***Fainting.*** Feet, cold. ***Flatulence.*** Gangrene. Hair, loss. Headache. Heart, diseases. ***Heartburn. Hemorrhages.*** Hemorrhoids. ***Hypothermia.*** Influenza. Intermittents. Intertrigo. Irritation. Laryngitis. Lungs, congested. Measles. Mumps. Nosebleeds. Esophagitis. Orchitis. Otorrhea. Pneumonia. Pregnancy, disorders. Purpura. Scabies. Scurvy. Shiverings. ***Shock.*** Sleep, disorders. ***Stomach, disordered.*** Stomatitis. Trachea, dryness. Tympanites. Typhus. Ulcers. ***Vitality, low.*** Yellow fever. ***Weakness.***

HOMEOPATHIC - Carb-v., or vegetable charcoal, is itself a product of ***imperfect oxidation*** and disintegration, which are the keynotes of this remedy. It contains small quantity of Kali-carb., potassium carbonate.

Provings with the crude Carb-v. and the potentized substances showed that the latter were much more powerful in their effect on the organism. These brought out the fact that there is an exact correspondence between the effect of crude charcoal and potentized Carb-v. Both are anti-septic and deodorant.

The deodorant and disinfectant properties of charcoal in bulk had already been discovered when Hahnemann was at work on the Materia Medica. Its a deodorant, disinfectant and anti-septic properties are more enhanced in potencies. The signs and symptoms of decay and putrefaction are the leading indication for its medicinal use.

Carb-v. antidotes the effects of putrid meats or fish, rancid fats, salt or salt meats, and also the pathogenic actions of Chin., Lach. and Merc. Decomposition of food in the stomach, putrid diseases and ulcerations, symptoms of imperfect oxygenation of the blood.

Carb-v. acts upon the ***venous circulation*** and capillaries. ***Hemorrhage,*** blood dark, oozing from shock after surgical operations, persistent for hours or days. Hemorrhage from any mucus surface.

The blood seems to stagnate, causing blueness, coldness and ecchymoses. ***Body becomes blue, icy-cold. Vitality becomes low*** from loss of vital fluids. Bacteria find a rich soil in the nearly lifeless blood stream and sepsis and typhoid states ensue. Putrid (septic) condition of all its affections, coupled with a burning sensation.

Very debilitated. ***Almost lifeless***, but the head is hot, coldness, breath cool, pulse imperceptible, oppressed and quickened respiration. ***Must have air, must be fanned hard, must have all the windows open.*** Cold, but wants air to be fanned or thirst for cold water. ***Faints easily, is worn out***. Tremulous.

Always ***weak, sick and exhausted,*** but those states may occur suddenly. ***State of collapse*** in cholera, typhoid or other grave diseases. When the patient is almost lifeless, cold body, breath cold, pulse imperceptible, respiration quickened.

Lack of reaction after some violent attack, violent shock, violent suffering. Never well since. Patient seems to be too weak to hold out. ***Persons who have never fully recovered from the effects of some previous illness.*** Weakness from grave or serious diseases, from effects of drug and disease, or from obstinate complications.

Septic conditions. Lymphatic glands, are swollen, indurated or suppurating. Gangrene, humid, senile. Thick, acrid discharges. Ulcerations, aphthous. ***Blueness and decomposition. Flatulence, fetor***.

Sensation of fullness. Sense of weight, as in the head (occiput), eyes and eyelids, before the ears in the stomach and elsewhere in the body. General bruised soreness, old catarrhs. Bedwetting, which is worse in morning after the first sleep.

Burning itching on skin. Frozen limbs. Chilblains, excoriations between toes. Numbness of parts lain on. Burning, sense of weight or heavy aching in bones, ulcers etc. Tinea capitis or scald-head. Scalp very sensitive, feels as if bruised.

Whooping cough with pain at base of brain. Excessive gagging cough in the morning, compelling him to vomit everything, immediately after breakfast (Dros.).

MIND - Confusion, which makes thinking difficult. Confusion better mental exertion. Torpor and indolence. Slow thinking, worse in morning on waking. Sudden loss of memory. ***Indifference to everything he hears or sees.*** Indifference, hears everything without pleasure or pain. Indifference to music which he loves.

Sluggish, slow, lazy. Peevish, irritable and inclined to anger. Anxiety in evening, could scarcely remain lying still. ***Anxiety in morning*** on waking. Anxiety on closing eyes. Restlessness in company. Indolent. Irritable. Dejected. Child wishes to vent itself in rage, strikes, kicks, bites, in worm affections.

Oversensitive to noise. Timidity about appearing in public. Aversion to presence of strangers. Fear of people. Easily frightened or startled. Aversion to darkness. Fear of ghosts. Fear of accidents. Sees frightful images in the dark.

Abdomen - ***Greatly distended,*** especially upper part, worse lying down, better passing wind. ***Flatulent colic***, forcing the patient to bend double. Obstructed flatulence, giving rise to complaints. Pain as from lifting a weight. Abdomen feels as if hanging down, walks bent. Cannot bear tight clothing around waist and abdomen. Epigastric region very tender. Ailments from intestinal fistulae. Abdominal sufferings, worse from the smallest portion of food.

Back - Severe pain in small of back, with a sensation of a plug, unable to sit down, had to put a pillow under it when lying. Burning behind shoulder.

Breasts - Lumps in breasts with indurations of axillary glands. Breasts, hard, swollen with impending abscess. Prostration after nursing.

Causations - Carbon monoxide poisoning. Blood loss. Shock. Surgery. Effects of alcohol, meat, fish, especially if tainted, ice-water, vegetables, salt or salt meats. Disorders from high living and especially butter-eating.

Chest - Heavy sore or weak chest, on awakening. Burning in chest with hemoptysis. Brown yellow spots on chest. Sore ribs.

Constitutions - Suited to atonic conditions where there is lack of reaction. The typical Carb-v, patient is fat, sluggish, lazy and has a tendency to chronicity of complaints. Complaints of old people. Persons who have never fully recovered from the effects of some previous illness. School girls and boys are sluggish, slow to learn, suffer from night terrors, will not sleep alone or go to bed in the dark.

Ears - Deafness or otorrhea, following exanthemata. Ears dry. Something heavy seems to lie before the ears. Deficient or badly smelling yellow wax. Mumps with metastases.

Eyes - As of heavy weight on eyes. Hemorrhages from eyes with congestion to head. Vision of floating black spots. Burning in eyes. Muscles of eyes painful when looking up. Pupils do not react to light. Asthenopia.

Face - Face blue, cold with cold sweat. Puffy, cyanotic, ***pale***, ***hippocratic,*** pinched (Cupr., Op.). Mottled cheeks and red nose. Twitching upper lip. Brown or black looking, cracked lips.

Female - Too early and too copious menses, pale blood. During menstruation, burning in hands and soles. Menorrhagia, burning across sacrum, passive flow. Leucorrhea, thick, greenish, milky, causing itching and burning, worse before menses. Feels best with a free leucorrhea. Sore, hot, itching, swollen, vulva. Vulva swollen, aphthae. Varicose veins on pudendum and vulva with burning, bluish ulcers. Vaginal fistula, burning pains.

Food - Aversion to ***fat things***, meat and milk, which causes flatulence. Aversion to the most digestible and the best kind of food. Desire for salty, sour things or sweet things, coffee. Worse from brandy.

Head - Cold sweat on forehead. Head hot with cold limbs. Takes cold in head easily. Dull, compressive, heavy. Headaches, worse occiput, worse overheating, lying or pressure of hat, ***over-indulgence.*** Pimples on forehead and face. ***Hair, sore, falls off easily*** in handfuls, after severe illness, after childbirth. Scalp itches when warm in bed. Hat pressed upon head like a heavy weight.

Heart - Continuous anxious palpitation, worse eating, sitting. Thread-like, weak and small, intermittent pulse. Burning around the heart. Pulsation throughout the body.

Kidneys - Albumin, protein in the urine. Nephritis, septic or from alcohol. Urine, copious, clear yellow or thick and whitish. Diabetes. Bedwetting at night. Urine, suppressed in cholera and retained from standing on the cold pavements.

Limbs - Heavy, stiff, feel paralyzed. ***Limbs go to sleep***. Want of muscular energy, joints weak. Burning pain in bones and limbs. Numbness when lying on limbs. Pain in shins. ***Cold from knees down***. Cramp in soles. Feet numb and sweaty. Foul foot sweat, worse walking. Toes red, swollen. Senile gangrene of fingers and toes with fiery burning vesicles, oozing bloody water. Paralytic weakness of the wrists and of the fingers, when seizing anything. Arms weary when writing.

Liver - Pain in liver. Jaundice from over eating or eating too rich food.

Lungs - ***Asphyxiation.*** Breathing, laborious, quick and short, worse walking. Wants to take a deep breath. Breath cold, ***must be fanned***. Cheyne-Stokes breathing in organic heart disease. Destructive lung diseases. Cough with itching in larynx, spasmodic with gagging and vomiting of mucus. ***Cough with burning in chest***, worse in evening, in open air, after eating and talking. ***Spasmodic cough,*** bluish face, offensive expectoration. Occasional spells of long coughing attacks. Wheezing and rattling of mucus in chest. Expectoration with retching. Expectoration is very thick, sticky, yellow and profuse. Hemorrhage from lungs. Neglected pneumonia. Whooping cough, especially in the beginning, with bluish face, and its complications. ***Asthma in aged with blue skin***. ***Hoarseness, worse evenings***, talking, evening oppression of breathing, sore and raw chest. Roughness in larynx with deep rough voice.

Male - Discharge of prostatic fluid, while straining at stool. Itching and moisture at thigh near scrotum. Seminal discharge too soon during sex, followed by roaring in head. Swelling of testes from metastasis of mumps.

Modalities - ***Better from belchings.*** Better elevating feet. Better cool air. Better from fanning. ***Worse from high living, rich food.*** Worse decayed food. Worse from poultry, fat food, butter, coffee, milk, ***Worse wine***. Worse icy drinks. ***Worse from warmth,*** warm, damp weather, humid, cooling off. Worse walking in open air. Worse cold night air, frosty, wind on head. Worse extremes of temperature. ***Worse from depletions. Worse exhausting diseases.*** Worse dissipation. Worse suppressions. Worse over lifting. Worse pressure of clothes. Worse old age. Worse reading aloud, singing.

Mouth - ***Breath cold.*** Bad smell from mouth. Bitter, sour, taste. Increased saliva. Tongue, cold, black, swollen, covered with white, yellow-brown mucus. Aphthae, bluish, black ulcers with burning. Loose teeth. Tooth pain while eating hot or cold things. Teeth very sensitive when chewing. Scorbutic gums. Blood oozes from gums when cleaning teeth. Gums retracted and bleed easily, painful while chewing. Gums black. Pyorrhea.

Nose - ***Nosebleed in daily attacks with pale face.*** Bleeding after straining, with pale face. Tip of nose red and scabby, itching around nostrils. Eruption in corner of nose. Varicose veins on nose. Descending colds. Nose cold, hay asthma. Coryza with cough, especially in moist, warm weather. Sneezing from irritation in larynx, worse blowing nose. Ineffectual effort to sneeze.

Rectum - Hot, moist offensive flatus. Itching, gnawing and burning in rectum and anus. ***Acrid, corrosive moisture from rectum.*** A musty, glutinous moisture exudes. Excoriation of anus. Soreness, itching, moisture of perineum, especially at night. Discharge of blood from rectum. Burning varicose veins (Mur-ac.). ***Bluish,*** white, burning hemorrhoids, pain after stools. Ineffectual urging, even soft stool passed with difficulty. Frequent, involuntary, putrid, cadaverous smelling stools, followed by burning. Feces escape with flatus. Painful diarrhea of old people.

Skin - ***Blue, cold and bruised***. Purpura. Wounds heal and break out again. Marbled with venous over-distention. Moist skin, ***hot perspiration***. Fine moist rash with burning. Burning in various places. Itching, worse on evening, when warm in bed. Bedsores, bleed easily. Foul ulcers, indolent, burning and bleeding. ***Varicose ulcers***, bleeding easily, pus smells like asafetida. Ulcers heal and break out again. Ichorous, offensive discharge. Tendency to gangrene of the margins. Senile gangrene beginning in the toes. Carbuncles (Ars., Anthr.). Varicose veins during pregnancy. Falling out of hair from a general weakened condition.

Sleep - Unrefreshing. Awakes often from cold limbs especially cold knees. Comatose sleep with rattling in throat. Frequent yawning and stretching which seems to agree. Horror during sleep.

Stomach - Burning in stomach, extending to back along spine, with coldness. ***Contractive pains extending to chest with distention of abdomen***. Epigastric region is very sensitive. Faint empty feeling in stomach, not relieved by eating. Loathes even the thought of food. Crampy pains forcing patient to bend double. ***Digestion slow, food putrefies*** before it digests. ***The simplest food distresses.*** Distress comes on a half-hour after eating. Rancid, sour or putrid ***belchings***. Belchings after eating and drinking, temporary relief from belching. ***Heartburn.*** Water brash, asthmatic breathing from flatulence. ***Heaviness, fullness and sleepiness***, tense from flatulence, with pain, worse lying down. Stomach ulcers, cancer. Vomiting of blood. Nausea in the morning. Stomach pain of nursing women.

Temperature - ***Icy coldness,*** unilateral of tongue, knees, legs, foot, at night. Coldness with thirst. Chill begins in forearm. Cold worse coughing. Alternate chill and heat. Warm head and cold limbs. Internal burning heat, at heart, chest with cold icy skin and cold sweat. Burning in various places. Yellow fever. Hectic fever, exhausting sweats. Sweats easily, on eating. Sweat sour on face.

Throat - Sensation as if closed. Aphthous, sore. Hawking of bloody, black mucus. Painful on swallowing food.

Vertigo - Vertigo with nausea and tinnitus.

COMMENTS - Suited to conditions where there is lack of reaction (Op.) to low states of the vital powers, where the venous system is engorged. Lack of reaction in pupils (Op.).

For near death states. "The corpse reviver." In India, they say it pulls back souls from the jaws of death. Comas (Op., Chin.). Diabetic comas. Usually given for the last stage of processes. Last stage of pneumonia, cyanotic, weak, debilitated, faint.

Shock from heart failure (Arn. first). Never well since a traumatic accident where they feel weak and sluggish. Hypo-oxygenation, with shortness of breath, varicose veins, hemorrhoids, gas and bloating. Weakness after hemorrhage.

Listless and indifferent. Feebleness. Collapse (Camph.), with short, shallow breathing. Collapse with cold knees. The patient sinks and breaks out in a cold sweat, faints and collapses from weakness and lack of air (Acon., Ign., or Gels. if from emotional trauma).

Debility of greater intensity than Carbo an. in children or old people after exhausting diseases. Great debility as soon as he makes the least effort. Debility following childbirth, causing falling out of hair.

Cannot be aroused, cannot think, so weak they cannot lift their head off the pillow (Stann. is weak in the chest, can barely speak).

Frequent hemorrhages. Nosebleeds or hemorrhage from throat in dysentery. Hemorrhage from the bowels, lungs. Dyspnea, from chronic aortitis. Congestive symptoms like those of poisoning by carbonic acid. Pulse thready, face pale, covered with cold sweat, desire to be fanned, anxiety without restlessness.

Fever, intermittent, hectic, typhoid, yellow fever and cholera. In intermittents of long standing where quinine has been abused. Thirst only during chill. Feet ice-cold up to knees. Heat in burning flushes. Sweat sour or offensive. Weak, befogged mind.

Characteristic coldness. Worse from warmth. Great desire for air, must be fanned. Cold breath (cholera), cold knees, cold, but wants to be fanned.

Dull headache in occiput with confusion of mind, proceeding from occiput to forehead, dull, heavy aching over eyes in warm room, buzzing in ears, very sensitive to pressure of hat. Hippocratic countenance. Vertigo from stomach with fainting, especially at meals.

Burning pains (Carb-an.), especially in the limbs, with varicose veins. Numbness of limbs. Lividity, mottled skin. Round ulcers. Indolent gangrene. Varicose veins of arms, legs, vulva.

Catarrh from warm, moist atmosphere. Cough is worse on entering cold air from a warm room. Hoarseness from damp air, worse morning or evening. Cough caused by a sensation as if sulphur fumes were in larynx.

Menorrhagia and metrorrhagia with burning pains across sacrum and spine. Corrosive menstrual discharge, strong pungent odor. Premature and profuse menses. Headache during menses. Preceded and followed by leucorrhea. Greenish yellow leucorrhea, worse in morning. Leucorrhea excoriates. Perineum moist, raw, oozing. Itching, burning soreness and smarting at vulva and anus. Hemorrhoids.

Excessive accumulation of gas in stomach and intestines. "Stomach feels full and tense from flatulence. Great pain in stomach on account of flatulence, worse especially on lying down." Weak digestion with much flatulence, better by eructation. Flatulence accompanies many other complaints, including asthma and heart disorders.

Heaviness in the stomach, full feeling and burning. Aversion to fat, meat, and milk, which causes flatulence. Desire for coffee (which does not relieve), for acids, for sweet and salt things.

Guernsey considered Carb-v. especially suited to cachectic individuals whose vital powers has become weakened. In cases where disease seems to have been engrafted on the system by reason of the depressing influence of some prior derangement.

A. H. Birdsall recorded a typical case of Carb-v. intermittent. "A man, 36, had fever eight months, partially suppressed by Arsenic and Quinine. Type, tertian. Headache for one or two hours before chill.

"Chill always from 9 to 10 a.m., beginning in feet and hands, spreading over body, nails very blue. Thirst with chill. Cold stage lasts two to three hours, followed immediately by hot stage, much heat in head and face, which is flushed red, thirstlessness. Sweating stage short, sweat sour.

"Apyrexia: Sweats easily, especially from least warmth, awakens in morning always with slight sour-smelling sweat. Weak, dispirited, flatulent. A single dose of Carb-v. cured. There were only three more attacks, each of diminished intensity."

A carbon ointment made by carbonizing a wine cork by plunging it into a clear fire and then, in its still glowing state, into Vaseline and mixing thoroughly is regarded as a sovereign remedy in anal irritation and hemorrhoid troubles.

RELATIONS - ***Antidoted by:*** Ars., Ambra, Camph., Coff., Lach., Nit-s-d., Ferr. (Teste). ***It antidotes:*** Effects of putrid meats of fish, rancid fats, salt or salt meats, Chin., Lach., Merc. ***Compare:*** (1) Raph. in flatulence. Caust., Lach., Eup-per., Phos. and Rumex in hoarseness, Rumex is worse 4 a.m. and

11 p.m. Caust. worse in morning from dry cold. Carb-v. worse evening from damp evening air. (2) Camph., China in hemorrhages intermittents, hectic disorders of alcoholics, Ip. in hemorrhages and intermittents, Meny. in intermittents with coldness of legs. (3) Op., Sulph. and Psor. in deficient reaction. (4) Sul-ac. in dyspepsia of alcoholics. Carb-v. has more putridity, Sul-ac. more sourness. (5) Phos. in easily bleeding ulcers, Puls., bad effect from fat food and pastry, Sulph. in acrid-smelling menses, erysipelas of breasts, Ars. and Bellis in effects of ice-cream and ice-water in hot weather. (6) Nux-v. in dyspepsia, easily angered, effects of debauchery. Nux-v. is thin, spare, yellow, wiry, Carb-v sluggish, stout, lazy. (7) Sec. in hemorrhages, cold breath, coldness worse by warmth. Calc., Carb-an. and Stram. in aversion to darkness. (8) Lach. in weak digestion. Lach. craves milk, Carb-v. has aversion to it. Intolerance of clothing around waist intermittent fever, flashes of burning heat without thirst. (9) Sep. in bearing-down in rectum and vagina. Carb-v. has strong odor of menses which Sep. has not. (10) Rhus-t. in strains in typhus, Colch. in cholera, cold breath, prostration. Cupr. (11) Carboneum - Spasms commencing in tongue, down trachea and limbs. Tingling sensation. (12) Lyc., Ars., Chin., Carb-v. contains potash. ***Complementary:*** Chin., Dros., Kali-c. - stitches in heart.

REFERENCES - Boericke. Clarke. Murphy.

CARBOLICUM ACIDUM

(Carbolic Acid)

PHARMACY - carb-ac. Carbolicum acidum. Carbolic acid. Phenolum. Phenol. Monoxy benzine. Phenic acid. Phenyl alcohol. Solution in rectified spirit. ***Historical dose:*** Trituration and all potencies.

CLINICAL - Acne. ***Allergic, reactions. Anaphylactic, shock.*** Backache. ***Bee stings.*** Belchings. ***Burns.*** Carbuncles. Cholera. Colds. ***Constipation.*** Diabetes. Diarrhea. Dysentery. ***Dyspepsia.*** Eczema. Erysipelas. Flatulence. Gangrene. Heartburn. Hydrocephalus. Influenza. Intermittent, fever. Irritation. Leprosy. Leucorrhea. Meningitis. Neuralgias. Pneumonia. Psoriasis. Pityriasis, versicolor. ***Prostration***. Scarlatina. Smallpox. Smell, disordered. Stomach, disorders. Toothaches. Ulcers. Uremia. Uterus, displacements. Vomiting.

HOMEOPATHIC - Carb-ac., like the Carbons, is a powerful anti-septic and its use as such in surgery has led, incidentally, to the poisoning of both patients and surgeons. These experiences have provided a number of the symptoms indicating its medicinal use.

Carb-ac. is a languid, painless, foul and destructive remedy. Acts primarily on the central nervous system. It affects the mucus membranes, heart, blood and respiration. Stomach symptoms are also important.

Marked ***prostration***, even paralytic with loss of sensation and motion. Collapse. Stupor. Paralysis of sensation and motion. Feeble pulse and depressed breathing. Death due to paralysis of respiratory centers.

Malignant and septic conditions. Physical exertion brings on abscess somewhere. Discharges are foul, burning. Putrid discharges (Bapt.). Bloody discharges. Scarlet fever with marked tendency to destruction of tissue internally and fetid odor.

Terrible pains coming and going suddenly. Pricking, ***burning sensation.*** Trembling with an uncertain, staggering walk. Arthritis.

Mental and bodily languor, disinclination to study with headache like a band.

Very marked ***acuteness of smell. Increased olfactory sensibility.*** Spasmodic coughs. ***Allergic reactions to bee stings*** (Apis). In cholera when Verat. is indicated but fails.

MIND - Mental and bodily languor. Disinclination to do any mental or physical work. Unfit for study, as reading aggravates all symptoms. Periods of mental abstraction. Mental exertion aggravates. Unconsciousness.

Absent minded, starts when spoken to. Difficulty of remembering passed events. Forgetful, can't remember anything, becomes easily confused. Starts to do something and forgets it. Entire disinclination to study, what he had accomplished seemed very trifling.

Very irritable. Fear of impending disease at night in bed. Sense of bewilderment. Mental and physical exhilaration. Constantly agitated, moaning continuously and occasionally uttering a piercing cry, recognizes no one, acute hydrocephalus.

Abdomen - Flatulence. Colic of nursing infants. Soreness of hypochondria worse motion. Abdominal muscles sore.

Back - Aching between scapula. Pains in loins, worse straightening up and better pressure. Stitching pain, in right side of neck. Drawing in muscles of neck. ***Severe pain, in lumbo-sacral region***. Soreness of muscles of back and limbs.

Bladder - Frequent urination. Irritable bladder in old men, with frequent urination at night, of prostatic nature. Straining on passing urine.

Eyes - Severe orbital neuralgia over right eye. Contraction alternating with dilatation of pupils in hydrocephalus. Neuralgic twitching in eyeballs. Photophobia during headache.

Face - Dusky face. ***Pale about nose and mouth.*** Face pale, pinched, with cold sweat. Face cyanotic. Lips covered with a white membrane. ***Swelling of face and tongue from bee stings.*** Twitching in cheeks and temples. Lupus.

Female - Discharges always offensive (Nit-ac., Nux-v., Sep.). Pustules about vulva containing bloody pus. Severe backache across loins with dragging down thighs, from uterine displacement. ***Painful swelling of left ovary***, worse walking in open air. Induration of cervix. Erosions of cervix, fetid, acrid discharge. Thick, irritating leucorrhea, causing itching and burning (Kreos.). Leucorrhea in children (Cann-s., Merc., Puls., Sep.). Puerperal fever with offensive discharge.

Food - Appetite lost. Cheerful while eating. ***Desire for stimulants and tobacco.*** Desire for whiskey. Nausea from cold water. Hiccough after dinner.

Head - Orbital neuralgia over right eye. Headache, better from green tea, while smoking. Headaches appearing at the time of menses. Tight feeling as if compressed by a rubber band (Gels.). As of a hot ball in forehead. Tender scalp.

Heart - Heart worse after indiscretion in eating. Stitches in region of heart. Palpitation, or violent action of heart at night. Bellows murmur over mitral valves. Organic valvular heart disease. Thready pulse. Pulse rapid, weak or intermittent, irregular.

Kidneys - Tired sensation in renal region. Urine, scanty, green. Urine alkaline. Urine scanty and red, in scarlatina. Urine dark, almost black. Albuminuria. Urine contained albumen in meningitis. Urinated freely an excessive quantity of saccharine urine. Diabetes.

Limbs - Cramps in fore part of leg, close to tibia, during walking. ***Stiffness of limbs, hydrocephaloid.*** Cold hands and feet. Gnawing pains in shin bones. Arthritis.

Modalities - Better from smoking. Better strong tea. Better rubbing, binding. There is intolerance of a warm room, but also sensitiveness to cold air which aggravate many symptoms. Worse from jar. Worse reading. Worse pregnancy. Worse combing hair.

Mouth - Intensely foul breath with constipation. Burning in mouth to stomach. Lips dry, cracked, painful or black.

Nose - ***Smell very acute***. Putrid discharge. Ozaena with fetor and ulceration. Influenza and resulting debility.

Perspiration - Profuse, cold sweat. ***Profound prostration, collapse and bathed in cold sweat.*** Clammy sweat on head, face and hands. Profuse sweat with restlessness. Sweats at night

Rectum - Constipation with retraction of abdomen. ***Constipation with very offensive breath***. Passes mucus from anus while urinating. Fetid, rice water diarrhea. Thin, black, putrid diarrhea. Bloody, like scrapings of intestines. Shreddy stools. Great tenesmus.

Skin - Burning, itching vesicles and pustules. Bloody vesicles or pustules. Burns tend to ulcerate. Erysipelas.

Sleep - Very sleepy.

Stomach - ***Fermentative dyspepsia*** with bad taste and breath. Heat rises up esophagus. Constant belching, nausea, ***vomiting***, heartburn. Flatulent distention of stomach and abdomen. Painful flatulence often marked in one part of the bowel. Nausea and vomiting during pregnancy, from seasickness, cancer. Dark, olive green vomit. Sore stomach.

Temperature - General chilliness and coldness of surface. Chills runs from head downward. Chilly sensation while in a warm room. Chilly in open air.

Throat - Glazed. Fauces red and covered with exudation. Uvula whitened and shriveled. Ulcerated patches on inside of lips and cheeks. ***Burning in mouth to stomach***. ***Putrid discharge***. Almost impossible to swallow. ***Diphtheria, fetid breath, regurgitation*** on swallowing liquids, but little pain (Bapt.). Face dusky red, white about mouth and nose. Rapid sinking of vital forces.

Vertigo - Vertigo, felt as if staggering, like a drunken man. Giddiness, not better closing eyes. Vertigo on going up and down stairs, better walking fast in open air, worse sitting down. Vertigo with fear of falling, trembling.

COMMENTS - Anaphylactic shock from bee stings (Apis, Hist.). The skin is inflamed, and other symptoms appear with burning, tingling, itching and numbness. Pains come suddenly. Burning, pricking, sticking pains. Numbness and twitching.

Profound prostration and fatigue, convulsions, collapse, cold, clammy sweat. Constant yawning. Palpitations of the heart at night. Putrid discharges.

The urine is very dark, black or black olive-green, grass or olive-green. Great flatulent distention of the abdomen with belching of wind. Desire for stimulants. Vomiting in alcoholic, in pregnant women, with violent frontal headache.

Many poisoning cases show pneumonia, single or double, affecting the bases principally. Gangrene has been caused by the application of 2 to 5 percent solutions, prescribed by Dr. Streintz.

Fahnestock observed a case of poisoning from inhaling the fumes. The patient, a woman, feeling ill, ran across the street to a neighbor's. Before reaching the house she fell prostrate, pale, gasping for breath.

When taken in, she had to be propped up in order to breathe, trembled all over, wanted her hands held, "pricking like needles," all over body, unable to raise right arm. Cold hands and feet. Wanted a drink of water every few minutes, nausea but no vomiting, pain in lumbar region. Symptoms lasted four hours.

Allen noted that it relieved cases of cancer of the stomach, and epithelioma of the cheek and nose with hemorrhages.

Deschere found Carb-ac. 30c of great service in uterine displacements with or without discharges but these, if present, are always offensive. The symptoms first relieved are the agonizing backache across the loins with a dragging sensation down the buttocks into the thighs.

Cooper regarded it as specific in influenza in the 3x for the attack and 30c for resulting debility.

Dr. Proctor recorded a brilliant cure of a double basal pneumonia with drop doses of the B. P. solution after failure of more commonly used remedies. Nervous dyspepsia of intensely painful character has frequently been cured by it.

R. K. Ghosh found it admirable in cases of cholera where Verat. seems indicated and fails. There is intolerance of warm room, but also sensitiveness to cold air which aggravates many symptoms.

Ghosh also reported great improvement in a case of diabetes when the remedy was given for something else.

Proell recorded his own case of idiopathic erysipelas affecting the back of the right hand, first three fingers and arm with violet-colored swelling and roughness. Rhus-t. removed the fever, but did nothing to stop the erysipelas. Carb-ac. 30c did so promptly.

RELATIONS - ***Antidote:*** Alcohol, Vinegar, Chalk, Iodine. Glauber's Salt in watery solution. ***Compare:*** (1) Apis, Gels. Merc. and Sulph. (2) In band-like headache, Ars., Carb-v., Chin. and Kreos. (3) in burns, uicers, unhealthy offensive discharges, Pic-ac. (4) Ant-t. and

Vario. in smallpox. (5) Chrysarobin, locally in ringworm of the scalp, 5-10 per cent. in glycerin and alcohol. Equal parts. (6) Ars., Kreos., Carbo, Guano. - Violent headache as from a band around head. Itching of nostrils, back, thighs, genitals. (6) Symptoms like hay fever, All-c, Ars. ***Incompatible:*** Glycerin and vegetable oils. In burns from carbolic acid, Elias Price found milk give immediate relief. He suggests A draft of milk in poisoning cases.

REFERENCES - Boericke. Clarke. Murphy.

CARBON TETRACHLORIDE

PHARMACY - carb-tcl. Carbon tetrachloride. ***Historical dose:*** Trituration and all potencies.

CLINICAL - Hookworms. Parasites. Worms.

HOMEOPATHIC - Carbon tetrachloride is a ***worm and parasite remedy*** of great potency. It has shown itself to be the best vermifuge for treatment of hookworm in a country where this disease predominates.

It gives little discomfort to the patient, is palatable, requires no preparation of the patient and, when pure, is apparently not toxic in homeopathic doses, all of which features are of advantage in a popular campaign.

COMMENTS - Dr. Lambert, in Suva, Fiji, noted the usefulness of Carb-tcl. for hookworms, he employed it in 50,000 cases.

W. G. Smillie and S. B. Pessoa of Sao Paulo, Brazil, also found Carb-tcl. to be extremely efficient in removing hookworms. A small dose given to adults has been proved to remove 95 percent of all the hookworms harbored.

REFERENCES - Boericke.

CARBONEUM

(Lamp-black)

PHARMACY - carbn. Carboneum. Lamp-black. Amorphous carbon obtained from the chimney of a coal-oil lamp. Trituration. ***Historical dose:*** Trituration and all potencies.

CLINICAL - Convulsions. Sore throats. Tetanus. Tongue, spasms.

HOMEOPATHIC - This substance was proved by Dr. Burt in the 1x trituration. Carbn. produced sore throat, a great craving for acids, and a peculiar convulsive attack.

The attack began with spasms, commencing on the tongue, passing down the trachea to the lungs which prevented him from breathing for about two moments, then gradually left and went to the stomach, arms, hands and legs. It took four persons to hold him, two at his hands and two at his feet.

Spasms both tonic and clonic. Lasted two hours then gradually ceased. The hands had no feeling in them, they were closed and could not be opened. Wrists perfectly pulseless, hands shriveled and cold. At 2 p.m., the spasms came on very suddenly, the same as the first time, but not so violent.

The spasms did not affect the lungs this time, but were much harder in the stomach. Lasted three hours then gradually ceased. He seemed at the point of death. The spasms left him so weak that he could not lift his hand to his head nor sit up.

RELATIONS - ***Compare:*** (1) Carb-an., Carb-v., Carb-h., Carb-o., Nux-v., Aeth., Oena.

REFERENCES - Boericke. Clarke.

CARBONEUM HYDROGENISATUM

(Carburetted Hydrogen)

PHARMACY - carbn-h. Carboneum hydrogenisatum. Carburetted hydrogen. Ethylene. Olefiant gas. Solution in alcohol. ***Historical dose:*** Trituration and all potencies.

CLINICAL - Eyes, convulsions. Strokes. Tetanus. Whooping cough.

HOMEOPATHIC - This carbon gas, which was experimented with by Sir Humphrey Davy, produces a condition almost resembling a stroke attack. Illuminating gas is a complex gas, carburetted hydrogen being the leading ingredient.

It was a popular custom to take children suffering from whooping cough to breathe the air at a gas-works. A case has been recorded in which an accidental escape of gas in a child's bedroom affected a prompt cure of its whooping cough.

Stupefaction, comatose, surface cold and completely insensible. Spasm as in lock-jaw. Arms flexed at elbows. Trismus. Involuntary stools and urine. Steady and extreme oscillation of the eyeballs. Eyes distorted. Lids half closed. Dark bodies moving before eyes. Pupils insensible to light.

MIND - Stupefaction. Extraordinary sensation of contentment. All thoughts appear in a moment as if seen in an inner mirror.

Back - Violent spasm in the extensors of the back.

Eyes - Eyes distorted, half closed. Eyeballs oscillate steadily, synchronously with breathing. Dark bodies moving before eyes.

Face - Staring look. Face turgid. Cheeks flap. Some degree of trismus, interrupted by yawning.

Head - Pressure in brain. Excruciating pain in forehead and between eyes.

Heart - Beating of the heart scarcely perceptible. Pulse strong, rapid, regular, or small and extremely weak.

Limbs - Spasmodic stitching and trembling of limbs, felt paralyzed.

Lungs - Voice feeble and indistinct. Paroxysms of cough. Dyspnea. Violent tearing pains in thorax.

Modalities - Better by open air (convulsions).

Rectum - Involuntary passage of stool and urine. Stools rice-water, thin feces mixed with dark blood and mucus.

Skin - Skin icy cold. Sweating copiously, sweat smells of gas.

Sleep - Sleep prolonged and very deep, interrupted by cramps in jaws and toes.

Stomach - Violent cramps in stomach. Nausea and vomiting.

Vertigo - Vertigo, worse going into open air. Vertigo with nausea, loss of memory and sensation.

RELATIONS - *Compare:* (1) Chloroform, Ether, Amyl-n., Carboneum.

REFERENCES - Boericke. Clarke.

CARBONEUM OXYGENISATUM

(Carbonous Oxide)

PHARMACY - carbn-o. Carboneum oxygenisatum. Carbonous oxide. Solution in water. ***Historical dose:*** Trituration and all potencies.

CLINICAL - Coma. Cramps. Headache. Herpes zoster. Paralysis. Pemphigus. Sciatica. Trismus.

HOMEOPATHIC - The effects of Carb-o. have been noted in persons poisoned by the gas. Carb-o. produces a state like intoxication. The person is confused, stupid. Loss of consciousness. Anesthesia, but the slightest touch with a hot iron recalls sensibility.

Great sleepiness lasting for several days interrupted by cramps in cheeks and toes. Convulsions and cramps. Great coldness of surface, hands icy cold. Marked improvement of symptoms, especially of chest in open air.

RELATIONS - *Compare:* (1) Carb-h.

REFERENCES - Boericke. Clarke.

CARBONEUM SULPHURATUM

(Carbon Bisulphide)

PHARMACY - carbn-s. Carboneum sulphuratum. Carbon bisulphide. Alcohol sulphuris. Alcohol lampadii. Solution in rectified spirit. ***Historical dose:*** All potencies.

CLINICAL - Acne. Amblyopia. Anemia. Burns. Clergyman's sore throat. ***Coal gas, effects.*** Color-blindness. Glandular, swellings. Goiter. Gout. Heartburn. Hemiplegia. Hernia. Herpes. Impetigo. ***Impotency.*** Lead, poisoning. Liver, disorders. Memory, lost. Meniere's disease. Muscular, atrophy. Noises, head. Rheumatism. Scabies. Scalds. Sciatica. Spinal sclerosis. Strokes. Tetanus. Tinnitus. ***Toothache.***

HOMEOPATHIC - Carbn-s. combines many characters of its two elements. It was first brought into notice by its effects on workers in rubber works. This remedy has a deep and disorganizing action and an immense range of action and symptomatology.

Lack of vital heat. Sensitive to warm, damp weather. Worse from warmth. Sensitive patients, worse cold, wasted muscles and skin and mucus membranes anesthetic. Tabes. Anesthesia of skin and mucus membranes.

Chronic rheumatism. Sciatica. Paralysis with intense congestion of nerve centers. Sensory difficulties in limbs. ***Diminished sensibility*** of arms, hands and feet. Peripheral neuritis. Tremor. Muscular weakness Ataxia. Strong increase of mechanical muscular irritability. A feeling of vibration and trembling in whole body, particularly in hands.

Burning, tearing, jerking, and stitching pains, apt to return at regular intervals for a long time. Pains come and go quickly.

Special affinity for eyes. Disturbance of sight and sensibility. Vision better in evening, in twilight, after eating. ***"Toothache brought on by warm food"*** (Carb-v., Sulph.). Ringing in the ears with poor hearing.

Eruptions of herpes and impetigo, discharges excoriating and producing violent itching. Herpetic diathesis.

Flatulency (Carb-v.) and abdominal soreness (Sulph.). Diarrhea every four to six weeks. Digestive disorders of extreme severity. Periodic diarrhea, comes every six weeks. Incontinence of urine.

Inability to sleep. Sleep is restless with tossing in bed. Giddiness. ***Impotence***. Chronic lead poisoning. Useful in patients broken down by abuse of alcohol.

MIND - Irritable, anxious intolerant, stupor. Sluggishness of mind. ***Confusion during headache.*** Memory lost. Dullness in children. Childish behavior. Idiocy and childishness.

Anxiety in morning, on waking. Anxiety in bed. Anxiety at night. ***Oversensitive to noise.*** Fear while walking in the dark.

Changeable mood. Extravagant gaiety or destructive anger. Dementia alternating with excitement. Great excitement at night has to be confined. Doesn't know what to do with things in the hands.

Hallucination of sight and hearing. Visions of magnificent grandeur. Delirium, with incoherent talking. Singing. Delusions, surrounded by enemies. Delusions he is about to receive an injury. Delirium talks of money.

Violent, vehement. Desire to strike. Biting. ***Sought for things lying before them.*** Cheerful, free from care, after wind passed. Suicidal disposition, throwing himself from a window.

Abdomen - Distention with soreness and rumbling. Flatulence, better after stool. Rumbling and flatulent complaint, twisting, rolling and rumbling as if diarrhea would set in. ***Cutting pain in bowels.*** Abdominal walls as if bruised and sore. ***Pain with wandering swellings as from flatus.*** Navel drawn inward, with pain. ***Strangulated hernia.*** Griping pain around navel with urging to stool. Liver troubles, with edema of feet.

Back - Rheumatic, with stiffness of neck. Pains in lumbar region and loins. Sensation of weight between scapula, compelling to bend forward. Sensation as if dislocated.

Bladder - Cramping, in bladder and neck of bladder. Urging to urinate, passes but few drops at a time. Urging to urinate with burning in urethra and tenesmus in neck of bladder.

Causations - Ill effects of coal gas.

Chest - Sharp pains under short ribs. ***Flying sharp pains and burning in chest***, quickly passing over, but frequently returning. Oppression and fullness in chest. Constriction, as if expiration were impeded, better deep respirations, better in open air, worse ascending steps. Warmth and fullness in chest with difficult breathing.

Constitutions - Broken-down, weak constitutions.

Coughs - Cough from irritability of larynx. Cough after lying down. Cough from tickling in posterior part of palate, straining the chest and making it sore. Cough from heartburn.

Ears - Sharp pain in ears after stool. Pain in left ear on swallowing. Sharp pain in right ear. Ears feel obstructed. Deafness, as if ears were obstructed by a fixed substance. Hearing impaired. ***Noises in head.*** Tinnitus aurium. ***Meniere's disease.*** Buzzing and singing noises like an Aeolian harp.

Eyes - Eyes sunken, fixed, expressionless. Sunken eyes, with gray rings. Itching. Inflammation, followed by atrophy of optic nerve. Asthenopia and dyschromotopsia. Myopia. Cloudiness and atrophy of optic disc. Central scotoma. Retinal congestion, optic disc pale. Optic neuritis advancing toward atrophy. Arteries and veins congested. Reading causes lachrymation. Lids heavy. Lids sore on moving, quivering.

Face - Face pale, with clammy sweat. Face pale, with flushes of heat. Expression bewildered and as of one demented. Eruption on nose and cheeks similar to acne of drunkards. Tetter-like eruption on left cheek, from scratching with fingernails; spreads and is covered with yellowish-brown scabs, disfiguring the face; almost unbearable on account of continued itching. Pushes the lower jaw far forward, and gnashes with it against the upper one. Lips dry and burning.

Female - Atrophy of ovaries. Labor-pains too weak.

Food - Ravenous appetite. Appetite lost. Hunger with aversion to eating. Great thirst. Desire for beer. Aversion to meat. Worse tobacco, wine and beer. Worse from alcohol. Drunken, unconscious from whiskey.

Head - Headache as from a tight cap. Dull muddled feeling in forehead. ***Noises in head.*** Constriction of forehead and occiput. Pressure pain in forehead. Violent pain, increasing till it causes confusion of mind. Brushing hair is painful. Itching on head. Head sinks forward in walking. Single nodules on head, sore to touch. Headache and dizziness.

Heart - Anemic murmur. Murmur of first sounds extended along great vessels.

Kidneys - Tickling in forepart of urethra and sensation as if something would run out. Cutting, smarting and burning during urination. Urination painful and slow, with tenesmus, even bloody urine. Can't retain urine long. Urine albuminous, turbid.

Limbs - Emaciation. Paralysis. Trembling. Sore, bruised limbs. ***Edema.*** Anesthesia of arms and hands. Sciatica. Cramps in limbs. Lighting-like pains with cramps. Flying pains, returning regularly for a long time. ***Progressive neuritis.*** Hemiplegia of right side. Formication, tingling as from electric currents. Pain in lower limbs with cramps and formications. Gait unsteady tottering, worse in dark. ***Tearing in limbs, coming and going, now in one and again in another limb.*** Feet insensible. Fingers swollen, insensible, rigid, stiff. Herpes on dorsal surface of hands.

Lungs - ***Breathing difficult.*** Emphysema. Asphyxia from alcohol or coal gas. ***Expiration hot.***

Male - Burning in urethra with erections. Atrophied testicles. Scrotum shrivelled and drawn up. Desire lost, parts atrophied. Frequent, profuse nocturnal emissions. At first, sexual desire increased, then lost. Impotence.

Modalities - Better in open air. Better warm drinks. Worse after breakfast. Worse at night. Worse from slightest motion. Worse walking. Worse bathing. Worse during and after eating. Worse at night. Worse from warmth.

Mouth - Anesthesia of mouth and tongue. Sweetish, foul, bitter, sour, pappy, metallic taste. ***Neuralgia of teeth.*** Toothache brought on by warm food. Hawking of salty mucus. Tongue cold. Tongue burning, stiff. Lisping, stammering speech like that of a child. Ulceration of the lips. Lips blue, moist, with convulsive movements.

Nose - Eruptions on nose. Sneezing with sensitiveness in chest. Tip of nose burns, as if raw, and is quite red. Tickling in point of nose with irritation to sneeze. Nosebleed. Smell is lost.

Perspiration - Sweats after much walking. Sweat, relieves the headache. Suppression of usual sweat.

Rectum - Itching and burning at anus. Constipation with belching. Constipation with herpes. Diarrhea. Fetid diarrhea alternating with constipation. ***Very offensive and frequent passage of flatus.*** After stool, headache, stitches in ears, pressure in stomach, burning pain, weakness and trembling. ***Stool not increased, but accompanied by tenesmus.*** Stool of yellow, frothy, sour-smelling fluid, nights. Stool with retraction of umbilicus and tenesmus. Stool thin, papescent and small.

Skin - Anesthesia. Burning, itching. Ulcers. Small wounds fester. Skin cancer. Furunculosis. Chronic skin diseases with much itching. Eruptions on face, red, elevated. ***Vesicles on a red, inflamed and swollen base.*** Vesicles contain an opaque, yellowish fluid, which forms thick, yellowish scabs, sometimes the discharge excoriates and produces violent itching.

Sleep - Sleep is restless with tossing in bed. Deep morning sleep with anxious, vexatious dreams.

Stomach - Sour eructations after coughing. ***Sour eructations and passage of much sour flatus***, better belching. Distension, better noisy eructations. Burning pains. Heartburn, worse pressure. Sensations of warmth in stomach. ***Flying sharp pains in region of stomach.*** Stomach as if tied together. Stomach painful to external pressure. Pressing, sharp pains of short duration, radiating to cardiac region. Loud belching. ***Nausea, with fainting spells***. Nausea, better eructations or vomiting. Vomiting of food with glairy mucus. ***Vomiting of bitter water.*** Inclination to vomit when entering a room or going into open air.

Temperature - ***Coldness, during headache.*** Feverish attacks, during headache.

Throat - Burning in throat extending to stomach. Tickling in back of palate after lying down, causes violent, dry cough. Sensation as if a hair has lodged in throat. As if a piece of bone has lodged in esophagus. Sharp, contracting pain. Scraping feeling in throat with fine stitches. Goitre. Voice feeble, of a deep tone. Hoarseness. Irritation to hawk. Heat in larynx, scratching and scraped feeling. Clergyman's sore throat.

Vertigo - Sudden attacks of vertigo while sitting.

Vision - Dim vision, objects fade away. Myopia. Loss of vision, progressive with central scotoma. Vision greatly impaired. Everything seems in a fog. Color blindness, red and green, not for white. Vision better evening, twilight, after eating.

COMMENTS - In the Medical Argus, H. H. Crippen collected, from several sources, instances of workers intoxicated with Carbn-s.

Carb-s. combines many characteristics of its two elements. It was brought to notice by its effects on workers in rubber works. Pains come and go quickly. The periodicity shows itself, as in diarrhea, which comes every six weeks.

The worse from warmth common to Carb-v. and Sulph. shows itself in Carb-s. A feeling of vibration and trembling in whole body, particularly in hands. Carb-s. has the flatulence of Carb-v. and the abdominal soreness of Sulph.

In many cases, the action on vision was very marked. Myopia, asthenopia, achromatopsia, dyschromatopsia. Cloudiness and atrophy of optic disc. Optic discs pale. Central scotoma for light and colors. Retinal congestion. Arteries and veins tortuous. Veins are distended and arteries contracted. Everything seemed in a fog, as if a spider's web over objects, green or red.

One patient had complete right side hemiplegia, following sudden loss of consciousness, blindness of right eye and great impairment of vision of left.

Loss of memory, especially for words, was a very frequent symptom. Delusions were common: "Heard voices and believed he had committed a robbery," "sensation of a hole close by into which he was in danger of falling."

One acute case concerned a girl, aged 15, who was employed in vulcanizing works, and was exposed to the fumes one whole day. Before this, she had, from smaller exposures to the fumes, frontal pains and heaviness of the head.

After this, the pains became more violent and were accompanied by painful contraction of masseters, then by stiffness of neck and vertebral column, finally of legs and arms. The contracture was generalized, but nowhere complete, though the jaws could not be separated. Ulcerative stomatitis ensued and tartar accumulated on the teeth.

E. Case cured with Carb-s. 30c in a slender, nervous woman, a "Sensation, as of a weight between the scapulae, compelling her to bend forward. Throbbing in the dorsal spine as if a heart were beating there. Constipation with ineffectual urging to stool. hemorrhage of bright blood from rectum after stool. Itching of anus after stool, also in the night. Feet swollen, hot and throbbing in the evening."

RELATIONS - ***Compare:*** (1) Kali xantate - Similar in action. Acts on cortical substance, loss of memory, marked blood degeneration, impotence and senility. (2) Tuberculinum, Radium, Carbo-v., Sulph., Caust., Salicyl. ac., Chin. (3) In eye symptoms, vision - Benz-d-n. (4) Thyr. - in progressive diminution of sight with central scotoma. (5) Caust., Chin., and Nat-sal. in Meniere's disease, Carb-v. in flatulence. (6) Sulph., Lyc. - sensitiveness of abdomen. (7) Anac. - hears voices. (8) Cann-i. - opening and shutting sensation in head. (9) Kali-bi., Sil. (10) Sulph. - hair sensation in throat.

REFERENCES - Boericke. Clarke. Phatak.

CARCINOSIN

(Cancer Nosode)

PHARMACY - carc. Carcinosin. Cancer nosode. Carcinosin Foubister. Carcinosin Burnett. Carcinosinum. Carcinosin was originally made from the discharge of a breast cancer. ***Historical dose:*** All potencies.

CLINICAL - Abuse. AIDS. ***Allergies. Anticipation.*** Arthritis. Asthma. Attention deficit syndrome. Autism. ***Breast, cancer. Cancer.*** Cirrhosis. Constipation. ***Diabetes.*** Down's syndrome. Dwarfishness. Emaciation. ***Fatigue, chronic.*** Fibromyalgia. ***Flatulence.*** Fright. Grief. ***Head, injuries. Hemophilia. Hemorrhoids***. Hepatitis. Hernia. Hodgkin's disease. Hormonal, imbalance. Humiliation. Hyperactivity. ***Immune, deficiency. Influenza. Insomnia. Keloids***. Lipoma. Lymphogranulomatosis. Mastitis. Melancholy. Moles. Mongolism. ***Mononucleosis***. Nightmares. ***Night-watching. Obsessive-compulsive disorder.*** Osteomyelitis. Osteoporosis. Ovarian, cysts. Pernicious, anemia. Pneumonia. ***Polyps.*** Rape. Rheumatoid, arthritis. Sexual, abuse. Sinusitis. Spondylitis. ***Thallasemia.*** Tuberculosis. ***Vaccination, effects. Whooping cough***. Worms.

HOMEOPATHIC - A nosode prepared from breast cancer by Foubister. Carcinosin acts favorably and modifies all cases in which either a history of cancer can be elicited or symptoms of the disease itself exist.

Carc. can be used as an ***intercurrent remedy.*** Indicated in constantly changing symptoms and states. ***Contradictory and alternating states.*** Many symptoms similar to AIDS, periodic high fevers, swollen glands, emaciation, chronic severe insomnia, diarrhea.

Cancers. Tumors, benign, cystic, fibroids. Lipoma. ***Cancerous affections,*** hereditary, breast cancer. Cancer of the breast glands with great pain. Induration of the uterus and cervix. History of cancer in the family. ***Keloids***. Prevents keloid formation. ***Polyps.***

Cancerous cachexia, emaciation. Emaciation from cancer or progressive muscular disease. Hodgkin's disease, lymphogranulomatosis. Osteitis, chronic osteomyelitis. ***Brittle bones*** (Calc-p.).

Childhood diseases too severe, absent or too late. Child's development is arrested. Dwarfishness. Malformations, mongolism. Down's syndrome.

Hemophilia. Hemorrhages from orifices of the body. Pernicious anemia or family history. ***Thallasemia.*** Ailments from blood transfusions. Retinal hemorrhage. Veins are prominent all over body. Varicose veins.

Chronic fatigue. Excessive ***weariness and fatigue***. Low blood sugar, causing fatigue, revived from sleep. Trembling in morning on waking. Chronic insomnia from no apparent cause (Coff.).

Complaints due to anticipation. Antidotes the ill effects of vaccinations (Thuj., Sil.).

Tendency to inflammation. Inflammation of joints, rheumatoid arthritis. Rheumatism. Physical exertion, aggravates or ameliorates. Pains, constricting, throbbing internally. Offensive discharges, hemorrhages and pain. Discharges, acrid, thick.

Mononucleosis, never well since. ***Pneumonia,*** never well since. ***Tuberculosis,*** prophylaxis, hereditary. Sycosis. Syphilis. Glandular fever. Glands are enlarged, tubercular, open. ***Multiple allergies.*** Allergy to foods, and chemicals.

Diabetes insipidus. ***Diabetes mellitus,*** hereditary. Indigestion, accumulation of gas in stomach and bowels. Worms. Obesity.

Phobias. Sea-bathing aggravates. Aversion to bathing or washing. Hot flashes of menopause with perspiration. Good health before the paroxysms. Annual periodicity. Symptoms on one side or alternating sides (Lac-c.).

MIND - Passionate people who ***over-extend themselves.*** Sympathetic. ***Desires dancing and music. Desire for travel.*** Restless, feel hurried. Bored easily. Difficult concentration. Autism. Mental retardation. Hyperactivity. Attention deficit syndrome. ***Fastidious.*** Obsessive-compulsive disorder.

Anxiety of what might happen. Fears of the unknown, death, dark, or being alone. Fears of failure, of exams, heights, crowds. Fear of not being able to accomplish their goals. Chronic nightmares and night terrors. ***Fear of getting cancer*** or that they have cancer. Fear that they have an incurable disease. Worry about health. ***Loves the excitement of thunderstorms*** (Sep.), or a fear of thunderstorms (Phos.).

Foubister observed that people who lived under ***severe fear for long periods*** of time often needed this remedy, chronic terror or fearful situations, never well since fearful time. ***Sexual abuse and for abusive relationships***.

History of emotional suppression and deep guilt (Staph.). History of ***nursing a loved one*** with some chronic, debilitating disease. Closed emotionally. Ameliorated from weeping, aggravated by suppressing tears. Worse reprimanded or reproached. Worse with consolation.

Abdomen - ***Flatulence.*** Inguinal, hernia in children. Chronic, ulcerative colitis. ***Burning pains like fire*** in the ascending colon. Right iliac region painful. Constrictive pain, better bending. Cramping pain, better bending double. Pains, worse from 4 p.m. to 6 p.m., better pressure and bending forward, hot drinks.

Back - Spondylitis. Eczema. Pustules. Formication. Itching, thoracic region, between scapula, while undressing. Pain, right side of neck on turning head. Pain, right lumbar region. Twitching of muscles.

Breasts - Violent tension in breasts, before menses. ***Swelling and tenderness before menses.*** Induration. Chronic mastitis. Breasts changes shape. ***Breast cancer,*** especially with a family history of cancer. Nodules. Retraction of nipples. Discharge from nipple like bloody water.

Causations - Family history of cancer. Loss of sleep, night-watching, nursing of loved ones. Overwork or exertion. Emotional shocks, grief, anticipation. Sexual abuse victims. Vaccinations. Ailments from windy weather.

Chest - Swelling of axillary glands. Constriction. Oppression of chest, on inspiration. Tuberculosis. Lipoma, left side, non-malignant. Acne. Eczema on sternum.

Constitutions - Cancer miasm.

Coughs - Morning cough while dressing, worse bathing. Coughs, worse from eating, inspiration, laughing, shaving, singing. Tickling in throat-pit causes cough. Coughs, on becoming warm, when entering a warm room from open air. ***Whooping cough,*** early in life, hereditary, ailments ever since.

Ears - Boils inside, alternately one ear, then the other. Eruptions in meatus. Otitis media. Inflammation, right lobe. Noises in ears. Stopped up sensation.

Eyes - Soreness in eyes. Weakness of eyes. ***Bluish tinge or spots on sclera,*** especially in children. Blueness of iris. Cornea ulceration. Retinal bleeding, diabetes. ***Blinking,*** frequent winking. Twitching of lower eyelids, eyebrows. Stinging pain, lids, upper. Stitching in upper lids. Recurrent styes. Eyelashes long and silken.

Face - Brown, ***cafe-au-lait spots***, copper colored, pale. Heat flushes in the face, during menopause. Bluish lips. Stiffness of lower jaws. Facial paralysis. Twitches, tics with frequent blinking of the eyes. Acne Herpes on upper lips and nose.

Female - Frequent menses, too early, too soon. Bleeding between menses. Imaginary pregnancy. Increased sex drive. Disposition to masturbation, too frequent or too early. Uterine bleeding after sex. Flatus from vagina. Ailments since menopause. Encysted tumors. Ovarian cysts. Uterine fibroids and tumors. Cancer.

Food - Capricious, changeable appetite. Ravenous or wanting appetite. Desires ***chocolate,*** coffee, sweets, sugar, ***fat,*** eggs, butter, cheese, cream, milk, ham fat, bacon, and smoked meat. Desires raw potatoes and onions, garlic, vinegar, fruit, soup, salt and pepper, ***spicy foods,*** farinaceous food, ***food that makes him worse***. Aversion to soup, sweets, fat, butter, eggs, ice cream, rich foods, alcoholic drinks, coffee, meat, salty food, and fruit. Aggravated from alcoholic drinks, wine, coffee, milk, eggs, fat, meat, fruit, rich food, salty things, sweets. Thirst for large quantities. Desires cold drinks, cold milk, warm drinks, alcoholic drinks, wine.

Head - Constriction and contraction sensation in brain. Heaviness in forehead. ***Head injuries*** (Nat-s.). Swelling of brain. Tired feeling with headache. Headaches on sides. Pressing pain in right side of temples. Headaches after excitement of emotions. Headache deep inside brain. Deep aching in brain. Headaches after injuries, after childbirth. Throbbing, pulsating in brain. Pulsating pain in forehead, extending to eyes, above the eyes or behind them. Worse windy, stormy weather and physical exertion.

Heart - Constriction, grasping sensation. Sighing breath, causing the heart to constrict. Palpitations, audible, tumultuous, violent and visible. Palpitations in the afternoon, 2 p.m. to 6 p.m.

Kidneys - Frequent urination, involuntary at night. Albuminous and bloody urine, contains granular casts. Nephritis. Kidney diseases.

Limbs - Weakness, numbness and aching, especially in the thighs. Twitching of limbs and individual muscles. Rheumatic pain in joints. Ganglion. Sciatica. Varicose veins in lower limbs. Weakness of thigh, better exertion. Pain in lower limbs, better warmth of bed. Aching pain in thigh, better exertion. Numbness of thigh, better exertion or nap. Pain in legs, better from heat, warmth of bed, gentle exertion, quick motion, after a short sleep. Warts on soles of feet, hands, palms. Crippled or distorted nails, hangnails. Itching eczema eruptions on hands. Abnormal hairiness of arms and legs. Sudden heaviness of upper arms. Twisting sensation in upper limbs.

Liver - Hepatitis infectious. Enlarged and weak liver. Cirrhosis of liver, hereditary.

Lungs - ***Deep desire to breathe.*** Yawning. Difficult breathing, after running. Asthma and recurring bronchitis. Asthma, after fright, wet weather, in morning, forenoon, 10 a.m. Chronic pneumonia in children. Cough, worse from talking, laughing, yawning, undressing or dressing, cold air, tickle in throat. Expectoration is bloody, spitting blood.

Male - Increased sex drive. Disposition to masturbation, in children. Troublesome or wanting erections. Condylomata.

Modalities - Better from open air. Better during thunderstorms. Worse from warm room. Worse weather extremes. Worse air at seashore. Worse full or new moon. Approaching storms can either ameliorate or aggravate.

Mouth - Aphthae. Patches of white discoloration. Putrid taste in mouth. Sensation of lumps on palate. Soreness in palate, worse hot drinks. Prickling in palate, worse in morning and evening. Papillae absent at tip of tongue. Ulcers on edges of tongue. Pressing in gums. Burning vesicles on gums. Stammering speech.

Neck - Hypothyroid. Goiter. Induration of glands. Swelling of thyroid. Clothing aggravates.

Nose - Recurring sinusitis. Catarrh of sinuses. Catarrh in cold weather. Hay fever, allergies. Frequent, recurrent coryza. Excoriating, thick, yellow discharge. Persistent, recurrent nosebleeds. Varicose veins.

Perspiration - Profuse, with an offensive smell. Sweat during sleep.

Rectum - ***Constipation*** and inactivity of the colon, without desire or urging. Inactivity of rectum. Constipation better at the seashore. ***Black, dry, hard***, tarry-looking stool. Pain like a splinter after stool. Pulsation sensation. Constriction, closure and general pain, better bending, pressing, warm drinks. Worse from itching and scratching. ***Hemorrhage*** from anus. ***Hemorrhoids***. Rectal fissure, fistula. Condylomatas. Prolapsed rectum in children. Diarrhea in children from excitement, emotions. Worm complaints in children.

Skin - ***Café-au-lait spots.*** Brown, liver spots. ***Moles and nevi.*** Boils. Warts. Excrescences. Itching, without eruptions, worse undressing. Psoriasis. Eczema in children. ***Keloids.*** Acne on face, back and chest. Ecchymosis. ***Wounds*** are slow to heal. Ulcers. Bed sores. Lupus, erythematosum. Purpura hemorrhagica.

Sleep - ***Chronic or acute insomnia,*** causeless. Insomnia from grief, mental activity. ***Sleeplessness from anticipation or anxiety. Sleeplessness from*** nursing loved ones. Child must be carried or rocked to sleep. Deep, heavy sleepers. ***Sleeps in the knee-chest position*** or on the right side. Sleeps on abdomen. Sleeps with arms over head. Genu-pectoral position during sleep, on knees with face forced into pillow. Children sleep on their knees and elbows. Restless sleep, but ameliorated from short naps (Phos.). ***Unrefreshing sleep***. Waking after midnight, 4 a.m., from dreams. Wakes early and frequent, as from a fright, from shocks through the body or twitching. Worse from interrupted sleep.

Stomach - Anxiety in pit. Pain on bending double, from coughing, worse hot drinks, better pressure. Indigestion. Belchings. Heartburn in children. Congenital stenosis. Stomach ulcers. Nausea, from motion, in the morning, at beginning of menses, during menses. Persistent nausea during pregnancy. Periodic vomiting, alternating with diarrhea. Vomiting from anticipation. ***Cyclic vomiting*** in infants, bulimia. Malnutrition due to effects of additives.

Teeth - Decayed, hollow teeth. Toothache. Grinding of teeth during sleep.

Temperature - High fevers of unknown origin. Influenza, constantly relapsing, never well since. Acute or chronic mononucleosis. Recurrent history of glandular fever. Rheumatic fever in childhood. Fever after vaccinations.

Throat - Sore throat, in morning, better cold drinks, worse warm drinks. Scraping in throat before able to speak. Chronic hoarseness. Clears throat before speaking. Lump sensation in larynx. Lump in throat, worse from empty swallowing, at night, on waking, and from heat, better cold. Pain on empty swallowing. ***Enlargement of tonsils***. Recurrent tonsillitis.

Vertigo - Rising from stooping.

COMMENTS - Phatak stated "A nosode prepared from Carcinoma is claimed to act favorably, modifying the cases in which there is a history of carcinoma or the disease itself exists. Can be used as an intercurrent remedy along with indicated."

Clarke used it more frequently than any other as a miasmatic remedy. Clarke had met with a suicidal tendency in several cancer patients, the cancer nosodes may be appropriate in mental cases, especially where the heredity points that way.

Burnett had a number of different cancer preparations and followed his instincts largely in their use and selection. He used Carc. in treating depraved inherited conditions in children, such as infantile self-abuse, with good effects, which Clarke later confirmed.

Kent used Carc. for cases of incurable cancer with sharp, burning, tearing pains. He claimed it would palliate the cancer for years, although it would not cure it.

Foubister studied 200 pregnant women who had cancer and, later, their children. The children had a tendency to birthmarks and to blue sclera, a blue spot in the white of the eye, or blue shading in the white of their eye. Useful fro deep pigmentations, strawberry angioma. Can prevent keloids.

There can be a cancer miasm if cancer is on one or both sides of the family. Useful for children with multiple miasms. Indicated remedies don't work, or there is a short amelioration and needs repeating, with a strong history of cancer, diabetes, tuberculosis or gonorrhea.

Etiology can include trauma, frights, grief, physical injuries, vaccinations and attacks on the immune system. Hormone use. Grimmer thought that cancer came from living or thinking wrongly.

Foubister made an observation that people who lived under severe fear for long periods of time often needed this remedy. Sexual abuse and abusive relationships, particularly if it leads to suppressed emotions. Chronic insomnia. Phobias. Glandular fever, mononucleosis and chronic fatigue.

Down's syndrome. History of severe acute infections in the child, especially whooping cough and pneumonia, and the child never totally recovered. Asthma in children, worse from vaccinations. Antidotes the ill effects of vaccinations (Thuj.). Worms.

Similar to many polycrest remedies. Better from naps (Phos.). Better or worse by the seashore. Better dancing (Sep.). Craves cold drinks (Phos.). Moles, birthmarks and freckles (Thuj.). Fastidiousness (Ars.). Enjoys thunderstorms (Sep.).

RELATIONS - Consider this remedy when other well indicated remedies don't work or the improvement doesn't last. ***Compare:*** (1) Tub., Thuj., Med., Syph., Sep., Nat-m., Calc-p., Dys-co., Lyc., Phos., Psor., Ars., Ars-i., Puls., Sulph., Op., Alum., Staph. (2) In cancer - Ars., Hydr., Bufo, Con., Phyt., Aster., Scirr. (3) Phos., Sep., Ars., Med., Thuj., Cocc.

REFERENCES - Foubister. Murphy. Phatak.

CARDIOSPERMUM HALICACABUM

(Balloon Vine)

PHARMACY - cardi-h. Cardiospermum halicacabum. Balloon vine. N.O. Sapindaceae.

CLINICAL - Allergies. Belching. Cramps. ***Exhaustion.*** Heartburn. Heat, flushes. Nasal, congestion. Nausea. Sinusitis.

HOMEOPATHIC - Excessive physical irritability and painful, sore muscles. ***Lassitude***. Tired, sore feeling in arms and legs and desire to stretch. ***Exhaustion, torpor, listless.*** Flushes of heat. Desire for open air.

Allergic skin eruptions caused by drugs, detergents, insect stings. Increased lachrymation. Burning pain in eyes, worse night. ***Congestion and obstruction of nose and sinuses.*** Copious discharge from nose. Nasal discharge clear, gray, bloody, or thick and yellow.

Nausea worse morning, worse after eating. Heartburn and eructations worse night (Rob.) Constricted sensation in chest, better lying down.

MIND - ***Great mental sluggishness and apathy.*** Mental dullness. Weakness of memory. Increased forgetfulness, particularly for things related to work.

Hurried in occupation. Nervous and restlessness. Desire to bite nails. Aversion to company. Desire for company. Causeless weeping.

Abdomen - Gurgling. Itching, umbilicus. Cramping pain in evening. Cramping at night, in bed. Cramping after eating.

Chest - Constriction in chest, better lying down. Pain in chest after drinking cold juice. Sore pain before menses.

Eyes - Itching better rubbing.

Food - Aversion to coffee. Desires potatoes. Worse strawberries.

Head - Headache in forehead. Headache in temple Pain in temple extending to root of nose. Pulsating.

Limbs - Coldness of hands; of feet. Cramps in toes. Offensive perspiration of feet. Pulsation in soles of feet. Swelling of feet before menses.

Mouth - Dryness. Chapped lips. Numbness of tongue. Pain in tongue, as if burnt.

Nose - Sneezing in morning on waking.

Sleep - Dreams of dogs. Strange dreams.

Vertigo - Vertigo better after eating. Objects seem to move.

Vision - Sees objects beside field of vision.

REFERENCES - Murphy.

CARDUUS BENEDICTUS

(Blessed Thisde)

PHARMACY - card-b. Carduus benedictus. Blessed thistle. Cincus benedictus. Centaurea benedicta. Carline thistle. N. O. Composite. Tincture of whole plant when in flower. ***Historical dose:*** Tincture and all potencies.

CLINICAL - Amaurosis. Asphyxia. Coma. Diarrhea. Dysphagia. Esophagus, stricture. Eyes, disorders. Fevers. Headaches. Hoarseness. Joints, cracking. Varicose, veins. Vision, disorders.

HERBAL - Indigenous to the Mediterranean region and brought to Central Europe as a medicine as early as the Middle Ages, where it is still cultivated. The Carline thistle has an enormous root and purple composite flowers surrounded by radical spinous leaves. Flourishes on dry stony ground and wasteland.

This thistle was used externally for wounds, especially burns. It is said to have obtained its name 'benedictus' from its high reputation as a heal-all, being supposed even to cure the plague. It is a basic ingredient of the Benedictine Liqueur and other bitter tonics, stomach bitters.

HOMEOPATHIC - The provings by Rückert showed a prominent sensation of contraction which occurs in many parts. Twitchings and disturbance of vision, flickerings, muscae volitantes. ***Blackness before eyes for a short time.*** Eyeballs feel larger.

The gastro-abdominal disturbances of Card-m. are observed in a less degree in Card-b. Disordered taste, dysphagia. Yawning and hiccough. Cutting pains in abdomen, vomiting and diarrhea.

Burning runs through the proving. ***Bitter burning*** in the stomach, as if it were much deranged. Burning in hands after sweat. Burning in the arms on exerting them. Tension in tendons. Cracking and aching in joints. Aching, cutting pain. Red, and afterwards, yellow, spots on the skin.

The respiratory sphere is strongly affected and there is pain and contractive sensation in the trachea with hoarseness. Inspired air feels cold. Feeling as if buccal cavity were contracted. Slight swelling of the veins.

Modalities - Worse by motion. Worse touch. Worse walking. Worse stretching the limbs.

COMMENTS - Two fatal cases of poisoning were recorded, a boy and a girl, from eating the thistle root. In the girl's case, there was stertorous breathing, drowsiness, retching without actual vomiting, asphyxia and coma.

After death the tongue protruded slightly between the lips, pupils were greatly dilated, there was evidence of general venous congestion. In the boy's case, the veins of the brain were extremely congested.

RELATIONS - ***Compare:*** (1) Card-m., Bell., Atro. - vision. (2) Chin. and Sal-ac. - noises in ears. (3) Agar. - twitching of eyelids.

REFERENCES - Clarke.

CARDUUS MARIANUS

(St. Mary's Thistle)

PHARMACY - card-m. Carduus marianus. St. Mary's Thistle. Silybum marianus. N. O. Composite. Tincture or trituration of the seeds. ***Historical dose:*** Tincture and all potencies.

CLINICAL - Alcohol, abuse. Asthma. ***Biliousness.*** Bronchitis. ***Cirrhosis.*** Constipation. Debility. Diaphragm, high. Dropsy. ***Edema.*** Fever. ***Gallstone, colic. Gallstones. Headaches.*** Heartburn. Hematemesis. Hemoptysis. Hemorrhages. Hemorrhoids. ***Hepatitis.*** Influenza. Intermittents. Jaundice. Kidney, stones. ***Liver, disorders.*** Melaena. Metrorrhagia. Nausea. Neuralgias. Nosebleeds. Pleurisy. Rheumatism. Salivation. Sciatica. ***Spleen, disorders.*** Tuberculosis. Typhlitis. Ulcers. ***Varicose, ulcers. Varicose, veins.*** Vomiting. Waterbrash.

HERBAL - Rademacher, the medical alchemist, found Card-m. to be a primarily liver remedy, all its manifestations originating in some disorder of the liver. Burnett agreed, noting that it is primarily a liver and spleen remedy.

HOMEOPATHIC - The action of this remedy is centered in the ***liver and portal system***, causing soreness, pain, and jaundice. It has a specific relation to the vascular system. Useful for a history of a toxic liver. It establishes a healthy flow of bile, and helps reduce the tendency for reformation of gallstones.

Chronic liver weakness and ***cirrhosis of the liver***, especially with ascites, a water-filled abdomen, and edema. Cirrhosis with swollen legs and varicose veins. Liver enlargement in the transverse direction (Chel. is more vertical). ***Gallstone colic.*** Jaundice. ***Hepatitis*** with hot flashes, flushing of heat.

Damaged liver (Nux-v.). May help liver cancer. Dropsical conditions depending on liver disease and when due to pelvic congestion. Hemorrhages, especially connected with hepatic disease. Bilious fever. Infection of the gallbladder.

Liver headaches (Sang., Chel.), migraines, often worse on the right side. Liver disorders associated with lung disorders. Influenza when liver is affected. Low blood sugar. Never well since mononucleosis or hepatitis. For the abuse of alcoholic beverages, especially beer.

Characteristic bitter taste in the back of the mouth. The tongue has white down the center with a red tip. ***Portal stasis.*** Hemorrhoids with itching, burning in the rectum, dark urine.

Spleen disease (Cean.). Associated with digestion problems and with a bitter taste in the mouth. Vomiting of bile-like substances. Chronic heartburn, fatigue after eating. Drawing pain up the abdomen, from the umbilicus to the solar plexus. Rumbling in the abdomen, clay-colored stools, blood in the stool.

Diseases of miners associated with difficult breathing, asthma (Sil.). Debility, fatigue, worse eating and riding with frequent yawning. ***Varicose veins and ulcers.*** Stitching, drawing, burning pains.

MIND - Melancholy with liver disorders. Joyless, apathetic. Despondency. Disposition to become angry. Hypochondriacal. Forgets what he has just intended to do.

Abdomen - Sluggish peristalsis in colon. Fullness and soreness in hepatic region, with moist skin. Distention with rumbling, cutting pains. Painless flatulence in small intestine. Pain in region of liver. Cutting pain in bowels, changing from place to place. Stitches in spleen, worse on inspiration, stooping. Stitches in small intestine, better pressure. Sensation of motion in intestines on expiration, around navel. Pressure with sensation of warmth in small intestine, on left side of abdomen. Pulsation in abdomen.

Back - Sensitiveness in dorsal and cervical vertebrae. Drawing pains in back. Drawing, tearing, burning in left shoulder blade.

Chest - Pain in chest going to shoulders, back, loins and abdomen with urging to urinate. Stitching pains in lower right ribs and front, worse moving, walking. Pain during breathing. Stitches in chest, from left nipple to right downward. Diaphragm high.

Constitutions - Choleric constitutions.

Eyes - Pressure as if eyeballs were pressed against side of orbits. Burning and pressure in eyeballs and lids.

Face - Earthy, yellowish-gray, dirty or florid complexion. Heat in face. Weak upper lip.

Female - Menses too profuse or suppressed. Metrorrhagia. Chronic uterine hemorrhage with portal derangement.

Food - Poor appetite. Voracious appetite. Aversion to salt meat. Abuse of beer. Great fatigue after eating. Low blood sugar. Soups salted as usual tasted insipid, at other times well salted food is repugnant.

Head - Headache better eating. Headache shortly before meals, disappearing after eating. Dull frontal headache with foul tongue. ***Liver headaches.*** Bilious headaches. Burning and pressure in head. Constriction, contractive feeling skull, over eyebrows. Pain in left parietal bone.

Heart - Pain, pressure, and stitches in region of heart. Oppression on deep breathing.

Kidneys - Urging to urinate. Pressure on bladder, producing dribbling of urine after unavailing urging to stool. Strangury. Burning at meatus, in urethra. Urine, cloudy, golden-colored, turbid. Kidney stones.

Limbs - Violent rheumatic pains in right deltoid, right arm. Pain in hip joint spreading through buttocks down the thighs, worse stooping, with difficult rising. Weakness felt in feet, especially after sitting. Drawing pain in muscles. Cramp-like pain in muscles of arms, hands, calves, and feet.

Liver - Liver, engorged, swollen laterally, painful to pressure. Hyperemia of liver. Pains in region of liver, with dizziness, bad taste in mouth and jaundiced skin. ***Cirrhosis of liver with general edema. Jaundice*** with dull headache, bitter taste in mouth, and white tongue. Left lobe is very sensitive. ***Gallstones.*** Gallstone diseases with an enlarged liver. ***Terrible attacks of gallstone colic.*** Swelling of gallbladder with painful tenderness. Stitches in liver, worse lying on left side. Liver disorders cause lung diseases, causing hemoptysis. Tension in liver when lying on right side, worse pressure. Crawling sensation.

Lungs - Asthmatic respiration. Asthma of miners. Cough with stitches in sides of chest with bloody sputum. Expectoration of pure blood, mucus mixed with blood. Splenic or hepatic cough.

Modalities - Better from bleeding. Worse from lying on left side. Worse motion. Worse touch. Worse eating. Worse beer. Worse cellars.

Mouth - Bitter taste. Collection of water in mouth. Smooth sensation of mucus membrane of palate, as though covered with fat.

Nose - Burning in right nostril. Tickling, first in right, then left nostril, with watery discharge. Habitual nosebleed. Sudden profuse nosebleed, relieving vertigo.

Perspiration - Sweat on forehead and back after meals. Sweats over whole body, with lassitude, on awakening.

Rectum - Burning pain in the rectum and anus, which interferes with sitting. Itching. Paste-like, clay stools. Bright yellow stools. Constipation. ***Stools hard, difficult, knotty, alternates with diarrhea.*** Bleeding hemorrhoids. Prolapse of rectum. Profuse diarrhea due to rectal cancer. Melaena. Stools either bileless or black.

Skin - ***Varicose veins and ulcers.*** Broken or hard thrombosed veins. Itching on lying down at night. Eruption on lower part of sternum.

Sleep - Restless sleep with frequent awakening and many dreams. Nightmares from lying on back. Fatigue with yawning. Uncontrollable yawning.

Stomach - Bitter taste. Sour eructations. Repeated belchings of air with burning in esophagus. Burning as of acidity. Sensation of emptiness. ***Pressure in the stomach.*** Griping pain. Colicky pain with waterbrash. Stitches in left side of stomach, near spleen (Cean.). Sour contents of stomach and intestines. ***Nausea, retching and vomiting*** of green acid fluid or blood. Nausea with salivation. Hematemesis. Tendency to attacks of bilious vomiting. Continual nausea with desire to vomit. Vomiting of pregnancy.

Temperature - Chill and fever with jaundice. Chilliness at night, worse uncovering. Chilliness on awakening with strong urge to urinate. Epidemic influenza. Bilious fever.

Throat - Irritation in posterior part of larynx causing cough. Fauces as if rough and dry, with scraping, causes coughing. Swallowing painful. Larynx as if dry. Pressing pain on speaking and swallowing.

Tongue - Tongue furred. Tongue white, white center, red tip and edges. Tongue white-coated on side, and weak.

Vertigo - Vertigo with tendency to fall forward, better by nosebleed.

COMMENTS - G. F. Laidlaw gave a condensed translation of Rademacher's remarks about Card-m.: "He regards hematemesis as most frequently due to chronic disease of the spleen, less frequently to disease of the liver. People who have long suffered from pains in the left hypochondrium are apt to vomit blood after which they are relieved.

"Rademacher regards the bleeding as often beneficial and says it should not be checked too soon. In the treatment of hematemesis he says it is best to use a remedy that acts on the epigastric region without irritating the stomach and interfering with the healing of the lesion. Such a remedy he found in a decoction of the seeds of Card-m.

"He used to give Opium before, but this, he says in some people 'produces an array of symptoms similar to those seen in severe hemorrhage and might aggravate and condition.'"

Rademacher added: "It is probable that many small hemorrhages of the stomach escape notice because there is no vomiting and that it is in this manner that obscure abdominal complaints are sometimes suddenly relieved or cured."

Burnett related the case of a girl of sixteen who had severe attacks of vomiting for three months with pains in abdomen. The vomiting was relieved by remedies symptomatically related, but the pains were not.

An examination showed the "liver and spleen both very much enlarged so that they seem to fill the abdomen." Card-m. tincture in 5 drop doses, night and morning soon cured the patient.

Dudgeon gave an account of Windelband and Kunze's experience with the remedy. Windelband, in treating a woman for chronic swelling of the liver with Card-m., incidentally cured at the same time some "colossal varicose ulcers."

This experience led Dudgeon to cure a large number of similar cases with the same remedy. He also cured cases of gastro-intestinal catarrh, nosebleeds, metrorrhagia, hemorrhoidal flux, dependent on portal congestion. Tenderness of the liver, bilious fever, symptoms resembling peritonitis and stitch-in-the-side have been cured by it.

Kunze commended the remedy in cases of stomach spasms, contractive pains, vomiting occurring at the climax, cold rising from precordium to throat, feeling of spasmodic constriction, pressive, shooting pain in right side of abdomen spreading to back or shoulder.

Kunze cured with it pains in the hepatic and splenic regions accompanied with hemoptysis, or expectoration of viscid, lumpy mucus, and evening fever. Even tuberculosis pituitosa has been cured by it. Local muscular rheumatisms dependent on liver disease.

E. A. Cook gave Card-m. 1c to a patient suffering from liver congestion, swollen veins of legs, hemorrhoids and headache with great benefit to all the symptoms.

On the second day the patient developed new symptoms, which she had never had before and which alarmed her greatly: "Great giddiness with inclination to fall forward and a sudden and profuse nosebleed followed by great relief."

A striking cure by Card-m. in "Miner's Disease" is recorded by Proell.: "An old miner in the gold mines of Bockstein suffered from the so-called *"Bergsucht"* (miner's disease). His chief symptoms were: earthy complexion, eyes dim, hardness of hearing, mucus coating on tongue, loss of appetite even for his favorite food and tobacco.

"Great dyspnea and palpitations on going up-hill, spleen and stomach distended, with much gas eructated, constant borborygmus, constipation alternating with diarrhea, but the latter more frequent, evacuations gray, urine scanty and pale, skin dry as if withered, great weakness, pulse slow and weak.

"Especially remarkable was the disposition of this man. Formerly cheerful, he is now joyless and apathetic, the most important events he took no notice.

"He was given the tincture of Card-m., a few drops four times a day. Unable to effect any alteration in his food, drink or regimen.

"A month after this he returned looking much better. On asking him how he was, he replied: 'You have made a new man of me.' Almost all the former symptoms had disappeared and given place to the opposite.

"His complexion was fresh, his eyes sparkled, he was cheerful, wished to live and work, had good appetite, motions brown, more urine passed, pulse normal. He said for the first time he knew what it was to be well and he remained so for many years."

Proell also recommended it in disorders of the liver, spleen and kidneys caused by abuse of alcoholic beverages, especially beer. He related two cases, one in a cook who had symptoms of cirrhosis of the liver and general dropsy which made her features unrecognizable, and one in a worker in a brewery who developed dropsy.

Both were cured by the tincture. The brewery man, thinking the remedy was intended to be purgative and thinking the 4 drops prescribed would not be sufficient took the whole amount, 2 1/2 drachms, at one dose, without markedly bad effects and was quickly cured.

Proell added that Card-m. is indicated where there is a relaxed state of the mucus membrane of the stomach. Evidenced by flatulence and diarrhea, especially when the stools are clay-colored. Much fatigue is experienced, worse after eating, when riding, on awaking, frequently accompanied by yawning.

Chilliness is prominent, on awaking, at night, worse uncovering. Coldness of knees. Head very sensitive to cold. Sweating of forehead and back after meals. Stitches, drawing pressure are prominent, also radiating paints, constriction, band-sensation and cramps.

RELATIONS - ***Compare:*** (1) Lyc., Chel. Chion., Nux-v., Podo. (2) Card. benedictus - strong action on eyes and sensation of contraction in many parts, stomach symptoms similar. (3) Merc., Bry., Aloe. (4) Bry. - nosebleed.

REFERENCES - Boericke. Clarke. Murphy. Phatak.

CARLSBAD AQUA

(Carlsbad Springs)

PHARMACY - carl. Carlsbad aqua. Carlsbad Springs. Karlsbad. The Waters of the Sprudel Springs and Muhlbrünnen Springs. It is a very complicated solution containing the sulphite, bicarbonate and chloride of sodium in preponderating quantity with carbonates, sulfates, phosphates, fluoride and oxides of calcium, magnesium, strontium, ferrum, manganum, potassium, aluminum, silicon and carbon, with traces of iodide and bromide of sodium of caesium, rubidium, lithium and boric oxide. Karlsbad, Dilutions. ***Historical dose:*** Tincture and all potencies.

CLINICAL - Blushing. Constipation. Cramp. Debility. Diabetes. Gout. ***Hot, flashes.*** Rheumatism. Sciatica. Sprains. Urination, urgings. ***Weakness.***

HOMEOPATHIC - Carl. is famous for its action on the liver and in the treatment of obesity, diabetes and gout. Clarke found Carlsbad in the potencies responded admirably to its indications.

General weakness with discomfort. General anxious sensation as if blood in artery would stagnate, with constant flushes of heat. Pains are dislocated and spraining, drawing, tearing, stitching, burning, dull shocks and jerks.

Sensation of weakness, prostration, so that she trembled and could hold nothing securely. Tired, dejected, sluggish, anxious trembling. Great liability to take cold. ***Hot flashes. Flushes of heat all over***. Periodicity, effects repeated after from two to four weeks (Ox-ac., Sulph.). Itching on various parts.

In homeopathic doses, Carl. is useful in weakness of all organs. Weakness of all organs of organs of speech. Weakness of bladder, stream weak and slow, only passed with assistance of abdominal muscles. Weakness of rectum, stool slow and only passed with help of distant parts of intestinal canal. Constipation.

MIND - General anxious state. Excited and peevish. Feels weak and incapable. Poor self confidence. Discouraged and anxious about domestic duties. Discouraged before menses. Homesickness. Irritability.

Absorbed, buried in thought. Anxiety in the house, better open air. ***Confusion better walking in open air.*** Excitement over trifles. Sympathetic, weeping from sympathy with others. Sensitive, affected to tears by the sorrows of others.

Difficult thinking, indisposition to all mental exertions. Absent-minded, forgets names. ***Aversion to reading.*** Difficulty writing, often omits letters.

Abdomen - Pressing, pinching in the hypochondria. Twitching in jerks. Burning pain in spleen. Sensation of ring stretched around abdomen.

Back - Drawing pain in nape of neck and shoulder blade. Stiffness, paralysis, pressure. Heat and burning and at times a shudder over back. Tensive and pressing pains from small of back.

Chest - Heaviness, fullness, oppression, anxiety. Peculiar sensation of oppression in lower part of chest, as if lung had not room enough to expand. Stitching in chest. Weakness in the chest while writing.

Ears - Increased warmth in ear, which itches. Fine twitching from Eustachian tube to tympanum. Humming, roaring, ringing. Transient loss of hearing.

Eyes - Heat streams from eyes with burning and pressing in them. Violent pressure above orbits. Twitching, quivering in upper lids. Excessive lachrymation, worse using eyes. Eyes weak, water, lids agglutinated. Cannot do fine, near work. Objects swim before sight. Appearance of black spots swimming about.

Face - Face yellow, sallow, changes color. Red and hot. Pain in zygomatic process, feels as if cobwebs were on it.

Female - Three days after cessation of menstruation, discharge of lumps of tenacious black blood. ***Hot flashes.*** Leucorrhea.

Food - Appetite and thirst much increased.

Head - Aches with swollen temporal veins (Sang.), better motion in open air. Rush of blood to head, with heaviness and confusion. Pressing, stupefying, tearing headache. Throbbing and beating in head. Hair falls out.

Heart - Painfulness in heart, frequent transient stitching and painful drawing. Tension and contraction in heart region.

Kidneys - Stream weak and slow, only passed by pressing abdominal muscles. Frequent urging with discharge of copious, watery urine. Brick red sediment. Tenacious, like frog-spawn. Urine stains linen dark yellow.

Limbs - Cracking in all the joints. Trembling and crawling. Restlessness of limbs, with yawning. Sensation of falling asleep, stiffness. Going-to-sleep sensation in finger-tips. Heaviness of the arms after writing, with coldness. Varicoses of superficial veins of lower limbs.

Lungs - Frequent hawking of mucus. Sensation of soreness, sensitiveness, scraping and tickling. Difficult breathing on ascending steps.

Male - Testicles swollen without sign of inflammation, pressive pain.

Modalities - Better in open air. Better on motion. Even the headaches are better by motion. Worse morning and evening. Worse after lying down in bed. Worse after eating and drinking. Worse on ascending.

Mouth - Offensive smell from mouth. Sour or salty taste. Clayey, pappy taste with salivation. Flow of saliva and frequent spitting. Dryness of whole mouth, especially roof, as if dried up, with increased thirst.

Nose - Catarrh of nose and throat, with hoarseness. Frequent sneezing, blowing out thick mucus. Swelling of nasal veins. Habitual bleeding of nose. Nosebleed on suppression of menses. Loss of smell after stoppage of nose.

Perspiration - Sweats more easily. Stains linen yellow.

Rectum - Burning in rectum with constant pressure. Feces held back. Stool slow and only passed by much abdominal pressure. Mucus diarrhea. Stools green, or dark green. Discharge of bloody mucus, with itching. Bleeding from hemorrhoids. Shooting pain. Gallstones passed.

Sleep - Constant yawning and sleepiness, worse after a meal. Frightful dreams with tossing. Dreams are not remembered.

Stomach - Sensation of emptiness. Pressure and heaviness after eating. Heartburn (Carb-v.). Frequent belching, sometimes smelling and tasting of the food, sometimes very bitter. Hiccough and yawning at same time, worse after drinking and eating. Nausea with salivation and shuddering.

Teeth - Thick, pappy mucus coating on teeth. Gums painfully swollen. Teeth loosen and fall out. Prominent teeth. Tearing in roots of upper molars, worse after every meal. Toothache, worse cold or warmth.

Throat - Hoarseness and roughness of voice. Constantly hawking up of much mucus.

Tongue - Tongue coated white, with offensive smell from mouth.

Vertigo - Dizzy confusion and heaviness, worse after eating, better open air. Momentary attacks of vertigo, had to hold himself up. Vertigo with turning as if in a circle, better open air.

COMMENTS - The action of Carl. has been observed on some healthy persons, but the bulk of the symptoms, many of which are strikingly peculiar, have been obtained from patients under treatment. They are, however, characteristic and have furnished the indications for many homeopathic cures.

W. J. Guernsey cured with it sciatica in an old man with a eramp in his left ankle. About a month after ceasing the remedy the patient complained that he felt paralyzed in the loins for several hours after rising from bed, better as the day advanced. This was a new symptom very like the Carlsbad effects.

Noted periodicity, effects repeated after two to four weeks. The skin has red spots and streaks, frequently burning like fire. Pimples and pustules. Crawling and prickling on various parts with sweat breaking out. Itching on various parts. Much itching and increased sweat of genitals.

Increased sensitiveness of the skin. Sensitiveness to cold air, great liability to take cold. Frequent alternations of shuddering, chilliness and heat. Flushes of heat all over, especially in face with sweat on forehead. Heat of head with redness of face and creeping shudders. Sweats more easily. Sweat stains linen yellow.

RELATIONS - ***Compare:*** (1) Nat-s. - sensitive to cold. (2) Carb-an. - sweat staining yellow. (3) All-c. - lachrymation, Nux-v. - worse after eating, Puls., Carb-v. - better in open air. (4) Bell., Glon. - headache. (5) Anac., Apis, Nux-m., Ph-ac. - absent-minded, Aloe. - cracking in head.

REFERENCES - Boericke. Clarke.

CARYA ALBA

(Shell bark)

PHARMACY - cary. Carya alba. Shell bark. Shag bark. Hickory. N. O. Juglandaceae. Tincture of nuts. ***Historical dose:*** Tincture and all potencies.

CLINICAL - Hemorrhages. Purpura. Scurvy.

HOMEOPATHIC - Like Juglans Regia and Juglans Cinerea, Carya alba appears to posses anti-scorbutic properties. An exclusive diet of the nuts for three or four weeks in a girl seven years old, produced pronounced symptoms of scurvy. Hemorrhages from all surfaces, on the least excoriation of skin, very dark blood gushed out. Blood gushed from gums, nose, ears and other parts.

RELATIONS - ***Compare:*** (1) Arn., Carb-v., Phos., Merc., Ham., Bry., Rhus-t. (2) Cit-l. and the Juglandaceae.

REFERENCES - Boericke. Clarke.

CASCARILLA

(Sweet Bark)

PHARMACY - casc. Cascarilla. Sweet bark. Croton eleuteria. N. O. Euphorbiacae. Tincture of dried bark. ***Historical dose:*** Tincture and all potencies.

CLINICAL - Anemia. Anus, bleeding. Backache. Colic. Constipation. Cough. Diarrhea. Dropsy. Hemoptysis. Hemorrhages. Intermittents. Vomiting.

HERBAL - Cascarilla has a family similarity to the other Euphorbian plants. Casc. acts prominently on the digestive tract, constipation.

HOMEOPATHIC - The leading symptoms include a sensation of swelling deep down in throat. Accumulation of mucus in throat. Hunger after meals and a feeling of emptiness. Aversion to the smell of tobacco smoke.

Abdominal symptoms are better by warm drinks. Feeling of movement in abdomen as if hot water undulating there. The concussion of every step is felt painfully in the stomach. Marked ***inclination to vomit***. Griping preceding morning stool. Boils in inguinal region. Constipation. Diarrhea with backache and lassitude.

Abdomen - Tension and pressure on the hypochondria. Movement in the abdomen as if hot water were undulating there. Flatulent, aching colic.

Back - Backache and weakness, muscles pained violently.

Chest - Hemoptysis. Stitch upwards on left side.

Ears - Buzzing in the ears. Internal and external heat of the ears.

Food - Desire for hot drinks. Aversion to tobacco smoke. Hunger after meals.

Mouth - Roughness of the tongue. Bitter taste in the mouth. Aversion to tobacco smoke.

Rectum - Constipation, stools hard, covered with mucus (Graph.). Bright blood with stool. Diarrhea alternating with hard, lumpy stool, with backache and lassitude, preceded by griping. Gnawing pain high up in rectum .

Stomach - Heat in the stomach and burning pain in the epigastrium. Pressure on the stomach, as if from fullness. Pain in the stomach as from concussion. Pain in stomach as from a shock. Nausea and vomiting. Pressing colic.

Throat - Sore throat on swallowing, as if from an internal swelling.

COMMENTS - Marked lassitude and muscular weakness. Backache and weakness. Inclination to lie down. Sleep with clear consciousness. Heat with thirst from warm drinks (intermittents). Short, dry cough from tickling in trachea. hemoptysis. Stitch upward in left side of chest.

Constant slight urging with gnawing pain high up in rectum. Constipation, stools hard in pieces, covered with mucus. Passes bright blood with or without stool in large quantities, causing weakness.

RELATIONS - ***Compare:*** (1) Crot-t. - better from warm drinks. (2) Chin. - effects of loss of blood intermittents. (3) Graph. - mucus with stools.

REFERENCES - Boericke. Clarke.

CASSIA SOPHERA

(Senna Sophera)

PHARMACY - cassi-s. Cassia sophera. Senna sophera. Senna esculenta. N. O. Leguminosae, Caesalpinioideae.

CLINICAL - Dyspnea. ***Knee, pain.*** Osteoarthritis.

HERBAL - Cassia sophera is indigenous to India and has been frequently used by ancient Indian physicians for its efficacy in respiratory disorders. Its Sanskrit name 'Kasamarda' which means 'Destroyer of Cough.'

An effective herbal laxative is made from the senna pods, and leaves. The purgative constituents are closely allied to those of Aloes and Rhubarb. The active substances are glycosides called sennosides. Senna pods have a milder effect and have fewer side-effects than Senna leaves.

The main effect is an increase in intestinal peristalsis and a reduction in the water absorption of the intestinal wall, which leads to accelerated stools.

Side effects, especially from fresh senna leaves, are intense cramp, excessive abdominal cramps, and irritation of bladder and uterus.

Senna should not be administered to people who suffer from hemorrhoids or enteritis. Their use during pregnancy or the lactation period is not recommended because of their excretion via the mother's milk.

HOMEOPATHIC - Two provings were undertaken by the Indian Central Council for Research in Homoeopathy. The first proving (1972-74) included 21 males and 9 females, the second (1974-76) 24 males and 13 females. Both provings were carried out with the mother tincture, 30th and 200th centesimal potencies.

MIND - Anxiety about future. Causeless anxiety. Anxiety and restlessness. Fear to go to sleep lest heart would stop beating. Anxiety and fear of losing his way home. Forgetful of duties and of facts. Forgets to lock his room.

Changeable moods. Intolerant of contradiction. Angry when contradicted. Desire to be alone. Desire to lie down quietly. Aversion to talk to others.

Abdomen - ***Flatulence and distension*** of abdomen, worse morning, evening, better after eating, drinking water. ***Intense abdominal cramps.*** Squeezing, crampy, colicky pain in right hypochondrium, worse after eating, worse fatty foods. ***Colicky pain*** worse changing position, bending forward. Colicky pain better fasting, gentle pressure and rest. Colicky pain worse lying on right side, better lying on left side.

Back - Backache in dorsal region, scapula, worse cold air, better heat of sun, pressure. Pain in lumbar region, worse bending forward, better pressure. Sensation of heaviness in cervical region, worse bending forward, better pressure. Perspiration at cervical region during fever.

Bladder - Irritation of bladder.

Chest - Chest pain with coughs. In the proving the chest pain was confined to the left side.

Cough - Dry cough worse lying on right side. Cough with pain in chest. Cough and thick, yellow expectoration. Cough worse in morning and evening. Cough better from warmth.

Ears - Aching pain in ears, worse eating. Heat flushes in ears during vertigo.

Eyes - Itching of upper lids, worse sunlight, better cold applications. Heaviness of eyelids, better cold open air. Burning pain in eyes, worse motion, pressure, warmth. Burning pain in eyes, better lying down, after sleep, cold applications. Pain in eyes, worse bending head forward, better closing eyes.

Food - Diminished appetite. Excessive hunger. Thirstlessness. Thirst for large quantities of water at frequent and long intervals. Thirst for small quantities of water at frequent intervals. Aversion to bread. Desires curd, eggs, pickles. Desires salty things, sweets. Desires warm drinks, warm food. Better milk. Better hot tea. Better cold drinks. Worse fatty foods.

Head - Dull pain in temporal and frontal regions. Headaches, worse heat, daytime. Headaches, better cold applications, tight bandaging. Bursting pain in forehead, worse motion, exertion, stooping, Bursting pain in forehead, better pressure, tight bandage, open air, lying down. Hammering pain in forehead, worse heat, better gentle pressure. Sensation of heat in forehead, worse sun, better cold bath. Heaviness sensation, worse talking, better keeping quiet. Heaviness in forehead, worse evening, exertion, stooping. Heaviness in forehead, better morning, lying down, pressure. Heaviness in occiput, worse exertion, warmth. Heaviness in occiput, better washing head with cold water, better lying down, pressure.

Limbs - ***Pain in knee joints,*** worse first movement, rising from seat, better continued motion, pressure.

Lungs - Difficult breathing, worse dust, smoke. Dyspnea, worse winter, change of weather. Dyspnea, worse cold drinks, walking. Thick, yellow expectoration.

Modalities - Better rest and pressure. Better lying quietly. Better cold, cold applications. Better cold air. Better cold drinks. Worse warmth. Worse motion (pains).

Mouth - Dryness of mouth and increased thirst. Excessive salivation and impaired taste.

Nose - Nasal obstruction at night, worse cold. Nasal obstruction, better daytime, warmth. Followed by watery nasal discharge. Profuse, thin, watery, bland discharge. Dryness of nose in morning, followed by watery discharge during daytime.

Perspiration - Profuse perspiration, face and axilla. Unclean smell from the body.

Rectum - Ineffectual urge to pass stool. Constipation, no urge for 3 to 4 days. Stool passed after great straining.

Skin - Eruptions, like ringworm on thighs. Itching, worse night, better scratching.

Sleep - Disturbed sleep. Sleeplessness before midnight.

Stomach - Excessive hunger and gnawing sensation in epigastrium, better eating, milk. Nausea preceded by vertigo.

Teeth - Pain in teeth and gums with earache worse eating, pressing teeth together.

Throat - Dryness better sipping cold water. Sensation of heat spreading over whole body, better cold drinks. Burning pain, worse cold air, cold applications, swallowing, better hot tea.

Vertigo - Vertigo better lying down. ***Vertigo with a tendency to fall forward or backward.*** Heat flushes in ears during vertigo. Dim vision during vertigo. Nausea preceded by vertigo.

Vision - Blurred vision during menses. Dim vision during vertigo, better cold applications.

COMMENTS - Clarke mentions for Senna: "a nasty unclean smell from the body."

"Of 16 patients presenting unspecific pain in the knee joints, with the modalities mentioned above, 15 were relieved after taking Cassia. This indicates its possible use in osteoarthritis." (Central Council).

"Although dyspnea was observed in a prover during the course of proving, the modalities have only been obtained and confirmed during the clinical studies." (Central Council).

"While proving the vertigo symptom was accompanied by a tendency to fall forward, the clinically confirmed symptom was accompanied by a tendency to fall backward." (Central Council).

RELATIONS - ***Antidotes:*** Nux-v., Cham. ***Compare:*** (1) Bry. Kali-c., Nux-v. (2) Senn., (Cassia acutifolia., Cassia angustifolia., Cassia obovata).

REFERENCES - Central Council. Clarke. Murphy.

CASTANEA VESCA

(Chestnut Leaves)

PHARMACY - cast-v. Castanea vesca. Chestnut leaves. Castanea vulgaris. N. O. Cupuliferae. Fagaceae. Tincture of leaves gathered in summer. ***Historical dose:*** Tincture and all potencies.

CLINICAL - Coughs. Diarrhea. Lumbago. ***Whooping cough.***

HOMEOPATHIC - Cast-v. has been proved by Dr. H. C. Houghton and three others. Cast-v. has cured whooping cough, early stage, violent, spasmodic, very dry ringing cough.

Slight acrid feeling in throat. Desire for warm drinks. Very thirsty. Very free sweat after drinking. Loss of appetite. Sensitive abdominal walls. Soft stools of short, small pieces like chopped tape, accompanied with severe pain and rumbling, pain better by stool. Diarrhea. Thick urine. Lumbago, weak back, can hardly straighten up.

RELATIONS - ***Compare:*** (1) Pertussin, Whooping cough - when symptoms return again after being allayed. (2) Am-br., Dros., Meph., Naph., Am-br.

REFERENCES - Boericke. Clarke.

CASTOR EQUI

(Rudimentary Thumbnail of the Horse)

PHARMACY - cast-eq. Castor equi. Rudimentary thumbnail of the horse. Triturations are made from the scales of rudimentary thumbnail of the horse. ***Historical dose:*** Trituration and all potencies.

CLINICAL - Breasts, swollen. Coccyx, pain. Fainting. Epilepsy. Nails, disorders. ***Nipples, cracked. Nipples, ulcerated. Psoriasis. Skin, disorders.*** Warts.

HOMEOPATHIC - This is a very ancient remedy and was proved and introduced into homeopathy by Hering. The clinical experience of Hering and his fellow-provers has shown this to be highly useful remedy in ***cracked and ulcerated nipples***.

Cast-eq. especially acts on the ***nipples, the nails and bones,*** causing pains in right tibia and coccyx. General action on thickening of the skin and epithelium.

Nails become brittle and fall off. Chapped hands.

Affects principally female organs, especially the nipples. ***Cracked and ulcerated nipples*** of nursing women, excessively tender, cannot bear the touch of clothing. Warts on forehead, breasts. ***Psoriasis of the tongue.*** Bones, especially tibia and coccyx are painful. Fainting. Epilepsy. Desire to smoke tobacco.

MIND - Unusual laughter about things not funny.

Abdomen - Colic with urging wakes him in the morning, followed by a very thin, watery, somewhat burning stool, with passage of offensive flatus. Pain in left inguinal region.

Back - ***Weakness of spine.*** Pain in coccyx, worse every evening, while sitting.

Breasts - Breasts swollen, sensitive, worse descending stairs. Nipples almost hanging. ***Cracked, sore nipples in nursing women***, excessively tender, cannot bear touch of clothing, even in neglected cases, ragged. Swelling of breasts. ***Violent itching in breasts.*** Reddened areola.

Chest - Burning pains on chest.

Ears - Sensation of dryness in left ear, compelling to scratch. Twitching, internally in left ear.

Eyes - Frequent twitching in right eyelid. Itching in canthi.

Face - Sensation as if trismus. Transitory, burning, prickling pain in face and also on body. Prickling and heat on both cheeks. Dry lips with thirst in evening.

Food - Sense of hunger, even after eating, during coryza. Lack of appetite during headache. Desire to smoke tobacco. Great accumulation of saliva, immediately after eating. Soon after pains in teeth, loud rumbling in abdomen.

Head - Sensation as if occiput had gone to sleep. Scalp goes to sleep, numb. As if something crawling in hair. Pressure in forehead. Pressive pain in temples. Deep pressure in occiput. Headache with vertigo and nausea, sour stomach and lack of appetite.

Heart - Peculiar sensation about heart as of something alive struggling.

Limbs - Repeated pain in right tibia. Arms and legs sore as if beaten. Pain in left elbow and right knee. Right wrist-joint as if sprained. ***Very brittle nails.*** Crumbling of fingernails from slightest knock against them.

Mouth - Burning, on front of tongue. ***Psoriasis of the tongue.*** Pain in hollow teeth of left side, must pick them.

Nose - Pressive pain in nasal bones. Coryza, fluent, with constant sensation of hunger, even after eating

Rectum - Urgent stool, preceded by colic and passage of flatus.

Skin - General action on thickening of the skin and epithelium. Warts. ***Psoriasis.*** Nails drop off. Brittle nails.

Sleep - Restless sleep with numbness of right arm. Sleepiness in early evening. Stretches arms up over head and cracks fingers during sleep. Restless sleep, with many dreams. In winter dreams of fresh fruit hanging on trees.

Stomach - Repeated empty eructations.

Throat - Disagreeable, sick feeling in larynx.

Vertigo - Vertigo, headache and nausea in mornings, sour stomach and lack of appetite.

COMMENTS - General action on thickening of the skin and epithelium. Principally affects the female organs. Cracked and ulcerated nipples (Sars., Sil., Petr., Calen.), especially of nursing women. Nipples excessively tender, cannot bear touch of clothing.

Chapped hands. Fainting. Epilepsy. Desire to smoke tobacco. Psoriasis of tongue. Warts on forehead and breasts. Burnett cured with it a case of wart on forehead.

RELATIONS - ***Compare:*** (1) Calc-ox., Hipp., Cast., Mosch. Graph. (2) Hep. relieves the sore nipples. (3) Thuj. has removed warts caused by Cast-eq.

REFERENCES - Boericke. Clarke. Phatak. Murphy.

CASTOREUM CANADENSE

(Beaver Secretion)

PHARMACY - cast. Castoreum canadense. Beaver secretion. N. O. Rodentia. Tincture of secretion, found in preputial sacs of beaver. Castoreum when fresh is yellow and of the consistence of syrup, when dry it is dark red or brown and of the consistence of hard wax. ***Historical dose:*** Tincture and all potencies.

CLINICAL - Amenorrhea. Chorea. Colic. Convulsions. Day-blindness. Digestion, disordered. Dysmenorrhea. Eclampsia. Epilepsy. Flatulence. Hernia. ***Hysteria.*** Ileus. Menstrual colic. Paralysis. Pregnancy, vomiting. Prostration. Reaction, deficient. Sexual, disorders. Sycosis. Tetanus. Typhoid. Typhus. Warts.

Yawning.

HOMEOPATHIC - Caspari proved Russian Cast., Nenning, that of Southern Europe. Teste remarked that Cast. has been regarded as a resinous substance and he observed, moreover, that the beaver feeds almost entirely on the resinous bark of pine trees. In Siberia, beavers feed on the bark of the birch, which may make a difference in the effects of Cast. from different countries.

Cast. is a great remedy for hysteria. ***Weakness and lack of reaction.*** Marked prostration. Nervous palpitations. ***Nervous women*** who do not recover fully, but are continually irritable and suffer from debilitating sweats. Constant yawning. Restless sleep with frightful dreams and starts.

Day blindness, cannot endure the light. Spasmodic disorders after debilitating diseases. ***Creeping, tingling sensation, worse sleep.*** Chorea. Epilepsy. Fibrillar twitchings. Heaviness of the whole body. ***Pains are better by pressure, rubbing.*** Reflex uterine effects, are nervous and spasmodic. Menstrual colic with pallor and cold sweat. Feeling of fullness in the stomach as if too much had been eaten.

MIND - Irritability. Easily sheds tears. Melancholic and full of anxious longings.

Abdomen - Colic or other abdominal complaints, accompanied with yawning. Colic with weakness, better pressure.

Back - Pain as from excoriation, in the sacral region and back. Drawing pains in nape of the neck.

Chest - Stitches in chest, heat as if fire were burning in it.

Constitutions - Suited to nervous women with pains, cramps, and weakness after severe illness. Hysterical individuals. Abdominal soreness. Nervous attacks when the aura starts from abdomen.

Ears - Acute dragging in the ears. Tinkling, buzzing, and gurgling in the ears, dispersed by boring the ear with the finger.

Eyes - Day blindness. Cannot endure the light.

Female - Pain commences in middle of thighs. Violent, cutting dysmenorrheal colic with a few drops of blood, then cold sweat. Amenorrhea with a painful tympanites.

Food - Repugnance to food and constant nausea. Violent thirst, could not drink enough.

Kidneys - Frequent emission of urine, with burning thirst, day and night. After the emission of urine, desire to vomit with disgust.

Limbs - Nocturnal dragging in shoulders and arms. Spasms of hands and feet. Hands hot with swelling of veins. Weakness of the lower limbs.

Lungs - Breathing is short, difficult. Short breath when ascending. Slow, deep inspiration with short expiration.

Male - Seminal emissions with great excitability.

Modalities - Better from pressure. Worse from emotions. Worse cold. Worse during menses. Worse debilitating diseases.

Mouth - Tongue, swollen, twitching. Round pea-like elevation in center of tongue with redness around. Tongue sensitive to touch or food, with drawing pain towards hyoid bone.

Nose - Obstruction of the nose. Flow of aqueous, acrid, corrosive mucus from the nose.

Rectum - Summer diarrhea with green, mucus stools.

Sleep - Constant yawning as accompanied symptom. Yawns in sleep. Restless sleep with frightful dreams and starts.

Stomach - Regurgitation of a bitter acidity. Vomiting of white, bitter mucus. Sensation of contraction and pain of ulceration.

Teeth - Toothache when eating, provoked by cold and mitigated by hot things. Toothache with acute drawing pains. Swelling of the gums at night, with acute pulling in the temples.

Temperature - Predominant chilliness. Chilliness with icy coldness in back. Exhausting sweats after fevers.

Throat - Hoarseness, with disposition to clear throat. Dryness of esophagus. Burning pain in the throat, as from heartburn.

COMMENTS - Cast. resembles Ambr., Mosch., Ign. and Valer. Teste placed Cast. in the Thuj. group with Plat. and Bism. Teste concluded from analogy that Cast. would be an anti-sycotic, and he proved his point by initiating with it the cure of a case of pedunculated vegetations around the anus in a hysterical young woman. Thuj. completed the cure.

Teste quoted from Trousseau and Pideux the following indications, which he confirmed:

(1) Amenorrhea, accompanied with painful and tympanitic swelling of the abdomen. We mean the cases where only a few drops of blood escape from the uterus with a sort of uterine tenesmus.

(2) The cases of colic to which Castoreum seems to be principally adapted are of the nervous kind, that seem to be particularly seated in the small intestine. They are accompanied with paleness and cold sweats, a sudden sinking of strength, as if the very principle of life had been struck down.

They are without any alvine evacuations, come suddenly after lively emotions, a cold on the bowels or by the feet, as after long exposure to a cold rain.

Cast. causes jerking in small groups of muscular tissues, a sensation of heaviness of whole body, trembling of limbs.

RELATIONS - ***Antidote:*** Colch. ***Compare:*** (1) Ambra, Mosch., Mur-ac., Valer.

REFERENCES - Boericke. Clarke.

CAULOPHYLLUM THALICTROIDES

(Blue Cohosh)

PHARMACY - caul. Caulophyllum thalictroides. Blue cohosh. Squaw root. Leontice thalictroides. N. O. Berberidacae. Tincture or trituration of root. ***Historical dose:*** Trituration, tincture and ali potencies.

CLINICAL - After-pains. Amenorrhea. Aphthae. Bearing-down, pains. Breast, pains. Chloasma. Cholera, morbus. Chorea. Dysmenorrhea. ***False, labor.*** Feet, disorders. Gonorrhea. Hands, disorders. Infertility. ***Labor, pains.*** Leucorrhea. Menopause. Menorrhagia. Menstruation, disorders. ***Miscarriages.*** Ovarian, neuralgia. Paraplegia. Pityriasis. Pregnancy, disorders. ***Premature, labor.*** Rheumatic, gout. Rheumatism. ***Thrush.*** Trembling. Uterine, spasm. ***Uterine atony. Weakness.***

HERBAL - Caul., the Blue Cohosh, is closely related in action to Cimic., the Black Cohosh, though they belong to different families of plants.

HOMEOPATHIC - Caul. has only had one proving, by Dr. Burt, the majority of the indications were derived from tradition and clinical experience.

Caul. acts most markedly on the female generative organs and on rheumatic states. ***Lack of tone of the uterus.*** Left ovarian and left infra-breast pains. Leucorrhea in young girls or during pregnancy. Complaints due to uterine disorders.

Bearing-down pains. Uterine spasms (Sep.). ***False labor pains.*** During labor, when the pains are deficient and the patient is exhausted and fretful. ***Labor pains are weak or irregular,*** they cease from exhaustion or they are too painful.

Internal trembling with weakness. Exhaustion and general debility. Reflex symptoms having a uterine origin, like headaches, hoarseness, rheumatism, vomiting, cramps and spasms. Hysterical or epileptiform spasms at puberty, during dysmenorrhea. Chorea at puberty.

A rheumatic remedy, especially acting on ***small joints. Erratic pains*** flying about from place to place, drawing, cramping, shooting, rheumatic in character, ending in neck which gets stiff. ***Thrush***, locally and internally. Paraplegia from disorders of the uterus. Paraplegia after childbirth.

MIND - Nervous. Excitable. Fretful, irritable and apprehensive. Easily displeased.

Abdomen - Drawing pains in the right side over the liver. Severe colic. Pain in the umbilicus.

Back - Rheumatic stiffness of neck. Severe drawing in sternocleidomastoid, drawing head to left. Dull pains in lumbar region.

Causations - Childbirth. Miscarriages.

Constitutions - Rheumatic constitutions.

Eyes - Drawing pains over the left eye. Eyes aching, with a feeling of something under the lids. Profuse secretion of tears.

Face - Moth spots on forehead, with leucorrhea. Heavy upper lid, has to raise them with fingers, with leucorrhea.

Female - ***Habitual or threaten miscarriage*** from uterine atony (Helon., Puls., Sep.). ***False labor pains. Labor pains are weak or irregular,*** they cease from exhaustion or they are too painful. Revives labor pains and furthers progress of labor. Spasmodic and severe pains, which fly in all directions, shivering without progress. ***Extraordinary rigidity of os*** (Bell., Gels., Verat-v.). After-pains. Profuse and prolonged lochia. Menorrhagia after hasty labor, flow very profuse. Profuse menses, late. Violent, intermittent cramping pains with little flow. Dysmenorrhea. Uterus retroverted. Irritable vagina, spasmodic intense pains. Leucorrhea with moth-spots on forehead. Profuse acrid leucorrhea, often in little girls. Needle-like pains in cervix. Placenta is retained.

Head - Headaches from uterine or spinal troubles. Headaches over left eye, pressure behind eye, severe by spells, worse stooping, from light, from noon until night.

Limbs - ***Rheumatism of small joints.*** Severe drawing, erratic pain and stiffness in small joints, fingers, toes, ankles, etc. Aching in wrists. Sore nodes on finger joints. Cutting pain in fingers joints on closing hands. Erratic pains, changing place every few minutes. Aching, sore lower limbs, before menses. Paraplegia after childbirth.

Lungs - Hoarseness and loss of voice. Panting breathing.

Male - Sharp, stinging pains in glans penis.

Modalities - Worse from pregnancy. Worse suppressed menses. Worse open air. Worse coffee.

Mouth - Aphthae. Thrush. Tongue coated white. Teeth feel sore and elongated.

Neck - Stiff, with head drawn to left.

Nose - Drawing pains in the nose.

Rectum - Stool, soft white. Watery stools, great quantity.

Skin - Chloasma, on neck. Discoloration of skin in women with menstrual and uterine disorder. Hot and dry skin.

Stomach - Cardialgia, spasms of the stomach. Dyspepsia with spasmodic symptoms. Frequent gulping of sour, bitter fluid, with vertigo. Vomiting of uterine origin.

Temperature - As if too full of blood. High fever.

Throat - Pain in the fauces. Frequent inclination to swallow.

COMMENTS - Threatened miscarriage due to uterine atony, with a history of habitual abortion or miscarriage. Weak, atonic uterus (Sep.). Inertia of the uterus. False conception or pregnancy. Sterility with a history of uterine atony or a prolapsed or weak uterus.

Can be used for tendency to miscarriage, long ineffectual labor, weakness after childbirth, postpartum depression, but not in general during pregnancy because it can stimulate labor.

Labor with a full feeling, bearing down with a rigid os, severe labor pains accompanied by severe exhaustion. Exhausting labor, weak pains. Ineffectual labor (Puls.), false labor, premature labor. Rigid os, will not dilate further during labor, with thirst (Gels. is not thirsty, Bell., Verat-v.).

Lack of expulsive power where the placenta is retained, internal trembling. White, milk-like vaginal discharge after childbirth that persists for weeks with exhaustion. Postpartum hemorrhage with passive oozing coupled with exhaustion, venous hemorrhage.

Cervical erosion with a milky white discharge and chorine fatigue. Cervicitis (yellow-green discharge, Thuj.), indurated cervix (Con.). Extreme fatigue and uterine weakness (Helon., keynote is they have a consciousness of the womb). Antispasmodic.

Menstrual cramps with severe fatigue and exhaustion, labor-like pains. Drawing pain in the thigh, feels heavy and tired. Vaginitis with bearing down pains in the uterus, acrid and burning leucorrhea. Exhausted with vaginitis, thirsty. Menopause and hot flashes with weakness (Sep.).

Chorea at puberty. Problems at puberty, including weakness, menstrual cramps that come since first menses (Puls.). Was given, with some success, for chloasma and pityriasis versicolor, curing dysmenorrhea at the same time.

Great nervous excitement, tremulous weakness over whole body. Sleepless and restless, but exhausted. Can scarcely speak. Sleepless, restless, nervous, recalling the effects of coffee, which is incompatible with it. Generally chilly and wants warm clothing.

Arthritis in the small joints, fingers, wrists, toes and ankles, especially if since childbirth or menopause, or since some problem with the uterus. Painful, swollen joints during pregnancy. Drawing pains in the joints with the menstrual cramps, as though the tendons had contracted.

Rheumatic disorders of the small joints and muscles. Pains are intermittent and paroxysmal and fly about from place to place, generally worse at night. Erratic, wandering pains from joint to joint, stiffness in the fingers. Joints are swollen and painful. Stiff neck.

Nash regarded "internal trembling" as a strong characteristic when associated with the weakness, he cured long-continued passive hemorrhage associated with these symptoms.

Nash prescribed Caul. 3c for a woman of forty, seven months pregnant, who was attacked with severe pain and swelling of all the finger joints, wrapping them in mustard was the only thing that relieved her sufficiently to allow her to get sleep.

Caul. relieved the finger pains, but caused such severe labor-like pains that it had to be discontinued for fear of causing miscarriage. The bearing-down then ceased and the finger pains returned and continued until delivery, when they ceased for a few days.

Then the lochia increased to a flooding, a passive, dark, liquid with great weakness and internal trembling. Now the terrible finger pains returned. Afraid to give Caul., other remedies were tried, but in vain. At last Nash gave Caul. 200c, which rapidly cleared up the whole case.

RELATIONS - ***Compare:*** (1) Viol-o. - rheumatic carpal and metacarpal joints. (2) Cimic., Sep. (3) Gels. in dysmenorrhea, it is like Gels. and follows it well. (4) Puls. in labor-pains, but the mental condition is opposite, Cimic. (5) Bell. in intermittent and paroxysmal pains, Calc. - leucorrhea in little girls. (6) Lil-t., Lach., Sulph., Ust. and Vib-od. in left ovarian and infrabreast pains. (7) Mag-m. in uterine spasms, Bry. in rheumatism. (8) Sec., Sep., Goss. ***Incompatible:*** Coffea.

REFERENCES - Boericke. Clarke. Murphy.

CAUSTICUM

(Caustic Potash)

PHARMACY - caust. Causticum. Caustic potash. Causticum Hahnemanni. Hahnemann's tincture of acris sine kali. Potassium hydrate. Obtained by distilling a mixture of slaked lime and a solution of potassium sulphate. Tincture with spirit. ***Historical dose:*** Tincture and all potencies.

CLINICAL - Acne rosacea. Amaurosis. Arthritis. ***Bell's palsy.*** Bedwetting. Bladder, disorders. Bronchitis. ***Burns.*** Cataract. Chorea. Coccyx, pain. Constipation. Convulsions. Cough. Deafness. Dentition. Diphtheria. Ears, otorrhea. Emaciation. Epilepsy. Eye, disorders. ***Facial, paralysis.*** Fistula. Goiter. Hemorrhoids. Headaches. Heart, disorders. Heel, blistered. Herpes, zoster. Hip, disease. Impotence. Influenza. Intermittent, fever. Intertrigo. ***Laryngitis.*** Lead, poisoning. Leucorrhea. Locomotor, ataxia. Meniere's, disease. Menstruation, disorders. ***Muscle, pains.*** Nails, crippled. Neuralgias. ***Paralysis.*** Pemphigus. Pregnancy. Prostatitis. Ptosis. ***Rheumatism.*** Scabies. Scrofula. Skin, eruptions. Smallpox. ***Stammering. Strokes.*** Syphilis. ***Tendons, contracted.*** Throat disorders. Tongue, paralysis. Ulcers. Urethritis. Urine, disordered. Varicose, veins. ***Voice, lost.*** Warts. Whooping cough.

HOMEOPATHIC - Caust. is one of the great polycrest medicines for chronic diseases. The chemical composition is still uncertain though it is considered to be potassium hydrate or caustic potash.

Caust. acts upon the nerves, motor and sensory and on muscles voluntary and involuntary of bladder, larynx and limbs.

Chronic rheumatic, arthritic and paralytic disorders. Characteristic ***burning, rawness and soreness***. Indicated in tearing, drawing pains in the muscular and fibrous tissues with deformities about the joints.

Chronic rheumatic disorders cause contraction of tendons and deformities about the joints. Stiff joints. Restlessness at night with tearing pains in joints and bones and faint-like sinking of strength.

Progressive loss of muscular strength, tendinous contractures. ***Weakness, loss of muscular strength***, causing increasing uncertainty of control over the muscles, finally ending in ***paralysis of single organs*** or parts. ***Local paralysis,*** vocal cords, muscles of swallowing of tongue, eyelids, face, bladder and limbs. Paralysis from exposure to cold. Post-diphtheria paralysis. Paralysis from lead poisoning. Cold water tones the paralysis.

Trembling. Convulsions. Chorea in nervous girls, worse during menses. Cramps here and there. Epilepsy, runs in circle, then falls down, at puberty. Restlessness at night, especially the legs are constantly on the go.

Catarrhal disorders of the air passages. Seems to prefer dark-complexioned and rigid-fibered persons. The skin is of a ***dirty white sallow*** with warts, especially on the face. Fissures from least provocation, about wings of nose, lips, anus etc.

Emaciation, due to disease, fright, worry, grief and of long lasting illness. Children are slow in learning to talk and walk. Awkward at talking, chewing, walking. Broken down seniles. Patient is susceptible to both cold and heat.

MIND - Timid, nervous, anxious. Reticent. ***Anxiety of conscience*** as if she had committed a crime. ***Night watching, nursing loved ones,*** keeping late hours and missing sleep from taking care of someone (Phos. and Cocc.). ***Over sympathetic.*** Lacks control, balance.

Melancholy. Sadness. Taciturn and distrustful inclined to fits of anger with scolding. Hopeless, despondent, wants to die. Whining mood. Looks on the dark side. Suspicious, mistrustful. Weeps. Laughs before, with or after spasms. Convulsions from suppressed eruptions.

Grief, feels betrayed (Ign.). Bitter, emotionally caustic. Holds grudges. Weakness, ailments from long-lasting grief, sudden emotions.

Foreboding. Fear of impending doom, that something bad is going to happen (Calc.). Full of fearful fancies, worse at twilight. Sees fearful images when closing eyes. Fear of the dark and fear of being alone (Phos.). Vexed with business worries.

Cannot tolerate to seeing injustice (Staph.). Affected by bad news, makes them angry and motivated. Obsessive motivation for a cause, politics and injustice. Idealistic, more focused than Nat-m. Disappointed easily and argumentative (Ign.). Ambitionless.

Absent-minded. Memory fails. Confounds letters and syllables. Mental fatigue and paralysis. Mental exertion causes symptoms, such as stitches in temples, tension in head and scalp, especially forehead to temples. Thinking of complaints aggravates them, especially hemorrhoids.

Children are overly concerned about other people and oversensitive. Inquisitive and intelligent. Can get frustrated and feel powerless. Child does not want to go to bed alone, least thing makes him cry.

Insanity with mental confusion. Very sensitive to light and noises, also better cold drinks (Phos.).

Abdomen - Enlarged abdomen in children. Colic, spasmodic. Pain radiates to back and chest, better bending double, worse least food. Painful swelling of the navel.

Back - Back pain goes forwards or to the thighs. Pain in spine, worse swallowing. Stiffness between shoulders. Pain in hips, worse coughing. Bruised, darting pains around coccyx. Cramps in lumbar region and buttock. Dull pain in nape of neck. Stiffness of neck or back on rising from a chair, could scarcely move the head. Torticollis.

Breasts - Disappearance of milk from fatigue, night-watching or anxiety. Nipples, sore, cracked, surrounded with herpes.

Sticking pain below left breasts, dysmenorrhea. Violent itching about breasts in nursing women.

Causations - Ill effects of burns and scalds, fright, grief, worry, sorrow, night watching.

Chest - Chest tight sore, vest seems tight. Mucus under sternum, which he cannot reach. Pain in chest with palpitations.

Constitutions - Anti-psoric, anti-sycotic and anti-syphilitic. It is one of Grauvogl's hydrogenoid remedies, hence is a chilly medicine. Suited to dark-haired persons with rigid tissue, delicate skins. Adapted to broken down, worn out senile persons. Lymphatic torpid temperament.

Ears - Ringing, roaring, pulsating, with deafness. Meniere's disease. Words and steps re-echo. Chronic middle-ear catarrh and great accumulation of earwax. Thick gluey purulent discharge. Burning in ears, they become red.

Eyes - Paralysis of ocular muscles after exposure to cold. Paralysis of one eyelid (right). Heavy drooping eyelids. Ptosis (Gels.). Weakness of recti muscles. Diplopia, better looking to right. Continuous eye pain with inclination to touch and rub the eyes, which seems to relieve the pressure in it. Profuse acrid tears. Vision obscured as from gauze, on blowing nose. Sparks and dark spots before the eyes. Objects look large. Cataract with motor disturbances. Rolling of eyes, epilepsy. Eyes remain open without winking, paralysis. Eyelids quiver. Inflammation of eyelids, ulceration. Warts on eyebrows. Fissures in canthi.

Face - Face yellow, sickly looking. Feels furry. Eruptions. Warts. Cramps in lips. Pain in facial bones. Pain in jaws with difficulty in opening mouth. Prosopalgia better cold water. ***Facial paralysis*** (right) worse opening mouth. Dental fistula.

Female - Menses cease at night, flow only during day (Cycl., Puls.). Menses late and profuse. Anxiety, sadness and weakness during menses. Dreams during menses. Dysmenorrhea with tearing pains in back and thighs. Leucorrhea, smelling like menses. Leucorrhea, profuse, flow during night with great weakness. ***Aversion to sex.*** Uterine inertia during labor. Smarting in the pudendum after urination.

Food - Feels hunger, but appetite vanishes at the sight of food, or with thought or smell during pregnancy. Aversion to sweets. Worse after eating fresh meat, smoked meat agrees.

Head - Painless commotion in the whole head. Pain in right frontal eminence. Sensation as of an empty space between the forehead and brain, better hot application. To and fro or nodding motions or turning to right. Tight scalp. Stitches in temples on mental exertion. Nausea and vomiting or blindness during headache, then paralysis. Small, soft, round nodes on scalp or glabella.

Heart - Palpitation with pain in chest, burning and languor.

Kidneys - Paralysis of bladder from long retention of urine and consequent incontinence. Retention of urine after labor after surgical operations. ***Involuntary passage of urine, on coughing,*** walking, blowing nose, sneezing. Involuntary during first sleep at night, or from slightest excitement. Insensibility of urethra while passing urine. Burning in urethra when urinating, worse after sex. ***Urine dribbles or passes slowly.*** Urine is passed better sitting. Urine, black, cloudy, white. Itching of meatus.

Limbs - Twisting and jerking in limbs, chorea. ***Paralysis of single parts.*** Paralysis of deltoid, cannot raise hand to head. Paralytic feeling in the right hand with paralysis of tongue. Heaviness and weakness. Dull, tearing pain in hands and arms. Unsteadiness of muscles of forearm and hand. Numbness of hands. Trembling of hands. Contracted tendons. Cracking and tension in knees, stiffness in hollow of knee. ***Burning in joints.*** Tearing joints. Arthritis deformans. Rheumatic tearing in limbs, better from the warmth, especially heat of bed. Disposition to stretch, bend or crack the joints. Cannot walk without suffering. Left-sided sciatica with numbness. ***Unsteady walking and easily falling.*** Weak ankles. Restless legs at night. Pain like electric shocks in legs. Itching on dorsum of feet. Cannot stand on heels. Cramps in calves, feet toes and Achilles tendon. Writer's cramp. Whitlow of great toes. Slow learning to walk.

Lungs - Wandering chest pains, better pressure, worse sneezing. Oppressive breathing while talking and walking. Tightness or scraping in chest. Cannot lie down at night. Purring in chest. Sore streak in larynx. Pain in the larynx, worse blowing nose. Aphonia or hoarseness with pain in chest, worse morning, stooping, better talking. ***Difficulty of voice*** of singers and public speakers (Royal). Short breath, before coughing. Cough, hollow, hard, dry, incessant. Cough from tickling in throat pit of larynx. Cough at night, morning, worse stooping, heat of bed, cold air, better sips of cold water. Cough during pregnancy. Cannot cough deep enough, expectoration, slips back again, scanty, greasy, ropy like soapsuds, must be swallowed.

Male - Increase of smegma about the glans. Semen bloody during sex. Red spots on penis. Bruised soreness in testes.

Modalities - ***Better from cold drinks*** (even chill). Better damp wet weather. Better washing. Better warmth of bed. Better gentle motion. ***Worse in clear fine weather. Worse dry cold air.*** Worse winds, drafts. Worse extremes of temperature. Worse change of weather. Worse 3 a.m. to 4 a.m. Worse evenings at 6 p.m. to 8 p.m. Worse twilight. Worse darkness. Worse exertion. Worse stooping. Worse motion of carriage. Worse taking hold of anything. Worse bathing in the river in summer. Worse after stool. Worse from suppressed eruptions. Worse coffee, fats, sour things.

Mouth - Bites inside of cheek from chewing. Fatty taste. Recurrent abscess in gums, dental fistula. Teeth, feel loose, elongated, ache, worse from cold or warmth. Swelling in side of cheek or induration. Swelling at root of tongue. Paralysis of tongue with indistinct speech, words seem to jerk out. Tongue, red in middle, sides coated. Painful vesicles on tip. Rheumatism of joint of lower jaw.

Nose - Coryza with hoarseness. Sneezing in the morning. Thick yellow or greenish-yellow discharge. Nostrils ulcerated. Nosebleed during spasms. Pimples on tip of nose. Scaly nose. Old warts.

Rectum - Sore and burns. Small hard pustules around anus. Large hemorrhoids impeding the stools worse walking, standing and when thinking of them. Fistula with pulsation and pain in perineum. Anus prolapses on coughing. Itching in anus better cold water. Partial paralysis of rectum. Cramps in rectum on stooping, with desire for urination. Rectum insensible to solid stool. Stools, hard tough, covered with mucous, shines like grease, soft and small, size of goose quill (Phos.). Stool passes easily when standing. Constipation with frequent ineffectual urging. Diarrhea from cold.

Skin - Old burns that do not get well. Ill effects from burns. Pain of burns. Cracks, ulcers. Soreness in folds of skin, back of ears, between thighs. Skin prone to intertrigo during dentition. Warts, seedy, large, jagged, bleeding easily, ulcerating. on fingertips, nose, lids, brows. Itching. Scars freshen up, old injuries reopen.

Sleep - Yawning, when listening or paying attention to others. Yawning and stretching. Very drowsy, can hardly keep awake. Sleeplessness with dry heat. Frequent movements of arms and legs during sleep. Laughs and cries during sleep. Wakes with slightest noise.

Stomach - Greasy, taste, belchings. Water brash, salty. Acid dyspepsia. Feels as if lime were burning in stomach. Pain in stomach from ice water. Sensation of a ball rising in the throat. Sour vomiting followed by sour belchings. Vomiting of blood at night. Fresh meat causes nausea, smoked meat agrees.

Temperature - Coldness, not better by warmth. Coldness, left sided of diseased part with pain. Flushes of heat. Sweat about 4 a.m., profuse, on slight exertion, open air. Heat from 6 to 8 p.m.

Throat - Urging to swallow continuously as if the throat were too narrow. Swallows the wrong way or comes through nose.

Difficulty in swallowing from paralysis of throat, unable to hawk out mucus, swallows it. Scraping, burning, rawness in throat. Throat symptoms worse stooping.

Vertigo - Vertigo during sleep, at night in the morning, while lying down, on stooping, from looking up, during menstruation.

COMMENTS - The weakening effect of potassium in allopathic overdosing is well known and was strongly brought out in the Causticum provings.

Caust. is good for neurological problems with the neck, degeneration of the nerves, vertebrae, with brachial neuralgia, stiffness, and muscle weakness in the neck. Bell's palsy. Facial paralysis. Parkinson's disease. Weakness resulting from long standing grief or disease.

Paralytic weakness. Paralysis of single nerves or single parts. Paralysis of both the voluntary and involuntary muscles. Ptosis, facial paralysis, paralysis of tongue of limbs of vocal cords of bladder of rectum, lead paralysis. Facial paralysis from cold drought, neuralgia of right cheekbones to mastoid process, worse at night.

Convulsions, cramps, starting, restlessness, twitching. Contraction of flexor tendons. Trembling. Torticollis, spasm of the neck (Lachn.). Dupuytren's contracture. Epilepsy, when fit occurs in sleep and urine escapes. Chorea, the right side is more affected than left, words seem to be jerked out. Restless legs at night.

Arthritis with burning and stiffness. Jaw joints affected with rheumatism. Carpal tunnel syndrome. Rheumatism tends to stiffen joints and contract limbs. Neuralgic and rheumatic affections, tearing, drawing pains. Tendons can be indurated and thicken. Stiffness of the joints and neck (Rhus-t.) Keynote pains are raw, burning, sore, and tender.

Headache that draws and tears through the body. Sensation as if there was an empty space between the bone of the skull and the brain, better by warmth. Headache, cannot keep upper eyelids up. Ptosis of the eyelids. Eyelids droop, weakness of the muscles (Gels., Sep.).

Vertigo, excitement of brain and spine incapable, tends to fall forward or sideways (locomotor ataxia) with anxiety, weakness in head, sight as if through a fog, skin dry and hot, constipation.

Intermittent fevers, "sweat coming after the chill without intervening heat." Marked periodicity. Periodic, paroxysmal attacks, twice a day to every two, three or four weeks an attack, at new moon.

Sickly, sallow, low-spirited expression. Skin is dirty-white. Eruptions on scalp behind ears. Weakened and emaciated appearance, especially about the face, the abdomen is large. Glandular indurations. Scrofulous children. Scrofulous inflammations about eyes, ears and scalp.

Nails are crippled. Old, large inflamed and indurated warts, on hands, close to the fingernails, face, and margins of eyelids. Burning itching on face, discharging acrid fluid which forms crusts. Burns due to caustic chemicals, chemical burns (Canth., Urt-u.).

Eustachian tubes with tinnitus and reverberation. Sounds re-echo unpleasantly, an ordinary voice sounds loud.

Hoarseness with dry cough and redness of fauces, the result of weather or catching cold, worse in morning. Dry, hollow cough with mucus on chest, patient cannot expectorate, must swallow the phlegm raised. Cannot cough deep enough for relief. Accumulations of mucus in larynx and fauces, catarrh of throat.

Rawness and burning down throat and trachea. Laryngitis, hoarseness and speech problems, especially stammering and stuttering in children (Nat-m.). Semi-paralysis of the tongue where the child stutters and stammers and cannot talk right (Merc.). Aphonia, paralysis of vocal cords. Difficult swallowing of liquids.

Constant sensation as if lime was burning in stomach with water brash. Pressure and fullness in abdomen as if it would burst, much worse by food. Griping, cutting, better by bending double, worse after least food or tightening clothes, menstrual colic (Coloc.).

Spasm of rectum prevents walking. "Passes stool best standing." Obstinate constipation (paralysis of rectum), stools covered with shiny coating of mucus. Hemorrhoids, unbearable by walking, thinking of them, touch. Well-marked aggravations of anal symptoms. Painful pustules near anus discharging pus, blood, serum.

Paralysis of bladder. Itching at orifice of urethra. Itching scrotum, cannot retain urine. Difficult, frequent urination with spasm of bladder. Tendency for urine to escape during the day from any extra exertion, laughing, walking. Bedwetting, especially during first sleep, worse winter, better in summer. Coughing expels urine. Dribbling of the urine. Urine is irritating and burning (Canth.) Prostatitis and urethritis.

Blood with semen. Sexual appetite in women is abolished (Sep.). Constant indifference, except after the period. Sadness during period. Menses too early, too abundant. After menses, a little blood passes occasionally, smelling badly. Nursing women lose their milk after exertion or loss of sleep.

Slow learning to talk and walk and stumbling on attempting to walk.

Nash cured a severe case of prosopalgia with Caust. The patient was emaciated and debilitated by long suffering, pains came in paroxysms and were of a drawing nature. She had suffered from eczema at times before the neuralgia appeared. Sulph. had been given in vain. Caust. 200c rapidly cured.

Guernsey commended Caust. in the after-effects of burns and scalds. Patients say, "I have never been well since that burn." Its caustic properties may be its "signature" here. Guernsey gave "sensation as if lime were being slaked in the stomach."

Macfarlan confirmed: "Sudden severe pains commence in the left hip joint, lasts a short time, feels as if it had been injured, legs very sore or rather the lower limbs ache and feel tired." "Forearms in front very sore to touch and pressure, muscles of limbs sore generally."

Kraft cured cases of incontinence following over-distention of the bladder owing to want of opportunity to attend to the call to urinate at the time, such as occurs in shop girls and schoolgirls, who cannot leave their tasks.

RELATIONS - ***Antidoted by:*** Asaf., Coff., Coloc., Dulc., Guai. - in rheumatic contractions, Nit-s-d., Nux-v. ***Antidote to:*** Asaf., Chin., Coloc., Euphr., Plumb. (Lead poisoning), type-poisoning, abuse of Merc., and Sulph. In scabies. ***Compare:*** (1) Rhus-t., Ars., Am-p. - facial paralysis. (2) Calc. - images on closing eyes. (3) Nat-m. and Sep. - Spurting of urine with cough. (4) Rhus-t. - rheumatism from damp and cold, but with Rhus-t. there is restlessness and better from motion. Caust. has restlessness at night only. (5) Eup-per. - hoarseness worse in morning, influenza with aching all over body, has more soreness on chest than Caust. (6) Sal-ac., Chin., Carb-s. - Meniere's disease. (7) Staph., Coloc. - anger and colic. (8) Bar-c. - mental weakness, paralysis, worse damp weather. (9) Sep. - Enuresis in first sleep, in deep sleep, Bell., Sulph. (10) Sars. - Urine, especially in women, is passed without patient's knowledge. (11) Bell., Hyos., Ign., Lach., Lyc. and Phos. - difficult swallowing of liquids. (12) Calc., Carb-an., Phos., Stroph. and Stram. - Fear of darkness. (13) Gels. - Ptosis, paralysis, faint-like weakness and trembling, blindness. (14) Acon. - paralysis from cold. (15) Kali-bi. - blindness with headache, Kali-bi. has blindness better, as headache worse. ***Complementary:*** Carb-v., Staph., Coloc., Petros. Merc. assists the action of Caust. and vice versa in smallpox, (Teste). ***Incompatible:*** Acids, Coff., Phos.

REFERENCES - Boericke. Clarke. Murphy. Phatak.

CEANOTHUS AMERICANUS

(Red Root)

PHARMACY - cean. Ceanothus americanus. Red root. New Jersey Tea. N. O. Rhamnacae. Tincture of fresh leaves. The fresh leaves are pounded to a pulp and macerated in two parts by weight of alcohol. ***Historical dose:*** Tincture and all potencies. Locally as hair tonic.

CLINICAL - Anemia. Bronchitis. Diarrhea. Dyspnea. Heart, disorders. Intermittent, fever. Jaundice. Leucorrhea. Leukemia. Menses, suppressed. Metrorrhagia. Neuralgia. Side, pains. ***Spleen, disorders***. ***Splenitis.***

HERBAL - This remedy has a special ***affinity to the spleen,*** which enlarges enormously.

HOMEOPATHIC - ***Enlargement of spleen*** and liver (Chin.). ***Deep-seated or cutting pains*** and fullness in region of spleen. Painful inflammation, enlargement of spleen, either alone or with other disorders.

Low spirits with splenic affection. Headache on the right side with spleen pain. Pain in left hypochondrium with dyspnea, diarrhea.

Ague cake of malaria. Marked blood pressure reducing powers. Active hemostatic, materially reducing the time for blood clotting. Anemic patients where liver and spleen are at fault. Leukemia.

Periodical neuralgia. Chilliness, principally down back, shivering, rigors, must sit over fire, worse in cold weather. Chronic bronchitis with profuse secretion. Weight loss. A left-sided remedy generally.

MIND - Apathy. ***Low-spirited, fears he will become unfit for work.*** Great nervous excitement with chilliness and loss of appetite. Felt as if nerves were shaken, at dinner could scarcely hold knife and fork. Don't care feeling all the time, cannot work.

Abdomen - Deep-seated pain in left hypochondrium. Unable to lie on left side. Pain in liver and back. Pain in left side, with leucorrhea and chilliness. Sensitiveness in umbilical region with desire to relax abdominal muscles. Whole abdomen moves with beat of heat. Bearing-down in abdomen, worse after eating.

Back - Carotids throbbing in neck. Pain under right scapula. Dull pain in lumbar region. Constant dull pain in kidneys and up back. Chilliness down back. Weakness in small of back and legs.

Chest - Soreness behind the sternum. Constricted feeling in chest.

Constitutions - Sanguine constitutions.

Eyes - Eyes feel too large, lids swollen. Dry sensation of cornea, with a dull pain in orbital region.

Face - Cheeks and ears feel hot with cold fingers.

Female - Profuse, thick, yellow leucorrhea, with pain under left ribs. Weakening leucorrhea. Menses, ten days too early and very profuse. Menses every two weeks. Metrorrhagia with spleen pain.

Food - Loss of appetite. Craving for something sour. Cannot eat pastry. Thirst for water, but it made him sick.

Head - Headache, right side with pain in region of spleen. Head seems to move with every beat of the heart. Head feels as if the brain were too large. Dull frontal headache, better lying down. Crackling sensation.

Heart - Palpitations and dyspnea with enlarged spleen. Pulse full and very strong, heart's pulsations visible through the clothes. Heartbeat so hard it shook him all over. Chest feels too small for heart.

Kidneys - Sharp pain above pubes in region of bladder, before urination. Constant urging to urinate. Urine is quite green, contains bile, strong odor, frothy. Urine is alkaline with increased phosphates, high specific gravity, trace of sugar. After urinating, feeling as if all had not passed. Pain in back and irritation of urethra.

Limbs - Pains down forearms and fingers. Weakness of knees, must lie down. Dull pains in anterior part of thighs.

Liver - Full feeling in region of liver. Pain in liver, worse lying on right side, beginning immediately after dinner.

Lungs - Congested feelings in lungs. Chest sore internally, worse deep inspiration. Violent dyspnea.

Male - Syphilitic complaints.

Modalities - Great weakness on walking or standing. Aversion to move, feels too weak. Worse from cold weather. Worse lying on left side. Worse motion.

Mouth - Aphthous disorders of mouth and fauces. Mouth dry. Tongue, white coat down center. Tongue looks dirty. Food tasteless, unless highly seasoned.

Rectum - Continual bearing-down in rectum with constricting sensation, particularly with diarrhea. Dysentery. Light brown stool with loud flatus.

Sleep - Awake all night. Sleeplessness. Dreamed of snakes, robbers.

Spleen - Chronic hypertrophy of spleen. Enormous ***enlargement of the spleen. Deep-seated or cutting pains*** and fullness in region of spleen. ***Splenitis,*** pain all up the left side. Severe pain in region of spleen with low spirits. Dull pain in region of spleen.

Stomach - Wanted to drink water, but it made him sick.

Temperature - Shivering, loss of appetite and nervous excitement. Rigors at frequent intervals. Intermittents with splenic enlargements. Cheeks and ears hot with cold fingers. At 4 p.m., six chills in succession with constant chilliness up and down back after chill very hot, fever, pulse 120, throbbing carotids.

Throat - Throat dry, raw sensation on swallowing.

Vertigo - Vertigo on turning in bed.

COMMENTS - Burnett, following Hale, is our chief authority for Cean. Great affinity for the spleen in tincture or in potency. Good for trauma to the spleen, enlarged spleen, painful spleen in any blood disease or dying patient. Stitching pains, sharp pains in the spleen. Large and painful spleen.

Diarrhea and dysentery (compare Cas-s. and other Rhamnee) have frequently been observed in patients taking Cean. for spleen disorders. Leucorrhea, profuse, thick, yellow, with pain in left side.

Malaria, intermittent fevers and chills, and for severe cases where the spleen will swell. Peripheral edema with swollen spleen. ***Leukemia with enlarged spleen.*** Blood diseases including anemia and platelet problems. Pain generally on the left.

Cean. was proved by I. C. Fahnestock, but its place had already been made clear by clinical use and definite clinical symptoms have been observed.

Fahnestock's two provers took repeated doses of the tincture and both had severe symptoms. One had malaria five years before, treated with quinine. This prover suffered more acutely than the other and in the end had to be treated. Nat-m. 30c soon put an end to his symptoms. The other prover had practically identical, but less severe, symptoms.

Commonly used during the American Civil War. Dr. Hale, a homeopathic surgeon, gave Cean. in tincture and potency for his many cases of ruptured spleens from bayonet wounds and gunshots.

Dr. Hale said, "During the late Civil War I used this plant for splenitis, and was so well satisfied that I've been using it for six years on every case. I do not remember using anything else for an enlarged spleen. I have used it in the worst cases I ever saw from infancy to old age. I've yet to hear of its failure. However serious, it will help the swollen, enlarged, infected spleen."

P. C. Majumdar cured with Cean. 3x a case which had been diagnosed as heart disease, there were palpitations and dyspnea on exertion. Majumdar found the spleen enormously large.

R. K. Ghosh cured many cases of suppression of menses and leucorrhea in patients from malarial districts. Menses too profuse and too early with pain in left side. Cannot lie down for pain in left side.

RELATIONS - ***Antidote:*** Nat-m. ***Compare:*** (1) Cedr., Myric., Bell-p., Agar., Berb., Chin., Nat-m. (2) Ox-ac. - pain in left side. (3) Casc. - diarrhea, syphilis. (4) Tinospora cordifolia - a Hindu medicine for chronic cases of fever with enlarged spleen. (5) Polymnia uvedalia, Bearsfoot - acute splenitis with tenderness over left hypochondriac region, spleen enlarged, ague cake. Vascular atony, tissues sodden, flabby and non-elastic. Enlarged glands influences all ductless glands. (6) Ceanothus thrysiflorus, California Lilac - pharyngitis tonsillitis, nasal catarrh, diphtheria. Tincture internally and as a gargle. ***Follows well:*** Cean. is followed well by: Berb., Con., Myric., Querc.

REFERENCES - Anshutz. Boericke. Clarke. Murphy. Phatak.

CEDRON

(Rattlesnake Bean)

PHARMACY - cedr. Cedron. Rattlesnake bean. Simaruba ferroginea. Simaba cedron. N. O. Simarubacae. Tincture of seeds. Tincture of pure bean scraped on wound. ***Historical dose:*** Tincture and all potencies.

CLINICAL - Ague. Cerebrospinal, meningitis. Ciliary, neuralgia. Chorea. Convulsions. ***Epilepsy, menstrual.*** Glaucoma. Gout. Hydrophobia. Hysteria. ***Intermittent, fever.***

Malaria. Neuralgias. Neuritis. Rheumatism. *Snakebites.* Stings. Toothaches.

HERBAL - Cedr. is particularly useful in tropical or in damp, warm, marshy countries. Malarial disorders of damp, warm, marshy countries. The seeds from Panama has accounts of ***antidoting snakebites*** when chewed immediately after being bitten. It also heals snakebites and the stings of insects, with tincture of pure bean being scraped on the wound.

HOMEOPATHIC - Petroz and Teste introduced Cedr. into homeopathic practice, because of its powers of ***antidoting snakebites*** and also of its traditional reputation in intermittent fevers.

Clock-like periodicity is the most marked characteristic of this remedy. It has been found curative in malarial affections, especially neuralgias. ***Neuralgias occurring at exact periodicity***. Hysterical spasms regularly night and morning. Chills in persons returned from tropical climates.

Mania. Complaints after sex, chorea in women, neuralgia in men. Trembling. Numbness of the whole body. Convulsions during menses. Chorea after menses. Lectophobia. Bluish-red face, forearm to elbow and hands and feet cold, sweat beneath axilla and on chest.

MIND - Nervous excitement, followed by depression. Restlessness, as driven from place to place. Lectophobia. Body heavy, mind depressed. Mental symptoms are worse at night.

Abdomen - Abdomen hard and distended. Stitches in spleen and liver. Flatulence, colic and cramp. Borborygmi (left side).

Back - Stiff neck, pains all along spine. Pain in neck and loins on rising in morning. Pain under scapula and in pelvis.

Causations - Antidotes the effect of snakebites and stings of insects.

Chest - Oppression. Sharp, darting-cutting pains under floating ribs and scapula.

Constitutions - Adapted to persons of an excitable nervous temperament, especially to females.

Ears - Tinnitus. Hardness of hearing at night.

Eyes - Eyes red. Burn like fire. Shooting over left eye. Severe pain in eyeballs with radiating pains around the eye, scalding lachrymation. Periodic supra-orbital neuralgia. Pain over the eye, worse sex. Iritis, choroiditis. Objects appear red at night and yellow by day.

Face - Animated red face. Flying heat of face alternating with chills. Tumid face, pupils much dilated. Prosopalgia (right). Wandering pains, spasmodic distortion of muscles. Lips cold, bluish, dry during menses.

Female - Many symptoms appear after sex and during the menses. ***Epilepsy during menses.*** Leucorrhea in place of menses. Ptyalism and leucorrhea after menses. Genital excitement at daybreak with discharge like leucorrhea and swollen breasts with pain. Puerperal eclampsia.

Food - Longing for cold drinks in some, for warm in others. Great thirst during menses. Loss of appetite.

Head - Orbital neuralgia. Roaring in ears produced by quinine. Stammers after sex. Crazy feeling from pain across forehead, worse working on black. Pain from temple to temple across eyes. Whole body feels numb during headache. Head feels as if swollen. Pain over whole right side of face, coming on about 9 a.m.

Heart - Palpitations and hurried breathing with headache. Irregular action. Pulse quick and full with animated, red face. Pulse uncountable.

Kidneys - Pain in kidneys. Burning along ureter and in urethra. Feeling as if a drop of urine in urethra or a constant dripping from it.

Limbs - Acute, sudden pain in ball of right thumb up arm to shoulder, same in right foot to knee, causing her to drop to the floor. Dropsy of knee joint. Sharp pain in joints, worse feet and hands. Pain in ball of right foot, extending to knee. Shingles with radiating pain.

Lungs - Difficult respiration with partial loss of voice, recurring at different intervals. Suffocative fits recurring regularly every day 10 to 12 o'clock. Suffocating fits, worse after sex, sleep, better by eating.

Troublesome cough every morning at six, lasting two hours. Respiration much affected after sex. Breath cold.

Male - After sex, pain over left eye. Gonorrhea-like discharge, lasting three days. Gleet with formication over whole body. Desire with firm erections, all night, on waking.

Modalities - Better from standing erect. Worse periodically. Worse at the same hour. Worse open air. Worse before a storm. Worse lying down. Worse after sleep.

Mouth - Prickling itching of tongue. Painful pricking of tongue with sensation of heat. Feels paralyzed. Difficulty of speech. Stammering after sex. Mouth and tongue dry, breath fetid during menses. Profuse ptyalism after menses.

Nose - Point of nose cold with chilliness and yawning, 9 a.m. Profuse secretion. Glassy-looking mucus or thin, clear, acrid.

Rectum - Involuntary stool during chorea attack. Ineffectual urging.

Sleep - Yawning and stretching. Drowsy, sometimes very profound sleep. Restless, frequent waking. Worse after sleep. Dreamed of pleasant social interviews with female acquaintances. Dreamed of quarreling with a dead sister and other dead friends, cried about it and awoke with sensation of a stone in the stomach.

Stomach - Nausea with distention of the stomach. Sensation as of a stone on stomach.

Teeth - Toothache every night during menses with bleeding gums. Sudden toothache in left upper molars. Sensation as if cold air touched the teeth on inspiration.

Temperature - *Malaria.* Quotidian or tertian fever with marked regularity. ***Regular paroxysms of fever, coming at same hour,*** commencing every day 6 p.m. by chills in back and limbs or cold feet and hands. Excitement before chill. Chill with congestion to head, hands, feet and nose remain icy cold. Shivering and chill, followed by profuse perspiration every evening. During sweat, coldness and heat irregularly intermingle. Hot stage, dryness, heaviness of head, redness of face, burning heat in hands, pulse full and accelerated, thirst with desire for warm drinks.

Throat - Larynx constricted and tender. Intermittent laryngitis. Burning and constriction, difficult swallowing. Prickling and tingling in throat and fauces, extending some way down esophagus. Pain on small spot next root of tongue, as of a foreign body, worse from pressure.

COMMENTS - Characteristic clock-like periodicity in the recurrence of the symptoms. Rapidity of action (Bell.).

Fevers of low, marshy regions in warm seasons and tropical countries. Chills in persons returned from tropical climates. Intermittent fever commencing the same hour every day or every other day. During the fever, there is a red face in the hot stage, thirst with desire for warm drinks. Profuse perspiration. Excitement before chill. General debility, languor and fainting. Malaise.

Predominance of nervous symptoms. Trembling. Accurately periodic neuralgias. Swollen sensations, numbness of the whole body. Enlarged sensation. Sensation as if paralyzed. Strong sexual excitement. Epileptiform convulsions during menses. Complaints after sex (chorea in women, neuralgia in men).

A large number of symptoms appear on left side, but right side of head, face, right elbow and right deltoid are affected. Worse after sleep, lying down, night, open air, before a storm. Better standing erect. Objects appear red at night, yellow by day.

Teste reported a case in which Hellert was bitten by a coral snake. "During the few seconds which it took him to take the antidote out of the little bag which he wore suspended around his neck, he was seized with violent pains at the heart and throat, but he had scarcely chewed and swallowed a small portion of Cedron of the size of a small bean, when the pain ceased as by magic. An oppression and general prostration remained.

"He chewed another portion of the same fruit and applied it to the wound externally and in another quarter of an hour all he felt was a slight colic, which disappeared after eating a little. This colic was followed immediately by a copious evacuation of a substance that looked like curdled milk, white with a slightly yellowish tint." Other cases were also reported.

Halbert related a case of malarial fever in a soldier. Chills and fever were clock-like in regularity of recurrence. Liver and spleen were much enlarged.

Anemia was extreme and there was this additional peculiarity: intermittent stomach pain occurring with the febrile crises.

In conjunction with these conditions there was a manifestation of chorea symptoms involving face and shoulders mostly, the twitchings being troublesome in the inter febrile state. Often there were debilitating hysterical spasms, the heart became irritable and sometimes irregular.

After other remedies had failed to make any impression, Cedr. cured in only three weeks, the improvement setting in immediately.

RELATIONS - ***Antidoted by:*** Lach., Bell. ***Antidote to:*** Lach. ***Compare:*** (1) Ars., Aran., Bell., (2) Cedr. removes roaring in ears of Chin. Bell. removes "Objects appear red at night, and yellowish by day" of Cedr., (3) Ars. and Sabad. - complaints return same hour every day. (4) Aran. - ague when chills predominates.

REFERENCES - Boericke. Clarke. Murphy. Phatak.

CEMENT

PHARMACY - cem. Cement. Cement rock. The preparation for possible use is made by triturating a good cement with sugar of milk on the decimal scale. ***Historical dose:*** Trituration and all potencies.

CLINICAL - Eczema. Cement maker's itch. ***Itching.***

HOMEOPATHIC - Cement maker's itch is an occupational disease, entirely distinct from ordinary itch, being neither parasitic nor contagious, but produced by the chemical or mechanical action of the cement upon the skin.

Some physicians have attributed the corrosive action to calcium carbonate and to sulphuric acid. Fresh cement, however, does not contain carbonate. It is questioned whether slaked lime or even partly slaked lime will produce this effect. Masons working with lime mortar are seldom, if ever, attacked with cement maker's itch. The quantity of sulphuric acid in cement is very small.

Cement maker's itch and ordinary itch have one symptom in common: ***intense itching, especially at night.*** The itching appears to be increased by the heat of the bed and also is more annoying in summer than in winter. Scratching may produce infected wounds and swelling. It is likely to be followed by eczema and other complications.

The managers of cement works should always require their workmen to wear cotton gloves and garments tightly fastened at the neck and at the wrists. Cement workers on arches or ceilings should wear masks. Both gloves and masks should frequently be washed.

REFERENCES - Anshutz.

CENCHRIS CONTORTRIX

(Copperhead Snake)

PHARMACY - cench. Cenchris contortrix. Copperhead snake. American copperhead. Ancistrodon mokeson. Ancistrodon contortrix. Agkistrodon piscivorus. N. O. Ophidians. Crotalida. North America. Solution of venom. ***Historical dose:*** All potencies.

CLINICAL - Amaurosis. Catarrh. Coma. Diarrhea. Dyspnea. Eyes, swelling over. Headaches. Heart, disorders. Lethargy. Leucorrhea. Menorrhagia. Nightmare. Ovary, pain. Palpitations. Restlessness. Throat, disorders. Vulva, eruption.

HOMEOPATHIC - Cenchris has the main features of all the serpent poisons. Cench. is a wonderful restorative and deep acting remedy. Like Ars., it has a dyspnea, mental and physical restlessness, thirst for small quantities of water. Needs clothing loose (Lach.).

Coma, semi-consciousness. Insensibility of cornea. Swelling of upper lip. General swelling, paralysis. Cold, clammy sweat. Increased sexual desire in both sexes. Ineffectual attempts to recline. Right ovarian region painful.

MIND - Forgetful. Memory lost. Dreamy, absent-minded. Marked alteration of moods, vivid dreams. Took the wrong car without realizing where she was going. When riding in the car, rode past the place she intended to get off at. ***Time passes too slowly.*** Lethargy.

Anxiety, feels she will die suddenly. Anxiety in evening in bed. Anxiety while lying. Presentiment of death. Fear of apoplexy. Jealousy. Quarrelsome from jealousy.

Suspicious, thinks her husband is going to put her in an insane asylum, every day, 3 p.m. to 8 p.m., for ten days, yet knew it was a delusion. Delusion of being in two places at the same time.

Abdomen - Intolerance of tight clothing.

Eyes - Swelling like bags over eyes and under brows. Redness of margins and twitching. Aching and itching in eyes. Left eye waters from cough. Dim vision. Insensibility of cornea.

Face - Expression bloated, besotted. Face sallow. Burning face. Blue circles around eyes.

Female - Increased desire. Yellow leucorrhea. Pain in right ovary. Herpetic eruption on labia. Menstrual flow very profuse, light with dark clots.

Head - Aching pain in left frontal eminence and left side of teeth. Swelling around eyes, aching and itching in eyes.

Heart - Feels as if heart were distended or swollen to fill the whole chest. Strongly conscious of heart. Palpitations. Hard aching and sudden sharp stitching in heart. Throbbing or fluttering under left scapula. At 3 p.m., sensation of fluttering followed by feeling that heart fell down into abdomen. Then, pulse feeble with heat lasting until after midnight.

Lungs - Hard, dry, tickling cough, worse 3 p.m., even causing escape of urine.

Male - Violent sexual desire.

Modalities - Worse on waking. Worse lying down. Worse pressure. Worse in the afternoon. Worse evening and all night.

Nose - Catarrh, scabs, obstruction.

Sleep - Vivid, horrible and lascivious dreams, cannot be shaken off during waking hours.

Stomach - Nausea better by ice, worse by water, causes vomiting.

Stool - Diarrhea early in morning, on waking. Stool, gushing, frequent, watery, at first without pain, after several hours, great pain before the motions.

Temperature - Chill or fever beginning in afternoon.

Throat - Accumulation of glossy, thick, tough mucus. Difficult empty swallowing, but easy swallowing of solids and liquids. Warm drinks grateful.

COMMENTS - Marked alternation of moods. Dreamy absentmindedness. Swelling above eyes, below brow like an over-hanging bag of water. Diarrhea with pain before stool, stool papescent, cold but not chilly. Yellow leucorrhea. Pain in right ovary. Herpetic eruption on labia.

Hard, dry, tickling cough, worse 3 p.m. Restlessness and sense of suffocation, palpitation, sensation of dying. Chokes, must lie with head drawn back. Tight clothing is unbearable.

Chill or fever beginning in afternoon. Feeling as if whole body were enlarged to bursting, worse in region of heart. "Awoke with throbbing in vulva and anus, followed by a dull aching in the sacral region, better by walking about."

RELATIONS - ***Compare:*** (1) Ars., Lach. (2) Clotho Arictans - Puff Adder - Should have a great sphere of usefulness in many conditions where excessive swelling in leading feature.

REFERENCES - Boericke. Clarke.

CENTAUREA TAGANA

PHARMACY - cent. Centaurea tagana. N. O. Compositae. Tincture of root. ***Historical dose:*** Tincture and all potencies.

CLINICAL - Coryza. Diarrhea. Eyes, inflammation. Fevers. Homesickness. Influenza. Intermittent, fever. Vision, vanishing.

HERBAL - The Centaurea are allied to the thistles. Dr. Chagon, Duc de Sorentino, experimented with the root of Cent.

HOMEOPATHIC - Marked symptoms of congestion. ***Blood surges painfully at every movement.*** The symptoms are worse at night, in the morning on waking, by movement, during and after urinating. Better by eating.

COMMENTS - Allen reported a case in which a bright servant-girl who took it seemed stupefied for several days. The earliest symptoms appeared a quarter of an hour after taking the medicine, viz., those of the arms together with dull pains in the hypogastrium, shiverings and general heat, especially on forehead, which was covered with sweat.

These were followed by a stupefying pain in temples, frontal protuberances orbital arches and eyes. Next came dimness of sight, appetite alternating with nausea, increase of salvia and vomiting, running of the nose, lachrymation, belchings, rapid sinking of strength, general uneasiness, confusion of mind, weariness, dull sunken eyes, spasmodic sweating, itching and pricking in the skin, drowsiness and thirst.

A state of reaction after four or six hours brought some quiet. Next day, in the forenoon or towards evening, the above symptoms reappeared but with less violence and some of them assumed a periodic form.

Then ensued coryza, colic, diarrhea, fevers of various types, pains in the arms, dry cough, etc. The action ended with the symptoms of catarrh of angina and of fever in the forenoon and with confusion and pain in the forehead. This gives a general idea of the action of this remedy.

RELATIONS - ***Compare:*** (1) Bell., Cedr., Card-b., Card-m., Glon., Chin.

REFERENCES - Clarke.

CENTAURY

(Bach Flower Essence)

PHARMACY - cent-b. Centaury. Centaurium umbellatum. Pick the flowers, put them in a bowl of water and let them sit in the sun for several hours. The water imbued with healing power is used as medicine. ***Historical dose:*** Take two drops from the stock bottle into a one ounce dropper bottle, (add brandy or alcohol, if this bottle will be used for days or weeks). This is the dosage bottle, take a few drops straight into the mouth or as needed in a little water or juice.

HOMEOPATHIC - Centaury belongs to Bach's group of ***Over sensitivity to Influences and Ideas,*** along with Agrimony, Walnut and Holly. Lack of stamina may be apparent, people may not seem fully invigorated or empowered. Weakness in the mind, emotions and body. The psychosomatic diseases of hypertension (Will-b.), hyperthyroidism (Verv-b.), insulin dependent diabetes, soft tissue rheumatism and rheumatoid arthritis (Chic-b.).

In a mental illness, when excessive submissiveness and attempts to please others are part of the underlying dynamic. Dependent personality disorder (Cer-b.). Over-compliance and disregard of one's own needs (Oak-b.). One gives others priority over oneself, seeing their needs first and de-emphasizing one's own.

MIND - The mind is easily impressed with the needs and demands of others, to the point of wishing to do good and be of service. The balance of perception is tilted in favor of others. Feelings of guilt and loyalty may further bind and narrow one's way.

Life may seem more drudgery than adventure. A mistake of the service-oriented person is to overlook growing personal weakness and exhaustion. As needs of others seem predominant, one's own needs assume less importance and one's health and strength may be undermined slowly. Serving others may be a refuge for some, a binding up of one's identity with a positive attitude, a way to build self-esteem and find approval by others.

Sadness due to unfulfilled potential or unanswered needs. Disappointment, resentment or frustration in the helpful person due to insensitivity and neglect.

Lacks the courage to make their needs known, or their ethical principles may prevent them from entertaining resentful impulses. Can't assert their needs to others.

REFERENCES - Bach.

CEPHALANTHUS OCCIDENTALIS

(Crane Willow)

PHARMACY - ceph. Cephalanthus occidentalis. Crane willow. Button bush. N. O. Rubiacae. The fresh bark of branches and roots is pounded to a pulp and macerated in two parts by weight of alcohol. ***Historical dose:*** Tincture and all potencies.

CLINICAL - Constipated. Intermittent, fever. Nightmares. Rheumatic, fevers. Sore, throat.

HOMEOPATHIC - The item given below was contributed to the American Observer, 1875, by Dr. E. D. Wright. "Cures of intermittent fever, quotidian and tertian fever, sore throat with quinsy it had very good effect. Rheumatic fevers with soreness of the flesh. A worker fell in the river. Cold and inflammatory fever was cured quickly.

"Proving of one-half ounce in a day. First day: raw, sore throat, nervous and excited. Felt light and easy, happy. The bowels were constipated.

"Second day: with the same dose. Dreams about fighting, quarreling. Sleep was restless and tossing over. Joints of the fingers lame. Griping pains in the lungs in body and limbs, especially in the joints toothache. Bowels loose, stool offensive. Hemorrhoids."

REFERENCES - Anshutz.

CEPHALANDRA INDICA

(Telakucha)

PHARMACY - cephd. Cephalandra indica. Telakucha. Bimba. N. O. Cucurbitaceae. Historical dose: Tincture and all potencies.

CLINICAL - Abscesses. Biliousness. Boils. Carbuncles. Cough. ***Diabetes.*** Dropsy. Dysentery. Fever. Glands, enlarged. ***Glycosuria.*** Headache. Hemorrhage. Jaundice. Skin, diseases.

HERBAL - Telakucha is a perennial creeping herb with long tapering tuberous roots and deep green leaves, It is found to grow abundantly in a wild state in Bengal and in other parts of India. It possesses a smooth green fleshy frui whose taste is very bitter.

When the fruit becomes ripe its color becomes scarlet and its taste becomes sweet and it is sometimes eaten as a vegetable. It possesses the reputation of being an excellent remedy in reducing the amount of sugar in the urine of patients suffering from diabetes mellitus and mitigating their other sufferings.

According to Dhanvantariya Nirghanta, it is a good medicine for fever, dropsy, hemorrhage of the stomach. Jaundice and flatulence. It suppresses urine.

According to Rajnirghanta, it is bitter, cures cough and vomiting, excellent remedy for blood poisoning, arrests hemorrhage of the stomach.

The Ayurvedic physicians of India use the extracted juice of the leaves to allay the burning pains of poisonous boils and carbuncles, and for general burning pains. It is also used by them in bloody dysentery and in biliousness. They also use it in diabetes mellitus.

HOMEOPATHIC - Dr. Sarat Chandra Ghose, introduced this remedy to homeopathy and he conducted the first provings. He found Cephalandra indica an effective remedy for ***diabetes mellitus*** and insipidus.

Over-sensitivity to noise and external impressions. Biliousness, bilious complaints. Septic boils, abscesses, and carbuncles. Burning pains all over the body, better cold applications. Profuse urination.

Giddiness. Dysentery with white and bloody stools. Headache from excessive exposure under sun's rays. Chronic fever associated with burning of eyes, face and other parts of body. Dropsy, jaundice, flatulence. Hemorrhage from the stomach. Blood poisoning.

MIND - Moroseness. Fretfulness. Disinclination to do any work. Gloomy disposition. Could not remember all events, memory partially gone.

Abdomen - Full of flatuence. Abdomen distended.

Eyes - Burning of eyes.

Face - Redness of face with burning.

Food - Loss of appetite.

Head - Headache from excessive exposure under sun's rays.

Kidneys - Passage of copious quantity of urine at a time, clear urine, exhaustion and weakness after urination. Glycosuria. Presence of sugar in urine.

Modalites - Better by cold or cold applications. Worse after urination.

Mouth - Excessive dryness of mouth with great thirst for large quantities of water at a time, worse after urination. Lips dry and parched.

Rectum - Greenish, mucus stools mixed or tinged with blood. Pain before and during stool. White and bloody stools.

Sensations - Burning sensation exists all over the body, ameliorated by anything cold or cold applications.

Skin - Sickly, yellow skin was marked.

Throat - Dryness of throat.

Vertigo - Giddiness, worse after urination.

COMMENTS - Dr. Ghose reports the following case: Babu Satish Roy fell a victim of diabetes mellitus and suffered from this disease for two years.

November 12, 1928. Ghose was called in to see the patient this day in the morning. The following symptoms were present: Gloomy, morose and fretful. Lost weight steadily.

Passed large quantities of urine every now and then which exhausted him greatly. Urine was examined and the tests show that there was sugar in the urine, quantity being 20 grains per ounce. Great thirst was present.

Burning sensation was present all over the body. Dryness of mouth and throat was present. Ghose prescribed Cephalandra indica 1x to be taken thrice daily.

Now 18, 1928. He saw the patient again this morning, and heard from him that he was faring much better than before. Passed urine not so often as before, burning sensation and thirst were considerably less than before; cheerfulness returned and he was feeling stronger than before.

Prescribed the same medicine in the same potency twice daily. Asked him to get his urine examined again.

Nov. 28, 1928. Ghose saw him this morning, The urine examination report indicated that sugar had lessened, quantity being 4 grains per ounce. Burning sensation and thirst practically disappeared. The same prescription was repeated.

Dec. 10, 1928. The report of urine examination indicated that there was no sugar in the urine. In other respects the patient was all right. Ghose advised him to take occasional doses of Cephalandra indica in 3x potency.

The patient made an eventful recovery and no sugar could be found in his urine later on.

RELATIONS - Compare: Uran-n., Phos.

REFERENCES - Ghose.

CERATO

(Bach Flower Essence)

PHARMACY - cer-b. Cerato. Ceratostigma willomottiana. Fresh flowers are put in a bowl of water and allowed to sit in the sun for several hours. The water imbued with healing power is used as medicine. ***Historical dose:*** Take two drops from the stock bottle into a one ounce dropper bottle, (add brandy or alcohol, if this bottle will be used for days or weeks). This is the dosage bottle, take a few drops straight into the mouth or as needed in a little water or juice.

HOMEOPATHIC - Cerato belongs to ***Bach's group of for those who suffer Uncertainty,*** along with Scler-b., Gent-b., Gors-b., Horn-b. and Wld-o-b. Lack of assertiveness may exist, the person is rather retreating and allows others to lead. In regard to uncertain, unsteady gait or posture, especially if caused by reluctance and inhibition, Cer-b. will give physical assurance. In diseases of the immune system, when it does not know how to achieve health, Cer-b. may aid in reviving inner strength and help the organism decide on a strategy of defense.

Internal agony, preoccupation with oneself, hampering self-observation and shyness are common (Mimul-b., Lar-b.). Speech problems arising from inner uncertainty. Useful during language development when inner certainty needs to be improved.

Further, it could assist in developmental disorders by helping the mind gain in certainty and enhancing learning potential (Ch-bd-b.). In other distortions of expression of personality, fixed ideas and irrational anxieties, inappropriate laughing and immature behavior.

In mental illness, this remedy can be of service in gender identity disorders, anxiety disorders, delusions, elimination disorders and sexual disorders (Cher-p-b. for the last two), or whenever there is an underlying uncertainty of consciousness expression.

MIND - Lack of self-esteem and easily stimulated feelings of inferiority. One is impressed by others' decisive demeanor, wants to measure up, wishes for recognition and approval by others. Continued doubting, uncertainty and lack of decisiveness and self-assurance.

Relies heavily on the advice of others, often admiring their decisive move through life and feeling less adequate themselves. Overly impressed with outward shows and trends, people in charge of themselves and the situation, while they feel hampered within, often blaming themselves for this uncomfortable state.

Mistrust in one's capacity to judge correctly and make the appropriate decision. Dependent personality disorder, addresses the excessive dependence on the approval and advice of others (Cent-b.).

Anxiety disorders. Delusions. For those lost in their own reality.

REFERENCES - Bach.

CEREUS BONPLANDII

PHARMACY - cere-b. Cereus bonplandii. A variety of Cactus grandiflorus. N. O. Cactaceae. Tincture of stems. The fresh green stems are pounded to a pulp and macerated in two parts by weight of alcohol. ***Historical dose:*** Tincture and all potencies.

CLINICAL - ***Eczema.*** Emaciation. Eyes, neuralgia. ***Heart, disorders.*** Insanity. Kidney, disorders. Neuralgia.

HOMEOPATHIC - Cereus bonplandii is a variety of Cactus grandiflorus. The principal symptoms of Cere-b. are in connection with the heart (Cact.).

Cere-b. was proved by John H. Fitch in substantial doses. The prover lost 7.5 pounds in weight. He felt weighed down by an incubus. When mental symptoms subsided, bodily symptoms increased and vice versa. Could not bear contact of clothes, felt better on undressing.

Fitch who regarded Cere-b. as an ***"anti-psoric of remarkable power"*** cured with it a case of eczema of both hands extending up to elbows. Deposits in urine. Dropsy of cardiac and kidney origin. Left intercostal neuralgia. Anterior crural neuralgia.

Fitch cured two cases of insanity, one in a young woman, gloomy, restless inclined to curse, swear and throw things at persons, if resisted. The other case was in a married women who had spiritual delusions that she had committed the unpardonable sin, etc. This came on originally after confinement.

Marked symptoms included a desire to be at work, doing something useful. Pains through globe of eyes and orbit. Pain through heart in left great pectoral muscle, left side of chest. Expanding sensation in chest followed by sudden collapse. The effect on the nervous system passed off in four or five days.

Pains have a tendency to spread to other parts. Most appear on left side. ***"Itching in right popliteal space"*** lasted eight or nine years after the proving. "Itching with roughness of the skin like eczema above left knee anteriorly." "Itching with eruption like herpes below left scapula remained permanent."

MIND - Gloomy and restless. Great desire to work and to be doing something useful. Inclination to curse and swear (Anac., Nit-ac.). Inclination to throw things (Staph.) at persons if resisted. Loathing of life before menses. Delusion is under a powerful influence. Mistakes in time. Praying.

Chest - Pain in chest through heart with pain running toward spleen. Pain in left pectoral muscle and cartilages of left lower ribs. Difficult, sighing respiration, as from some compression of chest.

Head - Occipital headache and pain through the globe of the eyes and orbits (Cedr., Onos.). Pain across the brain from left to right. Pain along right malar bone running to temple.

Heart - Convulsive pains at the heart, feels as if transfixed. Hypertrophy of heart. Sensation of a great weight on heart and pricking pain.

Limbs - Pain in neck, back, shoulders, down arms, hands and fingers. Pain in knees and joints of lower limbs.

Modalities - Better undressing. Worse at night. Worse from pressure of clothing.

Skin - Itching of skin (Dolich., Sulph.).

COMMENTS - Symptoms from the proving including a miserable feeling on retiring. Throws himself on bed without undressing. Great yawning fit. Feels not pleasant. Feels half sick. Very dull in the morning. Feels very badly, has an ill-defined bad feeling in the evening and at night. Easily chilled in a room, better on disrobing for bed.

Alternations of symptoms of mind and bodily pains. When pains of the body are noticed, symptoms affecting the mind are suspended. The most prominent symptoms are the catarrhal and gastric ones, while those affecting the chest, heart, eyes, brain and nerves are more slowly developed and are the ones that persist.

Remarkable anti-psoric. Some skin symptoms developed by it persisted off and on for year. Itching of the right popliteal space. Itching with roughness of the skin like eczema, above the left knee anteriorly. Itching with an eruption resembling herpes zoster below the left scapula. Sleeplessness.

The provings point in the direction of kidney troubles and deposits in the urine. Dropsy of heart and kidney origin. Intercostal neuralgia, worse on left side. Anterior crural neuralgia. Rheumatism. Eczema of both hands, extending to elbows. Albuminuria with great edema.

RELATIONS - *Compare:* (1) Cact., Spig., Kalm. (2) Cere-s. - very irritable with tendency to swear, wild anger and low morals. Disturbance in speech in writing leaves off the last syllable. Paralyzed feeling. Pains in heart and dwindling of sexual organs. Emissions, followed by pain in testicles.

REFERENCES - Anshutz. Boericke. Clarke

CEREUS SERPENTINUS

PHARMACY - cere-s. Cereus serpentinus. N. O. Cactaceae. Tincture of stems. ***Historical dose:*** Tincture and all potencies.

CLINICAL - Anger, fits. Bedwetting. Heart, pains. Impotency. Nosebleed.

HOMEOPATHIC - J. H. Fitch proved Cer-s., as well as Cere-b. Kunze also proved Cere-s. The heart was less prominently affected by Cere-s. than by the other cacti, but pains in head and a paralyzed feeling were experienced.

Paralyzed feeling. Pains in heart. A voluptuous feeling, dwindling of sexual organs. Impotency. Emissions, followed by pain in testicles. Worse on exposure to cold, to which there is great sensitiveness.

MIND - Prominent mental irritations. Very irritable with tendency to swear. Wild anger and low morals. Disturbance in speech, leaves off the last syllable. Mistakes in writing.

RELATIONS - *Compare:* (1) Cact., Cere-b., Con. (2) Psor. - sensitiveness to cold. (3) Anac. - inclined to swear.

REFERENCES - Boericke. Clarke.

CERIUM OXALICUM

(Cerium Oxalate)

PHARMACY - cer-ox. Cerium oxalicum. Cerium oxalate. Trituration. ***Historical dose:*** Trituration and all potencies.

CLINICAL - Cough, reflex, Dysmenorrhea. ***Morning, sickness.*** Seasickness. Vomiting.

HOMEOPATHIC - Originally introduced by Sir James Simpson as a remedy for the morning sickness of pregnancy and chronic cases of vomiting, which he supposed to be due to some eruption on the mucus membrane of the stomach, Cer-ox., has fairly maintained its reputation.

Hale found it of most use in cases of vomiting of half-digested food. It was mostly been given in lower triturations by homeopaths and in five to ten grain doses by allopaths. In the latter doses, it has produced decidedly narcotic effect in two cases.

Spasmodic coughs of nervous or reflex origin. Whooping cough with vomiting and hemorrhage. Spasmodic reflex vomiting. Seasickness. ***Morning sickness. Vomiting of pregnancy*** and of half-digested food. Dysmenorrhea in fleshy and robust women, scanty flow, pain coming before or at commencement with feeling of tenesmus, better when the flow is established (Lach.).

RELATIONS - ***Compare:*** (1) Ingluvin - made from gizzard of a fowl. Vomiting of pregnancy, gastric neurasthenia. Infantile vomiting and diarrhea. 3x trituration. (2) Amyg., Lac-ac., Ip.

REFERENCES - Boericke. Clarke.

CERVUS CAMPESTRIS

(Brazilian Deer)

PHARMACY - cerv. Cervus campestris. Brazilian deer. Cervus brasilicus. Triturations of the hide covered with hair. ***Historical dose:*** Trituration and all potencies.

CLINICAL - Sciatica. Taste, altered. Tongue, painful.

HOMEOPATHIC - Mure proved this substance. One symptom appears to be peculiar: "Taste of doughy bread in the mouth."

Abdomen - Pricking in navel when lying. Needle-like pain intermitting in right groin in direction of joint after walking.

Eyes - Sensitive to light, especially sunlight.

Face - Face mottled.

Limbs - Numbness of arm on which he lies of hand and legs. Frequent pain, now in left buttock now in thigh.

Mouth - Taste of doughy bread. Coppery taste with heat in throat when taking the drug.

Sleep - Drowsiness and yawning.

RELATIONS - ***Compare:*** (1) Carb-an.

REFERENCES - Boericke. Clarke.

CESIUM MURIATICUM

(Cesium Chloride)

PHARMACY - ces-mur. Cesium muriaticum. Cesium chloride. Triturations. ***Historical dose:*** All potencies.

CLINICAL - Backaches. Cancer, pains. Colic. Diarrhea. Headaches. Languor.

HOMEOPATHIC - Cesium has pain in the lumbar region and testicles. Headaches with a darting pain through the temples. Cancer, pains. Diarrhea and colic. Languor.

RELATIONS - ***Compare:*** (1) Ars., Hydr-s.

REFERENCES - Boericke.

CETRARIA ISLANDICA

(Iceland Moss)

PHARMACY - cetr. Cetraria islandica. Iceland moss. Lichen islandicus. N. O. Lichenes. Iceland. Decoction and tincture. ***Historical dose:*** Tincture and all potencies.

CLINICAL - Atrophy. Catarrh. Diarrhea. Emaciation. Lungs, weak. Scrofulous. Scurvy. Tuberculosis. Ulcers. Weakness.

HERBAL - The well-known Iceland Moss, growing in large quantities in Alaska, recommended to the Old School since 1674 by Olaf Borrichins, Hiaren and others. Cetr. has been used in decoction and as a food and has been found curative empirically. It is used as a decoction and boiled with milk as an expectorant and nutrient in bronchorrhea, catarrh, etc.

HOMEOPATHIC - Indications include a bitter, slimy taste, full and satisfied feeling after eating a little, and habitual vomiting. Weak lungs. Frequent catarrhs. Tickling and spasmodic feeling in windpipe on waking. Copious expectoration. Fetid taste and smell causing nausea.

All kinds of bloody expectoration. Emaciated people. Chronic diarrhea with bloody expectoration. Chronic diarrhea of tuberculosis patients. Scrofulous emaciation. Atrophy, depending on suppurative processes.

RELATIONS - ***Compare:*** (1) Stict., Iod.

REFERENCES - Boericke.

CHAMOMILLA VULGARIS

(German Chamomile)

PHARMACY - cham. Chamomilla vulgaris. German chamomile. Chamomilla matricaria. Matricaria chamomilla. N. O. Composite. Tincture of whole fresh plant. ***Historical dose:*** Tincture and all potencies.

CLINICAL - Acidity. Anger. Asthma. Belchings. Blepharitis. Blepharospasm. Catarrh. Coffee, habit. ***Coffee, abuse. Colic.*** Convulsions. Coughs. Cramps. Croup. ***Dentition.*** Diarrhea. ***Dysmenorrhea.*** Dyspepsia. ***Earaches.*** Eye, disorders. Erysipelas. Excitement. Excoriation. Fainting. Fevers. ***Flatulence.*** Gout. Headaches. Hernia. Hysterical. Influenza. Jaundice. Lienteria. ***Labor, disorders,*** after-pains. Mastitis. ***Menstruation, disordered.*** Menstrual, cramps. Miliary, eruption. Milk-fever. Miscarriage. Mumps. Neuralgias. Ophthalmia. ***Otitis, media. Pains, severe.*** Parotiditis. Perichondritis. Peritonitis. Rheumatism. Salivation. Sciatic, pain. ***Screaming.*** Sensitiveness. Spasms. Speech disorders. ***Toothache.*** Ulcers. Uterus, diseases. Whooping cough.

HERBAL - "Chamomile tea" has removed the night-sweats of tuberculosis.

HOMEOPATHIC - Cham. is particularly suited to diseases of children, pregnant women and nurses. Especially of frequent employment in diseases of children, where peevishness, restlessness and colic give the needful indications. Mental and physical symptoms appear in paroxysms, ***irritability,*** restlessness, ***colic,*** cough etc.

Cham. is for highly emotional, ***temperamental and oversensitive*** persons. The senses are too acute. ***Sensitive, irritable***. Cannot bear to be looked at. Cannot be civil to doctor. Impatient. Peevish. ***Very cross, cannot be appeased.*** Frantic irritability and snappish. Hard to please.

Hypersensitive to pain (Nux-v.), intolerance of pain, agony with pain. Pain out of proportion with problem. ***Pains unendurable***, associated with numbness. ***Pain is intolerable,*** becomes mad with pain or magnifies her pains and prostrated with pain. Tosses about. Cries out from pain or walks the floor. Worse thinking of their pain. ***Demands instant relief from suffering***, would rather die than suffer. Wandering pains (Puls.). Hot sweat with pains, thirsty.

Ill-humor, anger with rage, violence and heat. ***Bad temper and irritable*** (Nux-v. i malicious). ***Ill effects of anger. Colic,*** diarrhea, jaundice, twitching and convulsion after anger. Biliousness preceded by anger.

Repeated spasms of face, arms, legs etc. Cramps with bilious vomiting of muscles. Convulsion during dentition. During convulsions body becomes stiff, eyes roll about, face becomes wry, thumbs turn inwards.

Teething pains. Toothache when entering a warm room or from drinking anything warm. Fetor of breath and of discharges in general. Gastralgia, food eaten lies like load on stomach, hypochondria distended. Tongue yellowish white. Bitter taste. Colic better by drinking coffee. Hypersensitive from ***abuse of coffee*** and narcotics. Thirsty, hot.

Otitis media with severe ear pains. Very ***sensitive to the wind, can cause earache*** with fever and anger. Worse drafts and wind, fear of the wind. Stopped up colds with dripping of hot water from nose. Night-sweats. Hot sweat on head. ***One cheek red, the other pale.*** Face sweats after eating or drinking.

Child cries and must be carried about to be quieted. Relieved by being carried fast, walking while carrying. Worse from 9 p.m. to midnight. Worse stuffy rooms, warm (Puls.). Worse excitement (Coff.). Thirst for cold drinks. Nightmares.

MIND - ***Irritable, fussy, whining and moaning.*** Capricious. Child wants many things which he then refuses. ***Discontented and dissatisfied, demanding.*** They do not know what they want. ***Children want to be carried and held.*** Child can only be quieted when carried about and petted constantly.

Extremely sensitive to every type of pain, always complaining. ***Sensitive to music, noise.*** Aversion to talking. Can't bear anyone near him. ***Violent from the pains.*** Aversion to being touched. Kicks when carried and becomes stiff. ***Oversensitive after coffee***

Despair with the pains.

Obstinate. Fretful, peevish, a frenzy of irritability and sensitivity. Fussy (Nux-v.). Ugly behavior, ***cross and uncivil, quarrelsome.*** Spiteful, snappish. Whining restlessness. Fidgety, hyper. Hasty, hurried. Abrupt. Sensitive to reprimands. Sensitive nerves.

Complaints from anger and vexation. Anger can bring out Cham. state (Staph., Coloc.). Mistrust. Faint after intense emotions or intense pain. Averse to being spoken to, touched, or being looked at. Omits words while writing and speaking.

Excitement and confusion. Fear of wind. Anxiety with ineffectual urging to urinate, without much urine in bladder. Impatience, everything goes too slowly. Impatient, intolerant of being interrupted. ***Weeping during sleep.*** Cross and sleepless. Restlessness, driving out of bed.

Melancholia, with constant moaning and muttering to herself, walks all the time with downcast eyes. Women become suddenly ***capricious, quarrelsome, obstinate***, before menses. No consideration for feelings of others and will enter into a dispute or quarrel with them regardless.

Peevishness about everything, with dyspnea. Dwells on past disagreeable occurrences. Moaning on account of a very trifling offence, which has happened a long time ago. Indifference to pleasure. ***Irritability when spoken to during menses.*** Tries to get away from her friends if they seek to comfort her. Dissatisfaction with everything she undertakes. Irresolution. Thoughts of dying.

Abdomen - Distended abdomen. ***Spells of colic*** from time to time. ***Flatulent colic*** after anger, with red cheeks and hot perspiration. Pain from side to side or going upward after anger. ***Colic in infants, children. Colic during dentition.*** Griping in region of navel and pain in small of back. Cutting pains, wind colic, worse night, urinating, better warm applications. As if bowels were knotted and abdomen empty. Acute duodenitis.

Back - Insupportable pain in loins and hips. Lumbago. Stiffness of neck muscles. Severe pains in loins and hips, opposite to that on which patient is lying.

Breasts - Breasts sore, nipples inflamed and very tender. Infants' breasts tender. Cramps, when child nurses. Milk is spoiled, baby won't suck.

Causations - Ill effects of bad temper. ***Abuse of coffee*** or narcotics. ***Dentition.***

Constitutions - Suited to diseases of pregnant women, nurses and little children. Irritable, colicky babies, teething problems, earaches. Hypersensitive to pain. Arthritic diathesis. Neuralgic or gouty rheumatic diathesis.

Ears - ***Sensitive to cold wind*** or noise about ears. ***Earache with soreness, swelling and heat, driving patient frantic.*** Earache, sticking, better warmth. Stitching pain. ***Otitis media with fever and pain.*** Ears feel stopped up. ***Ears sensitive to touch and painful.*** Ringing after hemorrhages. Roaring in the ears as of rushing water. Music is insupportable. As if hot water was running out. Hear voices of absent persons, at night.

Eyes - Lids smart. Yellow conjunctiva. Spasmodic closing of lids. Bloody water from the eyes of newborn babies.

Face - Swelling or ***redness of the cheek.*** Red cheeks and hot sweat during colic. ***One cheek red and hot, other pale and cold.*** Face pale, sunken, distorted by pain. Neuralgia of the face with hot sweat about the head, pain extending into ear. Jerking of tongue and facial muscles. Jaws feel tired. Stitches in jaw extending to inner ear and teeth. Sweats after eating or drinking.

Female - Irregular labor-like pains, going up and down inner thighs, with profuse discharge of clotted, dark blood. ***Intolerable labor pains, sends the doctors and nurse away,*** then calls again. Lochia too profuse and bloody or suppressed. Puerperal convulsions after anger. Distressing after pains. Menorrhagia with black clots, profuse with coldness of limbs and much thirst. ***Menstrual cramps with alot of pain and irritability.*** Dysmenorrhea from anger or emotions. Membranous dysmenorrhea, specially at puberty. Yellow, and acrid leucorrhea. Oozing of dark, foul blood with occasional gush of bright, red blood.

Head - Throbbing headache in one half of the brain, inclination to bend head backwards. As if hair stood on end with shivering. ***Headaches, worse from coffee.*** Hot, clammy sweat on forehead and scalp during sleep, wetting the hair. Headache of delicate, over-fatigued women. Headache, better when mind is engaged, worse morning and 9 p.m.

Kidneys - Urine hot and yellowish. Stitches in urethra.

Limbs - Numbness and stiffness of hands, when grasping objects. Palms dry. Violent rheumatic pains drive him out of bed at night, compelled to walk about. Burning of soles at night (Sulph.). Feet as if paralyzed, cannot step on them, at night. Feel as if she is walking on the ends of bones of her legs. Cramps in calves. Ankles give way in the afternoon.

Liver - Hepatic colic.

Lungs - Spells of dry tickling cough. Hoarseness, hawking, rawness of larynx. Asthma from anger, worse dry weather, better bending head back. Irritable, dry, tickling cough, suffocative tightness of chest with bitter expectoration in daytime. Rattling of mucus in child's chest. Anger provokes a cough in children. Whooping cough, suffocating, then vomits. Cough worse 9 p.m. to 12 p.m. during sleep, does not wake up the child.

Modalities - ***Better from being carried.*** Better warm wet weather. Better heat. Better sweating. Better cold applications. Walking improves backache and rheumatic pains. ***Worse from anger.*** Worse touch, being looked at. Worse lying in bed. Worse covering. Worse belchings. ***Worse during dentition. Worse from coffee.*** Worse narcotics, alcohol, and stimulants. Worse noise, music. Worse heat, warm food. ***Worse at night.*** Worse cold air, damp air. ***Worse from cold, wind.*** Great dread of wind.

Mouth - Toothache, worse after warm drinks, coffee, at night. ***Worse during dentition.*** Toothache worse during pregnancy. Toothache drives to distraction. Teeth feel elongated. ***Distress of teething children*** (Calc-p., Ter.). Jerking in tongue. Thick, white, yellow fur on tongue. Nightly salivation of sweetish taste. Painful wisdom teeth. Bitter taste. Bad, sour breath.

Nose - Extremely sensitive to all smells. Crawling in nose, until eyes water. Hot coryza, with obstruction of nose, inability to sleep. Skin wrinkled.

Rectum - Diarrhea during dentition, from cold, or anger. Stools, hot, green, watery, fetid, slimy with colic. Stools, ***sour, slimy, hacked.*** Stools, yellow-green or ***lienteric***. Stools, smelling like bad eggs. ***Stools are grass green*** (Mag-c.). Stools, like chopped white and yellow mucus like chopped eggs and spinach. Anus swollen and pouting. Hemorrhoids with painful fissures.

Skin - Rash of infants and of nursing mothers. Jaundice after anger. Burning, smarting in ulcers, at night. Skin unhealthy, every injury suppurates.

Sleep - Drowsy, but cannot sleep. ***Sleeplessness due to pain, teething, colic, ear infections.*** Sleepless from abuse of stimulants, coffee, narcotics. Moaning, weeping and wailing during sleep. Anxious, frightened dreams with half-open eyes. Pain disturbs sleep. Sleeps with thighs separated.

Stomach - Belchings like bad eggs, foul. Acid rising, regurgitation of food. ***Colic in infants, children.*** Pressive pains, as from a stone (Bry., Abies-n.). Violent retching before vomiting. Severe, bitter, bilious vomiting with griping. Vomiting after morphine. Sweats after eating or drinking. Thirst, for cold water, sour drinks. Aversion to coffee, warm drinks. Nausea after coffee. Tongue yellow, tastes bitter.

Temperature - Chilly, yet gets easily overheated, hence takes cold. Coldness of one part with heat of another, worse uncovering. Alternate chill and heat. Feverish from suppressed discharges. Sweat on head. Thirst during fever.

Throat - Inability to swallow solid food when lying. Parotid and submaxillary glands swollen. Constriction and pain as from a plug.

COMMENTS - Kent differentiated Cham from Puls. by noting that you want to hug Puls., and spank Cham. For any childhood disease with Cham. picture.

Teste remarked on this that Cham. antidotes not only Coff., but also Caust. and most of the members of the Caust. group. Cham. may be a remedy in croup or croupy cough, if mental symptoms and time conditions correspond.

Earaches, teething and colic. Wisdom teeth in adults. Toothache worse drinking something warm, at night. Ear infections, ear is hypersensitive to the least touch. Fevers. Whooping cough. Dry, hacking cough.

Unbearable pains, drive to despair, the patient insists that the doctor shall cure them at once. Prostrating debility as soon as the pains begin. Hypersensitive with great irritability and crossness.

Sleeplessness due to teething, colic, ear infections. Insomnia of children, start in sleep, twitching of hands and face, hot sweat of head and face, one cheek red. Puts feet out of bed, soles burn. Aggravation from heat, worse by warm food. Nocturnal salivation.

Rheumatism compelling to get up and walk about, thirsty, hot, almost beside himself. Muscles of face and hands twitch. Intertrigo of children. Inflammation of the parotid glands. Infantile jaundice, neonatal jaundice, with sleeplessness, crying and screaming since birth.

Diarrhea is hot, slimy, watery, yellow-brown or yellowish-green stool like chopped egg. Stools are grass green (Mag-c.). Diarrhea with colic. Offensive, excoriation around anus. Wind colic. Worse belching of wind.

Threatened miscarriage caused by anger. The pain of labor or at menses is centered in the womb, bearing down, painful contractions, unbearable, they extend down thighs and are felt in the back. Leucorrhea is acrid, watery, corrosive, smarting. Menorrhagia dark clots, fetid, temper always worse before and during flow.

Guernsey noted that "there is in Chamomilla a little thread of symptoms and nearly always found running through it. This is a spiteful, sudden or uncivil irritability." In spite of its obvious analogies with Puls. Ip., Acon. and Con., it has marked and exclusive characteristics of its own.

"It increases the general nervous sensibility and stimulates the cerebral functions: a property that seems to give rise secondarily to the various organic alterations that Cham. is capable of producing and for which it has so often been given with success."

Hahnemann said, "It appears to diminish in a great degree, the excessive sensitiveness to pain and the violent derangements which pain occasions in the moral condition of the patient. This is the reason why it appeases a multitude of sufferings to which coffee drinkers and persons who have been treated with narcotic palliatives are subject. And this is likewise the reason why it ought not to be given to those who bear pain patiently and with resignation. I mention this rule here, for it is of very great importance."

W. H. Baker (Rochester) recorded such a case. A chubby boy, light hair, blue eyes has a croupy cough. Acon. and Spong. at first controlled it, but afterwards failed.

The cough became a loose, rattling, suffocating cough, the mucus came up in the throat and nearly suffocated him. Paroxysms at midnight. During the day he was hoarse, ever impatient, nothing seemed to suit him. Cham. 100,000c cured, improvement setting in within two hours.

Dr. Anderson of Dover, Delaware, related the case of a man who had to change three to five times every night due to excessive sweating. A cup of weak chamomile tea was ordered every night. The second night there was slight diminution, the third he only had to change twice, the fourth once and after that there was no more trouble.

The plant in this case was probably Anthemis cotula, or wild chamomile of the U.S. Dr. Anderson learned its use from "an old woman." But the sweats of Cham. are also very marked.

Nash mentioned a characteristic in the association of numbness or alternation of it with pains. He related the case of a man who had very painful rheumatism of left shoulder and who got no better from the usual remedies, but was speedily cured by Cham., the indication being "Numbness with the pains." Nash differentiated the restlessness of Acon., Ars. from that of Cham. by the absence in the case of the last of fear of death. The Cham. patient "would rather die than suffer so."

RELATIONS - Cham. antidotes: Coffee, and the narcotics. Especially opium as it corresponds to its secondary effects, useful in nerve storms when morphine is discontinued. ***Antidotes:*** Camph., Nux-v., Puls. ***It is antidoted by:*** Acon., Alum., Borax, Camph., Cocc., Coff., Coloc., Coni., Ign., Nux-v., and especially Puls. Puls. and Cham. antidote one another and precede or follow each other well. ***Compare:*** (1) Cina, Calc-p., Acon., Puls., Coff., Bell., Staph., Ign., Cypr., Anthemis. (2) in dentition, Bell., Borax, Calc., Terebe. (3) in oversensitiveness, Acon., Coff., Hep., Hyos., Ign. (4) toothache, Merc. Merc. has hard, pale swelling of face, Cham. red and hot), sour breath. (5) in coffee drinkers, Nux-v. Cham. has bad temper during menses, Nux-v. has malicious temper. (6) toothache worse in bed at night: worse from warmth, Sulph., Merc., Puls. (7) indignation and it's effects, Coloc., Staph., Nux-v. (8) Bry., aversion to be looked at, Ant-c., Chin., Stram. (9) better by moving about, Rhus-t., Ferr., Verat. has maddening pains compelling to walk about, but there is none of the feverishness and excitement of Cham. (10) Rubus villosus, Blackberry - diarrhea of infancy, stools watery and clay colored. ***Complementary:*** Bell. in diseases of children, Cham. acts more on nerves of abdomen, Bell. more on cranial nerves.

REFERENCES - Boericke. Clarke. Phatak.

CHAPARRO AMARGOSO
(Goat-bush)

PHARMACY - chap. Chaparro amargoso. Goat-bush. Chaparro bush. Bishirandi amargoso. Castila nicholsoni. Castella texana. N. O. Simarubacae. Fluid extract from bark of stem. A small, thorny bush, three to five feet high with a small, saffron-colored flower. ***Historical dose:*** Tincture and all potencies.

CLINICAL - Diarrhea. Dysentery.

HERBAL - Dr. M. J. Bleim of San Antonio, Texas, communicated to the North American Journal of Homeopathy of March, 1899, an article in praise of this Mexican plant. Chaparro is prized by Mexican doctors as a tonic and anti-periodic. Chronic diarrhea. Dysentery. Stools with little pain, but with much mucus Tenderness over liver.

COMMENTS - Dr. Bleim reported three case he cured with Chap. The first, Mr. A. of New Orleans, was eighteen months ill with dysentery and was sent to Dr. Bleim under suspicion of tuberculosis.

Before seeing the doctor, he met a stock man who said he could cure him, having been himself cured with the remedy afte a like experience. Chap. was the remedy, a teaspoonful of the extract three times a day After three doses there was considerable improvement. He took no more medicine and had no further trouble.

A boy, age 12, had been treated for several months by Dr. Bleim with indifferent results. Chap. was given, half a teaspoonful three times a day. In forty-eight hours the discharge ceased and the bowels became normal.

The third case was an acute case that had improved rapidly under Merc-c. and colon-douches, but came to a standstill a a certain point: three or four stools a day more or less pain, no appetite, very weak.

Chap. was ordered, at a teaspoonful dose three times a day. There was immediate general improvement, in forty-eight hour the bowels were normal, and within a few weeks strength was entirely restored.

Dr. R. T. Knox of Gonzales, noted hi own case. He had dysentery for three years Nothing gave more than temporary relief Discharge after discharge of quantities o bloody matter, accompanied with much pain. Ravenously hungry all the time in land of plenty.

Under the advice of a farmer he wa persuaded to drink freely of a tea made o the shrub before each meal. The infusio had the appearance of sparkling beer an was intensely bitter. In three days there wa great improvement. In two weeks the bowel were under control, stools consistent, partl molded, sleep good. Recovery was perfec

RELATIONS - ***Compare:*** (1) Kali-c., Cupr ar., Caps.

REFERENCES - Boericke. Clarke.

CHAULMOOGRA

(Taraktogenos)

PHARMACY - chaul. Chaulmoogra. Taraktogenos. Gynocardia odorata. Hydnocarpus kurzii. Oleum chaulmoograe, hydnocarpi. Tincture of the seeds. ***Historical dose:*** Tincture and all potencies.

HERBAL - The Chaulmoogra oil and its derivatives are to a certain extent effective in the treatment of ***leprosy,*** especially in early cases.

REFERENCES - Boericke.

CHEIRANTHUS CHEIRI

(Common Wallflower)

PHARMACY - cheir. Cheiranthus cheiri. Common wallflower. N. O. Cruciferae. A tincture is used made from a single dark-flowered plant. Tincture. ***Historical dose:*** Tincture and all potencies.

CLINICAL - Deafness. Wisdom-teeth.

HOMEOPATHIC - Our knowledge of the medicinal use of Cheir. is due to Dr. Cooper. He considered as a keynote of the remedy, ***"Nose stopped at night from irritation of cutting wisdom teeth."*** Cutting wisdom teeth.

COMMENTS - The cases Cooper cured with it included the case of a young man, who had deafness and otorrhea on his left side while cutting three wisdom teeth.

Cured by two doses of the tincture given at six weeks intervals.

Cooper's second case concerned a girl, 22, who became deaf after measles, cutting wisdom teeth. She was greatly improved. His third case concerned a girl, 20, who was used to taking purgative pills. She had pain in her lower back, jaundiced appearance, bilious feeling, sickness of stomach. Cheir. removed the symptoms at once.

Anshutz said "No proving of this remedy has come under my notice, yet I considered the following case worth reporting:

T. T., age twenty, a clerk, admission date 30th April, 1892, never heard well on the left side, but particularly deaf the last month and deafness increases: watch, hearing contact only. History of much earache in childhood, left ear discharge does run out. Wisdom teeth, left upper and right, lower and upper, breaking through.

"Gave Cheiranthus cheiri. 28th May, hears very much better in left ear. No medicine. 11th June, continues improving gradually in left ear. 25th June, continues to hear voices very fairly on the left side, but no improvement since last time. Gave Cheiranthus cheiri. 25th July, restoration of improving condition."

RELATIONS - ***Compare:*** (1) Armor., Sin-a., Brass., Raph. (2) wisdom teeth - Mag-c., Ferr-pic.

REFERENCES - Anshutz. Clarke.

CHELIDONIUM MAJUS

(Greater Celandine)

PHARMACY - chel. Chelidonium majus. Greater celandine. N. O. Papaveracae. Chelidoniae. Tincture of entire fresh plant, at time of flowering. ***Historical dose:*** Tincture and all potencies.

CLINICAL - Angina pectoris. Arthritis. Backaches. ***Bilious***. Bronchitis. Cancer. Chest, disorders. Chorea. Colic. Constipation. Coughs. Diabetes mellitus. Diarrhea. Dyspepsia. Eczema. ***Gallbladder, pains.*** Gallstones. Gonorrhea. ***Headaches.*** Hemoptysis. Hemorrhoids. ***Hepatitis. Hydrocele***. Hypoglycemia. Indigestion. Influenza. Intercostal, neuralgia. ***Jaundice.*** Lachrymal, fistula. Laryngismus. Leucorrhea. ***Liver, disorders. Liver, pains.*** Lung disorders. Morning, sickness. Nausea. Neonatal, jaundice. Nephritis. Neuralgias. Nosebleed. Pleurodynia. ***Pneumonia.*** Rheumatism. Scald-head. Stiff-neck. Taste, altered, Tumors. Vertigo. Vomiting. Warts. Whooping, cough. Worms. Yawning.

HERBAL - Chelidonium is a poppy and therefore allied to Op. and Sang. with which it has many features in common. Closely allied to Lyc., when Lyc. seems indicated but fails to act, Chel. should be considered.

The juice of Chel. causes vesication when applied to the skin. The juice is yellow, like bile. Probably based on the "signature" of the bile-like juice, it was recommended as a remedy for jaundice by Galen and Dioscorides.

Given on the broad ground of organ-therapy in tinctures, material or semi-material doses, it has achieved notable results in cases of ***liver disease***. An extract used locally in cancer cases has gained a reputation in the old school.

Chelidonium works very well in tincture for a weak liver with low blood sugar, morning fatigue, and a craving for sweets (also Card-m.).

HOMEOPATHIC - Chelidonium acts upon the liver, spleen, kidneys, portal system, right side of abdomen and right lower lung. Predominantly a ***right sided remedy*** (Sang., Lyc.), with right infrascapular pain and the action on the liver. Also an action on the cecum, right ovary and on the base of the right lung.

A major ***liver remedy***, covering many of the direct reflex symptoms of diseased conditions of that organ. Keynote a continued, bruised, ***sharp, aching pain at the inferior angle of the right scapula.*** Jaundice. ***Yellowness and bilious*** disturbances. Bilious complications during pregnancy, lung disorders. Paralytic drawing and lameness in single parts.

Neuralgia over the right eye and in right malar bone. Headaches over the right eye, ***"bilious headaches,"*** with a bad taste in the mouth and a yellow tongue, irritable, may vomit bile. Arthritis associated with liver problems.

Great lethargy and indisposition to make any effort. Horror of motion. Feels tired on little exertion. ***Serous effusions. Hydrocele.*** Stitching pains. Heavy, stiff, sore, paralyzed, dislocated or broken feeling. Numbness. Ailments brought on or renewed by change of weather.

MIND - Despondent. Restless, hence agile. Anxiety as if she had committed a crime. Sudden anxiety, with strong palpitations. Fear of going crazy. Fear he has ruined his health. Fear of her condition being observed. Delusions that he has an incurable disease. Restlessness, constantly moves from place to place.

Bilious temperament. Forceful, very obstinate. ***Cross, and irritable***. Domineering and sceptical, not impressed by authority. ***Irritable, upset easily.*** Desires to beat children. Vexed about every trifle and violent attacks of passionate outbursts of temper. Loses control, when she gets out of bed, couldn't explain why.

Feels like crying with ill humor or without any reason. Thinks she must die. Sudden excitement with confusion of intellect at night. Talked incoherently during fit of anxiety. Inclination to weep. Weeping when carried.

Confusion at night on waking. Stupid feeling on looking intently. Aversion to mental exertion or conversation. Great absence of mind, forgets what she wants to do or has done. Imagines she can't think and will lose her reason. Forgetful of shaving or dressing. Unconsciousness, better rubbing soles of feet.

Abdomen - Sensation of fullness. Abdominal pains better wine. Rumbling followed by diarrhea. Fatty liver with icterus. Epigastric region tender. Constriction across abdomen, as if by a string. Distention. Ascites with yellow palms. Burning pain in bowels. Sensation as if an animal wriggling in epigastrium. Navel drawn in during colic. ***Severe pain around umbilical region.*** Painful pressure over umbilicus. Numbness in muscles of hepatic region. Pinching and cutting pains in bowels, with rumbling and gurgling. Pain and rumbling in cecal region. Pot-belly, with worms. Swelling and ulceration of inguinal glands.

Back - Aching soreness in all vertebrae, worse motion and pressure on spinous processes. Burning pain in back. ***Fixed pain under inner and lower angle of the right scapula,*** which may extend into chest and stomach, causing nausea or vomiting. ***Pain beneath right scapula, worse inspiration and motion of right arm.*** Pain from neck to temple (right). Pressing pain in vertebrae, worse bending backwards and forwards. Occiput heavy with pain in right side of back. Pain in nape. Stiffness in back between shoulders. Stiff neck, head drawn to left. As if a string around the neck. Cervico-brachial neuralgia. Pain at lower angle of left scapula. Shivering running down back.

Bladder - Frequent urging. Catarrh of bladder, with sexual excitation. Discharge of pus from urethra. Strangury, lasting all day, with scanty urination. Dragging pain in bladder, with spasmodic trembling pains in inguinal region. Stabbing pain in region of bladder. Cutting pain in urethra on urinating and continuing after urinating. Burning pain in urethra on urinating.

Chest - Skin yellow on throat and chest. Pain in right side of chest and shoulder with difficult respiration. Constriction of chest. Oppression on inspiration after dinner. As if a tight girdle around chest, hindering breathing. Deep seated pain or nail sensation, deep in right chest. Pain in lower right ribs, worse bending towards left side. Stitches under left clavicle and in region of right breast. Pains in right side of chest and shoulder, with difficult respiration. Intercostal neuralgia.

Constitutions - Bilious constitutions.

Cough - Short, exhausting. Violent cough with pain behind sternum, at night. Cough with constant tickling in larynx. Cough with painful contraction of abdomen. Racking cough as in tuberculosis, with copious mucus expectoration. Cough, as from dust with much rattling, but little expectoration or it flies from mouth. Whooping cough, spasmodic cough, loose, rattling, expectoration difficult.

Ears - Coldness or burning of ears. One ear cold, the other warm. Itching in right concha. Hearing lost, during cough. Deafness with liver disorders. Neuralgic pains in and around ears. Long-continued stitch in right external ear, passing off gradually. Sticking in ears. Sensation in both the ears, as if wind were rushing out or something crawling out. Loss of hearing during cough. Ears feel stopped. Loud distant roaring. Sounds as from a distant storm of wind. Humming. Ringing in left ear while walking.

Eyes - Aching in eyeballs, worse moving eyes. ***Dirty yellow color of whites.*** Burning and shooting pain in eyes. Burning in lids. Soreness of eyes, worse looking up. Tears fairly gush out. Orbits as if bruised on moving eyes. Orbital neuralgia of right eye with profuse lachrymation, pupils contracted, relieved by pressure. Lachrymation, when looking intently, with pain in eyes or from tickling in larynx. Mucus in eyes. Could not open eyes with prosopalgia. Agglutination of lids in morning. Thick, yellow mucus discharge from eyes. Fistula lachrymalis. Hordeolum. Photophobia. Lens uniformly grey.

Face - Dark red or sallow, sunken. Face red and swollen. Dry lips. Lips burning, dry, chapped, scabby. ***Yellow face, worse nose and cheeks.*** Itching of whole face and forehead. Wilted skin. Right cheekbone feels as if swollen with tearing pain. Flushes of heat. Nodular eruptions. Violent tearing pains. Acne. Red pimples on different parts of face. Inflamed pimples on chin and cheeks. Itching herpes, mostly on chin. Facial erysipelas. Lower jaw drops.

Female - Menses, too late and too profuse. Menses too long duration. Irregular menses, with profuse flow. Acrid leucorrhea. Leucorrhea, white, stains linen yellow. Burning in vagina, recurs at the same hour during day. Longing for unusual articles of food during pregnancy. Breast milk diminished.

Food - Loss of appetite, with disgust and nausea. Loss of appetite, with great emaciation. Nausea, better drinking milk. Itching better eating. Aversion to meat, coffee. Aversion to cheese, spinach. ***Generally better after eating.*** Hypoglycemia. ***Generally better from hot drinks.*** Desire for very hot drinks. Desire cheese, strange things during pregnancy. ***Prefers hot food and drink.*** Fond of vinegar or sour wine. Craves milk, piquant or hot food and drinks. Bitter taste when not eating or drinking. Cold drinks disagree. Thirstlessness.

Head - ***Headache better after eating.*** Headache extends backwards. Occiput feels heavy as lead, icy coldness of occiput from nape of neck. ***Nausea and bilious vomiting with sick headaches.*** Heavy, lethargic, drowsiness, very marked with general numbness. ***Right-sided headaches***

down behind ears and shoulder blade. Neuralgia over right eye, right cheekbone and right ear with excessive lachrymation, preceded by pain in liver. Pressing headache. Pressure in brain, with burning over eyebrows. Outward pressing, in forehead. Cranium feels too small. Congestion to cerebellum. Falling out of hair. Scalp on crown painful. Severe itching on occiput.

Heart - Angina pectoris. Violent palpitation with tightness in chest. Periodic palpitations. Lancinating pain in heart. Stitches in cardiac region, must breathe short, followed by strong palpitations and anxiety. Periodic palpitations. Beating of heart so strong that clothing is lifted from chest. Pulse slow, small and quick. Pulse full and hard.

Kidneys - Kidneys are sensitive to pressure, even of clothing. Spasmodic pain in right kidney and liver. Violent paroxysms of pain in kidneys, with intense headache, vertigo and syncope. Violent pain in direction of ureters, preceding passing of turbid urine. Urine copious. Profuse, foaming, yellow urine, dark turbid, like beer (Chen-a.). Urine stains the diaper dark yellow. Urine yellow as gold. Urine smells acid or ammoniacal. Urine has a resinous odour. Diabetes mellitus. Urine red, cloudy, with chalky sediment.

Limbs - Whole flesh sore to touch. Limbs feel paralyzed. Heavy feeling in lower limbs. Rheumatic pain in hips and thighs. Paresis of lower limbs with rigidity of muscles. Burning and stiffness in right knee, worse moving. Intolerable pains in heels, as if pinched by too narrow a shoe, worse right. Ankles stiff. Feels paralyzed. ***One foot cold, other hot.*** Pain in arms, shoulders, hands, fingertips. Icy coldness of fingertips, wrists sore, tearing in metacarpal bones. Edematous swelling of limbs. Edema around ankles and feet. Wandering pains in joints.

Liver - ***Liver pains going backward***. Pains fixed at angle of right scapula. Liver enlarged, tender. Hypoglycemia. ***Jaundice due to hepatic and gallbladder obstruction.*** Jaundice, sometimes with clear urine, tongue white, stools dark, offensive urine. ***Gallbladder colic.*** Gallstones (Berb.). Pressive pain in region of liver. Dull throbbing pain in region of liver.

Lungs - Nightly attacks of asthma with sense of constriction in chest. Dyspnea, worse urinating. Very quick and short inspirations. Pressive pain on deep inspiration. Hemoptysis. Copious, mucus, in morning. Respiratory symptoms with liver symptoms. Bronchial pneumonia. ***Bilious pneumonia.*** Blood-streaked phlegm, or brownish-bloody sputum. ***Right sided pneumonia.*** Small lumps of mucus fly from mouth when coughing. In left lung soreness like a wound, by deep breathing, coughing and sneezing.

Male - Acne on genitals. Eczema rubrum on scrotum. Frequent erections, even during day. Pain in glans. Itching, creeping on scrotum and glans. Drawing pains in spermatic cords, testicles. ***Hydrocele***. Redness, heat and swelling of scrotum. Painful swelling of right testicle. Gonorrhea and secondary syphilis, with ulcerated buboes.

Modalities - ***Better after dinner, eating.*** Better lying on abdomen. Better pressure. Better bending backward. Better hot bath. ***Better hot food***. Better milk. Worse from motion. Worse looking up. Worse cough. Worse touch. ***Worse right side.*** Worse change of weather. Worse northeast wind. Worse 4 a.m. and 4 p.m. Worse very early in morning.

Mouth - Burning pain in mouth. Mucus in mouth and tough mucus saliva. Salivation with nausea, giddiness. Bitter, pasty taste. Bad odor from mouth. Taste acid, insipid, metallic. Bitter water collects in mouth. Mucus flies from mouth when coughing. Oozing of blood from mucus membranes of mouth.

Nose - Flapping of ala nasi (Lyc.). Red. Obstruction with liver complaints. Tip of nose swollen and red. Dryness. Delusions of smell. Soreness of nostrils and flow of water from nose, with eruption like measles. Fluent coryza with sneezing. Thick blood in mucus in morning when blowing nose. Itching of nose and tip of nose.

Perspiration - Sweaty with aversion to uncover and without relief. Sweat during sleep, after midnight, from slight exertion. Sweats from slight exertion. Awakes in morning perspiring, after many unremembered dreams. Watery, sour-smelling sweat. Copious sweat, in evening.

Rectum - Constipation. Alternation of diarrhea and constipation. Chronic diarrhea with liver affection. Diarrhea without pain, without urging. Crawling and itching in rectum. Burning and itching of anus (Rat., Sulph.). Burning and cutting pain in rectum. Frequent discharge of flatus. Fermentation and sluggish bowels. Sensation as if anus were contracted, alternating with itching, during stool. Round worms.

Skin - Burning pain like nettles, preceding an eruption like measles. Dry heat of skin, itches, yellow. Wilted, wrinkled skin. Skin cool and dry. Skin cool and rough. Sallow, cold, clammy. ***Jaundice. Yellow-grey color of skin.*** Neonatal jaundice (Phos., Cham., Chin.).Itching as in jaundice. Painful red pimples and pustules. Itching, better eating. Old, spreading, offensive ulcers. Sallow, cold, clammy. Veins swollen. Red, ring-shaped, confluent spots, skin seems mottled. Scabs, exuding moisture and scaling off.

Sleep - Lethargic. ***Drowsy and chilly.*** Sleepiness without being able to sleep. Falls asleep while speaking. ***Unrefreshing sleep.*** Frequent yawning, drowsy and sleepy during day. Can't sleep because of numbness and coldness of limbs. Sleeplessness during headache. Wakes up repeatedly, feels wretchedly. Dreams of bodies, corpses and funerals. Confused dreams. Vivid dreams about business matters, causes unrefreshing sleep. Unremembered dreams.

Stomach - Eructations, tasting like juniper berries. Constant eructation of wind. Heartburn with eructations. Anxiety and oppression at stomach. Pain through stomach to back and right shoulder blade. Pressure in pit on stooping. Gastric pains, gnawing scraping better eating. ***Nausea, vomiting, better very hot water.*** Nausea and vomiting, with feeling of heat in stomach, spreading over whole body. ***Nausea and bilious vomiting with sick headaches.*** Nausea and vomiting in pregnancy. Sensations of heat or coldness in stomach. As if a plug in stomach. Qualmishness better belching. Vomiting of tough, acid or greenish mucus.

Stool - Fluid feces, often escape unexpectedly. Stools, hard, round balls like sheep's dung. Stools bright yellow, pasty, clay-colored. Stools float in water. Stools like rice-water, tinged yellow. Deficiency of biliary coloring matter in stools. Yellow watery stool containing flakes of mucus.

Teeth - Gums pale and bleed easily. Drawing or tearing pains, better warmth, worse at night in bed. Drawing pain in upper incisors. Drawing pain, through middle incisors of lower jaw. Toothache, chiefly in whole left cheek, worse at night. Pressure or transient pain in teeth.

Temperature - General lack of vital heat, coldness of limbs. Chill and coldness of whole body. Chilliness, with cold feet, in morning on waking. Yawning and shivering before attack of neuralgia. Violent fit of shivering daily. Fluctuating temperature. High fever. Burning heat spreads from hands over the body.

Throat - Hoarseness in afternoon. Choking during bilious eructations. Choking, worse breathing, as from hasty swallowing or as if too large a morsel had been swallowed. Spasm of glottis on expiration, with cough. Pressure or heat in trachea. Pressure in larynx as if air could not pass through. Severe tickling in larynx. Irritation to cough in trachea. Shooting and burning pain in throat and larynx. Pricking pain in larynx, rendering loud speaking impossible. Left sided goiter. Tonsils ache. Shooting in tonsils. Venereal ulcers in throat.

Tongue - Tongue pale, moist, whitish. Tongue dried up, brown, cracked. ***Tongue yellow with imprint of teeth, large and flabby (Merc., Hydr.).*** Narrow, pointed tongue. Tongue red on edges and tip. Tongue red and sore, with raised papillae.

Vertigo - Vertigo with liver disturbance. Vertigo with inclination to fall forward. Vertigo, felt in vertex, worse closing eyes with bilious vomiting and pain in liver. Vertigo, worse rising from bed or sitting. Vertigo on closing eyes, as if turning in a circle. Vertigo with shivering over upper part of body.

Vision - Blackish-grey specks before eyes. Misty appearance. Amaurosis from rheumatic troubles, also after suppression of ringworm. Muscae volitantes. Dazzling spots. Blinding spot, lachrymation when looking at it. Dim vision. Diplopia. Sparks, during headache. Flickering, brilliant specks. Candlelight seems very small. Blackness, with sensation of fainting. When reading or writing, letters run together and seem blurred.

COMMENTS - Chelidonium is a major liver remedy and is also a venous medicine. According to Rademacher, Chel. acts on the center of the liver. Neonatal jaundice remedy (Phos., Cham., Chin.). Yellow tongue, yellow skin, yellow eyes. Hepatitis (Phos.). Yellowness of the skin, ulceration.

Prominent paralytic symptoms. Chills or creeps accompany the headache or the jaundice. Constipation with clay-colored stools or diarrhea with bright yellow stools. Nausea during pregnancy with desire for food, better by drinking milk. Desire for hot food and drinks, only water almost boiling will stay on stomach. "Aversion to cheese" in many gastric conditions. Eating ameliorates.

Desire to lie down after a meal. Great debility and drowsiness after eating and on waking. Aversion to move, feels tired on least exertion. Sleepiness and yawning (Op.). Better hot baths. Worse 4:00 pm or 4:00 am (Lyc.).

The dirty yellow complexion produced by Chel. along with other signs of cachexia, strongly suggests cancer. The action of Sang., its relative, in breast cancer is well known. Additionally, Op., in addition to its narcotic influence, is believed by Snow to have a retarding effect on cancerous growth.

Pneumonia with bilious symptoms. Fan-like movement of alae nasi in chest disorders (Lyc.). Numerous cases of pneumonia of right lung have been cured when associated with hepatic derangement, distressing pain under right scapula. Hepatization of upper half of right lung.

Bry. is very similar to Chel. in pneumonia but the pains go continually to the back in Chel. and esp. to the right scapula. Rattling in lungs, worse changing position after waking. Frequently useful in bronchitis of children, with dusky red face, oppressed breathing.

Strong action in the respiratory sphere. Characteristic cough is caused by a sensation of "dust" in the air passages.

St. Clair Smith related a case of a young woman, who had for several weeks a dry, racking, fatiguing cough night and day, worse at night, no expectoration and no pain. She looked completely worn out. The cough was excited by a sensation as if throat and larynx were full of dust.

Chel. 3c, a powder every two hours, was given. She only took three when the "dust" left the throat, and with it the cough, and never returned.

Carleton Smith cured a "Dry cough through day with pain and stitches right side, severe hoarseness 5 p.m., voice scarcely audible."

C. M. Foss recorded a typical Chel. case simulating cancer. A man, 45, had catarrh of the nose and, at the same time of the stomach. He had been told he had stomach cancer. Tenderness over stomach with sinking, gone feeling, at times reaching a state of painful anguish. Sickness at stomach. All symptoms better by eating. Chel. 6x cured at once.

Teste, who proved Chel., placed it at the head of a group which includes Caps. and Viol-o. He mentioned the analogy between the juice of Chel. and the juice of Garcinia morella, and Gamb. Both are bright yellow and change to orange and brown on drying.

Some authorities have recommended Chel. juice as a substitute for Gamb. as a hydragogue cathartic. Its ancient external uses ranged from an application in eye disorders to chronic ulcers and warts.

In Teste's proving he emphasized a dull and heavy, deep-seated pain in whole right side of chest and right shoulder, at 1:30 p.m., without cough, but with embarrassed respirations.

This pain, which is at times accompanied by dull beatings in the chest, does not allow him to draw a long breath, it is not perceptibly aggravated by the motions of the arm. The pain is particularly felt in the axilla and under the shoulder blade.

A sort of numbness of the muscles in the region of the liver and in the right side of the neck, face and head. Apprehension of threatening pneumonia. Great anxiety. Constant desire to stir and change one's position. "Extremely profuse emission of a whitish and foaming urine." "2 p.m.: drowsiness which is so marked, even in the open air, that she is near falling asleep while walking, lasts half an hour."

A large field in rheumatic disorders. Edema, heat, tenderness and stiffness are the leading indications. A baby girl had rheumatism of both ankles for a week, when it settled in the right one, which became greatly swollen, very tender, painful and hot. Constipated for two months previously, whitish stools. Chel. improved in twelve hours and cured entirely in a week.

In another case of acute rheumatism of feet and ankles, supervening on a slow, remittent fever, Chel. cured after the failure of Rhus-t. and Bry. The patient was a girl of six. Both ankles were affected, feet much swollen and extended. The slightest movement or touch extorted screams. The only relief was constant bathing with hot water.

W. A. Burr cured a case of right sciatic rheumatism of ten years' history in a very corpulent woman, age 55. In her case, there were aggravations coming on in the afternoon and evening of each day and lasting into the middle of the night.

During the paroxysms, the outer ankle and lower leg became cyanotic, swelling around ankle, constriction above, great sensitiveness to touch and motion. Very nervous during the spells. Great external sensitiveness, aversion to touch and worse from it.

RELATIONS - ***Antidoted by:*** Acon., Cham., acids, wine and coffee, Camph. It is antidote to: Bry. ***Compare:*** (1) In pain below angle of scapula, Jug-c., Chenop. - Lower than angle and nearer spine), Ran-b. (edge of left, through to chest, Lob-c. - inside edge right scapula, Ang. - Cutting from just beneath right scapula to breast, near nipple. (2) Nux-v., Sulph., Bry., Lyc., Op., Podo., Sang., Ars. (3) Chel. - Spasm of smooth muscle everywhere intestinal colic, uterine colic, bronchial spasm, tachycardia. (4) Boldoa fragrans. (5) Elemuy Gauterusa - Stone in kidneys and bladder, grain doses of powdered bark in water or 5 drops of tincture. Pellagra. (6) Ip., Led., Sulph. (7) Kali-c. - pneumonia in later stages, copious exudation into lungs, rattling with cough, worse 2-3 a.m. (8) Colch. - nausea with desire for food. (9) Acon., Ars., Bell., Calc., Caps., Chin., Gamb., Graph., Ign., Nit-ac., Nux-v., Phos., Podo., Puls., Rhus, Sep., Spig., Sulph., Viol-o. ***Complementary:*** Bry. is a close analog in many symptoms—yellow tongue, swelling of liver. Ars., Ip., Lyc., Sulph. often completes its work.

REFERENCES - Boericke. Clarke. Phatak.

CHELONE GLABRA

(Snake-head)

PHARMACY - chelo. Chelone glabra. Snake-head. Balmony. Turtle-head. N. O. Scrofulariaceae. Tincture of the whole plant. ***Historical dose:*** Tincture and all potencies.

CLINICAL - Cachexia. Debility. Dumb-ague. Dyspepsia. Jaundice. Liver, disorders. Malaise. Quinine. Worms.

HERBAL - Chelo. has been used by old-school practitioners and herbalists as a liver and worm remedy. Burnett used it as an organ-remedy in liver disorders.

HOMEOPATHIC - Burnett's indications are "pain or soreness of the left lobe of the liver and extending downwards." Chelo. acts in a line between the hilus of the liver and the fundus of the uterus.

Liver disorders with pain or soreness of the left lobe of the liver, extending downwards. Soreness of external parts, as if skin were off, debility. Dyspepsia with hepatic torpor. Jaundice. ***Round and thread worms***. Dumb ague. Malaise, following intermittents.

COMMENTS - According to some observers it antidotes the quinine cachexia and is a remedy for "dumb-ague," i.e., ill-defined paroxysms of aching and fever following severe malarial fevers. "Soreness of external parts, as if the skin were off, especially about elbow," has been confirmed as an indication. Hale noted "debility from loss of tone of digestive organs or liver or from exhausting diseases." One to five-drop doses of the tincture have been given.

RELATIONS - ***Compare:*** (1) Chin., Chenop., Cina, Helon., Hydr. (2) Card-m. - left lobe of liver. (3) Scrofularias, Grat., Dig., Tab., Scroph-n.

REFERENCES - Boericke. Clarke.

CHENOPODIUM ANTHELMINTICUM

(Jerusalem Oak)

PHARMACY - chen-a. Chenopodium anthelminticum. Jerusalem oak. Chenopodium ambrosioides. Wormseed. N. O. Chenopodiacae. North America. Central America. Tincture of fresh plant. Solution of seed oil. ***Historical dose:*** Tincture and all potencies. Oil of Chen-a. for hookworm.

CLINICAL - Aphasia. Asthma. Cerebral deafness. Convulsions. ***Deafness***. Dropsy. ***Ear, disorders.*** Epilepsy. Headaches. Hemicrania. Hemiplegia. Hookworm. Leucorrhea. Meniere's, disease. Menses, suppressed. Otitis, media. Paralysis. Roundworm. Scapula, pain. Strokes. ***Tinnitus.*** Tonsillitis. Vertigo. Worms.

HERBAL - Oil of Chenopodium has been used for hookworm and roundworm.

HOMEOPATHIC - Several cases of poisoning have been reported in which all the symptoms of a stroke and the consequent right hemiplegia with aphasia were reproduced. Stertorous breathing with the very peculiar rattle as of a ball rolling loose in the trachea. Heavy breathing with flapping of cheeks.

Vanishing of sight and roaring in ears with (right) hemicrania. Roaring in ears as of cannons going off, ringing, deafness. Meniere's disease. Affections of auditory nerves (Nat-sal.). ***Serous or bloody effusions in the labyrinth.*** Chronic otitis media. Buzzing noises. Absent or deficient bone conduction. A consciousness of the ear.

Hearing better for shrill, high-pitched sounds than for low ones. ***Deafness progressive for human voice*** but great sensitiveness to sound as of a passing vehicle or to distant sounds. Aural vertigo. ***Sudden vertigo***.

Characteristic dull pain below the angle of right scapula and nearer the spine than the similar pain of Chel. Chenopodii glauci aphis has a similar pain below angle of left scapula.

Paralysis with spasms of forearms and hand in flexion contraction of limbs. Right sided convulsion and paralysis. Staggering gait. Pains through heart, under right scapula and in right shoulder.

Sub-acute and chronic enlargement of tonsils in pale, scrofulous children. Caseous deposits with painful inflammation of tonsils. Rough, furry feeling in throat. Stertorous breathing (Op.). Fever after a fright. Jaundiced. Urine, profuse, foamy, yellow, burning. Menses suppressed, leucorrhea instead.

MIND - Constantly repeats an action. Weeping mood. Insensible, convulsed, foaming at mouth. Loss of memory of attack after it is over. Weeping mood, suppressed menses. Forgetful of words while speaking. Uses wrong words. Aphasia.

Back - Intense pain between angle of right shoulder blade near spine and through the chest. Pain beneath point of right scapula, with giddiness in forehead, ringing in ears and pale face.

Chest - Pains through heart, under right scapula and in right shoulder. Pain throughout right chest, beginning at attachment of 6th rib to its cartilage and extending to front of right scapula.

Ears - Torpor of auditory nerve. Hearing is better for the high-pitched sounds. Comparative deafness to sound of voice, but great sensitiveness to sound as of passing vehicles and also a shrinking from low tones. Buzzing in ears. Roaring in ears as of cannons, deafness. Tinnitus synchronous with heartbeats.

Eyes - Impaired movement of right eyeball, loss of sensitiveness. Vanishing of sight.

Face - Flapping cheeks with stertorous breathing.

Female - Menses is suppressed, has leucorrhea instead, with rough, furry feeling in throat.

Head - Pain in whole right side of head, with roaring in ears, dim sight or complete loss of vision. Dull, pressive pain in vertex extending through head.

Kidneys - Slight pain in region of kidneys. Involuntary urination. Copious, yellow, foaming urine with acrid sensation in urethra. Yellowish sediment (Chel.).

Limbs - Hemiplegia with contraction of limbs. Frequent twitching and stiffness of right limbs. Paralysis and spasm of right forearm and hand in flexion.

Lungs - Stertorous breathing with flapping cheeks. Dyspnea, peculiar rattle as of a ball rolling loose in trachea. Respiration embarrassed by a quantity of yellow frothy material which was constantly regurgitated.

Skin - Jaundice.

Stomach - Perversion of taste. Disagreeable belchings, nausea. Constant, profuse regurgitation of yellow, frothy material smelling of worm-seed.

Throat - Enlargement of the tonsils. Chronically enlarged tonsils, caseous deposits. Furry feeling in throat.

Vertigo - Aural vertigo. Vertigo with transient vanishing of sight.

COMMENTS - Complete aphasia in a patient who took 1 1/2 oz. of worm-seed oil and 30 drops of turpentine. Five days from taking the dose he died in profound coma with high temperature.

"Whatever he did he would keep repeating. When the doctor entered he arose and shook him heartily by the hand, and then sat down. In about a minute he arose, solemnly came forward and again shook hands. This he repeated twenty times in as many minutes. He then went through the performance of washing his hands in an empty basin and repeated this many times."

In poisoning cases, there was hemiplegia with contractions of limbs and certain epileptic seizures. When given as a vermifuge it frequently produces progressive and long-lasting deafness.

The peculiar deafness corresponds nearly to the "cerebral deafness" described by Cooper in which the watch-hearing is good while the voice-hearing is bad or absent.

Linnell cured with it two cases in which there was deafness to voice-hearing but sensitiveness to other sounds. In one case there was implication of left labyrinth with slight chronic otitis media of both ears, deafness in the left ear several years, no tinnitus, consciousness of the ear, sensitive to musical sounds, deaf for watch and voice, hearing diminished.

Linnell also cured a roaring tinnitus synchronous with heart. Sensitiveness to cold. Hearing better for high-pitched than low-pitched sounds.

Allen reported three cases of poisoning in which there was insensibility, convulsions, and foaming at the mouth. All remembrance of taking the poison was lost upon recovery.

Deep, heavy, stertorous breathing accompanied by a very peculiar rattle, as if there were a ball rolling loose in the trachea. Any attempt to swallow threatened instant suffocation. Pulse small, weak, frequent and feeble. Eyes insensible to light or external objects. Convulsive movements of right half of body. Limbs cold.

In one case, a patient took 1.5 oz. of worm-seed oil and 30 drops of turpentine. It produced disagreeable belchings and nausea. Staggering like a drunken man. Deafness to the sound of the voice, but exquisite sensitiveness to the sound of passing vehicles, they sounded like cannons in his ears, also annoying buzzing.

In smoking, he would scarcely light his cigar before he would lay it down again and take a fresh one, arguing perversion of taste. By afternoon the mantelpiece was strewn with cigars only partly used.

No disposition to engage in conversation. Aphasia, he clearly wanted his attendant to get or do something but could not make him understand. The attendant wrote, "Don't understand," showed it to him and gave him, paper and pencil. After great efforts he wrote distinctly words with no meaning.

The voice and hearing became progressively worse but he heard the tea-bell three stories below, promptly and to the astonishment of the family, got up and walked deliberately into the dining-room. He did not seem to know his accustomed seat and sat in the wrong place.

During the afternoon became completely aphasic. Finding himself unable to express his ideas, this seemed to amuse him much and he laughed heartily. Whatever he did he would keep repeating.

When the doctor entered he arose and shook him heartily by the hand and then sat down. In about a minute he arose, solemnly came forward and again shook hands. This he repeated twenty times in as many minutes. He then went through the performance of washing his hands in an empty basin and repeated this many times.

Sitting at tea, he ate with apparent relish, taking singly tea and bread. While grasping a piece of bread, there was a distinct spasm of right forearm and hand, fingers firmly clenched, hand forcibly flexed on forearm.

Assisted to his room, his walk was entirely natural, when put to bed showed some resistance, striking at the doctor. He at once commenced to groan. tossed from side to side of the bed, suggesting abdominal distress. Soon became unconscious, right arm paralyzed, dragging helplessly.

The next day, continued impairment of motion and sensation right side, right eyeball insensitive to touch. During the third day, there was frequent twitching and stiffness of the right limbs, culminating in a one-side convulsion during the early morning of the fourth day. At noon on the third day, copious involuntary urination in bed.

This continued to the end, except when drawn off. In the afternoon, heavy breathing and the flapping cheeks of a stroke appeared. Constant regurgitation of yellow frothy material from mouth, smelling of worm-seed, as also did the perspiration. This material was at times so profuse as to embarrass respiration.

During one of the attacks of dyspnea and while in drenching sweat, which suggested dissolution, he was gently turned in bed, immediately a general convulsion set in, markedly opisthotonic, lasting ten minutes, despite the use of chloroform. By this time jaundice appeared, having been only noticed the day before.

RELATIONS - ***Compare:*** (1) Aphis, Chel., Chen-v. (2) In strokes and puffing respiration, Chin., Op., Lyc. (3) In deafness, Chin., Chin-s., Chin-sal. and Salicylates in general.

REFERENCES - Boericke. Clarke. Murphy. Phatak.

CHENOPODIUM VULVARIA

(Stinking Goosefoot)

PHARMACY - chen-v. Chenopodium vulvaria. Stinking goosefoot. Stinkender Gänsefuss. Chenopodium olidum. N.O. Chenopodiacae. Europe. Tincture of fresh plant. ***Historical dose:*** Tincture and all potencies.

CLINICAL - Bedwetting. Constipation. Scapula, pain under. Spleen, pain.

HOMEOPATHIC - Chen-v. has an odor of decaying fish and contains Trimethylamine. It constantly gives off ammonia. Chen-v. seemed to affect the left side more than the right in provings.

Pain in middle of back on right side of spinal column (Chen-a.), increasing gradually to a pressing wedge-like pain, beneath right scapula, worse when sitting. Pain spine of left scapula.

Pressure on the left side of the head. Restlessness caused by pricking pains. Constipation with external hemorrhoids. Nocturnal cold saliva, cooling sensation in abdomen.

Modalities - Sitting aggravates the pain in back, better by bending backwards. Walking aggravates sharp pains in spleen and pain in right knee.

RELATIONS - ***Compare:*** (1) Am-c., Trimeth., Chen-a., Aphis.

REFERENCES - Clarke.

CHERRY PLUM

(Bach Flower Essence)

PHARMACY - cher-p-b. Cherry plum. Prunus cerasifera. Twigs of flowers are picked and boiled for half an hour. The boiled water is strained and used as medicine. ***Historical dose:*** Take two drops from the stock bottle into a one ounce dropper bottle, (add brandy or alcohol, if this bottle will be used for days or weeks). This is the dosage bottle, take a few drops straight into the mouth or as needed in a little water or juice.

HOMEOPATHIC - The remedy Cherry Plum belongs to the group ***For Those who have Fear,*** as classified by Bach. Further remedies in this group are Rck-r-b., Mimul-b., Asp-b., and Rd-ch-b. Cher-p-b. can help people suffering from diseases of the nervous system to find added peace in mind and body (Rck-r-b.). Extreme nervousness with a threatened nervous breakdown (Rck-r-b, Verv-b.). Nervous twitches, grimaces, and gestures are common in severe cases. The body expresses the mental struggle taking place within.

The remedy is of service in tic disorders, elimination disorders and sexual disorders (Cer-b.). Mounting tension can release suddenly in unpredictable outbursts of violence. Physical concomitant symptoms related to speech problems.

Phobias of all kind (Mimul-b, Rck-r-b.). Fear of sudden physical or mental failure, as in stammering, or in diseases such as epilepsy or repeated fainting. Fear of losing control over one's faculties, one feels helpless in the face of overwhelming stress.

Severe pain, when one feels almost unable to bear the strain and torture, when the mind is at the verge of breaking down. During drug rehabilitation, physical and emotional cravings can be reduced. In some cases, unbearable pain can lead to homicide or suicide.

MIND - The mind is over-strained and out of balance, after prolonged mental effort leading to failing nerve power and exhaustion. Delusions and psychotic states when the boundaries of consciousness are disintegrating and the mind becomes subjected to unconscious and primordial forces.

Nervousness, shyness and stage fright. Great anguish and distress, with intense fear of losing control. Fear that all balance will be lost and the impulsive, unwanted thoughts will win. Thrill or excitement from doing forbidden things.

Problems in regard to impulses (Imp-b., Holly-b, Verv-b.). Obsessive-compulsive, perfectionist or ritualistic behavior, with the intention to avoid succumbing to the dreaded impulses. Impulses dictating to carry out certain acts, dangerous to oneself or others, or socially unfit. Crimes and suicides.

REFERENCES - Bach.

CHESTNUT BUD

(Bach Flower Essence)

PHARMACY - ch-bd-b. Chestnut bud. Aesculus hippocastanum. The young twigs with shoots are boiled for half an hour, the water is strained and used as medicine. ***Historical dose:*** Take two drops from the stock bottle into a one ounce dropper bottle, (add brandy or alcohol, if this bottle will be used for days or weeks). This is the dosage bottle, take a few drops straight into the mouth or as needed in a little water or juice.

HOMEOPATHIC - Chestnut Bud, with Clem-b., Honey-b., Wld-r-b., Oliv-b. and Wh-ch-b., belongs to Bach's group of ***Not Sufficient Interest in Present Circumstances.*** These remedies help those not fully engaged in the here and now. Impulsive physical conduct and some degree of hyperactivity or restlessness can be concomitant physical features. One may bring the self and others in danger through recklessness, or disregard important physical needs.

Developmental problems, attention-deficit and hyperactivity disorder and disruptive behaviors. Ch-bd-b. helps the mind to settle into restful concentration and retain the learning material. Personality disorders marked by a refusal to change and acquire empathy for others, such as in antisocial, criminal and personality disorders (Vine-b.).

MIND - Restless and impulsive, easily distracted. Absent-minded, not set on learning in the factual and moral sense. Jumps from topic to topic, goes superficially through a text, rushes ahead impatiently. Learned material is not contained very well, although capacity for memory is usually present. Inappropriate laughing or gliding over reprimands. Do not learn readily from their experiences, are often heedless or careless.

Easily carried by positive as well as negative emotions. Unreasonable, easily swayed, naïve. Emotionally unstable, impulsive. Defiant and somewhat lacking in integrity or depth. People not willing to obey laws and adjust to a normal socialization process.

REFERENCES - Bach.

CHICORY

(Bach Flower Essence)

PHARMACY - chic-b. Chicory. Cichorium intybus. The flowers are picked, floated in a bowl of water and let sit in the sun for several hours. The strained water is used as medicine. ***Historical dose:*** Take two drops from the stock bottle into a one ounce dropper bottle, (add brandy or alcohol, if this bottle will be used for days or weeks). This is the dosage bottle, take a few drops straight into the mouth or as needed in a little water or juice.

HOMEOPATHIC - Chicory belongs to the group of ***Over-care for Others' Welfare,*** as classified by Bach. The other remedies in this group are Rck-w-b., Beech-b., Vine-b., Verv-b. This group deals with mental, emotional imbalances in regard to caring for or controlling others. The inactive Chic-b. type may show an unspoken need to be loved. (Scler-b.).

Self-pity, prone to pout or look hurt and withdrawn. Overly controlling and service-oriented, while suppressing hostile emotions and demanding attention when sick. Self-protective with an anxious attempt to hold in emotions. Ulcer patients, if prone to tyrannical outbursts, yet falling ill whenever affection is withdrawn.

Anorexia, vomiting, nausea, bulimia and over-eating, in an effort to draw attention and love. Bronchial asthma, with difficulty in expiring, can rest on emotional hurt and self-pity. Diseases of soft tissue, rheumatism and rheumatoid arthritis of a psychosomatic origin. Hypochondriasis, pain disorders. Chronic constipation.

MIND - Bent on taking care of others according to one's own design or idea, may be interpreted as being too forceful or unnecessary. Self-pity, a sense of not being appreciated for one's efforts.

Fairly rigid opinions and ways of working with others. Conviction that one's perceptions and opinions are correct and one assumes the right to enforce them on others. Tendency to be overly careful with details, one's daily duties and cleanliness. Possessiveness of people, as well as of goods.

Preoccupation with pain without physical findings. Personality disorders, based on attention seeking within the sexual sphere. Feigning sickness in order to gain attention (Ch-bd-b., Heath-b.). Eating disorders (Crb-a-b., Must-b.). Hysterical neurosis, when the body expresses through illness the unvoiced need for attention and love.

Need to be the center of attention and be appreciated. Self-pity, sullenness and pouting, if affectionate attention is not offered. Annoyance and persisted self-pity if consoled, as if to arouse even more sympathy in the other.

Manipulation, power play, pretense, threat, possessiveness, or feigning of sickness in order to convey that they feel hurt, offended, or overlooked. May reject being consoled, which increases their self-pity and may create further alienation in others.

REFERENCES - Bach.

CHIMAPHILA MACULATA

(Spotted Wintergreen)

PHARMACY - chim-m. Chimaphila maculata. Spotted wintergreen. N. O. Pyrolae, a tribe of the Ericaceae. Tincture of root and leaves. Tincture of fresh plant in flower. ***Historical dose:*** Tincture and all potencies.

CLINICAL - Angina pectoris. Diarrhea. Headache. Sore, throat. Tongue, stiffness. Toothaches. Worm-fever.

HOMEOPATHIC - Chim-m. has been proved independently of Chim. Some symptoms of Chim-rot. are included. Intense gnawing hunger. Burning fever, blood feels heated. The throat and tonsils are strongly affected. Headache, worse on lying down. Feels better in warm room.

Constitutions - Suited to mild, amiable, refined, sensitive intellectual persons.

RELATIONS - ***Compare:*** (1) Puls., Chim.

REFERENCES - Clarke.

CHIMAPHILA UMBELLATA

(Pipsissewa)

PHARMACY - chim. Chimaphila umbellata. Pipsissewa. Groundholly. Prince's pine. Pyrola umbellata. N. O. Pyrolae, a tribe of the Ericaceae. Europe. Asia. North America. Tincture of root and leaves or of fresh plant in flower. ***Historical dose:*** Tincture and all potencies.

CLINICAL - Acne. ***Bladder, disorders. Breast, disorders. Breast, tumors.*** Breast-feeding, disorders. ***Cancer.*** Cataract. ***Cystitis.*** Diabetes. Dropsies. Eczema. Fevers. Glands, enlarged. Gleet. Gonorrhea. Herpes. Intermittent, fever. Jaundice. ***Kidneys, disorders.*** Leucorrhea. Liver, disorders. Nephritis. Proctitis. ***Prostate, enlargement.*** Prostatitis. Pterygium. Ringworm. Scrofula. ***Skin, affections.*** Stricture. Syphilis. Toothaches. Tumors. Ulcers, malignant. Urinary disorders. Whitlow.

HERBAL - Chim. is a medicine used by many North American Indians for gravel and urinary disorders. It has also been used as a vulnerary.

Among the herbalists it is used as an ***alternative in skin affections***, e.g., acne, herpes, eczema in enlarged lymphatic glands in joint rheumatism. It is said by them to act mainly as an eliminative through the bowels and kidneys. They use it in cases of chyliferous urine, cystitis, strangury, smarting, burning pains on urination, turbid urine and frequent urination and diabetes.

HOMEOPATHIC - Chim. acts principally on the kidneys and bladder, producing gravel in kidneys and acute and chronic catarrh in the bladder (cystitis). ***Scanty urine loaded with ropy, muco-purulent sediment.*** Calculus. Hepatic and kidney dropsies.

Passive kidney, uterine and intestinal hemorrhages. Leucorrhea. Gonorrhea. Chim. also acts on the prostate and liver. ***Prostatic enlargement.*** Prostatic irritation. Catarrhal states with mucus, pus and blood, offensive or not.

Affects lymphatic and mesenteric glands and female breasts. Plethoric young women with dysuria. Women with large breasts. Chronic alcoholics. Incipient and progressive cataracts.

Abdomen - Aching pain below right hypochondrium while writing. Organic disease of the liver with ascites. Ascites. Scrofulous mesenteric gland.

Back - Sensation in region of kidneys, as if something were fluttering within.

Breasts - Suppression of milk. Rapid atrophy of breasts. Scirrhus tumors. Painful tumor of breasts, not ulcerated, with undue secretion of milk. Painful breast tumor in young unmarried women. Women with very large breasts and tumor in the breast gland with sharp pain through it.

Constitutions - Suited to cachectic, scrofulous individuals and broken-down constitutions. Abdominal and kidney dropsies in broken-drown constitutions and intemperate subjects. Women with large breasts or plethoric women with dysuria.

Eyes - Halo around the light. Stabbing pain in the left eye with lachrymation.

Face - Flushing of cheeks with some general heat and quickened pulse.

Female - Labia inflamed, swollen. Pain in vagina. Hot flashes. Prolapsed uterus or vagina. Leucorrhea.

Head - Pain in left frontal protuberance. Halo about the light. Itching of eyelids. Stabbing pain in the left eye with lachrymation. Tinea capitis.

Kidneys - Acute inflammation of the urinary tract. ***Nephritis.*** Suppressed urine in infants. Urging to urinate. Urine turbid offensive, containing ropy or bloody mucus and depositing a copious sediment. Burning and scalding during urination and straining afterwards. Must strain before flow comes. Scanty urine. Fluttering in region of kidney. ***Cystitis.*** Bladder tenesmus, worse sitting, better walking. Cannot pass urine without standing with feet apart and body inclined forwards. Clots of blood pass with urine. Sugar in urine.

Limbs - Feeling of a band above left knee. Acute rheumatism of shoulder. Pain in right arm, about upper half of biceps and shoulder joint. Fistulous ulcer on right forearm, with stinging and crawling. Paronychia.

Male - ***Acute prostatitis*** with retention and dysuria and feeling of a ball in perineum, as if sitting on a ball (Cann-i.). Gonorrhea and prostatitis. Smarting in urethra from neck of bladder to meatus, excessive itching. Gonorrhea, gleet, syphilis, prostatorrhea. Loss of prostatic fluid. Prostatic enlargement and irritation. Atrophy of testicles.

Modalities - Better from walking. Worse in damp weather, washing in cold water, sitting on cold stones or pavements, beginning urination, and on left side.

Mouth - Jaws feel stiff, cannot close mouth at night, sleeps with the mouth open. Vesicular ulcers in mouth.

Rectum - Sticking pain in left side rectum, deep in. Inclination to stool, either ineffectual or attended with great pain. Bloody mucus stools. Griping after stool. Diarrhea. Obstinate constipation, with hemorrhoids. Worms.

Skin - Scrofulous ulcers. Glandular enlargements. Redness, vesication or desquamation. Eruption of dark red spots without sensation. Malignant ulcers. Scarlet fever.

Teeth - Toothache, as if being gently pulled, worse after eating or from exertion, better by cold water.

Temperature - Hectic fever and night sweats. Flushing of checks with general heat.

Throat - Palate sore, very sensitive to warm drink or food. Rawness of upper and back part of palate.

Tongue - Tongue smarting, sore. Full of vesicles, great thirst and desire to cool the tongue. Tongue is furred, more towards root, no appetite.

COMMENTS - Chim. has been proved by Jean G. Bute and H. P. Gatchell. It causes flushing of cheeks with some general heat and accelerated pulse. Increase of appetite. Worse in cold damp weather, after washing in cold water, from sitting on a cold, wet stone.

Acute rheumatism of shoulder. Edema of arms (right). Inward trembling without mental disturbance.

Cannot close jaws at night, jaws feel stiff, sleeps with mouth open. Toothache worse after eating and from exertion, better by cold water. Palate sore, very sensitive to warm drink or food, rawness of upper and back part of palate.

Inflammation of liver with ascites, abdominal and kidney dropsies. Enlarged mesenteric glands. Gallstone colic. Particularly indicated for kidney and liver problems in conjunction (Berb., Lyc.). Constant pain in region of kidneys, as if something fluttering in kidney region, first one side, then the other.

Obstinate constipation and hemorrhoids. Deep-seated shooting pain in the left side of anus. "Sensation of swelling in perineum on sitting, as if a ball was pressing against it."

Pressing fullness in region of bladder. Bladder tenesmus, strangury. Constant desire to urinate, must rise several times in the night. Great quantities of thick, ropy mucus in urine. Blood in urine. Smarting pain, painful irritation from neck of bladder, whole length of urethra to meatus.

Prostatic disorders. Loss of prostatic fluid. Bruised pain in testicle, with stricture. Leucorrhea. Rapid atrophy of breasts or tumors.

In homeopathic practice, Coburn reported the cures in several cases. The first concerned a case of stricture in a man, 30. He had dysuria, severe pain, scalding and burning. At times urine voided in a large gush, at others in thready stream and towards the end, drained off drop by drop. Merc-c. and Canth. had temporarily relieved.

Coburn also noted a case of prostatitis after sitting on cold stone. There was pain and a sensation as if he had bruised one of the testicles.

The third case Coburn recorded concerned a case of breast cancer in a 21 year old patient. Tumor in left breast, hard, movable, sharp pains at site. For four months, under Arn., Ars., Cic., Thuj., the tumor increased, skin became contracted, nipple drawn in. In eight months, it broke out into an irregular ulceration with lacerated edges, fetid discharge. Axillary glands swollen.

Chim. 1c in 10 drops doses, every four hours was given and the same locally applied. The pains diminished. Swelling decreased, and in six months the patient was well.

RELATIONS - ***Compare:*** (1) Chim-m. - intense gnawing hunger, burning fever, sensation of swelling in arm pits. (2) Uva., Ledum, Epigea. (3) Apoc. - dropsy, Agnus - gonorrhea, breast-feeding, Con., Coff. - toothache better by cold water. (4) Rhod., Kalm., Uva., Sabal. (5) In pterygium Calc., Zinc. Ball in perineum, Cann-i.

REFERENCES - Boericke. Clarke. Murphy. Phatak.

CHINA BOLIVIANA

PHARMACY - chin-b. China boliviana. Cinchona boliviana. A variety of Cinchona calisaya growing further north. N. O. Rubiacae. Tincture of bark. ***Historical dose:*** Tincture and all potencies.

CLINICAL - Aphthae. Corns. Coryza. Flatulence. Mouth, ulcerated. Pneumonia. Wry-neck.

HOMEOPATHIC - China boliviana has the main features of Chin. off., but some are peculiar and deserve separate mention. Chin-b. was proved by Modiedo.

Chin-b. has ulceration of commissures of mouth. Cough with dagger-like pains in base of right lung. Rigidity of nape of neck. Hands red hot or cold and sticky. Sticky sweat about the anus. Flatulence. Disturbed and dream-filled sleep. Sensitiveness to touch.

MIND - Gloom alternating with serenity. Alternation of bad and good humor. Fits of rage, blasphemes. Cowardice.

Abdomen - Pain in both hypochondria and under ribs on waking in the morning. Pain in splenic region.

Back - Nape of neck rigid, cannot turn head to right, any sudden movement causes a snap or crack. Wry-neck. Pain in left shoulder, left buttock and also in right hip bone on sitting up in bed.

Ears - Detonation as of a cannon in right ear. Ringing, humming, whistling sounds.

Eyes - Violent pains like a stab in left eyes, followed by itching and tears.

Face - Aphthae on inner surface of lips, ulceration of commissures.

Food - Hunger or lack of appetite, repugnance to meat. After eating, feels a weight in stomach. Cold, sneezing, sleepy and desire to sleep in evening.

Head - Headache in morning on awaking, leaves during the day or lasts all day and leaves during sleep.

Limbs - Legs and feet icy cold, as if blown on by wintry wind. Painful corns.

Lungs - Cough with pain in right lung, as from a dagger buried there, at times makes breathing laborious, burning in eyes, limbs cold. Unbearable pain in right lung, extends to region of liver, sensitive to touch.

Male - Pollutions exceedingly weakening. Excoriation on inner and lower part of prepuce. Gleet and ulceration of prepuce.

Mouth - Mouth bitter in morning on waking.

Nose - Much sneezing on awaking with smell of fresh pus. Sensation of incipient cold with tight feeling and pain in throat. Violent cold in head. Mucus from posterior sinuses.

Rectum - Biting in anus as from worms, excoriated sensation. Viscous sweat on anus.

Sleep - Dreams of the sea, of fishes, swimming, bathing. Dreams of journeys by land and sea, Dreams of vomiting of worms.

Stomach - Much gas rises from stomach.

Throat - Constriction and burning in throat.

Vertigo - Vertigo as after a drunken fit, voracious appetite.

REFERENCES - Clarke.

CHINA OFFICINALIS

(Peruvian Bark)

PHARMACY - chin. China officinalis. Peruvian bark. China regia. Kina-Kina. Cinchona calisaya. Cinchona rubra. Cinchona succirubra. N. O. Rubiacae. Central and South America. Tincture of the dried bark. ***Historical dose:*** Tincture and all potencies.

CLINICAL - Abscesses. Albuminuria. Alcoholism. Amaurosis. Amblyopia. Anasarca. ***Anemia.*** Aphthae. Asthma. Back, weakness. ***Bedwetting.*** Bilious, attack. ***Blood, loss.*** Breast-feeding, disorders. ***Cachexia.*** Candida. Catarrhal, disorders. ***Chills.*** Chorea. ***Cirrhosis.*** Colic. Colitis. Coma, Constipation. Coughs. ***Debility. Dehydration. Delirium. Dermatitis.*** Diabetes. ***Diarrhea.*** Digestive, disorders. Dropsy. Dyspepsia. ***Dysentery.*** Dysmenorrhea. Ears, deafness. Ears, noises. ***Edema.*** Emaciation. Emissions. Empyema. Epilepsy. Erysipelas. Eye, disorders. Facial, neuralgia. ***Fainting.*** Fatigue. ***Fermentation. Fevers. Flatulence. Food, poisoning. Gallstone, colic. Gallstones.*** Gangrene. Headaches. Hectic, fever. Hematuria. ***Hemorrhages.*** Hemorrhoids. ***Hepatitis.*** Hip, joint, disease. Ichthyosis, Impotency. ***Indigestion.*** Infertility. Influenza. ***Insomnia. Intermittent, fever. Jaundice.*** Labor, pains. Leucorrhea. Lienteria. ***Liver, diseases. Malaria.*** Masturbation. Meniere's disease. Menstruation. Mercury, poisoning. Muscae, volitantes. Nausea. Neuralgia. ***Night blindness.*** Ovaritis. Paralysis. ***Parasites.*** Pemphigus. ***Pneumonia.*** Peritonitis. Perspiration. Pleurisy. Psoriasis. Pylorus. Rheumatism. ***Sleep, disorders.*** Spermatorrhea. ***Spleen, disorders. Stomach, disorders.*** Strokes. Suffocation, fits. Taste, disordered. Tea, effects. Thirst. ***Tinnitus.*** Tobacco, habit. Traumatic, fever. ***Traveler's diarrhea.*** Tropical, fever. Tuberculosis. ***Tympanitis.*** Ulcers. Varicose, veins. Vertigo. Vomiting. ***Weakness. Worms.***

HERBAL - Kina is the Peruvian name for *"bark,"* and *"Kina-Kina"* is the *"Bark of barks."* The story of its introduction into European medical practice is one of the romances of the Healing Art, as the story of its frightful abuse is one of its many tragedies.

The tincture of Chin., Cinchona rubra, is useful in removing the craving for alcohol in alcoholics who wish to reform. Ten to thirty drops two or three times a day is the usual dose for this. Where the general symptoms correspond, the potencies would probably do better.

HOMEOPATHIC - Cinchona bark was to Hahnemann what the falling was to Newton and the swinging lamp to Galileo. Dissatisfied with the explanations of the action of Bark in curing ague that were current in his time, Hahnemann took the powdered Bark himself, being in health and behold, a malaria attack ensured.

A repetition of the experiment produced the same result. Further experiments revealed that action of Bark which is the opposite of ***"tonic,"*** positively debilitating in fact, already referred to.

China affects the blood, making it thinner and impoverished. It weakens the heart and impairs the ***circulation,*** producing congestion and ***hemorrhages,*** anemia, relaxation and collapse. Gallbladder disorders. Gallstones. Worse since gallbladder surgery.

Debility due to ***profuse, exhausting discharges, loss of vital fluids,*** excessive suppuration, diarrhea, hemorrhages etc. Dropsy after loss of fluids, hemorrhages. ***Blood loss with weakness.*** Inflammation of bleeding organ after hemorrhages. Convulsions during the hemorrhages. ***Profuse hemorrhages,*** with loss of sight, faintness and ***ringing in ears.***

Weak digestion, fermentation, gas and diarrhea. ***Gas and bloating of the abdomen***. Post-operative ***gas pains***, no relief from passing it. Gout. Chronic suppurative pyelitis.

Traveler's diarrhea or tropical diseases. Hepatitis and severe diarrheas. ***Food poisonings,*** worse from bad water or fruit. from eating bad fruit, unripe fruit, bad meat, decomposing meat (Ars.).

Marked periodicity. ***Intermittent periodicity*** is very marked in fever and neuralgias. The patient becomes very weak, oversensitive and nervous, everything upsets him, light, noise, odors, drafts, pain etc.

bursting pain. Neuralgia. Wounds become black and gangrenous. Psoas abscess. Epilepsy, chorea, paralysis from loss of fluids.

Keynote gas and bloating, diarrhea, indigestion, irritability. Very sensitive to touch and pressure, especially around the abdomen. Intestinal candida. ***Fermentation in the bowels.*** Failure to thrive, malabsorption in babies (Aeth., Mag-c.). Emaciation, especially of children. Anemia. Hard swelling. Rheumatism. Sepsis.

MIND - Apathetic, indifferent, disobedient, taciturn, despondent. Lack of self-confidence. Dislike of all mental and physical work. Reluctant to speak. Unable to think. Slow flow of ideas, can't arrange his thoughts. Mental exhaustion (Sil.). Makes mistakes in speech or writing.

Mind constantly changing from one thing to another. Ideas crowd in mind, prevent sleep. ***Abundant ideas and clearness of mind in evening.*** Full of plans and projects, in evening and at night and reflects upon their execution. ***Insomnia from fantasies,*** builds air castles. Loss of control over mind.

Anxiety in morning on waking. Excessively anxious about trifles. Inconsolable anxiety. ***Oversensitive to noise.*** Fearful and apprehensive. Fear of dogs and other animals, at night. Excessive vividness of mind and imagination during headache.

Sudden crying and tossing about, when cheerful. ***Excitement after hearing horrible things.*** Dwells on past disagreeable occurrences at night. Cheerfulness alternating with gloom. Weeping about a fancied need.

Discontented mood. Disobedient, stubborn. ***Irritable, sensitive and very touchy***. Irritability, even if looked at. Irritability after sex. Contempt for everything. Peevish, ill-humored, easily angered. Ill humor, worse hugging and caressing. ***Reproaches others.*** Disposition to hurt other people's feelings. Aversion to be looked at.

Delirium from the loss of fluids. Sees faces and objects on closing eyes. Indifference, sad, no desire to live. Fixed ideas, that he is unhappy, persecuted by enemies. Runs about. Desire for suicide but lacks courage. "Intolerable anxiety about 8 p.m. and 2 a.m., springs out of bed and wishes to take his own life, but does not go near the window or take a knife (Alum.) with heat of the body without thirst."

Abdomen - Liver and spleen swollen and enlarged. ***Tympanitic abdomen.*** Abdomen distended, wants to belch, eructations afford no relief. Flatulent bloating, better motion. ***Much flatulent colic,*** better bending double. ***Dysentery with dehydration and weakness.*** Abdominal colic with hunger. Colic better bending double. Colic with shivering. Colitis. Constrictive pains from incarcerated flatulence. ***Post-operative gas pains***, no relief from passing it. ***Fermentation in instestines from eating fruit.*** Heat in abdomen as if hot water running down. Pain from rectum to genitals. Pain in right hypochondrium. Internal coldness of stomach and abdomen. Gastro-duodenal catarrh. ***Parasites, worms.*** Swelling, inflammation, induration of spleen. Strangulated hernia.

Back - Pressure as of a stone between scapulae. Inter-scapular spine painful. Sharp pains across kidneys, worse movement, at night. Knife-like pains around the back. Heavy pressure on sacrum. Backache as from sitting bent for long time. ***Intolerable pain in lumbar region.*** Lumbago, worse slight motion. Spinal affections with diminished sexual desire. Sweat on back and neck from least motion. Sharp pains in spine and shoulders.

Causations - Ill effects of ***dehydration, loss of vital fluids***. Masturbation. ***Blood loss.*** Ill effects of vexation, anger, cold, mercury, onanism, and suppressed coryza. ***Food poisoning.*** Ill effects of eating fish, fruit, bad meat or fish, impure water, milk, tea, beer, beer, sour wine, or alcohol.

Chest - Painful, sore chest with soreness between scapulae, cannot bear percussion or auscultation. Pressing, stinging pains in chest and trachea. Pressive drawing pains, across lower portion of chest while sitting, causes anxiety, disappearing while standing and walking. Oppression in chest as if from a lump. Sides of chest feel as if beaten. Sticking pain in small spot below last right ribs, worse slightest pressure or walking. Boils on chest.

Constitutions - Suited to persons of thin, dry, bilious constitutions. Leucophlegmatic persons with a disposition to dropsical disorders, catarrhs or diarrhea, to disorders of women.

Cough - Asthmatic cough, at 3 a.m., followed by frothy, badly tasting expectoration. ***Violent, hacking cough after every meal.*** Paroxysms, after eating or laughing, worse evening, night. Spasmodic coughs from irritation of larynx. Spasmodic coughs as from fumes of sulphur, at night and in mornings. Spasmodic coughs with bilious vomit. Cough causes cutting pain in lower abdomen. expectoration difficult, black. Cough with pain in larynx and sternum. Cough with pain throughout whole cavity of chest. Dry cough, with taste of blood. Cough during or after measles. Coughs worse talking, lying with head low or on left side. Cough worse lightly touching larynx. Coughs from draft of air, loss of fluids. Cough from laughing. Cough after eating, drinking.

Ears - External ear, sensitive to touch. Lobules red and swollen. Stitches in ears. Tearing pain worse least touch. Foul, purulent, bloody discharge. Hemorrhage from ears after prolonged suppuration. Hemorrhage from ear, offensive, bloody, purulent discharge. ***Tinnitus, then vertigo.*** Humming, roaring, or tickling. Meniere's disease. ***Ringing in ears with headache.*** Ringing in ears with debility. Noises in ears, with faintness, great weakness, trembling debility, after menses. Hardness of hearing. ***Hearing sensitive to noise.***

Eyes - Inflammation and itching of eyes and eyelids in persons debilitated by loss of vital fluids. Blue color around eyes. Hollow eyes. Yellowish sclerotica. Iritis from loss of blood after confinement. Night blindness, due to anemic retina. Amaurosis, scalding lachrymation. Lachrymation, with crawling pain in eyes. Photophobia, eyes sensitive to bright light. Distortion of eyeballs. ***Pressure in eyes as from drowsiness.*** Pressive, burning pains in eyes, much heat, redness of eyes. Eyes painful on reading and writing. Eyes smart as from salt. Motion of eyes painful. Stitching as from sand. Eyes as if filled with smoke. Sensation of foreign body in eye, with inflammation and heat, worse evening. Pupils dilated or contracted. Involuntary closing of eyelids from mere weakness. Intermittent ciliary neuralgia. Ulcers in course of pannus, with much pain in morning. Ulceration of cornea.

Face - ***Sallow, pale complexion.*** Red, hot face, with cold hands. Earthy, sickly, pale, hippocratic, bluish around the eyes. Lips, dry, black and shriveled. Lips deep blue. Bloated face. Swelling of veins. Face hot, when entering room from open air. ***Face flushed after hemorrhage, sexual excess or loss of vital fluids.*** Facial neuralgia. Faceache nervous or rheumatic. Prosopalgia worse touch or motion. Needle-like pains, in left face, left chest and left hand. Violent tearing, burning pains in face. Submaxillary glands swollen. Erysipelas of face and hairy portion of scalp.

Female - Dysmenorrhea. Menstrual colic. ***Menses dark, profuse.*** Profuse menses with anemia and pain. Menses too early. ***Menses clotted with abdominal distention.*** Suppression of menses from chagrin. Metrorrhagia, blood dark with fainting, convulsions. Painful heaviness in pelvis. Painful induration in the vagina. Dropsy of ovaries, uterus. Ovaritis from sexual excess. Ovaritis from hemorrhage. Leucorrhea, instead or before menses with spasmodic uterine contraction. Bloody leucorrhea, seems to take the place of the usual menstrual discharge. Leucorrhea with painful bearing down to vulva and anus. Discharge of bloody serum, alternating with pus. Congestion to uterus, fullness, pressing and heaviness, worse walking. Uterine spasms. ***Uterine hemorrhage, with ringing in ears, fainting.*** Desire too strong in lying-in women. Labor pains cease from hemorrhage. ***Anemia, exhaustion, blood loss since childbirth.*** Promotes expulsion of moles. Long-lasting lochia sometimes fetid, cheesy or purulent.

Food - Voracious appetite in emaciated children. Hunger and yet want of appetite, only while eating some appetite and natural taste for food return. Quick satiety. Anorexia, feels satiated all the time. Complete loss of appetite in people suffering from malaria. Aversion to all food. Aversion to food or canine hunger, during fever. ***Aversion to hot food, fats and rich food, fruit, meat.*** Aversion to bread, butter, coffee. Aversion to beer, coffee, milk. Craving, for dainties, sour or sweet things. Desires various things without knowing what, especially children. ***Desires highly seasoned food***, sour fruit, fruit, Desires wine, salt, coffee. Desires sour, cooling things, roasted coffee. ***Food poisoning from bad meat, impure water.*** Ill effects of tea. Milk disagrees. Bitter or sour eructations after milk, heartburn after milk. Diarrhea from fruit, milk, beer. ***Food tastes bitter, even water.*** Food tastes too salty. Fruit, tea causes flatulence. Warm drinks impede digestion. Thirst for cold water, worsens diarrhea. Thirst during abdominal colic. Thirst during apyrexia, before chill. Thirstlessness or thirst for cold drink only, during fever.

Head - Bursting, throbbing pain with throbbing of carotids. ***Intense throbbing of head and carotids.*** Congestion of blood to head during menses. As if skull would burst. Sensation as if brain were swashing to and fro, causing pain. Bruised pain in brain, worse temples. ***Congestive headaches.*** Head heavy. Dullness and confusion of head. Spasmodic headache in vertex. ***Headaches after hemorrhage.*** Headaches, worse in open air, current of air, sun, by contact, stepping. Headaches, better by hard pressure, rubbing, warm room, moving head up and down. Nosebleed relieves headaches. Sharp pains from temple to temple. ***Headaches from suppressed coryza.*** Burning in forehead with sweat on it. Supraorbital neuralgia. Sweats when walking in open air. Sore, sensitive scalp, worse touching or combing hair.

Heart - Movement excites palpitations. Irregular, with weak, rapid beats followed by strong heartbeats. Suffocative attacks, syncope, anemia and dropsy. As if blood flowed warm from the heart. Melancholy feeling about heart, with desire to take a deep breath. Pulse small, hard, rapid and irregular. Palpitations with distension of veins. Strong, violent palpitations with feeble pulse and cold skin. Pulse more quiet after meals.

Kidneys - Sharp pains across kidneys, worse movement and at night. Burning at meatus, worse rubbing of clothes. Urine turbid, dark, scanty. Pinkish sediment. Hematuria. ***Bedwetting of weakly children.*** Pressure in bladder follows frequent and ineffectual efforts to urinate. Frequent urination with pressure in bladder. Urine turbid, dark, scanty. Urine pale, becoming cloudy or depositing a dingy, yellow, loose sediment. Scanty, greenish-yellow, brick-dust sediment. Albuminuria. Diabetes.

Limbs - Great debility, trembling with numbness of limbs. Pain in marrow. Decay of bones with profuse sweat. Sensation as of a string around limb. ***Pains in limbs and joints.*** Paralytic stiffness in all joints on rising after sleeping. ***Pain as if sprained, worse slight touch,*** hard pressure relieves. Averse to exercise, sensitive to touch. Weariness of joints, worse mornings and when sitting. Joints as if bruised, worse rest, better motion. Joints swollen, very sensitive with dread of open air. Twitching in knees. As if heavy load on shoulders. Spasmodic stretching of arms with clenched fingers. Hands tremble while writing. As of a band about legs or arms. ***Cold hands and feet.*** One hand is icy cold other is warm. Emaciation of hands and feet. Swelling of veins of the hands. Nails blue.

Liver - Liver and spleen swollen and enlarged. ***Gallstone colic. Gallstones.*** Obstruction in gallbladder with colic, periodic recurrence, yellow skin and conjunctiva, constipation. ***Worse since gallbladder removed.*** Jaundice after leucorrhea, masturbation, sexual excess, diarrhea. ***Hepatitis with exhaustion.*** Swelling and induration of liver. Periodical liver symptoms. ***Cirrhosis and edema.*** Liver weakness due to alcohol or poor diet. Pain in hepatic region, as from subcutaneous ulceration, very sensitive to touch.

Lungs - Asthma, worse damp weather, autumn or after depletion. Wheezing, whistling inspiration, crowing, rattling, oppressed and painful breathing. Asphyxia of newborn, after great loss of blood by the mother. Dyspnea, sharp pain in left lung. Cannot breathe with head low. ***Suffocative catarrh, rattling in lungs***. Puffy, rattling, breathing. Every motion excites palpitation and takes his breath. Inclination to take a deep breath. Wants to be fanned but not too hard, for it takes her breath. Rattling in lungs, loud sounds through nose. ***Pneumonia after hemorrhages or with bilious symptoms.*** Pneumonia, and other lung affections, symptoms being worse every other day. Pleurisy in persons who have lost much blood. Pleuro-pneumonia with profuse exudation, prostration, emaciation and pallor during confinement. Suppurative tuberculosis. Tuberculosis in alcoholics. Hemoptysis. Hemorrhage from lungs. Asphyxia of newborn due to great blood loss by the mother.

Male - Swelling of testes and spermatic cord, after gonorrhea. Orchitis. Swelling of epididymis. Tearing pain in left testis and left side of prepuce. Cramplike, contractive pain in testes, evenings. ***Frequent emissions, followed by great weakness.*** Impotence from overindulgence. ***Lost of vital fluids.*** Morbid sexual desire with lascivious fancies. Sexual desire with craving for dainties.

Modalities - Better from hard pressure. Better bending double. Better open air. Better warmth. Better loose clothes. Worse from jar. ***Worse slightest touch***. Worse bending over. Worse during and after stool. ***Worse loss of vital fluids***. Worse noise. Worse cold, winds, drafts, open air. Worse mental exertion. ***Worse after eating***. Worse fruits, fish, milk. ***Worse impure water, spoiled meat.*** Worse tea, smoking. Worse at night, midnight. Worse increase of moon. Worse every other day, every fourteen days, every three months. Worse periodically. Worse from 1 a.m. to 10 a.m. Worse 12 p.m. or 1 p.m. Worse from 8 a.m. to 2 or 3 p.m. Worse in autumn, summer.

Mouth - Dryness of mouth. ***Food, water tastes bitter***, acute, or too salty, even water. Bitter taste in mouth for a while after eating. Gums swollen. Putrid taste in morning. Painful sensitive swelling of uvula. Salivation day and night, years after mercury.

Nose - Ill effects from suppressed coryza, headache. Checked catarrh causes headache. Pressive pain in root of nose. Hay fever, watery coryza with pain in temples. ***Violent, dry sneezing***. Sneezing, water discharge, coryza. ***Smell too acute.*** Sensitive to odor of flowers, cooking and tobacco. Cold sweat about nose. Nose, hot, red. Easily bleeding from nose, especially on rising. Nosebleed with paleness of face, fainting. Nosebleed with congestion of blood to head.

Perspiration - Debilitating night sweats. ***Debilitating sweats from weakness, depletions.*** Profuse sweats, caused by every little exertion. Profuse sweat during sleep, or on being covered up. ***Drenching sweats, at night,*** worse least motion. Greasy or oily sweat on side lain on. Cold and clammy sweat with hemorrhages. Copious sweat, exhausting, at night. Suppressed sweat. ***Debilitating sweats from malaria, fevers.*** Sweats after waking at 3 a.m., with thirst. Sweats on face and hands. Sweats on side lain on. Sweats after meals.

Rectum - Involuntary stools. ***Traveler's diarrhea.*** Difficult stools even when soft (Alum., Plat.). ***Diarrhea and dehydration.*** Diarrhea after weaning in children. ***Chronic diarrhea*** in children, who become drowsy, pupils dilated, body becomes cold especially chin and nose, with rapid respiration. ***Dysentery with dehydration and weakness.*** Constipation, large accumulation of feces. Sharp pain in rectum during stool. Accumulation of much flatus, which will pass neither up nor down. Bleeding hemorrhoids, burning and itching. Mucus discharge from rectum. Tingling in anus. Worm troubles, worse at night, fullness in abdomen, with heartburn and waterbrash.

Skin - Skin dry, flaccid. Waxy pale or yellow skin. Jaundice. Yellow color. Itching, bleeding after scratching. Cold and blue skin. ***Extreme sensitiveness to touch, but hard pressure relieves.*** One hand ice cold, the other warm. ***Coldness, with much sweat.*** Anasarca (Ars., Apis). ***Dermatitis***, erysipelas. Indurated glands, scrofulous ulcers and decay. Psoriasis and ichthyosis. Pemphigus. Humid gangrene. Ulcers flat, shallow, copious discharge.

Sleep - Drowsiness. Overpowering sleepiness during day, when sitting and after eating. Heavy, snoring sleep, especially in children. Snoring, blowing expiration moaning, whining, during sleep. Protracted sleeplessness. ***Sleeplessness from an overactive mind.*** Sleeplessness from hunger. Sleeplessness from pressive pain in head. Waking from pains, noise and when feet get cold. Unrefreshing or constant stupor. Wakens early. ***Unrefreshed sleep, wakes confused.*** Dreamy kind of reverie as soon as he falls asleep. Anxious, or frightful dreams with confused consciousness on waking, so that the dream cannot be rid of and fear of dream remains.

Stomach - ***Flatulence.*** Flatulence in stomach for a long time after a meal, as if he had just eaten. Bloated stomach. Fermentation after eating fruits. ***Indigestion. Digestion, weak and slow.*** Cold feeling in stomach. Pulsations and rumbling in epigastrium. Stomach sore, as if ulcerated. ***Gastric disorders from eating fish, tea, sour wine, new beer, impure water, fruit, milk.*** Weight after eating small quantity of food. Spasmodic pain in stomach. ***Belching of bitter fluid.*** Eructations, taste of food. ***Regurgitation of food,*** gives no relief, worse eating fruit. Pulsations and rumbling in pit. ***Hiccoughs***. Hematemesis. Darting pain crosswise in hypogastric region. ***Frequent vomiting of undigested food.*** Vomiting worse at night. Sour vomiting of water, mucus and food. Vomiting of food, in debilitated persons.

Stools - Involuntary stools. Very weakening stools, with much flatulence. Stools loose, brownish, painless with a feeling of debility. Stools, worse at night, after meals. Stools, very weakening with much flatulence. ***Stools with undigested food.*** Stools, frothy, yellow, dark, foul, watery. ***Stools bloody, painless***. Stools, worse during hot weather. Stools, worse from ***fruit***, milk, or beer. White stools with dark urine. Stool loose and green in children, with great flatulence.

Teeth - Teeth loose and painful only when chewing. Black coating of teeth covered with dark sordes. Painful numbness in decayed teeth. Gums swollen. Toothache, better by pressing teeth firmly together and warmth. Toothache during sweat. Toothache while infant sucks the breast. Toothache with sweat. Pressure as if blood were forced into teeth. Throbbing pain, better external warmth.

Temperature - ***Chills on alternate days.*** Chill, then thirst, then fever, then thirst. Chill generally in forenoon. Chill alternating with fever, in afternoon. Chill begins in the breast. ***Internal chills, violent, with icy cold hands and feet, and congestion of blood to head.*** Chills with headache, congestion of head, paleness of face, pain in liver. Can't get warm in evening in bed. Influenza with debility. ***Malaria.*** Stages of chill, heat and sweat well marked. ***Intermittent fever***. Typhoid and gastric fever. ***Periodic fever and chils.*** Fever returns every week. Hectic fever. ***Tropical fevers.*** Sepsis. Red hot face, with cold hands with cold body. General heat with distended veins. Fever with dryness of mouth and lips.

Throat - Difficult swallowing, as from contraction of esophagus. Enlarged tonsils. Throat feels rough, scraped, producing a sore sensation on swallowing. Gangrene of throat. Larynx and trachea as if sore. Hoarse, rough voice. Deep, husky voice when talking or singing. Sensation as if something adhering to larynx.

Tongue - Burning stitches on tongue. Cracked, black or yellow coated tongue. Burning as from pepper on tip of tongue, followed by salivation. Tongue, thick, dirty coated. Painful swelling posteriorly on side of tongue. Tongue parched or raw as if burnt. Tongue dotted here and there with yellowish vesicles, some of them broken and looking sore.

Vertigo - Vertigo, falls backwards. Dizzy when walking. Vertigo on waking at night. Vertigo can't sit upright. Head inclined to sink backward, worse motion and walking, better lying. Vertigc on waking at night. ***Vertigo from anemia.*** Vertigo on raising head. ***Vertigo after loss of vital fluids.*** Vertigo on rising as if he would fall backward. Vertigo in occiput, when sitting. Vertigo with heat in head, worse when lying.

Vision - Shortsightedness after typhus, with diarrhea. Letters run together and look like black spots on a white ground. Vision better in morning. Sudden blindness with violent pain in occiput extending into eyes. ***Night blindness in anemic retina.*** Amaurosis, scalding lachrymation. Transient blindness, with flickering before eyes. Focal distance of eyes unequal for near and far points. Amblyopia in alcoholics. Amblyopia after masturbation, surging of blood to head. Black specks, bright dazzling illusions. Weakness of vision and neuralgia above eye. Dimness and weakness of vision, can only distinguish outlines of distant objects. Letters pale, surrounded by white borders. Flame of candle seems to be of a dazzling sulphur color. Sees spots.

COMMENTS - Teste wrote, "According to Humboldt about 500,000 pounds of this bark are annually exported to Europe for the purpose of being converted into sulphate of quinine." Well could Teste add the exclamation. "Poor patients!" As with almost every other good thing that comes into its hands, allopathy has contrived to do an infinity of harm with quinine to make up for the good.

Ip. (as well as Gali. and Mit.) belongs to the same natural order of plants as Chin., and the relation of the two to intermittent fever, hemorrhages and gastro-enteric disturbances is very similar.

Coff. also belongs to the Rubiacae and is nearly allied in many of its nervous symptoms to Chin.

The tincture is anti-septic, destroying ameboid motion and retarding tissue change. It weakens the heart and impairs the circulation. Chin. helps with congestions and hemorrhages, anemia and complete relaxation and collapse.

The result of suppression is thus sketched by Hahnemann's master-hand: "True, he (the patient) can no longer complain that the paroxysms of his original disease occurs any more on regular days and at regular hours, but behold his earthy complexion, his bloated countenance, his languishing looks!

"Behold how difficult it is for him to breathe, see his hard and distended abdomen the swelling of the hypochondria, see how his stomach is oppressed and pained by everything he eats, how his appetite is diminished, how his taste is altered, how loose his bowels are and how unnatural and contrary to what they should be, how his sleep is restless, unrefreshing and full of dreams.

"Behold him weak, out of humor and prostrated, his sensibility morbidly excited, his intellectual faculties weakened, how much more does he suffer than when he was a prey to his fever !

"The number of patients who have been consigned to an early grave by quinine probably falls short only of the number that mercury can claim. When first introduced it was (as chloral and hundreds of other poisons have been since) declared on the highest authority to be incapable of harm "in whatever dose it may be taken."

Debility caused by an excessive drain of animal fluids, such as loss of blood, excessive suppuration, loss of semen, and after prolonged strain of overwork, mental or bodily. A "pumped-out" condition, and the sensitive, irritable state of mind that accompanies such.

Never well since blood loss, surgery, loss of fluids, especially if the liver, the colon or the digestive tract has shut down or been weakened since the blood loss.

Hemorrhages occur from every orifice of the body. Rectal bleeding, nosebleeds, menstrual blood, birthing.

Perspiration, dehydration from high fevers, from heat stroke. Loss of fluids from diarrhea, a history of dysentery or parasites with exhausting, debilitative diarrhea. Weakness from breast-feeding.

Terrible irritability, always worse at night. Sense of unhappiness. Believes he is pursued by enemies in business.

Intermittent fever from marsh miasm, tertian or quartan in type.

Chill and heat without thirst, thirst occurring either before or after chill. Chill followed by long-lasting heat, generally with desire to uncover, face fiery red, often delirium, profuse and debilitating, followed by sweat.

In the apyrexial period, the face is a sallow, dingy yellow, the spleen is enlarged and painful, the appetite is totally lost, or else there is canine hunger, the feet swell and as soon as the patient closes his eyes for sleep he sees figures.

Typhoid and gastric fever. Hectic fever. Lung conditions which are attended with hectic. Suppuration of the lungs, especially in alcoholics. Weakening night-sweats. Prostration, chilly, wants to be wrapped up but cannot bear the fire.

Periodicity in fever and in neuralgias. Characteristic worse every other day. Neuralgia is generally infra-orbital. Weak eyes and ringing in ears, such as follow depletion. Loss of sight, deafness, ringing in the ears. Humming, throbbing in ears. The nose, ears and chin are cold, complexion sallow, dingy, yellow.

Headache, congestive, throbbing like many hammers hammering on temples, ringing in the ears, worse from drought of air, open air, slightest contact, better by hard pressure. Scalp sensitive.

Asthma, wheezing, suffocative catarrh and paralysis of lungs in old people. Respiration labored, loud and stertorous with puffing, blowing out of cheeks on each expiration.

Rheumatism, characterized by soft swelling, pale red, very tender to touch. Great sensitiveness to touch. Flesh sore to touch. Even a current of air blowing on the part causes great pain (Plb.).

Cannot get wide awake, head remains confused and stupid. Cannot get rid of dreams, even after waking the impression continues. Saliva found on the pillow in the morning.

Thick, dirty yellow coating on tongue, bitter taste on waking. Aphthae of weakly people. Thirst for cold water. Everything tastes bitter, even water (everything except water, Acon.).

Canine hunger, especially at night. Hunger after meals with feeling of emptiness. If a meal is late, he is sure to suffer from it. Total loss of appetite. Craves spicy (Nux-v.) and wine.

Full feeling after the least food, but belching only better temporarily. After eating, a lump under mid-sternum. Stomach so weak it cannot tolerate any food at all. Very sour stomach. Slow digestion. Diarrhea after fruit. Dyspepsia after loss of fluids. Nausea, worse on sitting up. Stomach sore to touch.

Very flatulent. Guernsey described it as an uncomfortable distention of abdomen with a wish to belch up or a sensation as if the abdomen were packed full, not in the least better by eructation.

Gastric troubles of children who are always wanting dainties, irritable on waking, bad taste, white tongue. Tympany coming on early in a case. Spleen aching, sore. Liver swollen, sensitive. Feeling of subcutaneous ulceration.

Gallstone colic, duodenal, catarrh, jaundice. Fermentation in bowels, frothy, sour diarrhea. Yellow, watery, undigested diarrhea, with much flatus and no pain. Diarrhea of dark inky fluid, stools frequent at night, only after food during the day. Useful in cases where purgatives have been abused (Nux-v.).

Excessive seminal losses. Menorrhagia, metrorrhagia, post-partum hemorrhage. Leucorrhea before period, painful pressure towards groins and anus, fetid or bloody leucorrhea before period with contractions in inner parts.

Koch and others have attributed the hematuria of African intermittents to quinine.

Hering said Chin. is useful after abuse of chamomile tea when hemorrhage from uterus results.

Nash cured a case of acute rheumatism with Chin. on the modality "worse every other day."

E. Carleton related the cure of a case of spasm of the glottis in a middle-aged man. Sudden attacks. 3 a.m., suffocation seemed imminent. At length with one tremendous effort, while sitting bent forward, a little air would be forced into the lungs in spite of the epiglottis with a noise audible at a distance. After each succeeding expiration the inspiration would become less difficult. Chin. 200c cured.

A. Villers cured with Chin. 30c a girl, 20, who, after a chill, had a pain in her right hip worse by every movement and which she could only describe as being like the pain in the legs which occurred before the menses.

She was pale and had much hard nursing work. The menses were scanty and she was weak. Three days after taking Chin., the pain was gone after having persisted for five months.

Clarke removed with Chin. the dropsy and relieved all the other symptoms of a case of cirrhosis of the liver in a hard drinker. He remained at his work for many months, but in the end, his old habits proved too much for him and he died from an acute illness following a cold.

RELATIONS - ***Antidoted by:*** Ferr., Ars., Nat-m., Carb-v., Aran., Eup-per., Ip., Merc., Nux-v., Puls., Rhus, Sep., Sulph., Verat. ***Antidote to:*** Ars., Calc., Cham., Coff., Ferr., Hell., Iod., Merc., Sulph., Verat. Is useful in bad effects of tea-drinking and after abuse of chamomile tea, with uterine hemorrhage. ***Compare:*** (1) Ars. - prostration without pain, black stools. (2) Carb-v. - flatulence, diarrhea, great weakness, Chin. stool is caused by every attempt to eat and drink. (3) Coloc. - beer intoxicates easily. (4) Cedr., Caps., Cupr-ac. - black, thin stools. (5) Psor. - rapid exhaustion following acute diseases, Psor. has despair of recovery. (6) Puls. - bitter taste, worse eating at night. (7) Meniere's disease, Sal-ac. (8) Ph-ac. - lientery, seminal emissions, diarrhea, but this does not exhaust with Ph-ac. (9) worse from brandy - Ars., Carb-v., Nux-v. (10) diarrhea immediately after eating - Ars., Aloe., Lyc., Podo., Staph., Trom. (11) hepatitis with great tenderness - Phos., Acon., Ars., Lyc. (12) Cephalanthus - intermittent fever, sore throat, rheumatic symptoms, vivid dreams. (14) Ars., Cedr., Nat-s. ***Complementary:*** Ferr., Calc-p. ***Incompatible:*** after Dig., Sel.

REFERENCES - Boericke. Clarke. Murphy. Phatak.

CHININUM ARSENICOSUM

(Quinine Arsenite)

PHARMACY - chin-ar. Chininum arsenicosum. Quinine arsenite. Trituration or solution. ***Historical dose:*** All potencies.

CLINICAL - Angina pectoris. Anorexia. ***Asthma.*** Bright's disease. Chills. Coryza. Diarrhea. ***Diphtheria. Dyspnea.*** Epilepsy. Fever. Gastralgia. Headache. Hectic fever. Hemicrania. Hyperacidity. ***Intermittent, fever.*** Keratitis. ***Malaria.*** Nausea. Neuralgias. Ophthalmia. Palpitations. ***Prostration.*** Rheumatism. Scarlatina. Sleeplessness. Sore-throat, malignant. Spinal, irritation. Syphilis. Tobacco, effects. Tuberculosis. Vertigo. Vomiting. ***Weakness.***

HOMEOPATHIC - This is one of the salts of Chin. that combines the Chin. physical symptoms and Ars. mental symptoms. The Arsenite of Quinine combines many of the properties of its components, but having been proved, it can be treated as a separate medicine. Useful in diphtheria with great prostration, especially cases that are prolonged, and in malarial affections, neuralgia, etc.

Weariness and prostration, useful as a general tonic, often with very marked beneficial and prompt effect. Continuous fever with oscillating temperature. Profuse, exhaustive sweat, at night.

Stomach pain, pressure in solar plexus with tender spine just at back of it. ***Hyperacidity*** alternating with decrease of acidity. Anorexia. Eggs and fish produce diarrhea. Nausea and vomiting, followed by sleep. Sleeplessness due to nervous causes.

Periodic asthmatic attacks with great prostration. ***Shortness of breath on ascend-***

ing. Palpitations. Sensation as if heart had stopped. Icy skin. Coldness of hands and feet, knees and limbs.

The periodicity is intensified and this is especially noted in the neuralgias. An irritable mood precedes the headache, which is worse by mental and bodily exercise.

MIND - ***Great anxiety*** and nightly delirium. Anxiety, with unquenchable thirst, must sit up bent forward, if possible at open window. Fears at night. Fear of evil. Fear of ghosts. Child sits up when lamenting. ***Prostration and disinclination for mental work.*** Believes he can't long endure such utter prostration. ***Weakness and weariness.*** Desire to sit or lie in one place and not be disturbed.

Great irritability. Irritability precedes headache. Censorious with friends. ***Depressed spirits, wishes to be quiet and let alone.*** Thinking of complaints aggravates, chills brought on by thinking of them. Mental dullness with inclination to vomit. Memory impaired. Hemicrania from fright.

Abdomen - Pain in epigastrium, as from foul stomach. Pain as from flatus wedged into flexure of colon. Pressure in solar plexus. Aching around navel and in ilium. ***Colic from incarcerated flatus.*** Severe colicky pains in evening, better by pressure. Soreness, in a small spot, below and to right of umbilicus. Distension and rumbling in abdomen. Left hypochondriac region enlarged. Abdomen bloated, in intermittent fever.

Back - Pain in muscles between left shoulder and neck, as if sprained, on rising from sleep, 4 p.m. Back feels weak as after a long journey.

Causations - Ill effects of tobacco. Fright. Eggs and fish produce diarrhea.

Chest - Severe stitching pains in chest, later in precordia, worse on inspiration. Tightening sensation in mediastinum, in front at left of breastbone. Intercostal neuralgia. Aching in intercostal muscles, right side. Peculiar pain, dull with pressure, as if caused by flatulence, coming and going rapidly. Chest as if hollow or full. Paralysis of respiratory muscles on left side.

Ears - Ringing in ears like bells, with congestion towards head. Noise in ears and dullness of hearing.

Eyes - Flickering with pain and lachrymation. Keratitis. Intense photophobia and spasms of orbital muscles, gushing of hot tears. Scrofulous ophthalmia, worse after midnight.

Face - Pale, sallow and bloated face, intermittent fever. Trembling of facial muscles, especially orbicularis palpebrum. Swelling of submaxillary and parotid glands, in diphtheria. Dull pain in left temporal region at articulation of lower jaw. Face pale, sallow bloated. Blueness of lips, in tuberculosis.

Food - Anorexia. Appetite gone. Ravenous appetite. Aversion to meat. Desire for sweets. Indigestion from unripe fruit. Eggs or fish cause painless diarrhea at once. Gastralgia from ill-baked bread. Diarrhea after eating. Violent thirst for cold water, yet it disturbs. No thirst with fever. Aversion to cold water, during rheumatic headache. Water tastes bitter.

Head - Headache, worse mental and physical exertion. Tired feeling. Head feels too full. Throbbing. Dull, heavy headache, frontal and occipital. Darting pains running up into head. Bruised feeling all over head after fever and sleep. Hemicrania from fright, physical and mental exertion. Periodical headache in occiput, from noise or excitement. Neuralgic headache, in right temple and above eye. Furuncles and abscesses which relieve head.

Heart - ***Cardiac dyspnea***, circulatory weakness after acute infections, early myocardial degeneration. Short of breath on ascending, cardiac dyspnea. Palpitations. Sensation as if heart stopped. Suffocative attacks, occurring in periodical paroxysms. Must have open air. ***Circulatory weakness*** after acute infections, early myocardial degeneration. Trembling of heart, palpitations, on leaning against back. Pulse small, very frequent. Pulse irregular. Pulse can't be felt on left side.

Kidneys - Frequent, tiresome urging. Spasmodic retention of urine, better application of hot cloths to chest. Urine scanty or increased.

Limbs - Weak limbs. ***Coldness of limbs.*** Tearing pains. Pain in left wrist, stiffness of left arm. Pain of fatigue in right wrist. Burning pain as in periosteum of left elbow. Annoying feeling of fatigue in right shoulder. Sore, tired aching in joints, bones and muscles. Tearing pains. Coldness of hands and feet, knees and limbs. Limbs icy cold, tuberculosis.

Lungs - Periodic asthma attacks, with great prostration. ***Asthmatic breathing on ascending.*** Dyspnea on ascending. ***Suffocative attacks*** beginning in morning and lasting till noon. Must sit bent forward and, if possible, at an open window during attack of suffocation, worse any other position. Breathing unsatisfactory, wants more air than can take into his lungs. Respiration very free, as if thorax were hollow. Bronchial catarrh with periodical fever, worse at night. Cough with little expectoration. Slight cough, at long intervals, seems to come from full feeling in chest. Dyspnea with anxiety, in tuberculosis.

Male - Peculiar burning ache about bladder sphincter and throughout urethra.

Modalities - Better by motion (vertigo). Better by eating (gastralgia). Better yawning. Better pressure. Better bending forwards. Better open air. Better sitting up. Worse rest, morning, forenoon. Worse when stomach is empty. Worse looking up. Worse motion. Worse on ascending.

Mouth - Burning canker spot on inside of left upper lip. ***Fetid breath, in diphtheria and scarlatina.*** Tongue thickly furred. Yellow, slimy coating on tongue. Dryness in roof of mouth, gnawing and nausea. Sweetish taste after clearing throat and coughing. Metallic bitter taste in mouth. Tongue black, sore and swollen. Tongue coated thick and brown, diphtheria. Soreness and redness of tip of tongue.

Nose - Profuse coryza, better erect position and out of doors. Post-nasal catarrh, worse left side. Copious nosebleed. Fluent coryza, profuse limpid and watery discharge. Nose stopped up with a purulent and bloody substance, diphtheria. Corners of nose excoriated, diphtheria. Yellow discharge. Left nostril fills up when lying on that side. Nose clearer when in an erect posture and in open air.

Perspiration - Cold, clammy sweat. No sweat after fever, but weak, broken-up feeling in morning and no appetite for breakfast. Cold, clammy sweat, all over. Cold sweat after epileptic attack.

Rectum - ***Burning in anus after stool.*** Violent urging to stool. Diarrhea, in the morning, hardly had time to dress. Bad-smelling flatus. Diarrhea at night and after eating. Diarrhea from malaria. Stools thin, watery, offensive, with pain in bowels. Stool pappy, watery, fetid. Stool thin, brown, painless. Stool with mucus and blood, preceded and followed by tenesmus. Brown, liquid jelly-like lumps.

Skin - Goose bumps, especially of lower extremities. Dry skin, pallor of skin, with rapid exhaustion. Periodical furuncles and abscesses. Burning, erysipelatous redness and violent itching, worse by warmth, better by cold.

Sleep - Sleeplessness due to nervous causes. Deep sleep after suffocative attacks. Goes to sleep after tea and sleeps heavily all night. Sleep frequently interrupted. ***Restless sleep.*** Restless until 3 a.m., constantly changing position, particularly as soon as pillow becomes warm. Awakes from sleep exhausted and bathed in sweat after attack of dyspnea. Nervous restlessness, anxious dreams. Night full of visions, heavy sleep till morning.

Stomach - Burning, sore feeling in stomach, worse motion, going up stairs, better expanding chest. ***Hyperacidity*** (Rob., Arg-n.). Alternation of hyperacidity and decrease of acid. Sour bitter eructations. ***Regurgitation of food.*** Hiccough and belching, followed by urging to stool. Empty sensation. Nausea with waning strength, especially of lower limbs. Nausea and vomiting followed by sleep. Sensation from stomach through entire intestinal canal as if diarrhea would set in. Nausea and vomiting, followed by sleep, with hemicrania.

Temperature - General chill and cold. ***Chill comes in waves*** in evening, with restlessness, gooseflesh, worse moving hands and feet to a cool place in bed, also on motion, and by thinking of it. After the feverish cough in the chill, no reaction of warmth. Heat with nausea. ***Continuous fever with weakness.*** After chill, fever toward midnight, pulse full and strong, with inclination to throw off covers.

Throat - Throat feels sore and raw, worse coughing and sneezing. Constant hacking and clearing of throat. Malignant angina during scarlatina, with paleness of skin, and exhaustion. Hoarseness, with diphtheria. ***Diphtheria with great fetor oris***, submaxillary glands swollen and painful. Tonsils covered with a grey exudation. Swallowing of liquids very difficult.

Vertigo - Sudden attacks of vertigo. Vertigo is worse looking up.

COMMENTS - Bonino, who gave it a prolonged proving, found the chief effects were manifested on the stomach, solar plexus, ligaments and skin. According to him, it corresponds to tobacco intoxication and its effects, indigestion from unripe fruits, and stomach pain from coarse food or ill-baked bread.

Marked weakness, prostration and disinclination for mental exertion. Effects of severe and depressing influences on the mind to convalescence from long-lasting sickness. Slow circulation, relaxed limbs.

Chronic rheumatism of the joints without swelling. Tertiary syphilis of periosteum. Colic from incarcerated flatus intermittent fever with predominating chills. Little thirst and continuous almost convulsive yawning.

RELATIONS - ***Compare:*** (1) Chin., also Ferr-citric. in nephritis with great anemia, acid dyspepsia in chlorosis. (2) Chin-m. - in severe neuralgic pains around eyes with chills, exaggerated sensitiveness to alcohol and tobacco, prostration and restlessness. (3) Enothera - effortless diarrhea with nervous exhaustion incipient hydrocephaloid. (4) Macrozamia spiralis - extreme debility after illness, collapse.

REFERENCES - Boericke. Clarke. Murphy.

CHININUM MURIATICUM

(Quinine Muriate)

PHARMACY - chin-m. Chininum muriaticum. Quinine muriate. Trituration or solution. ***Historical dose:*** All potencies.

CLINICAL - Alcoholism. Eyes, neuralgia. Gastritis. Headaches. Intermittents. Iritis. Keratitis. Neuralgia. Pannus. Sclerotitis. Tobacco, effects. Trachoma.

HOMEOPATHIC - Chin-m. resembles Chin-ar. very closely. An excellent proving by old-school authorities was published in Virchow's Archives.

Chin-m. has been used for eye affections, especially when accompanied by severe intermitting neuralgic pains in and around the eyes. Eye affections with chills. Lachrymation. Photophobia. Ulceration of cornea of malarial origin.

Intermittent fever following bronchopneumonia, shaking chill 5 a.m. accompanied by fatiguing cough, rattling in bronchi without expectoration.

In one prover it caused an exaggerated sensitiveness to alcohol and tobacco. Two glasses of beer make him tipsy. Prostration and weakness are marked in all provers and accompany the headaches and other symptoms. Feeling of enlargement in eyeballs in tongue, head symptoms are better after a walk.

RELATIONS - ***Antidoted by:*** Ferr-o-r. ***Compare:*** (1) Chin-s., Chin-a. (2) Nat-m. - headaches.

REFERENCES - Clarke.

CHININUM SALICYLICUM

(Quinine Salicylate)

PHARMACY - chin-sal. Chininum salicylicum. Quinine salicylate. Trituration or solution. ***Historical dose:*** All potencies.

CLINICAL - Ear, disorders. Deafness. Hearing, impaired. ***Meniere's disease.*** Tinnitus.

HOMEOPATHIC - Cozzolino stated "Of all the preparations of Quinine the Salicylate is the most injurious to the structures of the internal ear and, therefore in all likelihood, the most powerful homeopathic curative."

REFERENCES - Clarke.

CHININUM SULPHURICUM

(Quinine Sulphate)

PHARMACY - chin-s. Chininum sulphuricum. Quinine sulphate. Trituration. ***Historical dose:*** Trituration and all potencies.

CLINICAL - Angina pectoris. Anorexia. Asthma. ***Black-water, fever.*** Brow, ague. ***Cachexia.*** Cancerous, ulcers. Cholera. Concussion. Deafness. Delirium. Diarrhea. Dropsy. Dysentery. Dysmenorrhea. ***Ear, disorders.*** Gangrenous, suppurations. Gravel. Headaches. Hearing, impaired. Hematuria. Hemorrhages. Hemorrhoids. Intermittent, fever. ***Malaria. Meniere's disease. Nephritis.*** Neuralgia. Noises, in head. Parotiditis. Pruritus vulva. Puerperal, convulsions. Pyemia. Rectum, prolapsed. Remittent, fever. ***Rheumatism.*** Scarlatina. Spinal, irritation. Spleen, enlarged. ***Tinnitus.*** Typhus, fever. Urticaria. Varicose, veins. Variola.

HOMEOPATHIC - Chin-s. closely resembles Chin. in its effects, but as it has been proved separately and as observations of the effects of over-dosing have supplied many additional symptoms, there is plenty of guidance in the selection of one in preference to the other.

In old-school practice, the Sulphate of Quinine has almost entirely taken the place of the crude bark as a remedy. A dose of Chin-s. in high potency sometimes arouses suppressed malaria and brings back the paroxysm. Aside from its undoubted influence over malaria, it is indicated whenever there is a marked periodicity and spinal sensitiveness.

Chin-s. acts on the nerves causing great sensitiveness to external influences. Periodical neuralgia (Cedr.). ***Tinnitus. Violent ringing, buzzing and roaring in ears.*** Deafness. Tinkling in the ears. ***Meniere's disease.*** Buzzing, especially in left ear, sometimes occasioning deafness on that side. Hardness of hearing, sometimes with violent headache.

Rapid decrease of red blood cells and reduction of hemoglobin with tendency to leucocytosis. Thready vessels. Weak and nervous, little exertion causes palpitations. Inability to remain standing. Falling in street. Wants to lie down.

Deathly sick and faint, felt as if she would sink through bed.

Acute joint rheumatism. Gout. Itching and congested conditions of the rectum. Symptoms of ***chronic interstitial nephritis.*** Retro-bulbar neuritis with sudden loss of sight. Hiccough.

MIND - Memory weak, thoughts not clear. Indolence on waking in morning. Indolence with lassitude. Indifference, stupid expression, vacant stare, aversion to answering questions. Discouragement, inclination to cry. Slowness of reflection. Lost power of naming objects. Speechless.

Despair. Melancholy. Morose, depression and ill-humor. Anxiety with fear. ***Anxiety about future.*** Nervous. Fits of anxiety. ***Fear of impending evil.*** Great anguish. ***Fear of misfortune. Loud sobbing and weeping.*** Buoyancy, excited state, later despondency. Clearness of mind, abundant ideas, at night. Making many plans in evening.

Semiconsciousness, partly insensible to pain. Decrease of imaginative faculty with inability to remain standing. ***Delirium during fever.*** Delirium with great restlessness, followed by stupor in morning. ***Delirium with humming in ears.*** Delirium with screaming and jumping out of bed. Delirium all night while lying quietly on back. Delirium as if from intoxication.

Abdomen - Distension of abdomen, with much rumbling and discharge of flatus. Flatulent colic of an intermittent type. Movement in the abdomen and emission of wind, after a meal, with violent risings. ***Pain in region of liver and spleen on bending, taking a deep breath, or coughing.*** Violent cutting, colicky pains in region of transverse colon, after eating. Pains in liver shortly before going to bed. Dull pain in region of spleen, disappearing on pressure. ***Painful enlargement of spleen after intermittent fever.*** Stitches in spleen.

Back - Periodical pains in back. ***Periodical cervical neuralgia.*** Cervical, dorsal spine aches or very tender with oppression of breath. Spine, great sensitiveness of the dorsal vertebrae, pain on pressure. ***Spine painful on pressure in all stages of fever paroxysm.*** Last cervical sensitive. Pain extends to head and neck.

Blood - An immediate and rapid decrease in red blood cells and reduction in hemoglobin with increase in elimination of chlorides. Tendency to polynucleated leucocytosis.

Chest - Oppression of chest, can scarcely breathe from weakness. Pain across the chest. ***Painful sense of pressure and weight on chest.*** Pressure on the left side of the chest. Intercostal neuralgia.

Ears - ***Meniere's disease.*** Noises in ears, worse during a chill. ***Noises in ears, worse during vertigo.*** Violent ringing, buzzing and roaring in ears. Tinkling in the ears. ***Tinnitus.*** Deafness. Deafness from concussion of brain. ***Hardness of hearing,*** sometimes with violent headache. Buzzing, especially in left ear, sometimes occasioning deafness on that side.

Eyes - Dryness of eyes. Eyes staring and lustreless. Eyes close from weariness. Conjunctiva injected. Lachrymation and conjunctivitis. Squint on alternating days (children). Sensibility of the eyes with lachrymation. Extreme photophobia. Violent stitching, throbbing pains. Orbital neuralgia. Pupils dilated or contracted. Twitching of eyelids. Lids red and swollen. Disc and retina very anemic.

Face - Flushed face. Redness of the face. Heat of the face. Pale anxious face. Earth-colored face. Dull and stupid expression. Complexion yellow. Sickly look, air of suffering with sunken eyes. Neuralgia under eye. ***Neuralgia pains return with great regularity, better by pressure.*** Brow ague. Bluish-colored lips. Eruption on the upper lip.

Female - Passive metrorrhagia, with diminished irritability. Violent uterine contractions sufficient to produce miscarriage. Labor pains appearing like tonic spasms. Labor pains with convulsive twitches, unconsciousness after childbirth. Violent uterine neuralgia, returning at same hour every afternoon, worse after confinement.

Food - Want of appetite, for many days. Anorexia. Indifference for food and drink. Hungry at night. Bulimia, sometimes at night. Hunger with faintness, as from fasting. Excessive repugnance to all food. Disagreeable taste of food. Bread appears bitter. Thirst, mostly only during sweat. Thirst during chill and apyrexia.

Head - Confusion feeling in head. ***Intermittent neuralgia at regular hours.*** Dull headache with debility or numbness. Violent headache, throbbing, pressive, or tearing pains in forehead and temples. Violent throbbing, with vertigo and heat in face and prostration. ***Beating, throbbing in vertex.*** Pain in forehead and temples, increasing gradually at noon, of malarial origin, with vertigo and pulsation, worse left side. Head as if enlarged. Sensitiveness and tightness of scalp. Soreness of roots of hair.

Heart - Precordial anxiety. Palpitations. Palpitation from slight exertion. Angina pectoris with marasmus. Heart weak and feeble, with prostration. Pulse full and large. Pulse weak, trembling, scarcely perceptible.

Kidneys - Burning in urethra during urination. Small amount of urea and phosphoric acid with excess or uric acid and abundance of chlorides. Excessive flow. Albuminuria. Deposit of straw yellow, granular or brick red sediment. Diminution of urine. Frothy urine. Sediment yellowish-white of a strong odor. Brick-dust sediment. Gravel. Profuse hemorrhage. Urine, bloody, turbid, slimy, clay-colored, greasy sediment. Hematuria and hemoglobinuria.

Limbs - ***Acute joint rheumatism.*** Joints very sensitive. Heaviness and aching in all limbs and joints. Paralysis of the limbs. Weakness, trembling of the limbs. Cracking of the shoulder joint. Tearings in the legs. Painful sensitiveness in the malleoli. Edematous swelling of the feet.

Lungs - Increased breathing. Slow, irregular breathing. [11] Dyspnea and anxiety with intercostal pain. Accelerated breathing, with abnormal rising and falling of thorax. Tickling at bifurcation of trachea. Irritation in the throat. Violent cough during the day. Dry, loose cough. Cough caused by a small, painful spot in the throat. On coughing, expectoration of gelatinous mucus. Hemorrhage from lungs with diarrhea, fever, cold sweat and prostration.

Male - Suppression or diminution of sexual desire. Forcing pain in the direction of the groins.

Modalities - Better from yawning. Better pressure. Better bending forwards. ***Worse from exact periodicity*** (Cedr.). Worse 10 a.m. to 11 a.m. Worse touch, cold. Motion causes chilliness. Stooping causes giddiness.

Mouth - Aphthae in weakly persons. Dryness with heat, thirst. Sensation of constriction in the mouth. Great paleness of the buccal cavity. Erosion of the gums. Accumulation of mucus in the mouth. Saliva increased. Nocturnal angina. Taste pasty, flat or bitter. Speech disturbed or difficult.

Nose - Frequent bleeding at the nose. Severe nosebleed in young people. Frequent sneezing.

Perspiration - Profuse sweat, worse but exhausts. Sweats with thirst. Sweats profuse, even while quiet. ***Sweats improves all symptoms but headache, which is aggravated.*** Sweats coming on gradually after heat. Sweats on least motion. Sweats in mornings in bed. Profuse, exhausting sweats with nightly diarrhea. Profuse sweat on back and neck, during sleep.

Rectum - Obstinate constipation. Constipation or soft stools, followed by weakness. Dysentery. Diarrhea. Evacuations exhale a gangrenous odor. Stools are white and pap-like. Stools hard, insufficient, indolent, sometimes in small fragments. Nightly diarrhea. Urgent inclination to evacuate. Involuntary stools. Many stools during the day. Hemorrhoids.

Skin - Itching, erythema. Jaundice. Vesication, pustules, purpura. Skin is flaccid or sensitive to the touch. Shrivelled skin. Petechiae. Urticaria. Red rash over whole body with severe stinging, followed by desquamation. Sudamina and red spots. Gangrenous inflammations. Formation of a thick scurf.

Sleep - Frequent yawning. Drowsiness during the day. Sleep profound and unrefreshing. Agitated, with debilitating sweats, tossings. Insomnia from fever and chills. Sleeplessness from overstimulation of nervous system. Extravagant dreams.

Stomach - Dyspepsia or heartburn, with nausea, loathing of food, eructations, bitter taste, vomiting of bile. Heartburn or burning in stomach and esophagus, and feeling of constriction and pulling sensation. Cramp in the stomach. Fullness in the stomach, and tension of the abdomen. Risings after a meal. Bitter hiccough and retching. Nausea with risings. Nausea, with inclination to vomit. Vomiting during an intermittent fever. Pressure, heat in the stomach.

Temperature - ***Malaria.*** Anticipating chills. Subnormal temperature. Painful swelling of veins during a chill. Shivering even in a warm room. Chill daily at 3 p.m. Clear apyrexia. ***Delirium during fever.*** Increasing fever and prostration with profuse night sweats. Thirst in all stages. Anguish with fever and chills. ***Stages of chill, fever and sweat well marked and distinct.*** Tertian or quartan fever with trembling of limbs, pain in spleen, spine sensitive, face pale, thirst, lips blue, ringing in ears. Typhus with great prostration.

Throat - Pains in the throat. Burning in the throat. Tickling in the larynx. Scraping in the throat. Sensation of dryness in the pit of the throat. Feeling as though a foreign body were lodged there.

Tongue - Bitter taste with clean tongue Tongue white. Tongue thick yellow fur Tongue yellow at root. Tongue white o yellow in centre, pale at margin. Drynes of tongue.

Vertigo - ***Vertigo with tinnitus.*** Vertigo wit twitching of the eyelids, and throbbin headache. Vertigo on stooping. ***Whirlin as if the head were falling backward***

As if intoxicated with buzzing in the ear and giddiness. Falling in street, inability to remain standing.

Vision - Can see objects only when looking sideways. Transient amaurosis. Amaurosis. Sparks before the eyes. Sight dimmed as by a fog with dryness of the eyes. Black spots. Obscuration of the sight, when looking fixedly at an object.

COMMENTS - Chin-s. is even more powerful as an anti-septic than Chin., and it is probable that it is in virtue of its property of antagonizing the malarial poison that it suppresses intermittent fever when it does not cure. It only cures when the fever corresponds to its own type. "Black-water fever" has been developed by Chin-s. in intermittents.

Koch deserves much credit for showing that the worst features of African fevers are due to over-dosing with Quinine and not to the disease.

When a fever is "suppressed" there is generally an unholy alliance between disease-force and drug-force, which is expended on some part of the organism, resulting at times in lifelong ill-health. The "Quinine cachexia" is well-known, including a sallow complexion, emaciation, deafness and singing in the ears, enlarged spleen, disposition to shiver and great debility.

Extremely well marked intermittents, the attacks returning at the same hour each day. The onset may anticipate. Great sensitiveness to external influences. Sleeplessness and over-stimulation of nervous system.

Skin flaccid and sensitive to touch. Red rash over whole body with severe stinging, followed by desquamation. Twitching of left eyelid, worse in the evening. Aphthae in weakly people. Tartar on teeth.

Debilitating discharges. Weak and nervous, a little exercise causes sweat from least exertion. Head gradually breaks into sweat when perfectly quiet. Headache extending from occiput to forehead. Whirling in the head like a mill-wheel.

Hunger at night. Prolapsed rectum, especially in children. Hematuria and hemoglobinuria. Arrhythmia. Palpitations. Painfulness and swelling of varicose veins during a chill. Julius E. Schmitt cured a case on this last indication.

E. W. Sawyer related this instructive history. He learned from his cook that her brother (age 16), could not take a particle of quinine without causing a profuse flow of blood with the urine, sometimes within half an hour, always without pain. This had followed every time his doctors had tried to break his ague with quinine.

A year later a farmer's wife, age 60, came to Dr. Sawyer to be treated for bloody urine unattended with pain or uneasiness. She attributed it to strain from walking two miles on a slippery road. She had been for months under Hygienic treatment without benefit and was alarmingly weak from loss of blood. Rhus-t. 200c, Ham. 1x, Erig. 1x, Chin. Ix, Ferr-m. 2x were given in succession in vain.

At last, calling to mind the case of the youth, he gave Chin-s. in 1/16 grains doses three times a day and a prompt cure was effected.

Tyrrell had a patient in whom in any potency it caused her to become "deathly sick and faint, thought she would die, could not raise her head, felt she would sink through the bed." Sinking sensation.

Sac-alb. produced in her the same symptoms and she accused the doctor of having given her quinine (Ars. has "sinking sensation, as if bed had gone from under her and she had alighted on the floor." Bell., Dulc., Rhus-t., Lach., have "sinking through the bed.").

RELATIONS - ***Antidotes:*** Parthenum, Nat-m., Lach., Arn., Puls. ***Compare:*** (1) Chin., Chin-sal. - deafness, tinnitus and Meniere's disease. (2) Ars., Eupat., Methyl blue. (3) Camph-br. is said to intensify the action of Quinine and render it more permanent. (4) Baja, an East Indian drug, said to be almost infallible in intermittent fever, quartan type, pulsating headache injected eyes, flushed face. Liver and spleen enlarged. Edema. (5) Also Pambotano, a Mexican remedy for intermittent and tropical fevers.

REFERENCES - Boericke. Clarke. Murphy.

CHIONANTHUS VIRGINICA

(Fringe-tree)

PHARMACY - chion. Chionanthus virginica. Fringe-tree bark. Chionanthus americana. N. O. Oleacee. The bark, which is the part employed, contains Saponin. Tincture. ***Historical dose:*** Tincture and all potencies.

CLINICAL - Cholecystitis. Constipation. Debility. ***Diabetes.*** Emaciation. ***Gallstone, colic. Gallstones***. Headaches. Jaundice. ***Liver, diseases***. Malaria. ***Migraines.*** Neurasthenia. Nursing women, complaints. Pancreatic, disease.

HERBAL - Chionanthus is useful for neurasthenia, periodical, sick, menstrual or bilious headaches. It has a powerful action on the liver and on the head. Taken for several weeks, in drop doses, will often break up the sick headache habit. Pain in the forehead, chiefly over eyes. Eyeballs very painful with pressure over root of nose.

HOMEOPATHIC - Chion. acts powerfully on the liver and is indicated in hypertrophy, obstructed liver in malaria districts. ***Enlarged liver***, constipation, clay-colored stool with jaundice and high-colored urine. Liver region sore. Liver derangement. ***Gallstones*** (Berb., Cholest., Calc.). Chronic jaundice. ***Jaundice,*** recurring every summer. Jaundice with arrest of menses.

Enlarged spleen (Cean.). ***Diabetes mellitus***. Paroxysmal, abdominal pain. Bruise, soreness is felt in various organs, liver, eyeballs etc. Pains ascend upwards from forehead, stomach etc. Sensation of contraction of stomach as if something alive moving in it with uneasy sensation in liver and spleen. Rheumatic pains in left ankle and tarsal bone.

MIND - Listless, apathetic. Feels worn out. No desire to do anything. Wants to be let alone. Hypochondriacal, inclined to look on the dark side.

Abdomen - Abdominal pains somewhat better by lying on stomach and abdomen. Cutting and twisting pains all through the abdomen. Sore abdomen, enlarged with jaundice and constipation. Gripping at navel. Aching in umbilical region, griping. Feels as if a string were tied in a ***"slip-knot"*** around intestines which was suddenly drawn tight and then gradually loosened. Pancreatic disease. Weakness in hypogastrium. Passage of offensive flatus.

Back - Sore, weak, bruised feeling all over small of back. Small of back exceedingly weak. Pain from seventh to tenth dorsal vertebra, on waking.

Constitutions - Suited to the bilious temperaments.

Eyes - Eyeballs feel bruised and sore. Yellow conjunctiva. Whites of eyes have a yellowish cast all over. Blood vessels of sclerotic very much enlarged.

Face - Face has a yellowish appearance. Perspiration on face during fever, while asleep.

Food - Complete loss of appetite. Tried to eat, but food nauseated. Eating and drinking relieved empty, weak feeling in stomach to some extent.

Head - Severe bilious, sick headaches, worse stooping, motion, jarring. Dull frontal headache, over root of nose, over eyes, through temples. Feels sore and bruised. Heavy, dull feeling in forehead. Forehead very hot and dry. Perspiration on head during fever, while asleep.

Kidneys - Bile and sugar in urine. Large amount of high specific gravity, frequent urination. Urine very dark, orange-yellow color, thick, black, syrupy.

Limbs - Cold sweat on the back of hands during stool. Rheumatic pain in left ankle and tarsal bones. Rheumatic pain in articulations of left thumb. Sore, aching, tired feeling in lower limbs.

Liver - Hypertrophy of liver. Hepatic region tender. Cholecystitis. Bilious colic. Gallstones. Obstruction of liver in malaria districts. Enormous liver, constipation, stools clay-colored, skin very yellow. Soreness in region of liver. Chronic cases of jaundice. Jaundice recurring every summer. Jaundice with arrest of menses.

Lungs - Astringent expectoration.

Modalities - Better from lying on abdomen. Worse from jarring. Worse motion Worse cold.

Mouth - Tongue heavily coated. Tongue, broad with thick greenish yellow fur, feels drawn up. Dry sensation not relieved by water, also profuse saliva.

Nose - Pressing at the root of nose or squeezing on bridge. Drawing or pressing at root of nose during headache.

Rectum - Constipation. Diarrhea. ***Clay-colored stool***, tarry, also soft, yellow and pasty. Stool copious, watery, dark brown. Stools undigested and showing an absence of bile. Stools terribly offensive, like carrion. Emission of flatus during stool. Hot, scalding sensation in anus during stool. Cold sweat on forehead and back of hand during stool.

Skin - Marked moisture of skin. Yellow, sallow, greenish, itching. Chronic jaundice, recurring every summer, caused by drinking too much cider.

Sleep - Could not go to sleep before midnight. Nervous and restless after going to bed. Feels very badly and sick all over on waking in the morning. Sleepy during the day, could hardly keep awake. Perspiration on head and face during sleep.

Stomach - Belching, nausea, and vomiting. Great nausea and retching with desire for stool. Bitter, sour, hot, bilious, ropy, gushing vomiting, sets the teeth on edge. Vomiting with colic and cold sweat on forehead and back of hands. Nausea and vomiting of pregnancy.

Temperature - Cold sweat on back of hands. Chill at noon. Chilly sensations darting through body from front to back. Aching in back or limbs before and during fever. Wants to be covered during chill and fever. No thirst during chill or fever. Headache and backache during fever, eyeballs very sore.

COMMENTS - A proving of Chion. was made by Dr. John Z. Lawshe and was communicated with additions to the Southern Journal of Homeopathy by H. C. Morrow.

One observer, who gave Chion. to a nursing woman who had liver disorder with jaundiced tint, noticed that while rapid improvement of the liver symptoms occurred, at the same time the milk disappeared and the menses returned.

The medicine was stopped and Sabal. given and the milk returned. Six weeks later Chion. was again given and identically the same result took place." Jaundice with arrest of menses" should be a strong indication.

Sherbino cured a case of neurasthenia in a clergyman who had complained of perspiration all summer. Weakness in arms and legs. Prostrated after preaching, mind ran on sermon and kept him awake. Stupid, drowsy all the time, appetite poor, all food gave distress.

RELATIONS - ***Compare:*** (1) Bry., Card-m., Cean., Chin., Euon., Chel., Lept., Merc., Podo. (2) In bilious vomiting, Bry., Eup-per., Iris. (3) Nux-v., in green frothy stools, Elat., Grat., Kali-bi., Mag-c., Iris., Merc. (4) in weakness, bruised and sore feelings, Arn., Bapt., Bry., Eup-per., Gels., Nux-v., Rhus-t. in headache, Bell., Bry., Caps., Gels., Nux-v. (5) sensation of something alive, Croc., Thuj.

REFERENCES - Boericke. Clarke. Phatak.

CHLORALUM HYDRATUM

(Chloral Hydrate)

PHARMACY - chlol. Chloralum hydratum. Choral hydrate. This gas is proved in the form of Chlorine water. Solution, trituration. ***Historical dose:*** Trituration, tincture and all potencies.

CLINICAL - Anemia. Angina pectoris. Asthma. Bedsores. Bedwetting. Bronchitis. Chorea. Conjunctivitis. Coughs. Dermatitis. Dropsy. Dysmenorrhea. ***Dyspnea***. Emaciation. Erysipelas. Eye, disorders. Hay, fever. Hemorrhagic, diathesis. Heart, disorders. Hydrophobia. Keratitis. Labor, abnormal. Laryngitis. Laryngismus, stridulous. Leucorrhea. Night-terrors. Palpitations. Paralysis. Ptosis. Puerperal, convulsions. Purpura. Spasms. Strokes. Urticaria.

HOMEOPATHIC - Chloralum hydratum was used in physiological doses is a powerful hypnotic and cardiac depressant. Introduced as hypnotic, Chlol. soon showed that it possessed wide powers of disturbing the organism and many people (including the late Professor Tyndall) were fatally poisoned by overdosing.

A person under the influence of Chlol. hears voices, sees visions of arches, etc., when in the dark or when the eyes are shut. Emotional excitability, hallucinations. Night-terrors in children.

Marked effect on the skin, producing rashes, erythema, ecchymosis, purpura etc. These symptoms have been used homeopathically with much success, especially in the treatment of allergic hives.

Marked action on respiratory organs. The brain, eyes, urinary and sexual organs and skin are most affected. Inflamed and ulcerated mucus membranes. Muscular prostration. Spasms of the glottis. Marked sensation of constriction. Patients rapidly emaciate.

MIND - Fears insanity or losing senses. Forgets names and persons. Night-terrors.

Constitution - Hemorrhagic diathesis.

Ears - Hears voices.

Eyes - Protruding eyes, blood-shot and watery. Conjunctivitis, burning in eye and lids, eyeball feels too large, everything looks white. Circles of light, black spots. Illusions of sight where eyes are closed or at night. Dim vision.

Face - Swollen with protruding eyes.

Head - Morning headache, worse in forehead, also in occiput, on motion, better in open air. Passive cerebral hyperemia. Feeling as if hot band were drawn from temple to temple.

Lungs - ***Sudden dyspnea*** from spasms of the vocal cords, with protruding eyes, blue face, cold sweat. Extreme dyspnea with sensation of weight and constriction of chest. ***Inspiration free but cannot exhale***. Asthma or hay fever with sleeplessness. As if air were forced into upper chest.

Modalities - Wants fanning, open air. Better from open air. Better motion. Worse from expiration. Worse evening, night, after midnight. Worse lying down. Worse after hot drinks. Worse stimulants. Worse eating.

Mouth - Putrid odor from mouth. Putrid aphthae. Tongue, dry, black.

Nose - Smoky or sooty. Coryza, acrid with headache, suddenly running in drops with lachrymation.

Skin - Red blotches like measles. Intense itching. Urticaria, worse spirituous liquors, hot drinks. Erythema aggravated by alcoholic drinks, with palpitation, causes pain in tendons and extensors. Surface of body stone-cold. Wheals come on from a chill, better warmth. Purpura (Phos., Crot-h.).

Skin - Sensitive, dry, yellow, shriveled.

Sleep - Insomnia, hallucinations, horrid dreams. Somnolence.

Temperature - Easy sweat.

Throat - Choking sensation inability to swallow. Laryngitis. Laryngismus stridulous. Aching tickling or whistling in throat pit.

COMMENTS - W. S. Gee cured with it a terrific headache of several days' duration. Dull, heavy aching in forehead, coming on each morning 8 a.m., worse sudden motion, lying down, better in open air.

The 6c gave great relief, though it aggravated at first, the aggravation occurring ten minutes after each dose. One dose of the 25x cured permanently.

The brain is congested, hard, full, pressing pains in head. Eyes injected, the eyeballs feel too large, lids swollen, heavy, can hardly lift them. Asthma and wheezing respirations, probably due to an urticaria condition of the lung tissue.

Insomnia due to over-fatigue. Snoring in sleep. When lying on back inspiration was through the nose, while expiration was blown from the lips as in a stroke.

The heart's action is increased with oppression. Palpitation, hypertrophy. Paralysis of heart. Heart dilated or weakened with peculiar fullness and lightness of chest and sense of emptiness in stomach. Marked sense of sinking and oppression at the pit of the stomach, and shows a profound action on the solar plexus.

RELATIONS - ***Antidoted by:*** Am-c., Atro., Dig. (heart), Mosch., Electricity. ***Compare:*** (1) Bell. and Op. in stertorous breathing and puffing out cheeks, Gels., Nux-v. (2) in urticaria, Astac. Bell., Chlf., Chin., Op., Apis. (3) Veronal - a dangerous drug made by the action of alcohol upon urea and contains the same radical that alcohol does. Makes a man just as drunk as pure alcohol. Staggers, cannot stand up. (Varney.) Confluent, reddish spots, dermatitis, itching of glans and prepuce, circumscribed dermatitis patch on first metacarpal phalangeal joint. (4) Luminal - sleeplessness with skin symptoms, migraine headaches and lethargy like epidemic encephalitis. (Royal).

REFERENCES - Boericke. Clarke. Phatak.

CHLORAMPHENICOLUM

PHARMACY - chloram. Chloramphenicol. Chloromycetinum. Antibiotic drug. Originally from cultures of streptomyces venezuelae. ***Historical dose:*** Trituration, tincture and all potencies.

CLINICAL - Anorexia. Aplastic, anemia. Cholera. Delirium. Glossitis. Hallucinations. Nausea. Stomatitis. Typhoid, fever. Vomiting. Weakness.

HOMEOPATHIC - Extracted initially from bacterial cultures of the streptomyces venezualae, chloramphenicol, or Chloromycetin, is obtained today by synthetic methods. Digestive absorption is good and rapid. The intestinal concentration of the antibiotic is active, causing a change in the intestinal flora, which is common to the wide spectrum antibiotics (tetracyclines).

Toxicology. Gray's syndrome can be seen in the new-born and nursing child, characterized by vomiting, meteorism, cyanosis and irregular respirations, terminating in death by the collapse of the vasomotor system. This syndrome can also be observed in children and adults.

Serious disturbances of the bone-marrow in adults, ending in aplastic anemia, hypoplastic anemia, reduction of the amount of blood platelets, reduction of granulous leukocytes, or consumption, occurring as long as 1 to 3 months after treatment.

The symptomatology was established by O. A. Julian, referring to the toxicology of chloramphenicol, and resulting in a homeopathic proving from January to March 1970 with the participation of six provers, including three women. The potencies used were 30c, 7c, 3x and a placebo.

Pronounced asthenia or weakness. Discouragement in the morning. Pallor. Euphoria. Anorexia, nausea, vomiting. Intestinal spasms with diarrhea. Aversion to sugar and sweets. Pains at different levels of the vertebral column and pelvis. Vesicular, papular, muscular erythema. Considerable axillary sweating.

MIND - Delirium. Mental confusion. Hallucinations. Agitation with the need to move a great deal. Apathy, extreme muscular weakness, depression. Feels sad, despairing, but the condition improves on rising.

Abdomen - Enterocolitis of the mucus membranes. Typhoid fever. Spasmodic infections of the colon. Infantile cholera. European cholera. Catarrhal icterus.

Back - Pain in the back and between the shoulder blades. Lumbar and sacroiliac pains on the right. Pain on the left side of the back. Pain in the lumbar region in sharp bouts. Iliac and lumbar pains lasting a fortnight.

Blood - Aplastic anemia, degeneration of the reticular system, of leukocytes, of blood platelets. Prolonged bleeding. Irreducible blood-clot.

Ears - Disorders of the cochlea.

Eyes - Paresis of accommodation, ciliary muscle. Optic neuritis.

Female - Vulvovaginitis.

Food - Aversion to sugar and sweets. Anorexia. Morbid hunger, causing pain in the morning. Thirst for large quantities of liquid, especially beer.

Head - Recurring headache.

Heart - Vascular hypertrophy with bouts of arterial tension. Pulse accelerated. Tachycardia not altered by changing position.

Kidneys - Dysuria. Frequent urination. Hematuria. Colicky pain in the left kidney.

Limbs - Muscular weakness. Polyneuritic pains. Pain in the patella. Chronic degenerative rheumatism. Dry arthritis of the knee. Progressive polyarthritis.

Lungs - Dyspnea without cause. Wheezing, not altered by changing position.

Modalities - Laterality predominantly right-sided. Better from pressure by the hands. Better holding the head high. Worse after meals.

Mouth - Mouth foul-smelling. Dull, bitter taste. Dryness of the mouth, with bad breath. Tongue black, hairy. Glossitis. Inflammation of the lips. Bleeding gums. Stomatitis.

Nose - Nosebleed.

Rectum - Constipation, vomiting. Cholera-type syndrome. Diarrhea. Colic and diarrhea, following the ingestion of sweet pies. Urgency, with tenesmus. Stools thin, dark, scanty. Stool soft with nauseating fetid odor. Anal burning. Inflammation of the anus and rectum.

Skin - Ecchymosis and petechial purpura. Vesicular, papular, muscular erythema. Rash like scarlet fever. Allergic syndrome with fever and edema. Considerable axillary sweating. Hair seems to grow darker. Hardened erythema. Urticaria.

Sleep - Extreme sleepiness after meals. Waking at night from 2 a.m. to 5 a.m. with a throbbing headache.

Stomach - Hematemesis.

Temperature - Hypothermia. State of collapse with cyanosis.

Throat - Redness with difficulty in swallowing.

Vertigo - Prolonged bouts of vertigo.

COMMENTS - Extreme sleepiness around 5 o'clock in the afternoon. In bed, at night, discomfort throughout the body. Restless, must move, gets out of bed, because he feels too hot, forced to uncover himself and walk. Heat or impression of heat over all parts of the body, compelling him to move.

RELATIONS - ***Compare:*** (1) Ars. - Prostration, agitation, fear of death, burning pains. Cadaverous smell of secretions. (2) Verat. - State of collapse with icy sensation over whole body: face pale, bluish, cold sweating. Cramping abdominal pains with diarrhea. (3) Rhus-t. - Aching and stiffness, agitation, need to change position, pain in the lumbar and sacral regions with stiffness, aching limbs, burning, stinging vesicular eruption.

REFERENCES - Julian.

CHLOROFORMUM

(Chloroform)

PHARMACY - chlf. Chloroformum. Chloroform. Methylene trichloride. Solution. ***Historical dose:*** Tincture and all potencies.

CLINICAL - Arachnitis. Asphyxia. Colic. Convulsions. Delirium, tremens. Flatulence. Gall-stones. Muscae, volitantes. Bladder, paralysis. Puerperal, convulsions. Sick, headache. Smell, lost. Taste, lost. Tetanus. Typhus. Vertigo.

HOMEOPATHIC - Chloroform is the well-known anesthetic, the general effects of which in arresting sensation need no description. Unlike ether and nitrous oxide, which must be administered without air, chloroform vapor must have an abundance of air inhaled with it or asphyxia results.

Its most noteworthy effect is the complete relaxation of all the voluntary muscles of the body. It may cause death by paralyzing the respiration or the heart. Its use is contraindicated where there is brain softening, fatty heart, alcoholism or albuminuria.

General anesthetic and anti-spasmodic. Complete muscular relaxation. Weak and quick pulse, shallow or stertorous breathing. Convulsions, nephritic or biliary colic, gastralgia. Great weakness, especially on right side. Limbs very tired from knees down.

Much perspiration all over face and chest. Drowsy and dizzy. Dry lips and throat, dry tickling cough at night. Flatulence, food regurgitates. Sore and bruised feeling in stomach. Catching pain around heart. Sharp pain in right chest when he takes long breath, shortness of breath on exertion.

MIND - Delirium where excitement and violence predominate. Wild excitement, followed by complete insensibility. Sings comical songs, could scarcely be persuaded to leave the piano. Obscene language used under its influence in two provers. Desire to kill.

Ears - Roaring in ears like boiling water.

Eyes - Conjunctiva insensible. Pupils dilated insensible to light. Eyes turned up. Sight gradually went out and returned gradually. Small black points, large black or gray spots, float a few inches before the eye, follow the motion of the eye. Bright and dark points, sparks, flashes of light, bright streaks.

Face - Face as if intoxicated, flushed, livid.

Head - Severe, bursting headache in forehead. Headache, with dizziness, roaring in the ears, excessive nausea and vomiting. Head drawn down upon the shoulders, eyes opened and closed rapidly, pupils contracted and rapid convulsive movements of face of muscles of limbs.

Heart - Constantly increasing retardation and weakening of action of heart and arteries.

Kidneys - Paralysis of sphincter of bladder after childbirth.

Lungs - Stertorous breathing.

Mouth - Teeth smooth, as after acids (fourth day). Soapy taste. Taste lost.

Nose - Complete loss of smell (lasted two months).

Stomach - Burning in stomach, alternating with chilliness. Much acidity and great distention of stomach and bowels with gas. Abdomen tense, rumbling. Belchings. Nervous hiccough. Nausea and vomiting. Seasickness or morning sickness.

Throat - Burning in throat, scraping. Violent scraping and coldness in fauces on inspiration.

Vertigo - Vertigo, rising from spine into occiput. Whirling in head as if he would fall forward. As if ground waving on closing eyes.

COMMENTS - Marcy cured with it a case of arachnitis ending in convulsions. It is especially indicated in delirium where excitement and violence predominate, desire to kill. Paralysis of voluntary and involuntary muscles and special senses.

Chloroform will dissolve gallstones and cases have been treated by the injection of Chloroform into the gallbladder. Symptoms were obtained by Dr. D. Macfarlan with the 6c potency.

ELATIONS - ***Antidoted by:*** Phosphorus is the remedy to give for narcosis of chloroform. Amyl-n, Ip., Brandy, Ice in rectum. ***It antidotes:*** Strychnine. ***Compare:*** (1) Chloralum., Phos. (2) Ether - post-operative bronchitis. (3) Spiritus Aetheris Compositus, Hoffman's Anodyne - Flatulence, angina pectoris.

REFERENCES - Boericke. Clarke. Phatak.

CHLORPROMAZINUM

(Chlorpromazine)

PHARMACY - chlorpr. Chlorpromazinum. Chlorpromazine. Marketed under the name Largactil. ***Historical dose:*** All potencies.

CLINICAL - Allergies. Aplastic anemia. Botulism. Chorea. Cushing's disease. Diabetes insipidus. Diabetes mellitus. Diphtheria. Encephalitis. Epilepsy. Genetic disorders. Hallucinations. Hypertension. Multiple sclerosis. Obesity. Parkinson's disease. Septicemia. Skin disorders.

HOMEOPATHIC - Chlorpromazine's properties are characterized by an action which is anti-spasmodic, anti-convulsive, hypnotic and sedative. Recent pharmacological research indicates that even in extremely weak doses, chlorpromazine induces abnormal changes in the form of the bacteria sometimes associated with increased pathogenic power, which alters cellular permeability and stunts the growth of the bacteria or kills them.

Clinically, chlorpromazine is used as an anti-emetic sedative and as a potentializer of the activity of several medicating agents (general anesthetic, hypnotics, analgesics). In psychiatry, Largactil is prescribed for cases of acute psychosis, maniacal excitability and for insomnia.

A proving was carried out from December 1963 to January 1964 by sixteen members of the "Association of Homeopathic Doctors," in Matunga, Bombay, under the direction of Dr. N. P. Pai. The potency was 30c. A toxicological summary was made by O. A. Julian, which concerned the toxic consequences of chlorpromazine treatment.

General slowing down of pace of life. Mobility in the face reduced, has a leaden look, tends to be silent. General feeling of failing with depression. Tubercular tendencies or recurrence of old lesions. Allergic, tubercular conditions with syphilitic complication. Hallucinations, disturbed sleep.

Hepatic, gastric intestinal complaints. Diabetes mellitus. Hypertension. Genetic disorders in both sexes. Virilism. Vesicular, bullous eruptions and pigmentation disorders. Skin disorders and abnormal hair growth. Obesity, predominantly of the lower regions of the body.

MIND - Irritability or apathy. Absent-minded, difficulty in concentrating. Amnesia, lasting only a short time. Loss of memory, gaps in the memory. Melancholy. Premonition of bad news. Extreme anguish at 10 a.m. Thoughts are automatic. Pre-senile insanity with cerebral atrophy. Hallucinations. Personality disorders and behavioral complaints in children.

Abdomen - Intestinal atony and colic. Flatulence. Painful pressure in the epigastric region.

Back - Rheumatism of the vertebrae. Lumbago. Stiff pains in the lumbar region.

Blood - Aplastic anemia. Diminution of blood platelets. Septicemia. Agranulocytosis with Vincent's angina of the mouth and toxic infectious conditions.

Breasts - Excessive milk. Gynecomastia.

Chest - Oppression and burning in the chest. Pain behind the sternum.

Constitutions - Allergic, tubercular conditions with syphilitic complexion and complaints of the thalamus.

Eyes - Burning of the eyelids aggravated at the end of the day. Spasms of the ciliary muscles. Brownish discoloration of the conjunctiva. Pigmentary accumulation of the cornea. Conjunctivitis. Blepharitis. Cataract. Intestinal keratitis. Visual hallucinations.

Face - Neuralgia of trigeminal nerve. Facial paralysis. Lips dry, grazed, scabby, cracked.

Female - Considerable leucorrhea like egg-white. Amenorrhea. Painful menses. Cervicitis. Vaginitis, trichomonas, mycotic. Cystic inflammation of the ovary. Vomiting during pregnancy. Stretch-marks. Sexual precocity. Diminution of sexual desire.

Food - Hypoglycemic condition, weakness, sweating, hunger-pangs, faintness.

Head - Epidemic encephalitis. Frontal and occipital headache, aggravated at the end of the day.

Heart - Hypotension. Rhythm disorders. Aneurysm of the aorta.

Kidneys - Dysuria. Polyuria. Urine red-brick color, like blood. Atony of the bladder. Enuresis in the adults.

Limbs - Muscular pains in the arms and calves. Phlebitis. Varicosity of the lower limbs. Post-diphtheria paralysis.

Liver - Viral hepatitis. Liver enlarged and sensitive. Infectious epidemic jaundice. Gallstones. Cirrhosis.

Lungs - Emphysema. Asthma. Cardiac dyspnea. Pneumothorax.

Male - Dysuria. Feeling of swollen prostate. Inflammation of the prostate gland. Adenoma of the prostate. Clear diminution of sexual desire. Impotence.

Modalities - Aggravation of most of the symptoms at the end of the day.

Mouth - Breath fetid. Mouth dry. Paresis of one side of the tongue. Tongue dry, thick, cracked. Pityriasis of the tongue. Thrush. Aphthous stomatitis and glossitis. Pruritus and sensitivity of the gums. Bleeding gingivitis. Pain in the upper molars.

Nerves - Parkinson's disease. Multiple sclerosis. Clonic muscular contractions. Convulsive epileptiform fits. Chorea with irregular jerking. Trembling, hypertony, stiffness. Catatonic with total immobility. Paresis of the cranial nerves.

Nose - Nose blocked. Rhinitis.

Rectum - Stubborn constipation.

Skin - Vesicular, bullous eruptions. Pigmentation disorders. Photo-sensitivity to sunlight with erythema and edema of the face and hands. Violent discoloration of the skin. Dermatitis caused by sensitivity to light. Acne. Eczema. Herpes zoster Chickenpox. Pemphigus. Dermatitis Melanosis. Wheals.

Sleep - Sleepy. Insomnia between 1 a.m and 3 a.m., with dreams of animals. Nightmares. Confused dreams. Wakes tired with sleepiness in the morning.

Stomach - Burning pain in the stomach Anorexia and nausea in the mornin Stomach and duodenal ulcers. Stomach ache, in the form of stiffness. Impressic that there is a stone lying on the stomac

Temperature - Feverishness, with feeling coldness. Feet cold and the cold creeps far as the thighs. Hypothermia or localiz hyperthermia.

Throat - Dysphagia with feeling of a lump in the throat.

RELATIONS - ***Compare:*** (1) Anhal. - Cortical, thalamic, visceral hyperesthesia. Audio-visual hallucinations. Schizophrenic condition. Loss of libido. (2) Cic. - Cataleptic state. Convulsions and muscular spasms. Pustular eruptions on the face and hands. (3) Phos. - Inability to think. Insomnia before midnight and vertigo on waking. Nightly hunger and vomiting, empty stomach. Constipation or diarrhea. Tendency to hemorrhage. Icteric condition. (4) Syph. - Premature aging, loss of memory, sadness, aggravation at night. Fear of madness and obsessions (needs to wash hands all the time). Desire for alcohol. Hardening of the spermatic cord and of the uterus. (5) Tub. - Hypochondriac. Bad-tempered. Headache with feeling of constriction as of an iron band, oppression, irritating cough. Thick sputum. Anorexia. Aversion to meat. Gastric cramps. Tenesmus of the bladder. Pains and bruising of the limbs. Itching eczema. Perspiration, straining the underclothes yellow.

REFERENCES - Julian.

CHLORUM AQUA

(Chlorine Water)

PHARMACY - chlor. Chlorum aqua. Chlorine water. Chlorine gas in water. Chlorine, the element. Solution. Chlorine water, when full strength is required, must be freshly prepared. ***Historical dose:*** Tincture and all potencies.

CLINICAL - Aphthae. Asthma. Catarrh. Chlorosis. Colds. Convulsions. Coughs. Croup. Dentition. Diphtheria. Gastritis. Hemoptysis. Impotence. Laryngismus. Pleurisy. Sore throat. Tuberculosis. Typhus. Ulcers.

HOMEOPATHIC - Chlorum has been proved in the form of *"Chlorine water,"* and has been tested clinically. Marked effect on the respiratory organs, producing spasm of the glottis as the chief symptom of the drug. Asthma to relieve the spasm of glottis. Useful externally and internally in gangrene.

Spasms and convulsions. Laryngeal spasm is especially pronounced, the chief difficulty is in exhaling, can draw in the air well enough. Coryza and catarrh.

Convulsive attacks on cutting eye-teeth. Mouth inflamed, ulcerated. Rapid emaciation. Acute rheumatic pains.

MIND - Irritability, inclined to anger. Marked loss of memory, especially for names. Apprehension. Fear of becoming crazy. Fear of poverty. Inclined to anger. Want of self-confidence. Effects of excitement. Quiet delirium, alternating with greatest restlessness and desire to run away. Coma, fainting with cold, viscous sweats.

Eyes - Running of tears, worse in open air. Suddenly numerous, fantastic images appeared before the eyes, disappearing with lightning-like rapidity.

Face - Face swollen with protruding eyes. Face pale, often greenish. Heightened color.

Head - Painful aching in vertex and down left side, with inclination to lie down. Warm sweat breaks out on forehead while coughing.

Heart - Increased action of the heart.

Lungs - Constriction with suffocation. Inspiration free with obstructed expiration (Meph.). Sudden dyspnea from spasm of the vocal cords with staring protruding eyes, blue face, cold sweat, pulse small. Spasm of the glottis. Irritation of epiglottis, larynx and bronchials. Coryza with sudden gushes of sharp, corroding fluid, making nose sore inside. Prolonged, loud, whistling rales. Loss of voice from damp air. Sooty, smoky nostrils, livid face.

Male - Sudden impotence and aversion to sexual intercourse.

Modalities - Chest affections better from open air, causes running of tears. Spasm of glottis worse from midnight to 7 a.m. Nasal complaints worse lying down. Inclination to lie down with headache. Restless, worse walking up and down. Sitting with sun shining on back causes shuddering. Damp air causes loss of voice.

Mouth - Mouth dry. Putrid odor from mouth. Very acid saliva. Aphthae. Tongue black, as if burnt.

Nose - Nose dry, smoky or sooty. Corrosive feeling in corners of nose. Violent sneezing, in the morning. Sudden running in drops of sharp corroding fluid with tears in eyes, dry tongue, palate and fauces. Coryza with headache. Thin coryza, soon changing to yellow, copious mucus. Loss of smell.

Stomach - Acid stomach and other gastric troubles (in workmen exposed to chlorine fumes and who eat chalk for it). Desire to vomit when coughing, without nausea.

Stool - Diarrhea in the morning, with dry mouth, after the eruption appears with typhus. Bright blood stools. Hemorrhage in typhus, blood black, coagulated or thin, smelling like carrion.

Teeth - Sensation as if teeth were too full, as if injured by acids. Black teeth.

Temperature - Chilliness and crawls, 10 a.m. to 2 p.m. Burning, dry heat with anxiety and raving. Genial glow all over with night-sweat. Cold sweat. Viscous sweat. Typhus.

Throat - Dry, sore from uvula to bronchi. Choking sensation, inability to swallow.

COMMENTS - Excessive sensitiveness of skin. Nettle rash with fever. Cutis anserina. Skin dry, yellow, shriveled. Malignant pustule and carbuncle. Typhoid state. Fears he will go crazy, that he won't be able to make a living. Cannot remember names of people he sees, or if he sees the names, cannot remember the person.

E. Z. Bacon recorded two cases of chlorine poisoning. The first case was in a boy of 5, who, after passing through diphtheria to apparent complete recovery, was suddenly seized with symptoms of croup. Loss of voice, crowing inspiration, prolonged expiration incessant dry cough, great restlessness, high fever, and profuse perspiration.

The symptoms were worse lying on a lounge by the fire, better when lying in his mother's lap and still more relieved by being carried about. During the previous illness, Platt's chlorides had been placed in the room as a disinfectant and it occurred to the doctor that chlorine vapor is much heavier than air. He himself lay down, and in a few minutes felt the irritating vapor and began to cough and hack. This soon passed away on sitting up.

The removal of the chlorides has a remarkable effect on the child, cough and respiration were greatly relieved. But the relief came too late, as the cause was not discovered for several days during which time the patient had become steadily weaker, and he died the same afternoon.

The other case was that of an old woman who suffered from chronic bronchitis and on January 2, 1892, developed an attack of laryngitis. In three days she was well, but in the two subsequent weeks, on exactly the same day, a fresh attack occurred. As the doctor soon discovered, his patient went to the back room, where chlorides were kept, every Monday to wash a few things she did not care to send to the laundry.

The chlorides were banished, and though the washing was continued, there were no more attacks of laryngitis. Dr. Bacon added, that since giving up the use of disinfectants, other than plenty of fresh air, he has never had laryngeal complications in scarlatina or diphtheria, though his neighbors have had plenty.

Whitman recommended chlorine water as a efficient palliative in a fit of asthma. He began with 10 drops, then in five minutes 20 more, and than in another five minutes, half a teaspoonful in a little water. It greatly facilitates expectoration.

In typhus fever, Goullon recommended chlorine water, five drops every two or three hours until the tongue is dry. Clarke had excellent results from the 12c and 30c in nasal catarrh and in breathlessness remaining after acute bronchitis.

RELATIONS - It is antidote to: Hydrocyanic acid and Sulfuretted hydrogen. Albumen. ***Compare:*** (1) Meph. - inability to exhale, closely resembles Bromine and Iodine. (2) Nat-m. - sore mouth and other chlorides. (3) Lyc. - impotence. (4) Plb-a. - blood-spitting and pleurisy. ***Follows well:*** Phos.

REFERENCES - Boericke. Clarke. Phatak.

CHOCOLATE

(Cocoa)

PHARMACY - choc. Chocolate. Cocoa. Theobroma cocoa. Theobroma cacao. N. O. Sterculiaceae. Tribe, Buettnerieae. Tropical America. Trituration of the seeds. ***Historical dose:*** Trituration and all potencies.

CLINICAL - Anxiety. Fears. Poor memory.

HOMEOPATHIC - "Theobroma" is Greek for "Food of the Gods." Mayan Indian legend has it that the cocoa tree was a gift from the gods. The Mayas believed the drink made from the cocoa seeds would nourish them after death. The Aztecs believed cocoa would relieve their fatigue and stimulate their mental and psychic abilities.

The Spanish invaders were surprised to find that the cocoa beans were valued more than any other substance, even more than gold. The Aztecs used a chocolate drink as a base in many of their medicinal formulas. The Aztec nobility used the chocolate drink favored with vanilla and spices as a pleasurable drink.

The main ingredients of chocolate are caffeine, phenyl ethylamine, theobromine and theophylline. Feeding with waste chocolate led to fatal poisoning in calves. The animals showed excitement, stared about in all directions, walked with exaggerated strides and had convulsions. One calf died, possibly from heart failure.

Sherr wrote "My 22 month old male Tibetan Terrier ate a large bar of Bourneville chocolate. He became extremely hyperactive, panting, restless, couldn't stay still in one place, ran up and down stairs. He came up and licked me, went away, came back, went outside, came inside and two hours after eating the chocolate, he gave a large moan, wail and died instantly, outside in the sun from a heart attack."

Scalp warm and itchy. Back of neck itchy. Under axilla itchy. Skin dry and rough. Skin burns easily. Gums bleeding while cleaning teeth. Catarrhal congestion in head. Catarrhal deafness ameliorated when ears pop. Ache in big toe joints.

Mind rushing and jumping from one thing to another. Irritability. Startled by sudden noises. Unease and discomfort with men. Anxiety before meeting people. Poor memory. Vivid and prolonged dreams. Dreams of fire. Desire for chocolate and ice cream.

MIND - Moods changeable. Emotional highs and lows, Very depressed. Activity alternating with lethargy. Slow mind, has to think before answering questions. Weepy during menses, took everything to heart. More sensitive to music. Selfish, impatient and intolerant. Irritable. Sarcastic, mocking people, aggressive in a joking way. Humorless, intolerant, almost cruel.

Anxiety that something would happen. Feels open and vulnerable. Fear of accidents, cars, being attacked. Fear of dogs. Fear of something happening. Paranoid. Anxiety about health. Apprehensive. Nervous thinks someone would notice.

Feels panicky about work things to do. Difficult concentration. Forgetful, absent minded. Reading is impossible. Aversion to writing. Mistakes in writing. Mind is repeating the same things over and over. Jumping from subject to subject while speaking. Nervous and stuttering.

Grief and despair. Lost interest in loved ones, feels totally indifferent. Self-conscious, anxious and vulnerable as if being watched. Feels rejected and oversensitive. Hid away from the world, feels life would fall apart. Felt isolated. Unsociable, averse company and conversation. Desire to be alone in the evening.

Abdomen - Bloated abdomen with belching, flatus and nausea, worse after supper. Rumbling and gas in the abdomen. Loud rumbling in abdomen while lying. Woke with pain from gas in upper abdomen. Pain dull, becoming sharper. Aching lower pelvic region when sitting. Sharp pain in liver.

Back - Shivers up spine with chill in evening. Strong itching at middle of spine, shoulder blade. Prickly feeling on the back of the neck. Stabbing pain in back, between spine and left shoulder. Tightness around thoracic vertebrae. Back pains.

Stiff feeling with painful neck, while sleeping on back. Feels very vulnerable in the base of the spine. Spine and back feel uncomfortable with a deep restlessness, uneasiness and irritability. Sensation that back is larger and wider.

Breasts - Breasts feel fuller. Desire to rub breasts. Stitching pains, sensation as if fine threads were being drawn through breasts. Painful breasts before menstrual period.

Chest - Feeling of a powerful explosion inside chest, taking breath away, as if diaphragm went into a spasm. Pain in chest with belching. Chest heavy, aches inside. Tenderness in sternum and lower ribs. Tightness in xiphoid. Left clavicle has itch and pain. Whole upper left quadrant of chest has some tight dull pain. Pain under the ribs. Stitching pains at base of right lung. Stabbing pain in back between spine and left shoulder, worse inhalation. Tingling in chest, creeping down from spine. Cold feeling in the lungs. Cough hurts chest and head. Catarrhal feeling behind the sternum.

Coughs - Cough from throat, from deep in center of chest by xiphoid of sternum. Painful cough, chest worse movement. Cough with nausea and a sensation of mucus behind the sternum. Sudden attack of a retching and gagging cough. Loose cough with thick, pale green mucus, from trachea and lungs. Dry coughs, in evening, after swallowing. Spasms of hard dry cough on going to bed, better cold water. Lying in bed coughing. Wakes coughing at 4 a.m.

Dreams - Dreamless sleep. Dreams are not remembered. Dreams are fragmented, confused, obscure. Dreams of familiar people, friends. Dream of selling fruit and vegetables in the market. Dreaming flying and jumping, being on a boat journey, falling from a window. Dreams of babies bathing, the babies were like helpless little animals, almost dead. Dreams of pain in the right ovarian/pelvic region. Vivid dream of worms.

Ears - Feeling of fullness, buzzing or fuzziness in both ears, worse left. Tingling sensation left ear, worse loud music. Ears feel blocked. Ears popped and buzzed while eating. Dullness of hearing until ears popped. Flushed and hot ears. Left ear burning and red. Ears burning, extending occasionally to mastoids. Sensitive feeling in ears. Intense pain behind right ear. Pulsations in ear and neck. Hearing more acute, especially for deeper tones which have more resonance.

Eyes - Right eye sticky and closed. Eyes tired and smarting, desire to clench lids together. Eyes inflamed with flushed face. Tension in the eyeballs. Eyes feel heavy, with dryness and pressure at the back of the eyes. Eyelids feel wider and higher. Eyes painful and feel swollen. Eyes ache, sensitive to pressure. Deep pain over right eye. Bruised feeling over right eye. Right eye felt lower than left eye. Eyes sore and stinging, better pressing lids with fingers. Heavy feeling over eyes. Pupils dilated during headache. Looking down when walking, ground seems further away. Dark specks falling down in profusion while reading. Tired feeling in artificial light. Photophobia.

Face - Skin of face dry, chapped, very thin, blotchy and wrinkly. Face flushed and hot, red after supper. Red and livid spot on left cheek. Skin on cheekbones tingles and burns. Twitching under right eye. Deep ache in left jaw, extending to ear. Numbness around lips extending to nostrils. Rash around mouth, worse left side. Lips dry and cracked. Cold sore on lips.

Female - Menses lighter then usual, then becoming very heavy. Menses heavier and longer than usual. No desire for sex. Sexual desire increased.

Food - Appetite improved. Wakes up feeling hungry. Lack of appetite and thirst. Averse food. Aversion to sweets, to usual tea. Desires hot drinks, but aggravates. Desire for hot, black currant juice, orange juice, soda water, cold water, refreshing things. Desires sweet food, sauerkraut, and fruit, especially citrus. Desire to eat red things, red peppers, red fruit, red grapes beetroot soup.

Head - Sensation of congestion in head. Sensation of tightness around head. Sensation of forehead protruding. Head feels big, worse right side. Head is heavy. Dull sensation between vertex and occiput on mid-line. Top of head feels sensitive, better after eating. Sutures feels more pointed, like the top of a roof. Sensation as if something loose in head, as if a string connected uvula to sinuses. Sensation as if a cold spot went through head. Frontal headache. Sharp pain at top of forehead. Headache like a band around head. Throbbing pain over left eye. Headache feels like rod pushing my head apart from inside. Pounding inside head. Headache behind eyes and throbbing pain around temples. Pressure over eyes, better lying down. Headache, worse coughing, better holding head. Headache with earache. Awake from severe headache. Vomiting with migraines. Dry, very large, flaky dandruff. Hair is very dry and lifeless.

Heart - Tightness in back of heart. As if back of heart pushing against back. Feeling of heart bulging through ribs, better when lying on left side. As if heart is beating more towards the back and sides between the scapulae. Feels heart banging and bulging through the ribs. Doesn't feel the heart at all. In the night, the heart stops beating.

Larynx - Sudden loss of voice during cold. Voice slides up and down the scale, high pitched to low and husky, breaks, almost lost. Lack of control over voice.

Limbs - Aching in joints. Wandering pain in hands and feet, in muscles, joints and small bones. Clumsy, drops things, bumps into things. Hands less capable of doing fine movements, such as writing. Wrists feel weaker and flatter. Aching muscles of arms, in bed. Sharp, deep pain in the legs, on the inside of the malleolus. Tightness in thigh muscle. Sharp, shooting, momentary pain up inside of right gluteal muscle. Feet feel like blocks of ice, so cold, bones are painful. Toes are like ice. Deep ache in joints of both big toes. Legs felt powerless and like heavy rubber. When legs are moved there is a time lapse between the thought and the action.

Lungs - More air going in with less effort, breaths much slower and further apart. On breathing in, chest felt tight. Breathing from lower down in the lungs. During cough, expectoration of very clear mucus mixed with saliva. Thick, pale green mucus on coughing from deep in chest. Cough of green sticky chunks.

Mouth - Dry mouth. Bad taste in mouth with thirst. Taste of nicotine in mouth, like an old ashtray. Tea tasted of nothing, just hot water. Tea or orange juice tasteless. Hollow feeling in mouth. Tenderness in left rear palate of mouth when touched with tongue. Salivation increased. Salivation when lying down, with heartburn. Ulcers on inside of mouth and cheeks and at corners of lips. Chewing lips.

Neck - Tension in the shoulders extending to the base of the neck, in the spine where dorsal and cervical regions meet. Back of neck stiff and tight. The muscles on either side of the cervical vertebrae feel as if they are being laced up tight together. Intense tension, bends the neck back, leads to a sensation as if the back of the head is horribly elongated.

Nose - Nose feels smaller or longer and face feels sharper. Nose is cold, wet and dripping. Nose blocked with thick mucus in warm indoors. Nose stuffy and runny. Awakes with runny nose, phlegm in throat. Clear discharge with itching at end of nostrils. Constant desire to blow nose. Green or yellow mucus, with small amount blood. Clear, white, bubbly discharge in evening. Sneezing, followed by coryza. Nosebleed. Pimple inside upper right nostril. Acute sense of smell, especially to flowers.

Perspiration - Perspiration increased. Woke in night feeling hot and sweaty. Sweet smell of perspiration at night. Restless and hot, sweat all night. Relieved by beginning to sweat.

Rectum - Profuse, watery, very smelly diarrhea, with a lot of rumbling. Explosive diarrhea with flatus. Light brown stools, worse as day went on. Stool difficult to pass, yet not very hard. Sour smelling flatus. Offensive flatus in the evening. Rectum sore.

Skin - Dry skin, itching. Itching scapulae, shins, forearms, pelvis and forehead. Scratching until it bled. Small, dry pimples. Lips very dry. Hands feel coarser and more leathery. Skin feels numb, less sensitive to touch. Feels crawly and "sensitive" to touch of clothes.

Sleep - Yawning a lot. Overcome with sleepiness. Deep sleep. Sleeps poorly, restless, waking often. Sleeps on back. Wakes with painful and stiff neck, needs to change positions. When on side, pain went away. Wakes at 2 to 3 a.m., feeling hot and sweaty, at 5 a.m. very alert and alive. Very tired on waking. Sleepiness during menses.

Stomach - Sensation of weakness in stomach and wooziness in the head with general weakness. Stomach feels aggravated and full. Dull pain like indigestion. Pain comes in waves and with big belches. Belching in evenings, followed by acid taste in mouth. Intense, frequent bouts of heartburn while sitting. Heartburn while smoking cigarettes and from hot drinks, but not from hot food. Heartburn worse 2 to 4 p.m. Feeling queasy after a cup of tea. Nausea with bad taste in mouth. Nausea and vomiting at midnight with migraines.

Stool - Stool hard and in very small pieces. Stool soft and less dry. Very loose, frequent stool, verging on diarrhea. Watery stools, smelly, light brown.

Teeth - Aching pain gums and around roots of teeth. Toothache in right upper canine tooth.

Temperature - Tired, as if a cold or flu would come on. Wakes with flue or cold symptoms. Tendency to take colds. Uncoordinated, feel heavy and slow (Gels.). Fever and chills, all night. Alternates between being chilled, feverish and sweating. Face hot, body chilled. Chilled easily. Shaking and trembling, teeth chatter when in bed. Restless and hot, sweat all night, desire to sleep in cold part of house.

Throat - Terrible dry feeling in throat on waking. Awakes with runny nose, phlegm in throat. Mucus plug in throat, coughs to dislodge it. Constant desire to clear throat because of a plug of mucus behind sternum. Hawking beige mucus from posterior sinuses. Raw and sore throat, peppery feeling, especially high in the fauces. Soreness and tenderness in throat and glands both sides. Dark red throat, internal, worse left side. Tingling in throat. Desire not to swallow, but very hungry. Difficult swallowing with sore left throat.

Tongue - Small, white, raised spots on tongue. Small, red spots on base of tongue. Tongue coated yellow brown at back, as if smoked many cigarettes. Whitish-yellow tongue. Tongue looks as if it is painted a beige color.

Vertigo - Faint buzzing all over head. Blurred, fuzzy feeling comes over head in waves, pleasant and relaxing. Thick and fuzzy head, like a hangover. Not quite with it, like looking through a cloud. Felt dizzy on rising, with nausea after drinking tea.

RELATIONS - ***Compare:*** (1) Cacao.

REFERENCES - Allen. Sherr.

CHOLESTERINUM

(Cholesterine)

PHARMACY - chol. Cholesterinum. Cholesterine. Gallstones. Trituration of gallstones. From the epithelium lining of gallbladder and the larger ducts. Sarcode. ***Historical dose:*** Trituration and all potencies.

CLINICAL - Cancer. Cirrhosis. Eyes, opacities. Fibroids. ***Gallstone, colic. Gallstones***. Insomnia. Jaundice. ***Liver, diseases.*** Tumors.

HOMEOPATHIC - Cholesterinum crystallizes in leaflets with a mother-of-pearl luster and a fatty feel. It is soluble in alcohol and ether. It occurs in the blood and brain, yolk of eggs, seeds and buds of plants, but most abundantly in the bile and gallstones.

Dr. Wilhelm Ameke of Berlin first mentioned this remedy. Dr. Burnett, at Ameke's suggestion, used the lower potencies with more or less success for several years, a description of which Burnett gives in his Diseases of the Liver.

Chol. was introduced by Swan. He appeared to have taken his hint from Burnett's work and potentized the remedy, using a gallstone for his preparations.

Swan affirmed, after much experience, that it is almost a specific for ***gallstone colic.*** It relieves the distress at once and this after failure with Nux-v., Chin., Card-m., Podo. and other apparently well-selected remedies.

Ameke recommended Chol. as a remedy in cancer of the liver. Chol. is the physiological opponent of Lec., both seem to play some unknown part in the growth of tumors. Benign tumors, uterine fibroids. Gallstones. Chronic jaundice. ***Obstinate hepatic engorgements.*** Opacities of the vitreous. Insomnia.

MIND - Irritable. Delirium. Moody.

Abdomen - Burning pain in side, on walking holds his hand on side.

Back - Itching of coccyx.

Eyes - Vitreous opacities of eyes.

Face - Discolored bluish.

Female - Tumors, benign, fibroids.

Limbs - Leg cramps.

Liver - Hepatic engorgements. ***Gallstones and gallstone colic.*** Jaundice. Liver cancer. Liver diseases.

Modalities - Worse from touch or jar. Worse lying on side. Worse bending or sudden motion.

Skin - Red, coppery spots after the desquamation.

COMMENTS - Potentized cholesterol gallstones. Gallstones and gallstone colic. Liver cancer, palliates dying liver cancer patients.

Yingling reported some cures of gallstone colic and other diseases of the liver in the Medical Advance, August, 1908 and noted that "In gallstone colic, the patient suffers so severely that it is almost impossible to obtain symptoms. In such a case, when one cannot give a well-selected remedy, give Cholesterinum and thus far it has never failed.

"It can be used instead of Morphine in cases where the symptoms cannot be obtained for the proper selection of a remedy. It is very improbable that a person suffering from gallstone colic will wait very long for the physician to study the case."

Ameke claimed to have derived great advantages from its use in cases diagnosed as cancer of the liver, or in such obstinate engorgements that malignancy was suspected.

Clarke cured a case in the last stage of liver disease. He had been given up by his medical attendant, who ordered him to make his will without delay.

Burnett claimed to have twice cured cancer of the liver with it and "in hepatic engorgements that by reason of their intractable and slow yielding to well-selected remedies make one think of cancer."

In such conditions, where the diagnosis is in doubt, especially if the patient has been subjected to repeated attacks of biliary colic, Chol., he claimed is very satisfactory and at times its action even striking. It has been used with success in the removal of opacities of the vitreous.

Burnett used the 3x or the 3c trituration and substantial doses. He commended it in "obstinate hepatic engorgements, which by reason of their obstinacy make one think interrogatively of cancer."

Also in "cases in which there appears to be a semi-malignant affection involving the left lobe of the liver and what lies between it and the pylorus and the pancreas." In such cases Burnett gave alternately Chol. 3x and Iodoform 3x.

RELATIONS - ***Compare:*** (1) Taurocholate of Soda.

REFERENCES - Boericke. Clarke. Murphy.

CHROMICUM ACIDUM

(Chromic Acid)

PHARMACY - chr-ac. Chromicum acidum. Chromic acid. Chromium sesquioxide. Anhydrous solution or Chromic oxide. Trituration. ***Historical dose:*** Trituration and all potencies.

CLINICAL - Angina pectoris. Brain, inflammation. Coughs. Diarrhea. Eyes, disorders. Gangrene. Gout. Hemorrhoids. Lumbago. Lupus. Ranula. Rheumatism. Stiff, neck. Syphilis. Throat, sore. Toothaches. Trismus. Tuberculosis, laryngeal. Ulcers. Warts.

HOMEOPATHIC - Chromic acid is a powerful antiseptic which has been used for disinfecting purposes to arrest fetid discharge and correct fetid odors. Offensive discharge. ***"Foul smelling, bloody lochia."***

Inflammation and destruction of epithelium and mucus membranes, a false membrane, gangrene. On the skin it has been used to destroy warts. Cutting pains in eyes. Cough, hard, sometimes deep, swallows sputa. Vomits breakfast. Diphtheria. Post-nasal tumors. Epithelioma of the tongue. ***Symptoms come and go suddenly*** and return periodically.

Limbs - Uneasiness in limbs. Pain in shoulder blades and back of neck. Pain in knees and balls of feet. Drawing pain in soles while walking.

Modalities - Worse least draft of air. Worse cold water. Worse at night and early in morning. Worse 2 a.m. to 6 a.m. Pain worse on left side.

Nose - Ulcer and scabs in nose. Offensive smell. Corrosive pain. Ozaena (Aur.).

Rectum - Frequent, copious water, with nausea and vertigo. Hemorrhoids internal and bleeding. Weakness in small of back.

Throat - Diphtheria, sore throat. Tough mucus with inclination to swallow it, worse causing hawking. Post-nasal tumors.

COMMENTS - Suddenness of many of the symptoms. Symptoms appear and disappear suddenly and return periodically. Disagreeable pricking and itching here and there with uneasiness in limbs. Pains suddenly shifting to various parts of trunk, on waking. On turning to right side, pain in left side goes off. Sensation of a vacuum at heart of emptiness in chest.

Well-marked rheumatic symptoms. Clarke frequently obtained good results in rheumatic cases with both preparations.

RELATIONS - ***Antidotes:*** Daph. has cured the rheumatic pains. Merc-c. in small doses has counteracted the general effects in workmen. The restlessness and relief from motion suggest Rhus-t. ***Compare:*** (1) Kali-bi., Rhus-t. (2) Chromium sulphate in locomotor ataxia, goiter, serve us as a remedy in cases of hypertrophy. Herpes preputialis. Wry neck. Also exophthalmia inhibits the vagus, relieving tachycardia. Acts like a nerve tonic where there is lack of nervous tone. Fibroid tumors. Infantile paralysis. Dose for adults, 3 to 5 grains after meals and at bedtime.

REFERENCES - Boericke. Clarke.

CHROMIUM KALI SULPHURATUM

(Chromic Sulphate)

PHARMACY - chrom-k-s. Chromium kali sulphuratum. Chromic sulphate. Chrome alum potassic. ***Historical dose:*** Trituration and all potencies.

CLINICAL - Catarrh. Hay asthma. Hay fever.

HOMEOPATHIC - Chrom-k-s. was introduced into homeopathic practice some years ago by Dr. Mersch of Brussels. Clarke used it on Dr. Mersch's indications in the 6x trituration and downwards. It sometimes succeeds in the 3x, and even the 1x, when higher numbers fail. There is no proving, but it can be used on general indications for coughs and catarrhs which its constituents will readily suggest. Valuable for hay fever.

RELATIONS - ***Compare:*** (1) All-c, Psor. Sabad., Naph., Sang. Kali-bi.

REFERENCES - Clarke.

CHROMIUM METALLICUM

(Chromium Metal)

PHARMACY - chrom. Chromium metallicum. Chromium metal. ***Historical dose:*** All potencies.

CLINICAL - ***Anemia.*** Arteriosclerosis. Cancer. Coma. Cystic fibrosis. Delirium. Diabetes. Diarrhea. Ear, infections. Epithelioma. Flatus. Headache. Heart, diseases. Hyper-cholesterolemia. Kidney, diseases. Meningitis. ***Mucus, secretions.*** Nausea. Pancreas, diseases. Paralysis. Ranula. Rheumatic, pains. Sciatica. Sinusitis. Stomach, complaints. Vertigo. Vomiting.

HOMEOPATHIC - ***Discharges thick, tough, stringy, sticky, green and yellow***. Pains changing place or in one spot. Boring, scraping pains. Cancer. Paralysis. Collapse, coma. Ear infections. Sinusitis. Heart diseases. Arteriosclerosis.

Anemia. Pain under the heart. Hypercholesterolemia. Stomach complaints. Vomiting blue or green. Affections of pancreas. Diabetes. Cystic fibrosis. Diarrhea, green or bluish. Flatus. Affections of kidneys. Blood and albumin in urine. Sciatica. Itching.

Suddenness. "Symptoms appear and disappear suddenly and return periodically." [Clarke]

Wandering pains. "Disagreeable pricking and itching here and there, with uneasiness in limbs, so that he was obliged to get up from sitting or lying and walk about." [Hering]

"The rheumatic pains shift suddenly from one part to another. This type of pains are felt in the eyes, when they are sudden, and momentary in both eyes." [Blackwood]

Mucus secretions increased, tough, stringy. At night sensation as if eyes were enlarged. Fetid, musty smell in posterior nares, chiefly perceived during expiration.

"Sensation during the eating of the food, which tastes well and natural, as if the exhaled air smelt putrid, almost causing nausea. He smells several times of the food, thinking that the stench might proceed from that." [Allen]

MIND - Weakness of memory, how to make several letters. Restlessness during pain. Restlessness in morning, better rising. Restlessness in morning before rising.

Delirium in meningitis cerebrospinalis or encephalitis. Scolding in meningitis. Delusion of being heavy. Comes across as a closed personality.

Have difficulty in expressing themselves. When answering, always considering whether they are revealing bad things about themselves.

Abdomen - Rumbling in morning, better emission of flatus. Rumbling in morning on waking.

Back - Pain in dorsal region, at inner angle of left scapula. Aching pain in lumbar region in morning in bed (Chr-o.).

Ears - Sensation of water in right ear, appearing and disappearing suddenly.

Eyes - Sensation of enlargement at night. Cutting pain in evening.

Face - Heat at 10 p.m.

Female - Offensive, fetid lochia.

Food - Worse cold drinks. Worse tea.

Head - Headache. Fullness at night, with peculiar sensation of lightness at the heart.

Heart - Sensation of emptiness at region of heart.

Lungs - Like fine twine threads.

Modalities - Better motion. Worse morning. Worse 5 a.m. to 9 a.m. Worse cold. Worse least draft of air. Worse cold water. Worse night and early morning. Worse 2 a.m. to 6 a.m.

Mouth - Epithelioma of tongue. Putrid odor while eating. Prickling of tongue. Ranula, periodic. Metallic taste during dinner.

Nose - Tumor, posterior nares.

Rectum - Sudden urging for stool. Diarrhea, green or bluish. Watery, stool.

Skin - Wounds, bites of rabid dogs.

Sleep - Waking with heart symptoms. Dreams of riding horses through a stream. Dreams of being poisoned. Dreams of urinating. Dreams that he had an attack of strangury, which the next morning proved to be the fact, he did not get over it for two hours. Dreams of crossing a stream of water on horseback, and water froze.

Stomach - Nausea better walking. Transient nausea when stomach is empty. Vomiting, breakfast.

Teeth - Pain extending to ear, extending to forehead.

Throat - Constant disposition to swallow from thick mucus.

Vertigo - Vertigo with inclination to fall to the right side. Vertigo while walking.

REFERENCES - Allen. Blackwood.

CHRYSANTHEMUM

(Ox-eye Daisy)

PHARMACY - chrysan. Chrysanthemum leucanthemum. Ox-eye daisy. Leucanthemum vulgare. Compositae. ***Historical dose:*** Tincture and all potencies.

HOMEOPATHIC - Chrysan. has a specific action on sudoriparous glands. Quiets nervous system (Cypr.). Right-sided tearing pain in bones of jaw and temple. Pain in teeth and gums, worse touch, better warmth.

Irritable and tearful. ***Insomnia and night-sweats***. Colliquative sweating and hyperesthesia of nervous system. Material doses of the tincture have been used in the past.

REFERENCES - Boericke.

CHRYSAROBINUM

(Goa Powder)

PHARMACY - chrysar. Chrysarobinum. Goa powder. Andira araroba. N. O. Papilionoideae. ***Historical dose:*** Tincture and all potencies.

CLINICAL - Acne. Blepharitis. Conjunctivitis. Herpes. Itching. Keratitis. Photophobia. Psoriasis. Ringworm.

HOMEOPATHIC - Chrysar. has been used successfully in skin diseases especially in ***ringworm, psoriasis,*** herpes, and acne rosacea. Vesicular or squamous lesions, associated with foul smelling discharge and crust formation, tend to become confluent and to give the appearance of a single crust covering the entire area.

Violent itching of thighs, legs and ***ears***. Dry, scaly eruption, especially around eyes and ears. Scabs with pus underneath (Mez.).

Ears - Eczema behind ears. Filthy, scabby condition with tendency to form thick crust. Whole ear and surrounding tissue appears to be one scab.

Eyes - Optical hyperesthesia. Intense photophobia. Blepharitis, conjunctivitis, keratitis.

COMMENTS - It contains chrysophan, which is rapidly oxidized into chrysophanic acid. This is also contained in Rheum and Senn. Acts as a powerful irritant of the skin.

RELATIONS - ***Compare:*** (1) Rhubarb and Senn.

REFERENCES - Boericke.

CHRYSOPHANICUM ACIDUM

(Chrysophanic acid)

PHARMACY - chrys-ac. Chrysophanicum acidum. Chrysophanic acid. An organic acid obtained from rhubarb and some lichens. ***Historical dose:*** Tincture and all potencies.

CLINICAL - Blepharitis. Conjunctivitis. Ophthalmia. Psoriasis. Ringworm.

HOMEOPATHIC - Chrys-ac. is a constituent of *"Goa powder."* Tried as a local application in the form of ointment in bad cases of psoriasis on one limb, Chrys-ac. has caused the disappearance of the eruption on the other limb as well, showing a constitutional action.

A. B. Norton used it successfully internally and externally in blepharitis, conjunctivitis and keratitis, the phlyctenular variety, also in eczema behind ears.

G. C. McDermott confirmed this. Used locally (grains 4 to grains 8 with Vaseline), internally, or both, it is a magnificent remedy in eye and ear cases where a filthy, scabby condition exists with a tendency to form thick crusts.

Cases in which the whole ear and surrounding tissue appeared to be one great scab from the center of which oozed the pus which came from a suppurative otitis media cleared up in two or three weeks under internal and external use of Chrys-ac. Also cases where a similar condition of eyelids and skin of face obtained. Clarke often saw a ringworm disappear rapidly from a few applications of the ointment.

It has been used with some success in the lower triturations internally for psoriasis, ringworm and other skin affections, also as a local application in ringworm.

COMMENTS - It is a powerful irritant of the skin and mucus membranes. Given internally in crude form it has caused nausea, vomiting and purging.

E. W. Beebe of Milwaukee related the effect on a friend, troubled with blepharitis, who applied to his eyelid a one-in-ten ointment made with Vaseline. The effect was immediate.

Marked conjunctiva inflammation of globe and eyelid, contraction of pupils, intense photophobia, the least ray of light producing great pain increased by a throbbing sensation synchronous with the pulse. This was accompanied with phosphorescent flashes of light.

On forcing eyes to look at objects, retinal impressions remained some time after closing them. Swelling of lids and irritation of skin around. After lasting a week there was marked improvement and a second, milder application completed the cure.

Beebe regarded the condition set up as one of "Retinal asthenopia." Graafe called it "optical hyperesthesia."

RELATIONS - ***Compare:*** Physostigma and Pilocarpine are its analogs.

REFERENCES - Boericke. Clarke.

CICHORIUM INTYBUS

(Chicory)

PHARMACY - cich. Cichorium intybus. Chicory. Endive. N. O. Composite. Tincture or trituration of dried root. ***Historical dose:*** Tincture and all potencies.

CLINICAL - Amblyopia. Constipation. Fatigue. Headaches.

HERBAL - Chicory is the well-known salad, the root of which is used for mixing with coffee. When taken in infusion like coffee, it acts as a gentle aperient. A chicory-roaster observed that he "could not read at night, not from any external irritation of the eyes, but from a feeling of deadness in them."

HOMEOPATHIC - Chicory has been proved and symptoms have been observed including a general heaviness and headaches. Weight at stomach and great indisposition to bodily and mental exertion. Want of energy. Bowels relaxed.

RELATIONS - ***Compare:*** Chicory, a Bach Flower Essence.

REFERENCES - Clarke.

CICUTA MACULATA

(Spotted Cowbane)

PHARMACY - cic-m. Cicuta maculata. Spotted cowbane. Beaver poison. N. O. Umbelliferae. Tincture of root gathered in summer. ***Historical dose:*** Tincture and all potencies.

CLINICAL - Coma. Convulsions. Epilepsy. Tetanus.

HOMEOPATHIC - The effects of the Cic-m. are very similar to those of the Cic. The most prominent symptoms include falls unconscious, tetanic or clonic convulsions, and body covered with sweat. Consider in epilepsy and tetanus.

RELATIONS - ***Compare:*** (1) Cicuta virosa.

REFERENCES - Clarke.

CICUTA VIROSA

(Water Hemlock)

PHARMACY - cic. Cicuta virosa. Water hemlock. Cowbane. N. O. Umbelliferae. Tincture of fresh root gathered at time of flowering. ***Historical dose:*** All potencies.

CLINICAL - Bladder, paralysis. Cancer. Catalepsy. ***Cerebrospinal, meningitis.*** Coccyx, pain. Colic. ***Concussions. Convulsions.*** Delirium. Delusions. Diarrhea. Eczema. ***Epilepsy.*** Epithelioma. Esophagus, stricture. Eyes, inflammation. Face, eruptions. Fever. Hallucinations. Headaches. ***Head, injuries. Hemorrhage. Hiccoughs***. Hysteria. Impetigo. Injuries. Mania. ***Meningitis.*** Myelitis. Nightmares. Numbness. ***Opisthotonos***. Paralysis. Psoriasis. Puerperal, convulsions. Screaming. Snow-blindness. Spasms. ***Strabismus.*** Stuttering. ***Suppressed, eruptions. Tetanus.*** Trismus. Twitching. Vomiting. Worms.

HOMEOPATHIC - Cicuta virosa is one of the most active of the poisonous umbelliferae. Chiefly acts on the brain, medulla oblongata, nervous system, the gastro-intestinal tract, and the skin. The action producing spasmodic affections including hiccough, trismus, ***tetanus and convulsions,*** and locked jaws.

Violent general action with frightful distortions. ***Bending of the head, neck and spine backwards***. Strange desires. Moaning and howling. Does absurd things. Sensation of internal chill. Dilated pupils. Shocks from head down body. Face bluish. Froths at mouth. Bites the tongue.

Violent spasmodic effects. Great agitation. ***Frightful contortions.*** Epilepsy. Gesticulations, odd motions. ***"Jerking of the left arm all day."*** Tremor when touched. Trembling palpitations. Spasms of diaphragm, hiccough of gullet.

Spasms move downwards with terrific violence with sudden shocks through body or head. ***"Head turned or twisted to one side"*** in convulsions. Convulsions followed by sudden rigidity, shrieks, then jerks and violent distortions, then prolonged unconsciousness.

Utter prostration follows the convulsive attacks. ***Opisthotonos*** and frightful ***facial distortions.*** Bloody foam from the mouth. ***Muscles become rigid.*** Catalepsy. Tearing, jerking in coccyx. Spasms are renewed by touch, by noise, loud talking.

Falls and the effects of concussions. Convergent strabismus from fall or blow. ***Concussion of brain.*** Cerebro-spinal meningitis. Sleeps and weeps on being aroused, distorts facial muscles and stares vacantly. Troubles arising from shaving. Marked action on the skin. Hungry immediately after a meal.

MIND - Dullness after injuries of head. ***Anxiety about future.*** Excitement and apprehension about future. Excessively affected by sad stories. ***Horrible things, sad stories affect her profoundly.*** Sad when seeing others happy. Worse from fright (Op., Ig.). Fright can cause epilepsy.

Suspicious. Mistrustful, shuns men. ***Aversion to presence of strangers.*** Despises others. ***Aversion to company.*** Desires to be alone during menses. ***Contemptuous.*** Melancholy with indifference. Sadness after concussion of brain.

Does not remember what has happened, does not recognize anybody but answers well. Feels as if he was in a strange place. Everything appears strange and terrible. ***Avoids the sight of people.*** Confounds present with the past, feels like a child. Memory blank, for hours or days. Thinking of complaints helps.

Falls to ground and rolls about with or without convulsions. ***Moaning, howling and weeping.*** Epilepsy with moaning and whining. Stupefaction between convulsions. ***Shrieking before convulsions.*** Delirium with gestures. Mania with dancing, laughing and ridiculous gestures. Sings, dances, shouts. Violent. Impulsive. Rash behavior. Childish behavior. Hallucinations and convulsions after typhoid.

Abdomen - Distended and painful. Rumbling in abdomen. Flatulence with anxiety and crossness. ***Colic with convulsions with vomiting.*** Heat and burning in abdomen. Sudden, sharp, pains from navel extending to neck of bladder. Tearing pain deep in abdomen.

Observed: Flatulence with anxiety and crossness. Rumbling in abdomen. Distended and painful. Chronic painful hernia.

Back - Spasms and cramps in muscles of neck. The head drawn backwards. Opisthotonos. ***Back bent backward like an arch***. Muscles of neck contract and become hard as wood. Weakness in muscles of back after standing only a short time. Jerking, tearing in coccyx, especially during menses. Right scapula as if bruised. Neuralgia at nape with dull occipital headache.

Causations - Bad effects from falls, blows and concussions. Tetanus. Splinters in flesh.

Chest - Chest feels tight, can hardly breathe. Heat or cold sensation in chest. Tonic spasm in pectoral muscles. Sensations as if something the size of a fist was lodged in chest and throat. Lower end of sternum as if sore or bruised, when walking.

Constitutions - Suited to nervous elderly people and children.

Ears - Ears hot or cold. Earache caused by filling teeth with gold. ***Hemorrhage from ears***. Sore behind ear as after a blow. Suppurating, burning eruption on and about ears. Oversensitiveness of hearing. Difficult hearing. Doesn't hear well unless one speaks loudly to her, and she pays attention. Sudden detonation, especially on swallowing. Roaring noises in ears.

Eyes - Pupils dilated in concussion of the brain, contracted in spasms. ***Strabismus,*** periodic, spasmodic after a fall or blow. Eyelids twitch. Spasmodic disorders of eyes. Eyes roll, jerk and stare. Stares persistently at objects. Objects recede, approach and seem double, black. Letters go up and down or disappear, when reading. Effects of exposure to snow.

Face - Ashy paleness of face, during convulsions. Flushed face, with headache and restless sleep. Red or pale face and drawn, sweaty. ***Face is distorted horrible or ridiculously.*** Trismus, disposition to grind teeth. Lockjaw. ***Twitching of facial muscles.*** Faceache caused by filling teeth with gold. Pustules which run together forming thick, yellow scabs on face and head. Dark red pimples on face. Epithelioma of lips. Painful ulcers on lips.

Female - Spasmodic states when menses do not appear. Coccyx painful during menses. Puerperal convulsions. Eclampsia during childbirth. Convulsions during pregnancy, delivery.

Food - Inability to distinguish between edible and inedible. Stomachache, sleepiness, feel satisfied immediately after eating. Great hunger soon after a meal. ***Craves coal, chalk and many other strange articles***. Longing for wine. Thirst, extreme, with convulsions.

Head - Headache on waking in morning. ***Convulsions from concussion of brain.*** Sudden, violent shocks through head. ***Head turned or twisted to one side.*** Congestion of head with vomiting and purging. Head retracted, spine rigid. ***Neck muscles are contracted.*** Headache alternating with pain in abdomen. Head symptoms relieved by emission of flatus. ***Cerebro-spinal meningitis.*** One-sided headache, stupefying, as from a rush of blood, better sitting erect. ***Cerebral diseases following suppressed eruptions.*** Sudden, violent shocks through head. Jerks the head. Thick, yellow scabs on head. Sweat during sleep.

Heart - Trembling palpitations of the heart. Feels as if the heart stopped beating with faint feeling. Heart's action weak. Rapid pulse. Pulse weak, slow, at times imperceptible.

Kidneys - Involuntary urination in old men. Urine is passed with great force. Stricture of urethra after inflammation, gonorrhea. Paralysis of bladder with great anxiety about it. Passes large quantities of urine or else none at all.

Limbs - Curved limbs which cannot be straightened, nor straight ones bent. Jerking and twitching in the arms and fingers. Jerking in left arm all day. ***Cramps and spasms.*** Trembling of left leg. Feet turned inward and toes turned upwards in spasms, while walking. Swings feet in half circle while walking. Forearms and legs as if bruised. Complete powerlessness of limbs after sudden jerks. Great weakness in arms and legs, after slight exertion. ***Rigid limbs.*** Trembling in upper and lower limbs. Cold limbs.

Lungs - Oppressed, can scarcely breathe, may arise from tonic spasm of pectoral muscles. Snoring. Interrupted, in spells. Want of breath the whole day. Difficult, chest feels too tight. Suspended, at times gasping.

Male - Testes drawn up towards external abdominal rings. Sharp pains in fossa navicularis, with nightly emissions. Sore, drawing pains in urethra, as far as glans, obliging one to urinate. Pollutions without lascivious dreams.

Modalities - Better from thinking of pain. Better warmth. ***Worse from concussions***. ***Worse from injury to brain and spine.*** Worse turning the head. Worse from cold, drafts. Worse tobacco smoke. Worse jar.

Worse noise. Worse slightest touch. Worse dentition. Worse suppressed eruptions. Worse from worms. Worse from splinters in flesh. Worse turning the head.

Mouth - Foam in and around mouth. Swelling of the tongue, speech difficult. Bites the tongue. Grinding of the teeth with lock jaw. Water brash, saliva flows from mouth with heat all over. Thirst, burning pressure. White, painful, burning ulcers on edges of tongue, painful to touch. Tongue coated, dry. Speech difficul. ***Stuttering.*** Couldn't speak from having no control over movements of tongue and mouth. Speechlessness from wounded esophagus. Speechlessness in cerebrospinal meningitis.

Nose - Slight touch causes it to bleed. Frequent sneezing without coryza. Nostrils seem stopped. Nostrils ulcerated, with yellow, purulent discharge from nose.

Perspiration - Sweats at night and in morning. Sweats on abdomen. Profuse sweats at night, without being able to sleep.

Rectum - Diarrhea in morning with irresistible desire to urinate. Itching in rectum with burning pain after rubbing. Diarrheic stool followed by constipation. Prolapsed rectum. Frequent liquid stools. Cholera when purging ceases, and congestion to brain and chest. Desire to urinate after stool. Stools thin, slimy. Stools expelled suddenly, sudden urging. Scarcely able to retain stool.

Skin - Eczema, no itching, exudation forms into a ***hard, lemon-colored crust***. Pustules coalesce into thick, yellow massive scabs, worse head and face. ***Suppressed eruption causes brain disease.*** Elevated eruptions, as large as peas. Barber's, baker's itch. Red vesicles on right scapula, painful to touch. Burning, itching of skin over whole body. Impetigo, honeycomb-like crusts, which fall off and leave a bright red smooth surface.

Sleep - Complete sleeplessness in hysterical spasms. Frequent waking, with sweat all over, from which he feels refreshed. Bites the tongue in sleep. Starting during sleep. Deep sleep. Dreams vivid, but not remembered. Vivid dreams about events of previous day. ***Nightmares after movies and sad stories.*** Nightmares of people being mutilated, attacked, tortured.

Stomach - Burning heat in stomach. ***Hiccoughs***. Loud hiccough with crying, alternating with thoracic spasms. Indigestion, with insensibility, frothing at mouth. Vomiting of bile of blood on stooping, on rising in pregnancy. Throbbing in pit of the stomach with distention. Pains with vomiting, painful distension of abdomen and spasm of pectoral muscles. Vomiting during convulsions. Vomit yellow, like mucus. Vomiting during headache.

Teeth - Toothache caused by filling teeth with gold. Grinding of teeth with pressing of jaws together like lockjaw.

Temperature - Chilliness, constant desire to be near a warm stove. Chill starts in chest and runs down legs and into arms with staring look. Cold internally and externally. Typhoid fever. Nervous fever, characterized by great stupidity. Worm fevers in children, with colic and convulsions.

Throat - Effects of swallowing sharp fish bones. Dry. Feels as if grown together. Spasms of esophagus, cannot swallow from injury of fish bone etc. Stricture of esophagus. Strangling on attempting to swallow. Danger of suffocation from swallowing sharp pieces of bone. Choking on attempting to examine the throat. Constriction of esophagus from intestinal irritation. Constriction with spasmodic contraction of muscles of neck, almost like tetanus.

Vertigo - Vertigo with stomach pain and muscular spasms. Objects move from side to side or approach and recede. Vertigo with desire to hold on to something when standing still. Vertigo with reeling, falling to the ground. Vertigo on stooping. Vertigo after injuries to head. Vertigo on rising from bed.

Vision - Momentary loss of vision. Frequent vanishing of sight. Letters disappear or go up and down. Colors of rainbow around letters. Letters seem to turn when reading. Objects appear black. Objects vacillate. Diplopia. Iris-like circles around candle.

Can scarcely see in sunlight.

COMMENTS - Characteristic twitching and spasmodic jerks. ***"Bending the head backward."*** Useful for residue from a trauma that included convulsions, or if current treatment masks residue symptoms.

Convulsions, epilepsy, severe neck and spinal trauma, head injuries. Keynote ***arching of the back***. Epilepsy, spasms, trauma cases, or spinal diseases with severe back spasms.

Contortions of the body. The body takes on strange postures and contortions of the limbs. Chorea (Caust.), involuntary contractions, jerking, and rigidity of the limbs. Mania, dancing, singing, grotesque postures (Hyos.). Moans and howls with great agitation, makes gesticulations, odd motions, head turned or twisted to one side.

Cataleptic after contortions, no recall of the attack, tranquil feeling (Op.). Utter prostration after the convulsions. Drug overdoses with convulsions, paralysis, respiratory failure, twitching and jerking of the limbs.

Cerebrospinal meningitis, the opisthotonos being the leading indication. Meningitis, where the neck goes back, eyes are glassy and body is twitching and jerking with spasms and a high fever (Bell, without the flushed face). Delirium in meningitis, pupils are fixed and staring.

Tetanus (Hyper., Led.), with violent spasms and severe lockjaw. Usually later stages of clinical tetanus. Head injuries that cause visual disturbances, twitchings of the eyes, double vision. Lazy eye, strabismus.

Eclampsia, toxemia. Convulsions during pregnancy. Convulsions due to uremia, too much uric acid in the blood or kidney failure. Strange desires, such as to eat coal.

Marked action on the skin, including the eruption of pustules which run together with yellowish honey-colored scabs, especially about mouth and matting the whiskers. Epithelioma, growths covered with honey-colored scabs.

Nash cured eczema capitis in a young woman with Cic. Her whole scalp was covered as with a solid cap.

Grimmer used it for cancers of the skin, epithelioma, convulsive violence as in cerebrospinal meningitis. Also in opisthotonos, strabismus, violent spasmodic jerks, paralysis, especially of the bladder, stricture of the esophagus.

Teste mentioned the case of a woman of 58 who ceased to menstruate at 30 in consequence of a fright, and who was of "robust constitution, irritable, nervous and excessively fanciful and odd." She had a chronic swelling of the left ovary. Cic. had a remarkably quieting effect for several weeks, and during that time the swelling diminished considerably. The patient had to leave Paris, so the treatment could not be followed up.

Dr. H. Von Musits treated a case of acute meningitis in J. N. R., 43, male, married, a user of alcohol and tobacco, bookkeeper.

After the intense summer heat, symptoms developed including convulsions, distortion of limbs, head turned backward. Trismus. Froth from mouth. Biting of the tongue. Oppression of breathing. Entire loss of consciousness and of power of swallowing. Convulsions, followed by complete exhaustion. Stupor. Swelling of face. Inability to move the tongue. The whole body seems to be of enormous size.

The patient had three convulsions during twenty-four hours, followed by the swelling of the tongue and body. Extreme trembling of the hands. Articulation difficult.

Next day, profuse watery diarrhea stools, worse by any noise, sudden entrance of any person into the room or loud talking. Better by rest and in a dark room. Several times previously he had symptoms of nervous exhaustion. His brother, a physician, died the previous spring from paresis in consequence of excessive use of alcohol and drugging.

After two doses of Cic. 200c there were no more convulsions and the patient was perfectly cured in two weeks. There was no relapse.

Banerjee recorded the case of "A lad, aged five years, had an attack of cholera three days before my visit. Had been treated by a homeopath from beginning of attack.

The patient was suffering from convulsions, when I first saw him on the fourth day. The convulsive fits were very severe since the third day of the attack of cholera.

"The symptoms were: eyes half turned, head drawn toward the left side and the hands and feet of the same side were contracted. He was given Bell., Hyos., Cina and Bryonia without effect. Cicuta virosa was then given. The first dose mitigated the severity of the fits, the second dose put the child to sleep and thus he was saved from imminent death."

RELATIONS - ***Antidoted by:*** Arn., Op., for massive doses tobacco. Antidote to: Opium. ***Compare:*** (1) Cicuta maculata. (2) Con., Enanth., Stry., Bell. (3) Con., Aeth., Oena. Croc., Hyper. - spinal concussion, Hyos. - twitchings, Hell, Hydr-ac. - body thrown back, cramps in neck. (4) Nux-v. and Stry. - tetanus, but with Nux-v. there is not the utter prostration and great oppression of breathing of Cic., Nux-v. is less epileptiform and has more excitability. ***Compatible after:*** Lach after Ars. and Con. (Cancer of lip), Cupr. (Aphasia in chorea).

REFERENCES - Boericke. Clarke. Grimmer. Murphy. Phatak.

CIMEX LECTULARIUS
(Bedbug)

PHARMACY - cimx. Cimex lectularius. Bedbug. Acanthia lectularia. N. O. Hemiptera. Tincture or trituration. ***Historical dose:*** All potencies.

CLINICAL - Chill. Colic. Constipation. Contractures. Cough. Fever. ***Hamstrings.*** Headaches. Hemorrhoids. Intermittent, fever. Liver, pain. Muscle, contractions. Seminal, emissions. Skin, disorders. ***Tendons, disorders.*** Yawning.

HOMEOPATHIC - Cimex is an ancient remedy for intermittent fever. Nash recorded the following cure by Dr. Brewster of Syracuse. After driving a fractious horse that tried to run away over a very rough road, a man was so bruised and sprained about the buttocks and legs that he was confined to the house for a long time.

It settled finally into what appeared likely to be permanent contraction of the lower limbs. No remedy relieved until Dr. Brewster remembered a case of intermittent fever that he had cured twenty years before, being guided by this symptom. Cimex 600c (Jenichen) promptly cured.

Characteristic weariness and ***inclination to stretch.*** The flexors are most affected, pains in all joints ***as if tendons were contracted and too short,*** every motion or stretching of arms or legs causes tightening pain in them. ***Hamstrings feel too short*** (Am-m.). Sensation of retraction of arm tendons. The whole right side is especially affected.

MIND - Anxiety, after chill. Clenching of hands with violent rage at beginning of chill. Sensation as if he could creep into himself and on that account could not sufficiently crouch together. His own sweat is disgusting to him.

Abdomen - Pain in the liver, as if it had been strained by bending the right side inward, the spot is painful when touching it or coughing. Colic, followed by emissions of flatulence or liquid stools.

Back - Pain in the small of the back, extending over the abdomen with distention of the abdomen, worse when sitting. Weariness in loins, must sit down.

Chest - Chest feels oppressed during chill. After chill, heaviness in chest, anxiety.

Female - Shooting pain from vagina up towards left ovary.

Head - Confusion of head as if headache would ensue. Pain like needle stitches in vertex with cough. Pain under right frontal bone. Violent headache, caused by drinking. Great rage, vehement at beginning of chilly stage. Would like to tear everything to pieces. Sweating on head, nose and chest.

Heart - Pulse feeble, intermitting.

Kidneys - Urine brown with a deposit of sediment (during the fever, when he drinks).

Limbs - ***Hamstrings feel too short, knees flexed,*** attempting to stretch them causes pain in thighs. ***Pains in all joints, as if tendons were too short***, especially knee joints. Knees feel cold, as from a cold wind. Pain in right shoulder and the anterior muscles of the chest, extending through the whole arm down to the nails, the finger feel as if they had gone to sleep.

Lungs - Dry cough with gagging, as if he would vomit with perspiration. Breathing oppressed after chill.

Modalities - Worse motion. Worse stretching or extending the part. Worse in morning. Worse from drinking. Weariness compels to lie down. Pain in small of back worse sitting. Sweat on nose during rest in morning.

Mouth - Tongue coated white. Swollen feeling of the tongue. Feeling as if burnt on the tongue in the region of the palate and the upper anterior gums.

Nose - Annoying dryness of nostrils. Fluent coryza with pressure in frontal sinuses. Constant sneezing in forenoon. Sweat on nose, morning during rest.

Rectum - Constipation, feces dry, hard, and in small balls (Op., Plum., Thuj.). Rectal ulcer.

Sleep - Great drowsiness, falls asleep when sitting in the morning. Irresistible sleepiness during chill. Frequent yawning with cold feeling on skin.

Stomach - Sour belchings.

Stool - Stools hard, in small balls. After the discharge of a small piece of white stool, the rectum closes firmly. Stools with hemorrhoidal sufferings.

Temperature - Chilliness of whole body, worse lying down. Thirst during apyrexia, but little during chilly stage, still less during hot stage and none during sweating. Before the cold stage, thirst, heaviness in the lower limbs. At the beginning of the chill, clenching of the hands and violent rage. The perspiration after the hot stage is accompanied by hunger. Perspiration mostly on the head and chest. Musty offensive sweat. During the intermittent fever, constipation, stools dry.

Throat - Dryness, causing him to drink all day. Esophagus becomes constricted during the hot stage.

COMMENTS - Tertian and quartan intermittents. Musty smelling sweats. Night-sweats. Heat with gagging, esophagus feels constricted. Before chill, thirst and heaviness in legs, less thirst with chill, still less with dry heat, none with sweat.

Chill commences with clenching of hands and violent raging. Pains in all joints as if tendons contracted during chill. Sensation as of a cold wind blowing on knees. After the chill, thirst, but drinking causes violent headache, tickling in larynx causing dry, continuous cough. Gagging and belching at end of cough.

Urging to stool. Hard stool, in small balls. Discharges of a small piece of white stool, then rectum closes firmly. Stools with hemorrhoidal sufferings. Incontinence of urine. Hot urine, brown or red sediment.

Urticarious eruption. Irresistible sleepiness. Frequent yawning. Frequent erections in morning, seminal emissions.

A. W. K. Choudhury related a case of intermittent (quotidian) cured with Cimex 30c, the chief indications being: "Chill slight, thirst some days, none other days, shiverings, passed water twice during chill, chill worse by lying down increase of cough if he drinks water during chill."

RELATIONS - ***Compare:*** (1) Nat-m. - headache lessens in the sweating stage. (2) Ars. - headache remains or increases in the sweating stage. (3) Bell. - throbbing of the head in intermittents. (4) Ars. and Bry. - gagging at end of cough.

REFERENCES - Boericke. Clarke.

CIMICIFUGA RACEMOSA
(Black Cohosh)

PHARMACY - cimic. Cimicifuga racemosa. Black cohosh. Actea racemosa. Macrotys racemosa. Actea monogynia. Cimicifuga serpentaria. Black snakeroot. Botroflus serpentaria. N. O. Ranunculacee. North America. Tincture of the root. ***Historical dose:*** Tincture and all potencies.

CLINICAL - Abortion, tendency. Angina, pectoris. Appetite, disordered. ***Back, pains.*** Breast, disorders. Cerebrospinal, meningitis. Chest, pains. Chorea. Colic. ***Cramps.*** Delirium, tremens. Diaphragm. Dyspepsia. Epilepsy. Faintness. Fevers. Gout. Headaches. Heart, disorders. ***Hot, flashes.*** Hysteria. ***Labor, pains***. Lumbago. Melancholy. Meningitis. ***Menopause. Menstruation, disorders.*** Miscarriage. Muscle, pain. Neuralgia. Ovaries, disorders.

Perichondritis. Pleurodynia. Pregnancy, disorders. ***Puerperal, fever.*** Puerperal, mania. ***Rheumatism.*** Sciatica, pains. Sleeplessness. Spinal irritation. Stiff-neck. Tinnitus. Tremors. ***Uterus, disorders.*** Vomiting.

HOMEOPATHIC - Wide action upon the cerebrospinal and muscular system, as well as upon the uterus and ovaries. The generative organs in the female are particularly affected. Uterine and ovarian pains are very marked. Infra-breast pains. Tenderness of the uterine region. ***Pain across pelvis from hip to hip.*** Left ovarian pains.

Leucorrhea with feeling of weight in uterus. Painful and irregular menses. Menses with backache, nervousness, irregular in time and amount, more flow, more pain. Labor-like pains. ***Displaced labor pains to hips, thighs or back.***

Pains are violent, aching, shooting, wander here and there. Compressive pains. Pains like electric shocks, with cries, faints etc.

Pains go upwards or side to side, up the neck, about the throat from ovary to ovary. Belly of the muscles feel bruised, sore, heavy aching. ***Muscular and crampy pains,*** primarily of neurotic origin, occurring in nearly every part of the body. Sore and tender along the tract of pain.

Trembling, twitching in various organs or of part lain on. Alternating clonic and tonic spasms. Nervous shuddering. Spasms of cerebro-spinal fever. Chorea, at puberty with delayed menses, cardiac. Hysterical and epileptic convulsions at the time of menses.

Agitation. General sick feeling with exhaustion. Many of the symptoms are irregular, changeful or they alternate in groups, alternation of physical and mental effects. Alternate mental and rheumatic symptoms. Symptoms referable to the pelvic organs prominent.

Lumbago. Muscle pain. Useful in rheumatic, nervous subjects with ovarian irritation, uterine cramps and heavy limbs. Children during dentition. Influenza. Cold air seems to penetrate the system, very sensitive to it. Headache is better in open air, worse in warm room. Migraine.

MIND - Melancholy. Depression with low spirits and exhaustion. ***Gloom and dejection, as if there was a black cloud over everything.*** Forebodings of death, insanity, impending evil etc. Fear of death. Fear of riding in a closed carriage. Fear that those in house will kill him. Fear of rats. ***Thinks she is going crazy.*** Vision of rats, mice, various colors and forms.

Nervous, fidgety, excitable and jerky. Incessant talking, changing from one subject to another, as in delirium tremens (Lach.). Desire to wander from place to place. Hysteria. Mania, before menses. Mania, alcoholic, tries to injure himself. Puerperal mania, following disappearance of neuralgias.

Weak will. Indifferent. Suspicious. Oversensitive, especially for pain. ***Hypochondriasis.*** Sits and mopes in great sadness, when questioned breaks into tears. Mental symptoms are better by diarrhea or menses, worse after rheumatism.

Abdomen - Colic better bending double and after stools. Sharp pains across hypogastrium.

Back - Rheumatic pains in muscles of back and neck. ***Stiffness and contraction in neck and back.*** Stiff neck, sensitive, worse pain or pressure, causes nausea and retching. Neck aches, throws the head back. Pain in the angle of left scapula. Spine very sensitive, especially upper part. Pain in lumbar and sacral region, down thighs and through hips. Crick in back.

Breasts - Burning in breasts. Infra-breast pains, worse left side. Presses breasts as though in pain.

Causations - Ill effects of anxiety, fright, disappointed love, overexertion, business failures, or childbirth.

Chest - Intercostal rheumatism. Sharp stitches in left chest, motion exhorting cries. Left-sided infra-breast pain. Pleurodynia.

Constitutions - Suited to the menopausal period, to nervous persons, to children during dentition, diarrhea. Nervousness from anxiety or overexertion. Rheumatic persons. Plump, delicate, sensitive, nervous, chilly women who complain of aching pain in back, neck, here and there.

Many of the complaints are dependent upon uterine or ovarian irritation.

Ears - Tinnitus. Sensitive to least noise with spasmodic labor pains. Violent noises in ear with deafness.

Eyes - Eyes feel big, wild look. Asthenopia associated with pelvic trouble. Deep-seated throbbing and ***shooting pains*** in eyes. ***Intense aching in eyeballs*** or behind them, better pressure, worse slightest motion. Pain from eyes to vertex. Ciliary neuralgia. As if a needle were run into the eyeballs, worse closing eyes. Photophobia from artificial light. Sees red flashes with dark borders.

Face - Pale, hot. Wild, fearful expression. Neuralgia affecting malar bones, better night, reappears the next day. Facial blemishes in young women. Forehead feels cold.

Female - Menses are profuse, dark, coagulated, scanty with backache, nervousness, irregular in time and amount, more flow, more pain. Menses suppressed from emotions, cold. Hysteric or epileptic spasms at the time of menses. Great debility between menses. Amenorrhea. Leucorrhea with a sensation of weight in the uterus. ***Pain across pelvis from hip to hip.*** Ovarian neuralgia, pain across pelvis from ovary to ovary or goes upwards or downwards along the thighs. Uterine atony. Mania. Slow labor pains with nervous shivers. ***Puerperal fever.*** After-pains with great sensitiveness and ***intolerance to pain***, worse in groins. Lochia suppressed by cold or emotions.

Food - No thirst, slight feeling of hunger in stomach, rumbling in abdomen. ***Great thirst.*** Appetite variable. No appetite for dinner, wants to drink cold water, little at a time suffices.

Head - Waving or wild sensation in brain. Head retracted (meningitis). ***Opening and shutting*** sensation in brain. Brain feels too large. Shooting, throbbing pains, headache after mental worry, over-study or from reflex uterine disease, better open air. ***Pressing outward pain.*** Feeling as of a blow or as if a bolt has been driven from occiput to vertex up to the eyes (left).

Heart - Heart's action ceases suddenly, impending suffocation. Sore, as if swollen or enlarged. Pulse weak, irregular, trembling, drops every third or fourth beat. Tremulous action. Numbness of left arm, feels as if bound to side. Needle-like pains at heart. Angina pectoris, pain spreads all over the chest to the back and down the left arm which feels numb and as if bound to the side. Cardiac neuralgia in childbirth.

Kidneys - Profuse clear urine, causing weakness, with yellow sand. Nervous urination.

Limbs - Alternation of rheumatic and mental symptoms. Uneasy and restless feeling in the limbs. Chorea movements, accompanied by rheumatism. Rheumatism affecting the belly of muscles, especially large muscles. Aching in limbs and ***muscular soreness***. Jerking of limbs. Numbness of limbs. Cramps. Left arm feels as if bound to the side, constant irregular motion of left arm (chorea). Hands tremble while writing. Cold sweat on hands and feet. Soles itching. Cramps in calves. Stiffness and contracted Achilles tendon. Trembling of legs, can scarcely walk.

Lungs - Tickling, short, dry, constant cough worse at night, speaking. Cough when secretion is scanty-spasmodic, dry, with muscular soreness and nervous irritation. Nervous cough.

Modalities - Better from warm wraps. Better open air. Better continued motion. Better pressure. Better grasping things. Better rest, and eating. Worse from damp, cold air. Worse change of weather. Worse heat and cold, draft. Worse alcohol, especially wine. Worse from motion. Worse sitting. Worse puberty. Worse during menses, labor, menopause. Worse emotions. Worse in the morning, and at night (malar neuralgia better at night). Pains in arms and Achilles tendon worse as evening approaches.

Mouth - Saliva thick. Coppery taste. Hawks up viscid coppery tasting mucus. Thick mucus on teeth. Cannot speak a word though she tries. Tongue and mouth feel warm. Tongue pointed and trembling, swollen.

Nose - Sensitive to cold air, every inhalation seems to bring the cold air in contact with the brain.

Rectum - Frequent thin, dark offensive stools. Alternate diarrhea and constipation. Morning diarrhea of children.

Sensations - As of lifting up of skull, as if top of head would fly off, as of a bolt through from base of skull to vertex. Inspired air seems to penetrate skull and into brain, causing a cold sensation. Intense pain in and around the eyes (lancinating), worse moving head or eyes.

Skin - Locally and internally for ivy poisoning.

Sleep - Sleeplessness. Sleeps with arms overhead or yawning. Comatose, as if drunk. Brain irritation of children during dentition.

Stomach - Sinking in the epigastrium (Sep., Sulph.). ***Gnawing pain***. Nausea and vomiting from pressure on spine and cervical region, pregnancy, alcohol. Vomits green substance, groans, raves and presses the head with both the hands for relief. Belchings with nausea, vomiting and headache.

Throat - Burning. Thyroid aches before menses.

COMMENTS - Frontal, vertical or occipital headache, accompanied by great pain in the eyeballs, better pressure, worse slightest motion. Headache with a feeling as if going crazy. Headaches reflected from pelvic organs. Depression as if a black cloud has settled over them.

Rheumatism affecting the vertebral joints and especially in the neck. Cerebrospinal meningitis, head and neck retracted. Clarke found a pain at the nape of the neck very characteristic.

Sciatica with sharp, shooting pains down the limbs with back spasms. Hip and lumbosacral problems that affect uterus and other organs (Aesc.). Back spasms from injury to the spine (Mag-p.). Arthritis that came on with menopause, large joints (small joints, Caul.).

Pains in the joints and limbs. Pains like electric shocks, here and there, sharp in various parts, chest and uterine pains shoot from side to side. A general bruised feeling all over as if sore, worse by touch.

Malar neuralgia, ceasing at night. Bad taste and breath. Coated tongue, sticky saliva, viscid mucus in throat. Disordered digestion. Marked sinking at epigastrium.

Dry, teasing cough, worse at night and from every attempt to speak. Sharp pains in the heart and chest. Pains down left arm, which is numb (Acon., Puls., Rhus-t.), as if bound to the side. Palpitation from the least motion. Heartbeat ceases suddenly.

Premenstrual syndrome with cramps. Backache with painful menses, muscle spasms in the back with the period. Pain in the hip with menstrual cramps, hip can lock up. Symptoms worse during the period. Depression with menses. Menopausal depression.

Painful prolapse of the uterus with cramps, spasms, backaches and hip aches, because pelvis is out of alignment (Sep. has prolapse due to weakness and lack of tone).

Labor pains felt in the back or thighs. Muscle contractions in their thighs with labor pains, or they feel as if their back will break (Kali-c., Cham.). Puerperal mania. According to Lippe a characteristic indication is: "The recently delivered uterus becomes actually jammed in the pelvis with great pain."

Cimic. should be given in daily doses in low 1x potency two months before term, when indicated. It ensures living births in women who have previously borne only dead children without any discoverable cause. If given before the term, it renders labor easier, cures sickness of pregnancy, and prevents the after pains.

In cases of tinnitus aurium it has proved curative in old-school practice in 15 to 30 drops of the tincture, whether due to direct or reflex irritation.

Clarke greatly relieved an inveterate case of epilepsy in which the aura was a "waving sensation in the brain," which is a leading symptom of the remedy.

A patient who was taking 6-drop doses of the tincture complained of a feeling as if his heart had stopped.

RELATIONS - ***Compare:*** (1) Rham-cal. - muscular pains, lumbago, pleurodynia, acute rheumatism. (2) Derris pinnata - neuralgic headaches of rheumatic origin. (3) Aristolochia milhom. - pain in achilles tendon, diabetes. Caul., Puls., Lil-t., Agar. (4) Macrotin - especially for lumbago.

REFERENCES - Boericke. Clarke. Murphy. Phatak.

CINA MARITIMA

(Wormseed)

PHARMACY - cina. Cina maritima. Wormseed. Cina artemisia. Artemisia maritima. Artemisia cintra. Semen cine. Flores cine. Tartarian southernwood. N. O. Composite. Tincture. Cina is the source of the alkaloid Santonin. ***Historical dose:*** Tincture and all potencies.

CLINICAL - Abdomen, distended. Anemia. ***Anal, itching.*** Asthenopia. Asthma. ***Bedwetting.*** Bronchitis. Borborygmi. Cachexia. ***Chorea. Colic.*** Constipation. Convulsions. ***Coughs. Dentition.*** Diarrhea. Emaciation. Eyes, disorders. ***Grinding, teeth***. Headaches. Hiccough. Hydrocephaloid. Hypoglycemia. Indigestion. Intermittent, fever. Itching. Leucorrhea. Malassimilation. Nausea. Neuralgia. Nosebleed. Paraplegia. ***Parasites. Pinworms***. Remittent, fever. ***Roundworms***. Scarlatina. ***Spasms.*** Strabismus. ***Threadworms. Twitchings.*** Urine, milky. Vision, disorders. Vomiting. ***Whooping cough. Worms***.

HERBAL - This remedy is a preparation of Artemisia cintra, Tartarian southernwood or wormseed. The Artemisiae held a prominent place among the drugs of the ancient physicians from Hippocrates to Serapion. They were recommended as febrifuge, stomachic and anthelmintic.

Cina is the source of the alkaloid Santonin which has a very strong anti-helminthic action. Cina is a powerful remedy for the elimination of round worms.

HOMEOPATHIC - Cina is preeminently a ***worm remedy,*** as it causes all the symptoms which characterize worm infestation, both mental, nervous and bodily. It corresponds more to the effects of lumbrici then to those of other worms.

Reflex symptoms from abdominal irritation. ***Extreme sensitiveness of mind and body***: offended by the slightest thing, peevish and obstinate, aversion to be caressed. Child cannot bear to have hair combed or brushed.

Irritation of the nose, causing constant desire to rub, prick or press into it. ***Grinding teeth during sleep***. Restless sleep, tossing all about the bed. Child lies on belly or on hands and knees during sleep. ***Nocturnal bedwetting,*** urine white, turbid, at times fetid.

Over-sensitiveness of skin, cannot endure to be approached touched or pressed upon. Whole body is painfully sore to motion and touch, bruised soreness. Hair is sensitive to touch.

Touch induces or aggravates spasms. ***Twitching, spasms.*** Convulsions with screams and violent jerkings of the hands and feet. Convulsions with consciousness. Chorea. Unilateral. Children throw arms from side to side during spasms. Paraplegia with unnatural hunger.

Variable appetite. ***Greater the hunger, greater the emaciation***. Scrofulous. ***Sour smell of body*** especially children. Children during dentition.

Pain comes in shocks. Jumps suddenly as though he felt pain. Trembling with shivering, when yawning. Complaints concomitant to yawning, which comes on whenever someone yawns.

MIND - Extreme ill-humor and naughtiness in children. Wants to be carried, but carrying gives no relief. Wants to be rocked. Irritability better rocking fast. ***Very touchy,*** irritable, petulant and dissatisfied. ***Child is very cross***, does not want to be touched or carried. ***Hard to please.*** Desires many things, but rejects everything offered. Nervous.

Child can't be quieted. ***Irritability of temper.*** Irritability during dentition. Violent screaming attacks at night. Child lying on the back and striking and kicking with hands and feet. ***Screaming, striking and biting.*** Nothing pleases them for any length of time. Crying out as if in delirium.

Morose in daytime. Indisposition to play, in children. Convulsions in children when they are scolded or punished.

Dislike of strangers (Bar-c.). ***Indifference to caresses.*** Worse if being looked at (Ant-t.). Unreal feeling of having done something wrong, abnormal consciousness. Unconscious with frothing at mouth.

Sensitive, nervous women who get pain in head and eyes from sewing (Ruta). Irritability during menses. Earnest and sensitive, offended at the slightest joke. Fear of evil while walking in open air, in evening. Throws things away. Causeless weeping.

Starting from sleep. Complaining on waking. Frightened easily on waking. Hallucinations of sight, smell and taste. As if frightened, jumps out of bed, sees imaginary objects, screams, trembles, talks hurriedly, anxious in evening and before midnight.

Abdomen - Bloated and hard abdomen. Abdomen as if empty. ***Twisting pain about the navel,*** better pressure (Spig.). Pressing outward in belly. Pain on pressing upon navel. ***Colic with cutting, pinching pains from worms.*** Unpleasant, warm feeling. Pinching or cramplike pressure transversely across epigastric region after a meal.

Back - Drawing, tearing pains down along whole spine. Tearing, jerking pain in middle of spine. Paralytic feeling in nape. Bruised pain in lumbar region, not worse motion. Lancinating pain in upper part of spinal column extendind to right scapula.

Causations - Ill effects of parasites, worms.

Chest - Sternum as if lying too close to back. Cramplike, contracted sensation. Constriction of right side, with difficult breathing. Chest as if pressed together from both sides. As if chest was full of mucus. Sharp pain in left side. Burning and soreness in chest. Two dull piercing pains in quick succession near sternum.

Constitutions - Generally hungry, cross, ugly and wants to be rocked. Children who are big, fat, rosy and scrofulous, they stiffen out, when looked at, during cough or when they become cross.

Cough - Gagging cough in the morning. ***Whooping cough.*** Violent cough recurring paroxysms, as of down in throat. Cough ends in spasm. Cough so violent as to bring tears and sternum pains, feels as if something had been torn off. Child is afraid to speak of move for fear of bringing on paroxysm of coughing. Periodic cough, returning spring and fall. Swallows after coughing. After coughing, moaning, anxious, gasps for air and turns pale.

Ears - Cramplike jerking in external ear, like earache. Digging and scratching in ears. Dull stitches below mastoid process. Hearing impaired.

Eyes - Dark rings around the eyes. Dilated pupils. Photophobia. ***Pulsation of ciliary muscle.*** Eyestrain, especially when presbyopia sets in. Strabismus from abdominal irritation, from worms. Eyebrows twitch when staring at any object. Drooping and heaviness of lids. Fatigue of eyes from sewing. ***Eyestrain with headache.*** Pain in eyes when reading or staring. Sensations as if sand had got into eyes, worse when reading. Lachrymation during cough. Spots on cornea. Itching of inner canthus.

Face - Face alternately pale and cold, or red and hot. Face puffy. ***Bluish white*** about the mouth. ***Pale with dark rings around eyes.*** Pale with sickly look during cough. Pale streak down centre of face. Cold perspiration. Grinds teeth during sleep. ***Chorea movements of face*** and hands. Tearing pain, in malar bones, worse touch and pressure. One cheek red, the other pale. Twitching of muscles about eyes and face, with disordered stomach and bowels.

Female - Child refuses breast. Aversion to mother's milk. Uterine hemorrhage before puberty. Menses too early and profuse. Labor-like pains frequently recurring, as if menses would appear. Labor-like pains during pregnancy. Spasmodic yawning in amenorrhea.

Food - ***Hunger voracious after eating.*** Gets hungry soon after a meal with feeling of emptiness. Indigestion. ***Canine hunger. Hunger during or before intermittent fever.*** Aversion to mother's milk. Bread tastes bitter. Desires many and different things. Craving for sweets, bread. Refuses ordinary food and desires dainties. ***Eats***

alot but doesn't gain weight. Malassimilation. Children are hungry, the greater the hunger the greater the emaciation. Hypoglycemia. Thirst for cold drinks. Difficult swallowing of liquids.

Head - Headache, alternating with pain in abdomen, relieved by stooping (Mez.). Headache from straining eyes. Headache from sewing. Pain in head when reading or staring. Headache, before and after epileptic attack. Turning the head from one side to other. Child leans his head sideways all the time. Women must let hair down during headache. ***Children cannot tolerate to have their hair combed.*** Anemic headache, better stooping, worse mental exertion. Weak, hollow, empty sensation in head with inclination to vomit. Stupefying headache. Meningeal irritability, from worms.

Heart - Trembling beating of heart. Anguish about heart when working in open air. Pulse fast, 136 beats. Pulse intermitting every seventeenth beat. Pulse small, but hard and accelerated.

Kidneys - Urine, turbid, ***white, milky.*** Urine, turns milky on standing. Involuntary at night. ***Bedwetting,*** worse every full moon. Frequent urging with passage of much urine, all day. ***Involuntary urination.*** Urine becomes turbid immediately.

Limbs - Child throws arms from side to side. Stretches out feet spasmodically, especially children. ***Twitching and jerking*** distortion of limbs, trembling. ***Sudden inward jerking of fingers of right hand.*** Left foot in constant spasmodic motion. Sudden paraplegia, with unnatural hunger. Paralyzed shocks, patient will jump suddenly, as though in pain. Nocturnal convulsions. Sensation of constriction around loins. Loins fatigued, as if he had stood a long time.

Lungs - Capillary bronchitis in children and loss of breath. Rattling in lungs and throat with excessive nervous irritability. Suffocative attacks. Expectoration difficult. ***Gurgling from throat to stomach after coughing***. Catching and painful breathing. Short, interrupted breathing. Short breaths, with omission of some inspirations. Breathing as from spasms in chest. Very short breath, as if he had much mucus in chest, without being obliged to cough. Difficult, loud breathing. Short breaths, moaning, with open mouth. Loud whistling whoop in trachea while inspiring, not audible on expiration. Inhalation broken into two.

Male - Bad effects on masturbation, weakness of sight. Itching of genitals.

Modalities - Better from lying on abdomen. Better wiping eyes. Better motion, shaking head. Better from rocking. ***Worse from worms.*** Worse vexation. Worse being looked at. Worse staring. Worse yawning. ***Worse during sleep***. Worse external pressure. ***Worse from touch.*** Worse open air, cold air, cold water. Worse sun, summer. ***Worse full moon.*** Worse at night. Worse before midnight child wakes up frightened. Worse yawning.

Mouth - Sensitiveness of teeth to cold air and to cold drinks. ***Grinds teeth at night during sleep.*** Chews and swallows in sleep. Much frothy saliva with rattling mucus on chest. Foul breath. Bitter taste before chill. Dryness and rawness of mouth, palate. Clean tongue. Whitish sore place on margin of tongue, very painful to touch. Tongue coated brownish-yellow.

Nose - Itching of nose all the time. ***Picks and bores at nose,*** until it bleeds. Wants to rub nose and pick at it. ***Child picks its nose and cries out in sleep.*** Sneezing with whooping cough. Nostrils drawn in. Violent sneezing with stitches in temples. Slimy discharge from nose. Bleeding from nose and mouth, with burning in nose. Nosebleed, dark blood, with pain in forehead. Stoppage of nose in evening.

Perspiration - Cold sweat on forehead, nose and hands. ***Sour smell of body*** especially children. After the sweat or before the chill, vomiting of food, with canine hunger at the same time.

Rectum - ***Worms*** (Naph., Sabad., Nat-p.). ***Itching of anus. Roundworms or threadworms.*** Stools white, watery. Involuntary stools. Stools reddish mucus. Stools greenish slimy. Constipation. Stool rather hard and black. White mucus like small pieces of popped corn, preceded by pinching colic.

Skin - Skin affections of infants and scrofulous children. Itching unchanged or lessened by scratching. Rubbing of face, ears, nose and perineum. ***Itching and irritating spots on skin associated with worms.*** Furuncles or red pimples. Ulcers with scanty discharge.

Sleep - Restless sleep, tosses about, with cries and lamentations. Turns over, kicks off bedclothes. ***Troubles while yawning***. Trembling of body, with shivering sensation, while yawning. Gets on hands and knees or on abdomen in sleep. Child flops over on its belly, sleeps better that way. Screams and talks in sleep. ***Grinds teeth at night during sleep.*** Chews and swallows in sleep. Grits teeth. ***Night terrors of children, cries out, screams, wakes frightened.*** Sleeps erect, with head leaned backward or to right side. Child never sleeps long at a time. Hiccough during sleep. Child will sleep only when violently rocked.

Stomach - ***Voracious hunger, digging, gnawing sensation, after eating.*** Frequent hiccough. Indigestion. Epigastric pain, worse first waking in morning and before meals. Constant pressure in stomach at night, causes restlessness. Digging in pit, with feeling of crawling of numberless worms. Pain or uneasiness below sternum. Vomiting and diarrhea immediately after eating and especially drinking. ***Vomiting of lumbrici and ascarides.*** Vomiting with a clean tongue. Nausea and vomiting of mucus or food, followed by chill, heat and thirst.

Temperature - Daily chill at same hour, then heat without thirst. Chill with shivering and shaking, even near warm stove, with hot cheeks, no thirst. Chills ascends from upper part of body to head, or from back upward. Chills not better external warmth, mostly in evening and with great paleness of face. Chills in evening and fever all night. ***Chills in nursing children.*** Chills with vomiting of bile or food. Hunger, colicky pains, and chilliness with thirst. Hungry before chill and after sweat. Fever, face is cold and hands warm. Fever with clean tongue. After remittent fever excessive prostration with irritability and involuntary urination.

Throat - Dryness of throat. Difficulty swallowing liquids, noisy swallowing. Clucking, gurgling noise from throat to stomach after coughing or convulsions. Constant involuntary motion of swallowing. Sensations as if there is a ball rising in throat. Pains on attempting to talk, with peculiar, hoarse, soundless cough. Mucus collects in larynx in morning after rising, and soon again after expectoration. Hoarseness with much mucus in larynx and trachea. Paralysis of vocal cords from catching cold and difficulty of breathing at every fit of coughing. Titillation low down in trachea, causes cough.

Vertigo - Vertigo with faintness and tottering. Vertigo on rising from bed, better lying down. Vertigo with blackness before eyes.

Vision - When looking at a thing steadily, reading, he sees it as through a gauze, which better wiping eyes. Yellow, blue, violet or green vision. On rising from bed, black before eyes, with dizziness in head, and faintness, totters to and fro, better lying down. Vision of colors is altered, blue seems green, red, yellowish brown, white, yellow, etc. Weak sight from masturbation.

COMMENTS - General reflex irritation. The child may chew or scratch a certain part of the body habitually. Grinding the teeth (Tub.). Picking the nose so much that it bleeds and gets irritated, nerves feeling flaming hot. Biting and picking the lips. Biting fingernails. Twitching of the eye or face, lazy eye. Boring itch in the ear. Cough. Sensitive scalp.

Malassimilation. Voracious appetite with lack of weight gain (Iod.). Sinking, gnawing immediately after a meal, unsatisfied. Hypoglycemia. Craves sweets. Severe hunger at night. Bulimia. Difficult swallowing of liquid, clucking noise from throat to stomach. Foul, putrid breath, wormy. Itching of the anus and lips.

Foul and putrid diarrhea. Diarrhea, green or white stool, slimy. Colic, indigestion, gas and diarrhea with bad smelling stools. Diarrhea when upset or angry. Sour stomach, sour eruption. Fermentation, sour gas and regurgitations. History of dysentery, with chronic fatigue. In the cachectic who have pains in the belly and deranged abdominal functions and suffer nervously.

Poor sleep. Yawning. Night terrors (Calc., Tub., Syph.). Bedwetting. Irritation to the bladder, a small amount of urine will cause the urge to urinate. During sleep, grinding of the teeth, bedwetting, and muscle jerking.

Hypersensitive to touch. Better pressure on the abdomen, may sleep on stomach (Med.). Muscle twitching, especially of head or face. Desire to rub their head against something, as if an itch deep in their brain, meningeal irritation. Headache. Motions in legs, especially the left.

Larynx extremely sensitive, touching it causes suffocative spasm. Cough excited by sensation of feather down in throat. Reflex cough, caused by writing or reading (to oneself).

Spasmodic asthma after food that disagrees. Sensation as if sternum lies too close to back, embarrasses breathing and causes anxiety and sweat. Stomach and intestinal pain with fevers when the leading symptoms are present.

Fever, with thirst, chill, face pale and cold, hands warm, nausea or vomiting of bile or food. Periodic high fevers, often from digestive or colon problems.

Aversion to the light. Strabismus with sickly look and dark circles around eyes, yellow vision. Asthenopia, defective accommodation, yellow vision. Asthenopia from onanism, when reading by artificial light is next to impossible. Eyes feel veiled, need constant wiping. Spasmodic strabismus from abdominal irritation. Prosopalgia of supra and infra-orbital region and zygoma chiefly, pains pressing, screwing with hyperesthesia.

Sunken face, blue or gray rings around the mouth, glassy-eyed. Whole face is red and flushed but around their mouth is pale. Blue circles around the eyes.

Cross and ugly children. Touchy. Capricious (Cham.). Fretful with an ugly disposition, irritable. Hyperactive children with a lot of anger, fear and obstinacy. Rages of anger and bingeing. Better steady and passive motion, being rocked.

Charles Mohr commended it for anemic persons suffering from indigestion and non-assimilation of food or after acute illness when they have headache, vertigo and neuralgia.

Sherbino found "getting on hands and knees in sleep" to be a strong indication (Med.).

Guernsey said it is suited to complaints which are concomitant to yawning, which come on whenever one yawns.

Nash mentioned two cases of typhoid in which Cina. proved curative, the indications being "Intense circumscribed redness of the cheeks and frequent and violent rubbing of the nose."

S. C. Ghose recorded a striking cure by Cina. 6c and 200c of a case of infantile remittent fever in which the classical symptoms of the drug were present, the fever came on very irregularly.

RELATIONS - ***Antidoted by:*** Camph., Caps., Chin., Pip-n. ***Antidote to:*** Caps., Chin., Merc. ***Compare:*** (1) Santon. (2) aversion to be touched - Ant-c., Ant-t., Hep. Cham., Thuj. (3) gurgling along esophagus when swallowing fluids - Hell., Cupr., difficult swallowing liquids, Bell., Caust., Hyos., Ign., Lach., Lyc., Phos. (4) in cough worse by reading or writing - Mang., Meph., Nux-v., Plat. in white stools, Dig. (5) ravenous hunger - Ars., Calc., Iod., Sil. Staph., aversion to be caressed, Ars., Lach. in squint, Alum. (6) asthenopia and defective accommodation - Art., but Art-v. has dizziness from colored light and Cina is better from rubbing. (7) Helmintochortos, Worm-moss - acts very powerfully on intestinal worms, especially the lumbricoid. (8) Teucr., Ign., Cham., Spig. ***Follows well:*** Dros. and Ant-t.

REFERENCES - Boericke. Clarke. Murphy. Phatak.

CINERARIA MARITIMA
(Dusty Miller)

PHARMACY - cine. Cineraria maritima. Dusty miller. Senecio cineraria. N. O. Composite. Corybiferae. Tincture or succus of the fresh plant, growing wild, gathered just before the flower-buds open. ***Historical dose:*** Tincture and all potencies.

CLINICAL - *Cataract.* Corneal, opacity. Eye, injuries.

HERBAL - This is an unproved drug, but it has been used with a good deal of success in cases of ***cataract*** as an external application. The method adopted is to instill one drop four or five times a day into the affected eye, for several months.

HOMEOPATHIC - Most effective in traumatic eye cases. ***Traumatic cataract and corneal opacities,*** as well as senile cataract. No reports of cures by internal use of the remedy alone, but in some cases it was given internally as well as used externally. Generally, the patients have received specific homeopathic treatment internally at the same time.

RELATIONS - ***Compare:*** (1) In cataract, Calc-f. Phos., Platanus, Cann-i., Caust., Naph., Led., Nat-m., Sil.

REFERENCES - Boericke. Clarke. Phatak.

CINNABARIS
(Red Mercuric Sulphide)

PHARMACY - cinnb. Cinnabaris. Red mercuric sulphide. Mercuric sulphide. Mercurius sulphuratus ruber. Hydrargyrum sulphuratum rubrum. Trituration. ***Historical dose:*** Trituration and all potencies.

CLINICAL - Albuminuria. Bubo. Catarrh. Chancre. Cystitis. Dysentery. ***Eye, infections.*** Gleet. Gonorrhea. Gout. Leucorrhea. Nose, sensitive. Priapism. Rheumatism. Sciatica. Scrofula. Sleep, abnormal. Sycosis. Syphilis. Tapeworm. ***Ulcers. Warts.***

HOMEOPATHIC - Cinnb. corresponds to sycosis as well as to syphilis and to combinations of the two. Warts on the prepuce (Thuj.), especially for fan-shaped warts. General nervous, uneasy sensation. Weariness, languor. Tired and prostrated, worse before eating, better when riding in the open air.

General sensitiveness to touch, bones of skull, scalp, roots of hair, bridge of nose, warts bleed when touched. Sensation on bridge of nose as if touched with metallic substance. Uneasy creeping and pressing sensation about nasal bones as from wearing spectacles when not used to them. Headache with nosebleed.

Frequent jerkings and pullings. Certain forms of ciliary neuralgia and ulceration upon a syphilitic base. Cold and chilly in warm room. Symptoms intermit in severity.

MIND - Indolence and indisposition to mental labor. Forgetful. Fretful, easily provoked. Sleepless during night. Sensation of fullness in the head from mental application. Desire to be alone.

Abdomen - Flashes of heat confined to the abdomen with great flatulence, worse in the forenoon.

Back - Pain in back part of neck when head is thrown back, extending to occiput. Wrenching pains in the vertebrae of the neck. The muscles of the neck seem as if contracted. Tearing in the side of the back. Aching in the small of the back, as if bruised. Pain all over the back down to the loins.

Chest - Chest oppressed, feels contracted, relieved by stretching. Pain running over the ensiform cartilage from the seventh rib on the right side diagonally through the chest. Pulsating and shooting pains in the chest, especially when walking.

Constitutions - Anti-sycotic and anti-syphilitic.

Ears - Roaring in the ears with swelling of the face, after eating. Scurfy eruption in right external ear. Itching in right ear.

Eyes - ***Redness of whole eye. Eye infections.*** Lids granulated, canthi and lids red. Severe shooting pain in bones of orbit, especially running from inner to outer canthus in the bone. ***Pains from lachrymal duct around eye to temple*** from inner canthus across brows to ear.

Face - Heat and swelling, mostly about the eyes.

Female - Leucorrhea, discharge with a feeling of pressure in vagina.

Head - Congestion to head, face purple red. Congestion of blood to the head, worse after eating. Violent and frightful attack of headaches, better by compression of the head. Intense headache, he cannot raise his head from the pillow, relieved by external pressure. Dull pain in the forehead, which is cold, relieved by heat. Shooting pain in the left side of the head. Painful sensitiveness of the cranium and of the hair on being touched. Stupefying buzzing in the head.

Heart - Heart flutters, then rushes of blood to the head.

Kidneys - Frequent and increasing emission of watery urine, also during the night. Pain, as if from a sore in the urethra, when urinating, this pain wakes him up at night.

Limbs - Sensation of lameness in all the limbs. Pulling and shuddering in the arms and legs. Pain in long bones when barometer lowers. Cold knees or joints. Left leg feels shorter than the right, while walking. Cramp in calves after walking. Pain in Achilles tendon and os calcis when walking. Nodes on shin bones. Pain in forearm from elbow down, including hands.

Lungs - Dyspnea with heat. Cough from tickling in the throat. Dry cough in single shocks, when lying down, better by sitting up. Hoarseness in the evening.

Male - Jerking in penis during sleep. Foul acrid sweat between scrotum and thighs. ***Warts on prepuce***, fan-shaped and bleed easily. Small red pimples on glans. Itching of corona glandis. Redness and swelling of prepuce, testicles enlarged, buboes, angry looking chancres. Syphilis, squamous and vesicular. Old hard chancres.

Modalities - Better from rest. Better open air. Better sunshine. Better after dinner. Worse from light. Worse summer. Worse dampness. Worse walking. Worse night. Worse touch. Worse lying on right side, feels as if contents of body were being dragged over to that side. Sweat worse at noon. Headache worse after sleep.

Mouth - Dry mouth and throat, wakes from sleep, must rinse the mouth Both corners of the mouth are chapped. Tongue coated white with a putrid, bitter taste in the morning. Burning, constrictive sensation in the palate. Salivation and increased flow of urine.

Nose - Nasal catarrh. Hawks stringy mucus from throat or lumpy mucus drops from the posterior sinuses. Discharge from the nose is acrid, foul, burning, watery or dark lumps. Coryza with lumps of dirty, yellow mucus are discharged from the posterior sinuses. Violent, fluent, burning coryza. Itching of the nose, with bleeding after blowing it. Pain about root, extending into bones on each side (Aur.).

Rectum - Formication in the anus, as from a large worm. Little pimples around the anus with burning and itching. Bloody dysentery. Tenesmus. Evacuations, soft and frequent. Thin, white stools. Green mucus diarrhea, which stains the skin about anus and scrotum a copper color.

Sleep - Sleepiness in the daytime and sleeplessness at night, unconquerable desire to sleep after dinner, early in the evening. Restlessness and sleeplessness at night from a constant flow of ideas changing from one thing to another. Restless sleep with vivid dreams and much talking. Nightmares after midnight.

Skin - Red eruptions. Violent itching and pricking. Honeycombed ulcers. ***Very fiery-red looking ulcers***. Condyloma, easily bleeding. Buboes. Nodes on the shin bones. Sweat on nose.

Stomach - Soreness in the stomach, with dizziness and lightness in the head and tightness in the temples. Nausea, alleviated by belchings. Nausea with water brash, in the evening.

Temperature - Pulse slower in the forepart of the day, accelerated in the evening. Coldness and chilliness in the warm room. Heat of the body during the whole night. Profuse perspiration between the thighs. Perspiration most at noon.

Throat - Stringy mucus passed through posterior sinuses into throat. Dryness of mouth and throat, must rinse the mouth. Fiery-looking ulcers in mouth and throat.

Vertigo - Giddiness in the morning after rising, when stooping with nausea.

COMMENTS - The skin is much affected. Redness predominates (the color of the drug). Red spots. Heat, redness and swelling of face, especially about eyes. Eruption on posterior cervical region, on inner and lower part of thigh with itching.

Warts, pimples, pustules, ulcers, violent itching and pricking, especially about joints. Glands enlarged. The back of the neck is affected. Pain extending to occiput when head is thrown back. Pain right side of neck on turning head. Muscles seem contracted.

Leucorrhea, discharge causes a pressure in the vagina. Jerking in penis, occurring during sleep. Tearing stitches in glans. Burning, stinging, itching of corona glandis. Frequent hemorrhages, nosebleed, bleeding hemorrhoids.

Dysenteric symptoms. Obstinate constipation, stools hard and too large. Protrusion of anus during stool. Formication as from a large worm. Little pimples around anus with burning and itching.

Berridge reported this symptom cured: "Left leg feels shorter than right while walking."

Guernsey said "We are led to use this for very red and very fiery-looking ulcers, which may occur in the throat or on any other part of the body. Ulcers in the mouth, on the legs, particularly if there be nodes on the shin-bones. In very angry looking chancres."

RELATIONS - ***Antidoted by:*** Hep., Nit-ac., Opium and Sulphur. ***Compare:*** (1) Hep., Camph. (red spots), Lach., Merc., Nit-ac. (2) Thuj. - Cinnb. is better than Thuj in warts on prepuce. (3) Sep. - warts on margin of prepuce, Ant-t. - warts at back of glans. (4) Seneg. has better bending head backward, Clem. has headache worse from same, Clem. also has vertigo on lifting head up or moving head, Cinnb. has pain in back of neck when head is thrown back.

REFERENCES - Boericke. Clarke. Phatak.

CINNAMONUM CEYLANICUM

(Cinnamon Tree)

PHARMACY - cinnam. Cinnamonum ce lanicum. Cinnamon tree. Cinnamomu zeylanicum. Cinnamomum cassia. N. Lauracae. Tincture. ***Historical dose:*** Tinctu and all potencies.

CLINICAL - Ascites. Decay. Cancer. Chil ness. Constipation. Diarrhea. Exhaustio Forgetfulness. ***Hemorrhages.*** Headache Hoarseness. ***Hysteria.*** Leucorrhea. ***Meno rhagia. Metrorrhagia.*** Nausea. ***Post-partur hemorrhage***. Vomiting.

HERBAL - Cinnam. has been used in lar doses by the old school in cases of uteri cancer and some success has been claim for it. Cancer where pain and fetor a present.

For cancer, use a strong decoction, one-ha pint a day. Oil of cinnamon in water soluti is the best local disinfectant. 3-4 drops two quarts of water as a douche, wherever germicide and disinfectant is needed. Thr drops on sugar for hiccough.

HOMEOPATHIC - A leading feature of Ci namon is hemorrhage, and has had abunda clinical verification. ***Hemorrhage*** is brig red and clear, worse by any physical exe tion. Nosebleeds.

Hemorrhage during the pregnancy, ***threa ening miscarriage***. A strain in loins or fal step brings on a profuse flow of bright bloo ***Post-partum hemorrhage***. Hemorrhag from bowels, hemoptysis, etc.

Great weakness as after loss of fluic Hysterical attacks, going off with belchin with nausea or vomiting. Talking causes hy terical attacks. Feeble patients with langu circulation. Gastric disturbances. Flatulen and diarrhea. Pains in bones and muscle

Symptoms are worse while riding, exe tion, talking, afternoon, and evening up midnight.

MIND - Forgetfulness. Anxiety. Child screar and weeps until midnight. Delusion left si of body is diminished, smaller. ***Hyster*** Great stupor in hysteria. Hysteria wh nothing brings on the attacks more surely than talking.

Abdomen - Much flatulence with colic and pain in uterus. Metastasis of gout to stomach and intestines.

Chest - Pain in chest. Anxiety and oppression in precordial region, causing constriction of chest.

Constitutions - Lymphatic, feeble, cachectic women with lax tissues and languid circulation. A women advanced in years, hysterical convulsions.

Ears - Heat around left ear.

Eyes - Pain from left eye up to vertex in a line along the middle. Itching of the eyes. Improves weakness of vision.

Face - Whole face turned red.

Female - ***Menses early, profuse, prolonged, bright red.*** Menorrhagia, with itching at nose, bright red blood, worse after false step or strain. Bearing-down sensation. Uterine hemorrhages caused by overlifting. Repeated small hemorrhages during pregnancy and puerperal state. Metrorrhagia. Sleepy. Fingers seem swollen. No desire for anything. Worse on any exertion, lifting, straining, over-stretching arms, false step.

Food - Canine hunger with nausea and debility when passing the meal hour. Want of appetite with diarrhea and acidity of stomach.

Heart - Great cardiac anxiety and loss of pulse with attacks. Heart weakness. Strengthens the heart. Hysteria.

Kidneys - Retention of urine.

Liver - Obstructions or induration of liver.

Lungs - Oppressed breathing, with vertigo and weakness.

Male - Excessive irritability of sexual organs, causes erections. Impotence, sensation of weakness in legs.

Mouth - Toothache. Offensive taste in mouth. Ptyalism, particularly with pain in back.

Nose - Frequent attacks of nosebleed. Tough mucus from nose.

Sleep - Profound sleep with attacks.

Stomach - Tonic effect on stomach. Pressure and cramps in stomach. Hiccough with diarrhea, want of appetite and acidity of stomach. Belching with colic. Nausea while riding with gagging and vomiting of mucus. Nausea and retching every day at same hour for four days. Chronic vomiting. Paroxysms subside as soon as vomiting sets in. Vomiting of pregnancy.

Stool - Long continued constipation, stool in hard balls. Diarrhea, worse after drinking with acidity. Hemorrhage from bowels, bright red and clear blood, occurring especially after any physical exertion.

Temperature - Chilliness with trembling of limbs. Great fever in evening. Transient heat with sweat. Nervous and typhoid fevers with great impairment of digestion, vomiting, diarrhea and exhaustion.

Throat - Sore throat. Hoarseness with cough. Clears the voice when muffled by secretions, scatters the phlegm and is useful for tickling in larynx.

Vertigo - Vertigo with weakness and oppression of breathing. Fainting.

COMMENTS - Particularly useful for hemorrhage. Uterine hemorrhage, bleeding fibroids, any emergency hemorrhage. Profuse diarrhea. Can be used easily as a home remedy, either in potency or as a tea in an emergency.

Boericke said "a profuse flow of bright blood." One case documented a woman who had a uterine hemorrhage after childbirth and she craved cinnamon, Cinnam. helped.

RELATIONS - ***Antidoted by:*** Acon. ***It antidotes:*** Opium. ***Compare:*** (1) Ip., Phos., Sil., Trill.

REFERENCES - Boericke. Clarke. Murphy.

CIPRO

(Ciprofloxacin)

PHARMACY - cipr. Cipro. Ciprofloxacin. Cipro is a fluorinated quinolone, belonging to a class of fluorinated antibiotics. ***Historical dose:*** All potencies.

CLINICAL - Abdominal pain. Acid, reflux. Acidosis. Allergies. Anemia. Angina pectoris. Agranulocytosis. Antrax. Ataxia. Blisters. Blood, clots. Convulsions. Diarrhea. Diplopia. Dyspnea. Edema. Headaches. Heart, disorders. ***Heartburn.*** Hematuria.

Hepatitis. ***Hives.*** Hyperpigmentation. Insomnia. Itching. Jaundice. Liver, disorders. Kidney, disorders. Kidney, stones. Musculoskeletal, disorders. Nausea. Nephritis. Nightmares. Nosebleed. Palpitations. ***Rhabdomyolysis. Sun, allergy.*** Sunburns. Swelling. ***Tendon, rupture.*** Tendonitis. Thrush. Tinnitus. Tremors. Vaginitis. Vertigo. Vomiting. Weakness.

HOMEOPATHIC - Cipro is a very toxic antibiotic drug used for the treatment of antrax and other infections. As many as 20% of people taking Cipro have reported severe side effects. The most common side-effects reported are gastrointestinal in nature such as nausea, diarrhea, vomiting, and abdominal pain.

Ciprofloxacin administration results in elevated serum fluoride levels. Cipro can cause musculo-skeletal disorders such as rhabdomyolysis. ***Tendonitis and tendon rupture.*** Achilles tendon rupture was shown to even after withdrawal of the drug.

Other fluoroquinolones are now withdrawn from the market because they had caused ***severe liver and kidney damage*** and even deaths. Fatal liver failure associated with ciprofloxacin has been reported. Ciprofloxacin has been implicated in several cases of acute kidney failure and dysfunction. Respiratory distress is a side-effect of ciprofloxacin.

Photosensitivity can result when light interacts with chemical agents in the skin and eyes. This process can produce undesirable clinical consequences, such as phototoxicity, ***exaggerated sunburn, sun allergy or sun-carcinogenicity.*** People receiving Patients taking Cipro are warned not to expose themselves to direct sunlight. Rashes develop on the areas exposed.

This medication may stimulate the central nervous system, which may lead to tremors, restlessness, light-headedness, confusion, depression, and hallucinations. Other central nervous system reactions include nervousness, agitation, insomnia, anxiety, nightmares, and paranoia.

Cipro can cause increased pressure within the brain. Convulsions have been reported in people receiving the drug. Seizures. Sluggishness. Tingling sensation. Vague feeling of illness. Weakness.

Swelling of the face, lips, neck, eyes, or hands. Agranulocytosis, potentially fatal condition where the white blood cell count goes extremely low. Blood and albumin in the urine, elevated serum potassium, glucose, and albumin. Elevation of triglycerides and cholesterol.

MIND - Abnormal dread or fear. Anxiety. Nervousness. ***Agitation and restlessness.*** Mental confusion. Depersonalization. Loss of sense of identity. Depression. Irritability. Delirium. Hallucinations. Manic attacks. Paranoia. Toxic psychosis.

Abdomen - Bleeding in the intestines. Flatus. Intestinal inflammation. Intestinal perforation. Swelling of the pancreas.

Back - Back pain. Neck pain.

Blood - Acidosis. Anemia. Agranulocytosis. Swelling of the blood vessels or lymph system.

Ears - Hearing loss. Ringing in the ears.

Eyes - Eye pain. Yellow eyes. Involuntary eye movement. Blurred vision. Double vision. Decreased vision. Change in color perception. Sensitivity to light.

Face - Swelling of the face.

Female - Vaginal inflammation.

Food - Lack of appetite. Loss of appetite.

Head - Headache. ***Light-headedness.*** Blood clot to the brain.

Heart - Angina pectoris. Cardiopulmonary arrest. Irregular heartbeat. Palpitations. Pounding heartbeat. High blood pressure. Heart attack. Heart flutters.

Kidneys - Inability to urinate. ***Kidney damage.*** Large volumes of urine. Kidney failure. Urinary retention. Urethral bleeding. Acidosis. Nephritis. Increased urinary output. Kidney stones. Dark urine. Blood in urine.

Limbs - Achiness. Joint stiffness. Joint pain. Gout flare-up. Convulsions. Ataxia, lack of muscle coordination. Tendon, rupture. Achilles tendon rupture. Tendonitis.

Liver - Hepatitis. ***Liver damage.*** Jaundice. Liver failure.

Lungs - Dyspnea. Respiratory distress. Labored breathing. Blood clots in the lungs. Coughing up blood. Difficult breathing.

Bronchial spasms.

Male - Burning in penis. Prostatitis.

Mouth - Mouth sores. Bad taste in mouth. Thrush. Oral fungal infection.

Nose - Nosebleed. Loss of sense of smell.

Rectum - Diarrhea. Constipation. Pale or dark stools.

Skin - Blistering of skin. Burning sensations. Severe allergic reaction. ***Skin hypersensitivity.*** Cuticle candidiasis (yeast). Skin peeling. Itching. ***Hives.*** Redness. Red bumps on skin. ***Skin sensitivity to sunlight.*** Sunburns. Hyperpigmentation. Unusual darkening of the skin. Yellow skin.

Sleep - Drowsiness. Inability to fall or stay asleep. Insomnia. Nightmares.

Stomach - Acid, reflux. ***Heartburn.*** Indigestion. Bleeding in the stomach. Hiccoughs. Nausea and vomiting.

Temperature - Chills. Fever. Heat flushing.

Throat - Difficulty in swallowing. Swelling of the throat. Speech difficulties.

Vertigo - Dizziness. Light-headedness. Fainting.

RELATIONS - ***Compare:*** Calc-f., Fl-ac.

REFERENCES - Murphy.

CISTUS CANADENSIS

(Rock Rose)

PHARMACY - cist. Cistus canadensis. Rock rose. Helianthemum canadense. Ice-plant. Frost-weed. N. O. Cistacae. Tincture of whole flowering plant. ***Historical dose:*** Tincture and all potencies. Locally as a wash to arrest fetid discharges.

CLINICAL - Bone disorders. Breast, cancer. ***Cancer.*** Diarrhea. Erysipelas. ***Glandular swellings.*** Herpes zoster. Hip joint disease. Hospital gangrene. Leucorrhea. Lupus. Mastitis. Ophthalmia. Panaritium. Parotiditis. Pharyngitis. ***Pyorrhea.*** Scorbutus. Scrofula. Sore, throat. Ulcers.

HOMEOPATHIC - Cistus is a very ancient remedy for scrofulous disorders, in scorbutic states, and for gangrenous ulcerations. The provings and homeopathic uses confirm its suitability in these respects and bring out clearer indications.

Affects the glands, especially of naso-pharynx, neck and breasts (left). ***Malignant disease of the glands of the neck.*** Indurated glandular swelling of the neck and throat. Suppuration of the glands of the neck. Breast cancer, hardness of the breasts.

Cancer of the lower lip. Scorbutic, swollen gums separating from the teeth, gums bleed easily, putrid, disgusting. Cold tongue. Decay of the lower jaw. Desire for acid food and fruits. Saliva in throat. Belchings in stomach.

Affinity for the naso-pharynx, aborts colds that center in posterior nose. Sniffling. Mucus discharges are thick, yellow, foul, leave a painful rawness. Worse sweating, discharges. Scrofulous ophthalmia.

Herpetic eruptions, scorbutic states, chronic swellings and gangrenous ulcerations. Poisoned wounds, bites, phagadenic ulcers. Suppurations. Lupus. Internal and external itching. Burnings. Formication through the whole body with anxious, difficult breathing. Indurations. Callosities with cracks.

Extreme sensitivity to cold. Sensation of coldness in various parts. Inhaled air feels cool. Cold breath.

Grimmer said "This patient is extremely sensitive to cold and all complaints become worse after exposure to cold." All mental excitement aggravates.

MIND - Fear. Bad effects from vexation. All mental excitement aggravates (stitches in throat, cough).

Abdomen - Stitches in left hypochondrium. ***Cool feeling*** in abdomen. Pain in groin coming from back.

Back - Hard, swollen glands in the neck. Neck is studded with tumors. Burning, bruised pain in the coccyx, preventing sitting, touch.

Breasts - Induration of breasts, sensitive to cold air. Mastitis. Breast cancer.

Causations - Bad effects from anger, vexation.

Chest - Coldness in chest. Chest feels raw after expectoration. Trachea feels narrow. Hemorrhage from lungs.

Constitutions - Suited to scrofulous subjects who are very sensitive to cold air.

Ears - Watery discharge, fetid pus, after eruptive diseases. Discharge of water and bad-smelling pus. Tetter on and around ears, extending to external meatus. Inner swelling of ears with discharge.

Eyes - Feeling as if something passing around the eye. Weight above eyes. Scrofulous inflammation. Canthi cracked. Stitches in eyes.

Face - Decay of the lower jaw with suppurating glands on neck. Swelling of parotid glands. Open, bleeding, cancer on lower lip. Lips cracked. Tip of nose painful. Itching, burning and crusts, on zygoma. Vesicular erysipelas. Lupus.

Female - Sensitive to cold air. Bad smelling leucorrhea. Cancer.

Food - Desire for acid food and fruits, cheese, pungent things.

Head - Head drawn to one side by swelling. in the neck. Forehead cold, and sensation of coolness inside forehead, in a very warm room. Pressive pain at root of nose with headache. Headache from missed meals, better eating.

Limbs - Sprained pain in wrist. Cold feet. Cracked finger tips, sensitive to cold. Workmen develop hard place on their hands with cracks. Tetter on hands. Syphilitic ulcers on lower limbs with hard swelling around. White swelling.

Lungs - Asthmatic after lying down. Larynx and trachea feel cool on inhaling cold air. Trachea feels narrow and breathing becomes difficult, preceded by formication. Expectoration of quantities of glairy, tenacious mucus, on lying down. Chest feels raw after expectoration.

Male - Itching on scrotum.

Modalities - Better from eating. Better swallowing. Better expectoration. Great sensitiveness to touch. Worse from touch. Worse slightest exposure to cold air. Worse drafts. Worse cold water. Worse evening, night, morning. Worse mental exertion. Worse excitement. Worse touch. Worse motion. Diarrhea worse from drinking coffee.

Mouth - Scorbutic, receding gums, easily bleeding, putrid. ***Pyorrhea*** (Merc-c., Caust., Staph., Kreos.). ***Mouth feels cold***, putrid, impure breath. Tongue feels cold. ***Hurts to protrude the tongue.*** Breath cool. Saliva cold.

Nose - Cold feeling or burning in nose. Tip painful. Eczema of the nose. As of a lump in naso-pharynx. Pressing pain at the root of the nose with headache. Chronic nasal catarrh, frequent violent sneezing.

Rectum - Chronic dysentery. Stool, thin, yellow, urgent, worse in morning. Diarrhea from coffee and fruit, with goiter and nausea. Chronic diarrhea in wet weather in scrawny scrofulous children.

Skin - General itching which prevents sleep. Itching, crawling all over without eruptions. Small, painful pimples. Skin of hands hard, thick, dry, fissured, deep cracks. Itching of swollen hands and arms. Mercurio-syphilitic ulcers. Hemicrania. Lupus. ***Glands inflamed and indurated***.

Sleep - Very restless at night. Sleepless from coldness or dryness in throat. Night sweats.

Stomach - ***Cool feeling*** in stomach before and after eating. Empty and cool belching. Frequent nausea with diarrhea. Diarrhea after drinking coffee.

Temperature - Chilliness, followed by heat with trembling. Heat with thirst, causing to drink frequently. Sweats easily. Night sweats.

Throat - Soft, spongy feeling, itching in the throat. Heat and itching in throat. Small, dry spot in throat, must sip water frequently. ***Throat, very dry*** and becomes ***sore on inhaling least cold air.*** Breath, tongue, and throat feel cold. Uvula and tonsils swollen. Glands swollen and suppurating. Goiter with frequent diarrhea. Head drawn to one side by swellings in neck. Pains when coughing. Hawking of mucus.

COMMENTS - "Sensitive to cold air" and feelings of coldness. Cold feelings in larynx, in abdomen. "Inhaling the slightest cold air causes sore-throat, which he has not when inhaling in a warm room."

Indurated glandular swelling of the neck and throat. Trembling with the fever. Sensation as if ants were running through the whole body (in evening with anxious difficult breathing). Prominent stitches. Characteristic soft or spongy feeling.

Clarke cured with Cist. a case of sore throat that had lasted for years under allopathic treatment with local swabbings. There was an accumulation of thick yellow, leathery phlegm that had to be cleared away by a local means. The patient complained of a "spongy" feeling in the throat and the led him to the remedy.

RELATIONS - ***Antidoted by:*** Rhus-t., Camph. and Sep. ***Compare:*** (1) Con., Calc., Arg-n., Bell., (2) Carb-v. - cold breath. (3) Sulph. - morning diarrhea. ***Compatible:*** Magnesium - the plant grows on a magnesium soil.

REFERENCES - Boericke. Clarke. Grimmer.

CITRICUM ACIDUM

(Citric Acid)

PHARMACY - cit-ac. Citricum acidum. Citric acid. ***Historical dose:*** Tincture and all potencies.

HOMEOPATHIC - All forms of ***dropsy*** and swellings are benefited with Citric acid and lemon juice, tablespoonful every 3 to 4 hours. ***Scurvy***. Chronic rheumatism and hemorrhages. Pain from tongue cancer.

RELATIONS - ***Compare:*** (1) Citrus limon, Citrus vulgaris.

REFERENCES - Boericke.

CITRUS DECUMANA

(Grape-fruit)

PHARMACY - cit-d. Citrus decumana. Grape-fruit. Citrus paradisi. Shaddock. N. O. Rutacae. Expressed juice. ***Historical dose:*** Tincture and all potencies.

HOMEOPATHIC - Citrus decumana has tinnitus, ***head noises*** and ringing in ears. Sensation of pressure in the temporal region.

RELATIONS - ***Compare:*** (1) Citrus limon, Citrus vulgaris.

REFERENCES - Boericke.

CITRUS LIMONUM

(Lemon)

PHARMACY - cit-l. Citrus limonum. Lemon. Citrus medica. N. O. Rutacae. Expressed juice. ***Historical dose:*** Tincture and all potencies.

CLINICAL - Cancer. Colic. Constipation. Convulsions. Diarrhea. Dropsy. Dysentery. Dyspnea. Eruptions. Faintness. Headaches. Hemorrhages. Herpes. Rheumatism. Scurvy. Splenitis. Sunstroke.

HERBAL - Lemon juice and citric acid are traditional remedies for and preventives of sea-scurvy. It can be used as a local application (in one part of citric acid to eight of water).

HOMEOPATHIC - That their action is homeopathic has been proved by the occurrence of scurvy from the excessive use of the acid when taken for other purposes.

Cit-l. has a powerful effect on the circulation and on the blood itself. Faintness, a weak pulse, hemorrhages and swellings. Excessive menstruation.

Inflammation and painful enlargement of the spleen, dyspnea. Stiffness in the joints, particularly in the fingers, bruised feeling, particularly in the feet. Herpetic eruptions. Cancer pains. Sore throats. Daily headache.

RELATIONS - ***Antidoted by:*** Acon., Asarum, Datura, Euphorbia, Hep., Sepia. ***It antidotes:*** Acon., Euphorb., Stram., snakebites and all animal poisons. It increases the curative effects of Bell. ***Compare:*** (1) It should be compared with Acetic acid and the ***"bruised pain in the joints"*** recalls the action of its congener, Ruta, Bell., Lach. (2) As an antidote against Stram. It has been employed with great success, the juice of the fruit being administered by the teaspoonful.

REFERENCES - Boericke. Clarke.

CITRUS VULGARIS

(Bitter Orange)

PHARMACY - cit-v. Citrus vulgaris. Bitter orange. Aurantium amara. Aurantii cortex. N. O. Rutacae. Tincture of Seville orange peel. ***Historical dose:*** Tincture and all potencies.

CLINICAL - Choking, sensation. Faintness. Headache. Metrorrhagia. Neuralgia. Palpitations. Pleurodynia. Scarlatina. Throat, rising in.

HERBAL - The tincture of the_orange peel is used as a pleasant bitter tonic in old-school practice. On sensitive individuals, oranges in any form produce pathogenic effects. Boiled dried orange peel excites the intestine in a manner similar to other forms of cellulose or agar.

There is an increased flow of bile which continues for hours. It unites both a cholagogue action with a mechanical stimulus to peristalsis. An orange eaten before breakfast is said to destroy the craving for alcohol in alcoholics.

HOMEOPATHIC - One patient could never eat an orange without experiencing a fearful taste at the back of the nose and throat. This lasted many days and caused choking sensations and faintness.

For diseases of the elderly with coldness and chilliness. Neuralgias and skin symptoms. Facial neuralgias, mostly right-sided. Itching, redness and swelling of hands. Headache with nausea, vomiting and vertigo.

Frequent and irresistible yawning. Disturbed sleep. Great excitement, quick motions. Pains in kidneys and bladder. Too copious menses. Pleurodynia. Palpitations. Thoracic oppression.

Face - Neuralgia of face, shooting, gnawing pains, in temples, especially right side.

Head - Right sided headache.

Skin - Itching, general or more often only in upper limbs, with redness and swelling of hands. Eruption and other symptoms like scarlatina.

Teeth - Constant toothache. Teeth become decayed, wear off.

Throat - Something seems to rise in thro and choke. Fearful taste at back of nos and throat, lasting for days and causin choking sensation and faintness.

RELATIONS - ***Compare:*** (1) Ruta, Angustur (2) Citrus limonum. (3) Citric acid. (4) Citru decumana.

REFERENCES - Boericke. Clarke.

CLEMATIS

(Bach Flower Essence)

PHARMACY - clem-b. Clematis. Clemati vitalba. Flowers are picked with the stalk placed in a bowl of water and allowed to si in the sun for several hours. The water i strained and used as medicine. ***Historica dose:*** Take two drops from the stock bottl into a one ounce dropper bottle, (add brand or alcohol, if this bottle will be used fo days or weeks). This is the dosage bottle take a few drops straight into the mouth o as needed in a little water or juice.

HOMEOPATHIC - This remedy belongs to th group of ***Not Sufficient Interest in Presen Circumstances,*** as classified by Bach. Th additional remedies of this group are Honey b., Wld-r-b., Oliv-b., Wh-ch-b., Must-b. and Ch-bd-b.. This group of remedies helps thos not fully engaged in the here and now. Shocke by sudden noise and startles easily whe touched. Sleepiness, drowsiness, fainting and vertigo. In some comatose states, Clem-b. may restore consciousness. The body may seem a if not "inhabited," as the mind draws to futur dream castles or removes due to exhaustion o emotional hardship. Out-of-body experiences

MIND - Hazy reality. Passive. Tendency t suddenly lose touch and become drowsy o sleepy. Lightheaded or vacant feeling. Lack o concentration. Prevalent absent-mindedness interrupted by spurts of interest.

Delusions with ecstatic content (Verv-b.), pleasant visions and reveries. Set on dreams of future fulfillment, rather than seeing the present as promising and trying to find happiness therein. States from daydreaming about future happiness, fatigue, strenuous or saddening daily routines. Hopeful.

Happy when dreaming, reality seems harsh, void of meaning, lonely or sad.

REFERENCES - Bach.

CLEMATIS ERECTA

(Virgin's Bower)

PHARMACY - clem. Clematis erecta. Virgin's bower. Upright virgin's bower. Flammula jovis. N. O. Ranunculacee. Europe. Tincture of leaves and stems. ***Historical dose:*** Tincture and all potencies.

CLINICAL - Acne. Arthritic, nodosities. Blepharitis. Cancer. Conjunctivitis. ***Eyes, disorders.*** Face, pimples. ***Gonorrhea.*** Headaches. Homesickness. Nausea. Orchitis. Rheumatism. Skin, rashes. ***Testicles, infections. Toothache.*** Urethra, stricture.

HOMEOPATHIC - Clematis, like other Ranunculi, is a direct irritant of the skin producing inflammation and vesication. In the provings, the external head (left), eyes, teeth (left), skin, urinary and male sexual organs show the greatest number of symptoms.

Acts especially on the skin, mucus membranes of eyes and urethra, ***glands,*** breasts, ovaries and genito-urinary organs, especially the testicles. Glands become ***very hard and painfully*** swollen. Herpes, stricture of the urethra, cancer of the breast and testes. ***Inflammation of eyes,*** worse left, smarting, burning, stitches, redness, lachrymation, photophobia. Sensation as if fire were streaming from eyes.

Neuralgic pains in various parts. Pains relieved by perspiration. Burning, itching, stinging, crawling. Muscles flaccid or twitch. Distant pulsation in whole body. Vibrating sensation through the body after lying down. Strictures. Emaciation. ***Great sleepiness***. Great debility from 3 p.m. to 5 p.m. Aversion to be washed.

MIND - ***Confused feeling, better in open air.*** Peevish, dissatisfied without any cause. Melancholy, preoccupied with sad thoughts. General sadness and dread of misfortune. Sadness better after eating. Cheerful alternating with sadness, followed by irritability and prostration.

Homesick (Caps.). Ailments from homesickness. Memory weak. Indifference. Aversion to talking. Indolence in morning, better evening. Aversion to reading, desires to be read to. Irritable, taciturn, doesn't want to go out. Low sex drive. Fear of being alone, but disinclined to meet even agreeable company. Sleepy, dreamy.

Abdomen - Pain from abdomen to chest, worse breathing and during urination. Swelling of inguinal glands with jerking pains, with scirrhus or suppressed gonorrhea, rheumatism of joints.

Back - Itching pustules around the neck, with excoriation after scratching. Humid tetters from the nape of the neck to the occiput. Eruption of pustules in the lumbar region.

Breasts - Breast and uterine cancer. Swelling and induration of breasts. Glandular induration and tumors of breast. Breast cancer with stitches in shoulders and uterus. Shooting pain in breast, worse urinating. Full, heavy, sensitive breasts.

Causations - Homesickness.

Constitutions - Suited to light-haired people with torpid, cachectic conditions, swellings and indurations of the glandular system. Syphilitic taint. Scrofulous, rheumatic, gonorrheal and syphilitic patients.

Ears - Burning pain in exterior of the ear. Tinkling, ringing in the ear.

Eyes - Complaints from bright sunlight. Chronic conjunctivitis. Pustular conjunctivitis with tinea capitis, eyes inflamed and protruding. Chronic blepharitis with sore and swollen meibomian glands. Iritis with great ***sensitiveness to cold***. Heat in eyes, ***sensitive to air***, must close them. Burning, as if fire were streaming out and smarting, worse closing eyes. Lachrymation. Flickering before eyes.

Face - White blisters on face and nose, as if sunburned. Pain in right side of face to eye, ear and temple, better holding cold water in the mouth. Swelling of the submaxillary glands with hard tubercles, throbbing, aggravated on being touched. Lip cancer.

Female - Menses too early. Swelling and induration of the mammary glands. Breast and uterine cancer.

Food - Weakness, nausea and sleepiness after eating. Prolonged satiety, though the food continues pleasant to the taste. Increased thirst, with desire for ice. Aversion to beer. Nausea on smoking tobacco, with weakness of the legs.

Head - ***Confused feeling, better in open air.*** Hammering and strokes in the head. Boring pain in temples. Headaches, worse bending head backward. Head feels full and heavy, hanging down. Eruption on occiput at base of hair, moist, pustular sensitive. Itching on the hairy scalp.

Heart - Sharp stitches at heart, from within outwards.

Kidneys - Urethra feels constricted, like a large whip-cord painful on pressure. Stricture of urethra. Frequent, scanty urination, burning at orifice. Burning in urethra during urination. ***Urine stops and starts***, emitted drop by drop. Must strain to pass a few drops, then full stream follows. Inability to pass all the urine, dribbling after urinating. Last drops of urine cause violent burning. Tingling in urethra lasting some time after urinating. Pain along the spermatic cord, worse at night.

Limbs - Arthritic nodosities in the joints of the fingers. Axillary glands swollen. Weakness in limbs after eating or with nausea on smoking tobacco. Scaly tetters in the thigh.

Lungs - Breathing impaired, worse ascending the hill or walking over uneven road. Barking, dry cough with stitches in chest. Expectoration of bloody saliva.

Male - Orchitis. Testes hang heavy or retracted. ***Testicles indurated with bruised feeling.*** Swelling of right half of the scrotum. Ilio-scrotal neuralgia. Swelling of the spermatic cord with burning and soreness, extending to abdomen. Violent erections with stitches in urethra. Burning in penis during seminal discharge during sex. Aversion for sex.

Modalities - Better from sweating. Better open air. ***Worse from gonorrhea.*** Worse touch. Worse motion. Worse moist poultices. Worse from heat of bed. Worse night. Worse cold washing or air, cold water. Worse during increasing and new moon, better during the waning moon. Monthly aggravations. Headache and toothache are worse lying down in evening.

Mouth - Breath offensive to others. Dryness of the tongue in the morning. Dull shootings and piercings in the root of the tongue. Small blisters on the tongue and in the throat, which soon become ulcers.

Skin - ***Glands*** hot, painful, ***swollen***, worse inguinal glands. Vesicles, pustules. Red, burning, scaly, scabby. Corroding eruptions, ending in flat eating ulcers with thick crusts and eczema worse occiput and lower legs. Varicose ulcers. Herpes zoster. Itches terribly, worse washing in cold water, worse face and hands and ***scalp around occiput***.

Sleep - Sleepiness. Restless, dreamy sleep with vibratory sensation throughout the body.

Stomach - Disagreeable sensation of coldness in the stomach. Weakness in all the limbs after eating with pulsation in arteries. Nausea on smoking tobacco with weakness of legs.

Teeth - Toothache, ***worse at night and from tobacco***, temporarily worse from heat of bed. Toothache in a decayed molar tooth, much better by cold water. Shooting pains or successive pullings in the teeth. Sensation as if the decayed tooth were too long. The least contact is exceedingly painful.

Temperature - Pulse accelerated. Quartan fever, characterized by shuddering, followed by sweat. Sweat on waking, and sensitiveness of the skin, which the patient cannot bear to be uncovered. Dry heat, with sensation of general heat.

Throat - Heat and burning in the mouth and throat. Sensation of roughness in the throat.

Vertigo - Giddiness if he lifts his head up, or when moving the head.

COMMENTS - Clematis was used by Stoerck before Hahnemann's time in cancerous and other foul ulcers, inveterate skin eruptions, syphilis and rheumatism.

Affections of the urethra, penis in general, prepuce in particular. May have to wait a long time before he can urinate with intense pain along fore part of urethra. Flow of urine by fits and starts. Mucus in the urine, but not pus. Beginning of inflammatory stricture. Stricture of the urethra

Swelling of inguinal glands. Painful inflamed, swollen testicles. Great affinity for the testes. Useful for cases of undescended testicles, painful, partially descended testicles, and hydroceles where the scrotum swells with fluid (Con., Spong.). Indurated testicles. Testicular cancer. Gonorrhea that goes to the testes. Herpes. Breast cancer.

Generally a right-sided remedy. Great debility, twitching of muscles, vibrating sensation through body. Giddiness when lifting up head or when moving head.

Useful for poison ivy and poison oak. Vesicles and weeping of yellow, acrid fluid on body (Rhus-t.). Fluid stings, worse bathing. Impetigo, fluid seeping from beneath the scabs.

RELATIONS - ***It is antidoted by:*** Bry. (Toothache, urinary symptoms), Camph. ***Antidote to:*** Merc. ***Compare:*** (1) Clematis vitalba - varicose and other ulcers. (2) Sil., Staph., Petr., Oleand., Canth., Phos. acid. (3) Ars. - skin, Clem. has more redness is worse from washing, has moist, alternating with dry scabs. (4) Puls. - gonorrheal orchitis, testicle tender and hard as a stone. (5) Bell., Bry., Calc., Canth., Con., Caust., Dulc. (syphilitic ulcerations), Graph., Merc. (iritis sensitive to cold), Petr. (impetigo on neck and occiput). (6) Sars. - syphilitic ulcers. (7) In "aversion to be washed," compare Ant-c., Hep., Phos., Sep., Spig., Sulph. (8) In bending head back, Cinnb., Cobalt. has worse bending head forward. ***Compatible:*** Sil.

REFERENCES - Boericke. Clarke. Murphy. Phatak.

COBALTUM METALLICUM

(Cobalt Metal)

PHARMACY - cob. Cobaltum metallicum. Cobalt metal (Co. At. Wt. 58.6). Trituration. ***Historical dose:*** Trituration and all potencies.

CLINICAL - ***Backaches***. Constipation. Eye, disorders. Fatigue. Gonorrhea. Hemorrhages. Headaches. Impotency. Liver, disorders. Lumbago. Masturbation, effects. Neurasthenia. Sexual, disorders.

HOMEOPATHIC - Cobaltum is useful for neurasthenic states of spinal origin with sexual disturbances. Affects the spine, lumbar region, genitals, kidneys and bones. Fatigue, agitation and bone pains, worse in morning. Aching in bones. Soreness.

Characteristic ***very severe backache,*** worse sitting, better rising up, walking or lying down. Backache with seminal emissions. Discharges frothy. Sourness of taste, stomach, foot, sweat etc. Fatigue.

MIND - Great exhilaration of spirits, vivacity and rapid flow of thoughts. All mental excitement increases suffering. Constant interchange of mental moods. Sense of guilt. Thinks too little of himself. Delusion he is a criminal and others know it. Confusion from motion. Reproaches himself. Desire for mental work.

Abdomen - Empty feeling at navel. Yellow spots on abdomen. Sharp pains in the region of spleen, worse taking deep breath.

Back - Backache in lumbar region and weak legs. ***Pain in back and sacrum, worse while sitting, better*** walking or lying. Weakness in legs and backache after emissions. Aching pain in lumbar, worse sex, sitting, better on rising, walking or lying down with weak knees, cannot straighten up. Pain along the spine and from the sacrum down through the legs into the feet.

Eyes - Photophobia in spring. Darting pain in the eyes on coming into sunshine. Spring catarrh.

Face - Disposition to keep jaws tightly closed.

Head - Headache, worse stooping, jarring. Sensation as if the brain went up and down, on stepping. Headache, worse bending head ***forward***. Itching of hairy scalp and beard.

Kidneys - Smarting at the meatus at the end of urination. Albuminuria. Urine has a strong pungent smell.

Limbs - Trembling of limbs especially legs, aching when sitting. Flushes of heat along legs. Shooting into thighs from liver. Sudden weakness in left hip, worse walking. ***Weak knees***. Tingling, pricking in feet. Foot sweat, mostly between the toes, smelling sour. Aching in wrist joints.

Liver - Shooting pains in the region of the liver. Shooting from liver region down into the thighs.

Lungs - Cough with copious, frothy, sweetish white mucus with lumps in it.

Male - Pain in end of urethra, greenish discharge, brown spots on genitals and abdomen. Pain in right testicle, better urinating. Discharge of semen without erections. Frequent nocturnal emissions with lewd dreams, headache and backache. Impotency. Yellow-brown spots on genitals.

Modalities - Better from hawking mucus. Better continued motion. Better walking. Worse from sexual losses. Worse lying down. Worse rising from sitting. Worse sitting. Worse morning. Worse heat of bed or sun. Cold air causes lachrymation and aggravates pain in teeth. Warmth of bed causes itching all over. Jarring aggravates headache.

Mouth - Teeth feel too long. Tongue coated white (Ant-c.), with cracks across the middle. Sour taste.

Rectum - Desire for stool, while walking, worse on standing, followed by diarrhea. Constant dropping of blood from the anus, no blood from the stools.

Skin - Pimples about buttocks. chin, hairy scalp. Itching all over when getting warm in bed.

Sleep - Wakeful, can do with less sleep. Drowsy and can hardly get enough sleep. Unrefreshing. ***Disturbed by lewd dreams***.

Stomach - Sour or bitter water rises up with pain in stomach.

Vertigo - Vertigo with feeling as if head grows large, worse stools.

COMMENTS - Frequent nocturnal emissions with lewd dreams, with partial or no erections. Impotence. Drowsiness, unrefreshing sleep. Headache worse bending head forward. Pimples on the head and elsewhere, itching of the skin when warm in bed at night.

Smarting and darting pains in eyes. Lachrymation in open air. Pain in hollow tooth, which feels too long and is sensitive to touch. Tongue thickly coated white, cracks across middle. No appetite for supper. Urine has strong pungent smell.

RELATIONS - ***Compare:*** (1) Cann-i., Sep., Sel. (2) Zinc. - in pain in back worse sitting. (3) Agn. - impotency, Nux-v. (4) effects of masturbation, Sel., Titan., Thallium. (5) Nitrate of Cobalt is a perfect antidote to Cyanide of Potassium, the two forming an insoluble compound.

REFERENCES - Boericke. Clarke. Phatak.

COBALTUM NITRICUM

(Cobalt Nitrate)

PHARMACY - cob-n. Cobaltum nitricum. Cobalt nitrate. A chemically pure product. Trituration. ***Historical dose:*** Trituration and all potencies.

CLINICAL - Amenorrhea. Anemia. Arthritis. Blood, tumors. Chlorosis. Conjunctivitis. Deafness. Emaciation. Encephalitis. Fatigue. Fibroids. Hemiplegia. Infertility. Meningitis. Metrorrhagia. Miscarriage. Neuritis. Orchitis. Paralysis. Paraplegia. Pericarditis. Pleurodynia. Sterility. Syphilis.

HOMEOPATHIC - Cobalt has been known since ancient times and it was introduced for used in the manufacture of blue china, Dutch delftware, Moutier and Gien's crockery and Sévre porcelain. A great deal of research is carried out on it in industry and agriculture including experiments concerning the toxicity of cobalt and its salts.

In 1899, Pettini and Messina, by administering cobalt chloride in the food of dogs cats and rabbits, noticed an increase in th level of hemoglobin.

More recently, Polonowski, Sutter and Briska, showed an increase of red corpuscles due to cobalt. Canjolle pointed to the complaints of pulmonary ventilation with a fall in arterial tension. According to Zarone, this hypotension is linked to a toxic attack on the myocardium.

In occupational medicine, Desoille, Merklen and Cotteril reported cases of poisoning of workers in which the clinical symptoms noted respiratory complaints and an increase in the level of red corpuscles.

A lack of fertility and miscarriage due to bleeding under the placenta. Emaciation, bluish-red coloring of the muscles and viscera, serous effusion. The thyroid gland is the location for pseudo-carcinomatous changes.

The homeopathic proving was re-evaluated by G. Maring in 1955 with fifteen provers, seven men and eight women. He used the 3x, 6x, 12x, and 30x potencies.

Symptoms included general fatigue in the morning, immediately on waking, lasting through the day with the feeling of being sleepy and heavy. General lassitude. Face pale, discolored. Frontal headache, vertigo. Nervous.

General emaciation. Irregular appetite, diarrhea. Better during the afternoon. Trembling hands. Loss of libido. Heaviness of the limbs. Pains in the bones. Pleurodynia on the left side. Cardiac pain. Metrorrhagia.

Syphilitic hemiplegia and paraplegia. Syphilitic radicular neuritis. Tabes. Diffuse meningitis and encephalitis or general paralysis. Spasmodic dorsal tabes. Thyroid problems. Every morbid manifestation developing either from hereditary or acquired syphilis. Hardening processes.

MIND - Anxiety. Excitability and over-activity, followed by inhibition and general depression. Depressive state with difficulty in concentrating as a result of a persistent headache. Sullen. Sadness on waking. Memory poor on first waking.

Abdomen - Chronic enteritis. Intestinal rumbling, ameliorated by belchings. Pressing abdominal pains, low, spreading towards the back.

Back - Vertebral growth dystrophy in children. Dorsal pain accompanied by a sensation of heat and headaches.

Blood - Chlorosis, anemia in young girls. Biermer's anemia. Increase of red blood corpuscles, hemoglobin. Acceleration of the sedimentation rate.

Chest - Pain on the left side of the chest, aggravated by respiration.

Ears - Noise like roaring in the ears. Deafness. Edema of the ear.

Eyes - Purulent conjunctivitis. Interstitial keratitis. Iritis. Inflammation of the choroid and retina. Eyelids heavy, swollen. Sensation of sand in the eyes. Boring pain around the left eye. Sensation of a veil over the eyes, when writing. Vision complaints, cannot focus for close work.

Female - Metrorrhagia. Secondary amenorrhea. Kraurosis of the vulva. Stenosis and atresia of the neck of the uterus. Hemorrhagic metritis. Uterine fibroids. Sclera-cystic inflammation of the ovary. Recurring miscarriage. Sterility. Frigidity. Lack of libido.

Food - Appetite diminished. Desire for fried potatoes and fluids.

Head - Frontal pressing headache with feeling of the skull sunken above the eyes. Itching of the scalp. Head numb, as though tied by a band. Sensation of heat in the head with icy cold feet.

Heart - Palpitations with sensation of rolling below the ribs. Pericardial effusion. Shivering in the evening, exhausting fever and nightly perspiration. Cyanosis of the limbs of the hands and feet. Pericarditis. Aortitis (syphilitic). Arteritis (syphilitic).

Kidneys - Pain in the kidneys. Bladder sensitive with urging and involuntary urination. Urine dark, odor of garlic.

Limbs - Arthritis. Charcot's joints. Pseudotabes from arthritis of the vertebral joints. Legs heavy, painful, especially in the morning. Limping with numbness of the legs as after walking or from exercise. Feet icy cold.

Lungs - Cortical pleurisy.

Male - Sexual asthenia. Impotence. Absence of spermatozoa in the semen. Orchitis and syphilitic orchi-epidydimitis. Blood tumors.

Modalities - Better in the afternoon and evening. Better from eructation. Worse in the morning, on rising.

Mouth - Vesicles around the lips. Mouth and throat dry. Need to clear the throat. Difficult swallowing. Sensation of swelling and inflammation of the gums. Pain in the gums and around the sockets of absent teeth.

Nose - Snuffling with frequent sneezing and tickling feeling in the nose. Purulent coryza. Sudden nosebleeds.

Rectum - Diarrhea in the morning with tenesmus. Stools soft, yellow and copious or hard in balls.

Skin - Vesicular eruption, palms of the hands. Urticarial eruptions, aggravated after midnight. Skin discolored. Skin has cancerous tendency. Dryness of the palms. Sudamina. Vitiligo.

Sleep - Sleep deep, but unrefreshing. Troubled dreams of falling from a height or obscene or unpleasant. Wakes tired with the need for more sleep.

Stomach - Nausea in the morning with eructation and headache. Sensation of acidity and emptiness in the stomach after eating. Gastric pains.

Vertigo - Vertigo on rising, cannot stand up, aggravated by moving the head.

RELATIONS - ***Compare:*** (1) Ferr. - Congestive headache, paleness of mucus membranes, pains in the bones, amenorrhea with vicarious hemorrhage, nosebleeds, or hemoptysis. (2) Merc. - Slow thinking with bad memory for names. Weakness with trembling hands. Alveolar pyorrhea. Menses profuse with blood and large clots. Nightly pains in the bones. (3) Syph. - Memory complaints and difficulty in concentrating. Nightly lightning pains in the bones. Hardening of the genital organs. Frequent need to wash the hands.

REFERENCES - Julian.

COCA ERYTHROXYLON

(Coca leaves)

PHARMACY - coca. Coca erythroxylon. Coca leaves. Erythroxylon coca. N. O. Linee, suborder Erythroxylee. Tincture of leaves. Solution or trituration of the alkaloid, Cocaine. The alkaloid Cocaine is the well-known local anesthetic. ***Historical dose:*** All potencies.

CLINICAL - ***Altitude sickness.*** Angina pectoris. Aphonia. ***Asthma.*** Bedwetting. Chorea. Colic. Constipation. Cough. Deafness. Debility. Delirium tremens. Diabetes. Diplopia. Dysentery. Dyspepsia. Dyspnea. Emaciation. Emphysema. Fainting. Fever. Flatulence. ***Headaches***. Heart, disease. Hemorrhoids. ***Hoarseness. Insomnia.*** Marasmus. Migraine. ***Mountain sickness.*** Neuritis. Nervousness. ***Nosebleed. Numbness.*** Nymphomania. ***Palpitations***. Photophobia. Rheumatism. Satyriasis. Scrofula. Scurvy. ***Sleeplessness.*** Tinnitus. Trembling. Tuberculosis. Vertigo. Voice, weakness.

HERBAL - The Divine Plant of the Incas, Coca. has been used for centuries by natives of Western South America as an intoxicant and also as a remedy for "veta," the condition induced in persons on coming to live in highlands that is characterized by faintness, throbbing heart and head, and dysentery. Coca is like tea and coffee in arresting tissue-change and enabling those who take it to undergo unusual fatigues.

HOMEOPATHIC - Complaints related to mountain climbing. ***Altitude, mountain sickness.*** Palpitations, dyspnea, anxiety and insomnia. Dizziness, dyspnea and exhaustion on going to high altitudes, mountain climbing, airplane flying etc.

Exhaustion of the brain and nervous system from physical and mental strain. Muscle exhaustion. Ringing in the ears, deafness and also fever (Chin.). Tooth decay. ***Voice loss***. Nocturnal bedwetting. Emphysema (Queb.). Characteristic ***sensation as if a worm or small foreign bodies were under the skin***, moving away when touched.

Cocaine poisoning causes a sensation ***as if small foreign bodies were under the skin***, generally like grains of sand or else as of a worm under the skin.

It is known as Magnan's Symptom, after the neurologist who first described it. His description is "a sensation as if foreign bodies were under the skin, generally small round substances like grains of sand."

Korkasoff reported a case of multiple neuritis in which this symptom was present. The patient was a woman who was being treated for a uterine affection by means of vaginal tampons containing cocaine. A discontinuance of these caused the disappearance of the symptom.

MIND - Lively mood, inclination for mental work. ***Clearness of mind at night.*** Hurry in movements. Timidity. Bashful, ill at ease in society. Craves solitude, obscurity and darkness. Irritability on waking in morning. Confusion of mind. Personal appearance neglected. Deceitful. Sense of right and wrong abolished.

Melancholy from nervous exhaustion. Mental prostration alternating with exhilaration. Mental depression and drowsiness. Muddled feeling in brain. Want of will power. Forsaken feeling. Loss of energy. Unpleasant feeling about himself. Slow in finding words to express oneself.

Loquacious excitement with blissful visions. ***Great mental excitement.*** Exhilaration, before menses. Wonderful visions. Hallucinations of hearing. Very changeable mood. Pleasant fancies. Loquacious excitement with blissful visions. Sense of impending death. ***Overpowered by indescribable anxiety.*** Nervousness and nightly restlessness of children during dentition. Fear of falling when walking.

Abdomen - Tympanitic distention of abdomen. Pressure and tension in hypochondria after meals. Violent pains with bloated distention. Colic. Passage of much flatulence. Violent bellyache, better frequent discharges of inodorous flatus.

Causations - ***Ascending, high altitudes.***

Chest - Sudden attack of cramp in chest, became cold and unable to continue the ascent. Intense oppression in chest. Rush of blood to chest with slight headache. ***Heaviness and oppression of chest.*** Pain under clavicles, worse under left. Transient, shooting, in chest, between third and sixth ribs, worse during deep inspiration.

Constitutions - Suited to old people. Short-breathed people, weakly, nervous, fat, plethoric people. Children with marasmus.

Ears - Tinnitus. ***Noises in ears.*** Ringing, buzzing, and humming in ears with fever. Acute and painful hearing.

Eyes - Pressure and pain in eyes. Aching pain behind eyes causing feeling as if squinting inwards. Diplopia. Intolerance of light with dilated pupils. White, dark and fiery spots before the eyes. Flickering before the eyes. Dark cloud before eyes. Indistinct vision soon followed by headache and nausea. Pupils dilated with great photophobia. Heaviness of lids.

Female - Menses flow in gushes, awakening her from sound sleep. Nymphomania during menses and after childbirth.

Food - Retards hunger and thirst. Very little need of nourishment, even during heavy work and remarkable vigor. Great satiety for a long time. No appetite except for sweets. Aversion to solid food. Desires stimulants. Craving for alcohol and tobacco. Ailments from salt food. Can't eat salty food. Great thirst. Bad effects of stimulants, alcohol and tobacco.

Head - Fainting fit from climbing mountains. ***Headaches of high altitudes***. Headache with vertigo, preceded by flashes of light. Shocks coming from occiput with vertigo. Like a band across forehead. Migraine, worse coughing, better eating, sunset. Pressive pain in occiput. Sensation as if brain was muddled. Fullness and pressive pain in forehead. Occiput painful and tender to touch, worse coughing. Occipital headache with chilliness. Violent headache, just over eyes with low ringing in ears.

Heart - ***Angina pectoris from climbing mountains or over-exertion.*** Violent and audible palpitations with flushing. ***Violent palpitations from overexertion.*** Rapid pulse with violent sweating. Pulse extremely slow and intermittent, loses one beat in four. ***Palpitations with weak heart and dyspnea.*** Pulse weak and accelerated, increased arterial tension. Throbbing of heart against ribs audible. Exhaustion of heart with irregular action.

Kidneys - Fine stitches in female urethra before urinating. Frequent desire, with increase, flow. Film on urine. Urine smells like sweat. Yellowish red flocculent deposits, oily scum on surface. Nocturnal bedwetting. Pains in perineum at end of urination. Decrease of solids in urine. Urine turbid on standing and covered with a light pellicle.

Limbs - Weakness of limbs. Feeling of internal cold with numbness of hands and feet. Crawling, numbness of arms. When walking, takes involuntary quick steps, head inclined forward with vertigo. Rheumatism, coming from slightest cold.

Lungs - Oppressed breathing at night. ***Altitudes sickness.*** Rapid breathing. ***Want of breath, worse ascending, high altitudes.*** Cough from cold air or fast walking. ***Short of breath***, especially in aged athletes. Dyspnea of those who use tobacco or whiskey to excess. Emphysema. ***Asthma***, ***spasmodic variety.*** Senile asthma. Obstructed breathing and heaviness in chest oblige him to walk slowly. ***Incessant dyspnea***, with desire to take a deep breath. Hawking of small, transparent pieces of mucus. Expectoration of small limps like boiled starch, after rising in morning. Hemoptysis. Upper portion of both lungs as if constricted, during whole day.

Male - Diabetes with impotency (Ph-ac.). Sensation as if penis were absent. Emissions. Spermatorrhea and partial impotence. Nervous prostration from sexual excess. Satyriasis. Weakness, seminal emissions with voluptuous dreams.

Modalities - Better from wine. Better after dinner. Better lying on face. Better quick motion. Better open air. Better after sunset. Worse from cold air. ***Worse ascending, high altitudes. Worse climbing mountains.*** Worse mental or physical exertion. Worse walking. Worse sitting. Worse salty food.

Mouth - Mouth dry, especially on waking. Peppery sensation in the mouth. Tongue furred. Tooth decay. Lips blue, swollen, chapped. Lips and gums pale. Dryness of lips and mouth. Ulceration at corners of mouth. Taste salty, slimy, bitter. Taste lost in morning. Fetid breath.

Nose - Sense of smell greatly diminished. ***Nosebleed from high altitudes.*** Nosebleed passing from right to left. Sneezing, and running of clear water from nose. Heat and irritation in nostrils.

Rectum - Dysentery of high altitudes. Sphincters relaxed. Flatus from bowels, smells like burnt gunpowder. Constipation from inactivity of rectum, stools dry, like walnuts. Hemorrhoids, painful on walking or sitting. Urging to stool, followed by natural evacuation. Constipation. Constant desire to stool after gonorrhea.

Skin - Itching and prickling under the skin. ***Like a worm or insects crawling under the skin***, moving away when touched. Scarlatina-like rash over body. Increased heat of skin.

Sleep - Nervousness with nightly restlessness during teething. ***Chronic sleeplessness.*** Inclination to sleep, but can find no rest. Great drowsiness. Awakens with a shock in brain. Can find no rest anywhere, but sleepy. Awakes with a shock in brain when lying on back.

Stomach - Empty feeling or full feeling in stomach. Incarcerated flatus, rises with noise and violence, as if it would split the esophagus. Dyspepsia, especially in hypochondriacs. Hiccough after supper. Active digestion. Frequent eructations. Weak and difficult digestion.

Temperature - Sense of flushing, especially up the back with palpitations. Chilliness and headache in afternoon. At night, heat and sleeplessness, with throbbing in arteries. Night sweats. Flushes of heat on the back and burning in abdomen. Extreme weariness accompanies the fever.

Throat - ***Hoarseness***, worse after talking. Voice loss. Weak vocal cords. Uvula feels swollen, swallowing difficult. Dryness early in morning. Tuberculosis of larynx. Belchings, rise with noise and violence, as if it would split the esophagus. Tickling in fauces and pharynx. Hawking of small, transparent lumps of mucus, chiefly in morning.

Vertigo - Fainting fit from climbing mountains. Vertigo and fainting after exertion. - Vertigo with shocks coming from occiput. Vertigo with involuntary quick stepping when walking.

COMMENTS - Dr. J. W. Springthorpe described a variety of this symptoms experienced by himself and recorded in a paper entitled "The Confessions of the Cocainist." He called it "Hunting the Cocaine bug." "You imagine," he says, "that in your skin are worms or similar things, moving along.

"If you touch them with wool and especially with absorbent wool, they run away and disappear, only to peep cautiously out of some corner to see if there is any danger. These worms are projected only on the Cocainist's own person or clothing. He sees them on his linen in his skin, creeping along his penholder, but not on other, people or things and not on clothes brought clean from the laundry."

Cooper cured a case of chronic rheumatism in an aged woman who had this symptom with the fraction of a grain of cocaine given in single doses at long intervals.

In a case reported in Lancet, June, 1886, a man who had a 4 percent solution of cocaine applied to a tooth swallowed twenty to thirty drops of the solution. Half an hour after, he was seized with a feeling of faintness and giddiness followed by an attack of palpitation with a sense of flushing, especially up the back.

There was a marked diminution of smell, great difficulty in producing vomiting, a scarlatina-like rash over the body, especially about the neck, dimness of vision, relaxation of sphincters and weakness of limbs. The mind remained clear, but the pulse was fast, weak and intermittent.

A striking case was recorded in the British Medical Journal of December 13, 1890. At a meeting of the Paris Academie de Medecine on December 2nd, M. Hallopeau presented a communication after distinguishing two forms of cocaine poisoning: the acute in which the symptoms are produced immediately after a dose and speedily pass off, and the chronic in which they are due to the prolonged use of the drug.

He then related a case that in his opinion showed that the poisonous effects, while coming on acutely, might last for a considerable time. On March 7, 1890, a man had about eight milligrams of hydrochlorate of cocaine injected into his gum as a preliminary to the extraction of a tooth. Toxic symptoms at once supervened.

There was intense precordial oppression with thready pulse and extreme excitement and loquacity. The patient walked about the room, hitting out at random with his fists and crying out that he was dying. In ten minutes he became quiet and the tooth was extracted after which he was able to walk home, but arrived there in a state of extreme prostration.

Then ensued a train of nervous symptoms, such as continual headache, intractable sleeplessness, a bad taste in the mouth with attacks of excitement accompanied by giddiness, faintness, and a sense of impending death.

All brain work was impossible, the patient could not do the simplest sum in arithmetic and was in a state of profound depression. A sense of formication and numbness in the hands and forearms was almost incessant. This condition lasted four months. It was two months after the injection before the least improvement was observed, and then progress towards recovery was very slow.

M. Hallopeau thought the symptoms indicated a poisonous action of cocaine on the nervous centers and especially the brain. As it is impossible to suppose that so small a quantity of the drug should have remained in the circulation, he was driven to conclude either that it was stored up in the cells of certain nervous centers or that it produced in them persistent lesions.

Among other effects observed from its use in dentistry are "mental depression and drowsiness and intense oppression in chest, dilatation of pupils, acceleration of pulse and breathing and mental excitement."

W. J. Guernsey quoted in H. P., November, 1888 from Med. Register, August 11. 1888, the experience of J. E. Shadle who applied pledgets of a 4 percent solution of cocaine to the nasal cavities of a man of 35, preparatory to operation.

On each occasion he complained of a "cold, gone, relaxed feeling about the external genitals and a sensation as if he penis were absent. Towards the end of treatment he noticed a permanent weakness of the sexual organs and finally seminal losses and impotence set in and continued until the Cocaine was entirely withheld."

R. K. Ghosh noted experiences with Coca (which he finds in drop doses act better in such cases than in the potencies) in palpitation and dyspnea on ascending, when arising from nervous causes, especially in complaints from self-abuse generally.

After the invigorating effects of cocaine have passed off, including the sense of lightness and ability to climb a mountain without fatigue, or when the intoxication has been carried to a further degree, there is a sense of heaviness, numbness and drowsiness with a disinclination to move.

Extreme weariness, especially weakness of the legs. Extreme affects from altitude sickness. Fatigue. Characteristic headache, headaches of high altitudes. Tight headache, as if a rubber band were stretched across the forehead.

After affects from altitude sickness (Carb-v., Sil., Calc.). Can be used prophylactically if there's a history of altitude sickness or lung weakness. Asthma aggravated by altitude. Effects of cold, cough from cold air, rheumatism from slightest cold.

Excessive secretion of urine with or without sugar. Nocturnal bedwetting. General affect of relaxing the sphincters. Sensation as if the esophagus would be rent by force of rising flatus. Nymphomania after childbirth during menses, from irritation of eczema or other disorders of the vulva in satyriasis.

RELATIONS - ***Antidoted by:*** Gundlach discovered the best antidote to be Gels. ***Compare:*** (1) Ars., Guar., Cypr., Cham. (2) Arn., Calc., Ars. - effects of climbing. (3) Stram. likes company and light, Coca likes solitude and darkness. (4) Scutel., Valer., Cann-i., Thea, Coffea, Tab.

REFERENCES - Boericke. Clarke. Murphy. Phatak.

COCAINUM HYDROCHLORICUM

(Cocaine)

PHARMACY - cocain. Cocainum hydrochloricum. Cocaine. An Alkaloid from coca leaves. ***Historical dose:*** Tincture and all potencies.

CLINICAL - ***Altitude sickness.*** Angina, pectoris. Asthma. Chorea. Constipation, chronic. Cough. Deafness. Debility. Delirium tremens. Dyspnea. Fever. Glaucoma. Heart, disease. ***Hemorrhages***. Hemorrhoids. ***Mountain sickness.*** Parkinson's disease. Paralysis. Rheumatism. Scrofula. Scurvy. Trembling. Voice, weakness.

HOMEOPATHIC - The symptoms of Coca. and Cocain. are mostly similar. Besides the great usefulness of cocaine as a local anesthetic, it has specific homeopathic uses, though the symptoms are mainly clinical. ***Sensation as if small foreign bodies or worms were under the skin***. Chorea. Parkinson's disease. Delirium tremens. Alcoholic or senile trembling. Glaucoma. Paralysis.

MIND - Cerebral activity. Talkative. Insomnia. ***Irrational jealousy***. ***Moral sense blunted.*** Constant desire to do something great to ***undertake vast feats of strength. Sees and feels bugs and worms.*** Frightful persecutory hallucinations. Hallucinations of hearing. Thinks he hears unpleasant talk about himself. Personal appearance neglected.

Eyes - Glaucoma, increased tension, decreased corneal sensibility. Eyes staring, expressionless.

Head - Throbbing and bursting sensation. ***Pupils dilated***. Hearing greatly increased. Roaring and noises in head.

Nerves - Parkinson's disease, chorea, alcoholic tremors and senile trembling. Local sensory paralysis. Formication and numbness in hands and forearms.

Sensations - As if a small foreign body or a worm under the skin, seeing and feeling of bugs on his own person and on his clothes and as if parts of the body were absent (more pronounced in Cocain. than Coca.).

Sleep - Restless, cannot sleep for hours after retiring.

Stomach - Loss of appetite for solid food, ***likes sweets. Hemorrhages*** from bowels, stomach.

Temperature - Coldness with intense pallor.

Throat - Dry, burning, tickling, constricted, paralysis of muscles of deglutition. Speech difficult.

RELATIONS - Antidote to disagreeable effects occasionally resulting from injection of cocaine into skin or gums, drop doses of nitro-glycer. 1% sol. ***Compare:*** (1) Coca. (2) Stovain - an analgesic, a vaso-motor dilator.

REFERENCES - Boericke.

COCCINELLA SEPTEMPUNCTATA

(Lady Bug)

PHARMACY - cocci-s. Coccinella septempunctata. Lady bug. Coccinella. Ladybird. Sun-chafer. N. O. Coleoptera. Tincture of freshly crushed beetles. ***Historical dose:*** All potencies.

CLINICAL - Dyspnea. Face, neuralgia. Headache. Heartburn. Hiccoughs. Hydrophobia. *Neuralgia.* Tic douloureux. ***Toothaches.***

HOMEOPATHIC - Neuralgias in teeth, gums, mouth. Uvula feels too long. Awakened by profuse accumulation of saliva, vomits and complains of sore throat. Hydrophobia (Canth.). Worse by any bright object.

Back - ***Pain in region of kidneys and loins.***

Eyes - Cannot open eyes during paroxysm.

Face - Rush of blood to face. Cheeks red, especially right. Face ache. Pressure and heaviness, especially over right eye.

Food - Appetite lost.

Head - Dull headache, as from an enlargement of the brain towards the occiput. Tearing and shooting pains. Pain in forehead over right eye, sensitive to touch from superior molars to forehead. Aching in temples and occiput. Periodical attacks of frontal neuralgia. Pain worse from any bright object, better sleep.

Heart - Subdued, ***intermittent pulse***, with remission of pain in face. Contracted pulse, during toothache.

Limbs - Icy cold limbs during neuralgia.

Lungs - Dyspnea. Oppressed breathing with disappearance of pain in face.

Modalities - Worse by any bright object.

Mouth - ***Cold sensation*** in teeth and mouth (Cist.). Tobacco aggravates the tongue severely. Swollen gums.

Sleep - Nocturnal attacks of pain entirely preventing sleep, but could not sleep even when pain did not appear. Pain ends in a general heat and sleep of two or three hours, from which he wakes without any pain.

Stomach - Hiccough and burning in stomach.

Teeth - Chronic pain extending from superior molars to forehead. ***Throbbing toothache.*** Sensation of coldness in all the teeth. Painful sensation in back teeth as if they were hollow and air were forced into them. Pulsative jerking in back teeth.

Throat - Sensation in the throat as though the uvula was too long (Nux-v., when the uvula is bluish and inflamed).

Vertigo - Vertigo after cessation of toothache.

COMMENTS - Most of the symptoms appear in the teeth and nerves of the face and mouth. Neuralgia, worse at night, accompanied by icy cold limbs and cold, moist skin, the right side is most affected. Pains extend from one part to another and may jump from side to side.

Attacks recur periodically, often of brief duration but quickly recurring. Attacks are generally worse at night, but may be entirely absent in the night. Returning every eight, ten, twelve, fourteen or twenty days.

RELATIONS - ***Compare:*** (1) Canth., Mang. (2) in tic douloureux, Spig., Thuj.

REFERENCES - Boericke. Clarke.

COCCULUS INDICUS

(Indian Cockle)

PHARMACY - cocc. Cocculus indicus. Indian cockle. Anamirta cocculus. Menisperma cocculus. N. O. Menispermacae. A tincture is prepared from the powered seeds, which contain a crystallizable principle picrotoxine, a powerful poison. ***Historical dose:*** All potencies.

CLINICAL - Amenorrhea. Anger, ill effects. Anorexia. Asthma. Bones, disorders. Bulimia. Cerebro-spinal, meningitis. Chills. Choking. Chorea. Colic. Convulsions. Coryza. Cough. ***Cramps. Debility.*** Dysmenorrhea. Dyspnea. Faintness. ***Fatigue, chronic.*** Fevers. ***Grief.*** Hangovers. Headaches. Hemorrhoids. Hernia. Hiccoughs. Influenza. Intermittent, fever. ***Insomnia. Jet, lag.*** Knee, weakness. Memory, weakness. Meniere's disease. Meningitis. Mental, excitement. Menstrual, problems. Menstruation, painful. Mononucleosis. Morning sickness. ***Motion sickness. Muscles, weak. Nausea. Night-watching.*** Numbness. ***Nursing, others***. Overexertion. Palpitations. Paralysis. ***Paralytic, pain***. Parotiditis. Rheumatism. ***Seasickness. Sleep, deprivation. Sleep, loss.*** Somnolence. ***Spasms.*** Spinal, irritation. ***Sympathetic.*** Tympany. Ulcers. ***Vertigo. Vomiting.***

HERBAL - Cocculus has been used from ancient times as a poison for stupefying fish and making them easy to catch. It produces great disturbance of the sensorium and the symptoms of intoxication in human beings. Commonly used as an adulteration of beer to heighten its intoxicating properties. A decoction of cocculus is a domestic remedy used locally for destroying head or body lice.

HOMEOPATHIC - Paralysis of face tongue, pharynx, paraplegia with numbness and tingling. Numbness. ***Sensation of hollowness or emptiness,*** head, chest, abdomen. As if single parts had gone to sleep. Too weak to hold up head, stand or even speak. Feels too weak to talk loud.

Symptoms are worse riding in a cars, airplanes, trains or on shipboard, hence its use in ***motion sickness, seasickness***. Sleep loss and fatigue from travels.

Vertigo and dizziness with nausea and vomiting. Ailments from ***loss of sleep or nursing of loved ones.*** Speech difficult at beginning of attacks of vertigo, afterwards, difficulty in reading and thinking.

Alternating symptoms. Unilateral disorders. Sensitive to cold. Falls down to ground unconscious. Senses acute. Slowness in moving, answering, wants plenty of time to do everything. Adenitis with cold, hard glandular swellings. Valuable remedy in hernias, both umbilical and inguinal, is particularly indicated when abdominal muscles are weak and it seems as if a hernia would easily take place.

Shuddering. ***Painful contracture*** of limbs and trunk, tetanus. Tremors of head, lower jaw from excitement, exertion, pain. Intentional tremors. Twitching of isolated groups of muscles. Spasms, through the body like electric shocks. Cramps in muscles, in masseters, in abdomen, dysmenorrhea in the heart. Convulsions from non-appearance or suddenly checked menses.

MIND - Mind benumbed with vertigo, nausea. ***Mental fatigue from sleep deprivation.*** Heavy and stupid feelings. ***Ailments from loss of sleep.*** Spacey. Dazed. ***Night-watching.*** Things seem unreal. Slowness of comprehension, must read a passage over several times in order to understand it. Memories are bad or blank out at times. Memory lost. Distracted easily forgets what he has just thought. When her mind is turned away from herself her sufferings are forgotten.

Generally very sympathetic to others. ***Ailments from the nursing of loved ones.*** Thoughts fixed on one unpleasant subject. ***Profound grief and sadness***. Sadness as if from insult. Depression. Despair feels as if incurable. Mild, indolent and despondent in the face of difficulties.

Sits as if absorbed in deep and sad thoughts and observes nothing about her. Indulges in sad reveries. Dwells on past disagreeable occurrences. Answers slowly reflects long. Tearful chagrin about least trifle. Weeping spells, especially if they can't function and do the things they want to.

Mental confusion after drinking and eating. Very anxious about health of others, but little concerned as to his own health. ***Sudden great anxiety.*** Anxiety before menses. Anxiety from night-watching. Anxiety during sleep. Mind is worse from suppressed menses. Weeping during menses.

Fear of not getting proper amount of sleep. Fear of death. Fears the unknown, danger. Especially fear surrounding health and illness of others. Fear of ghosts and specters. Excitement after hearing horrible things. Frighten easily from noises. Fear of sudden noises.

Oversensitive to everything. Very sensitive to fear, anger, grief and all mental disturbances. Sensitive moods, everything worries and offends. Startles very easily. Easily offended, cannot bear contradiction. Sentimental. Sensitive to noise and touch. ***Intolerance of noise.*** Intolerance of any disturbing influence. Sensitive to insults, slights and disappointment.

Capricious. Vacillatory, doesn't accomplish anything at her work. Excessive irritability, excited by loud talking or least increase of temperature. ***Anger from any interruptions.*** Anger from contradiction. Enlargement of liver after anger. Starting, with trembling all over body, from slight noise or slight unexpected touch.

Irresistible inclination to sing. Absorbed in reveries. Sensitive to all external impressions. Speaks hastily. Talkative, witty, joking, dancing, gesticulating. Sees something alive on walls, floor, chair etc. ***Time passes too quickly.*** Alcoholics, reeling, roaring, quarrelsome, singing. Loud cries of despair and irritation, alternating with stupefaction of brain. Feeling as after committing a wicked deed, with desire to escape.

Abdomen - Bloated with intestinal gas. Great rumbling in bowels. Colic, flatus, twisting pain with faintness and salivation. Flatulent colic in pregnancy. Cramps in epigastrium with difficulty in breathing. Cramps deep in abdomen, instead of menses. ***Abdominal muscles weak***, as if a hernia would take place. Inguinal hernia is apt to protrude and become incarcerated. Umbilical hernia, with obstinate constipation. ***Pain in abdominal ring,*** as if something were forced through. Pains in region of spleen. ***As if full of sharp stones,*** on every movement. Emptiness and sensation of hollowness in abdomen. Sensation as if bowels would fall out. Hypochondria as if beaten. Ulcerative colitis.

Back - Drawing, lacerating or boring pains. Pressure in scapula and nape. ***Pain in shoulder and arms as if bruised.*** Stiffness on moving shoulders. Stiffness in cervical muscles, with great weakness. ***Paralytic pain in small of the back.*** Paralysis from lumbar region downward. Spinal weakness in lumbar region, worse walking. Weak neck, cannot hold up head. Trembling in back. Cracking or stiffness of vertebrae.

Breasts - Shivering over breasts.

Causations - Ill effects of anger, fright, grief, anxiety, disappointment. ***Sleep loss. Nursing loved ones. Ill effects of night-watching***. Overstrain mental and physical, traveling. ***Motion sickness.*** Noise. Hot or cold air. Sun. Tea-drinking.

Chest - Sensation of emptiness or of cramps in chest. Audible rumbling in chest (left side), as from emptiness, worse walking. Hysterical cramps in chest with sighing and moaning. Cramping, in chest during menstrual period. Pressure under ribs, better belching. Fine stitches in various parts of chest. Contractive tension of right side of chest, taking away the breath. Oppression in chest, better after vomiting of green mucus.

Constitutions - Suited to light haired, timid, nervous, persons, bookworms, unmarried, childless women. Sensitive, romantic girls. Light-haired females, especially during pregnancy, causing much nausea and backache.

Cough - Cough from choking in throat. Fatiguing, from oppression of chest. Cough worse indulging disposition to cough. Spasmodic cough, in anemic and hysterical women. Cough from choking in throat.

Ears - Sensitive to hearing, dreads sudden noise. Feel closed (right). Noises as from rushing water. Hardness of hearing. Pain as if ears torn out of head with headache. Meniere's disease, ringing in the ears, oozy and loss of balance. Roaring or ringing in ears.

Eyes - Pain as if eyes torn out of head, during headache. Eyes open and immovable. Eyes dull and glassy. Eyes closed with the balls constantly rolling about in spasms. Protruding eyes. Jerking of eyelids. Pressure as from dust in eyes. Eyelids inflamed. Dryness of lids. Eyelids feel as if paralyzed. Bruised pain in eyes, with inability to open lids at night. Sharp or shooting pains in eyes from within outward. Pupils, contracted or dilated.

Face - Bloated, distorted and cold to touch. Blue margins around eyes. Flushed hot face and head during vertigo or unconsciousness. Countenance devoid of any signs of mental activity. Heat in face, and redness of cheeks, even in a cold room. Earthy countenance, with painful expression. Paralysis of facial nerve of one sided. Lines of face deepened, it seems drawn. ***Cramp-like pain in masseter muscle, worse opening the mouth.*** Prosopalgia in afternoon with wide radiations of pain. Tearing pains. Swelling of parotid glands. Swelling and induration of submaxillary glands.

Female - Amenorrhea causes mental alienation. Sudden cessation of menses. Menses, too early, profuse. Menses too often. Menses gushes out in stream when rising on feet on tiptoe. Menses clotted, with spasmodic colic. Cutting, cramping pain in region of uterus and ovaries, on appearance of menses. ***Weak during menstruation, scarcely able to stand.*** Dysmenorrhea with profuse dark menses. As if uterus were distended, during dysmenorrhea. Dysmenorrhea followed by hemorrhoids. Clutching in uterus. Purulent, gushing leucorrhea between menses or in place of menses. ***Leucorrhea very weakening***, can scarcely speak. Leucorrhea gushing, when squatting and stooping during pregnancy with frequent urging to urinate. Discharge of bloody mucus from uterus during pregnancy. Hour-glass contraction of uterus with terrible pain in lumbar region. Labor pains spasmodic and irregular.

Food - All symptoms and affections, worse eating or drinking. Loss of appetite. Loathing of food and drink. Disgust for smell of food (Colch.). ***Nausea when merely looking at the food, at the thought or smell of food.*** Aversion to beer, acids, sour things. ***Aversion to food***. Aversion to drink, tobacco. Desire for cold drinks, but eating or drinking anything cold causes tearing in limbs. Desires beer. Worse from coffee. Thirst, without desire to drink. ***Confusion and vertigo after drinking, eating.*** Will eat nothing but bread and water, at other times eats ravenously. Bulimia. Food tastes as if salted too little, tobacco tastes bitter. Thirstless.

Head - Congestion of blood to head, with mental derangement. ***Sick headache from carriage riding***, cannot lie on back part of head. ***Pain in occiput*** and nape worse lying on it, better bending backwards, worse coffee. Migrain headaches. Headaches unable to bear least light, noise causes nausea and vomiting. Headaches from working in sun. Headache as if skull would burst. Headache returning at each menstrual period. Sensation of emptiness or hollowness in head. Opening and shutting sensation, especially in occiput. Dullness and confusion of head, worse reading. Heavy head. Convulsive trembling of head from weakness of muscles of neck. Cramps in left temporal muscles. Trembling of the head. Throbbing in forehead. Tossing of head and incessant trembling of hands.

Heart - Palpitations, worse quick motion, mental excitement, with vertigo and faintness. Endocarditis. Nervous palpitations. Palpitations after rheumatism. During an attack of palpitation has vertigo and sensation as if about to faint. Pulse small, hard and frequent. Pulse often imperceptible, weak. Pulse seldom hard and somewhat accelerated. Feels pulse beat through whole body during heat, at times palpitation.

Kidneys - Frequent desire to urinate with small discharge in pregnant women. Watery urine. Tensive, aching pain in orifice of urethra, between acts of urination. Itching and stinging near fossa navicularis. Involuntary urination during epileptic attack. Diuresis, during prosopalgia.

Limbs - Limbs go to sleep. Lower limbs are very weak, numb and unsteady. Lameness, worse by bending. Paraplegia. One-sided paralysis, worse after sleep. ***Painful stiffness in all joints.*** Acute rheumatism, pain springing from joint to joint, with redness, swelling and stiffness. Limbs straightened out, painful when flexed or vice versa. ***Trembling and pain in limbs.*** Clumsy gait. Edema of feet with paralysis of lower limbs. ***Knees crack on motion***. Humerus feels broken. Soles numb, while sitting. Involuntary motion of right arm and right leg, better during sleep. Alternation of pain between arms. Pain in shoulder and arms as if bruised. Hands, numb or hot and cold alternately become numb on grasping objects, trembles while eating. Hands and feet become cold after change of position. ***Violent spasms of arms and legs.*** Takes hold of things awkwardly and drops them. Bones feel as if they were broken.

Liver - Liver more painful after anger, worse least jar. Enlargement of liver after anger. Sharp pains in liver region. Pressive pain in hepatic region worse coughing and bending over.

Lungs - Dyspnea as from constriction of trachea, as if irritated by smoke. Choking constriction in upper part of esophagus, oppressing breathing and inducing cough. Hysterical asthma. Dyspnea, oppressing breathing and inducing cough. Shortness of breath, on account of tension in abdomen. Quick, anxious and oppressed breathing. Slow, heavy and laborious breathing. Panting. Dyspnea from pain in bowels during diarrheic stool, in amenorrhea.

Male - Drawing, sore pain in testes when touched. Genitals sensitive with desire for sex. Sexual desire increased alternating with decreased. Seminal emissions at night. Itching of scrotum.

Modalities - Better from sitting. Better lying quiet, on side. Better in a warm room. Worse eating or drinking. ***Worse from motion of trains, boat, cars.*** Worse from motion. Worse exertion. Worse rising from bed. Worse bending over or stooping. Worse kneeling, walking. Worse swimming. Worse swallowing saliva. ***Worse from loss of sleep.*** Worse from touch, pressure. Worse jar, pain. Worse emotions, anxiety. ***Worse from nursing others.*** Worse at menses. Worse eating. Worse noise. Worse sun, cold, open air. Worse evening, night. Worse midnight and 1 a.m. Worse warmth of bed.

Mouth - Dryness and burning of mouth and throat. Dryness of mouth at night, without thirst. ***Metallic taste with loss of appetite.*** Coppery, metallic, sour taste after coughing. Taste, sour, offensive. Taste like sulphur, putrid, nauseous. Food tastes as if salted too little, tobacco tastes bitter. Tremor of lower jaw and chattering of teeth, when attempting to speak. Foamy phlegm from mouth. Salivation during nausea and vertigo. Thick saliva. Corner of mouth, wing of nose and tip of tongue distorted. Lips parched and dry. Corners of mouth sore.

Nose - Swelling of the nose. Coryza, with ulcerated nostrils. Very acute sense of smell. Worse from strong odors. Sense of smell weak. Ulcerated nostrils. Discharge from nose bloody, pus-like.

Perspiration - Sweat from slight exertion, on affected part. Cold sweat now of one, now of the other hand. Cold sweat only on face. Sweat stands out in drops on face, is now cold and then again hot. Exhausting sweat over whole body. Sweat in morning, principally on chest. Sweat from pain in bowels. Sweat during diarrheic stool.

Rectum - Burning pain in rectum with soft, loose stool, sometimes yellow. Diarrhea brought on by riding in cars or carriage. Diarrhea is better lying on sides. Diarrhea with bilious vomiting. Constipation, with ineffectual urging to stool on account of lack of peristaltic motion. Bleeding hemorrhoids. Prolapsed rectum after stool. After stool, violent tenesmus, even unto fainting. Contraction of rectum, during too early menses.

Skin - Skin feels soft, is white and moist. Paleness of skin, wretched color. Itching of skin from warmth. Burning and itching as from nettles. Great itching, especially in the evening, worse undressing, in a feather bed. Ulcers very sensitive to touch. Red pimples, like grains of millet. Miliary eruptions or red spots, worse undressing. Induration, cold swelling of the glands, with stinging pains. Red irregular spots on chest and behind ears. Pimples filling with pus, and then drying up and disappearing.

Sleep - *Loss of sleep,* complaints from night-watching, nursing. ***Slightest loss of sleep aggravates.*** Coma vigil. ***Insomnia.*** Sleepless from mental or physical exhaustion. Constant drowsiness, after loss of sleep, night-watching, nursing. ***Sleep deprivation.*** Spasmodic yawning with hiccough. ***Sleepless from nursing of others.*** Sleeplessness from business thoughts, from anxiety and restlessness. Anxious frightful dreams. Sleep frequently interrupted by waking and starting. Sleep unrefreshing. Maniacal sleeplessness. Dreams are anxious, frightful.

Stomach - Esophagus is dry, burning. Putrid eructations. Gastralgia from suppression of menses. Violent cramp in stomach, griping, squeezing, lacerating sensation. Cramps in stomach with flatulence and much saliva. ***Motion sickness.*** Seasickness. Sensation of hunger or emptiness, even to fainting. ***Nausea and vomiting from riding in cars, boats or looking at boat in motion.*** Nausea with faintness and vomiting, worse on becoming cold or taking cold. Nausea, rising to head or felt in head. Retching. ***Vomiting of sour bitter.*** Bad odor, of vomit, with profuse flow of saliva. Vomiting with headache, pain in bowels. Vomiting on taking cold, with syncope. Vomiting from cerebral tumors. Vomiting from loud talk. Cramp in stomach during and after meal. Hiccough and spasmodic yawning. Chronic dyspepsia from prolong study. Morning sickness.

Stool - Small, frequent stools with flatus. Foul-smelling stool, during colic. Hard stool every other day, expelled with great difficulty. Watery stools, none in night, but comes on directly after rising from bed. Simultaneous with vomiting, sudden, thin, black, slimy, very fetid stool. Disposition to stool, but peristaltic motion in upper intestines is wanting. Thin, whitish-yellow watery stool. Fetid or hot flatus, emission of hot flatus before stool.

Teeth - Teeth feel chilly. Teeth as if long and loose. Pain in teeth, better when biting with empty mouth. Toothache in hollow tooth, pains only when chewing, even soft food. Toothache in upper incisors. Toothache with headache and ringing in ears. Drawing pain in dental nerves. Fine drawing pain in borders of teeth.

Temperature - Chills alternating with fever. Chills in evening and shivering. ***Chilliness with perspiration and heat of skin.*** Chills with flatulent colic, nausea, vertigo, coldness of lower limbs and heat of head. Chills with great disgust at even smell of food. Internal chill with great trembling of head. Upward and downward shaking chills. Chills running down back, in evening. ***Nervous form of low fever from fits of anger.*** Dry heat, the whole night through. Flushes of heat, with burning heat of cheeks and cold feet. Heat in head, chilliness in body. Burning heat and redness of cheeks.

Throat - Constriction in throat, with difficult breathing and inclination to cough. Paralysis of the muscles preventing swallowing. Tickling in throat with lachrymation. Tightness in larynx. Voice whimpering and tremulous. Speech difficult, during vertigo. Sensation of constriction. Pressive pain in tonsils, worse when swallowing saliva than when swallowing food.

Tongue - Bitter taste at root of tongue. Complains of dryness of tongue, which is moist and clean. Dry, rough tongue. Dry tongue, with whitish-yellow coat, without thirst. Tongue coated white and dry upon edges. Pains at base of tongue when stretching tongue out. Tongue, as if paralyzed, speech difficult or hasty, pains at the base when protruded. Root of tongue as if swollen.

Vertigo - Vertigo, nausea when riding or sitting up. ***Seasickness and motion sickness*** (Tab.). Vertigo and dizziness, with nausea and vomiting. ***Vertigo when riding in a car or train.*** Vertigo on sitting up. ***Vertigo worse watching moving surroundings.*** Vertigo with palpitations, worse in morning, raising head, felt in forehead. ***Vertigo from loss of sleep.*** Constant sensation as if about to faint. Vertigo as if intoxicated.

Vision - Dim vision with black spots before eyes. Dark spots before eyes, though objects appear clearly. While reading, can only see left half of line of writing. Black spots seen after reading.

COMMENTS - Chiefly affects the right hypochondrium (especially liver), inner hypogastrium, inner forehead, back, upper arm and the bones of the arm. Irritable weakness. Slowness and numbness over their body (Calc., Alum.).

Vertigo and dizziness, with nausea and vomiting. Attacks of vertigo with confusion as if they are lost. Nauseated with whirling sensation. Sensation as if drunk because everything spins (Con., when turning in bed). Seasickness and motion sickness (Tab.). Motion sickness brought on by trying to read while riding in a car or train, or from looking out the window at things going by, from seeing a moving object. Jet lag.

Nerve exhaustion, weakness. Too tired to sleep. Chronic fatigue since loss of sleep or stress. Twilight sleepers, chronic insomnia with no recollection of sleeping, although they sleep for small amounts. Wake unrefreshed. excited nervous system (Coff.), worse coffee. All symptoms worse from loss of sleep. Conditions caused by loss of sleep and night-watching. May be used prophylactically to prevent conditions arising from loss of sleep.

Stinging pains, stitches, constriction in the hands, a pithy feeling. Sensitive to touch. The least jar is unbearable. Keynote empty, hollow feeling in the body, lungs, stomach, legs. Hollow weakness. Sensation of hollowness or emptiness in the head or other parts. Sense of lightness of the body. Opening and shutting sensation, especially in the occiput. Sinking feeling.

Paralytic pains or pains as of dislocation. Paralytic weakness, lax muscles. Weakness of neck muscles with heaviness of head. Migratory numbness. Sensation as if single parts have gone to sleep. Neurological problems, locomotor ataxia, incoordination, stumbling, lack of control, and the knees tend to give out.

Immovability of parts affected. Ataxia, staggering gait. Paralytic rigidity. Limbs become very painful to flex, but they often continuously bend them to obtain relief. Rigid limbs, chorea, involuntary motions (Caust.). Cramp, spasm, etc., coupled with electric-like shooting pain. Faintness from the pain. Joint rheumatism, ulcers, neuralgic disorders of bones.

Esophageal spasms. In the elderly, spasms can cause food to get stuck, inability to swallow (Caust.). Sensation of worms crawling in the stomach, pinches and scrapes in the stomach (Coloc.). Inguinal hernias (Nux-v., Lyc.). Hemorrhoids during menses. Metallic, bitter taste in the mouth. Desires beer. Drunkenness and hangovers (Nux-v.).

Meniere's disease, ringing in the ears, oozy and loss of balance. Poor vision with weak eye muscles. Dimness of eyesight. Severe occipital headache, sense that head opens and closes. Flu or mononucleosis with loss of sleep.

Morning sickness, when they can't stand the sight, thought and smell of food, especially when they are in the car (Colch.). Amenorrhea, may have vaginal discharge instead of period. Symptoms may be worse with menses.

Cocc. cured a case of delirium at onset of menses during first and second days, the patient said, "I always see something alive, on wall, floor, chairs or anywhere, always rolling and will roll on me."

A case of "spasmodic, flatulent colic, about midnight, flatus passed without relief," recurring several nights, was cured by Cocc. 3x. Lippe cured a case of enlargement of the liver after childbirth, the indication being "the liver was more painful after anger."

RELATIONS - ***Antidotes:*** Coff., Nux-v. ***Compare:*** (1) Picrotoxin - alkaloid of Cocculus - epilepsy, attacks in the morning on leaving horizontal position, hernia, locomotor ataxia, night-sweats. (2) Symphoricarpus - morning sickness. (3) Petr., Calad., Puls., Ign.

REFERENCES - Boericke. Clarke. Murphy. Phatak.

COCCUS CACTI

(Cochineal)

PHARMACY - coc-c. Coccus cacti. Cochineal. Dactylopius coccus. N. O. Hemiptera. An insect infesting cactus plants. The tincture is prepared from the dried bodies of the female insects. They also constitute a well-known dye. ***Historical dose:*** Trituration and all potencies.

CLINICAL - Anasarca. Anuria. Ascites. Asthma. Backache. Dysuria. Catarrh. ***Coughs.*** Gonorrhea. Gravel. Hemorrhages. Heart, disorders. Impotence. Irritation, nerves. Labia, inflammation. Menorrhagia. Nephritis. Spasms. Tinnitus. Tuberculosis. Uric acid, diathesis. ***Vomiting. Whooping, cough.***

HOMEOPATHIC - Coccus Cacti has sometimes been confounded with the Coccinella septempunctata, both are insects known as "Cochenille" in French.

Coc-c. causes a catarrhal condition and irritation of the throat, respiratory and genito-urinary organs. Affects the mucus membranes. Spasmodic morning cough. ***Whooping cough attacks end with vomiting of tough mucus***. Regular paroxysms or violent tickling, ***hacking cough*** ending in vomiting or raising ***much clear ropy mucus,*** hanging from mouth.

General lassitude. The least exertion causes lassitude and tendency to perspire or cough, worse during exercise. Pain in occiput is worse mental exertion. Intolerable internal itchings, burning like pepper. Pulsation in different organs. Sensation as of a fluid forcing its way during pain. Spasms.

Spasmodic pains in kidneys with visceral tenesmus. Catarrhal conditions of the bladder. Anuria. Ascites. Anasarca. ***Discharges are stringy,*** including hemorrhages, which are apt to be in large, black clots. Rising up causes hemorrhage with passage of large clots from uterus. Periodic symptoms.

MIND - Confusion, better open air. Apprehensive, irritable, fretful. Anxiety after eating. Anxiety from irregular action of heart. Lively, talkative mood. Excitement after beer. Delusions of being enlarged. Sadness, early morning on waking. Sadness afternoon 2 p.m. to 3 p.m.

Abdomen - Excruciating pain from left iliac region, extending to the groins half way down the thighs, as if fluid were forcing its way there.

Back - Coldness in back.

Constitutions - Uric acid, gouty, rheumatic diathesis.

Cough - Cough from rawness in air-passages. Short paroxysms, followed by easy expectoration of globules of mucus. Suffocative cough, worse first waking, with tough, white mucus, which strangles. ***Whooping cough attacks end with vomiting of tough mucus.*** Spasmodic cough in morning, worse 6 a.m. or 7 a.m. Spasmodic cough on first rising. ***Regular attacks of violent, tickling, racking coughs ending in vomiting or raising much clear ropy mucus.*** Periodical coughs, slowly increasing then gradually decreasing in its intensity, better cold air or cold drinks. Cough worse warm room. Violent cough, caused by brushing teeth, by rinsing mouth, by trying to clear throat of viscid mucus. Coughs of alcoholics.

Ears - Cracking in ears, when swallowing.

Eyes - Sensation as of a foreign body between the upper lid and the eyeball.

Face - Crawling sensation. Becomes purple, red worse coughing.

Female - Menses too early, profuse, ***black*** and thick, ***dark clots*** with dysuria. Large clots escape from the vagina when passing urine, when quiet or when rising up. Intermittent menses, flow only in the evening or at night. ***Inflamed labia.*** Vulva sensitive, worse when urinating.

Head - Throbbing pain with sensation as if fluid were forcing its way. Suboccipital soreness, worse after sleep and exertion. Headache, worse from lying on back, better with the head high. Dull pain over right eye in morning. ***Sensation of a foreign body between upper lid and eyeball.*** Distress from cinders in eye.

Heart - Sensation as if everything were pressed toward the heart.

Kidneys - Region of kidneys painful to pressure. Constant urging to urinate, better after passing blood clots from the vagina in females. Sticking pain along ureters. Lancinating, violent pain from kidneys to bladder with dysuria. ***Urine, brick-red sediment. urinary stones, hematuria, urates*** and uric acid. Deep-colored, thick urine. Nephritis. Nephritic colic.

Limbs - Sensation as if a fine splinter were under the fingernails.

Lungs - Fauces very sensitive. Walking against wind takes breath away. Shortness of breath. Chronic bronchitis complicated with gravel, large quantities of albuminous, tenacious mucus, are expectorated. Constant hawking from enlarged uvula, coryza with inflamed fauces.

Male - Pulsation in glans.

Modalities - Better from washing in cold water. Better cold drinks. Better walking. Worse left side. Worse after sleep. Worse touch, pressure of clothing. Worse slightest exertion. Worse periodically, from heat, cold exposure, lying down, night and early morning, awakening, brushing teeth, irritation of throat, rinsing mouth. Cough worse on waking.

Mouth - Tip of tongue burns like pepper. Sweetish, metallic taste. Salivation, constant desire to spit. Loud speaking or brushing of teeth causes cough.

Nose - Burning as of pepper in nostrils. Accumulation of thick viscid mucus in naso-pharynx.

Sensations - As if a ball or stone lying in stomach. Raging pain as though a fluid were injected into a small blood vessel. As if something ascending towards stomach. As of mucus ascending and descending trachea, as of a plug of mucus moving in chest. As if head would split.

Stomach - Irritation of throat, hawking, brushing of the teeth causes retching and vomiting. Thirst, drinks water often and in large quantities.

Temperature - Burning, as of pepper.

Throat - Sensation as of a thread hanging down the back of the throat. Sensation as if uvula is elongated. ***Tickling in larynx***. Any irritation in throat causes cough, retching and vomiting. Constricted throat or as of a plug lodged in it. Profuse post-nasal discharge. Accumulation of much viscid mucus, hawking it, excites cough, retching and vomiting.

COMMENTS - Coc-c. acts especially on mucus membranes, kidneys (Canth.), and in causing hemorrhages in disturbing the heart (Cact.). Hemorrhages are apt to be in large black clots, especially hemorrhages from kidneys and uterus.

Sensation as if a hair or crumb were lodged behind the larynx and as if a thread were hanging down the back of the throat causing a cough. "Cough, worse in morning, the child awakens and is immediately seized with a paroxysm of coughing ending in vomiting clear, ropy mucus hanging in long string from the mouth."

Rapid, spasmodic coughs in periodic attacks. Constant irritating cough. Sense of dry spot or tickle. Hoarseness. Fatigue of vocal organs. Violent tickling in larynx. Stitching and ulcerating pains below clavicles, especially left. Whooping cough (Dros., Cupr.), bronchitis.

Lancinating, stitching and pricking sensations. Itching, sticking and biting in various parts of the skin, red spots and itching pimples. Sharp pains and itching of glans penis, symptoms of the passage of small stones.

General sensitiveness to touch and pressure, rinsing mouth or brushing teeth causes cough and vomiting. Most symptoms worse from warmth, cough worse entering warm room, throat worse by warmth of bed. Tickling in trachea and cough better open air. Teeth very sensitive to cold. Catarrh worse on slightest exposure. Catarrh from autumn until warm weather.

Berridge cured with Coc-c. a case of gonorrhea, guided by the symptom "excruciating pain in left iliac region extending to groin and halfway down thigh, as if a fluid were forcing its way there."

Kunkel recorded the case of a man, 75, who suffered from nocturnal bedwetting up to the age of seven. When almost 20 he frequently passed large quantities of uric acid and at the same time he began to have symptoms of chronic catarrh of the colon, frequent scanty stools, much mucus, cross humor, itching anus, threatening of hemorrhoids but no bleeding.

Insomnia soon followed. Coc-c. 2c and 3c was given without benefit. Aqua calcis did some good, but not much. In three successive years he was sent to Carlsbad with good results to the intestinal catarrh, the sleeplessness was untouched.

Gradually all kinds of arthritic symptoms developed, especially in knees. There was occasionally a considerable flow of urine and the more copious it was the better the patient slept and the less pain in the joints. The same relief followed an attack of diarrhea.

Four weeks at Assmanhausen caused the excretion of large quantities of uric acid one year, but had no effect the next and the knee got worse. Wiesbaden helped one year but not the next.

Half a tumbler of Kronenquelle water drunk every morning helped the knee and enabled him to walk better than he had for a long time. In three or four years, the excretions of uric acid had ceased and the patient's state grew worse, insomnia recurred, diarrhea became much more frequent.

A fortnight previous to such attack, the patient noticed he had great aversion to butcher's meat. Coc-c. 30c morning and evening was given. Gradually sleep returned. There was almost daily excretion of uric acid, sometimes in the form of large shot, the diarrhea ceased and the patient went about his work with pleasure.

RELATIONS - ***Compare:*** (1) Canth., Cact., Oci., Sars. (2) apices of lungs sore, tenacious mucus, Kali-bi. (3) Many Cactus symptoms, like the pricking and sticking pains, heart disturbances, reappear in the pathogenesis of this Cactus-fed insect.

REFERENCES - Boericke. Clarke. Murphy. Phatak.

COCHLEARIA ARMORACIA

(Horse Radish)

PHARMACY - coch. Cochlearia armoracia. Horse radish. Armoracia sativa. Armoracia rusticana. N. O. Crucifer. Tincture of root. ***Historical dose:*** Tincture and all potencies.

CLINICAL - Albuminuria. Aphonia. Asthma. ***Backache***. Cataract. ***Colic.*** Cornea, spots. Coryza. Eruptions. Eyes, disorders. ***Flatulence***. Gonorrhea. Gravel. Headaches. Impotency. Leucorrhea. Lungs, edema. Rheumatism. Scurvy. Strangury. Toothache. Ulcers. Urinary, disorders.

HERBAL - Cochlearia and Cochlearia officinalis (Coch-o), are old-world anti-scorbutics, and the homeopathic provings have confirmed the old experience. Coch. has the anti-scorbutic properties of the other Cruciferae and is specially efficacious in scurvy from eating salt. The essential oil is said to be identical with that of Sinapis.

Coch. is useful as a condiment in enfeebled states of the stomach. Raises the vital forces. An infusion of the root in cider, for dropsy, causes copious diuresis. Locally cures dandruff. Used as a gargle in scorbutic gums and sore throat. Hoarseness and in relaxed conditions of the fauces.

HOMEOPATHIC - Affects the mucus membranes. Frontal bone and sinus, antrum and salivary glands are specifically affected by this remedy. Mucus stools. Bloated sensation. Gonorrhea. Leucorrhea. Asthma and tuberculosis.

The peculiar symptoms are in connection with the teeth. Some violent abdominal pains were experienced. ***Colic with backache.*** Wandering chronic rheumatism. Tearing pains from the belly through to back, down the back and settling in sacrum.

MIND - Anxiety, driven to despair by pain Difficult thinking in evening. Irresolution Melancholy alternating with merriness Worse from nervous excitement. Worse from vexation.

Abdomen - Spasms through to back and loins. Borborygmi in morning. Crampy tensive pain above epigastrium apparently in diaphragm, better by bending forward

Back - Pain in back as from ***incarcerated flatulence*** from abdomen through to back and down into sacrum.

Causations - Checked foot sweat. Nervous excitement. Cold.

Chest - Chest painful to touch.

Eyes - Traumatic inflammation of eyes and cataract. Lachrymation. Swelling of eyes. ***Sore and scrofulous***. Spots on cornea. Copious running from eyes. Obscuration of sight for some minutes. Styes. Rheumatic ophthalmia.

Face - Twitching of left corner of mouth, 4 a.m. Soreness of upper lip.

Female - Stringy black blood passes from the vagina when urinating, also during the night. Menses every ten or fifteen days. Menses suppressed with chlorosis. Leucorrhea. Since menopause, cramp in stomach.

Food - Unnatural craving for food with profuse, painless diarrhea.

Head - Pressing, boring pain as if frontal bone would fall out. Violent headache with vomiting. Headache, now one side now the other, worse opening the eyes (wide), but not on reading or motion. Violent headache with nausea, worse sitting up. Aching, boring pains in head, as if brain bursting. Impaired hearing.

Kidneys - Burning and cutting at glans penis before, during, and after urination. Frequent urination. Increased desire and increased secretion. Urination difficult, causing burning, tenderness and inflammation of urethra as in first stage of gonorrhea. Strangury. Gravel. Albuminuria. Uneasiness in region of kidneys.

Limbs - Twitching in limbs. Towards morning, pain in all joints when lying still, worse lying on side, better on motion and when getting up. Suppressed foot sweat.

Lungs - Promotes expectoration and relieves cough, increases activity of respiratory organs. Dry, hacking, laryngeal cough, also after influenza cough, dry or loose, worse lying down. Coryza with hoarseness. Mucus asthma and tuberculosis. Edema of lungs. Throat feels rough and hoarse. Aphonia with blood-spitting, oppressed breathing.

Male - Burning or cutting at glans before, during or after urination. Gonorrhea. Impotence.

Modalities - Bending forward better. Touch or slight pressure aggravates many symptoms. Worse evening and night.

Mouth - Paralysis of tongue. Biting sensation on tongue. Tongue furred white. Very offensive odor from mouth and lungs.

Rectum - Tenesmus all night until morning, sometimes discharging a little blood. Profuse painless diarrhea with craving for food. Diarrhea after great nervous excitement. Mucus stools. Involuntary passage of mucus from anus. Itching and burning at anus.

Sleep - Very refreshing, awoke with clearer mind than usual.

Stomach - Belching and cramps. Belchings of sulphurous odor like garlic. Bilious regurgitations. Pain towards back, worse pressure on dorsal vertebrae. Colic with backache. ***Violent cramp from stomach through both sides around to back***. Gripping around navel. Cramp in stomach, pain drives to despair.

Teeth - Dull sensation in teeth, as if they were soft and became bent and moved in their sockets on chewing. Scurvy of salt-eaters. Dental fistula.

Throat - Dryness of pharynx, larynx and posterior sinuses. Scraping in throat with nausea. Hawking thick, viscid mucus.

RELATIONS - ***Compare:*** (1) The Cruciferae generally. (2) Canth., Caps., Rhus-t, Sin-n. (2) Arg-n. - diarrhea from nervous excitement.

REFERENCES - Boericke. Clarke.

COCOS NUCIFERA

(Coconut Oil)

PHARMACY - coco-n. Cocos nucifera. Coconut. N. O. Palmae. ***Historical dose:*** Tincture and all potencies.

CLINICAL - Abscess. Asthma. Baldness. Bronchitis. Bruises. Burns. Colds. Colitis. Constipation. Coughs. Dermatitis. Diarrhea. Dropsy. Dysmenorrhea. Dysentery. Earache. Eczema. Fever. Gingivitis. Gonorrhea. Influenza. Jaundice. Kidney, stones. Lice.

Malnutrition. Measles. Nausea. Parasites. Rash. Scabies. Scurvy. ***Skin, disorders.*** Sore throat. ***Stomach, disorders.*** Swelling. Syphilis. Toothache. Tuberculosis. Tumors. Typhoid. Ulcers. Weakness. Worms. Wounds.

HERBAL - Early Spanish explorers called it coco, which means "monkey face" because the three indentations (eyes) on the hairy nut resembles the head and face of a monkey. Nucifera means "nut-bearing."

Coconut oil is of special interest because it possesses healing properties far beyond that of any other dietary oil and is extensively used in traditional medicine among Asian and Pacific populations. Pacific islanders consider coconut oil to be the cure for all illness.

Coconut oil does not form harmful by-products when heated to normal cooking temperature like other vegetable oils do. It has no harmful or discomforting side effects. It is non-toxic to humans.

Root - In Java, a concoction from the root is used to treat dysentery.

Leaves - In India, the hairs on the lower surface of the leaves are used to stop bleeding.

Bark - In Ghana, the bark is used as an antiseptic, to clean the teeth and the ashes are used to treat scabies.

Milk - In Mexico, the milk is considered to be diuretic and is used to combat intestinal worms.

Oil - The Tahitians use the oil of coconut with perfumed flowers to apply to their hair. It is also used to heal wounds and sprains.

Husk - It is also said in Tahiti that for skull fractures, the husk was used to cover the head and it would fit nicely and hold the head injury in place until complete healing had occurred. This way the patient was protected against any further shock to his head.

MIND - Feeling trapped. Feeling like she is losing her freedom.

Abdomen - Feel bloated.

Breast - Breast soreness. Feels like a pin being pushed through breast. Stabbing, burning pain.

Chest - Tightness of chest. Burning stabbing pain in the intercostal area.

Food - Malnutrition. Craving for sweet foods. Weakness.

Lungs - Gasping for air. Need for fresh air.

Modalities - Worse in cold weather. Worse after vaccinations. Worse after antibiotics.

Rectum - Severe constipation. Diarrhea, explosive. Yellow stools.

Skin - Skin very soft. Dermatitis. Eczema. Jaundice. Rash. Wounds. Skin of fingers sore, burning and cracked.

Stomach - Nausea. Ulcers.

Throat - Dry throat. Feel like something is stuck in the throat, like a piece of shredded coconut. Croaky voice.

Vertigo - Dizziness before meal time. Vertigo in the morning, on waking. Vertigo after eating. Vertigo feeling of swaying, feels like going to fall. Vertigo feel drunk. Vertigo with no sense of balance, has to hold on. Vertigo, with nausea.

COMMENTS - Nutritional studies show that coconut and coconut oil, in one form or another, may provide a wide range of health benefits.

Kills bacteria that cause ulcers, throat infections, urinary tract infections, gum disease and cavities, pneumonia, and gonorrhea. Kills fungi and yeasts that cause candidiasis, ringworm, athlete's foot, thrush, diaper rash, and other infections. Expels or kills tapeworms, lice, giardia, and other parasites.

Provides a nutritional source of quick energy. Boosts energy and endurance, enhancing physical and athletic performance. Helps relieve symptoms associated with chronic fatigue syndrome.

Improves digestion and absorption of other nutrients including vitamins, minerals, and amino acids. Reduces problems associated with malabsorption syndrome and cystic fibrosis. Improves calcium and magnesium absorption and supports the development of strong bones and teeth. Helps protect against osteoporosis.

Supports thyroid function. Promotes loss of excess weight by increasing metabolic rate. Is utilized by the body to produce energy in preference to being stored as body fat like other dietary fats. Helps prevent obesity and overweight problems.

Improves insulin secretion and utilization of blood glucose. Relieves stress on pancreas and enzyme systems of the body. Reduces symptoms associated with pancreatitis. Helps relieve symptoms and reduce health risks associated with diabetes. Helps protect against kidney disease and bladder infections. Dissolves kidney stones. Helps prevent liver disease.

Helps relieve symptoms associated with gallbladder disease. Relieves symptoms associated with Crohn's disease, ulcerative colitis, and stomach ulcers. Improves digestion and bowel function. Relieves pain and irritation caused by hemorrhoids.

Reduces inflammation. Supports tissue healing and repair. Supports and aids immune system function. Functions as a protective antioxidant. Helps to protect the body from harmful free radicals that promote premature aging and degenerative disease. Does not deplete the body's antioxidant reserves like other oils do.

Helps protect the body from breast, colon, and other cancers. Relieves symptoms associated with benign prostatic hyperplasia (prostate enlargement). Reduces epileptic seizures. Helps prevent periodontal disease and tooth decay.

Applied topically helps to form a chemical barrier on the skin to ward of infection. Reduces symptoms associated the psoriasis, eczema, and dermatitis. Supports the natural chemical balance of the skin. Softens skin and helps relieve dryness and flaking. Prevents wrinkles, sagging skin, and age spots.

Promotes healthy looking hair and complexion. Provides protection form damaging effects of ultraviolet radiation form the sun. Helps control dandruff.

RELATIONS - ***Compare:*** (1) Aloe vera. Calen.

REFERENCES - Murphy.

CODEINUM

(Codeine)

PHARMACY - cod. Codeinum. Codeine. Codeine purum. Codeine phosphoricum. Codeine sulphuricum. Alkaloid from Opium. Papaveraceae. ***Historical dose:*** Trituration and all potencies.

CLINICAL - Blepharospasm. Chorea. Constipation. ***Cough.*** Diabetes. Eczema. Numbness. ***Pruritus***. Restlessness. Spasms. Stomach pain. Twitchings. Vomiting, pregnancy.

HOMEOPATHIC - Codeine possesses many of the properties of opium, from which it is derived, but it is sufficiently distinctive to entitle it to a separate description. Cod. seems to possess in great degree the exhilarating properties some persons experience when taking opium, though it is not without strong soporific effects as well.

Disorders of sensation, notably troublesome itching. Marked sensitiveness of surface. ***Itching*** with feeling of warmth, numbness and prickling. Characteristic "Itching with warmth. Itching and heat of face and head. A sensation of agreeable warmth."

Trembling of whole body. Chorea. Involuntary twitching of muscles of arms and lower limbs. Convulsive twitchings of muscles and limbs and especially of orbital muscles, are very marked. Twitchings prevent sleep at night. Numbness and prickling.

Extreme restlessness. Symptoms are periodic, paroxysmal, at times sudden. Diabetes.

MIND - Great exhilaration of spirits. Depression with desire to sleep, frightful dreams and dull headache on awaking. Increased or diminished power of fixing attention or applying mind. Confusion of the mind. Depression with dull headache. Inability to apply mind. Lascivious thoughts. Bewildered on waking.

Back - Neuralgic pains from occiput to back of neck. Convulsions in muscles of back. Sharp pains extending from stomach and chest through to back, between shoulders, worse on right side.

Bladder - Semi-paralysis of bladder. Quantity of urine increased. Sugar in urine.

Causations - Fatigue and excessive mental excitement causes headache.

Eyes - Involuntary twitching of eyelid (Agar.), sometimes better by rubbing. Pupils contracted. Sudden failure of vision. On blowing nose sparks before eyes.

Food - Great thirst with desire for bitter substances.

Head - Pain from occiput to back of neck. Skin of face and scalp sore after neuralgia. Dull headache in morning, gradually diminishes towards noon, when it disappears. Headache with dry lips and constant desire to moisten them. Headache from fatigue and excessive mental excitement.

Heart - Uneasy feeling about heart. Fluttering and oppression, with great desire to walk in open air. Violent pulsations of heart and carotids. Painful pulsation when attempting to study or write.

Limbs - Paralytic weakness in arms and legs. Spasmodic twitches in arms and legs. Numbness of hands and feet, prickling and numb sensation in various parts of the body.

Lungs - Dry cough worse at night. Tickling in larynx and coughing. ***Short and irritating cough***, worse at night. Copious, purulent expectoration. Night cough of tuberculosis. Troublesome cough with copious mucus and sometimes purulent, expectoration with nervous excitability.

Male - Sexual excitement during the night, leading to pollutions.

Modalities - Worse by motion and better by rest. Headaches are worse in morning. Restlessness and cough worse at night.

Mouth - Mouth dry. Unable to articulate.

Nose - Mucus discharge with irritation of the Schneiderian membrane. Entire loss of smell for several days.

Rectum - Constipation with tenderness of bowels, especially transverse and descending colon, with some flatulence.

Skin - Itchy, dry and prickling. Eczematous eruption with troublesome itching. Itching with feeling of warmth.

Sleep - Sleepy and drowsy. Cough disturbing sleep. Twitchings in sleep. Frightful dreams.

Stomach - Spasmodic pain at pit of stomach. Belchings. Empty belchings with acute pains in stomach. Nausea and vomiting, sometimes preceded by an agreeable glow at epigastrium. Violent spasmodic pain at pit of stomach (solar plexus).

Throat - Strong pulsations in both carotids Tickling sensation in throat in afternoons and evenings.

Vertigo - Dizziness on blowing nose. When closing eyes objects appear to turnaround.

RELATIONS - ***Compare:*** (1) Agar., Hyos., Am-be. (2) Op. in sickness, pains in stomach and region of solar plexus, constipation, sexual excitement. (3) Agar. - twitching of eyelids. (4) Ars. - pains in legs, nightly restlessness. (5) Hyos. - twitching of eyelids after reading. (6) Lach. - sensitiveness of surface. (7) Rhus-t., Sulph., Sul-ac. - trembling. (8) Culex - vertigo on blowing nose.

REFERENCES - Boericke. Clarke.

COFFEA CRUDA

(Unroasted Coffee)

PHARMACY - coff. Coffea cruda. Unroasted coffee. Coffea arabica. N. O. Rubiacie. Tincture from raw berries. Tincture of dried seeds. ***Historical dose:*** Trituration and all potencies.

CLINICAL - After-pains. Anxiety. Asthma. Chills. ***Colic.*** Convulsions. Delirium tremens. Dentitions. Diarrhea. Ear, neuralgia. Ecstasy. ***Excitement.*** Fainting. Fever. Flatulence. Fright. ***Headaches.*** Heart, disorders. Hernia. ***Hyperactivity***. Hypertension. Hyperesthesia. Hysteria. ***Insomnia. Labor, pains.*** Leucorrhea. Metrorrhagia. Neuralgias. Nymphomania. Over-sensitiveness. Pain, severe. Palpitations. Prosopalgia. Sciatica. Shocks. ***Sleeplessness.*** Strokes. ***Toothaches. Unconsciousnes.*** Vertigo. Vomiting.

HERBAL - The effects of Coffea cruda have to be considered separately from those of Coffea tosta, since the roasting converts much of the caffeine into caffeone or methylamine, which gives coffee its aroma. But the effects are very similar.

HOMEOPATHIC - The provings of Coff. were made with the raw berries. Coff. belongs to the same family as Chin. and Ip., and like these remedies has many symptoms like intermittent fever. It has been noticed that coffee-drinkers with malaria are more difficult to cure than those who do not drink coffee.

Over excitable and over sensitive nerves, special senses become ***over acute***. ***Hyperactivity of mind and body***. Sudden emotions, especially joy and pleasurable surprise, can produce dangerous symptoms.

Severe insomnia. Great nervous agitation and restlessness. Hysteria, screaming weeping. Convulsions of teething children with grinding of the teeth and coldness of the limbs. Convulsions from excessive playing or laughing in weakly children.

Skin hypersensitive. Touch, noise, odors, pain become intolerable. Neuralgia in various parts, always with great nervous excitability. ***Intolerance of pain, driving to despair.*** Nervous palpitations.

Stimulates the functional activity of all organs increasing the nervous and vascular activity. Sensation of warmth.

Coffee drinking is likely to increased production of uric acid, causing irritation of kidneys, muscle and joint pains, and should be curtailed or careful watching in the elderly as they are more susceptible to the stimulating action of coffee or tea.

Clarke noted that although it is believed that coffee antidotes almost all homeopathic medicines, it is doubtful whether it could do so, especially when remedies are given in high potency. Experience shows that correctly selected homeopathic remedies act in spite of taking coffee.

MIND - ***Clearness of mind*** in evening, at night. Unusual activity of mind and body. Full of ideas, quick to act. Easy comprehension, irritability, excited, senses acute. Sentimental. Faints easily. ***Fright from sudden pleasant surprise.*** Complaints from fright. Ailments from disappointed love. Ailments from excessive laughing and playing. Trembles.

Clinging to persons or furniture. Confusion during paroxysm of pain. ***Tossing about in anguish*** (Acon.). Throws things about. ***Pains seem intolerable, driving to despair with weeping.*** Fear of death during labor or after-pains. ***Fear of death from pains***. Fear of danger on falling asleep. Fear of fresh air. Pangs of conscience. Weeps, laments and tosses about, over trifles.

Immoderate activity and vigour. Increased feeling of energy and health. Ecstasy. Buoyancy. Great loquacity, brain feels clear and is active, he feels strong enough to do anything. Hasty eating and drinking. Hurried in movements. Memory becomes very acute. ***Memory active until midnight.*** Wakeful, full of ideas. Lively fancies, full of plans for the future. Theorizing. Weeping from delight.

Capriciousness. Cry and laugh easily. Now joyous now gloomy. Mental and physical exhaustion. Delirium tremens, with trembling of hands. Thinks that he is not at home, restlessness. Annoyed by voices. Resents sympathy. Weeping during headache, during menses.

All senses more acute, reads fine print easier. Hearing, smell, taste and touch acute. Excitement as if hurried. ***Sensitive to noises,*** even if anyone walks across the floor. Fear of least noise. Impressionable to pleasurable impressions. ***Unconsciousness, fainting after strong emotions.*** Unconsciousness during childbirth.

Abdomen - Flatulence. Intolerance of tight clothing. Clothes are oppressive. ***Abdominal pains with despair.*** Tension of epigastric region, with sensitivity to touch. ***Colic, which seems to be unendurable.*** Pains as if abdomen would burst. Pressure in abdomen as from incarcerated flatus. Distended abdomen, extreme emaciation. Incarcerated hernia.

Back - Small of back as if lame, while sitting or standing.

Breasts - Agalactia. ***Emaciation of breasts.*** Breast cysts from coffee drinking.

Causations - Effects of sudden emotion, especially pleasurable ones. Ill effects of fear, fright, disappointed love, over fatigue, excessive laughing, long journey. Wine. Slight passive movements are perceived as enormous, children at times cannot bear to be carried about.

Chest - Sharp pains in sides during cough.

Constitutions - Complaints during infancy and dentition. Suited to tall, lean, and stooping persons with dark complexions. Sanguine choleric temperament.

Cough - Short, dry cough of measles in nervous, delicate children. Short, dry, hacking, constant, [5] as from constriction of larynx. [4] Cough and sleeplessness after measles. Feels exhausted after coughing. [5] Irritable, nervous, at night, with anxiety and sleeplessness. [11] Irritation to cough, with coryza, worse open air. Single, sudden shocks, quickly following each other. From irritation in throat, phlegm in back part of throat. When falling asleep or soon after. Dry, hacking, like whooping cough, with this difference, that the spasms are principally experienced during inspirations, not during expirations.

Ears - ***Sensitive hearing***. Noise is painful, even footsteps. ***Sensitive to noise, music, voices***. Hearing acute, overhears distant sounds. Hardness of hearing with buzzing as of a swarm of bees. Noises and singing in ears, with nervous people. Crackling noise in head, synchronous with pulse, worse mornings and in open air, better indoors.

Eyes - Burning in eyes and throbbing in temples, during sick headache. Eyes half open during sleep, with convulsive motion of eyes when awake. Eyes reddish and shining. Pupils dilated. Bright eyes. Can read fine print more distinctly. Power of vision increased, esp. in open air. Scintillations. Dim vision during cough.

Face - Shining red face with much fever. Flushed face during sick headache. Transitory flushes in face. One cheek hot and red, with constant shuddering. Dry heat with red cheeks. ***Aching, sharp, radiating pains.*** Prosopalgia extending to molar teeth, ears, forehead and scalp. Sweat on face with internal chilliness.

Female - Menses too early and long lasting. Profuse menses with excessive sensitiveness of organs and voluptuous itching. Dysmenorrhea, large clots of black blood, with extreme sensitiveness of genitals. Toothache during menses. Bearing down in genitals with frequent urination. Metrorrhagia. Severe after pains or labor pains with fear of death. Voluptuous itching in the vulva. ***Hypersensitive vulva and vagina.*** Vagina and vulva are too sensitive to rub or scratch, aversion to sex. Leucorrhea like mucus, or milky, worse while urinating. Severe after-pains or labor pains, with fear of death. Labor-pains ceasing, with loquacity. Irregular, ineffectual labor-pains. Puerperal fever from mental excitement. Nymphomania.

Food - Diminished appetite. Hasty eating and drinking. Excessive hunger. Aversion to coffee. Bad effects from wine and liquor. ***Bad effects from drinking too much wine.*** Thirst increased, esp. at night. ***Worse from drinking too much coffee.*** Thirst during sweat. Headache from eating too much.

Head - Headaches from mental overexertion, thinking or talking. Sensation as if brain were torn to pieces. ***As if a nail were driven into the head.*** Sensation as if brain is shattered or crushed. ***Headaches worse motion, noise, music or light.*** Tight pain, worse from noise, smell, narcotics. Head feels too small. Feels and hears a cracking in vertex. ***Coffee and caffeine headaches*** (Cham.). Temples throbbing with burning in eyes. ***Pains driving to despair***, patient runs wildly about room. Rush of blood to head, after exhausting joy. Threatening apoplexy. Hyperemia of brain after abuse of Bell.

Heart - Violent irregular palpitations, especially after excessive joy or surprise. Nervous palpitation with trembling of limbs, worse sun, heat. Hypertension. Sudden rise of blood pressure and urinary suppression. Pulse full and frequent. Pulse intermitting. Pulse more frequent, but less vigorous, even small and weak.

Kidneys - Suppression of urine. Frequent, profuse urination of colorless urine. Pressure on bladder. Urine passes off drop by drop.

Limbs - Trembling of hands, cannot hold the pen. Twitching of limbs. Crural neuralgia, worse motion afternoon and night, better by pressure. Pain in limbs, worse noise. Coldness of limbs, hands and feet. Sciatica, worse motion, afternoon and night with restlessness and sleeplessness at night.

Lungs - Short, dry cough of measles in nervous, delicate children. Asthmatic attacks in morning, wants to move continually. Short inspiration, chest heaves visibly. Suffocative fits.

Male - Hypersensitiveness of sexual organs. Scrotum relaxed. Hot, itching genitals. ***Emissions at night, followed by great languor and irritability of temper.*** Greatly excited sexual desire, with dry heat of body.

Modalities - Better warmth. Better from lying down, sleep. Better cold drinks. Better holding ice in mouth. ***Worse excessive excitement. Worse strong emotions, joy.*** Worse mental exertion. Worse overeating. Worse alcohol, wine, narcotics. ***Worse from strong odors, noise.*** Worse open air. Worse cold, wind. ***Worse from touch***, would like to rub the part but it is too sensitive. Worse at night, sleeps until 3 a.m. Warm drinks aggravate toothache.

Mouth - Excessive dryness of mouth at night. Hot breath. Taste more acute. Delicate taste. Taste sweetish. Loss of taste. Salivation during pregnancy. Hasty eating and drinking.

Nose - ***Acute, sensitive smell.*** Nosebleed with heaviness of head and ill humor during straining at stool.

Perspiration - Cold, clammy sweat, over whole body, but chiefly on palms of hands. Slight sweat, mostly in face.

Rectum - Constant alternations of constipation and diarrhea. Constipation and hemorrhoids. Constipation in sick headache. Diarrhea, watery, painless all day. Diarrhea in housewives from too much care about domestic affairs. Diarrhea during dentition, after the use of chamomile tea. Hemorrhoidal conditions. Spasmodic contraction of sphincter, with burning and itching in anus. Fetid flatus. Liquid, fecal, offensive stools, from sudden joy or taking cold in open air.

Sensations - As if head too small, as if something hard pressing on surface of brain, as if head would burst and fly to pieces if she moved. As if intestines were being cut. As if body would burst. Tight pains and sensations. Sensation of warmth.

Skin - Skin very sensitive, eruptions become extremely irritable. Painfully sensitive. Itching, scratches until it bleeds. Itching of eruption changes into burning. Measly spots on the skin, with dry heat. Purple miliary eruptions all over. Scarlet fever, may aid in bringing out the eruption in cases of extreme wakefulness and nervous excitement. Scarlet rash with overwhelming pains and lamenting. Varicella, smallpox. Dryness of skin, but not in febrile diseases. Stinging and smarting on skin.

Sleep - Restless sleep, frequent, sudden starting and waking. ***Nervous sleeplessness. Insomnia.*** Sleeplessness, before or after midnight, from nursing the sick. Sleeps until 3 a.m., after which only dozing. ***Sleeplessness from excessive use of coffee.*** Wakes with a start, sleep disturbed by dreams. ***Sleepless, on account of mental activity, flow of ideas.*** Disturbed sleep from itching of anus. Sleeplessness after pleasurable excitement. ***Sleepless with nervous excitability.*** Sleepless so long as any noise or light continues, at night. Sleeplessness after acute diseases. Long and vivid dreams. Pleasant dreams, even merry.

Stomach - Intolerance of tight clothing. Bilious vomiting and restlessness at commencement of variola. Gastric derangements of infants. ***Anguish and pressure in stomach pit.*** Burning in stomach during vertigo. Stomach feels over loaded during colic. Burning, sour eructations. Hiccoughs. Eructation like rotten eggs. Violent spasmodic eructations, with rising of the ingesta. Continual nausea during headache. Constant inclination to vomit, felt in throat. Vomiting of mucus during violent attacks of megrim.

Teeth - Dentition of anemic, sensitive children. Convulsive grinding of teeth. Toothache during menses. ***Toothache,***

better holding ice water in mouth, worse as it warms. Severe toothache, ***intolerant of the pain*** with restlessness, anxiety and weeping.

Temperature - Chilliness worse every movement. Internal chills with external heat of face and body. Chills with heat of head and sweat of face. Chills running down back. Running all through limbs. Shivering, from least exposure to cold air. Chills without thirst. Traumatic fever. Even with mild fever patient is very nervous and sensitive. Ague, paroxysms every fourth day, two well days intervening. Intermittent fever. Feverish with pain and always ready to weep.

Throat - Sore throat, worse cold air. Sore throat, parts very sensitive. Swelling and painfulness of throat, worse swallowing. Pain as from a plug with constant desire to swallow. Uvula too long, swollen. Larynx as if covered with dry mucus. Trachea as if raw. Roughness and hoarseness in larynx, in morning on waking. Spasm of glottis, starts from sleep with short inhalation or gasping.

Vertigo - Dizziness and confusion in the head. Vertigo with blackness before eyes. Vertigo when stooping. Vertigo during cough. Vertigo with whirling sensation in head, occasionally a general faint feeling, worse thinking. Vertigo with burning in stomach. Vertigo during sick headache, worse change of position or from moderate outdoor exercise.

COMMENTS - Teste grouped Coff. with Caust. He remarked that potentized Coff. prevents or neutralizes in many persons the effects of roasted coffee. Teste noted that this quasi-isopathic action is by no means confined to Coff., potentizations of many other drugs being antidotal to secondary effects of the crude substances.

Hahnemann described the migraine of coffee-drinkers thus: "It comes in the morning after waking increasing little by little. The pain becomes intolerable and sometimes burning integument of head very sensitive and painful on slightest touch. Body and mind excessively sensitive. Patients look exhausted, retire to dark places, close their eyes to avoid light of day, remain seated in an armchair or stretched on a bed.

"The least noise or motion excites the pain. They avoid talking, being talked to or hearing others talk. The body is colder than usual though no chills are experienced, the hands and feet are especially cold.

"They loathe everything, especially food and drink, on account of a continual sickness at the stomach. If the attack is very violent a vomiting of mucus takes place, which, however, does not relieve the headache. There are no alvine discharges. This kind of megrim scarcely ever leaves before evening.

"If the paroxysm is less violent, a little strong coffee which was the first cause of such a headache will produce a temporary palliation of the pain, but the disposition to relapse becomes so much greater.

The attacks come irregularly, every fortnight or every few weeks without any apparent cause and quite suddenly, so much so that the patient often does not feel a single unpleasant symptom the evening preceding the attack. Such a headache has never been seen by me except in real coffee-drinkers."

More recently, Dr. Gilles de la Tourette (Lancet, July 20, 1895) has described the effects of coffee. In his opinion they are very frequently mistaken for the effects of alcohol.

"Morning vomiting of glairy mucus, pain in the pit of the stomach, thickly-coated tongue, loss of appetite. The disgust excited by even the idea of solid food is such that these patients eat nothing else but bread soaked in their poison—coffee. There supervene then nausea, vomiting and painful acid belchings."

The effects of coffee are less deep than those of alcohol and quickly disappear when the habit is discontinued.

Characteristic exaltation of the senses and sensibility in general (Acon.). Sight is improved, fine print can be read easily, hearing is more acute and noises are intolerable and are accompanied with fear of death. The mental activities are exalted. Great sensitiveness to touch or contact.

Nervous energy, anxious, wide awake, and hypersensitive to all light and noise, any stimulus. Ailments due to over-excitement (Arg-n., Phos.), pleasant surprises, joy. Happy excitement. Very sensitive to the cold and the wind.

Over excitement from severe pain, hypersensitive to the pain. Frets over the pain. Cannot stand the pain, pain out of proportion. Pain leads to sleeplessness and over excitability. An emergency remedy for amputation pain and severe nerve pain with burning.

Tendency to be intellectual, very quick minded, clear thinkers with brilliant memories, but can't turn their sensitivity off, an increased nervous system. Voracious mental appetite (Sulph.). Hyperactivity.

Severe insomnia from an overactive mind. Sleep is disturbed by terrifying dreams. Slowed pulse. Headaches (Cham. for coffee headache). One-sided headaches with the sensation as if a nail was being pounded in (Ign., Thuja, Anac., Nux-v.), usually right over the eye. Sense of lightness of movement, the head feels light, full of vigor.

Ringing in the ears or a roaring sensation in the head. For teething and toothache. Tendency to colic. Diarrhea in housewives who have much care and trouble in managing their households. Labor pains.

RELATIONS - ***Antidotes:*** Nux-v., Coff., Tab. Strong black coffee, drunk as hot as possible is indispensable as an antidote in a large number of poisons, especially narcotics. Hot coffee by rectum in cases of extreme collapse. ***Compare:*** (1) Coff-t. (2) Cypr. - ecstasy. (3) Bry. and Cham. - toothache better by cold. (4) Acon. - predicts hour of death. Coca, Codeine. ***Complementary:*** Acon. ***Incompatible:*** Camph., Cocc.

REFERENCES - Boericke. Clarke. Murphy. Phatak.

COFFEA TOSTA

(Roasted Coffee Berries)

PHARMACY - coff-t. Coffea tosta. Roasted coffee berries. N. O. Rubiacae. Infusion of the well-roasted berries. ***Historical dose:*** Trituration and all potencies.

CLINICAL - Antidote, poisons. Chills. Cholera. Delirium tremens. Diarrhea. Fainting. Fever. ***Headaches.*** Heart, disorders. Hemorrhoids. Hyperesthesia. ***Insomnia. Labor, pains.*** Migraine. Nervousness. Neuritis. ***Pains.*** Palpitations. Seminal, emissions. ***Toothaches.*** Urinary, disorders. Vertigo. Vomiting.

HERBAL - The roasting of coffee develops certain vitamin-like substances. Pigeons which had developed *"deficiency"* neuritis and paralysis on diet of polished rice lost their disabilities on the addition of 8 cc to a 5% infusion of coffee to their food. Unroasted coffee was useless.

HOMEOPATHIC - The symptoms of Coff-t. have been principally obtained from sensitive persons on whom strong coffee has acted injuriously and the clinical uses have been mainly based on these. But there is a definite and extensive proving of Coff-t. given in Allen. While it is often given in the form of black coffee, it is also available for use in the potencies.

Coff-t. is serviceable against both cold and heat. Beneficial to persons who live in the open air. Toothache, better by cold (Coff.), ***"cold water better intense pain in sound teeth of right lower jaw."*** Clarke has several times cured a toothache like this with Coff. 30c.

Heart disorders with troublesome palpitations from heart-irritability and in general nervous excitement. Tense arteries. Periodic headaches in hysterical women. Nervous and gastric headaches.

Vomiting on least exertion. Diarrhea from overwork and too much care. Gout and rheumatism with tendency to form chalkstone. ***Labor pains are intolerable.*** Useful in confinements to relieve the excess of suffering which some women experience.

Body and mind excessively sensitive. Looks exhausted, retires to lonely and dark places and closes eyes in order to avoid light. Least noise or motion excites pains. Avoids talking or being talked to or hearing others talk. Body colder than usual, although no chills are experienced. Hands and feet very cold.

MIND - Increased intellectual activity and perception of sounds, motion. Great excitement. Full of apprehension of terrible things happening. Depression and despair. Thinks she will die during labor. Begs that some one might end her life. Strange feeling in her head with palpitations, trembling and chilliness. Doesn't know where she is. Delirium tremens.

Abdomen - Cramplike drawing pains in umbilical region with severe pains in lumbar region. Pains in abdomen during labor.

Ears - Ringing and noises as if falling rain, during vertigo.

Eyes - Shining bright eyes during labor. Sees dazzling colors, principally blue and yellow, before eyes.

Face - Pale face during vertigo with fainting. Face hot and deeply flushed, during labor. Excruciating facial neuralgia from decayed teeth.

Female - ***Very severe labor pains***. Patient becoming greatly excited, constant tossing about with violent movements of limbs, she complains of the severity of pains and is sure she will die. After rupture of bag of waters, very severe pains in lumbar region.

Food - Loathes all food and drinks on account of continual nausea.

Head - Nervous and gastric headaches. ***Periodical headaches of hysterical women.*** Migraine coming on in morning shortly after awaking. Pains increasing little by little. Pains become intolerable. Burning pains. ***Coffee and caffeine headaches*** (Cham.). Scalp sensitive, hurts when touched ever so slightly. Headaches come on irregularly, without premonitory symptoms. If headache attack is very violent, vomiting of mucus, which doesn't diminish the pain. Headaches worse least noise or motion.

Heart - ***Palpitations from irritable heart.*** Small and frequent pulse, during labor. Arteries tense.

Kidneys - Assists the passage of gravel and small urinary calculi, and impedes their further formation in bladder. Catarrh of bladder, especially of old debauchees. Diabetes mellitus.

Limbs - Gout and rheumatism, where there is a disposition to the formation of chalk-stones in joints. Pains in left shoulder-joint. Trembling of hands. Iliac pains. Pains in left foot and joint of big toe.

Lungs - Spasmodic asthma. Asthma thymicum. Whooping cough.

Male - Seminal emission at 3 a.m. Seminal emission with voluptuous itching, followed by chill and cold, clammy sweat.

Modalities - Worse least noise. Worse light. Worse motion.

Rectum - Diarrhea from overwork or too much worry. Obstinate diarrhea of elderly people occurring after an attack of cholera. Chronic diarrhea. Hemorrhoidal complaints.

Sleep - Nervous and restless sleep. Obstinate sleeplessness. ***Insomnia from overactivity of the mind.*** Sleepless from sensitivity to noise, light.

Stomach - Tight feeling in stomach after eating. Cramp of stomach. Vomits without least exertion. Epidemic cholera, particularly against the weakening vomiting and tormenting thirst, and it was useful in subduing the premonitory symptoms.

Teeth - Intense pain in sound teeth of right lower jaw nearly driving him crazy. No application relieves except cold water in mouth. Toothache returns as water becomes warm. Premature decay of teeth in children.

Temperature - Feels chilly, without being cold, and trembles. Intermittent fever. Continued fever with disposition to diarrhea. Inflammatory fever in children with excitability, starting and twitching in sleep, restlessness and crying.

Vertigo - Vertigo comes in attacks. Vertigo with obscured vision, unable to distinguish surrounding objects. Vertigo with ringing in ears and noise as of falling rain. Vertigo, suddenly falls to the ground insensible. Vertigo with palpitation of heart. Vertigo with easy vomiting and paleness of face during paroxysms.

COMMENTS - Its value is well known as an allopathic antidote to opium and its derivatives in poisonous doses. Additionally, it counteracts the effects of Nux-v., Bell., Coloc., Valer., Cic., Cham., Phos, Ph-ac., lead, Salts of Antimony, narcotic mushrooms, poisonous sumac, tobacco, bitter almonds, and prussic acid.

On account of its extensive antidotal properties coffee has largely been condemned by homeopathic practitioners, but it should be remembered that it does not antidote all remedies.

RELATIONS - ***Antidoted by:*** Caps., Cham., Coff. Crud., Nux-v. ***Compare:*** (1) Coff. crud., Caffeine. (2) Cham., Nux-v., Valer.,

REFERENCES - Clarke. Murphy.

COLCHICINUM

(Colchicine)

PHARMACY - colchin. Colchicinum. Colchicine. Alkaloid of Colchicum autumnale. Trituration. ***Historical dose:*** Trituration and all potencies.

CLINICAL - Arthritis. Convulsive, jerkings. Diarrhea. Exhaustion. Fevers. Gout. Intestinal, catarrh. Pleurisy. Prostration. Rheumatic, fever. ***Rheumatism.*** Sleeplessness. Spasms.

HOMEOPATHIC - This colchine alkaloid has been proved and the symptoms are sufficiently distinctive. The symptoms point strongly to its use in that form of intestinal catarrh characterized by the appearance of shreddy membranes.

Arthritis deformans in early stages. ***Intense pain of rheumatism.*** Rheumatic fever, gout. ***Convulsive jerkings of right hand.*** Endocarditis and pericarditis. Pleurisy. Very great exhaustion increasing to feverish excitement.

Abdomen - Distention and sensitiveness. Frequent rumbling.

Eyes - Pupils widely dilated.

Face - Tearing pains in face.

Kidneys - Urine turbid, depositing a copious white sediment.

Limbs - Convulsive jerkings of right hand.

Mouth - Increased secretion of saliva.

Pulse - Pulse during the first two hours sank about eleven beats.

Rectum - Urging, causing him to leave the bed. Copious pasty evacuation. Stools with tenesmus and consisting of a thin fluid with numerous flakes looking like cooked egg white in pieces from two to four inches long. Stools thin, yellowish green, slimy, accompanied by pain. Liquid stools.

Sleep - Awakened from sleep soon after midnight by uneasy dreams. Somnolency and collapse.

Stomach - Pains and sensitiveness in epigastrium. On rising from bed, at night, nausea suddenly increased and was followed by vomiting of undigested food, and afterwards of a bitter greenish fluid. Vomiting early in the morning. Vomiting of blood for nine or ten days.

Temperature - Chill about noon on first day, followed by violent heat lasting several hours with increased thirst, very rapid pulse, confusion of the head, uneasiness and sleeplessness.

RELATIONS - ***Compare:*** (1) Ars., Caust., Colch.

REFERENCES - Boericke. Clarke.

COLCHICUM AUTUMNALE

(Meadow Saffron)

PHARMACY - colch. Colchicum autumnale. Meadow saffron. N. O. Melanthacae of the Liliaceae. Colchicaceae. Tincture of the bulb dug in spring. The flowers of the plant appear in autumn, the leaves not until the following spring. ***Historical dose:*** All potencies.

CLINICAL - Albuminuria. Appendicitis. ***Arthritis.*** Ascites. Asiatic, cholera. Asthma. Backache. Bright's disease. Cataracts. Cholera. ***Colic.*** Colitis. Coryza. Coughs. Cramps. Debility. Dehydration. Delirium. Diabetes. ***Diarrhea.*** Dropsy. Dyspnea. ***Dysentery.*** Eye, disorders. Feet, painful. ***Flatulence. Gout.*** Headache. Heart, disorders. Hydrothorax. Ileus. Intermittent, fever. Intestinal, catarrh.

Iritis. ***Joint, pains.*** Lumbago. Memory weak. ***Morning sickness.*** Muscle, pains. ***Nausea.*** Nephritis. Night-watching. Nosebleed. Pericarditis. Pleurodynia. Proctalgia. Prostatitis. ***Prostration.*** Rectum, prolapsed. ***Rheumatism. Smell, acute.*** Sneezing. Stiffneck. Styes. ***Suppressed sweat.*** Tongue, sensation lost. Torticollis. Typhlitis. Typhoid, fever. ***Uric acid diathesis.*** Urticaria. Vertigo. ***Vomiting.***

HOMEOPATHIC - Colchicum is best known as a remedy for ***gout and rheumatism***. It markedly affects muscles, fibrous tissue, serous membranes, and joints, especially the small ones.

Colch. relieves gouty paroxysms. Red, hot and swollen parts. Tearing pain, worse in the evening, at night, and from touch. Stubbing the toes hurts exceedingly.

Many joints are affected at the same time. Small, rapidly shifting areas of severe pain, but little swelling. Pains are tearing, digging, drawing. Tingling, crawling. Stitching, jerking, drawing pains in muscles, periosteum and joints. Pains worse from mental exertion, emotions, slightest touch and vibrations.

There is the irritability and aversion to touch so common in gout, pain in small joints and especially the great toes. Affects the periosteum and synovial membranes of joints.

The stomach is acutely disordered, nausea and vomiting. ***Nausea at thought, sight or smell of food, especially of cooking***. Dysentery. ***Uric acid diathesis,*** pale yellow sediment like fine flour. Urine black as ink. Urine loaded with albumen and casts.

Extreme relaxation of the muscular system, the head falls forward on the chest or falls back when the patient is raised from the pillow, arms fall helpless by the side. ***Great prostration, internal coldness***.

Tendency to collapse. Moist collapse, due to dehydration, as after repeated vomiting or purging. Cardiac and arthritic disorders. Dropsy. Hydropericardium, hydrothorax, ascites, hydrometra. The patient must rest and lie down. Cannot lie on left side.

Effects of night-watching and over study. Shocks as from electricity through one half of body. Bad effects from suppressed sweat. Dreams of mice.

MIND - Mind befogged, but answers correctly. Intellect beclouded, though he gives correct answers. Mind generally distracted. Can read, but cannot understand a short sentence. Memory weak. Weakness of memory from fatigue. Deficiency of ideas. Disorders in comprehension and association of ideas. Lacks words to express ideas. When writing, forgets syllables and entire words. Confounds objects.

Very irritable with the pains (Cham.). Pains worse mental exertion or by emotions. Intolerant of pain, his suffering seem unendurable. ***Depressed, irritable and sensitive.*** Peevish, nothing satisfies him. Discontented, not satisfied with anything. Misdeeds of others make him quite beside himself.

Extreme impressions such as bright light, strong odors, contact aggravate him. ***Sensitive to all external impressions.*** Hatred of odors. Frequent starting and trembling are felt through body.

Delirium during headache. Starting during sleep. Delusions, sees mice, hears noises. Vision heightened, but intellectual faculties dulled. Carphologia. Sardonic laughing. Indifference, doesn't complain unless questioned, then says nothing of his condition. Absence of apprehension, no fear of death.

Abdomen - Mucus colitis, after dysentery. Pain in transverse colon. ***Distention of abdomen.*** Distended cecum and ascending colon. Fullness and continuous rumbling. Borborygmi. ***Colicky pains.*** Colic, worse eating, after flatulent food, with great distension, better bending double. ***Icy coldness of abdomen with colic.*** Ascites with fold over the pubic region. Surface of abdomen hotter than rest of body and extremely sensitive to touch. Pulsation in abdomen. Pain over liver. Tearing pain about sigmoid flexure of colon, worse pressure and at night. Griping pains.

Back - Backache, better rest and pressure. Lumbago. Aching in lumbar and lumbosacral region. Ache better pressure and rest. Tension in neck muscles felt even on swallowing. Violent pain in region of kidneys, better lying on back only. Dull pain across loins. Spot on sacrum feels sore and bruised as if ulcerated, very sensitive to touch. Stinging and tension between scapulae. Torticollis.

Breasts - Breast full, skin hot, pulse strong. Tearing, lancinating pain, deep in right breast, extending to back. Nipples dark, brownish-red, protruding. Nipples, unbearable pain on slightest touch by child.

Causations - Bad effects of grief, night-watching, over study. Misbehavior of others. Getting wet. ***Suppressed sweat.*** Complaints from getting overheated.

Chest - Violent cutting pains, interrupting breathing. Stinging and tearing pains in muscles of chest. Chest as if squeezed by a tight band. Tensive feeling in chest. Sharp pain in chest on inspiration and coughing. Lacerating, tearing pain in chest. Lancinating pain, as with a knife, in right side of chest. Dull stitches in posterior part of thorax during expiration. Pleurodynia from catching cold or from living in damp dwellings. Serous effusion in chest with rheumatic and gouty persons. Hydrothorax, with marked dyspnea and edema of limbs. Spitting blood after chest injuries. Rheumatism of pectoral muscles.

Constitutions - Complaints of old people, asthmatic people. It corresponds to the ***gouty constitution***. Leuco-phlegmatic and melancholic, venous constitutions, uric acid diathesis.

Cough - Frequent, short, dry cough from tickling in larynx. Cough at night, compelling him to sit up, excited by scraping in chest, with much expectoration. Cough at night, with involuntary spurting of urine. Slight cough with coryza.

Ears - Itching, crawling in ears. Dryness of ears. Ears feel stopped up with roaring. Tingling of ears as after being frosted. Sharp, shooting, below right tragus. Earache with lacerating pains. Earache with discharge. Hearing very acute.

Eyes - Eyes sunken, staring, hollow, congested, protruding. Diffused inflammation and congestion. Pain in and around the eyeball extending to occiput. Eyes half open. Visible contraction in lower lid. Acrid tears, worse in open air. Violent tearing pain in eyes. Edges of lids red and burning. Soft cataract. Kerato-iritis, with pus in anterior chamber of eye. Rheumatic iritis with great soreness of eyeballs. Stye on left lower lids. Ulceration of meibomian glands. Pupils unequal, left pupil contracted.

Face - Edematous swelling, cheeks red, hot, sweaty. Edema of lids and face. Pinched, sunken as in collapse. Sickly, sad, suffering expression. Pain in facial muscles, moving about. Tingling and edematous swelling, cheeks red, hot, sweaty. Pain behind angle of right lower jaw. ***Very irritable with the pains*** (Cham.). Tingling in face as after being frozen. Cheeks, lips and eyelids purple. Risus sardonicus. Blotchy papular rash on face.

Female - Menses too early and scanty. Itching of genitals. Sensation of swelling in vulva and clitoris. Coldness of thighs after menses. Feverish restlessness in last month of pregnancy. ***Intense boring or tensive pain in ovary***, must bend double, with great restlessness. Dropsy of uterus from suppression of menses. Hemorrhage of uterus. ***Morning sickness*** with sensitivity to the smell of food (Sep.). Puerperal fever.

Food - ***Gags from mere mention of food.*** Craving for various things but averse to them when smelling them. ***Loathes the smell or sight of food***, better lying quietly. Nausea and anxiety from smell of cooking, or from fat food. ***Nausea from odor of fat meat, eggs, fish.*** Eggs disagree cause derangement of stomach. Tastelessness of food. Thirst for effervescent, aerated waters, alcoholic beverages. No thirst.

Head - Difficulty in moving head. Creeping in forehead and over head. Pressive headache, better supper, warmth, lying quiet. Headache chiefly frontal and temporal, but also occipital and in nape of neck, worse afternoon and evening. Aching in occiput, worse mental effort. Neuralgic, tearing pain in scalp in small spots. Headache over left eye, worse open air. Hemicrania, either of right or left side, changing about.

Very violent headache, coming in evening and lasting until morning. Hot forehead. Forehead covered with cold sweat. Great falling off of hair.

Heart - Cardiac dyspnea. Heart disease, following rheumatism. Anxiety in region of heart. ***Violent palpitations with oppression of chest.*** Pressure and oppression in the region of the heart, better walking. Cutting or stinging at heart, weak heart. Trembling in precordial region, with sticking pains. Sound of heart becomes weaker, pulse of low tension. ***Heart disease and rheumatism.*** Hydropericardium. Pericarditis, with severe pain, oppression and dyspnea. Effusion into pericardium. Weak heart. Pulse not felt. Pulse is thready, imperceptible.

Kidneys - Kidney failure with high uric acid. ***Uremia.*** Burning in urinary passages before urination. More urging, more discharge of urine. Diabetes. ***Nephritis with extreme pain*** in region of kidneys. Burning in urethra, as if urine were very warm. Tickling burning in urethra and discharge of a few drops, after urination. Raw pain, in urethra during urination.

Limbs - Limbs, lame, weak, tingling, cold. ***Arthritic pain, patient screams with pain on touching a joint.*** Joints stiff and hot, shifting rheumatism, pains worse at night. Rheumatic pain in joints of fingers, toes, wrists and ankles. ***Painful gout in big toe, cannot bear to have it touched or moved.*** Pain worse in evening and warm weather. Tearing in limbs during warm weather, stinging during cold. Sharp pain down left arm. Pins and needles in hands and wrists, fingertips numb. ***Tingling in finger-nails.*** Finger joints distorted, fingers flexed but in constant motion. Knees knock together, can hardly walk. Buttocks hot. Right plantar reflex abolished. Edematous swelling and coldness of legs and feet. Bloating of hands and feet with dysentery. Rheumatism in spring.

Lungs - Chest seems squeezed by a hand. Night cough with involuntary spurting of urine. ***Great dyspnea.*** Cardiac dyspnea. Dyspnea with palpitations of heart from 11 a.m. to 3 a.m. ***Lies in bed gasping for breath***, with pericarditis. Difficult breathing, better bending forward. Accelerated and audible breathing. Slow, irregular breathing. Asthmatic breathing with moist sound. Asthma with hydrothorax or hydropericardium. Asthma with dropsy of lower limbs. Hurried breathing with groans. Rapid and short, quick breathing.

Male - Edema of scrotum. Tearing in glands and left spermatic cord. Itching at prepuce and orifice of urethra. Chordee after gonorrhea.

Modalities - Better from warmth. Better rest. Better doubling up. Better sitting. Better stooping. Better after stools. Better lying quietly. Better open air. Oppression and colic better bending forward. ***Worse from motion*** (Bry.). Can't lie on left side. Worse touch, vibrations. Worse stubbing toes. Worse bodily or mental exertion. Worse from stretching. Worse checked sweat. Worse vomiting. Worse loss of sleep. ***Worse from smell of food.*** Worse at night, evening. Worse sundown to sunrise. Worse from changing weather. ***Worse cold, autumn.*** Symptoms generally ***worse cold damp, worse getting wet, bathing, living in damp dwellings***, changes to damp weather. Worse from rising up in bed.

Mouth - Sensation of warmth and dryness in mouth. Cracked lips. Thick, brownish coating on lips, teeth and tongue. Taste, flat, bitter. Flow of saliva with a sense of dryness. Mouth hangs open. Heat in the mouth with thirst. Profuse salivation with dryness of throat. Affection of salivary glands in Bright's disease. Cold breath. Loss of speech. Inflammation and redness of palate and fauces.

Nose - Nostrils dry and black. ***Smell morbidly acute. Odors of eggs, meat nauseate even to fainting.*** Strong odors make him quite beside himself. ***Smell so acute that he smells odors others can't smell.*** Obstinate coryza, discharge thin, tenacious, never watery. Sore pain in septum. Nosebleed, evenings. Sneezing, with crawling sensation in nose.

Perspiration - Copious, cold sweat, without relief. Copious sour sweat suddenly coming and going with rheumatism. Sweat cold on face. Sour sweat, nightly. Clammy sweat on whole surface, with low temperature of skin, in acute rheumatism. Acid reaction of sweat and urine. Suppressed sweat.

Rectum - Mucus colitis after dysentery. ***Autumn dysentery,*** when days are warm and nights are cold. Hemorrhage from bowels in autumnal, cold, damp weather. Very offensive flatus, in evening. Diarrhea, then gouty effects. Ineffectual pressing, feels feces in rectum, but cannot expel them. Pain, as if anus were torn open with prolapse. ***Agonizing pains remain long after stool.*** Spasmodic constriction of sphincter, followed by urging to stool. Unsatisfactory urging to stool, better passing flatus. Tingling, itching, burning and tearing in anus. Protrusion of rectum. Obstinate constipation in ileus.

Skin - Skin dry, sweat suppressed or profuse. Blotchy papular rash on face. Pink spots on back, chest and abdomen. Urticaria. Stitches in skin. Tingling here and there, as after being frozen. Skin dry and pale, swollen, parts cold and glistening. Dryness of skin. Itching as in nettle-rash, unchanged by scratching. Erysipelas, smooth. Purple efflorescence on face, neck, and upper anterior part of thorax, inside of thighs, scrotum and groins in patches.

Sleep - Falls asleep while reading. Lies prostrate on back. ***Sleeplessness from restlessness of limbs.*** At night, disturbed sleep or driven away by pains. Irresistible sleepiness, drowsiness, when not in too much pain. Drowsiness during day. Starting, jerking in sleep. Frightful dreams, awakening from sleep.

Stomach - Gastric affections before and during an attack of rheumatism. Burning pains. Eructations, with burning in stomach. ***Icy coldness of stomach with colic.*** Pain in stomach and flatulence. Dry mouth, tongue burns, gums and teeth pain. Profuse salivary secretion. Gouty gastralgia. Gastralgia from sudden suppressed sweat. Stomach as if full and swollen, as if he had eaten too much. ***Nausea and retching.*** Nausea and inclination to vomit, caused by swallowing saliva. ***Nausea from odor of fat meat, eggs, fish.*** Vomiting of mucus, bile and food, worse any motion. Vomiting of the water he drank. Vomiting and purging of rice-water stools, with thirst. Vomiting first food, then fluid.

Stools - ***Changeable stools***, greenish, reddish, excoriating, slightly sour smelling, copious, frequent, watery or bilious. Stools are painful, scanty, transparent, jelly-like mucus. ***Bloody stools.*** Stools scanty, discharged only by hard straining, even if soft, with pain in lumbar region. ***Stools contain white shreddy particles in large quantities.*** Stools frequently orange-yellow, slimy with bright-yellow flakes. Scanty stool with tenesmus, salivation and copious urination. Stools pass insensibly, involuntary. Feces mixed with light blue matter. Profuse watery stools in hot, damp weather.

Teeth - Gums and teeth painful. Teeth very sensitive when pressing them together. Grinding of teeth. Teeth feel too long. Tearing pain in roots of teeth and gums. Toothache, worse cold and immediately after warm things. Toothache, worse at night.

Temperature - Chilliness and coldness running through all limbs down back. Shuddering and creeping chills in isolated parts. Chills even near warm stove, intermingled with short flushes of heat. Cold sensation of head and limbs, in acute rheumatism. Dry heat at night with excessive thirst. Dry heat of whole body, constantly increasing and palpitations, thirst. Body hot, limbs cold. Intermittent, fever.

Throat - Much greenish, thin mucus in the throat, comes involuntarily in the mouth. Voice hoarse, or deeper than usual. Hoarseness in morning, with roughness of throat. Itching in larynx and trachea. Throat as if dry. Constriction of esophagus. Tickling as if coryza were setting in, inducing cough and clearing throat. Tonsils inflamed and swollen, spots covered with pus, swallowing difficult. Heat in pharynx and whole length of esophagus.

Tongue - Glossitis. Tongue burns. Tongue, bright red, heavy, stiff and numb, protruded with difficulty. ***Brown tongue.***

Loss of sensibility in tongue. Tongue cold. Tearing, burning and sticking pain in tongue. Tongue coated white.

Urine - Urine, hot, highly colored, watery, black sediment. Albuminuria. Profuse secretion of urine. Urine of sour smell and acid reaction. ***Dark, scanty or suppressed urine.*** Pale yellow, greenish urine. Urine turbid, leaves an orange-colored ring in vessel. Bloody, brown, black, inky urine. Whitish sediment in urine.

Vertigo - Vertigo while sitting, after walking. Vertigo on rising.

Vision - Spots before eyes. Variations in visual acuity. Dim vision after reading. Lost vision, for a minute or two on getting out of bed.

COMMENTS - Coldness in the abdomen, stomach, and limbs. Profuse cold sweat, marked chills with or without periodicity. Burning in the cavities, especially the abdomen. Sensation of icy coldness or burning in stomach. Bloated abdomen.

Diarrhea. Cholera. Dysentery with bloody stools and mucus. Autumn dysentery, Spring rheumatism. Dysentery and rheumatism are exceedingly painful. Stools have jelly-like mucus, membranous shreds. Rice-water stool, with hippocratic face, coldness, cramps, prostration. Stool accompanied by violent tenesmus. Protrusion of rectum.

Affinity for the kidneys. Kidney failure with high uric acid. Effective for gout and joint conditions. In gouty diabetes, the uric acid reappears as the sugar disappears. Rheumatism can appear on disappearance of uric acid from urine.

Arthritis in the small joints. Stiffness that's better with motion (Rhus-t.). Arthritis, worse motion (Nux-v., Bry.). Conditions worse in the autumn, damp weather and change of weather (Dulc., Rhus-t., Nat-s.). Cold and chilly, dampness penetrates. Ailments from getting wet and chilled, changes to damp weather.

Oppression and anxiety in the heart, better by walking. Stitches about heart and loss of consciousness. Pericarditis on the disappearance of symptoms from limbs.

All functions, mental and bodily, are slow. Nutrition and digestion are at a stand and yet the patient does not emaciate rapidly.

Great prostration, debility from loss of sleep, the prostration of typhoid fever and typhoid states. Extreme disinclination to move, worse from motion. Convulsions, cramps and restlessness. Pains are very acute and unendurable.

Very sensitive and irritable. Cannot endure strong smells. Smell of food nauseates. Morning sickness with sensitive to the smell of food (Sep.).

Nash recorded a striking cure by Colch. 200c. The patient was an old woman who was vomiting blood and passing as many as sixteen bloody stools in the day. The doors of the room had to be most carefully kept closed to prevent any smell of cooking reaching her as that immediately provoked nausea.

Guernsey noted that "after evacuation, as in dysenteric, there is generally relief but in typhus fever, sometimes a terrific spasmodic pain of the anal sphincter comes on after stool. This may occur in diarrhea."

The rice-water stool, hippocratic face, coldness, cramps, and prostration, led Salzer to use it for certain epidemics of Asiatic cholera.

J. R. Simson of Tonawanda, N.Y., cured a very bad case of typhoid presenting symptoms including "his left pupil was contracted so as to be almost imperceptible, while the right was dilated to the full extent." This is peculiar to Colch. and no remedy relieved the patient until he received this.

B. Simmons called attention to the powerlessness of the affected parts, especially when occurring in leuco-phlegmatic subjects and when there is edematous swelling of the parts.

He cured a woman, 36, mother of two children, of leuco-phlegmatic temperament, who complained of rheumatism of the hands, which were swollen, joints stiff and powerless, pain as if bruised, the arms being affected but in less degree. "She was unable to brush her own hair, not so much from the pain as from the extreme weakness and powerlessness of the parts affected."

T.F. Allen gave ***"Tingling in finger-nails"*** as characteristic of Colch., no other remedy has it as strong.

RELATIONS - ***Antidotes:*** Thuj., Camph., Cocc., Nux-v., Puls. ***Compare:*** (1) Colchicinum - intestinal catarrh and shreddy membranes, convulsive jerkings of right hand, rheumatic fever, gout, endo and pericarditis, pleurisy, arthritis deformans in early stages intense pain of rheumatism 3x trituration. (2) Carb-v., Arn., Lil-t., Ars., Cocc., Kali-c., Verat.

REFERENCES - Boericke. Clarke. Murphy. Phatak.

COLIBACILLINUM

(Escherichia coli)

PHARMACY - coli. Colibacillinum. Escherichia coli. ***Historical dose:*** All potencies

CLINICAL - Anorexia. Backaches. Bradycardia. Chills. Colitis. Constipation. Cystitis. ***Dehydration. Diarrhea.*** Dysentery. Epididymitis. Fever. Flatulence. ***Food poisoning. Gastroenteritis.*** Headaches. Hematuria. Hepatitis. Hypotension. Indigestion. Insomnia. Leucorrhea. Menorrhea. Metritis. ***Nausea.*** Nephritis. Prostatitis. Puerperal fever. Rheumatism. Salpingitis. Septic fever. ***Traveller's diarrhea.*** Typhoid fever. Vaginitis. ***Vomiting.*** Weakness. Worms.

HOMEOPATHIC - The bacteria species, E. coli, occurs normally in the intestines of man and other vertebrates. It is widely distributed in nature, and is a frequent cause of ***food poisoning and infections*** of the urogenital tract and of diarrhea in infants.

In babies and young children, ***profuse weakening diarrhea*** with hypothermia, bradycardia, ***dehydration.***

Hypotension, tendency to weakness, even collapse. Paleness, anxiety, vertigo, sweats, sound of the heart become muffed, and lowering of the blood pressure.

General fatigue and depression which goes on aggravating with digestive and urinary troubles. Progressive asthenia. ***Mental and physical weakness.*** Permanent worn out condition.

MIND - Mental weakness. ***Great timidity.*** Irresolution and lack of self-confidence. Always hesitating, cannot decide on anything. Constant mental confusion because of the loss of memory. Forgets proper names. Loss of memory. Amnesia of recent events. Weakness of memory with great difficulty to find out the right word. Uses very often one word for another.

Depressive melancholia. ***Sadness and weariness.*** Obsessional neurosis. Confused deliriums. Schizophrenic states, loss of contact with his environment and with his own reality. Catatonic condition with somnolence and dreams.

Abdomen - Bloating after eating. Slow intestinal transit. Flatulence, intestinal spasms. ***Gastroenteritis.*** Heaviness and drawing in the intestines. Rumbling. Expulsion of putrid gas. Spasmodic colitis.

Back - Backaches. Lumbar pains.

Eyes - Swelling of the upper eyelids, sometimes left, sometimes right.

Female - Salpingitis, metritis, vaginitis. Vaginitis with burning pains. Leucorrhea. Heaviness of the lower abdomen with ovarian pains. Menorrhea. Yellow leucorrhea, sightly irritating. Sexual relation becomes difficult, with vulvo-vaginal burning sensation.

Food - Capricious appetite or anorexia. ***Food poisoning.*** Worse dairy products, milk. Worse eggs. Worse from eating undercooked meat, fish.

Head - Empty feeling in the head. Frontal and suborditary headache, worse by humid coldness. Headaches after contrariety and strong emotions.

Heart - Bradycardia. Hypotension. Sound of the heart become muffed.

Kidneys - Nephritis. Heat and burning after urination. Cystitis. Painful sensation in the region of kidney. Frequent urination of little quantity. Painful urination with the sensation of burning at the end of the flow. Sensation as if he must go again to pass urine immediately after urination. Urine smells bad. Hematuria. Aggravation of urinary troubles in cold humid weather.

Limbs - Polyarticular pains. Swelling of small joints of legs and hands. Rheumatism. Chronic degenerative rheumatism.

Liver - Hepatitis. Enlarged sensitive liver. Gall bladder, painful.

Male - Erection and ejaculation sometimes painful, with the sensation of burning in the urethra after sex. Cystitis, prostatitis. Relapsing epididymitis.

Modalities - Better by heat. Better warmth. Worse by cold. Worse humid cold. Worse by the sea. Worse after rest. Worse milk. Worse slightest mental or physical exertion. Worse cold, damp weather.

Rectum - ***Infants with diarrhea and dehydration.*** Diarrhea. ***Profuse weakening diarrhea.*** Constipation. ***Traveller's diarrhea.*** Alternating diarrhea and constipation. ***Bloody, foul smelling stools.*** Worms.

Sleep - Deep and heavy sleep. Insomnia.

Stomach - ***Nausea and vomiting*** after eating spoiled foods. Very slow digestion with the sensation of the stomach remaining heavy for a long time.

Temperature - Chilly, specially after eating. Nocturnal chill. Sensation of intense coldness with chill immediately after meals. ***Fever with great weakness.*** Typhoid fever. Septic fever. Puerperal fever.

Tongue - Tongue, coated yellowish-white. Tongue with a red clear stripe down the center. White tongue.

RELATIONS - ***Compare:*** (1) Pyrog., Chin., Ars., Lyc., Sepia, Psor., Med., Thuj. (2) Bowel nosodes. (3) Thymol., Folliculium. Cynodon dactylon.

REFERENCES - Julian.

COLLINSONIA CANADENSIS

(Stone-Root)

PHARMACY - coll. Collinsonia canadensis. Stone-root. Horse balm. Richweed. N. O. Labiate. Tincture of fresh root. Trituration. ***Historical dose:*** Trituration, tincture and all potencies.

CLINICAL - Atony. ***Catarrh.*** Colic. ***Constipation. Cough.*** Diarrhea. Dropsy. Dysentery. Dysmenorrhea. Dyspepsia. Hemorrhages. Heart, disorders. ***Hemorrhoids.*** Hoarseness. Labor. Pregnancy, disorders. Proctitis. Pruritus, vulvae. Rheumatism.

HERBAL - Collinsonia is native to North America. It has a very tough, hard, knotted root. As a domestic remedy, it is known for chronic catarrhal conditions, especially of the stomach, bowels and bladder. Also of the nose, pharynx and larynx and in tubular and capillary bronchitis.

HOMEOPATHIC - Congestion in pelvic organs, especially anus, rectum and uterus, resulting in ***hemorrhoids and constipation,*** especially in females. ***Constipation of children from intestinal atony.*** It is said to be of special value when given before operations, for rectal diseases.

Sense of weight and constriction. Venous engorgement. Depressed arterial tension, general atony of muscular fiber. ***Chronic nasal, gastric and pharyngeal catarrh***, due to portal obstruction. Pruritus in pregnancy with hemorrhoids.

Irritation of cardiac nerves, palpitation, faintness, oppression. Dropsy from cardiac disease. Heart disorders that alternate with suppressed bleeding hemorrhoids. Sensitiveness about the heart, fullness, oppressed breathing, faintness.

MIND - Gloomy. Sullen. Excitable. Irresolution.

Abdomen - Distended abdomen. Colic with flatulence and nausea. Heavy, digging ache in pelvis. Sharp, cutting pain in hypogastric region. Severe pain in lower part of abdomen. Congestion of portal system and of pelvic viscera. Flatulent rumbling in stomach and bowels.

Chest - Chest pains alternating with hemorrhoids. Fullness and oppression of chest.

Face - Yellow discoloration around the eyes.

Female - Genitals considerably swollen and inflamed. Amenorrhea from pelvic congestion. Dysmenorrhea, swelling and dark redness of genitals, pain on sitting down. Membranous dysmenorrhea. Terrible dysmenorrhea, with hemorrhoids, diarrhea and loss of appetite. Cold feeling in thighs after menses. Sensation of swelling of labia and of clitoris. Lancinating pain in ovaries, worse right side. Prolapsed uterus, hemorrhoids during pregnancy. Leucorrhea with pruritus. Itching of vulva with hemorrhoids during pregnancy.

Food - Loss of appetite. Excessive appetite with spasms of stomach and flatulence. Loss of appetite with dysmenorrhea.

Head - Dull, frontal headache with constipation or hemorrhoids. Headache from suppressed hemorrhoidal discharge. Headache with frequent flying pains in legs, tearing in knees.

Heart - Palpitations, rapid but weak. Dropsy after heart symptoms are relieved, hemorrhoids or menses return. Palpitations in patients subject to hemorrhoids and indigestion. Rapid pulse. Heart's action rapid, regular or irregular, slightest motion or excitement aggravates. Valvular heart disease, following a severe and prolonged attack of acute rheumatism.

Kidneys - Chronic nephritis and cystitis. Catarrh of bladder. Urine increased.

Limbs - Sensation as if limbs were enlarged. Lower limbs seem not to belong to him. Tearing pain in arms, hands and legs. Cold feeling in thighs after menses. Tearing pain in both knees, extending down inside of legs to feet, while sitting.

Liver - Dull pain in liver region. Portal vein congestion.

Lungs - Difficult breathing and faintness. Severe attacks of dyspnea with great weakness. Oppression, faintness and dyspnea (Acon-f.). ***Cough from excessive use of voice.*** Harassing, dry cough. Chest pains alternate with hemorrhoids. Spitting of blood after suppression of hemorrhoids. Dark, tough coagula, enveloped in viscid mucus. Hemorrhage from lungs.

Male - Varicocele with rectal symptoms. Spermatorrhea kept up by hemorrhoids and constipation.

Modalities - Better from heat. Better morning. Worse during hemorrhoids or from suppressed hemorrhoids. Worse from the slightest emotion. Worse excitement. Worse during pregnancy. Worse at night. Worse from cold.

Mouth - Tongue yellow with bitter taste (Coloc., Bry.).

Nose - Chronic catarrh. Sinus congestion.

Rectum - Sensation as if rectum is ***full of sharp sticks.*** Chronic hemorrhoids, alternating with heart, chest or rheumatic symptoms. ***Painful bleeding hemorrhoids.*** Vascular engorgement of rectum. ***Sense of constriction***. Rectum, aches, burns. Rectum seems dry and full of sand, with cardiac pain. ***Most obstinate constipation*** with protruding hemorrhoids. Constipation during pregnancy with dysmenorrhea, following labor. ***Alternate constipation and diarrhea*** and great flatulence. Prolapsed anus. ***Itching of anus*** (Teucr., Rat.). Dysentery with tenesmus.

Sensations - Constriction and feeling of enlargement in various parts and organs of the body, limbs, vulva, clitoris etc.

Sleep - Disposition to sleep during day. Sleep disturbed by hypogastric pains.

Stomach - Constant heaviness in stomach. Cramplike pains in stomach with nausea. Sharp, cutting pains in stomach, every five minutes while sitting. Nausea with obstinate constipation, during pregnancy. Vomiting with pain and heat in stomach.

Stools - Sluggish stool with distended abdomen. Chronic diarrhea of children. Diarrhea after delivery. Acrid diarrhea. Light colored stools, lumpy with hard straining, mucus or black stools. Dry feces.

Temperature - Flushes of heat with oppressive breathing, with hemorrhoids.

Throat - Hoarseness. ***Speaker's sore throat,*** sharp pain in larynx.

Vertigo - Vertigo with gastric and hemorrhoidal troubles. Periodical spells of faintness.

COMMENTS - It has been proved twice, first by Burt and later by Dowla. The former took the tincture, the latter the powder. Both experienced headache, the former in connection with abdominal and rectal disturbance. The latter with flushing, sensation of heat, numbness, feeling of enlargement. The legs felt light, as if he could run like a deer.

Nux-v. relieved the sensations, the symptoms passing off from above downwards. In Dr. Burt's case, the symptoms generally passed from above downwards.

The greatest number of Dr. Burt's symptoms were experienced in the bowels and rectum, including pains in umbilicus and hypogastrium, constipation with hard light stools, great straining, faintness, stools of mucus and blood.

These symptoms suggested the use of the remedy in cases of hemorrhoids, where it has proved most efficacious. Hemorrhoids during the menses. Prolapse of the rectum with hemorrhoids. It reduces complications when given before operations on rectal disease.

It is, according to Hammond, "a stimulant, a most valuable tonic, a positive diuretic and mild laxative." Hammond commended it in the palpitations of the menopause. Irritation of cardiac nerves, palpitation, faintness, oppression.

F. S. Smith mentioned that it has a domestic reputation in rheumatism. He recorded a case (sub-acute) in a woodsman of 30. It began in the foot and ankle and traveled over nearly every joint in the body. A few drops of Coll. tincture was mixed in a tumbler of water and a teaspoonful given every two hours. Rapid cure resulted.

Dewey mentioned that it cured a case in which there was severe constrictive pain about the heart in a man who habitually passed blood by stool, the heart symptoms coming on when the bleeding ceased and disappearing when it was re-established. Coll. cured both.

Nash cured cases of the most obstinate constipation with Coll. In one there was severe colic, which had recurred for several years, the concomitant symptoms being great flatulence and hemorrhoidal troubles.

He differentiated between Aesc. and Coll., in that Aesc. has a sense of fullness in the rectum, which Coll. does not, and Aesc. hemorrhoids do not bleed as a rule, while those of Coll. bleed persistently.

Aesc. has pain, soreness and aching in the back. Coll. has more persistently constipation with colic on account of it. Aesc. may have constipation or may not. Coll. has shown marked power of disturbing the circulation and causing hemorrhages and also of disturbing cutaneous sensation.

Symptoms are worse in the evening and night, better in the morning. Worse by slightest emotion or excitement.

Inveterate cases of dyspepsia with a weight in epigastrium and hemorrhoids. Neuralgia and rheumatic pains were experienced by the provers in many parts: upper jaw, arms, hands, knees, joints. Sensitiveness about the heart, fullness, oppressed breathing, faintness. Heart disorders alternate with suppressed bleeding hemorrhoids.

RELATIONS - ***Antidote:*** Nux-v. ***Compare:*** (1) Aesc., Aloes, Ham., Lycopus, Negundo, Sulph., Nux-v.

REFERENCES - Clarke. Murphy.

COLOCYNTHINUM

PHARMACY - colocin. Colocynthinum. N. O. Cucurbitaceae. Colocin. is an active glucoside of Citrullus colocynthis. Dilutions in alcohol. ***Historical dose:*** All potencies.

CLINICAL - Colic. Cough. Debility. Diarrhea. Feet, burning in. Genitals, congestion, pain. Headaches. Neuralgia. Spinal pains. Traveling, effects.

HOMEOPATHIC - Having had a separate proving, Colocynthinum must be considered apart from Coloc., from which it is derived, although the symptoms of the two bear a close resemblance.

Prominent neuralgic symptoms. Stitches and sensations of heat are found in many parts. Pulsation in the pit of the stomach, with prickling stitches on back in neighborhood of middle thoracic vertebrae.

Diarrhea and colic, better bending forward. Congestion to male genital organs and pain in them. Burning pains in soles of the feet.

Modalities - Better by bending over, black coffee. Worse by motion, better by rest, herein appears the relationship of the glucoside to Bry., the botanical relative of Coloc. Worse evening. Worse riding in cars.

REFERENCES - Clarke.

COLOCYNTHIS

(Bitter Cucumber)

PHARMACY - coloc. Colocynthis. Bitter cucumber. Cucumis colocynthis. Citrullus colocynthis. Bitter apple. N. O. Cucurbitaceae. Turkey. Tincture of pulp of fruit. ***Historical dose:*** All potencies.

CLINICAL - Cataract. Ciliary, neuralgia. ***Colic.*** Colitis. Coxalgia. ***Cramps.*** Delirium. Diabetes. Diarrhea. Dysentery. ***Dysmenorrhea.*** Gallbladder, colic. Glaucoma. Headaches. Hoarseness. Humiliation. Kidney, colic. Lead, poisoning. ***Menstrual, pains.*** Nausea. ***Neuralgias. Ovarian, cysts.*** Ovary, disorders. ***Pains, severe.*** Phimosis. Peritonitis. Rheumatism. ***Sciatica.*** Toothaches. Tumor. Uterus, pains. Vaginal, pains. Vomiting.

HOMEOPATHIC - Colocynth was used as a drastic purgative in allopathic practice. Coloc. should be compared to Bry. as they both have the same general features.

Pain in muscles, nerves and joints, gastroenteric disturbance and the same condition in regard to rheumatic joints, worse by movement. Great irritability and ailments from mental emotion, though the latter feature is more marked in Coloc.

Coloc. is useful in acute disorders of digestive tract and intestines. It develops most of its symptoms in the abdomen and head, causing intense neuralgias. ***Neuralgic pains are cutting,*** pinching, clamping, gnawing or boring. Neuralgic pains followed by numbness, ***better by pressure***. Long-lasting action on large nerves, especially ***tri-facial, sciatic and spinal nerves.***

Agonizing pain in abdomen. Colic causing patient to bend double. Cries out from pains, wriggles for relief, or must bend him double. ***Sudden, atrocious, crampings, tearing pains*** which make the patient ***twist and turn.*** The patient will press something hard against the abdomen.

Sensations of cutting, twisting, grinding, contracting and bruised pains. ***Pains as if clamped with iron bands***. Pains are accompanied by nausea and diuresis and the patient vomits from intensity of pain. Faints with pain and with coldness. Rheumatic pain in the limbs is better by discharge of flatus.

Cramps and twitching and shortening of muscles. Constrictions and contractions. Formication in affected part. Bladder cramps or spasms following operations on orifices (Hyper.). Urine odor of perspiration (Berb., Nit-ac.). Prostration, as if all his strength was failing.

Especially suitable for ***irritable persons easily angered*** and ill effects there from. Women with painful, profuse menstruation and of sedentary habits.

MIND - ***Anger with indignation*** (Staph., Cham., Bry., Nux-v.). ***Extremely irritable***. Impatient. Anger, easily vexed during pain. Humiliation caused by offense. ***Ailments after anger, with silent grief.*** Children are worse when reprimanded (Cham.). Easily offended, aggravated when questioned (Bry.).

Morose, becomes offended at everything. ***Greatly affected by the misfortunes of others.*** Want of religious feeling. Wants to be alone, even friends irritate. Offended at everything. ***Screams with pain***, wants to walk about. Restlessness before menses. Restlessness, anguish, agony, suppressed rage.

Depressed and joyless. Disposition to weep and cry. Complaining bitterly day and night. Walks about room in great agony from headache. Delirium alternating with sopor, with constant desire to escape, eyes half closed. Disinclined to talk, to answer. Becomes angry when questioned. Confusion from beer, wine.

Abdomen - ***Agonizing cutting pain causing patient to bend over double*** and pressing on the abdomen. Violent, cutting, gripping, grasping, clutching pains. ***Radiating, colicky pains.*** Cutting pain in abdomen after anger. Colic with cramps in calves. Cutting pains in bowels at navel. ***Colic pains, come in waves, better doubling up, hard pressure.*** Pains are worse least food or drink, except coffee and tobacco smoking. ***Colic from drinking while overheated.*** Pressure improves the pain in abdomen in acute stage but when pain remains for a long time, parts become tender and pressure aggravates the pain. ***Intestines feel squeezed between stones.*** Intestines feel as if bruised. Flatulent colic.

Colic with cramps in calves. During colic, infant lies on abdomen and screams when he is slightly moved.

Back - Pain under right scapula, better pressure. Lumbar ache, better pressure. Bruised pain in lumbar region. As of a heavy weight in lumbar-dorsal region, better lying on left side. Cramp like pains in the hips, better lying on the affected side. Neck stiff, worse moving head. Muscles of nape as if stiff when moving head.

Bladder - Tenesmus of bladder. Bladder catarrh, discharge like fresh white of egg, ***viscid*** (Ph-ac.). ***Pains on urinating over whole abdomen***. Burning along urethra during stools. Itching at orifice. Bladder spasms after operation on the orifices. Sudden violent pressure upon bladder, which was full, passed off suddenly on emission of flatus. Retention of urine.

Breasts - Painful nodes in breasts. Sharp pains.

Causations - Ill effects of anger indignation, chagrin, grief, catching cold, or excessive venery.

Chest - Oppression of chest. Pain in intercostal muscles. Stitching, in right or left side of chest. Swelling and suppuration of axillary glands.

Constitutions - Suited to easily angered, irritable persons with tendency to corpulence. For women of sedentary habits with copious menstruation. To blondes, persons of choleric temperament and those liable to cramps and colic from fruit, lead poisoning or excessive venery.

Ears - ***Sounds re-echo in ears.*** Crawling, itching, stitching, aching, better by putting finger into ear. Roaring and throbbing, especially in left ear.

Eyes - Pain and twitching in eyelids. Burning eyelids. Severe burning, sticking and cutting pains. Pains sharp, boring, ***better from pressure***. Violent pain in eyeballs which precede the development of glaucoma. Sensation as if eye would fall out on stooping. Gouty disorders of eyes. Smarting in eyes, with pain in eyeballs. Great itching in right eyeball, must rub. Discharge of acrid fluid. Bluish-white ring around cornea, in rheumatic form of iritis. Redness and lachrymation. Dimness of vision. Region around eye very sensitive to touch, during headache. Conjunctivitis, with tendency to ulceration.

Face - ***Face distorted from pains.*** Cheeks cold. Tearing, shooting and swelling of face, left side great soreness, relieved by pressure (Chin.). Prosopalgia with eye symptoms. ***Neuralgia with chilliness***. Pain anywhere is reflected on the face. Sensation as if left side of face were being torn from right side. Deathly color of face, during colicky pains in bowels. Face red and purple. Pimples on face.

Female - Amenorrhea and chronic diarrhea. Suppression of menses or lochia from indignation. Menses copious in women with sedentary habits. Menses increased and too frequent. Dysmenorrhea, worse eating and drinking. Bearing-down cramps, causing her to bend double (Sep.). Metritis from indignation. ***Boring pain in ovary. Must bend over double with great pain and restlessness***. Uterus prolapsed. Clutching pain in ovarian region. Ovarian tumors, cysts. Ovaritis. Round, small cystic tumors in ovaries or broad ligaments. ***Ovarian cysts*** with pain better flexing thigh on pelvis. Wants abdomen supported by pressure. Puerperal fever brought on by indignation or grief because of unkind treatment. Swelling of labia with dragging pain and heat in vagina. Yellow, thick, offensive leucorrhea between menses.

Food - Appetite variable, mostly poor. Canine hunger. Food and drink taste bitter. Aversion to food. ***Coffee helps the colic, headache.*** Desires for bread and beer. Potatoes and starchy food disagree. Potatoes causes bellyache. Confusion from beer, after wine. Constipation from cheese. Very thirsty. Drinks much, without thirst.

Head - Head hot, red face, glistening eyes. Dullness of head and giddiness at beginning of colic. Lateral cutting pains with nausea, vomiting. ***Headache better coffee.*** Pains, better pressure and heat. Burning pains, digging, rending and tearing. Headache with nausea and vomiting. ***Headache with soreness of scalp***. Roots of hair painful. Head pains worse stooping. Headache worse lying on back and moving eyelids. Heaviness in forehead with stupefaction. Pressure in both temples.

Heart - Strong throbbing in all blood vessels. Heart feels pushed up by a distended stomach. Stitches in cardiac region. Pulse generally hard, full, accelerated. Pulse small and weak.

Kidneys - Kidney colic with diuresis. Fetid, small quantities of urine with frequent urging. Diabetes.

Limbs - Rheumatic pains in limbs and joints, after catching cold. ***Contraction of muscles***. Cramps in muscles during sex. All the limbs are drawn together. Stiffness of joints and shortening of tendons. ***Cramp-like pain in hip***, lies on affected side, pain from hip to knee. Heaviness of limbs during headache. Spontaneous luxation of the hip joints. Sciatic pain, left side, drawing, tearing. ***Sciatic pain, better pressure and heat***, worse gentle touch. Pain in right deltoid. Pain down right thigh, muscles and tendons feel too short, numbness with pains (Gnaph.). Icy coldness of hands and feet. Cold hands with warm feet. Knees feel stiff, cold. Pain in left knee joint. Feet cold with colic.

Liver - Gallbladder, colic.

Lungs - Short cough when smoking tobacco. Difficulty breathing during menses, ovarian tumor. Asthmatic attacks at night with slow, difficult breathing, which provokes cough. Anxious and oppressed, sensation as if about to smother. Tickling cough frequently during night. Dry cough from tickling in throat.

Male - Sensation as if everything were flowing towards genitals from both sides of the abdomen, causing seminal emission. Pain and swelling of testicles and spermatic cord. Retraction of testicles and priapism, with retention of urine. Paraphimosis. Retraction of prepuce behind glans during sleep. Strong sexual desire with erections. Impotency.

Modalities - Better coffee, smoking. Warmth ameliorates most pains. Better lying with head bent forward. Better lying on abdomen. ***Better bending double.*** Better rest, motion. ***Better hard pressure, warmth.*** Better after stool or flatus. Worse from emotions, chagrin. ***Worse anger, vexation and indignation.*** Worse from lying on painless side. Worse before and after urination. Worse drafts, taking cold. Worse at 4 p.m. Worse lying in bed, evening and night. Worse eating, drinking.

Mouth - ***Persistent bitter taste.*** Teeth feel too long. Offensive smell from mouth from decayed teeth. Bitter taste of food and drink. Offensive or metallic taste. Stinging in velum palati. Burning on the tip of the tongue. Tongue rough, as from sand. As if tongue had been scalded. Burning on anterior surface of tongue.

Nose - Throbbing, burrowing pains from left side of nose to glabella. Nose stopped up. Purulent nasal discharge. Fluent coryza, worse open air, better indoors. Sense of smell impaired during headache.

Perspiration - Sweats at night. Cold sweat. Sweat smelling like urine. Sweat causes itching of skin. Sweats mainly on head and limbs. Profuse, warm sweat on forehead and neck.

Rectum - Constipation, hard stools, as if passing stones. Diarrhea from pain, from anger, with indignation. Ineffectual urging to stool, followed by sudden stool. ***Burning pain in anus***, after green, yellowish, slimy, watery discharges, streaked with pure blood. Slippery bubbles escape from anus. Pricking at anus, with constant discharge of mucus. Painful swollen hemorrhoids. Musty odor.

Skin - Itching, prickling, crawling, formication. Desquamation over whole body. Dryness and heat of skin. Smarting, itching, followed by perspiration. Itching, burning ulcers. Carbuncles, with continuous burning pain. Boils on neck and face. Corns. Herpes on face. Itch-like eruptions.

Sleep - Sleepless and restless, with pains after anger. Yawning and sleepiness. Sleeps badly, often wakes tired and irritable. Dreams disturb sleep. Vivid, anxious, voluptuous dreams.

Stomach - Burning pain in stomach. ***Violent cutting, tearing pains.*** Feeling in stomach as if something would not yield, drawing pain. ***Cramps in stomach*** at night, better eructations. Sensation of fullness in epigastric region. Pain in stomach with toothache or headache. ***Sharp pains before menses***, with extreme nausea and vomiting. Nausea, with greenish vomiting. Retching and bending body forward. Vomiting and diarrhea from anger, with indignation. Vomiting of food without nausea. Vomits from pain. Vomiting of bitter water.

Stool - Chronic watery diarrhea, worse in the morning. Bloody diarrhea with violent pain in bowels. ***Jelly-like stools***. Stools frothy, watery, shreddy, yellow. ***Dysenteric stool renewed each time by the least food or drink.*** Stools sour or gelatinous. Stools with flatulence and pain. Stools, sourish, with flatulence and pain.

Teeth - Teeth feel too long. As if nerves were compressed or stretched. Neuralgic pains, on one side, recurring daily. Drawing pain. Throbbing, first in one, then in another tooth.

Temperature - Coldness of hands and soles, rest of the body warm. Chill and shivering with pains. Cold sweat at night, smelling like urine. Feeling of coldness in whole body. Internal chill with external heat. Chill proceeding from abdomen. Chill during headache. Chill with inclination to perspire. Partial coldness and partial heat of skin. Bilious fever with cardialgia, spasmodic colic, diarrheic stool.

Throat - Cramps in gullet, with empty belchings and palpitation of the heart. Throat as if constricted, with empty eructations and palpitation of heart. Dryness, rawness, roughness or scraping in throat. Sensation of constriction of larynx, better open air. Frequent tickling and irritation in larynx induces cough at night.

Urine - Urine, gelatinous, sticky, stringy. Tough mucus sediment in urine which can be drawn out into strings. Urine milky white. Urine coagulates on standing. Red hard crystals adhering to the vessels. Urine like brown beer, becoming turbid as soon as cold, depositing copious sediment.

Vertigo - Vertigo when quickly turning head. ***Vertigo when turning head to the left***. Vertigo with nausea. Vertigo with slight delirium and deafness. Vertigo from stimulants.

COMMENTS - Guernsey wrote "The strongest characteristic calling for the use of this remedy is an agonizing pain in the abdomen causing the patient to bend over double. Relief is obtained by motion, such as twisting, turning and wriggling around and the motion is kept up steadily while the pain lasts.

The pain is worse by eating or drinking the least amount. This pain may occur alone or in the dysentery, cholera, etc. The doubling over the patient is the chief characteristic."

The patient bends double or presses something hard against the abdomen, leans over chairs, the table or bed-posts to get relief. The characteristic griping, forcing the patient to bend double, may be accompanied by cramps in other parts, with or without stool. If a stool occurs it gives immediate relief (Nux-v. the opposite), worse any attempt to eat or drink.

Griping, cutting, tearing and spasmodic pains in the body, burning pains, pulsations through the body, sensation as of hard stones or potatoes in the body. Pains accompanied by stiffness and retarded motion of the affected parts, especially the hip joints. Pains affecting joints are worse from motion.

Sciatica. Arthritis and gouty headaches with ophthalmia. Facial neuralgia with pains extending to eye. Neuralgic pains are better by rest.

Cramps occur in the legs, uterus and ovaries. A sensation as if clamped with iron bands is very characteristic in coxalgia and dysmenorrhea. Dragging in uterus and vagina. Suppressed lochia from indignation.

Diabetes with milky, gelatinous or colloid urine. Perspiration may smell like urine. Bitter taste in mouth, strong aversion to food. Worse raw fruits or something cold on a hot day (Bell-p., Ruta.). Worse tobacco, better coffee. Easily intoxicated by any stimulants.

Diarrhea from grief, indignation, or chagrin. Severe, painful dysentery. As if hard stones are rubbing the intestines, or hot knifes stabbing the intestines. Vomiting yellow, bitter fluid. Tension of the bowels as they are forced inward right below the navel, forcing the person to bend double.

Babies with colic may have severe pain radiating from the umbilicus. According to Nash, Mag-p. comes nearest to it in colic and neuralgic disorders. Cham. is also very close, both having colic from disturbing emotions, but the Cham. child does not double up, they toss about.

The Staph. patient is likely to have black or decayed teeth and sore eyelids and there is a chronic tendency to colic. Verat. has colic better bending double, but it has also cold sweat. Dioscorea has wind colic, but is better by stretching out. The Stann. child wants to be carried with the abdomen on the mother's shoulder.

Chilly, sensitive to cold and damp, cold winds. Better heat. Affections of the left side generally. 4 p.m. aggravation (Lyc., Hell., Caust.). One prover experienced that "at 4 p.m. the colic came on, six days in succession."

RELATIONS - ***Antidoted by:*** Camph., Caust., Cham., Coff., Op., Staph. Large doses are counteracted by tepid milk, infusion of galls, Camph., and Op. ***It antidotes:*** Caust., Magnes. Also Coloc. is the best antidote to lead poisoning. (Royal). ***Compare:*** (1) Lobelia erinus - violent cork-screw-like pains in abdomen. (2) Dipodium punctatum - writhing. twisting like a dying snake. Intractable insomnia. (3) Dios., Cham., Cocc., Merc, Plum., Mag-p. (4) Merc. - dysentery with much tenesmus). (5) Bry. - nearest analog. (6) Elat., Cucurbita pepo. (7) Dios. - griping, tearing, cutting, spasmodic pains in body, but better stretching body and motion. (8) Caust. - joint rheumatism, follows Coloc. in colic. (9) Canth., Cham., Chel., Chin. (beer intoxicates easily), Cocc., Gamb., Lyc., Merc., Nux-v. (10) Plb. - inclination to assume strange attitudes in bed. (11) Staph. - anger with vexation, abdominal pains, neuralgia—they follow one another well. (12) From emotions, Cham., Bry., Gels., Ph-ac. Ign. ***Compatible:*** Staph., Cham., Caust.

REFERENCES - Boericke. Clarke. Murphy. Phatak.

COLOSTRUM

PHARMACY - colos. Colostrum. The human milk first secreted after childbirth. Solution. ***Historical dose:*** Tincture and all potencies.

CLINICAL - Colic. Dentition. Diarrhea. Emaciation. Fever. Nausea. Vomiting.

HOMEOPATHIC - The symptoms of Colostrum are purely clinical. Its use in diarrhea was probably suggested by the purgative effect of Colos. on the infant.

Colicky pains in hypogastrium. Green, watery, yellow, watery, mucus, bilious stools. Profuse, sour-smelling, excoriating stools.

Great nervous irritability or listlessness. Fever. Pale face. Tongue coated white or yellow. Vomiting of sour or bitter substances. Loss of appetite. Emaciation. The whole body smells sour.

Abdomen - Colicky pains in the hypogastrium during stool.

Face - Pale face.

Food - Loss of appetite.

Modalities - Worse in nursing infants during dentition. ***Worse during stool.***

Mouth - Tongue coated white or yellow.

Perspiration - The whole body smells sour.

Rectum - Aggravation of the diarrhea in nursing infants. Diarrhea during dentition.

Stomach - Nausea. Vomiting of sour or bitter substances.

Stools - Green, watery stools. Yellow stools. Watery stools. Mucus stools. Bilious stools. Profuse stools. Sour-smelling stools. Excoriating stools.

REFERENCES - Clarke.

COMOCLADIA DENTATA

(Guao)

PHARMACY - com. Comocladia dentata. Guao. N. O. Anacardiacae. Cuba. Tincture of leaves and bark. ***Historical dose:*** Tincture and all potencies.

CLINICAL - Antrum of Highmore, disorders. Breasts, disorders. Ciliary, neuralgia. Ears, disorders. Eczema. Erysipelas. Eyes, disorders. Glaucoma. Herpes, zoster. Leprosy. Neuralgia. Skin, malignant inflammations. Toothaches. Ulcers.

HOMEOPATHIC - Comocladia shows its affinity with the Rhus family by the virulence of its effects on the skin, the slightest contact, and at times even walking in the neighborhood of the growing tree, being sufficient to cause violent inflammation. Both are irritant poisons.

The trunk and branches of the tree contain a milky fluid, turning black on exposure to sunlight, discoloring the skin, linen, etc. Compare with Anacardium. The plant causes tormenting itching, swelling, redness, vesication, ulceration.

Important eye and skin symptoms. Malignant skin inflammation with enormous swelling or edema of left leg and foot. Deep ulcers with hard edges. Skin red all over. Recurrent eczema. Leprosy.

Throbbing pains, worse by heat. Sacro-iliac and abdominal pain. Wandering rheumatic pains. Pain in joints and ankles.

Burning, itching of the eyes, which feel too large. Right eye very painful, feels large, protruded than left. Ciliary neuralgia. Burning itching of the nose with violent sneezing. Affections of antrum. Pain under the left breast or nipple extending to left scapula, when coughing.

Abdomen - Severe flatulent pain in abdomen preceding and during a diarrhea stool, followed by a feeling of weakness and perspiration on face and neck.

Back - On moving head, sense of fullness, rigidity and lameness of muscles of neck. Rheumatic pains and stitches in back, stitches leave a burning.

Breasts - Sharp pain in left breast, about one inch above nipple, leaves a burning sensation. Sloughing ulcer on right breast.

Chest - Pain from right side of chest down arm to fingers. Cough with pain under left breast, going through to left scapula.

Ears - Heat and fullness in right ear. Left ear cracked and desquamating a substance like powered starch.

Eyes - Glaucoma, sense of fullness, ***eyeball feels too large***. Ciliary neuralgia with eyes feeling large and protruded, ***worse right eye***. Eyes are ***worse near warm stove***, feels as if pressed outward. Sees only glimmer of light with left eye. Motion of the eyes aggravates.

Face - Swollen, with projecting eyes.

Limbs - Sharp pains through right shoulder to scapula. Painful burning on arms. Crampy sensation in muscles of right upper arm. Drawing, cramping in fingers. Vesicular eruption on arms and hands. Herpes on legs.

Lungs - Spasmodic, dry cough at night. Soreness in left lung. Cannot draw a long breath on account of sharp pain at center of thorax on left side.

Male - Intense itching on lower part of penis, also on inner side of prepuce. Continued tingling, itching of scrotum during night.

Modalities - Better from open air. Better motion, scratching. Better pressure. Worse from touch. Worse warmth. Worse rest. Worse at night (Rhus-t.). Rheumatic pains are better by motion and worse by rest (Rhus-t.). Heat aggravates and open air ameliorates most of the symptoms (opposite Rhus-t.).

Mouth - Mouth dry. Tongue coated dirty yellow. Sensation as if a tooth were being drawn out of its socket. Pain in teeth better by pressure. When toothache stops, head feels large. Gums of lower jaw inflamed.

Skin - Itches, red and pimples. ***Redness*** all over like a scarlatina. Red stripes on skin (Euph.). Erysipelas. Pustular eczema of the trunk and limbs. Deep ulcers with hard edges. Leprosy.

Sleep - Dreamy, refreshing sleep with pleasant dreams, almost clairvoyant.

COMMENTS - Peculiar eye symptoms, including a pain in the right eye, the sensation as if it were larger and more protruded than the left. Throbbing pains as if the eyeballs are bulging or would burst. Glaucoma (Jab.). Ciliary neuralgia, eye pains. Eye symptoms are worse warm rooms, heat, even that of the sun.

Cough with pain under the left breast going through to the left scapula. Sacroiliac pain (Aesc.).

Hale quoted from Navarro about cures of ulcers "Sloughing ulcer of right breast. An indolent ulcer, in the lower third of right leg, deep, discharging bloody fetid pus. Inflammation of left leg and foot with enormous swelling and fever."

RELATIONS - ***Compare:*** (1) Rhus-t., Anac., Euphor.

REFERENCES - Boericke. Clarke. Murphy. Phatak.

CONCHIOLINUM

(Mother of Pearl)

PHARMACY - conch. Conchiolinum. Mother of pearl. Mater perlarum. Triturations. ***Historical dose:*** Trituration and all potencies.

CLINICAL - Bone, disorders. Fever. Lung, disorders. Osteitis. Pyemia.

HOMEOPATHIC - Conch. has a wide range of action in disorders of bones, especially when the growing ends are affected. Calc-p. and Calc. are its nearest analogs.

Observations made on workers in mother-of-pearl factories showed that inhalation of the dust produces catarrh of the respiratory organs and, later on inflammation of the ends of bones. This begins in the diaphyses, but may spread to the epiphyses. It attacks young subjects.

First there is a more or less intense pain in the bone, comes suddenly, at first continuous, later intermittent. Soon after the appearance of the pain there is fever, thirst, loss of appetite, sleeplessness, dark-colored urine with sediment.

Then swelling occurs, developing on one or the other end of a diaphysis, never in the middle of it nor in the epiphysis. The swelling has a clear, sharp margin.

Swelling is very painful to the slightest touch, at first soft, elastic and slightly fluctuating. It may become as hard as a bone. Suppuration may occur. The bones that have been affected are lower jaw, scapula, humerus, radius, ulna, tibia, fibula, tarsal and metatarsal bones.

COMMENTS - Clarke cured with Conch. 3c a delicate boy who at three different times had had pain in his left knee. The left inner condyle was swollen and tender. The cure was rapid and the general health much improved at the same time.

REFERENCES - Clarke.

CONIUM MACULATUM

(Poison Hemlock)

PHARMACY - con. Conium maculatum. Poison hemlock. N. O. Umbelliferae. Coniinum. Tincture of fresh plant in flower. ***Historical dose:*** All potencies.

CLINICAL - Abstinence. Asthma. Arteriosclerosis. Belching. Bladder, disorders. ***Breast, cancer.*** Bronchitis. Bruises. ***Debility. Cancer.*** Cataract. ***Cervicitis.*** Chorea. Coughs. Cysts. Depression. Diphtheria, paralysis. Dysmenorrhea. Emaciation. Erysipelas. Eye, disorders. Galactorrhea. ***Heartburn.*** Herpes. Hypochondriasis. ***Indurations.*** Infertility. ***Injuries***. Jaundice. Liver, disorders. Melancholia. Menstruation, disorders. ***Multiple, sclerosis. Muscular, weakness. Nerve, disorders.*** Neuritis. Numbness. Ovaries, disorders. ***Paralysis.*** Peritonitis. Photophobia. Pregnancy, disorders. ***Prostate, cancer.*** Ptosis. Scrofula. Spermatorrhea. Stomach, disorders. Testicle, disorders. Tetters. ***Trembling***. Trismus. Tuberculosis. ***Tumors.*** Ulcers. Uterine, cancer. Vertigo. Vision, disorders. ***Weakness.***

HOMEOPATHIC - An ancient remedy, rendered classical by Plato's graphic description of this poison given to the Greek philosopher Socrates to cause his death. The ascending paralysis it produces, ending in respiration failure, shows the ultimate tendency of many symptoms produced in the provings.

Con. has difficult gait, trembling, sudden loss of strength while walking, painful stiffness of legs, urinary troubles, weakened memory, sexual debility, etc. Affects the nerves and muscles, causing incoordination and paralysis, uncertain gait, difficult speech. ***Patient becomes gradually weak***. Irregular, action, and development of symptoms.

Progressive debility. Great debility in the morning in bed. General feeling as if bruised by blows. ***Weakness of body and mind. Trembling*** of all the limbs, with palpitations. Suddenly sick and weak with numbness. Paroxysms of hysteria and hypochondriasis from sexual abstinence or sexual excess. Hysterical convulsions. Faints at stool.

Glands, especially breasts and ovaries, are affected with engorgement and ***stony indurations.*** Alters glandular structure to scrofulous and cancerous conditions. Sensation as of a lump in brain, in epigastrium. Tearing, stabbing pains. New growths. Cancerous diathesis.

Ascending symptoms, paralysis after diphtheria. Arteriosclerosis. Decay of sternum. Insomnia of multiple neuritis. Easily intoxicated (Zinc.). Sensation as of a hoop or band or something tight around the part. Desire for warmth, especially that of sun. Great liability to take cold. Night and morning sweat with offensive odor and smarting in skin or offensive odor without sweat.

Often found in old age, a time of debility, weakness, languor, local congestions and sluggishness. Useful in old age or for those persons who become old early. Troubles at the change of life, old maids, bachelors. For youths who suffer from ill effects of masturbation. Tumor growth invites it. Tonic after influenza.

MIND - Slow, impaired comprehension. Difficulty in understanding what is read. Difficulty concentrating. Cannot think after using eyes. Poor memory, symptoms similar to Alzheimer's disease. Benumbed sensation. Inability to sustain mental effort, tired sensation in brain, imbecility. Senility, weakness.

Timid. Indifferent. ***Depression.*** Grief, especially from loss of personal property (Aur.). Grief after death of a loved one, after a prolonged illness. Consolation aggravates (Nat-m.). Sad, dissatisfied with herself and surroundings. As if great guilt weighed upon him.

Excitement causes mental depression. Feel as if they were to cry and swallow and choke as from a lump in the throat. Tired of life. Discouraged. Broken down feeling. Trifles seem important. Cares very little for things. No inclination for business or study. Makes useless purchases, wastes or ruins them. Sensation of unreality, as if in a dream.

Insanity, periodical or alternating. Superstitious. Worse when idle. Averse to society, yet fears being alone, especially during menses. Ill effects of ***repressed sexual desire.***

While walking on the road wants to grab and abuse somebody. Likes to wear his best clothes. Thinks that animals are jumping on his bed.

Abdomen - Abdomen hard and distended. Distention, worse after taking milk. Cutting pain before passing flatus. Trembling of whole abdomen. Tremulous weakness, palpitation of heart after every stool. Hypogastric pain goes down legs. Sensitive, bruised, swollen, knife-like pains. Painful tightness.

Back - Spinal injuries. Ill effects of bruises and shocks to spine. Coccyodynia. Dull aching in lumbar and sacral region. Pain between shoulders. Drawing pain in the lumbar vertebrae worse standing. Coccyx pain. Neck cold. Enlargement of neck. Pediculated tumor at the center of back. Small, flat wart like growths on buttocks.

Breasts - ***Breasts enlarge and become painful*** before and during menses (Calc., Lac-c.), worse at every step. Wants to press breast hard with hand. ***Breast cancer with hard tumor. Tumors after injury.*** Breasts lax and shrunken with or without sexual desire. ***Hard tumors*** in breasts with stitches or piercing pain. ***Stitches in breasts and in nipples,*** on taking deep breath or walking. Too much milk before menses.

Causations - The effects of blows, contusions or falls. Effects of bruises and shocks to spine. Over straining, over work, over study. Grief. Sexual excess, sexual abstinence.

Chest - Sharp pain from sternum to spine. Decay of the sternum. Tightness of chest better by coughing. The clothes lie like a weight on chest and shoulders.

Constitutions - Corresponds to elderly persons, old, feeble men, old maids and bachelors. Persons of strong, sedentary habit more than to lively. Persons who are easily intoxicated with stimulants (Zinc.). Slender persons and children. Scrofulous constitutions, cancers and glandular enlargements. Cancerous diathesis.

Ears - Accumulation of ear wax like paper pulp or blood. Red, hard wax, causing hardness of hearing. Ears feel stopped on blowing nose. Oversensitive to noise. Parotid gland swollen and hard.

Eyes - Paralysis of ocular muscles (Caust.). Feel crossed. Lids, heavy, droop worse outside. Ptosis of eyelids. Conjunctivitis and keratitis. ***Photophobia and excessive lachrymation*** without inflammation or from slightest abrasion or ulceration of the eye. Burning in eyes. Sweats on closing eyes. Corneal pustules. Cataract after eye injury. Diplopia. Myopia. Dim-sighted, worse artificial light. Vision colored, red. As if fringe falling over eyes. Black spots before eyes with vertigo. Vision becomes more blurred when vexed.

Face - Moist and spreading herpes on face. Cancer of the lip from pressure of pipe. Sub-maxillary glands are swollen and hard.

Female - Menses, irregular, too late, scanty. Dysmenorrhea with drawing down thighs. Rash before menses. Small, red, burning pimples appear with scanty menses and disappear after menses. Itching around pudenda or deep in vagina. Leucorrhea, white, acrid, preceded by griping in abdomen after urination. ***Cervicitis. Induration of os and cervix.*** Ovaritis. Ovary enlarged, indurated. Cutting pain in ovaries and uterus. Prolapse of uterus from straining at a hard stool. Ill effects of ***repressed sexual desire*** or suppressed menses or from excessive indulgence. Motion of child painful during pregnancy.

Food - Craving for salt, coffee and sour things. Aversion to bread. Amelioration from eating and aggravation a few hours after meals.

Head - Stupefying headache, with nausea and vomiting of mucus with a feeling as of foreign body under the skull. Temples compressed, worse after meals. Sensation as of a lump in right half of brain. Sick headaches with inability to urinate. Pain in head from sinciput to occiput, better stooping and moving the head. Bruised, semi-lateral pains. Dull occipital pain on rising in morning. Sensation of fullness, bursting in brain during headache. One side numb and cold. Hot spots on head.

Heart - Palpitations, worse exertion, drinking, at stools, etc. Pulse unequal, irregular.

Kidneys - Difficulty in passing urine in the beginning even when standing, then it flows freely. Interrupted urination, ***urine stops and starts,*** better standing. Dribbling in old men (Cop.). Urine feels very hot. Interrupted discharge (Clem.). Cutting and burning after urination.

Limbs - Shoulders feel bruised, clothes lie like a weight on them. Axillary glands enlarged. ***Axillary glands pain with numb feeling down arm***. Hands, weary, heavy, trembling, unsteady. ***Perspiration of hands.*** Nails yellow. Fingers and toes numb. Heels, as if bone would push through them. Shooting in heels. ***Putting feet on chair relieves pain***. Cracking in knee joint. ***Muscular weakness***, especially of lower limbs. Can walk straight and steadily with eyes closed, but staggers, becomes giddy, is nauseated when walking with open eyes.

Liver - Severe aching in and around the liver. Chronic jaundice and pain in right hypochondrium.

Lungs - Shortness of breath on taking the least exercise, oppressed breathing, constriction of chest, pains in chest. Constant tormenting cough from dry spot in the larynx or tickling in chest and throat pit, worse when lying down, laughing, talking and during pregnancy, has to sit up. Cough seems to come from abdomen. Cough on taking deep breath. Loose coughs without expectoration, has to swallow what he coughs up.

Male - Ill effects of ***suppressed sexual desires.*** Desire increased, power decreased. Sexual desire without erection. Sexual nervousness with feeble erection. Erections imperfect and of too short duration. ***Impotence.*** Seminal discharge, provoked by mere presence of a woman or contact. Cutting in urethra while semen passes. Sexual nervousness, dejection after sex. ***Prostatitis.*** Dribbling of prostatic fluid, worse stools, emotions, etc. ***Prostate cancer.*** Testicles hard and enlarged. Itching in prepuce.

Modalities - Better while fasting. Better from letting limbs hang down. Better walking bent. Better sitting down. Better stooping. Better walking. Better motion. Better pressure. Better sun. Better dark. ***Worse from seeing moving objects.*** Worse sexual abuse or excess. ***Worse from celibacy***. Worse before and during menses. Worse old age. ***Worse alcohol.*** Worse pressure of tight clothing. Worse raising arms. Worse standing. Worse lying down with head low. ***Worse turning in bed***. Worse jar. Worse after exertion. Worse bodily or mental injury. Worse at night. Worse cold, taking cold. Worse snowy air. Worse spring. Worse dry, hot air.

Mouth - Toothache, worse cold food, but not cold drinks. Tongue cancer. Sour saliva. Soreness about the root of tongue. Distortion of tongue and mouth. Speech difficult from paralysis of tongue.

Nose - Polyps. Bleeds easily, becomes sore. Picks nose constantly. Frequent sneezing. Obstinate obstruction of nose. Acute smell.

Rectum - Ineffective urging to stool. Involuntary stools while sleeping. Constipation on alternate days. Burning or coldness in rectum during stool. Cold flatus, stool. ***Tremulous weakness after every stool*** (Verat., Ars., Arg-n.).

Sensations - Sensation as if a hoop, band or something tight was around the parts. Deficiency of irritability of the body, the body has very little sensation. Darting from within outwards, tension in inner parts, also in outer parts, pricking in the bones.

Skin - Greenish, like an old bruise. Yellow skin with papular eruption, yellow fingernails. Red spots turning yellow or green. ***Glands enlarged and indurated,*** also mesenteric. Flying stitches through the glands. Tumors, piercing pains, worse at night. Induration after contusions. Foul, eczematous eruptions. Chronic ulcers with fetid discharge. Gangrenous ulcers. Urticaria from violent bodily exertion. Anesthesia or inactivity of the skin. Night and morning sweat with offensive odor and smarting in skin.

Sleep - ***Sweat as soon as one sleeps***, even when closing eyes. Drowsiness by day. Sleeps after midnight. Inclination to sleep in the evening, with falling down of the eyelids. Disturbed and unrefreshing sleep. Starting of the limbs during sleep. Anxious and frightful dreams, of disease, mutilation, death, danger, and quarrels. Nightmares.

Stomach - ***Attacks of sick feeling.*** Painful spasms of the stomach. Distention of stomach after taking milk. Better from eating, aggravation a few hours after meals. ***Acrid heartburn*** and acid belchings, ***worse on going to bed***. Acidity and burning, painful spot the level of the sternum. Cancerous ulcers. Terrible nausea. Vomiting of coffee grounds, chocolate colored lumps or clear sour water. Nausea and vomiting during pregnancy. Heartburn in pregnant women where an excessive heartburn comes on, when going to bed at night.

Temperature - Coldness of nape, of calf, etc. Hot flushes or sweat, on dropping to sleep or when closing the eyes. Sweat, under the eyes, on chin, cold on nape and palms offensive causing smarting of skin.

Throat - As if a round body were ascending from stomach (globus). Food goes down the wrong way and stops. Paresis of esophagus. Constant inclination to swallow as from a lump in the throat worse walking in open air. Tonsils enlarged.

Vertigo - ***Vertigo, when lying down and when turning over in bed,*** when turning head *sidewise* or turning eyes, worse shaking head, slight noise or conversation of others, especially towards the left.

COMMENTS - Hahnemann noted that it is exceedingly difficult to distinguish between the primary and secondary effects of Con. He thought that the primary action is one of "rigidity, condensation and constriction of the tissues with swelling of the glands and diminution of the senses."

Teste concurred, adding that the action is primarily inflammatory and that this accounts for its suitability for "persons of a lively, quick, sanguine disposition with a marked development of the glandular system." It is characteristically adapted to painful glandular affections, "principally such as result from a strain or blow, but the precise cause of which may have escaped our recollection."

Teste placed Con. at the head of the analogs of Acon. Con. is to the glands and capillary system what Acon. is to the heart and arterial system. In many cases Con. may be regarded as the "Aconite of chronic diseases." The other Acon. analogs, according to him, are Cham., Seneg., Canth. and Ph-ac.

Scirrhus tumors, ulcerating and otherwise. Chronic or sub-acute inflammation with bloody engorgement of the parenchyma, induration, and even subsequent ulceration of the tissues.

Induration and inflammations of the breast and nipples. Useful for treating indurated, precancerous tissues. Breast cancer with a history of trauma to the breast. Hard lumps in breast, induration, can be painless. Breast can shrivel, atrophy (Iod.). Effects of hurts to the breast by falls or blows.

Pains in breast before menses, worse by every step. Scanty menses, especially in old maids. Checked lochia. Indurated cervix, cervical cancer. Prostate and testicular cancer.

Sexual conditions including hypertrophy or atrophy of glands, excess of function or abrogation. Unsatisfied sexual desire, ailments from suppressed sex drive. Hysteria and hypochondriasis from abstinence from sexual intercourse.

Pronounced constipation or diarrhea. Weakness, tremulousness and palpitation after every evacuation. Faintness after stool. Burning or coldness in the rectum. Flatulent tendency (Ammc., Asaf.). Pancreatic cancer (Calc-ar., Phos.).

Photophobia, ptosis. Red vision. Sweat on closing the eyes. Eye symptoms are worse night and early morning. Accumulation of earwax. Hot spots on the head. Erysipelas, pain piercing to brain.

Numbness and deadness of limbs. Stabbing pains. Weak-spells, faintness, sudden loss of strength while walking. Ascending paralysis. Multiple sclerosis.

Vertigo, particularly in the elderly, worse on turning in bed or sudden turns from side to side. Symptoms worse when idle.

Grimmer noted its usefulness in breast cancer after bruises or injuries. Sterck used Con. and made some notable cures of scirrhus tumors, ulcerating and otherwise.

A. H. Birdsall reported a case of contusion of the testicle. He found the patient writhing in agony, the pain complained of being "sharp, cutting, running up spermatic cord to lower part of back and also through scrotum to root of penis." Con. 200c relieved in five minutes and at the end of twenty minutes the pain was gone.

Clarke used the remedy with success in many cases of weakness from masturbation in men and youths. "Emission on the slightest stimulus, such as merely being in the society of a woman."

Goodno cured a girl of 25 of severe dysmenorrhea with scanty, almost arrested flow, which had existed since the periods commenced. She also had nosebleed, cough and stitches through the left lung at times. Two years previously, after unusual excitement, she had bearing-down pains, prolapse and ante-version.

The dysmenorrhea pains were relieved by Sepia and other remedies, but the prolapse increased with bearing-down as though the womb would be forced from the vulva, worse standing and walking, before and during menses. Intermittent flow of urine. Cutting pain after urination.

Obstinate constipation of long standing. Stool (once in seven days) large, hard, followed by tremulous weakness, she must lie down. Dull pain below left breast. Prompt relief and speedy cure were effected by Con. 1,000c.

Proell mentioned excellent results with Con. 10c in strangury and ischuria, when the urine cannot be discharged from nervousness or swelling of the prostate (Nat-s. 5c trituration was effective where the bladder could not be entirely emptied.).

Sircar recorded a striking case of a patient who had severe diarrhea, for which he was about to give Sulph., when he asked if the stools were hot. "On the contrary, they are cold," replied the patient. Sircar found "cold flatulence" under Con. and gave it on analogy with brilliant effect.

Guernsey wrote "This remedy is characterized by a great dizziness, brought on when lying down and moving the head ever so slightly or even the eyes—all the contents of the room appear to whirl around, patient wishes to keep the head perfectly still. In urinating the water flows at first in a full stream, then stops, flows again, again stops."

Nash thought "turning the head sideways" is the most characteristic form of the modality "worse by moving the head." Some give it is as "lying down in bed and turning over," but he regards the "lying down" as the least important part. Nash cured a patient who had all the symptoms of locomotor ataxia and who could not, when walking, turn the head the least bit sideways without staggering or falling.

A case of lumbago was cured with Con. in six days after seven months' suffering. Symptoms include an inability to turn over in bed without being dizzy, worse ascending, by exercise. Feeling of ball pressing into back over left hip. Pain shooting down left leg, ending in a spot that felt as though pricked by a bunch of hot needles. Yellow nails.

Nash mentioned the characteristic "Sweats day or night, as soon as one sleeps or even on closing the eyes." This enabled Lippe to cure a man of 80 of hemiplegia.

R. C. Markham cured with Con. 1,000c. an obstinate cough, dry, hard, frequent with asthmatic wheezing or fine rattling in chest on deep breathing, worse slightest exposure to cold air, getting into cold bed or out of a warm one or even putting arms out was sufficient to bring on severe coughing.

The guiding symptom which appeared last and led to the remedy was a pain in the apex of the left lung with soreness in a small spot midway between neck and shoulder just back of the clavicle. The pain, cutting and stitch-like, ran downward and inward toward the sternum.

RELATIONS - ***Compare:*** (1) Bar-c., Hydr., Iod., Kali-p., Hyos., Cur. (2) Scirr. a cancer nosode - cancerous diathesis, enlarged glands, cancer of breast, worms.

REFERENCES - Boericke. Clarke. Grimmer. Phatak.

CONVALLARIA MAJALIS

(Lily of the Valley)

PHARMACY - conv. Convallaria majalis. Lily of the Valley. N.O. Liliaceae. Convallariaceae. ***Historical dose:*** Tincture and all potencies.

CLINICAL - ***Anasarca***. Angina pectoris. Aneurysm. Diarrhea. ***Dyspnea.*** Endocarditis. ***Heart, disorders.*** Herpes. Morning, sickness. Orthopnea. Pruritus, vulvae. Tobacco, heart. Venous, stasis. Vomiting.

HERBAL - Convallaria is a popular remedy in Russia for heart disorders and it has been introduced into old-school medicine principally as a heart remedy. It compares closely in its action with Lil-t.

Conv. also resembles its other botanical relatives, Aloe., All-c. and All-s. It is strongly purgative and causes morning vomiting. The symptoms from its proving show that its nearest analog is Lilium tigrinum.

HOMEOPATHIC - Increases energy of heart's action, renders it more regular. It is of use when the ventricles are over distended and dilatation begins, and when there is an absence of compensatory hypertrophy and venous stasis is marked.

Dyspnea, dropsy, aneurysm tendency ***Anasarca***. Sensation as if heart ceased beating, then starting very suddenly. Tobacco heart. Soreness of uterine region with palpitation of heart. Movement in abdomen as from a fist of a child.

MIND - Dull intellect, can hardly think. Mind wanders from subject when reading. Irritable, when asked a question. Depression. Grieves easily. Hysterical manifestations.

Abdomen - Sensitive. Colicky pains. Gurgling and pain on taking deep breath. Clothes feel too tight. Movement in abdomen like fist of a child.

Back - Pain and aching in lumbar region.

Face - Hydroa in nose and lips, raw and sore. Nosebleed. Sees imaginary gray spot about three inches square.

Female - Great ***soreness in uterine region with sympathetic palpitations of heart.*** Pain in sacro-iliac joints, running down leg. Itching of urinary meatus and vaginal orifice.

Head - Dull headache, worse ascending, hawking. Scalp sensitive.

Heart - Heart disorders. Extremely rapid and irregular pulse. Feeling as if heartbeat throughout the chest. ***Sensation as if heart ceased beating, then starting very suddenly.*** Palpitation from the least exertion. Endocarditis with orthopnea. Angina pectoris. Tobacco heart, especially when due to cigarettes.

Kidneys - Aching in bladder, feels distended. Frequent, offensive urination, scanty urine. Dropsy, anuric tendency.

Limbs - Aching of legs and big toe. Trembling of hands. Aching in wrists and ankles.

Lungs - Pulmonary congestion. Orthopnea. ***Dyspnea*** while walking. Hot feeling in throat.

Modalities - Better in open air. Worse from lying on back. Worse in warm room (All-c.).

Mouth - Grating of teeth in the morning. Coppery taste. Tongue feels sore and scalded, broad and thick with heavy, dirty coating.

Temperature - Chilly in back and down spine, followed by fever, little sweat. Thirst and headache during chill. Dyspnea during fever.

Throat - Raw feeling in back of throat when inspiring.

COMMENTS - Nash used it in the 30c with very satisfactory results in women complaining of great soreness in uterine region with sympathetic palpitation of the heart. He also removed cardiac dropsy when this uterine soreness was present.

Berridge credited it with this symptom: "Movement in the abdomen as from the fist of a child," like Sulph., Thuj., and Croc. In the case of Conv., the symptom occurs when lying on the back. Sleepiness accompanies many symptoms.

RELATIONS - ***Compare:*** (1) Dig., Crat., Lil-t. (2) Adonis - feeble heart action due only to functional disturbance.

REFERENCES - Boericke. Clarke. Phatak.

CONVOLVULUS ARVENSIS

(Bind-weed)

PHARMACY - convo-a. Convolvulus arvensis. Bind-weed. N. O. Convolvulacae. Tincture of whole flowering plant. Tincture of root. ***Historical dose:*** Tincture and all potencies.

HOMEOPATHIC - Very few experiments have been made with this plant, and in those the resinoid of the root and pure Convolvulin were used.

The few symptoms recorded are all in the gastro-intestinal sphere. Eructation after eating. Colic and diarrhea, liquid stool. Stools are soft, semi-fluid evacuation, preceded by flatulence and violent colic. Stools with pain.

REFERENCES - Boericke. Clarke.

CONVOLVULUS DUARTINUS

(Morning Glory)

PHARMACY - convo-d. Convolvulus duartinus. Morning glory. Ipomoeabona. N. O. Convolvulacae. Tincture of flowers. ***Historical dose:*** Tincture and all potencies.

CLINICAL - Colic. Constipation. Eye, inflammation. Headaches. Numbness. Rheumatism. Vertigo.

HOMEOPATHIC - Convo-d. was proved under Mure. Recorded symptoms include reveries in the daytime, dreams of dead persons, and numbness in limbs. Symptoms are worse in morning and better after cold bath.

MIND - Moral weakness. Reveries in the daytime.

Abdomen - Pain in abdomen with internal heat. Violent colic with drawings.

Eyes - Inflammation of the left eye.

Head - Burning in frontal region, ceasing after a cold bath. Pain in frontal region with heat at root of nose. Pain in left temple (corresponding to inflamed left eye).

Kidneys - Red urine. Yellow sediment in urine.

Limbs - Numbness of arms, worse when hanging down. Pains in left shoulder in left wrist. Numbness of right index and middle fingers. Sharp pain in right knee. Pain fore part of left leg for four days. Deep-seated pain in calves.

Sleep - Drowsiness in daytime. Dreams about quarreling, about dead persons, falling out of his front teeth, of flying along a lighted street, appearance of a ghost. Wakes with a start.

Stool - Constipation.

Throat - Heat and dryness at anterior and upper part of esophagus.

Teeth - Toothache. Swelling of gums. Tongue feels swollen.

Vertigo - Vertigo with faintness.

REFERENCES - Clarke.

COPAIVA

(Balsam of Copaiva)

PHARMACY - cop. Copaiva. Balsam of copaiva. Balsamum copaivae. Copaifera officinalis. Copaifera reticulata. N. O. Leguminosae. Caesalpinioideae. Tincture of the balsam. ***Historical dose:*** Tincture and all potencies.

CLINICAL - Acne. Anus, itching. ***Bladder, catarrh.*** Blenorrhagia. ***Bronchitis.*** Catarrh. ***Colitis***. Coughs. Cystitis. Dysentery. Dysuria. Fistula. Gastritis. Gonorrhea. Headaches. Hemorrhoids. ***Hives***. Measles. Nosebleeds. Prostatitis. Pruritus. Roseola. Urethritis. Urticaria. Vulva, inflammation.

HERBAL - Copaiva is an old world remedy for gonorrhea and it has been used for other blennorrhagic conditions. It has been proved and observations have also been made on patients who have overdosed with the remedy.

A. P. Bowie verified the indication "In old persons, (men) who from cold or other causes cannot urinate or where there is frequent desire and only a few drops pass with much straining. Frequently with a mucus discharge from the bowels with much rumbling and rolling in the bowels."

Bowie gave 5-drop doses of the first dilution. He also recommended an ointment of 10 drops of the balsam in vaseline, "to relieve the burning and itching at the anus caused by hemorrhoids."

HOMEOPATHIC - The chief action is on the genito-urinary organs and rectum. Irritation accompanying thickening of bladder. Burning at neck of bladder and in urethra, discharge milky, corrosive, meatus tumid and inflamed.

Affects the mucus membranes of the respiratory organs and the skin, producing a well-marked nettle-rash. ***Chronic bronchitis***, with profuse, greenish-gray, disgusting-smelling sputa. Colds and catarrhs. Excessive discharge. Foul, ***blenorrhea,*** bronchorrhea, suppuration.

MIND - Weeps on hearing a piano.

Bladder - ***Catarrh of bladder***. Dysuria. Retention with pain in bladder, anus and rectum. Burning pressure, painful urination by drops. Constant desire to urinate. Urine acrid, scanty, bloody, odor of violets. Greenish, turbid color, peculiar pungent odor. Swelling of orifice. Urethra feels wide open. Suppuration, ascends urinary tract. Purulent or acrid milky gonorrhea.

Constitutions - Suited to the irritable bladder of elderly women.

Ears - Excessive sensitiveness to sharp sounds.

Face - Acne, disfiguring the face. Face red, flushed.

Female - Itching of vulva and anus with bloody purulent discharge. Profuse, strong-smelling menstrual discharge with pains radiating to hip bones, with nausea

Food - Tastes too salty.

Head - Flushes of blood to the head and face. Scalp sensitive. Excessive sensitive ness, pain in occiput. Occipital headache, better gentle hand pressure. Dull, frontal headache, passes to occiput and back again with throbbing. Worse right side and motion.

Lungs - Bronchial catarrh with profuse, greenish, offensive discharge. Bronchiectasis. Tickling in larynx, trachea and bronchials. Painful cough with heat and oppression of chest. Burning in lungs. Cough with profuse, gray, purulent, greenish, offensive sputum. Foul bloody expectoration.

Male - Prostatitis. Testicles sensitive and swollen. Blenorrhagia. Pulsations in penis.

Modalities - Worse from morning. Worse taking cold.

Mouth - Teeth cold.

Nose - Rawness and soreness of nostrils with stopped-up feeling, dryness of posterior sinuses. ***Burning and dryness***, crusts on turbinated bones. Profuse, thick, fetid discharge from nasal passages, running down throat at night. Marked catarrhal condition in upper respiratory tract. Nosebleed, lasting several days in small boys.

Rectum - *Mucus colitis*. Stools covered with mucus with colic and chilliness. Burning and itching of anus, caused by hemorrhoids.

Skin - *Hives* with fever and constipation. Roseola. Erysipelatous inflammation, around the abdomen. Bullous eruptions. Circumscribed, lenticular patches with itching, mottled appearance. Chronic urticaria in children.

Stomach - Food seems too salty. Gastric troubles during menstruation or following urticaria. Gas and intestinal flatulence, urging to stool and difficult passage with pain.

Throat - Chronic catarrh of the throat.

RELATIONS - ***Antidote:*** Bell., Merc. ***Compare:*** (1) Santalum - aching in kidneys. (2) Cann-i., Canth., Barosma, Cub., Apis, Vespa, Erig., Senecio, Sepia.

REFERENCES - Boericke. Clarke. Phatak.

CORALLIUM RUBRUM

(Red Coral)

PHARMACY - cor-r. Corallium rubrum. Red coral. Gorgonio nobilis. N. O. Gorgoniaceae. Trituration. ***Historical dose:*** Trituration and all potencies.

CLINICAL - Asthma. Catarrh. Chancre. Constipation. Colds. Coryza. ***Coughs.*** Eruptions. Glands, inflamed. Headaches. Hoarseness. Hysteria. Measles. Nosebleed. ***Post-nasal, catarrh.*** Psoriasis. Purpura. Sore, throat. Syphilis. ***Whooping cough.***

HOMEOPATHIC - Red coral, the product of a coralligene zoophyte, contains calcium carbonate and iron oxide (the origin of its color), gelatin and other elements. In medical alchemy, red coral was considered to have *"strengthening tonic properties,"* and to be astringent, sudorific, diuretic and absorbent.

Cor-r. affects the mucus membranes, especially of respiratory organs. The provings of coral develop much coryza, nosebleed and even ulceration within the nostrils.

Eruptions, which are for the most part of its own color, coral-red. Red spots on the palms of the hands, at first coral, then darker, and finally coppery. Coral-red chancres.

Whooping and spasmodic coughs, especially when the attack comes on with a ***very rapid coughs*** and the attacks follow so closely as to almost run into each other. ***Violent coughing attacks***. Coughs often preceded by sensation of smothering, followed by exhaustion. ***Coughs with expectoration of blood.*** Congestion of face, purple colored face, after dinner.

Ulcerations in the respiratory organs with a stringy discharge. Feeling as if cold air were streaming through skull and air-passages. Too cold when uncovered and too hot when covered, better by artificial heat.

MIND - Peevish, inclined to scold and swear at his pains. Irascibility and ill-humor. Wine has a natural taste, but immediately stupefies him.

Delusion, feels as if newly born in the world and overwhelmed with wonder at the novelty of his surroundings. Stupefaction after wine. Confusion after beer. Confusion from spirituous liquors. Fear of suffering.

Back - Stiffness in nape of neck. Pain as if the small of the back were broken. Pressing pain in scapulae during cough. Neck stiff.

Chest - Sensation as if cold air were streaming through air-passages in morning on deep inspiration, with provocation to cough. Difficult hawking of bronchial mucus. Pain in sternum during cough.

Cough - ***Dry, spasmodic, suffocative cough.*** Very rapid cough. Short, barking cough. Nervous cough. ***Reverberating machine-gun like cough.*** Continuous hysterical cough. Violent spasmodic cough. Coughs begins with gasping for breath. ***Almost continuous paroxysms of violent spasmodic cough.*** Cough as soon as he eats. Coughs with a purple face, followed by vomiting of stringy mucus and exhaustion. Cough with bleeding from mouth and nose. ***Cough followed by vomiting of stringy mucus and by exhaustion.*** Isolated cough at regular intervals throughout the day. Feels suffocated and greatly exhausted after whooping cough. Whooping cough when attacks comes on with a very rapid cough, and attacks follow so closely as to almost run into each other. Coughs and coughs until patient falls back as limber as a rag.

Eyes - Hot and painful eyes, bathed in tears on closing. Sensation of compression in the orbit. Pain, as from excoriation in the eyes. Eye pain, violently worse during every motion. Sensation of burning in the eyes. Burning of eyes from candlelight. Pressure as from sand in reddened eyes in evening. Enlarged pupils in whooping cough. Extremely sensitive drawing pain in left orbit.

Face - Grows purple and black with coughing. Heat in the face, worse on bending head forward, by stooping. Pain, as from dislocation in the maxillary joint. Left zygoma painful, as if bruised, worse touch. Left articulation of lower jaw as if sprained, when moving jaw. Painful swelling of left submaxillary gland worse swallowing or bending head forward.

Food - No appetite. ***Violent thirst.*** Insipidity of food. Food tastes like sawdust. Bread, farinaceous foods tastes like straw. Sweetish taste of beer. ***Craves salty foods and acids.*** Intoxication after drinking very little wine.

Head - Hot cheeks and forehead with cold feet, after dinner. Confusion in the head, feels empty, hollow, very large. ***Congestion of blood to head on stooping.*** Violent pain as if parietal bones were forced apart, worse stooping. Headache with severe pain in back of the eyeballs, worse inhaling cold air. ***Pressing pain in forehead.*** Pain aggravated by breathing cold air through nose. Head feels large, empty, hollow. As if cold air were blowing through, when head is moved quietly or shaken. As if forehead were flattened. Meningeal inflammation threatening in yellow fever.

Heart - Pulse full and hard. Quick pulse; in whooping cough.

Kidneys - Loam or clay-colored urine, with similar sediment. Burning urine.

Limbs - Great lassitude in all limbs after a short walk in evening. Smooth spots of a deep-red color. Pressive pain in the shoulder blades, aggravated by coughing. Pain in the wrists, as if he had been writing much and rapidly. Pain in the knees, tibia and tarsal joint, as if he had walked a great deal. Red, itching, miliary eruption rough, feeling like a grater to the touch, on both elbows.

Lungs - Crowing during inspiration. Asthma. Smothering sensation before paroxysms of cough. ***Air passages feel cold on deep inspiration*** (Cist.). Hawking of profuse mucus. Difficult, oppressed breathing. ***Profuse secretion of mucus dropping through posterior sinuses.*** Feels suffocated and greatly exhausted after whooping cough. Cold expectoration.

Male - Balanitis. Ulcers on glans and inner prepuce with yellow ichor. Very red flat ulcers, on glans and under surface of prepuce. ***Ulcers very sensitive to touch.*** Emissions and weakened sexual power Swelling of prepuce. Margin of prepuce feels sore when linen touches it. ***Frenum painful, as if pricked by needles.*** Profus sweat on genitals. ***Involuntary seminal emissions during sleep.***

Modalities - Better - covering. Worse from inhaling air. Worse open air. Worse changing from a warm to cold room. Worse eating. Worse towards morning. Worse stooping. Worse after dinner. Worse touch. Worse uncovering.

Mouth - Food tastes like sawdust. Bread tastes like straw. Beer tastes sweet. Pain in articulation of left lower jaw. ***White coated tongue in whooping cough.*** Lips cracked and painful. Lips chapped, painful and swollen.

Nose - Great dryness of mucus membrane of nose and throat. Nosebleed at night. Bleeding from one nostril at a time. Bleeding of the nose from one nostril at a time. Nose stopped up and ulcerated. ***Post-nasal catarrh.*** Fluent coryza. ***Profuse secretion of mucus dropping through posterior sinuses***. Violent fluent catarrh of odorless mucus. Dry coryza, nose stopped up and ulcerated. Smells odors of smoke, onions, etc. Inspired air feels cold (Cist.). Painful ulcer in nostrils.

Perspiration - Profuse sweat on genitals.

Rectum - ***Constipation, followed by copious papescent stool.*** Profuse discharge of mucus from anus at night.

Skin - Psoriasis of palms and soles. Coral-colored, then dark red spots, changing to copper-colored spots. Red, flat ulcers. Psoriasis smooth, copper-coloured spots.

Sleep - Yawning, violent, frequent and in rapid succession. Great sleepiness, falls asleep while standing. Sleeps with head under covers. If he uncovers himself, he feels too cold, and when covered, feels too hot. Can't sleep before midnight, tosses about. Starts as soon as she falls asleep, from a frightened dream.

Stomach - ***Nausea, with dryness of the tongue and violent headache***, worse when sitting up. Vomiting of quantities of tough, ropy, stringy mucus. Vomiting with loose cough.

Teeth - Every tooth on the left side ***feels as if set on edge.*** As if the teeth were too close to one another or as if a tenacious body were lodged between them.

Temperature - Chill, but skin of usual warmth. Chill with headache and violent thirst. Chill better by external heat. Febrile shivering, with burning thirst. Dry heat internally and externally, with full and hard pulse. Dry heat without thirst, and not followed by perspiration. Hot parts feel cold when uncovered.

Throat - Great dryness of fauces. Throat very sensitive, ***especially to cold air,*** causes coughing. Great dryness of the palate, fauces and throat. Constant hawking, from the accumulation of mucus in the posterior sinuses. Sensation of excoriation on swallowing. Laryngismus stridulus resembling whooping cough. Hawking of profuse mucus. Left submaxillary glands swollen and painful, worse swallowing or bending head forward.

COMMENTS - Cor-r. corresponds to a combination of syphilis and psora. Cough like whooping cough. Cough in machine-gun paroxysms. Crowing inspiration, sensation as if inspired air was icy cold. May cough up blood. Useful for chronic bronchitis. Smothering sensation before cough, after, great exhaustion. Change of air causes coughing.

Sensation of emptiness or hollowness in the head. Head feels very large. Sensation as if forehead were flattened. Feels cold when uncovered and too hot when covered. Very sensitive to cold air and drafts. Much drowsiness, many symptoms appear during sleep.

J. N. Lowe cured with Cor-r. an infant, a year old, suffering from laryngismus stridulus, the indications being worse during sleep and after waking. Lach., given first, failed to relieve.

Guernsey's indication is "Whooping cough or any other kind of cough when the attack comes on with a very rapid cough and the attacks follow so closely as to almost run into each other." Found most effective in the nervous "machine-gun" cough where the patient gives an isolated cough at regular intervals through the day.

Nash found it the most useful of all remedies in post-nasal catarrh. Guernsey's other indication is "red, flat ulcers on the glans and inner surface of the prepuce with secretion of a quantity of yellow ichor."

RELATIONS - ***Compare:*** (1) Bell., Dros., Meph., Caust. ***Complementary:*** Sulph.

REFERENCES - Boericke. Clarke. Murphy. Phatak.

CORALLORHIZA ODONTORHIZA

(Crawley Root)

PHARMACY - corh. Corallorhiza odontorhiza. Crawley root. N. O. Orchidaceae. ***Historical dose:*** Tincture and all potencies.

HOMEOPATHIC - Intensely nervous and restless, burning of palms and soles, no thirst, chill or perspiration. Can bear only slightest covering. Hectic fever, coming on 9 a.m. to 10 a.m., and lasting until midnight.

REFERENCES - Boericke.

CORDYCEPS

(Caterpillar Fungus)

PHARMACY - cordy. Cordyceps. Caterpillar fungus. Cordyceps ophioglossoides. Deer fungus. Club-head fungus. A Tibetan mushroom. ***Historical dose:*** Tincture and all potencies.

CLINICAL - Altitude sickness. Alzheimer's disease. Anemia. Asthma. Bronchitis. ***Chronic, fatigue.*** Drug, withdrawal Dyspnea. Emaciation. Emphysema. Exhaustion. Hepatitis. Impotence. Lung, cancer. Lymphoma. Mental, weakness. Metrorrhagia. ***Mountain, sickness.*** Nerve, weakness. Senility. Sexual, weakness. ***Shortness of breath.*** Tuberculosis.

HERBAL - Cordyceps is used for a wide range of conditions including fatigue, sexual dysfunction, coughs. It is an adaptogen or immune stimulant. Over a thousand years ago, Tibetan herdsman in the Himalayas observed their yaks became vitalized after eating this fungus. Cordyceps is an energy and stamina booster.

Cordyceps is a renown star of the Chinese tonic herbal system, and is an extremely effective and powerful health enhancing agent, equal to Ginseng and Reishi. This rare and precious fungus is considered to be an tonic of the highest stature.

Cordyceps is used to strengthen the body and mind at a constitutional level. It is thought to be able to increase the "vital force for all activities." It restores the energy reserves consumed by excessive exertion, adaption to stress or aging. It is said to build sexual and physical power, mental energy, the immune system and is universally believed in Asia to prolong life.

Cordyceps is considered in Asia to be a powerful tonic for athletes. It greatly improves performance and muscle building capability. It can be used to strengthen respiratory power in those who require extra energy in order to perform physical work, labor, sports or exercise.

Cordyceps is also ***a major lung tonic.*** It can be used by those who suffer from lung weakness. It is especially beneficial to those who suffer chronic lung problems with cough, wheezing or shortness of breath.

Cordyceps is highly regarded in China as a tonic for those who are recovering from an illness or an operation, or after giving birth. In these cases, the Cordyceps helps the patient recover their physical power, to improve their appetite, and to protect the body from infection.

It is used for backache due to injury, fatigue, stress or simple aging. Long term use of Cordyceps helps to strengthen the skeletal structure, and specifically benefits the lower back region, the knees and ankles.

HOMEOPATHIC - Mental and physical exhaustion due to over work. Nerve weakness. ***Chronic fatigue.*** Mountain sickness. ***Shortness of breath.*** Lack of strength and endurance.

Weak stamina. It increases athletic and general performance, especially in long distance races. Alzheimer's disease. Antidotes opium and narcotic withdrawal symptoms (Aven.).

Back - Backache due to injury, fatigue, stress or simple aging. Lumbar weakness.

Female - Metrorrhagia, abnormal menstruation. Sexual frigidity and infertility. Loss of sexual drive.

Food - ***Increased appetite.***

General - Tiredness. Chronic fatigue syndrome. Debility. Immune weakness. Anemia. Hypercholesterolemia. Lymphoma.

Heart - Arrhythmias. Weakness of heart.

Liver - Chronic obstructive hepatic diseases. Prevention of liver and spleen atrophy.

Lungs - ***Difficult breathing, worse exertion.*** Constricted bronchials. Asthma. Persistent cough. Shortness of breath. Mountain sickness. Emphysema. Lung cancer. Tuberculosis.

Male - Sexual hypofunction. Loss of sexual drive. Impotence. Seminal emissions with aching of loins and knees.

Nerves - Sedative and hypnotic action, tranquilizer.

Skin - Fungus infections.

COMMENTS - Cordyceps is one of the primary herbal substances used daily as an anti-aging agent and for the purposes of rejuvenation.

Cordyceps as a sexual tonic is considered to have a profound long range strengthening capacity. It is commonly used for impotence, sexual debility, frigidity and infertility. Sexual debility.

Cordyceps helps the body resist a wide range of pathogenic bacteria, fungi and viruses. It is used in Asia to help treat fungus and yeast infections. Intensive research is being conducted in China and Japan relating to Cordyceps and treating certain varieties of cancer.

REFERENCES - Murphy.

CORIARIA RUSCIFOLIA

(Toot Berry)

PHARMACY - cori-r. Coriaria ruscifolia. Toot berry. Tupa-kihi or Tutu. New Zealand. N. O. Coriarieae. Tincture or trituration of the berries. ***Historical dose:*** Trituration, tincture and all potencies.

CLINICAL - Delirium tremens. Mania. Memory, lost. Vomiting.

HOMEOPATHIC - A prover who ate 1 1/2 grains of the resin experienced a disagreeable, irritating sensation in throat, extending to the stomach with pain across region of stomach, accompanied by nausea (in five min.).

In a quarter of an hour, vomiting came on, continuing more or less for two hours. Very unpleasant sensations continued for two hours more when, after great flushing of the face with all but intolerable heat, the effects passed away.

Coriaria produces intoxication very like that of alcohol. Great muscular activity as in acute mania, requiring several persons to hold a person when under the influence of the drug. Complete loss of memory, after coming out of the acute stage of the poisoning.

REFERENCES - Clarke.

CORNUS ALTERNIFOLIA

(Swamp Walnut)

PHARMACY - corn-a. Cornus alternifolia. Swamp walnut. Alternate-leaved cornel. N. O. Cornaceae. North America. Decoction or tincture of leaves. ***Historical dose:*** Tincture and all potencies.

CLINICAL - Eczema. Emaciation. Eruptions. Fever. Insomnia. Intermittent fever. ***Skin, cracked.***

HERBAL - F. H. Lutze communicated to Hom. Recorder, a Long Island farmer's cure for eczema using a decoction of the leaves of this tree. His method was to give a wine glassful three times a day for three days.

Then, for the next three days, apply it locally or wash the part with it, then administer it internally for another three days and so on. He cured, with this method, all his cases in eighteen days. This was the first acquaintance Lutze had with the remedy.

HOMEOPATHIC - Later on he made a proving on himself and another, eliciting symptoms of fever, restlessness and insomnia. Disturbed sleep. Weak and tired. Cold feeling in chest, as if full of ice. Skin eruptions with emaciation. Eczema, ***skin cracked.***

Modalities - Symptoms better after walking in open air. Better after supper.

RELATIONS - ***Compare:*** (1) In the skin effects it compares more closely with Cornus circinata. (2) In fever with drowsiness and gastro-enteric disturbance it is practically identical with the other Cornels. All three have greatly disturbed sleep.

REFERENCES - Clarke.

CORNUS CIRCINATA

(Round-leaved Dogwood)

PHARMACY - corn. Cornus circinata. Round-leaved dogwood. Green osier. N. O. Cornaceae. Infusion of tincture of fresh bark. ***Historical dose:*** Tincture and all potencies.

CLINICAL - Aphthae. Bilious, headache. Coryza. Diarrhea. Dysentery. Eczema. Hepatitis. Intermittent, fever. Jaundice. Liver, derangement. Mucus membranes, ulcers. Pruritus vulvae. Urticaria.

HERBAL - A popular remedy for aphthous and ulcerated conditions of the mucus membranes. Hale said he had seen it cure chronic ulceration of the mouth and throat, which had recurred for many years. A remedy for old malaria.

HOMEOPATHIC - Corn. has had an extensive proving. The fever symptoms are identical with those of Cornus f.

Liver derangement with aching eyeballs. Chronic malaria, hepatitis, jaundice. Pain in pit of stomach with distended abdomen. Dark, foul stools with burning in anus. Diarrhea, dark bilious offensive with sallow complexion.

Vesicular eruption associated with liver disease or aphthous stomatitis. Vesicular eczema of face of infants with nursing sore mouth. Sleepy before chill, with heat after meals. Disturbed sleep. Weakness in morning. Weak and depressed.

MIND - Forgetful. Unable to concentrate attention. Indolence with loss of mental and physical energy. Mind confused on rising in the morning. Indifferent, with drowsiness. Depression and petulance.

Abdomen - Chronic hepatitis and bilious derangement. Borborygmus. Distention, better after loose stool. Griping in umbilical region, worse during stool. Constant working in bowels as if all in motion.

Back - Drawing pains at nape of neck. Dull pains in back. Sore pains in lumbar region, worse bending forward.

Chest - Choking sensation in upper part of thorax. Soreness of chest. Stitches, bruised feeling, in chest and back. Dragging down on each side of chest. Intermittent shooting pains in chest and abdomen. Rheumatic or neuralgic pains. Fine, scarlet rash on chest with itching.

Ears - Ringing in ears.

Eyes - Eyes sunken, hollow, as after a debauch, dark circles under them. Conjunctiva tinged yellow. Soreness of eyeballs, aching pains through them. Eyeballs and lids heavy. Herpes of lids.

Face - Heat and burning in face, without redness. Countenance yellow, or pale, sallow, and sunken, indicating suffering and debility.

Female - Leucorrhea. Pruritus.

Food - Thirst for cold drinks, desire for sour drinks.

Head - Dullness and weight in head, especially temples, better by coffee. Heaviness of head, with nausea. Aching and throbbing pain over left eyebrow. Dull pains over eyeballs, unusual pulsation extending to back of head. Pulsating headache in temples.

Heart - Perceptible pulsations in chest. Palpitations of heart. Circulation accelerated.

Kidneys - Frequent desire to pass water. Urine scanty and high-colored.

Male - Increased desire, but lack of power. Frequent strong and persistent erections during the night. Pruritus.

Modalities - Better by coffee. Worse from taking cold. Worse summer heat. Worse at night. Worse on waking. Worse motion of any kind.

Mouth - Ulceration of tongue, gums and mouth. Aphthae. Burning in mouth, throat and stomach.

Limbs - Weakness of limbs. Legs weak and tremulous, particularly when ascending. Pain in right hip while lying in bed. Itching on legs and thighs, burning sensation in feet. Coldness of hands and feet after a loose stool. Burning and itching sensation in hands and arms.

Lungs - Frequent inclination to expand chest by taking a long breath. Cough with sharp stitches in chest. Dry, spasmodic cough, or tedious, chronic cough, with mucus expectoration.

Nose - Prickling in nose and nasal bones. Coryza early in morning.

Rectum - Burning in anus. Dysentery and diarrhea with inactivity of liver. Loose, dark stool, immediately after dinner. Ulceration of rectum. Dark, bilious offensive diarrhea with sallow complexion. Diarrhea with excessive debility and nervous irritability. Urgency to stool, early in morning in bed.

Sleep - Drowsiness with entire loss of mental and physical energy, heavy feeling in head, depression of spirits. Sleep unrefreshing and disturbed by unpleasant dreams. Tendency to perspire.

Stomach - Acid heartburn, painful and slow digestion. Sense of faintness and emptiness in stomach and bowels. Distention, burning, oppression. Pulsating pain in stomach. Belchings. Gagging as if to vomit in morning. Nausea, with confused and heavy pain in head. Nausea with bitter taste and aversion to all kinds of food.

Skin - Yellow or earthy appearance of skin. Itching, burning or prickling sensations, worse by scratching or rubbing. Eczema, pruritus and similar disorders of external genitals. Vesicular eczema of face in infants with nursing sore mouth.

Temperature - Chilliness with nausea, dull pain in head, debility, and languor. Chilly sensation, followed by transient flushing. Flushes of heat and coldness in alternation, followed by cold perspiration. Transient flushes of heat pervading whole body, with shooting pains through brain. General clammy sweat, with headache, nausea, pain in back, lassitude, and confusion of ideas.

RELATIONS - ***Compare:*** (1) Cornus alternifolia.

REFERENCES - Boericke. Clarke. Phatak.

CORNUS FLORIDA

(Dogwood)

PHARMACY - corn-f. Cornus florida. Dogwood. N. O. Cornaceae. Tincture of fresh bark. ***Historical dose:*** Tincture and all potencies.

CLINICAL - Chills. Dyspepsia. Headache. Heartburn. Intermittent fever. Malaria. Neuralgia. Pneumonia.

HOMEOPATHIC - Hale commended Corn-f. in obstinate intermittents where quinine had been abused and where there was sleepiness for days before chill, a sluggish flow of ideas, and a dull, heavy headache.

Intermittent fever with drowsiness. Feels cold, but is warm to touch. Great exhaustion in intervals. General clammy sweat. Chill is preceded by drowsiness, heat is associated with drowsiness. Headache after quinine.

Hale also commended it in old cases of dyspepsia where the chief symptom is acid heartburn. Chronic malaria indigestion and distressing acid heartburn.

Paroxysms attended with nausea, vomiting and sometimes with watery or bilious diarrhea. Chills, with cold, clammy skin. Violent headache with throbbing, stupor, confusion of intellect and vomiting.

General debility from loss of fluids and night sweats. Neuralgic pains in arms, chest and trunk. Sensation as if broken in two. Pneumonia, with stitches in the chest.

RELATIONS - ***Compare:*** (1) Other Cornels. (2) Eup-per., Nux-v., Chin., Kali-c., Abies-n., Abies-c.

REFERENCES - Boericke. Clarke. Hale.

CORTISONE

PHARMACY - cortiso. Cortisone. Cortisone is used in an acetate form and is prepared today by synthesis. It is a cortico-suprarenal hormone, belonging to the group of 11 steroids or 11-oxycorticosteroid hormones. ***Historical dose:*** Trituration and all potencies.

CLINICAL - Acne. Addison's disease. Allergic, rhinitis. Amenorrhea. Cataract. Conjunctivitis. Constipation. Cushing's syndrome. Depression. Dyspepsia. Edema. Goiter. Hay fever. Heatstroke. Hypertension. Hypothyroidism. Lupus, erythematosis. Memory weak. ***Moon-faced***. Muscular, atrophy. Obesity. Ophthalmic, migraine. Osteoporosis. Osteo-necrosis. Psoriasis. Styes. Sunstroke. Ulcers. Virilism.

HOMEOPATHIC - The Corticoid are a group of synthetic bodies whose action is analogous to that of Cortisone, but with greater power at equal weight and theoretically with greater tolerance.

All corticoids can have side effects including the perforation of gastric and duodenal ulcers, gastric and duodenal hemorrhaging, psychological complaints, virilism, acne, osteoporosis, diminution of resistance to infections and to tuberculosis, amenorrhea and Cushing's syndrome.

Prednisone and prednisolone cause less retention of water and salt and less potassium reduction in the blood than cortisone, but on the other hand, can be the cause of myopathy.

The homeopathic proving of cortisone was carried out during May and June 1963 by W. L. Templeton on eight provers and five controls, using the potencies 6c, 12c and 30c, prepared by A. Nelson and Co. Ltd.

Symptoms included a general lack of reaction and decrease of the organic reactional capacity. Slowness of the body and of the mind with irritability. Bradycardia torpor.

Rhythmic disorders of glands, especially the pituitary, adrenal, pancreas. Dysthyroidism with tendency to hypothyroidism. Inhibition of secretion of ACTH. Goiter. Hypercorticism, moon-faced. Virilism.

Polydipsia. Morbid hunger. Tendency to obesity with retention of water. Acrid dyspepsia, which can lead to gastric ulcers. Vomiting.

Headache. Intra-cranial hypertension. Right frontal and orbital pain, aggravated by the heat in a room, by pressure and in the afternoon. Impaired vision. Dryness of nasal and pharyngeal mucus membranes with coughing and dry, sticky eyes. Vertigo. Convulsions, the back of the eye reveals papillary edema.

Skin discolored, vesicular eruption, dryness and cracking of the skin on the face and hands with exfoliation of the nail beds. Face round, puffy, ***moon-faced***. Legs swollen with edema. Sacroiliac pain, as if the back were about to break.

MIND - Unstable mood, alternating between euphoria, melancholy and excitement. Excitability with increased activity. Action calms him. Fatigue with weariness. Loss of willpower.

Heavy, confused, irritable, impatient. Memory weak, mental effort arduous, aggravating the general condition. Difficulty in concentrating. Melancholic state. Thoughts of death. Depressive conditions.

Abdomen - Hepatic deficiency. Spasmodic entero-colitis.

Back - Dorsal pain, under the ribs on the left side, spreading to the anterior sacroiliac, ameliorated by movement and pressure, as if broken, aggravated in a sitting position, by bending down and in the morning. Pain between the bones.

Blood - Increased production of the thrombocyte. Erythroid hyperplasia. Polymorphism of the leukocytes.

Chest - Skin of the thorax discolored. Red rash on the lower part of the sternum.

Constitutions - Psoric and allergic constitutions. Slow, irritable subjects with a dull mind. Suitable especially, but not exclusively, for carbonic type and for Bernard's fat Sulphur types. Subjects fleshy with round face, sad, weeping for no reason.

Ears - Ringing in the ears.

Eyes - Tension behind the eyeballs. Eyeballs painful, dry, edges of the eyelids agglutinated. Inflammation of the inner canthus. Allergic conjunctivitis. Styes. Cataract. Accommodation difficult. Foggy vision.

Face - Acne of the face, shoulders, and back.

Female - Amenorrhea in young girls. Menses copious, blood thick. Pelvic congestion. Heaviness in the lower abdomen. Sensation of repletion in the stomach, ameliorated by menstrual flow and by walking. Vulvar eczema.

Food - Insatiable appetite, has butterflies if he does not eat. Milk and fats provoke nausea.

Head - Headache, as from a band around the head. Pulsating headache around the right eye, the vertex and the left side of the occiput. Sensation of frontal and occipital rending. Pain stronger around the right eye and forehead. Pain aggravated by pressure, heat, movement, sun. Ameliorated in the open air.

Heart - Arterial hypertension. Purpura. Ecchymosis.

Kidneys - Nephrotic syndrome. Frequent, pressing urination. Urination at night, oliguria. Edema.

Limbs - Osteoporosis. Painful post-traumatic osteoporosis. Osteo-necrosis of the hip in particular. Painful joints. Muscular atrophy of the quadriceps of the lower limbs. Legs restless, not ameliorated by movement in bed. Drawing pain behind the knees. Pain in the loin, worse when seated or lying down. Sacroiliac pain, as if it were about to break. Vesicular eruption on the backs of the hands, itching with round marks. worse with the heat. Dryness and irritation of the back of the hands.

Lungs - Dyspnea, aggravated in a warm room. Heaviness behind the sternum, respiration difficult. Short of breath, from nervous irritation, from warming himself and when in a hot room. Respiratory allergies, hay fever. Bronchitis with much sputum. Gray, gelatinous sputum. Laryngeal cough with sneezing in the morning. Cough aggravated by laughing, becoming excited, by walking, by physical fatigue, worse by undressing and by shaving.

Male - Diminution of sexual desire.

Modalities - Better from menstrual flow. Better walking. Better in the evening. Worse in the morning. Worse from external heat. Worse immobility. Worse scratching. Worse coughing. Worse pressure. Worse predominantly on the left side.

Mouth - Dryness of the mouth, especially in the morning. Dryness of the throat and pharynx, worse with swallowing, ameliorated by eating warm honey. Uvula red.

Nose - Allergic rhinitis. Hay fever. Sneezing, worse in the morning, better by washing.

Rectum - Diarrhea on rising in the morning, after breakfast, after a meal. Constipation and incomplete evacuation of hard stools in balls.

Skin - Eczema with puffiness of the face. Round, raised marks, slightly hard, on the hands, ankle, cheek and left side of the neck. Itching rash on the legs, feet and hands. Red rash at the nail beds and on the backs of the fingers. Rash worse with heat. Red streaks on the skin, streaked with weals. Face and hands rough, chapping. Slow healing of wounds. Increased growth of hair in the usual places.

Sleep - Sleep light. Agitated, easily disturbed, cannot sleep. Does not refresh, wakes tired.

Stomach - Amelioration by empty swallowing, aggravated in the morning and by hot drinks. Gastric ulcer.

Urine - Loss of potassium, calcium, phosphorus. Diminution of ascorbic acid. Retention of chloride and sodium. Increase of creatinine, cholesterol, uric acid. Glycosuria. Proteinuria. Tubular casts in the urine.

Vertigo - Vertigo, aggravated in a warm room.

COMMENTS - Its fundamental properties are promotion of the formation of glycogen, diminution of the use of glucide by the tissues, negation of the nitrogen balance, elevation of urinary elimination of uric acid of creatine (without any change in the level of creatinine in the urine) and of potassium, sodium retention, varying action on the urinary elimination of phosphorous and calcium.

Degeneration of the lymphoid organs with lymphocytopenia. Increase of globulins in the plasma and inhibition of conjunctival inflammatory reactions. Inhibits the production of ACTH and produces atrophy of the suprarenal cortex. It gives the impression of well being and euphoria, but there is the possibility of maniacal or depressive psychological complaints.

RELATIONS - ***Compare:*** (1) Ars., Sep., Sulph. - Impatient, quarrelsome, has grandiose ideas, pain and burning eruptions. (2) Psor. - Sad, periodic migraines, anxious, scabby, weeping eruptions, weakness of the back and limbs as if dislocated. (3) Puls. - changing, variable, weeps at the slightest trifle, alternation of smiles and tears. Erratic pains, dry cough, congestion of the veins.

REFERENCES - Julian.

CORYDALIS CAVA

(Fumaria cava)

PHARMACY - cory-c. Corydalis cava. Fumaria cava. N. O. Papaveraceae. ***Historical dose:*** Tincture and all potencies.

CLINICAL - Dyspnea. Headaches. Palpitations. Rheumatic pains. Stomach pain.

HERBAL - Catharral and inflammatory affections of mucous membranes with burning pains. Furunculosis.

MIND - Anxiety and dyspnea. Sadness without cause. Indifference.

Food - Desire for sour and pungent. Voracious appetite, waking at night from hunger. Aversion to wine.

Head - Right-sided headache. Pain in forehead, temple, occiput. Pressing or shooting pain. Headaches, worse motion. Headaches, better open air. Heat of head.

Heart - Palpitations, paroxysmal, worse lying on left side. Palpitations, worse ascending, worse 3 a.m.

Limbs - Rheumatic pains, especially in hands and fingers, worse motion, better warmth.

Lungs - Anxiety and dyspnea. Dyspnea, anxiety, palpitations, cold sweat on forehead.

Modalites - Worse rest. Worse warmth.

Nose - Obstruction of nose. Yellowish mucus discharge.

Stomach - Pressing pain in stomach. Stomach pain, worse after eating, coffee, bending double. Pressing pain, better stretching. Nausea, retching and diarrhea. Epigastrium sensitive to pressure.

Throat - Swollen sensation in throat when lying down. Sensation as if thyroid were enlarged.

Vertigo - Vertigo, as if ground gave way. Vertigo worse closing eyes.

REFERENCES - Murphy.

CORYDALIS FORMOSA

(Wild Turkey Pea)

PHARMACY - cory. Corydalis formosa. Wild turkey pea. Dicentra canadensis. Stagger weed. N. O. Fumariaceae. Papaveraceae. Tincture of bulbous root gathered when plant is in flower. Trituration of the dried root. Triturations of Corydalin. ***Historical dose:*** Trituration, tincture and all potencies.

CLINICAL - Cachexia. Cancer. Gastric, catarrh. Scrofula. Syphilis. Ulceration. Ulcers.

HERBAL - Hale commended Corydalis in scrofulous discrasia, obstinate skin diseases, and cachexia of intermittents with enlargement of the liver and spleen.

In massive doses it has cured, according to herbal authorities, "A derangement of the stomach, attended with profuse morbid secretion of mucus, there being always a coated tongue with fetor of the breath and loss of appetite and digestion."

Cory. is therefore indicated, as Hale remarked, in gastric catarrh, being an analog in this respect of Hydr. It has not been used in the potencies, a usual dose has been ten drops of the tincture four times a day.

HOMEOPATHIC - It is an unproved remedy, but clinical experience has revealed a specific relation of the manifestation of syphilis, including Hunterian chancre, syphilitic nodes, falling of the hair, and syphilitic ulcerations of scalp. Dry, scaly scabs on the faces of old people. Swollen lymphatic glands.

Pronounced cancer cachexia. Gummata and night-pains. Chronic diseases with atony. Tongue clean, broad and full. Tissues flabby, doughy, cold. Gastric catarrh (Hydr.) Syphilitic and non-syphilitic ulcerations of fauces. Ulcers of mouth and fauces.

RELATIONS - ***Compare:*** (1) Nit-ac., Kali-i., Fl-ac.

REFERENCES - Boericke. Clarke. Hale.

COTO

(Coto Bark)

PHARMACY - coto. Coto. Coto bark. N. O. Lauracae. Bolivia. A bark of Nectandra coto. Tincture. Trituration of the alkaloid Cotoin. ***Historical dose:*** Trituration, tincture and all potencies.

CLINICAL - Diarrhea. Tubercular, diarrhea.

HERBAL - The bark has been used in medicine as a diarrhea remedy, probably from aboriginal tradition. Hansen says it is especially valuable in "chronic tubercular, watery diarrhea, very copious stools and exhausting." Only drop doses of the tincture have been used.

REFERENCES - Clarke. Hansen.

COTYLEDON UMBILICUS

(Pennywort)

PHARMACY - cot. Cotyledon umbilicus. Pennywort. Navelwort. Kidneywort. Umbilicus pendulinus. Le Nombril de Venus. N. O. Crassulaceae. House-leek-family. Tincture of the plant. ***Historical dose:*** Tincture and all potencies.

CLINICAL - Epilepsy. Headache. Heart, disorders. Hysteria. Sciatica. Sinuses. Spleen, disorders. Rheumatism.

HOMEOPATHIC - Cotyledon has had a considerable proving. Cooper considered it a cancer remedy. He cured with it sinuses in buttock. A patient to whom he gave it for polyps said it made him stagger as if drunk.

Marked action on the heart, oppression of the chest, and fullness in the throat. Oppressed breathing, disturbed heart. Catarrh of larynx and trachea. Well-marked pains through the breast to scapula. Pains in the region of the spleen.

Rheumatic symptoms. Sciatica. Hysterical joint. Numb aching in muscular and fibrous tissue. Weak, faint feeling.

Stitching, pricking, jerking pains are predominant sensations.

A feeling as if some part of the body, like a foot or the head, were absent. The senses of sight and hearing are dulled. A yellow patch follows the eyesight. Disagreeable surging in ears, ears feel stuffed. Pressing vertex headache. Epilepsy.

MIND - Lost and confused feeling. Could not articulate for some time on awaking. ***Feeling as if a part of the body were absent.*** Ailments from suppressed emotion.

Abdomen - Long stitching in left hypochondrium. Dull pains in left hypochondrium. Dull pushing in region of spleen recurring at intervals.

Back - Pain through to scapula from region of left breast. Pain at angles of scapulae.

Breasts - Pain under left nipple and aching in right breast.

Chest - Full, bursting feeling, as if from obstruction at heart.

Head - Headache, causing desire for open air, which ameliorates. Dull headache with cold feet. Dull, heavy, stupefying pain in forehead and vertex, shifting suddenly between them.

Heart - Heat about heart. Uneasiness. Clawing, dragging pain on riding, better by compressing side.

Kidneys - Calls to urinate frequent. Increased flow of clear urine.

Limbs - Aching in back and thighs. Aching in all joints. Skin sensitive, rubbing of trousers causes an acute sting. Aching in left thigh followed by numbness. Stinging pain under left gluteus maximus in region of sciatic nerve. Legs and arms feel heavy and sore. Between attacks of headache, gnawing, rheumatic pain in right shoulder. Aching, bruised pain in wrists. Aching, tingling in hands, especially at night, preventing sleep, tingling down arm when the nerve is struck.

Lungs - Oppressed breathing. Tickling in larynx with dry cough. Shooting in all directions in chest, particularly under right scapula and left nipple during evening. Stitches below both nipples.

Modalities - Worse morning and evening.

Rectum - Bowels freely opened, later, constipation.

Stomach - Pain at epigastrium through to shoulder, with nausea. On swallowing, the morsel seems to pass and press against some swelling in cardiac region.

Throat - Constant choking in throat, feeling as if he would burst into tears. Back of throat feels as if covered with thick mucus.

RELATIONS - ***Compare:*** (1) Ambr., Asaf., Hepat., Ign., Lach., Sedum acre.

REFERENCES - Boericke. Clarke.

CRAB APPLE

(Bach Flower Essence)

PHARMACY - crb-a-b. Crab apple. Malus pumila. Pyrus malus. Small twigs with whole clusters of flowers are boiled for half an hour. The water is strained and used as medicine. ***Historical dose:*** Take two drops from the stock bottle into a one ounce dropper bottle, (add brandy or alcohol, if this bottle will be used for days or weeks). This is the dosage bottle, take a few drops straight into the mouth or as needed in a little water or juice.

HOMEOPATHIC - The remedy Crab Apple, together with Oak-b., Will-b., Star-b-b., Sw-ch-b., Elm-b., Pine-b., and Lar-b., belongs to the group of ***For Despondency or Despair,*** as classified by Bach. States of severity. Burdening condition, without sufficient power or possibility to grow above.

Unclean skin, acne. Accumulated wastes in the blood stream. Cleansing of digestive tract. Long-lasting viral infections. Chronic poisoning due to environmental hazards. Helps draw out impurities from a wound, if applied to the bandage.

Chronic diarrhea. Feelings of disgust or repulsion. Strong repulsion toward the food consumed with the urge to vomit. Vomiting, nausea and emaciation (Chic-b., Must-b.). Anorexia and bulimia, tendency to obsess with weight problems.

MIND - Self-centered. Concentrates on the unclean, shameful, bothering and burdensome. Obsessive preoccupation with beauty flaws or states of sickness considered unclean and unbecoming. Fear of contamination, by germs or unclean surroundings.

Obsessive-compulsive disorder with deep shame (Cher-p-b., Pine-b.). Shame about appearance or inner guilt and uncleanness. Regrets sinful or shameful behavior. Feels soiled or dirty after abuse or molestation. Intense craving or desire to be cleansed and purified. Feels helpless in regard to the problem. Unable to shake off or overcome the condition. Minor problems assume disproportionate importance. Despair.

REFERENCES - Bach.

CRATAEGUS OXYACANTHA

(Hawthorn Berries)

PHARMACY - crat. Crataegus oxyacantha. Hawthorn berries. Crataegus monogyna. Crataegus laevigata. N. O. Rosacea. The fresh berries are pounded to a pulp and macerated in two times their weight of alcohol. Tincture of the ripe fruit. ***Historical dose:*** Tincture and all potencies, fluid extract or tincture, one to fifteen drops.

CLINICAL - Anasarca. Anemia. Aneurysm. Angina pectoris. ***Arteriosclerosis. Dropsy. Dyspnea.*** Dyspepsia. ***Dyspnea***. Edema. ***Heart, disorders.*** Heart, failure. Heart, hypertrophy. ***Heart, weakness.*** Hemorrhages. ***High blood pressure.*** Insomnia. Myocarditis. Nausea. Weakness.

HERBAL - Crat. is a great ***positive heart tonic.*** It has produced some heart symptoms and doubtless has a homeopathic relation, but it is not a heart-poison like digitalis and has no cumulative action. In tonic, it works very slowly, may palliate long term.

For recovery from heart attacks. Increases heart strength. Congestive heart failure, heart weakness, enlarged heart. Chronic heart disease with extreme weakness. Heart-failure threatened from slightest exertion. ***Irregularity of heart.***

HOMEOPATHIC - Produces giddiness. Shortness of breath with a slow pulse. Weak, rapid, and lowered pulse. Slow and irregular pulse. Air hunger. ***High blood pressure***, also useful for low blood pressure.

Very feeble and irregular heart action. Weakness in the valves, regurgitation, valve prolapse. Dyspnea and dropsy, from failure of heart-power whether from valvular affection or from anemia. Hypertrophy, dilation, nervous palpitation, arrhythmia. Insomnia. Aortic anemia, edema, cutaneous chilliness. Myocarditis. General anasarca.

Arteriosclerosis, said to have a solvent power upon crustaceous and ***calcareous deposits in arteries.*** Cardio-hemorrhagic or lithemic cases. Dyspepsia and nervous prostration with heart failure. Heart problems after rheumatism. Alcoholic heart. A sedative in cross, irritable patients with cardiac symptoms.

Oppression of the chest. Pain under the collarbone, chest pain in general. Stitching pain. Nervous with pain in back of head and neck. Weakness, exhaustion. Sudden weakness. Cold limbs. Pallor. Nervous palpitations. Collapse from typhoid. Hemorrhages from bowels.

MIND - Irritable, cross and melancholic. Apprehensive, despondent. Despair, feels weak and fragile. Mental dullness. Makes mistakes. Confused feeling, followed by a feeling of quiet and calmness mentally.

Anxiety with palpitations. Hurried feeling with rapid action of heat. Very nervous and irritable, with pain in back of head and neck. Irritable, cross and despondent.

Morose and sulky. Ailments from grief. Despair about recovery. Irritability with heart disease. Cross, ill-humor, peevish. Sadness, depression.

Chest - Painful sensation of pressure in left side of chest below the clavicle.

Eyes - Conjunctival irritation, with nasal discharge.

Head - Very nervous and irritable with pain in back of head and neck.

Heart - Circulatory weakness. Angina pectoris. Anxiety with palpitations. Palpitations, tumultuous, violent, vehement. Heart muscles seem flabby, worn out. ***Heart weakness*** with oppression, stitches and insomnia. Fatty degeneration. ***Hypertrophy of heart.*** Aortic disease. Aneurysm of the aorta. Aortitis. ***Cardiac dropsy***. Cardiac dyspnea. Pain in region of heart, ***under left clavicle***, and under left scapula. ***Heart dilated, first sound weak.*** Incompetent valves. Valvular murmurs. Valvular incompetence. Myocarditis. Pericarditis. Sustains the heart in infectious diseases. Neurosis cordis. Fatty degeneration of heart.

Kidneys - ***Diabetes***, especially in children. Urine diminished. Urine contains traces of albumen and an excess of phosphates.

Limbs - Limbs cold and edematous. Coldness of fingers. Blueness of limbs. Swelling of lower limbs. Swelling of feet.

Lungs - Cough with an albuminous expectoration. ***Extreme dyspnea on least exertion*** without much increase of pulse.

Nose - Nasal discharges.

Perspiration - Excessive sweat. Palms sweaty. Perspiration of limbs.

Pulse - Pulse accelerated. ***Pulse irregular, feeble, intermittent***.

Modalities - Better fresh air. Better quiet and rest. Worse in warm room. ***Worse least exertion.*** Worse at night. Worse from rheumatic affections.

Skin - Skin eruptions. Burning, smarting eruptions on back of neck, axillae and chin, worse heat and sweating, better washing. Excessive perspiration. Fingers and toes blue. Coldness of skin. Blueness of fingers and toes, worse exertion or excitement. Great pallor of skin, with rush of blood to head.

Sleep - Insomnia of heart patients. Sleeplessness in aortic disease.

Stomach - Nausea. Dyspepsia and nervous prostration with heart failure.

Temperature - Cutaneous chilliness. Blueness of fingers and toes, all aggravated by exertion or excitement. Chilliness in heart disease.

Vertigo - Faintness and collapse.

COMMENTS - Crat. was introduced into medicine as a heart remedy by Dr. Greene of Ennis, Ireland, and it has been used empirically with much success in cases of heart failure. It has usually been given in drop doses of the tincture.

Dr. Green had a reputation for the cure of heart disease that caused patients to flock to him from all parts of the United Kingdom. He cured the majority of them and amassed considerable wealth by means of his secret medicine. Contrary to the code, he, though a physician in good standing, refused to reveal the remedy to his professional brethren.

After his death, his daughter, a Mrs. Graham, revealed that the remedy her father had used so successfully was crataegus oxyacantha.

Halbert in Clinique, March, 1899, recorded the case of "Mr. S., a young man sixteen years of age, had worked hard at manual labor since his twelfth year to support a widowed mother. He had in fact, done a man's work before his physical maturity would permit it. For some time he has shown signs of cardiac hypertrophy and had been cautioned by physicians to take good care as to his heart.

"About a year ago during some gymnastic extreme in the nature of sport, he was suddenly admonished that something had 'given way,' and for relief was obliged to take to his bed. When I first saw him he was obliged to lie down, respiration was labored and irregular and the heart's action was greatly exaggerated and erratic.

"There was decided precordial bulging, the apex beat was considerably displaced, downward and to the left and the whole cardiac dullness was greatly extended, the impulse was heaving in character with considerable mitral systolic blowing and the corresponding diastolic intensification, there were also signs of considerable pulmonary engorgement and some pain in the chest region.

"The patient was put into a warm bath for twenty minutes and then carefully returned to bed. Aconite 3x was administered every half-hour and continued hourly for a day or two afterward until he was somewhat relieved.

"Crataegus, five-drop doses of the tincture, was then administered five times daily for a long time. The effects of this remedy were most remarkable, the cardiac irritation gradually lessened, the area of dullness decreased and the rhythm improved, at the same time all the general symptoms improved rapidly.

"He has now been using the remedy for several months and the result is most satisfactory. I have every reason to expect a cure of the extreme symptoms and believe the heart will be reduced to a safe hypertrophy, will virtually be a cure."

A girl of twelve had a sudden collapse in the third week of typhoid. Crat. five drops, every two hours was given on the indications of a great pallor with irregular breathing, cold limbs, pulse 120, very weak and irregular. Strychnia, Dig. and Cact. had failed to give more than temporary relief. Under Crat. she rallied at once.

T. C. Duncan gave complete relief in a case of angina pectoris, the pain being above and to the left of the stomach. Strong pulse and forcible indications of hypertrophy were found. A very tender spot on the left side of the spine. Crat. removed at the same time "a hurried feeling" and the anxious expression on her face.

Dr. Duncan produced a "hurried feeling" in himself when proving Crat., which he attributed to the rapid action of the stimulated heart.

Anshutz reported that Dr. Jennings procured for himself some of the remedy and his experience with it explains Dr. Green's national reputation.

Dr. Jennings wrote of the case of a Mr. B., aged seventy-three years. "I found him gasping for breath when I entered the room with a pulse-rate of 158 and very feeble, great edema of lower limbs and abdomen.

"A more desperate case could hardly be found. I gave him fifteen drops of Crataegus in half a wineglass of water. In fifteen minutes the pulse beat was 126 and stronger and breathing was not so labored. In twenty-five minutes pulse beat 110 and the force was still increasing, breathing much easier.

"He now got ten drops in same quantity of water and in one hour from the time I entered the house he was, for the first time in ten days, able to lie horizontally. I made an examination of the heart and found mitral regurgitation from valvular deficiency with great enlargement." For the edema, he prescribed Hydrargyrum cum creta, Squill and Digitalis.

"He received ten drops four times a day of the Crataegus and was permitted to use some light beer to which he had become accustomed at meal time. He made a rapid and apparently full recovery until in three months, he felt as well as any man of his age in Chicago.

"He occasionally, particularly in the change of weather takes some of the Crataegus which, he says, quickly stops shortness of breath or pain in the heart. His father and a brother died of heart disease."

In another case, a woman "was suffering from a compensatory enlargement of the heart from mitral insufficiency," was taken with dyspnea when Dr. Jennings was called and was nearly dead.

Under Crataegus, and some other indicated remedies, she made an excellent recovery. "In a letter from her, three months afterward, she said she was feeling well, but that she would not feel fully secure without some of the Crataegus."

"The forty other cases ran courses somewhat similar…all having been apparently cured. Yet I am not satisfied beyond a doubt, that any of those patients were completely cured except those whose troubles of the heart were functional. And it is possible and even probable that in weather of a heavy atmosphere or when it is surcharged with electricity or if the patient be subjected to great excitement or sudden or violent commotion or exercise he may suffer again therewith.

"Cardiac impulse after a few days' use of the Crataegus is greatly strengthened and yields that low soft tone so characteristic of the first sound, as shown by the cardiograph. The entire central nervous system seems to be influenced favorably by its use, the appetite increases and assimilation and nutrition improve.

"Also a sense of quietude and well-being rests on the patient and he who before its use was cross, melancholic and irritable after a few days of its use shows marked signs of improvement in his mental state.

"I doubt if it is indicated in fatty enlargement. The dose which I have found to be the most available is from ten to fifteen drops after meals or food. If taken before it may in very susceptible patients, cause nausea. I find also that after its use for a month it may be well to discontinue for a week or two, when it should be renewed for another month or so.

"Usually three months seem to be the proper time for actual treatment and after that only at such times as a warning pain of the heart or dyspnea may point out."

Dr. T. C. Duncan contributed the case of Mrs. A., a printer, who "came to me complaining of some pain in the side as if it would take her life. She did not have it all the time, only at times, usually the last of the week, when tired.

"I prescribed Bryonia, then Belladonna without prompt relief. One Saturday she came with a severe attack, locating the pain with her right hand above and to the left of the stomach. The pulse was strong and forcible.

"On careful examination I found the heart beat below normal indicating hypertrophy. I examined the spine and to the left of the vertebra about two inches I found a very tender spot (spinal hyperemia). She told me that when a girl she had several attacks and that her own family physician gave her a remedy that relieved her at once.

"She had tried several physicians, among them an allopath, who gave hypodermic injections of morphine without relief. Hot applications sometimes relieved. I now recognized that I had a case of angina pectoris and that her early attacks were due, I thought to carrying her heavy brother. Now the attacks come when she becomes tired holding her composing stick, at the same time she became very much flurried, so much so that she had stop work because she was confused.

"I now gave her a prescription for Cactus, but told her I would like to try first a new remedy, giving her Crataegus, saturating some disks with tincture. I directed her to take two disks every hour until relieved and then less often. If not relieved to take the Cactus.

"She returned in a week reporting that she was relieved after the first dose of Crataegus. More, that hurried, flurried feeling had not troubled her this week. Her face has a parchment skin and the expression of anxiety so significant of heart disease was certainly relieved. I have not seen her since."

The proving of this remedy produced a flurried feeling due, to the rapid action of the stimulated heart. A nervous female medical student who also proved it had "an unusual rush of blood to the head with confused feeling," followed later by "a feeling of quiet and calmness mentally."

RELATIONS - *Compare:* (1) Aven., Heliant., Alfa., (2) Stroph., Dig., Iber., Naja, Cact.

REFERENCES - Anshutz. Boericke. Clarke. Murphy. Phatak.

CRESYLOLUM

(Cresol)

PHARMACY - cresol. Cresylolum. Cresol. The cresols are phenols (ortho, meta, para) derived from toluene. They are extracted from tar, coal-tar, wood-tar. They are also prepared synthetically. ***Historical dose:*** Trituration, tincture and all potencies.

CLINICAL - Allergies. Anemia. Anorexia. Atherosclerosis. Emaciation. Maniac, depression. Muscular, atrophy. Paralysis. Premature, senility. Schizophrenia.

HOMEOPATHIC - The word "cresol" is derived from "creosote" and the suffix "-ol," which means phenol. The cresols are powerful antiseptics, soluble in soap, but their use is restricted, owing to their strong odor. They are used, however, as primary material in the manufacture of bakelites, they form cresolins.

The homeopathic proving was established by O. A. Julian in 1958 on five provers, three men, two women and a dog, as well as by the study of cases of chronic poisoning. The potencies 5c, 7c and 9c were used.

Sclerosis of the cerebral, nervous and vascular systems. Muscular atrophy, especially of the small muscles in the hands. Paresis or atrophic paralysis of the lower limbs. Quivering beneath the skin of the entire body. Pigmentation disorders, melanosis. Papular erythema.

Hypertensive kidney sclerosis. Allergic conditions from a cancerous evolution. Anemia with thrombocytopenia and leucopenia. Asthenia, anorexia and emaciation.

MIND - Schizophrenia with euphoria and volubility. Manic depressive psychosis. Euphoria, with abundant gesticulation, can lead to ecstasy. Loquacious mood. Schizophrenia in children.

Anguish in the evening. Indifference. Distracted, gives the impression of being deep in thought. Unhappy visions. Hears bells. Irritable. Often repeats himself. trembling of upper limbs.

COMMENTS - A long-standing experiment and numerous clinical observations by O. A. Julian and several of his colleagues allow the confirmation that Cresol. is a very valuable remedy, especially with regard to neuro-psychological, cardiovascular and cutaneous infections.

It is almost a homeopathic phenobarbital in cases of epilepsy. It's particularly effective in a large number of epileptic cases if one is the first doctor to see the patient. If, on the other hand, allopathic treatment has already been prescribed, it is essential to know how to combine homeopathic remedies with a slow and progressive reduction of the previously prescribed classical remedies.

Clinical observation, plus electro-encephalogram readings are used to direct this reduction of the allopathic dosage. By contrast, the number of Cresol. drops of 7c can be increased, which results in a better sedation of cortical irritability.

RELATIONS - *Compare:* (1) Arg-m. - Subject thin, sad, agitated and loquacious. Loss of memory, paretic state of lower limbs with trembling. (2) Plb. - Rapid emaciation, cortical and somatic weakness, gradual paralysis of the limbs. Abdomen hard retracted. (3) Caust. - Mental failing, melancholic, critical, paretic weakness.

REFERENCES - Julian.

CROCUS SATIVUM

(Saffron)

PHARMACY - croc. Crocus sativus. Saffron. N. O. Iridaceae. Tincture of dried stigmas. Tincture of the fresh young shoots. ***Historical dose:*** Tincture and all potencies.

CLINICAL - Abortion, threatened. After-pains. Anger. Asthenopia. Blepharospasm. Brain, congestion. Chorea. ***Constipation***.

Dysmenorrhea. Fainting. Gastric disorders. Hemoptysis. ***Hemorrhages.*** Headaches. Heart disorders. Hysteria. Lachrymation. Leucorrhea. Mania. Menorrhagia. Menstruation, heavy. Metrorrhagia. Miscarriage. Nosebleeds. Ophthalmia. Pregnancy, disorders. Surgery, after effects. Tumors. Ulceration. ***Uterine, hemorrhage.*** Wounds.

HOMEOPATHIC - Characteristic ***hemorrhage*** from various parts when the ***blood is black, stringy, clotting,*** forming itself into long black strings hanging from the bleeding orifice. Viscid blood, dark. Clotting. Tumors. Lipoma. Encephaloma.

Symptoms rapidly change sides or mental and physical symptoms alternate. Rapid alternation of mental conditions. Jerking or spasmodic contraction of single sets of muscles. Chorea and hysteria. Chorea every seven days with hilarity, singing and dancing.

Sensation as if something alive were moving internally in abdomen, chest etc. with nausea, faintness and shivering or jumping about various parts. Drowsiness, better by literary occupation. Prostration, weariness, fainting with nosebleed, metrorrhagia.

MIND - Mind very much distracted. Forgetful. Impressionable, affectionate and moody. Loss of ideas on attempting to write anything down. Childish behavior. Confusion, better open air. Industrious. Irritability, takes everything in bad part. Mistakes in time, confounds present with past. Uneasy, anxious, sorrowful mood.

Happy and affectionate, then angry. ***Changeable disposition.*** Rapidly changing or alternating mental disposition, opposite to each other. Anger with violence, rapidly followed by abject repentance.

Remorse, repents quickly. Laughter quickly followed by tears. Cheerful at night. Cheerful, alternating with sadness, violence.

Hysterical laughter, laughing mania. Involuntary laughter and weeping, worse music. Jesting. Loquacious. Vivid recollection from music heard (Lyc.). Singing in sleep. Sings on hearing a single note sung. Jumping, dancing, laughing, whistling, wants to kiss everybody.

Delusion he is unfit for business.

Abdomen - Abdomen swollen, feeling of something heavy. ***Sensation as if something living were jumping about*** in the stomach and abdomen (left side) (Thuj.).

Back - Sudden feeling of coldness in back, as if cold water were thrown over him, with icy-cold limbs.

Breasts - Jumping pain in left breast, as if drawn towards the back, as if jumping alive in right breast. Jerking pain in interior of left breast, as if drawn toward back by means of thread (Crot-t.).

Causations - Effects of blows.

Constitutions - Suited to women and hysterical men.

Ears - Noises in ears with hardness of hearing, worse stooping.

Eyes - Dry, burning, ***as after weeping***. Asthenopia with extreme photophobia. Pupils enlarged and react slowly. Threatened glaucoma, embolism of central retinal artery. Ciliary neuralgia, pain from eyes to top of head. Lachrymation when reading. Must wipe eyes as if mucus or water were in them. Sensation as if she had been looking through too sharp spectacles. ***Feels as if smoke in eyes. Sensation as if cold air was rushing through eye*** (Fl-ac., Syph.). Electric sparks or jumping spots before eyes. Twitching of the upper eyelid. Lids heavy.

Face - Hot, red, or alternating with paleness.

Female - Menses dark, viscid, too frequent and copious, ***black and slimy***. Urging of blood to genitals. Uterine hemorrhage, ***clots with long strings***, worse from least movement, worse during full or new moon. Threatened miscarriage, especially when hemorrhage is ***dark and stringy***. False pregnancy. Movements of fetus are violent and painful.

Food - Great thirst for cold drinks.

Head - Throbbing, pulsating headache at menopausal period, during menses, or instead of menses, better pressure.

Heart - Sensation of heat ascending to the heart impeding breathing, better yawning.

Dull stitches in the left chest. Anxious palpitation, worse ascending stairs.

Limbs - Spasmodic contractions and twitchings of single set of muscles. Chorea and hysteria with great alteration of feeling. Upper limbs fall asleep. Weakness in knees and legs. Cracking in hip joint and knees, worse stooping. Pain in ankles and soles. Cold as ice with metrorrhagia, nosebleed.

Lungs - Heaviness in chest, must take deep breath. Dry cough, better laying the hand on the pit of the stomach. Wheezy cough with frothy expectoration, containing threads like fine twine, worse lying down. Expectoration stringy like thread.

Male - Excitement of sexual desire.

Modalities - Better after breakfast. Better in open air. Better yawning, desire to take a long breath. Worse from motion. Worse lying down. Worse reading. Worse looking fixedly at an object. Worse from puberty. Worse pregnancy. Worse fasting. Worse during new and full moon. Worse hot weather. Worse heat, warm room. Worse in morning.

Mouth - Unusual warmth in mouth. Sour taste. Foul, offensive, sickly breath.

Nose - Nosebleed, ***strings of dark blood*** hanging down the nose, with faintness and cold sweat on forehead. Nosebleed at puberty of young girls

Rectum - ***Obstinate constipation*** due to portal stagnation. Constipation in infants. Stools contain dark stringy blood. Crawling and stitches in anus. Useful after operations for hemorrhoids.

Skin - Prickling and crawling. Scarlet redness or spots on the skin. Old scars open and suppurate. Lipoma. Encephaloma. Disperses tumors.

Sleep - Deep sleep. Sings in sleep.

Stomach - Gastric troubles, bloatedness, belchings, vomiting etc.

Temperature - Flushes of internal heat with prickling and crawling in skin. Sweat only on the lower half of the body. Continuous, foul smelling sweat, worse debility, hemorrhages after childbirth.

Throat - Feeling as if uvula were elongated, during and when not swallowing in hysteria. Feeling of nausea in throat and chest.

COMMENTS - Cooper and Culpepper agreed in thinking that Croc. is very similar to Calen. in its action. It is a vulnerary and corresponds to the effects of blows (deafness, tumors, etc.).

Dark hemorrhage. Uterine hemorrhage of dark, black, stringy blood, often associated with miscarriages or cancer of the uterus (Sec.). Painful suppuration of bruised parts, old scars re-open and suppurate.

Lipoma and encephaloma of scalp. Used externally to scatter indolent tumors and ecchymosis. Tumor with ulceration and characteristic bleeding. A warm sensation ascending to the heart, impeding breathing, better by yawning.

Tingling, crawling, pricking and itching occur in the skin. Scarlet redness of the whole body or scarlet spots on the skin. A domestic remedy for bringing out measles eruptions.

Stitches, shocks, throbbings, broad thrusts. Cuttings and jerkings. Twitchings of single sets of muscles (chorea). Sensitive to music, involuntarily joins in on hearing anyone sing.

Croc. has been successfully given to pregnant women who have complained of violent fetal movements, as well as in cases of imaginary pregnancy.

Clarke once cured a young artist who had become subject to violent outbursts of rage. He would take up a knife to throw at his mother, with whom he lived, and almost immediately after would be abjectly repentant. The household was on the point of being broken up when the trouble was completely removed by Croc.

On one occasion in a hospital, Clarke happened to see a young girl who was desperately ill with heart failure and valvular disease in a fit of hysterical laughter. This made him think of Croc.

The only definite sensation she complained of in the heart region was a "jumping" sensation. Croc. 30c was given and very soon she was able to lie down flat (after having been propped up for weeks) and from that time she made a rapid recovery.

Cooper gave single doses of the tincture in a case of malignant disease of the side following extirpation of a cancerous kidney. The result was an arrest of progress after an initial aggravation and complete relief of pain.

The patient was a woman, who had formerly had hemorrhages with dark clots during her periods and feeling of weight towards womb. She had also the sensation of something moving in the abdomen.

Teste cited from Murray the case of several children "who were seized with an extraordinary laughing mania from having, smelled of leather bottles that had contained essence of saffron."

RELATIONS - ***Antidote:*** Op., Bell. ***Compare:*** (1) Ip., Trill., Plat., Chin., Phos., Ust., Sabin.

REFERENCES - Boericke. Clarke. Murphy. Phatak.

CROTALUS CASCAVELLA

(Brazilian Rattle-snake)

PHARMACY - crot-c. Crotalus cascavella. Brazilian rattle-snake. Crotalus durissus. N. O. Crotalide. Middle and South America. Trituration of the venom with Saccharum lactis. ***Historical dose:*** All potencies.

CLINICAL - Goiter. Hallucinations. Headache. Mania. Metrorrhagia. Nosebleed. Paralysis. Poliomyelitis. Uterus, pains.

HOMEOPATHIC - The poison of Cascavella is an deadly as that of the other Crotalide and the general symptoms are like those of the other members of the group, but the mental symptoms are more pronounced and peculiar. The proving was done by Mure, with additional effects reported by Higgins.

Crot-c. has frequent sharp pains, worse by cold washing. Symptoms are worse at night. Pains in bones. Paralysis of articulation. Embarrassed, stertorous breathing and semi-consciousness. Hallucinations, a magnetic state is induced, with a cutting sensation all around the eyeball. Thoughts and dreams of death. Headache after sleep (Lach.).

MIND - Restlessness worse drinking. Answers monosyllabic, "no" to all questions. ***Clairvoyance.*** Fear at night. ***Fear of being alone.*** Fear that someone is behind him. ***Thoughts of death when alone.*** Hurried. Loquacity. Moaning during sleep. Starting during sleep.

Delusions that the eyes were falling out. Delusions hears footsteps behind him. Fancies he hears groans. Sees spectres, ghosts, spirits. Death appears as a gigantic black skeleton. Hears voices that he must follow. Insanity alternating with metrorrhagia.

RELATIONS - ***Compare:*** (1) Crot-h., Lach., Naja, Vip.

REFERENCES - Clarke.

CROTALUS HORRIDUS

(Timber Rattlesnake)

PHARMACY - crot-h. Crotalus horridus. Timber rattlesnake. N. O. Crotalide. North America. Trituration of sugar of milk saturated with the venom. Solution of the venom in glycerin. ***Historical dose:*** All potencies.

CLINICAL - Abscesses. Amblyopia. Appendicitis. Bilious, fever. Blindness. Boils. ***Bubonic plague.*** Cancer. Carbuncles. Chancre. ***Ciliary neuralgias. Cirrhosis.*** Convulsions. Delirium tremens. Dementia. Diphtheria. Dysmenorrhea. Dyspepsia. Ears, discharges. Ebola. Ecchymosis. ***Edema.*** Epilepsy. Eyes, disorders. Erysipelas. Face, distortion. Hematuria. Hepatitis. ***Hemorrhages.*** Heart, disorders. Herpes. Hydrophobia. Intestinal, hemorrhage. ***Jaundice.*** Keratitis. ***Liver, disorders.*** Lungs, disorders. Malaria. Mania. Mastitis. Measles. Melancholy. Meningitis. Milk-leg. Ovaries, disorders. Ozaena. Palpitations. ***Paralysis***. Peritonitis. Phlebitis. ***Plague.*** Psoriasis, palms. ***Purpura, hemorrhagica***. Pyemia. Remittent, fever. Rheumatism. Scarlatina. Senile, dementia. ***Septic, blood.*** Sleeplessness. Smallpox. Stings. ***Strokes.*** Sunstroke. Syphilis. Tetanus. Tongue, inflammation. Tongue, cancer. Typhlitis. Ulcers. Urticaria. Vaccination, effects. Varicose, veins. Varicocele. Vomiting, bilious. White-leg. Whooping cough. ***Yellow, fever***.

HOMEOPATHIC - Crotalus horridus, the rattlesnake venom, affects the blood, heart and liver. It produces profound nervous shock with deathly sickness, trembling and prostration. Easily tired by slight exertion. Profound nutritional action, nutritional troubles in old age.

Low septic states. General disorganization of the blood, hemorrhages and jaundice. ***Hemorrhages from every part of the body.*** Hemorrhages are slow, oozing dark thin blood, not clots. Hemorrhages from all the orifices and surfaces, especially from the pharynx. Hemorrhages from the pores of the skin. Bloody pus, sweat.

Tissues rapidly decompose producing putrid and ***malignant conditions.*** Dark or bluish parts. ***Septic conditions*** in the tonsils, goiter, ulcers, abscesses, blood boils. Moldy odors of secretions. Fetor of evacuations and discharges. Tendency to carbuncles. Petechiae. Neuralgia as a sequel to sepsis.

Gangrene. Malignant scarlatina, ***yellow fever***. ***Bubonic plague.*** Cholera. Stroke victims with bloody eyes. Chronic biliousness. Metastasis of erysipelas to brain. Menopausal conditions.

Fainting. Easily tired by slight exertion. Paralysis, post-diphtheria of the insane. Progressive muscular atrophy. Convulsions, epilepsy with trembling of the limbs, foaming at the mouth, violent cries, delirium. In epilepsy, the average rate is far greater than in normal conditions. Sleeps into his symptoms.

Pains alternate rapidly with each other and frequently recur, also appear and disappear suddenly after lasting some time (except headache). General burning. Swelling of whole body. Edema in general or of affected part. More ***right-sided*** in its action. Great periodicity.

MIND - Clouded perception, impaired memory. Timid. Aversion to his family. Weak memory, cannot express himself correctly. Loss of memory, for words and figures. Mistakes in writing. Connected thoughts difficult. Senile dementia incipient, forgets figures, names and places or suspicious about his friends.

Weeping mood, agony, despair. Melancholy. Sadness during headache. Readily moved to tears. Weeping, tearful mood, while reading. Marked indifference. Thoughts dwell on death continually. Fears of evil. Sensitive to certain persons.

Nervous agitation, anxious, pale, with cold sweat. Irritable, cross. Impatient. Irritable, cross, infuriated by least annoyance. Suspicion and snappishness, or quiet indifference. Plaintive speech. Intense restlessness, twitching and nervous agitation.

Loquacious with desire to escape. Delusions of cerebral decay. Feels as if surrounded by foes or hideous animals. Delirium, with wide open eyes. Delirium, muttering, mumbles, jumbles and stumbles over his words. Delusions awakes struggling with imaginary foes. Delirium tremens with constant drowsiness, but with inability to sleep. Mania in zymotic diseases and when connected with puerperal or ovario-uterine disease. Insanity with coldness of skin.

Abdomen - Burning pain in abdomen. Swollen, hot, tender. Inguinal glands enlarged. Bubo. Intestinal hemorrhage. Violent pain in left side near last ribs as if in diaphragm. Heat and tenderness of abdomen, can scarcely bear clothes on. Coldness in the stomach or abdomen as from a piece of ice. Violent pains in colon. Violent pain in region of appendix. Appendix feels large. Peritonitis. Typhlitis.

Back - Tearing pains from right shoulder to neck, worse on moving arm. Pain on top of shoulder and in ascending aorta. Aching in right kidney and in stomach. Drawing, tensive pain from right shoulder along neck, as from a tense tendon, worse pressure and moving arm. Softening of spinal cord. Carbuncles, boils, pustules, pimples or bed sores.

Breasts - Inflamed breasts.

Causations - Ill effects of fright, alcohol, sun, lightning, foul water, insect stings, noxious effluvia, or vaccinations.

Chest - Excessive oppression of chest. Burning in chest with heat in forehead. Stitches in right chest near sternum. Oppression in old people. Hydrothorax in fever and ague. Left axillary glands swollen and tender.

Constitutions - Broken-down constitutions. Chronic bilious, menopausal or albuminuric conditions. Hemorrhagic diathesis. Septic toxemic or even miasmatic disease.

Cough - Cough from external pressure on larynx. Cough as if from salt or pepper. Cough on awaking from sleep. Cough with stitch in left side. Dry cough on speaking, worse in dry or cold air. Nervous cough. Whooping cough, with blueness or pallor which is long in passing off. Cough with bloody sputum of moldy odor. Cough from tickling in throat. Cough with stitch in left side and bloody expectoration.

Ears - Otorrhea after scarlatina, offensive and bloody, with deafness. Otorrhea, result of alcoholism. Blood oozes from ears. Feeling of stoppage in right ear. Full sensation in ears. Erysipelas of external ear. Deafness, illusions of hearing. Auditory vertigo. Sensitive to noises.

Eyes - Dry and burning sensation. Yellow color of eyes. Burning, red with lachrymation. ***Ciliary neuralgia***, tearing, boring pain, as if a cut had been made around eyes. ***Retinal hemorrhages.*** Bleeding eyes after strokes. Blood exudes from eyes. ***For absorption of eye hemorrhages*** into the vitreous. Photophobia, worse during menses. Very sensitive to light, especially ***lamp light***. Ptosis. Keratitis. Exopthalmic goitre.

Face - ***Sallow***. Dark, besotted face. Face yellow, death like pallor. Distorted on waking. Lips, swollen, stiff and numb. Lockjaw. Acne of masturbators. Small blisters around eyes. Eruption around mouth. Frequently recurring erysipelas of face. Face swollen and red during delirium tremens and fever. Swelling of submaxillary and parotid glands.

Female - Uterine hemorrhage with faintness at stomach. Sensation as if the uterus would drop out. Prolonged menses. Dysmenorrhea with pain in hypogastrium, down the thighs with aching in the region of the heart. Painful drawing in uterine ligaments. Puerperal fever. Offensive lochia. Phlegmasia alba dolens, worse touch. Alcoholics with delayed menses. Ovarian neuralgia. Ovarian abscess. Vicarious menses. ***Menopausal flushings, sweat.*** Fungoid cancer of uterus. Cauliflower excrescences. ***Miscarriage during course of septic or zymotic disease.*** Miscarriage from other blood-poisoning causes.

Food - Hunger with trembling, weakness, and occipital headache. Aversion to meat. Craves pork. Desires stimulants, sugar. ***Diseases caused by abuse of alcohol.*** Unquenchable burning thirst.

Head - Dull, heavy occipital pain, on right side and right eye. ***Pain in occiput, as of a blow.*** Headache in waves from spine. ***Severe pain at the center of forehead.*** Headache with pain in heart, on lying on left side. ***Sick headache with vertigo.*** Headache worse jarring, must walk on tiptoe. Dull headache before attack of uremic coma. Bilious headache every few days. Throbbing headache with nausea before menses. Meningitis. Violent itching of scalp, eruptions, pustules. Falling off of hair, as a result of toxemia. Soreness in back of head on pressure.

Heart - Aching in region of heart. Weak, trembles, action feeble. Heart beats rapidly, but feebly. Trembling feeling of heart. Heart tender when lying on left side. Much pain in heart, through left shoulder and down left arm. Palpitations with sore pain in and about heart. Palpitations as if heart tumbled about. Palpitation during menses. Pulse rapid and weak, scarcely perceptible. Pulse feeble and quick, then slow. Pulse fluttering, frequent. Pulse small, quick, threadlike. Pulse wavy, or slow.

Kidneys - Nephritis. Inflamed kidney. Suppression or painful retention of urine. Urine scanty, dark and red with blood. Nephritis albuminosa in pregnancy. Albuminuria in course of typhoid, diphtheria. Albuminous, dark, scanty (Merc-c.). Dark, bloody urine, green-yellow. Casts. Hematuria with bronchitis. Hematuria with bladder or prostate cancer. Hemorrhage from kidney after scarlet fever. Hemorrhage from urethra. Urine copious and light colored. Yellow or reddish-yellow urine, from much bile.

Limbs - Phlebitis, varicose veins and varicocele. ***Right-sided paralysis***. Paralysis of left hand and leg. Arms and legs become numb, first one and then the other.

Lower limbs go to sleep easily. Cannot keep legs still. Pain in top of shoulders. Hands tremble, swollen. Hands feel dead when sewing. Heaviness as if bones were made of heavy wood. Bruised pain in joints and bones. Numb pain as after cramp, in anterior of fingers and in toes. Right-sided paralysis. Limbs inflamed, swollen and gangrenous. Contraction of flexors. Gonorrheal rheumatism. Cannot keep legs still.

Liver - ***Jaundice, malignant with hemorrhage.*** Stitches in region of liver on drawing a long breath, worse by pressure. Aching in liver, vomiting, coldness. Pain in region of liver and top of shoulders.

Lungs - Asthma with cardiac disease. Asthma, with great debility and prostration, blue, puffy countenance, cold sweat. Anxious, labored breathing. Oppression in old people. Tickling from a dry spot in larynx. Difficult breathing, as if lungs would not expand. Embarrassed breathing with constriction of throat. Quick, labored breathing with weak pulse and nervous agitation. Bronchiectasis, putrid bronchitis, chronic bronchorrhea. Edema or gangrene of lungs. Pneumonia with tendency to gangrene or haemorrhage.

Male - Prostate cancer, painful (Con.). Sexual instinct increased with entire relaxations of penis. Sharp cutting in glans.

Modalities - Better from rest, motion, light. Head and stomach symptoms better from open air. Worse in morning, on waking or wakes the patient up in the night. Worse right side. Worse lying. Worse falling asleep. Worse jar. Worse exertion. ***Worse from alcohol.*** Worse open air. Worse damp, wet. Worse evening and morning. Worse in spring. Worse changing to warm weather. Worse yearly. Cold air aggravates the throat and respiratory symptoms. Dry air aggravates cough.

Mouth - Complete loss of taste. Fills up with saliva. Saliva bloody, frothy. Salivation at night. Stiff palate. Cannot speak on account of sensation of constriction around tongue and throat. Fetid breath. Putrid, sore mouth. Moldy smell of breath.

Nose - Nosebleed especially during diphtheria or other septic diseases. ***Nosebleed, blood black and stringy***. Ozaena after exanthemata or syphilis. Nosebleed with flushes of face, vertigo or fainting. Bloody discharge. Tip of nose swollen and cold. Tip of nose, blue and red.

Perspiration - Bloody sweat. Sudden attacks of cold sweat. Colored sweat.

Rectum - Constipation with headache. Shuddering with diarrhea, aphonia. Diarrhea with nausea, thirst and anxiety. Diarrhea from septic matter in food or drink. Dysentery, septic. Hemorrhoids in pregnant women, and with menstrual irregularities. Hemorrhoids connected with heart disease or liver disease. Rectal hemorrhage, blood dark, fluid, non-coagulable. Rectal hemorrhage when of hepatic, splenic or cardiac origin. Bleeding from anus when standing and walking. Violent purging, with disagreeable sensation through whole body and nauseous taste. Perineal abscess.

Sensations - As from a blow on occiput. As if tongue and all around throat were tied up. As of a plug in throat to be swallowed, of choking. As if the heart turned over like a tumbler pigeon.

Skin - Skin cold and dry. Skin dry, stiff, like thin parchment. ***Lymphangitis and septicemia,*** from dissecting wounds. Skin, cold and dry. Yellow color of the whole body. Jaundice. ***Purpura hemorrhagica***. Great sensitiveness of skin of ***right half*** of body. Sore sensation relieved by pressure. Pustular eruptions. Blood boils, carbuncles, felons. ***Hemorrhages from every part of body.*** Chilblains, felons. Boils, carbuncles and eruptions are surrounded by purplish, mottled skin and edema. Anthrax. Vesication. Dissecting wounds. ***Edema*** about the affected part. Petechial spots. Old scars break open again. Old ulcers. Bloody sweat. Post-vaccination eruptions. Stings of insects. Gangrene with diarrhea. Pemphigus.

Sleep - Drowsy, but cannot sleep. ***Sleeplessness from nervous and mental distress***. Sleepless from nervous agitation. Starting in sleep. Smothering sensation when awaking. Symptoms worse after sleep. Dreams of dead persons. Travelling dreams. Dreams of quarrels. Horrible dreams. Yawning.

Stomach - Atonic dyspepsia. Trembling, fluttering below the epigastrium. Heartburn. Intolerance of clothing about epigastrium. Faintness and sinking at stomach. Ulceration of the stomach. Gastritis in chronic alcoholism. ***Cancer of stomach*** with vomiting of bloody, slimy mucus. Constriction of pylorus. Nausea on movement. Unable to retain anything. Violent vomiting of food. Constant nausea and vomiting every month after menstruation. Cannot lie on right side without vomiting dark-green matter. Black or coffee-grounds vomiting. Bilious vomiting. Vomiting of blood. Ulceration of stomach. Vomiting on least exertion.

Stool - White stools. Stools, black, dark green, thin, offensive, like coffee-grounds. Stools followed by debility. Liquid stools, with colic. Involuntary stool.

Teeth - Gums white. Bleeding of gums. Gums swollen, painful, borders reddened. Grinding of teeth during sleep.

Temperature - Chill alternating with heat. Severe chills. Malignant fevers of a ***hemorrhagic or putrescent character***. Low bilious remittents. Plague fever. Black water fever. Yellow fever. Cerebrospinal meningitis (Cic., Cup-a.). High fever. Bloody sweat, cold sweats. Pyemia. Hectic fever with burns, compound fractures, lacerated wounds, dissection wounds, cellulitis, erysipelas, stings of insects.

Throat - Dry, swollen, dark red with thirst. Spasm of esophagus, cannot swallow any solid substance. Gangrenous with much swelling. Tickling from a dry spot in larynx. Tight constriction of throat. Hoarseness, with weak, rough voice. Sore throat. Fauces sensitive to dry or cold air. Quinsy with much venous congestion. Tonsils bulge and are tender. Laryngismus stridulus. Edema glottidis. Paralytic aphonia. Ulceration from necrosis of cartilages of larynx. Acute laryngitis from burns. Laryngitis from stings of insects.

Tongue - Glossitis. Tongue numb and stiff. Tongue, yellow, enormously swollen, protruded to the right. Tongue red and small, but feels swollen. Tongue fiery red, dry in center, smooth and polished. Cancer of tongue with hemorrhage. Tongue very foul, with red tip. Tongue swollen to nearly twice the normal size. Edema of tongue after sting of insects.

Vertigo - Vertigo with pale face. Auditory vertigo. Menière's disease. Vertigo with faintness, weakness and trembling. Fainting on assuming upright position. Dizziness and fainting with occipital headache. Anemic vertigo, better resting head. Vertigo from fright. Vertigo with dilated pupils. Vertigo from lightning or sunstroke.

Vision - Amblyopia from hemorrhage, debility and exhaustion. Amblyopia from grief or from over use of vision. Diplopia. Illusions, blue colors. Dim vision for distant objects. Dim vision when reading. Lost vision with lethargy and coldness. Momentary disappearance of vision with profuse lachrymation. Muscae volitantes and various colored flames. Weak vision after an attack of keratitis or kerato-iritis.

COMMENTS - Crot-h. produces profound nervous shock and prostration with trembling, mental alienation and disorganization of the fluids and tissues. Bleeding from all orifices and surfaces. Hemorrhagic diathesis caused by previous low states of system, by zymotic or septic poisoning, by abuse of alcohol, etc.

Low, typhoid states with oppressed nervous system and degraded blood-supply. Neuralgia occurring as a sequel of septic toxemic or even miasmatic disease or chronic bilious, menopausal or albuminuric conditions. Broken-down constitutions. Sleepy, but cannot sleep. Grinds teeth.

Predominantly a right-side medicine (Lach. is left). Acts strongly on the liver and corresponds to jaundice and yellow fever. Used as a prophylactic against yellow fever. For this inoculation with diluted virus has been practiced.

The cobra poison (Naja.) coagulates blood into long strings. Crotalus poison is acid, the Viper neutral. The Rotton-snake ("Birri") causes more sloughing than any other.

Hering wrote that Crot-h. is preferable in fluid hemorrhages, with yellow skin, hence in yellow fever with black vomit, and nosebleed of diphtheria. Naja. has more nervous phenomena. Lach. has cold, clammy skin, rather than cold and dry, hemorrhage with charred-straw sediment, and more markedly ailments of the left side. Elaps is preferable in otorrhea and in disorders of the right lung.

Hayward observed that sloughing is a strong indication for Crot-h. and the cure with this remedy of his own daughter of scarlatina maligna with gangrenous-looking sore-throat was a dramatic outcome of his researches. Symptoms of Crotalus Durissus as well as Crotalus Horridus are included in the pathogenesis.

A case of rattlesnake bite and its isopathic cure, related by Dr. J. S. M. Chaffee in Hom. News, Sept., 1892, gives a good general idea of the action of the venom.

"I was called to see James Wright, aged 54 years, who, while binding wheat, was bitten on third finger of right hand by a rattlesnake. I found him bleeding from the bitten finger and from eyes, nose, ears, mouth, rectum and urethra, pulse 110, small, wiry, respiration 40, temperature 105, haggard expression, whole body bathed in hot perspiration, delirium.

"This patient had the regular routine treatment of whisky, quinine and carbonate ammonia for ninety-six hours, when the attendants withdrew and pronounced the case beyond the reach of medical aid. A marked characteristic symptom was a moldy smell of breath with scarlet red tongue and difficult swallowing. Great sensitiveness of skin of right half of body, so much so that the slightest touch would produce twitching of muscles of that side.

"I prescribed Crot-h. 30c trituration, 30 grains in four ounces of water, a teaspoonful every hour, until my return visit, twenty-four hours later, when I found marked improvement.

Temperature normal, pulse full, soft and regular, delirium gone, saliva and urine slightly tinged with blood, appetite returning, he having asked for food for the first time since the accident. The medicine was continued for two more days, when recovery was practically complete."

RELATIONS - ***Antidote:*** Lach., Alcohol. Radiant heat, Camphor. ***Compare:*** (1) Both., Naja - more nervous phenomena. (2) Lach. - more markedly worse on left side. (3) Elaps - preferable in otorrhea and disorders of right lung. (4) Crotalus cascavella - poliomyelitis.

REFERENCES - Boericke. Clarke. Phatak.

CROTON TIGLIUM

(Croton Oil Seeds)

PHARMACY - croto-t. Croton tiglium. Croton oil seeds. Tiglium officinale. N. O. Euphorbiacae. Tincture of the oil from the seeds. ***Historical dose:*** All potencies.

CLINICAL - Blisters. Cholera, infantum. Colic. Diarrhea. Eczema. Eruptions. Herpes, zoster. Neuralgias. Ophthalmia. Otorrhea. ***Poison ivy***. Pustules. Rashes. ***Rhus, poisoning. Skin, disorders.*** Vesicles.

HOMEOPATHIC - Croton Tiglium was used as a powerful purgative and irritant of the skin in ordinary practice, therefore causing watery discharges.

Croto-t. has a strong affinity for skin, face and external genitals. It is one of the ***antidotes to rhus poisoning,*** as is evident from its wide and intense action upon the skin and mucus surface, causing irritation and inflammation with formation of vesicles and mucus discharges.

Croto-t. is a valuable remedy in diarrhea, summer complaints and ***skin disorders.*** Skin symptoms alternating with internal symptoms, diarrhea etc. Many symptoms spread from below upwards.

Peculiar feeling as if parts were drawn backwards, eyes, nipples, etc. Skin feels hide-bound, tight all over. ***Burning in the esophagus***. Marked eye symptoms include purulent ophthalmia, ulceration and hypopion.

Affects the mucus membranes of the intestines. Colic before stool, constant urging, worse from eating, drinking, and every movement. Stool is yellowish or yellowish green. Characteristic sudden evacuation in one gush, like a shot, followed by great prostration.

MIND - Morose, dissatisfied. Cannot think outside himself. Feels all spent up. Feeling of anxiety, as though some personal misfortune would befall him. Not disposed to work.

Abdomen - Pressure on the navel causes pain in the rectum or urging for stool. Colic, better hot milk.

Breasts - Nodes in breasts with pain from nipple to scapula. Breast hard, swollen. Inflamed breasts. Nipples very sore to touch. ***Pain from nipple to back*** when child nurses.

Chest - ***Drawing-pain through the left chest into the back.***

Constitutions - Psoric and allergic constitutions.

Ears - Otorrhea, with great itching.

Eyes - Purulent ophthalmia, red and raw appearance. Pustules on cornea with eruptions around eyes. Granular lids, pustules of cornea. ***Eyes feel drawn backward. Tensive pain above right orbit.***

Face - Pustular eruptions on the face. As though insects were creeping.

Female - Intense itching of genitals, better by gentle rubbing.

Head - Pressing pain in forehead, especially orbits. Weight of hat causes headache.

Kidneys - Night urine, foaming, dark orange colored, turbid on standing, greasy particles floating on top. Day urine is pale with white sediment.

Limbs - Neck and shoulders painful.

Lungs - Asthma with cough, as soon as he touches the pillow, must sit up. Could not expand the lungs. Feels as though he could not inhale deeply enough. Sensitive to deep breathing.

Male - Eczema of scrotum. Vesicular eruptions on scrotum and penis. Left testes retracted, right pendent.

Modalities - Better after sleep. Better gentle rubbing. Many symptoms are worse at night. Worse least food or drink. Worse during summer. Worse night, morning. Worse receding eruptions. Worse washing. Worse touch, pressure. Worse motion, and when sitting or crouching. Dizziness and faintness are worse in open air. Drinking cold water while heated causes complete loss of voice. Colic worse hot milk. Diarrhea is worse in summer.

Mouth - Neuralgia of the tongue. Burning in esophagus.

Rectum - Swashing sensation in intestines. Pain in the anus as if a plug were forcing outwards. Constant urging to stool, followed by sudden evacuations. Copious, watery stools with much urging, ***then profuse sudden gushing stools of yellow water.*** Diarrhea worse drinking the least quantity or while eating, followed by prostration. Summer diarrhea. Cholera infantum.

Sensations - As if the skin were hide-bound. Mentally hide-bound, can't think outside of himself. As of a string pulling from one part to another, from eyeball to back of head, from nipple to back, with pain in nipple when the child nurses. Cutting, sticking, stinging, stitching pains and burning stitches. Writhing in transverse colon. As if a plug were forcing outwards at anus.

Skin - ***Rhus poisoning, poison ivy and oak.*** Eczema. Herpes zoster, stinging, smarting pains of the eruption. Vesicular erysipelas. Confluent, oozing, vesicles. Pustular eruptions, clustered blisters, which burst and form crusts, especially on ***face and genitals*** with fearful itching, followed by painful burning. ***Intense itching, but scratching is painful***. Violently itching, burning, red skin, sore if scratched, better gentle rubbing. ***Feels hide-bound.***

Stomach - Excessive nausea with vanishing of sight.

Vertigo - Vertigo, worse drinking.

COMMENTS - On the skin, Croto-t. produces erythema, erysipelas, eczema, and herpes pustules. Large, copper-colored spots almost like liver-spots. Small, red blotches that are not very apparent in thighs, abdomen and genitals, all accompanied with intolerable itching. Useful to antidote poison ivy and poison oak, particularly on the face and groin. Croto-t. antidotes Rhus-t. and the antidote to Croto-t. is Ant-t.

Guernsey gave the skin indications as "in any skin disease which itches very much, but the patient cannot bear to scratch very hard as it hurts, a very slight scratch, a mere rub suffices to allay the itching. Erysipelas that itches exceedingly." He also gives "otorrhea when there is much itching."

Teste, who was among the first to use Croto-t. homeopathically, gave a very interesting account of it. He quoted Trousseau and Pidoux as saying that it often happens that eruptions are developed on parts not touched by the remedy in those who have been engaged in making Croto-t. ointments on patients.

The face and the scrotum especially have been thus attacked. The itching which it causes, according to Teste, is at first more tingling than burning (the contrary taking place with Rhus-t.). The itching changes to burning (like Rhus-t.).

Teste recorded the case of a delicate, cachectic, psoric girl of four who had suffered for two years without interruption from a fetid discharge from the nose, less in winter, more in summer. Before this, she had a vesicular eruption on chest and neck, which disappeared by itself, followed in three or four days by the discharge.

After the failure of Sulph., Merc., Calc., on the indication of the previous eruption. Teste gave Croto-t., and in less than a fortnight the disease lost three-fourths of its intensity, although it was in mid-summer. Six months completed the cure, the only other remedies given during the time were Lob. and Kreos.

A second case from Teste records a man of forty, very fleshy, who for fifteen years had been subject to attacks of gout returning every spring, except on two occasions when a most fatiguing and obstinate rash appeared instead.

This consisted of an intense redness of the whole body, accompanied with a burning itching, especially in the hollow of the hands, at the chest, and behind the ears.

These parts were the seat of a yellowish, plastic exudation, emanating from a multitude of small vesicles in close contact with each other. They were only distinctly perceived in places where they were less numerous and where a greater degree of resistance on the part of the epidermis imparted to them a certain persistence.

Each time this eruption broke out, it lasted three months in spite of purgatives and the baths of Bareges and Aix les Bains. When Teste saw the patient, he had neither gout nor eczema, but a dry, racking, almost convulsive and unceasing cough.

Skin was rather hot, there was thirst, a little headache, heat in the chest, no dyspnea. Sometimes, especially in the evening, but only for a few days, he showed a tendency to syncope.

At the end of three weeks, having received no benefit from Teste's treatment, the patient took of his own accord three tablespoonfuls of the "Syrup of White Poppy," at bedtime. The cough ceased entirely for some hours and then returned in its old intensity.

But during the intermission the malady had come out on the skin, and at daybreak the patient found himself covered from head to foot with his old horrible eczema. He was almost unrecognizable and in a state of the deepest anxiety and despair. He expected three or four months of it.

Teste then gave Croto-t. The itching disappeared the same day. Within five or six days there remained not a trace of either cough or eruption. As the patient left Paris, Teste was not able to follow the case in subsequent years.

Conrad Wesselheft cured a case of proctalgia in a woman of thirty with Croto-t. 3x. The attacks came on after stool, lasting half a day and preventing her from fulfilling her duties as a teacher. There were no hemorrhoids, only sensitiveness of rectum to touch.

He was led to the remedy by having previously had another patient who suffered from a similar pain after using Croton pills. Pain in the rectum came on with extreme intensity after straining at stool and the patient (also a woman) was in agony for three hours afterwards with frequent tenesmus.

The pills were stopped and Nux-v. given, and she was well in a week.

RELATIONS - ***Antidote:*** Ant-t. ***Compare:*** (1) Rhus-t., Anagallis, Anac., Sepia. (2) Momordica charantia - has marked drastic properties, producing colic, nausea, vomiting, cholera-like symptoms, abdomen seems full of fluid discharged explosively, thin, watery, yellow. Great thirst.

REFERENCES - Boericke. Clarke. Murphy. Phatak.

CUBEBA OFFICINALIS

(Cubebs)

PHARMACY - cub. Cubeba officinalis. Cubebs. Piper cubeba. N. O. Piperaceae. Tincture of dried unripe fruit. ***Historical dose:*** Tincture and all potencies.

CLINICAL - Albuminuria. Aphthae. Bedwetting. Catarrh. Croup. Cystitis. Diarrhea. Dysentery. Gleet. Gonorrhea. Hernia. Leucorrhea. Orchitis. Prostatitis. Rheumatism. Roseola. ***Urethritis.*** Urticaria.

HOMEOPATHIC - Cubeba is an old-world remedy for gonorrhea and gleet. It affects the mucus membrane of the nose, air passages, intestines, and the uro-genital tract. It acts well in persons of bilious temperament with tendency to constipation.

Burning, rawness is felt in the throat in stomach, abdomen, rectum, urethra, fossa navicularis. Catarrh. Discharges are thick, acrid, yellow, pus like, green, offensive after violent inflammation. Frequent urination of a nervous origin. Leucorrhea in young girls.

MIND - Weakness of intellect. Frequent absence of mind. Loss of memory. Is unable to accomplish anything. Waking reveries. All his ideas are confused and wandering. Cannot find words to express himself. Exaltation of temper and mental faculties. Starting from noises. Uneasiness, anxiety, can't remain in bed.

Madness, with sorts of beastly extravagances. Impatient, irritable, a mere trifle provokes him. Furious insanity, with wickedness. Breaks everything within his reach, out of sheer malice. Mania, desire to strike and to kill. Impulse to swear at people. Impulse to strike them and spit in their faces, even to bite them.

Proneness to debauchery and every species of excess. Shamelessly indecent in thoughts, words, and gestures, especially towards evening. Delirium. Lascivious words and thoughts, with violent priapism. Lewd talk. Incoherent speech during sleep.

Paroxysms of foolish gaiety, with great loquacity, or silent weeping, towards evening. Want of decision and will-power. Fits of dejection, apathy, insensibility. Indifferent to everything.

Regards himself as more of an invalid than be really is. Delusion he is unfortunate. Disturbed about his health and social position. Paroxysms of anxiety, suffocation and fainting. Excessive nervous excitement; he is very easily frightened.

Abdomen - Distended and very sensitive. Burning in stomach and abdomen. Burning and pressure about navel. Cutting pain in hypogastrium before stools. Sensation of weight, pressure and pain.

Constitutions - Suitable to persons of bilious constitution with tendency to constipation.

Cough - Cough seems to tear bronchi. Cough in bronchitis. Incessant cough, bronchial. Barking and croupy cough with feeling as of a foreign body in larynx. During and after cough cold sweat upon breast and back, burning in abdomen. Cough with coryza and hoarseness.

Ears - Obstinate otorrhea. Offensive discharge.

Eyes - Rheumatic or gonorrheal ophthalmia. Fullness in eyes, turgid and watery.

Face - Fullness of face or red and pale by turns. Lips puffed, dry and shining. Twist of mouth to one side.

Female - Urethritis. Vaginitis, chronic with profuse discharge. Acrid leucorrhea in young girls. Leucorrhea, profuse, acrid, offensive, yellow or green, with pruritus. Leucorrhea with erythema at inner surface of thighs. Menses too soon, often preceded and followed by leucorrhea. Menses scanty, and consisting mostly of leucorrhea.

Food - Increased appetite. Craving for oranges, onions, almonds and nuts. Desires delicacies, acid fruits. Desires brandy, spirits, fresh bread. Mucus diarrhea worse fruit, acids. Unquenchable thirst with feeling of dryness of mouth and burning in throat.

Head - Veins of the forehead and temples are distended. Contractive and pressive pains with drowsiness, but without sleep. Deep-seated pains. The hairs becomes white. Falling off the hair, especially in the evening. Pustules on the scalp, forming scabs like those of small-pox. Intolerable itching of the head, with burning ulcers.

Kidneys - Burning and itching in fossa navicularis. Hematuria. Cystitis. ***Urethritis with much mucus***, especially in women. Cramp, cutting, burning in urethra after urination, with constriction. Stringy gonorrhea. Sensation as if bladder still contained water. Last drops of urine passed with pain. Urine frothy. Urine copious, dark. Urine, odor of violets. Nocturnal enuresis.

Limbs - Sensation of heat in palms and soles. Numbness of fingers and toes. Wrists stiff and thicker about joints. Acute, deep-seated pains.

Lungs - Dyspnea. Catarrh of nose and throat with fetid odor and expectoration. Mucus trickles from posterior sinuses. Rawness of throat and hoarseness. False membrane in larynx, danger of suffocation. Hurried and noisy breathing. Impeded breathing with crepitant rales. Dyspnea and sense of suffocation.

Male - Pale, copious, slimy discharge from urethra after use of alcohol. Prostatitis with thick yellow discharge. Pressure and heaviness in penis. Sexual excitement. Gonorrhea with profuse discharge and scalding pain during urination. Pale, copious, slimy discharge, causing soiled linen to become stiff. Thick, yellowish-green discharge with frequent obstruction of urethra.

Modalities - Better from getting up and walking about. Worse from night, in bed.

Mouth - Aphthae of lips and gums. On attempting to smile or speak his mouth seems to twist to one side. Mouth as if dry, though moistened with an oily saliva, great thirst. Tongue furred and moist or very white.

Nose - Post-nasal catarrh. Mucus trickles from nose into throat with rawness of throat and hoarseness. Nasal catarrh, with fetid odor and catarrh of throat. Nasal catarrhwith greenish-yellow expectoration.

Rectum - Constipation with hemorrhoids and tenderness of perineum. Burning and itching of anus. Relief of pains after stool. Loud flatus during stool. Long-continued tenesmus. Gelatinous stools of transparent mucus mixed with whitish, shining particles like rice, worse night, in bed, better getting up and walking about. Diarrhea with rumbling and cutting in abdomen and burning in rectum. Stools cold.

Skin - Eruption all over body like urticaria. Roseolous papules without fever or itching. Intense itching. Skin diseases with kidney affections. Skin diseases with catarrh of bladder and urethra.

Stomach - Burning in stomach and abdomen. Uneasiness, heat at pit with fever. Sour eructations. Nausea and vomiting.

Throat - Swallows saliva constantly to relieve burning and dryness of the throat. Catarrh.

Vertigo - Frequent giddiness, so that he is afraid of falling.

COMMENTS - Burning in throat with dryness, constant need to swallow saliva. Burning in stomach, abdomen, rectum, urethra and fossa navicularis. Prickling in soles of feet. Sensation of downward weight and pressure in region of femoral ring, worse on walking, riding or lifting.

Stools and colic are worse at night in bed, better getting up and walking about. Urine foaming. Albuminous, bloody. Acrid leucorrhea in children. Skin diseases with kidney disorders.

Nash defined its place in gonorrhea as "After the inflammatory stage is passed under the usual remedies for that stage, if there still remains burning in the urethra after urination and the discharge remains thick, yellow or pus-like (with Puls. the discharge is bland with Merc. all symptoms are Worse at night). Thin (gleety) discharge does not correspond to any of the three."

RELATIONS - Cop. with which it is compatible. *Compare:* (1) Cucurbitas. (2) Cop., Santa. (3) Piper methyst. Piper nigrum and Matico. Caps, Canth. (4) irritable bladder in females. Terebe., Cann-s. (5) Iod. - membranous croup.

REFERENCES - Boericke. Clarke. Phatak.

CUCURBITA CITRULLUS

(Watermelon Seeds)

PHARMACY - cuc-c. Cucurbita citrullus. Watermelon seeds. N. O. Cucurbitaceae. Cucurbita. ***Historical dose:*** Tincture and all potencies.

CLINICAL - Backache. Coryza. Diuresis. Dysuria. Rheumatism. Sneezing. Sinusitis.

HERBAL - Infusion of watermelon seeds for painful urination with a sense of constriction and backache.

HOMEOPATHIC - All those with hydrogenoid constitution and suffering from rheumatic problems were found to be affected most. Tendency to suppuration. Tendency to catching cold. Internal heat but external coldness. Increased perspiration.

MIND - Irritable, on the slightest provocation or controversy. Irritable, esp. with children. Violent anger. Wants to fight, but lacks the physical strength, so cannot. Depressed feeling in the morning. Desires death.

Abdomen - Fullness, bloated feeling. Pain in abdomen worse milk, worse coffee. Pain in left side of abdomen. Abdomen pain, worse pressure. Abdomen pain, better lying on right side, passing flatus, warmth.

Face - Swelling of face in morning. Swelling of left cheek in morning.

Food - Increased appetite. Must eat, cannot remain hungry which she could before. Hungry at night and also in the morning. Appetite increased after stools. Aversion to sweets. Desire for sweets decreased. Desires cold drinks. Desires ice cream, spicy food. Worse coffee, milk. Better warm drinks.

Headache - Left-sided headache. Bursting pain. Heaviness. Headaches worse after 4 p.m., evening. Headaches worse pressure, motion of head. Headaches worse sun, reading, lying down. Headaches better warm bath, open air, rest, night, sitting.

Modalities - Worse left side. Worse Sun. Worse travelling.

Mouth - Salivation increased. Stringy saliva.

Nose - Sneezing. Coryza. Watery, acrid discharge, followed by sticky, greenish discharge. Sinusitis maxillaris.

Perspiration - Profuse perspiration at the nape of neck at night.

Rectum - Sudden urging for stool in early morning, worse 3 a.m. to 6 a.m.

Sleep - Drowsiness. Increased sleep with drowsiness.

Stomach - Retching of stringy mucus.

Throat - Sore throat, with pain in spots mainly left side, worse Empty swallowing.

Vertigo - Faint feeling and vertigo.

RELATIONS - ***Compare:*** Equisetum.

REFERENCES - Boericke.

CUCURBITA PEPO

(Pumpkin Seeds)

PHARMACY - cuc-p. Cucurbita pepo. Pumpkin seeds. Cucumis macrocarpus. N. O. Cucurbitaceae. Cucurbita. Tincture of fresh plant. ***Historical dose:*** Tincture and all potencies. ***Historical dose:*** Tincture and all potencies, two ounces of seed, yielding one of pulp. May be mixed with cream and taken like porridge.

CLINICAL - Gonorrhea. Morning, sickness. Nausea. Roundworm. Seasickness. ***Tapeworm.*** Urinary, disorders. Vomiting. ***Worms.***

HERBAL - Cucurbita pepo is of service in strangury and urinary affections, also in gastritis, enteritis, and febrile diseases. A tincture of the vines and of the seeds has been prescribed with alleged benefit in vomiting of pregnancy. It also has cured vomiting of food and salivation in non-pregnant women. Intense nausea immediately after eating.

Vomiting during pregnancy. Seasickness.

One of the most efficient and least harmful of vermifuges, which may be given safely to children. An infusion of the seeds has also been found effectual in removing tapeworm. After a few hours, a purgative, like castor oil, may be administered to aid in the expulsion of the worm. This is also effectual in removing the roundworm.

HOMEOPATHIC - Hansen mentioned that missionaries found the mother tincture of great use in seasickness and vomiting during pregnancy. Bonino recorded that Cuc-p. 3c cured salivation and vomiting in a woman in whom the menses were absent and who was erroneously supposed to be pregnant.

Grist recorded a case in which a woman, four months pregnant, vomited almost from conception and for six weeks had not retained a meal. "I am almost starved to death," she said, was pale, haggard, tongue clean. Soon after eating or drinking anything she became intensely nauseated.

The doctor got a fresh pumpkin stem, cut it into thin slices and covered them with alcohol. At the end of half an hour he poured off a little and made a 1x dilution and directed half a drachm to be put in half a tea cupful of water, a teaspoonful every two hours. There was no further vomiting.

Dr. Griste's indication was *"Intense nausea immediately after eating."*

COMMENTS - For treatment, the seeds should be scalded, the softened outer skins peeled off as the green, inner pulp is used. Use two ounces of the seeds, yielding an ounce of pulp, for each patient. The pulp should be rubbed in a mortar or some other vessel to make a smooth mass.

The seed^ may be mixed with milk or cream, and sweetened and taken like porridge. It should be taken in the morning after a twelve to sixteen hour fast, and be followed in two hours by a castor-oil purge.

The infusion may be drank freely. The expressed oil of the pumpkin seeds, in doses of 6 to 12 drops, several times a day, is said to be a most certain and efficient diuretic, giving quick relief in scalding of urine, spasmodic affections of the urinary passages, and has cured gonorrhea.

Half a fluid ounce of oil of pumpkin seeds, taken upon a fasting stomach, repeated in 2 hours, and in another 2 hours followed by a dose of castor oil containing 1/2 fluid ounce of the pumpkin-seed oil, has been effectual in removing tapeworm.

Hale's method of using this remedy was to have the patient eat only a little of the lightest food all day, taking no supper and, on going to bed, to eat one ounce of the peeled seeds, bruised with milk or cream.

In the morning on waking, he had them take a tablespoonful of castor oil, mixed with half a teaspoonful of pure sulfuric ether. No breakfast was taken, only a cup of tea or coffee. In two or three hours the oil would operate, expelling the worm.

RELATIONS - ***Compare:*** (1) Filix, Cina, Cuprum oxid. nig., Spig.

REFERENCES - Boericke. Clarke.

CULEX MUSCA

(Mosquito)

PHARMACY - culx. Culex musca. Mosquito. N. O. Culicide. Insecta. Tincture. ***Historical dose:*** All potencies.

CLINICAL - Cramps. ***Edema.*** Flatus. Vertigo.

HOMEOPATHIC - Kent wrote "When this remedy is needed your patient will present to you a picture of something on fire, he burns like something he would like to mention and perhaps does mention the place, the itching and burning are present every where in this remedy, he rubs and scratches wherever the eruptions appears."

Edematous swelling. Sensation as of cold air blowing through a hole in clothes on the chest or back. Strange feeling of having been poisoned. Menses stain indelibly. Generally a right-sided remedy.

Sharp, stinging pains all over the body like needles, lightning-like. Pain, itching, burning, worse in a warm room and better in the open air. Pains darting here and there, aggravated by light pressure and ameliorated by hard pressure. Griping pain down over hips, then into the womb.

Vertigo on blowing the nose. Tired and weak. Can scarcely move, cannot walk straight, with soreness and aching all over the body. Nervous, finds it impossible to keep still, almost constant motion of the hands and feet (Zinc.).

MIND - Busy scratching to relieve the itching, and walking to relieve the restlessness, any interruption makes him impatient and ready to quarrel. Anxiety and fear of death. Poor memory and a disinclination for all work.

Abdomen - Cramps in the abdomen during stool, with rumbling and the passing of much offensive flatus. Colicky pairs come on about 10 a.m. and last from one to three hours. Blotches on the abdomen the size of a twenty-five cent piece. Itching, burning, with little pimples on the blotches.

Back - Dull pain in the right side in the region of the kidney, extending up the back to the occiput.

Chest - Cutting pains in the right pectoral muscles. Right side of the neck is swollen.

Ears - Swelling of the parotid glands and soreness on pressure, pain as if he were going to have mumps. Sharp pains in both ears followed by sticky, watery discharge.

Eyes - Inflamed eyeballs. Stye-like ulceration. Rending pains in the eyeballs, could not keep his eyes open, yet it pained to keep them shut. Eyes feel tired. Feeling of fullness in the right eye, extending to the parotid gland, to the sub-lingual, and finally involves the right side of the face and head. Margins of the lids are sore and crusted over. Inflammation of the lids, worse in the morning with a discharge of sticky fluid.

Face - Swollen sub-maxillary gland, tender on pressure. Eruption on the face and between the eyes, contains a colorless fluid, with swelling and puffiness under the eyes. Heat and redness of the right side of the face, with a sore bruised feeling.

Female - Menses, too soon, with a profuse dark clotted flow. Violent pains in the uterus, compelling her to go to bed. Itching and burning in vagina, so intense that she feels as if she could tear it to pieces, can return at intervals for years.

Food - Ravenous appetite, feels faint if supper is late. Especially hungry and faint in the morning, cannot wait for breakfast to be prepared.

Head - Dull, frontal headache, begins on waking at 5 a.m. and passes away after lying awake for a while. Headache, worse from the least motion. Headache followed by intense vertigo in the afternoon, located in a spot over the right eye. Head pains go from the cerebellum to the forehead or right temple. Boring pains in the temples, several times a day. Pain comes and goes across the forehead just above the eyes. Rending pain in back of the eyeballs. Itching and stinging of the scalp.

Limbs - Hands and fingers are hot and burning, as if fiozen with severe pain. As if he must tear the flesh for relief while the back of the hands felt cold and benumbed. Right hand is cold, left hand is warm. Lower limbs feel heavy and restless. Feet are tired all day. Soles tender while walking. Intense itching on the tops of the feet.

Lungs - Oppression and anxiety in the chest. Apex of the right lung sore, aggravated by deep breathing or raising the right arm. Deep sighing breathing, with constant desire for a deep breath. Constant desire to sneeze and cough. On rising, hawking and coughing dark green scabs and strings of tough mucus tinged with dark blood. Cough caused by burning in the chest. Whistling, strangling, choking cough, with red face and water running from the eyes. Dry hacking cough with the feeling as if he would vomit. Small amount of yellowish white expectoration.

Male - Burning of the glans penis. Strong smelling discharge from the glans. Itching of the scrotum from swollen, burning spots, like bee stings. Rubbing aggravates itching, stinging, and burning.

Mouth - Dryness and burning. Constant wetting of the lips. Saliva leaves the lips sticky. Whitish saliva, leaves a bad taste in the mouth in the morning. Sickish taste as if he had been drinking warm mineral water. Periodical attacks of salivation, at night the pillow is wet and the daytime the saliva accumulates and causes continued swallowing (Merc.). Foul breath, seemed as if he could smell it himself.

Nose - Itching, stinging and tickling. Rubs and scratches because his nose itches inside and out, but rubbing increased burning. Shining redness on top of nose. Nose is swollen. Eruptions contain a clear colorless fluid. Nosebleed, morning and night on blowing the nose. Head feels stuffed. Ineffectual desire to sneeze. Watery discharge with bloody scabs on the inside, dry or moist and bloody. Copious discharge, greenish or light-colored.

Rectum - Usual desire for morning stool is absent. Stool is scanty, lumpy and expelled with effort. First part of the stool is hard and scratches the anus, followed by a soft stool. After stool, sensation that he has not finished so he sits and strains until blood comes (Merc.). Itching and burning of the anus, scalding hot and raw as from a bite.

Skin - ***Tormented by itching, burning, heat.*** Must scratch to relieve the constant itching, but aggravates. No comfort in or out of bed.

Sleep - Restless, unrefreshing sleep, much tossing about. Dreams of quarrels, fights and of the dead. Heat of the bed causes him to waken frequently, must rise early in the morning to move around for relief.

Stomach - Thirst for cold water which causes burning in the stomach with urging to stool, followed by loose, dark brown, offensive stool, much tenesmus lasting several days and gradually subsiding into painless diarrhea. Sickening pains and belching of much offensive gas. Nausea, day and night from even the thought of food. Nausea with gagging and retching and inability to vomit.

Stomach - Increased appetite. Undigested food sours in the stomach.

Temperature - Hot flushes as if a chill would follow, followed by warm, sticky, strong smelling perspiration.

Throat - Burning and dryness of the throat. Soreness in throat and in the posterior sinuses on swallowing solids or fluids. The right side of the throat is always sore. Hoarseness, could scarcely speak a word, in the morning.

Tongue - Tongue is coated white, dry, swollen, thick on waking. Edge of the tongue is covered with a double row of small, painful vesicles. Tongue numb, with ulceration at the tip following scarlet fever.

COMMENTS - Culex was proved by Kent, but the only verification Clarke found was of the symptom "vertigo every time he blows his nose."

W. P. Wesselheft cured a man, 40, stout, thick-set, light brunette, who had swelling on upper jaw over first right tricuspid. Slight redness of cheek. Abscess threatened with paroxysmal throbbing, dull pain better by warm applications. This came on after exposure to wet weather.

Merc. and Rhus-t. did no good. The patient then said that whenever he blew his nose he had vertigo with a sense of fullness in the ears. Culx. promptly relieved the pain and in forty-eight hours the swelling had gone.

RELATIONS - ***Compare:*** Apis.

REFERENCES - Clarke. Kent.

CUNDURANGO

(Condor Plant)

PHARMACY - cund. Cundurango. Condor plant. Condurango. Gonolobus cundurango. Marsdenia cundurango. N. O. Asclepiadacae. Ecuador. South America. Tincture and trituration of the dried bark of the stem. ***Historical dose:*** Tincture and all potencies.

CLINICAL - Anus, cracks. Breast, tumors. ***Cancer. Cracks.*** Eczema. Epithelioma. Fistula. Headaches. Locomotor, ataxia. Lupus. Rodent, ulcer. Smallpox. Stomach, cancer. Stomach, disorders. Syphilis. Tumors. ***Ulcers.*** Varicose, ulcers.

HOMEOPATHIC - The Condor plant was first introduced into medicine as a ***cancer remedy*** by Dr. Bliss of Washington. Cundurango belongs to the Milk-weed family and is thus related to Asclepias Syriaca and Tuberosa and also to Calotropis.

Cancer, especially for those originating in epithelial structures. Scirrhus cancers. Cancer of the breasts with retraction of the nipples and sharp pains emanating from the tumor over the whole breast. Jagged ulcers of the tongue. Tumors, strictures of the esophagus.

Cancer of the stomach with constant burning and vomiting, food seems to stick behind the sternum. Allays the stomach pain accompanying cancer of stomach. Stimulates the digestive functions and thus improves the general health. Modifies secretions of digestive glands. Chronic stomach catarrh.

Cutting, stinging, burning, tingling, constrictive and piercing pains. Cracks at muco-cutaneous orifices and warty excrescences. ***Painful cracks in corner of mouth***. Blotches. Eczema, pimples, pustules. Indolent ulcers. Varicose ulcers. Lupus. Syphilitic affections.

The active principle (Condurangin) produces locomotor ataxia. This remedy is worth trying when other seemingly indicated remedies fail to effect the disease.

MIND - Depressed, miserable. Irritable.

Abdomen - Pain in right hypochondrium.

Back - Dull, heavy, continuing pain in left scapula.

Breasts - Tumor of breast on either side. Cracked, painful, suppurating nipples. Retraction of the nipples. Hard, painful swellings around nipple, ranging in size from pigeon's to hen's egg. Axillary glands swollen, emaciation.

Chest - Cancer-like ulcers on false ribs, as large as hand.

Constitutions - Cancerous diathesis. Broken-down constitution. In Burnett's opinion, it is anti-psoric.

Eyes - Flat epithelioma on lower eyelid. Appearance of objects before eyes.

Face - ***Deep crack in corner in corner of mouth,*** warty growths occupying edges. Ulcer on chin, right side perforating to gums.

Head - Severe dull headache all day. ***Violent pain in left temple***, cutting in left temple and through ball of left eye. Sensation as if forehead were broad and high, as if left half were bigger than right. Left half feels heavy, right half feels clear.

Heart - Constrictive pain. Sharp, distinct pain in heart on rising in morning, followed by passage of flatus.

Kidneys - Incontinence of urine. Urine scanty, high-colored, loaded with phosphates.

Limbs - Soreness all over body like rheumatism, worse through left shoulder and under left scapula (burning). Cracks on hips and in bends of knees.

Mouth - Slight pain in left half of tongue. Small, painful pustule on right side of tip of tongue, on upper surface towards edge. Cracks at angles of mouth. Tongue cancer.

Nose - Much glairy mucus from nose, alternating with unusual dryness. Stiffness in nose. Pressive full feeling in bridge. Flat epithelioma left side of nose. Nasal sound to voice.

Rectum - Constipation. Cracks at anus, terrible pains when bowels are moved.

Skin - Fissures form about the muco-cutaneous outlets. Epithelioma of lips or anus. Ulcerative stage of carcinoma when fissures form. Some small congenital warty excrescences enlarge and look fresh. Blotches, pimples and boils.

Stomach - Anorexia. Painful disorders of the stomach, ulceration. Stomach cancer. Vomiting of food with indurations and constant burning pain. Stricture of esophagus with burning pains behind sternum, where food seems to stick.

Throat - Aching in throat, extending to stomach with great burning in stomach. Persistent sore throat, with burning, aching and a husky feeling which causes a dry, hacking cough.

Vertigo - Great dizziness on stooping, or turning head.

COMMENTS - Burnett, who proved it and whose symptoms were of a severe nature, observed that it produced "a painful crack in the right corner of the mouth." These cracks were produced in several patients who were taking the drug and Burnett cured similar cracks with it. He regarded them as a keynote indication and has cured patients of tumors, some undoubtedly cancerous, who had that symptom as a concomitant.

Clotar Muller cured with Cund. several cases of old, obstinate, foul-smelling, ichorous ulcers. Carcinoma of the lips, an unclean and sinus ulcer.

Dudgeon recorded a cure with Cund. first dilution of an undoubted case of cancer of left breast in a women of sixty-nine. The nipple was so retracted as to be invisible.

A hard tumor the size of an egg on the outer side of the nipple was the center of sharp pains radiating from it, the whole breast was very tender to touch. The tumor increased steadily under Hydr. and Phyt. and was only checked temporarily by Con. Under Cund., it entirely disappeared.

Burnett considered it to have a strong affinity for the tongue. He cured a jagged ulcer of the tongue (doubtful whether cancerous or syphilitic), where the tongue and lips were red.

One prover had a slight creeping pain along the periosteum of the right humerus and Clarke observed "a creeping sensation up the back and headache in right temple" in a patient taking it in the 1x tincture.

An old-school authority, Dr. Guyvenot, credits Condurango with causing a "veritable locomotor ataxia." It appears late and he thinks it is due to the formation of some toxic substance by the splitting up of the alkaloid in the organism.

RELATIONS - ***Compare:*** (1) Aster. Con., Hydr., Ars.

REFERENCES - Boericke. Clarke. Phatak.

CUPHEA VISCOSISSIMA

(Flux-weed)

PHARMACY - cuph. Cuphea viscosissima. Flux-weed. Lythrum petiolatum. Waxweed. Red pennyroyal. N. O. Lythraceae. Decoction or tincture of fresh plants collected in July or August. ***Historical dose:*** Tincture and all potencies.

CLINICAL - Acidity. ***Cholera infantum.*** Diarrhea. Dysentery. Fever. Sleeplessness. Tenesmus. Vomiting.

HERBAL - Cuphea viscosissima is a popular remedy in some parts of the U.S. for summer diarrhea and dysentery, as one of its names, ***"Flux weed,"*** would imply. The entire plant has a clammy, sticky feel. It contains a large percentage of tannic acid and seems to possess decidedly tonic properties, as children rally rapidly under its use.

HOMEOPATHIC - Vomiting of undigested food. ***Cholera infantum***, much acidity. Frequent green, watery, acid stools. Tenesmus and great pain. Obstinate constipation. High fever, restlessness and sleeplessness.

COMMENTS - Cuphea viscosissima was first introduced to homeopathic practice by Dr. A. Roth of Frederick, Maryland, who was induced to try it in his practice by a female patient. His experience was confirmed by S. G. A. Brown.

Dr. Roth gave from 5 to 10-drop doses, according to age. He considered in to have "tonic" properties. Roth found it to be highly successful in two chief forms, but useless in diarrhea from cold.

The first form consists of cases arising from acidity of milk or food. There is vomiting of undigested food or curdled milk with frequent green, watery, acid stools, varying in number from five to thirty a day. Children are fretful and feverish, can retain nothing on stomach, food seems to pass right through the child.

In the second form, stools are decidedly dysenteric, small frequent, bloody with tenesmus and great pain, high fever, restlessness and sleeplessness.

Brown said "If you have a child that is fretful and feverish, vomits curdled milk from a hyperacidity of the stomach, has frequent green, watery, acid stools or even if the stools are dysenteric with great tenesmus and colic, high fever and restlessness, give Cuphea."

RELATIONS - ***Compare:*** (1) Aeth. (2) Coto Bark - intestinal catarrh, chronic, copious, exhausting diarrhea and dysentery, colliquitine sweats of tuberculosis and chronic diarrhea. (3) Typha latifolia, Cat-tail flag - diarrhea, dysentery, summer complaint of children. Tincture and first potency.

REFERENCES - Anshutz. Boericke. Clarke.

CUPRESSUS AUSTRALIS

PHARMACY - cupre-au. Cupressus australis. N. O. Coniferae. Tincture of fruit and leaves. *Historical dose:* Tincture and all potencies.

HOMEOPATHIC - Cupre-au. has had a proving, which, though not extensive, is sufficient to show the analog of its action with that of Thuj. Sharp, piercing and pricking pains are prominent. General feeling of warmth. Headaches. Rheumatism. Gonorrhea.

RELATIONS - ***Compare:*** (1) Abies-n., Sabin., Thuj.

REFERENCES - Clarke.

CUPRESSUS LAWSONIANA

PHARMACY - cupre-l. Cupressus lawsoniana. N. O. Coniferae. Tincture of berries and leaves. *Historical dose:* Tincture and all potencies.

CLINICAL - Keloids. Lipoma. Tumors. Warts.

HOMEOPATHIC - Cupre-l. has been proved in a fragmentary way by Burnett, who had to relinquish the proving on account of the "terrible pains it caused in the stomach."

Burnett concluded from his experience that the action of Cupre-l. is like that of Thuj. He successfully used it as a variant of that remedy and of Sabin. in the cure of tumors like cocks-comb growth in the mouth, lipoma of the thigh, and keloids.

REFERENCES - Clarke.

CUPRUM ACETICUM

(Copper Acetate)

PHARMACY - cupr-acet. Cuprum aceticum. Copper acetate. Verdigris. Solutions. *Historical dose:* Trituration and all potencies.

CLINICAL - Angina pectoris. Brain disorders. Brow ague. Cerebrospinal meningitis. Cholera. Chorea. Croup. Diarrhea. Eruptions. Erysipelas. Hallucinations. Hydrocephalus. ***Labor*, *pains.*** Leprosy. Mania. Measles. Paralyzes. Psoriasis. Scarlatina. Smallpox. Strabismus. Stroke. Tapeworm. Uremia. Vertigo. Whooping cough.

HOMEOPATHIC - Burnett cured with Cupr-acet. a case of left-sided brow ague of many years' standing. He used Rademacher's Tincture of Copper. The pain was described as boring, screwing and was spoken of by the patient as "awful."

Burnett was unable to say whether the cure was strictly homeopathic or whether the Cuprum acted on the basis of the Paracelsus's Universalia, of which it is one.

Cupr-acet. produces the leading features of Cupr., including cramps, griping pains, spasms, paralytic disorders and convulsions. Attacks come on suddenly and periodically. ***Protracted labor***.

Facial neuralgia in cheekbone, upper jaw and behind the ear better by chewing, pressure and hot applications. Chorea, periodical with melancholy and dread of society. In epilepsy, aura begins in the knee and ascends to hypogastrium.

Chronic psoriasis and leprous-like eruption over whole body in spots of various sizes without itching. It corresponds to the results of repelled eruptions. Hay fever with burning excoriation. Paroxysmal cough with tough, tenacious mucus and fear of suffocation.

Constitutions - Suited to the carbo-nitrogenous constitution.

Face - Collapsed, hippocratic. Facial neuralgia in cheekbone, upper jaw and behind right ear. Better by chewing, pressure and external warmth.

Head - Neuralgia with heaviness of head, burning, stinging and stitching in temples and forehead. Violent throbbing and sharp pains in forehead. Left-sided brow ague. Brain seems void. Inclined to gape and cry. Loses consciousness, ***head reels when in large room***. Constant protrusion and retraction of tongue (Lach.).

Lungs - Spasmodic constriction of the chest. Violent spasmodic cough. Short, difficult respiration. Dyspnea. Attacks of angina pectoris coming on when excited.

Modalities - Better chewing. Better pressure. Better night. Better lying on affected side and warmth. Worse from heat. Worse motion. Worse emotions. Worse touch.

Skin - Leprous-like eruption over whole

body in spots of various sizes, without itching.

Stomach - Violent spasmodic pains in stomach and abdomen. Vomiting. Violent tenesmus. Slimy brown diarrhea. Cholera.

Vertigo - Head reels when in a high-ceilinged room.

COMMENTS - A man, 50, was cured with Cupr-acet. 5c trituration. of a tonic spasm of the toes of the right foot, very painful, lasting for hours, brought on by friction, standing on cold floors, etc. There was no traceable cause and no other derangement of health. Complete cure in five days after months of previous suffering.

Petroz recommended its use in smallpox and verified his induction in practice. As pointed out by General Phelps, the "Crimson Cross Ointment" which was used successfully by Fielden in the Gloucester epidemic of smallpox owes its virtue to the Cupr-acet. which it contains.

In epilepsy, the aura begins in the knees and ascends to hypogastrium, when patient becomes insensible. The symptoms are worse by heat and motion. The patient frequently changes posture.

RELATIONS - Acts similarly to Cupr. but is more violent in action. In poisoning cases it is ***Antidoted by:*** sugar or white of egg, given freely. Homeopathic antidotes: Bell., Chin., Con., Cic., Dulc., Hep., Ip., Merc., Nux-v. ***Compare:*** (1) Calc., Gels. - overworked brain. (2) Cic. and Solanaceae - mental symptoms. (3) Zinc. - hydrocephalus and convulsions from suppressed exanthems.

REFERENCES - Boericke. Clarke. Phatak.

CUPRUM ARSENICOSUM

(Copper Arsenite)

PHARMACY - cupr-ar. Cuprum arsenicosum. Copper arsenite. Scheeles green. Trituration. ***Historical dose:*** Trituration and all potencies.

CLINICAL - Boils. Carbuncles. Cholera. Cholerine. Chorea. ***Convulsions. Cramps***. Diabetes. Diarrhea. Gangrene. Gastro-enteritis. Enteralgia. Headaches. ***Nephritis***. Neuralgic, pains. Paralysis, left sided. Ulcers. ***Uremia.*** Uterine, neuralgia. Vomiting.

HOMEOPATHIC - Cupr-ar. combines the characters of its two metallic components. J. N. Majumdar noted the great characteristic of Cupr-ar. in choleraic conditions after B. L. Bhaduri pointed it out to him. Majumdar noted "icy-coldness of the whole body with cramps and an obstinate hiccough."

Various intestinal affections. Cholera morbus and infantum. Rice water stools. Entero-colitis, diarrhea and dysentery. Gastro-intestinal disturbances of influenza or typhoid. Inflammation of the digestive tract with violent colic, vomiting, diarrhea and uremia, with obstinate hiccough and icy cold body.

Deficient kidney action. Urine of garlicky odor. ***Uremic convulsions***, headache, vertigo and unconscious conditions resulting from brain edema. Uremic convulsions preceded by gastro-intestinal symptoms. ***Nephritis of pregnancy***.

Awful distress in epigastric region, burning along esophagus and in urethra. Numbness, creeping, itching and chilly sensations. Intense neuralgic pains in abdomen. Visceral neuralgia, sharp shooting abdominal pains.

Painful neuroses, enteroptosis. ***Violent cramps*** in chest, fingers, calves toes etc. Delirium and tremor cordis. ***Leg cramps,*** better pressing foot on the floor. Numb paralyzed feeling in the legs. Trembling of the whole body when attempting to walk. Chorea after fright.

Bronchial asthma and with emphysema. Chlorosis. Weak heart. Purulent endocarditis (Royal). Cold, clammy intermittent sweat.

Abdomen - Gastro-enteritis. Violent abdominal pain. Rumbling and sharp, cutting pain.

Back - Persistent lameness. Pain in lumbar region, lower left shoulder blade, chest tight.

Heart - Cardiac rhythm and force altered due to defective elimination.

Kidneys - Diabetes. Kidney inefficiency and uremia. ***Garlic odor of urine***. Urine of high specific gravity increased, acetones and diacetic acid.

Limbs - ***Cramps in calves of legs***, worse after midnight, only relieved by getting out of bed and standing. Gangrene ulcers.

Male - Perspiration of scrotum is constantly damp and moist. Boils on scrotum. Purulent discharge of a ***white color*** from urethra, tingling and burning in urethra. Pain in prostate, pains in penis.

Modalities - Better rest and worse motion, but stiffness of back and tingling of hands are better from motion. Damp weather causes neuralgia of abdomen.

Mouth - Tongue thickly coated, dirty brown, white, metallic taste, thirst. Dry mouth.

Rectum - Rice water stools. Cholera infantum, cholera (Verat., Camph.). Rumbling and sharp, cutting pain. Dark liquid stools. Diarrhea in tuberculosis.

Skin - Icy cold sweat and skin even when dry. Cold, clammy perspiration of an intermittent nature. Acne, pustules on face and in the genital region, ulcers look like chancre. Gangrene, carbuncles.

COMMENTS - Salzer showed that "cold, clammy perspiration of intermittent nature" is unique and characteristic. He found it most valuable in the collapse stage of cholera, where intermittent cold, clammy sweat was noted. The skin is very sensitive to touch and pressure worse all symptoms. Weakness and restlessness. Periodicity in the symptoms.

RELATIONS - ***Compare:*** (1) Ars. and Cupr. preparations (2) Acon., Cimic. - angina pectoris, numbness of left side of body, paresis of left arm. (3) Merc-c. - diarrhea and tenesmus. (3) Iris-v.

REFERENCES - Boericke. Clarke. Phatak.

CUPRUM METALLICUM

(Copper Metal)

PHARMACY - cupr. Cuprum metallicum. Copper metal, (Cu, At. Wt. 6). Trituration. ***Historical dose:*** Trituration and all potencies.

CLINICAL - After-pains. Angina pectoris. Asthma. Asthma miller. Bronchitis. Cardialgia. Catarrh. Chlorosis. ***Cholera. Chorea. Convulsions. Colic. Coughs. Cramps.*** Croup. Cyanosis. Dentition. Dyspnea. Emissions. ***Epilepsy.*** Eruptions. Erysipelas. Fainting. Gout. Hematemesis. Herpes. Hyperesthesia. Hysteria. ***Larynx, spasms.*** Mania. Measles. Meningitis. Neuralgias. Palpitations. Paralysis. Pneumonia. Psoriasis. Ringworm. Sleeplessness. ***Spasms.*** Spinal irritation. Tapeworms. Ulcers. ***Whooping cough.*** Worms. Yellow fever.

HOMEOPATHIC - Metallic copper is one of the most important remedies where the diseased conditions "appear" on account of the non-appearance or suppressions of eruptions and the discharges.

Skin eruptions and foot-sweat. Effects of suppression of eruptions, exanthems and foot-sweat, whether these effects are internal pains or spasms or oppression of the brain and mental disturbance.

Affects the nerves of the cerebro-spinal axis and muscles, causing ***spasmodic effects, convulsions and cramps of violent form. Cramps in toes, fingers, calves*** where the muscles are knotted, better stretching. Cramps beginning in fingers and toes, violent, contractive and intermitting pain.

Cramps may occur in the chest (angina pectoris), behind the sternum. Cramps in the limbs in elderly people, particularly leg cramps (Calc., Mag-p., acutely). Cramps before sex, preventing sex, in the calves, soles and feet.

Spasms with blue face and clenched thumbs. Jerking during sleep. Restless tossing all night. Stupor with jerking of muscles. Paralysis of isolated muscles. ***Chorea from fright,*** periodical. Chorea from suppressed eruptions.

Convulsions of children during dentition, children lie on abdomen and jerk the buttock up. ***Convulsions are tonic or clonic***. With convulsions, the eyes roll upward, out, or inward (Aeth.).

Convulsions start in the knees, toes, or fingers and radiate over the whole body with piercing ties. Twisting of the head to one side. Trismus followed by headache. Spasmodic laughter. Shivering. Deathly exhaustion with cold perspiration.

Epilepsy, at night, during menses. Violent epilepsy, legs may shoot out and lock in spasm. Epilepsy after suppressed eruptions, especially on the head (Zinc). Epilepsy after fright.

In epilepsy, aura begins at knees, ascends to hypogastrium, then unconsciousness, foaming and falling. The patient falls with a shriek, passes urine and feces. Headache follows after spasms or a group of symptoms. Followed by the appearance as if the patient were dead or in a state of ecstasy.

Pains like knife-thrusts, worse on least motion, that take away the breath. Patient thinks that he must die if they last. The thrusts go through to the back from the umbilicus. Pains worse touch and motion. Pressive pains, as from a blow being broken, racking darts through the whole body.

Cholera (Verat., Camph.). Gushing watery stools, with blue, cold extremities and jerking and cramping. ***Tape-worms.*** Complaints from scarlet fever, including excessive vomiting, stupor, and convulsions. Nausea. Meningitis. Chlorosis.

Hypersensitive, every drug overacts without curing. Easy relapses. Symptoms disposed to appear periodically and in groups. Complaints begin in left side (Lach.).

MIND - Nervous. Uneasy. Fixed ideas, malicious and morose. Sullen, tricky, alternating yielding and head-strong. Imitates, mimics. Speaks in a whisper because of pain. Uses words not intended. Sense of losing consciousness.

Attacks of rage, wants to bite the bystanders. Mania, bites, beats, tears the things. Delirium, cold sweat. Piercing shrieks. Weeps violently. Convulsive laughter. Fearful. Confusion, afraid of everybody who approaches him. Loquacious, then melancholy with fear of death. Fear of society, shuns everybody.

Abdomen - Tense, hot and tender to touch. Neuralgia of abdominal viscera. Spasmodic movements of abdominal muscles. ***Frightful colic*** with contraction of the abdomen. Better pressure, worse raising arms. Intussusception, with fecal vomiting.

Back - Paralysis of all the muscles up to the neck. Sensation of heaviness in the axillary glands. Swelling of the glands of the neck. Hyperesthesia of spinal column. Backache top of sacrum.

Causations - Ailments from emotions, anger, fright, suppressions, loss of sleep, mentally and bodily over-work. Chorea from fright. Getting wet causes epileptic attacks.

Chest - ***Spasm and constriction*** of chest. Painful constriction of the chest (lower). Loud rattling in chest. Round balls moving to and fro under the ribs, better tight clothing and lying quiet.

Constitutions - Suited to fair-haired people. Carbo-nitrogenoid constitution. Women who have borne many children (after-pains).

Eyes - Aching over eyes. Fixed, staring, sunken, glistening, turned upwards. Eyeballs rotate quickly behind closed lids or roll from side to side. Bruised pain in the orbits, worse moving the eyes. Lids spasmodically closed, twitching of lids (left). Photophobia.

Face - Distorted, ***pale bluish***, livid, sunken, pinched. Icy cold. Lips blue. Chewing motion of the lower jaw. Lockjaw. ***Contraction of jaws*** with foam at mouth.

Female - Menses too late, protracted. Menses absent due to suppression of foot sweat. Violent cramps in abdomen extending into the chest before or during menses, or from suppressions of the menses ,or from suppressed foot sweats (Sil.). Convulsions before menses. Puerperal convulsions with open mouth and opisthotonos. ***After-pains***, especially in women who had borne many children. Ebullition of blood, and palpitations. Chlorosis.

Food - Desire for ***cold drinks***, which ameliorate. Milk causes belching. Food tastes sweetish, or metallic, acid, or salt, watery. Desire for cold food in preference to hot.

Head - Meningitis, cannot hold head erect or bores into the pillow. Pulls her hair. Shakes the head from side to side. Strange tingling, crawling in the vertex (suppressed menses). Headache after epilepsy. Sensation as if water were poured over the head with headache. Empty feeling with pain. Purple, red swelling of head with convulsions. Bruised pain in brain and eyes on turning them.

Heart - Palpitations, precordial anxiety and pain. Palpitations before menses. Fatty degeneration (Phos.). Angina pectoris with asthmatic symptoms and cramps. Slow pulse or hard, full and quick.

Kidneys - Suppression of urine in cholera, uremia. Urgent desire to urinate with scanty emission. Frequent emission of fetid, viscid urine. Passes clear, watery urine during or after spasms. Burning shootings in the urethra, during and subsequent to the emission of urine. Bedwetting.

Limbs - ***Cramps in calves, soles***, and palms. Jerking, twitching of muscles in hands and feet. Clonic spasms, beginning in fingers and toes. ***Clenching of thumbs in palms***. Joints contracted. Great weariness of limbs. Knees double up involuntary when walking, bringing him down. Ankles painfully heavy. Ankylosis of shoulder joint. Coldness of hands. Epilepsy, aura begins in knees, feel as if broken.

Liver - Cirrhosis of liver.

Lungs - Dyspnea with epigastric uneasiness. Dyspnea, cannot bear anything near the mouth, worse coughing, laughing, bending backwards, before the menses. Hoarseness, worse breathing cold air. Cough in violent paroxysms, coughs herself out of breath, ***better cold drinks,*** worse deep breathing, bending backwards with cramps, lachrymation. Cough has a gurgling sound. Suffocative attacks, worse 3 a.m. (Am-c.). Trembling after coughing. Whooping cough, better swallowing water with vomiting, spasms and purple face. Asthma, hiccough before, alternating with spasmodic vomiting. Angina with asthmatic symptoms and cramps.

Male - Cramps in calves prevents sex, especially in old or nervous young men.

Modalities - Better during perspiration. ***Better drinking cold water***. Better being mesmerized. Better laying hand on affected part. Better pressure over heart. Headache better wrapping head. Worse from emotions, anger, fright. Worse loss of sleep. Worse suppression. Worse bodily and mental over work. Worse from motion. Worse raising arms. Worse touch. Worse pressure. Worse before menses. Worse evening and night. Worse cold air, cold wind. Worse hot weather. Worse at new moon.

Mouth - ***Strong metallic, slimy taste*** with flow of saliva. Froth from mouth. Grinds the teeth. Food tastes like clear water. Stammering speech, loss of speech. Paralysis of tongue. Firmly closed or open with tongue darting in and out like a snake in convulsions.

Nose - Stoppage of the nose. Sensation of violent congestion of blood to nose (Meli.). Violent, fluent coryza.

Rectum - Cholera with cramps in abdomen and calves. Cholera, summer diarrhea in children. Diarrhea, profuse, spurting out of green water. Black, painful, bloody with tenesmus and weakness. Constipation with great heat of body. Round, tapeworms or threadworms.

Skin - ***Bluish***, marbled skin. Suppressed or undeveloped eruptions. Severe itching without eruptions. Chronic psoriasis. Ulcers, itching spots and pimples at the folds of joints. Yellow scaly eruptions (bend of elbow). Leprosy.

Sleep - Lethargic sleep. Profound sleep, with shocks in the body and starting in the limbs. Constant rumbling in abdomen during sleep.

Stomach - Painful crampy pressure in epigastrium, worse touch and movement. Lies on stomach and jerks the buttocks up (colic, convulsions). ***When drinking, the fluid descends with gurgling sound*** (Laur.). As if something bitter were in stomach. Hiccough, before vomiting, convulsions, spasms or asthma. Pronounced nausea. Periodical attacks of vomiting. Vomiting, violent tormenting with agonizing colic, diarrhea, shrieks or convulsions, ***better cold drinks.*** Vomits always on waking up in morning, on least motion.

Temperature - Chilly. Icy coldness of skin. Sweat, cold, clammy, at night, sour smelling after convulsions.

Throat - Swelling of the glands of the neck. ***Spasms of throat.*** Unable to talk on account of spasms of throat. Dryness of the throat, with thirst. Inflammation of the pharynx. Audible sound of drinking (gurgling), while swallowing it. Intermittent aphonia in professional singers.

Vertigo - Giddiness accompanies many ailments, head falls forward on chest. Vertigo with internal tremors, head sinks forwards on the chest, better stool, lying down, worse looking up.

COMMENTS - Metallic copper is an anti-psoric remedy, working from within outwards. It is one of the most important remedies that relieve states arising from the "striking inward" of diseases or the failure of eruptions or discharge to appear. Suppressed discharges that lead to spasms and convulsions.

Relieve internal spasms which renders it appropriate to the collapse stage of cholera (Sulph.). A prophylactic either when worn next the skin or when taken internally.

Maliciousness and a desire to injure. Screaming with cerebral or mental symptoms. Loquaciousness. Violent head pains that are worse over the left eye. Brain seems paralyzed. Over-sensitiveness of the skin, especially in the region of the stomach and fourth and fifth dorsal vertebrae.

Cramps, spasms, twitches, and convulsions. Twitches of little muscles spread into the major muscles and can ultimately go into a convulsion. Face will turn blue, fingers and toes cramp, thumb will go into the hand and lock. Back arches, neck goes back. Drawing in the fingers. Sudden and severe flexion and extension of the limbs.

Cramps and convulsions in meningitis, cholera, whooping cough and spasmatic asthma. Spasms of the stomach that lead to nausea and vomiting. Severe spasms after a vexation or a fright (Op.). Vomiting, hiccoughs and spasms better by drinking cold water.

Whooping cough. Violent, spasmodic coughing, worse cold air (Rumx.). Wheezing and spasm. Spasmodic breathing with rattling in the chest. Asthma with bluish lips and spasms and constriction of the chest. Constriction pains with stress of asthma (Cact.). Constriction below the xiphoid process. Feels as if stuck with the knife from the xiphoid to the back.

Cramps at puberty, better bathing in cold water. Convulsions during menses. Dysmenorrhea associated with cramps in the fingers, severe cramps and spasms In the uterus. Labor pains are so severe they start convulsing. Or they feel the labor pains and their hands and feet start cramping up or spasms outside the uterus. Sudden blindness during labor.

Senile gangrene with the toes and fingers due to poor circulation, with cramps and spasms in the fingers and toes (Ars., Sec., Agar.). Chlorosis from abuse of iron.

J. C. McLaren noted "Cramps or spasms beginning in hands and feet, extending to belly."

Guernsey said that "a slimy metallic taste in the mouth" is one of the strongest indications for Cupr. (Rhus-t.). Paralysis of the tongue, stammering (Caust., Merc.). Grinds teeth at night. Thirst for cold drinks and ameliorated by cold drinks. Worse inhaling cold air.

Mackechnie made a brilliant cure of psoriasis in a young girl with Cupr. The leading features of its symptomatology are cramps, convulsions, violent spasms, coming on from disappearance of pains, discharges, eruptions, mental derangement. Patient screams with suppression of menses. Tonic spasms of thumbs. Eyeballs turn up. Opisthotonos. Tonic and clonic spasms.

Convulsions during pregnancy. Puerperal convulsions which begin in the fingers or toes and spread all over the body. Can also have a great restlessness between the attacks, either filling up the entire interval or only a part of the time.

Mossa regarded Cupr. as one of the remedies for the effects of fright, and relates the case of a girl who after a fright was affected by involuntary motions of left arm and leg developing into pronounced general chorea. Cupr. brought about slow but decided recovery.

Another girl, 12, who had recovered from whooping cough got a kind of chorea from repeated frights on seeing an epileptic. To the muscular movements was added silly behavior including a heavy tongue, slow speech and unwieldy gait. Frightened at night. Greediness in eating and drinking.

Ign., Stram., Sulph., did little good. She became ill-natured. Cupr. every four days cured completely in three months.

Mackechnie reported the case of a boy who became epileptic after being locked up in school. Very great improvement followed the administration of Cupr.

Schwencke cured a case of epilepsy of forty years' standing with Cupr. 6c after Bell. and Hyos. had done little good. The patient was a man aged 45. The fits began suddenly towards morning with chewing motion of lower jaw, gnashing of teeth, becomes upright and rigid in bed, shrieks, limbs convulsed. After giving way to violent anger, attacks become more severe, arms and legs were thrown outwards and trunk arched upward.

Cupr. was given. For a time the attacks continued, but gradually improvement set in and in less than three months they ceased altogether. The "anger" in this case and the "ill-humor" in Mossa's are noteworthy as maliciousness is an indication for Cupr.

In a second case cured by Schwencke, that of a man, 38, epileptic seven years, a pressive headache preceded the attacks, ascending from nape to forehead, then there was profuse salivation, head turned to left, eyes closed tongue in active motion in open mouth, trunk arched upward, slight spasms of right arm outward. After the attack, there was a dullness in the head and a feeling in the body as if beaten.

Cupr. first removed the fits and then the dullness of the head.

RELATIONS - ***Antidotes:*** Bell., Hep., Camph. Copper is found in Dulc., Staph., Con. and some other plants. Also in the king-crab, Limulus. ***Compare:*** (1) Cupr-s. Cupr-cyan. - meningitis basilaris. (2) Cholas terrapina - cramps in calves and feet, rheumatism with cramp-like pains, Plb., Nux-v, Verat.

REFERENCES - Boericke. Clarke. Murphy. Phatak.

CUPRUM OXYDATUM NIGRUM

PHARMACY - cupr-o. Cuprum oxydatum nigrum. ***Historical dose:*** Trituration and all potencies.

CLINICAL - ***Hookworms.*** Parasites. Tapeworms. Trichinosis.

HOMEOPATHIC - Cuprum oxydatum nigrum has cured all kinds of worms including ***hookworm,*** tapeworms and trichinosis according to Zopfy's 60 years' experience.

RELATIONS - ***Compare:*** (1) Filix, Cina, Spig. Carbon tetrachlor.

REFERENCES - Boericke.

CUPRUM SULPHURICUM

(Copper Sulphate)

PHARMACY - cupr-s. Cuprum sulphuricum. Copper sulphate. Trituration. ***Historical dose:*** Trituration and all potencies.

CLINICAL - Alopecia. Conjunctivitis. Diarrhea. Dysentery. Eyes, granular lids. Scabies. Syphilis. Trachoma.

HOMEOPATHIC - Sulphate of Copper is a well-known emetic and caustic. It is a well-known application in allopathic practice for stimulating flabby granulations and it has cured itching eruptions and manifestations of syphilis. Pains better rest.

Cupr-s. causes forcible vomiting and much nausea. ***Burning at vertex.*** Paleness of face or jaundiced appearance, pale skin generally. Tongue and lips bluish. Granular eyelids. Catarrhal and purulent conjunctivitis. Incessant, spasmodic cough, worse at night. Diarrhea. Enlarged liver.

J. D. Tyrrell mentioned the case of a woman who could not use Cupr-s. for "stamping" fancywork because it "made her face hurt and swell so she could scarcely see and her lips became everted, turned inside out, she said."

RELATIONS - ***Antidoted by:*** Milk, eggs, pure yellow prussiate of potash. ***Compare:*** (1) Kali-bi. - cough and Merc.

REFERENCES - Clarke.

CURARE WOORARI

(Arrow Poison)

PHARMACY - cur. Curare woorari. Arrow-poison. Curara. Woorara. Woorali. Hoorali. Oorari. N. O. Loganiacae. Tincture. ***Historical dose:*** Tincture and all potencies.

CLINICAL - Cancer. ***Catalepsy.*** Cirrhosis. Corns. Coughs. Debility. Diabetes. Dysmenorrhea. ***Dyspnea.*** Ear, disorders. Eczema. Emphysema. Epilepsy. Facial, paralysis. Faintness. Headache. Leprosy. Liver, spots. Locomotor, ataxia. Nervous, debility. Neuralgias. Otitis. Ozaena. ***Paralysis.*** Ptosis. Rabies. ***Reflexes, weak.*** Scrofula, disorders. Tetanus. Tuberculosis. Ulcerations. Uterus, disorders. Vaginitis. Whooping cough.

HOMEOPATHIC - An arrow poison used by South American Indians, Curare affects the muscles and brain. It is a muscular poison, causing paralysis of muscles without impairing the sensations and consciousness.

Muscular paralysis without impairing any sensation or consciousness. It causes death by paralysis of the respiratory muscles. ***Reflex action is diminished or abolished.*** In many ways, its action is opposite that of Nux-v.

Paralysis, facial, mouth, threatening respiration. Catalepsy. Trismus. Nervous debility. Sensation as if the brain were full of fluid. As of a heavy weight hung to the limbs. Weakness, heaviness, numbness, numbness with tingling. Piercing, sharp pains. Throbbing pains.

Debility of the aged (Bar-c.) and from loss of fluids. Glycosuria with motor paralysis. Diabetes mellitus. Decreases the output of adrenalin. Vomiting of bile in cirrhosis of liver. Fetid discharges. Leprosy. Many symptoms appear on right side.

MIND - Indecision, no longer wishes to think or act for herself. Inability to think or study, forgetful, stupid, sleepy, indolent. Excited, hurried feeling. Depressed, desire to be alone.

Abdomen - Weary ache from throat to left hip. Neuralgic pain in hypogastrium with pressure in vagina. Pain in groin low down with heaviness in limbs while walking. Bowels feel sore and bruised.

Back - Tired pain up and down spine. Stiffness in neck, head drawn back. Stiffness of muscles or right neck and shoulder. Dull, tired ache in shoulders and across back, numb. Chills running up back and all over body.

Chest - ***Sore to pressure or touch.***

Constitutions - Suited to scrofulous children, producing scrofulous eruptions on skin, eczema, especially of face and behind ears, and yellow brown liver-spots.

Ears - Otitis interna, driving crazy. Noises, unbearable earache. Purulent discharge. Swelling of lobes of ear. Sharp pains start from ears, extending down to legs.

Eyes - Sharp, stitching pains over right eye. Ptosis of right side. Heavy eyes, lids can hardly be kept open. Eyes haggard, sunken. Feel as if full of sticks. Red, hot, sensitive to light. Black spots before vision, especially worse from reading.

Face - Facial and mouth paralysis. Paralysis of muscles of expression. Aching right side of face. Tongue and mouth drawn. Red face.

Female - Menses too early. During menses, colic, headache and kidney pain. Dysmenorrhea. Leucorrhea, thick, purulent offensive, in clots. Bearing-down, dragging, tired, in all pelvic organs. Vaginitis. Griping in right ovary. Ulcerations of os uteri, scirrhus. Aversion to sex.

Food - Thirst and great hunger with fever. Sudden hunger almost to faintness. Better after first mouthful of food. Aversion to bread. Great thirst especially evening and night. Craves acids.

Head - Head drawn backward. Rush of blood to head. Brain feels full of fluid. Head confused, great weight in vertex. Head beats like a hammer, with vomiting of bile. Nervous headache. Sharp pains all over head. Falling out of hair.

Heart - Precordial pain, anguish with palpitations and stinging pains in heart.

Kidneys - Digging, crampy pain in kidneys, dry mouth, great thirst. Urine copious, urgent, bladder feels distended. Clear and frequent urine. Sugar in urine, great emaciation (acute diabetes).

Limbs - Paralysis of limbs, burning with

heat and chills. Aching in all the limbs and body. Numbness and tingling. Debility, paralysis. Catalepsy. Reflexes lessened or abolished. ***Arms weak, heavy.*** Cannot lift the fingers. Weakness of hands and fingers in pianists. Legs tremble, give way in walking. Favors development of corns.

Lungs - Severe pains in lungs, especially left. Shortness of breath. ***Threatened paralysis of the respiration*** on falling asleep. ***Very distressing dyspnea***. Dyspnea, stitching pains right side. Dyspnea, worse ascending. Short, dry, hacking cough, provokes vomiting, followed by fainting. Dry cough with soreness of chest walls. Cough, worse breathing cold air, laughing, moving, eating. Cough troublesome in morning.

Modalities - Worse from motion. Worse walking. Worse ascending, 2 a.m. and 2 p.m. to 3 p.m. Worse from dampness. Worse cold weather, cold wind. Worse change of weather.

Mouth - Mouth dry. Tongue and mouth drawn to right. Tongue coated. On waking, tongue yellowish at base, papillae raised, light pink anteriorly, yellow-white, bitter or bloody taste.

Nose - Nasal catarrh. Ozaena, fetid lumps of pus. Tubercles on nose.

Rectum - Extreme watery diarrhea. Diarrhea with constant urging, fetid, thin mush-like feces. Excessive pain in hemorrhoids.

Skin - Leprosy. Dirty-looking skin. Itching, with hunger. Eczema. Liver-spots. Boils. Tubercles on nose. Blood oozes through.

Sleep - Drowsy, cannot keep awake. Nights restless, always desiring to put feet out of bed, especially towards morning.

Stomach - Empty, gone feeling in stomach. Sharp pain in pit of stomach, followed by nausea. Shooting in stomach. Heartburn, pain and distention after eating ever so little. Chill after eating. Nausea in morning after eating. Vomits green bile all night. Frequent and annoying hiccoughs.

Temperature - Chill, creeping up back without thirst. Body blue, and yet fever. Heat worse at night and in open air. Sweat with every exertion. Sweat, cold and bloody, especially at nights.

Throat - Burning heat in throat with sensation of distention.

Vertigo - Instant giddiness, falling in swoon while standing or walking. Dizzy when looking at near objects or at water.

COMMENTS - Causes death by paralysis of the respiratory muscles. Reflex action is diminished or abolished (opp. Nux-v.). Catalepsy, immobility with fixed gaze on waking. Indicated by debility short of paralysis, the debility of the aged and nervous, and debility from the loss of fluids.

Fetid odor of secretions and discharges. It favors the formation of corns. Its relation to hydrophobia and tetanus is probably antipathic. Used allopathically in tetanus treatments.

A cure of a pseudo-hypertrophic paralysis by the 200c was recorded. Two cases of diabetes in middle-aged men have been cured by Burkhardt with Cur. 4c. Diabetes mellitus.

Grimmer noted that it is useful for cancer with weakness and a tendency to faint, extreme debility, difficult breathing, vertigo with fainting. States of catalepsy, worse by exercise, walking, etc., worse in dampness. Cold air, cold weather, worse 2 a.m. and 2 p.m. to 3 p.m.

RELATIONS - ***Antidote to:*** Strychnia and to the poison of rabies. In cases of poisoning artificial respiration must be resorted to. Bromine and Chlorine antidote its effects. If the poisoning is due to a punctured wound, rubbing in tobacco or salt will neutralize it. ***Compare:*** (1) Cystisin - motor paralysis. (2) Con., Caust., Crot-h., Nux-v. (3) Aran. - fever worse in damp weather. (4) Ferr. - hammering pains in head. (5) Crot-h. - blows in region of cerebellum. (6) In yellow-brown spots on skin, Sep., Lyc., Nux-v., Sulph. ***Compatible:*** After Arn. (paralysis from injury) after Bell. (paralysis after nosebleed). ***Follows well:*** in debility of the aged: Bar-c.

REFERENCES - Boericke. Clarke. Murphy. Phatak.

CURCUMA LONGA

(Turmeric)

PHARMACY - curc. Curcuma longa. Turmeric. Curcuma rotunda. Southern Asia. N. O. Zingiberaceae. Rhizome. ***Historical dose:*** Tincture and all potencies.

CLINICAL - Atherosclerosis. Cancer. Gastritis. Indigestion. Liver, problems. Osteoarthritis. Parasites. Skin, diseases. Stomach, disorders. Uveitis. Worms. Wounds.

HERBAL - Turmeric (Curcuma longa), a flowering plant in the ginger family, is widely used as a food coloring and is one of the principal ingredients in curry powder. Turmeric is fragrant and has a bitter, somewhat sharp taste.

The aboveground and underground roots, or rhizomes, are used in medicinal and food preparations. These are generally boiled and then dried, turning into the familiar yellow powder. Curcumin from turmeric, as well as other substances in this herb, have antioxidant properties.

Turmeric has long been used in both Ayurvedic and Chinese medicine as an anti-inflammatory, to treat digestive disorders and liver problems, and for the trea:ment of skin diseases and wound healing.

Curcumin has been shown, to stimulate the production of bile and to facilitate the emptying of the gallbladder. It has also demonstrated a protective effect on the liver, anti-tumor action, and ability to reduce inflammation and fight certain infections.

Turmeric is for a variety of digestive disorders. Curcumin, for example, one of the active ingredients in turmeric, induces the flow of bile, which helps break down fats. Stomach upset, gas, abdominal cramps.

Extracts of turmeric root can reduced secretion of acid from the stomach and protected against injuries such as inflammation along the stomach (gastritis) or intestinal walls and ulcers from certain medications, stress, or alcohol.

Because of its ability to reduce inflammation, turmeric may help relieve the symptoms of osteoarthritis. Early studies suggest that turmeric may prove helpful in preventing the build up of atherosclerosis (blockage of arteries that can eventually cause a heart attack or stroke) in one of two ways.

Turmeric may also prevent platelet build up along the walls of an injured blood vessel. Platelets collecting at the site of a damaged blood vessel cause blood clots to form and blockage of the artery as well.

Curcumin has potential in the treatment of various forms of cancer, including prostate, breast, skin, and colon. Roundworms and Intestinal worms. Turmeric, may reduce the destructive activity of parasites or roundworms.

Turmeric's volatile oil functions as an external antibiotic, preventing bacterial infection in wounds. Turmeric applied to wounds hastens the healing process.

Inflammation of the uvea, and the retina. The uvea contains many of the blood vessels that nourish the eye. Inflammation of this area, therefore, can affect the cornea, the retina, the sclera, and other important parts of the eye.

REFERENCES - Potter.

CYCLAMEN EUROPAEUM

(Sow-Bread)

PHARMACY - cycl. Cyclamen europaeum. Sow-bread. N. O. Primulacae. Tincture of the root gathered in spring. ***Historical dose:*** Tincture and all potencies.

CLINICAL - Anemia. Bone, pain. Chlorosis. Coryza. Diplopia. Dyspepsia. Enteralgia. Eye, disorders. Headaches. Heel, pain. ***Hiccoughs.*** Menstruation, disorders. Menopause. Pregnancy. Prostatitis. Rheumatism. ***Sleepiness***. Strabismus. Thirstless. Urethritis. Vertigo. Weaning, complaints. Writer's spasm.

HOMEOPATHIC - Cyclamen has a traditional reputation as a remedy for disorders of the uterus and appendages. Later provings affirmed this reputation. Large doses produce violent purging and vomiting, disturbed digestion with very salty saliva.

Cycl. is in many ways similar to Puls., from which it differs mainly in having no relief from open air and in not having thirstlessness as so frequent an accompaniment of other conditions.

Anemic and chlorotic conditions. Affections of uterus. Gastro-intestinal and genito-urinary tracts affected inducing secondary anemia and various reflexes. Cough, at night while asleep without waking, especially in children (Cham., Nit-ac.). ***Sleepiness, morose and lassitude***.

MIND - Dull, sleepy and morose. Depression, with weeping desire to be alone. Silent weeping. Grieves, sadness as if he had committed a bad act or not done his duty. Self-reproaches. Terrors of conscience. Tearful and broods over imaginary grief.

A joyous feeling alternating with irritability. Hallucinations as if two persons were lying in her bed. The room seems too small. Thinks she is alone and persecuted.

Abdomen - Fullness and pressure. Uneasiness in the abdomen with nausea. Painful on the slightest touch. Sudden attacks of griping, with pinching. Borborygmi in the abdomen, immediately after a meal. Running in bowels as if something alive.

Back - Excoriation in the nape of the neck. Aching, with paralytic weakness, or traction in the nape of the neck and in the neck. Dull stitches in the region of the kidney, worse when drawing a long breath.

Breasts - Air seems to stream from the nipples. Milk in virgin breast or non-pregnant women. Swelling of breast with milky secretion after menses.

Causations - Ill effects of inward grief and terror of conscience.

Constitutions - Suited to the blonde leuco-phlegmatic subjects with chlorotic conditions, disinclined for labor and easily fatigued. Special senses enfeebled or their functions suspended.

Ears - Itching in the ears with increased wax. Drawing in the ears. Diminution of hearing, as if the ears were stopped.

Eyes - Disturbance of vision, associated with gastric disturbances. Dim vision with headache, worse on waking with spots before eyes. Diplopia. ***Flickering of various colors***. Hemiopia. ***Sees countless stars***. Fluttering, glittering or black spots. Squint, especially connected with menstrual irregularities. Convergent squint after convulsions, left eye drawn inwards.

Face - Pale, anemic. Upper lip, as if numb or indurated.

Female - Menses changeable, ***profuse, black***, membranous, ***clotted too early, with labor-like pains*** from back to pubes. The flow is less when moving about. Dysmenorrhea. Menstrual irregularities with megrim and blindness or fiery spots before eyes. Suppression of menses after excessive dancing or being over heated. Leucorrhea with retarded or scanty menses. ***Hiccough during pregnancy***. Post-partum hemorrhage with colicky bearing-down pains with relief after gush of blood.

Food - Desire for lemonade, sardines, inedible things. Aversion to bread, butter, fat, beer. Disgust for meat, especially pork. Loss of appetite after taking beef tea or a cup of tea. No thirst all day.

Head - Prolonged migraine. One-sided headache. Headaches in morning with ***flickering before eyes***, better cold water. Pain in left temple. Brain as if wrapped up in a cloth. As if brain wobbled about while walking, menses absent or scanty. Frequent sneezing with itching in ears.

Heart - Pressure on the heart, as from congestion of blood. Sensible palpitations of the heart, stitches in the region of the heart. Frequent palpitations from suppressed menses.

Kidneys - Frequent desire to urinate with abundant emission of whitish urine. Shootings in the urethra, followed by a sudden discharge of a dark red urine. Urine profuse, watery and frequent.

Limbs - Pains in parts where bones lie near the surface. Pains in periosteum. Shooting pains in the loins. Weakness of knees. ***Burning, sore heels,*** better walking, worse sitting, standing. Chilblains. Cramp-like slow contractions of the right thumb and index finger, they have to be extended by force. Writer's spasms.

Lungs - Scraping and dryness in the pharynx, causing a suffocative cough. Coughing without waking.

Male - Prepuce and corona glandis feel sore after slight rubbing. Stitches and pressure in prostate with urging to stool and urination.

Modalities - Better from moistening diseased parts, bathing. Better rubbing parts. Better moving about, walking. Better warm room. Better during menstrual flow. Better weeping. Better lemonade. Worse cold, cold water. Worse open air. Worse night, evenings. Worse eating at night. Worse standing. Worse sitting, rest. Worse fats. Menstrual flow worse sitting. Worse drawing shoulders forward or backward.

Mouth - Taste lost or salty, which is communicated to all food. Saliva salty. Tongue loaded with a white coating. Fine stitches on the surface of the tongue. Burning on the tip of the tongue. Dryness of the lips, without thirst.

Nose - Fluent coryza, with sneezing. Sneezing with itching in the ear. Loss of smell.

Rectum - Drawing pressure in the anus. ***Pain about anus and perineum***, as if a spot were suppurating, when walking or sitting. Pressure in the rectum. Discharge of blood from the rectum. Evacuations hard and frequent. Diarrhea after every cup of coffee.

Skin - Gnawing itching in several parts of the skin. Itching, in the evening in bed. Acne in young women. Pruritus better scratching and appearance of menses, worse at night in bed.

Sleep - Great inclination to lie down, and to sleep. Nightmares when falling to sleep. Unrefreshing sleep, with terrible, frightful, lascivious dreams.

Stomach - Satiety after a few mouthfuls, loathing and nausea from the least food afterwards. Nausea felt in throat. ***Salty taste***, hiccough-like eructation, worse fat food. Hiccough, worse pregnancy, with yawning. Vomiting of pregnancy.

Temperature - Attacks of chilliness in the morning or evening. During the evening, chill and great sensitiveness to cold air or to being uncovered. Chilly all over, not better by covers. Febrile shivering and cold, followed by heat. Offensive sweat.

Throat - When reading aloud the voice is weak. The tonsils and palate are shriveled and white. Dryness in the throat. Burning and scraping in throat. Sensation of painful constriction in the throat. Nausea in throat.

Vertigo - Vertigo, objects turn in circles or look pale, worse open air, better in a room and sitting.

COMMENTS - Debility, torpidity of mind and body. Dullness of senses. Flickering before the eyes, squint, especially in connection with menstrual irregularities or fevers. After convulsions, convergent squint, left eye drawn inwards. Amblyopia, diplopia, hemiopia.

Digestive disturbances. Saliva has a salty taste, which is communicated to all food eaten. After eating but little, satiety, aversion to food with nausea in palate and thirst. Aversion to bread, butter, meat, fat, beer and ordinary food. Craving for lemonade, sardines, inedible things. Frequent vomiting in morning.

Prostatic troubles with stitches and pressure, urging to stool and urination. Menstruation too early, with some relief of melancholy mood and heaviness of feet. Scanty or suppressed menstruation with headache and vertigo. During pregnancy, hiccough, loathing and nausea in mouth and throat, complaints after weaning.

Pressing, drawing or tearing pains at parts where bones lie near surface. Chilliness. Itching leaving a numb sensation. Chilblains, itching and pricking, worse at night in bed.

Eidherr of Vienna gave the best account of this remedy. He noted the more copious menstruation, more frequent, too early, with severe abdominal pains. Accompanied with labor-like pains, flow is excessive, black and lumpy. Commencement of menses after protracted cessation.

Eidherr's clinical experience illustrates in a remarkable way Cycl.'s sphere of action. In one instance a higher potency of the same remedy antidoted this effect. He found the remedy especially suited to blonde leucophlegmatic subjects.

The "Sleepiness, morose and lassitude," and also the vertigo noted by Hahnemann, are prominent in many of Eidherr's cases.

J. K., 24, blonde, pale delicate skin, pale lips and gums, had menstruated normally until 22, when she got wet at a picnic just as menstruation was starting. It stopped at once and did not reappear until ten months later after vigorous use of all kinds of domestic remedies.

The periods were then accompanied by terrible abdominal, labor-like pains, lasting eleven hours. Menses recurred every two or four months, always with the pains, starting from sacrum, extending along both sides of abdomen to pelvis.

They were periodical, every one, two or five minutes during which time there was no flow, the blood appearing after these attacks was somewhat watery.

Other symptoms included slightly edematous eyelids, pressing pain in the forehead and vertigo frequently changing into syncope. Chilliness of the whole body. Disturbed, unrefreshing sleep interspersed with terrible dreams. Continued loathing for meat. Longing for salt fish. Frequent vomiting in morning. After partial relief from Puls., Cycl. made a complete cure.

The ocular symptoms which developed were remarkable. The vertigo and headache were untouched by Puls., but quickly subsided under Cycl. 15x.

On their disappearance she saw fiery flames dancing before her eyes, on awakening at night and in the morning she saw everything double. And she had the hallucination as if two persons lay in her bed and that the body of the other overlapped hers by half.

Cycl. was discontinued and in two days her sight was normal.

Anna F., 20, blonde, menstruated since her tenth year. In her seventeenth year she suffered from chlorosis, ever since, menstruation was regular, but lasting only one or two days in a moderate degree. Troubled at other times by vertigo and pressing pain in forehead and temples, which attacks were ameliorated by foot baths with ashes.

Appetite poor, little thirst, stool regular, sleeps too long, always sleepy, dejected mood, morose. All movements, as well as speech, were languid, palpitation. Puls. made no change, Cycl. 3x quickly improved the headache, vertigo and spirits. After three days, sight became obscured and there was glimmering before eyes.

A case of hemicrania was cured with Cycl. Theresa F., 37., had menstruated sparingly and irregularly (often at two or three months' intervals). For four years suffered from violent headache affecting right side of head and face, coming every 8-14 days, spells lasting 12-36 hours.

During menstruation, the attacks were extra severe. Patient was emaciated, skin, gums and lips pale. Right eye closed owing to cramps in eyelids. When forcibly opened, a stream of hot tears gushed out, otherwise the eye was normal.

Under Cycl. 3c the symptoms diminished, but there appeared "glittering sparks before the eyes" and these remained after all symptoms of headache had gone. Cycl. was given persistently, the periods became regular and rather copious, and the headaches entirely ceased.

Another case (in a wet-nurse who had just weaned her baby) presented unceasing, violent, stitching pain in temporal region extending to vertex. Throbbing temporal arteries. Bell. diminished the pain, but vertigo came on.

Under Cycl. 3x, the headache and vertigo disappeared altogether, but the patient complained of her sight having become so weak that she did not dare to walk alone. This passed off when the medicine was discontinued and her headache did not recur.

Cycl. cured a boy of violent squinting. Six months before, he had a fall from a table, convulsion followed and after the second attack the squinting came on. Arn. was given and the convulsions did not recur, but the squinting remained. Cycl. 15x was given and after a few weeks the squint entirely disappeared.

Wurmb cured a case of squint in a coachman with Cycl.

RELATIONS - ***Antidoted by:*** Camph., Coff., Puls. The modalities of Cycl. are in general opposite to those of Puls., the menstrual flow of Cycl. is more profuse while at rest with Puls. the opposite is the case. ***Compare:*** (1) Puls., Ign., Ambr. (2) Ferr. and Chin. resemble it in chlorosis. (3) Crocus and Thuj. in sensation of something alive in abdomen. (4) Am-m. - menses worse at night. (5) Iris-v. and Kali-bi. (migraine with scintillations, headache worse as sight returns, Kali-bi. (6) Coc-c. - leucorrhea worse sitting better walking, Cycl. menses worse sitting better walking. (7) Rhus-t. (enteralgia), Gels. and Seneg. (diplopia), Arn. (falls), Bar-c., Calc., Canth. (chilly and fever), Cocc. (8) In speedy satiety, Lyc., Nux-v., Sep. (9) In prostatitis and urethritis, Lith-c., Dig., Sel., Caust., Lyc., Apis in squint, Alum., sudden vanishing of sight with menses, Sep., Puls. (Puls. scanty, Cycl. profuse and dark). (10) nausea in throat, Sep. Berb., pain in heels on standing. Desire for lemonade, Bell., Sabin.

REFERENCES - Boericke. Clarke. Phatak.

CYNODON DACTYLON

(Doorba)

PHARMACY - cyn-d. Cynodon dactylon. Doorba. Grantha doorba bhargavi. N. O. Graminaceae. A grass from India. Tincture of the whole fresh plant. ***Historical dose:*** Tincture and all potencies.

CLINICAL - Amenorrhea. Anasarca. Cholera. Conjunctivitis. Diarrhea, summer. Dysentery. Flatulence. Headaches. Hematuria. Scabies. Ulcerative, colitis.

HERBAL - The Cynodon dactylon grows throughout India, and is used in some of the religious ceremonies of the country. Popularly known as doorba, the Sanskrit name for this plant is grantha doorba bhargavi. It is an elegant perennial plant that flowers throughout the whole year.

The freshly extracted juice of the grass is useful for hematuria, vomiting and as an application for conjunctivitis. A decoction of the plant is used as a diuretic and can be useful for dropsy and anasarca. Chakradatta mentioned it as being an excellent remedy for scabies and amenorrhea.

HOMEOPATHIC - Jugal Kishore carried out a homeopathic proving on three provers, two men and one woman. The potencies used were the mother tincture, 6x and 200c. The stock of Cyn-d. was supplied by the Hahnemann Publishing Co. of Calcutta.

General weakness, more marked in the hands, with difficulty in writing. General lassitude, laziness, aversion to work. The least physical effort causes pain all over. Mental work causes frontal headaches. Aversion to noise, but desires jolly company.

Elective action on the gastro-intestinal passages and urinary system. Flatulence and abdominal cramps. Stools irritating with acrid odor and noisy expulsion. Urgent need to stool. Urethral pain after urination.

Pain in the upper or lower limbs, ameliorated by a tight bandage or by walking. Heat in the soles of the feet with the need to take the feet out from beneath the covers.

MIND - Irritable, quarrelsome, flies into a rage. Angry without cause. Aversion to noise and does not want to be spoken to. Desire jolly company.

Abdomen - Flatulence and abdominal distention after 4 p.m. Cramping abdominal pains, with an urge to go to stool. Pain in the right hypochondrium, which disappears after resting. Heaviness around the umbilicus. Impression of a ball below and around the umbilicus.

Eyes - Conjunctivitis. Conjunctiva are painfully sensitive. Swelling of the upper right eyelid, worse in the morning. Eyelids stuck together in the morning. Pain in the eyes in morning after a bath or washing the face.

Food - Loss of appetite, which returns on eating.

Head - Forehead hot and heavy. Pain on the right side of the head and in very localized areas of the body. Headache after mental exertion or anger.

Kidneys - Involuntary urination while sneezing. Frequent and copious urination. Urethral pain after urination with feeling of not having finished.

Limbs - Sudden, shooting pain in the back of the left forearm. Feeling of great weakness in the forearms and hands. Aggravation from typewriting. Pain in the upper part of the body, especially in the back. Pain and restlessness in the legs when lying down at night, better by rising from the bed or by tight bandaging. Sensation of heat in the soles of the feet, desire to put the feet outside the covers.

Modalities - Better from heat, eating. Worse in the afternoon, evening. Worse from physical or mental exertion. Worse predominantly on the right side.

Mouth - Increased salivation with insipid taste. Loss of sense of taste. Dryness of the palate, cannot take sour or spicy food, better by taking something cold. Red patch on the palate and small red granules in the pharynx.

Rectum - Urgent need to go to stool when rising with a feeling of colic. Urgent need to go to stool continues during the day. Stools hard, difficult to evacuate. Stools semi-solid, then soft with irritating mucus. Stools, irritating, yellow and soft. Offensive, acrid stools with noisy expulsion. Much gas passed with stools.

Sleep - Sleepiness after meals. Heavy sleep. Sleep disturbed by pains in the legs.

Stomach - Sensation of heaviness in the stomach after lunch.

Temperature - Feverish, needs to cover himself. Sensation of heat in tips of toes.

RELATIONS - ***Compare:*** (1) Podo. - Diarrhea in the morning, fetid stools, expelled in a rush, tenesmus general weakness, rumbling and feeling of emptiness in the abdomen. (2) Verat. - Copious diarrhea, abdominal colic, extreme weakness with cold sweating. (3) Aloe - Abdominal distention, hot stomach, heavy with expulsion of burning irritating gases. Diarrhea after resting, urgent need to go to stool. Involuntary passing of stools when urinating or when expelling wind.

REFERENCES - Julian.

CYPRIPEDIUM PUBESCENS

(Yellow Lady's Slipper)

PHARMACY - cypr. Cypripedium pubescens. Yellow lady's slipper. N. O. Orchidaceae. Tincture and infusions of fresh root gathered in autumn. ***Historical dose:*** Tincture and all potencies.

CLINICAL - ***Brain, disorders.*** Chorea. Convulsions. ***Debility.*** Delirium, tremens. Ecstasy. Epilepsy. ***Insomnia.*** Mental, despondency. Nervous, debility. ***Nervousness.*** Neuralgias. Post-influenzal, debility. Rhus, poisoning. ***Sleeplessness.*** Spermatorrhea. Styes.

HERBAL - Lady's slipper has great repute as a ***"nervine"*** among eclectics and in domestic practice. It ranks with Scut. and Valer. Hale noted a strong infusion causes exhilaration followed by calmness and is much resorted to by women whose nerves are shattered by long illness or excessive indulgence in green-tea or coffee.

HOMEOPATHIC - Indicated in the brain-hyperesthesia of children who wake in the night lively and full of play. Epilepsy from reflex irritation. Trembling and twitching of limbs. Nervousness in children from teething and intestinal troubles. Debility after gout. The skin symptoms correspond to those of Rhus-t. poisoning, for which it has been found an efficient antidote.

MIND - Sleeplessness and agitation. Irascibility. Throws emotional fits. Hysterical symptoms. Ecstasy, preliminary to incipient brain disorder. Indifference.

Constitutions - Suited to nervous disorders from mental over-excitement or reflex nervous excitement. Nervous weakness after influenza.

Eyes - Stye on right lower lid.

Female - Amenorrhea with hysteria. Great nervous debility and despondency. Irritable vagina, hysterical symptoms, sleeplessness and agitation.

Head - Child cries out at night, is wakeful and begins to laugh and play. Brain hypersensitivity in young children often the result of over stimulation of brain. ***Hydrocephaloid*** symptoms, result of long, exhausting diarrhea, sleeplessness.

Headaches of elderly people and during menopausal.

Male - Spermatorrhea with great nervous prostration and dejection of spirits.

Sleep - Sleeplessness with desire to talk. A constant crowding of pleasant ideas with restlessness of body. Ecstasy, children awaken in night from sleep ***"wide-awake,"*** unnaturally playful, with no desire to go to sleep again.

Vertigo - Vertigo followed by heaviness and dragging of left foot.

RELATIONS - ***Antidote to:*** Rhus poisoning. ***Compare:*** (1) Aven., Kali-br., Scut., Valer., Ign. (2) Skin relations: Grind., Anac. (3) Ambra. Coca, Guar., Thea, Zinc. (4) In ecstasy, Coffea.

REFERENCES - Boericke. Clarke.

CYSTISUS LABURNUM

(Laburnum Anagyroides)

PHARMACY - cyt-l. Cystisus laburnum. Laburnum anagyroides. Cystisus aubour. N. O. Leguminose. Tincture or trituration of seeds. Tincture of fresh bark. The tincture is prepared from the essences of the flowers and young leaves. ***Historical dose:*** Tincture and all potencies.

CLINICAL - Abdominal typhus. Angina, pectoris. Convulsions. Cramps. Cyanosis. Diarrhea. Dyspepsia. Eyes, disorders. Heart, anomalies. Heat-stroke. Hydrocephalus. Hypertension. Influenza. Meningitis. Migraines. Morning sickness. Motion sickness. Nausea. Raynaud's disease. Spasms. Sunstroke. Thyroid disorders. Typhoid. Vertigo. Vomiting, pregnancy. Writer's cramp.

HOMEOPATHIC - The proving was done by Joseph Schier in 1900-1901 on sixteen provers using the low potencies and the mother tincture. J. Mezger made a clinical re-proving with it.

Cystisus Laburnum, or wild laburnum, is a member of the leguminosae family. Cystisus Aubour is a shrub or small tree, growing naturally or cultivated as an ornamental plant with trifoliate leaves. It has pale, yellow flowers which hang in clusters with long pods and which are hairy when yellow.

All parts of this well-known ornamental tree are poisonous, especially the flowers and seeds, owing to the presence of cytisin. This oxygenated, unsaturated alkaloid is toxic to the glands, which it first arouses and then paralyzes. It causes convulsions and can lead to death by asphyxia. The toxicity of cytisin is allied to that of nicotine.

Knowledge of it is derived chiefly from the accidental poisoning of children who have eaten the pea-like seeds and pods.

A typical case can be seen in that of W. G., et. 10, who ate eight to ten seeds. Five or ten minutes later, began to sweat, but soon became cold and shivering, skin pale, pulse scarcely perceptible, general collapse.

Pupils dilated. Drowsy and giddy, without pain. Emetics and brandy were given, but after an hour of this there was no improvement. An enema of hot, strong coffee was then given, the patient was wrapped in blankets and hot bottles applied. The collapse then gradually passed off.

Cyt-l. acts on the central and sympathetic nervous system causing cramping spasmodic conditions. Hyperesthesia of the peripheral nerves. Cerebral shock. Epidemic cerebral and spinal meningitis. Migraine. Nausea, pallor, cold sweating. Vertigo. Face pale. Dryness of the mouth tongue and throat. Sunstroke. Heatstroke. Travel sickness (air, sea and car).

MIND - Intense uneasiness, anguish. Depressive and irritable condition. Maniacal depressive conditions. Oppression. Insomnia. Sleepiness to the point of being in a stupor. Comatose condition.

Abdomen - Chronic gastro-duodenitis. Spasmodic colon afflictions. Mesenteric irritation.

Back - Muscular cramps. Drawing pains starting at the nape of the neck, spreading towards the occiput.

Chest - Angina pectoris. Feeling of tightness in the chest.

Eyes - Pupils dilated.

Female - Dysmenorrhea. Menopausal complaints. Copious leucorrhea.

Head - Neuralgic pains in the head of a migraine type. Pulsating headaches Pressing frontal pain. Pricking pain i the left temple.

Heart - Hypertensive attack with state of collapse, pale, livid face and cold sweating. Palpitations with accelerated pulse. Arterial pulsation in all limbs. Rhythmic anomalies. Raynaud's disease.

Limbs - Weakness and numbness of the limbs. Sensation of breaking in all the limbs. Stiffness and drawing pains in the limbs. Muscular cramps.

Lungs - Respiration rapid at first, then slower and difficult. Wheezing respiration. Whooping cough.

Male - Strong erections.

Modalities - Better after passing wind, after going to stool. Worse from the cold. Worse in the afternoon, evening. Worse predominantly on the left side.

Mouth - Dryness of mouth, tongue and back of throat. Burning, mouth and pharynx.

Nose - Nosebleeds.

Rectum - Diarrhea with painful abdominal colic, intestinal rumbling and anal tenesmus. Cholera-type diarrhea.

Skin - Skin cold, cold sweating. Cyanosis. Pruritus. Vesicules around the cheek.

Sleep - Insomnia with delirium. Worrying dreams.

Stomach - Gastric heaviness, burning pains in the stomach. Acrid dyspepsia. Nausea with vertigo and vomiting.

Temperature - Discomfort, accompanied by a feeling of coldness.

Throat - Feeling of constriction in the throat. Tickling sensation in the throat with the need to clear it.

Vertigo - Vertigo and absent feeling. Constant vertigo, even while lying, if she attempted to sit upright, she immediately fell back again.

COMMENTS - In one case of poisoning by Cyt-l., the head was hot and rigidly thrown back. Muscular twitchings about the face. Convulsions, insensibility, drowsiness and mental indifference.

Two boys who were poisoned by the root of an old tree had very strange waving motions of the arms and convulsive drawing up of the legs, first one leg then the other. Pupils equally dilated.

A boy who ate the green twigs of Cyt-l. was seized with vomiting, pain in the stomach and collapse, there was no diarrhea but tenesmus and erections. After a few hours he passed 300 grams of grass-green urine, after which he felt better. Soon after passing, the urine assumed a natural color.

RELATIONS - Antidoted by: Coffee and stimulants, hot and cold douches to chest. ***Compare:*** (1) Nux-v. (2) Gels. - better by copious urination. (3) Tab. - Prostration, nausea, vomiting, general coldness and cold sweating, vertigo and pallor. (4) Verat. - State of discomfort, collapse, coldness of the limbs, cyanosis, prostration, vomiting, cold sweating and tiring diarrhea. (5) Bapt. - Intense nervous depression, extreme agitation, impression that the body is double, sensation of breaking in the bones, putrid breath, fetid diarrhea.

REFERENCES - Clarke. Julian.

D

DAMIANA APHRODISIACA

(Turnera Aphrodisiaca)

PHARMACY - dam. Damiana aphrodisiaca. Turnera aphrodisiaca. N. O. Turneraceae. Tincture of fresh plant. Tincture of dried leaves. ***Historical dose:*** Tincture and all potencies.

CLINICAL - Amenorrhea. ***Chronic, fatigue***. Dysmenorrhea. Gonorrhea. Headaches. Infertility. ***Impotence. Incontinence.*** Leucorrhea. Migraines. Prostate, disorders. ***Sexual, weakness.*** Spinal, injury. Spermatorrhea. Syphilis. Urinary, disorders.

HERBAL - Damiana is the local name of the herb Turnera aphrodisiaca. It has long been a domestic medicine in Mexico, where it is used to ***"invigorate the system."***

Indians discovered that a decoction of it was a great invigorator after wearisome journeys and dispels fatigue. They also found in it a remedy for the inability to exercise the reproductive functions in both sexes.

Back - Spinal injury.

Bladder - Urinary disorders. ***Incontinence.***

Female - Dysmenorrhea. Amenorrhea. Leucorrhea. Sexual weakness. Infertility.

Head - Headaches, migraines.

Male - Prostate disorders. Spermatorrhea. Gonorrhea. Syphilis. ***Impotence.*** Sexual weakness.

COMMENTS - Hale collected a great deal of experience concerning this remedy from old-school sources, showing its power over the genito-urinary system.

Douglass reported three cases of incontinence of urine, including the case of a man, age 63, who had dribbling of urine day and night for four years. He was given Dam. 2x in water, four times a day, and was cured in two months.

History of curing cases of severe migraines. One or two doses given within an hour would cause the headache to cease and induced sleep, from which the patient woke free from headache and with good appetite.

Spinal injury from a fall. Sexual excess. Syphilis or gonorrhea. Amenorrhea, dysmenorrhea and leucorrhea.

RELATIONS - ***Compare:*** (1) Impotence, injuries, over-exertion, fatigue, Bell-p., Arn., Agn. (2) Prostatic affections, Sabal., Solid. (3) Migraines, Bry., Epipheg.

REFERENCES - Clarke. Murphy.

DAPHNE INDICA

(Spurge Laurel)

PHARMACY - daph. Daphne indica. Spurge laurel. Daphne odora. Sweet-scented spurge laurel. N. O. Thymelaceae. Tincture of fresh bark. ***Historical dose:*** Tincture and all potencies, esp. the first to sixth potencies.

CLINICAL - Amaurosis. Amblyopia. Constipation. Coughs. Exhaustion. Eyes disorders. Exostosis. Fever. Gastralgia. Gonorrheal rheumatism. Gout. Halitosis. Leprosy. Mercurio-syphilis. Prostatorrhea. Rheumatism. Splenitis. Sleeplessness. Syphilis. ***Tobacco, craving.*** Toothache.

HOMEOPATHIC - Daphne indica was proved by G. Bute. It, like its relative Daph. mezereon, produces disorders of the muscles, bones and skin, hence its relation to syphilis and the anti-syphilitic remedies Aur., Merc., and Staph. Clammy skin. Red rash in spots on legs in evening. Itching. Daph. oleoides is credited by Hering with relieving leprosy.

Daph. acts on the tissues, muscles, bones and skin. ***Fetid breath***, urine, sweat. Erratic and electric-like pains. Sudden, lightning jerks in different parts of the body. Exostoses with stitching, pressing or dull pain, worse at night. Bruised pain. Exhaustion. Parts of the body feel separated (Bapt.).

Burning in stomach. Gastric symptoms, worse from alcohol. For the ***craving for tobacco*** (Calad.). Prostate discharges, worse from tobacco.

MIND - Despondent and sad. Mental dejection. Timidity. Exhaustion. Absent-minded. Indecisive, walks about room and can't make up his mind to anything.

Agitated. Irritability. Over-excitement and trembling, during the pains.

Any effort at thinking causes pain or soreness in brain. Fearful and trembling, from pain about heart.

Abdomen - Colic with chilliness. Pain in the abdomen, with shiverings. Contraction of the abdomen. Shootings and pains in the region of the spleen. Arthritic pains which pass rapidly from the limbs to the abdomen. Trembling in abdominal muscles.

Back - Pain in the nape of the neck with headache. Screwing pain from the ear to the shoulder. Sensation as though the cervical glands were much swollen. Sharp pain beneath left scapula. Burning itching in the back. Painful pulling along the spinal marrow, worse by stooping.

Ears - Burning about ears and on vertex with constant inclination to yawn. Buzzing, roaring in ears. Roaring and humming.

Eyes - Scraping in the eyes. Violent pains in the eyeballs, in the evening, with great nervous excitement. Painful sensation as if the eyes were pushed outwards from the head. Sensation around the eyes and eyelids with dryness and heaviness of eyelids. ***Contraction of the pupils.*** Eyes inflamed, weak, dull, as it were swimming in tears.

Face - Heat and burning sensation in the cheeks, around the ears, and in the vertex, sometimes with constant inclination to yawn. Sensation of swelling. Stiffness and tension in the temporo-maxillary joint, with burning, smarting in the skin.

Food - Loss of appetite, moderate thirst. Craving to smoke tobacco. Gouty pains worse alcohol.

Head - Headache, provoked by all kinds of intellectual labor. ***Bursting pain on rising in bed.*** Heat in head, especially in vertex. Feels as if skull would burst. ***Sensation as if head were separated from body***. Soft nodular swellings on bones about vertex, pain worse at night and touch. Itching on scalp. Painful pulsation in temples with soreness when touched.

Heart - Palpitations and starting of the heart, with inability to remain lying on the left side. Acute pains in the region of the heart, with discouragement and trembling.

Kidneys - ***Frequent and abundant emission of urine.*** Pain, as from excoriation in the urethra, when urinating. Urine fetid, turbid, thick, yellowish like rotten eggs. ***Reddish sediment, which adheres to the side of the vessel.*** Frequent bedwetting at night.

Limbs - Shooting pains, shift rapidly, worse cold air. Pains shift upwards towards the abdomen and heart. Bone-ache, piercing pains in the bones and acute shooting pains in the fingers. Excessive itching on the arms and hands. Rheumatic pains in thighs and knees. Buttocks cold. Right toe swollen, painful.

Lungs - Cough, fatigues and hinders sleep. Thin, slimy, copious, and bloody expectoration. Cough, with vomiting, and yellowish frothy expectoration, mixed sometimes with streaks of blood. Suffocative feeling with throat complaints. ***Yellow, often frothy, blood-streaked expectoration.*** Copious, thin, slimy mucus. Suffocating fits at night.

Male - Toothache with erections, after sex. Sweating of scrotum. Discharge of prostatic fluid, after making water. Prostatic discharge worse smoking.

Modalities - Worse from cold air. Worse touch, pressure. Worse evening in bed. Worse at night. Worse waning moon. Cold air aggravates wandering gout. Lying down aggravates gouty pains, backache. Pains are worse from warmth of bed. Stooping or bending aggravates pains in spinal cord. Walking aggravates rheumatic pains in thighs. Gastric symptoms worse alcohol. Pains worse warmth of bed.

Mouth - Dryness of mouth as if burnt, after sleep. ***Tongue coated on one side only*** (Rhus-t.). Fetor of the tongue. Dryness of the tongue after sleep, as if it had been burned. Saliva, hot. Foul smelling breath. Salivation, with toothache.

Nose - Nose scurfy, with some heat.

Perspiration - Clammy, offensive sweat, with a putrid smell. Viscid sweat over the whole body.

Rectum - Stools scanty, bloody at end. ***Constipation.***

Sleep - Inclination to sleep with inability to accomplish it. Sleeplessness from aching in bones. Starting on falling to sleep, with fright, with chilliness, shivering, clamminess and viscid sweat. Agitated, unrefreshing sleep. Nightmares. Dreams of black cats. Dreams of fire.

Skin - Clammy skin. Red rash in spots on legs, in evening.

Stomach - ***Burning in stomach and sensation of soreness after each meal.*** Pressure in stomach after drinking. Sensation of fullness and ebullition in the precordial region. Aching in the stomach after drinking. ***Heartburn and sour vomiting.*** Frequent cramps in the stomach. After each meal, burning pain and sensation of excoriation in the stomach, with frequent risings of flatus, the pains extend to left hypochondrium and to the back. Nausea and vomiting after breakfast.

Teeth - Pulsation in the teeth and gums. Acute drawing pains in all the teeth. Toothache, with and without salivation. Toothache with fits of shivering, or disposition to perspire. Toothache with erections, after sex.

Temperature - Chilliness with stretching and yawning. Fever, similar to typhus, with excessive shivering, followed by continued heat, and complete loss of appetite. Fever with gastric and nervous suffering.

Throat - Soreness in left side of throat on pressure. Inflammation of throat and suppuration of tonsils. Feeble voice.

Vision - Floating black spots. Weak sight, with confusion of the letters when reading. While reading, the letters fade and appear as a black line. Diplopia.

COMMENTS - Tongue coated on one side only (Rhus-t.). Foul-smelling tongue. Ptyalism with hot saliva. Fetidity is a marked feature of breath, urine, sweat. Sensation that parts of the body are separated from one another.

Sudden pains, wander suddenly from limbs. Pain shoots into the region of the heart or abdomen. Sudden stitch in region of spleen. Ball of right great toe swollen and very painful. Cold feeling on buttocks.

RELATIONS - ***Antidoted by:*** Bry., Dig., Rhus-t., Sil., Sep., Zinc. ***Antidote to:*** Chr-ac., Merc. ***Compare:*** (1) Fl-ac., Aur., Mez., Staph. (2) Thuj. - effects of suppressed gonorrhea. (3) Benz-ac. - fetid urine, Puls., Chin., (4) Taxus - erratic pains, Verat. - lightning pains, Bapt. - limbs seem scattered about the bed, Ars. - body seems divided at waist. (5) Dirca belongs to the same family.

REFERENCES - Boericke. Clarke.

DATURA ARBOREA

PHARMACY - dat-a. Datura arborea. Brugmansia suaveolens. Brugmansia candida. N.O. Solanaceae. Tincture of the flowers. ***Historical dose:*** All potencies.

CLINICAL - Brain, disorders. Clairvoyance. Confusion. Spinal, irritation. Vertigo.

HOMEOPATHIC - According to Froriep, the juice instilled into the eye causes amaurosis. The odor of the flowers, left in a room for two days, caused many remarkable symptoms including spasms.

While cutting and handling the flowers, there was depletion of the nervous circulation in the medulla oblongata. Cerebellum and a spinal irritation.

Sensation as if forehead were expanded. Headache. Heartburn. Burning sensation around cardiac end of stomach, extending to esophagus, with sense of constriction. Heat and fullness over liver region.

MIND - Confusion of ideas with nervous irritation. Can't concentrate thoughts. Floating sensation as if ideas were floating outside of brain. Brain floats in thousands of problems and grand ideas.

Strange feeling of pleasant and easy comfort, as if he scarcely touched earth with his feet and had to gather ideas from afar. Sensation as if they were floating in the clouds. Involved in a most beautiful atmosphere, bright and calm as the sunlight at noon.

RELATIONS - ***Compare:*** (1) Stram.

REFERENCES - Clarke.

DATURA FEROX

(Chinese Datura)

PHARMACY - dat-f. Datura ferox. Chinese datura. N. O. Solanaceae. Trituration of seeds. Tincture of unripe fruit. ***Historical dose:*** All potencies.

CLINICAL - Delirium. Mania.

HOMEOPATHIC - Poisoning with this drug causes raving madness.

A girl who ate half an unripe fruit was completely out of her mind in a quarter of an hour, dizzy. Sleepy, slept with eyes open. If disturbed, she sprang up raving and uttered unintelligible words, if one sang she began to dance in the Favanese fashion.

This symptom may prove a keynote in certain cases of mental alienation. Dryness of the mouth was also noted in this case, as with Bell. and other Solanaceae.

REFERENCES - Clarke.

DATURA METEL

(Indian Datura)

PHARMACY - dat-m. Datura metel. Indian datura. N. O. Solanaceae. Trituration of seeds. ***Historical dose:*** All potencies.

CLINICAL - Convulsions. Delirium. Epilepsy. Eye disorders. Mania. Timidity.

HOMEOPATHIC - Dat-m. causes a sleepy condition and later delirium and spasms. The soporose state may be absent. Delirium may be vociferous or merely garrulous. Patient usually manifests excessive timidity. Picks at real or imaginary objects. Performs ridiculous antics.

Several movements appear due to perverted vision and inability to judge distances. After the delirium, patient remembers nothing of what has occurred. Extreme dilatation of pupils. Flickering before eyes with sensitiveness to light. Pulse and temperature undergo extremes of exaltation and depression.

RELATIONS - ***Compare:*** (1) Other Solanaceae.

REFERENCES - Clarke.

DEOXYRIBONUCLEIC ACIDUM

(DNA)

PHARMACY - des-ac. Deoxyribonucleic acidum. DNA. ***Historical dose:*** All potencies.

CLINICAL - Allergies. Amnesia. Cancer. Down's Syndrome. ***Emaciation.*** Epilepsy. Fatigue. Hypersensitivity. Hyperthyroidism. Insomnia. Manic, depression. Neuralgia. Neurosis. Premature senility.

HOMEOPATHIC - The proving of DNA, following the method indicated by Hahnemann, was conducted from 1970 to 1972 by O. A. Julian. Thirty people took part in this proving, four of whom were women, and all were doctors. Using the single blind method, the 30c, 7c, and 3x potencies were used, along with a placebo.

The symptoms of that proving were incorporated with indications given by some Belgian homeopathic authors, who carried out some clinical research using potencies of DNA.

Symptoms include a sense of general well being, more so in the morning. Difficulty in assembling thoughts, poor powers of concentration. Does not want to be idle, need to work. Difficulty working, but better when body fatigue wears off. General hypersensitivity, with asthenia. Tendency to hyperthyroidism.

MIND - Hot-tempered, nervous disposition. Bad-tempered. Extremely irritable, with general feeling of discomfort in the morning. General feeling of uneasiness. Personality disorders, periods of dual personality. Narcissistic neurosis. Neurosis from anguish. Manic depression psychosis.

General amnesia. Lack of willpower. Physical and psychological slowness, backwardness. Impossible for him to work, cannot concentrate. Mental slowness from the after effects of poliomyelitis. Down's syndrome.

Abdomen - Pain in the epigastrium. Distention, not eased by food. Flatulence and rumbling. Disorders of the liver, pancreas. Biliary sycosis.

Back - Pain in the left shoulder, in the acromion and the clavicular joints. Torticollis. Arthrosis of the neck and back. Intercostal neuralgia.

Blood - Peripheral circulatory complaints: hands cold during the day, hot in the evening. Leucopenia. Hemorrhage. Nightly acroparesthesia.

Constitutions - Psoric and allergic constitutions. Cancerous condition.

Eyes - Persistent bilateral conjunctivitis. Asthenopia. Extreme ocular fatigue, difficulty in seeing things in the distance clearly. Myopia. Bright spots before the eyes, which disappear when closed, appearing around 10:30 a.m., and last for an hour.

Female - Anal and vulvar pruritus.

Food - ***Increases the appetite.*** Hunger pangs between meals. Anorexia.

Head - Neuritis and neuralgia of the brain. Headache and nausea after drinking a little wine. Pulsating headache over the whole head. Headache concomitant with need to go to stool, which does not provide relief. Ophthalmic migraine.

Kidneys - Painful urination. Urinates, especially about half an hour after meals. Irregular diuresis, sometimes copious, with yellow urine, sometimes copious and pale. Oliguria.

Limbs - White spot on the left index finger. Arm very painful, aggravated by pressure. Nightly recurring cramps in the calves. Osteomyelitis. Fractures repair slowly. Peri-arthritis of the scapula and humerus. Arthrosis of hips and shoulders. Patches of sclerosis.

Male - Sexual mania. Diminution of libido. Hypertrophy of the prostate. Eczema of the scrotum.

Modalities - Better from rest. Better lying in the dark. Better laterality left side. Worse from movement.

Mouth - White coating over the whole tongue reaching even the edges, not removed easily by brushing. Burning sensation in mouth mucus membranes, with sensitive gums. Gingivitis. Angina. Gums bleed when brushing the teeth.

Nose - Frontal sinusitis.

Rectum - Tendency to constipation, with dry, dark stools. Tendency to diarrhea after meals, with flatulence. Anal eczema, with burning and oozing.

Skin - Burns. Psoriasis. Eczema. Marginal and eczematous rash, with burning and oozing. Reappearance of an eczematous dermatitis. Inflammatory folliculitis of the thighs. Alopecia. Seborrhea.

Sleep - Twilight sleep. In the evening, irresistible desire to sleep, once in bed, no longer wants to sleep. Insomnia. Disturbed sleep. Sleepwalking. Erotic dreams at the end of the night. Dreams of dead bodies.

Stomach - Acid dyspepsia. Burning in the stomach and esophagus. Chilliness after meals, with a cold feeling between the shoulders and feeling of heat on the face, disappearing with movement.

Throat - Laryngitis. Splinter-like feeling in the throat in the morning on waking. Raw feeling in the throat. Feeling of a foreign body, especially on the left side, ameliorated by cold water and by swallowing. .

RELATIONS - ***Compare:*** (1) Plat., Nep., Arg-n.

REFERENCES - Julian.

DERRIS PINNATA

PHARMACY - der. Derris pinnata. N. O. Leguminosae. Papilionoideae. China. Tincture of plant. ***Historical dose:*** Tincture and all potencies.

CLINICAL - Asthma. Blepharospasm. Diarrhea. Dysentery. Eyes, inflammation. Locomotor ataxia. Mania. Ozaena. Smell, affected. Tic douloureux.

HOMEOPATHIC - Dr. X. Roussel is the authority for this plant. Peculiar symptoms include "He walks as if stepping on down," Painful and convulsive tic douloureux. Electric shocks and cramps.

Exalted sense of smell. "He perceives celestial odors," also "intolerable smells after frequent sneezing." Heat helps toothache. Viscid urine and viscid saliva. Many symptoms, including diarrhea, come on at night. Worse from touch.

MIND - Delusion that he is seasick. Fear of falling on turning head. Censorious with dearest friends. He is afraid of killing some one with a knife. Singing alternating with weeping.

RELATIONS - ***Compare:*** (1) Anac. - sense of smell. (2) Stict. - levitation. (3) Ign. - ball in throat, hysteria.

REFERENCES - Clarke.

DESMODIUM GANGETICUM

PHARMACY - desm-g. Desmodium gangeticum. N. O. Leguminosae. India. Tincture of plant. ***Historical dose:*** Tincture and all potencies.

CLINICAL - Asthma. Catarrhal. Cough. Dropsy. Fever. Headache. Heat, flushes. Intermittent, fever. Meningitis. Neuralgia. Pleurodynia. Rheumatism. Typhoid, fever. Ulcers. Vomiting. Wry-neck.

HERBAL - It is a small tree growing in the forest and is found throughout the plains of India, also the lower Himalayan regions.

The Hindu physicians have highly extolled it as an alternative, tonic, and bitter remedy. They have found it efficacious in vomiting, fevers, dropsy, ulcers, cough, respiratory troubles and affections due to worms.

It is a bitter tonic and febrifuge. It is also digestive and anti-catarrhal. It is one of the principal ingredients of Dashamula, an ayurvedic decoction of reputation successfully used in many diseases, namely typhoid fever, cough, asthma, pleurodynia.

HOMEOPATHIC - Desmodium gangeticum can safely be used in typhoid fever and cerebro-spinal meningitis when the patient feels pain all over the body, there is sleepiness, or comatose sleep, headache is present, and there is feeling as if the head is bound up with a tape or rope.

In intermittent or remittent fevers of children it can be used when there are sleepiness or drowsiness and pains over the body. In this respect it bears a close resemblance to Gelsemium and in place of which it may be given.

It may be employed in remittent and typhoid fevers and cerebro-spinal meningitis associated with pains over the whole body, specially over the spine, headache and sleepiness with a feeling as if a tape lay around the head.

The fever comes on in the morning generally at 7 a.m. There is slight chilliness, lasting for 2 or 3 hours. From the onset burning sensation is felt over the face and eyes and in the hands and feet. Flushes of heat come out of the face.

There is remission of fever with perspiration over forehead and back part of the hands and in feet. The fever indicating this drug is quotidian in character, regularly returning daily. The pains all over the body and headache and other symptoms may also be present.

The above are the characteristic symptoms in which Desmodium gangeticum will be found an excellent remedy in intermittent fevers. It is also a valuable remedy for wry-neck.

COMMENTS - The late Dr. Aghore Ch. Bhaduri. with his three pupils made a proving of this drug. The result of the proving is given below.

He felt pains all over the body. Nervous pain, specially in the legs and neck. Burning sensation was felt in the hands and feet. Sleepiness.

Pains like rheumatism and neuralgia were felt in hands, feet, legs and the rest of the body. Could not sit straight on account of spinal pain. Burning sensation was felt in the eyes, face hands and feet and flushes of heat ignited from the face.

Neuralgic pain was felt in the stomach. Pain was felt in knee joint. Headache associated with a sensation as if all sides of the head are bound up with a tape. The above were the symptoms which were noticed by Dr. Bhaduri during the course of the proving.

RELATIONS - ***Compare:*** In burning sensations, it can be compared with Azadirachta, Kalmegha, Rohitaka, Sulphur, etc.

REFERENCES - Ghose.

DICHAPETALUM THUNBERGH

PHARMACY - dicha. Dichapetalum thunbergh. Dichapetalaceae or Chailletiaceae family. The flower inhabits tropical the regions. Tincture of leaves and bark. ***Historical dose:*** Tincture and all potencies.

CLINICAL - Arthrosis. Cellulitis. Duodenal, ulcer. Eczema. Hernia. Joint, pain. Lichen planus. Migraines. Neuralgias. Rhinitis. Sinusitis. Tonsillitis. Vertigo.

HERBAL - Dicha. is a dicotyledonous family with super-ovarized dialypetals, growing as trees or shrubs with simple alternate leaves, flowers in clusters or corymbs. The fruit is a drupe with a pendant seed, which has no albumen.

HOMEOPATHIC - Dicha. was brought to Europe by Dr. Willmar-Schwabe of Germany. The symptomatology was established by G. Maring on a group of four women and three men, all doctors. Using a double blind method, the 3x, 4x, 6x, 15x, and 30x potencies were used, along with a placebo.

General fatigue of the body, despite a state of euphoria when working. Sudden lack of energy with fatigue and a feeling of hunger, ameliorated by food and alcohol. Sullen mood. Inner trembling. Snuffles. Sensation of trembling inside the entire body.

Stiffness at the nape of the neck, back, loins and sacrum. Occipital headaches. Migraines. Vertigo, buzzing in the ears, visual and psychosomatic complaints. Radicular neuritis. Chronic infection of the mucus membranes. Cervical and brachial neuralgia. Lichen planus.

MIND - Sullen moods. Mental fatigue. Disinterested, must make an effort to work.

Abdomen - Rumbling and pinching feeling in the abdomen, ameliorated by eating and expelling wind. Passage through intestines accelerated with more frequent stools. Duodenal ulcer. Diaphragmatic hernia.

Back - Pain between the shoulders. Pain in the right shoulder, spreading towards the neck. Dorsal pain and stiffness like ankylosis. Severe pain and stiffness in the lumbar region, when seated or when walking. Pain in the lumbar region with drawing pains around the thighs. Drawing pains in the sacrum, ameliorated by urinating or expelling wind, worse when standing. Cellulitis of the nape of the neck.

Chest - A retro-sternal pain, worse when swallowing.

Female - Premature, too frequent menses. Amelioration of rheumatic pains at the beginning of menses.

Food - Low blood sugar. Fatigue is ameliorated by food and alcohol.

Head - Migraines. Occipital headaches. Pounding headache on all sides of the head, better by rest and fresh air. Diffuse, dull head pain with numbness of the head. Pain and stiffness at the nape of the neck.

Heart - Pain in the precordial region with palpitations, followed by ascending hot flushes. Cardiac anguish with feeling of uneasiness and difficulty in falling asleep.

Limbs - Fatigue and rheumatic pains in the limbs. Joint pain. Arthrosis. Legs feel like rubber. Heaviness in the calves.

Modalities - Better from fresh air. Better resting. Better eating. Better from menses. Worse on right side. Worse from standing. Worse walking.

Mouth - Dryness, formication and tension at the lips. Quick, short, drawing pains in the teeth of the lower jaw.

Nose - Itching of the nose and face. Feeling of having a cold with blocked nose. Painful drawing sensation at the root of the nose, especially when the eyes converge to read. Sinusitis. Rhinitis.

Rectum - Bleeding hemorrhoids.

Skin - Deep eczematic fissure on the palm of the hand, stretching along the 'lifeline,' with scaly eruption at the edges. Herpes-type eruptions, which itch, on the inner side of the left ankle with burning and scratching. Lichen-type eczema, in cement workers and bakers. Lichen planus.

Temperature - Shivering and sensation of cold, even when in a warm room. Rising heat, as if about to have a fever.

Throat - Tonsillitis. Painful pulling on the right tonsil. Feeling of a grating lump in the throat. Fit of laryngeal coughing. Aphonia, ameliorated after speaking for a long time. Swallowing painful on the right side of the throat. Dysphagia.

RELATIONS - ***Compare:*** (1) Rhus-t. - Aching, stiffness, ameliorated by prolonged movement, vesicular eruptions, burning and itching. (2) Tub. - Joint pains with stiffness, dragging, worse on waking and after meals. (3) Zinc - Occipital pain with heavy feeling on the vertex or the root of the nose. Nose blocked, burning pains in the back, fidgety feet.

REFERENCES - Julian.

DICTAMNUS ALBUS
(Fraxinella)

PHARMACY - dict. Dictamnus albus. Fraxinella. Dictamnus fraxinella. N. O. Rutacae. Tincture of whole plant. ***Historical dose:*** Tincture and all potencies.

CLINICAL - Constipation. Flatulence. Leucorrhea. Metrorrhagia.

HOMEOPATHIC - Dictamnus acts on the female organs. Increased secretions. Early menses, of black clots, preceded by blindness. Profuse, corrosive leucorrhea with tenesmus. Bearing down with bilious vomiting, worse standing. Cramps from anterior thighs into the uterus before the menses.

Sensation of milk flowing into breasts. Increased flow of urine. Frequent emission of copious, offensive flatus. Sensation of a lump rising in the throat. Worse from standing. Sleepwalking. Dreams of piecing bodies of her children together.

REFERENCES - Clarke.

DIGITALINUM

PHARMACY - digin. Digitalinum. Active principle, glucoside of Digitalis purpurea. N. O. Scrophulariaceae. Trituration. ***Historical dose:*** Trituration and all potencies.

CLINICAL - Asthma. Diarrhea. Emissions. Exophthalmus. Fainting. Heart disorders. Palpitations. Spermatorrhea. Vertigo. Vision, hallucinations.

HOMEOPATHIC - Digin. is a poison of great activity. It produces a profound effect on muscular tissue, both voluntary and involuntary, more especially on the heart. Irregular and intermittent action.

Digin. causes profound prostration, even to inability to move a muscle. The heart is slowed or else its action is made rapid and feeble. ***Sensation as if the heart stood still***. Paralytic weakness, numbness, tremulousness of the limbs. Cold, clammy surface. Goose-flesh.

A sinking, faint sensation at the epigastrium. Shivering. Diarrhea, the stools are not characteristically white as are those of the plant. Nausea and vomiting of egg yolk matter. Drinking causes nausea and vomiting. Symptoms are better after dinner.

Sensitiveness of eyes to light and nose to odors. Disorders of vision and hearing. Confusion of the head, better walking in open air. Chilliness and fever worse in afternoon and evening. Heart pains are worse lying on left side. Pains in trunk worse during rest. Many symptoms appear on waking in the morning.

COMMENTS - According to Hale, Digin. is indicated in cases of "overburdened heart where it is constantly laboring."

Digin. cured the case of Mrs. X, who had for over a year swelling of her right hand and fingers, which she thought to be rheumatic. Digitalis has the symptoms, "swelling of right hand and fingers," and this would have been given, but only Digin. was at hand. It was given in 4x potency. After the second dose the swelling began to subside, and in two or three days was completely gone.

One prover noted "frontal headache, dazzlings, loss of appetite, sinking at epigastrium with intestinal flatulence, borborygmi, eructation. Slight abdominal pains, urine abundant, great fatigue, painful heat in evening but no thirst."

For a whole day pressure in supra orbital region towards frontal sinus and when walking a feeling as if the ground gave way under his feet. Sexual weakness is shown in "Deep sleep in which an emission occurs without waking him." "Sexual power diminished or quite abolished temporarily."

RELATIONS - ***Compare:*** (1) Dam., Dig., Con., Grat., Tab., Gels., Sec.

REFERENCES - Clarke.

DIGITALIS PURPUREA

(Foxglove)

PHARMACY - dig. Digitalis purpurea. Foxglove. N. O. Scrofulariaceae. Tincture from the leaves of the second year of the plant. ***Historical dose:*** Tincture and all potencies.

CLINICAL - Amaurosis. ***Angina pectoris.*** Aphthae. Ascites. Asthma. ***Balanitis.*** Bright's disease. Cataract. Collapse. Congestive heart failure. Coryza. ***Cyanosis.*** Cystitis. Delirium tremens. Diplopia. Dropsy. ***Dyspnea.*** Emphysema. ***Faintness.*** Fevers. Gonorrhea. Headache. ***Heart, disorders. Heart, weakness.*** Hepatitis. ***Hot, flushes.*** Hydrocele. Hydrocephalus. Hydrothorax. Impotence. Jaundice. ***Liver, disorders.*** Lungs, congestion. Melancholy. Memory, lost. Meningitis. ***Mitral valve, disease. Nausea.*** Nephritis. ***Neuralgias.*** Noises, in head. Pericarditis. Phimosis. Pleurisy. Pneumonia. ***Prostate, enlarged.*** Prostration. Pulmonary, edema. ***Pulse, slow.*** Ptyalism. Spermatorrhea. Stomatitis. Toothache. Uremia. ***Urethritis.*** Urinary, disorders. Vertigo. Vision, disorders. Vomiting. ***Weakness.***

HOMEOPATHIC - Digitalis is a ***heart remedy***, but also affects the liver, lungs, stomach and genito-urinary organs. Dig. should be considered in all diseases where the heart is chiefly involved with abnormally ***slow, irregular or intermittent pulse***, along with indefinite and causeless symptoms.

Weakness and dilation of the myocardium. Indicated in failure of compensation. Auricular flutter and ***fibrillation***, especially when subsequent to rheumatic fever. Useful for people with side effects from the digitalis drug.

Symptoms of organic heart disease, such as great weakness and sinking of strength, faintness, coldness of skin and irregular respiration, cardiac irritability. Faint, as if dying. ***Bluish*** appearance of face. ***Cardiac muscular failure*** when systole is present. Stimulates the heart's muscles, increases force of systole, increases length.

Heart blockage with a very slow pulse. The ***pulse is weak, irregular intermittent, abnormally slow*** and dropsy of external and internal parts. Slow pulse in recumbent posture, but irregular and dicrotic on sitting up. Irregular pulse. Pulse can be slow or it can be intermittent. Slow pulse with menopause, puberty, or after sexual abuse.

Congestive heart failure, especially in elderly people with dizziness and ringing in the ears. Tightness of the chest and weak heart. Constriction of the chest (Cact.). Weary feeling and their limbs feel heavy (Gels., Con.). Fluttering of the heart (Nat-m.). High blood pressure, with kidney involvement or prostate problems.

Sense of suffocation, a fear of suffocation relating to a weak heart. Sinking feeling in the stomach with heart palpitations. ***Faintness.*** Sensation as if he would die if he moves during the palpitations. ***Great weakness,*** can hardly talk, sinking of strength. Collapse. Prostration from slight exertion.

As of an electric shock going through the body. ***Cyanosis.*** Must walk about, with precordial anxiety, with urging to urinate. Dropsy with suppression of urine. Jaundice from induration and ***hypertrophy of the liver***. Jaundice with heart disease. Tongue is blue and clean, thick and flabby. Eye troubles after tobacco.

MIND - Great anxiety, as from troubled conscience. Reproaches himself. ***Great guilt, better weeping.*** Anxious, low-spirited and tearful. Extreme anxiety related to the heart. ***Anxious about the future***. Excitement, stammers when talking to strangers. Excitement at night.

Suspicious. Fearful. ***Fear of suffocation at night.*** Fear of insanity. Fear from music. Fear of death while walking. Feels as if he would fly to pieces. Every emotional shock strikes in epigastrium. Fear arising from stomach. Hurried, abrupt speech.

Deep sighing and grief with heart problems (Ign., Calc-p.). Arrhythmias and palpitations that are worse since grief (Nat-m). Despair. Despondent. ***Sadness from unhappy love.*** Sadness, great depression, with sleeplessness. ***Weeping improves symptoms.*** Weeping from music. A broken heart with the sensation that the heart will fly to pieces.

Melancholy, dull lethargic with ***slow pulse***. Excessive desire to be alone. Tries to escape if others force themselves on her. Stammers when talking to strangers. Converses with absent people. Unsympathetic.

Dullness of senses. Thinking difficult. Weak memory. Forgets everything immediately. Insane obstinacy and disobedience, with desire to escape. ***Suspicious.*** Irritability after sex. Lascivious thoughts in old men with enlarged prostate.

Abdomen - Ascites. Severe abdominal pains. Pain in left side apparently in descending colon and under false ribs. ***Tenderness of epigastrium***. Pulsation in the abdominal aorta and epigastric constriction. After a meal, pressure and inflation of the abdomen and of the stomach. Sensation as if intestines were twisted. Griping pain. Incarcerated hernia. Bowel symptoms alternating with chest symptoms.

Back - Stiffness and tension of the muscles of the neck and of the nape of the neck. Drawing pains in the back and in the loins, as after a chill. Bruise-like pains in the loins on blowing the nose. Tearing, sharp, aching and cutting pains, in neck. Lacerating, and sharp pains in lumbar region.

Bladder - Cystitis, after passing a few drops the desire to urinate is increased and the patient walks about in great distress. ***Urethritis,*** phimosis, strangury. Full feeling after urination. Urine, suppressed. ***Sharp cutting or throbbing pain*** at neck of bladder. Difficult urination. ***Pain, as if a straw was being thrust back and forth,*** worse at night. Constriction and burning, as if urethra was too small. Dragging in bladder as if distended, not better frequent urination. Contractive pain in bladder, during urination. Urine more easily retained in recumbent position. After urination pressure in bladder and burning in urethra.

Breasts - Shuddering at the breasts.

Causations - Ill effects of high living, sexual abuse or excessive alcohol intake.

Chest - ***Angina pectoris.*** Great weakness in chest, can't bear to talk. ***Suffocative painful constriction of chest***, as if internal parts were grown together. Creeping all over skin. Smarting in the chest. Tension in the chest with necessity to breathe deeply. Contractive, pressing pain in the chest, when sitting with the body bent. Sensation of soreness. Congestion in the chest. Raw, sore feeling in chest, with cough. Trembling in chest.

Constitutions - Nervous lymphatic constitutions. Children with very pale complexions, light hair, scrofulous.

Cough - Dry cough, on deep inspiration. Cough followed by great prostration. Cough after eating, with vomiting of food. Cough causes pain in shoulders and arms or sore, raw feeling in the chest. Cough from suppressed menses. Hemoptysis with weak heart or from chronic bronchitis, before menses. Hollow, deep, spasmodic cough, excited by roughness and scratching in palate and in trachea.

Ears - Otalgia with contractive pains in the ears. Swelling of the parotids and behind the ear. Veins distended on ears. Single stitches behind the ears. Hissing before the ears like boiling water, with hardness of hearing.

Eyes - Yellowish, red eyes. Both the eyes turned to left. Burning in eyes and stitches darting through them. Lachrymation, worse in bright light or cold air. Veins distended on eyes. Blueness of eyelids. Swelling of lower lid. Mydriasis. Lid margins red, swollen. Agglutinated lids in morning. Catarrhal inflammation of eye. Meibomian glands inflamed. Chronic conjunctivitis. Detachment of retina. Cataract. Painless obscuration of lens. Irregular pupils. Pupils dilated and insensible.

Face - Paleness of the face. ***Cyanosis.*** Blue color of the lips and eyelids. Bluish swelling of the lips. Dryness of the lips. Eruptions on the lips. Eruptions with gnawing itching in the cheeks and in the chin. Cramp-like and drawing pains in the cheekbones. Distended veins. Pores of the face black and suppurating.

Female - Menses scanty and too late. Labor-like pains in abdomen and back before menses. Menorrhagia. Uterine hemorrhage. Dropsy of uterus. Bleeding from lungs instead of menses. Menopausal period, sudden flushes of heat followed by great debility, least motion causes palpitations. Leucorrhea. Lascivious state of fancy day and night. Nymphomania.

Food - Want of appetite, sometimes even with a clean tongue. Smell of food causes violent nausea and gagging. ***Desire for bitter things.*** Desire for beer. Bread tastes bitter. Continuous thirst with dry lips. Thirst for acid, sour, cold drinks. Cough worse cold drinks. Worse after meals. Worse cold food or drinks, alcohol. Worse after drinking. Worse from spirituous liquors. After cold water or ice cream, sharp pain in forehead extending to nose.

Head - Face bluish. Dullness of head as from intoxication, with increased mental activity. Heaviness of head with sensation as if it would fall backward. ***Brain feels fatigued and weak, from weak action of heart.*** Confusion, fullness and noises in head. Crashes, cracking in head, on dropping to sleep. Bores head in the pillow. Pulls the hair. Violent, lancinating pains, in vertex and occiput. Spastic hemicrania. ***Throbbing, in forehead.*** Sharp, shooting pains in forehead, after drinking cold water or eating ice cream. Pressure in forehead when exerting mind or thinking of it. Sharp pains in temples, evening and night.

Heart - Sinking feeling at heart. ***Sudden sensation as if heart stood still.*** Sensation as if heart would cease beating if he moves, must hold the breath and keep still (opposite of Gels.). Precordial anxiety, with sensation of weakness in forearm. Audible throbbing of heart. Metallic sounding heart-beat. The least movement causes violent palpitations. Palpitations with depression from grief. ***Angina pectoris.*** Attacks of angina, worse raising arms with tingling in arm and fingers. ***Constant pain or anguish in region of heart.*** Frequent sharp pains in heart. ***Irregular heartbeat especially with mitral valve disease.*** Cardiac failure following fevers. Heart tired after sprains. Hypertrophy with dilatation. ***Cardiac failure following fevers.*** Cardiac dropsy. Pericarditis, copious serous exudation. Rheumatism of heart with irregular pulse. ***Pulse weak and quickened by least movement.*** Pulse small, weak and excessively slow, irregular, intermitting. ***Very slow pulse.*** Especially slow when at rest, every other beat intermits, but accelerated by the slightest movement. Thready pulse.

Kidneys - Nephritis after scarlatina. Uremia. Contracted kidneys. Profuse and frequent emission of clear pale urine. Frequent urination at night. Continued urging, urine in drops, dark, hot, burning. Suppressed urine. Ammoniacal and turbid urine. Brick-dust sediment. Urine thick, turbid, yellowish-brown, blackish, acrid. Diminished secretion alternating with copious secretion of watery urine.

Limbs - Rheumatic pain in joints. Swelling of the feet. ***Sensation as if a red-hot wire suddenly darted through legs.*** Stinging pains in muscles of upper and lower limbs. Piercing pains in joints. Shining, white swelling of joints. Muscular debility. Numbness, heaviness or paralytic weakness, worse left arm. Fingers become numb easily and frequently. Coldness of hands and feet. One hand hot, the other cold. Nails blue. Fingers swell at night.

Liver - ***Enlarged, sore, painful liver.*** Soreness over region of liver, with jaundice. ***Liver, hard and painful.*** Jaundice from induration. ***Hypertrophy of the liver***. Jaundice with heart disease.

Lungs - Cardiac asthma. Slow, asthmatic attack early in morning. Great weakness in the lungs. Lungs feel compressed. ***Dyspnea, constant desire to breathe deeply.*** Breathing irregular, difficult. ***Deep sighing.*** Breathing slow, worse talking, walking, drinking cold things. ***Cannot bear to talk*** (Stan.). ***Suffocates when he drops to sleep,*** fear of suffocation at night. ***Can only breathe in gasps***, each one seeming as if it would be the last. Chronic bronchitis, passive congestion of the lungs, giving bloody sputum due to failing myocardium. Expectoration, sweetish like boiled starch, mixed with bloody mucus. Yellow, jelly-like mucus, difficult expectoration. Cannot expectorate without vomiting. Moist rales, yet cough dry. Senile pneumonia. Emphysema with heart disease. Edema of lungs. Hydrothorax.

Male - Dropsical swelling of genitals (Sulph.). ***Prostate enlarged, in elderly men.*** Hydrocele (left), scrotum looks like a bladder filled with water. Testicles swollen. Bruise-like pain in testes with swelling. Contusive pain in right testicle. ***Balanitis with edema of prepuce.*** Gonorrhea (Med.). Profuse, thick, yellow-white gonorrheal discharge. As if something were running out in urethra after emission. Irritation of sexual organs, with painful erections, night and day. Desire strongly excited, frequent erections and pollutions. Atonic nightly emissions after sex. Spermatorrhea. Pollutions always with lewd dreams and subsequent pains in penis. Early morning erections. Sexual desire without ability.

Modalities - Better when stomach is empty. ***Better from weeping.*** Better lying flat on back. Better sitting erect. Better rest. Better in open air, cool air. Worse from lying on left side. Worse sitting erect. Worse being raised up in bed. Worse touch, pressure. Worse motion. Worse exertion. Worse sexual abuse or excess. Worse from food. Worse smell of food. Worse cold food or drinks, alcohol. Worse after meals. Worse music. Worse from cold air, cold weather. Worse changes of weather. Worse heat. Worse night. Worse waking in the morning.

Mouth - Soreness of mouth, gums and tongue. Aphthae. Stomatitis. Bitter taste. Taste flat, clammy, slimy. Sweet taste, with constant salivation. Copious salivation. Salivation after smoking tobacco. Scraped feeling in mouth. Severe toothache in a hollow tooth.

Nose - Coryza with hoarseness. Pain at the root of the nose, after vomiting. Nosebleeds.

Perspiration - Cold, clammy sweat. Copious sweat at night. Perspiration after the chill, no heat intervening. Sweats on upper part of body, on face. Sweats during cough. Covered with copious perspiration, without relief of heart symptoms. Cold sweat, on body, warm on palms of hands.

Rectum - Evacuation forcible. Constipation. ***White, chalk-like, ashy, pasty stool.*** Diarrhea during jaundice. Watery diarrhea. Stool mixed with mucus. Frequent, distressing and exceedingly offensive stools. Stools, perfectly flat and shaped like a boat. Renewed desire and urging in rectum after stool.

Sensations - As if the heart would stand still if he moved, must hold the breath and keep still (Gels. has "must keep moving or the heart would stop"). As if heart had torn itself loose and were swaying to and fro by a thin thread. As if the lungs were constricted and tied up in bundles. As if the stomach would sink into abdomen. As if something were running out of urethra, as of a weight attached to stomach, as if the internal parts were grown together. As if the brain were loose, as if something fell forward in the head on stooping, as if the brain were made of fine glass and shattered at a blow.

Skin - Dry, arid heat of skin. Paleness of the skin. Cyanosis. Bluish skin particularly at the eyelids, lips tongue and nails. Blue distended veins. Cold skin. Dropsy. Elastic white swelling of whole body. ***Itching and jaundiced.*** Gnawing itching increasing to intolerable burning pricking. Corrosive itching. Erythema, deep red, worse on back like measles. Measly eruptions on back. Sebaceous follicles ulcerate. Skin painful to touch. Desquamation of the skin.

Sleep - Lethargy. Continuous sleepiness. Drowsy in the day. Unrefreshing, agitated sleep. Somnolency interrupted by fits of convulsive vomiting. Uneasy sleep at night on account of constant desire to urinate. Frequent waking, as from anxiety. Nightmares. ***Starts from sleep*** in alarm that he is falling from a height in a dream. Dreams of falling from a height or into water. Dreams with jerking and electric-like sensations through the body.

Stomach - Discomfort in stomach, even after a small quantity of food, or from mere sight or smell. Burning in stomach and into esophagus. ***Faintness, great weakness in stomach.*** Extreme anxiety in pit, causing frequent deep sighs. Epigastric region tender. ***Neuralgic pain in stomach***. Stomach burning, extending to esophagus. Gulping up of an acrid or tasteless fluid. ***Deathly nausea, with faint sinking in stomach.*** Persistent nausea and vomiting with clean tongue (Ip.). ***Excessive nausea, not better vomiting.*** Nausea before and after urination. The mere sight or smell of food excites nausea. Nausea early on rising, with thirst. ***Faintness*** and vomiting from motion. Nausea and vomiting of pregnancy. Vomits easily, on taking anything into stomach. Vomiting, with extremely feeble and irregular pulse. Vomiting of bile, mucus.

Temperature - Chills alternating with heat. Coldness in the hands and in the feet with cold perspiration. Chilliness and shivering of the whole body. Chills with head and redness of the face. Internal chills with external heat. Chilliness before stool. Frequent and sudden flushes of heat, followed by nervous weakness, at menopausal period. ***Sudden hot flushes, with palpitation from least motion.*** Heat of body with cold sweat of face. During cough. General violent heat, with swollen veins and rapid pulse. Fever with profuse sweat. Heat of one hand and coldness of the other.

Throat - Scraped feeling in throat. Stinging in throat between acts of swallowing. Choking when he tries to swallow. Spasm of glottis with diarrhea and thirst. Edema of larynx. Frequent painless hoarseness. Hoarseness in early morning.

Tongue - Blue tongue and lips. Tongue blue, thick, flabby. Tongue clean with nausea and vomiting. Veins distended on tongue. Tongue pale. Tongue coated white.

Vertigo - Constant dizziness with ringing in ears. Vertigo, when walking or riding. Vertigo with trembling. Vertigo on rising from sitting, with very slow pulse. Vertigo from cardiac or hepatic disorders. Vertigo with anxiety and faintness. Vertigo as if faintness would occur.

Vision - Diplopia. Dim vision. Dark bodies like flies, before eyes. ***Change in acuteness of perception of shades of green.*** Objects appear green and yellow. Sees hairs before his eyes. Loss of vision and many symptoms with anemia of retina and optic nerve. Hemiopia, as if upper part of field of vision were covered by a dark cloud. Optical illusions in bright or prismatic colors.

COMMENTS - Slow, weak, irregular and intermittent pulse. Acute cyanosis (Carb-v.). Palpitations, with hot flashes. Prostration from slight exertion. Restlessness with a great nervous weakness. Lassitude, mental and bodily. Faintness. Convulsions with retraction of head, syncope and collapse. History of helping reduce or control aneurysm. Vertigo, dizziness as if intoxicated.

Pneumonia and pleurisy. Senile pneumonia. Asthmatic sufferings as from hydrothorax. Respiration is painfully restricted at night, when lying down or in the day, when walking or seated. In the morning, suffocating constriction of the chest, forcing the patient to rise up in the bed.

Delirium tremens in high livers, stomach and liver diseases with the mental state of the drug. Enlarged, sore, and painful liver. Deathly sinking in the epigastrium. Every shock, like bad news, strikes her in the epigastrium. Portal engorgement. White, pasty stools. Constant irritation or urge to urinate. Urine can be dark brown. Dribbling of the urine.

Nausea and vomiting, worse from smell of food, not better by vomiting. Violent nausea with clean tongue. The food eaten comes up by mouthfuls, cannot expectorate without vomiting. Terrible pain at root of nose after vomiting. Thirst for water.

Enlarged prostate in elderly men, with lascivious thoughts. Prostate enlargement and weaknesses with concomitant heart disease. Impotence. History of gonorrhea. Yellow-white urethral discharge. People with a history of excess, particularly sex and alcohol, with weakened heart or liver.

Discharged blood coagulates slowly or not at all. Distended veins in eyes, ears, lips and tongue. Blue skin. Absence of fever.

Teste classed Dig. with Bry. and Ign. He noted that there is an "anxious and concentrated sadness with sleeplessness at night, owing to pains at the heart: for instance from unhappy love, especially in women of brown complexions, firm and obstinate dispositions. In such cases far preferable to Ignatia."

Ross regarded the indications as being: "dry cough with mucus rales and no expectoration or only 'prune juice' expectoration, cyanosis, cold limbs, feeble intermittent pulse, deathly nausea or gone sensation at epigastrium."

Malcolm Macfarlan reported Dig. having produced severe urethritis, phimosis and strangury. He cured with it many cases of gonorrhea.

Ballard cured a man of headache and dizziness, originating probably in gonorrhea suppressed several years before. He complained of feeling bad about the head after drinking and this keynote symptom was elicited: "after drinking cold water the pain would seat itself in the forehead and extend down the nose."

RELATIONS - *Antidotes:* Camph., China. *Compare:* (1) Crat. - a true heart tonic. (2) Adon., Kalm., Spig., Liatris, Serum ang. (3) Nerium odorum - resembles in heart effects Digitalis, but also has an action like Stry. on spinal cord. Spasms appear more in upper part of body. Palpitations, weak heart will be strengthened by it. Lock-jaw. (4) Digitoxinum. Nit-s-dulc. increases action of Dig. (5) Convallaria - heart disease with vertigo and digestive disturbances. *Compatible:* Bell., Bry., Cham., Lyc., Nux-v. *Incompatible:* China.

REFERENCES - Boericke. Clarke. Murphy. Phatak.

DIGITOXINUM

(Digitoxin)

PHARMACY - digox. Digitoxinum. Digitoxin. "Crystallized digitaline" of Nativelle. Neither a glucoside, nor an alkaloid. N. O. Scrophulariaceae. Trituration. *Historical dose:* All potencies.

CLINICAL - Faintness. Phlegmon. Suppuration. Vision disordered. Vomiting.

HOMEOPATHIC - Digitoxinum is made from Digitalis dissolved in chloroform. The most active principle of Digitalis, Digox. has yellow vision, phlegmonous inflammation going on to suppuration, and very marked and distressing nausea, ***aggravated by champagne and aerated waters.*** Faintness, rapid loss of power. Prostration, limbs refuse their service, cannot rise from bed without assistance.

Chest - Oppression and anxiety in chest. Heartbeat and intermissions plainly felt.

Eyes - Weak sight. Features of friends seemed to swim and become indistinct. Objects in room run together without any outlines, can only distinguish some very dark or bright, or large or small images in the field of vision. All objects, especially bright ones, seem in a slightly yellow light.

Face - Paleness and collapsed appearance of face.

Food - Aversion to food.

Limbs - Prostration. Limbs refuse their service, cannot rise from bed without assistance. Phlegmonous inflammation going on to suppuration.

Pulse - Slow, intermittent pulse. Pulse at first normal and regular, then markedly slow, intermittent, dicrotic and then tricrotic. Pulse easily excited by the slightest excitement or physical exertion.

Sleep - No rest on account of distressing nausea and weakness. Restless sleep with partial sleep, interrupted by confused, anxious and frightful dreams.

Stomach - Faint feelings, nausea and discomfort. Carbonated waters and ordinary drinking water aggravated the nausea. Violent vomiting, bilious-colored masses of mucus, preceded, accompanied and followed by retchings.

Vertigo - Faintness, rapid loss of power. Slight vertigo with nausea and faintness.

COMMENTS - Digitox. was proved by Kopfe, who took a single dose of 2 mg. at 10 a. m. It began to take effect in an hour, producing faintness, nausea and slight vertigo, which increased until he was obliged to hurry home at 1 o'clock to avoid vomiting in the street. He was too weak to walk and had to take a carriage. He went to bed immediately and remained in bed three days and part of the fourth. The pulse had remained regular and at the usual rate, 80 to 84, but at 2 o'clock was 58 and intermitting.

Constant excessive nausea preventing sleep. Vomiting dark greenish masses of mucus gave instant relief, which only lasted a short time. Then, the pulse went down to 42 intermitting after every two beats, the heart-beats and intermission being plainly felt in the chest. The limbs refused service in spite of the greatest exertion of will power.

Sight became weak, faces of friends were indistinguishable and he knew them only by their voices. Objects ran together without outlines, so that he could only distinguish some very dark or bright, or large or small images in the field of vision. All objects, especially bright ones, seemed in a slightly yellow light.

Yellow vision was persistent, lasting eight days. The nausea continued and was aggravated by drinking champagne, aerated waters and ordinary water. The second night was very restless with partial sleep interrupted four times in an hour by confused, anxious dreams and frightful fantasies. In the evening of the third day he was able with effort to eat a little and did not vomit.

On the fourth day he was up a little and felt better, was able to eat a little meat and drink as much water as he wished. On the fifth day he was able to walk out a little, leaning on the arm of another. During the three succeeding days the symptoms gradually disappeared. With sound sleep and extraordinary appetite, physical strength and normal vision returned.

In some experiments made on dogs, it was noted that subcutaneous injections were invariably followed with phlegmonous inflammation proceeding to suppuration.

RELATIONS - ***Compare:*** (1) Dig. - worse from drinking is marked in both. (2) Digitalinum, Cina and Santonine in yellow vision.

REFERENCES - Clarke.

DIOSCOREA VILLOSA
(Wild Yam)

PHARMACY - dios. Dioscorea villosa. Wild yam. Dioscorein. N. O. Dioscoreaceae. ***Parts:*** Tincture of fresh root or trituration of resinoid, Dioscorein. ***Historical dose:*** Tincture and all potencies.

CLINICAL - Abdomen, pains. Acne. Angina pectoris. Biliousness. Chorea. Colds. ***Colic, pains.*** Constipation. Coughs. Cramps. Diarrhea. Dysentery. Dysmenorrhea. Dyspepsia. Dyspnea. Enteralgia. Felons. Flatulence. ***Gallstone, colic.*** Gallbladder, disorders. Headaches. Hemorrhoids. Knee, pain. Leg, pain. Liver, disorders. Lumbago. Mental, disorders. ***Menstrual, cramps. Neuralgias.*** Paronychia. Parotiditis. Pregnancy, heartburn. ***Kidney stone. Kidney colic.*** Rheumatism. Sciatica. Spinal irritation. Spleen, pains. Smell, disordered. Spermatorrhea. Stomach, pain. Tea, effects. Toothache. Whitlow.

HOMEOPATHIC - Burt, who made a proving of this remedy, said "The grand sphere for the use of Dioscorea is among colic of the intestines and stomach, where the celiac and umbilical plexuses are in a state of great hyperesthesia, the pain and spasm being unbearable."

Dios. resembles Coloc. in colicky pains, but is better by stretching out and by moving about, while Coloc. is better bending double and worse by motion. ***Colic pain, better from bending backwards. Gallstone colic.*** Kidney colic.

Pains are remittent and paroxysmal. ***Pains are unbearable, sharp, cutting, twisting, griping, grinding,*** that dart about or radiate to distant parts. Pains suddenly cease in one part, then start in another part. Nervous shuddering from pain.

Pain in the bowels, spasmodic, twisting, writhing, drawing, lancinating, pulsating, burning. Pains radiate upwards and downwards. Frequent sharp, darting pains from one part to another. Pains spread, especially from abdomen to distant parts.

Flatulence after meals in stomach or bowels. Violent colic from fasting, some excess in eating, or some dietary error, as eating old cheese or uncooked fruit, pastry, etc., especially if they are great tea drinkers.

Acts on the nerves, abdominal, sciatic and on spinal cord. Chorea with seminal emissions. Painful disorders of abdominal or pelvic viscera. Persons of feeble digestive powers, tea-drinkers with much flatulence. Useful for whitlow.

MIND - Cross, nervous and easily troubled. Depressed after seminal emissions. Uses wrong words, opposite, putting right for left or vice versa. Calls things by wrong names.

Conversation aggravates. Fear in a crowd. Fear of people. Aversion to women. Restlessness better walking. Feels tired, yet still keeps walking around room.

Abdomen - Colic, pains radiate from abdomen to back, chest, arms. ***Colic, worse bending forwards*** and while lying. ***Colic, better bending backwards***, walking about. Twisting and sharp, cutting pains in bowels. Excessive flatulent colic, after excess in eating, errors in diet, or in tea drinkers. Flatulent distension after meals in persons of weak digestion. Rumbling with emission of much flatus. Side pains. ***Pains suddenly shift to different parts, appear in remote localities, as fingers and toes***. Pains in a small spot. Griping, cutting in hypogastric region with intermittent cutting in stomach and small intestines. Bowels sore and tender on pressure. Abdomen tympanitic and very sensitive to pressure. Pressure causes rumbling.

Back - Lameness in back, in morning. Lameness worse stooping. Dull pain in back of neck, stiff. ***Severe backache.*** Sharp pains in the back. Spinal cord feels bruised all the way up and down. Spinal hyperesthesia. Itching over right scapula. Drawing pains in sacrum, sacroiliac joint.

Breasts - Pain in region of nipples.

Causations - Ill effects of excessive eating, tea drinking, fasting. Masturbation. Errors in diet.

Chest - Angina pectoris with labored breathing and feeble action of the heart. Chest pains radiate to both the arms. ***Pain along sternum and extending into arms***. Tight feeling all along sternum. Chest doesn't seem to expand on breathing. Burning behind top of sternum.

Constitutions - Suited to persons of feeble digestive powers, old or young.

Cough - Hacking cough from irritation and tickling low down in throat. Cough with pain in epigastrium. Cough with dull pain in temples, brownish-yellow tongue, weak knees.

Ears - Dull, pressing pains in front of both ears. Both ears feel suddenly stopped up, and are sore to touch. Sharp pain in front and behind the ears. Pains in ears, worse blowing nose or coughing. Itching in internal ears, worse right. Nausea felt in ears. Small balls of wax fall out. Buzzing noise in head. Ringing, buzzing, during headache.

Eyes - Eyes weak, sore and smarting. Sharp pain from right eye to occiput. As if a round ball or stick in the eyes. Hot air steaming out of them. Lachrymation, hot tears, smarting, wants to keep lids closed. Eyelids stiff in morning. Agglutination of the lids mornings.

Face - Full, grinding, drawing, digging or sharp, darting pains at angle of left lower jaw. Spasmodic closing of jaws, biting tongue when neither eating nor drinking. Lips dry, commissures sore. Little pimples with black heads. Corners of mouth sore. Soreness and sharp aching pain in both parotid glands.

Female - ***Violent dysmenorrhea, pains radiate from the uterus.*** Dysmenorrhea, spasmodic uterine colic, pains suddenly fly to distant parts. False labor pains. After-pains. Cramps in fingers and toes alternating with uterine pains. Pregnancy with severe pain with cramps in fingers and toes, alternating with false labor pains.

Food - Disgust for food, with flat, clammy, bitter or sweet taste. Flatulence after meals. Very sleepy after dinner. Thirst during pain in bowels. After eating, nausea and faintness. Colic, after excess in eating, errors in diet, or in tea drinkers.

Head - Dull pain in both the temples. Temples as if squeezed in a vice, better pressure but worse afterwards. Sharp pain in temples. Head feels as if tied with a band. Sensation as if head were crushed down. Digging, cutting pain in the temples in occiput, over eyes. Buzzing in head. Confused, full head. Fullness in head speedily followed by spasmodic pains in abdomen.

Heart - Angina pectoris, pain back of sternum into arms, labored breathing, ***Feeble action of heart.*** Pain through chest and tightness across, especially with flatulence. Sharp pain in region of heart, arrests breathing, worse lying left side. Pulse intermitting.

Kidneys - Kidney colic, pain extending to testicles and the limbs. ***Writhing with crampy pains with passing of kidney stone***. Spasmodic stricture of urethra with pain about navel, better by pressure, pressure on rectum, paroxysmal colic. Constant desire to pass urine.

Limbs - Aching and stiffness in joints. ***Cold limbs during colic.*** Sciatic pain (right) shoot down the thighs with burning or numbness worse motion, sitting up, better standing on toes, lying still. Limbs feel weak, especially knees, after seminal emission. Hamstring seems too short (Cimx.). ***Cramps in flexors of fingers and toes.*** Numbness of left hand. Pain in left shoulder. Grinding in elbows. Panaritium, early stage, pain, pricking, sharp, agonizing. Paronychia. ***Felons*** in beginning, when pricking is first felt.

Liver - ***Sharp pains from liver, shooting upward to right nipple.*** Gallbladder colic, pain extending to the chest, back and arms. ***Gallbladder colic worse bending forward, better bending backwards***.

Lungs - Tight feeling all along sternum. Chest does not seem to expand on breathing. Short-winded. Dyspnea from slight exertion. Hacking cough from irritation and tickling low down in the throat. Cough, with pain in region of umbilicus and temples, brown tongue, weak knees. Dull, aching or sharp, cutting pains in both lungs from front to back or vice versa. Sharp cutting pain from left axilla to nipple and down side deep in lung.

Male - ***Relaxation and coldness of organs***. Pains shoot into testicles from region of kidneys. ***Strong smelling sweat*** on scrotum and pubes. Pain and spasm of spermatic cord. Erections lasting all night. Diminished sexual desire. Emission of semen during sleep. Seminal emission without erection, then weakness, especially in the knees. Constant excitement of genitals.

Modalities - ***Better from stretching out***. Better standing erect. ***Better bending back.*** Better motion, hard pressure. Better open air. Worse from tea. Worse eating. Worse night. ***Worse lying down.*** Worse evening. ***Worse bending forwards***. Worse seminal emissions.

Mouth - Mouth dry and bitter in morning. Bitter, bad taste. Dry mouth, but full of sticky mucus, no thirst. Saliva runs out while asleep. Soreness of gums and roof of mouth. Spasmodic closure of the jaw.

Nose - Soreness of nostrils. Irritation of nasal passages with much sneezing. Nose stopped up, dry. Discharge of bright red blood from left nostril. Watery discharge. Any bad smell remains in the nose for a long time. Offensive, bad smell in nose as if bilious.

Perspiration - Sweats easily when chilly. Sweat, cold, clammy or of strong odor, on genitals. Sweats from least exertion. Cold, clammy sweat, all over, in angina pectoris.

Rectum - Burning at anus, after loose morning stool. Burning in rectum during stool. Frequent, urgent, hurried desire for stool. Loose stools with much straining. Constipation. Diarrhea, worse in morning, driving out of bed, followed by exhaustion and weakness. Yellowish diarrhea, followed by exhaustion, as if flatus and feces were hot. Very offensive flatulence. ***Alternate constipation and relaxation during pregnancy.*** Stools do not relieve the pain in abdomen. Darting from anus to liver. Itching in rectum. Hemorrhoids with darting pains to liver. Hemorrhoids look like bunches of grapes or red cherries, protrude after stool with pain in anus. Involuntary discharge of slimy mucus from anus. Stools slimy, dark-colored, bilious, very offensive, light mushy. Black, hard, dry, lumpy stool.

Sensations - As if top of head was lifted off. As if temples were in a vice. As if head tied with a band (also neck). As if sticks, etc. in eyes, as if hot air streamed out of them. As if tongue burnt. As if a stone were in stomach. In a small spot in abdomen sensation as if drawn forcibly upward and backward to spine.

Skin - Itching and burning of various parts. Little pimples with black heads. Panaritium, early when pains are sharp and agonizing or when pricking is felt. Brittle nails.

Sleep - Sleeplessness from too intent thinking. Restless after 2 a. m., must move, yet it hurts, he is so sore. First sleep late, wakes early. Many symptoms are worse after sleep, bitter mouth, pains in bowels, hard beating of heart. Aroused suddenly with slow, but hard beating of heart. Vivid dreams. Dreams of women. Dreams all night. Dreams with seminal emissions.

Stomach - Dyspepsia of a flatulent character, resulting from tea, after excess in eating, errors in diet. Belching of large quantities of offensive gas, sour, bitter gas. Heartburn. Burning in the stomach. Burning, aching pains in stomach during pregnancy. Heartburn in pregnant women. ***Violent, colicky pains, causing desire to bend double, which makes him worse, must walk erect.*** Painful cramps in stomach. ***Hiccoughs***. Neuralgia of stomach. Faint, uneasy feeling at stomach. ***Sinking at the pit*** of the stomach. Sensation as if a stone in stomach. Sharp cramping pain in the pit of the stomach, then belching, hiccough and passing flatus, better standing erect. Gastrodynia. Nausea. Vomiting, heartburn and gastralgia during menses. Vomiting and purging.

Teeth - Pains in front teeth. Sharp aching pain in an upper right molar. Toothache, as if the bare nerve was touched. Soreness of gums. Gums on inner side of front upper teeth swollen.

Temperature - Chills with bitter mouth. Chills with aching bones, backache. Chills pains in lungs, sore throat, etc. Chills commences over left scapula, spreading over back. Chills running down back. Chill on rising. Chills, couldn't get warm.

Throat - Irritation, burning and smarting in throat and fauces. Fauces rough, dry, frequent inclination to swallow, but it causes nausea and shudderings. Belching gas, but throat so dry it prevents the escape of gas. Constricted feeling as from something tight about neck, makes breathing difficult. Itching in left tonsil. Sharp pain in tonsil up to ear. Left tonsil smarts and itches, with inclination to cough. Constant desire to swallow, but it causes nausea and irritated feeling in throat, left side.

Tongue - Heavy brown coating on the tongue, in mornings, no thirst. Sides of tongue sore as if burnt. Bites the tongue, when not eating or drinking. Tip of tongue sore and brown, worse morning.

Vertigo - Vertigo and dizziness, goes to right while walking. Vertigo inclined to fall backward. Faintness, worse sitting up in bed. Vertigo with numbness, worse lying down. Vertigo from onanism. Vertigo with heat in head, with sharp pains in forehead extending to ears.

COMMENTS - Hale considered as a characteristic: "A constant pain, aggravated at regular intervals by paroxysms of intense suffering." Any kind of colic or neuralgia with these characteristics may indicate Dios., which stands in the highest rank among stomach and abdominal remedies with important actions in many other spheres.

Great faintness at stomach. Morning diarrhea. Pains worse at meals, better moving about, cannot sit still. Seminal emissions (passive) with weakness of knees.

According to Cushing's proving, the primary effect of Dios. was to cause strong-smelling perspiration of the genitals, constant excitement with strong and frequent erections day and night, amorous dreams with emissions. Afterwards came relaxed genitals, absence of desire and emissions without erections.

In the female sphere it has frequently cured dysmenorrhea, uterine colic and after-pains, also gastric disorders during pregnancy and the menses.

J. B. Bell pointed out how closely the throat symptoms of Dios. resemble the initial stage of a cold when it has attacked the fauces and before it has spread to the nose or chest.

RELATIONS - ***Antidotes:*** Cham., Camph. Tamus belongs to the same N. O. Verat. relieved pain in right temple. ***Compare:*** (1) Coloc. - differs in modalities. (2) Bism., Bry. (3) Nux-v. - stomach, Cham., Coloc., Ip., Kali-bi., Podo., Rhus-t., Rum., Stann., Sulph., (4) Aesc., Aloe., Coll., Nux-v. (hemorrhoids), Sars. (urinary symptoms). (5) Calc., Cann-i. Gels., Calad., Agn., Nux-v. Phos. (sexual organs), Cimic., Aesc., Aloe., Bry., Nux-v. (headache), Sil. (whitlow). Verat., (6) Caps. - pain in ears on coughing.

REFERENCES - Boericke. Clarke. Murphy. Phatak.

DIOSMA LINCARIS

(Buku)

PHARMACY - diosm. Diosma lincaris. Buku. N. O. Rutaceae. Buku from Cape of Good Hope. ***Historical dose:*** Tincture and all potencies.

CLINICAL - Cirrhosis. Diarrhea. Fright. ***Gastro-enteritis.*** Headache. Hematuria. ***Hepatitis. Hysteria.*** Insomnia. Liver, atrophy. Nausea. Night sweats. Splenitis. ***Stomach, pain.*** Vertigo.

HOMEOPATHIC - Diosm. has been used in convulsive or epileptiform attacks and ***hysteria***. Cerebral disorders with dullness or stupefaction. Mental disorders in nervous or ascetic individuals, particularly where there is constant fear of death or erotic or maniacal attacks.

Stomach pain. Gastro-enteritis. Splenitis (Cean.). ***Hepatitis***, cirrhosis or liver atrophy. Hematuria with ovarian or uterine lesions. Sudden fright with trembling and weakness of the legs (La Rota).

COMMENTS - Somnolence, nervous insomnia, night sweats. Violent vertigo. Erratic pains with bad humor, desire to weep or fear of sickness. Headache, chiefly frontal, radiating to the occiput.

Eyes brilliant with lachrymation or itching. Stupefaction with hardness of hearing or noises from aural pressure. Earthy face with disseminated rosaceous eruption.

Crampy pains on ingesting food. Nausea, fetid breath with sensation of emptiness. ***Sensation of meteorism with stinging pains in the spleen***. Painful sensation in the abdomen with pubic pressure, the pressure of clothing becomes insupportable with emission of high-colored, bloody urine. Frequent yellow diarrhea, worse at night.

Sensation of heat or of cold in the hands with convulsive movements of the fingers. Weakness of the legs, aggravated by sitting down. Menses abundant, anticipating, sometimes metrorrhagic in type.

REFERENCES - Boericke.

DIPHTHERIA, PERTUSSIS, TETANUS

(DPT Vaccine)

PHARMACY - dpt. Diphtheria, pertussis, tetanus vaccine. DPT vaccine. Nosodes. ***Historical dose:*** All potencies.

CLINICAL - ***Anorexia.*** Asthma. Attention deficit. Autism. ***Brain, damage.*** Cerebral, palsy. Colds. Colic. ***Coma. Convulsions.*** Coughs. ***Cri, encephalique.*** Delirium. Diabetes. Dyslexia. Emaciation. ***Epilepsy.*** Fevers. ***Flaccid, paralysis.*** Hemolytic, anemia. Hives. Hyperactivity. Hypoglycemia. Infantile, spasms. Influenza. Insomnia. Learning, disabilities. Meningitis, viral. Nasal, congestion. Otitis, media. ***Respiratory, distress. Spasms.*** Speech, disorders. Thrombocytopenia. ***Tremors.*** Tumors. ***Vaccination, reactions.***

HOMEOPATHIC - In addition to the DPT, this vaccine contains formaldehyde, a mercury derivative and aluminum phosphate, and was incubated in animal entrails. Can attack and damage the immune and nervous systems.

DPT vaccinations have been linked to sudden infant death syndrome, brain damage, autism, blindness, epilepsy and death. Learning disabilities and hyperactivity in children. Fevers, febrile convulsions, seizures, and diarrheas. Tendency to colds, flus, earaches, sore throats, etc.

Terrible screams, rigid body with head bent back, eyes open. High pitched, inconsolable crying. Cri encephalique, thin high-pitched eerie wailing.

Persistent crying, continues for hours or days. Brief periods of sleep interrupted by long bouts of screaming.

Insomnia and emaciation. Profound prostration. Anorexia and weight loss. Hemolytic anemia, yellow skin, colorless lips. Respiratory distress, asthma, coughs, etc.

Brain damage, comas, seizures and blindness. Dyslexia. Visual perception problems, auditory processing deficit, fine motor delay, and an attention span deficit. Learning disabilities. Cerebral palsy. Viral meningitis.

MIND - Brain damaged children. Learning disabilities. Autism. Dyslexia, visual perception problems, auditory processing deficit. Hyperactivity, restless. Explosive, out of control emotions. Unable to sit still for more than a few minutes, cries easily without warning. Screaming temper tantrums. Cri encephalique.

Timid, nervous trembling fearful child. Passive, in a daze as if sleepwalking. Doesn't want to be held, rocked or fed. Screaming as if afraid of being dropped. Runs around the house and hid as if was frightened to death. Sudden fear while playing, with desire to be held. A great feeling of anxiety and doom. Hallucinations. Periods of unconsciousness. Coma.

Back - Arches back when crying, especially if being held.

Blood - Hypoglycemia. Hemolytic anemia. Thrombocytopenia.

Causations - Vaccinations. ***Reactions to the DPT vaccine.***

Constitutions - Delicate and sensitive children with a weak, damaged or undeveloped immune system.

Ears - Chronic ear infections. Auditory processing deficit. Deafness.

Eyes - Eye twitching. Visual perception problems. Hallucinations. Blindness.

Food - ***Anorexia*** and chronic weight loss. Pushes the food away. Hypoglycemia. Allergies to milk.

Head - Head bent back with a rigid body. Viral meningitis.

Limbs - Loss of muscle control. Spasms of lower limbs. ***Flaccid paralysis.*** Hemiplegia. Hemiparesis. Paresis.

Lungs - ***Respiratory distress.*** Pneumonia. Bronchial asthma. Dyspnea. Spasmodic coughs day and night. Prolonged coughing attacks. Croupy hard cough with vomiting, must sit up. The coughs are like whooping cough.

Modalities - Worse at night. Worse during sleep. ***Worse after vaccinations.***

Mouth - Speech disorders.

Nose - Nasal congestion. Allergies, worse spring and fall. Constant runny nose, clear discharge. Nosebleed.

Rectum - Chronic diarrhea, yellow, curdy, strange smelling, offensive, and curdish. Dark green, almost black diarrhea, with clumps of mucus. Violent, explosive gas every few minutes.

Skin - Local reaction to injection, pain, redness. Hives. Red, purple, hot, swollen, walnut-size lump. Induration. Abscess. Swelling of face hands and feet.

Sleep - Excessive sleepiness. Deep stuporous sleep, unable to be awakened. Brief periods of sleep interrupted by long bouts of high pitched screaming.

Stomach - Projectile vomiting. Anorexia and chronic weight loss.

Temperature - Fever occurring rapidly. Fever with hallucinations, convulsions.

Throat - Sore throat.

COMMENTS - Harris Coulter recorded some reactions to DPT vaccines in his book *A Shot In The Dark*: "Child collapses with white or ashen skin, and death-like unconsciousness. She'd turn blue and didn't appear to be breathing. She'd start breathing on being shaken with white skin and blue or purple blue around the mouth going to death. Nonresponsive, limp, flaccid, with screaming eyes rolled back in his head.

"Sitting, staring ahead with eyes dilated and mouth open, her lips were blue and her body stiff. The right side of her body would tremble and she'd occasionally make sucking sounds. Brief 'generalized bending' or 'jack knife' spasms with sudden forward dropping of the head with adduction and flexion of the arms.

"After a short period of staring, dropping head to chest and falling asleep with eyes open, progressed to starring and sudden violent jerking of upper body forward. Her hands would go straight up in the air, her feet would go straight out, she would clench her fists and hold her breath for 2 to 3 seconds, and then cry a high shrill cry."

"Tremor of intensity" in the hands and feet. "Opens eyes and mouth and utters a brief shout shortly after falling asleep" with or without fever. "Generally tonic-clonic, resistant to routine anticonvulsant therapy, and with poor intellectual prognosis." Difficult or impossible to control with medication. Chronic seizures, grand mal, petit mal and localized.

RELATIONS - To antidote the bad effects of DPT shots consider one of the following: Acute reactions - Ledum, Apis, Hyper., Bell., Cic., DPT in potency. Chronic reactions - Sil., Thuj., DPT in potency. ***Compare:*** (1) Diphtherinum., Pertussin. (2) Silica, Thuja. (3) Cham., Bell., Mosch., Nat-m., Apis, Cicuta, Cupr., Zinc.

REFERENCES - Coulter.

DIPHTHERINUM

(Diphtheria Nosode)

PHARMACY - diph. Diphtherinum. Diphtheria nosode. Trituration of diphtheric membrane. Dilutions of diphtheria toxin. ***Historical dose:*** All potencies.

CLINICAL - Anorexia. ***Bronchitis***. ***Colds***. Croup. ***Diphtheria. Diphtheria, paralysis.*** Emaciation. Myelitis. Nosebleed. ***Paralysis.*** Polyneuritis. Prostration. ***Sore, throat***. Tachycardia. ***Tonsillitis. Vaccination, effects.***

HOMEOPATHIC - Diphtherinum is useful as a prophylactic in diphtheria, post-diphtheria complications like ***paralysis***, or when the ***diphtheria vaccination*** was used. Adapted to scrofulous individuals and patients prone to catarrhal disorders of respiratory organs.

Diphtheria, laryngeal diphtheria. ***Post-diphtheria paralysis***. Painless diphtheria, symptoms almost or entirely objective. Patient too weak, apathetic or too prostrated to complain. Sopor or stupor, but easily aroused when spoken to (Bapt., Sulph.). Relapsing diphtheria.

Patients with weak or exhausted vitality, hence are extremely susceptible to the virus, when the attack from the onset tends to malignancy (Lac-c., Merc-cy.). Glands swollen, tongue red and swollen, breath and discharge very offensive. Diphtheria membrane is thick, dark. Nosebleed, profound prostration. Swallows without pain, but fluids are vomited or returned by the nose.

Tendency to colds and bronchitis, palpitations. ***Severe sore throats, and inflamed tonsils.*** Catarrhal disorders of the respiratory passage. Offensive discharges. Internal trembling. Emaciation and chilliness. Jerking in single muscles. Drawing in muscles, then sudden snap. Carphology.

MIND - Prostrated, yet restless without any pain. Wants to be held. Sees imaginary objects. Carphology. Sopor, stupor, but easily aroused when spoken to.

Abdomen - Pain in the epigastric region.

Constitutions - Adapted to strumous diathesis, scrofulous, psoric or tubercular persons, prone to catarrhal disorders of throat and respiratory mucus membranes.

Eyes - Troubles of accommodation. Short sight. Sees visions.

Face - Pale. Flushed, center of cheeks purple.

Food - Anorexia.

Head - Moisture at the margin of hair.

Heart - Paleness with palpitations. Tachycardia. Hypotension, adyamia.

Limbs - Polyneuritis. Paralysis. ***Post-diphtheria paralysis***. Paresis of the lower limbs. Sensitive motor nerves of the lower limbs.

Lungs - Dyspnea. ***Bronchitis***. ***Colds***. Croup. Harsh cough, voice lost. Persistent, humid cough with bad smelling, fetid expectorations. Difficulty to expectorate, worse at night, especially in children and old persons.

Modalities - Better from heat. Better in bed. Better cold. Better drinking milk in sips. Worse from lying down. Worse movement.

Mouth - Moist, red and swollen tongue, with red tip or dark red spot. Red papillae.

Nose - Mucus coryza. Yellow thick nasal discharge. Bad smelling, nasal crusts with fetid secretion. Reflux of liquids by the nose or while vomiting. Nosebleeds. Fanning of the alae nasi with snoring.

Rectum - Constipation.

Skin - Dry, hot palms, feel withered. Dry skin.

Sleep - Talks in sleep with open eyes.

Stomach - Faintness, better sips of milk.

Temperature - Low temperature, chilliness with palpitations, hypotension. Chilly, then hot. Subfebrile state.

Throat - ***Painless diphtheria***. Relapsing diphtheria. ***Obstinate tonsillitis***. Throat is red, swollen, dark. Big tonsils with false membranes. Thick, gray membrane, on tonsil (left). Swallows without pain, but fluids are vomited or returned through the nose. Wants cold air down the throat or craves cold drinks.

COMMENTS - The potencies of this nosode are prepared either from the diphtheria bacteria or membranes from an affected patient. It was first made from the membrane from a case of malignant diphtheria, triturated with milk sugar to the 6c, then potentized by Swan.

Diphtherinum has cured of diphtheria and post-diphtheria disorders to its credit. These potencies have been very effective not only in malignant diphtheria but in many cases of post-diphtheria paralysis and nervous disorders following the use of anti-toxin.

Clarke wrote that, in diphtheria, the malignancy is present from the start. The well-known features of diphtheria must be the guide to the use of this nosode. He noted that it will, most likely, be found useful in the paralysis of diphtheria and other similar spinal affections.

O. A. Julian described his own research and clinical experiences as a practicing doctor in his village between 1935 and 1939 where he had to treat cases of diphtheria.

The indications he gave are chiefly clinical, including a fluctuating temperature, very little pain, membrane in vertical folds on posterior wall of throat. When the membrane first appeared, it spread forward as far as the border of the tonsils and began to fade and disappear first from the center of posterior pharynx.

Diphtheria (Apis., Lac-c.). Ailments from the diphtheria vaccination, especially extreme exhaustion or weakness. Can be used prophylactically during an epidemic, for someone who has been exposed to diphtheria. Can be useful in severe sore throats, strep throat.

Dark red swelling of tonsil and palatine arches. Parotid and cervical glands greatly swollen. Offensive breath and discharges from throat, nose and mouth. Tongue swollen, very red, with little coating. Diphtheria membrane is thick, dark gray or brownish black. Swallows without pain, but fluids are vomited or returned by the nose.

Temperature low or subnormal, pulse weak and rapid. Limbs cold with marked debility. Patient lies in a semi-stupid condition, eyes dull, besotted (Apis., Bapt.). Nosebleeds or profound prostration from very onset of attack (Ail., Apis., Carb-ac.), collapse almost at very beginning (Crot., Merc-cy.). Pulse weak but rapid, vital reaction very low.

RELATIONS - ***Compare:*** (1) Diphtherotoxin - chronic bronchitis with rales. Cartier suggests it in the vago-paralytic forms of Bronchitis of the aged or in toxic bronchitis after grip. (2) DPT vaccine.

REFERENCES - Boericke. Clarke. Murphy. Phatak.

DIRCA PALUSTRIS

(Leatherwood)

PHARMACY - dirc. Dirca palustris. Leatherwood. Moosewood. Wicopy. N. O. Thymelaceae. Tincture of inner bark of branches. ***Historical dose:*** Tincture and all potencies.

CLINICAL - Colic. Constipation. Cough. Debility. Diarrhea. Dyspepsia. Eyes, disorders. Flatulence. Headaches. Heart, disorders. Neuralgia. Rheumatism.

HERBAL - Dirca palustris belongs to the same family as Daphne Indica and Mezereum and is the only American member of the family. Dirca has symptoms showing its relationship to the other two, but it has not been used extensively in practice.

HOMEOPATHIC - Dirc. is a gastro-intestinal irritant inducing salivation, vomiting and purgation. Cerebral hyperemia, neuralgic pains with depression, palpitations and dyspnea.

MIND - Time seemed to pass slowly. Absent-minded.

Abdomen - Burning below umbilicus. Lancinations in the left hypochondrium with tympanites. Dull ache low down in pelvis, bearing down, not better by sitting or lying. Rumbling in bowels. Burning and uncomfortable sensation in bowels. Colic better bending forward and better by stool, but smarting in anus remains.

Back - Heavy pain across back and through loins in region of kidneys.

Bladder - Pain and soreness in region of bladder.

Eyes - Eyes sore and painful to touch. Photophobia on waking, continuing all day, especially from gaslight. Lids heavy. Sensation as if brows corrugated and as if brain were also drawn down.

Face - Face red, full and bloated in morning.

Female - Uterus seems too low and as if it would prolapse during stool. Menses two days too early, less copious and prolonged than usual.

Food - No thirst.

Head - Pains all through the head, extending down into spine. Headache in temples extending inwards, better by hard pressure. Headache, throbbing and beating, worse by coughing or moving. Scalp feels dry and tight.

Heart - Excitability of heart's action from least motion. Palpitations on going up slight elevation. Pulse suddenly becomes weak and irregular.

Limbs - Dull, neuralgic pain in both shoulders, cannot keep them still. Neuralgic pains in legs. Muscles of thighs sore and stiff.

Lungs - Sharp pain in right thorax running down into abdomen and up into left shoulder. Great dyspnea from exertion, from walking up a slight elevation. Cough, worse morning, raising offensive, sweetish-tasting mucus.

Modalities - Colic better by bending forward, headache better by pressure. Pains in the bowels are better by stool. Motion aggravates most symptoms, walking aggravates vertigo and pain in bowels.

Mouth - Tongue coated smoothly and evenly white, dirty. Sour taste.

Rectum - Throbbing, stitching pains in anus. Soreness and smarting, worse after stool. Tenesmus and straining. Constipation, urgent desire, but passes only frothy mucus. Dry, sticky feces. Diarrhea stools, sudden, gushing, watery, thin, yellowish fecal.

Sleep - Sleepy, but unable to sleep. Dreams of dead bodies.

Stomach - Empty belchings. Uneasy feeling as if a lump or weight in stomach.

Throat - Stinging pains in larynx from without inwards, very sharp pricking pain and sensation of suffocation. Throat red, raw, acrid feeling, hurts to swallow food or liquids.

Vertigo - Vertigo on walking, seems as if he would fall to left.

COMMENTS - Vital depression, neuralgic pains in the head, trunk and limbs, many of the pains proceeding from without inward. Oppression and pains in the chest. Excitability of the heart's action from the slightest motion.

Disordered digestion. Weight at the stomach. Moist, white coated tongue. Sweetish expectoration. Rumbling of flatulence, colic better by bending forward, diarrhea and tenesmus, later constipation. Hot and restless at night, cannot sleep, dreams of dead bodies.

RELATIONS - ***Compare:*** (1) Cann-i. - time passes slowly. (2) Ant-c. - tongue, Lyc. - constipation and flatulence. (3) Bry., Puls., Abies-n. - weight at stomach. (4) Stann. - sweet expectoration.

REFERENCES - Clarke.

DOLICHOS PRURIENS

(Cowhage)

PHARMACY - dol. Dolichos pruriens. Cowhage. Mucuna pruriens. Cow-itch. N. O. Leguminosae. Papilionoideae. Trituration or tincture of whole pod. ***Historical dose:*** Tincture and all potencies.

CLINICAL - Bedwetting. ***Bloated, abdomen.*** Colic. ***Constipation***. Cough. Dentition. Gums, pain. ***Hemorrhoids.*** Hepatitis. Herpes, zoster. Hodgkin's disease. ***Itching***. Jaundice. Jaw, pain. Neuralgias. ***Pruritus. Senile, pruritus. Sore, throat.*** Worms.

HOMEOPATHIC - General ***intense itching without eruption,*** worse by scratching. Itching of the skin without the appearance of a rash or swelling. Itching is better from cold water, but it burns the skin and causes trembling. ***Senile pruritus.*** Itching excessively at night.

Neuralgia following herpes zoster. Exalted nervous sensibility, as in dentition. Gums intensely sensitive, seem to itch. Pain in the throat on right side below angle of jaw as if a splinter were embedded vertically in it. Yellow spots all over. Jaundice. Hemorrhoidal diathesis. A right-sided medicine with pronounced liver and skin symptoms.

Abdomen - ***Bloated***, swollen abdomen with constipation. Colic from getting feet wet. Pain in abdomen in right lumbar region. Bruised pain below umbilicus. Bruised pain left inguinal region. Pains in spleen with gravel.

Back - Pain over right carotid artery, as if a splinter was sticking there. Pain in muscles on right side of neck. Pain under left scapula continuing until herpes zoster breaks out.

Chest - Pains through the apices of both lungs. Eruption on left axilla, spreading in rings forward to sternum and back to spine with much burning and smarting. Herpes zoster.

Constitutions - Psoric and allergic constitutions.

Ears - Sudden dart of pain in right ear, later in left.

Eyes - Eyes yellow. Pain in right eye. Eruption on margin of eyelids.

Face - Face yellow. Circumscribed redness of one cheek. Swelling of face, especially of lips. Prickling, itching of face. Pain in right maxilla.

Kidneys - Bedwetting with gravel. Small stones pass away. Ischuria with or without gravel.

Limbs - Dry, tettery eruptions on arms and legs, resembling herpes zoster. Aching pain in right arm and shoulder. Pain on the top of right shoulder. Aching soreness in last phalanx of right middle finger. Pain at root of nail of right index finger.

Liver - Hepatitis. Jaundice. Swelling of liver, pain goes through from left lobe. Liver problems with itching.

Lungs - Coughs on lying down at night, with wheezing and dyspnea.

Male - Impotence.

Modalities - Worse at night. Worse scratching. Worse right side. Warmth aggravates itching at night. Cold water burns on the itching skin. Colic from getting feet wet.

Mouth - Strong taste of blood in mouth with cough. Gums irritated, wants them continually rubbed, dentition. Pain in gums prevents sleep. Soreness and tenderness of gums, even in teething children. Dull aching in a carious tooth, right side.

Pregnancy - Intolerable itching all over body in pregnant women, worse at night, preventing sleep, worse from scratching, no perceptible eruption on the skin.

Rectum - ***Constipation with intense itching***. Constipation with liver complaint, during teething or pregnancy. White stools. Tenesmus with looseness of bowels. Pain in anus with stool. ***Hemorrhoids*** with burning sensation. Worms, threadworms.

Skin - Violent itching all over body without any visible eruption, swelling or rash, worse across shoulders, about elbows and knees, and hairy parts. Itching excessively at night. Skin burns at night in bed. Herpes zoster. Jaundice, skin yellow in spots or all over.

Sleep - Burning in skin is intolerable at night in bed. Sleepless.

Stomach - Noisy movement of flatus in stomach. Flatulent eructation. Vomits bile.

Throat - ***Pain in throat,*** worse swallowing, below right angle of jaw, ***as if splinter were imbedded vertically***. Pain in right throat, a subdued, contraction sensation, went to left side. Sudden sensation of a choking lump in throat. Slight fullness just behind posterior palatine arch. Roughness of throat.

COMMENTS - Dry skin with severe itching without eruption, can scratch until they bleed (Alum.). Scratching increases the itching. Violent itching that prevents the person from sleeping at night. Restless. Severe idiopathic pruritus. Senile pruritus, yellow spots on the skin. Shingles, and pain after shingles (Mez., Rhus-t.). Herpes zoster.

Itching with jaundice, hepatitis, liver involvement. Hepatitis. Jaundice. Gas and bloating (Lyc.), rumbling in the abdomen. Constipation, hemorrhoids. Worms. Ailments from a food allergy that aggravated the liver. Hodgkin's disease. Worse tight clothing (Lyc., Chin.), at night, in the heat of the bed. Generally a right sided remedy.

Kraft recorded a striking cure with Dol. 1,200c of a woman who had symptoms of jaundice, white stools and desperate itching, preventing sleep at night. There was in addition, enormous distention of abdomen with continuous rattling of gas, intolerance of anything tight around neck or body intense restlessness, unable to sit still a minute.

RELATIONS - Aconite antidotes it, and in "cases of dentition with fever Aconite should be given before Dolichos to prevent convulsions" (Hering). Dolichos follows Rhus-t. in herpes. ***Compare:*** (1) Rhus-t. cured herpes zoster after failure of Rhus-t. (2) Fago., Bell. - dentition. (3) Arg-n., Hep., Nit-ac. - throat. (4) Cann-i. - time passes slowly. Ant-c. - tongue. (5) Lyc. - constipation and flatulence. (6) Bry., Puls., Abies-n. - weight at stomach. (7) Stann. - sweet expectoration.

REFERENCES - Boericke. Clarke. Murphy. Phatak.

DORYPHORA DECEMLINEATA

(Colorado Potato-bug)

PHARMACY - dor. Doryphora decemlineata. Colorado potato-bug. Leptinotarsa decemlineata. Colorado Beetle. N. O. Coleoptera. Insecta. Tincture prepared by covering the crushed live beetles with alcohol. ***Historical dose:*** Tincture and all potencies.

CLINICAL - Backache. Delirium. Diarrhea. Diphtheria. Dysentery. Erysipelas. Fevers. Gastric, disorders. Gleet. Gonorrhea. ***Kidneys, disorders.*** Myxedema. Parotiditis. Spleen, pain. Typhoid. Ulcerations. Urethritis.

HOMEOPATHIC - Doryphora in its general effects bears a strong resemblance to Cantharis. An extensive proving has been made and to this have been added the effects of poisoning from handling the insects and from inhaling the vapor when they have been burned or scalded.

Two children inhaled vapor from a kettle in which some beetles had been placed, one died and the other recovered after a serious illness resembling typhoid fever. Local application causes ulceration.

The blood will not coagulate, blood globules disorganized, enormous swelling of the whole body, swelling of the feet with burning, elastic swelling of whole body which will not pit on pressure (suggesting its applicability in myxedema).

Acts on the urinary organs. ***Burning sensations.*** Burning and inflammation of glans penis. Burning in mouth, throat, gullet, stomach, abdomen, rectum and urinary passages (Canth.), strangury with urethritis and itching. Urethritis in children from local irritation. Gonorrhea and gleet.

Swelling of body. A feeling of weight or heaviness. Great trembling in limbs. Fainting, weakness, prostration, collapse. Weakness, worse by talking (Stan.). Prostration after typhoid and diphtheria have been cured.

MIND - Irritability. Bad temper. Delirium, talkative. Stupor with muttering and loud rumbling in bowels.

Abdomen - Abdomen feels heavy, sore and tender, burning. Pain in spleen. Pain in bowels, worse by eating and drinking and by deep inspiration. Rumbling in bowels (with stupor).

Back - Pain in lumbar region.

Chest - Soreness and oppression of chest with sore throat.

Eyes - Eyes red, sore, protruding, pupils much dilated, sight much impaired.

Face - Face bloated and red, giving appearance of a confirmed drunkard.

Food - Loss of appetite, great thirst. Craving for something sour, symptoms worse by smoking.

Kidneys - Difficult urination. Retention of urine. Dysuria with burning, stinging pain. Urethritis. Urethra inflamed with excruciating pain when urinating. Pain in back and loins. Gonorrhea.

Limbs - Severe trembling in limbs, especially right arm and leg.

Male - Itching and burning of glans penis, which is swollen and bluish red. Urethra inflamed with severe pain, especially when urinating.

Modalities - Better in open air. Worse from smoking. Worse warm room. Worse motion. Worse pressure aggravates (pain in kidneys).

Mouth - Violent heat in mouth. Dark brown coating on tongue. Offensive taste. Parotiditis.

Rectum - Morning diarrhea with pain in abdomen and burning in rectum. Bloody, slimy stools. Heaviness, intense pain in rectum.

Skin - An abraded surface on the wrist of one engaged in picking the bugs became painful, a deep sloughing ulcer developed and the bones were laid bare.

Sleep - Sleepless until 12 a.m., then restless sleep with terrifying dreams. Tossing about all night. While sleeping, wild dreams, screams as if in great distress.

Stomach - Nausea and vomiting. Vomits dark, grumous acrid matter of dirty brown fluid with diarrhea.

Temperature - Skin alternately cold, clammy and hot with fever. Coldness of hands and feet. High fever during night, restless and sleepless. Violent fever 8 a.m. to 2 p.m.

Throat - Dry feeling in throat with desire to swallow. Throat raw and constricted. Burning in throat and down esophagus with stomachache and cough.

RELATIONS - The local effect is ***antidoted by:*** earth, other antidotes are: vinegar and other vegetable acids, Stram. ***Compare:*** (1) Agar., Ail., Apis, Canth., Crot-h., Lach. (2) The Solanaceae. generally, as the beetle partakes of the properties of the plants it infests. (3) In non-coagulation of the blood, Hirudo.

REFERENCES - Boericke. Clarke.

DROSERA ROTUNDIFOLIA

(Round-leaved Sundew)

PHARMACY - dros. Drosera rotundifolia. Round-leaved sundew. Drosera longifolia. N. O. Droseraceae. Tincture of active fresh plant. ***Historical dose:*** Tincture and all potencies.

CLINICAL - Amblyopia. Anxiety. ***Asthma. Bronchitis.*** Catarrhs. Colic. ***Coughs.*** Coxalgias. Delusions. Epilepsy. Fears. Hemorrhage. Headaches. Hoarseness. ***Laryngitis.*** Measles. Nausea. Sciatica. ***Tuberculosis.*** Vomiting. ***Whooping, cough***.

HOMEOPATHIC - Teste, who placed Drosera in his Zincum group of medicines, mentioned that it grows in damp prairies, along the border of marshes and is avoided by animals. Barrich stated that when eaten by sheep it gives them a fatal cough.

Hahnemann noted Dros. was the principal remedy for ***whooping cough***. It was recommended by German physicians of the eighteenth century as a panacea for hoarseness, chest disorders and even for tuberculosis.

Markedly affects the respiratory organs. Spasmodic, catarrhal and hemorrhagic effects. ***Spasmodic cough resembling whooping cough.*** Whooping cough, spasmodic cough of tuberculosis. Frequent spells of barking cough, worse evening and after midnight, where the patient holds his side. Every effort to raise a little phlegm ends in retching and vomiting, vomits if he cannot get up phlegm.

Spasmodic and constricting pains in the abdomen, larynx, throat, chest, and hypochondria. Crawling in larynx. Feeling as if a soft substance were lodged in larynx, as a feather. Difficulty swallowing solids. Voice fails.

Hemorrhages of bright red blood from nose and mouth (bloody saliva). Hemorrhages with vomit, stool, or expectoration. Bleeding, burning ulcers, cutting pains. Prickling, burning, itching eruptions, worse undressing, better scratching. Lancinations in brain. Convulsions. Epileptic attacks with rigidity, after, twitching limbs, hemoptysis and sleep.

Sticking sharp pains. Gnawing, stinging pains in joints and long bones. Pains about hip joints. Sciatica with "pressing pains, worse from pressure from stooping from lying on painful part, better after rising from bed." Stitches from left loin into penis, itching stitches in glans.

MIND - Self-willed, obstinate, insists upon carrying out his plans. Pertinacity in executing resolutions. Very irritable. Easily angered, a trifle makes him besides himself. Impatience. Restlessness. Extremely uneasy. Can't concentrate on one subject, must change, changes to something else.

Anxiety when alone. Anxiety with flushes of heat. Anxiety respecting the future. Anxiety in evenings. Dread of the night. Fear of ghosts. Fears being alone, but suspicious of friends. Great mistrust.

Depressed mood, with gloomy forebodings. Homesickness. Discouraged. Sadness when alone in daytime. Delusions of persecution. Imagines he was being deceived by spiteful, envious people. Inclination to drown oneself. Anxiety in evening, as if it would impel him to commit suicide by drowning.

Abdomen - Colic after taking acids, sour foods. Anxious feeling in hypochondria. Pains in the hypochondria, on coughing and on being touched. Must press on pain with the hand when he coughs.

Back - Stiffness at the nape of the neck with pains during movement. Bruise-like pains in the back, particularly early in the morning. Itching stitch in coccyx when sitting. Nape painful to touch. Neck stiff and painful on motion.

Chest - Pains, like a subcutaneous ulceration in the sternum, on pressing upon chest. ***Pains in the chest on coughing*** and on sneezing, has to press his chest with the hand (Bry.). Stitches below axilla. ***Sharp pains in chest when sneezing or coughing.*** Constriction of chest, worse talking, singing. Oppression of the chest, as if something stopped the voice on coughing or speaking, or as if the breath could not be expelled. ***Tightness of the chest on coughing.*** Black pores on chest and shoulder.

Constitutions - Tubercular constitution.

Coughs - Coughs takes breath away. ***Whooping cough.*** Spasmodic, dry irritative cough. ***Attacks follow each other very rapidly***, can scarcely breathe. Cough very deep and hoarse, worse after midnight. ***Deep barking or choking coughs.*** Cough and chokes, worse singing, talking. ***Periodical fits of rapid coughing.*** Harassing and titillating cough in children, not during the day, but commencing as soon as the head touches the pillow at night. ***Prolonged and incessant coughs.*** Cough with violent tickling in larynx arouses one from sleep. Hemoptysis after convulsions. Yellow sputum, with bleeding from nose and mouth. Coughs followed by retching, vomiting.

Ears - Shootings and squeezing in the ears, especially on swallowing. Right internal ear as if painfully pressed together. Sharp pain in ears. Hardness of hearing with buzzing, roaring, humming and drumming in the ears.

Eyes - Eyes very dry. Prominent from coughing, during measles, in convulsions. Shooting in the eyes towards the outside, especially on stooping. Severe sharp pains, from within outward, in eyes. Presbyopia and weakness of the eyes. Photophobia. Suspension of the sight or confusion and paleness of the letters while reading. As if gauze before the eyes. Dazzling by candlelight and daylight. Contraction of the pupils. Pupils first contracted, later dilated.

Face - Cold sweat on forehead. Pale with hollow cheeks and sunken eyes. ***Coldness of left half of face*** with stinging pains and ***dry heat of right half***. Faceache worse pressure and touch. Burning and pricking sensation in the skin of the cheeks, below the eyes. ***Face hot and red with cold hands.*** Pressure in the cheekbones towards the outside, aggravated by pressure and contact. Lips cracked and constantly dry. Small pustules here and there on face with fine stitching sensation, worse when touched. Black pores in the chin.

Female - Delay of first menses. Menses too late. Menses too scanty. Dark blood. Suppressed or retarded menses. Leucorrhea with labor-like pains, spasmodic pains in the abdomen.

Food - Food seems tasteless. Bitter taste of food, especially of bread. Bitter taste of all food during pregnancy. Aversion to pork. Aversion to acids and sour foods. Thirst in the morning. Worse acids and sour foods. Worse after fatty food. Worse tobacco smoke.

Head - Pressive pains in the head, especially in the forehead and cheekbones, sometimes with nausea and dizziness. Painful perplexity of the head, as after loud speaking. Pressing headache with stupefaction and nausea. Headache worse when stooping, better from motion and cold air. Beating and hammering in the forehead. Brain painfully affected by stepping. Pains, as if excoriation in the scalp. Smarting, burning pain in scalp. Corrosive itching on scalp. Itching, gnawing on forepart of scalp, better rubbing.

Kidneys - Frequent, profuse urination. Frequent urging with scanty emission, often drop by drop. Emission of urine at night. Brownish urine of a strong smell. Watery, inodorous urine with fetid stool of white mucus. Urine dark and of strong smell.

Limbs - All limbs feel lame. Bed feels too hard. Limbs feel as if beaten. ***Pain in the long bones.*** Pain in humerus at night only. Paralytic pains in the coxo-femoral joint and thighs. Laming pain in right hip joint and thigh with pain in ankle, must limp when walking. Stiffness in joints of feet. Fingers contract spasmodically with rigidity when grasping anything. Writer's cramp.

Lungs - ***Asthma when talking.*** Asthma with contraction of the throat at every word uttered. Severe dyspnea threatening suffocation. Dyspnea with blueness of face and lips. Dyspnea with cold sweat on forehead. Dyspnea with vomiting of tough mucus. Oppressed breathing, as if holding back the breath. ***Yellow expectoration with bleeding from nose and mouth, retching.*** Bitter, or offensive expectoration. Salty expectoration. Bloody and purulent. Black clotted or bright red frothy blood.

Male - Itching stitches in glans.

Modalities - Better from pressure. Better open air. Better motion. Better sitting up in bed. Better remaining quiet. Worse towards evening. Worse after midnight. Worse on lying down. Worse getting warm in bed, warmth. Worse drinking, cold food. Worse sour things, acids. Worse vomiting. Worse laughing, talking, singing. Worse stooping. Worse after measles. Worse during rest. Worse weeping.

Mouth - Putrid taste. Offensive breath during cough. Bleeding of the mouth. Bloody saliva. Profuse flow of watery saliva. Small round painless swelling in middle of tongue. Shooting pains in teeth from hot drinks. Fine prickings on dorsum of tongue. Stitching, smarting, in right side and tip of tongue. Loss of taste. Ulceration of velum palate. Ulcers on tongue. Whitish ulcer on tip of tongue.

Nose - Profuse fluent coryza, in morning. Constant dryness of the nose. Black pores on the nose. Nosebleed, in the evening. Bleeding from coughing, stooping, on blowing the nose. Painful sneezing. Fluent coryza with sneezing. Sensitive to sour smells.

Perspiration - Warm perspiration at night. Copious sweat all over body. Sweats with cough bringing on violent retching. Cold sweat, on forehead, face, abdomen and feet. Warm sweat, at night. Sweats after midnight and in morning hours. Perspires immediately on waking from sleep.

Rectum - Frequent evacuations of bloody mucus, with cutting pains after the stool in the abdomen and small of the back. Outward pressing in rectum, independent of stool. Frequent stool with colic. Stools, soft fluid. Stools, white, slimy and stinking. Stools, with watery, odorless urine. Discharge of bloody mucus.

Skin - Eruption with painful soreness or stinging. Violent itching, while undressing. Itching better by rubbing or wiping with hand. Prickling, stinging, itching, gnawing in skin. Skin readily peels off when scratching. Measles. Black pores on chest and shoulder. Bleeding, burning ulcers.

Sleep - Sleepless, feels too wakeful. Sleep at noon and in the evening at sunset. Snoring during sleep and when lying on the back. Frequent starts with fright during sleep. Frequent waking with perspiration. Great weariness on waking. Vivid dreams. Anxious dreams. Dreams, over the wrong-doings of others. Dreams of thirst and drinking, awakes, is thirsty and must drink.

Stomach - Shootings and beatings in the pit of the stomach. Clawing sensation in the pit of the stomach. Difficulty in swallowing solid foods. Water brash. Bitter belching. Frequent hiccough. Nausea after fatty foods. Nausea at night or before dinner. Nausea with stupefying pressure in forehead. Vomiting at night and after dinner. Vomiting of blood. Vomiting of bile in the morning. Vomiting of slimy matter and of food during the cough.

Temperature - Too cold, even in bed. Chilliness during the day, heat during the night. Shivers when at rest, better moving. Fever with headache and convulsive cough. ***Fever with whooping cough.*** Measles. Intermittent fever with nausea and inclination to vomit and other gastric sufferings, or with sore throat. Hot face and cold hands with shivering. Thirst in the morning during the hot stage of the fever and not during the cold stage.

Throat - ***Clergyman's sore throat*** with rough, scraping, dry sensation deep in the fauces. ***Hoarseness***, laryngitis. ***Deep, hoarse voice***. Voice, hollow, toneless, cracked, requires exertion to speak. Difficulty swallowing solid food, as from contraction of the throat. Stinging in throat when swallowing. Sensation in the throat, as if crumbs of bread had been stopped in it. Sensation as if a feather in larynx. Hawking of yellowish or greenish mucus. Ulceration of soft palate. Laryngeal tuberculosis with rapid emaciation.

Vertigo - Vertigo when walking in open air. Vertigo with inclination to fall to the ***left side.***

Vision - Farsighted. Weakness of eyes when looking carefully at small things. Quivering before eyes. Dazzling, worse light, daylight or candlelight. Light or glare of fire dazzles before eyes. When reading, letters run together. Frequent vanishing of sight, when reading. Letters look pale and blurred.

COMMENTS - A strong history of use in whooping cough. Spasmodic coughing at night ending in vomiting or nosebleeds. Choking, suffocating cough. Coughing spasms, worse lying down. Patients hold their chest when coughing (Bry.). Hoarseness. Worse after sleep, lying down, and stuffy rooms, better open air.

Indications in the premonitory stage by pallor, weakness, anemia. Pallor of larynx, dry cough. Loss of appetite, emaciation.

Chronic bronchitis, especially in the elderly. Difficulty swallowing during bronchitis or whooping cough, especially solids. Spasmodic croup (Acon., Spong., Hep.). Redness and swelling of mucus membrane covering and between the arytenoid cartilages. Speaker's sore throat (Rhus-t., Arg., Arg-n.).

Raises the resistance against tuberculosis, useful for tuberculosis of the lungs, larynx and bones in the joints. Laryngeal tuberculosis. Tuberculosis with vomiting of food from coughing, with gastric irritation and profuse expectoration. Tubercular glands. Tuberculosis with swollen glands, spasmodic coughing, and coughing up blood.

Dr. Serrand of Paris maintained that Dros. has an important place in the prophylaxis of tubercle.

He noted that sheep eating Drosera leaves acquire a nocturnal cough and die, and that the pleura of cats to which Drosera had been administered were found studded with tubercles. He commended it in cases of declared tuberculosis as well. He gave it in the low potencies.

Buchmann of Alvensleben agreed with Hahnemann that Dros. in high potency should not be often repeated. Buchmann had a bronchial catarrh which used to attack him every spring and fall, characterized by a violent tickling cough, which almost drove him to distraction at night.

Buchmann cured himself with Dros. 1x. and tincture. A single dose as soon as the tickling in the larynx commenced sufficed to allay it at once and allowed him to rest and it was only repeated when the tickling returned.

RELATIONS - ***Antidoted by:*** Camph. ***Compare:*** (1) Bell., Cor-r., Cupr., Hyos., Ip., Samb., Meph., Op., Coc-c. (2) In inability to expectorate, Caust., Sep., Arn., Kali-c. (3) Teste considers Meny. the closest analog. (4) Fluoroform, 2 per cent. watery solution, 2 to 4 drops after paroxysms, considered specific for whooping cough. (5) Ouabain from leaves of Carissa schimperi, an arrow poison - respiratory spasm, whooping cough is cut short in first stage and reduced in frequency of attacks and hastens convalescence. (6) Chel., Corall., Cupr., Cast., Arg-n., Meny. ***Complementary:*** Nux-v. ***Compatible:*** Calc., Puls., Verat., Gnaph.

REFERENCES - Boericke. Clarke. Murphy. Phatak.

DUBOISINUM

PHARMACY - dubin. Duboisinum. Corkwood tree alkaloid. Duboisia myoporoides. Duboisia hopwoodii. N. O. Solanaceae. Queensland. Tincture and solution of alkaloid prepared from extract of the leaves. ***Historical dose:*** Tincture and all potencies.

CLINICAL - Delirium. Drowsiness. Eye, disorders. Locomotor, ataxia. Mouth, dryness. Paralysis. Presbyopia. Pupils, dilated. Throat, dryness. Vertigo. Vision, disorders.

HOMEOPATHIC - Duboisia belongs to the same order as belladonna, and its alkaloid, sulphate of duboisia, has been used as a substitute of atropine. Its application to the eye has caused marked constitutional symptoms of fever, delirium, stupor and dry mouth.

Characteristic dryness of mucus membranes. Cool feeling in the eyes. Feeling of largeness in eyes, tongue. Inability to stand with the eyes shut, locomotor ataxia. Sensation as if stepping on empty space.

COMMENTS - Dubin. has been proved. A symptom which may prove a keynote is " a red spot floating in the field of vision." Guided by this, C. H. Helfrich cured a case of hyperemia of optic nerve with Dubin. 3c.

RELATIONS - ***Antidoted by:*** coffee, lemon juice. ***Compare:*** (1) Bell., Atro., Dulc., Stram. (2) Anhal. - colored vision.

REFERENCES - Boericke. Clarke.

DUBOISIA MYOPOROIDES

(Corkwood Tree)

PHARMACY - dubo-m. Duboisia myoporoides. Corkwood tree. Corkwood elm. N. O. Solanaceae. Queensland. Tincture from the leaves. ***Historical dose:*** Tincture and all potencies.

CLINICAL - ***Conjunctivitis.*** Delirium. Drowsiness. Exophthalmic goiter. Eyes, dilated pupils. Locomotor, ataxia. Mouth, dryness. ***Mydriasis***. Paralysis. Pharyngitis. Presbyopia. Scarlet, fever. Throat, dryness. Vertigo. Vision, disorders.

HOMEOPATHIC - Duboisia acts chiefly on the nervous system, eyes, upper respiratory tract. Recommended in pharyngitis with black, stringy mucus. Palliative for exophthalmic goiter. Dilated pupil. ***Red spot floats in the field of vision.*** On the eye it acts more promptly than Atropine, much stronger as a mydriatic.

Dry mouth. Checked perspiration. Scarlet fever. Headache and drowsiness. ***Vertigo with pale face***, not gastric in origin. Sensation as if stepping on empty space. Locomotor ataxia.

MIND - Memory impaired. Absent-minded. Incoherent. ***Silly and nonsensical.***

Eyes - Acute and chronic ***conjunctivitis***. Hyperemia of retina. Fundus red, blood vessels full and tortuous. Paralysis or weakness of accommodation. ***Mydriasis***. Pupils dilated with dim vision. ***Pain over eye***, between it and brow.

Head - Impossible to stand with eyes shut, tendency to fall backwards.

Limbs - Trembling, numbness and weakness. Loss of power in limbs, staggers, feels as if he stepped on empty space.

Lungs - Larynx dry, hoarse voice, difficult phonation. Dry cough with oppressed breathing.

Vertigo - ***Vertigo with pale face***, not gastric in origin.

RELATIONS - ***Antidotes:*** Morphine, Pilocarp. It antagonizes Muscarine. Hystero-epilepsy. Motor restlessness of insane. It has been used as a substitute for atropine. ***Compare:*** (1) Bell., Stram., Hyos.

REFERENCES - Boericke.

DULCAMARA

(Woody Nightshade)

PHARMACY - dulc. Dulcamara. Woody nightshade. Bitter-sweet. Solanum dulcamara. N. O. Solanaceae. Not to be confounded with "Deadly Nightshade," Belladonna, nor with "Climbing Bitter-sweet," Celastrus. Dulcamara tincture prepared from fresh green stems and leaves, gathered just before flowering. ***Historical dose:*** Tincture and all potencies.

CLINICAL - ***Adenitis.*** Anasarca. Aphonia. Bladder, disorders. Blepharophthalmia. ***Catarrh.*** Cholera. ***Colds.*** Crusta, lactea. Diarrhea. Dropsy. Dysentery. Emaciation. Exostoses. Fevers. ***Glands, swollen.*** Hemorrhages. ***Hay fever.*** Headaches. Hemorrhages. Hemorrhoids. ***Herpes.*** Influenza. Irritation. Lichen. Lumbago. Measles. Meningitis. ***Mononucleosis.*** Muscle, pain. Myelitis. Nettle-rash. Neuralgias. Ophthalmia. Paralyzes. Pemphigus. ***Rheumatism.*** Scarlatina. Scrofula. Stammering. ***Sore, throat. Stiff-neck.*** Tibia, pains. Tongue, disorders. Tonsillitis. Tumor. Typhoid. Urination, difficult. ***Urticaria. Warts***. Whooping cough.

HOMEOPATHIC - The leading indication for Dulcamara is found in its modality, ***worse from cold and damp***. Effects of lying on damp ground (e.g., paralysis), conditions which are worse in cold, damp weather or from changes from hot to cold weather.

Effects of damp weather, colds after exposure to wet, especially diarrhea. Results from sitting on cold, damp ground. Hot days and cold nights toward the close of summer. Patients living or working in damp, cold basements (Nat-s.).

Rheumatic troubles induced by damp cold are aggravated by every cold change, somewhat relieved by moving about. Stiffness, numbness, aching and soreness of muscles on every exposure to cold especially of back and loins.

Tearing pains. Dropsy, anasarca. One-sided spasms with speechlessness. Paralysis of single parts, vocal cords, tongue, etc. Paralyzed parts icy cold. Congestive headache with neuralgia and dry nose.

Adenitis, glands, swollen and indurated. Enlarged glands. Exostoses. Hemorrhages, blood watery or bright red. Eruptions on hands, arms or face around the menstrual period. Griping in bowels around the umbilicus in testes.

MIND - Mental confusion, cannot concentrate. Difficult speech, cannot find the right word. Dullness and painful stupefaction of head. Dullness of senses. Rejects the things asked for. Haughty. Domineering, strong-minded and possessive. Scolds without being angry. Quarrelsome without anger.

Depression. Easily becomes delirious with pain. Restless and impatient. Weeping after hallucinations. Delusions as if bed were sinking. Sees spectres on waking. Impatience in morning. Irritability during daytime. Starting on falling asleep. Throws things away in morning.

Abdomen - Dropsy of abdomen. Eruptions or pain about the navel. ***Cutting pain at navel*** followed by painful, green, slimy stools. Colic from cold. Cold feeling in bowels. Cutting pain about navel, followed by painful, green, slimy stools. Swelling of inguinal glands (Merc.).

Back - Heat and burning in back. ***Pain in small of back***, as after long stooping. ***Backache, worse damp cold weather.*** Lumbar region and sacrum feel cold. Spinal meningitis during scarlatina or measles, eruption doesn't develop. Myelitis after taking cold during menses. Hyperemia of spinal cord. ***Rheumatic affections of spinal cord.*** Swelling of glands of neck. Stiffness and lameness across neck and shoulders after getting cold and wet. Stiff neck.

Bladder - Cystitis. Catarrh of bladder from taking cold. Bladder wall thickened. ***Must urinate when getting chilled***. Frequent urination. Strangury, painful urination. Retention of urine from cold or cold drinks. Involuntary urination from paralysis of bladder. Ischuria from wading with bare feet in cold water. Strangury, painful urination.

Breasts - Breasts, engorged and sore, delicate, sensitive to cold. Sore nipples after weaning. Breasts, swollen with absent menses or leucorrhea. Herpes on breasts in nursing women. Breasts, engorged, hard, sore, with amenorrhea or leucorrhea. Eruptions on skin after weaning. Suppressed milk from taking cold.

Causations - Damp with cold, wading, washing. Injuries. Checked eruptions or perspiration. Complaints of workers in ice factory. People who are exposed to a constant change of temperature, air conditioning.

Chest - Great oppression of the chest, especially when breathing. Pain in left chest as if lung moved in waves. Dull shooting, as from blows in and upon the sides of the chest. Sharp pains, here and there in chest. Small pimples on chest and abdomen.

Constitutions - Suited to phlegmatic, torpid, scrofulous patients, who are restless and irritable and who take cold on damp changes.

Coughs - Coughs in infants and elderly people. Whooping cough with excessive secretion of mucus. Panting cough, like whooping cough, worse each deep inspiration. ***Cough after physical exertion.*** Hoarse, spasmodic cough. ***Loose, rattling cough, worse cold, wet weather.*** Dry, teasing, winter coughs. Cough, caused by tickling in the back of throat in prolonged fits with much loose easy expectoration. Must cough a long time to expel phlegm. Copious mucus with loose cough. Barking cough, after a deep breath.

Ears - Child very susceptible to earache. Stitching earache with nausea, whole night, preventing sleep. Buzzing in ears. Swelling of parotids after measles. Middle-ear catarrh (Merc-d., Kali-m.). Earache with nausea. Impaired hearing with humming in ears and dull pain.

Eyes - Every time he takes cold it settles in eyes. Aching pain when reading. Aching with dimness of sight. Ophthalmia neonatorum. Chemosis of conjunctiva. Ophthalmia from catching cold. Hay fever with a profuse, watery discharge, worse in open air. Thick, yellow discharge, granular lids. Twitching of eyelids in cold air. Jerking in muscles of eyes. Paralysis of upper lid. Pupils much dilated. Idiopathic iritis after exposure in damp weather. Threatened amaurosis in scrofulous children. Dim vision. Sees as through a gauze. Sees sparks.

Face - Face bloated. Faceache and asthma, after disappearance of tetters in face. Facial neuralgia, ***worse from the slightest exposure to cold***. Tearing in cheek extending to ear orbit and jaw, ***preceded by coldness of parts and attended by canine hunger***. Twitching of lips in cold air. Humid eruptions on cheeks and face generally. Thick, brown, yellow crusts on face. Swelling of parotids after measles. Pimples and little ulcers around mouth. Warts. ***Herpes about lips.*** Cold sores on lips (Nat-m.).

Female - Rash appears on the skin before menses. Menses watery. Menses delayed and too short. Dysmenorrhea with blotches all over. Menses, milk, suppressed by cold or dampness. Suppression of menses from cold or dampness. Herpetic eruptions on vulva, worse every cold change of weather, or by exposure in cold, damp situations. Lochia suppressed by cold or damp. Threatened miscarriage induced by exposure in a damp, cold place. Pruritus with heat and sexual desire.

Food - Hunger without appetite. Hunger after fever. Aversion to food. Aversion to coffee. Great thirst for cold drinks.

Head - Congestion to head with buzzing in ears. Headache, relieved by conversation. Headache with great uneasiness, depressed spirits. Occiput feels large, cold. Occipital pain ascending from nape of neck. Back part of head chilled, heavy, aching during cold weather. Sensation as if a board were pressing against the forehead. Sensation as if hair stood on end. ***Tinea capitis,*** crusta lactea and dandruff, worse change of weather. ***Scald head,*** thick brown crusts, bleeding when scratched, causing hair to fall out. ***Ringworm of scalp.***

Heart - Palpitations at night. Pulse hard, small and tense, worse at night. Pulse soft, full, slow, bounding. Pulse slower than beat of heart. Pulse frequent at night, slow during day. Pulse collapsed.

Kidneys - Burning in meatus while urinating. Must urinate when getting chilled. ***Nephritis from cold.*** Ischuria from wading with bare feet in cold water. Pain in region of kidneys, with dropsy and albumen in urine. Urine increases with every little cold. Cloudy, slimy or foul urine. Urine with thick, ***mucus***, purulent sediment. Urine offensive, turbid when passed, and excoriating the skin.

Limbs - Rheumatic symptoms alternating with diarrhea or acute eruptions. ***Rheumatism after exposure to wet.*** Paralyzed limbs. ***Feet icy cold***. Cold feeling in bones. Sudden swelling of body and puffiness of limbs. Swelling of calf of leg. Pain in shinbones. Exostosis on arms after suppressed scabies. Trembling of arm (right) with urinary difficulty. Perspiration on palms of hands. Warts on hands and fingers.

Lungs - Asthma with dyspnea. Asthma with faceache after disappearance of tetters in face. Oppressed breathing from a cold. Dyspnea with accumulation of mucus. Impending paralysis of lungs. Copious mucus. Easy expectoration of tasteless mucus, often streaked with blood. Rheumatic pleuritis and pleuro-pneumonia, with tough, difficult, discoloured sputa. Hydrothorax, worse wet weather. Bronchitis with offensive smelling night sweat. Tuberculosis, worse in changes from warm to cold. Tuberculosis, sputum tough, green.

Male - Enlarged testes with griping pain. Impotence. Herpes. Eruptions, brown, dry, humid or furfuraceous. Eruptions, red, pale red. Eruptions with a red areola. Eruptions, round, scaly and small. Eruptions, suppurating, yellow.

Modalities - Better lying on side. Better moving the affected part. Better external warmth. Better dry weather. ***Worse from being chilled while hot***, Worse hot days and cold nights. Worse sudden changes of temperature. ***Worse cold wet, damp, rainy weather***. Worse cellars. Worse getting wet. Worse using water. Worse autumn, night. ***Worse from damp ground***. Worse cold drinks, ice cream. Worse cold to feet, Worse suppressed discharges. Worse eruptions or sweat. Worse beds, and rest. Worse getting feet cold. Worse injuries. Worse before storms.

Mouth - Mouth and tongue dry. Distorted, drawn to one side. Bitter taste. Saliva, tenacious. Saliva, ropy with toothache. Cold sores on lips. Putrid sore mouth with salivation and swollen cervical glands. Mucus membrane of mouth greatly swollen and very red. Holds cold water constantly in mouth, as pain and heat is better thereby. Scurvy from cold.

Nose - ***Hay fever, profuse, watery discharge***, worse open air. Hay fever, sensitive to newly mown grass. Hay fever in August. Discharge suppressed from least contact with cold air. Complete stoppage of nose. ***Nose stuffs up when there is a cold rain.*** Wants nose kept warm, least cold air stops the nose. Aching pain. Thick, yellow mucus, bloody crusts. ***Severe coryza with hot, dry skin, limbs cold, stiff, numb and painful; general offensive sweat.*** Dry or profuse coryza. Coryza of the newborn. ***Summer colds with diarrhea.*** Nosebleed in place of menses. Nosebleed blood bright red, and hot, with pressure above nose.

Perspiration - Foul sweat. Sweats with skin diseases. Sweats with copious limpid urine. Sweats at night, over whole body, often offensive. Offensive sweat, night and morning. Sweats in axilla and palms. Suppressed sweat. Conditions arising from sudden cooling of body whilst sweating.

Rectum - Itching of rectum. Burning in anus after stool. Biting pain in rectum as from salt. Constipation and painful strangury. Cutting pain at navel followed by painful, green, slimy stools. Profuse thin stools in morning. Diarrhea of green, sour, watery. Diarrhea slimy, bloody, ***mucus***, worse at night. Diarrhea especially in the summer. Diarrhea when the weather suddenly becomes cold. ***Diarrhea from damp, cold weather***. Diarrhea from repelled eruptions. Diarrhea after suppression of eczema. Watery, slimy, lienteric stool after eating. Green, watery, slimy, bloody, mucus stools. Sour, watery stools, worse at night, summer, damp cold weather. Yellow diarrhea, alternating with greenish.

Sensations - As of a board pressing against forehead, as if head were enlarged, as if hair stood on end. As if fire were darting out of eyes. As if worms were crawling up and down in abdomen, biting in rectum as from salt. As if lung moved in waves. As if arms were of wood, as of needles over whole body. Crawling, tickling itching of various parts, tip of tongue.

Skin - ***Pruritus, worse in cold, wet weather***. Herpes zoster, pemphigus. Eruptions, scaly, thick, crusty, moist, bleeding or herpetic, worse before menses. Humid eruptions on face, genitals, hands etc. ***Urticaria***, red spots, brought on by exposure or sour stomach. Nettle-rash over whole body with violent itching. Thick, brown-yellow crusts, bleeding when scratched. Sensitive bleeding ulcers. Little boils. ***Warts***, large, smooth, on face and palmar surface of hands. Small furuncles on places hurt. Eczema, rash of infants. Red spots, as from fleabites. ***Ringworm in the hair in children.*** Anasarca. Impetigo, little boil-like eruptions that spread. Skin callous.

Sleep - Uneasy, restless sleep, with confused dreams, frequent sweat, tossing from side to side. During sleep mouth open, snoring. Falling asleep in evening, starting as if frightened. Sleep worse after 3 a.m. Fearfully confused dreams.

Stomach - Indigestion with chilliness from every cold change of weather. Belchings with shuddering. Heartburn. Nausea with desire for stool. Vomiting of white, tenacious mucus. Shivering, chilliness while vomiting. Vomiting of mucus after cold drinks. Vomiting of greenish, yellow, slimy substances.

Teeth - Teeth thickly coated with tenacious, foul mucus. Teeth deeply imprinting cheeks and edges of tongue. Toothache from cold with diarrhea. Toothache with confusion in head, profuse salivation. Teeth feel blunt, or numb. Receding, spongy gums with salivation.

Temperature - Chill alternating with heat. Icy coldness with pains. Coldness in different parts, icy of paralyzed parts. Chill starts in the back, not better by warmth, worse evening. Chill with urging in stool and urination. Chilliness with thirst. Dry, burning heat all over.

Throat - Adenitis. Pressure as if uvula were too long. ***Tonsillitis from every change of weather.*** Much mucus in fauces. Rough, hoarse voice. Continual hawking up of very tough saliva, with much rawness in fauces. Constant titillation in larynx, with desire to cough. Trachea full of mucus, tough, greenish sputum with moderate cough. Swelling and indurated glands from cold.

Tongue - Tongue, swollen, hindering speech, paralyzed inarticulate or difficult speech. Dry, rough tongue, rough scraping in throat after taking cold in damp weather. Itching, crawling on tip of tongue. Tongue and jaw become lame if cold air or water chills him.

Vertigo - Vertigo on waking in morning. Giddy and dizzy. Vertigo with trembling and weakness. Momentary vertigo, when walking, with darkness before eyes.

COMMENTS - Sensitiveness to cold and damp runs through the Solanaceae. and is marked in Bell. and Caps., but it is supreme in Dulc. This feature among others renders them all good antidotes to Merc.

Bar-c. is the complement of Dulc. in "worse from cold weather, especially in scrofulous children." Every cold settles in the eyes, throat or affects the bladder, respiration or bowels.

In poisoning cases, Dulc. produces hard, griping pains in the bowels, unconsciousness, tetanic spasms, trismus, loud, rattling breathing, and death. One-sided spasms. Convulsions beginning in the face. Trembling, especially of the right arm.

Paralysis, of the tongue, lungs, and heart (pneumogastric paralysis). Paralysis of the bladder. Rheumatic paralyzes. Paralyzed part feels icy cold. "Paralysis of vocal cords (aphonia) from sleeping over a damp cellar."

Scrofulous-looking eruptions. Moist or dry, red, tettery eruptions, especially on the face. Furfuraceous, herpetic. Urticaria. Small furuncles appear on places hurt by concussion. Skin callous. Warts, fleshy or large, smooth. Painless ulcers. Skin eruptions are sensitive to touch, pressure better.

Dropsical disorders. Catarrhal troubles. Dry mucus membranes. Offensive sweat, effects of sudden cooling while sweating. Results of suppressed eruptions.

Diarrhea, vomiting with the stool. Bladder infections. Mucous-like sediment in the urine. Mucopurulent urine is often associated with general one-sided sensitiveness, especially of the abdomen.

Dulc. 30c cured in two doses a rash like mosquito-stings appearing every month before the menses, worse when warm, compelled to sit where it is cold.

Clarke gave Dulc. 30c with complete relief to the pain in a case of sarcoma of the bones at the base of the skull in which there were stabbing pains in the front of the head and partial paralysis of the tongue. It was the latter symptom that determined the choice of the remedy.

McLaren cured with a single dose the following case, which was the result of a wetting. Facial paralysis, following neuralgia, the eye having remained unclosed for eight months. Red rash with itching worse in damp weather. After a slight aggravation improvement began in two weeks and continued steadily.

RELATIONS - ***Antidoted by:*** Camph., Cupr., Ip., Kali-c., Merc. Follows well: Bry., Calc., Lyc., Rhus-t., Sep., Verat. ***Compare:*** (1) Acon., Ars., Cham., Hell., Nit-ac., Puls., Staph., Sulph. (2) In faintness during stool, Crot-t., Verat. (3) Effects of cold, moist winds, Ars., Calc., Nux-v. m. (cold dry, winds, Acon., Bry.). (4) Effects of exposure to wet and better by motion, Rhus-t. Rheumatic paralysis, Rhus-t., Caust. Hasty speech and actions, Hep., Bell., Lach., Sulph. Paralysis of lungs, Solanum. (5) Pimpinello - Bibernell - respiratory mucus membrane sensitive to drafts, pain and coldness in occiput and nape. Whole body weak, heavy head and drowsiness, lumbago and stiff neck, pain from nape to shoulder, chilliness. (6) Rhus-t., Cimic., Calc., Puls., Bry., Nat-s. ***Complementary:*** Baryta c. ***Incompatible:*** Bell., Lach.

REFERENCES - Boericke. Clarke. Murphy. Phatak.

DYSENTERY BACILLUS

PHARMACY - dys-co. Dysentery bacillus. Dysentery co. Bacillus dysenteriae. Shigella dysenteriae. A Bowel nosode. ***Historical dose:*** All potencies.

CLINICAL - Anemia. ***Anxiety.*** Arthritis. Backache. Blepharitis, ***Bruises***. ***Colitis. Diarrhea.*** Duodenal, ulcer. Dysmenorrhea. ***Colitis. Fears.*** Fibrositis. Flatus. ***Headaches. Heartburn. Indigestion. Migraines.*** Nausea. Osteoporosis. Otorrhea. Pharyngitis. Pleurodynia. Rheumatism. Spondylitis. Styes. Tachycardia. Thyrotoxicosis. Tonsillitis. Ulcers. ***Vomiting.***

HOMEOPATHIC - This is the nosode prepared from Bacillus dysenteriae. Dys-co. affects every tissue of the body and is suitable for many slow and insidious chronic states. Dys-co., patients are typically the Arg-n. type.

Fearful and phobic, abdominal symptoms due to apprehension. ***"Anticipatory"*** nervous tension. Inhibition and insecurity. Mental aberrations and nervous symptoms precede and are associated with myocardial and circulatory disease.

Least excitement exhausts and aggravates symptoms. "Anxiety and excitement felt in the epigastrium," "nausea from excitement" and "diarrhea from excitement." Excitement, anxiety or any agitation causes palpitations, flushing, perspiration, breathlessness and even pain in the heart region.

Involuntary movements, tics or twitching (like chorea). Instability of the capillary circulation, causing blushing, frontal headaches from excitement. Dry skin, scaly, with circinate lesions.

Dilation of stomach. Spasm in the pylorus. Retention of digested contents. ***Indigestion pain*** with distention and discomfort. ***Heartburn.*** Cyclical vomiting in children. Diarrhea or indigestion from eating sweets and fat, which they are fond of.

MIND - High strung and very sensitive to all impressions. Tense and nervous. ***Easily excited and flustered.*** Forgetful, especially after interruptions. Full of worries about little things. ***Anticipating fear of difficulties*** that might arise (Arg-n.). ***Full of fears.*** Claustrophobia. Shy, lacks confidence.

Abdomen - Distention and flatus. ***Colitis.*** Pain and tenderness over gallbladder.

Back - Fibrositis, rheumatism of neck and shoulders. Backache. Spondylitis.

Chest - Pleurodynia. Pain in chest on exertion. Tightness in lower ribs.

Constitutions - Tense facial expression, not fearful but alert and ready to react. Anxious, restless, fidgety, timid and uneasy among strangers, easily upset by criticism.

Ears - Otorrhea. Sudden swelling of ears, blue, red, thin, scalding.

Eyes - Blepharitis, styes. Conjunctivitis with photophobia. Twitching of eyelids. Sensation of floating bodies, woolly spots before eyes. Yellow color vision.

Face - Both children and adults show a marked anemia, watery, bluish pallor with puffiness of eyelids and cheeks. Veins frequently dilated and bluish lips that are apt to get dry and cracked. Neuralgia, supra and infra orbital. Twitching of muscles of face.

Female - Menses irregular. Dysmenorrhea. Throbbing pelvis and perineum. Infantile masturbation.

Food - ***Fond of sweets, salt, milk and fat.***

Head - Headache, frontal, over the eyes or in vertex, brought on by excitement. ***Blinding headaches*** with looseness of bowel. ***Migraines***, more headache than vomiting. Headaches often occur at regular time periods of 7 to 14 day cycles. Fuzzy head. Scalp is painful to comb. Dry, scaly painful spots.

Heart - Tachycardia, palpitations, extra systoles. Palpitations before important events. Anticipatory discomfort in the cardiac area. Heart rate is fast and may be irregular.

Limbs - Osteoporosis. Arthritis and periostitis. Pain in knees, ankles.

Lungs - Shortness of breath. Bronchial catarrh. Pertussis-like cough. Blood stained sputum.

Modalities - Worse from 3 a.m. to 6 a.m. Patients feel the cold, chilly and want warmth, yet are easily heated up by the exertion and warm room. Feels cold, chilly and rapidly perspire from excitement and mental exertion. Nausea and faintness in warm room, relieved by open air. Desires air and space.

Mouth - Bad taste. Tongue raw and burning. Lips are dry and cracked. Rheumatism of jaw.

Nose - ***Hay fever.*** Vasomotor rhinorrhea. ***Frequent coryza.*** Pain at the root of nose.

Rectum - Constipation and diarrhea. Weak expulsion of hard knotted stool with mucus. Loose morning diarrhea, stools forcibly expelled and acrid, burning. ***Looseness,*** frequent motions 5 or 6 per day. Diarrhea on excitement or worry. Throbbing rectum with sense of block or cork. Hemorrhoids and anal fissures. Hemorrhoids come down when walking.

Sleep - Insomnia, from crowding of thoughts, excitement, and palpitations. Sudden shocks through the body on falling to sleep, awakening with fear, palpitation and breathlessness. Wakes at 2 or 3 a.m. with pain and discomfort in epigastrium.

Stomach - ***Pain, worse from eating***, better lying down. Ptosis stomach, dilation, splashing. Emptiness between meals and sometimes nausea in the morning on awakening relieved by eating. Sinking emptiness during day with relief from rest and food. ***Chronic indigestion***. Eructation, heartburn, some hours after food. Acrid vomiting burning up throat, bilious vomiting. Thirst and desire for cold drink, but worse afterwards. Mental strain reacts on stomach and aggravates the stomach stasis.

Throat - Enlarged thyroid. Recurrent tonsillitis. Pharyngitis. Dry throat.

Urine - Urge to urination in tram or train.

COMMENTS - Selective action on cardiac muscles. Cardiac disorder. Function disturbance of heart action, associated with nerve tension. Affects the venous circulation. Walls of veins get thin and veins dilated. Varicose veins. "Bruises very early and bleeds easily." Stasis of abdominal circulation.

Tendency to blush, with pallor. Flabbiness. Limbs, cold, bluish and perspiring. Rheumatism. "Growing pains," associated with valvular heart disease. Weak reaction.

Hypotonic stomach. Delayed digestion with pain, relieved by eating. Duodenal ulcer, with nervous tension felt in stomach and heart area (Prot., has unperceived tension). Ulcers (Lyc., Nux-v.).

Dry skin. Ribbed brittle nails, dandruff and dry brittle hair. Cracked fingertips. The cracks and fissures are deeper with an indurated base. Eruptions are dry and sluggish, come out slowly. Tendency to scale and crust, gummy discharge (Graph.).

Herpes on face, neck, chest. Blisters between fingers. Scaly eruptions on flexures. Dermatitis of hands and palms, dry, cracked and painful. Flat warts on hands. Psoriasis. Urticaria attacks.

Brain fatigue. Little power of concentration. "Loses train of ideas from interruption." "Forgets what he was going to say." "Forgets what she went for." Lack of initiative, easily deflected.

Hypersensitive, expressed as shyness or timidity. Unsociable. Aversion to meeting strangers. Tense around strangers, alert. Fear of being alone. "I desire to be left to myself, but have a fear of being alone."

Mental uneasiness, physical restlessness, fidgets, chorea movements of facial muscles or limbs. Nervous tension, constant, triggered by anticipation. Impatience, hurry. Restless, desire to go from place to place (Tub.).

Depression, from tiredness, constant tension. Anxiety. "Feels miserable from the fear that she can not accomplish what she was to do." Desire to be left alone, and indulge in tears. Consolation aggravates the weeping and brings out irritability.

Burdened with over conscientiousness. Easily upset by criticism. Fear, in train, tram, bus and church, afraid in theater, lift office etc. Fear of the future, dark, thunder and storms.

RELATIONS - ***Compare:*** (1) There is close relationship between Dys-co., Arg-n. and Ars. (2) It is also related to Kalm., Nux-v. and Lycopodium also follow it well in gastric disorders. (3) Proteus.

REFERENCES - Bach. Paterson.

E

ECHINACEA ANGUSTIFOLIA

(Purple Cone-flower)

PHARMACY - echi. Echinacea angustifolia. Purple cone-flower. Echinacea rudbeckia. N. O. Composite, allied to Rudbeckia. (Echinacea angustifolia, is the western species not to be confounded with Echinacea purpurea, or Black Sampson, the eastern species.) Tincture of whole fresh plant. The whole plant including the root is pounded to a pulp and macerated in two parts by weight of alcohol. ***Historical dose:*** Tincture and all potencies. Locally, as a cleansing and antiseptic wash.

CLINICAL - Abscess. Aphthae. ***Appendicitis.*** Auto-infection. ***Bites. Blood, disorders. Blood, poisoning. Boils.*** Canker sores. Carbuncles. Colds. Cramps. Diarrhea. Diphtheria. Enteric, fever. ***Erysipelas.*** Fevers. ***Gangrene***. Goiter. Gonorrhea. Hemorrhoids. Hepatitis. ***Impetigo. Immune, disorders.*** Influenza. Leucorrhea. ***Lymphangitis.*** Meningitis. Ozaena. ***Poisoned, wounds***. Post-partum infections. Pustules. Pyemia. Rheumatism. Rhus, poisoning. Scarlatina. ***Septicemia. Snake, bites.*** Sore, throats. Struma. Syphilis. Tonsilitis. Typhoid, fever. Ulcers. ***Vaccinations, effects. Wounds.***

HERBAL - Echi. is a blood and immune tonic. This well-known drug came to notice as "Meyers's Blood Purifier," the proprietor did not know the name of the drug used and sent a whole plant to Professors King and Lloyd of Cincinnati, who identified it as Echinacea angustifolia.

Echi. has long been used by herbalists in typhoid conditions, diphtheria, malignant scarlatina, carbuncles and boils. Also as a septic remedy in snake, animal or insect bites.

Dr. H. W. Felled noted in the Eclectic Medical Journal, that "if any single statement were to be made concerning the virtues of Echinacea it would read something like this: 'A corrector of the depravation of the body fluids' and even this does not sufficiently cover the ground."

Antiseptic, anti-fermentative and anti-zymotic. Tissue alterations as are exhibited in boils, carbuncles, abscesses or cellular glandular inflammations. Locally useful for cleansing and as an antiseptic wash for wounds (Calen.).

Potency is not well proven, so it is used primarily in tincture to stimulate the immune system. Homeopaths have generally followed the herbalists in using substantial doses of the tincture (5 to 40 drops), adjusted to the particulars of the case.

HOMEOPATHIC - ***Blood poisoning or weak blood.*** Septicemia from a cut or wound, or after surgery (Pyrog.). Acute auto-infection, ***septic conditions, bites of poisonous animals, lymphangitis***. Tendency to malignancy in acute and sub-acute disorders. ***Gangrene*** (Rhus-t., Ars.).

Snakebites, insect bites and stings. ***Venomous infection***. Lymphatic inflammation, after crushing injuries. Foul discharges with emaciation and great debility. Cerebro-spinal meningitis. Post-partum infections. Infections at the site of a vaccination.

Ear infections. Fetid ozaena. Recurring strep throat. Beneficial in some cases of leucorrhea with bright yellow discharge, as from a suppurating surface.

Boils, do not suppurate. Carbuncles, bluish-red color and intense pain. ***Erysipelas*** and foul ulcers. Goiter with exophthalmic symptoms. Pustules. Hemorrhoids. Diarrhea in typhoid. Gonorrhea.

Asthenia, adynamia. Weak and tired, aching in muscles. Weakness felt more in stomach, bowels, heart, in knees, with vertigo. Useful in the last stages of cancer to ease pain (Ars.).

MIND - ***Prostration of mind.*** Slowness in every action, speech, pace. Confused, cannot exert mind. Depressed or cross. ***Brain fag and vertigo.*** Very nervous could not study. ***Aversion to thinking.*** Does not wish to think or study. ***Dullness from headache***, with cross, irritable feelings. Becomes angry when corrected, does not wish to be contradicted.

Abdomen - Abdomen tender, sensitive and tympanitic. Pain in right hypochondrium. ***Appendicitis.*** Pain about umbilicus, better by bending double. ***Cramping pain better passing flatus.*** Sharp, cutting, pains coming and going suddenly. Full feeling with borborygmus.

Back - Chills up the back. Pain in back of neck. Dull pain in small of back over kidneys. Pain in lumbar region, worse from stooping.

Chest - Pain as of a lump in chest and under sternum. Sharp, burning pain in sternum. Pain in pectoral muscles, diaphragm, right lung. Full feeling in upper part of lungs. Sore feeling.

Constitutions - Broken-down and weak constitutions.

Ears - Shooting pain in right ear.

Eyes - Brows twitch. Feel hot on closing them. Lachrymation from cold air. Sharp pains in eyes and temples. Pains back of right eye. Eyes pain on looking at an object and will fill with tears, better by closing them. Eyes ache when reading. Sleepy sensation in eyes, but cannot sleep.

Face - Bluish. Face flushed. Red flushes from pain in head. ***Pale face with headache***, vomiting. Fine eruptions on forehead and cheeks. Neuralgic pain in left upper branch of fifth nerve. Numbness of lips.

Female - Discharges suppressed. Mucus from vagina in evening. Excoriating leucorrhea. ***Puerperal septicemia***. Pain in right iliac region, which seems deep, lasting but a short time.

Food - Loss of appetite. Nausea, could not eat. ***Desire cold drinks.*** Desire for cold water.

Head - Headaches with a peculiar, periodical flushing of the face, dizziness and profound prostration. ***Enlarged sensation in brain.*** Sharp pain deep in brain, seems too large. ***Fullness in temples.*** Pain in temples on motion. Pulsating headache. Throbbing through the temples. Hot burning forehead. ***Dullness in head*** with cross, irritable feeling. Pain in forehead on sneezing (Nat-m.). Headache over eyes with sneezing.

Heart - Anxiety about the heart. Increasing but variable pulse. Rapid beating of heart. Slight pain over heart. Stitching pain in left chest (apex of heart). ***Tongue, lips and fauces tingle*** with sense of fear about heart (Acon.). Accelerated full pulse.

Kidneys - Desire for frequent urination. Involuntary urination. Albuminous, scanty, dark urine. Urine increased, pale and copious. Sense of heat while passing urine. Pain and burning on urination.

Limbs - Rheumatic pain after tonsillitis. ***Aching in limbs*** and general lassitude, weakness. Pain between shoulders, which extends to axilla and down the arms. Sharp pain in left elbow. Pain in wrists and fingers. Pain in right thumb. Cold hands and feet. Hands are alternately numb or restless, on awakening. Chilliness in right leg. Left hip and knee pains. Pain in right leg.

Liver - Hepatitis. As if a load in back part of liver.

Lungs - Pain as of a lump under the sternum. Burning under the left scapula.

Male - Seminal emissions. Soreness, pain in perineum. Perineum seems stretched. Pain in right spermatic cord. Testicles drawn up and sore. Pain in meatus while urinating.

Modalities - Better from lying down. Better rest. Pains come and go suddenly and are better by bending double. Worse after physical or mental exertion. Worse injury, operations. Worse cold air. Worse evening. Worse after eating.

Mouth - Biting, tingling on lips. Corners of mouth and lips crack. Canker sores. Aphthae. Gums recede and bleed easily. Dry sensation in back part of mouth. Metallic taste. Bad taste in the mouth in the morning. Burning, peppery taste when taking remedy. Promotes the flow of saliva.

Nose - Stuffiness of nostrils with mucus in sinuses and pharynx. Foul smelling discharge, membranous formations protruding. Post-nasal catarrh with ulceration and fetor. Nose feels stuffed up. Right nostril raw, bleeding. Nostrils sore.

Perspiration - Sweat chiefly on upper part of body. Sweats on forehead.

Rectum - Griping pains followed by passing offensive flatus or a loose yellowish stool, producing great exhaustion. Diarrhea following pain in stomach, going through bowels. Blood flows after stools.

Skin - Dry skin. Intense itching and burning of skin on neck. ***Blackness of external parts.*** Little papules on skin with redness, feeling like nettles. Small red pimples on neck and face. Recurring boils. Carbuncles. Irritations from insect bites and poisonous plants. ***Dissecting wounds.*** Lymphatics enlarged. Gangrene. Old tibial ulcers.

Sleep - Drowsy, could not read, with yawning. ***Sleepiness with confusion and weakness.*** Sleep disturbed, wakes often. ***Sleepiness after eating.*** Dreams about difficulties, laborious or quarrelsome, about exciting things, about dead relations.

Stomach - Sense of something large and hard in stomach. Dull pain in stomach. Distension, eructations do not relieve (Chin.). Pain in stomach, going down through bowels, followed by diarrhea. Nausea with chilliness, better lying down. Sour, bloody vomit like coffee grounds. Nausea with eructation of gas. Sour belching, burning the throat, or tasteless. Heartburn.

Teeth - Teeth sensitive to draft of air. Darting pains in the teeth, worse on right side. Neuralgic pains in superior and inferior maxilla. Dull aching of the teeth.

Temperature - Irregular, chills, rise of temperature and sweat. ***Chilliness with nausea***. Cold flashes all over back. Chill in left occiput. Temperature raised a degree with flushed face and fullness of head. ***Malarial fever***.

Throat - ***Sore throat***, ***worse left side.*** Ulcerated sore throat. Mucus in throat with raw sensation. Constant clearing of mucus from throat. Frothy mucus, hawks from throat. Tonsilitis. Tonsils purple or black, gray exudation extending to posterior sinuses and air-passages. Irritation of larynx. Voice husky.

Tongue - Tongue dry and swollen, sores, dirty brownish. White coating of tongue with red edges. ***Tongue, lips and fauces tingle*** with sense of fear about heart (Acon.). Slight burning of tongue. Tongue, numb, with a peppery taste.

Vertigo - Vertigo with weakness, dizziness and profound prostration. Vertigo when changing position of head.

COMMENTS - J. C. Fahnestock extensively proved the remedy, and additional symptoms were contributed by T. C. Duncan. With one exception the provers were males.

The first symptom noticed was a biting, tingling sensation on the tongue, lips and fauces (Acon.), with a sense of fear and pain about the heart. Febrile symptoms, full head, flushed face and accelerated pulse followed.

Languor was experienced by many provers, and neuralgic, sharp, darting, shifting pains. Marked drowsiness. Catarrh of the digestive and respiratory tracts. Griping pains, offensive flatus and loose, yellowish stool.

In two provers there was found a diminution of red blood corpuscles after the proving. Chilliness (coldness of right leg) and sensitiveness to cold, worse from exposure to cold air.

A remarkable case of vaccination poisoning is recorded in a man, 45, cured mainly by Echi. in 20-drop doses. The symptoms included an ebbed vitality. He became so weak he could not sit up, his hair fell out, and an eruption of psoriasis appeared on his limbs that extended to his body.

The disease advanced rapidly, the nails fell off. Left iritis supervened and then keratitis of the right eye. Under Kali-i. and phospho-albumen as a food, the hair ceased to fall out, but other symptoms became rapidly worse. Echi. was now given, and slowly the disease was arrested, then gradual improvement and an ultimate cure ensued. The report does not mention if the patient recovered sight in the left eye.

RELATIONS - ***Compare:*** (1) Cench., Both., Ars., Lach., Bapt., Rhus-t., Cistus, Hepar. (2) the vulnerary Composites, Arn., Calen. and Bell-p. (3) The closest analog is Bapt. (4) In snakebites it compares with Lobelia purpurascens. (5) in boils with Anthr. (6) Head feels enlarged, Arg-n., Bapt., Bov., Glon., Nux-v. Mosch., Nux-v. (7) Cases of Rhus-poisoning have been cured with Echin. a.

REFERENCES - Boericke. Clarke. Murphy.

ECHINACEA PURPUREA

(Black Sampson)

PHARMACY - echi-p. Echinacea purpurea. Black Sampson. N. O. Composite. Eastern States of America. Tincture of fresh root. ***Historical dose:*** Tincture and all potencies.

CLINICAL - Boils. Carbuncles. Diphtheria. Fatigue. ***Furuncles***. Impetigo. Putrid fevers. Pyemia. Scarlatina. Septicemia. Suppuration. Vaccination, effects. Wounds.

HERBAL - Echinacea purpurea is a popular remedy in the eastern states because it has been used in place of Echi. Echi-p. has probably a very similar action and the root causes the same pungent sensation on lips and tongue as the tincture of Echi.

HOMEOPATHIC - Echi-p. treats changes in the blood, simulating typhoid, pyemia, diphtheria, scarlatina, septicemia, and the effects of vaccination (Thuj.). Tendency to suppuration. Offensive discharges (Arn., Bapt.). Biting, tingling sensations.

Listless feeling, worse evening. High fever and flushed face (Bapt., Bell.). Marked chilliness. The black root has been taken as a ***"signature"*** of the remedy in cases of low fevers where a black tongue was observed.

MIND - Mental confusion. Tired, drowsy.

Fever - High fever, with fatigue. Typhoid fever. Low fevers where a black tongue was observed.

Modalities - Better from rest in bed. Better pressure. Better bending double. Worse in the evening. Worse stooping.

Skin - Infected wounds. Lacerated wounds. Impetigo. Dry skin. Boils, carbuncles and ***furuncles***.

COMMENTS - George Royal wrote of his experiences with Echi-p. He used it for ***furuncles*** with a dry skin. Small boils ("catboils"), very sensitive and seemed to come in crops, more about the neck and shoulders. Carbuncles with profuse sanguino-purulent discharge, marked large sloughing, coming in crops mostly about the neck, sometimes on perineum.

Royal would usually give such patients five drops of the 1st every three hours and apply a hot solution of 1 part of the tincture to 9 of water; changing the application often. He noted that it could be used in a similar manner to treat bruised or lacerated wounds.

It cured a case of a strumous, young bricklayer whose hand and fingers were to be amputated because of symptoms of sepsis (i. e., enlargement of the glands under the arms and temperature).

Echinacea 1c internally and tincture locally checked the sepsis and saved the fingers. In this case the skin and muscles were brought as nearly as possible to normal position and the Echinacea applied and changed every hour for 48 hours.

Royal used it successfully, only once, for suppurative appendicitis, i.e., after pus had formed and evacuated into the intestines. Merc. and Hepar had both failed to heal but Echinacea 1c, five drops every night and morning for three weeks, cured.

Used with success in recurring attacks of chronic inflammation about the cecum, and in a few cases of typhoid when the tired feeling was the ranking symptom.

RELATIONS - ***Compare:*** Echi., Bapt., Pyrogen.

REFERENCES - Clarke, Royal.

ELAEIS GUINEENSIS

(Palm Oil)

PHARMACY - elae. Elaeis guineensis. Palm oil. Aouara. Avoira. N. O. Palmaceae. Triturations of the fruit. ***Historical dose:*** Trituration and all potencies.

CLINICAL - Diarrhea. Elephantiasis, arabum. Gastric, disorders. Headaches. Leprosy. Scleroderma. Sight, defective. Skin, disorders. Sore, throat.

HOMEOPATHIC - Elae. was proved by Mure. Notable symptoms of leprosy and of scleroderma appear in the provings including anesthesia, and swelling and hardening of the skin.

Aching, lancinations, burning, bruised and throbbing pains. Sensation as if a peg stuck in false ribs. Swelling of parts.

The greatest number of symptoms appeared on the lower limbs and skin.

MIND - Merry mood. Disobedient.

Abdomen - Colic after a cold drink. Pain with bruised sensation in abdomen.

Chest - Pain in middle of chest as if pricked by needles. Lancinations every five minutes in right chest.

Eyes - Swelling of eyes. Unable to look steadily at an object. Sight weak, confused vision by candlelight. He makes letters much too large.

Kidneys - White urine.

Limbs - Staggering gait. Weakness of legs. Swelling of right leg. Throbbing in calves. Hammering in tibia, nape of neck and right foot. Soreness of soles of feet when walking and when touched. Swelling of left arm. Beating in left arm. Insensibility of head to heat, but an hour after he feels it badly.

Lungs - Breathing embarrassed. Pricking in larynx on breathing. Cough with lancination in sides.

Modalities - Better from rest. Worse from cold drinks. Colic worse from descending stairs. Lancinations worse from deep breathing.

Mouth - Burning in tongue, has to stop eating. Bad odor from mouth.

Neck - Constrictive pains around neck as if from tight string. Throbbing in nape.

Rectum - Frequent diarrhea. Black stools.

Skin - Skin seems thicker. Swelling, roughness and itching of skin on left leg. Small vesicles appear on swollen right leg and left arm and on other parts without swelling. Itching all over, preventing sleep.

Stomach - Foul belchings. Vomiting of a cake immediately after eating it.

Throat - Lancinations in throat when swallowing, stinging when swallowing saliva.

RELATIONS - ***Compare:*** (1) Anac., Rhus-t.

REFERENCES - Clarke.

ELAPS CORALLINUS

(Brazilian Coral snake)

PHARMACY - elaps. Elaps corallinus. Brazilian coral snake. Micrurus frontalis. Micrurus corallinus. N. O. Elapidae. Poison pressed from the venom-sac of the living snake and triturated with sugar of milk. ***Historical dose:*** All potencies.

CLINICAL - Acidity. Amaurosis. Axilla, itching. ***Black, discharges.*** Cancer. Deafness. Ear disorders. Ear, wax. ***Hemorrhages.*** Headache. Hemiplegia. Knee, pain in. Metrorrhagia. ***Nasal, catarrh***. Naso-pharyngitis. Nosebleed. Ozaena. ***Paralysis***. Pneumonia. Throat, ulcerated. Tuberculosis.

HOMEOPATHIC - Like other snake poisons, the poison of the coral snake disorganizes the blood, producing ***black discharges***, especially hemorrhages. Characteristic pre-eminent blackness of its discharges and hemorrhages. Sensation as if all the blood were collected in head. Black earwax.

Adynamic sepsis. Spasms, then paralysis. Oscillatory movements. ***Right-sided paralysis***. The right side feels weak insensible or even paralyzed. Must have oscillatory motion. Sensation of ***internal coldness***. Twisting sensation. As of a heavy load or weight on the affected part.

Sudden pain in stomach. ***Cold feeling in stomach***. Acidity of stomach with faint feeling. Spasm of esophagus, pharynx constricted, food and liquids suddenly arrested and then fall heavily into stomach. Spasms followed by paresis.

Cold things disagree. Fruit and cold drinks lie like ice on stomach and cause a cold feeling in chest. Desire for sweetened buttermilk. Nausea and vomiting. The prostrating diarrhea of tuberculosis.

Ear, nose and throat symptoms. Sudden deafness at night with roaring and cracking in ear. Mucus membranes wrinkled. Dreams of dead people. Shuddering from least contradiction, with pricking.

MIND - Depressed. Absorbed, buried in thoughts in daytime. Absent minded. Angry about one's self, does not wish to be spoken to. Desire to strike. Shuddering from least contradiction. Can speak, but cannot understand speech. Imagines he hears someone talking.

Fear as if something horrible might happen. ***Fear of the rain***. Never feels happy in wet weather. Fear of having a stroke. ***Fear of getting a fatal disease.*** Fear being left alone. Fear causes chattering of the teeth and trembling.

Aversion to company. Avoids the sight of people, wants to get into the country away from people. Desire to travel. ***Hysteria before menses.*** Taciturn during menses. Playful. Delusion he is being beaten. Delusion he is falling forward. Delusion of being injured.

Abdomen - Colic with urging to stool. Bowels feel twisted together in a knot. Painful pressure in right side of liver. Lancinating pain from both groins to symphysis pubis.

Back - Stiffness in the right side of neck. Lancinations in left side of neck. Lancinations in the whole spinal marrow from occiput to sacrum. Pressure between the shoulders. Coldness in back. Pain in the back with chilliness, cold feet and strangury.

Chest - Oppression of chest on going upstairs. Feeling of a heavy load on chest. ***Coldness in chest after drinking***. Itching eruption in axilla. Rush of blood to chest in morning. ***Sharp pain and soreness to touch across chest.*** Soreness from right to left axilla

Constitutions - Rheumatic constitutions.

Ears - Crusty eruption on ear. Earwax, ***black*** and hard with difficult hearing. Offensive, serous ***greenish*** discharge. Intolerable itching in ear. Otorrhea. ***Watery, yellow or yellow-green discharge with deafness.*** Sudden attack of nightly deafness with roaring and crackling in ears. Cracking in ears on swallowing. ***Buzzing noise.*** Illusions of hearing.

Eyes - Eyes red and inflamed. Watery eyes. Eyes look glassy. Stye on left eye, with lancinating pain. Bloated around the eyes in the morning. Burning and dryness in both eyes on waking. Burning in lids. ***Eyeballs feel sticky under lids.*** Violent itching in left eye. Aversion to light, desire to close eyes.

Face - Bloated around eyes in morning. Red spots on face. Red blotches on bloated face. Dull, yellowish color. Crusty eruption on cheek. Redness and swelling of right cheek. Swelling of face.

Female - Itching of vulva and vagina. Dysmenorrhea with a flow of black blood. Discharge of black blood between menses. Sensation as if something burst in the womb, then continuous stream of dark colored blood, better when urinating. Itching of vulva and vagina. Weight at uterus and vagina after an hysterical attack.

Food - Canine hunger, yet unable to eat. Acidity after every mouthful. Aversion to meat. Aversion to bananas. Desire for ice. Desires milk, whipping-cream. Desire for sweetened buttermilk. Desires sweets. Desires salads. ***Cold drinks and fruit feel like ice in stomach, and cause coldness in chest.*** Worse fruits. Thirst during fever.

Head - Congestion of blood to head on stooping. Violent headache, extending from ***forehead to occiput***. Headache pain in one eye, then the other. Fullness in head. Rushes of blood to the head. ***Pain in occiput, worse mental exertion.*** Weight and pain in forehead. Lancinating pain, left then right side. ***Severe sharp pain in forehead, with heaviness of head.*** Stinging pain with sleeplessness.

Heart - Sensation of laceration in region of heart. Palpitations with anxiety and trembling of hands.

Kidneys - Urine red. ***Discharge of mucus from urethra.*** Red urine with cloudy sediment. Thick urine with red sediment. Suppression of urine. Strangury.

Limbs - Soreness of limbs worse at night. Arms weak. Arms and hands swollen bluish. Pricking under the nails. Skin peeling off on palms and finger tips. Vesicular eruptions on feet. Icy cold feet. Knee joints feel sprained.

Lungs - Air hunger. Pneumonia. Each inspiration causes a crackling sound in lungs. ***Cough with terrible pain through lungs.*** Hemoptysis. Hemorrhage from lungs, black as ink and watery. ***Sharp pain in apex of lungs***, better walking. Stitches in apex of right lung. Sharp pain in left side of chest, worse breathing. Lungs feel forcibly separated. Worse right lung and expectoration of black blood.

Modalities - Better from rest. Better lying on abdomen. Walking relieves nosebleed, pain in abdomen and chest. ***Worse cold drinks, food, air.*** Worse drafts, wind. Worse night. ***Worse wet weather.*** Worse dampness. ***Worse approach of storms.*** Worse exertion. Worse touch. Worse warmth of bed. ***Cold things disagree***.

Nose - Coryza from least draft of air. White and watery nasal discharge. Mucus membrane wrinkled. ***Chronic nasal catarrh with fetid odor and greenish crusts***. Ozaena with a yellowish-green discharge. Nostrils plugged up with dry mucus. ***Nosebleeds, black like ink*** after a blow. Sudden, profuse nosebleed while walking. Pain at root of nose. Pains from nose to ears on swallowing. Eruptions about nose. Sneezing at night.

Perspiration - Sweats on forehead and neck. Profuse sweat. Cold perspiration all over.

Rectum - Constipation. Constriction of sphincter after bloody stools. Cholera. Diarrhea, copious liquid stools, watery, frothy. Diarrhea of an olive green color. Stools of black, frothy blood. Prolapsed anus. Formication at anus as from worms.

Skin - ***Skin hot, dry.*** Glands and skin of axilla affected. Itching with tetters, eruptions. Yellow spots on hands and fingers. Small blisters, on limbs. Fingertips peel off. Red pimples on fingertips. Little pimples, followed by desquamation. Typhoid when ulcers have eaten into tissues and black blood is discharged.

Sleep - Drowsy all day, no sleep at night. Sleeplessness from sharp headache. Bites hand during sleep. Dreams of business. Dreams of dead people.

Stomach - ***Stomach feels cold.*** Sensation as if food turned like corkscrew on swallowing. Burning in stomach. Acidity after every mouthful. Sinking, faint feeling in stomach. ***Pain in stomach better lying on abdomen.*** Paralysis of esophagus. Sensation of a sponge in esophagus. Spasmodic contractions of esophagus and pharynx, food and liquids are suddenly arrested and then fall heavily into the stomach. Sour eructations. Vomiting followed by diarrhea. Vomiting of mucus. Vomiting of green bile.

Temperature - Terrible coldness after drinking, as if ice water were rising and falling through left lung. ***Feels cold, cold things disagree***. Shivering after cold drinks. Coldness in back. Shaking chill, felt internally as if in bones. Dry heat and burning redness of face. Skin hot, dry, but complains of feeling cold. Fever with thirst. Heat alternating with chill. Heat flushes, in evening.

Throat - Tonsils swollen. Sides of throat sore to touch. ***Red blotches in throat.*** Painful, difficult swallowing of solids and liquids. Pressure pain in throat. Thick, very offensive, dry, greenish-yellow crusts upon the posterior pharyngeal wall and extremely foul breath. Ulceration of throat, worse left side.

Vertigo - Fainting caused by stooping. Vertigo with tendency to fall forward. Faints with vomiting or on stooping.

Vision - Letters run together when reading. Veil before eyes. Large red fiery spots before eyes. Red bar before eyes when opening them. Dirty red spot before eyes. Black rings before eyes (left).

COMMENTS - Rumbling in ears as of thunder. Sensation in brain as if shaken. Sensation as if food turned like a corkscrew on swallowing, as if intestines were twisted by a cord and strung together in a knot. Fluids roll audibly into stomach.

Marked pains in the lungs (especially right). Sensation within chest and at sternum as if pleura were pulled off and the lungs violently drawn apart. Sensation as if a heavy load, iron bar or weight on parts. Marked periodicity.

Affects the glands and skin of axilla. Clarke cured with Elaps. 200c a very old-standing case of irritating rash in axilla, (right) with recurrent suppuration of axillary glands.

E. V. Moffatt found Elaps 6c almost a specific in chronic naso-pharyngeal catarrh with greenish crusts and subjective disagreeable odor.

RELATIONS - ***Antidoted by:*** Radiated heat, Alcohol, Ars. ***Compare:*** (1) Dr. Higgins used the gallbladder of the coral snake, Fel Elapidis Corallini. (2) Ars., Carb-v., Crot-h., Lach., Mur-ac., Nit-ac., Rhus-t. (3) red spot before sight, Dub., (4) effects of cold, wet weather, Dulc. (5) Eucal. rostrata - offensive dark discharge from right ear. (6) Crot-h., Alumn., Carb-v., Ars., Lach.

REFERENCES - Boericke. Clarke. Phatak.

ELATERIUM OFFICINARUM

(Squirting Cucumber)

PHARMACY - elat. Elaterium officinarum. Squirting cucumber. Ecballium elaterium. Momordica elaterium. N. O. Cucurbitaceae. Tincture of unripe fruit. Trituration of Elaterinum, ***Historical dose:*** Trituration and all potencies.

CLINICAL - Abscesses. ***Beriberi.*** Bilious, fever. Bladder, disorders. Boils. ***Cholera.*** Colic. Cramps. ***Diarrhea.*** Dropsy. Dysentery. Erysipelas. Intermittent, fever. Jaundice. Liver, disorders. Measles. Nettle rash. Neuralgias. Rheumatism. Sciatica. Scurvy. ***Vomiting. Yawning***.

HOMEOPATHIC - Characteristic explosion, as how the ripe fruit scatters its seeds. Profuse watery stools, coming out with a gush. Violent vomiting and purging with copious forceful watery, olive green, bilious or frothy evacuations.

Dull, olive-green discharges and frothy stools. ***Cholera***, cholerine and infantile diarrhea. Jaundice of newborns, with bilious stools, urine staining the diaper.

Causes tissues to drain of their watery contents. Used in the absorption of dropsical fluids, minute doses will often affect this. Promotes the opening of abscesses and boils. Urticaria, better rubbing.

Chilliness with much yawning and stretching. Gaping and yawning, with fever before the chill or before the chill of cholera. Yawning throughout the chill. For the effects of damp weather or standing on damp ground, worse by damp. Irresistible desire to wander from home to home.

MIND - Depression of spirits. Fear of some approaching disaster. Mental disorders coming on as a consequence of suppressed malaria. Desire to leave home. Irresistible desire to wander from home at night.

Abdomen - Abdomen retracted. Feeling of stricture or oppression at the epigastrium. Dull pain in the epigastrium. Dull pain in the right of hypochondrium. Cutting, griping pains in the bowels. Rumbling of flatus in the course of the cecum and colon.

Back - Pains in the left sterno-mastoideus muscle, near its insertion into the sternum. Pains under the right shoulder blade. Sticking pains in the lumbar region. Aching pain in the region of the left kidney.

Causations - Effects of damp weather.

Chest - Sharp pains at the lower part of the sternum, passing through to the spine.

Ears - Sticking pain near the rim of the cartilage of left ear.

Eyes - Sticking, as of a splinter, in the inner canthus of left eye.

Food - Loss of appetite.

Head - Confusion of the head, followed by headache. Violent headache with sensation of constriction of the temples and forehead. Dull pain, pain in the temples.

Kidneys - Increased flow of limpid urine.

Limbs - Arthritic nodules. Pain in limbs, darting into fingers and toes. Pain extends down limbs, pain in hip joints with diarrhea. Shooting, also dull aching pains in the course of left sciatic nerve to the instep and toes. Sharp pains in fingers and thumbs, knees, toes and instep. Gouty pain in great toes.

Modalities - Worse from damp weather. Worse standing on damp ground.

Mouth - Tongue coated with a dirty-brown fur. Bitter taste in the mouth, with salivation. Unpleasant smell to the breath.

Nose - Nosebleed.

Rectum - Bleeding hemorrhoids. Soreness of the anus. Discharges from the bowels of frothy water, coming out with a gush. Stools are ***watery, copious, forceful. Squirting diarrhea***, frothy, dull, olive green with cutting in abdomen.

Sensations - As if a splinter in left eye. As if posterior sinuses and upper part of esophagus were enlarged.

Skin - Dropsical. Orange-colored skin. Smarts, stings and burns. Urticaria from suppressed intermittent.

Sleep - Incessant gaping. Much yawning and stretching.

Stomach - Pain in the pit of the stomach. Griping pains in bowels. Belching of gas. Nausea and vomiting with great weakness. Vomiting a dark brown fluid mixed with food.

Temperature - Chill comes on with much ***yawning and stretching***, lasting all through chill. Chills and fever with spurting diarrhea. Perspiration relieves all the symptoms. If the intermittent fever is suppressed, urticaria break out all over the body.

Throat - Pain in the back of the throat, as if scalded. Scraping in the throat. A feeling as if the choana and upper part of the esophagus were enlarged.

COMMENTS - According to Cooper, Beriberi has been greatly helped by Elat. Used with good effect in scurvy where gushing diarrhea is a marked symptom.

RELATIONS - ***Compare:*** (1) Crot-t., Gamb. (2) Bry. and Coloc. (sciatica), Verat. (neuralgia), Colch., Crot-t., Verat. - choleraic affections, Sec. - olive green diarrhea., Canth. - dysenteric diarrhea with painful urination. (3) Apis, Hep., Ign., Rhus-t. - urticaria during intermittent fever.

REFERENCES - Boericke. Clarke. Phatak.

ELECTRICITAS
(Electricity)

PHARMACY - electr. Electricitas. Electricity. Potencies are made from sugar of milk saturated with the current. ***Historical dose:*** Tincture and all potencies.

CLINICAL - Chorea. Headaches. Hysteria. Paralysis. Rheumatism.

HOMEOPATHIC - While Caspari is the authority for the symptoms caused by electricity, the powerful effect exercised on some by the approach of a thunderstorm and the influence of an electric current is well known.

In those who have been electrified, there is shaking of the whole body, commencing in the maxillary bones, tingling in the parts electrified, and violent burning. Effects of atmospheric electricity and static electricity. Dreads approach of thunderstorms.

General relaxation, sometimes with moral depression and headache. Anxiety, nervous tremors, restlessness, palpitations. Relaxation of the nerves and muscles. Lassitude and stiffness of the limbs. Heaviness of limbs, swelling of parts. Heat in the whole body.

Loss of the weight of the body, weakness of the parts shaken. Dragging sensations in all the limbs, as far as the ends of the fingers and toes, nocturnal shootings in parts that are paralyzed. St. Vitus' dance. Epileptic fits hastened and aggravated.

MIND - Intense nervous anxiety. Nervous tremors. Restlessness, anxiety and anguish. ***Fear on the approach of a thunderstorm.*** Anxiety, restlessness with palpitations and headaches. Internal anguish. Violent agitation. Timidity. Sighs and screams through nervous fear. Weeps in paroxysms.

General depression after a meal. Depression and weariness, sometimes with giddiness or drowsiness. Ill-humor. Furor. Errors in the perception of time. Loss of memory. Involuntary laughter. Insensibility, foolish actions. Loss of consciousness.

Abdomen - Spasmodic tension and contraction in the abdomen. Aching in the abdomen. Colic. Cutting pains, on the approach of a storm, or with diarrhea. Darting pains from left to right side. Shivering in the abdomen or else burning, sometimes with tension. Inflation of the abdomen, borborygmi in the abdomen, sometimes with fermentation.

Back - Difficulty in moving the neck. Tingling in a muscle shortened by suppuration. Tingling in the vertebral column. Darting pains in an enlarged gland of the neck. Furunculi on the back and nape of the neck. Drawing pains across the shoulder blades, as by a thread. Burning in the shoulder.

Chest - Constriction of the chest. Pains in the chest, sensation of coldness in the left side. Chest and shoulders feel like marble.

Ears - Pains in the ear. Drawing pains from the jaws to the ears. Lancinations in right ear, proceeding from the neck. Pulsations in the ear. Redness and heat of the ear. Swelling of the interior of the ear. Suppuration and a small pustule in the auditory duct. Vesicles full of acrid serum behind the ear. Augmented secretion of wax. Murmuring, sometimes with a sensation as if a flock of wool were before the ears.

Eyes - Haggard eyes. Wandering and haggard looks. Gnawing sensation in left eye or violent drawing pains, extending to forehead. Sensation as if the eyes were much sunken. Sensation as if something were passing out of the eye. Aching in the eyes, as from dryness. Redness of conjunctiva. Inflammation of the eyes. Swelling of edges of eyelids, at the external angle. Lachrymation, especially of right eye. Contraction of pupils, which were abnormally dilated.

Face - Bright red. Expression of terror. Increase of sweat on the face. Swelling of the face. Violent drawing pain above left eyebrow. Contraction of the muscles of the face, especially of the mouth. Scabby eruption on the face, on the arms and over the body. Eruption about the mouth and on the chin. Large blisters on the cheeks. Lips cracked, the upper lip puffed out.

Female - Copious menses, sometimes with pressure in the rectum. Black and thick blood of the menses. Appearance of the menses (in the electric bath).

Food - Increased appetite, great inclination to eat between meals. Thirst during febrile shivering.

Head - Pains in the head, sometimes drawing. Bruise-like pain in occiput. Crushing pressure in forehead, as from a stone. Shootings in right side of head or from vertex to the temple and right side of forehead. Tearings in the occiput from the nape of the neck to the forehead. Painful cramps in the head. Violent pulsations (beatings), or else heat throughout the head. Disagreeable shaking, most frequently from behind.

Heart - Palpitations, especially at the approach of a storm. Palpitations with fever, headache, or with restlessness and vivid redness of the face. Disposition to fall in syncope. Painful and rapid, sharp pain proceeding from the heart across the chest.

Kidneys - Sensations as though the bladder were going to burst. Augmented secretion of urine. Very frequent emission of urine. Involuntary emission of urine. Orange-yellow urine in the morning; during the day, like water in which meat has been washed. Urine thick, deep-colored, red like blood, abundantly charged with mucus. White sediment. Discharge of blood with the urine. Leucorrhea, at first serous, afterwards thick in pieces of the size of a hazelnut.

Limbs - Grievous pains in the limbs, pains in old wounds or in enfeebled bodies from a change of temperature. Stiffness of the limbs. Paralysis, especially of the inferior limbs. Trembling of the limbs, chiefly of those which have been shaken, general trembling. Springing up of the tendons. Convulsions of the limbs.

Lungs - Respiration accelerated. Feeble and faint respiration. Respiration arrested. Dyspnea. Oppression of the chest. Asthma, with palpitations and disposition to syncope. Cough, with much tickling in throat, or pressure in forehead from within outwards. Short, irritable cough. Spitting of blood. Rough larynx.

Mouth - Great dryness of the mouth. Augmented secretion of saliva, foam at the mouth. Increased excoriation, painful, in the interior of right cheek. On the palate, vesicles with desquamation of the epidermis. Dumbness, inability to utter a sound.

Nose - Tingling or outward pressure in the nose. Sneezing. Augmented secretion of nasal mucus. Discharge, on blowing the nose of a liquid like milk, aggravation of preexisting coryza. Nosebleed. Loss of smell.

Perspiration - Increased perspiration. Excessive nocturnal sweat, in gouty persons without mitigation, with anxiety during a storm.

Rectum - Fruitless inclination. The stools are at first facilitated and afterwards restricted. Tenesmus and cutting pains. Violent pressure in the rectum during the stools. Burning in the anus. Hemorrhoidal flux.

Skin - Itching or tingling over the whole body. Eruption of small nodosities on the spots touched by electrical sparks, eruption like miliary or measles, white vesicles, itch-like eruption at the joints of carbuncles, which proceed to suppuration. The skin becomes black, wheals on the skin. Violent pains and swelling of one of the feet which had been frozen twelve years before.

Sleep - Great drowsiness. Yawning and stretching, sometimes with shuddering over the whole body. Profound sleep. Sleeplessness, with tossing, for long periods. Confused and disquieting dreams.

Stomach - Fullness of the stomach after eating the least thing. Loathing. Abundant saliva. Sour taste. Heartburn. Nausea, after a meal. Retching and vomiting with inflammation of throat and cough. Vomiting of blood.

Stool - Diarrhea, with colic, or at the approach of a storm. Diarrhea with retraction of the testicles. constriction in anus with dry stools after diarrhea. Frequent stools, liquid, hot, black, yellow and fetid.

Teeth - Tearing pains in upper teeth, proceeding from the head. Drawings in the gums, proceeding from right ear. Quick, darting pain, as of subcutaneous ulceration, in places once occupied by molar teeth. Quick growth of the teeth in children.

Throat - Constant tickling in the throat. Pressure on swallowing. Difficult deglution. Inflammation of the gullet.

Tongue - Sensitiveness of the tongue, at the point, which is also red. Papillae very prominent. Dry tongue, charged with a yellow coating. Swelling, thickness of the tongue. Vesicles on the tongue with excoriation pain.

Vertigo - Giddiness, especially on stooping. Confusion of head. Syncope and tendency to fall down.

Vision - Clouded vision. Objects all appear yellow to the sight. Everything appears pale. A dark room appears to be illuminated. Little black spots before right eye. Blindness. Sight improved (curative symptom).

COMMENTS - Dr. Seward related a number of cases in which the injudicious use of electric baths brought on tuberculosis. In another case, the chest and arms became stiff and paralyzed. A young married woman, who had general and local (uterine) electric treatment, complained after it of feeling very heavy, as if she weighed a ton.

One patient after a bath, said his chest and shoulders "felt like marble." He became tubercular and died. The paralysis caused by electricity was in several cases quickly relieved by Morph-acet., both in the solution and in the potencies.

RELATIONS - ***Antidoted by:*** Morph-acet. Electr. antidotes Merc. ***Compare:*** (1) Phos. is the best antidote to the effects of storms. (2) Rhod. is worse before a storm. (3) Galvanismus and Magnetismus.

REFERENCES - Clarke.

ELM

(Bach Flower Essence)

PHARMACY - elm-b. Elm. Ulmus procera. Boil twigs and blossoms for half an hour, strain the water and use as medicine. ***Historical dose:*** Take two drops from the stock bottle into a one ounce dropper bottle, (add brandy or alcohol, if this bottle will be used for days or weeks). This is the dosage bottle, take a few drops straight into the mouth or as needed in a little water or juice.

HOMEOPATHIC - Elm belongs to Bach's group of ***Despondency and Despair,*** along with Crb-a-b., Oak-b., Will-b., Star-b-b., Sw-ch-b., Pine-b. and Lar-b. The group deals with states of cppressive, burdening hardship. Tendency to exhaustion in mind, emotions and body. Listlessness and lethargy. Unresolved, overwhelming conflicts or over work leading to the formation of chronic diseases (Wh-ch-b.).

MIND - High expectations for self. Strong sense of duty. Difficulty planning. Overwhelmed by duty. Feeling of being lost in details, lack of progress. Anxiety over future challenges or duties. Dread, anxiety, intimidation. Internal exhaustion, feelings of inadequacy. Disillusionment and despair. Sadness over unrealistic goals.

REFERENCES - Bach.

EMBELIA RIBES

(Krimighna)

PHARMACY - emb. Embelia ribes. Krimighna. N. O. Myrsineae. The medicine was prepared from the seeds. ***Historical dose:*** All potencies.

CLINICAL - Constipation. Diarrhea. Dyspepsia. Flatulence. Indigestion. Rheumatism. Worms.

HERBAL - The pulp is purgative. The fresh juice is cooling, diuretic and laxative. The fruit is carminative, anthelmintic, alternative and stimulant. It is employed in habitual constipation of children and in acute capillary bronchitis. As a carminative the fruit is given dyspepsia and flatulence. As an alternative in skin diseases and rheumatism. If taken for a long time, it is found to turn the urine acid and red. (R. N. Khory: Materia Medica of India, Vol. II, p. 426.).

Charaka states that it is a grand medicine to kill worms. It is also called Krimighna which literally means killer of worms. Sushruta says it is good for piles and worms. If it be regularly used in special seasons it will increase longevity.

The seeds of this plant are used as an anthelmintic. Powdered seeds in doses of one to two drams are administered with sugar or honey in an empty stomach to expel tape worms. (R. N. Chopra: Indigenous Drugs of India, p. 577.)

Clinicaly it is very useful in diseases of children associated with or proceeding from worms. It is a grand medicine in diarrhea, dyspepsia and flatulence owing to worms.

If Nux vomica, cina, santonine and other remedies for worms be ineffective, Embelia ribes will be found to be a sovereign remedy in those complaints. In this new remedy, the urine becomes pungent and blood colored and this is one of the characteristic symptoms for the administration of this remedy.

Other symptoms are fretfulness, moroseness and irritability of the patient. Grinding of the teeth. Patient always picks his nose. Tongue is dry, nausea exists. The abdomen gets distended. Stools are undigested. Urine is blood colored and pungent. Patient shrieks during sleep. Itching in the rectum, itching in the nose, and worms come out with the stool.

HOMEOPATHIC - Name of the Prover - Babu sris Chandra Ghose, age 28, or robust physique and of excellent health.

MIND - Became morose. The prover became fretful and irritable.

Nose - Itching sensation was felt in both the nostrils.

Rectum - Itching sensation was felt in the rectum. Large number of worms came out of the rectum and was expelled with the stool. Passed three undigested stools in quick succession. Worms were expelled with the stools.

Stomach - There was distension of the stomach.

Urine - Urine became red colored and strong smelling.

COMMENTS - Case 1 - The son of Babu srish Ch. Roy, B. A., was suffering from remittent fever continued with unabated fury for six days without any remission.

I was called in to treat the son, aged 6 years, on the 6th March, 1931. I continued to treat the boy with Gelsemium and Bryonia for four days, but unfortunately no improvement took place.

10th March - I went to see the boy this morning and gathered the following symptoms:

The patient was morose and fretful. Patient always picked his nose. Tongue was dry. There was terrible nausea. Abdomen was greatly distended. Passed undigested stools. Urine red colored and pungent. The boy was found to shriek out during sleep. Fever in the morning it was found to be 101° and it generally rose up to 103° in the evening.

I gave Cina 20 and 200 for two days on account of the predominance of worm symptoms. Cina did no good.

At last I gave him Embelia ribes 1x thrice on the 12th March. It acted very nicely to bring down the temperature to 99° in the morning next day.

13th March - At 11 a.m. temperature rose, but again fell down to 99° at 4 a.m. on that day and complete remission took place at eleven PM

14th March - There was no fever. Urine was clear, fretfulness was gone, there was no distension of abdomen, no loose stools passed and the patient was cured within 3 days. All along these days he took 2 doses of the new remedy. And since that time the patient did not suffer from worm troubles any more.

Case 2 - The daughter of Babu Ram Ratan Chatterjee, B. L., aged 4 years, suffered off and on from worm troubles. Ordinary homeopathic remedies were given by a homeopath, but there was no perceptible improvement. I was sent for on the 2nd November, 1932.

I marked the following symptoms: The child was ill-humored and restless. There was great hunger soon after a meal. Could not be quieted by any persuasion. The patient always bored her finger into the nose. The abdomen was distended. Always disturbed sleep. Loose stool with undigested particles of food. Grinding of teeth. Blood colored urine.

As the above were clear-cut symptoms of the presence of worms in the system, I prescribed Embelia ribes 1x twice daily. After using this remedy for a fortnight, the patient was perfectly cured.

I prescribed this new drug in 1x potency in several cases suffering from worm troubles and I am glad to say that all of those patients were radically cured.

REFERENCES - Ghose.

EMERALD

(Gemstone)

PHARMACY -emer. Emerald. Gemstone. Triturations. ***Historical dose:*** All potencies.

CLINICAL - Allergies. Alzheimer's, disease. Amenorrhea. Asthma. Cancer. Cataract. Chronic, fatigue. Dyslexia. Endometriosis. Epilepsy. Fainting. Glaucoma. Grief. Hemorrhages. Nursing, others. Senility. Stammering. Sycosis. Tinnitus. Trauma. Weakness.

HOMEOPATHIC - Useful for conditions of exhaustion and debility due to an overtaxed nervous system. Alzheimer's disease, senility. Epilepsy. After strokes and brain injuries. Encourages regeneration of nervous tissue.

Desire to sleep, to give up the struggle, for "all the problems to go away." Useful in desperate cases when the patient seems to be giving up. Feeling of being "not in the body," when the body has been so injured that it is no longer a wholly viable vehicle.

Chronic fatigue. Post traumatic stress, with disorientated. Weeps, especially at night, when alone. More cheerful during the day. Inhibition and lack of confidence. Allergy to peanuts.

MIND - Arrogance and haughtiness. Negative, bitter thoughts. Frustration. Resentment and bitterness from the past. Inability to forgive. Envy and jealousy. Hatred for those who have done well or better. Great negativity. Wakes with vengeful feelings.

Easily manipulated, or becomes manipulative. Addictive personalities, do not see the threat of their addiction, particularly in relationships. Fosters the strength to face deep issues that otherwise would lie buried.

Grief after sustained traumas or sadness. Rekindles imagination and intuition after emotional distress. Distracted and hard to concentrate. Calms the mind and improves memory.

Fearful accepting their fate. Indecisive and changeable. Mistakes and misinterprets meanings. Poor moral judgment. Encourages the id over the ego.

Back - Pain in the spine, especially after injuries. Tightness of the shoulders and cervical vertebrae. Lumbar and sacral areas are painful, worse menstrual problems.

Ears - Tinnitus comes and goes. Hardness of hearing.

Eyes - Glaucoma and cataract. Watering eyes when sneezing and laughing. Long or short sight becomes exaggerated.

Female - Uterine problems after grief or trauma. Endometriosis. Hemorrhages. Amenorrhea. Cancer of the uterus or the ovaries. History of frequent miscarriages. Useful for anxiety, weakness and debility during pregnancy. Useful for reducing the side effects upon ending hormone treatment.

Food - Poor assimilation of food.

Head - Headaches at night, worse left side. Light headed and dizzy. Stroke, affecting the left side of head and body.

Intestines - Bowel cancer, especially if it is secondary to cancer of the generative organs or from suppressed sycosis (i.e. polyps or warts).

Kidney - Kidney pains, worse right.

Limbs - Legs and feet very cold, but upper part and hands can be hot. Feels draft on the lower half of the body. Stiffness of the joints, especially hands and wrists.

Lungs - Difficulty breathing, worse night. Pressure on the chest, mediastinal region. Left side of chest most affected. Shallow breathing. Useful as a support or intercurrent remedy in asthma.

Heart - Sluggish circulation with cold extremities, especially the feet and lower legs, worse night. Can become too hot in the daytime.

Nose - Frequent need to blow nose, but little mucous.

Skin - Dryness of complaints, hot, burning itching (Apis.). Recurrent abscesses.

Stomach - Throat, esophagus and stomach all feel connected in discomfort (Ign., Nux-v.). Indigestion with painful trapped wind in the chest. Nausea, comes in waves. Better from limes and bitter fruit. Allergy to peanuts. Unable to lose weight in spite of dieting.

Throat - Dryness of throat and mouth. Sensations of constriction and of lump in the throat. Allergies that cause swelling of the throat. Throat cancer.

COMMENTS - Sycotic, syphilitic and tubercular. Useful in treating pathology (Cars.), especially for cancer of internal organs (given 30c or higher once a week). Cleanses the lymph system. Improves circulation.

Useful to support the action of heart remedies (Carb-v., Ars., Phos., and the snake poisons). Angina, where indicated remedies do not work. For drainage in cancer and blood problems (in the x potencies).

Radiation exposure. For emotional distress after general anesthetics. Mood or temperature swings.

Relates to the heart chakra. Encourages verbal expression of what would otherwise not be expressed due to grief (Nat-m., Aur., Lach., Caust.). Useful for deep grief. Works well when given repetition.

REFERENCES - Murphy.

EMETINUM

(Emetine)

PHARMACY - emetin. Emetinum. Emetine. It is the principal alkaloid of Ipecac. In physiological doses must be carefully watched. ***Historical dose:*** Trituration and all potencies.

CLINICAL - ***Amebiasis***. Colic. Diarrhea. Dysentery. Hematemesis. Hemorrhages. Pneumonia. Psoriasis. Pyorrhea.

HOMEOPATHIC - Emetin. is a powerful amebicide, but is not a bactericide. Specific for ***amebiasis.*** Useful for the treatment of amebic dysentery. Diarrhea with colic pains and nausea.

May produce hepatization of lungs, rapid heart action, and lobar pneumonia. Tendency to fall forward. Pyorrhea. Psoriasis.

RELATIONS - ***Compare:*** (1) In hematemesis and other hemorrhages, compare Gelin., which has a marked effect on the coagulability of the blood. Hypodermically or if by mouth, a 10 per cent. jelly, about 4 oz., three times a day.

REFERENCES - Boericke.

EOSINUM

(Eosin)

PHARMACY - eos. Eosinum. Eosin. ***Historical dose:*** Trituration and all potencies.

CLINICAL - Arthritis. Cancer. Vertigo.

HOMEOPATHIC - Proved in potencies by Dr. B.C. Woodbury. Eosin is a remedy for cancer. Polyarthritis. Peculiar sensation of being very tall with tendency to vertigo.

Burning in various parts on skin. Shifting location after scratching, which relieves. ***Burning*** under fingernails and toenails, on soles. ***Itching*** and redness of kneecaps. ***Redness*** of palms. Redness, burning and ***numbness*** of tongue.

REFERENCES - Boericke. Woodbury.

EPHEDRA VULGARIS

(Ma Huang)

PHARMACY - ephe. Ephedra vulgaris.Ma huang. Ephedra distachya. N. O. Gnetacee. Ephedraceae. Tincture of branches and flowers. ***Historical dose:*** Tincture and all potencies.

CLINICAL - Asthma. Exophthalmic goiter. Headaches.

HOMEOPATHIC - Ephedra has been proved in Russia by Dr. B. H. Mouravow. Ephedra produced symptoms when twenty drops of a strong alcoholic extract were taken five times a day, fifteen drops four times a day were taken without apparent effect.

General weakness from early morning, great fatigue. Extreme apathy. Asthma. Stiff-neck and backward pulling of whole body on turning the head. Starting of the eyes from the orbits as if pushed out.

To Mouravow, these symptoms suggested exophthalmic goiter. He also considered that the remedy acted on the ganglions of the sympathetic nerve and caused congestion of the spinal cord.

MIND - Extreme apathy and fatigue.

Abdomen - Dull pain in region of spleen (Cean.).

Back - Stiffness of neck with exophthalmos. Stiffness of neck and backward pulling of all the body on turning head, with a dull pain in region of spleen.

Eyes - Heavy eyes. Pain in the eye. Starting from their orbits, as if pushed out.

Head - Violent headache, nausea, general weakness, with a slow pulse. Left side hemicrania with numbness of entire left arm.

Heart - Abatement of the pulse, increases rapidity of action of heart. Strong heartbeat with weakening of pulse, respiration is accelerated.

Kidneys - Retention of the urine (fourth day).

Limbs - Heaviness in all the limbs, in evening. Numbness of entire left arm with left-side hemicrania.

Sleep - Longing for sleep.

RELATIONS - ***Compare:*** (1) Ferr., Iod., Lycopus v., Spong., (2) Thyroid. - exophthalmos.

REFERENCES - Clarke.

EPIGEA REPENS

(Gravel Weed)

PHARMACY - epig. Epigea repens. Gravel weed. Trailing arbutus. N. O. Ericaceae. Tincture of fresh leaves. The fresh leaves are pounded to a pulp and macerated in two parts by weight of alcohol, ***Historical dose:*** Tincture and all potencies.

CLINICAL - Bladder, disorders. ***Cystitis.*** Dysuria. ***Gravel.*** Kidney, stones. Pyelitis. Stones, urinary. Strangury. ***Uric acid.***

HERBAL - Epigea has long had a reputation in urinary difficulties and even in calculous disorders. The common appellation of "gravel root" shows that the popular belief points in the direction of its use.

Hale mentioned Epig. as having been a popular remedy in kidney stones throughout the United States ever since the settlement. It has been successful in removing dysuria and strangury as well as urinary tenesmus.

HOMEOPATHIC - Chronic cystitis with ***dysuria***. Pyelitis with incontinence of urine. ***Mucus, pus and uric acid deposit***, gravel, kidney stones. Fine sand in urine of a ***brown color***. Burning in neck of bladder while urinating. Tenesmus after urination. Croaking noise and rumbling in bowels.

COMMENTS - Hale gave ten drops of the tincture six times a day to a patient who had a bloody muco-purulent sediment in the urine with intense dysuria. A copious deposit of fine brown sand was observed and all symptoms were relieved.

RELATIONS - ***Compare:*** (1) Mitch., Chim., Cann-i., Calc. ren., Urt-u., Uric acid. (2) Uva, Lyc. Pareira. (3) Epigea contains Arbutin, Formic acid. (4) Arbutus, Uva ursi.

REFERENCES - Anshutz. Clarke. Hale.

EPILOBIUM PALUSTRE

(Willow Herb)

PHARMACY - epil. Epilobium palustre. Willow herb. Epilobium linears. N. O. Onagraceae. Tincture of fresh rhizome. ***Historical dose:*** Tincture and all potencies.

CLINICAL - Dysphagia. Fever. Larynx, disorders. Ptyalism. Throat, sore.

HOMEOPATHIC - A boy poisoned with the flowers of Epil. hirsutum had strong epileptiform convulsions in rapid succession. Epil. was proved by Dr. J. S. Wright using a tincture of the root.

Headache. Red face. Ptyalism, chokes on saliva. Feeling of throat filling up, could not swallow water. Larynx sore to pressure, swollen on outside, with hard lumps on both sides of larynx. Cannot swallow liquids, can fly out of nose. Loose stools, red urine.

Hard chill beginning at 11 a.m., lasting an hour. High fever, with aching all over and severe headache, lasting through the night, could not sleep. Fever and headache passed off, but returns in the afternoon and evening more severely, lasting all night. Dull and sleepy, but could not sleep.

REFERENCES - Allen. Clarke.

EPIPHEGUS VIRGINIANA

(Beech-drop)

PHARMACY – epip. Epiphegus virginiana. Beech-drop. Epiphegus americana. Cancer root. Orobanche virginiana. N. O. Orobanchaceae. Tincture of whole fresh plant in full flower. ***Historical dose:*** Tincture and all potencies.

CLINICAL - Cancer. Diarrhea. Gonorrhea. ***Headaches.*** Neurasthenia. Palpitations. Salivation. ***Sub-involution, uterus.***

HOMEOPATHIC - Epip. is a remedy for sick, neurasthenic and ***nervous headaches***, especially in women, brought on or made worse by exertion, nervous strain, etc.

Headaches with pressive pain, as if fingertips were pressing into the temples inwards or compressive pain going backwards, worse until 4 p.m., then better with spitting of viscid saliva and nausea.

Neurasthenia. Languid feeling. Drowsy after meals. Tongue coated yellow, bitter taste. Loose stools. ***Sub-involution of the uterus*** with painful menstruation and congestion.

MIND - Confusion of mind, makes wrong letters or words in writing. Fears death from heart palpitations, injury to her health from the drug.

Causations - Physical or nervous overstrain. Any unusual exertion or excitement, as going on a visit or doing a day's shopping.

Eyes - Smarting. Could not read because the words seemed to be blurred.

Female - ***Subinvolution of uterus***, with painful menses and congestion.

Head - ***Nervous headaches. Pain, worse left side.*** Pressing pain in temples from ***without inwards***. Headaches from nervous strain caused by mental or physical exhaustion, ***preceded by hunger.*** Sick headache coming on when deviating from ordinary pursuits, weekly sick headaches. ***Viscid salivation***, constant inclination to spit.

Heart - Palpitations, causing weakness.

Limbs - Pain in left shoulder, left knee.

Modalities - Better from sleep. Worse from fatigue. Worse nervous strain. Worse eyestrain. Worse working in open air. Worse rising up in bed.

Mouth - Tongue coated yellow, bitter taste. Saliva viscid, almost constant desire to spit. Sticky viscid, bitter taste in mouth.

Rectum - Loose stools. Stool passed with difficulty, though feces soft.

Stomach - Nausea.

Teeth - Tartar on teeth.

COMMENTS - Grimmer noted skin cancers, palpitations with weakness, and a constant desire to spit viscid saliva. Severe headache brought on by exertion, relieved by a good sleep. Symptoms travel right to left.

RELATIONS - ***Compare:*** (1) Iris, Meli., Sang. (2) Fagus - beech-nuts - headache and salivation, swelling on mouth, dread of water. (3) It is allied to the Scrofulariaceae. (4) Phos. - in better from sleep, Lach., Sulph. and Nat-m. have the opposite, worse from sleep in the most marked degree.

REFERENCES - Boericke. Clarke. Grimmer.

EPIPHYSTERINUM

PHARMACY - epih. Epiphysterinum. Epiphysterin. A nosode. ***Historical dose:*** All potencies.

CLINICAL - Fibroids. Menorrhagia. Tumors. Uterine, hemorrhage.

HOMEOPATHIC - One of Dr. Burnett's nosodes, he used it in cases of hemorrhage in a patient suffering from a fibrous tumor, possibly with malignant elements.

COMMENTS - Clarke found Epih. of great value in controlling uterine hemorrhage, whether connected with fibrous growth or not. He used it in the 30c and higher potencies, giving one or two doses weekly.

RELATIONS - ***Compare:*** (1) The cancer nosodes, Carc. (2) in the fibroid tumors and uterine hemorrhages, like Thlaspi., Fraxin., Hydr. and its alkaloids.

REFERENCES - Boericke. Clarke. Phatak.

EQUISETUM HYEMALE

(Horse-tail)

PHARMACY - equis. Equisetum hyemale. Horse-tail. Scouring-rush. N. O. Equisetaceae. A rush growing in damp soil in Europe and America. Tincture of fresh plant chopped and pounded to a pulp. ***Historical dose:*** Tincture and all potencies.

CLINICAL - Albuminuria. ***Bedwetting.*** Bladder, disorders. ***Cystitis.*** Diabetes. Dropsy. Dysuria. Gleet. Gonorrhea. Gravel. Hematuria. Involuntary, urination. ***Kidney, disorders. Kidney, weakness.*** Paralysis. ***Polyuria.*** Urinary, retention.

HERBAL - Equisetum contains silica in an appreciable quantity. Horsetail tea is widely know as a ***kidney and bladder tonic***. It is a natural and soothing diuretic used for polyuria and urinary retention.

Teaspoonful doses of the decoction or the tincture in hot water is found useful to allay irritability of the urinary tract, kidney stones, dysuria, pleuritis effusion and dropsy.

HOMEOPATHIC - Affinity for the urinary organs. ***Pain in the kidneys*** (especially right), in the bladder and urinary passages. Irritation of the bladder and kidneys.

Urinary retention and dysuria, especially in women during pregnancy and after confinement. ***Constant desire to urinate*** and ***passes large quantities of clear, light-colored urine*** without relief.

Cystitis. Severe, dull pain that does not lessen after urination. Aching, full, tender bladder, not better after urinating. Pain in bladder as from distention. Pricking, burning, cutting pain in urethra while urinating.

Dribbling urine in old women with involuntary stool. Much mucus in urine. Bedwetting (Lyc., Nat-m., Sil., Sep.). ***Nocturnal bedwetting of children*** without causes except habit. Bedwetting when he dreams, he always sees a crowd of people. Pain in sacroiliac joints.

MIND - Very irritable and easily fatigued.

Abdomen - Distended feeling. Sharp pains on either side of hypogastrium, extending to middle line. Dull, heavy pains in either side of lower abdomen and bladder with frequent desire to urinate, not better by urinating. Severe pain in lower abdomen with passage of fetid flatus.

Back - Pains in back, especially while sitting, better lying on back and walking. Right lumbar region painful. Heavy sensation like a lump in right lumbar region. Severe rheumatic pains in region of sacral-lumbar joint and through left hip joint extending down outer side of left leg, ending in front three inches above knee.

Bladder - ***Frequent, profuse urination of clear, watery urine.*** Urgent desire to urinate with prickling, biting, itching, and soreness of meatus from contact and pressure, worse scratching. ***Retention of urine after childbirth.*** Retention and dysuria during pregnancy. Pricking in urethra a short distance back from meatus. Severe, dull pain in bladder. ***Feeling of fullness in bladder, not relieved by urinating.*** Profuse urination with burning in urethra and sharp pain at root of penis. ***Sharp, burning***, cutting pain in urethra while urinating. Involuntary urination during daytime. Bedwetting, nocturnal and diurnal. ***Bedwetting in children*** with dreams or nightmares when passing urine. ***Obliged to rise several times at night to urinate.*** Incontinence in old women, with involuntary stools.

Breasts - Sharp stitch in left breast, one inch to left and over nipple.

Ears - Dull, transient pain and stiff feeling behind left mastoid. Confused feeling in ears. Confusion of sounds, confused noises, fearful rumbling.

Eyes - Severe pain in roof of right orbit. Sharp pain in outer angle of right eye.

Face - Face flushed, feeling of heat. ***Disposed to frown.*** As if blood pressed into face. Heat and burning without redness.

Head - Severe headache with intense pain in upper part of eyes or roof of orbit. Headache with heat of face without redness. Constrictive feeling across forehead. Sticking and darting pains, changing locality. Constriction of whole scalp, as if drawn tightly over whole skull. Feeling of skin continuing to contract, continual desire to wrinkle up forehead.

Heart - Sharp pain in region of heart, worse by inspiration.

Kidneys - Nephritis. Diabetes insipidus. ***Weak and sensitive kidneys from abuse of diuretics.*** Slight pain in right kidney, then in left, extending down left side of sacrum. ***Frequent urination at night.*** Deep pain in region of right kidney, extending to lower abdomen with urgent desire to urinate. Polyuria associated with diabetes. Frequent urging, with ***severe pain at the close of urination***.

Limbs - Pain in upper part of shoulders and in region of vertebra prominence, worse by least motion or contact. Pain in right shoulder to middle of upper arm. Pain in left shoulder with shivering over body and great heat of head. Pain in right hip joint and near knee joint. Knees very weak on least exertion. Dull, heavy pain under left patella. On awakening, sharp pain inner side of left knee, better after moving about a short time.

Male - Violent erections in the afternoon. Soreness of testicles and cords, worse left.

Modalities - Better in afternoon. Better lying down. Better continued motion. Worse right side. Worse movement. Worse touch. Worse pressure. Worse contact. Worse sitting down. Worse at close of urination.

Rectum - Smarting in anus during and after stool. Stool with aching in anus and feeling as if rectum would protrude. Feeling as if some feces still remained. Sticking-like pains in anus (11 a. m.). Stool with great flatulence.

Sleep - Very sleepy, heavy eyelids. Sleep disturbed by tiresome dreams. Dreams of many persons, places and things. ***Dreams of crowds of people.*** Nightmare when passing urine.

Stomach - Excessive hunger, appetite greatly increased.

Temperature - Creeping chills beginning below and creeping up back.

Throat - Sharp sticking in throat.

Urine - Copious amounts of watery urine. Urine flows only drop by drop. ***Profuse urination of clear, watery urine.*** Passes large quantities of clear, light-colored urine without relief. Albuminuria. Urine cloudy. Great excess of mucus on standing.

COMMENTS - Equis. is a deep anti-sycotic. Pain in the kidneys, especially the right. Pain in the bladder and urinary passages, as from distention. Retention and dysuria, especially in women during pregnancy and after confinement.

Severe cystitis. Acute bladder infections, especially when passing large amounts of pale urine. Polyuria. Frequent urination or lack of urination. Paralysis of the bladder, urinary retention (Acon., Apis., Caust.).

Constant desire to urinate, passes large quantities of clear, light-colored urine without relief. Severe, dull pain that does not lessen after urination, irritation of the bladder, especially in women. Burning pain at the end of urination (Sars.).

Diabetes with frequent urination. General paralysis with loss of control over bladder and rectum. Multiple sclerosis cases with incontinence of the urine. For the side effects of strong diuretics.

Loss of hair, and weak nails. Mending broken bones, can help retain calcium and prevent osteoporosis. Hot flashes. The tincture is a natural diuretic and tonic for weak kidneys, and is also good for hemorrhoids.

Farrington noted the bedwetting with frequent painful urging to urinate, causing the patient to rise at night. According to Grimmer, this remedy cured a case of uterine cancer.

RELATIONS - ***Compare:*** (1) Sars., Apis, Berb., Hydrang., Ferr-p., Linaria, Chim. (2) Cann-i., Puls., (3) Canth. comes closest, there is less bleeding, tenesmus, scalding and fibrinous flakes than with Canth., but more mucus.

REFERENCES - Boericke. Clarke. Murphy. Phatak.

ERECHTHITES HIERACIFOLIA

(Fireweed)

PHARMACY - erech. Erechthites hieracifolia. Fireweed. Senecio hieracifolia. Erechthites praealta. N. O. Composite. Tincture of whole fresh plant. ***Historical dose:*** Tincture and all potencies.

CLINICAL - Diarrhea. Eczema. Gonorrhea. ***Hemorrhages.*** Herpes. Metrorrhagia. Nausea. Nosebleeds. Psoriasis. Orchitis. ***Rhus poisoning***. Ulcers.

HERBAL - Erechthites belongs to the composite and closely allied to erigeron and the groundsel family (Senec.). *"Fireweed"* is so called because it grows abundantly in clearings which have been burnt out.

According to Hale, *"Oil of Fireweed"* is also extracted from erigeron and is said by alchemists to be similar to turpentine. All three cause active and passive hemorrhages, the former being the primary and the latter the secondary action.

HOMEOPATHIC - Erech. is indicated in hemorrhages of bright red blood from nose, mouth, bowels, kidneys, uterus and especially the lungs. ***Hemorrhage from any part***, always attended by excitement of the circulation. Passive hemorrhages of dark fluid blood. Nosebleed of bright blood.

Metrorrhagia. Flashes of heat that suddenly give way to coldness. Scanty urine, edema of the limbs. Useful as a local application in skin affections, herpes, eczema, psoriasis and indolent ulcers. Increased appetite. Increased feeling of strength and desire for exercise.

Hale commended it in gonorrhea and orchitis.

Back - Stitches in middle of back. Aching across small of back.

Female - Premature and profuse menses. Metrorrhagia.

Head - Giddiness with nausea. Dull frontal headache. Throbbing of temporal arteries with flushes of heat running across the back from one shoulder to the other. The sensation of heat suddenly gives way to that of coldness.

Kidneys - Increased flow of urine. Slight burning at meatus during urination.

Limbs - Cold feeling in back of legs. Legs feel stiff and painful.

Male - Prolonged erections with dreams of nudity, towards morning. Orchitis from suppressed discharge. Gonorrhea with scanty discharges and great pain.

Rectum - Griping followed by three copious discharges of semi-solid, yellow fecal matter.

Skin - ***Symptoms like rhus poisoning***.

Sleep - Dreams of nudity and shame.

Stomach - Enormous appetite. Feeling in stomach as if it would be dissolved after drinking cold water. Belchings and heartburn after eating warm bread and coffee (cured).

Throat - Sore throat.

RELATIONS - ***Compare:*** (1) Rhus-t. Senec., Erigeron, Ham. Mill., Calc., Canth., Terebe., Puls., Clem.

REFERENCES - Boericke. Clarke.

ERGOTINUM

PHARMACY - ergot. Ergotinum. Ergotin. Alkaloids of Secale cornutum. Trituration. ***Historical dose:*** Trituration and all potencies.

CLINICAL - Alopecia. Anal, incontinence. Bedwetting. Dysmenorrhea. Faintness. Gangrene. Heart, paralysis. Hemorrhages. Menorrhagia. Migraines. Miscarriage. Neurological, disorders. ***Pre-menstrual, migraines.*** Sphincters, paralysis. Urticaria.

HOMEOPATHIC - Ergotinum is the total extract of the ergot Claviceps Purpurea. The ergot is the intermediary stage through which this mushroom passes in order to complete its development. Claviceps Pupurea, otherwise known as Secale Cornutum, is widely used in homeopathic medicine, with its own indications.

This Ascomycetes Pyrenomycetes is a parasite on the ears of rye, as well as on other grain such as wheat or oats, and on other plants such as Cypetaceae and palm trees.

The toxicity of ergot has been known for a long time, manifested by the medieval epidemics of Saint Anthony's Fire due to the consumption of contaminated flour. Its oxytocic and abortive powers are also well known.

The insoluble polypeptide alkaloids are stimulants of smooth tissues, especially uterine and vascular. Affects the sympathetic system, counteracts the effects of adrenalin. Ergotinine, the extract of ergot of rye, is used in allopathic medicine, as a constrictor of blood vessels to encourage hemostasis, as in uterine and pulmonary hemorrhages.

Ergot. acts by causing contraction of the arterioles and its effect is produced most promptly when it is administered by subcutaneous injection. Its homeopathic use are in the main identical with those of Sec., but Ergot. will sometimes succeed when Sec. fails.

Ergot. is primarily a female remedy, functional complaints of the female genitalia. ***Pre-menstrual migraines.*** Menstrual complaints. Vulvar itching.

General ill-defined discomforts, head feeling empty, misty vision, noise in the ears, vertigo, nausea, occasional vomiting.

Nervous system disturbed, anxiety, faintness. Nerve attacks with sudden strokes, abrupt clouding of consciousness, both psychological and physical. For cases with a loss of consciousness.

Certain forms of alopecia or allergy. Urticaria. Bedwetting in both sexes with no anatomical lesion or any urinary infection, with an increase in the level of neurosis from anguish.

MIND - Anxious, hyper-emotiional state. Instability of the character. Slowing down of mental processes. Chronic mental depression. Depressive state, particularly before menstruation. ***Sadness and weeping before menses.*** Loss of consciousness.

Breasts - Premenstrual swelling of the breasts and abdomen.

Ears - Buzzing, intermittent deafness.

Eyes - Visual complaints such as mistiness, cloudy vision, luminous spots before the eyes. Black patches, black or glinting spots across the field of vision.

Female - ***Pre-menstrual syndrome***. Painful menstruation with no clinically discernible lesion. Dysmenorrhea with red, non-clotting blood. Menorrhagia in young virgins from the beginning of menses in the young woman. Vulvo-vaginal itching, congestion, redness, dryness of the mucus membranes. Hyper functioning of the pituitary and ovaries.

Head - Migraines. Habitual headaches. ***Premenstrual migraines.*** Diffuse alopecia. Round patches of alopecia.

Skin - Alopecia-type areas. Urticaria. Pruritus. Edema.

Sleep - Insomnia, especially in women.

Vertigo - Attacks of faintness.

COMMENTS - "Wide-open anus sensation" (Sec., Phos.). Koeck of Munich recorded a case of a patient who suffered from diarrhea since the Franco-German war and latterly had lost all power of retention. The rectum had lost all sensation, so that the patient had no warning and was never clean.

Old school treatment had failed to relieve him. He was about to be pensioned by his employers and had thoughts of suicide. Sec. 3x ameliorated slightly, the 2x had the same result.

"Remembering Kafka's advice to use the alkaloid when the indicated drug did not seem to act, he prescribed Ergotin 2x." After taking this for four days the patient regained control.

Demange recorded the case of a young woman suffering from typhoid fever and threatened with heart paralysis. Stimulating injections of ether and of rum and frictions completely failed to rally her.

Cyanosis increased rapidly and threatened the trunk. Fainting spells occurred in rapid succession, pulse filiform. Ergot. was then injected and the pulse rose and the symptoms of collapse disappeared. Most of the symptoms of this patient may be found under Sec.

RELATIONS - ***Compare:*** (1) Sec. - Dysmenorrhea with blood clotting and black blood. (2) Folliculinum - Pre-menstrual syndrome with swelling, headaches, hypermenorrhea. (3) Thyr. - Depressive condition, anxious with hyperthyroid tendency, trembling and pigmentation, especially of the eyelids. (4) Ign. - Nervous, paradoxical instability, anguish with feeling of constriction in the throat and the epigastrium. (5) Lil-t. - Complaints in the uterus and ovarian region, heaviness of the lower abdomen.

REFERENCES - Boericke. Clarke. Julian.

ERIGERON CANADENSIS

(Fleabane)

PHARMACY - erig. Erigeron canadensis. Fleabane. Leptilon canadense. N. O. Compositae. Canada. Tincture from the fresh plant when in bloom. ***Historical dose:*** Tincture and all potencies.

CLINICAL - Black, eye. Bruises. Coughs. ***Dysentery.*** Dysuria. Gleet. Gonorrhea. Hematocele. ***Hemorrhages.*** Hemorrhoids. Injuries. ***Leucorrhea***. Metrorrhagia. Miscarriage. Placenta, previa. Proctalgia. Spermatorrhea. ***Tympanites***. Uterus, weak. Wounds.

HERBAL - Native Americans used Erigeron as an application to wounds. It compares as a vulnerary with Arn. Erig. is chiefly known as a remedy for hemorrhages and congestions in all parts of the body. Bright red hemorrhages.

HOMEOPATHIC - Erig. has been proved by Burt and others. Wilmot Moore gave it with success in three cases of placenta previa. He gave the 1x trituration (of what part of the plant is not mentioned) on the tongue.

Hemorrhagic remedy, especially when hemorrhages are ***profuse, bright red***, gushing. Persistent hemorrhage from the bladder. Uterine hemorrhage with painful urination. Pain in left ovary and hip. Chronic gonorrhea with burning urination, continual dribbling. Gleet.

Burning congestions. Hard aching. Sensation as if something had lodged in upper part of esophagus.

Dysentery with soreness and burning in the bladder. ***Tympanites***. Prominent pains in umbilical region. Feeling as if anus had been torn. Urination is painful or suppressed, sharp stinging pains in region of left kidney.

MIND - Great despondency. Excessive fatigue in morning, all day with great depression. No ambition to move in afternoon and evening. Sadness with feeling of great languor. Weeping during urination.

Abdomen - Abdomen distended. Frequent distress in umbilicus with hard, aching distress in whole dorsal region. Frequent dull pain in umbilical region, can be severe, cutting, with a feeling in anus as if it had been torn.

Back - Dull, aching distress in whole dorsal region. Dull pains in lumbar and sacral regions. Severe sticking, stabbing pain in region of left kidney, passing to right kidney.

Bladder - Frequent desire. Dysuria of teething children. Urination painful or suppressed. Crying when urinating. Urine profuse, with strong odor. External parts (female) inflamed or irritated with considerable mucus discharge.

Ears - Loud singing in right ear.

Eyes - Smarting, burning, in afternoon or evening. Ecchymosis around from below. Slight agglutination of lids in morning.

Face - Congested, red face.

Female - Miscarriage, because of exertion. ***Pregnant women with a weak uterus.*** Bloody discharge on slight exertion. Metrorrhagia with violent irritation of rectum and bladder and prolapse uterus. Metrorrhagia after miscarriage with diarrhea or dysentery after least motion. Uterine hemorrhage, bright-red flow (Phos.). ***Bloody lochia returns after least motion,*** comes in gushes, between periods. Bleeding hemorrhoids, nosebleed instead of menses (Bry.) ***Leucorrhea with urinary irritation***, profuse.

Head - Congestion of the head, red face, nosebleed, febrile action. Awakened with dull headache, with aching distress in all the large joints. Dull frontal headache with smarting in eyes.

Heart - Palpitations.

Kidneys - Persistent hemorrhage from the bladder. Bladder, rectal tenesmus with metrorrhagia. Aching in bladder. Retention of urine. Dysuria during dentition, crying when urinating.

Limbs - Aching dullness in all the joints and limbs. Hard aching in all the limbs.

Lungs - Cough, bloody expectoration. Incipient tuberculosis.

Male - Sticky sweat on genitals. Gonorrhea and gleet. Blue, black spots on genitals. Pain in right lumbar region passing down to testicle.

Modalities - Worse from exertion. Worse rest. Worse left side. Worse rainy weather. Every movement aggravates flow, causes bloody lochia to return.

Mouth - Bad taste in mouth.

Nose - Nosebleed of bright red blood. Increased secretion of mucus all forenoon. Nosebleed.

Rectum - Hemorrhages from the bowels. Burning in the bowels and rectum, hard lumps of feces mixed with the discharges. Hemorrhoids, bleeding with a hard, lumpy stools, burning in the margin of anus, it feels as if torn. Rheumatic pains in abdominal muscles. Stools small, streaked with blood. Mushy stools.

Skin - Ecchymosis. Slightly elevated, sharply defined vesicles on skin.

Stomach - Sharp cutting pains in epigastric region every few minutes followed by dull pains. Burning in stomach and abdomen. Belchings of air. Violent retching and burning in the stomach. Vomit or stool of pure blood.

Throat - Increased secretion of mucus in nostrils all forenoon. Feeling of roughness of pharynx. Sensation as if something had lodged in the upper part of the esophagus that caused frequent inclination to swallow.

RELATIONS - *Compare:* (1) Ip., Phos., Ham., Arn., Canth., Cop., Sabin. (2) Terebinthina similar. (3) It is related to Senec., Erech.

REFERENCES - Boericke. Clarke. Phatak.

ERIODICTYON CALIFORNICUM

(Yerba Santa)

PHARMACY - erio. Eriodictyon californicum. Yerba santa. Eriodyction glutinosum. N. O. Hydrophyllaceae. Tincture of whole plant. ***Historical dose:*** Tincture and all potencies.

CLINICAL - Asthma. Bronchitis. Catarrh. Coryza. ***Coughs***. Influenza. Nausea. Night-sweats. Tuberculosis. Wheezing.

HERBAL - Yerba Santa, the holy plant, is a popular expectorant remedy in Mexico and California. Allen said "Eriodyction has a strong terebinthine taste and abounds in a resinous matter which sometimes exudes so copiously that in drying, the specimens stick firmly together and to the paper."

HOMEOPATHIC - Erio. is a remedy for asthmatic and bronchial disorders. Asthmatic breathing with accumulation of mucus, relieved when the mucus is cleared. Coryza and catarrh. ***Coughs after influenza***. Whooping cough. Furthers absorption of effusion in pleural cavity.

Tubercular conditions, especially bronchial tuberculosis. Tuberculosis as the result of frequent bronchial catarrhs. Impaired digestion, poor appetite, intolerance of food. Wasting, night-sweats.

Ears - Pain in ears. Sharp, shooting pain in right ear, at intervals or on suddenly changing position of head to right or left, changing to just below external ear.

Head - Pressure outwards, worse occiput. Aching at base of cranium, 8 a.m. Sensation of pressure outwards on all sides of head, greatest at cerebellum upwards. Intense, dull, heavy pain in back of head and over eyes. Burning in occiput, heavy pain as if occiput was being pressed out.

Lungs - Asthma, coryza and ***mucus secretions***. Wheezing. Chronic bronchitis, bronchial tuberculosis with profuse, easily raised bronchial secretion, giving relief. Wheezing voice, at 5 p.m. Dull pain in right lung, front.

Male - Sore, dragging, tender feeling in testicles, worse left, could not bear any pressure, better gentle support. Dreaded to move because of its tenderness. Slight fluttering at intervals at bottom of testicles.

Modalities - Worse in afternoon. Nausea, worse on running. Symptoms come at intervals or on any sudden changes of position.

Mouth - Foul mouth in morning. Burning in fauces.

Nose - Coryza with dizziness and sneezing. Yellowish-green catarrh.

Stomach - Great appetite. Nausea. Deathly sickness, worse by running.

Temperature - Slight fever, cheeks flushed and burning.

Throat - Burning sensation in fauces and throat.

Vertigo - Dizziness and a sense of intoxication.

COMMENTS - G. M. Payne's proving brought out marked preference for the right lung. Foul mouth in the morning on rising. J. Perry Seward gave it with great success in two cases of cough remaining after influenza.

RELATIONS - ***Compare:*** (1) Grind., Aral., Eucal., Ip. (2) Balsam of Peru, Pix liquida, Stann. (3) afternoon aggravation. Lyc., Grind., Phos., Hep., Rumex, Caust., Dros.

REFERENCES - Boericke. Clarke.

ERODIUM CICUTARIUM

(Hemlock Stork's Bill)

PHARMACY - erod. Erodium cicutarium. Hemlock Stork's bill. N. O. Geraniaceae. Tincture of fresh plant. ***Historical dose:*** Tincture and all potencies. Decoction of half ounce of the herb to six ounces of water.

CLINICAL - Hemorrhages. Menorrhagia. Metrorrhagia. Uterine, polyps.

HOMEOPATHIC - Erodium is a popular hemostatic remedy in Russia, and is especially used for metrorrhagia and menorrhagia. Uterine hemorrhage with polyps. Has controlled hemorrhage after Sec. failed.

Komorowitch cured with it numbers of cases in which Ergot. and Hydr. had failed, including a case of cervical polyps. After three day's use of the decoction, the polyps were found lying free in the vagina.

RELATIONS - ***Compare:*** (1) Ger.

REFERENCES - Boericke. Clarke.

ERYNGIUM AQUATICUM

(Button Snake-root)

PHARMACY - ery-a. Eryngium aquaticum. Button snake-root. N. O. Umbelliferae. Tincture of fresh root. ***Historical dose:*** Tincture and all potencies.

CLINICAL - Anus, prolapse. Conjunctivitis. Constipation. Cough. Diarrhea. Dropsy. Gleet. Gonorrhea. Hemorrhoids. ***Influenza.*** Laryngitis. Leucorrhea. Kidney, colic. Prostate, weakness. Sclerotitis. Sexual, weakness. Strabismus. Spermatorrhea. Urine incontinence. Wounds.

HERBAL - Eryngium is a remedy for urinary disorders. The English Eryngo, the E. Maritinum, is noted as an aphrodisiac and is very similar in appearance to the Eryngium aquaticum.

HOMEOPATHIC - Acts on the mucus membranes, producing ***thick yellow mucus discharges*** from eyes, ears, nose, mouth, bowels, urethra and vagina. Cough with a sense of constriction. Hemorrhages from stomach and bowels. Influenza.

It is a vulnerary, antidoting the effect of blows. Headaches, expanding sensation in forehead, dull, dragging pain in occiput, neck and shoulders. ***Seminal and prostate weakness.*** For spermatorrhea properly so called or emission of semen without erections. Strangury with nervous weakness. Sweat smells like urine, in evening.

MIND - Thoughts are confused. Very sober and depressed in spirits. Very dull at night. Not able to think steadily on any subject. Cannot concentrate on any subject, the effort causes heavy full, pain if persisted at.

Abdomen - Severe colicky or cramping pains in small intestines. Severe pain in left groin and testicle.

Back - When headache is less severe, it is worse in neck and shoulders. Weakness and heavy dragging pain in lumbar region.

Chest - Oppression of chest, feeling of fulness, inability to take a full breath.

Ears - Bruised tearing pain, as if ears being torn off. Inflammation of Eustachian tube, left ear swollen in and out, tender to pressure, constant aching, bleeding readily, thick white, bloody, foul-smelling pus. Continued singing and ringing with creaking sound in left ear.

Eyes - Purulent inflammation of left eye, sticking discharge causing gumming of lids, conjunctiva granular and rough. Muscles of eyes feel stiff, pain on moving them quickly. Burning, sensitive to light. Effects of exposure to strong light, squinting, sclerotitis, watery or purulent discharges.

Female - Leucorrhea.

Head - Sharp, shooting pain over left eye, when sitting in stooping posture leaves eye, passes into neck and along muscles of shoulder and beneath scapula. Shooting in coronary region and in right side of face from eyes to teeth in morning. Dull, dragging pain in occiput, neck and shoulders, when less severe in head is worse in shoulder. Scalp sore, combing hair causes pain (Cina.).

Kidneys - Congestion of kidneys with dull pain in back, running down the ureters and limbs. Pain behind pubes. ***Kidney pain, colic*** (Berb., Pareir., Calc.). Spasmodic stricture. Tenesmus of bladder and urethra. Difficult and frequent urination. Must urinate every five minutes, urine dropping away all the time and burning like fire. Stinging, burning pain in urethra, behind glans during urination. Irritable bladder from enlarged prostate gland or from pressure of uterus.

Lungs - Oppression of chest, feeling of fullness inability to take a long breath. Short, hacking cough. Cough with sensation of constriction in throat. Smarting in throat and larynx.

Male - Discharge of prostatic fluid from slight causes. Desire suppressed, then excited with lewd dreams and pollutions. Seminal emissions without erections, with lassitude (Dios., Phos-ac). Emissions without erections, day and night, followed by great lassitude after injury to testicles. Gonorrhea with painful erections. Gleet.

Modalities - Better from heat. Worse from motion, mental exertion. Bending head forward aggravates head symptoms. Turning eyes causes pain in them. Most symptoms occur on left side and extend or move from part to part.

Mouth - Thick, tenacious, disagreeable mucus in mouth.

Nose - Profuse, thick, yellow mucus discharge.

Rectum - Constipation. Tenesmus at stool, with a sensation of cutting as they pass through anus. Stools dark leaden color, dry and very hard. Mucus diarrhea of children. Hemorrhoids and prolapsed anus.

Stomach - Partial anorexia. Hollowness or emptiness in stomach with heavy, dragging pain. Nausea, followed by acrid belchings. Spitting of bright arterial blood, mixed with black clots, with burning in epigastrium after a blow on the stomach. Burning in stomach or esophagus after taking the drug.

Throat - Chronic laryngitis. Smarting, raw pain along left side of throat, dry tongue. Intense redness, slight swelling without pain, profuse secretion of thick whitish mucus.

Vertigo - Vertigo with an expanding sensation in frontal region above eyes, worse stooping, causing dimness of sight.

COMMENTS - Ery-a. has two remarkable cures, reported by Dr. Parks. In the first, a married man injured his testicles by jumping upon a horse, this was followed by discharge of what was considered semen for fifteen years during which time he was treated by allopaths and homeopaths.

The emissions were without erections, day or night, and followed by great lassitude. Dr. Parks tried a number of the usual remedies without permanent benefit. He then gave a half grain dose, three times a day of the third decimal trituration of the "Eryngium aquaticum." In five days the emissions were entirely suppressed and did not return.

The second case concerned a married man who was not conscious of having sustained any injury, who was troubled for eight to ten years with emissions at night with erections The semen also passed by day with urine. The loss of semen was followed by great lassitude and depression, continuing from twelve to forty-eight hours. There was also partial impotence. He had been treated allopathically.

Dr. Parks gave him Ph-ac. for two weeks without material benefit. He then the Ery-a., as above with the same excellent and prompt result.

J. Whitfield cured three cases of kidney colic with stones (two left side, the other not stated) with Ery-a.

Hale found it useful in epidemic influenza when there was raw, smarting burning in throat and larynx, with constant irritating cough and expectoration of yellow mucus. Loss of energy and nervous weakness.

W. K. Leonard reported the following case of a young Methodist minister, apparently healthy, who was just over his twelfth attack of kidney colic.

The attacks had recurred at intervals of two to four weeks and lasted from one to three days. They were so weakening as to keep him incapacitated in the intervals.

He had old-school treatment including morphine and quinine, without benefit. The attacks were accompanied with severe nervous chills and it was for these that the quinine had been prescribed. Ery-a. tincture, five drops three times a day, put an end to the trouble.

RELATIONS - ***Compare:*** (1) Con., Cann-i., Dios., Oci., Clem.

REFERENCES - Boericke. Clarke.

ERYNGIUM MARITIMUM

(Sea Holly)

PHARMACY - ery-m. Eryngium maritimum. Sea holly. N. O. Umbelliferae. Tincture of whole plant including root. ***Historical dose:*** Tincture and all potencies.

CLINICAL - Cough. Debility. Fever. Herpes. Sexual weakness. Skin eruption.

HERBAL - The maritime Eryngium is a beautiful plant growing on sand-hills by the sea with holly-like leaves of a pale blue color with metallic luster, in general appearance much more resembling a thistle than an Umbelliferae.

HOMEOPATHIC - Ery-m. was proved by one prover only, E. B. Ivatts, but the symptoms showed considerable resemblance to those of Ery-a.

Pains in the eyes, groins, larynx, nape of neck, sinking at epigastrium and weakness of the male sexual organs appear in both. Ery-m. has its symptoms more prominently on the right side. Circulation deadened or as if stagnated, but great determination of blood to surface.

MIND - Light and unusually cheerful. On awaking in the morning feeling so merry commences to sing in bed (usually heavy and drowsy).

Abdomen - All viscera seemed prostrated and as heavy as lead. Dull, continuous pain in bowels. Pain in one spot in right groin.

Back - Pain at nape, compelling the support of head on hand or against something. Occasional shooting pains under left scapula.

Eyes - Pain at back of right eye, left eye feeling weak. Inclination to close eyes to shut out moving objects.

Fever - Chills commencing at nape, going down shoulders and back. Chills predominate, little fever heat

Limbs - Veins of hands at back appear contracted and depressed so as to be hardly visible, though generally full and prominent. Sore pain in muscles inside right thigh just above knee.

Lungs - Occasional darting pains through lungs to back. Occasional stomach cough during the day, sending a spasmodic pain to the head.

Male - Insensibility of corona glandis. Absence of desire (secondary action), power of erection quite gone.

Skin - Patch of eruption half the size of palm of hand came out in cluster where pain had been the day previous like fine pin-heads, points feeling rough to fingers, died away next day leaving red areola.

Stomach - Loss of appetite. Sinking feeling at pit of stomach.

Throat - Voice low, larynx feels weak. Great dryness of throat, larynx and lips.

Urine - Increased flow of urine, very red, thick on standing.

RELATIONS - ***Compare:*** (1) Phel., Con. and other Umbelliferae.

REFERENCES - Boericke. Clarke.

ERYTHRINUS

(Red Mullet Fish)

PHARMACY - eryth. Erythrinus. Red mullet fish. N. O. Erythrininae. South America. Tincture of the whole fish. ***Historical dose:*** Tincture and all potencies.

CLINICAL - Pityriasis rubra. Syphilis.

HOMEOPATHIC - Dr. Burnett is the authority for this medicine. He based his use of it on an account of its effects on some sailors who ate the fish and came out with a peculiar red rash which became chronic and which the doctors took for a form of syphilis.

COMMENTS - Burnett cured with it a case of pityriasis rubra appearing in a large patch on the chest, and benefited other cases. He believed this form of skin affection to be a manifestation of syphilis in the second generation, the father of the patient he cured having had syphilis.

RELATIONS - Aur-m. is the complementary remedy.

REFERENCES - Clarke.

ESCHSCHOLTZIA CALIFORNICA

(California Poppy)

PHARMACY - esch. Eschscholtzia californica. California poppy. N. O. Papaveraceae. Tincture of the whole plant. ***Historical dose:*** Tincture and all potencies.

CLINICAL - Insomnia. Paralysis.

HERBAL - A harmless soporific herbal remedy (Aven.), experiments showed it to act like morphine. It has been used as a nerve sedative to help induce a peaceful sleep.

Esch. causes general weakness torpor, accelerated respiration, complete paralysis of the limbs. Slowing of the circulation. Nervous and restless. Insomnia due to anxiety and worry.

REFERENCES - Boericke.

ESERINUM PHYSOSTIGMINUM

(Eserine)

PHARMACY - esin. Eserinum physostigminum. Eserine. Physostigmine. The alkaloid of Physostigma venenosum, Calabar Bean. Trituration or solution. ***Historical dose:*** Trituration and all potencies.

CLINICAL - *Astigmatism*. Blepharospasm. Ciliary, spasm. Glaucoma. Headaches. Heart, weakness. Pupil, contracted. Salivation. Sweat, excessive. Vision, blurred. Vomiting.

HOMEOPATHIC - Eserine, the alkaloid of physostigma, is best known as used by oculists to procure contraction of the pupils in glaucoma. Esin. contracts the pupils dilated by atropine, but not those by Gels. It slows the action of the heart and increases arterial tension.

Ciliary spasm and spasmodic ***astigmatism*** due to irregular action of ciliary muscles. Blepharospasms with ***pupils contracted***. Twitching of lids, soreness of eyeballs. ***Blurred vision after using eyes.*** Pains around eyes and head.

Eyes - Contraction of pupils. Spasm of accommodation. Ciliary spasm. Blepharospasm. Pain and irritation of eyes on continued reading. Used locally to contract the pupil.

Face - Pale color.

Head - Violent headache with repeated vomiting.

Heart - Signs of cardiac weakness increased, after repeated vomiting. Pulse small and thready.

Mouth - Saliva, first increased, later arrested.

Perspiration - Face and upper part of the body covered with profuse perspiration.

Stomach - Vomited profusely, with headache. Repeated vomiting with signs of cardiac weakness.

COMMENTS - A remark of Mittendorf that "spasm of the accommodation is also produced artificially by Eserine," led R. B. Leach to prescribe successfully the 6x trituration in cases of ciliary spasm and of astigmatism due to irregular action of the ciliary muscles. Esin. has also produced blepharospasm.

A solution of one grain to the drachm (mixed in mistake for a grain to the ounce) was instilled into the eye of a woman of 60 suffering from cataract. Sweating and lachrymation followed and, as these passed off in a quarter of an hour "clonic spasm of the eyelids" set in, "the upper lid falling down on the lower every few seconds."

Spasmodic feeling in lips and the same sensation under jaw of left side followed. Feeling of tremor and spasm without retinal movement, followed in an hour. Pupils contracted to small point.

RELATIONS - ***Compare:*** (1) Phys., Jab., Opium.

REFERENCES - Boericke. Clarke.

ESTROGEN

PHARMACY - estro. Estrogen. A female hormone. ***Historical dose:*** All potencies.

CLINICAL - Allergic reaction. Amenorrhea. Blood, clots. Breast cancer. Breast, disorders. Candida. Depression. Dizziness. Dryness. Fibroid. Fluid retention. Gallbladder, disease. Gynecomastia. Hair loss. Heart, disease. Hemorrhage. Hepatitis. High blood pressure. Hot, flashes. Migraine. Menopause. Nausea. Pancreatitis. PMS. Rash. Strokes. Tumors. Twitching. Weight, loss. Vaginitis. Vomiting.

HOMEOPATHIC - More common side effects may include: Back pain, headache. Skin redness and irritation at the site of the patch.

Less common or rare side effects may include: Abdominal cramps, bloating. Breakthrough bleeding. Breast enlargement. Breast tenderness. Change in cervical secretions, Change in menstrual flow. Change in sex drive. Change in weight. Darkening of skin.

Dizziness. Fluid retention. Growth of benign fibroid tumors in the uterus. Intolerance to contact lenses. Migraine. Nausea. Rash. Severe allergic reaction. Vaginal bleeding.

Other side effects reported with estradiol include: Abnormal withdrawal bleeding. Certain cancers. Cardiovascular disease. Excessive growth of hair. Gallbladder disease. Hair loss. High blood pressure. Reddened skin. Twitching. Vaginal yeast infection

Menopausal symptoms. Atrophic vaginitis. Dizziness. Mild headaches. Myocardial infarction. Pulmonary embolism. Thrombophlebitis.

MIND - Depression.

Abdomen - Pancreatitis. Abdominal cramping or bloating. Abdominal pain, tenderness, or swelling.

Breasts - Breast pain. Breast tenderness. Breast enlargement. Breast tumors. Breast lumps. Discharge from breast.

Chest - Pain in your chest or calves.

Eyes - Vision changes. Yellowing of the eyes.

Female - Amenorrhea. ***Breakthrough bleeding.*** Heavier vaginal bleeding between regular menses. ***Menopausal symptoms.*** Menorrhagia, prolonged or heavier menses. ***Vaginal dryness.*** Spotting, lighter vaginal bleeding between regular menses. Endometrial atrophy. ***Libido decreased.*** Abnormal bleeding of the vagina.

Food - Anorexia. Loss of appetite.

Head - Migraine headaches. Severe headache, dizziness, or faintness.

Limbs - Peripheral edema. Weakness or numbness of an arm or leg. Thrombophlebitis.

Liver - Gallbladder obstruction. Hepatitis.

Lungs - Sudden shortness of breath. Coughing up blood. Pulmonary embolism.

Male - Gynecomastia. Libido decreased.

Rectum - Diarrhea.

Skin - ***Dryness of skin.*** Skin irritation, redness, or rash. Darkening of skin. Yellowing of skin.

Stomach - Nausea. Vomiting.

Temperature - Hot flushes and sweats.

Throat - Difficulty with speech.

RELATIONS - ***Compare:*** (1) Sep., Foll., Lach., Puls.

REFERENCES - Murphy.

EUCALYPTUS GLOBULUS

(Blue Gum-tree)

PHARMACY - eucal. Eucalyptus globulus. Blue gum-tree. Fever-tree. N. O. Myrtacae. Tincture of fresh leaves. Essential oil, Eucalyptol. ***Historical dose:*** Tincture and all potencies.

CLINICAL - Aneurysm. Aortitis. ***Asthma.*** Bladder, disorders. Bronchitis. Cachexia. ***Coryza.*** Diarrhea. ***Dysentery.*** Dyspepsia. Dysuria. Fistulae. Gonorrhea. Gout. ***Influenza***. Intermittent, fever. Kidney, disease. Migraines. ***Nephritis***. Ophthalmia. Quinine, cachexia. Rheumatism. Spleen, affection. Strychnine, poisoning. Syphilis. Toxemia. Tumors. ***Typhoid.*** Urethra, stricture. Urethral, caruncle. Varicose, ulcers. Worms.

HERBAL - Eucalyptus, the gum-tree, is a native of Australia. It was transplanted to marshy districts in mild climates on account of its capability of absorbing water and its alleged power of destroying malarial poisons.

Eucal. became well-known during the influenza epidemic as a prophylactic and disinfectant. Eucalyptus is a powerful antiseptic and disinfectant.

Merrel noted that the volatile oil possesses in common with other terpenes, the property of converting water in the presence of air and sunlight into hydrogen peroxide or to convert oxygen into ozone.

Used locally in catarrhal affections, especially when of a suppurating or putrid nature. Enlarged, ulcerated tonsils and inflamed throat. Use the tincture locally as a gargle.

HOMEOPATHIC - Eucal. affects the mucus membranes, producing profuse acrid and foul catarrhal discharges, with aching, stiffness and weariness, as from taking cold. Marked effects on catarrhal processes, malaria and intestinal disturbances.

Relapsing or intermittent fevers. ***Typhoid fever***. Malaria. Useful in convalescence from intermittents. Odorous sweat. ***Influenza*** (Gels.), said to be a preventive for influenza. Coryza, headache of a dull, congestive character, sore throat.

Hemorrhages internally and locally (Ham.). Exhausted with toxemia and hemorrhage. Sticking, jerking pains at night. Remarkable bodily exhaustion, no desire for any motion, unable to do any real mental work, study, etc. Rheumatism.

Atonic dyspepsia, gastric and intestinal catarrh. Indigestion with excessive development of fetid gas and fever. Slow digestion. A gastro-intestinal irritant with pain in stomach and upper intestines several hours after eating. Diuresis and increase of urea.

MIND - Mental exhilaration. Exhilaration with feeling of buoyancy and increased strength. Desire for exercise, to move about. Intoxication followed by mental depression and exhaustion. Dull and drowsy.

Abdomen - ***Gastrointestinal derangements*** with sleeplessness and restlessness. Burning in epigastrium and umbilical regions. As if a weight in bowels. Sharp aching in the hypogastrium, worse after dinner. Flatulent distention. Spleen hard and contracted.

Breasts - Swellings in different parts of body, one below nipple in right side, size of filbert with stabbing, darting pains.

Ears - Tinnitus. Ringing in ears.

Eyes - Eyes hot, burning, smarting. Eyes smart and burn. Catarrhal ophthalmia. Eyelids heavy. Gonorrheal ophthalmia. Dim vision.

Face - Flushed, congested face.

Female - Acrid, fetid leucorrhea. Ulcer around orifice of urethra. Vascular tumors of urethra.

Food - Increased appetite, tormenting thirst.

Head - Cerebral congestion with much excitement. Dull and congestive headache. Migraine. Sick headache. Nervous headache, and other pains in head, not exactly periodical. Headache in anemic persons. Eucal. relieves the pain and causes sleep.

Heart - Painful palpitation. Strong beating of abdominal aorta. Aneurysms pressing on vagus nerve. Sudden flushing of face with much flatulence, in women at menopause.

Kidneys - Suppurative inflammation of kidneys. ***Acute nephritis,*** complications from influenza. ***Urethral caruncle***. Bladder feels loss of expulsive force. ***Catarrh of bladder***. Spasmodic stricture, gonorrhea. Burning and tenesmus. Diuresis. Hematuria. Urine contains pus and is deficient in urea. Urine has the odor of violets.

Limbs - Rheumatic pains, worse at night, walking or carrying anything. Stiff, weary sensation. ***Pricking sensation, followed by painful aching.*** Nodular swellings over metacarpal and metatarsal joints.

Lungs - ***Asthma with great dyspnea and palpitations.*** Breathing is quickened. Cardiac asthma. Moist asthma. ***Bronchial asthma. Bronchitis in elderly, feeble persons.*** Bronchorrhea (Bals-p.). Fetid form of bronchitis, bronchial dilatation and emphysema. Irritative cough. ***Coughs of influenza.*** Profuse expectoration of offensive muco-pus. Expectoration is white, thick with frothy mucus. Whooping cough in rickety children.

Male - Increased sexual appetite. Subacute and chronic gonorrhea. Recent chancres.

Modalities - Worse periodically. Worse night.

Mouth - Aphthae. Mouth burns. Mouth feels full. Relaxed aphthous condition. Excessive secretion of saliva. Slightly burning taste extending into throat and esophagus with thirst. Tongue pasty.

Nose - ***Coryza***, sore throat. ***Stuffed-up sensation***. Thin, watery coryza, nose does not stop running. ***Chronic catarrhal, purulent and fetid discharge***. Ethmoid and frontal sinus involved. Tension across the nose, tightness across the bridge.

Rectum - ***Dysentery*** with rectal heat, tenesmus, hemorrhage. Typhoid diarrhea. Aching pains in bowels with feeling of impending diarrhea. ***Acute diarrhea.*** Chronic diarrhea, mucus and bloody. Stools thin, watery, preceded by sharp pains. Fetor of stools and flatus. Condition of mucus membrane favoring worms.

Sensations - Burning pains and sensations predominate, but also pricking, stabbing, and sharp aching.

Skin - Glandular enlargements and nodular swelling over joints. Foul and indolent ulcers. Herpetic eruptions.

Stomach - Hot, burning sensation in stomach. Strong smelling, burning eructations. ***Slow difficult and painful digestion*** with much fetid gas. Pain in epigastrium and upper abdomen ameliorated by food. Beating and emptiness with pulsation in epigastric arteries. Throbbing in stomach. Fullness, pressure and weight in stomach. Malignant disease of stomach with vomiting of blood and sour fluid. Cancer. Nausea and vomiting with chill.

Temperature - Chill, then nausea and vomiting. Fever with aching. Continued and typhoid fevers. Scarlet fever.

Throat - Aphthous condition of throat with burning. Burns, feels full. Excessive secretions of saliva. Constant sensation of phlegm in throat. Enlarged, ulcerated tonsils and inflamed throat.

Vertigo - Vertigo during all stages of intermittent fever.

COMMENTS - Vascular conditions including a distinct beating in stomach region, accompanying a sense of emptiness, one prover referred this to the abdominal aorta. Vascular tumors of the female urethra. Glandular enlargements and nodular swellings over joints.

Marked periodicity. Most pains occur at night. It has an intoxicating effect and produces a desire for exercise. Discharges show a tendency to foulness, high temperature, accelerated but not strong pulse. Largely used for bronchitis and bronchial asthma.

It cured a tumor, the size of a filbert with stabbing pains below left nipple.

C. E. Fischer cured many case of dysentery with it.

Dr. Arthur Dalzell related two striking cases of bronchial asthma promptly relieved with five-drop doses of Oil of Eucalyptus given in a tablespoonful of water. The dose was given last thing at night. It also relieved the dyspnea in a case of mitral insufficiency.

RELATIONS - *Compare:* (1) Eucalyptus tereticoris - menstrual cough and prostration. (2) Eucalyptol - depresses temperature of healthy body more than Quinine, acts on kidneys like Ter., Anac., Hydr., Kali-s. Eucalyptus neutralizes ill effects of Stry. (3) Angophora, Red Gum - dysentery, pains, tenesmus, better lying flat on face, obstinate constipation. Eucalyptus rostrata, Kino.

REFERENCES - Boericke. Clarke.

EUGENIA JAMBOSA

(Rose-apple)

PHARMACY - eug. Eugenia jambosa. Rose-apple. Jambosa vulgaris. Eugenia vulgaris. Malabar, Plum-tree. N. O. Myrtacae. A tree native to the tropics, never without flower or fruit. Tincture of fresh seeds. ***Historical dose:*** Tincture and all potencies.

CLINICAL - Acne rosacea. Catarrhal, fever. Catarrhs. ***Comedones.*** Constipation. Coryza. Cough. ***Cramps***. Diarrhea. Diplopia. Hernia. Hiccough. Impotence. Influenza. Nausea. Otitis. Pimples. Throat, sore.

HOMEOPATHIC - Eug. like Eucal., produces a state of intoxication similar to alcohol. Talkative, but indolent. Excitement soon changing to depression. Characteristic ***better after urination***, becomes more cheerful, exhilarated, but passing into gloominess again soon after. ***Nausea, better from smoking.***

Acne rosacea. Acne, simple and indurated. ***Comedones***. The pimples are painful for some distance around. Sufferings occur especially in the evening and at night. An old wound from a thrust became painful again. Rheumatic pain wanders from place to place with catarrh.

MIND - Quite talkative but indolent. Prefers to do nothing but smoke all day. Remarkably changed, mentally, after urination. Sadness better urination, but soon everything became gloomy again.

Constant desire to sit alone and reflect. Everything seems wrong. Nothing seems right. Restlessness, constantly changing positions. Forgets all his business. Delusion, all things seem beautiful after urination.

Abdomen - Flatulence, rumbling in bowels. Colic, with labor-like pains, pressing downward, much urging to stool and to urinate. Burning pain in abdomen. Drawing about navel. Inguinal hernia from a fall.

Back - Burning, itching in a small spot on back, worse after scratching. Sticking pains in back. Pain in small of back and in calves. Aching in sacrum and knees.

Ears - Catarrhal otitis.

Eyes - Eyes look sleepy and drunken. Burning pain, in the afternoon. Suddenly biting in the eyes as from pepper. Needle-like stitches in inner canthus right eye. ***Hot lachrymation***. Lachrymation with burning and gnawing pains. Whirling before right eye.

Face - Pimples on the face with painful sensibility of their circumferences.

Food - Appetite increased. Great thirst. Great desire to smoke tobacco (Calad., Daph.). Agreeable taste, of tobacco, of food and drink when smoking.

Head - Headache as if a board were lying on right side. Dullness and slight sticking pain. Pressive, pinching pain, in small spot deep in forehead. Pressive pinching pain, on vertex. Neuralgia in left forehead over eye. Headache in evening nausea, vomiting. Nocturnal headache, with burning in eyes, great thirst and much urination.

Kidneys - Burning during urination. Frequent urination at night. Shuddering or sudden increase of brightness and of light before the eyes after urinating. Deep-colored urine.

Limbs - ***Nightly cramps in soles of feet*** (Calc., Cupr., Mag-p.). Fissures between toes. Skin recedes from the nails, forming pus. Cramp-like and paralytic pains in the tibia and in the heels. Hot hands.

Lungs - Catarrh with much mucus and rheumatic pains. Rattling in lungs. Moist cough without yellowish, bloody expectoration in the evening and at night.

Male - Impotence. Emission of semen too slow or entirely wanting during sex. Perspiration and thirst after sex.

Mouth - Abundant accumulation of frothy and viscid saliva in the mouth, especially before a meal and when talking.

Nose - Mucus goes from nose into throat.

Perspiration - Sweats when walking.

Rectum - Cramp or pinching pains in rectum. Constipation. Urging to stool and colic. Tenesmus, urging to stool. Loose evacuation, followed by vomiting. ***Hemorrhoids bleed copiously for days with great relief of mind and body.*** Scanty evacuation of stool, the consistence of pap and sandy, spurting and fetid. Very scanty, pasty, gritty stool. ***Scanty, hard stool after much pressing***, followed by spasmodic closure of anus. Offensive, sputtering stool, without much urging.

Sensations - Headache as if a heavy board were lying on right side. As of cramp in orifice of stomach, as if a ten-pound weight were hanging on rectum and as if everything below would fall out.

Skin - Acne rosacea. Acne, simple and indurated. ***Comedones***. Desquamation and suppuration of the skin around the nail of the thumb. Skin cracks about toes.

Sleep - Profound sleep. Stupefying sleep, even at noon with confused dreams. Yawning while walking in open air. Difficult waking.

Stomach - Heartburn at night. Cramp in orifice of stomach, causing nausea. Contractive, pinching sensation deep in stomach. Sensation as of cramp in orifice of stomach, which results in nausea. Nausea rising up from end of esophagus.

Temperature - Shiverings run over him after urination. Coldness, as if the body were naked. Perspiration in the morning with burning thirst. Hot hands. Fever, heat before midnight with little thirst and much sweat.

Throat - At night, violent thirst from dryness low down in throat, so that he did not feel the drink, which also did not better the dryness. Pain in small spot in region of left corner of hyoid bone. Inflamed throat (in catarrhal fever).

Vertigo - Whirling in head while sitting. Vertigo after rising from lying down. Vertigo caused by rush of blood to head. Dizzy and nauseated, in evening.

COMMENTS - Effects the eyes and vision. Darkness and double vision, on looking intently double vision disappears. Whirling before right eye as if it would become dark. Whirling in the head while sitting, houses at a distance seem to turn bottom upwards.

Inflamed eyes. As though fire came out of eyes and tears ran out in streams in evening and night. Worse by sun, causes eyes to fill with water. Burning worse by closing eyes, prevents sleeping at night. Burning not better from cold water.

Pain in small of back and calves. Aching in sacrum and knees. Sticking pain in back as if something were sticking in spine, better by bending back. Rheumatic pain wanders from place to place with catarrh.

An old wound from a thrust became painful again. Skin disease, worse during menses. Open air causes much exhaustion, yawning while walking in morning.

RELATIONS - ***Antidoted by:*** Coffee, by smoking tobacco. ***Compare:*** (1) Myrtus chekan - chronic bronchitis. (2) Ant-t., Berb-a. (3) Eucal. a myrtaceous tree in catarrhal conditions, Laur. and drugs containing Hydrocyanic acid, Puls. - fugitive rheumatic pains.

REFERENCES - Boericke. Clarke.

EUONYMINUM

PHARMACY - euonin. Euonyminum. A concentrated extract, so-called active principle from the bark of Euonymus Americana, E. atropurpurea and other American species of Euonymus. Celastraceae. ***Historical dose:*** Tincture and all potencies.

CLINICAL - Albuminuria. Bright's disease. Cholera. Diarrhea. Dropsy. Dysentery. Gallstones. Indigestion. Liver, disorders. Nausea.

HOMEOPATHIC - Euonyminum is largely used by herbalists in cases of constipation, indigestion, and torpid liver. It has not been proved, but Hale quoted the following account of its effects, which do not seem to differ much from Euon.

"In very large doses, it proves a drastic cathartic, its operation being attended with a death-like nausea, excessive tormina and cold sweats. The dejections from the bowels are profuse, violent and accompanied by much flatus."

COMMENTS - Lutze recorded a case of albuminuria of pregnancy with dropsy cured with the 1x, and also a case of albuminuria and dropsy in a young man of seventeen. This patient had eczema and was cured by Lutze with Ars. 200c. Later he got a chill from standing in the water fishing. He suffered from malaise and finally dropsy developed.

After a week of treatment, he was indifferent, drowsy, sleeping most of the day and night, sometimes with heavy breathing. Anasarca general, chiefly in face and limbs. Pulse full, slow, 50 to 60.

Occasionally dull frontal or occipital headache, face sallow, sclerotics yellow, temperature 102 to 103. Urine scanty, 1,017 (later 1,009), containing large quantities of albumen, epithelial casts and granular debris, no bile or chlorides. Stool grayish. He had no pains or subjective symptoms.

There were all the evidences of a fully-developed case of acute Bright's disease. He was given Euonymus 1x, 2 grains in half a tumbler of water, a spoonful every hour. In three days there was evident improvement. The treatment was continued for a month, when he was nearly well, the cure being completed with Puls., Calc., Sulph. at long intervals.

REFERENCES - Boericke. Clarke.

EUONYMUS ATROPURPUREA

(Burning Bush)

PHARMACY - euon-a. Euonymus atropurpurea. Burning bush. Wahoo. N. O. Celastraceae. Tincture of fresh bark and root. ***Historical dose:*** Tincture and all potencies.

CLINICAL - Albuminuria. Bilious fever. Biliousness. Cholera morbus. Constipation. Diarrhea. Gallstones. Gout. Heart, weakness. Headaches. Hemorrhoids. Levitation. Liver disorders. Rheumatism. Vertigo.

HOMEOPATHIC - Euon-a., like Euonin. and Euon., is a favorite liver remedy among herbalists. It has not been proved, but clinical experience shows that its action is very like that of its botanical relatives.

Migraines. Headache, mental disturbances and much distress in hepatic and kidney region. Bilious headache, coated tongue, bad taste, constipation.

Passive congestion and torpor of liver. Chronic catarrhal disorders of stomach and intestines. Profuse stools, varying or of several colors. Albuminuria. Chronic rheumatism and gout. Weak heart.

MIND - Mental confusion. Loss of memory, unable to recall familiar names. Despondent, irritable.

Abdomen - Flatus and pain. Pain about umbilical region, navel.

Back - Crawling in back. Dull pain between shoulders and about kidney and splenic region, pain in lumbar region better lying down.

Constitutions - Brunettes more easily affected.

Head - Bilious headaches, pressure over brows, compressing eyes. Heavy frontal headache. Sore, tired feeling, bruised feeling of scalp. Pain over right eye extending back through the head.

Kidneys - Urine scanty, high-colored. Acidity increased. Urine poured out rapidly.

Limbs - Aching in all joints, especially ankles. Feet feel swollen and tired.

Liver - Liver engorged. Gallstones.

Modalities - Better from cool air. Better pressure. Worse from eating. Worse evening.

Mouth - Dry, pasty taste.

Rectum - Anus very sore and burning. Constipation with hemorrhoids and severe backache. Diarrhea, stools variable and profuse, bloody.

Stomach - Thirsty. Feels full and uncomfortable.

Vertigo - Vertigo, obscure vision and gastric derangement, associated with albuminuria. Vertigo in forehead, as if drawn up and pitched forward.

COMMENTS - A woman who tasted the juice of the bark related her experience to Hale: "I felt immediately a sick weakening feeling all through the nervous system, dull, heavy pain through upper portion of head together with enlarged blurred feeling. I seemed so drawn up from the floor, that is seemed difficult to place my foot down when walking with sufficient firmness to stand up, a tipping over sensation when sitting and walking."

She also had a deathly sickness at her stomach with perspiration and heat in her face, in alternation with chills in the back and back part of the arms. Some of the symptoms returned the next day, but were dissipated by vinegar, which must be looked upon as its antidote.

RELATIONS - ***Compare:*** (1) Euonymus Europoea. Spindle-tree - liver disorders, biliousness, lumbago, gastric derangements with albuminuria. (2) Cutting pains in malar bones tongue, penis up to bladder, Podo. (3) Am-pic., Chel., Euonymin 1x trituration. albuminuria.

REFERENCES - Boericke. Clarke. Phatak.

EUONYMUS EUROPAEA

(Spindle-tree)

PHARMACY - euon. Euonymus europaea. Spindle-tree. N. O. Celastraceae. Trituration of dried seeds. Tincture of fresh seeds. ***Historical dose:*** Trituration and all potencies.

CLINICAL - Albuminuria. Backaches. ***Bilious.*** Cholera. Collapse. Constipation. Convulsions. Diarrhea. Gallstones. Gastric, derangements. Headaches. Hemorrhoids. ***Liver, disorders.*** Lumbago. Pustules. Vertigo.

HERBAL - The Celastraceae, to which Euonymus belongs, are closely related to the Rhamnacae which include the well-known purgative Cascara sagrada.

HOMEOPATHIC - Euon. has been used successfully in cases of engorgement of the liver, ***biliousness,*** headache, coated tongue, bad taste, and constipation. Passive constipation with hemorrhoids or severe pain in back like lumbago.

Diarrhea, profuse stool, variable in color. Gastric derangements with albuminuria, headache, weakness, vertigo and obscuration of sight. Liver disorders, biliousness, lumbago.

COMMENTS - Allen recalls the effects of Euonyminum in a case of poisoning with the seeds. "A man, forty-three took eighteen seeds one morning and as many the following evening. He was seized with frightful abdominal pain and profuse diarrhea, eventually bloody.

"He was not seen until the evening, when he was in a state of profound collapse with involuntary evacuations of blood and mucus. On lifting him up tetanic convulsions were induced which immediately preceded death."

In its proving, cutting, sticking and drawing pains predominated. The left side is more affected than the right. Cutting pains in the malar bones in the tongue. Cutting in the penis extends up to the bladder.

Pains compel lying down and are then relieved or reappear in other parts. Violent shivering chill over whole body. Pains in chest, head and abdomen, worse after eating. Tingling in the skin which provokes scratching, followed by a burning sensation. Eruption of small dry pustules.

RELATIONS - ***Compare:*** (1) Podo., Rham., Iris, Euon. atrop.

REFERENCES - Boericke. Clarke. Phatak.

EUPATORIUM AROMATICUM

(White Snake-root)

PHARMACY - eup-a. Eupatorium aromaticum. White snake-root. Eupatorium urticifolium. Deer-wort. Pool-root. N. O. Composite. Found in low woods from Massachusetts to Louisiana. Flowers are white and aromatic. Tincture of root. ***Historical dose:*** Tincture and all potencies.

CLINICAL - Ague. Aphthae. Chorea. Gravel. Hysteria. Neurasthenia. ***Sore, nipples***. Stomatitis. Vomiting.

HERBAL - Eupatorium aromaticum, when chewed, produces in the mouth a warm, aromatic, pungent sensation and is regarded as a "warm, stimulating tonic."

Hale quoted herbal authorities as commending this plant in "aphthous stomatitis" in women and children. Also for burning in the stomach with "nursing sore mouth," before and after confinement. Locally it is useful as a mouthwash.

Eup-a. is a "nervine," like Scutellaria and Cypripedium for "restlessness and morbid watchfulness, morbid irritability of the nervous system, tremors, chorea and hysteria." Like Eup-pur., it has been used for gravel. The Native Americans used it as a cure for ague.

HOMEOPATHIC - Eup-a. is doubly indicated where nervous weakness and aphthous disease are combined. Nervous weakness, restlessness and morbid watchfulness.

Hysteria and chorea. Low fevers with extreme restlessness. Aphthous disease. ***Sore nipples***. Sore mouth in infants.

Vomiting of bile, pain in stomach, headache and fever.

COMMENTS - In a case of sore mouth in a man, 57, recorded by P. S. Duff, Eup-a. caused soon "a general aggravation like a cold or catarrh, annoyed by pain in left shoulder, posterior scapular region, pulse 94 unnatural, tight in left bronchia, felt ill, dull and oppressed."

RELATIONS - ***Compare:*** (1) Lapsana communis - useful in sore nipples and hemorrhoids. (2) Hyos., Passi., Hydrin-mur.

REFERENCES - Boericke. Clarke. Phatak.

EUPATORIUM PERFOLIATUM

(Bone-set)

PHARMACY - eup-per. Eupatorium perfoliatum. Bone-set. Thoroughwort. N. O. Composite. Tincture of whole plant. ***Historical dose:*** Tincture and all potencies.

CLINICAL - Anus, herpes. Back, pain. Bilious, fever. ***Bones, pains.*** Cachexia. ***Chills.*** Cough. ***Dengue, fever.*** Diarrhea. Fractures. ***Fever.*** Gout. Headaches. ***Hiccoughs. Hoarseness.*** Indigestion. ***Influenza.*** Intermittent, fever. Jaundice. Liver, pain. ***Malaria.*** Measles. Mouth, cracks. Nausea. Ophthalmia. Relapsing, fever. Remittent fever. Rheumatism. Ringworm. Spotted fever. Syphilitic pains. Thirst. Vomiting. Wounds.

HERBAL - Eupatorium perfoliatum is an herbal remedy recommended by Dioscorides for ill-conditioned ulcers, dysentery, stings of reptiles, chronic fevers and obstructed livers.

It is known as "Boneset" from the prompt manner in which it relieves pain in limbs and muscles that accompanies some forms of febrile disease like malaria and influenza. Eup-per. is a boon in miasmatic districts, along rivers and marshes. Clarke found Eup-per. most useful in ***epidemic influenza***.

HOMEOPATHIC - Characteristic ***violent aching, bone-breaking pains.*** Bone pains, general soreness and fevers. ***Distressing bone pains*** and muscle pains, with ***malarial fevers and influenza***. Dengue fever. Colds.

Conditions where there is a great deal of bone pain. Muscles of chest, back and limbs feel bruised, sore aching. Inability to lie on the left side. Sluggishness of all organs and functions. Weakness.

Acts upon the gastro-hepatic organs and bronchial mucus membrane. Bilious effects. Restless, chilly and nauseated. Cachexia from old chronic, bilious intermittents. Useful in old broken down constitutions of inebriate. Marked periodicity (Ars., Chin., Cedr.), changing periodicity, chill in the morning one day, in the evening the next.

MIND - Feels at night as if going out of his mind. Anxiety, despondency. Very restless, cannot keep still, though wishes to. Sadness during heat. Moaning during chill. Moans with aching pains.

Abdomen - Abdomen distension and tympanitic. Avoids tight clothing. Colicky pains in upper abdomen with headache and other pains. Cramps. Griping pain worse after stool, with tenesmus. Tightness in left hypochondrium.

Back - Backache before and during chill. Chill spreads from back. Pain in back of neck and between the shoulders. Intense backache. Pain as if beaten, pain ascends. ***Aching pain in back.*** Beating pain in nape and occiput, better after rising. Trembling in back during fever. Weakness in small of back. Deep-seated pains in loins, with soreness from motion. Trembling in back during fever.

Breasts - Aching, under left breast, can't lie on left side. Pain through right nipple, when breathing.

Causations - Ill effects of the ice-house.

Chest - Great oppression of chest. Raw, hot, sore chest and bronchi. Muscles of chest are sore, worse from inspiration. Soreness in chest, can't twist when standing, sitting or lying. Pain and soreness behind sternum.

Constitutions - Worn-out constitutions from inebriety.

Cough - ***Hoarseness and cough with soreness in chest,*** must support it. Cough after eruptive stage of measles. Cough preceding or following measles. ***Cough with influenza.*** Chronic, loose cough, chest sore, worse at night. ***Cough better getting on hands and knees.*** Cough lying on back. Loose cough, at night. ***Cough from laryngeal tickling.*** Cough with soreness and heat in bronchi, flushed face, tearful eyes. Hectic cough from suppressed intermittent fever. Cough worse from 2 a.m. to 4 a.m.

Ears - Buzzing in ears with heat on vertex. Could hear everything while seemingly in profound sleep, but couldn't speak.

Eyes - Eyes glistened. Yellow eyes. Painful soreness of eyeballs, lids. Sore aching eyeballs with headache. Great aversion to light. Intense, darting pain through eyes, as from needles. Increased lachrymation, during cough. Redness of margins of lids. Glutinous secretion from meibomian glands.

Face - Sudden, severe contraction of muscles of right cheek. Yellow face. Sallow, sickly in intermittent fever. Pale face, during catarrhs. Flushed face during cough or fever.

Female - Itching of the mons veneries. Herpes on thighs.

Food - Canine hunger during or before ague. Anorexia of alcoholics. Food has no taste. Thirst for cold water, before and during chill. Great thirst for cold water, but after drinking shuddering and vomiting of bile. Craving for ice cream. Desire for acid drinks.

Head - Head pains alternating with gouty pains. ***Occipital pain after lying down with sense of weight.*** Headache with soreness internally. Throbbing, sore pain. Sensation as of a metal cap on head. Top and back of head with painful. ***Headaches with soreness of eyeballs***. Headaches better by vomiting of bile, by conversation. Sick headaches every third and seventh day. ***Headaches with influenza.*** Lifts head with hands during headache. Headache and nausea every other morning, when awaking. Violent headache, comes on before the chill and lasts through all the stages, worse during the sweat.

Heart - Pressure as if heart is in too small a space. Pain, soreness in cardiac region, worse by least motion or turning body around.

Kidneys - Dark-colored, clear urine. Watery urine, during intermittents. Urine profuse, pale, with gout. Urine alternately profuse and scanty. Dark-brown, scanty urine, depositing a whitish, clay-like sediment.

Limbs - ***Bone aches with influenza.*** Swellings of limbs with the debility. ***Aching in bones with soreness of flesh.*** Painful gouty nodes, associated with headache. ***Bone aches with fever and chills.*** Gouty soreness and inflamed nodosities of joints, associated with headache. Dropsy of legs, feet and ankles. ***Aching in arms and wrists***. Bruised pain in calves. Swelling of left great toe.

Liver - Liver problems on the use of alcoholic drinks. ***Soreness and sharp pains*** in region of liver on moving or coughing.

Lungs - Dyspnea, must lie with head and shoulders high. Difficulty of breathing, with perspiration, anxious countenance, sleeplessness. Sharp pain through right lung on deep inspiration, at night, disturbed breathing frightens him.

Male - Itching of the groin. Herpes on scrotum and thighs.

Modalities - Better by conversation. Better by getting on hands and knees. ***Better vomiting bile.*** Better lying on face. Better sweating. ***Worse from cold air.*** Worse night. ***Worse periodically.*** Worse every third or fourth day. Worse lying on part. Worse morning. ***Worse at 7 a.m. to 9 a.m.*** Worse coughing. Worse motion. Worse smell or sight of food.

Mouth - Taste bitter. Breath smells moldy, sourish. Paleness of the mucus membrane of the mouth. Cracks in corners of mouth. Soreness of the corners of the mouth. Tongue yellow, covered with white fur.

Nose - Coryza with sneezing, with aching in the bones. Sneezing with influenza. Nose very dry and stopped up.

Perspiration - Coldness during night sweats. ***Sweat, relieves all the symptoms except the headache.*** Sweat scanty. Skin bathed in sweat. Sweats at night, with chilliness. Sweats from moving or uncovering. Profuse sweat at night in old cases of intermittent fever. Copious sweats, in rheumatism.

Rectum - Cramps. Constipated with sore liver. Stools, frequent, whitish, green, watery. Constipation with catarrh. Purging stools with smarting and heat in anus. Morning diarrhea.

Skin - Jaundice. ***Skin pale and sensitive during fever.*** Eruptions develop late, especially in measles. Ringworm. Herpectic eruptions.

Sleep - Stretching and yawning, before chill. Sleepiness with difficult breathing. Has to lie with head high. Headache on awaking.

Stomach - Tight clothing is oppressive. ***Hiccoughs.*** Indigestion from alcohol of old people. Great thirst for cold water, but after drinking shuddering and vomiting of bile. Distressing pain in the stomach not better until all is vomited. Indigestion consequent on the use of alcoholic drinks. Nausea from smell or sight of food. Nausea, vomiting of bile at close of chill or hot stage, throbbing headache. ***Vomits water or food that has been taken.*** Vomiting and purging of bile of green liquid several quarts at a time. Vomiting preceded by thirst.

Temperature - ***Chill preceded by thirst, with great soreness and aching of bones***. Pain all over, in the bones as if broken, before the chill. Chill between 7 a.m. and 9 a.m. At the conclusion of the chill, vomiting of bile or after every draft. Thirst continues during the chill and heat. ***Influenza with weak pulse, prostration, bones sore.*** Influenza in inebriates and with old people. Great weakness and prostration during the fever. Burning heat. Intermittent fever paroxysm generally commences in the morning.

Throat - Hoarseness, worse morning. Hoarseness and cough, with soreness in chest; must support it. Soreness in trachea and bronchia. Fauces sore, dryness of throat. Throat dry, at times becomes hoarse and loses her voice.

Vertigo - Vertigo, sensation of falling to left, worse lying on right side, better vomiting. Early in morning whirling around in brain as if he had been whirled in cool screen: repeated after a short cessation.

COMMENTS - Characteristic soreness, painful aching in the bones. Bruised feeling, especially in old injuries. Useful for residual bone pain, after the flu. Aching in limbs, throughout the body. Parietal protuberances, sore with pain.

Pains come and go quickly (Bell., Coloc., Mag-p.). Pain and extreme tenderness of left glutei muscles. Aching in the right scapula (similar to Chel., Phos., Gels.). A right-sided remedy, difficult to lie on the left side (Phos.). Swelling of the limbs.

Headaches with internal soreness. Migraine headaches, severe pain at the base of the brain. Congestive headache (Bell.). Headache with nausea and vomiting. Sleepiness and yawning. Dizzy with a tendency to fall to the left.

Influenza, periodic flus (Bry., Ip., Nux-v., Ars.). Winter colds, with sneezing in the back of the head. Bursting, severe headaches and a thirst for cold water (Bry., Oscilloc. has the headache and bone pains). Eyeballs are sore and achy. Dizziness (Gels.). Runny nose (All-c.). High fever, alternates with chills.

High fever with bone ache (Merc., Aur.). Bilious fevers. Edema with intermittent fever or malaria. Yellow fever. History of malaria. Periodic attacks of fever, colds, infection. High fever with increased aching, followed by scanty or profuse sweat. All pains better with sweat except headaches, which are worse. Headache is better rising up. Prostration.

Chilliness predominates, wants to be covered, better in the house, worse in open air. Chills with a shudder down the back. Chills begin in the small of the back with aching in the limbs as though every bone in the body were being broken. Difficulty getting comfortable because of a bruised feeling, restless (Ars.).

Prominent catarrhal symptoms. Sore throat, hoarseness in the morning.

Hoarseness with aching soreness of the trachea. Hoarse, rough, dry, hacking cough with scraping in bronchia. Desire for something cold to relieve the throat.

Sternal pains, especially when coughing. Bruised feeling with cough, desire to hold the chest (Bry.). Cough with extreme soreness down trachea. Painful cough. Nocturnal, loose cough. Cough better by getting on hands and knees, kneeling with face towards pillow, worse lying on back.

W. P. Defriez reported a case in which, every winter for several years, the patient had been annoyed by a dry, hacking cough with paroxysms lasting some time, only relieved by getting on hands and knees. Eup-per. cured.

Cough arising from irritation of the liver. Bilious vomiting and diarrhea, bilious sick headaches. Liver pain, soreness, may desire to rub the liver which is enlarged and tender. Hepatitis. Jaundice, clay-colored, white stools. Bile in the urine, mahogany colored urine. Gout.

Bitter, bile taste in the mouth. Intense thirst, but drinking cold water causes shuddering and vomiting of bile. Eating causes violent, distressing pains which are relieved only by vomiting. Can be disgusted by food, nausea from smelling food (Colch.).

RELATIONS - ***Compare:*** (1) Bry., Sep., Nat-m., Chel. (2) Nyctanthes arbor-tristis - bilious fever insatiable thirst, bitter vomiting at close of chill, also constipation of children.

REFERENCES - Boericke. Clarke. Murphy. Phatak.

EUPATORIUM PURPUREUM

(Gravel Root)

PHARMACY - eup-pur. Eupatorium purpureum. Gravel root. Queen of the meadow. Joe Pye weed. Trumpet weed. N. O. Composite. Tincture of the root. ***Historical dose:*** Tincture and all potencies.

CLINICAL - Albuminuria. Bedwetting. ***Bladder, irritable.*** Chills. Cystitis. ***Diabetes, insipidus.*** Dropsy. Dyspnea. Dysuria. Enlarged, prostate. Fever. Gravel. Headache. Hematuria. Homesickness. Hysteria. Impotence. Indigestion. Infertility. Intermittent fever. Leucorrhea. Miscarriages. Kidney colic. Metritis. Nausea. Rheumatism. Sciatica. Stones. Strangury. Throat, sore. Urine, retention. Vomiting.

HERBAL - The common name, "gravel root," indicates the traditional use of the drug and in the hands of the eclectics it has well in cases of irritable bladder, diabetes insipidus, incontinence of urine, and kidney stones. Hale mentioned that impotency has been cured in the male and infertility and uterine atony in the female. It is similar in action to Cimic. and Helon. here.

HOMEOPATHIC - Eup-pur. was well proved by a Mrs. Dresser; she experienced a feeling of homesickness even when living in her own house. Distressing dyspnea from dropsy.

Kidney dropsy. Albuminuria, diabetes, strangury, ***irritable bladder***. Cystitis in pregnant women from riding over rough roads. Enlarged prostate. Impotency and infertility.

Bone pains, nausea and vomiting accompany fever. Sweat is slight. Restless tossing, moaning, unable to lie down. General soreness (Eup-pur.). Chills and pains run upwards, beginning in the back, with shaking and comparatively little coldness.

MIND - Homesick, even though at home and among family. Sighing. Depressed and sleepy. Hysterical, low-spirited state. Great fear of sickness. Talkative, exclamations.

Stupid, dull mind. Delusions of sight and hearing. Delusion that heels were crowding through boots. Delusion so marked that she felt compelled to look and see if it was really the case.

Abdomen - Pain and soreness of abdomen, much worse left side. Hypogastric region swollen and hot. Rumbling, rolling and twisting pain in bowels. Severe colic after voiding urine.

Back - Weight and heaviness in back and loins. Cutting pain in neck running from left shoulder to occiput. Between shoulder-blades chilly feeling. Pains running upward from sacrum into kidneys from left side of back and hip. Distressing pain in lumbar region before chill.

Bladder - *Cystitis* in pregnant women on riding on rough roads. ***Bladder irritability in women.*** Strangury. Burning in bladder and urethra on urinating. Constant desire, even after frequent urination, the bladder feels full. Soreness and pain in bladder. ***Smarting and burning pain very intense in bladder and urethra.*** Cutting, aching pain in bladder, with constant desire to urinate.

Chest - Grating sensation in chest at every deep inspiration.

Cough - Hacking cough in evening. Cough with soreness and heat in bronchia. Dry, hacking cough in spells. Cough before attack of intermittent fever. Cough continuing throughout paroxysm.

Ears - Ears feel full. Illusions of hearing. Crackling, worse on swallowing.

Eyes - Staring. Red and swollen, with headache. Lachrymation.

Face - Face flushed. Lips blue.

Female - Profuse leucorrhea, caused by exhaustion and chronic metritis. Numbness, worse in groin. External genitals, vulva feels as though wet. Quick, jerking pain in left ovary. Tense, cutting pain above left ovary. Sterility from ovarian atony. ***Threatened miscarriages.*** Habitual miscarriage at third or fourth month. Inefficient labor-pains.

Food - No appetite. Loss of appetite during fever, desire to eat immediately after. Desire for warm drinks. Desires lemonade. Desires cold drinks during chill. Thirst during chill and heat. Thirst before chill, none during. Thirst with dropsy. Longing for hot drinks.

Head - Sick headache beginning in morning, worse afternoon and evening, worse in cold air. Left sided headache with vertigo, as if falling to the left side. Pain from left shoulder to occiput.

Heart - Violent palpitations. Fluttering in heart and throat. Pulse accelerated and full.

Kidneys - ***Nephritis, with severe pain in back, after taking cold.*** Chronic nephritis. Deep, dull pain in kidneys. Cutting pains. ***Diabetes insipidus.*** Dysuria. Insufficient flow, milky. Urine smells sweet. Urinary stream smaller. Hematuria. Incontinence of urine, in children. Frequent effort with passage of but a few drops of urine. Weak, tired and faint after urinary symptoms. Kidney and bladder stones.

Limbs - Tired, weak, uneasiness in limbs with numbness and gnawing pains. Rheumatic pains shifting from place to place, always from below upward. Soreness of bones, aching of limbs as if bones were broken. Pains come and go suddenly, very restless, but not better by motion. Pains in arms and legs before chill, limbs cold during fever. Neuralgia of right shoulder or right knee, passing over to left.

Lungs - Dyspnea with dropsy. Sighing every few minutes. Strong desire to inflate the lungs, which she continued to do from time to time without noticing particularly that she was doing so.

Male - Impotency from exhaustion or abuse.

Modalities - Worse from motion. Worse left side. Changing position ever so little causes chilliness down back. Sensation as if falling to left side (Eup-per.).

Mouth - Tongue furred, brown along center. Tongue, prickling and stinging in tip, on back. Numbness of tongue. Saliva abundant.

Nose - Coryza. Hoarseness. Hacking cough, in evening. Cough with soreness and heat in bronchi.

Perspiration - Sweats about forehead. Sweats on upper portion of body.

Rectum - Bilious diarrhea. Pressure and weight on rectum. Feeling as if bowels must be moved immediately, without being able to do so. Bowels loose, during ague.

Sleep - Yawning, gaping and sighing. Sleepy and depressed. Sleep restless and mind disturbed, frightful dreams.

Skin - Skin hot and dry with fever, hot to touch in face.

Stomach - Wants lemonade or cold drinks during chill. Much wind in stomach, belchings almost constant. Nausea at smell or sight of food or cooking. Great nausea but no vomiting, with chill. Vomiting with fever with sick headache. Griping, crampy pain.

Temperature - ***No thirst*** during chill, but much frontal ache. ***Chill commences in back***. Violent shaking with comparatively little coldness. Fever with protracted bone pains, nausea and vomiting, followed by slight sweat, mostly about forehead and head.

Throat - Choking fullness, must swallow often. Burning, as if had swallowed some hot substance, most at back of throat, worse swallowing. Pain left side of throat, causing pain on swallowing, before chill. Fluttering in throat pit.

Vertigo - Light headed, dizzy, as if flying round and round. Vertigo as if falling towards left side. Vertigo worse morning. Vertigo with illusions of sight and hearing.

RELATIONS - ***Compare:*** (1) Senec., Cann-s., Helon., Ph-ac, Triticum, Epigea. (2) Apoc. - dropsy., Apis., Cann-s., Canth., Cop., For., Hydrc., Mit., Senec., (3) Vespa - kidney symptoms. (4) Caps., Ph-ac. in homesickness. (5) Eup-per., Colch. - nausea at smell of food.

REFERENCES - Boericke. Clarke. Phatak.

EUPHORBIA AMYGDALOIDES
(Wood Spurge)

PHARMACY - euph-a. Euphorbia amygdaloides. Wood spurge. Euphorbia sylvatica. N. O. Euphorbiacae. Middle and Southern Europe. Tincture of plant. ***Historical dose:*** All potencies.

CLINICAL - Antrum, pain. Anus, spasms, prolapse. Debility. Diarrhea. Dysentery. Hemorrhoids. Skin, eruptions. Smell, illusion. Spleen disorders. Throat, soreness.

HOMEOPATHIC - Produces irritation and burning sensations of the intestinal tract with vomiting and diarrhea. Dark brown, watery, mucus stools, sometimes mixed with solid feces. Sometimes offensive with blood, mostly in afternoon. Diarrhea, stools difficult with painful anal spasm.

If stool lasts two or three days there is prolapse returning very gradually, if replaced within half an hour the bowel generally prolapses again. If the diarrhea lasts longer, external hemorrhoids appear, not returning with the prolapse.

Rheumatic pains come on when heated. Malaise, tired weak feeling during and after walking. Restlessness all night, turning about half awake and half asleep. Pain in antrum. Sense of taste blunted. Cold water relieves burning in back of throat (Caps., burning worse from cold water). Skin disorders. Symptoms go from right to left.

Abdomen - Tightness, stitch in region of spleen. Sensation as if a long worm writhing in region of transverse colon or duodenum. Throbbing in groins.

Liver - Severe stitches in liver, when walking up a hill.

Lungs - Heat in chest, radiating from stomach. Feeling as if lungs remained partly inflated. Hoarseness.

Modalities - Better after eating. Worse evening. Worse from walking.

Rectum - Feeling or action of the liver, followed by griping and passing of offensive flatus. Offensive diarrhea, followed by slight prolapse rendering sitting uneasy, going off gradually. Stool difficult from painful spasm of anus, continued after the evacuation.

Sensations - Illusion of smell, ***"odor of mice."*** Seething sensation in the head and thigh.

Stool - Dark brown, watery, mucus stool, sometimes mixed with solid feces, sometimes offensive. Feces small, lumpy, slimy with prolapse, though there had been no straining. Diarrhea returns at lengthened intervals.

Stomach - Nausea, worse moving about indoors, better sitting still, from supper.

REFERENCES - Clarke.

EUPHORBIA COROLLATA
(Large Flowering Spurge)

PHARMACY - euph-c. Euphorbia corollata. Large flowering spurge. N. O. Euphorbiacae. North America. Tincture and triturations of the root. ***Historical dose:*** All potencies.

CLINICAL - Cholera. Cholera, infantum. Cholerine. Dehydration. Diarrhea. Gastritis. Nausea. Seasickness. Vomiting.

HOMEOPATHIC - Euph-c. is a diaphoretic, expectorant and cathartic of the old school. It produces gastro-enteric disturbances like other Euphorbias, but with peculiarities especially in the sequence and character of the vomit.

Deadly nausea, sudden and powerful vomiting of food in stomach. Vomits large quantities of water mixed with mucus, then of clear fluid like rice-water. Copious watery evacuations of the bowels.

Gastro-enteric disturbances with great anxiety, deadly prostration and cold sweat. Attacks recur after short intermissions. Dehydration. Feeling of clawing in stomach, cold sweat (Verat.).

COMMENTS - Grimmer remarked "Euphorbia tends to particularly affect the gastrointestinal tract, copious vomiting, rice water stools, cold sweat, prostration, wants to die, intermittent attacks."

REFERENCES - Clarke. Grimmer.

EUPHORBIA CYPARISSIAS

(Cypress spurge)

PHARMACY - euph-cy. Euphorbia cyparissias. Cypress spurge. N. O. Euphorbiacae. Europe, North Africa. Tincture of fresh plant. ***Historical dose:*** All potencies.

CLINICAL - Erysipelas. Miliaria. Vesicles.

HOMEOPATHIC - The effects of Euph-cy. have been observed on persons pulling the plants and getting the juice on hands and face. Acts as an intense irritant of the skin and produces a feeling of chilliness.

REFERENCES - Clarke.

EUPHORBIA HETERODOXA

(Alveloz)

PHARMACY - euph-he. Euphorbia heterodoxa. Alveloz. N. O. Euphorbiacae. A soft resin insoluble in alcohol or water. Trituration. ***Historical dose:*** All potencies.

HOMEOPATHIC - The resin has been used allopathically as an external application in cases of cancer and has produced the most terrible pains. Euph-he. has been found to alleviate the ***burning pains of cancer*** in homeopathic potencies.

RELATIONS - ***Compare:*** (1) Euphorbium.

REFERENCES - Clarke.

EUPHORBIA HYPERICIFOLIA

(Large Spotted Spurge)

PHARMACY - euph-hy. Euphorbia hypericifolia. Large spotted spurge. N. O. Euphoribiaceae. Tincture of whole plant. ***Historical dose:*** All potencies.

CLINICAL - Constipation. Headaches.

HOMEOPATHIC - Dr. True took the infusion and tincture of Euph-hy. and obtained symptoms from both. Symptoms include headache in fore part of head, pain centering at crown with heat above the eyes and fullness and oppression at epigastrium, followed by languor and drowsiness. Constipation.

REFERENCES - Clarke.

EUPHORBIA IPECACUANHAE

(Ipecacuan Spurge)

PHARMACY - euph-ip. Euphorbia ipecacuanha. Ipecacuan spurge. N. O. Euphorbiacae. Trituration of the powdered root. ***Historical dose:*** All potencies.

HOMEOPATHIC - Euph-ip. is a more active emetic than Ip. Long-continued vomiting with a sense of heat, vertigo, indistinct vision and prostration. Gastritis.

REFERENCES - Clarke. Grimmer.

EUPHORBIA LATHYRIS

(Caper Spurge)

PHARMACY - euph-l. Euphorbia lathyris. Caper spurge. N. O. Euphorbiacae. A tincture of the whole plant is made. ***Historical dose:*** All potencies.

CLINICAL - Cholera. Diarrhea. Dysentery.

HOMEOPATHIC - The fresh, milky juice is exceedingly acrid when applied to the skin and the fruit is highly purgative and poisonous. The juice causes redness, itching, pimples, sometimes gangrene.

Poisoning from the seeds produces symptoms including retching, vomiting, and bloody stools with brilliant eyes, flushed face. The abdomen is drawn inward.

The whole body is stiff and icy cold. Uneasiness. The symptoms point to its use in erysipelas, poison oak, etc. Rheumatic pains during rest. Paralytic weakness in joints.

MIND - Delirium and hallucinations. Stupor, coma.

Eyes - Almost closed from ***edema of eyelids***.

Face - At first ruddy glow on cheeks, afterwards death-like pallor. Cold perspiration in beads on forehead. Red, puffed face and in spots suppurating. Erythema, beginning on face, gradually extending into the hair parts and then spreading over whole body. Glossy eruption, rough edematous with burning and smarting, aggravated by touch and cold air, ameliorated by close room and sweet-oil applications. Bran-like desquamation. Stinging, smarting and burning of face when touched. Sensation of cobwebs.

Heart - Weak and fluttering.

Kidneys - Copious flow of urine.

Lungs - Labored breathing. Cold breath, musty odor. Cough, first hacking, as from inhalation of sulphur, later on, regular paroxysms like whooping cough. Cough ending in diarrhea and vomiting, with sleepiness between each paroxysm.

Male - Inflammation of scrotum, resulting in deep acrid ulcers with intense itching and burning, worse touching the parts, or from washing.

Modalities - Better close room. Better sweet-oil application. Worse touch. Worse cold air.

Mouth - Tongue coated, slimy, acrid taste. Breath cold, musty odor.

Nose - End of nose very much inflamed externally. ***Very sensitive and edematous*** mucus membranes with ulceration.

Pulse - 120 beats, full, bounding, somewhat irregular.

Rectum - Drastic purgation from large doses, mild laxative condition from smaller doses, followed several weeks afterwards by obstinate constipation. Stools of white, transparent, gelatinous mucus, later mingled with blood.

Skin - Erythema, beginning on uncovered parts and face, and spreading over whole body, glossy, rough, edematous with burning and smarting. Fine bran-like desquamation following in the wake of the erythema. Eruption rough, scaly, smarting and burning, when scratched forms deep, ragged ulcers. Ulcerated skin remains red.

Sleep - Restlessness at night. Sleep disturbed, anxious dreams.

Stomach - Nausea and vomiting of copious, clear water intermingled with white, gelatinous lumps.

Temperature - Body bathed in profuse perspiration, standing out like beads on forehead. Cold, clammy perspiration on forehead. Temperature increased.

RELATIONS - ***Antidoted by:*** Rhus-t. - skin symptoms. Verat. - vomiting, purging, cough and coma.

REFERENCES - Clarke.

EUPHORBIA PEPLUS

(Petty Spurge)

PHARMACY - euph-pe. Euphorbia peplus. Petty spurge. N. O. Euphorbiacae. Effect of juice and local application of leaves. ***Historical dose:*** All potencies.

CLINICAL - Ecthyma. Erysipelas. Sore, throat.

HOMEOPATHIC - The application of the juice and leaves sets up intense and painful inflammation, erysipelatous, phlegmonous, pustular with intense burning pain.

COMMENTS - In one of the cases observed, the juice of the stem was applied to an inflamed gum. In another, a boy applied the leaves as a poultice to a black eye.

Burnett produced a sore throat in himself by chewing the herb. He cured with the 3x a case of simple sore throat with swelling and painful swallowing.

REFERENCES - Clarke.

EUPHORBIA PILULIFERA

PHARMACY - euph-pi. Euphorbia pilulifera. Euphorbia hirta. N. O. Euphorbiacae. Tincture. ***Historical dose:*** All potencies.

CLINICAL - Asthma. Bronchitis. Dyspnea. Gonorrhea. Hay fever. Leucorrhea. Sunstroke. Traumatism. Urethritis.

HOMEOPATHIC - In the Medical Press of May 3, 1893, Dr. George Foy gave an account of this medicine. Gray, in 1817, mentioned it as a remedy for syphilis and for venomous bites.

In gonorrhea, when there are intense pains at each urination, burning pains which oblige the patient to sit down or to keep quiet, and violent desire to pass water (Cann-s., Canth.). Humid asthma with prostration and restlessness. Hemorrhages caused by sunstroke or traumatism.

None of the irritant effects common to most of the Euphorbias were produced, but there was a powerful action on the heart. First, an alarmingly quick pulse, and then a sudden chill.

Cardiac dyspnea, hay fever and bronchitis. Urethritis with intense pain on urinating and much urging. Acrid leucorrhea, worse least movement. It has been used by the old-school practitioners in asthma, hay asthma and bronchitis, chiefly in considerable doses.

COMMENTS - In the Universal Homeopathic Annual, Dr. Cartier gave this account: "Euphorbia pilulifera has given excellent results in cases of acrid leucorrhea, aggravated by the least motion, especially useful for pale, delicate and sensitive women" (Facaranda).

REFERENCES - Clarke.

EUPHORBIA POLYCARPA

(Golondrina)

PHARMACY - euph-po. Euphorbia polycarpa. Golondrina. Euphorbia golondrina. N. O. Euphorbiacae. ***Historical dose:*** All potencies.

CLINICAL - Snakebites.

HOMEOPATHIC - An antidote to snake poison, its use also renders the body immune to the influence of the snake venom and thus acts as a prophylactic.

RELATIONS - ***Compare:*** (1) Cedron., The Euphorbias. (2) Euphorbia prostata - Used by Indians as an infallible remedy against bites of poisonous insects and snakes, especially the rattle-snake. (3) Plumeria celinus Tincture internally and locally every 15 minutes for snake poisoning, (Dr. Correa). (4) Micania guacho, a Brazilian snake cure. (5) Selaginella - Macerate in milk, locally and internally for bites of snakes and spiders. Iodium, tincture for rattle snake bites externally and one drop doses every 10 minutes. (6) Gymnema sylvestre will abolish the taste of bitter things, sense of taste altered, powdered root for snakebite, (7) Sisyrinchium - Ten to fifteen drop doses of tincture for rattlesnake bites.

REFERENCES - Boericke. Clarke.

EUPHORBIUM OFFICINARUM

(Gum Euphorbium)

PHARMACY - euph. Euphorbium officinarum. Gum euphorbium. Euphorbia resinifera. The resinous exudation or juice of Euphorbia resinifera exported from Morocco. Euphorbia resinifera is a cactus-like plant of the Euphorbiacae. N. O. Euphorbiacae. ***Historical dose:*** All potencies.

CLINICAL - Blisters. Bone, disease. Cancer. ***Cancer, pains.*** Cataract. Coccyx, pain. Coughs. Crusta, lactea. Diplopia. ***Erysipelas.*** Eyes, inflammation. ***Gangrene.*** Hay fever. Headache. Heartburn. Influenza. Peritonitis. Sciatica. Syphilis. Teeth, disorders. Toothaches. Ulcers. Vision, disorders. Warts. Writer's cramp.

HOMEOPATHIC - Euph. is an irritant to the skin and mucus membranes, causing much secretion with a sense of dryness. ***Terrible burning pains, as if a live coal were on or in the part.*** Burning pain in bones. Burning pain in internal parts. ***Burning pains of cancer.***

Pains in limbs and paralytic weakness in joints. Rheumatic pains of a tearing, pressing, and stinging character, but only during rest.

Slow inflammations. Blisters. Gangrene of old persons. Everything appears larger than it really is. Convulsions with loss of consciousness. Congestion of blood to head.

MIND - Acute mania with symptoms of violent cerebral congestion. Melancholy. Anxiety and apprehension. Starting at night while lying awake in bed. Wants to be by himself and in silence. Quiet, reflective mood. Inclination to work.

Temporary attacks of madness. Delusion he sees the same man walking after him that he sees walking before him. Insists upon saying his prayers at the tail of his horse. Everything seems larger than it really is.

Abdomen - Excessive colic and tympanites. Spasmodic, flatulent colic. ***Burning like fire in abdomen and stomach.*** Griping through whole intestinal canal, followed by thin stool, with burning itching about rectum. Much rumbling, followed by emission of flatus. Anxious sore aching in lower abdomen. Sunken. Feels hollow.

Back - Coccyx sensitive to touch. Pain in coccyx, worse on rising from sitting, worse after stool. Feeling of pressure in muscles of back. Sensation in lumbar region or joints, as if paralyzed.

Chest - Burning and sharp pains in left side of chest, during rest, better motion. Stitch-like pressure upon sternum while sitting and standing. Warm feeling in chest, as if hot food had been swallowed. As if left lobe of lung was adhering. Heaviness in pectoral muscles, when turning body to right side.

Ears - Ringing in ears, also when sneezing. Roaring at night. Buzzing in right ear, can't sleep at night.

Eyes - Pale-red inflammation of eyelids with nightly agglutination. Swelling of lids. Heaviness of upper lids. Biting in eyes, with lachrymation. Great dryness in eyes with profuse discharge. Eyes inflamed and agglutinated in morning. Intolerance of light. Chronic ophthalmia. Eyelids itch severely, are wet and agglutinated. Purulent discharge.

Face - Red swelling of cheeks. Burning in cheek, worse left. Eyes inflamed and agglutinated in morning. ***Erysipelas.*** Yellow blisters.

Food - Great hunger. Thirst for cold drinks.

Head - Stupefying frontal headache. Constrictive headache in occiput. Violent, pressive headache. ***Erysipelas of head and face, with digging, boring and gnawing pains***. Sore pain as if beaten, in occiput, worse morning. ***Bruised pain in head***, in occiput and forehead.

Heart - Irregular, hurried pulse.

Limbs - Paralytic pains. Hip-joint as if sprained. Pain in hip joint and coccyx. Paralytic tightness in shoulder joint, mornings, from moving arm. Cramp in muscles of right hand when writing. Paralytic pain in wrist on moving it. Great weakness of legs. Cold sweat on legs in morning. Burning, at night in bones of hip and thigh. Numbness of feet when sitting. Sciatica.

Lungs - Breathing oppressed as if chest were not wide enough. Violent, fluent coryza with burning and cough. Spasmodic, dry cough, day and night with asthma. Constant cough with stitches from pit of stomach to sides of chest. Croup, dry, hollow, cough. Warm feeling in chest, as if hot food had been swallowed.

Modalities - Better from application of oil. Better cold application. Better motion. ***Worse from sitting.*** Worse rest. Worse beginning of motion. Worse mercury. Worse touch.

Mouth - Dryness of mouth without thirst. Mouth feels coated with rancid grease. Profuse saliva. Saliva tastes salty. Mouth feels coated with rancid grease. Flat taste in mouth, after breakfast. White coated tongue. Much tenacious mucus in mouth, after midday sleep. Salivation preceded by shivering. Teeth as if screwed together, brittle, crumbling, decay.

Nose - Nasal itching with mucus secretions from naso-pharynx. Much abortive sneezing. Coryza with swelling. Acrid ozaena. Violent, fluent coryza, with burning and cough. Coryza with watery discharge from eyes and nose.

Rectum - Burning, sore, around anus. Constipation from inactivity of bowels, hard stool, difficult to pass. Griping pain followed by thin stool. Violent burning itching of rectum. Profuse diarrhea and vomiting. Diarrhea with tenesmus, burning at anus and soreness in abdomen. Stools like glue, painful and flatulent, preceded by itching of rectum. Stool first thin, then knotty. Stools fermented, profuse, clay.

Skin - Erysipelatous inflammation, especially of the cheek. Biting, stinging, red, swollen. ***Vesicular erysipelas***. Pustules, vesicles filled with yellow lymph or liquid. Carbuncle. Old, torpid, indolent ulcers with biting, sharp pain. ***Gangrene*** (Echi., Sec.). Ulcerating carcinoma and epithelioma of the skin. As if thin cord lay under skin.

Sleep - Sleepiness during day. Sleeplessness with tremulous tossing about before midnight, roaring in ears, unable to close eyes. Sudden starting up as from an electric shock at night, while lying awake in bed. Anxious, vivid dreams at night, causing him to cry out, whereupon he awakes.

Stomach - Burning like fire in stomach and abdomen. ***Inflammation of stomach.*** Eructations. Frequent hiccough. ***Erysipelatous gastritis.*** Profuse empty eructations. As if stomach were hanging loose. Nausea with shuddering. Vomiting with diarrhea. Waterbrash.

Temperature - Chilliness and shivering over whole body, in morning. Chilliness while walking in open air. Shivering over back with glowing cheeks and cold hands. Constant chilliness with constant sweat. Coldness of body with internal burning heat. Great heat. Fever with aversion to be dressed, clothing feels too heavy. Heat only on head. High fever.

Throat - Burning as from hot coal in throat with pain and anxiety. Scraping and rawness in throat. Burning in throat and stomach as if flame were rushing out. Burning pains with pain and anxiety.

Vertigo - Violent vertigo, when standing. Vertigo walking in open air.

Vision - Diplopia. Dim or feeble vision. Cataract. Lens milk white. Sees better on a dark day.

RELATIONS - ***Antidoted by:*** Camph., Op., large quantities of lemon juice. ***It antidotes:*** Ars., Nux-v. v. ***Compare:*** (1) Euphorbia marginata, Snow on the mountain - Honey from the flowers is poisonous, detected by the hot, acrid taste. The milky juice produces skin symptoms like Rhus-t. (2) Psoralea - A Columbian plant - pains of cancer, ulcers. Leucorrhea fetid. Pruritus. Uterine tumors. (3) Crot-t., Jatr. (4) Colch., Elat., Ant-t., Verat. (5) Euphorbiacious plants Acal., Crot-t., Jatr., Mancin., Mercurialis., Ricinus, Yucca fil. ***It follows:*** Graph., Lach., Puls., Sep., Sulph.

REFERENCES - Clarke.

EUPHRASIA OFFICINALIS
(Eyebright)

PHARMACY - euphr. Euphrasia officinalis. Eyebright. N. O. Scrofulariaceae. Tincture of whole plant. ***Historical dose:*** Tincture and all potencies.

CLINICAL - ***Allergies.*** Anus, prolapse. Blepharitis. Cataract. Colds. Colic. Condylomata. ***Conjunctivitis.*** Coryza. Cough. ***Eye, disorders.*** Glandular swellings. Granular, eyelids. ***Hay fever.*** Influenza. Iritis. ***Lachrymation.*** Lips, stiffness. ***Measles.*** Nasal, catarrh. Nose, cancer. Parotiditis. Phlyctenule. Pimples. Ptosis. Prostate gland, disorders. Scrofula. Staphyloma. Sycosis.

HERBAL - The common name of "eyebright" gives the indication for the use of this remedy. According to Grauvogl, the plant has a "signature of a black spot in the corolla which looks like the eye's pupil."

HOMEOPATHIC - Produces inflammation of the conjunctiva membranes and profuse lachrymation. It affects the mucus membranes of the ***eyes,*** nose and chest, producing acute catarrh with free, acrid, watery secretions. Irritation extends to the skin around the eye and nose, disorders of the external nose.

Allergies and hay fever. Tears are acrid, nasal discharge is bland, worse in the evening. Sensation ***as if sand in the eyes.*** Acrid pus. Catarrh in the chest, producing hoarseness and cough with profuse expectoration. Hawking up of offensive mucus, may cause vomiting.

Cough after the disappearance of hemorrhoids. Colic, hemorrhoids and condylomata at anus. Drowsiness without being able to sleep, frequent waking in the night as from fright. Symptoms are better in open air. ***Frequent yawning when walking in the open air.***

MIND - Taciturn and repugnant to conversation. Aversion to answering. Disinclined to talk. Hypochondriacal mood, takes no interest in his surroundings. Indolence. Melancholy.

Abstraction of the mind. Weakness of memory. Confusion better cold bath, better washing face. Inclination to sit. Starting from sleep.

Abdomen - Frequent colic. Pinchings in abdomen by short fits. Pressive squeezing and burning across abdomen. Colic, alternately with disorders of eyes.

Back - Cramp-like, pressive pains in back. Swelling of cervical glands.

Chest - Pressive pain beneath sternum. Transient sticking here and there in chest. Sharp pains under the sternum during an inspiration.

Cough - Cough with easy expectoration, in daytime only, better lying down, better at night. Cough caused by irritation in larynx. Cough with profuse expectoration of mucus. Cough from smoke of wood. Cough after disappearance of hemorrhoids. Cough can be suppressed by a sip of water. Cough after influenza. Whooping cough only in daytime, with profuse lachrymation.

Ears - Otalgia with piercing pains in the region of the tympanum. Earache. Impaired, during catarrhal fever. Ringing in ear.

Eyes - Hay fever with watery eyes. ***Catarrhal conjunctivitis,*** discharge of acrid matter. ***Eyes water all the time.*** Conjunctivitis with measles. Conjunctivitis instead of the menses. ***Acrid lachrymation, bland coryza*** (All-c., opposite). Thick, acrid, yellow discharge from the eyes (Merc.). ***Profuse hot or acrid tears,*** worse open air, lying or coughing. ***Sensation as if sand in the eyes.*** Little blister on cornea. Sticky mucus on cornea, must wink to remove it. Frequent inclination to blink. Photophobia with spasms of the lids. Sharp pains in eyeballs from bright light. Ptosis (Gels., Caust.). ***Burning and swelling of the lids.*** Burning, sharp pains in eyes. Pressive, cutting pains in the eyes. Pain in the eye, alternating with pain in abdomen. Pressure in eyes. Chronic sore eyes. Rheumatic iritis. Cataract with watery eyes. Opacities of cornea after injury.

Face - Redness of the face. Rash on face, itching in warmth, becoming red and burning when moistened. Miliary eruption on the face with sensation of burning and redness, on wetting the face. Stiffness of left cheek, tongue. Upper lip stiff as if made of wood. Shootings in the lower jaw and chin.

Female - ***Menses late, painful, flow lasts only an hour or day***. Menses scanty, and short. ***Amenorrhea with ophthalmia*** and ulcer on right side of the nose. Stitching pains and itching when walking in open air. Condylomata.

Food - Better from coffee. Nausea and bitterness after smoking. Cough better eating. Tickling in trachea worse tobacco smoke.

Head - Headaches with coryza. Pressive headache with photophobia and heat, chiefly in the forehead. Sensation as if the head would burst. ***Catarrhal headache*** with profuse discharge from eyes and nose. Shootings pain in the temples and in the forehead. Pulsations of head. Beating in the head, perceptible on the outside. Dullness of head with pressure on vertex. Sharp pains in brain.

Kidneys - Frequent and copious emission of clear urine. Nocturnal irritability of bladder. Dribbling urine. Urine too often and copious.

Limbs - Numbness in the arms and hands. Cramp-like pressive pains in the hands and the fingers. Fits of (painless) swelling in the joints of the hand or of the fingers on moving them. Cramp pain in the metacarpus. Torpor of the fingers. Shootings in the legs during repose. Stitches in the hip and knee joints when walking. Tension, as from contraction of the tendons, Achilles tendon, on walking. Cracking in the outer ankle of left foot, when stepping.

Lungs - Difficulty of breathing, shortness of breath, even when seated. Cough with suspension of respiration. Cough with much, easy expectoration in day, less on lying down, at night. Frequent yawning when walking in open air. Cough in the morning with copious expectoration of mucus and fluent coryza. Whooping cough only in day with profuse lachrymation.

Male - Spasmodic retraction of genitals with pressure above the pubic bone. Retraction and tingling of the testes. ***Prostatitis***. Nocturnal irritability of bladder, dribbling urine. Lancination and voluptuous itching in the glans and in the prepuce. Condylomata and sycotic growths, itching, stinging with sore and burning pain when touched.

Modalities - ***Better from open air.*** Better winking. Better wiping eyes. Better dark. Better in bed or getting out of bed. Better from coffee. ***Worse wind.*** Worse south winds. Worse warmth. ***Worse from sunlight.*** Worse room, indoor. Worse evening. Worse after sleep. Lying down aggravates coryza, better cough. Cold air and wind causes lachrymation. Walking in open air causes yawning.

Mouth - Paralytic stiffness of the tongue and of the cheeks, making speech difficult. Stammering and frequent interruptions in the speech. Sensation of clucking, which mounts into the throat. Shooting pains in lower teeth. Copious bleeding of gums. Nausea and bitterness in the mouth after smoking.

Nose - ***Hay fever and allergies.*** Profuse bland, fluent coryza, with scalding tears and aversion to light. ***Profuse, bland fluent coryza.*** Fluent coryza by day, obstruction of the nose at night. Violent irritation to sneeze, without cold or apparent cause. Excoriation and painful sensibility of the nostrils. Nosebleeds. Purulent pimples on the ale nasi. Small red spots, like pimples, on upper right side of nose. Eruption on wings of nose. Flat cancer on the right side of the nose.

Perspiration - Copious nocturnal sweat. Sweats, mostly on chest, at night during sleep. Sweat often has a strong odor. Very offensive sweat and most copious on front of chest.

Rectum - ***Constipation***. Hard and scanty evacuations. Dysentery. Prolapse anus. Pressive in anus while sitting with hemorrhoids. Old flat condylomata at anus with severe burning, worse at night. Daily stool, but it is hard and scanty.

Sensations - As if dust or sand in eyes, as if a hair hung over eyes. As if upper lip were made of wood, stiffness of left cheek and tongue.

Skin - First stage of measles, eye symptoms marked. In measles with watery eyes and fluent coryza it is sometimes the best remedy. Condylomata, itching when walking, burning when touched. Touching skin produces aggravation. Consequences of blows, bruises and contusions. Fine eruption around eyes and on nose. Warts.

Sleep - Usually worse after sleep. Yawning when walking in open air. Sleepy during the day. Frequent waking (as from fright) at and after 3 a.m., lasting until 6 a.m., when he falls in a stupor from which he wakens with many complaints. Frightful dreams with frequent waking and starting with fright. Dreams of fire, lightning, flames, etc.

Stomach - Hiccough. Risings with taste of food. Nausea and bitterness after smoking. Vomiting from hawking mucus.

Temperature - Chilly and cold. Chill in the forenoon. Descending fever. Attacks of heat during day. Fever with redness of face and cold hands.

Throat - Gagging when clearing throat in morning. Catarrhal hoarseness, mornings. Irritation of larynx impelling him to cough, followed by tensive pressure beneath sternum.

Vertigo - Vertigo with heaviness of head. Vertigo with tendency to fall.

Vision - Dim vision hysterical. Everything seems enveloped in a mist and to move. Blurred vision, better wiping. Dim vision, as through a veil, in evening. Dim vision by candlelight, the light seems to vary. Light of candle seems to be dark and to flicker, during headache. Obscuration of vision for distant objects, while walking in open air.

COMMENTS - Great affinity for the eyes. Nonspecific organ remedy for the eyes. Good for concomitant symptoms relating to the eyes, particularly tearing or watery eyes, unrelated to current condition. Great value as an eye-lotion, can remove corneal opacities.

Allergy infections where the eyes are prominently involved, where the eye swells and waters. Watery, runny eyes, the whites of the eyes are red. Copious tearing, hot, acrid tears that irritate the skin. Eyes smart.

Conjunctivitis (Arg-n., Puls.). Conjunctivitis with measles, eye problems since measles. Pink eye, with yellow discharge, better walking around slowly (Puls.). Acute bacterial infections. Sensation that sand or gravel is under the eyelid, constant irritation or itchiness.

For dry eyes or blocked ducts. Migraine headaches with eye symptoms. Whooping cough with lachrymation. Photophobia. Colds, hay fever. Sneezing attacks. Coryza worse lying down, at night and in the open air. Worse windy weather. Chilly.

Hering noted a cure of "flat cancer on right side of nose."

Ames of Rockland, Ohio, recorded the case of an old man of 79 to whom he gave Euphr. 3x for lachrymation and sneezing. It relieved him of those symptoms in addition to prostatic trouble he had for some years, which compelled him to rise frequently in the night to urinate. This led Ames to give Euphr. in other cases of prostatic trouble with good results.

RELATIONS - ***Antidoted by:*** Camph., Puls. ***Compare:*** (1) Hydrophyllum, Burr-flower, (catarrhal inflammation of eyes, hot lachrymation with itching, swollen lids, dull headache, also for effects of Poison-Oak). (2) All-c., Ars., Gels., Kali-hp., Sabadilla. (3) Aeth., All-c. - tears bland of Euphr., corrosive. (4) Apis, Arg-n., Ars., Hep., Kali-bi., Kali-i., Merc., Merc-c. (5) Puls., Grat., Dig., Tab. ***Compatible:*** Acon., Calc., Con., Nux-v., Phos., Puls., Rhus-t., Sil., Sulph.

REFERENCES - Boericke. Clarke. Murphy. Phatak.

EUPIONUM

(Wood tar)

PHARMACY - eupi. Eupionum. Wood tar. On distilling wood tar of the rubber tree a volatile oil is obtained which separates into a lighter and heavier oil, the heavier oil is Kreosote, the lighter is Eupion. ***Historical dose:*** Tincture and all potencies.

CLINICAL - Amenorrhea. Cough. ***Cramps.*** Dreams. Glandular swellings. Groin, pains. Hemorrhages. Headache. ***Leucorrhea.*** Menorrhagia. Neuralgia. Nosebleed. Night-sweats. Ovarian, pain. Pruritus. Toothache. Tuberculosis. Tumors. ***Uterine, displacements***. Vicarious, menstruation.

HOMEOPATHIC - Eupionum is a lighter volatile oil obtained from distillation of wood tar. It was proved by Wahle in Rome, who also proved paraffin. The effects of Eupi. bear a close resemblance to those of Kreos., but are by no means identical with them.

Eupi. has a large number of symptoms centered in the female sexual organs. ***Uterine displacements***. Pain in back, followed by a bland leucorrhea. Menses too early and copious, thin flow.

Sacrum pains as if broken, backache extends to pelvis, better leaning against anything for support or bending backwards. Cramps in calves at night. ***Intense sweat from slightest exertion.*** A sense in the feet as if walking on needles. Sensation as if whole body were made of jelly. Disgusting dreams.

MIND - Cheerful, joyous disposition. Irritable, angers easily. Frightened on waking. Great weakness of memory.

Abdomen - Stitches when walking in left anterior crest of ilium. Squeezing, pressing pain in left groin when quiet. Pains better passing flatus. Contracting pain and twisting better by bending over, day before menstruation. Cutting pains during menstruation, when the pains cease discharge is always copious, blood red and very thin.

Back - Sacrum pains as if broken. Pressive heaviness in lumbar vertebrae. Severe backache, must lean against something for support. Pains extend into pelvis. Backache alternating with leucorrhea. Backache during menses.

Breasts - Breasts increase in size with pressive pains in them, as if something painful were drawn through them, with oppression. Stitches under right breast.

Chest - Heaviness, oppression, stitches and tickling in chest. Stitches and pressure in sternum.

Ears - Pressing in ears as if the wind was blown forcibly into them for a long time, the external parts being equally affected. Shooting and tearing in left ear, extending to external temporal region.

Eyes - Eyes weak, as if she had cried. Pressure above eyes as if the globes would be pushed out. Burning, pressive pains in eye, copious lachrymation. Lachrymation worse in fresh air, better in room. Everything appears pale, as if a thin veil were before eyes.

Face - Hard nodule, the size of a pea, on lower portion of inner side of right cheek. Upper lip fissured and painful, as if raw. Lips and throat always dry, yet without thirst. Lips painful as if sore.

Female - Menses too early and copious, irritable. During menses, irritable and disinclined to talk, burning and stitches in chest and heart. ***Gushing leucorrhea***, yellow, staining. Leucorrhea with severe backache after menses, when pain in the back ceases, leucorrhea gushes out. Sore pain between labia during urination. Pruritus pudendi, labia swollen. ***Burning in right ovary.*** Chronic tubal disease. Uterine flexions. Uterine displacements.

Head - Heat at vertex, stitches from vertex down limbs into abdomen and genitals. Sore painful spots on head. Painful pulsation in forehead.

Heart - Palpitations with slow pulse, believes her heart must be heard some distance away. Severe palpitations before menses, ceasing when the flow begins.

Kidneys - Frequent inclination, scanty discharge, worse when standing than sitting. Copious urine, lemon color, chestnut brown before menses. Hot urine passed without pain.

Limbs - ***Cramps in the calves***, worse at night. Paralytic, dislocation pain in right knee. Stitches in either knee. Tearing in limbs and restlessness in legs preventing sleep. Dislocation pains in joints of right hand. Heads of bones of fingers feel too large. Hands go to sleep easily.

Lungs - Crawling in upper bronchi causing dry cough. Rough, scraping, metallic, dry cough. Hard, suffocating, dry cough with stitches in chest, returning every winter. Cough better by warm drinks, by sitting up on bed with breaking out of perspiration.

Modalities - Bending forward ameliorates pain in abdomen. Bending backwards ameliorates backache. Rest ameliorates headache and pains in abdomen, aggravates other symptoms. Coughing and sneezing aggravates pains in abdomen. Cough returning every winter. Hot drink aggravates toothache. Worse morning and night. Worse blowing the nose.

Mouth - Whole tongue red, covered with raised pimples like herring roe. Tip of tongue dry, back covered with thin, dirty white coating. Anterior part of tongue rough like a grater. Insensible feeling in mouth, as if scalded by fat. Pappy and sticky in mouth, early in morning. Sour, putrid taste after eating.

Nose - Sneezing, each time he blows his nose the sneezing reappears. Sneezing with fluent coryza in morning. Left nostril cracked, bleeding. Bleeding, blood thin and fluid, when blowing nose. Menstrual flow intermits with nosebleed. Soreness in upper nose on drawing air through nostrils in evening.

Rectum - Itching after stool. Ineffectual inclination and straining. Tenesmus, better when blood is passed, this weakens her. Constipation, stool every three or four days with great straining and prolapsed uterus. Hard, dry stools with great straining. Dark blood in painless stools.

Sensations - As if dislocation of joints. As if muscles torn from bones, as if skin and muscles were too short. Soles of feet numb as if walking on needles, sticking in heels.

Skin - Nodule on left forearm. Itching, biting in skin, in genitals, penetrating whole body, worse night, better during motion.

Sleep - Yawning with chilliness and shivering. Sleepiness towards noon. Dreams of disgusting things, of naked persons, anxious dreams of her child falling into the water. Frightful dreams, the same dream repeated, that she is pursued, or falling into an abyss. Wakes bathed in perspiration.

Stomach - Region of stomach feels internally sore and distended, pains under both short ribs. Bloated and sensation of fullness of stomach with internal chilliness in evening. Belchings tasting of food. Vomiting of food. Vomit emanating from lower abdomen, dark green, tasteless mucus.

Teeth - The teeth stick together when the jaws are closed. Teeth painful as if loose, gums swollen, scorbutic, worse by hot soup. Toothache-like numbness in carious molars, coming on immediately on lying down, better on rising and moving about. Sensation as if gums swollen and teeth would drop out. Gums swollen. Painful jerking-tearing in gums.

Temperature - Chilliness, with headache, stitching, better by warm drink. Dry heat towards noon. Foul smelling sweat on least exertion, when eating, all night. Copious night-sweat towards morning.

Throat - Sensation below larynx as if something was sticking there, with a short, dry, hacking cough. In morning, much white bad-tasting mucus in throat, expectorated after slight paroxysms of coughing. Sensation of mucus in throat without being able to expectorate. Sensation of dryness of uvula.

Vertigo - Everything turns around on sitting up in bed.

COMMENTS - Menstruation is too early and too copious, thin and fluid flow. Cutting in abdomen ceases when flow comes on. Nosebleed, when menstrual flow intermits. Yellow leucorrhea after menses, staining yellow.

Leucorrhea with severe backache, has to lean against something to give relief, when the backache ceases the discharge gushes out.

Palpitation with slow pulse. Painless pulsation in the head. Pulsations all over body while sitting quietly. Sticking pains in head and other parts. Cramps in the calves when accompanying uterine or chest complaints.

Weak eyes and obscured vision. Pressing in ears as if wind were blown in with force and for a long time. Teeth stick together when jaws are closed in morning sensation as if teeth were embedded in some soft matter. Tongue covered with raised nodules. Pain in inguinal region.

Nodules appear on inner side of right cheek, left side of neck and left forearm. Painful glandular swellings in groins. Spasmodic, periodic pain an inch up rectum. Bloody stool.

Headache and chilliness. Coldness of whole right side of the body. Colliquative perspiration. Perspires from least exertion, when eating, all night (with tuberculosis). Wobbling sensation in upper part of body, everything becomes dark to her. Great irritability.

RELATIONS - Graph. antidoted the effects on eyelids. ***Compare:*** (1) Kreos. and the Carbons. (2) Lach. - pain ceases when discharges appear.

REFERENCES - Boericke. Clarke. Phatak

EYESENHARDTIA POLYSTACIA

(Orteaga)

PHARMACY - eys. Eyesenhardtia polystacia. Orteaga. Eyesenhardtia adenostylis. N. O. Anonaceae family. Central America, western Texas. Tincture of the hardwood of the trunk. ***Historical dose:*** Tincture and all potencies.

CLINICAL - Cystitis. Headaches. Kidney, colic. Kidney, diseases. Neuralgias.

HERBAL - A small tree, belonging to the Anonaceae family, found in Guatemala and West Texas. Central American natives used it for kidney diseases.

HOMEOPATHIC - The symptomatology was established by Egee in 1932, on seven provers, using the 6x potency.

Slow and difficult concentration. Sleepiness in the afternoon and evening. Neuralgia of the forehead and eyes. Dull aching in the head, localized especially on the forehead and above the eyes. Eyelids heavy. Throat dry. Burning pain in the thighs. Cystitis. Urination frequent, late and scanty. Kidney colic. Worse between 4 p.m. and 6 p.m. Worse in the evening.

REFERENCES - Julian.

F

FABIANA IMBRICATA

(Pichi Pichi)

PHARMACY - fab. Fabiana imbricata. Pichi pichi. N. O. Solanaceae. A South American shrub cultivated in Southern California. Tincture of the juice. Fluid extract. ***Historical dose:*** Tincture and all potencies.

CLINICAL - Bladder, weakness. Cystitis. Dysuria. Gallstones. Gonorrhea. Jaundice. Kidney, stones. Liver, disorders. Prostate, disease. ***Prostatitis.*** Uric acid, diathesis.

HOMEOPATHIC - Fabiana imbricata has been used as a terebrinthine diuretic. It has tonic and chologogue properties, and is used in the treatment of nasal catarrh, jaundice, dyspepsia. Albert Schneider noted that it increases the secretion of bile.

Liver disorders. Gallstones. Uric acid diathesis, cystitis, ***prostatitis***, and dysuria. Bladder tenesmus and burning after urination. Excoriating urine and kidney stones. Bladder catarrh with suppurative prostatic conditions. Gonorrhea. Post-gonorrheal urinary conditions.

REFERENCES - Boericke. Clarke.

FAGOPYRUM ESCULENTUM

(Buckwheat)

PHARMACY - fago. Fagopyrum esculentum. Buckwheat. Polygonum fagopyrum. N. O. Polygonacae. Tincture of the whole mature plant. The fresh mature plant is pounded to a pulp and macerated in two parts by weight of alcohol. ***Historical dose:*** Tincture and all potencies.

CLINICAL - Arteries, throbbing. Belching. Depression. Diarrhea. Eczema. Eyes, disorders. Genitals, sweat. Granular, eyelids. Hands, sweat. Headache. Heart, disorders. Heartburn. Intertrigo. ***Itching. Leucorrhea.*** Liver, disorders. Mumps. Nausea. Nose, crusts. Ophthalmia. Palpitations. Pruritus, pudendi. ***Pruritus, vulvae***. Rheumatism. Skin, eruptions. Styes. Taste, altered. Throat, sore.

HOMEOPATHIC - Fagopyrum, commonly known as buckwheat, acts upon the skin and the digestive organs. It has had an extensive proving. Though there is little clinical experience with this herbal remedy on record, some features are sufficiently well marked to justify their being classed as characteristics.

Itching, felt in different parts of the body, eyes, posterior sinuses, anus, deep in hands, legs etc. Intense an ***itching of the arms and legs***, becoming worse toward evening. Senile itching, ***pruritus***.

Itching erythema. Blotches like fleabites, sometimes all over the body, sore to the touch and are multiplied by scratching. Persistent eruptions. Large blind boils.

The ***itching of the face*** is especially marked about the roots of the whiskers. Persistent itching of the hands which is ***"deep in,"*** being supposed to be the result of irritation of the coats of the arteries.

Offensive excretions. Fluent coryza. Post-nasal catarrh, dry crusts, granular appearance of posterior sinuses with itching. Pain in streaks. Visible pulsation of the carotids and other arteries.

MIND - Depressed and irritable. Irritable, cross. Exceedingly happy. Inability to fix attention, study or to remember what has been read. Aversion to being spoken to. Confusion of mind better after eating. Restlessness during mental labor, when attempting to study.

Abdomen - Abdomen distended with flatulence, worse by pressure of clothes. Soreness in hypogastrium.

Back - Stiffness and bruised feeling in the muscles of the neck with sensation as if nape would not support the head.

Breasts - Breast less painful than usual before period.

Chest - Heavy feeling, bruised pains and stitches in chest. Twinges of pain up and down left breast, outer side. Sharp, stitch-like needle prick in right breast on inspiration. After retiring, severe sticking through breast from nipple backward, better by pressure.

Constitutions - Weak constitutions.

Ears - Itching in and around ears. Heat, itching and neuralgic pains in external ears. Itching along Eustachian tubes.

Eyes - Eyes swollen, red, hot, itching, as if sand in eyes. ***Itching*** and smarting, swelling, heat and soreness. Itching in the margins. Aching deep in eyeballs. As if eyeballs were pushed out. Lachrymation, worse by reading. Pain along lachrymal duct. Meibomian glands of left lower lid inflamed.

Face - Face flushed. Soreness of left malar bone, also of temporal region. Lips dry and cracked, vertical crack on upper lip.

Female - Itching, better by cold water. ***Pruritus vulvae with yellow leucorrhea***, worse rest. Leucorrhea staining yellow. Burning in right ovary. Pains in right ovary, on walking in afternoon.

Head - Itching in and around eyes and ears. Pains deep in head with ***upward pressure***. Headaches with a tired neck, better bending backwards. Head hot, better bending backward with tired neck. Occipital headache. Bursting pains. Cerebral hyperemia.

Heart - Pain around heart, better lying on back, extending to left shoulder and arm. Palpitations with oppression. Pulse irregular intermittent, rapid. Light feeling in chest. ***Throbbing in all arteries*** after retiring.

Kidneys - Stitching pains in region of right kidney. Cutting in urethra. Difficulty in voiding last drops of urine, several drops pass after he thinks he has finished.

Limbs - Stiffness and bruised sensation in the muscles of the neck, with sensation as if nape of neck could not support head. Pain in shoulder with pain along fingers. ***Itching in arms and legs***, worse towards evening. Itching deep in hands. Streaking pains in arms and legs. Feet numb and pricking.

Liver - Pain in region of liver on stooping. Bruised, sore feeling at 10 a.m., worse lying on right side. Sharp sticking through liver from the back.

Lungs - Touching the neck occasions a cough with a smarting sensation extending to the ear and throat, under lobe of right ear. Breath very offensive.

Male - Profuse offensive sweat of genital organs.

Modalities - Better coffee. Better cold water. Better cold applications. Better cold air. Better sitting still. Better in a warm room. Better pressure and motion. Worse in the afternoon. Worse from sunlight. Worse walking. Worse in bright sunlight. Worse from motion. Worse deep inspiration. Worse stooping. Worse ascending. Worse writing. Worse scratching. Worse riding in cars. Worse lying on right side. Worse after retiring.

Mouth - Soreness of teeth on closing them, worse by cold water. Gums sore and bleed easily. Swelling in roof of mouth. Bad taste in mouth in morning. Taste of ingesta after dinner, with belchings.

Neck - Parotid and submaxillary glands swollen, sore and painful. Stiffness of neck and soreness of all neck muscles. Neck tired, as if unable to support head. Dull pain in back of neck, at base of occiput, better bending head backwards.

Nose - Itching in posterior sinuses. Postnasal catarrh. Fluent coryza with sneezing, followed by dryness and crust formation. Nose red and sore externally. Septum deeply cracked.

Rectum - Itching in anus. Burning in rectum after stool, creeping, urging, tenesmus. Diarrhea with tenesmus, stools watery or pappy with flatulence, very offensive.

Skin - Eczema. Erythema. Intertrigo. Blind boils. Skin hot, swollen. ***Severe itching, better by bathing in cold water***, worse scratching, and touch. ***Itching of hands, deep within***. Itching of knees, elbows and hairy portions. ***Senile pruritus***. Sore, red blotches. Vesicular, pustular and phlegmonous dermatitis.

Sleep - Constant desire to yawn and stretch, 5 to 6 p.m. Restless night, wakes 5 a.m. and sleeps again, many dreams.

Stomach - Bruised, sore feeling in stomach. Uneasy, empty feeling in stomach. Belchings of ***scalding, hot***, acid, watery substance, better coffee. Drooling. Persistent nausea, better eating.

Temperature - Chills along back in afternoon. Cold, clammy sweat at night, very profuse. Sweat of hands, though cold. Hands and feet alternately hot and cold. Soles of feet moist, disagreeable odor in axilla. Face, head and hands burn in afternoon. Heat and restlessness after retiring.

Throat - Soreness and a feeling of excoriation deep down pharynx. Uvula elongated, tonsils swollen. Thick mucus collects in throat on rising. Badly-smelling cheesy mass coughed up. Feeling as if a lump in esophagus, painful on swallowing. Throbbing of carotids.

COMMENTS - Berridge recorded two cases in which Fago. was of service. The first case concerned a dull, bruised pain in top of left shoulder, rather posteriorly, extending up neck, worse on moving the part, appearing on waking, going off after breakfast and returning later in the day.

Constipation. Nausea a little before 11 a.m., afterwards dull pain in left temple and a feeling of heat all over. After aggravating the pain in the shoulder, Fago. removed the symptoms.

In the second case, Fago. permanently removed, after a week's aggravation, sinking in the stomach about 6 p.m. or 7 p.m., and temporarily removed a chronic diarrhea about 6 p.m. or 7 a.m. The diarrhea was later increased and was met by Lach.

Hale mentioned that there was a popular belief that indulgence in buckwheat cakes is a prolific cause of skin eruptions. He found it curative in cases of eczema, erythema and intertrigo.

Deep-seated and persistent effects upon the head. Vertigo, confusion. Severe pressive or bursting pain in many parts of head with upward pressure. Pain in forehead, back of eyes, through temporal region on either side. Congestive headaches (Bell., Glon., Nux-v., Sep.).

Itching, smarting, swelling, heat and soreness in the eyes. Soreness in the ears. Erysipelas, frostbite (Agar.). Swollen, red, inflamed and sore nose. Fluent coryza with sneezing, followed by fullness, dryness and the formation of crusts. Burning, soreness and persistent pain from even gentle pressure.

The face is pale or unevenly flushed with dark semicircles below the eyes. Swollen, hot and dry, as though severely sunburned, with cracked and sore lips. The mouth feels dry and hot and yet saliva is not wanting. Soreness and swelling of roof of mouth. Tongue is red and fissured along its edges. Bad taste in the morning (Puls.).

Soreness with pain in throat, just back of the isthmus of the fauces. Feeling of excoriation and soreness extending deep down in the pharynx. Elongated uvula, swollen and red tonsils. Sensation of rawness in the throat (Phyt.). Scarlet redness of the neck below the mastoid process. Throbbing of the carotids. Neck feels tired, the head heavy. Parotid glands are swollen and painful.

Persistent morning nausea, vomiting of pregnancy. Appetite improved by eating (opposite of Lyc., Nux-m.). Empty or "all-gone" feeling at the stomach (Sep.). Fullness and pain in the abdomen, but no rumbling. Frequent discharges of flatus. The region of the liver is painful, tender, worse from pressure, compelling the patient to lie on the left side. Stools are pappy or watery, profuse, offensive, followed by tenesmus.

Scalding urine, pain extends from testicles to abdomen. Profuse, offensive smelling perspiration on the male genital organ. Bruised or burning pain in the right ovary, particularly when walking. Pruritus with slight yellow leucorrhea, more when at rest than when exercising.

Persistent, heavy, pulsating pain in chest, worse from deep inspiration. Dull pains around the heart, with oppression and occasional sharp pains passing through the heart. Pressure with the hand increases the oppression. Increased pulse, extremely variable.

Stiffness and soreness of all the muscles of the neck, with pain and a feeling as if the neck would hardly support the head. Dull pains in small of back with stitching pains in the region of the kidneys. Pains with occasional sharp stitches extend from the arms to muscles of both sides of chest.

Dull, aching, rheumatic pains in the shoulder. Stinging and burning pains extend the whole length of fingers, aggravated by motion. Streaking pains pass through arms and legs with sharp pains extending to feet. Pains extend from hips to small of back, frequently run down to the feet.

Sleepiness in the evening, stretching and yawning. Easily wakened when the mind is diverted, but soon falls again into sleepiness. Sleep is disturbed by troublesome dreams and frequent waking.

RELATIONS - ***Compare:*** (1) Dolichos, Bov., Psor., Sulph., Urtica. (2) Rhus-t. - better by motion, Senega - better bending head back. (3) Lyc. - hours of aggravation 3 to 6 p.m. (4) Puls., Polygonum. (5) Coffee relieves stomach symptoms.

REFERENCES - Anshutz. Clarke.

FAGUS SILVATICA

(Beechnut)

PHARMACY - fagu. Fagus silvatica. Beechnut. Fagus farfara. N. O. Cupuliferae. Fagaceae. Tincture or trituration of the nuts. The beech-nuts are pounded to a pulp and macerated in five parts by weight of alcohol. ***Historical dose:*** Tincture and all potencies.

CLINICAL - Convulsions. Epilepsy. Headaches. Hydrophobia. Rabies. Vertigo.

HOMEOPATHIC - Knowledge of this remedy is derived from the ill effects of eating the nuts, among which are dread of liquids and salivation, suggesting its use in hydrophobia or rabies. John Bauhin said that the nuts would disorder the head like darnel; hogs grow stupid and drowsy by feeding on them. Ray and Mangetus agree.

Trembling, convulsions with periodic spasms, stiffness and coldness have been observed, pointing to nerve irritation. Swelling of the mouth and headache were noted in one case. In some instances, death has resulted from the effects of the nuts.

COMMENTS - Dr. E. Berridge contributed a case in which "a boy aged 13 had eaten four days ago a large quantity of beech nuts. I found him in great pain, languid and terrified. Also, with apprehensions of present death. Pulse very unequal, sometimes extremely quick, sometimes languid and intermittent, skin burning violently, mouth flowing with froth and saliva.

"Intolerable thirst, entreating for drink, but so soon as any liquid was brought he seemed to shudder with equal horror, as if he had been eating unripe grapes. Soon after eating the nuts he had been seized with torpor, gloominess and dread of liquids. He had not been bitten by any rabid animal.

"Next day, early in the morning, he was the same, but seemed to talk more in his wildness and perturbation of mind and his mouth flowed with foam more abundantly, the urine he had voided by night was red and fiery, depositing a copious turbid white sediment, resembling an emulsion of beech nuts, subsiding as deep as the breadth of the finger at the bottom of the vessel.

"A few hours before he died he vomited a porraceous bile after which he died quietly."

RELATIONS - ***Compare:*** (1) Epiphegus in headache and salivation, Epiphegus which grows on the beech and partakes of its properties. (2) Rabies - Bell., Lyssin.

REFERENCES - Anshutz.

FEL TAURI

(Ox bile)

PHARMACY - fel. Fel tauri. Ox bile. Ox gall. Bilis bovina. Bilinum. N. O. Ruminantia. Impissated gall triturated with sugar of milk or lower dilutions may be made with water. ***Historical dose:*** Tincture and all potencies.

CLINICAL - Asthma. Catarrh. Cirrhosis. Constipation. Diabetes. Diarrhea. Flatus. Gallstones. Headaches. Indigestion. Jaundice. Rheumatism.

HOMEOPATHIC - Ox gall is a remedy of very ancient use. It is used in the old school mostly as a purgative, for preventing putrefactive changes in the intestines, and for increasing peristalsis. It was proved by Buchner.

Disordered digestion, diarrhea, constipation. Chronic gastric and intestinal catarrh. Much flatus, ascites. Diabetes. Obstruction of the gall ducts. Gallstones. Jaundice.

Cirrhosis of liver. Increases the duodenal secretion, emulsifies fats and increases the action of the intestines. Liquefies bile and acts as a purgative and chologogue.

Nape of neck pains. Pains in joints and cramps. Headache. ***Tendency to sleep after eating.***

MIND - Peevish, irritable mood. Greatly inclined to all kinds of business, unpleasant impression did not affect him.

Abdomen - Violent peristaltic movements. Rumblings and motions in abdomen.

Back - Tension in nape.

Chest - Anxiety in chest. Constriction, on walking at 3 a.m. cannot sleep again for tightness of breath and cannot remain lying, it seems as though something in throat prevented free passage of the air, better by deep inspiration and sitting upright.

Food - Increased thirst.

Head - Confusion. Violent headache in morning, on pressure upon right temple, extending to occiput and nape of neck.

Kidneys - Urging. Offensive urine.

Limbs - Some tearings in left shoulder joint, extending up to nape of neck. Cramp in right toe.

Male - Scrotum itching, moist.

Rectum - Stool with urging and sensation of warmth in anus. Stool thin, pasty, followed by pressing, although with crumbling feces.

Stomach - Gurgling in stomach and epigastric region. Odorless and tasteless belchings.

Sleep - ***Tendency to sleep after eating***. Sound sleep in morning with some perspiration.

RELATIONS - ***Compare:*** (1) Merc-d. (2) Chol. in gallstones. (3) Calcul-b. - triturate Gallstones up to 10 to 12x.

REFERENCES - Boericke. Clarke.

FELDSPAR

PHARMACY - feld. Feldspar. Mineral varieties, containing alumina, silica and oxygen.
Historical dose: All potencies.

CLINICAL - Arteriosclerosis. Fainting. Otosclerosis. Weakness.

HOMEOPATHIC - It is a silicate compound containing potassium, sodium and aluminium. Kaolin is a disintegrated feldspar which has lost its potassium and sodium but has retained the silicate of aluminium. It is not similar to feldspar in its use.

The chemical composition suggests a use in arteriosclerosis and those illnesses showing sclerosis and fibrosis of the tissue.

COMMENTS - Two cases of otosclerosis were cured clinically, both occurring in patients forty-one years old. Both were nervous, disposed to tremble, and complained of weakness.

One said he felt if he had been struck on the head and was about to faint. He had sensations of heat on hands and feet. His head pained on moving.

Both cases recovered after many weeks of treatment. These symptoms are common to silica and the kalis, hence, the weakness is characteristic of Feld.

A woman age 38, had had varicose veins for many years. Her skin injured easily. Under Feld. she was freed of the pains in the legs. The tendency of the skin to injure disappeared at the start of treatment, the varicose veins remained.

A woman age 48, was given Feld. for retinal hemorrhages five months after the attack. At times she showed glycosuria and was very nervous. After two months treatment, the nervousness and eye affects improved fifty percent, and she experienced a feeling of general well being.

A woman age 53, received Feld. for fainting spells resulting from an arteriosclerotic heart. She suffered from incipient arcus seniles; by resting in bed she regained normalcy, at least concerning her domestic work.

A man age 70, with an arteriosclerotic kidney, suffered from hematuria. Under Feld. he was on his feet again as an ambulatory patient.

A woman age 84, with marked arteriosclerosis, cardiac decompensation and edema received Feld. and a decoction of Apoc. The dropsy disappeared.

Several weeks later the dropsy returned, gangrene of the foot developed, and she died.

A man age 70, with severe dropsy of both feet, received Feld. and Apoc. He recovered in two months. We can only guess what the future holds in store for him.

A woman age 50, with high arterial pressure, spells of weakness, and nervous exhaustion, received Feld. in a series of doses. Her complaints disappeared. Chronic cases improve slowly, quick results should not be expected in these cases.

RELATIONS - ***Compare:*** (1) Sil., Calc-f., Calc.

REFERENCES - Thompson.

FERRUM ACETICUM

(Iron Acetate)

PHARMACY - ferr-acet. Ferrum aceticum. Iron acetate. ***Historical dose:*** All potencies.

CLINICAL - Asthma. Cough. Hemoptysis. Nosebleeds. Tuberculosis. ***Varicose, veins.*** Vomiting.

HOMEOPATHIC - Especially adapted to thin, pale, weak children who grow rapidly and are easily exhausted. Alkaline urine in acute diseases. ***Varicose veins of the feet.*** Pain in right deltoid.

Copious expectoration of greenish pus, asthma. Tuberculosis, constant cough, vomiting of food after eating, hemoptysis. Nosebleeds. Worse sitting still, or lying down.

REFERENCES - Boericke.

FERRUM ARSENICOSUM

(Iron Arseniate)

PHARMACY - ferr-ar. Ferrum arsenicosum. Iron arseniate. Tri-ferric diarsenate. Trituration. ***Historical dose:*** All potencies.

CLINICAL - Albuminuria. ***Anemia.*** Bright's disease. Chilly. Chlorosis. Constipation. Debility. Diarrhea. Eczema. Headache. Impetigo. Leucorrhea. Liver, enlargement. Psoriasis. Spleen, enlargement.

HOMEOPATHIC - Hale was the first to use Ferr-ar., giving the 2x with a promptly curative result to an anemic girl who had been given iron and arsenic separately, under old-school treatment, in vain.

P. C. Majumdar put Ferr-ar. to excellent use in cases of enlarged liver and spleen with fever. When there is no fever Ferr-i. is better.

Enlarged liver and spleen with high fever of a continued type. During fever the face is flushed and sweaty, but during the intermission the face is pale. No thirst during any stage of the fever, heat intense and prolonged with slight burning of the whole body, emaciation and debility.

Undigested stool. Constipation, sometimes, colliquative diarrhea, the stools consisting of undigested matter and mucus. Albuminuria. Skin dry. Eczema, psoriasis, impetigo. Simple and pernicious anemia and chlorosis. Disinclination to work, even to leave his bed.

MINDS - Conscientious about trifles. ***Restlessness at night,*** driving out of bed. ***Sensitive to noise.*** Fear in a crowd. Fear of evil. Fear of people. Tossing about in bed.

COMMENTS - Majumdar reported two cases. The first, concerning a robust, healthy man, 25, who went into a malaria district of Bengal and had his first attack of fever. He was given large does of quinine, which suppressed the paroxysms for a time, but they continually recurred.

After four years he returned home a changed man: pale, jaundiced, emaciated, abdomen filled with enlarged and indurated liver and spleen, slighly tender to pressure. His organs left no room for food. Obstinate constipation. High fever generally appearing in afternoon, no chill or thirst, but copious sweat without much relief to fever.

Ferr-ar. 6c, twice daily, made an improvement in three days. It was continued for a month and a half with occasional stoppages and in six months he was completely restored to health.

The second case concerned a boy, 15, who suffered from fever and enlarged spleen. The liver was not enlarged.

Voracious appetite, but no digestion, undigested diarrhea stools. Continued fever, 102 to 104, burning of body. Some thirst. Great emaciation.

Ferr-ar. 6c was given night and morning. He was cured perfectly in a year.

RELATIONS - ***Compare:*** (1) Ferr-i., Ferr., Ars., Calc-a., Chin.

REFERENCES - Clarke.

FERRUM BROMATUM

(Iron Bromide)

PHARMACY - ferr-br. Ferrum bromatum. Iron bromide. Trituration. Solution. ***Historical dose:*** All potencies.

CLINICAL - Anemia. Diarrhea. Headaches. Leucorrhea. Numbness. Spermatorrhea. Uterus, prolapsed.

HOMEOPATHIC - Dr. Sarah N. Smith of New York proved Ferr-br., using the sixth dilution, made by Boericke and Tafel. Ferr-br. Produced, in this order, were very distinct symptoms in the head and eyes, dry mouth and nose, relieved by coryza, a feeling that she might die, diarrhea, burning in urethra when urinating, sticky, excoriating leucorrhea, and weight and discomfort in uterus.

The symptoms that made the most impression on the prover were the ***"dead, numbness"*** feeling of the scalp, the unconscious moaning after stool and the sticky, excoriating leucorrhea. Heaviness and discomfort in the uterus was so severe that she declined to continue the proving as it interfered with her work.

COMMENTS - Hale mentioned this remedy as having been highly commended in cases of spermatorrhea with anemia, debility and depression.

RELATIONS - ***Compare:*** (1) Heavy eyes. Con., Caust., Gels. (2) Smarting while urinating, Cann-s. - has burning while urinating and after.

REFERENCES - Clarke.

FERRUM CYANATUM

(Iron Cyanide)

PHARMACY - ferr-cy. Ferrum cyanatum. Iron cyanide. ***Historical dose:*** All potencies.

CLINICAL - Cardialgia. Chorea. Constipation. ***Epilepsy.*** Flatulence. Nausea.

HOMEOPATHIC - Neuroses with irritable weakness. Hypersensitiveness, especially of a periodical character. Chorea. ***Epilepsy.*** Cardialgia with nausea and flatulence. Constipation, alternating with diarrhea.

REFERENCES - Boericke.

FERRUM IODATUM

(Iron Iodide)

PHARMACY - ferr-i. Ferrum iodatum. Iron iodide. Trituration of freshly prepared crystals. Solution. ***Historical dose:*** All potencies.

CLINICAL - Albuminuria. Alcohol, effects. Amenorrhea. ***Anemia.*** Boils. Breast, tumors. Bronchorrhea. Cancer. Catarrh. Coryza. Debility. Diabetes. Dyspepsia. Exophthalmic, goiter. Eyes, scrofulous. ***Glands, enlargement.*** gonorrhea. Heartburn. Impetigo. Kidneys, disorders. Leucorrhea. Liver, enlarged. Nephritis. Pneumonia. Scoliosis. Scrofula. Spleen, enlarged. Tuberculosis. ***Uterus, prolapsed.*** Writer's cramp.

HOMEOPATHIC - Ferrum iodatum has been independently proved, and corresponds more particularly to scrofulous affection, glandular enlargement and tumors.

Grimmer used Ferr-i. for breast tumors, cancer, exophthalmic goiter inflammation and enlargement of glands, symptoms and conditions based on the tubercular diathesis. Berridge removed with Ferr-i. "Morning catarrh, hot and restless in bed, sweet smell of urine."

"Food seems to push up to throat as if it has not been swallowed," somewhat like the Ferr. symptom "as if something rolled into throat and closed it like a valve." Sharp or cutting pains in the eyes, ears and root of nose to occiput. Sensation as if lying in a cramped position.

Anemia. Body emaciated. Debility following drain upon vital forces. Impetigo of the cheek. Crops of boils. Acute nephritis following eruptive diseases. Exophthalmic goiter following suppression of menses. ***Uterine displacements.*** Breast tumors, cancer and conditions based on the tubercular diathesis.

MIND - Dullness of mind and confusion in head worse when reading aloud. Anxiety. Aversion to company. Conscientious about trifles.

Confusion worse putting hat on. Confusion while reading. Confusion after smoking. Confusion while writing.

Abdomen - Abdomen bloated after food or drink. Fullness, even after a little food, stuffed feeling, as if she could not lean forward. Abdomen swollen. As if a cord were drawn connecting the navel and anus.

Back - Small of back as if broken. Pain as if lying in a cramped position. Neck sore when touched or on moving. Dull pain in back. Stiffness on getting up from bed, better during day.

Chest - Oppression of chest with inclination to lie on back. Pressure beneath sternum.

Constitutions - Suited to scrofulous or mercurial diathesis to subjects of relaxed tissue (tuberculosis in the third stage, bronchorrhea, pneumonia).

Cough - Hemoptysis. Short, hacking cough with yellowish-white, thick expectoration.

Ears - Roaring in ears.

Eyes - ***Eyes shut on account of pain.*** Lids swollen, discharging copious quantities of pus when forcibly opened. Exophthalmic goiter, after menses suppressed. Burning in eyelids. ***Photophobia.*** Trachoma. Bright objects floating before eyes, like sparks of fire, after breakfast.

Face - Red, chlorotic look. Itching of right cheek, reddening when rubbed. ***Submaxillary and cervical glands swollen and hard.*** Vesicles, when rubbed, become raw.

Female - Amenorrhea. Menses is absent with exophthalmic goiter. Menses suppressed or scanty. Constant bearing down. When sitting, ***a feeling as if something pressed upward in vagina***. Retroversion and prolapse of uterus. Prolapsed uterus, difficult to retain the urine. Itching and soreness of vulva and vagina. Leucorrhea like boiled starch.

Food - No appetite. Craving for sardines or salty fish. Great thirst.

Head - Headache with a confused sensation. Headache with feeling of heaviness and pressure. Sharp pain from below eye up through head to vertex. Cutting pain from bridge of nose to occiput. Headache on going to bed. Throbbing pain in head on right side and forehead. Headache worse smoking.

Heart - Palpitations at night. Heartbeats seems to go into stomach, and cause a nervous, trembling feeling. Bloodvessels throb all over, even when quiet. Violent beating of heart on rising or when turning in bed.

Kidneys - Difficulty in retaining urine. Incontinence in anemic children. ***Crawling sensation in urethra and rectum.*** Sensation as if urine were stopped at fossa navicularis. Urine, sweet smelling. Urine, dark colored. Urine, depositing thick white sediment.

Limbs - Weak, trembling feeling in limbs on using hands and on walking. Paralyzed and bruised feeling in all limbs, with great aversion to moving about.

Lungs - Bronchorrhea. Chronic pneumonia. Shortness of breath, obliged to take a deep breath. Greenish, purulent, containing small, cheesy particles. Grayish-white, rather tenacious mucus drawn out in threads.

Male - Nocturnal emissions with violent pain and burning in urethra. Inability to urinate. Tenesmus of neck of bladder. Prickling itching in urethra, with frequent urging to urinate, but scanty flow. Gonorrhea.

Modalities - Better from open air. Worse from motion. Worse touch. Worse warmth. Worse at night and in the morning.

Mouth - Salivation. Sudden bleeding of gums. Offensive taste. Metallic, bitter taste. Flat, insipid taste. Taste of peppermint. Dryness of mouth and throat. Mucus membrane of mouth bright red or dotted with red.

Nose - Nose dry, stopped up. Blowing nose gives no relief. Coryza. Scrofulous swelling of nose, with ulcers and crusts inside. Discharge of mucus from nose, trachea, and larynx. Discharge all day, with stuffed-up feeling at night. Discharge thick, yellow or green.

Perspiration - Sweat at night is cold and copious, and comes from the least exertion.

Rectum - Crawling in rectum. Constriction in rectum and anus. Sensation as if worms were in it. Small, hard stool, with sticking pain. Constipation then loose stools, preceded by griping pain.

Sensations - As if anus were compressed. As if worms were in anus. As if something twisted around about in a circle, as if a cord were drawn connecting navel and anus, as if a screw were boring in anus.

Skin - Pale skin. Eczema. Lichen. Short-lasting skin eruptions. Eruptions like urticaria.

Sleep - Frequent starting in sleep and waking with feeling as if paralyzed. Restless sleep with frequent waking. Dreams of long past events. Dreams of thieves. Dreams of fighting with them.

Stomach - Dyspepsia with nausea and headache. Impaired digestion. Food seems to push up in the throat, as if it had not been swallowed. Violent eructations. Sour and bitter risings. Stomach full of gas.

Throat - Sore pain, as if of a splinter, shooting in different directions. Hoarse. Violent scraping and tickling in throat and nose. Frequent rattling of mucus in throat.

Tongue - Burning on tongue. Tongue coated thickly yellow.

Vertigo - Dizziness worse moving.

COMMENTS - P.C. Majumdar used Ferr-i. with success in cases of enlarged liver and spleen when unaccompanied by fever. When fever is present Ferr-ars. is the better remedy.

"Feels as if she has eaten too much, a sort of upward pressure. Stuffed feeling in abdomen as if she could not lean forward, costiveness," especially in cases of enlarged spleen. "Sweet-smelling urine."

RELATIONS - ***Compare:*** (1) Alum. - anemia, leucorrhea, prolapse uterus. Alumn. - swollen vagina, prolapse uterus. (2) Caul. - prolapse uterus and leucorrhea from atony, fitful, crampy pains. (3) Helon. - pruritus, prolapse, leucorrhea. albuminuria. (4) Hydr. - debility and atony, tenacious, profuse leucorrhea, palpitations. (5) Graph. - chlorosis, leucorrhea profuse, hot, watery. (6) Iod. - red face, irritability, corroding leucorrhea, emaciation marked. (7) Kali-bi. - has stringy, albuminous leucorrhea, stringy expectoration. (8) Thyr. - palpitations, exophthalmic goiter. (9) Ferr-br. - leucorrhea, prolapsed uterus. (10) Ferr-a. - enlarged liver and spleen.

REFERENCES - Boericke. Clarke. Phatak.

FERRUM MAGNETICUM

(Magnetic Ferric Oxide)

PHARMACY - ferr-ma. Ferrum magneticum. Magnetic ferric oxide. Loadstone. Iron sesquioxide. A black oxide of iron. ***Historical dose:*** All potencies.

CLINICAL - Amaurosis. Diarrhea. Flatus. Ganglions. Paralysis. Rheumatism. Vision, disorders. Warts. Weakness. Whitlow.

HOMEOPATHIC - Caspari is the authority for Ferr-ma. Teste, who put Ferr-ma. in the Arnica group along with Led., Crot-t., Rhus-t. and Spig., had some experience with it. Indicated for the sycotic constitution. Small warts on hands.

Ferr-ma. produces paralytic weaknesses like the other iron preparations, of which this is the most peculiar: after perspiring during a moderate walk, weakness and lassitude, which seem to proceed from the abdomen. Difficulty of movement and relaxation of muscles.

Prickings, lancinations, tingling and itching in different parts. Pains and itchings, some of which reappear at intervals of four weeks. Pain in nape of neck. Trembling in the legs and arms. Excessive lassitude. Fatigue on taking the slightest exercise.

Worse during a meal, flatulency, grumblings, movements in abdomen with urgent diarrhea after a meal (Ferr.). Abdominal sufferings are felt more on the left side. Very abundant and frequent emission of fetid wind.

MIND - Indecision and long reflection before undertaking anything. Indolence, slowness of movement. Air of importance and self-sufficiency. Irascibility.

Abdomen - Movements and grumbling in abdomen. Loose evacuations with much flatulency, especially left side, with pullings in legs. Abundant and frequent emission of fetid flatus.

Chest - Tearing and lancination in the left side of the chest, when breathing. Sensation of emptiness in the chest.

Ears - Tingling in the ears. Itching, wringing and cold lancinations in the auditory duct. Pullings in the ears and the pharynx when swallowing.

Eyes - Pricking itching in the canthi. Painful sensibility of the lachrymal sac with profuse lachrymation. Pressive pain on the eyelid, which impedes the sight. Swelling of the lower lid, which makes the eye appear smaller. Darkness before the right eye, causing it to wink.

Face - Face dejected with general heat, followed by redness of the face. Itching and tingling in the face and on the lips. Eruptions on the forehead in the eyebrows, at the root of the nose, on the cheeks, the lips and the chin.

Head - Pulsative headache, by fits. Circumscribed headache in the morning, generally on right side. Headache on stooping, on moving the arms, and on going up stairs. Itching in the scalp. Small, painful eruption on the scalp. Falling off of the hair.

Kidneys - Urine red and copious, which becomes the color of clay after having stood some time.

Limbs - Cramp-like, paralytic pullings or jerking pullings in the forearms and hands. Paralytic pulling in the right arm. Pain, as from dislocation in the wrist. Dryness and tension in the hands. Small warts on the back of the hands and on the wrist. Whitlow. Acute lancination in the knee. Ganglion of the foot. Tingling and pricking in the heels. Starting in the soles of the feet. Painful little toe.

Lungs - Frequent hawking of mucus. Dry cough after dinner, proceeding from an irritation in the trachea, as if one had swallowed dust.

Male - Itching and lancination in the scrotum and in the extremity of the glans. Increased sexual desire, with and without erection, or absence of all sexual desire, yet without importance.

Mouth - Accumulation of water and saliva in the mouth. Itching sensation in the posterior part of the palate.

Neck - In the morning, pain in the nape of the neck, as if from having lain in an inconvenient position.

Nose - Sneezing, with stoppage of one nostril and catarrh.

Rectum - Urgent want to evacuate with expulsion of flatus only. Small, liquid evacuation when expelling flatus. Itching and shooting in the anus. Tingling and itching in the rectum.

Skin - Itching and tingling in different parts, especially in the evening, mitigated by scratching, but appearing in other parts. Red spots, sometimes of a bright red or bluish red, some disappear on being pressed. Small warts on the hands.

Sleep - Violent and noisy yawnings with accumulation of water in the mouth. Drowsiness with prompt sleep on lying down or even when seated. Absurd dreams at night. Dreams immediately after lying down, waking with a start, coldness causing trembling. Inclination to remain in bed in the morning. After rising, weakness in the knees.

Stomach - Flatulence during a meal, afterwards fatigue and burning pain in epigastrium, especially on breathing. Nausea. Abortive risings.

Teeth - Bleeding of the gums, when slightly pressed upon. Painful sensibility of the teeth during mastication.

Temperature - Shivering and cold in the side opposite to that on which the patient has lain. Heat, as if a catarrh were developing itself with lassitude and downcast eyes.

Internal heat with perspiration and slow pulse after washing the body. The pulse is slow and small. Perspiration on the slightest exercise. Sweat in the morning on the body and on the occiput. Sweat of an acid smell, as in measles.

Throat - Bitter and rancid taste in the pharynx, on hawking. Sensation as if mucus were adhering to the uvula. Lancinations in the throat. Pressure in the esophagus, as if too much had been swallowed at one time.

COMMENTS - Ferr-ma. relieved, after Spig. failed, in an old man suffering from chronic rheumatism of the nape of the neck with irritable disposition.

Cured a case of compound capsular cataract in a gouty patient. A third patient had rheumatism of both thighs, coming on after violent exercise. This patient was treated in two attacks. In the first attack he received Arn. first and then Ferr-ma. In the second, Ferr-ma. was given at once and the effect was speedy and marked.

Teste noted the case of a patient who had a very unpleasant experience with the medicine. He suffered from a mercurial neurosis and was very sensitive to medicines. Teste was led to give the medicine due to a painful contraction of the posterior cervical muscles, against which no remedy he had tried had produced any effect.

Teste gave Ferr-ma., four globules in a tumbler of water, two tablespoonfuls every day. The first tablespoonful, taken in the morning, seemed to produce a sensible improvement. A quarter of an hour after the second dose, taken at 4 p.m., the sight became dim, a halo of fire, red and violet, was seen first in front of the right eye, and afterwards in front of the left eye.

Soon after, this halo, which formed a circular zigzag-shaped line, became narrower and narrower. Finally produced such a complete blindness, that the patient assured Teste he was unable to distinguish night from daylight. This lasted one hour and did not pass off entirely until after a meal.

Much more distressing phenomena followed towards 8 p.m. The pain in the nape, which first was seated on the left side, passed to the right invading the whole extent of the trapezoid muscle, where it became literally frightful.

"For two days and nights the patient, who was a brave and strong man and whom I had seen bear the most painful surgical operations without uttering a sound, suffered to such an extent that he uttered heart-rending cries."

Camph., Puls. and Bry failed to relieve, the first rather aggravated. Rhus-t. effected some relief. But it did not prevent the recurrence, for eight days in succession of the visual phenomena, though with less intensity then the first time, at irregular intervals, generally 6 or 7 a.m. and sometimes even at night in perfect darkness.

RELATIONS - ***Compare:*** (1) Ferr., Elect., Galv., Magn. arct., Magn. aust.

REFERENCES - Boericke. Clarke.

FERRUM METALLICUM

(Iron Metal)

PHARMACY - ferr. Ferrum metallicum. Iron metal (Fe, At. Wt. 56). Includes symptoms of the acetate and the carbonate. Triturations of the pure metal and of the carbonate, solution of the acetate. ***Historical dose:*** All potencies.

CLINICAL - ***Anemia***. Aphonia. Asthma. Biliousness. ***Blood, disorders. Blood, loss. Bruises.*** Cachexia. Catalepsy. Chlorosis. Chorea. ***Constipation.*** Cough. Cramps, ***Debility.*** Diarrhea. Bedwetting. Fever, intermittent. Goiter, exophthalmic. Gonorrhea. ***Hemorrhages.*** Heart, disorders. Hectic, fever. Hydrocephalus. ***Iron, poisoning.*** Jaundice. Kidneys, disorders. Lienteria. ***Morning, sickness.*** Menstruation, disorders. ***Miscarriages.*** Nausea. Neuralgia. Paralysis, viscera. Pregnancy, disorders. Rectum, prolapsed. Rectum, weak. ***Rheumatism.*** Shoulder, pains. Spasms. Syphilis. Toothache. Tuberculosis. Urinary, incontinence. Varicose, veins. Vertigo. Vomiting. ***Weakness.***

HOMEOPATHIC - Ferr. is one of the prominent constituents of the animal body, present in considerable quantity in the blood. It is present in many articles of daily food and, when given in excess, its first effect is to increase the amount of iron in the blood.

Ferr. is adapted to young, weakly persons, anemic and chlorotic with pseudo-plethora. ***Over-sensitive***, weakness, but looks strong. Delicate girls, constipated, with low spirits. Red-faced old men.

Iron poisoning, symptoms including nausea and vomiting, varicose veins (Sep.), easy bruising, nosebleeds of pale blood, swelling of the limbs, anemia, and sensitivity to smell. Bad affects of iron pills, particularly during pregnancy.

Anemia with weakness. Anemia in those subject to irregular distributions of blood, particularly the young. Flushed cheeks, pallor of lips and mucus membranes, fatigue and breathlessness, and any motion will set up the symptoms. Useful in anemia of cancer and syphilis as a secondary remedy.

Hemorrhages, bright blood or with small clots. Veins dilate during neuralgia, menses or fever. Irregular distribution of blood. Congestions, surgings of blood and pulsations. Orgasms of blood to face, chest, head and lungs. Flushes easily, worse after any active effort. Chlorosis, worse in winter. Hemorrhagic tuberculosis, but it may aggravate.

Dropsy or paralysis after loss of vital fluids, hemorrhages. Rapid emaciation. Cachexia. Pressure, on chest, stomach etc. Cold limbs, muscles relaxed and flabby. Catalepsy. Red parts become pale. Cracking in joints. Softening of bones. Nightly pains that compel motion of part.

Ferr. stimulates the appetite, augment the heart's beats and the bodily vigor. Dryness of mouth, vagina. Exophthalmic goiter from suppressed menses. Spleen, digestion and left deltoid are also affected.

MIND - Mind confused. Can't collect his thoughts. Confusion better washing face. Brain-fag. Always in the right. Proud and haughty. Excitement after menses.

Sensitive, excitable. ***Slight noises unbearable***. Irritability from noise. Oversensitive to pain. ***Ailments from anger.*** Irritable mind and body. Excited from slightest opposition. Anger from contradiction. Intolerant of contradiction.

Changeable mood. Nervous, hysterical. Great alternations of mood, excessively lively, then sad and melancholic. Weeps and laughs immoderately.

Restlessness, must walk about slowly. Anxiety from slight causes. Anxiety as after committing a crime. Fear of having a stroke. Great anxiety about family. ***Restlessness, driving out of bed***, wants to go from one bed to another.

Despondent after menses. Desire for solitude. Aversion to friends. Sadness better exertion. Conversation aggravates. ***Occupation relieves.*** Great indifference. Not inclined to talk or study, from nervous restlessness. Constant thoughts of death.

Abdomen - Colic with watery diarrhea. Rumbling in bowels. Flatulent colic at night. Bowels feel sore to touch. Hard, distended, sore, bruised when walking. Soreness of abdominal walls. ***Soreness all over abdomen, better warmth.*** Sharp pain in abdomen. Sensation as if bowels were bruised, or weakened by cathartics. Shooting pain in left hypochondrium. Cramp-like in region of spleen.

Back - Neck and shoulder painful. ***Rheumatism of the neck and shoulder.*** Neck sore and stiff. Lumbago all night, goes off on rising. Lumbago, better slow walking. Stitch-like jerks in small of back when walking. Pain between scapula.

Blood - Blood diseases, with exhaustion. ***Anemia with exhaustion.*** Anemia with pregnancy. Chlorosis. Hemorrhages. Ailments from blood loss. ***Bleeding, pale or watery blood and weakness*** (Chin., Phos.). Weak blood. Hemophilia. Throbbing pains, the blood vessels all over the body throb violently. Hemorrhages from over-fullness of blood vessels Hemorrhages from vasomotor paralysis, Hemorrhages from delicacy of the blood vessels themselves.

Chest - Anxiety in chest. ***Chest oppressed, breathing difficult.*** Constriction of chest, worse walking. Flying stitches in the chest. Feeling of dryness in chest. Surging of blood to chest. Rush of blood to chest and head, with cold hands and feet. Pressure under sternum, with catarrh and cough. Sharp pain in chest when coughing. Burning pain in sternum after coughing.

Constitutions - Sanguine temperament. Adapted to young, anemic, pseudo-plethoric persons, who though looking strong are so weak that they are unable even to speak or walk, want to lie down.

Coughs - Cough dry, spasmodic. ***Dry, tickling cough, worse moving, better lying down.*** Cough with pain in the occiput. Breath fails at end of coughing fit. Cough, worse abuse of tea, quinine, brandy. ***Cough after loss of fluids.*** Tickling cough in trachea, worse moving, better lying down. ***Cough from tobacco smoke.*** Cough after eating. Cough, must sit up to raise sputum. ***Hemoptysis*** (Mill.). Dry, tickling cough with blood spitting. Spasmodic whooping cough at once better eating a small quantity of food.

Ears - Sharp pain in ears in morning. Ulcerative pain of outer ear. Fetid discharge from left ear. Oversensitive to noise. Noises in ears better leaning the head on table. Ringing in the ears, worse before menses. Ringing in right ear. Singing, humming.

Eyes - Eyes cloudy, watery, dull with blue rings around them. Eyes red with burning pain. Swelling and redness of the eyelids. Puffy eyelids. Pain over eyes (left). Exophthalmic goiter after suppression of menses. Photophobia. Weakness of eyes with lachrymation. Pupils contracted. Suppurating stye on upper lid.

Face - ***False plethora.*** Face feels as if bloated. ***Blushes easily.*** Pale face and ***flushes red from least pain, emotions or exertion.*** Florid. Lips pale. Face pale with red spots on each cheek. Neuralgia after cold washing and overheating. ***Red parts become white, bloodless and puffy.*** Blue rings around eyes, which are dull and lustreless. Distended veins. ***Easy flushing of face, after drinking wine.*** Face fiery red during vomiting.

Female - Women who are weak, delicate, chlorotic, yet have a fiery-red face. Amenorrhea. ***Suppression of menses with extreme nervousness.*** Menses, pale, watery. Passive flow, dark, clotted. Menses too early, too profuse and protracted. ***During menses, must keep perfectly still, least movement greatly worse flow.*** Menses with labor-like pains. Menses remit a day or two and then return. Dysmenorrhea with scanty discharge of pale blood with violent colic. Sticking, shooting pains in uterus. Discharge of long pieces of mucus from uterus. Uterine hemorrhage with labor-like pain in abdomen and small of back. Leucorrhea, milky, acrid, watery, at puberty. Leucorrhea resembling watery milk, smarting and corroding when first appearing, not afterward. Itching of vulva. Sensitive vagina. ***Vagina too dry, pain as if raw.*** Swellings and indurations in vagina. Vagina insensible during sex. Prolapse of vagina. Promotes expulsion of moles. Sexual desire diminished. Sterility. ***Tendency to miscarriage.*** Uterine hemorrhage with threatened premature labour, at end of eight month. ***Morning sickness, constipation, nausea, worse from iron pills.*** Eruption on genitals or inflamed. Ascarides in vulva. Gonorrhea.

Food - Appetite good and bad alternately. ***Voracious appetite.*** Loss of appetite. All food tastes bitter. Unquenchable thirst or thirstlessness. Aversion to eating and drinking during headache. Aversion to meat, children accustomed to meat suddenly become disgusted with it. Aversion to beer. Aversion to sour things, sour fruits. Aversion to accustomed tobacco. Desire for raw tomatoes. Desire for sweets. Desire for bread and butter. ***Worse from eggs.*** Worse abuse of tea, quinine, brandy. Worse tobacco smoke. ***Intolerance of eggs.*** Worse tomatoes. Worse hot things. Worse fat food. Worse drinking milk. Worse sour fruit. Worse after drinking beer. Bread tastes dry and bitter. Wine agrees, if not acid. Meat and acids, sour fruit, as well as beer, causes nausea.

Head - Head hot, feet cold. ***Rush of blood to head with flushes of heat in face.*** Congestion of head with pale face. Headache after menses, with hot head and cold feet. ***Hammering, pulsating, congestive headache***, pain extends to teeth with cold limbs. Severe, frontal headache with cold feet. ***Pain in back of head*** with roaring in neck. Sudden pain over left eye. Stinging headache. ***Long continued headache, often lasting 2 to 3 days.*** Headache during coryza. Feeling of an iron band around head, better external pressure, with red face. Writing causes headache to reappear. Scalp and hair painful to touch. Must take down the hair. Falling out of hair. Hydrocephalus with open fontanels and great anemia.

Heart - Anemic murmurs. Hypertrophy of heart. Fatty degeneration of heart. Endocarditis with chlorotic symptoms. Sense of oppression. Throbbing in all blood vessels. ***Heart suddenly bleeds into the blood vessels*** and as suddenly draws a reflux, leaving pallor of surface. ***Palpitations, worse least motion, better walking slowly.*** Palpitations with fear, has to move about, can neither sit nor stand. Palpitations of masturbators after loss of fluids. Constrictive pain in region of heart. ***Pulse full, but soft and yielding.*** Pulse increased by exertion. ***Pulse small and weak.***

Kidneys - Chronic nephritis. Albuminuria. Diabetes. Kidney pain with desire to urinate. Involuntary urination, especially during the day, when standing, from sudden movement, walking in children. Copious urination with nervousness. Tickling in urethra extending to bladder. Chronic catarrh of bladder and gleet. Burning in urethra during urination, as if urine were hot. Urine hot with menorrhagia. Urine clear as water, in anemia.

Limbs - ***Dropsy after loss of vital fluids.*** Swollen hands and feet. Sudden cramps or tearing pains in the limbs. ***Restlessness in limbs.*** Contraction of limbs. Cracking in joints. Pain in hip joint, tibia, soles and heel. Heels pain, worse lying on back. ***Rheumatism of the shoulder. Rheumatism of the left deltoid muscle***. Tearing pains in deltoid, worse at night, driving him out of bed, and motion diminishes the pain. Difficulty raising the arm. ***Deltoid muscle soreness and pain.*** Irresistible desire to bend the arm with intense pain. Hands tremble when writing, better when writing fast.

Liver - Tightness and fullness in region of liver. Liver enlarged. ***Neonatal jaudice in child from mother taking iron pills during pregnancy.*** Liver sensitive to pressure.

Lungs - Asthma worse after 12 p.m., must sit up, worse sitting still, better walking slowly about. Catarrhal asthma every morning from 10 a.m. to 11a.m. ***Dyspnea better walking slowly and talking.*** Dyspnea after midnight, also when sitting up. ***Suffocative fits in evening in bed.*** Slowly increasing dyspnea, in pneumonia. Shortness of breath from tension in abdomen. Difficult inspiration, as from heaviness of chest. Neglected pleuro-pneumonia, absorbs exudation. ***Hemoptysis*** (Mill.). Spitting of blood in tuberculosis. Spitting of blood, of masturbators. Pneumonia.

Male - Nightly emissions, with backache after over-exertion. Impotency. Increased sexual desire. Erections night and day, Sterility, low sperm count. Discharge of mucus from urethra after a cold. Gleet, copious, painless, milky.

Modalities - Better in summer. Better solitude. ***Better moving about slowly***. Better from gentle motion. Better slight bleeding (Puls.). Better from leaning head on something. Better after rising. ***Worse at night, midnight***. Worse heat. Worse cold. Worse while sitting still. Worse after cold washing. Worse overheating. Worse from sudden motion. Worse raising arms. ***Worse loss of vital fluids.*** Worse eating, drinking. ***Worse from emotions, anger.*** Worse violent exertion. Worse while sweating. Worse during menses. Worse noise. Worse conversation.

Mouth - Breath hot. Dry mouth in morning. Canker sores. Mouth dry, food seems too dry, all solid food tastes dry and insipid. Sweet or bitter taste. Earthy, pasty taste, like rotten eggs. Taste of blood. Toothache from tea. Toothache better icy cold water. ***Pain in teeth, relieved by icy-cold water***. Numb, pithy feeling of tongue, as if burned. Burnt sensation on back and middle portion of tongue. Tongue coated white.

Nose - Nostrils dilated during expiration. ***Nosebleed in anemic patients***. Nosebleed alternating with hemoptysis. ***Nosebleed in anemic children, with changing of color of face.*** Nosebleed in mornings when stooping. Clots of blood constantly accumulate in nose, during coryza. Mucus membranes relaxed, boggy, anemic, pale. Dripping of fluid from posterior nares or frontal sinuses, with headache. Bloody, purulent, greenish, slimy, acrid discharges. Scabs come out of nose or are coughed up every few weeks.

Perspiration - ***Profuse, debilitating sweats.*** Profuse sweats at every motion. Anxious, cold sweat, during cramps of different parts. Cold sweat during convulsions. Clammy, yellow, cold, acrid sweats. Worse while sweating. Sweats often confined to lower part of body. Sweats preceded by headache. Nausea during sweat. Sweats lessened while speaking. Fetid sweats on going to sleep. Sweat at night of a very strong odor.

Rectum - Chronic constipation with easily flushed head and face, cold hands and feet. ***Constipation from taking iron pills.*** Constipation during pregnancy. Contractive pain in rectum. Cramping, in rectum, after stool. ***Prolapsed rectum in children.*** Hemorrhoids, copious bleeding or ichorous oozing. Hemorrhoids with itching and gnawing, tearing pains. ***Itching of anus due to ascarides or worms in children.*** Evacuation of mucus, with worms. Attempts to eat bring on diarrhea. Diarrhea, painless, worse while eating. ***Summer diarrhea of children with emaciation.*** Nightly, gushing and spluttering of undigested food, alternating with constipation, worse if nervous or tired. ***Diarrhea during pregnancy.*** Frequent diarrhea, stools watery, with or without tenesmus. Rice-water discharges. Stools, hard difficult, followed by backache or cramps in rectum, prolapsed rectum. Acrid, watery diarrhea, excoriating anus.

Skin - ***Pale skin. Flushes easily.*** Skin pits on pressure. Skin withered, flabby. Dry skin in pneumonia. Jaundice. Yellow-brown spots, sore to touch. Black or dark violet spots. Burning, with pain as if excoriated when touched. Scarlatina during desquamation. Skin peels off on shoulders and left hand. Ulcers pale, edematous. Warts on fingers and backs of hands.

Sleep - Falls asleep from debility, while sewing, sitting and studying. ***Must lie on back at night.*** Sleepy at night with inability to sleep. Sleeplessness. Child doesn't sleep because of itching from worms. ***Restless sleep at night. Anxious tossing in bed.*** Sleep disturbed by dreams; much weariness in morning. Vivid dreams. Nightmares. Confused, unpleasant dreams. Dreams of being engaged in war. Dreams of falling into water.

Stomach - Stomach won't tolerate any food, causes distention and pressure. Heat and burning in stomach. ***Spits up food by the mouthful*** (Phos.). Belchings of food. Bitter eructations after fat food. Flatulent dyspepsia. Cramp-like pain in stomach. Hemorrhage from stomach. Nausea during headache. ***Nausea and vomiting after eating.*** Vomits after eggs. Easy vomiting without nausea. ***Vomiting after midnight***. Vomiting during pregnancy. Vomiting in morning after breakfast. Vomiting of everything eaten without being digested. Vomiting of food after exertion.

Temperature - ***Chill with red face and thirst.*** General coldness of limbs, head and face hot. Chilly every evening. Frequent short attacks of chilly shivering, ***Chill at 4 a.m.*** Chills with great thirst, preceded and succeeded by headache. Chills with trembling all over. Heat with distended veins. Heat in palms and soles. ***Heat flushes over body*** as if sweat would break out. Hectic fever. Sensation of heat all over body, which is cold to touch. ***Heat with very red face*** and inclination to uncover. Fever abating when moving about. Intermittent fever.

Throat - ***Sore throat with burning pains.*** Burning in larynx and tracnea after talking. Sensation as if a lump (left side), worse swallowing empty. As if something rolling in the throat and closing it like a valve. Sensation as if something was in larynx, which he wished to remove by hawking or coughing. Aching, pressing pain in throat while swallowing. ***Hoarseness, with sense of roughness in larynx.*** Voice changeable. Complete aphonia, causes much anxiety. Speaking causes general weakness. Exophthalmic goiter.

Vertigo - Vertigo on suddenly rising. Vertigo as if balancing to and fro. Vertigo on seeing flowing water. Vertigo on crossing a bridge over water. Vertigo during headache. Vertigo during headache. Vertigo with nausea, prostration, lethargy. Vertigo with disposition to fall forward. Vertigo on descending. Giddy as if drunk, when walking.

Vision - Letters run together when reading or writing. At night can see in the dark, hysteria. Darkness before eyes, giddy. Darkness before eyes in evening, with aching pains and slight nosebleed. Attacks of blindness.

COMMENTS - Hahnemann described the effects of iron on persons who habitually drink chalybeate waters: "In such localities there are few persons who can resist the noxious influence of the continued use of such waters and remain quite well, each being affected according to his peculiar nature."

"There we find more than anywhere else chronic disorders of great gravity and peculiar character, even when the regimen is otherwise faultless.

"Weakness, almost amounting to paralysis of the whole body and of single parts. Some kinds of violent limb pains. Abdominal disorders of various sorts, vomiting of food by day or by night. Tuberculosis. Tubercular pulmonary ailments often with blood spitting, deficient vital warmth.

"Suppression of the menses, miscarriages, impotence, in both sexes infertility. Jaundice and many other rare cachexias are common occurrences."

Blood diseases, especially if with exhaustion. Anemia, hemophilia. Hemorrhages from over-fullness of blood vessels, from vasomotor paralysis, or from delicacy of the vessels themselves. Throbbing pains, the blood vessels all over the body throb violently.

Bleeding, pale or watery blood, (Phos.) and weakness (Chin.). Uterine hemorrhage. Weakness and tiredness since hemorrhage (Chin.). Irregular distribution of blood in chlorotics.

Abnormally pale mucus membranes. Bruises easily, nosebleeds. Palpitations, worse least exertion, excitement. Face flushes. Varicose veins. Legs swell and bruise easily. Hands and feet swell.

Anemia, chronic fatigue since blood loss, chemotherapy or radiation. Lack of stamina. Menses that cause anemia and weakness. Paralytic weakness. Restlessness. Tremor. Rheumatic symptoms, especially of left shoulder and deltoid.

Neuralgia, brought on by washing in cold water, especially after being over-heated. Hammering headache, pain worse after midnight. Pain in os on lying down. Feeling of dryness in vagina.

Gastralgia, heavy pressure in the region of the stomach. Walls of abdomen are sore. A feeling as if something rolled into the throat and closed it like a valve. Frequent spells of nausea, periodic vomiting. Intolerance of eggs.

Marked cramps. Irritability of the bowels causing diarrhea while eating. Diarrhea coming on when the patient beings to eat. Constipation. Irritability of the bladder, causing incontinence of urine when standing. The liver and spleen are affected. Neonatal jaundice. Good for over-dosing from quinine.

Kunkel noted the case of a patient about forty-five, who had repeated attacks of joint rheumatism. Kunkel cured the case based on the symptom "intolerance to eggs" after he had been dosed for three weeks with salicylate of soda by allopaths.

RELATIONS - ***Antidotes:*** Ars., Hep. ***Compare:*** (1) All Ferrums. (2) Rumex - similar in respiratory and digestive sphere and contains organic iron. (3) Graph., Mang., Cupr. ***Complementary:*** Chin., Alum., Ham.

REFERENCES - Boericke. Clarke. Murphy. Phatak.

FERRUM MURIATICUM

(Iron Chloride)

PHARMACY - ferr-m. Ferrum muriaticum. Iron chloride. Sesquichloratum. Ferrous chloride. Ferrous dichloride. Tincture consisting of 25 parts of crystals to 225 parts of alcohol. ***Historical dose:*** All potencies.

CLINICAL - Anemia. Anorexia. Cramps. ***Diarrhea.*** Diphtheria. Erysipelas. Hemoptysis. Insomnia. ***Malaria.*** Nephritis. Pyelitis. ***Shoulder, pain.*** Spleen, enlarged. Vertigo.

HOMEOPATHIC - This remedy has been employed in enlargement of the spleen due to ***malaria***. There is great pain in the left hypochondrium which is worse at night. The face is pale and anemic. Vertigo, anorexia, sleeplessness and a sensation of coldness alternating with heat and lasting for several hours

It is also of service in ***chronic diarrhea***, with loss of appetite, pain and tenesmus. The passages consist of blood and membranous shreds.

Phlegmonous erysipelas. ***Pain in right shoulder,*** right elbow. Marked tendency to cramps. Round red spots on cheeks. Hemoptysis of dark, blood clot.

Suppressed menstruation. Chronic interstitial nephritis. Pyelitis. Bright crystals in urine. Copious urination at puberty. Diphtheria. Very dark and watery stools. Painful sexual intercourse. Tendency to seminal emissions.

COMMENTS - Useful for anemia, given in the 3x after meals. For chronic interstitial nephritis, 1 to 5 drops of the tincture, 3 times daily.

RELATIONS - ***Compare:*** Cean., Ferr.

REFERENCES - Blackwood. Boericke.

FERRUM PERNITRICUM

(Iron Pernitrate)

PHARMACY - ferr-pern. Ferrum pernitricum. Iron pernitrate. Dilutions of the Ferri Pernitratis Liquor of B. P. ***Historical dose:*** All potencies.

CLINICAL - Diarrhea. Eyes, affection. Glands, disorders. Lienteria.

HOMEOPATHIC - Ferr-pern. has been used by old school practitioners with good effect for diarrhea. Diarrhea of tuberculosis. Diarrhea in feeble and nervous female or in scrofulous children with enlarged glands and obstinate ophthalmia.

COMMENTS - Cooper, who gave much attention to the iron preparations, gave as a characteristic, "Cough with florid complexion." In cases presenting marked features of Ferr. and Nit-ac., Ferr-pern. should be helpful.

REFERENCES - Clarke.

FERRUM PHOSPHORICUM

(Iron Phosphate)

PHARMACY - ferr-p. Ferrum phosphoricum. Iron phosphate. Ferric phosphate. Ferroso-ferric phosphate. White phosphate of iron (Schüssler's). This is said to be a true ferric phosphate as contrasted with the ordinary phosphate of iron, which is a ferrous-hydric phosphate. ***Historical dose:*** All potencies.

CLINICAL - ***Anemia.*** Anus, prolapse. ***Bedwetting***. Bladder, paralysis. Bronchitis. Bright's disease. Bruises. Chills. Colic. ***Colds.*** Conjunctivitis. Contusions. Coryza. ***Coughs.*** Croup. Cystitis. ***Debility.*** Delirium tremens. Diabetes. Diarrhea. Dyspepsia. Dysentery. Ear, disorders. Erysipelas. ***Fevers.*** Frostbite. Gastritis. Gonorrhea. Hematemesis. ***Hemoptysis. Hemorrhages.*** Heart, palpitations. Hyperemia. Inflammation. Influenza. Injuries. ***Iron, poisoning. Fevers.*** Kidneys, weak. Mastoiditis. Measles. Mumps. Nevus. Neuralgias. ***Nosebleeds.*** Otitis, media. Pleurisy. Pneumonia. Raynaud's disease. Rheumatism. Sprains. Styes. Tarsal, cysts. ***Throat, sore.*** Tuberculosis. Urinary, incontinence. Veins, varicose. Vomiting. ***Weakness.*** Whooping cough. Wounds.

HOMEOPATHIC - Knowledge of Ferr-p. comes from Schüssler's work and the clinical experience of those who have used it on his indications. It has also been proved by Dr. John Moffat.

Early stages of febrile conditions, it stands midway between the activity of Acon. and Bell., and the sluggishness and torpidity of Gels. Marked prostration, face more active than Gels. The superficial redness never assumes the dusky hue of Gels. Pulse soft and flowing, no anxious restlessness of Acon.

Typically not full blooded and robust, but nervous, sensitive, anemic with false plethora and easy flushing (Ferr.). Pale, anemic subjects with violent local congestions.

Anemia. Hemorrhages and disorders of the veins. Passive congestions and hemorrhages due to hyperemia. Bright hemorrhages from any orifice. ***Increases hemoglobin.*** Discharges are blood streaked or like meat-water. Fresh wounds, pains, contusions, and sprains.

Inflammation, induration, and enlargement of blood vessels. ***First stage of all inflammatory disorders.*** Inflammation of the soft parts. Acute inflammatory rheumatism, especially of the right shoulder (Ferr-m.). Rheumatic paralysis. Bruised soreness on the chest, shoulders, muscles.

Emaciation. Great prostration, can hardly move about. Great physical and mental lassitude, indisposed to physical exertion. Nervousness. Burning rawness. Generally right-sided.

Takes cold easily. Susceptibility to chest troubles. Bronchitis of young children. Acute exacerbation of tuberculosis.

MIND - Anger and apathy. Keeps quiet. Averse to company. Fear of going into a crowd. Very talkative, hilarious and excited. Transient mania from cerebral irritation. Indifferent to pleasurable things.

Abdomen - First stage of peritonitis. Distended intolerance of clothes. Colic before stool. Pain in abdomen with watery diarrhea. Abdominal hernia in persons otherwise robust. Inflamed and incarcerated hernia.

Back - Crick in neck and back. Stiff neck.

Blood - *Anemia.* Blood disorders. Hemorrhages. Chlorosis. ***Iron poisoning.*** Hematochromotosis. Hyperemia, congestion of blood. Hemorrhages, uterine hemorrhages, nosebleeds. Bright red blood (Phos.). ***Ailments from loss of blood, debility.*** Ailments from blood transfusions (Ferr., Chin.).

Causations - Ill effects of checked sweat, blood loss, mechanical injuries.

Chest - Chest heavy, sore or congested. Pleurisy, stitching pain worse coughing and deep breathing.

Constitutions - Suited to nervous, sensitive, anemic persons. ***Sanguine constitutions.*** To the leuco-phlegmatic temperament to young persons with varicose veins. The inflammatory, febrile, emaciating, wasting tuberculosis. Corresponds to Grauvogl's oxygenoid constitution.

Cough - ***Short, painful, tickling cough.*** Hard, dry cough, with sore chest. Cough worse at night, with much rattling of mucus in chest. Hacking, tormenting, spasmodic cough, worse morning and evening. Cough worse going into open air. ***Paroxysmal cough, mostly at night or during day when asleep.*** Whooping cough with retching and vomiting. Tormenting cough, when bending head forward or touching larynx.

Ears - ***First stage of otitis.*** Ear canal inflammed, red, and swollen. ***Acute otitis media*** (Bell.). Throbbing pains. Eardrum red and bulging. Otitis media, with muco-purulent discharge. Eustachian tubes inflamed. Catarrhal affection of eustachian tube and ear. ***Prevents suppuration.*** Mastoid process swollen and sore. Noises, tinnitus worse lying. Deafness from colds, worse during menses. Sensitive to noise. Roaring or buzzing from rush of blood to head.

Eyes - ***Acute conjunctivitis*** without suppuration or discharge of mucus. ***Traumatic conjunctivitis*** (Acon.). Measles with conjunctivitis and photophobia. Red, inflamed with burning sensation. Feeling of a tiny particle in upper eyelid. Feeling as of sand under lids. Ophthalmia, first stage, marked redness with great pain, and without mucus or pus. Encysted tumors of the eyelids. Eyes suffused, cannot see on stooping. Eyes inflamed during dentition. Hyperemia of optic disc and retina with blurred vision. Stye on lower lid.

Face - ***Paleness alternating with redness.*** Florid complexion. Face earthy, pale, sallow. Heat and redness of face during pain. Flushed, cheeks sore and hot. Hot cheeks during toothache. ***Facial neural-***

gia, with stinging, pressing or throbbing pains, worse shaking head, stooping and all motion. Facial neuralgia, better cold applications. Painful red swelling of parotids.

Female - Menses, with bearing-down sensation and headche. Menses every three weeks. Dysmenorrhea, with sacral pain, headache. Dysmenorrhea, frequent urging to urinate, pain in left ovary. Dysmenorrhea with vomiting and indigestion. Bearing down pain in uterus. Constant dull pain in either ovarian region. Vagina sensitive, can't bear examination. Vaginismus, pain during sex. Vagina dry and hot.

Food - Loss of appetite. Chills while eating at table. Aversion to meat and milk. Desire for stimulants. Desire for sour things. Better drinking tea. Worse by eating. Worse meat, herring, cake. Worse tea and coffee.

Head - Rush of blood to head. Soreness to touch, cold, noise, jar. Headache, shooting, aching from vertex down over the sides of the head with earache, better nosebleed, cold application. ***Headache with stinging, pressing or throbbing pains, worse shaking head, stooping and all motion.*** Throbbing headache with sensitive scalp. ***Headache better cold applications***. Head often feels as if pushed forward while walking with vertigo. Empty sensation in the head during menses. ***Vertex sensitive to cold air, noise and any jar***. Congestion to head with epilepsy.Blind headache. Headache during pregnancy. Ill effects of heat of sun.

Heart - First stage of cardiac diseases. Palpitations from congestion. Pulse rapid. ***Short, quick, full, soft.*** Flowing pulse.

Kidneys - Frequent desire to urinate. ***Diurnal bedwetting,*** better lying down. Incontinence. Urine spurts with every cough. Polyuria. Urinates after every drink. Irritation at neck of bladder. Urine retained in children during fever.

Limbs - Fractures at beginning of injury to soft parts, adjacent parts red, hot and painful. ***Acute rheumatism.*** Rheumatism attacking one joint after another, worse slightest motion. ***Rheumatic pain in shoulder***, pains extend to chest and wrist. Jerking in limbs. Sore, bruised pain in shoulders, extending to chest and wrist. ***Sprains of the elbows.*** Wrists ache with loss of power to grasp. Hands swollen and painful. Fingers contracted by acute articular rheumatism. Palms hot, in children. Whitlow. Varicose veins.

Lungs - First stage of all inflammatory affections. Acute bronchial catarrh affecting larger and smaller bronchi. ***Bronchitis of young children.*** Congestions of lungs. Croup. Short, painful, tickling and hacking, tormenting, spasmodic cough, worse morning and evening. Hard, dry cough with sore chest. Pneumonia, the first stage. ***Hemoptysis of pure blood,*** in pneumonia, after concussion or fall (Mill.). Hemoptysis after concussion or fall. Pleurisy, sharp pain, right side, worse coughing and deep breathing.

Male - Seminal emissions. Inflammatory stage of gonorrhea.

Modalities - ***Better cold applications.*** Better bleeding. Better lying down. Better from rest. Better from gentle motion. Worse at night. Worse 4 a.m. to 6 a.m. Worse cold air. Worse open air. Worse checked sweat. Worse right side. Worse touch. Worse jar. Worse motion. Worse noise. Worse cold drinks and sour food. Worse meat, herring, coffee, and cake. Worse right side.

Mouth - Mouth hot, fauces red inflamed. Toothache, better cold. Ranula in vascular. Tongue swollen and dark red. Inflammation of tongue, fauces and tonsils. Redness, pain without exudation.

Nose - ***Predisposition to colds and sore throats.*** Acute coryza and sore throat. ***First stage of colds, influenza.*** Nosebleed in children. Nosebleed with blood-spitting. ***Nosebleeds***, bright red blood (Phos.). Controls soreness and bleeding after operations. Watery discharge with colds.

Perspiration - Night sweats of anemia or tuberculosis. Copious night sweats, does not relieve pains of rheumatism. Sweats driving out of bed. Sweats between 4 a.m. and 6 a.m. Sweats with increase of pains.

Rectum - Diarrhea worse midnight till morning. Habitual constipation. Constipation caused by atony of muscular fibres of intestines. ***First stage of dysentery with much blood in discharges.*** Hemorrhoids with obstinate constipation. Hemorrhoids with catarrh of stomach and bowels. Summer diarrhea with red face and soft pulse. Chronic diarrhea. Disposition to prolapse rectum. Stools of yellow water. Stools watery, bloody, undigested.

Skin - Pale, flushed skin. ***Bleeds easily.*** Bruises easily. Acne. Measles with conjunctivitis and photophobia. Measles in beginning. Acne. ***Capillary congestion with burning of skin***, worse violent exertion or warm room. Erysipelas with intense fever and inflammatory symptoms.

Sleep - Restless and sleepless. Drowsiness. Restless sleep followed by great depression in morning. Night sweats of anemia or tuberculosis. Sleepless from severity of pains. Anxious dreams.

Stomach - Dyspepsia. ***Sour belchings***. Chill while eating. Catarrh of stomach and bowels. Pain in stomach worse after eating. Acute and chronic gastralgia worse eating and pressure on stomach. Gastralgia with vomiting of food. Sudden attacks of deathly nausea. Persistent vomiting of food in morning, before eating. ***Vomiting of undigested food***. Vomiting green matter. Vomiting of bright red blood. Vomiting during pains.

Teeth - Toothache better cold. Toothache always appearing after eating food. Toothache worse warm drinks, better cold drinks. Congestive or inflammatory toothache. Decayed teeth. Complaints during dentition. Dentition with fever.

Temperature - Chill with desire to stretch, at 1 p.m. First stage of catarrhal and ***inflammatory fevers. Fevers of unknown origin.*** Continued infectious fevers. Intermittent fevers. Fever and sore throat. Pneumonia fever. Hemorrhagic fevers. Measles fever. Heat with sweaty hands.

Throat - ***Predisposition to colds and sore throats.*** Sore throat with colds, pain worse empty swallowing. Fauces red, inflamed. Ulcerated sore throat. ***Tonsils red and swollen.*** Inflamed eustachian tubes. First stage of diphtheria. ***Hoarseness from overstraining voice.*** Laryngitis with hoarseness of singers. Laryngitis with fauces inflamed and red. ***Sore throat of singers.*** Ranula in vascular, sanguine constitutions. ***Much mucus in throat and rattling in chest.*** After operations on throat and nose to control bleeding and relieve soreness. Feeling of nausea in throat. Croup.

Vertigo - Vertigo with rush of blood to head. ***Fainting from the sight of blood.*** Vertigo from anemia, weakness. Vertigo with constant feeling as if head were being suddenly pushed forward, with danger of falling. Great dizziness, everything swims around him, muscles seemed so weak he could hardly move about. Vertigo caused by congestion to various parts of brain or head.

COMMENTS - Hematochromotosis. Hyperemia, congestion of blood. Hemorrhages, uterine hemorrhages, nosebleeds. Tendency to bleed. Bright red blood (Phos.), thicker than Ferr. Ailments from loss of blood, debility. Ailments from blood transfusions (Ferr., Chin.). Fainting from the sight of blood or from weakness.

Coughing up of blood, in pneumonia cases. Vomiting blood. Blood in the stool, bleeding hemorrhoids, blood in the urine, with no symptoms. Fainting spells, weak with circulatory problems. Great emaciation.

Fevers of unknown origin. Early stage of acute diseases. Nonspecific convalescent remedy. Nonspecific inflammation.

Nondescript sore throats and colds. Flus. Bronchitis with a short, painful cough. Acute coryza (Ars., Acon., All-c.). Earaches, with redness. Otitis media with throbbing (Bell.). Mastoiditis (Caps., Bell.), with inflammation as the only symptom. Eye infections, bloodshot and red eyes with no other symptoms. Conjunctivitis (Euph.).

Red face that feels cool, flushed but weak. Face goes red when child is picked up. Teething in children with a fever and a hot, red face (Bell.). Toothaches or inflammation of gums. Toothache, better cold (Mag-p. better heat).

Acute arthritis, hands swollen and red. Neck stiff from being out in the cold. Cold hands and feet. Chilly. Sensitive to open or cold air. Results of checked perspiration on a warm summer day (peritonitis). Pains go from below upward. Thirsty for ice cold drinks. Desires sour things.

Similar to Phos., where Ferr. is more similar to Puls.

In Schüssler's therapy Ferr-p. takes the place filled by Acon., Bell., Gels., Verat-v., Arn. and other remedies which correspond to disturbed states of circulation, irritation and relaxation of tissue.

Schüssler noted "The pains which correspond to iron are increased by motion, but relieved by cold in the muscle-cells iron is found in the form of a phosphate, we should therefore in therapeutics use Ferrum phosphoricum."

Nimier and Parenteau cured several cases of right-supra-orbital neuralgia with morning aggravation with Ferr-p. 6x. The morning aggravation appeared to be the distinctive indication.

Nash said the hemorrhages are bright red, but occur not in the plethoric subjects of Acon., but rather in pale, anemic subjects liable to sudden local congestions.

Cooper cured with Ferr-p. a case of tuberculosis in a patient "of the transparent-skin type, the hemoglobin shining through."

According to Cooper, Ferr-p. antidoted "violent dysuria, night and day," caused by Stront-br. "Painless irritability of tissue" is Cooper's keynote, as exemplified in diurnal bedwetting.

Halbert cured a case of Raynaud's disease of the fingers and toes in which amputation seemed inevitable. He affected a complete cure with Ferr-p. 6x trituration.

Ferr-p. can be used as a nutritional supplement for anemia in the 6x potency. Schüssler generally used the 12x trituration.

RELATIONS - ***Compare:*** (1) Oxygenoid constitution. (2) Acon., Chin., Ars, Graph., Petr. (3) Ferrum pyrophosph. - congestion of brain and headache following great loss of blood, tarsal cysts. (4) Gels. - more flowing pulse, Caust. and Puls. - cough with spurting of urine. (5) Kali-m. - croup, pneumonia, palpitations, typhus, Kali-p. - colic, threatened gangrene. (6) Calc-s. - hip joint disease, Calc-p. - chlorosis, hemorrhoids, Calc-f. - hemorrhoids, Nat-s. - diabetes, Ant-t. - capillary bronchitis.

REFERENCES - Boericke. Clarke. Murphy. Phatak.

FERRUM PICRICUM

(Iron Picrate)

PHARMACY - ferr-pic. Ferrum picricum. Iron picrate. Trituration. Tincture. ***Historical dose:*** All potencies.

CLINICAL - Albuminuria. Bilious, disorders. Corns. Deafness. Dyspepsia. Ears, diseases. Fatigue. Gout. Headache. Indigestion. Jaundice. ***Liver, disorders.*** Lupoid, warts. Lupus. ***Nosebleeds***. Polyuria. ***Prostate, enlarged.*** Rheumatic, arthritis. Rodent, ulcer. Tinnitus. ***Vasculitis.*** Voice, loss. ***Warts.***

HOMEOPATHIC - Ferrum picricum is considered a great remedy to complete the action of other medicines. Indicated by the functional failure of an organ under exertion.

This is an unproved medicine, but Dr. Cooper gave the leading indications for its use and these are so clear that it has taken a definite position in the Materia Medica.

Ferr-pic. is a liver medicine and is particularly suited to persons with dark hair and eyes and bilious-looking patients. A dirty appearance about the joints indicates it, the stain due to bile pigments.

Senile hypertrophy of the prostate gland, with frequent urination at night, with full feeling and pressure in rectum. Smarting at neck of the bladder and penis. Meatus dry. Retention of urine.

Warts and epithelial growths, corns with yellowish discoloration. ***Nosebleeds***. Chronic deafness and tinnitus due to gout. Pseudo-leukemia. Failed voice after public speaking.

MIND - ***Prostration of mind.*** Irritable and sensitive.

Back - Pain in right side of neck and down right arm.

Causations - Overwork, exertion. Fatigue, overpowering effects of fatigue.

Constitutions - Suited to dark-haired, plethoric people.

Ears - Tinnitus. Humming in ears as from telegraph wires. Crackling in ears and low-pitched voice. Vascular deafness. Deafness before menses. Dental neuralgia, radiating towards ears and eyes.

Face - Lupoid wart on face.

Food - Loss of appetite. Indigestion.

Head - Headache after meals, especially in bilious, dark-haired persons. Bilious headaches. Giddiness with disturbance of cerebral circulation, pain in occiput, and inability to walk.

Kidneys - ***Frequent urination*** at night with full feeling. Retention of urine. ***Smarting at neck of bladder*** and penis (Baros.). Pain along entire urethra.

Limbs - Chronic gout. Dirty appearance about joints. Pain in right side of neck and down right arm. Locomotor ataxia, ocular stage. Hands covered with warts.

Liver - Liver and bilious disorders. Jaundice. Liver weakness. Liver sensitive, some jaundice.

Male - Prostate gland enlarged.

Modalities - Worse from fatigue.

Mouth - Dental neuralgia, radiating towards ears and eyes. Furred tongue.

Rectum - ***Pressure in the rectum.*** Constipation.

Skin - Warts, multiple, pedunculated. Sensation as if a wart were growing on thumb. Corns. Jaundice. Dirty looking skin about joints.

Sleep - Restless sleep with unpleasant (often erotic) dreams.

Stomach - Dyspepsia.

COMMENTS - Acts best in plethoric people with sensitive livers. Burnett cured with it rheumatic arthritis in a dark-haired subject.

Effects of fatigue (Pic-ac.), unusual fatigue. Cooper described it as the failure of an organ under exertion which would not ordinarily strain it, e.g., failure of the voice in public speakers.

Noises in the ears. Nervous deafness, "diffused vasculitis."

Dr. Cooper was led to give Ferr-pic. in cases of warts by a symptom produced in a patient to whom he was giving it for deafness, "sensation as if a wart were growing on the thumb."

Cooper observed that warts, especially old pedunculated warts, frequently accompany chronic deafness. He considered it especially indicated for multiple warts on the hand, and noted a case of lupoid warts cured by it.

P. C. Majumdar cured a student suffering from anemia and malarious fever off and on for a year. The student had impaired hearing of both ears, buzzing, hissing, and vertigo. Indigestion, headache and tired feeling after bodily or mental exertion. Majumdar considered Ferr-pic. suited to the results of malarious fever, sexual excesses and blood loss.

It has a specific action in the prostate gland. Puller cured with it a case of albuminuria. Dudley Wright confirmed Cooper's observation that it will frequently control senile prostate hypertrophy.

Dr. Mende considers Ferr-pic. almost specific in nosebleed.

Ferr-pic. is apt to aggravate if given too low.

RELATIONS - ***Compare:*** (1) Pic-ac., Nit-ac., Thuj. Am-pic., Calc-pic. (2) the Ferrum preparations. (3) Buchu, Sulph.

REFERENCES - Boericke. Clarke. Cooper. Phatak.

FERRUM SULPHURICUM

(Iron Sulphate)

PHARMACY - ferr-s. Ferrum sulphuricum. Iron sulphate. Ferrous sulphate. Iron vitriol. Green vitriol. Copperas. Trituration of the pure crystals. ***Historical dose:*** All potencies.

CLINICAL - Aphthae. Bulimia. Cardialgia. Chorea. Constipation. Diarrhea. Eczema. Gallbladder, pain. Gastritis. Gonorrhea. Hemorrhages. Headache. Helminthiasis. Menorrhagia. Nettle rash. Scrofula. Spasms. Toothache.

HOMEOPATHIC - Ferr-s. has the leading features of the other Ferrums, but many of the Sulphur characters appear, especially in the modalities. There is worse from warmth or warm room, better from cold air, ice, or fresh air.

Acidity and belchings of food in particles (Sulph.). Watery and painless stools. Sensation of fermentation or purring in stomach. Pain in gallbladder. Toothache. Basedow's disease.

Passive hemorrhages. Pallor or flushing. Sensation as if all the blood were rushing into head and face. Menorrhagia. Pressing, throbbing between periods with rush of blood to head.

Muscular pains or contractions. Weakness. Local atony, disposition to congestions. Nettle rash, aphthae, eczema with sluggish liver. Feeling of general heat and disposition to sweat with sensation in skin of back as if he wore a stout woolen shirt.

COMMENTS - This remedy has been employed in diarrhea when the stools are watery, reddish-brown. Stools, odorless and painless. There is great pallor of the skin, emaciation, anemia. Edema of the lower limbs. Affects the blood-vessels and heart. Anemic murmurs.

Also in menorrhagia, when the flow is of long duration and is profuse. There is a pressing, throbbing between the periods, with ringing in the ears and a sensation as though the blood were rushing to the face. Face is scarlet red. The bowels are constipated, and there is loss of appetite.

RELATIONS - ***Compare:*** (1) Phos. - regurgitation of food in particles. (2) Cina - worms. (3) Bapt. - pain in region of gallbladder. (4) Ferr., Meli.

REFERENCES - Boericke. Clarke.

FERRUM TARTARICUM

(Iron Tartrate)

PHARMACY - ferr-t. Ferrum tartaricum. Iron tartrate. ***Historical dose:*** All potencies.

HOMEOPATHIC - Ferr-t. has heart pain, heat sensation at cardiac orifice of stomach.

REFERENCES - Boericke.

FERRUM VALERIANICUM

(Iron Valerianate)

PHARMACY - ferr-val. Ferrum valerianicum. Iron valerianate. A dark brick-red, amorphous powder. Triturations, and dilutions. ***Historical dose:*** All potencies.

HOMEOPATHIC - This remedy is indicated in cases of ***hysteria, chorea and nervous disorders***.

Also indicated in those suffering from ***chlorosis and anemia***. Insomnia, nervousness and anemia. Sleeplessness from anxiety and worry.

RELATIONS - ***Compare:*** Valer., Ign.

REFERENCES - Blackwood.

FERULA GLAUCA

(Bounafa)

PHARMACY - ferul. Ferula glauca. Bounafa. Ferula neapolitana. N. O. Umbelliferae. Tincture of plant. ***Historical dose:*** Tincture and all potencies.

HOMEOPATHIC - Ferul. has been proved. Heat and burning are produced in parts and sensations of coldness in others. Prominent stiffness and constriction. Aphthae. Cough, worse in damp or cold weather. Slow digestion. Diarrhea. Hemorrhoids. Nymphomania, pruritus vulvae. Violent sexual excitement in women.

RELATIONS - ***Compare:*** (1) Other Umbelliferae, tongue as if burnt, Sang.

REFERENCES - Boericke. Clarke. Phatak.

FICUS INDICA

(Banyan Tree)

PHARMACY - fic-i. Ficus indica. Banyan tree. Vata. N. O. Moraceae. India. Tincture of the bark. Tincture of the hanging roots and buds.

CLINICAL - Colic. Diabetes. Diarrhea. Dyspepsia. ***Dysentery.*** Enteroptosis. Gonorrhea. Hematuria. ***Hemorrhages.*** Hemorrhoids. Leucorrhea. Nausea.

HOMEOPATHIC - The banyan tree is planted throughout India. It grows to a height of about a hundred feet and is a common roadside tree.

Ficus Indica has being used successfully in all kinds of ***hemorrhages.*** Pure red blood. It possesses greater anti-hemorrhagic properties than Ficus religiosa.

Hemorrhage from the throat or mouth. Dysentery and piles mixed with blood. Hemorrhage before evacuations. Acute or chronic bloody dysentery associated with great urging, colic and tenesmus (Merc-c.).

Diarrhea, with nausea. ***Feels as if bowels were settled down in lower abdomen.*** Enteroptosis with loose and frequent evacuations. Sick feeling in lower third of abdomen.

Copious hemorrhages during menses. Bloody leucorrhea. Nervous weakness due to seminal discharge. Gonorrhea and diabetes associated with burning sensation during urination and in hematuria.

COMMENTS - Proving by Dr. O. N. Banerjee, Calcutta, India, in the Homoeopathic Recorder, July, 1891.

Dr. O. N. Banerjee wrote "In June, 1888, while visiting a patient in the country I saw in the garden a large tree of the variety known as Ficus Indica. As the tree is considered sacred I regarded it and its branches, which were ladened with ripe, yellow fruit, with the greatest interest, and plucking one of the fruits, ate it upon an empty stomach.

"To my great astonishment there occurred one hour thereafter an unusual frequent desire to urinate, I did not relish my breakfast, there was loss of appetite and sour belching; in the afternoon the urine became phosphatic and I suffered from headache; in the evening I felt an itching of the thighs, heaviness of the head, dullness of the mind, and a burning heat over the body; there was but a scanty discharge of urine during the day.

"After gathering a large quantity of fruit I returned to Calcutta and made an alcoholic tincture thereof. This was distributed among nine provers and two drops of the mother tincture were taken every morning before breakfast for eight days.

"As a remedy it has been used successfully in every case presenting the following conditions: Frequent, at times unsatisfactory discharge of amber-colored or phosphatic urine with discharge of seminal fluid. Headache, heaviness of the head. Itching of the limbs. Thirst. Dyspepsia. Ill humor. Irregular stool. Disturbed sleep."

RELATIONS - ***Compare:*** (1) Merc. cor., Chin., Phos.

REFERENCES - Boericke. Ghose.

FICUS RELIGIOSA

(Ashwathya)

PHARMACY - fic. Ficus religiosa. Ashwathya. Bo-tree. Pakur. N. O. Moraceae. India. Tincture of juice of fresh leaves mixed with equal parts of alcohol. ***Historical dose:*** Tincture and all potencies.

CLINICAL - ***Bloody, discharges.*** Dysentery. Hematemesis. ***Hemorrhages.*** Hemorrhoids. Menorrhagia. Nosebleed. Typhoid. Vomiting.

HOMEOPATHIC - Dr. Sarat Chandra Ghose of Midnapore made the first proving and thereby discovered its power to cause and cure ***hemorrhages*** of many kinds. Ghose related some striking cases cured with the remedy in cases of dysentery, hematemesis, hemorrhage of typhoid, bleeding hemorrhoids and nosebleed.

General hemorrhages. Vomiting of a bright red blood. Hemoptysis. Menorrhagia. Profuse discharge of bright red blood, bearing-down pains in lower abdomen. Bloody urine. Very weak and restless. Headache, burning at the top of the head. Sight dim.

MIND - Quiet and disinclined to move. Sad and melancholic.

Abdomen - Bearing-down pains in lower part of abdomen.

Eyes - Sight dim.

Face - Face became yellow.

Female - Menorrhagia, bright red blood, bearing-down pains in lower abdomen.

Head - Burning at vertex, vertigo and slight headache.

Kidneys - Frequent desire to urinate. Urine contains much blood.

Lungs - Difficult breathing, cough with vomiting of blood, pulse very weak.

Nose - Nosebleed.

Rectum - Dysentery with menorrhagia. Dysentery, bright red blood.

Stomach - Pain and sick feeling in stomach. Nausea, vomiting of bright red blood.

COMMENTS - Dr. Ghose participated in his own proving, along with his wife and a dog. The dog, which was perfectly strong and healthy, received 40 drops of the tincture one morning. No result followed that day and the dose was repeated the next morning.

The animal commenced and continued to vomit blood of a bright red color. It kept very quiet and was unwilling to move. After three doses of five drops of the tincture given in quick succession, the vomiting ceased. The same treatment (minute doses of the remedy) was effectual in arresting the effects of the drug throughout the provings.

Mrs. Ghose took the tincture in 20-drop doses repeatedly throughout two days. On the third day dysentery and menorrhagia set in simultaneously. The blood was bright red.

Other symptoms included a headache, very weak and restless, sight dim, burning at the top of the head. The face became yellowish, breathing difficult. She became sad and melancholic. With the profuse discharge of bright red blood there were bearing-down pains in the lower abdomen.

Dr. Ghose took 40 drops in one dose. The result was a frequent desire to pass water, which gradually became bloody, containing much blood. Inclination to cough, causing him to spit blood. Slight headache, giddiness and nausea. Sight dim. Very weak and restless. The tincture was taken three drops every two hours, and after the third dose the symptoms vanished.

RELATIONS - ***Compare:*** (1) Acalypha, Ip., Arn., Mill., Phos., Hirudo, Cact., Ferr. Thlaspi.

REFERENCES - Boericke. Clarke.

FILIX MAS

(Male Fern)

PHARMACY - fil. Filix mas. Male fern. Aspidium filix-mas. N. O. Filices. Dryopteridaceae. Tincture of fresh root or fresh root grated. Maceration of fresh root. ***Historical dose:*** Tincture and all potencies.

CLINICAL - Abdomen, bloated. Abortion. Blindness. Infertility. Miscarriage. ***Tapeworm***. Worms.

HERBAL - The male fern has been recognized as a vermifuge from the time of Galen. For worm symptoms, especially with constipation. Dioscorides credits it with the power of causing infertility and abortion.

HOMEOPATHIC - A fragmentary proving in Allen's Appendix records a case in which 15 to 20 drops of the tincture given three times a day to a woman suffering from bloated abdomen with more or less pain caused diminution of the bloating. Also, severe prolapse of vagina. Pain and tenesmus of bladder with copious and frequent emission of urine, with intense pain.

Filix was then discontinued and Chim. relieved the symptoms. They did not return afterwards, except after much walking or standing.

The leading symptoms include a pale face with blue rings around the eyes, and blindness from atrophy of the optic nerve. ***Torpid inflammations of lymphatic glands.*** Pulmonary tuberculosis in young patients, no fever with limited, ulcerated lesions. Gnawing, boring pains in abdomen, worse after sweet things. ***Tapeworms.*** Soporific conditions.

Abdomen - Bloated. Gnawing and boring in bowels, worse eating sweet things. Great pain in abdomen with diarrhea and constant vomiting. ***Worm colic*** with itching of nose, pale face, blue rings around eyes. Painless hiccough.

Eyes - Blindness, monocular amblyopia. Blindness, first mydriasis and amaurosis with normal fundus, eight days later, atrophy of optic nerve. Immobility of pupil.

Face - Pale face, blue rings around eyes.

Female - Menstruation stimulated. Prolapse

of vagina with pains and tenesmus of bladder and copious frequent emission of urine with internal pains. Abortion. Sterility.

Limbs - Numbness of right wrist.

Nose - Itching of nose.

Rectum - Violent vomiting and diarrhea. Ineffectual urging to stool. Pappy stools. Worm symptoms with constipation. Worm colic.

Sleep - Soporific condition. Restless and sleepless at night.

Stomach - Nausea. Sick after taking food.

Temperature - Violent rigor, fever, great pain in abdomen with diarrhea and constant vomiting.

COMMENTS - C. S. Spencer recorded this effect from taking capsules each containing ten minims of the oil of male fern for tapeworm:

"A feeling of nausea, abdomen became painfully distended with colicky pains. Menses returned after only one week's absence and continued profusely for three weeks. Very sick after taking her food. The worm was got rid of and the capsules stopped when these symptoms passed away."

Hering said the best time to give the drug for expulsion of tapeworm is in the summer when the fresh root can be obtained. If an ounce of the grated root is given in the forenoon, usually the tapeworm comes away in the afternoon.

Teste used it successfully in a case of violent dyspnea without cough, with stitches in region of heart and obscure symptoms of pericarditis. The patient was a young woman of lymphatico-nervous temperament and was much weakened by long sickness.

RELATIONS - ***Compare:*** (1) Aspidium alhamanticum. Panna - 3 doses, 2 grams each, all in half hour, fasting in a glass of milk. Tasteless and will remove tapeworm. (2) Cina, Gran., Kousso.

REFERENCES - Boericke. Clarke.

FLAVUS BACILLUS

PHARMACY - flav. Flavus bacillus. Neisseria pharingis flava. Neissericeae. Micrococcales. A non-pathogenic bacterium found in the upper respiratory passages but was also found in cerebrospinal fluid during meningitis. ***Historical dose:*** All potencies.

CLINICAL - Arthritis. Arthrosis. Brachial, neuralgia. Coughs. Dysmenorrhea. Dysphagia. Dyspnea. Endometriosis. ***Headaches.*** Intoxication. Otitis. Palpitations. Premenstrual syndrome. Rhinitis. Sciatica. Sinusitis. Thyroid, problems.

HOMEOPATHIC - Flavus is a bacterium called Neisseria Phringis Flava, belonging to the Neisseria family of the Micrococcales order. These microbes are in the shape of shells arranged in pairs like coffee beans. They are Gram-positive. Neisseria Flava is an aerobic saprophyte found in the upper respiratory passages.

Flavus is not considered to be pathogenic. Nevertheless, it was isolated from the cerebrospinal fluid of several children suffering from meningitis. It owes its name to the formation of a yellow pigment in the middle of the culture colony.

Flav. shows signs of irritation in the eyes, nose and pharynx which can lead to spasmodic rhinitis. Sensation of a lump in the throat. Feeling like feathers in the throat (Kali-bi.). Feeling of gravel in the larynx after speaking for a long time. Thyroid problems.

Headaches. ***Peri-orbital headaches***, localized on the right side (Sang.). Pain at the level of the frontal and maxillary sinuses. Discharge from the eyes and nose. Tendency to colds, coughs and expectorates. Slight localized trembling, particularly in the fingers. Intoxication.

MIND - Low morale, exaggerates difficulties. Sensitive to others' emotions and being contradicted.

Back - Arthrosis of the cervical column with cracking. Neck pains. Cervical-brachial neuralgia. Pain in the back, spreading to both arms.

Constitutions - Psoric, sycotic and tubercular constitutions.

Ears - Frequent attacks of otitis, recurring. Pain in the right ear.

Eyes - Per-orbital headache, localized on the right side. Eyes red in the evening, when tired. Eye fatigue. Eyes swollen in the morning, on waking, eyelids heavy. Conjunctivitis.

Female - Menses irregular, too early, of varying quantities with pale blood. Menses too frequent. Menses late with premenstrual syndrome. Loss of blood at ovulation. Dysmenorrhea. Endometriosis. Hot flushes, worse at night.

Food - Complaints aggravated by wine (Zinc, Nux-v.).

Head - Peri-orbital headaches, localized on the right side (Sang.).

Heart - Palpitations at night with feeling of fever, worse after drinking wine.

Limbs - Arthrosis, rheumatic arthritis. Sciatica. Pain in the joints with cracking situated at the knees, wrists, shoulders and fingers. Pain in the left hip, left arm. Slight localized trembling, particularly in the fingers.

Lungs - Dyspnea, worse at night, worse around 2 a.m., with waking and suffocation. Coughing in the morning for 1 hour, on waking.

Modalities - Better in the autumn. Better spring. Better from hot baths. Worse from cold. Worse heat. Worse at night. Worse in the morning. Worse on the left side. Worse after drinking wine.

Mouth - Arthritis of the jaw with loose teeth.

Nose - Nose dry with dry scabs. Nasal discharge of greenish pus (Kali-bi.). Sinusitis. Sneezes easily. Spasmodic coryza. Nasal congestion at night, one nostril becomes blocked. Bleeding from the nose in the morning on waking.

Skin - Perspiration from the palms. Dry eczema of the palms. Ecchymosis occurring regularly from the slightest shock.

Stomach - Digestion bad. Digestive complaints after moist food. Frequent nausea after meals.

Throat - Red, sore throat. Sore throat after having had wet feet. Throat dry with slight discomfort at night. Throat inflamed. Frequent loss of voice. Dysphagia. Tickling sensation in the right side of the larynx. Dry cough, aggravated in the morning. Feeling that the hard palate is touching the tongue.

RELATIONS - ***Compare:*** (1) Kali-bi. - Coryza and sinusitis with sensation of blocked nose and tickling in the nostrils. Thick yellow or greenish discharge, viscous or running, forming greenish elastic lumps, sticky, which leave the mucus membranes raw and burning. (2) Zinc - Also shows aggravation from wine, but the depressive condition is infinitely more accentuated. General weakness. Cannot keep his legs still.

REFERENCES - Julian.

FLOR DE PIEDRA

PHARMACY - flor-p. Flor de piedra. Lophophytum leandri. Balanophoraceae. South America. Tincture of whole dried plant. ***Historical dose:*** Tincture and all potencies.

CLINICAL - Cholecystitis. Colic. Colitis. Diabetes. Dysthyroidism. Emaciation, Epilepsy. Exophthalmus. Goiter. Headache. Hyperthyroidism. Hypothyroidism. Rickets. Vertigo.

HERBAL - Flor de Piedra grows in the tropical forests of Argentina, Paraguay and Brazil. This plant is used by the natives for stomach and liver disturbances. In Pio Carrera's book on Brazilian phototherapy, rickets and epilepsy are also indicated.

HOMEOPATHIC - W. Schwabe brought back the plant from Brazil. In collaboration with others, he carried out a proving on sixteen provers (10 women and 6 men), using the 6x, 4x, 3x, and 2x potencies, on February 21, 1964.

J. R. Reside undertook another proving in 1966-67. Finally, Juliette Fourmon undertook an extremely thorough clinical proving.

Emaciation from the pituitary or the thyroid gland. Neuro-endocrine complaints. Congestion of the thyroid with vago-sympathetic disharmony. Pituitary diabetes. Cardiac complication of hyperthyroidism.

Pain in the heart and liver. General nausea. Distention and spasmodic diarrhea.

Constriction of the neck. Feeling of tightness around the neck. Headache, vertigo. Sudden tiredness, especially in the morning.

MIND - Increase in general activity. Mentally alert, clear-headed. Bright, then slow. Confused, lacking focus. Depressed.

Abdomen - Wakes at 2 a.m. with abdominal pains, ameliorated by going to stool. Heavy, full feeling and abdominal distention. Pressure in the right iliac region. Cannot bear the pressure of underclothes.

Back - Pain in the right shoulder on lifting the right arm.

Blood - Disorders of the basal metabolism. Hypo-cholesterolemia.

Chest - Right subcostal pain. Feeling of oppression in the thorax, rather more to the right that the left side. Thoracic pain, worse by movement and deep respiration.

Constitutions - Suited to tubercular, nervous, phosphoric or phospho-fluoric types.

Ears - Pruritus of the auditory canal.

Eyes - Eyes bloodshot. Stye on the lower right eyelid. Orbital pain of a pressing type, when reading. Diminution in visual activity.

Female - Menses infrequent, abundant, but late by five days. Greenish vaginal discharge.

Food - Extreme thirst.

Head - Left frontal or temporal headache, ameliorated in the open air, increased in the evening. Headaches, as though the brain would burst with visual disturbances and zigzags at the edge of the field of vision.

Heart - Palpitations.

Kidneys - Abundant urine.

Limbs - Painful drawing and pricking feeling in the left arm, elbow and hand, with formication in the left hand. Drawing pain in the right thigh down to the calf and heel. Sharp, cutting pain in the left knee, worse when walking. Heaviness in the legs. Right foot slightly edematous and sensitive to pressure. Feet cold.

Lungs - Irritating, dry, hacking cough.

Modalities - Better from open air, Better heat. Worse in the evening. Worse from exertion.

Mouth - Mouth dry with difficulty in swallowing. Ulcers in the mouth and on the lips and tongue. Heartburn. Diminution in sense of taste.

Nose - Dryness in the nose. Fits of sneezing.

Rectum - Tendency to diarrhea with grayish or pale yellow stools.

Skin - Generalized pruritus, but particularly the ears, scalp, arms and face, abdomen and anal region. Marks on the thighs and lower limbs. Perspiration.

Sleep - Sleep disturbed. Fiery, hot feeling in bed.

Stomach - Acrid dyspepsia. Nausea and epigastric discomfort.

Temperature - Profuse sweating and hot flushes.

Throat - Throat dry, empty swallowing to clear the throat. Feeling of a lump in the back of the throat. Stabbing pain in the throat, worse during the morning.

Vertigo - Vertigo and tendency to fall to the left.

COMMENTS - Freiwald reported favorable results in thyroid infections, using the potencies 3x and 6x and in infections of the liver and bladder, using 4x and 6x. Juliette Fourmon reported some clinical successes in goiter cases, hyperthyroidism, and in a case of bilateral degenerative labyrinthitis.

M. Tetau made a general review of thyroid disorders and their homeopathic and biotherapeutic treatment, noting the value of Lophophytum Leandri.

RELATIONS - *Compare:* (1) Iodum - Anxious, cannot stay still, emaciation, hoarseness, diarrhea. Precordial anxiety with palpitation at the slightest exertion. (2) Hedera Helix. (3) Nat-m. - Emaciation of the upper part of the body, headache, dryness of the mouth and fissure on the middle of the lower lip. Abnormal desire for salt. (4) Tuberculinum - Asthenia, emaciation, erratic pains, constant need to move, diarrhea in the morning, sweating at the least physical or mental effort.

REFERENCES - Julian.

FLUORICUM ACIDUM

(Fluoric Acid)

PHARMACY - fl-ac. Fluoricum acidum. Fluoric acid. Hydrofluoric acid. Made by distilling pure fluorspar (Calcium fluoride) in a state of fine powder with sulphuric acid. Solution. ***Historical dose:*** All potencies.

CLINICAL - Abscess. Alcoholism. Alopecia. ***Bedsores.*** Birthmarks. ***Bone disorders.*** Brain, atrophy. Coccyx, pain. ***Dental, fistula. Dropsy. Edema.*** Exostosis. Eyes, disorders. Felon. Fistula. ***Fluoride, poisoning.*** Gleet. ***Goiter.*** Gonorrhea. Hair, loss. Headaches. Hemorrhoids. Hydrocele. Keloids. Liver, induration. Locomotor ataxia. Nevi. Nose, inflammation. Nymphomania. Otorrhea. Peritonitis. Perspiration. Pityriasis. Satyriasis. Scars. Spleen, pains. Strokes. Suppuration. Syphilis. ***Teeth, decayed.*** Toothaches. Tongue, ulceration. ***Ulcers.*** Varicocele. ***Varicose, ulcers. Varicose, veins.*** Veins, diseased. Whitlow.

HOMEOPATHIC - Fl-ac. acts on the lower tissues of the body much like Sil., which it follows and precedes well, although their modalities differ, Fl-ac. is better from cold applications. Useful after the abuse of Sil.

Slow, deeply destructive effects. ***Decay of long bones, ulcerations, bedsores, varicose veins***. Necrosis of the bones, favors the expulsion of the necrosed part. Acts especially upon lower tissues.

Teeth are deficient in enamel, black, rough, unsightly-looking. Early ***decay of teeth.*** Calcareous degeneration. Nails grow rapidly. Felon. Nevus, flat.

Edema. Tissues are puffy indurated and fistulous. Dropsy with numbness or without. Old scars, scars become redder and itch. Red blotches on body which tend to desquamate. Small red spots here and there, worse by warmth, better in cool place. Discharges are thin, foul, acrid or salty, causing itching.

Increased sensitiveness of vision and hearing. ***Glabella region bloated***. Numbness of the part not lain on in brain diseases, spinal disorders. ***Goiter.*** Affinity for rectal, dental and lachrymal fistulas. Suffering if the call for evacuation is not immediately attended to.

Old cases of nightly fevers, coming on periodically. Always feels too hot, wants to bathe in cold water. Patient is compelled to move about energetically.

Hob-nailed liver of the alcoholics. Complaints of old age or the prematurely aged with weak, distended blood vessels. Especially adapted to chronic diseases with syphilitic and mercurial history. Secondary syphilis.

MIND - Absent-mindedness. Forgetful in evening, better morning. Great loss of memory. Forgets almost everything. Forgets dates. Mistakes right for left.

Opinionated, strong-minded. ***Domineering behavior.*** Irritability, sends the nurse home. ***Abuses and reproaches others.*** Irritability with absent persons. Sensitive to noise. Conversation aggravates.

Depression of mind. ***Aversion to his own family.*** Aversion to those loved best (Sep.). Sits silently, does not utter a single word, nor answers anyone when questioned. Inability to realize responsibility. ***Shuns responsibilities.*** Indifference to business affairs. Indifference to loved ones, to relations.

Anxious ideas. Apprehensive, causes sweat, better morning than evening. Fear of having a stroke. Sensation as if danger menaced him, but without fear.

Impulse to walk fast, necessity to be always on the move. Becomes interested and converses pleasantly with strangers. Buoyancy of mind. Mentally elated and excited. Fears nothing and is self-satisfied. Cheerful during menses. Cheerful when walking in open air.

Delusion, marriage must be broken. Thinks he must drive children out of the house, must dissolve marriage. Thinks he must get rid of servants. Stands on the street looking at women as they pass by, so great is his lust. Nymphomania.

Abdomen - Ascites from hepatic disorders. Induration, enlargement and portal congestion. Flatus and belchings. Sensation of emptiness at the region of navel with a desire to draw a deep breath, better bandaging. Burning, pinching, about navel.

Back - Pain in third cervical vertebra. Coccyx pain worse motion and exercise. Bruised, in sacrum. Aching in sacrum and lumbar region, better stretching and bending backwards, esp. by pressure. Stiffness of nape. Lameness in back, hips and legs.

Breasts - Nipples sore, cracked, itching. Itching on left breast.

Chest - Oppression in chest, difficult breathing, great dyspnea, better bending backwards. Hydrothorax. Upper part of chest seems most affected. Scaly eruption on chest and arms. Itching under ribs left side.

Constitutions - Suited to complaints of old age or the prematurely aged. Suited to the weakly constitutions, sallow skin, emaciation. Pale, miserable, cachectic, flabby and broken down patients. ***Dropsy of limbs*** in old, feeble constitutions.

Ears - Intolerable itching in ears. Itching momentarily better scratching, but followed by burning. Profuse otorrhea. Otitis externa. Great sensitiveness in morning to little noises. Difficulty in hearing human voices, with numbness of bones around ear. Deafness, better bending head back. Singing, ringing.

Eyes - Burning in eyes. Increased lachrymation. Chronic inflammation of lachrymal sac, worse cold air. Lachrymal fistula, worse] cold air. Violent itching of inner canthus. As if sand in eyes. As if something in the eyes, that could not be rubbed off, must wink. ***Sensation as of a cold wind*** blowing through the eyes. Left eye smaller than right.

Face - Heat in face, wants to wash it in cold water. Pale. Exostoses of bones of face. Heat in face, wants to wash it in cold water. Crusta lactea, dry, scaly, itches very much. Suppurating tubercles in skin of forehead and face. Sweats on face. Right lower jaw swollen.

Female - Menses, blood thick and coagulated. Menses too early, copious, frequent, too long. Feels distressed if the flow is slightly delayed. Metrorrhagia with difficulty of breathing. Copious and excoriating leucorrhea, itching. Acrid leucorrhea, causes itching. Ulceration of uterus and os. Nymphomania.

Food - Hungry. Averse to coffee. Desire for pungent, spicy, highly seasoned food. Desire for fancy dishes. Craves refreshing drinks. Craving for cold things. Craves cold water. Warm drinks produce diarrhea. Desire for wine. Worse from sweet things. Worse from coffee.

Head - Atrophy of brain. Stunning headache, better urinating. Pressure on sides of head from within outward. Compressing pain in temples. Pressure in occiput. Pain along the sutures. Numb sensation in forehead. Puffy glabella. Congestion of blood to head during pregnancy. Decay of ossicles and mastoid with copious discharge, worse warmth (Sil.). Decay of skull bones. ***Exostosis.*** Decay of skin. Itching of head. Brittle hair. New hair dry and breaks off. Falling out of hair after fevers. Alopecia areata. Baldness. Scaly eruptions on head.

Heart - Sore pain in heart. Pulse somewhat accelerated, only during exercise. Small, frequent pulse.

Kidneys - Involuntary urination at night. Increases urine in dropsy, with great relief. Burning in urethra during and after urination. Upward drawing in the urethra. Whitish or purple colored sediment. Urine pungent and fetid. Urine alkaline. Urine, scanty, dark.

Limbs - ***Dropsy of limbs*** in old feeble constitutions. Limbs go to sleep. Osteitis. Decay and necrosis, especially of long bones. Constant redness of the hands, especially the palms. Hot, sweaty palms. Inflammation of joints of fingers. Feeling of hair on back of fingers. Soreness between toes. Nails distorted. Nails crumble. Nails grow rapidly. Felon. As of a splinter under the nail. Nails corrugated lengthwise. Corns are sore. Necrotic bones. Ulcer over tibia.

Liver - Ascites from hepatic disorders. Degeneration of liver in consequence of alcoholism. Soreness over liver. Hepatic disorders with ascites.

Lungs - Difficulty of breathing with, or alternating with, metrorrhagia. Great dyspnea, better bending backwards. Wheezing. Difficult breathing, in afternoon and evening. Great dyspnea, has to be propped up in bed.

Male - Burning in urethra. Oily pungent smelling sweat on genitals. Dropsical swelling on penis. Gleety discharge at night, staining linen yellow. Varicocele. ***Swollen scrotum.*** Violent erections at night. Increased sexual desire in old men. Overwhelming sexual desire, keeping him awake at night. Enjoyment excessive. Gonorrhea. Sensation of fullness in spermatic cords. Sudden loss of sexual power. Impotence. Yellow drop from urethra in morning.

Modalities - Better cold. Bending open air. ***Better cool bathing***. Better walking. Better rapid motion. Better bending head back. Better short sleep. Better sitting. Better eating. ***Worse heat of room.*** Worse night. Worse morning. ***Worse warmth.*** Worse warm drinks. Worse alcohol, red wine. Worse sour foods. Worse rest. Worse rising. Worse coffee. Worse standing.

Mouth - Mouth coated with mucus in morning. Painful ulcer in right angle of jaw. Affects teeth and bones of upper jaw. Increased flow of saliva, with sneezing. Viscid, tasteless saliva in mouth. Syphilitic ulceration of mouth, which is very sensitive to cold.

Nose - Red, swollen, inflamed nose. Fluent coryza during sleep. Sneezing with salivation. Chronic nasal catarrh with ulceration of the septum. ***Sudden copious watery discharge from eyes, nose and mouth.*** Nose obstructed and dull heavy pain in forehead. Itching on right side of nose. Cold water causes coryza. Posterior nares feel expanded, during a walk.

Perspiration - Profuse and sour, offensive perspiration. Feels as if hot vapor were emitted from all the pores. ***Acrid, eroding sweat, excites itching.*** Sweat on diseased part. Sweats on hands and feet. One-sided sweat (left). Sweats in afternoon. Sweats during exercise. Sweat relieves. Excessive sweat on feet. Sweat promotes excoriation and bedsores.

Rectum - Flatus and eructations with constriction of anus. Constipation. Itching and burning at anus. Bilious diarrhea with aversion to coffee. Diarrhea worse on alternate days. Warm drinks and salmon produce diarrhea. Itching in perineum. Very loose, bright yellow stools, with much mucus, preceded by considerable griping. Stools frequent and hard. Stools pappy, yellowish brown, fetid, with tenesmus and prolapsed anus.

Sensations - Sensation as of a cold wind blowing under lids, even in warm room, as of air passing down from shoulder joint to fingers. Numbness of limbs even when not lain on. Increased ability to exercise his muscles without fatigue. Less affected by excessive heat in summer or cold in winter.

Skin - Dry, harsh, itching or cracked skin. Burning pains on small spots of skin. ***Itching, especially of the orifices.*** Itching in spots, worse warmth. Itching of scars. Keloids. Scars, surrounded by pimples, become red around the edges. Bedsores, worse warmth. ***Varicose veins***. Atony of capillary and venous system. Tissues bloated. Nevus or birthmarks on children. Nails grow rapidly. ***Ulcers, red edges and vesicles.*** Ulcers on ankles. Syphilitic tubercles. Syphilitic rupia. Periosteal abscess. Hard, dry warts. Frequent small boils, carbuncles.

Sleep - Sudden sleepiness. Drowsy and sleepy in early evening. Sleeplessness without inclination to sleep. A short sleep suffices and refreshes him. Sleep disturbed by accumulation of mucus in fauces. Sensation as if sleeping on side not lain on. Sleeplessness in evening from crowding of thoughts. Dreams towards morning. Dreams of fire. Dreams with amaurosis.

Stomach - Frequent eructations and discharge of flatulence. Sour eructations. Stale eructations. Burning, pinching pain in stomach, before stool. Heaviness and weight in stomach. Heat in stomach before meals. Gnawing hunger, is always eating which temporarily relieves. Sour or stale belchings. Bilious vomiting on slightest errors in diet. Stomach symptoms, better tight clothes.

Teeth - Affects teeth and bones of upper jaw. Great sensitiveness of teeth. Late dentition. ***Teeth, decay rapidly, worse at roots***. Thin enamel. Teeth feel warm, heavy, rough. ***Dental fistula with bloody, salty discharge.*** Acrid, foul taste from roots of teeth. Teeth coated with mucus in morning. Wisdom teeth come late. Toothache worse cold drinks. Toothache better until water becomes warm in mouth.

Temperature - Nightly fevers coming on periodically. Ebullitions of heat with pain in bones. Feels as if burning vapor were emitted from pores. General heat with nausea, with inclination to uncover. Face constantly hot, wants to bathe it continually in cold water.

Throat - Excessive pain, when swallowing or talking. ***Sore throat, worse inspiring cold air.*** Throat sensitive to cold. slightest exposure resulting in sore throat, with increase of pain and impeded swallowing. ***Constriction in throat, with difficult swallowing.*** Hawking of phlegm, mixed with blood. Red blotches, over palate and sides of cheek, bleeding easily. ***Throat intensely red and much swollen, with fetid breath, nasal voice.*** Goitre. Trachea sore and raw. Weak voice. Dryness in larynx and trachea. Itching in larynx, causes hawking and swallowing. Soreness and increased irritability in larynx with impeded respiration and wheezing. Syphilitic ulceration of throat.

Tongue - Tongue, fissured in all directions, painful when talking. Ulcer on and under tongue. Tongue as if stiff, with restricted mobility. Tongue vivid red at tip and edges. Tongue coated yellow in centre. Tongue whitish and dry. Numbness and tingling of tongue. Pricking sensation of tongue.

Vertigo - Vertigo with nausea, must sit down. Feeling as if in an earthquake.

Vision - Amaurosis. Dark spot before eye, worse reading. Flashes like lightning. Red photopsia, due to retinal excitement.

COMMENTS - Severe bone diseases and ulcers, where the bones decompose instead of healing. Necrosis of the bones, bone abscesses. Bone pains (Merc., Calc-f.). For syphilis, when it causes ulcers and goes to the bones.

Tendency to form ulcers on the skin and in the mouth that do not heal well, particularly in the elderly. Ulcers can have a red edge. Bedsores. Keloids that ulcerate or don't heal well (Sil.).

Varicose veins that swell and ulcerate with severe burning pain, worse heat (Sec., Lach.). Varicose veins with itching, swelling and burning pains. Varicose veins or ulcers aggravated after each childbirth.

Hot blooded. Worse heat. Better from cold washing and walking in the open air (opposite Sil.). Constant desire to walk in the open air, and does not fatigue. Hungry. Symptoms seem to move from below upward.

For children with weak tooth enamel (Sil., Calc-f.), or whose teeth erupt rotten and abscessed (Kreo., Calc-f.). Generally a woman's remedy. Hate between spouses.

Guernsey noted that it tends to affect the right ear, the left teeth, left hypochondrium, left side of the abdomen, right side and nape of the neck, and the right side of the back.

McLachlan added that the left hand is affected rather than the right, and the pus tends to point on the dorsum of the finger. T. F. Allen noted its use for whitlow.

RELATIONS - ***Compare:*** (1) Thiosin. - action on scar tissues, adhesions, strictures, tumors. Calc-f., Sil. (2) Coca - fatigue, Coffea - toothache. (3) Cit-ac. and Sep. - aversion to one's family. (4) Ox-ac. - diarrhea worse from coffee. (5) Rhus-t. and Ruta - Coccyx, pain. (6) Sil. - fistula, onychia, bone diseases, Coccyx, pain. (7) Brom., Iod., Spong. and Kali-c. - goiter. (8) Staph. - teeth. ***Complementary:*** Sil. ***Compatible:*** after Ars. in ascites from gin-drinker's liver after Kali-c. in hip disease after Ph-ac. in diabetes. ***Followed well by:*** Sulph., Nit-ac.

REFERENCES - Boericke. Clarke. Murphy. Phatak.

FLUORIDE

PHARMACY - fluor. Fluoride. ***Historical dose:*** All potencies.

CLINICAL - ***Bone, disorders.*** Cancer. Collagen, diseases. Constipation. Decayed, teeth. Faintness. Miscarriages. Nausea. Skin, rash. Stomach cramps. Rash. ***Teeth, disorders.*** Ulcers. Vomiting. Weight loss. Wrinkles.

HOMEOPATHIC - In a number of small villages in Sicily, Turkey and India there is naturally occurring fluoride in the water ranging from 0.7 to 5.4 ppm. Here the villagers and their livestock are chronically ill, while neighboring villages with no fluoride have no such illnesses. Premature aging is the overall effect.

Children have brown decaying teeth; young adults often have none. Young men are bent over and crippled with pain in their joints and hips. Their skin is wrinkled and they look 60 at age 30 to 40.

There is premature hardening of the arteries. Loss of appetite and sex drive by age 30. The rate of stillborn miscarriages by 4 months is extremely high.

Fluoride damages enzymes which results in a wide range of chronic diseases. Fluoride causes breakdown of collagen. It also leads to irregular formation of collagen which serves as a major structural component of skin, ligaments, tendons, muscles, cartilage, bones and teeth.

Female - Miscarriages.

Limbs - ***Bone, disorders.*** Tremors. Aching bones. Stiffness.

Rectum - Constipation.

Skin - Skin rash. Wrinkled, skin. Ulcers.

Stomach - Stomach cramps. Nausea. Bloody vomit.

Teeth - Deformed teeth. Decayed teeth. Brown or black discoloration of the teeth.

Vertigo - Faintness.

RELATIONS - ***Compare:*** (1) Fl-ac., Calc-f.

REFERENCES - Murphy.

FOENICULUM SATIVUM

(Fennel)

PHARMACY - foen. Foeniculum sativum. Fennel. Foeniculum vulgare. N. O. Umbelliferae. Tincture of seed. ***Historical dose:*** Tincture and all potencies.

CLINICAL -

HERBAL - The fruit (seeds) are quite fragrant, and are among the most relaxing and least pungent of all the aromatics. They are eminently carminative, and quite diffusive; and are usually better received by the stomach than are cummin or dill seeds, being also more relaxing than these, but more stimulating than anise seed. Their principal use is in combination with senna, rhubarb, juglans, rhamnus, and other cathartics. The oil may be made into essence.

From a very early period of medical history, fennel seed has been credited with the power of increasing the secretion of milk, (galactagogue.) Its use for this purpose is most extensive in Germany; but leading physicians of many countries ascribe to it excellent power in this direction. The infusion of the seed may be used without limitation.

Huefeland employed it in the following combination: Fennel seeds, one drachm; sweet orange-peel, half a drachm; carbonate of magnesia, three drachms; sugar, two drachms. Mix the powders, and give a teaspoonful three times a day. This preparation is greatly extolled through Germany. Others have given formulas combining the fennel with anise seed, parsley root, licorice root, etc., and using an infusion freely.

HOMEOPATHIC -

The whole plant has an aromatic odor and taste, owing to a volatile oil by which it is pervaded.It is cultivated largely in Italy and Sicily for the sake of the shoots, which are eaten raw, or in salad, or boiled as pot-herbs.

The odor of fennel-seed is fragrant, its taste warm, sweet and agreeably aromatic. It is among our most grateful aromatics, and in this country much employed in the old school as a carminative and as corrigent of other less pleasant medicines, especially senna and rhubarb. In infants it is employed as a tea, or injection, to produce the expulsion of flatus.

In most of the ancient books on the practice of medicine we find it in common use as a modifier and corrective of cathartic infusions, to prevent griping, and to obviate flatulence. As far back as Hippocrates can its employment be traced.

Pressure in the left upper jawbone, which soon ceases. Pungent pain in the right elbow joint, it recurs often during several days. Diarrhea. Increased secretion of urine. Excites the vascular system and the respiratory organs.

REFERENCES - Murphy.

FOLLICULINUM

(Ovarian Follicle)

PHARMACY - foll. Folliculinum. Ovarian follicle. Oestron. Estrone. Hormone secreted by the ovaries. Trituration. ***Historical dose:*** All potencies.

CLINICAL - Acne. Alopecia. Amenorrhea. Backache. Cystitis. Headaches. Leucorrhea. Mastitis. Metrorrhagia. Migraines. Palpitations. ***Premenstrual, syndrome.*** Seborrhea. Tachycardia. Vaginal, pruritus.

HOMEOPATHIC - A female remedy, affecting primarily the female hormonal system. Foll. in a homeopathic dilution could be indicated in premenstrual syndrome, as well as for all the functional symptoms present in a patient.

Premenstrual syndrome. Weight gain without excessive eating, worse before menses or during ovulation. Premenstrual migraines. Congestive headaches, either with redness of the face or the opposite with pallor, but still with the sensation of chilliness at the limbs.

Frequent ecchymosis, bruises very easily. Acne on the face and seborrhea of the nostrils. Hypersensitive to heat, noise and contact.

Foll. in low potencies of 3x and 4c is an arouser to be given in cases of amenorrhea and insufficient menstruation. In 7c, it is a regulator.

In 9c, it is a restrainer and a dose should be given either towards the tenth day of the cycle, when the pains predominate on the 14th day or 5 days before the beginning of menstruation, when the discomforts are predominant before the arrival of menses.

MIND - Alternation of excitability and depression, worse before menses. Irritable and sensitive before the menses. Extreme instability with anguish, worse at nightfall. Sexual hyper-excitability. Fixed ideas of a sexual nature.

Abdomen - Abdominal meteorism, worse three or four days before menses. Liver swollen, soft and hypertrophic.

Back - Lumbar pains, worse during ovulation. Backache before menses.

Bladder - Recurring cystitis in women.

Breasts - Breasts enormous, swollen, cannot bear being constricted or touched. The pain is ameliorated or disappears with menses. Congestive mastitis.

Eyes - Swelling with edema of the conjunctiva tissue.

Face - Acne on the face and seborrhea of the nostrils.

Female - Congestion, uterine, and premenstrual pains. Vaginal, vulvar pruritus, worse before menses. Menses prolonged, blood bright red with clotting. Menses painful for the first few days. Leucorrhea. Yellow or brownish discharge, sometimes blood streaked, between menses, especially during ovulation. Small losses of blood during ovulation. Uterus is fibrous with metrorrhagia.

Head - Alopecia in women.

Heart - Tachycardia. Palpitations with faintness. Sensation of constriction around the heart with feeling of a bar in the precordial region, spreading to the left arm.

Lungs - Need for fresh air, takes large breaths of air and sighs deeply. Fitful cough, worse when in company, with sensation of constriction around the heart.

Modalities - Better after the third day of menses. Better with movement. Better fresh air. Worse before menses. Worse during ovulation. Worse from heat and resting.

Nose - Coryza with headache and profuse discharge. Hay fever.

Rectum - Feeling of heaviness in the rectum. Chronic constipation, sometimes alternation of constipation and diarrhea.

Skin - Dry eczema, worse during ovulation, before menses. Dry eruption of the fingers with splitting and chapping of the skin.

Stomach - Indigestion. Nausea with vomiting. Premenstrual pain in the right hypochondrium.

Throat - Swallowing of liquids very painful. Cannot bear pressure on the pharynx.

RELATIONS - ***Compare:*** (1) The closest remedy is Lach. Like this remedy, it has: Alternating excitability and depression, extreme sensitivity to contact, amelioration by menstrual flow. But, unlike Lachesis, we do not find: Laterality or aggravation from sleep, but, on the contrary, aggravation during ovulation. (2) Sepia, Lac-c., Puls., Kali-c.

REFERENCES - Julian.

FORMALINUM

(Formaldehyde)

PHARMACY - formal. Formalinum. Formaldehyde. Formaldehydum solutum. Aqueous solution (35 percent) of Formaldehyde gas. ***Historical dose:*** All potencies.

CLINICAL - Anuria. Albuminuria. Catarrhal, disorders. Chills. ***Dyspnea.*** Eczema. ***Forgetfulness. Laryngismus, stridulus.*** Ptyalism. Tuberculosis. ***Vertigo. Whooping cough.***

HOMEOPATHIC - Formalinum is a powerful disinfectant and deodorant, as well as a potent poison. Prevents growth and kills almost any pathogenic microorganism. It seems to have the peculiar property of eating into malignant tumors, leaving the surrounding healthy tissue uncharred an unchanged.

MIND - Anxiety. ***Forgetfulness.*** Dullness of mind. Unconsciousness.

Head - Coryza, eyes water.

Kidneys - Anuria, albuminous urine.

Lungs - ***Dyspnea. Whooping cough.***

Mouth - Ptyalism, thick saliva. Loss of taste.

Rectum - Intense urging to stool, watery stools.

Skin - Puckers skin like leather, wrinkles, scales off. Eczema in neighborhood of wound. Damp sweat most marked on right upper extremity.

Stomach - Food feels as if it were a ball in stomach. Burning in mouth and stomach.

Temperature - Chills in forenoon, followed by long fever. Bones ache during whole paroxysm. During fever forgets where he was.

Throat - ***Laryngismus stridulus.***

Vertigo - ***Severe vertigo.***

COMMENTS - A plug of cotton wool soaked in a 20 percent solution of formaldehyde and applied for a few hours, will produce a necrotic slough, which must be scraped away before the next application, otherwise it hardens.

Formal., in hot water as vapor, is a most valuable therapeutic agent in whooping cough, tuberculosis and in catarrhal disorders of the upper air-passages.

RELATIONS - ***Antidote:*** Ammonia water. ***Compare:*** (1) Ammonium formaldehyde, known commercially as Cystogen. Dose, five to seven grains two to four times daily, dissolved in hot water after meals. Prevents the decomposition of urine in the bladder, kidneys and ureters. Turbid urine rendered clear and non-irritating, phosphatic deposits dissolved and growth of pyogenic bacteria arrested. (2) Also, Urotropin - A diuretic and solvent of uric acid concretions, relieves cystitis associated with putrefaction. Three grains well diluted. When administered it invariably appears in the cerebro-spinal fluid and therefore advised in threatened meningeal infection.

REFERENCES - Boericke.

FORMICA RUFA

(Red Ants)

PHARMACY - form. Formica rufa. Red ants. Myrmexine. Contains formic acid. N. O. Hymenoptera. Tincture from crushed live ants. Contains formic acid. ***Historical dose:*** Tincture and all potencies.

CLINICAL - ***Arthritis.*** Brain disorders. Bruises. Chorea. Cough, ***Diarrhea.*** Dislocations. Dropsies. Eyes disorders. Facial, paralysis. Foot-sweat, checked. Gout. Hair, loss. Headaches. Nodes. Over-lifting, complaints from. Paralysis. ***Polyps. Rheumatism.*** Spinal, disorders. Spleen, pain. Stroke. Tapeworm. Throat, sore. Vision, disorders.

HOMEOPATHIC - Formica rufa causes many rheumatic and gouty pains. Pains appear suddenly and dart from place to place: left, then right, then left. Pains are worse from motion, better pressure.

Arthritis with sudden rheumatic or gouty pains. Chronic gout and stiffness in joints. Acute outbursts of gouty poisons, especially when assuming the neuralgic forms. The spinal cord is affected, paralyzes and spasms occurring. It affects the liver, kidneys and right side.

Influence on the formation of polyps. Tuberculosis. Carcinoma, cancer. Apoplectic diseases. Lupus. Chronic nephritis. Atrophy of wounds. Takes cold easily. Clammy skin, disagreeable sweat during night, sweat without relief. Chorea from checked foot sweat. Complaints from over lifting.

MIND - Indisposed, morose. Fearful, apprehensive. Exhilarated after pain. Remarkable and unexpected activity of the mind during the day with absence of usual dullness and sleepiness. Forgetful in the evening.

Abdomen - Flatulence. Drawing pain around navel before stools. Dull pain in region of spleen. Hardening of mesenteric glands.

Back - Soreness in neck and up into head. Severe pain in left side of neck while chewing. Severe pain across sacrum and dorsum of each hand. Affection of spinal cord.

Breasts - Violent penetrating pain in region of right nipple. Lack of milk in nursing women.

Causations - Complaints from over-lifting. Checked foot-sweat. Wounds. Great liability to take cold, consequences of cold and wet, cold bathing, damp weather.

Chests - Pleuritic pains.

Coughs - Cough tedious and long-lasting, worse at night and worse motion. Cough with aching in forehead and constrictive pain in chest. Cough, mostly at night. Violent attacks of cough with vomiting, day and night.

Ears - Ringing and buzzing. Deafness. Cracking in left ear with headache. Polyps. External sensitiveness of right ear and temple. Parts around ear feel swollen.

Eyes - Pain in the eyes on waking, better washing. Rheumatic iritis. Rheumatic ophthalmia. Macule and ulcers on cornea. Dim sight. Flickering before eyes. Pterygium. Spasmodic twitching of upper eyelid.

Face - Entire left side of face and cheek feel as if paralyzed.

Female - Menses scanty and pale with bearing-down pain in back. Menses appear eight days too soon. Ovarian cysts containing water or blood.

Head - Brain feels too heavy and large. As if bubbles bursting in forehead. Headache with cracking in left ear. Headache better after combing hair. Vertigo.

Heart - Uneasy pain in region of heart. Fluttering palpitations.

Kidneys - Paralysis of bladder. Quantity of urine increased, urates. Urine like saffron, bright yellow, no sediment, passed frequently. Bloody, albuminous urine with much urging.

Limbs - Rheumatic pains, stiff and contracted joints. ***Rheumatism comes on with suddenness and restlessness.*** Muscles feel strained and torn from their attachment. Stiffness and contraction of joints. Hard nodes around joints in and out. ***Weakness of lower limbs.*** Paraplegia. Pain in hips. Itching in armpits in morning. Hands numb.

Lungs - Nervous asthma. Hoarseness with dry, sore throat, with aching in forehead and constrictive pain in chest, pleuritic pains.

Male - Seminal emissions, weakness. Long-lasting erections after urinating in morning. Scanty ejaculation with incomplete erection. ***"Slothful to venery."***

Modalities - Better warmth. ***Better pressure***. Better rubbing. Better combing hair. Better after midnight. Worse motion. Worse sitting. Worse dampness. Worse cold washing. Worse cold. Worse before snowstorms.

Mouth - Water tastes sweetish.

Neck - Pain in neck when chewing, especially on closing jaws.

Nose - *Nasal polyps*. Coryza and stopped up feeling.

Rectum - Constriction in the anus. Drawing pain ***around navel*** before stool. Pain in bowels before stool with shuddering chilliness. In the morning, difficult passages of small quantities of flatus, afterwards diarrhea-like urging in the rectum. Light, foaming stools.

Skin - ***Red, itching and burning***. Nettle-rash. Hives in flat plaques. Nodes around joints. Wounds that atrophy. Profuse sweat without relief.

Sleep - Could get to sleep if she could get the right position. All night dry throat, woke her out of sleep. Disagreeable sweat during night, awoke with clammy skin. Wakes early and feels she has had sufficient sleep. On awaking, headache, vomiting with headache, pain in eyes, stitches in ears.

Stomach - Constant pressure at the cardiac end of the stomach, with burning pain. Pains shifts from stomach to vertex. Gas cannot be passed. Nausea with headache and vomiting of a yellowish bitter mucus.

Temperature - Profuse sweat without relief.

Throat - Sore throat in morning with much mucus, worse left side. Hoarseness with sore throat. Pain in neck when hawking or gargling.

Vertigo - Vertigo, all things seem to move to and fro, reeling of body. Pain in left supra-orbital region when going to bed with dizziness, blackness before eyes, better by sitting down.

COMMENTS - Sensation as if brain too heavy and large. Sensation as if a bubble burst in forehead. Hering noted its use "in all kinds of apoplectic diseases. It strengthens the brain." Cooper gave the 3x with success in cases of weakness of the lower limbs.

J. W. Thomson reported the case of a man, aged 84, who had severe neuralgic pains between posterior of right ear and center of occiput. He apparently recovered, but returned eighteen months later with a steady, sore and burning pain in the same region, swollen and tender around, but especially behind right ear.

He could only sleep in one comfortable position, which he could not describe, but only knew when he found it and he must be covered up warmly behind right ear and between that and occiput and neck. All on the right side. Better from taking right hand and rubbing gently behind right ear. Sweat afforded no relief, the whole head seemed to sympathize with the distress. He had dribbling of urine.

Form. was given, six doses, one before each meal. On the second day towards evening, he felt worse, and on the third day there were twinges and spasms of severe pain in addition to the sore pain that he had experienced before. These gradually got better and on the fourth day even the soreness was much better.

The main thing, however, was that he felt mentally better, said his mind and head felt stronger and from feeling depressed he had become cheerful and life did not seem the burden it had for some time past.

RELATIONS - ***Compare:*** (1) Formic acid. Ars., Bry. (2) Dulc. - Rheumatism. (3) Urt-u. - nettle-rash, gout, rheumatism. (4) Frag-v. - lack of breast secretion. (5) Trom. - Diarrhea. (6) Caps. - Burning pains worse by cold water. ***Compatible:*** after Cham.

REFERENCES - Boericke. Clarke. Phatak.

FORMICICUM ACIDUM

(Formic Acid)

PHARMACY - form-ac. Formicicum acidum. Formic acid. ***Historical dose:*** Tincture and all potencies.

CLINICAL - Arthritis. Catarrh. Gout. Polyps. ***Tremors***. Varicose veins. ***Vision, weak.***

HOMEOPATHIC - Form-ac. is known to the homeopathic Materia Medica only in the preparation of Formica rufa, a tincture made of ants that contain the acid. Apis and other insects contain formic acid, as well as Urtica urens and many other plants.

Form-ac. in small doses increases muscular strength and resistance to fatigue. Feels stronger and more fit in ordinary walking.

Chronic muscular pains and soreness.

Tremors. Gout and joint rheumatism, which appear suddenly. Pains usually worse on right side, motion and better from pressure.

Chronic arthritis following an attack of acute rheumatic fever. Chronic arthritis in connection with gouty diathesis. Marked diuretic effect, greater elimination of products of disassimilation, particularly urea. ***Failing vision***.

Hering gave as an indication for Form-ac.: "Burning pain, burning from washing, renewed burning from cold washing."

In prescribing it for varicose veins, polyps, catarrh, Clarke ordered an ounce or two of a solution of formic acid to the proportion of one part of the acid to eleven of distilled water. Of this, one teaspoonful is taken in a tablespoonful of water after food once or twice daily.

COMMENTS - Mr. R. Wallace Ellison of Richmond, sent three letters to Anshutz concerning his experiences with formic acid.

"About two years and nine months ago I added to my daily diet from one to two grains of Formic Acid with the result that it has produced the following results in my body: Polyps and fibrous matter absorbed from my nose. Nose tongue, lips and some other parts greatly reduced in thickness.

"Chronic catarrh of nose, throat and intestines practically cured. Stiff joints throughout the whole body have become loose. Short sight diminished by fifty percent. Eyes have changed in color from light slate gray to a darker shade.

"Varicose veins in left leg and others at base of neck now of no consequence. Facial and bodily appearance so altered that even my mother is puzzled and I can meet and converse with people who formerly knew me very intimately without my identity being discovered.

"I have also tried its effects upon a sickly and scabby pony and found it quickly restored the animal to health as well as giving it a beautiful, healthy crop of hair. Anyone who cares can produce this result in the case of an old pony. I hasten to add what I would have mentioned before, that the quantity taken during the last two years was not much over 1 grains daily.

"I found that 2 grs. daily was too much for regular use, though it served the purpose. If my theory be correct, perhaps 1 grains daily would be the proper thing and best to be taken in the form of honey, raw juice of sugar cane, etc.

"When I first commenced I used to drink about a pint of water with it, but now I just put the teaspoonful of acid into a very small quantity of water and drink it. It has a pleasant, 'fruity' sort of taste. I add a little citric acid and sugar to it and I believe this improves the effect.

"Chronic arthritis of traumatic nature can be cured by formic acid. In the latter case Formic acid 6x showed quicker and better results than 12x or 30x which are indicated in the previous cases. In general the disappearance of the stiffness of the joint is the first sign of improvement. Then the pain and swelling cease gradually in 1-6 months time."

In the Homeopathic World of April, 1902, Dr. Dudgeon gave an account of the work of Dr. Edward Krull of Gustrow, who was led to think of formic acid as a remedy from its constant occurrence in the internal organs and soft parts of the body.

He found it constantly present in the sweat of healthy persons, but very much diminished in or entirely absent from the sweat of persons affected with tuberculosis. He thought to supply the defect in tubercular subjects by introducing it into the system in material doses.

He found no benefit when he gave considerable doses by the mouth, so he used hypodermic injections of the watery solution. After two years of experiments he found to his surprise that the more dilute his injections were, the more powerful the effects and he ended by giving injections of a dilution which corresponds to our 3c or 4c and waiting five or six months before repeating the injection.

Dudgeon noted "He treated in this way with success external and internal tuberculosis, chronic nephritis and malignant tumors.

It was necessary for the success of the treatment that the nutrition of the body should be well maintained. In cachectic states the treatment is not indicated. It will be remembered that Hering mentions the case of an anemic woman who died from the effects of an ant-vapor bath.

"The general effects which were observed in all the cases treated by Krull's method were: Immediate increase of nutrition, the appetite improved, the weight increased, all this without any material change in the diet.

"In all the patients during the first months, sometimes every two or three days, sometimes at an interval of weeks, there occurred slight transient attacks of pain in the abdomen, on the right and left of the umbilicus, sometimes accompanied by urging to stool.

"If several copious fecal evacuations occurred, this had no bad effect on the patient, they seemed to have a critical character. After the injection the menses came on earlier and were more copious, all diseased organs and parts showed greater activity.

"In the first and second stages of tuberculosis cure is the rule. In the third stage the treatment only does harm, rapidly diminishing the strength.

"The action is most remarkable in lupus. During the first days after the injection the effected part commences to grow vividly red, rises up somewhat and discharges moderately and is the seat of shooting pains occasionally. Curative action usually begins in the third week.

"In carcinoma of the breast and stomach, the tumor first increases in size and becomes very sensitive and the skin over it feels warmer. The shorter the term the tumor has existed and the stronger the constitution, the sooner does reaction occur and the consequent cure of the disease."

In the concluding words of Dudgeon's article, "Tuberculosis, chronic nephritis and carcinoma are not diseases in which we can claim a great amount of success. So where other remedies fail or cannot be discovered we may take Solomon's advice and 'Go to the ant!'"

RELATIONS - ***Compare:*** Formica rufa., Apis., Urtica urens.

REFERENCES - Anshutz. Boericke. Clarke.

FRAGARIA VESCA

(Wood-Strawberry)

PHARMACY - frag. Fragaria vesca. Wood-strawberry. N. O. Rosacea. Tincture of the ripe fruit. Infusion of the root. ***Historical dose:*** Tincture and all potencies.

CLINICAL - Anasarca. Biliousness. Chilblains. Convulsions. Erysipelas. Faintness. Gonorrhea. Sprue. Strokes. Tapeworm. Tongue, strawberry, swollen. Urticaria. Weaning.

HERBAL - An infusion of the root diminishes the size of the breasts and dries up the milk, useful in women who wish to wean their children.

In ancient medicine, Fragaria vesca was used in decoctions of leaves, roots or fruit, ripe or unripe, or combinations of these. Fragaria vesca is commended by W. Salmon as a wash for sore-mouth, as a hemostatic arresting the menses and stopping ***"bloody-flux,"*** swelling of the spleen, many forms of skin eruption and for ***"clearing the complexion."***

HOMEOPATHIC - The allergic effects from those who are sensitive to strawberries have been utilized in homeopathy. The well-known ***"strawberry tongue"*** is an indication for its use. Dr. Burnett gave it as ***"pippy tongue."*** Faintness, suffocation like a stroke, convulsions and death have resulted, general anasarca and especially swollen tongue. Profuse viscid sweat.

Lippe mentioned "Tapeworm. Pain in chilblains in hot weather." In two instances Clarke noted the indulgence in strawberries to revive symptoms of gonorrhea in men who thought themselves cured. A number of cases of sprue or pilosis have been cured by a diet of strawberries ad libitum.

RELATIONS - ***Compare:*** (1) Hydr-ac., Apis, Ars. Crat.

REFERENCES - Boericke. Clarke. Phatak.

FRANCISCAEA UNIFLORA
(Brazilian Manaca Root)

PHARMACY - franc. Franciscaea uniflora. Brazilian manaca root. Brunfelsia hopeana. Manaca. N. O. Scrophulariacae. Allied to Brunfelsia. Tincture of fresh root. An alkaloid, Franciscein, is also used. ***Historical dose:*** Tincture and all potencies.

CLINICAL - Headaches. Pericarditis. Rheumatism. Syphilis. Vomiting.

HERBAL - Franciscaea uniflora is a Brazilian remedy of great local repute as an anti-syphilitic and anti-rheumatic.

HOMEOPATHIC - It is called *"vegetable mercury."* In large doses it is a poison, causing violent purgation and emesis. Many cases of acute, sub-acute and chronic cases of rheumatism have been reported cured with the tincture, also pericarditis complicating rheumatism.

Hansen noted characteristic symptoms including an intense headache like a band around the head, and lancinating, sticking pain in occiput, neck and spine. Terrible aching all over with great heat, followed by profuse sweat, which relieves all symptoms.

Chronic stiffness of the muscles. Gonorrheal rheumatism. Syphilis and rheumatism, great heat over body, much aching, better sweat. Pericarditis with rheumatism. Rheumatic pains in feet and lower part of legs.

REFERENCES - Boericke. Clarke.

FRANKINCENSE
(Olibanum)

PHARMACY - Frankincense. Olibanum. Frankincense is an aromatic gum resin obtained from the trees: Boswellia thurifera, Boswellia sacra, Boswellia carterii. N. O. Burseraceae. ***Historical dose:*** Tincture and all potencies.

CLINICAL - Acne. Anxiety. ***Arthritis.*** Asthma. ***Bronchitis. Coughs.*** Dysentery. Fevers. Fungal, infections. Joint, pain. Laryngitis. Leprosy. Scars. ***Skin, disorders.*** Stretch marks. Tumors. Ulcers. Vomiting. Wounds.

HERBAL - Frankincense remedies appear in the Syriac Book of Medicine, ancient Arabic texts, and in Ayurveda and Chinese medical writings. Greek and Roman physicians used Frankincense in the treatment of a great variety of diseases. It is stimulant, but seldom used now internally, though formerly was in great repute. Pliny mentions it as an antidote to hemlock.

The famous eleventh-century Arabian physician, Avicenna, recommended its cooling effects as a remedy for infections and illnesses that increase the body's temperature. Avicenna used it for tumors, ulcers, vomiting, dysentery and fevers. In China it is used for leprosy.

Recently, the Frankincense boswellic acids that are a part of the resin it produces have shown some promise as a treatment for asthma and various inflamatory conditions. The inhalation of steam laden with the volatile portion of the drug is said to relieve bronchitis and laryngitis.

The essential oil of Frankincense has been used for anxiety, stress, asthma, bronchitis, severe coughing, scars and stretch marks. This oil is rejuvenating to the skin, treating acne, bacterial and fungal infections, and to treat wounds and scars.

Thus, it is used in cosmetics, soaps, and perfumes. The anti-inflammatory properties of frankincense very effective as a treatment for joint pain and arthritis.

COMMENTS - Frankincense is used in incense and perfumes. Its principal use now is in the manufacture of incense and pastilles. It is used in plasters and might be substituted for Balsam of Peru or Balsam or Tolu.

It is also a natural insecticide and was used in ancient Egypt to fumigate wheat silos and repel wheat moths. In Arabia, the smoke of burning frankincense resin is used to repel mosquitoes and sand flies.

Researchers have found that burning frankincense indoors improves the acoustic properties of the room. In ancient Egypt the resin was a key ingredient for embalming the dead.

RELATIONS - ***Compare:*** Myrrh, Camphor.

REFERENCES - Murphy.

FRANZENSBAD AQUA

(Franzens-quelle)

PHARMACY - franz. Franzensbad aqua. Franzens-quelle. Salz-quelle. Wiesen-quelle. The alkaline-saline springs of Franzensbad, near Eger in Bohemia. ***Historical dose:*** Tincture and all potencies.

CLINICAL - Chlorosis. Constipation. Debility. Diarrhea. Dyspepsia. Nervous, derangement.

HOMEOPATHIC - The waters of each of the three springs, Franzens-quelle, Salz-quelle and Wiesen-quelle, have been proved by Dr. Watzke. Sodium sulphate is by far the most predominant ingredient in each, the chloride and carbonate of soda coming next. The waters are also highly charged with carbonic acid gas.

The Franzensbad waters are resorted to for their tonic effect, especially in chronic derangement of the digestion, obstinate constipation and inertia of the lower bowel. Anemia following passive hemorrhage. Chlorosis and nervous disturbances caused by debility.

Great physical or mental weakness. Increased sensitiveness to the cold. General sensitiveness of the surface. Contractive sensations. Contractive pain in whole forehead, sensation of contraction of skin of forehead between eyebrows. Many symptoms of disordered stomach and bowels occurred and some peculiar symptoms in the penis and generative organs.

RELATIONS - ***Compare:*** Nat-s., Kali-i. - diffused sensitiveness.

REFERENCES - Boericke. Clarke. Phatak.

FRAXINUS AMERICANA

(White Ash)

PHARMACY - frax. Fraxinus americana. White ash. N. O. Oleaceae. Tincture of the bark. ***Historical dose:*** Tincture and all potencies.

CLINICAL - Cramps. Depression. Dysmenorrhea. Eczema. Fever, sores. ***Fibroids.*** Hot, flashes. Leucorrhea. ***Menopause. Uterus, disorders.*** Uterus, prolapse. Uterus, tumors.

HOMEOPATHIC - Frax. had a fragmentary proving, but the chief clinical authority for its use is Dr. Burnett, who regarded it as a uterine tonic in all heavy states of the uterus with prolapse, bearing-down and relaxed ligaments. Burnett called it "the medicinal pessary." Clarke repeatedly verified these indications.

It is an organ remedy of the first rank. A ***uterine tonic,*** especially useful for nervous females. ***Uterine tumors, especially fibroids with bearing-down sensations.*** Uterine displacements. Enlargement of the uterus. Subinvolution and prolapse. Fever sores on lips. Cramps in feet. Cold creeping and hot flashes. Infantile eczema.

MIND - Depression with nervous restlessness and anxiety. Must talk.

Abdomen - Heavy bearing-down pain, extending to the thighs or falling out sensation with fibroids. Tenderness in left inguinal region.

Female - Profuse menses. Dysmenorrhea. Profuse leucorrhea. Watery, non-irritating leucorrhea. ***Uterus is enlarged, heavy and prolapsed.*** Uterine tumors. Subinvolution. Sensitive left ovary. ***Fibroids*** with bearing-down sensation, cramping in feet, worse in afternoon and night.

Head - ***Hot spot*** or dryness on vertex. Headache, with vertigo, followed by fever. Throbbing pain in back of head and neck.

Kidneys - Urine scanty and brown.

Limbs - Cramps in feet after midnight.

Lungs - Pain through the lungs.

Modalities - Worse injury, sprains. Worse lifting.

Mouth - Fever sores on the lips.

Rectum - Bowels constipated.

Skin - Infantile eczema.

Sleep - Wakefulness the first part of the night. Dreamed that two rough men came into house, awoke breathing quick, with a fearful feeling.

Temperature - Fevers. Cold creeping and hot flushes.

COMMENTS - Burnett writes: "A maiden lady, forty-three years of age, came under my observation on January 19th, 1892, telling me of her painful nerves and flushes that ave troubled her ever since she changed. She gets gouty swellings of the feet, and has leucorrhea. Is much given to sleeping draughts. The womb is somewhat large, the pain in the feet considerable, depriving her of sleep."

"On condition that she abjures sleeping draughts once and for all, I undertake her case. This is an invariable condition with me, as it is quite impossible to really cure people who take hypnotics."

"I gave Fraxinus Americanus tincture. Ten drops in water at bedtime. March 3rd. Has done her much good, womb is lighter, and she is better able to do her work. She sleeps now quite well without any sedative, a sure proof that the neurasthenia was here primarily a womb ailing."

RELATIONS - ***Compare:*** (1) Sep., Lil-t., Sec. (2) Epiphegus, Nat-hyperchlor., Hydr. (3) Galega - Goat's Rue.

REFERENCES - Boericke. Clarke.

FRAXINUS EXCELSIOR

(European Ash)

PHARMACY - frax-e. Fraxinus excelsior. European ash. Common ash. N. O. Oleaceae. Tincture of the leaves. The fresh leaves are pounded to a pulp and macerated with two parts by weight of alcohol. ***Historical dose:*** Tincture and all potencies.

CLINICAL - Arthritis. Gout. Joint, disorders. Rheumatism.

HERBAL - Ash leaves were highly recommended by the medical alchemist Dr. Rademacher and were extensively used in Germany on his suggestion. In the Union Medical for Nov. 27, 1852, two French physicians, Drs. Pouget and Peyraud, detailed several case of gout and rheumatism cured by an infusion of ash-leaves in boiling water. Dr. Peyraud himself was one of those relieved.

A commercial traveler, who had been gouty for twenty years and had saturated himself with the syrup of Boubee and other vaunted specifics, consulted Dr. Pouget. At this time he was almost constant prisoner in his room successive attacks. After eleven days' use of the infusion he was able to walk two kilometers (one and a quarter miles), in fifteen days he resumed his journeys and was able to travel without suffering from Bordeaux to Quimper.

Acute and chronice painful gout and rheumatism. Joint rheumatism in numerous instances.

COMMENTS - Anshutz recorded the case of Dr. Peyraud. In 1842, Peyraud had his first attack of gout, which was severe and lasted for twenty-five days. During the three following years the attacks increased in frequency and severity.

Having derived little benefit from the remedial means that he had resorted to, he listened to the suggestion of one of his patients, an inhabitant of the department of Dordogne in France, who advised him to try an infusion of ash leaves. Informing Peyraud, at the same time, that his forefathers had been cured by this prescription and that many of the country people got rid of "their pains" by employing it.

Dr. Peyraud took the infusion of ash leaves and from 1845 to 1849 had no fit of gout. He then had an attack, which yielded in five days to the infusion of ash leaves, used under the observation of Dr. Pouget.

Dr. Pouget recalled that when he was a physician at Soreze in 1824, the peasants of that place had spoken to him of the great power which an infusion of ash leaves had in driving away pains. He afterwards discovered that it had been used forty years ago as a gout specific by the peasants of Auvergne.

RELATIONS - ***Compare:*** (1) Colch., Rhus-t.

REFERENCES - Anshutz. Clarke.

FUCHSINUM

PHARMACY - fuch. Fuchsinum. Rosanilin hydrochloride. A coloring substance used in adulteration of wine, magenta. Onagraceae. ***Historical dose:*** Tincture and all potencies.

CLINICAL - Albuminuria. Gum, disease. Kidney, disorders. Nephritis. Salivation.

HOMEOPATHIC - Fuchsinum produces redness of ears, deep red discoloration of mouth, swollen gums with burning and tendency to salivation. Deep red urine, albuminous and light red. Cortical nephritis with albuminuria. Profuse diarrhea with abdominal pains. Cortical substances of kidneys degenerated.

REFERENCES - Boericke.

FUCUS VESICULOSUS

(Bladder-wrack)

PHARMACY - fuc. Fucus vesiculosus. Bladder-wrack. Sea-wrack. Sea-kelp. Kelp-ware. N. O. Algae. Phaeophyceae. Rich in iodine. Tincture and trituration of the dried plant. The fresh alga gathered in May or June are pounded to a pulp and macerated in two parts by weight of alcohol. ***Historical dose:*** Trituration, tincture and all potencies.

CLINICAL - Constipation. Dyspepsia. Flatulence. ***Goiter.*** Obesity. Thyroid, enlargement.

HERBAL - In the American Eclectic Dispensatory, John King stated "Fucus vesiculosus, sea wrack or bladder-wrack, has a peculiar odor and a nauseous saline taste. The charcoal of this plant has long had the reputation of the deobstruent and been given in goiter and scrofulous swelling.

"The dose is a teaspoonful of the tincture twice or three times daily in a well-developed case. Half a teaspoonful twice a day will answer in recent cases. Smaller doses seem not to produce any effect. The medicine is very unpleasant to the taste, but causes no disturbance after it has been taken. It ought to be taken, each dose in a few ounces of water and preferably between meals."

HOMEOPATHIC - Fuc. is a tissue remedy of great power and must be compared with Iod., of which it contains a large proportion. Digestion is improved and flatulence diminished. Obstinate constipation, forehead feels as if compressed by an iron ring.

Very weak and restless. Thyroid enlargement in obese subjects. ***Obesity and non-toxic goiter***, also exophthalmic. Goiter has been cured with it in teaspoonful doses of the tincture given two or three times a day.

Abdomen - Flatulency diminished and then disappears. Bearing-down pains in lower part of abdomen.

Eyes - Sight dim.

Face - Face became yellow.

Female - Menorrhagia, bright red blood, bearing-down pains in lower abdomen.

Head - Intolerable headache, forehead felt as if compressed by an iron ring. Headache with hemorrhages. Burning at vertex. Nausea, vertigo, and slight headache.

Kidneys - Frequent desire to urinate. Urine contains much blood.

Lungs - Difficult breathing. Sense of suffocation, especially during menses. Inclination to cough, causing him to spit blood.

Nose - Nosebleed.

Rectum - Obstinate, chronic constipation. Dysentery, blood bright red. Dysentery with menorrhagia.

Stomach - Vomiting of bright red blood.

COMMENTS - Anshutz wrote "The following letter, by Dr. J. Herbert Knapp to the Homeopathic Recorder, was published in 1896: 'After treating many cases of exophthalmic goiter, I have come to the conclusion that I have found a specific for that disease in Fucus vesiculosus, (sea-wrack). I might record one case.

" 'Mrs. Mary B., age 24 years, German, came into my clinic at the Brooklyn E. D. Homeopathic Dispensary to be treated for swelling of the neck of several years duration. I gave her the tincture of Fucus ves., thirty drops three times a day. The treatment began December 1, 1895 and patient was discharged cured, on October 2, 1896. Would be pleased to hear from any others who have had any experience with Fucus vesiculosus.'

"So far as I now remember, this is the only hint I ever receive which led me to try in goiter. At the same time, I do not feel sure of this. I had met in some medical journal a statement respecting the relation of this drug to goiter, which fact led me to look it up in the 'Eclectic Dispensatory.' But if so, I cannot recall the authority.

"At all events, I was led to try the remedy in a pronounced case of goiter with such goods results that I have never since given any other remedy for that disease either in the exophthalmic or in the uncomplicated form.

"What is more, I have never known it to fail to cure when the patient was under thirty years of age. After that time of life or about that period, it seems to be no longer efficacious.

"I have now used it on more than twenty-four cases with the same unvarying result and never with any other result-that is, no unpleasant consequences have ever accompanied or followed its use.

"I published this fact in the medical investigator after I had used it in a few case and again announced it in the Chicago Homeopathic Medical Society still later and again have frequently repeated it with growing confidence and of greater numbers of cases in medical societies in colleges and in private conversation with physicians.

"And yet the fact is so utterly unknown that your journal published Dr. Knapp's inquiry respecting it, which shows how easily a good thing may be forgotten. Also how readily a genuine specific may be superseded by a host of abortive procedures right under the eyes of the profession. It is most probable that more real good remedies have been forgotten or cast aside in medicine.

"Respecting this Fucus vesiculosus and its use in goiter, I would like to add a few words. The drug is of variable quality. If one specimen fails to give satisfaction it ought to be discarded and another tried. The pharmacist must be importuned to make special efforts to give us an article that is not inert, but contains all the activity that belongs to the drug.

"Time is required for effecting a cure. This varies according to the age and size of the goiter. Three months may suffice for a small goiter of one year's growth. Six months may be required for one twice as large and of longer standing. A year and a half is the longest period during which I have had to continue the medicine. But during all that time the goiter was manifestly diminishing."

RELATIONS - ***Compare:*** (1) Phyt., Thyr., Bad., Iod.

REFERENCES - Anshutz. Boericke.

FULIGO LIGNI

(Soot)

PHARMACY - fuli. Fuligo ligni. Soot. ***Historical dose:*** Trituration and all potencies.

CLINICAL - ***Cancer.*** Eczema. Metrorrhagia. Pruritus, vulvae. Tetters. Ulcers. Uterine, hemorrhage.

HOMEOPATHIC - Fuligo ligni acts on the glandular system, and mucus membranes. Chronic irritations of mucus membranes of mouth. Obstinate ulcers, epidermis, tetters, eczema.

Cancer, especially of the scrotum. Chimney sweeper's cancer. Epithelial cancers. Cancer of womb with metrorrhagia. Uterine hemorrhage. Pruritus vulvae. Sadness. Thoughts of suicide.

RELATIONS - ***Compare:*** (1) Kreos.

REFERENCES - Boericke.

FUMARIA OFFICINALIS

(Fumitory)

PHARMACY - fum. Fumaria officinalis. Fumitory. Earth smoke. The mother tincture is prepared from the whole fresh plant in flower of Fumaria officinalis. N. O. Papaveraceae. ***Historical dose:*** Tincture and all potencies.

CLINICAL - Backache. ***Bloating.*** Constipation. ***Cramps.*** Diarrhea. ***Flatus.*** Gallbladder, disorders. Headache. Jaundice. Leucorrhea. Liver, disorders. Migraine. Nausea. Sinus, congestion. Sneezing.

HERBAL - The Fumaria plant contains an alkaloid, fumarine, that brings about hyposthenia and, when applied externally, as with other Papaveraceae, has an anesthetic effect.

It also has a regulating effect on a disturbed gallbladder function.

In herbal medicine, therefore, it is prescribed for jaundice and bilious migraines.

The high content of potassium salts means that the herb also has diuretic, sweat-inducing and laxative characteristics.

"Physicians and writers from Dioscorides to Chaucer, and from the fourteenth century to Cullen and to modern times value its purifying power. French and German physicians still prefer it to most other medicines as a purifier of the blood. Sometimes the dried leaves are smoked in the manner of tobacco, for disorders of the head. A decoction makes a curative lotion for milk-crust on the scalp of an infant." (Grieve).

HOMEOPATHIC - The main indications are blood cleansing and detoxification. Disturbances in liver function. Tuberculosis.

Sensation of heaviness in body. ***Tired and fatigued, weary.*** Chilliness and "goose bumps."

Tightening sensation in forehead. Pain behind the eyes, better pressure. Congestion of sinuses. Sneezing. Heaviness of eyes, difficult to keep them open. Tight sensation in throat.

Fluctuations in appetite, sometimes increased, sometimes decreased. Desire for sweets and chocolates. Thirsty for small sips. ***Abdomen bloated with gas.*** Cramping pain. Sweet odor to the stools. Stools long and thin.

MIND - Alternating mood, high and low energy. Nervous, better company. Frantic feeling, with agitation of the mind, worse night. Fear of the future. Fear of heart attack.

Frustrated. Negative thoughts. Sadness, feels like crying. Aversion to company. Desire to curse. Delusion of earthquake.

Confusion and great difficulty concentrating. Spaced out feeling. Delusion she is standing outside of herself and watches life. Sense of shame about sexual identity.

Abdomen - ***Gas and bloating.*** Sulphur odor to flatus. ***Cramping pains.*** Sharp pains in the abdomen, particularly in the solar plexus.

Back - Backache. Lower back pain. Eruptions, red bumps. Stiffness unrelieved with exercise. Tension in cervical region, worse right side. Cervical pain radiating to temples. Sharp pain in right flank.

Chest - Sharp pain in left side of chest.

Eyes - Heaviness of eyes, cannot keep them open. Stinging pain in the eyes. Swelling of eyes.

Female - Menses, delayed. Cramps and heavy flow with the onset of menses. White leucorrhea. Clear or white vaginal discharge.

Food - Fluctuations in appetite, sometimes increased, sometimes decreased. Desires sweets and chocolate. Thirsty for small sips.

Head - Headache, better pressure. Headache behind eyes. Tightening in forehead. Head pain extending to the neck then radiating to the temples.

Kidneys - Increased frequency of urination. Urine, strong odor.

Limbs - Pain in right shoulder and arm. Sensation of pins and needles in upper limbs. Cramping pain in the elbow.

Male - Nocturnal seminal emissions.

Modalities - Worse many things. Worse light, sunlight particularly. Worse lying down. Worse at 4 p.m.

Mouth - Sore pain in tip of tongue. Metallic taste in mouth.

Nose - Congestion in the sinuses. Sneezing.

Rectum - Constipation and diarrhea. Diarrhea, gushing like water. Flatus smelling like sulphur. ***Loose stools.*** Increased urge for bowel movements. Increased bowel movements, 3 to 4 times per day. ***Long and thin stools.*** Stools, odor sweet. Sticky stools.

Skin - Dry, scaly skin. Skin is sore to touch.

Sleep - Sleeping for longer periods of time. Waking unrefreshed. ***Vivid dreams.*** Dreams of fighting, violence. Dreams of dead bodies. Sexual dreams.

Stomach - Nausea.

Throat - Scratchy and sore throat. ***Tightness in throat.***

RELATIONS - ***Compare:*** (1) Kreos.

REFERENCES - Riley. Schwabe.

G

GADUS MORRHUA

(Cod Fish)

PHARMACY - gad. Gadus morrhua. Cod fish. N. O. Gadide. Trituration of first cervical vertebra of the fish. ***Historical dose:*** Trituration and all potencies.

CLINICAL - Asthma. Bladder, disorders. Bone disorders. Coughs. Hands, hot. Tuberculosis.

HOMEOPATHIC - Knowledge of this remedy comes mostly from Petroz. Like Ol-j., Jac., Gadus has a powerful action on the respiratory apparatus.

Frequent breathing with flapping of alae nasi. (Lyc.). Rush of blood to chest. Pain in lungs and cough. Dry heat in palms of hands. Affects the bones.

MIND - Hopelessness and desire for death are prominent.

RELATIONS - ***Compare:*** (1) Ol-j., Calc., Calc-p., Conch.

REFERENCES - Clarke.

GAERTNER BACILLUS

(Bowel Nosode)

PHARMACY - gaert. Gaertner bacillus. Bacillus gaertner. Salmonella enteritidis. A bowel nosode of Bach. ***Historical dose:*** All potencies.

CLINICAL - ***Acidosis. Celiac, disease.*** Blisters. Cachexia. Colitis. Dentition. Emaciation. Eye, disorders. Fibrositis. Gastro-enteritis. ***Growth, disorders.*** Hypersensitive. Indigestion. ***Ketosis. Malnutrition.*** Marasmus. ***Neurasthenia.*** Otorrhea. Smallpox. Urticaria. Tabes mesenterica. Threadworms. Urticaria. ***Vomiting.*** Worms.

HOMEOPATHIC - This organism was first isolated from a case of food poisoning and, when identified by Gaertner, was given the title B. Enteritidis, the bacillus of the intestine.

The keynote is nutrition, and this nosode might suitably be named "the children nosode." Clinically useful for the nutritional disorders common to children.

For children fed on artificial food who have poor digestion.

Affects the digestive tract. Inability to digest fat, ***celiac disease, ketosis intestinal infantilism. Malnutrition***, either from lack of adequate diet or failure to metabolize, e.g. in steatorrhea, celiac disease or following gastric operations and in some cases of colitis.

Indicated by marked emaciation, marasmus, especially in children, the elderly, or with malignant disease. ***Growth disorders.*** Poorly nourished bodies and poor muscular development, but with active minds. Restless, lack of attention. Hypersensitive to physical or psychological impressions. Fear of the dark and of being alone. Urticaria.

MIND - Hypersensitive to all impressions. Restless. Mental uneasiness. Pessimistic, lack of confidence. Fear of heights, of the dark and of being alone.

Abdomen - Chronic gastro-enteritis, tabes mesenterica.

Back - Severe pain in hip and back.

Chest - Bronchial colds. Nocturnal coughs.

Constitutions - Fair hair, blue eyes, freckles. Pale, thin. Long, black eyelashes.

Ears - Otorrhea, worse when teething.

Eyes - White sclerotics. Styes.

Female - Profuse, offensive leucorrhea. Pruritus vulvae.

Food - Desires oatmeal, cheese, eggs, milk, pudding, sugar and sweets. Averse to bread, butter, butcher meat, and fish.

Kidneys - Blood and mucus with urine. Burning in urethra.

Limbs - Fibrositis. Sciatica. Shoulder rheumatism, worse at night. Rheumatism hands and feet. Chilblains on hands in winter. Bites nails. Pes planus. Soles of feet covered with blisters, itch and are worse at night.

Male - Hydrocele.

Mouth - Herpes. Dry, scaly eruption. Salivation. Deep fissures in tongue. Teeth black.

Nose - Polyps. Catarrh.

Rectum - ***Constipation.*** Blood and mucus in stool. ***Diarrhea offensive,*** attacks every few weeks. Itching of anus. Worms, threadworms (Cina).

Skin - Urticaria, heat spots. Circinate eruption on sternum. Eruption on back, head and neck. Boils on arms and legs. Perspiration, worse at night.

Sleep - Desires light in room. Desires company, especially mother. Late in falling to sleep. Sleep walking. Restless sleep, night terrors.

Stomach - Pain in stomach. Dilated stomach. ***Vomits everything,*** worse after sweets. Headache and vomiting. ***Acidosis attacks*.**

COMMENTS - Ghosh noted "Gaertner in 30c potency may be used in extensive suppuration with intestinal disorders in small-pox."

E. Paterson thought that Gaert. may help in teething troubles where Cham. fails. Defective digestion of fat as of Puls. has a worthy trial of this remedy. "In all varieties of neurasthenia, I know of no single remedy to compare with the Gaertner nosode."

Wheeler noted: "For cases of children who get a discharging ear every time they cut a tooth, give one dose of Gaertner 30, followed the next day by the dose of Silica 30c and repeat the Gaertner as soon as there is any sign of a further out break of this ear discharge."

Griggs indicated that "it is helpful to make a comparison and to remember the Dys-co. child whose nervous tension expressed itself by an uneasiness of the muscular system. Although fidgety and uneasy, the shyness of his temperament would prevent him from leaving his chair while you are taking the preliminary notes in your consulting room.

"The Gaertner child has mental uneasiness. He must know the reason for everything you do and for what purpose you use this or that article lying on you desk or somewhere in the room. Furthermore, he will proceed to make close inspection of it, but you will notice that his attention is not held long on any subject."

RELATIONS - ***Compare:*** (1) The remedies most closely associated with this nosode are Dys-co., Phos., Sil. and Merc.

REFERENCES - Bach. Boericke. Paterson.

GALANTHUS NIVALIS

(Snowdrop)

PHARMACY - gala. Galanthus nivalis. Snowdrop. N. O. Amaryllidaceae. ***Historical dose:*** Tincture and all potencies.

CLINICAL - Faintness. Heart, disorders. Mitral, insufficiency. Murmurs. ***Myocarditis.*** Sore, throat.

HOMEOPATHIC - Proving by Dr. A Whiting. Therapeutically decided benefit in cases of mitral regurgitation with broken down compensation. Faintness and sinking sensations.

Myocarditis with some degree of mitral insufficiency. Systolic murmur at apex. Heart weak with sensation of collapse, as if she must fall. Pulse very irregular, rapid and uneven, violent palpitations. Sore dry throat with dull headache. Half conscious and worried feeling during sleep.

REFERENCES - Boericke.

GALEGA OFFICINALIS

(Goat's Rue)

PHARMACY - galeg. Galega officinalis. Goat's rue. N. O. Leguminose. Papilionoideae. Aqueous extract, infusion or tincture of whole fresh plant. ***Historical dose:*** Tincture and all potencies.

CLINICAL - Anemia. Backaches. Breastfeeding. Breast, disorders. Debility. Kidney, pain. Malnutrition.

HERBAL - Galega, as its name implies, has an ancient reputation as a milk-gland stimulant. The Galege are nearly related to Glycyrrhiza, the source of licorice.

Increases the quantity and quality of the milk in nursing women, it also improves the appetite. An excellent tonic in cases of anemia and impaired nutrition. Backache and debility.

Dorretta gave Galeg., in liquid extract of the leaves, for a common form of backache, which he located in the kidney though it is unaccompanied by any sign of kidney disease.

Carron de la Carriere tested its action on the milk glands of nursing women. He found it rapidly increased the quantity and quality of the milk and increased the woman's appetite.

RELATIONS - ***Compare:*** (1) Agn-c., Calc. in kidney pain, Sant.

REFERENCES - Clarke.

GALIUM APARINE

(Cleavers)

PHARMACY - gali. Galium aparine. Cleavers. Goose grass. N. O. Galiacae, considered by some a sub-order of Rubiacae. Tincture and infusion of fresh plant. Extract. Poultices. ***Historical dose:*** Tincture and all potencies.

CLINICAL - Bladder, irritability. Calculus. Cancer. Cystitis. Dysuria. Gravel. Kidney, stones. Psoriasis. Tumors. Ulcers.

HERBAL - Galium has had no proving, but it is a popular remedy for cancer given internally and used externally, and also for scrofulous swellings and ulcers. It is further used as a diuretic and as a solvent for gravel and stone.

HOMEOPATHIC - Gali. acts on the urinary organs as a diuretic. Dysuria and cystitis. Gravel and kidney stones. Dropsy.

Gali. has clinical confirmation of its use in cancerous ulcers and tumors. Suspends or modifies cancerous action. Favors healthy granulations on ulcerated surfaces. Inveterate skin disorders and scurvy.

COMMENTS - Grimmer said this remedy cured a case of nodulated tumor of the tongue diagnosed to be cancer. A case of psoriasis of the left hand was also reported cured. Substantial doses were given in each case, and in the later poultices of the herb were used as well.

REFERENCES - Boericke. Clarke.

GALLICUM ACIDUM

(Gallic Acid)

PHARMACY - gall-ac. Gallicum acidum. Gallic acid. Trituration. ***Historical dose:*** Trituration and all potencies.

CLINICAL - Asthma. Constipation. Debility. Delirium. ***Heartburn***. Hematuria. Hemophilia. Hemorrhages. Kidneys, pain. ***Pulmonary, hemorrhage***. ***Tuberculosis.*** Urticaria.

HOMEOPATHIC - Gallic acid is the well-known astringent, derivative of tannic acid, obtained from galls or oak-apples. It is used in old-school practice as a local application to arrest hemorrhages and in popular practice to check excessive menstruation.

A case is recorded in which the application of an ointment containing gallic acid or the insertion of a tannin suppository for hemorrhoids caused an attack resembling hay asthma with an eruption of urticaria. The experience was repeated several times before the cause was discovered.

This is sufficient to show that Gall-ac. is homeopathic to pulmonary cases in which it has been largely used by the old school as well as the new. Pulmonary hemorrhage, excessive expectoration, and the night-sweats of tuberculosis.

Tuberculosis. Weakness with irritability. Excessive dryness of mouth and throat. Sense of contraction of anus. Jerking of limbs. Itching of skin.

MIND - Wild delirium at night, very restless, jumps out of bed, sweats. Rude, abuses every one. Cursing. Strange speech. Jealousy. Afraid to be alone.

Eyes - Photophobia with burning of lids.

Head - Pain in back of head and neck.

Kidneys - Kidneys painful. Distress along ureters into bladder. Dull heavy pain in bladder, directly over pubis. Urine loaded with thick, cream-colored mucus. Hematuria.

Lungs - Pain in lungs. ***Pulmonary hemorrhage***. Excessive expectoration. Much mucus in throat in the morning, dry at night.

Nose - Thick, stringy discharge from nose.

Rectum - Copious stool, anus feels constricted. Chronic mucus discharges. Faint feeling after stool.

Throat - Much mucus in throat in morning. Dry throat at night.

COMMENTS - Marcy, of New York, recorded the case of a young woman who had a cavity in the left lung with purulent expectoration, night-sweats, evening fever, pulse 130. Under the prolonged use of Gall-ac. 1x she recovered her normal health except that the left lung remained dull and she had great shortness of breath on the slightest exertion. Her flesh, strength and general appearance were as when she was in perfect health.

Bayles said Gall-ac. rapidly checks secretions, give general tone to the stomach, increases appetite, and removes constipation. ***Heartburn***. Hematuria. Hemophilia. Passive hemorrhages when pulse is feeble and capillaries relaxed, cold skin.

RELATIONS - ***Compare:*** (1) Querc., Tann-ac., Bac., Ars-i., (2) Phos. relieved pain in right lung. (3) Ars., Iod.

REFERENCES - Boericke. Clarke.

GALPHIMIA GLAUCA

PHARMACY - galph. Galphimia glauca. N. O. Malpighiaceae family. Mexico. The tincture is prepared from the dried leaves and flowers. ***Historical dose:*** Tincture and all potencies.

CLINICAL - Allergies. Dermatitis. Eczema. Edema. Gastritis. Hay fever. Herpes. Hypersensitivity. Mycosis. Neurodermatitis. Sneezing. Sudamina. Urticaria.

HERBAL - Galphimia glauca is a wild plant, belonging to the Malpighiaceae family and growing in Mexico.

HOMEOPATHIC - There is no existing Homeopathic proving but it was used in clinical experimentation by a group of German doctors from 1964 to 1966, using the 3x, 4x, 6x, and 12x potencies, for a variety of allergic infections.

Allergic vasomotor afflictions of the nose. Hay fever. Sneezing. Bronchial asthma. Allergies with hay fever, asthma, sensitive skin. Skin allergies. Urticaria, herpetic dermatitis. Allergic eczema, mycotic eczema.

Recurring herpes of the lips or genitalia. Hypersecretion from the nasal and ocular mucus membranes. Edema of the eyelids. Vesicular, papular eruptions. Sudamina. Neurodermatitis. Shooting pains in the stomach. Gastritis or gastric complaints. Hypersensitivity to weather changes.

RELATIONS - ***Compare:*** (1) Ars., Psor., Nat-m.

REFERENCES - Julian.

GALVANISMUS

(Galvanism)

PHARMACY - galv. Galvanismus. Galvanism. Potencies are made by triturating sugar of milk which has been subjected to the influence of either electric pole. ***Historical dose:*** All potencies.

CLINICAL - Asthma. Brain-fag. Diarrhea. Epilepsy. Fevers. Headache. Hemorrhoids, Hydrocephalus. Paralysis. Rheumatism. Salivation. Tetanus. Tongue disorders. Toothache. Vision, illusions.

HOMEOPATHIC - Farrington noted a "benumbed feeling at the back of the head in brain-fag, the positive pole being applied to the cervical region, the negative to the vertex."

Muscular contractions, shuddering, shivering. Burning or cold-water sensation on skin. Disorders of sight and hearing, with confusion of the head and headache. Putrid smell before nose. Many sensations appear in the tongue. Salivation. Copious menses.

RELATIONS - ***Compare:*** (1) Kali-br., Gels., Electr., M-arct., M-aust.

REFERENCES - Clarke.

GAMBOGIA MORELLA

(Gummi Gutti)

PHARMACY - gamb. Gambogia morella. Gummi gutti. Garcinia morella. Gamboge. N. O. Guttifere. China. Tincture of the resinous gum obtained from the tree. ***Historical dose:*** Tincture and all potencies.

CLINICAL - Anus disorders. Backache. Blows, effects. Burning, pains. Coccyx, pain. Colic. ***Diarrhea.*** Dysentery. Eyes, inflammation. Flatulence. ***Food, poisoning.*** Lienteria.

Rheumatic, pains. ***Sneezing***. Sore, pains. Throat, sore. Typhlitis. Vomiting.

HOMEOPATHIC - Affects the stomach and bowels, chiefly known as a remedy for a diarrhea similar to Crot-t.

Burning in anus after stool, anus sore and excoriated. ***Profuse watery diarrhea,*** particularly with elderly people. Stool preceded by excessive cutting about navel. Stool is expelled all at once after considerable urging and is followed by a feeling of great relief. Stools are yellow, green, bloody, lienteric.

Frightful vomiting and purging with fainting. Burning in the liver. Pain in small of back, as if bruised or sprained. Pain in sacrum, resulting from a blow. Gnawing pains in the coccyx. Burning pains. General soreness. Rheumatic symptoms. Periodic symptoms.

MIND - Irritable in morning on waking. Despondency, sadness. Cheerful and talkative. Feeling of ease, great lightness of all his motions.

Abdomen - ***Gurgling in abdomen, as of fluid running from a bottle.*** Rushing sounds in abdomen as from motions of air. Tenderness in epigastrium. Pain and distention of abdomen from flatulence after stool. ***Rumbling and rolling.*** Ileo-cecal region sensitive to pressure. Pinching pain in abdomen immediately after eating.

Back - Pain in coccyx. Small of back as if bruised or sprained. Gnawing pain in coccyx. Pain and itching between scapula. Cutting pain across top of sacrum and in left hip. Cutting pain in muscles just above sacroiliac symphysis on left side.

Chest - Congestion of blood to chest. Chest, sore and raw. Pressure and weight in chest. Pressure pain in middle of chest. Sharp pains in sternum. Sharp pains going from both sides of chest towards each other.

Cough - Dry, with hoarseness and hawking of mucus. Severe cough, at night, compelling him to sit up, with easy expectoration of mucus. Cough better sitting up.

Ears - Ringing in left ear all the time. Lancination pain in ears.

Eyes - Burning in eyes. Itching and burning in eyes. Itching of eyelids, he rubs them. ***Eyelids stick together with sneezing***. Eyes as if sticky and dry. Nightly agglutination of lids, burning in morning. Violent burning of eyes with photophobia. Smarting of eyes with lachrymation. Very severe pain in eyeballs.

Face - Swelling of face. Swelling of eyelids, nose and lips. Upper lip swollen. Itching, smarting on right cheek, chin and upper lip.

Female - Menses too early and too profuse. Menses long-lasting. Congestion to sexual organs. Leucorrhea.

Food - Aversion to food. Violent thirst in evening. Appetite good, but a little food satisfies. Thirst after dinner. Thirst during chill. Great thirst, in chronic diarrhea. Worse after drinking ale.

Head - Gastric headaches. Head hot, face red, during attacks of diarrhea. Heat rises to head, with sweat. Heavy sensation with inertia and drowsiness. Sensation of great coldness in left temple as from a wet cloth. Vertex as if bruised, in forenoon, better open air. Oppressive pain with heaviness in forehead. Compressive pain. Pain in coronal suture.

Kidneys - Sharp pain in left kidney. Infrequent urination. Increased secretion of urine. Urine smells like onions. Urine diminished in dropsy.

Limbs - Stinging and numb feeling in ball of right thumb. Tearing pain in shoulders. Sharp pain, in upper limbs. Itching blisters on both hands, at first pale, afterwards red. Severe aching deep in hip, and severe cutting pain about trochanter major. Aching pain in knees. Cramp in calf with contraction of toes. Heaviness and languor of feet.

Liver - Burning in liver.

Lungs - Expectoration of blood.

Male - Gleety discharge agglutinating orifice of urethra.

Modalities - Better by motion. Better in open air. Better after stools. Better sitting up. Worse evening and at night. Worse motion. Worse in open air. Worse after stools. Most symptoms come on while sitting, and go off during motion in open air.

Mouth - Aphthae. Deep ulcers in mouth, inner side of lips and cheeks. Bitter taste in mouth. Feeling of coldness at the edge of teeth. Burning vesicles on inner side of lips. Dryness of mouth. Clammy, adhesive state of mouth.

Nose - ***Violent chronic sneezing,*** in daytime only. Smarting as if a sore pimple existed immediately below right nostril. Dryness of right nostril. Much mucus in nose, smelling like pus. Tendency to hemorrhages from nose and lungs.

Perspiration - Sweats all over, at night. Sweats on awaking at 4 a.m. Cold sweats on limbs, during stool.

Rectum - Burning and heat in anus during stool. ***Tenesmus after stool with burning in anus.*** Pinching, gurgling in bowels, then sudden yellow or green. Diarrhea alternating with constipation. Hard, insufficient stool, with strong urging. Dysentery, with retained stool, with pain in sacral region. Frequent emission of flatulence. ***Thin stools*** coming out in prolonged gushes with burning at anus. ***Diarrhea with sudden and forcible ejection of bilious stools.*** Diarrhea after drinking ale. Profuse, watery diarrhea in hot weather, particularly old people. Yellow and green diarrheic stool, mixed with mucus. Stools of dark green mucus, offensive, corrosive. Infantile diarrhea.

Skin - Violent itching in various parts of body, burning after scratching, worse evening and night. After scratching, burning and ulcerative pain, with swelling and redness of parts, worse evening and night. Biting as of ants over whole body, worse evening and night. Itching on various parts of surface pleasantly better gentle friction. Itching and formication here and there all night. Pemphigus.

Sleep - Sleepiness, great inclination to sleep. Sleeplessness from weight on chest. Anxious, vexatious dreams. Dreams with broken sleep.

Stomach - Frequent violent empty eructations. Gulping up of sour water. Gnawing pain in stomach. Emptiness in stomach and abdomen. Great irritability of the stomach. Pain in the stomach after food. Acute darting, stitching pain in stomach. Nausea, inclination to vomit with accumulation of saliva in mouth. Frightful vomiting and purging, with fainting. Ulcerative pain in stomach, better after eating. Vomiting and purging with fainting.

Temperature - Violent chill, beginning in back. Chill with empty eructations. Internal and external coldness from 7 p.m. to 8 p.m. Violent shaking chill at 7 p.m., beginning in back. Sudden shaking chill at night, waking him from sleep, and suddenly disappearing. Chill with chattering of teeth and violent thirst. Increased heat with anxiety.

Throat - Swollen sensation. Violent stitches in right side of throat. Pain as from soreness in throat. Rawness and burning in throat, causes constant hawking. Sore, in throat. Scratching sensation in larynx. Tickling in larynx and trachea from epiglottis to pit of throat.

Tongue - Burning, smarting and dryness of tongue and throat. Burning of anterior half or only tip of tongue, which feels hard. Raw, rough feeling in fauces and at root of tongue.

Vertigo - Vertigo during rest or motion. Vertigo in morning. Vertigo on rising. Confusion of head with feeling of reeling or motion from side to side.

COMMENTS - Gamb. painted on the chest in lung tuberculosis was considered by Abrams a specific. Also incipient diarrhea cases were symptomatically cured in several weeks.

RELATIONS - ***Antidoted by:*** Camph., Coff., Coloc., Kali-c., Op. ***Compare:*** (1) Crot-t., Aloes, Podo., Puls. - cough better sitting up, better open air. (2) Apoc. - stool expelled all one, but Gamb. has cutting before and better after stool. (3) Crot-t. has stool in one gush, but Gamb. is not worse from least food or drink like Crot.

REFERENCES - Boericke. Clarke. Phatak.

GASTEIN AQUA

(Gastein Springs)

PHARMACY - gast. Gastein aqua. Gastein springs. The hot springs of Wildbad Gasterin in Salzburg, Austria. Dilutions. ***Historical dose:*** Tincture and all potencies.

CLINICAL - Amenorrhea. Callosities. Colds. Constipation. Debility. Diarrhea. Dysmenorrhea. Gout. Hemorrhoids. Paralysis. Rheumatism. Scars. Sexual, weakness. Stones. Strokes. Typhlitis. Varicose ulcers.

HOMEOPATHIC - The hot springs of Wildbad Gasterin in Salzburg, Austria, contain sodium sulphate predominantly, but also silicic acid, potassium sulphate and carbonate, lithium chloride, magnesium carbonate, ferrum carbonate, aluminium phosphate and traces of calcium fluoride, strontium, arsenicum, titanic acid, rubidium, cesium, also free carbonic acid. Lapis albus is a kind of gneiss found in the spring. It is a silicofluoride of calcium.

Constantin James described the effects of the baths as a "General unpleasant sensation. Instead of expanding (as would be expected in a warm bath) the skin is drawn up upon itself as if by a tight astringent. There is slight dyspnea, the abdominal walls draw together, the testicles rise to the inguinal rings.

"Soon an unusual warmth, accompanied by shocks and tremors, spreads throughout all the limbs. The pulse becomes hard and vibrating, the face becomes suffused, there is humming in the ears. It is now time to leave the bath to stay longer is attended with danger.

"Then after the seventh to the fourteenth bath the thermal influence tends to concentrate itself entirely on the nervous system. Thus it seems to the patient that an increase of vitality spreads through his whole being, he feels more active then before, the longest walks cause hardly any fatigue and that is promptly repaired by sleep.

"Among individual symptoms noted are diminished secretions. Activity of all the veins, excitement of the circulation. Weakness and weariness with dragging sensation in the abdomen, as if it were too heavy. Exhaustion and inclination to sleep.

"Takes cold very easily, which was caused then cured. Pulsation in the body, especially in the arms with jumping in them. Contractive sensations predominate. Scar tissues and callosities are affected. Worse before a storm."

COMMENTS - The baths affect phlegmatic patients in an increase of force and tone, causing the disappearance of involuntary losses of semen. In irritable temperaments it will provoke erotic dreams and unwanted excitement, in such cases the waters are aphrodisiac.

Sensation of indescribable mental and physical comfort runs through all the tissues during the bath. Predominantly influences the sexual system.

RELATIONS - ***Compare:*** (1) Lap-a., Fl-ac. Sil., Canth., Phos.

REFERENCES - Clarke.

GAULTHERIA PROCUMBENS

(Wintergreen)

PHARMACY - gaul. Gaultheria procumbens. Wintergreen. N. O. Ericacae. The oil contains methyl salicylate and is one of the sources of salicine. Tincture of fresh leaves, oil obtained from the leaves. ***Historical dose:*** Tincture and all potencies.

CLINICAL - Cystitis. Gastritis. Kidney, inflammation. ***Neuralgias.*** Pleurodynia. Rheumatism. ***Sciatica.*** Vomiting.

HERBAL - An evergreen trailing vine found in cool, damp woods. The oil contains methyl salicylate and is one of the sources of salicine.

HOMEOPATHIC - Several cases of poisoning with the oil have been recorded in which symptoms of acute gastritis appeared. Prolonged vomiting, set up afresh by the least thing taken, as a cup of water. Severe pain in epigastrium. Slow, laborious breathing.

Insensibility and hot skin. Inflammatory arthritis, rheumatism, ***sciatica*** and other neuralgias. Pleurodynia. Bladder and prostatic irritation. Kidney inflammation. Undue sexual excitement.

Abdomen - Very severe pain in epigastrium and inferior part of the hypochondria, greatly worse by pressure of finger.

Chest - Pleurodynia with pain in anterior mediastinum.

Ears - Marked dullness of hearing.

Food - Inordinate, uncontrollable appetite for food. Irritability of the stomach, everything, even cold water, is immediately rejected.

Head - Neuralgia of head and face.

Skin - Smarting and burning. Intense erythema, worse cold bathing, better olive oil and cool air blowing on part.

Stomach - Acute gastritis, severe pain in epigastrium, ***Prolonged vomiting.*** Uncontrollable appetite, with irritable stomach. Stomach pain from nervous depression.

Tongue - Tongue dry, smooth and slightly swollen. Speech rather indistinct from the swelling.

COMMENTS - B. F. Lang related his experience with material does in ciliary neuralgia, facial neuralgia, gastric, ovarian, uterine and menstrual neuralgias, sciatica and inflammatory rheumatism.

Anshutz wrote on the action of Gaultheria: "My attention was first called to its use about ten years ago southern Ohio, where I received most pleasing results in the treatment of inflammatory rheumatism. Afterwards to complaints in form of neuralgia."

"While I am not a champion of any specific, I want to say that this drug has given me the quickest and most satisfactory results of any remedy in the Materia Medica. If there is anything that a person wants relief from quick and now, it is from these excruciating pains."

"Often was I called to treat some obstinate cases of ciliary neuralgia or facial or in fact nearly every form of neuralgia and found my skill taxed to its utmost to bring out the balm. Did I find it in the homeopathic indicated remedy? I trust so, but not in any Materia Medica. I don't say but what I got some results from them, but I found it in this a "helper", it came to my relief immediately and to the great comfort of the patient."

"In severest cases of neuralgia of the head and face it would do its work quick and well.

Equally well has it served me in very severe cases of neuralgia of stomach and bowels, while for the past few years it has done faithful work in ovarian and uterine neuralgia following or preceding difficult menstruation. I have many a dear friend today whose relief from suffering was found in this remedy. I am satisfied that it should be given a prominent place in our Materia Medica."

"Lest this article should become tedious, I will cite a few cases. Mr. A., traveling man from Chicago, a few years ago called on me for temporary relief of a severe case of ciliary neuralgia. He had suffered for many years with it, every spring especially and that he had consulted great numbers of physicians of Chicago, Milwaukee and Cincinnati. He said, "had taken bushels of drugs, both old and new school," with only temporary relief."

"So he expected nothing more, as he was told he must wear it out. I told him I thought I could give him relief. I furnished him one-half ounce of Gaultheria with directions to take, did not see him again for two years."

"When he came into my office one day and greeted me by saying I was the only man that could ever give him any permanent relief from his sufferings, that he never had any return after first day taking medicine."

"Miss B., dressmaker, came to me suffering terribly with facial neuralgia and greeted me similar to No. 1, that she expected nothing but temporary relief, as she had been afflicted for a long time. Gave her 2 drachms of oil of Wintergreen told her to take one dose immediately and another in two hours if the pain did not quiet down."

"She was careful to ask if it was an opiate, as she objected to that. I assured her it was not, saw her next day, said that pain disappeared and had not returned. I was acquainted with the lady for three and one-half years and she only had one return of the disease, which the same remedy relieved immediately. Many cases more could I cite in which it never has failed me."

"Another case: Mrs. G., I was called to relieve a severe case of neuralgia of stomach and bowels this last summer, who had been under the care of two of my worthy competitors. They had exhausted their pill case and for about three weeks the poor woman had suffered everything but death itself."

"After diagnosing the case I put her on this remedy and in two hours she was relieved. After two days was able to be about and cured shortly by no other remedy than it. I want to say you will find a true friend in this remedy in all forms of neuralgia and only give a few suggestions now, but if it should be necessary could give scores to prove its value. I mentioned in the beginning that it had been of great value in inflammatory rheumatism."

"A word as to the best way of giving the drug. I have found that the dose should never be less than five drops and if pain is severe fifteen drops repeated in half hour afterwards two hours apart. For adult it may be necessary to give twenty drops at first. It always should be dropped on sugar and taken."

"One suggestion: I would like to have it put in a tablet of about two to five drops pure oil, as I think it could be taken more satisfactorily. While the crude oil is very pleasant to take at first, yet, on account of its strong odor, will nauseate after awhile if not removed from room. I am confident that if you make this into a tablet and place it among your remedies you would have a weapon that you could place into the hands of doctors of untold value in these troubles."

RELATIONS - ***Compare:*** (1) Bry., Rhus-t., Salol., Nat-sal., Kalm., Led., Spirae. (2) Gaultheria contains Arbin., Sal-ac. (3) Methy-sal. - an artificial Gaultheria oil for rheumatism, especially when the salicylates cannot be used. Itching and epididymitis, locally. (4) after Canth. in burns.

REFERENCES - Anshutz. Clarke.

GELSEMIUM SEMPERVIRENS

(Yellow Jasmine)

PHARMACY - gels. Gelsemium sempervirens. Yellow jasmine. Gelsemium lucidum. Yellow jessamine. Gelsemium nitidum. Bignonia sempervirens. N. O. Loganiacee. Tincture of the bark of the root. ***Historical dose:*** All potencies.

CLINICAL - Amaurosis. ***Anxiety.*** Aphonia. Astigmatism. ***Bad, news.*** Bilious fever. Brain, disorders. ***Chills.*** Choroiditis. ***Chronic, fatigue. Colds.*** Coma. Constipation. Convulsions, Deafness. ***Debility.*** Dengue, fever. Diarrhea. Diphtheria. ***Diplopia. Drug, overdose.*** Dupuytren's contraction. Dysentery. Dysmenorrhea. ***Emotional, shock.*** Epilepsy. Esophagus, stricture. Eyes, disorders. ***Fatigue. Fevers. Fright.*** Gonorrhea. Hay fever. Headaches. Heat, effects. Heart, disorders. Hysteria ***Influenza.*** Intermittent, fever. Jaundice. Labor, pains. Liver, disorders. Locomotor, ataxia. Measles. Meningitis. Menstruation, disorders. Metrorrhagia. Multiple sclerosis. Muscle pain. ***Muscular, weakness***. Neuralgias. Nystagmus. ***Paralysis.*** Parkinson's disease. Paraplegia. Pregnancy, toxemia. ***Ptosis.*** Puerperal, convulsions. Remittent, fever. Retina, disorders. Rheumatism. Salpingitis. Sexual, excesses. Sleep, disordered. Spasms. Sun, headaches. Sunstroke. Teething. Tic douloureux. Tobacco, effects. Tongue, disorders. Toothache. ***Tremors.*** Uterus, disorders. ***Vertigo. Viral infections.*** Voice, loss. ***Weakness.*** Writers' cramp.

HOMEOPATHIC - First introduced by Hale, Gelsemium belongs to the same order of plants as Nux-v. and Cur., and ranks among the vegetable polycrests. Like its botanical relatives, Gels. is a great paralyzer. Mental and bodily paresis. Sluggish mind. Relaxed muscular system, limbs feel so heavy he can hardly move them.

Functional ***paralysis*** of all descriptions, of various groups of muscles. Various degrees of ***motor paralysis***. Ptosis in the eye muscles and diplopia. Loss of the ability to swallow. Diarrhea from depressing emotions or bad news. Post-diphtheria paralysis.

Muscular weakness, lack of muscular coordination. In muscles, especially in the limbs, it causes overpowering ***aching, tiredness, heaviness, weakness and soreness***. General prostration and complete relaxation.

Dizziness, drowsiness and trembling. ***Tremors*** or twitchings of single muscles, face, chin tongue etc. Hysterical convulsions. Chorea of pregnancy. Parkinson's disease. Body feels light in nervous, hysterical subjects.

Mental prostration, ***anxiety.*** Lassitude (Mur-ac.), but the patient does not express it. Slow pulse, tired feeling. ***Apathetic and dull.*** Circulation becomes sluggish, causing arterial or venous congestion with sense of fullness and heaviness in different organs.

Coma and strokes. Alternate pelvic organ symptoms with head symptoms. Debility after seminal discharges, great prostration from irritability of seminal vesicles. Catarrh of mucus membranes with watery discharges. ***Influenza with malaise***. ***Never well since influenza.*** Measles. Pellagra.

Wants to lie down quietly, half reclined, wants to be held. Children have a fear of falling, they can grab the nurse or crib (Bor.).

General depression from heat of sun. Cold and dampness brings on many complaints. Effects of bad news, anger, grief when accompanied by trembling and fatigue. ***Drug overdose.*** Nervous disorders from tobacco.

MIND - ***Mental dullness, dizzy, drowsy and droopy***. Dazed mind. Answers slowly. Weak, tired, delicate, timid. Desire to be quiet, to be left alone. ***Apathy, regarding their illness.*** Mental exertion cause a sense of helplessness and weakness.

Mental exhaustion. Dullness, languor, listless. Incapacity to think or fix the attention. Vacant feeling on attempting to concentrate. Stupefaction during vertigo. Vanishing of thoughts on mental exertion.

Great depression with confusion of mind and exhaustion. Depression of spirits. ***Desire for be alone.*** Apathy and indolence. Indifference to business affairs. Inability to attend to anything requiring thought.

Wants to be quiet. Irritability, doesn't wish to be spoken to. Nervous, irritable, easily angered.

Excitable, easy to anger, especially in children and adolescents. ***Bad effects from fright, fear, bad news. Fear of falling***, especially in children (Bor.). ***Fear of doctors and dentists. Stage fright.*** Emotional excitement, fear, etc., lead to bodily ailments. Effects of grief, cannot cry, broods over her loss.

Ailments from anticipation. ***Nervous dread of appearing in public.*** Fear of upcoming ordeals. Dread of ordeals, pain. ***Lack of courage.*** Anticipation of any unusual ordeal, preparing for church, theatre, or to meet an engagement, brings on diarrhea. ***Fear of going to doctor or dentist.***

Anxiety about present and future. Anxiety about health. Anxiety during thunderstorm. Apprehensive feeling at approach of thunderstorm. Overpowering fear, with fatigue, exhaustion and drowsiness. Fear from traumatic shock.

Fear of losing self-control. Fear that unless on the move the heart will cease beating. Fear of falling. Child starts and grasps the nurse, and screams as if afraid of falling (Bor.). Fear of death. Fear of pain. Fear of injury.

Confusion, acts as if crazy. Delirious on falling to sleep. Delirium with incoherent talk. Sensation of intoxication during diarrhea. Acute mania after melancholy. Absolute lack of fear. High places aggravates. Impulse to jump from a height, from window. Cataleptic immobility with dilated pupils, closed eyes but conscious.

Abdomen - Rumbling in abdomen with discharge of wind above and below. ***Acute catarrhal enteritis during damp weather.*** Gnawing pain in the transverse colon. Sudden spasmodic pains in upper part of abdomen, compelling him to cry, leaving a sensation of contraction. ***Soreness in abdominal walls.*** Tenderness in right iliac region during typhus. Periodic colic with diarrhea, yellow discharges. Neuralgia of intestines periodic, malarial. Intestinal obstructions. Strangulated hernia.

Back - Backache with occipital pains. Backache day before appearance of menses. Complete relaxation of the whole muscular system. ***Chilliness up and the down back.*** Languor, muscles feel bruised. Every exertion causes fatigue. ***Dull aches, heavy pains, up and down in spine, better walking.*** Pain in muscles of back, hips and lower limbs, mostly deep-seated. Dull aching in lumbar and sacral region, passing upward. Pains under scapula. Pain in neck, especially upper sternocleido muscles. Lameness and stiffness of neck. Neck feels bruised, unable to hold the head. Spinal congestion, with incipient aphasia. Paralytic condition of lumbar and sacral muscles.

Bladder - Partial paralysis of bladder, intermittent flow (Clem.). Bladder paralysis following diphtheria. Bladder paralysis in elderly people. ***Retention of urine***. Dysuria. Frequent urging, with scanty emission and tenesmus of bladder. ***Incontinence from excitement.*** Incontinence from paralysis of sphincter. Constant dribbling of urine, but not a drop flows on making the greatest effort. Alternate dysuria and bedwetting. ***Bedwetting in nervous children at night.*** Bladder spasm in women, often combined with uterine spasms. Bladder spasm in men, with colic. Bladder distended up to navel.

Causations - Ill effects of fright, depressing emotions, anger, bad news, unpleasant surprise, traumatic shock. Sun, heat, warm or cold damp weather. Alcohol, drugs. Masturbation.

Chest - Oppression about chest. Heaviness in middle of chest. As if a lump behind the chest. Burning in chest, when coughing. Periodical pain in pectoral muscles. Constrictive pain around lower part of chest. Stitches in chest from above downward.

Constitutions - Suited to children and young people, to persons of a nervous, weak, hysterical temperament. Suitable to irritable, sensitive, excitable people.

Cough - Dry cough, with sore chest and fluent coryza. Cough from tickling in eustachian tube. Cough from tickling or roughness of fauces. Croupy cough in measles. Convulsive, spasmodic cough. Spasmodic cough in hysterical women. Irritative cough without expectoration. Coughs a good deal during the night.

Ears - Catarrhal inflammation, at beginning of head cold and closure of eustachian tube. Ear pain while swallowing. ***Earache from cold.*** Earache and sore throat. Neuralgic otalgia. Great sensitiveness to all sounds. Impaired hearing from cold. Sudden loss of hearing for a short time, rushing and roaring in ears. Catarrhal deafness with pain from throat into middle ear. Deafness and loss of speech from quinine.

Eyes - Dullness, sleepy look of eyes. Eyes, red sore aching, suffused. Eyes red and watery. ***Heavy, drooping eyelids.*** Ptosis, can hardly open eyes. Ptosis due to congestion of brain, exhaustion. ***Orbital neuralgia with contraction and twitching of muscles.*** Bruised pain back of orbits. Disturbed eye muscular apparatus. ***Serous inflammations***. Eyeballs sore when moving them. Eyeballs oscillate laterally when using them. Deep inflammations with haziness of vitreous. Photophobia worse sun or gaslight. Asthenopia. Glaucoma. Blepharitis and conjunctival hyperemia. Descemetitis. Retinitis. Detached retina from injury or myopia. Serous choroiditis. One pupil dilated, the other contracted. Yellow color of eyes.

Face - Face looks fatigued, droopy. ***Hot, heavy, flushed, besotted-looking*** (Bapt., Op.). Dusky hue of face with vertigo and dim vision. Neuralgia of face. Facial muscles contracted, especially around the mouth. Trigeminal neuralgia after exposure on a cold damp day. Chin quivers. Lower jaw dropped, wags sideways. Shooting pains in jaws. Facial paralysis. Erythema of face and neck. Sore, acute, red pimples on face.

Female - Menses retarded, pain extends to back and hips. ***Dysmenorrhea with scanty flow.*** Dysmenorrhea preceded by sick headache, vomiting, bearing down in abdomen. Menorrhagia, almost continuous flow, without any pain. Suppressed menses with nosebleeds. Epileptiform convulsions at menstrual period or from suppressed menses (Oean.). Uterus heavy sore, feels as if squeezed (Cham., Nux-v.,

Ust.). Cramps in abdomen and legs during pregnancy. Threatened miscarriage from sudden depressing emotions. False labor-pains, pains pass up back. ***Inefficient labor pains or none at all.*** Labor pains go up, backward or down the thighs. Nervous chills during first stage of labor. ***Rigidity of os during labor*** (Bell.). As if a wave from uterus to throat with choking feeling, impedes labor. Severe after-pains. Twitching of muscles of the whole body with drowsiness, before puerperal convulsions. Deep yellow leucorrhea with aching across lower part of the back. White leucorrhea, with fullness in uterine region. White leucorrhea with aching across lower part of back. Leucorrhea in gushes, day and night. Leucorrhea with constipation. Sex difficult from contraction of the vaginal muscles. Vaginismus.

Food - Low appetite and thirst. ***Thirstlessness with trembling***. Thirst with sweat, but not with fever. Difficult swallowing of warm food. Vertigo worse smoking. Sleeplessness from smoking. Headache worse wine. Eye symptoms worse wine.

Head - ***Dull headache with influenza.*** Headache coming on suddenly, with dimness of sight or diplopia. ***Sensation as if a band*** around head with occipital headache. ***Dull, heavy ache with heaviness of eyelids***. Bruised sensation. Sick headache. Headache worse mental exertion, heat of sun, lying with head low. ***Nervous headaches from emotional excitement.*** Headache better pressure and lying with head high. Wants to have head raised on pillow. ***Pain in temple, extending into ear*** and nose, chin. Headache with muscular soreness of neck and shoulders. Headache preceded by blindness. ***Headache better profuse urination.*** Headache with faintness. Hemicrania preceded by great sensitiveness to noise. ***Occipital headaches.*** Delirious on falling asleep. Meningitis, congestive stage, pain at the back of head and dilated pupils. Fontanels pulsate strongly. Swollen feeling in head. Scalp sore to touch. Threatened or actual stroke, with stupor, coma and paralysis.

Heart - Feeble heart, slow heart's action with cold hands and feet. As if blood had ceased to circulate. ***A feeling as if it were necessary to keep in motion or else heart's action would cease***. Pain in heart on rising from seat. Palpitations and oppression of heart, worse when thinking of it. Hysterical palpitations. Sore pain in heart. Sharp pains in region of heart. Pulse soft, weak, full and flowing. Slow pulse (Dig., Kalm., Apoc.), greatly accelerated on motion. ***Weak, slow pulse of old age.*** Pulse slow, full, soft, compressible.

Kidneys - Pain in region of kidneys, as if produced by pressure of a blunt instrument. Kidney pain during fever. Constant urination, hysterical. Spasmodic affection of ureters from passage of calculi. ***Urine profuse, clear, watery, with chilliness and trembling.*** Urine much increased in quantity. Urine stream intermittent. Albuminuria.

Limbs - Fatigue of limbs after slight exercise. ***Deep-seated, aching, in bones and joints.*** Myalgia from overexertion. Loss of power of muscular control. ***Excessive trembling and weakness of all the limbs.*** Heavy sensation in lower limbs. Knees weak worse descending tottering gait, cannot direct his legs. ***Muscle aches, chills and fatigue with influenza.*** Hard aching in humerus (right). Feeling of partial luxation of patella when walking. ***Numbness and weakness of limbs.*** Wandering, rheumatic pains. Cramps in muscles of the forearm. Coldness of wrists and hands. Hot, dry, numb hands, especially palms. Wants hands in cool water. Neuralgic pains in limbs, after scarlatina. Professional neurosis. Writer's cramp.

Liver - ***Hepatitis with chronic fatigue.*** Passive congestion of liver with vertigo, dim sight and fullness of head. Griping pain in gall bladder. Deficient secretion of bile. Jaundice with prostration and clay-colored stools.

Lungs - Heavy, labored breathing. Tiresome, slow breathing. Slow breathing with great prostration. Acute bronchitis. ***Dyspnea and great chilliness.*** Respiration quickened. Spasmodic disorders of lungs and diaphragm. Spasmodic asthma. Oppressed breathing with cold hands and feet. ***Sudden sensation of suffocation.*** Extreme restlessness from threatened suffocation, demands for fresh air. Sudden and severe attacks of dyspnea, with crowing noise, profuse sweat and dark flushed face. Scanty expectoration of mucus.

Male - Genitals cold, relaxed (Ph-ac.). Continually profuse warm sweat on scrotum. Dragging pain in testes. Gonorrhea, in first stage, discharge scanty, tendency to corrode, much heat, smarting at meatus. Whitish discharge in gonorrhea. Suppressed gonorrhea, with fever, rheumatism, orchitis. Excitable sexual desire. ***Spermatorrhea without erections***. Spermatorrhea during stool. Too early ejaculation during sex. Sexual power exhausted, slightest caress causes an emission.

Modalities - ***Better from profuse urination.*** Better alcoholic drinks, stimulants. Better mental efforts. Better open air. Better sweating. Better shaking. Better bending forwards. Better continued motion. Better reclining. Better with head held high. Better in afternoon. ***Worse emotions or excitement.*** Worse surprise, anxiety. Worse shocks, ordeals. ***Worse bad news.*** Worse from tobacco smoking. Worse dentition. Worse motion. ***Worse from anticipation.*** Worse thinking of his ailments. Worse damp weather. ***Worse humid weather, spring.*** Worse fog. Worse before a thunderstorm. Worse heat of sun. Worse summer. Worse at 10 a.m. Worse periodically.

Mouth - Dryness of mouth, must swallow frequently. Putrid taste and breath. Bitter taste. Taste, clammy and feverish during the sweat. Saliva yellow as from blood. Muscles of mouth seem contracted. ***Speech thick, as if drunk, he can hardly speak.*** Sore mouth, with febrile and catarrhal states, intermittent or remittent type. Roof of mouth feels, as if swollen.

Nose - Disposition to catch colds and influenza, with every change of weather. Spring and summer colds. ***Acute coryza with dull headache and fever.*** Coryza with thin acrid watery discharge. Stuffed nose. ***Coryza with influenza.*** Sneezing, fullness at root of nose. ***Sneezing, early morning.*** Swelling of turbinates. Nosebleed with suppressed menses. Sensation as if hot water flowing from the nostrils. Hay fever. Watery, excoriating discharge. Nasal catarrh, with prostration, with sore throat. Nasal voice. Coryza in changeable weather. Itching and tickling in soft palate and naso-pharynx. Dryness of nose.

Perspiration - Sweats freely from slight exertion. Cold sweat. Sweat coming gradually and moderately, always relieves pains. Sometimes profuse, with languor and prostration. Sweats at night. Night sweats of tuberculosis. Most profuse sweat on genitals. Sticky sweat.

Rectum - Partial paralysis of rectum and sphincter. Paralysis of the anal sphincter. Prolapse rectum. Rectal pains after labor. Passage of flatus before stool. Diarrhea, painless in nervous persons. ***Diarrhea after sudden emotions as grief, fright, bad news.*** Diarrhea during dentition. Urging to stool caused by exciting news. Disposition to go to stool whenever anything startles her. ***Diarrhea from anticipation of an unusual ordeal*** (Arg-n., Ph-ac.). Painless or involuntary stools. Copious yellow stools. ***Stools, cream colored.*** Stool papescent, dark yellow. ***Stools, tea-green***. Stools yellow, bilious, clay-colored.

Sensations - Lightness of head or body. As if the head were enlarged. As if there were a tape around the head. As if the skin were contracted in the middle of the forehead. As if a lump were in throat which could not be swallowed. As if a lump were in the esophagus. Load in stomach. As if stomach were quite gone. As if the uterus were squeezed by a hand. As if he would die, as if the blood ceased to circulate, as if the heart would stop unless he kept moving. As if a knife were thrust through from occiput to forehead. As if eyes were jumping out of head.

Skin - Papular eruption, like measles. Itching of skin, without eruption, worse at night and from warmth. Hot dry, moist, yellow, itching, measles-like eruption. Erysipelas.

Measles, catarrhal symptoms, aids in bringing out eruption. Measles with cerebral symptoms. ***Retrocedent measles, with livid spots***. Livid spots. Scarlet fever with stupor and flushed face. Erythema of face and neck. Pimples on forehead and neck. Pimples like small cutaneous indurations. Rubeola.

Sleep - Sleepless from nervous irritation (Coff.). ***Insomnia from mental excitement***, uncontrollable thinking or tobacco. ***Insomnia from exhaustion.*** Sleepless from itching. Sleeplessness during dentition. Sleeplessness in delirium tremens. ***Heavy, stupid sleep.*** Cannot get fully to sleep. Restless sleep, worse toward morning. Starts on falling to sleep. ***Drowsiness with influenza.*** Delirious on falling asleep. Incoherent talking during half awake state. Sleepiness of students. Languor and drowsiness when trying to study. Sudden shrill cries on awaking in meningitis. Awakens from sleep with headache or colic. Yawning. Night terrors from nose being stopped up and dry. Unpleasant dreams after midnight. Sexual dreams with nocturnal emissions. Dreams followed next day by great languor and irritability. Dreams with pain at base of brain.

Stomach - Sour eructations. ***Feeling of emptiness or weakness in the stomach***. Flatulence of stomach. Rumbling and dull pain. Cramps in stomach, worse riding or sitting erect. Hiccough, worse evening. Tenderness of stomach with vomiting.

Teeth - Toothache from a cold. ***Toothache with nervous excitement.*** Toothache with a weak and trembling condition. Toothache, purely nervous. Pains from teeth extend to temple. Pains come in paroxysms. Neuralgic pains and darts through jaws and face. Toothache with congestion of head and face. ***Dentition, child frantic, awakens with sudden screams.*** Gums swollen and tender. Child frantic at times, when gums are examined.

Temperature - Chills, without thirst, along spine. ***Influenza with chills, muscular soreness, great prostration and headache.*** Chill with aching and languor, mixed with heat or alternating with heat. ***Chills up and down back.*** Wave-like chills, extending upward from sacrum to occiput. ***Wants to be held, because he shakes so much***. Cold hands and feet. Coldness so severe as to be painful. ***Nervous chills***. Nervous, shuddering, chills, preceded by visual disturbances. ***Nervous chills during labor.*** Heat and sweat stages, long and exhausting. ***Fever with drowsiness.*** Bilious remittent, malarial, typhoid, cerebro-spinal fevers. ***Fever and thirstlessness.*** Measles, influenza and colds. ***Fever with a stupor, dizziness, faintness, and weakness.*** Fever with nervous restlessness. Fever with intense burning. ***Wants to lie still and rest with influenza.***

Throat - Throat feels rough, burning. ***Pain from throat to ear***. Swallowing causes pain in ear (Hep., Nux-v.). Difficult swallowing. Inability to swallow or speak. ***Feeling of a painful lump in throat*** that cannot be swallowed. Sore throat during menses. Tonsils swollen and very red. Tonsillitis from acute catarrh. Tonsillitis, shooting pain into ears. ***Post-diphtheria paralysis***. Paralytic dysphagia, especially worse from warm food. ***Spasms of glottis,*** long crowing inspiration, sudden and forcible expiration. Dryness of throat with hoarseness. Hoarseness after depressing emotions. Hoarseness during menses. Burning pain in larynx and chest, when coughing. Larynx raw, as if ulcerated. Aphonia. ***Loss of voice from fright.*** Loss of voice, with dryness and burning in throat.

Tongue - Thick, yellow coating on tongue. ***Tongue numb and trembles while protruding.*** Edges of tongue red, centre white. Tongue inflamed in middle. Tongue brown, nearly clear. Tongue thick, coated, yellowish, paralysed.

Vertigo - Vertigo on rising, lightheaded, worse by sudden movement of the head and walking. ***Dizziness and blurred vision***. Vertigo spreads from occiput, as if drunk with visual symptoms. Staggering as if intoxicated when trying to move, worse from smoking. Vertigo with loss of sight, chilliness, accelerated pulse, dullness of vision, double vision. Vertigo of child on being carried.

Vision - ***Dim vision.*** Dim vision during pregnancy. Blurring and discomfort in eyes even after accurately adjusted glasses. ***Slow accommodation of vision.*** Vision blurred, smoky (Cycl., Phos.). ***Blurred vision with pain above eyes.*** Obscured vision on stooping. Blind spells. Blindness with dilated pupils. ***Double vision***, when looking sideways. Diplopia during headache. Diplopia during pregnancy. ***Diplopia with multiple sclerosis.*** Affections of vision before migraine. Pupils dilated and insensible to light. ***Hysterical amblyopia***. Amaurosis after stroke. Amaurosis from masturbation. Astigmatism. Vision dim, can neither read nor write, words run together. Sees swimming black specks. Misty or glimmering appearance. Distant objects seem indistinct, when riding or walking.

COMMENTS - Overall fatigue with a sense of fright. Ailments due to bad news and fright (Op.), fright causes weakness. Acute shock, shaking and trembling. Trembling with fear. Incontinence with fear. Fear of failure, acute fear or panic (Acon.). Anticipatory anxiety.

Convalescence. Chronic fatigue ever since a viral infection (Ph-ac.), especially if the limbs feel heavy, exhaustion. Ailments from flu shots. For the elderly who become weak, frail, and lose confidence after infections.

Viral infections, particularly influenza, mono, meningitis, and hepatitis, with tiredness and weakness. Sore throats, worse swallowing. Coryza and hay fever with early morning sneezing and streaming colds. Catarrh generally occurs in warm, moist, relaxing weather.

Major influenza remedy. Influenza epidemics and for prevention. Dizzy drowsy, droopy and dumb. Slow onset of flu symptoms. Influenza infections with tiredness and weakness. Apathy and indifferance during the flu. Wants to be alone and quiet when sick. Sore throats and colds. Fever without thirst. Muscle aches and weakness. Influenza with dull headaches. Never well since influenza, chronic fatigue. Worse since flu vaccinations.

Paralysis. Excessive weakness and trembling. Weakness and paralysis of the limbs, the limbs feel heavy, with trembling. Keynote tremors. Multiple sclerosis. Neuralgic problems. Epileptic attacks beginning with a throbbing headache.

Headaches with a heavy feeling, dizziness. Sensation of a band around their head. Throbbing headaches, particularly in the occiput and forehead. Nondescript headache with dullness. Headache begins in the occiput and spreads over the whole head, settling down over the eyes.

Migraine headaches with double vision, weakness, and nausea. Violent headache may occur if needing to urinate at night and not doing so. Headache with stiff neck, worse morning, better urinating, with irregular action of the eye muscles. Double vision, dimness of vision. Ptosis of the eyelids.

Vertigo. Dizziness from weakness, especially during viral infections, flus, and colds. Drowsy. Sense of dullness, apathy. Low stamina. Aversion to the least effort. Neurotic symptoms in cigar-makers, with impotence, palpitations. Drug overdose resulting in a stupor or coma.

Paralysis of the tongue, trembling of the tongue, particularly in typhoid cases. The tongue is thinly coated. Dry lips. Face is flushed (less that Bapt.). Itching of the skin, measles-like eruptions. Measles and eruptive disorders with drowsy state, suffused face, and convulsions.

Thirstlessness with low fevers. Cold extremities. Chills up and down the spine. Trembling and shaking, can be from extreme exhaustion. Euphoria followed by weakness. Generally a slow onset, with aches and pains, especially after exerting themselves.

Nervous diarrhea due to stress, worry and anxiety. Stools generally yellow, whether diarrhea or constipation. Nervous heartburn and colic. Hysterical dysphagia or aphonia after emotions.

Dysmenorrhea, epileptiform convulsions during menstrual period, rigid os in labor, chill, beginning in hands or feet and running up back. Aggravation before, during, and after menses.

Aversion to noise and light, desire to be left alone. Desires fresh air (Bry., Lyc., Ars.).Wants to lie down and rest. Wants to be held, that he may not shake. Must be covered in all stages of the paroxysm.

Worse thinking about their symptoms. Complaints from sudden changes of weather, particularly from hot or dry to damp air. Worse sunlight, heat of the sun, summer, damp weather, cold, damp atmosphere, fog. Great distress and apprehensive feeling at approach of a thunderstorm.

Symptoms may be better urinating. Better from stimulants, especially alcoholic. Cold drinks are vomited immediately, but warm or spirituous drinks can be swallowed. Pain at the back of the head is better from hot applications.

Motion aggravates most symptoms, but alleviates muscular heart pains. Rising from a seat causes pain in the heart. Heaviness of the head is better from shaking the head. Lifting the arms causes trembling of the hands. Playing the piano causes a tired sensation in the arms.

J. H. Nankivell drank two ounces of tincture of Gels. instead of a glass of sherry. He walked a few feet with assistance and in another minute his legs were paralyzed. He dragged himself to the bedside with his arms, but they were unable to help him to bed into which he had to be lifted.

As long as he lay quiet there was no trouble, but on the least exertion there were excessive tremors. Vomiting occurred during the next twenty-four hours. Temperature rose to 101.5° F. Heart's action very violent and intermittent.

All the muscles of the eyes were affected, but, of voluntary muscles, those of the right side suffered most. Prolonged conversation involved paralysis of upper lip. There was somnolence, absence of mental excitement and good appetite.

The effects passed away in the order of occurrence from below upwards, but after the arms had recovered, vision was not perfect for twenty-four hours.

A patient of Clarke once took a drachm of the tincture for a headache. On going out, he could not tell which side of the street he was on. He was near St. Paul's Cathedral and saw two cathedrals instead of one.

J. G. Blackley pointed out the suitability of Gels. to writer's cramp and professional paralyzes. Clarke relieved with it cases of Dupuytren's contraction.

Erskine White cured an infant born in convulsions three weeks after its mother had been terribly frightened by seeing her little brother nearly burnt to death.

The only guiding symptom was "the child's chin quivered incessantly." In thirty seconds after the dose the quivering ceased, in three minutes the convulsions were at an end.

White had to ride twelve miles over mountains to reach the patient after receiving the summons, so the convulsions must have lasted a considerable time.

RELATIONS - ***Antidotes:*** Atrop, Chin., Coff., Dig., Nux-m. Coff., Dig., Alcoholic stimulants relieve all complaints where Gels. is useful. In cases of poisoning, artificial respiration and faradization of respiratory muscles. Foy found Nitro-glycerine a perfect antidote in one case. Jephson antidoted his case with Strychnine. ***It antidotes:*** Mag-p. It antagonizes: Atrop., Op. ***Compare:*** (1) Bell - labor, Caul., Caust. - complaints of women, Cocc., Con., Cur. - paralysis. (2) Ferr-p. - fever, Phos. - effect of thunderstorms, Ol-an., Verat. - headache, Bor. - sense of falling. (3) Bry. - typhoid, dreads movement, Gels. because he is so weak, Bry. because movement worse pains. (4) Hyper. worse from fog. Ign. - gastric disorders of cigar makers, Bapt., Ip., Acon., Cimic., Mag-p. (5) Culx. - vertigo on blowing the nose with fullness of the ears. ***Compatible:*** Bap. (in typhoid influenza), Ip. (in dumb ague).

REFERENCES - Boericke. Clarke. Hale. Murphy. Phatak.

GENISTA TINCTORIA

(Dyer's Weed)

PHARMACY - genist. Genista tinctoria. Dyer's weed. Dyer's greenweed. N. O. Leguminose. Papilionoideae. Contains scopolamine. Tincture of whole plant. ***Historical dose:*** Tincture and all potencies.

CLINICAL - Diarrhea. Earache. Headache.

HOMEOPATHIC - Genista was proved by E. B. Cushing. It has been used for frontal headaches and vertigo, worse motion, better open air and eating. Dry throat. Awakes with waterbrash. Promotes diuresis in dropsical conditions. Urgent desire for stool, which is expelled suddenly.

Sharp, piercing pains in the head and ear. Brain feels loose. Sensitive feeling in brain, eye and throat. A peculiar eruption of dark, red, confluent spots. Itching eruption on elbows, knees and ankles.

Modalities - Better in the open air. Better cool rooms. Better by eating (headache). Worse from rising. Worse turning quickly. Worse shaking head. Worse walking.

RELATIONS - ***Compare:*** (1) Brain feels loose, Cic-v., Nat-s., Bar-c., Rhus-t.

REFERENCES - Clarke.

GENTIAN

(Bach Flower Essence)

PHARMACY - gent-b. Gentian. Gentiana amarella. Flowers are picked, floated on to a bowl of water and left standing in the sun for several hours. The strained water is used as medicine. ***Historical dose:*** Take two drops from the stock bottle into a one ounce dropper bottle, (add brandy or alcohol, if this bottle will be used for days or weeks). This is the dosage bottle, take a few drops straight into the mouth or as needed in a little water or juice.

HOMEOPATHIC - Gent-b., together with Cer-b., Scler-b., Gors-b., Horn-b., and Wld-o-b., belongs to Bach's group of ***For Those who Suffer Uncertainty***. Doubts and uncertainties over daily affairs. Doubtful and discouraged about the slow process of cure. Lack of physical stamina.

MIND - Easily discouraged. Weakened capacity for perseverance. Lack of courage, inner stamina and faith. Disheartened as soon as hindrances arise. Lack of centeredness, self assurance, willpower. Tendency to give up. Lack of interest. Tendency to exaggerate, especially small setbacks. Sadness or depression.

REFERENCES - Bach.

GENTIANA CRUCIATA

(Cross-leaved Gentian)

PHARMACY - gent-c. Gentiana cruciata. Cross-leaved gentian. Kreutz-Enzian. N. O. Gentianacae. Tincture of root. ***Historical dose:*** Tincture and all potencies.

CLINICAL - Belching. Diarrhea. Dyspepsia. Dysphagia. Hernia. Hoarseness. Stiff neck. Stomach, affection. Throat, sore.

HERBAL - The Treasury of Botany stated "Gent. cruciata has been invested with imaginary virtues, because its leaves grow in the form of a cross, it has been recommended in hydrophobia."

HOMEOPATHIC - Gentiana cruciata's reputation as a remedy for hydrophobia is partly justified in the provings. It also has throat and stomach symptoms. Dysphagia, vertigo with headache, pressing inward sensation in eyes. Constricted of the throat, head and abdomen. Distention, fullness and tightness in abdomen. Creeping over body as from fleas.

MIND - Weeping mood with disinclination to talk. Very peculiar anxiety, acceleration and difficulty of breathing, swelling of the temporal veins and feeling of pressure in the temporal region. On reading, print seemed indistinct and as if covered with a veil.

Abdomen - Sensitive, griping, sore sensation in umbilical region, better sitting and lying, worse after dinner or smoking, standing, or walking, obliging him to bend forward, therewith umbilicus seemed to be drawn inward. Distention, fullness, tightness and constriction. Dragging in right inguinal region with feeling of protrusion, very sensitive.

Back - Drawing and jerking along right side of neck, extending to shoulder. Drawing in cervical muscles, extending to ears, worse by turning head, an uneasiness so that he could not remain long in one position. Tension in lumber region.

Eyes - Sensation as though eyes were lying deep in orbit, piercing inward sensation in right eye. Print indistinct, as if covered with a veil.

Female - Menstruation three days earlier than usual, during which there was a headache as if head too full with feeling of distention in the skull, better during rest and worse by motion, preventing sleep for a long time.

Food - Appetite increased or lost.

Head - Sensitiveness of whole head and brain after dinner, worse by violent motion of the head. Swelling of temporal veins and feeling of pressure in temporal region. Sudden stitch through left temple. Distressing tension and at times transient jerking in region of vertex, tension soon became a very acute constant pressure, worse by exerting eyes or constant thought.

Limbs - Distressing drawing in right shoulder lasting several minutes. Cramp-like pains in soles of feet.

Modalities - Better from drinking fresh water. Better warm soup. Better open air. Worse after eating.

Mouth - Two aphthous ulcers on margin of lower lip on either side of frenum. Increased flow of saliva.

Rectum - Movings about in intestines with slight headache, followed by copious pasty evacuation. Constant violent urging, followed by watery evacuations. Pasty diarrhea and stools without the usual itching in anus.

Stomach - Burning, fullness, pressure in stomach. Pressure in stomach as if a stone were in it with inclination to vomit. Sensation of pressing inward in pit of stomach. Acid belchings, watery vomiting. Great nausea with inclination to lie down. Vomiting with some difficulty, a small quantity of mucus of an acid odor intensely bitter, leaving a scraping and rawness in throat.

Throat - Frequent attacks of hoarseness and sensitiveness of the throat. Weak voice. Slight redness and distressing sensation of constriction within the throat, swallowing is very difficult. Rawness and scrapings, causing frequent hawking with constriction when swallowing. Intermittent, deep redness of fauces. Stitches in tonsils.

Vertigo - Confusion and whirling.

COMMENTS - The proving developed a number of striking symptoms in the throat and digestive tract. Movings about in stomach and abdomen. Pressure in the stomach as if a stone was in it with inclination to vomit.

All the symptoms of right inguinal hernia occurred in one prover. A peculiar sense of anxiety, faintness, uneasiness. One prover felt as if all the nerves were tense, so that walking was difficult. Creeping over the body as from fleas in the evening.

RELATIONS - ***Compare:*** (1) Gent-l., Lyc. - better from warm drink. (2) Bry., Puls. (3) Abies-n., - pressure in stomach as from a stone. (4) Kali-bi. - tenacious mucus in throat. (5) Gent-q. (6) Hydr., Nux-v. (7) Epip. - thick saliva.

REFERENCES - Boericke. Clarke.

GENTIANA LUTEA
(Yellow Gentian)

PHARMACY - gent-l. Gentiana lutea. Yellow gentian. N. O. Gentianacae. Tincture of root. ***Historical dose:*** Tincture and all potencies.

CLINICAL - ***Anorexia.*** Biliousness. Colic. Debility. Diarrhea. Dyspepsia. Fever. Gout. Headaches. Stomach, disorders. Throat, constriction.

HERBAL - The yellow gentian is the source of the well-known tonic of herbal practice; it may cause increased the appetite in the healthy.

HOMEOPATHIC - Chief symptoms from the provings were in the alimentary sphere, including ***ravenous hunger*** as well as ***a diminished appetite.*** Marked stomach symptoms. Aching in the eyes and throat. Dry, thick saliva. Dry mouth, bitter or earthy taste, nausea, vomiting, colic. Diarrhea with yellow stools, rheumatic pains, sensations of constriction are marked and common. Febrile conditions.

MIND - Dull feeling of whole body. Morose mood, general dejection. Confusion while writing.

Abdomen - Inflation and tension of stomach and abdomen (Poth.). Colic, umbilical region sensitive to touch. Flatulence.

Back - Pain in the back and bowels, much worse by motion, better by sitting. Sensation of a cord or pressure and weight around the loins.

Chest - Oppression of the chest, fullness in the chest, sometimes with pressure and difficulty of respiration. Pressure on left side near the throat.

Eyes - Pressure in eyeballs. Frequent aching in the eyes. Redness of the conjunctiva. Obscuration of the sight for some moments, so that objects immediately before the eyes cannot be distinguished, could not see the person with whom he was talking for a few moments.

Head - Frontal headache, better eating and open air. Brain feels loose, head tender.

Limbs - Rheumatic tension and dragging in the right hand, with inflammatory redness of two articulations of the fingers, spasmodic symptoms and pain of the part during movement.

Modalities - Worse in the afternoon. Worse after eating. Worse on motion.

Mouth - Dryness of the month and throat, saliva thicker than usual. Intensely bitter, earthy taste. Swelling, fine sticking in throat, mostly in posterior portion of plate.

Nose - Irritation in nose, as in coryza, followed by a watery discharge.

Rectum - Urgent inflation to evacuate, sometimes sudden, with abundant stools, followed by painful sensitiveness of the abdomen, pressure on the anus while wanting to go to stool. Dragging towards anus with tenesmus. Sudden urging with copious evacuation.

Sleep - Yawning. Inclination to sleep without power to go to sleep. Uneasy sleep disturbed by abdominal symptoms and fever. Sleep impeded by colic, which obliges the patient to turn in bed, sometimes on one side and sometimes on the other.

Stomach - Acid risings, ravenous hunger, nausea, weight and aching in stomach.

Stool - Stool soft, yellow, preceded by colicky pains, which become so severe after the stool that they force the patient to bend double. Soft stools, immediately after rising. Bilious diarrhea in afternoon.

Temperature - Febrile shuddering, as from electric shocks, followed by lassitude, depression and tension in the limbs. Increase of natural heat in head, cheeks and whole body. Heat originating in the lumber vertebrae. Pulse accelerated.

Throat - Frequent hawking of mucus, which is difficult to loose. Rawness, roughness of the throat. Hoarseness.

Vertigo - Vertigo is worse from rising or motion. Vertigo better in the open air.

RELATIONS - ***Compare:*** (1) Gent-q. (2) Gent. l., Hydr., Nux-v., Epip. - thick saliva.

REFERENCES - Boericke. Clarke.

GENTIANA QUINQUEFLORA

(Five-flowered Gentian)

PHARMACY - gent-q. Gentiana quinquefolia. Five-flowered gentian. Gall of the earth. N. O. Gentianacae. Decoction of the herb. Tincture of fresh plant in flower September, October. ***Historical dose:*** Tincture and all potencies.

CLINICAL - Anorexia. Cholera infantum. Dyspepsia. Intermittent fever. Weakness.

HERBAL - Gent-q. is a pleasant bitter and appears, like the other Gentians, to be a positive tonic. It has a popular reputation in Ohio and other parts of the United States as an anti-periodic and tonic. Valuable tonic for old cases of dyspepsia and torpid liver.

Dr. Yelvington of Susquehanna, who said he learned its value from a tribe of Native Americans, said it has succeeded in obstinate intermittents where quinine and other anti-periodics had failed. He used the decoction of the herb, but a fluid extract or the saturated tincture is a better form for administration in fever.

Yelvington also used it in cases of infantile fever and cholera infantum. "As a tonic in enfeebled patients and in chronic diseases, it is a remedy par excellence, appearing to exert an action over organs of nutrition and assimilation, as well as being a stimulant to the excretory organs."

REFERENCES - Boericke. Clarke.

GERANIUM MACULATUM

(Wild Cranesbill)

PHARMACY - ger. Geranium maculatum. Wild cranesbill. N. O. Geraniaceae. Tincture and triturations of root. Infusion of the plant. ***Historical dose:*** Tincture and all potencies.

CLINICAL - Diarrhea. Diplopia. Dysentery. Headaches. ***Hemorrhages.*** Leucorrhea. ***Migraines.*** Ptosis. Stool, ineffectual. Throat, sore. ***Ulcers.*** Vomiting.

HERBAL - Geranium maculatum, in the herbal tinctures and lower potencies, has been used successfully in cases of hemorrhage from various parts, nose, stomach and lungs. It has also been used for chronic diarrhea and leucorrhea.

Locally in ulcers, it will destroy the pyogenic membrane.

HOMEOPATHIC - Under the use of the drug, the blood in hemorrhages becomes darker, clots more easily and is much less in quantity. The root contains both tannic and gallic acids.

There are two fragmentary provings of Ger. one made with root preparations, one with infusion of the plant. The chief symptoms observed have been diplopia and other disorders of vision and a constant and ineffectual desire for stool.

Migraines, habitual sick headaches. ***Profuse, hemorrhages,*** pulmonary and from different organs. Vomiting of blood. ***Ulceration of stomach. Atonic and foul ulcers.*** Summer complaints.

Breasts - Sore nipples (Eup-a.).

Eyes - Ptosis and dilated pupils. Fullness in the eyes. Great difficulty in walking with eyes open, though he could walk with them closed.

Female - Menses too profuse. Post-partum hemorrhage.

Head - Giddiness with diplopia, better closing eyes. Sick headache. Slight pain in occiput, low down.

Mouth - Dry mouth. Tip of tongue dry and burning.

Rectum - Constant desire to go to stool with inability to pass anything for some time. Chronic diarrhea with offensive mucus. Constipation.

Stomach - Catarrhal gastritis with profuse secretion. ***Lessens the vomiting in gastric ulcers.*** Tendency to ulceration and passive hemorrhage.

Throat - Pharyngitis.

Vertigo - Vertigo with diplopia. Vertigo better closing eyes. Vertigo with blurred vision and constant ineffectual urging to stool.

RELATIONS - ***Compare:*** (1) Ger. - Constant hawking and spitting in elderly people. (2) Erod. - a popular hemostatic in Russia and especially used for metrorrhagia and menorrhagia. (3) Hydrin., Cinch., Sabin. (4) Ham., Hydr., Hematoxylin., Rat., Fic., Erod.

REFERENCES - Boericke. Clarke.

GERMANIUM METALLICUM

PHARMACY - germ. Germanium metallicum. ***Historical dose:*** All potencies.

CLINICAL - Amyloidosis. Anemia. Arthritis. Bronchitis. Cancer. Diabetes. Headaches. Hypertension. Kidney, failure. Malaria. Palpitations. Paralysis. Pneumonia.

HOMEOPATHIC - Severe illnesses with dysfunction of nerves, liver, kidney. Demyelinisation of the nerves. Numbness. Ataxia, cerebellum. Chronic fatigue. ***Extreme weakness, as if the vital force is leaving the body.*** Feeling of heaviness, present throughout the pathogenesis.

MIND - Absent minded. Mentally slow and confused. Forgetful. Cannot adapt. Inept. Incapability. Makes mistakes in writing and speaking. Dyslexia. Difficulties with concentration, confusion. The answer is there but it can not come out.

Moody. Feels weak, dull, empty, flat. Indifferent. Everything appears unreal. Lack of romantic feelings. Hopeless. Feels helpless. ***Guilty feelings.*** Self reproach, hates himself. Disgusted with himself. Gloomy. Doomed feelings. Restlessness.

Fear of responsibilities. Fear of being criticized. Fear of being a total failure. Fear of being unmasked. Fear of falling. Fear of paralysis.

Irritable when having to answer questions. Feeling of isolation. Feels like a stranger in society. Does not feel connected. Feels invaded, somebody has entered their territory. Feels trapped.

Emotions are strong but cannot come out or are kept under strict control. Suppressed anger or outburst of anger. ***Holding anger inside, aggravates.*** Such outburts are very quickly forgotten with no feeling of remorse.

Delusion, that he is a prisoner. Delusion that the world is shabby. Delusion that she estranged, isolated. Delusion, everything looks smaller or lower. Time going more slowly, Hearing voices. Delusions, hands don't belong to him.

Abdomen - Feels as if a lump in the solar plexus.

Back - Back spasms. Ache lower sacrum, left side, better stretching and deep pressure. Tension in neck as if nerve was trapped. Aching back of neck extending to right side of occiput, tender to touch, better massage. On waking, intense pain between last cervical and first thoracic vertebrae. Twinges of pain. Muscles feel sore on pressure. Sudden sharp pains appear and disappear quickly. Sharp pain on waking, like a sharp point in shoulder, worse turning head to right. Sharp pain, left scapula. Spasm, left lumbar region, extending to leg.

Bladder - Cutting, pressing pain in the right side of the bladder.

Blood - Hemolysis. ***Anemia.*** High blood pressure. Amyloidosis.

Breasts - Tenderness in breasts. Wart on right breast with cheesy discharge. Sharp pain in right nipple. Sharp pain in right breast pulling from inside to outside. Sharp pain in left lower breast while walking in the open air. Sensation in right breast as if something is trying to come out through the duct.

Chest - Constriction in chest on coughing with clear expectoration. Pain on left side when coughing. Twinge, both breasts, lateral. Aching pain in lateral side of left breast. Aching pain in right breast. Aching on inspiration, worse bending, moving forward, lifting arm. Cramping lateral side right breast. Sensation of a lump in chest on waking. Tightness in the chest in a small spot. Tickling behind sternum.

Cough - Cough in evening. Cough better hot drinks. Dry cough, with tickle in throat while lying in bed, worse cold water. Dry cough in pairs, with irritation in throat. Dry, racking cough better lying down, with no expectoration. Dry, tickling cough. Hard, dry cough waking from sleep at night. Hollow, barking cough in bed. Sharp, tickling, barking cough, worse evening, cold drinks, better warm drinks. Spasm across lower abdomen with cough.

Ears - Aching pain moved into ear with pressure in both ear drums. Cracking in the ears from yawning. Pain, throbbing behind the ears. Sharp pain in right ear. Tightness in ear drum. Noises in ear. Ringing noise. Low, whispering sounds. Humming vibrating sound in head. Sensitive to noises.

Eyes - Burning pain with lachrymation and discharge from nose. Dry, gritty eyes. Burning and itching of eyelids. Cold sensation of the eyes. Eyes cold and watery as if exposed to a cold draft. Stiffness with swelling upper eyelids and below eyebrows. Cannot open eyes properly.

Face - Whole face swollen. Rash then extends behind ears. Face more greasy than usual. Purulent eruptions. Pain on cheekbone and above gum like sinusitis. Submaxillary glands swollen and sore to touch.

Female - Menses early. Pain-free menses. Menses started with brown-black discharge followed by red blood. Menses with protracted heavy flow. Dark clotting flow. Bright heavy clots on rising. Tiredness with ovulation. Tiredness during and after period. Leucorrhea thick and yellow. Vaginal discharge offensive. Internal itching with slight yellow discharge turning slightly pink. Itching in vulva. Irresistible itching around vagina. Itching bump on clitoris. White discharge from bump on clitoris. Flatus from vagina. Intense, tearing, bearing down pains in vagina and anal before menses. Sharp pain like hot needles lower abdomen and ovaries. Cramp-like labor pains. Pain before the flow starts, pacing and restlessness. Bleeding very scanty but clotted. Sudden stabbing pain right ovary. Twinge of pain in left ovary. Soreness in opening of vagina, worse by touch. Sexual desire increased. Heightened sexual sensations.

Food - Appetite increased.

Head - Headache with sharp, stabbing pains. Headache, worse moving. Head feels loose inside. Headache over left eye better cold bathing on waking. Head congestion with catarrhal symptoms. Heaviness sensation, occiput. Pressing pain in temples. Dull pain between the temples. Crawling sensation, right side of head. Light-headed, better eating. Slight dizziness in head with throbbing pain in temples. Dandruff and itchy scalp.

Heart - Palpitations. Palpitations could start at any moment, as if with anxiety in the chest.

Kidneys - Sudden stabbing pain, right kidney while sitting. Kidney injuries. Kidney failure. Diabetes. Frequent urination. Frequent urging for small amounts. Feeling of heat while passing urine. Stabbing sudden pain right kidney while sitting. Aromatic odor of urine. Powerful stream. Copious urine. Very dark urine with reddish hue and very strong smell. Concentrated, urine, with acid quality.

Limbs - Paralysis. Legs trembling. Inflammation of joints. Cold hands. Cold, wet, clammy feet. Feet very sweaty, odorless. Warm sensation of arms. Incoordination. Hands very dry rough and papery, palms red. Blood blister on finger, sore to touch. Itchy eruptions on shins, better in hot water. Rash slightly raised and a bit itchy, extending down arms. Itchy eruptions on right shin after shower or bath. Pimples on right buttock and thigh. Pain, aching in right shoulder as if bone is sensitive. Pain, aching, left hand near bone. Sciatic pain, leg, right, while standing. Aching in thigh muscles in bed. Knee pains, when walking, worse descending. Dragging pain in knee. Tension in knees when sitting. Stiffness, and soreness calves. Cramping pain in the right big toe. Prickling sensation in arms and hands.

Liver - Liver injuries.

Lungs - Pneumonia. Bronchitis. Soreness with slight wheeze in bronchi. Slow, deep respiration. Out of breath on climbing one flight of stairs. Sighing. Restriction in lungs with coughing. Funny sensation on breathing. Once the air passed through the throat felt fluttering sensation in chest and bronchi. Can't breathe deeply, air can't get through properly.

Male - Coldness in the whole penis with formication in the prepuce. Desire for sex with strong erection which remained long after emission. No sexual interest. Desire absent. Shooting pain in right testicle. Intense sharp pain in the tip of the prepuce of very short duration. Emissions smelling of fish. Emissions profuse.

Mouth - Dry mouth. Metallic taste in mouth, better glass of water. Greenish-white coating on the tongue and inside of upper lip. Salivation increased. Pain aching in jaw as if chewing something. Tingling in the middle of lower lip.

Nose - Itching of nose, external and internal, better rubbing. Abundant sneezing during coryza. Sneezing with watery coryza. Sneezing with mucus on waking. Head congestion with catarrhal symptoms. Nasal discharge clear and bland. Clear discharge following chest cough. Discharge thin watery pale and yellow. Nasal discharge salty.

Perspiration - Perspiration absent at night. Sweats during eating. Sweats with hot flushes. Perspiration from smelling soap.

Rectum - Itching of the anus. Constipation, difficult stool. Stools on alternate days. Stools alternating between hard and soft. Explosive flatulence. Flatulence offensive. Diarrhea and flatulence. Diarrhea with thirstlessness. Diarrhea, followed by increased energy. Intense pain in rectum from sexual excitement. Pressing tearing in rectum after stool, extending towards genitals. Sharp pain in rectum extends to ovaries, worse stool.

Skin - Rash on chest. Very fine itchy rash behind ears, worse left side. Inflamed pimples on skin of back. Molloscum contagiousum. Eruption red, soft, tender. Right palm very dry and flaky. Skin feels as if an ant were rapidly crawling, then biting. Tingling. Itching on the right side of the chin. Biting, prickling and itching after bath or shower. Swelling, on waking. Eyes swollen virtually shut, rash and swelling now extending to right side of face with red blotches and terrible burning, worse water, worse scratching and rubbing. Skin very oily all over. Skin greasy, and sticky, better washing.

Sleep - Sleepy, must lie down and sleep. Waking 3.30 a.m. Wakes at 5 a.m. Couldn't sleep. Sleep interrupted by cold feeling in the stomach. Stays awake in spite of sleepiness because of pain in the head and eyes. Sleep interrupted by splattering sound inside head. Sleeping on right side impossible with aching in kidney. Yawning constantly with sleepiness. Yawning, paroxysmal. Yawning, which provokes crackling in the ears. Yawning throughout day. Dreams of being pursued. Dreams of accidents. Dreams of war. Dreams of being raped. Dreams of burglars. Dreams of invasion.

Stomach - Eructations while eating. Eructations very bitter and sour. Stomach feels cold, better warm drinks. Stomach feels bloated and full of air during and after eating. Tightness in the stomach. Heaviness and bubbling pain in stomach after eating. Sore pain if pressed. Nausea, wobbly queasy feeling worse after eating. Nausea after drinking beer. Nausea better lying down. Vomits suddenly with extra salivation. Vomiting in morning. Vomiting after alcohol.

Stools - Stool yellow, loose and offensive, alternating with hard stool. Stool scanty, dry dark brown, with mucus. Loose stools. Stools frequent. Stools, frequent.

Teeth - Sharp cutting pain in all gums. Pain in teeth from cold water. Sharp pain in teeth. Sudden nerve pains in teeth and gums.

Throat - Sore throats, with much mucus. Sore and prickling throat on waking. Rasping, grating feeling in trachea while coughing and sneezing. Sore throat started in top of pharynx, worse eating oranges. Difficulty speaking.

Vertigo - Vertigo on turning head. Vertigo on writing and studying. Vertigo on going to bed, as soon as head hit the pillow. Vertigo worse closing eyes and opening again. Dizziness after massage.

Vision - Black in front of eyes on rising up from lying in the evening.

RELATIONS - ***Compare:*** (1) Gallium., Ferr.

REFERENCES - Sherr.

GETTYSBURG AQUA

(Gettysburg Mineral Spring)

PHARMACY - get. Gettysburg aqua. Gettysburg mineral spring salt from Gettysburg, Pennsylvania, USA. Trituration. ***Historical dose:*** Trituration and all potencies.

CLINICAL - Bone, disorders. Hip, disease. ***Ligaments, rigid***. Potts' disease. Scrofula. Ulcers.

HOMEOPATHIC - Magnesium sulphate is the predominant ingredient of Gettysburg aqua, but the water contains many salts of alkalis and earths with a number of metals. Contains lithium and silica, which it is similar to. Gettysburg aqua is indicated in the decay of vertebrae or the hip, ulceration of joints, when the discharge excoriates. Scrofulous children.

Sub-acute and chronic rheumatism. Sensation of rigidity. ***Ligaments rigid***. Worse stiffness of muscles on moving. Cannot remain long in one position. Stiffness of muscles on moving. Joints weak. Cannot lift things. ***Pain not perceived when quiet***. Pain in ligaments relieved by rest.

Stringy mucus from throat and posterior sinuses. ***Rawness***. Neck muscles rigid. Subacute gouty state. White coated tongue. High colored urine with red sandy sediment.

Modalities - Better rest. Worse in the morning. ***Worse from moving***, especially in lumbar region and joints of hips, shoulders and wrists.

RELATIONS - ***Compare:*** (1) Lyc., Phos. Rhus-t. (2) Puls., but modalities differ.

REFERENCES - Boericke. Clarke.

GEUM RIVALE

(Water Avens)

PHARMACY - geum. Geum rivale. Water avens. N. O. Rosacea. Tincture of the plant in flower. ***Historical dose:*** Tincture and all potencies.

CLINICAL - Bladder disorders. Penis, pains.

HOMEOPATHIC - Hering is the authority for this medicine. Disorders of bladder with pains in penis. Relaxed mucus membranes with excessive and depraved secretions. Worse eating, imperfect digestion and assimilation.

Tearing, jerking pains, which instantly unfit him for everything, seem to shoot from deep within the abdomen, below the umbilicus to the end of the urethra. They are like electric shocks, excessively severe and always occur twice in succession. As soon as he eats anything they return, then he is obliged to lie down.

REFERENCES - Clarke.

GINKGO BILOBA

(Maidenhair Tree)

PHARMACY - gink. Ginkgo biloba. Maidenhair tree. Galisburin adiantifolia. Ginkgo is a tree belonging to the Taxaceae family in the Conifer group. The tincture is prepared from the fresh leaves gathered in spring. ***Historical dose:*** Tincture and all potencies.

CLINICAL - ***Absent-minded.*** Asthma. Alzheimer's disease. Attention, weak. Brain, disorders. Concentration, poor. Dyslexia. Influenza. ***Memory, weak.*** Mental, weakness. Mumps. Laryngitis. Senility. Tonsillitis.

HERBAL - Gingko is indicated for the circulatory system and the brain. It is a well-known brain tonic that improves the cerebral blood flow and helps treat and prevent problems with memory, senility and mental dullness.

HOMEOPATHIC - The proving was carried out by E. A. Maury in 1933, with the mother tincture on seven provers (five men and two women), and with the 6th potency on two male provers.

Early stage of influenza. General numbness and shivering. Pain above the left orbital nerve. Burning pain in the pharynx and stomach. Urinary complaints. Vesicular, itching eruption.

MIND - Mental weakness. Exhausted. Sensation of mental fatigue (Sil.). Mental work is an effort to carry out. Poor concentration. Dullness of mind. ***Absent-minded and forgetful***. Senility. Alzheimer's disease. Loss of memory and inability to solve mental tasks.

Nebulous condition with the impression of unreality. Irrational fears with rapid speech. Needs to criticize others and himself. Suppressed anger with desire to tear up something (Staph.).

Abdomen - Abdomen tense and swollen. Pain in the region of the bladder and loins. Colic, followed by diarrhea-like stools. Intestinal diseases caused by worms.

Back - Pains at the nape of the neck, at the tips of the scapulae.

Ears - Buzzing noises.

Eyes - Eyeballs painful, especially on looking up and to the right. Sensation of impaired vision with a veil in front of the eyes. Ophthalmic migraine.

Female - Premature menses. Premenstrual lumbar pains. Leucorrhea.

Head - Frontal headache. Heaviness in the frontal region. Orbital neuralgia. Pain above the left orbital nerve. Sweating on the nape of the neck. Vertigo.

Limbs - General cramps and writer's cramp. Clenching of the right hand with trembling. Legs feel like jelly, feet feel icy.

Lungs - Difficult expectoration of thick sputum. Dyspnea. Laryngitis. Laryngeal irritation with cough. Asthma.

Male - Urethral discharge of yellowish pus. Diminished sex drive.

Modalities - Better from the heat, rest. Worse from cold. Worse walking. Worse drinking. Worse looking up and to the right. Worse right side. Worse around 2 a.m. to 3 a.m.

Mouth - Dry. Tongue yellow towards the root. Swallowing difficult with scraping sensation in the pharynx.

Rectum - Diarrhea-like stools. Worms. Sensation of heat in the anus.

Skin - Transient smallpox-like eruption. Vesicular, burning, itching eruption. Eczema.

Sleep - Heavy sleep with nightmares, dreams of corpses. Insomnia between 2 a.m. and 3 a.m.

Stomach - Sensation of emptiness in the stomach. Heaviness and burning in the stomach. Dyspepsia.

Throat - Pharyngitis. Congestion of the parotid glands. Rising pain along the line of the lower maxilla. Prickling pains in the left tonsil with need to clear the throat regularly.

COMMENTS - Useful during the early stages of influenza. Pale face with drawn features. General numbness and shivering. Pain above the left orbital nerve. Burning pain in the pharynx and stomach. Urinary complaints. Vesicular, itching eruption. Irrational fear and volubility.

RELATIONS - ***Compare:*** (1) Rhus-t. - general aching with constant need to move. Vesicular, burning, itching eruptions. (2) Canth. - burning in the mucus membranes. Eruption of burning vesicles. Dysuria. (3) Com. - Right ciliary neuralgia.

REFERENCES - Boericke. Clarke. Murphy.

GINSENG

(Wild Ginseng)

PHARMACY - gins. Ginseng. Wild ginseng. Panax quinquefolia. Panax ginseng. Aralia quinquefolia. Schinseng. N. O. Araliacee. Trituration and tincture of the root. ***Historical dose:*** Trituration, tincture and all potencies.

CLINICAL - Appendicitis. Backache. Borborygmi. Debility. Flatus. Headaches. ***Hiccough***. ***Lumbago.*** Memory, weak. ***Rheumatism.*** Sciatica. Sexual excitement. Typhlitis.

HERBAL - The symptoms of the Chinese and the American Ginseng are taken together, as the two are probably identical. The root is forked like that of the mandrake. The name ginseng is said to signify "the resemblance of a man" or a man's thigh. The shape of the root might indicate an action on the pelvis and lower limbs.

HOMEOPATHIC - Lembke and others have proved it. It is an aromatic stimulant and removes feelings of fatigue, imparting a joyous sense of vigor and elasticity to the limbs, especially the upper limbs, and clearness of mind.

Malaise. Yawning. Drowsiness with headache. Feeling of extreme heat and intense coldness, longing to expose the body to cool air. Stimulates the secretory glands, especially salivary. Dry mouth, tongue and lips. Mouth and throat are sensitive to the ordinary air of room. ***Hiccoughs***. Affects the respiratory organs.

Acts on the lower part of the spinal cord, ***lumbago, sciatica and rheumatism***. Paralytic weakness. Skin symptoms, itching pimples on neck and chest. The right side of the body is most affected. Pain in right side of hypogastrium, extending into groin.

MIND - Mood quiet and contented with good courage. Calm, but impatient impulses. Disposition to weep. Anxious about the future. Fear of misfortunes. Fear of accidents. Thinking is difficult. Memory weak.

Abdomen - Tense, painful, rumbling. Pain in right side. Loud gurgling in ileo-cecal region. Dull borborygmi in the abdomen, tension and feeling of inflation, emission of wind, uneasiness and yawning. Peri-typhlitis.

Back - Stiffness in back. Coldness in back and spine. Pressure in dorsal vertebrae. Frequent cracking in upper cervical vertebrae on moving head. Heaviness and stiffness in nape. Drawings in neck muscles. Weight in nape of neck with contusive pain along back of sacrum. Pulsation in vessels of right side of neck. Painful lassitude along back with bruised feeling down to and in sacrum. Deep lancinations around loins, between the shoulder blades, extending to right shoulder.

Chest - Aching and oppression in the chest with great difficulty of respiration. Oppression of the chest with anxiety and lancinations in pit of stomach and lumbar region. Prostration of strength and lassitude in the limbs.

Eyes - Pressure on the eyes. Pupils alternately large and small. Unpleasant sensation of coldness on surface of eyeball. Great difficulty in opening the eyelids, which are heavy and painful, itching of the eyelids. Biting and itching in margins of lids. Vision indistinct. Sensation of fatigue when exposed to the light. Objects appear double when looked at fixedly in reading, the characters become confused.

Face - Alternation of redness and paleness. Burning erythematous redness on right cheek, alae nasi, chin. Lips red, dry, rough, thick, cracked and bleeding, especially the lower lip. Drawing in jaws and bones of face.

Head - Head seems at times enlarged and to sway to one side. Pressure in longitudinal sinuses. Drawing pains. Painful sensitiveness of the head. One-sided head pain. Lancinations from right side of the forehead as far as the orbit with heaviness of the eyelids. Sudden shock in occiput, followed by pains, as of a bruise.

Heart - Severe pain, cutting, dagger-like lancinations and stitches in precordia. Some violent beats while sitting and followed by sensation of floundering of heart with rapid, small indistinct pulse. Pulse very irregular.

Kidneys - Sticking and voluptuous twitching in navicular fossa. Pruritus and burning in urethra with frequent urging to urinate. Yellowish lemon-colored urine, depositing a red sediment.

Limbs - Skin feels tight, contracted. ***Stiff, contracted joints***. Much cracking in joints on moving. Bruised pain in limbs alternating in different parts. Heaviness of lower limbs. Bruised pain in small of back and thighs, nightly digging in right lower limb to toes. Eruption on upper inner thighs. Hands feel swollen. Violent burning heat in fingertips.

Lungs - Short anxious respiration or slow and deep with exertion. Frequent deep inspiration and tightness of chest as if he could not get enough air, better while walking. Contractive pain across lower thorax. Dry cough in paroxysms. Voice rough and hoarse.

Male - Voluptuous tickling at end of urethra. Pressure in testicles. ***Weakness of genital organs.*** Sexual excitement. Nocturnal erections without pollutions. Painful erections while sitting at engrossing business. Rheumatic pains after frequent emissions.

Modalities - Better at dinner. Worse in open air. Worse night. Worse from talking. Worse bending, turning. Worse descending stairs. Worse sitting.

Mouth - Tongue red and smarting with thirst. Tongue white, dry with large glistening papilla. Green saliva. Swallowing of saliva, very difficult on account of dryness. Mouth, lips and teeth very dry, voice rough and scraping.

Rectum - Evacuation difficult. Sticking in rectum. Tenesmus and lancinations. Hard stool, which is not emitted without efforts, followed by burning in the anus. Thin stools preceded by short violent pain, extending from within the pelvis to the thighs, as though one must sink to the ground. Liquid stools in the evening, preceded by colic.

Skin - Itching pimples on the skin of the neck and of the chest. Itching below right foot.

Sleep - Much yawning and drowsiness. Vivid, lascivious dreams, of which the recollection remains. Awakens with difficulty or else with a start.

Stomach - Pressure on the stomach. Oppression and pressure of clothing intolerable. Painful drawings in the stomach, as from hunger. Swelling and pulsation of the stomach. Contractive pain in the stomach with anguish, difficulty of respiration. Drawing pains in the stomach and lancinations in right side, which stop respiration. Inclination to vomit.

Temperature - Coldness, numbness, trembling of hands, fingers white. Chilliness through the back extending into arms, into bones of back, cold hands, blue nails.

Throat - Tonsillitis (Bell.), in dark-complexioned people.

Vertigo - Vertigo, cloudiness, confusion, giddiness and heaviness of the head. Vertigo on going down winding stairs. Vertigo while standing, the ground seems to waver. Vertigo with gray spots before eyes. Vertigo with semi-lateral headache, occipital. Vertigo difficult opening of eyelids, objects appear double.

COMMENTS - Very valuable herb in China, the wild ginseng of Siberia is said to be the best. Natives along the Ussuri river use it boiled for headaches, colds, fevers, and stomach pains. In America, it is a domestic remedy for the after pains of labor.

J. H. Henry said it acts on the lower part of the spinal marrow. He noted that it is also useful for "bruised pains in small of back and thighs (on rising from bed). Great languor with paralytic, rheumatic pains in lower limbs. Arthritic swelling of the foot, which had been exerted a long time. Violent pain in big toe."

Henry also mentioned a "nightly digging in right lower limb from hip to big toe, cramp, pains from right hip to toes, lancinating, tearing in right tarsal joint." He considered it specific in lumbago, sciatica and chronic rheumatism that are accompanied by a frequent desire to urinate and sexual excitement.

RELATIONS - ***Compare:*** (1) Aral., Coca. (2) Hed. - depression and skin irritation antidoted by Gunpowder. (3) In ***"Drowsiness with headache"*** Bruce., Hera., Gels., Nat-s. (4) Nux-m. and Sulph. in dry lips, Bry.

REFERENCES - Boericke. Clarke. Murphy.

GLONOINUM

(Nitroglycerine)

PHARMACY - glon. Glonoinum. Nitroglycerine. Spirits glycerinus nitrate. Dilutions with alcohol. ***Historical dose:*** All potencies.

CLINICAL - ***Angina pectoris.*** Aphasia. Brain, congestion. Bright's disease. Colic. Convulsions. Epilepsy. Fright. Goiter. ***Headaches. Heart, disorders.*** Hypertension. Mania. Meningitis. Menses, suppression. Migraines. Neuralgias. Nosebleeds. ***Palpitations.*** Paralysis. Rheumatism. Sciatica. Seasickness. Snow-headache. ***Strokes. Sun-headaches. Sunstroke.*** Toothache. Trauma.

HOMEOPATHIC - Hering said that Sobrero discovered nitroglycerine in 1847, but none could be obtained for physiological experiment until Morris Davis, after long and laborious trials, and under Hering's own direction, succeeded in producing the substance in sufficient quantities for a proving.

Nitroglycerine is an explosive substance, therefore its action is quick and violent, a tempestuous remedy. The signature of this potent explosive may be said to be ***"bursting"*** and ***"expansion."***

The keynote action is the tendency to sudden congestion and violent irregularities of the circulation. ***Sudden vascular congestion***. Surges of blood. ***Violent pulsations, ebullitions*** and irregular congestions. ***Blood rushes upwards, to head and heart.*** Small, wiry pulse, pallor, arterial spasm, anemia of brain.

Collapse, feeble heart, syncope, dicrotic pulse. Affinity for the arteries (Ham., for veins). Stimulates the heart and circulatory system, usually going to the head and chest producing violent pain. Throbbing and pulsation in the area. Quick and violent action.

Arterial tension, in chronic interstitial nephritis. Strokes. General pulsations throughout body, often with numbness. ***Pulsating pains***. Pains that come long after injuries. Burning in small areas or in a single parts.

Congestive headaches, hyperemia of the brain from excess of heat or cold. ***Bursting and expansion sensations.*** Great vertigo on assuming an upright posture from rising up in bed, rising from a seat, etc. Heat in the head, throbbing headache. Violent convulsions, associated with cerebral congestion.

Extreme irritability, easily excited by the slightest opposition, ending in congestive head symptoms. Intercranial, menopausal disturbances or due to menstrual suppression. Convulsions, epileptiform from cerebral congestion or suppressed menses. Eclampsia.

Sciatica in atheromatous subjects with cold shriveled limb. Itching all over body, with later acne and furuncle formation. Old scars break out again. Clothing seems tight. Seasickness. Bulimia. Ailments from sunstroke or heat, can't bear heat about the head, the sun, the heat from a stove.

MIND - *Confused,* bewildered. ***Mental confusion with dizziness.*** Confusion on waking, at night, better open air. Conversation difficult, with confused ideas. Forgetful during headache. Worse mental exhaustion. Great lassitude, no inclination to work. Disinclined to speak.

Ailments from mental excitement, fright, fear, mechanical injuries and their later consequences. Desires death during headache. Suicidal, attempts to jump from window during headache.

Shock, sudden attacks of terror. ***Fear from sensation of swelling of throat.*** Apprehensive of approaching death. Fears she has been poisoned. Fear of having a stroke on waking. Shudders and weeps during intermissions of pain. Frantic with pain, attempts to run away or jump out of a window.

Very irritable. Dwells on past disagreeable occurrences, recalls old grievances. ***Aversion to husband, dislikes her own children.***

Dare not go out into the street. Sits with head on hands and elbow on knees. Familiar places seemed strange after headache. Cannot recognize localities. Recognizes nobody. Loses senses, sinks down unconscious.

Delusion house is not in right place, while walking in street after headache. As if in a dream, doesn't know where he is. ***Time passes too slowly.*** Delusion distances are enlarged.

Insanity from long continued heat of sun. Exalted ideas, thinks she is God and everyone her inferior. Unusually bright and loquacious, with great flow of ideas. Desires room perfectly still, is worse noise.

Abdomen - Rumbling in lower part of the abdomen, principally when lying on left side. Rumbling in hypogastrium. Gallstone colic. Colic, cutting pain principally below the navel, waking in the morning, before and after loose stools.

Back - Burning heat between the shoulder blades. Hot sensation down back, along the spine. Burning between scapula. Pain in the whole spinal column or heat and chilliness. Stiffness, tightness around the neck, clothing seems to be too tight. Neck feels weak and tired, cannot support the head. Sensation of fullness, tension, pulsation. Stiffness of neck during headache.

Breasts - Throbbing pain begins in left breast, darts suddenly to head, worse motion.

Causations - Ill effects of sun, heat, bright snow, fear or fright, and jarring injuries.

Chest - Congestions to chest alternating with congestions to head. Oppression of the chest, alternating with headache. Heat, rising from chest to face and head. Chest feels screwed together. Constriction. Numbness moves upwards in chest and down left arm. Sweats on the chest.

Constitutions - Suited to florid, plethoric, sensitive women. Nervous, sanguine, readily affected persons.

Ears - Ears red. Sharp shooting pain behind ears. Throbbing, piercing from within outward in right ear, each beat of heart is heard in ears, full feeling. Ringing, singing or cracking in the ears. Deafness, paralysis of auditory nerve. Ears sensitive to jarring. Sensation of fullness in and around the ears. Mastoiditis. Menière's disease.

Eyes - Eyes sunken, dry. Red, lower eyeballs or lids. Eyes protrude, look wild, upturned or rolled outwards and upwards in convulsions. Sharp pain, soreness or pressure in eyeballs. Lids stick to ball. Photophobia. Pupils dilated, eyes rolled upward and outward. Pupils contracted in sunstroke.

Face - ***Redness of face, which comes and goes.*** Flushed face alternating with pale. Flushed, hot face. Dusky face. Face bluish. Faceache with twitching of facial muscles. Pain at the root of the nose. Neuralgia of face with pulsating pains. Chin feels too long. Trigeminal neuralgia, left side of face. Periodical attacks of facial neuralgia. Lower lip feels swollen or numb. Jaws clenched in sunstroke. Pain in malar bones, ending in headache. Veins of temples swollen. Cold sweat on face during congestion to head. Sweat on face.

Female - Delayed menses. ***Sudden cessation of menses with congestion to head and chest, with headache and fainting.*** Menses scanty. Menses with lumbar pain. Headaches after profuse menses. Since menarche, congestion to head, with loss of consciousness. ***Menopausal flushing.*** During pregnancy, headache, congestions of blood to the head and chest. Eclampsia, unconscious, face bright-red, puffed, pulse full, hard, urine copious and albuminous.

Food - Loss of appetite. Abnormal hunger. Wants cold water, dry parched feeling. Increased desire to smoke. Alcoholic stimulants cause delirium, congestion, stupor, sleepiness and subsequent depression. Wine aggravates all symptoms.

Head - Rush of blood to head. Cerebral congestion. ***Throbbing and bursting headache.*** Sudden, violent congestion to head, throbbing felt with every pulse, at every step. As if blood were surging back and forth. ***Waves of terrible, pounding pain.*** Cracking, snapping, shocks, explosions or soreness deep in brain. ***Head heavy, but cannot lay it on pillow.*** Headache, before, during, after, or in place of menses. Headache with nausea. Shocks in head, synchronous with pulse. Headache better from sleep. Holds the head tightly. ***Throbbing in temples, worse walking.*** Veins of temples distended. Neuralgia of head and face. Head feels large, as if skull were too small for brain. ***Headache with protrusion of eyeballs.*** As if standing on the head with expanding and contracting sensation. Headache and pulse increase and diminish together. ***Threatened strokes.*** Meningitis. Cri encephalique. Knocks head against wall, during frightful bursting headache. ***Sun headache,*** increases and decreases with the sun. ***Sunstroke.*** Effects of sunstroke, heat on head, as in type-setters and workers under gas and electric light. Headache from injury to spine.

Heart - ***Angina pectoris.*** Anxiety in precordia. Cardiac pain radiates to all parts. Heart pain, worse from wine. Sharp pain in heart on stooping. Laborious action. ***Violent palpitations with throbbing carotids.*** Palpitations with dyspnea with heat in face. Heart seems full, quivers. Boiling sensation in the region. Fluttering of heart. Pressure in heart as if it was being contracted. ***High blood pressure and headaches.*** Throbbing in the whole body to the fingertips. Purring noise at the region of the heart. ***Any exertion brings on rush of blood to heart and fainting spells.*** Cannot go uphill because of heart pain. Full, tense pulse. Venous pulse. Pulse rapid when walking. Pulse rapidduring headache. Pulse rises and falls alternately. Pulse low and feeble in sunstroke.

Kidneys - Acute and chronic interstitial ***nephritis with high blood pressure.*** Tubal nephritis with headache, brought on by walking in sun, numbness in arms and hands alternating with intense tingling. Profuse pale, albuminous urine, more frequent at night. Increased secretion of pale urine, has to rise frequently during the night. Urine high-colored, burning while passing. Red sediment and muddy, reddish-yellow slime.

Limbs - Itching all over, worse limbs. Drawing pain in all limbs. Limbs feel bloated. Weak and tremulous feeling in limbs. Numbness in left limbs. Sciatica better flexing legs on abdomen. Unsteady gait. Knees give way. Thighs and knees weak and knock together during headache. Pain in left biceps. Trembling hands. Fingers and toes spread apart during convulsions.

Lungs - Heavy, labored breathing. Desire to take a long, deep inspiration. Sighing. Numbness moves upwards in chest and down left arm. Oppression of chest alternating with headache. As if a load on chest. Frequent, expectoration of thick mucus.

Modalities - Better from open air. Better cold things, cold application. Better elevating head. Better lying still (opposite Bell.). Worse bending head backward. Worse stooping. Worse left side. ***Worse motion, shaking, jarring***. Worse stimulants, wine. Worse fruits, peaches. Worse gaslight. Worse cutting hair. Worse weight of hat. Worse suppressed menses. Worse lying down. Worse from 6 a.m. to noon. ***Worse in sun***. Worse open fire. ***Worse heat on head.*** Worse becoming overheated. ***Worse hot weather***. Worse from injury.

Mouth - Saliva increased, thick in a.m. Froth at mouth. Bitter taste with nausea. Aromatic, sweet, warm things, leave a fatty taste. Lower lip feels swollen. Throbbing pain in teeth, teeth feel elongated. Pulsating toothache. Itching of soft palate and throat. Hard palate sensitive as if swollen.

Nose - Nosebleeds on going out into the heat of the sun, face flushed, hot, red. Pain at root of nose. The headache extends into the nose. Sudden sneezing, fluent coryza.

Pains - ***Bursting, throbbing,*** pulsative, tearing, piercing, stabbing, gnawing. Sensation of fullness.

Perspiration - Perspiration, principally in the face, after sleeping. Perspiration on forehead. Profuse sweat, mostly on face and chest. Sweats principally on face, after sleeping. Sweats on hands. Perspiration relieves the nausea. Sweats alternates with chilliness. Feeling as if sweat would break out all over. Cold sweat on face, during congestion to head.

Rectum - Constipation with itching, painful hemorrhoids, with pinching in abdomen before and after stool. Diarrhea, copious black, lumpy stools. Diarrhea with sudden stoppage of menses. Morning diarrhea with sharp burning with rumbling. Diarrhea evening and night after eating peaches. Stools, loose, scanty, with much rumbling. Diarrhoeic stools with rumbling and discharge of flatus. Frequent passage of flatus during stools, with a loud, sharp noise.

Sensations - Brain as if expanding, as if moving in waves, as if hanging with head downwards, as if something were pumped into vertex, as if everything were crowded out at forehead. Sensation as if warm water were running upwards from nape of neck. As if the neck were held by a hand. Sensation as if some one were pulling eyes from within outward. Noise in left ear as if it came from heart. As if heart would rise to throat. Sensation as if chin feels too long.

Skin - Itching all over, the limbs. Old scars break out again.

Sleep - Weakness as from loss of sleep. Yawning with the headache, congestion of blood to the head. Sleepiness early in the evening. Difficult to waken. Awakes with fear of having a stroke. Confused dreams. Dreams of homesickness. Dreams with tears.

Stomach - Gastralgia in anemic patients with feeble circulation. Faint, gnawing and empty feeling at pit of stomach. Stomach pain in anemic patients with feeble circulation. Horrible faint feeling at the pit of stomach with throbbing. Rumbling in hypogastrium, worse lying on left side. Nausea with faint feeling. Nausea and vomiting in brain congestions or during sunstroke. Spasmodic vomiting in hydrocephalus. Seasickness.

Teeth - Gums swollen and sensitive to touch. Teeth feel elongated. Throbbing pain in the teeth. Pulsating toothache with headache. Toothache from taking cold, after having been overheated. Stabbing pains in gums right side passing to left, worse from hot, better from cold applications. Toothache after hitting, in chewing a hard substance, a bad tooth. Teeth decay after mercury.

Temperature - Chill after getting heated, alternates with sweat, vomiting. Intermittent fever. Fever with hot sweat. Heat in face, ascending from pit of stomach to head. ***Heat flushes.*** General warmth, flushes of heat, waves of heat upward.

Throat - Throat feels full. Sensation as if the throat were swelling. As if string were tied around neck, which prevented blood from returning to head. Collar must be opened. Chokes and swells up under ear. The soft palate feels contracted and dry. Itching of the soft palate and throat. In the throat tickling, heat, soreness.

Tongue - Tongue is milk-white without coating. Tongue coated heavily at back. Tongue, heavy, cannot protrude straight. Tongue numb. Tongue as if burnt. Tongue prickling, smarting, and stinging. Tongue feels swollen and raw with spasmodic twitchings.

Vertigo - Vertigo on assuming upright position. ***Vertigo with confusion.*** Vertigo, worse from stooping or moving head.

Vertigo in open air. Vertigo with nausea. Vertigo with dim vision. Vertigo with black spots before eyes. Vertigo with headache. Vertigo with nausea. Vertigo in sunstroke. Vertigo after a head injury.

Vision - Dim vision during vertigo. Impaired vision during raging headache. Letters appear smaller. Sparks before eyes. Spells of blindness. Black spots, during headache, when turning quickly. Black specks, sparks, flashes, before eyes. Objects dance with every pulsation. Black floating spots on attempting to stoop.

COMMENTS - Guernsey recorded that Glon. is suited to troubles of the head in type-setters and in men who work under a gaslight steadily, so that the heat falls on the head.

Severe, painful palpitations and sudden rushes of blood to the head with a threatened stroke. Palpitations with trembling limbs. Heart attack (Acon.). High blood pressure. Panic attacks when the blood rushes to the head, can get painful palpitations and a fear of having a heart attack. Cardiac neuralgia (angina pectoris) with radiating pains.

Vascular headache, with pounding, throbbing and a red face. Violent action of the heart, rush of blood to the head. Vascular headaches due to high blood pressure with flushed face, dilated pupils, palpitated heart. Bursting and throbbing headaches. Worse light touch to the head.

Sensation of waves in the blood with headache. Headaches ever since heat stroke or from exposure to the sun. Sense of constriction in the throat with headache, throbbing carotid arteries. Headaches after having hair cut (Bell.). Meningitis. Nausea and vomiting of cerebral origin.

Great sensitivity to the least motion. Will carry his head very carefully in order to avoid any motion (Bry.). The headache is in the whole head, worse with exposure to the sun, better with pressure.

Pains appear in occiput and at the base of the brain. Gnawing in occiput, sore pain, pressure, severe pain extending to the eyes and temples. Pains move from within outward, from front to back. Sensation of expanding in head and body.

Sensation as if something were moving in the nerves from the back of the neck upward to the head. The eyes may be fixed or protrude. Aversion to bright light, black spots before sight. Both hands and feet are cold.

Flushes of heat rising from the chest to the head, then throbbing pain in head (Bell.). Heat stroke. For ailments from working under strong lights or the sun. Faint from hot place.

Neuralgias are accompanied with throbbing, often worse at night, preventing sleep. Supra-orbital neuralgia, pulsating, retinal congestion from exposure to strong light. Facial neuralgia, extending through head. Violent, stabbing, neuralgic pains, so violent as to make patient frantic, he wants to escape to jump out of window.

Menopausal disturbances. Hot flashes with pulsation, heat, severe palpitation with wave sensation resulting in headaches. Face is flushed or pale. Fainting, sudden unconsciousness, convulsions, especially during labor.

Horrible apprehension, fear of being poisoned. Ailments from fear. Loss of a sense of location. Bad effects of having hair cut, of exposure to heat from the sun or fire. Ailments from too much riding or driving, seasickness. Sensitive to alcohol (Zinc). Cannot bear weight of hair, clothing seems too tight.

RELATIONS - ***Antidoted by:*** Acon. Camph., Coff., Nux-v. ***Compare:*** (1) Op., Stram., Verat-v. (2) Amyl-n. (3) Cimic. - waving in brain. (4) Petr. and Crot-h. - loss of location. (5) Bell. - cephalic cry but not as marked in Bell., also Bell. has better bending head back and better covering head. (6) Glon. - better uncovered, Apis. (7) Hyos. - fears being poisoned. (8) Gels. - inclination to jump out of window. (9) Stram., Sang. - headache with the sun, ear sensitive to jar. (10) Nit-ac. and Bell. - sensitiveness to jar. (11) Meli. - headache with crimson face. (12) Lyc. and Phos. - burning between shoulders. (13) Dig. and Dios. - headache extending into nose. (14) Sec. - fingers spread apart.

REFERENCES - Boericke. Clarke. Murphy. Phatak.

GLYCERINUM

(Glycerine)

PHARMACY - glyc. Glycerinum. Glycerine. ***Historical dose:*** Tincture and all potencies. Pure glycerine in teaspoonful doses, 3 times a day with lemon juice for pernicious anemia.

CLINICAL - Carbuncle. Diabetes. Influenza. Pneumonia. Pernicious anemia. Rheumatic pains. Weakness.

HOMEOPATHIC - Glycerine is a liquid obtained by the decomposition of vegetable or animal fats or fixed oils, containing not less than 95 percent of absolute glycerol, a triatomic alcohol existing in fats and fixed oils in combination with the fatty acids.

Dr. Wm. B. Griggs noted that potentized glycerine seems to act deeply and long, building up tissue, hence of great use in marasmus, mental and physical debility, diabetes, etc. It disturbs nutrition in its primary action and, secondarily, seems to improve the general state of nutrition. Builds tissue. Seems to affect most of the organs and tissues of the body.

General sense of exhaustion. Neurasthenia. Headache with a sense of fullness in the head and throbbing, aggravated by motion. Dullness of the mind, a sense of mental and physical weakness, restless sleep and dreaming, much physical languor, almost to a state of utter prostration.

Balances the general metabolism. Loss of appetite, constipation, profuse urination with traces of sugar. Gastro-intestinal disease. Senile debility. Acute catarrhal conditions of the mucus membrane of the naso-pharynx and nephritis in the aged. Influenza, pneumonia.

Chest - Chest seems full.

Female - Profuse, long-lasting flow, with bearing down heaviness in uterus.

Head - Feels full, throbs, especially occiput. Mentally confused. Severe headache two days before menstruation.

Kidneys - Profuse and frequent urination. Increased specific gravity and sugar. Diabetes.

Limbs - Rheumatic pains of a remittent type. Feet painful and hot, feel enlarged.

Lungs - Hacking cough with sense of weakness. ***Influenza pneumonia.***

Nose - Stopped up, sneezing, irritating coryza. Sensation of crawling on mucus membrane. Post-nasal dripping.

Stomach - Fermentation, burning in stomach and esophagus.

COMMENTS - Anshutz reported three cases. The first concerned a homeopathic physician in Philadelphia, aged 61 years. He was refused insurance on account of albumen casts and sugar in urine, and had been under his own care for months.

He developed a severe infection on his neck, six inches in diameter, a carbuncle was operated on by Dr. Herbert S. Leopold very successfully. He had extreme nervousness, profuse urination with a specific gravity of 1.030. Sugar, etc. in urine examined by a Philadelphia chemist, extreme debility, prostration, etc. Glyc. in 30c and 200c eliminated sugar and albumin in three months and the patient gained fifteen pounds.

The second case concerned Mr. S., baker, age 66 years. Diabetes for years, weakness, dyspnea, headache, urine with sugar, acetone, great debility. No albumin or casts. He was placed on strict diet and given Sulph., Ph-ac., Uran-n., Ars., Syzyg. and potentized blood. Glyc. was then given with the result that the urine cleared up, a good appetite developed and after a period of two years sexual vigor returned.

Finally, the third case was C. H., a baby two years old. Drs. Yeager and Macfarlan assisted in the case. Influenza pneumonia. Profuse coryza and dyspnea. Consolidation in both lungs, weakness and debility after twelve days. Glyc. 200c was given and a complete recovery ensued with improvement at once.

RELATIONS - ***Compare:*** (1) Lac-ac., Lec. Gels., Calc.

REFERENCES - Anshutz. Boericke.

GLYCYRRHIZA GLABRA

(Licorice Root)

PHARMACY - glyc-g. Glycyrrhiza glabra. Licorice root. Liquiritia officinalis. Sweet-wort. Europe and Asia. N. O. Leguminosae. Papilionoideae. ***Historical dose:*** Tincture and all potencies.

CLINICAL - Addison's disease. Allergies. Athlete's foot. Arthritis. Asthma. Baldness. Bronchitis. Bursitis. ***Canker sores.*** Catarrh. Chronic fatigue. ***Colds. Coughs.*** Dandruff. Dyspepsia. Eczema. Emphysema. Gastritis. Gingivitis. Gout. Fungal, infections. ***Heartburn.*** Herpes. Hoarseness. Indigestion. Influenza. Liver problems. Lyme disease. Menopause. ***Mouth, ulcers. Peptic ulcers.*** Prostate, enlargement. ***Psoriasis.*** Shingles. Stomach, ulcers. ***Sore throat.*** Tendonitis. Tooth, decay. Tuberculosis. ***Ulcers.*** Viral, infections. Yeast, infections.

HERBAL - Liquorice his one of the most commonly used herbs in herbal medicine and has a very long history of use, both as a medicine and also as a flavoring to disguise the unpleasant flavor of other medications.

Liquorice was known to the ancients as far back as the third century B. C. for its efficacy in the case of dry coughs. The Greeks, recommended it for the treatment of gastric and peptic ulcers. Later, Arab physicians used Licorice to relieve coughs and side effects associated with laxatives.

It is a very sweet, moist, soothing herb that detoxifies and protects the liver and is also powerfully anti-inflammatory, being used in conditions as varied as arthritis and mouth ulcers.

The root is alterative, antispasmodic, demulcent, diuretic, emollient, expectorant, laxative, moderately pectoral and tonic. The root has also been shown to have a hormonal effect similar to the ovarian hormones.

Liquorice root is much used in cough medicines and also in the treatment of catarrhal infections of the urinary tract. It is taken internally in the treatment of Addison's disease, asthma, bronchitis, coughs, peptic ulcer, arthritis, allergic complaints. Externally, the root is used in the treatment of psoriasis, herpes, eczema and shingles.

Licorice root has an impressive list of well documented uses and is probably one of the most over-looked of all herbal remedies.

It is used for many ailments including asthma, athlete's foot, baldness, body odor, bursitis, canker sores. Chronic fatigue, depression. ***Colds, coughs and influenza.*** Dandruff. Emphysema. Gingivitis and tooth decay. Gout. Heartburn. Viral infections. Fungal infections. Ulcers. Liver problems, Lyme disease. Menopause. Psoriasis. Shingles. ***Sore throats.*** Tendonitis. Tuberculosis. Yeast infections. Prostate enlargement. Arthritis.

Other uses of the plant include the treatment of hormone imbalances and menopausal symptoms in women.

RELATIONS - ***Compare:*** Ulmus fuva, Melaleuca alternifolia.

REFERENCES - Murphy.

GNAPHALIUM POLYCEPHALUM

(Cud-weed)

PHARMACY - gnaph. Gnaphalium polycephalum. Cud-weed. Old balsam. Gnaphalium dioica. Gnaphalium uliginosum. Sweet-scented everlasting flower. N. O. Composite. Tincture of fresh plant. ***Historical dose:*** Tincture and all potencies.

CLINICAL - Anterior crural neuralgia. ***Chills.*** Cholera. Cholera, infantum. Colic. Diarrhea. ***Dysmenorrhea.*** Gout. Lumbago. Neuralgia. Night-sweats. ***Numbness***. Polyuria. Prostate gland. Rheumatism. ***Sciatica.***

HOMEOPATHIC - Gnaph. has been used mainly in disorders of the ***sciatic nerve***, but it also has an action on the abdominal organs, causing vomiting, colic and diarrhea, thus comparing with Coloc. in both spheres.

Sciatica and lumbago with numbness alternating with the pain. ***Intense sciatic pain*** (Mag-p., Rhus-t., Coloc., Hyper.), alternating with or followed by numbness. Lumbago with numbness of part. Rheumatism. Anterior crural neuralgia.

Pain in joints as if they lacked oil. Pain worse lying down, motion, stepping, by sitting in a chair, better by flexing the limbs on abdomen (Colo.). Sticking pain and numbness. Sharp, shooting pains, or electric-like sensation down the backs of the legs.

Offensive diarrhea with colic, worse in the morning. Polyuria. Weight and heaviness in the pelvis. ***Dysmenorrhea*** with scanty menses, very painful during the first day.

MIND - Very irritable for two or three days after the diarrhea.

Abdomen - Colic, pain in various parts of the abdomen. Cecum is sensitive. Borborygmus with emission of much flatus.

Back - Chronic backache in lumbar region, better resting on back. Lumbago with numbness in lower part of back and weight in pelvis.

Face - Intermittent pains of superior maxillary of both sides. Dull, heavy, bloated appearance. Neuralgic pain of an intermittent from in both upper maxillary bones.

Female - ***Dysmenorrhea*** with scanty and painful menses. Sensation of weight in pelvis. Sensation of fullness in pelvis.

Kidneys - Pains in kidneys with frequent slight pain in prostate gland. Sensation of pain and fullness in bladder, even when just emptied.

Limbs - Rheumatic pain in ankle joints and legs. ***Intense pain along the sciatic nerve, numbness alternates with pain.*** Feeling of weakness, as if incapable of raising the slightest weight. Rheumatic pains in elbows and shoulders. Frequent pains in calves and feet. Cramps in calves of legs and feet when in bed. Gouty pains in big toes. Gouty concretions. Anterior crural neuralgia (Staph.). Chronic muscular rheumatism of back and neck. Pain in joints as if they lacked oil. Better drawing limbs up, flexing thigh on abdomen.

Male - Irritation of prostate gland. Increased sexual passion.

Modalities - Better from flexing limbs. Better sitting in a chair. Worse from walking. Worse lying. Worse cold damp.

Mouth - Mouth feels parched and tastes badly. Flat, sweetish, sickening taste. Tongue covered with long white fur, better by thorough washing with cold water.

Rectum - First stage of cholera infantum, vomiting and purging. Rumbling in bowels with stool before breakfast. Looseness of bowels with passage of pale-colored feces. Diarrhea discharge in morning and during day with irritable temper. Dark-colored, liquid offensive stool in morning afterwards pain in bowels all day, in children.

Stomach - Vomiting and purging like cholera morbus in the night and all next day. Flatus, windy belchings, nausea and hiccough.

Vertigo - Giddy, especially after rising from recumbent position.

COMMENTS - Cramps in calves and back of thighs, hamstrings. Sciatica pain in worse on lying down, by motion, by stepping, better when sitting in a chair, better drawing up the limb.

Diarrhea is watery and offensive, occurs in the morning and is repeated during the day. Rumbling in the bowels, colicky pains and the patient is cross and irritable. Urine is scanty. Appetite and taste are lost.

Dr. W. McGeorge recorded that Gnaph. has a reputation for colds, fevers and night-sweats. The last was caused in one of the provers. It cured one case of chills. The periodicity appears in the intermittent neuralgia of the upper jaws.

McGeorge noted a sense of "weight and fullness in the pelvis" for dysmenorrhea. Dysmenorrhea when the menses are scanty and very painful during the first day.

Sexual excitement in male provers, pain and irritation in the prostate gland. Headache better by washing in cold water. Fur on tongue removed by thorough washing with cold water.

McGeorge cured a very aggravated case of sciatica in a man, resulting from a strain. The left leg was cramped and drawn up, worse in cold and damp weather.

Dr. George Shelton recorded two cases. The first, a clergyman, 27, had sharp cutting pains, starting from inner side right thigh, just below Poupart's ligament, extending down course of anterior crural nerve to a point about its lower third.

The pains were paroxysmal, came on when walking, occasionally when lying down. He had one or two attacks in the pulpit. In several instances the pain had extended down the right cord into the testicle and caused him to draw up the leg, flexing the thigh on the abdomen. This condition was also present in Dr. McGeorge's case. A few doses of Gnaph. 1c cured him completely.

The second case occurred in a widow, 68, who had severe pains in the outer side of her right thigh for six years, part of which she had been confined to bed. The pains were paroxysmal, cutting, tearing, extending down the course of the sciatic nerve.

Attacks were worse at night and more frequent, causing her to roll about the bed and cry out with the pain. All the resources of allopathy had been in vain. Rhus-t., Coloc., Sulph., gave no help. Bell. relieved slightly. Gnaph. 1c wrought gradual improvement, and in eight weeks the cure was complete.

Clarke had a case, cured with Gnaph. 30c., of a very gouty man, with the alternation of numbness with pain.

RELATIONS - ***Compare:*** (1) Xanth., Cham., Coloc., Ip., Merc., Puls., Lyc., Caul.

REFERENCES - Boericke. Clarke. Murphy. Phatak.

GORSE

(Bach Flower Essence)

PHARMACY - gors-b. Gorse. Ulex europaeus. Flowers from the bush are placed in a bowl of water and allowed to stand in the sun for several hours. The strained water is used as medicine. ***Historical dose:*** Take two drops from the stock bottle into a one ounce dropper bottle, (add brandy or alcohol, if this bottle will be used for days or weeks). This is the dosage bottle, take a few drops straight into the mouth or as needed in a little water or juice.

HOMEOPATHIC - This remedy belongs to Bach's group ***For Those who Suffer Uncertainty,*** along with Cer-b., Scler-b., Gent-b., Horn-b. and Wld-o-b. For those suffering from doubt, hopelessness, uncertainty and lack of clarity of purpose in daily affairs.

Will raise spirits in cases of true hopelessness, such as terminal illness. Lowered vitality and sinking of strength. Sense of resignation to a hopeless situation.

MIND - Deep-hopelessness (Aur.). Calm, with underlying sadness and a sense of misfortune and suffering. Denial and recurring disappointment. Negativity. Uncertainty about the future.

REFERENCES - Bach.

GOSSYPIUM HERBACEUM

(Cotton Plant)

PHARMACY - goss. Gossypium herbaceum. Cotton plant. N. O. Malvaceae. Tincture of fresh inner root bark, chopped and pounded to a pulp. ***Historical dose:*** Tincture and all potencies.

CLINICAL - Amenorrhea. Chills. Dysmenorrhea. Fibroids. Infertility. Labia, abscess. Miscarriage. Morning sickness. Nausea. Ovaries, pains. Pregnancy, vomiting. Retained, placenta. Tumor. Uterus, bearing down.

HERBAL - In herbal practice, Gossypium was used as a powerful emmenagogue.

HOMEOPATHIC - Goss. has been mainly used in affection of the female generative organs. It has been taken in the form of the extract stimulate the uterus and ovaries.

Nausea with flow of saliva and inclination to vomit in the morning, before breakfast with sensitive uterine region. Sensitive stomach with much gas. Vomits on motion or raising up. Morning sickness of pregnancy. Hyperemesis.

Menses, late, scanty, watery. Tardy menses, with sensation that the flow is about to start and yet does not. Bearing down pains in the uterus. "Intermittent pains in the ovaries," extending towards uterus. Sterility from uterine torpor. Sensitive womb. Subinvolution. Fibroids. Tumors in breast with swelling of axillary glands.

Pain in neck. Sympathetic symptoms of stomach, heart, bowels and nervous system arising from disturbance of uterine functions. Stinging, drawing, tearing and sometimes burning pains.

Pains extend from one place to another, jumping from one place to another. Move from above downward.

Abdomen - Sharp pain in right hypochondrium, lasting for a few minutes. Drawing pain from both hypochondriac regions extending to stomach.

Back - Pain in back. Pain in cervical region with tendency for head to draw backward, with nervousness. Backache, weight and dragging pain in pelvis.

Breasts - Tumor of the breast with swelling of axillary glands.

Constitution - Tall, anemic patients with nervous chills.

Eyes - Drawing pain over eyes with stinging pain in pupils.

Female - Labia swollen and itching. Suppressed menstruation. Menses too watery. Backache, weight and dragging in pelvis. ***Intermittent pain in ovaries***. Uterine subinvolution and fibroids with gastric pain and debility. Retained placenta. Morning sickness with sensitive uterine region.

Food - Anorexia with uneasy, depressed feeling at scrobiculum cordis at time of menses.

Head - Pain in cervical region with tendency for head to draw backward with nervousness. Pain, first burning, then stinging, extending from both temporal bones to middle of frontal bone.

Kidneys - Frequent desire to urinate with burning pains.

Limbs - Heavy feeling in both hands, better hanging them down, worse in warmth of bed.

Modalities - Pains are generally worse by motion, better by rest.

Nose - Nostrils swollen and inflamed.

Sleep - Caused her to sleep a great part of the time.

Stomach - Nausea with accumulation of saliva in mouth inclination to vomit before breakfast. Rotating pain in pit of stomach.

Temperature - General external chilliness, with internal heat.

Throat - Tonsils swollen, worse right side.

RELATIONS - ***Compare:*** (1) Action similar to Ergot when made from fresh green root. (2) Lil-t., Sabin., Cimic., Apis. Asar., Bell., Bry., Puls., Sec., Sep., Ust.

REFERENCES - Boericke. Clarke.

GRANATUM POMEGRANATE
(Pomegranate)

PHARMACY - gran. Granatum pomegranate. Pomegranate. Punica granatum. N. O. Granatee. Lythraceae. Homeopathic provings were made with a tincture or trituration of bark of root. ***Historical dose:*** Trituration, tincture and all potencies.

CLINICAL - Ascarides. Emaciation. Gastralgia. Heart, weakness. Hernia. Jaw, cracking. Nausea. Tapeworm. Toothache. ***Salivation***. ***Vertigo***. Worms.

HERBAL - Pomegranate is a well-known vermifuge, especially used for the expulsion of tinea. For this a decoction of the rind of the fruit is used in the following manner: An alkaloid, Pelletierine, discovered by Bertrand Pelletier, is obtained from the rind of the fruit.

After a mild purge the previous night in the morning, 30 grams of Sulphate of Pelletierine is administered in a solution containing 50 grams of tannic acid. This is followed by a glass of water in ten minutes and a brisk purge in half an hour.

Granatum is used as a vermifuge for the expulsion of tapeworm. ***Salivation*** with nausea and vertigo. Spasm of the glottis.

HOMEOPATHIC - The provings bring out many symptoms of helminthiasis, including pale blue rings around eyes, and itching, crawling and tickling of the nose. Ravenous hunger, craving for sour or juicy things, fruit, coffee. Loss of appetite. Emaciation.

Swelling of navel. Nausea, fermenting in abdomen, griping, dragging in inguinal region as if hernia would protrude. Itching and tickling in anus frequently during the day. Discomfort. Great weariness and exhaustion, scarcely able to keep upright.

Trembling. Convulsive movements. Itching of the skin of various places, face and body, as if pimples would break out.

Biting and itching in palms of hands. Yawning. Great sensitiveness.

MIND - Great sensitiveness and impressibility. Fear, dread of work during headache. Confusion of mind after a carousal. Stupefaction and intellectual embarrassment. Hypochondriacal.

Dejection and discouragement. Quarrelsome humor. Melancholy, gloomy temper. Irritability and arrogance. Censorious. Reproaches others.

Abdomen - Pain in stomach and abdomen, ***worse about umbilicus*** (Cocc., Nux-m., Plum.). Ineffectual urging. Dragging in vaginal region, as if hernia would protrude. Swelling resembling umbilical hernia.

Back - Pain between shoulders, even clothing is oppressive. Pain around shoulders, as if heavy load had been carried.

Chest - Oppressed with sighing. Pain between shoulders, even clothing is oppressive.

Eyes - Sunken eyes, pupils dilated, weak sight.

Food - Ravenous hunger, craving for sour or juicy things, fruit, coffee. Loss of appetite. Great thirst for water.

Head - Feels empty. Stupefying pain and painful heaviness in the head, forehead. Pressure on the forehead and the occiput. Acute drawing pains chiefly on right side of head shooting in forehead.

Limbs - Pain around shoulders, as if heavy load had been carried. Pain in all finger joints. Tearing pain in knee joint. Convulsive movements.

Modalities - Better after dinner. Pain in abdomen is better after drinking cold water.

Rectum - Burning, itching in the anus, on the buttocks and perineum, scrotum and thighs. Diarrhea with frequent stools. Evacuation of fecal matter and mucus. Pressure in rectum afterwards. Burning heat in rectum. Prolapsed rectum during the stool. Shooting pains in anus and rectum.

Skin - ***Itching in the palms***. Sensation as if pimples would break out. Jaundiced complexion.

Stomach - ***Constant hunger***. Poor digestion. Loses flesh. Vomiting at night.

Vertigo - ***Vertigo very persistent.*** Vertigo during intellectual labor or in the morning on rising. Vertigo with obscuration of the eyes. Vertigo with nausea and aching in the stomach.

RELATIONS - ***Compare:*** (1) Pelletierine - one of its constituents - an anthelmintic, especially for tapeworm. (2) Cina, Kou. Ars., Iod., Teucr., Cuc.

REFERENCES - Boericke. Clarke.

GRAPHITES NATURALIS

(Black Lead)

PHARMACY - graph. Graphites naturalis. Black lead. Plumbago. Trituration of prepared from finest English drawing-pencils. A modification of carbon. ***Historical dose:*** Trituration and all potencies. Locally as a cerate in sore nipples.

CLINICAL - Acne. Amenorrhea. Anus, disorders. Blepharitis. Breasts, cancer. Breasts, indurated. Cancer. Catarrh. Chaps. Chlorosis. Colic. Constipation. Deafness. Dropsy. Dysmenorrhea. Ears, disorders. ***Eczema. Erysipelas.*** Eye, disorders. Face. Erythema. Feet, disorders. ***Fissures. Gastro-intestinal disorders.*** Glandular, swellings. Gleet. Gravel. Headaches. Hemorrhoid. Herpes. Hydrocele. ***Indurations.*** Influenza. Irritation. Lachrymal duct, inflamed. Leucorrhea. Lips, cracked. Liver, indurated. Menstruation, disorders. ***Leucorrhea. Nails, disorders***. Noises, head. Nose, disorders. Nosebleeds. ***Obesity.*** Ovarian, tumors. ***Palpitations.*** Paralysis. Parotiditis. Pityriasis. Priapism. Pruritus, vagina. ***Psoriasis.*** Ptosis. Rectum, disorders. Rhus, poisoning. ***Scars.*** Scrofula. Seminal, emission. ***Skin, disorders.*** Smell, disorders. Stomach, cramps. Stomach, pain. Sycotic, diathesis. Syphilis. Trichinosis. Tumors. Ulcers. Urine, disordered. Uterus, cancer. Vaccination, effects. Wens. Whooping, cough. Worms.

HOMEOPATHIC - Graphites is a mineral carbon, related to Carb-an. and Carb-v. It contains a small percentage of iron, and so is also related to Ferr.

S. Weinhold first thought of using this substance as a drug. He was led to it by seeing workmen in a mirror-factory use it as a local application for tetters. Ruggeri followed him, using it both internally and locally.

Tendency to produce ***excoriations, cracks or fissures,*** at muco-cutaneous junction of eyes, nostrils, mouth, anus, nipples, finger-tips, folds of skin. Mucus membranes are cracked and fissured and have scanty secretions. Excoriations between toes.

Thickening and induration of skin, glands, tarsi, nail, scars. Thick crusts on the skin. Tendency to callosities.

Aids the ***absorption of scar tissue*** (Thiosin.). ***Cancerous diathesis in old scars.*** Recrudescence of scars. Syphilitic and ***constitutional*** ulcers. Tendency to grow cystic tumors, wens. ***Eradicates tendency to erysipelas***.

Watery hemorrhages. Dropsy. Edema. Paralysis or sensation of paralysis. Contractions of muscles. Cramps and burning in different places. Offensive discharges and secretions. Discharges are, thin, foul, scanty and acrid. Sweat stains are yellow, sour, offensive. Gushing leucorrhea. Swollen genitals.

Alternating digestive and skin symptoms. Gastro-intestinal disorders alternating with acne and erythema of face, herpetic lesions or scrofulous hypochondriasis. Sourness of taste, belchings, stools, urine, blood about teeth etc.

Frequently feels faint with partial loss of senses. ***Sensitive to cold.*** Cold aggravates bone pains, coryza and stomach. Emanation of suffering parts. Sensation of burning, numbness and deadness. Pains go to parts not lain on. General sense of uneasiness, tremulousness, which elicits groans. Sudden sinking of strength.

Cancer of pylorus. Duodenal ulcer. Infiltrations. Weakness, then a relaxed condition, anemia, and chlorosis. Lymphatic glands are swollen. Take colds easily. Anemia with redness of face. Tendency to obesity.

MIND - Mentally sluggish. poor memory. Forgetful, makes mistakes in speaking and writing. Remembers all the events of youth, recent events are forgotten. Fatigue from scientific labor. Dread of work.

Fidgety while sitting at work. Energized from work, followed by apathy, anxiety. Very irritable and fretful. ***Obstinate and moody.*** Miserable and unhappy. Impulse to groan. Insolent. Offended easily. ***Periodic depressions.*** Anxiety about spiritual welfare. Full of fear in morning.

Ailments from grief or fright. Sad, fearsome, irresolute, hesitates at trifles. Grief about slightest occurrences. Internal grief and despair. Despair over trifles. Thinks of nothing but death.

Weeping ameliorates symptoms. Weeping alternating with irritability and laughter at trifles. Weeps without cause. ***Weeping from music.*** Weeping during menses.

Apprehensive, despondent. Fear of insanity. ***Fears are better after weeping.*** Great tendency to start. ***Anxiety in morning on waking.*** Excitement at night. Intense restlessness, which drives him out of bed at night. ***Anxiety better warmth***. Restlessness better walking in open air.

Persistent thoughts, haunted by unpleasant subjects, better walking in open air. ***Restlessness while working.*** Dwells upon past disagreeable occurrences at night.

Slowness of purpose. Dullness in morning. Dullness after a siesta. ***Inability to think from weakness in brain. Indolence***, better open air. Feels indifferent to everybody and everything, from exhaustion.

Absent-minded. Unable to decide. Timid. Child impudent, teasing, laughing at reprimands. ***Anguish before menses.*** Cataleptic conditions, consciousness but without the power to move or speak.

Abdomen - Abdomen distended, as from incarcerated flatus. ***Cannot bear tight clothes around the waist.*** Flatulence. Very fetid gas preceded by colic. Pain of gas opposite the side on which he lies. Intestinal torpor. Pain as if intestines were torn. Nauseous feeling in abdomen. Cramp like pain in abdomen with deficient secretion of urine, at night. Inguinal region sensitive, swollen.

Back - Spinal pains. Pain in small of back with great weakness. Pain in the nape of neck and shoulders, worse looking up and stooping the head. Sacral pains with crawling. ***Painless swollen glands on side of neck.*** Numbness of sacrum, down the legs. Pain in the lumbar region as if vertebrae were broken.

Breasts - Induration of breasts and ovaries. Breasts swollen and hard. ***Cracks in nipples.*** Breast cancer from old scars, remaining after mammary abscess. Nipples, sore, cracked and blistered.

Causations - Ill effects of grief, fear, over lifting, surgery.

Chest - Constriction of chest, as if too narrow. Feels as if about to suffocate when falling asleep, jumps out of bed, takes hold of something and must eat something, worse after midnight. Cramps in the chest. Pain in middle of chest with cough, scraping and soreness.

Constitutions - Suited to persons who have a tendency to put on unhealthy fat. Fat, relaxed, chilly and costive. Defective animal heat from defective oxygenation, always cold indoors or out. Chlorotics. Affections of glands, skin and mucus membranes, especially at orifices. Syphilitic and "constitutional" ulcers.

Coughs - Dry cough, troublesome with sweat on face. Cough at night, caused by deep inspiration. Loose cough from tickling deep in chest. Cough with strangling, red face, watery eyes, straining all over. Fatiguing cough, before and during menses.

Ears - ***Moisture and eruptions, fissures in and behind the ear.*** Thin, white scaly membrane covering the eardrum. ***Eczema behind the ears.*** Briny otorrhea. As if hard body behind ear. ***Cracks and fissures behind the ears.*** Feel stuffed at full moon. As if air inside, as if filled with water. ***Dryness of inner ear***. Snapping after every eructation. Hardness of hearing. ***Hears better in noise***. Tinnitus. Hissing in the ears. Detonation in ear like report of a gun. Cracking in ears when eating.

Eyes - Recurrent keratitis. Blepharitis. Ophthalmia with intolerance of artificial light. Hot tears. ***Eyelids, red and swollen***. Dryness of the lids. ***Eczema of lids, fissured***. Eyelids, heavy and falling. Cystic tumors on eyelids. Sore or cracked outer canthi. Ingrown lashes. Phlyctenae. Sight vanishes during menses. ***Shuns daylight.*** Photophobia. Letters appear double, when writing, seem together when reading.

Face - ***Flushes of heat in face.*** Pale, bloated, haggard, flushed. Feels as if cobwebs were on it. Acne before the menses. ***Itching pimples, moist after scratching.*** Moist eczema around the mouth, chin and nose. Erysipelas, burning and stinging. Lips cracked and sore. Formication on lips during menses. Painful nodules on the lower jaw. Barber's itch. Facial paralysis with distortion of muscles and difficult speech. Falling of hair from chin.

Female - ***Menses, too late.*** Menses scanty, pale, irregular, painful. ***Sighing during menses.*** Hoarseness, coryza, cough, morning sickness, sweats, swelling of feet or headache during menses. ***Leucorrhea, pale, thin, profuse, white, excoriating in gushes*** with weakness in back. Leucorrhea worse before and after menses. Leucorrhea in place of menses. ***Acrid, excoriating leucorrhea in gushes day or night, before and after menses.*** Swelling and hardness of ovary (left) worse after menses. Induration of ovaries, uterus and breasts. Pain in the uterus when reaching high with arms. Retro-version of uterus, heaviness in hypogastrium with cutting pain down thighs. Uterus feels as if coming out through vagina. Vagina, dry, hot or cold. Eczematous eruptions around the vulva. Great aversion to sex.

Food - Excessive hunger or no appetite, worse when hungry. Aversion to meat, fish. Aversion to cooked food, salt. Aversion to soup. Sweets nauseate. Better warm milk, worse cold drinks. Desires chicken, beer, sweets. ***Worse sweets.*** Worse boiled meat. ***Hot drinks disagree.***

Head - Rush of blood to head, with flushed face, nosebleed or distention and flatulence. ***Burning on vertex, in a small spot.*** Headache in morning on waking, mostly on one side with inclination to vomit. Headache with nausea during menses. Heavy weight or dull pressure at the occiput, as if head is drawn back. ***Pain as if constricted in occiput***, which pains as if broken on looking up. Desolate, empty feeling in head. Rheumatic pains on one side of head, extending to teeth and neck. ***Pressive pain or burning spot on vertex***. Sensation of cobweb on forehead. Skin of forehead as if drawn into folds. Brain feels numb. Humid, itching eruption on hairy scalp, emitting a fetid odor. ***Much scaliness on head, causing distressing itching, becomes scurf***, which disappears on washing, and is then humid. Hair, matted, brittle or falling out of hair, worse vertex and sides. Milk crusts. Eczema capitis, scabs sore to touch. Bald spots. Herpes. Hair falls out, even on sides of head.

Heart - As if an electric shock from heart to neck. Strong pulsations in the whole body. Palpitations of heart with anxiety with nosebleeds. ***Palpitations from least exertion.*** Cold feeling in precordium. Pulse slows during day, fast in the morning

Kidneys - Burning between acts of urinating. Biting pain in urethra after urination. Stricture of urethra. Pain in sacrum or coccyx while urinating. Nocturnal bedwetting. Frequent urination at night. Dark brown urine. Urine, sour smelling, turbid, stream slender. Urine turbid, with white sediment. Sour smelling urine.

Limbs - ***Edema of legs.*** Paralyzed feeling in the limbs. Cannot stretch enough. Burnings, cramps, jerking. Arms and legs go to sleep. ***Excoriation of thighs while walking.*** Bunions worse fire heat, better pressure. Burning in soles and heels. Feet cold, wet. Acrid, foot sweat, chafes the toes. Stiffness and contraction of toes. Foul excoriating sweat, worse evening. Burning pressure beneath the armpit. Hands or feet either hot or cold. Pain in thumb joint as if sprained. ***Nails, brittle and crumbling.*** Nails deformed, painful, sore, thick and crippled. ***Nails, thick, rough ingrown.*** Horny callosities on hands with cracks. Cracks and fissures in fingertips. Swelling of feet.

Lungs - Spasmodic asthma, suffocative attacks wake from sleep, must eat something. Dry, troublesome cough with sweat on face. Lachrymation, worse taking deep breath.

Male - Herpetic eruption on organs. Hydrocele. Sexual debility with increased desire. Priapism. Ejaculation too early or failing during sex. Cramps in calves during sex. Averse to sex, lack of sexual enjoyment. Impotence from excessive indulgence or masturbation.

Modalities - Better in the dark. Better from wrapping up. Better after walking. Better in open air. Better hot drinks, especially milk. Better eating. Better belchings. Better touch. Worse from cold. Worse drafts. Worse warmth of bed. Worse night. Worse wet feet. Worse light. Worse motion. Worse scratching. Worse suppression of eruptions or secretions. Worse during and after menses. Worse empty swallowing. Worse fats. Worse hot drinks.

Mouth - Angles of the mouth ulcerated. Taste, sour like rotten eggs. Rotten, sour, foul odor from mouth. Breath smells like urine. Salivation, at night. Dots of thick, white fur on tongue. Burning blisters on tongue. Teeth on edge. Blood from teeth, tastes sour. Easy bleeding and swelling of the gums.

Nose - Stuffed coryza. Coryza from cold. Colds at menses. Chronic catarrh. Sore on blowing it is painful internally. Discharge offensive especially during menses. Excoriated. ***Scabs and fissures in the nostrils.*** Painful internally. Eczema of nose. Sneezing on opening the eyes. Smell acute, cannot bear the smell of flowers. Dryness with loss of smell. Nosebleed with rush of blood to the head, worse before menses.

Perspiration - Profuse sweat at night. Profuse sweat during menses. Sweats often on front of body only. Offensive, sour sweat, stains yellow. Cold sweat. Entire inability to sweat. Sweats from slightest motion.

Rectum - ***Fissures of anus,*** cutting pain during stool, followed by constriction and aching for hours. Fissures bleed and ulcerate. Constipation, large, difficult, knotty stools united by mucus threads. Chronic diarrhea, brownish, liquid, undigested ***offensive***. Stools, large, difficult, slimy coated or loose, brown, lienteric and very foul. Lump of stool, conjoined with threads of mucus, masses of mucus. Stools are slender, pasty. Diarrhea from slightest indiscretion in eating. Burning hemorrhoids, pain on sitting down or on taking a wide step. Anus and pudenda, smarting, itching, sore, on wiping anus, before menses. Prolapse of rectum. Varicose veins of the rectum. Tapeworms.

Sensations - As if skin of forehead was drawn into folds. As if a skin were before ear. As if a hard body as large as an egg were behind ear. As of a cobweb over the face. As of a lump in stomach with beating as of two hammers. As if intestines were torn, croaking as of a frog in abdomen. As if everything would be torn to pieces during menstruation.

Skin - ***Dry, rough skin,*** irritable. Skin breaks easily and exudes a gluey honey like moisture, worse in folds and slow to heal. ***Unhealthy skin, every little injury suppurates.*** Eruptions worse from heat. ***Eczema.*** Pimples and acne. Wandering or recurrent erysipelas. ***Moist, crusty eruptions, oozing out a sticky exudation***. Phlegmonous erysipelas of face, burning and stinging pain. Rawness in bends of limbs, groins, neck, behind ears. Cracks in nipples, mouth, between toes, anus. ***Old scars ulcerate.*** Burning pain in old scars. Old scars with indurated base and margins with burning. ***Wens***. Chronic poison oak. Psoriasis. Gouty nodosities. Swelling and induration of the glands. Ulcers discharging a ***glutinous*** fluid, thin and sticky.

Sleep - Excessively tired and sleepy. Sleepy during day. Sleeplessness until midnight. Constant talking during sleep. Nightly pains felt in sleep. Amazingly weary and sleepy. Does not feel fresh in the morning. Amorous dreams with emissions. Horrible dreams. Dreams about fatal accidents.

Stomach - Gastralgia with burning pains radiating through abdomen. Sour or foul belchings. Frequent eructations, tasting of ingesta. Eructation of sour green water. Eructations while walking. Pressure in stomach. ***Constrictive pain in stomach***. Recurrent stomach pain with vomiting of food immediately after eating, stomach worse by cold. Burning in stomach, causing hunger, better from eating or hot drinks especially milk, lying down. Periodical gastralgia, with vomiting of food immediately after eating. Morning sickness during menses. Nausea like faintness, prevents sleep. Nausea with spasm in throat. Nausea during headache. Nausea with sour vomiting. Vomiting of sour of food. Vomiting and purging and icy cold sweat with headache. Cancer of pylorus.

Temperature - Chill in the evening worse eating better open air and drinking water. Chill with coldness of whole body. Chill in morning in bed. Chill during menses. Wants covers in all stages of fever. Recurrent periodical fever. Fever with restlessness, unable to sleep, or remain in bed on account of it. Flushes of heat. Dry heat every evening and night. Burning heat in hands and soles and feet. Heat when riding in a carriage.

Throat - Chronic sore throat. Chronic hoarseness with skin disorders. Tonsils enlarged. Nodulated goiter. ***Choking, on swallowing from goiter.*** As of a lump in throat worse empty swallowing, urging to swallow from constant spasms. As if food would not go down from spasms. Hoarseness as soon as he starts singing. Voice lacks control, better using it. Ulcerative pain in throat when swallowing.

Vertigo - Vertigo, worse looking upwards, reading or sewing. Vertigo with nausea and sour vomiting. Vertigo with hyperesthesia of eyes. Vertigo from overexertion of eyes. Vertigo from venous stagnation. Confusion and vertigo in morning on waking.

COMMENTS - Hahnemann was quick to perceive that Graph. was much more than a mere remedy for skin disorders, it proved to be a leading anti-psoric, similar to Sulph. Hahnemann's provings and observations defined its powers over skin disorders.

The skin of Graph. is rough, hard and dry. Eczematous and herpetic eruptions predominate. Poor healing of the skin, tendency to scarring, keloids. Impetigo, eczema. Psoriasis.

Cracks between fingers and toes (Petr.), behind the ears, in the bends of joints, folds of skin, around the lips and anus, and margin of the hair. Intertrigo, infection in the folds of the skin, can fester and form pus. Yellow, sticky, honey-like discharge underneath the scabs.

Pimples, acne. Wens. For the results of repelled eruptions of any kind. Fungal infections that deform the nails, tend to split. Brittle, crack and split down the middle. Pus and infection under the nails (Ant-c.).

The circulation is at first excited, then there is a loss of energy and consequent venous hyperemia. Irregularities in the distribution of the blood occur, leading to pallor of skin and mucus membranes.

Fainting readily occurs with great anxiety, motion is impaired and the tissues relaxed, but paralysis is not complete. Characteristic rush of blood to the head with a flushed face. Hemorrhages.

Strong affinity for the breasts. Cracked nipples (Petr., Sars.). Blocked milk ducts, abscess of the breast. For cancer, particularly of the breast, where the cancer occurs on the site of a scar, where the cancer regrows in the scar of a lumpectomy. Also if there is a history of cracked nipples and abscessed breasts.

Pain under left breast at menstrual period, often waking patient in the night. Scanty menses, with headache, skin-affection. Getting feet wet causes delayed menses. Hysterical melancholia with occipital headache. Profuse, gushing leucorrhea, excoriating.

Cracks along the labia. Moist itching excoriation around anus and fissures. Very low sex drive (Sep.). Uncontrollable sexual excitement with violent erections. Priapism. Impotence.

Clean tongue. Fishy taste in the morning, disappearing later in the day. Milk agrees, especially when hot. Roasted, but not boiled meat or potatoes. Diarrhea, thin offensive, partly digested stools. Constipation, stools coming in lumps coated with mucus and with mucus shreds. Anal fissures, can pass blood and painful stools.

Weak, exhaustion of whole body. Spasms, contractions of muscles, twitching of eyelids. Cataleptic condition. Sensitiveness of internal parts, numbness in various parts, drawing pain in whole body. Bathing after measles causes paralysis of face. Attacks occur during summer and autumn. Suffering parts emaciated.

General obesity with a thick, white, profuse irritating discharge. Suffocative spells which arouse the patient from sleep, he must jump out of bed, worse after midnight (Lach., worse after sleep).

General condition is not sensitive (opposite of Hep.). Abnormally acute senses, cannot tolerate the smell of flowers. Music causes weeping. Sadness. Ears feel stuffed during the full moon. Hardness of hearing is better when riding in a carriage. Easy to over-lift.

Teste classed Graph. in the Puls. group with Sil., Calc., Hep. and Phos. It affects the nutrition in a peculiar way, it is a remedy for those persons who have a tendency to put on unhealthy fat or for those who begin to emaciate. Graph. is an anti-psoric.

Typically *"fat, chilly and costive."* Especially active in patients who are rather stout, of fair complexion with a tendency to skin disorders and constipation, with a delayed menstrual history.

Hufeland related the cure of a lady, 41, by the internal and external use of Graph. of an acne rosacea which had defied all other modes of treatment.

Kent and Grimmer noted cases of late stage breast cancer that they treated with high potencies. Graph. caused the tumors, and in one case the entire breast, to slough off and heal.

Nash recorded a case of a child who was relieved of an eczema capitis under old-school treatment, whereupon entero-colitis set in and became so alarming that it was pronounced "tuberculosis of the bowels."

Nash found the child greatly emaciated with little or no appetite, very restless, passing "stools of brown fluid mixed with undigested substances and of an intolerably fetid odor." Graph. 6,000c cured promptly.

Goullon cured two notable cases of cramps in the stomach with "improvement of the cramps by eating."

Clarke cured two very severe cases of nosebleed in elderly people. In one case, there had been flushing of head and neck for many months previous to the attack, and flushing preceded and accompanied each occurrence of the bleeding.

In the other case, the patient said the precursory flush seemed to come up from his toes. He had his nostrils plugged without avail. Graph. in a high potency, cured promptly in both instances.

When giving Graph. internally in cases of anal eruption, the external use of an ointment made with a drachm of the 3x trituration to an ounce of Cetacean ointment is of great service.

Hirsh or Prague used Graph. locally in cases of disease of the nails with very good results.

RELATIONS - ***Antidoted by:*** Acon., Ars. Nux-v. ***Antidote to:*** Ars-i., Rhus-t. ***Compare:*** (1) Petr., Lach., Carb-v., Carb-a., Caust., Nit-ac., Rhus-t. - erysipelas, left then right, Graph., right then left. Ant-c., Rat., Peon, Nit-ac., Sil. (2) In priapism. - Pic-ac. (3) In disorders of right ovary, Pall. (4) Aur, Puls., Lyc. Stram., Alum. (5) hears better in cars - Nit-ac. (6) Obesity, Calc-a. Trichiasis, Borax. Fat constitutions, Calc. (7) Sulph. has margins of lids reddened with Graph. they are paler then usual, Euphr. has thick, purulent discharge, Graph. has thin. (8) Graph. is a chronic or overgrown Puls. - but Puls. has Worse and Graph. has better from milk. (9) The associated constipation with mucus-covered stools and gastric flatulency should be taken into consideration and differentiate it from such remedies as Petr. and Lyc. ***Complementary:*** Arg-n. - follows well in gastric derangements, Caust., Hep., Lyc., Ars., Tub. ***It follows:*** Calc., Calc-f., Lyc., Puls., Sep., Sulph.

REFERENCES - Boericke. Clarke. Phatak.

GRATIOLA OFFICINALIS

(Hedge Hyssop)

PHARMACY - grat. Gratiola officinalis. Hedge hyssop. Herb of Grace. N. O. Scrophulariacae. Grows in moist places. Tincture of fresh plant before flowering. ***Historical dose:*** Tincture and all potencies.

CLINICAL - Brain disorders. Cholera. Coccyx, pain. Colic. Constipation. Cramps, Diarrhea. Dropsy. Eye disorders. Gout. Headaches. Hemorrhoids. Hydrocephalus. Hysteria. Mania. Masturbation. Mesenteric glands. Nausea. Neuralgias. Nymphomania. Palpitations. Rheumatic pain. Stomach pains. Tetanus. Vision, disordered.

HERBAL - Gratiola, "the Herb of Grace," is one of the most important members of the great Scrophularian group, which includes Dig., Euphr., Tab., Scroph., and should be carefully studied with these.

Cooper used it with great success in a case of gouty acidity with great constipation and in the constipation of cancer. He regards it as "the vegetable antacid." It is said to have formed the basis for a once famous nostrum for gout, "Eau Médicinale."

HOMEOPATHIC - Symptoms of a fully developed, rapid attack of Asiatic cholera are produced. A large proportion of the effects of Gratiola are expended on the gastro-intestinal tract. It is an inodorous plant of bitter taste and very poisonous, causing violent colic, bloody stools, enteritis, jaundice.

Affection of the solar plexus. Constant sinking but cannot eat, bitter taste. Cramps beginning at pit of stomach; pains radiating from stomach. Urine is diminished, reddish, turbid.

Diarrhea, yellowish, gushing, watery, as though rushing from a hydrant. Vomiting of yellowish fluid. Summer diarrhea from excessive drinking of water whether cold or hot. Soreness, burning or irritation of anus follows the stools.

Teste considered Grat. the Cham. of chronic diseases. Teste saw four cases of nymphomania in females to whom herb doctors had given injections of a decoction of freshly gathered Gratiola. Burnett considered it specific in female masturbation and nymphomania.

Especially useful in females, Nux-v.-like symptoms in females. Chronic catarrhal conditions, leucorrhea and gonorrhea. Obstinate ulcers.

Trembling in limbs, convulsions, cramps, excitement and disordered condition of the sexual powers. Paralytic pains and feeling of coldness especially in the abdomen. Cerebral disorders without fever. Nervous prostration. Neuralgia due to abuse of coffee.

MIND - Anxiety, gnawing, empty feeling, rolling about in epigastric region. Peevishness. ***Confusion when lying down.*** Ill humor, tired of life. ***Mental troubles from overweening pride.*** Answers, reflects long. Taciturn.

Great depression and disinclination to do anything. Weak will. Lack of perseverance. Ill-humor. Irresolution.

Violent anger from contradiction. ***Delirium tremens.*** Hysterical. Loquacity and gaiety. Delusion being diminished, smaller. Absorbed in reveries. Nymphomania.

Apprehensive about the future. Fear of eating when hungry. Hypochondriasis and hysteria arising from abdominal troubles.

Abdomen - Shooting pains in the abdomen. Inflation of the abdomen. Rumbling with nausea, eructation and vertigo. Flatulent and pressive colic with nausea and disagreeable risings. Feeling of coldness in abdomen, lasting half an hour.

Back - Pain in coccyx after stool. Neck as if seized by hands.

Breasts - Darting pain in breasts. Shootings in right breast, worse on rising during menses.

Causations - Coffee causes neuralgia.

Chest - Heat in the chest, then the head and hands with redness of the face. Pressure on the chest. Shootings in the chest on breathing. Pimples on the chest, which burn after having been scratched.

Ears - Itching of ears.

Eyes - Eyes feel dry as if sand were in them. Dry, burning eyes. Itching about eyelashes.

Face - Burning heat and redness of the face. Sensation of tension in the face, it feels swollen. Swelling of upper lip. Tearing on one side of face. Painful crack in left side of chin. Tingling, burning in malar bones.

Female - Menses too profuse, premature and too long. Persistent leucorrhea. Tendency to masturbation. ***Nymphomania***. Irritable condition of sexual organs with congestions.

Food - Hunger after a meal with feeling of emptiness. Craves nothing but bread. Worse during and after eating, vertigo during and after a meal.

Head - ***Rush of blood*** with vanishing of sight. Sick headache. Tightness in forehead with wrinkles in skin. Sensation as if brain was contracting and head became smaller.

Heart - Palpitations after stools, with oppression of the chest. Pulse small, intermittent.

Kidneys - Burning in the urethra during and after urination. Diminished secretion of urine. Scanty and reddish urine, which becomes turbid on standing with cloudy sediment.

Limbs - Limb gives way with sciatic pain. Rheumatic pains in the shoulders, arms, fingers, particularly in elbow and wrist joint. Itching in the palm of the hand.

Lungs - Dry cough, excited by a sensation of roughness in the chest in the morning or at night. Nocturnal cough with pain as from excoriation in trachea, oppression of the chest and shivering.

Male - Painful rigidity of the penis after seminal emission, nightly. Stitches in left spermatic cord, ascending though the abdomen up to the chest. Drawing pain in glans.

Modalities - Better from open air. Better rest. Worse from eating. Worse drinking too much water. Worse hot or cold. Worse abuse of coffee. Worse dinner. Worse warm room. Worse summer. Worse motion.

Mouth - Accumulation of much saliva in the mouth. Mouth bitter or clammy. Fetid breath in the morning after waking. Tongue rough, covered with mucus. Sensation of cold in the teeth. Nocturnal tearing or piercing in the molars.

Nose - Frequent sneezing. Stoppage of the nose. Smarting, itching in left nostril. Pressure at upper part of nose.

Perspiration - Constant vaporous exhalation from body.

Rectum - ***Diarrhea, green, frothy water***, followed by anal burning. Diarrhea, ***forcibly evacuated without pain.*** Summer diarrhea from drinking of excess of water. Rectum constricted. ***Constipation*** with gouty acidity. Hemorrhoids with hypochondriasis.

Sensations - As if brain contracted, as if head grew smaller, as if brain would fall forward. As if sand in eyes, as if throat contracted. As if a stone rolling from side to side in stomach.

Skin - Itching with burning after scratching. Running and corrosive eruptions, which resemble scabies. Small boils. Miliary pimples with yellow tips.

Sleep - Insomnia. Irresistible drowsiness with yawning and involuntary closure of eyes. Great sleepiness and lassitude after meals. Deep sleep, like stupor.

Stomach - Dyspepsia with much distention of the stomach. Emptiness after eating. Cramps and colic after supper and during night with swelling of abdomen and constipation. Dysphagia for liquids. As of a cold water or loose, heavy load in stomach.

Temperature - Tendency to chilliness. Chilliness in a warm room during sleep, after an evacuation, with the hair standing on end. Heat ascending to the face with redness and increased external warmth.

Throat - Pressure in throat, as from thick mucus. Accumulation of mucus in throat. Phlegm in throat with inability to throw it off. Pain in throat obliging one to swallow constantly. Stinging in throat. Tingling, roughness and scraping in throat.

Vertigo - Vertigo during and after meals, hunger and feeling of emptiness after meals.

Vision - Myopia. Shortsightedness with burning heat in face. All objects seem white, even green trees. Mist before eyes when reading or writing. Sudden vanishing of sight while writing or looking at light objects, better closing eyes, but constantly returns.

COMMENTS - Two excellent cures with Grat. have been recorded by C. W. Sonnenschmidt. The first case, Mrs. C., 53, was attacked in June with diarrhea, yellow, watery, frothy stools gushing out with force. Severe cutting pains in abdomen, rumbling of flatulence. Occasional nausea and vomiting. Coloc. and Ip. failed to relieve. Then on close inquiry it was elicited that "a cold feeling in the abdomen" had been a feature throughout. Grat. off. 3c, cured promptly.

In the second case, a three-weeks' old infant was attacked with diarrhea and colic. There were two or three stools in quick succession and then an interval of an hour or two. Stools, green or yellow watery, frothy, expelled suddenly. Nausea and vomiting. Severe pain before stools, relieved afterwards, for a short time. Cham., Coloc., and Verat. failed, then Grat. rapidly cured. It also removed "redness around anus and on the side an abrasion of half an inch in extent, which caused some oozing of blood."

E. E. Case cured a woman, age 50, of hemorrhoids with Constipation, difficult stools. External hemorrhoids from any exertion and after stool. Biting, stinging tension in tumors. During stool, a sensation as if the rectal membrane was torn.

After stool, all the nerve of the pelvis seem in a high state of tension, the flesh on the perineum feels as if torn from the bone. Sleepless before midnight, peevish, melancholy. Grat. 200c cured.

The left side is more affected than the right. The head and eye symptoms are of the first importance. Rush of blood to head with vanishing of sight is a keynote. Heat ascending to face with redness and increased external warmth. A number of pains are experienced in the coccyx. Chilly, shuddering on entering a warm room. Constant vaporous emanations from body.

RELATIONS - ***Antidoted by:*** Caust., Bell., Euph., Nux-v. ***It antidotes:*** Iod. ***Compare:*** (1) Dig., Euph., Tab., Cham., Am-c., Nux-v. Apis, Bell., Hell., Cham., Nux-v., Elat., Podo. (2) Hunger after meals with feeling of emptiness, Lauro., Calc., Casc., Chin., Cina, (3) Emptiness after stool, Petr. (4) Vanishing of sight and headache, Gels. (5) Dig., Tab., Euphr., Scroph.

REFERENCES - Boericke. Clarke. Phatak.

GRINDELIA ROBUSTA

(Rosin-wood)

PHARMACY - grin. Grindelia robusta. Rosin-wood. Grindelia squarrosa. N. O. Composite. A tincture is made of the leaves and unexpanded flowers. Bundy's proving of G. squarrosa was made with a tincture of the dried plant. ***Historical dose:*** Tincture and all potencies. Tincture in 1 to 15 drop doses.

CLINICAL - ***Asthma.*** Bites. Blisters. Bronchitis. Burns. Cheyne-Stokes. Conjunctivitis. Emphysema. Erythema. Eyes, pains. Flea-bites. Glaucoma. Heart, disorders. Herpes, zoster. Hyperchlorhydria. Iritis. Itching. Liver, pain. ***Lung, disorders.*** Malaria. Nausea. Ophthalmia. Pruritus, vulvae. Pruritus, vagina. Rash. Rheumatism. ***Rhus poisoning.*** Roseola. Skin, disorders. Spleen, disorders. Stings. Ulcers.

HERBAL - The Grindelia are a genus of asteroid composites growing on the Pacific coast and inland on the mountains. The terminal heads of yellow flowers and the leaves are usually covered with a viscid balsamic secretion, after which they have been called *"gum plants."*

There is practically no difference in the action between Grindelia robusta and Grindelia squarrosa, although G. squarrosa is credited with more spleen symptoms. Following Hering, Clarke did not think it necessary to separate the two Grindelias. Several species have been used in cased of asthma, bronchitis, rhus poisoning, and heart and skin disorders.

HOMEOPATHIC - Grindelia produces paresis of the pneumo-gastric nerve, interfering with respiration and producing profuse secretion in bronchial tubes. Dull pains and fullness in left hypochondrium, chronic malaria, gastric pains associated with spleen congestion.

Induces paralysis, beginning in the limbs. Its action is shown on the heart, first quickening, then retarding it. Raises the blood pressure. Acts on the cardio-pulmonary distribution of the pneumo gastric in dry catarrh (Ant-t. in muco-purulent).

Smothering after falling asleep or on awakening. Asthmatic conditions, chronic bronchitis. Bronchorrhea with tough, tenacious, whitish mucus. Asthma and emphysema with dilated heart. Rattling breathing. Cannot breathe when lying down.

Cheyne-Stokes respiration. Hyperchlorhydria when attended with asthmatic and other neurotic symptoms. Hyperemia of gastric mucus membrane with difficult respiration.

Nausea and retching of gastric ulcer. Sugar in urine. Cutting sore pain in the region of spleen extending to hips. Spleen enlarged. An effective antidote to Rhus-poisoning, locally and internally, also for burns, blisters, vaginal catarrh and herpes zoster.

MIND - Longing for sunshine, light and company.

Abdomen - Unbearable pain in region of liver and spleen, so severe he cannot lie still a moment. Cutting pain in region of spleen, extending to hips. Spleen enlarged (Cean., Card-m.). Soreness like that of acute rheumatism.

Eyes - Conjunctiva injected. Pupils dilated. ***Pain in eyeballs,*** running back to brain, worse moving eyes. Purulent ophthalmia and iritis. Iritis, traumatic, or arising from cold or a metastasis of rheumatism. Pain in left eye and right knee joint like rheumatism.

Face - Face livid. Burning in chin.

Female - Pruritus of vagina and vulva, whether from leucorrhea, aphthae or of venous origin.

Head - Terrible fullness in head, as though he had taken ten or more grains of quinine.

Heart - Weak heart and respiration.

Limbs - Legs greatly swollen, especially about ankle-joint. Severe pain, can hardly get about. Large ulcers over tibia. Chronic ulceration of leg.

Lungs - Acts on the pulmonary circulation. Wheezing and oppression in bronchitis patients. ***Bronchitis with heart disease.*** Asthma with a profuse tenacious expectoration, which relieves. ***Stops breathing when falling asleep, wakes with a start*** and gasps for breath. Must sit up to breathe, ***cannot breathe when lying down.*** Whooping cough with profuse mucus secretion (Coc-c.). Rales are disseminated with foamy mucus, very difficult to detach. Sibilant rales. Cheyne-Stokes respiration. Bronchorrhea with tough, whitish, mucus expectoration. Tough, muco-purulent expectoration, after pneumonia or in chronic bronchitis.

Modalities - Sitting position in bed on account of difficult breathing. Worse from falling asleep. Worse motion. Worse in the dark.

Skin - Bites of insects, fleabites. Itching and burning. Rash-like roseola with severe burning and itching. Vesicular and papular eruptions. ***Poison oak*** (locally as a wash). Herpes zoster. Ulcers with swollen, purplish skin.

COMMENTS - In the clinical experiences recorded, it is Grindelia robusta that is chiefly mentioned, though sometimes it is not specified.

History of results for asthma and emphysema with a dilated heart. Good in tonic for asthma, particularly in cases with a great deal of previous medication (Lob.). Chronic bronchial asthma and spasmodic bronchial cough, with profuse, tenacious expectoration, which gives relief.

Cheyne-Stokes respiration. The breath stops when the patient goes to sleep and awakes with a start, gasping for breath. Irregular heart action and hay fever when associated with difficult breathing.

Sense of suffocation on falling asleep (Lach.). Symptoms are worse by movement, worse in the dark, worse on falling asleep. It removed aversion to darkness in one patient who wanted a light in the room all night.

One writer obtained excellent results from "Grindelia" in a number of cases of asthma and emphysema with dilated heart.

H. W. Foster reported the cure of a case of asthma with G. robusta that shows that Dr. Bundy's proving of G. squarrosa is good for both remedies. Dr. Foster's patient was awakened by asthmatic attacks, the room seeming too small. After getting quiet, just as he would commence to lose himself in sleep he would suddenly awaken again because he seemed to have forgotten to breathe. Grin. 30c relieved at once.

Gatchell recommended an external application of a lotion, one part Grindelia robusta in ten parts water, for itching and painful erythematous eruptions. It is also useful for bites and stings of insects. Used locally and internally as an antidote for Rhus toxicodendron skin rashes.

The only proving is by Dr. T. H. Bundy, who took a teaspoonful of a tincture of the dried plant of G. squarrosa and in half an hour followed it by another. The result was that he produced some intensely severe pains in head and eyes (left, then right), and symptoms in liver, spleen, nervous system and lungs. Altogether, he passed "the most terrible night of his life."

The proving is remarkable for the number of peculiar symptoms induced. First there was "fullness in head as after a heavy dose of quinine." Then, intense pain in the left eye and right knee joint exactly like acute rheumatism. The knee pain lasted only half an hour, and then the third teaspoonful was taken. The eye pain became agonizing, the pupil became widely dilated. It was two hours before the right eye became affected.

At this time, unbearable pain in whole of liver and spleen came on. It was so severe it was impossible to lie still. There was intense soreness of the region, like that of acute rheumatism.

The eye pains were in the eyeballs running directly back into the brain, worse by movement.

There was a kind of paralysis of the vagus nerve. On falling asleep, the respiratory movement would cease and would not be resumed until he woke up from the resulting suffocation.

RELATIONS - ***It antidotes:*** Rhus-t. ***Compare:*** (1) Tart-emet. Erio., Lach., Sang. (2) Am-m., Ant-t., Kali-bi. (3) Lach. - worse from sleep, left then right. (4) Gels. - worse from sleep. Gels. has waking up feeling the heart has stopped, must keep moving to keep it going, Grind. feels respiration has stopped. (5) Stram. - fear of the dark. (6) Op., Lach., Carb-an. - fears to go to sleep. (2) Dyspnea on falling asleep: Am-c., Ant-t., Arum-t., Bad., Bry., Cadm-s., Carb-an., Carb-v., Graph., Lach., Nux-m., Op. (8) Ran-b. and both the Grindelias.

REFERENCES - Boericke. Clarke. Phatak.

GUACO

(Climbing Hemp Weed)

PHARMACY - gua. Guaco. Climbing hemp weed. Mikania guaco. N. O. Composite. Tropical America. Tincture or decoction of leaves. ***Historical dose:*** Tincture and all potencies.

CLINICAL - ***Bulbar, paralysis.*** Cancer. Cholera. Deafness. Diarrhea. ***Dysentery***. Hydrophobia. Leucorrhea. Paralysis. Phosphaturia. Rheumatism. Spine, disorders. Strokes. ***Syphilis***. Tongue, paralysis.

HERBAL - Mikania guaco is a climbing composite of tropical America. Guaco has a local repute as a remedy for the bites of serpents, hydrophobia, cholera and cancer.

HOMEOPATHIC - Gua. acts on the nervous system and female organs. ***Bulbar paralysis. Spinal irritation. Syphilis***. Cancer. Cholera. ***Diarrhea and dysentery with aching in sacrum and loins***. Deafness. Tongue heavy and difficult to move. Beer drinkers threatened with strokes.

Abdomen - Pain and rumbling in bowels, followed by watery stools.

Back - Pain between scapulae, extending to forearm. Burning in nape of shoulders. ***Pain along spine***, worse from bending. Weariness through hips and lumbar region.

Causations - Antidote to bites of scorpions and snakes (Golondrina).

Ears - Deafness.

Female - Copious, corroding, putrid, debilitating leucorrhea. Itching and smarting at night, as if fire were running out of parts.

Head - Headache, red face. Heaviness and difficulty in moving tongue.

Kidneys - Unusual flow of urine with excess phosphates. Pain over region of bladder and weight and weariness through hips and loins.

Limbs - Pain in deltoid, shoulders, elbows, arms and fingers. ***Paralysis of lower limbs***. Legs heavy. Pain about hip joint. Pain in ankle-joints and soles.

Modalities - Worse from motion. Worse bending. Worse at night.

Mouth - Tongue heavy, difficult to move.

Throat - Larynx and trachea constricted, difficult deglutition.

COMMENTS - In the homeopathic provings, rice-water stools occurred along with difficult swallowing, as in hydrophobia. One proving also showed an action on the bladder and urinary organs, producing excess phosphates.

A woman who took a decoction for four moths steadily was obliged to discontinue because it produced copious, corrosive, putrid leucorrhea, causing great debility, tanning the inside of the thighs and staining linen yellow. She felt as if fire was running out of her. Terrible itching and smarting.

Another prover had severe spinal and occipital pains, paresis of tongue and difficult deglutition. Burning and tearing in soles. Pain as if beaten. Pains extend to other parts, mostly from above downwards.

RELATIONS - ***Antidoted by:*** Kreos. and Sulph. (leucorrhea). ***Compare:*** (1) Ox-ac., Lathyr., Caust. Alum. (2) Bell. - menstrual flow feels hot. (3) Ph-ac. - Phosphaturia. (4) Leucorrhea staining yellow, Carb-an., Kreos., Nit-ac.

REFERENCES - Boericke. Clarke.

GUAIACUM OFFICINALE

(Lignum Vite Resin)

PHARMACY - guai. Guaiacum officinale. Lignum vite resin. Lignum sanctum resin. Gum guaiacum. N. O. Zygophyllaceae. The gum resin of a large tree growing in West Indies. Tincture of the gum resin. ***Historical dose:*** Tincture and all potencies.

CLINICAL - Abscess. Amenorrhea. Aneurysm. Bones disorders. Bronchitis. Decay. Cholera, infantum. Constipation. Contraction. Cough. Diarrhea. Diphtheria. Dysmenorrhea. Earache. Emaciation. Fever. Gout. ***Growing, pains.*** Headache. Hernia. Membranous, dysmenorrhea. Mercury, effects. Neuralgia. Osteomalacia. Otitis. Ovaries inflammation. Pleurisy. Rheumatism. Sciatica. Stomach disorders. Syphilis. Throat, disorders. Tonsillitis. Toothaches. Torticollis. Tuberculosis. Vomiting.

HOMEOPATHIC - Guai., which is one of Hahnemann's anti-psorics, is best known as a remedy in gout and rheumatism and as a diuretic, but it has also taken a place in old-school therapeutics as a remedy for tuberculosis. Guai. was first recommended by Brinton in the Lancet in 1857 for quinsy, was given in full doses and produced a crisis of sweat and profuse urination.

Homeopathic provings developed and defined the sphere of its utility in these respects and many more. It acts on mucus membranes, muscles, fibrous tissue, joints and bones. Arthritic diathesis. Acute rheumatism. Gouty nodosities on joints. Nodes. Exostosis. ***Growing pains.*** Tonsillitis with rheumatism. Secondary syphilis.

Contraction of limbs, stiffness and immobility. Muscles and tendons are contracted, resulting in pain, rigidity and swelling of the joints, and deformity. Muscles and tendons seem too short or feel sore. Contractions between scapulae, palms etc., causing distortions and immobility.

Unclean odor from whole body. Promotes suppuration of abscesses. ***Free foul, secretions,*** expectoration, sweat, etc. Bones become spongy or suppurate. Burning heat in affected part. Sensitiveness and aggravation from local heat.

Gnawing or sticking pains in chest. Pains often end in stitch, especially head. Contractive pain between scapula. Violent pains in limbs after a cold. Feeling that he must yawn, stretch with uneasy feeling in the whole body.

Violent, spasmodic inflammatory disorders of windpipe and larynx with palpitation, preventing motion or calling for help, feels suffocating. Cough dry or with copious bloody or purulent expectoration of very offensive odor.

Heat, swelling and blotchiness of face. Prosopalgia every day from 6 p.m. to 4 a.m. Toothache when biting jaws together.

Progressive emaciation. Desire for apples, which helps the gastric symptoms, and a general aversion to milk and food. "Violent hunger afternoon and evening," similar to the "sinking" sensations of Sulph. and the anti-psorics. Nausea from sensation of phlegm in throat.

Marked flatulence. "Every morning vomits a mass of watery phlegm with great exertion, followed by great exhaustion." Morning diarrhea with dry skin and chilliness. Cholera infantum, the face is like that of an old person. Constipation, dry, hard, crumbling and very offensive stool.

Continuous urging even after urination with profuse fetid urine. Stitches in neck of bladder after ineffectual pressure to urinate. Cutting while urinating.

General ill feeling, better yawning and stretching, worse from the least motion. Clothes feel damp. Perspiration on head on walking in open air. Chilly crawls over breasts. Chilliness in back. Cannot bear heat with pains in limbs. Marked periodicity. Stomach illness returns every summer.

MIND - Indolent, obstinate, fretful. Disinclination to labor. Sad and depressed. Weak memory. Forgetful, thoughtless, staring. Forgetful of names. Slow to comprehend. Delusion everything seems narrow.

Strong desire to criticize and despise everything. Inclination to blame everybody and scold. Defiant. Disobedience. Shrieking during sleep. Weeping after nightmare.

Abdomen - Distention, flatulent. Intestinal fermentation. Sensation of constriction or stoppage in epigastrium, causing cough, dyspnea.

Back - Pain from head to neck. ***Aching in nape. Stiff neck and sore shoulders.*** Contractive pain between scapulae. Stitches between scapulae to occiput. One-sided stiffness of back from neck to sacrum.

Breasts - Cold crawling over breasts. Shuddering in breasts with goose bumps.

Chest - ***Pleuritic stitches.*** Chest pains in articulations of ribs, with shortness of breathing until expectoration sets in. Pain in the chest while riding in the open air, better pressure and walking, worse sitting and standing.

Ears - Aching in left ear.

Eyes - Exophthalmos. Pupils dilated. Eyeballs seem too big to be covered by the eyelids, or eyelids appear too short. Hard pimples around the eyes.

Face - Neuralgia of the left side of the face, daily from 6 p.m. to 4 a.m. Face like an old person.

Female - Ovaritis in the rheumatism, with irregular menstruation, dysmenorrhea and irritable bladder.

Food - Aversion to milk, to all food, could not eat anything. ***Desire for apples*** and other fruits, which relieve gastric symptoms.

Head - ***Gouty and rheumatic pain in head and face, extending to neck***. Tearing pain in skull, worse cold, wet weather. ***Pains often end in a stitch,*** especially in head. Head feels swollen and blood vessels distended. Brain feels loose. Headache better walking and pressure, worse sitting and standing.

Kidneys - Continuous urging, even after urination. Sharp stitches during or after urination.

Limbs - ***Growing pains*** (Calc-p.). Arthritis deformans. Arthritic lancinations followed by contraction of limbs. Sciatica and lumbago. ***Gouty tearing pains with contractions.*** Immovable stiffness. Joints swollen, painful and intolerant of pressure, can bear no heat. Stinging pain in the limbs. ***Feeling of heat*** in the affected limbs. Rheumatic pain in shoulders, arms and hands. ***Rheumatic pain in wrists.*** Pricking in buttocks, as if sitting on needles. Hamstrings too short. Ankle pain extending up the leg, causing lameness.

Lungs - ***Feels suffocated***. Recurrent pleurisy. Pleuritic stitches, worse deep breathing. Stitching in apex of (left) lung. Tuberculosis. Dry, tight cough. Fetid breath after coughing.

Male - Seminal emissions without dreams. Discharge from urethra.

Modalities - Better external pressure. Better apples. Better yawning and stretching. Better from cold locally. ***Worse from heat.*** Worse cold, wet weather. Worse touch. Worse motion. Worse exertion. Worse rapid growth. Worse mercury. Worse puberty. Worse 6 p.m. to 4 a.m.

Mouth - Tongue furred.

Nose - Pains in bones of nose. Nose swollen. Fluent coryza.

Perspiration - Profuse sweat on single parts, face, etc. Sweats at night. Much sweat, especially on head and face. Sweats on walking in open air. Sweat is usually offensive.

Rectum - Cholera infantum, face like an old person, emaciation. Diarrhea.

Sleep - Yawns and stretches for relief of general ill feeling. Frequent waking from sleep, as if from falling.

Stomach - Thick, white fur on tongue. Constricted epigastric region. Burning in stomach. Vomits a mass of watery mucus, then exhaustion. Stomach disorders return in summer.

Temperature - Sweat profuse on single parts, face etc. Night sweats. Burning of body. Hot palms. Burning fever with hot face and dry cough. Fever with chill in the evening.

Throat - Dry, burning, swollen. Sharp stitches towards the ear on swallowing, cannot swallow without a drink. ***Acute tonsillitis***, painful to touch. Recurrent tonsillitis followed by rheumatism. Syphilitic sore throat. Rheumatic sore throat with weak throat muscles.

Vertigo - Vertigo on rising.

COMMENTS - Affected parts are very sensitive to touch, worse from heat. Offensive secretions. Rheumatism in syphilitic and mercurial patients. Growing pains in children.

Acute tonsillitis, simple or rheumatic. Syphilitic sore throat. "Burning in the throat." Erythematous or inflammatory angina with bright redness (Bell.). Edema (Apis.). Phlegmon with tendency to suppuration of tonsils (Bar-c., Apis.).

Burning sensations in mouth, throat and stomach. Stitches in chest going from front to back or from below upward in region of apex, worse from motion and deep inspiration. "Sharp pain about mid-day under right breast to shoulder."

Neuralgia of left side of head and face, extending to neck. Sharp stitches in brain. Sensation as if the brain were loose. External headache with sensation as if blood vessels were over-filled, extending to face and neck. Tearing pains in skull. Swelling and sensation of swelling in eyes and nose. Eyes feel protruded.

Ozanam gave it in the 1c, 2c and 3c dilutions and found that he got the curative effects without crisis, which was an unnecessary effect of the drug. Guai., said Ozanam, seems to combine the properties of Bell., Apis and Bar-c.

Houghton cured with Guai. 3x a case of gouty inflammation of the meatus of the ear and tympanum after failure with Ferr-p. Concomitant rheumatic lameness and soreness led him to Guai.

Verwey treated a woman, who for several years had a frequently recurring gouty inflammation of the knees. After Chin. 30c had failed to relieve, Guai. 30c was given without obvious benefit. Guai. 1c was then given, and after a few hours the swelling broke and the pains quickly subsided.

A short time after, the same patient accidentally injured the same knee. Under Guai. 1c the swelling soon broke and the pain was relieved, but an abscess formed at the same time on the upper thigh. The pain became unbearable and the patient's husband "begged for more of the drops that had twice before made the swelling break."

It was again given and in six hours the abscess evacuated. On two later occasions Dr. Verwey saw Guai. act in the same way on scrofulous and gouty abscesses. This is probably analogous to its action in quinsy.

RELATIONS - ***Antidoted by:*** Nux-v. ***Antidote to:*** Caust., Rhus-t. ***Compare:*** (1) Merc., Caust., Rhus-t., Mez., Rhod. (2) Ph-ac. - growing pains. (3) Cimic. - pleurodynia and tuberculosis. (4) Bry. - chronic rheumatism when the joints are distorted, worse motion, pleurisy in second stage of tuberculosis. (5) Coloc. - contractions after rheumatism. (6) Caust. - Guai. is better than Caust., which it follows well, when either gout or rheumatism causes distortion of limbs. (7) Araceae - late tuberculosis, pleuritic pains left apex. (8) Kali-i., Phyt., Still. ***Compatible:*** After Merc. - Rheumatism, gout and syphilis, after Sulph. in cholera infantum, after Caust. in torticollis. ***Follows:*** Sep.

REFERENCES - Boericke. Clarke.

GUARANA

(Brazilian Coca)

PHARMACY - guar. Guarana. Brazilian coca. Paullinia sorbilis. N. O. Sapindaceae. Alcoholic solution of dried paste made from seeds. ***Historical dose:*** Tincture and all potencies.

CLINICAL - Alcohol. Chlorosis. Cholera infantum. Coffee. Depression. Diarrhea. Eyelids, twitching. Headache. Insomnia. Neuralgia. Spasms. Urticaria. Tuberculosis.

HERBAL - Guarana is a climbing shrub of Brazil, the seeds of which contain caffeine and are used by the natives for making a stimulating beverage.

HOMEOPATHIC - Guar. is used in conditions of nervous exhaustion, sick headache in those who have abused tea and coffee. Headache followed by vomiting and excited by any error in diet or depression of mind. Throbbing, congestive headache after excessive use of liquor.

Neuralgia. Persistent twitching of eyelids. Paralysis. Restlessness, nervousness, weariness. Reduced vital powers, with grief, depression of spirits, loss of appetite. Debility after prostrating diseases. Chlorosis. Diarrhea.

MIND - Intellectual excitement, mental hyperesthesia. Extravagant behavior. Grief, depression of spirits.

Bladder - Spasm of bladder.

Causations - Ill effects of alcohol or coffee.

Eyes - Persistent twitching of eyelids.

Head - Sick headache from excess of tea or coffee. Throbbing, congestive headache after excessive use of alcohol.

Rectum - Cholera infantum. Stools profuse, bloody, bright green, mucus, flakes intermixed, odorless. Diarrhea of tuberculosis.

Skin - Chloasma on temples and arms. Urticaria (Dulc., Apis, Chlol.). Prurigo.

Sleep - Uncontrollable sleepiness and heaviness of head, with flushed face after eating.

RELATIONS - ***Compare:*** (1) Agar. - Twitching of eyelids. (2) Ign., Nux-v. (3) in sick headache, Coff., Coca., Thea.

REFERENCES - Boericke. Clarke.

GUAREA TRICHILOIDES

(Ballwood)

PHARMACY - guare. Guarea trichiloides. Ballwood. Redwood. N. O. Meliacee. Caribbean. Central America. Tincture and trituration of dried bark. ***Historical dose:*** Tincture and all potencies.

CLINICAL - Asthma. Bones disorders. ***Chemosis.*** Dysphagia. Eyes disorders. Hernia. Intermittent fever. Liver spots. Lupus. ***Pterygium.*** Ptosis. Strokes. Tongue disorders. Tonsils, swollen. Vertigo. Whooping cough.

HOMEOPATHIC - Petroz is the authority for this remedy, which produces a number of symptoms in the eyes. R. K. Ghosh cured a number of cases of chemosis and pterygium. He found a lotion of Guarea tincture of great assistance.

Lupus of an ochre-red color. Eye symptoms alternate with diminished hearing. A number of symptoms were experienced in the umbilicus and inguinal rings. Flow of blood between menses.

On the skin there were liver spots and an eruption with burning vesicles. Aromatic-smelling sweat. Sweat during or after eating. Suppuration of glands. Steatoma, hot swelling, swelling of affected parts.

Sensation of constriction. Sudden shocks of whole body. Bruised pains. Pains in periosteum. In the head there is a sensation as if the brain were falling forward and a sensation as of a blow on the head leaving numbness and diminished thinking power.

MIND - Anxiety during fever. Irresolution. Loquacity. Indifference. Fear of losing reason.

Abdomen - Hardness at umbilicus. Abdomen distended with lancination in groins and inguinal ring. Bruised pain externally.

Chest - Sensation of hollowness and dilatation of chest.

Ears - Swelling of periosteum behind ears. Sensation in ears as of a peg of a worm, pushing-out feeling. Roaring in ears.

Eyes - Conjunctiva inflamed, swollen. Tearing pain in eyeballs, tension, forced-out feeling. Objects appear gray, upside down. Eye symptoms alternate with diminished hearing.

Face - Suppurating swellings on face. Swelling of upper lip.

Female - Fetid leucorrhea after menses. Flow of blood between menstrual periods. Itching of pudenda. Labor pains suppressed. Lochia is scanty.

Food - Canine hunger in evening, speedy satiety. Aversion to milk, fish and hot, greasy, cooked food.

Head - Sensation as if brain were falling forwards, as from a blow on head.

Limbs - Jactitation of limbs. Cracking in joints. Nightly pains in bones. Bruised pain in bones. Caries.

Lungs - Cough with sweat, pain and tightness of chest, larynx irritated. Cough dry barking, violent, deep-seated. Breathing, sobbing, difficult during chill. Respiratory symptoms worse from putting hand to throat.

Modalities - Better hot drinks. Better wrapping warmly. Acids and cold water aggravates. Bone pains worse at night.

Mouth - Mouth smells of cheese. Sweet taste, food tastes insipid.

Nose - Coryza with hardened secretion with heat. Nose stuffed, ineffectual desire to sneeze, constriction at root of nose.

Rectum - Constriction of anus and rectum. Urging to stool. Constipation.

Skin - Yellow spots on temples. Liver spots on arms. Eruptions behind ears. Herpes. Itching. Lupus of ochre-red color.

Sleep - Sleepy in open air. Dreams, anxious, melancholy, full of strife.

Stomach - Constriction in stomach, bruised. Sour belchings with tension and pressure at stomach. Inclination to vomit during fever. Vomiting, sour, green.

Temperature - Coldness followed by heat with sweat. Heat of upper part of body, coldness of bones. Sweat chiefly during and after eating. Sweat aromatic.

Throat - Tonsils swollen. Esophagus has raw pain, sensation of contraction and burning heat. Swallowing difficult.

Tongue - Tongue coated during the fever, grayish yellow, swollen, paralyzed, bleeding. Tongue feels cold and dry. Lancinations in tongue.

RELATIONS - ***Compare:*** (1) Bov. - flow of blood between menses. (2) Crot-h. - as if had a blow on the head. Anac. - peg in ear. Gels - vertigo, ptosis. Aza., Apis - chemosis, asthma millari. Arn. - injuries. Phos. - steatoma. Ign. - nerves. Merc. and Sil. - Bone-pains, suppuration.

REFERENCES - Boericke. Clarke.

GUATTERIA GUAMERIA

(Elemuy)

PHARMACY - guat. Guatteria guameria. Elemuy. Yumel. N.O. Anonaceae family. Central and Southern America. Tincture from the dried bark of the plant. ***Historical dose:*** Tincture and all potencies.

CLINICAL - Anorexia. Belching. Jaundice. ***Gallbladder, disorders.*** Gallstones. Hematuria. Hepatitis. Leucorrhea. ***Liver, disorders.*** Nausea. Palpitations. Pneumonia. Tachycardia.

HOMEOPATHIC - Described in 1790 by J. B. Guatteria and in 1906 by G. F. Gaumer. The symptomatology was established by Castro on seventeen adults of both sexes, using 3x and 6x, in 1944.

There are grounds for thinking that Guat. will take one of the first places among the homeotherapeutic remedies for liver conditions, alongside Chlorpr.

Guat. acts on the liver, gallbladder, kidneys and pancreas. Digestive complaints with liver and biliary manifestation. Predominantly on the right side, lungs, scapulae, shoulders, kidneys.

MIND - Irresolute, weak memory. Sad. Obsessive ideas.

Abdomen - Epigastric pain, spreading towards the right hypochondrium, right kidney and the base of the right lung. Abdominal distention, ameliorated by belching.

Constitutions - Allergic, psoric or sycotic constitutions.

Eyes - Conjunctival jaundice with photophobia, myosis and itching, ameliorated by rubbing.

Female - Excoriating, white leucorrheal discharge.

Food - Extreme thirst. Anorexia, nausea. Aggravated by hot foods, condiments and sweets.

Head - Occipital pain, aggravated in a warm room and by lying down. Frontal pulsating headache.

Heart - Palpitations and tachycardia, worse after eating.

Kidneys - Hematuria, urine thick with muddy deposits of calcium oxalate. Urinary density increased. Urinary urea diminished.

Limbs - Pain and joint aching, especially of the fingers, knees and shoulders, predominantly on the right, with stiffness.

Liver - Congestion of the liver. Liver deficiency. Jaundice from hepatitis or gallstones. Gallstones. Inflammation of the gallbladder.

Lungs - Lung infections on the right side, bronchitis. Viral pneumonia. Dry cough with blockage in the base of the right lung, linked with congestion of the liver, aggravated by lying on the right side. Painful cough, with palpitations and tachycardia, worse after eating.

Modalities - Better from rest. Better food, if administered in small, repeated quantities. Worse in a warm room. Worse movement. Worse on right side. Worse after meals.

Mouth - Tongue dirty, yellow, furred, especially at the root. Bad breath, mouth tastes bitter. Excessive, thick salivation.

Rectum - Diarrhea with cramping colic or constipation, followed by burning and tenesmus after stools passed. Stools bright green or bright yellow, hard or liquid, mucous, with a nauseating odor.

Skin - Skin dirty, especially on the face, discolored, pigmented with brown spots on the forehead and cheeks. Brownish stains on the arms and backs of the hands. Perspiration stains underwear yellow. Eruptions with itching, yellowness, aggravated by eating, ameliorated by prolonged rest. Vesicular tension disorders.

Stomach - Acrid dyspepsia. Bilious yellow and green vomiting, aggravated by hot food, movement. Burning in the esophagus and stomach, aggravated by condiments and sweets.

Vertigo - Vertigo with headaches, heavy head.

RELATIONS - ***Compare:*** (1) Chel. - Same side and located on the right, stools golden yellow. (2) Chin. - Extreme abdominal distentions, aggravation from loss of fluids, diarrhea. (3) Lyc. - Melancholy, irritable, dyspepsia, hepatic disorders, aggravated from 4 p.m. to 8 p.m. (4) Lac-c. - Perspiration stains the underwear yellow, symptoms move from right to left.

REFERENCES - Julian.

GUNPOWDER

(Black Gunpowder)

PHARMACY - gunp. Gunpowder. Black gunpowder. Carbon-Sulphur-Kali-Nitricum. ***Historical dose:*** Trituration and all potencies.

CLINICAL - ***Abscesses.*** Acne. Bites. ***Blood, poisoning.*** Boils. Carbuncles. Cuts, poisoned. Dyspepsia. Eczema. Fistula. ***Food, poisoning. Foot-rot.*** Glands, disorders. ***Gonorrhea.*** Gunshot, wounds. ***Herpes.*** Herpes, zoster. ***Infections.*** Injuries. Ivy, poisoning. Leucoderma. Methane, poisoning. Ophthalmia. Osteomyelitis. Ptomaine, poisoning. Pyorrhea. ***Septicemia.*** Shingles. Syphilis. Tonsillitis. Toxicity. ***Ulcers.*** Vaccinosis. ***Worms. Wounds.***

HOMEOPATHIC - Gunpowder was first published in the Homeopathic World, London in 1914 by Clarke. A combination remedy of carbon, sulphur and potassium nitrate. Useful for all kinds of blood poisoning, for septic wounds and ptomaine poisoning.

Strong history of use in wartime, particularly useful in World War I and II. Gunshot wounds, surgical septicemia, boils. Methane poisoning. Wartime ailments.

Blood disorders. ***Blood poisoning*** from pyorrhea alveolaris. Septic suppurations. Infected wounds. Wounds that refuse to heal. Abscessed bites, infections and wounds, antiseptic. Swollen and abscessed glands. Osteomyelitis.

Poisoning from bad food or water. Poisoning from meats that have been unsuccessfully tinned. Acute infections, boils, abscesses, carbuncles, and bites. Antidote to ivy and primula rash.

Antidoting the ***ill effects of vaccinations***. Preventative for various kinds of inoculations. Gonorrhea and syphilis. Shingles of the face and eyes.

In some country districts a decoction of gunpowder is given to children for worms with much success.

Blood - Blood disorders. ***Blood poisoning.***

Causations - Bites. ***Blood poisoning.*** Vaccinations. Wounds. Gonorrhea. Herpes zoster. ***Worms.***

Glands - Swollen and inflamed. Swollen axillary glands. Abscessed glands.

Male - Gonorrhea and syphilis.

Mouth - Sores, boils. Gum abscesses. Pyorrhea.

Skin - Boils, abscesses, carbuncles and bites. Fistula. Infected wounds. Shingles.

COMMENTS - Dr. Clarke referred to the old fashioned gunpowder that was in use before the era of high explosives and smokeless powder. Black gunpowder is a mixture and not a chemical compound. It contains three remedies, two of them polycrests.

Nitre with sulphur and charcoal forms gunpowder. A teaspoonful of this in hot water was a favorite remedy for gonorrhea among soldiers when black powder was used. In the lower triturations, gunpowder has cured ascarides in adults.

The London Police Force also knew it as a boil remedy. "Get six-penny worth of gunpowder from an oil store and take as much as would lie on a sixpence night and morning for four days and then leave it off for the same time and resume if necessary" is one such prescription.

Canon Roland Upcher noted that Norfolk shepherds rubbed gunpowder onto the sheep's wounds made during sheep-shearing, and took it to cure or prevent ill effects from handling sheep who suffered from "foot-rot."

Upcher published cases of skin eruption mistaken for scabies, actually caused by handling ivy. Cured with Gunp. 3x.

Clarke experimented with Gunp. 2x and developed severe herpes facialis involving the right eyebrow and the right side of the nose.

Clarke confirmed the proving by curing shingles. He heard of a case of lumbrici cured with an infusion of Gunpowder by the patient.

A woman, who had a very sensitive skin, was bitten by a gnat on the foot, resulting in swelling inflammation and suppuration. There was a ring of inflammation around the bite, constantly spreading and detaching the epidermis as it spread. After the failure of several remedies, Gunpowder 3x rapidly cured.

A man had a bad cut with a knife on the left index finger. The wound refused to heal. An inflammatory ring stripped off the epidermis and spread more and more. Lachesis and other remedies failed to make any impression. Gunp. 3x rapidly cured.

Another woman was very severely poisoned by sewer-gas. There followed swelling of the right arm and axillary glands of the right side. Three months after the accident the right arm was almost fixed at the elbow-joint with swelling. It threatened suppuration above and below. The axillary glands were as large as a hen's egg.

Gunp. 3x gradually resolved the trouble and, though the cure was interrupted by an attack of measles, the motility of the arm was fully restored.

Canon Upcher found that occasional doses of Hep. highly increase its effects.

RELATIONS - Calen. externally is also complementary. ***Compare:*** Thuja, Sil., Bar-c. - septic tonsils.

REFERENCES - Boericke. Clarke. Murphy.

GYMNEMA SYLVESTRE

PHARMACY - gymne. Gymnema sylvestre. N. O. Asclepiadacae. Tincture of leaves. ***Historical dose:*** Tincture and all potencies.

CLINICAL - Hives. Snakebite. Taste, altered

HERBAL - This plant, which grows in the Deccan peninsula, Assam and some parts of Africa, is a woody climber with long, slender branches. The powdered root has a reputation among the natives as a remedy for snakebite.

HOMEOPATHIC - The leaves have a bitter, astringent and slightly acid taste. Immediately after chewing them, the sense of taste for sugar and for bitters were lost, the effect lasting some hours.

Sense of taste altered. Everything else could be tasted, for instance, the ginger in gingerbread, but not the sweet. Quinine tasted like chalk.

REFERENCES - Boericke. Clarke.

GYMNOCLADUS CANADENSIS

(American Coffee-tree)

PHARMACY - gymn. Gymnocladus canadensis. American coffee-tree. Chicot. Gymnocladus dioica. N. O. Leguminose. Tincture of fresh pulp of the pods. ***Historical dose:*** Tincture and all potencies.

CLINICAL - Erysipelas. Fever. Headache. Spleen, pain in. Throat, sore. Tongue, blue. Toothache. Whitlow.

HOMEOPATHIC - Gymn. causes numbness and blueness, especially of the tongue. ***Bluish-white coating of tongue.*** Sore throat, dark livid redness of fauces.

"Erysipelatous swelling of face and head, hot face, it feels swollen is compelled to rub the eyes." Hives.

Headache, throbbing in forehead, temples and over eyes. Full, tight headache, with sensation as if the eyes were pushed forward. Burning in eyes. Full sensations and burning pains. Desire for heat and quiet.

C. T. Bingham cured a man of headache following influenza "a constant severe pain in front part of head, especially under eyebrows and upper part of nose."

It lasted over two weeks, never ceasing and at times intolerable. Bones of eye-sockets were sore to touch. Tongue was covered all over with bluish-white coat, did not enjoy food. Very weak. Gym. 2x cured.

Epidemic fevers of typhoid character have been cured by it.

MIND - Forgets everything. Slow grasp, cannot think, comprehend or study. Indifference to what happens around him.

Abdomen - Pain in left side as if spleen were swollen. Soreness and tenderness of abdomen. Stitches in bowels and umbilical region.

Bladder - Pressure on bladder. Frequent desire to urinate, urine passed in a small stream.

Chest - Pressure on chest and sternum.

Eyes - As if were pushed forward, wants to rub them. Pain under brows into the nose.

Face - Erysipelatous swelling. Crawling as of flies over the face.

Head - Tight feeling, as if bound.

Limbs - Violent pain in left forearm, in radius, as if bones were crushed and broken. Pulsation in left index finger, as if panaritium were forming.

Male - Itching of gland and prepuce.

Modalities - Better from rest. Better rubbing eyes. Better leaning against something. Worse from cold. Worse cold drinks. Worse drafts. Worse walking. Aversion to motion, easily fatigued.

Mouth - Great sensibility of teeth, especially to cold air. Toothache from slightest cold air or drink.

Lungs - Tickling with dry, hard, racking cough. Tickling in throat in morning causing cough, increasing through day.

Stomach - Hot, sour belchings. Burning spot in stomach.

Stool - Constipation with ineffectual desire. Aching fullness in rectum after stool.

Throat - Sore throat, dark livid redness of fauces and tonsils. Smarting in larynx. Sticking pain. Mucus in throat and hawking.

Tongue - ***Bluish, white tongue.***

COMMENTS - Fever symptoms. Desire for heat, wants to be near the fire. Cold chills and pains in bowels. Perspiration in axillary regions and palms. Toothache from slightest cold air or drink. Violent pain in left forearm as if the bones were crushed.

RELATIONS - *Compare:* (1) Lachn., Lach., Ail., Rhus-t. (2) Nux-v., Agar. Aeth., Bell., Cic., Hyos., Sol-n., Stram.

REFERENCES - Boericke. Clarke.

H

HAEMATOXYLON CAMPECHIANUM

(Logwood tree)

PHARMACY - haem. Haematoxylon campechianum. Logwood tree. N. O. Leguminose. Caesalpinioideae. Central America. Tincture of the heart wood. ***Historical dose:*** Tincture and all potencies.

CLINICAL - Angina pectoris. Borborygmi. Colic. Diarrhea. Dysmenorrhea. Eyes, disorders. Headaches. Herpes zoster. Indigestion. Leucorrhea. Melancholy. Ptosis. Throat, sore.

HOMEOPATHIC - Logwood is a well-known dye of commerce. The tincture was proved by Jouve in 1939 and some very distinctive symptoms were produced including general uneasiness with anxiety arising from the stomach, and colic. Weak digestion accompanies and complicates most other conditions.

General sensitiveness. Painful sensibility of the limbs with lassitude. ***Constriction*** in many parts, culminating in the stomach and abdomen. Colic with chest symptoms like angina pectoris. ***Sensation as if a bar lay across chest.*** Chilliness predominates, but the symptoms are better in open air.

MIND - Ill humor, sadness, melancholy. Inclination to repose, desire to weep. Difficulty when reflecting and expressing one's ideas. Vexation. ***Anxiety at night.*** Anxiety arising from the stomach. Mistakes in speaking.

Abdomen - Tympanitic distention of the abdomen and rising of air. Tension and digging in the abdomen. Pain in the abdomen with yawning inclination to vomit and stretch. Borborygmi. Colic with painful sensibility of the abdomen to the touch, inflation. Colic and diarrhea in morning. After the colic, general cold with burning heat in the palms of he hands.

Back - Pain and chilliness between the shoulders.

Chest - ***Sensation as if a bar lay transversely across chest*** from region of heart to right side with acute pain in left upper portion of chest. Constriction, extending from the chest to the epigastrium, with smarting and burning pain increased by the touch. Angina pectoris.

Ears - Violent pain in right ear, extending to throat.

Eyes - Redness of the conjunctiva. Redness of the eyes with blue margins. Eyes downcast and surrounded by a livid circle. Heaviness in the eyes. Heaviness of the eyelids, compels them to close. Painful pressure on the eyes with sensation of constriction. Sensation as if sand were introduced into the eyes. Pupils contracted and sight confused. Mist before the eyes, on reading, the letters vanish. Amelioration of the symptoms when in open air.

Face - Face pale, dejected and changed, discomposed. Pain in face.

Female - Colic, as if the menses were going to appear with slimy, whitish discharge from the vagina. ***Weak feeling with painful bearing down sensation at menstrual period.*** Pain in hypogastrium, attended with slimy, whitish leucorrhea.

Head - Head feels constricted, heavy, hot, painful. Constriction in the forehead and in the occiput with burning heat in the head. Headache at night, as from indigestion, with swelling of the stomach and abdomen, anxiety, inclination to vomit, sour risings of food. Headache in the forehead with inclination to vomit on stooping. Pain in left forehead, spreading over face and affecting left teeth.

Heart - Convulsive pain in heart region with oppression. Great soreness in the region of the heart with anguish, redoubled throbbing, small pulse, burning in the hands and shivering of the body. Palpitations of the heart with diminished perspiration of the feet.

Kidneys - Urine red, scanty and burning.

Limbs - The limbs are painful and languid. Pain in left shoulder, as if inflamed. Suppression of the habitual sweat of the feet.

Modalities - Worse at night. Worse on stooping. Worse pressure. Worse touch.

Rectum - Borborygmi. Colic and diarrhea in morning.

Skin - Dry skin. Herpes zoster.

Sleep - Irresistible drowsiness. Frequent yawning.

Stomach - Painful digging from abdomen to throat, causing pain in region of heart with oppression. Painful swelling in the stomach with pressure at the epigastrium and risings of flatus. Colic, tympanitis. Borborygmi and diarrhea. Inclination to vomit, sour risings of food.

Temperature - Chilliness predominates, shuddering, goose flesh.

Throat - Lower jaw with stinging in teeth and cheek. Throat feels contracted with burning pain during swallowing. Sore throat with difficult swallowing, inclination to swallow, salivation and smarting. Sensation of a foreign substance in the throat with yawning and stretching.

Vertigo - Vertigo, so as to occasion falling and dullness of ideas.

COMMENTS - Sensation as if a bar lay transversely across from region of heart to right side with acute pain in left upper portion of chest. Haem. cured a case of herpes zoster with agonizing pain as if a bar lay across the chest, arresting the breathing.

RELATIONS - ***Antidoted by:*** Camph. ***Compare:*** (1) Cact. (2) in compressive pains, Cact., Lil-t., Coloc., Aur., Naja.

REFERENCES - Boericke. Clarke.

HALCION
(Triazolam)

PHARMACY - halc. Halcion. Triazolam. An allopathic drug. ***Historical dose:*** All potencies.

CLINICAL - ***Amnesia.*** Apnea. Coma. Constipation. Convulsions. Delusions. Diarrhea. ***Disorientation.*** Dizziness. Fainting. Fatigue. Hangover. Headaches. Incontinence. Impaired, coordination. ***Insomnia.*** Nausea. Nervousness. Nightmares. Sleep, apnea. ***Sleep, disorders.*** Sleepwalking. Tinnitus. Vomiting.

HOMEOPATHIC - Halcion is a drug used for short-term treatment of insomnia. It is a member of the benzodiazepine class of drugs, many of which are used as tranquilizers.

It's homeopathic used can be surmised from the side effects of this medication.

Coordination problems. Dizziness, drowsiness. Nervousness. Changes in sexual drive. Chest pain. Congestion. Cramping pains. Dreaming and sleep abnormalities. Tendency to fall, stumble. Chronic fatigue. Impaired urination. Morning "hangover" effects. Tiredness and weakness.

MIND - ***Mental confusion.*** Perceptual problems. Loss of sense of reality. ***Disorientation.*** Anxiety and depression. Increased anxiety during the daytime. Inappropriate behavior. Irritability. Aggressiveness, agitation. Behavior problems. Restlessness.

Memory impairment, memory loss. ***Traveler's amnesia*** has been reported by patients who took Halcion to induce sleep while traveling. ***Anterograde amnesia***, forgetting events after an injury. Nervousness. Sense of well-being, excitement. Hallucinations and delusions. Coma.

Back - Muscle spasms in the shoulders or neck.

Ears - Ringing in the ears.

Eyes - Visual disturbances. Yellowing of the whites of the eyes.

Female - Menstrual irregularities. Changes in sexual drive.

Food - Loss of appetite. Worse from alcohol. Worse grapefruit juice.

Head - Headaches. Light-headedness.

Heart - Rapid heart rate.

Male - Changes in sexual drive.

Kidneys - Incontinence.

Limbs - Stiff awkward movements. Tingling or pins and needles.

Lungs - Shallow or difficult breathing.

Mouth - Dry mouth. Burning tongue. Inflammation of the tongue and mouth. Slurred or difficult speech. Taste changes.

Rectum - Diarrhea. Constipation.

Skin - Skin inflammation. Itching. Yellowing of the skin.

Sleep - Sleep disturbances including insomnia, sleepwalking. Drowsiness during the daytime. Insomnia. Rebound insomnia in patients who have stopped taking the Halcion drug. Sleep apnea. Nightmares.

Stomach - Nausea and vomiting.

Vertigo - Fainting. Dizziness and impaired coordination.

COMMENTS - The drug Halcion has been associated with the following withdrawal symptoms: Convulsions, cramps, tremors, vomiting, sweating, feeling ill, perceptual problems, and insomnia.

Symptoms of the Halcion overdose may include: Apnea (temporary cessation of breathing), coma, confusion, excessive sleepiness, problems in coordination, seizures, shallow or difficult breathing, slurred speech

RELATIONS - ***Compare:*** (1) Cocc., Coff.

REFERENCES - Murphy.

HALL AQUA

(Salt Springs)

PHARMACY - hall. Hall aqua. Salt springs of Hall in upper Austria. Containing chlorides, iodides, bromides, carbonates of the alkalies, alkaline earths and iron. The main ingredient is chloride of natrium. Dilutions. ***Historical dose:*** Tincture and all potencies.

CLINICAL - Anemia. Breast, disorders. Exophthalmus. Glands, enlarged. ***Goiter.*** Night-sweats. Weakness.

HOMEOPATHIC - The salt springs of Hall contains chlorides, iodides, bromides, carbonates of the alkalies and alkaline earths and iron, but by far the largest ingredient is chloride of sodium. Provings have been made of this water, many of them on patients suffering from goiter.

In the provings, many marked symptoms appeared in the breast glands. Great weakness and exhausting night-sweats were produced, and all the symptoms of cold in the head and chest.

A number of symptoms occured after sleep and some of them woke the provers in the night. One prover had a sensation as if her stomach would fall out and as if her breasts would fall off. In many cases the pains were transient, acute and returned after a short interval.

RELATIONS - ***Compare:*** (1) Nat-m., Sil-mar. - stitches shooting out of nipple. (2) Ol-an.

REFERENCES - Clarke.

HALOPERIDOL

(Haldol)

PHARMACY - halo. Haloperidol. Haldol. An allopathic drug. Halo. is a butyrophenon used as an anti-psychotic. ***Historical dose:*** All potencies.

CLINICAL - Allergies. Backache. Catatonia. Conjunctivitis. Dermatitis. Headaches. Heart, disorders. Hypotension. Impotency. Liver, disorders. Memory, weak. Nausea. Neurosis. Paresthesia. Parkinson's disease. Pseudo-bulbar, syndrome. Raynaud's syndrome. Sclerosis. Schizophrenia. Tachycardia. Vertigo.

HOMEOPATHIC - A butyrophenone drug used as an antipsychotic, also used in Huntington's chorea and Gilles de la Tourette's disease. The present symptomatology is the result of the examination of the toxicology record of the side effects of Haloperidol, and of a homeopathic proving.

The proving was done by O. A. Julian who used Haloperidol in 30c, 7c, 3x and placebo, with twenty-eight collaborators in 1974-75. Out of twenty-eight provers, there were six women, and most of the provers were also doctors or students of medicine.

Instability of the mind and body. Weariness, fidgets in the lower limbs, buzzing in the ears, dizzy feeling on rising. Constant need to move when in bed, resulting from sensation of formication in all the joints of the body. Physiological slowness.

Disturbances of synthetic processes of the mind. Sensation of constant stress. Dawdles. Mumbles. Sensation of unreality, of being outside self, particularly in morning. Loss of notion of time. Frequent forgetfulness of everyday tasks. Confused. Difficult concentration.

Desire to stay lying down and do nothing. Strong need to sleep. Talkative, especially in the evening after 9 p.m., with need to relate stories. Excited. Tendency to philosophical speculation.

Sensation of constricted throat, of chest being in a vice, respiration difficult, thorax painful. Tachycardia. Respiratory rhythm disorders. Excess salivation. Nausea in the morning. Desires salty foods. Empty urging and constipation. General sweating. Legs give way.

MIND - Extreme difficulty in concentrating and in intellectual thought. Forgetfulness and loss of sense of time. Impression of being behind a cloud. Great waves of pessimism for no reason. Depression. Neurosis from anguish. Anxious, restless. Very talkative.

Depersonalization of the self. Impression of disintegration of personality, especially after 9 p.m. Catatonia with attitudes, gestures, words, all strange and stereotyped. Schizophrenia and schizophrenic conditions. Euphoric state in the evening. Feeling of living "outside of myself," and returns to himself a few hours later.

Abdomen - Rumbling and belching. Painful contractions of the abdominal muscles.

Back - Backache. Stiffness at the nape of the neck, trembling, shaky walk.

Bladder - Retention in the bladder. Dysuria. Urinary and fecal incontinence.

Constitutions - Allergic, cancerous conditions with psychopathic tendency.

Ears - Earache in the left ear.

Eyes - Conjunctivitis. Cataract. Vision misty. Deep, burning sensation in the eyes, rising to the surface with tingling in the eyelids, appearing slowly, gradually between 11 a.m. and noon.

Face - Face expressionless of fixed expression. Fixed gaze.

Female - Disturbed libido.

Food - Hypoglycemia. Desires salty foods, which relieve. Loss of appetite, especially at midday.

Head - Headache in the morning, localized at the frontal region.

Heart - Tachycardia. Faintness and syncope. Hypotension. Rapid pulse. Circulatory complaints, formication of the ankle, knee, wrist, elbow, scapular and humeral regions.

Limbs - Arthralgia. Muscle pain. Raynaud's syndrome. Pains in the bones, especially left metatarsal bone, wrists, elbows, and knees. Painful cramps in the afternoon in both thighs. Cramps in the calves. Pain in the right elbow with appearance of a few red spots. Pains in the wrists and right thumb. Hands hot, fingertips freezing.

Lungs - Asthmatic wheezing. Irregular respiration, either rapid and superficial or short inhalation following very slow exhalation followed by an arrest of pulmonary ventilation for a few seconds.

Male - Total impotence. Diminished or disturbed libido.

Modalities - Better from closing the eyes. Better hot water. Better walking in company. Better salty food. Worse in the morning.

Mouth - Excessive salivation. Bad breath in the morning and after each meal.

Perspiration - Profuse perspiration. Sweating from the hands, more intense between 1 p.m. and 3 p.m. Fairly intense sweating from the whole body. Hands and axilla extremely wet. Palms of hands very hot, despite the fingertips being frozen.

Rectum - Frequent desire to go to stool, then expelling nothing. Persistent constipation, slightly ameliorated by eating prunes. Spasmodic constipation. Fecal incontinence. Anal pruritus, lasting for four days.

Skin - Skin yellowish, blotchy, pink cheeks. ***Abnormal hair growth.*** Hyperhidrosis. Dermatitis in brown patches on the legs.

Sleep - Insomnia. Sleep disturbed. Fear of cancer-type dreams. Sleeps better on the stomach. Frequent desire to sleep. Rises with feeling of not having slept enough, even after a good night's sleep. Difficulty getting started in the morning. Sleepy during the day.

Stomach - Quickly satisfied. Acrid dyspepsia. Nausea, vomiting, digestive discomfort. Nausea in the morning or during the day.

Temperature - Fever and chilliness. Overheated.

Throat - Constricted throat.

Vertigo - Vertigo with stumbling gait. Dizzy sensation with visual fog, on rising.

COMMENTS - Difficult concentrating, feeling as if in a fog, as if dead. Headache in the morning. Short headaches localized in the frontal region. Headache behind the right eye, better by closing eyes, lasting only a few seconds.

Heaviness of the head, starting at the nape of the neck and spreading to the occiput and rising to the top of the head, ameliorated by lying down, closing the eyes and placing the hands over the eyes. Difficulty in moving, grimacing and protrusion of the tongue. Very severe spasms of the ocular rotary muscles.

Muscular stiffness and contracture. Painful contractions of the abdominal, brachial and lumbar muscles. Fleeting torticollis when stretching. Constant restlessness of the lower limbs, cannot stay sitting or lying down. Extreme trembling, stumbling gait. Raynaud's syndrome.

Hysterical stitch. Paresthesia. Extreme sensitivity to touch. Symptoms better by stretching out the hands perpendicularly to the axis of the body and by bending the legs. Sleeps lying on stomach.

Tachycardia. Faintness and syncope. Hypotension. Rapid pulse. Circulatory complaints including formication of the ankle, knee, wrist, elbow, scapular and humeral regions. Proliferation of hair.

RELATIONS - ***Compare:*** (1) Phos. Lyc. Puls. Zinc. Med. Cocc. Hydrog. (2) Anh. - Hyperesthesia of the cortex, thalamus and organs, visual hallucinations, loss of contact with surroundings, accommodation difficult and perception disorders. (3) Chlorpr. - Melancholy, difficulty in concentrating, loss of memory, had to make great effort for intellectual work, trembles, hypertonia, stiffness. (4) Agar. - Vertigo in the morning, clumsy hand movements, frontal headache, spreading to the nose with pains as if pricked by icy needles, head moves constantly, spasmodic jerking in the limbs.

REFERENCES - Julian.

HAMAMELIS VIRGINIANA

(Witch-hazel)

PHARMACY - ham. Hamamelis virginiana. Witch-hazel. Hamamelis macrophylla. Hamamelis dioica. N. O. Hamamelidacee. A shrub growing in all parts of U. S. in damp woods or along streams, flowers in autumn, flowers yellow, the seeds ripen the year following. Tincture of fresh bark of twigs and root. A resinoid, Hamamelin is also prepared. ***Historical dose:*** Tincture and all potencies.

CLINICAL - ***Aching, pains.*** Ankles, weak. Black eye. ***Bruises. Burns.*** Cancer. Chilblains. Edema. Enteric, fever. Gastric, ulcers. Hematemesis. Hematocele. Hematuria. Hemoptysis. ***Hemorrhages. Hemorrhoids.*** Leucorrhea. Menstruation, disorders. Miscarriage, threatened. Nipples, sore. Noises, head. Nosebleeds. Orchitis. Ovaries, disorders. Ovaritis. ***Phlebitis.*** Phimosis. Phlegmasia alba dolens. Purpura. Rheumatism. Scurvy. Smallpox. ***Sore, pains.*** Tuberculosis. Ulcers. Uterus, disorders. Vaginismus. Varicocele. ***Varicose, ulcers. Varicose, veins.*** Wounds.

HERBAL - The deep red color of the tincture may be taken as the ***signature*** of its therapeutic action. No remedy has a wider sphere of usefulness in cases of hemorrhage and disordered blood vessels.

It has also a decided relation to the effects of mechanical injuries including first-degree burns. As a local application it takes rank with Arn. and Calen. in the materia medica.

HOMEOPATHIC - The principle action of this remedy is on the veins especially of rectum, genitals, limbs and throat, producing ***venous congestion, varicose veins, hemorrhoids and hemorrhages.***

Acts upon the coats of the veins causing relaxation with consequent engorgement. Passive venous hemorrhages from any part. ***Phlebitis.*** Veins, painful, varicose, sore, cutting, swollen inflamed. Painful, hard, knotty.

Hemorrhages cause great exhaustion, out of proportion to the amount of loss. Hemorrhages, capillary, dark, fluid, relieves or causes undue weakness.

Hemorrhoids with much bleeding and marked soreness of the part, the back feels as if it would break (Aesc. has little or no bleeding). Tense, bursting feeling in hemorrhoids, joints or lower limbs.

Bruised, soreness of the affected part from which blood flows, in blood vessels, abdomen etc. Great value in ***open, painful wounds*** with weakness from blood loss. Relieves the pain after surgery (Calen.), supercedes the use of morphine. Prickling, stinging pain in veins, muscles, skin.

MIND - Forgetful of words when talking. No desire to study or work. Averse to being spoken to. Irritable, gloomy, depressed, stupid. Feels unappreciated. Wants respect due to him. Hemorrhages with tranquil mind.

Reverence for those around him. Anxiety at night. Sadness better evening. Depressed after emissions with regretful mind. Sadness from masturbation. Felt as if he was going out of his mind during headache over left eye. Thinks constantly of his ailment. Wandering thoughts while studying.

Abdomen - Burning in the epigastrium and umbilicus. Pain all around lower abdomen. Cramps in stomach and transverse colon two hours after a hearty dinner. Varicose veins of abdomen. Flatulence. Inguinal glands tender and enlarged.

Back - Sore pain down cervical vertebrae. Breaking backache. Painful scapulae. Severe pain in lumbar and hypogastric region, extending down legs. Rheumatism of scapula. Chilliness in back and hips, extending down legs.

Breasts - Sore nipples, bleeding.

Causations - Burns. Injuries.

Chest - Chest feels sore and constricted, worse by a long or deep breath. Stitches in lower part of lungs. Dull, aching pain constantly in muscles of left chest, worse using arms afternoon and evening.

Constitutions - Venous constitutions.

Coughs - Tickling, with taste of blood on awakening. Dry cough, severe stinging in the uvula, as if it would break. Hemoptysis, tickling cough with taste of blood. Dry, short, with sensation of dryness in throat. Cough from a varicose condition of throat.

Ears - Deafness in right ear, passes off by noon. Buzzing, ringing in ears. Bleeding at right ear, also nosebleed, which clears her head, relieving her.

Eyes - Traumatic effects. ***Sore pain*** in eyes, eyes painful under slight pressure. Painful weakness. ***Black eye.*** Iritis, conjunctivitis. Blood shot eyes. Hastens absorption of intra-occular hemorrhage. Eyes feel forced out, better pressure of finger. Eyes inflamed, vessels greatly injected, caused by a foreign substance. Intense soreness after operations.

Face - Burning in right cheek. Muscles feel sore and stiff. Occasional shooting pains along right superior maxillary to malar bone. Lips are dry, sore, cracked.

Female - Vicarious menstruation. ***Menses dark, profuse with soreness in abdomen.*** Jolting brings on menses. Bleeding, midway between menstrual periods, only in daytime. Inter-menstrual pain. Leucorrhea, bloody with soreness of vagina. Uterine hemorrhage, bearing-down pain in back. Ovarian congestion and neuralgia, feel very sore. Ovaritis after a blow or after abortion with soreness over the whole abdomen. Vagina very tender, sore. Vulva itches. Vaginismus. During pregnancy, legs become painful, can neither stand nor walk. Milk leg.

Food - Appetite good. No appetite for breakfast. Nausea from pork. Considerable thirst, better by small quantities of water. Very thirsty in afternoon and evening, throat dry. Averse to water, makes him sick to think of it.

Head - Feeling as of a bolt from temple to temple. Numbness over frontal bone. Hammering headache, over left eye, left temple, as if he would go out of his mind. Stupid feeling in head. Stupor, dullness, headache, crowding fullness in head and neck, also in forehead. Fullness of head, followed by a nosebleed. Bursting headache on waking. Headache after an emission.

Heart - Pulse accelerated, full. Palpitations. Pricking pain in region of heart and superficial veins of both arms.

Kidneys - Dull ache about kidneys. Hematuria with increased desire for urination. Hematuria, passive congestion of the kidneys, dull pain in kidney region. Dull ache about kidneys. Urine clear copious. Scanty high-colored urine. Irritation of the urethra, followed by a discharge and ardor urine.

Limbs - Great lassitude and weariness of the limbs and elsewhere. Tense, bursting feeling in limbs and joints. Very sore muscles and joints. Rheumatism with great soreness of the muscles. Tired feeling in arms and legs. ***Phlebitis. Varicose veins.*** Varicose ulcers with bloody bases. Neuralgia of internal saphenous nerve. ***Milk-leg, hemorrhoids and sore nipples after childbirth.***

Lungs - Smothering sensation when lying. Expectoration thick, yellowish or greenish gray, tasting putrid. Hemoptysis, tickling cough with taste of blood.

Male - Severe neuralgic pains in testicles. Pain running down the spermatic cords into the testes. Orchitis, intense soreness and swelling, worse touch. Testicles enlarged, hot and painful. Epididymitis. Varicocele. Hematocele. Emission at night without being aware of it. Profuse cold sweat on scrotum, capillary stasis.

Modalities - Worse from injuries. Worse bruises. Worse pressure. Worse jar, touch. Worse motion. Worse exertion. Worse warm, moist air. Worse open air. Worse humid, rainy weather. Worse cold. Worse during day (pains).

Mouth - Burns of tongue and lips, or feels burnt. Blisters on sides of tongue, canker spots near the tip. Tongue coated white. Bloody, metallic taste. Passive hemorrhage from gums after tooth extraction with soreness.

Nose - Over-sensitive sense of smell. Bad smell from the nose. Nose feels stopped up. Sneezing spells, watery, excoriating, burning discharge. ***Nosebleeds***, flow passive, non-coagulable, with tightness at the bridge of the nose. Profuse nosebleed, idiopathic or vicarious. Nosebleeds with hemiplegia in old men. The nosebleed clears head and relieves.

Rectum - Anus feels sore and raw. Itching at the anus. Pulsation in rectum. ***Hemorrhoids, bleeding profusely with soreness.*** Costive, hard stools, coated with mucus. Large quantities of a tar-like blood in stools, particularly with typhoid or dysentery.

Perspiration - Sweats freely at night, after lying down.

Skin - Burns. Ecchymosis. Purpura. ***Bruises,*** traumatic inflammations (Arn.). Bluish chilblains. ***Varicose veins and ulcers***, very sore. Varicose ulcers with bloody bases.

Sleep - Restlessness at night. Uneasy, restless morning sleep. Emissions of semen during sleep.

Stomach - Blisters on side. Pain and heaviness at the back of stomach. Throbbing and pain in stomach. Cramp in stomach after eating. Belchings after a meal, taste of the food. Nausea, headache in frontal bone on awaking. Nausea and inclination to vomit after a meal. Vomiting of black blood. Hematemesis, black blood.

Teeth - Sharp pain along the molar teeth, extending to the malar bone, also in temporal region. Teeth ache, can scarcely sleep, yet not decayed. Pains worse in warm room. Gums sore, painful, swollen, bleed easily, dark fluid. Passive venous hemorrhage after extraction of teeth.

Temperature - Cold creeps in the open air, chills run up the legs, head stopped up, dull pain over orbit. Chilliness over back and hips, extending down the limbs. Chilly on going to bed, dreading an attack of fever. Fever at night, hands hot, burning in the eyelids on closing them.

Throat - Hoarse on waking. Sore throat, worse right side, right tonsil more swollen, reddened, with distended veins. Sore throat in those predisposed to fullness of the veins, worse in warm, moist air. Mucous membrane distended and bluish, varicosis of throat. Stinging, breaking pain in uvula, while coughing. Hawks considerably.

Vertigo - Swimming sensation on rising. Vertigo when stooping. Nausea and vertigo with desire to lie down.

COMMENTS - Hering, who learned its properties from Mr. Pond of "Pond's Extract" fame (Pond was a patient of Hering's), made the first provings and introduced the remedy into homeopathy. He defines its position as being between Acon. and Arn.

"Pond's Extract" is an aqueous distillate prepared from the leaves. A number of interesting superstitions are associated with the shrub, and shoots of it are used as "divining rods" for discovering water and metals.

It is tonic, astringent, sedative and hemostatic. Applied topically to varicose veins. May help relieve the pain from burns (Canth.). It has been used as a mouthwash with spongy, bleeding gums.

Hale gave a very full account of the remedy, noting that conditions likely to require Ham. include phlebitis and varicose veins, hemorrhoids, venous hemorrhages. The local application of Ham. to a sprained knee has been known to set up inflammation in the veins of the part and the provers who had varicose veins experienced increased sensitiveness and unusual sensations in them, a number were cured.

Passive hemorrhages (Chin.), with intense soreness. The part from which the flow of blood proceeds feels sore and bruised. Fullness, soreness, and a bruised feeling. Hemorrhages are mostly dark and may occur from any orifice.

Bruising and bleeding under the skin (Arn., Sul-ac.). Ecchymosis. Bruising from a puncture wound. Lack of ligament tone. Laxed ligaments, tendons, or tissues. Tired, aching, feeling in the back and lower limbs. Rheumatic symptoms with characteristic soreness.

Congestion, inflammation and bleeding of hemorrhoidal vessels, with marked action in the throat (Aesc.). Phlebitis and varicose veins with soreness. Varicose angina, where the veins of the pharynx are large and blue. Taste of blood in the mouth.

Headache, chiefly in the temples, throbbing, hammering, especially over left eye. Black eye (Symph., Led.). History of use in painful tumors, especially ulcerated malignant tumors where there is bruised, dark bluish or purplish color.

Pricking pain in the rectum, anal itching. Dysentery, when the amount of blood is unusually large, dark, small clots or patches through the mucus. Constipation. Hemorrhoids.

Metrorrhagia, menorrhagia, vicarious menstruation and hemorrhages between the period, particularly if it's dark red blood. Stagnant blood in the uterus. Ovulatory bleeding. Orchitis, ovarian disorders, phlebitis and varicose veins. Venous stasis (Bell-p., Sep.), particularly after childbirth. Ovarian disorders, orchitis, with soreness

Thirst. Toothache worse in warm room, from touch. Takes cold easily from every exposure, but especially to warm, moist air.

Dr. Ward noted a case in which he cured inter-menstrual pain. Allen mentioned in the provings an inter-menstrual flow and Dr. Ward observed that if his patient has had the flow, the soreness so distinctly felt might not have been realized.

Hughes gave Ham. to a young woman suffering from a daily nosebleed and throbbing headache. The first dose was followed by a flushing of the face and most distressing throbbing, aching and sense of fullness in the head.

The second dose brought back all the symptoms in the head and a feeling as if it would burst. Some days later, the 3x was given and again the dilatation of the cerebral vessels occurred, through the symptoms were not so severe.

The scapular pain bears on the experience of Dr. Koech, who cured with Ham. many cases of scapular rheumatism. He regarded it as a specific in disorders of the last five cervical nerves.

Bree said it will relieve the excessive thirst that most patients with heart troubles complain.

RELATIONS - ***Antidoted by:*** Arn., Camph., Chin., Puls. - toothache. ***Compare:*** (1) Arn., Calen. is better than either in hastening the absorption of intra-ocular hemorrhage. (2) Chlor., Sec., - purpura. (3) Fl-ac., Lach., Puls., Nux-v., Aesc, Nit-ac. - in varicose veins and hemorrhoids. (4) Spong., Puls. - orchitis. Ham. has more soreness. (5) Cimic. - abdominal soreness after labor, Ham. is an excellent external application. (6) Bry - vicarious menstruation. (7) hemorrhage in typhoid, Nit-ac. light. Ham. dark. (8) Bell., Euphor., Rhus-t., Tereb., - as an application in burns of first degree. (9) Hirudo - hemorrhages. (10) in hemorrhoids: Fl-ac., Aloe, Mur-ac. (11) in varicose veins, Mangifera indica. ***Complementary to:*** Ferrum in hemorrhages.

REFERENCES - Boericke. Clarke. Phatak.

HEATHER

(Bach Flower Essence)

PHARMACY - heath-b. Heather. Calluna vulgaris. The flowering stems are placed in a bowl of water and allowed to sit in the sun for several hours. The water is strained and used as medicine. ***Historical dose:*** Take two drops from the stock bottle into a one ounce dropper bottle (add brandy or alcohol, if this bottle will be used for days or weeks). This is the dosage bottle, take a few drops straight into the mouth or as needed in a little water or juice.

HOMEOPATHIC - Heath-b., with Wat-v-b. and Imp-b., belongs to Bach's group of ***Loneliness.*** For suffering from inner loneliness as a result of being too centered within their own selves and losing the connection with others.

Overbearing and agitated. Sleep-like disorders (see Chic-b., Ch-bd-b.) or obsessively fixated ideas (Wh-ch-b.). Feigning or unconscious production of sickness, urge to talk about symptoms.

MIND - Self-centered. Worry over self. Feeling that one deserves sympathy and regard. Stuck on personal affairs. Attaches importance to experienced hardships and dilemmas.

Craves attention and sympathy. Attention-getting behavior. Talkative over seemingly unimportant details, to get attention, feel special or show self-pity. Feigning sickness, hypochondriasis (Chic-b., Mimul-b.).

REFERENCES - Bach.

HECLA LAVA

(Volcanic Ash)

PHARMACY - hecla. Hecla lava. Volcanic ash. Lava Heclae. Volcanic ash from Mount Hecla in Iceland. The finer ash falling in distant localities. The ash of this volcano contains silica, alumina, lime, magnesia with some oxide of iron. Trituration. ***Historical dose:*** Trituration and all potencies, lower triturations.

CLINICAL - Abscess, gums. Antrum of Highmore, tumor. Arthritis deformans. Arthritic nodosities. Boils, gums. ***Bone, deformities. Bones, disorders. Bones, spurs. Bone, tumors.*** Breast, tumors. Dentition, difficult. ***Exostoses***. Facial, neuralgia. Glands, disorders. Hallux vulgus. Hip joint, arthritis. ***Jaw, pain. Jaw, tumors.*** Milk, deficient. Neuralgias. Nodosities. ***Osteitis.*** Osteomalacia. ***Osteosarcoma.*** Paget's disease. Periostitis. Rickets. Syphilis, bones. Teeth, decay. ***Toothaches***. ***Tumors.*** Varicose, veins. Warts. White, swellings. Whitlow.

HOMEOPATHIC - When traveling in Iceland, Garth Wilkinson noticed that the sheep in the vicinity of Hecla had immense ***bony growths on the jaws***. Another effect noticed was the drying up of the milk both in sheep and cows. The finer ash which feel on pastures at a distance was the most deleterious, the gross ash near the mountain was inert.

Wilkinson added that he used Hecla. with excellent effect in toothache, gum abscess, swellings about the jaws and in difficult dentition.

Hecla. affects mostly the bones of the head, jaws, ***jawbones***, teeth and legs. ***Osteosarcoma, exostosis and osteitis,*** arrests development and prevents recurrence.

Clinical experience has shown the power of Hecla. to arrest many forms of bone disease including osteosarcoma, scrofulous and syphilitic osteitis and exostoses. Painful swellings, sensitive to touch, worse from touch and pressure.

Exostosis, gum abscess, ***toothaches,*** difficult teething. Nodosities, decay of bone, etc. Bone necrosis. Necrosis and sinus after mastoid operation. Facial neuralgia from decayed teeth and after extraction.

Induration and infiltration of cervical glands, studding the neck like a row of pearls. ***Tumors*** in general. White swellings. Whitlow and gumboils. Syphilis. Predominantly affects the right side.

Mind - Irritability. Nervousness in the morning. Sensitive to criticisms. Outburst of violent anger and feeling of helplessness. Indignation. Suppression of anger. Ailments from shock.

Back - Induration and infiltration of the glands. Neck glands are enlarged and indurated, like a row of pearls

Bones - Necrosis and destruction of bone. Bone inflammation. ***Bone spurs, tumors*** or exostoses, especially of the head, jaws, leg. Benign bone cysts, tumors. Painful bone tumors or nodosities after injury. Exostoses of fingers. Tumors of the tibia with severe continuous pain. Osteomalacia, rickets. Osteitis, periostitis. Osteitis deformans. Osteosarcoma.

Breasts - Breast tumors or nodules. Diminished milk while nursing. Dried up, no breast milk.

Causations - Injury to bone.

Chest - Muscle pain, especially of intercostal muscles.

Ears - Caries of mastoid bone. Exostosis in external meatus of ear.

Face - ***Facial neuralgia from decayed teeth*** and after extraction. Polyps, commencing in Antrum of Highmore. Tumor, deforming face, forcing eyeball upward, obstructing nostrils, extending downward into the mouth, impeding breathing and chewing, nosebleed, headache.

Head - Chronic headache, from dental or bone disease. Headache from injury of dental nerves. Tumors of the skull.

Jaws - ***Abscess or enlargement of bone*** remaining after a tooth extraction. Violent pain in upper jaw. ***Enlargement of maxillary bone***, from injury to jaw. Painful to touch, ***upper jaw, swelling*** under right alae nasi sensitive. Right cuspid of upper jaw sensitive to slight pressure.

Limbs - Severe, continuous pain in lower limbs. Swollen and bulging thighs and legs. Varicose veins. Arthritic nodosities. Exostoses of tibia, severe continuous pain incapacitating from work. Hip joint disease. Hallux vulgus. Deformity or nodules of the fingers, toes.

Modalities - Worse from touch. Worse pressure. Worse beginning of motion. Worse sitting, rest. Worse left side.

Mouth - Neuralgia from decayed tooth in cavity from which tooth has been extracted. Pain in wound, where tooth has been extracted. Abscess of gums. Difficult dentition in scrofulous and rickety children.

Neck - Swollen cervical glands, like a string of pearls.

Nose - Nasal polyps or tumors. Ulceration. Destructive, syphilitic ulceration of nasal bones.

Skin - Black warts. Actinomycosis. White swellings.

Teeth - ***Toothaches,*** especially of teeth that are very sensitive to pressure with swelling about jaws. ***Dental abscess*** with swelling, pus worse pressure on teeth. ***Decay of teeth.*** Pain or neuralgia after extraction. Chronic dental or jaw abscess. Chronic gingivitis. Fistula. Gumboil. Delayed or difficult dentition in malnourished children.

Vertigo - Vertigo everything goes up, down and sidewise.

COMMENTS - Affinity for bone deformities, bone spurs and tumors (Calc-f.), bone diseases. Calcium deposits in the joints that cause deformities, deforming or rheumatoid arthritis. Spinal curvatures. Hypertrophied bone. Bone cancer. Osgood-Schlatter.

Bone lesions, osteitis, periostitis, exostosis, tumor, often follow an injury to the bone. Painful and tender lesions. Enlarged and indurated cervical nodes, sometimes likened to "a string of pearls."

Decomposition and necrosis of the sinus and nasal bones, or for a history of damage or surgery in the area. Severe toothache, where the jawbone aches, boring and digging pains in the bone. Bony lesion after a dental abscess. Late state syphilis where the nasal bones deteriorate. Facial neuralgias after tooth extractions. Damage to the jawbone from dental surgery. Ulcerations of the bone.

Burnett noted "On July 3, 1880, a young lady, age 15, came under my observation with an exostosis on her right os calcis, somewhat smaller an a little flatter than half a walnut shell. It was at times painful.

"Patient was in other respects in good health and well nourished, but her teeth were not very sound. She goes blue in winter, and suffers also very badly from chilblains both on hands and feet, worse on hand.

"Hecla lava 2c given six grains three times a day. July 17th. The exostosis is decidedly smaller; it never pains now. September 25. The exostosis has entirely disappeared; the two heels being compared, no difference between them now can be discovered."

Burnett stated "I have cured several bony tumours of the jaws with the same remedy, and that very promptly: they were all of recent origin."

RELATIONS - ***Compare:*** (1) Calc-f., Calc., Merc., Phos., Sil. Still., Sulph., Kali-i., Symph., Ruta. (2) Conch. - diaphysis of bone affected, parts extremely sensitive to touch. (3) Amph. - great affinity for the jaw bones, worse by air and dampness. (4) Slag - great itching of parts.

REFERENCES - Boericke. Clarke. Murphy. Phatak.

HEDEOMA PULEGIOIDES

(Pennyroyal)

PHARMACY - hedeo. Hedeoma pulegioides. Pennyroyal. American pennyroyal. N. O. Labiate. The British Pennyroyal is Mentha pulegium. Tincture of whole fresh plant. ***Historical dose:*** Tincture and all potencies.

CLINICAL - Amenorrhea. Dysmenorrhea. Gastritis. Flatulent, colic. Leucorrhea. Miscarriages. Nausea. Poison oak. Vertigo. Vomiting.

HERBAL - Hedeoma puleg. is also known as the common English Pennyroyal, the German Poley, the Arabic Alnam, and the ancient Greek Glachon. Hedeoma belongs to that large class of mints and common herbs that have been cast aside by the medical profession as worthless.

Hedeoma is one of the oldest remedies known, a common household herb long before the time of Hippocrates. Hippocrates and the ancient physicians used it as a tea for increasing the flow of urine, for kidney stones, and as a uterine stimulant. Popularly believed to be valuable for treating miscarriage in weak, cachectic women.

HOMEOPATHIC - Marked female symptoms, often associated with nervous disturbances. Bearing-down pains, worse by any movement and accompanied by almost paralytic weakness of the legs.

Nervous symptoms, jerkings and twitchings. Weak, faint, better lying down, inability to sit up. Pains in abdomen, worse after eating or drinking, touch and pressure. Flatulent colic. ***Pain along ureter***. Red sand in urine. Antidotes effects of poison oak (Grin.).

Abdomen - Distended, sore and sensitive. Flatulent colic.

Female - Leucorrhea with itching and burning. Ovaries congested and painful, bearing-down spasmodic contractions. Bearing-down pains with much backache, worse least movement.

Head - Dull, heavy feeling in morning. Sore pain, as from a cut. Weak, faint, better lying down.

Kidneys - Dragging pain from kidney to bladder. Dull burning pain over left kidney. Frequent urging, cutting pains. Pain along left ureter. Burning irritation at neck of bladder causing frequent, intense desire to urinate and inability to retain urine for more than a few minutes, better urinating.

Limbs - Pain, coldness and paretic conditions. Twitchings, jerkings, soreness. ***Pain in thumb joint***. Achilles tendon painful, as if sprained and swollen, walking painful.

Stomach - Gastritis. ***Everything taken into stomach causes pain***. Tongue coated thin white. Nausea.

COMMENTS - Anshutz wrote "Hedeoma contains three bodies peculiar to the plant, three different oils, also formic and acetic acid and likewise ischeptoic acid. There are on record seven cases of poisoning. Two provings have been made by myself. Several of the poisoning cases are very meagre and of little value.

"One teaspoonful of the oil, three drachms of the essence, seems to be almost a fatal dose in one case only was abortion produced and that from one ounce of the oil, followed by collapse and death.

"The leading symptoms of the cases of poisoning are briefly: Vertigo. Dimness of vision. Dilated pupils. Nausea and vomiting. Persistent severe bearing-down pains from the upper part of the sacrum and the region of the kidney to the uterus like true labor paints. Frequent painful, scanty, burning urination. Small, rapid pulse. Nervous weakness. Cold clammy limbs."

Dr. Toothaker reported a case in which the bearing-down labor-like pains and the scanty, painful urination lasted for many days and were very severe.

Clarke prescribed this remedy in two cases. In the first, a woman of gouty, rheumatic tendency, who had dragging burning pains in the left ureter going to the bladder and was passing quantities of "red sand." The pain lasted for ten days. Hedeo. 1c, on discs, was given, one disc every two hours. Complete relief was obtained after two doses.

The second case concerned a man of 60, very fond of champagne, who was bothered by constant burning irritation at the neck of the bladder, which caused frequent, intense desire to urinate and an inability to retain his urine for more than a few minutes. He always had marked relief on urinating. Urine retained in the bladder increased this irritation at the neck of the bladder and also caused an uneasy pain in the right testicle.

These symptoms had been more or less persistent for months and the attacks always lasted days at a time. Complete relief was obtained after one or two doses of Hedeo. 1c.

RELATIONS - *Compare:* (1) Menth., Sep., Lil-t. (2) Oci. - uric acid diathesis, pain in ureters. (3) Hed.

REFERENCES - Anshutz. Boericke. Clarke. Phatak.

HEDERA HELIX

(Common Ivy)

PHARMACY - hed. Hedera helix. Common ivy. Ground ivy. Glechoma hederacea. N. O. Araliacee. Tincture of young shoots. Tincture of flowering twigs. ***Historical dose:*** Tincture and all potencies.

CLINICAL - Angina pectoris. Anxiety. Arterial sclerosis. Arthrosis deformans. ***Cataract.*** Cerebro-spinalis. Cirrhosis. Convulsions. Cough. Delirium. Diarrhea. Emphysema. Gallstones. Gastritis. Hay fever. Hemorrhoids. Herpes. Hydrocephalus. Insomnia. Leucorrhea. Menorrhagia. Myocarditis. Raynaud's syndrome. Rhinorrhea. Rickets. Sinusitis. Tachycardia. Whooping cough.

HERBAL - Hedera helix, or Ivy, is a shrub that grows all over Europe. It is a creeper, which fixes itself by clinging roots. The leaves are cadiform at the base and more separated in the higher parts of the plant.

The fruit is bluish-black in color, equal to a pea in size. Historically, the wood was used for coughs as an anti-spasmodicl; the leaf was used internally as an emmenagogue and externally as a topical anti-neuralgic. The fruit was used for intoxication, digestive and nervous complaints, delirium, and convulsions. The mother tincture is used for coughs and is prepared from the flowering twigs.

HOMEOPATHIC - The symptomatology was established by Mezger in 1932 on seventeen people, using the 1x, 6x, and 15x potencies, for a period of twelve weeks. Easily tired, ameliorated by fresh air or noticeable increase in physical ability.

Dr. Cooper's experience has shown it to have a relation to rickets and rickety conditions. Rhinorrhea cerebro-spinalis. Hed. has been used for "clearing the sight" and Cooper said it has cured cases of cataract.

Joint pains and circulatory complaints, especially in the middle of the night. Cardiac palpitations. Acts on blood vessels, menorrhagia. Menses reduced, vesicular eruption on the face and body.

Swelling of the thyroid glands. Glandula sub-mentalis inflamed. Extreme anxiety with the feeling of constriction of the throat. Cough with laryngeal and tracheal irritation. Morbid hunger, gastric cramps. Diarrhea. Anus feels raw and sore. Hemorrhoids with rectal irritation and bleeding.

Delirium and convulsions. Chronic hydrocephalus, rhinorrhea, and cerebro-spinalis. General improvement in fresh air, but extreme sensibility to catching cold and to chills. Symptoms start on the left side and spread towards the right.

MIND - Constant state of unrest and worry. Anxiety, which grows all the more as he feels incapable of mastering it. Insomnia. Psychological symptoms improve in fresh air.

Abdomen - Pancreatitis.

Constitutions - Tubercular conditions, especially in phosphoric types.

Ears - Pain and buzzing.

Eyes - Feeling of sand in the eyelids. ***Cataract.*** Muscae volitantes.

Female - Premenstrual leucorrhea. Acrid, scorching discharge. Menses late, shorter and less copious. Infrequent menses. Feels better during menses. Amenorrhea in young girls. Pain in the Fallopian tubes and left ovary. Sclera-cystic ovaritis, especially on the left side. Genital tuberculosis.

Food - Lack of appetite or strong hunger pangs.

Head - Catarrhal inflammation of the frontal sinuses with headache. Headache, especially in the left side of the forehead and nape of the neck. Neuralgic pains in the head, ameliorated by fresh air.

Heart - Angina pectoris. Needle-like pains in the precordial region. Palpitations and anguish with swelling of the thyroid gland. Myocarditis. Arterial sclerosis. Rhythmic anomaly, accompanied by tachycardia. Thyrotoxic tachycardia. Extrasystole or paroxysmal tachycardia, in a young subject with a normal heart.

Kidneys - Frequent, abundant urination.

Limbs - Pain in the arms, legs, back and sacral region, sometimes ameliorated, sometimes aggravated by movement. Muscular rheumatism. Joint rheumatism. Tubercular inflammatory dislocating rheumatism. Arthrosis deformans. Nocturnal paresthesia pains in the arms. Raynaud's syndrome.

Liver - Inflammation of the gallbladder. Gallstones. Pain in the region of the gallbladder. Cirrhosis of the liver with cardiac decompensation.

Lungs - Irritated cough with grayish or yellow sputum. Whooping cough. Bronchial asthma in children. Emphysema.

Modalities - Better from fresh air. Better cold baths. Better in a room. Better movement. Better friction, massage. Better in the afternoon and evening. Worse in the middle of the night. Worse 3 a.m.

Mouth - Transparent vesicles on the lips and on inside of cheeks in a group, circumscribed by a red ring. Toothache from hot and cold. Dental neuralgia.

Nose - Hay fever. Acute and chronic rhinitis. Sinusitis (frontal, ethmoidal). Pharyngitis. Nasal discharge, worse in a warm room. Pain in the ethmoid and frontal sinuses. Chronic tracheitis, caused by a lesion in the nasal mucous membrane.

Rectum - Stools copious, either diarrhea or constipation.

Skin - Pruritus. Eruption of small pustules on the skin of the face and body. Prurigo. Urticaria. Labial and genital herpes.

Sleep - Wakes around 3 a.m., falls asleep again after eating a little.

Stomach - Pain on empty stomach, ameliorated by eating. Nausea, gastric heaviness, stomach cramps. Gastritis. Stomach and duodenal ulcers.

Temperature - Peripheral circulatory complaints. Feet and hands icy, red. Shivering and chilliness with bouts of perspiration and palpitations. Shivering and nausea in the evening until 4 a.m.

Throat - Chronic tracheitis. Pain around the tonsils and throat on swallowing. Hoarseness and inflammation of the larynx. Cough with a cold and inflammation of the pharynx, aggravated by heat and by speaking.

Vertigo - Vertigo on bending down and from rapid movement of the head.

COMMENTS - Cooper published case of a woman of twenty, who was cured of chronic hydrocephalus with a single dose. When she was brought to Cooper, the circumference of her head was 27.5 inches, rendering her an object of wonder and ridicule and reacting on her disposition and nervous state.

The condition had existed from childhood and was apparently growing much worse. There were two large edematous swellings on the nape of the neck, one on either side and immediately below the occiput, evidently the result of intra-hydrocephalic pressure.

One drop of Hed. tincture was placed on her tongue. The next morning, clear fluid began dripping from the nostrils, a "cerebrospinal rhinorrhea" in face.

This continued for three weeks, between twenty and thirty pocket-handkerchiefs were used in a day. Simultaneously the swellings began to diminish and had completely disappeared when the discharge ceased.

Thirteen months later, when being measured for a hat, it was found that the size of the head was reduced to 25 inches and no longer occasioned remark.

When, later on, some symptoms of brain pressure seemed to threaten, a second dose of Hed. completely dispelled them. The disposition of the patient was completely changed from being nervous, unhappy and diffident, she became lively, cheerful and active.

RELATIONS - ***Compare:*** (1) Aral-r., Gins., Sil., Nat-m. (2) Iodum - is the remedy, whose symptomatology is very similar. Iodum shows more emaciation inflammation and hardening of the lymphatic glands. Ovarian pain on the right and menses more abundant. (3) Calc-f. - Fear that his way of life will collapse. Pains aggravated by humid or cold weather. Menses copious. Hardening of the breasts, ovary or uterus. (4) Nat-m. - Depressed and sad, prefers solitude. Emaciation. Fissure in the middle of the lower lip. Chronic, periodic headaches with strong pulsating, as though the head would burst. Dryness of the mouth with extreme thirst.

REFERENCES - Clarke. Julian.

HEDYSARUM ILDEFONSIANUM

(Brazilian Burdock)

PHARMACY - hedy. Hedysarum ildefonsianum. Brazilian burdock. Hedysarum desmodium. Barba de Roy. Carapicho. N. O. Leguminose. Papilionoideae. ***Historical dose:*** Tincture and all potencies.

CLINICAL - Gonorrhea. Ophthalmia. Penis, inflammation.

HERBAL - This plant is named by Mure, who gave an account of it in his book and described it as "The brownish ligneous stem of this plant is about three feet high, it is ramose, pubescent, especially above. Leaves alternate, pinnate, trifoliate, folioles oval and slightly tormentose, on a hairy, bi stipulate petiole.

"The flowers, which are small and seated on filiform unifloral peduncles, form loose, terminal spikes. Fruit oval, hairy, on bent peduncles and attaching itself very intimately to clothes and to hairy skin of animals.

"The chief effect of Hedysarum was inflammation of the penis and of the eyes, which should indicate it in some cases of gonorrheal ophthalmia."

REFERENCES - Clarke.

HELIANTHUS ANNUUS

(Sunflower)

PHARMACY - helia. Helianthus annuus. Sunflower. N. O. Composite. Tincture of mature flower-heads. Tincture of ripe seeds. ***Historical dose:*** Tincture and all potencies.

CLINICAL - Colds. Constipation. Coryza. Hemorrhoids. Intermittent fever. Nasal obstruction. Nausea. Nosebleeds. Spleen, disorders. Throat, sore. Urticaria. Vomiting. Wounds.

HOMEOPATHIC - Helia. is a spleen remedy (Cean.). Spleen disorders. Chronic cases of intermittent fever. Coryza, catarrh, nasal hemorrhage and thick scabs in nose. Rheumatic pain in left knee. Externally, used as a vulnerary like Arn. and Calen.

In the provers there were marked effects on stomach, with nausea and vomiting. Congestion and dryness of mouth and pharynx.

Dry mouth. Redness and heat of skin, worse external warmth. Black stools (Lept.), soft, with an emission of semen; stools become black, hard, occurring every other day. Hemorrhoids.

Abdomen - Spleen enlarged and painful.

Eyes - Slight redness on margin of left upper lid with smarting in inner canthus. Eyes suffused. Weakness of the eyes.

Face - Anxious, countenance. Face deeply flushed.

Food - Thirst, nausea.

Head - Headache.

Limbs - Rheumatic pain in left knee on descending stairs.

Lungs - Cough in forenoon with gelatinous expectoration streaked with blood. Breath rather difficult and hurried.

Modalities - Better after vomiting. Worse from external heat, especially the skin.

Mouth - Tongue and fauces very red and inclined to dryness. Unusually hot taste when eating. Difficulty in articulation. Sticking in upper back teeth.

Nose - Coryza, catarrh. Nosebleeds and thick scabs in nose.

Rectum - Hemorrhoids. Stools soft, black, hard, every other day, with emission of semen.

Skin - Skin generally of scarlet redness and very hot. Tingling of skin. Many urticaria-like pimples. Groups of red pimples on inner side of knee with slight itching. Small red tetter to right of navel. Measles.

Stomach - Vomiting, increasing in severity.

Throat - Voice hoarse. Stiffness and dryness of the throat. Sensation of glowing in the throat and stomach. Severe burning in fauces, esophagus and epigastrium.

COMMENTS - Dr. Cessoles proved the expressed juice of the flowers, some observations have also been made on the effects of eating the seeds. In some parts of America the Native Americans use the seeds as an article of food.

Hansen said it equals Arn. and Calen., also yellow-flowered composites, as an application to wounds. Burnett regarded Helianthus as a great spleen remedy.

RELATIONS - ***Compare:*** (1) Lept. - black stools. (2) Arn., Calen., Hyper. - wounds. (3) Cean. - spleen.

REFERENCES - Boericke. Clarke.

HELIOTROPINUM

(Heliotrope)

PHARMACY - helio. Heliotropinum peruvianum. Heliotrope. Cherry pie. N. O. Boraginaceae. Tincture of whole fresh plant when in flower. ***Historical dose:*** Tincture and all potencies.

CLINICAL - Backaches. Clergyman's, throat. Dysmenorrhea. Headache. Hoarseness. Leucorrhea. Sore, throat. Uterus, displacement.

HOMEOPATHIC - Helio. has been slightly proved. Cooper used this remedy clinically and considered hoarseness and ***"thick voice"*** a great indication. He cured clergyman's sore throat with it.

Helio. has an action in uterine displacement, leucorrhea, backache. There is a bearing down from heavy, waterlogged condition of the uterus.

Symptoms of pressure and tension were produced in many parts: pressure on the sternum impeding breathing, pressure on the head, on mons veneries, pain as if beaten in leg muscles.

Chest - Pressure and oppression of external parts of chest, without affecting breathing.

Eyes - Feeling of tension in left inner canthus extending down into nasal bone. As if a swelling were there. Eye seems drawn together and smaller.

Female - Membranous dysmenorrhea. Leucorrhea. Pressure on mons veneries only when sitting. Uterine displacements with backache, especially if subject to loss of voice.

Head - Headache in forehead like a pressure and drawing pressing pain, better walking in open air.

Limbs - Pain, as if beaten above ankle, extending up the muscles, even when sitting. Itching on tibia, with sensations as if there was an eruption.

Modalities - Head symptoms better on walking in the open air. Other symptoms were worse after resting. Worse on inspiration.

Stomach - Pressure in pit of stomach, worse on inspiration. Epigastric region is sore to touch, most violent after eating and in evening.

Throat - Voice thick, clergyman's sore throat.

COMMENTS - Cooper gave Helio. to a woman who had been advised by several surgeons to have various organs either braced up surgically or removed. She described the effect as having made her "feel just as if braced up" six hours after taking the dose.

Helio. is especially indicated if there is also a tendency to loss of voice. It has also cured membranous dysmenorrhea.

RELATIONS - ***Compare:*** (1) Bor. - membranous dysmenorrhea., (2) Symph. - bruised pain in leg.

REFERENCES - Clarke.

HELIX TOSTA

(Toasted Snail)

PHARMACY - helix. Helix tosta. Toasted snail. N. O. Helicide. Trituration. ***Historical dose:*** Trituration and all potencies.

CLINICAL - Dyspnea. Hemoptysis. Hemorrhage. Hoarseness. Tuberculosis.

HOMEOPATHIC - Snails have a tradition for curing tuberculosis.

COMMENTS - W. H. Leonard reported two cases cured with Helix 100,000c. In the first, a man had frequent hemoptysis. Continuous hoarseness with a dry tickling cough, worse at night, preventing sleep. Dyspnea, worse from ascending stairs. He had already had all the usual remedies.

Helix 100,000c., three powders were given. There was no more hemorrhage. A few weeks later a return was feared and a few more doses were given. Four months later the patient was greatly improved in health and remained well.

In the second case, a woman of tubercular diathesis developed the disease after confinement. Several well-indicated remedies failed to check its progress. At length, hemorrhage set in.

Helix was given, as in the other case, with prompt effect. Hemorrhage ceased, cough and expectoration gradually improved, and in eight months the patient was well and remained so.

REFERENCES - Clarke.

HELLEBORUS FOETIDUS

(Bears Foot)

PHARMACY - hell-f. Helleborus foetidus. Bears foot. N. O. Ranunculacee. Tincture of the root. ***Historical dose:*** All potencies.

CLINICAL - Cholera. Hair, loss. Nails, brittle. Scarlatina. Skin, peeling. Stiff-neck.

HOMEOPATHIC - The effects of Hell-f. have been observed on several persons. It is a violent narcotic-acrid poison and in fatal poisoning cases death has taken place in convulsions.

The vision is disordered, choleraic symptoms occur, skin, hair and nails exfoliate. "Profuse discharge from ulcerated surfaces." Anxiety, better after vomiting.

RELATIONS - ***Compare:*** (1) Verat. - copious liquid stools. (2) Hell., Hell-v., Colch.

REFERENCES - Clarke.

HELLEBORUS NIGER

(Black Hellebore)

PHARMACY - hell. Helleborus niger. Black hellebore. Snow-rose. Christmas rose. N. O. Ranunculacee. Central Europe. Tincture of dry powdered root. Juice of fresh root mixed with equal parts of alcohol. ***Historical dose:*** All potencies.

CLINICAL - Albuminuria. Amenorrhea. Apathy. Aphthae. Ascites. ***Brain, disorders.*** Cholera. ***Coma. Concussions.*** Convulsions. Cough. Cystitis. Depression. Diarrhea. Dropsical, swellings. Dullness. Epilepsy. Fevers. Headaches. Head injury. Hernia. Homesickness. Hydrocele. Hydrocephalus. Hydrothorax. Hysteria. Kidneys, congestion. Mania. Melancholy. ***Meningitis. Night -blindness.*** Post-partum, convulsions. Scarlatina. Strokes. Stupor. Tetanus. Typhoid, fever. Ulcers. Uremia. Wounds.

HERBAL - "Black" hellebore receives its name from the external color of its root. It is commonly known as the Christmas Rose or black hellebore. Black hellebore was one of the drugs used to produce the "Helleborism of the ancients," a subject of Hahnemann's famous writings.

HOMEOPATHIC - ***Low states of vitality*** and serious diseases, when everything around the patient looks dark and dusky. Patient's face, lips, hands etc. become dark, nostrils sooty. Parts that are usually red can turn white. Feeble and delicate.

Sensorial depression. Senses become blunt and responses are sluggish, sees, hears, and tastes imperfectly. Mania of a melancholy type.

Muscles do not obey the will, can stagger, drops things etc. General ***muscular weakness***, which may go on to complete paralysis, accompanied by dropsical effusions Convulsions and twitching of muscles, automatic acts, automatic motion of one arm and leg.

Epilepsy with consciousness, followed by deep sleep. Convulsions with extreme coldness in nursing children. Noise arrests the paroxysms of convulsions. One side is paralyzed, the other keeps up automatic motions.

Sinking sensation. Gradual onset of the disease with progressive weakness. Lies on back with knees drawn up or with legs spread apart. State of effusion in hydrocephalus. Serous effusions. Characteristic aggravation from 4 p.m. to 8 p.m. (Lyc.).

MIND - Dull, stupid, slow perception. Slow in answering. Answers confusedly as if thinking of something else. Inattention. Sensorial apathy and constant thoughtless staring at one spot alternating with unintelligible muttering. Gloomy, dismal, despair.

Irritable, worse consolation, does not want to be disturbed. Aversion to company, better when alone. ***Indifference to loved ones, relations. Indifference to pleasures***. Indifferance to everything. Indifferance to sufferings. Envious seeing others happy.

Ailments from disappointed love. Homesickness. Worse or better from thinking of complaints.

Fixed ideas. Just sits and says nothing, does nothing. Hysterical mania from self-accusation. Drops things when attention is diverted, as when being spoken to. Things look new and different. Melancholy during puberty. Sensitive to noise.

Involuntary sighing. Picks at lips and clothes, ends of fingers. His mind seems to have lost all control over his body. Stubborn silence. Would not eat or speak. Never expresses desire for anything. Idiocy after a stroke. ***Complete unconsciousness.*** When aroused he talks about spirits and says he sees devils.

Fear of dying. Believes she is doing wrong. Thinks she is going to die on a certain day. Delusions, sees devils. Delusions sees images in the dark. Delusions pursued by enemies. Fancies at talking with dead people.

Abdomen - Distended. Swollen, painful to touch. Coldness in abdomen. Inflation of the epigastrium with pain of ulceration and impeded respiration. Ascites. Griping, pinching colic with weakness. Griping, pinching about navel, in the abdomen, followed by gelatinous stools. Rumbling and borborygmi in the abdomen, gurgling, as if bowels were full of water. Severe, hard pressure on middle of os pubis.

Back - Gnawing and obtuse lancinations of the spine. Pain, as from a bruise, between the shoulder blades. Neck rigid (meningitis). Stiffness and painful sensibility of the neck and the nape of the neck during movement. Swelling of the glands of the neck.

Bladder - Cystitis. Constant desire to urinate, causing spasms, passing very little. Urination suppressed. Child can't urinate. Bladder overdistended. Bladder becomes paralyzed and greatly distended during pregnancy. Uremia. Dropsy. Frequent urging, with scanty discharge. After great pressure he passes, with much pain, a few drops of blood.

Breasts - Pain under left nipple, pains all over her, forced her menses on, had to get up at night to pass water.

Causations - Ill effects of checked exanthemata, blows, disappointed love.

Chest - Constriction of the throat, nose and chest. Heat in the chest. Tension in region of left short ribs during cough. Sharp cutting pain in region of lower ribs across chest, from within outward, worse inspiration. Chest constricted, gasps for breath with open mouth, propped up in bed.

Coughs - Short, dry cough, worse at night, smoking or suddenly appears while smoking. Dry cough with gagging. Sudden cough, constant hacking.

Ears - Shootings in the ears, day and night with searching piercing. Roaring and ringing. Apparatus of hearing intact, yet hears nothing distinctly nor comprehends.

Eyes - Eyeballs red, glassy. Eyeballs turn upwards, squinting, vacant look. Contraction alternating with dilatation of pupil. Eyes wide open, sunken. Blue edges. Stupid staring or tired look. Night blindness. Photophobia without inflammation. Squinting of eyes with insensibility to light. Sensation as if eyelids were pressed down, difficult to open them. Lids sticky, dry. Loss of hair from eyebrows.

Face - Face flushes red and then becomes pale. Pale, sunken, edematous, red hot or cold. Wrinkled. Neuralgia on left side, parts so tender he cannot chew. Face distorted, yellowish. Constant chewing motion of the lower jaw, hangs open. Cold sweat on face, icy-cold.

Female - Suppression of the menses. Amenorrhea from disappointed love, from damp feet and getting wet through. Pains all over her body forces her menses on. Uterine dropsy with piercing pain in limbs. Puerperal convulsions, arrested by sudden noise.

Food - Anorexia, with brain complaints. Speedy satiety with repugnance as to rest of meal. Organs of taste in working order, yet finds not the proper taste in anything. Nausea, can't take food, though hungry. Aversion to vegetables, meat, sauerkraut. Thirst absent in most complaints or thirst with disgust for drinks. Violent thirst and usually canine hunger during fever. Greedily swallows the cold water, then bites the spoon, while unconsciousness, with hydrocephalus. Children nurse greedily.

Head - Concussion of the brain from blow on the head (after Arn. has failed). ***Rolls the head constantly with moaning.*** Hydrocephalus. Dropsy of brain. ***Bores into pillow***. Meningitis. Strikes the head. Forehead wrinkled in folds in brain disorders. Brain feels too large. Cold sweat. ***Stupefying headache, worse stooping.*** Headache ends in vomiting. Shooting pains, causing sudden screams. Dull pain in occiput with sensation of water swashing inside. Electric shock passes through brain before spasms. Heat deep within head. Pain in vertex as if a nail were driven in. Humid scurf on scalp. Hair falls off with pricking on scalp.

Heart - Palpitations. Heart's action weak. Anxiousness about heart which prevents him resting anywhere. Pulse, small, slow, soft, almost imperceptible. Slow, small, soft pulse, often slower than beating of heart. Pulse intermittent in hydrocephalus.

Kidneys - Congestion of kidneys with extensive effusion of serum in abdominal cavity and tissue of lower limbs. Nephritis causing dropsical symptoms. Uremia. Large quantity of pale, watery urine. Urine scanty, dark with floating, dark specks. ***Coffee-ground sediment***, especially during pregnancy. Passes blood and slime, with burning and stinging.

Limbs - Limbs heavy and painful. Stretching of limbs. Edema of legs. Shiverings, alternating with shooting pains in the limbs. ***Automatic motion of one arm and leg,*** except when asleep. Thumb drawn into palm (Cupr.). Legs drawn up with every attempt to change the position. Contractive pain in the loins. Vesicular eruption between fingers and toes.

Lungs - Suffocating constriction in the lungs, throat and nose. Sighing respiration. Accelerated or deep and slow respiration. ***Gasps for breath but can't inhale.*** Hydrothorax (Merc., Sulph.). Breathes easier lying down.

Male - Hydrocele from suppressed eruption, on either side. Suppression of sexual desire with flaccidity of the genital parts.

Modalities - Better when mind is diverted. Better in warm air. Better by wrapping up. Breathing easier when lying down. Worse from cold air. Worse uncovering. Worse evening until morning. Worse 4 p.m. to 8 p.m. Worse from puberty. Worse dentition. Worse suppressions. Worse exertion. Worse motion. Worse touch. Worse stooping. Worse when thinking of ailment.

Mouth - Lips dry and cracked. Mouth dry, also palate, with cutting and scraping in palate on moving mouth to swallow. Meaningless picking of lips. ***Chewing motion***. Greedily swallows cold water, though unconscious. Child nurses greedily with disgust for food. ***Horrible smell from mouth.*** Apthous, lienteria. ***Falling of lower jaw***. Ptyalism, with sore corners of mouth. Mouth, gums and tongue full of flat yellow ulcers, with elevated grey edges, or red, swollen edges. Salivation. Will take no food except drink. Eruption of blisters around mouth.

Nose - Dirty, dry nostrils. Nostrils, sooty, dilated. Nose pointed. Fluent coryza with confusion of head, as if bruised. Sneezing. Smell diminished. Rubs nose in hydrocephalus.

Perspiration - Nocturnal sweat towards the morning. Cold, clammy perspiration. Sweats temperature unchanged. Sticky sweat. Sweat relieves. Sweats less after sleep.

Rectum - Constipation alternating with mucous diarrhea. Feeling as if intestines had no power to evacuate feces, during soft stool. Diarrhea with pain in the abdomen and nausea. Diarrhea preceded by colic, which is better after every stool. Diarrhea during acute hydrocephalus, dentition or pregnancy. Stools, involuntary, loose, watery, like frog-spawn, of white jelly-like mucus. Watery and frequent evacuations. Burning, smarting, at anus, after stools. Hemorrhoids.

Skin - ***Pale***, ***dropsical***, itching. Anasarca. Angio-neurotic edema. Sudden, watery, swelling of skin. Livid spots on skin. Military eruptions. Falling off of hair and nails. General desquamation of the skin.

Sleep - Stuporous, cannot be fully aroused. Sleepiness with eyes half open and pupils turned upwards. Confused, anxious dreams, the remembrance of which is not retained. Tossing in the bed. Sleeps with shrieks and starts. Sudden screams in sleep. Muscles twitch during sleep. ***Cri encephalique*** (Apis.).

Stomach - Heaviness, fullness of the stomach. Pit of stomach sunken. Burning and scraping in the stomach, which extends to esophagus during pregnancy. Nausea, sometimes with excessive hunger, rising up from pit of stomach. Nausea during pregnancy, before and during stool. Nausea and violent vomiting, with much heat in stomach. Vomiting of greenish-black substance with colic. Anorexia with brain complaints.

Teeth - Grinds the teeth. Toothache at night with shooting and tearing pains, worse by cold and heat.

Temperature - Coldness of the body, especially the limbs. Chill spreads from arms. Goose bumps. Chill with fever, sweat and aversion to uncover. Chilliness predominates during the day with heat of the face and drowsiness. Heat followed by chill with colic.

Throat - Bitter taste in the throat, worse by eating. Water rattles down throat. Scraping feeling on back of palate. Tiresome dryness on palate and cutting and scraping pain on moving the parts in swallowing. Aching, sore throat on swallowing, feels excoriated.

Tongue - Tongue, numb, trembling, covered with yellow ulcers. Tongue red and dry, white in morning. Pimples on tip. Bitter taste, worse eating.

Vertigo - Vertigo with nausea, watery vomit and loose bowels, worse stooping, better becoming erect.

Vision - Early stage of amaurosis. Night-blindness. Vision unimpaired, nevertheless sees imperfectly and doesn't regard the objects he sees.

COMMENTS - Hahnemann wrote "I conclude from various observations that one of the first effects of Black Hellebore is a kind of stupor, a dullness of the sensorium commune, a condition where with sight unimpaired, nothing is seen very fully and the patient does not pay any attention to anything.

"The hearing is perfectly sound, but nothing is heard distinctly. With perfectly constituted gustatory organs, everything seems to have lost its taste. Where the mind is often or always without ideas. Where the past is forgotten or little remembered. Where nothing gives one any pleasure. Where one's sleep is very light and a really sound, refreshing sleep is not to be had and where one desires to work without having the necessary strength or attention required for it."

Cooper, who studied the Hellebores very closely, noted that they produce the "sinking sensation" more intensely than any other drugs. The winter aconite (Eranthis hyemalis), a close ally of Hell., "acts on the solar plexus and works upwards, causing dyspnea."

Cooper quoted from Flora Historica an interesting account of how French prisoners of war at Norman-cross were suffering from an epidemic of night-blindness (nyctalopia), when for lack of snuff they took to using powdered black hellebore with the result that they were cured of their blindness in a few days.

Teste grouped Hell. in the Chamomilla class with Grat. and Viol-t., all of which cause "a joint derangement of the cerebral functions and even of the whole nervous system, a painful increase of the sentient action, followed by a considerable depression of the vital forces and a certain disorder of the mental faculties."

Impaired mental functioning. Functional shut-downs of various parts of the brain, particularly since fever, trauma, drug overdoses. Fluid buildup in the brain. Loss of memory.

Stupor or coma since head injury (Arn., Nat-s.). Hydrocephalus. Strokes followed by idiocy. Brain symptoms during dentition. May help for autism.

Lack of response to sensations, mumbling. Pupils are fixed and dilated, or fixed and contracted (Op.). Craves cold water. Mouth chews, bites, while unconscious. Constantly picks the lips or bedding while unconscious. Grinding teeth, the head bores into the pillow. Pulse is slow and feeble, the respiration is slow and the temperature low. Torpidity and apathy (Op.).

From a purely nervous derangement, it can go on to inflammatory states of the brain and its meninges. Keynote drowsiness, particularly in meningitis or fever. Effusion from the inflamed membranes. Dropsical conditions, post-scarlatina dropsy.

The forehead is wrinkled, there are automatic movements of one arm and leg, while the other is paralyzed. The head rolls from side of side with screams. Chewing motion of jaws. Greedy drinking of water.

Stupefying headaches, as though contents of head were bulging at forehead and eyes. Shocks pass through the brain like electricity. Boring and shaking in forehead and occiput, bruised pain, heat in brain. Pains in occiput and nape of neck.

In fever, sooty appearance of the nostrils, dry, yellow tongue with red edges, horribly offensive breath, drinks roll audibly into stomach. Pale, cold face. Pulse is faint, imperceptible. Fever is worse 4 to 8 p.m.

Suppressed urine in high fevers (Apis). Scanty or entirely suppressed urine, sometimes with sediment like coffee grounds. Urine symptoms in general conditions, will increase the flow. Vomiting and purging, the vomit is apt to be green and the stools jelly-like.

Hydrocele from suppressed eruptions. Ulcers with dropsical conditions (Cooper treated with Hell. and Hell-v. given internally). History of use as an application to drain the tissues of ulcers. Hell. fet. is noted for "profuse discharge from ulcerated surface."

Clarke frequently cured with Hell. a headache which the patient could only describe as a "stupid headache."

Teste cured with Hell. a case of epilepsy in a little girl five weeks old after the failure of Cham. Cham. was given to the nurse, Hell. directly to the patient.

History of a case of brain concussion resulting from a blow on the head (after Arn. failed). One pupil was larger than the other, the patient was drowsy, answered questions slowly, one leg dragged on walking.

RELATIONS - ***Antidote:*** Camph., Chin. ***Compare:*** (1) Threatening effusion, Tub., Apis, Zinc., Op., Chin., Cic., Iodof. (2) Hell-f. - Acts especially on spleen (Cean.), also rectum and sciatic nerve. Splenic pains extend to scapula, neck and head, worse left side and evening, chronic ague cake, hypertrophied uterus, glandular enlargements, hair and nails falling off, skin peeling.

REFERENCES - Boericke. Clarke. Murphy.

HELLEBORUS ORIENTALIS

PHARMACY - hell-o. Helleborus orientalis. N. O. Ranunculacee. Tincture of root. ***Historical dose:*** All potencies.

CLINICAL - Apathy. Diarrhea. Exhaustion. Indigestion. Salivation.

HOMEOPATHIC - This was proved by V. Schroff on Lederer, and produced symptoms like those of the other Hellebores. Particular to Hell-o., there was accumulation of water in the mouth with a clean tongue. Bad taste with clean tongue. Prostration, exhaustion and disinclination to work, burning in stomach, diarrhea. Symptoms better from coffee.

REFERENCES - Clarke.

HELLEBORUS VIRIDIS

(Green Hellebore)

PHARMACY - hell-v. Helleborus viridis. Green hellebore. N. O. Ranunculacee. Tincture of root of young shoots. ***Historical dose:*** All potencies.

CLINICAL - Colic. Diarrhea. Epilepsy. Sore throat. Ulcers.

HOMEOPATHIC - Hell-v. was proved by Schroff. It produced roaring in the ears, itching in the nose and prickling of the tongue, diarrhea of liquid stools, a condition of sopor.

Cooper cured with it ulcers of the leg, near the ankle after the failure of Hell. Also a case of epilepsy in a child, the concomitant symptoms being head sweats before the fit, diarrhea for four days, and sleepiness.

REFERENCES - Clarke.

HELODERMA SUSPECTUM

(Gila Monster)

PHARMACY - helo. Heloderma suspectum. Gila monster. Heloderma horridus. N. O. Helodermide of the Lacertilia. Trituration of sugar of milk saturated with the venom. Solution of the venom in alcohol. ***Historical dose:*** All potencies, thirtieth potency.

CLINICAL - Brain, affected. Cerebrospinal meningitis. Coldness. Cyanosis. Depression. Headache. Heart failure. Locomotor ataxia. Melancholy. Neuralgia. Numbness. Paralysis. Paralysis agitans. Parkinson's disease.

HOMEOPATHIC - The first notice of the remedy is from Dr. Charles D. Belden, who supplied Boericke and Tafel with a living specimen and poison he obtained.

Heloderma is sluggish and slow of movement when kept in the dark, but may develop great activity when brought into the sunlight. The only vulnerable part seems to be at the junction of the head with the spine, a blow on which will kill it.

Belden noted that this animal does not bite frequently, but when it does it is understood that the result is a benumbing paralysis similar to Parkinson's disease or to locomotor ataxia. There is no tetanic phase, a condition almost reverse in objective symptoms to Hydrocy. acid or Strychnia.

Helo. is indicated in many forms of disease characterized by ***great coldness, "an arctic"*** coldness as the ***intense icy coldness*** is the most peculiar symptom of the poison. Cold waves from occiput to feet or ascending, as if frozen from within outwards.

Breath and tongue are cold, cold feeling in lungs and chest, coldness across scapula, burning in the spine. Cold, creeping ring around the body.

The eyeball becomes more prominent and the cornea shows opacities. Boyd noted that the exophthalmus is due to the pressure of the blood behind the eyeball.

Steps high and puts heel down hard, sensation as if walking on a sponge or as if with swollen feet. Turns to right when walking. Stitch pains going from left to right. Weak, giddy, making it difficult to stand. Unable to balance himself. Patient staggers while walking. Movement does not increase the pain. Throbbing all over body. Bone pains.

MIND - Melancholy with weeping. Depression. No inclination for exertion in any way. Passively indifferent. Forgetfulness. Difficulty in remembering the spelling of simple words. Unable to confine mind to any object. Startling easily with trembling, on slight noise. In spite of very severe symptoms, not alarmed.

Abdomen - Sensation of constriction about the whole abdomen. Throbbing, rumbling in bowels. Sharp, shooting, stitching pain in bowels, more on left side. Pain across pubic bones, extending down into left testicle.

Back - Stiff neck, aching in bones of neck. Painfulness of upper neck. Chill in back from base of brain downwards. Coldness across scapulae. Pain in back, pain in lumbar muscles awakening him. Burning along spine.

Chest - Cold feeling in lungs and in heart. Sharp stitch through right nipple to inside of the right arms.

Ears - Pressure behind left ear, pressure in ear from within outward. Copious flow of wax. Ears dry and scurfy. Ringing in ear like night-bell.

Eyes - Itching of eyelids, heavy, hard to keep open. Eyeballs become more prominent and the cornea shows opacities. Lachrymation.

Face - Cold, crawling feeling, from temple down right cheek, as if facial muscles were drawn tight over the bones. Stiffness of jaw. Dry lips. As if pricked with points of ice. Sensation of heat. Flushes of heat.

Female - Burning and dryness of the vagina.

Food - Dislikes sweet things, worse from taking them.

Head - Cold pressure within the skull. ***Cold band around head.*** Heat on vertex. Benumbed feeling all over head. Soreness and stiffness in occiput. Throbbing on vertex. Pain beginning in right ear, extending around back of head to left ear. Sensation as if head would fall to right side. As if scalp were drawn tight over skull. Bores head in pillow. Awakes suddenly with jerk in head.

Heart - Palpitations and dyspnea from slight exertion. Slow labored thumping of heart. Pressure at heart. Tingling, trembling, oppression and coldness around heart. Sticking pains, shooting from left to right. Stitches in heart. Soreness in heat, more under left nipple.

Kidneys - Aching, stitching in right kidney. Bladder irritable, frequent urging to pass urine. Tenderness in urethra with sensation of discharge. Urine not as free as usual, muddy. Intermittent flow. Urine is greenish-yellow, fetid like decaying fruit. Burning in the urethra during and after urination.

Limbs - Stretching relives pains in muscles and limbs. Numbness and trembling. Coldness. Numbness of the arms from the hands to the elbows. Cyanosis of hands. Tingling, creeping sensation on the legs as if from insects. Leg is insensible to an electric battery. Leg is wasting away, skin very dry and inelastic. Ankle turn easily when trying to walk. Sensation as if walking on sponge and as if feet were swollen. Staggering gait. Cock's gait. When walking, lifts feet higher than usual and puts down heel hard. Feet cold as ice or burn.

Lungs - Slight, hacking cough with pain in the left scapulae. Fullness in chest, requiring an effort to inflate the lungs. Oppressed for breath from least exertion.

Male - Cold penis and testicle with gluey discharge. Pain and enlargement of left testicle.

Modalities - Better from stretching. Better warmth. Worse when thinking of her ailments. Worse being cheered by company. Worse from cold. Worse exposure to cold air. Worse stormy weather. Worse lying in bed at night. Worse after sleep.

Mouth - Breath cold. Tongue dry and cracked in the morning. Tongue cold, tender and dry. Very thirsty. Swallowing difficult. Dryness of lips. Soreness.

Nerves - Startled easily. Tired feeling, very weak and nervous. Trembling, of left side, hands shaky, can be controlled with effort. Intense aching in bones and all parts of body.

Nose - Left nostril sore, ulcerated. Dry, itching scurfs in nostrils. Severe attack of sneezing. Fluent discharge.

Pulse - Full and jerky.

Rectum - Constipation from torpor of the rectum. Loose, copious stool, lumpy, mushy, preceded by stitches in abdomen, with considerable flatus. Stool soft, dark, difficult to expel. Hemorrhoids, swollen, itch and bleed. Itching of the anus.

Skin - Yellow skin. Itching, as from insects.

Sleep - Drowsiness, but inability to sleep. Restless sleep, awakens at 3 a.m. Awakened from sleep by jerking in head, trembling of limbs, pain in lumbar muscles.

Stomach - Empty belchings, especially before breakfast. Empty, gone sensation in the stomach. Acid burning in stomach.

Temperature - ***Internal coldness***, as if frozen to death. ***Temperature subnormal*** (Camph.). ***Cold spots***. Cold rings around body. ***Arctic coldness***. Severe chill ran down back. Cold waves (Abies-c., Acon.), ascend from feet or downward from base of brain. Hot flushes and burning in head and along spine.

Throat - Swallowing difficult. Dryness, parched sensation. Tingling. Soreness, tenderness to touch. Stinging, sore feeling in right tonsil.

Vertigo - Sensation as if would fall to right side.

COMMENTS - The Gila monster is a native of Arizona, New Mexico and Texas. It is smaller than the Mexican variety, called Heloderma horridum, the "Crust lizard" or the "Gila monster," which is generally regarded as harmless.

Belden described it as "an ugly, disagreeable-looking creature, the head long and blunt, eyes black and bead-like, tail half the length of the body, thick-set and club-like. The entire body cased in a thinly coated armor, marked curiously with yellow and black." Its skin is studded with nail or tubercle-like heads.

The venom is alkaline in reaction. A number of cases of bites are on record. A dog bitten in the nose "uttered fearful howls and when after great difficulty, he was released, had symptoms like 'blind staggers,' began turning around in a circle and died in twenty minutes."

A young miner bitten in the leg, through in robust health at the time, at once began to lose flesh, became melancholic and died in a few months like a person with rapid tuberculosis.

A Native American woman bitten in the leg survived, but the leg shriveled and she became a semi-idiot, though she lived over thirty years after. The writer of an article quoted by the Recorder from the New York Sun related her case, describing the effect as:

"Where the person survives an hour or two after the bite, the agony is described as awful to witness. The poison goes through the human system with rapidity and causes unspeakable pain and excruciating agony from head to foot.

Though paralyzed, every muscle, bone, sinew and nerve is keenly alive to intense pain. The sufferer's head seems as if it would split open. Very few persons bitten can speak after the first fifteen minutes, but unconsciousness seldom comes until a few minutes before death."

Belden noted its reputation of being fatal to drinkers and to affect non-drinkers less severely. This is borne out somewhat by the recovery of Mr. Vail of Tucson, a man of temperate habits, after a bite; and the death of a man bitten while drunk, after lingering several months.

This lingering nature of the poison is markedly different from snake poisons, which generally kill quickly, if at all.

Mr. Vail said his suffering was intense, the pain proceeding from the wounded part to the head and back. Immediately after receiving the wound, which was on his index finger, both wrist and finger were tightly bandaged.

Two hours later, the wound was cleansed and dressed and the bandages reapplied. For three days those intense pains would shoot toward the head and spine on loosening the bandages in the least degree.

After three months the only perceptible result was a swollen tongue that seemed then unwilling to resume its proper size. The treatment he received was profuse sweating by administration of Jab.

This much was known when Dr. Robert Boocock made his proving. His first experience was with three or four drops of a solution of the 6x trituration, one drachm in four ounces of alcohol.

He was seized with an internal coldness from the heart as if being frozen to death internally and had no way of warming himself. "Coldness from within outward." The coldness of this remedy is more intense than that of any other. The prover called it "arctic coldness."

The coldness was at times followed by sensations of heat and burning. Dr. Boocock's observation of the cold sensations of Helo. was confirmed by a young clerk in the employment of Messrs. Boericke and Tafel, who took six doses of Helo. 6c out of bravado.

The second night he awoke and felt a cold sensation creeping down his body and legs and was in a very cold clammy sweat. This lasted all the rest of the night and he could get no more sleep. It began to pass off by morning, and he felt no more of it.

Helo. produced the constricting sensations of the serpent venoms as well as the numbness, darting pains and the sensitiveness to external pressure. Many of the symptoms came on in the night waking the prover from sleep (Lach. is "worse from sleep").

Tremors, spongy feeling of feet on walking. Pains in back and limbs. Belden recommended it for locomotor ataxia and Parkinson's disease (Merc., Rhus-t., Ars., Zinc), particularly with depression. Raynaud's disease. Polyneuritis, peripheral neuralgias. May be useful for hypothermia.

Dr. Boocock gave great relief with the medicine in a case of Parkinson's disease.

E. E. Case effected great improvement in a case of locomotor ataxia in an auburn-haired woman, 55. She had the classical symptoms of the complaint and "tingling, creeping sensations in legs as if from insects. She was worse lying in bed at night, worse from exposure from touch. Arms numb. Legs insensible to battery. Tongue dry and cracked. Swallowing difficult."

Under Helo. 900c and later, 45,000c after the appearance of an eruption, she recovered a fair degree of health and usefulness.

C. E. Johnson reported to Dr. Boocock the relief of a woman who had many of the symptoms of the proving (and had been pronounced incurable), complaining especially of the intense coldness. She received Helo. 200c and the coldness disappeared almost completely.

Boocock cured a case of "blue hands," remaining long after diphtheria paralysis and he restored two patients apparently moribund. In one case the breathing was slow, "tongue cold and slate-colored, breath cold."

The other case was that of a woman, 65. In the act of dressing, strength suddenly left her, mouth fell open tongue and breath cold and she was apparently dying and felt so. There was intense pain at the back of the head. Helo. 200c was given, as in the other case, and she made a good recovery.

Dr. Boocock compared the weakness he experienced in the proving to that of Gels., only Gels. did not dry up the mouth and secretions as Helo. did.

RELATIONS - ***Compare:*** (1) Lacer. - skin eruptions. Vesicles under tongue. Increased mental acumen. Difficult swallowing. Constant accumulation of saliva in the mouth. ***Nausea,*** violent pressure in stomach. Camph., Lach.

(2) Crot-h., Camph. - coldness. (3) Arg-n., Alum. - locomotor ataxia. (4) Ant-t. and Merc. - Parkinson's disease, Gels., Con., Lyss.

REFERENCES - Anshutz. Boericke. Clarke. Murphy. Phatak.

HELONIAS DIOICA

(Unicorn-root)

PHARMACY - helon. Helonias dioica. Unicorn-root. Helonias lutea. False unicorn. Devil's Bit. Blazing Star. N. O. Melanthacee. Tincture of the root. Triturations of the resinoid Helonin. ***Historical dose:*** Trituration, tincture and all potencies.

CLINICAL - Albuminuria. Amenorrhea. Anemia. ***Atony, uterus.*** Backaches. Breast, disorders. Chlorosis. Cramps. Debility. Depression. Diabetes. Dysmenorrhea. Impotency. Kidney, pains. ***Leucorrhea.*** Lochia, prolonged. Menopausal, disorders. Menorrhagia. Metrorrhagia. Pruritus vulva. Rheumatism. Splenalgia. Infertility. ***Uterus, disorders.***

HERBAL - Helonias has been called a ***uterine tonic.***

HOMEOPATHIC - Helonias has an extensive range of action, as its provings show, but it predominantly affects the uterus. One of the keynote indications for its use is a ***"consciousness of the womb."*** Relaxation of the uterine ligaments, misplacements and prolapse (Sep.). Exhaustion from the least mental or physical exertion.

Emaciation or chronic fatigue since childbirth (Sep., Caul.), or multiple abortions or miscarriages. Tendency to ***prolapse and other malposition of the womb***, from ***uterine atony.*** Uterine reflexes. Dropsy after uterine hemorrhage.

Toxemia of pregnancy with great fatigue. Premenstrual syndrome with fatigue, swollen breasts, and metrorrhagia. Suppressed menses. Congested kidneys, as if the monthly congestion, instead of venting itself through the uterine vessels, had extended to the kidneys.

Bearing down pain, and chronic vaginal infections since childbirth. Sensation of weakness, dragging in the sacrum and pelvis with great languor and ***prostration***.

Tired backaches in females. Constant aching and tenderness over kidneys. Muscles, heavy, sore, aching, burning. Sleepless, with a worn out feeling. Diabetes mellitus and insipidus. Anemia.

MIND - Extreme depression, gloom. ***Profound melancholia***. May have a preliminary feeling of wellness depression. Irritable, cannot endure the least contradiction. Finds faults with everyone. Conversation unpleasant, desires to be left alone. ***Better when busy***. Patient must be doing something to engage mind. ***Consciousness of the womb***.

Abdomen - Burning in the lower third of abdomen. Pain in left side, as if in spleen, which feels as if distended, causing a dull ache. Colic-like pains in hypogastric region off and on all day. Motion and rumbling in abdomen, as if diarrhea would come on, cramps in the stomach.

Back - ***Pain and weight in back***, tired and weak. Aching and burning across the lumbar region, ***can trace outlines of kidneys by constant burning***. Boring pain in lumbar region, extending down legs. Aching between scapulae. Weakness, weight and dragging down in sacrum, down to buttocks. Great languor, better exercising.

Bladder - Frequent desire and urging. Involuntary discharge of urine after the bladder feels empty. Profuse urine, clear, ***albuminous***, saccharine, phosphatic. Strangury. Burning, scalding when urinating. Diabetes mellitus and insipidus.

Breasts - Breasts swollen, nipples painful and tender, worse pressure of clothes.

Chest - Chest sensitive to the air. Aching, as if the front of chest had been compressed in a vice, as if squeezed.

Constitutions - Suited to nervous, run-down females, easily fatigued by any work, who complain of a tired backache, a tired feeling extending into the limbs. Some of this passes off after commencing to work.

Face - Pale, earthy. Sallow, having an expression of suffering.

Female - ***Conscious of womb.*** Uterus, ***weak***, heavy, sore, tender, ulcerated or prolapsed or other malpositions. Weight and soreness in womb. Dragging in sacral region with prolapse, especially after a miscarriage. Backache after miscarriage (Kali-c.). Heavy dragging in pelvis. ***Menses too frequent, too profuse***. Menses, suppressed, kidneys congested. Foul, lumpy or curdled leucorrhea. Albuminuria during pregnancy. Debility attending menopause. Hemorrhage from atony of dark, foul blood. ***Pruritus vulvae***. Parts hot, red, swollen, burn and itch terribly. Vulva, aphthous inflamed. Loss of sexual desire and power with or without sterility.

Food - Loss of appetite, food tasteless. Belchings, cramps. Fullness and painful congestion of the stomach. Bilious, sleepy during the day.

Head - Burning sensation on top. Heat or upward pressure in vertex, as if skull were too full. Headache, better mental exertion.

Heart - Palpitations.

Kidneys - Burning sensation at the kidneys. Constant aching, extreme tenderness of kidneys. Dull ache and heat in region of the kidneys instead of menses. Nephritis of pregnancy with obstinate vomiting.

Limbs - Severe pains in right hip joint, worse during motion. Sore pain in outer side of thighs. Sensation as if cool wind streamed up calves. Feet feel numb, when sitting.

Male - Sexual desire and power increased. Erections unusually strong and frequent. Impotence.

Modalities - Better if busy. Better from diversion. Better holding abdomen. Worse from fatigue. Worse pregnancy. Worse stooping. Worse motion. Worse touch, pressure of clothes. Worse pressure on breasts, nipples or kidneys.

Mouth - Salivation of pregnant women and teething children. Aphthae during pregnancy. Bitter taste in early a.m.

Rectum - Stool loose, yellow in the morning, lumps of feces in the evening.

Skin - Pale, earthy, sallow. Epidermis of the labia peels off thin, transparent exfoliation.

Sleep - Drowsy, heavy. Sleepy during the day.

Stomach - Cramp-like pain in the stomach. Burning in stomach, belchings. Irritable stomach with general dropsy.

Temperature - Feels hot when tired. Flushes of heat pass over him with every movement while in a room. Chills, seemingly radiating from solar plexus all over body, caused by motion of arms.

COMMENTS - Alternate sensations of heat and cold. Burning sensations, particularly at the epigastrium. Useful for menopausal temperature disturbances.

Irritation in mucous membranes, sore mouth, irritable stomach, burning and scalding when urinating, irritated vaginal mucous membrane.

Backache in the lumbar region, over the kidneys or in the sacrum. Pains are worse on commencing to work, better after working a little (Rhus-t.). Pain from the kidneys, especially the right. Generally scanty urine.

Marvin A. Custis reported a case. "Mrs. L, 28, has two children, both living. Has prolapse of uterus, ulceration of cervix, dark offensive leucorrhea. Her system is worn out and her expression one of great distress.

"Irritable, finds fault with every one and cannot bear contradiction. Restless, wants to move around, as she feels better when mind and body are employed.

"She had a severe backache and a sore and heavy feeling in the womb, she said she was always 'conscious of her womb.'

"Helon. 30c every three hours for two days, and then every night, was prescribed with a warm water injection night and morning. At the end of three weeks the leucorrhea had almost ceased, the womb was in the first position and she 'forgets that she has such an organ.'"

L. L. Danforth treated Mrs. W., who had intense pruritus, vulvar and vaginal, for several weeks. "She could tear the flesh out" it was so intense. There was vulvovaginitis, the labia and adjoining skin were red, swollen and covered with thin, white, curdy deposits.

Further examination showed a thin, albuminous leucorrhea pouring from a congested cervix, evidently the cause of the pruritus. The leucorrhea coagulated on the vagina, forming small curds covering the mucous membrane of vagina and vulva. Helon. tincture on tablets speedily relieved.

S. A. Jones found that Helon. turned an alkaline urine acid, and increased the amount of urea as well as the amount of urine secreted. Jones considered this the result of a condition of debility, venous paresis, the result of previous arterial tonic contraction.

RELATIONS - ***Compare:*** (1) Alet., Lil-t, Puls., Senec., Stann. (2) Agri. - painful kidneys, indigestion and menstrual difficulties, bronchorrhea and catarrh of bladder. Cough with profuse expectoration attended with expulsion of urine. Tincture 1 to 10 drops.

REFERENCES - Boericke. Clarke. Murphy. Phatak.

HEPAR SULPHURIS CALCAREUM

(Calcium Sulphide)

PHARMACY - hep. Hepar sulphuris calcareum. Calcium sulphide. Calcarea sulphurata Hahnemanni. An impure Sulphide of Calcium prepared by burning in a crucible the white interior of oyster shells with pure flowers of sulphur. Trituration. ***Historical dose:*** Trituration and all potencies.

CLINICAL - ***Abscess.*** Amaurosis. Angina, pectoris. Asthma. Axilla, abscess. Beard, eruptions. Blepharitis. ***Boils.*** Breast, disorders. Bronchitis. Bubo. Burns. ***Carbuncle.*** Decay. Chilblains. Chlorosis. ***Colds.*** Constipation. Cornea, ulceration. Cornea, opacity. ***Coughs. Croup.*** Diaphragmitis. Diarrhea. ***Ear, infections.*** Ears, polyps. Eczema. Emphysema. Erysipelas. Eyes, disorders. Glandular, swellings. Headaches. Hectic, fever. Hemoptysis. Hemorrhoids. Herpes. Hip joint disease. Hoarseness. Jaundice. Joints, disorders. Laryngitis. Leucorrhea. Lips, swollen. Liver, disorders. Lungs, disorders. Lupus. Marasmus. Menorrhagia. Mouth, sore. Nipples, sore. Ovaries, disorders. Pleurisy. Pneumonia. Pylorus, disorders. Quinsy. Rheumatism. Scarlatina. Scrofula. ***Skin, disorders.*** Spinal, irritation. Syphilis. Styes. Suppuration. Syphilis. Tenesmus. Throat, sore. Tuberculosis. Ulcers. Urticaria. Wens. Whitlow. Whooping, cough

HOMEOPATHIC - *"Liver of Sulphur"* is a name given by the old alchemists to several sulphur compounds whose color was supposed to resemble that of the liver. Before Hahnemann's time, Hep., Sulfuret of lime, was used as an external remedy for itch, rheumatism, gout, goiter and scrofulous swellings.

Hahnemann prepared Hep. with oyster shells instead of ordinary lime. As it is a chemical combination of Calc. and Sulph., it has some of the properties of both, but is very different from either and though it is useful to compare them, Hep. must be studied as a separate entity.

Material doses were used in pellagra. The higher potencies may abort the suppuration, the lower promote it. If it is necessary to hasten it, give 2x. Hep.; 1x will often start secretions and profuse drainage in stuffy colds.

In 1794, Hahnemann proposed to use it internally to arrest mercurial salivation. A few years later it was tried for asthma and pulmonary tuberculosis, with success.

It acts on the mucous membranes, causing croupy, ***catarrhal*** process with a tendency to hemorrhage and ulceration. ***Tendency to suppuration***. Lesions spread by the formation of small papules around the side of the old lesions.

The catarrh may be in the throat, stomach, uterus, or urethra, and is characterized by ***thick, yellow, acrid, ropy discharge***. Mucus in the stools, the urine, and is hawked up. Easy perspiration with mucus. Infected sinus with pus formation.

Great ***sensitiveness to all impressions***. Hypersensitiveness. Chilliness. Sweating, but desire to pull blanket around him. ***Feeling as if wind were blowing on some part***. ***Splinter-like pains.*** The side of the body on which he lies at night becomes gradually insufferably painful, he must turn. Craving for sour and strong things.

Syphilis after gross medication. For the abuse of mercury.

MIND - Mental dullness. Forgetful. Weak memory. Depression. Dejected and sad. Remorse. Bitter crying. Dissatisfaction with one's self and others. Anguish in the evening and night with thoughts of suicide.

Delicate, ***oversensitive to impressions***, people and places. Hypersensitive. Hasty speech and hasty drinking. Restlessness, desires a constant change. Hurried. Child does not laugh, and is not inclined to play or to amuse itself in any way. Children who lose their tempers and hit, kick and scream (Cham., Cina.).

Quarrelsome. ***Extreme irritability, peevishness***. Abusive and vehement. Ferocious. ***Slightest upset irritates him***. Everybody disturbs him. Bad tempered. Angry because of pain, at the least trifle. ***Impulsive.*** Impulse to do violence and to destroy, to start fires. Impulse to kill, to stab with a knife, especially if annoyed. Insanity and mania.

Abdomen - Distended, tense, chronic abdominal disorders. Pain in the groins as if sprained. Atrophy, cancer of liver.

Back - Neuralgia of neck. Dull, dragging, heavy pain across lumbar region, uses arms to raise himself from a seat.

Breasts - Pain in right breast on sneezing. Breasts cancer. Retracted, sore nipples, cracked in nursing women.

Causations - Cold, dry winds. Injuries. Suppressed eruptions. Abuse of mercury.

Chest - Constriction and tightness, oppression. Anxiety and heat in chest. Burning, sharp, sore, pressing pains, worse motion. Weakness of the chest, preventing talking. Pleuritis. Empyema. Angina pectoris. Inflammation of diaphragm. Axilla abscessed, offensive perspiration. Boils, eczema, herpes, pimples.

Constitutions - Slow, torpid constitutions with lax tissue and light hair, great sensitiveness to slightest contact of ulcers, eruptions and affected parts. Suited to the psoric, scrofulous, diathesis. Debilitated subjects. Tendency to suppurations. Cross children. Torpid, lymphatic constitutions, persons with light hair and complexion, slow to act, muscles soft and flabby.

Cough - Loose cough, bloody or thick, yellow, tenacious sputum, raises much mucus. ***Cough from exposure to cold, especially to dry, cold air, west or north-west winds.*** Dry, hoarse, rattling cough. ***Croupy, choking cough***. Croup with loose, rattling cough, worse in morning. Suffocative attacks, has to rise up and bend head backwards. Cough worse whenever any ***part of the body gets cold or uncovered*** or from eating anything cold. Loses voice and coughs when exposed to dry, cold wind. Cough troublesome when walking. Cough ameliorated by wrapping up, keeping warm.

Ears - ***Otitis media, painful*** (Cham.). Ears are ***sensitive to touch, wind***. Discharge of fetid pus from the ears. Pustules in auditory canal and auricle. Scurfs on and behind the ears. Mastoiditis. Whizzing and throbbing in ears with hardness of hearing. Roaring. Deafness from Eustachian catarrh after scarlet fever.

Eyes - Purulent conjunctivitis with chemosis, profuse discharge, great sensitiveness to touch and air. Iritis with pus in anterior chamber. Ophthalmia, thick mucous discharge. ***Corneal ulcers***. Eyes and lids red and inflamed. Pain in the eyes, as if pulled back into the head. Boring pain in upper bones of the orbits. Eyeballs sore to touch. ***Hypopion***. Yellow. Photophobia. Vision obscured by reading, field reduced one-half. Bright circles before eyes. Objects appear red and too large.

Face - Yellowish, sunken complexion. Vesicular erysipelas with pricking in parts. Cancer on lips. Middle of lower lip cracked. Ulcers in corners of mouth. Shooting in jaw on opening mouth. Neuralgia of right side, extending in streak into temple, ear, ale and lip. Pains in bones of face, especially when being touched.

Female - Menorrhagia and metrorrhagia with fibroids. Menses late and scanty. Pruritus vulvae with profuse leucorrhea with sexual excitement. Thick, acrid, yellow, ropy leucorrhea. ***Leucorrhea smells like old cheese*** (Sanic.). Vagina sore during sex, bleeding after. Itching of pudenda and nipples, worse during menses. ***Abscesses***

of labia with great sensitiveness. Profuse perspiration at the menopause (Til., Jab.). Erosion of cervix. Removes the tendency to habitual adherent placenta. Hot, watery, discharge from uterus.

Food - Desire for acids, pickles, vinegar, sour food. Desires wine, fruit, spicy and strong-tasting food, warm drinks. Better from spicy foods. Aversion to fat food, butter, cheese, which aggravate. Worse from alcohol, brandy, whiskey, tea, sweets, cold food, drinks and ice.

Head - Boring pain in the right temple and in root of nose every morning. Eczema on forehead along the line of hair, worse after washing. Scalp sensitive and sore. Humid scald-head itching and burning. Cold sweat on head.

Heart - Anxiety in heart. Enlarged heart. Murmurs. Violent palpitations, with anxiety, worse after fright, eating. Palpitations from a slowly progressing weakness. Palpitations in the morning on waking. Angina pectoris. Stenocardia. Pericarditis. Gouty heart.

Kidneys - Bladder difficulties of elderly men (Phos., Sulph., Cop.). Voided slowly without force, drops vertically, weak bladder. Seems as if some urine always remained. Mucus, greasy pellicle on urine. Gleety discharge, thick, yellow. Putrid odor of urine.

Limbs - Finger joints swollen, tendency to easy dislocation. Nail of great toe painful on slight pressure.

Liver - Jaundice. Hepatitis, hepatic abscess. Stitching in region of liver when walking, coughing, breathing or touching it (Bry., Merc.). Cutting pain from liver to right scapula worse lying on back or right side.

Lungs - Bronchiectasis. Bronchitis of elderly, exhausted people. Emphysema. Pleuritis. Breathing difficult worse lying on left side. Anxious, wheezing, moist breathing. Asthma worse in dry cold air, better in damp. ***Pneumonia in suppurative stage*** with fever. Lobar pneumonia. Chronic pneumonia, with profuse purulent expectoration. ***Empyema.*** Sputum varies from scanty to tenacious mucopurulent. First stage of pulmonary tuberculosis. Sputum pus-like, bloody tuberculous masses, or small balls, when crushed, emit a carrion-like odor. Paralysis of lungs.

Male - Obstinate gonorrhea "does not get well." Herpes, sensitive, bleed easily. Figwarts of offensive odor. Ulcers externally on prepuce similar to chancre (Nit-ac.). Suppurating inguinal glands. Humid soreness on genitals and between scrotum and thigh. Itching of glans, frenum and scrotum. Excitement and emission without amorous fancies.

Modalities - Better in damp weather. Better warmth, wrapping head up. Better pressure, after eating. Worse inhaling air. Worse cold air, dry winds. Worse slightest draft. Worse open air. Worse single parts of the body getting cold. Worse from touch. Worse motion. Worse washing. Worse slight bleeding. Worse blowing the nose. Worse on waking. Worse at night.

Mouth - Tongue, white, yellow, dirty, swollen, large, tabby, slimy, with imprints of teeth, feels as if scalded. Bitter taste. Aphthae. Ptyalism. Gums and mouth painful to touch and bleed readily. Bleeding painful cancerous growth on hard palate. Stomatitis of nursing mothers or weakly children.

Nose - ***Hay fever.*** Sinusitis after coryza. Sneezes every time he goes into a cold, dry wind with running from nose, later, thick offensive discharge. Stopped up every time he goes out into cold air. Ozaena. Offensive discharge, ***smells like old cheese.*** Post nasal dripping. Sore, bleeds, bloody crusts. Soreness of nostrils with catarrhal troubles. Air feels cold in nose.

Perspiration - Clammy, cold sweat. Constant offensive exhalation from the body. ***Offensive sweats.*** Sour, fetid, cheesy odors. ***Profuse sweat***, sour, sticky, offensive, debilitating. Sweats day and night without relief, better from warmth, covers, worse from eating, exertion, uncovering. Night-sweats with tuberculosis. Perspiration with menopause.

Rectum - Loss of power to expel even a soft stool. Clay-colored, soft, ***sour***, white, undigested, ***fetid*** stools. Lumpy stools, coated or mixed with mucus. Raw smarting in the rectum during stools, remaining long afterwards. Obstinate constipation of pregnancy, after purgatives. Hemorrhoids, even slight bleeding exhausts.

Skin - ***Unhealthy skin, every little injury suppurates*** (Psor., Sil.). ***Boils and abscesses.*** Suppurating glands. ***Chronic and recurring urticaria***. ***Ulcers very sensitive to contact***, burning, stinging, easily bleeding. Cancerous ulcers. Atonic ulcers, following removal of tumors. Putrid ulcers, ***surrounded by little pimples***. Ulcers with bloody suppuration, smelling like old cheese. ***Papules, pimples*** prone to suppurate and extend. Acne in youth, suppurate with prickly pain, bleeds easily. Cold-sores, ***very sensitive***. Ringworm. Smallpox. Chapped skin with ***deep cracks on hands and feet***. Great sensitiveness to slightest touch. Cannot bear to be uncovered, ***wants to be wrapped up warmly***. Sticking or pricking in afflicted parts. Angio-neurotic edema.

Stomach - Stomach ulcers and cancer. Painful epigastric tumors with pulsations. Distention of stomach, compelling one to loosen the clothing. Burning in stomach. Heaviness and pressure in stomach after a slight meal. Gone feeling in stomach with loathing of food or as of a sharp lump in stomach. Weak digestion. Frequent belchings without taste or smell. Apt to vomit all food, retaining only milk or water, mixed. Cannot eat bread or vegetables.

Temperature - Chilly in open air. ***Chilly from slightest draft***. Chills and shiverings. Heat alternating with chill. Hectic fever. Dry, burning heat at night. Intermittent fever. Malaria. Typhoid, yellow fever. Catarrhal fever. Eruptive fever, measles, smallpox. Fever with teething.

Throat - Follicular pharyngitis. Hawks up yellow tenacious mucus. Quinsy with ***impending suppuration***. Stitches in throat extending to the ear when swallowing. When swallowing, sensation as if a plug. Sensation of ***a splinter in throat.*** Hoarseness with loss of voice.

Vertigo - Vertigo, with headache, nausea, with a tendency to fall. Vertigo in mornings. Worse on rising, when shaking the head, from motion.

COMMENTS - Guernsey noted the effects on the skin and touch, "any trouble occurring on the skin where there is a great sensitiveness to the slightest touch, patient can't bear to have even the clothes touch the part or have it touched in any way. Exanthema like nettle rash, sore to the slightest touch. Skin hard to heal, inflammation, sensitive soreness of skin."

Teste added that the sensitiveness is not confined to touch. There is excessive sensitiveness to the air, patient can't bear the least draft and if a hand accidentally gets outside the bedclothes it brings on an aggravation.

Characteristic over-sensitiveness. Sensitivity to touch, to pain, can suffer intensely (Cham.). The slightest pain causes fainting. Sensitive to the stimulation of light, noise and odors. Desires constant change, can't adjust to find comfort.

Very chilly, particularly when sick. Very sensitive to drafts, even uncovering a hand or foot can bring on a coughing spasm (Rumx., Rhus-t.). Worse from air conditioning, better warmth and heat. Sensitiveness to cold, dry air (Acon., Bry.).

Restlessness and anxiety (Ars.). Anxious about pain (Ign.), and worse pain, can overreact and become hysterical or violent (Nux-v., Cham.). Frenzy because of pain, impulsive. Very irritable, abusive. Can have an impulse to kill or throw someone in a fire or out the window. Can have a desire to set fires, desire to kill her child. Swears and curses, fears they may do something violent.

Painful, inflamed sores and wounds, slow to heal. Painful, hypersensitive boils (Bell., Tarent.), with sticking pains. Tendency to boils, painful eruptions, ulcers, abscesses and pus. Suppuration, inflammation and severe pain from foreign bodies under the skin or in eye (Sil.).

Sensation of foreign body under the skin or in the eye. Abscesses anywhere in the body, with sensitivity. Throbbing, stabbing pains, splinter-like sensations. Splinters under the nail that abscess (Sil., Myris.). Sticking pains in the nails.

Itching, particularly in affects the bends of the elbows and popliteal spaces. Itching in connection with jaundice. Pruritus, especially when of mercurial origin. Inflammations, especially of respiratory organs, bowels and kidneys and the skin.

Colds and flus from exposure to drafts or cold dry winds (Kali-c.). Chronic sinusitis or bronchitis from exposure to cold winds, drafts or cold dry weather. Sinusitis with yellow, thick discharge (Puls.) with irritability. Coryza, nose swollen and sore to the touch, especially inside the ale. Boring at root of nose with catarrhal symptoms or headaches. Suffocative attacks in the respiratory organs. Asthma.

Whooping cough. Croup that's worse from dry cold (Acon., Spong.). Yellow discharge. Dry, painful, hacking cough, as though a feather were in the throat. Loose cough with wheezing and rattling, as if mucus would come up but it does not. Choking cough. Cough, worse drafts, more often in the early morning (Acon. in evening).

Inflammation of the throat. Painful, swollen tonsils. Abscessed tonsillitis. Discharge from the tonsils. Quinsy, with throbbing pains, where suppuration is imminent (Calc-s. after it breaks). Sore throats with pain on swallowing, as though a splinter or fish bone were caught in the throat. Sticking pains. Hoarseness.

Earaches in children, with night sweats that don't relieve (Merc.). Tearing and pressure as though it would burst. Pus. Side of face is sensitive, hypersensitive to noise. Sensitive to the least touch or draft (Caust.). Abscess in the ear with bloody, yellow, or pus-like discharge from the ear. Ear canal is very painful. Sticking pains in the ears. Eye disorders, likes to have eyes tightly covered.

Toothaches, especially if there is an abscess or boil. Very irritable because of the sharp, dental pain. Food or drink aggravates. Drinking water goes to the bone. Desires acids and sour things.

Semi-paralytic condition of the rectum and bladder (Alum.). Stools are passed with great difficulty even when clay-like and soft. Diarrhea with sour stools. Fetid stools with a sour body smell in children.

Impeded urination, obliged to wait before urine passes, then flows slowly for many days. Never able to finish urinating, seems as if some always remains in bladder. Urine drops vertically down. Acrid urine. Complaints during urination and after.

Nocturnal emissions. Escape of prostatic fluid at any time and at stool. Affections of the sexual organs occurring on the right side. Vaginitis with thick, cheesy, fetid discharge, with a bad odor like rotten cheese (Kali-p., Kreos.).

Anti-psoric. Marked periodicity, everyday, every four weeks (attack of paralysis). Every four months (scabby eruptions on head). Whitlows every winter. Bilious attacks in the spring and autumn.

In Hahnemann's article, "Medicine of Experience," he speaks of the itch-like eruptions caused by Hep. and its corrective properties in wool-workers' itch.

Guernsey noted that there is respiration with mucous rattle, expiration in the morning, none in the evening, cough with expectoration during the day, none in the night (in croup no expectoration at night but only in the daytime with the suffocative coughing spells, low, weak voice).

P. Foster distinguished between Hep., Calc-s. and Kali-s. in their action on tissues. Kali-s. acts on the epidermis, Hep. on lymphatic glandular system, skin and respiratory mucous membrane, Calc-s. acts much as Hep., only more deeply. Hep. acts on abscesses before they open, Calc-s. after.

Foster cured a woman with Calc-s. of "several large ulcers in the gluteal region 3 inches in diameter and 3/4 inches deep, exposing the bone." The pain ceased immediately and the cure was completed in two months.

The relation of Hepar to the suppuration process is very marked. It meets the hectic condition generally and the process locally.

Clarke once cured with Hep. 6c a case of axillary abscess with a large collection of pus. The whole was absorbed without breaking.

A case of pustular ophthalmia of the left eye was cured after Sulph. and Calc. had failed. It was better keeping the eye closely covered with some soft fabric, worse mornings, better as the day advanced. Pimples surrounded affected eye.

In a case of eczema pudendi in a young girl, 11, three months after puberty, the parts red and itching, Merc. was given and the whole body became covered with the rash. Hep. was then given and removed all symptoms immediately. "Sweats day and night without relief."

It antidotes the sensitiveness of Merc. to atmospheric conditions. In the old days of mercurialization, one of the chief things to be avoided by a patient under the "course" was exposure to chill.

RELATIONS - ***Antidoted by:*** Acet-ac., Bell., Cham., Sil. ***It antidotes:*** Metals and especially mercurial preparations, Nit-ac., Calc., Iod., Kali-i. ***Compare:*** (1) Croup - Acon., Spong. (2) Sil., Calc-s., Calen., Sulph., Staph., Myris. (3) Hep. antidotes bad effects from mercury, iodine, potassium, (4) Cod-liver oil removes the weakening effects of ether. ***Compatible with:*** Acon., Arn., Bell., Lach., Merc., Nit-ac., Sil., Spon., Zinc. ***Complementary to:*** Calen. in injuries.

REFERENCES - Boericke. Clarke. Murphy. Phatak.

HEPATICA TRILOBA

(Liverwort)

PHARMACY - hepat. Hepatica triloba. Liverwort. Hepatica nobilis. Anemone hepatica. N. O. Ranunculacee. Tincture of full-grown leaves. ***Historical dose:*** Tincture and all potencies.

CLINICAL - Bronchitis. Catarrh. Dyspepsia. Hoarseness. Nosebleeds. Pneumonia. Throat, sore.

HERBAL - Hepatica is an ancient remedy which received its name from a fancied resemblance of its leaves to the shape of the liver.

HOMEOPATHIC - Definite knowledge of Hepat. began with an experiment made by Dr. D. G. Kimball, who chewed the leaves every day for a chronic irritation of the throat and lungs.

Tickling irritation in the throat and sensation about epiglottis as of particles of food remaining. ***Scraping and rough sensation.*** Pharyngeal catarrh with profuse, serous sputa and hoarseness. Accumulation of viscid, tenacious phlegm with frequent hawking. Sputa sweet, profuse, creamy. Induces free and easy expectoration. Soreness at the nostrils.

Eyes - Eyes somewhat sensitive to light. Itching and smarting eyes. Slightly agglutinated in morning.

Lungs - Some pain and constriction of right chest. Irritation of the fauces. Bronchitis with circumscribed pneumonia. Sputa bloody, purulent, profuse, yellow, creamy and exceedingly sweet. Free and easy expectoration.

Nose - Nosebleeds. Bloody mucus frequently blown from left nostril, for three or four days in succession. Soreness of end of nose at entrance of nostrils.

Stomach - Aids digestion.

Throat - Rough scraping, irritative and tickling sensation in throat and fauces. Pharyngeal catarrh with profuse serous expectoration and hoarseness. Irritation of fauces, tickling, itching, scraping, almost constant, worse by eating or inhalation of dust.

COMMENTS - Hale experienced an attack of circumscribed pneumonia with bloody expectoration or else, profuse, yellow, creamy, exceedingly sweet. Some pain and constriction in right chest, tickling in fauces, worse by eating or from inhalation of dust. Hale chewed the dry leaves and in a few days was well.

Wegge of Copenhagen confirmed its value in pharyngeal catarrh with profuse serous sputa and hoarseness.

RELATIONS - ***Compare:*** (1) Stann., Cist., Caust., Hydr., Phos., Sang., Rumx., Lach., Kali-bi.

REFERENCES - Boericke. Clarke.

HERACLEUM SPHONDYLIUM

(Hogweed)

PHARMACY - hera. (bran.). Heracleum sphondylium. Hogweed. Branca ursina. Bears breech. N. O. Umbelliferae. Tincture of whole plant. ***Historical dose:*** Tincture and all potencies.

CLINICAL - Colic. Debility. Diarrhea. Dyspepsia. Epilepsy. Gout. Headaches. Migraines. Seborrhea, capitis. Skin, disorders. Spleen, pain. Vomiting.

HOMEOPATHIC - Hera. was found to exercise a pronounced action on the digestion, producing hunger with inability to eat, nausea, vomiting, colic, diarrhea and pain in the spleen. It also affected the sexual organs and the skin.

Headache with drowsiness, worse on moving in open air, better tying up the head with a cloth. Exhaustion indolence and weakness. Recommended as a spinal stimulant in epilepsy with flatulency, gouty and skin symptoms.

MIND - Hypochondriac troubles. Fretfulness and ill-humor, taciturn.

Abdomen - Abdominal and splenic pain. Throbbing and pain in the region of the spleen. Flatulence and colic, with nausea and offensive eructations. Sticking and griping colic, obliging him to bend up.

Chest - Oppression of the chest, with palpitation. Oppression of the chest and chilliness. Sharp pain in the chest on inspiration.

Eyes - Lachrymation and weakness of the eyes while reading.

Female - Transient sticking pain in the labia.

Food - Hungry but unable to eat. Hunger, with nausea, and dread of all food. Increased thirst.

Head - Migraines. Sick headaches. Headaches with drowsiness, worse moving in open air, better tying up head with cloth. ***Much perspiration on head,*** and violent itching. Seborrhea capitis. Excessive oily secretion on the head.

Limbs - Gouty, tearing pains in the limbs. Sticking and burning in the feet.

Lungs - Dry, hacking cough, with feeling of soreness and transient stitches in the chest. Arrest of breathing on ascending a mountain.

Male - Drawings in the penis. Sharp pain in the glans penis. Emissions.

Mouth - Bitter taste in the mouth.

Nose - Frequent sneezing, with stitches in the region of the spleen.

Rectum - Slimy, offensive diarrhea. Stool delayed, with urging and pain in the anus.

Skin - Violent itching on the skin, and moist eruption, like the itch. Dry eruption on the chest, burning after scratching. Itching and biting on the scrotum.

Stomach - Pain with inclination to vomit. Bitter risings and taste. Sweet and bitter eructations, with gulping up of bitter fluid. Qualmish nausea, bitter, bilious vomiting, with pains in the stomach, and violent congestion of the head. Pressive in the stomach, with nausea and pressure in the pit of the stomach, after eating, as from a stone.

Temperature - Chilliness, with frequent yawning and inclination to sleep in afternoon.

Throat - Increased collection of mucus, crawling, rawness and scraping in the throat. Pressure in the throat, as from tenacious mucus.

Vertigo - Vertigo while reading and sitting.

RELATIONS - ***Compare:*** (1) Con., Abies-n. (2) Cean. in headache with drowsiness. (3) Bruc., Gins., Gels., Nat-s., Nux-m., Sulph.

REFERENCES - Allen. Boericke. Clarke. Murphy.

HEROINUM

(Heroin)

PHARMACY - herin. Heroinum. Heroin. Diamorphine. Papaveraceae.

CLINICAL - Addictions. Amenorrhea. Belching. Blisters. Coma. Constipation. Coryza. Cramps. Diarrhea. Drug, addiction. Drug, overdose. Eczema. Emaciation. Euthanasia. Faintness. Headaches. Heartburn. Insomnia. Mania. Narcotic, abuse. Nausea. Numbness. Sinusitis. Stiffness. Tinnitus. Tobacco. Urticaria. Vertigo. Vomiting. Warts. Wounds.

HOMEOPATHIC - Addiction to drugs, allopathic medicines. Ailments from narcotics. Desire for narcotics. Physical euphoria. Drug overdose.

Lack of reaction, with weakness. Faintness. Weakness, accompanied by nausea. Weariness, in the afternoon. Sluggishness of the body. Emaciation. Sore, aching, bruised pain in joints, muscles. Stiffness. Wounds. Inflammation of sinuses. Pulse frequent. Coma.

Desire to be in the wind, near a warm stove. Trembling, externally with coldness, better warmth, eating. Aversion to smell of tobacco, sensitive to tobacco.

MIND - Confusion, difficult concentration. Weak memory. Dullness. Mentally absorbed. Abstraction of mind. Depersonalization. Awkward, drops things. Spaced-out feeling. Everything seems unreal. Apathy to external impressions. Activity alternating with lassitude. Indifference.

Mental shock. Ailments from embarrassment, wounded honor. Ailments from mortification. Drug addiction and alcoholism. Morphine abuse. Disposition to become a criminal.

Euphoria alternating with sadness. Contentment. Full of desires for unattainable things. Fearless in spite of danger. No sense of danger, reckless. Frightened easily. Anxiety, alternating with indifference. Anxiety about his family, when alone, about the future. Fear of losing control, that something bad will happen. Claustrophobia.

Self-destructive. Insecure. Critical of oneself, feels underappreciated. Despair of life, of social position. Childish behavior. Forsaken feeling. Irresolution and indecision. Discontented. Restlessness. Antisocial behavior. Desire for solitude. Aversion to company, to answering questions. Unfeeling, hardhearted with his family. Dictatorial. Fastidious.

Abrupt, rough behavior. Impatience. Irritability when disturbed. Offended easily. Violent anger. Rage, fury with cursing. Anger from contradiction. Anger alternating with tranquility. Chaotic behavior. Knocking his head against wall and things. Mutilates his body.

Manic depression. Lascivious, lustful. Sexual mania. Religious affections, too occupied with religion. Feels doomed. Delusions that he is accused of committing a crime, betrayed. Delusions of being alone in the world. Thinks he is a criminal and others know it. Delusions of being double, of having two wills. Sees faces in the air around her. Imagines that he has been poisoned.

Abdomen - Distension, elongated. Cramping, griping, pressing, sore pain. Tension, pressure, better bending double. Sore pain in iliac region, worse pressure. Stitching pain in umbilicus, sides, especially on right. Restlessness, uneasiness. Eczema.

Back - Thoracic pain, between or under right scapulae. Tearing pain below left scapulae. Stiffness in lumbar region, pain, worse exertion, on right side.

Breasts - Sensitive breasts. Softness of breasts. Breast swelling and pain. Burning pain, under left breast.

Breathing - Respiration impeded, arrested, obstructed with anxiety. Respiration difficult if hurried.

Causations - Drug addiction. Alcoholism. Mental shock. Ailments from embarrassment, mortification, wounded honor.

Chest - Anxiety in chest. Internal coldness. Heat flushes. Constriction, extending to throat, on left side, with sighing, after sex. Burning pain under left breast. Cutting pain on coughing, on inspiration. Chest pain, during cough or fever, worse inspiration. Griping pain on left side. Pain lying on side, worse motion. Pain in sides, on motion. Stitching pain in sternum on waking. Axillary glands inflamed, especially right.

Coughs - Dry cough from tickling in larynx. Tickling cough, worse lying down. Cough on first lying down. Cough from talking, in the afternoon, 3 p.m.

Ears - Heat in right ear. Ear pain, on the left. Stopped sensation. Tinnitus. Noises in ear, humming, singing, especially on the right. Hearing impaired, as if from cotton in ear, in right ear. Acute hearing.

Eyes - Itching, lachrymation. Sore pain in left eye. Tired sensation. Photophobia. Pupils contracted to a pinpoint. Heavy eyelids, difficult to open.

Face - Urticaria. Red eruptions on cheeks, right. Herpes about upper lips. Painful lips, as if excoriated. Swollen lips. Tingling of lips, extending to nose. Sore, bruised pain, in lower jaws, lips. Corners of mouth cracked, especially left. Stitching pain, lower jaws. Heat flushes.

Female - Amenorrhea. Menses, too frequent, copious, dark, painless, scanty. Traces of menses between the periods. Ovarian pain during menses, at ovulation. Sore pain in ovaries, uterus. Sexual desire, increased, in morning in bed. Sexual desire, diminished, wanting. Orgasm, wanting.

Food - Appetite diminished. Ravenous appetite, accompanied by nausea, after eating, on waking, during perspiration. Thirst on waking. Desires cold water, wine, warm or hot drinks, coffee, soda water, carbonated drinks, fruit juice. Desires carrots, raw food, fruit, meat, bacon, pastry, sweets, spices, ginger. Desires alcohol, but aggravates, excessive hangover. Aversion to meat, dairy, chocolate, sweets, and tea.

Head - Congestion. Constriction, band or hoop sensation, from forehead, extending to neck. Sensation of contraction, fullness, heavy, light. Numbness in the forehead, extending to nose in the evening, or in the vertex. Pain, with nausea, when bending head forward, after sex. Pain better lying down, in the morning, rising from lying, worse from motion. Cutting pain in the temples, right side. Pinching pain. Pressing, like a cap, in the vertex, extending to forehead. Sore pain on vertex. Shaking, tingling, pulsating sensation, on vertex extending to ears. Headache, above left or right eye, behind the eyes, in temples, vertex extending to ear, eyes. Headache from riding in a carriage, from exposure to sun. Headache better from vomiting.

Heart - Conscious of heart's action. Cutting pain. Palpitations, extending to throat, in the morning after breakfast.

Larynx - Cold sensation. Constriction. Voice, croaking.

Limbs - Awkwardness. Weakness, especially in lower legs, in afternoon. Aching pain, in lower limbs, ankles, feet, heels, knees, and hips. Aching in the morning. Burning pain, in joints. Sensation of heaviness in the lower limbs. Hip pain when ascending stairs, knee pain on motion, while sitting, particularly the left. Shooting pain in leg, stitching pain in thigh. Twitching in the lower limbs, foot and thighs. Tingling in hands, legs, feet while standing, upper limbs. Sensation that legs will buckle. Lower limbs itch. Warts and heat on the feet, soles. Stiff ankles. Coldness on the hands and feet. Hands hot and dry, finger joints inflamed. Pains in first joints of fingers. Brittle fingernails, felon. Hands drop things. Pain in upper arm, in shoulder, followed by pain in right shoulder, better pressure.

Kidneys - Stitching pain in right kidney.

Male - Sexual desire diminished, wanting, or increased.

Modalities - Better open air. Better after rain. Better hot bathing. Better after sex. Worse in afternoon.

Mouth - Burning pain, heat. Burning pain inside of lips. Painless ulcers, inside of lips. Cool, frothy, sour saliva. Itching, sore pain in palate. Biting cheek when talking or chewing. Spongy gums. Bleeding gums when cleaning them.

Neck - Stiffness in cervical region, when bending forward. Pain in neck region, extending to right scapulae. Pain and swelling in cervical glands.

Nose - Coldness, heaviness. Perspiration on nose. Sinus complaints. Catarrh. Obstruction or coryza in the morning. Sneezing after rising. Tip of nostrils itching, tingling. Burning, smarting pain in root of nose. Acute sense of smell.

Rectum - Constipation, ineffectual urging and straining. Insufficient bowel movements. Lack of peristaltic action. Painful urging. Diarrhea. Cutting pain, when sitting, extending to ovaries.

Sensations - Internal knotted sensation. Analgesia. Insensibility. Heaviness in the afternoon. External numbness. Tingling of affected parts.

Skin - Contraction, as if skin would burst. Itching blisters, eruptions, worse from soap. Eruptions from sun. Urticaria. Itching without eruptions. Stinging pain, as from needles and pins. Bitten, as if by an insect, like fleabites. Sensitiveness to touch. Warts. Radiant skin unnaturally.

Sleep - Sleepiness in afternoon, evening, while driving. Insomnia from anxiety, from coldness. Anxious, restless sleep. Disturbed sleep, from anxiety, by cough. Unrefreshing sleep. Heavy or light sleep. Prolonged sleep. Sleeps curled up. Frequent waking with anxiety. Waking after midnight from chill. Waking too early.

Stomach - Cramping, pressing pain, extending to abdomen, into chest. Sensation of a ball. Empty sensation, without hunger, during nausea. Fullness, after eating, with oppression of breathing. Belching. Heartburn. Nausea while riding in a carriage. Nausea before eating, better from eating. Easy, painless vomiting. Vomiting after eating, late at night. Hernia, hiatus.

Teeth - Chattering teeth. Sensitive, tender teeth, from brushing. Sore, bruised pain. Corroded sensation.

Temperature - Heat sensation, alternating with sensation of cold. Lack of vital heat. Chilly in general, especially in afternoon. Icy coldness of the body. Flushes of heat, with perspiration, in evenings, in room.

Throat - Choking. Narrow sensation. Constriction. Lump sensation. Pain on empty swallowing. Thick, yellow mucus, with constant disposition to swallow. Coated. Sensation of mucus. Inflammation, right side. Aching pain, better from warmth. Sore pain in esophagus. Sore throat, better eating, warm drinks. Heat in throat, after cough, extending to stomach. Cold sensation in throat, esophagus. Dryness.

Tongue - Burning pain. Burnt sensation on sides of tongue. Pain on right side. Tongue yellow, white, heavily coated. Acute, metallic, sour taste. Loss of taste.

Urine - Pale color.

Vertigo - Vertigo accompanied by heaviness in head. Vertigo while lying, standing, on rising. Vertigo with nausea.

Vision - Blue colors before the eyes. Blue halo of fire. Rays. Swimming of objects. Vision foggy, better from closing eyes.

RELATIONS - ***Compare:*** (1) Nux-v. Anac. (2) Op. Cann-i. Hyos.

REFERENCES - Snowdon.

HIPPOCAMPUS KUDA

(Yellow Seahorse)

PHARMACY - hippo-k. Hippocampus kuda. Yellow seahorse. Spotted Seahorse. ***Historical dose:*** All potencies.

CLINICAL - Claustrophobia. Headaches. Heartburn. Nausea. Numbness. Tinnitus.

HOMEOPATHIC - Hippocampus kuda is found along the eastern coast of India and in the waters surrounding all of Indonesia up into the Sea of Japan.

Alternating states. Desire to go outside, amelioration from open air. General fatigue and heaviness sensation. Oversensitive to noise, odors, and tastes.

MIND - Mood swings. Alternating emotions. Aversion to company, yet aversion to being alone. Feels trapped. Claustrophobia.

Back - Back pain, with heaviness in the back and neck. Stiffness in cervical region.

Ears - Roaring, ringing noises in the ear, vibrations. Ears feel clogged, as if filled with water, or as if under water (Kali-m.).

Food - Desires fruit, juicy things, particularly melons. Worse from salt, salty foods and coffee.

Head - One sided headaches.

Hearing - Muffled sounds. Hearing acute or impaired.

Limbs - Heavy, aching, tired, feeling in the extremities. Aching and cramping pains. Numbness.

Male - Sexual desire diminished.

Rectum - Involuntary stool, sudden urging to stool.

Sleep - Difficulty going to sleep. Light and very restless sleep, with lots of waking at night. Wakes earlier in the morning. Wakes unrefreshed. Daytime sleepiness. Strong desire or need to nap. Short naps ameliorate (Phos.).

Smell - Sensitive to strange or unpleasant odors.

Stomach - Nausea, comes in waves. As if seasick. Heartburn.

Vertigo - Light headed feeling.

RELATIONS - ***Compare:*** (1) Sep. Kali-m.

REFERENCES - Sonz. Stewart.

HIPPOMANES

(Horse Meconium)

PHARMACY - hipp. Hippomanes. Horse meconium. A meconium deposit out of the amniotic fluid taken from the Colt. Trituration of the dried substance taken from the tongue of a newly-born filly. ***Historical dose:*** All potencies.

CLINICAL - Chills. Chorea. Headaches. Melancholy. Prostatitis. Rheumatism. Twitching. Wrist, paralysis.

HOMEOPATHIC - A famous aphrodisiac of the Greeks. Hering said it is soft, glutinous mucous substance of a urinous odor, which floats in the allantois fluid or is attached of the allantois membrane of the mare or cow, chiefly during the last months of pregnancy.

Melancholy. Weakness, restlessness. Chilliness, better from being covered. Violent pain in wrists. Paralysis of wrist, in morning. Weakness of hands and fingers so that nothing can be held.

Desire to lie down, but no relief on doing so. Headache, better lying on painful side, worse walking in sun. Sensation as if the head would fall forward on walking. As if a plug in the throat. Icy coldness in stomach. Sensation as if a swelling retarded the flow of the urine.

MIND - Melancholy, has no use for the world. Doesn't want to have anything to do with the world. Homesickness in evening. Fear from noise. Desire to travel. Restlessness, must move from place to place.

Aversion to being approached. Aversion to company. ***Inclination to sit.*** Sits in a corner. ***Sits still.*** Sits as if wrapped in deep sad thoughts and notices nothing. Averse to being spoken to. Wants to be let alone.

Chest - Sharp pains in left side of chest.

Eyes - Sharp pains in eyes. Painfulness of eyes when moving them with headache. Light of the candle looks blue.

Face - Involuntary twitching of under lip.

Female - Menstruation too early.

Food - Confusion better from coffee. Desire for acids. Aversion to sweet things.

Head - Pressive pain in temples. Violent headache, better when lying on painful side, worse when walking in sun. Head feels so heavy that it falls forward if he raises himself. Sensation of lightness. Dry hair, falling off of hair.

Kidneys - Frequent discharge of watery urine. Urine discharge in a small stream with straining, feels as if a swelling retarded it, prostatitis. Drawing pain from anus through urethra.

Limbs - *Chorea.* Weakness in joints of feet, knee, soles, hands and fingers. Paralysis of wrists. Violent pain in wrist. ***Sprained sensation in wrist***. Weakness after growing too fast. Heaviness in limbs.

Lungs - Barking cough during sleep.

Male - Sexual desire increased. Prostatitis. Drawing pain in testicles.

Mouth - Bitter taste in mouth. Tongue coated white with red tip. Increased secretion of saliva with headache or sore throat.

Nose - Sensation of coldness when drawing the air in. Nosebleed in morning.

Rectum - Spasmodic contraction of anal sphincter. Hard stool in balls. Soft stool with vomiting, discharge of prostatic fluid after urination.

Skin - Itching as from flannel on skin, worse on chest and between shoulders.

Stomach - ***Icy coldness in stomach.*** Nausea, in a draft of air. Sensation of emptiness in stomach and head. Nausea during headache.

Temperature - Chill, beginning in back, better being warmly covered in bed. Heat in evening with dull headache.

Throat - Larynx feels, raw, as if air were too cold. Tickling in throat when breathing. Painfulness of left tonsil. Sensation of plug in throat, left side.

RELATIONS - ***Antidoted by:*** Coffee. Caust. relieved the paralysis of wrist. ***Compare:*** (1) Caust. (2) Anac. - plug sensation.

REFERENCES - Boericke. Clarke. Grimmer.

HIPPOZAENINUM

(Glanders Nosode)

PHARMACY - hippoz. Hippozaeninum. Glanders nosode. Glanderinum malleinum. Farcin. The nosode of glanders or farcy. Triturations of sugar of milk saturated with the virus. ***Historical dose:*** All potencies.

CLINICAL - Abscesses. Bedsores. Boils. Bronchitis. Cancer. Carbuncles. Decay. Catarrh, chronic. Cold, chronic. Diphtheria. Elephantiasis. Erysipelas. ***Glanders.*** Glands, inflamed. Hip-disease. Liver, enlarged. Lupus. Nasal, cartilages, ulceration. Edema. Ozaena. Parotiditis. Phlegmasia alba dolens. Phlegmon. Plague. Pustules. Putrid, fever. Pyemia. Scrofula. Smallpox. Syphilis. Tuberculosis. Ulcers. Whooping cough.

HOMEOPATHIC - Hippoz. is a powerful nosode introduced by Dr. Garth Wilkinson. The disease is called ***"Glanders"*** when the catarrhal symptoms are pronounced, ***"Farcy,"*** when these are not noticeable, the skin being chiefly affected with deposits in the lungs. Homeopathic preparations of both have been made.

In horses, glanders affects the lungs and the upper respiratory tract, causing coughs and disseminated ulcerations and deposits throughout the lungs. Mallein, a toxin prepared from glanders, was used in veterinary practice as a test injection for deciding whether a horse suspected of glanders actually has the disease or not. If the horse reacts it is concluded there is glanders.

In a number of cases in which animals reacted to the first injections, repetition of the test has failed to elicit reaction, thus suggesting that Mallein is curative as well as diagnostic.

The nosode has been used by homeopaths, at the suggestion of Wilkinson, on the phenomena of the disease as guides. It has been used in a large number of cases involving low forms of suppuration and catarrh. Malignant ulcerations and swellings, abscesses and enlarged glands and also in conditions similar in kind, but less in severity.

Weakness, fatigue, general discomfort. General prostration with considerable emaciation. Numerous ecchymoses in internal organs. Inflammation of lymphatic vessels and swelling of glands. Phlegmasia alba dolens. Pyemia, erysipelas. Chronic rhinitis, bloody secretion.

Symptoms suggesting tuberculosis, cancer, syphilis, etc. It promises useful service in the treatment of ozaena, scrofulous swellings.

Abdomen - Gastro-intestinal catarrh, indigestion, constipation in later stage, diarrhea. Spleen enlarged, filled with blood, softened and liquefied, of a grayish or dark color. Wedge-shaped abscess in spleen. Swollen inguinal glands.

Coughs - Cough and obstructed respiration, resulting from scar contraction of mucous membrane of nose and larynx. Whooping cough. Severe cough with profuse expectoration.

Ears - Tinkling sounds in ears. Hoarse and deafness. Inflammation of parotid gland.

Eyes - Full of tears or slime. Pupils dilated with collapse. Papules on choroid coat of eye.

Face - Maxillary gland swollen, firmly attached to the maxilla, uneven, rugged, mostly painless, burning at times. Submaxillary and sublingual glands swollen and painful at times, abscesses are formed which open externally.

Female - Slimy discharge from vagina. Uterine phlebitis. Miscarriage.

Food - Loss of appetite. Thirst excessive, especially with diarrhea.

Head - Fainting turns with headache. Inflammation of membranes of brain. Scattered abscesses in brain substance. Purulent collections between bones of skull and dura mater. Tubercles may appear in periosteum of skull in dura mater in plexus choroides. A diffused myelitis malleolus, attributable to infiltration. Bones of skull and face (frontal most) decayed. Hair loses its glisten.

Kidneys - Tubercles and abscesses in kidneys. Albumen in urine, also leucine and tyrosine.

Limbs - Obscure pain in limbs, mostly in muscles and joints. Swollen arm with sore finger. Phlegmonous and erysipelatous with pustules and ulcers. Hip-disease. Psoas and lumbar abscesses. Old, bad leg ulcers. Anasarca of lower limbs.

Liver - Enlarged liver, signs of fatty degeneration. Hepatitis with gangrenous and ulcerative inflammation of gall-ducts.

Lungs - Papules and ulcerations in frontal sinuses, pharynx, larynx and trachea. Bronchitis, especially in elderly persons, where suffocation from excessive secretion is imminent. Noisy breathing. Loud, snoring respiration before fatal termination, breath fetid. Tubercles, size of millet seed to a pea, of a gray, yellowish or reddish color. Tuberculosis, diminishes expectoration and recurring aggravations and checks liability to catarrhal disorders. Lung disease of cattle.

Male - Tubercles and abscesses of glans penis, testicles.

Mouth - Difficulty speaking. Tongue dry, thickly covered with a black, sooty deposit. Gums covered with a black, sooty deposit. Bleeding gums. Breath putrid. Ulcers in mouth. Buccal passages filled with tenacious lymph and mucus. Scrofulous swelling of left parotid gland in a child.

Nose - Cartilage exposed and decayed. Decay of nasal bones. Nose and mouth ulcerated. Swelling and redness of nose and adjacent parts, with severe pain. Discharge often one-sided, albuminous tough, viscous, discolored, gray, greenish. Bloody and offensive, acrid, corroding discharge. Obstinate catarrh. Chronic ozaena.

Pulse - Frequent and small pulse, 110 to 120. Retarded pulse.

Rectum - Colliquative diarrhea with a general cachexia and exhaustion precede the fatal termination. Constipation.

Skin - Erysipelatous erythema. Malignant erysipelas, particularly if attended by large formations of pus and destruction of parts. Confluent smallpox. Abscesses, pustules and ulcers over all of body. Ulcers have no disposition to heal, livid appearance.

Sleep - Insomnia and great restlessness. Nocturnal delirium.

Temperature - Frequent chilliness. Chills and fever in cases of abscesses and ulcers. Skin becomes cool with collapse. Fever when a series of abscesses follow in rapid succession. Putrid fever. Plague. May be tried in scarlatina, where odor of breath is putrid, mouth filled with tenacious lymph and mucus tonsils greatly swollen.

Throat - Hoarseness. Swollen tonsils closing posterior channels. Ulcerations on velum of palate. Upon mucous membrane of pharynx ecchymoses, redness, swelling, eruptions and foul ulcers.

COMMENTS - Clarke used Hippoz. with excellent effects in cases of inveterate nasal catarrh and of glandular enlargement. The nasal affection may go on to ozaena, ulceration of nasal cartilages and bones.

Papules and ulcerations in frontal sinuses, pharynx, larynx and trachea. Hoarseness. Old cases of bronchitis, especially in old persons where suffocation from excessive secretion seemed imminent. Bronchial asthma. Whooping cough. Long-lasting coughs.

RELATIONS - ***Compare:*** (1) Bacil., Syph., Variol. (2) The serpent poisons. (3) Aur., Cadm-s., Kali-bi., Hep., Psor.

REFERENCES - Boericke. Clarke.

HIPPURICUM ACIDUM

(Hippuric Acid)

PHARMACY - hip-ac. Hippuricum acidum. Hippuric acid. ***Historical dose:*** All potencies.

CLINICAL - Arthritic pains. Backaches. Blepharitis. Chemosis. Cirrhosis. Dacryocystitis. Diarrhea. Diphtheria. Gastritis. Headaches. Jaundice. Laryngitis. Menorrhagia. Migraine. Pimples. Premenstrual syndrome. Vincent's angina.

HOMEOPATHIC - Hippuric acid is present in urine, very rarely as an amorphous and crystalline deposit. The proving was carried out in 1952-53 by Dr. W. B. Griggs on seven men and three women over a period of forty-five days using potencies ranging from 1x to 6x.

Its chief action is on the external tissues of the eyes and naso-pharynx, joint surfaces, liver and mucous membranes. Nasal secretion viscous, yellow evil-smelling. Inflammation of the throat with a dry cough, especially at night.

Pain in the liver with bouts of nausea and a jaundiced complexion. Hyper-productivity of the ovarian follicles. Eruption of pimples on back, chest, legs. Severe headache on the right side, aggravated by heat and ameliorated in the open air.

General muscular soreness and tenderness. Muscular and joint pains in the shoulders, back, lower limbs. Right side is especially affected. Rheumatic and poisoned subjects. Allergic mesenchymatic with arthritic tendencies. Arthritic and tubercular conditions in elderly patients. Weak exhausted types.

MIND - Concealed anxiety. Irritability.

Abdomen - Pain and heaviness in the liver. Entero-colitis. Abscess beneath the diaphragm. Infectious epidemic jaundice. Cirrhosis. Acute cholecystitis.

Back - Lumbar aching, especially at the end of the day. Backache extending down hips.

Breasts - Breasts painful during menses.

Chest - Pain on the right side of,the chest when coughing.

Ears - Buzzing in the ears.

Eyes - Eyelids inflamed and swollen, edema. Jaundiced, yellow conjunctiva. Painful inflammation, especially of the lower lid, on the right side. Dacryocystitis. Blepharitis. Chemosis. Visual complaints.

Female - Premenstrual syndrome. Menstruation prolonged yet scanty. Menstrual flow for three weeks with complete relief of muscular and joint pains. Menorrhagia. Hyper-productivity of the ovarian follicle.

Head - Dull, constant pain over right eye, worse in warm room. Dull aching, aggravated in warm room, ameliorated by fresh air. Occipital headaches, vertigo. Migraine.

Kidneys - Hot, pungent urine, smelling strongly.

Limbs - Pain in shoulders and limbs. Pain in middle of thigh posteriorly shooting down right leg. Sore, swollen joints. Tired, grating sensation in the joints.

Lungs - Cough dry, irregular, gasping, worse at the end of the day. Dry right-sided pleurisy.

Modalities - Better in the open air. Better with pressure. Worse in a warm room, heat. Worse with movement. Worse in late afternoon or at night.

Mouth - Offensive breath.

Nose - Sensation of a blocked nose. Swelling over lower ethmoid bone. Sinusitis. Secretion thick, viscous, yellow, evil-smelling. Acute rhinitis. Adenoids. Nasal polyps.

Rectum - Diarrhea with watery, fetid stools.

Skin - Itching, burning, tingling and shuddering sensations. Yellow coloring of the skin. Eruption of spots and pimples, on the back, chest and legs. Papules looking like goose flesh on chest. Erythema.

Stomach - Feeling of a lump in the pit of the stomach. Lump in pit of stomach. Soreness and pressure over liver. Acid rising. Acrid belching. Nausea, vomiting, hepatic pains, especially when pressure is applied.

Throat - Acute laryngitis. Dry throat. Pain and difficulty in swallowing. Sore, raw, dry, foul odor, gummy exudate, thickness and infiltration of tissues around throat. Eructation with a lump in the throat.

Exudation thick and membranous around the tonsils and the back of the throat. Gangrenous inflammation of throat.

RELATIONS - ***Compare:*** (1) Benzoic acid seems to be an analog. Benz-ac. - A uremic type with brown, strong urine, whitish, fetid diarrhea, joint pains especially in the big toe and Achilles' tendon. (2) Merc-cy. - Infectious, weak conditions. Diphtheria. Inflammation of the anus and rectum. Bad breath and cervical inflammation. (3) Guai. - Red, burning tonsillitis. Pleurodynia with a dry cough. Diarrhea resembling that of cholera. Joint pains. (4) Rhus-t. - Erythematous and vesicular rash. Muscular and joint pains, worse during rest, ameliorated by a change of position or by continued movement.

REFERENCES - Boericke. Clarke. Julian.

HIRUDO MEDICINALIS

(Leech)

PHARMACY - hir. Hirudo medicinalis. Leech. Sanguisuga officinalis. N. O. Hirudinea. Tincture of the animal. ***Historical dose:*** All potencies.

CLINICAL - Aerophagy. Alcoholism. Angina. Anal, bleeding. Aneurysms. Cervicitis. Colic. Conjunctivitis. Headaches. Hemiplegia. Hemoptysis. ***Hemorrhages.*** Hepatitis. Jaundice. Leucorrhea. Myelitis. Ovarian, cysts. Paraplegia. Thrombophlebitis.

HOMEOPATHIC - Burnett was the first to use Sanguisuga or Hirudo medicinalis as a homeopathic remedy for hemorrhages. Dangerous hemorrhages have frequently followed the application of leeches and it has been ascertained that the leech does not merely bite, it poisons the bitten part in such a way as to render the blood in it watery.

The symptomatology was established by members of the International Homeopathic League, following the Congress in Amsterdam in 1961-62. Members of the British, American and Chilean leagues participated in the proving. The group from London, whose report was made by Reside, was made up of eighteen people, nine men and nine women.

Hir. caused the provers to feel lively and energetic, then exhausted suddenly, shivers, felt depressed. Alternating well being and depression. Throbbing frontal or occipital headache. Progressive lacunar cerebral sclerosis. Syphilitic hemiplegia and paraplegia. Myelitis, tabes. Transverse, myelitis, preceded by intermittent claudication.

Tendency to bleed. Bleeds easily from all the orifices. Irregular heartbeat and congestion of the veins. Menses irregular and burning leucorrhea. Gastro-intestinal malfunctioning with nausea, vertigo, diarrhea or constipation (stools streaked with bright red blood).

MIND - Lively spirit, alert, animated with sense of well being. Condition alternates with lack of energy, sleepiness and tires easily. Depressed, sad, sluggish. Weary with a heavy head and difficulty in concentrating. Irritable, angry or tearful. Fear of falling backwards when looking up.

Abdomen - Severe abdominal distention. Acute pain in the epigastric region and hypochondrium. Wakes at 2 a.m. from abdominal colic, worse after defecation. Colic with nausea and diarrhea around 10 a.m. Alcoholic hepatitis. Aerophagy, accumulation of air in the colon.

Blood - Hemorrhage. Jaundice caused by destruction of red corpuscles. Disease due to a change in the quality of blood platelets, prothrombin deficiency, thrombocyte dystrophy and capillary weakness. Skin and mucous purpura. Thrombophlebitis.

Chest - Angina pectoris.

Constitutions - Allergic and psoric constitutions. Phosphoric, syphilitic and neurobiliary types. Hemophiliac types.

Ears - Outer ear hot. Left ear red and burning. Boil in the auditory canal.

Eyes - Red, painful photophobia. Difficulty focusing. Nervous twitching of the lower eyelid. Conjunctivitis.

Face - Neuralgic pains on the left or right of the face.

Female - Left-sided ovarian pain like being stabbed. Brownish leucorrhea two days before menses. Menses, too early or late, heavy or light, painful or less painful than usual. Feeling in the pelvis as if menses would come on two weeks before due. Cervicitis. Endometriosis. Incoordination of the hypophysis, thalamus and ovary. Ovarian cysts. Pre-cancerous condition of the neck and body of the uterus.

Food - Thirst for cold drinks in large quantities. Indigestion from fatty foods with consequent anorexia.

Head - Hot, heavy head, with pulsations going from the occiput towards the forehead, with dizziness. Headache at the vertex, accompanied by nausea. Pulsating frontal and occipital headache, especially in the evening. Feeling as though the head were in a vice. Wakes during the night from a constrictive headache located around the occiput.

Heart - Extra systolic rhythm anomaly. Irregular heartbeats when lying down. Heart irregular with dull, diffuse pain in the precordial region when going to bed. Pain in the region of the heart when sitting, when bent forwards, ameliorated by sitting up straight. Rheumatic endocarditis. Aneurysm of the aorta. Syphilitic aortitis.

Limbs - Pain in the left arm. Sharp pain in the joints of the hands, elbows and shoulders. Transient pains in the legs. Hands and feet cold in a warm room. Swelling of the left ankle. Feet swollen and painful.

Lungs - Hemoptysis.

Modalities - Better from sitting. Better coughing. Worse after defecation. Worse left side, but not exclusively.

Mouth - Mouth painful with bleeding gums. Small ulcerous swelling on the uvula. Ulcerations on the soft palate, roof of the mouth and tongue.

Nose - Nosebleed, slight bleeding on wiping nose. Pimples and boils on the nose. Pustule on the left side of the nose. Swelling on the nose.

Rectum - Proctitis. Anal pruritus. Rectal pain after passing stool. Bright red blood seen in stools, caused by painful constipation. Bacillary or protozoic dysentery.

Skin - Spots on the nose and face with pustules and boils, small wounds. Rough patch on chin. Burning spot on upper lip. Boils. Anthrax. Axillary adenitis of sweat glands. Sycosis of the beard.

Sleep - Sleep disturbed by disordered dreams or nightmares, thinks he is being followed.

Stomach - Nausea, flatulence, general weakness, worse in the morning. Alcoholic gastritis. Discomfort in the stomach after lunch with nausea and burning acridity and a tart taste. Nausea before eating with diarrhea. Vomiting around 4 a.m. Gastric and duodenal ulcer (hemorrhaging type).

Temperature - Cold shivers coming suddenly without apparent cause.

Throat - Swallowing painful. Throat painful with sensation of a ball stuck in it. Tonsils, neck glands swollen. Tonsillitis, glandular fever, infectious mononucleosis.

Vertigo - Vertigo after exertion or when sitting down. Fear of falling backwards when looking up.

COMMENTS - Burnett had a case of persistent bleeding from the rectum, the blood was watery and all the usual hemorrhagic remedies failed to arrest it. Burnett thought that Hir. might prove a similar remedy. He had a tincture made and attenuated, gave the 5c potency and cured the case.

To make Hir., macerate the end of a leech's head for twenty minutes in a mixture of sand and a physiological serum. Centrifuge the liquid and a green liquid residue is obtained, which is dried after the addition of thymol. The substance obtained forms the stock for the preparation of the potencies. W. Schwabe of Stuttgart, who prepared this stock, called it "Hirudin."

RELATIONS - ***Compare:*** (1) Lat-m. (2) Naja - Weakness and cardiac complaints with coughing and choking. Left-sided ovarian pain. Sudden desire to commit suicide. (3) Crot-h. - Skin or cellulitic inflammations. Hemorrhaging of black, clot less blood. Infectious or adynamic conditions.

REFERENCES - Clarke. Julian.

HISTAMINUM MURIATICUM
(Histamine)

PHARMACY - hist. Histaminum muriaticum. Histamine. Imidazolethylamine. Histamine hydrochloricum. ***Historical dose:*** All potencies.

CLINICAL - ***Allergic, reactions.*** Angina pectoris. Arteritis. Asthenia. Asthma. Bee stings. Blepharitis. Bronchitis. Cancer. Cervicitis. Colitis. Conjunctivitis. Cystitis. Dysthyroidism. ***Edema.*** Emphysema. Gastric, duodenal ulcers. Headaches. ***Hives.*** Insomnia. ***Itching.*** Ovaritis. Pericarditis. ***Pruritus.*** Pyelonephritis. ***Rashes.*** Typhoid fever. ***Urticaria.*** Vertigo. Whooping cough.

HOMEOPATHIC - Histamine is a capillary vessel dilator, an arteriole vessel constrictor, and a hypertensive. It constricts the bronchi and stimulates the tissues of the intestine, the uterus, and the gastric and pancreatic salivary secretions. It is normally used in the form of histamine bi-chlorhydrate, which serves as the stock for homeopathic preparations.

The symptomatology was established in 1950 by J. Gringuaz of Buenos Aires, on thirty-nine provers, using the potencies 30c, 200c, 1000c, then 12c, 6c and 3c.

Hist. has general asthenia as after physical exertion. Feeling of constriction in different parts of the heart. Quivering and cramping contracture of the muscles. Irritable, susceptible, impatient, with need to walk up and down.

All symptoms of the skin and mucous membranes in allergic types. Dryness of the mucous membranes. Redness and burning sensation in circumscribed areas of the skin. Red, itching papules.

Burning, cramping, spasmodic pains in the joints and muscles. Headaches and vertigo with sensation of heat and burning on the head and face. Loss of sense of taste. Feeling that the teeth are loose.

Pruritus and burning in the nose, throat, ears and vagina. Burning pains in the scrotum and left ovary. Oliguria with burning and pain on urination. Burning epigastric and abdominal pains. Burning precordial pain. Burning thoracic pain, fitful coughing.

MIND - Sensitive to the slightest trifles. Impatient, restless with need to move from place to place aimlessly. Nervous when waiting. Quarrelsome. Slowness and difficulty in understanding. Cannot find correct words, forgets proper nouns.

Melancholic with anguish and reduction of mental faculties. Sad, prostration which disappears by forced walking. Pain and gastric constriction when receiving news or remembering a painful experience. Psychogenic allergy.

Abdomen - Acrid dyspepsia. Gastric and duodenal ulcers. Painful contractions. Sensation of constriction at belt-level. Spasmodic enterocolitis. Hemorrhagic rectocolitis. Ulcerous membranous colitis. Typhoid fever and paratyphoid fever.

Chest - Stinging pains in various parts of the thorax. Thoracic pain, as if caused by contusion or crushing. Angina pectoris. Feeling of anguish in the chest, which necessitates deep breathing.

Constitutions - Allergic and psoric constitutions. Tubercular types with dysthyroidism.

Ears - Pain in one or other of the ears, spreading to all the sense organs. Pain in the mastoid. Feeling of blocked ears with ringing and heaviness in the ears. Alternating sensation that the ear is blocked, then clear.

Eyes - Contracture and muscular twitching of the eyelids and around the eyes. Spasmodic closing of the eyelids. Allergic conjunctivitis. Blepharitis. Feeling of a foreign body in the eyes. Stinging pain, as if a nail were being driven into the eye, better from cold, aggravated by a draft. Edge of the eyelids red, edematous. Feeling of heat and pruritus at the edge of the eyelids. Yellowish secretion from the eyelids or dryness of the mucous membranes.

Face - Facial pains on one side of the face, spreading towards the upper and lower maxilla and the teeth. Unilateral heat on the face.

Female - Left-sided ovarian pain, spreading to the leg and left hypochondrium. Menses too early or late. Diminution in quantity of menstrual flow. Menses extremely foul-smelling. Leucorrhea with smell of "burnt" blood. Cystitis. Ovaritis and salpingitis. Cervicitis. Cervical cancer.

Head - Frontal pain, at the temples and nape of the neck, spreading towards the front and back of the head. Heavy, compressive headaches, better by cold, pressure and fresh air, aggravated by movement, bending the head, and sun. Sensation of tension of tightness at the scalp with pruritus. Sensation of heat and itching in localized places.

Heart - Precordial pain as if produced by a needle. Pericarditis. The heartbeat is irregular with an extra systole with compensatory intervals. Pain in the heart region with constrictive feeling, drawing, dull pains. Heart pain that alternates with or accompanies a toothache. Feeling of heart "caught up," and need to hold it with the hand. Heart feels too large. Feeling as if drops of icy water were flowing through the heart.

Kidneys - Cystitis. Pyelonephritis. Unbearable feeling of heat in the bladder, all the time, needs to urinate, but can only pass a few drops at a time. Urinary retention with urination only in drops, feeling of having to strain and accompanying the hemorrhoid congestion. Despair at inability to urinate. Urine burns like fire. Needle-like pain in the bladder towards the urethral canal.

Limbs - Arteritis of the lower limbs. Allergic rheumatism. Muscular and joint pains, burning, stinging, drawing, dull, crushing pains. Involuntary spasms and muscular contractions. Feeling of exhaustion, does not want to make the slightest movement. Formication, tickling, pruritus in the muscles. Feeling of heat, as if he had been burned. Sensation of an electric current across the arms. Sensation as if band were tied around the stomach and around the limbs.

Lungs - Lack of air, feeling of oppression, constriction in the chest. Coughing fits which almost choke him with tickling in the throat preventing speech. Persistent, dry, fitful cough, coming from the throat or the supra-sternal cavity. Yellowish, white-yellow, or greenish-yellow sputum, tasting of cheese. Dilatation of the bronchi. Chronic bronchitis. Asthma. Emphysema. Whooping cough.

Male - Hydrocele. Epididymitis and orchitis. Prostatic adenoma. Burning, stinging, drawing pains. Pain travels from one side to the other. Pain moves in the scrotum with occipital headache.

Modalities - Better from pressure. Better fanning. Worse from heat. Worse movement. Worse nervous irritation, and deep breathing.

Mouth - Mouth dry. Loss of sense of taste. Wine smells of perfume. Salivary secretion sometimes profuse, sometimes dried-up. Heat and itching in the mouth. Dares not open mouth too wide, as a result of pains arising from the passing of cold air. Accompanying dental and precordial pains.

Nose - Pruritus in the nose with feeling that the skin on the nose is shrinking. Feeling that nasal orifices are enlarged. Feeling of painful dryness in the nostrils. Inspiration difficult and painful in cold air. Nose blocked on one or both sides. Head cold with blocked nostril on one side and feeling of heat and prickling. Spasmodic rhinitis.

Rectum - Painful contractions, followed by diarrhea. Black stools with a nauseating odor. Tenesmus and feeling of not having finished, when expelling stools.

Skin - ***Urticaria.*** Red, itching papules, the size of a pea, all over the body, better scratching, worse bathing. Redness and heat on the skin of the face, as after a first degree burn. Sensation of heat and burning, hyperasesthesia. Formication and tickling with numbness on different areas of the skin. Lichen planus. Prurigo strophulus. Hair becomes dry. Alopecia, hair loss from the head and body.

Sleep - Insomnia until 2 to 3 a.m. Insomnia with abundance of ideas. Dreams of insects.

Stomach - Nausea when eating or thinking about eating. Stomach heavy, distended, as though it would burst. Stomachache, as if he had eaten indigestible food. Tense, anguishing pain, caused by a weak feeling in the pit of the stomach, worse when recalling unpleasant memories or receiving news. Sensation of fire in the stomach.

Teeth - Dull or drawing pains in the teeth and cavities of extracted teeth. Alveolar, dental pyorrhea. Teeth feel loose, dares not chew for fear of losing teeth.

Temperature - General chills, shivering, alternating with feeling of heat. Feeling of great heat with sweating and weakness.

Throat - Painful dryness of the pharynx, worse swallowing or heat, better from cold. Dry throat. Feeling of a lump or a foreign body in the throat. Feeling of pressure, constriction in the throat, as if tied by a band.

Vertigo - Vertigo, as if on a swing with nausea and misty vision.

RELATIONS - ***Compare:*** (1) Apis - Acute inflammations with rosy edema, prickling, burning pains, as if produced by red-hot needles. (2) Ars. - Anxiety, agitation. Burning pains. Cadaverous odor of the secretions. (3) Sec. - Tendency to hemorrhage. Burning pains and chilliness all over the body, putrid diarrhea, cramps, especially in the lower limbs, chilliness, pallor and burning pains at the limbs, worse in the cold.

REFERENCFS - Julian.

HOITZIA COCCINEA

(Colibri flower)

PHARMACY - hoit. Hoitzia coccinea. Colibri flower. Loeselia coccinea. N. O. Polimoniaceae. Mexico. The tincture is obtained from the entire fresh plant. Tincture of the dried root. ***Historical dose:*** Tincture and all potencies.

CLINICAL - Aching. Blepharitis. Chickenpox. Conjunctivitis. Diphtheria. Encephalitis. Eye, disorders. Gastric, typhus. Hematuria. Iritis. Keratitis. Measles. Meningitis. Miliary, fever. Myocardia. Paratyphoid, fever. Pericarditis. Photophobia. Scarlet fever. Smallpox. Typhoid fever. Typhus. Vaccinations, effects. Valvulitis.

HERBAL - Hoitzia coccinea grows in the valley of Mexico. Its common name Colibri flower comes from the feeling on touching it. It seems to be covered with small thorns.

HOMEOPATHIC - Hoit. has high temperature from the start and increases in intensity. Stifling feeling of heat, general aching. Shivers at every movement. Red appearance, high and steady temperature. Acute infectious conditions.

Nervous and circulatory over-excitability. Uneasiness, fear, exaltation. Heavy sleep. Congestion of the head, eyes, stomach intestines and genital organs. Pains in the throat, neck and ears. Thirsty, anorexia, frequent and scanty urination.

Scarlet fever, anasarca-type and urticarial eruptions. Post-vaccination encephalitis. Anti-smallpox and anti-diphtheria. Encephalitis following measles, chickenpox. Serous meningitis in young subjects.

MIND - Fearful, anguished state of mind. Nervous excitability, groaning. Hallucinations.

Abdomen - Pains in the epigastric and intestinal regions. Acute inflammation of the gallbladder and biliary passages. Acute enterocolitis. Crohn's disease, terminal ileitis. Abdominal muscles painful.

Chest - Constrictive oppression as after running a race. Sensation of tightness in the thorax, as if in a breast-plate.

Ears - Sensation of blocking in the auditory canal. Crackling noises with dryness of the ear. Acute congestive otitis.

Eyes - Bloodshot and burning, conjunctiva red. Blepharitis. Conjunctivitis. Iritis. Keratitis. Edges of eyelids red, edematous. Eyelids heavy, swollen, tend to close, half closed. Gaze is fixed and vague. Photophobia, weeping.

Face - Face red, swollen.

Female - Copious menstruation, which improves the general condition. Menses late by two to three months, then menorrhagia with intense bilateral ovarian pains. Profuse metrorrhagia with acute, burning pains, tearing pains, black blood with clotting and a putrid odor. Lochia, very copious. Burning and itching leucorrhea. Heat in the low abdomen, painful with feeling of a foreign body in the abdomen.

Food - Thirst for water, which repulses, followed by vomiting.

Head - Head heavy with sensation of fullness. Congestive beating in the temples with dizziness. Acute frontal headache, stupefying, soothed by holding the painful area tightly.

Heart - Strong and rapid heartbeats, resounding in the head and audible. Pericarditis. Myocardia. Valvulitis.

Kidneys - Urine red, frothy, blood-streaked. Pain and burning in the urethra. Tenesmus of the bladder. Slow difficult, painful urination, as a result of prostatic congestion.

Limbs - Acute joint rheumatism. Muscular rheumatism. Limbs are painful, aching. Ameliorated by lying in a curled-up position.

Lungs - Frequent, deep inhalation, provoking a slight cough. Frequent, short, persistent coughing. Sputum like egg-white, foamy, profuse. Pneumonia. Bronchopneumonia.

Male - Prostatic adenoma.

Modalities - Better lying in a curled-up position. Worse from movement.

Mouth - Mouth dry, burning. Swollen gums and tongue. Saliva thick, sticky, difficult to spit. Breath fetid.

Nose - Nose swollen, painful. Vesicles and scabs on the edges of the nostrils. Nosebleed frequent, but lasts only a short time. Maxillary and frontal sinusitis. Ethmoiditis.

Rectum - Stools hard, dry, round, burning, followed by a dysentery-like pressing need to evacuate with tenesmus.

Skin - First and second degree burns. Erythema. Solar erythema (phlyctena). Scarlet fever-type and anasarca-type eruption with itching and burning. Urticaria eruptions on the feet, hands and face with a bluish complexion. Edema. Seborrheic alopecia. Anthrax.

Stomach - Acute pain in the stomach with vomiting of mucus and bile. Phlegmonic gastritis.

Temperature - Congestive fever, high, steady, even after appearance of eruption.

Throat - Throat red, swollen, burning.

COMMENTS - Hoitzia is a voracious plant belonging to the Polimoniaceae family. It grows up to 1 meter in height with a tap-root, gnarled with fine isolated rootlets, which in turn give out other smaller rootlets. It has a straight, cylindrical stem, "sub-ligneous," covered with small whitish hairs, alternated, oval, spear-shaped leaves and axillary flowers.

In herbal medicine, it is used as a sudorific remedy. The Mexican cowherds use it for fevers and eruptions in their cattle. The women use a decoction of the plant for washing their hair as it prevents hair from falling out.

Twenty drops of the mother tincture in a half-liter of boiled water can be used as a compress for irritations of the scalp resulting from the use of hair dyes. The mother tincture is obtained from the entire fresh plant and it was Manuel De. Legarreta who established its homeopathic proving.

RELATIONS - ***Compare:*** (1) Bell. - Active congestion with nervous and vascular excitability. Dryness of the mucous membranes. Photophobia. Hyperthermia. (2) Euphr. - Irritating, excoriating weeping from the eyes. Non-irritating coryza. Amenorrhea. Frequent urination. (3) Ars. - Agitation with fear of death. Burning pains. Cadaverous odor of secretions. (4) Rhus-t. - Agitation of the body. Stiffness of the limbs. Skin red, swollen with vesicular, burning, itching eruptions.

REFERENCES - Julian.

HOLLY

(Bach Flower Essence)

PHARMACY - holly-b. Holly. Ilex aquifolium. Flowering twigs are boiled for half an hour, the water strained and used as medicine. ***Historical dose:*** Take two drops from the stock bottle into a one ounce dropper bottle (add brandy or alcohol, if this bottle will be used for days or weeks). This is the dosage bottle, take a few drops straight into the mouth or as needed in a little water or juice.

HOMEOPATHIC - The remedy Holly-b. belongs to the group of ***Oversensitivity to Influences and Ideas,*** as classified by Bach. Additional remedies in this group are Agri-b., Cent-b. and Waln-b., all helping those suffering from vulnerability to disturbances from outside.

The Holly-b. state can be a state of exhaustion, frazzled nerves and over stimulation by environmental impact. Urge to "fight" oneself free of excessive noise and turmoil. Internal suffering and agony, stifled feeling.

Nervousness, physical irritability. Tension headaches or migraines after annoying experiences. Suppressed anger. Psychosomatic illness (Will-b.). Antisocial personality disorders (Ch-bd-b., Vine-b.). Disorders with aggressive or jealous features.

Prone to outbursts of anger, rage or violence which can also lead to injuries for oneself and others. Impulse control, when rage is not bridled (Ch-p-b., Imp-b., Verv-b.). Persecutory or paranoid delusions, heightened accusation and antagonism against the imagined threat of others (Beech-b, Will-b.).

MIND - Over sensitivity to minor occurrences. Irritable, easily annoyed. Prone to vexation. Strong emotions. Agitated, aggressive state. Overly suspicious, envious, jealous. Revengeful, angry, wounded pride. Perceives disturbances or other people as threats to peace and well-being. Urge to be free of the annoyance, even to the point of violence.

REFERENCES - Bach.

HOMARUS GAMMARUS

(Lobster Digestive Fluid)

PHARMACY - hom. Homarus gammarus. Lobster digestive fluid. N. O. Crustacea. Triturations of sugar of milk saturated with the digesting fluid of the lobster, a thick, reddish offensive liquid contained in a sac situated at the back of the mouth. ***Historical dose:*** Tincture and all potencies, sixth potency.

CLINICAL - Back, pains. Bones, pains. Coryza. Diaphragm, pain. Dyspepsia. Eyes, disorders. Flatulence. Granular, throat. Headaches. Liver, pains. Edema. Paralysis, nervous. Pruritus. Sleep, disordered. Spleen, pains. Throat, sore. Wrist, pain.

HOMEOPATHIC - A. M. Cushing studied the affect of lobster poison, noting the specific affect eating lobster has shown on specific occasions. Noting that persons have been known to die after eating lobster and then drinking milk, Cushing put a little of the poison into warm milk. In ten minutes it was a hard mass. Cushing found that milk aggravated his symptoms during the proving.

"Worse from milk." Other prominent symptoms from his proving included a severe sore throat, dry, inflamed throat with large, granulated blood vessels. Throat burns with tough mucus.

Headaches, chiefly frontal and temporal pain, with soreness in eyes. Pain in stomach and abdomen, better after eating. Deranged digestion. Belching. Disturbed sleep, waking at night with flatulence.

Chilliness. Itching of the skin. Sharp and sudden pains, all day and after retiring. Back pains. Strange, dull feeling all over, not dizzy. Sick feeling, unable to move, but better moving. Nervous feeling, restlessness, but dread of moving. Sexual excitement.

MIND - Frightened feeling. Dullness of mind. Nervous, but with dread of moving.

Abdomen - Pain in diaphragm and hypochondria. Pain in liver and spleen.

Back - Aching just below diaphragm in center of right scapula, in morning, inside of scapula, worse right. Sharp pain at superior spinous process of left ilium. Sharp pain, transient, sudden in right side near kidney, forcing him to sit down.

Causations - Milk.

Chest - Sharp pain in back side of left lung. Burning distress at right of lower end of sternum in both sides, with difficult breathing.

Ears - Frequent stabbing through lower lobe of left ear, had to pinch it.

Eyes - Aching, smarting in eyes. Aching pain in left ball. Profuse lachrymation. Lids stuck together in the morning. Edema of lids.

Head - Headache in morning, sharp at times, mostly in temporal region, worse left. Dizziness.

Limbs - Grinding pain just above elbows. Pain in left wrist in afternoon. Pain in right thigh and leg. Knees weak and trembling, worse right, worse afternoon. Lame pain in right knee. Left foot lame through toe joints at times.

Liver - Pain in lower part of liver. Sharp pain in region of left lobe of liver, worse drawing a long breath.

Lungs - Intense edema of throat rendering breathing almost impossible. Difficult breathing after retiring.

Male - Long-continued excitement every morning and in night.

Modalities - Better from motion. Better inhaling cold air. Better eating. Better passing wind. Weakness worse walking. Worse from drinking milk. Worse after sleep. Worse at night. Worse on drawing a long breath.

Mouth - Profuse salivation.

Nose - Stinging and burning in nasal passages extending to throat after rising. Sensation of mucus in left nostril. Nose stopped in morning. Discharge from the nose, watery from left nostril. Sneezing often.

Pulse - Pulse full, rolling.

Rectum - Frequent inclination to stool during the day. Alternate diarrhea and constipation, changing every three or four days. Large, long tenacious stool after much effort.

Skin - Sore pimple on left thigh, outside. Itching in various parts, frequently, day and night, before and after retiring, better scratching, but appearing in another place. Itching sudden, worse night, in limbs, frequent sudden darting, on various parts, worse legs.

Sleep - Restless at night. Sleepless. Woke early and could not go to sleep on account of pains all over, worse epigastric region, back, arms and legs.

Stomach - Belching tasteless wind in the morning. Pain in morning with occasional hot flashes. Sharp pain after a light breakfast. Burning in stomach.

Temperature - Chilliness all over with trembling. Feet cold and damp, afterwards burning.

Throat - Pain near left ear, sharp, sudden, transient. Burning in throat, right side and in esophagus, stomach and bowels. Edema of throat, can hardly breathe.

COMMENTS - During the proving, Cushing noted that he "Felt as though could not move, on moving no pain, felt better by moving." On this indication with others, he cured a case with Hom. 4x.

The patient had headache, sore throat, loss of appetite and when she awoke in the morning felt as if she could not move at all. On receiving Hom., there was a speedy restoration of keen appetite, both for food and work and loss of headache and sore throat.

Another cured case had "No appetite, distress in stomach, restless sleep, very tired in morning." A case of frequent "bilious spells" was also cured in a man who had Nux-v. and Dios. with only temporary relief.

L. H. Hallock related a personal experience in which, an hour after eating a small amount of lobster salad, general pruritus commenced, worse in lower limbs, especially the calves. The itching was of a biting, burning character, not better by rubbing or scratching, almost unendurable.

It lasted two hours in spite of bathing with hot and cold water, fresh and salt. No sooner had the itching abated than his lips, nose, eyes began to swell, until the eyes were closed and lips almost completely inverted.

Throat swollen and edematous so that it was almost impossible to breathe, profuse salivation.

Eight hours after the meal he had the appearance of a severe and protracted debauch. In twenty-four hours was as well as ever. Once subsequently he had a similar experience after eating lobster.

RELATIONS - ***Compare:*** (1) Sep., Murx., Aster., Astac. (2) in cold damp feet, Calc. (3) Lach. - worse after sleep. (4) Hydr., Phyt., Pic-ac. (5) Worse from milk, Calc., Chin., Con., Nit-ac., Sulph., Mag-c., Aeth.

REFERENCES - Boericke. Clarke.

HOMERIA COLLINA

(Cape Tulip)

PHARMACY - home. Homeria collina. Cape tulip. N. O. Iridaceae. Tincture of bulbs. ***Historical dose:*** Tincture and all potencies.

CLINICAL - Collapse. Constipation. Nausea. Vomiting.

HOMEOPATHIC - Homeria is a violent narcotic-acrid poison very like Colchicum in its effects. Collapse, almost insensible, cold limbs. Severe nausea and vomiting. Obstinate constipation. Pulse is irregular and the pupils are dilated.

In one case of toxic poisoning, a Malay woman with her three grandchildren, ages 12, 8 and 6, ate a small basinful of the bulbs with their supper (between 7 p.m. and 8 p.m.). About 1 a.m. the woman woke with severe nausea and vomiting and found the children similarly affected.

She tried to call for help, but found herself too weak to leave her bed and when, by five o'clock, assistance arrived the eldest girl was found moribund and expired almost immediately.

The boy of 8 died an hour later. The youngest child was found in collapse, almost insensible, cold limbs, pulse scarcely 50 and irregular, pupils much dilated. The grandmother's symptoms were similar, but lesser in degree, accompanied by constant efforts at vomiting. By using stimulants she and the child eventually recovered.

REFERENCES - Clarke.

HONEYSUCKLE

(Bach Flower Essence)

PHARMACY - honey-b. Honeysuckle. Lonisera caprifolium. The flowering heads are picked with a few leaves and boiled for half an hour. The water is strained and used as medicine. ***Historical dose:*** Take two drops from the stock bottle into a one ounce dropper bottle (add brandy or alcohol, if this bottle will be used for days or weeks). This is the dosage bottle, take a few drops straight into the mouth or as needed in a little water or juice.

HOMEOPATHIC - Honeysuckle belongs to Bach's group of ***Not Sufficient Interest in Present Circumstances,*** along with the remedies Clem-b., Wld-r-b., Oliv-b, Wh-ch-b., Must-b., and Ch-bd-b. These remedies are for those not fully engaged in the here and now and consequently not living to the fullest.

Dwells on the past. Homesickness, lost love, loss of beauty or position in life. Sentimental visions of the past. Delusions, visions, or voices of lost loved ones after unresolved trauma or severe grief (Star-b-b.). Lethargy, sleepiness and diminished vitality. Often occurs in the elderly.

MIND - Dwells on past memories, nostalgic. Sadness, with sense of loss. Longs to relive former happiness. Believes the happiness of the past cannot be repeated in the future. Hopeless and resigned to future.

REFERENCES - Bach.

HORNBEAM

(Bach Flower Essence)

PHARMACY - horn-b. Hornbeam. Carpinus betulus. Collect twigs with both male and female flowers, the males are the catkins, whereas the females are smaller and actually look more like flowers and grow at the end of the twig. Boil for half an hour, strain the water and use as medicine. ***Historical dose:*** Take two drops from the stock bottle into a one ounce dropper bottle (add brandy or alcohol, if this bottle will be used for days or weeks). This is the dosage bottle, take a few drops straight into the mouth or as needed in a little water or juice.

HOMEOPATHIC - Hornbeam, together with Cer-b., Scler-b., Gent-b, Gors-b. and Wld-o-b., belongs to Bach's group of ***For Those who Suffer Uncertainty.*** For those suffering from lack of certainty or strength of purpose in their daily affairs.

Lethargy in mind and body. Mild depression. Diminished concentration and easy fatigue after head injuries (Scler-b., Must-b, Wld-o-b.). Useful for prolonged mental work, revitalizes clarity and concentration and gives perseverance. Developmental, learning disabilities and retardation (Ch-bd-b., Must-b., Wld-o-b.).

Brain dysfunction due to physical causation. Physical fatigue, with a devitalization of the body (Wld-o-b.). Avoidance of work and procrastination due to fatigue. Work does not appeal, one feels lax in fiber.

MIND - Fatigued and listless, with bodily lethargy. Dullness, difficulty concentrating due to lack of energy. Lack of interest, boredom. Frustration, overwhelmed feeling. Irritable, occasional resentment and unkindness.

REFERENCES - Bach.

HUMAN GROWTH HORMONE

(H.G.H.)

PHARMACY - hgh. Human growth hormone. H.G.H. Sarcode.

CLINICAL - Acromegaly. Bones, weak. ***Carpal tunnel syndrome.*** Cellulite. Constipation. Depression. Diabetes. Edema. Emaciation. Fatigue. ***Gynecomastia.*** Hair, loss. Impotency. Indigestion. Malnutrition. Menopause. Muscle, weakness. Osteoporosis. Pituitary, disorders. Sexual, weakness. Wrinkled, skin.

HOMEOPATHIC - Growth hormone is known to be critical for tissue repair, muscle growth, healing, brain function, physical and mental health, bone strength, energy and metabolism.

Organ health and integrity. Joint pains and fluid retention. Bone strength. Integrity of hair, nails, and skin. Tissue growth and repair, cell replacement, poor wound healing. Conversion of body fat to muscle mass. Enzyme production. Growth retardation. Premature aging. Energy level. Brain and sexual functions.

MIND - Forgetful, weak memory. Depression.

Bones - Weak bones. Osteoporosis.

Face - Wrinkled skin.

Female - Irregular menses. Menopause, hot flashes. Low sex drive.

Head - Hair loss.

Male - ***Gynecomastia.*** Sexual weakness, low sex drive. Impotency.

Limbs - Weak bones and muscles. Osteoporosis. Brittle nails. Joint pains. ***Carpal tunnel syndrome.***

Rectum - Constipation.

Skin - Dryness. Brown spots. Wrinkled skin. Cellulite.

Sleep - Disturbed, unrefreshing sleep.

Stomach - Indigestion.

RELATIONS - ***Compare:*** (1) Pituitary gland. Thyroid.

REFERENCES - Murphy.

HURA BRASILIENSIS

(Assaku)

PHARMACY - hura. Hura brasiliensis. Assaku. N. O. Euphorbiacae. Tincture of milky juice. *Historical dose:* Tincture and all potencies.

CLINICAL - Blindness. Hysteria. Leucorrhea. Leprosy. Sinuses disorders. Skin disorders. Spine, pains.

HOMEOPATHIC - The milky juice called Assaku by the Brazilians of Hura is as powerful as that of the better-known Euphorbians. Hura. has been used in leprosy when the skin feels as if it were hide bound.

Two of the provers had been affected with leprosy, but under homeopathic treatment they seemed to have recovered. During the proving, one of them had symptoms of compression of the spinal marrow with very great suffering.

Skin of forehead feels drawn tight. Tense vesicles. Stiff neck, pain in back. Throbbing in fingertips. Sensation of splinter under thumbnails. Itching, pimples on all projecting portions of bone, malar bones, etc.

MIND - Excited and oppressed as if by some misfortune. Causeless weeping followed by laughter. Laughing followed by chilliness. Laughing from every paroxysm of pain. Flow of sad thoughts. Imagines she will lose some one dear to her. Thinks he is about to lose a friend. Exaggerated conscientiousness. Irritable. Indisposed to work.

Fear of fever on going to bed. Weeping when singing. Biting hands, himself. Desire to break things. Forsaken feeling, Sensation of isolation. Impatience from pain. Mistakes in localities. Mistakes in time. Reproaches himself. Weeping in open air.

Delusions that she is alone in the world. Delusions that he is despised. Delusions has lost the affection of friends. Delusions his friends have lost all confidence in him. Delusions floating in air. Delusions that he is unfortunate. Delusions on falling asleep.

Abdomen - Frightful colic with diarrhea and shivering. Throbbing in left side of abdomen. Twisting pain in left side with very painful, shooting, extorting cries. Stitch in ileo-cecal region, worse on movement.

Back - Stiff-neck, right side, least motion is painfully felt in nape. Dislocated and tearing pain in dorsal region, on sitting down. Severe pains in lumber region, weakness. Excruciating pain in lumbo-sacral region, when trying to lift a weight.

Breasts - Sensation of small ball under right breast. Sharp pain shifting from shoulder to left breast. Stitches, throbbing in breasts.

Chest - Lancinations in chest preventing deep breathing. Throbbings in chest. Nervous shivering all over chest. Suffocative sensation, especially when thinking of anything that has gone wrong.

Ears - Pain behind and in right ear. Stoppage in ears. Loud whizzing and whistling sound in ears.

Eyes - Prickling and burning in eyes, sensation as if sand in them. Eyelids red. Vision dim. Blindness. Sparks and zigzags before the sight when walking.

Face - Face weary-looking as after a debauch, rings around eyes. Face dull and dark-looking with paleness mottled with red. Face scarlet and bloated. Heat rising to face. Swellings on upper part of right cheek. Lips red. Small pimples inside lower lip.

Female - Pain in uterus as if compressed, as if a sharp instrument were thrust into it, followed by lancinations in vagina. Menses scanty, eight days too early, profuse with leucorrhea.

Food - Hunger, sometimes immediately after a meal.

Head - Rush of blood to the head. Heaviness, numbness of the head. Painful lancinations through head. Constriction in back of head. Skin of forehead feels drawn tight.

Heart - Constant pain at heart, sometimes very sharp, arresting breathing.

Kidneys - Acute pain in right kidney while walking, with great urging to urinate. Urine light green, clear, deposits a white sediment.

Limbs - Weariness of limbs. Lancinations, throbbing, rheumatic pains, numbness in upper and lower limbs. Dislocated pains in joints. Throbbing in fingertips. Heat in nails, sensation as if part of nail had been torn off. Pain as from splinter under thumbnail.

Lungs - Feeling of suffocation. Sighs and yawns much. Dryness of glottis causing cough. Considerable yellow, thick, frothy sputa. Expectoration rusty-colored, foul, bloody, like milk-chocolate.

Male - Intolerable erections. Amorous dreams with erections, lemon-colored semen. Weight in testicles when walking.

Mouth - Tongue white, pain at tip. Fleshy excrescence on inside of lips. Clammy mouth, foul smell. Taste of copper, blood, clammy, smoky.

Nose - Redness of (left) wing of nose. Constriction, throbbing at root of nose. Coryza, nosebleed. Sense of smell very acute.

Rectum - Constriction at anus. Frequent, ineffectual urging to stool. Diarrhea succeeded by great weakness of chest. Stools are liquid, painless, flowing constantly, offensive containing thread-worms. Constipation, hard, difficult stools.

Skin - Large pimples, itching, painful to touch on face. Cluster of pimples or vesicles on various parts. Red vesicular pimples, the vesicles break on pressure and water squirts out with great force. Small vesicular pimples with itching. Itching on forehead, eyelids, chin, beard, back, legs, sleep disturbed by it.

Sleep - Yawning and drowsiness. Nightly restlessness. Dreams of traveling, swimming, yellow water, corpses, or assassins.

Stomach - Great hunger with pain in stomach, satisfied immediately on eating. Qualmishness. Stomachache, as from hunger.

Teeth - Lancinations in teeth and gums, passing to ear. Pimples on gums.

Temperature - Feet and body constantly cold and damp. Heat and transient perspiration. Flushes of heat in face. Cold sweat on face and all over body.

Throat - Irritation of throat with dryness. Spitting of blood in morning.

Vertigo - Confusion. Dizziness.

COMMENTS - Mure's provings were made with single doses of the 5c potency. All the provers had symptoms of nervous excitement, twitching and irritability. The gastro-intestinal irritation of the other Euphorbians was marked.

Farrington noted that the vesicles are so tense that when pricked they eject their contents. Sensation of a splinter under thumbnails. Eruptions tend to occur on the skin covering projecting portions of bone or the malar bones. He compared it with Canth.

A case of leprosy was reported cured with Assaku, which led to its extensive use in this disease, though Mure noted it had not cured any others.

RELATIONS - ***Antidoted by:*** Camph., Op. ***Compare:*** (1) Crot-t., Ric., Euphor., Hura-c. (2) Calo. - Leprosy, livid and gangrenous tubercles, thickening of the skin. (3) Urin.

REFERENCES - Boericke. Clarke.

HURA CREPITANS

(Monkey's Dinner-bell)

PHARMACY - hura-c. Hura crepitans. Monkey's dinner-bell. Sand-box. N. O. Euphorbiacae. Tincture of seeds. ***Historical dose:*** Tincture and all potencies.

CLINICAL - Blindness. Burning, pains. Diarrhea. Headache. Sore, throat. Vomiting.

HERBAL - The Treasury of Botany only recognizes one species of Hura, H. crepitans. But Mure compared his Hura with H. crepitans and they are probably varieties of the same species as the properties of the milk are the same.

The rounded, hard-shelled fruits are about the size of an orange and have as many deep furrows as there are cells, each cell containing a single flattened seed.

When the fruit is ripe and exposed to a dry atmosphere, it bursts with great force, accompanied by a loud, sharp crack like the report of a pistol, for which reason it is often called the Monkey's Dinner-bell.

HOMEOPATHIC - The Hura-c. seeds are emetic, in a green state violently purgative, but when dry, according to Lunan, they lose this property.

An oil is extracted from them and sometimes used as a purgative, about twenty drops of it equal in action to a tablespoonful of castor oil.

A venomous milky juice is abundant in all parts of the plant and causes almost immediate blindness if applied to the eye.

The observed effects of Hura-c. were found from eating the seeds. Burning in throat, vomiting and purging, suffocation, headache, were the main symptoms complained.

RELATIONS - ***Antidoted by:*** Camph., Op. ***Compare:*** (1) Hur-br., Ric., Crot-t. (2) Caps. - burning in throat not better by water.

REFERENCES - Boericke. Clarke.

HYDRANGEA ARBORESCENS

(Seven-barks)

PHARMACY - hydrang. Hydrangea arborescens. Seven-barks. N. O. Hydrangeacee or Saxifragaceae. Tincture of fresh leaves and young shoots. Fluid extract. ***Historical dose:*** Tincture and all potencies.

CLINICAL - Bladder, catarrh. Bladder, stones. Cystitis. Diabetes. Dizziness. Gravel. Gout. ***Kidney, colic. Kidney, stones.*** Nephritis. Prostatic, disorders. ***Prostate, enlarged.*** Pyelitis. Rheumatism. Urinary, incontinence.

HERBAL - Like some other members of the Saxifragaceae, Hydrangea has a traditional reputation as a *"stone-breaking"* remedy as it was used in calculous diseases for many years.

Hansen noted that Hydrang. arrested the tendency to formation of calculus in the bladder and relieved distress from renal calculus, with soreness over the region of the kidneys and bloody urine.

HOMEOPATHIC - Hydrang. is a remedy for gravel, profuse deposit of white amorphous salts in urine. ***Kidney stones, kidney colic, bloody urine.*** It appears to act strongly on the neck of the bladder and on the ureters. Gout and rheumatism. Oppression of the chest. Pain in lumbar region. Dizziness.

Mind - Nervous and worried. Violent attacks of anger. Outbursts of anger due to pains.

Abdomen - Colic. Abdominal symptoms and enlarged prostate. ***Sharp pain in loins,*** especially left side.

Bladder - Bladder catarrh, stones. Urinary incontinence. Frequent urination. Spasmodic stricture. Cystitis. Burning in urethra and frequent desire, but hard to start. Stitching pain during urination.

Food - ***Great thirst*** with abdominal symptoms.

Male - Prostate hypertrophy. ***Enlarged prostate*** (Ferr-pic., Sabal.).

Kidneys - Pyelitis. Nephritis. Calculus in the ureter with prostate enlargement. ***Kidney stones, kidney colic.*** Sore kidneys. Pain in left kidney, ureter. Radiating pains (Berb.).

Urine - Profuse deposit of white amorphous salts. Gravel deposits. Yellow sand. ***Bloody urine.*** Heavy deposit of mucus.

COMMENTS - Dr. Nottingham of Lansing said that in physiological doses it produces giddiness, oppression of the chest and acts as a cathartic, diuretic, sialogogue and narcotic.

Nottingham used it with brilliant results in the case of Mr. B., 71, tall, slender, dark. He was exceedingly irritable and frequently subject to violent paroxysms of anger. For many years he had been accustomed to make the most reckless use of drugs and was always requesting his homeopathic doctor to give him *"something stronger."*

For eight years he had suffered from bladder sphincter irritation with dribbling of urine, severe spasms of prostate, kidney catarrh, yellow sand in urine and even small stones. After persistent use of the best indicated remedies with no effect, the fluid extract of Hydrangea was given, a teaspoonful every three or four hours. The symptoms disappeared in a very short time.

Cooper has also used this remedy (which, he says is the thirstiest plant known) with good effect in diabetes in cases presenting great thirst with abdominal symptoms and in enlarged prostate.

Hansen added that it is particularly useful for profuse deposits of white amorphous salts in the urine.

Hydrang. has arrested the tendency to formation of stones, relieves distress from kidney stones with soreness over region of kidneys and bloody urine.

RELATIONS - ***Compare:*** (1) Lyc., Chim., Berb., Pareir., Uva., Sabal., Oxyd., (2) Geum. (3) Polytr. - according to Dr. Cushing in tincture or infusion for enlarged prostate or prostatitis.

REFERENCES - Boericke. Clarke.

HYDRASTINUM MURIATICUM

(Hydrastia Muriate)

PHARMACY - hydr-m. Hydrastinum muriaticum. Hydrastia muriate. An alkalolid of Hydrastis canadensis. Trituration of the crystals. ***Historical dose:*** Trituration and all potencies.

CLINICAL - Aphthae. Digestive, disorders. Fibroid, tumors. Hemorrhages. Metrorrhagia. Ozaena. Sore, throat. Stomach, dilatation. Ulcers.

HOMEOPATHIC - The alkaloids of Hydrastis have been largely used in the allopathic school for internal hemorrhage. Hydr-m. was found to be inconvenient by reason of its irritant properties. Its use in fibroid tumors was advocated by Dr. Burford and others in the homeopathic school.

Locally used in aphthous sore mouth, ulcers, ulcerated sore throat, ozaena, etc. Hydr-m. is a uterine hemostatic and also a vaso-constrictor. ***Hemorrhages in dilatation of the stomach*** and chronic digestive disorders. Metrorrhagia, especially from fibroid tumors.

COMMENTS - A case of central uterine fibroid tumor, about the size of a large orange, and pressing on the bladder, causing bladder symptoms, was quickly reduced in size with the disappearance of all symptoms by Hydr-m. 3x.

REFERENCES - Boericke. Clarke.

HYDRASTIS CANADENSIS

(Golden Seal)

PHARMACY - hydr. Hydrastis canadensis. Golden seal. Orange-root. Yellow Puccoon. N. O. Ranunculacee. Tincture of the fresh root. ***Historical dose:*** Tincture and all potencies.

CLINICAL - Alcoholism. Asthma. Backaches. ***Breast, cancer. Cachexia. Cancer.*** Catarrh. Chancroids. ***Colon, cancer.*** Constipation. Corns. Dyspepsia. Eczema. Ears, disorders. ***Emaciation.*** Fainting. Fistula. Gastric, catarrh. ***Goiter***. Gonorrhea. Hemorrhoids. Jaundice. ***Leucorrhea. Liver, cancer.*** Liver, disorders. Lumbago. Lupus. ***Malnutrition.*** Menorrhagia. Metrorrhagia. Mouth, sore. Nails, disorders. Nipples, sore. Nursing, women. Placenta, adherent. Post-nasal, catarrh. Pruritus, vulvae. ***Rectal, cancer.*** Rectum, disorders. Sciatica. Seborrhea. ***Sinusitis.*** Smallpox. ***Stomach, cancer. Stomach, disorders.*** Syphilis. Taste, disordered. Throat, deafness. Throat, sore. Tongue, disorders. Typhus. ***Ulcers.*** Uterus, disorders.

HERBAL - Hydrastis, the Golden Seal plant, is the only specimen of its genus among the Ranunculacee. It grows in shady woods in rich soil and damp meadows. The fruit is like a raspberry and the plant is sometimes called ground raspberry in consequence. The root, from which the tincture is made, is really a perennial underground stem, thick, knotty and yellow.

The yellow color is very intense and has been used as a dye by Native Americans. The first mention of it in medical literature is by Rafinesque. Hale quoted him as saying that it is "tonic, ophthalmic, detergent," and that "it is said to enter into compound remedies for cancer, acting as a detergent tonic and the Cherokees are supposed to use it in that disease."

HOMEOPATHIC - Later experience agreed with this reputation and Hydr. won its chief fame through its use in cancer cases. Clarke thought it may fairly be said that more cases of cancer have been cured with Hydrastis than with any other single remedy. ***Cancer and pre-cancerous states***, before ulceration with pain.

Shallow ulcers. Small wounds bleed and suppurate. Tendency to hemorrhage and ulcerations. Modifies the course of ***smallpox*** internally and topically. Garth Wilkinson noted the modification of smallpox, abolishing its distressing symptoms, shortening its course, lessening its danger and greatly mitigating its consequences.

Catarrh characterized by ***thick, yellow, acrid, ropy discharge***. Mucus is found in the stools and in the urine. Hawks up mucus. Sense of raw burning. Poor digestion and obstinate constipation. Marked action on the liver. ***Goiter*** of puberty and pregnancy. Clothing feels uncomfortable about groins. Lumbago.

Weak muscular power. Emaciation and prostration. Frequent fainting spells with profuse perspiration. Prominent cerebral effects, feels his wits sharpened, head cleared, facile expression.

MIND - Absent-mindedness, forgetful. Dullness of memory. Forgetful. Weakness of memory. Can't remember what he is reading or talking about. Disturbed by least noise. So nervous that to hear any one speak is unbearable. Averse to conversation.

Apathetic. Indifference to everything. Moody. High-spirited. Extreme restlessness. Cheerful on rising in morning. Nervous and sensitive.

Gloomy, taciturn and disagreeable. Hopelessness. Depression and gloom, sure of death and desires it. Discouragement incidental to long suffering and weakness. ***Irritability after dinner.*** Irritable, disposed to be spiteful. Malicious. Desire to strike. Moaning with occasional outcries from pain.

Abdomen - Burning pain in umbilical region with goneness, faintness in epigastrium. Gastro-duodenal catarrh. ***Colon cancer.*** Flatulent colic with faintness. Loud rumbling with dull aching, worse moving. Abdominal walls painful on pressure, during flatulent colic. Cutting, colicky pains, better after passing flatus. Sharp pain in the cecal region. Sharp pain spleen region. Pains in the groin as if he had strained himself. Griping pains with the stools. Groins as if sprained. Severe pain in bowels from getting feet wet during menses. Gurgling in ileocaecal region, with bloated abdomen. Intestinal catarrh, followed by ulceration.

Back - Dull, heavy, dragging pain and stiffness, particularly ***across lumbar region, must use arms in raising himself from seat.*** Neuralgia of neck. Muscles of neck feel sore. Tired aching across small of back and in limbs, knees ache, better by walking about. Chronic suppuration and swelling of cervical glands with great weakness. Debility and weakness in back and lower limbs better walking about. Excoriation in folds of skin of neck.

Breasts - ***Cracked and sore nipples*** of nursing women. Pain in breast (right) on sneezing. Pain in right breast and down arm. ***Breast cancer***, pains like knives thrust into part. ***Nipple retracted.*** Hard, irregular tumor of left breast, glands in axilla enlarged and painful, cachectic appearance.

Chest - Chest raw, sore, burning. Pain from chest to left shoulde with numbness of arm, and palpitations. Thoracic or intercostal myalgia. Axillary glands tender and swollen. Excessive offensive sweat of axilla.

Constitutions - It produces atonic cachectic, degenerative conditions, hence suitable in old, easily tired, weak persons with great debility and emaciation. Emaciated, broken-down constitutions. Cancer and precancerous states. Cancerous diathesis.

Coughs - Dry, harsh cough. ***Loose cough, bloody or thick, yellow tenacious sputum.*** Loose cough, raises much mucus. Dry, harsh, rattling cough from tickling in larynx. Catarrhal cough of long standing. Cough with febrile symptoms in evening and night. Cough with debility in children. Cough with rawness of larynx. Cough with tingling and smarting in throat.

Ears - Ears red, thickened and covered with scales. Pain in right ear. Otorrhea, thick mucus discharge (fetid). Fissures behind ears, where ears connect with head. Membrana tympani purplish and bulging. Perforation of eardrum. ***Eustachian catarrh*** with high-pitched voice. Roaring in the ears like machinery. Tinnitus from catarrh of inner ear. Deafness from eustachian catarrh. Deafness after scarlet fever. Throat deafness. Thick, offensive, irritating, catarrhal and purulent discharges from external auditory meatus.

Eyes - Chronic inflammation of eyes. Dark greenish-yellow conjunctiva. Yellow eyes. Opacity of the cornea. Ophthalmia with thick mucus discharge. Scrofulous ophthalmia, with or without ulceration. Profuse secretion of tears, smarting and burning of eyes and lids. Lids agglutinated. Lids greatly swollen and excoriated. Large painful stye on left lid. Blepharitis. Conjunctivitis without discharge. Conjunctivitis with sensation of dryness and scratching.

Face - Thin, yellow, sunken face. Expression weary, dull, skin pale, or yellow-white. Erysipelatous eruption following flushes of heat. Tenacious mucus hangs in shreds from mouth. Epithelioma of face, nose and lips. Aphthae on lips with swelling of tongue. Comedones.

Female - Endometritis. Profuse menses, flowing ten days or more. Menorrhagia and metrorrhagia with fibroids. Congestive dysmenorrhea. Leucorrhea, worse after menses (Bov., Calc.). ***Thick, acrid, yellow, ropy leucorrhea***. Pruritus vulvae with profuse leucorrhea (Calc., Kreos., Sep.). Hot, watery, discharge from uterus. Fibroid tumors at menopause. Uterine hemorrhage. Uterine complaints better recumbent position. Removes the tendency to habitual adherent placenta. Erosion and excoriation of cervix. Inflammation of cervix, with heat and itching of vagina. Vagina sore during sex, bleeding afterwards.

Food - Poor appetite with constipation. ***Irritability after dinner.*** Indigestion from atony of the stomach, especially in elderly people. Bread or vegetables cause acidity, weakness, indigestion. ***Worse by excessive use of alcohol.***

Head - ***Frontal headache arising from catarrh.*** Headache from gastric difficulties. ***Sinusitis after coryza*** (Kali-bi.). Neuralgia of the scalp and neck. Dull, pressing frontal pain, especially connected with constipation. Eczema on forehead along the line of hair, worse after washing. Eczema of scalp with thick crusts.

Heart - Heavy beating of heart with dyspnea. Intermittent heartbeats. Heart agitated. Palpitations from a slowly progressing weakness. Palpitations with faintness. Palpitation; irregular, and at times laboured action of heart. Violent long-continued palpitation in morning. Pulse slow during the chill.

Kidneys - Dull aching in region of kidneys. ***Gleety discharge, thick, yellow.*** Mucus in urine. Difficult, painful urination. Suppression of urine. Incontinence. Catarrh of bladder, with thick, ropy mucous sediment in urine. Urine smells decomposed, putrid. Chronic cystitis. Symptoms of ulceration of bladder. Urine increased and of neutral reaction. High colored urine which deposits a cloudy sediment when standing. Constant desire to urinate.

Limbs - Rheumatic pains. Limbs tired, ache, feel weak, with coryza. Sharp, shifting pain, in right arm and leg, then left leg. Pain from right hip to knee while walking. Aching in sole of left foot, no relief from change of position. Irritable, indolent, atonic or scrofulous ulcers on the legs.

Liver - Cutting pain from liver to right scapula, worse lying on back or right side. Jaundice, with catarrh of stomach and duodenum. Jaundice from structural disease of liver. ***Liver cancer.*** Atrophy of liver. Torpor of the liver, with pale, scanty stools. Gallstones. Catarrhal inflammation of mucous lining of gall bladder and biliary ducts.

Lungs - Asthma and edema of lungs. Cancer of right lung. Laryngeal and bronchial catarrh, later stages. ***Bronchitis in old, exhausted persons with thick, yellow, tenacious, stringy expectoration***. Breathing difficult, worse lying on left side. Frequent fainting spells with cold sweat all over. Feels suffocating when lying on left side. Tuberculosis with emptiness in stomach, emaciation, loss of appetite. Bloody, or thick, yellow, tenacious.

Male - Gonorrhea, in second stage, discharge thick and yellow. Gleet, debility, copious, painless discharge. Debility after spermatorrhea. Hydrocele. Dragging in right groin to testicle, then to left testicle, then to left groin. Long lasting gonorrhea, with great moral and physical depression.

Modalities - Better dry weather. Better warm covering. Better from pressure. Better rest. Worse from inhaling air. Worse cold air. Worse dry winds. Worse open air. Worse at night. Worse slight bleeding. Worse washing. Worse touch. Worse old age. Worse motion. Skin symptoms are worse from warmth, washing. Catarrhal symptoms are worse from harsh, dry winds, out of doors. Worse abuse of wine. Worse abuse of drugs.

Mouth - Aphthae. ***Stomatitis during course of eruptive fevers.*** Stomatitis of nursing mothers or weakly children. ***Bitter taste.*** Peppery, flat taste in mouth. Excessive secretion of thick, tenacious mucus. Bleeding, painful cancerous growth or tumor on hard palate. Aphthae on the lips. Cancer of lips. Epithelial cancer of lip. Bleeding painful cancerous growths on hard palate.

Nose - Burning pain in nose. ***Thick, tenacious yellow-green mucus. Coryza watery, excoriating,*** burning, smarting and rawness. Sneezing, with fullness over eyes. ***Sinusitis after coryza*** (Kali-bi.). Post-nasal dripping. Constant discharge of thick white mucus, sinus headache. ***Thick, white or yellow, tenacious nasal discharge.*** Secretions so profuse as to be removed in long tenacious shreds or pieces. Ozaena, with bloody, purulent discharge. Ozaena, with ulceration of septum. Blows nose all the time. Tickling, like a hair in right nostril. Air feels cold in nose. Nosebleed with burning rawness, followed by itching. Nosebleed before menses.

Perspiration - Profuse, offensive sweat on genitals. Profuse cold sweat all over. Sweats during frequent sudden attacks of fainty spells. Tendency to profuse perspiration and unhealthy skin (Hep.).

Rectum - Contraction and spasms. Constipation alternating with diarrhea. No desire for stool. ***Obstinate constipation of pregnancy***. Constipation after purgatives. ***Constipation with a sinking feeling in stomach.*** Constipation from sluggish state of bowels. Raw smarting in the rectum during stools, remaining long afterwards. ***Constipation with hemorrhoids.*** Proctitis. Fistula of anus. Prolapsed, anus fissured. Fissures and excoriations of anus. Prolapse of rectum. Hemorrhoids, even slight bleeding exhausts. ***Fetid flatus.*** Noisy discharge of flatus. Exhaustion and fainting after stool. Ulceration of rectum, after bad cases of dysentery.

Skin - Jaundice, dark greenish-yellow color. Cancerous ulcers. Atonic ulcers, following removal of tumors. Lupus. Hot, dry skin, with fever. Burning heat and itching in skin. ***Erysipelatous rash on face, neck, palms, joints of fingers and wrist, with maddening, burning heat, later skin exfoliates.*** Nettle rash, hives, worse from scratching, worse at night. Scarlet raised nodular eruption. Infantile intertrigo. Eruptions like smallpox. ***Smallpox, all stages, itching tingling of the eruption.*** Smallpox with great redness, swelling and itching. Obstinate excoriations of skin. Yellowish looking vesicles, filled with a limpid fluid.

Sleep - Awakened by backache and dull pains in navel and hypogastric region. Restless sleep. Difficulty in awaking. Dreams wearisome.

Stomach - Belchings of sour fluid. Sore feeling in stomach more or less constant. Faintness at the stomach, sinking, gone feeling in stomach with loathing of food or as of a sharp lump in stomach. Atonic dyspepsia. Chronic gastritis. ***Weak digestion with debility.*** Acute, distressing cutting pains. Chronic gastric catarrh, ulceration. Painful epigastric tumors with pulsations. ***Stomach ulcers with emaciation.*** Marasmus. Ulcers and cancer. ***Stomach cancer with emaciation.*** Regurgitation of food by mouthful, without nausea. Vomits all she eats, except milk and water mixed.

Stools - Feces in form of hard balls coated over with yellowish, tough mucus. Slimy, tenacious discharges with tenesmus. Stools hard and knotty, of a gray or brown color. Scanty stools alternating with discharge of membranous casts. Stool light colored, soft, acrid, greenish. Stool lumpy, covered with yellow mucus. Greenish stools.

Temperature - Chills at night. Chill morning or evening. Chilliness, especially in back or thighs, with aching, pulse slow. Heat in flushes. Great heat of whole body. Constant dull burning pains all the evening. Gastric, bilious or typhoid forms of fever, with gastric disturbances, jaundice and great debility following. Heat alternating with chill. Influenza in cold, weak, debilitated persons.

Throat - Throat dry, raw, sore, smarting. Throat as if excoriated, on swallowing. Scraping in larynx. Uvula sore and relaxed. ***Hawking of yellow, thick mucus from posterior sinuses*** (Kali-bi.). Follicular pharyngitis. Ulcers in the throat, especially after mercury. ***Post-nasal dripping**, **waking from sleep.*** Cancerous ulcers. Goiter of puberty and pregnancy. Roughness in throat in morning on waking. Smarting and tingling in throat. Sore throat from gastric derangement. Sore throat, with increased mucus, with burning and rawness.

Tongue - Tongue raw, with dark red appearance and raised papillae. ***Tongue yellow, dirty.*** Tongue white, swollen, large, flabby, slimy. Tongue coated with thick white fur. Tongue coated with a yellow stripe. ***Tongue shows imprint of teeth*** (Merc.). Ulceration of tongue, fissures toward the edges. Tongue as if burned or scalded, later a vesicle forms on the tip. Tongue cancer. Tongue and lips parched, red and dry.

Vertigo - Feeling as if intoxicated.

Vision - Lack of accommodative power of eyes. Asthenopia. Sparks and light spots on closing eyes.

COMMENTS - Grimmer noted that Hydr. has been proven highly effective in liver cancer. Even in advanced cases it has been of great assistance in the relief of pain, permitting the patient to retain consciousness to the end without the need of narcotics or analgesics.

Affinity for stomach, liver and colon cancer (Cadm.). Skin adheres to the tumor, mottled, bluish. Burning pains, knife-like pains at the site of tumors, especially rectal tumors. Colon cancer with severe constipation and lumpy mucus in the stools. Blood and yellow, stringy mucus in the stool with a knife-like cutting pain in the rectum every time they have a bowel movement.

Cancer at the emaciation stage, the last stages of cancer. Loss of appetite with severe constipation. Tonic can revive appetite (Alf.). ***Cachexia, emaciation*** associated with chronic disease with yellowish tinge to the skin and sunken features. Weakness and faintness spells with sudden attacks of loss of energy and weakness. Cold sweats. Excessive sweat, especially of the armpits or genitals.

Offensive ulcers, chancroids, fissures. Ulcerations of the mucus membranes, especially the stomach. Malignant ulcers, with vomiting of ropy, sticky mucus. Useful in pre-cancerous stage, a period of undefined ill-health without any discernible new growth. Never well since cancer, emaciated and weak. Used in both potency and tincture for cancer treatment, commonly used as a supportive remedy in addition to primary treatment.

Yellow or white, tough and stringy catarrh of almost all mucous surfaces, nasal catarrh, pharyngeal, bronchial, gastric, duodenal intestinal, urethral (gonorrhea, gleet), vaginal.

Sinusitis with yellow, thick, stringy, lumpy mucus. Chronic lung disease, coughing up thick, yellow globs. Asthmatic states. Chronic dry, harsh, rattling coughs. Chronic weakness and obstruction.

Dull, heavy, sodden-looking facial expression, yellow-white in color. Large, flabby and slimy-looking tongue, bluish-white under the fur, which is yellow, slimy and sticky. Tongue is indented by the teeth.

Little appetite. Weak digestion of bread and vegetables. Sour, putrid belchings. Fullness and weight at stomach. Characteristic empty, aching "gone" feeling, worse after a meal. Jaundice and liver enlargement. Gall-bladder attacks. Bitter taste in the mouth.

Bowel movements are either infrequent and constipated or frequent with loose, soft, light-colored stools. Torpor of the bowels, stools lumpy, covered with yellowish, tough mucus. Continual pain in the head and a bad taste in the mouth with constipation. Severe backache, wakes in the night, worse damp weather.

Hard, indurated cancer of the breast or cervix (Con.), with yellow, stringy mucus. Scirrhus of uterus or breasts. Breast abscesses, or abscessed glands. Sore mouth nursing-women, sore nipples. Vaginitis with yellow, stringy discharge. Metrorrhagia, leucorrhea. Pruritus vulva. Retained placentas.

Garth Wilkinson found it an excellent remedy for smallpox taken externally and topically. Eczema, drying into crusts and burning like fire, has been cured with an application of one part Hydr. tincture to nine parts of glycerine. The burning was removed.

Clarke once saw a woman, 60, who had been given Hydr., 5 drops of tincture in water three times a day. After a week she developed a scarlet rash, raised and nodular, exceedingly irritable, especially at night. It was on every part of the body except the face and was worse on her buttocks and elbows. It remained a week. At the same time, the patient became very ill with sickness and general digestive disorder.

Weiss gave a woman, 31, who had adherent placenta in several confinements in succession, Hydr. 3x three drops daily from the fourth month during her last three pregnancies.

Each terminated without adherent placenta. Four other cases of habitual adherent placenta were successfully treated in the same way.

Clifton noted that the dyspepsia occurred frequently in tubercular families and in cases of actual tuberculosis, the loss of appetite and "goneness" being especially prominent. He found that the tincture and lower potencies worked best in dyspepsia, while the higher potencies were better in catarrh of nose and fauces.

RELATIONS - ***Antidote:*** Sulph. Useful after too much Chlorate of Potash for sore throat. ***Compare:*** (1) Hydr-m., Xanrhi., Kali-bi., Con., Ars-i., Phyt., Aster., Stann., Puls. (2) Gali. - cancer of the tongue. (3) Manz. - diarrhea, gonorrhea, gleet, leucorrhea, catarrhal conditions. (4) Hydrastine sulphate 1x - hemorrhage of bowels in typhoid. (5) Marr. - a stimulant to mucous membranes, especially laryngeal and bronchial, chronic bronchitis, dyspepsia and hepatic disorders, colds and coughs.

REFERENCES - Boericke. Clarke. Grimmer. Murphy. Phatak.

HYDRAZINUM SULPHURICUM

(Hydrazine Sulphate)

PHARMACY - hydr-s. Hydrazinum sulphuricum. Hydrazine sulphate. ***Historical dose:*** Tincture and all potencies.

CLINICAL - ***Anorexia.*** Arrhythmias. ***Cachexia. Cancer. Emaciation.*** Hodgkin's, disease. Hypoglycemia. Hypotension. ***Liver disorders.*** Lymphoma. Melanoma. Nausea. Neuritis. ***Numbness***. Tumors. Vertigo. Vomiting. ***Weakness.*** Weight, loss.

HOMEOPATHIC - Dr. Joseph Gold, in 1968, wrote a paper for the Oncology Journal called "A proposed treatment of cancer by inhibition of gluconeogenesis" in which he noted that Hydr-s., dramatically reverses ***cachexia***, the wasting-away process that kills many cancer patients.

"This inexpensive chemical, with little or no side effects, also has a clinically documented anti-tumor action. It causes malignant tumors to stop growing, to reduce in size, and, in some cases, to disappear.

"A number of cancer patients diagnosed as terminal have experienced tumor stabilization and remission through hydrazine sulfate therapy. About half of all patients who take hydrazine sulfate experience weight gain, restored appetite, extended survival time, and a significant reduction in pain and suffering.

"Many patients report an increase in vigor and strength and the disappearance of symptoms of the disease, along with feelings of well-being and optimism.

"The common types of cancer most frequently reported to benefit from hydrazine sulfate therapy are recto-colon cancer, ovarian cancer, prostatic cancer, lung cancer, Hodgkin's disease and other lymphomas, thyroid cancer, melanoma, and breast cancer. Some rare types of cancer also benefit.

"Hydrazine sulfate is known to produce excitement, lethargy, convulsions, hypotension, arrhythmias, fatty changes in the liver, hypoglycemia and weight loss.

"Toxicity. If inappropriately high doses of hydrazine sulphate are taken, numbness, nausea, vomiting, drowsiness and nerve inflammation may occur. Side effects may include nausea, some pruritus, dizziness due to low blood sugar, or peripheral neuritis.

"The following toxic symptoms have been reported: nausea, vomiting, anorexia, abnormal sensations affecting both upper and lower limbs, impaired fine motor functions (writing), confusion, abnormal electromyograms."

COMMENTS - In one case, a sixty-two-year-old woman with widely disseminated cancer of the cervix, in a very debilitated condition, was put on Hydr-s.

After one week, a secondary tumor the size of an orange had completely disappeared, much to the amazement of the woman's doctors, and her neck nodes had become markedly smaller.

After three weeks on the therapy, the patient had gained weight and was active and in good spirits. The woman was discharged from the hospital a short time later.

RELATIONS - ***Compare:*** (1) Cachexia - Alf., Cadm-s., Ars., Hydr.

REFERENCES - Gold. Murphy.

HYDROBROMICUM ACIDUM

(Hydrobromic Acid)

PHARMACY - hydrobr-ac. Hydrobromicum acidum. Hydrobromic acid. ***Historical dose:*** All potencies.

CLINICAL - Tinnitus. Vertigo.

HOMEOPATHIC - Seems to have a specific effect on the inferior cervical ganglion increasing the action of the sympathetic nerves, promoting vaso-constriction. Relieves headache, tinnitus and vertigo, especially in vaso-motor stomach disturbance.

Dry and puckering throat. Constriction in pharynx and chest. Waves of heat over face and neck. Pulsating tinnitus with great nervous irritability. Vertigo with palpitations, arms heavy, seemed as if parts did not belong to him.

REFERENCES - Boericke.

HYDROCOTYLE ASIATICA

(Gotu Kola)

PHARMACY - hydrc. Hydrocotyle asiatica. Gotu kola. Indian pennywort. Centella asiatica. N. O. Umbelliferae. India and South Africa. Tincture of whole fresh plant. ***Historical dose:*** Tincture and all potencies.

CLINICAL - Acne rosacea. Constipation. Elephantiasis, arabum. Favus. Gangrene, amputation. Gonorrhea. Gout. Ichthyosis. ***Leprosy.*** Leucorrhea. Liver, contraction. ***Lupus.*** Neuralgia orbitalis. Skin disorders. Syphilis. Uterus, follicular inflammation. Vagina, pruritus.

HERBAL - Hydrc. has been long known as an Indian remedy. Gotu Kola is known as Indian Pennywort. It produces hypertrophy and induration of connective tissue. Curative in disorders that exhibit interstitial inflammation and cellular proliferation in any part. Hypertrophy and induration of connective tissue. Boileau was the first to use it as a remedy in leprosy.

HOMEOPATHIC - Hydrc. has a considerable reputation in ***leprosy and lupus***, when there is no ulceration. Elephantiasis. Excessive thickening of skin and marked exfoliation of skin.

Copper colored eruptions in various places.

Intolerable itching especially of soles, vagina. Very copious perspiration. Ulceration of the womb. Pains of cervical cancer. Difficulty in maintaining an upright posture.

MIND - Weak concentration. Forgetful. Poor memory. Indifference. Gloomy thoughts, inclination for solitude. Misanthropy. Gaiety, loquacity.

Abdomen - Borborygmi in different parts. Flatus. Heat in hypogastrium. ***Wind colic.*** Rumbling in different parts. Violent contractions of intestines. Pain, every five minutes, worse transverse colon. Constriction. Sensation as if all the organs were in motion.

Back - Renewal of old rheumatic pains in left rhomboid, worse pressure. Bruised pain in loins. Obstruction in region of kidneys with heaviness. Swelling of cervical glands.

Chest - Pustules on chest.

Ears - Pain in left internal meatus. Throbbing in right ear, ringing in left with stoppage. Confused noise in left, blowing sound.

Eyes - Eyes look unsteady. Injection of palpebral conjunctiva. Pricking in eyes. Vision dim, dazzling. Tumours of eyelids. Epithelioma.

Face - Intoxicated expression. Intermittent pain in left cheekbone and about orbits. ***Neuralgic affections of supra and infra-orbital nerves.*** Ulcer irregular and livid. Papular eruption. ***Copper colored eruption on face***. Large tubercle on right alae nasi. Tubercles, as large as lentils, near root of nose at both sides and painless.

Female - Menses too early. ***Profuse leucorrhea.*** Pruritus of vagina. Shooting and itching in vagina. Vulva, vagina and cervix red. ***Heat and redness of vagina and vulva.*** Dull pain in ovarian region. Uterus feels heavy. Pain in whole uterus, left side. Severe labor-like pain in uterus and appendages. ***Granular ulceration of womb***. Partly fungus, partly granular ulcer on upper lip of neck of uterus, with profuse leucorrhea.

Food - Loathing of food. Anorexia, then strong appetite. Aversion to tobacco smoking.

Head - Headache with general lassitude and prostration. Congestion of blood to the head, heaviness. Painful drawing in almost all cranial nerves. Neuralgic pain in external frontal nerve. Intense pain with some swelling in posterior part of skull. Occiput acutely sensitive to touch. Constriction of back part of skull and scalp. Tinea favosa.

Heart - Cardiac spasm. Stenosis of aorta. Constriction of heart with quiet and regular pulse or with a few separate beats in certain arteries or with hot flushes in different parts of the face. Irregular beating of heart. Pulse stronger and fuller.

Kidneys - Slight formication in kidney. Constriction of bladder. Inflammation, irritation of neck of bladder. Irritation of urethra. Frequent desire to urinate, urine increased. Urine becomes brown on cooling. Urine turbid without sediment.

Limbs - Bruised feeling in the muscles. Rheumatic disorders. Gout with very severe paroxysms. Contractions of forearms and legs. Irresistible inclination to stretch. Pain in all joints, muscles, worse left. Sensations as if hot water ran through marrow of bones. Yellowish spots on legs. ***Insupportable itching of soles of feet.*** Back of right foot was covered with small indurations, having a large thick crust.

Liver - Cirrhosis of liver. Pain in upper part of liver. Obstruction in hepatic region.

Lungs - Pricking in vicinity of glottis. Dryness of windpipe of ventricles of larynx. Oppression of chest, which suddenly ceases and then returns at longer or shorter intervals. Breath short. Speaking soon fatigues. Irritation of air-passages. Difficult expectoration of bronchial mucus.

Male - Drawing in spermatic cords, worse left. Feeling of weight in prostate gland. ***Acute and secondary gonorrhea.*** Suppressed gonorrhea. Scrotum relaxed. Indifference to intercourse. Impotence.

Mouth - Stomatitis aphthosa. Syphilitic patches in mouth. Whitish spots on left upper and under sides of tongue. Impediment in speech. Redness of velum palati with pain on swallowing, worse by food. Hyperemia of mucus membrane. Saliva increased. Insipid or bitter taste, unpleasant in morning.

Nose - Dry coryza. Stoppage of nose. Swelling of nose. Tickling, worse left nostril. Feeling as before bleeding. Bleeding. Lupus excedens of nose.

Perspiration - Profuse sweat.

Rectum - Weight in rectum. ***Constipation.*** Burning, itching in anus. Ineffectual desire for stool. Stools dry, dark, increased, easier.

Skin - Dry eruptions. Erysipelatous redness. ***Pemphigus benignus.*** Eczema. Copper-colored eruptions in various places. ***Great thickening of epidermoid layer and exfoliation of scales.*** Psoriasis on trunk and limbs, palms and soles. ***Intolerable itching.*** Syphilitic disorders. ***Acne***. Leprosy. ***Elephantiasis*** (Ars.). Lupus non-exedens. Pustules. Circular spots with dry scaly edges. Yellowish spots. Pricking on different parts.

Sleep - Yawing and stretching. Sleepiness in the daytime. Heavy, dreamless sleep. Persistent dreaming.

Stomach - Anxiety in region of stomach. Belchings frequent, acid. Swelling of stomach. ***Cramping pain in stomach, without nausea.*** Contraction, cramp like pain. Sensation as if gases collected into a ball. Heat in stomach region spreading out like a bar. Nausea.

Temperature - Shivering in afternoon. Cold hands and feet with general condition resembling precursory stage of fever without alteration of pulse. Febrile movements. Heat of skin.

Throat - Voice weak. Tonsils red. Esophagus is dry and rough. Burning and pricking in esophagus and pharynx. Disorder of constrictor muscles of pharynx.

Vertigo - Vertigo with torpor. Vertigo with congestion and heaviness.

COMMENTS - The skin and the female generative organs are the chief seats of the drug's action, though the liver, the nerves and the mucus membranes are also powerfully acted upon.

Skin disorders including acne, eczema, pemphigus, lupus, copper-colored eruptions, papular eruptions on face and intolerable itching in various places. Granular ulceration. Gouty and rheumatic disorders. Bruised feeling in all the muscles. Affections of the trigeminus nerve.

Aphthous and syphilitic stomatitis. Irritation of the neck of the bladder increased secretion of urine. Heat and itching in vagina. Weight in uterus. Weight in the ***"male uterus,"*** the prostate gland.

A patient who was taking Hydrc. for eczema with advantage complained of persistent dreaming all the time he was asleep and an unpleasant mouth on waking in the morning.

Auduit cured the case of a girl, 20, weak and sickly-looking, who was troubled with glandular swellings since childhood, and for eight years had lupus excedens of nose. Her mother had a coppery eruption on her face.

On the right of her nose was a button the size of a sixpence covered with a thick crust covering yellow pus mixed with blood. Margins were irregular and livid. Five other buttons the size of lentils were near the root of the nose on both sides.

Hydrc. was given in 6c, 3c, tincture and the 18c potencies in succession with intermissions and completely cured in five months.

RELATIONS - ***Compare:*** (1) Elaesis - South American Palm - scleroderma, elephantiasis, leprosy, skin thickened, itching and hardened. Anesthesia. (2) Hura, or Trychnos Gaultheriana - bites of serpents, ulcers and cutaneous disorders generally. Hoang-na. (3) Chaulomoogra oil, Hydr., Ars., Aur., Sep.

REFERENCES - Boericke. Clarke. Phatak.

HYDROCYANICUM ACIDUM

(Prussic Acid)

PHARMACY - hydr-ac. Hydrocyanicum acidum. Prussic acid. Dilutions. ***Historical dose:*** All potencies.

CLINICAL - Angina pectoris. Anorexia. Asthma. Catalepsy. Cholera, asiatica. Colic. ***Collapse.*** Coma. ***Convulsions.*** Cyanosis. Delirium. Dyspepsia. Epilepsy. Hemiplegia. Hiccoughs. Labor, pains. Narcolepsy. Nausea. Paralysis. Stings. Stomach, catarrh. Strokes. Sun-stroke. Tetanus. Uremic, convulsions. Vomiting. Whooping cough.

HOMEOPATHIC - The pathogenesis of Hydr-ac. is mainly composed of symptoms observed in poisoning cases and those clinically verified, but it has also been proved by Joerg and his pupils.

Hydr-ac. is one of the deadliest and most rapidly acting of poisons. Hence its applicability in cases of critical intensity, such as the collapse stage of cholera, when it supervenes on sudden cessation of all discharges, convulsions during severe attacks of illness.

Convulsions and paralysis are the leading keynotes of the medicine's action. In the convulsions, the body is stiffened and thrown back, cramp in nape of neck.

Paroxysmal breathing, jaws set, foaming at mouth, face flushed, bluish tint. Lightning like jerks from head to feet.

Coldness is a strong feature with the remedy, marble coldness within and without. ***Blue tinge of the skin*** is also characteristic. Sudden effects, spasms, strokes. Collapse (Ars., Verat.), due to a pulmonary condition. Spasmodic constriction in larynx, feeling of suffocation, pain and tightness in chest, palpitation, pulse weak, irregular. Cyanosis.

Hysterical and epileptic convulsions. Epileptic attacks preceded by nausea and vomiting or water brash. ***Sinking sensation at the epigastrium.*** Evacuations cease suddenly, sinks down unconscious. Cholera. Intestinal cramps and colics. Tetanus, narcolepsy. Prolonged faints. Catalepsy. Lack of reaction.

MIND - Concentration difficult. ***Confusion, better open air.*** Senses acute. Speech incoherent. Inability to think. Anxious feeling and fretfulness. She asks no questions and returns no answers.

Fear of imaginary troubles. Fear of death. Fear of house falling. Fear of horses, cars. Fear of crossing the street, even when the vehicle is at a considerable distance.

Gestures, involuntary motions of hands. Insanity from excessive excitement. Loud involuntary screams, just before the convulsions. ***At times is forced to scream out suddenly, she knows not why.*** Wild delirium. Laughing, loudly.

Frequently rises in bed, ***gazes vacantly about for a minute***, then throws herself forcibly upon pillow, or flings herself from one side to the other. Seems to notice no person, unless they interfere with her plans. Unconscious.

Abdomen - Coldness of abdomen alternating with burning. Cold feeling in abdomen with sharp pains. Burning from navel to esophagus. ***Enteralgia with distension of abdomen.*** Region of navel sensitive to touch, and upon deep pressure a sensation as from a resistant body. Abdominal muscles firmly contracted and hard as a board. Yellow or brownish spots on abdomen.

Back - Muscles of the dorsal region are contracted.

Chest - Angina pectoris. Torturing pain in chest. Tightness in chest, sensation of suffocation. Brownish spots on chest and abdomen.

Cough - Dry, spasmodic, suffocative cough. Dry tickling cough at night. ***Dry, tickling cough in consumptives.*** Whooping cough with convulsions. Violent paroxysms, or frequent cough excited by a pricking sensation, which begins in larynx. Coughing with much rattling of mucus.

Ears - Roaring and deafness in ears.

Eyes - Distorted and half open eyes. Protrusion of eyes. Paralysis of lids. ***Eyes turned towards right and upwards, followed by general spasms.*** Eyeballs fixed. Pupils motionless or dilated. Dim vision gauze before eyes.

Face - Pale or bluish, looks old. Sallow and gray complexion. Lips pale or bluish. Jaws clenched in rigid spasm. Frightful contortion of muscles. Froths at mouth. Distorted, bloated and bluish face.

Food - Loss of appetite from nervous exhaustion, the result of overwork and anxiety. Anorexia. ***Drinks rumble through throat and stomach***. Absence of thirst, with heat of whole body, or violent thirst. Can drink during epileptiform attacks, but can't eat.

Head - Headaches with blindness. Headaches with protruded, half open eyes. Violent stupefying headache. Confusion of head. ***Intense cerebral congestion,*** preceded by vertigo, weight and great pain in back of head. Brain feels on fire. ***As if a cloud were going over his brain*** in a case of sunstroke. Supra-orbital neuralgia with flushing on same side of face. ***Sudden and desperate cases of cerebrospinal meningitis.*** Violent pressure in occiput and forehead, worse right side.

Heart - Cardiac asthma. Angina pectoris with feeling of suffocation and torturing pains in chest. Angina pectoris, severe pain (Ox-ac., Spig.). ***Clutches at the heart as if in distress.*** Irregular, feeble beating of heart. Violent palpitations. Heart failure, compression at heart. Blood vessels distended, writhing in them. Occasionally utters a groan or a sigh, and ***presses hand forcibly over region of heart***, as if suffering pain there. ***Pulse, failing, weak, irregular.*** Pulse unequal with occasional strong beats.

Kidneys - Retention of urine. ***Uremia with diminished action of heart.*** Copious emission of watery urine. Involuntary urination.

Limbs - Cold limbs. Hands icy cold. Languor and weakness of limbs. Loss of sensation in limbs, with stiffness of limbs. Paralysis first of lower, then of upper limbs. ***Varicose ulcers.*** Staggering and trembling.

Lungs - ***Asphyxia.*** Breathing slow, rattling, irregular, gasping. Noisy and agitated breathing. Asphyxia. Dry, spasmodic, suffocative cough. ***Asthma with choking, contraction of throat.*** Asthma, with with puffy face and feeble action of heart, or heart's action may be violent. Convulsions with whooping cough. ***Paralysis of lungs*** (Queb.). Arrest of breathing from stitches in larynx. Hurried and labored breathing, during severe spasms of all muscles, worse at night, on falling asleep. Feeling of suffocation during torturing pains in chest. Marked cyanosis, venously congested lung. Threatened pulmonary apoplexy.

Modalities - Worse from full moon. Worse suppressions. Worse storms. Indigestion, which is worse after eating. Headache is worse at night. Vertigo worse open air.

Mouth - Froth at mouth, forming large bubbles. Salivation. Loss of speech. Dry mouth. Distortion of corners of mouth. Pus, metallic, astringent taste. Taste acrid, sweet or fetid. Grinding of teeth during convulsions.

Nose - Dryness of nose. Discharge of greenish brown looking fetid pieces of hardened mucus, with stinging high up in nose. Enlarged, bluish wings of nose. Increased secretion of saliva.

Perspiration - Body covered with sweat.

Rectum - Cholera. ***Involuntary stools with hiccough and great prostration.*** Involuntary stool in bed. Sudden cessation of all discharges. Last stage of Asiatic cholera, when diarrhea has ceased and vomiting has decreased, when there is anguish with pressure on chest, and the patient becomes cold, with gradual extinction of pulse.

Skin - Bluish eruptions. Bad cases of smallpox. Scarlet fever, the eruption is dark colored and soon becomes livid. Paleness with a bluish tinge. Dryness. Itching. Formication. Erythema.

Sleep - Drowsiness. Yawning with shivering. Coma vigil. Irresistible drowsiness. Lies like one dead. Lies with head fixed and thrown backwards, and legs fixed and rigid. Lies in an apparently unconscious state, limbs and jaws rigid, forearms fixed on arms, which are firmly pressed on side. Prolonged sleeplessness or very heavy sleep. Vivid incoherent dreams.

Stomach - Acidity and heartburn. ***Stomach pain***, worse when stomach is empty. ***Drinks, rumbles through throat and stomach.*** Burning from navel to esophagus, chronic dyspepsia. ***Great sinking at pit of stomach***. Pulsative pain in precordial region. Intense pain in stomach and intestines, with much flatulence. ***Dyspepsia*** from chronic inflammation of stomach and bowels. Vomiting of a black fluid.

Temperature - Icy coldness, especially hands. General coldness with heat in head. ***Coldness within and without, like marble.*** Frequent hot flushes at menopause. ***Heat in bed with coldness of limbs.*** Heat and sweat over whole body.

Throat - ***Noisy swallowing drink rumbles through throat and stomach.*** Spasms or paralysis of esophagus. Scraping sensation in throat, followed by secretion of mucus in bronchia. Swollen sensation. Burning and scraping. Tickling and scraping in larynx and bronchial tubes with expectoration of yellowish or whitish mucus.

Tongue - Tongue cold. Tongue paralyzed and protruded. Tongue coated white. Tongue feels cold and burns at tip. Tongue lame, stiff.

Vertigo - Vertigo with feeling of intoxication. Vertigo with frequent headaches, stupefaction and falling down. Sudden feeling as if everything about him moved slowly. Dizzy without reeling. Vertigo during headache. Cloudiness of senses, objects seem to move. Vertigo from insufficiency of arterial contraction.

COMMENTS - A. H. Croucher cured a boy, 3 1/2, of convulsions with Hydr-ac. The first attack occurred six months previously. His father's sister had died of epilepsy.

Before the fits came on he could walk well, but could not afterwards. The fits occurred at intervals of about three weeks when a succession of them occurred, each lasting about five minutes during two or three days. During the intervals between the fits he would generally scream.

In the morning on awaking, the patient cried out, then convulsions occurred, body and limbs convulsed, eyelids twitched but remained open, eyeballs turned up and to right. Seemed quite unconscious.

Hydr-ac. 2x, one drop three times a day increased afterwards to two drops and continued for a fortnight. No more convulsions, but three months later a rash developed all over him.

The characteristic blue tint of Hydr-ac. is apparent after death in some poisoning cases. Livid spots on limbs, nails violet. In one case there was a brilliant violent hue all over. The heat is greatly disturbed, blueness and coldness of surface. Marble coldness within and without.

It acts on the medulla and through the vagus nerve on heart and respiration. Irregular and gasping breathing. Dry tearing cough, worse at night. Cough in tuberculosis. The pulse is feeble, imperceptible. The patient clutches at the heart as if in distress. Profound prostration.

Persistent and tonic tetanic spasm, without any reflex excitability (unlike Nux-v.). Paralysis attacks first the lower, then the upper limbs. Acts powerfully on the muscles of face, jaws and back. Pronounced risus sardonicus. Lividity, frothing.

Disturbed digestion, worse after eating. Drinks roll audibly into the stomach. It cured a boy, 4, of a fever with the symptom: "when swallowing a teaspoonful of liquid it sounds like water rolling into an empty barrel."

Headache, worse at night and vertigo, worse in the open air. In a case of sunstroke, Cash removed the symptom "Feels as if a cloud were going over his brain."

RELATIONS - ***Antidoted by:*** Camph., Coff., Ip., Nux-v., Op., Verat. ***Compare:*** (1) Camph. - cholera, coldness, Helod. - coldness. (2) Cic. - spinal cord, cramp in nape. (3) Con. - paralysis spreading from below upward. (4) Oena. - epilepsy. (5) Lauro. - dry tickling cough, Lauro. has also a cough with jelly-like sputa dotted with bloody points. (6) Lach., Tab. (asphyxia), Hell. (7) Solania - paralysis of lungs and heart. (8) Nux-v. - tetanus, but of different type.

REFERENCES - Boericke. Clarke. Phatak.

HYDROGEN

(The Element)

PHARMACY - hydrog. Hydrogen. The element. ***Historical dose:*** All potencies.

CLINICAL - Acidosis. Alkalosis. Aphthae. Backaches. Congenital deformities. Cystitis. Diarrhea. Fainting. Fistula. Headaches. Hemorrhoids. Insomnia. Nevi. Rash. Sprains. Stomach, pains. Ulcers. Weakness.

HOMEOPATHIC - Hydrogen was the first element to be formed. This primordial element begins Mendeleev's Periodic Table. It has a positively-charged proton as its nucleus and a negatively-charged electron-cloud around it.

Hydrogen was proved by Jeremy Sherr and his team of provers in England. They used modern hydrogen with its increased tritium content as it is now.

Symptoms included sudden manifestations. Sensation of heat on waking. Excessive weakness, fainting weakness, with nausea. Tremulous weakness. Headache with sensation of heat. Burning, cutting, stinging, stitching pains. Fever with thirst.

Aphthae and profuse saliva; dry mouth and throat. Desire and inclination to lie down. Lassitude after eating. Ulcers, fistula, nevi. Accidents and sprains. Symptoms on one side, better left side. Annual periodicity.

MIND - Difficult concentration. Mistakes in speaking, spelling, writing. Mistakes the left and right sides. Trouble explaining the mental state. Absent-minded in morning, evening. Confused. Disjointed and jumbled thoughts. Tendency to lose things, accident prone. Hurry, industrious. Interested in esoteric subjects. Averse to studying.

Ailments during full moon. Ailments from quarrels. Causeless anger. Indisposed to talk when angry. Throws things away when angry. Feels grubby. Difficulty coping with stress.

Tendency to panic, nervous apprehension. Anxiety about money and fear of poverty. Desire to be alone. Aversion to being touched. Bites fingers. Ennui. Irresolution about what to do with life. Blames self. Confusion about identity, especially sexual.

Emotional confusion. Strong alternation of moods. Vulnerable, weepy. Love, lovesick, overflowing love for humanity. Sighing. Sympathetic. Everything seems ludicrous. Laughed at serious things. Loquacious. Talking to self. Singing. Suspicion, paranoia. Angry, irritable. Causeless anger, tendency to throw things, to not talk. Ailments from quarrels.

Depression, especially during full moon. Silent, morose, introverted. Self-pity. Insecurity. Thoughts of death. Thoughts of dead bodies. Suicidal tendency. Despair, hopelessness. Apathetic, bored. Resignation. Distant and detached, indifferent to loved ones, emotionally numb. Religious tendency. Near-death experiences.

Altered perception. Sense of unreality, of separation from the world, detached (Granit-m.). Spacey feeling. Sensation of universal consciousness and enlightenment.

Delusion body is enlarged. Delusion he is diminished, smaller than normal. Delusion he is dirty. Delusion he is despised. Delusion he is detached (Granit.). Delusion there is a division between himself and others. Delusion as if being pulled downward. Delusion has insects on back of head. Delusion that he is persecuted. Delusion fancied body was too small for soul or that it was separated from soul.

Abdomen - Sunken feeling. Achy pain in the right iliac in the late morning. Sharp pain, left lower abdomen, feels like movement of gas. Stabbing pain in right, lower abdomen, groin. Pain in the abdomen after stool, better bending double. Aversion to tight clothing around waist with nausea.

Back - Coldness in back. Sensation of dry, radiating heat at the sacrum through the night. Itching on back below scapula on coughing. Tiredness in back with aching. Weakness in back. Twinges of pain across back. Stabbing pains. Sharp neuralgic pain shooting from left shoulder near neck, like an electric shock. Aching and weakness in lower and mid-back. Aching pain in sacrum making him want to rock backwards and forwards. Lumbar pain, better hot bath. Aching pain, right lower inside angle of scapula. Deep, bruised pain between left scapula and vertebral column. ***Back pain on motion.*** Backache, better lying on the painful side. Tension of cervical region during headache.

Breasts - Breasts enlarged. Shooting pain in the right nipple.

Chest - Constriction on waking, with wheezing. ***Tickling in chest.*** Feeling of anxiety in chest. Hard pain in the chest like someone was squeezing it. ***Tickling behind sternum.*** Short, sharp pains lower end of sternum. Sensation of dryness.

Coughs - Coughs on waking. Cough worse in morning, better through the day and worse at night. Middle of the night, cough with catarrh at back of throat, better after a drink. Deep barking cough, with no expectoration, compelled by tickling in throat. Barking cough with lachrymation and nose running with clear fluid. Cough with wheezing, has to lean forward. Dry tickling cough from behind the sternum, aggravated by smoking and drinking. Cough from swollen sensation in throat. Cough relieves diarrhea, swallowing.

Dreams - Confused, unremembered dreams. Frightening dreams. Dreams of death. Dreams of dead people. Dreams of crimes. Dreams of murder. Dreams of suffering animals. Dreams of children. Dreams of being busy. Dreams of high places. Dreams of journey by car. Dreams of escape. Amorous dreams. Dreams of loved ones dying. Dreams of their children. Dreams that she was pregnant. Headache in the dream and woke up with a headache.

Ears - Blocked sensation in ears, worse swallowing. Eustachian tube blocked, like in an airplane. Aching in right ear, with a cold sensation as if blowing on it. Deep aching pain in right ear. Sharp inward stabbing pains in left ear, followed by ringing in ear. Sharp pain in left ear after waking. Left sided earache coming in waves. Pulsing in ears. Ringing noise, with headache. Very conscious of sounds and noises. Right ear feels cold. Ears felt rough and itchy. Formication sensation. Itching behind ears and in left external meatus on waking.

Eyes - Lachrymation, pain in nose. Stinging pain. Pain, as from sand. Bloodshot and watery. Watery eyes during cough, after yawning. Sensation as if grit in left eye at night. Prickly and tired. Eyes feel heavy. Green-yellow crust around left eye on waking. Blinking a lot. Left eye twitches. Desire to close eyes with headache. Swelling of upper eyelids. Bright red pustule on rim of right upper lid with sticking, pricking pain, worse by blinking. Sharp pain above left eye. Ecchymosis. Eyesight deteriorated. Photophobia.

Face - Face looks pale and drawn with black circles under eyes and chin down. Looks older. Flushed, hot face with red cheeks, weakness. Flushed face with headache after anger. Red spots on cheeks. Dry, scaly skin under chin. Very rough, chapped lips. Crack appeared in corner of mouth, left side. Skin flaking on waking. Pimples right side of chin. Aching facial bones with a cold. Twinge in jaw joint, worse motion and opening mouth. Aching, morning on waking, especially the teeth. Stiffness and pain right jaw. Left side tender and aches. Sensation of coldness. Numbness of lips. ***Numbness, tingling lips, worse on left***, as if anesthetized. Tingling in left side. Growth of hair on upper lip.

Female - Menses, three days earlier. Menses up to two weeks late with slow onset of intermittent bleeding. ***Menses, clotted, copious.*** Menses, intermittent, commence on waking. Black blood to begin with, later in the day it became more red with dark clots. Menses, heavier or lighter than usual, starts and stops with more clotting. Pain between ovaries, extending to just above the pubic bone. High sexual energy. Itching of genitalia, better scratching. Brown vaginal discharge.

Food - Appetite increased. Hungry as if nothing will fill the emptiness in stomach, better eating bread. Appetite diminished, with weight loss. Complete loss of appetite with weeping. ***Very thirsty for cold drinks***. Thirstlessness during headache. ***Aversion to spices***, highly seasoned food. Aversion to coffee, tea. Aversion to tobacco. Aversion to hot drinks and hot food. ***Craving***

for spicy foods. Desires cold drinks. Desires carbonated drinks. Desires pineapple, sweets, alcohol. Desires to smoke tobacco. Better from warm drinks. ***Nauseous after a cup of tea***. Worse smell of garlic, causes nausea. Worse tea. Worse smell of vinegar.

Hands - Hands feel icy cold to touch. Cold sweat on palms with apprehension. Warm, glowing hands on waking. Fingers of left hand feel cold and numb. Fingernails swollen, hot, very sensitive to touch, suppurating yellow water or pus under the skin.

Head - Head feels hazy, unpleasant, too heavy for the neck. Band around the skull. Tenderness at the base of the skull. Dull ache in vertex and behind eyes. Attack like a stroke, worse moving head. Slight humming in head. Tingly sensation over head and face with vertigo. ***Formication, crawling like insects.*** Formication which moves about on the scalp. Sensation as if something is crawling on head, on the back of the head. Sweating on forehead. Profuse perspiration in bed at night, soaking the pillow. Hair sticky after washing.

Headaches - Headache better talking, better writing. Headache, worse sudden movement, reading, traveling in a car. Frontal headache. ***Aching deep in brain.*** Pain in small spot. ***Throbbing headache extending to root of nose.*** Constant piercing pain in the center of the skull. Skull bones aching. Headache with a feeling of a line across the top of the head from side to side. Pain in spots that can be covered by a finger. Burning, throbbing pain, left side of head and face. Sharp, piercing pains. Headache over right eyebrow. Headache all day before period, left side. Headache prevents work, better from a short nap.

Heart - Conscious of heartbeat. Feeling of anxiety. Single thump in the heart. Palpitations, pounding. Palpitations while lying on left side, with a sensation of buzzing as if nerves firing in the heart. Thudding palpitations, frightened him, thought he was having a heart attack. On climbing the stairs, three or four heavy beats of the heart with stiffness of the legs.

Kidneys - Bladder feels full, but little passes. After just one cup of tea at breakfast, urination three times in twenty minutes. Urinate frequently due to nerves. Woke at midnight to pass urinate. Bladder fuller than usual on waking. Urine escaped with cough. Urine smelled strong. Stinging, burning pain along the urethra at the end of and after urination.

Larynx - Voice deep, with roughness and lots of phlegm in the throat. Weak and rough voice. Voice lower as if getting a cold, as if something stuck at the bottom of larynx. Tickling between larynx and sternum with dryness.

Legs - Heaviness and restlessness of legs at night (Caust.). Legs feel weak, wobbly when walking. Calves feel heavy and tired. Stiffness of legs on climbing stairs. Tingling in legs, feet. Formication on the inside of the lower right leg. Hot thighs with cold feet. Lower legs feeling numb and cold as if dead. Coldness of right leg, right foot. Feet cold with hot flushes, while walking outside. Soles of feet felt numb when walking. Felt as though shoes too tight. Athlete's foot.

Limbs - Heaviness of legs at night (Caust.). ***Heaviness of lower limbs as from fatigue.*** Clumsy. Muscles in right buttock very sore. Pain in back of right knee. Aching in shin bones. Soreness and tenderness in soles of feet. Burning sensation of soles of the feet. Shooting pain in right heel. Throbbing pain in the big toe of right foot. Broken skin and redness between toes. Sharp neuralgic pain shooting from left shoulder like an electric shock. Splinter-like pain, right elbow. ***Numbness and tingling in arms.*** Aching shoulders and arms extending to fingers. Left arm aches. Pain in wrist after writing. Hands shaking while trying to write or after anger. Feeling cold, especially hands and lower legs. ***Coldness of right leg, right foot.*** Nails brittle. Piercing pain as if stuck with a piece of wood. Feels as if the skin is trying to burst out from swelling. ***Restlessness of legs at night.*** Cuts become slightly septic, tender to touch and swollen.

Lungs - Breathing difficult on inhalation. *Sighing*, needing air. Wheezing on waking with itching in the back. Cough with difficult expectoration of very small amounts of thick, yellow mucus. Clear, white and bubbly expectoration hawked up from throat. Coughs, bringing up egg-white mucus, or a dark phlegm. Mucus difficult to cough up.

Male - Crack, split on the foreskin and a red rash on the end of the penis. Burning, aching sensation at the base of the penis on the left.

Modalities - Better open air. Worse becoming cold and tendency to take cold. Worse night. Worse sleep. Worse morning on waking. Worse daytime. Worse from 9 p.m. to 9 a.m.

Mouth - Bitter taste in mouth. Food tastes dry, like sawdust. Water tastes metallic. Sensation of dryness on mouth and lips. Dry mouth with thirst. Swelling mouth and lips. Small ulcer behind the teeth, bottom left side. Ulcer right side of lower jaw under lip. Gums bleeding. Salivation at night, with toothache. Metallic taste in mouth. Burning peppery sensation in the mouth, throat, extending into ears and nose, with watery eyes.

Neck - Stiffness in neck. Neck feels enlarged, numb. Feeling as if tendons in back of neck too short. Neck feels as if been struck a blow. Pain in right side, on swallowing cold liquids. Tension in neck with headache. Gland in neck on right side swollen, painful and hard to touch. Sensitive to cold, wanted a scarf. Red spots on left side.

Nose - Dryness in morning on waking. Sneezing on waking, during daytime. Coryza worse eating. Sneezing during daytime. Sneezing in cold air. Sneezing during chill. Sneezing and feeling cold, followed by a warm feeling. Sneezing with acrid, itchy sensation. Sneezing and thin coryza. Tingling in nose, as if about to sneeze. Sharp peppery sensation behind left nostril. Pain root of nose, with obstruction. Raw pain from constantly blowing the nose. Nose stuffy with clear, fluid coryza, worse eating. Nose running white, clear fluid like a tap, while eating. Slight catarrh and much sneezing in the evening. Thick green mucus congestion in nose, difficult to swallow. Mucus streaked with blood on blowing the nose. Mucus of an egg-white consistency. Flakey yellow-green catarrh with bits of blood. Pale green crusts from nose. Itching inside nose. Tip and wings of nose throbbing during headache. Sensation of movement, "as though worms moving." Sensation of large bump at the end of the left nostril. Acute sense of smell.

Perspiration - Cold sweat with paranoid anxiety. Clammy sweat in bed at night during sleep, with fever feeling. Waking from frightening dream in a cold sweat. Perspiration with heat and odor on waking. Cold sweat on waking from nightmare. Perspiration during chills (Verat.).

Rectum - Diarrhea after headache. Sensation of a ball in the rectum. Feeling of fullness in rectum. Pain in rectum when sitting, as if forcing back a stool. Urging to stool absent all day. Urgent desire for stool in the morning. Constipated, strains to pass a stool, with hard stool. Fast expulsion of diarrhea-like stool. Flatulence smelling of putrid eggs. Anus sore during and after stool. Bleeding hemorrhoids and fissures around anus. Moisture with fishy odor (Sanic.).

Skin - Herpetic eruptions. Sunburned mainly on the left side of the back, although the whole of him was in the sun.

Sleep - Sudden sleepiness. Unable to get to sleep. Couldn't sleep with irritability. Insomnia. Sleepless from thoughts at night. Sleep deep and refreshing. Wants to sleep propped up on pillow because of sore throat and stuffy head. Painful to move from one position to another. Restless at night. Waking several times in the night. Woke in the night with a terrible fright, shaky, about to scream. Very warm in bed at night on waking. Perspiration all over. Uncovers limbs to cool down. Waking early. Very sleepy in morning, needed frequent short naps during the day. Attacks of yawning. Sleepy at noon could not stop yawning, much better after lunch.

Stomach - Anxious, queasy feeling, with apprehension. Wobbly feeling in stomach, constant feeling of nausea, worse bending over, better breathing deeply and standing still. Stomach feels distended and bloated one hour before evening meal. Sensation of wind in stomach with belching. Retching after bending over. Retching after tea. Retching while preparing food. Retching from the thought or smell of food. Nausea in epigastrium and umbilical region. Nausea with weakness, headache, flushing and trembling. Nausea better movement, walking about, and eating. ***Nausea from the smell of food***, garlic. Nausea coming on while lying in bed. Nausea in the morning on waking. Nausea on driving the car. Nausea worse bending forwards, better breathing deeply.

Stool - Diarrhea from fermentation, with sour, acrid, watery stools. Diarrhea after headache. ***Forcible, sudden, gushing stool.*** Spurting out with much flatus. Clay-colored, pale, yellowish soft stool, in the morning. Stool slender, small and loose, long and soft. Small, hard stool which felt large. Small, lumpy stool. ***Light-colored stool***. Stool with lots of mucus. Flatus with discharge of gray, white mucus. Fishy odor.

Teeth - Severe stabbing tooth pain throughout whole mouth. Pains unbearable. Pressing pain in lower incisors. Aching pain in teeth on right side, extending to right ear and top of right eye. Toothache on upper right side. Severe toothache, left lower side, with left sided earache, worse eating. Toothache at night. Woke with severe toothache, better drinking cold water.

Temperature - Shivery feeling. Chilly with the influenza. Chill followed by heat. Fever during the night with vivid nightmares, with perspiration. Felt hot internally and externally with red cheeks. Slight fever on waking.

Throat - Throat painful and dry, not better by drinking. Rawness of throat and roof of mouth. Right side of throat painful on swallowing. Sore throat with blocked nose, worse sneezing. Sore throat on waking in morning, and inspiring cold air. Sore throat better warm drinks. Pain moved from the left to the right. Burning sensation on roof of mouth, at back of throat. Post-nasal catarrh, worse from swallowing. ***Mucus drawn from posterior nares.*** Phlegm in throat. Sensation of mucus (Rhod.). Catarrhal feeling, back of throat. Sensation of a film over the throat, with difficulty in breathing. Throat feels furry with a furry taste. Sensation of a hair on the right side of the throat. Sensation of a lump in the throat. Tickle, deep in throat causing coughs. Frequent swallowing. Choked on a piece of food.

Tongue - Tongue white, more in center. Small white spot to the left of the middle of the tongue, feels sharp, worse touch and eating. Tongue feels numb and smooth. Numbness of tip of tongue. Spot on the right side of the tongue with sharp pain, worse moving tongue. Feels like tongue has been cut.

Vertigo - Dizzy on getting out of bed in morning. Lost balance slightly towards the right. Vertigo in waves, all day. Vertigo, worse on rising from sitting, moving head. Vertigo during headache. Nausea and vertigo.

Vision - Specks of light, black spots floating across the vision. Lights in front of eyes when jumping up quickly. After looking away from a picture on the wall, retained white image on the vision.

COMMENTS - Other remarks from the provers of Hydrog. include: Time sense seems warped. Time is different on this level, its moving very quickly. A lifetime is a very short space of time. Confused about what happened when and where, about what happened in the past. Problems assimilating the notion of time. Felt stuck in time.

Relaxed attitude to work (curative). Concentration improved (curative). More efficient than usual. Ready to fill in odd spaces of time with odd jobs (curative). Felt alert and mentally active in the evening and night. Memory improved.

Have given up my normal planning and making lists. I used to organize all the time (curative).

Confidence is improved before and during teaching (curative). Less procrastination than usual (curative). Less nervous with strangers (curative). Usual tendency to bite and tear thumbs much better (curative). Mood better in the evening more cheerful and positive.

Although feeling very tired, not feeling irritable or snappy as usually would when tired (curative). Felt emotionally 'stretched out', but calm. Irritations don't make me so cross. The 'stretchiness' absorbed the daily irritations, they didn't peak up enough to a point where I felt irritated and cross (curative).

Dreams were vivid. Revolting dreams. Dream of a girl at school who committed suicide. Dream of participating in a play about death. Dream of my dead grandmother in the afternoon. Several erotic dreams.

Difficult to pass stool. Usual diarrhea after headache or eating gone (curative). Expected diarrhea from anticipation and eating a full tea cake did not materialize (curative). Menses started again during the menopause after an absence of six months. Noticed mustache seemed less and hair was finer in a woman, observers agreed. Mustache in a woman (disappeared).

Scalp less dry, less dandruff, less itchy (curative). Spot on hairline at the base of the neck, very itchy. Sore pimple on the back of the head. Usual itching of scalp has been absent (curative). Usual flatulence is improved (curative).

Less stiffness and aching in the back on waking that usual (curative). Back much less strained on physical work than usual (curative).

RELATIONS - ***Compare:*** (1) Cann-i., Phos., Sulphur., Lyc. Calc. Kali-s., Ferr-ar. Nat-ar. Nat-phos.

REFERENCES - Sherr.

HYDROGEN PEROXIDUM

(Hydrogen Peroxide)

PHARMACY - hydro-p. Hydrogen peroxidum. Hydrogen peroxide. Hydrogen dioxide.

CLINICAL - Abscesses. Diabetes. Diarrhea. Dyspepsia. Fever. Rheumatism. Tumors. Ulcers.

HOMEOPATHIC - Hydro-p. is a stimulant, antiseptic and disinfectant. Atonic dyspepsia. Low forms of fever. Chronic rheumatism. Scrofulous, syphilitic or non-specific ulcers. Scrofulous tumors.

Infants suffering from diarrhea were allowed to drink freely of cold water containing a few drops of the solution of hydrogen peroxide. This agent is used extensively in surgery as an antiseptic.

RELATIONS - ***Compare:*** Ozone.

REFERENCES - Murphy.

HYDROPHIS CYANOCINCTUS

(Sea serpent)

PHARMACY - hydro-c. Hydrophis cyanocinctus. Sea serpent. Pacific Islands, Australia, India and China. The tincture is made from the venom of the sea serpent. ***Historical dose:*** Tincture and all potencies.

CLINICAL - Blepharitis. Cervicitis. Conjunctivitis. Depression. Earache. Enterocolitis. Headache. Polyneuritis. Poliomyelitis. Menorrhagia. Myopathy. Styes. Vaginitis.

HOMEOPATHIC - Hydrophis cyanocinctus is a venom of a sea serpent whose habitat is along the coasts of the Pacific islands, Australia, India and China.

J. R. Reside carried out a double blind homeopathic proving from January to June 1958, on ten provers, eight men and two women using the potencies 6c and 30c.

Hydro-c., from a toxicological point of view, attacks the peripheral nerves, giving a symptom table similar to that of poliomyelitis. Paresis, paralysis without sensory disorders. Stinging pains in the limbs and thorax. Dry throat.

MIND - Depressive, clouded mental state, weepy, especially during menopause. Disgust for life. State of euphoria, followed by a period of sadness with tears, ameliorated by consolation. Irritable. Lethargic, sleepy, lacks initiative. Forgetful and unable to concentrate. Anxiety with clairvoyance.

Abdomen - Enterocolitis. Rectocolitis. Violent, sharp, stinging pains with feeling of tension along the colon, worse in the morning and on the left side.

Ears - Earache. Pains in the left earlobe. Deafness in the left ear.

Eyes - Conjunctivitis. Burning, especially on the left side. Troubled vision. Blepharitis. Pruritus of the eyelids. Eyelids heavy. Styes, especially on the left.

Female - Menses abundant. Menorrhagia. Blood-streaked vaginal discharge. Vaginitis. Cervicitis. Salpingo-ovaritis. Pre-neoplastic conditions.

Head - Headache with beating in the temples and sensation of a tight band. Headache with heavy head, worse on the left, at the front. Headache worse in the morning, from heat, better in fresh air. Pruritus of the scalp.

Heart - Pain in the precordial region, spreading to the left hemi-thorax, worse when lying flat. Feeling of dryness and burning in the thorax. Extra systole. Arrhythmia. Valvular disease. Coronary arthritis. Angina pectoris. Septicemia.

Limbs - Paretic and paralytic syndromes of the lower limbs. Painful paresthesia. Numbness, heavy feeling in the limbs. Stinging pains in the limbs and the left hip. Pain in the thumbs and arms, especially the left. Feet cold.

Lungs - Dyspnea. Tracheitis and bronchitis.

Modalities - Worse at night. Worse after nightmares. Worse on waking. Worse in the morning. Worse lying flat. Worse on the left side. Worse before menses. Worse from heat. Worse speaking.

Mouth - Dry, worse in the morning. Left maxillary pain, which prevents mastication. Toothache in the molars, on the left side.

Nose - Burning catarrh, ameliorated in the fresh air. Coryza.

Rectum - Constipation and acute pains after going to stool. Painful, swollen hemorrhoids. Anal pruritus.

Skin - Spots on the face and nape of the neck. Skin dry with chapped hands. Skin itching at different parts of the body.

Sleep - Sleep disturbed, woken by nightmares between 2.30 and 4.30 a.m. with feeling of anguish, heat and feels very ill. Wakes with a feeling of thoracic oppression. Calls out in his sleep. Worse at night and after nightmares.

Stomach - Nausea, thirsty for cold drinks. Epigastric pains and pain in the right hypochondrium, worse after meals.

Temperature - Profuse sweating without a temperature. Fever with shivering, inflammation of the throat.

Throat - Dry, burning. Tonsils sore. Tonsillitis. Pharyngitis. Hoarseness worse in the morning and after speaking. Laryngitis. Tickling cough and dryness in the larynx.

RELATIONS - ***Compare:*** (1) Lach. - worse after sleep and when lying down with localization on the left side and pain in the precordial region with constriction. (2) Lath. - paresis of the limbs.

REFERENCES - Julian.

HYDROPHYLLUM VIRGINICUM

(Virginian Waterleaf)

PHARMACY - hydro-v. Hydrophyllum virginicum. Virginian waterleaf. N. O. Hydrophyllaceae. Tincture of fresh plant in flower. ***Historical dose:*** Tincture and all potencies.

CLINICAL - Eyelids, swollen. Eyes, inflammation. Rhus, poisoning.

HERBAL - The Hydrophyllaceae are nearly allied to the Borages. They grow among moist, shady rocks and derive their name from the small quantity of water held in the cavity of each leaf in spring.

Hydro-v. should prove to be a good adjunct to Euphrasia. The older writers speak of it as an antidote to rhus poisoning. Eye inflammation.

HOMEOPATHIC - The only homeopathic experience on record is that of Dr. Hoyt of Indiana, recorded by Hale.

Ten minutes after gathering a cluster of the blue flowers, Hoyt noticed his eyes began to water and burn with slight itching. By the time he reached home he was suffering severely, eyelids swollen, fiery red, some sensitiveness to light.

The symptoms continued through afternoon and evening and kept him awake some time. In the morning, the lids were agglutinated and eyes sensitive to light. The burning and smarting were less, but lachrymation remained and it was a week before the eyes were quite right.

Dr. Hoyt tested the remedy in one case of catarrhal inflammation of the eyes, which it cured.

REFERENCES - Clarke. Hale.

HYOSCINUM BROMHYDRICUM

(Scopolamine hydrobromide)

PHARMACY - hyosin. Hyoscinum bromhydricum. Scopolamine hydrobromide. Crystalline alkaloid of Hyoscyamus, ($C_{17}H_{23}NO_3$). Bromines. Hyosymous. Solanaceae. ***Historical dose:*** All potencies.

CLINICAL - Chorea. Insomnia. Mania. Nervous, exhaustion. Parkinson's disease. Shock. Tremors. Tuberculosis. Uremia.

HOMEOPATHIC - Hyosin. corresponds to the effects of strong poisons introduced into or generated within the body. It is similar in its effects to alcohol, both recent and remote.

Shock. Acute nervous exhaustion. Mania and chorea. Insomnia. Nervous agitation. Paralysis agitans. ***Tremors of disseminated sclerosis***. Dry cough in tuberculosis. Uremia.

REFERENCES - Boericke. Clarke.

HYOSCYAMUS NIGER

(Henbane)

PHARMACY - hyos. Hyoscyamus niger. Henbane. Stinking Roger. Hog-bean. Hyosymous. N. O. Solanaceae. Tincture of fresh plant. ***Historical dose:*** All potencies.

CLINICAL - ***Alcoholism.*** Alzheimer's disease. Amaurosis. Angina, pectoris. Bladder, paralysis. Bronchitis. Chorea. Coma, vigil. Convulsions. Coughs. ***Delirium.*** Delirium, tremens. Diarrhea. Dysmenorrhea. Eclampsia. Enteric, fever. Epilepsy. Eyes, disorders. Fevers. Hemoptysis. Hemorrhages. Hiccough. ***Hydrophobia.*** Hypochondriasis. ***Hysteria. Insanity.*** Lochia, suppressed. ***Mania.*** Manic depression. Meningitis. ***Mental, disorders.*** Neuralgias. Night-blindness. Nosebleeds. ***Nymphomania.*** Paralysis. Parkinson's, disease. Parotiditis. Pneumonia. Puerperal, mania. Rage. Schizophrenia. ***Senility.*** Sexual, mania. Sleep, disordered. Stammering, speech. Syphilophobia. Tetanus. ***Toothaches.*** Tympanites. Urine, retention. Vision, disorders.

HERBAL - Hyoscyamus, "Hog-bean," is nearly allied to Belladonna botanically, and in pathogenetic action the two drugs are much alike in their main features. Hyos. is found growing on old rubbish heaps, near ruins, on roadsides and sometimes by the seashore.

Hyos. is one of our best remedies in toothache, having well-defined symptoms. Hyos. is also an ancient domestic remedy for toothache, the application being peculiar. A penny is made hot in the fire and when taken out a pinch of Henbane seeds is dropped on it and fumes come away. A wineglass is inverted over it and this is soon filled with the fumes and applied to the mouth, when the fumes are inhaled.

The popular idea is that the fumes expel the "worms" of toothache, but, as Lauder Brunton showed, the supposed "worms" are the embryos of the seeds forcibly expelled on the rupture of the seed coats by the heat.

HOMEOPATHIC - Hyos. disturbs the mind, brain and nervous system profoundly, preventing functions. ***Mania of a quarrelsome and obscene character***. Inclined to be unseemly and immodest in acts, gestures and expressions. Persists in undressing herself or uncovering genitals. Is jealous and afraid of being poisoned. Talkative.

Weakness and ***nervous agitation***. Typhoid and other infections with ***coma vigil. Tremulous weakness and twitching of tendons***. Subsultus tendinum. Non-inflammatory cerebral activity. ***Toxic gastritis.***

Gestures, carphology, picks at bed clothes, with fingers. When lying on back, suddenly sits up and lies down again. Convulsions, trembling, jerks, twitchings, cramps are very marked features. Muscular twitchings, spasmodic affections, generally with delirium.

Active mania or convulsions, alternate with or ends in deep sopor. Motions of the arms are clutching or angular, throws arms about, misses what is reached for, totters while walking. Paralysis after spasms.

Epilepsy, vertigo before the attack. Falls suddenly to the ground with cries. Child sobs and cries without waking. Eclampsia. Chorea, local, twitchings of solitary muscles, squinting, stammering. Sensation as if walking on and through air.

MIND - Confused mind, as if intoxicated. ***Alcoholism***, drug addictions. Bouts of drinking or intoxicated rages. Sings, recites poetry, talks, babbles, quarrels. Great hilarity, inclined to laugh at everything. Obscene gestures, exposes himself. Does foolish things, behaves like a mad person.

Muttering delirium. Low, speech with ***constant carphologia, deep stupor.*** Violent outbreaks of delirium with weakness. ***Very suspicious, jealous***. Restless, jumps out of bed, wants to escape. ***Hallucinations and delusions.*** Rage with desire to strike, bite, fight insult, scold and to kill. Tendency to maniacal activity.

Erotic mania, exposes genitals. Exaggerated sexual behavior, especially touching and petting themselves constantly (Plat.). Entire loss of modesty. Fondles the genitals. ***Nymphomania***, lascivious mania. Talkative, obscene. Sings amorous songs.

Senility. Alzheimer's disease with bizarre, ludicrous behavior. ***Passive insanity***. Mental confusion. Picking at the air, the bedclothes. Chewing the lips. Incessant talking to themselves. Talks with imaginary persons to dead ones. Imagines things are animals. Thinks he is in the wrong place but doesn't want to go home.

Fear with delirium. ***Fears to eat or drink,*** of being poisoned. Fears being alone, being bitten by wild animals, being pursued. Hydrophobia, anxiety on hearing running water. Syphilophobia.

Speechless from fright. Ailments from grief, disappointed love. Manic depression after grief. Unconsciousness, can barely be aroused. Involuntary passage of urine and feces. Coma.

Abdomen - Distention. Cutting pain in lower portion of abdomen. Colic, as if abdomen would burst, presses fists into sides. Colic with vomiting, belchings, hiccough and screaming. Colic better vomiting. Abdominal muscles seem strained or bruised. Red spots on abdomen. Umbilicus open, urine oozing through. Gastritis or peritonitis with hiccough. Tympanites.

Back - Pains in the back, especially the lumbar region, with swelling of the feet. Lancinations in the loins and shoulder blades. Stiff neck, contracted to one side. Stiffness of cervical muscles, with tension as if too short, on bending neck. Spinal meningitis, with convulsions, jerks of muscles. Pains after injury. Herpetic spots on nape. Abscesses on left side of neck.

Bladder - ***Involuntary urination.*** Bladder paralyzed. Prolapsed bladder and retention of urine. No urge to urinate (Caust.). Frequent, scanty, painful, nightly urination. Retention of urine after childbirth. Enuresis, in children with brain troubles. Prostate slightly enlarged.

Brain - Brain feels loose, fluctuating. Brain seems to shake about when walking and on stooping. Inflammation of brain with unconsciousness, head is shaken to and fro. Stupor after concussion of the brain.

Breasts - Soreness in spots to left of nipple, alternating with stitches.

Causations - Ill effects of suppressed lochia or milk. Grief, unhappy love. Jealousy. Fright, disappointed love.

Chest - Spasms, forcing bending forward. Spasms of chest with shortness of breath, forcing him to bend forward. Tight feeling across chest, as from overexertion, running. Stitches in sides. Muscles of chest sore. Atelectasis pulmonum. Red spots on chest.

Chill - Whole body cold, with burning redness of face. Chills with cold limbs. Chill alternating with heat. General shivering, coldness, sudden chills. Chills from feet upwards, up back from small of back. Chills at night, can't get warm in bed.

Constitutions - Suited to nervous, irritable, excitable, sanguine, light-haired people.

Cough - ***Dry, hacking spasmodic cough*** from a dry spot in larynx at night. Paroxysmal coughs, short, rapid, frequent, shaking chest, abdomen, whole body, like whooping cough. Cough from itching in the throat, as if uvula were too long. Exhausting cough with sweat. Cough worse lying down, eating, drinking, talking, singing, better sitting up. Hemoptysis of bright red blood with spasms.

Ears - Deafness from paralysis of auditory nerve. Impaired hearing, as if stupefied, especially after apoplexy. Buzzing, singing, rushing noises.

Eyes - Pupils dilated, sparkling, fixed and insensible. Tearing pain in right eye, which waters. Shooting pain from eyes into nose and head. Eyes roll about in orbits. Quivering of eyeball. Strabismus. Eyelids open and close with a sudden force. Spasmodic closing of lids. Eyes open but does not pay attention. Constantly stares at surrounding objects. Diplopia, hemeralopia, myopia. Objects, seem red, large or with colored borders (yellow). Aversion to light.

Face - Red, hot and swollen face (Bell.). Flushed, dark red. Face cold and pale. Distorted face. Stupid expression. Dry lips. Muscles twitch, when protruding the tongue. Grimaces and ***makes ridiculous gestures.*** Lower jaw drops with muttering. Lockjaw with consciousness. Face dark colored and bloated after epileptic attack. Face becomes red during paroxysms of cough.

Female - Hysterical or epileptic spasms before menses. Irregular menses. Profuse flow of menses. Headache, nausea and profuse sweat during menses. Pale flow, with convulsions. Convulsive trembling of hands and feet during menses. Bedwetting during menses. Metrorrhagia. Hemorrhage, bright red blood. Colds that settled in the uterus and cause labor-like pains. ***Excited sexual desire, nymphomania.*** Lasciviousness, uncovers sexual parts. Convulsions during pregnancy. Milk and lochia suppressed. Spasms of pregnant women. Puerperal mania. Painless diarrhea in lying-in women.

Fever - High fever with delirium, stupor, sopor. Fever with cerebral symptoms. Burning heat all over, without external redness. Heat in face and head, on skin. Blood burns in veins. Throw bedclothes entirely off, not because they are too warm, but they will not remain covered.

Food - Loss of taste. Bulimia with violent thirst with inability to swallow. Thirst with drinking but little at a time. Aversion to water. ***Fears to eat or drink*** from fear of being poisoned. After a meal, headache intoxication, great anguish and sadness. After drinking, convulsions. Vomiting of food and drink.

Head - Aching, lightness and confusion of head. Rolls or shakes the head to and fro, when bending forward, in stupor, after concussion of the brain. Heaviness of head and violent pains, alternating with pains in nape of neck. Constrictive, stupefying pain in forehead. Pulsating headache. Violent pulsations, like waves, head shakes. Pressure in vertex, better heat.

Heart - Pressure, tightness and anxiety in precordial region. Violent stitch in precordial region. Oppression of heart with transient stitches. Sensation as if heart and chest were torn to pieces. Tearing, sticking in heart. Soreness, tightness of heart region. Heart's action violent, tremulous, irregular. Carotids beat violently. Inflammation of blood vessels. Chronic palpitations with anxiety, fear. Unable to move body without anxiety, apprehension of suffocation or swooning.

Kidneys - Nephritis with delirium. Frequent emission of urine as clear as water. Urine turbid, with muco-purulent sediment. Red, sandy sediment.

Larynx - Hysterical aphonia. Hoarseness, with dry and inflamed throat. Voice rough on account of mucus in larynx and trachea. Constriction of larynx during cough.

Limbs - Lancinating pains in almost all joints, worse on motion. Great restlessness, every ***muscle twitches***. Cold hands and feet. Will not be covered. ***Picking at bedclothes***, plays with hands, reaches out for things. Spasms and convulsions. Alternate convulsions of upper and lower limbs. Cramps in calves and toes. Trembling of hands and feet. Fists clenched with retraction of thumbs during convulsions (Cupr.). Epileptic attacks ending in deep sleep. Child sobs and cries without waking.

Lungs - Pneumonia with cerebral symptoms, delirium, sopor. Slow, rattling breathing. Hemoptysis, bright red, mixed with clots. Salty mucus. Suffocating fits. Paroxysms of dyspnea at night on lying, must jump up. Loss of breath, panting. Difficult breathing, alternating with anxiety or oppression of chest. Suffocating spells and convulsions during labor.

Male - Impotence. Excessive sexual desire. Lasciviousness, ***exposes his genitals.*** Plays with genitals during fever. ***Desire to expose himself, take clothes off.***

Modalities - Better from sitting up. Better motion. Better warmth. Better stooping. ***Worse from emotions.*** Worse jealousy. Worse fright. Worse unhappy love. ***Worse from touch***. Worse cold, cold air. Worse evening and night. Worse before, commencing and during menstruation. Worse when lying down. Worse after eating.

Mouth - Foams at mouth. Offensive odor from mouth. Putrid or salt taste. Saliva, bloody with salty taste. Dryness of mouth, fauces and lips. Soreness of soft parts between gums and cheeks. Sordes on teeth, closes tightly. Mouth closed tightly. Lower jaw drops.

Neck - Tettery spots on the nape of the neck. Stiff, contracted to one side.

Nose - Dryness of nose. Cramp-like pressure at the root of the nose and the zygomata. Sudden jerks at root of the nose. Pressing pinching pain at root of nose and malar bones. Nostrils sooty, smoky. Nosebleed, bright red, with salivation. Colds from dry, cold air. Loss of smell and taste.

Perspiration - Warm or cold sweat. Sour and weakening perspiration. Violent sweats after thirst. Perspires during short naps. Clammy during sleep.

Pulse - Pulse is full, hard, strong, rapid intermitting. Pulse slow, small, scarcely perceptible.

Rectum - Rectal sphincter is weak causing great difficulty in retaining feces. Frequent desire for stool, with small discharges. Involuntary stools, worse mental excitement or during sleep. Involuntary stools during fevers. Diarrhea, colicky, pains, aggravated by mental excitement or during sleep. Loose stools. Stools involuntary, bloody, yellow, watery or although hard, worse mental excitement during sleep during fevers, while urinating. Diarrhea after childbirth. Constipation with epilepsy. Hemorrhoids bleed profusely.

Skin - Skin and muscles lax. Skin usually dry and hot. Pale, with delirium. Brittle skin, lack of sensation. Scarlet-like rash spreads over whole body, which becomes purplish. Scarlatina with marked mental symptoms. Red rash. Miliary eruptions. Chickenpox with vesicles in crops. Large pustules in clusters. Large blood boils. Brown spots. Gangrenous spots. Pustules around ulcers. Ulcers bleed and become painful. Eruption of dry pimples. Anthrax. Suppressed eruptions with diarrhea.

Sleep - Sleeplessness all night, with restlessness, twitching and starting. ***Starts out of sleep,*** frightened. Sleeplessness after serious disease. Nervous wakefulness. Coma vigil. Sopor with convulsions. Epileptic attacks ending in deep sleep. Falls asleep while answering. Sits up and then goes to sleep again. Laughs during sleep. Child sobs and cries in sleep without waking. When sleeping, carphologia or smiling countenance or starts with fright. Profound, comatose sleep with convulsions and involuntary movements of the limbs. Sleeps days without interruption.

Speech - Stammering and stuttering. Low, muttering speech. Speech impaired, difficult and unintelligible. Speech loss from suppression of urination or fright.

Stomach - Burning in stomach. Cramps in stomach, better after vomiting, worse after irritating food. Bitter, empty belchings. Gastritis or peritonitis with hiccough. Hiccough from concussion of brain. Hiccough of nursing children. Retching and vomiting, of bloody mucus. Nausea, vomiting with vertigo, convulsions. Hematemesis, violent cramps, relieved by vomiting, epigastrium tender.

Temperature - Low fever with hot, pale skin. Warm sweat. Subsultus during fevers. Septic fevers. Slides down in bed.

Teeth - Children grind teeth during convulsions. Grinding of teeth, so that they become loose. Pressing of gums together during dentition. Teeth feel loose, too long, when chewing. ***Toothaches***, after taking cold or in open air. Toothache, driving to despair. Violent pain in teeth with twitching of muscles of hands, face, etc. Tearing in teeth. Pain in gums after extraction of tooth. Teeth covered with sordes.

Throat - Spasmodic constriction of throat, inability to swallow liquids, better from solid and warm food. Difficult swallowing, as from constriction. ***Elongation of uvula.*** Fluids come out of the nose or go into larynx. Dread of liquids. Stinging dryness. Throat dry, burning, shooting, pricking pains.

Tongue - Tongue dry, red, cracked, stiff and immovable. Tongue clean, parched, looks like burnt leather. Tongue covered with blood. Tongue as if numb and lame. Tongue protruded with difficulty, can hardly draw it in. Tongue rattles in mouth. Tongue shaken to and fro, with a trembling movement. Bites the tongue while talking. Speech impaired.

Vertigo - Vertigo, before spasms, from smell of flowers, gas etc. Vertigo as if intoxicated. Vertigo, as if water swashing in head. Vertigo, worse walking, usually with obscured vision.

Vision - Diplopia. Farsighted. Incipient amaurosis. Dim vision, as if veil were before eyes. Night blindness. Perversion of vision. Deceptive vision. Objects have colored borders. Objects appear smaller or larger. When reading, the letters move about, from mydriasis. Momentary loss of sight.

COMMENTS - Low, muttering delirium (Bell. tends to be violent and furious). Fits of ungovernable rage (less sustained than Bell.). Face is pale or bluish (Bell. is red). Hyos. corresponds to a great variety of cases of melancholia than Bell., with the characteristic "suspicion," so frequently met with in cases of insanity (Lach.).

One patient, a clever lawyer, suffered from a nervous breakdown and had to abandon his business entirely. He then had a kind of fit and became cold and senseless, his face working much. After that he fell asleep, and had another attack an hour and a half later.

After this he was suspicious and said that his wife was poisoning him. He took a single dose of Hyos. 1,000c, given in food or drink without his knowledge. It was repeated once a week. He began to improve and in a few months was restored to health, though some other medicines were given later on.

Characteristic twitching throughout the body. Clonic spasms, twitching of groups of muscles. Twitchings, subsultus tendinum and picking at the bedclothes. Chorea. Spasms with unconsciousness. Convulsions followed by coma and stupor. Convulsions in children from frights, worms. Epilepsy with erratic behavior and gestures before the attack.

Sensorium so clouded that if the patient is roused to answer he falls back into a stupor again. Sight is disordered, sees things too large or too near and grasps at them. Picks the bedclothes and mutters. Drowsy, but restless. Insomnia, patient lies awake for hours. Children twitch in sleep, cry out, tremble and awake frightened.

Dry and unwieldy tongue. Teeth covered with sordes. Pulmonary conditions.

Cough is worse on lying down, almost completely removed by sitting up, worse at night, worse after eating, drinking or talking. Cough from elongated uvula. Parotiditis with metastasis to brain.

Useful for influenza when it takes the typhoid form. Clarke rapidly cured a boy in whom influenza attacked the meninges of the brain with pains in the head, especially forehead, piercing to the brain.

RELATIONS - ***Antidotes:*** Bell., Camph., Stram. ***Compare:*** (1) Bell., Stram., Agar., Gels. (2) Hyosin. (3) Scopolia, the Japanese Belladonna, is chemically identical with Hyoscine. - Joyous delirium, licking of lips and smacking of mouth, sleepless, tries to get out of bed, sees cats, picks imaginary hairs, warms hands before imaginary fire, etc.

REFERENCES - Boericke. Clarke. Murphy. Phatak.

HYPERICUM PERFORATUM

(St. John's Wort)

PHARMACY - hyper. Hypericum perforatum. St. John's-wort. N. O. Hypericacee. Guttiferae. Tincture of whole fresh plant. ***Historical dose:*** Tincture and all potencies.

CLINICAL - After-pains. Asthma. ***Bites. Blood, poisonings.*** Bone, fractures. Brachial, neuralgia. Breast, disorders. Brain, concussion. Bruises. Bunions. ***Coccyx, injury.*** Corns. ***Depression.*** Diarrhea. Fingernail, injuries. ***Gunshots.*** Headaches. Hemorrhoids, bleeding. Hypersensitiveness. Impotency. ***Injuries.*** Labor, effects. ***Lacerations.*** Meningitis. Mental, disorders. ***Neuralgia. Neuritis.*** Panaritium. Paralysis. ***Punctures.*** Rabies. Rheumatism. Scars. Sciatica. Spasms. ***Spinal, concussion. Spinal, injections. Spinal, injury.*** Stiff-neck. Surgery, effects. ***Tailbone, pain. Tetanus.*** Toenail, injuries. Ulcerations. Vaccination, reactions. Whooping, cough. ***Wounds.***

HERBAL - The leaves of various species of Hypericum are sprinkled with pellucid dots and black glands that contain an essential oil. These, which are most conspicuous in Hypericum perforatum, have evidently given the signature which has led to the chief use of the plant in medicine, that is for wounds or puncture of the tissues.

The leaves, moreover, are lance-shaped.

HOMEOPATHIC - Hyper. has been used for general depression, especially nervous depression following wounds, effects of shock and fright. Nerves are severely sensitive. Excessive painfulness. ***Injury to nerves,*** especially fingers, toes, nails.

Puncture wounds. Wounds are more tender than appearance would indicate.

Penetrating wounds. ***Infected wounds. Bites of animals and insects***. Gunshot wounds. Relieves pain after operations (Calen.). Neuralgia of the stump. ***Crushed fingers, especially tips***.

Tetanus, lockjaw. Dental work, nerve pains. Neuritis, tingling, burning and numbness. Neuritis of head or chest in epigastrium inter-scapular spine, fingertips etc. Brachial neuralgia. ***Tailbone pains from injury***. ***Brain and spinal cord injuries***. ***Spinal taps***, injections, severe pains. Spinal concussion. Whiplash.

Lacerations, with intolerable, violent, shooting and sharp pains. ***Shooting pains from injured part.*** Pain in old scars. Joints feel bruised. Pains extend towards the trunk or down sides with crawling and numbness.

Spasms after every injury. Shuddering. Jerks in the limbs. Convulsions after knocking the body against anything. Lies on back, jerking head backwards. Spasmodic asthmatic attacks with changes of weather or before storms, better by copious expectoration. Constant drowsiness. Hemorrhoids.

MIND - Brain fag and neurasthenia. Weak memory. Forgets what she wanted to say. Mistakes in writing, omitting letters. ***Mistakes in speaking***, using wrong words, saying right for left or vice versa. Irritable, inclined to speak sharply.

Depression. Melancholy. Seasonal Affective Disorder. Great nervous depression after shock. ***Complaints from fright.*** Mental effects of injury, fright and shock. Mental dullness after head injuries, surgical operations. Head injury (Nat-s.).

Mental excitement as after drinking tea. Mental symptoms before thunderstorm. Delirium. Talking nonsense. Sees spirits.

Feels lifted high in air or anxiety lest he fall from a height. Singing followed by weeping and loud screaming, with gasping for breath.

Abdomen - Bubbling at navel. Cutting pain in region of navel. Tympanitic distention, better after stool. Sticking pain in right hypochondrium. ***Effects of surgery, laparotomy.*** Pinching pains during menses. Colic. Pains after operation for incarcerated hernia. Awakes with distended abdomen, better stool.

Back - Radiating, shooting pains up spine and down limbs. ***Coccyx injury from fall***. Coccyx pain radiating up spine and down limbs, inability to walk or stoop after. After a fall, slightest motion of arms or neck extorts cries. ***Pressure over sacrum***. Aching pain and sensation of lameness in the small of the back. ***Pinched nerves in back. Violent, sharp pain*** and inability to walk or stoop. Sharp pains in the small of the back. ***Spinal concussion. Painfully sensitive spine.*** Spinal tenderness, with paroxysms of terrible pain, screaming if approached. Cervical vertebrae very sensitive to the touch. Pain in nape of neck. Pain in hips, small of back and coccyx after labor. Jerking and twitching of muscles. Lies on back jerking head backward.

Breasts - Scirrhus of breast from injury. Painful scar after mastectomy. Stitches from within outward, through left breast and sternum, worse from motion.

Causations - Ill effects of fright, shocks. Injections, punctures, bites, gunshot wounds, stab wounds. Lacerations, surgery. Dental work. Bruises. Worse after forceps delivery, as a complication of injury.

Chest - Anxiety in chest in forenoon with short breath. Sharp pains between or under breasts. Pressure and burning in the chest. Tightness in the chest, worse in foggy weather. Stinging in left chest, worse when moving. Cutting pain in upper right chest, then in lower left. Continual sharp pains from within outward, through left breast and sternum, worse motion.

Constitutions - Nervous constitutions.

Coughs - Frequent, dry, hacking cough. Spells of short barking cough. Coughs in meningitis. Hacking cough from irritation in throat, worse heat and cold air. Dry cough and prostration in morning. Whooping cough, worse 6 p.m. to 10 p.m.

Ears - Ears hot. Scurf on ear. Sticking through the right ear in evening. Itching in right meatus. Sensitiveness of hearing during menses. Shooting pain through ear.

Eyes - Disturbed look, stares at people. Eyes fixed. Sticking pain through (right) eye. Burning stinging in tarsi. Stye on left lower lid. Pains in eyes and ears. Pupils dilated.

Face - Expression of suffering. Hot and bloated in meningitis. Eczema of face, eruptions seem to be under the skin. Intense itching. Tension, tearing in cheek, in left zygoma. ***Facial neuralgia and toothache.*** Right side of face aches. Eruption around mouth and on right ear. Yellowish green scabs with cracking and moisture.

Female - Menses increased in quantity. Menses too late, headache, sickening pain in abdomen, sensitive to noises. Leucorrhea with delayed menses, palpitation, pressure in small of back, and heaviness in lower bowels. Leucorrhea in a child, milky, but corroding. Tension in region of uterus, as from a tight bandage. Afterpains violent in sacrum and hips, with severe headache. Afterpains after forceps delivery. Labor pains tardy. Scirrhus of breast caused by injury.

Food - Appetite increased morning and evening. Tastelessness of food. Thirst with feeling of heat in mouth. Great thirst. Desire for pickles. Desire for warm drinks in meningitis. Craving for wine. Smoking tobacco doesn't taste well.

Head - Head hot, with throbbing of carotids. Headache as if brain would be torn to pieces. Curling sensation on vertex. Tearing, sharp pains in the brain. ***Head injury.*** Headache and meningitis depending upon an injury to the nervous system. ***Fractured skull, bone splinters.*** Heaviness or formication in brain. Pulsation, heat and burning in the vertex. ***Throbbing***

pains. Head feels as if touched by icy cold hand. Head feels larger, drawn to a point. Sensation as if the head became elongated. Brain feels loose. ***Dull pain, on vertex.*** Headache, extending into zygoma or cheek. Headache with sore eyes after a fall. Hair moist, rest of body burning hot. Falling of hair after injury.

Heart - Hard beating of heart. The heart feels as though it would fall down in the evening. Palpitations. Local congestions and capillary weakness with or without hemorrhages and nervous depression, following wounds. Pulse quick, hard, accelerated.

Kidneys - Nightly urging to urinate with vertigo. Desire to urinate with violent tearing in the genital organs. Swelling and hardness of female urethra with burning soreness and sensitiveness. Retention of urine. Dribbling away of urine without being aware of it, after concussion of spine. Urine much diminished. Urine bloody, turbid. Urine of peculiar odor.

Limbs - Articular rheumatism. ***Neuritis*** with tingling, burning pain, numbness and flossy skin. ***Amputation pains.*** Traumatic neuralgia and neuritis. Compound fractures of hands and feet, with great laceration of soft parts. Aching in sciatic nerve (left) after prolonged sitting. Joints feel bruised. Hysterical joints. ***Tetanus*** (Phys., Kali-br.). Limbs as if they were numb. Limbs feel detached. Sharp pain in upper and lower limbs. ***Violent pain and inability to walk or stoop after a fall on coccyx, tailbone.*** Darting pain in shoulders. Pressure along ulnar side of arm. ***Crawling in hands and feet***. Pain in toes and fingers, especially in tips. Cramp in calves. Panaritium. Tingling of feet when lying in bed.

Lungs - Asphyxia after a fall. ***Asthma after injury of spine.*** Spasmodic asthmatic attacks with changes of weather from clear to damp, or before storms. Asthma, worse in the foggy weather and better profuse expectoration. Hoarseness, scraping and roughness in larynx, upper part of pharynx and sinuses in foggy weather. Pneumonia in persons who have hemorrhoids.

Male - Tearing pain in genitals, with desire to urinate. Sexual functions excited.

Modalities - Better from lying on face. Better bending head back. Better rubbing. Better lying quietly. ***Worse from injury.*** Worse after forceps delivery. ***Worse from punctures. Worse from bites, stings.*** Worse concussion of spine or coccyx. Worse shock. ***Worse from cuts, surgery.*** Worse exertion. ***Worse jar***. Worse motion. Worse change of weather. Worse fog. Worse cold damp weather. Worse in a close room. ***Worse touch, pressure.*** Worse before a storm. Worse at night.

Mouth - Dry, burning heat in mouth. Mouth and lips dry and burning. Insipid taste, of blood. Thirst with feeling of heat in mouth. Craving for wine with feeling of heat in mouth. Old ulcers or sores in mouth when very sensitive. Lips dry, feel hot.

Nose - Pain in bridge of nose on rising. Sore within nose, itching, continually picking it. Dryness of nose with sneezing of left nostril, with crusts in it. Smell very acute.

Perspiration - Moist hair on the head. Hyperhidrosis, sweating of scalp, worse morning after sleep.

Rectum - Burning, biting and feeling of dryness in rectum. Severe urging, dry, dull, pressing pain. Constipation, violent tenesmus with discharge of a hard little ball with nausea. Constipation with nausea. Diarrhea driving out of bed in morning. Summer diarrhea with eruptions on the skin. Summer diarrhea, slimy stools. ***Hemorrhoids with pain, bleeding and tenderness,*** use tincture externally and internally. Loose, bilious, yellow stools evening or morning.

Skin - ***Stings of insects and insect bites.*** Burns. ***Punctures, stab wounds. Lacerated wounds*** with much prostration from loss of blood. ***Painful scars in tissues rich in nerves.*** Old ulcers or sores in mouth when very sensitive. ***Dog and animal bites.*** Skin rough as if full of small knots. ***Cat scratches.*** Eczema of hands and face. Intense itching, eruption seems to be under the skin. ***Pains from surgical cuts.*** Great itching when undressing. Herpes zoster.

Smarting eruption like nettle-rash, on the hands. Falling of hair after injury. Pimples on forehead, throat, back, hips. Hard, dry, yellow crusts form on healing wounds or open sores. Foul, torpid and phagedenic ulcers. Tetters, beginning with sore places, and forming hard, yellow crusts, with violent itching.

Sleep - Constant drowsiness. Talks wildly in night after 4 a.m. while asleep, apprehensive, gasped for air. Spasmodic jerks in arms or legs on going to sleep, twitching. Wakes 4 a.m. with sense of levitation. Feels refreshed or weary on waking. Active, vivid, distressing dreams. Dreams of traveling. Laborious dreams.

Stomach - Belches while drinking water. Pressure at the stomach on eating but little. Feeling of lump in stomach (Abies-n., Bry.). Sticking pain in stomach. Eructations, tasteless, bitter, preventing sleep at night. Nausea, weakness every morning. Nausea, abdomen distended, cracking pains in bowels, awaking in the night. Nausea and inclination to vomit.

Teeth - ***Nerve pains after dental work.*** Toothache better lying on affected side quietly. ***Injuries to dental nerves.*** Pains after root canals. Teeth sensitive and painful after dental surgery.

Temperature - Shuddering over whole body with desire to urinate. Chill followed by heat, with sweat on hands and feet. Heat with delirium, wild, staring look. Hot head, throbbing of the carotids, bright-red, bloated face. Burning heat of the skin, great oppression and anguish.

Throat - Raw, sore feeling in throat, after sneezing. Sensation as of a worm moving in throat. Hot risings in esophagus after a fright or with anxious feeling. Hoarseness, scraping and roughness in larynx, upper part of pharynx and nares, in foggy weather.

Tongue - Tongue coated white or dirty yellow, at base, tip clean. Great soreness of tongue, from lacerated wounds, with inability to speak, not from stiffness or swelling, but extreme soreness. Tongue, white at the back, tip clean. Tongue coated white, or yellow, with great thirst.

Vertigo - Confusion, vertigo and heaviness. Vertigo at night, with urging to urinate. Vertigo with loathing on waking. Vertigo with pain in temples. Vertigo with feeling of weakness and trembling of limbs.

COMMENTS - Müller, and others, proved Hyper., relating the drug to wounds, the consequences of wounds, tearing, rheumatic, shaking pains, and paralytic weakness. Crawling sensations in hands and feet, fuzzy feeling, sticking in them as from needles.

One of the provers had, on waking at 4 a.m., a feeling as though she were suspended and not lying in bed, at another time as though she were lying very heavy in bed. The former condition led to cures in effects of accidents attended with the sensation "as if being lifted high into the air and great anxiety lest she should fall from this height."

For ***acute traumas***. ***Puncture wounds, animal bites, lacerations*** (Led.). Gunshot and stab wounds, cuts from glass. Spinal taps, vaccinations. Trauma from a pinched nerve with needle-like pains that shoot from the area.

Head and nerve injuries, spinal shock injuries. Tetanus. Specific for ***tailbone injuries and whiplash***. Injuries to the spine that lead to epilepsy, paralysis or depression. Neuritis. Trauma from dental work (Arn.). Amputations, phantom pains.

Characteristic sharp, shooting, radiating pains, burning, tingling. Wounds are very sensitive to touch (Led. punctures are not particularly sensitive). Ulceration and sloughing of wounds. Hard, dry, yellow crusts form on healing wound. Exalted sense of pain, as well as hearing and smell.

Affinity for wounds of parts rich in nerves, particularly the brain, spine (spinal irritation from falls), coccyx, and finger-ends. Great nervous depression following shock or wounds. Old scars that flare up.

Bunions and corns when the pain in excruciating. Violent labor-pains and after-pains. Tympanitic distention of abdomen, cutting pains. Summer diarrhea with eruption. Palpitation and local congestions with or without hemorrhage.

Asthma, worse in foggy weather, attacks were better by copious expectoration. Whooping cough that is worse 6 to 10 p.m. Tightness of the chest, stinging that is worse on moving.

W. J. Guernsey related the case of a nine-year-old boy who was bitten by a pet rat on the first finger of his left hand. Nothing was observed at the time, but some time after, he became ill and his state was alarming when Dr. Guernsey was called.

The boy could talk with great difficulty, teeth firmly locked, conscious, neck so stiff the head could scarcely be moved. There was more tenderness about the wound than the appearance would indicate, hence Hyper. was preferred to Led.

It was given (8 p.m.) in the 500c, dissolved in water, at first every fifteen minutes, later every two hours. At 3 a.m. there was improvement, he fell asleep and the next morning was practically convalescent.

Gilchrist said Hyper. 3x, given at intervals of twenty minutes for twelve hours or longer, seems to control perfectly the pain following laparotomy.

Roehrig considered Hyper. externally and internally the nearest thing to a specific in bleeding hemorrhoids. He gave it to pneumonia patients who have hemorrhoids, it cured the pneumonia and prevented the arrest of the flux.

Usher confirmed this, "pain, bleeding and tenderness" were his indications. "It seems to suit the plethoric with great soreness." He used the 1x.

RELATIONS - ***Antidotes:*** Ars., Cham., Led. ***Compare:*** (1) Led. - puncture wounds and bites of animals. Plan. (2) Calen., Arn., Staph., Plan., Ruta, Coff.

REFERENCES - Boericke. Clarke. Murphy. Phatak.

HYPOTHALAMUS GLAND

PHARMACY - hypoth. Hypothalamus gland. The mother tincture is prepared from the hypothalamus of the ox. ***Historical dose:*** All potencies.

CLINICAL - Amenorrhea. Anorexia. Anxiety. Asthma. Baldness. Bedwetting. Constipation. Dysmenorrhea. Dyspnea. Epilepsy. Flatulence. Hemorrhoids. Insomnia. Thyroid, disorders.

HOMEOPATHIC - Hypothalamus glands are made up of pure hypothalamic hormones, (vasopressin and oxytocin, combined with a transporting protein). These hormones are liberated in their active form, under such stimuli as pain and modifications in the blood biochemistry, as well as changes in the volume of the blood.

The posterior hypophysis is therefore subject to a direct nervous control. There are no neurosecretory tissues going from the hypothalamus to the adenohypophysis, however, the blood irrigation of this gland is completely assured by the vessel gates which form in the median protuberance and which traverse the pituitary stem to flow into the sinusoid of the anterior hypophysis.

Neurons, notably those from the median protuberance, secrete substances which travel down from the neurons and accumulate at the end of the tissues. When the cells of the median protuberance are stimulated, these agents penetrate the vessel gates and the sinusoid and instigate the liberating of the anterior hypophyseal stimulants.

The usage of hypothalamus in homeopathy is clinical in nature; there is no homeopathic proving.

Clinical symptoms include physiological and nervous instability. Epileptic vertigo with almost complete loss of consciousness for a few minutes with extreme paleness of the face. Epileptiform convulsions, especially during puberty.

Occipital headaches, accompanied by an intense feeling of sadness, aggravated in the evening. Circulatory complaints with livid color of the lower limbs. Feeling that the heart has stopped and then started again, faster. Congested veins.

Malfunctioning of the thyroid with a fall in the basal metabolism. Disorders of the appetite and of the water metabolism. Water retention with obesity. Sensation of intense heat, as if sitting on a very hot furnace. Baldness during the menopause.

MIND - Depression, linked to psychological or physical stress. Likeable, extremely sensitive. Cries about trifles. Alternating smiles and tears. Easily discouraged. Sad, melancholic.

Mental fatigue, feeling that the brain is cluttered with ideas which are constantly changing. Anxiety, aggravated by darkness. Fear of falling asleep lest he should not wake again.

Lack of ability to make decisions, which can lead to loss of willpower. Sexual impulses take him by surprise, either morbid dread of the opposite sex or irresistible attraction. Morbid hunger-pangs, alternating with periods of anorexia.

Abdomen - Flatulence with extremely noisy rumbling, located principally on the right side of the abdomen.

Constitutions - Tubercular constitutions.

Female - Epileptiform complaints during puberty, especially in young girls. Menstrual cycle irregular, sometimes too short, sometimes too long. Menses copious, bleeding ameliorated by lying position. Menstrual blood very dark, congeals easily. Blood clots. Amenorrhea after physical or psychological stress. White discharge, aggravated during ovulation.

Food - Appetite disorders. Mental anorexia. Cannot bear either raw or sweet foods.

Head - Occipital headaches, accompanied by an intense feeling of sadness, aggravated in the evening.

Heart - Circulatory complaints with livid color of the lower limbs and acrocyanosis of the limbs. Feeling that the heart has stopped and then started again, faster.

Kidneys - Complaints of the water metabolism with water retention and obesity. Tenesmus of the bladder. Burning during and after urination. Urinary incontinence when lying down, walking or coughing. Bedwetting in the young.

Limbs - Inflammation of the skin beneath the nails.

Lungs - Bronchial asthma. Heavy cough, causing shooting pains in the clavicles, sternum and occiput. Cough aggravated when lying down, ameliorated by standing up. Asthma occurring after end of menses. Dyspnea with oppression and shooting pains in the left arm, not aggravated by exertion.

Male - Sexual deviations. Drawing sensation, pains going from the knee towards the testicle, especially on the right side. Inflammation of epididymis, evolving into a chronic state.

Modalities - Aggravation from cold. Tendency to evening rise of temperature, occurring irregularly but may last for several months.

Mouth - Tongue covered with a whitish coating. Loss of taste.

Nose - Thick, irritating, yellowish coryza, better heat, worse cold.

Rectum - Stubborn constipation. Stool black, very difficult to expel in small, caked balls. Hemorrhoids, bleeding easily.

Skin - Papular and pustular skin diseases. Attacks of acne during puberty, large pimples, purplish in color with itching, aggravated by scratching. Small varicose veins, very noticeable, violet in color. Nails break and have white spots. Baldness in women with thinning of the hair at the hairline.

Sleep - Insomnia or sudden, irresistible need to sleep, usually lasting only a short while, but occurring several times in one day.

Stomach - Gastric pains two hours after eating.

Temperature - Tendency to evening rise of temperature, occurring irregularly but may last for several months. Temperature fluctuations.

Vertigo - Epileptic vertigo with almost complete loss of consciousness for a few minutes with extreme paleness of the face.

RELATIONS - ***Compare:*** (1) The closest remedy is Puls., but unlike Puls., Hypoth. is aggravated by the cold, ameliorated by the heat. (2) Also note Bac. and Tub.

REFERENCES - Julian.

I

IBERIS AMARA

(Bitter Candytuft)

PHARMACY - iber. Iberis amara. Bitter candytuft. Lepidium iberis. N. O. Crucifer. Tincture of seeds. ***Historical dose:*** Tincture and all potencies.

CLINICAL - Angina pectoris. Asthma. Bradycardia. Bronchitis. Debility. Dropsy. ***Dyspnea.*** Fatigue. ***Heart, disorders. Heart, enlarged***. Heart, weakness. Liver, pain. Numbness. ***Palpitations.*** Rheumatic myocarditis. Tachycardia. Vertigo.

HERBAL - The genus was named by Dioscorides from Iberia, Spain, its supposed original habitat. Ancient authorities mentioned Iberis as useful in the treatment of hypertrophy of the heart. This led Hale to have the remedy proved. Hale considered Iber.'s primary depressing action a transient one, the secondary, exciting action is more persistent.

HOMEOPATHIC - Iber. has a marked action on the heart and is useful in heart diseases. Sylvester observed that Iber. controlled the violence and sharp action of the heart and softened the pulse. Hale's provers confirmed this observation, the pulse being softened even during palpitations.

Controls vascular excitement in hypertrophy with thickening of the heart's walls. ***Heart enlarged with thickening of the heart walls***. Infarction of the myocardium. Paroxysmal tachycardia. ***Conscious of heart's action***. State of nervous excitement and fright.

Dull or stitching pains. "On turning on left side a sharp sticking pain is felt as if a needle were crosswise in the ventricles and pricked at each contraction." Sharp, stinging pains, through the chest. Pains down the left arm and numbness with an intermittent pulse.

Palpitations with vertigo and choking in the throat, worse slightest exertion, laughing, coughing. Palpitations and breathlessness on slightest exertion. Dyspnea and palpitations on going up the stairs (Calc.).

Darting pains through heart. Weakness of heart after influenza (Crat.). Cold hands and feet.

Numbness and tingling in left hand and arm. Feeling of lameness and soreness through whole body, as from a cold. Fullness and heat in head and neck, vertigo, nausea. Liver region full and painful. Choking sensation in the throat. White stool (Dig.). Desire for stimulants.

MIND - Nervous and irritable, especially on rising in the morning. Frightened, indefinable fear with trembling. Excited, cold sweat on face. Fear of taking too much medicine. Depression. Sad, down-hearted, oppressed with desire to sigh. Aware of heart's action.

Bad-tempered. Very irritable with dullness of mind and lack of memory. Inability to fix mind on any one thing. Diminution in intellectual capacity with poor powers of concentration. Trouble in remembering recent events, but can remember past events.

Abdomen - Heaviness and pain in the hepatic region. Fullness with oppression in right hypochondriac region. Fullness and distention of bowels. Intestinal process accelerated with painful cramps, eased by the elimination of gas.

Back - Sensation of fullness in neck and head.

Chest - Fullness in chest with fullness and heat in head and neck and flushed face. Continued feeling of weight and anxiety in chest. Slight pain under sternum, at articulation of third rib. Fullness and constriction under sternum with sharp pain through chest.

Ears - Dullness of hearing and comprehension, labored breathing. Roaring in ears with heaviness of head, slight nausea and palpitation of heart.

Eyes - Red eyes with flushed face. Feeling in eyes as if being forced outward. Flashes before eyes with dull headache and palpitations of heart.

Face - Sick looking. Flushed hot face and red eyes with palpitations. Cold sweat on face, with fearfulness.

Food - Loss of appetite with feeling of indigestion. Desire for stimulants. Ameliorated by eating.

Head - Headache with nausea and loss of appetite. Dull headache, with vertigo and feverish chilliness. Sensation of heaviness and fullness in the head with buzzing in the ears. Congestion and headache, ameliorated by fresh air.

Heart - Conscious of heart's action. Heart's action weak and fluttering, with small weak pulse. ***Pulse full, irregular intermittent***. Pulse has peculiar double beats, which seem to run into each other. Pulse full, soft and easily compressed. ***Enlarged heart.*** Dropsy with enlarged heart. Dilation of heart. Hypertrophy of heart. ***Tachycardia***. Palpitations with vertigo and choking in throat. ***Violent palpitations induced by slightest exertion or by laughing or coughing.*** Wakes with palpitations about 2 a.m. On turning on left side, stitching pain as of needles through ventricles felt at each systole. Darting pains through heart. Stabbing pain in heart with constriction in throat. Sharp pains in cardiac region. Sensation of weight and pressure with occasional sharp, stinging pains.

Kidneys - Frequent but scanty urination. Excessive evacuation of urine. Frequent presence of bile pigment in the urine.

Limbs - Cold feet and hands. Numbness and tingling in left hand and arm. Whole body sore, lame and trembling.

Lungs - Dyspnea and palpitations on going upstairs. ***Heart dyspnea, shortness of breath***. Constant desire to draw breath without relief (Carb-v.). Respiration more frequent and labored. Pulmonary rattle with viscous, stringy sputum. Constant hawking of thick, stringy mucus until after a meal. Cough causes redness of face.

Modalities - Better by eating, belching, expelling gas, cold. Worse lying down, on left side, on turning in bed, motion, exertion, sitting still. Worse from heat, warm room, at night, morning, on rising.

Mouth - Dryness of the mouth with bitter or peppery taste.

Rectum - Pain in region of liver with large, clay-colored stool. Tenderness of bowels with thin, whitish stool.

Sleep - Sleep disturbed with aggravating dreams. Restless turning in bed with ludicrous dreams.

Stomach - Heavy and full sensation in the gastric region. After eating, sour belching, better hawking of stringy mucus. Nausea with cold, chilly feelings over body. Heartburn, nausea with belching, which eases the condition.

Temperature - Cold, chilly feeling with nausea. Feverish chilliness. Quickly passing febrile symptoms. Heat and fullness in neck and head with flushed face and cold feet and hands.

Throat - Dryness in the throat and larynx with feeling of constriction. Tickling in throat. Throat as if filled with dust. As if both tonsils were enlarged. Throat and trachea fills up with mucus. Constant hawking up of thick, viscid, stringy mucus better after a meal. Choking sensation in throat with fullness and heat, just above cricoid cartilage. Constrictive sensation in throat with stabbing pains in heart, dyspnea and palpitations.

Vertigo - Vertigo and pains around heart. ***Vertigo, as if occiput were turning around***. Vertigo, eyes feel forced outwards. Vertigo on standing, ameliorated by lying down. Vertigo with dull pain and chilliness.

COMMENTS - Proctor related his own experience with this remedy. After an attack of influenza of moderate intensity in 1890, he suffered from cardiac weakness for over two years. Every waking moment was attended with cardiac distress.

On the least agitation the weakness developed into irregular palpitation with great anxiety. Worse from tobacco, which had to be discarded. Worse from wine, except port. After all the usual remedies had been taken in vain, he took Iber., one drop in a powder on the tongue, two or three times a day.

After about ten days the heart suddenly fell almost into its perfect, regular, unconscious beat and retired at once and finally from further observation. Proctor repeatedly gave Iber. since then in similar cases with the same success.

RELATIONS - *Compare:* (1) Aml-n., Lepi., Spig., Dig., Cact., Bell., Crat., Phase. (2) Spig. - Palpitations, violent contraction of the heart with oppression and anxiety. (3) Cact. - Sensation of constriction in the heart like a vice. Constriction of the head and chest. (4) Aur. - Palpitations with hot flushes, forcing the patient to remain seated with the body bent forwards.

REFERENCES - Boericke. Clarke. Julian.

ICHTHYOLUM

PHARMACY - ichth. Ichthyolum. Ammonium ichthyol sulphonate. Solution. The most important of the salts are the ichthyosulphonic acids, prepared from a bituminous mineral of Tyrol, which is rich in fossilized remains of fish. A clear, reddish-brown viscid liquid. ***Historical dose:*** Tincture and all potencies.

CLINICAL - Acne, rosacea. Alcoholism. Arthritis. ***Boils.*** Bronchiectasis. Bronchitis. Chilblains. Coryza. ***Cough.*** Eczema. Gonorrhea. Gout. Hay fever. ***Hives. Nausea.*** Neuralgias. Polyarthritis. Pruritus, vulvae. Psoriasis. Rheumatism. Scabies. Skin disorders. ***Tuberculosis. Uric acid.*** Urticaria.

HOMEOPATHIC - Ichthyolum is an unproved remedy which has been used in old-school therapeutics as an external application and internally in skin affections, rheumatism, scrofula, nephritis and gonorrhea.

Ichth. is a powerful antiseptic. It has achieved marked results as an external application to rheumatic joints. A solution of equal parts of Ichthyol and water is warmed and applied to the affected joint on calico and covered with heated cloths, outside of which is an impervious fabric to prevent evaporation.

Pure Ichthyol or an ointment of Lanoline and Ichthyol may be used instead with Lanoline making up 20 to 50 percent of the ointment. Externally, it is used as an ointment for chronic eczema, psoriasis, acne rosacea, gouty joints, chilblains and scabies. Rectal suppositories for senile prostate. Its action on skin, mucus membranes and kidneys is prompt and useful.

It is strongly anti-parasitic, redness, pain and inflammation, and decreases tension. Polyarthritis. Chronic rheumatism. ***Uric acid diathesis***. Gouty joints. Alcoholism, when nothing will stay on stomach.

Hay fever. ***Chronic hives.*** Excellent in winter coughs of old people. ***Tuberculosis, helps nutrition.*** Scarpa claimed to have used it with excellent effect in a large number of cases of tuberculosis.

MIND - Irritable and depressed. Forgetful, lack of concentration.

Abdomen - Griping in umbilical and left hypogastric region.

Eyes - Burn, red, worse any change of temperature.

Face - Skin feels dry and itches. Acne on chin.

Female - Fullness in lower abdomen. Nausea at time of menses.

Food - ***Increased appetite***.

Head - Dull aching, better cold, pressure. Dull frontal and supra-orbital headache, worse moving eyes, cold air, better warmth.

Kidneys - Burning pain in meatus. Increased in quantity and frequency. Uric acid deposits.

Limbs - Lameness in right shoulder and right lower extremity.

Lungs - ***Dry, teasing cough***. Bronchitis, especially of the aged. Bronchiectasis and tuberculosis.

Mouth - Disagreeable taste, burning sensation, very thirsty.

Nose - Bland coryza, stuffed feeling, feels sore inside. Irresistible desire to sneeze.

Rectum - Disposition to soft, shapeless stools. Early morning diarrhea.

Skin - Heat and irritation, ***Itching***. Scaly and itching eczema. Psoriasis. ***Hives.*** Acne rosacea, erysipelas. ***Crops of boils***. Itching during pregnancy.

Stomach - ***Nausea.***

Throat - Irritated, pain to ears, sore, dry with hawking and expectoration.

COMMENTS - Anshutz wrote: "The principal action of Ichthyol in the following proving seems to have been on the mucus membranes of the nose and throat, on muscle tissue, producing rheumatic pain, on the skin and on the urine.

"The blood count was not conclusive, only two cases being tested and in one a diminution of red blood corpuscles before after taking the drug) was noted. No marked change in the number or character of the leucocytes and lymphocytes was noted.

"Most of the provers had increased appetite and after taking the drug for some time a marked feeling of well-being. Stool became free in some cases diarrhea and offensive.

"A languid, tired feeling with mental torpidity while actively taking the drug was usually followed by a feeling of improved, vigorous health when the drug was left off to be again repeated upon renewed administration of the remedy.

"The skin showed many interesting changes worthy of further proving, pruritus, acne and urticaria being produced. Rheumatic pains in different parts of the body were also noted.

"The urine showed valuable changes: Increased urination was noted in all cases with a change in color from the usual straw to a dark straw or reddish tint. The solids were increased, as were the sulphates.

"In many cases uric acid was deposited in the form of brick-dust or red sand, which microscopically proved to be the lozenge, plate and gravel form of uric acid crystals.

"Calcium oxalate crystals were also found in a few cases and in several instances the passage of the crystals produced a mild inflammation of the pelvis of the kidney (mild catarrhal pyelitis) which in the writer's case disappeared after six months, when the urine had again become normal.

"Therapeutically it would seem that in Ichthyol we have a potent remedy for the uric acid diathesis with its various manifestations and symptoms. Lithemia, as indicated by the urinary proving, should prove amenable to the drug if given in potency.

"Hay fever symptoms were also prominent in the proving of the drug and its application in this intractable affection is awaited with interest, local applications of Ichthyol having been used by a number of physicians in cases of hay fever with quite satisfactory results for some time.

"The lachrymation, coryza and the dry, teasing cough of measles seems also well pictured in some of the symptoms produced by this drug. Whooping cough tonsillitis and tiresome intractable cough of the aged suffering from bronchial disorders would also appear to offer a chance for trial with this remedy.

"It was prescribed it in several cases of gonorrhea with frequent urination and burning in the anterior urethra with some success. Some have seen the remedy act beneficially in dry, hacking coughs such as were developed by the provers.

"The 3x, 6x and 8x potency, especially the latter, were employed."

RELATIONS - ***Compare:*** (1) Hep., Calc., Sil., Sulph., Ars., Petr. (2) Ichth. belongs to the Petroleum class of remedies. (3) Carb-ac. (4) Caust. - lime-water compresses to allay inflammations. (5) Plantago - anodyne application.

REFERENCES - Boericke. Clarke. Phatak.

ICTODES FOETIDA

(Skunk Cabbage)

PHARMACY - ictod. Ictodes foetida. Skunk cabbage. Skunk-weed. Dracontium foetidum. Pothos foetidus. Symplocarpus foetidus. N. O. Orontiacee, Calliacee orontoide, allied to Araceae. Tincture of whole fresh plant including root. The root loses its pungent taste and appears to be nearly inert a few weeks after it is gathered. ***Historical dose:*** Tincture and all potencies.

CLINICAL - Amenorrhea. ***Asthma.*** Catarrh. Coughs. Dropsy. Dyspnea. Epilepsy. Headaches. Herpes. Hysteria. Nausea. Pertussis. Rheumatism. Scurvy. Ulcers. Vertigo. Vomiting. Whooping cough. Worms.

HERBAL - The smell from spathe and Ictod. flowers is pungent and very subtle. The seeds are said to afford more relief in asthmatic cases than the root, for they are remarkably active, pungent and exhale the odor of asafetida.

An acrid principle resides in the root, even when perfectly dry, producing an effect like that of the Arum and the Ranunculi. When chewed in the mouth, the root is slow in manifesting its peculiar taste, but after some moments a pricking sensation is felt, which soon amounts to a disagreeable smarting and continues for some time.

This acrimony is readily dissipated by heat and the decoction retains none of it. The distilled water is impregnated with it, if the process is carefully conducted, but loses it on standing a short time. To insure a tolerably uniform activity of this medicine, the root should be kept in dried slices and not reduced to powder until it is needed.

The bruised leaves are frequently applied to ulcers and recent wounds with good effect. They are also used as an external application in cutaneous disorders and the expressed juice has been successfully applied to different species of herpes. The leaves are also used to dress blisters with the view of promoting their discharge.

The Treasury of Botany explains the traditional uses of this plant in medicine: "The roots in cases of asthma, the leaves as an application to ulcers. The seeds are also considered to be anti-spasmodic and useful in coughs."

Skunk cabbage is not only a good antispasmodic in all cases where such are indicated, but it is also a powerful emmenagogue, antihelmintic and a valuable remedy in dropsy in spasms, rheumatism, palpitations, etc.

HOMEOPATHIC - Hering, and others, proved Ictod. and largely confirmed its popular reputation, and also its clinical relationship to the Arum family. Ictod. is a powerful anti-spasmodic, expectorant, vermifuge, menagogue, sudorific, etc.

Spasmodic asthma and coughs. ***Asthmatic complaints worse by inhalation of dust*** and relieved by stools. Burning sensations from fauces down throat, enlarged glands of throat, swelling of nose and sneezing, spasmodic cough and skin disorders. Pertussis. Pain in throat while sneezing.

Hysterics. Epilepsy. Erratic and spasmodic pains. Dropsy. Chronic rheumatism. Headache in small spots with throbbing in temporal arteries. Red swelling across the nose. Tongue numb. Abdomen distended. Inclined to smoke, but it does not taste good.

Used in childbed to promote birth. Erratic and spasmodic pains with childbirth. Worms, the pulverized root should be administered in molasses for a sufficient length of time, following it up with a purgative. Scurvy.

MIND - Absence of mind. Inattention, enters sick-room without knocking, does not listen to patient. Irritable, cross. Impetuous, inclined to contradict.

Abdomen - Expansion and tension in abdomen. Pain in abdomen here and there in single spots. When walking, sensation as if the entrails were hanging loose and flabby without any pain.

Chest - Pain in chest and in axilla, seems to have a connection with burning in esophagus. Pressing pain in sternum.

Face - Swollen submaxillary glands.

Female - Amenorrhea.

Food - Inclined to smoke, but it does not taste good.

Head - Headache in single places, lasting a short while, then changing place. Dullness, pressing pain in temples, now more in one, then more in the other, with violent pulsation of arteries. Drawing in forehead in two lines from protuberances to glabella, where it draws outward as from a magnet.

Kidneys - Great urging, urine dark.

Limbs - Aching along right tibia.

Lungs - Spasmodic asthma, cough. Asthma, worse or caused by dust. Heaves in horses from dusty hay. Inclined to take a deep breath. Hollowness of chest with constriction in fauces and chest. Senile catarrh. Sudden anxiety with dyspnea and sweat, followed by stool, which relieves.

Male - Titillation, voluptuous but painful, around corona glandis.

Modalities - Better in open air. Motion aggravates.

Mouth - Scurvy. Numbness of tongue, cannot touch teeth with it. Papilla elevated. Tongue red and sore on tip and edges.

Nose - The nose is swollen as far as the nasal bones extend, red like a saddle, sore to touch, worse left side. Cartilage cold and bloodless with red spots on cheeks and small pimples on left side of face. Violent sneezing with pains in palate, fauces and esophagus to stomach, hurting for a while after in cardiac end of stomach.

Skin - Herpes and skin affections.

Stomach - Nausea and vomiting. With every firm step, pain in pit of stomach as from something breaking loose.

Throat - Burning from fauces down through chest. Esophagus is painful on sneezing.

Vertigo - Vertigo and dimness of sight.

COMMENTS - Anshutz reported: "a young woman, about eighteen years of age, was harassed by severe convulsive and hysteric paroxysms, almost incessantly in so much that her friends estimated the number at seven hundred in the course of a few weeks, her abdomen was remarkably tumefied and tense and there was a bloatedness of the whole surface of her body and the slightest touch would occasion intolerable pain.

"At length her limbs became rigid and immovable and her jaw was so completely locked that she was unable to articulate and liquids could only be introduced through the vacuity of a lost tooth. She had been treated with a variety of antispasmodic and other medicines, by an experienced physician without relief. Having prepared a strong infusion of the dried root of skunk cabbage, Anshutz directed half a tea cupful to be given every few hours without any other medicine.

"The favorable effects of which were soon observable and by persisting in the use of it about ten days the muscular contractions were removed, the jaw was relaxed and her faculty of speech and swallowing with the use of all her limbs, were completely effected.

"Another young woman had the most distressing attacks of hysteria for several days without obtaining relief by the medicines prescribed. When the skunk cabbage infusion as so successfully directed that her fits were immediately arrested and in a few days a cure was completely affected.

"The brother of this patient was seized with violent convulsions of the whole body in consequence of a cut on his foot, the skunk cabbage was administered and he was speedily restored to perfect health.

"A woman was affected with violent spasmodic pains, twenty four hours after childbirth, six doses of skunk cabbage entirely removed her complaints. A number of cases catarrhal disorders of the old people in which a syrup prepared from the root in substance has alleviated and removed the complaint.

"In delicate stomachs it occasion vomiting even in a small quantity. In several cases of gastrodynia, where it was given with a view to its antispasmodic effect, it was ejected from the stomach more speedily than common cathartic medicines.

"In a dose of thirty grains to bring on not only vomiting, but headache, vertigo and temporary blindness. The root is a pungent antispasmodic in colics and griping of the bowels. Leaves when bruised relieve painful swellings, whitlows, etc.

"In chronic cough attended with a cold phlegmatic habit of body, the powdered root of this plant was employed with the most decided benefit. In an old man who has been for many years afflicted with a very troublesome cough and difficulty of breathing. In cases of chronic catarrhal and asthmatic disorders."

RELATIONS - ***Compare:*** (1) Arum t., Asaf., Meph.

REFERENCES - Anshutz.

IGNATIA AMARA

(St. Ignatius Bean)

PHARMACY - ign. Ignatia amara. St. Ignatia's bean. Strychnos ignatia. Strychnos multiflora. Faba indica. N. O. Loganiacae. Philippine Islands. The seeds of Ign. contain a larger proportion of strychnine than those of Nux vomica. Tincture of dried seeds. Tincture and trituration of the seeds. ***Historical dose:*** All potencies.

CLINICAL - ***Amenorrhea.*** Anger, effects. Anguish. Anorexia. Anus, disorders. Anxiety. Appetite, disordered. Ascarides. ***Asthenopia***. Back, weakness. Belching. Bulimia. Catalepsy. Chilblains. Chills. Chorea. Ciliary neuralgia. Clavus. ***Colic.*** Constipation. ***Convulsions. Cramps.*** Croup. Coughs. Debility. Dentition. ***Depression.*** Diarrhea. Diphtheria. ***Disappointment. Dysmenorrhea.*** Dyspepsia. ***Dyspnea. Epilepsy.*** Esophagus, disorders. Fainting. Fever. Flatulence, obstructed. ***Fright, effects.*** Glands, enlarged. ***Globus, hystericus. Grief***. Headaches. Heart, disorders. Hemorrhoids. Hiccoughs. Hydrocephalus. ***Hysteria***. Hysterical-joint. ***Insomnia.*** Intermittent, fever. Lockjaw. Locomotor ataxia. Melancholy. Meningitis. Menopause. Metrorrhagia. Monomania. Nausea. Neuralgia. Nightmares. Nosebleed. Numbness. Ophthalmia. Opisthotonos. ***Palpitations.*** Paralysis. Plague. Premenstrual syndrome. Rectum, pain. Rectum, prolapsed. Rheumatic, fever. Sciatica. ***Sensitiveness. Shock, emotional. Sighing.*** Sinking. Sleep, disordered. ***Spasms.*** Spinal, irritation. Tenesmus. Throat, sore. ***Tobacco, allergy. Tonsillitis.*** Toothaches. ***Tremors. Twitching.*** Ulcers. Urine, abnormal. Vagina, spasm. Vertigo. Voice, lost. Vomiting. Yawning. Whooping cough. ***Worms. Worry.***

HOMEOPATHIC - Ignatia seeds contain a larger proportion of strychnine than those of Nux vomica, yet there is a great difference between the characteristic features of the two drugs, pointing to the importance of considering the medicines apart form their "active" principles. Ign. has been called the "feminine" of the "masculine" Nux-v.

Ignatia is adapted to persons of nervous temperament, especially women of a sensitive, easily excited nature and mild disposition, who are quick to perceive and rapid in execution.

Marked hypersensitivity of all the senses and a tendency to clonic spasms. ***Effects of grief and worry. An emotional state of grief or frustration***. For emotional shock, conflict, disappointment, fright and grief.

Characteristic ***changeable and erratic character*** of its symptoms. It causes erratic, contradictory, paradoxical mental and physical effects, which change rapidly and are opposite each other. Alert, nervous, apprehensive, rigid, trembling patients who suffer acutely in mind or body. Worse by drinking coffee. ***Cannot bear the smell of tobacco smoke***.

Violent spasmodic effects, with rigidity, twitching and tremors. Spasms with cries or involuntary laughter. Spasms alternating with oppressed breathing. Hysteria.

Convulsions of children during dentition after punishment after fear or fright, return at the same hour daily. Chorea after fright from grief worse after eating, better lying on back. Catalepsy with opisthotonos (Nat-m. will follow in some chronic conditions). Paralysis after great mental emotions or night watching.

Pain in small, circumscribed spots (Ox-ac.), worse close attention. Pains change their locality, come gradually, abate suddenly or come and go suddenly. ***Oversensitive to pain.*** Nervous shuddering with pain.

Hiccoughs and hysterical vomiting. ***Sensation of lump,*** foreign body or sharp pressure. Globus. Symptoms pass after profuse urination. Preventative and curative for plague. Clavus.

MIND - ***Suppressed or deep grief with long-drawn sighs. Sobs in long drawn-out sighs.*** Anguish, shrieks for help. Melancholic, sad, tearful. ***Sadness and sighing with empty feeling in pit of stomach.***

Ailments from grief, emotional shocks and disappointments. Ailments from hearing bad news, ***from fright,*** vexation with reserved displeasure, shame or embarrassments.

Disorders of the mind, particularly if actuated by grief, sadness, hopelessness, hysterical variableness, fantastic illusions.

Much unhappiness, cannot sleep, entirely absorbed in grief. Inward weeping. Broods, sometimes over imaginary troubles. Introspective. Narrating her symptoms aggravates. ***Worse from consolation.*** Desire to be alone, to smother grief. Full of suppressed grief, seems weighed down by it. Indifference. Aversion to every amusement.

Oversensitive and nervous. Intolerant of contradiction or reprimands. ***Constantly frustrated.*** Irritable. Everything irks her. ***Quarrelsome.*** Angry at self. Sense of neglected duty. ***Internal conflicts.*** Anger, followed by quiet grief or sorrow.

Capricious, changeable, ***rapid alternation of moods. Highly emotional and moody. Oversensitive to pain. Joking and laughter changing to sadness and tears.*** Uncontrollable emotions. Hysteria. Globus hystericus. Every little emotion disturbs.

Spasms and insanity after grief or fright. Epilepsy after grief or fright. Delights to bring on her fits and produce a scare or a scene. Rages and tears clothes, can scarcely be restrained. Looks about the bed as if to find something. Childish behavior. Monomania. Obsessive compulsive disorder. Bulimia. Anorexia.

Anxiety, as if something terrible had happened. Fearfulness, terror, alternating with irresolution and inertness. Fear of trifles, of things coming near, of robbers at night on waking. Fear of being hurt and disappointed. Fear he will never sleep again.

Mild, gentle, yielding, whimsical and introverted. ***Idealistic, sentimental and romantic.*** Sensitive, impressionable. Delicately conscientious. Faints, falls easily in love, with married men (Nat-m.). ***Love sick,*** homesick. Aversion to being alone. Jealousy from disappointed love. Inclined to be very secretive and passive. Fixed ideas. Perfectionist.

Delusion she is breaking her vow. Imagines her soul can't be saved and cries. Imagines that she might go crazy, with suppressed menses.

Believes herself married and pregnant. Hatred of men. Suicidal thoughts and desire to escape.

Mistakes in writing and talking and awkward motions. Incapacity for thought in evening. Very great weakness of memory. Forgets everything except dreams. Hurried in mental work. Sensitive to noise.

Abdomen - ***Abdominal spasms and cramps.*** Periodic cramp-like pains in the abdomen. Weak feeling in upper abdomen. Throbbing in abdomen (Aloe, Sang.). Twisting pain around navel. Colicky, griping pains in sides of abdomen. ***Abdominal colic pains worse brandy, coffee and sweet things. Flatulent colic, especially at night.*** Flatulence presses on the bladder. ***Extreme flatulence with hysteria.*** Rumbling in bowels. ***Fullness and distension, causes inability to breathe.*** Sensation as if the intestines were going to burst. Sensation of hardness and swelling in region of spleen. Sensation of protrusion in umbilical region. Anxious feeling rising from abdomen, after breakfast. Distension of abdomen after eating, during pregnancy.

Back - Convulsive bending backwards of the spine. Back is bent forward. ***Back spasms and cramps.*** Cutting, sharp pains from small of back. Backache during chill. Weak back with sciatica. ***Twitching of muscles.*** Aching pain in the glands of the neck. Stiffness of the nape of the neck. Pain in the os sacrum in the morning, when lying on the back. Violent sacral pains. Spinal disease with gressus gallinaceus.

Breasts - Sharp pains in nipples on deep inspiration. Milk diminished. Infantile colic after taking breast of mother or nurse, who suffers from grief.

Causations - Ill effects of disappointed love, grief, fright, worry, jealousy, old spinal injuries.

Chest - Sharp pain in left chest. Sharp pains in chest from flatulent colic. ***Constriction of the chest***. Chest feels as if too small. Throbbing, aching in the chest. Shootings in the chest and in the sides, excited by flatulency. Oppression of chest, with severe choking sensation from stomach up into throat, better eructation.

Constitutions - Suited to sensitive, excitable, nervous temperament, women of a sensitive, easily excited nature, dark hair and skin, but mild disposition, quick to perceive, rapid to execute. Romantic, idealistic and overworked. Suitable to persons who had been starving either from want or other causes.

Coughs - Nervous cough and oppression frequently accompanying catarrhal affections in young people and women. Dry, hoarse cough. ***Dry, hacking, spasmodic cough in quick successive shocks, shutting off the breath.*** Hollow spasmodic cough, worse in the evening, little expectoration, leaving pain in trachea. Coughing increases the desire to cough. Cough, every time he stands still during a walk. Cough after warm drinks. Cough, as from dust or sulphur fumes. Cough as from feathers in pit of throat. Sleepy after each coughing spell. ***Reflex coughs from more remote affections of womb, ovaries and with worms.*** Whooping cough.

Ears - One ear red and hot. Tugging pain in ears. Obstinate itching in auditory canal. Intolerance of noise. Noise causes headache. Loud talking aggravates headaches. Roaring noises, better by music. Sound before ear, as from a strong wind. Hardness of hearing. Deafness, except for the human voice. Worry takes away hearing and intensifies the noises.

Eyes - Inflammation, redness of the eyes. Acrid tears in eyes, during day. Lachrymation with much mucus and burning in eyes during headache, especially in the brightness of the sun. Fixed look with dilated pupils. Photophobia, can't bear the glare of light. Sunlight causes headache (Nat-m.). Photophobia during menses. Ophthalmia of newborn infants. Herpes in cornea. ***Asthenopia*** with spasms of lids and neuralgic pain about eyes (Nat-m.). Ciliary neuralgia. Stabbing pain deep in eyes. Convulsive movements of the eyes, and of the eyelids. ***Twitching of eyelids.*** Swelling of upper lid. Eyelid turned upward. Eyelids seem dry. Sensation as if sand were under upper lids. Sensation of pressure and heaviness. Sensation as if eye would fall out, worse reading, sewing, etc.

Face - Face changes color when at rest. Flushing of face on emotions. Redness and heat of one cheek, red and pale alternately. Face clay-colored and sunken, with blue rings around eyes. Eruption on the face. Lips dry, cracked, and bleeding. Scabs on the commissure of the lips, and on the lips. Ulceration of the corners of the mouth. Perspiration on the face alone. Sweats on face while eating. Pains in the submaxillary glands. Swelling of the parotids, with shooting pain. ***Twitching of muscles of face and lips.*** Twitching of corners of mouth. Masseters stiff and hard. Facial muscles distort on attempting to speak. ***Spasmodic clenching of the jaws.*** Emotional trismus. Lockjaw. ***Pain in the lower jaw, as if dislocated.*** Prosopalgia due to presence of ascarides. Prosopalgia during pregnancy. Prosopalgia due to prolonged nursing.

Female - ***Suppressed menses from grief.*** Amenorrhea. Premenstrual syndrome. ***Sighing before menses.*** Constant burning heat in vagina, worse before menses. Menses, irregular, too early, too profuse, or scanty. Menstrual blood black, of putrid odor, in clots. Menses with great fatigue, spasmodic pains in stomach and abdomen. ***Menstrual cramps.*** Dysmenorrhea, with great pressure. Metrorrhagia from chamomile tea. ***Uterine hemorrhages from grief or emotional excitement.*** Cramp-like and compressive pains in the region of the uterus. Violent labor-like pains followed by purulent acrid leucorrhea. Bearing-down pains with leucorrhea. Corrosive and purulent leucorrhea, preceded by contractive pressure in the uterus. Pruritus of young girls, with leucorrhea and ascarides. Chronic leucorrhea with sexual desire. Sexual frigidity. Intensely sore pain at entrance of vagina during sex, almost driving her frantic. Nausea, weakness, sinking in stomach, better eating, during pregnancy. ***Threaten miscarriage after emotional upset, fright or grief.*** Labor pains, spasms amounting almost to convulsions. Labor doesn't progress.

After pains with much sighing, sadness and despondency. Puerperal convulsions with vomiting.

Food - Loss of appetite before and during menses. Loss of appetite from deep grief. Food has a bitter, repulsive taste, or no taste. Refuses to eat. Averse to ordinary diet, longs for great variety of indigestible articles. Appetite for various things, but when offered appetite fails. Hunger and nausea at same time. Hunger after fever. ***Aversion to fruit,***, warm food, meat, milk, alcohol, brandy, ***tobacco***. Nausea from smoking, ***repugnance to smelling tobacco smoke.*** Craving for acid things, acid fruit, sour things, raw or indigestible things, cheese, bread, sweets, chocolate. Desires cold food, which is digested, warm food causes indigestion. Milk taken in the morning leaves an after-taste for a long time. Worse tea, coffee, brandy. Beer tastes bitter or putrid. Diarrhea from fruit.

Head - Periodic, weekly, fortnightly or monthly headaches. ***Nervous headaches in hysterical women, suddenly appearing and disappearing.*** Congestive headaches following anger or grief. ***Headache, worse smoking or smelling tobacco.*** Inclines head forward. Throws the head backwards from weight at occiput or during spasms. Headache alternating with backache. ***Headache as if a nail were driven out through the side.*** As if a needle were pushed through over right eye into brain. Headache, worse or better by stooping. Head feels hollow, heavy, worse stooping. Throbbing pains, with every beat of arteries, worse stooping. Severe throbbing in forehead and over eyes, worse light. ***Headache from abuse of snuff, tobacco, smoking, alcohol, coffee.*** Headache from close attention. Headache, as if bruised or beaten in morning on waking. Headache as if temples would be pressed out. Lancinating, boring pains deep in brain with nausea. Cramp-like pain over root of nose. Trembling and shaking of head. Hydrocephalus. Meningitis, cerebrospinalis with rapid alternation of symptoms. Loss of hair.

Heart - Anxious feeling in heart region. Uncertain, weak, weary sensation in heart, after excessive anxiety followed by sudden joy. ***Constriction at heart, with anxiety and disposition to cry.*** Palpitations at night, with shootings in the heart. ***Palpitations while engaged in deep thought***, during menses, in morning in bed. Sticking in precordial region on expiration. Cardiac hyperesthesia. Pulse hard, full and frequent, with throbbing in blood vessels. Pulse variable, frequent in morning, slower during day and evening.

Kidneys - Sudden, irresistible desire to urinate. Continual urge to urinate after taking coffee. Constant urination after coughing. Urging to urinate with inability to pass urine. Involuntary emission of urine. Burning and smarting pain in urethra when urinating. Painful pressure, with scraping sensation in neck of bladder, worse walking. Itching in the fore part of the urethra. Frequent, profuse, watery urine (Ph-ac.). Urine clear, lemon-colored, turbid, scanty, dark and acrid.

Limbs - ***Cramps, twitching and spasms in the limbs.*** Jerking in limbs. Painfulness of limbs on going to sleep. Tingling and sensation as if limbs had gone to sleep. Sciatica, worse in winter, better in summer. As if flesh was loose on bones from a blow. ***Joints as if dislocated.*** Lancinating, cutting pain in the shoulder joint, when bending the arm forward. Trembling of hands when writing. Warm sweat on the palms. Knees are involuntarily drawn upwards, when walking. Knees hot with cold nose. Cramps in calves. Pain in Achilles tendon and calf. Burning in heels on placing them near one another, when they come in contact they are cold to touch, worse at night. Heavy sensation in feet. Ulcerative pain in soles. Corns painful as if sore.

Lungs - ***Dyspnea***, as from a load on chest. Catching respiration. ***Takes deep breath,*** for relief. ***Much sighing***. Sighing and sobbing continue long after crying. Loses breath when running. Oppressed breathing, alternating with convulsions. Oppressed breathing, at night, worse after midnight. Snoring inspiration during sleep. Inspiration slow, expiration quick. Expectoration tasting and smelling like old catarrh. Difficult expectoration, in evening. Choking, spasms of glottis (Cupr.). Sleepy after coughing.

Male - Sweat on scrotum. Itching about genitals, in bed. Much itching in the penis, removed by scratching. Soreness and ulcerative pain, with itching at margin of prepuce. Pain in penis, during cough. Penis, contracted, becomes small. Lasciviousness and weakness of genital power, without erections. Absence of sexual desire. Sexual desire with impotence. Erections with painful uneasiness, and aching at the pubis. Erection before and during stool with emission of prostatic fluid.

Modalities - Better while eating, swallowing, sour things. Better change of position, lying on affected part, lying on back, pressure, deep breathing, near a warm stove, urination, being alone. ***Worse shock, grief, worry, fright, chagrin, emotions, after losing persons or objects*** that were very dear. Worse from open air, cold, external warmth, at the same hour and day, in the morning. Worse odors, after meals, liquids, ***coffee, stimulants, tobacco smoke***. Worse yawning, stooping, walking, standing, slight touch.

Mouth - Foam at the mouth. Putrid odor from mouth. ***Sour taste***. Accumulation of acid saliva in the mouth. Constant flow of saliva prevents sleep. Mouth constantly full of white, frothy mucus. Constant spitting. ***Spasmodic closing of the jaws.*** Bites inside of cheeks when talking or chewing. Redness and inflammation of the mouth and of the palate. Sharp pains in palate, extending to the ear. Swelling of orifices of salivary glands. Inner surface of lower lip seems raw. Lips dry, cracked, bleeding.

Nose - Fluent coryza. Stoppage of one nostril, dry coryza, with dull headache, and excessive nervous excitement. Dry catarrh, with crawling and itching in nostrils, which are sore, sensitive or swollen. Nostrils excoriated and ulcerated, with swelling of the nose. Pain over the root of the nose. Dryness of the nose. Cold, with hot knees. Sensitive to inspired air. Sneezing attacks. Nosebleed.

Perspiration - Sweat at times cold, but generally warm and somewhat sour-smelling. Sweat, worse on eating, often on a small spot on the face. Feeling as if sweat would break out, but does not. Warm sweat, on palms of hands. Slight sweat only on face. Sweats with fainting. Sweats in children during dentition.

Rectum - Constipation from taking cold. Constipation from riding in a carriage. Constipation with constant, ineffectual urging to stool. Diarrhea alternating with constipation. Diarrhea from fruit. Diarrhea from fright. Diarrhea from emotional excitement, grief. Painless diarrhea with rumbling of gas. Prolapse of rectum from moderate straining at stool. ***Painful constriction of anus after stool.*** Painless contractions of anus. Hemorrhoids, better sitting, worse coughing. Sharp pain in hemorrhoids during cough. Sharp pain from anus deep into rectum. Hemorrhage and pain, worse when stool is loose. ***Pressure as if a sharp instrument from within outward***. Contraction of the anus. Spasmodic tension in rectum. Discharge of blood from the anus. Blotches at anus. Itching, crawling and tingling in the anus. Threadworms in rectum. Ascarides in the rectum.

Skin - Itching, nettle-rash. Nettle rash over the whole body with violent itching during fever. Itching on becoming warm in the open air. Great sensitiveness of the skin to a draft of air. Excoriation of the skin, especially around vagina and mouth. Fine pricking like flea bites. Ulcers, painless, discharge scanty. Ulcers, burning, generally worse slight touch, better hard pressure. Chilblains.

Sleep - Violent spasmodic yawning with running from eyes. Sleepy after coughing. ***Insomnia from grief, worries***. Sleeplessness from anxious thoughts, depressing emotions, overstraining mind, ***relationships or business cares.*** Jerking of limbs on going to sleep. Very light sleep, hears everything that happens around him.

Frequent changing position at night in bed. Whimpering while sleeping. Children with hiccough, chewing motions of mouth during sleep. Sleepwalking from wounded pride, honor. Profound and comatose sleep with a stertorous breathing. Nightmares, over and over again. Dreams about grief, death of loved ones, broken relationships. Child awakes from sleep with piercing cries and trembles all over.

Stomach - Periodical attacks of cramps in the stomach, worse slightest contact. ***Sinking feeling in stomach,*** relieved by taking a deep breath. Gnawing, cutting pains in stomach. All-gone sensation in stomach. Feeling in stomach as from fasting, with physical exhaustion. Trembling in stomach. Catarrh of stomach from grief or worries. ***Much flatulence***. Dyspepsia with great nervous prostration, caused by mental depression. Hiccough after emotions, from smoking. Hiccough with belchings empty or bitter after eating, drinking. Sour eructation. Hunger with nausea. Nausea with agitation and anguish. Nauseous feeling in pit during cough. Nausea while standing, better sitting down. Nausea or vomiting, better indigestible things. Vomiting of bile and mucus. Regurgitation of food, or of bitter serous matter.

Stool - Stools, whitish, yellowish white, slimy, thin, pasty. Stools, mucus, bloody mucus, mucus with colic, acrid. Stools large and soft, pass with difficulty.

Teeth - Looseness of the teeth. Toothache, as if the teeth were broken. Boring pain in front teeth. Soreness in all teeth. Toothache, towards the end of a meal, worse after its conclusion, worse after drinking coffee and smoking. Toothache from cold. Difficult dentition with convulsions.

Temperature - External chills with internal heat, or external heat with internal chill. Chill or heat of single parts only. Chill with thirst, not relieved by external heat. Chill with red face. Shaking chill. Chill during pains. Chills begins as soon as back is least uncovered. Chills proceeding from abdomen. Fever with itching, nettle-rash all over body. Fever with aversion to uncover but no thirst. Febrile shivering, especially in the back and arms. Fever with thirst for cold water, and sometimes with nausea and vomiting. Fever with cold feet. Frequent heat flushes with sweat. Fever with fainting. Fever with coldness of feet and spasmodic twitching of limbs.

Throat - ***Hysterical spasm of throat***, result of suppressed grief, can't swallow either liquids or solids. Spasm of glottis (Calc.). Tendency to choke. Choking sensation from stomach up to throat. Cramps in gullet. ***Globus hystericus. Sensation as if a lump in throat,*** that cannot be swallowed. Sore throat, as if there were a plug in it, when not swallowing. Sore throat, sharp pain when not swallowing, better eating something solid. Sharp pain extending to ear, between acts of swallowing. Constrictive sensation in larynx and trachea. As if a foreign body were lying over larynx. Sore larynx. Laryngismus that can be heard all over the house. Crawling sensation in throat. Tonsillitis. Inflamed, hard swollen tonsils. Small ulcers on tonsils. ***Follicular tonsillitis.*** Whitish tough mucus in spots on tonsils, simulating diphtheria. Putrid throat, seldom painful. Hoarseness from cold. Whispering voice, can't speak loudly. Voice trembling. Submaxillary glands painful when moving the neck. Goiter.

Tongue - Tendency to bite the tongue, on one side, when chewing or speaking. Moist, white, flabby tongue, loaded with a white coating, shows marks of teeth. Anterior half of tongue as if numb. Tongue trembles when protruded.

Vertigo - Vertigo with sparks before the eyes, gastric symptoms and yawning. Vertigo, worse slightest motion of head, stooping. Vertigo as if swung to and fro in a swing or cradle.

Vision - Flashes of light from violent coughing. Sparks before the eyes. Flickering zigzags and serpentine white flickering at one side of field of vision. Dimness before one eye while reading, as if tears were in it, which is not the case. Amblyopia and asthenopia in females, due to onanism or ciliary neuralgia.

COMMENTS - Sudden shock and grief (Staph., Caust., more anger with the grief). ***Hysteria from grief. Shock from frights (Op.), bad news, and from disappointment***. Since shock, sleepless, irritable, angry. Crying with the inability to control themselves, choking, spasmodic crying.

Alternate moods, contradictory behavior. ***Conflicted emotions***, love/hate relationships (Staph., Nat-m.). Acute, unrequited love (Nat-m.). Generally idealistic and romantic, leading to disappointment and unfulfilled hopes. Perfectionist, obsessive, chronic or acute frustration. Dislikes consolation (Nat-m.). Characteristic sighing respiration. Sentimental.

Fear of being trapped, of being possessed, changed. Fear of being embarrassed, of losing control. Frigidity, due to desire for control, often cannot orgasm. Can shut down sex drive. Women may become masculinized, stoic, after disappoint in love.

Confident, but also low self esteem. Overly concerned with appearance. Hard on themselves in terms of weight, have an ideal body image and a drive for perfection. Anorexia, bulimia.

Hard, critical. Tendency to argue when hurt. Internal conflicts, particularly over sense of dependency. Complains of a communication problem in relationships. Reactive (Nat-m. is more introverted). Sense of irresolution.

Physical paradoxes, strange behavior. Ulcer and heartburn that is better hot, spicy foods. Sore throat, better swallowing solid foods. Painful, inflamed joints that are better pressure.

Neurological problems since grief or shock. Lump in the throat, tight feeling, empty feeling in the chest or the stomach since a grief. Neurological diseases after grief, especially choreas, spasms, or epilepsy. Convulsions, spasms from fright. Epilepsy from emotional conflict. Hysterical paralysis.

Cramps and spasms (Nux-v.). Spasms and convulsions, ending in long-drawn sighs. Nervous twitchings and convulsions. The child stiffens and bends backward. Half-unconscious state, thumbs clenched, face blue. Distortion of the facial muscles whenever the patient attempts to speak. Severe numbness down the legs. Back spasms.

Excessive pains rapidly alternate in character. Exaggerated and outlandish symptoms. Pains change their locality, come gradually and abate suddenly or come and go suddenly. Pains in small, circumscribed spots. Pressure as of a sharp instrument from within outward. Sensations of formication and numbness.

Headache as if a nail were driven out through the side of the head, better by lying on it. Headaches terminate with a profuse flow of urine. Migraines. Dentition. Toothache, worse after a meal, not so bad while eating.

Hoarse hacking, irritable and irritating cough. The longer the cough lasts, the more the irritation increases. Kent described it as "hack, hack-et-hack, ending in sobbing." Cough every time he stands still during a walk. Hollow, spasmodic cough as from sulphur fumes. Cough as from inspired feathery dust. Hysterical aphonia. Laryngismus stridulus, patient sits up in bed.

Knots in the stomach, colitis. Sour saliva and sour taste in mouth. Craves cheese, sweets and chocolate. Strong aggravation from tobacco, coffee. Sensitive to stimulants. Pronounced "goneness" or sinking at the stomach, often at night. Sensation as if the stomach were relaxed.

Regurgitation of food. Hiccough, worse by eating, smoking or emotional disturbances (especially in children). Empty retching better by eating. Vomiting at night. Hysterical vomiting.

Painful conditions of the anus and rectum, including hemorrhoids and prolapse. Especially when characterized by "sharp, stitching pains shooting up the rectum," or "constricting pain at anus worse after stool, better while sitting."

Dysmenorrhea, labor-like bearing-down in hypogastrium, better by pressure, lying down, change of position. Flow is black, putrid, clotted if profuse.

Sudden loss of function in any organ. Insomnia, with conflict. Tendency to chilliness. During intermittent fever, thirst occurs only during the chill stage.

Teste placed Ign. in his Ip. group as nausea and vomiting, reversed peristalsis, congestive headaches and engorgements resulting from vomiting, tenesmus, and intermittent fevers are the leading characteristics of the group.

Clarke once gave instant relief with Ign. 30c in the case of a woman who had just heard of her brother's death (not unexpected) and who complained of an intense pain in the head just over the root of the nose.

Dr. Nash related a case of puerperal convulsions in which this feature led to a cure.

Clarke astonished himself once by curing rapidly with Ign. a severe case of rheumatic fever, which had been making no progress under Bry.

B. Simmons explained the sciatica pains as "lancinating, cutting pains, beating, bursting pains, chilliness with thirst, flushes of heat, chiefly face without thirst." The limb is swollen and thigh knotty and she cannot get up or lie down without pain, generally left side.

RELATIONS - ***Antidoted by:*** Puls. (chief antidote), Arn., Camph., Cham., Cocc., Coff. ***It antidotes:*** Brandy, coffee, chamomile tea tobacco, Sel., Zinc. ***Compare:*** (1) Nat-m., Phos-ac. - grief, especially for chronic condition. (2) difficult swallowing of liquids, Bell., Caust., Cina, Hyos., Lach., Lyc., Phos. (3) Globus hystericus - Lach., Lyc., Plb. (4) Worry and its effects, Nux-v., Sulph. (5) Jealousy, Apis, Lach., Hyos. (6) Disappointed love, Nat-m., Ph-ac. (7) Zinc., Kali-p., Sep., Cimic. (8) Panacea arvensis - sensitiveness over gastric region with hunger but an aversion to food. (9) Croc. - irresistible fits of laughter, rapidly alternating mental states. (10) Lyc. - sinking sensation at night, preventing sleep, canine hunger at night, also Chin. (11) Sep. - sinking, gone sensation, with Ign. it is attended with sighing. (12) In functional paralysis from fatigue, emotions or worms, Stann., Cocc., Phos. (13) Hysteria, Cupr., Plat., Hyos., Asaf., Mosch., Valer., Nux-m. (14) Spasms in delicate women, Bell., Hyos. (15) Sudden effects of emotions, Staph., Op. (16) In uterine spasms, Cocc., Cham., Mag-m., Cimic. (17) Extreme sensitiveness to pain, Coff., Cham. ***Compatible:*** Ars., Bell., Calc., Chin., Lyc., Nux-v., Puls., Rhus-t., Sep., Sulph., Zinc. ***Incompatible:*** Coff., Tab., Nux-v.

REFERENCES - Boericke. Clarke. Murphy. Phatak.

ILEX AQUIFOLIUM

(American Holly)

PHARMACY - ilx-a. Ilex aquifolium. American holly. Ilex opaca. N. O. Aquifoliacee. Tincture of fresh leaves, berries and young shoots. ***Historical dose:*** Tincture and all potencies.

CLINICAL - Colic. Coughs. Diarrhea. Eye, disorders. Gout. Intermittent, fever. Jaundice. Pleurisy. Rheumatism. Spleen, pain. Staphyloma.

HERBAL - The best-known members of the Ilex genus are the common Holly and the Ilex Paraguayensis, or Paraguay tea, from which the drink called mate is made. The leaves of Ilex-aq. are reputed to be equal to cinchona in the treatment of intermittent fever.

Haller commended the juice of the leaves in jaundice, the berries are purgative and emetic. Hale quoted Rafinesque as saying, "The decoction and wine have been used for cough, pleurisy, colic, gout and rheumatism."

HOMEOPATHIC - Ilx-a. has been used in coughs, pleurisy, colic, gout and rheumatism. Infiltration of cornea, staphyloma, nightly burning in orbits, rheumatic inflammation of eye. Intermittent fever. Marked eye symptoms, spleen pain. All symptoms better in winter.

COMMENTS - Cooper cured spleen pain with it. His keynote indication for it is ***"symptoms better in winter."*** He improved with it a bad case of chronic deafness having that peculiarity. A feeling of irritation in the urethra with constant dripping from orifice, probably from prostate, in a man about 50, disappeared after a drop of the tincture.

Cooper said the diarrhea of Ilx-a. is accompanied with mucus flux and he suggests that it may be useful in pilosis (sprue).

Hale quoted an article by Dr. Hendricks on the affect of Ilx-a. on the eye. With 5-drop doses of the 1x, given four times a day. Dr. Hendricks cured several cases of "rheumatic inflammation of the eye with periostitis of the frontal bone, which often leads to staphylomatous degeneration of the cornea."

Hendricks noted the case of a girl, 17, who had been under the most renowned oculists since her fifth year. She had great infiltration of cornea, staphyloma, eyeball looked like a lump of flesh. Nightly burning pains in orbits. Ilx-a. cured completely in six days.

RELATIONS - ***Compare:*** (1) Ilx-p. Ilx-v. (2) Ilx-c- Excellent diuretic and substitute for tea.

REFERENCES - Boericke. Clarke.

ILEX PARAGUARIENSIS

(Yerba Mate)

PHARMACY - Ilx-p. Ilex paraguariensis. Yerba mate. Ilex mate. ***Historical dose:*** Tincture and all potencies.

CLINICAL - Anorexia. Depression. Headaches. Heartburn. Hemicrania. Kidney, colic. Neurasthenia. Sunstroke.

HERBAL - Yerba mate is said to be of use as a prophylactic against sunstroke, being a stimulant to the circulation as a diaphoresis and diuresis herb.

HOMEOPATHIC - Persistent epigastric pain, sense of dryness of mouth and pharynx. Anorexia, heartburn with nervous depression, neurasthenia. Somnolence, incapacity for work. Diminution of urinary secretion. Headaches and pruritus, itching. Kidney colic. Hemicrania.

RELATIONS - ***Compare:*** (1) Ilx-a. Ilx-v. (2) Ilx-c- Excellent diuretic and substitute for tea.

REFERENCES - Boericke. Clarke.

ILEX VOMITORIA

(Yaupon)

PHARMACY - ilx-v. Ilex vomitoria. Yaupon. N.O. Aquifoliaceae. ***Historical dose:*** Tincture and all potencies.

CLINICAL - Gout. Nephritis.

HOMEOPATHIC - Ilx-v. has emetic, tonic and digestive qualities, with no sleepless effects. Its active principle is said to act as a powerful diuretic employed in nephritis and gout.

REFERENCES - Boericke.

IMPATIENS

(Bach Flower Essence)

PHARMACY - imp-b. Impatiens. Impatiens glandulifera. Impatiens balsamina. The mauve flowers are picked and floated on to a bowl of water which is left in the sun for several hours. The water is strained and preserved as medicine. ***Historical dose:*** Take two drops from the stock bottle into a one ounce dropper bottle, (add brandy or alcohol, if this bottle will be used for days or weeks). This is the dosage bottle, take a few drops straight into the mouth or as needed in a little water or juice.

HOMEOPATHIC - Together with Heath-b. and Wat-v-b., this remedy belongs to the group of ***Loneliness,*** as classified by Bach. All three remedies bring healing to those suffering from inner loneliness mostly due to self-centered reasons.

Nervous tension and cardiovascular strain. High blood pressure, heart trouble. Internal agitation and impatience. Useful for increasing patience and forbearance. Sudden explosions of temper with possible violence. Threatened nervous breakdown.

MIND - Restlessness. Internal agitation. Frustrated, dissatisfied, irritable. Impatience, short of temper. Easily feels despair or feels overwhelmed. Sense of urgency. Feels driven to do one thing after another. Efficient. Self-centered. Problems with impulse control (Cher-p-b., Holly-b., Verv-b.).

REFERENCES - Bach.

IMPERATORIA OSTRUTHIUM

PHARMACY - imp. Imperatoria ostruthium. Peucedanum ostruth. N. O. Umbelliferae. Tincture or infusion of root. ***Historical dose:*** Tincture and all potencies.

CLINICAL - Skin, disorders. Stomach, disorders.

HOMEOPATHIC - Imperatoria, like Athamanta, belongs to the genus Peucedanum. Kleemann observed the effects of the infusion of the root, a teaspoonful every two hours. A few symptoms were noted, including "diminished secretion of mucus in intestines and air passages."

RELATIONS - ***Compare:*** (1) Atha. and Umbelliferae.

REFERENCES - Boericke. Clarke.

INDIGO TINCTORIA

PHARMACY - indg. Indigo tinctoria. An oxidation product from the juices of several plants, chiefly Indigo tinctoria. N. O. Leguminose. Papilionoideae. Trituration. ***Historical dose:*** Trituration and all potencies.

CLINICAL - Acne. Amenorrhea. Anus, prolapse. ***Belchings***. Brachial neuralgia. Constipation. Cough. Diarrhea. ***Epilepsy.*** Face, pimples on. Headache. Hysteria. Kidney, colic. Melancholy. Neurasthenia. Nosebleed. Pinworms. ***Sciatica***. Skin, disorders. Toothache. Urethra, stricture. Worms.

HERBAL - Indigo was introduced into medicine as a remedy for epilepsy. Pure powdered Indigo placed on the wound cures snake and spider poison (Kali-perm., Golondrina, Cedr.).

HOMEOPATHIC - It has been extensively proved by homeopaths and observations have also been made of its effects on epileptic patients who were receiving large doses from old-school practitioners.

Marked action on the nervous system. ***Epilepsy***, when the attacks are preceded by a furious excitable disposition followed by melancholy, timidity and mildness. Undulating sensation in the brain with obscuration of vision or sensation as if the brain were frozen, before the attack.

Neurasthenia and hysteria. Excited mood and desire to be busy. Pain in the limbs worse after every meal. ***Sciatica pain*** from middle of thighs to the knee. Stricture of esophagus, blue color (Cupr.).

Back - Sharp pain between the scapula. Sharp pain in the small of the back, going off after an evacuation.

Breasts - Shooting pains in and around the breasts. Stinging in the breasts, going off momentarily by rubbing. Burning in the breasts during the menses.

Chest - Rumbling and grumbling in the chest at every inspiration.

Ears - Pressure and roaring.

Eyes - Convulsive twitching and quivering of the eyelids, impeding the sight. Pressure in the eyeball. Inflammation of the meibomian glands on the lower lids.

Face - Tearing, piercing and gnawing pains in bones of the face and especially of lower jaw. Pricking in right malar bone. Pain in the submaxillary glands extending to the teeth. Congestion in the face with burning cheeks.

Female - Menstruation too early. Acts as an emmenagogue.

Head - Convulsions. Undulating sensation through whole head. Sensation of a band around forehead. Sensation as if brain were frozen. Hair feels pulled from vertex. Gloomy, cries at night.

Kidneys - Catarrh of bladder. kidney colic. Stricture of urethra. Frequent desire to urinate with burning in the fundus of the bladder. Urine turbid.

Limbs - ***Pain in limbs worse after every meal.*** Drawing in the muscles, in deltoid. Convulsive startings in the arms. Weakness of arms. Veins of the hands red, inflamed and tense. ***Sciatica***. Aching, stinging, bruised pain in sciatic nerve. Tearing in the lower limbs, especially in the toes. Pain from middle of thigh to knee. Boring pain in knee joint, better walking.

Lungs - Violent, suffocating cough inducing vomiting, bleeding of the nose, in the evening, before and after lying down.

Male - Depressed sexual desire. Itching of the urethra, glans and scrotum.

Modalities - Better pressure, rubbing, motion, walking. Worse during rest and sitting, in afternoon, evening. Worse after eating and after evening meal. Warmth rushes to head on entering a warm room after walking in cold air.

Mouth - Sensation of burning on the tongue and in the bottom of the palate. Vesicles on the tip of the tongue. Metallic taste in tongue with contracted feeling in pharynx. Spitting of bloody saliva. Numbness of interior of mouth in the morning after waking.

Nerves - Excessive nervous irritation. Epilepsy, flashes of heat from abdomen to head, fit begins with dizziness. Aura from a painful spot between shoulders. Hysterical symptoms where pain predominates. Reflex spasms from worms.

Nose - Excessive sneezing and bleeding from nose. Nosebleed with vanishing of sight. Tearing and incisive pains in the bones and cartilages of the nose.

Rectum - Obstinate constipation, stool scanty, hard, retained. Diarrhea, stool liquid with flatulence and colic. Prolapsed anus after each stool. Falling of rectum. Dull sticking in rectum. Aroused at night with horrible itching at anus. Pinworms.

Skin - Face and whole body covered with pimples. Fine heat-rash, especially left side of face extending from forehead to throat. Boils on ribs and various parts. Itching in face and various parts of body, better by rubbing. Itching of skin with constipation.

Sleep - Sleepiness in the evening and disturbed sleep at night. Children aroused at night with horrible itching at anus. At night, anxious waking with a start. Anxious dreams. Nervous irritation. Predominance of cold. Sudden convulsions. Illusory sensations.

Stomach - Tingling pain in the pit of the stomach. Bloated stomach. Flushes of heat rising from stomach to head. ***Belchings***. Empty risings. Retching and vomiting of watery fluid. Vomiting of glue-like mucus. Anorexia.

Teeth - Drawing, gnawing, tearing pains in teeth (right). Teeth as if being pulled out.

Temperature - Chilliness with cold hands and violent headache with constant desire to urinate, urine turbid. Great heat, particularly in the face with increased secretion of urine.

Vertigo - Vertigo with nausea. Vertigo with headache, better in evening and worse in open air.

COMMENTS - Neuralgic and nervous symptoms. Brachial and sciatic neuralgia, worse while sitting, better by moving about. Catarrhal cough, coming in long paroxysms in evening. Dry suffocative cough in evening and after going to bed. Cough with nosebleed.

Whitish, moist tongue. Sour or foul breath. A large but soft abdomen. Diarrhea of two or three stools in twenty-four hours like grayish paper, sour. Ascarides in rectum, even crawling out during sleep.

Epilepsy with great melancholy or a furious excitable disposition before the attacks and mild and timid after. Sudden attacks, apparently originating in the solar plexus from which flushes of heat arise to the head, induced by cold or fright.

Undulating sensation in the brain (which Clarke also observed in a case of epilepsy benefited by Cimic.), with obscured vision. Chilliness.

Nash noted the case of a hard-working man, over 70, who gradually became unable to work. Weak, stiffness all over, especially right side, arm and leg. Pain in right hip running down leg, worse beginning to move after resting. Could hardly turn over in bed.

Appetite poor, stomach distressed, four or five hours after eating, if he ate more than a very little. Pains in the limbs decidedly worse after every meal. Indg. cured promptly.

Teste tried Indg. in cases of epilepsy, but with little success, except in cases arising from the presence of worms. In cases of worm fever he used it with great effect. The patients were children from ten to twelve years old, lymphatic, apathetic, peevish, who ate a great deal.

Teste also used Indg. with success for semi-liquid diarrhea (three to four stools a day, coming on especially after exercise in a stout old man, frequently given to excess of eating). Chronic catarrh of the bladder. Stricture of urethra after old gonorrhea with Plb. and Sep.

RELATIONS - ***Antidoted by:*** Camph., Bry., Nux-v. ***Compare:*** (1) Cupr. (2) Sulph. - epilepsy, sinking sensation, hot flushes, worm fever. (3) Kali-br. - epilepsy, acne. (4) Cimic. - epilepsy with waving sensation in brain. (5) Rhus-t. - worse by rest, better by motion. (6) Ind., timid, sad, low-spirited, Bufo, vehement or excitable, Bufo - epilepsy. (7) Lyc. - worse in afternoon. (8) Ign. - sad introverted. (9) Bapt. and other Leguminose.

REFERENCES - Boericke. Clarke. Phatak.

INDIUM METALLICUM

(Indium Metal)

PHARMACY - ind. Indium metallicum. Indium metal. At. Wt. 113.7. Trituration of the pure metal. ***Historical dose:*** Trituration and all potencies.

CLINICAL - ***Backaches.*** Chronic fatigue. Depression. Dyspepsia. Foot-sweats. Headaches. Megrim. Migraine. Nausea. Nosebleeds. Paralysis, sphincters. Pollutions. Sexual, perversion. Sore throat. Throat, ulceration. Uvula, enlarged, ulcerated.

HOMEOPATHIC - Indium received its name from the indigo blue line in the spectrum through which its presence was discovered in Zinc-blend. It is a rare metal, nearly like lead in appearance and softness.

Indium was proved under the direction of Bell, and the symptoms mark it out as allied in action to Sel. and Titan. in its general action. Affects the ***male sexual sphere***. Diminished power and control, frequency of nocturnal emissions, sexual dreams of perversion. Sexual psychopathy. Seminal emissions.

Restlessness, compelling to move about. Headaches and migraines, with sleepiness and nausea. ***Backaches.*** Throat conditions, worse in evening, better by eating, drinking cold water. The urine is horribly offensive after standing a short while.

MIND - Depression. Sleepy and irritable with pain in the occipital region. State of indifference. Psychologically exhausted, cannot work. Sexual psychopathy.

Back - ***Backaches.*** Stiffness at the nape of the neck, neck and shoulders.

Chest - Burning pain behind the sternum. Pain in the left side of the thorax and towards the left axilla.

Constitutions - Tubercular types.

Ears - Painful pustules on the outer ear. Helix red and feels sharp, needle-like pains.

Eyes - Uncertain sight in the evening. People seem pale or yellow.

Face - Painful suppurating pimples. Corners of mouth cracked and sore (Cund.).

Female - Menses prolonged. Drawing pains in the low abdomen with marked irritability.

Head - Sudden violent or beating headaches, especially in the right occipital region. ***Bursting pain in head when straining at stool.*** Dull pains in temples and forehead with ***nausea***, weakness, ***sleepiness***. Pruritus of the scalp with internal head pains.

Kidneys - Horribly offensive smell of urine after standing a short time.

Limbs - Pains in the limbs, especially in left arm. Jerking in the legs. Muscular shuddering. Pain in the muscles, especially in the right ankle, then moving to the left ankle and spreading over the whole foot. Weakness of the legs, feels particularly tired after walking, becomes restless and needs to move again. Toes itch (Agar.).

Lungs - Must breathe deeply.

Male - Drawing pains along spermatic cord. Testicles tender. Testes soft, heavy. Increased sexual desire, nocturnal discharge followed by insufficient erection, premature ejaculation. Emissions too frequent. Diminished power.

Modalities - Better out of doors, in cold air, drinking or washing in cold water. Worse in a warm room, motion, early morning, 3 a.m. to 4 a.m., afternoon, 3 p.m. to 6 p.m. Faintness at 11 a.m.

Mouth - Pharyngeal muco-viscous secretions, sticky and yellow.

Nose - Violent attack of sneezing.

Rectum - Loses control of the anal sphincter when urinating. Headaches during difficult evacuation of the bowel.

Sleep - Hallucinatory dreams.

Stomach - Acrid dyspepsia. Nausea with headaches at breakfast. Weakness in the stomach around 11 a.m.

Throat - Uvula enlarged, ulcerated. Thick, tough mucus in back part of pharynx. Generally worse in evening.

COMMENTS - Depressed. Headaches, violent pain in the head when straining at stool.

Berridge reported the case of a boy, 10, who was constipated five or six years. Stool about once a week, dark and short, sometimes with blood, anus sore after stool. He had to strain much, seizing his thighs with his hands and straightening himself forcibly, the effort makes his face red and the head feels as if it would burst. Ind. in high potencies cured.

RELATIONS - *Compare:* (1) Sel., Titan. - male sexual organs. (2) Bell. (headache, menses), Aspar. - urine, Sang. - headache, rheumatism. (3) Phos., Nat-c., Sulph. and Zinc. - faintness, 11 a.m., (4) Ferr. - headache, ebullitions, lameness of shoulder muscles. (5) Bruc., Lach., Nux-m., Op., Stann. and Stry. - Headache with sleepiness. Ind. has nausea as well as sleepiness. (6) In throat symptoms better from eating and drinking. Ind. resembles Esch., Benz-ac., Cist., Lach. (7) Mur-ac. - Adynamic types, red face, dry tongue, cannot urinate without evacuating the rectum. (8) Tub. - Constant need to move about, changing, erratic pains, has to make an effort to urinate during the stool.

REFERENCES - Boericke. Clarke. Julian.

INDOLUM

(Indol)

PHARMACY - Indol. Indolum. Crystalline compound from Indigo or as a product of putrefaction of proteins. ***Historical dose:*** Trituration and all potencies.

CLINICAL - Auto-intoxication. Constipation. Delusions. Dullness. Fatigue. Headaches. Nervous. ***Sleepiness***.

HOMEOPATHIC - Indolum's primary action is to increase the elimination of Indican. Auto-intoxication. Persistent desire to sleep, dull, discontented mental state. Delusions. Nervousness, constant motion of fingers and feet. Intestinal putrefaction.

Food - Great thirst. Hungry sensation after full meal.

Head - Dull occipital and frontal headache in afternoon. Dull sensation over eyes. Eyeballs hot and hurt when moved. Pupils dilated with headache.

Limbs - Very tired and sore in lower limbs. Feet burn. Sore knee joints.

Sleep - ***Sleepiness***. Continuous dreaming.

Rectum - Constipation.

Stomach - Bloated feeling.

RELATIONS - ***Compare:*** (1) Skat.

REFERENCES - Boericke.

INFLUENZINUM

(Influenza Nosode)

PHARMACY - influ. Influenzinum. Influenza nosode. The nosode of influenza virus of the Asian and common flu. ***Historical dose:*** All potencies.

CLINICAL - ***Aching, pain.*** Anorexia. Bronchitis. Bronchial, asthma. Bronchopneumonia. Cardiac neurosis. Catarrh. ***Chills.*** Chronic ***Colds.*** Conjunctivitis. Coryza. Depression. Diarrhea. Encephalitis. Enterocolitis. ***Fatigue. Fever.*** Hyperthermia. Hypotension. ***Influenza.*** Laryngitis. Meningitis. Mononucleosis. Otitis. Pharyngitis. Sinusitis. Sycosis. ***Weakness.***

HOMEOPATHIC - With many practitioners, Influenzinum has taken the place of Baptisia as the routine remedy in epidemics.

It can be given in the 12c or 30c potency, either in the form of tincture, pills or ten pellets may be dissolved in six ounces of water. Of this a dessert spoonful may be given for a dose. It may be repeated every two hours. This will be found sufficient to control a large proportion of the cases.

Clarke directed his patients that when ***"colds"*** appear in their family, have those who are unaffected take Ars. 3c three times daily, and have the patients take Influ. 30c every hour or two.

This generally prevents the spread of the trouble and clears up the colds, whether they are influenza or not.

Influ. has the ability to develop old troubles and thus it takes a variety of forms in different persons. It need not be expected to cure all cases unaided or indeed to be appropriate to every case.

Influenza. Influenza encephalitis. Entero-colitis of influenza. Diarrhea of influenza. Meningitis. Measles. Weakness and fatigue. General ill feeling with chill, headache, diffused pains. Neurotic, depressive persons. Stiffness. Tendency to hypotension. Hyperthermia. Sycosis. Anorexia.

MIND - Apathy and indifference. Mental dullness. Brain fatigue. ***Post-influenza depressive neurosis.*** Weak memory.

Abdomen - Gastro-intestinal pain.

Blood - Leucopenia with mononucleosis.

Ears - Otitis with influenza.

Eyes - Eyes are heavy and sensitive to movements. Stiffness of eyes. Blepharitis. Conjunctivitis of influenza.

Head - Meningitis. Encephalitis with vomiting. Headache of influenza.

Heart - Hypotension. Cardiac neurosis. Weakness of the myocardia.

Limbs - Aches and pains. Rheumatism. Rheumatoid pains during humid and cold weather. Intermittent lameness. Venous stasis of lower limbs. Venous and arterial congestion of the lower limbs. Varicose veins and ulcers (Oscilloc.).

Lungs - Dry painful cough. Bronchial asthma. Bronchitis. Bronchopneumonia of influenza. Sub-acute edema of babies.

Nose - Acute or chronic coryza. Acute and chronic rhino-pharyngitis. Nasal congestion. Coryza of influenza. Sinusitis. Nasal polyps. Chronic atrophic rhinitis.

Rectum - Weakness of the anal sphincter. Weakening diarrhea.

Throat - Pharyngitis. Chronic laryngitis. Stridulous laryngitis of children. Nasal voice. Laryngitis of influenza.

RELATIONS - ***Compare:*** (1) Gels., Oscilloc.. (2) Mim-p. - inflammation of the eyes and nasal mucosa. Headache, worse by movement, better while closing eyes. Diarrhea with colic and irritating stools. (3) Galph. - Hypersensitiveness to change of weather, Hypersecretion of nasal and ocular mucous. (4) Luf-op.: fronto-occipital headache. Acute or chronic inflammation of the nasal mucosa. ***Compatible with:*** Gels., Cimic., Ars., Bell., Bry., Hep., Merc. and many others.

REFERENCES - Boericke. Clarke. Julian.

INONOTUS OBLIQUUS

(Chaga Mushroom)

PHARMACY - inon. Inonotus obliquus. Chaga mushroom. ***Historical dose:*** All potencies.

CLINICAL - Asthma. Bronchitis. ***Cancer.*** Chronic fatigue. Diabetes. Hypertension. Influenza. Tuberculosis. Tumors.

HERBAL - Chaga mushroom is a black parasitic fungus produced on the living trunks of mature birch that resembles burnt charcoal. It causes the tree's death in 5-7 years, and in fact, Chaga mushroom is called "birch cancer" in Russia. The shape of the mushroom also resembles that of cancer in the human body. Since the 16th century, Chaga mushroom has been used as a remedy for cancer and diseases of the digestive system.

This wood-rotting fungus has been used as a folk medicine in many East European countries including Russia, to treat gastritis, ulcers, tuberculosis (TB) of the bones, and cancer. The inner brown layer closest to the tree is the portion of the fungus most often used.

Medical research has shown Chaga to be effective as an anti-tumor agent. In 1958, scientific studies in Finland and Russia found this mushroom provided an epochal effect in uterine, liver, breast, and gastric cancer, and hypertension and diabetes.

Most often consumed in a hot tea mixture, Chaga has been used as a traditional folk medicine in Russia and Eastern Europe since at least the fifteen hundreds for a variety of diseases, including stomach pain, ulcers, asthma, bronchitis, liver problems, and even cancer.

Chaga is currently enjoying a resurgence as a possible treatment for a wide variety of diseases and health problems, including chronic fatigue syndrome, the flu, stomach problems, and even HIV and certain types of cancer.

Recent studies in the U.S., Russia, and other countries have shown Chaga to have anti-tumor benefits related to the mammary glands and female sex organs. Japanese research not only found similar antiviral activity, but also discovered that Chaga shows activity against HIV (protease inhibition).

COMMENTS - The Chinese Monk Shen Nong proclaimed Chaga as a superior class medicinal herb, for its diverse and complete homeopathic properties, in his work Shen Nong Ben Cao Jin; the first of the three ancient medical books that serve as the foundation of Traditional Chinese Medicine.

Since then, Traditional Chinese Medicine practitioners have applied Chaga as a remedy for viral diseases such as influenza, anti-inflammatory treatment of stomach ulcers, the arrest and reversal of tumor growth, balancing the endocrine system in the treatment of diabetes, anti-oxidant uses in detoxifying the body, and as a daily supplement for the overall balancing of the body's immune system and anti-aging properties increasing longevity of life.

Documented as early as 4600 years ago, ancient Asian folk medicine practitioners relied upon Chaga, a medicinal mushroom, to maintain a healthy life energy balance ("Chi"), preserve youth, promote longevity, and boost the body's immune system to fight viral, bacterial, fungal and parasitic maladies.

As a folk medicine, Chaga was ingested by the local people of the Siberian mountain regions in tea or powder form, inhaled from smoke, and applied to the skin for healing of injury or rash. Indigenous people from that area have been documented to live beyond 100 years of age.

REFERENCES - Murphy.

INSULINUM
(Insulin)

PHARMACY - insulin. Insulinum. Insulin. An aqueous solution of an active principle from the pancreas which affects the sugar metabolism. Triturations. ***Historical dose:*** All potencies.

CLINICAL - Abscesses. Acidosis. Acne. Bedsores. Boils. Cancer. Carbuncles. Dermatitis. ***Diabetes.*** Diarrhea. Dysentery. Eczema. Fatigue. Glycosuria. Gout. ***Hepatitis.*** Hypoglycemia. Insulin, effects. ***Liver, enlarged.*** Marasmus. Mastoiditis. Otitis. Otorrhea. Pancreas, disorders. Pneumonia. Polyuria. Septicemia. Typhoid. Ulcers. Varicose, ulcers. Weakness.

HOMEOPATHIC - This pancreatic hormone plays an important part in the process of sugar metabolism in the body. Its capacity to burn sugar into carbon dioxide and water, thereby helping the body with fat combustion, has made it very useful in the hands of the allopathic school saving patients from death in cases of diabetic acidosis.

If Insulin. is administered at suitable intervals in diabetes mellitus, the blood sugar is maintained at a normal level and the urine remains free of sugar. Restores the ability to oxidize carbohydrates and to store glycogen in the liver.

It was proved by Dr. William F. Baker, and Dr. S. K. Ghosh of Calcutta. Some use of Insulin. homeopathically has been made by Baker, showing its applicability in acne, carbuncles, and erythema with itching eczema.

Insulin is indicated for persistent cases of skin irritation, boils or varicose ulceration with polyuria. For gouty patients with glycosuria when skin manifestations are persistent, give three times daily after eating.

Dr. Ghose used it in potency for overdoses of insulin, followed by weakness, fatigue and tremulousness with profuse sweating. Patient is debilitated. Asthenia. Emaciation with loose bowels. Craving for sweets.

Chronic intestinal troubles with diarrhea and enlarged liver. Enlarged liver with chronic sepsis or chronic suppurative otitis.

Chronic diarrhea of children with enlarged liver and debility. Infantile liver without jaundice.

Abdomen - Duodenal ulcers. Chronic intestinal troubles with diarrhea and enlarged liver.

Blood - Hypoglycemia. Septicemia.

Constitutions - Broken down constitution from infectious or suppurative diseases.

Ears - Chronic suppurative otitis. Chronic otorrhea and mastoiditis.

Food - Desires sugar and sweets, but aggravated by them.

Liver - ***Hepatitis.*** Chronic functional derangement of liver. Enlarged liver associated with many complaints.

Modalities - Worse after typhoid or pneumonia.

Rectum - Chronic diarrhea. Prolonged greenish diarrhea continuing after an attack of dysentery.

Skin - Acute dermatitis with chronic diarrhea and liver trouble. Eczema, allergic eczema. Acne, erythema with itching eczema. Boils and abscesses. Ulcers and suppurative ailments with enlarged liver.

Tongue - Tongue is coated white.

COMMENTS - Dr. Ghose wrote: "But from the dynamic standpoint, it will be observed, that Insulin in potency has even greater utility where glycogenic balance of the liver is disturbed.

"In cases of hepatitis and hepatic enlargement where the liver is embarrassed by long continued toxic process, it has a very great scope. Thus in cases where liver is enlarged towards the end of acute infectious diseases, such as Typhoid, Pneumonia, etc., a few doses of Insulin 30 will restore normal balance and enhance the process of re-generation rapidly."

Chronic intestinal disorder, especially with looseness of bowels with enlarged liver. Chronic otorrhea and mastoiditis in emaciated children where the pus is thin, especially when combined with enlarged liver and chronic diarrhea or as aftereffects of acute infectious diseases.

Ulcers, boils, bed sores, hypopyon as aftereffects of acute infectious diseases with disordered liver.

Eczema with chronic liver troubles. Allergic eczema. Suppuration of the scrofulous glands in the neck. General suppuration.

RELATIONS - ***Compare:*** (1) Calc-ar., Chin., Phos., Caps.

REFERENCES - Boericke. Ghose.

INULA HELENIUM

(Scabwort)

PHARMACY - inul. Inula helenium. Scabwort. Elecampane. N. O. Compositae. Tincture of fresh root dug in autumn of the second year. The juice of the root was proved. ***Historical dose:*** Tincture and all potencies.

CLINICAL - Backache. Bronchitis. ***Cough.*** Cramp. Diabetes. Dyspepsia. Dysmenorrhea. ***Dry, cough.*** Erysipelas. Leucorrhea. Rectum, pain in. Sciatica. Toothache.

HERBAL - Inula is a perennial plant with a stem from three to four feet high, large saw-toothed leaves tapering to a stalk, and large heads of yellow flowers.

The root has an aromatic camphor-like taste due to the presence of a crystalline substance called helenin, allied to the chemical constitution to kreosote. It also contains a quantity of starchy material, inulin, which differs from ordinary starch in being colored yellow by iodine.

The Treasury of Botany noted that elecampane was formerly much used as an aromatic tonic and as a stimulant of all the secreting organs, likewise in coughs, dyspepsia. A popular tradition credits it with the cure of facial erysipelas, and certain symptoms in the provings seem to confirm this.

HOMEOPATHIC - Fischer proved the root juice. Clinical experience added to and confirmed many of the traditional symptoms, including the old reputation of the remedy in coughs.

A pronounced effect was observed in the pelvic organs, pressing and dragging towards the rectum and genitals. ***Bearing-down sensation in pelvic organs.*** Affects the mucus membranes.

Marked ***bronchial symptoms. Violent tickling in larynx, producing a dry cough,*** worse lying down, worse at night, larynx painful. ***Dry cough*** with constant tickling in throat-pit, difficult breathing and sensation as if hoarseness would occur. Sub-sternal pain. Diabetes.

MIND - Excessive anxiety and trembling of the whole body, chattering of teeth from cold, during menstruation.

Abdomen - Violent motion beneath right hypochondrium, as though something living were moving about. Sticking as with two pins to right of umbilicus. Sensation as if a knife between umbilicus and right groin. Stitches in left side of abdomen towards left groin.

Back - Pain through back and chest, on inspiration. Transient pain in right scapula. Violent backache during menstruation.

Chest - Stitches behind sternum and beneath left seventh and eighth ribs. Throbbing and jerking pain as from suppuration, in middle of chest.

Ears - Dull stitches in left ear, with transient sticking above right eyebrow in evening.

Eyes - Twitching in upper lids. Burning in left eyeball. Swimming before eyes and pressure in temples and forehead.

Face - Left side of face red and hot, a white spot near nose. Flushes of heat, left cheek glowing.

Female - Menses too early and painful. Itching of legs during menses, chattering of teeth from cold during menstruation. Chronic metritis. Moving about in abdomen, stitches in genitals, followed by yellowish leucorrhea. Labor-like pains, urging to stool, dragging in genitals with violent backache.

Head - Rush of blood to head with sleeplessness. Throbbing after eating, pressure in temples and forehead. Jerking, tearing pain in occiput. Headache in right side, afterward in left. Sticking headache in right side. Burning headache in left temple, in a spot as large as a silver dollar in evening.

Kidneys - Urging to urinate ten times in one hour, urine passes by drops. Urine smells of violets (Terebe.).

Limbs - Coldness, shaking in bed, cold, blue hands and nails. Pain in right shoulder and wrist. Tearing, jerking in right arm. Upper arms as far as elbows fall asleep. Tearing in left palm, unable to double fingers. Pain in lower limbs, feet and ankles. Tensive drawing in hips. Sticking in right hip. Cramp in calves during sleep.

Lungs - Chronic bronchitis. Difficult breathing with dry cough, constant tickling in throat. Dry cough, worse at night and lying down, larynx painful. Teasing cough with much thick expectoration, with fatigue and weak digestion.

Modalities - Worse from motion, after eating, at night, lying down (except the uterine pain, which compels patient to remain lying).

Mouth - Dryness of mouth with scraping and tickling in throat, swallowing difficult. Pain in decayed teeth, worse at night.

Nose - Stitches in right side of middle of nose. Sticking, crawling in root of nose, extending to eyebrows.

Rectum - Pressing, dragging towards rectum and genitals, as if substance would come out, occurring repeatedly.

Skin - Itching as from fleas, violent on legs during menses, with burning after scratching in bed.

Sleep - Sleep restless, starting and crying out. Dreams are lascivious, disgusting.

Stomach - Sticking pain in epigastric region. Twisting as of a ball in epigastric region, above umbilicus. Nausea in morning coming from stomach.

Throat - Violent tickling in larynx, producing dry cough. Palliative in tubercular laryngitis.

Vertigo - Vertigo on stooping. Confusion of head with nausea in evening.

COMMENTS - Headache and labor-like pains. Sensation as of something alive moving about internally, also twisting as of a ball in umbilical region, as if a substance would come out of rectum and genitals.

Sensation as though some one was poking him with a finger in various parts of the body, especially in diaphragm, so painful he awoke with clenched teeth. Numerous sticking pains as with pins or a knife. The majority of the symptoms occurred on the right side.

RELATIONS - ***Compare:*** (1) Croc., Ign. (2) Arum-d. - loose cough worse at night on lying down. (3) Sep. - forcing in genitals and rectum. (4) Croc. and Thuj. - sensation of something alive. (5) Terebe. - urine smelling of violets. (6) Ign. - cough worse lying down and in evening. (7) Sulph. Psor. - worse at night in bed.

REFERENCES - Boericke. Clarke.

IODOFORMUM

(Iodoform)

PHARMACY - iodof. Iodoformum. Iodoform. Trituration. Solution. ***Historical dose:*** Triturations, tincture and all potencies, second trituration. Three grains on the back of the tongue will relieve attack of asthmatic breathing.

CLINICAL - Breast, pains. Chancre. ***Cholera, infantum.*** Coughs. Delirium. Diplopia. Diarrhea. Eczema. Enteric, fever. Eye, disorders. Headaches. Heart, disorders. Hydrocephalus. Locomotor, ataxia. Mania. ***Meningitis.*** Paralysis. ***Tuberculosis.***

HOMEOPATHIC - Iodof. was proved by Underwood and Haines. The proving symptoms were supplemented with recorded effects observed on patients treated with it in old-school practice, as well as cases of fatal poisoning.

In some instances, the symptoms of acute meningitis have been produced. Based on this, W. J. Martin cured two cases of tubercular meningitis with Iodof. 2x. He put 4 grains in half a tumbler of water and gave a teaspoonful every two hours.

One case was that of a child, fourteen months old, the symptoms including sleeping too much, constant movement of the mouth as though chewing or sucking, boring head back and rolling it from side to side. Had been ill twelve days.

Violent convulsions followed, face distorted, eyes squinting, head retracted, neck and back stiffness. Automatic movement of one arm and leg. The child was expected to die that night, but Iodof. was given and improvement set in. Fever abated, and in one week all symptoms had passed away.

Tuberculous conditions, especially tubercular meningitis (Bac.). Chronic diarrhea, stools, greenish, watery, undigested with irritable temper, due to suspected tuberculosis. Sub-acute and chronic diarrhea of children.

Failed sight due to retro-bulbar neuritis, central scotoma, partial atrophy of the optic disc. Pupils dilated, contract unequally. Cannot stand or walk with eyes closed. Sleep interrupted by sighing and cries. Mesenteric glands enlarged.

MIND - Apathetic. Irritable. Weak-minded. Forgetful. Amnesia for recent events. Did not recognize persons. Nightly restlessness. Melancholia. Excitement. Anguish. Fear of death, bemoans her approaching death. Drowsiness developing into perfect coma.

Hallucinations of sight and hearing, delusions. Screams out, leaves her bed but falls down after walking a few steps. Talks nonsense. Excessive talkativeness. Sees double. Dresses himself in strange costumes. Imagined he had the best tenor voice in the world and proceeded to hire a large concert hall.

Abdomen - Flatulent colic. Rumbling in abdomen. Scaphoid abdomen. Abdomen distended, mesenteric glands enlarged. Cutting in abdomen. Warmth in abdomen. Right inguinal region, sharp pain, cutting, with desire for stool, sore pain.

Back - Contraction of muscles of neck. Bruised sensation in nape. Spine sore, does not wish it touched. Pain along spine, along right side of dorsal vertebrae, in lumbar region, with weakness and straining. Sharp pain in angle of scapula.

Chest - Sore pain in apex of right lung. Feeling of a weight on chest. Pain in left breast like a hand grasping at the base of the heart.

Ears - Sticking in right ear, sticking, then fullness. Ears feeling dry and feverish, and full. Neuralgic pains in left ear. Dull hearing.

Eyes - ***Pupils, dilated***, contract unequally, react poorly. Eyes bloodshot and painful. Sensitive to light. Vision double. Failing sight due to retro-bulbar neuritis, central scotoma-partial atrophy of optic disc.

Face - Drawing, pressing pains in malar-bones, in zygomatic muscles, worse motion and bending forward. Stiffness of zygomatic muscles. Twitching of facial muscles. Aching in right lower jaw. Lips and throat dry, lips dry and stinging.

Head - *Meningitis*. Sharp, neuralgic pain. Head feels heavy, as if it could not be lifted from the pillow. Stitching in temples. Frontal pain, worse from descending stairs. Headache on waking. Itching of occiput.

Heart - Sticking through heart.

Kidneys - Urine very yellow, smelling like saffron. Albumen and casts in urine.

Limbs - Legs weak. Weakness of knees when going upstairs. Cannot stand and walk with eyes closed.

Lungs - Cough and wheezing on going to bed. Cough from the dryness of throat. Hemoptysis. Asthmatic breathing. Respiration irregular, deep inspirations alternating with apnea. Smothering sensation.

Modalities - Better by uncovering. Worse at night, warmth, touch, motion, riding in cars.

Mouth - Metallic taste. Sharp pain in upper teeth. Aching in teeth. Teeth feel sore and too long.

Perspiration - Sweats easily from motion. Sweats on head.

Rectum - ***Cholera infantum.*** Chronic diarrhea. ***Stools greenish, watery, undigested.*** Diarrhea with suspected tuberculosis. Stool delayed, with feeling as if anus were drawn up into rectum.

Skin - Red rash over loins, back of arms and elbows. Fine eruption of macules, papules and vesicles. Diffuse redness with edema. Horrible irritation all over body.

Sleep - Sleepiness. Very drowsy. Sleep interrupted by sighing and cries. Jerks and shocks in nerves when trying to sleep. Wakefulness. Restless sleep, full of dreams. Confused dreams, of accidents.

Stomach - Nausea, at times.

Temperature - Susceptible to hot weather. Heat at night, keeps laying off covers. Temperature may be elevated to 104 F° or more.

Throat - Aphonic disturbance of voice. Stitching in right side of throat. Dryness of throat, with bitter taste, dryness with rawness on swallowing.

Vertigo - Sudden giddiness. Confusion with nausea. Feeling as if he had been intoxicated. Vertigo on sitting up in bed.

COMMENTS - A boy of 10 had Iodof. thickly applied to a point on an amputated limb at which the stitches did not hold well. On the third day he was sleepy after a restless night with frequent sighing. The dressing was renewed and on the same day, not having eaten anything since the day before, he had several attacks of vomiting, bilious and easy.

All these symptoms increased during the next few days. The child was constipated and seemed to suffer from his head. Nights very restless, sleep interrupted by sighing and cries like those of meningitis. Drowsiness during the day. Pupils unequally contracted, reacted slowly to light. He was perfectly indifferent and did not recognize those about him.

Later, nightly agitation was replaced by tranquil delirium. Pulse rapid and small. On the sixth day the dressing was changed, on the seventh day the symptoms began to abate and disappeared after the ninth.

In one case of poisoning, a woman, 26 who had taken 42 grains of Iodoform in eighty days, suddenly after a hot bath felt very dizzy and weak in the legs, felt unable to knit and diplopia set in. Symptoms of mania followed, weakness, staggering on closing the eyes. For twelve days she was unable to walk alone.

In one case, that of a soldier who had Iodoform applied to his arm, a scarlatina-like rash appeared, spreading from arm over the body and ending in desquamation.

Scarlatina was actually diagnosed, but some doubt was raised and suspicion being thrown on the Iodoform, a piece of silver was placed in the mouth. Immediately a garlic taste was experienced, showing the presence of Iodoform, which other tests confirmed.

In cases of medicinal poisoning, the symptoms sometimes come speedily and sometimes only after a long period of medication. Symptoms set in with great suddenness and intensity. Symptoms are worse from heat and damp.

Depression. Marked drowsiness. Malaise, loss of strength and of appetite. Occasional vomiting. Moderate fever, rapid pulse. Eczema.

RELATIONS - ***Antidoted by:*** Hep., Sang. (skin). ***Compare:*** (1) Iod., Kali-i., Merc.

REFERENCES - Boericke. Clarke.

IODUM PURUM

(Iodine)

PHARMACY - iod. Iodum purum. Iodine. At. Wt. 126.53. An element. Halogens. Tincture. ***Historical dose:*** Tincture and all potencies.

CLINICAL - ***Adenoids. Appetite, disordered.*** Arthritis, deformans. Atrophy. Brain, atrophy. Breast, disorders. Cancer. Cachexia. Chilblains. Chyluria. Constipation. Coryza. Cough. Croup. ***Debility.*** Diabetes. Diarrhea. ***Emaciation.*** Enteric, fever. Galactorrhea. ***Gland, disorders. Goiter.*** Headaches. Heart, disorders, hypertrophy. Hemorrhoids. Hiccough. Hydrocephalus. ***Hyperactive.*** Infertility. Iritis. Jaundice. Joints, disorders. Laryngitis. Leucorrhea. Liver, disorders. Lymphatic, swellings. ***Malnutrition.*** Melancholy. ***Metabolism, disorders.*** Myocarditis. Ovaries, disorders. Ozaena. ***Plague. Pneumonia.*** Prostate gland, enlarged. ***Restlessness.*** Rheumatic, gout. Rheumatism. Salivation. Scars. Seborrhea. Synovitis. Syphilis. Tabes mesenterica. Tachycardia. Throat, disorders. ***Thyroid, disorders.*** Tonsils, disorders. Tremors. Tuberculosis. Uterus, disorders. Voice, disorders. Vomiting. ***Weight, loss.*** Worms.

HOMEOPATHIC - Ioduretted solution of Kali-i. is said to expels tapeworms dead. Iodine tincture is an allopathic skin disinfectant. Locally, it is an effective and easily managed microbicide. Ideal agent to keep wounds clean and disinfected (Calen.). For gunshot wounds (Hyper.). and compound fractures. Bites of insects, reptiles, etc.

Great absorption action, rapid and intense absorption. Useful as a paint in all kinds of swellings, particularly swollen glands. Given internally, the absorbents are stimulated to fresh activity; muscles, fat, tissues and glands waste away and general emaciation is the result. New growths and hyperplasia are affected before the normal tissues.

Especially affects all glandular structures, respiratory organs, and the circulatory system. ***Glands,*** thyroid, testes, mesenteric and mammary, first ***swell, hard and heavy***, then dwindle, atrophy. ***Goiter***. Facial paralysis or epilepsy from suppression of goiter. Atrophy or induration of testes, ovaries, uterus. ***Plague. Adenoid vegetations***.

Rapid metabolism. Loses flesh, yet hungry and eating well (Abrot.). ***Emaciation, weight loss*** with good appetite, glandular atrophy. Hungry with much thirst. Better after eating. ***Great debility, the slightest effort induces perspiration***.

Wasting diseases of scrofulous patients. Patients are generally exceedingly thin, dark complexioned, enlarged lymphatic glands, with a voracious appetite but remains thin. Tubercular type. ***Feels always too hot***, craves cold air.

Capillary congestion followed by ecchymosis, edema, hemorrhages and nutritive disturbances. Abnormal vaso-constriction. Acute disorders of the respiratory organs. ***Pneumonia***, rapid extension. Tuberculosis. Acute catarrh of all mucus membranes.

Arthritis deformans. ***Acts prominently on the connective tissue. Acute exacerbation of chronic inflammations.*** Trembling of limbs or body. Pancreatic diseases. Lead poisoning. Sluggish vital reaction. Chronicity.

MIND - ***Anxiety when quiet***. Anxiety about the present, no reference to the future. Anxiety during cough. ***Intolerably cross and restless***, excited, worse warm room. Hurried while walking. Feels better if busy. Inclined to move about, not permitting to sit or sleep, but motion aggravates and exhausts. Desire to travel.

Forgetful. Constantly feels as if he had forgotten something, and doesn't know what. Fixed, immovable thoughts. Does not understand why he has done something. Tendency to do some strange things without any cause. ***Impulsive behavior.*** Sudden impulse to run and do violence, to himself or others, but worse motion, which exhausts. Impulse to kill somebody, himself.

Anxious and worried if he does not eat (Cina., Sulph.). Anxiety as if going crazy.

Anxiety better eating, when hungry, better walking in open air. Fear of people, of physicians, when anyone comes near. Apprehends an accident from every trifle. Fear of evil. Fear with overcarefulness.

Melancholy. Depression, dejected with tendency to weep. Suicidal tendency. Irritability, with sadness. Disappointed love. Aversion to company, to strangers. Shuns everyone. Can't bear to be looked at. Cheers up in open air. Heart palpitations when thinking of real or imaginary wrongs. Thinks he is well.

Abdomen - Swelling and distension, or emaciation and sinking in of abdomen. Cutting pain in abdomen. Trembling in abdomen. Incarcerated flatulence. Pancreatic disease. Region of spleen very painful. Enlarged spleen, with salivation. Liver and spleen sore and enlarged. Violent throbbing of aorta abdominalis. Mesenteric glands enlarged. Swelling of inguinal glands.

Back - Back pains like rheumatism. Sharp pain in small of back. Pain in sacrum and coccyx. Spinal complaints with gressus vaccinus. Large boil between scapulae, with gangrene of legs. Swelling and induration of cervical glands. Swelling of the neck when speaking, grows thick. Yellow spots on neck. Redness on neck and chest as if ecchymosed.

Breasts - Breasts hyperesthesia. ***Dwindling of breasts***. Atrophy of breast glands. Breasts heavy, as if would fall. Nodosities in the skin of breasts with black points. Tumors in breast. Excessive flow of very thin, watery milk with great weakness and rapid emaciation. Suppression of milk with atrophy and relaxation of breasts.

Causations - Ill effects of nervous shock, disappointed love.

Chest - Burning, stinging tension in skin of chest. Sharp, quick, piercing pains. Tickling all over chest. Raw sensation in bronchi. Great weakness about chest. Difficult expansion of chest. Clavicular region, on right side, sunken. Pleuritic effusions. Swelling of axillary glands.

Constitutions - Suited to persons of dark hair and complexion, dark, yellow, tawny skin. Over-grown boys with weak chest and aged persons.

Cough - Short, dry, irritating cough, worse at night, followed in morning by sweat. Dry cough in morning. Cough from tickling in larynx. Cough as from a feather in throat. Croupy cough with difficult respiration, wheezing. Wheezing, metallic cough. Cough from every effort to expand chest. Cough causing glowing heat in head and face. Suffocating cough can hardly get her breath. Can't lie down from cough, sits bent forward.

Ears - Sensitiveness to noise. Reverberations in head. Buzzing. Hearing first sensitive, then dull. Catarrhal deafness. ***Eustachian deafness***. Chronic deafness with adhesions in the middle ear. Indolent ulcers of membrana tympani.

Eyes - Pain in eyes. Protrusion of eyes. Dark rings. Dirty yellowish color of sclera. Staring with wide open eyes. Pupil dilated. Constant motion of eyeballs. Convulsive movements and quivering of the eyes, of lower eyelids. Trembling of lids. Edematous swelling of lids. Eyelids seem to be retracted. ***Acute dacryocystitis***. Acute inflammation of lachrymal duct. Smarting pain, as from excoriation. Violent, profuse lachrymation.

Face - Face pale, sometimes yellowish or greenish, alternating with red. Withered, brownish, sallow or dusky. Bluish lips. Coldness of face in fleshy children. Miserable look. Twitching of facial muscles. Facial paralysis after reduction of goiter. Swollen submaxillary glands. Suppurating ulcer on left cheek.

Female - Chronic amenorrhea. Sudden appearance of menses, very profuse and with severe abdominal pains. Great weakness during menses (Alum., Carban., Cocc.). Menses irregular. Menses, brown, renewed after every stool. Violent dysmenorrhea with very scanty discharge. Uterine hemorrhage. Metrorrhagia, with acute pain in breasts. Leucorrhea, acrid, eroding thighs and linen, worse during menses. Thin, yellow leucorrhoea in scrofulous women, with induration and swelling of os uteri, and swelling of vagina. Leucorrhea alternating with cough. ***Ovaritis with leucorrhea*** (Apis., Bell., Lach.). Ovarian cysts. Dropsical swelling of ovaries with pressing down toward genitals. Great sensitiveness of right ovarian region during or after menses. ***Wedge-like pain from ovary to uterus.*** Miscarriage. Sterility from atrophy of ovaries and breasts. Cancerous degeneration at neck of uterus.

Food - Variable appetite. ***Ravenous hunger with great thirst.*** Loses flesh, yet hungry and eating well (Abrot.). Only feels well while eating in any diseased condition. Gets anxious or worried if he does not eat. Food doesn't nourish or strengthen. Desire for meat, spirituous liquors, acid things. Drinking cold milk helps constipation. Milk causes vomiting. Heartburn after indigestible food.

Head - Dull pressure in frontal sinuses, during coryza. Headache at root of nose and frontal sinus. Reverberations in head. ***Throbbing in head*** and all over body. Feeling of a tight band. ***Rush of blood to head.*** Headache so violent it almost makes him crazy. Chronic, congestive headache of elderly people (Phos.). Headache of elderly people, worse in warm air, fatigue, walking fast, riding in car. Brain as if stirred around with a spoon. Atrophy of brain. Apoplexy. Falling off of hair. Scald head.

Heart - Great precordial anxiety, obliging him to constantly change his position. Violent heart action. Feeling of vibration or purring over heart. Feels as if squeezed by an iron hand (Cact.), followed by great weakness and faintness. Myocarditis, painful compression around heart. Tachycardia. Pericarditis in complication with pneumonia. Mitral insufficiency. Dilatation of heart, after scarlatina. Palpitations, with faintness, worse least exertion, warm bath, better cold bath. Intermittent action of heart. Pulsation in large arterial trunks. Pulse rapid, small, weak, tumultuous, irregular, large, hard and accelerated.

Kidneys - Obstinate retention of urine. Stoppage of urine, or it flows, stops, and flows again. Stricture of urethra. Uremia. Urination frequent and copious. Incontinence in old people. Urine dark, thick, ammoniacal. Urine, dark, yellow-green (Bov.), sediment like red pepper. Urine milky with variegated cuticle on its surface. Milky white fluid runs from urethra after stool.

Limbs - Trembling and weariness in limbs and debility. Pulsation in large arterial trunks. Chronic arthritic affections, stiff and enlarged joints. ***Joints inflamed and painful.*** Synovitis. ***Rheumatic pain in joints.*** Rheumatic pains, nightly pains in joints and bones. Constrictive sensations, white swellings. Gonorrheal rheumatism. Rheumatism of nape and upper limbs. Cold hands and feet. Subsultus tendinum of hands and feet. Back of hands, brown, as if swollen, painful when turning hand, not when closing fingers. Acrid sweat of feet (Sil.). Edema of the feet. Painful corns.

Liver - Pains in region of liver with jaundice, emaciation. Hepatitis, with fever, dry tongue, restlessness, etc. Jaundice, eyes, skin, nails yellow. Cirrhosis of liver. Liver and spleen sore and enlarged.

Lungs - Asthma, breathes heavily when quiet. Hay asthma. Shortness of breath at least exertion or talking. Inspiration difficult. ***Raw and tickling feeling provoking a dry cough.*** Difficult expansion of chest, blood-streaked sputum internal dry heat, external coldness. Pleuritis effusion. ***Pneumonia.*** Right-sided pneumonia with high temperature. Hepatization spreads rapidly with persistent high temperature, absence of pain in spite of great involvement, worse warmth, craves cool air. ***Croupy cough with difficult respiration, wheezy.*** Croup in scrofulous children with dark hair and eyes. Dry, morning cough from tickling in larynx. ***Cold extends downwards*** from head to throat and bronchials. Cough is worse indoors in warm, wet weather and when lying on back. Large quantities of transparent mucus. Tough, sweetish, yellow, tasteless mucus. Frequently blood-streaked mucus, with cough. Gluey, rusty yellow expectoration, mingled with blood streaks, dislodged with difficulty and sticks fast to handkerchief.

Male - Testicles swollen and indurated. Painless swelling of testicles with offensive sweat. Offensive sweating of genitals. ***Orchitis.*** Hydrocele. Sarcocele. Twisting pain in spermatic cord. Senile hypertrophy and induration of prostate. Prostate gland swollen and indurated. Incontinence in old men with prostatic enlargement. Atrophy of testes with loss of sexual power. Hypertrophy of testicles, with sexual excitement.

Modalities - ***Better from cold, air***, walking about in open air, bathing, eating. Worse sitting up, ascending, exertion, touch, pressure, right side. Worse from warmth, ***heat of room***, wrapping up, rest, night, when quiet in warmth, talking, fasting. Worse during certain moon phases.

Mouth - Offensive odor from mouth. Profuse, fetid, soapy, sweet saliva. Metallic, salty, soapy, sour taste, with purulent stools. Mouth filled with mucus on waking in morning, with putrid taste, not better washing mouth with water. Aphthae with putrid smell and profuse, fetid salivation. Foul ulcers and salivation. Glands on inside of cheeks intensely painful as if sharp vinegar in mouth. Little blisters on gums. Gums loose and bleed easily.

Nose - Red and swollen. Profuse, sudden sneezing with dripping of hot water. ***Nasal catarrh thin, excoriating.*** Sneezing with sudden, violent influenza. Acute influenzas with hot, watery discharge, pain at root of nose and over frontal sinuses. Dry coryza becomes fluent in open air. ***Fluent, hot coryza*** with general heat of skin. Blowing of much yellow mucus from nose. Chronic fetid discharge. Discharge of mucus from posterior nares. Pain at the root of the nose and frontal sinuses. Nose stopped up. ***Acute nasal engorgement with high blood pressure.*** Descending colds. Tendency to ulceration. Nosebleeds. Loss of smell. Alae nasi as if spread wide apart.

Perspiration - Debilitating, sour-smelling sweats. Cold, viscid sweat. Sweats easily. Sweats with inclination to uncover. Profuse night sweats with great emaciation and debility. Sweats, better in early morning.

Rectum - Burning and itching in anus. Hemorrhoids protrude and burn, worse heat. Constipation with ineffectual urging, better by drinking cold milk. Constipation alternating with diarrhea (Ant-c.). ***Chronic diarrhea of an exhausting character.*** Chronic morning diarrhea of emaciated, scrofulous children. Fatty diarrhea from pancreatic affections. Dysenteric mucus stools without feces. Stools, whitish, frothy, whey-like, fatty, cheesy or lienteric, pancreatic disorders. Stools of watery, foaming, whitish mucus. Stools hard, knotting, dark-colored, blackish. Hemorrhage at every stool.

Skin - Clammy, moist, hot, dry, dirty, skin. Yellow and withered skin. Brown spots on skin. Skin turns brown in Addison's disease. Thickening of epidermis. Nodosities on skin. Tendency to papulae, small boils and abscesses. Acne. Urticaria. Impetigo scrofulosa. Herpes. Ringworm. Fungus articularis after measles. Syphilis with ulceration of skin. Bleeding ulcers. Ulcers with copious pus, bloody and corroding. Anasarca of cardiac disease. Itching and pimples in old scars. ***Scars break open.*** Glands enlarged.

Sleep - Restlessness, prevents sleep. Sleeplessness after midnight. Restless sleep with vivid or anxious dreams. Dreams of eating.

Stomach - Gastric derangement with constipation. Pulsation, throbbing in the pit of the stomach. Bitter taste to solid food, not drinks. Hiccough. Sour eructations with burning. Empty belchings, as if every particle of food were turned into gas. Sharp pains in stomach. Nausea, with spasmodic pain in stomach. Vomiting of bile with violent pain in stomach. Vomiting of first water, then food. Vomit tasting salty, oily. Vomiting greasy substances.

Teeth - Gums swollen, red, inflamed, softening, receding from teeth. Gums loose and bleed easily. Absorption of gums and alveolar processes. Small ash-colored ulcers on gums. Teeth yellow and covered with mucus in morning.

Temperature - Shaking chilliness, in warm room. Cold chills run up back. Hands, nose, feet icy cold. Cold feet the whole night. Chill alternating with heat. Flushes of heat all over the body, heat waves to head. Marked fever, restlessness, red cheeks, apathetic. Hyperpyrexia or external coldness with anxiety or stupor. Hectic fever. Internal heat, with coldness of skin. Heat with inclination to uncover.

Throat - Great hoarseness or complete aphonia. Constriction, impeding deglutition. Burning and scraping in throat. Raw and tickling feeling provoking a dry cough. Uvula swollen. Edema of glottis. Larynx feels constricted. ***Pain in larynx***. Laryngitis with painful roughness, worse during cough. Child grasps throat when coughing (Samb.). ***Croup caused by long-continued damp weather.*** Ulcers in throat, with swelling of glands of neck. Enlargement of tonsils and of glands of neck. Submaxillary glands swollen. Hypertrophy of thyroid gland. Goiter, hard with sensation of constriction. Diphtheria. Rough voice. Voice has a deep, hoarse, rough sound, becoming continually deeper.

Tongue - Tongue covered with thick brown, leather-like coating. Tongue brown in center, white at edges. Tongue moist, with mucus streak at sides. Tongue, hypertrophied, painful, nodular or fissured. Sweetish taste on tip of tongue.

Vertigo - Vertigo, worse from stooping, in warm room. Vertigo on active exertion. Vertigo with throbbing headache, with throbbing all over body. Rising aggravates, and causes faintness. Confusion in head, with aversion to earnest work. Very weak and tremulous.

Vision - Obscured vision like a veil before eyes. Optical illusions in bright colors. Small sparks, while sewing. Flimmering. Diplopia.

COMMENTS - Scrofulous and syphilitic indurations, effusions, tumors and goiters. Affinity for the glands and thyroid. Hypertrophy of the glands, and emaciation of the body. Hyperthyroidism. Goiters of the thyroid, exophthalmic goiter (Grave's disease), where the eyes bulge out. Indurated goiters, thyroid cysts, swollen thyroid. Facial paralysis and epilepsy, following suppression of goiter.

Tumors with keynote hardness and atrophy. Emaciation or enlargement of the glands. Hyperactivity with swollen glands. Affinity for salivary glands and pancreas, especially when there is a diarrhea of milky, whey-like stools.

Indurations or atrophy of testes, ovaries and uterus. Ovarian, uterine and cervical cancer. Atrophy of the breasts. Characteristic one breast larger than the other. Failure to thrive in infants with emaciation and swollen glands, always hungry. Emaciation of single parts.

Keynote ravenous eating, yet emaciation. Increases or decreases appetite. Severe hypoglycemia. Canine hunger. Severe ranges of blood sugar, with erratic, manic behavior. Can get violent and angry when hungry. Burning pains, better eating.

Produces atrophy of nerve and brain tissue, as well as of other tissues. Acute hydrocephalus. Pleuritic effusions. Tubercular disease, tabes mesenterica, pulmonary tuberculosis. tuberculosis of rapidly-growing young people, thin and dark.

Pneumonia and tubercular disorders with lung consolidation. Dyspnea, cough with blood-streaked expectoration, tickling all over chest, weakness and emaciation. Symptoms worse in a warm room. Croup or for a croupy cough (Spong., Brom.).

Heart disorders. Palpitation from the slightest cause, like lightning. Sensation as if being squeezed. Hypertrophy. With the heart symptoms there is a "gone," exhausted feeling and the patient is scarcely able to breathe or walk.

Excessive weakness. Nervousness, restlessness, twitching, subsultus tendinum. Sense of trembling in inner parts. Fainting on going upstairs.

Vertigo with throbbing in the head, agitated, vivid dreams and restless sleep. Nocturnal sweat, pulse quick, small, and hard.

Rheumatism. Growth defects, curvature of bones, in children's ailments (follows Calc. well). Characteristic hot-bloodedness. Sensitive to heat.

Irritable, cross. Anxious, apprehensive. Extremely restless, hurried, must move about. Tearful and sad. Shuns persons. Effects of amorousness and disappointed love. Averse to all intellectual labor.

Excessive mental excitement. Panic attacks. Irresistible impulse to run. Feels she will fall if she walks. May be useful for AIDS when there is psychosis with swollen glands and emaciation. Impulse to murder.

Clarke saw it given with excellent effect in the lower potencies when swollen and deformed joints have been left behind after an attack of acute rheumatism.

He used it with excellent effect in the case of a young woman who had a nervous shock and had lost all appetite and desire to live. She was much emaciated and had quietly made up her mind to starve herself to death.

Clarke gave five drops of Iod. 3x in a wineglass of water half an hour before meal-times and her appetite returned with such vigor she could not choose but eat and was soon restored to a normal mental and bodily state.

C. S. McKay noticed lumbrici passed by an infant who had tasted iodine accidentally and used the experience in another case, giving a dilute solution (one part of the tincture to three of water of this three drops every three hours) and produced the expulsion of lumbrici when Sant. had completely failed.

Grimmer wrote that when it is indicated it cures cancer of the breast and uterus.

Nash noted that Iod. is one of the remedies affected by the moon's changes. In cases of goiter where it is indicated, he gave a powder of Iod. 100,000c. every night for four nights after the full moon.

RELATIONS - ***It antidotes:*** Merc. ***Follows well:*** Merc., Hep. (croup), Ars. ***Followed well by:*** Arg-n., Calc., Merc. Phos., Puls. ***Complementary:*** Lyc., Bad. ***Compare:*** (1) Thyr., Hep., Merc., Phos. (2) Abrot., Nat-m., Sanic., Tub. (3) Brom. has light hair and complexion, Iod. dark. (4) Bor. - carrion-like odor of ulcers. (5) Chlor., Nat-m. - ravenous appetite yet gets thing - Nat. m. especially about the neck. (6) Kali-i. - talkative as if from alcohol. (7) Bar-c. - tabes mesenterica, extreme hunger, emaciates, talkative, averse to strangers, Bar-c. suited to dwarfish persons, has not the intolerable crossness of Iod., which is worse than that of Ant-c. (8) Alum. - apprehensive, fears. (9) Apis - in joint effusions, sensitiveness, hydrocephalus. (10) Cact. and Spig. (11) Hydr. - uterine affections.

REFERENCES - Boericke. Clarke. Murphy. Phatak.

IPECACUANHA

(Ipecac Root)

PHARMACY - ip. Ipecacuanha. Ipec root. Cephaelis ipecacuanha. Psychotria ipecacuanha. Uragoga ipecacuanha. N. O. Rubiaceae. Tincture and trituration of the dried root. ***Historical dose:*** Trituration, tincture and all potencies.

CLINICAL - Anemia. Anorexia. Asthma. Bronchitis. Catarrh, Chills. Cholera. Cholera, infantum. Colic. Convulsions. ***Coughs. Cramps.*** Cyanosis. Deafness. Diarrhea. Drug, addictions. ***Drug, poisoning.*** Dyspepsia. ***Dyspnea. Dysentery.*** Enteric, fever. Eyes, disorders. Fever. ***Food, poisoning.*** Gallstone, colic. Gastric, ulcer. Gastritis. ***Gastroenteritis.*** Hematemesis. ***Hemorrhages.*** Hemorrhoids. ***Hemoptysis.*** Hysteria. Indigestion. Intermittent, fever. Menstruation, disorders. ***Migraine***. Miscarriage. ***Morning, sickness. Nausea.*** Nosebleeds. ***Opium, habit.*** Opisthotonos. Pityriasis. Pneumonia. ***Poisonings.*** Pregnancy, disorders. Remittent, fever. Salivation. Spasms. ***Stomach, disorders.*** Tetanus. Toothache. Tuberculosis. ***Uterine, hemorrhage. Vomiting. Whooping, cough.*** Worm fever. Yellow fever.

HERBAL - Ipecac is likely to be of help wherever ailments are associated with the presence of constant nausea. Ipecacuanha wine has a well-known emetic effect. Mixed with oil, powdered ipecac has been used to vesicate the skin and, diluted, the tincture is used for the bites of insects, bee and wasp-stings.

In material doses, it produces violent irritation of the skin and, between the acts of vomiting, an uncontrollable desire to scratch.

HOMEOPATHIC - ***Persistent nausea and vomiting***. Profuse salivation with nausea. Constant desire to vomit. Disgust for food, empty vomiting, vomiting of bile or blood. Not better by vomiting. Immediately after vomiting, instead of relief, there is the desire to vomit again. Characteristic feeling "as if the stomach were hanging down relaxed." Tongue is clean, or not very dirty.

Affinity for the pneumo-gastric nerve, producing gastro-intestinal disturbances and respiratory disorders with ***continuous nausea.*** Nausea and shortness of breath usually accompany most of the complaints. ***Bright red, gushing hemorrhages with nausea***. Discharges are foamy and profuse.

Spasmodic disorders. Opisthotonos and emprosthotonos. Body rigid, stretched out, followed by spasmodic jerking of arms towards each other. Awkward, stumbles against everything. Tetanic spasms from swallowing tobacco. Infantile convulsions. Convulsions in whooping cough from suppressed exanthema from indigestible food.

Oversensitive to heat and cold. Faints suddenly in summer or hot room. ***Morphine or heroin addiction*** (Aven.). Especially indicated in fat children and adults, who are feeble and catch cold in relaxing atmosphere, warm, moist weather.

MIND - Mental depression. Sad, morose. Dejected mood. Peevish, irritable, scornful mood. Impatient, fretful. Full of desires, but do not know what they want. Hard to please. Holds everything in contempt. Disgust with everything. Haughty. Censorious, critical. Intolerance of noise.

Wrapped in thought, taciturn. Moaning and sighing with the fever. ***Anxiety during fever.*** Restlessness during the fever. Awkward and stumbles against everything. Shrieking before convulsions. Child cries and screams violently and incessantly.

Delusion he is unfortunate. Hypochondriasis. Disposition to slander. Ailments from anger, mortification, vexation and reserved displeasure. Irascible, restless, angry in suddenly appearing spells.

Abdomen - ***Cramps with nausea and vomiting.*** Flatulent colic with frequent loose stools. Colic of children with diarrhea, restlessness, screaming and tossing about. Cold drinks or ice cream causes colic. Abdominal colic after sour or unripe fruit, beer, etc. Clawing pains as from a hand clawing intestines. ***Cutting pain worse around the navel***. Inguinal hernia. Griping, drawing or cutting pain about the navel. Pinching pain. Sharp pain from navel to uterus. Diaphragm, as if pressed between two stones.

Back - Tetanic spasms of back which bends the back backwards or forwards. Pain in back, during urination. Shooting from kidney region into thighs. Cramps between scapulae during motion.

Causations - Ill effects of vexation, reserved displeasure. Injuries, loss of blood, suppressed eruptions. Morphine, opium and heroin addictions. Quinine. ***Food poisoning.*** Indigestible food, rich food, pork, pastry, fruits, candy, ice cream.

Chest - Constant constriction in chest and larynx, worse least motion. Chest seems full of phlegm, but does not yield to coughing.

Constitutions - Suited to stout persons of lax tissue, to fair people, to women and children, to emphysematous persons, to persons who have a history of nosebleed or other blood loss. Indicated in fat children and adults who are feeble and catch cold in warm wet weather.

Cough - Suffocative, paroxysmal cough. ***Cough incessant and violent with every breath***. ***Cough with nausea and vomiting***, or vomiting without nausea. Dry cough caused by tickling in upper part of larynx. Dry, spasmodic cough, after coryza. Cough producing sonorous and bubbling rales. Suffocative, strangling cough with much mucus accumulated in bronchia. ***Hemoptysis.*** Cough with spitting of blood, worse from least effort. Cough during fever. Whooping cough with nosebleed and bleeding from mouth. Child becomes stiff and blue or red in face, stiffens out with cough. Cough in teething children. Dry, spasmodic coughs of elderly persons, coming on in fits.

Ears - Cannot endure the least noise. Coldness and chilliness of the ears, during the fever.

Eyes - Inflamed, red eyes. Red circle around cornea. Yellow sclera. Dilated pupils. Eyes fixed and turned to right. Conjunctivitis. Ulcers of cornea or conjunctiva. Pustular inflammation of cornea and conjunctiva. Cornea dim. Profuse, gushing lachrymation with nausea. Shooting pains through the eyeball. Twitching of eyelids. Lids red and swollen after catching cold. Eyes tire from near vision. Cannot move eyes without nausea. Nausea from looking at moving objects. Photophobia without redness of eyes. Light, candlelight aggravates.

Face - Puffed or sunken. ***One side of face hot, the other cold.*** Pale, blue about the eyes or lips, white linea nasalis. Redness of the skin around the mouth. Lips blue during chill. Lips covered with small aphthae and eruptions. Rash in the face. Pityriasis. Periodical orbital neuralgias with some lachrymation, photophobia and smarting eyelids. Convulsive startings of the muscles of the face.

Female - Menses too early and too profuse. ***Menses with cramps and constant nausea.*** Scanty menses with great weakness. Menses return every two weeks. Prolapsed uterus worse during menses. Great debility and leucorrhea during intervals of menses. ***Uterine hemorrhages, profuse, bright red,*** steady flow or gushing with nausea and gasping with each gush of blood. ***Pain from navel to uterus.*** Cutting pain in uterus from left to right. Dragging sensation towards uterus and anus. ***Nausea and vomiting during pregnancy. Threatened miscarriage***, often with sharp or pinching pain around umbilicus. Hemorrhage following labor or after miscarriage. Hemorrhage from placenta previa. Arterial bleeding from partial separation of placenta. Labor pains spasmodic, cutting across from left to right with nausea and clutching about navel. Labor pains running downward.

Food - General loss of appetite as from weakness of stomach. ***Great disgust and loathing of any sort of food.*** No appetite, earthy taste, stomach feels relaxed, nausea. ***Nausea from smell of food.*** Violent hunger when nausea is over. Thirstlessness. No thirst during chill, but much thirst all through fever. Stomach disordered by rich food, pork, pastry, fruits, candy, ice cream. ***Food poisoning.*** Desires or adverse to sweets and dainty things. Worse cold drinks, black coffee, sour beer, smoking tobacco. Worse from fats, ice cream, pastry, pork, unripe fruit, salads. Cold drinks or ice-cream causes colic. Cold water worsens spasmodic cough.

Head - Cold sweat on forehead. Heat and throbbing in head, with red cheeks. Aching pain, pressure in forehead. Throbbing in forehead. ***Migraine or gastric headaches with nausea and vomiting. Headaches with nosebleed.*** Headache as if brain compressed. Bones of skull feel crushed or bruised. Pain, bruised feeling in brain. Pain in occiput, worse vomiting during chill. Shooting pain in vertex. Pain in the occiput and the neck. Headache over left eye. Pain extends to teeth and root of tongue. Stinging pain with heaviness of head. Hydrocephaloid, fontanels open.

Heart - Pain in heart, followed by dryness of mouth and great thirst. Pulse large and soft. Pulse accelerated but weak, sometimes imperceptible.

Kidneys - Shooting pain from kidney, down the thighs to the knees. Ineffectual urging to urinate. Burning in urethra during urination. Red, scanty urine. Urine turbid, with red sediment. Hematuria with nausea and cutting in abdomen and urethra, with oppression in chest and short breath.

Limbs - ***Pains in limbs during chill.*** Numbness, as if joints had gone to sleep. Shocks in limbs on falling asleep. Body stretched stiff, followed by spasmodic jerking of arms towards each other. Pains as if bruised in all the bones and joints. Femur as if dislocated on sitting down. Cold hands and feet. Coldness of one hand, other is hot.

Lungs - Cyanosis. ***Dyspnea with constant constriction in chest.*** Attacks of difficult shortness of breathing. ***Gasps for air at open window.*** Difficult expiration. Sighing. Shortness of breath as from inhaling dust. Suffocative attacks from foreign substance in wind pipe. Threatened suffocation from accumulation of mucus. Asthma with skin disease. Humid asthma from damp or sudden changes in weather. Spasmodic asthma after suppressed eruptions. Croup. Bronchopneumonia. Pneumonia. Bubbling rales. ***Loose, coarse rattle in chest without expectoration.*** Suffocative cough, child becomes stiff and blue in the face. Continued sneezing, coryza, wheezing cough. ***Bleeding from lungs with nausea***, feeling of constriction, rattling cough. Hemoptysis from slightest exertion (Mill.).

Modalities - Better from open air, rest, pressure, closing eyes, cold drinks. ***Worse from drugs, morphine.*** Worse after overeating, vomiting, lying down, motion. Worse from mixed or rich foods, ice cream, pork, veal, candy, fruits, berries, raisins, salads, lemon peel. Worse cold, winter, dry weather, ***warmth, damp***, external heat, periodically. Catarrh, asthma and chill are worse in warm, moist wind. Summer heat or hot room causes fainting.

Mouth - Mouth moist with much saliva. Saliva increased. Earthy, bitter, sweetish, bloody taste. Smarting pain in mouth and on tongue. Child thrusts its fists into the mouth and screams during dentition.

Nose - ***Nosebleed, bright red blood.*** Nosebleed during cough, headache, every time the patient takes cold. Coryza with stoppage of nose and nausea. Discharge of thin mucus with cough and expectoration. Sneezing. Itching of nose. Loss of smell.

Perspiration - Cold, clammy. Hands and feet drip cold sweat. Very profuse sweats, mostly during night. Sweats with redness of one cheek and paleness of the other. Hot sweats, sudden attacks in room. Sour sweat with turbid urine. Sweat stains yellow. Profuse perspiration after quinine.

Rectum - Rectal pain so great that it nauseates. Itching at anus. Hemorrhoids bleeding very profusely. Diarrhea after overloading stomach with sweets or fat pastry. Diarrhea from taking cold, due to chill or from emotions. Amoebic dysentery with tenesmus, while straining. Dysentery with head hot and cold legs. Cholera infantum. Beginning cholera infantum, with nausea, vomiting, colic, diarrhea. Autumn diarrhea. Diarrhea of teething children, yellow, white or green discharges. Worm and parasites.

Skin - Pale, lax. Miliary rash. Erysipelas. Itching, unchanged by scratching. Itching with nausea, scratches until he vomits. Suppressed rash or eruptions. Delayed eruption in scarlatina. Rash in lying-in women. Herpetic eruptions.

Sleep - Sleeplessness. Shocks in all limbs on going to sleep (Ign.). Restless, unrefreshing sleep. Eyes half open during sleep with moaning and groaning. Starting during sleep. Loss of sleep that causes nausea and fatigue. Frightful dreams, with frequent starts and terror during sleep. Yawning and stretching.

Stomach - Stomach feels relaxed, as if hanging down. ***Sinking sensation in stomach.*** Pressing pain in stomach. Indescribable pain and sick feeling in stomach. Violent clutching and cramping pains. Attacks of cramps. Dyspepsia. Gastritis, inveterate cases, not even a drop of water will stay down, continuous gagging. ***Gastroenteritis.*** Eructations with rumbling in abdomen. Hiccoughs. ***Food poisoning***. Loss of appetite and frequent nausea. ***Horrid nausea, not better vomiting.*** Nausea, copious salivation, violent itching in the skin and empty risings. ***Constant nausea and vomiting*** with pale, twitching of face. Incessant retching with vomiting of watery fluids and cutting pain in belly. ***Vomits blood, bile, food, mucus***, grass-green mucus, black matter like pitch. Hematemesis of children. Bilious vomiting. Vomiting with thirst, sweat, and bad breath. ***Nausea and vomiting with menses, cramps, during pregnancy.*** Nausea from smell of food, from looking at moving objects, from slightest motion or cough. Retching, especially after drinking anything cold or after smoking. Constant nausea and retching of hysterical women. Vomiting of infants at the breast. Morning vomiting in weakly persons who are affected by worms.

Stools - Mucus fetid diarrhea, worse at night. Stools, brown, grass or yellow green, lemon colored. Stools, painless, fermented frothy or bloody, slimy, pitch-like. Stools covered with red, bloody mucus, or lumps of mucus. ***Stools like frothy molasses*** with griping at navel. Stools spurting out with much flatus. Stools very offensive, putrid smelling.

Teeth - Teeth chatter, with chill. Toothache, with a jerk radiating to temples, better while eating. Toothache in a hollow tooth as if it would be torn out.

Temperature - Chill alternating with heat. Short chill with long heat. Internal chill, with external heat. Chill and much heat, nausea, vomiting, and dyspnea. ***Chill with nausea, vomiting,*** great lassitude, weariness, oppression of the chest. Chills, up and down back. Coldness of upper part of body. Anxious dry heat in evening. Heat with or without thirst. ***Fever with nausea and vomiting.*** Catarrhal or gastric fevers. Intermittent fever, irregular cases after quinine. Infantile remittent fever. Suppressed of mixed intermittents, nausea in all stages. Relapses with improper diet.

Throat - Sore throat, as from swelling of the pharynx. Difficult swallowing, as from paralysis of the tongue and of the gullet. Fauces, stinging, rough, sore, and dry. Pressure in throat with pains in diaphragm. Deep red color of tonsils and pharynx. Tickling in upper part of larynx. Croup. ***Gagging and choking.*** Spasms of vocal cords. Spasm of glottis, with blueness of face and coldness of limbs. Spasmodic contractive sensation in the throat. ***Hoarseness***, especially at end of a cold. Complete aphonia. Voice hollow.

Tongue - ***Tongue clean, not coated.*** Tongue, dry, yellow, white, pale. Red, pointed tongue. Tongue coated in middle, edges red. Flat taste, with white, thickly coated tongue. Smarting pain on tongue.

Vertigo - Vertigo with tottering and staggering. Vertigo when walking, when turning around, during pregnancy.

Vision - Obscuration of vision. State of vision constantly changing. Blue and red halo around light. Optical illusions in bright colors. Spasm of accommodation from weakness of ciliary muscle.

COMMENTS - The stomach disgust of the remedy is depicted on the countenance, which expresses nausea. Sickly, disgusted appearance. The corners of the mouth are drawn down. Blue rings around the eyes.

Deathly nausea (Tab.). Constant nausea, not ameliorated by vomiting. Can vomit blood. Salivation and vomiting of white, stringy mucus. Vomiting can lead to shudders with a chill, severe spasms, convulsions. Can be sleepy after vomiting.

Desire for fresh air, thirstless while nauseas (Puls.).Any condition with concomitant nausea and vomiting. Vomiting after pregnancy. Sensation as if the stomach is hanging down (Sep.).

Corresponding mental state, "moroseness and contempt for everything," "disdainful humor." Irritability in adults, crying and screaming in children. Restless and exhausted (Ars.). Disgust. Sensitiveness (Chin.), over sensitive to heat and cold. Better by touch.

Exhaustion and an achy, bruised feeling. Sore pain in the shoulder blades. Bone pains in the head and elsewhere. Pains as if bones were all torn to pieces. Keynote cutting pains in the left side of the abdomen over to the right. Peripheral neuritis. Generally a left sided remedy.

Intermittent headaches. Migraine headaches. Bruised feeling, severe prostration. Headache "as if bruised, all through the bones of the head and down into the root of the tongue." Pain extending to roots of teeth.

Headache with nausea. Gastric headache, originating in the stomach, nausea precedes the headache and persists throughout. Desire to lie perfectly still. Meningitis with vomiting and a high fever. Tetanus, lockjaw with severe spasms and retching.

Marked periodic action. Intermittent fevers (Eup-per.). Characteristic nausea through all the stages. Stages can be completely mixed up, short chill, followed by long fever. Can have a pain in the upper back between the shoulder blades with fever (Gel. has a chill).

Violent dyspnea with wheezing and great weight and anxiety about the precordia. Threatened suffocation from accumulation of mucus. Loss of breath, pale, stiff and blue. Strangling with gagging and vomiting of mucus, bleeding from nose or mouth. Coughing up mucus, gagging. Must stand by the window to get oxygen. Worse damp weather and changes in weather.

Pneumonia and bronchitis with severe shortness of breath with rattling mucus (Ant-t.). For bronchitis in infants with coarse rattling in the chest. Concomitant respiratory and gastric symptoms. For emphysema in the elderly. Suffocative respiration (Spong.), but wet.

Asthma with a breathless feeling, nausea and vomiting, with thick, yellow mucus (Lob., Ars., Ant-t., Ant-c.). Dry, spasmodic, constricted, asthmatic cough. Whooping cough. Characteristic spasmodic rigidity in whooping cough.

Sub-acute inflammation of the cornea with intense pain. Pustular conjunctivitis, especially in children. Inflammation with tearing pain and gushing of tears. Photophobia. Violent neuralgia of eyeballs, shooting in the head with gushes of tears, nausea, etc.

Hemorrhage with bright, red blood (Phos.). Gushing blood, with sinking feeling and nausea (Ferr. is weak and flushed with gushing). Nosebleeds with a sensation of nausea and sinking, or nosebleeds from coughing and sneezing attacks.

Uterine hemorrhage. Threatened miscarriage, with a sharp pain around the umbilicus, running downward to the uterus. Miscarriage due to spasmodic vomiting. Spotting blood before contractions. Hemorrhage after childbirth with bright red blood, nausea, disgust and weakness.

Metrorrhagia after confinement with a low pulse, nausea. Steady flow of bright red blood, which may soak through the bed to the floor or may run over the foot of the bed. Constant nausea and discharge of blood before the proper period. Menstrual cramps with nausea and vomiting, must lie still in bed. Copious menses.

Bloody diarrhea associated with nausea and vomiting. Constant urge to stool, tenesmus. Stools can be bloody, burning, offensive, watery. Severe colic that is associated with dysentery. Suppressed skin eruptions that go to the stomach and bowels and cause severe colic.

Stomach symptoms worse from ice cream, pork, and rich, fatty foods (Puls.). Bad taste in the mouth. The thought, smell or idea of food causes patient to gag and choke. Anorexia.

Heroin withdrawal symptoms. J. R. Haynes used Ip. as an antidote to the opium and morphine addiction. He gave five drops of Ip. tincture for every grain of morphine, or its equivalent in heroin or opium, which the patient has been accustomed to take.

Jahr recommended that in all cases of intermittents in which no other remedy is particularly indicated Ip. should be given. It will either cure the case or bring out more indications for another remedy.

Clarke frequently found this advice useful. As most intermittents have been treated with quinine, it is thought the antidotal properties of Ip. may have good effects.

Allen noted that Ip. dilutions have helped granulations of the eyelids.

Cooper cured an immense uterine fibroid with persistent painful irritation of the skin. There was constant retching and vomiting, made worse by eating. Vaginal irritation with thick leucorrhea and a feeling of desperation.

Dr. Nancy T. Williams cured several cases of gallstone colic on the symptom "external chilliness with internal heat," with Ip. 6c. The relief was prompt and lasting.

Dr. Edwin Muskett noted its specific use for malignant pustule and anthrax, used locally and internally.

Hahnemann considered it a short-acting medicine.

RELATIONS - ***Antidoted by:*** Arn., Ars., Chin., Copper fumes, Dulc., Ferr., Laur., Op., Sul-ac., Tab., Ant-t. ***Compare:*** (1) Lob., Emetin., Ars., Tab., Cham., Puls., Ant-t., Squil, Conv. - colic and diarrhea. (2) In asthma, Lob., Blatta. (3) Typh. - dysentery, diarrhea and summer complaint. (4) Euph-hy. - very similar to Ipecac. Irritation of the respiratory and gastro-intestinal tracts and female organs. (5) Lip. - persistent dry, hard, bronchial cough-asthma and chronic bronchitis. ***Complementary:*** Cupr., Arn.

REFERENCES - Boericke. Clarke. Murphy. Phatak.

IPOMOEA PURPUREA

(Morning Glory)

PHARMACY - ipom. Ipomoea purpurea. Morning glory. Convolvulus duartinus. Bind-weed. N. O. Convulvulaceae, family. The mother tincture is prepared from the dried bark. ***Historical dose:*** Tincture and all potencies.

CLINICAL - Anorexia. Backache. Bilious, vomiting. Catatonia. Cholecystitis. Delirium. Epilepsy. Fever. Flatulence. Headache. Insomnia. Jaundice. Kidney, colic. Kidney, disorders. Worms.

HOMEOPATHIC - Ipomoea is used solely as a drastic purgative in allopathic medicine; not one homeopathic treatise mentions it as a remedy for constipation.

Castro carried out a proving in 1940, using the potencies 1x, 2x, 3x, at the rate of 1-200 drops per day in progressive doses.

Symptoms included fever, agitation and mental confusion. Delirium with hallucinations, excitability, and mumbling. Predominant irritation of the brain. Epilepsy. Catatonia. Insomnia and delirious dreams.

Neuromuscular and arthritic pains. Aching in top of right shoulder, in small of back and limbs. Pain in left lumbar muscles on stooping. Kidney disorders with pain in back. Kidney colic. Much abdominal flatulence. Bilious vomiting.

MIND - Desire for solitude. Sadness, tears, hypersensitive to noise. Intense anxiety with palpitations. Prostration. Loss of memory. Delirious dreams. Nocturnal terror in children, especially in the worm-ridden.

Abdomen - Abdomen distended. Sharp cutting pain in abdomen above umbilicus. Rumbling and grumbling in epigastric region and lower bowels. Rumbling of flatus with pain in the colon. Sensation of heat in the epigastrium before passing stools. Cholecystitis. Biliary sycosis syndrome.

Back - Heaviness of the back and neck, aggravated at night, on going to bed. Pain, aching in lumbar region. Pain in first dorsal vertebrae. Itching over left scapula.

Chest - Thoracic spasms. Feeling of laryngeal and pectoral constriction.

Constitutions - Suited to neuro-bilious, hypersensitive types, prone to epileptiform fits. Useful for phospho-fluoric types, syphilitic.

Ears - Buzzing noise in ears.

Eyes - Smarting pain in eyes. Itching of internal canthus of left eye. Pupils dilated.

Food - Anorexia. Aggravated by and aversion to fatty foods, meat and milk.

Head - Great heaviness of head. Headache first in right, then in left temple. Headache with a unilateral perspiration. Itching of scalp.

Heart - Palpitations with anxiety and hysterical spasms. Pulse accelerated with extra systole.

Kidneys - ***Severe pain in left kidney with nausea and occasional vomiting.*** Kidney pain spreading towards the left ureter. ***Kidney stones.*** Kidney disorders or gravel with pain in back. Kidney colic, predominantly on the left side.

Limbs - Limbs cold, sweating, heavy. Joints painful. Muscular spasms with fatigue. Pain in the left lumbar muscles on bending down. Aching in top of right shoulder. Pain in left shoulder and arm.

Lungs - Irregular breathing. Disposition to cough with sneezing.

Modalities - Better from lying down. Worse in the morning, at night, from fatty foods.

Mouth - Mouth discolored, with a bad taste. Feeling of swallowing his tongue.

Nose - Smarting and dryness in nostrils. Purulent discharge from nose. Very acute sense of smell.

Rectum - Rectal tenesmus. Stools soft, orange-yellow in color.

Skin - Skin discolored, yellow, dry, despite cold sweating. Viral jaundice.

Sleep - Nocturnal aggravation, forcing him to get up.

Stomach - Acrid dyspepsia. Hiccoughs, thirsty for cold water. Yellow-green vomiting.

Temperature - Chilliness alternating with backache. Flushes of heat, followed by copious sweat. General fever with total insomnia, cold sweats and contracture of the jaw muscles.

Throat - Pain in left tonsil. Throat dry, constant need to swallow, but swallowing difficult.

Vertigo - Vertigo with nausea, ameliorated by lying down.

RELATIONS - ***Compare:*** (1) Cresol. (2) Stram. - hallucinations, delirium with talkativeness. (3) Hyos. - delirium, strips himself. (4) Agar. - muscular jerks in the lower limbs. (5) Nux-v. - abdominal distention, neuromuscular over excitability.

REFERENCES - Boericke. Julian.

IRIDIUM METALLICUM

(Iridium Metal)

PHARMACY - irid. Iridium metallicum. Iridium metal. At. Wt. 193.10. Trituration. ***Historical dose:*** Trituration and all potencies.

CLINICAL - Abscesses. Amenorrhea. ***Anemia.*** Axilla, abscess. Bronchitis. Cancer. Cerebral, hemorrhage. Cramps. Eczema. Epilepsy. ***Exhaustion***. Gout. Headache. Heart, disorders. Hemiplegia. Lupus. Multiple sclerosis. Nephritis. Neuralgias. Numbness. Paralysis. Parkinson's disease. Rheumatism. Septicemia. Spinal, paresis. Trembling. Urticaria. ***Uterine, tumors. Weakness.***

HOMEOPATHIC - Iridium is a rare metal of the platinum group, found in platinum ore. It is one of the heaviest known substances. It shares with Osm., Pall. and Plat. a place in the treatment of rheumatism and gout.

Boring, contracting pains. Sensations of being swollen, blown up, heavy, full. Shocks and twitching. Epilepsy, clonic, tonic, tetanic. Spinal paresis. Numbness and paralysis. Trembling. Parkinson's disease. Multiple sclerosis. Lupus.

Anemia with decreased red corpuscles. ***Exhaustion after disease***. Weakness, nervousness and restlessness. ***Weakness after influenza.*** Cerebral hemorrhage. Congestion of blood. Affections of bones, necrosis and inflammation. Abscesses. Septicemia. Intestinal putrefaction. Trypanosoma infections.

Glands swollen, inflamed, indurated. Problems with testes and ovaries, inflammations, cancer, cryptorchism. ***Uterine tumors.*** Sterility, amenorrhea, metrorrhagia. Nephritis of pregnancy. Children who are puny, weak-limbs and grow too fast.

MIND - Facilitates mental labor. Forgetful. Difficult concentration. Sensation as if mind were void. Confusion, loses his way in well-known streets. Feeling of self confidence.

Anxiety on waking, as if something bad is going to happen. Clinging to persons. Bites nails. Averse to being disturbed. Irritability from noise. Weeping after anger. Sadness, better walking in open air.

Abdomen - Dragging pain as if menses would come in abdomen.

Back - Spinal paresis, especially for the aged and after disease. Weariness in back and limbs. Weakness of cervical region, as if it could not support weight of head.

Breasts - Piercing, gnawing pains in breasts.

Chest - Sensation of iron band around chest.

Ears - Feeling of numbness in ears and throughout the body lasting a short time. Heat of ears when lying down. Sounds seem distant.

Eyes - Eyes red, heavy. Eye inflammations. Itching in morning on waking. Desire to close the eyes. Feeling as if eyes were being affected from below upward. Ingrown eyelashes. Far sighted. Visual disturbances.

Face - Face swollen. Sensation of swelling in morning on rising. Sensation of elongation of left side of face. Numbness of lips. Stinging pain in the left malar bone. Pain, pressure in right malar bone. Animated expression.

Female - Swelling of ovaries without dropsy. Corroding and suppurating ulcers of uterus, bluish patches on uterus. Uterine tumors with suppuration. Sterility. Amenorrhea, metrorrhagia.

Food - Desire for carbonated drinks. Aversion to brown bread. Worse from cold drinks, oranges.

Head - Right side of scalp sensitive. "Wooden" feeling in right side of head. Heaviness of head like liquid lead. Swashing sensation. Numbness in occiput. Pains in middle of occipital bone. Open air and noise seem to bruise the head. Pain, like cold metal pressing across forehead. Neuralgia of head especially temples, drives one crazy.

Heart - High blood pressure. Heart weakness, infarction. Heart failure, pain. Pulse, too fast, too slow, full, weak, irregular. Sensation as if an iron rod is standing straight in the heart region.

Kidneys - Weakness in kidney region. Nephritis during pregnancy.

Limbs - Neuralgia of the limbs. Dislocated feeling in left hip joint and dull pain toward left gluteal region. Pressing in groin and left thigh. Tension in both thighs, especially left. Achilles tendon painful, aggravated by walking. Achilles tendon torn from jumping.

Lungs - Difficulty breathing deeply. Short of breath, aggravated from climbing the stairs. Hoarse cough, worse talking. Profuse, thick, yellowish discharge. Chronic laryngeal catarrh.

Mouth - Increased saliva, with sensation in malar bones, which is more perceptible on left side. One-sided white discoloration of tongue.

Stomach - Cramps in stomach.

Nose - Posterior sinuses feel raw inflamed. Bridge of nose painful, feels too narrow. Profuse, watery coryza, better indoors. Ozaena. Profuse, thick, yellowish discharge.

Vision - Colors look brighter. Everything looks golden. Zigzags, in shape of circle.

COMMENTS - A. J. Tafel took 20 grains of the 3c trituration. He experienced a number of symptoms, all within two hours of taking the dose.

Prominent among them were a sensation of numbness in ears and throughout the body. A feeling as if they eyes were being affected from below upward. A feeling as of a triangle in face, the based formed by the two malar bones, the apex in the vertex. Cramp-like contractions in the right calf. The majority of symptoms appeared on the left side.

Laboucher said it is "admirable in all cases of anemia." He claimed it was better than Chin. for the aged and persons exhausted by disease, for puny, weak-limbed children and for those who grow too fast. He mentioned a particular alternation of symptoms or reaction. Painful weakness of lower limbs and kidney region, followed by a favorable reaction, self confidence and facilitated mental labor.

Laboucher gave Irid. in the 4c potency, Pall. in the 3c, Plat. in 2c and Osm. in the 1c. He said Irid. is superior to Pall., Plat. and to Osm. in uterine tumors.

RELATIONS - ***Compare:*** (1) Plat., Pall., Osm.. (2) In uterine diseases, Aur. and Aur-mur. (3) In exhaustion after disease, Chin. Irid-m.

REFERENCES - Boericke. Clarke.

IRIDIUM MURIATICUM

(Iridium Chloride)

PHARMACY - irid-m. Iridium muriaticum. Iridium chloride. ***Historical dose:*** Trituration and all potencies.

CLINICAL - Headache. Salivation.

HOMEOPATHIC - Irid-m. produces salivation and stiffness of the jaws followed by head and nervous symptoms. Congestion of sinuses and bronchials. Headache worse right side, heavy feeling as of liquid lead. Dragging pain in lower back.

REFERENCES - Boericke.

IRIS FLORENTINA

(Orris Root)

PHARMACY - iris-fl. Iris florentina. Orris root. White flag. N. O. Iridaceae. Tincture of fresh rhizome. ***Historical dose:*** Tincture and all potencies.

CLINICAL - Convulsions. Delirium. Diarrhea. Headache. Hemiplegia (r.).

HOMEOPATHIC - Iris-fl. gives an odor of violets to the breath and communicates to vinegar a flavor of raspberries, hence is used in the manufacture of raspberry vinegar.

Powdered orris root has been used as an application to the hair and in some young girls has produced violent symptoms.

Headaches and giddiness occurred on waking in the morning. Complete paralysis of the right side. In one case, convulsions and delirium from which complete recovery did not take place for three months.

RELATIONS - ***Compare:*** (1) Verat., Sabad., Iris.

REFERENCES - Clarke.

IRIS FOETIDISSIMA

PHARMACY - iris-foe. Iris foetidissima. N. O. Iridaceae. Tincture of root. ***Historical dose:*** Tincture and all potencies.

CLINICAL - Headaches. Hernia.

HOMEOPATHIC - Iris-foe. was proved under Berridge's direction. One prover, Dr. Crocker, chewed a piece of the root, another took the tincture, one experienced symptoms from potentizing the drug and later the 14c dilution. The rest took very high potencies.

The prover who chewed the root experienced a burning feeling in mouth and fauces extending to stomach, not relieved by cold water or anything else. A number of pains were felt in the head.

RELATIONS - ***Compare:*** (1) The arums and the other irises.

REFERENCES - Clarke.

IRIS GERMANICA

(Blue Garden Iris)

PHARMACY - iris-g. Iris germanica. Blue garden iris. Root also used to make orris root. N. O. Iridaceae. Tincture of fresh rhizome. ***Historical dose:*** Tincture and all potencies.

CLINICAL - Diarrhea. Dropsy. Freckles.

HERBAL - The fresh root of Iris-g, Iris-fl. and the common yellow iris, Iris pseudo-acorus, have been much used in dropsies and violently cathartic. Diarrhea. The juice has also been used for the removal of freckles from the skin.

REFERENCES - Clarke.

IRIS TENAX

PHARMACY - iris-t. Iris tenax. Iris minor. N. O. Iridaceae. Oregon. Tincture of the lower or bulbous stems. Tincture of the whole plant. ***Historical dose:*** Tincture and all potencies.

CLINICAL - ***Appendicitis***. Fever. Headache. Homesickness. ***Ileo-cecal, pain.*** Intermittents. Mania. Peri-typhlitis. Sleeplessness. Stomatitis. Vomiting. Xerostoma.

HERBAL - The herb Iris tenax "grows very luxuriantly in the clay ground and on the hillsides of Oregon." The tissue of the plant is so strong that it was used by Native Americans for making cord and weaving into bags, etc.

HOMEOPATHIC - Dr. George Wigg of Portland, Oregon proved Iris-t. in the later part of 1885. He published the proving under the name of Iris minor. This, as Heath later showed, is a local name only, its true botanical name is Iris tenax.

Dr. Wigg particularly noted the absence of saliva with dry mouth. Burning in eyes without tears. Pain in one tooth only. Itching and burning of scalp without eruption. Chill at 2 p.m. ***Painful spot in ileo-cecal region.*** Bilious vomiting, burning sensations (Iris.). Deathly sensation at point of stomach. Appendicitis. Gloomy, cast-down, homesick feeling.

MIND - Gloomy, cast-down, homesick feeling.

Abdomen - Appendicitis. ***Pain in ileo-cecal region.*** Pains from adhesions after surgery.

Modalities - Sweet oil and camphor ameliorates burning in mouth and throat. Worse by sucking in cold air, (burning in mouth and throat). Hot applications aggravates pain in bowels. Cup of tea aggravates vomiting. Worse on waking.

COMMENTS - Dr. Wigg, age 44, took 5 drops to 1x of the strong tincture. A female prover took repeated doses of Iris-t. 2x and 3x. The order in which the symptoms occurred in Dr. Wigg's case is roughly as follows:

In the first fifteen minutes, there was burning in the mouth and throat. This passed off in the night, but was intensified by each fresh dose. After the second dose, taken early the next morning, the burning was reproduced, followed two hours later by dry mouth and absence of saliva.

This was followed by a mental gloom and homesick feeling, increasing towards midnight. Headache in temples. Itching and burning of the scalp. Toothache. Sinking, all gone feeling. Abdominal pains, diarrhea. Desperate exhaustion compelling him to keep in bed. Hard chill followed by rise of temperature.

Wigg noticed the all-gone feeling particularly on standing up, on walking in the morning. Cold water did not improve the burning in mouth and throat. A cold pillow improved pain in the temples.

The acute pains in the bowels passed off in the night, but for fourteen days there was a tender spot over the ileo-cecal region and the bowels did not act normally for ten days.

In the female prover, it produced a strange sensation in her mind: she though some of her friends had died, the next day she was unusually cheerful.

The most remarkable symptoms were the "fearful pain in the ileo-cecal region and the hard chill at 2 p.m." These indications led to the cure in the two following cases:

The first case concerned Miss A., a schoolteacher, who had for several years a pain beginning in right eye, extending to the right half of her head. When the pain was most severe, she vomited a quantity of green bile. When she did not vomit she had nausea and chill between 2 and 3 p.m. The pain passed off in sleep at night. It always began on Saturday, before rising.

Iris-t. 30x every six hours commencing on Friday morning, was given and quickly cured after Iris., Aloe, Cimic. and Kali-bi. had failed to give much relief. The relief from Iris-t. was so marked the patient thought she had received morphine.

The second case concerned Mr. E., who drank a large quantity of buttermilk while in a state of perspiration after walking thirty miles over a mountainous country in August. Four hours after, he was taken with fearful pain in ileo-cecal region. This caused a deathly sensation at his epigastrium. Finally he vomited much dark green bile without relief.

An old school doctor was called in and diagnosed obstruction with probable death in four days. He lingered three weeks and was brought home to Portland where Dr. Wigg saw him and diagnosed typhilitis, badly treated. Pressure on the ileo-cecal region caused the death like sensation at stomach pit. Pain continued until he vomited a cupful of dark green bile. He was somewhat constipated.

Under Iris-t. 15x every three hours he commenced to improve at once and in two weeks was back at his business.

RELATIONS - ***Compare:*** (1) Effect on cecal region - Arn., Ars., Lach., Sil. (2) Headache - Gels., Grat., Iris., Kali-bi., Ign. (3) Burning not worse by cold, Caps. (4) Homesickness - Caps., Ph-ac.

REFERENCES - Clarke.

IRIS VERSICOLOR

(Blue Flag)

PHARMACY - iris. Iris versicolor. Blue flag. Iris hexona. N. O. Iridaceae. Tincture of fresh root collected in early spring or autumn. Trituration of the resinoid. Irin or Irisin. ***Historical dose:*** Trituration, tincture and all potencies.

CLINICAL - Cholera. Colic. Diabetes. Goiter. ***Headaches.*** Indigestion. Leucorrhea. ***Migraines.*** Morning sickness. ***Nausea.*** Neuralgia. Pancreas, disorders. Rheumatism. Sciatica. Thyroid, disorders. ***Vomiting.***

HOMEOPATHIC - Sick headaches. ***Gastric or hepatic sick headaches*** with blur before the eyes at the beginning. ***Migraine headaches***.

Great nausea and vomiting. ***Vomiting sour or bitter substances***, excoriates the throat. Vomiting of stringy, glairy, ropy mucus, hangs in strings down to receptacle on the floor.

Burning of mouth, tongue, and throat, can go into stomach, even the anus if there is diarrhea. Affinity for the digestive tract, gastro-intestinal mucus membranes, thyroid, ***pancreas,*** and salivary glands.

Liver and pancreas affected, producing profuse secretions, which are sour, acrid and burning. Increases the flow of bile. Oily nose, greasy taste and fatty stools. Cholera infantum and cholera morbus. Symptoms set in suddenly, with a rapid elimination.

MIND - Mental depression. Despondency. Low-spirited. Dullness of mental faculties. Weak memory. Inability to fix the mind on any subject. Wandering thoughts while writing. Muttering. Laughs at own actions.

Ill humor. Censorious. Easily vexed. Irritable mood, disposed to find fault, particularly in morning. ***Restlessness at night.*** Nervous fretfulness. General appearance of anguish. Fear of approaching illness.

Abdomen - Cutting pain. ***Burning in epigastric region, with tenderness, vomiting of food. Awful burning in region of pancreas.*** Sharp griping pains in the bowels. Flatulent colic. Colicky pain before each spell of vomiting and purging. Colic, better by bending forward, better by discharge of flatulence. Pain in the abdomen, better by discharge of flatus.

Back - Stiffness in the back, increasing on sitting down. Crampy, in right lumbar region.

Chest - Rheumatism in muscles of chest, with acid indigestion. Cutting pain in left side as if ribs were pressing against lung.

Cough - Dry cough caused by tickling in larynx with a dry, smarting or burning sensation in throat.

Ears - Roaring, buzzing. ***Ringing in ears with deafness***. Aural vertigo with intense noises in ears.

Eyes - Sunken with blue circles. Redness of conjunctiva. Inflammation of eyelids, from cold. Burning in internal canthus. Violent supra-orbital pains. Periodic visual disturbances, blindness, hemiopia, with headache.

Face - General appearance of anguish. Pustular eruptions on face, around nose, lips and cheeks, secreting a bloody, irritating matter. Dry, cracked lips. Neuralgia after breakfast, beginning in infra-orbital nerve and involving whole face. Neuralgic pains in right side of face.

Female - Neuralgia and rheumatism of uterus. Menses regular, but excessive. Leucorrhea. Morning sickness of pregnancy, vomits sour or bitter, with protracted nausea, profuse ropy saliva, tenderness over stomach.

Food - Hunger with inability to eat. Loss of taste and appetite. Bitter, putrid taste. Nausea and empty belchings, from irregularities of diet. Chronic indigestion of milk. Intense and urgent thirst during diarrhea.

Head - Dullness of the head. ***Chronic pain in forehead. Dull throbbing or shooting pains in right side of forehead.*** Tired headache from mental exhaustion (studying, sewing), worse coughing, cold air, better gentle motion. Headache begins with blurring of vision, after relaxing from a mental strain. ***Frontal headache over left eye with nausea. Headache alternating sides.*** Headache as if a band around head. Severe pains, through temples and over eyes, with vertigo, nausea and vomiting. Shooting pain in temples with contractive feeling of the scalp. Scalp feels constricted. ***Sick headaches*** with diarrhea, in bilious subjects, worse rest, begins with a blur before eyes. Reflex headache from acid stomach or irritation of stomach from acid secretion. ***Neuralgic pain usually begins over one eye.*** Neuralgic pain, one-sided, with gastric symptoms. Right temples affected. Pustular eruption on scalp. Scabs, yellow matter oozing from under crust, with matted hair.

Heart - Accelerated pulse.

Kidneys - Burning along the length of urethra after urination. Cutting and pricking pain in urethra while urinating. Urine very high colored and scanty. Profuse, clear urine with headache. Diabetes.

Limbs - Sharp tearing, shifting, in joints. Shooting, laming pains along limb. Sciatica, as if left hip joint were wrenched. Pain extends to popliteal space. Gonorrheal rheumatism.

Liver - Liver sore. Pain in the region of the liver, worse from motion.

Male - Coldness and itching of parts. Coldness and relaxation of scrotum. Excitement of genitals reflex from excessively acid stomach. Nocturnal emissions with amorous dreams. Secondary gonorrhea or gleet.

Modalities - Better from gentle, continued motion. Worse in evening, night, after midnight, 2 a.m. to 3 a.m. Worse from mental exhaustion, rest, hot weather. Worse periodically, weekly, spring and autumn.

Mouth - Burning in mouth and fauces as if on fire. Feels greasy, burnt or scalded. Stomatitis, with burning pain in mouth and fauces. Tongue burns or feels cold. ***Greasy or sweetish taste.*** Flat taste. Loss of taste. Profuse flow of saliva (Merc., IP., Kali-i.).Ropy saliva, drops when talking. ***Profuse salivation during headache.*** Salivation after diphtheria, with swelling of parotids. Saliva tastes greasy, slimy. Mouth and tongue feel scalded. Slight toothache in a warm room. Ulcers on mucus membranes of cheeks.

Nose - Oily. Constant sneezing.

Perspiration - Perspiration over the whole body, but principally in the hypochondria. Sweat smells of vinegar.

Sleep - Sleeplessness. Starting in sleep.

Stools - Stools watery, with burning at anus and through intestinal canal. ***Stools, bilious, acrid, watery, burn like fire.*** Stools thin, tinged with bile, copious, in a continuous stream. Stools, green, undigested, mushy, pappy with fetid flatus. Stools, fatty, fetid or coppery smelling.

Rectum - Acute mucus enteritis. ***Constipation*** with gastric derangement. Constipation succeeded by thin, watery diarrhea. ***Sudden attacks of diarrhea. Painless cholera morbus.*** Periodical night diarrhea with pain and green discharges. Summer diarrhea occurring in hottest part of season. Urging to stools with headache, facial neuralgia and pain in teeth. Burning at anus during stool. Burning after stool. Anus feels sore as if sharp points sticking in it. Distressed feeling as if rectum is prolapsed. Hemorrhoids.

Skin - ***Great itching at night.*** Fine eruption, showing black points after scratching. Eczema with nightly itching. Herpes zoster and gastric derangements. Psoriasis, irregular patches with shining scales. Psoriasis on knees, elbows and body. Pustular eruptions on scalp and face, around mouth.

Stomach - ***Burning of whole alimentary canal***, not better by cold drinks. Burning distress in stomach and pancreas, with watery diarrhea and great prostration. Sour, bitter belchings. ***Continuous nausea.*** Nausea from riding, overexertion. ***Vomiting with burning pain.*** Vomiting of sweetish water, sour, bloody, bile. ***Bitter, acrid, watery, sour vomiting. Vomiting during headache.*** Periodic vomiting spells, every month, six weeks, lasts for two or three days. Protracted nausea and vomiting during pregnancy. Vomiting of sour milk in children.

Temperature - Chills with sleepiness. Chilliness during the whole night. Chills over whole body, even when well covered. Head and face cold. Fever followed by chill, with cold hands and feet. Bilious and typhoid fevers. Fever with muttering delirium and bilious diarrhea.

Throat - Heat and smarting in throat. Burning from fauces to stomach, better inhaling cool air or drinking cold water. Shooting pains in tonsils extends to ears. Vomit excoriates throat. Thyroid disorders. Goiter.

Vertigo - Aural vertigo with intense noises in ears. Immediate dizziness with pressure in forehead. Slight giddiness, coming on suddenly while walking within doors.

COMMENTS - Migraine headaches, worse on the left side, over the left eye (Thuj., Anac.). Sick headaches, associated with dietary allergies. Sensation of a nail over the left eye, pain as if being driven into supraorbital arch (Thuj., Sang. on right). Constipation preceding the migraine (Bry.). Buzzing and ringing in the ears associated with the headaches.

Affinity for the pancreas (Spong., Con., Phos.). Diabetes. Characteristic burning. Stomach troubles accompanied by burning of tongue, throat, esophagus and stomach, and burning of the anus if diarrhea is present.

Nausea and vomiting, loss of appetite, constipation. The vomiting is not always sour, but may be bitter or sweetish. Profuse saliva. Vomit or saliva may be white, stringy, or ropy (Ip.).

Nash once had a case of stomach trouble in a middle-aged woman. She had frequent attacks, vomiting a stringy, glairy mucus which was very ropy. The vomit would hang in strings from her mouth to the receptacle on the floor.

Then the vomit became dark colored, like coffee, she became very weak, vomited all nourishment. She also had profuse secretion of ropy saliva.

Thinking she had cancer of the stomach, she made her will and set her house in order to die. Kali-bi. was given with no benefit, but Iris cured her completely in a short time and she remained well.

RELATIONS - ***Antidote:*** Nux-v. ***Compare:*** (1) Iris-fl. - delirium, convulsions and paralysis. (2) Iris-fa. - headache and hernia. (3) Iris-g. - Blue Garden Iris - dropsy and freckles. (4) Pancreat. (5) Pep. (6) Ip., Podo., Sanguin., Ars., Ant-c.

REFERENCES - Boericke. Clarke. Nash. Murphy. Phatak.

ITU

PHARMACY - itu. Itu. Resina itu. Brazil. Solution in alcohol of the resin. ***Historical dose:*** Tincture and all potencies.

CLINICAL - Ears, noises. Hernia. Muscae, volitantes. Stiff-neck. Toothache. Vulvitis.

HOMEOPATHIC - Itu is one of the remedies proved by Mure. All he tells about the source of it is that "This resin, which comes to us from the province of St. Paul is used empirically for hernia."

Symptoms include a sudden report in the ear, with frightful pain extending to teeth for several minutes, repeated as many as eight times in a day, profuse sweat after the reports. Earache when the least dampness sets in. Toothache worse after a cold drink. Chilliness at hypogastrium, especially in evening.

REFERENCES - Boericke. Clarke.

J

JABORANDI

(Pilocarpus Jaborandi)

PHARMACY - jab. Jaborandi. Pilocarpus jaborandi. Pilocarpus pennatifolius aut microphyllus. The alkaloid is pilocarpine. N. O. Rutaceae. Tincture of fresh leaves. Tincture of dried leaves and stems. ***Historical dose:*** Tincture and all potencies, third potency.

CLINICAL - Alopecia. Asthenopia. Baldness. Bronchitis. Burns. Cataract. Ciliary, spasm. Diarrhea. Dysmenorrhea. Erysipelas. ***Exophthalmic, goiter***. Eye, disorders, Eye, surgery. ***Eye-strain. Gland, disorders. Glaucoma***. ***Hair, loss***. Heart, disorders. Hot, flushings. Hypermetropia. Leucorrhea. Menopause. Miliaria. ***Mumps***. ***Night-sweats. Perspiration, excessive***. Pregnancy, salivation. ***Salivation, excessive***. Scalds. Snakebites. Strabismus. Tuberculosis. Worms.

HERBAL - Jaborandi is a South American tree growing up to twenty feet high. It is used by South American natives as an antidote to snakebites of the Trigonocephalus group.

HOMEOPATHIC - A few minutes after a dose of Jab., the face, ears and neck become deeply flushed and drops of perspiration break out all over the body, the mouth waters and saliva pours out in an almost continuous stream.

A single dose often produces enormous amounts of sweat and saliva, not infrequently half a pint. The observation of its action on the skin and salivary glands led to extensive provings.

A powerful glandular stimulant, it produces hypersecretion from upper respiratory tract and salivary glands. Increases lachrymal, nasal, bronchial and intestinal secretions to a lesser degree.

Abnormal sweats, perspiration, salivation. Heavy night sweats, hot flushes. ***Night sweats*** of tuberculosis patients. Sweat only on the left side, dry on the right. Drawing pain in joints during perspiration.

Exophthalmic goiter with increased heart's action and pulsation of arteries, tremors and nervousness, heat and sweating, bronchial irritation. Acts upon the thyroid and its sudorific action may be due to it.

Limits the duration of mumps. Mumps when metastasized to the testes, causing infertility, metastasized to the breasts. Never well since mumps (Morbill., Parot.).

Pronounced action in the eyes, it has been found to be useful in many conditions of eye weakness, especially hypermetropia, ciliary spasm, convergent strabismus and after operations for strabismus. Mydriatic properties. Miosis. Glaucoma.

Headaches, more on the left side. Headaches worse at noon every day. Pains appear gradually and disappear gradually. Symptoms are generally more on the left.

Kidney disease, especially with uremia, eliminating both water and urea. Nausea. Stomach distress, better from eating. Scarlatinal dropsy. Contra-indicated in heart failure, in post-puerperal uremia, and in senile cases.

MIND - Mental confusion. Dullness of mind. Cheerfulness, gaiety. Very nervous and tremulous. Disinclination to speak. Desire to kill loved ones. Fixed idea that she will murder all her family with a hatchet.

Abdomen - Empty, gone feeling. Cutting in lower abdomen. Severe pains over pubes with strong desire to pass water, which relieved. Ailments of the pancreas.

Breasts - Milk absent or deficient. Milk increased, too profuse.

Chest - Sticking in chest. Pain in chest and around heart. Pressure on chest with anxiety, palpitation and pain in region of heart. Anxiety in chest with oppression, preventing sleep.

Ears - Serous exudation into tympanic cavity. Tinnitus. Nervous deafness, better in noise. Noises and vertigo.

Eyes - Tension in eyes. ***Pupils contracted, do not react to light.*** Glaucoma. Atrophic choroiditis. Vitreous opacities. ***Eyestrain*** from whatever cause (Ruta.). ***Eye pain from exertion of vision at fine work.*** Eyes easily tire from slightest use. Sensation of heat and burning in eyes during exertion.

Smarting pain in eyes. Lachrymation during coryza, headache. Irritation from electric or other artificial light. Staring eyes. Irritability of the ciliary muscle. Periodic strabismus. Spasms of the accommodation while reading. ***Near-sighted***. Hyperopia. Exophthalmos, protrusion of eyes. Squints, convergent after surgery. Lids twitch.

Face - Redness of face and of ears. Pallor with heat of face and throbbing of temporal arteries. ***Mumps***, especially when metastasis to the testes. Inflammation of parotid gland.

Female - Menses, start with coldness, throbbing in head and pelvis, and backache. Menses scanty, congested head, dry skin. Leucorrhea. Edema of pregnancy. Puerperal convulsions in a stupor, threatened suffocation from inability to swallow excessive quantity of saliva. Heat and dryness of vagina during labor. Labor pains ceasing or sluggish. Flushing at menopause.

Food - Good appetite. Hunger disappeared and he could not eat. Urgent thirst.

Head - Empty, hollow sensation in head. Headache every day about noon. Headache from straining eyes. Headache with smarting and pain in eyeballs. Pulsating in temporal vessels, at vertex. Throbbing pain in vertex and front of head. Pain in lower part of occiput. Light hair turns black. Baldness.

Heart - Pain in heart region. Oppression of chest. Nervous cardiac disorders. Violent ebullitions to heart and chest. Palpitations, during perspiration. Pulse is irregular, dicrotic. Irregularity, weakness and rapidity of action. Cyanosis, collapse.

Kidneys - Scanty, pain over pubes with much urging. Burning in urethra with urging to urinate. Urine dark. Urine increased during the sweat.

Lungs - Edema of lungs. Breathing difficult, hurried. Slow, sighing respiration. Bronchial mucus membrane inflamed. Loose cough. Much inclination to cough and difficult breathing. Frothy or profuse, thin, serous expectoration.

Male - Orchitis from metastasis of mumps. Orchitis with incipient bronchial trouble.

Modalities - Worse left side, exertion of eyes, exhaustion, start of menses, cold. Nausea worse motion of eyes.

Mouth - Tension in salivary glands. ***Profuse salivation with profuse sweating***, with dry skin. Saliva viscid like egg white, or stringy but not viscid. Constant spitting of alkaline saliva. Saliva contained a notable quantity of urea. Salivation during pregnancy. Dryness of mouth.

Nose - Copious nasal discharge. Coryza and perspiration (Merc.).

Perspiration - ***Excessive perspiration from all parts of the body***. Sweat on forehead, then over whole body, then chiefly on face, legs and feet. Sweat breaks out on the face and upper part of the chest. Sweats with palpitations, general pulsations and tremors. Copious sweating with chilliness, with salivation, with diarrhea (Verat.). Nervous sweats. Semi-lateral or unilateral sweat. ***Night-sweats.*** Perspiration in bed. ***Hot flushes and sweats.*** Perspiration during menopause. Sweat contains urea. Perspired easily before taking, but did not sweat during the proving.

Rectum - Constipation. Hard stools. Diarrhea with flushed face and profuse perspiration. Diarrhea during daytime. Stools are watery, yellow. Frequent, undigested, gushing, weakening, papescent, and large and painless stools. Passage of threadworms.

Skin - Redness of skin. Persistent dryness of skin. Dry eczema.

Sleep - Sleepiness. Profound sleep in daytime. Fell asleep while sitting reading. ***Night-sweats.*** Perspiration in bed. Did not sleep well on account of restlessness, with pressure on chest and hurried breathing. Distressing dreams towards morning. Dreams of accidents and fights, waking him twice a night.

Stomach - Thirst in morning on waking. Hiccough, before vomiting. Nausea, sudden and retching often with hiccough Vomiting after supper. Nausea worse motion of eyes. Nausea on looking at objects moving, vomiting, pressure and pain in stomach. Stubborn vomiting of pregnancy. Nausea during menopause.

Temperature - Chilly up and down back at 7 p.m. Shivering. Chilliness with sweat. Cold limbs. Heat flushes, at menopause, with profuse sweat, nausea and vomiting.

Throat - Exophthalmic goiter with increased heart's action, pulsation in arteries, tremors and nervousness. Swelling of submaxillary glands (Merc., Calc.). Dryness at back of throat. Soreness and smarting of throat.

Vertigo - Headache with vertigo. Vertigo with nausea after exertion of vision. Vertigo as if head were too light, on moving or looking at objects.

Vision - ***White spots before eyes.*** Everything at a distance appears hazy. Vision becomes indistinct every few moments. Focal distance changes while reading. Dim vision, better looking sideways (Chin-s.). Retinal images retained long after using eyes.

COMMENTS - Sandesberg noticed that the internal use of Jab. and pilocarpine in cases of detached retina and choroiditis seemed to occasion opacity of the crystalline lens. He treated a horse for iridochoroiditis and large opacities of the vitreous with infusion of Jab. leaves and injections of Pilo. The disease was quickly arrested, the vitreous cleared up completely, but during the first week the crystalline lens became opaque.

Jab. has been used as a remedy for baldness and it forms the principal ingredient in some of the popular hair restorer tonics. In a number of patients taking it, white hair and blonde hair have been observed to turn black.

Jab. has a reputation for stimulating breast secretions. A case is quoted from the Lancet in which a woman whose milk had ceased for a fortnight received ten drops of the fluid extract every four hours. The secretion of milk was re-established, but the patient began to suffer from extreme nervous excitement accompanied by a fixed idea that she should murder her family with a hatchet.

The drug was stopped and these symptoms disappeared, and with them, the activity of the breast glands.

Bell commended it in diarrhea with gushing, painless stools, flushed face, profuse salivation and sweat, and intense thirst with dark urine that is scanty or profuse.

Cooper saw Jab. cause violent leucorrhea as well as a discharge of threadworms. He noted its use in relieving "a feeling of coldness and faintness and neuralgic throbbings in head and pelvis with a backache" when the period begins. He suggested treating with a drop or two of Jab. in hot water.

The Hom. News, February, 1900, quoted an incidental cure of dysmenorrhea in a woman, age 23, who received five-drop does of Jab. for increased eye-tension which rapidly disappeared. The patient noticed that she passed the next menstrual period without pain though she usually had to spend two to four days in bed. The drug was continued in smaller doses and the improvement was maintained.

Hale commended its use in women or young girls who always have dry skin, scanty menses and a tendency of blood to the head.

Duncan aborted erysipelas by painting the tincture on the part four to five times daily. A sharp smarting is the first effect, followed by a more agreeable, soothing sensation. For burns, scalds and some forms of eczema and psoriasis.

One patient, after having been injected with pilocarpine, complained of great sensitiveness to cold, constantly taking cold and bronchitis, the skin became irritable.

Dudgeon recorded a case of a man, 45, who rose at an early hour and went to the other side of his bedroom to get a dose of Nux-v. 3c for some fancied derangement of his stomach. On coming back to bed he was seized with a sudden, violent, crimson flushing of the face followed almost immediately by profuse perspiration, beginning in the face and head and extending all over the body.

This was followed by extreme coldness of the limbs and sickness terminating in the vomiting of sour mucus.

The attacks recurred every quarter of an hour throughout the day. Not only was he unable to get out of bed, he could not raise himself up in bed or lie otherwise than on his right side without the most distressing giddiness and a feeling "as if he should die." Pulse 60, regular and strong, temperature below normal.

Ten drops of Jab. 1c were mixed in half a tumbler of water and a dessert spoonful given immediately and repeated every half hour. After the second dose the attacks ceased and he was able to take bread and milk without sickness. He had a good night's rest and was perfectly well the next day.

RELATIONS - ***Compare:*** (1) Amyl-n., Atrop., Phys., Lyc, Ruta. (2) Piloc. - Meniere's disease, rapidly progressive tuberculosis with free hemorrhages, profuse sweating, 2x trituration. (3) Atropine is the antagonist to pilocarpine in dose of one one-hundredth grain for one-sixth of pilocarpine.

REFERENCES - Boericke. Clarke. Murphy.

JACARANDA CAROBA

(Brazilian Caroba Tree)

PHARMACY - jac-c. Jacaranda caroba. Brazilian caroba tree. Caroba tree. Jacaranda procera. Bignonia caroba. Jacaranda Brasiliensis. N. O. Bignoniaceae. Jacarandae. Tincture of fresh flowers. ***Historical dose:*** Tincture and all potencies.

CLINICAL - Anal, itching. Balanorrhea. Chancre. Chordee. Coryza. Gonorrhea. Morning sickness. Muscular, rheumatism. Phimosis. Rheumatism. Syphilis.

HERBAL – "There are several species of Jacaranda," especially Jacaranda procera, "that have the reputation of being curative in syphilis" notes the Treasury of Botany. Mure proved Jacaranda caroba, and the symptoms of the proving certainly confirmed this.

HOMEOPATHIC - Jac-c. has a reputation in venereal diseases and rheumatism. The urinary and sexual symptoms are important. Rheumatic symptoms, pains in the limbs. Lancinations in the heart. Morning sickness. Itching at anus.

Hering confirmed symptoms including tearing pains affected the whole organism when urine contacts a chancre. Prepuce much swollen, could not be drawn over glans, on attempting to do so, copious discharge of yellowish green pus. Chordee in gonorrhea. Dull pain under sternum on raising head and drawing breath.

Abdomen - Painful stitch in the right and left side of navel. Acute pain at the hypogastrium when pressing upon it. Swelling of the right groin, painful to touch.

Back - Pain in nape. Neck so painful that the head cannot be turned to right. Stiffness in loins.

Chest - Dull pain under the sternum on raising head and drawing breath. Prickling under the sternum.

Ears - Flapping in the ears, as of wings. Stoppage and heat in the left ear, with burning, digging pain extending to the left nostril.

Eyes - Eyes pain, are inflamed and watery.

Food - ***Food tastes insipid, nausea while eating.***

Head - Fullness in the head. Pain, as if a plug were pressing on the right side of the forehead. Dull pain between the forehead and right temple. Coryza with heavy head.

Heart - Sensation as if the heartbeat was in the pit of the stomach. Sharp pain in region of heart. Painful stitch at the heart, extending to the right side. Stitch at the heart, which seems to beat slowly.

Kidneys - Urethra inflamed, discharge of yellow matter.

Limbs - Morning soreness and stiffness of muscles. Weakness of lumbar region. Gonorrheal rheumatism. Gonorrheal and syphilitic arthritis. Rheumatic pain in right knee. Itching pimples on hands.

Male - Heat and pain in penis. Painful erections. Chordee. Itching pimples on glans and prepuce. Discharge of yellowish white liquid from the prepuce. Prepuce painful and swollen. The prepuce cannot be drawn back. Phimosis. Suppuration between the glans and prepuce. Acute pain in the left testicle when walking. Heat and swelling of the scrotum. Syphilis. Chancroid.

Mouth - Dry mouth in the morning in bed. Mouth dry and clammy. Raw pain at the left side of tongue. Food tastes flat or acid.

Nose - Sneezing and fluent coryza. Coryza, with heaviness and weariness at the vertex, forehead, and eyes.

Rectum - Constipation. Acute pain with lancinations in the anus. Prickling around the anus. Itching at the anus while sitting. Excrescence at the anus.

Sleep - Restless sleep with frightful dreams.

Stomach - Fullness at the pit of the stomach, with hurried breathing. Pressure at the pit of the stomach. Painful stitch between the pit of the stomach and the umbilicus. Nausea when eating.

Temperature - Internal chill. Dry, prickling heat all over.

Throat - Sore and dry. Vesicles in pharynx. Sore throat with constrictions of the pharynx and difficult swallowing. Constrictive sensation at the throat.

Vertigo - Vertigo on rising with heavy forehead.

COMMENTS - Mahony confirmed symptoms including "Food tastes insipid, nausea during eating." Motion aggravates. Symptoms come on when walking, raising head, sitting.

J. S. Whittinghill cured several cases of muscular rheumatism characterized by a peculiar soreness and stiffness of muscles in the morning.

RELATIONS - ***Compare:*** (1) Thuj. - gonorrhea, rheumatism. (2) Cor-r. - red and sensitive chancre and chancroids. (3) Jac-g.

REFERENCES - Boericke. Clarke.

JACARANDA GUALANDAI

PHARMACY - jac. Jacaranda gualandai. N. O. Bignoniaceae. The dried leaves are crushed and macerated in five parts by weight of alcohol. ***Historical dose:*** Tincture and all potencies.

CLINICAL - Diarrhea. Ophthalmia. Rheumatism. Syphilis. ***Ulcers.*** Vertigo.

HERBAL - Dr. J. S, Whittinghill contributed the following from the Eclectic Medical Journal concerning Jacaranda: "Of this South American remedy the Dispensatory says it is used in Brazil and other South American countries for syphilis, sometimes under the name Carroba."

HOMEOPATHIC - Jac. has syphilitic symptoms, especially of the eyes and throat. Chancroids. ***Atonic ulcers.*** Dark, painless diarrhea. Weakness of memory and inability to study.

Back - Weakness of the lumbar region.

Eyes - Pains and inflammation of the eye with redness, more marked in the left eye. Sensation of sand in the eyes. Ophthalmia, which begins in the left eye with lachrymation and night agglutination of the eyelids. Syphilitic-like ophthalmia. Weakness of sight.

Male - Pain in the penis. Increased secretion of urine. Gonorrhea with a discharge which stains the linen a dirty yellow color. Chancroids.

Rectum - Diarrhea with dark mulberry-colored stools without pain or tenesmus, but with mucus.

Throat - Pain and burning of the larynx, when laughing or reading aloud. Small vesicles in the pharynx.

Vertigo - Vertigo on rising after stooping, with momentary loss of sight and sensation of heaviness in the forehead.

COMMENTS - Dr. J. F. Convers, of Bogotá, found Jac. to be useful in certain kinds of rheumatism. He noted the case of one patient who suffered from rheumatism for about 10 years, and never became serious. Sometimes she was nearly relieved from it. She lost a good deal of sleep due to it.

Her wrist would become painful and very weak from ordinary labor. She complained of being stiff and had pain from any motion, particularly in the morning. She needed assistance dressing. Upon sudden motion, she had the sensation of the muscles tearing and being bruised, painful on pressure.

Convers gave her different remedies as they seemed to be indicated with no result. He thought there could be nothing lost by trying Jac. and did so. In a few days, she was entirely relieved of muscular pains.

Six weeks after, her symptoms returned, but a second dose again relieved and the pains did not return.

Convers tried Jac. on three other patients with the same peculiar morning stiffness and soreness. All were relieved in a few days and experienced no further muscular pains.

Convers used the mother tincture at 5 drops per dose and the 3x dilution of it in the treatment of gonorrhea and chancroids with the great success.

Anshutz noted that it is a complementary and antidote to Merc.

REFERENCES - Anshutz. Boericke. Clarke.

JADE

(Nephrite)

PHARMACY - jad. Jade. Nephrite. Jadeite. Jade is found in two varieties. Jadeite and Nephrite and comes in a wide range of colors including white, lavender, red, brown, yellow, orange, blue, and green, each color said to relate more specifically to certain ailments or organs. ***Historical dose:*** The gem mother tincture diluted can be applied externally and given internally. Four to Eight drops of Jade Essence in a cup of pure water. Repeat as needed.

CLINICAL - Asthma. Detoxification. Eye, disorders. Gastric, pains. Heartburn. Kidney, disorders. Kidney, stones.

HOMEOPATHIC - The Portuguese, who brought home jade pieces from their settlement in Canton, China, called jade *piedre de ilharga*, or stone of the loins, because they believed it to be strong medicine for kidney ailments. Jade objects brought back to Spain from the new world were called by the Spanish version of this phrase *piedra de hijada*. This became the French *ejade* and then, finally, jade. Jadeite is from the Spanish, piedra de ijada, "stone of the side," because its supposed to cure kidney ailments if applied to the side of the body.

Suggested healing properties common to all colors of Jade include, ability to mellow one's existence, rid negative thoughts and energy, soothe the mind. Thus making tasks seem easier and less complicated. Strengthen the body's filtration and cleansing systems. Develop a greater capacity for love, and assist in the removal of toxins. Also said to be a very protective stone.

Jade was known as the kidney stone, and it was widely employed as a remedy for renal disease. It was worn over this organ to break up kidney stones. Powdered and mixed with gold and silver, jade strengthened the lungs, the vocal organs, and the heart and prolonged life.

A potion of jade, rice, and dew was employed to harden bones, make muscles more supple, calm the mind, and purify the blood. Taken regularly, this prescription eliminated hunger and thirst as well as sensations of heat and cold.

Believed to protect the body from decay, jade was used for embalming. When worn around a child's neck jade would guard against infantile disease. It also was worn to relieve gastric pains and heartburn, to calm asthma, and to aid childbirth. Four grains, dissolved in wine, relieved bile.

Suggested healing properties common to all colors of Jade include, ability to mellow one's existence, rid negative thoughts and energy, soothe the mind making tasks seem easier and less complicated, strengthen the body's filtration and cleansing systems, develop a greater capacity for love, and assist in the removal of toxins. Also said to be a very protective stone.

Health, wealth, longevity stone. Ancient Chinese used also for courage, wisdom, justice, mercy, emotional balance, stamina, love, fidelity, humility, generosity, peace, harmony. Lungs, heart, thymus, immune, kidney and blood detoxification, nervous system. A gentle, steady energy.

Increases fertility, longevity. Provides wisdom when evaluating issues or problems. Brings needed energy. Improves concentration. Encourages education. Considered a "Dream Stone." Benefits eye disorders, kidney stones and female discomfort.

COMMENTS - The ancient jade carved in China was what we today call nephrite jade: an amphibolite mineral. In the 19th Century

, it was discovered that the material from the new world was not the same mineral as the jade from China. The mineral from Central America, a pyroxene, was called jadeite to distinguish it from the original nephrite.

Because of its smooth even texture, jade has long been a preferred material for carving. The most common shape is the flat donut-shaped disc called a pi, which is commonly worn as a necklace. The Emerald Buddha, the sacred image that is enshrined at Wat Phra Kaeo in Bangkok, Thailand, is actually beautiful green jadeite.

Good fortune, prosperity. A peaceful stone for centuries of primary importance to the people of the Orient (where it is considered to be one of the most importance symbols of purity and serentiy). The Chinese referred to jade as the musical stone, because of the melodic tones it makes when struck.

For centuries, jade was thought to be a single gemstone, but in 1863 two types were recognized: jadeite and nephrite. Jade, Venus: Chinese Stone of Heaven. Since at least 2950 BC, jade has been treasured in China as the royal gemstone, yu. The character for jade resembles a capital I with a line across the middle: the top represents the heavens, the bottom the earth, and the center section, mankind.

The word yu is used in Chinese to call something precious, as in English we use gold. Jade was thought to preserve the body after death and can be found in emperors' tombs from thousands of years ago. One tomb contained an entire suit made out of jade, to assure the physical immortality of its owner. For thousands of years, jade was a symbol of love and virtue as well as a status symbol.

RELATIONS - ***Compare:*** Aurum Met. Nat. Mur. Rose Quartz.

REFERENCES - Murphy.

JALAPA

(Ipomoea Jalapa)

PHARMACY - jal. Jalapa. Ipomoea jalapa. Ipomoea purga. Exogonium purga. Concolvulus purga. N. O. Convolvulacae. Mexico. Trituration of dried root. ***Historical dose:*** Tincture and all potencies.

CLINICAL - Anus, soreness. ***Colic.*** Coryza. ***Diarrhea.*** Gout. Fainting. Restlessness.

HOMEOPATHIC - Jalapa, the well-known purgative of old school practice, had a short proving by Jeanes. Allen cured a case of "coryza in an infant, violent attacks of crying and intense pain, quiet during the day, but screaming all night."

Colic and diarrhea. Severe abdominal pain, ***"as if the abdomen would be cut to pieces,"*** severe griping, cutting pains. Pain is better by belchings of frothy matter and flatulence.

Cutting colic before and during the stool. Stools are watery, sour smelling and bloody. Stools, watery, muddy or sour, bloody. Infantile diarrhea with general coldness, blueness of face. Pain in sigmoid flexure.

General coldness and blueness of the face. Restlessness and anxiety. Great weakness with fainting fits, excessive uneasiness and tossing about of limbs. Symptoms are worse at night. A child may be quite ***quiet all day, but screams and tossed about all night.***

MIND - Great restlessness with anxiety. Fainting fits, weakness. Quiet all day, but screams and tossed about all night. Weeping in sleep, good during day. Screams and restless all night. Shrieking in children.

Abdomen - Abdomen distended. Pain in middle of abdomen and in region of left superior flexure of colon. Pain in right hypochondrium. Pain in cecum. ***Colic,*** violent pain in small intestines, as if abdomen would be cut to pieces. Inflammation of intestines. Severe griping, cutting pain in bowels, worse at night. Flatulent rumbling in bowels. Flatulence and nausea.

Back - Severe pain about superior margin of left scapula.

Ears - Humming in ears.

Head - Violent headache. Pain in head, smarting in skin of forehead.

Kidneys - Pain and pressure in region of bladder.

Limbs - Excessive uneasiness and tossing about of limbs. Aching in arms and legs, mostly right side. Pain in thighs. Pain in large joint of great toe. Smarting on inside edge and at root of left great toenail with heat, tearing and pulsation. Burning of soles of feet.

Male - Thrilling sensation in urethra while urinating.

Modalities - Worse night, belchings.

Mouth - Dryness of lips. Tongue, smooth, glazed, dry, smarting and biting. Stinging on tongue and in fauces.

Perspiration - Great disposition to perspiration of head and superior parts of body.

Rectum - Pinching and griping. ***Severe cutting, griping pain in bowels.*** Cutting colic before and during stool. Watery diarrhea, thin, muddy stools. Stools, violent, excessive, bloody, watery, with weak pulse, sour smelling, with great restlessness and anxiety. Infantile diarrhea, general coldness, blueness of face. Pain in sigmoid flexure of colon. Soreness of anus.

Stomach - Flatulent and frothy belchings with abatement of pain. Nausea.

Temperature - General coldness and blueness of face. Febrile attacks.

COMMENTS - Nash cured with Jal. 12c a desperate case of enterocolitis in which there was screaming all day as well as all night. With the screaming there was constant body contortions, bending forward, backward and sideways alternately.

RELATIONS - ***Antidotes:*** Elat., Cann-s. ***Compare:*** (1) Camph. - diarrhea with coldness. (2) Coloc. - colic. (3) Iris-t. - pain in cecum.

REFERENCES - Boericke. Clarke.

__JASMINUM OFFICINALE

(White Jessamine)

PHARMACY - jasm. Jasminum officinale. White jessamine. N. O. Jasminaceae. Some botanists include jasmine in the Oleaceae. Jasminum should not be confounded with Gelsemium, the "Yellow Jessamine," or "Carolina Jessamine," which belongs to a different order of plants. Tincture of red berries. ***Historical dose:*** Tincture and all potencies.

CLINICAL - Coma. Convulsions. Lockjaw. Tetanus. Vomiting.

HOMEOPATHIC - W. H. Hull recorded the case of a boy who ate the red berries, causing vomiting, convulsions, tetanus and a comatose state. Symptoms went from above downwards and from left to right.

Muscular movements were observed first about the eyes and face, especially on the left side, towards which eyes and facial muscles were directed. The movements became generally more severe, going from head to left arm, then to left lower limbs, until finally the whole body was thrown into violent convulsions.

At one time the spasms were chiefly opisthotonos, when the whole surface was congested almost to a blackened hue, most marked about the muscles of the head and throat, jaws locked, trismus complete, better by a bath. The body was weak and almost helpless for a few days. Lay on the floor in a fainting fit. Perfect insensibility. Surface cool.

MIND - Comatose condition. Perfect insensibility.

Eyes - Pupils immoderately dilated.

Face - Face pale. Muscular movement first above eyes and face, especially left side towards which eyes and facial muscles were directed.

Lungs - Breathing somewhat bronchial but of unusual frequency.

Pulse - Slow and feeble.

Stomach - Vomiting. Slight emesis after first sleep.

COMMENTS - The Treasury of Botany stated that the bitter leaves of Jasminum floribundum are used in Abyssinia against tapeworms. In India, the bitter root of Jasminum angustifolium, powdered and mixed with the powdered root of Acorus calamus, is considered an excellent application in ringworm.

REFERENCES - Boericke. Clarke.

JATROPHA CURCAS
(Purging Nut)

PHARMACY - jatr. Jatropha curcas. Purging nut. Atropha curcas. Physic nut. N. O. Euphorbiaceae. West Indies. Tincture and trituration of seeds. ***Historical dose:*** Trituration, tincture and all potencies, third to thirtieth potency.

CLINICAL - Blepharospasm. Borborygmi. ***Cholera.*** Cholerine. Constipation. Cramps. ***Diarrhea.*** Eyelids, inflamed. ***Food, poisoning.*** Heels, sensitive. Hiccough. Mouth, ulceration. Skin, disorders. Tympanites. Vomiting. ***Worms.***

HOMEOPATHIC - Jatr. is one of the most active of the Euphorbians and strongly resembles Croto-t. in its action, especially in the urgent gushing stools and the irritation and pimples of the skin. It is also an active purgative, affecting the stomach and intestines.

Kent described the sphere of Jatr. in cholera, noting that "The characteristic is rice water discharge, it has vomiting and purging, more or less sweat, more or less cramps. Suppression of urine, the great prostration, syncope and rapid onset peculiar to cholera and it has this to differentiate it from all other remedies. The vomiting and purging and evacuations are thick, albuminous, lumpy instead of thin and watery."

Jatr. corresponds more to the earlier stage than to the collapse stage of cholera. Predominant cramps, gripping cutting pains, sensation as if balls were rolling together in abdomen. Violent cramps that draw the muscles of calf flat. The patient writhes about in bed with pain.

Sudden desire for stool and constant noise of liquids in abdomen, especially left side. Marked and peculiar gurgling, like water. ***Much noise in the abdomen as if a bottle was being emptied,*** followed later by a thin stool or by profuse gushing stools. Rice water stools.

Vomiting, easy, albuminous. Hiccough followed by copious vomiting. Unquenchable thirst. ***Food poisoning.*** Icy ***coldness*** of the whole body, especially lower limbs.

MIND - Apathy. Indifference to pain. Anxiety and anguish, with burning in stomach and coldness of body.

Abdomen - Abdomen swollen and sore to touch. Tympanites. Pain in hypochondria, deep in abdomen, behind the navel. Gripping, sticking, in abdomen. ***Lancinating, stinging pain with the colic.*** Colic with rumbling in abdomen, better walking in open air. ***Distended with gurgling noises.*** Much noise in abdomen, as if a full bottle was emptied, followed by thin stool. ***Noise like the gurgling of water*** during the fecal discharge. Sensation as if balls were rolling together in abdomen.

Back - Stiffness of muscles of nape of neck and forehead. Bruised feeling muscles of back and chest. Stiffness in lumbar region.

Chest - Constriction in chest with anxiety, preventing sleep. Violent aching pain in left clavicle. Sticking from above downwards, deep in chest behind sternum. Pain in region of left third rib inside the nipple.

Ears - Burning hot ears with heat in the back part of the head.

Eyes - Itching and smarting of margins of lids. Twitching of left upper lid. Bright and dark spots before eyes. Black points before eyes.

Face - Hot face and head, chilliness in the back. Pale face with blue margins around the eyes. Painful cracked lips.

Female - Vomiting during pregnancy.

Food - Great thirst. Violent, unquenchable thirst, not satisfied by drinking water. Dreads to drink on account of nausea. ***Food poisoning.***

Head - Heat and heaviness of the head. Heat in head, face and ears. Stupefaction with yawning and nausea. Headache with nausea and vomiting. Violent pressing pain in the temples, ceasing in open air and reappearing when entering a room. Stiffness of muscles on forehead and neck.

Heart - Feeling of sinking and nausea in the precordial region, followed by soft stool. Violent palpitation, shaking the chest, when moving slowly about the room. Pulse is irregular, small thready and intermittent, greatly slowed. Almost pulseless.

Kidneys - Violent urging to urinate. Urine pale yellow, frothy.

Limbs - Muscles of limbs contracted by violent spasms. Pain in the limbs and joints. Cramps in muscles, especially calves, legs and feet. Pain in ankles, feet and toes. Heels sensitive.

Liver - Pain in region of liver and under right scapula to shoulder.

Lungs - Painful pressure right side of larynx at night, waking him, not worse by touch. Respiration quick, panting, difficult. Short, hacking, persistent cough. Hollow cough.

Male - Aching in genital as after excessive sexual intercourse. Drawing in genitals, extending along inner side right thigh to navel.

Modalities - Better by placing hands in cold water. Worse summer, walking in open air, morning, pressure, touch, covering. Patient seeks to cool himself by throwing off covers and lying on ground. Headaches are worse in a room.

Mouth - Metallic, bloody taste with much spitting of saliva. Increased accumulation of thin saliva. Long continued pain and burning of the tongue. Numbness of tongue with heat and dryness of mouth. Mouth feels as if scalded.

Nose - Ulcers in the nose and mouth. Itching of the nose while eating.

Rectum - ***Loud noise in abdomen like gurgling of water***, associated with coldness, cramps, nausea and vomiting. First stage of cholera, before collapse. ***Diarrhea, forced discharge.*** Sudden, profuse, watery, rice-water stool, gushes from him like a torrent. Very copious, mushy stools with quantities of lumbrici and threadworms. Constipation. Stitches in anus and rectum.

Skin - Pimples on wrist, back of hand, cheek, back of neck, bend of right thigh. Itching and slightest tension around mouth. Itching between fingers in palms, between toes in bed at night, first worse then better by rubbing.

Sleep - Excessive drowsiness. Restlessness at night on account of rush of thought and palpitations. Attacks of anxiety at night, not permitting sleep.

Stomach - Heat and burning in stomach with crampy, constrictive pain in the epigastrium. ***Food poisoning.*** Belchings of air. Hiccough, followed by copious vomiting. ***Very easy vomiting***, of a large mass of dark green bile, with acrid feeling from throat. Nausea and vomiting, brought on by drinking water. Vomiting during pregnancy.

Temperature - Chilliness and clammy perspiration. Coldness of the whole body, mottled blue. Chilliness in the back, cold hands, blue nails, with heat in the mouth, throat, face and head.

Throat - Burning in the mouth and throat, followed by dryness. Spasmodic constriction in throat, ascending from stomach.

Vertigo - Giddiness, followed by unconsciousness and delirium.

COMMENTS - Diarrhea associated with coldness, mottled blue surface, cold sweat. Sudden desire for stool. Diarrhea accompanied by copious and easy vomiting of watery, albuminous, ropy liquid. Water is almost immediately vomited. Cholera. Suddenly occurring summer diarrhea.

Mouth dry, itching between toes, at night. Profuse, watery diarrhea after midnight. In the morning, stools, headache, are worse. Metallic bloody taste, much spitting of saliva. Farrington noted that it is useful in cases of suppressed measles.

RELATIONS - ***Compare:*** (1) Camph., Verat., Gamb., Crot-t. (2) Jatr-u., Sponge nettle - edema and cardiac paresis.

REFERENCES - Clarke.

JATROPHA URENS

(Spurge Nettle)

PHARMACY - jatr-u. Jatropha urens. Spurge nettle. Tread softly. N. O. Euphorbiaceae. Southern United States. Tincture of fresh plant. ***Historical dose:*** Tincture and all potencies.

CLINICAL - Cardiac, paresis. Edema.

HOMEOPATHIC - According to Allen, this is the most poisonous plant known. He quoted, from the Kew Gardens Quarterly, the experience of Mr. Smith, who touched his wrist against the fine bristly stings of the plant while reaching over it. He experienced numbness and swelling of the lips. His circulation stopped and Smith soon fell unconscious, the last thing he remembered were cries of "Run for the doctor!"

COMMENTS - Other Jatropha include Jatr. glauca, or Jatr. glandulifera, of the East Indies. It has a curious nodulated, gouty looking stem. When crushed, the seeds yield an oil that is used as an external application against rheumatism.

REFERENCES - Clarke.

JOANESIA ASOCA

(Ashoka Bark)

PHARMACY - joan. Joanesia asoca. Ashoka bark. Jonosia asoca. Saraca indica. Bark of an Indian Tree. N. O. Caesalpinioideae. Tincture of bark or seeds. Dried bark. ***Historical dose:*** Tincture and all potencies.

CLINICAL - ***Amenorrhea.*** Constipation. Dysmenorrhea. Emaciation. Fibroids. Headache. Hemorrhoids. Hysteria. Leucorrhea. Menopause. Menorrhagia. Metrorrhagia. Nausea. Palpitations. Uterine, disorders. Vomiting.

HERBAL - Joanesia is a noted plant in India and its therapeutic properties in curing and alleviating all sorts of menstrual troubles and uterine disorders date back from antiquities. Long-lasting costiveness, occasional headache and vertigo associated with uterine derangements are some of the marked symptoms of the drug.

Joanesia is a sovereign remedy for amenorrhea or scanty menses with intolerable pain and burning sensation during the passage of urine. In dysmenorrhea its efficacy has been verified by several homeopaths of our country.

The Ayurvedic physicians prize it as an uterine tonic. It imparts a healthy tone and an all round strength to the uterus which has been weakened by long-lasting disorders of the uterus.

In the cure of leucorrhea its action can never be questioned and upon bloody leucorrhea, whether acute or chronic, it exerts an exhilarating and permanent curative action which sometimes appears to be a miracle. It removes weakness and physical emaciation to the females suffering from long - lasting uterine complaints, or due to those causes.

It is generally considered to be an astringent medicine and uterine sedative. It is said to possess a stimulating effect on the endometrium and on the ovarian tissue.

Joanesia is extensively employed in uterine ailments especially menorrhagia which is the outcome of uterine fibroids and other causes.

In cases of bloody leucorrhea its efficacy is sure and pronounced. Menstrual flow appears too soon, is copious and lasts long and this sort of flow makes the female very weak, anemic and bloodless, she experiences burning sensation all over the face and eyes suffers from pain in the lumbar region and constipation.

Joanesia is considered by competent authorities to be an excellent remedy for the eradication of the above complaints. Asoka will be found to be a grand medicine if the menstrual flow be stopped for any cause and for which colicky abdominal pains supervene.

HOMEOPATHIC - Joanesia was introduced by Dr. N. D. Ray, of Calcutta. Extensive sphere of action on female organs. Amenorrhea and metrorrhagia.

The remedy is principally used by the native physicians of India for menorrhagia, metrorrhagia, leucorrhea from delayed menses or in the place of menses. Infantile leucorrhea, child getting thin and emaciated in spite of getting usual nourishment.

Joanesia has been found to be an excellent medicine for the complaints appearing at the time of menopause. For barrenness it is generally used with success.

In bleeding piles, its efficacy has been verified. In bleeding piles, the color of the blood is red, the patient experiences severe pain and stiff feeling in the back and suffers from constipation, there is burning sensation while passing urine, and there is also burning of the hands, feet and eyes in the evening.

MIND - The patients are generally affectionate, nervous, sentimental, gloomy and religious. Good-natured, affectionate. Absentminded. Timid. Easily weeping, easily excitable, easily fatigued. Disinclination to work. Not very imaginative.

Changeable thoughts. Satisfied with small things. Slow to understand. Disposition to take cold easily, feels better in the open air. Impatient. Cannot bear sufferings. Hysterical exaggerates sufferings.

Abdomen - Hard distended abdomen, pain on pressure, passage of foul-smelling wind, eructation, flatulent colic, worse in the evening, soreness in lower abdomen or pelvis.

Back - Coldness between shoulders. Pain along spine, radiating to abdomen and thighs. Pain at the ape of the neck along the spine. Pain in sacrum and in back radiates on both sides of the abdomen and down the thighs.

Bladder - Irritable bladder. Bladder irritable, desire for frequent passage of urine. Tenderness of bladder.

Chest - Tight feeling across the chest.

Ears - Pains in ear. Hardness of hearing especially after catarrhal or severe cold.

Eyes - Pain in the eyeballs. Redness of the conjunctiva. Burning and itching sensation. Styes on upper lids. Profuse lachrymation. Short-sightedness. Great sensibility of eyes to light. Supra-orbital pains on one or both sides. Great photophobia. Tired feeling in the eyes with least exertion, such as reading and staring at an object.

Face - Paleness of the face, alternately with heat and redness of the cheeks. Pimples on the face.

Female - Menses suppressed and irregular. Headache due to suppression of menses. Severe headache due to scanty flow of menses with severe pain all over the lower parts of the abdomen, pain in back and thighs. Menstrual colic. Delayed and irregular menses. Menstrual discharge scanty, pale and watery, sometimes bad odor and blackish, slightly clotted and painful. Leucorrhea. Amenorrhea at puberty with headache, palpitation, hysteria, loss of appetite, constipation. Pain in ovaries before the flow. Congestive feelings in pelvic organs as before menses. Pain in both ovarian regions. Pain in the sacral region, better on the appearance of menses with free flow. Menorrhagia.

Food - Want of appetite and dislike for food. No desire for food, eats little. Thirsty. Desire for sweets. Desire for acid and sour things. Drinks large quantities of water. Disinclined to take milk, which when taken agrees well.

Head - Stupefying headache, frontal headache, worse sometimes on right temple and sometimes on the left. Unilateral headache. Reflex uterine congestive headache, with scanty menstrual discharge relieved by free flow, nausea, vertigo, disinclination for food or drink, periodical headache, better after bathing, sweat of forehead, relieved of all symptoms in the open air, heaviness of the whole head. Congestive headache, better open air and by free flow.

Heart - Palpitations. Pain in the region of the heart. Pulse quick, full and hard. Accentuated first sound. Palpitations, worse on movement or walking or bending forward.

Kidneys - Urine scanty, bloody, passes frequently. Involuntary urination at night in bed. Profuse emission of watery urine, pain in loin.

Limbs - Weakness in limbs. Shifting pain from place to place. Pains in small joints. Numbness of the limbs. Pain along the thighs.

Lungs - Respiration hurried. Difficulty in breathing when walking, worse in the afternoon and evening. Hacking throat cough.

Male - Testicles swollen, drawing pain in the spermatic cords, itching in the scrotum, discharge of prostatic fluid, emission at night with or without dreams.

Mouth - Dryness of the mouth, excessive thirst, drinks large quantities of water at a time, tongue coated with thick, white or brown coating, bleeding of the gums, toothache.

Nose - Nasal catarrh, sneezing, profuse watery discharge from the nose. Nostrils sore. Obstruction of the nose. Loss of sense of smell. Ulceration of the nostrils. Profuse bleeding from the nose of red color.

Rectum - Hemorrhoids. Obstinate constipation. Feces are hard. Large stool and passed every third or fourth day. Evacuation difficult, pain before stools. Stools are covered with slime or mucus. Pains on the back. Soreness in anus. Blind or bleeding piles. Protrusion of hemorrhoids with itching, smarting and pain.

Sleep - Disturbed sleep. Sleeplessness. Fearful dreams. Dreams of traveling.

Stomach - Excessive nausea, sometimes vomiting. Vomiting of bile. Biliousness. Pain in epigastrium. Colicky pain.

Temperature - Chilliness without thirst. Dry heat with restlessness. Redness of cheeks. Flushed face, running from the nose, catarrhal symptoms.

Throat - Redness of the throat, tonsils and uvula, sore throat, easily takes cold, troublesome throat cough.

REFERENCES - Boericke. Clarke. Ghose.

JUGLANS CINEREA

(Butternut)

PHARMACY - jug-c. Juglans cinerea. Butternut. Juglans cathartica. N. O. Juglandaceae. North America. Tincture of bark of root. Triturations of the resinoid Juglandin. ***Historical dose:*** Tincture and all potencies, tincture to third potency.

CLINICAL - Acne. Angina pectoris. Axilla, pain. Chest, pain. Gallstones. Coryza. Dropsy. Eczema. Erysipelas. Erythema nodosum. Gallstones. ***Headaches.*** Herpes. Hydrothorax. Impetigo. Lichen. Migraines. Pemphigus. Ringworm. Rodent ulcer. Scapula, pain. Scarlatina. Tetters. Vision, lost.

HOMEOPATHIC - The butternut and the black walnut (Juglans nigra) are the American representatives of the walnut family. It has a reputation as a mild cathartic. Applied to the skin, the juice causes reddening and blistering. It was successfully used in camp diarrhea and dysentery in the early American wars. The green rind, rubbed on tetters and ringworm, has a reputation for curing them.

Jug-c. and Jug-r., or Nux Juglans, have both been proved and studied. With both, the digestion is disordered, accompanied with other acute symptoms, including headaches. These are followed by chronic skin disorders.

Sharp, ***occipital headache***, usually associated with liver disturbance. Pain in chest, axilla and scapula with suffocative sensation. Feeling as if all internal organs were too large, especially those of left side. Gallstones. ***Faulty elimination*** that produces jaundice and various skin eruptions. Itching is worse when overheated from exercise.

MIND - Absent-minded. Confusion. Difficulty concentrating. Dull feeling, cannot remember anything that was read. Depression of spirits. Aversion to company. Want to do nothing but eat and sleep.

Abdomen - Soreness in region of liver. Stitches in hepatic region, and under right scapula. Pain in the hypochondrium. Heavy pain in umbilical region. Flatulent pain in different parts of abdomen. Burning in abdomen after stool.

Back - Muscles of neck rigid, lame. Pricking up and down spine. Pain in lumbar vertebrae. Pain between scapula. Sticking under right scapula on stooping.

Chest - Pain in left chest. Retro-sternal pain. Angina pectoris. Oppression at chest, hindering long breathing with cutting pains in lungs. Tuberculosis with great emaciation. Dropsy of chest, of rheumatic origin.

Eyes - Eyes red and swollen. Inflammation, with pustules on lids and around eyes. Eyes burning in afternoon. Feeling in eyes as if drawn together. Loss of vision on sudden motion, with faint-like giddiness.

Face - Pallor. Erythematous redness with dry, burning sensation.

Food - Ferocious appetite. Thirsty, wants to drink all the time.

Head - Dull, full head. Head feels enlarged. Dull headache, better when getting up. ***Sharp*, *occipital headache***. Severe headache, can hardly see. Eruption on scalp. Itching of scalp, intense, must scratch constantly. Pustules on lids and around eyes.

Kidneys - Frequent and copious urination, with burning, smarting, with a headache.

Limbs - Aching pains in the limbs. Sharp, rheumatic pain in shoulders and wrists. Pain in right axilla in afternoon. Pain in elbows and knees. Cramp-like pain in hip at night. Pain in thighs and left knee in forenoon. Occasionally sharp pain in calves.

Lungs - Expectoration of very tenacious mucus, raising a quantity of dark blood.

Modalities - Better getting heated, exercise, scratching, rising in the morning. Worse walking, chest pains. Going up hill causes retro-sternal pain. Stooping causes pain in scapula and back.

Mouth - Acrid feeling in mouth and throat. Coppery taste. Tongue coated white, yellow in the morning. Dryness of root of tongue and fauces. Burning and pricking in mouth and throat. Swelling of submaxillary glands, worse right. Soreness in region of tonsils, externally.

Nose - Tingling in nose, sneezing. ***Coryza, preceded by pain under sternum,*** with threatening suffocation. Copious, bland, thick mucus discharge.

Rectum - Constipation, with griping in umbilical region. Constipation preceded by diarrhea. Diarrhea with burning in anus before and after stool. Yellowish-green stools with tenesmus and burning at anus. A drastic purge, producing irritation and inflammation of mucus membrane of bowels. Bilious, copious, frequent, painless stools. Loose stool, smelling like onions. Camp diarrhea.

Skin - Jaundice with pain about liver and right scapula. Red-like flush of scarlatina. Erythema and erysipelatous redness. ***Itching and prickling when heated.*** Eczema, especially on lower limbs, sacrum and hands. ***Pustules***.

Sleep - Constant yawning, without sleepiness. Sleepiness. Sleeplessness after 3 a.m. Sleep restless, light, unrefreshing. Dreams are vivid, frightful.

Stomach - Burning in stomach. Sinking in stomach extends to abdomen, with headache. Atonic dyspepsia with much belchings and flatulent distention. Nausea in morning. Nausea worse at night.

Temperature - Chilliness, alternating with flashes of heat. Chilliness along spine, beginning in back when near the fire, without coldness of flesh.

Throat - Sore throat in forenoon with roughness on swallowing. Fauces dry. Pain in right side of fauces. Burning in pharynx.

Vertigo - Vertigo with slight nausea. Slight vertigo with sinking faint feeling in stomach extending to abdomen.

COMMENTS - Scrofulous and scorbutic conditions. Rheumatic pains. Characteristic sharp shooting pain in occiput. Headache, with frequent urination and burning. Morning headaches (Nux-v., Bry., Chel., Iris.).

Disturbance of the digestive organs (Iris.). Pains in liver and right scapula. Epigastric sinking, extending to the abdomen, with a headache. Acute diarrhea.

Dark, clotted hemorrhage from the lungs (Jug-r., from the uterus). Acute pains and numbness in the axilla (Jug-r. affects the skin and glands of the axilla).

Eruptions. Scarlatina. Rodent ulcer. One patient who was taking Jug-c. for acne developed all the symptoms of angina pectoris.

RELATIONS - ***Compare:*** (1) Juglin. - duodenal catarrh, bilious diarrhea. (2) Chel., Bry., Iris.

REFERENCES - Boericke. Clarke.

__JUGLANS REGIA

(Walnut)

PHARMACY - jug-r. Juglans regia. Walnut. Nux juglans. N. O. Juglandaceae. Tincture of leaves and of rind of green fruit. ***Historical dose:*** Tincture and all potencies.

CLINICAL - Acne. Anus, burning. Axillary glands, suppuration. Chancre. ***Eruptions.*** Exhaustion. Eyes, pain. Favus. Flatulence. Headaches. Herpes. Levitation, sensation. Menorrhagia. Purpura. Ringworm. Skin, disorders. Scurvy. Spleen, pain. ***Styes***. Syphilis.

HERBAL - The Treasury of Botany noted, "Its plantation should not be too near dwellings, as some persons are affected by the powerful aroma of its foliage. It was said that in the golden age, when men lived upon acorns, the gods lived upon Walnuts and hence the name of Juglans, Jovis glans or Jupiter's nuts".

HOMEOPATHIC - Excited, as if intoxicated in the evening in bed and a feeling as if the head were floating in the air, or as if flying. Sharp pains in the forehead (Jug-c. in the occiput). Muscles relaxed. ***Prominent skin eruptions.*** Exhaustion and disinclination for the usual business.

MIND - Mental indolence. Disinclined to talk or argue. Inattention when reading and disinclination to work. Peevishness. Discontented in evening. Excited in evening in bed as if intoxicated. Feeling as if the head were floating in the air.

Abdomen - Fullness, bloated, tension and heaviness in the abdomen. Pain in epigastric region with distention of abdomen. Drawing with pressure in region of spleen. Pain above umbilicus.

Back - Stitches in sacral region. Violent stitches in the small of the back, causing one to tremble.

Chest - Oppression. Sticking in lungs not dependent on motion or respiration. Itching on the sternum.

Ears - Aching and fullness in right, then left ear, followed by a discharge of pus from both ears. Burning in left ear, then redness and swelling. External ear inflamed, with painful sores. Eruption behind ears of children.

Eyes - Burning in eyes. Pressive pain above eye (left) worse by motion. ***Styes.*** Feeling of coryza.

Face - Swelling of left cheek and upper lip.

Female - Menses preceded by pressive drawing pains in the abdomen, worse by motion, accompanied with general exhaustion and loss of appetite. Menstruation early, too profuse, discharge of a large quantity of black, pitch-like clots.

Food - Unusually great appetite without increase of thirst. Thirstlessness while eating and aversion to wine. Appetite lost. Thirst increased. Aversion to tobacco smoking in the evening.

Head - Confused, feels as if head were floating in air. ***Occipital sharp pain.***

Kidneys - Frequent desire to pass water from loss of tone of sphincter. Constant urging and involuntary dribbling. Copious urine, but no thirst. Urine scanty, clear, dark red.

Limbs - Drawing pain, as if sprained. Paralyzed feeling in legs and knees with weakness. Sticking and itching in right leg and right fingers.

Male - Frequent erections day and night. Burning in penis after sex.

Modalities - Worse by motion. Worse after fat food, evening, at 9 p.m. and after 9 p.m. Migraine worse by speaking. Pain in abdomen worse by laughing. Warmth of bed aggravates toothache. Itching, worse at night. Rash aggravated by undressing, washing.

Mouth - Tongue coated white in morning with bitter, slimy taste. Salivation. Tearing in hollow teeth, worse warmth of bed.

Rectum - Stool twice a day, preceded or accompanied by pain in abdomen. Thin, soft, large, hard, difficult, scanty stool. Large stool, then burning pain and pressure in anus. Stool delayed. Constipation. Itching at the anus in the evening, with stitches, compelling one to walk about.

Skin - Comedones and acne of the face. Itching and eruptions of small red pustules. Pimples on face, red pimples on face, neck, shoulders and back. Scalp red and itches violently at night. Crusta lactea with soreness around ears. Chancre-like ulcer. Axillary glands suppurate.

Sleep - Yawning in afternoon with stretching. Sleepiness. Inability to sleep after dinner, though inclined to do so earlier than usual. Restless sleep with frightful dreams.

Stomach - Fullness and bloated of the stomach. Burning in stomach. Hiccough more violent after eating. Belchings are violent, frequent, loud, tasting as after eating fat. Nausea at 6 a.m. and after supper. Vomiting, woke suddenly vomited food eaten four hours before, then slept without further trouble.

Throat - Aphonia or great hoarseness. Hawking of much mucus.

COMMENTS - Severe flatulence and bloating of the abdomen. Affects the spleen more than the liver (opposite of Jug-c.). Diarrhea and many rectal and anal symptoms. Hemorrhagic, black and clotted blood (Jug-c., Cary.), particularly uterine hemorrhages. Inflammation and ulceration in the male sexual organs.

Pronounced skin symptoms. Scrofula. Scabs on the arms and in axilla. Symptoms go from the right axilla to the left.

Farrington said Jug-r. is one of the best remedies in "tinea favosa, especially in the scalp behind the ear, itching is intense at night so that the patient has difficulty in sleeping."

Clotar Müller, who experienced the axillary skin symptoms in his own person, had never suffered from a skin affection before. One of the provers was cured of an itching eruption of the legs from which he had suffered in winter for four years, the itching commencing as soon as he began to undress.

Many of the symptoms closely resembled syphilis and the affection of the cheek in one of the provers was actually diagnosed as syphilitic by a doctor who saw him in Müller's absence. The left side of head, face and abdomen were mostly affected. Axillary symptoms proceed from right to left.

In one case, a nurse poisoned her left arm some years before from septic and possibly syphilitic cause, inflammation of the axillary glands ensued, first of the left then of the right, leaving an eczematous itching condition. The glands of the groin also became affected.

Elaps. 200c relieved the bulk of the conditions, but there was still a little irritation occasionally in the axilla and Jug-r. 2c three times a day was given.

Five days after beginning the Jug-r., an eruption of minute vesicles appeared on her back, itching a great deal. It extended up the center of her back from sacrum to mid-dorsal region, spreading out below, tapering above. She had scratched holes in two places.

The rash was worse after washing. All soreness and irritation had gone from the arms and axilla. The rash was antidoted with Rhus-t. 2c. She had no more trouble with her glands.

Müller observed, "In the digestive organs it causes derangement and irritation, which simultaneously call forth abnormal symptoms in other organs, especially in the head. After this action, which is brief, appear various exanthematous symptoms, which appear late and run a chronic course."

RELATIONS - ***Antidoted by:*** Rhus-t. ***Compare:*** (1) Jug-c., Cary. (2) Rhus-t. - skin. (3) Graph. - tinea favosa behind ears. (4) Rumex - rash worse undressing. (5) Mez., Merc. (6) Cean. - spleen. (7) Lyc. - flatulence. ***Follows well:*** Elaps. - axillary affections, black hemorrhages. Sulph. - head hot, cold limbs. Grind. - pain over left eye.

REFERENCES - Boericke. Clarke.

JUNCUS EFFUSUS

(Soft Rush)

PHARMACY - junc. Juncus effusus. Soft rush. Common rush. Juncus communis. N. O. Juncaceae. Tincture of root. ***Historical dose:*** Tincture and all potencies.

CLINICAL - Asthma. Backache. Calculus. Catarrh. Dropsy. Dysuria. Flatulence. Headache. Kidney, diseases. Rheumatism. Scars disorders.

HERBAL - According to Nowack and Rinks, Juncus is a diuretic and has been used in dropsical, kidney stones and kidney diseases. Hartmann used the tincture with success in dysuria, strangury and ischuria. In Livonia, a decoction is used for stone and gravel.

HOMEOPATHIC - Junc-e. was proved by Dr. Whale, producing a number of symptoms. The exact preparation used in the proving was not recorded. Fresh plant tinctures should be used in any further experiments.

The most notable symptoms were ***bubbling sensations*** in various parts. A number of pressive and sticking pains were noted in the chest. Pulling in cervical vertebrae in neck muscles. Rumbling of flatus in abdomen; abdominal symptoms were markedly better when flatus was emitted.

Rheumatic pains worse by rest, on left side, appeared or were worse at night and came on again in morning and evening. Worse flexing parts, bending sideways. Better stretching out arm. Chilliness worse on uncovering. Better by motion.

RELATIONS - ***Compare:*** (1) Rhus-t. - worse rest and uncovering, better stretching. (2) Berb. - bubbling sensations. (3) Sil. - scars.

REFERENCES - Boericke. Clarke.

JUNIPERUS COMMUNIS

(Juniper Berries)

PHARMACY - juni-c. Juniperus communis. Juniper berries. N. O. Gymnosperm of the Conifer. Cupressaceae. Juniperus. Tincture of fresh ripe berries. ***Historical dose:*** Tincture and all potencies.

CLINICAL - ***Allergies.*** Cedar, fever. ***Coryza. Coughs.*** Dropsy. Dysmenorrhea. ***Hay fever.*** Hemorrhages. Nephritis. Pyelitis.

HERBAL - Gin owes its distinctive properties to the oil of juniper berries, perhaps explaining why the spirit is in such popular repute as a remedy for dysmenorrhea. It has a very powerful action on the kidneys and has cured cases of kidney dropsy.

HOMEOPATHIC - Juni-c. has not been proved, but sufficient is known of its action to warrant its inclusion and to show the analogy between its action and that of Sabina.

Hale commended it in certain coughs with scanty, loaded urine. He said German doctors used juniper in gastric affections, abdominal flatulence and colic. Catarrhal inflammation of kidneys. Dropsy with suppression of urine. Elderly persons with poor digestion and scanty secretion of urine. Chronic pyelitis.

Chest - Painful ribs and sternum from coughing attacks (Bry.).

Kidneys - Nephritis. Strangury, bloody, scanty urine, violet odor (Tereb.). Weight in kidney region. Pyelitis. Kidney hyperemia (Eucal.).

Lungs - Severe, painful coughs. Cough with scanty, loaded urine.

Male - Prostatic discharge.

Nose - Coryza. Hay fever. Allergies. ***Violent sneezing from cedar pollen.***

Comments - Hale wrote, "I have known cases of dysmenorrhea and uterine hemorrhage cured by the common Juniper, and I have treated some kidney and bladder difficulties with Juniper. The popularity of pure gin in dysmenorrhea is owing to the effects of the oil of Juniper berries which it contains.

"In domestic practice, an infusion of Juniper leaves and berries is used successfully in amenorrhea and dysmenorrhea, as well as retention, suppression, and other urinary troubles.

"In some cases of dropsy, a tincture of the berries, or the oil of Juniper, will act on the kidneys favorably after the failure of other medicines.

"We ought to have provings of the common Juniper, and give it a place in our Materia Medica. I would also suggest that the tincture be made from equal parts by weight of the fresh berries and green leaves. The Oil of Juniper of commerce is made from the berries alone.

"German physicians make much use of Juniper in gastric complaints, in abdominal flatulence, colics, and even in some hepatic affections. I know that the 3x of Oleum juniperus is useful in certain coughs, with scanty urine, loaded with solid matters."

RELATIONS - ***Compare:*** (1) All-c., Wye., Sabin., Tereb.

REFERENCES - Boericke. Clarke. Hale. Murphy.

JUNIPERUS VIRGINIANUS

(Red Cedar)

PHARMACY - juni. Juniperus virginianus. Red cedar. N. O. Gymnosperm of the Conifer. Tincture of fresh twigs. Tincture of twigs and berries. Tincture of the oil. ***Historical dose:*** Tincture and all potencies.

CLINICAL - Chilliness. Comatose. Convulsions. Cystitis. Delirium. Dropsy. Dysuria. Eyes, twitching. Fever. Nausea. Pyelitis. Strangury. Strokes. Tetanus. Uterine, hemorrhage. Vomiting.

HOMEOPATHIC - The effects of Juni. have been largely observed on women who have taken it to stimulate the uterus or bring on the menses. A number of fatal cases have occurred from overdose of the herb.

The patients passing into violent convulsions, followed by an apoplectic or stroke condition, insensibility and collapse. Hands at times clenched. Jaws firmly fixed. Staggering. Comatose sleep. Chilliness. Rigors followed by fever. Considerable fever and pain, similar to labor pains. Sweats. Pulse very irregular.

Persistent dragging pain in back. Hyperemia of kidneys. Pyelitis and cystitis. Dropsy of the aged with suppressed urine. Violent tenesmus of bladder. Constant urging to urinate. Dysuria, burning, cutting pain in urethra when urinating. Uterine hemorrhage.

Mind - Emotional during the paroxysm of fever. Fright. Raved incoherently. Delirious. Insensible state. Moaning.

Abdomen - Abdomen swollen and hot. Complained of intensity of pain in abdomen. Pain in the bowels. Thirst.

Bladder - Cystitis. Violent tenesmus of bladder. Constant urging to urinate. Dysuria, burning, cutting pain in urethra when urinating.

Eyes - Eyes bloodshot. Sclerotic congestion. Pupils dilated. Eyes glare and twitch. Eyes felt as if bursting from their sockets.

Face - Very red, swollen and livid face. Veins of the face, head, and neck fully distended. Ecchymosis.

Female - Uterine hemorrhage.

Food - Great thirst.

Head - Head felt as if enclosed with an iron band.

Kidneys - Hyperemia of kidneys. Pyelitis. Great difficulty in passing urine.

Rectum - Violent purging. Bowels loose.

Skin - Skin dry and parched.

Sleep - Deep, comatose sleep.

Stomach - Considerable distension and tenderness at pit of stomach. Stomach pain. Sick and distressed in stomach. Nausea and vomiting a black and then a greenish matter. Heartburn.

Throat - Fauces in spots denuded of their mucus covering.

REFERENCES - Allen. Clarke.

JUSTICIA ADHATODA

(Malabar Nut)

PHARMACY - just. Justicia adhatoda. Malabar nut. Adhatoda vasica. Vasika. Singhee. An Indian Shrub. Acanthaceae. Tincture of the fresh leaves. ***Historical dose:*** Tincture and all potencies.

CLINICAL - ***Allergies***. Appetite, loss. Asthma. Blood, spitting, Bronchitis. Colds. Constipation. ***Coryza.*** Coughs. Depression. ***Dyspnea.*** Fevers. ***Hay fever.*** Jaundice. Pneumonia. ***Sneezing***. Thirst. Tuberculosis. Vomiting. Whooping cough.

HERBAL - The Ayurvedic physicians of India prize justicia. They are so very sure of its efficacy that they call it Vaidyamata, i.e. mother of physicians. They claim that no death can occur from cough of any kind if Vasika can play its role and find time to display its healing virtues.

HOMEOPATHIC - Dry, spasmodic, constricted cough. Violent ***dyspnea*** associated with the cough. Threatened suffocation. Whooping cough, with breath loss, pale, stiff and blue, and rigidity of the body. Cough with tightness of chest, as if it would burst with bronchial rattle, obstruction of breath and sneezing.

Vomiting with the cough, no food or drink is retained. Dry mucus membranes, especially of the mouth and throat, with thirst. Tough expectoration. Acute catarrhal conditions of the respiratory tract, particularly in the beginning. Colds.

Coryza, fluent, acrid with violent sneezing, coughing or asthmatic attacks. ***Fits of sneezing*** with lachrymation and loss of smell and taste. ***Allergies and hay fever.*** Bronchitis, pneumonia. First stages of tuberculosis, with spitting of blood. Hoarseness.

Functional derangements of the liver. Jaundice. Thirst. Great loss of appetite. Obstinate constipation.

Stiffening out, trembling and convulsions with cough or fever. Puffy hands and feet in morning. Chilliness. Fever. Marked oversensitiveness to external impressions.

MIND - Irritability, easily angered. Bad humor. Anxious and discouraged. Depression of spirits. Averse to conversation. Sensitive to external impressions.

Chest - ***Tightness across chest,*** as if it would burst.

Coughs - ***Cough with sneezing.*** Dry cough from sternal region all over chest. ***Paroxysmal cough*** with suffocative obstruction of respiration. ***Whooping cough***.

Eyes - Lachrymation.

Head - Hot, full and heavy head.

Limbs - Puffy hands and feet in morning.

Liver - Jaundice. Liver weakness. Liver pains.

Lungs - Acute catarrhal conditions of the respiratory tract. ***Severe dyspnea with cough.*** Obstruction of breath and sneezing. Asthmatic attacks, cannot endure a close, warm room. Bronchitis and pneumonia. ***Rattling in bronchi.*** Tough mucus. Tuberculosis.

Modalities - Worse in a close room, from dust, noise, eating.

Mouth - Mouth is dry. Loss of taste.

Nose - ***Allergies and hay fever.*** Profuse, fluent coryza, with constant sneezing. ***Coryza with cough***. Fits of sneezing with lachrymation and loss of smell and taste.

Stomach - Nausea and vomiting.

Throat - Hoarseness, larynx painful. Dry and painful during empty swallowing. Tenacious mucus.

COMMENTS - Blackwood wrote, "This one of the most ancient drugs in India, the most highly valued by Ayurveda. Its field of use is in colds, coryza, cough of any kind, vomiting, bronchitis, pneumonia, tuberculosis, spitting of blood. Fevers, jaundice, loss of appetite, and constipation. These ailments are what the ancient physicians use it for."

It was proved by two men, twenty-seven and thirty-two years of age; their symptoms were later clinically verified. Proving symptoms included catarrh, violent sneezing, watering eyes, profuse coryza, loss of appetite, vomiting, liver pains, hoarseness and very painful suffocative cough with blood streaked mucus and high temperature.

Ghose recorded a case of coryza. "My son had an attack of cold. He had fluent coryza, with constant sneezing; there was hoarseness with swollen nose; there was stoppage of nose at night; there was also thirst; no appetite existed; there were occasional coughing fits, but no expectoration ensued.

"I prescribed Justicia 1x every three hours. After administration of the third dose he fell asleep. He came round within three days. From the second day there was no hoarseness."

Ghose also recorded another case of coryza. The son of Babu Bhupati Choudhuri, of Bhowanipore, suffered from a severe attack of cold. Copious fluent coryza, accompanied by violent coughing, the eyes were somewhat swollen and watered all the time; he was feverish. Ghose prescribed Just. 1x every three hours, and he was fully cured within two days.

RELATIONS - ***Compare:*** (1) Seems to come between All-c. and Euphr.

REFERENCES - Anshutz. Blackwood. Boericke. Clarke. Ghose.

K

KALI ACETICUM

(Potassium Acetate)

PHARMACY - kali-acet. Kali aceticum. Potassium acetate. Acetate of potash. Kali acetas. Solution in distilled water. ***Historical dose:*** Tincture and all potencies.

CLINICAL - Diabetes. Diarrhea. Dropsy. Headaches. Hemorrhoids. Urine, alkaline.

HOMEOPATHIC - Kali-acet. is well known in allopathic practice as a diuretic and, to a lesser degree, as a cathartic. Derivatives have been used in cases of dropsy, chiefly ascites and hydrothorax. The homeopathic uses are chiefly in cases of over-secretion of urine and in diarrhea.

The provings have brought out a preponderance of abdominal and urinary symptoms. Great disturbance in the circulation of fluids in the tissues (Acet-ac.). Griping diarrhea. Increased flow of urine, which was more watery and alkaline. Bleeding of hemorrhoids.

Weakness, trembling, profuse perspiration, especially about the head. Trembling and anxiety in whole body of transient duration. Symptoms generally worse in morning, but there was a headache, worse 4 p.m.

Abdomen - Unnatural distention of abdomen after dinner. Griping. An indefinite gnawing pain lasting an hour. Gnawing sensation in abdomen which lasted until evening. Pains in region of umbilicus, lasting until going to bed, when they suddenly disappeared.

Head - Dull headache in morning. Headache about 4 p.m. Much perspiration of head.

Kidneys - Urine very much increased in quantity and very watery. Urine strongly alkaline, sweetish odor, yellow color, ammoniacal.

Limbs - Extreme weariness and trembling in all limbs in morning. Great weariness of all limbs, with some headache, disappearing half an hour after an afternoon nap.

Rectum - Bleeding hemorrhoids, several times during day. Diarrhea. Two stools in evening.

Stomach - Constrictive, dull pain in stomach, extending to low down in abdomen, gradually disappearing after two hours. Dull, pressive, pinching and constrictive pain in epigastric region, coming on a few minutes after each dose and lasting an hour.

Temperature - Much perspiration on head, especially from 11 a.m. to 1 p.m. Profuse perspiration, very offensive during exertion.

RELATIONS - ***Compare:*** (1) Acet-ac., Kali-c., Am-a. (2) Lyc. - worse at 4 p.m.

REFERENCES - Clarke.

KALI ARSENICOSUM

(Potassium Arsenite)

PHARMACY - kali-ar. Kali arsenicosum. Potassium arsenite. Fowler's solution (the form in which Kali-ar. has been tested, consists of 1 part arsenious acid, 1 part carbonate of potash, 3 parts compound tincture of lavender, and 95 parts distilled water). Dilutions should be made from this. ***Historical dose:*** All potencies.

CLINICAL - ***Anxiety, attacks. Asthma.*** Bright's disease. Cancer. Deafness. Diarrhea. Dropsy ***Eczema.*** Emaciation. Epithelioma. Exophthalmus. Eye, disorders. Faintness. Herpes, zoster. Jealousy. Measles. Melancholy. Miliary, rash. Lung, disorders. Neuralgias. Neurasthenia. ***Palpitations. Panic, attacks. Psoriasis.*** Skin, disorders. Tongue, neuralgia. Tremors. Varicose, veins. Ulcers.

HOMEOPATHIC - It is not possible to separate entirely the pathogenesis of Kali-ar. and Ars. Kali-ar. is the favorite form in which arsenic is prescribed by the allopaths, consequently the bulk of observations from over-dosing are due to this preparation, named *Liquor arsenicalis*, considered arsenic and nothing else.

Much of our knowledge relating to this remedy comes to us from the effects of overdosing and protracted use of the medicine on patients suffering from chronic skin and blood diseases. The arsenic symptoms predominate.

Epithelioma developed in a patient after prolonged treatment with allopathic Kali-ar. for psoriasis.

During treatment for right-sided herpes, patients noted color changes in their eyes and skin. Sclerotics became thick and yellow instead of clear and bluish. The iris, which was blue, became gray. Skin, instead of being fair and florid, became muddy and older looking.

Tendency towards ***anxiety and skin diseases.*** Restless, nervous. Great weakness. Emaciation, anemia. Faintness. Neurasthenia. ***Chilly and sensitive to cold.*** Cannot get too warm even in summer. Tremors. Sudden noise or touch throws the whole body into a tremor.

Inveterate skin diseases, malignant tendency. Intolerable itching, worse undressing, walking, warmth. Chronic eczema. Psoriasis. Herpes zoster, measles, miliary rash. Epithelioma. Numerous small nodules under the skin. Gouty nodosities. Rheumatic, gouty and syphilitic pains. Varicose veins. Dropsy.

Cauliflower-like excrescences of os uterus with flying pains, foul smelling discharges and pressure below the pelvis. Black leg ulcer running bloody, foul water with cutting, burning, itching and dyspnea. Phagedenic ulcers, deep base and turned up edges.

Burning in throat. The tongue burns, numb. Tongue neuralgia. Exophthalmos, eye affections. Deafness. Aching in stomach. Passes much gas, then diarrhea. Bright's disease. Palpitations with nephritis. All the sufferings are worse at night.

MIND - Morose and quarrelsome. Scolding, retired and discontented. Jealous. Anguish. Face looks frightened and anxious. Startled, fixed look, protruding brilliant eyes. ***Anxiety and panic attacks. Anxiety about health.*** Anxiety on going to bed. Anxiety with difficult breathing. Hysteria.

Fears felt in the stomach. ***Fear of getting a life threatening disease,*** of high blood pressure, of having a stroke, ***of heart disease,*** of getting cancer. Fear in a crowd, of being alone, of death, dying, of being murdered, poisoned. Fear of thieves, burglars, at night, of evil. Fear that something bad will happen. Superstitious.

Mental and physical restlessness. Excitable. Great nervousness. Oversensitive to noise, especially to voices. Starting from noises. Timidity. Capriciousness. Concentration difficult. Confusion. Weak memory.

Depression, melancholy. Sadness when alone. Despair of recovery. Suicidal disposition. Apathy. Indifferent to everything, scarcely answered questions addressed to her or replies to them in a peevish tone. Aversion to answering questions. Behaves like a mad person. Delusion head is enlarged. Sudden impulse to kill.

Abdomen - Burning pain in bowels, unquenchable thirst, belly tense and painful involuntary watery stools with sense as if a red-hot iron were in anus. Frequent griping pains in bowels and constant desire for stool, considerable tenderness in whole abdomen, which is distended.

Back - ***Backache with sciatica***, worse pressure. Much pain and tenderness down spine.

Ears - Otorrhea. Ear discharge bloody, fetid and yellow.

Eyes - Startled look with protruding, brilliant eyes, pale face and sunken cheeks. Eyes red. Whites of eyes look thick and yellow. Jaundice. The blue iris becomes gray. Dark discoloration around orbit. Inflamed, itching of conjunctiva. Conjunctiva glassy. Right eye weaker, watery, as after weeping. ***Swollen lower eyelids.*** Heat and itchiness of lids, followed by swelling and tenderness. Eye sensitive to light.

Face - Face pale and waxy. Complexion muddy. Puffy under eyes. Old looking. Nodular eruption on face, boils. Furfuraceous eruption on beard.

Female - Cauliflower excrescences of uterine cervix with flying pains, foul smelling discharge and pressure below pubis. Menses absent. Milk entirely arrested.

Food - Appetite lost. Aversion to fat, meat. Intense thirst. Drinks in small sips. Desires sweet, sour, vinegar, fruits, lemon, refreshing food. Desires mustard, spices, milk, coffee, warm food, fat. Worse from milk, ice cream, sour, fruits, melon, strawberry, alcohol, spoiled food.

Head - Headache from gastric causes or catarrh. Headache in left parietal bone, as if it was sore and pressed upon by hand. Headaches worse after eating, lying, motion and noise. Headaches better sitting, external heat, hot drinks and wrapping up head. Head as if heavy and enlarged. Constricted feeling in head, as if there was a wound in the bone that was being scratched. Crusta lactea. Behaves like a crazy person.

Heart - Heart attacks with anxiety and fear. ***Palpitations with anxiety and fear.*** High blood pressure from worry and fear. Weak heart. Pulse weak and contracted, small, scarcely perceptible, rapid.

Kidneys - Urine scanty with pellicle.

Limbs - Gouty nodosities, worse change of weather. Crampy feeling of lower limbs with partial loss of motion and sensation, livid in places, tending to slough. Aching pain in right shoulder and elbow, followed by herpetic eruption. Knees bent up so he could not move his feet. Swollen ankles. Palms and soles speckled over with corns. Varicose veins of legs. Ulcers on legs with general psoriasis. Black ulcer on leg, running bloody, foul water, with cutting, burning, itching and dyspnea.

Lungs - Anxiety with difficult breathing. Asthma with panic attacks. ***Asthma, rapid, anxious breathing, worse 2 a.m. to 3 a.m.*** Asthma better from sitting, worse lying down. Pneumonia with stitching pains in pleura.

Modalities - Better on rainy days. Aversion to open air. ***Worse touch***, lying down, warmth of bed, warmth, cold feet, noise. Worse after midnight, from 1 a.m. to 3 a.m.

Mouth - In middle, towards tip of tongue, a smooth, red spot with troublesome burning and numbness. Toothache, better heat, worse eating, cold drinks and during menses. Pulsating and tearing pain, radiates to ears, head and temples. Gums swollen and tender.

Nose - Colds. Hay fever. Sneezing. Watery, acrid discharge. Sinusitis. Chronic nasal catarrh. Nasal discharge bloody, burning, excoriating, offensive, greenish, thick or yellow.

Perspiration - Sweats when walking.

Rectum - Discharge of much gas, followed by diarrhea. Violent diarrhea. Cholera. ***Diarrhea worse after midnight,*** from milk. Stools white, watery, frothy. Foul odor, with cramps. Sensation as of a red-hot iron in anus. Hemorrhoids, bleeding, external and internal, worse walking.

Sensations - The head feels larger. Protrusion of eyeballs. Burning and numbness of tongue. Tongue feels too large. ***Anxiety felt in solar plexus***. Sensation of a ball rising from the pit of stomach to throat causing suffocation. As if a red-hot iron were in anus.

Skin - ***Dry, scaly, wilted skin.*** Acne, pustules worse during menses. ***Chronic eczema, intolerable itching, worse from warmth***, walking, undressing. ***Psoriasis***, lichen. Psoriasis in numerous patches, with great itching. Discoloration of skin after psoriasis. Numerous small nodules under skin. Phagedenic ulcers. Fissures in bends of arms and knees. Skin cancer, where suddenly an alarming malignancy without any external signs sets in.

Sleep - Restless and anxious sleep. Sleeplessness, worse 1 a.m. to 4 a.m. Sleeps with hand over the heart. Nightmares, vivid dreams.

Stomach - Anxiety feeling with palpitations from pit of stomach. Empty feeling in stomach. Sinking at epigastrium with faintness. Weight in stomach after eating. Sensation as of a ball rising from pit of stomach to larynx threatening suffocation, better by loud belching. Nausea and vomiting. Constant pain and nausea after food, frequent vomiting of ingesta.

Temperature - Cold temperature on skin. Fever with lassitude.

Throat - Some gastric cough and frequent raking of throat and fauces of a mucopurulent secretion mixed with specks of blood. ***Burning in throat.*** Sensation in throat and larynx as if forced asunder.

Throat dry and sore. Throat constricted with copious flow of saliva. Complete aphonia, following skin affection.

Tongue - Tongue clear, whitish, red like raw beef. Tongue coated on edges only with mucus stripes. Tongue swollen, felt too large in mouth, numb. Neuralgic or burning in tongue. Smooth red spot in middle of tongue toward tip that burns and is numb.

Vertigo - Vertigo while walking in the open air.

COMMENTS - Cases of Kali-ar. poisoning with massive doses present nothing to distinguish them from cases of other arsenical preparations, but Kali-ar. has had a short proving and a number of cases of allopathic provings are on record.

Jonathan Hutchinson recorded a number of cases of right-sided herpes. One of his patients observed that, while taking Kali-ar., her sclerotics became thick and yellow instead of clear and bluish. The iris, which was blue, became more gray. Her skin, instead of being fair and florid, became muddy and older looking.

This was a mystery to Hutchinson as he usually gave Kali-ar. to make the skin clearer, but he was compelled to record the fact, though he did not apparently perceive the homeopathic solution of the mystery.

Hutchinson also noted cases of epithelioma developing after prolonged medication with Kali-ar. for psoriasis. In another case, an attack of measles was almost exactly mimicked.

Useful as a backup for Ars., particularly if Ars. palliates or stops working.

Skin symptoms with a tendency toward malignancy. Psoriasis. Herpes. Itching, worse at night, on undressing, and by warmth. Lupus. Indicated for the burning pains of dying cancer patients. Deafness associated with constant sickness.

Asthma, worse 2 a.m. to 3 a.m. (Ars. worse 11 p.m. to 2 a.m.). Sinus problems. Shortness of breath, hyperventilate with panic. Weak from going up stairs (Calc., Sil.).

Fainting spells and fear of fainting (Gels., Arg-n.). Pulsations in the body followed by shaking and trembling. Sinking sensations. Fevers and shaking chills. Migraines, or fear of getting migraines, causing panic.

Panic stricken (Acon.). Panic attacks, fear of having a panic attack. Chronic hypochondriacs, fear of heart attack, high blood pressure, stroke or cancer. Fear of death. Agoraphobia, claustrophobia. Superstitious (Arg-n., Zinc, Rhus-t., Ars.). Suspicious of others. Periodic rushes of adrenaline, pheochromocytoma. Ailments after fright.

Panic with a burning or energy in the solar plexus area (Kali-c., Ign., Calc., Carc.). Better when distracted from panic attacks or fears. Despair over recovery. Desires company, insecure (Ars.). Hypersensitive to surroundings (Phos.). Chilly, sensitive to drafts.

Restless and sleepless. Anxiety about dead people or dreams about dead people. May dream of fire and wake up in a panic that the house is on fire. Can lie on their left and hold their heart when they sleep. May get palpitations when sleeping on the right.

Lump rising from the stomach to the throat. Thirsty, but aggravated by cold drinks. Desires sweets, warm drinks.

Marked periodicity (Ars.), symptoms were worse every other day in the morning, mind symptoms worse every third day. Worse after midnight, on right side. The right-sidedness of Ars. was reproduced in the right-sided herpes, repeatedly noticed by Hutchinson, but there was a left-sided headache.

RELATIONS - In some cases of overdosing, Kali-i. proved antidotal. For other antidotes see Ars., which it greatly resembles and with which it must be compared. ***Compare:*** (1) Ars., Lev., Nat-a. and other arsenic compounds. (2) Chin. - periodicity. (3) Cic., Op. - fixed eyeballs. (4) Rumx. and Jug-r. - worse when undressing. (5) Iod., Kali-bi., Merc-c., Kali-c.

REFERENCES - Boericke. Clarke. Grimmer. Murphy. Phatak.

KALI BICHROMICUM

(Potassium Bichromate)

PHARMACY - kali-bi. Kali bichromicum. Potassium bichromate. Red Chromate of Potash. Bichromate of Potash. Potassium dichromate. Potasse bichromas. Solution in distilled water. Trituration. ***Historical dose:*** All potencies.

CLINICAL - Acne. Anemia. Asthma. Blotches. Bone, disorders. Bronchitis. Burns. Cachexia. ***Catarrh.*** Coccyx, pain. Conjunctivitis. Constipation. Cornea, opacities. ***Colds. Coryza. Descemetitis.*** Duodenum, ulcers. Dyspepsia. Ears, inflammation. Emaciation. Epilepsy. Eyes, inflamed. Farcy. Gastric, ulcer. Glanders. Gleet. Gonorrhea. Gout. Hay fever. ***Headache.*** Intermittent, fever. Intestines, ulceration. Iritis. Keratitis. Leucorrhea. Lumbago. Lupus. Measles. Menopausal, flushes. ***Migraines. Mucus, plugs.*** Mumps. ***Nasal, congestion.*** Neuralgia. Nightmares. Nodes. Nosebleeds. Nose, soreness. Obesity. Ophthalmia. Ozaena. Polyps. ***Post-nasal, catarrh.*** Pruritus, vulvae. ***Rheumatism.*** Rhinitis, atrophic. Sciatica. Scrofula. ***Sinusitis.*** Smell, illusions. Sun-headache. Sycosis. Syphilis. Throat, sore. Tobacco, intolerance. Trachea, disorders. Ulcers. Urethritis. Warts. Whooping cough.

HOMEOPATHIC - Kali-bi., with the other chromium preparations, Chr-ac. and Chr-ox., was introduced into the Materia Medica by Dr. J. Drysdale. All chromium salts are derived from potassium bichromate, which is manufactured in large quantities from chrome-iron-ore. The association of chromium with ferrum is noteworthy.

The bichromate is largely used in dying, calico-printing, wood staining, photography and as a solution for producing the current in electric batteries. Many symptoms were obtained from workmen engaged in the preparation of the salt, some of which had been noted before Drysdale studied the drug.

Drysdale published his first proving in 1844 in the British Journal of Homeopathy. The Austrian Society proved it the following year.

Kali-bi. has an affinity for the mucus membranes of the air passages, nose, pharynx, stomach and duodenum. Keynote ***thick, sticky, ropy, stringy, tough, yellow***, ***green mucus*** discharges. The mucus adheres to the part and can be drawn out in strings. Formation of crusts on mucus membranes and skin. Membranes look furred.

Catarrh of pharynx, larynx, bronchi and nose and a ***tough, stringy, viscid secretion*** is produced. ***Perforation of the nasal septum***. Chronic atonic catarrh. Ozaena. Shooting from root of nose to external angle of eye, begins in the morning, increases to noon, and ceases toward evening.

Itching in vagina, ear, lungs etc. ***As if a hair on tongue,*** in nostrils etc. Sore throat. Yellowness of discharges, eyes, vision tongue etc. Keratitis and iritis. Epilepsy, ropy saliva from mouth during convulsions. Dilatation of stomach and heart.

Ulcers on the skin, mucus membranes and bones. Ulcers with dark dots, deep, perforating, round, punched out with over-hanging edges or thick crusts. Septic or peptic ulcers. Stubborn suppurations, inflammations. Polyps. Bone-pains and nodes.

Pains wander from part to part. Diagonal pains. ***Pains migrate quickly*** from place to place and finally attack the stomach. ***Pains occur in small spots***. Pains appear and disappear suddenly. Sharp stitching pains. Neuralgia, daily at the same hour. Weakness and weariness after pains. Cracking of joints.

Alternating and shifting conditions. Headache alternates with blindness. Rheumatic pains alternate with gastric symptoms or with dysentery. Ascending symptoms, gastric pains, chills, heat etc. Plastic or fibrous exudations spread downwards. Sensation of heaviness in different parts.

Indolent or sluggish reaction in many conditions. Diseased conditions progress slowly but deeply, causing great weakness bordering on paralysis but little fever. More adapted to sub-acute rather than the violent acute stage.

Sickly, chilly and cachetic. Affections of autumn and spring. Complaints of hot weather. "

Great liability to take cold in open air," and " moderately cold air is felt very unpleasantly." Eruptions begin in warm weather (opp. Rhus-t.). Sun headaches.

Secondary and tertiary syphilis. Syphilitic rheumatism. Kali-bi. as "chrome-water" was also remarkably successful. It been used as a local application for ulcers in very weak solutions, about 1 to 2,000.

MIND - Mentally ill-humored and low in spirit. Listless. Indifference to business affairs. Indolent, aversion to mental and physical exertion. Weak memory, vanishing thoughts. ***Impatience.*** Irritability, ***sadness, better after eating.***

Anxiety arising from chest. Anxiety before menses. Anthropophobia. Avoids human society. Doesn't recognize his relatives. Senseless staring at an object. Feeling as if losing their reason. ***Talks to himself***.

Abdomen - Stitches in region of liver and spleen, through to spine. Feeling of constriction from liver to shoulder (right). Cutting pain in abdomen, soon after eating. ***Cutting pains to loins***, cannot walk, extends to groins. Chronic intestinal ulceration with vomiting and emaciation. Painful retraction, soreness and burning. As if something eating in bowels.

Back - Violent aching. Stiffness of neck worse bending head forward. Stabbing pain from third cervical to fifth dorsal vertebra. Stitches at lower angle of left scapula. Aching in back and down left side into hip. As if something cracked across sacrum, worse stooping. Pain in coccyx and sacrum extending up and down, worse walking, sitting and touching it. Coccyx pains before urination, better after. Cutting through loins, cannot walk.

Bladder - Continuous desire to urinate during day. Frequent discharge of watery urine, of strong smell, awaking him at night. Burning in urethra. Stitches in urethra after urinating. ***After urinating a drop seems to remain which cannot be expelled***. Urethra becomes clogged up. Suppression of urine following cholera.

Breasts - Milk is stringy, watery.

Causations - Ill effects from indulgence in beer and malt liquor.

Chest - Pressure and heaviness on chest, as from a weight. Stitches in sides of chest. Pain at trachea bifurcation, on coughing from mid-sternum to back. Burning, pain at sternum. Rawness under sternum. Itching behind sternum, causes violent, racking, paroxysmal cough.

Constitutions - Adapted to fat, fair, fleshy, light complexioned persons, subject to catarrhs or with syphilitic or scrofulous history. Suited to sluggish people and fair-haired, fat persons, especially fat, chubby children.

Ears - Redness. Eruption covering both ears. Violent tickling in ears. Sharp stitches in ears. Swollen ear with tearing pains. Pulsating in ears at night, external meatus swollen and inflamed. Stinging from external meatus into internal ear. Lancinating pain, chronic suppuration. Thick, yellow, stringy, fetid discharge. Tympanum perforated. Ulcers upon tympanum. Stitches in left ear and left parotid gland, during headache.

Eyes - ***Descemetitis*** with only moderate irritation of eye. Dense opacities of cornea. Ulcers on cornea, no pain or photophobia. Conjunctiva, yellow, puffy, covered with yellow-brown spots. Conjunctivitis, granular lids with pannus. Iritis with punctate deposits on inner surface of cornea. Slight pain with severe ulceration or inflammation (Con. opposite.). Ropy and yellow discharge. Eyelids, swollen, winking during convulsions, itching, granular. Eyelids twitch on opening. Supra-orbital neuralgia, right side. Photophobia only by daylight.

Face - Pale, yellowish, blotchy, red, florid. Acne (Kali-br., Kali-ar.). Mumps on the right side. Sweat on upper lip. Bones sensitive, especially beneath orbits.

Female - Menses too early, with vertigo, nausea and headache. Menses with suppression of urine or red urine. Membranous dysmenorrhea. ***Yellow, green tenacious leucorrhea.*** Leucorrhea, acrid, yellow, ropy with pain across sacrum. Leucorrhea that can be drawn out in long strings. Subinvolution of uterus. Prolapsed uterus, worse hot weather.

Pruritus of vulva, with great burning and excitement. Itching, burning of vulva with sexual excitement. Soreness and rawness in vagina. Swelling of genitals. Vomiting during pregnancy.

Food - Desire for acid foods and drinks. ***Desires beer*** and malt liquors, but they aggravate. Dislikes water. Cannot digest meat. Overeats.

Head - Periodical headaches with vertigo and nausea. ***Headaches, over eyebrows***, preceded by blurred vision. Headache with persistent retching and vomiting of food, bile. ***Migraines in small spots and from suppressed catarrh.*** Violent headache from occiput to forehead if nasal discharge ceases. Blindness, followed by violent headache, over eyebrows or outward along the brows. Headache, worse from cold, sinus congestion. Headache better pressing at the root of the nose, better from warm soup. Sensation as if a solid block in forehead. ***Sinus headache with stopped-up sensation in nose.*** Violent shooting pains from root of nose. ***Aching and fullness in glabella***. Sharp pains in bones. ***Bones of head feel sore.*** Frontal pain, usually over one eye. Dull, heavy throbbing above eyes, as if head would burst. Supraorbital neuralgia, right side. Eczema of scalp, raw and oozing a thin moisture which dries into yellow scabs. Eruption of painful small boils on back of head.

Heart - Weak heart. Dilated with kidney lesions, insufficiency of aortic valves. Pricking in region of heart. Cold feeling around heart (Kali-n.). Pressure on heart after eating. Pulsation felt in all the arteries. Palpitations with rattling in throat, during cough. Pulse irregular, small, contracted, with nosebleed.

Kidneys - Heaviness sensation in kidneys. Constant aching. Shooting in kidney region with suppressed urine and prostration. Sharp shooting, first in left then right kidney. Congestion of kidneys. Nephritis with scanty, albuminous urine and casts. Pyelitis, urine with epithelial cells, mucus, pus or blood.

Limbs - Pain, swelling, stiffness and crackling of all joints. Pains fly rapidly from one place to another (Kali-s., Puls.). ***Pains in small spots*** (Ox-ac.). Wandering pains along the bones, worse cold. Bones feels sore and bruised. Tearing pains in tibia. Shin bones, painful, periostitis from blow. ***Very weak limbs.*** Paralytic weakness of hands. Syphilitic rheumatism (Mez.). Rheumatic pains worse eating. Rheumatic pain in hip joints and knees. Heaviness of legs. Left-sided sciatica, better motion and flexing the leg, worse standing, sitting or lying in bed. Pain in tendons of muscles of calf, as if stretched, causes lameness. Achilles tendon swollen and tender. Left ankle as if dislocated. Pain along border of the foot. Soreness of heels when walking.

Liver - Soreness in right hypochondrium, fatty infiltration of liver and increase in soft fibrous tissue.

Lungs - Acute capillary bronchitis. Chronic bronchitis. Bronchial dilatation with fetid breath and expectoration. Dry, metallic, hacking cough. Cough with pain in sternum, extending to shoulders, worse when undressing. ***Profuse, yellow expectoration, very glutinous and sticky***, coming out in a long, stringy and very tenacious mass. Cough better expectoration. Membranous croup, extending to larynx and sinuses. Asthma worse from sex. Wheezing, panting on awaking, then cough which forces him to sit up, bent forward. Wheezing at night after whooping cough. Wheezing with retching and expectoration of tough mucus, which can be drawn in strings to the feet.

Male - Pricking and itching at glans penis. Itching and pain of penis with pustules. Ulcers with paroxysmal stitches, aggravated at night. Syphilitic ulcers with cheesy, tenacious exudation. Chancres ulcerating deeply. Constriction at root of penis, at night, on waking. Gleet with stringy or jelly-like profuse discharge, clogging the urethra. Prostatic fluid escapes during stool. Stitches in prostate when walking, must stand still. Erections (Pic-ac.). Sexual desire absent in fleshy persons.

Mouth - Dry mouth, better by drinking cold water. Sticky mouth. Dry, viscid saliva. Sweet, metallic, taste. Tongue glistens, cracked, ***red, dry, shining,*** smooth or heavy, lemon yellow, furred in dysentery. Tongue thickly coated, broad, flat, indented. Tongue pains at the root when protruded. As of a hair on back part of the tongue, not better by eating or drinking. Aphthous ulcers deeply corroding. Toothache, radiating with swelling of the glands.

Modalities - Better from heat, wrapping up, pressure, motion, short sleep. Skin symptoms better cold weather. Open air ameliorates, especially vertigo, but aggravates the gastric complaints and chilliness. Worse from cold, damp, open air, spring, hot weather. Worse from undressing, stooping, sitting, after sleep, morning, 2 a.m. to 3 a.m. ***Worse from suppressed catarrh,*** protruding tongue, ***alcohol, beer.*** Worse by eating, causes cough, weight in stomach.

Nose - ***Pressure and pain at root or bridge of nose.*** Nose feels heavy, dry. ***Sinusitis*** with distress and fullness at root of nose. Chronic rhinitis. Profuse, watery nasal discharge. ***Nasal discharges, thick, stringy, ropy, lumpy, sticky, greenish, yellow,*** acrid. ***Post-nasal drip of thick mucus*** (Hydr.). Much hawking of thick mucus. ***Coryza with obstruction of nose.*** Ozaena. ***Suppressed catarrh.*** Fetid smell from retention of discharge in nose. ***Loss of smell.*** Violent sneezing, worse in the morning. Tickling as from a hair in left nostril. Inability to breathe through nose. ***Large mucus plugs.*** Tough, elastic plugs, leave a raw surface. Clinkers in nose. Snuffles, especially in overweight children. ***Nasal septum ulcerates***, round ulcer. Abscess. Thick, dark red blood from nose. Nasal polyps. Sensation as if two loose bones were rubbing together on blowing the nose. Nasal diphtheria. Expired air feels hot.

Perspiration - Cold sweat on forehead, hands, feet and thighs. Perspiration on back during effort at stool. Profuse sweats while sitting quietly.

Rectum - Sensation of a plug in anus. Periodic constipation with pain across the loins and brown urine. Dysentery, tenesmus, stools are brown, frothy. Stools, jelly-like, gelatinous, ***worse mornings***.

Skin - Skin is hot, dry and red, better cool air. Brown spots. Acne. Lupus with burning. Burning, tingling in skin. Herpes zoster. Blisters on soles. Skin eruptions, worse summer. Dryness of skin, with itching of whole body. Itching with vesicular eruption. Papular eruptions. Pustular eruption, resembling smallpox with burning pains. Pustules with black tops. ***Ulcers with punched-out edges.*** Ulcers with tendency to penetrate and tenacious exudation. Ulcers painful in cold weather. Depressed, round scars after healing of eruptions or ulcers.

Sleep - Drowsiness in open air. Great inclination to stretch and yawn. During sleep frequent starts, incoherent talk, tossing of arms. Unrefreshing, feels debilitated in limbs. Wakened by dyspnea, palpitation. Wakened with desire to urinate. Worse on waking.

Stomach - Dilatation of stomach. Gastritis. Sore spot in stomach or food lies like a load. Feels as if digestion had stopped. ***Round ulcer of stomach***. Nausea with heat in the body, better eating and open air. Nausea with burning in anus and erections. Nausea and vomiting after beer. Regurgitates liquids. Vomiting more than he drinks of bright, yellow water. Gastric symptoms are relieved after eating, and the rheumatic symptoms reappear.

Temperature - Hot flushes, followed by sticky sweat, then chill. Burning of upper part of body and face with internal chilliness and violent thirst. Chilliness alternating with flushes of heat. Chill with sweat. Cold sweat on hands and feet. Attacks of chilliness from feet upwards, and sensation as if skull on vertex became contracted, in frequently returning paroxysms. Chilliness in back, with sleepiness. Chills with giddiness and nausea, followed by heat. Sensation of coldness and trembling.

Throat - Dry, burning and rough. Burning, extending to the stomach. Fauces red and inflamed. Tickling in larynx with cough and belchings, then vertigo, worse eating, better heat. Fissured pharynx. Aphthae. Something sticks in with pain into neck and shoulders. Throat pains when putting the tongue out. Voice is hoarse, worse evening. Catarrhal laryngitis, cough has a brassy sound. Hawks up thick mucus, must wipe it away. Diphtheria with profound prostration and soft pulse. ***Tough and stringy discharge from mouth and throat.*** Sensation of choking on lying down. ***Uvula relaxed, edematous,*** bladder-like. Pseudo membranous deposit on tonsils and soft palate. Parotid glands swollen. Tonsils swollen with deafness in children.

Urine - Scanty, high-colored urine, with a white film and copious whitish sediment and pain in back. Urine alkaline and ropy. Ropy mucus in urine. ***Hematochyluria***. Bloody urine and pain in back.

Vertigo - Vertigo in many complaints, on stooping or when rising from a seat. Vertigo with nausea and inclination to vomit. Vertigo followed by vomiting of acid, white mucus fluid. Vertigo better from walking in open air.

Vision - Dim vision, confused, during vertigo. ***Blindness before headache***, sight returns with the increasing headache. Vision seems crossed, better looking with one eye. Sees double. Figures vanish on looking at them. All objects seem to be enveloped in a yellow mist. Yellow sight. Sees various colors and bright sparks.

COMMENTS - Characteristic formation of large mucus plugs or clinkers on membranes, especially in the nose. This may be regarded as an advanced stage of the stringy mucus secretions. Formation of false membranes in croup and diphtheria with hoarse, metallic cough. Formation of casts of the bronchial tubes in fibrinous bronchitis.

Sinus infections, sinusitis, nasal discharges. Sinusitis after a cold, particularly if a history. Keynote of thick yellow-green mucus that can be so thick that they may not be able to blow it out. Viscous, sticky, lumpy, stringy mucus (Hydr., Puls., Merc.). Mucus in lumps, can have blood. Jelly-like mucus. Loss of smell.

Severe pain at the root of the nose when the discharge stops. Sinusitis with bone pains in the face. Very severe sinus headaches. Headaches over the eye or at the root of the nose. Severe headaches with suppressed discharge. Blinding migraine headaches, severe pain (Iris, Nat-m.). Pains over either eye, often followed by sinus congestion.

Mucus in the chest, difficult to expectorate (Caust., Ant-t.). Copious mucus in the lungs, especially in the bronchioles. Gelatinous mucus in the elderly, coughed up in the morning, dark green, jelly mucus.

Cough with stringy, difficult expectoration, worse early morning. A pain from mid sternum through to back. Brassy cough. Coughs up sticky mucus. Cough caused by eating. Sensation as if a hair on the back part of the tongue or in the left nostril.

Wet asthma (Kali-c., Puls., Ant-t.). Asthma in children, stringy mucus that relieves. Otitis media with a discharge (Merc.). Stringy vomit. Vaginitis with stringy discharge. Stringy breast milk.

Circular ulcers, as if someone punched them out of the skin. Ulcers from burns. Sores and ulcers that don't heal with ropy mucus. Internal and external ulceration.

Shifting pains and sudden pains (Lac-c.). Pains appear and disappear suddenly. Diagonal pains. Localized pain. Stinging pains all over. Pains in short jerks as if a nerve were suddenly pulled. Cramps in various parts. Twitches in hands and feet.

Arthritis with wandering pains or pains in small spots. Joints crack with arthritis. Rheumatic-like or shooting and pricking pains. Rheumatic pains were worse and the gastric pains better after eating.

Great prostration, discomfort, debility and desire to lie down. Neuralgic attacks, recurring every day, at the same hour. Epilepsy with a flow of tough, stringy fluid from the mouth during the attacks. Vertigo with many complaints, on stooping or rising from a seat.

Mentally ill-humored and low in spirit. Listless, aversion to mental and physical exertion. Weak memory, vanishing of thoughts. Anxiety arising from chest.

Swollen abdomen immediately after a full meal. Food lies like a load, as if digestion were suspended. Weight in pit of stomach immediately after eating, flatulence. Severe diarrhea, stools are lumpy, mucus and jelly-like substances. Odorless stools.

Painful vomiting, sour, mixed with clear mucus, may be bitter from the presence of bile. Vomiting from attempt to eat or drink, with distress and burning rawness about the stomach. Vomiting in alcoholics, especially beer-drinkers. Gastric ulcers.

Aversion to meat, desires for beer, acid drinks. Beer and malt liquors aggravate, more pronounced in hot weather, autumn, and spring. Chronic effects of drinking too much malt liquor, especially lager beer.

Some of the workmen found they could not drink coffee as it made them worse and they were obliged to take to tea instead. This bears out Hering's dictum that "wine-drinkers should take coffee and beer drinkers should take tea." Coffee antidotes wine and tea antidotes beer.

W. J. Pierce recorded the case of James S., 40. For four months past, as soon as he swallowed food (not liquids), a tickling in the throat excited a severe cough, which stopped only on vomiting and was followed by a watery coryza. This was so distressing that for two months he had eaten only two meals a day.

There was pharyngeal catarrh with stringy mucus hanging from naso-pharynx. Kali-bi. 1c, a tablet every two hours, was given. He had no more vomiting and only coughed twice in the next five days and was soon quite cured.

J. B. Garrison recorded the rapid action of Kali-bi. in two cases of intermittent fever on an indication given to him by Martin Dischere. Dischere once mistakenly took an overdose of Kali-bi., which was followed by vomiting of a large quantity of bright yellow water, tasting very bitter.

Garrison's first case was that of a laborer, ill a month with fever, pains and paroxysm at 1 p.m. Just before Garrison saw him he had vomited "a large quantity of bright yellow water." Kali-bi. 1x, one grain dissolved in a tumbler of water, a teaspoonful every two hours, cured at once.

The second case was that of a woman who had been nine months under allopathic treatment. She had not been out of the house for two months and had been told she could not recover. Among other symptoms, she vomited much more than she drank. In the morning, she vomited a large bowlful of bright yellow fluid.

Goullon gave the case of an enormously fat man of "formless colossal body" who complained of chronic accumulation of phlegm. He seemed fairly filled up with it, especially in the morning, for which all domestic remedies and mineral waters had been given in vain.

Kali-bi. 2x was ordered, a few grains in hot water every evening. In two weeks, the patient could resume his walks. He felt easy on his chest, the accumulation of phlegm disappeared, his bowels became regular instead of constipated. Kali-bi. is particularly suited to fat people.

Storer cured with Kali-bi. a case of asthma in a man who noticed that the attacks were caused by and always followed sex. Kali-bi. was prescribed on other indications, but this symptom must be noted. Marked worse from sex and from emissions.

Nash related a cure with Kali-bi. 30c, in which a women had deep, punched-out ulcers with regular edges. One of them had perforated the soft palate and threatened the whole palate. It had a syphilitic appearance and also a stringy discharge, but not to a great amount. In three weeks, the local condition entirely healed and the patient's general state improved correspondingly.

H. W. Champlin cited a case of chronic rheumatism in a woman over 70. She was restless and sleepless at night and Rhus-t. relieved this somewhat. Closer investigation brought out that the pains changed rapidly from one place to another and that they occupied small spots that could be covered with the point of a finger. Kali-bi. cured rapidly.

Grimmer noted that the anemia and cachexia in its pathogenesis, together with the fact that it has cured lupus, puts this remedy in the anticancer group. It affects the skin and mucus membranes (the internal skin) markedly. Catarrhal and rheumatic states are prominent features calling for its use.

RELATIONS - ***Antidotes:*** Ars., Lach. ***Compare:*** (1) Ant-t., Brom., Hep., Ind., Calc., Ant-c. (2) In the production of false membranes: Brom., Caust., Sul-ac., Ip. (3) Oxyg., Caust., Kali-c. - fat subjects. (4) Kali-i., Nit-ac. - syphilis. (5) Bor. - croup, fair subjects. (6) Mez., Sil., Phyt. - bone diseases. (7) Hydr. and Iris. - viscous, tough secretions. (8) Sep. and Teucr. "clinkers." (9) Puls. - wandering rheumatism, gonorrheal rheumatism, pains worse in warm room, measles, catarrhal deafness, swelling of salivary glands. (10) Coc-c., whooping cough, mucus, clear stringy, Kali-bi. yellow stringy. Rhus-t. - better of pain on moving affected part, Rhus-t. has better by warmth, eruptions of Kali-bi. begin in hot weather, those of Rhus-t. in cold. (11) Sulph. - sensation of hair in throat.

REFERENCES - Boericke. Clarke. Grimmer. Murphy. Phatak.

KALI BROMATUM

(Potassium Bromide)

PHARMACY - kali-br. Kali bromatum. Potassium bromide. Solution. Trituration. ***Historical dose:*** Trituration and all potencies.

CLINICAL - ***Acne.*** Albuminuria. Alcoholism. ***Amnesia. Aphasia.*** Asthma. Backache. ***Cholera, infantum.*** Chorea. Chordee. Colic. ***Convulsions.*** Delirium. ***Delusions. Depression.*** Diabetes mellitus. ***Epilepsy.*** Erythema nodosum. Headaches. Hemorrhoids. Imbecility. Impotency. Insanity. ***Insomnia.*** Laryngeal, spasms. Laryngismus. Locomotor, ataxia. Mania. Manic depression. Melancholy. Memory, weakness. Menorrhagia. Metrorrhagia. ***Nightmares. Night-terrors.*** Nose, eruption. Numbness. Nymphomania. Ovaries, disorders. Paralysis. Parkinson's disease. Pityriasis. Polyps, rectal. Prostration. ***Psoriasis. Schizophrenia.*** Screaming. Sebaceous, cysts. Seborrhea. Self-abuse. ***Senility.*** Sensibility, loss. ***Sleeplessness.*** Sleepwalking. Speech, disorders. Sterility. ***Strokes.*** Syphilis. Tabes dorsalis. Tetanus. Uremia. Urine, incontinence. Uterine, fibroids. Vaginismus. Vertigo.

HOMEOPATHIC - Like all potash salts, this weakens the heart and lowers temperature. Causes brominism. Symptoms of allopathic overdoses are added to the proving symptoms and the clinical experience of homeopaths.

Alberton noted that Kali-br. has been given allopathically in epileptic and other convulsive disorders with the idea of overwhelming the disease rather than of curing it. The effect has been to reduce or prevent the recurrence of epileptic attacks at the expense of keeping the patient constantly under the influence of the drug and producing a state of mental imbecility, ***"decreasing the excitability and power of the motor cells of the brain."***

Hare noted that the keynotes for the bromides include general weakness and feebleness of the nervous system, post-typhoid and post-puerperal insanity, senile softening of the brain and irritation of the gastro-intestinal mucus membrane.

Kali-br. affects the mind and nerves, producing ***failure of mental power, loss of memory***. Melancholy. General numbness and anesthesia of mucus membranes especially of eyes, throat and skin.

Skin eruptions, psoriasis. ***Acne***, especially at puberty and at the menstrual period. Clarke knew of no remedy of such universal usefulness in cases of simple acne as in Kali-br. 30c. Moist eruptions and pityriasis of the scalp. Seborrhea. Erythema nodosum.

Epilepsy, associated with sexual excess or abuse in men and with menses in women. Attacks during the new moon, followed by headaches. Onset of diseased condition is slow without any pain. Convulsions. Parkinson's disease. Numbness of whole body. ***Symptoms of strokes***. Paralysis. Aphasia, somnolence and stertor. Loss of sexual desire. Sexual fantasies, satyriasis and nymphomania. Uremia. Albuminuria. Nodular form of chronic gout.

MIND - Brain fag from grief and anxiety. Failing brain-power (Anac., Bar-c., Phos.). ***Loss of memory.*** Forgetful on waking in morning. Senile softening of the brain. Weak memory, confused thoughts. Perception slow, answers slowly.

Mistakes in speaking or writing. Confusion as to his identity, over daily affairs. ***Amnesic aphasia.*** Aphasia, from embolism of middle cerebral artery. Forgets how to talk, has to be told the word before he can speak it.

Ailments after emotional excitement. Nervous irritability from severe illness or death of a friend, loss of property or reputation. ***Wrings hands, hands and fingers in constant motion.*** Feeling of helplessness, in afternoon. Fits of uncontrollable weeping.

Extremely sensitive to pain. Fidgety, busy hands, fumbles in his pockets. Hurried when eating. Moves arms about wildly. Headstrong and haughty when sick. Domineering. Loss of self-confidence.

Constant fear of breaking down under stress. Constant worry, fears to see people or to be spoken to. Fear of being alone, of his own shadow, to walk past certain corners, of a ringing doorbell. Fear of new people. Fear of insanity. Fear of being poisoned (Hyos.).

Sadness in morning on waking. Melancholy, much concerned about health, complains without cause. ***Deep depression with painful delusions and persistent insomnia.*** Profound indifference and disgust for life. Suicidal depression, mania with trembling. Manic depression. ***Schizophrenia.***

Religious depression. Feeling of moral deficiency; want of moral feeling. Imagines he is singled out as an object of divine wrath. Dread of impending destruction of all near to her. Remorse, wrings hands, bursts into tears.

Active delirium. Delirium with delusions. ***Paranoid delusions, thinks he is pursued***. Suspicious, delusions of conspiracies, that his life is threatened. Delusion he will commit some great crime, that she will murder her children or husband, that her child is dead. Delusion that he is a devil.

Hallucinations of sight and sound, with or without mania, precede brain and paralytic symptoms. Horrible visions, can't be comforted by friends. Mental symptoms after a stroke. Chronic alcoholism.

Abdomen - Abdomen sunken, almost stuck to vertebral column. ***Retraction of abdomen*** with spasms. Prostration. Ascites of hepatic or splenic origin. Flatulent colic. Colic in young children. Cutting colic. ***Internal coldness*** of abdomen during painless diarrhea. Sensation as if bowels were falling out. Trembling sensation in bowels. Enlargement of liver and spleen. Small tumor in region of spleen.

Back - Backache, tired lameness of legs. Tabes dorsalis from sexual excesses.

Causations - Ill effects of worry, anger, fright, emotional disturbance. Chorea from fright. Loss of business, reputation and embarrassment. Illness or death of a near friend. Sexual excess, sexual abuse.

Chest - Burning in chest. Tightness of chest when breathing.

Constitutions - Nervous constitutions. Children who can swallow solids with ease from birth, yet choke when they try to drink.

Cough - Cough dry, hard and almost incessant. Dry, fatiguing, paroxysmal cough. Dry, spasmodic cough in weak, nervous children. Dry cough due to reflex action from stomach, intestines or uterus. Hacking cough at night. Whooping cough. Nervous cough during pregnancy.

Ears - Hardness of hearing. Ringing in ear. Sounds echo in ears, headache. Roaring synchronous with pulse, at night.

Eyes - Eyes sunken, lusterless, gaze fixed. Eyeballs move in every direction. Squinting after night terrors of children. Vision dim. Pupils dilated, with heavy lids and drowsiness. Vessels of fundus enlarged, conjunctiva congested.

Face - ***Acne in young people.*** Acne worse before menses. Pimples on face, cheeks and forehead. Bluish-red eruptions. ***Itching pimples, pustules leave scars.*** Complexion yellow, cachectic. Face flushed. Face pale, appeared as one drunk with hallucinations. Expression wearied, anxious, dull, stupefied, imbecile, expressionless. Papular rash.

Female - Menses scanty. Epileptic attacks at or near menstrual periods. Menorrhagia with strong sexual desire. Headache, insomnia, and heat in genitals after menses. Metrorrhagia. Flooding in young women with sexual desire. Sterility from excessive sexual indulgence. Sexual feeling lost. Aversion to sex (Sep.). Excessive sexual desire during menses. Nymphomania during puerperal state. Pruritus of external genitals. Voluptuous itching, tingling and irritation in external genitals. Ovarian neuralgia, with great nervous uneasiness from ungratified sexual desire. Cystic tumors of ovaries. Ovarian swelling, tenderness of left ovary. Uterine fibroids. Induration of uterus. Enlargement of uterus. Subinvolution. Vaginismus. Convulsions during labor. Painful heat flushings and congestion to head during menopause.

Food - Taste foul, salty, lost. Intense thirst with dry mouth. Dysphagia of liquids (Hyos.). Troublesome pressure at stomach after diner, lassitude. Anorexia.

Head - Heaviness of head, confusion, slow speech, staggers as if drunk. ***Numb feeling in head,*** worse occiput. Severe throbbing, aching, in occipital region. Headache from concussion of brain. Headache after epileptic attack. Migraine with flushed face, throbbing temples, injected conjunctiva, photophobia. ***Congestive headaches.*** Mercurial headache. Brain irritated. Anemia of brain from loss of fluids. ***Symptoms of apoplexy.*** Constrictive sensation in brain as if too tight. Drooping of head, cannot hold it erect. Incipient meningitis. Hydrocephalus. Scalp feels tight. Seborrhea. Pityriasis.

Heart - Weakens the heart and lowers temperature. Feeble heart with intermitting action. Action of heart slow and fluttering. Heart's beat weak, sounds distant and feeble. Pulse, accelerated, later becomes slower and small. Cardiac neuroses from spinal or uterine irritation.

Kidneys - Diabetes mellitus (Ph-ac.). Urethra numb, sensibility diminished. Incontinence of urine. Involuntary nocturnal emissions of urine. Neuralgia of neck of bladder. Urine profuse with thirst. Urine copious, pale, abundance of phosphates. Urine scanty, even suppressed in collapse. Urine dribbling a few drops at beginning of every stool.

Limbs - Jerking and twitching of muscles. ***Fidgety hands***, busy twitching of fingers. Hands and fingers in constant motion. Trembling of hands during voluntary motion. Unsteady gait. Cannot stand erect, legs weak.

Lungs - Asthma with dry cough, tosses arms about wildly. Asthma of nervous origin. Spasmodic asthma of children. Infantile capillary bronchitis with severe dyspnea. Pneumonia in alcoholics. Great dyspnea, breath hot, hurried. Spasmodic croup. Cough dry, fatiguing, hacking cough at night. Copious, whitish expectoration in torpid cases of bronchitis. Reflex cough during pregnancy.

Male - Spermatorrhea. Chordee during gonorrhea. ***Effects of sexual excesses***, especially loss of memory, impaired co-ordination, numbness and tingling in limbs. Lessened desire, debility and impotence, with melancholy, epilepsy, nervous prostration. Lascivious fancies and dreams. Erections at night, with backache, uncontrollable fidgetiness. Impotence with melancholy, loss of memory, nervous prostration, epilepsy. Excessive sexual desire with constant erections at night. Satyriasis. Sexual excitement during partial slumber.

Modalities - Better when busy mentally and physically. Skin better in cold weather. Worse from mental exertion. Worse from emotions, anger, fright, worry, grief. Worse at night. Worse at 2 a.m. Worse periodically, new moon. Worse at summer, hot weather. Worse from puberty. Worse before, during and after menses. Worse unsatisfied sexual desire. Worse sexual excess. Cough worse lying down.

Mouth - Fetid breath, a peculiar sickening odor, profuse saliva. Suppressed salivation in teething children. Foul, salty taste. Loss of taste. Numbness. Difficult speech, stammering.

Nose - Smell impaired. Erythematous swelling of nose. Coryza with tendency to extension into throat. Thick mucus and yellow scabs in nostrils.

Perspiration - Sweat abundant, viscid, all over, long lasting and exhausting (ague).

Rectum - Asiatic cholera, first stage, vomiting, cramps, rice-water discharges. ***Cholera infantum*** with reflex cerebral irritation, jerking and twitching of muscles. Persistent diarrhea, much blood expelled. Painless diarrhea, with great chilliness, even in a hot room. Constipation, stools very dry, hard and infrequent. Painful hemorrhoids. Blind hemorrhoids, intensely painful varices with black stools. Fissure of rectum and painful growths. Spasmodic stricture of sphincter ani. Rectal polyps.

Sensations - Parts feel as if growing large. Paroxysms of numbness, feels as if needles were pricking him. Trembling sensation.

Skin - Anesthesia of skin. Skin cold, clammy. ***Acne simplex*** and indurate, bluish red, pustular, worse on face and chest. Acne of face, cheeks and forehead. Pimples leave scars. Itching, worse on chest, shoulders and face. ***Psoriasis***, syphilitic psoriasis. Moist eczema of legs. Moist eruptions, scars remaining after eruptions. Eruption of small boils in successive crops with troublesome itching. Large indolent, painful pustules, boils. Seborrhea. Pityriasis. Rose-colored eruption on lower limbs. Long lasting scrofulous ulcerations. Sebaceous cysts. Scars remaining after eruptions.

Sleep - Extreme drowsiness. ***Insomnia.*** Sleeplessness due to worry, grief and sexual excess. Sleeplessness in anemic patients or nervous persons. Sleepless, restless can only calm herself by incessant occupation. Sleeplessness during convalescence from acute diseases. Restless sleep. Deep, profound sleep. Grinding teeth in sleep. ***Night terrors in children, awake screaming, unconscious, recognizes no one,*** followed by squinting. Sleepwalking in children. Waking with severe headache in a child. Horrible dreams.

Stomach - Dyspepsia. Weakness of stomach. ***Persistent hiccough*** (Sul-ac.). Vomiting of all drinks and intense thirst, with cholera infantum. Vomiting with intense thirst after each meal. Vomiting of mucus. Hysterical vomiting after exciting emotions. Vomiting of alcoholics after a debauch. Morning sickness.

Stool - Green, watery, rice-water stools with rapid collapse, painless. Frequent, green, water stools, with violent abdominal spasms. Bloody mucopurulent diarrhea. Stools painless.

Teeth - Odontitis of children. Difficult dentition in children, with vomiting and diarrhea. Gums as if numb. Grinding teeth in sleep with moans and cries.

Temperature - Body cold, skin corrugated and mottled. Cold limbs. Shivering with cold and cold skin. Heat like cold stage, not very strongly marked. Head hot, feels as if in a furnace with coldness and chills. Chilliness in a hot room and itching during high fever. Painful hot flushing of the face during menopause.

Throat - Congestion of uvula and fauces, then edematous. ***Anesthesia*** of fauces, pharynx and larynx. Hoarseness, extremely painful and disagreeable. Dryness of throat. Dysphagia of liquids, can swallow only solids, especially in children (Hyos.). Laryngismus stridulus, uncomplicated, from neurosis or reflex irritation. Spasmodic croup. Chronic catarrh. Diphtheria with quick pulse, fever, dry tongue, and offensive breath.

Tongue - Tongue protrudes with a jerk, chorea. Tongue is red, brown, dry, enlarged, tender. White tongue.

Vertigo - Vertigo, as if ground gave way, worse stooping. Vertigo with palpitations, nausea and even unconsciousness. Dizziness, noises in ear, nervous excitement, sleepless. Staggering gait.

COMMENTS - Kali-br. has a very profound action on the generative organs and the mental side of the generative sphere causing sensual, lascivious fancies, satyriasis and nymphomania, and finally impotence and wasting of the sexual organs.

Epilepsy, particularly cases associated with sexual excess or abuse in men and those in which the fits occur during or near the menstrual period in women. Epilepsy after fright, anger, or childbirth. Can be affected by phases of the moon. Headache after the attack.

Spasms from fright, anger or emotions. Spasms in nervous, plethoric persons during childbirth. Staggering gait, ataxia, numbness and tingling in legs and spine with increase in sexual appetite.

Paralysis with twitchings of the limbs. Fidgeting of the hands and feet (Hyos.). Reflexes are diminished and there is loss of general sensibility and also of certain parts, particularly fauces, larynx and urethra. Benumbed sensation of the brain.

Schizophrenia, manic depression. Suicidal depression. Depressed, melancholic, uncontrollable weeping. Laughing and crying fits. Disordered faculties. Fear of going insane, fear of losing mental or emotional control. Memory loss, amnesia (Anac.). Aphasia.

Chronic insomnia, especially in the elderly (Calc., Ars.). Insomnia due to worry, mortification, grief, financial shock and loss (Aur.). Restlessness and sleeplessness from worry. Drowsiness.

Deep sleep may be broken by a start, though waking is very difficult. Confused dreams. Night terrors in children where they scream, without recollection of the terror (Tub., Calc.). Grind teeth and moan while sleeping. Sleepwalking.

Cholera infantum with hydrocephalic symptoms. Dentition. Whooping cough. Bright's disease. Acne, particularly relating to hormonal changes. Sebaceous cysts and wens. Growths.

Ovarian cysts, fibroids and fatty tumors. Uterine hemorrhage, with ovarian tumors. Metrorrhagia or menorrhagia, may arise from reflected irritation and may be accompanied with sexual excitement.

Hering noted that Kali-br. is useful for "flooding, especially in young women."

Amory Hare noted that pulmonary edema or suffocative bronchitis may develop in the lungs. The patient may become cachectic and the condition can resemble typhoid fever.

Wenzel Heyberger recorded a case of diabetes in a woman, 68, cured with Kali-br. The patient had been ill five months and was reduced to a skeleton. She first noticed a remarkably good appetite, but after meals had heartburn and belchings.

She had polyuria and frequent disturbances at night to pass water. Weak in the head, confused, memory impaired. Vision was almost gone. Rushing and roaring in ears. Tormenting thirst. Stools difficult and delayed. Powders medicated with Kali-br. 2c were given, one every six hours.

The first night the patient slept without disturbance and the quantity of urine and proportion of sugar diminished. After about six weeks, the improvement seemed to stop and Kali-br. was given in allopathic doses, but this aggravated the condition. Kali-br. 2c was resumed and the case went to a cure.

Hale cured with Kali-br. many cases of cholera infantum and one case of "violent periodic umbilical colic, leaving tenderness on pressure." The characteristic hour of recurrence was 5 p.m.

Buford used it extensively in such cases and in potencies approaching the crude form. Kali-br. is more particularly adapted to persons inclined to obesity, to children, and to nervous women. More symptoms have been noted on the right side than on the left.

RELATIONS - Kali-br. is ***Antidoted by:*** Vegetable acids, oils, Camp., Nux-v., Zinc. ***It antidotes:*** Lead poisoning. ***It follows well:*** Acon. and Spong. in croup, Eug. in acne. ***Compare:*** (1) Camph. Am-br., Aur. (2) Bor. - night-terrors. (3) Kali-c. - persons inclined to obesity. also Am-c., Calc., Graph. (4) Kali-i. - acne, syphilis, Kali-p. and Calc. - night terrors. (5) Hyos. - mania, excited sensorium without inflammation of brain, fears being poisoned, sees ghosts, sexual excitement. (6) Plat. - sees ghosts, demons. (7) Arg-n. - fearful apprehensive mood, imagines cannot pass a certain point. (8) Glon. - fears being poisoned, also Rhus-t. (9) Staph. - mental depression, weakness of legs from masturbation. (10) Gels. - incoordination of muscles. (11) Con. - nervous cough during pregnancy. (12) Bov., Stram. - slow, difficult speech, stammering. (13) Ip. - cholera infantum. (14) Zinc. - fidgety restlessness, Zinc. of feet, Kali-br. of hands. (15) Tarent. - reflex symptoms, any little irritation such as dentition or indigestion may causes convulsions. Fidgety hands.

REFERENCES - Boericke. Clarke. Murphy. Phatak.

KALI CARBONICUM

(Potassium Carbonate)

PHARMACY - kali-c. Kali carbonicum. Potassium carbonate. Potassic carbonate. Salt of Tartar. Solution. Trituration. ***Historical dose:*** Trituration and all potencies.

CLINICAL - Amenorrhea. Anemia. ***Asthma.*** Axilla, perspiration. ***Backaches.*** Biliousness. ***Bronchitis.*** Catarrh. Chilblains. ***Colds. Coughs.*** Debility. Dropsy. Dysmenorrhea. Dyspepsia. Ear, inflammation. Eyes, inflammation. Face, blotches. Fears. Freckles. Hair, disorders. Headaches. Heart, disorders. Hemorrhage. Hemorrhoids. Hip joint disease. Hydrothorax. Hysteria. Kidneys, disorders. Larynx, catarrh. Leucorrhea. Liver, disorders. ***Lumbago.*** Lungs, disorders. Menopause, disorders. Menorrhagia. Metrorrhagia. ***Pleurisy.*** Pleurodynia. ***Pneumonia.*** Pregnancy, disorders. Premenstrual, syndrome. Sciatica. Sleeplessness. Spinal, irritation. Stomach, disorders. Stomach, pain. Throat, sore. Toothaches. Tuberculosis. Typhoid. Urination, frequent. Urticaria. Uterus, cancer. Wens. Whooping cough.

HOMEOPATHIC - Kali-c. is potassium carbonate, sometimes called "vegetable alkali," and existing in all plants. It was originally obtained from the ashes left after burning wood and vegetable structures, although it is not limited to vegetable structures.

Kali-c. is typical of the Kali group of remedies. The potassium salts have an affinity for solid tissues and blood corpuscles. The fibrous tissues and ligaments of the joints, uterus and back are particularly affected. Tissues are often relaxed, joints give way, the back feels as if broken, the patient feels compelled to lie down or lean on something.

Goullon specifically mentioned Kali-c. usefulness in chronic laryngeal catarrh and knee conditions. Useful for conditions of the uterus, heart, lungs, pleura, bronchi and larynx.

Keynote sweat, backache and weakness. Weakness of the muscles, heart, the back, limbs, weakness of intellect. Useful for patients with vague symptoms, or for those who withhold their symptoms. Soft pulse, coldness. General depression. Soporific.

Sharp stitching, cutting pains. Jerking, stabbing or catching pains, better by motion, worse during rest and lying on affected side. Stinging pains from within out, in muscles and internal parts. Throbbing pains, numbness or coldness of single parts, abdomen, fingers. Pain in small spot, on left side, on uncovered parts. Parts lain on are painful or go to sleep.

Twitching of the muscles, rigidity and atony of the muscles. Convulsions, seems to pass off with belchings. Tendency to start with a loud cry, when touched, even lightly, especially in the soles, which leads a thrill throughout the whole body. ***Giving-out*** sensation.

Tendency to dropsy. Bag-like swellings over the eyes, between the eyebrows and the upper lids. For fleshy, elderly people with dropsical and paretic tendencies. Fatty degeneration. Hypothyroidism.

Tuberculosis. Tubercular diathesis. Old gouty cases, advanced Bright's. Discharges are profuse and acrid. Sudden unconsciousness. Closing of ulcers or fistulous openings, catching cold and over strain. Disposition to phlebitis.

Goullon noted the importance of this polycrest in female complaints. It is similar to Sep., although it differs in having pains and trouble before protracted and frequent menses. Menopausal flushings, associated with disturbance of the heart, violent palpitations. Miscarriage, and the consequent debilitated states. Useful after labor.

Sensitive to every atmospheric change and ***intolerance of cold weather***. Early morning aggravation. Generally worse 2 a.m. to 4 a.m.

MIND - ***Obstinate and dogmatic.*** Narrow-minded, rigid, strong imprinted beliefs. Deep desire for routine, propriety. Impractical, stoic. Refusal to admit to sickness. May mislead others by acting healthier than they are.

Antagonism with herself. Quarrels with family. Peevish and irritable, after sex. Impetuous. ***Desire for company, yet treats them outrageously*** and worse from consolation.

Alternating mood, at one time good and quiet, at another excited and angry at trifles. Frequently hopeful, frequently despondent. Indifference with bodily exhaustion. Sadness in open air. Great depression. Want of self-confidence.

Mental dullness. Weakness of memory for expressing oneself. Impaired intellect. Absentminded, forgetful. At a loss to know how to say what she wishes. Sudden attack of unconsciousness. Sensation as if bed were sinking. Desire to be carried.

Full of fear and imaginations. Frightened from touch. ***Fear of death when alone.*** Imagines himself sick. Fears of the future, of the unknown, of ghosts. Fear of losing control. Kleptomania.

Anxiety, in stomach. Anxious about his own diseased condition. Anxiety from flatulence when lying on right side. Anxiety, excitement when hungry. Nervous excitability, hysteria, sudden shrieking.

Hypersensitive to pain, noise touch. Easily startled, starts when touched especially on feet, on dropping to sleep. ***Starting from noise.*** Never quiet or contented. Admonitions causes weeping. Weeping when telling of her sickness. Weeping with headache.

Abdomen - Yellow, scaly spots on abdomen. ***Distension and coldness of abdomen.*** Hard, tympanitic and cold. ***Abdomen feels as if it would burst.*** Hard distension of abdomen with painfulness of umbilical region. Throbbing at navel. Much flatulence. Incarceration of flatus with colic. Pain from left side through abdomen, must turn on right side before he can rise. Cutting pain as if intestines were torn. Feeling as if a cold fluid passed through intestines during menses. Sensation of a lump rising from the abdomen, to throat and on coughing. Swelling of inguinal glands.

Back - Backache as if broken. ***Severe backache before and during menses, during pregnancy, labor or after a miscarriage.*** Stiffness and paralytic feeling in back. Backache with weak feeling, must lie down. Backache, must rise in order to turn over in bed. ***Lumbago*** with sudden sharp pains extending up and down, back and down the thighs. ***Lower back feels weak***. Burning in spine (Gua.). Spine painful while eating. Pulsations in back. Gnawing pain in coccyx. Pain in buttocks and thighs and hip joint. Sharp pain in region of kidneys and right scapula. Tearing pain in lumbar region, impeding respiration. Swelling of cervical glands.

Breasts - Fine stitches in breasts. ***Swollen, sensitive and painful breasts***, before menses.

Causations - Ill effects of suppressions of eruptions in childhood. Never well since pneumonia, catching cold, overstrain.

Chest - Angina pectoris. ***Stabbing, stitching pains.*** Cutting pain in chest, worse lying on right side. Sore pain in chest. ***Coldness of chest.*** Lungs seem to stick to the ribs. ***Whole chest very sensitive during coughing.*** Weakness of chest from rapid walking, also tightness and oppression. Dull, painful stitches in chest. Pressure in the chest. Small pimples on chest and back. Painful swelling of axillary glands. Sweat in axilla. Hydrothorax. Pleurisy.

Constitutions - Suited to dark haired, aged persons of lax tissue, inclined to be fat. To diseases after childbirth or after loss of fluids. Suited for those who are thin blooded, cold, sensitive to atmospheric changes to every draft of air, always shivering with dropsical and paralytic tendency. Tubercular diathesis.

Coughs - ***Dry, hard, suffocative, choking cough about 3 a.m. with sharp pains***. Tormenting cough, wakens from sleep. Cough with acute pain in chest. Cough with relaxed uvula. Incessant, hard retching or choking, futile cough, then vomiting. Spasmodic cough with gagging or vomiting of ingesta and sour phlegm. Cough after measles, worse eating or drinking.

Ears - Stitches in ears from within outwards. Itching in ears. Purulent discharge from ears. Discharge of yellow liquid cerumen. Right ear is hot, left is pale and cold. Itching, cracking, ringing and roaring. Noises in ear with headache. Noise is disagreeable. Intolerance of human voice.

Eyes - Asthenopia. Sharp pains in eyes. Pressure in and above eyes. Eyes as if pressed inward, while reading. Soreness of external canthus, with burning pain. Small round ulcers on cornea. Painful sensation of light penetrating the brain on shutting the eyes. Deep pain in eyes, with lachrymation and photophobia. Lachrymation when yawning. Lids stick together in morning. ***Swelling of eyelids.*** Enormous bag-like swelling under and over eyes. Swelling of glabella between brows. Cold eyelids.

Face - Haggard, exhausted look. Bloated in morning. Pale, sickly, sallow with sunken eyes. Freckles. Light brown spots, old warts, papulous eruptions. Pimples on face and eyebrows, with redness and swelling. Inflammation and swelling of parotids. Swelling of lower jaw and submaxillary glands. Tearing stitches in cheek. Cramps in jaws. Drawing pain in face. One cheek hot, the other cold. Scurf on upper lip. Lips peel, chapped.

Female - Amenorrhea with backache. Difficult first menses. Menses, delayed in young girls with chest symptoms and ascites. Suppressed menses with anasarca or ascites. Itching of vulva before menses. ***Premenstrual syndrome, swollen breasts, water retention.*** Menses irritating, pungent odor. Violent colicky pain before menses. Menses, early with profuse discharge (Calc.). Menses too late, pale, scanty with soreness about genitals. Profuse and long-continued menses of bright red blood. Menorrhagia, better taking bath. Uterine hemorrhage, constant oozing after copious flow with violent backache, relieved from sitting and pressure. Hemorrhages after curetting or other treatments. Leucorrhea with labor-like pains causing itching and burning, better washing. Soreness of genitals during sex and during menses. Uterine tumors, cysts. Eclampsia, better belchings. Impending miscarriage with pains from back into buttocks and thighs. ***Labor pains inefficient. Labor pains felt in back,*** down the hips and thighs. ***Complaints after childbirth or miscarriage.*** After miscarriage, when there is great weakness of back. Puerperal fever with cutting pain in hypogastrium with black and scanty urine. Promotes expulsion of moles.

Food - Disgust for food or ravenous appetite. When hungry, feels anxious, nauseated, nervous, tingling, palpitation etc. Wants to eat frequently but least food oppresses her. Disgust for food. Milk and warm food disagree. Diarrhea worse milk. Ice water disagrees. Aversion to meat. Desire for sweets or acids.

Head - Burning in top of head and soles of feet. ***Headache from riding in cold wind.*** Headache comes on with yawning. Wakes from headache. Headache into eyes, worse motion, sneezing, coughing, stooping, yawning. Headache better when raising the head and pressing the forehead. Headache on riding in carriage. ***Catarrhal, congestive headaches***, better free discharge from nose. One-sided headache with nausea. Throbbing and humming. Sensation as if something loose in head, turning, twisting towards the forehead. Aching in occiput. Sharp pains in forehead, temples. Pressing as of a stone in forehead and vertex. Pressure and drawing tearing in forehead. ***Great dryness of hair***. Hair, dry, falls out (Fl-ac.) from eyebrows, temples and beard. Painful tumors on scalp. Wens on scalp.

Heart - Angina pectoris. ***Tendency to fatty degeneration of heart***. Dyspnea with violent and irregular beating of heart. Threatened heart failure. Insufficiency of mitral valves. Pulse is small, soft, variable, intermittent or dicrotic. ***Weak, rapid pulse intermits***, due to digestive disturbance. Heart's action intermittent, irregular, tumultuous, weak. ***Arrhythmia.*** Palpitations, then weakness, in valvular disease. Palpitations and burning in heart region. ***Palpitations on slightest effort.*** Violent palpitations, shakes the whole body, throbbing extending to fingertips and toes. Sensation as if heart were suspended, seems to hang by a thread. Sharp pains about heart and through to scapula.

Kidneys - ***Sharp pain in kidneys,*** going from buttocks to thighs. Burning in left kidney. Nephritis from exposure to cold or injury. Pressure on bladder long before urination, the more it is pressed less the urine flows. Slow urination with burning in urethra. ***Urine, foamy with thick red sediment.*** Rises several times at night to urinate. Nocturnal bedwetting of adults. Involuntary urination when coughing, sneezing, etc.

Limbs - ***Arthritis.*** Deformative arthritis, worse in small joints. Rheumatic joint pains. Nightly rheumatic pains. Sharp, aching pains in the joints and tendons. Pressive pain in joints. Limbs go to sleep easily. ***Back and legs give out***. Limbs feel numb and heavy. Uneasiness, heaviness, jerking, tearing and swelling in limbs. Limbs sensitive to pressure. Jerks the limbs, especially when the feet are touched. ***Cold hands and cold feet in bed.*** Sciatica, tearing pain in the thighs with jerking of muscles. Paralysis of elderly people and dropsical disorders. ***Hip joint disease.*** Weakness in arms, feel numb, cold. Tearing in arms from shoulder to wrist. Lacerating in wrist joint. ***Pain from hip to knee.*** Knees painful, worse going downstairs or upstairs. White swelling of knees. ***Soles very sensitive***. Itching of great toes with pain. Spasmodic contraction of fingers and toes. Tips of toes and fingers painful. Burning like fire in fingers.

Liver - Sharp pain or soreness. Chronic liver troubles, with soreness. Jaundice and dropsy.

Lungs - Shortness of breath in morning. Dyspnea, as if no air could get into lungs. Labored breathing, after paroxysms of cough. ***Arrest of breath awakens at night.*** Leaning forward relieves chest symptoms. ***Asthmatic, wheezing***, worse least motion or walking. Asthma, worse from 2 a.m. to 4 a.m. Asthma, alternating with diarrhea with vertigo. ***Asthma, better when sitting up or bending forward.*** Asthma, better from rocking back and forth. Asthma with loss of appetite. ***Tendency to colds, better in warm climate.*** Bronchitis, whole chest very sensitive. Pneumonia. Pneumonia, after measles. ***Never well since pneumonia.*** Pleurisy, Pleuritis with violent palpitations. ***Hydrothorax***. Tendency to tuberculosis. Whooping cough. Expectoration must be swallowed, cheesy taste, copious, offensive, lumpy. Expectoration scanty and tenacious.

Male - Copious, painful pollutions with painful erections. Strange, uneasy feeling in genitals. Chronic gonorrhea, painful scanty discharge, burning during and after urination. Complaints after sex. ***Excessive emissions, followed by weakness***. Prostration after sex, often with shuddering. Sleeplessness and uneasiness for 2 or 3 days after sex. Aversion to sex.

Modalities - Better in warm weather, warmth, open air, moving about, sitting with elbows on knees. ***Worse from cold air,*** cold weather, draft, change of weather, after overheating. ***Worse 2 a.m. to 4 a.m.,*** lying on left side, ***lying on painful side***. Worse exertion, sudden or unguarded motion, touch, stooping, sex. Worse soup, coffee, water, loss of fluids. ***Worse since pneumonia.*** Worse before menses, ***after childbirth, miscarriage.***

Mouth - Offensive odor from mouth every morning, like old cheese. Much saliva constantly in mouth. Bad, slimy taste. Mouth covered with painful, burning vesicles. Aphthae. General dryness of mouth without thirst, with stricture of esophagus in gastritis. Sticking and biting in posterior portion of palate. Burning, soreness or painful pimples on tip of tongue. Gums separate from teeth. Itching in gums, pus oozes out.

Nose - Swollen, hard, red, covered with pimples. Itching, burning in nose. Sore, scurfy, crusty nostrils. ***Ulcerated nostrils.*** Dryness of nose alternating with obstruction. Chronic catarrh. Chronic colds. Breathes through mouth. Obstruction better walking in open air. ***Stuffs up in warm room***. Descending coryza. Coryza during menses. Post-nasal dripping (Spig.). Fetid, thick, fluent, yellow-green, crusty discharge. Bloody nasal mucus. Nosebleed on washing face in morning. Ulcerative pain in right nostril.

Perspiration - Offensive or sour smelling sweat. Scanty sweat, foul on feet. Perspires on slightest exertion. General inability to sweat. Sweats on painful part, on affected part. Sweats mostly on upper parts. Sweats at night, without relief, with cough. Perspires on every mental exertion, reading, writing. Perspires after pneumonia. Perspires after eating. Easily sweats, excited by exercise during day. Warm drinks aggravates.

Rectum - Discharge of much flatus. Ascarides. ***Constipation,*** after or during menses, in women after frequent miscarriages or multiple and difficult childbirths (Sep.). Constipation alternating with diarrhea. Ineffectual urging to stool, rectum feels too weak to expel it. Chronic diarrhea of dyspeptics, only during the day. Painless diarrhea with rumbling in abdomen and burning at anus. Stitching like fine needles during pregnancy or red-hot poker in rectum, better cool bathing. Burning in rectum and anus. Itching of rectum (Ign.). Itching, ulcerated pimples around anus. Easy prolapse of rectum (Graph., Podo.). Anal fistula. Hemorrhoids, large, swollen, painful, burn like fire, Hemorrhoids ***extremely sensitive to touch***, inflamed, bleeding. Pain in hemorrhoids when coughing.

Sensations - Sensation as if bed were sinking. Sensation of a lump rolling over on coughing, rising from right abdomen to throat. Pulsative pains and throbbings. Burning sensation and burning pains. Whole body as if it were hollow.

Skin - Skin dry, sensitive, itching, better scratching. Eczema eruption dry at first, but when scratched exuding moisture. Burning as from mustard plaster. General itching or hives during menses. Nettle rash before menses. Itching of warts. Tension, pressure, rending in scars. Herpetic spots on face. Ulcers bleed at night.

Sleep - Yawns with headache. Sleepiness during forepart of day and during day. Drowsy after eating, falls asleep while eating. ***Sleeplessness from cough.*** Nocturnal restlessness before menses. Restless, dreamful sleep during menses. Twitching of limbs, grinding of teeth, crying while sleeping. Talks in sleep. Wakes at 1 a.m. or 2 a.m., cannot sleep again. ***Wakes at about 2 a.m. to 4 a.m.*** with nearly all complaints. Horrid, anxious dreams with frequent awaking and desire to urinate. Dreams of water, thieves, misfortunes, diseases, dead people. Erotic, imaginative, fantastic, sentimental.

Stomach - ***Anxiety felt in stomach.*** Easy choking when eating. Gagging. Fullness even after little drink or food. Feeling of lump in pit of stomach. ***Stomach feels as if it would burst.*** Constant feeling as if ***stomach were full of water***. Epigastric pain to back. Epigastrium is very sensitive externally. Gastric disorders from ice water. Dyspepsia of old people, burning acidity, bloating. ***Everything eaten seems to turn into gas.*** Flatulence, distended and sensitive. Salty, sour regurgitation. ***Sour belchings.*** Sour eructations before menses. Nausea on every inward emotion. Nausea with faintness and anxiety. ***Nausea, better lying down.*** Nausea at sight of food, in morning. Vomiting of sour mucus, ingesta and slime. Nocturnal vomiting of food. Nausea during pregnancy.

Stools - Stools, difficult, large, hard lumps, with sharp pains. Stool like sheep's dung. Large discharge of blood with natural stool. Stools followed by burning or torn feeling. Insufficient soft stool after much pressure most of it remains.

Teeth - Tearing, lancinating pains. Drawing pains. Tearing pain in teeth, jaws. Stitches in teeth with swelling of cheeks. Toothache only while eating. Toothache, alternating with stitching pains in left breast, only while eating. Looseness of teeth. Gums separate from teeth. Pyorrhea. Itching in gums, pus oozes out.

Temperature - Chills with dyspnea, hot hands and sleepiness in open air. Frequent shuddering during day. Chilly in morning. Internal heat with external chilliness. Internal burning. Fever with surging of blood or throbbing in blood vessels. Fever with dyspnea.

Throat - Dry, parched, rough. Hoarseness and loss of voice. Stricture of esophagus. ***Swallowing difficult,*** food slowly descends, remains halfway in esophagus with gagging and vomiting. Small particles of food go easily in windpipe. Sticking pain as from fish bone or splinters. Stinging pain when swallowing. ***Sore throat, always takes cold and the cold settles in throat.*** Throat feels as if squeezed, as if lungs came into throat. Catarrhal aphonia with violent sneezing. Scratching and stinging in throat and chest during cough. Hawks up tough mucus in morning. Tonsils enlarged. Swelling of cervical glands.

Tongue - Tongue, gray-white. Tip of tongue burns as if raw. Burning, soreness or painful pimples on tip of tongue. Tongue covered with painful, burning vesicles. Tongue coated gray, in sick headache.

Vertigo - Vertigo on turning around, when rapidly turning head or body, when walking. Vertigo from riding in a carriage. Vertigo, as if proceeding from stomach. Must lie down as soon as vertigo comes on, otherwise he is thrown down. Vertigo, as after intoxication.

Vision - Vision weak after measles, miscarriage, ***after sex***. Spots, gauze and black points before the eyes. Bright sparks, blue, green spots, drops. Muscae volitantes while reading or looking at a bright light. Sees sparks, during cough. Can't fix sight of any object steadily without water running from eyes and feeling of dizziness.

COMMENTS - Generally very sensitive to changes in weather, particularly sensitive in affected area. Chilly, tendency to take cold. Symptoms worse when body temperature is low, aversion to open air. Very sensitive to drafts, will catch a cold at every little draft. Cannot tolerate drafts (Nux-v., Calc., Hep., Sulph.).

Easily startled by any noise, especially if unexpected. Cannot bear to be touched, starts when touched ever so lightly, especially on the feet. Generally right sided, particularly the base of the right lung, and the apices, according to Goullon. Worse exertion.

Characteristic sweat, backache and weakness, particularly in conditions of debility from loss of fluids. Keynote bag-like swellings or puffiness around the upper eye, eyebrow, can be between the eyebrows. Alternating symptoms. Organ pathology due to suppressed mental symptoms.

Constant backache, with a giving out feeling in the back and legs, or as if the back was broken. The pain may extend downwards to the buttocks and even to the knee. Pain from hip to knee (more especially if right sided). Lower backache, especially during labor, menstrual cramps.

Lumbago. Hip joint disease. Spasms, puerperal convulsions and paralysis. Twitching of muscles, rigidity of muscles, muscular atony. Disposition to over lifting.

Stitching pains, pulsations, better by pressure and by lying flat on the back. Sharp, stabbing pains that are worse motion. Sticking, burning, sharp pains like knives or needles. Sharp pains, wandering and stabbing, especially with arthritis.

Osteoarthritis, deformative arthritis and migratory arthritis, pains that go from joint to joint. Burning and stabbing pains in the fingers and toes. Gout, gouty arthritis. Stiffness in neck and shoulders. Pain worse motion, with sharp pains. Edema. Peripheral edema, varicose veins.

Affinity for tissues. Tumors, cancers and fibroids. Affects the blood and circulation. Anemia with great debility, skin watery, milky white. Hemorrhages.

Dropsical disorders. Ulcers, bleeding at night.

Throbbing of blood vessels all over body and to ends of fingers and toes. Irregular heart. Fatty degeneration of the heart and other muscles. Sensation as if the heart were suspended by a thread. History of heart attack.

Great affinity for the lungs. Pneumonia and pleurisy (Bry.), worse coughing or movement, better pressure. Chronic respiratory problems in the elderly (Phos.). Sharp, stabbing, and stitching pains in the lungs. Oppression of breathing. Shortness of breath. Asthma, better sitting up in bed or on all fours. May sit up in bed with pillows (Ars.), may sleep sitting up.

Coughs worse from 2 a.m. to 4 a.m. Dry, paroxysmal cough, loosens viscid mucus or pus which must be swallowed. Spasms with gagging or vomiting of ingesta. Expectoration of hard, white or smoky masses, which fly from the throat when coughing, with globules of pus.

Tendency to sinus headaches. Useful for sick headaches. Violent headaches about the inner temples, violent stitching or jerking pains, on one side of the head or both. One-sided headache with nausea. Pressure and drawing in forehead extending into eyes and root of nose. Congestion to head and heat of face often accompany the headaches.

Toothache, only when eating. Easy choking, food easily gets into windpipe. Difficulty swallowing. Pain in the back when swallowing. Fish bone sensation in the throat, general tendency to stitching pains.

Disordered digestion, flatulence, distention, constipation. Gas, bloating, craving for sweets (Lyc.). Intolerance for milk, aversion to brown bread. Colic pains, severe colitis. Lack of muscular control especially with urologic things. History of diabetes.

Premenstrual syndrome with bloating, water retention. Very sensitive breasts, painful before the period. Backache with period, or preceding period. Insufficient labor pains, transferred labor. Labor pains felt in back (Cimic., felt in thighs).

Insomnia, cannot relax, without reason. Unrefreshed sleep. Drowsiness, while eating. Worse after sex, feel weak and prostrated (Sil., Calc.), sleepless after sex. Complaints after sex in males, especially complaints of the eyes.

One case of a headache that Clarke cured was better by lying down, better by a tight band around the head.

A man had an ulcer of the right leg with swelling of the ankle and he complained of waking at 2 a.m. Kali-c. 30c cured, but in the meantime he developed a great weakness of the right thigh, as if it would give out when walking.

The symptom "pain from the hip to the knee" led to a cure in a woman, 73, stout, short, pale and of very soft tissue, who had for four months suffered from rheumatic pains, and an offensive vaginal discharge.

A local practitioner was consulted and pronounced it cancer of the womb in an advanced stage and gave her four months to live. She described to Clarke the pain as being all around the lower abdomen and a "dull, heavy, depressing, dead pain, commencing at the inner part of the top of the right hip, iliac crest and extending to the knee."

The pain was so severe it made her feel quite sick and faint. The discharge was very offensive like decaying meat. Great weakness and trembling accompanied the discharge. Urine was almost like blood at times, and had a sandy sediment.

Kali-c. 1,000c. was given and at once improvement set in. In a few months all the bad symptoms had disappeared and never returned. The patient lived ten years after this episode.

Id of Stettin, Germany, recorded the case of a woman, 65, who suffered from chronic bronchial catarrh and emphysema. In November, 1886, she had asthmatic complaints, depriving her of sleep with cough and mucus expectoration difficult to raise.

She was so weary when eating that she fell asleep and could not finish her meal.

Tired after eating. In the morning, passed much flatulence. Kali-c. 10c removed the condition in a few days.

The following March after a cold there was a recurrence, but without the weariness, and Kali-c. failed. Ars. 15c rapidly cured.

The same patient also had a toothache alternating with tearing, stitching pain in left breast and under left false ribs. The side pains were worse at night, especially in evening as soon as she lay down, worse lying down, particularly worse lying on the right (painless) side. Not influenced by pressure or motion.

RELATIONS - ***Antidotes:*** Camph., Coff. ***Compare:*** (1) Kali-sal. - vomiting, especially of pregnancy, arteriosclerosis with chronic rheumatism. (2) Kali-sil. - gouty nodosities. (3) Kali-acet. - diabetes, diarrhea, dropsy, alkaline urine, very much increased in quantity. (4) Kali-cit. - Bright's disease-1 grains to wineglass of water. (5) Kali-ox - lumbago, convulsions. (6) Kali-pic. - jaundice, violent belchings. (7) Kali-t. - paraplegia. (8) Kali-tel. - garlicky odor of breath, salivation, swollen tongue. (9) Calc., Am-p., Phos., Lyc., Bry., Nat-m, Stann., Sep. ***Complementary:*** Carb-v. - lowness of vitality may suggest a preliminary course of Carb-v. to nurse up recuperation to the point that Kali-c. would come in helpfully. ***Follows:*** Nux-v. often in stomach and bladder troubles.

REFERENCES - Boericke. Clarke. Murphy. Phatak.

KALI CHLORICUM

(Potassium Chlorate)

PHARMACY - kali-chl. Kali Chloricum. Potassium chlorate. Potassic chlorate. Trituration. Solution. ***Historical dose:*** All potencies.

CLINICAL - ***Albuminuria.*** Anemia. Aphthae. Asthma. Cancrum oris. Clumsiness. Colic. Convulsions. Crusta lactea. Cystitis. Dysentery. Edema. Epithelioma. Facial, paralysis. Hangnails. Hematuria. Hemorrhages. Hemorrhoids. Hepatitis. Mercurial, poisoning. Mouth, inflammation. ***Nephritis.*** Neuralgias. ***Noma.*** Paralysis. Pharyngitis. Pimples. Proctalgia. Purpura. Scurvy. Stomatitis. Syphilis. Tic douloureux. ***Toxemia.*** Ulcers.

HOMEOPATHIC - Kali-chl. is not to be confused with the chloride that constitutes Schüssler's Kali-m. Hering amalgamated the symptoms of the two under the heading Kali-m., but Clarke kept them separate. Kali-chl. is an exceedingly active poison. It has long been used in the old school in solution as a wash for sore mouth and foul ulcers.

Hutchinson observed a number of cases in which it produced the very condition that it was give to cure, the "most acute ulceration and follicular stomatitis. The whole mucus surface was red and tumid and in the cheeks, lips, etc., were numerous gray-based ulcers."

Fatal poisoning has occurred, death occurring in convulsions. The blood is disorganized and after death, the liver, spleen and kidneys are found softened and filled with disorganized blood, this should give it a place in cases of lardaceous and fatty degeneration of solid viscera. The mouth, hypochondria and rectum are the most affected.

Profound prostration, coldness in different parts and organs. Easy hemorrhages, nosebleed, bloody stools etc. Hemoglobinuria. Anemia. Septicemia. ***Noma.*** Discharges are fetid. Gray, white, plastic exudates.

Chronic nephritis. Parenchymatous nephritis with stomatitis. Acute ulcerative and follicular stomatitis. Scurvy. Hepatitis. Lardaceous and fatty degeneration of liver, spleen and kidneys and other solid organs. ***Toxemic conditions of pregnancy*** with urinary symptoms.

MIND - Cheerfulness alternating with sadness. Confusion while walking in open air. Confusion from wine. Delusion he must starve. ***Refuses to eat.*** Desires death during chill.

Abdomen - Griping colic with shifting of flatulence and diarrhea, followed by continuous rectal pain.

Chest - Constriction of chest, as from sulphur fumes.

Face - Swollen, she can hardly see in the morning. Neuralgic pains, worse talking, eating or slight touch, followed by numbness.

Heart - Coldness in precordial region. Right pulse full, left small. Coldness in blood.

Kidneys - Nephritis. Urine albuminous, scanty, suppressed. Albumin and bile, high phosphoric acid with low total solids. Hematuria, diuresis.

Limbs - Ankles swell in the evening. Arms, feet cold.

Modalities - Better from nosebleed, mental symptoms. Worse from cold, coughing, sneezing, a jar, mercury.

Mouth - Whole mucus surface red, tumid with gray-based ulcers. ***Stomatitis,*** aphthous and ***gangrenous.*** Fetor. Noma. Scurvy. Salivation, profuse secretion of acid saliva. Tongue, swollen, cold. Mercurial stomatitis (as a mouth wash).

Nose - Bleeding at night, only from right nostril.

Rectum - Diarrhea, profuse, greenish mucus. Griping colic with shifting of flatulence and diarrhea, followed by continuous rectal pain. Dysentery, much blood passing with mucus, profuse greenish. Cries with violent cutting pain in the rectum in dysentery and diarrhea.

Skin - Cold. Jaundice. Discolored, chocolate tint. Pimples between lip and chin. Itching miliary or papular eruptions.

Stomach - Sudden, incessant vomiting of all food, of offensive dark green mucus. Stomach cold. Sensations of a weight in the epigastric and umbilical regions. Flatulence.

Throat - Cold feeling in throat.

COMMENTS - Rushmore recorded a proving of Kali-chl. in an unmarried woman, 50, short, brunette, who had goiter in early life, which disappeared under the application of iodine. Later on, a fibroid tumor developed in the uterus. For this the patient was advised to take crude potassium chlorate, dissolved in water, daily.

Symptoms observed included an increased moral irritability. Felt dreadfully dull and stupid. Dizzy on stooping and rising. Slight headache over eyes, objects appear double, beside each other. Face swollen so she could hardly see on rising in morning. Smarting of tongue.

Kali-chl. took away her desire for acids. Diminished appetite. Much commotion and flatulence in abdomen. Increased urine. Dreams of terrible things never thought. Great coolness, shivering on cold days, seemed as if it cooled off her blood. Clumsiness. General bloated feeling.

In the provers, great weakness manifested. Rheumatic and neuralgic pains, many occurring in the facial nerves. Facial paralysis. Pimples in various parts, between lip and chin. The heart was the seat of much disturbance, and a coldness was felt about the precordia. Disordered stomach and bowels. Excited sexual organs.

Allen credited Kali-chl. with the cure of "Dysentery with most violent cutting pains as from knives, frequent stools, tenesmus, making the patient cry out, evacuations very small, almost pure blood, great prostration."

Allen noted that it cured epithelioma of the face and of the great toe.

RELATIONS - ***Antidote to:*** Merc. ***Compare:*** (1) Especially Kali-m. (2) Caust. - facial paralysis. (3) Kali-bi. - follicular pharyngitis. (4) Zinc., Cadm-s. and Cact. - asthma with great constriction of chest. (5) Graph., Kali-n. and Nat-m. - cold feeling about heart.

REFERENCES - Boericke. Clarke. Phatak.

KALI CHLOROSUM

(Javelle Water)

PHARMACY - kali-chls. Kali chlorosum. Javelle water. Bleaching fluid. Formula variable, contains potassium hypochlorate principally, chloride and some carbonate. Solution. ***Historical dose:*** All potencies.

CLINICAL - Aphonia. Asthma. Coryza. Diphtheria.

HOMEOPATHIC - The observations with Javelle water are from poisoning cases. The most notable symptoms were watery eyes, pale, puffy face, and constriction of the throat and chest. Much sensitivity. Sensitiveness of epigastrium and especially of larynx and whole anterior portion of neck. Cramps and restlessness.

RELATIONS - ***Compare:*** (1) Kali-chl., Calc-m., Chlor., Nat-hchls.

REFERENCES - Clarke.

KALI CITRICUM

(Potassium Citrate)

PHARMACY - kali-cit. Kali citricum. Potassium citrate. Citrate of potash. Solution. Trituration. ***Historical dose:*** Trituration and all potencies.

HOMEOPATHIC - Kali-cit. has been used in solution (eight to ten grains to a wineglass of water) to assist the action of the kidneys in sufferers from Bright's disease who were under the absolute skim-milk dietary. It has also been used in the same way in old school practice, as a solvent for gouty concretions about joints.

COMMENTS - Kali-cit. has not been proved, but "Agricola" recorded the effect of a large dose given by an allopath to a patient suffering from suppressed kidney action after influenza.

In three days the kidneys acted freely, but new symptoms were set up including tympanites, a constant flow of mucus from the anus. Awful gastric and abdominal pains, "as if a machine were at work inside, skinning the inside of the stomach and the whole length of the intestinal tube" (Nit-ac.). Flatus was constant and in great amount, producing a pain of its own, which was a prominent feature.

REFERENCES - Clarke.

KALI CYANATUM

(Potassium Cyanide)

PHARMACY - kali-cy. Kali cyanatum. Potassium cyanide. Cyanide of potash. Kali cyanidum. Kali cyanuretum. Solution. Trituration. ***Historical dose:*** All potencies.

CLINICAL - Aphasia. Asthma. Cancer. Cheyne-Stokes. Chills. Ciliary, neuralgias. Convulsions. Epilepsy. Eye, disorders. Facial pain. Headaches. Memory lost. Neuralgias. Rheumatism. Sciatica. Speech, lost. Strokes. ***Tongue, cancer.*** Vertigo.

HOMEOPATHIC - Commonly used in photography. As it is easily accessible, many cases of suicide and attempted suicide have occurred by its means. It is from the symptoms observed in such cases, as well as the provings by Lembke and others, that this remedy is understood.

Agonizing neuralgias, especially of orbital and supra-maxillary with screaming and loss of consciousness. Neuralgic pains are unbearable, more common in the temporal and facial regions involving the trigeminal nerve.

Ciliary neuralgia, trifacial neuralgia, tic douloureux. Epilepsy. General convulsions. Sudden convulsive action of whole body, about ten minutes after heart ceased to beat. Sphincters rigidly contracted.

Sudden sinking sensation. Sick headache. Stroke. Prolonged stupor. Intense vertigo, objects seem to be moving around him. Head drawn backwards, unable to tolerate any covering on head. Convulsive motion of eyelids and eyeballs. Pupils largely dilated and insensible to light. Obscuration of vision.

Cheyne-Stokes breathing. Asthma. ***Cancer of the tongue*** with indurated edges. Speech loss. Rheumatism. Sciatica, unsteady gait.

MIND - Gentle disposition. Irritability with absent persons. Crossness almost uncontrollable on entering room, but cold, open air produces good mood. Aphasia, inability to recollect certain words for several days. Lies on floor in a deep stupor.

Abdomen - A feeling as if bowels were about to act. Pains in abdomen and groin in afternoon.

Back - Vague pain in neck. Marked weakness in lumbar regions with dull pain and weakness of iliac region, while walking and in afternoon.

Chest - Anxious feeling in the chest. Oppression of chest.

Ears - Rushing in ears.

Eyes - Eyes fixed. Eyelids began to open and shut alternately, eyeballs stared in different directions. Eyes closed, but on raising lids the eyeballs were seen to be in uninterrupted convulsive motion. Swelling of upper lids. Pupils largely distended and insensible to light. Obscuration of vision. Loss of sight, then double vision as sight returns. Diplopia.

Face - Severe neuralgia in temporal region, recurring daily at same hour. Pain in orbital and supra-maxillary region, with screaming and loss of consciousness.

Head - Head drawn backwards. Gnawing pain across temple. Sharp pains in occiput. Soreness of scalp over parietal regions. Unable to tolerate any covering on head, whether in the cold or warmth, because it causes a headache for months after.

Heart - Stitches in heart and lungs. Jerking stitches in heart on respiration. Palpitation of heart. Pulse at times fifteen beats slower than usual.

Kidneys - Bladder distended by a large amount of urine, which has to be evacuated by a catheter. Urine came away involuntarily.

Limbs - Unsteady gait. Limbs icy cold, rigid and convulsed. Limbs are flaccid with occasional convulsions more like a shuddering than anything else. Tetanic spasms of muscles of arms and legs.

Lungs - Cough prevents sleep, respiration weak, cannot take deep breath. Hoarse voice. Loud mucus rattle. Superficial respiration, slow and difficult breathing. Respiration nearly suspended, but thorax convulsively raised, at irregular intervals, far apart.

Modalities - Better from motion in open air. ***Worse from 4 a.m. to 4 p.m.***

Mouth - *Cancerous ulceration of tongue* with indurated edges. Tongue has peculiar dark ground seen through heavy, white coating. Lips and mucus membrane of mouth pale. Slight frothing at the mouth. Difficult speech, power of speech lost but intelligence intact.

Nose - Inside of nose is parched, hot and dry. Expelling blood, blood drying quickly in nose.

Rectum - Bowels obstinately constipated, feces came away involuntarily.

Sleep - Sleepiness during day. Restless, dream filled sleep all night, could not lie on one side for any length of time. Dreams very lively, especially towards morning, can be horrid, exciting.

Stomach - Copious vomiting, followed by return of consciousness. Severe burning in stomach. Sharp gastric pains. Great sensitiveness of epigastric region. Pain at epigastrium of a griping intermittent character.

Temperature - Hands and face covered with cold perspiration. Surface of whole body cold and moist. Shivers. Coldness of limbs, pendulous and without muscular power. Chill on waking from naps, or wakes him before he can get soundly asleep, followed by a very slight sweat. Wakes 6 a.m. with heat and disagreeable feverish perspiration over whole body, except legs below the knees with flushed face.

Throat - Astringent sensation in throat with nausea, lasting until after midnight. Feeling of constriction about fauces, with muscular tremors about throat, great stiffness in throat after. Patient was able to swallow as soon as a large amount of fluid filled the pharynx, after every swallow the whole body was seized with convulsive tremors and flushes of redness spreading over the face. Had no sensation of act of swallowing.

Vertigo - Intense vertigo, so that all objects seemed to be moving around him.

COMMENTS - Stroke and epileptic symptoms (Hydr-ac.), with pronounced, slow breathing. Strong tetanic convulsions. Loss of consciousness and vision, vision returns doubled when consciousness returns. The chief clinical uses have been in epithelioma of the tongue, apoplectic and epileptic conditions, respiratory disorders, rheumatism of the joints and neuralgias.

In one poisoning case, the fingers were stretched out and spasmodically contracted.

In another case, after the failure of all efforts to restore the patient (a photographer) with ether injections and repeated washings out of the stomach, he was placed in a hot bath and icy-cold water was poured over his head and nape.

Each time water was poured on his head, the patient drew deep inspirations which gradually grew deeper and more regular until consciousness was restored.

He complained of sharp occipital and gastric pains. Convalescence was rapid, but a general muscular weakness and impairment of speech lasted a long time.

Cattel recorded in the early volumes of the Brit. Jour. of Homeopathy several remarkable cases of neuralgia cured by Kali-cy. He followed Hering's guiding symptoms, "agonizing attacks of neuralgic pains between temporal regions and ciliary arch and maxilla with screaming and apparent loss of sensibility, as if struck with a stroke, pulse 84, face flushed."

"Severe neuralgia in temporal region and left upper jaw, daily at 4 a.m. increasing until 10 and ceasing at 4 p.m. in the interval, anorexia, fever, headache." The symptoms were worse in a room, worse immediately after meals (fullness), and better by motion in open air.

E. T. Adams treated an inveterate whiskey-drinker, 55, for a swelling on the right side of the tongue, excavated so deeply that the first joint of the thumb could be laid in it. It had been pronounced cancerous.

The patient could take no solid nutriment and fluids only with great pain. Under Kali-cy., he recovered rapidly, was able to walk and to eat dry bread and cooked beef with comparative ease. Persuaded by his former attendants to undergo operation, he died nineteen days after.

Pertroz was the first to give Kali-cy. 1,000c in cases of this kind. A woman had cancerous ulcer of right side of tongue involving the root. With a view of relieving the woman's sufferings, Petroz gave her Kali-cy. 1,000c once in four days.

In two weeks the suffering was much diminished, the tongue appeared less thick and speech easier. In another fortnight the patient's countenance had lost its gray hue and drawn features and she could eat a crumb of bread. The case went on to complete and permanent cure.

RELATIONS - ***Compare:*** (1) Plat., Stann., Cedr., Mez. (2) Mur-ac. (3) Hy-ac., Camph. (3) In periodic ciliary neuralgia, Cedron. (4) Neuralgia gradually increasing and decreasing, Stann., Plat. (5) Also, according to Cooper, Sulph. (6) Sudden onset, gradual decline, Sul-ac. (7) Fingers spread out, Sec.

REFERENCES - Boericke. Clarke. Grimmer. Murphy.

KALI FERROCYANATUM

(Potassic Ferrocyanide)

PHARMACY - kali-fcy. Kali ferrocyanatum. Potassic ferrocyanide. Prussian blue. Yellow prussiate of potash. Kali ferrocyanidum. ***Historical dose:*** All potencies.

CLINICAL - Heart, disorders. Leucorrhea. Neuralgias. Pulse weak.

HOMEOPATHIC - Prussian blue has physical and mental prostration following an infectious disease. Inability to sustained routine work. Neuralgic disorders depending on impoverished blood and exhausted nerve centers, especially spinal.

Fatty and functional heart troubles. Pulse weak, small, irregular. Uterine symptoms with a bearing-down sensation (Sep.) and gastric sinking. Profuse, pus-like leucorrhea with a passive hemorrhage.

REFERENCES - Boericke.

KALI HYPOPHOSPHORICUM

(Potassium Hypophosphate)

PHARMACY - kali-hp. Kali hypophosphoricum. Potassium hypophosphate. ***Historical dose:*** Trituration and all potencies.

CLINICAL - Anemia. Tea, effects.

HOMEOPATHIC - Great ***debility with atrophy of muscular tissue.*** Phosphaturia with general anemia or leucocythemia. Chronic bronchitis where the expectoration are ***thick and fetid***, sometimes ***scanty and tough***. Effects of excessive tea drinking.

REFERENCES - Boericke.

KALI IODATUM

(Potassium Iodide)

PHARMACY - kali-i. Kali iodatum. Potassium iodide. Kali hydroiodicum. Solution. Trituration. ***Historical dose:*** Trituration and all potencies.

CLINICAL - ***Acne, rosacea***. Actinomycosis. Allergies. Aneurysm. Anhidrosis. Arteriosclerosis. Asthma. Boils. Bright's, disease. Bubo. Bunions. ***Cancer.*** Cachexia. Colds. Condylomata. Coryza. Coughs. Croup. Debility. Decay, bones. Dropsy. Ears, pain. Edema, glottidis. Emaciation. Erythema, nodosum. Eyes, disorders. ***Facial, neuralgias***. Fibroids. ***Gland, swellings.*** Goiter. Gonorrhea. Gout. Hemorrhages. Hay fever. Housemaid's knee. Influenza. Inter-menstrual, hemorrhage. ***Iritis***. Joints, disorders. Laryngitis. Liver, diseases. Locomotor, ataxia. Lumbago. Lungs, disorders. ***Meningitis***. Menstruation, disorders. Neuralgias. Nodes. Noises, ears. Nystagmus. Odor, body. Pancreatitis. Paralysis. Pleurisy. ***Pleuritic, effusion.*** Prostate, disorders. ***Radiation, poisoning. Rheumatism.*** Rickets. Rupia. ***Sciatica.*** Scrofula. Smallpox. Spine, curvature. Spleen. ***Syphilis. Thyroid, disorders.*** Tic, douloureux. Tinnitus. Tongue, neuralgia. Tuberculosis. Tumors. Ulcers. Wens.

HOMEOPATHIC - Potassium iodide was used as anti-syphilitic remedy and is also antidotal to mercury. Kali-i. is perhaps more anti-scrofulous than anti-syphilitic. It acts best in scrofulous patients, especially if syphilis or mercurialization, or both, are added. It also causes infiltration, edema and dropsy of various kinds. The blood is acted upon and hemorrhage occurs, and purpura hemorrhagica.

Grimmer said Kali-i. cured many types of tumors and cancers generally based on a syphilitic or tubercular miasms, and often there is a combination of both these in many cases of malignancy. Nightly aggravations of complaints.

Hering spoke of Kali-i. as having been curative in pneumonia and Bright's disease. Specific for aneurysm. Has been commended as a protective against foot and-mouth disease in cattle. In material doses, for fungoid disease (thrush, ringworm, etc.) and bacterial diseases like tuberculosis.

Syphilis. In acute form with evening, remitting fever, going off in nightly perspiration. Second stage, mucus membranes and skin ulcerations. Tertiary symptoms, nodes.

Glandular swellings. Glands enlarged and indurated. Glands are swollen or atrophied. Dropsy from pressure from swollen glands. Infiltrations, edema. Profuse, watery, acrid coryza, especially when associated with pain in frontal sinus. Discharges are copious, watery, acrid, salty, thick, green or foul. Spitting blood.

Exostosis, swelling of the bones and rickets. Feels used up. Crushing or sharp stitching pains. Diffused soreness after pains of affected part. Pains long after injury. Coldness of painful part in bones.

Purpura and hemorrhagic diathesis. ***Diffused sensitiveness,*** of glands, scalp, etc. ***Rheumatism in neck, back***, and feet, especially heels and soles. Rheumatism, worse cold and wet. Contraction of muscles and tendons, chronic arthritis with spurious ankylosis.

Weakness, emaciation. Arteriosclerosis. Cachexia. Actinomycosis. Fungoid diseases. Tea-taster's cough due to inhaling the fungus. Craves motion in open air. Brings about often favorable reaction in many chronic ailments even when not clearly symptomatically indicated.

MIND - Always troubled. Despondent. Trivial details of life seem insupportable. Nervous, must walk. Troublesome impressions easily become fixed ideas. Loss of memory. Cannot find words at the moment wanted, cannot write, play music, or think.

Anxious. Fright at every trifle, ***starting from noise***. Inclined to sadness and weeping, especially in the evening. Half-mad all night, talkative and full of jokes. Dreads the return of dawn.

Restlessness during headache. Abusive, bad temper. Harsh tempered and cruel. Irritable, irascible, especially towards his children, his family. Indifference to her children. Aversion to being touched.

Abdomen - Flatulence with air hunger. Squeaking or clucking noise in abdomen. Sudden painful bloating of abdomen. Cutting and burning pain around navel. Swollen spleen after intermittent. Inguinal glands swollen.

Back - Small of the back as if in a vice. Bruised pain in lumbar region worse sitting bent. Pain in coccyx, as from a fall. Sharp pain in small of back when sitting. Chronic rheumatism of chest and back. Chills from sacrum up over back.

Breasts - Atrophy of breasts. Tumor of breast. Galactorrhea.

Chest - Air-passages raw. Chest pains go backwards. Pain from sternum to back.

Constitutions - Hemorrhagic diathesis. Gouty, rheumatic, syphilitic diathesis.

Cough - Violent cough, worse morning. Dry, morning and evening, with soreness of larynx, or rawness in throat. Deep, hollow, with whitish and greenish sputum, and tearing pain starting from ensiform cartilage. Hoarse, with pain through chest.

Ears - Tearing pain in right ear. Boring pain in the ears. Otitis media. Membranae tympani depressed with adhesions. Noises in ear. Tinnitus. Deafness.

Eyes - Sunken eyes. Conjunctiva red. Puffy, burning, watery eyes. Profuse lachrymation. ***Syphilitic iritis***. Pustular keratitis and chemosis. Glaucoma. Pustules on cornea. Constant oscillations of the eyeballs. Winking is painful. Photophobia. Bony tumors of the orbit. Edema around eyes. Edema of eyelids with lachrymation. Lower lids twitch.

Face - Red face, with anxiety and restlessness. Blotches on cheeks. ***Facial neuralgias***. Sharp pain in upper jaw. Tight pain at zygomata. Glutinous mucus on lips in a.m. Dry, chapped lips. Swelling and suppuration of submaxillary glands.

Female - Menses late, profuse. Menses too scanty. Dysmenorrhea with great urging to urinate. Uterus feels as if squeezed during menses. Leucorrhea, corrosive like meat washing. Leucorrhea watery, acrid, milky white, green or yellow, purulent. Mucus discharge from vagina. Fibroid tumors. Metritis. Severe burning, tearing and twitching, in ovarian region. Swelling and congestion of ovaries.

Food - Aversion to all food, to broth. Much thirst. Cold food and drink aggravate. All symptoms worse by drinking cold milk.

Head - Headache and heaviness in head. Severe headache with lachrymation. Bilateral headaches. Violent headaches, as if screwed, through sides of head, worse warmth and pressure. Hard painful lumps on cranium with headache. Congestive headache. Aching pain in sinuses. ***Intense pain over eyes and root of nose.*** Sharp pain in forehead on stooping. Brain feels enlarged. Big head and small jaws, rickets. Pain in scalp on scratching, as if ulcerated. Meningitis. Hydrocephalus. Scalp fissured and sore. Tender spots on head. Hair changes color and falls off.

Heart - Heart feels very weak. Fluttering of heart with nervousness. Palpitations and darting pains worse when walking. Aneurysm. Endocarditis. Valvular defects after repeated endocarditis. Pulse weak, slow, soft.

Kidneys - Darting pains in kidney region. Nephritis with pains in back. Urine increased with unquenchable thirst. Painful urging to urinate, better appearance of menses. Frequent urination of copious, clear, urine, worse before menses, at night. Nocturnal bedwetting.

Limbs - Severe bone pains. Contraction of joints. Periosteum thickened, especially tibia, sensitive to touch (Kali-bi., Asaf.). Chronic arthritis. Rheumatic pains at night and in damp weather. ***Rheumatism of knees with effusion***. Pain in small of back and coccyx. Pain in hip, forcing limping. ***Sciatica,*** worse lying, on the affected side, sitting, standing, wakes him at night, better walking and flexing legs. Formication of lower limbs when sitting, better lying down. Tip of thumb ulcerates and turns yellow.

Lungs - Whistling asthmatic breathing. Asthma, of young people. Dyspnea on ascending with pain in heart. Difficult breathing on waking at night, with loss of voice. Air hunger with flatulency in a.m., wakes choking. ***Colds travels downward to chest.*** Dry bronchitis. Air passages raw. Violent cough, worse in morning. ***Expectoration like soap suds, greenish***. Pneumonia, when hepatization commences. ***Pneumococcic meningitis***. Stitching pains through lungs to back. Pulmonary edema with pneumonia. Pleuro-pneumonia. Lobular pneumonia. Hydrothorax (Merc., Sulph.). ***Pleuritic effusion.*** Tuberculosis, exhausting night sweats and loose stools. Sputum like soap-suds, green.

Male - Enlargement of prostate, with retention of urine. Chronic gonorrhea, discharge thick, green. Excoriation by least friction. Penis swollen, inflamed. Paraphimosis. Spermatic cords thickened. Atrophy of testes with diminution of sexual desire. Syphilis with indolent, swollen glands.

Modalities - Better from motion, cold, open air. Worse from heat, warm clothing or warm room, damp weather, changing weather. Worse pressure, touch, jarring, mercury, seaside, sunset to sunrise. Worse cold foods, especially milk.

Mouth - Offensive odor from mouth. Bitter taste, salty on waking. Increased saliva, bloody with a sweetish or disgusting taste. Saliva smells like onions. Viscid, salty saliva during pregnancy. Heat in whole mouth with swelling. Numbness of mouth, in morning on waking. Ulcers in mouth, as if coated with milk.

Nose - Red, swollen, especially the tip. ***Nasal catarrh involving frontal sinus.*** Burning, throbbing in nose and sinuses. Tightness at the root of the nose. Violent sneezing. Takes cold from every damp day. Coryza, descending, with salivation and dyspnea. ***Profuse, acrid, hot, watery discharge, worse cool air.*** Profuse, greenish, non-irritating discharges. Discharge of watery, cool, greenish, irritating, corroding mucus. Stuffiness and dryness of nose without discharge. ***Ozaena with perforated septum***. Takes cold from every damp day. Accumulation of very tenacious mucus in nostrils. Loss of smell.

Perspiration - Profuse night sweats, which relieve.

Rectum - Diarrhea with pain in lumber region, as if broken or as if menses would appear. Early morning diarrhea of tuberculosis. Frequent stools. Light-green or yellow watery stools. Constipation. Stools scanty, hard, difficult. Serous mucus from rectum. Cancer of rectum. Fissured anus of infants.

Sensations - As though head were enlarged, as if it were screwed in, as if a large quantity of water were forced into brain, as if it would be forced asunder. As if a leaflet were at root of nose, as if a worm was crawling at root of nose. Back as if in a vice. As of a tumor in ovaries. Pain in chest as if cut to pieces. Bruised feeling in coccyx.

Skin - Acne, hydroa. ***Acne rosacea***. Hives. Giant urticaria. Erythema nodosum. ***Rough nodules***. ***Small boils***. ***Itching eruptions worse heat.*** Itching, generally better scratching, worse at night. Itching herpes on face. Purple spots, worse on legs. Tendency to edematous swellings, eyelids, mouth, uvula, etc. Furuncular eruption. Pustular eruption, leaving scars. Rupia syphilitica. Vesicular eruptions. Vesicles from exposure to sun. Condylomata.

Sleep - Restless sleep. Frequent yawning without drowsiness. Sleeplessness from anguish. Weeps loudly during sleep, unconscious of it. Horrid dreams.

Stomach - Faintness at epigastrium. Emptiness and qualmish feeling, not better eating. Heartburn with flatulence. Throbbing, painful burning. Hiccough in evening. Sensation as if water brash is occurring. Nausea and vomiting with salivation. Violent vomiting with copious salivation. Rumbling and shrill noises in stomach. Flatulence.

Teeth - Toothache nagging, as if a worm were digging in it. Toothache at roots of teeth. Jerking toothache worse at night, better warmth. Teeth as if elongated. Teeth decayed. Gnawing pains. Gums recede from loose teeth. Gums swollen. Gumboils.

Temperature - Chilly in bones. Chilly in painful parts. Uncovers, then chilly. Chills with drowsiness. Alternate heat and chill. Heat with shudders. Fever in evening. Hot and dry, then drenching sweat. Fever with shuddering. Flushes, with dullness of head.

Throat - Dryness and itching in throat. Stinging pain when swallowing or talking. ***Larynx feels raw***. Laryngeal edema. Loss of voice. Sore throat of speakers. Hoarseness with pain in chest. Nasal, catarrhal voice. Choking sensation from increased mucus. Uvula swollen and elongated. Enlarged tonsils. Goiter sensitive to contact.

Tongue - Epithelioma of tongue. Blisters on tip of tongue, with burning pain. Tongue white, swollen, shows impressions of teeth. Severe pain at root of tongue, at night.

Vertigo - Vertigo in the dark. Vertigo, worse railway traveling. Vertigo with reeling, after meals. Vertigo on awaking, giddy, fluttering, must get up or smother.

Vision - Dim and foggy vision, after scrofulous ophthalmia. Blurred vision and diplopia, only notices when looking to left. Complete blindness from effusion of water in brain. Blindness with dilated pupils, staring, watery eyes.

COMMENTS – Kali-i. is used in both potency and the crude salt, the general explanation is that the solvent action of the drug is most powerfully excited on new tissues.

Cancer. Tumors of the breast and uterus. Condylomata. Glandular swelling. Thyroid problems or goiter, with green discharge. Enlarged lymphatic glands, syphilitic nodes.

Neuralgic or inflammatory conditions where there is heightened and diffused sensitiveness of the affected part. Serous effusion on the brain, secondary to hepatization of the lungs. Relieves the throbbing, pulsative noises, especially when the heart is hypertrophied and inclined to fatty degeneration.

Laryngeal and pulmonary tuberculosis. Deep, hollow, hoarse cough with pain through breast. Stitches through the lungs in the middle of sternum, through sternum to back or deep in chest while walking. Chest symptoms worse in early morning 2 a.m. to 5 a.m.

Expectoration is greenish, copious and looks like soapsuds. Chronic sinusitis. Thick, green mucus. Coryza recurs repeatedly from every little cold and makes the nose red and swollen.

Coryza, discharge is acrid, watery, the eyes smart and are puffed. Lachrymation. Iritis, keratitis and chemosis. Thick, green offensive discharge, ozaena and perforation of the bones may occur.

Scrofulous and syphilitic eruptions. Papular and pustular eruption, especially on scalp and down back, the pustules leaving scars when they heal. Tinnitus aurium, sharp, shrill, hissing and piercing noises.

Terrible pain at the root of the tongue. Disordered digestive tract. Loss of appetite and indigestion with flatulence and bloating (Lyc.). Loose stools at 5 a.m. (Merc.). May crave or be aggravated by milk.

Headache worse 5 a.m., worse after a night's rest, heat. The chill of intermittent fever is not better by warmth, but many symptoms of the teeth and scalp are alleviated by warmth.

Rickets. Sciatica (Naphtin.). Burning, better slow walking, worse sitting, at night, lying on painful side, rest, standing, heat (Rhus-t., better heat). General aversion to heat.

Motion aggravates, especially walking, after the first movement in the lower limbs it is more bearable. Sitting hurts and flexing limbs helps some of the pains. Worse from touch. Great sensitiveness to atmospheric changes, better in open air.

Especially suitable for pale, delicate subjects who flush easily and are manifestly plethoric. For a diffused arterial vasiculosis or venous state. Warm-blooded, violent, destructive people.

Several cases of abdominal tumor were successfully treated with Kali-i. in 3x, 10c and 15c triturations. Two of these had been unsuccessfully treated with the crude salt. Patients could not tolerate it on account of loss of appetite and irritation of the mucus membrane of mouth and throat.

One of these patients had a large tumor on the level of the great curvature of the stomach extending on both sides, plunging into the abdominal cavity and extending into the pelvis, it was adherent and difficult to define.

She had a jaundiced, dirty-looking skin and loss of appetite and vomited most of her food. A suspicion of latent syphilis led Gaudy to the remedy, which was perfectly tolerated in potency, though not in the crude. Health rapidly improved and in three months there was hardly any tumor to be discovered.

Cooper reported a second case in which a patient's womb was packed with fibroids and there was pain in the right inguinal region on exertion. Spirits were depressed, tinnitus like the buzzing of flies, constantly tired, sleepy feeling down the limbs, hot burning feet, though sometimes intense shivering all over. Pains in the breasts, which were tender.

Patient was unable to go long without food, constant distention as from flatus, sinking at scrobiculus cordis at 11 a.m., dreamy sleep. Kali-i. 30c left the patient in absolute comfort.

Cooper pointed out the characteristic diffused sensitiveness over affected parts that appeared in the provings. Hartlaub and Trinks noted the provers' experience of the painful scalp on scratching, as if ulcerated (after eleven days). Swelling of the whole thyroid gland increasing very rapidly with some sensitiveness to touch and pressure.

RELATIONS - ***Antidoted by:*** Hep., also Nit-ac. ***Antidote to:*** Merc., Lead poisoning. ***Compare:*** (1) Iod., Merc., Sulph., Mez. (2) Chopheenee - a Hindu remedy for syphilitic eruptions, ulcerations and bone-pains, used in tincture. (2) Iod. - goiter, heart affections, worse from warmth, tuberculosis. (3) Caust. - worse by touch, syphilis. (4) Kali-c. - worse from sex, worse 2-4 a.m., extreme sensitiveness. (5) Lach. - smothering sensation on waking and has hard lumps on scalp. (6) Kali-i. causes infiltration of bones as well as soft tissues. (7) Psor. and Gels. - in hay fever, Gels. has more sneezing. (8) Merc. - syphilis, catarrh, sensitiveness to weather, stitching pains through lungs. Merc. in different directions, Kali-i. through sternum to back. (9) Erio. "Yerba Santa" - catarrhal tuberculosis. (10) Ant-t. - threatened paralysis of lungs. (11) Ars. - catarrhal symptoms, wasting, restlessness. (12) Bell. - brain congestion. (13) Apis - dropsy, worse by heat. (14) Lyc. - flatulent distention. (15) Mez., Puls., Sil., Sulph., Cimic., Chin., Nat-s. (16) Carb-s. - nisus in the ears. ***Follows well:*** Merc. ***Followed well by:*** Nit-ac.

REFERENCES - Boericke. Clarke. Grimmer. Murphy. Phatak.

KALI MURIATICUM

(Potassium Chloride)

PHARMACY - kali-m. Kali muriaticum. Potassium chloride. Kali chloratum. Not to be confounded with Chlorate of potash, Kali chloricum. Trituration. Solution. ***Historical dose:*** Trituration and all potencies.

CLINICAL - Acne. ***Allergies.*** Aphthae. Breasts, cysts. Bubo. Bunion. Burns. Cataract. Chilblains. ***Colds.*** Constipation. ***Coryza.*** Croup. Cystitis. Diarrhea. Diphtheria. Dropsy. Dysentery. ***Ear, disorders.*** Eczema. Embolisms. ***Eustachian, congestion***. Eye, disorders. Glands, swollen. Hay fever. ***Hemorrhoids.*** Hodgkin's disease. Ingrown, toenails. Jaundice. Joints, stiff. Leucorrhea. Measles. Morning, sickness. Mumps. ***Nasal, congestion.*** Rheumatism. Scorbutus. Shingles. ***Sinusitis.*** Smallpox. Sycosis. Tendons, creaking. Thread-worms. Vaccination, effects. Warts.

HOMEOPATHIC - Schüssler introduced Kali-m. into homeopathy. His account of it is "it is contained in nearly all the cells and is chemically related to fibrin. It will dissolve white or grayish-white secretions of the mucus membrane and plastic exudations."

When the cells of the epidermis lose molecules of Kali-m. due to a morbid irritation, the fibrin comes to the surface as a white or whitish-gray mass. When dried, this forms a mealy covering. If the irritation affects the tissues under the epidermis, then fibrin and serum are exuded, causing the affected spot on the epidermis to rise in blisters. Similar processes may take place in and below epithelial cells.

Useful in ***catarrhal disorders*** in the subacute inflammatory states, fibrinous exudations and glandular swellings. ***Whiteness of secretions***, exudations, eruptions of tissues. Tough, fibrinous exudations and discharges. ***Milky white,*** viscid, sticky, thick, slimy or lumpy discharges. ***White or gray coating of base of tongue*** and expectoration of thick, white phlegm.

Blood clots too readily. Embolism, indurations, hard swellings. Hard deposits. glandular swelling. Sore, cutting or sticking, shifting pains. Bursitis, patellar. Crawling and numbness. Crosswise symptoms. Slow reaction. Stubborn infiltration.

MIND - Discontent, discouraged. Sadness alternating with cheerfulness. Fears evil. Sits in silence. Imagines he must starve. Irritable and angry, at trifles.

Abdomen - Abdominal tenderness and swelling, fullness after eating. Flatulence. Tensive pressure in region of liver, better emission of flatus. Pressing pain in region of spleen. Colic with shifting of flatulence. Colic with diarrhea. Colic in pelvic region. Catarrh of duodenum from chill. Peritonitis. Suppurating buboes.

Back - Heaviness under right shoulder. Buzzing under right scapula. Lightning pains from small of back to feet. Backache better lying down. Must get out of bed and sit up.

Bladder - Cystitis. Inflammation of bladder with violent fever. Acute cases of inflammation of bladder, when swelling has set in and discharge is thick, white mucus. Acute and chronic catarrh of bladder. Dribbling urination. Discharge of white, thick mucus. Itching in urethra.

Breasts - Breasts cysts. Soft, tender nodes or growths in breasts. Painful breasts before or at menses.

Causations - Ill effects of vaccination, sprains, burns, blows, cuts.

Chest - Rawness in chest. Flushes of heat in chest. Constriction of chest as from vapors of sulphur. Oppression of chest with violent palpitations.

Cough - Loud, noisy stomach cough. Cough short, acute, and spasmodic. Whooping cough. ***Sputum thick and white.*** Violent cough during coryza.

Ears - Otitis media. Swimmer's ear infection. Earache with swelling of glands. ***Eustachian tube blocked***. Soreness of Eustachian tube. ***Glue ear.*** Great effusion about the auricle. ***Catarrhal conditions of the middle ear***. Deafness from catarrhal condition and occlusion of Eustachian tubes. Deafness from swelling of internal ear. ***Sensation of a plug in ears.*** Snapping, popping noises in ear. Crackling noises on blowing nose or swallowing. Swollen glands about the ear. Threatened mastoiditis.

Eyes - Trachoma. Cataract. Corneal opacities, pustules. Exudation in retina. Scintillations on coughing. White mucus, purulent scabs. Superficial ulcer. Congestion to eyes, irritated. Redness with some pain. Sensation of sand in eye. Edges of eyelids scabby. Yellow crusts of pus on edges.

Face - Bluish, sunken. Cheeks swollen and painful. Lips hot, swollen. Chapped lips from cold. Eruptions around mouth. Pimples on forehead, face, lips and chin. Barber's itch. Swollen glands about jaw and neck. Face aches with swelling of gums or cheek. Mumps without fever. Paralysis, following pain in face. Paralysis of right facial nerve. Muscles of face twitch and tremble, worse eating, speaking or coughing. Lightning-like attacks of pain in face.

Female - Menses too late or suppressed, checked or too early. Excessive discharge, ***dark, clotted*** or tough. Menses black blood like tar (Plat.). Leucorrhea, discharge of milky-white mucus, thick, non-irritating, bland. Morning sickness with vomiting of white phlegm. Threatened miscarriage.

Food - Habitual loss of appetite or refuses food. ***Fatty or rich food causes indigestion***. Worse cold drinks.

Head - Confusion in head, also in occiput, with peculiar sensation in cervical muscles. ***Sick headache with white-coated tongue***. Headache with vomiting of white phlegm. ***Sinus headache with thick white discharge.*** Headache with sneezing and coryza. ***Catarrh of frontal sinuses.*** Aching pain in temple. Stunning shock in or a leaden load holds down occiput, better letting hair down and warmth. Brain feels loose. Meningitis. Crusta lactea. Copious white dandruff. Perspiration on head.

Heart - Heart disease causing dropsy. Coldness in region of heart. Pericarditis. Palpitations from excessive flow of blood to heart. Pulse accelerated, or soft and sluggish. Pulse not synchronous with beats of heart.

Kidneys - Kidney disease with dropsy. Catarrhal nephritis. Dribbling urine. Discharge white thick mucus. Turbid urine, with dirty yellow sediment. Diabetes. Albuminuria during pregnancy.

Limbs - Rheumatic fever. ***Swelling around joints***. Exudation and swelling around the joints. Rheumatic pains felt only during motion or increased by it. Nightly rheumatic pains, worse from warmth of bed. Lightning-like pains from small of back to feet, must get out of bed and sit up. ***Cramps in limbs.*** Twitching thighs. Tension in leg alternating with tension in arm. Cutting in bones. Bursitis. Cold foot sweat. Cold hands and feet. Chilblains on hands or feet or any part. Cracking of tendons in the back of the hand. Hands get stiff while writing or knitting.

Liver - Liver disease with dropsy. Jaundice, caused by a chill, resulting in catarrh of duodenum. Sluggish action or complete torpidity of liver. Pain in right side.

Lungs - Difficult or oppressed breathing. Asthma with gastric derangements, mucus white and hard to cough up. Rattling sounds of air passing through thick, tenacious mucus in the bronchi, difficult to cough up. ***Catarrhal pneumonia.*** Bronchitis. Croupy inflammation of lungs. ***Mucus white, thick and hard to cough up.*** Yellowish green mucus. Expectoration sticky, milky or flies from the mouth. Hemorrhage from lungs.

Male - Chronic syphilis. ***Gonorrhea.*** Gleet combined with eczema, visible or latent. Soft swelling of buboes, soft chancre. Condylomata. Hydrocele. Itching of scrotum. Orchitis from suppressed gonorrhea. Violent emissions with voluptuous dreams. Violent erections with emissions. Sexual desire diminished, with chilliness and apathy.

Modalities - Better from cold drinks, rubbing, letting hair down. Worse from open air, drafts, dampness, night. Worse cold drinks, fatty, rich food or pastry. Worse motion, sprains, lying, during menses. Rheumatic symptoms worse from warmth of bed.

Mouth - Aphthae. Thrush, white ulcers in the mouth. Eruptions around the mouth. Breath excessively fetid, in ulceration and diphtheria. Profuse and acid saliva. Accumulation of mucus. Salty, bitter taste, with coldness of tongue. Heat and dryness in mouth. Swollen glands about jaw and neck. Scorbutic gums. Gumboil before matter forms. Toothache with swelling of the gums and cheeks.

Nose - Nasal catarrh. Stuffy cold in head. Hawking of mucus from posterior sinuses. Phlegm or catarrh, ***white and thick discharges***. Vault of pharynx covered with adherent crust. Nosebleeds (Arn., Phos.).

Perspiration - Sweating of head.

Rectum - Constipation, light-colored stools. Diarrhea after fatty food. Dysentery, purging with slimy stools. ***Hemorrhoids***, bleeding, blood dark and thick, fibrinous, clotted. Anus sore, worse walking or after stools. Itching or crawling in anus after stools. Threadworms, causing itching at anus.

Skin - Chickenpox. Smallpox. Blisters arising from burns. Acne. Pimples on face, neck, etc. Erythema. Herpes zoster. Vesicular erysipelas and shingles. Eczema from suppressed or deranged uterine functions. ***Vesicles containing thick, white contents***. Itching of whole body, in bed. Dry, flour-like scales on the skin (Ars.). Greenish, brownish, yellow crusts. Branny. Proud flesh. Carbuncles. Condylomata. Warty excrescences. Eruptions connected with stomach or menstrual disorders.

Sleep - Restless sleep, startled at least noise. Anxious dreams, towards morning. Somnolence.

Stomach - Dyspepsia and indigestion, with a whitish-gray tongue. Cutting pain in stomach. Eructations alternating with pains in chest and abdomen. Empty, sour eructations. Empty feeling in stomach. Pain in the stomach with constipation. Bulimia, hunger disappears by drinking water. Sick feeling after taking fat. ***Fatty or rich food causes indigestion***. Morning sickness with vomiting of white phlegm. Nausea with eructations. Nausea with shivers. Stomach heavy, at night. Vomits food. Vomiting of white, opaque mucus, blood.

Stools - Pale, light-colored, hard or flocculent stools. Stools clay-colored, white, or slimy. Painful stools, passing nothing but mucus. Bloody stools, or bloody mucus. Stools so dry it almost crumbles.

Temperature - Shivering all over, or over back and neck, with warm feet. Continual chilliness with stiffness of hands, with vomiting of white (not transparent) mucus, in open air.

Throat - Chronic sore throat. ***"Hospital"*** sore throat. Croup, membranous exudation. Loss of voice, hoarseness. ***Follicular tonsillitis***. Tonsils swollen, inflamed, swallowing excessively painful. Tonsils enlarged, can hardly breathe. Grayish-white, ulcerated throat. Adherent crusts in vault of pharynx. Pharynx feels cold. Eustachian catarrh. Hawks out thick, white mucus, cheesy.

Tongue - ***Grayish-white, sticky, thick, slimy,*** or dry coating on tongue. Tongue mapped, gray or white at base. Tongue white, or only in middle. Coating of tongue after diarrhea. Coldness of tongue. Sensation as if a tumor were growing on the tongue. Glossitis. Burning, stinging blisters on tongue.

Vertigo - Vertigo after violent exercise. Vertigo with congestion to head. Vertigo during headache.

Vision - Scintillations on coughing or sneezing. Smoky and misty vision. Letters appear smaller when reading.

COMMENTS - Chronic catarrhal condition of the middle ear. Eustachian tube catarrh (Merc-d.). Closed Eustachian tubes. Pain in ears during pressure changes. Snapping and noises in the ear.

Common cold with yellow or watery mucus. A milky, white, thick discharge, can be lumpy or stringy. Grayish white, dry or slimy tongue. Bleeding hemorrhoids, dark, fibrous, clotted blood. Diphtheria. Rheumatic fever with exudation and swelling around the joints. Better from cold drinks.

It is said to have cured cataracts after Calc-fl. helped. Clarke cured with it rheumatism affecting mostly the left shoulder and the elbow, worse in the morning on rising. There is some clinical evidence of helping breast cysts.

Boericke and Dewey noted the "protruded appearance of eyes, white tongue, croupy, hard cough, harsh barking."

Hering added "cough, noisy with protruded appearance of eyes." In one case, it caused a severe aggravation in which the patient felt "as if eyes would be forced out of head with cough."

Similar to Kali-chl, which has the keynote symptom "tendency to rush of blood to both eyes and light before both eyes on coughing and sneezing."

RELATIONS - ***Antidoted by:*** Bell., Calc-s., Hydr., Puls. ***Compare:*** (1) Bell., which Kali-m. follows well in the catarrhal and hypertrophic conditions. (2) Kino - otorrhea with stitches in right ear. (3) Bry., Merc., Puls., Sulph. (4) Kali-chl. in tough secretions, Kali-bi., Kali-c., Hydr. (5) in rheumatic affections, Bry., Rhus-t., Sulph. (6) Merc-d. in the Eustachian tube and in inflammations of ear. (7) Graph., Nat-m., Nit-ac., Sil., Apis, Thuj. (8) Puls. in worse from fatty food, worse from warmth. ***It follows well:*** Calc-p. Calc-fl., Ferr-p.

REFERENCES - Boericke. Clarke. Murphy. Phatak.

KALI NITRICUM

(Potassium Nitrate)

PHARMACY - kali-n. Kali nitricum. Potassium nitrate. Saltpetre. Nitre. Trituration. Solution. ***Historical dose:*** Trituration and all potencies.

CLINICAL - Asthma. Bedwetting. Chest, pain. Colic. Debility. Diabetes, insipidus. ***Dropsy.*** Dysentery. Dysmenorrhea. Gastritis. Headaches. Heart, disorders. Hemorrhages. Herpes. Meniere's disease. Menorrhagia. Nephritis. Nosebleeds. Peritonitis. Pleurisy. Pneumonia. Polyps. Rheumatism. Tuberculosis. Vertigo.

HOMEOPATHIC - The Saltpetre of the Alchemists, Kali-n. is known in old-school practice principally as a "refrigerant diuretic" and as the active agent in the well known "nitre papers," which are burnt, producing fumes to allay attacks of asthma.

A solution of saltpetre as an application was an old remedy for inveterate mange in cats. Nitre with sulphur and charcoal forms gunpowder. A teaspoonful of this in hot water was a favorite remedy for gonorrhea among soldiers in the days when black powder was used.

Affects the respiratory organs, kidneys, heart and blood vessels. Secretions are increased into cavities. Sudden ***dropsical swellings over the whole body***. Pains are dull stitching, throbbing. Wooden, numbness. Very weak.

Asthma and cardiac asthma. Relapsing tuberculosis. Hemorrhagic tendency. Rheumatism. Gastro-intestinal inflammation with much debility and relapse in tuberculosis. Suppurative nephritis. Incontinence of urine in children.

MIND - Peevish, fretful. Bored. Mental weariness from lack of occupation or interest. Discouragement. Sadness when alone. Aversion to thinking in morning. Fear of death. Anxiety and congestion to chest. Anxiety during headache.

Abdomen - Excessive distention of abdomen. Griping about umbilicus. Stitching and sticking pains. Violent pain in right side after eating veal. Peritonitis. Incarceration of flatus, especially in afternoon and evening. Very loud rumbling in abdomen.

Back - Aching in lumbar region. Pains in back on stooping. Shootings in and between scapula. Pains extend into the chest. Shooting pains in sacral region. Violent pains in loins on waking. Feeling in back as if kidneys engorged.

Chest - Chest feels constricted. Oppression on chest, when ascending. Contractive pain in chest. Sticking in left side near sternum. Inflammation of lungs.

Constitutions - Suited to asthmatic constitutions and chest complaints.

Ears - Shooting in ears. Inflammation and swelling of lobe of right ear. Chronic deafness from paralysis of auditory nerve. Vertigo and tinnitus. Tinkling and ringing in ears.

Eyes - Burning in eyes, with lachrymation and photophobia. External angle of right eye twitches, worse chewing. Vision becomes clouded. Turbid corpus vitreum (Arn., Ham., Phos.). Transient blindness. Colored circles before eyes. In evening, candles appear surrounded by a rainbow-like halo.

Female - ***Profuse menses, black like ink.*** Menses too early, profuse, preceded and with violent backache. Burning pains in the ovarian region only during menses (Zinc. after menses). Leucorrhea.

Food - Better hot food. Aversion to beef, eggs, meat, veal. ***Worse from eating veal,*** causing headache, diarrhea. Worse from cold food, fats, rich food, milk. Worse from beef, fish, lobster, oysters. Worse from beer, wine, bread, coffee, rice, soup, watery fruits and vegetables.

Head - Headache with vertigo, as if falling to right side and backwards, worse stooping. Head pain, better motion of carriage. Pains in occiput, better letting hair down. Scalp very sensitive.

Heart - Violent stitch in precordia and beating of heart. Palpitations, worse lying. ***Pulse is weak, small*** and thready.

Kidneys - Diabetes insipidus. Dull kidney pains. Burning in urethra while urinating and greatly diminished urine. Frequent and profuse emission of clear urine.

Limbs - Drawing in limbs with paralytic weakness. Rheumatic pains and stitches in limbs and joints. Stitches between shoulder blades. Tearing and sticking in shoulders and joints. Hands and fingers seem swollen.

Lungs - Rapid gasping breathing, sits upright. Congestion of right lung. Dyspnea so great that breath cannot be held long enough to drink, though thirsty. ***Asthma*** with excessive dyspnea, nausea, dull stitches and burning in chest. ***Spasmodic croup***, paroxysm of crowing. Bronchitis with sharp, short, dry, hacking cough. Acute exacerbations in tuberculosis. Dry, morning cough with pain in the chest and bloody expectoration. Sour-smelling expectoration. Expectoration of clotted blood after hawking mucus.

Modalities - Better lying down, lying on right side, uncovering head, gentle motion, drinking water in sips. Worse cold, damp, taking cold, morning, afternoon. Worse lying with head low, walking, breathing, eating veal, coffee, wine, beer.

Mouth - Tongue loaded with a white coating. Tongue red with burning pimples. Burning blister at tip of tongue. Crawling on tongue. Taste disagreeable, nauseous, disgusting, sour. Fetid breath. Throat constricted and sore.

Nose - Violent coryza with obstruction of nose, and loss of smell. Sneezing. Swollen feeling, worse in the ***right nostril***. Burning in nose with digging and clawing pain. The nasal bones are painful, especially to the touch. Swelling of interior of nose. Ulcers in the nostrils covered by a scurf. Nosebleed with acrid blood. Polyps (Thuj., Sang-n.). Point red and itching.

Perspiration - Profuse perspiration every alternate night (Nit-ac.).

Rectum - Frequent pressing in rectum. Urgent want to evacuate with tenesmus. Dysentery with much cutting pain, great thirst and icy coldness of feet. ***Diarrhea from eating veal***. Membranous shreds with tenesmus. Thin, watery dark, bloody stools. Feces difficult, and retarded, evacuated with much effort. Hard like sheep's dung.

Skin - Lancinations in skin. Pricking like needles, followed by burning. Tubercles, size of a pea. Burning vesicles filled with yellowish serum, which break when scratched. Sudden dropsical swelling.

Sleep - Drowsiness during day. Disturbed sleep at night, constant dreaming, with frequent awakening. Anxious and uneasy dreams about dangerous situations. Nightmare. Coma.

Stomach - Faint-like weakness at stomach pit. Epigastric or sub-sternal pains go towards axilla. Gnawing, spasmodic weakness, and pressure on epigastrium. Burning in stomach. Severe pain after every meal. Nausea, as if about to vomit worse at night. Ineffectual retching. Vomiting of mucus, mixed with blood.

Teeth - Toothache, with sharp drawing, or tearing pains in teeth and head. Shooting in carious teeth, when touched. Pulsative toothache, at night, worse by cold things. Swelling of gums, of an inflammatory or scorbutic character, they bleed readily.

Temperature - External coldness, chin, skin. Extraordinary shiverings not better by hot drinks or coverings. Coldness in afternoon with thirst, or coldness, preceded by headache. Quotidian fever, with drawing pains in limbs. Profuse and colliquative sweat. Sweat in morning, especially on chest. Internal burning.

Throat - Laryngeal diphtheria. Sore throat with shooting pain. Nocturnal pain in throat, as if it were contracting. Impeded swallowing from tension and cutting in the larynx. Hoarseness. Loss of speech.

Vertigo - Fainting fits with vertigo in morning, worse on standing, better sitting down. Vertigo and tinnitus.

COMMENTS - Kali-n. has been extensively proved by homeopaths and symptoms have been added from cases of poisoning, so that its characteristics are well defined. It is almost equal to Kali-c. in producing stitching pains and it is similar to it in having a cough at 3 a.m.

Severe stitching, cutting, lancinating, tearing and pressing pains. As with many other Kalis, there is external sensitiveness of scalp, of abdomen, of testes.

Diabetes insipidus. Bedwetting. Painful colic. Diarrhea and dysentery. Sexual excitement. Pain in testes and cords. Menorrhagia with flow of ink-like blackness.

"The pain-like contraction in the eyes, forehead and face concentrates in the tip of the nose. Swollen feeling in right nostril, which is painful on pressure, sore pain in upper part of right nostril with external sensitiveness," these two last symptoms led to the cure of large nasal polyps in a girl.

In a poisoning case, during the recovery there was intense vertigo with tinnitus, which should indicate Kali-n. in some cases of Meniere's disease. Easy intoxication by wine or beer was noted by several provers. A peculiar symptom is a sour taste in the throat.

In the asthmatic state the breathlessness is so great that the patient, though thirsty, can only drink a sip at a time between the breaths. Allen defined the asthma of Kali-n. as asthma with excessive dyspnea, faintness and nausea with dull stitches or with burning pain in chest, rather free expectoration.

RELATIONS - ***Antidotes:*** Op., Nit-s-d. It antidotes opium or morphine poisoning, 8 to 10 grains to glass of water. ***Compare:*** (1) Cann-s. which contains a large amount of Kali-n. (2) Lyc., Sang., All-s., Ant-i.

REFERENCES - Boericke. Clarke. Phatak.

KALI OXALICUM

(Potassium Bioxalate)

PHARMACY - kali-ox. Kali oxalicum. Potassium bioxalate. Kali oxalas. Salts of sorrel. Trituration. Solution. ***Historical dose:*** All potencies.

CLINICAL - Convulsions. Cramps. Eyes inflamed. Lumbago. Vomiting.

HOMEOPATHIC - Only cases of poisoning have been observed with this salt. The main symptoms of Kali-ox. are those of violent irritation. Convulsions. Violent and continuous vomiting. Throbbing in the head with great thirst. Cramps. Severe pains in the back (Ox-ac., Rumx-a.). Coldness and collapse. One patient became insane.

MIND - Extreme depression. Insanity.

Abdomen - Violent pains in abdomen and convulsions. Scalding sensation extended over abdomen with tenderness on tolerably firm pressure.

Back - Pain in back. Severe lumbar pain.

Bladder - Urination accompanied by a sensation of scalding.

Eyes - Great soreness of eyes with dim vision. Conjunctive injected, pupils dilated.

Face - Countenance flushed. Face pale, anxious-looking and covered with a cold sweat. Face and lips pale with continual riggers over whole body.

Food - Great thirst and throbbing pain in head.

Head - Swimming in head, heaviness, throbbing pain and great thirst.

Kidneys - Urination accompanied by a sensation of scalding.

Limbs - Spasmodic contractions in hands. Great weakness in lower limbs. Cramps in legs. Muscular weakness. Falls and utters loud cries. Tendency to faint. Lying on the floor quite faint. Nails and fingers blue.

Mouth - Tongue and fauces red and irritable. Very strong acid taste of poison lasting two days.

Skin - Cold and clammy.

Stomach - Vomiting and faintness. Vomiting, continuing at intervals of ten minutes to an hour for nearly a week. Very severe burning pain in stomach and bowels. Excruciating pain, followed by violent convulsions and death.

Temperature - Sensations of coldness, succeeded by burning heat in chest and stomach and general muscular weakness. Continued rigors affecting whole body.

Throat - Scalding sensation in throat and stomach.

REFERENCES - Clarke.

KALI PERMANGANICUM

(Potassium Permanganate)

PHARMACY - kali-perm. Kali permanganicum. Potassium permanganate. Permanganate of potash. Kali manganicum. Kali hypermanganicum. Solution in distilled water. Trituration. ***Historical dose:*** Trituration and all potencies.

CLINICAL - ***Bites.*** Cough. ***Diphtheria.*** Gastritis. Opium poisoning. Ozaena. Salivation. ***Snakebites.*** Throat, sore. Uvula, swollen. Warts.

HOMEOPATHIC - Kali-perm. is a well-known disinfectant and has been chiefly used in medicine as a local application in diphtheria and other conditions where there are fetid discharges. Kali-perm. counteracts the effects of alkaloids of many poisonous plants owing to its oxidizing powers, if given before the alkaloid has been absorbed.

A case of opium poisoning is reported in which an ounce of laudanum had been swallowed by mistake. Kali-perm. in dilute solution (2 grains to the pint) was given repeatedly and acted promptly. The next day, only dryness of mouth and throat was felt. Intense irritation of nose, throat and larynx.

Kraft, who used it largely in ***diphtheria***, dissolved a few grains in a tumbler of water, sufficient to make it very red. A teaspoonful of this was put into another tumbler of water and a teaspoonful out of the second tumbler was given every hour or two.

Various septic conditions, the tissues are infiltrated with tendency to sloughing. ***Bites of snakes and for other animal poisons*** (Led.). Dysmenorrhea.

Diphtheria, with extreme fetor of the breath and bloody discharges from the nose and intense prostration. Intense irritation of nose, throat and larynx with bloody and bloody discharges and constant inclination and constant flow of ropy mucus from the stomach. The uvula was swollen and red.

Back - Muscles of neck feel sore.

Chest - Aching in region of cricoid cartilage, worse every attempt to swallow.

Ears - Sharp pricking pains extending from throat to left mastoid process, apparently along Eustachian tube.

Eyes - Profuse lachrymation.

Face - Face hot.

Food - Appetite lost. Thirst, inability to drink.

Head - Head feels full.

Kidneys - Compelled to urinate frequently. Urine copious, clear, watery.

Limbs - Legs feel as though he could not move them, tremble on attempting to stand.

Lungs - Short, hacking cough, with a constant, painful urging to swallow, with blood-streaked sputa.

Mouth - Fetor of breath. Mouth and lips very dry, lips smart when exposed to cold air. Increased flow of saliva runs constantly out of the mouth. Swollen uvula. Speech painful, difficult, hoarse.

Nose - Posterior sinuses painful. Nasal discharge smart and irritates. Bloody discharge, nose feels stuffed and full as in catarrh. Profuse bleeding from nose.

Rectum - Obstinate constipation.

Skin - Profuse sweat.

Sleep - Restless at night. Sleepless.

Stomach - Hot, burning pain in stomach. Sickening pain in stomach. Nausea and constant inclination to swallow. Nausea and vomiting.

Throat - Constrictive, smarting sensation in throat. Swollen and painful. Larynx feels raw. Everything hawked up streaked with blood. Constant inclination to swallow.

COMMENTS - Potassium permanganate is recognized as being the most effective chemical antidote in cases of morphine or opium poisoning, acting directly on the morphine and oxidizing it to less toxic substances.

To be effective, the permanganate must come in direct contact with the opium or morphine in the stomach. The treatment is administration of two to five grains of potassium permanganate in dilute aqueous solution as soon as possible after the poison is taken, this amount to be increased if very large doses of the poison have been taken.

Washing out the stomach with a quantity of 1 to 500 solution of permanganate is also recommended, using at least a pint of this solution either by a stomach pump or by enforced vomiting.

RELATIONS - Kali-perm. antidotes opium. ***Compare:*** (1) Other oxidizing salts, especially Kali-bi., also Mang., Caust., Kali-c. (2) in edematous uvula, Mur-ac., Apis. (3) in diphtheria, Diph., Merc-cy., Arum-t., Kali-bi., Kali-m., (4) in thick, ropy mucus, Kali-bi.

REFERENCES - Boericke. Clarke.

KALI PHOSPHORICUM

(Potassium Phosphate)

PHARMACY - kali-p. Kali phosphoricum. Potassium phosphate. Trituration. Solution in distilled water. ***Historical dose:*** Trituration and all potencies.

CLINICAL - Agoraphobia. Alopecia, areata. Amenorrhea. Anemia. Aphthae. Asthma. Atrophy. Bedwetting. Brain, concussion. ***Brain-fag.*** Brain, softening. Cancrum oris. Carbuncle. ***Cerebral, anemia***. Chilblains. Cholera. Constipation. Coughs. Diarrhea. Diphtheria. Dysentery. Dyspepsia. Emaciation. Enterocolitis. Erysipelas. Face, neuralgia. ***Fatigue.*** Feet, fidgety. Gangrene. Hay fever. ***Headaches.*** Hernia. Hypochondriasis. Hysteria. Impotency. ***Insomnia.*** Leucorrhea. Leukemia. Melancholia. ***Memory, weak.*** Menstrual, disorders. Miscarriage. ***Nervous, prostration***. ***Neurasthenia. Night-terrors.*** Noma. Nosebleeds. Nymphomania. Ozaena. Palpitations. Paralysis. Pemphigus. Pneumonia. Ptosis. Puerperal fever. Puerperal mania. Pulmonary, edema. Seasickness. Sciatica. Scurvy. Stomach, ulcer. Typhoid fever. Typhus fever. Ulcers. Urticaria. Vertigo. ***Weakness.*** Whitlow. Whooping cough.

HOMEOPATHIC - Schüssler used this remedy for conditions arising from want of nerve power. According to Schüssler, Kali-p. is contained in the cells of the brains, nerves, muscles, blood (corpuscles and plasma) and intercellular fluids.

A disturbance in the motions of its molecules produces despondency, anxiety, fearfulness, fearfulness, homesickness, suspiciousness, agoraphobia, and weak memory. There is at first a small and frequent pulse, later it is retarded.

Pain with sensation of paralysis in sensory nerves. Weakness of muscles and nerves even to paralysis. Retarded nutrition, even total arrest in a limited area of cells and then a softening.

Cases in which there is increased sensitivity to all impressions from a weakness of the vital resistance or control. In weakened states from mental or physical shock, from over strain or over drain of the system.

H. T. Doge noted that it is indicated for worn-out nursing mothers, tired to distraction by nervous babies. Worn-out business and professional men or women, or students. Doge recommended the higher potencies where indications are close.

Characteristic low, nervous condition. Generally ***nervous, sensitive, weak and easily fagged*** by slight causes like pain, worry, mental fatigue etc. Conditions arising from ***lack of nerve power***, neurasthenia, and mental and physical depression. ***Nervous prostration***. Weak and tired.

Marked disturbance of the sympathetic nervous system, usually from excitement, overwork and worry. Convalescence after exhausting diseases. Muscular weakness after acute diseases. States of ***weakness and decay***, gangrenous conditions. Suspected malignant tumors. Delayed labor.

Putrid, carrion like odor of secretions, foul odor of the body. Foul breath, with brownish mustard-like coat on the tongue. ***Secretions are golden yellow.*** Emaciation, wasting diseases. After surgery, when in the healing process ***the skin is drawn tight*** over the wound, especially cancer.

Stitching pains. Dull, heavy ache between the shoulders. Paralytic weakness or pain with sensation of paralysis. Paralysis infantile during dentition. Nervous, restless, fidgety feeling in feet, trembling sensation in muscles of legs. Numb sensations.

Sexual excitement from indulgence or suppression. Irregular, menses, pulse, etc. Seasickness without nausea. Especially adapted to the young.

MIND - ***Mental and physical prostration*** caused by a combination of ***overworking*** and psychological factors like excitement, worry and vexation. Mental fatigue from over study or overwork. ***Brain fatigue. Mental exertion aggravates.***

Ailments from strong emotions, fright, grief, care. Extreme lassitude and depression, lethargy, gloom. Morose. Great despondency about business. ***Slightest labor seems a heavy task***. Dullness of mind. Weak memory. Forgetful, loss of memory.

Shyness, disinclined to converse. Indisposition to meet people or to talk with them. Sighing or moaning. Homesickness. Sadness on waking. Weariness of life and fear of death. Negative, dark forebodings.

Very nervous, starts easily. Anxiety and worry. ***Anxiety with nervous dread***. Apprehensive about future. Fear of being alone, open spaces, crowds. Fear about his health, of death.

Angry. Irritability when spoken to. Impatience about trifles. Gloomy moods. Dwelling upon grievances. Suspicious. Obstinate. Perverted affections. Aversion to own family, cruel to husband, baby.

Easily frightened. Starting from noise, when touched. Sensitive to light and noise, especially during menses. Disposition to feel bodily pains too acutely. Oversensitive children. Children cry and scream, fly into passion, can hardly articulate. ***Night terrors***. Shyness, excessive blushing, from undue sensitiveness.

Hysterical fits of laughter and crying. Weeping about trifles. Religious melancholy, believes she is eternally and irretrievably damned. Continually weeping and crying. Wringing hands. Tears things. Pulling to pieces and tearing her clothing, as well as bed covering. Doesn't recognize her surroundings.

Abdomen - Abdomen feels cold, better covering. Cutting pain in abdomen. Affections of spleen. Splenic leukemia. Enterocolitis. Hernia. Flatulence with distress about heart.

Back - Stiffness of back after rest, better gentle motion. Paralytic lameness of back, must lean on a chair. Rheumatic pains and weakness. Spinal irritation. Creeping sensation and intense pain along spine, relieves the headache.

Constitutions - Weak nervous system and brain. Suited to pale, sensitive, irritable persons.

Causations - Ill effects of mechanical injuries, grief, or vexation. Mental overwork.

Chest - Pain in lower part of left chest, worse coughing. Axillary sweat smells of onions.

Ears - Ulceration of the eardrum and middle ear suppurations, with foul discharge. ***Sensitive hearing, cannot endure noise.*** Noises in ears from nervous exhaustion. Noises in head on falling asleep. ***Humming and buzzing*** in the ears. Deafness from atrophic condition of nerve.

Eyes - Burn, sting, with a lot of tears. Yellow-gray milky secretion. Retinitis. Drooping of eyelids, especially the left (Caust.). Squint after brain diseases. Weakness of vision. Loss of perceptive power, after diphtheria from exhaustion. Black spots before eyes.

Face - Sad, careworn look. Livid and sunken with hollow eyes. Neuralgia of face followed by great weakness. Right-sided neuralgia, relieved by cold applications. Sharp pains from riding in cold air. Brown stripe at the edge of hair.

Female - Delayed menses with depression. Menses irregular. ***Menses too late or too scanty*** in pale, irritable, sensitive, lachrymose females. Menses, too profuse discharge. Menses, deep-red or black-red, thin and not coagulating. Menses, sometimes with offensive odor. ***Horribly foul leucorrhea.*** Periodical discharge of copious orange colored fluid from vagina and rectum. Intense sexual desire for days after the menses. Tired, worn out, nervous women, subject to miscarriage. Feeble and ineffectual labor pains. Puerperal fever with absurd notions or mania.

Food - Hungry soon after eating. Wants to eat almost every hour. No appetite except for sweets. Craves ice cold water, cold drinks, vinegar, sweets. Aversion to food, bread and meat.

Head - Excruciating nervous headache with great sensitiveness to noise. ***Headache of students, worse mental exertion.*** Occipital pain, better after rising. Pains and weight at back of head, with feeling of weariness and exhaustion. ***Cerebral anemia***. Headache with weary, empty, gone feeling at stomach (Ign., Sep.), with hunger. Headaches worse before and during menses. Headache are relieved by gentle motion.

Heart - Sluggish circulation in sensitive, nervous subjects. Weak action of heart causes fainting. Palpitations with shortness of breath, with nervousness, anxiety, sleeplessness Palpitations, worse slightest motion or ascending stairs. Intermittent action of heart from violent emotions, fright, grief, care. Pulse irregular.

Kidneys - Nocturnal bedwetting, in nervous, excitable children and in old people. Incontinence of urine. ***Very yellow urine***, saffron yellow or milky. Bleeding from urethra. Urine comes in stops and starts.

Limbs - Paralytic lameness in back and limbs. Paralyzing pain in limbs, better motion and external warmth, worse during rest. Exertion aggravates. Pains with depression and subsequent exhaustion. Prickling in hands and feet. Numb fingertips. Feet fidgety. Chilblains. Foot feels frostbitten. Pains in soles.

Lungs - Nervous asthma, least food aggravates. Short breath, worse going upstairs. ***Cough with yellow expectoration***. ***Whooping cough*** in highly nervous patients with great exhaustion. Frothy, expectoration with pulmonary edema.

Male - Nocturnal emissions. Sexual excitement. Impotency. Sexual power diminished. Prostration and weak vision after sex or after nightly emissions (Kali-c.).

Modalities - Better from warmth, rest, sleep, gentle motion, leaning against something. Better from nourishment, eating, when menses comes. ***Worse mental and physical exertion, anxiety and worry.*** Worse from slight causes. Worse from cold, dry air, cold drinks, eating. Worse puberty, sex, excitement, touch, pain, early morning.

Mouth - Aphthae. ***Breath offensive, fetid***. Palate feels greasy. ***Mouth excessively dry***, in morning. Gums, spongy, receding, with bright-red seam. Noma. Slow speech, becoming inarticulate. Nervous, chattering of teeth.

Nose - Hay fever with nervous irritability. Hay fever, as a prophylactic. Itching in posterior sinuses. Violent sneezing with symptoms of fresh cold, at 2 a.m. Ozaena. Nasal disease with offensive odor. Fetid discharge. Nosebleeds.

Perspiration - Excessive, exhausting, strong-smelling sweats. Axillary sweat smells of onions.

Rectum - ***Diarrhea, foul, putrid odor.*** Diarrhea caused by fright. Diarrhea with depression and exhaustion. Brain affection with diarrhea smelling like carrion. Diarrhea, at night and after eating. Dysentery, stools consist of pure blood, patient becomes delirious, abdomen swells. Cholera, rice water stools (Verat., Ars., Jatr.). Hot, golden yellow stools. Painless stools. Prolapse rectum (Ign., Podo.). Paretic condition of rectum and colon after removal of hemorrhoids.

Sensations - As if tongue would cleave to root of mouth, as if a ball were rising in throat, as if a rocket had passed through head.

Skin - Skin diseases with bad smelling discharge. Greasy, offensive smelling crusts or scales. Ulcers, ichorous, bad smelling. Vesicles with bloody, ichorous contents. Pemphigus. Urticaria. Erysipelas bordering on gangrene. Gangrene. Blue spots on skin. Skin inactive. Cold skin. Jaundiced.

Sleep - Drowsy. Yawning. ***Sleeplessness from worry, over study, business troubles.*** Sleeplessness from overactive mind. Restlessness and heat during sleep. Sleepwalking. Sighing and moaning during sleep. Amorous dreams. ***Night terrors.*** Awakening with fright and screaming. Loss of sleep.

Stomach - Indigestion with great nervous depression. Gastritis with failing strength. Nervous, gone sensation at the pit of stomach, better eating (Ign., Sep., Sulph.).

Hungry soon after eating. Feels seasick without nausea. Nausea, better belchings, worse coughing.

Teeth - Nervous chattering of teeth. Toothache, with easily-bleeding gums. Gums spongy and receding (Caps., Ham., Lach.). Toothache of highly nervous, delicate, pale, irritable, sensitive persons.

Temperature - Subnormal temperature. Yellow fever.

Throat - Aphonia. Paralysis of vocal cords. Hoarseness from overexertion of voice. Croup, last stage. Sensation as if a ball rising in throat. Gangrenous sore throat.

Tongue - Tongue coated brownish, yellow like liquid mustard. Sensation as if tongue would adhere to roof of mouth from dryness of mouth. Creeping paralysis of the tongue.

Vertigo - Vertigo from fatigue, from lying down, when facing the sun, on standing up from sitting, when looking upward (Gran.).

COMMENTS - Chronic fatigue from excessive mental work or over-exertion of the mind; the mind and nervous system become weak. Mental fatigue. Headaches from over studying. Nervous insomnia (Aven.). Memory loss and difficultly concentrating in the elderly. Pain in the back of neck and head. General irritability, great despondency.

Depressed states of mind and body. Hypochondriasis, hysteria. Neurasthenia. Great lassitude, emaciation. Nervous, hot, restless, easily startled. The least touch causes starting. Trembling of hands from nervousness. Stitching pains. Numb fingertips.

Spasms of irritable weakness, paralysis. Progressive muscular atrophy, around ulcer of stomach. Typhoid, typhus fever. Septic states, septic fevers and hemorrhages. Phagedenic chancre, carbuncles. Toothache alternating with headache. Alopecia areata. Scurvy.

Menstrual headaches, backaches with menses. Severe vaginitis with yellow-brown, offensive discharge (Kreos.). Worse after sex and sensitiveness to touch. Aching in sacrum. Frequent urination, passing large quantities night and day, containing phosphates.

H. C. Allen noted the indications of waking in the early morning, the peculiar mouth and the severe action on the skin. Characteristic golden or orange-yellow color. Urine is very yellow. Allen gave the remedy for sleeplessness, and cured an old pelvic abscess with orange colored discharge.

W. T. Laird pointed out that Kali-p. cures a nervous dyspepsia almost identical with that of Anac. The Kali-p. patient is more decidedly neurasthenic than the other and the relapses, which are frequent in both, are mostly due to dietetic errors in Anac. cases and to excitement or worry in the Kali-p. cases.

H. M. Rean reported cures in cases of amenorrhea. One young woman, who was very nervous, pale blonde, skin rather waxy, cross and snappish, but cried easily, had a constant dull headache, yet was very drowsy all day.

Fidgety, at times could not control herself, and called her mother to hold her hands. Menses did not appear until eighteen and were scanty then and since. Kali-p. 3x four times daily caused great improvement at next menstrual period. In three months the menses were regular and normal, and in five months the patient was perfectly well.

J. C. Nottingham considered a leading indication of Kali-p. "nervousness arising from excessive sexual excitement, whether indulged or suppressed." He has cured impotence and seminal losses on these indications.

RELATIONS - ***Compare:*** (1) Zinc., Gels., Cimic., Lach., Mur-ac. (2) Kali-hp. (3) Macroz.- extreme debility after severe illness, collapse. Macroz., weariness from no assignable cause, no pains. Boring pain at vertex, vomiting and retching all night, impossible to eyes, giddiness and cold. (4) Genist.

REFERENCES - Boericke. Clarke. Murphy. Phatak.

KALI SILICICUM

(Potassium Silicate)

PHARMACY - kali-sil. Kali silicicum. Potassium silicate. Silicate of potash. ***Historical dose:*** Trituration and all potencies.

CLINICAL - Backache. Chilly. Constipation. Diarrhea. Eczema. Emaciation. Flatulence. Headaches. Leucorrhea. Nasal catarrh. Nausea. Photophobia. Vertigo. Warts.

HOMEOPATHIC - Kali-sil. is a deep acting remedy. Marked lassitude. Desire to lie down all the time. Absent-minded, anxious indolent, timid. Feeble will power. Emaciation. Head congested, blood surges from body to head. Nasal catarrh, discharge ***bloody***, excoriating offensive. Nose, swollen, ulcerated.

Stiffness over body and limbs. Creeping sensation over limbs. Twitching of muscles. Weak and weary. Weight in stomach after eating, nausea, pain, flatulence. Pain in liver region. Constipation. Construction of anus during stool. Vertigo, coldness of head, photophobia.

MIND - Absent-minded. Confusion from mental exertion. Anxious. Indolent. Timid. Feeble willpower. Mental troubles worse consolation. Irritability and irresolution, after sex.

Eyes - Eyes better from heat. Photophobia.

Female - Backache during menses. Leucorrhea, excoriating, yellow, worse after menses. Eruptions on vulva. Itching of vulva.

Head - Head congested. Blood surges from body to head. Coldness of head. Headaches, worse from cold air. Headaches worse after sex, mental exertion, stooping and exerting the eyes. Headaches better warmth and wrapping head up.

Limbs - Creeping sensation over limbs. Stiffness of body and limbs. Twitching of muscles. Weak and weary limbs. Gouty nodosities. Offensive sweat on feet and between toes.

Liver - Pains in liver region.

Modalities - Better heat, summer. Worse open air, drafts, cold, winter, uncovering, bathing. Worse exertion, motion.

Nose - Nasal catarrh. Discharge bloody, excoriating, offensive. Nose swollen, ulcerated. Discharge and breath offensive.

Rectum - Constipation. Diarrhea, after midnight and at night. Painful diarrhea, during menses. Stools insufficient and difficult even though soft. Stools bloody, frequent, offensive, purulent and watery. Constriction of anus during stool. Itching of anus after stool.

Skin - Injuries and small wounds that suppurate and refuse to heal. Eczema. Warts, painful, stinging, suppurating, withering.

Stomach - Nausea, pain, flatulence. Weight in stomach after eating. Aversion to meat.

Temperature - Chilly, weak, wants to keep still and rest.

Vertigo – Vertigo while sitting and stooping.

REFERENCES - Boericke.

KALI SULPHURICUM

(Potassium Sulphate)

PHARMACY - kali-s. Kali sulphuricum. Potassium sulphate. Trituration. ***Historical dose:*** Trituration and all potencies.

CLINICAL - Arthritic nodes. Asthma. Bronchitis. Cataract. ***Catarrh.*** Chorea. Colds. Constipation. ***Dandruff.*** Diarrhea. Dyspepsia. ***Eczema.*** Epithelioma. Eustachian catarrh. Gleet. Gonorrhea. Headache. Hemorrhoids. Intermittent fever. Leucorrhea. Metrorrhagia. Nails, diseased. Nasal, catarrh. Nettle-rash. Ophthalmia. Orchitis. Otorrhea. Ozaena. Palpitations. Pneumonia. Polyps. ***Psoriasis.*** Rheumatism. Rhus poisoning. Scabies. Scaldhead. Seborrhea. ***Sinusitis.*** Skin, disorders. Suppurations. Toothache. Vertigo. Whooping cough.

HOMEOPATHIC - Kali-s., introduced by Schüssler, affects respiration, mucus membranes and skin where it causes desquamation. Schüssler explains that Kali-s., in reciprocal action with iron, effects the transfer of the inhaled oxygen to all the cells and is contained in all the cells containing iron.

When a sulphate and any oxide of iron come into contact with decomposing organic substances they surrender their oxygen and form sulphate of iron. With more oxygen added, this may be further decomposed into sulphuric acid and an oxide of iron.

A deficiency of Kali-s. causes a sensation of heaviness and weariness, vertigo, chilliness, palpitations of the heart, anxiety, sadness, toothache, headache and pain in the limbs. Symptoms are worse in a warm room and towards evening, better in open, cool air.

Catarrh of larynx, bronchi, nostrils, etc., with yellow discharges. Catarrh of the stomach where the tongue has a yellowish mucus coating. ***Profuse and deep yellow discharges,*** thin or sticky.

Ailments accompanied by profuse desquamation. Suppurations. ***Yellow, mucus and serous discharges,*** profuse and intermittent. Later stages of inflammation. ***Wandering pains***, wandering rheumatism (Puls., Kali-bi.). Stitching, tearing, festering pains that shift about.

Torpid processes. Lack of reaction. ***Warm-blooded.*** Oxaluria. Facilitates the formation of new epithelium. Epithelial cancer. Interrupted growth of nails. Gonorrhea and ophthalmia neonatorum (Puls.).

MIND - Always hurried. Irritable. Timid. Confusion and restlessness, worse in a warm room. Mental exertion aggravates. Desires and then rejects things. Desire to lie down, but lying aggravates so must walk for relief.

Anxiety, better in the open air. Anxiety in evening. Frightened at trifles. Fear of falling, of losing her reason. Claustrophobia with fear of suffocation.

Abdomen - Colicky pains, abdomen feels cold to touch. Abdomen cold and distended after eating. Hard, ascites, in whooping cough. Empty feeling in hypogastrium, better passing flatus.

Back - Pain in nape. Stiff neck, head inclined towards left. Rheumatic pains in back and limbs, worse in warm room, better cool open air.

Causations - Ill effects of chill when over heated. Injuries.

Chest - Anxiety in chest.

Ears - Eustachian deafness. Stinking otorrhea. Brown offensive secretion from right ear. Offensive discharge with polyps. ***Discharge of yellow matter*** (Hydr.). Watery, sticky, thin discharge.

Eyes - Purulent yellow mucus in eye diseases. Sticky, watery discharge from eyes. Thin, yellow crusts on eyelids. Cataract. Ophthalmia neonatorum.

Face - Aches in heated room, better cool open air. Epithelioma.

Female - Menses too late, scanty. Menses with a feeling of weight in the abdomen. Metrorrhagia. Leucorrhea, yellowish, watery.

Food - Burning thirst. Craves sweets, cold food, cold drinks. Dread of hot drinks. Averse to and worse from eggs.

Head - Rheumatic headache, beginning in evening. Headaches worse warm room, better open air. Headache during menses. Great pain on moving head from side to side or backwards. ***Dandruff yellow, moist and sticky.*** Scaldhead. Bald spots, after gonorrhea.

Kidneys - Albuminuria after scarlatina. Oxaluria. Pyelitis.

Limbs - Rheumatism. Rheumatic pains, worse heat, evening, better cold weather or cold applications. Pain in back and limbs, worse in a warm room. ***Shifting, wandering pains***. Arthritic nodes. Cold hands and feet. Scaly eruption on arms, better hot water. Diseased condition of nails.

Lungs - Asthma with yellow, slimy expectoration, easily expelled. Coarse rales in lungs. Bronchitis, mucus is distinctly yellow and slimy, thin, or watery matter and profuse. ***Rattling of mucus in lungs*** (Ant-t.). Post-influenza cough, especially in children. Cough, worse in evening and in hot atmosphere. Croupy cough (Hep., Spong.). Pneumonia with wheezing. ***Yellow, loose rattling mucus is coughed up with difficulty.*** Sputum consists of watery matter. Whooping cough.

Male - Gonorrhea, slimy, yellowish, green discharges. Gleet. Orchitis after suppressed gonorrhea.

Modalities - Better from walking, fasting, discharge of flatus, cool, open air. Worse in evening (Puls.), noise, consolation. ***Cannot stand warm rooms or other forms of heat***. Worse warm air, warm wraps, warm weather, heated room.

Mouth - Mouth breathing, snoring. Insipid, pappy taste. Loss of taste and smell. Tongue coated yellow and slimy. Yellow mucus coating on tongue. Painful gums. Toothache, worse warm room and toward evening, better cool open air. Blistered lips and mouth. Lower lip swollen. Epithelioma on lip.

Nose - ***Colds with a yellow, slimy discharge***. Yellow, thick discharge, alternating with watery discharge. ***Sinusitis*** with thick yellow, green discharges. Nose obstructed. Loss of smell and taste (Nat-m.). Swelling of the ***nasal pharyngeal mucus membrane***, remaining after removal of adenoids.

Perspiration - Profuse, easy sweat.

Rectum - Constipation with hemorrhoids (Sulph.). Stools large like sheep's dung. ***Black, thin, offensive stools.*** Stools light-colored and bilious. Yellow, slimy diarrhea.

Skin - Dry skin. Itching, worse heat. Peeling, flaking of skin. ***Psoriasis*** (Ars., Thyr.). Intertrigo. Eczema, burning, itching, papular eruption. ***Desquamation of skin.*** Promotes desquamation after erysipelas. Accelerates removal of scabs in smallpox. Nettle rash. ***Yellow scales.*** Favus. Yellow skin, jaundice. Skin affections with yellow, slimy discharge. Ulcers, ooze thin ***yellow water.*** Polyps. Epithelioma. ***Suppressed rash of measles or other eruptive diseases, with harsh and dry skin.*** Seborrhea. Scabs with yellow pus. Ringworm of scalp or beard with abundant scales. Scabies. Rhus poisoning.

Sleep - Sleeplessness from heat, warm room. Vivid, terrifying dreams of ghosts, death, robbers, murder. Dreams with violent struggling in their sleep.

Stomach - Burning thirst. Pressure and feeling of fullness in stomach. Sensation as if a heavy load on stomach. Sensation of faintness in stomach with befogged feeling in head. Catarrh of stomach and duodenum. Nausea, and vomiting.

Temperature - Chilliness. Cold hands and feet. Intermittent fever. Temperature rises at night.

Throat - Croupy hoarseness (Hep., Spong.). Constant scraping. Sore throat and hoarseness after catching a cold. Every cold settles in larynx.

Vertigo - Dreadful vertigo on rising from lying, on standing from sitting. Vertigo when looking upwards. Vertigo with a fear of falling.

COMMENTS - Useful for chronic Puls. conditions, recurring earaches, asthma, respiratory problems, when Puls. doesn't cure completely. Yellow discharges, thick and bland, especially from the sinuses and lungs. Rattling mucus (Ant-t.). Wandering arthritis, worse hot applications and hot baths.

Desquamation. Skin conditions with flaking and peeling. Psoriasis, eczema, dandruff. Scabs with yellow pus. Ulcers ooze yellow, watery fluid. Skin cancer. Tongue can be yellow with a slimy coating. General sluggishness.

Modalities similar to Puls. Worse in warm, stuffy rooms, at twilight, better fresh air. Thirstless. Better walking in the fresh, open air. Mood changes and can weep easily. Claustrophobic with fear of suffocation.

M. E. Douglass reported an asthma case with a lot of thick, yellow expectoration. Much rattling in chest, with labored breathing and talking almost impossible, this was cured with Kali-s. 3x, five grains every hour in the attack.

Hansen cured with Kali-s. a case of psoriasis beginning on the right leg, later attacking the left elbow and left leg. Eruption, papular, oval and annular with paler centers, covered with whitish scales, skin beneath red and smooth. The guiding symptom was "great desquamation of the epidermis."

RELATIONS - ***Antidote to:*** Rhus poisoning. ***Compare:*** (1) Kali-s., Puls., Kali-bi., Nat-m. (2) Puls., Kali-bi. (3) Hydr. - dyspepsia, epithelioma. (4) Chr-ac. 3x. - produces in the nasal passages very fine threads from the septum to external wall, disorders of nasal fosse and hay fever. Chronic colds. Sneezing, red, watery eyes, irritation of mucus membrane. *Compatible:* Acet-ac. (itching and redness of skin), Calc., Hep., Puls., Rhus-t., Sep., Sil., Sulph.

REFERENCES - Boericke. Clarke. Murphy.

KALI TARTARICUM

(Potassium Tartrate)

PHARMACY - kali-t. Kali tartaricum. Potassium tartrate. Cream of tartar. Tartrate of potash. Trituration. Solution. ***Historical dose:*** Trituration and all potencies.

CLINICAL - Colitis. Debility. Diarrhea. Emaciation. Flatulence. Paraplegia. Vomiting. Weakness.

HOMEOPATHIC - A few symptoms of this well-known substance are collected in Allen's works. Among them, pain in loins and paraplegia are very noticeable. Emaciation. Extreme weakness, can scarcely walk. Vomiting of black-green fluid. Feces look like coffee-grounds. Pain in umbilical region with great thirst.

Abdomen - Pain in umbilical region with thirst. Flatulence and griping. Pain in loins.

Limbs - Thighs and legs paralyzed.

Mouth - Tongue brown and dry.

Pulse - Pulse feeble.

Rectum - Diarrhea and violent vomiting. Feces like coffee-grounds.

Stomach - Great thirst and pain in umbilical region. Inflammation of stomach and intestines. Violent vomiting and diarrhea. Vomits a black-green fluid.

REFERENCES - Clarke.

KALI TELLURICUM

(Potassium Tellurate)

PHARMACY - kali-tel. Kali telluricum. Potassium tellurate. Trituration. Solution. ***Historical dose:*** All potencies.

CLINICAL - Insomnia. Salivation. Tongue, swelling.

HOMEOPATHIC - A few symptoms of Kali-tel. have been observed, of which the garlicky odor of the breath was the most noticeable and persistent. Offensive breath. Tongue coated white and swollen, with salivation. Appetite increased at first, later diminished, finally lost.

Heart - Oppression in cardiac region.

Mouth - Tongue coated white and somewhat swollen. Offensive garlicky odor in mouth. Copious secretion of saliva.

Sleep - Sleepiness during first days.

Stomach - Inclination to vomit.

RELATIONS - ***Compare:*** (1) Tell., Phos. and Kali-p. - garlicky odor.

REFERENCES - Clarke.

KALMIA LATIFOLIA

(Mountain Laurel)

PHARMACY - kalm. Kalmia latifolia. Mountain laurel. Ledum floribus bullatis. American laurel. Calico bush. Cistus chamerhododendros. N. O. Ericaceae. Rocky sterile hills, near water in New England States. Flowers May and June. Tincture of fresh leaves when the plant is in flower. ***Historical dose:*** Tincture and all potencies.

CLINICAL - ***Albuminuria***. Angina, pectoris. Arthritis. Blindness. Bright's disease. Coryza. Dropsy. Dysmenorrhea. Gastralgia. Globus hystericus. Gout. Headache. ***Heart, disease.*** Hoarseness. ***Locomotor, ataxia.*** Lumbago. Nausea. ***Neuralgias. Palpitations.*** Ptosis. Pregnancy, albuminuria. ***Rheumatic, fever. Rheumatism.*** Retinitis. Scleroderma. Sun-headaches. Syphilitic, sore throat. Tachycardia. Tinnitus. Tobacco, effects. Tobacco, heart. Vertigo. Vomiting.

HERBAL - Kalmia is the name of a genus of heath worts native to North America. Kalmia latifolia, which has large and showy flowers, is found in the northern parts of the United States.

Its flowers yield a honey said to be deleterious, and its leaves and shoots certainly are so to cattle. Dr. Meadows says cattle eat Kalmia in the latter part of the winter when they are in want of something green.

K. angustifolia, probably for the same reason, has the name of lamb-kill. The powdered leaves are used as a local remedy in some skin diseases. The hard wood of K. latifolia is used in the manufacture of various articles. The Treasury of Botany noted that the Canadian partridge is said to become poisonous to humans after feeding on Kalmia berries.

HOMEOPATHIC - Hering introduced Kalm. into homeopathic practice, and he, and some friends, completed the first proving. The head, including the eyes and face, shows the majority of its action, followed by the heart. A number of skin symptoms confirm the popular use of the leaves, among them a ***stiffness*** of the skin, especially of the eyelids.

A heart, nerve, circulation and ***rheumatic remedy.*** In small doses, it accelerates the heart's action, in larger doses, it moderates it greatly. Nausea and slow pulse frequently accompany conditions.

Neuralgic pains, ***shoot downwards with numbness***, tingling, trembling or paralytic weakness. ***Neuralgia*** after the disappearance of herpetic eruptions. Great weakness with neuralgia. ***Pains of locomotor ataxia.*** Protracted and continuous fevers with tympanites. ***Albuminuria***. Paralytic sensations, pains and achings in the limbs.

Pains shift rapidly, shooting outward along the nerves with much nausea and slow pulse. Aching, bruised, stiff feeling. Dull tearing, crushing pain, moving downwards. Pain alternating with cardiac symptoms or between upper and lower limbs. Rheumatism, syphilitic. Motion brings on complaints.

MIND - Confusion of brain. Memory and mental faculties are perfect in a recumbent posture, but vertigo on attempting to move. Anxiety and palpitations. Irritable, cross. Talk of others aggravates.

Abdomen - Incarcerated flatus with nausea. Sensation of weakness in abdomen extending to throat, better by eructation. Sudden pains in paroxysms, across abdomen, above umbilicus. Neuralgia of bowels.

Back - Pain from neck down arm, brachialgia. Pain down back, as if it would break. Pain in localized regions of spine, through the shoulders. Sharp pain in lower part of left scapula. ***Lumbar pain of nervous origin,*** with heat and burning. Sensation of lameness in small of back. Drawing or sharp pain in spine.

Chest - Angina pectoris with dyspnea and pain. Feverish heat with great pain in chest, worse when breathing and from slightest motion. Pain in chest as from a sprain. Sharp pain in lower chest. Shooting through chest above heart into shoulder blade. Pain in left arm. False pleurisy of winter season. Rheumatism of muscles of thorax and back, worse from every motion.

Ears - Sharp pain in and behind right ear, at night. Acute inflammation of meatus. Sound like blowing a horn after cracking in head. Meniere's disease.

Eyes - ***Stiff, drawing sensation when moving eyes. Pains increased by moving the eye.*** Pressure in and above right eye. Paralysis of upper lids. Stiff eyelids. Retinitis, albuminuria especially during pregnancy. Rheumatic iritis. Scleritis. Itching in eyes, stinging when rubbing them. Eye symptoms worse evening and in open air.

Face - Anxious expression. Flushing with vertigo. Redness of face during throbbing headache. ***Neuralgia, worse right side.*** Neuralgia from exposure to cold, better eating, worse from worry or mental exertion. ***Trigeminal neuralgia.*** Facial neuralgia after herpes zoster. Sharp and tearing pains in bones of jaw and face. Itching of face at night. Tired feeling in masseters. Cracked lips with dry skin.

Female - Menses too soon. Menses regular but painful. Suppressed menses, with severe neuralgic pains throughout whole body, with pain in limbs, back and inside of thighs. Leucorrhea, one week after menses, aggravating other symptoms.

Head - Cracking in head, sounds like a horn blowing in the ears, frightens him. Headache worse and better with sun. ***Headache begins at sunrise, worse at noon and leaves at sunset.*** Headache worse bright sunlight. Headache better profuse urination. Shooting pain from nape to vertex and face. Maddening supra-orbital pain (right). Pain in front and temporal region from head, to nape, and to teeth, from cardiac origin. Aching in forehead.

Heart - Angina pectoris with empty eructations. Heart disease, after frequent attacks of rheumatism, or alternating with it. Tumultuous action, rapid and visible. Paroxysms of anguish around heart. Fluttering of heart with anxiety. Pains, sharp, burning shooting, stabbing, radiating to left scapula and arm. ***Sharp pains take away the breath***. Tachycardia with pains (Thyr.). Severe palpitations with constriction of throat, worse motion. ***Palpitations, worse leaning forward***, better sitting erect. Gouty and rheumatic metastasis of heart. Shooting through chest above heart into shoulder blades. ***Tobacco heart.*** Hypertrophy, valvular insufficiency. Aortic obstruction. Pulse slow, weak, tremulous (Dig., Apoc.). Frequent pulse.

Kidneys - Frequent urination of large quantity of yellow urine, with sharp pains in lumbar region. Frequent urination of scanty, hot urine. Profuse urination, better headache. Post-scarlatinal nephritis. Albuminuria with pains in lower limbs, dropsy. Albuminuria during pregnancy.

Limbs - ***Pains affects a large part of a limb*** or several joints and pass through quickly. Weakness, numbness, pricking and sense of coldness in limbs. ***Joints red, hot, swollen.*** Pains from hips to knees and feet. ***Pains along ulnar nerve,*** goes into third or fourth fingers. Tingling and numbness of left arm (heart pains). Deltoid rheumatism, especially right.

Liver - Pains in region of liver.

Lungs - Dyspnea and pressure from epigastrium toward the heart. Short-breathed, must breathe quickly, involuntary. Difficult and oppressed breathing, throat feels swollen, nausea, with palpitations and anxiety. Noise as from spasm of glottis when breathing. Hoarseness with coryza. Tickling in trachea. Frequent cough caused by dryness or scraping in the throat. Expectoration easy, smooth, gray, tasting putrid, salty.

Male - Frequent, spontaneous, lasting erections without desire. Pain in the right testicle in morning, in the left testicle in afternoon.

Modalities - Better from eating cloudy weather, continued motion, sitting, or standing upright. ***Worse looking down***, turning eyes, stooping, ***bending forward***, motion, lying on left side. Worse from heat of sun, open air, becoming cold, from sunrise to sunset. Worse during leucorrhea.

Mouth - Tingling in salivary gland. Sublingual salivary gland inflamed. Bitter taste with nausea, better eating. Tongue white, dry. Sharp pain in tongue. Tongue, sore left side, hurts when talking. Teeth tender, during facial neuralgia. Pressing in molars, late in evening. Tired feeling in chewing muscles. Lips, stiff, dry, swollen.

Nose - Coryza, with increased sense of smell. Coryza with sneezing, dullness, headache and hoarseness. Tearing in root of nose and nasal bones, with nausea.

Perspiration - Cold sweat.

Rectum - Diarrhea with dullness, dizziness, weariness, nausea and bellyache. Stools like mush, easily discharged. Stools as if glazed, followed by pressure on rectum.

Sensations - As if something loose in head diagonally across the top. As if the body was surcharged with electricity, as shuddering without coldness. As if something was being pressed away from under sternum.

Skin - Stiff, dry skin. Sensation of rigidity. Pricking sensation in skin with moderate sweat. Erysipelatous on hand with oppressed breathing. Scabies-like eruptions. Red inflamed places here and there, exceedingly painful, as if boils would form. Scleroderma.

Sleep - Sleepless. Restless sleep, turns often. Periosteal pains prevent sleep. While sleeping, stands up and walks about. Talks in sleep. Fantastic dreams. Dreams of murder. ***Wakes very early in morning***.

Stomach - Crampy pain with eructation of gas. Pain in pit of stomach, ***worse by bending forward, relieved by sitting erect***. Sensation of something being pressed under the epigastrium. Warm, glowing sensation in epigastrium. Gastralgia with empty eructations. Bilious attacks with nausea, vertigo and headache. Nausea and vomiting. Wine relieves vomiting.

Temperature - Shivering and coldness. Shaking chill in cold air; chills run over back. Protracted and continued fevers with tympanites. Fever with burning and pain in back and loins.

Throat - Throat feels swollen. Sensation as of a ball rising. Pressure in throat, stitches in eyes and nausea. Dryness in throat with aching pains, causing cough, difficult swallowing and thirst. Chronic syphilitic sore throat. Tickling in trachea. Noise as from spasm in glottis when breathing. Hoarseness during coryza.

Vertigo - Vertigo with headache, nausea, blindness, pains in the limbs and weariness. Vertigo worse from motion (Bry.), worse stooping, looking down. Vertigo with blindness.

Vision - Impaired vision. Vision becomes black on looking downward. Diplopia, from paralysis of ocular muscles. Glimmering vision, with dimness.

COMMENTS - For paralytic weakness and trembling. Neuralgias in almost all regions, generally on the right side. Wandering arthritis, sharp, shooting pain jumps from joint to joint. Arthritis with heart conditions or neuralgias. Wandering rheumatic pains that travel from above downwards. Rheumatic fever.

Pain, followed by numbness in the joints (Naphtin. with sciatica). Joints can swell, become red, hot and throbbing (Bell.). Pains worse sunrise to sunset (Nat-m., Spig.). Painful facial neuralgias (Spig., Mag-p.). Neuralgic pains are better from food.

Pain in the back, shuns all exertion, can hardly go up stairs. Pains in the periosteum preventing sleep. Pain between shoulders coming up over the head. Pain with nausea and slow pulse. Pain during the early part of the night or soon after going to sleep. Pain from a sudden chill or exposure to a sudden wind.

Tumultuous action of the heart and slow pulse. Every heartbeat has a strumming as if it would burst, along sternum to throat. Palpitations are better lying on back and breathing, worse on left side, from mental effort.

Generally acts on the right side of the head, the left side of the chest and the left arm. Vertigo from least motion, worse from motion (Bry.), even motion of eyes and eyelids is painful. Vertigo is worse on stooping, on looking down, on rising from a seat.

Headache comes on in the morning, worse again in evening. Headache, worse heat, better cold. Sun headache, worse or better with the sun. Headache and eye symptoms are worse in evening, from open air. Rubbing eyes causes stinging in them.

Scleroderma. Cheek roughness every summer. Much external sensitiveness, face, pit of stomach, muscles of neck sore, worse by touch.

Dry throat. Feeling as if a ball was rising in the throat. Dry, stiff, swollen, cracked lips. Tingling in the salivary glands immediately after eating. Stitches in the tongue.

Sensation of weakness in abdomen extending to throat. Vomiting with ruminating action, without the least nausea, better with wine. Pressure on rectum after stool. Symptoms worse during leucorrhea.

Vonder Luhe cured with Kalm. 200c an intercostal neuralgia of the left side, so intense that the patient could not lie down or sleep at night. The chief guiding symptom was a concomitant numb sensation of the whole left arm.

Lambert recorded the case of a gatekeeper, age 54, who had smoked since he was seven years old. He suffered from "tobacco heart" palpitations, occurring on the least exertion or fright and sometimes awakening him in the night. Intermittent pulse, no valvular lesion, tingling in the left arm and leg and sensation as if the blood did not circulate in them.

He could walk, but not far. The chief complaint was a sharp pain in the right temple like pins and needles, of eighteen months' duration. It was induced by touch and turning the head quickly. Kalm. 3x cured the temporal neuralgia and greatly alleviated all the other symptoms.

Proell cured with Kalm. 1c, 2c and 3c headaches and weak memory in a boy of 13 that were preventing him from continuing his studies. He also had insufficiency of the mitral value.

RELATIONS - ***Antidoted by:*** Acon., Bell. ***Antidote to:*** Tab. ***Compare:*** (1) Kalm. contains Arbutin. (2) Der. of great service in neuralgic headaches of rheumatic origin). (3) Spig., Puls. ***Complementary:*** Benz-ac. ***Follows well:*** Nux-v., Thyr., Spig.

REFERENCES - Boericke. Clarke. Murphy. Phatak.

KAMALA

(Spoonwood)

PHARMACY - kam. Kamala. Spoonwood. Croton coccineus. Rottlera tinctoria. Mallotus philippinensis. N. O. Euphorbiacae. India, South Arabia, Australia. A red mealy inflammable powder, obtained from the tri-lobed capsules of the plant. Tincture. Solution in ether. Trituration. ***Historical dose:*** Tincture and all potencies.

CLINICAL - Leprosy. Pustules. Skin, affections. ***Tapeworm. Worms.***

HERBAL - Kamala is best known in medicine as a remedy for tapeworms. It is given in doses of half to two drachms. The Treasury of Botany noted that "Among the Arabs of Aden it is given internally in leprosy, and used in solution to remove freckles and pustules, while in this country it has been used successfully in treating the eruption known as 'wildfire' (Strophulus volaticus) in children, by rubbing the powder over the affected part with moist lint.

"Kam. appears, however, to be most valued as an ***anthelmintic***, and has been extensively used with much success in India in cases of ***tapeworms***, three drachms being sufficient for a robust person, and half that quantity for one of feeble habit."

RELATIONS - ***Compare:*** (1) Kam. shows by its clinical uses it relationship with Croton and the other Euphorbians.

REFERENCES - Clarke.

KARAKA

(Kopi Tree)

PHARMACY - kara. Karaka. Kopi tree. Corynocarpus levigatus. N. O. Myrsinacee, Allen puts it in Anacardiacae. New Zealand. Tincture or Trituration of fresh seeds. ***Historical dose:*** Trituration, tincture and all potencies.

CLINICAL - Convulsions. Pains. Paralysis.

HOMEOPATHIC - The Treasury of Botany noted that karaka seeds contain a tasteless farinaceous substance and are eaten in times of scarcity. The raw seeds are poisonous and produce spasmodic pains, giddiness and partial paralysis. To render them edible, they are steamed for twenty-four hours and then either buried in the ground or allowed to soak in water for some days.

G. Bennett recorded a few symptoms observed in the case of a Maori chief poisoned with the seeds. Spasm with pains. Violent pain lasting a week. Partial paralysis. Heat anesthesia, when warm water was applied he did not feel any warmth from it. Violent spasms and convulsions of whole body, arms and legs stretched violently and rigidly out. Permanent rigid distortion.

COMMENTS - C. F. Fischer proved Kara. and used it clinically in cases of convulsions. He recorded an account of its effect from the proceedings of the New Zealand Institute.

"Violent spasms and convulsions of whole body, arms and legs stretched violently and rigidly out, great flushings of heat, protrusion of eyes and tongue, gnashing of jaws. The poison proves rapidly fatal if the patient is not attended to immediately and the limbs are permanently and rigidly distorted if they are not fixed in proper positions until the crisis is passed.

"The general treatment is to bind the patient (generally a child) with the limbs in right positions, dig a pit and place him in it, standing, buried up to the chin with a gag in his mouth.

"The writer described a youth, age 12, who had recovered after being poisoned, but whose limbs had not been properly secured and were ever after absolutely useless.

"One leg was curved up behind his loins, the other bent up with the foot outwards. One arm inclined behind his shoulder, the other slightly bent and extended forward and all, as to muscles inflexibly rigid. He could not move himself or even drive away the flies."

REFERENCES - Clarke.

KARWINSKIA HUMBOLDTIANA

PHARMACY - karw-h. Karwinskia humboldtiana. N. O. Rhamnacae. Found in Mexico and Southern North America. The seeds, crushed and macerated are used for the preparation of the tincture. ***Historical dose:*** Tincture and all potencies.

CLINICAL - Acute poliomyelitis. Acute bulbar paralysis. Amyotrophy. Bedsores. Dyspnea. ***Encephalitis. Paralysis.*** Paresis. ***Poliomyelitis.*** Quadriplegia.

HERBAL - The plant Karwinskia belongs to the Rhamnacae family, it is found in the northern states of Mexico. It is known locally under different names including Tullidora, the "little coyote," "wild capuli," "little black rod," and "cacachila."

It is a small shrub, but can grow up to 9 meters in some places. The leaves are elliptical or oblong, rounded at the end, the flowers are small, yellow-green in color. The fruits are small in clusters from 6 to 9 mm in diameter, dark violet in color, usually containing four seeds of which only two are reproductive.

The seeds are toxic, causing paralysis of the limbs, which becomes generalized and can terminate in death. They contain a fatty acid, a yellow substance and a glucoside, which is the cause of the paralysis of the motor nerves.

HOMEOPATHIC - The clinical observation of the mass intoxication of one hundred and six soldiers constitutes the first Memoirs of Dr. Castillo Najeros, published in Mexico in 1918. A homeopathic proving of Karw-h. was carried out by Luis de Legarreta and published in 1961 in his Materia Medica of Mexican Plants.

Karw-h. is a remedy with neurotrophic action, paralyzing the motor nerves. Flaccid paralysis, which increases, ending in quadriplegia.

Ascending progressive paralysis, flaccid and painless, predominantly on the left side, with amyotrophy of the lower limbs. Acute spinal paralysis, sub-acute atrophic spinal paralysis. Chronic anterior paralysis. Loss of contractility and mobility of the leg muscles. Reduction of tendons reflexes and skin.

Paresis of paralysis, rising to the upper limbs and muscles of the thorax and diaphragm. Paralysis of the lips, tongue and larynx. No diminution of reflexes of the bladder and intestines. Poliomyelitis. Acute and sub-acute, polioencephalitis. Bedsores.

Abdomen - Lack of intestinal inactivity, partial obstruction.

Back - Cramping pains in the back.

Ears - Buzzing in both ears.

Head - Severe headache. Constant headache with feeling of heaviness.

Heart - Pulse slower with fever.

Limbs - Progressive paralysis. Cramping pains in the arms and legs. Loss of contractility and mobility of the leg muscles.

Lungs - Dyspnea, which becomes worse and can end in respiratory paralysis. Bronchopneumonia, paralytic alveolitis, which can cause fatal asphyxia. Difficult speech.

Rectum - Diarrhea in the first 48 hours, followed by intestinal paralysis with difficulty in evacuating.

Skin - Bedsores.

Stomach - Nausea with vomiting.

RELATIONS - ***Compare:*** (1) Lath. - Weakness, then paralysis of the lower limbs with exaggerated reflexes and complaints of sensitivity. (2) Hydroph. - Paralysis with muscular dystrophy. (3) Plb. - Rapid emaciation, progressive paralysis of the limbs with amyotrophy and starting in the extensor muscles.

REFERENCES - Julian.

KEROSOLENUM
(Kerosene)

PHARMACY - keroso. Kerosolenum. Kerosene. One of the lighter products, obtained by distillation from the crude oil. Kerosolene being the trade name given by the "Downer Kerosene Oil Company," nearly identical with gasoline. Solution in rectified spirit. ***Historical dose:*** All potencies.

CLINICAL - Anesthesia. Asphyxia. Convulsions. Delirium. Ecstasy. Laughter.

HOMEOPATHIC - The effects of Keroso. have been observed on workmen, and experiments have been made with it for the purpose of testing its anesthetic properties.

Keroso. causes a pleasurable kind of intoxication, but too much muscular rigidity, asphyxia and intermittent pulse to render it a safe anesthetic. Moderate convulsions.

Laughter was noticed in two cases and this should prove an indication in some kinds of delirium and insanity. Partially or wholly insensible, but rapidly recovers when brought into open air. Insensibility complete, though eyes not closed.

MIND - Sense of complete loneliness. Insensible, with inclination to laugh. Cannot keep still

Chest - Breathing checked during convulsions due to rigid contraction of chest muscles.

Eyes - Eyes a little unnaturally open and staring.

Face - Momentary dusky redness of face at each convulsion (as in epilepsy).

Head - Peculiar lightness of head. Slight headache.

Limbs - Weakness of the limbs.

Modalities - Better in open air.

Pulse - Accelerated intermittent, volume diminished during insensibility.

Temperature - Some sweating.

RELATIONS - ***Compare:*** (1) Petr., Paraf., Benzin.

REFERENCES - Clarke.

KISSINGEN AQUA
(Saline Springs)

PHARMACY - kiss. Kissingen aqua. Saline springs. Cold, chlorinated, gaseous, saline Springs of Kissingen in Bavaria. Dilutions. ***Historical dose:*** Tincture and all potencies.

CLINICAL - Albuminuria. Constipation. Corns. Diabetes. Diarrhea. Gallbladder, disorders. Gout. Hemorrhoids. Liver, disorders. Mesenteric glands, disorders. Noises, ears. Rectum, disorders. Spleen, disorders. Warts.

HOMEOPATHIC - Kissingen water has been proved by Carl Preu and observations have been made on its general effects. Nat-m. is the leading solid ingredient, existing in the proportion of 5.82 out of a total of 8.55 in the 1,000. It compares with Nauheim, Kreutznach and, to some extent, with Vichy.

Useful for abdominal affections, especially a catarrhal condition of intestinal atony. Convalescence from typhoid and gallbladder affections. Disorders of the liver, spleen and intestinal glands.

Gout where the asthmatic principle appears to be repercussed upon the abdominal viscera, for then the waters draw it out to the joints. The dosage must be managed with extreme prudence, too much can bring on a true attack of gout.

Modalities - Worse in the forenoon, at night, on waking, while reading and writing. Vertigo worse while eating. Toothache worse during menstruation.

COMMENTS - Constantin James, recorded in Allen, noted that the dose is from three to six glasses of the water in the morning and two glasses at 4 p.m., but the general rule is that no more it to be drunk than the stomach can digest without difficulty.

In the first days, appetite and force is increase, but as the water is absorbed the effects become general. Then an eliminatory "crisis" comes on. The stools become brownish, loose, bilious. The urine is turbid, depositing a sediment which rapidly putrefies.

The secretion of the bronchial, genital, and ocular mucus membranes, as well as the skin, is increased and changed in character. Moral and physical prostration, old and long-forgotten troubles reappear. This crisis, which appears in the first or second week, soon disappears of itself and the cure proceeds.

In one case, a patient vomited blood after the disappearance of a hemorrhoidal flux. Kiss. restored the latter, and the blood-vomiting ceased.

Trembling, pulsation of the whole body. Weariness. Stitches here and there. Muscle volitantes. Noises in the ears. Chills, heat and perspiration. Tearful disposition, especially at 10 a.m. "If he only looks at any one he must weep."

RELATIONS - *Compare:* (1) Nat-m. - weeping disposition, chill at 10 a.m., catarrh, constipation. (2) Ant-c. - saburral condition. (3) Urt-u. - gout. (4) Ferr-pic. - warts and corns.

REFERENCES - Clarke.

KOLA NUT

(Sterculia Acuminata)

PHARMACY - kola. Kola nut. Sterculia acuminata. Nux colae. Cola acuminata. Tincture of the ripe nuts without their shell containing caffeine and theobromine. N.O. Sterculiaceae. ***Historical dose:*** Tincture and all potencies.

CLINICAL - Alcoholism. ***Asthma.*** Diarrhea. ***Neurasthenia.***

HERBAL - Kola regulates the circulation and the heart rhythm. Weak heart. ***Asthma***. ***Neurasthenia.*** Promotes the appetite and digestion. Diuretic and anti-diarrhea. Lessens the craving for ***alcohol***.

Kola nuts give the power to endure prolonged physical exertion without taking food and without feeling fatigued.

RELATIONS - *Compare:* (1) Querc., Coca. (2) Alf. (3) Aven., Lach., Nux-v., Kudzu.

REFERENCES - Boericke.

KOUSSO

(Brayera Anthelminthica)

PHARMACY - kou. Kousso. Brayera anthelminthica. Hagenia abyssinica. Kuso. Cosso. N. O. Rosacee. Abyssinia. Infusion of dried flowers. Tincture of flowers. ***Historical dose:*** Tincture and all potencies.

CLINICAL - Miscarriage. Tapeworm. Worms.

HERBAL - The flowers of Kousso are a favorite remedy for tapeworm with the natives of Abyssinia. The use of them in European practice for that purpose has led to the observation of the few recorded symptoms, among which thirst, nausea and vomiting are prominent. In one case miscarriage was caused.

To use as a vermifuge, take a quarter of an ounce of the dried flowers and boil in four ounces of distilled water. Infuse for fifteen minutes without straining. The powder is to be taken with the infusion in the morning, fasting. Two such drafts may be given. It is best to give a purgative before and an hour or two after the draft.

Nausea and vomiting. Vertigo. Precordial anxiety, slowing and irregular pulse, delirium and collapse. Rapid and extreme prostration.

HOMEOPATHIC - Alexander Milne remarked "Though Kousso leads to the expulsion of the worm, it seems not to improve the morbid condition which favors its production." The prostration caused by the treatment is so great that Milne advises a course of Cinch. and Ferr. to follow.

RELATIONS - *Compare:* (1) Cuc-c., Gran., Fil. (2) Kam., an efficient remedy for tapeworm in 30-60 minims of tincture taken in cinnamon water.

REFERENCES - Clarke.

KREOSOTUM

(Beech wood Kreosote)

PHARMACY - kreos. Kreosotum. Beech wood kreosote. Carbo pyroligneus. A product of distillation of wood tar from Fagus sylvaticus. This remedy is a mixture of phenols obtained from distillation of wood tar. Solution in Rectified Spirit. ***Historical dose:*** Tincture and all potencies.

CLINICAL - Abscess. Acne. Amenorrhea. Bedwetting. Belchings. ***Blood, poisoning. Cancer.*** Carbuncles. ***Cholera infantum.*** Coccyx, pain. Colic. Congenital syphilis. Constipation. Dentition. Diarrhea. Ear, disorders. Epithelioma. Eruptions. Flushings. ***Gangrene.*** Hemorrhages. Herpes. ***Hoarseness.*** Hysterical, vomiting. Impetigo. Irritations. ***Leucorrhea.*** Lupus. Menopause. Menstruation. Neuralgias. Ovary, disorders. Prostate, irritation. Pregnancy, vomiting. Pustules. ***Putrid, odor.*** Rheumatism. Seasickness. Septic, wounds. Stomach, disorders. Syphilis. Syphilitic deafness. Tongue, inflammation. ***Toothache, decay.*** Tuberculosis. ***Ulcers.*** Urine, incontinence. Uterus disorders. Vaginitis. Vomiting. Whooping cough. Yawning.

HOMEOPATHIC - The preservative principle of smoke was discovered by Reichenbach, a Moravian alchemist, early in the nineteenth century. Reichenbach discovered Kreosotum, and introduced it into medical practice and there was a rush for the new remedy. Its name, derived from the Greek, means "flesh-preserver." For a short time, it was a panacea and then fell into neglect, except among homeopaths.

Meredith proved on himself "the first heavy distillate from hard green wood," obtained at charcoal works in the 4x potency. The symptoms observed were so similar to those of Kreos. that they need not be separated, including a great thirst in the evening, enormous appetite, stabbings here and there, eyes feel as if in a woody smoke, sneezing, nasal pus, and spleen pain.

Teste grouped Kreos with Ars., Merc-c. Plb., Stann., Nit-ac., Sul-ac., Croc. and Arg-met. in his Merc. group.

He noted that several members of this group, while preserving dead organic matter from decomposition, have just the opposite effect on living tissues.

The entire group shows symptoms including suppressed or, more frequently, increased secretions with putridity. Foul breath, bloating, decay of teeth and bones. Cadaverous coldness. Ravenous hunger, to anorexia. Predominant left-sidedness. The group favors the production of intestinal parasites and all are therefore anthelmintic.

Teste added that Kermes of Weinsberg had collected 135 cases in which death has occurred apparently from eating smoked food. The leading symptoms in all were a burning pain at the epigastrium, bloody vomiting, meteorism, violent colic with constipation, slow breathing, sinking of pulse and dilatation of pupils.

Kreos. is the most active of the carbons, producing rapid ulcerations and destructions of tissues. Disorganizes the blood. Pulsations all over the body and profuse bleeding from small wounds. Very severe, old neuralgic affections, pains aggravated by rest. Great debility with miserable feeling.

Inflammatory ulcerations, ***cancers***, epitheliomas. Useful in treating cancerous ulcers of the gastrointestinal tract and uterus. Affinity for the glands and mucus membranes, particularly the digestive tract and genitals.

Tumefaction, puffiness, gangrene. Rapid decomposition of fluids and secretions and burning pains. ***Excoriating***, burning and offensive discharges. ***Profuse, acrid, hot, foul, discharges,*** belchings, sputum etc., that redden the part. Lumpy discharges, menses etc. Hemorrhages, passive, brown, dark from small wounds. Blackness of teeth, leucorrhea, lochia.

Fullness. Heaviness. Rapid emaciation. Scurvy. Complaints accompanying yawning. Pulsations all over the body. Congenital syphilis. Overgrown, poorly developed children. Ailments of teething children. Post-menopausal diseases.

MIND - Deep, nervous and mental derangement, violent oscillation of symptoms. Ailments from strong emotions. Stupefaction, dizziness and vacancy in head with complete loss of thought, sight and hearing. Vanishing of thoughts. Stupid, forgetful.

Cross, willful and obstinate. Peevish, fretful, irritable, especially during headache. Dissatisfied, with everything. Child wants everything but throws it away when given. Apprehensive. Starting from fright. Fear at the thought of sex in women. Fear of fasting. Shrieking in children during stool.

Dwells on past disagreeable occurrences. Longs for death. Delusions, visions of fire, things seem taller. ***Says he is well when very sick.*** Sensitive. Music causes weeping and palpitations.

Prostration and restlessness. Restlessness at night, after midnight. at 3 a.m. Children scream at night. Children would not sleep unless caressed and fondled. Child moans constantly or dozes with half open eyes, or is cross and sleepless during dentition. Restlessness before menses. Excitement before menses. Weak minded with suppressed menses.

Abdomen - Burning pain in bowels. Pressure in region of spleen. Griping pain about navel before menses. Inflation and tension of abdomen. Contractive pain in abdomen. Shooting pain in abdomen. Pain, as from ulceration in abdomen, when breathing and moving. Painful sensation of coldness in abdomen with too scanty emission of urine. Violent abdominal cramps, worse in groins. Colic, resembling labor pains. Obstinate flatus in old abdominal disease. Tabes mesenterica.

Back - Great debility with backache. Sharp pain from small of back. Burning in sacrum. Scapulae as if bruised. Dragging pain in back extending to genitals and down the thighs. Sensation as if everything would come out (in women), with urging to stool and urination, with leucorrhea. Burning in back before menses. Glands of neck swollen.

Breasts - Sharp pain in breasts. Dwindling of breasts with small, hard, painful lumps. Breast cancer with hard, bluish red, and covered with little, scurfy protuberances.

Chest - Anxious feeling of heaviness and oppression in chest. Deep pain in chest. Sharp pain in chest, just over heart. Raw burning in chest, as if a hot coal. Sensation as if sternum were being crushed in.

Constitutions - Dark complexion, slight, lean. Livid complexion, sad and irritable disposition. Old women with post-menopausal disease. Torpid, leuco-phlegmatic temperament. Old-looking children, hard to awaken. Blondes. Over grown, and poorly developed children with marasmus. Hemorrhagic diathesis.

Cough - Cough, worse evening, with efforts to vomit, with pain in chest. Dry, spasmodic cough in morning, causes retching. Cough after influenza (Erio.). Cough during dentition. Winter coughs of old people with ***heavy pressure on sternum***. Fatiguing cough with old people, with copious sputa, thick, yellow or white. Cough with little sputum.

Ears - Heat, burning, swelling and redness of left outer ear. Eruption around and pimples within. Itching in ears. Difficult hearing. ***Difficult hearing during menses, buzzing and roaring.*** Buzzing in head before menses. Sharp pain in ears. Humid tetter on ears.

Eyes - Eyes sunken with blue rings around. Eyes protruding. Hot, acrid, smarting tears. Heat in eyes with ulceration. Burning heat with lachrymation, worse bright light. Salty lachrymation. Lids red and swollen. Agglutination of eyelids. Constant quivering of eyelids. Uncontrollable twitching. Intense itching of margins of eyelids. Suffering of eyes alternating with limbs.

Face - Sick, suffering expression. Face hot, cheeks red. Yellow pallor with red blotches during chill or heat. Burning pains, worse talking or exertion, better lying on affected side. Lips red, bleeding. Upper lip sore and cracked. Moistens lips frequently without being thirsty. Scaly herpes on eyelids, cheeks and around mouth. Acne.

Old looking children.

Female - Premenstrual syndrome with irritability, headache, nausea, etc. Before menses looks swollen as if pregnant. Menses too early, prolonged,, worse lifting, overexertion. ***Menstrual flow intermits*** (Puls.), ceases on sitting or walking, reappears on lying down. Profuse, lumpy menses. ***Discharge of clots of blood having a foul smell.*** Vaginitis. Yellow, acrid leucorrhea, smells like green corn, worse between periods. ***Offensive, corrosive leucorrhea***, gushing like bloody water, staining the linen yellow. Milky leucorrhea following pain in coccyx. ***Leucorrhea during pregnancy.*** Vomiting of pregnancy with salivation. Lochia blackish, lumpy and very offensive. Hemorrhage after sex. Violent pain during sex, burning in parts, followed by discharge of dark blood the next day. Sharp pain in vagina. Burning and soreness in external and internal parts. ***Awful burning, as of red hot coal in pelvis.*** Corrosive itching within vulva, between labia and thighs, burning and swelling of labia. Scirrhus of vagina, painful to slight touch. Warty or cauliflower excrescences of cervix. ***Cancer, erosion of cervix. Uterine cancer.***

Food - Loss of appetite, everything tastes bitter. Aversion to meat. Craving for smoked meat. Disgust of food during convalescence. Better warm food, worse cold food, fasting.

Head - Heaviness or pressure in various parts of head. Pressing outward in forehead. Buzzing in head. Pulsation in forehead and vertex. Dull pain as from a board pressing against the forehead. Occipital pain (Gels., Zinc-pic.). Headache with sleepiness. Severe headache before and during menses. Scalp sensitive, worse combing hair. Falling of hair.

Heart - Anxiety at heart with oppressed breathing. Sharp pain in heart region. Pulsation in all arteries when at rest. Pulse small, hard, slow. Pulse soft, weak, quick and trembling.

Kidneys - ***Must hurry when desire comes to urinate.*** As if a lump pressing down on bladder. Hurried, involuntary urination when lying, on coughing. Can urinate only when lying. ***Bedwetting in the first part of night.*** Frequent urination with copious urine during day. Diabetes. Drinks much but passes little at a time. ***Urine offensive.*** Urine chestnut brown, clouded, reddish. Urine with red or white sediment. Urine colorless. Violent itching of vulva and vagina, worse when urinating.

Limbs - Skin on limbs dry and rough. Bruised pain in limbs. Paralytic sensation in limbs on waking. Boring pain in hip and knee joints, with sensation as if leg was too long when standing. Sharp pain in joints. Swelling of knee joints and wrists alternating with sensation of numbness and rigidity of limbs. Pain in left thumb as if sprained. Burning in soles. Ecchymosis, dorsal surface of fingers and hands eczematous. Sore scapulae.

Liver - Shooting and pressive pains in hepatic region. Sensation of fullness and pain as from contusion in liver.

Lungs - Raw burning in lungs, pains and oppression. Sternum feels pressed in. Shortness of breath with sensation of heaviness in chest. Difficult breathing with anxiety. Gangrene of lungs. ***Copious, purulent expectoration***, after every cough. Hemoptysis, periodic attacks. Black, coagulated blood expectorated. White mucus, easily detached. Neglected tuberculosis. Bronchitis with heavy pressure on sternum. Bronchial irritation during dentition.

Male - Burning in genitals during sex from coming in contact with acrid vaginal discharge, penis swells next day. Prepuce, bluish black with hemorrhage and gangrene. Sexual desire too weak. Impotence during sex.

Modalities - Better from warmth, hot food, motion, pressure, after sleep. ***Worse from dentition,*** pregnancy, during and after menses, sex. Worse when lying down, rest, touch, sprains, eating. Worse in summer, open air, cold, 6 p.m. to 6 a.m., bad smells

Mouth - Aphthae or salivation during pregnancy. Bitter, flat taste, low down in throat. Putrid odor. Tongue coated white, sometimes dry. Pus, bluish, spongy, bleeding gums. ***Very painful dentition***, child will not sleep. Intolerable toothache during pregnancy. Lips red, bleeding.

Nose - Offensive smell and discharge. Frequent sneezing in morning. Chronic catarrh of old people. Nasal secretion thick. Catarrh, fluent or dry, with much sneezing. Nasal catarrh, fluent, with acrid rawness in air-passages. Nosebleed thin, bright red blood. Nosebleed with heaviness and throbbing in forehead, with sleepiness. Lupus on nose and face, with burning (Ars.).

Perspiration - Cold sweat, feels weak. Sweats with heat and redness of cheeks. Sweats after coughing. Scanty sweat, only during morning.

Rectum - Diarrhea during menses. Diarrhea in nursing infants. Dysentery with nausea and vomiting. ***Cholera infantum,*** with painful dentition, green stools, nausea, dry skin, exhaustion. Constipation, evacuation very difficult, with burning. Cramp-like pain in rectum during stool. Sore pain, worse deep breathing. Child struggles and screams during stool, as if it would go into a fit. Constriction of rectum with uterine cancer. Burning hemorrhoids.

Sensations - As if a board was across forehead. As if brain would force through forehead. As if something floating before eyes. As if a hard twisted ball was lying in umbilical region, burning as of hot coals deep in pelvis, as if small of back would break. As if scapula and other parts bruised. As if tendon of elbow joint too short. As if hip dislocated, as if leg too long when standing.

Skin - Dry, scaly eruptions, like psoriasis. Violently itching, moist or scruffy eczema on eyelids, face, joints, back of hands. Itching, worse towards evening. Nodosities and blisters like bug bites. Pustules and herpes. Wheals like urticaria. Urticaria after menses. Herpetic eruptions, better warmth. Old ulcers, painful, putrid. Ulcers break out and heal. Ulcers bleed after sex. Small wounds bleed freely (Crot-h., Lach., Phos.). Senile gangrene.

Sleep - Great desire to sleep, with frequent yawning. ***Sleeplessness, worse before midnight.*** Children would not sleep unless caressed and fondled. Starting, when scarcely fallen asleep. Disturbed, restlessness of the whole body or sensation of fatigue and pains in all limbs. Tosses about without any apparent cause. Laughing during sleep. Child very difficult to waken out of sleep. Anxious dreams of pursuit, fire, falling from a height, being poisoned. Dreams of urinating, erections.

Stomach - Stomach cancer. Coldness, like ice water, in the stomach. Soreness or burning in epigastric region, temporarily better eating. Painful hard spot. Bitter taste after swallowing water. Hot, frothy belchings. Belching and hiccough. Nausea, vomiting food several hours after eating. Seasickness. ***Nausea and vomiting before menses.*** Nausea during pregnancy, with constant inclination to vomit without doing so. Sympathetic vomiting. Vomiting sweetish water in the morning during pregnancy. Vomiting undigested food with uterine ulcer. Vomiting of large quantities of sour, acrid fluid or of white, foamy mucus. Hematemesis.

Stools - Diarrhea, bloody, fetid, dark, brown, lienteric. Stools grayish or white, chopped. Very fetid, offensive, cadaverous-smelling stools. Bloody stools. Green stools during dentition.

Teeth - ***Very painful dentition***, ***child will not sleep.*** Pegged teeth. Black spots on teeth. ***Teeth dark and crumbly*** (Staph., Ant-c.). ***Very rapid decay of teeth*** with spongy, bleeding gums. Toothache from decayed teeth. Intolerable toothache during pregnancy. Gums puffy, bluish. Bleeding of gums and nose, blood dark, quickly coagulating. Protruding gums infiltrated with dark watery fluid. Persistent oozing of dark, slightly coagulated blood after extraction of tooth.

Temperature - Predominance of cold, tendency to shiver. Thirst after shiverings. Transient chill without thirst. Chilly while at rest. Chill with great bodily restlessness.

Always feels chilly at menstrual period. Coldness of face and hands. Feverish sensation over whole body, with good appetite. Flushes of heat with circumscribed redness of the cheeks.

Throat - ***Putrid odor.*** Bitter taste when swallowing food or drinking water. Burning pain with inflammation. Burning, choking sensation. ***Hoarseness with pain in larynx,*** better sneezing. Scraping in throat with roughness and dryness.

Vertigo - Vertigo on turning around quickly, with staggering. Vertigo in morning, in open air, passes off in a room. Must hold on to something.

Vision - Confused, as when looking through a veil. Dim vision, as if something was floating before eyes, obliging to wipe them constantly. Dim vision during vomiting.

COMMENTS - A remedy for decomposition of tissue or rotting away of flesh (Pyrog., Carb-an.). Discharges are brownish, yellow, and very offensive, a carrion-like odor, cadaver-like odor, putrid, like rotten flesh. Tendencies toward bacterial infections. Tendency to hemorrhage.

Stomach and uterine cancers, gangrene, and injuries where the tissue decomposes and smells putrid. Breath or discharges that smell of rotting flesh. Cadaverous-smelling stools. Emaciation with decomposition. History of use in typhoid.

Intermittent fevers, marked periodicity. According to Grauvogl, Kreos. has a short period of action, one or two days. He noted the incompatibility in intermittents. Chin., which has a period of two to three weeks, may be given after Kreos., but not Kreos. after Chin.

Marked burning and stitching pains. Lupus of nose with burning pains. Chronic pneumonia with pain like red-hot coals in the chest. Pain and stiffness across hips and sacrum, at 7 a.m. sitting up in bed, continuing through the day. Knees give way and joints crack, particularly in the overweight.

Guernsey noted that Kreos. particularly affects the inner temples, external ears and lobe of the ear. Chronic headache accompanied with great drowsiness, with moaning in their sleep.

Intense itching. General sensitiveness to touch and contact. Large purulent blisters on concha of both ears with a red base like smallpox pustules. Small warts on the scalp after a headache. W. P. Wesselheft noted the indication of coarse, red, elevated acne pimples.

Clarke used it for toothache cases where the teeth are decayed, especially if the gums are scorbutic. Foul breath. Useful for infections, abscesses and a bad taste after a pulled tooth. Teeth decay, fall out, with swollen gums that bleed easily (Staph., Merc.). Gums are dark red or blue and very painful. Pyorrhea.

Nash noted the specific action on children, especially during dentition. Painful dentition. Useful for teeth that come in rotten and brown, then break. Teste observed that it acted well on infants in the cradle, particularly for congenital syphilis.

Teste emphasized a discharge of fetid pus from the nostrils. Hoarseness is better by sneezing. Cough compels sitting up all night, causes involuntary urination. Eye symptoms alternate with drawing in the limbs.

Incessant vomiting, due to stomach weakness, inability to digest and rejection of a meal hours after it was eaten. Vomiting sweetish water during pregnancy, with ptyalism. Incessant vomiting with cadaverous stools in malignant disease of the stomach. Cholera infantum.

Nocturnal bedwetting from too profound sleep, child cannot be awakened when taken up. Bedwetting when the urine smells foul, offensive (Benz-ac.). Prostate and bladder irritation during night. Frequently rises to pass very little urine, urine comes in a spray. Sudden, great urging, the patient cannot go quickly enough. Copious, pale urine.

Complaints after menstruation or menopause. Foul smelling vaginitis where the chief complaint is the odor and not itching or burning. Guernsey notes the putrid leucorrhea, especially when it's fetid and exhausting.

Discharge stains the clothing yellow or brown. Leucorrhea is better sitting, worse standing and walking. Foul and offensive lochia after childbirth.

Sufferings from the non-appearance of menses, at menopause. General symptoms are worse after menstruation, during leucorrhea, when yawning.

Grauvogl cured with Kreos. 3x a young woman, 20, of suppression of menses with a concomitant state of imbecility.

In another woman who had suppressed menses with tertian intermittent fever, the intermittent was cured with Chin-s. one grain four times a day and then Grauvogl, hearing for the first time of the suppression of the menses, gave Kreos. 3x with the result that the fever returned in full force.

Quinine was again given and the fever again disappeared. Before the next period, as the patient was of the Nux-v. type, that remedy was given and the period was re-established.

Gentry recorded a case of a woman, 45, on visiting a friend ill with dysentery, was struck by the odor, went home, commenced to vomit, and vomited all food or drink and continued without ceasing, vomiting or retching for three weeks, being fed by the rectum all the time. She was greatly emaciated and had to be held up by the nurse.

One dose of Kreos. 200c was given. In twenty minutes the retching ceased. The patient fell asleep, had no more vomiting and rapidly recovered. Up to this time she had been under allopaths, who advised that homeopathy should be tried, as they could do no more.

James H. Freer cured a woman, over 80, who suffered from incontinence of urine during bronchial attacks, which compelled her to keep to bed.

Villers had reported a case of incontinence, worse when lying down, that was cured by Kreos. This led Freer to the remedy, which rapidly cleared up the case, bronchitis and all. Freer also cured incontinence in a case of locomotor ataxia in a man, 74, with Kreos. 6c.

An allopathic authority, Vladimir de Holstein of Paris, accidentally cured aggravated constipation in a chlorotic girl with 6 drop doses of Kreos., given in beer or milk. He gave it with the idea of "disinfecting" the intestines.

Meredith cured with it a young woman, 17, of intense urethral scalding after urination.

Cooper cured with Kreos. 30c a case of auditory vertigo in a patient with pegged teeth. No other medicine would touch the case. It is also frequently called for in acquired syphilis, especially in the skin manifestations. Kreos. cured at the same time constipation of ten to twelve days' duration.

Harmar Smith cured a girl, 10, of very frequent and violent eructation, she was apparently healthy in other respects. Bell. and Puls. did no good. Arg-n., aggravated. Kreos. 2x at once did good and cured in a few days.

RELATIONS - ***Antidote:*** Antidoted by: Acon. (vascular erethism), Nux (violent pulsations in every part of body), according to Teste, Ferr. is the best antidote. ***Compare:*** (1) Fuli., Carb-ac., Iod., Lach. (2) Guajol. - is the principal constituent of Kreosote and similar in action, used in pulmonary tuberculosis. (3) Piper augustifolia - gonorrhea, hemorrhage from lungs, catarrhal condition of genitor-urinary organs and gastro-intestinal tract. Topically a hemostatic. Difficult, dry, deep, winter cough. Use the tincture. (4) Eupi. and Kreos., have many similar symptoms, hemorrhages, pulsations and menstrual disorders. (5) Pix. - in tuberculosis. (6) Kali-c. - product of burning wood, stitches, worse after sex. (7) Sep. - intermittent menses, outward pressure in genitals, painful sex, vomiting of pregnancy. ***Complementary:*** in malignant diseases: Ars., Phos., Sulph. ***Followed well by:*** Sulph., Ars. (in malignant disease), Bell., Calc., Kali-ca., Lyc., Nit-ac., Rhus., Sep. ***Incompatible:*** Carb-v., also after Chin.

REFERENCES - Boericke. Clarke. Grimmer. Murphy.

L

LAC CANINUM

(Dog's Milk)

PHARMACY - lac-c. Lac caninum. Dog's milk. Dilutions. ***Historical dose:*** All potencies.

CLINICAL - Arms, varicose. ***Arthritis.*** Backache. Bedwetting. Breast infections. ***Breasts, painful.*** Chancre. Colic. Croup. Cough. ***Delusions.*** Depression. Diarrhea. ***Diphtheria.*** Dysmenorrhea. Epulis. Eye, disorders. Fatty, degeneration. ***Galactorrhea***. Gonorrhea. ***Headaches.*** Hematuria. Hemorrhages. Hysteria. Ichthyosis. Leucorrhea. Mastitis. ***Migraines.*** Menses, disorders. Nephritis. Neuralgia. Nosebleeds. Otitis. Ovarian, disorders. Photophobia. Polyuria. ***Prostration***. Ranula. ***Rheumatism.*** Sciatica. Scurvy. Spinal, irritation. Stomach, disorders. Syphilis. ***Throat, sore. Tonsillitis.*** Toxemia. Tumors. Ulcers. ***Uterus, disorders.*** Vaccinosis. Varicose, veins. Warts. ***Weakness.***

HOMEOPATHIC - Sammonicus and Sextus praised Lac-c. for photophobia and otitis. Pliny claimed that it cures ulceration of the uterine cervical os. Historically, it was considered an antidote to deadly poisons.

The Lac-c. provings were made with the 30c and upwards, and were published by Swan and Berridge. As in the cases of Bufo., Cast-eq., and other historical remedies, homeopathy has confirmed the accuracy of older observations. Disorganizes the blood and affects the throat, breasts, kidneys and rectum.

Great lassitude. ***Great weakness and prostration***. Sinking spells every morning. Feels as if walking on air or of not touching the bed when lying down. Keynote ***erratic pains, alternating sides***, often very rapid.

Diphtheria, both as a curative and as a prophylactic. Mouth and throat covered with aphthous yellowish-white ulcerations, easily bleeding. Sore throats, that cease entirely, only to commence on the opposite side, and often returning to its first location. Sore throats apt to begin and end with the menses.

Headaches where there is a sharp pain over the left eye, alternates to the right, then back again, with photophobia. Headaches, better cold compresses. Violent frontal and occipital headaches, migraines.

The pains moves from side to side. Sensitive to light and noise, the least touch aggravates. Cannot bear one part of the body to touch another, must keep even the fingers separate. The spine aches and is sensitive to the touch (Agar.).

Arthritis (Puls., Led.), particularly when moving crosswise. ***Arthritis***, better with ice on the joints, worse motion and heat (Apis.). ***Wandering rheumatic pains.*** Sciatica, pains alternating from the left to the right. Swelling of the joints with wandering pains.

Coldness in different parts and organs, in blood. Easy hemorrhages, nosebleed, bloody stools. Fetid discharges. Gray, white, plastic exudates. Fatty degeneration of liver, spleen and kidneys and other solid organs. Scurvy. Toxemia of pregnancy. Breast infections. Decided effect in drying up milk in women who cannot nurse the baby.

MIND - ***Alternation of moods.*** Mental symptoms worse before menses. Fixed ideas. Feels weak, nerves out of order. Paroxysms of nervousness. Very nervous, easily startled. ***Oversensitive, can't bear anything to touch her***.

Very restless, cannot concentrate her thoughts or mind to read, wants to leave everything as soon as it is begun. Absent-minded. Very forgetful, makes mistakes in writing, speaking. Makes purchases and walks away without them.

Pessimism. Severe hopelessness. ***Despondent***. Want of self-confidence. Self loathing, especially of the body. Feeling of disgust and horror. Fits of weeping two or three times a day. Depression, doubts ability and success. Thinks himself of little consequence. Undertakes many things, perseveres in nothing.

Feels she is not herself. Feels that everything she says is a lie, that she is full of strange, peculiar feelings. Imagines that he wears someone else's nose. Desire for company, light.

Hysteria, delusions, fears. Hysteria at height of sexual orgasm.

Cross and irritable, with headache. Hatred. Insolent. Intense hatefulness. Attacks of rage, cursing and swearing at the slightest provocation. Child cross and irritable, screams all the time, especially at night, will not be pacified in any way.

Anxiety about health. Fear of disease, of tuberculosis, heart disease, heart attacks, dying. Fears she will become unable to perform her duties. Fear of going insane because of tormenting thoughts. ***Fear of fainting***, of falling down the stairs. Fears to be alone. ***Fear of snakes*** (Calc., Lach.).

Delusions while sitting and thinking ***Delusions, dreams of snakes***, vermin, insects, spiders. Sees big eyes and creeping things. Sees faces, worse in the dark. Delusion that the air surrounding her is full of hovering spirits. Delusion that she wears someone else's nose. Delusions of having a horrible disease, that her whole body is filled with pus.

Abdomen - Extreme heat in abdomen. ***Abdomen very swollen and hard.*** Abdomen very sensitive, can't bear it touched. Bearing-down pains in abdomen. ***Pressure from within outwards, as if contents of abdomen would be forced outwards.*** Severe shooting pains in abdomen. Severe burning, in right hypochondriac and iliac region. Griping colic with shifting of flatulence and diarrhea, followed by continuous rectal pain. Feeling of tension in left groin, does not want to walk or stand.

Back - Backache, nearly all day between scapula, worse after becoming warm. Cold creeping down back. Spine aches from base of brain to coccyx. Spine very sensitive to touch or pressure. Sharp neuralgic pain under right scapula. Lameness and cutting pain under left scapula, worse turning in bed. ***Stiffness of neck***. Aching in neck, wants to bend head forwards.

Breasts - Breasts seem very full ***Breasts swollen, painful before menses*** (Calc., Con., Kali-c.. Puls.). and better on appearance of menses. ***Breasts sensitive to touch, pressure.*** Breasts sore when going up or down stairs, during menses. ***Mastitis, worse from the least movement.*** Breasts very painful with sharp, darting pain in right ovarian region. Constant pain in breasts, nipples. Breasts feel as if full of hard lumps. Breasts tumors and cancer. Tumors re-appear in opposite breast after being surgically removed. Knots and cakes in breasts, after miscarriage. ***Galactorrhea***. Loss of milk while nursing without any known cause. Milk scanty. ***Dries up the breast-milk***.

Causations - Result of fall. Diphtheria.

Chest - Constriction of chest, as from sulphur fumes. Clavicles sore to touch. Feeling of oppression and tightness behind sternum, with desire to draw a deep breath. Stabbing pain in right chest, just below nipple. Trembling, jerking and fluttering through chest. Fetid sweat in axilla, staining linen brown. Herpetic eruption in axilla with brownish scab.

Cough - Cough from tickling under middle of sternum. Cough from constant tickling in throat. Hard, metallic cough. Croupy, dry cough. Hoarse barking cough. Cough with pain and oppression of chest.

Ears - ***Ear infections that alternates from ear to ear.*** Green odorless discharge. Sensation as if ears were full. Intense pain in right ear. Very sharp pain in right middle ear, must cover ear when walking in wind. Wakened at night by aching pains in the ear of the side she is lying on. Noises in ears. ***Reverberation of voice, as if speaking in a large empty room.*** Ringing in the right ear, buzzing at night. Sounds seems very far off. Deafness from hereditary syphilis.

Eyes - Dark brown ring under eyes. Eyes dull and lusterless. Eyes sensitive to light, cold air. Heaviness in eyeballs, with outward pressure. Eyes slightly swollen, profuse lachrymation with catarrh. ***Eyes watery and discharging.*** Agglutination of eyelids. Sharp pain in back of socket or right eye. Intense darting pain around left eye. Upper eyelids very heavy, can scarcely keep eyes open, very sleepy.

Face - Burning, flushing of face. Face very red, and then suddenly pale. Pale, careworn, anxious. Marked pallor of face. Swollen, she can hardly see in the morning. Neuralgic pains, worse talking, eating or slight touch, followed by numbness. Cracking of jaw while eating (Nit-ac. Rhus-t.). Swelling of submaxillary glands. Swelling of parotid passes from right to left.

Female - Menses too early, profuse. Menses scanty at first with pain in left ovary. ***Menses flow in gushes.*** Dysmenorrhea, abdomen sensitive even to weight of clothing. Membranous dysmenorrhea, pain in left groin. Leucorrhea all day, but none at night, even after taking a long walk. Foul smell from genitals. Intense painful soreness of vulva. Itching of vulva. Herpes. Raw and bad smelling sores between labia and thighs. Sexual organs easily excited. Flatus from vagina. Bearing down pains as if everything would fall out through vagina. ***Sharp pains in ovaries, alternating sides. Pain in left ovarian region***. Heat in ovarian and uterine region. Retroverted uterus. Very severe after pains, shooting down into thighs.

Food - Great hunger for large quantities, cannot satisfy her hunger. No appetite. Considerable thirst. Drinks little and often. Pain in throat better warm or cold drinks. Aversion to liquids, water, anything sweet, fat, greasy food. Desire for highly seasoned foods, salt, pepper, mustard, pungent things. Desires warm drinks, whiskey. ***Craves milk and drinks much of it, aggravates.*** Thought of milk makes sick, during sick headache.

Head - ***Headache with blurred vision, nausea and vomiting.*** Sick headaches. ***Headaches that alternates sides.*** Headaches over left eye on first awaking. Occipital pain with shooting extending to forehead. ***Migraines.*** Sensation as if brain were alternately contracted and relaxed. Severe pressure on brain. Pains and throbbing in temples. Constant noise in head. Head very sore and itches almost all the time. Sore pimples on scalp, discharging and forming scabs.

Heart - Coldness in precordial region, in blood. Heart beats rapidly from slight causes. Pulse rapid, quick. Full right pulse, small on the left. Palpitations of heart, irregular, causing shortness of breath. Violent palpitations when lying on left side, better turning on right. Pains when going up and down stairs.

Kidneys - Nephritis. Constant desire to urinate, passing large quantities frequently, or scanty urine. Urination causes intense pain in urethra, soon passing off. Urine albuminous, scanty, infrequent, suppressed. Urine dark, heavily loaded with thick reddish sediment. Hematuria. Sensation after urinating as if bladder still full. Dreams of urinating and wakes with urgent need. Nocturnal bedwetting.

Limbs - ***Alternating pains.*** Pain in limbs as if beaten. Aching pains in limbs and back. ***Rheumatic pains, flying from joint to joint and side to side.*** Rheumatism, better cold and cold applications. ***Wandering pains from joint to joint.*** Sciatica, right side. Pain in arms to fingers. Arms, feet cold. Burning of hands and feet at night. Ankles swell in the evening. Legs feel numb and stiff, cramps in feet.

Lungs - Very labored breathing, couldn't lie down flat. Lungs feel as though fastened to chest. Profuse, sticky, tough, white mucus in masses, with coryza.

Male - Right spermatic cord, low down, sore to touch. Red, smooth, glistening, cauliflower-like chancre on prepuce, left side of frenum, penis greatly swollen. Buboes and chancres. Gonorrheal with intermittent pains in the urethra. When gonorrhea is better, nasal catarrh sets in. Marked sexual desire.

Modalities - Better cold, cold drinks. Better open air, walking. Better turning on right side. Better from nosebleed, mental symptoms. Worse from cold, drafts, sharp winds. ***Worse touch***. Worse pressure, motion. Worse a jar. Worse coughing, sneezing. Worse empty swallowing. Worse from rest. Worse at night. Worse after sleep. Worse during menses. Worse mercury. Worse morning of one day and in the evening of next.

Mouth - Mouth very dry without thirst. Putrid taste increased by sweets. Breath very offensive, putrid. Profuse salivation, slightly viscid, ran from mouth during sleep. Mouth constantly full of mucus, constant inclination to swallow, which causes pain. Drooling in diphtheria. Roof of mouth sore with blisters. Fetor. Acute ulceration and follicular stomatitis, aphthous and gangrenous. Nursing sore mouth. Noma. ***Jaw cracks while eating*** (Nit-ac, Rhus-t.). Dry and peeling lips. Scurvy. Stutters when talking fast, has to speak slowly.

Nose - Fluids escape through nose, while drinking. Profuse, purulent nasal discharge at night. ***Discharge acrid, nose and lips raw.*** Watery discharge, followed by dry sensation in nose. Coryza, one nostril stuffed up, the other free, alternating sides. Stuffed feeling in nose and throat. Bones of nose sore to pressure. ***Coryza with discharge of thick white mucus.*** Fluent catarrh from tubal nasal discharge like gonorrhea, staining pillow greenish yellow. Discharge of bloody pus. Nosebleed when speaking or swallowing. Nosebleeds at night, only from right nostril. Alae nasi and corners of mouth cracked. Smell of flowers seems to send chill over her.

Perspiration - Bathed in warm sweat, about face, neck and hands. Clammy sweat all over. Copious sweat of rank smell. Exhausting sweat after sleep, at night.

Rectum - Dysentery, blood with profuse, greenish mucus, cries with violent cutting pain in the rectum. Profuse diarrhea with colic pain. Diarrhea coming out with great force. Obstinate constipation. Great tenesmus, rectum as if it could not expel feces because they are soft. Urgent desire for stool, but passes only wind. Mucus yellow liquid stools. Stools large, whitish, rough, scaly, hard.

Skin - Dry, hot skin. Pimples between lip and chin. Herpetic eruption in both axilla. Ichthyosis with bran like desquamation of skin. ***Very small blotches like fleabites.*** Shining, glazed and red appearance of ulcers on shin and wrist. Crusts on skin, grayish yellow matter formed underneath and squeezed out.

Sleep - Great desire to sleep. Sleeplessness from emotional strain, with entire nervous debility, crying. Can't find any comfortable position in bed. Cries out and talks in sleep. ***Dreams of snakes***. Dreams of urinating, of going on a journey. Wakes at night with a sensation as if bed were in motion. ***Symptoms worse after sleep.***

Stomach - Stomach tender and bloated. Coldness in stomach. Burning in epigastric region, feeling of a weight and pressure of a stone in stomach. Weak, sinking feeling at stomach-pit, with nausea, on waking. Gnawing, hungry feeling, not better eating. Severe throbbing in region of solar plexus. Nausea on waking, with headache. Nausea at beginning of diphtheria. Nausea better by belchings of wind. Sudden, incessant vomiting of all food. Frequent attacks of severe vomiting. Vomiting of offensive, dark green mucus.

Teeth - Pain in left upper molars, coming from left temple through left ear. Teeth sensitive to cold water. Teeth loose, caused by defective nutrition and exposure. Gums swollen, ulcerated, retracted, bleeding.

Temperature - Chilly feeling lasting all day. Internal chilliness with external warmth. Fever and chills for a few days, up and down every few hours. Heat alternating with chill. Intense fever on waking, with perspiration. Exhausting sweats after sleep. Wakes at night in cold perspiration with fearful foreboding.

Throat - ***Sore throat,*** from constant inclination to swallow saliva. Painful swallowing, pain extends to ears. Sore throat and cough with menstruation. Sensitive to touch. Swelling of throat, worse after sleep. Throat cold, feels burned raw. Sensation as if throat were closing and he would choke. ***Shining glazed*** appearance of deposit, ***pearly-white*** or like white porcelain. Throat glistens like fish scales. ***Uvula coated.*** White ulcers on tonsils. Both tonsils swollen and covered with spots of exudation. Tonsils swollen as almost to close throat. ***Tonsillitis, diphtheria, symptoms change repeatedly from side to side.*** Larynx sensitive to pressure.

Lump in throat. Wakes with mouth and throat painfully dry. Throat feels stiff as a board. Pricking sensation in throat. Tickling sensation causes constant cough. Hoarseness during menses.

Tongue - Dryness of tip of tongue. Tongue, swollen, cold, stiff, looks patched. Tongue coated white with bright red edges, profuse salivation. ***Tongue coated whitish gray***, brown, yellow.

Vertigo - Dizzy sensation with slight nausea. Sensation of walking or floating in air (Stict.). Waking at night with sensation as if bed were in motion. Vertigo before menses.

Vision - Blurred vision, nausea and vomiting at height of attack of headache. Sensation of a film before eyes. ***Tendency in retina to retain the impression of objects and colors,*** or the old image is projected into the next. Difficulty in distinguishing objects. Colored spots before the eyes. ***Difficulty in reading, letters run together***, page doesn't look clear.

COMMENTS - Hering stated that "Dioscorides, Rhasis, Pliny and Sextus recommended it for the removal of the dead fetus." Hering added that the remedy was revived by Dr. Reisig of New York, who used it successfully in the treatment of diphtheria. After Dr. Reisig, the remedy was used by Bayard and Swan. Swan's potencies were prepared from Reisig's 17c.

Lac-c. was one of the major remedies for the diphtheria epidemics in the United States. Diphtheria with fetid discharges. Diphtheria paralysis. For the affects of diphtheria. Glistening, inflamed membranes, particularly of the throat.

Glistening, ulcerated tonsils. Tonsillitis. Swollen mucus follicles, covered with cream-colored mucus. Glossy throat, may have white patches on the tonsils. Sore throats, worse on the left, alternates sides. Sensitive, externally and internally (Hep.). Difficult swallowing, sharp pain that shoots to the ear (Phyt.). Tickling sensation in the throat or a lump in the throat.

Corners of the mouth and alae nasi are cracked. Hay fever and sinusitis where the discharges alternate.

Ozaena. Discharges of the upper palate. Bloody pus discharges several times a day. Crusts, under which gray matter forms. Bones of the nose are sore to pressure.

Hormonal and breast problems. Premenstrual syndrome with irritability, impulsiveness. Premenstrual syndrome with swollen, hypersensitive breasts, so sensitive the clothes cannot touch the breasts (Calc., Con.). Hysteria, especially before menses, can get violent (Lach.). Crying and weeping spells. Sore throats and headaches before menses. Menses ameliorate symptoms.

Ovarian cysts (Thuj.). After a rupture or surgery of an ovarian cyst, cysts appear on other side. Breast cancer after surgery that metastasized to the other breast. Mastitis, worse least motion (Bry.).

Hypersensitive nipples in nursing mothers, cannot continue nursing. More milk in one breast than the other, or pain in one breast while the baby nurses the other. For conditions causing milk to dry up, or to dry up milk. Lack of milk (Urt-u.).

Restless, nervous and prostration. Vertigo (Con., Phos., Cocc, Asar.). Sensation of lightness or levitation, seemed to walk on air (Asar., Calc.), as if they are floating up off the bed. Makes mistakes in writing and speaking, poor memory.

Periodic symptoms, worse in the morning of one day and in the afternoon of the next. Generally left sided, but will often move to the right. Alternating sides. Worse after sleep (Lach.). Very sensitive to the cold and cold wind, but better cold applications, worse heat. Desire milk and spicy foods.

The modality "alternation of sides" once led Clarke to the cure of an eczematous condition of the eyelids in a child. The child's aunt, who brought her to him, causally remarked that it often left one side entirely and went to the other and then back again. Lac-c. cleared it up in a very short time.

E. T. Balch asked for advice in the case of Maud, age 10, a brunette of healthy parents. She had fallen forward and hurt her chest while playing one and a half years earlier.

Nothing was thought of it at the time, but when brought to Dr. Balch, she was pale, emaciated, capricious, with no desire for play.

Her sleep was disturbed by frightful dreams. During the day, piteously begged her mother to take her, she was so afraid. She felt as though snakes were on her back. In response to advice, Balch gave one dose of Lac-c. 50,000c. dry, and in twenty-four hours the child became more lively and cheerful and very soon all abnormal sensations disappeared.

RELATIONS - ***Compare:*** (1) Lach., Cong. (2) Lac-v. - headache, rheumatic pains, constipation. (3) Lac-v-c., curds - nausea of pregnancy. (4) Lac-v-f. - diphtheria, leucorrhea, menorrhagia, dysphagia. (5) Lac-ac.

REFERENCES - Boericke. Clarke. Murphy. Phatak.

LAC CAPRINUM

(Goat's Milk)

PHARMACY - lac-cpr. Lac caprinum. Goat's milk. Dilutions. N. O. Bovidae. ***Historical dose:*** All potencies.

CLINICAL - Arthritis. Backache. Headache. Hoarseness. Indigestion. ***Joint, pains.*** Leucorrhea. Palpitations. Rheumatism. Sexual, disorders. Vertigo.

HOMEOPATHIC - ***Joint, pains. Wandering pains. Sharp, stitching pains***. ***Cracking*** in joints. Stiff, painful neck, worse turning head, worse draft, cold with dull, heavy sensation in head. ***Chilliness.*** Digestive disturbances. Pain in stomach, very tense, gurgling around 11 a.m. to 12 a.m. Sensation as if passage is obstructed.

Headache above left eye, disappearing quickly, later on the right side. Icy cold feet in bed preventing sleep. Worse after eating, as if stomach expands. Fetid odor from axilla, genitals, or feet. Vertigo better lying. Palpitations, worse coffee, fright, fear of heart disease.

MIND - Anticipatory anxieties. Anxiety in chest. Impatience. Restlessness, nervousness, driving from place to place. Hurry, haste, everybody moves too slowly. ***Startled easily.*** Fear of being taken by surprise or attacked. Fear of sharp things. ***Fear of having a heart attack.*** Fear of heights. Oversensitive to noise. Sensitive to odors.

Capricious. Sadness, melancholy, especially during headache. Weeping, tearful mood, with headache. Homesickness. Desire for company, worse when alone. Averse to company with head pain. Aversion to music. ***Strong sexual desires.*** Fear of own sexual impulses. Contemptuous. Indifference to opinion of others. Censorious. Suspicious, mistrustful. Indignation. Sulking. Indolence, aversion to work.

Irritability from trifles. Easy anger, lying down ameliorates. Anger, on waking. Anger from being interrupted. Uncontrollable anger, rage. Shrieking, screaming, desire to strike. Quarrelsomeness, scolding. Malicious. Threatening. Complaining. Rudeness.

Abdomen - Heaviness.

Back - Backache. Pain, between scapulae.

Chest - Anxiety, in chest.

Dreams - Anxious dreams of quarrels, being pursued. Dreams of old friends, animals, goats, vegetables, fruits, flowers. Amorous dreams with pollutions.

Eyes - Pain in the morning. Winking.

Female - Leucorrhea, curdy. Scanty menses with sensation of profuse flow.

Food - Desires fried foods, cold milk, cold tea, spices, sweets.

Head - Headache above left eye, disappearing quickly, then on the right side. Fullness in the forehead. Heaviness in the forehead, above the eyes, better from pulling hair. Headache in the morning, 10 a.m. until 3 p.m. Pain accompanied by eye-blinking, sneezing, compelled to close eyes. Pain in forehead, left temple, better after sleep. Pressing pain in vertex, from exposure to sun, worse slightest motion.

Heart - Palpitations, worse from coffee, fright.

Limbs - Arthritis. ***Joint, pains.*** Rheumatism. ***Wandering pains. Sharp, stitching pains.*** Pain in left thigh.

Male - Sexual, disorders. Sexual perversions. Night dreams with pollutions.

Modalities - Desire for cold bathing with intolerance for warm bathing. Warmth aggravates.

Neck - Stiff and painful, worse turning head, draft, cold.

Nose - Pain at root of nose. Acute smell. Sneezing.

Perspiration - Fetid odor from axilla, genitals, or feet.

Sleep - Icy cold feet in bed preventing sleep. Unrefreshing sleep.

Stomach - Appetite diminished, from anxiety. Burning pain, after eating, better bending double.

Throat - Hoarseness.

Urine - Burning, hot.

Vertigo - Vertigo, as if everything were turning in a circle, better lying down.

RELATIONS - ***Compare:*** Lac-c., Kali-c., Lac-f., Lac-h., Lac-v., Lac-v-c., Lac-d.

REFERENCES - Sankaran.

LAC DELPHINUM

(Dolphin's Milk)

PHARMACY - lac-del. Lac delphinum. Dolphin's milk. Dilutions. ***Historical dose:*** All potencies.

CLINICAL - Aphthae. Constipation. Diarrhea. Flatulence. Headaches. Heartburn. Hemorrhoids. Numbness. Photophobia. Pneumonia. Vertigo.

HOMEOPATHIC - Delirium during chill.

MIND - Feels he is alone. Sensation of isolation. Insecurity. Introverted. Spaced-out feeling. Desire for company. Wants to be watched constantly. Conscientious about trifles. Irritability. Clairvoyant.

Tranquility. Affectionate. Amorous disposition. Communicative, expansive. Jesting. Antics, plays. Laughing easily. Desire for amusement. Sentimental with music. Desires bright colors. Love for animals. Loss of self-control. Impelled to touch things.

Fearlessness. Ailments from fright or fear. Anxiety about his family, children. Anxiety after eating. Fear of impending danger, of accidents, robbers. Fear in a crowd. Oversensitive to noise, on going to sleep.

Abdomen - Flatulence.

Back - Dull pain, on lying down.

Bladder - Burning, sore pains. Frequent urging to urinate, morbid desire. Urine odor strong, offensive.

Chest - Gurgling sounds. Sensation of a bubble, sides. Rib pain.

Ears - Redness. Sensation of dryness. Stopped sensation. Hearing acute.

Eyes - Photophobia. Burning pain, redness. Eye pain during fever. Burning eyes from reaction to perfume.

Face - Pressing pain. Maxillary sinus pain.

Food - Appetite diminished, enjoyment lost. Increased, hunger in morning. Thirst for cold drinks.

Head - Headaches, occiput, temples. Dull pains, worse right side.

Limbs - Numbness, better motion, rubbing, walking. Numbness in upper limbs during sleep. Numbness in leg, in morning. Cramp-like pains. Throbbing pain. Heavy feeling. Swelling of lower limbs, ankles. Sensation as if blister on toe. Foot perspiration. Eruption on foot. Itching on thigh, forearm, palm, in spots.

Lungs - Tickling in the air passages. Dry, short coughs. Expectoration grayish. Pneumonia.

Male - Sexual desire increased.

Mouth - Aphthae. Discoloration of tongue, red edges.

Nose - Nasal catarrh. Coryza with fever. Post-nasal discharge, watery. Sense of fullness. Pressing, pain.

Rectum - Inactive bowels. Constipation. Diarrhea. Stools dark, dry, infrequent, loose, small and watery. Flatus after dinner. Burning, smarting hemorrhoids.

Sleep - Light, restless sleep, turning left to right all night. Sleep interrupted. Position changes frequently. Sleep, semi-conscious, hears everything. Unrefreshing sleep. Anxious to wake up on time.

Stomach - Gnawing, pressing, burning pain, pressure, better warm applications, worse lying down on back. Burning pain, heartburn, after eating, coffee. Nausea in the morning.

Throat - Dryness, painful on swallowing, worse morning. Burning pain. Sore throat, left side. Lump in throat. Voice loss.

Vertigo - Vertigo during chill. Vertigo, with spaciness, obscurity of vision. Vertigo swaying toward left. Vertigo turning in a circle to the right. Vertigo as if floating.

Vision - Blurred, foggy vision. Acute vision for small objects. Objects seem large.

RELATIONS - ***Compare:*** Lac-c., Lac-f., Lac-h., Lac-v., Lac-v-c., Lac-d.

REFERENCES - Herrick.

LAC EQUINUM

(Horse's Milk)

PHARMACY - lac-eq. Lac equinum. Horse's milk. Lac equorum. Dilutions. ***Historical dose:*** All potencies.

CLINICAL - Backache. Constipation. Convulsions. Fatigue. Flatulence. Herpes. Insomnia. Weakness.

HOMEOPATHIC - Convulsions on waking. Convulsions followed by paralysis. Convulsions during the fever. Tonic, clonic convulsions. Convulsions on right side of body. Convulsions in children. Intolerance of clothes. Fatigue. Evening or twilight, amel. Worse alcohol. Pulse, frequent, motion aggravates. Tension of muscles. Weakness after warm bathing. Weakness from warm weather. Weakness after menses.

MIND - Impatient, hurried. Irritable. Restless. Desire to travel. Industrious. Anger in traffic. Sensitive to noise. Easily offended. Complaining, quarrelsome. Discontented. Indignation, frustration. Cannot support injustice. Critical, censorious. Cursing. Dictatorial.

Forgetful. Memory weakness. Mistakes, transposes letters and numbers. Fuzzy sensation of mind. Wandering thoughts. Anticipatory anxiety, better lemonade. Anxiety of conscience. Anxiety after menses. Delusions of neglected duty. Insane delusions. Desire to escape.

Abdomen - Distension. Flatulence, after eating. Cramping pain, pressure.

Back - Backache, worse rising from a seat. Pimples. Backache, lumbar region. Aching pain lumbar region.

Bladder - Urination frequent.

Dreams - Vivid dreams, difficult to remember. Dreams of unsuccessful efforts. Dreams of fights, police, being pursued, animals, restrained by collars. Dreams of difficulties during journeys, foreigners. Amorous dreams, of being naked.

Eyes - Dry eyes.

Female - Decreased sex drive. Menses, early. Pains during menses. Ovary pain alternating sides, after menses. Left ovary pain after menses. Sexual passion, diminished or increased. Tingling voluptuous in left ovary, after menses

Food - Appetite increased. Desires lemonade. Aversion to chocolate.

Head - Headaches, worse forehead. Tension, constricted feeling.

Heart - Tachycardia.

Limbs - Cold feet. Sore knee on rising, ascending stairs. Pain in right shoulder. Hip pain, right side on walking. Hip pain, right side after rising from a seat. Hip pain, right side, extending to knee. Hip pain, alternating sides. Cramps, hands, legs. Blotches. Discoloration of toenails. Urticaria. Itching. Heaviness sensation while walking. Numbness right hand. Restless, hands, feet. Stiffness of knees, in morning on rising.

Lungs - Dry cough. Dyspnea. Difficult, taking a deep breath. Breath stops at epigastric area. Asthmatic, wheezing respiration. Difficult breathing.

Male - Decreased sex drive.

Mouth - Gums bleed easily.

Nose - Coryza, in open air, better cold.

Perspiration - Profuse sweats.

Rectum - Constipation. Incomplete evacuation. Urge to stool, with insufficient results. Loose stools. Mucus and flatus with stool.

Sleep - Insomnia. Sleepless after midnight. Wakes 3 a.m. to 5 a.m. Bad sleep. Sleeplessness, from full moon. Waking, frequent. Waking, 12 a.m. - 1 a.m. Waking, 2 a.m. Waking, 3 a.m. or 4 a.m. Waking as from a fright. Unrefreshing sleep.

Skin - Acne. Herpetic eruptions, itching, pimples. Skin discolored blackish, bluish. Eruptions, circinate.

Stomach - Belching. Burning pain. Nausea.

Throat - Constriction of throat.

Vertigo - Vertigo on waking.

RELATIONS - ***Compare:*** Lac-c., Lac-f., Lac-h., Lac-v., Lac-v-c., Lac-d.

REFERENCES - Herrick.

LAC FELINUM

(Cat's Milk)

PHARMACY - lac-f. Lac felinum. Cat's milk. Dilutions. ***Historical dose:*** All potencies.

CLINICAL - ***Asthenopia.*** Breast, nodules. ***Ciliary neuralgia.*** Depression. Dysmenorrhea. Eye, disorders. Headaches. Keratitis. Leucorrhea. Mouth, inflammation. Neuralgias. Photophobia. Styes. Throat, catarrh. Trembling.

HOMEOPATHIC - Lac-f. was introduced by Swan; the full pathogenesis appears in Medical Visitor, Aug., 1893. The greatest number of the symptoms were experienced in the head and eyes, and many of them have been confirmed.

Lac-f. has eye symptoms, ciliary neuralgia, photophobia, ***asthenopia*** and dysmenorrhea. The clinically verified symptoms include a morbid conscientiousness, heaviness in forehead. Scalded sensation on tongue. Absence of appetite.

Eye disorders are mostly accompanied by shooting pains from eye backwards. Styes were present in some cases. Constant nervous trembling, especially of hands, as in alcoholics.

MIND - Great depression of spirits. Cannot weep, although sad. Feeling of helplessness. Contempt of self. ***Morbid conscientiousness,*** every little fault appeared a crime. Very irritable and cross to everyone. Aversion to men. Desire to travel.

Fear of pointed, sharp things, pins. Fear of falling downstairs, without vertigo. Mental illusion that the corners of furniture or any pointed object near her, were about to run into eyes.

Delusion she looks wretched on looking in mirror.

Abdomen - Pain in abdomen and back, as if menses about commencing. Pain in bowels. Sensation of a cold bandage over lower part of abdomen.

Breasts - Induration of breasts, nodules in breasts, pain, before menses. Milk, disappearing.

Chest - Oppressed breathing, continuing for several days. Difficulty in drawing a long breath, seems as if the breathing was done by upper part of lungs alone.

Eyes - ***Asthenopia.*** Sharp pain through center of left eyeball. Shooting pain from eyes backwards. Eye pains causing profuse lachrymation. ***Ciliary neuralgia.*** Heavy pressure downwards of eyebrows and eyelids, as if the parts were lead. ***Sensation as if eyes were drawn backward.*** Inclination to keep eyes shut. Eyes feel as if sunken in head and left eye occasionally waters. Twitching of outer end of left upper lid inside. Styes.

Female - Menses copious, too frequent, painful. Menses suppressed. Voluptuous itching. Itching of vulva inside and out, yellow leucorrhea. Leucorrhea ceased on third and reappeared on fourth day. Great weight and bearing down in pelvis like falling of the womb, worse when standing. Dragging pain in left ovary.

Food - No appetite. Great desire to eat paper. Craving for milk, salty things, fish. Aversion to milk, fats.

Head - Dull pain in forehead, in region of eyebrows. Heaviness in forehead. Heavy pressure in sides of head and vertex. ***Sharp pain over left eye.*** Acute pain on vertex, frontal region. Pulsations in head with sensation of heat in forehead and constriction across bridge of nose. ***Formication at vertex.*** Sensation of looseness of brain.

Kidneys - Frequent desire to urinate, urine very pale. Obstruction in urinating, has to wait.

Limbs - Numbness. Pain in right side of left wrist when using index finger. Legs ache. Left foot feels cold when touched by right foot. Coldness of foot, one cold the other hot. Sensitive feet. Touching feet.

Modalities - Worse lying on left side, on painful side.

Mouth - Loss of taste. Brassy taste in mouth. Salivation during sleep. Dryness of mouth. ***Sensation as if tongue were scalded by a hot drink.*** Redness under tongue, on gums and mouth. Very sore mouth. Soreness and sensation of ulcers on tongue and roof of mouth. Small white ulcers covering tongue and mouth. Tongue enlarged and serrated at edges by teeth.

Nose - Cannot bear the smell of clams of which she is normally very fond and cannot eat them. Icy coldness before headache.

Sleep - Dullness, sleepiness, gaping. Heavy, profound sleep, not easily awakened. Dreams of earthquakes, of being pursued.

Stomach - Great soreness and sensitiveness of epigastric region. After eating feels swollen, has to take off her dress and loosen clothes. Stomach sore all around just below the belt, worse left side. Occasionally very slight nausea. Heat in epigastrium.

Stool - Natural stool, but very slow in passing, at 2 a.m. Stool long, tenacious, slipping back when ceasing to strain, seeming inability of rectum to expel its contents.

Teeth - Pains in all the teeth as the hot pain from head touched them.

Temperature - Cold and heat alternately, each continuing but a short time.

Throat - Tough yellow mucus in pharynx, cannot hawk it up and has to swallow it. Mucus in pharynx and throat is thick, yellow tough, stringy, expectorated with difficulty and has a sickish sweet taste. Sensation of lump in throat.

COMMENTS - Many eye cases are on record. Swan wrote, "Terrible headache penetrating the left eyeball to center of brain with pain in left supra-orbital region extending through brain to right vertex."

In another case, Swan recorded "Pain in eyes back into head, extremely sharp with a sensation as if the eyes extended back. Great photophobia, any continued glare causes the pain."

Berridge reported the case of "Mr. H. 37. Left eye inflamed three weeks, deep red, photophobia, on left segment of cornea as ulcer. For three nights, pain like a knife running from left eye to left occiput, on lying down, especially on left side. Burning in left temple, near eye, worse at night.

"Lac-f. 40,000c. every four hours. Eye was better next days and steadily got well. The pain ceased first."

RELATIONS - ***Compare:*** (1) Lac-c., Lac-d. (2) In eye affections, Spig. (3) Styes - Staph., Puls., Hep.

REFERENCES - Clarke.

LAC HUMANUM

(Human Breast milk)

PHARMACY - lac-h. Lac humanum. Human breast milk. Milk from one nursing mother. Dilutions. ***Historical dose:*** All potencies.

CLINICAL - Addictions. Belching. Breast, disorders. Conjunctivitis. Coryza. Eating, disorders. Flatulence. Headache. Heartburn. Herpes. Hot flushes. Leucorrhea. Nausea. Pre-menstrual, syndrome. Rashes. Sciatica. Vertigo. Vomiting.

HOMEOPATHIC - Lac-h. is made from human breast milk, proved in 1993 by Jacqueline Houghton and Elisabeth Halahan in England. In folk medicine, mother's milk was used as a remedy for infant conjunctivitis.

Hormonal disturbances. Pre-menstrual syndrome. Breast disorders. Swollen breasts, before the menses. Sadness during menses. Addictions, eating disorders. Huge fluctuations in body weight, changes easily. The senses are more sensitive. Flushes of heat upward. Conjunctivitis.

MIND - Detached feelings. Indifference. Lack of feeling. Feels relaxed and tranquil. Absent-minded. Difficult trying to concentrate. Thoughts are disconnected. Sense of isolation. Automatic conduct. Unconsciousness

Changeable moods. Fastidious. Irresolution. Anxiety. Irritable. Discontented. Cursing. Wringing the hands. Lack of self confidence. Averse to company.

Abdomen - Distention, worse eating. Stitching in the hypochondrium. Flatulence. Sore abdomen during menses, worse from pressure.

Back - Stiffness of back. Neck stiff and cracking on turning the head.

Breasts - Swollen breasts, before the menses. Stitching in breasts. Sensation as if milk is coming.

Chest - Constriction and oppression. Pain from sternum to back.

Ears - Ache, stitching in left ear. Noises in the ears.

Eyes - Bloodshot. Conjunctivitis. Eyes feel tired. Lachrymation in the wind. As if sand is in the eye.

Face - Cracks in corner of mouth. Herpes about the lips. Rash, better after menses. Jaw feels dislocated.

Female - Sadness during menses. Menses is black and dark, clotted blood, prolonged. Bearing down pains. Leucorrhea like cream, clear, ropy and stringy. Sharp pain in ovaries. Sex drive increased.

Food - Appetite increased. Desires sweets, starches, chocolate, ginger, bacon, salt. Aversion to sour foods, milk. Increased thirst. Thirstless. Likes warm drinks. Worse from alcohol.

Head - Pressure and constriction. Headache. Bursting sensation, worse left side. Hammering pain.

Heart - Constriction and oppression. Cramp in heart.

Kidneys - Copious urination during menses. Strong, offensive odor, dark yellow urine.

Limbs - Drops things, awkward. Sciatica on right side. Knees are stiff, feel lame. Numbness of soles.

Lungs - Barking, dry cough. Loose cough with thick, white expectoration, difficult to expel, with a metallic taste.

Modalities - Better from eating, sex. Worse from alcohol, eating, before menses.

Mouth - Bleeding gums. Sore tongue. Vesicles.

Nose - Nasal congestion on waking. Coryza with clear, bland, one-sided discharge. Sneezing. Itching in posterior nares.

Rectum - Stools are first hard, then soft. Stools, ball like, offensive and soft.

Skin - Rashes and eruptions, worse before the menses. Itching. Goose bumps.

Sleep - Dreams about babies, children and family. Dreams about disaster, falling, war and death.

Stomach - Sour rising. Belchings, heartburn, nausea and hiccough, worse from eating. Nausea from the smell of food. Vomiting during headache.

Temperature - Lack of vital heat. Flushes of heat upward and a great feeling of relaxation.

Throat - Dryness and irritation. Sensation of a lump. Tenacious mucus in throat. Sore and raw throat. Tingling.

Vertigo - Vertigo as if intoxicated. Vertigo during headaches.

RELATIONS - ***Compare:*** Lac-c. Luna., Anac., Sep., Phos., Sulph.

REFERENCES - Assilem. Halahan. Houghton.

LAC LEONINUM

(Lion's Milk)

PHARMACY - lac-leo. Lac leoninum. Lion's milk. Lioness milk. Dilutions. ***Historical dose:*** All potencies.

CLINICAL - Awkwardness. Backache. Constipation. Dysmenorrhea. Headaches. Insomnia. Lumbago. Numbness.

MIND - Dictatorial, domineering, dogmatic, despotic. Ailments from anger, vexation. Anger from contradiction. Anger from reproaches. Fear of hearing bad news. Anxiety on waking from frightful dreams. Anxiety about future. Anxiety on waking. Awkwardness. Full of cares, worries for nature, animals, plants etc. Aversion to company yet aversion to be alone. Aversion to company. Company agg., fond of solitude. Desire for company. Comprehension, easy. Concentration, active. Contemptuous. Coquettish, too much.

Delusions of floating in air. Delusions that he is light, incorporeal, immaterial.

Forgetfulness. Forgetfulness, leaves behind his possessions. Forsaken feeling. cannot handle things anymore.

Overwhelmed by stress. Haughty. Impatience. Indignation.

Indolence aversion to work. Industrious, mania for work. Industrious, mania for work: evening. Irritability. Jealousy. Kleptomania.

Laughing when sad. Love for animals. Love for nature. Alternating moods. Changeable, variable moods. Music amel. Desire to play, playful. Quiet disposition. Rage, fury. ***Resentment to husband.*** Strong responsibility. Sadness, despondency, depression, melancholy. ***Oversensitive when hearing of cruelties.*** Sensitive, oversensitive to nature, surroundings. Suspiciousness, mistrustfulness. Sympathetic, compassionate.

Indisposed to talk, desire to be silent, taciturn. Clearness of thoughts. Tranquillity, serenity, calmness. Tranquillity in morning on waking. Unsympathetic, unscrupulous to friends and family, even towards closest. ***Unsympathetic, acts as if she cares.*** Violence, vehemence. Helpless feelings. Weeping, amel. Weeping, tearful mood in morning on waking. Weeping because she could not sleep. Aversion to mental work. Desire for mental work.

Back - Itching, scratching amel. Backache, dorsal region. Right scapulae pain extending to shoulder. Lumbago pain on turning. Lumbago pain bending backward agg. Aching drawing pain, cervical region. Stiffness. Tension, forenoon. Back tension extending to neck. Tension dorsal region.

Bladder - Bladder pain during urination. Pain after urination. Burning pain during urination. Burning pain after urination.

Chest - Pain, right ribs. Pain in false ribs. Aching pain in false ribs. Pinching pain. Stitching pain in ribs.

Dreams - Dreams of adolescence. Dreams: alone on earth, he is. Dreams of accidents. Dreams of crash of airplane. Amorous dreams. Dreams of animals. Dreams of cats, felines. Dreams of animals snakes. Anxious dreams. Dreams full of cares. Dreams about children. Dreams of childbirth. Dreams of death. Dreams of old friends. Dreams of monsters. Dreams of pursued, of being. Restless dreams. Dreams of urinating. Dreams of war.

Eyes - Swelling of eyelids. Discoloration of eyes, redness. Redness of eyelids. Swelling, eyes, eyelids.

Female - Menses, dark like pitch. Frequent menses. Menses, too early, too soon. Menses seven days too early. Menses painful. Dysmenorrhea. Menses too short. Sexual desire diminished or increased.

Food - Appetite diminished. Thirst for large quantities. Desires fruit, juicy things. Desires cold drinks, cold water. Desires cucumber. Desires indistinct, knows not what. Desires meat. Desires milk. Desires potatoes. Desires salads. Desires salt or salty food. Desires spinach. Desires vegetables. Desires yogurt.

Head - Pulsating and throbbing pains. Headaches, worse evening, 6 pm. Headaches, evenings 6 pm. until 4 am. Headaches, lying agg. Forehead pain evening agg. Occiput pain, extending to neck region. Temple pain. Pulsating, throbbing, evening. Pulsating, throbbing in forehead.

Heart - Heart pain. Pinching pain.

Kidneys - Pain in left kidney. Kidney pain in afternoon, 5 p.m. until 7 pm. Kidney pain, drinking amel. Pinching pain. Twitching.

Limbs - Awkwardness. Numbness, insensibility. Numbness during sleep. Numbness, upper limbs. Numbness, hands at night. Stiffness of joints, motion, amel. Tingling, prickling, upper limbs. Tingling, prickling, forearms, hands. Tingling, prickling hands at night.

Limbs pain - Tendons. Hips, while walking agg. Pinching pain, walking agg. Sore, bruised pain. Sore, bruised feet while walking amel.

Modalities - Better seashore air. Better being fanned. Better undressing. Better weeping. Worse warm clothes. Intolerance of clothing.

Mouth - Dryness of mouth.

Neck - Clothing agg. Aching pain in cervical region, bending head back amel. Aching pain in cervical region after supper, amel. Drawing pain, right side. ***Neck pain, extending to shoulders.*** Tension, neck. Stiffness on turning head.

Nose - Sneezing, evening agg.

Perspiration - Night sweats at 11 p.m. Fever agg. Acrid sweat. Odor acrid. Strong smelling sweat.

Rectum - Constipation. Flatus, offensive odor like spoiled eggs. Rectal pain in morning, 7 am. Cramping pain. Stool, dark color. Stool, odor like sulphur. Slender stool.

Skin - Itching, scratching amel.

Sleep - Refreshing sleep. Restless sleep. Short sleep. Sleepiness, afternoon agg. Sleepiness, afternoon: agg. Sleepiness, 1 p.m., after 3 p.m. Insomnia, at night. Sleeplessness from activity of thoughts. Sleeplessness from restlessness. Sleeplessness from thoughts. Unrefreshing sleep. Waking after midnight. Waking after 2-3 a.m. Waking with pain in throat. Waking from dreams, pain. Frequent waking.

Stomach - Belching, worse after eating.

Temperature - Sensation of heat.

Throat - Sore, bruised throat pain. Sore, bruised pain, morning, on waking.

Tongue - Pain, tip of tongue. Sore, bruised pain.

RELATIONS - *Compare:* Lac-c., Lac-f., Lac-h., Lac-v., Lac-v-c., Lac-d.

REFERENCES - Herrick.

LAC LOXODONTA AFRICANA

(African Elephant's Milk)

PHARMACY - lac-lox-a. Lac loxodonta africana. African elephant's milk. Dilutions. *Historical dose:* All potencies.

CLINICAL - Brain, fag. Coryza. Cramps. Depression. Diarrhea. Flatulence. Headaches. Itching. Nausea. Palpitations. Vertigo.

HOMEOPATHIC - Heavy sensation. Stoop shouldered. Lassitude, must lie down before dinner, at 5 p.m. Weariness, in the afternoon, from 8 p.m. to 9 p.m. Cramping pains. Shivers, as if air blew over body. Aversion to exercise. Better from playing in the water. Worse morning, on waking.

MIND - Changeable, variable mood. Loquacity, alternating with detachment. Euphoria, alternating with weariness. Light-hearted. Quick to act. Loss of conception of time. Time, passes too quickly, appears shorter. Theorizing about proven substance.

Difficulty thinking and comprehending. Makes mistakes when talking, uses wrong words. Makes mistakes in writing, confounding letters. Spaced-out feeling. Brain fag. Dullness, sluggishness mind. Mental exhaustion. Prostration. Torpor. Tranquility, calm.

Quiet disposition. Despair. Weeping, tearful mood. Sadness, depression. Awkwardness. Anxiety from pains. Quarrelsome. Scolding. Cursing, swearing.

Abdomen - Distention. Emptiness sensation. Drawing upward pain.

Back - Pain in cervical region, dorsal region, scapula. Crampy pains, in scapula, sacral region. Pain on straightening of the back.

Chest - Constriction. Pressing pain when sitting stooped, worse standing. Awareness of heart's beating. Palpitations, after tea. Perspiration in right axilla.

Cough - Dry cough. Cough with tightness in chest.

Ears - Ears, itching.

Eyes - Staring, tired sensation. Squinting. Swelling of eyelids. Discharge is yellow, on eyelids, morning. Acute vision, sees colors, green, stripes.

Face - Expression scowling. Pain in malar bones.

Female - As if bubble of water or air in vagina. Menses, early, heavy, with clots. Sexual desire decreased.

Food - Capricious appetite, diminished or increased. Desires alcohol, wine, sweets, chocolate, fresh fruit, melons, vegetables, yogurt, fish. Indistinct desire, know not what he wants. Averse to spices, tea, salmon.

Head - Headache moving from left to right. Headache in forehead, extending to neck. Headache with vertigo. Head pain on waking, with chilliness and shivering, 3 a.m. to 6 p.m. Headache, with perspiration on forehead, 3 a.m. to 6 p.m.

Kidneys - Pain in right kidney, morning, 5 a.m. to 8 a.m.

Limbs - Sensation in hand as if in puddle of water. Pain in finger joints. Restless hands, feet. Trembling, weak legs, in the afternoon. Cramps in thigh.

Modalities - Worse morning, on waking.

Mouth - Itching of palate.

Nose - Coryza. Itching.

Rectum - Diarrhea, loose stool. Flatulence.

Sleep - Sleepiness, on waking, in the afternoon, 3 to 4 p.m. Catnaps refresh, in the afternoon. Falling asleep difficult, because of flow of thoughts. Restless. Frequent waking, 3 a.m., in the morning. Deep, refreshing sleep.

Stomach - Anxiety on waking. Emptiness sensation, in the afternoon. Belching after breakfast, dinner. Nausea. Burning pain, after waking. Drawing pain, upward. Stomach tension.

Throat - Itching. Sore pain in the evening. Tension on the left side.

Vertigo - Descending vertigo, with headache. Vertigo from looking downward.

RELATIONS - ***Compare:*** Lac-c., Lac-f., Lac-h., Lac-v., Lac-v-c., Lac-d.

REFERENCES - Herrick.

LAC LUPINUM

(Gray Wolf's Milk)

PHARMACY - lac-lup. Lac lupinum. Gray Wolf's milk. Dilutions. ***Historical dose:*** All potencies.

CLINICAL - Awkwardness. Backache. Chest pain. Chills. Delirium. Dysmenorrhea. Fevers. Nausea. Sleeplessness. Typhoid. Typhus.

HOMEOPATHIC - Heavy sensation. Burning sensation, internally. Stiffness, rigidity of muscles. Internal tension. Weakness, enervation, in the daytime, from slight exertion. Weariness in the afternoon. Increased endurance.

Coldness in general. Chill at night. Fever with chill. Continued fever, typhus, typhoid. Relapsing fever. Worse becoming heated.

MIND - Alert mind. Clear thoughts. Heightened awareness of the body, skin surface. Cheerfulness, gaiety, happiness in company. Excitement, desire for fun. Contented with himself. Relaxed feeling. Quiet disposition and calm. Serious.

Disordered, wandering thoughts. Distracted, hurried. Impatience, alternating with patience. Excessive mind chatter. Confusion. Disoriented. Disorganized, losing things. Poor planning, roaming around, unsure. Errors of perception.

Heedless, careless. Indolence. Aversion to work. Neglects his business. Daydreaming. Indifference, apathy. Feels detached. Inclination to sit. Stupefaction, as if intoxicated. Desire to be silent, taciturn. Careless what others think.

Industrious, efficient. Wants to help others less fortunate. Sympathetic. Love and openness for friends. Appreciation for fatherly love, between younger and older men.

Sudden anxiety, with feeling that control over senses is lost. Anxiety as if something needs to be done but knows not what. Anxiety about business, about her condition. Fearful dreams.

Righteous feeling. Censorious, critical. Argumentative. Blames others in her family. Disposed to find fault. Quarrelsome. Scolding. Irritability. Everything causes feeling of isolation. Anger, irascibility, morning on waking. Anger with himself. Discontented, dissatisfied with everything, everyone.

Offended easily. Trifles aggravate, seem important, especially in the evening. Oversensitive to criticism. Sensitive to noise. Sentimental. Dwells on past disagreeable occurrences. Feeling of loss. Despair of life. Weeping, tearful mood from a story, music, church music, from offense. Whimpering from pain, everything aches.

Desires danger, to run everywhere, to run down hill, to kill. Suspicious, mistrustful, paranoid. Attempts to escape, looking for angles of escape. Aversion to company, better when alone. Desire for company.

Delirium during fever. Loss of self-control. Uncoordinated, in and out of consciousness.

Abdomen - Cramping, griping pain. Dragging, bearing down pain. Pressing pain.

Back - Backache dorsal region, right scapula. Spinal pains. Pain in lumbar region, night. Pain in right lumbar region, extending to abdomen. Neck stiffness, worse right side.

Chest - Chest pain, worse motion, better pressure. Chest weakness. Pain in the forenoon, 11 am. Cutting, stabbing pain in sternum. Pain during inspiration.

Ears - Discoloration, redness, especially in right.

Eyes - Sensation as if eyes wide open. Vision acute.

Face - Discoloration, red with heat. Redness in cheeks, around mouth, worse from cold weather, eating. Pimples on lower jaw. Lower jaw projects.

Female - Menses copious, frequent, too early, scanty. Dysmenorrhea. Sharp pain in ovaries. Uterus painful after menses. Sexual desire diminished.

Food - Appetite diminished. Increased hunger. Desires creamy food, fish, meat, spices, condiments, wine. Worse green or red chilies, apples. Aversion to apples. Desire to drink, without thirst. Thirst for small quantities, often. Thirst unquenchable, constant.

Head - Constriction in forehead. Forehead pain, behind eyes, especially on left. Pain on left then right. Forehead pain, extending to vertex. Pressing pain in temples. Swollen, distended feeling. Tension. Burning pain, redness, warm sensation. Tired sensation in head.

Kidneys - Aching pain in right. Pain in afternoon, 2 p.m.

Limbs - Awkwardness. Heaviness, tired limbs. Pain upper limbs, left. Trembling in upper limbs, hands. Coldness of hands, feet, hands turn blue. Cracking of right shoulder. Pain in right shoulder, extending to chest. Cramping pain in lower limbs, knees.

Mouth - Dryness in evening, with thirst, worse talking. Copious saliva. Cracked, dry lips. Sensitive gums. Worse from cold drinks.

Rectum - Stool, tenacious. Urging, for bowel movement at night.

Sleep - Sleeplessness from thoughts. Tossing about during sleep. Light, restless sleep. Waking from dreams. Waking 4 p.m. to 5 pm. Sleepiness in morning on waking.

Stomach - Nausea from odors of fish. Stomach pain after eating, in evening, while standing or walking, better lying down. Cramping, griping pain. Nausea during stomach pain.

Throat - Scraping, painful dryness. Throat pain in evening, on swallowing. Mucus difficult to detach.

RELATIONS - ***Compare:*** Lac-c., Lac-f., Lac-h., Lac-v., Lac-v-c., Lac-d.

REFERENCES - Herrick.

LAC MATERNA HUMANUM

(Mother's Milk)

PHARMACY - lac-mat. Lac materna humanum. Mother's milk. Milk from multiple nursing women. Dilutions. ***Historical dose:*** All potencies.

CLINICAL - Backache. Chest, pain. Chill. Delirium. Dysmenorrhea. Fever. Headache. Kidney, pain. Nausea. Sleeplessness. Typhoid fever. Typhus. Uterine pain. Vertigo.

HOMEOPATHIC - Continued fever, relapsing fever. Typhus, typhoid fever. Delirium during fever. Fever with chill. Attempts to escape, concern about strategy. Stupefaction, as if intoxicated. Tossing about during sleep.

MIND - Heightened awareness of body, skin surface. Aware of being looked at. Oversensitive to criticism. Offended easily. Sensitive to noise. Mind active with little things. Excessive mind chatter. Rushed flow of thoughts. Thoughts disordered, distracted, hurried, wandering. Clear, logical thoughts.

Heedless, careless what others think. Indecision. Impatience. Hurry, haste. Alternating impatience with patience. Industrious, efficient. Cheerfulness, gaiety, happiness in company. Calm under stress. Contented with himself. Quiet and calm. Serious. Relaxed.

Confusion, poor planning. Disorganized. Errors of perception. Dazed. Daydreaming. Indifference, apathy. Detached. Loses things. Indolence, aversion to work. Neglects his business.

Anxiety with feeling that control over senses is lost. Anxiety about business. Sudden anxiety, as if something needs to be done but knows not what. Fear of terrible dreams. Suspicious, mistrustful, paranoid.

Censorious, critical. Disposed to blame others. Quarrelsome. Scolding. Irritability. Argumentative. Anger, irascibility, especially in the morning. Anger with himself. Discontented, displeased with others. Feels righteous. Dwells on past disagreeable occurrences. Irresolution.

Aversion to company, better being alone. Isolation. Feelings of loss. Despair of life. Sentimental, sympathetic. Weeping, tearful mood from a story, movie, church music. Weeping from offense. Whimpering, tearful from pains. Trifles aggravate.

Desire for company. Desire for fun, excitement. Desires to help others less fortunate. Desires to run everywhere. Desires danger, pain, to kill. Desire to be silent, taciturn. Inclination to sit. Loss of self-control.

Abdomen - Flatulence. Griping, cramping pain in the abdomen. Dragging, bearing down, pressing sensations. Cramping pain precedes diarrhea. Distension after eating.

Back - Backache in spine, lumbar region, extending to abdomen. Pain in right scapulae. Stiffness in right cervical region. Intermittent pain. Sore pain after physical exertion. Stabbing pain, left side. Pain, cervical region after physical exertion. Stiffness, cervical region, bending forward aggravates.

Chest - Weakness. Chest pain, better pressure. Chest pain during inspiration, worse from motion. Cutting pain in sternum. Pain in forenoon, 11 a.m.

Ear - Redness. Vision acute. Congested, in eustachian tube.

Eyes - Dry eyes, afternoon. Itching, morning. Sensitive to light, squinting ameliorates. Sore eyes. Stinging pain, early morning after walk.

Face - Discoloration, red with heat. Redness in cheeks, around mouth, worse cold weather, eating. Pimples on lower jaw. Projects lower jaw.

Female - Menses, intermit. Menses copious, painful, frequent, too early, scanty. Dysmenorrhea. Sharp pain in ovaries. Uterine pain after menses. Sexual desire diminished.

Food - Appetite, diminished or increased. Desire to drink, without thirst. Thirstlessness. Thirst, unquenchable, constant, for small quantities. Desires chocolate. Desires fruit, mango, mandarins. Desires meat, seafood, salmon, mussels. Desires water with headache. ***Worse alcohol.***

Head - Constriction. Burning pain, redness. Tired sensation. Sensation as if head open wide. Swollen, distended feeling. Sensation of warmth. Tension headaches. Headache in forehead, behind eyes, in sides, left then right. Pressing pain, temples. Pain in forehead, extending to vertex.

Kidneys - Aching pain. Kidney pain, especially in right, in afternoon, 2 p.m. Urine color, yellow-brown. Urine odor, strong, offensive.

Limbs - Awkwardness. Heaviness, tired limbs. Coldness in hands and feet. Pain in fingers. Trembling hands. Pain in upper limbs, on left. Cracking and pain in right shoulder. Shoulder pain, extending to chest. Cramp-like pain in lower limbs, knees. Dislocation, left arm from socket. Aching pain, shoulders, left, then right.

Male - Sexual desire increased.

Mouth - Dryness with thirst, when talking, in evening. Copious saliva. Cracked, dry lips. Sensitive gums, worse cold drinks.

Nose - Coryza. Discharge, bland. Itching, posterior nares. ***Obstruction***, nasal, deep breathing ameliorates. Sensitive to putrid smells. Sensitive to pleasant, floral smells. Sneezing, dust aggravates.

Rectum - Diarrhea, after eating. Sudden urging to stool.

Skin - Bleeding ulcers, right side of nose. Bleeding, constant trickle from small cut in leg will not clot, slightest touch aggravates. Dry, red, itching spots, in folds of elbows. Dry, red, scaly, around elbow.

Dry, scaly in creases of elbows.

Sleep - Sleeplessness from thoughts. Light, restless sleep. Waking 4 p.m. to 5 p.m., from dreams. Sleepy in morning. Unrefreshing sleep. Difficult sleep, due to obstructed nose. Sleepiness, afternoo, evening. Waking early. Sleeplessness, before midnight.

Stomach - Cramping, griping pain. Pain after eating, while standing or walking, in evening, better lying down. Pain during nausea. Nausea from odor of fish. Relaxation.

Stool - Forcible, sudden gushing. Lumps and liquid stool. Stool odor, burnt. Odor, pungent, like fermented herbs. Offensive stool. Reddish-brown stool. Small stool, ill-formed chunks. Thin, lumpy and liquid stool. Thin, red stool. Watery stool, with red lump.

Temperature - Coldness in general. Chill at night.

Throat - Dryness painful. Irritation of throat. Mucus difficult to detach. Scraping. Throat pain, on swallowing, in evening. Sensation of a lump. Gagging, cold water ameliorates. Throat pain, breathing dry air aggravates. Sore pain when swallowing.

Vertigo - Vertigo with confusion of mind. Vertigo, while driving, ameliorates. Vertigo with rising and falling sensation. Vertigo during headache. Vertigo as if intoxicated. Light headed. Vertigo lying on back, ameliorates. Vertigo with nausea. Vertigo with incoherent speech. Vertigo with staggering. Standing while, aggravates. Sudden vertigo. Walking while, aggravates. Vertigo with vomiting.

RELATIONS - ***Compare:*** Lac-c., Lac-f., Lac-h., Lac-v., Lac-v-c., Lac-d.

REFERENCES - Hatherly. Smits.

LAC VACCINI FLOS

(Milk Cream)

PHARMACY - lac-v-f. Lac vaccini flos. Milk cream. Lactis vaccini flos. Cream from cow's milk. Dilutions. ***Historical dose:*** Tincture and all potencies.

CLINICAL - Diarrhea. Diphtheria. ***Dysmenorrhea.*** Flatulence. Hoarseness. Leucorrhea. Menorrhagia. Throat, sore.

HOMEOPATHIC - Swan proved this remedy; as with the other Lac preparations, a large number of the symptoms manifested in the throat and female sexual organs.

Dry throat and extreme difficulty of swallowing. Painful, frequent and profuse diarrhea. Feels very cold and, although well clothed, cannot get warm. Albuminous leucorrhea like white of egg, from exertion, standing. Sexual desire easily excited.

Abdomen - Tendency to flatulence in lower intestines.

Female - Menses seven days too soon. ***Menses profuse, cramps*** in and above region of navel, bending her double during the cramps. Albuminous leucorrhea like egg white. Sexual desire easily excited when the hand touches the bosom.

Food - Food tastes as if it lacked salt.

Kidneys - Urine appears to stain more yellow.

Limbs - Rigidity on posterior side of lower legs, just below knees, while walking, very unpleasant, but not painful.

Lungs - Sensation of shallow breathing, has to take a deep respiration to relieve.

Male - Soreness of end of prepuce, as if there were longitudinal cracks there, though none could be discovered.

Rectum - Painful, frequent and profuse diarrhea.

Skin - Itching of body above pubes and hips, on abdomen, chest and back without eruption.

Sleep - Wakefulness without restlessness. Drowsy and sleepy, head feels heavy. Constant talking during sleep. Slept and dreamed the same dreams, feels stupid, does not care to speak. Horrible dreams, saw a dead person in a coffin.

Temperature - Feels very cold and, although well clothed, cannot get warm.

Throat - Dry, red, sore upper part of pharynx in the morning, pain runs up to ears. Throat worse night and morning. Difficult swallowing, at night had to take hold of throat to assist in swallowing. Yellow mucus with a sickish sweet taste. Hoarseness after singing.

RELATIONS - ***Compare:*** (1) Lac-c., Lac-f., Lac-h., Lac-v., Lac-v-c., Lac-d. (2) Ars. stopped abruptly the excessive menses and accompanying pain, Lac-d. restored the flow and then they ceased naturally.

REFERENCES - Clarke.

LAC VACCINUM

(Cow's Milk)

PHARMACY - lac-v. Lac vaccinum. Cow's milk. Dilutions. ***Historical dose:*** All potencies.

CLINICAL - Albuminuria. Blindness. ***Colds.*** Constipation. Diabetes. Fever. Headaches. Leucorrhea. Milk, intolerance. ***Otitis media.*** Rheumatism. ***Sinusitis.*** Sternum, pains. Tongue, ulcers. Vertigo.

HOMEOPATHIC - Lac-v. was proved by J. C. Boardman of Trenton, New Jersey. Swan's 200c potency was used. The headaches, biliousness and constipation frequently induced by milk are well known.

The keynote of Lac-c. is alternation of sides, in Lac-v., the ***symptoms appeared on both sides at once***. Pains in chest, abdomen, hips, thighs and knees were all felt on right and left sides simultaneously. Headache. Great thirst and excessive flow of urine. Diabetes.

Burnett observed that children who drink much milk after their teeth are grown become ***very labile to catch colds and get ear infections.*** Milk frequently aggravates rheumatism.

MIND - General nervousness with depression of spirits, feeling as though about to hear bad news. Mental confusion.

Abdomen - Pain proceeding from sternum, extending across abdomen about an inch below umbilicus.

Back - Pains in sacrum.

Chest - A sharp pain on each side of sternum and about middle of chest with a sense of suffocation. Burning sensation. Sharp pains in left lower chest, beginning in right chest.

Ears - Ears felt stopped up, felt deaf in both ears, although she could hear as before. ***Otitis media, worse drinking milk.***

Eyes - Dull pain over eyes, more on right. Blurred, dimmed or obscured sight, off and on for a few moments at a time. Blindness of both eyes, comes and goes.

Female - White, watery leucorrhea, pain in sacrum.

Food - Thirst for cold water in quantities, drank three glasses during evening.

Head – Headache, heavy, dull, aching, drowsy, wants to go to sleep. Creeping sensation. Screw-like or vertical motion, beginning over left eye. Woke in morning with an aching pain all over head, most severe in occiput. Sensation like a fire-ball in each temple simultaneously.

Kidneys - Urinates every 15 minutes. Frequent discharge of profuse, clear urine, nearly colorless, no sediment. Urine not increased in morning, dark red without sediment.

Limbs - All the joints of body, especially knees, feel weak and powerless, as when half drunk. Aching pains in bones from hip joints to feet, with burning in both feet. Rheumatic pains in knee and ankles. Clammy, sticky coldness in hands and feet simultaneously.

Lungs - Asthma, worse drinking milk.

Mouth - Dirty, yellow coated tongue, parched. Acid saliva staining handkerchief yellow. Sore taste. ***Sores in mouth.*** Ulcers on tongue.

Nose - Nasal congestion, from allergies, worse drinking milk. ***Sinusitis***.

Rectum - Obstinate constipation.

Sleep - Must force herself to keep awake, to keep her eyes open, to avoid falling backwards. Sleepy and could have fallen asleep at any time during the whole day. General restlessness and bad dreams. Dreams of trying to lay out a corpse.

Stomach - Swelling or bloating. Contractive, pressing pain in stomach, better by external pressure. Sour taste, nausea, but no rising or vomiting.

Temperature - Slight fever over the entire body with moist hands and aching in legs from thighs to knees. Hands became hot and dry. Pain on left side of head with a chilling sensation.

Throat - Sensation of plug in throat or larynx.

Vertigo - Vertigo, falls backwards if she closes her eyes.

COMMENTS - Swan gave reported cures including short, rheumatic pains in knee and ankles on walking, passing fetid flatus. Belchings and passing of much flatus.

Fever at night followed by profuse sweat all over, the fever was preceded by chilly feeling, beginning at shoulders, then running up from feet to head, headache. Fullness of head, as if too large and heavy. Vertigo.

Flat white ulcers on tongue, sensitive, covered with white slimy mucus, extending to sides of cheeks. Brown crusts, having greasy appearance, especially in corners of mouth like "butter-sores."

RELATIONS - ***Compare:*** Lac-c., Lac-f., Lac-h., Lac-v., Lac-v-c., Lac-d.

REFERENCES - Clarke.

LAC VACCINUM BUTYRICUM

(Buttermilk)

PHARMACY - lac-v-b. Lac vaccinum butyricum. Buttermilk. Buttermilk made from cows milk. Dilutions. ***Historical dose:*** All potencies.

CLINICAL - Canker, sores. Coryza. Diarrhea. Dysentery. Flatulence. Hoarseness.

HOMEOPATHIC - Dullness of hearing, as if ear were filled with water. Sinus affections. Adherent nasal and postnasal mucus. Nose runs while eating. Stitches through chest on drawing deep breath or stooping. Canker sores. Scab at inner commissure of eye.

Diarrhea and dysentery. Loose stools, lumpy like small peas. Flatus from uterus and vagina, feels like marbles passing down. Itching of thumb and middle finger.

MIND - Great depression of spirits, the future looks dark and hopeless.

Abdomen - Rumbling in abdomen with loose stools. Flatulence, passes involuntarily.

Breasts - Sharp pain in left breast above nipple, on stooping or drawing deep breath.

Chest - Sensation as if an adhesion between lung and pleura. After stooping, sensation as if anterior mediastinum were filled with tenacious substance that stuck parts together; must throw shoulders back and separate parts. Sharp pain in left side below and to left of nipple on drawing deep breath. Painful stitch on right side between 6th and 7th ribs, to right of nipple. Tightness under sternum above center. Lameness through chest.

Ears - Dullness of hearing as if right ear were filled with water, or as if there were a thin film of wax on membrana tympani. Throbbing, beating in right ear.

Eyes - Pain around right eye. Eyeball sensitive to pressure. Sharp, hot pain passing into left eyeball leaves a sense of heat. Sore spot on inner commissure of left eye on which scab formed, on removing scab a raw, sore place remains. Burning in both lids of left eye with redness of the meibomian glands and dull pain in superior arch of orbit.

Face - Pain in bone beneath right eye, pressive as with point of a finger.

Female - Menses early. Flatus can be felt passing, like marbles, into and down uterus and vagina, expelled with a puff.

Head - Heat in head. Dull pain in coronal region with fullness. Creaking sound as head is turned, with throbbing in base of occiput. Pain in forehead over and in outer end of right eyebrow. Dull heavy pain over eyebrows, with sensation of heat in forehead.

Kidney - Urine scanty, dribbling. Extremely slow in passing urine. No power to urinate.

Limbs - Shoulder pain as if dislocated. Right elbow itches. Hands very hot. Painful numbness in upper side of left thumb, slight sensation of heat. Itching on bones of thumbs, no eruption. Violent itching on dorsal surface of right middle finger, spot slightly red. Rough skin inside left thumb. Painful transverse fissure, slight bleeding. Pain glutei medius and minimus, a tired aching makes sitting very uncomfortable. Moist itching, rough eruption, in left popliteal space.

Lungs - Irritation and coughing. Sensation as if an adhesion between lung and pleura.

Male - Painful throb to right testicle, as if in epididymis and extending up the spermatic cord, with slight sinking sensation at stomach. Nocturnal emission, generally unconscious and without dreams, next day glans congested, hard as during an erection, the rest of penis flaccid.

Mouth - Tickling, itching and stinging sensation on left edge of tongue. Canker sores on inside of cheeks and lips.

Nose - Great heat and dryness in nostrils. Coryza and hoarseness, sneezing. Water runs from nose on eating. Profuse watery mucus from right nostril, then sharp pain in forehead over eyes. Tough adhesive mucus, posterior nares, difficult to hawk. Frequent swallowing. Hard plugs of mucus. Inflamed pimple on point. Small, white vesicles on sides.

Skin - Skin hot and dry. Dry skin of hands, with or without heat, must wet fingers to hold anything or turn pages. Musty smell from body with moisture of skin, no sweat. Pimples in groups slightly itching, painless. Pimples sore, cannot be rubbed. Pimples on abdomen, nates, folds of nates, thighs.

Sleep - Sleepy during day. Yawning. Great drowsiness, could hardly keep eyes open. Wakes at 4 a.m. with no further desire for sleep. Dreams of the bodily appearance of the devil.

Stomach - Slight sinking sensation at stomach, as if he would faint, with throbbing in testicle.

Stool - Loose, lumpy, painless stool. Lumps the size of small peas, with pressure on anus as if rectum protruded. Soft stool, very offensive.

Temperature - Slight rise in temperature.

Throat - Dryness of posterior fauces. Mucus surfaces of throat and nose hot and dry. Great dryness of larynx worse at region of glottis. Irritation and coughing. Coryza and hoarseness.

RELATIONS - ***Compare:*** Lac-c., Lac-f., Lac-h., Lac-v., Lac-v-c., Lac-d.

REFERENCES - Roberts.

LAC VACCINUM COAGULATUM

(Milk Curds)

PHARMACY - lac-v-c. Lac vaccinum coagulatum. Milk curds. ***Historical dose:*** All potencies.

CLINICAL - Morning sickness.

HOMEOPATHIC - The only use that Clarke knows as having been made of Lac-v-c. is in the nausea of pregnancy, the indication is ***nausea of pregnancy*** with desire for food and better by drinking milk (Chel.).

RELATIONS - ***Compare:*** Lac-c., Lac-f., Lac-h., Lac-v., Lac-v-c., Lac-d.

REFERENCES - Clarke.

LAC VACCINUM DEFLORATUM

(Skimmed Cow's Milk)

PHARMACY - lac-d. Lac vaccinum defloratum. Skimmed cow's milk. Dilutions. ***Historical dose:*** All potencies.

CLINICAL - ***Albuminuria.*** Anemia. Appendicitis. ***Asthma.*** Breast, disorders. Bright's disease. Chilly. Colds. ***Constipation.*** Coryza. Cramps. Delusions. Depression. Diabetes. Dropsy. Dyspnea. Eczema. Fainting. ***Flatulence.*** Gastroenteritis. ***Headaches.*** Heart, disorders. Herpes. Leucorrhea. Lumbago. ***Malnutrition.*** Memory, lost. Menses, suppressed. ***Milk allergy. Migraines. Morning sickness. Motion sickness.*** Nausea. Obesity. Osteoporosis. Otitis media. Palpitations. ***Photophobia. Pimples.*** Sciatica. ***Sick headache.*** Sinusitis. Sore, throat. Tonsillitis. Vertigo. Vomiting.

HOMEOPATHIC - The idea of potentizing skimmed milk originated with Swan upon reading Donkin's "Skim Milk Treatment for Diabetes and Bright's disease." Milks contain an essence of all the tissues and salts of the animal that secretes it.

Lac-d. contains Nat-m., so it shares a thirst for large quantities, nausea and vomiting, and depression with crying and palpitations.

Lac-d. is useful in diseases with ***malnutrition*** and anemia. Feels completely exhausted, whether she does anything or not, great fatigue when walking.

Sick headaches with profuse flow of urine during pain. Headache ceases at sunset.

Sufferings from loss of sleep (Cocc.). ***Motion sickness.*** Dropsy from organic heart disease and from chronic liver complaints. Obesity. Osteoporosis. Sensation as if cold air was blowing on her, even while covered up, as if sheets were damp. Most symptoms occur in the morning.

Particularly useful for the symptoms caused by milk in some sensitive people, especially the violent headache and constipation. For those who become sick on taking milk.

MIND - ***Vacillation of mind.*** Listlessness. Disinclination for bodily or mental exertion. Doesn't want to see or talk to any one. Aversion to company. Loss of memory. ***Sadness before and during menses.*** Claustrophobia. Unconsciousness on raising arms above head.

Depression with crying, palpitations and fainting spells. Despondent, better conversation. No fear of death but is sure he is going to die. Suicidal disposition. Imagines all her friends are dead or will die. Delusions, thinks she will have to go to a convent.

Abdomen - Abdomen sore and sensitive to touch, worse pressure. ***Heaviness as of a stone in abdomen.*** Drawing pain, across lower part of abdomen. Severe pain across umbilicus, during headache. Chronic gastroenteritis, with chronic diarrhea and vomiting. ***Flatulence.***

Back - Constant pain in lumbar region. Lumbago. ***Hard pressive pains***, at fourth cervical vertebra. Chills creeping along back between scapulae. Herpetic eruptions on sides of neck, with itching and burning after scratching.

Breasts - ***Scanty flow of milk***, restores the milk. Decrease in size of breasts during pregnancy.

Chest - ***Soreness of chest with great pressure.*** Tuberculous deposit in apices of both lungs.

Ears - Otitis media, worse from drinking milk.

Eyes - ***Eyeballs intensely painful.*** Photophobia, even candlelight unbearable. Great pain in eyes on first going into light, soon passing off. Upper eyelids very heavy. ***Edges of eyelids feel contracted.*** Sensation as if eyes were full of little stones during headache.

Face - Pale, sickly look. Dark stains beneath eyes. Flushes of heat in left side of face. Sallow complexion with eczema. ***Pimples on face and forehead.*** Painless swelling of the face.

Female - Menses, delayed in girls who drink much milk. ***Menses delayed, with congestion of blood to head, coldness of hands, nausea and vertigo.*** Menses irregular, sometimes very dark and scanty, sometimes colorless water. Menses suppressed by putting hands in cold water. ***Pressing, bearing down pain in ovarian region.*** Drawing pain across uterine region. Sensation of weight and dragging in left ovarian region. Slight yellowish leucorrhea.

Food - ***Loss of appetite.*** Can neither eat nor drink during headache. ***Malnutrition.*** Great thirst for large quantities, often intense. Drinking cold water causes nausea. ***Aversion to milk,*** causes sick headache. Smell or thought of food causes nausea, during headache.

Head - Persistent headaches for years. ***Migraines***, cease at sunset. Pain begins in forehead to occiput, in morning on rising. ***Intense throbbing pains*** with blindness, nausea, vomiting and obstinate constipation. Headache preceded by blindness. Throbbing frontal headache with much pale urination, worse noise, light, motion. ***Sick headache, with icy coldness all through body. Sick headache*** with gastric symptoms, from drinking milk. ***Headache over left eye and in left temple with profuse lachrymation, photophobia.*** Headaches better cold applications, while generally better from heat. Head becomes sore on coughing. Headache during menses, better by bandaging, conversation. Headache alternating with tonsillitis. Head as if bruised, after headache. Distress in head after injury.

Heart - ***Pressure around heart*** with dyspnea, feeling that he is going to die. ***Sharp pain in apex of heart***, as if a knife was cutting up and down. Palpitations of heart and flushes of heat.

Kidneys - ***Constant pain in kidney region.*** Boring, sore pain in kidneys. Frequent and profuse urination with headache or other pains. ***Frequent but scanty urination.*** Lack of sensation when the bladder is full. Urination involuntary, while walking in cold air, while riding or when hurrying to catch a train. ***Albuminuria.*** Urine very pale, can't retain it. ***Urine very dark and thick.*** Urine comes away drop by drop, or gushes out. Urine with a sensation of very hot water passing over parts. Bed-wetting at night.

Limbs - Osteoporosis. Weak bones. Fingertips icy cold, rest of the hands warm. Aching, in wrists and ankles. Cold hands or feet during headache. Numbness and loss of sensation over outer and anterior surfaces of thighs. Weakness and aching in ankles, puffiness. Skin thickened at edges of feet.

Lungs - ***Asthma attacks***, so that he could scarcely breathe, accompanied by bloating in epigastric region. ***Asthma worse from drinking milk.*** Short, dry cough with difficult expectoration of a small lump of mucus, which ameliorates cough.

Modalities - Better from rest. Better pressure. Better bandage. Better conversation. Better profuse flow of urine. ***Worse from cold.*** Worse least draft. Worse wet. Worse hands in cold water. ***Worse milk. Worse in morning.*** Worse loss of sleep. Worse weekly. ***Worse motion.*** Worse walking. Worse sitting down. Lying down aggravates the vertigo, headache, and urinary pain.

Mouth - ***Offensive breath.*** Mouth very dry. Mouth clammy and frothy during conversation. Grinding of teeth during sleep.

Nose - ***Painful pressure or tightness at root of nose.*** Sinusitis. Colds. Children suffer from coryza from drinking milk. Nasal catarrh, worse drinking milk.

Perspiration - Profuse, staining yellow, difficult to wash out. Sense as if sheets were damp.

Rectum - Constipation with ineffectual urging. ***Persistent constipation,*** better only by purgatives or enema, with violent attacks of sick headaches. Large, hard stools, with great straining, painful, lacerating anus.

Sensations - As though a knife was cutting up and down through the heart. As if head would burst. As if top of head was lifted off. As if a ball of pain in center of forehead. As if eyes full of little stones. As if flesh was off bones and edges were separated and sticking out. As if sheets were damp, as if a cold air blowing on her.

Skin - Very sensitive to cold. Face, neck, arms and body generally flush color of a red rose, with swelling, but no itching or burning. Symmetrical patches, causing itching and burning after scratching. Skin thickened at the edges of feet.

Sleep - Sleepy all day long. Great restlessness, extreme and protracted suffering from loss of sleep at night. Worse from loss of sleep.

Stomach - Violent pain in stomach from fatigue. Cramps in epigastric region. ***Sour eructations.*** Nausea and vomiting, with sensation of deathly sickness. Nausea from a recumbent position. Incessant vomiting with no relation to eating. Vomiting first of undigested food, sour, acid, then of bitter water. Vomit looks like coffee grounds. ***Morning sickness. Motion sickness.***

Temperature - ***Always feels chilly.*** Very sensitive to cold. Very chilly when constipation is most persistent. Hectic fever, malignant typhoid. Hot fever continues until near morning, wakes in profuse sweat, which stains linen yellow. Sensation as if the sheets were damp.

Throat - ***Sore throat, worse when swallowing.*** Sore throat with slight, hacking cough. Sensation of a large ball rising from stomach to throat, causing distressing sense of suffocation. Globus hystericus.

Vertigo - Vertigo, worse lying on left side. Vertigo when moving head from pillow, opening eyes while lying, turning while lying, must sit up. Faintness on extending arms overhead. ***Cannot stand, but falls backwards.*** Light-headed with throbbing in temples.

Vision - Dim vision, as if a cloud before eyes, can only see lights, no objects, preceding headache.

COMMENTS - The first proving was made by a woman in New York whose headache and nausea with constipation were strongly marked. A subsequent, more extensive proving was made under Swan by Dr. Laura Morgan. Hering noted that with but few exceptions the symptoms have received clinical verification.

Migraines, especially for people allergic to milk. Hormonal migraines. Throbbing, blinding headaches with nausea and vomiting. Headaches, better pressure and bandaging. Periodic sick headaches in anemic women, nausea, vomiting and obstinate constipation. Loss of sleep (Cocc.). Periodic symptoms, every eight days.

Intense thirst and emaciation with diabetes. Diabetes and nephritis, especially when aggravated by milk (Nat-c.). Obstinate constipation. Nutrition is perverted. Weight loss or obesity. Dropsy. Fatty degeneration.

Severe vomiting with no relief (Ip.). Morning sickness with severe nausea and vomiting, acidic, bitter taste in the mouth. The menses are irregular, sometimes very dark, scanty, sometimes colorless water.

Lac-d. cured a case in which menses were suppressed suddenly from putting hands into cold water. Great pain in uterine region. Intense headache. Pains flew all over. Flushed face. The patient slept after first dose, the next morning a slight flow appeared. A second dose brought back flow profusely and patient felt well and the flow continued.

Burnett maintained that excess of milk in the dietary of children after they have cut their first teeth renders them susceptible to colds. It may be well to recall that milk is one of the articles forbidden to hydrogenoid or chilly patients.

RELATIONS - ***Compare:*** (1) Colos. - diarrhea in infants. Whole body smells sour. Colic. (2) Nat-m., Lac-c., Lac-v-c., Lac-ac., Sac-l. (3) Vac., a cow nosode. (4) Nat-m. - diabetes, headache, constipation, heart. (5) Cocc. - menstrual sick-headaches. (6) Cact. - heart, but Lac d. has not the ***"grasp"*** of Cact. (7) Nux-m. - head heavy, tends to fall to left. Lac-d. to right.

REFERENCES - Boericke. Clarke. Murphy.

LACERTA AGILIS

(Green Lizard)

PHARMACY - lacer. Lacerta agilis. Green lizard. Sand lizard. Large green spotted lizard. N. O. Lacertilia. Europe. Tincture of whole animal. A separate preparation of the spotted lizard should be made. ***Historical dose:*** All potencies.

CLINICAL - Blisters. Delirium. Indigestion. Skin, eruptions. Paralysis. Tongue, vesicles.

HOMEOPATHIC - The green lizard is usually considered to be non-poisonous, but Baldelli, who ate a lizard cut into small pieces, developed some decided symptoms of indigestion, blisters under the tongue and skin eruptions.

Lacer. has pain, swellings, numbness, left-sided paralysis, rigidity of the neck and jaw on the left side and tender muscles. Motion causes excruciating pains in bitten limb. Touch aggravates. Symptoms of the proving were better by drinking frequently vinegar and water.

MIND - Delirium with an alternating state of greatly increased mental acumen during intervals of reason.

COMMENTS - A girl, bitten on the sole of the left foot by a "large green spotted lizard," died of the effects of the bite after twenty-one days of suffering. This is recorded in Allen's Appendix and comes from an American source, so it is probably an American variety of Lacerta that is accountable for this.

RELATIONS - ***Antidote:*** vinegar. ***Compare:*** (1) Amph., Helo.

REFERENCES - Boericke. Clarke.

LACHESIS MUTA

(Bushmaster Snake)

PHARMACY - lach. Lachesis muta. Bushmaster. Surukuku. Trigonocephalous lachesis. N. O. Ophidia. Crotalida. South America. Dilution of the venom. Trituration. Dilutions. ***Historical dose:*** All potencies.

CLINICAL - Albuminuria. ***Alcoholism.*** Amblyopia. Aneurysm. Appendicitis. Asthenopia. Asthma. Atheroma. ***Bedsores. Boils.*** Bubo. Bubonic plague. Cancer. Carbuncles. Catalepsy. Cecum, inflammation. Cellulitis. Chancre. Chilblains. Ciliary neuralgia. Cough. Cyanosis. ***Delirium tremens.*** Delusions. Diphtheria. Dog, bite. Dropsy. Dyspepsia. Ears, disorders. Epilepsy. Erysipelas. Eyes, disorders. Fainting. Fistula lachrymalis. Flatulence. Gallstones. Gangrene. Glanders. Gums, bleeding. Hay fever. Headaches. ***Heart, disorders.*** Heartburn. Hemiplegia. ***Hemophilia. Hemorrhages.*** Hemorrhoids. Hepatitis. Hernia. Herpes. ***High blood pressure.*** Hoarseness. ***Hot, flushes.*** Hysteria. Injuries. Intermittent, fever. Jaundice. Labor, pains. Laryngismus. Laryngitis. Leprosy. Liver disorders. Locomotor, ataxia. Malignant, pustule. ***Mania. Manic depression.*** Measles. Meniere's disease. ***Menopause.*** Mercury, effects. Morvan's disease. Mumps. Neuralgias. Nymphomania. Otorrhea. Ovary, disorders. ***Paralysis.*** Perspiration. Phlegmasia alba dolens. Plague. Pneumonia. ***Premenstrual syndrome.*** Puerperal fever. Pulmonary, edema. Purpura. Pyemia. Quinsy. Rabies. Scarlatina. ***Schizophrenia.*** Sciatica. Stings. ***Strokes.*** Syphilis. ***Throat, sore.*** Trachea, disorders. Traumatic, fever. Tumors. ***Ulcers.*** Varicose, veins. Vertigo. ***Vicarious, menstruation.*** Warts. Whitlow. ***Wounds.***

HOMEOPATHIC - Lachesis was first introduced to homeopathy by Dr. Hering. His first experiments were made when he was studying the botany and zoology of the Upper Amazon for the German government. With the exception of his wife, all those around him were natives, who told him so much about the dreaded Surukuku that he offered a good reward for a live specimen.

One was brought in a bamboo box. Those who brought it immediately fled, along with his native servants. Hering stunned the snake with a blow on the head as the box opened, then, holding its head in a forked stick, he pressed its venom out of the poison bag upon milk sugar.

Handling the venom and preparing the lower potencies threw Hering into a fever with tossing delirium and mania, much to his wife's dismay. He slept through the night and woke with a clear mind.

He drank a little water to moisten his throat and asked his wife "What did I do and say?" His wife remembered and the symptoms were written down as the first installment of the proving. The natives crept back one by one next day and were astonished to find Hering and his wife alive.

The snake grows up to seven feet in length. It has fangs nearly an inch long, with a reddish brown skin marked along the back with black brown rhomboidal spots. Nearly all the provings of Lachesis were made with the 30c and higher potencies.

Like other snake venoms, it decomposes the blood, rendering it more fluid. It has a marked ***hemorrhagic tendency***. ***Hemorrhages*** are thin, containing dark particles like charred straw.

Vicarious hemorrhages, nosebleed, bloody urine etc. Small wounds bleed a great deal. Hemophilia. ***High blood pressure. Flushes of heat,*** rushes of blood. Useful during menopause and for those of a melancholic disposition.

Malignant or septic states, gangrene, diabetic, traumatic, cancer, carbuncle, diphtheria, erysipelas. Purpura, diphtheria and other low forms of disease, when the system is thoroughly poisoned with profound prostration.

Cellulitis with burning and blue color of the skin. Dropsy from liver and spleen diseases after scarlatina. Discharges are acrid and offensive. The ill effects of suppressed discharges.

Intensively rapid onset of the disease with great prostration. Intense nervous irritability with restless tossing and moving about.

Hysteria. ***Manic-depression.*** Hard throbbing or hammering pains. Neuralgic pains change locality with palpitations. As of thread drawing the part or spreading over.

Epilepsy, comes on during sleep from jealousy, onanism, loss of fluids. Chorea from piercing the ears. ***Delirium tremens*** with much trembling and confusion. Trembling of the whole body of hands, tongue, etc. Catalepsy. Diphtheria paralysis and other disorders (Botul.). Diphtheria carriers.

Great physical and mental tension. Nerves become very sensitive, especially the cutaneous and vasomotor ones. Excessive sensitiveness of the surface with intolerance of touch or constriction. ***Cannot bear anything tight anywhere***. ***Sensation of constriction*** or tension, in the throat, abdomen, head. Sensation as if a skullcap.

Ascending sensations in throat, from hot flashes, chills. ***Sensation of a lump*** in throat, abdomen, liver, rectum, etc. As if a lump rolls about in bladder. Blueness of the affected parts of hands. Excessive painfulness of throat, ulcers, spots on body. Drawing sensations in vertex, jaws, in the rectum.

Symptoms appear on left side, then go to the right, especially in the throat and ovaries. ***Left sided paralysis*** after a stroke or cerebral exhaustion. Awkward gait, left side weak. Symptoms can develop in sleep and the patient wakes up from symptoms, at any time, day and night.

MIND - Profoundly disturbed mind. Mental symptoms worse after sleep. Ill effects of grief, fright, vexation, anger, jealousy, disappointed love, masturbation. Ailments from night watching, over-fatigue, loss of fluids, over-study.

Rapidly alternating states, exalted mind, rapid succession of ideas. ***Mental confusion.*** Weak memory. Frequent mistakes are made in writing and speaking. Very imaginative. Nervous, excitable. Restless, uneasy, does not want to attend to business, wants to be off somewhere all the time. Undertakes many things, perseveres in nothing.

Great loquacity, rambling, with mocking, jealousy, mistrust, haughtiness, satire and ridiculous ideas.

Frequently jumping from one subject to another, then sadness. Repeats the same thing over and over. ***One word often leads into another story.***

Irritable, irascible, peevish. Mischievous. Disposed to be morose or to quarrel. Complains of trifles. Irritability alternating with loquacious delirium. ***Malicious, wants to get revenge.*** Passion, leading to anger. Hateful. Malice. ***Violent anger and behavior.***

Selfishness, possessive, jealousy, suspicion and violence. ***Insane jealousy and suspiciousness*** (Hyos.). Quarrelsome from jealousy. ***Jealousy, as foolish as it is irresistible.***

Chronic depression from long-lasting grief or sorrow. Intense sadness and anxiety. Weeps from anecdotes. ***Grief and jealousy.*** Forsaken feeling in the morning. Sadness in girls before puberty. ***Depression worse before menses***, better during menses. ***Depression since menopause.*** Aversion to company during pregnancy. Weary of life, suicidal depression.

Manic depression. Mania. Great mental activity, ideas crowd rapidly. Desire for mental work in evening. Mania from over study. ***Mania for work, shopping, spending money.*** Necessity to do everything rapidly.

Schizophrenia. Paranoid schizophrenia. Persecuted feeling, thinks herself pursued, hated and despised. Delusion of being followed by enemies who are trying to harm him.

Mental confusion or alienation. Feels as if he had two wills. Derangement of sense of time. ***Hysteria after suppression of discharges***. Memory active from suppressing sexual desire. Persistent erotic ideas without ability.

Superstitious. ***Fear of snakes.*** Hydrophobia. ***Fear of being poisoned,*** refuses medicine. Fear of suffocation (Puls.), that heart will stop, of death, of going insane. ***Fears going to sleep***, lying down.

Delirium. Delirium and convulsions from night watching, over fatigue and anxiety. Visions and delirious talk as soon as he shuts eyes. ***Ecstasy.***

Talks, sings or whistles constantly, makes odd motions with arms. Incoherent speech, talks as it were in a strange language. Crawls on the floor, spits often, hides, laughs or is angry during spasms.

Delusions and hallucinations. Feels full of poison. Nightly delusion of fire. Delusions of floating in the air. Thinks there are robbers in the house and wants to jump out of window.

Religious insanity (Verat., Stram.). or mania. ***Religious affections in children.*** Continually moaning that she was lost. Fear of being possessed. Thinks herself under super-human control. Persistent thoughts of evil. Prophetic perceptions, predicts the future correctly. Thinks she is dead and preparations are being made for her funeral.

Alcoholism. Violent alcoholism. Intoxicated state with fear, violence and mistrust. Intoxicated with jealousy, accusations. Delirium tremens.

Abdomen - Abdomen hot, sensitive, painfully stiff front loin down thighs. ***Cannot bear anything around waist***. Tympanitic, sensitive, painful (Bell.). Cutting pain in right side of abdomen causing fainting. Burning like fire in hypogastric and lumbar region. Shooting pain in region of spleen, worse walking. Acute cutting, stinging, radiating from navel. Intussusception, threatening sloughing. Swelling in cecal region, must lie on back with knees drawn up, appendicitis. Pain from anus to navel. Strangulated umbilical hernia. Appendicitis. Peritonitis. Spasmodic colic, better bending forward. Incarceration of flatus.

Back - Backache with great restlessness. Small of back as if lame and weak, or as if sprained. Backache with abdominal cramps and throbbing headache before menses. Neck sensitive to the least pressure. Neck stiff, moves jaws with difficulty. Stiffness in sacrum. ***Neuralgia of coccyx, worse rising from sitting***. Feels as if sitting on something sharp, must sit perfectly still. Myelitis. Sensation of threads stretched from back to arms, legs, eyes, etc.

Breasts - Swelling of breasts. Breasts inflamed, bluish with blackish streaks. Fungus hematodes on right breasts. Nipples swollen, erect, painful to touch. Extreme sensitiveness of nipples. Child doesn't want to nurse. Milk, thin, blue.

Causations - Ill effects of suppressed discharges, injuries, sprains, puncture wounds, bites. Ailments from night watching, over-fatigue, loss of fluids, over-study. Ill effects of grief, fright, vexation, anger, jealousy, disappointed love, masturbation. Never well since menopause. Alcohol, delirium, tremens.

Chest - Burning, stinging, like coals of fire from chest through to scapulae. Chest feels constricted. Oppression of chest during sleep. Sensation as if a plug (Anac.), which moves up and down, with short cough. Blueness of skin of outer chest. Scarlet, shining, herpetic eruption under breasts, worse scratching. Swollen glands in axilla. Garlic odor of sweat in axilla.

Constitutions - Especially suited to alcoholics.

Cough - Tickling, dry cough, suffocative fits. Cough causes stitching pains in affected parts. Cough during sleep without being conscious of it. Very exhausting cough, sometimes causing vomiting. Cough as if some fluid has gone the wrong way. Cough after rising from lying position. Cough from smoking.

Ears - ***Earache with sore throat.*** Tearing pain from zygoma into ear, with sore throat. Pulsations in ear. ***Ears sensitive to wind.*** Numbness about ear and cheek. Polyps. Earwax too hard, dry. Earwax like chewed paper. Hardness of hearing with lack of earwax. Blockage of Eustachian tube (Kali-m.). Sensitivity to sounds. Roaring and singing, better putting finger in ear and shaking it. Whizzing noise, as from insects. Cracking, whizzing, drumming, with reverberation.

Eyes - Eyes watery from pain. Feels as if eyes were forced out on pressing the throat. Sensation as if eyes were drawn together by cords which were tied in a knot at root of nose. ***Intra-ocular hemorrhages. Detached retina. Retinal bleeding.***

Apoplectic retinitis, absorbs hemorrhage. Cellulitis of orbit. Conjunctiva yellow. Unsteady look, eyes roll vacantly. Pupils at first contracted, then dilated. Photophobia. Pterygium. Fistula lachrymalis with eruptions on face.

Face - Blue circles around eyes. Purple, mottled, puffed, looks swollen, bloated. Jaundiced, chlorotic during heat. Pale. One cheek flushed, the other pale. Flushes of heat. Pain in facial bones. Trigeminal neuralgia, left side, heat running up into head (Phos.). Tearing pain in jaw bones (Amph., Phos.). Lower jaw drops during coma. Itching of face. Enormous swelling of lips. Septic mumps. Submaxillary and cervical glands swollen.

Female - Acts especially well at beginning and close of menstruation. ***Premenstrual syndrome.*** Menses too short, too feeble. Menses, black, scanty, lumpy, acrid, vicarious from nose. ***The less flow, the more pain.*** Dysmenorrhea, on first day. Dysmenorrhea with pain in left ovary. Labor-like pains during menses. ***Uterine and ovarian pains, all relieved by the flow*** (Eupi.). Menorrhagia with chills at night, flushes of heat by day. Leucorrhea before menses. Leucorrhea, copious, smarting, staining and stiffening the linen greenish. Leucorrhea thick yellow, milky. Ovarian tumors. Left ovary, swollen indurated, painful. ***Violent pain in left ovary.*** Uterus feels as if the os is open. Sexual desire excited. Nymphomania. ***Menopausal troubles***, like palpitations, hot flashes, hemorrhages, headaches, fainting spells. Prolapsed uterus during menopause.

Food - Hungry, cannot wait for food, or loss of hunger alternately. Better after eating, after fruit. Craving for coffee, which agrees. Desires alcohol, wine, oysters, farinaceous food, pickles, sour foods. Worse tobacco, wine, alcoholic drinks, acids and sour drinks. Throat symptoms are worse by hot drinks. Thirsty but fears to drink.

Head - Headache, heavy, bursting pain, down to nose. ***Congestive headaches, rush of blood to head.*** Bursting or throbbing, in temples. Headaches with flickerings, dim vision, very pale face. Pain through head on waking. Pain at root of nose. ***Weight, pressure or burning of the vertex.*** Waves of pain, worse after moving. One-sided headaches. Migraine, pain extending to neck and shoulders. ***Sun headaches.*** Sick headache, worse left side. ***Headaches before menses. Headaches during menopause.*** Burning of vertex with menopause. ***Left-sided stroke, after abuse of alcohol.*** Perforating tumor of the skull. Does not want hair touched. Sensitiveness of scalp. Falling of hair, especially during pregnancy.

Heart - Anxiety about heart. Visible palpitations of heart. Palpitations with pain. Palpitations with fainting spells, during menopause. ***Palpitations, worse warm room.*** Palpitations after sudden excitement. ***Palpitations in morning on waking.*** Constricted feeling causing palpitations with anxiety. Heart seems to stand still and then starts with a tremendous bound. Irregular heartbeats. Pulse, weak intermittent, slow, irregular. Restless, trembling. Weak heart, turns over or too big. ***High blood pressure.*** Carditis. Pericarditis. Senile arteriosclerosis. As if heart were hanging by a thread.

Kidneys - Sharp pains from kidneys through ureters. Small tumor in urethra causing retention. As if a ball rolling in the bladder when turning over. Pressure in bladder, with frequent urging. Inefficient urging. Violent burning during urination. No urine, no stool. Black, scanty urine with edema. Urine, frequent, foamy, dark, strong odor. Dark urine, with brown, gravelly sediment, like coffee grounds. Bloody urine. Albuminuria with hydrothorax. Dribbling after urination.

Limbs - ***Paralysis after stroke.*** Joints as if sprained, in morning on awaking. Bluish swelling of joints, after sprains. Erratic pains in joints. ***Pain in tibia*** after sore throat. Shortening of tendons. Sciatica, right side, better lying down. Sciatica, must lie still, worse by least motion. Rheumatism, with swelling of wrists and ankles. Knees cold or as if hot air is going through. Cramps in calves from fear. Toes feel broken. Foot sweat, foul or cold. Nightly burning in palms and soles. Tingling, pricking in left hand. ***Trembling of hands in alcoholics.*** Cracks in skin at the corners of nails. Felon, bluish swelling. Left arm numb, fingertips numb. Boils on thighs and fingers. Phlegmasia alba dolens.

Liver - ***Liver region sensitive, can't bear anything around waist.*** Sore, festering, throbbing deep in liver. Acute, in liver extending to stomach. Inflammation of liver with abscess. Hepatitis and abscess. Septic gallbladder. Liver complaints of alcoholics. Cirrhosis. Nutmeg liver. Liver complaints at menopause or after ague.

Lungs - ***Sensation of suffocation and strangulation*** on lying down, worse ***when anything is around throat***, compels patient to spring from bed and rush for open window. Wants to be fanned. ***Feels he must take a deep breath***. Cramp-like distress in precordial region. ***Breathing almost stops on falling asleep*** (Grind.). Can only breathe in upright position. Sensation as of a plug (Anac.), that moves up and down with a short cough. Large quantities of ropy mucus. Difficult expectoration, frothy, purulent, bloody with excessive perspiration. Watery, salty mucus, which has to be swallowed again. Hay asthma. Asthma, suffocating dyspnea. Asthma after scabies, if the itching ceases. Pneumonia. Hepatization, of left lung. Last stage of pneumonia. Bronchial attacks with cyanosis and cardiac disease. Cyanosis. Cyanosis neonatorum. Dropsy of lungs after scarlatina. Abscess of the lungs.

Male - Sore pain in urethra, in forepart of penis. Prepuce thickened. Scrotum swollen to enormous size. Buboes suppurating a long time. Sycotic ulcers, with bluish areolae. Gangrene of glans. Strong sexual desire, ideas, without physical power. During sex, the emission is tardy or does not occur at all. Semen with pungent odor. Cheerful after night emission. Ill effects of masturbation.

Modalities - ***Better with the appearance of discharges,*** warm applications, bathing affected part, ***open air***. Better hard pressure, sitting bent, loosening clothes. ***Better cold drinks,*** eating, especially fruits, belchings. Worse spring, summer, sun, cloudy weather, extremes of weather, heat of room. ***Worse from empty swallowing, liquids, hot drinks***, alcohol. Worse morning, ***after sleep***. Worse from motion, standing or stooping, closing eyes, slight touch, pressure of clothes, around neck, waist. ***Worse from suppressed discharges,*** at start and close of menses, ***menopause***.

Mouth - Copious, tenacious, thick, pasty saliva. Peppery, sour, coppery, nauseous taste. Bad odor from mouth. Cannot bear anything before mouth. Burning, in mouth with swelling of lips and gums. Gums, bluish, swollen, spongy, bleed easily. ***Aphthous and denuded spots*** with burning and rawness. Nursing sore mouth with swelling of tongue and lips. Stammering. Thick, blundering speech, cannot open mouth wide. ***Speechless after having a stroke.***

Nose - Pain at root of nose. Cannot bear anything before nose. Hay asthma, paroxysms of sneezing (Sil., Sabad.). Stopped up coryza, preceded by headache. Complaints after suppressed coryza. Postnasal discharge of mucus. Discharge with every cough. Offensive, bloody discharges, corroding nostrils and lips. Blood and pus from nose. Nosebleed on blowing the nose. Nosebleed, blood thick, black. ***Nosebleeds with amenorrhea.*** Nostrils sensitive. Vesicular eruption about nose. Red pimples on nose of alcoholics.

Perspiration - ***Hot flushes and hot perspiration.*** Bloody, sweat staining blackish, yellow. Garlicky odor of sweat. Profuse sweats with most complaints. Copious sweats at night, about neck, wakes him from sleep. Sweats in axilla.

Rectum - ***Constipation, offensive stool.*** Constipation, very hard stools, between menses. Constipation of pregnancy. Diarrhea alternating with constipation. Diarrhea in hot weather, from fruits and acids.

Diarrhea after menses, during menopause. Diarrhea with frothy urine. Constant urging in rectum, not for stool. Hemorrhage from bowels like ***charred straw, black particles***. ***Anus feels tight***, as if nothing could go through it. Spasmodic pains in anus before and after stool. Burning in anus during and after stools. Burning, cutting, in rectum worse standing. Darting pain up rectum every time he sneezes or coughs. Itching at anus, worse after sleep. Discharge of blood or mucus from anus, during menses. Beating in the anus as from hammers with menses. As if a ball rolling when turning over. Fistula in anus. ***Hemorrhoids protrude, become constricted, purplish.*** Hemorrhoids with sharp pains on sneezing or coughing. Hemorrhoids with scanty menses, in menopause.

Sensations - As if frightened by visions behind him. Feeling as if knives were being thrust into brow, as if tongue bound or tied up, as if a part of right side of head cut away. As if neck constricted with a cord. As if heart hanging by a thread and every beat would tear it off, as though heart turned over and ceased beating for a moment, as if heart hadn't room to beat.

Skin - Dilated capillaries. ***Bluish, purplish appearance***. Blue-black swellings. Cellulitis. Miliary eruptions. Purpura with intense prostration. ***Senile erysipelas***. Black measles. Scarlet fever and scarlet eruptions. Pustular eruptions become black. Boils, carbuncles, ulcers with bluish, purple surroundings. Burning in ulcers at night. Varicose ulcers. Fungoid ulcers. Ulcers sensitive to touch. Dark blisters. Bedsores with black edges. Wens. Small wounds bleed much. Pyemia, dissecting wounds. Scars, redden, hurt, break open and bleed.

Sleep - Afraid to go to sleep for fear he will die before he wakes. Sleepiness, yet cannot sleep (Bell., Op.). Wide awake in evening. Sleeplessness from cerebral irritation, burning soles, anxiety. Sleeplessness of alcoholics. Sudden starting when falling asleep. Children toss about moaning in sleep. Waking in fright at a trifle. Short naps disturbed by frightful dreams. Restless sleep, with many dreams and frequent waking, in morning is heavy and out of sorts. ***Frightful dreams of snakes.*** Amorous dreams. ***Sleeps into aggravation.***

Stomach - ***Can bear nothing tight over stomach, must loosen clothes.*** Pit of stomach painful to touch. Soreness or cramp in epigastrium. Trembling movement in the epigastric region. Nausea from anything tight on throat. Nausea after drinking ice water, after going to bed. Nausea with great flow of saliva. Any food causes distress. ***Gnawing pressure, better by eating,*** but returning in few hours, especially with cancer. Belchings, before epilepsy, at menses. Vomiting of food, bile, greenish matter, mucus, pus, blood. Vomits during menses with headache.

Stools - Stool lies close to anus without passing and without urging. Thin, offensive stools. Stools watery, light yellow, dark, chocolate-colored, grayish, like potter's clay. Stools hard like sheep dung, scanty and insufficient. Cadaverous-smelling stool of decomposed blood. Stools mixed with blood and slime, worse at night, after acid fruits.

Teeth - Teeth as if wedged. Chattering of teeth. Crumbling of teeth. Teeth feel too long in hollow teeth. ***Toothache, pain extends to ears***. Toothache from getting wet. Toothache during menses. Gums swollen, spongy, bleed. Gums dark purples during dentition. Periodontitis with swelling of cheek.

Temperature - Chills begin in small of back, runs up back. Chills worse drinking. Chills with sweat. Numbing coldness. Feet icy cold. Chills at night, flushes of heat by day. Internal heat, with cold feet. Shivering without coldness. Shivering during fever. ***Heat flushes with menopause,*** on vertex, on waking, on falling to sleep. Fever with violent headache, great loquacity. Intermittent fever every spring. Paroxysm returns after acids.

Throat - Throat very painful, worse slightest pressure, touch. ***Sore throats, worse left side, swallowing liquids.*** Chronic sore throat with much hawking, mucus sticks. Throat pain extends to ear. ***Collar and neckband must be very loose.*** Constriction, better eating. Throat pit feels swollen or sore spot back of pit. Feeling as if something was swollen which must be swallowed. As if a lump in throat, ascending and is swallowed back again. As if hot lump or soft body or crumb of bread. ***Worse from swallowing saliva or liquids.*** Cannot swallow sweet or acrid things. Choking. Tonsillitis. Tonsils purplish. Quinsy. Purple, livid color of throat. Diphtheria, dusky, black membrane, ***pain aggravated by hot drinks***. Septic parotiditis. Upper part of windpipe very sensitive to touch. Laryngismus stridulus. Larynx painful to touch. Loss of voice from paralysis of vocal cords or edema.

Tongue - Tongue red, dry and cracked at tip. Tip red, center brown. Tongue mapped, dry, black and stiff. Dry stripe in middle of tongue. Anterior half of tongue red, smooth and shining. Ulcers on sides of tongue. Blisters on tip of tongue. As if tongue was going to peel. Tongue swollen, burns. Tongue trembles when protruded. Tongue catches on teeth. Sudden forcible protrusion and retraction of tongue. Tongue as if bound or tied up. Sharp, in root of tongue, when yawning.

Vertigo - Fainting with pain in heart, nausea, pale face, vertigo. Vertigo on closing eyes, from walking in open air, before menses, and at menopause. Vertigo looking at the one and same object. Vertigo, relieved by onset of a discharge (menses or nasal catarrh). Vertigo, worse turning to right.

Vision - Paralysis of accommodation, causes asthenopia. Flickering vision, as from threads, or rays of sun. Dim vision with black flickering, often makes reading difficult. Blue ring about lights, with fiery rays. Glimmering vision, in sun, with headache. Sees zigzag figures during headache. Flickering vision with congestion of head. Defective vision, after diphtheria, extrinsic muscles too weak to maintain focus. Blindness with lung or heart affections.

COMMENTS - Characteristic aggravation from sleep. Nash noted the case of an old, syphilitic patient who suffered from obstinate constipation and was taken with severe attacks of colic. The pains seemed to extend all through the abdomen and always came on at night.

The man was not making any progress when, one day, he remarked to Nash, "Doctor, if I could only keep awake I would never have another attack." And in response to an inquiring look from the doctor, he added, "I mean that I sleep into the attack and waken in it." One dose of Lach. 200c cured the colic and the constipation too.

High blood pressure. Hemorrhages contain flakes of decomposed blood, looks like charred wheat straw. Hemorrhagic diathesis. Hemophiliacs, bleeding easily (Sabin., Phos.). Nosebleeds or heavy menses. The heart feels too large, cramp-like pain in precordia. Constriction. Palpitations with numbness down the arm. Cyanosis. Varicose veins.

Dark red eruptions, purplish swellings, black and blue spots. Small ulcers, sensitive to least touch. Buboes, plague (Naja.). Snakebites and infected wounds. Rabies, with thirst, spasms, sensitiveness and nervous prostration.

Excessive sensitiveness of the skin with intolerance to touch or constriction. Sensitive because of uneasiness from pain. Pain as if burnt or scalded on different parts. Pain in the shinbones. W. J. Guernsey pointed out that such pains often occur concomitantly with throat affections, worse or began on the left.

Sun-headaches. Headache with very pale face. Rush of blood to head. Throbbing headaches in temple with heat of head. Headache extending into nose, better when nasal catarrh comes on. Headaches, feels like the head will explode with blood.

Fainting fits and vertigo on closing eyes, on looking intently at any object in morning on waking. Fainting accompanying other complaints, with pain at heart, with nausea, with vertigo and pale face. Catalepsy. Awkward gait, weak left side. Gressus gallinaceus.

Low, muttering delirium. Intermittent fevers. Torpid state with cold limbs, tremor of body and hands, tremor of tongue. Tongue trembles, catches in the teeth or lower lip when the patient attempts to put it out. Numerous disturbances of sight and hearing. Clarke cured noises in the ears when worse after sleep.

Tickling, irritating cough. Diphtheria, mercurial and syphilitic sore throat. Sore throats, worse after sleep, from touch. Dark, bluish, purple color, with burning pains that are worse heat. Worse drinking liquids and better eating solids. Sensation of a lump in the throat (Ign.).

Touching the throat can cause suffocative spasms, cannot bear any pressure about neck. Pain from empty swallowing, liquids slightly easier, solid foods swallowed without pain. Prostration out of proportion to the appearance of the throat. Symptoms are worse on the left side or proceeding from the left to right.

Threatened paralysis of lungs. Asthma aggravated by sleep, can wake up choking. The least thing coming near mouth or nose interferes with breathing. Hay fever with a headache extending into nose, worse on suppression of the discharge. Sore nostrils and lips. Pus and blood from the nose. Red nose of alcoholics. Sensitiveness of the respiratory parts to touch, constriction and worse by anything tight around the neck.

Sinking feeling in the stomach, cannot go long without food. Symptoms are better after eating, especially after fruit. Unquenchable thirst, but nausea after drinking, worse by hot drinks. Desires oysters, wine, and coffee. Alcohol aggravates. Everything sours, heartburn. Fetid breath. Acute pain in liver extending towards stomach. Appendicitis.

Stitches in kidneys. Pain in the bladder and rectum. Desire to lift clothes up to prevent contact with the lower abdomen. Sensation as if a ball were rolling loose in the bladder or abdomen on turning over.

H. N. Martin noted that the urine has little black spots or flakes like soot floating in it. Urine is almost black, frequent, foaming, dark.

Urge to urinate after lying down, day or night, especially after sleep, more frequent in the night.

Constipation. Atony of the rectum. Painful constriction of anus followed by collapse. Visible spasmodic tenesmus in paroxysms from two to five minutes, extorting cries, passes blood and mucus. Diarrhea is fetid, cadaverous.

Tugging upward sensation. Full feeling in rectum and sensation as of little hammers beating. Burning in rectum. Stitch in rectum (upwards) when coughing or sneezing. Painful hemorrhoids, with scanty menses.

Severe premenstrual syndrome, energy before menses. Water retention and weight gain. Very sensitive, to light and noises, cries easily and becomes irritable. All symptoms ameliorated from menses.

Violent menstrual problems (Sep., Med.). Severe menstrual bleeding, dark blood with clots. Become weak and worn out from menses. Menses regular but scanty, pains better when flow is established. Symptoms occurring in connection with menses. In a case of Clarke's, Lach. 12c postponed the menses for a week.

Lochia are thin, ichorous insufficient. Swelling, induration of the ovaries, especially on the left. Tumors. Menopause, sensation of pulsating energy. Hot flashes. Varicose veins, the whole leg is swollen and aches, sore and burning. High sex drive, or suppressed drive.

Breast cancer, with a bluish appearance. Obstinate and distressing eruptions on the nipples and areola. Milk is thin and blue, nipples extremely sensitive to touch.

Better from the onset of a discharge or blood, worse from non-appearance of an expected discharge, as in menopause. Suppressions, particularly suppressed discharges.

Sensation as if a ball, lump or plug. Dislikes pressure or touch around the abdomen (Lyc., Chin.). or neck. Warm-blooded, worse heat. Symptoms begin on the left side and either remain there or proceed to the right.

Particularly suited to persons who have peculiar sensitiveness of the surface of the body. Debilitated, weakened persons. Children and elderly people. Thin rather than fat persons, persons who have been changed both mentally and physically by their illness. Women who have never been well since menopause.

Sufferers from effects of masturbation. Alcoholics. Persons who have been overdosed with mercury and for syphilitic disorders. Persons who cannot stand the sun and who are worse in summer weather.

RELATIONS - ***Antidote to venom:*** Ars., Merc., Radiate heat outwardly, alcohol inwardly, salt on the effects of bite. ***Antidotes to potencies:*** Alum., Bell., Cocc., Coff., Hep., Merc., Nit-ac., Nux-v., Ph-ac., to the visible spasmodic tenesmus of rectum, Sep. According to Teste the chief antidote is Cedron. ***It antidotes:*** Bufo, Crot-h., Rhus. ***Compare:*** (1) Puls. - menstrual cough, menses scanty, but pain worse as flow increases. (2) Con., Graph. - scanty menses. (3) Anthr. - carbuncles, boils. (4) Terebe., Kali-bi. - tongue glazed and shining, Apis, Lach. (5) Phos., Sulph. and Mur-ac. - piles during menses. (6) Bell. and Dulc. - paralysis of lungs. (7) Iris-t. - appendicitis. (8) Ph-ac. - disappointed love. (9) Lyss., Sabad. - throat affected left to right, Sabad., more chronic. (10) Cot. - menopausal troubles. Nat-m., Nit-ac., Crot-h. (11) Amph., snake lizard - right jaw swollen and painful, sharp pains, headaches, sharp pains. Eruption of vesicles and pimples. (12) Naja, Elaps., Crot-h., Lepi. (13) Nux-m. - cough of pregnancy, Lach. has a cough at menstrual period when it is going off. (14) Staph. - on swallowing, pain runs externally along parotid gland to the ears, perspiration impossible. (15) Sil., Caul., Sul., Ust. and Vib. - left ovarian and left inframammary pain. ***Complementary:*** Crot-c. often completes curative work of Lach. Also Lyc., Hep., Salam. ***Incompatible:*** Acet-ac., Am-c., Carb-ac.

REFERENCES - Boericke. Clarke. Murphy. Phatak.

LACHNANTHES TINCTORIA

(Spirit-weed)

PHARMACY - Lachn. Lachnanthes tinctoria. Spirit-weed. N. O. Hemodoracae. Tincture of whole plant. ***Historical dose:*** Tincture and all potencies.

CLINICAL - ***Chilliness.*** Cough. Delirium. Diphtheria. Headaches. Heart, pains. Nosebleeds. Pneumonia, typhoid. Rheumatism. Sore, throat. ***Stiff-neck. Torticollis. Tuberculosis.*** Typhoid fever. ***Wry neck.***

HOMEOPATHIC - Lachnantes grows in sandy swamps near the coast. The root is red and fibrous, sword-shaped leaves, hairy stem, and yellow, woolly flowers. It belongs to the same order as Aletris and is allied to the irises. A curious observation is that the white pigs and sheep of Virginia lose their hooves if they feed on Lachnantes, while the black varieties eat it without inconvenience.

A remedy for rheumatic symptoms about neck. ***Spasmodic torticollis***, painful torticollis (Caust., Mag-p., Rhus-t). Wry neck. ***Stiffness of neck***, drawn over to one side in sore throat. Pain in nape as if dislocated, when turning the neck or bending the head back.

Body icy cold, face yellow, tendency to sweat. Bubbling and boiling about the heart, rising to head. Bridge of nose feels pinched. Feeling of icy coldness in mid scapular region. Successfully used for diphtheria, typhoid fever, and typhoid pneumonia. ***Tuberculosis***. Affinity for the head, chest and circulation. Very restless, throws herself about, feels weak.

MIND - Restlessness, tosses about, with perspiration. Tossing about and whining. Ill-humored and sleepy. Despondent, bitter crying spells during headache. Sees images, while dozing through day.

Great loquacity, afterwards stupid and irritable. Loquacious delirium with brilliant eyes and circumscribed red cheeks, at night between 1 a.m. to 2 a.m.. Great hilarity, especially in the evening. Excited over a trifles.

Abdomen - Rolling of wind in abdomen and discharge of flatulency. Sensation of heat through abdomen.

Back - Burning in right scapula, in spine above sacrum. Burning in region of left kidney, extending towards right side. Pain and stiffness in back. ***Chilliness between the shoulder blades.*** Sensation between the shoulder blades as if wet with cold perspiration. Pain in nape, as if dislocated. ***Spasmodic torticollis.*** Rheumatism of the neck. ***Drawn over to one side*** in sore throat. Stiff neck, the head is drawn to one side. ***Wry neck.***

Bladder - Pressure on bladder while urinating.

Chest - Sensation of fullness in chest. Stitches on left side of chest, under right breast and under clavicle. Compelled to inhale deeply.

Ears - Singing in ear when walking in open air. Tearing in ears. Crawling and itching in ears, better by boring with the finger, but immediately returning and feeling as if something had closed the ear. Almost complete deafness during fever.

Eyes - Looks with fixed eyes. Bright, sparkling eyes with delirium. Pressing in eyes as from dust. Secretion of white mucus from eyes. Violent lachrymation and burning of eyes, sensation of dryness. Obscuration of sight, as if a cloud were before the eyes. Yellow spots before eyes. Eyes feel heavy, as if they could not be kept open. Sensation of twitching in upper eyelids.

Face - Swelling with redness and blueness under eyes. Pale, sickly countenance, face and lips bluish, eyes dull, feel thick and cold. Circumscribed redness of face with violent delirium and brilliant eyes. Yellow face. Sensation as if something were crawling over face.

Female - Menses too early, viscid blood mixed with mucus. Profuse, bright red menstrual blood. During menses, sensation of distention of abdomen, it feels as if it were boiling.

Food - Aversion to meat. Much thirst.

Head - Head feels heavy. ***Head feels enlarged***, worse least noise. Circumscribed red cheeks, scalp feels sore, as if hair was standing on end, burning in palms and soles. Bridge of nose feels as if pinched. Right-sided pain, extending down to jaw. Scalp painful.

Heart - Stitches in heart with anxiety. Frequent violent pulsations of heart, each beat is double, one hard and full, the other soft and small. Trembling of heart with great debility. Sensation of heat, bubbling and boiling around heart region, rising to head.

Male - Violent burning in left half of the scrotum, drawing toward right side. Tingling and itching of scrotum. Perspiration of scrotum and penis.

Mouth - Saliva of tough mucus. Sensation if the mouth were sore and thick. Swelling and tension of the lips. Lips red.

Limbs - Tearing from the shoulder, extending to finger joints. Tearing in elbow joints. Tearing in knuckles of the middle fingers of the right hand. Thumb and index finger feel as if sprained. Burning of palms and soles. Cramps in the feet during night.

Lungs - Cough worse in bed and after sleeping. Dry cough, as if it came from larynx with sore throat. Expectoration streaked with blood with severe pain in chest. Pneumonia.

Nose - Profuse nosebleeds, pale blood. Bridge of nose feels pinched.

Perspiration - Sensation the skin is moist and sticky. Perspires freely after midnight. Sweats during cold. Sweats with dizziness. Sweats in morning.

Rectum - Continuous stitch in rectum. Frequent unsuccessful desire to evacuate. Frequent stool, passes much wind.

Sensations - As if head or vertex enlarged, as if split open with a wedge, as if hair standing on end. As if a cloud before eyes, pressing as from dust in eyes. As if something had closed ear. Bridge of nose as if pinched. As of something crawling over face.

Skin - Sensation in skin as if an eruption would appear. Pimples appear here and there, containing a watery fluid. Itching and burning in the skin all night, worse after scratching. Stinging, itching and tingling on thighs, legs, feet, arms.

Sleep - Sleepiness with yawning, eyes feel so heavy that she cannot keep them open. Cannot go to sleep easily. Sleepless or restless sleep with distressing dreams. After waking and stretching, a shock followed by chilliness and goose bumps all over.

Stomach - Sensation of qualmishness above navel, when walking in open air. Fullness in pit of stomach, beating as from a pulse, as if a hammer were beating on an ulcerated spot.

Teeth - Pain in all the teeth when eating or drinking warm things. All the teeth feel loose and too long, worse in bed.

Temperature - Continuous chilliness. Icy coldness of body, perspiration, principally on forehead. The skin is cold, damp and clammy during the chills. Feels hot, but the chills run all over before the heat can develop itself. Flashes of heat alternating with chilliness. Fever with violent delirium and brilliant eyes. Fever with somnolency.

Throat - Great dryness in throat, especially on waking in the night with much coughing. Sore throat with short cough. Itching when swallowing. Sensation of swelling in pharynx with stiffness of neck and head drawn to one side (diphtheria).

Vertigo - Giddiness in the head with sensation of heat in chest and around heart and perspiration. Vertigo with icy coldness of the forehead.

COMMENTS - Hering said the Native Americans chewed the plant when they met the "white man" to give them a flow of language. Remarkable loquacity. Produces a desire to talk a flow of language and the courage to make a speech.

Strong affinity for the head, chest and circulation. Sharp stitches in quick succession in the right side of the chest below mamma. Sensation of heat, bubbling and boiling in chest and region of heart, rising to head, giddy, breaks out into perspiration. Trembling of the heart.

Tuberculosis when the neck is drawn over to one side. Rheumatism of the neck and stiffness of the neck. Stiffness of the neck with the head twisted to one (right) side, especially when occurring with a sore throat. Much dryness of throat, worse on waking in the night with coughing.

Headaches of great intensity, generally right-sided. Sensation as if the head is split open with a wedge, with icy coldness of the body, crying spells, worse by vomiting. Toothache, worse eating and drinking warm things.

Continued chilliness. Sensation as if a piece of ice was lying on back between shoulders, then a shock followed by coldness over the whole body with goose bumps. Cold attacks occur on moving, better after going to bed. During the cold sensation, the skin is damp and clammy.

Fever with loquacious delirium, brilliant eyes and circumscribed red cheeks. Blueness about face, under eyes, and lips. Burning of palms and soles, under nail of left toe.

Arthur Dalzell reported the case of Mrs. B., 43, who had fibroid tuberculosis of both lungs, collapse of right lower lobe. Great prostration and night-sweats. The bowels were alternately relaxed and confined. Pain and stiffness in the back, bruised all over, dry cough, roughness of throat, weak heart-sounds. Bad sleep owing to a cough.

Lachn. tincture, three drops every four hours, was given. In three days the prostration was diminished and the cough was much better, night-sweats and bruised feeling gone. From this time an emulsion containing cod-liver oil, liquor pancreaticus, eggs, cream, hypophosphites and eucalyptus oil were given in addition. The case went on to recovery.

Dalzell also recorded the case of Mrs. R., 45, who was in the last stage of tuberculosis. Right lung consolidated, left in cavities. This patient had circumscribed flush on face, brilliant eyes, throat felt rough, overall bruised feeling. Remittent fever. Skin dry, except at night, when she had profuse perspiration. Constant dry cough. Muco-purulent expectoration.

Lachn. tincture, five drops every three hours, relieved all the symptoms and procured euthanasia, the patient dying quite easily twelve days later.

RELATIONS - *Compare:* (1) Dulc., Bry., Puls. (2) Fel. - nape of neck pains and great tension there.

REFERENCES - Boericke. Clarke. Murphy. Phatak.

LACTICUM ACIDUM

(Lactic Acid)

PHARMACY - lac-ac. Lacticum acidum. Lactic acid. Milk acid. Lactis acidum. Dilutions. *Historical dose:* All potencies.

CLINICAL - ***Acidity. Aching, pain.*** Aphonia. Belchings. Bones, swelling. ***Breasts, disorders.*** Canker, sores. Coryza. Cough. ***Debility. Diabetes.*** Foot sweat. Gastroenteritis. ***Glands, enlarged.*** Hoarseness. Indigestion. Leucorrhea. Morning, sickness. ***Nausea***. Nosebleed. Pregnancy, sickness. Rheumatic, pains. Rheumatism. Sciatica. Throat, constricted. Throat, sore. Trembling. Vomiting. ***Water brash.*** Weakness.

HOMEOPATHIC - Hering noted that lactic acid was discovered by Scheele in sour milk, the result of the spontaneous fermentation of sugar of milk under the influence of casein. It is also met with in many vegetable products which have turned sour.

Reisig first introduced it into homeopathy. Lactic acid has been proved in both the lower and higher potencies, but many valuable observations have been made on patients taking substantial doses for diabetes as it was often given for diabetes in the past.

In these cases, the symptoms of rheumatic fever were directly traced to the acid. Pain, swelling, stiffness and tenderness of joints, worse by motion (as with Bry., which antidotes Lac-ac.). Flying pains about limbs.

One prover had pain along the right sciatic nerve. The well-known effects of milk that has soured on the stomach and remained undigested were produced. Nausea, vomiting, burning and sense of weight.

Weakness, as if from exercise, aversion to exercise. Rheumatic affections. Rheumatic pains in joints, knees, worse by motion. Trembling of whole body, while walking. ***Debility***, weariness of the limbs.

Acidity. Hot acrid belchings, worse smoking. Salivation, water brash. Morning sickness. Fullness or lump like puff ball in throat.

Frequent passing of large quantities of saccharine urine. ***Diabetes***. Sweaty feet. ***Breast troubles***.

MIND - Confusion. Forgetful, can't remember a thing an hour after it has happened. Dislikes to read or think. Lazy. Aversion to business or what formerly was pleasant to do. Contemptuous. Sarcastic. Finds fault, very exacting. Believes all she says is a lie. Great discouragement during pregnancy.

Abdomen - Pains across bowels and lower right side. Bearing down pain in upper part of abdomen. Sharp pain across lower abdomen before stool. Left hypochondrium sensitive to touch. Sharp cutting pains and jerking in muscle. Dull pain in left groin over hip bone.

Back - Pain in small of back, extending into shoulders. Sore aching in lower part of back, worse when walking. Stiff neck. Stiff down between scapulae and across shoulders.

Breasts - Pain in breasts with ***enlargement of axillary glands***.

Chest - Left side of chest sore and painful. Cutting or sticking pain in upper third of right side.

Constitutions - Suited to anemic, pale women. Large doses disagreed with melancholic, choleric constitution, dark hair and eyes.

Cough - Hoarse, hard, dry cough with dryness of glottis. Spasmodic, ringing cough from irritation in throat. Cough from hot eructations. Cough with nausea and constricted feeling in throat. Constant cough worse spring and fall, with foot sweat. Cough worse from smoking.

Ears - Disturbed and troubled by noise. Roaring in left ear on rising, in afternoon. Singing, snapping in left ear. Pain from parotids into ear, stiff feeling in parotids.

Eyes - Sensation of fullness in eyes with headache. Eyes feel tired. Eyes feel as if they would burst. Marked protrusion of eyes. Hyperesthesia of retina, steady aching in and behind eyeball. Pupils dilated.

Photophobia, direct light painful. Jerking of left upper lid.

Face - Face flushed or congested from headache. Erysipelatous redness on left cheek and side of nose. Small vesicles on nose in morning. Parotids feel stiff. Pains from parotids into ear.

Female - Menses scanty, more profuse than usual. Itching of vulva during flow. Leucorrhea, staining linen yellow, when checked, nasal catarrh ensues. Pain as if menstruating, sitting with feet high lessens uterine soreness. Pain in small of back and lower abdomen. Aching pain in region of right ovary, worse by rapid walking or exercise. ***Morning sickness*** with salivation, nausea and vomiting, water brash better by breakfast.

Food - Appetite impaired. Voracious appetite and great thirst. Eating generally improves symptoms. Nausea on waking, better by eating in diabetes or pregnancy.

Head - Congestion of head, painless with strong pulsation of vessels of neck. Head feels very large. Headache with sensation of fullness in vertex. Dull pain in forehead, just over eyes and extending into eyes. Pain in head and back all night. Pain in occiput and alternating between there and forehead. Head sore to touch. Fine miliary eruption on scalp.

Heart - Sharp pains around heart, causes palpitations.

Kidneys - Frequent pain in kidneys. Frequent desire to urinate large quantities. Urinates day and night, the attempt to retain it causes pain. Copious urine, deep brownish red, with much reddish sediment. Sugar in urine. Morning urine contained a large amount of salt, in evening a large excess of sugar.

Limbs - Limbs feel chilly. Debility, weariness of the limbs. Weakness as if from exercise with rheumatic pains in the bones, aversion to exercise. ***Rheumatic pain in joints and shoulders, wrists, knees,*** with much weakness. Joints swollen, not tender, stiff. Severe, sharp pains in joints, stiffness. All pains worse by movement. Trembling of whole body while walking.

Lungs - Saw-like rasping sound. Frequent deep sighing inspirations and expirations. Spasmodic, ringing cough, caused by irritation in throat.

Male - Annoying erections in morning, but loins ache too much to attempt sex. Seminal emissions three successive nights.

Modalities - Smoking aggravates all symptoms.

Mouth - Mouth and fauces very dry and hot. Much saliva in mouth, tasting salty. ***Copious salivation and water brash,*** especially during pregnancy. Acrid taste with nausea. Sour, coppery taste. Very sore mouth. Roof of mouth dry, feels burnt. Canker sores.

Nose - Great sensitiveness of smell. Severe coryza. Stopped nose. Sneezing. Thick, yellow mucus from head to throat. Dryness of posterior nares, with hawking of mucus. Nosebleed every morning.

Perspiration - Copious perspiration. Unusual perspiration of feet.

Rectum - Aching pain in anus. Soft, mushy stool, diarrhea. Greenish yellow stools with tenesmus. Very costive, stool once a week, hard, black.

Skin - Skin harsh and dry, no sweat. Itching and burning, worse by cold. Red spots or blotches on various parts of the body, particularly thighs and lower limbs.

Sleep - Stupid, drowsy all day, restless all night. Sleeplessness from vertigo, from backache. Dreams of sexual intercourse, with erections, no emission. Horrible dreams, of abysses.

Stomach - Burning and weight in stomach. Burning, hot gas from stomach to throat, causing profuse secretion of tenacious mucus, worse ***smoking***. ***Hot, acrid belchings.*** Food sours. Uneasiness in stomach after food and drink. Nausea with water brash or vomiting, better from eating. ***Nausea, morning sickness***, especially in ***pale, anemic*** women. Nausea on rising in morning. Nausea after breakfast, not severe, but very persistent. ***Nausea like seasickness.*** Constant nausea, persisting for days.

Temperature - Cold and chilly at times, mostly on limbs. Flushes of heat with headaches.

Throat - ***Dryness of throat with hoarseness.*** Dryness and rawness, extending to larynx. Sensation of a plug in the throat. Excessive hawking with or without nausea. Keeps swallowing. Difficulty of swallowing solids, liquids more easily. Fullness or lump like a puffball. Sense of constriction low down in throat, rough and dry. Intense burning in throat, fauces and esophagus worse by eructation. Fauces hot, dry and swollen. Aphonia. Hoarseness.

Tongue - Tongue dry, parched, red and raw. Thick yellow coating on tongue with bad taste in morning. Tongue sticky, coated thick white. Tongue sore on left side.

Vertigo - Vertigo when turning head suddenly, on stooping, on rising. Vertigo at night. Vertigo worse with heat. Vertigo as if tossed on a rough sea. with nausea like seasickness.

COMMENTS - Cartier noted its use for acute gastroenteritis, six to ten drops in a small glass of water. It was used locally in the tuberculous ulceration of vocal cords.

Nash regarded the concomitance of rheumatic pains as the chief guiding symptom here. He recorded a case of diabetes with rheumatic fever supervening, cured with Lac-ac. 200c.

Constant nausea, nausea on awaking, before rising. Nausea in diabetes, pregnancy, or rheumatism. Nausea, better from eating, belchings, worse from smoking. Smoking aggravates the belchings. Diabetes.

Severe pains in muscles and joints after exertion. Chronic fatigue with flu-like symptoms since physical over-exertion. Chronic fatigue with muscle aches. Inoffensive, copious foot-sweat (Sil.).

RELATIONS - ***Antidoted by:*** Bry. (relieved sharp pains upper third right side, but soreness remained). ***Compare:*** (1) Sarcol-ac. (2) Lith., Ph-ac. Lac-c., Lac-v-c., Lac-d., Sac-l. (3) In nausea of pregnancy, Nux-v., Puls., Ph-ac., Colch., Lyc., Lac-d. (4) Ip. - excessive hawking with or without nausea. (5) Caust. - phlegm in throat, cannot be hawked up, causing nausea. (6) Diabetes, Ph-ac., Acet-ac., Lac-d., Uran-n. (7) Flying rheumatism, Puls., Rhus-t. (8) Great discouragement, Psor. ***Incompatible:*** Coffee worse symptoms.

REFERENCES - Boericke. Clarke. Murphy. Phatak.

LACTUCA VIROSA

(Acrid Lettuce)

PHARMACY - lact. Lactuca virosa. Acrid lettuce. Poison lettuce. Opium lettuce. "Lactucarium" or Lettuce opium. N. O. Compositae. Genus, Cicoracee. Tincture of fresh flowering plant. Specimens of both Lactuca vir. and Lactuca sat. might be included in the tincture. Tincture of impissated juice. ***Historical dose:*** Tincture and all potencies.

CLINICAL - Angina pectoris. Anus, disorders. Ascites. Asthma. ***Breast-feeding, disorders.*** Constipation. Cough. Cramps. Diarrhea. Globus, hystericus. Gonorrhea. Headache. Heartburn. Hemiopia. Hysteria. ***Insomnia.*** Levitation. Liver, disorders. Musca, volitantes. Noises, ears. Pylorus, pain. Sleep, excessive. Smell, illusions. Spinal cord, pains. Spleen, disorders. Whooping cough. Yawning.

HERBAL - The leaves of garden lettuce, Lactuca sativa, when too old and going to seed, have a bitter taste and the stalk contains a milky juice which is intensely bitter. This juice contains Lactucin and is common to all lettuces, but is especially virulent in Lact. vir. from which (as well as well as from Lact. sat.) Lactucarium or "Lettuce Opium," is prepared.

HOMEOPATHIC - Brunton noted that Lact. has a soporific action and is used "instead of Opium to allay cough, quiet nervousness and induce sleep in cases where from idiosyncrasy, Opium is not borne." This use of lettuces has been known from very remote times and has not been added to by old-school observers. The sleep-provoking power of Lact. is recognizable in sensitive persons who eat ordinary garden lettuce in salad.

Boericke specified Lact. as a "true galactagogue," as it ***increases the milk in breasts.*** This remedy also acts upon the brain and circulatory system. Delirium tremens with sleeplessness, coldness and tremor. Hydrothorax and ascites.

Impotence. Sense of lightness and ***tightness*** affecting whole body, especially chest. Marked action on limbs.

MIND - Stupefaction of sense. Difficulty in thinking. Loss of memory. Anxiety and disturbed sleep. Great restlessness. Fear driving him from place to place. Negative thinking. Contrary. Excessive ill humor, provoked by slightest contradiction. Repulsive mood.

Prolonged emotional suffering, resulting in emotional deadness or coldness. Forsaken feeling. Disposition melancholy, fretful. Sadness with extravagant and exaggerated notions. Headache after grief.

Foolish behavior. Plays antics. Jumping. Singing or sighing. Delusions, sees soldiers on his bed. Delusions, that he would be murdered. Vivid, exaggerated fancies.

Abdomen - Sensation of weight, fullness. Movements in abdomen. Borborygmi, abundant emission of wind. Colic in early morning, tense abdomen, relieved somewhat by evacuation and passing of wind. Cramping pain, better passing flatus. Dull shocks or else lancinations in right hypochondrium. Contusive pain in liver region, in morning.

Back - Tension in muscles of neck or right side, sometimes spasmodic. Lancinations under right armpit. Pains in spinal marrow, as far as the cauda equina and extending to sacrum. Contusive pain in lumbar region. Drawing pains in loins towards the groins.

Breasts - Milk absent. ***Increase of milk in breasts*** (Asaf.).

Chest - Constriction. Sense of oppression of chest. Squeezing sensation in lower chest. Sensation of warmth. Pain on bending forward. Shaking of chest during cough.

Cough - Cough as from dust. Must hold chest with both hands.

Ears - Drawing pains in ears, shootings followed by tension in left ear. Buzzing in ears, ringing sound before ears, in evening, in bed.

Eyes - Biting in the eyes. Burning in eyes, especially in the lids. Redness of conjunctiva with increased mucus secretion in elderly persons. Pupils dilated. Cloudiness of vision, weakness of sight. Hemiopia. Flying insects before eyes, on stooping after a meal. Itching above the eyebrows.

Face - Pale. Heat of face with trembling and sensation of swelling of lips. Quivering in lips. Tingling with a feeling of tightness on face. Lancinations in chin at extremity of sub-maxillary nerve. Swelling of the lymphatic glands.

Female - Promotes menses. Menses too early. Bearing down and weak feeling about pelvic organs and general relaxed feeling. Painful gonorrhea.

Food - Want of appetite, food is repugnant, no appetite for bread and meat. Food tastes sickly, bitter. Appetite and thirst increased. Desires milk, pickles, sour. Aversion to bread, meat, wine. Better from bread, coffee, vegetable acids, worse from milk.

Head - Empty sensation. Sensation of looseness of brain. Dull, heavy, confused, dizzy. Heat of face and headache with general coldness. Pain, stupefying headache, after grief. Headache with disorders of respiratory organs.

Kidneys - Dragging pressure in region of bladder, as from urgency to urinate. Burning in urethra. ***Urine smells of violets.*** Urine clear as water, copious. Sensation as of a drop continuously passing along the urethra when seated.

Limbs - Cramp-like pains. Rush of blood to lower limbs. Sensation as if circulation in legs were suspended. Numbness while sitting. Coldness and numbness of feet and legs. Lame hip down left side, worse walking. Cramps in shin bones, extending to toes and side of leg involving calves. Tension in hollow of knee on rising from a seat, while walking. Tremor of hands and arms.

Lungs - Difficult breathing. Suffocative breathing from dropsy of the chest. Irritating, suffocating cough. Constant tickling cough. Incessant, spasmodic cough, as if chest would fly to pieces.

Male - Drawing pains at root of penis, in right spermatic cord and along internal surface of thigh. Diminished sexual appetite, chases away lasciviousness and voluptuous fancies. Painful erections during morning sleep. Swelling of a lymphatic vessel in penis, following morning erections.

Modalities - Better in open air, bending, sitting up. Worse from touch, crossing legs, sneezing, in a warm room. Yawning and stretching helps pressure in chest.

Mouth - Dry mouth, without thirst. White coating on tongue, thick mucus, sore, as if burned at tip. Contraction under tongue. Sharp pain in molars on left side of lower jaw, as if they were being twisted. Soreness of gums, on an empty socket on masticating.

Nose - Sensation as though end of nose were distended. Peculiar smell before nose and a similar taste in mouth. Coryza, followed by excoriation and dryness in nose. Frequent sneezing.

Rectum - Constipation, no stool the first day or else a tardy and hard evacuation (habitual constipation diminishes). Stool only after urgent calls and griping.

Sensations - As if chest would fly to pieces. As if circulation in legs was suspended. Coldness of stomach, throat, chest, feet.

Skin - Subcutaneous lancinating and pinching in various places. Inflammation and eruptions.

Sleep - Irresistible drowsiness in daytime. Frequent yawning and stretching of limbs. Restless, impossible to get to sleep. ***Insomnia.*** Disturbed sleep from anxiety, cough. Position, lying on back impossible. Sound, refreshing sleep. Deep, comatose sleep.

Stomach - Sensation of icy coldness in stomach. Sensation of retraction. Pains in stomach with contraction of pit of stomach, worse by pressure. After a meal, sensation of fullness in stomach with pressure downwards. Pain better passing flatus. Loathing, nausea, vomiting, sometimes with uneasiness at pit of stomach.

Temperature - Slight shivering chill. Frequent coldness over back and head, with heat in face. Chilliness in a warm room with coldness of hands and feet. Dry heat of upper part of body, with icy coldness of feet.

Throat - Slight burning in throat. Difficult swallowing with sensation as if uvula were raw with burning. Sensation of coldness in esophagus from eructations. Accumulation of mucus in throat, viscid mucus in throat in morning.

Vertigo - Vertigo with heaviness of head and lower limbs. Vertigo with blackness before eyes. Vertigo with sensation as if head were too large and expanded.

COMMENTS - There are several recorded instances of poisoning. A man, 25, ate Lact. in a salad, 7 p.m. and went to bed at 9. He woke at 11 with sharp, colicky pains, soon followed by nausea and vomiting that lasted all night. He fell asleep at 5 a.m., but in the morning was astonished to find himself unable to distinguish objects clearly.

A boy of 10 who ate the same meal became affected with lively delirium at midnight that lasted until morning. He jumped about on the bed, played all sorts of pranks and nobody could quiet him. He had no colic or vomiting.

His pupils were dilated until the iris was a mere rim. Trying to read he mistook M for P and O for V. In his delirium, he had hallucinations, saw on his bed a soldier, an inkstand, etc. Both these patients as well as another had liquid stools. The dilated pupils persisted some time.

Keynote indescribable sensation of tightness, affecting the whole body, but especially the chest. Intolerance to touch and pressure. Pain in spinal marrow even to cauda equina, streaming along coccyx. Right arm is much affected.

Much yawning and stretching to relieve the squeezing of the lower chest. Squeezing in left breast. Feeling as if a hundredweight on chest. Feeling of relaxation in the chest. Angina pectoris.

Asthma. Spasmodic cough in frequent paroxysms with feeling of suffocation. Attacks come suddenly without any apparent cause, induced by a violent tickling in pharynx and roof of mouth. Whooping cough, paroxysms preceded by anxiety. Antispasmodic. Chest symptoms are better sitting up.

Tightness in the liver region. Enlargements of the liver with tightness. Stomach pain, better bending. Pinching in umbilical region, better crossing the legs.

Constipation and diarrhea with many concomitant anal symptoms. Sensation as of a drop continually passing along the urethra when seated. Urine smells like violets. Hering noted "painful gonorrhea in females." Used as a galactagogue (Aven., Alf.).

Extraordinary lightness of body, more pronounced in open air. Feels as if swimming in bed. Dreams of swimming in the air or of walking above the ground. The head feels light, empty. Sensation as if head too large, as if brain loose. Sensation as if looking through gauze. Mild sedative.

Cured a case of hypertrophy of the ovaries in a woman of fifty as a consequence of a miscarriage twenty-five years before. The tumor was excessively large and the patient could get no rest because of the pain from the pressure. The rectum was contracted and feces evacuated with great pain.

"Fatigue during stool," and also "sleepiness during stool" were peculiar and may prove characteristic. Ebullitions rising up from abdomen suggest globus hystericus.

RELATIONS - ***Antidoted by:*** Vegetable acids and coffee. (In a proving of Lact., Acet-ac., aether and hoch. were more effectual than coffee). ***Compare:*** (1) Drowsiness, dryness and constipation - Op., Nux-m. (2) levitation, Stict. Puls., Ph-ac., Lac-c., Asar., Thuj., etc. (3) intolerance of anything tight around neck, Lach. (4) gonorrhea, urine smells of violets, Terebe. (5) squeezing in left breast, Bor. (6) Bor. has empty feeling. Coldness. (7) Helo., pain in soles as if he had jumped on a stone. (8) Bor., heart symptoms, Kali-c. and Kali-i., cough Dros. (9) Nabal. (10) Lach., Kali-c., (11) Spira. - galactagogue.

REFERENCES - Boericke. Clarke. Murphy. Phatak.

LAETRILE

(Amygdalin)

PHARMACY - laetr. Laetrile. Amygdalin. Pangamic acid. Vitamin B-17. Anti-cancer drug. ***Historical dose:*** All potencies.

CLINICAL - Anemia. Cancer. Cyanosis. Dizziness. Fatigue. Hair, loss. Headache. Hypotension. Liver, damage. Muscular, weakness. Nausea. Ptosis. Rheumatism. Tumors. Vomiting.

HOMEOPATHIC - Laetrile formula is laevo-D-mandelonitrile-B-glucoronide. Laetrile is a decomposition product resulting from the hydrolysis of amygdalin. This compound is chemically related to amygdalin, a substance found naturally in the pits of apricots and various other fruits.

The term "laetrile" was first proposed by Ernest T. Krebs, Jr. in 1949. Most proponents of laetrile for the treatment of cancer use the terms "laetrile" and "amygdalin" interchangeably. Amygdalin is one of the first and best known cyanogenic glycosides. Neither amygdalin nor laetrile contain free cyanide.

Amygdalin is a herbal constituent derived from the kernels of various fruits of the Genus Prunus (synonym amygdalus) , which includes the plum, prune, cherry, peach and apricot. It is among the most ancient herbal remedies used against cancer.

Apricot kernels have been in medical use since the days of Pen T'sao (an herbalist), in 2800 B.C., in China. The great Persian master of pharmacy, medicine and natural sciences, Avicenna (980-1037), recommended the use of apricot bitter oil in the treatment of tumors of the spleen, uterus, stomach and liver.

Some doctors believe that laetrile ***relieves the pain of cancer***. Experimental results show effects of amygdalin on breast tumors. Adenocarcinomas. Stoppage of growth of small tumors. Prevents the development of lung cancer metastases. Other reported uses have been in the treatment of high blood pressure and rheumatism.

Toxicities are generally mild when patients adhered to treatment schedules. The side effects associated with treatment mirror the symptoms of cyanide poisoning, including nausea, vomiting, and headache. Fatigue, muscular weakness, pain. Respiratory difficulties. Decreased blood cell counts. Hair loss and mouth sores.

More severe side effects are experienced when laetrile is given by mouth than when it is given by injection, including mental confusion, dizziness. Cyanosis, anemia, hypotension. Liver damage. Ptosis.

Ataxic neuropathies, difficulty walking due to damaged nerves. Coma.

RELATIONS - ***Compare:*** Ars., Cadm-s., Hydr.

REFERENCES - Murphy.

LAMIUM ALBUM

(White Nettle)

PHARMACY - lam. Lamium album. White nettle. Lamium levigatum. Lamium maculatum. Dead Nettle. N. O. Labiatae. Tincture of entire fresh plant while in flower and seed. ***Historical dose:*** Tincture and all potencies.

CLINICAL - Blisters. Chills. ***Headaches. Hemorrhoids.*** Hemoptysis. Hernia. Leucorrhea. Menstruation, early. Ulcers.

HOMEOPATHIC - Lamium was proved by Hahnemann and others, including Stapf. Affinity for female and urinary organs. Sensation in urethra as though a drop of water were flowing through it. Hemoptysis. ***Hemorrhoids*** and hard stool with blood.

Menses appeared too early and were scanty. Much leucorrhea with biting sensation or without sensation, white mucus.

"Deep-in" headache (Bac.), tightness of scalp and a backward and forward motion of the head. ***Headache with backward and forward motion of head.***

Much uneasiness of mind and body, trembling of limbs, weakness during the chill. Tearing and drawing in the limbs. Blisters on heel from slight rubbing. Ulcers on heel (All-c.).

MIND - Whining mood, inclination to weep, feels as if abandoned (Puls.). Great sadness with lachrymose humor. Great agitation and anxiety, which permit no rest.

Modalities - Better on rising, sitting. Worse while lying down in bed, in morning, rising from stooping. Worse in open air, drinking, eating.

COMMENTS - Farrington said, "Lamium has been recommended for external hemorrhoids. ***'Hard stool with blood'*** is the nearest symptom bearing on this."

RELATIONS - ***Compare:*** (1) Puls., All-c. (2) Members of the Mint tribe - Hedeo., Oci., Orig., Menth. (3) "Deep-in" headache, Bac. (4) Head moves backwards and forwards - Arn., Cham., Lyc.

REFERENCES - Boericke. Clarke.

LAPATHUM ACUTUM

(Common Dock)

PHARMACY - lapa. Lapathum acutum. Common dock. Lapathum sylvestre. Rumex obtusifolius. N. O. Polygonacae. Tincture of fresh root. ***Historical dose:*** Tincture and all potencies.

CLINICAL - Headache. Kidneys, pain. Leucorrhea. Nosebleed. Uterus, atony. Weariness.

HERBAL - Lapathum is the old name of the docks, now generally named rumex. The word is of Greek origin and signifies, according to Gerarde, "to soften, ease or purge the belly," and the name was given to "herbs used in pottage and medicine, very well known to have the power of cleansing."

HOMEOPATHIC - Lapa. was proved by Widenhorn. It produced some rather severe headaches and nosebleeds. Hansen said it is indicated in nosebleed following headache. Weight in stomach. Pain in kidneys with pressure from without inwards. Weak feeling in genitals. Leucorrhea with uterine bearing down pain. Weariness.

MIND - Sadness and morose, alternating with gaiety.

RELATIONS - ***Compare:*** (1) Rumx., Rheum., Phyt. (2) Sep., Lil-t. (3) Kidney pain, Santa.

REFERENCES - Boericke. Clarke.

LAPIS ALBUS

(White Stone)

PHARMACY - lap-a. Lapis albus. White stone. Calcarea silico-fluorica. Trituration. ***Historical dose:*** All potencies.

CLINICAL - Abscesses. Anemia. Bronchocele. ***Cancer. Cretinism.*** Dyspepsia. Dysmenorrhea. Epithelioma. Fibroids. Fibroma. ***Glands, disorders. Goiter.*** Growths. ***Hemorrhages***. Leucorrhea. Lipoma. Otitis media. Pruritus, vulva. Sarcoma. Scirrhous. Scrofula. Sores. Tuberculosis. Tumors. Ulcers.

HOMEOPATHIC - Lapis albus is silico-fluoride of calcium. A kind of gneiss, it was found by Grauvogl in the mineral springs of Gastein, Germany. These waters flow over gneiss formations into the valley of the Achen, where goiter and cretinism abound. The mineral waters have a reputation for curing ulcers, cancers and tumors.

Grauvogl cured with it a case of carcinoma and he and others have cured cases of goiter and scrofulous glands. ***Uterine cancer.*** Fibroid tumors with ***intense burning*** pains through the part with ***profuse hemorrhage***. Pre-ulcerative stage of carcinoma. Sarcoma. Lipoma. Growths.

Glandular disorders, glands are elastic and pliable (Calc-f. and Cist. have a stony hardness). ***Goiter***. Especially affects the connective tissue about the glands. Glandular swellings where no glands are usually found. Scrofulous affections, except in malarial cases. Fat, anemic babies with a ravenous appetite.

Burning, shooting, stinging pains in the stomach, pylorus, in the breasts and uterus. Severe menstrual pains causing weakness and swooning.

Chest - Persistent pains in breast region. Glandular hardening.

Ears - Suppurative otitis media.

Face - Opening in cheek as large as a silver dollar, in carcinoma. Epithelioma of lip, crusts coming off leave raw surface. Tumor of lower lip with burning, stinging pains, that make him jump off his feet.

Female - Painful menses, suddenly taken with pain so severe that she swoons. Severe pain preceding the flow. Pruritus vulva. Burning, shooting, stinging pains in breasts and uterus. Uterine carcinoma.

Food - Ravenous appetite.

Head - Sick headache.

Skin - Scrofulous abscesses and sores. Pruritus. Enlargement and induration of glands, ***especially the cervical glands***. Lipoma, sarcoma, carcinoma.

COMMENTS - In two cases of cervical glands cured by Lap-a. 6c, Dewey related that a ravenous appetite developed while the remedy was being taken. He also noted that the swelling of the glands was elastic rather than of stony hardness.

In one patient, the swelling was as large as a goose-egg in the right sternoclavicular region. This patient, a young woman, was a blonde, as also was a woman of thirty-five whom he cured of goiter with the remedy.

Whiting recorded a fragmentary proving of Lap-a. Mrs. Smith., 40, fair, stout, no children, had a large bronchocele. Averse to all animal food, craved sweets. Craved and drank much ice-water in all seasons since a child. Feet and legs cold to knees.

Lap-a. 6x was given, 2 grains, powders, one four times a day. She reported in a month that the tumor was rapidly diminishing in size, but she was having much pain in it. No further medicine was given.

Two months later, the tumor had diminished to one-half, and the patient stated that since taking the powders she had had no pain at her menstrual period, no dyspepsia and no sick-headaches. She had experienced severe dysmenorrhea since the menses first appeared. Since leaving off the medicine, the pain in the tumor ceased and also the decrease in size.

Lap-a. 6x was again given and again the pain in the tumor came on and in addition, itching of the external genitals. The 30c and 200c caused such intense itching that the patient refused to take any more medicine of any kind.

Since then, Whiting cured many cases of pruritus and also of dysmenorrhea with Lap-a. The pains come on before the flow and cause swooning.

One patient, 19, had dysmenorrhea from the first. Pain so severe she would fall unconscious wherever she might happen to be, the swoon lasting half an hour at times. Better when flow established. Lap-a. 200c cured.

Miss X., 34, normal until she had measles at age 20; since then, pain at commencement of menstruation, so severe as to cause fainting. "This severe pain would continue less for a day or until the flow was established." Lap-a. 200c cured in six months.

W. P. Wesselheft, discussing Whiting's paper, narrated the cure of a case of epithelioma of the lip in a man of seventy with Lap-a. 12x in water.

Dr. Gregory cured a young man of a tumor of the lip with Lap-a. 30c. It recurred two years later with "burning, stinging pain, which made him jump off his feet." More Lap-a. 30c was given and cured in a year. There was in further recurrence.

Bellows noted that where Sil. is indicated, progress is hastened by Lap-a.

RELATIONS - *Compare:* (1) Sil., Bad., Ars-i., Calc-i., Con., Kali-i., Aster. (2) Gast. - effect on scar tissues. (3) Ars., Calc., Cund., Iod., Kali-c., Spong.

REFERENCES - Anshutz. Boericke. Clarke.

LAPIS GRANITES MURVEY

(Granite Rock)

PHARMACY - lap-gr-m. Lapis granites murvey. Granite rock. Murvey granite from near Barna, Co. Galway, Ireland. Triturations. *Historical dose:* All potencies.

CLINICAL - Chronic fatigue. Constipation. Dandruff. Diarrhea. ***Exhaustion.*** Fevers. Flatulence. Headache. Influenza. Nausea. Rheumatism. ***Weakness.***

HOMEOPATHIC - Lap-gr-m. was first used as a medicine by ancient Egyptian physicians and it is mention in many of the medical scrolls. It has recently been proved in England by Nuala Eising.

Connemara granite of Ireland has one of the highest levels of radioactivity of the granites found in Britain and Ireland. The pink granite has a particularly high level of radioactivity. Granite in Ireland is considered responsible for a higher rate of cancer and Down's syndrome in that country.

Eising obtained a sample of the granite by breaking through a rock and taking a piece from the center which was previously not exposed. This was sent to the Galen Pharmacy and was potentized to the 30c potency, which was used by the provers.

Extreme exhaustion and weakness. Inability to move. Drags oneself around the place, having to lie down, sleep often. No inclination to do anything, pleasurable. Profound introversion and withdrawal. Occasional bursts of energy or nervous high energy.

Heavy and painful limbs. Rheumatic pains. Pressure, bruised and sore feeling. Headaches, frontal pain, or in temples. Delirious fevers or milder, recurring fevers, with profuse sweating.

Marked effect on the liver and digestive system, with nausea. Yellow skin. Lost or diminished sexual energy. Pain and discomfort in genital areas generally. Disturbed menstrual cycle and menstruation.

MIND - Apathy and weakness. Making decisions was a great effort. Spaced out all day and very giddy. Lack of concentration, very forgetful. Deep feeling of sadness and worthlessness. Weepy. Self-pity. Vulnerable feeling. Self-doubt, poor self-confidence.

Restlessness. Easily startled by sudden noises. Great fear for no apparent reason. Fear or panic attacks. Claustrophobia. Feeling of anticipation. Uneasy feelings as if something were about to happen or as if she had something to do and couldn't remember what.

Extremely introverted, detached and indifferent. Lonely. ***Introversion with arrogance.*** Believes that others are trivial or petty. ***Aversion to company***, to socializing. Contempt for others. Insolent and rude. Suspicious of motives of others. Outbursts of anger. Irritability or anger at being invaded or disturbed by others.

Abdomen - Dull, heavy, dragging pain in lower abdomen, has to bend double. Pain radiates down thighs. Tension in the solar plexus. Spluttery and full of gas with cramps in abdomen.

Back - Neck felt tense and painful. Aching, dull, heavy pain in the lower back. Pain in kidney region.

Breasts - Breasts sore and swollen.

Ears - Ear infections. Ears itchy inside and a thick discharge following. Eruption like a cold sore appeared on the left ear lobe, scabby, pus, itching. Ears felt like they were stuffed with cotton wool. Pressure and popping in ears, affecting hearing. Difficult hearing, voices and sounds seemed distant.

Eyes - Eyes were stinging, burning and watering. Burning sensation and pressure behind eyes. Eyelids felt heavy all day. Short-sighted.

Face - Pale. Face looks strained, frowns a lot.

Female - Disturbed menstrual cycle and menstruation, with pain and discomfort. Menses with severe pain in lower abdomen and lower back. Sharp pain in right ovary. Sexual urge diminished or lost.

Food - Appetite lost, with nausea. Hungry but couldn't find any food that interested her. Nibbling at food all the time out of boredom. Craving for sweets. Thirsty most of the time.

Head - Frontal pressure. Temples felt bruised and sore. Headache as if a tight band. Frontal headache, in morning. Head hot, scalp and forehead very itchy. Dandruff. Scalp scaly, itching with hair falling out.

Kidneys - Sharp, stabbing pains over kidneys. Aching pain in back over kidneys. Pressure on bladder. Frequent urination.

Limbs - Limbs sore and achy. Rheumatic pains, in right arm and left thigh at night. Sore, bruised type in left shoulder, over left kidney and in left hip. Arms were very heavy, had no power in them, lifting things was very difficult.

Lungs - Cough, like she was clearing her throat all the time. Short, phlegmy cough.

Male - Sexual energy lost or diminished.

Modalities - Better lying down, from alcohol. Worse from cold, even when hot. Worse from tobacco, particularly the weakness and nausea.

Nose - Acute sense of smell.

Rectum - Constipation and diarrhea. Chalky colored diarrhea, in the morning. Diarrhea with pains like premenstrual pains in her lower abdomen.

Skin - Very yellowish skin. Skin generally itchy, particularly the scalp. Pimples on neck and back. Eruptions, red patches of dry skin, intensely itching and burning. Must scratch, scratching brings up little lumps.

Sleep - Confused, exhausted on waking. Unrefreshing sleep. Dreams about the past, grandparents, mother, elderly relatives dying. Very aggressive dreams, attaching people, being in a war, being raped, dead babies.

Stomach - Nausea with lost of appetite.

Temperature - Fever with sweat. Hot and feverish, sweating on palms and back. Sweating in bed.

Throat - Throat sore and raw. Tickling in throat causing a cough.

Vertigo - Feels giddy and exhausted.

COMMENTS - Occasional desire for the company of one close friend, where no social effort was necessary, marked during anxiety. Assertive. Fear or panic attacks. Anxiety rising suddenly without apparent cause. Restlessness, have to keep moving. Trembling all over, particularly hands. Easily startled by sudden noises or while driving.

Eruptions. Red patches on skin, dry itching with aggravations from dairy products. Skin and scalp symptoms. Inner ear infections, with pressure and popping. Weakness and nausea aggravated by smoking.

One case concerned a man who had moved to Galway two years earlier and was having recurring panic attacks since then. He was very introverted, with profound feelings of loneliness and isolation. He was prone to outbursts of anger. Granite 200c cured.

A second case concerned a woman who suffered from severe headaches, pain from her eyes. She had been diagnosed as near-sighted and needed glasses. She was tired all the time and had difficulty getting out of bed in the morning.

Introverted, strong feelings of hatred and jealousy. Enjoyed trying to provoke her passive husband into fighting. Granite 200c cured. She has had her eyes tested again since the remedy and her sight became perfect.

RELATIONS - Sulph. antidoted one proving and Zinc. the other. ***Compare:*** (1) Sil., Sep., Staph., Plat., Nat-m.

REFERENCES - Eising. Watson.

LAPIS LAZULI

(Gemstone)

PHARMACY - lap-laz. Lapis lazuli. Gemstone. ***Historical dose:*** All potencies.

CLINICAL - Acne. Boils. Anal, itching. Conjunctivitis. Coryza. Diarrhea. Flatulence. Glands, swelling. Hair, loss. Headaches. Heartburn. Hemorrhoids. Hoarseness. Itching. Lachrymation. Leucorrhea. Meniere's, disease. Nausea. Night-sweats. Nosebleeds. Palpitations. Thyroid swollen. Tinnitus. Trembling. Vesicles. Weakness.

HOMEOPATHIC - The name lapis lazuli originated from Arabic "lazaward," meaning blue, and developed into azul, meaning blue sky. It is a combination of natrium-alumina-silicea with the golden lines and spots of pyrite.

In folk medicine, lapis lazuli was used to treat cataract, headache, laryngitis, pharyngitis, and to regulate the thyroid gland. Neuritis, neuralgic pains, cramping pains, joint pains, dysmenorrhea. Melancholy, fever, apoplexy, epilepsy. Spleen diseases. Respiratory tract.

MIND - Absent-minded. Difficult concentration. Mistakes in speaking. Awkward, drops things. Weariness, worse in morning. Apathy, with sleepiness.

Mind active. Fretful. Vexation. Anger, bad temper. Irritable. Offended easily, takes everything in a bad light. Conscientious about trifles. Haughty. Indifferent. Averse to company, presence of other people aggravate symptoms.

Tranquility, serenity, yielding disposition. Forsaken feeling. Sense of isolation. Despondent, depressed, gloomy, melancholy. Causeless sadness. Taciturn, desire to be silent. Cannot cry, though sad. Weeping suddenly.

Full of indefinite desires. Desire for retirement. Fear of rain, water. Fear of being hurt, of impending disease. Anxiety from the pains in the heart. Presentiment of death. Delusions eyes are falling out, that she is pregnant. Dreams of water, churches, witches. Prophetic dreams. Clairvoyance.

Abdomen - Distended. Flatulence, rumbling. Cutting, drawing and sharp pains.

Back - Backache in lumbar region. Lancinating, sharp, and pressing pains. Eruptions like flea bites. Itching.

Bladder - Urging to urinate. Burning pains.

Chest - Constriction, tension, tightness, on waking. Oppression of chest. Axillary glands swelling. Stitching pain in axilla.

Ears - Heat sensation. Ear pain on blowing nose. Tinnitus. Noises in ears, rushing, whistling.

Eyes - Conjunctivitis. Itching. Lachrymation from eye pain. Dim vision. Tired expression and sensation.

Face - Acne rosacea. Pale or red color. Boils. Crusty, scabby eruptions.

Female - Brown leucorrhea.

Food - Thirstless. Desires chocolate, alcohol.

Head - Hair, loss. Headaches. Itching of scalp.

Heart - As if heart would cease to beat. Pressing, stitching pain. Sore, bruised pain. Pain in heart, better walking. Palpitations with vertigo.

Kidneys - Drawing pains in kidneys.

Limbs - Numbness, upper limbs. Tottering gait. Cracking joints. Joint pains, burning, stitching. Trembling, worse after anger. Weak knees. Felon, onychia, paronychia, panaritium.

Male - Increased sexual desire.

Mouth - Dryness. Cracked, dry lips.

Neck - Swelling glands.

Nose - Nasal obstruction. Coryza. Fluent discharges. Nosebleeds, during headache or vertigo, on blowing the nose.

Rectum - Flatus, offensive like rotten eggs. Diarrhea. Stools, bloody, thin, liquid. Putrid odor of stool. Stools like balls. Anal itching. Rectal bleeding. Hemorrhoids.

Skin - Acne rosacea. Dry and itching. Night-sweats. Boils. Eruptions, crusty, scabby. Vesicles.

Sleep - Disturbed, during the full moon. Wakes after midnight. Wakes from vertigo.

Stomach - Nausea. Heartburn.

Throat - Cold sensation. Sore throat. Burning in throat. Sharp pains, on empty swallowing. Hoarseness. Nasal voice. Thyroid swollen.

Tongue - Burning sensation. Vesicles on tip. Metallic taste.

Vertigo - Vertigo in morning, on waking, with nosebleed, during headache. Vertigo and tinnitus like Meniere's disease.

RELATIONS - ***Compare:*** (1) Chin-s., Thios.

REFERENCES - Schadde.

LAPPA ARCTIUM

(Burdock)

PHARMACY - lappa. Lappa arctium. Burdock. Arctium lappa. Lappa major. Lappa officinalis. Arcion. Gobo. Great clote burre. N. O. Composite. Tincture of fresh root. ***Historical dose:*** Tincture and all potencies.

CLINICAL - Acne. Backache. Belching. Boils. Bunions. Diarrhea. Dupuytren's contraction. Dyspepsia. Eczema. Eruptions. Flatus. Glands, disorders. Gonorrhea. Gout. Impotency. Infertility. Leucorrhea. Phosphaturia. Prolapsed, uterus. Rheumatism. Ringworm. Scrofula. ***Sour, stomach.*** Styes. Ulcers. Uterus, prolapsed. Vaginitis. Vertigo.

HERBAL - A writer in the Amer. Homeopath recommended the local use of the seedling roots in acne. The roots are softened by soaking in water for two hours, then the blunt end is rubbed on each individual pimple. It is not to be repeated more often than once a week.

HOMEOPATHIC - Lappa arctium has been extensively proved, notably by Dr. Jeanes and Dr. S. A. Jones. The provings generally confirm older teachings.

Lappa chiefly affects the skin, liver, joints and uterus. Historically, it was given for prolapsed uterus, infertility, milky urine and sores about the joints. It was one of Culpepper's remedies for fetid sweat of axilla. Useful in skin therapeutics.

A large number of symptoms were observed upon the skin and mucus membranes. Acne, eczema, especially of the scalp, with discharge. Eruptions on the head, face and neck. In skin disorders, it has been used externally as a glycerol, as well as internally.

Styes and ulcerations on the edge of the eyelids. Crops of boils and styes (Anthr.). Profuse and frequent urination. Heavy, sore aching, as if lying uncomfortably. Numbness, lumbar region of aching calves. Constriction.

Abdomen - Flatulent dyspepsia, belching inodorous gas.

Back - Pains in back about eighth dorsal vertebra.

Chest - Trembling in chest. Acute tingling, cutting pain under middle of sternum, extending across breast.

Eyes - Redness about eyes. Crops of styes. Feeling as if the eye was small and constricted.

Face - Inveterate acne, worse touch. Spreading vesicular eruption, great tearing and itching. Herpetic eruption on right ala nasi.

Female - Uterine displacement, worse standing, walking, sudden jar. Bruised, sore, heavy feeling in uterus with great relaxation of vaginal tissue. Prolapsed uterus with much bearing down pain. Leucorrhea.

Head - Weight on vertex. Pain in head. Eczema of scalp.

Heart - Pain in heart with indescribable movement under sternum. Exceedingly rapid pulse with frequent intermissions.

Kidneys - Profuse and frequent urination. Milky phosphatic urine.

Limbs - Eruption on limbs. Soreness of muscles. Pain in all joints. Old sores about joints. Rheumatic and gouty pains. Rheumatic pains entirely relieved by onset of diarrhea. Sharp, darting, fugitive pains in tendons. Dupuytren's contraction. Front of thigh weak. Pain in hands, knees and ankles extending downward to fingers and toes. Bunion.

Lungs - Tickling in glottidis, loose-sounding cough, no expectoration. Short breath on exertion.

Male - Cutting, squeezed pain in whole length of urethra, scalding on urination. Ringworm-like patch of eruption on thigh beside testicles, groins raw. Loss of sexual desire.

Modalities - Better from cloudy weather. Worse cold, wet, shaking, violent exertion, lying on right side.

Nose - Red discoloration across the nose.

Rectum - Frequent yellow stools in forenoon, with some nausea. Diarrhea alternating with rheumatic symptoms.

Skin - Eruptions, sticky on head, face. Many small painful boils. Moist, offensive eruptions, grayish white crusts, especially when glands are swollen. Moist, foul eczema of infants. Old sores, about joints. ***Axillary sweat cold***, runs down chest, foul.

Stomach - ***Sour stomach,*** sour taste, all food turns sour, vomits it. Diarrhea alternating with rheumatic symptoms.

Vertigo - Vertigo with nausea and vomiting.

RELATIONS - ***Compare:*** (1) The composites, Arn., Calen., Cina. (2) Bry. - rheumatism. (3) Frax., Lil-t. and Sep. - in uterine prolapse. (4) Calc-p. - phosphaturia. (5) Vinc., Viol-t. - skin.

REFERENCES - Boericke. Clarke. Phatak.

LAPSANA COMMUNIS

(Nipple-wort)

PHARMACY - laps. Lapsana communis. Nipple-wort. N. O. Composite. Genus Cicoracee. Tincture of infusion of whole fresh plant. ***Historical dose:*** Tincture and all potencies.

CLINICAL - ***Hemorrhoids.*** Nipples, sore.

HERBAL - As the common name of Lapsana would imply, it is a popular remedy for sore nipples, a decoction of it being used as a lotion for that purpose. Cooper published documents in proof of its efficiency in hemorrhoids.

Three ounces of the green plant (or four of the dry) are boiled in three pints of thin water gruel until it is reduced to a pint and a half. The decoction is then strained. Half a pint is to be drunk on three mornings following, fasting immediately on getting out of bed.

One patient who was cured in this way said he had no swallowed the draft more than a few minutes before he felt his stomach as warm as if he had drunk hot brandy and water.

Only three doses were ordered and the patient was told, if not cured, to wait a fortnight before repeating the treatment.

HOMEOPATHIC - Laps. is a remedy for sore nipples and hemorrhoids. Cooper confirmed the power of Laps. over hemorrhoids, using single doses of the tincture.

RELATIONS - ***Compare:*** Calen.

REFERENCES - Clarke.

LARCH

(Bach Flower Remedy)

PHARMACY - lar-b. Larch. Larix decidua. Twigs with young leaves and flowers are picked and boiled for half an hour. The water is drained and used as medicine. ***Historical dose:*** Take two drops from the stock bottle into a one ounce dropper bottle (add brandy or alcohol, if this bottle will be used for days or weeks). This is the dosage bottle, take a few drops straight into the mouth or as needed in a little water or juice.

HOMEOPATHIC - Bach grouped Lar-b. under ***Despondency and Despair,*** with Crb-a-b., Oak-b., Will-b., Star-b-b., Sw-ch-b., Elm-b. and Pine-b.. States of low self-confidence. Lack of energy, drooping sensation, weary limbs and reluctant posture. Withdrawn.

MIND - Anticipates failure, feels that one cannot quite measure up to the challenges of life. Avoids new opportunities for growth and advancement. Sense of suppression, limitations. Feelings of inferiority, compares oneself with others. Fear of failure.

Bad self image. Focused within oneself (Cer-b., Mimul-b.). Worries about oneself. Sadness, regret, despondency, despair. Shy, lack of personal strength. Lonely, alienation from others. Lax and dampened, without energy or incentive.

REFERENCES - Bach.

LATHYRUS SATIVUS
(Wild Vetch)

PHARMACY - lath. Lathyrus sativus. Wild vetch. Lathyrus cicera. Lesser chick-pea. "Jesse," "Jarosse." N. O. Leguminose. Papilionoideae. Trituration of seeds. Tincture of the flower. Tincture of the green pods. Trituration of the dried pea. ***Historical dose:*** Tincture and all potencies.

CLINICAL - Amyotrophic lateral sclerosis. Athetosis. Beriberi. Constipation. Cramps. Depression. Diarrhea. Dysentery. ***Emaciated, limbs.*** Emaciation. Heartburn. Impotence. ***Infantile, paralysis.*** Locomotor ataxia. Lumbago. Multiple sclerosis. Nausea. ***Paralysis.*** Paralysis, spinal. Paraplegia. Parkinson's disease. ***Poliomyelitis.*** Rheumatic, paralysis. ***Rheumatism.*** Roaring (in horses). Spinal, sclerosis. Urine, incontinence. Vertigo. Vomiting.

HOMEOPATHIC - Lathyrus is a vetch, a member of the Leguminosae family that grows in India. Lathyrus contains variable amounts of a toxin that, when ingested, may cause lathyrism, a paralytic affection. Produces a perfect picture of certain spinal affections.

In Christison's Toxicology, it is stated that Lath. causes paraplegia, dragging gait, turning-in of the toes, stiffness and semi-flexion of the knee joints.

The clinical record of Lath. indicates that it may prove useful in numerous cases of bedridden paraplegias and infantile spinal paralysis, as well as in certain forms of myelitis. In 1877, Clarke published cases relieved by Lath., two of paralysis, one of multiple sclerosis, one of rheumatic paralysis with stiff knees.

Affects the anterior and lateral columns of the cord, causing paralytic disorders of lower limbs, spastic paralysis, lateral sclerosis, beriberi. ***Infantile paralysis***. Athetosis. Trembling of arms, worse on attempting to do anything. ***Increased reflexes***. Lack of pain. Wasting, exhaustive diseases with weakness and heaviness, slow recovery of nerve power. Sleepy, constant yawning.

MIND - Depressed, hypochondriacal. Lack of inner strength. Sense of being trapped by circumstances. Suppressed emotions.

Abdomen - Colic. Sensation as if a damp cloth around waist.

Back - Lumbago. Pain in back so severe as to prevent movement, worse or excited by touch.

Bladder - Increased bladder reflexes. Frequent urge to urinate, must hurry, or else voided involuntarily.

Ears - Singing in ears.

Kidneys - Pressure on bladder, if not immediately satisfied, urine, rushes out with great force. Incontinence of urine. Increased bladder reflex.

Limbs - Polio myelitis with marked spastic symptoms. Rheumatic paralysis. ***Excessive rigidity of legs, spastic gait.*** Tremulous, tottering gait. Knees knock together when walking. ***Knee jerks exaggerated.*** Cannot extend or cross legs when sitting. Sits bent forward, straightens up with difficulty. Stiffness and lameness of the ankles and knees. Heels do not touch the ground when walking. Feet are dragged or put down suddenly and forcibly while walking. While lying down legs can be moved from side to side but cannot be lifted. Legs blue, swollen, if hanging down. Cramps in legs, worse cold and cold feet. Legs are cold during day, become hot and burn at night better uncovering. Gluteal muscles and muscles of ***lower limbs are emaciated.***

Male - Impotence. Occasional erections and pollutions.

Modalities - Better uncovering, lying down (lower limbs move freely). Worse from cold, damp weather, touch, movement.

Mouth - ***Burning pain, tip of tongue.*** Tingling and numbness of tongue and lips, as if scalded.

Rectum - Diarrhea, with urgent pressure on intestines. Dysentery. Constipation.

Sensations - Sensation as of a damp cloth around the waist.

Sleep - Continuous yawning and sleepiness.

Stomach - Weight in stomach and indigestion. Heartburn. Nausea and vomiting. Vomiting of blood.

Vertigo - Vertigo when standing with eyes closed.

COMMENTS - The two varieties of Lathyrus that have occasioned poisonings are Lath. sativus and Lath. cicera. The peas are very alike in appearance. Those of Lath. cicera are rather smaller than Lath. sativus, more square, and are a lighter brown. Except for this brownish color they could easily be mistaken for ordinary peas. Lath. cicera has red flowers, Lath. sativus, bluish. Both are cultivated for food and are sometimes cut green for fodder.

In the British Journal of Homeopathy there is an account of a wheat famine in India, where the peas of the plant were substituted for wheat and used as a food. Those who subsisted on it were taken, even during sleep, with sudden paralysis of the lower limbs. This occurred without warning in young men more than in young women, and was never recovered from.

Another observer recorded fifty cases of people who had eaten the lathyrus bread and all stated that they became paralytic during the wet season of the country. They went to bed quite well and woke with stiff legs, unsteady gait and aching, but no severe pain. The upper limbs were free.

Another saw the disease in Algeria and described the symptoms in ten cases. Symptoms came on suddenly in damp weather with some pains in the loins, trembling, motor paralysis and exaggerated reflexes. He attributed these phenomena to an acute transverse myelitis with degenerative changes in the cord.

Polio (Gels.). Post-polio neuralgia syndrome (Rhus-t, Gels.). Guillain-Barre syndrome, ascending paralysis. Multiple sclerosis. Amyotrophic lateral sclerosis. Characteristic increased reflexes. Weak and lame joints. Severe muscle cramps in the calves. Pain induced by touch. Emaciation of the paralyzed muscles (Plb., Caust.).

Burning pain on the tip of the tongue. Weak bladder with sudden urgencies to urinate.

Never well since an influenza or a virus. Symptoms may be brought on or be made worse by cold or damp wind. Burning heat, better uncovering.

O'Connor found that marked benefit followed its use in old cases of myelitis with marked spastic symptoms. Bartlett recommended Lath. for excessive knee jerk and rigidity.

Hart spoke of it as a remedy for locomotor ataxia, but the absence of sensory symptoms and the presence of exaggerated reflexes would seem to contraindicate it in this disease. He also spoke of Lath. in spinal anemia, giving as symptoms "numbness, followed by pain in the lower limbs, sensation of a band around the body, unable to step or distinguish one limb from another."

In a case related by Bojanus, the general symptoms were the same. Lath. was the cause of the trouble, arising during the great Russian famine. Horses fed with Lath. along with oats manifested symptoms of paralysis of the limbs and also of the throat and wind-pipe, setting up the condition called "roaring." Some died of suffocation.

Clarke relieved several cases of spastic paralysis, including Miss R., 25, who had been ill four years with the usual symptoms of spastic paralysis. Excessive constipation and violent urging to pass water, if she attempted to retain it, it passed of itself. The muscles were hard and unyielding.

She was heavily drugged under allopathic treatment before coming under his care. Hyper. was first given with considerable benefit. As the improvement went no further, Lath. 1c and 30c were given and then the improvement was much more marked.

W. A. Dewey recorded a cure with Lath. 3x in a case of spastic paralysis in a man of twenty-eight. The attack had been coming on six months. The patient was a hunchback, having been deformed since the age of five, but this had given no more than the usual inconvenience.

On admission to the hospital (December 1, 1898), he was unable to make the slightest movement of the lower limbs, even of the toes.

The adductors were in a constant state of irritable contraction, so that the thighs were constantly crossed. Reflexes greatly exaggerated. No pain. Spine not tender. General health was normal. The only other symptom was a girdle sensation, as if he had a cold, damp cloth around his waist.

Three weeks after commencing Lath., there was slight lessening of rigidity. On April 5, 1899, he could raise his limbs and move his toes. On July 2nd he walked out of the hospital without difficulty, the abnormal irritability of the muscles having disappeared.

RELATIONS - ***Compare:*** (1) Oxyt., Sec. (2) Peti., a South American plant. - paralysis, paraplegia with numbness. Sensation of internal coldness. (3) Agrostema githago - burning sensation in stomach, through esophagus into throat in lower abdomen and anus, nausea, bitter vomiting, impaired locomotion, difficulty in remaining erect, vertigo and headache, burning from lower jaw to vertex.

REFERENCES - Anshutz. Boericke. Clarke. Murphy. Phatak.

LATRODECTUS HASELLTI

(Black Spider)

PHARMACY - lat-h. Latrodectus hasellti. Black spider. N. O. Arachnida. New South Wales. ***Historical dose:*** All potencies.

CLINICAL - ***Blood poisoning. Delusion***s. Edema. Emaciation. Memory, loss. Paralysis. Septicemia. Tinnitus. Vertigo.

HOMEOPATHIC - Long lasting effects seem to indicate Lat-h. for ***chronic blood poisoning***. Arrests intense pain in pyemia. Great edema near wound. Paralysis of limbs with great wasting of muscles. Violent, darting, burning pains preceding paralysis.

Septicemia conditions, blood poisoning. Tinnitus. Roaring noises. Loss of memory. Vertigo, tendency to fall forward. ***Delusion of flying***.

REFERENCES - Clarke.

LATRODECTUS KATIPO

(Red-back Spider.)

PHARMACY - lat-k. Latrodectus katipo. Red-back spider. N. O. Arachnida. New Zealand spider. Tincture of living spider. ***Historical dose:*** All potencies.

CLINICAL - Chorea. Delirium. Depression. Edema. Faintness. Heart, slow. Lymphangitis. Nettle-rash. Twitchings.

HOMEOPATHIC - Lat-k. is a venomous spider found in New Zealand and some parts of California. The symptoms recorded are the effects of bites. The seat of a bite becomes immediately painful and swelling occurs. In some cases, the swelling does not come on until some days after the bite.

In one case, five days after the bite, a scarlet papulous rash appeared on both limbs, burning like fire. The symptoms were somewhat slow in evolution. In a fatal case, that of a girl bitten on the abdomen, death did not occur until six weeks after the bite.

Lassitude, faintness, twitchings and trismus. Scarlet and burning eruptions. Lymphangitis with nervous twitchings. Long suffering, wasting. Loss of energy. Faint and pale.

MIND - Delirium, half smothered by imperfect intoxication. Semi-intoxicated state. Nervous depression.

Abdomen - Very severe drawing or cramping sensation in abdomen.

Face - Anxious expression. Extreme pallor changing to blue tint of face and body. Jaws stiff, could not open mouth to eat and could scarcely articulate.

Food - Loss of desire for food.

Heart - Almost pulseless. Pulse slow, scarcely more than twelve or fourteen beats to the minute.

Limbs - Severe shaking, burning pains ran from the bite on the foot up the limbs to back, with nervous twitching all over body. Pain felt almost equally in both limbs and seemed to center about heel. Feet felt as if rudely lacerated by dull instrument, walking him from sleep.

Lungs - Breathing almost ceased.

Skin - Small, red spot like flea-bite. Bitten surface raised, the raised part white with red halo with swelling and pain. Swelling size and shape of hen's egg. The bite remained a small purple point for nine days, on the tenth began to swell and turn white like a bee sting, pain and swelling rapidly increased, dorsum of foot and ankle like a puff-ball, red streak running up leg. A bright scarlet, papular eruption on both lower limbs, which stung and burned like fire.

Temperature - Limbs cold and flaccid. Cold, clammy sweat covered left lower extremity in morning.

RELATIONS - ***Compare:*** (1) Lat-m., Tarent., Mygal., Aran. (2) Apis, Vesp. and serpent poisons.

REFERENCES - Clarke.

LATRODECTUS MACTANS

(Black Widow Spider)

PHARMACY - lat-m. Latrodectus mactans. Black widow spider. N. O. Arachnida. Southern North America, South America. Tincture of living spider. ***Historical dose:*** All potencies.

CLINICAL - ***Angina pectoris.*** Chest, pains. Colic. Cramping, pain. ***Heart, attacks. Heart, disorders.*** Hematuria. Hemorrhages. Idiopathic thrombocytopenia. Infectious, purpura. Proteinuria.

HOMEOPATHIC - S. A. Jones and A. J. Tafel introduced Lat-m. into the Materia Medica. The bite produces tetanic effects that last several days. From the time a man was bitten he took 3 1/2 quart bottles of the best rectified whisky without any sign of intoxication.

Affects the heart, producing ***angina pectoris. Heart attacks.*** The precordial region seems to be the center of attack. ***Restless with heart pains*** and prostration. Constriction of chest muscles with radiation to shoulders and back. Fear of suffocating or dying.

Blood becomes thin, watery. Lowered coagulability. Inflammation of the coronary arteries. Pain in the solar plexus. Infectious purpura. Chronic hemorrhaging endothelial plasmatic condition. Chronic idiopathic thrombocytopenia.

Itching and redness of the part bitten, at first without pain, but violent pain soon commenced there (back of left hand), and extended in a short time up forearm and arm to shoulder and then to precordial region. Painful sensations extended up arm to shoulder, along neck to back of head, later, pain in precordia and apnea, screaming fearfully. Nervous tremors.

MIND - Speech hesitant with tears. Apparently moribund. Depression. Mental fatigue. Amnesia. Memory gives no answer to logical deduction. Reading impossible. Staring up at ceiling, vague, in a stupor. Emotional disturbances. Very nervous.

Acute and enormous anxiety, with sensation of imminent death. ***Anxiety about the heart.*** Intense anguish with the sensation of severe thoracic constriction. Screams fearfully with pain, exclaiming that she would lose her breath and die. ***Thinks he will suffocate.*** Fear of dying. Lamenting helplessly. Wailing.

Agitation. Mental irritability and restlessness. Sensitive to noise. Writhing and rolling in pain. Extreme state of nervous irritation with fear of going mad. Psychosis, becomes mad and psychotic, with hallucinations.

Abdomen - Severe abdominal pain with nausea and a sinking sensation at epigastrium. Colic and hardness of the abdominal wall. Chronic cramp of the abdominal muscles without painful tenderness on palpation.

Back - Dorsal and lumbar cramps, going from the nape to the loins.

Chest - ***Angina pectoris.*** Violent, precordial pain extending to the axilla and down the arm and forearm to fingers, with numbness of the extremity. Sinking sensation. Cramping pain from chest to abdomen.

Ears - Pain in the right middle ear.

Eyes - Constant pulsating pain in the eyes.

Face - Expression of deep anxiety.

Food - Extreme thirst, vomits what he drinks.

Head - Pain in neck to back of head. Occipital pain. Headache, aggravated between 2 p.m. and 3 p.m.

Heart - Precordial anxiety. ***Angina pectoris.*** Pain in precordia with a loss of breath. screaming fearfully, exclaiming that she would lose her breath and die. ***Violent heart pains, sharp, extending to shoulders or both arms to fingers with numbness. Restless with cardiac pain*** and prostration. Pulse feeble and rapid.

Limbs - Left arm partially paralyzed, or feels paralyzed, with pain. Hard, aching pain in axilla. Stinging in right wrist with itching and redness of bitten spot. Paresthesia of lower limbs. Weakness of legs followed by cramps in the abdominal muscles.

Kidneys - Burning pains on urinating in the urethra. Urine red, albuminous with casts. Proteinuria, hematuria, glycosuria, diminution in the level of nitrogen eliminated through the urine.

Lungs - Bronchial rales. Cough with hawking, yellow, thick, acrid sputum. Pulmonary edema. ***Gasping for breath***. Extreme apnea. Respiration only occasional, gasping. Respiration very slow, thinks he will suffocate. Fear of losing breath and dying.

Male - Frequent erections. Testicular pains, aggravated by movement. Very acute pains in the right testicle. Perspiration in the genital regions. Itching of prepuce with a little redness of the part.

Modalities - Better by sitting quietly. Worse from the slightest movement, even of the hands, exertion.

Mouth - Labial fissure. Copious salivation. Trembling of the tongue. White coloring of the tongue. Hypertrophy of the lingual papillae.

Nose - Nose blocked, thick, yellow discharge.

Pulse - Pulse, feeble and rapid. Pulse so frequent it could not be counted and so feeble it could scarcely be felt. Left pulse extinct, right pulse doubtful.

Rectum - Constriction of the anus with tarry stools. Copious evacuations similar to the black vomit.

Skin - Skin cold like ice, marble-white. Blue coloring. Heavy, cold perspiration. Skin very painful at the slightest touch. Burning of the soles of the feet. Eruption, which itches. Formication and extreme sensitivity. Loss of hair.

Sleep - Insomnia. Sleep disturbed, anxious. Dreams of flying.

Stomach - Eructation and loss of appetite. Nausea, then abdominal pains. Vomiting of black blood, which soothes the condition. Transfixation of pain or sinking at epigastrium. Feeling of weakness in epigastric region.

Throat - Throat red, dry. Tonsillitis with glairy deposit on tonsils. Pain on swallowing.

Vertigo - Vertigo and constrictive headache.

COMMENTS - Heart attack (Cact.), with sharp, shooting pains. Chest pain. Gasping for breath, difficulty breathing with a fear of dying.

Semple recorded a case of a man bitten on the prepuce. At first there was itching, in less than half an hour nausea, followed by severe abdominal pains. Soon after, violent precordial pains, extending to axilla and down left arm and forearm to fingers with numbness of the limbs and apnea. Dry cupping was resorted to and the blood that flowed was thin, florid and un-coagulable.

When Semple arrived, he found violent precordial pains, the left arm almost paralyzed, pulse 130, very feeble, Skin cold as marble, countenance expressive of deep anxiety. At eight the next morning, in spite of stimulants, the symptoms were worse and continued to increase until 2:30 p.m.

The pulse was uncountable and scarcely felt. Vomited black vomit, a quart or more. Soon after, reaction set in and the man gradually recovered. He had two copious stools like the black matter vomited earlier, and after that felt quite well.

Jones noted that the precordial region is the chief locus of attack. He considered the order of the occurrence of these symptoms of great importance.

Linnell recorded a case of angina pectoris, pain in precordial region and left arm, brought on by the slightest exertion, that was cured with Lat-m. 3c.

RELATIONS - ***Compare:*** (1) Lat-k. and other Arachnida. (2) Helo. - coldness. (3) Lach., Spig., Cimic., Cact., Kalm., Lycps. in angina pectoris. (4) Hir. - non-coagulating hemorrhages. (5) the Aran., Mygal., Ther., Lat-h., Lat-k. spider venoms. (6) Triat., Kissing bug - swelling with violent itching of fingers and toes. A smothering sensation and difficult breathing succeeded by fainting and rapid pulse. (7) Helo. - Intense chill, going from the inside to the outside. Vertigo with tendency to fall backwards. Numbness of the limbs. (8) Kalm. - Palpitations, aggravated when lying on the left side, pulse slow. Lightning pains, suddenly changing place. (9) Cact. - Feeling of constriction of the heart, as if a vice, spreading to the left arm, which feels numb. Hemorrhaging of black blood. (10) Spig. - Violent contractions of the heart with oppression, anxiety. Feels soothed when lying on the right side with head raised.

REFERENCES - Anshutz. Boericke. Clarke. Julian. Murphy.

LAUROCERASUS OFFICINALIS

(Cherry Laurel)

PHARMACY - laur. Laurocerasus officinalis. Cherry laurel. Common laurel. Aqua laurocerasi. Cerasus laurocerasus. Prunus laurocerasus. N. O. Rosacea. Tincture of young leaves. Dilutions of Aqua Laurocerasi. ***Historical dose:*** Tincture and all potencies.

CLINICAL - ***Asphyxia, neonatorum.*** Asthma. Breathing, difficult. Cholera. Cholera infantum. Chorea. Convulsions. Coughs. Cramps. ***Cyanosis. Debility.*** Diarrhea. Dysmenorrhea. Epilepsy. Heart, disorders. Hemorrhages. Liver disorders. Lock-jaw. Memory, lost. Menopause. Metrorrhagia. Palpitations. Pneumonia, typhoid. Strokes. Tetanus. Tumors. Twitchings. Whooping cough.

HOMEOPATHIC - Laurocerasus, the so-called "Laurel" of our gardens, is not a member of the Lauracae, though the Bay Laurel, Laurus nobilis, is. The Aqua Laurocerasi, prepared by distilling the fresh leaves, contains hydrocyanic acid and is supposed to owe all its medicinal virtue to this fact.

Symptoms accompanied by ***sudden debility*** and ***lack of reaction***, especially in chest and heart disorders. ***Asphyxia neonatorum. Cyanosis***, of heart disorders. Suffocating spells about heart compel him to lie down. General coldness not ameliorated by warmth. Coldness and blueness with epileptiform convulsions.

Hemorrhages of thin, bright blood mixed with gelatinous clots. Dry, tickling cough. Cough with jelly-like expectoration dotted with bloody points. Spasmodic tickling cough in cardiac patients.

Internal burning. Nervous collapse. Long lasting faints. Sensation of falling down in brain, in abdomen, in heart etc. Bluntness of special senses.

Strokes. Spasm of facial muscles and esophagus. Epilepsy, clonic spasms of all limbs with paralytic weakness. Chorea, emotional with constant jerks, cannot keep still. Twitchings. Gasping, before during and after spasms.

The speech indistinct after every excitement, gasping for breath. ***Drink rolls audibly through esophagus and intestines***. Weak sphincters. Violent pain in stomach with loss of speech.

MIND - Insensibility and complete loss of sensation. Loss of consciousness, with loss of speech and motion. ***Sudden loss of memory*** from fright, pain etc. Forgetful on motion. Dullness of special senses.

Angry when not understood. Want of moral feeling. Feels unloved. Cries easily when criticized. Sadness with impeded respiration.

Fear and anxiety about imaginary evils. Fear of insanity. Delusions, sees old men with long beards and distorted faces. Thinks she is accused, that she is criticized. Sees distorted faces on lying down during day. Visions of fire.

Abdomen - Falling down sensation of a lump in abdomen from above the navel to small of back, worse talking or overexertion. Gurgling flatulence.

Back - Painful stiffness in left side of neck and nape. Compressed feeling in shoulders and nape.

Causations - Effects of fright.

Chest - Constriction of chest. Burning in chest on taking inspiration. Dyspnea with sensation that he is unable to raise the chest walls, better lying down.

Ears - Hardness of hearing. Tingling, itching in ears.

Eyes - Dry eyes. Eyes widely open or half-closed, convulsed, prominent and fixed. Burning pain in eyes. Pupils dilated and immovable. Eyes distorted. Objects look larger. Darkness before the eyes, with obscuration of sight.

Face - Blue with gasping. Lock-jaw. Twitching of the muscles of face. As if flies and spiders are crawling over the skin.

Female - Pain in uterus with cancer, with oozing of bright blood with gelatinous clots, better sleep. Faints with coldness during menses. Burning and stinking in and below breasts.

Head - Head pain worse 11 a.m. to 1 p.m. Nightly tearing in vertex. As if a cold wind were blowing on head. As if brain were falling. Brain feels contracted and painful.

Heart - Clutching at heart, folds hands over the heart, as if there were some trouble there worse by any exercise. Pains in the region of heart. Pulse, weak, variable, slow or irregular. Mitral regurgitation. Palpitations.

Kidneys - Urine, retained, suppressed, involuntary, with palpitations, suffocation and fainting.

Limbs - Skin blue. Veins of hands distended. Clubbing of fingers. Toes and fingernails become knotty. Cold clammy feet up to the knees in chorea, heart disease. Feet numb on crossing the legs. Sprained pains in hips, thighs and heels.

Liver - Pain in the liver as though abscess were forming. Liver indurated, atrophied.

Lungs - Shallow breathing. ***Gasping for breath***, clutches at heart. Suffocation, gasps for breath, on sitting up. Exercise causes pain around heart. Small and feeble pulse. Threatening paralysis of lungs. Asphyxia neonatorum. ***Cyanosis neonatorum***. Cough with valvular disease. Tickling, ***dry cough***, with a copious, jelly-like, bloody expectoration.

Modalities - Better sitting up. Better lying with head low. Better sleep. Better eating. Better open air. Worse sitting up. Worse stooping. Worse exertion. Worse cold. Worse fright. Worse in the evening and night.

Mouth - Tongue, stiff, cold, burnt or numb. Speechlessness from pain in stomach. Foam at the mouth, with convulsions.

Rectum - Paralysis of anal sphincter, involuntary stools. Rectal cancer, with bleeding of bright red blood.

Sensations - Coolness of forehead as from draft of air. Weight on top of head. As if brain loose and falling into forehead when stooping. As if a veil before eyes. As if lungs could not be sufficiently expanded. As if lungs pressed against spine. As if mucus membranes were dry. Stitches are very prominent, also stiffness and pressure, especially pressure outward.

Skin - Cool, livid.

Sleep - Frequent yawning. Coma vigil. Sleeplessness from over-excitement and sudden heat. Fearful anxiety and restless, cannot fall to sleep. Spells of deep sleep with snoring and stertorous breathing. Troublesome and agitated dreams.

Stomach - Disgust for food during pregnancy. ***Drinks roll audibly*** through esophagus and intestines. Violent pain in stomach with loss of speech. Stomach pains during urination. Persistent hiccough. Bitter belchings. Nausea near a hot stove. Vomiting of food during cough.

Temperature - Coldness, chills and heat alternate. Shuddering, followed by burning heat. Heat running down the back. Thirst with dry mouth in afternoon.

Throat - Spasmodic contraction of throat and esophagus. Larynx and trachea raw. Low voice.

Vertigo - Vertigo with sleepiness.

COMMENTS - Laur. has a peculiar "gasping," gasping without really breathing. Blueness and twitching of the muscles of the face. Cyanosis, particularly in newborns (Acon., Carb-v.). Valvular problems, regurgitation, weak hearts.

Suffocative spells about the heart, worse by sitting up, the patient is compelled to lie down (Psor.). Some heart symptoms compel the patient to sit up. Blue around fingertips. Clubbing of fingers, common in cyanosis and tuberculosis.

Guernsey gave these leading symptoms, "gasping for breath, the patient puts his hand to the heart as if there was some trouble there, this may result from running a short distance, which puts him completely out of breath, going upstairs, walking or any exercise may bring the gasping on."

Cough with valvular heart disease, incessant cough, especially on lying down, fluttering in heart and gasping with cough. Spasmodic cough of later stages of whooping cough, when patient is much prostrated and has nervous spasmodic symptoms. Dry, harassing cough of tuberculosis. Alternation of chill, fever and sweat in tuberculosis.

Long-lasting faints (Camph. has sudden fainting), seems to have no reactive power, face pale, blue, cold surface. Prostrate before getting up in the morning with difficulty opening the eyes. Nervous disorders with constant jerks, cannot keep still. Allen noted an extremely nervous, excitable condition accompanying ailments.

Attacks of indigestion and pains across lower abdomen that come suddenly in the morning and generally disappear on getting up. Gnawing pain in lower abdomen, with occasional looseness of stool, particularly in old men. Green mucus diarrhea, with suffocative spells about heart.

Fluids roll audibly into the stomach. Digestion is weak, bowels confined. Low-spirited with flatulence and burning in chest after food. Audible and gurgling flatus, rolls about the upper abdomen. Constricted sensations in gullet, in rectum. Symptoms worse before eating.

Inclined to lose flesh and hemorrhages that are small in quantity and bright in color. Menorrhagia and dysmenorrhea. Eruptions are livid after pressure with the finger, the skin is long in regaining its color.

Constant tired and sick feeling. Sleepless with a great desire for sleep.

Coldness, internal coldness and external heat. Cold tongue. Heat of single parts. Warmth on center of forehead, then a coldness as from a draft of air lasting a long time. The left chest is most affected.

Pains start from the lower part of the spine and extend either around the pelvis or up to the head. Pains are accompanied with a sense of suffocation, a sick feeling with drowsiness, and a great desire to sleep that generally brings relief.

Cooper, in his work in Cancer and Cancer Symptoms, offered cases emphasizing the uterine symptoms. The indications of Laur., according to Cooper, are a sense of fatigue that pervades the whole system with a very painful condition of the hard and indurated tissue of the parts affected. Pain is much better by sleep.

Tendency to ooze blood, which is generally bright and mixed with gelatinous clots. This applies to the chest as well as to uterine and rectal symptoms, only the blood comes painlessly into the mouth, but with great pain in the vagina.

E. Wigg related the case of May S., 7, who had been troubled for some time with an almost incessant cough, for which many remedies were given without benefit. At last Wigg came to the conclusion that Laur. was the remedy and put ten drops of Laur. 200c into five tablespoonfuls of water ordering a teaspoonful of this to be taken every two hours when the child was awake.

This was at 4 p.m. After the third dose she fell asleep. At 3 a.m. she awoke in a very excited condition. Her mother asked her if she had not been dreaming, but her tongue was so stiff she could not answer. Suddenly she began to tremble all over as if in a chill.

After ten minutes she began to twitch and jerk. Wigg was sent for and found her in this convulsed state. She could not articulate for the thickness and heaviness of the tongue. The mind was clear. Recognizing the action of Laur., Wigg antidoted it with camphor, and later a cup of coffee, and symptoms ceased in a few hours. She had no more of the cough.

RELATIONS - ***Antidotes:*** the effects of digitalis given in crude doses. ***Antidoted by:*** Camph., Coff., Ip., Op. ***Compare:*** (1) Hydr-ac., Camph., Sec., Am-c., Ambr. (2) Amyg., Prun., Prun-v., and other Rosacea. (3) In hunger after meals with feeling of emptiness, Calc., Chin., Cas-s., Chion., Grat. (4) after meals and after stool, Petr. (5) in semi-lateral swelling of tongue, Calc., Sil., Thuj. Laur. has loss of speech with it. ***Compatible:*** Bell. Phos., Puls., Verat.

REFERENCES - Boericke. Clarke. Murphy.

LAURUS NOBILIS

(Bay Leaf)

PHARMACY - laur-n. Laurus nobilis. Bay leaf. Bay laurel. Sweet bay. Grecian laurel. Laurel tree. Bay tree. N. O. Lauraceae. Tincture. ***Historical dose:*** Tincture and all potencies.

CLINICAL - Amenorrhea. Arthritis. Bacterial, infections. Blood, sugar. Bronchitis. Bruises. Cancer. Colic. Flatulence. Fungal, infections. Headaches. Indigestion. Influenza. Migraine. Rheumatism. Sprains. Stomach, ulcers.

HERBAL - The bay tree is indigenous to Asia Minor, from where it spread to the Mediterranean and then to other countries with similar climates. Bay leaves and berries have been used for their astringent, carminative, diaphoretic, digestive, diuretic, emetic and stomachic properties.

It has a long history of folk use in the treatment of many ailments, particularly as an aid to digestion and in the treatment of bronchitis and influenza. It has been used to treat various types of cancer.

Bay leaf has been used as an herbal remedy for headaches. It contains compounds called parthenolides, which have proven useful in the treatment of migraines. It has also been shown to help the body process insulin more efficiently, leading to lower blood sugar levels. Reduces the effects of stomach ulcers.

Bay leaves also contain eugenol, which has anti-inflammatory and anti-oxidant properties. They are also anti-fungal and anti-bacterial. The leaves have been used to treat rheumatism, arthritic aches and pains. Upper respiratory tract disorders. Hysteria. Amenorrhea. Flatulent colic.

Bay oil, Oleum Lauri, has been used in liniments for bruising and sprains. The essential oil has narcotic, antibacterial and fungicidal properties. An infusion has been used to improve the appetite and as an emmenagogue.

The fruit is antiseptic, aromatic, digestive, narcotic and a stimulant. It has been used in making carminative medicines and was used in the past to promote digestion. It has a tonic effect, stimulating the appetite and the secretion of digestive juices.

COMMENTS - Bay Laurel is the source of the bay leaves which are used for their flavor in cooking. It was also the source of the laurel victory wreath of ancient Greece, and therefore the origin of the expression of "resting on one's laurels."

According to legend, the Delphi oracle chewed bay leaves, or sniffed the smoke of burning leaves to promote visionary trances. In the Middle Ages it was believed to have many magical qualities.

It has also been used to keep moths away; the leaves' lauric acid content gives it insecticidal properties.

RELATIONS - ***Compare:*** Cham., Catar., Mag-p.

REFERENCES - Murphy.

LAVANDULA VERA

(Lavender)

PHARMACY - lav-v. Lavandula vera. Lavender. Lavandula angustifolia. N. O. Lamiaceae. Tincture of the flowers. ***Historical dose:*** Tincture and all potencies.

CLINICAL - Backache. Belching. Burns. Constipation. Flatulence. ***Headaches.*** Indigestion. ***Insomnia.*** Lice. ***Memory, weak.*** Nausea. Palpitations. Toothache. Wounds.

HERBAL - Although lavender is a native of southern European hillsides, where it thrives in the sparse soil and burning sunshine, it has been grown in Britain for decades. The Romans would certainly have introduced a herb they esteemed so highly, and possibly it had been introduced before their days.

Historically, lavender has been used not only for its fragrance but also as a disinfectant, vulnerance (useful for healing wounds), sedative, stimulant, tonic and caiminative (a medicine that expels flatulence). The herbal history of lavender can be traced back to ancient Greece.

Dioscorides (an army doctor) mentioned French lavender, which seems to have been used only medicinally by the Greeks. He attributed to it certain laxative and invigorating qualities and recommended its use in a tea-like infusion for chest complaints.

The Romans used lavender to perfume their public baths (its name derives from the Latin "lavare," meaning to wash). Roman soldiers carried their own first aid kits of herbs, and whenever the armies settled herbs would be grown, including lavender.

The Romans were aware of lavender's healing, soothing and insect repellent properties, and used its oil in massage. They also burnt lavender in honor of their gods. Galen (129-199 AD) added lavender to the time honored antidotes, theriac and mithridate, and Nero's physician used it for anti-poison pills and in uterine disorders.

Abbes Hildegarde (1098-1180) from a monastery in the diocese of Malinz in Saxony, made some of the earliest mediaeval references to lavender in her writings. She realized its practical effect in getting rid of lice and prescribed it for cleaning eyes. She also thought it could drive away evil spirits.

The first original work on gardening written in English, a treatise by Jon Gardener (1440), mentions "lavyndull" growing in English gardens. From this date on, lavender is mentioned often in manuscripts and books, and it is clear that it became a popular herb valued for its medicinal virtues and scent.

HOMEOPATHIC - ***Insomnia.*** Memory, weak.

MIND - ***Lack of focus.*** Disorientated. Distracted, restless. Overwhelmed by responsibilities. Anxious, better alone. Worried feeling during the day. Active thoughts, prevents sleep.

Poor short term memory. Forgetful. Difficulty recalling events and conversations that occurred only days or even hours before. Difficult concentrating. Particularly tired when trying to communicate. Muddled up words or even forgot them altogether. Could not string a sentence together.

Disinclined to talk. Crossness and irritability. Jumpy, nerves on edge. Intolerant of others. Short tempered. Irritated by noise. Woke up feeling slightly headache and cross without reason. Does not feel comfortable but cannot say why.

Miserable and depressed. Negative outlook, fatalistic. Weeping. Felt insignificant and unlovable. Sensation that every thing feels far away. Indifferent to loved ones. Bored with life.

Abdomen - Constant burning indigestion, mid-abdomen. Bloating in abdomen.

Arms - Right arm painful. Burning sensation under right arm. Left elbow, bone pain as if sitting in damp. Elbow to hand felt numb, slight pins and needles. Right wrist, weak, difficulty in writing. Left hand, itchy at base of fingers, especially center finger.

Back - Backache. Lower back pain, in lumbar region. Lower back pain almost unbearable, better stretching. Dull aching pain over left kidney, right side of lumbar region. Pain better lying, worse sitting, bending down drawing up the knees. Dull nagging lumbar pain, worse lying, better sitting. Sharp, pulling ache. Unbearable pressing pain in lumbar region, feels as if internal organs are squeezed by hands, better bending down, drawing knees up, rest, worse movement, moving causes clinching pain, tighter and tighter.

Bladder - Slow urination.

Breasts - Sensitive breasts. Sharp tingling pain in right breast. Severely painful breasts.

Heart - Palpitations on climbing stairs.

Chest - Burning sensation in chest. Constant stinging pain in right breast. Tightness in chest muscles.

Ears - Severe stabbing pain in left ear. Loud sound like musical instrument in left ear.

Eyes - Heavy eyes through exhaustion, difficulty keeping the eyes open, the eyelids very heavy. Tiredness between and behind eyes. Painful left eye, wakes at night.

Generals - Immune system feels weak.

Female - Feels physically lighter before period. Menstrual flow heavy, stops abruptly.

Food - Appetite and thirst diminished. Appetite increased, no desire to eat. Increased thirst, evening. Wakes up with thirst. Thirsty with dry mouth. Desires for tea, orange juice. Desires green salad, fruit. Desires savory food. Averse to bread.

Head - ***Headaches.*** Congested feeling. Head feels clogged up, thick. Brain feels loose, floating, soft, spongy. Sensation of blood pulsating around brain. Dull headache on right side with stiff neck. Slight headache in forehead, above eyes. Throbbing frontal headache with pressure above eyes, better drinking water. Throbbing temples. Itching on right temple, red with white flakes.

Limbs - Uncoordinated movement. Constant dragging, painful ache in joints. Severe nagging aching in legs, thighs. Tingling, cramping limp in left leg. Pulling pain in right thigh. Aching pain in left calf muscle. Feet cold. Pain along side of big toenail on left foot.

Lungs - Breathing labored, better drinking

Mouth - Dry mouth with a slightly sensitive tongue, thirsty. Less saliva than usual. Increased saliva. Sticky saliva not better by washing mouth, eating or drinking. Thick saliva, better drinking. Dull aching in bottom right side of jaw. Toothache in carious teeth. Sharp pain upper incisor, better hot soup, worse cold butter.

Neck - Aching, painful neck.

Nose - Sense of smell increased. Slight running nose.

Rectum - Painless, sudden diarrhea. Constipation. Offensive stools. Sore rectum. Flatulent at night.

Shoulders - Stiff, aching pain in left shoulder. Painful right shoulder.

Skin - ***Dry skin***, itching, worse scratching, after hot water, better in water, particularly on hands. ***Burns.***

Sleep - ***Insomnia.*** Could not get to sleep even though tired. Restless, tossed around all over the place, constantly changing position. Disturbed sleep. Once asleep awakes early and find it difficult to get back to sleep. Heavy and unrefreshing sleep. Moaning in sleep.

Stomach - Stomach pains with hunger, even after eating. Stomach upset, burning indigestion. Indigestion, better milk, small meals. Slight dull ache, covering size of frying pan. Cramping pains with bloating and belching, better sitting up, worse lying down. Nausea. Upset stomach followed by constipation.

Throat - Sore, dry throats that persist, better drinking water, hot drinks. Sore throat only at night. Spasms, better drinking.

Tongue - Taste diminished. Unpleasant taste in mouth. Burning sensation on the tongue, sensitive, sore. Tip of tongue feels burnt, sore. Yellow coating on tongue.

Vertigo - Dizzy with flushed feeling, felt heat on top of head. Dizzy when turning suddenly, on driving car.

Vision - Diminished vision. Double vision, as if looking through frosted glass.

RELATIONS - ***Compare:*** Kali-p., Gink-b.

REFERENCES - Murphy.

LECITHINUM
(Lecithin)

PHARMACY - lec. Lecithinum. Lecithin. Prepared from the egg yolk or soybeans. ***Historical dose:*** Tincture and all potencies.

CLINICAL - Anemia. Convalescence. ***Fatigue.*** Impotency. Insomnia. ***Malnutrition. Neurasthenia.*** Ovarian, insufficiency. Tuberculosis. ***Weakness.***

HOMEOPATHIC - Lecithin is important in the vital processes of plant and animal organisms. It is prepared from the yolk of egg, a phosphorus containing complex organic body. Causes an immediate decrease in the excretion of phosphates.

Favorable influence upon the nutritive conditions and especially upon the blood. Marked improvement in nutrition and general improvement in tuberculosis.

Galactagogue, it renders breast milk more nourishing.

General weakness. Anemia. ***Neurasthenia.*** Useful for convalescence. Tired, weak, short breath, loss of flesh. Insomnia. Ovarian insufficiency. Sexually weak. Impotency.

MIND - Mental exhaustion and impotency. ***Prostration of mind.*** Forgetful, dull, confused, worse mental exertion. Concentration difficult. ***Confusion of mind, as if in a dream.*** Insomnia. Excitement in company. Fear of impending disease.

Ears - Pulsating and ringing in ears.

Face - Pain in zygoma, face pale.

Head - Aching, especially in occiput-pulsating and ringing in ears. Pain in zygoma, face pale.

Kidneys - Scanty with phosphates, sugar or albumen.

Limbs - Soreness, aching, lack of energy. Tired and weak.

Sexual - Anaphrodisia and ovarian insufficiency. Male power lost or enfeebled. Impotency.

Stomach - Loss of appetite. Thirsty, craves wine and coffee. Bloated feeling. Sore pain in stomach rising toward throat.

RELATIONS - ***Compare:*** Agn., Phos.

REFERENCES - Boericke. Phatak.

LEDUM PALUSTRE

(Wild Rosemary)

PHARMACY - led. Ledum palustre. Wild rosemary. Marsh tea. Marsh cistus. Labrador tea. N. O. Ericaceae. Tincture of dried small twigs and leaves collected after flowering begins. Tincture of whole fresh plant. ***Historical dose:*** Tincture and all potencies.

CLINICAL - Alcoholism. ***Anal, fissure.*** Ascites. Asthma. Bedsores. ***Bites. Black-eye.*** Boils. ***Bruises. Carbuncles***. Colic. Deafness. Ear, inflammation. Eczema. Erythema nodosum. Face, pimples. Feet, pains. ***Gout.*** Hemoptysis. Hands, pains. Joint, disorders. Lice. Meniere's disease. Priapism. Prickly, heat. ***Punctured, wounds.*** Rheumatism. ***Rhus, poisoning***. Skin, eruptions. ***Stings. Tetanus.*** Tinnitus. Tuberculosis. ***Vaccinations.*** Varicella. Whitlow. ***Wounds.***

HERBAL - Teste, who was one of the chief clinical authorities on Ledum, mentioned that it is native to damp regions of the North of Europe, and that no animal except the goat eats it on account of the strong, resinous smell of its leaves, which "keeps off lice and prevents flour from getting moldy."

Merat said Ledum cures the itch and scald-head, which Teste explained by its parasiticide action. This anti-parasitic action led Teste to think of Led. as a remedy for bites and punctured wounds, especially as certain symptoms of the proving seemed to agree with it.

The success which has attended this use of Led. in mosquito bites, stings of bees and wasps, rat bites, and needle pricks resulting in whitlows, confirmed the observation. Wesselheft noted that Led. aborted a felon in a few days, "Redness, swelling and throbbing in point of index finger from prick of a needle."

HOMEOPATHIC - Led. affects the fibrous tissue of joints, especially ankles, tendons, heels and skin, hence it can be called a rheumatic remedy, where rheumatism begins in the feet and travels upwards. Affected parts become purple puffy and then emaciate.

Punctured wounds, produced by sharp-pointed instruments or bites, particularly if the ***wounded parts are cold***. Insect stings, animal bites. ***Helps prevent tetanus*** (Hyper. if tetanus develops). ***Tetanus with twitching*** of muscles near wound.

Rheumatic diathesis, functional pain, altered secretions, deposits of solid, earthy matter in the tissues. Rheumatism begins in feet and travels upward. Painful, cold, edematous joints. Shifting, tearing pains. Weakness and numbness of the affected parts. Dropsy.

Rushes of blood. Abscess and septic conditions, better by cold. Petechia. ***Cold all the time,*** in bed in the house. ***General lack of body heat,*** heat of bed is intolerable. Pale, delicate persons. Alcoholism. Eruption, like poison-oak and is antidotal to it.

MIND - Absent-minded. Mental dullness. Sluggishness. Difficult thinking and comprehending. ***Confusion of mind, as if intoxicated,*** after eating. Anxiety. Timidity. Ennui, boredom.

Discontented in daytime. Morose and peevish humor. Vehement angry mood. Tendency to anger and rage. Violent. Misanthropy. Dissatisfied, hates his fellow beings. ***Hatred of men. Aversion to friends,*** company. Avoids the sight of people. Desire for solitude.

Frightened easily. Fear in a crowd. Fear he will die if he goes to sleep after nightmare. Delirium on closing eyes. Ideas abundant on closing eyes. Dementia. Moaning, groaning. Suicidal disposition. Unconsciousness, coma.

Abdomen - Pain in abdomen as if intestines were bruised. Sensation of fullness in upper part of the abdomen. Ascites. Drawing pain. Colic as if diarrhea would set in from umbilicus to anus. Dysenteric bellyache. Frequent discharge of flatus.

Back - Lumbago. Stiffness, cramps in back, worse rising from sitting.

Causations - Ill effects of punctured wounds, recent or chronic injuries, animal and insect bites, stings, bruises. Ill effects of alcohol, hair cutting or suppressed discharges.

Chest - Oppressive constriction of chest. Chest hurts when touched. Pain along trachea.

Constitutions - Sanguine temperament. Adapted to full-blooded, plethoric, robust people. Suited to pale, delicate persons. Complaints of people who always feel cold and chilly. Rheumatic, gouty diathesis, constitutions abused by alcohol.

Ears - Hardness of hearing, as if the ears were stuffed up with cotton, worse cutting the hair, wetting the head.

Eyes - Bloodshot or bruised. ***Black eye from injury.*** Hemorrhage into the anterior chamber after an iridectomy. Ptosis of eye (right) from injury. ***Contused wounds.*** Aching in eyes. Cataract with gout. Tears acrid, make the lower lids and cheeks sore.

Face - Mottled. Facial eczema. ***Red pimples on forehead and cheeks***, stinging when touched. Crusty eruptions around the nose and mouth. Swollen submental glands.

Female - Bleeding fibroids. Great coldness during menses, yet desires cold air. Menses too early and too copious, the blood is bright red. Leucorrhea.

Food - Violent thirst for cold water. Want of appetite and speedy satiety.

Head - Raging, pulsating headache, worse least covers. Blood boils on forehead. Itching as of lice. Misstep causes concussion in the brain. Affected after getting wet.

Kidneys - Urine often stops during the flow. Copious, clear, colorless urine, deficient in salts. Much uric acid and sand in urine.

Limbs - ***Gouty pains*** shoot all through the foot and limb and in joints, but especially in small joints. Gouty nodosities. Cracking in joints, worse warmth of bed. Cramps over hip joint. ***Rheumatism begins in lower limbs and ascends*** (Kalm., opposite.). Swollen blotchy ecchymotic legs and feet. Easily sprained ankles. Ankles swollen. ***Soles painful, can hardly step on them.*** Heels sore. Feet itch by night and are stiff in morning. Ball of great toe swollen (Both-l.). Feet held to earth as by a magnet, when attempting to move. Trembling of hands when moving them or grasping anything. Throbbing in right shoulder, on raising arm.

Lungs - Dyspnea, chest feels constricted. Suffocative arrest of breathing. Bronchitis with emphysema of the elderly. Whooping cough, spasmodic ***double inspiration*** with sobbing. Yellow, purulent, sputum. Cough with bloody expectoration. Hemoptysis, alternating with rheumatism or coxalgia.

Male - Inflammatory swelling of penis, the urethra is almost closed. Increased sexual desire. Violent and prolonged erections. Pollutions of bloody or serous semen.

Modalities - Better by application of ice water, bathing, cold, air, reposing. Worse in evening, night, heat of bed, warmth of covers, stove, air. Worse injury, motion of joints, spitting, eggs, wine.

Mouth - Bitter taste in the mouth, moldy when coughing. Sudden flow of watery saliva during colic. Musty taste with catarrhal affection.

Nose - Persistent nosebleed (Meli., Bry.). Soreness of the nose with violent burning.

Rectum - *Anal fissure.* Blind, smarting hemorrhoids.

Sensations - Pricking, biting sensations. Sensation of torpor of tissues, especially after suppressed discharge from ears, eyes and nose. Sensation as if something was gnawing in temples, occiput and ears. As if sand in eyes. As if eyeball would be forced out. Noises in ear as from ringing of bell or from a wind-storm, as if ear was obstructed by cotton. Itching as from lice on chest, as of lump in throat. As of boiling in hip joint. As if muscles of thigh in wrong position. As if knee beaten.

Skin - ***Puncture, stab wounds. Animal bites and insect stings.*** Ecchymosis. ***Long discoloration after injuries, injections, vaccinations.*** Twitches, from bites, nails, stings, with foul pus. Red spots and rash. Eruptions on only covered part. Acne on forehead, with sticking pain. Itching of feet and ankles, worse scratching and warmth of bed. ***Carbuncles*** (Anthr., Tarent-c.). ***Antidote to rhus poisoning*** (Grind., Cypr., Anac.). Bedsores. Edematous swelling.

Sleep - Great inclination to sleep during day, drowsiness with great wish to lie down. Sleeplessness with restless tossing, jerking, fantastic visions and images on closing eyes. Agitated, anxious dreams. Uneasy dreams in which he changes from place to place and from one subject to another. Lascivious dreams with emission of semen.

Stomach - Nausea with the inclination to vomit, on expectorating. Dry, retching with eructation. Contractive pain in sternum when eating quickly. Water brash with cramp-like pains in abdomen.

Temperature - Coldness, want of body heat. ***Coldness of parts,*** worse in limbs with the pain during fever, as if in cold water. Sensation as of cold water over parts, general coldness with heat of face. Foul sweat. Profuse night sweat.

Throat - Sore throat with shooting pain, during and after deglutition. Tormenting cough from tickling in larynx with nosebleed, then sobbing respiration, worse receding eruptions. Sensation as if there were a plug in the throat.

Vertigo - Vertigo when walking, with tendency to fall to one side. Distress when head is covered.

COMMENTS - Puncture wounds, stab wounds, animal bites and insect stings (Hyper.), particularly if septic in appearance. After affects of punctured wounds. Preventative for tetanus. Side effects of vaccinations.

Dental work with punctures (Hyper., Arn.). Bedsores. Sore, achy and bruised injuries (Arn.). Injured part feels cold. Wounded area can emaciate. Wounds are better with cold applications.

Red, gushing hemorrhages. Hemoptysis alternating with attacks of rheumatism. Lengthy discoloration of contused parts. Slight injuries cause ecchymoses. Ecchymosis from blood transfusions or IVs.

Marked eye symptoms. Nash says Led. 200c is unequaled as a remedy for "black-eye" from a blow (Symph., if there is pain in the eyeball). Ecchymoses of conjunctiva. Inflammation of ear with deafness from getting cold (as having hair cut).

Sticking, tearing, throbbing pains. Pain in ankle as from sprain; limbs as if beaten and bruised. Hot, tense, hard swellings. Hering noted that "Ledum has often been given to horses when they go lame and draw up their legs. The pains move upward."

Led. occupies the second place in Teste's Arn. group, in which are also Crot-t., Ferr., Mang., Rhus-t., and Spig. According to him, the sphere of Led. is frequently identical with that of Arn.

However, Led. has a special action on the capillary system in parts where cellular tissue is wanting and where a dry, resisting texture is present, as in the fingers and toes. "It is, perhaps for this reason that it acts better on the small joints than on the large joints," hence its appropriateness in gout.

Rheumatism and gout that migrates from joint to joint, generally from feet upward. Pains shoot upward (Kalm., downward). Symptoms are worse from warmth, better by sitting with feet and legs in cold water. The warmth of the bed is intolerable, he must get up and walk about.

Teste describes the characteristic skin affection of Led. as a sort of bluish or violet-colored tuberosities, especially on the forehead. Eczematous eruptions with a tingling itching, that spreads over the whole body, penetrating into the mouth, probably also into the air-passages and occasions a spasmodic cough (Rhus-t. and Crot-t.).

Teste reported "In a gouty subject I have seen cough precede by days the breaking out of vessel on the which could not fail to suggest the use of Led. These vesicles, which had existed on the bronchial membrane, before showing themselves in the face, on the shoulders, etc., became quite apparent on the tongue, where they might be traced to its root."

Eczema concentrated on one leg, less frequently on both at once. Ingalls commended a light paste of Led. (equal parts of Led., alcohol and water) as an application for carbuncles, giving Led. 1x internally at the same time.)

For hangovers from drinking hard liquor (Nux-v. is for wine and beer). For rhus poisoning.

Teste related a case of a puncture wound in which a young woman fell with an embroidery needle in her hand and the hand was pierced through, giving a serious wound. There was no hemorrhage, but Teste noticed the intense cold that accompanies and characterizes Ledum fever. Within a week, Led. cured the patient.

Yingling recorded a parallel case, A. J. M., 38, drove a rusty spike through his left foot near the arch of the instep, glancing to the inside of the foot without passing through the bone. This was at 5 p.m. At 8 p.m. a report was brought to Yingling relating the events.

A few moments after the accident the patient felt stiffening pains in the foot, running up the leg and rapidly increasing in severity. Great chilliness with chattering of teeth followed. The lower jaw became somewhat stiff, general shivering, the neck felt stiff.

The patient reported that he "can't endure it much longer." Led. 3x was sent and rapid improvement took place from the first dose. A compress of Calen. 3x. was also applied, an attack of tetanus being evidently aborted.

Teste recorded the case of an octogenarian who had rheumatism of his left arm, chiefly in the elbow and wrist, coming on in the night or early morning. There was no more sleep for him unless he rose and took a cold bath after which he could sleep. Cured with Led. 30c.

E. Carleton completed the cure of a case of primary syphilis in which Aur. had done well, where the feet were held to the earth as by a magnet when attempting to move, when moving felt as if pricked with needles.

The pain rising gradually from feet to head, every joint and muscle of body and limbs stiff and sore, sore night-sweats, great emaciation with loss of appetite. Led. 200c in water, cured completely and speedily.

Dr. R. Hilbert, a German physician, obtained very satisfactory results from the use of an infusion of the leaves of Led. as an expectorant in bronchitis. He stated that the feeling of pain along the trachea, which is characteristic of the early stages of acute bronchitis, disappeared after a few doses of the remedy.

The fever rapidly subsided, especially in the case of children. In chronic bronchitis, the infusion facilitates expectoration and lessens cough.

Particularly useful in bronchitis with emphysema of the aged, because of its action in rendering the bronchial secretion less viscid in these cases. It lessens dyspnea and stimulates the circulation. Whooping cough.

Lembke offered the indication that before the paroxysms there is an arrest of breathing. During attacks, there is nosebleed, a shattered feeling in head and chest, and rapid respiration. After, there is staggering, spasmodic contraction of diaphragm, and sobbing respiration. Worse in the evening.

RELATIONS - ***Antidoted by:*** Camph. according to Teste, Rhus-t. is the best antidote. ***It antidotes:*** Effects of alcohol, Apis. ***Compare:*** (1) Led. and Hyper. antidote spider poisons. (2) Ruta, Ham., Bell-p., Arn. (3) Kalm. - bot., Kalm. pains shoot down, Led. pains shoot up. (4) Arn. - trauma. Led. follows Arn. when it fails to relieve soreness, punctured wounds. (5) Crot-t. - skin cold. (6) Ham. - traumatic ecchymosis, black-eye. (7) Ruta - bruises, Ruta, especially of periosteum, Symph. of bone, Hyper. of nerve. (8) Apis - nightly itching of feet. (9) Am-m., Nat-c. (blistered heels), Zinc., Rhus-t., Nux-v., Sel., Fl-ac., Ant-c., Puls., Bov. (10) Sil. - worse from wine, Sil. - chronic rheumatism, extending from feet upwards, Sil. better covering up, Led. better uncovering. ***Compatible:*** Acon., Arn., Bell., Bry., Nux-v., Puls., Rhus-t., Sulph.

REFERENCES - Boericke. Clarke. Murphy. Phatak.

LEMNA MINOR

(Duckweed)

PHARMACY - lem-m. Lemna minor. Duckweed. N. O. Lemancee or Pistiacee. The fresh plant is pounded to a pulp and macerated in two parts by weight of alcohol. Tincture of the whole fresh plant. ***Historical dose:*** Tincture and all potencies.

CLINICAL - Asthma. ***Atrophic rhinitis***. Catarrh. Coryza. Diarrhea. Influenza. Nose, disorders. Ozaena. ***Polyps. Rhinitis.***

HOMEOPATHIC - Lindley noted Dr. Robert Cooper's description in the Homeopathic Monthly, "The lowest form of phenogamous vegetation. It consists of lenticular floating fronds, composed of stem and leaf together and bearing the flowers in slits in the edge."

It forms the green scum found on stagnant ponds and dikes. It is found in two varieties, Lemna minor and Lemna gibba.

Nose blocked with polyps. ***Nasal polyps, swollen turbinates. Atrophic rhinitis***, crusts and muco-purulent discharge very abundant with fetor. Asthma from nasal obstruction, worse in wet weather. Excessive catarrh with frequent sneezing attacks. Foul smell in nose or loss of smell.

Dr. Burnett noticed that Lem-m. patients have their nasal symptoms aggravated in damp and rainy weather. Lem-m.'s symptoms aggravated in heavy rains, Calen., when heavy clouds are about, Rhod. in thunder storms, and Dulc., in damp surroundings and in foggy weather.

Nasal polyps in a man, 60, that were markedly worse in wet weather took Lem-m. 3x at 5 drops three times a day for a month, and said "That is the best tonic I have ever taken," he could breathe quite comfortably.

Abdomen - Rumbling and disturbance in bowels. Twisting pains in bowels, followed by diarrhea.

Ears - Hearing impaired.

Face - Pale, dull, sickly look.

Head - Flitting pains about head and legs with pains in eyes during heavy rain. Drowsy by day, restless at night.

Lungs - Asthma with nasal obstruction. Asthma, attacks coming on in rainy weather. Snoring inspiration.

Modalities - Worse in damp. Worse rainy weather. ***Worse heavy rains.***

Mouth - ***Putrid taste*** on rising in the morning. Foulness of mouth, putrid teeth. Dry pharynx and larynx.

Nose - ***Polyps*** which swell in wet weather. Nostrils plugged by swollen turbinates. Nasal obstruction from an edematous condition. Coryza and catarrh. Ozaena. Discharge profuse, thick, purulent, viscid, yellow, white. Post-nasal dripping, ulceration. Crusts and muco-purulent discharge very abundant. Pain like a string from nostrils to ear. ***Foul smell from the nose and foul taste in the morning on waking.*** Dryness of naso-pharynx.

Rectum - Diarrhea, worse wet, damp weather. Disposition to noisy diarrhea. Diarrhea with pains across bowels as from flatus, worse after eating with very putrid teeth. Bowels acted freely with much heat in anus. Morning diarrhea.

Sleep - Snoring, cured after an aggravation of diarrhea.

Smell - Odors, imaginary and real. ***Putrid smell***. Loss of smell.

Throat - Sensation of intense dryness in pharynx and larynx. Dryness with atrophic rhinitis. Dropping of foul secretion from posterior sinuses.

COMMENTS - Nasal polyps (Sang., Thuj.), nostrils plugged by swollen turbinates and other causes. Chronic atrophic rhinitis. Putrid smell in the nose, or loss of sense of smell. Nasal symptoms are worse in wet weather.

Putrid taste in the mouth, especially on rising in the morning with a general foulness of mouth, due to postnasal dripping. Disposition to "noisy diarrhea."

Clarke recorded a case of a woman, 47, who had, two years previously, met with an accident, a sign board fell on her head when she was out walking in the street. Seven days after, she was taken with sneezing attacks, suffered from nasal catarrh with little intermission until March, 1893, when she came under his care.

Psor. 30c relieved her trouble, which had made her life almost unbearable, as she never dared make an appointment for fear of an attack coming on, and she discontinued treatment. That winter, a sharp attack of influenza brought back the catarrh and it proved less amenable to treatment.

Fears of polyps distressed the patient, though Clarke could not discover any. However, she again made progress, when he thought of giving her Lem-m. on indications given by Dr. Cooper.

On February 15, 1894, Clarke gave Lemna 3x, one tablet four times a day. February 22, she felt very much better, freer in the head than at any time during the last ten years, spirits braced up. She steadily progressed to cure, and by March 15 could endure the smell of strong scented flowers, which before - was impossible.

Captain B., aged forty-four, consulted Clarke on February 29, 1894, for violent neuralgia on the right side of the neck, the part being exquisitely sensitive to touch. He had a cough and cold for a month. On getting up in the morning, he filled two pocket handkerchiefs with yellow effusion before he got his nose clear.

Clarke gave him Bell. 12c to take until the neuralgia was better and then told him to take Lem-m. 3x, three times a day. On March 9 he reported that the Bell. speedily took away the neuralgia and that then the Lem-m. cleared off the catarrh in a most astonishing fashion. He never had a medicine act so magically before.

A man of sixty years of age with nasal polyps only moderately developed, yet of many years duration, was much troubled by the chronic nasal obstruction that was markedly worse in wet weather. Clarke gave him Lem-m. 3x, five drops in water, night and morning.

Returning in a month, he exclaimed, "That is the best tonic I have ever taken, I have never taken any medicine in my life that has done me so much good. I feel quite comfortable in my nose and can breathe through it quite well."

RELATIONS - ***Compare:*** (1) Dulc. - damp surroundings and foggy weather. (2) Calc., Teucr., Calen., Nat-s. (3) All-c., Agra., Chlor., etc., (4) in nasal catarrh, Teucr., Calc. and Thuj. in nasal polyps. (5) Psor., Cadm-s., Aur., Kali-bi. and Syph. in ozaena. (6) Anac. in bad smell in nose. ***Follows well:*** Calc., Merc., Psor.

REFERENCES - Boericke. Clarke. Murphy.

LEONURUS CARDIACA

(Motherwort)

PHARMACY - leon. Leonurus cardiaca. Motherwort. N. O. Labiate. Tincture or infusion of fresh plant. ***Historical dose:*** Tincture and all potencies.

CLINICAL - Dysentery. Hemorrhages. Miscarriages. ***Suppressed, lochia. Suppressed, menses.*** Vomiting.

HOMEOPATHIC - The popular name of this plant sufficiently indicates its traditional virtues. The only experience with it is an involuntary proving recorded by Clarence Bartlett.

A married woman, 40 took an infusion to produce miscarriage. Twenty-four hours later Bartlett saw her and found her vomiting and retching, passing bloody stools, suffering severe abdominal pains.

The pains were provoked by drinking anything more than a small quantity of water, which she did to allay her great thirst. Dry conjunctive, and a dry, cracked tongue were noted. The bowels symptoms were worse midnight to 3 a.m. Ars. 3x relieved all symptoms. She did not miscarry.

Influences pelvic organs, allays spasm and nervous irritability. Promotes secretions and reduces febrile excitement. ***Suppressed lochia*** and menses. Dysentery, with vomiting, frightful pains in abdomen and violent thirst. Tongue dry and cracked.

Abdomen - Very severe abdominal pains with soreness to touch. When lying on side, better drawing up legs; when on back, better with legs out straight.

Eyes - Conjunctive looked as if wiped dry.

Female - ***Suppressed lochia*** and menses. Tends to miscarriages.

Food - Intense thirst, yet drinking more than a very slight quantity of water, warm or cold, provokes epigastric pains.

Mouth - Tongue dry, coated or brownish white, covered with cracks in arborescent arrangement, main crack down center.

Rectum - During the night, frequent calls to stool. Stools dark brown, then bloody.

Stomach - Vomiting and retching.

RELATIONS - ***Antidoted by:*** Ars. ***Compare:*** Hedeo.

REFERENCES - Boericke. Clarke.

LEPIDIUM BONARIENSE

(Brazilian Cress)

PHARMACY - lepi. Lepidium bonariense. Brazilian cress. Lepidium mastruco. Senebiera pinnatifida N. O. Crucifere or Brassicacee. Tincture and trituration of fresh leaves. ***Historical dose:*** Tincture, trituration and all potencies.

CLINICAL - Breasts disorders. Cough. Headaches. Heart, disorders. Indigestion. Rheumatism.

HERBAL - Lepidium is a Brazilian cress. Mure noted that "It is very common in the neighborhood of Rio, where it is found along the roads and in stony regions." It is a great remedy in domestic practice in Brazil and is used for purposes similar to those for which Arn. is used.

All the Lepidium are anti-scorbutic and Lepidium oleraceum, the New Zealand variety, was eagerly sought after as a remedy for scurvy by the early voyagers.

HOMEOPATHIC - Disorders of breasts, heart. Heart symptoms with numbness and pain in left arm, sensation of sinking in pit of stomach. Sensation of a tight girdle around chest, as of a knife piercing the heart.

Sharp pain in left side of head, face, chest, hip to knee. Pain in neck, back and limbs. A streak of pain from the temple to the chin, as if the face were cut with a razor. Burning in the throat, roaring in ears.

MIND - Sad and quarrelsome. Inability to think. Imagined the floor sinking under her. Imagines herself pursued by a phantom in a churchyard, cries with loss of voice next morning.

COMMENTS - Mure's proving of Lepi. brought out some distinctive symptoms on the left side of the head, in the limbs, and especially in the heart.

Heart symptoms with numbness and pain in the left arm. Sinking feeling in the pit of the stomach indicating an action in the solar plexus. Darting pains. Sharp, throbbing pains. Worse from stooping, turning head to the right, when covered.

RELATIONS - ***Compare:*** (1) Arn., Lach. (2) Brass., Cheir., Thlaspi., Armor. sat., Raph., Sinap. (3) Spig., Kalm., Lycps. - heart problems.

REFERENCES - Boericke. Clarke.

LEPROMINIUM

(Leprosy Nosode)

PHARMACY - lepro. Leprominium. Leprosy nosode. ***Historical dose:*** All potencies.

CLINICAL - Acne, vulgaris. Alopecia. Aphonia. Dermatitis. Edema. Erythema multiforme. ***Flatulence***. Gingivitis. Glaucoma. ***Immune, disorders.*** Iritis. Kaposi's, sarcoma. Leprosy. Leucoderma. Leukemia. Lichen, planus. Lipoma. Lupus, erythematosus. ***Lupus, vulgaris***. Lymphoma. Molluscum, contagiosum. Neuritis. Neurofibromatosis. ***Numbness.*** Osteoarthritis. Pityriasis. ***Psora. Psoriasis.*** Rhinitis. Ringworm. Sarcoidosis. Scleroderma. ***Skin, disorders.*** Tinea versicolor. ***Urticaria.***

HOMEOPATHIC - Leprosy is a disfiguring, crippling disease prevalent in tropical countries. Dr. Vakil introduced Leprominium, using signs and symptoms collected from 100 patients suffering from various types of leprosy.

There are two preparations. The first, Leprominium H, was prepared from a leprous nodule from the ear of a patient where the presence of lepra bacilli was microscopically demonstrated.

The second, Leprominium A, is used for ascertaining the reactivity of the patient, and was prepared from the lepra bacilli cultured on the foot web of an armadillo.

MIND - Meticulous. Mild or irritable. Brooding. Weeping. Attributes disease to fate. Hopeful of recovery. Fearless. Aversion to begging.

Feels rejected. Likes company. Desires sympathy, yet secludes self to hide early stages of disease. Religious melancholy. Desire to put on white colored clothes, aversion to black colored clothes. ***Loathes life***, but not suicidal.

Abdomen - ***Flatulence*** in lower part of abdomen. Passing flatus ameliorates.

Cough - Chronic cough in some smokers with emphysematous changes.

Ears - Chronic otorrhea. Thickening and nodulation of the ear. Appearance as if had rat-bite.

Eyes - Swelling, puffy, baggy under eyes. Ectropion. Cannot close the eyes completely, sleeps with eyes half open. Eyelashes drop off. Red, painless discoloration. Sensation of heat. Xerophthalmia. Dryness, with bland or acrid lachrymation, worse from light, sun. Itching and agglutination. Photophobia. ***Squints.*** Conjunctivitis. Scleritis. Interstitial keratitis. ***Iritis***, iridocyclitis. Trachoma. Corneal opacity. Herpes simplex on cornea. Glaucoma. Cataract formation, left to right. Blindness.

Face - Anesthesia of the face, anesthetic patches. Numbness and cobweb sensation. Deformed, leonine, prematurely old appearance. Thickened skin of the face with permanent wrinkling. Nodules on the face, nodulation and ulceration of nose and lips. Edema, angioneurotic. Palsy. Paralysis. Trigeminal neuralgia. Waxy or oily look. Outer one third of eyebrows lost. Eyelashes lost. Mustache hair lost in the middle.

Female - Menopause early. Sexual desire absent.

Fever - Scanty perspiration. Rigors with fever. Remittent or intermittent fever with infections. Malaria giving rise to lepra reaction.

Food - Thirst increased. Desires green chilies, meat, fish, spicy, sour, ice cold water. Aversion to milk, sweets, worse from sour food.

Head - Alopecia areata. Hair loss on hypopigmented patches. Hair turns gray prematurely. Hemicrania.

Kidneys - Glomerulonephritis. Nephritic syndrome. Urination frequency increased in some patients. Intermittent flow. Urination painful, from walking in sun.

Limbs - Anesthesia of hands, feet. ***Heat in palms, soles.*** Ascending coldness. ***Hands and feet icy cold.*** Sensation of ice in limbs, better warm clothes. ***Numbness and tingling.*** Ascending numbness. Peripheral neuritis. Paralysis, paraplegia. Edema of the feet, worse evening, walking, hanging feet down. Wrist drop, foot drop. Pain in limbs, massaging ameliorates. Pain in knee joints, worse initial motion, better continued motion. Osteoarthritis. Nodules like neurofibromatosis. ***Deformities of limbs***. Patches hypopigmented, well defined, thickened, raised. Sensation loss on hypopigmented patches. Non-healing ulcers. Gangrene. Maggots.

Lungs - Tendency to catch cold. Pulmonary tuberculosis. Difficulty breathing.

Male - Gynecomastia. Sexual desire absent. Desire increase, with nocturnal emissions. Enlarged testes. ***Impotency***. Aspermatogenesis. Oligospermia.

Mouth - Swelling lips. Flat-topped nodules on tongue, lips. Deep fissure in tongue. Glossitis. Adherent uvula to soft palate. Uvula ulceration. Infiltration and nodules on uvula and soft palate. Small ulcers. Gums bleed easily. Gingivitis. Turgid and swollen gums, shiny purplish in color.

Nose - ***Nasal obstruction.*** Clinkers and scabs. Offensive scabs from nose but patient cannot smell. Waxy nose. Flattened tip. Collapse of the nose. Depressed nose. Atrophic rhinitis. Atrophy of the anterior and inferior turbinate. Perforation of septum. Nosebleeds, worse cold, wet on head, washing face, or sneezing.

Rectum - Constipation. Semi-solid stools with mucous, without pain in abdomen.

Skin - ***Lupus vulgaris***. Anesthesia, hypoesthesia or thickened erythematous anesthetic patches. Neurofibromatosis. Discoloration, ***dark pigmentation. Dryness of whole body***, in many patients with scanty perspiration. Cracks deep in palms and soles. Erythema multiforme, ulcerous lesions. Nodules, small, pedunculated. Eruptions bullous, macules, flat, hypopigmented or erythematous. Pemphigoid ***scabs,*** dark brown small, scaling, resembling exfoliative dermatitis. Ichthyosis. ***Psoriasis, itching all over.*** Ringworm. ***Urticaria.*** Scabies. Pellagra. Skin sticking to the bones giving a shiny appearance like scleroderma.

Sleep - Eyes remain half open during sleep. Dreams frightful, unremembered. Dreams of dead people, dead relatives. Refreshed on waking.

Teeth - Loose teeth, because of changes in the bones which secure the teeth. Upper central and lateral incisor dropping out.

Throat - Cicatrices, laryngeal and pharyngeal constriction. ***Sensation of something stuck in throat***. Hoarseness of voice. Loss of voice, complete aphonia.

Vertigo - Weak feeling, blackout. Vertigo with nausea, worse opening eyes, sun.

COMMENTS - Vakil concluded that Lepro. should prove to be a useful nosode on the basis of symptom similarity and also as an intercurrent remedy to clear the miasmatic background.

He noted that leprosy resembles many skin conditions, including leucoderma, nutritional discolouration of the skin, macular syphilides, tinea versiclour, lupus erythematosus, and lupus vulgaris. Neurofibromatosis, cutaneous sarcoidosis, leukaemia cutis, Kaposi's sarcoma, subcutaneous phycomycosis, lymphoma.

Seborrheic dermatitis, erythema multiforme, alopecia areata. Ringworm of the skin, psoriasis, lichen planus, pityriasis rosea, urticaria, scleroderma. Lipoma, acne vulgaris, molluscum contagiosum etc.

Leprosy can resemble progressive muscular atrophy, ainhum, gangrene, mango-toe, peripheral neuritis, Bell's palsy, Dupuytren's contracture, nasal deformities, maralaga paresthetica, carpal tunnel syndrome, syringomyelia, tabes dorsalis, and spina bifida. Leprosy also resembles syphilis to a great extent.

Leprosy affects the reticuloendothelial and immune system. The disease traumatizes the mind of the individual, and gives rise to symptoms resembling anxiety neurosis, depression and melancholia.

As it resembles many diseases, some of them chronic and intractable, and as this disease was widespread in many countries, “lepra” can be considered as a separate miasm. For complaints that develop slowly but give rise to irreversible pathological changes.

Vakil suggested that as Bac. and Tub. have separate spheres of action, Leprominium H and Leprominium A should have separate spheres of action.

Vakil noted the case of a female child, 6, came to the out-patient department of the Government Homeopathic Hospital with a rough patch of skin just near the right cubital fossa since she was 2. It was roughly 2 inches by 4 inches and itched slightly. There was thick scab formation with a raw surface underneath.

Mez. 30c was prescribed on the symptoms chilliness, possible bad effects of vaccination, and itching from touch. A small scab came off within a week, but there was no further improvement.

Vakil waited for 2 months, and was considering repeating the Mez. in a higher potency when he noticed an anesthetic patch on the back of the woman who accompanied her, who turned out to be the girl's neighbor.

Additional symptoms included a religious feeling, desire for white clothes, sympathetic and desiring sympathy for herself, tendency to catch cold, desire for green chilies and an obstinate skin condition.

Vakil prescribed Lepro. A 30x, single dose. To the surprise of all, the scabs started coming off within a week. By the end of the month she was 80% better. It was noticed that immediately after the administration of the nosode she had semi-solid stools with mucus and running of the nose for a week.

RELATIONS - ***Compare:*** Psor., Sulph. Mez.

REFERENCES - Vakil.

LEPTANDRA VIRGINICA

(Culver's Root)

PHARMACY - lept. Leptandra virginica. Culver's root. Veronica virginica. Black root. Culver's physic. Tall speedwell. N. O. Scrophulariaceae. Tincture of resinoid Leptandrin. Tincture of fresh root of second year. Trituration of dried root. A fresh plant tincture should also be made and tested. ***Historical dose:*** Trituration, tincture and all potencies.

CLINICAL - Ascites. Bilious, attack. Bilious, fever. ***Black, stools***. Constipation. Diarrhea. Dysentery. Dyspepsia. Headaches. ***Jaundice. Liver, disorders.*** Remittent fever infantile. ***Typhoid, fevers.*** Yellow fever.

HOMEOPATHIC - Leptandra, in the form of the resinoid Leptandrin, was proved by Burt. As one of the grand characteristics of it relative Digitalis is white stools, so the grand characteristic of Leptandra is ***black stools***.

Great varieties of stool, in the later stages of the proving it became dysenteric and mixed with shreds. Constipation with hard black stool, followed by softer stools.

Liver symptoms, with a dull, heavy, frontal headache. These symptoms confirm the use of the drug by eclectics as a kind of "vegetable calomel." Sensation as if something was passing out of rectum.

Farrington noted the dull aching in the right hypochondrium, gallbladder and back of liver, accompanied by soreness. Burning distress in and about liver after spreading to stomach and bowels, with drowsiness and despondency. Bilious and typhoid fevers with black, tarry stools.

Eye symptoms (Euphr.). Generally right-side. Chilly sensation along the spine and down right arm. Pains in right shoulder and arm. Symptoms are worse by motion, rising causes nausea and faintness. Weakness, so great he is hardly able to stand.

MIND - Hopeless, despondent and drowsy. Sadness with liver troubles. Irritable. Anxiety in abdomen after stool. Sensitive to penetrating noises. Weary, can hardly walk.

Abdomen - Sore or dull, burning ache over liver or near gall bladder, extending down over bowels to navel or towards left scapula or along spine, which feels chilly. Constant dull aching in umbilical region. Great distress in stomach and intestines with desire for stool.

Back - Chilly sensation in shoulders and down back. Sore, lame feeling in small of back. Constant distress with very sharp pains by spells in lumbar region.

Eyes - Smarting and aching in eyes with dull pain in eyeballs. Profuse lachrymation. Lids agglutinated.

Female - Menses, suppressed or retarded with liver affection. Warm, watery leucorrhea, runs down the limbs, from ulceration of the os.

Food - Canine hunger. Craving for cold food and drinks, raw food, salads. Worse fats, rich foods, meat and vegetables.

Head - Dull pain, vertigo, drowsiness and depression. Dull frontal headache, with aching in navel. Smarting and aching in eyes.

Heart - Soreness in heart. Pulse slow and full.

Kidneys - Red or orange colored urine with dull aching in lumbar region.

Limbs - Pain in sciatic nerve (left), worse on sitting. Nails very thin, soft and splitting.

Liver - Acute liver conditions. Dull, burning aching in liver, worse near gallbladder. Sore or dull pain, worse from touch or pressure. Burning distress in back part of liver and spine. Liver swollen transversely. Periodical liver derangement, every two or three months. ***Bilious states.*** Gallstones. ***Jaundice.*** Hepatitis. Portal vein congestion.

Modalities - Better from lying on abdomen, on side. Worse from cold drinks, exposure to wet weather, motion, periodically.

Mouth - Tongue, yellow or black down center. Flat taste.

Rectum - Prolapse of rectum with hemorrhoids. Bleeding hemorrhoids. Rectal hemorrhage.

Skin - Jaundice. Dry, hot skin.

Sleep - Sleepiness with liver troubles. Sound sleep. Sleep restless after midnight, feels very ill next day.

Stomach - Craving for cold drinks, which aggravate burning and aching in stomach. Sinking at the pit of stomach. Great distress in stomach and small intestines with immediate desire for stool. Nausea and deathly faintness on rising. Bilious vomiting. Vomiting of bile, yellow tongue, shooting pains about liver, black stools.

Stools - Jaundice with clay-colored stools. Stools, muddy, watery, worse in morning. ***Stools, tarry or black, foul*** with pain at umbilicus. ***Typhoid stools turn black and look like tar.*** Stingy, waxy or spurting stool in the morning with pain at navel.

Temperature - Chilly along the spine and down the arm. Shivering or dry, hot skin, limbs cold and numb tongue black down center. Bilious typhoid fever.

COMMENTS - Affects the right side and liver. Bilious states. Enfeebled portal circulation. Hemorrhages due to liver disorders. Jaundice and black, tarry stools. Conditions with black, tarry stools. Melanotic stools. Hepatitis.

History of cirrhosis, hepatitis, jaundice or colon cancer with dried blood in the stools. Colon cancer. Weakness, hardly able to stand or walk. Typhoid. Malarial conditions. Useful as an herbal tonic for the liver.

Hale noted the order of the different kinds of stools in the proving. First there are black, thick, tar-like, fetid stools. This is followed by thinner, brownish, often fetid stools. Then stools of mixed mucus, flocculent and watery matter with yellow bile or blood. Finally, there is mucous, bloody stool mixed with shred-like substances, often pure blood.

Hale said it is only in cases of dysentery that have developed in this way that Lept. is curative, not in cases primarily dysenteric. Cases due to sudden climatic changes have been cured by it.

Neidhard observed a periodicity in cases cured by him. Periodical, occurring every two or three months, yellow-coated tongue, constant nausea with vomiting of bile. Shooting or aching pains in region of liver, loss of appetite, urine brownish or very dark, often pain in transverse colon, giddiness. Characteristic very dark, almost black stools.

RELATIONS - ***Compare:*** (1) Podo., Iris, Bry., Merc., Ptel., Myric. (2) Like Dig. and Tab. it has sinking at the pit of the stomach.

REFERENCES - Boericke. Clarke. Murphy.

LEVICO AQUA

(Tyrol Mineral Springs)

PHARMACY - lev. Levico aqua. Tyrol mineral springs. An arsenical mineral water of the South Tyrol. Containing iron and copper with other elements. Dilutions. ***Historical dose:*** Tincture and all potencies.

CLINICAL - Anemia. Debility. Chorea. Skin, diseases.

HOMEOPATHIC - Levico has a high reputation among health resorts for nervous and skin cases, favoring assimilation and increasing nutrition.

Burnett is the only homeopathic authority. He said "Levico in 5 to 10 drop doses is a valuable intercurrent to help in grave cases where there is much debility. Notably after the searching remedies such as Bacillinum."

Lev. is supplied in two strengths, the strong and the weak. Either may be used in the doses indicated by Burnett, which is much smaller than that usually prescribed.

Chronic skin diseases. Chorea minor, spasms in scrofulous and anemic children. Debility. Favors assimilation and increases nutrition.

REFERENCES - Clarke.

LEVOMEPROMAZINE

PHARMACY - levo. Levomepromazine. Allopathic drug. ***Historical dose:*** All potencies.

CLINICAL - Agoraphobia. Alcoholism. Allergies. Anorexia. Athetosis. Chorea. Epilepsy. Hypotension. Hypothyroidism. Mental, disorders. Myoclonia. Parkinson's disease. Tachycardia. Wilson's Disease.

HOMEOPATHIC - Symptoms of the toxicologic iatrogenic effects of the drug. The salt, used therapeutically, is the maleate.

Depressive action, anti-convulsive, sedative, anti-emetic, anti-histaminic. It is used in psychiatry for maniacal cases, conditions of agitation, delirium and hallucination in the form of tablets of 5 mg and 25 mg.

Symptoms result from the toxicology of the product, the clinical case of a female patient in Brussels, from self-observation by a pharmacist, and from the proving by O. A. Julian, on a group of sixteen provers, nine men and seven women during the winter of 1968-69, using the 3x, 7c, 9c, 15c, 30c potencies and placebo.

Mental complaints of a depressive and schizophrenic nature. General apathy with nausea. Mental laziness with agitation. Morning lassitude. Fatigue, sleepiness around 5 p.m. with slow heartbeat.

Clear diminution in attention and ability to concentrate.

Hypotension and tachycardia. Multiple allergic sensitivities. Intestinal, hepatic and gastric malfunctioning. Increase in weight.

MIND - Disinterested state. Anxiety from anticipation. Premonition of an indefinable imminent event. State of panic with desire to cry out for help. Anguish, aggravated in a room with light and people. Neurosis from anguish.

Instability. Desire to weep. Fear of going mad, nervy, on edge. Agoraphobia. Desire to harm someone. Anorexia. Schizophrenia. Hallucinations in chronic alcoholics.

Abdomen - Distention after eating starchy food. Hypertrophic cirrhosis of the liver. Entero-hepatic syndrome. Gastric and intestinal dyspepsia.

Back - Pains in the shoulder.

Blood - Rise in the sedimentation rate.

Chest - Oppression of chest.

Constitutions - Suited to phospho-fluoric or tubercular types with psychomotor depression, hypotension and disinterest in the environment, listless with morning fatigue.

Ears - Diminished hearing.

Eyes - Feeling of eyes enlarged.

Food - Anorexia, alternating with bulimia and desire to eat anything. Progressive loss of appetite. Desire for alcoholic drinks which are badly tolerated. Cannot digest milk, milk products, crustacea.

Head - Diffuse, dull headache.

Heart - Acrocyanosis. Tachycardia neurosis, on exertion in anxious types. Postural hypotension. Heart constricted with anguish in the morning. Palpitations at the slightest effort.

Kidneys - Oliguria.

Limbs - Twisting spasms. Cramps, in the toes. Arthritis of the scapula and humerus. Clumsiness, drops things. Circulatory disorders at the periphery, the limbs of the limbs take on a purple color with mauve or white patches.

Lungs - Tachycardia with asthma. Dyspnea on effort. Dyspnea from anguish. Nervous asthma.

Male - Urinary retention. Diminished libido. Neurotic impotence.

Modalities - Better from gentle heat, coffee, tobacco. Worse from light, a crowd.

Mouth - Dryness in the mouth. Bitterness and bad breath. Tongue whitish-gray with absence of thirst.

Nose - Diminished sense of smell.

Rectum - Diarrhea with liquid stools around 8 p.m. with 4-5 successive stools. Constipation.

Skin - Pruritus sometimes accompanied by small urticaria patches. Prurigo strophulus. Painful skin hardening without suppuration, following intra-muscular injections of Levomepromazine.

Sleep - Yawning with sleepiness after meals. Unpleasant, anguished dreams, about the death of dear people.

Stomach - Gastric and intestinal dyspepsia.

Vertigo - Feeling of faintness.

RELATIONS - ***Compare:*** (1) Sep. - Apathy, sadness, headache with pressing pains. Feeling of emptiness in the stomach. Yellowish mark across the nose. Desire to be alone. (2) Tub. - Weakness with constant need to change place. Headache from mental exertion. Anxious, glum, melancholic. Morning diarrhea. (3) Chlorpr. - Disorders of the body of the endocrine system and the thalamus of an introverted psychopathic nature. Hallucination, genetic troubles. Thermal and hepatic disorders. General slowing down and dumbness. Catatonic syndrome. Vesicular, bullous rashes and pigmentation disorders.

REFERENCES - Julian.

LIATRIS SPICATA

(Colic Root)

PHARMACY - liatr. Liatris spicata. Colic root. Liatris serratula. Dense button-snakeroot. Gay feather. Devil's bit. N. O. Composite, tribe Cicoracee. Tincture of powdered fresh root. ***Historical dose:*** Tincture and all potencies.

CLINICAL - ***Anasarca.*** Colic. ***Diarrhea.*** Dropsy. Headache. Indigestion. Kidney, dropsy. Ulcers.

HERBAL - Liatris is an old herbal remedy for indigestion and colic. T. C. Duncan explained that it is called "Devil's bit" as a piece is missing from each tube, as if it had been bitten out.

Liatris has the reputation of being "aromatic, stimulant, diaphoretic, diuretic, anodyne and carminative," particularly useful in colic, headache and flatulency.

HOMEOPATHIC - ***General anasarca*** due to heart and kidney disease. Colic. ***Diarrhea*** with violent urging and pain in lower part of back. Suppressed urine. Dropsy from liver or spleen diseases. Kidney dropsy.

Applied locally to ulcers and unhealthy wounds. A prompt diuretic. Vascular stimulant. Increases functional activity of the skin, mucus membranes.

COMMENTS - Liatr. was introduced to homeopathic medicine because of its action in two cases of dropsy under eclectic treatment. The first was a case of dropsy from material enlargement of liver and spleen, the second was a case of dropsy with almost total suppression of urine. After other remedies had failed, Liatr. was given and, on the second day, the patient passed a gallon and a half of urine.

A. E. White wrote that it has a popular repute as specific in chronic diarrhea following exposure in camp life, and also as an application to non-granulating ulcers. For this purpose the root is to be chewed and then applied.

White was invited to chew a piece, which he did. In six or eight hours he had three successive calls to stool, very urgent, a little griping in lower back and some straining at stool. He has confirmed its use in camp diarrhea, but says it acts better if Sulph. or Merc-c. is given first.

White reported the case of Mr. X, 56, who had chronic diarrhea since the war. He had tried treatment of all kinds, homeopathic included. He had twelve to sixteen stools a day and had loss much weight. He was run down and had made up his mind he had only a short time to live.

He was given Sulph. 30x two doses, one each night, then Merc-c. 3x, a dose each night for five nights, then Liatr. 1x, four pellets each night for five weeks, by which time he was completely cured.

REFERENCES - Boericke. Clarke. Phatak.

LILIUM TIGRINUM

(Tiger Lily)

PHARMACY - lil-t. Lilium tigrinum. Tiger lily. N. O. Liliaceae. Tincture of fresh stalk, leaves and flowers. Some of the provings were made with tincture of the pollen alone. ***Historical dose:*** Tincture and all potencies.

CLINICAL - Angina pectoris. Arthritis. Asthenopia. ***Astigmatism.*** Dementia. ***Depression.*** Diarrhea, Dysentery. Eyes disorders. Fibroma. ***Heart, disorders.*** Hysteria. ***Ovarian disorders.*** Pruritus vulva. Sexual, disorders. Spinal irritation. Urination, frequent. ***Uterus, disorders. Uterus, prolapsed.***

HOMEOPATHIC - The tiger lily, which was introduced into the West from China and Japan, was first suggested as a remedy by W. E. Payne. Carrol Dunham urged Payne to have it proved and assisted by having it proved on a woman under his supervision. The account of this case is given in Dunham's Science of Therapeutics. Some of the provings were made with the tincture of the pollen alone.

The provings showed symptoms of increased activity, things went more easily. Ill humor, drowsiness, sleep but with unpleasant dreams. Sweetish nausea without inclination to vomit. Abnormal fullness worse after eating ever so little. Bloating more pronounced and chiefly across hips, in uterine region.

Darting pains in head and lower abdomen, from ovaries down thighs. Knees ache. Pressure in vagina, pain at of sacrum extending to hips. Increased sexual instinct. Crazy feeling with thoughts of suicide, head grows wild after being quiet for a short time. Increased depressing weight, worse evening.

During the provings, Lil-t. was given for 10 days, then stopped, but the symptoms continued to develop and increase in intensity for eight weeks longer, when it had to be put an end to by an antidote.

Lil-t. manifests its chief action upon the venous circulation, the ***heart and female organs,*** ovaries and uterus. Useful for reflex conditions dependent on pathological conditions of these organs.

Uterine reflex states, dependent on pathology of uterus or ovaries. Utero-ovarian sagging. Symptoms of sexual over excitement. Women exhausted by sexual excess. Often indicated in unmarried women.

Pain in small spots (Ox-ac.). Rheumatic arthritis. Burning palms and soles accompany complaints. ***Full, heavy or forced out feeling*** in uterus, ovaries, heart etc. Wandering, flying, shooting pains or opening and shutting pains, radiating from ovary to heart, to left breast, down the legs etc. Backward pains, about eyes to occiput, from nipples through chest, from heart to left scapula.

Affects the bladder and rectum. Pulsations, ebullitions, gurglings and burnings. Nervous tremors in hypogastrium in spine, knees etc. Venous congestion. Acrid discharges. Nervous, hysterical. Faints in warm room or after standing for a long time. Rheumatism.

MIND - ***Mental and physical symptoms alternate.*** Mental and uterine symptoms alternate. Mental and heart symptoms alternate. ***Hurried, wants to do several things at once***, walks fast, does not know why. ***Restlessness and nervousness.*** Must keep busy.

Haughty and proud. Capriciousness. Abrupt. ***Snappish.*** Censorious, critical. Irritability and sensitivity. Indifferent to anything done for her. Apathy, indifference to love ones. Averse to amusement. Very timid. Prefers company.

Anxiety with palpitations. ***Anxious, fears some organic and incurable disease***. Delusions that she has ***an incurable disease***. Anxiety about business, the future, health. Dementia from business worries. ***Fear of going insane,*** impending disease and suffering, being incurable. Fear of falling, from faintness, worse close warm room. Fear of evil.

Discontented. Dissatisfied, envious of others. Sentimental. Sits alone and broods over imaginary troubles, dwells on past. Grief, sighing. Constant inclination to weep. Grief, hunting for something to grieve oneself. ***Profound depression***, worse consolation. ***Post-partum depression***. Desires death. Suicidal disposition by poison.

Disposed to curse, strike, think obscene things. Cursing, swearing, blasphemy, and profanity. Feels as if she must scream out. Desire to pull the hair out. Hysteria. ***Wild, crazy feeling.*** Stupefaction, as if intoxicated. Religious affections and sadness. Tormented about salvation. Delusions that she is doomed.

Strong sexual desire, lessened by keeping busy. Confusion of mind from sexual excitement. Sexual excitement, alternating with apprehension of religious ideas, or despair. Nymphomania. Erotic, sexual fantasies. ***Dementia from sexual excesses,*** uterine problems.

Abdomen - Abdomen sore, distended, can't bear weight or covers. Skin of abdomen feels stretched and stiff. Abdomen sensitive to pressure or jarring. Trembling sensation in abdomen. ***Heavy dragging down feeling*** of whole abdominal contents with dysuria. Bearing down pain in lower part of abdomen, worse walking. Sharp pains, better gentle rubbing with warm hand, doubling up.

Back - Neck pain and aches, worse if tired. Glands on left side of neck swollen and painful. Broken feeling between scapula. Sensation of pulling upward from tip of coccyx. Spine sore, with stiffness, worse in loins. Dull pain in sacrum. Cold feeling across loins and sacrum. Back as if drawn backwards, after heart attack.

Breasts - Cutting pain in left breast, with sighing and shortness of breath. ***Pains in left breast and left ovary.*** Cramp like pain, in left breast, shoulder and fingers. Sensation as if a rivet or ball under left breast.

Causations - Ailments from being alone, celibacy, being unmarried. Ailments from sexual excesses, childbirth, menopause.

Chest - Constricted feeling in left side of chest. Oppressive load on chest. Tight, hot, congested feeling. Sharp, quick pains in left side of chest, with fluttering of heart. Chest feels as if too full of blood. As if a lump in the center of chest moving up and down on empty swallowing.

Ears - Neuralgia in right ear. Rushing sounds in ears after going to bed.

Eyes - ***Wild look in eyes.*** Biting and burning sensation, worse reading. Pain, extending back into head, lachrymation and impaired vision. Sensitive to light. Photophobia during pain in forehead. Hyperesthesia of retina. Weakened ciliary muscle (Arg-n.). Feel sprained.

Face - Heat and bloated feeling of face and head. Chilly feeling in face in afternoon.

Female - Amenorrhea with cardiac distress or burning stinging ovarian pains. Menses, early, scanty, dark, clotted offensive. Flow only when moving about. Menses cease when resting (Bell., Lac-c., Sep.). Dysmenorrhea with sensation of constriction from back around hips, ending in pubes. Offensive leucorrhea and great weakness during menses. Acrid, brown, thin leucorrhea, stains brown, worse after menses. Smarting in labia, worse after menses. ***Ovarian pains with palpitations, mental symptoms.*** Ovarian pain down thighs or up below the left breast. Sharp pain in region of ovaries and in back. Pains in left ovary and left breast. ***Stinging pain in left ovarian region.*** Bloated feeling in uterine region. Neuralgic pains in uterus, cannot bear pressure of clothes. ***Bearing-down pains*** with urgent desire for stool. Sub-involution. ***Congestion of uterus***. Prolapse uterus. Anteversion and retroversion of uterus. ***Sensation as though all organs would escape*** (Sep., Lac-c., Bell-p.), especially uterus. Constant desire to support parts externally, afraid to move. Nymphomania. Sexual desire increased, obscene, must keep herself busy. Sexual excitement, ending in orgasm. Voluptuous itching in vagina. Pruritus pudendi. Slow recovery after labor.

Food - Hungry, craving for meat, sour or sweet dainties. Aversion to coffee to bread. Thirsty, drinks often and much, before severe symptoms.

Head - Hot, dull, heavy, with morning diarrhea. Faint in warm room. ***Wild feeling in head, as though she would be crazy.*** Headache burning, dependent on uterine disorders, worse before and after menses, better at sunset. Headache over left eye to vertex with vertigo and visual effects. Sick headache every few days, much worse at menses. Drawing hot pain through head and eyes, better frequent sneezing. Sharp neuralgic pains over eyes, worse motion and evening. Stinging, burning pains in forehead.

Heart - ***Sensation as if heart were grasped in a vise*** (Cact.). Heart as if alternately grasped and relaxed. As if heart is hanging by a thread. Heart feels full to bursting. Cold feeling about heart. Heaviness in region of heart. Sensation as if heart stopped, followed by rush of blood to heart and palpitations. Palpitation from excitement, worse lying on either side. ***Palpitations during pregnancy.*** Pain in cardiac region with feeling of a load on chest. Angina pectoris with pain in right arm. Pulse irregular, very rapid. Pulsations all over the body.

Kidneys - Frequent urging. Constant pressure on bladder with constant desire to urinate, with a sensation as of a ball in rectum. Frequent urination, almost every fifteen minutes, with scanty discharges, followed by irritation and smarting in urethra. Urine, milky and scanty, ***hot like boiling oil.*** If desire is not attended to, feeling of congestion in chest.

Limbs - Pain in back and spine with trembling, often of a pressing-down character. Limbs feel cold, clammy, worse when excited or nervous. As if a cool wind blowing on legs. Staggering gait, cannot walk straight, or on uneven ground. Pain from hip to hip. Joints feel dry. Trembling of knees. Legs ache, cannot keep them still. Pain in right arm, hip, ankle joint. Burning in palms and soles. Paralytic stiffness of fingers. Pricking in fingers.

Lungs - Air hunger, takes long, deep breath. ***Suffocates in a warm or crowded room***, theater or church. Shortness of breath. Oppressed breathing with sighing. Sharp pain through right lung, worse in open air.

Male - Increased sexual desire. Lascivious dreams and emissions, followed by irritability, difficulty in fixing one's mind, selecting wrong words.

Modalities - Better from pressure, support, rubbing, lying on left side, crossing legs. Better from cool, open, fresh air, during the day, when busy. ***Worse from warmth of room***, sunset, evening, night, afternoon, from 5 p.m. to 8 a.m.. Worse from motion, walking, standing, jarring, lying on left side, pressure of bed clothes, rubbing. Worse after miscarriage. ***Worse from consolation.*** Diarrhea worse early morning.

Mouth - Sweet taste in back of mouth. Foul taste, better eating. Taste of blood, during congestion to chest. Saliva abundant. Mouth and throat feel coated on waking in the night. Tongue, coated yellowish, white in patches. Darting pain from teeth to ear.

Nose - Sneezing, better pain in head and eyes. Discharge thin, clear, yellow mucus. Nose stopped up. Stoppage of right nostril with pain in right side of face. Rubbed her nose violently. Constant desire to pick nose.

Rectum - ***Constant desire to defecate from pressure in rectum***, worse standing. Pressure downwards and backwards against rectum and anus. Weak, tremulous feeling extending to anus. Diarrhea, directly after dinner, sudden and peremptory. Early morning diarrhea after rising, urgent, cannot wait a moment. ***Sensation as if diarrhea would come on***, passing off by urinating. Dysentery, mucus and blood with tenesmus, especially in plethoric and nervous women at menopause. Stool preceded by griping pains or great urging, with pressure on rectum. Stools, small, frequent with tenesmus. Tenesmus of the rectum and bladder. Hemorrhoids after childbirth.

Sensations - With nausea, a lump in center of chest which could be moved down by empty swallowing. As if an electric current in fingers and hands. As if cool wind blowing on lower limbs.

Skin - Tingling, formication, burning in various parts. Irritation of upper chest and arms and a fine rash about forehead and around borders of the hair with much itching. Skin of abdomen feels stiff and stretched.

Sleep - Yawning, stretching, drowsy. Unable to sleep on account of wild feeling in head. Slept soundly, but suddenly waked by desire to evacuate bladder. Restless sleep, wild feeling in head, everything seems too hot. Unrefreshing sleep with bad dreams, half-awaking, labored. ***Frightful,*** unpleasant dreams. ***Amorous, lewd,*** voluptuous dreams.

Stomach - Hollow, empty sensation in stomach and bowels. As if a hard body rolling around, during day only. Hunger, as if from spine. Flatulence. Nausea with sensation of lump in stomach. Nausea with pressure in vagina and pain at top of sacrum. Nausea with morning diarrhea. Morning sickness with frequent, copious urination. Retching, but no vomiting. Feels like vomiting when touching epigastrium. Vomiting from displacement of uterus.

Temperature - Chilly in cool open air, otherwise better. Chilly sensation running down face, head and back. Chills with violent beating of heart and constriction. Great heat and lassitude in afternoon with throbbing throughout body.

Throat - Soreness and dryness. Hawking of mucus with constant nausea. Enlargement of right tonsil, with exudation. Feeling of lump, with pulsations when lying.

Vertigo - Vertigo feeling as if intoxicated, head confused and heavy. Vertigo when walking, staggering forward. Vertigo better in fresh open air, worse in close room.

Vision - ***Myopic astigmatism***, has to turn head sideways to see clearly, with frontal headache. Farsightedness. Presbyopia. Blurred vision with heat in eyes and lids. Blurred vision with prolapsed uterus. Dim vision after seminal emissions. Muscae volitantes.

COMMENTS - Characteristic downward dragging from shoulders, from thorax, from left breast, from epigastrium down to pelvis and out at the vagina as if everything would be forced through. Downward pressure in the rectum, bladder and loins.

General pelvic distress, affecting the bladder, rectum and back. Increased sexual instinct, more intense affect on female organs. High sex drive with bearing down pains (Sep., Murx.), and sharp, stabbing pains in the uterus. Consciousness of the ovaries as distinct, painful, burning spots with pains radiating from them down the thighs. Pains in the uterus and ovaries as if they were squeezed.

Premenstrual syndrome, worse consolation, very irritable before menses. Hurried and restless before menses (Arg-n., Sep.). Fatigue. Can have palpitations of tightness in the chest associated with menses or premenstrual syndrome.

Severe menstrual cramps (Sep.), as if squeezed with sharp, stabbing pains. Regular menses, flows only as long as she moves. Menses too soon, leucorrhea after menses. Intermittent, thin, brown leucorrhea, leaving a brown stain.

C. Sigmund Raue observed excellent results from Lil-t. 3x and 30c in cases of uterine fibroid presenting the characteristic symptoms of the remedy.

Another prover, a woman, 53, who had ceased to menstruate took a drop of Lil-t. 30c. She had a feeling of exhaustion as if the blood were pushed outward and later a blinding headache "as if all the blood were pressing outward through every aperture." Felt hurried and driven, without knowing why.

Sudden fluttering sensation in the heart, better if busy, with faintness, as though she could make no exertion but must sit still. Contractive pain in the heart, intermittent pressure. Alternate spasm and relaxation. Sharp pain in apex of heart. Pain and numbness in the right arm along with the heart pain. Alternation of heart pain with uterine or ovarian pains.

Intermittent action of the heart, every intermission is followed by a violent throb, causing an involuntary catching of the breath. At the same time, the blood rushes up through the carotids to the head, producing great heat and crowded feeling of head and face. Fever and sweat during the night.

Wandering pain, flying, shooting, squeezing and relaxing, opening and shutting, burning and radiating.

Pain radiates from ovary to heart, to left breast, down legs (especially left), across to opposite ovary, through left breast, to back from ilium, across sacrum. Pulling up sensation from the tip of the coccyx. Convulsive contractions of the muscles of the body. Backache. Generally left sided.

Intense restlessness, irritable nervous system, weak, trembling, aimless hurry, walks to and fro. Obscene thoughts. Disposition to strike and swear. Feeling as if she would be crazy if she did not hold tightly upon herself, feeling as if she must scream. Fear of dying.

One prover, who was astigmatic, had much suffering in the eyes during the proving, and found her astigmatism gone when the proving was over.

S. Lilienthal had among his symptoms "a sensation as if a rubber band were stretched tightly from temple to temple, as if a skullcap were crushing the head, as if the brain was being pushed through eyes and ears."

A patient to whom Clarke gave Lil-t. 30c said it caused a sensation in the abdomen as if the contents were "tied up in knots."

H. C. Allen noted the symptom "cannot walk on uneven ground."

Berridge cured a woman, 50, of heart pain, with a sensation as if the heart was grasped with a hand, with a cold feeling from apex of heart to under left scapula, excited by worry, worse lying on right side, better lying on left side and when busy at work.

RELATIONS - ***Antidoted by:*** Plat., Helon. (ante-version), Nux-v. (colic), Puls. ***Compare:*** (1) Cact., Helon., Murx., Sep., Plat., Pall. (2) Sep. - very like in most respects, but Lil-t. better by diverting mind and busying about, Sep. better by violent exertion, leucorrhea of Lil-t. is more excoriating, Lil-t. worse afternoon, Sep. better afternoon, Lil-t. pressure in anus, Sep. weight like a heavy ball. (3) Puls. - worse in warm room, venous stasis with taste of blood in mouth, weeping mood, Puls. quiet weeping. (4) Nat-m. - heart, uterus, coldness about heart. (5) Helon. - profound melancholy with consciousness of womb. (6) Cact. - heart constricted by iron band, constriction continuous, Lil-t. intermittent, uterine and ovarian pains. (7) Sulph. - early morning diarrhea, burning palms and soles. (8) Zinc - heart symptoms better by lying on left side. (9) Pall. over-sensitive Plat., hauteur. (10) Aur. - prolapse, Aur. from weight of organ, Lil-t. from relaxation of ligaments. (11) Rhus-t. - pain and numbness of left arm with heart disease, Lil-t. more characteristic, right.

REFERENCES - Boericke. Clarke. Murphy. Phatak.

LIMULUS CYCLOPS

(King-crab)

PHARMACY - lim. Limulus cyclops. King crab. Limulus polyphemus. Polyphemus occidentalis. Xiphosura. Horse foot. Saucepan. N. O. Merostomata or the pecilopoda of the Crustacea. Coast of North America. Triturations of the dried blood. ***Historical dose:*** Tincture and all potencies.

CLINICAL - Cholera. Colic. Constipation. Coryza. Diarrhea. Dyspnea. Fever. Hemorrhoids. Sea-bathing, effects. Skin, affection. Strokes. ***Vesicles.***

HOMEOPATHIC - Lim. was introduced by Hering, and partially proved by him and Lippe. Hering was surprised to see that the blood of the King crab he dissected was blue, and on investigation was found to contain copper. He thought it would prove to be another medicine for cholera.

The most notable symptoms include a rush of blood to the face with heat of the face and over whole body (Aster.). Bodily and mental exhaustion. Painful fullness of whole right side of body. Gastro enteric symptoms. ***Drowsiness after sea bathing***.

MIND - Mental depression. Weak memory. Forgetful, difficult to remember names. Confusion with heat of face, rush of blood to face, worse when meditating.

Abdomen - Abdomen hot and constricted. Colic with heat. Cramp-like pain with watery stools.

Chest - Oppression of chest.

Eyes - Pain behind left eyeball.

Face - Flushing of face, worse in afternoon. Rush of blood to face. Heat in face alternating with confusion in head.

Head - Headache from straining at stool.

Limbs - Crural neuralgia. Pain in right hip joint. Soles of feet ache, feel numb. Heels sore. Burning in palms.

Lungs - Husky voice. Dyspnea after drinking water. Oppression of chest.

Nose - Fluent coryza. Constant nasal dripping. Sneezing, worse drinking water. Pressure above nose and behind eyes.

Rectum - Hemorrhoids, constriction of anus.

Skin - ***Itching spots and vesicles on face and hands***.

Throat - Husky voice.

COMMENTS - The only italicized Lim. symptoms in Allen are "Frequent rush of blood to the face and painful fullness of the whole right half of the body, especially here and there and in the lower limbs" and "heat, burning and constriction in abdomen."

Gastrointestinal disturbance, a choleric condition. Headache caused by straining at stool. Dyspnea, worse drinking. Coryza worse drinking cold water. Flushing of the face, worse in afternoon. Heat in face alternated with confusion in head.

RELATIONS - ***Compare:*** (1) Aster., Hom., Cupr. (2) Ferr. - flushing. Ind. - pains in head from straining at stool. Ars. - ill-effects of sea-bathing.

REFERENCES - Boericke. Clarke.

LINARIA VULGARIS

(Snap dragon)

PHARMACY - lina. Linaria vulgaris. Snap dragon. Toad-flax. N. O. Scrophulariaceae. Tincture of fresh plant. ***Historical dose:*** Tincture and all potencies.

CLINICAL - Apathy. Bedwetting. Diarrhea. ***Fainting.*** Hemorrhoids. Ophthalmia. Tongue, roughness. Tongue, prickling.

HOMEOPATHIC - In domestic practice, Linaria has long been used as a lotion for inflamed eyes and as an application for painful hemorrhoids. It is said to be purgative and diuretic. Lina. was proved by Muller, Raidl and others.

Farrington commended it for cardiac fainting, "faints dead away without apparent cause"; and also in bedwetting, "bedwetting with frequent painful urging to urinate causing patient to rise at night." Carleton saw it produce "Fainting feeling three or four times a day, fainted away completely once."

Marked enteric symptoms. Pressure on stomach. Jaundice, splenic and hepatic hypertrophy. Salivation. Constriction of the throat. Thirst with rough tongue. Belchings. Nausea, vomiting. Bedwetting. Rectal symptoms. Diarrhea, with profuse urination. Better by taking tea with milk.

Great tiredness. General prostration. ***Irresistible sleepiness. Fainting from heart weakness***. Confusion in the head. Coldness. Oppression of the breathing and stitches in the chest. Symptoms worse walking in open air.

MIND - Peevish mind. Indifferent. Confusion, stupid feeling in the head.. Ill-humor with dull pain in forehead, with fever, after the sleep, lasting until midnight.

RELATIONS - ***Antidoted by:*** Tea in milk. ***Compare:*** (1) Dig. - fainting and other Scrophularia. (2) Caust., Eup-per., Equis. - bedwetting.

REFERENCES - Boericke. Clarke.

LINUM CATHARTICUM

(Purging Flax)

PHARMACY - linu-c. Linum catharticum. Purging flax. N. O. Linacee. Tincture of whole plant. ***Historical dose:*** Tincture and all potencies.

CLINICAL - Amenorrhea. Bronchitis. Cough. Diarrhea. Hemorrhoids. Laryngitis. Rheumatism.

HOMEOPATHIC - Proved by Stokes and Gaston, Linu-c. has marked colic and diarrhea of loose, bright yellow stools and also of slender stools.

Nasal and respiratory catarrh, stuffed-up condition of nose and chest. Troublesome cough and difficult expectoration of frothy, yellow mucus. Menses omitted or delayed. Depressed sexual functions in men, absence of desire in women.

MIND - Dullness and depression. Irritable.

Modalities - Cough, worse walking in open air. Headache, better in open air and from eating.

RELATIONS - ***Antidoted by:*** Sulph. (headache). ***Compare:*** Linu-u.

REFERENCES - Clarke.

LINUM USITATISSIMUM

(Flax-seed)

PHARMACY - linu-u. Linum usitatissimum. Flax-seed. Linseed. Common flax. Source of Linseed or Flax-seed. N. O. Linacee. Trituration and tincture of seed, meal, oil or freshly made poultice. ***Historical dose:*** Tincture and all potencies.

CLINICAL - Asthma. Convulsions. Hay fever. Headaches. Tongue, paralysis. Trismus. Urticaria.

HERBAL - Linseed-tea and linseed poultices are among the most innocent of domestic remedies, but occasionally the application of a linseed poultice has produced severe respiratory disturbances such as asthma, hives, etc. It has been found to contain a small quantity of hydrocyanic acid, which may account for this intensity.

The ***"soothing"*** effects of linseed-tea and linseed poultices are really of a specific and homeopathic nature. A teaspoonful of whole linseed, steeped in warm water for half an hour and then taken, acts as a laxative.

HOMEOPATHIC - Linu-u. is marked by ***intense irritation***. The decoction is of service in inflammation of the urinary passages, cystitis, strangury, etc. Diseases of the intestinal tract. Trismus and paralysis of the tongue. Asthma, hay fever and urticaria.

MIND - Perfectly conscious, but only able to express herself by signs.

Eyes - Unpleasant heat, burning, dryness. Intense conjunctivitis. Chemosis. Swelling of lids, completely closes eye in one hour, edema persisted three days.

Face - Face red and slightly moist. Violent, dull pain in cheeks and temples. Jaws immovably clenched.

Head - Heavy frontal headache. Violent pain in cheeks and temples. Rigid and prominent temporal muscles, jerk rapidly. Head shakes spasmodically in measured time.

Limbs - Upper limbs shaken by spasms, but pliable and uncontracted.

Lungs - Bronchial asthma. Livid, struggles for breath.

Mouth - Tip of the tongue turned upwards and backwards so as to touch the velum palati. Tongue drawn down into her throat. Complete paralysis of tongue. Could not articulate a syllable.

Nose - Irritation rapidly extended through lachrymal duct to nose. Heat, burning dryness with indescribably scraping. Itching sensation, nearly driving him wild. Nasal passage completely closed, compelled to breathe through mouth.

Skin - Herpes. Urticaria. One complete blotch from crown to toes, smarting, stinging, burning.

Stomach - Great weight in stomach. Fullness in stomach and precordial uneasiness, followed by convulsions. Severe colic. Vomiting with copious stools.

Throat - Irritation continued from eyes and nose down into throat. Throat filled with large white blisters.

COMMENTS - Clarke quoted the case of a woman in which the application of a linseed poultice to an ulcer over the right shin-bone produced an attack of asthma which nearly proved fatal. It was not the first time this had happened to her and she protested, but in vain, against the doctor's order. If a linseed poultice even come near her she felt constriction of the chest.

The doctor who ordered the poultice and reported the case, was speedily summoned to witness the worst attack of asthma he had ever seen. The patient was livid and struggling for breath. When the poultice was removed the symptoms gradually subsided. A crop of herpes appeared where the poultice had been and an eruption of urticaria over back, chest and arms.

Dr. A. G. Towner related his own experiences, noting that when he lived in New York state he could handle linseed in all forms freely, but after moving to Illinois, it affected him powerfully.

Once he rubbed his eye while preparing a poultice; intense conjunctivitis came on at once, chemosis, and in an hour the eye was closed and did not come right again for three days. The irritation passed along the lachrymal duct and the same burning and irritation took place in the nose, nearly driving him wild.

The swelling closed the nostrils and he had to breathe through his mouth. The irritation still spread, affecting the throat, which was covered with large white blisters and a desperate attack of bronchial asthma supervened, slightly relieved by large doses of Ip.

In two hours, the skin became affected with an attack of "hives" (urticaria). "I was one complete blotch from the crown of my head to the end of my toes, a complete bodily eruption, smart, sting, burn." He had five of these attacks.

The steam of a poultice would cause coryza, the dust would occasion a complete attack. One was caused by inadvertently eating a lozenge containing linseed.

An entirely different set of symptoms was recorded by Allen in which a girl, 19, drank a cupful of milk into which she had poured by mistake some spoonfuls of linseed oil. Immediately she felt a fullness in her stomach and precordial uneasiness. She vomited profusely and had copious stools. She went to bed, where she was seized with spasms.

Head shook spasmodically in measured time, the eyes and prominent temporal muscles jerked rapidly. Jaws clenched. Tongue paralyzed and drawn down into throat. All the time the brain was quite clear.

A clyster of Asaf. gave temporary relief, but the symptoms recurred for a time with renewed violence. On the third day she was quite recovered, but her health was not good for some time.

RELATIONS - ***Antidoted by:*** Ip., Asaf. ***Compare:*** (1) Linu-c. - in asthma and skin disorders. (2) Ars., Chloral., Apis.

REFERENCES - Boericke. Clarke.

LIPPIA MEXICANA

PHARMACY - lip. Lippia mexicana. N. O. Verbenacae. Tincture of whole fresh plant. ***Historical dose:*** Tincture and all potencies.

HOMEOPATHIC - The leading indication for Lip., as noted in the Chicago Medical Times, is a cough occurring every winter, especially in women. Hoarse ringing or barking chest coughs, without expectoration.

REFERENCES - Clarke.

LIPPSPRINGE AQUA

(Lippspringe Springs)

PHARMACY - lipp. Lippspringe aqua. Lippspringe springs. The waters of the mineral spring in Lippspringe, Westphalia. Containing the sulphates of sodium and calcium, the chloride of magnesium and other salts in smaller proportion with carbonic acid, nitrogen and oxygen gases. Dilutions. ***Historical dose:*** Tincture and all potencies.

CLINICAL - Diarrhea. Hemoptysis. Hemorrhoids. Jaundice. Leucorrhea. Menorrhagia. Urinary stones. Urticaria. Worms.

HOMEOPATHIC - Lipp. is a cold, sulphurated, saline spring, very gaseous, with a saline and piquant taste. James wrote, "It is used in drink and bath as a refreshing and laxative medication. It is vaunted above all against commencing tuberculosis complicated with hemoptysis, when the subjects are plethoric, irritable and liable to pulmonary congestion."

The homeopathic data on Lipp. are derived partly from provings and partly from observations on patients. Marked purging or diuretic effect. Increased quantity of urine, with great urging. Urinary stones.

In one case, there was "a peculiar feeling of comfort" after urination. Alternation of bloody stools with hemoptysis occurred in one case. "Itching of nose and anus" suggests Lipp. as a worm remedy.

Jerking of the limbs, uneasiness, cramps in calves. Sneezing, palpitation, cramp and restlessness were worse evening. Perspiration and diarrhea were worse at night.

Heaviness of chest, worse after sex and from smoking. Worse by walking, better after urination.

MIND - Depressed, sad. Irritable. Apprehensive, worse riding in carriage, a kind of anxiety in the heart of impending misfortune with homesickness. Weak memory. Great desire to write.

RELATIONS - ***Compare:*** (1) Calc-s., Nat-s., Mag-m. Restlessness, Rhus-t., Zinc., Caust. (2) better by urination, Gels., Eug., Lith-c. (3) worse after sex, Kali-c.

REFERENCES - Clarke.

LITHIUM BENZOICUM

(Lithium Benzoate)

PHARMACY - lith-be. Lithium benzoicum. Lithium benzoate. ***Historical dose:*** All potencies.

CLINICAL - Gallstones. Uric acid, deposits.

HOMEOPATHIC - Hale quoted T. O. Summers as saying that Lith-be. had great effect in diminishing uric acid deposits and increasing the free hippuric acid of the urine. "It acts upon the urine before it leaves the blood."

Deep-seated pains in loins in small of back. Uneasiness in bladder. Frequent desire. Bladder irritation. Diminishing uric acid. Gallstones.

REFERENCES - Boericke. Clarke.

LITHIUM BROMATUM

(Lithium Bromide)

PHARMACY - lith-br. Lithium bromatum. Lithium bromide. Trituration. Tincture. ***Historical dose:*** All potencies.

CLINICAL - Cerebral congestion. Epilepsy. Insomnia. Speech, thick. Strokes. Vertigo.

HOMEOPATHIC - Weir Mitchell gave thirty grains to a man (who had a previous attack of stroke and was hemiplegic) for numbness, vertigo, headache and thickness of speech. The one dose removed them in half an hour.

Mitchell gave Lith-br. in epilepsy when other bromides were not borne. Hale mentioned that it removed flushed face, insomnia and intense pain between the shoulder after any prolonged mental exertion. Cerebral congestion, threatened strokes, insomnia and epilepsy.

REFERENCES - Boericke. Clarke.

LITHIUM CARBONICUM

(Lithium Carbonate)

PHARMACY - lith-c. Lithium carbonicum. Lithium carbonate. Trituration. ***Historical dose:*** Trituration and all potencies.

CLINICAL - Albuminuria. Aneurysm. Angina pectoris. ***Barber's itch.*** Bubo. Coryza. Cystitis. ***Depression.*** Dyspepsia. Eye disorders. Gallstones. Glands, swelling. ***Gout. Headaches.*** Heart disorders. Hemiopia. Hernia. Kidney, disorders. ***Manic, depression.*** Menstruation, disorders. Nose disorders. Obesity. Ossification of arteries. Prostatitis. Retina, anemia. ***Rheumatism.*** Spleen disorders. Stomach pain. Syphilis. Urethritis. ***Uric acid diathesis.*** Urinary disorders.

HOMEOPATHIC - Hering introduced and made the first provings of Lith-c. It affects the entire organism, but notably the head and eyes, urinary organs, heart and joints. ***Uric acid diathesis.*** Gout and tophi. Acidity.

Chronic rheumatism connected with heart lesions and asthenopia. Rheumatism connected with heart or eye lesions. Rheumatic nodes. Arthritic complaints accompanied with heart or eye symptoms. Recurring attacks of acute inflammation of the small joints.

Whole body feels sore and heavy. Pressing from within outward in head, abdominal ring, perineum, chest. Pain as of a dull point. Violent sharp pains, as from red hot needles. Paralytic stiffness of the whole body. Prostration. Increase of bulk and weight.

Dry and harsh skin. Hot water aggravates the itching. Effects of bruises and falls. Bruised spots from falls and blows. Open air causes post-nasal dripping from nose and constriction of chest. Inspired air feels cold even into lungs.

MIND - Absent-minded. Slow, confused mind. Concentration difficult. Difficulty in remembering names. Makes mistakes while talking, omitting words, mispronounces, words. Want of self confidence. Timidity, bashful.

Restless, nervous. Anxiety and hopelessness at night, about future. Startled easily. Oversensitive. Easily irritable. Impatient. Quarrelsome, scolding. Averse to being spoken to, to being touched. Wants to be left alone.

Depression. Sadness, despondency. Disposed to weep about his lonesome condition. Staring, thoughtless. ***Manic depression. Obsessive compulsive disorders.*** Claustrophobia. Fear in narrow places.

Abdomen - Feels swollen as if distended with wind. Cannot endure slightest pressure of clothes from fullness in epigastrium (Lach., Lyc.). Pressure, pain in hepatic region. Pain in left abdominal ring like a pressing from within outward. Indurated inguinal glands. Syphilitic bubo in left groin.

Back - Pressure as from a dull point, here and there. Sticking pain in sacral region. Soreness in right side, extending to sacrum. Prostration in sacrum at night.

Bladder - Tenesmus of bladder, while and after urinating. Soreness of bladder with frequent urination. Pain in bladder extending to spermatic cord after urination. Flashes of pain in region of bladder, more towards right, before urination. Burning in urethra. Sub-acute and chronic cystitis.

Breasts - ***Pain in breast glands, which extends into the arms and fingers.***

Chest - Constriction of chest when walking in open air, after breakfast. Pressure in middle of chest from within outward, towards sides.

Constitutions - Gouty constitutions. Uric acid diathesis.

Ears - Pain behind left ear, extending to neck.

Eyes - Pain over eyes. Photophobia. Eyes sensitive after using them by candlelight. Eyes pain after reading. Dry lids.

Face - Prosopalgia. Both cheeks are covered with dry, bran-like scales. Glandular swellings on left side of face, throat and neck, some suppurating.

Female - Menses late, scanty. Menses cease suddenly and headache comes on.

Food - Appetite diminished. Appetite satisfied on beginning to eat. Worse after fruit or chocolate.

Head - Tension, as if bound, better sitting and going out. Constriction of forehead. Pains over the eyes. ***Headache, better while eating,*** but returns and remains until food is again taken. Headache from sudden suppression of menses. Head feels too large. Externally sensitive. Trembling and throbbing. Head pain, better rubbing.

Heart - Trembling and fluttering of the heart, extending to back, worse vexation. Throbbing, dull stitch in cardiac region. Sudden shock in heart. Rheumatic soreness in heart region. Heart pain, extends to head. ***Sore pain in heart, with eye symptoms.*** Heart pain associated with bladder pains, better after urinating. ***Heart symptoms, worse bending forward and better after urinating.*** Pressure in heart while urinating. Heart pain before menses.

Kidneys - Pain in right kidney and ureter. ***Uric acid diathesis.*** Frequent, copious urination disturbing sleep. While urinating, pressure in heart. Urine scanty with much thirst. Urine with red brown sediment. Urine less in spite of taking normal drinks. Urine, free and colorless. Turbid urine with mucus. Urine scanty and dark, acrid, sandy deposits.

Limbs - Paralytic stiffness all over. ***Uric acid diathesis.*** Arthritis and gout. ***Gout with pains in joints.*** Rheumatic pains throughout shoulder joint, arms, fingers and small joints. ***Pain in joints, relieved by very hot water.*** Nodular swellings in joints. Ankle joint pains while walking. Pain in hollow of foot, extending to the knee. Swelling and tenderness of finger and toe joints, better hot water. Itching about joints, feet and hands. Soreness of fingers, better grasping.

Lungs - Air feels cold on inspiring, even into lungs. Violent cough when lying down. Cough from irritation in throat. Expectoration of much mucus.

Male - Pain in testes. Sharp pain in penis when sitting. Erections after copious urination at night. Erections disturbing sleep, better urinating. Gonorrhea with hemorrhage, alternating with thick, profuse discharge.

Modalities - Better from rest, eating, urinating. Better motion, rising and moving about outside. Worse in morning, at night, motion, on right side. Worse during menses, after menses suppressed.

Mouth - Teeth feel numb, dull and loose, can't bite on them.

Nose - Swollen and red nose, especially right side. Nose internally sore and dry. Soreness of tip of nose. Nose obstructed, worse morning and forenoon. Coryza, dripping from nose in open air. Mucus discharge in evening.

Perspiration - Copious sweats.

Rectum - Violent, painful, dull stitch in perineum near anus, from above downward, from within outward. Emission of much offensive flatus on awaking from sleep. Diarrhea, stools light-yellow, offensive, worse from fruits or chocolates.

Sensations - Temples as if bound. Head too large. Eyes dry. As if veil before eyes. Lancination as from red-hot needles in bubo. Arm as if paralyzed. Border of foot and soles as if gouty, itching.

Skin - Dry, harsh skin. Rough rash all over body, much loose epithelium tough, dry, itchy skin. Dull stitch, ending in itching. Eczema. Scabby, tettery eruption on hands, head and cheeks, preceded by red, raw skin. ***Barber's itch.***

Sleep - Sleepless the whole night with anxiety and feeling of helplessness. Restless sleep. Sleep disturbed by pains in joints, sacrum and feet. Sleep disturbed from copious urination, followed by erections. Voluptuous dreams, disturbing sleep.

Stomach - ***Acidity of stomach.*** Sticking, burning pains. ***Gnawing pain in stomach, better by eating*** (Anac.). Nausea with gnawing in stomach.

Temperature - General feeling of heat in body. Fever with sweat on back of hands. Shuddering starting from chest.

Throat - Soreness of throat, extending to ear. Lumps of mucus drip into throat. Hawking up mucus in large quantities.

Vertigo - Vertigo with ringing in the ears. Vertigo during headache. Vertigo as if floating. Dizzy states.

Vision - Asthenopia. Hemiopia with pain over eyes, invisible right half, worse during menses. Black motes. Sunlight blinds him. Sensation as if a veil before eyes.

COMMENTS - Keynote soreness. Bones, joints, muscles, whole body sore as if beaten. Prostration of whole body, especially knee joints and sacrum. Paralytic stiffness of whole body. Pressing from within outward, in head, abdominal ring, perineum, chest. Bruised spots from falls or blows.

Rheumatic soreness in heart region. Heart symptoms, worse bending forward and better after urinating, though worse on rising to urinate. Heart pain before and during menses. Menses cease suddenly and headache comes on.

Heaviness, better while eating, worse after. Confusion in the head. Eyes pain as if sore. Red and inflamed nose, dropping of solid lumps down the back of the nose. Acidity of the stomach.

According to Allen, lithium lactate has been found valuable for sub-acute rheumatism of the shoulder joint.

RELATIONS - ***Compare:*** (1) Lyc., Am-p., Benz-ac., Calc. (2) Lithium benzoicum, Lithium bromatum, Lithium lacticum, Lithium chlor.

REFERENCES - Boericke. Clarke.

LITHIUM LACTICUM

(Lithium Lactate)

PHARMACY - lith-lac. Lithium lacticum. Lithium lactate. ***Historical dose:*** Trituration and all potencies.

CLINICAL - Joint, pains. Rheumatism.

HOMEOPATHIC - A chemist, while preparing a combination of lactic acid and lithium carbonate, experienced rheumatic pains in the small joints. On this hint, Berghaus used Lith-lac. in local sub-acute rheumatism with good effect.

Allen said it especially affects the shoulder. Rheumatism of the shoulder and small joints, relieved by moving about, worse resting.

REFERENCES - Boericke. Clarke.

LITHIUM MURIATICUM

(Lithium Muriate)

PHARMACY - lith-m. Lithium muriaticum. Lithium muriate. Dilute muriatic acid was saturated with the caustic and carbonate of lithium and evaporated. Solution. ***Historical dose:*** Trituration and all potencies.

CLINICAL - ***Blurred, vision.*** Heartburn. Heart, pains. Nose, sore. Tongue, numb. Vertigo. ***Weakness.***

HOMEOPATHIC - Hering, who proved Lith-c., also proved this salt. He put one drop on his tongue, it had a fatty-salt taste. The tongue became numb as if fat were on it. Pains in the head, back teeth and heart.

Gohrwisch, who took the third dilution, had pains in the heart region and a hot, burning uprising in the throat and pit of stomach like heartburn. He also had pains in his teeth. The tip of the nose was red, sore and somewhat swollen.

Lith-m. has the symptoms of quinine poisoning. ***General weakness,*** marked muscular and general prostration, no gastrointestinal effects.

Nose sore, heartburn, pain in teeth. ***Dizziness.*** Head feels full. ***Blurring of the vision.*** Ringing in ears, marked tremors.

RELATIONS - ***Compare:*** (1) Lith-c.

REFERENCES - Clarke.

LOBELIA CARDINALIS

(Red lobelia)

PHARMACY - lob-c. Lobelia cardinalis. Red lobelia. Cardinal flower. N. O. Lobeliacee. Campanulaceae. Tincture of fresh plant. ***Historical dose:*** Tincture and all potencies.

CLINICAL - Anorexia. Debility. Headache. Sore throat.

HOMEOPATHIC - S. D. Dubs proved Lob-c., taking ten drops of the tincture in one dose. Dubs' symptoms were confirmed by a second proving by Kopp.

Burning in mouth and throat. Sticking and pricking sensation in various parts, especially left chest and left hypochondrium. Oppression of breathing.

Headache at base of occiput worse by motion and shaking head, stiffness in nape. Throbbing and weakness in lower limbs.

Most of the effects of Lob-c. lasted two weeks and it was three weeks before the appetite returned. Thirst for cold water, relieving the burning in tongue and fauces. Many symptoms occurred at 8 a.m. Sleepy, but difficulty in sleeping.

COMMENTS - A woman, to whom Cooper gave one dose of Lob-c., had "flashes of light before eyes every day for a week." Cooper said it seemed to have an action distinct from that of other lobelias, since a dose of it brought back pains which had been relieved by Lob-d.

RELATIONS - ***Compare:*** (1) Lob., Lob-s. (2) Caps. - burning in mouth and throat, but Caps. is worse by cold water, Lob-c. better.

REFERENCES - Boericke. Clarke.

LOBELIA DORTMANNA

PHARMACY - lob-d. Lobelia dortmanna. N. O. Lobeliacee. Campanulaceae. Tincture of fresh plant. Principal indigenous British species, found in shallow lakes. ***Historical dose:*** Tincture and all potencies.

CLINICAL - Ears, noises. Headache. Indigestion. Pylorus, affections.

HOMEOPATHIC - Cooper observed the Lob-d. symptoms on patients after single doses of the tincture were allowed to exhaust their action. According to him, Lob-d. has much in common with Lob-e. and Lob-i.

RELATIONS - ***Compare:*** (1) Lob-i., Lob-s.

REFERENCES - Clarke.

LOBELIA ERINUS

PHARMACY - lob-e. Lobelia erinus. N. O. Lobeliacee. Campanulaceae. Tincture of fresh plant. ***Historical dose:*** Tincture and all potencies.

HOMEOPATHIC - Great dryness of skin, nasal and buccal mucus membranes. Dry patches of eczema, covering points of first fingers.

Malignant growths, extremely rapid development. Malignant disease of the face. Epithelioma. Skin cancer.

Cancer of the omentum. Cork-screw like pains in abdomen. Aversion to brandy.

Breasts disorders with tenderness of axilla, large, soft swelling. Left breast indurated and discharging. Left breast with scattered indurated nodules over adjacent tissues, burning and stinging pains, left arm swollen.

RELATIONS - ***Compare:*** Plb.

REFERENCES - Boericke.

LOBELIA INFLATA

(Indian Tobacco)

PHARMACY - lob. Lobelia inflata. Indian tobacco, Puke weed. N. O. Lobeliacee. Campanulaceae. Fields and roadsides from Canada to Southern U. S. Tincture of fresh plant when in flower and seed. Trituration of dried leaves. Acetum. ***Historical dose:*** Tincture and all potencies. Locally the tincture is antidotal to poison oak.

CLINICAL - Alcoholism. Allergies. Alopecia. Amenorrhea. Angina pectoris. ***Asthma.*** Bronchitis. Cardialgia. Coughs. Croup. ***Deafness.*** Diarrhea. Dysmenorrhea. ***Dyspepsia.*** Dyspnea. Emphysema. Faintness. Gallstones. Gastralgia. Hemorrhoids. Hay-asthma. Heart disorders. Hysteria. Meningeal headaches. Miller's, asthma. Morning sickness. Morphine, effects. ***Nausea.*** Palpitations. Pleurisy. Psoriasis. Rigid os. Seborrhea. Shoulders, pain. Stomach, disorders. Tea, effects. ***Tobacco, habit. Tobacco, effects.*** Urethra, stricture. Vagina, discharge. ***Vomiting,*** pregnancy. Wens. Whooping cough.

HERBAL - Matthew Lobe, whose name is given to this family of plants, was a physician and botanist attached to the court of James I. There are two British species, Lobelia dortmanna, found in shallow lakes, and Lobelia urens, which grows in healthy places.

Lobelia inflata, the North American variety, is the most important medically. According to Hale, this plant was used by the Indians as an emetic detergent in the same way as Verat. was used by the ancients to produce "Helleborism."

Samuel Thompson of New Hampshire, who founded the modern Botanical School, used chiefly lobelia, cayenne pepper and the vapor bath. Often the acetum lobelia acts better than any other preparation.

In veterinary practice, it is said to have proved curative in the tetanus of horses, a disease it is also said to produce.

Lobelia probably obtained the name of "Indian Tobacco" from the similarity of its action to that of tobacco in producing intense nausea, vomiting, profound depression at the epigastrium and collapse. Treatment should always begin with a single dose if the symptoms permit, as in some cases it produces violent depression.

It must be kept in mind when studying lobelia that the herbalists used it in two forms: the decoction to produce emesis and through which they seem to have obtained its antidotal action or by virtue of which they aborted acute gout, and the acetum tincture, which they gave in chronic diseases and in moderate doses."

HOMEOPATHIC - Lobelia is a vaso-motor stimulant, increases the activity of all vegetative processes. It spends its force mainly upon the pneumogastric nerve, producing a depressed, relaxed condition with oppression of chest and epigastrium, impeded respiration, nausea and vomiting.

Asthma and gastric disorders with fatigue, relaxation of muscles, ***nausea, vomiting and dyspepsia***. ***Asthma*** and labored breathing. Asthma with stomach disorders. ***Nausea and vomiting*** with nearly all the lung troubles or stomach disorders. ***Deathly sickness all over*** with oppressed rattling respiration. Diphtheria.

Increased secretions, relaxation and weakness with sweat. ***Catarrhal jaundice*** (Chion.). ***Suppressed discharges*** (Sulph.). Sits with elbows on knees. ***Cannot bear the odor of tobacco***, though addicted to its use. Bad effects of drunkenness.

MIND - Great depression and exhaustion. Despondent. Sobbing and weeping like a child. Presentiment of death and dyspnea. Fear of death. Felt he was dying with distress at chest. Felt he was dying, but was unconcerned.

Mentally restless. Confusion after eating, from motion. Lost his reason and became convulsed, it required several men to hold him. Violent raving with flushing of face and palpitations.

Abdomen - Abdomen distended with shortness of breath. Cutting and drawing pains in abdomen, worse after eating with headache. Sudden sharp pain, in left side of abdomen. Violent and painful constriction in epigastrium. Griping and twisting with nausea, violent risings and emission of foul flatus. Borborygmi. Rumbling in bowels and passage of flatus downward. Intussusception of bowels. Incarcerated hernia.

Back - Pain in sacrum, cannot bear slightest touch. Sits leaning forward. Swelling and pain left side of neck. Rheumatic pain between the scapula. Dull pressure between scapula. Pain under right scapula worse bending forward. Burning, in back, as if in posterior wall of stomach.

Breasts - Pain in the breast. Burning feeling in breast, passing upward. A tightness of the breast with heat in forehead. Drawing in left breast from nipple to axilla.

Causations - Alcohol, tea, tobacco, smoke. Wetting feet. Suppressions. Foreign bodies.

Chest - Burning, pricking in air passages. Burning feeling in the chest, passing upwards. Constriction or oppressive fullness in chest. ***Sensation of pressure or weight in chest, better by rapid walking***. Violent pains in chest, worse on breathing deeply. Tension in chest on turning body. As if band about chest with irresistible desire to cough. Rattle in chest, but does not expectorate.

Constitutions - Suited to persons inclined to be fleshy. Weak lungs.

Cough - Cramping, ringing cough, short breath, catching at throat. Spasmodic cough with sneezing, belching or gastric pain, worse motion. Single cough with a feeling of narrowness in chest. ***Cough with vomiting,*** yawning. Whooping cough, violent, racking, followed by expectoration of ropy mucus. Third stage of whooping cough, when expectoration ceases, or when relapses occur. Inflammatory condition of mucus membrane of larynx, trachea and bronchi. Irritation provokes coughing and expectoration.

Ears - Aching in left ear. Constantly recurring earaches. Sudden shutting up of right ear, as if stopped by a plug. Profuse discharge from the ear. Shooting pain extending into left ear from painful spot in throat. ***Deafness due to suppressed discharges,*** otorrhea or eczema.

Eyes - Burning pain in eyes. Pain and soreness in right eye. Itching in angles of eyelids. Pressing pain in eyeballs, most in upper part. Pupils dilated. Hemiopia. Vision dim.

Face - Sudden pallor. Bathed in cold sweat. Sweat on face with nausea. Heat of face. Chilly feeling in left cheek extending to ear. Neuralgia of face with retarded menses.

Female - Suppressed menses. Menses too early, too profuse. During menstruation violent pain in sacrum. Labor pains with shortness of breath, rigid os and perineum. Pain in her sacrum and a sense of weight in genitals. Violent pain in the sacrum with fever.

Head - Dull, heavy pain. Pressive pain on left side of occiput, worse at night and from motion. Sudden shocks through the head. ***Gastric headache with nausea, vomiting and great prostration. Sick headache with vertigo.*** Headaches, worse afternoon until midnight, coughing, ***from tobacco or tobacco smoke.*** Brain racked by cough which causes intolerable pain. Heaviness in head with lassitude in back. Wens. Seborrhea.

Heart - Deep-seated pain in region of heart. Precordial anxiety. Sensation of weakness and pressure in epigastrium rising to heart. Pulse, weak or soft, flowing. Sensation as if heart would stand still.

Kidneys - Sticking pain in region of right kidney. Urine suppressed or infrequent. Increased secretion of urine, sometimes with want to urinate. Urine cloudy, deep red, with loose deposit, dull red or brown sediment, soon becoming turbid.

Limbs - Shooting pains through whole body, into fingertips and toes. Rheumatic feeling in right shoulder joint, goes to left upper arm and around elbow joint. Fine crawling stitches inside of right deltoid. Rheumatic pain in right elbow joint. Sweat of palms, backs of hands dry and cool, fingertips cold.

Lungs - ***Asthma preceded by prickling all over.*** Asthma, attacks with weakness, felt in pit of stomach. Sighing. ***Hyperventilation.*** Short inhalation and long, deep exhalation. ***Panting, threatened with suffocation, fear of death. Dyspnea from constriction of chest, worse any exertion.*** Dyspnea from short exposure to cold. Dyspnea, with sense of a lump in stomach rising into mouth. Rattling in chest but no expectoration. Difficult breathing during labor pains. Emphysema with very dry tracheal and bronchial catarrh. Senile emphysema.

Male - Fatiguing heaviness, weight, in genital parts. Smarting of the prepuce.

Modalities - Better in afternoon, toward evening. Better from rapid walking, eating a little, warmth. ***Worse tobacco or tobacco smoke.*** Worse afternoon, evening and night, after sleep, cold, cold bathing. Worse slightest motion, exertion, touch, tea, suppressions, foreign bodies. Warm food causes vomiting.

Mouth - Acrid, burning taste in mouth, bitter, with foul tongue and thirst. ***Mercurial taste***. Sharp, disagreeable taste in mouth at tip of tongue and back of throat. ***Profuse salivation with good appetite***. Flow of clammy saliva in mouth with nausea. Tenacious mucus. Tongue white with a thick coating, on right side only. Dull, pressing pain in last left molar and temples.

Nose - Nosebleeds. Tip of nose very cold. ***Cannot bear smell or taste of tobacco.***

Perspiration - Profuse sweat and prostration. Sweats towards evening or at night. Copious sweats at night. Cold sweat. Sweats after fever. Sweats with sleep. Sweats after vomiting, breaks out all over with sweat. Sweats followed by a sensation as if thousands of needles were piercing her skin from within outward.

Rectum - Discharge of black blood right after stool. Copious hemorrhages from hemorrhoidal vessels. Stools like pap, soft, green, diarrhea, sometimes with frequent evacuations and confusion of head. Soft, whitish stool.

Sensations - As if foreign body in throat. As if lump in pit of throat. As if esophagus contracted from below upward. As if a lump rose up to meet food and obstruct its descent. As if a lump or heavy load in stomach. Fullness in trachea as if from chest. As if a lump in larynx. As if the heart would stand still. As if a band about chest. As if blood stagnated in chest (better moving about). As if thousands of needles were pricking her skin from within outward.

Skin - ***Prickling, itching all over body, with nausea.*** Vesicular itch-like pustules with tingling itching. Vesicular eruption on skin. Eruption between fingers, on dorsum of hands and on forearms. Plaques of edema with ecchymoses.

Sleep - Yawning, followed by crawling in nose and sneezing. Yawning and belching of gas. Disturbed sleep with many dreams, sometimes anxious, painful dreams. Dreams are many without intermediate awakening, cold sweats. Dream that arm was amputated, of being wounded by a shot. Wakened early by very vivid dreams.

Stomach - ***Faintness and weakness of epigastrium.*** Sensation as if esophagus were contracted from below upward. As if a lump or heavy load in stomach. Acrid, burning taste, acidity with contractive feeling in stomach. Acidity, flatulence, shortness of breath after eating. Frequent gulping up of a burning, sour fluid. Profuse flow of saliva with retching, hiccough, dyspnea with good appetite. Heartburn with profuse flow of saliva. Hiccough followed by drowsiness. ***Extreme nausea and vomiting***. Deathly nausea with vertigo, better by a little drink or food, worse night and early morning. ***Nausea with prickling itching of skin.*** Nausea and vomiting with profuse sweat, on face with respiratory symptoms. Morning sickness, suddenly disappears better by a little food and drink.

Temperature - Chilliness, coldness, of whole body, better near fire or from heat, worse after drinking. Thirst before the chill and through the whole fever. Intermittent fevers, commencing at noon with great paleness and anorexia. Heat with tendency to perspire.

Throat - Burning in throat, dryness of fauces. Dryness and pricking in throat, not better drinking. Sensation as if a lump in throat, impeding swallowing and respiration. Tickling in larynx with frequent fits of short coughing. Sensation of fullness in trachea. Spasmodic croup, with nausea, vomiting and threatening suffocation.

Vertigo - Vertigo with fear of death, nausea. Vertigo as if starting from left eye. Cerebral suffering, giddiness. Headache with slight giddiness.

COMMENTS - In Walter Besant's Life of Edward Henry Palmer, Palmer's own account of his cure by lobelia is recorded. In 1859, he was seized with pulmonary disease, which rapidly increased until he was told he had probably only a few months to live.

On the advice of a herbalist named Sherringham, he took a single large dose of lobelia and experienced a violent attack of vomiting, a cold chill mounting up from his feet, to hands, which he could no longer move, to his heart, which ceased to beat, to his throat, which ceased to breathe.

A doctor was sent for. "I felt myself dying," he said afterwards, describing the experience, "I was being killed by this dreadful cold spreading all over me. I was quite certain that my last moments had come. By the bedside stood my aunt, poor soul, crying. I saw the doctor feeling my pulseless wrist, watch in hand, the cold dews of death were on my forehead, the cold hand of death was on my limbs. Up to my lips, but no higher, I thought I was actually dead. I could see and hear but not speak, not even when the doctor let my hand fall on the pillow and said solemnly, 'He is gone.'"

Palmer said there was no pain, he was in no concern except about a book he wanted to finish. He recovered suddenly.

New strength came to him. The tuberculosis was arrested and was no more trouble to him for the rest of his life.

Symptoms concomitant with hereditary syphilis. Childhood tuberculosis. Childhood bronchopneumonia. Imperfect recoveries from chest affections, especially where tubercle threatens. Severe inflammatory conditions existing along with anthrax or with malignant deposits in different regions, useful in repeated as well as in single doses.

Whooping cough with dyspnea threatening suffocation. Must keep mouth open to breathe. Asthma with dryness of the throat and mouth, and a constricted feeling as if a band across the chest. Asthma with stomach nausea and vomiting (Ip.).

Pressive headaches, at the occiput, less frequently at the forehead, sometimes one-sided (left), worse by motion, in evening, and especially at night. Continual periodic headache in the afternoon and increasing until midnight, every third attack being alternately more or less violent. Headache following intoxication, worse afternoon until midnight, worse from tobacco.

Brain racked by a cough, causing an intolerable pain. Heat and sweat about the head and face. Persistent earaches and headaches due to suppressed discharges, where the lips are dry and hot and continual feverish colds are prominent (Ars-i.).

Semi-lateral coating of the tongue. Continuous nausea with constant flow of saliva and sensitivity to the smell of food or tobacco, especially during pregnancy (Ign., Sep, Colch.).

Gastric derangements, extreme nausea and vomiting. Vomiting, face bathed in cold sweat. Sudden pallor with profuse sweat. Morning sickness, effects of suppressed or missed menstrual periods.

Exfoliating rash, psoriasis. Faulty secondary digestion. Thin, poor, without appetite. Tabes mesenterica. Pediculi corporis.

Conditions due to suppression, including cases of tuberculosis. Ailments that never finish, whether beginning from acutely inflammatory causes or not, it also fights with symptoms occasioned by mechanical irritants, e.g., where a spicula of bone presses on the brain (compression) or where a bone is lodged in bronchus.

H. M. Broderick recorded the case of a young woman, 18, who was ill for two years under allopathic treatment. Her symptoms included labored breathing, and a sense of tightness across the chest compelling her to take deep inspirations, which caused pain in heart region.

Pulse full, very rapid, a cough after each deep breath. She was unable to lie down because of the oppression and pain. Facial muscles twitched. Menses never regularly established, would go several weeks over time and then would last only a day.

Lob. 3x was given in water. After the second dose she went to bed and slept. The remedy was repeated just before her next menstrual period. She had no more attacks and menstruation became normal.

An elderly woman who had not menstruated in two years had pain in her shoulders. Lob. relieved the pain and brought on the menses.

Cooper recorded the case of a young woman, 23, with a family history of tuberculosis on both sides. She had, when 14 to 15 years old, severe pain in the left and sometimes the right side and around her lower abdomen with a faint feeling. This lasted until the monthly period came on regularly and then she was well until 20, when diarrhea came on, which nothing was able to check and which kept her in bed for months at a time.

The symptoms were pains all around abdomen and up the back, much worse after undressing, feeling of exhaustion or falling to pieces inside and out, and she could not bear anything to touch her. Four or five bowel movements daily when taking medicine, if she leaves it off, continual movements all day, it literally runs from her, watery, sometimes light-colored, sometimes dark, never bloody.

Menses very irregular, sometimes five to six weeks in between. All the symptoms, especially diarrhea, worse then, much tenderness all over abdomen, especially in ovarian regions, legs ache fearfully, pains all over body, faints continually. Since the illness began, she was subject to neuralgia of the face, one or the other side, or both, extending to chest, coming and going suddenly at any time.

In spite of treatment of all kinds, including that of a skillful repertorian, she grew worse. She went into a hospital and there a small pile was removed with but temporary benefit, and after this the vagina as well as the rectum began to copiously discharge an excoriating fluid.

Lob., eight drops three times a day, was now given. She began to improve at once and in a few weeks was quite well. In this case, the difficulty first showed itself when the menstruation was commencing. It was relieved when the flow was regularly established, reappeared simultaneously with menstrual irregularity. In other cases there is an analogous history.

The nausea has been used in the same way as that of Tab. and other emetics to produce relaxation of muscles, as, for example, rigid os. Sometimes this is affected by direct physiological action, but it may be homeopathic as in this cured case, "with every uterine contraction violent dyspnea, which seems to neutralize labor pain, rigid os and perineum."

Cutler experienced a characteristic prickling sensation. Keynote tenderness of the sacrum.

Cooper noted a symptom recorded by Jahr, "violent pain in the sacrum with fever supervening upon suppression of the menses during their flow." Alongside this symptom may be placed another, also vouched for by Cooper, the power of eliminating foreign substances (Sil.).

In one case, a woman got a piece of mutton-bone down her windpipe and into one of the bronchials. She was taken to the London Hospital, but the idea of operation was abandoned as hopeless and she was sent out. Lob. tincture was given, five drops three times a day. Soon a most violent cough was set up in the course of which the patient coughed up a large quantity of fetid pus, and finally the bone.

Teste classed Lob. with Sulph., and though the provings and clinical experience do not fully bear out what he says about its skin action, the results of botanical practice, confirmed by Cooper, show that it has an anti-psoric action and relieves morbid states due to the suppression of discharges.

P. H. Hale said that with the intense nausea it causes, there is sometimes a prickling itching of the skin, and he thinks he has seen benefit from its use in suppressed urticaria with nausea and vomiting.

Teste gave the symptom "eruption between the fingers, on the dorsum of the hands and on the forearms, consisting of small vesicles accompanied by a tingling itching and resembling the itch pustules exactly." As with Sulph. "faintness at the stomach" is a grand characteristic which will be found in a large proportion of the cases calling for the remedy.

Hale quoted Dr. Cutler's account of his own case. He had been asthmatic for ten years, liable to very severe and prolonged attacks. During the intervals the patient scarcely ever passed a night without more or less of it and as often as not was unable to lie in bed.

In the middle of an attack he had a tablespoonful of a fresh plant tincture. In three or four minutes his breathing was quite free, but there was no nausea and, thinking that necessary, he took another spoonful ten minutes after the first and this occasioned sickness.

Ten minutes later he took a third spoonful, and this produced a sensible effect on the stomach coats and a very little vomiting and "a kind of prickling sensation through the whole system even to the limbs of the fingers and toes. The urinary passage was perceptibly affected, by producing a smarting sensation in passing urine, which was provoked by stimulus on the bladder."

But all these symptoms very soon subsided and vigor seemed to be restored to the constitution that he had not experienced for years.

Cooper recorded the case of a girl, 9, who was seized with a very bad headache affecting the whole head and continuing night and day for two days, Merc. and Verat-v. were given in vain. Lob. acet., two or three drops in a little water given in the morning after a bad night, gave immediate relief and restored the appetite.

Cooper considered it a meningitis headache and he finds Lob. and Kali-i. 30c especially useful in these. Excessive sensitiveness is a leading indication for the latter. A headache with "dull, heavy pain passing around the forehead from one temple to the other, immediately above eyebrows."

G. W. Boskowitz related the case of a man, 40, who had twice had gonorrhea, the second attack, three years before, having left him with a gleety discharge. For a year the stream had been diminishing until at last it took him half an hour to empty the bladder. Many surgeons had tried to pass an instrument and had failed.

Boskowitz also failed several times, until one day he dropped fifteen drops of Lob. tincture into the urethra and held the meatus to retain it, for five minutes. It produced a smarting which soon passed away and then the sound passed with ease. Boskowitz has used Lob. in similar cases with success.

Guernsey noted that the "urine has a deep red color and deposits a copious red sediment." Dyspnea, as well as nausea, occur in connection with imperfect menstrual cycles may indicate Lob.

Dr. Coffin professed to cure children and adults whose lives were despaired of from poisoning by various substances by decoctions of Lob., but whether by directly evacuant action or not it was not stated.

There is some clinical experience of a few drops mixed in water curing a baby of severe convulsions caused by taking in Chlorodyne.

In tincture, Lob. causes evacuation of the bowels and is an emetic. It is of service locally as in an enema, and in cases of difficult catheterism. A few drops of Lob. in boiling water takes away the pain and tension of inflamed hemorrhoids, the patient sits on a utensil thus filled.

The necessity of taking Lob. in doses sufficient to cause pathogenic symptoms was insisted on by Thompson and, though it led to some disasters, seems to have been the means of saving some lives.

Thompson tells how, as a boy, he chewed this herb and so learned practically its effects. He used to give it to other boys out of sport. One day while mowing he gave a sprig of it to a companion.

By the time they had got six rods the man said he thought the sprig would kill him: he never felt so ill in his life before. He was in a profuse perspiration, trembled all over and was as pale as a corpse.

Unable to walk, he lay down and vomited "two quarts." He was helped to his house, ate a good dinner and returned to work in the afternoon. After this he "felt better than he had for a long time." This gave Thompson his first notion of the medicinal virtues of Lob.

In a paper read before the Brit. Hom. Society, November 1, 1888. Cooper explained that he got no good out of Lob. until, under the advice of a herbalist, he used a solution made with common vinegar.

RELATIONS - ***Antidote:*** Ip., Tab. ***Compare:*** (1) The other lobelias, Dig. and Tab. - heart affections, vomiting, worse by motion, sudden pallor with profuse sweat. (2) Ars. - asthma, hay fever, gastric troubles. (3) Verat. - gastric troubles. (4) Ip. - asthma, gastric troubles. (5) Nux-v. - morning sickness, gastric troubles of alcoholics. (6) Bry. - worse by movement, cough causes headache. (7) Abies-n. and Thuj. - effects of tea. (8) Lac-ac. - vomiting with profuse salivation. (9) Kali-i. - meningitis headaches. (10) Ign. - worse tobacco or tobacco smoke.

REFERENCES - Boericke. Clarke. Murphy. Phatak.

LOBELIA PURPURASCENS

(Purple Lobelia)

PHARMACY - lob-p. Lobelia purpurascens. Purple lobelia. N. O. Lobeliacee. Campanulaceae. Tincture of whole fresh plant. ***Historical dose:*** Tincture and all potencies.

CLINICAL - Blood poisoning. Heart, paralysis. Influenza, headache. Lichen tropicus. Lungs, paralysis. Snakebites. Tongue, paralysis. Typhoid fever. Vertigo.

HOMEOPATHIC - The first mention of this plant was made by Erskine C. White under the name Lobelia rubra, corrected later by F. Kopp and White himself to Lob-p.

Lob-p. grows profusely in the Australian bush, preferably in moist places and most profusely, noted Kopp, where snakes most abound. White added that it prefers loose sandy soils. This is interesting since James S. Bray, quoted by White and Kopp, observed that the iguana after a fight with a snake, whenever it happened to be bitten, ate this Lobelia.

Bray once found a number of sheep dead and from their appearance he at first thought they had been bitten by snakes. But on examining their stomachs he found the leaves and stalks of Lob-p. and he came to the conclusion that this was the cause of their death.

Lob-p. acts very like Bapt. in low typhoid conditions and seems to neutralize the poison of influenza. Intense prostration, vital and nervous. Paralysis of lungs and resultant poisoning with carbonic acid gas, vomiting and coma. Deadly chill without shivering, but overpowering the system.

MIND - Hasty disposition. Confused and depressed. Dejection.

Causations - Blood poisoning. Snakebites.

Eyes - Can't keep eyes open. Spasmodic closure of lids.

Head - Headaches with nausea, vertigo. Headaches with pain between eyebrows.

Heart - Heart feel paralyzed. Heartbeats sound to him like boom of a drum.

Lungs - Respiration slow. Lungs feel paralyzed.

Modalities - Worse from movement, in damp weather.

Mouth - Decay of teeth, in nervous persons.

Skin - Liable to boils. Sweats copiously.

COMMENTS - White gave a short pathogenesis in which symptoms like the effects of snake-poison are prominent. His symptoms, together with those of Kopp, who crushed with his teeth and swallowed a leaf, will be found arranged in the Schema. They bear a strong family resemblance to those of Lob.

White gave a clinical experience of his own which is important. "This plant, if only touched carelessly with the teeth, produces overwhelming giddiness. I had noticed that the sickening stupor and headache it produces exactly resembled those of La Influenza, before I knew the name of the plant.

"My headache disappeared like magic under Lob. purp. tincture and I used to notice that all chest symptoms were avoided under its sway. The influenza breaks out in wet weather. This plant with its tiny gem-like white blossoms, always carpets the earth after each rain throughout the year."

Growing on sandy soil, it contains flint; like Sec., Staph. and the common carrot, it agrees especially well with patients who are deficient in silica and who are nervous, liable to boils of a hasty disposition, perspire profusely and whose teeth are always decaying.

RELATIONS - ***Compare:*** (1) Lob., Tab., Lach. and other snake-poisons. (2) Bapt. - influenza, typhoid. (3) Sec., Staph. - teeth.

REFERENCES - Clarke.

LOBELIA SYPHILITICA

(Great Blue Lobelia)

PHARMACY - lob-s. Lobelia syphilitica. Great blue lobelia. Lobelia cerulea. N. O. Lobeliacee. Campanulaceae. Grows in low grounds in U. S. Tincture of fresh plant. Acetum. ***Historical dose:*** Tincture and all potencies.

CLINICAL - Acidity. Adenoids. Asthma. Back, pains. Borborygmi. Cartilages, pains. Catarrh. Coryza. Cough. Diarrhea. Dyspepsia. Dyspnea. Eustachian catarrh. Flatulence. Hay fever. Influenza. Kidneys, pains. Lumbago. Melancholia. Post-nasal catarrh. Pylorus, pain. Sciatica. Spine, pains. Spleen disorders. Stomach cough. Throat, sore.

HOMEOPATHIC - The symptoms of the Lob-s. proving, while in many points like those of the other lobelias, do not bring out the emetic properties of Lob. There is, however, epigastric sinking, flatulence, dyspepsia and diarrhea. Lob-c., Lob. and Lob-s. all have a milky juice.

Lob-s. gives a perfect picture of sneezing influenza involving the posterior sinuses, palate and fauces. Eustachian catarrh. Internal nose painfully sensitive to cool air. Dull, aching pain over root of nose. Breathing difficult.

Depressed. Flushing after dinner better somewhat in open air. ***Great oppression in lower part of chest,*** as if air could not reach there. Dry, hacking cough. ***Pain in chest under short ribs of left side.***

Pain in forehead over eyes, pain and gas in bowels, followed by copious watery stools with tenesmus and soreness of anus. Pain in posterior part of spleen. Pain in knees. Prickling in soles.

MIND - Depressed, unhappy. Constant disposition to cry, with sadness and dejection. Bad effects from grief. ***Mental exertion aggravates.*** Brain weakness and exertion of mind intolerable. Frequent mistakes in spelling and writing. Confused feeling and slight aching in head. Seemed as if he would go wild.

Abdomen - Pain in posterior aspect of spleen.

Back - Pain in back on left side.

Causations - Grief. Suppressions.

Chest - Pain about and under short ribs.

Head - Reading and writing aggravates pain in forehead.

Lungs - Deep inspiration or inhaling moderately cool air aggravates.

Modalities - Soreness of ischium worse from touch. Worse motion, mental exertion, at dinner, at night.

Stomach - Drinking cold water relieves gastric symptoms.

COMMENTS - Hale quoted Rafinesque as saying that the analysis of Lob-s. shows it to contain silex, iron and muriate and phosphate of lime.

The marked action of Lob-s. on the posterior sinuses led Cooper to use it with success in cases of deafness arising from an "unhealthy, soft, swollen, easily bleeding catarrhal" condition of the nose-pharynx. This is emphasized by another symptom: "Dull aching pain in center of forehead, over root of nose."

Cooper, who used an acetic preparation, considered that with this, as well as with the Inflata, a history of suppression is a leading indication. There are many notable symptoms in the back, back of chest and about the lower ribs.

Some of these led Jeanes (the first prover) to make a very fine cure of melancholia in an educated intelligent man. "Great depression of spirits, unhappy state of mind, always associated with pain about and under short ribs in back on left side, extending outward nearly to left side, posterior aspect of region of spleen."

Pain on inside of right scapula. Farrington added, "Pain under (not below) inner border of left scapula, worse after weeping." Pain in right maxillary joint with pain in middle of right lung, breast, larynx, left side of chest near axilla with aching in left shoulder and arm.

Pains travel about, from right to left, from left tonsil to right, from back down legs, from eighth rib downward, aching from back of head down nape.

RELATIONS - ***Compare:*** (1) Other lobelias. (2) Puls. - mental depression and weeping. (3) Chel. and Ran-b. - scapular pains. (4) Hydr. - post-nasal catarrh. (5) Cean. - spleen. (6) Lob. has one-sided coating of tongue. Lob-s. has left half of palate dry. (7) Podo. relieved the diarrhea of Lob. s., but not the acute abdominal pains.

REFERENCES - Clarke.

LOLIUM TEMULENTUM

(Darnel)

PHARMACY - lol. Lolium temulentum. Darnel. Loleum temulentum. N. O. Graminee. Tincture of ripe spikelets. Tincture of ripe seeds. Trituration of the dried seeds. ***Historical dose:*** Tincture, trituration and all potencies.

CLINICAL - Convulsions. Delirium tremens. Paralysis. Parkinson's disease. Tremor. Writer's cramp.

HOMEOPATHIC - The name Darnel means "stupefied," and the plant's evil reputation is of very ancient date. The symptoms are the result of observations made on persons poisoned by eating a meal containing an admixture of Lolium tem.

Allen mentioned an assertion that Lolium is much infested with ergot and that it is to this that the poisoning symptoms are due, the unaffected grain being inert. Allen noted in support of this that the poisonings have been most frequently observed in low, wet districts and during wet seasons.

Tightness in the calves, violent pain in the calves as if bound with cords. This tightness affects the rest of the legs in less degree. Writer's cramp. Paralytic conditions. Tremors and convulsions, Parkinson's disease.

Nausea and vomiting of the bread containing it and mucus with it. Cold rigors internal chilliness, cold sweat. Delirium tremens. Prostration and restlessness. An Italian physician, Fantoni, tried it in headaches and meningitis.

Bonino cured a carpenter, ,29, who had trembling of the for hands eleven years, worse in the morning. The legs had also begun to tremble. His father and brother were similarly affected. Merc-v. and Agar. only relieved temporarily. Lol. cured.

MIND - Anxiety and general uneasiness. Depressed. Comprehension slow and difficult, distracted, confusion and stupefaction. Difficult speech. Mania. Slight delirium.

Ears - Noises in ears.

Head - Head feels heavy.

Limbs - Cold limbs. Gait unsteady. ***Trembling of all limbs***, cannot write, cannot hold a glass of water. Spasms of arms and legs. Violent pain in calves, as if bound by a cord.

Modalities - Worse damp, wet season.

Mouth - Tongue tremulous. Speech difficult, cannot pronounce the whole word.

Rectum - Severe purging.

Stomach - Nausea, vomiting.

Temperature - Cold rigors, especially in limbs.

Vertigo - Vertigo, must close eyes.

COMMENTS - Anshutz stated, "The use of the drug by Dr. Bonino was truly homeopathic for the short proving of it. Allen Encyclopedia reports trembling of the limbs and hand so great that 'he could not hold a glass of water.'

"A carpenter aged twenty-nine years, had been suffering ever since his eighteenth year of trembling in both hands, especially in the morning of late also his legs began to tremble. It is remarkable that both his father and his brother were subject to the same ailment, while no definite cause could be indicated.

"He was first given Mercurius, then Agaricus, which brought a partial but only transitory improvement. Finally Bonino prescribed Lol., which in a short time effected a cure."

Dr. Mossa commented that the pathogenic effects of this remedy which has not yet been proved at all are only known to some degree from its effects when it has been mixed with grain and baked into bread.

Lol. has caused chest troubles, vertigo (hence the name darnel-grass in German Taumellolch), trembling, paralysis with anguish and distress, vomiting, failing of the memory, blindness, headache, epileptic attacks, deep sleep and insanity.

RELATIONS - ***Compare:*** (1) Anan., Sec. (2) Lath. - paralysis, worse wet seasons. (3) Op. - sleep.

REFERENCES - Anshutz. Clarke.

LOMATIUM DISSECTUM

(Indian Carrot)

PHARMACY - lom-d. Lomatium dissectum. Indian carrot. Biscuit-root. N. O. Apiaceae. Tincture of fresh plant. ***Historical dose:*** Tincture and all potencies.

CLINICAL - AIDS. Bacterial, infections. ***Bronchitis.*** Candida. Chronic fatigue. Colds. Hepatitis. Herpes. HIV. Immune, weakness. ***Influenza. Lung, disorders. Pneumonia.*** Sinusitis. Sores. Tuberculosis. Viral, infections. Wounds.

HERBAL - Botanists named it Leptotaenia dissecta until 1942 when it was renamed Lomatium dissectum, a slightly different classification. One of the many Lomatium species is often called "Biscuit-root", as the pulp was pounded into cakes. Its large taproot and its kinship with common carrots, also gave it the name "Indian Carrot."

The root of the Lomatium dissectum plant is a natural medicine with extensive traditional use by the Native Americans of the Pacific Northwest and Northern Nevada where it grows. It was used primarily for upper respiratory infections, colds, and influenza although a great many other uses have been noted.

Anti-microbial especially in the lungs and upper respiratory tract. Traditionally used to treat all cases of colds and flus. It can be employed for quick acting relief in all cases of viral or bacterial infection, particularly where there is a large amount of thick or sticky mucus and where infection is deep seated and persistent. Specific for pneumonia, infective bronchitis and tuberculosis. Some research has indicated a greater activity against gram positive bacteria.

Its action of limiting infection makes Lomatium valuable as a mouth wash and gargle for oral and throat infections, as a douche for bacterial and viral infections as well as for Candida, as a skin wash for infected cuts or wounds, and in many other 'first aid' situations.

The anti-viral and anti-bacterial properties of Lomatium dissectum have attracted the interest of herbalists and Naturopathic physicians who are utilizing it in the treatment of today's most difficult viral diseases. It may be part of a protocol in the treatment of Hepatitis-C, Influenza, HIV, AIDS, Chronic-fatigue, Pneumonia, Bronchitis, Herpes simplex, Sinusitis, and common Colds.

COMMENTS - When the influenza epidemic hit Northern Nevada in 1918, Ernst Krebs MD of Carson City was surprised to see the local Washoe people recovering, and he inquired as to their medicine. They called it "Toh-sa" or "Do-sa". Dr. Krebs called it Balsamea, due to its biting odor of balsamic resins.

The Indians gather this root in the late fall, November being considered the proper month for gathering. The root is used in the fresh or dry state. It is cut up and a decoction is made by boiling the root in water, skimming off the top and giving large doses of the broth. A pound of root is considered about the proper dose to treat a case of fever for three days, which is the longest time needed to break up a fever due to influenza or a pulmonary disease, although the Washoes used it as a panacea.

Whether a coincidence or not, there was not a single death in the Washoe tribe from influenza or its complications, although Indians living in other parts of the State where the root did not grow died in numbers. It was such a remarkable coincidence that the root was investigated by a practicing physician who saw apparently hopeless cases recover without any other medication or care of any kind.

A preparation was prepared and employed in a great many cases among the whites, from the mildest to the most virulent types of influenza, and it proved, among other things, that it is the nearest approach we have today to a specific in epidemic influenza and the accompanying pneumonia. Where used early it proved itself to be a reliable agent in preventing pulmonary complications.

Other physicians were induced to give it a trial, with the same results. It is beyond the experimental stage, as its therapeutic action in this direction is established and beyond any doubt. The cases in which it has been used run into the hundreds. There is probably no therapeutic agent so valuable in the treatment of influenzal pneumonia and, as far as being tried, in ordinary lobar pneumonia if started early.

REFERENCES - Krebs. Murphy.

LONICERA PERICLYMENUM

(Wild Honeysuckle)

PHARMACY - lon-p. Lonicera periclymenum. Wild honeysuckle. European honeysuckle. Serotina. Woodbine. Goats' leaf. N. O. Caprifoliacee. Tincture of fresh plant. ***Historical dose:*** Tincture and all potencies.

CLINICAL - Anger. Asthma. Constipation. Dyspnea. Fevers. Hiccoughs. Irritability. ***Lung, disorders.*** Mouth, ulcers. Spasms. Ulcers. Vomiting.

HERBAL - The plant has expectorant and laxative properties. A syrup made from the flowers has been used in the treatment of respiratory diseases, shortness of breath and asthma. A decoction of the leaves is considered beneficial in treating diseases of the liver and spleen. It is used as a mouthwash for ulcers and is considered to be a good ingredient in gargles.

The flowers are antispasmodic, astringent, diuretic, expectorant, febrifuge and sudorific. The fruit is emetic and cathartic. The herbage is used as a cutaneous and mucus tonic and as a vulnerary. It is also diaphoretic. The leaves are laxative and slightly astringent. The seed is diuretic. The bark is anti-catarrhal, depurative, diuretic and sudorific.

HOMEOPATHIC - Cooper cured with Lon-p. irritability of temper with violent outbursts and has seen it produce the same (Croc.).

RELATIONS - ***Compare:*** (1) Lon-x., Vib., Op. Samb., Sym-r. (2) Nux-v., Staph., Hyos., Croc. - outbursts of temper.

REFERENCES - Clarke.

LONICERA XYLOSTEUM

(Fly Woodbine)

PHARMACY - lon-x. Lonicera xylosteum. Fly woodbine. N. O. Caprifoliacee. Trituration or tincture of berries. ***Historical dose:*** Tincture, trituration and all potencies, third to sixth potency.

CLINICAL - Albuminuria. Coma vigil. Convulsions. Syphilis. Uremia. Vomiting.

HOMEOPATHIC - Lon-x. is known from the effect of poisoning by its berries. Trembling and jerking of the limbs, violent convulsions. Abdomen retracted, especially in umbilical region. Vomiting and purging. Uremic convulsions. Albuminuria.

Syphilis. Contraction of one pupil and dilatation of the other. Seemed neither to hear nor see, unable to make answer. When raised from bed, limbs and head fall over as if paralyzed. Coma.

MIND - Dullness of the mind. Stupefaction. Coma.

Abdomen - Abdomen retracted, especially in umbilical region, soft. Violent colic.

Eyes - Contraction of one pupil and dilatation of the other. Pupils dilated. Conjunctiva red. Everything foggy and indistinct to vision for half an hour. Photophobia.

Face - Red face. Pale. Lips dry.

Food - Excessive thirst.

Head - Congestion of head and chest.

Heart - Violent impulse of heart. Pulse slow, small, soft, irregular.

Limbs - Jerking of limbs. Trembling of whole body. Violent convulsions. Limbs and head fall over as if paralyzed. Limbs cold.

Lungs - Respiration rapid and deep.

Mouth - Tongue moist, coated with mucus.

Rectum - Bloody stools.

Sleep - Sleepy. Constant deep sleep with half-open eyes, red face. Coma.

Stomach - Profuse vomiting, and purging.

Temperature - Limbs are cold. Profuse, cold perspiration. Fever.

RELATIONS - ***Compare:*** (1) Lon-p. (2) Dig. - slow pulse. (3) Cadm-s. and Rhod. one pupil contracted, the other dilated.

REFERENCES - Boericke. Clarke.

LOXOSCELES RECLUSA

(Brown Recluse Spider)

PHARMACY - loxo-r. Loxosceles reclusa. Brown recluse spider. Loxoscelidae. ***Historical dose:*** All potencies.

CLINICAL - Abscess. Alcoholism. Anorexia. Aphthae. Backache. Belching. ***Bites.*** Chronic fatigue syndrome. Cold, sores. Constipation. Coryza. Coughs. Depression. Diarrhea. Dyslexia. Ecchymosis. ***Erythema.*** Fibromyalgia. Gangrene. Headaches. Heartburn. Hoarseness. Incontinence. Insomnia. Leucorrhea. Nausea. Palpitations. Rheumatism. Sciatica. Suicidal. ***Ulcers.*** Warts. ***Wounds.***

HOMEOPATHIC - The victim is often not aware of the spider bite until two to six hours later, unless, and this is rarely the case, he witnesses the spider in the act. The first symptoms after the bite include a stinging sensation with mild to intense pain. The immediate local effects of envenomation are a transient erythema, which produces a dusky or mottled appearance to the skin. Sometimes a blister quickly follows.

During the first several hours the dusky hue expands, traveling downward from the site of the bite, along the forces of gravity. The pathologic process is fully established within six hours, and within 24 hours the area where necrosis is taking place is indeed striking.

The zone of erythema is replaced by violaceous discoloration, and subsequently an irregular zone of necrosis develops ranging in measurement from a few centimeters to more than 30 cm.

Aseptic necrosis proceeds to dry gangrenous slough and black eschar formation. Open ulcers form as the necrotic area breaks away from surrounding healthy tissue. Thus the venom diffuses through subcutaneous tissue until the supply is exhausted. In some cases it extends through the fascia, exposing the underlying muscles.

Healing of such ulcerous wounds can require months, and often a sunken scar endures. If the quantity of venom is small, no necrosis occurs and only the local erythema appears.

MIND - Cries easily. Oversensitive. Sentimental. Sighing. Forsaken feeling. Despair of recovery, in morning on waking. Sadness, despondency, depression, melancholy. Silent grief. Morbid thoughts. Suicidal depression. Thoughts of throwing himself from a height, hanging. Anxiety from pains.

Apathy. Awkwardness. Mental prostration. Forgetfulness. Memory weakness. Concentration difficult. Spaced-out feeling. Confusion. Lost conception of time. Tendency to lose things. Mistakes in spelling, time, writing words.

Industrious, mania for work. Conscientious about trifles. Reproachful. Indisposed to talk, desire to be silent, taciturn. Lack of self-confidence. Easily offended. Obstinate, headstrong. Rude. Rage, fury. Anger, alternating with quick repentance. Fear of dark, animals, bats.

Abdomen - Distension. Tingling. Cramping pain. Pains, better bending double.

Back - Backache, worse lumbar region. Numbness. Stiffness in neck and back.

Bladder - Incontinence in bed, at night. Urine bright yellow, strong odor, scanty.

Breasts - Stitching pain. Sore and bruised pain.

Coughs - Dry coughs. Coughs from mucus in throat.

Ears - Sharp, shooting pains. Noises in ears, hissing and ringing. Hears high-pitched noises.

Eyes - Ecchymosis. Pupils dilated. Yellow eyes. Bloodshot eyes in the morning. Burning pains.

Female - Menses frequent, too early, too late. Leucorrhea yellow, greenish. Pain in right ovary. Sexual desire increased.

Food - Desires eggs, meat, onions, tea, sweets, ice cream, sour foods. Aversion to seafood, spicy foods.

Head - Headaches, throbbing and pulsating. Frontal headaches, with burning, pressure in the eyes. Constricted feeling. Tingling.

Heart - Pulse frequent, accelerated. Palpitations after frightening dream.

Limbs - Joint pains, aching, cutting and burning. Shoulder pain and stiffness. Neuralgic pains. Sciatica, better walking. Numbness, insensibility. Tingling. Warts on feet.

Lungs - Accelerated breathing.

Modalities - Better at night. Bathing, better washing. Worse evening, morning on waking.

Mouth - Dry, cracked and fissured. Aphthae, on lips. Cold sores. Abscess of gums.

Nose - Coryza. Clear discharges. Acute sense of smell.

Rectum - Formication, burning in anus. Constipation. Diarrhea in morning, driving out of bed.

Sensation - Alternating heat sensation with cold. Body feels heavy. Emptiness, hollow sensation right side of body.

Skin - Cracks, fissures. Warts.

Sleep - Sleeplessness after waking.

Stomach - Emptiness, weak feeling. Faintness, goneness, hungry feeling. Stomach cramps. Heartburn. Belching. Nausea.

Stools - Stools acrid, corrosive, excoriating, bloody. Stools light-colored, yellow.

Throat - Sore throat. Hoarseness. Sensation of phlegm in throat.

RELATIONS - ***Compare:*** Tarent., Tarent-h., Lat-m.

REFERENCES - Klein.

LUFFA OPERCULATA

PHARMACY - luf-op. Luffa operculata. Esponjilla. Cabacinha. N.O. Cucurbitaceae. Columbia. South America. Tincture of the dried seeds. ***Historical dose:*** Tincture and all potencies.

CLINICAL - Asthma. Breathlessness. Bronchial, asthma. Coryza. Emaciation. Headaches. Laryngitis. Nasal polyps. Pharyngitis. Rhinitis. Sinusitis. Tachycardia.

HOMEOPATHIC - Luf-op. is an exotic plant which comes from Columbia and was introduced to Europe by W. Schwabe. The symptomatology was undertaken by him on eleven people (six men and five women), using the 5x, 3x, and 2x potencies. Each potency was used for one week.

Lassitude and physical fatigue. Frontal and occipital headache. Acute or chronic inflammation of the mucus membranes in the nasal cavities. Hypertrophy or atrophy of the nasal mucus membranes. Hypothyroid.

MIND - Lack of reaction with indifference and prostration.

Eyes - Musca volitantes.

Food - Extreme hunger with emaciation. Painful feeling of thirst and hunger, difficult to satisfy.

Head - Violent headaches going from the forehead towards the nape of the neck. Pain in the occipital region. Frontal pains with vertigo and musca volitantes.

Heart - Tachycardia.

Lungs - Breathlessness from the least effort. Bronchial asthma.

Modalities - Better in fresh air, worse in a room in dry air.

Mouth - Dryness of the tongue, back of the throat and pharynx. Burning sensation at the tip of the tongue.

Nose - Acute rhinitis and pharyngitis. Purulent sinusitis. Chronic atrophic rhinitis. Head colds with pale or yellow nasal secretion, especially in the morning. Dryness of the nasal mucus with sticky scab formations. Nasal polyps.

Rectum - Tendency to constipation.

Skin - Formation of small purulent, itching pimples on the face, lower lip and chin. Loses hair in abundance.

Stomach - Diffuse gastric pains. Empty feeling in the stomach.

RELATIONS - ***Compare:*** (1) Merc-i-r. - Coryza with hoarseness. Abundant discharge with post-nasal mucus, aggravated in the open air, ameliorated by heat. (2) Cinnb. - Pressing pains in the bones of the skull and nose with discharge of thick mucus and often nosebleed. (3) Hep. - Sour, fetid secretions with blocked nose immediately on going out into the cold air. Ameliorated in a warm room.

REFERENCES - Julian.

LUNA
(Moonlight)

PHARMACY - luna. Luna. Moonlight. Moon's rays. Sugar of milk is exposed on a glass plate to the moon's rays and stirred with a glass rod meanwhile. The sugar of milk so charged is dynamized in the usual way (Fincke). Higgins made a preparation by exposing pure water to the moon's rays for three or four hours in South America and then dynamizing the water so charged. ***Historical dose:*** All potencies.

CLINICAL - Acidity. Colic. Edema. ***Epilepsy.*** Female, disorders. Headaches. Heartburn. Inter-menstrual flow. Insomnia. Menses, problems. ***Nightmares.*** Ovary, pain. Scabies. ***Sleep, disorders.*** Sleepwalking. ***Somnambulism.*** Sycosis. ***Worms.***

HOMEOPATHIC - Goullon contributed to the Rev. Hom. Belge, January, 1897, a notable article on "The Influence of the Moon on the Human Organism," in which he mentioned, among other interesting facts, that sleepwalking is a lunar effect, that worm disorders are most troublesome at the full noon, and that goiter changes more or less with the moon.

Epilepsy worse at full moon may need Luna (Sil.). Scabies and worm disorders, worse at full moon. Nervous affections, especially in subjects of sycosis, influenced by the moon.

Excessive edema of face, neck and hands with neuralgic pains in the swollen parts. Skin diseases. Sour belchings, especially if tasting of ingesta. Acrid yellow leucorrhea through the day with backache. Pain in right ovary.

MIND - Mental faculties, especially ability to receive, retain and express ideas, are most powerfully affected by the full rays of the moon. ***Worse from exposure to moonlight.*** Worse from certain moon phases. Worse the day before the full moon. ***Ailments from full moon.***

Confusion of mind. Difficult concentration. Absent-minded. Forgetful. Mistakes in spelling, talking. Mind not clear. ***Spaced-out feeling.*** Feeling ***detached***, disconnected. Apathy, lack of motivation. Disinclined for mental or physical labor. ***Somnambulism.***

Mood changeable, worse before and during menses. Sensitive, emotionally. Depressed and anxious. Dwells on past disagreeable occurrences (Nat-m.). Irritable and impatient, easily angered, worse before menses.

Abrupt. Anger, in outbursts. Temper tantrums. Resentment, indifferent towards husband or partner. Irritable towards own children. Weeping after anger. Irritability on being spoken to. Wants to be let alone.

Abdomen - Faint feeling in stomach on awaking. Sensation of great distention. Colic, commencing two inches above umbilicus and seeming to pass directly upward to stomach, causing desire to bend forward. Pain around umbilicus, better by belchings. Pain through liver and spleen, worse 3 p.m.

Back - Very severe pain in sacral region in evening.

Chest - After ascending stairs, a peculiar heating sensation, beginning at lower extremity of sternum and extending outwards. Attachment of diaphragm on each side to a point under each arm, at same time warm glow down arms to fingertips, most in left.

Eyes - Swollen eyes that burn and sting (Apis). Sharp stinging sensation, leaving a smarting. ***Stinging in right eye.*** Weakness of eyes and feeling of sand. Swelling of eyelids and profuse discharge of purulent matter with a painful smarting and profuse lachrymation without heat or change of color.

Face - Edema of face.

Female - Menstrual cramps with bearing down pains. Menses less free, strings of dark blood, colic pain above umbilicus better by eructation. ***Menses flow heavier.*** Menses returned two days after ceasing. Uterine hemorrhage. Bearing-down sensation. Sharp pain left side vagina, then grows suddenly sharper, again returning to vagina and passing through to rectum. Sharp pains fly from vagina through abdomen, ceasing in stomach-pit. Pain better by passing flatus from vagina. Cramp-like pains in pelvic region, as if uterus were being contracted by a strong electric current.

Food - No appetite, slight nausea. Desires something, does not know what. Immediately ejected cup of tea during headache, the tea tasted sour.

Head - Slight giddiness with slight bitter taste on left side of tongue with increased saliva. Sharp pain just above root of nose. Congestion of blood to head with sensation of great fullness. ***Migraine headaches.*** Pain in occiput, changing to lame feeling on retiring. ***Headache before menses.*** Woke with very severe headache. Headache better by magnetic passes. Severe frontal headache during menses.

Heart - Pulse rapid. Suffocative sensation around heart. On retching, peculiar feeling around heart as though it stopped beating, better by belchings, worse by lying down.

Kidneys - Urine profuse, clear and watery, at times darker.

Limbs - Swollen feeling. Slight rheumatic pains in shoulders, especially left. Sharp, quick pain in left cervical nerve, intermittent every few seconds. Great lameness in anterior tibial region from walking. After retiring, aching in bones of lower limbs with pain in lumbo-sacral region. Sensation as if tightly bound in right calf and in hypochondria. Pain like growing-pain above left knee, better walking. Sharp pain in left great toe.

Modalities - Better by cold application. Pains, better in open air, belchings and by passing flatus from vagina. ***Worse before and after full moon, during increasing moon, exposure to moonlight.*** Worse after sleep, from milk.

Mouth - Bitter taste on the left side of tongue with increased flow of saliva. Increased saliva, all day, on waking, with faint feeling in stomach, with stinging in right eye.

Nose - Sensation of a cold in head. Coryza, sneezing and pain in occiput. Discharge of yellowish-green mucus from nose. Sensation of heavy cold in head with lachrymation, at 4 p.m.

Rectum - Urgent desire for stool, immediately better by passing flatus.

Skin - Unbearable itching. Stinging, itching right side of body as if an insect was biting the parts, felt most on foot, leg and forearm. Eczema.

Sleep - ***Insomnia***, worse moonlight. ***Somnambulism. Nightmares after exposure to moonlight***, particularly in children. Dreams of murder, death. Wakes after frightful dreams. Symptoms worse on waking. Felt as if had not slept enough.

Stomach - Burning, worse after drinking milk. Flatulency with burning in stomach. Sour belchings, tasting of ingesta. Woke at midnight with severe heartburn and great distress in stomach, had to get out of bed.

Temperature - Woke 6 a.m. with severe chill, after which he had headache, felt sick and weak all day, at night had horrible dreams of death.

Throat - Some soreness in throat.

COMMENTS - Conditions affected by the moon, particularly epilepsy, migraine headaches, insomnia, emotional and hormonal changes, neuralgic pains, and swelling of the hands and face. Conditions worse during full moon (Calc., Sil., Arg-n.). Dreams and nightmares, particularly in children. Dreams of dying. Irritable, unclear mind.

Increased worm activity. Growing pains in children, better walking. Swollen eyes that burn and sting (Apis). Sensation of sand or grit in the eyes (Euphr.). Pain in the occiput. Menstrual cramps with bearing down pains. Symptoms better in open air and cool air. Worse from sleep, milk.

According to Menuret, skin diseases are frequently influenced by the moon. He noted a case of eczematous affection which increased with each waning moon and was at its maximum intensity at the new moon when it covered the whole face and chest and was accompanied by unbearable itching. Then there was gradual improvement and the face became smooth, but scarcely had the full moon passed when all began again.

Moritz Hoffmann observed a young girl (daughter of an epileptic mother) whose whole body became swollen at every new moon, the swelling disappearing as the moon waned.

Mead told of a child who was subject to convulsions at each waning moon. Gale remarked that with weakly persons' excitability is most pronounced at the new moon and the full moon.

Swan communicated a proving of Luna 1,000c. made on a female physician, Dr. S. J. W. The prover was menstruating at the time the proving was commenced, but was otherwise in good health. Repeated doses were taken for two days. The effects lasted four weeks. Swan cured, with Luna, a case of excessive edema of face, neck and hands with neuralgic pain in the swollen parts.

Goullon quoted a remarkable case of sleep-walking from the Cercle Medical. "A youth of fifteen in good health in other respects, had been withdrawn from his apprenticeship, on account of his nightly promenades on roofs. He was put in a private asylum. Although his room was oriented so that no actual moon-rays could reach it, the moon nevertheless exercised a potent influence upon him.

"As soon as it reaches the horizon he gets out of bed and carefully with closed eyes, moves towards a window, so high that he has to jump in order to reach and open it. As it is barricaded with an iron trellis he gets down and, crossing the corridor, goes to the outer door, above which is a window.

"With cat-like agility he climbs up to this, when he is seized by three warders, who take him back to his room, where, only after the moon has set, can he lie down and go to sleep. In the morning he remembers nothing. At full moon the symptoms are still more extraordinary."

RELATIONS - ***Compare:*** (1) Aeth., Mag-c. - worse from milk. (2) Worse at new moon: Alum., Am-c., Bufo, Calc., Caust., Clem., Cupr., Daph., Lyc., Sabal., Sep., Sil. (3) Worse at full moon: Alum., Calc., Cycl., Graph., Kali-n., Nat-c., Nat-m., Sabin., Sep., Sil., Spon., Sulph., Teucr. (4) Worse during ***increasing moon***: Arn., Clem. (5) Worse during waning moon - Dulc., Thuj.

REFERENCES - Clarke. Murphy. Swan.

LUPULUS HUMULUS

(Hops)

PHARMACY - lup. Lupulus humulus. Hops. N. O. Cannabinacae of the Urticacee. Tincture of the seeded spikes. Trituration. Tincture of Lupuline, small resinous granules covering the scales. ***Historical dose:*** Tincture and all potencies.

CLINICAL - Alcoholism. Delirium. Diuresis. Dyspepsia. Dysuria. Excitement. Faintness. Gonorrhea. Headaches. ***Insomnia. Jaundice.*** Nausea. Paralytic, weakness. ***Sexual, weakness.*** Vertigo. Vomiting.

HERBAL - The "hops pillow" as a remedy for sleeplessness is well known, and this sleep provoking effect passes into delirium and stupefaction.

HOMEOPATHIC - Lup. has had a somewhat extensive proving, to the symptoms of which have been added the effects of working with hops and of sleeping in rooms where hops were stored.

Giddiness and stupefaction. Drawing and twitching in almost every muscle. Nervous tremors, wakefulness and delirium of alcoholics. Unstrung condition of the nervous system attended with nausea, dizziness, headache following a night's debauch. ***Infantile jaundice***. Urethral burning. ***Slow pulse***.

MIND - Morbid vigilance. Highly excited. Confusion. Frequent starting from deep sleep with violent delirium from which he could only be aroused with great difficulty, immediately lapsing again into stupor. Delirium of alcoholics. Mental functions remained indolent several months.

Abdomen - Fermentation and dull pains in abdomen. Dull griping in lower abdomen with nausea.

Eyes - Pupils remained dilated for several months.

Female - Diminishes and allays sexual appetite.

Food - Appetite lost. Great thirst.

Head - Dull, heavy headache with dizziness. Rush of blood to head and eyes. Heat in head and face with confusion and dull headache. Violent pulsating of temporal arteries. Drawing and twitching in every muscle.

Heart - Slow pulse.

Kidneys - Diuresis. Urine retarded, dark brown, clear. Burning in urethra during urination, not better by coffee.

Limbs - Great twitching of tendons. Paralytic weakness.

Lungs - Respiration is deep, almost stertorous.

Male - Diminishes and allays sexual appetite. Painful erections. Emissions, depending on ***sexual weakness and after onanism***. Spermatorrhea.

Neck - Strong pulsation of carotids.

Perspiration - Perspiration profuse, clammy, greasy.

Rectum - Stool softer than usual with urging so great he could hardly reach the closet. Stool retarded.

Skin - Scarlatina-like eruption on face. Feels like insects crawling under skin, feels chapped, skin peels.

Sleep - ***Drowsy*** during the day. Sopor. ***Insomnia.***

Stomach - Sensation of increased warmth in stomach. Nauseating eructations, tasting of hops. Nausea, vomiting.

Tongue - Tongue thickly coated, dry.

Vertigo - Vertigo, stupefaction.

COMMENTS - A child of twelve, who remained several days in a room where hops were being picked, experienced frequent starting up from deep sleep with violent delirium from which he could only be aroused with great difficulty, when he recognized the bystanders, but immediately fell backward into stupor.

It was months before he recovered. The effects which remained included dilated pupils, mental indolence, unsteady movements, and erythema.

Other symptoms are a turning sensation in stomach, fermenting in abdomen. Burning in urethra during urination. Nausea and vomiting. Faintness better in open air. Twitching of tendons.

RELATIONS - ***Antidotes:*** Coff., vinegar. ***Compare:*** (1) Urt-u., Cann-i., Cann-s., Nux-v., Op.

REFERENCES - Boericke. Clarke.

LYCIUM BARBARUM

(Goji Berries)

PHARMACY - lyci-b. Lycium barbarum. Goji berries. Chinese wolfberry. English wolfberry. Matrimony vine. Chinese boxthorn. N. O. Solanaceae. ***Historical dose:*** Tincture and all potencies.

CLINICAL - Anemia. Arthritis. Cancer. Cough. Diabetes. Nosebleeds.

HERBAL - The term "Goji" is the common name given to the Lycium barbarum berry by the Tibetans. Goji usually refers to varieties of Lycium called in English wolfberry, matrimony vine, or Chinese boxthorn.

The berries flourish in the tranquil valleys that are naturally protected by the Himalayan Mountains, and have been treasured for centuries by the Himalayan people.

Traditionally it has been used to treat inflammations, skin irritations, nosebleeds and aches and pains, and has also been used as a sedative. The fruit is the main source of medicinal extracts, although the leaves are also sometimes consumed as food.

In China, it is often used in combination with other botanicals to treat poor vision, anemia, and cough. In the tests, a polysaccharide isolated from Lycium has been shown to have anti-cancer effects. It also has some immune enhancing properties.

COMMENTS - An evergreen shrub that is often spiny and grows in temperate and subtropical regions, the two species most commonly used in folk medicine are Lycium chinense or Lycium barbarum, both in the nightshade (Solanaceae) family.

One legend recounts that during the Tang Dynasty (around 800 AD), a well had been dug beside a wall near a famous Buddhist temple that was covered with goji vines. Over the years, countless berries had fallen into the well.

Those who prayed there had the ruddy complexion of good health, and even at the age of eighty they had no white hair and had lost no teeth, simply because they drank the water from the well.

RELATIONS - ***Compare:*** (1) Crat., Sabal serr.

REFERENCES - Murphy.

LYCOPERSICUM ESCULENTUM

(Tomato)

PHARMACY - lycpr. Lycopersicum esculentum. Tomato. Solanum lycopersicum. Love apple. N. O. Solanaceae. Tincture of ripe fruit. Tincture of fresh flowering plant. ***Historical dose:*** Tincture and all potencies.

CLINICAL - Backache. Catarrh. Coryza. Deltoid rheumatism. Diabetes. Diarrhea. Eyes disorders. Gout. Headache. Leucorrhea. Lupus. Metrorrhagia. Obesity. Polyuria. Rheumatism. Throat sore.

HOMEOPATHIC - Clarke knew of one instance in which the slightest indulgence in tomatoes brings on an attack of gout. Cooper commended the use of tomatoes in cases of obesity. Cooper gave Lycpr. in a case of rodent ulcer and caused sharp pain and temporary spread of the disease.

Coryza, worse out of doors (All-c., better out of doors). Polyuria, with great thirst. Diabetes. Marked action on deltoid and pectoral muscles, pain is better lifting arm upward and outward. Pains leave after influenza. Right side principally affected, symptoms proceed from right to left.

MIND - Peevish about trifles. Very irritable, noises greatly annoy. Unusually mentally active for short periods, followed by longer periods of mental dullness. Weak memory, forgetful. Thoughts disappear, worse when leaning head against anything. Cannot keep mind fixed on work.

Abdomen - Great flatulency of abdomen.

Back - Cannot get into a comfortable position. Backache in lumbar region, making them gloomy and depressed. Rheumatic pain near attachment of trapezius muscle to spine. Heavy dragging in right scapula.

Breasts - Sore and tender scirrhous breast.

Chest - Slight sticking beneath left side of sternum, without difficulty of respiration. Oppression in chest in lower lobe of right lung.

Eyes - Dull, heavy, ache. Sore and burning. Pupils minutely contracted. Twitching in left inner canthus. Eyes water on close work. Letters run together when reading. Keeps wiping eyes to see clearly. Light painful. Lids feel heavy and swollen.

Face - Face flushed, pale. Pressure in right or left zygoma.

Female - Profuse leucorrheal discharge. Too frequent menstruation, brought on by free use of canned tomatoes, the flow would return whenever this food was eaten for a few meals.

Head - Intense throbbing, bursting headache. Bursting pain in head, especially vertex and when coughing. Dull, heavy pain in occiput. Headache in the occiput, spreads all over the head and settles with great violence in temples, worse tobacco smoke.

Heart - Fine, stitching pains at base of heart. Lame pain in region of heart. Pulse 100, full and flowing.

Kidneys - Increase of watery constituents of urine, not of total solids. Must rise at night to urinate. Constant debility when in open air, not at all in warm room.

Limbs - Intense aching, rheumatic pain in muscles of all limbs. Lame, tired feeling in all limbs with great exhaustion. Intense aching pain in lower limbs. Sharp sticking pain along course of right crural nerve. Painful sticking behind articulation of left hip. Sharp pain in right deltoid and pectoral muscles, worse lifting arm upward and outward. Lameness of left wrist, hand and fingers, where it is painful even when not moving it.

Lungs - Coughs are deep, harsh, starting from irritation in lower chest. Explosive cough. Dry, hacking cough coming on at night and keeping him awake. Expectoration white and in lumps, early in morning.

Modalities - Better in warm room, from external heat. The headache in one instance was completely better by tobacco smoke. Worse by noise, motion.

Mouth - Itching and tickling in roof of mouth. Tongue coated thick, yellow, white, more in center. Foul breath, taste.

Nose - Stopped catarrh. Profuse watery coryza excoriating ale, drops down posterior sinuses, salty taste, markedly worse out of doors.

Skin - Erythematous lupus much relieved (Cooper).

Sleep - Unable to fall asleep in evening tosses about, every position uncomfortable. Very restless sleep. Frequent waking and tossing, limbs when pressed feel paralyzed. Confused, disagreeable dreams. Wakened by insignificant dreams.

Stomach - Thirst for large quantities of water. Violent belchings of gas with taste of food. Great flatulency between 10 a.m. and 11:30. Burning sensation in stomach towards evening and during evening.

Stool - Brownish, watery diarrhea, yellow, frothy, no urging, painless.

Temperature - Chilliness towards night, preceded by thirst for large quantities of water. Chilliness and sweat. Sweat on awaking confined to a strip about four inches wide along whole length of back. Temperature from 100.5° to 101°F.

Throat - The throat slightly sore on swallowing. Mucus membrane of pharynx pale, tip of uvula and arches of pharynx red and inflamed. Burning raw feeling right side of throat, changing to left. Swelling of left tonsil. Constant desire to clear throat. Husky voice. Hoarseness with constant tickling in pit of throat. Hoarseness towards night.

Vertigo - Giddiness, with inclination to faint on attempting to walk.

COMMENTS - Gross made a proving of Lycpr., noting peevishness and loss of memory, sticking and pressing pains, a sense of paralysis, pressing and boring pains in head, and stopped catarrh. Some women cannot eat tomatoes without getting backache, leucorrhea or metrorrhagia.

In Gross's proving, the headache was worse in evening, she was obliged to rise in the night to urinate. The mind symptoms were worse and the headache better by leaning the head against something.

Dr. Herbert H. Roberts of Derby, Conn., published provings made by himself, two with the 3x and two with the 30x tinctures. "The original tincture was made from the thoroughly ripened fruit, great pains being taken to thoroughly macerate the seeds as well as the pulp." The rheumatic and congestive symptoms were mostly produced by the 3x, the nervous symptoms mostly by the 30x.

Roberts remarked that the natives of Mexico and California eat quantities of the ripe fruit to prevent rheumatism. The right deltoid was very markedly affected and should make Lycpr. a companion to Sang. in shoulder pains.

Headaches were intense and characteristic in some, great soreness remained after the pain had gone.

Dark-complexioned people seem to be suited to its action from two cases recorded by Roberts.

The first case concerned a widow, 50, dark complexion, large, stout, gray eyes. Sudden attack of grip. Very severe aching pains all over, up and down back, limbs, head. Beating, throbbing in head, beginning in occiput, spreading all over head, settling with great violence in temples.

Excruciating pain back of eyes and in balls as if they would burst with the pressure. Light causes pain. Delirium. Severe, deep, racking cough. Thirst for large quantities. Pupils contracted.

Lycpr. 3x every hour cleared away the fever and acute symptoms by the following morning and rapidly cured the remaining cough.

The second case was a man, 40, dark complexion, black hair and eyes, tall, thick-set. Severe bursting, throbbing pain beginning in occiput and settling with great force in temporal and frontal regions, eyes painful, worse from light, pupils contracted. Thirst for large quantities. Temperature 104° F. Pulse full flowing.

Lycpr. 3x every hour given in evening removed the headache before midnight. The next day, the right tonsil was swollen and inflamed, sore on swallowing, feeling of a lump there. Temperature 101°. He recovered rapidly.

RELATIONS - ***Antidoted by:*** Tobacco smoke. ***Compare:*** (1) Bell., Hyos., Dulc., Caps., Sol-t., Sol-n. (2) Ant-t. - weakness of cervical muscles. (3) In coryza, All-c. but All-c. has better open air, Lycpr. worse open air. (4) Contracted pupils, Op. (5) Deltoid rheumatism, Sang. (6) Diabetes, Uran-n. (7) Headache, sore throat, right side, Bell. (8) Headache worse on coughing, worse in open air, Caps.

REFERENCES - Boericke. Clarke. Phatak.

LYCOPODIUM CLAVATUM

(Club Moss)

PHARMACY - lyc. Lycopodium clavatum. Club moss. Muscus terrestris repens. Pes ursinus. Wolf's claw. Lycopodii pollen. N. O. Lycopodiacee. Hilly pastures and heaths in Central and Northern Europe, Russian Asia and North America. Common in Great Britain, especially the North. Its medicinal properties are disclosed by trituration and succussion of the spores. Tincture of fresh plant. Etherial tincture of spores (ether dissolves the spore cases). ***Historical dose:*** All potencies.

CLINICAL - Abdomen, weak. ***Acidity***. Albuminuria. ***Aneurysm.*** Angina pectoris. Aphasia. Asthma. Axilla, perspiration. ***Belching.*** Biliousness. Borborygmi. Bright's, disease. ***Bloating.*** Cachexia. Cancer. Cataract. Colic. ***Colitis.*** Constipation. Corns. Coughs. Cramps. Cystitis. Day-blindness. Debility. ***Diabetes.*** Diarrhea. Diphtheria. Dropsy. Dysentery. ***Dyslexia.*** Dysmenorrhea. Dyspepsia. Ear, eczema. Eczema. ***Emaciation.*** Epithelioma. Excoriation. Eye, inflammation. Face, eruptions. Feet, perspiring. Fibroma. ***Flatulence. Food, allergies. Gallstones.*** Glands, swelling. Goiter. Gout. Gravel. Hematuria. Hair, loss. Hands, chapped. Heartburn. Heart, diseases. ***Hemorrhoids. Hepatitis. Hernia.*** Hypochondriasis. ***Hypoglycemia.*** Hysteria. Impotence. ***Indigestion.*** Influenza. Intermittents. Intertrigo. Jaundice. Labor-pains, abnormal. Lip, cancer. ***Liver, derangement.*** Liver-spots. Locomotor, ataxia. Lumbago. Lungs disorders. ***Malnutrition.*** Menstruation, disorders. Metrorrhagia. Miscarriages. Nosebleeds. Nymphomania. Otorrhea. Panaritium. Paralysis. Parkinson's disease. Peritonitis. Phlegmasia, dolens. Plica polonica. Pneumonia. Polyps. ***Pre-senility***. Proctalgia. Prostatitis. Pylorus, disorders. Quinsy. ***Kidney colic. Kidney, disorders.*** Rheumatism. ***Sciatica.*** Skin, cracks. Sleep, abnormal. Speech, disordered. ***Stage-fright.*** Strains. Sunstroke. Taste, abnormal. Throat, sore. Tongue, coated, cramps. Tuberculosis. Typhoid, fever. Urine, abnormal. Varicose, veins. Warts. Water brash. Whooping cough. Worms. Yawning.

HOMEOPATHIC - The Lycopodiums stand between the mosses and the ferns. Fossils show that in past eras they occupied an important place in the world's vegetation. This remedy is inert until the spores are crushed. The spores from which the potencies are made have been called "vegetable sulphur" (probably on account of their use for producing stage-lightning at theaters).

In the old school the function of Lyc. has dwindled into its use as an "inert" coating for pills and an "inert" powder dusting on excoriated surfaces. Earlier practitioners did not consider it by any means inert.

Lyc. ranks with Sulph. and Calc. in the central trio around which all the rest of the Materia Medica can be grouped. Teste puts Lyc. at the head of a group containing Nat-m., Viol. tric. and Ant-c.

Lycopodium is adapted more especially to gradually developing ailments, functional power weakening with failures of the digestive powers, where the function of the liver is seriously disturbed. Deep seated, progressive chronic diseases. ***Pre-senility***. Cancer. Erectile tumors. Boils, recurring periodically.

Malnutrition, due to ***weakness of digestion***. Affinity for the urinary organs, throat, chest, and ovaries. Symptoms characteristically run from ***right to left***. It acts especially on ***right side*** of body and are ***worse from about 4 p.m. to 8 p.m***. Descending symptoms.

Primary action on digestive organs and adjoining glands, on liver and larger intestines rather than stomach. Aversion to bread, worse from eating bread, fermented foods and fermentable dough. Frequent and painful belchings. Sour belchings, vomiting, distention. Alternate diarrhea and constipation.

Pains come and go suddenly. Oversensitive to pain, patient is beside himself. Sense of internal paralysis. One side of the body hypertrophied at menopause. Atrophy of infants. The patient is thin, withered and ***full of gas and bloating.***

Acidity, sour, taste, belchings. Dropsy, ascites in liver diseases. ***Lithic acid diathesis.*** Kidney affections, with ***red sand in urine***, backache in kidney region, worse before urination. ***Stones, gallstones, gravel.***

Emaciation and debility from loss of fluids, in morning. Marked regulating influence upon the glandular (sebaceous) secretions. Hemorrhages, dark blood. Poor circulation, cold limbs. Lacks vital heat, intolerant of cold drinks, ***craves everything warm.*** Sensitive to noise and odors.

MIND - Failing brain-power (Anac., Bar-c., Kali-p.). ***Weak memory,*** confused thoughts. ***Dyslexia.*** Weakness of memory for names of letters. ***Spells or writes wrong words*** and syllables. Cannot read what he writes. Brain fag after influenza.

Concentration difficult during conversation. ***Confusion in warm room, better walking in open air.*** Confused thoughts. Confused about common words. Hears wrong words and syllables. Speech indistinct, stammers the last word. Lack of aptitude for finance and math.

Indecision. Timidity. ***Loss of self confidence.*** Loss of confidence in physician and remedies. ***Poor self-esteem.*** Anticipation. Averse to undertaking new things, yet goes through with ease.

Great anxiety, in pit of stomach. Anxiety, as if about to die. ***Anxiety in house,*** with company, during stormy weather, ***while walking in open air***. Conscientious about trifles. Apt to worry about the future. Hurried when eating.

Panic attacks (Ars., Phos., Kali-ar., Med.). Constant fear of breaking down under stress, ***fear of failure, public speaking, stage-fright.*** Fear of men, strangers, ***to be alone***. Fear of the dark, ghosts. Agoraphobia. Fear of being unable to reach his destination. Frightened of everything.

Melancholy. Resignation. Sadness in morning. Ill-humor and disposition to weep before menses. Extremely sensitive. Weeps all day, when thanked or meeting a friend. Sad, or cheerful, on hearing distant music. Excessively merry and laughs at simplest things, alternating with melancholy and low-spirited.

Awakes, irritable, angry, sad and anxious. Defiant, arbitrary. Headstrong and haughty when sick. ***Domineering.***

Reproaches others. ***Love for power.*** Hateful. Miserly. Easily aroused to anger. Quarrelsome. Fault finding. Suspicious. Distrustful. Hates being watched when at work.

Misanthropic, flees even from his children. Religious aversion to opposite sex. Aversion to company, yet dreads solitude. Childish fantasies. Delusions that he has neglected his duty. Delusion of being in two places at the same time. Delusion hears music in evening that was heard in the day.

Baby cries all day, sleeps all night. Cranky. Kicks, screams and very cross, on awaking from short, restless naps. Indisposition to play in children. Child desires to be carried. Oversensitive to pain. Feels as if she would die from weakness, when lying in bed.

Ailments from domineering parents or siblings. Ailments from abuse, mortification, anger or vexation. Ailments from fright. ***Looks older than he is.***

Abdomen - ***Bloated abdomen.*** Tympanitic distension with cold feet. Ascites. Brown spots on abdomen. ***Food allergies.*** Gastroenteritis from fright. Epigastric anxiety, pressure. Sensation as if a band about waist. Sensation of something moving up and down or as of a hard body rolling, when turning to the right side. Shooting pain across lower abdomen from right to left. Tension and pain in abdomen from incarcerated flatus. Hot pains flash across bowels. Bursting pain in abdomen, during stool. ***Fermentation in intestines*** like yeast. ***Much noisy flatulence,*** pressing out, worse lower abdomen. ***Immediately after eating, abdomen is bloated and full***. Flatulence before and after stool. ***Colic in babies*** with gas and bloating, worse evening. ***Diabetes.*** Inactive intestinal tract. ***Hernia, right side.*** Colon cancer.

Back - Pain and stiffness in back. Bubbling sensation. Throbbing and pulsating in back. Rising of warmth along spine. Lumbago, worse slightest motion, worse sitting erect, better urinating. Tensive pain in nape. One side of the neck stiff and swollen. Emaciation about the neck. ***Burning, as from hot coals*** between the scapulae. Pain in the back and right side from congestion of liver. Back as if broken during stool. Stitches in small of back. Darting in right cervical muscles from below upward. Swelling of cervical glands.

Bladder - ***Involuntary urination.*** Frequent urging to urinate, after taking cold, better riding in cars. Bearing down over bladder. Stitches in neck of bladder. Urging to urinate, must wait long before it will pass. Urine frequent and copious at night, scanty by day. Urine suppressed, retained.

Breasts - Stitches and burning pains in nipples, with discharge of blood and water. Hard burning nodosities in breasts with stitching, aching pains and soreness. Rawness of nipples, sore, fissured, bleed easily. Delayed menses with undeveloped breasts at puberty. Milk in breast without being pregnant. Child vomits blood after sucking bleeding nipples.

Causations - Ill effects of fear, fright, abuse, anger, anxiety, embarrassment. ***Ailments from sugar, sweets***, tobacco chewing, wine. Ailments from fevers, overlifting, masturbation, riding in a carriage.

Chest - Tensive, constrictive, burning pain in chest. Feeling of tightness in chest with burning. Itching on chest. Tension as of a hoop on chest. Constriction from right side all around short ribs. Difficult respiration due to hydrothorax and hydropericardium. Stitches in left side with inflammation of lungs. Dilatation of air tubes. Tearing and tension under clavicles. Foul, viscid sweat in axilla like onions. Swelling of axillary glands. Axillary abscess. Hydrothorax. Boils. Brown yellow spots on chest.

Constitutions - Grauvogle's carbo-nitrogenoid constitutions. Suited to persons of keen intellect, but feebler muscular development, upper part of body wasted, lower semi-dropsical, lean and predisposed to lung and hepatic conditions, herpetic and scrofulous constitutions. Weak muscular power, lack vital heat, circulation poor, it seems to stand still with cold, numb limbs or numbness may appear in spots. Hypochondriacs subject to skin diseases, lithic acid diathesis, much red sediment in urine, urine itself transparent, sallow people with cold limbs, haughty disposition, when sick, mistrustful, low of comprehension, weak memory. Weak children with well-developed heads but puny, sickly bodies, irritable, nervous and unmanageable when sick after sleep cross, pushing every one away angrily. Old women and children. Persons of dry temperament and dark complexion. Undernourished states. Old persons or who become old early, where the skin shows yellowish spots, or to precocious weakly children.

Cough - Cough is deep, hollow. Tickling cough. Dry cough in puny boys with emaciation. Cough, worse eating and drinking cold things, worse going down hill. Loose cough in daytime and suffocative fits at night. Night cough, tickling as from sulphur fumes.

Ears - Sensation as if hot blood rushed into ears. Itching in ear. Polyps. Thick, yellow, offensive discharge with deafness. Otorrhea and deafness with or without tinnitus. Otorrhea after scarlatina. External meatus excoriated by offensive discharge. Eczema, humid scurfs about and behind ears.

Eyes - Eyes sunken, blue rings. ***Eyes feel cold, hot, seem too large.*** Eyes painful as if bruised, and dazed by light. Stinging and smarting, worse evening, in light. ***Photophobia.*** Sparks before the eyes in the dark. Dilated pupils before menses. Cataract with suppressed menses. ***Inflammatory affections of eyes.*** Ophthalmia neonatorum during suppurative stage. Lachrymal fistula. ***Nocturnal agglutination and lachrymation by day.*** Ulceration and redness of lids. Smarting and burning of eyelids. Polyps on external canthi. Recurring styes. Styes on lids near internal canthus. Eyes half open during sleep.

Face - Freckles. Silly expression. Face withered, shriveled and emaciated. Yellowish, pale, gray with blue circles around the eyes. Grayish-yellow color of face with blue circles around eyes. Flushes of heat. Edema of face. Itching, scaly eruptions. Herpes on face and corner of mouth. Small, white, pedunculated warts on chin. ***Submaxillary glands swollen.*** Tearing pain in bones of face. Drawing or lacerating pain in lower jaw. ***Dropping of lower jaw, in typhoid fever*** (Lach., Op.). Twitchings. Twists face and mouth.

Female - Delayed menses with undeveloped breasts at puberty. Depressed mood and indigestion before menses. Menses too late, with sadness. Menses protracted, too profuse. Menses partly black, partly bright red. Menses of clots and serum. Menses suppressed for months, from fright. Chronic suppression of menses from tuberculosis or cancer. ***Dysmenorrhea, violent with fainting.*** Labor-like pains during menses with fainting. Discharge of blood from genitals during stools. Leucorrhea, acrid, with burning in vagina. Leucorrhea, periodical, milky, worse before full moon. ***Pains in right ovary, from right to left.*** Ovarian tumors. Ovarian dropsy. Dropsy of uterus. Cramps in uterus after stool. Flatus from vagina. Vaginitis. Serous cysts in vagina. Vagina, dry, burning, worse during and after sex. ***Aversion to sex.*** Sex painful. Nymphomania. Fetus seems to be turning somersaults. Disposition to miscarriage, moles.

Food - ***Malnutrition.*** Excessive hunger, canine hunger. Hurried when eating. ***Hypoglycemia,*** headache when not eating regularly. Loss of appetite. Bulimia, with much bloating. ***Diabetes.*** Likes to take drink and food hot. ***Desire for sweets,*** delicacies, pastries, alcohol. Food tastes sour. ***Food allergies, wheat. Worse from breads, fermented foods*** and fermentable dough. Aggravated from alcohol, wine, tobacco, ***flatulent food, cabbage, beans, oysters and onions. Aversion to sweets,*** bread, ***fermented foods,*** soup, meat, coffee. Averse to boiled food, warm food, cold drinks or food.

Head - ***Right-sided headaches. Pain begins on one side goes to other where it is worse.*** Headaches over eyes in severe colds. ***Headache with ravenous hunger, better eating.*** Frontal headache after breakfast. ***Headache, worse if not eating regularly***, lying down, stooping, better uncovering. Pulsating pain in occiput, at night, worse when hot. Pain in temples as if screwed together, worse menses. Catarrhal headache, worse when discharge from nose is slacked up. Hydrocephalus. Meningitis, tubercular. Incipient paralysis of the brain. Shakes head without any apparent cause or involuntarily, slow first, then rapid. Deep furrows on forehead. Eczema, moist oozing behind ears. Dandruff. ***Hair becomes gray early. Hair loss,*** premature baldness after abdominal affections, childbirth.

Hearing - ***Humming and roaring with hardness of hearing***, every noise causes peculiar echo in ear. Oversensitive hearing, to musical sounds and noise. Ringing, during stool. Singing noises as from boiling water. Noise is intolerable after distension of abdomen. Impaired of lost hearing, with otorrhea, with or without tinnitus. Deafness after scarlatina. Tearing pain in right or left meatus.

Heart - Aortic disease. ***Aneurysm*** (Bar-c.). Angina pectoris. Hypertrophy. ***Hydropericardium.*** Sensations as if circulation stood still. Pulsating tearing in region of heart. Ebullitions of blood. Accelerated pulse with cold face and feet. Pulse, fast, worse after eating, evening. Palpitations from overeating. Palpitations on turning over in bed at night. Cannot lie on left side.

Kidneys - Aching in kidney, worse before and better after urinating. Kidney colic in ureter (right) to bladder. Renal colic in ureter. Pain in back before urinating, ceases after flow, ***slow in coming***, must strain. Retention. Hot urine. ***Heavy red sediment***. Disposition to calculi. Hematuria. Urine bloody with paraplegia or sometimes with constipation. Child cries before urinating (Bor.). ***Polyuria during the night.*** Involuntary urination in fever or from fright during sex.

Limbs - Limbs go to sleep. Numbness, drawing and tearing in limbs. Twitching and jerking. ***Cannot lie on painful side***. Rheumatism. ***Stiffness of all joints.*** Chronic gout with chalky deposits in joints. Pain in bones at night. Curvature and decay of bones. ***Sciatica, worse right side***. Varicose veins on legs. Cramps in calves and toes at night in bed. Emaciation of one hand or one leg. Painful callosities on soles, toes and fingers contracted. Pain in heel on treading as from a pebble. Profuse sweat of the feet. ***One foot hot, the other cold.*** Corns. Chilblains. Hands and feet numb. Heaviness of arms. Tearing in shoulder and elbow joints. Axillary abscess.

Liver - Weak liver and poor digestion. Atrophic, nutmeg liver. Sensitive, congested liver. Sore, pressive, bruised, in region of liver, on breathing, worse touch. Liver painful to pressure in spots. Liver complaints after mortification. ***Chronic hepatitis***. Hepatitis with pneumonia. Hepatitis of children. ***Jaundice with flatulence***, retarded stool, weariness and drowsiness. ***Violent gallstone colic.*** Dropsy, due to hepatic disease, after abuse of alcohol. Ascites from liver diseases.

Lungs - Dull aching all over lungs. Craves air but is chilled by it. ***Shortness of breath***. Difficult breathing due to hydrothorax. Dyspnea, worse lying on back, during sleep. ***Short, rattling breathing***, worse lying on back. Neglected or unresolved pneumonia with great dyspnea. Catarrh of the chest in infants, seems full of mucus rattling. Senile catarrh. Bronchocele on right side. Flying of ala nasi and presence of mucus rales. Expectorations gray, thick, bloody, purulent, ***salty.*** Expectoration greenish-yellow, lumpy or foul expectoration. Abscess of the lungs, tuberculosis. Wheezing and asthma.

Male - Cutting pain in glans penis on urinating. Soreness between scrotum and thigh. Discharge of prostatic fluid without an erection. Chronic orchitis. Enlarged prostate. Tumor behind corona glandis. Condylomata. ***Sexual desire too strong. Performance anxiety.*** Premature seminal emission (Agn., Calad., Sel.). Exhausting pollutions. Falls asleep during sex. Sexual exhaustion, weakness. ***Impotence***. No erectile power, penis small, cold, relaxed. Loss of sexual desire after gonorrhea or cystitis.

Modalities - ***Better by motion***, belchings, urinating, after midnight. ***Better from warm food and drink,*** on getting cold, being uncovered, cold applications. ***Worse***

right side, from right to left, from above downward. ***Worse warm room,*** hot air, bed, warm applications, except throat and stomach which are better from warm drinks. ***Worse from pressure of clothes***, eating, ***oysters***, milk, vegetables, ***cabbage, beans***, bread, pastry. Worse wind, wet, stormy weather, 4 p.m. to 8 p.m., awakening. Worse before or from suppressed menses.

Mouth - Mouth hangs open. Sore lips. Bad odor from mouth. Dryness of mouth and tongue without thirst. Speech indistinct, stammers the last word. Saliva dries on palate and lips. ***Dropping of lower jaw in typhoid fever*** (Lach., Op.). Mouth waters. Gums bleed when touched or cleaning teeth. Taste too acute, sour, bitter, moldy. Blue lips. Ulcers on lips. Small tumors in mouth in various places.

Nose - Nasal troubles from childhood. ***Nose stopped up,*** snuffles, breathes through mouth, child starts from sleep rubbing the nose. ***Fan like motion of alae nasi in brain***, lung and abdominal troubles. Feeling of dryness. Sore pimples on tip of nose. Crusts and elastic plugs (Kali-bi.). Ulcerated nostrils. Acrid ozaena. ***Violent catarrh, with swelling of nose.*** Catarrh of nose and frontal sinuses. Discharge yellow and thick. Thick yellow discharge, copious and fatty. Fluent coryza. Chronic coryza, blows nose often. Scanty excoriating, discharge. Obstruction of nose during influenza. Sense of smell very acute.

Perspiration - ***Viscid and offensive perspiration.*** Cold, sour sweats. Foul sweat, smelling like onions, of axillary, feet. Sweats from least exertion. Clammy sweats at night with coldness of face. Perspiration on chest and trunk, face, about scalp and temples.

Rectum - Sharp pains and cramps in rectum. Aching and pressure in rectum, worse at night. Itching and tension at anus. Chilliness in rectum before stools. Biting and burning pain in rectum during and after stool. Rawness, ***great excoriations about anus,*** bleed easily, itching and moist. ***Hemorrhoids, aching, painful to touch*** (Mur-ac.). Hemorrhoids, painful when sitting, better hot bathing. Inactivity of bowels. Ineffectual urging from contraction of sphincters. Cramps in rectum and small of back, like labor pains. Feeling as if much remained unpassed after stools. Alternating diarrhea and constipation. Constipation, when away from home or traveling. Constipation of children, since puberty, since childbirth. Constipation or diarrhea during pregnancy. Diarrhea after suppression of skin eruptions.

Sensations - As if everything was turning around. As if brain vacillating to and fro. As if temples being screwed together. As if head would burst. As if head opened. Pain in head as if caused by wrong position. As if esophagus was being clutched and twisted. As if steam rising from stomach to head. As if something were moving up and down in stomach. As if stomach would fall down. As if suspensory ligament of liver would tear. As if drops of water were falling down. As if heart hung by a thread. Tension as from a cord in diaphragm. As if chest constricted with tight waistcoat. As if gimlets were running into spine. As if dogs with sharp teeth were gnawing her.

Skin - ***Dry skin, shrunken, especially palms.*** Skin becomes thick and indurated. Dropsy. Rawness in folds. Ulcerates. Ulcers fistulous. Fissured eruptions. Offensive secretions. Scabs do not separate. Abscesses beneath skin. Skin hot, burning, itching when warm. Eczema associated with urinary, gastric, hepatic disorders. Chronic eczema. Psoriasis. Hives, worse warmth. Acne. Blood boils, remain blue. Varicose veins. Brown spots, freckles worse on left side of face and nose. Nevi, erectile tumors. Lice, itching violently.

Sleep - Drowsy during day. Irresistible drowsiness after eating. Child sleeps all day and cries all night. Starting up on falling asleep. Restless sleep. Laughs and weeps in sleep. Soporous sleep in typhoid and exanthematous fevers. Confused, anxious, vivid dreams. Horrid dreams, of sickness, of fatal accidents. Frightful dreams frequently awaking him. ***Wakes at night feeling hungry.*** On waking, the child starts, becomes cross kicks, scolds or holds his mother. Awakes terrified. ***Unrefreshed in morning.***

Stomach - Sensation as if fasting after meals, but without hunger. Pressure in stomach with difficult breathing. Churning sensation. Coldness in stomach. Wakes at night feeling hungry. Nausea in morning before eating, with salivation. Hunger, but quick satiety. ***Eating ever so little creates fullness.*** Gastralgia and chronic gastritis. ***Great weakness of digestion with much bloating.*** Dyspepsia due to farinaceous and fermentable food, cabbage, beans, onions. Derangement of stomach from sweets and pastry. Cramps in stomach from eating fruit. Constrictive pains. Burning pain. Gnawing pain in stomach, better drinking hot water. Stomach pains better rubbing abdomen. Rumbling of flatulence (Carb-v., Chin.). Hiccoughs. Sour eructations, belchings. ***Belchings rise only to pharynx***. Vomiting of dark greenish masses, after eating and drinking. Vomits, food and bile, coagulated blood, dark greenish masses after eating and drinking. Stomach cancer. Perforating ulcer.

Stools - Diarrhea from cold drinks, cold food, beer, milk, fruit, vegetables. ***Stool hard, difficult, small incomplete.*** Stools, first part is hard is difficult to expel, last part is soft or thin and gushing. ***Stools pale, putrid, thin, brown.*** Stools mixed with hard lumps, sand. Stools thin, yellow, or reddish yellow fluid. Stools shaggy, reddish mucus, green, stringy, odorless mucus. Discharge of blood during stool.

Teeth - Teeth yellow. Front teeth feel loose. Teeth excessively painful to touch. Sensations as if teeth too long. Grinding of teeth during heavy stupor, as when fully awake. ***Toothache when chewing.*** Toothache with swelling of cheek, better warm application, warm drinks. Toothache at night, keeps her awake at night. Swelling of gum above front teeth, with swelling of upper lip. Gumboils. Gums and soft palate covered with a lardaceous coating. Gums bleed when touched or cleaning teeth. Fistula dentalis.

Temperature - Chill between 3 p.m. and 4 p.m., followed by sweat. Icy coldness, feels as if lying on ice. One chill followed by another (Calc., Sil., Hep.). Body becomes cold during cough. Chill alternating with heat. Periodic recurrence of chill. Fever, continuous, remittent intermittent. ***Fever and sweat every afternoon from 4 p.m. to 8 p.m.*** Old, broken down cases of malaria. Typhoid fever. Febrile attacks during tuberculosis.

Throat - ***Sore throat, better warm drinks, worse cold drinks, after sleep***. Stitching pain in throat. Throat feels cold. Dryness of throat without thirst. Inflammation of throat with sharp pain on swallowing and coughing, begins on right side. As if a hard body in esophagus. Sensation as if a ball rose up in throat. Chronic enlargement of the tonsils. Swelling and suppuration of tonsils. Tonsils covered with lardaceous ulcers. ***Ulceration of tonsils, beginning on right side***. Ulceration of vocal bands. Diphtheria, ***deposits spread from right to left***, worse cold drinks. Tubercular laryngitis, especially when ulceration commences. Food and drink regurgitates through nose.

Tongue - Tongue dry, black, cracked, swollen, stiff and heavy. White coated tongue with a dry line down center. Dryness of tongue, without thirst. ***Blisters on tongue.*** Tongue burning and thick, as after much smoking. Tongue feels scalded and raw. ***Vesicles on tip of tongue, ulcers on and under tongue.*** Convulsions of tongue. Tongue oscillates to and fro, trembles.

Urine - Urine, scanty, cries before urinating, must strain. Urine, milky, turbid, pale and clear, burning hot. Heavy red sediment in urine, thick, purulent, nauseating smell. Hematuria from gravel or chronic catarrh.

Vertigo - Vertigo when looking at anything turning. Vertigo in morning on rising. Vertigo reels back and forth. Vertigo in hot room. Gets hot during vertigo, face reddens, eyes water and become dim.

Vision - Day-blindness (Both.). Black, floating spots before eyes. Hemiopia, sees only one-half of an object. Must wipe mucus from eyes in order to see clearly. Letters run together or become indistinct while reading or writing, must vary distance of page. Impaired vision seems as if one was looking through fine lattice. Flickering and dim vision after a nap in afternoon. ***Night-blindness.*** In artificial light all objects tremble. Sees sparks in the dark.

COMMENTS - Lyc. was praised by Wedel, Lantilius, Gesner and others in cardialgia and flatulent colic of children and young girls, diseases of children, and nephritic colic and stones. Merat and de Lens spoke of its internal use in rheumatism, retention of urine, nephritis, epilepsy and pulmonary diseases. Diabetes, arthritis, hypoglycemia, depression, and dyslexia. Useful for early stage alcoholics.

Teste mentioned that it is recorded that a decoction of the plant caused vomiting. The use of the powder in intertrigo was not regarded as a physical one but as medicinal. In Poland it was used for powdering the hair in "plica polonica," a decoction being used internally and also externally at the same time.

Apprehensiveness. Anxiety about performance, particularly sexual. Fear of public speaking, failure, success, new situations, commitments and responsibility. Fear of being alone, of men, of his own shadow. Agoraphobia. Hypochondriacs. Panic attacks (Ars., Phos., Kali-ar., Med.). Susceptible to causes of fear that make a profound effect on bodily organs.

Profound sadness and inclination to weep. Poor confidence and low self-esteem. Forgetfulness. Peevish. Avaricious. Imperiousness. Miserliness. Overly concerned with image. Love of power. Dictatorial tendencies. Attracted to politics (Ign., Nat-m., Calc., Lyc., Nux-v.), for the power and the stature, the ego, the class, society. Can be domineering, aggressive.

Headaches, worse from 4 p.m. to 8 p.m., eating, warmth of bed, becoming heated during a walk, heat in general, mental exertion, better in open air, in cool place, by uncovering. Rush of blood to the head. Falling of hair with crusty scalp eruption.

Face is pale and yellow, deeply furrowed, looks elongated. Inflammation of eyes and lids. Ophthalmia, conjunctiva looks like red flesh. Sordes in teeth.

Facial neuralgias. Nodding and side to side movement of the head. Spasmodic movements of facial muscles, angles of mouth alternately drawn up and relaxed and spasmodic movements of tongue.

The tongue cannot be protruded, rolls from side to side like a pendulum. Cramp in the tongue when speaking, cutting off the end of every sentence. Rapid, fan-like movement of ale nasi occurring in cerebral, pulmonary and abdominal complaints, not synchronous with breathing.

Sciatica, cannot bear to lie on painful side it is so sensitive, especially if on right side. Paralysis and paralytic weakness of limbs, of brain. Heaviness of the arm. Contraction of the tendons, especially hamstrings. Right foot hot, left foot cold.

Cutting pains shooting from right to left in any part (opposite of Lach.). Burning pains better by heat, burning like hot coals between scapula. Burning stinging in breasts. Dryness of parts, of mucus membranes, of vagina, of skin, especially palms. Suppurative conditions, even gangrene.

Characteristic suddenness, sudden flashes of heat, lightning-like pains, sudden satiety. Pains and symptoms come and go suddenly (Bell.). Sensation as if a hand were in the body clutching the entrails (Bell.). Restlessness, better by motion (Rhus-t.).

Keynote worse from 4 p.m. to 8 p.m. In one case cured by Lyc. it was "bad from 4 p.m. to 6 p.m., better at 8 p.m., gone at 9 p.m." Characteristic right to left movement. Better from uncovering, particularly headaches (opposite Sil.). Better from loosening garments. Better from warm drinks, worse from cold food and drinks. Desires fresh air (Puls.).

Excessive sensitiveness, worse touch and pressure. All soft parts are sensitive, gums, epigastrium, abdomen, right side of chest, eruption around anus. Cannot bear any strong smells. Cannot endure noise. In the evening she continues to hear the music she has heard during the day.

Deficiency of vital heat. Puerperal fever with sensation as though hot balls dropped from each breast through to back, rolling down back, along each leg and dropping off heels, this alternates with a sensation as it balls of ice followed same course. Phlegmasia dolens.

Respiratory disorders. Salt sputa, milky, greenish yellow, thick yellow mucus, pus. Dry burning catarrh of nose, larynx, throat, chest. "Dry teasing cough in emaciated boys." Cough provoked by irritation from deep breathing, stretching out throat and by empty swallowing. Cough worse on waking.

Affects the blood vessels from the heart to the capillaries. Nevus, aneurysm, disordered heart. Varicose veins.

Weak digestive tract. Easy satiety. Sleepy after meals. Diabetes and hypoglycemia. Sinking sensation at epigastrium, worse in the night, waking up the patient or worse in afternoon. Cord-like tension across hypochondria. Great sensitiveness in liver region.

Borborygmi under left ribs in front. Sour stomach, sour taste, sour vomiting. Often thirsty, for small amounts, but drinking cold water causes nausea. Great weakness with the vomiting. Craves sugar and starch (Kali-c, Chin., Nat-c.). Aggravated by or averse to onions and garlic (Thuj.). Worse from flatulence foods, cabbage, broccoli, and beans.

Kidney colic with stinging, tearing, digging pain in right ureter to bladder, as if some small calculus was tearing its way to the bladder. Aching in back, kidneys, before urination, better after urinating. Pale, whitish, cloudy mucus, urine often fetid.

Child cries before urinating, red sand is found in diaper.

Gas and bloating. Incarcerated flatulence, more in intestines than in stomach, painful with better by belchings. Flatulence pressing outward, on rectum and bladder, sensation as if something moving up and down in the bowels.

Pushing out in right inguinal ring. Right inguinal hernia, especially in children. Spasmodic constriction of rectum. For constipation where purgatives have been abused. Constipation of infants.

Extreme sadness and irritability before menses, ceasing with the flow. Menses are too early and too profuse. Ill-humor. Bearing-down pains and headache. Intolerance of tight clothing. Left ovarian pain, dull aching, worse on raising the limb or turning in bed. Nausea, varicose veins and excessive fetal movements during pregnancy. Unsatisfactory labor pains.

Impotence, from masturbation, sexual excess, or age. Desire is strong but the power is absent, penis small, cold, relaxed.

There was an involuntary proving of Lyc. from inhalation of the fumes in the course of a chemical experiment, Lyc. powder being added to a boiling mass. The writer (apparently a medical man) had at times, while engaged in the experiments, frightful headaches (occiput, vertex and through right eye).

S. A. Jones called attention to the irritability of Lyc. and noted the cure of a boy with typhoid with excessive tympanites when the case seemed almost hopeless. The guiding symptoms were "when awake exceedingly cross, irritable, scolding, screaming, behaving disagreeably," which was quite different from his usual nature. Lyc. 30c was given.

The "fan-like movement" of the ale nasi led Halbert to the cure of a case of nervous asthma. Mrs. S., 28, had periodic attacks of spasmodic asthma, always ushered in by unusual excitement and attended by peculiar mental depression. The attack for which Halbert saw her was induced by a violent fit of anger and persisted longer than usual. Extreme despondency and melancholy, would have nothing to do with her friends.

Constriction of throat like globus, but always induced by regurgitation of food. Excessive appetite easily satisfied. Fullness of abdomen with flatulence. Constipation, dry, hard stools. Dyspnea. Slight cough with chest constriction, better in open air. All symptoms worse 4 p.m. to 8 p.m. Lyc. 6x cured.

A patient of Clarke's took Lyc. 30c and developed a "pain under sternum as if food lodged there and she could not breathe through it."

Loosvelt found that "half-open condition of the eyes during sleep" is a strong indication for Lyc. and led him to make cures in cases of bronchitis, pneumonia and typhoid when other remedies have failed.

Majumdar recorded the case of a boy, 14, who had general dropsy and anasarca consequent on the subsidence of an enlarged spleen under allopathic medication. There was afternoon fever (worse 4 to 8 p.m.), slight chilliness, but no thirst, difficult breathing on lying down, urine scanty and high colored, bowels constipated, heart's action weak but regular.

Apis caused the urine to be more free, but a troublesome diarrhea set in. Apoc. 6x removed the diarrhea, but had no effect on the dropsy. Lyc. 30c was then given purely on the symptoms and quickly cleared up the case.

H. Goullon cured a case of cystitis in a man, 55, subject to attacks of enteralgia. He was seized two days after such an attack with a severe cystitis with fever and palpitation of the heart. The calls to urinate were increased and he could hardly reach the vessel quick enough to prevent premature escape of the urine, so severe and sudden was the urging.

During, and sometimes after the passage, there was intense burning pain, "as if molten lead were flowing through the urethra." During the height of the pain he grasped his penis to obtain relief.

The urine, which was discharged in very scanty quantities, looked turbid, almost loamy, had a dirty brownish-red color and a peculiar odor of malt. Lyc. 12c was given, six drops in half a wine glassful of water, a teaspoonful every three hours. Cured in twenty-four hours.

Drysdale recorded the cure of a young woman whose hands were covered with warts. One 2 grains tablet of Lyc. 6c trituration was given at bedtime. The warts soon began to shrivel and in less than six weeks were all gone.

Clarke gave Miss E. Lyc. 30c for constipation. Soon after taking it she had pains in upper abdomen in all directions, urging to stool without ability to pass it, much flatus which could neither be got up nor down.

Lyc. 1,000c. was now given, a few globules dissolved in water, a teaspoonful at bedtime. All symptoms vanished. On rising, a second teaspoonful was taken and after this the bowels were well relieved.

On another occasion she took Lyc. 1,000c. in the evening and immediately felt her throat tight and uncomfortable, but this passed, and she went to bed. At 5 a.m. she woke with choking and had the greatest difficulty in getting her breath. She managed to reach a bottle of Bell. 3c and a dose of this relieved her at once.

A patient for whom Lyc. 5c had, to her great delight, reduced the gouty swellings about her finger joints. Now she could get rings on she had not been able to wear for years, but she was obliged to discontinue it on account of the distressing headaches it caused.

RELATIONS - ***Antidotes:*** Camph., Puls., Caust. ***Compare:*** (1) Alum. - Lyc. is the only vegetable that takes up aluminum (Allen). (2) Ant-c., Nat-m., Bry., Nux-v., (3) Both. - day-blindness, can scarcely see after sunrise, pain in right great toe. (4) Plumbg. - a Brazilian plant, Costive with red urine, pain in kidneys and joints and body generally, milky saliva, ulcerated mouth. (5) Kali-c., Nat-c., Calc-c., China, Sulph. ***Complementary:*** Lyc. acts with special benefit after calc. and Sulph., Iod., Graph, Lach., Chel., Hydr. follows Lyc. in indigestion.

REFERENCES - Boericke. Clarke. Murphy. Phatak.

LYCOPUS VIRGINICUS

(Bugle-weed)

PHARMACY - lycps. Lycopus virginicus. Bugle-weed. Virginia horehound. N. O. Labiate. Shady and wet places in North America. Tincture of fresh plant in flower. Tincture of the whole plant by macerating one part by weight of the fresh plant in two parts by weight of alcohol. ***Historical dose:*** Tincture and all potencies.

CLINICAL - Aneurysm. Bright's disease. Cough. Diabetes. Exophthalmos. ***Hemoptysis.*** Headache. Heart, diseases. Hemorrhoids. Malaria. Menorrhagia. Metrorrhagia. Pericarditis. Reptile, bites. Snakebites. Tarantula bites. Tuberculosis. Typho-malarial fever.

HOMEOPATHIC - According to Hale, Lycps. is mentioned by Rafinesque as "partaking of the properties of Digitalis, Sang., Cimic. and Spig." and as being "one of the mildest and best narcotics in existence."

Hale commended Lycps. as a substitute for Dig., having the advantage over it of being non-poisonous, as useful in hemoptysis and "wherever it is required to quell inordinate motions of the blood."

Briggs of Fort Lovell, related the cure of a patient of tarantula bite by application of a liquid made of Lycps. He said the Cherokee Indians allow themselves to be bitten by rattlesnakes, centipedes and tarantula, chewing as an antidote large quantities of lycopus and swallowing the juice.

H. W. Felter, an eclectic, is quoted as commending Lycps. in passive lung hemorrhage, wild, tumultuous beating of heart, which often precedes the lung hemorrhage, cough of tuberculosis. Lycps. does not disorder the stomach, he says, but acts a tonic and appetizer.

Morrisson made an extensive proving of Lycps. and developed unmistakable heart symptoms. Lowers the blood pressure, reduces the rate of the heart and increases the length of systole to a great degree (Adren.).

Diseases with tumultuous action of the heart and more or less pain. Feeble heart, with distress and weak pulse.

Cardiac irritability with depressed force, with or without organic disease. ***Hemoptysis due to valvular heart disease***. Passive hemorrhages.

Pulmonary complaints associated with loose stools. Hemorrhoidal bleeding. Characteristic cough with hemoptysis associated with feeble heart action. Violent cough at night. Lying down causes cardiac depression and lying on right side aggravates constriction of thorax.

Pains shift generally right to left. Exophthalmic goiter. Beneficial in toxic goiter used in the pre-operative stage. History of suppressed discharges.

MIND - Increased mental and physical activity in evening. Nervous, hurried and tremulous. General wakefulness and morbid vigilance. Instability. Irritability, unless spoken to very softly.

Mind wanders from one thing to another. Slow comprehension. Slight dullness of intellect with headache. Stupefaction, as if intoxicated, during menses.

Abdomen - Tugging pain in spleen. Tenderness in left hypochondrium. Aching in inguinal canal, bearing down as from hernia. Flatulence and rumbling. Severe colic followed by profuse, forcible diarrhea.

Back - Severe aching down spine. Acute pain at seventh cervical vertebra. Slight rheumatoid pain in left supra-scapular muscles.

Bladder - Tenderness in bladder. Bladder feels distended when empty.

Causations - Suppressed hemorrhoidal flow.

Chest - Constriction across lower half of thorax. Pulmonary disease associated with looseness of bowels.

Ears - Burning in right ear.

Eyes - Protrusion, pressing outward, with tumultuous action of heart. Eyes feel weak, as if fatigued. Neuralgic pain in right supra orbital region. Supra-orbital pain with aching in testicles.

Female - Menorrhagia and metrorrhagia. Menses intermit for ten or twelve days. Vagina very hot, os uterus engorged and swollen. Puffing of parts on and around pubes and vulva, dilated condition of vagina.

Head - Frontal headache, worse frontal eminences, often succeeded by labored heart. Pressure in forehead, worse left portion. Noise and throbbing in head preventing sleep after suppressed hemorrhoids.

Heart - Precordial pain, constriction, tenderness. Rheumatoid, flying pains, associated with heart disease. Cyanosis. Heart's action is tumultuous and forcible. Pulse, weak, irregular intermittent, tremulous, rapid. Palpitation from nervous irritation with oppression around heart. Cardiac asthma (Sumb.). Rapid heart action of smokers.

Kidneys - Profuse flow of liquid, watery urine, especially when the heart is most irritable, also scanty urine. Urine is scanty, thick, muddy. Diabetes mellitus, great thirst and emaciation.

Limbs - Muscular rheumatoid pains. Rheumatoid pains in forearm and wrists with trembling of hands. Hands unsteady, writing difficult. Rheumatoid pains in knees, legs, thighs, wandering to back. Slight lameness, unsteady gait.

Lungs - Asthma. Wheezing. Breathing oppressed. ***Cough with hemoptysis***, bleeding small but frequent. Cough and irritation of lungs with irregular action of heart.

Male - ***Pain in testicles***. Neuralgic pain in testicle with supra-orbital pain.

Modalities - Worse motion, exercise, walking, ascending. Worse at sunset, evening, morning, with aching down spine, better after rising.

Mouth - Toothache in lower molars.

Nose - Nosebleed. Sneezing and slight nasal catarrh.

Rectum - Constipation. Diarrhea in jaundice from weakened heart. Diarrhea with griping and rumbling. Bleeding from rectum. Hemorrhoids.

Skin - Prickings as if bitten by insects. Troublesome urticaria on left forearm and right leg, before retiring.

Sleep - Wakeful on retiring, though fatigued. Sleep restless, full of troublesome dreams.

Stomach - Circumscribed pain and compression in region of stomach. Indigestion with pain and distress in gastric region. Gastritis, enteritis. Nausea with faintness. Diarrhea, dysentery.

Throat - Rawness at back of right palate, extending to left. Burning in spot on soft palate, following headache.

Vertigo - Vertigo, tends to stagger to right.

COMMENTS - The association of Lycps. with Dig., Cimic. and Spig. particularly shows a very clear insight into the action of the remedy, which an experience of Clarke's seems to confirm.

Miss S., 25, came to him in October, 1899. About three years ago she had the first symptoms of exophthalmos, which was ascribed by her mother to a prescription of Macrin. in low potency, taken for pains in the eyes and continued for a long period.

The first symptoms were sore throat with ulcerations, then the goiter appeared and the heart became painful, its action intermittent with breathlessness and inability to take exertion.

After a course of Thyr. and later of Thuj. 30c (she had been vaccinated), Lycps. 12c was given and this took away all the heart pains. Attacks of influenza complicated the case and other remedies had to be given. The patient then did well under Spig. 30c, as far as the heart is concerned, though no impression was made on the goiter, which was small. The heart sounds were normal.

Characteristic shifting symptoms. Pains shift from heart to eyes, from head to heart, from heart to left wrist and right calf, and back to wrist and heart. Proell noted two of his cases in which there was a shift from rectum to heart and head.

Proell's two cases concerned suppression of hemorrhoidal flux. The patients were each 60 years of age, a man and a woman, both fair with light eyes, tall, very irritable with weak innervation of the heart without decided organic disease.

Both had, years before, hemorrhoidal flux which stopped suddenly. Both were hypochondriacal and had noise in their left ear.

This last symptom was the chief thing the man complained of, along with throbbing in the head preventing sleep.

Neither Cact., Kalm., nor Gels. helped radically. The night after taking Lycps. 1x, the man was a little better and in the forenoon bled from the rectum (about three table spoonfuls after defecation) with great general relief.

The woman had glycosuria, cataract of left eye and every third night was restless. Lycps. 1x, one drop in the evening. The following night she was excellent, and in the morning came an abundant bleeding from the rectum with great relief.

Morrison noted a case cured with Lycps. in which the sufferings were associated with the menstrual period, which was exactly regular but intermittent in flow. The first symptoms appeared within three or four hours of the onset of the flow and was a deep-seated pain with heat in occiput. Then followed a train of symptoms, among them nausea, and when the nausea came on the occipital pain was better.

Stanley Wilde cured a desperate case of pericarditis associated with bronchitis with Lycps. tincture, as well as a case of palpitation with darting pain in the heart in a young woman, following an attack of acute rheumatism two years before.

RELATIONS - ***Antidote to:*** Cimic. ***Compare:*** (1) Lam. - hemorrhoids, Oci. (2) Iber., Kalm., Spig., Crat., Cact., Dig., Hydr-ac., Laur., Prun., Spig. (heart). (3) Sang. (4) Ephedra Teamster's Tea - in exophthalmic goiter, eyes feel pushed out with tumultuous action of heart. (5) Fuc., Spartein, Crat., Adren.

REFERENCES - Boericke. Clarke. Phatak.

LYSIDINUM

(Methylglycoxalidine)

PHARMACY - lysid. Lysidinum. Methylglycoxalidine. Ethylene-Ethenyl-diamine. Lysidin. Lysidinum occurs in red-white crystals. The solution is a thick pink colored liquid. Trituration. Solution. ***Historical dose:*** Trituration and all potencies.

CLINICAL - Gout. Kidney stones. Oxaluria. Uric acid diathesis.

HOMEOPATHIC - Clifford Mitchel gave the 50 percent solution in ten-drop doses well diluted in aerated water, thrice daily in two cases of oxaluria. One case was in a young man, recent, and one in an old man, long standing. In the second case, the distressing lumbar pain was removed by a few doses though it had persisted for a number of days.

RELATIONS - ***Compare:*** (1) Nit-m-ac., Ox-ac., Sars., Urotrop.

REFERENCES - Clarke.

LYSSINUM

(Rabies Nosode)

PHARMACY - lyss. Lyssinum. Rabies nosode. Lyssin. Hydrophobinum. Trituration of sugar of milk saturated with the saliva of a rabid dog. Triturations might also be made of the cultured microorganisms. ***Historical dose:*** All potencies.

CLINICAL - Anxiety. Bubo. Clairvoyance. ***Convulsions.*** Corns, painful. Diarrhea. Dysentery. Esophagus, stricture. Fever. Hair, oily. Headaches. ***Hydrophobia.*** Hypersensitiveness. Hysteria. Insanity. Leucorrhea. Lyssophobia. Mania. Nervousness. Neuralgias. Paralysis. Pregnancy, convulsions. ***Rabies.*** Respiratory, paralysis. Salivation. Sciatica. Sunstroke. Tetanus. Toothache. Ulcers. Uterus, prolapse. Vaginismus. Wounds.

HOMEOPATHIC - Hering, in 1833, was the first to prove and to suggest the employment of this nosode in medicine. Later, it became notorious from the experiments of Pasteur. The pathogenesis of Lyss. is made up partly of symptoms observed in rabid animals and human patients, but chiefly of symptoms developed in the provings.

The remedy has been extensively used in practice, not only in cases of hydrophobia, but in many disorders in which the keynote symptoms have been present. The effects of bites of non-rabid dogs have been removed by this nosode.

Dysentery with pain and tenesmus on hearing water running from a tap. Copious viscid saliva. Thirst with inability to swallow. Suffocating feelings. Sighing and sighing respiration.

Trembling or quivering sensation throughout the whole body.

Sensitiveness to breath of air, to bright objects, especially the surface of water, to sounds, and, most of all, to the sound of running water. ***Convulsions brought on by dazzling light or sight of running water.*** Thought of light or water is enough to bring on an aggravation or a convulsion.

Aching in bones. Bluish discoloration of wounds. Complaints from abnormal sexual desire. Senses become over-acute. Noticeable rapid speech and impatience. Irritable, violent temper. Cannot bear the heat of the sun. Symptoms are better from sweating.

A number of cures of hydrophobia have been reported from forced perspirations, especially from prolonged and repeated use of the Turkish bath. This is known as the Buisson treatment from Dr. Buisson who originated it.

MIND - Hyperactivity of the mind. ***Hypersensitiveness of all senses***. Heightened awareness. ***Empathetic to others pain***. Clairvoyance. Emotions and bad news aggravate. History of physical or sexual abuse. Feelings of isolation and of being ridiculed or tormented.

Anxiety, restlessness, with great prostration. Rapid speech. Roams about. ***Anxiety from hearing church bells***. Indecision even in small matters. Thoughts of something terrible going to happen come into his mind against his will. ***Fear something bad will happen.*** Feels he cannot physically endure his fears much longer.

Lyssophobia, fear of insanity. Fear of driving, airplanes, injury, suffocation, choking, being bitten by dogs. Fear of being alone. Claustrophobia. Agoraphobia. ***Hydrophobia***. Fear of mirrors in room. Fear during pregnancy. Strange notions and apprehensions during pregnancy.

Worse thinking of water, fluids, brings on convulsions. ***Irritability on hearing or seeing water.*** The sight of water is intolerable. ***Wants water but can't drink it. Worse shining objects, mirrors.*** Copper metal, if in his room, makes him restless and full of pains. ***Never well since having a dog bite.***

Weary and incapable of mental exertion. Dullness and stupidity, at night restlessness. Depressed, as if something would happen. Felt as if she was going to die, as if she was going to sink away. Loss of consciousness.

Ill-humor. Irritable and critical. Impatient. Violent temper, impelled to do reckless things. ***Rude, abusive, bites and strikes***, bites or stabs himself. Growls. Cursing. Insane ideas enter his head. Thinks he is insulted, has suffered a wrong, that he is tormented. Anger followed by remorse.

Compulsive disorders. Ritualistic behavior. Excitement from hearing conversation. Can't bear to hear others sing, or eat apples. Does not hear or see persons around him. Doesn't answer questions. Clairvoyance.

Abdomen - Distension of abdomen, every evening. Rigidity of muscles of abdomen. Swelling of inguinal glands. ***Soreness in whole of lower abdomen.*** Pressing pain in right side, near last ribs with breathing in hypochondria after quick walking. ***Throbbing pains.*** Tearing pain from left hypochondriac region to right. Shooting pains in right side of abdomen. Drawing pain below navel. Colicky pain in abdomen.

Back - ***Great weakness in back, as if it would split and fall apart.*** Back extremely sore, as if beaten. Severe backache with numbness of hands. Shooting pains through small of back. ***Weakness in back, during copious menses.*** Considerable pain in lower part of back with soreness felt through to pubic region. ***Stiffness in joints of back.*** Hyperesthesia of skin along vertebral column. Pressing in neck and up back of head. Backaches with headaches. Pain in neck better bending head backwards. Stiff neck with shooting pains. Muscles of neck contract spasmodically. Sternocleidomastoid muscle on each side stands out like a thick cord.

Breasts - Both breasts swollen when waking in morning.

Causations - Ill effects of dog bites, rabies vaccinations.

Chest - Burning, surging through chest. Burning, stinging in left side of chest, with palpitations. Chest and abdomen feel expanded. Chest as if beaten, in evening. Rheumatic pains across chest when drawing in a breath. Weakness of chest. Lump in right axilla.

Ears - Ears feel stiff. Itching of ear. Itching in a small spot in upper part of both ears, better scratching. Sharp pains passing into in ears. Buzzing in right ear. Conversation in vicinity of patient may throw him into a most violent agitation. Hearing water poured out in next room makes him very irritable and nervous. Clairaudient.

Eyes - Eyes are wild, rolling, staring and livid. Dilatation of pupils. Eyes bloodshot. Eyes congested and painful. Itching heat in eyes. Burning of eyeballs. Stinging pain in left eye. Great weakness in eyes, without pain. Sensitive to light. Eyelids feel paralyzed on awaking. Pain in small in spot over right eye brow, worse writing.

Face - Face pale and yellowish. Bluish pimples on face. Heat and redness of face. Face sweats with sensation of heat with flushes. Countenance changes its aspect frequently. Quivering in face. Facial muscles become contorted. Spasms with froth before mouth. Gnawing and crawling sensation in zygoma. Lower jaw stiff and painful with inclination to yawn. Jawbones feel stiff, sore, aching in lower jaw.

Female - Menses frequent, protracted, dark, and at times fetid. ***Menses with hemorrhoids***, pulsations in anus and weakness of back. Menses with prolapsed uterus. ***Severe leucorrhea with pains in back*** and lower part of bowels, sore vagina. Slimy leucorrhea, profuse, running down the legs. White discharge like leucorrhea, weakening. Uterine sensitiveness, conscious of womb (Helon.). ***Uterus prolapsed.*** Uterine displacements. Any change of position that would tilt or rotate os uterus would cause much pain. Sharp pain in uterus, shooting down to labia. Pain in left ovarian region. ***Vagina sensitive, rendering sex painful*** (Berb.). Since childbirth, more pain with sex and a dislike to it.

Food - Voracious appetite, swallowed wheat without chewing. Inability to take solid food or it is consumed with greatest difficulty. Excessive desire for salt. Craves chocolate. Strange notions, desires or cravings during pregnancy. ***Wants water but can't drink it, aversion to water.*** Warm drinks, such as milk, soups and wine, are more easily taken than water. Aversion to apples, fat food. Worse after mutton. Excessive sensibility to smell of tobacco.

Head - Headache from bite of dog, whether rabid or not, worse by noise of running water, bright light. Chronic headaches from mental emotion or exertion. Sharp pain above eyebrows. Boring pain in forehead. ***Maddening outward pressing pain in forehead, sensation as if head would burst. Severe pressing in left side of head.*** Headaches with general weariness. Headaches with salivation. Headaches alternating with hot flushes in face. Rush of blood to head, while lying down. Throws the head back when sneezing. Very sensitive scalp. Dry hair becomes oily.

Heart - ***Heat and burning in heart.*** Violent pain in heart, as if it would burst or had needles running into it. ***Sharp pains in heart while walking.*** Dull pain in heart all day. ***Heart pains with sighing.*** Feels beating of pulse through whole body. Heart palpitated violently and felt as if it was coming up into throat. Palpitations causes anxiety.

Kidneys - Dull pressure in region of left kidney. Flying pains in urinary organs, causes difficulty and heat in urination. Desire to urinate on seeing running water, cannot urinate unless he hears water run. ***Urine too scanty and high-colored.*** Urine dark, brownish, with whitish sediment. Profuse watery urine, in evening.

Limbs - All muscles feel bruised in morning. Drawing in back and limbs. Severe twitching in arms and legs, resembling chorea. Weight and heaviness of legs and shoulders. Weakness in arms. Cramp in arms. Left hip aches in bone. Along left sciatic nerve a dull pain. Weakness in legs when going up stairs.

Lungs - Spasmodic contraction of respiratory muscles. ***Difficult breathing and spasmodic sensation in trachea. Dyspnea with flatulency, cough and rattling in chest.*** Breathing held for a time. Oppression in breathing. Breathing, gasping, irregular and quite rapid. Barking cough with gagging. Sighing, groaning respiration from cardiac pain. Frequent sighing and sobbing. Voice altered in its tone.

Male - Burning and itching on corona glandis. ***Strong erections, without sexual excitement or thoughts.*** Complaints from abnormal sexual desire. Painful erection of penis and frequent seminal emissions. Semen is discharged too late or not at all during sex. Pain in testicles after sex. Atrophy of testicles. Scrotum tightly drawn up. Hydrocele. Discharge of prostatic fluid, smelling salty and musty.

Modalities - Better gentle rubbing, bending backwards, steam or hot water bathing. ***Worse glistening objects, dazzling or reflected light,*** mirrors. ***Worse from sight or sound of running water,*** thinking of fluids, pouring water. Worse from heat of sun, wind, drafts. Worse stooping, riding in a carriage, mental exertion, bed news.

Mouth - Bitter taste in morning on awaking. Sore mouth, feels as if there were lumps in it. Feeling of coldness in mouth like essence of peppermint. Saliva tough, ropy, viscid, frothy. Constant spitting. Froths at mouth. ***Speech impeded from spasms of throat.*** Feeling of general malaise.

Nose - Nose stiff. Nose feels bruised. Itching in nose all day. Sneezing from tickling in nasal cavity. Frequent sneezing, as if a coryza would begin and from every little dust. Coryza with tickling in roof of mouth. Fluid nasal discharge. Great sensibility to smell of tobacco. Strong odors may start spasms.

Rectum - Darting pain into anus causes contraction. Difficult passage of flatus as if anus resisted expulsion. Desire for stool on hearing or seeing running water. Tenesmus during and after stool. Straining to evacuate, causes violent pain in small of back and in rectum. Constipation, stools very dark. Difficult stool, hemorrhoids protrude. Passage of bright red blood, with terrible burning and pricking in anus. Passes blood from anus during menses. ***Diarrhea worse hearing running water.*** Profuse, watery stools with pain in bowels, worse evening.

Skin - Biting, itching in various parts of body, worse by scratching. Itching as soon as beginning to get warm in bed. ***Malignant ulcers from bite of a dog.*** Bluish discoloration of bitten place (Lach.). Dark, livid-marks where inoculations were made. Pustules. Cancerous sores.

Sleep - Inclination to yawn and stretch, with stiffness of lower jaw. ***Yawns frequently without sleepiness***, especially when listening to others. Insomnia, sleepless in spite of narcotics. Sleeplessness from excitement or despair. Starting in sleep. Dreams of dogs, of high places, of insane asylums, churches. On waking, is morose and inclined to be angry.

Stomach - Aching pain with coldness in stomach. Hiccough. ***Gagging when he forcibly attempts to swallow water.*** Nausea with giddiness, headache and pale face after diarrhea. Nausea and vomiting, after diarrhea. Nausea and vomiting of a foamy, mucus, dark-colored substance resembling coffee grounds. Vomiting of food or fluid while drinking. Vomiting at night in sleep.

Stool - Tenesmus during and after stool. Dysenteric stools with tenesmus, renewed as soon as he hears or sees water run. Diarrhea with much pain, followed by nausea as if she would have to vomit. Stools of bloody mucus. Involuntary stools.

Teeth - Grinding of teeth. Teeth as if on edge. Painful sensation of coldness shooting into teeth. Frequent shooting pains in teeth. Toothache during pregnancy. Drawing pains in gums. Aching in swollen gums.

Temperature - Paroxysms of intense coldness, with pain in spine. Chilly feeling. Chills mixed and followed by heat and cold sweat. Cannot bear heat of sun. Intermittent fever. Fever every evening commencing at dusk and lasting until bedtime. Fever during headache.

Throat - Sore pain, constant desire to swallow. ***Difficult swallowing, gagging when swallowing water from spasms.*** Burning and stinging pain when swallowing water. Slight redness of palate and throat with spasm of esophagus and difficult speech. Sensation as if uvula were too long. Cooling sensation in esophagus. Voice altered in tone tones much suppressed. Hoarse, rough, harsh and weak voice.

Tongue - ***Tongue large, pale and flabby.*** Tongue coated with foam, with thin layer of yellowish white fur, in center. Tongue dark red on sides. ***Pricking sensation under tongue.*** Cool feeling on tongue like after peppermint. Pain or tickling in root of tongue. Root of tongue as if swollen.

Vertigo - Vertigo as if something was drawing around in a circle. Vertigo as if she could not hold her head straight. Vertigo with inclination to fall to right when stooping. Vertigo with dim sight while walking and sitting. Vertigo with chill and intolerable snappish headache. Vertigo with nausea, cramps in abdomen. Violent vertigo during morning. Vertigo temporarily better by return of diarrhea.

Vision - Sees sparks. Something moves to and fro before eyes while sewing. Vanishing of sight. Impaired vision with dilatation of pupils. Couldn't read longer than a few minutes at a time, when she would see letters double.

COMMENTS - Lyss. is a close analog of many of the animal poisons, especially Lach. Rabies (Bell., Stram., Canth.). It has been used as a prophylactic to prevent the development of rabies. Also, for the side effects of rabies shots.

For the effects of bites from non-rabid dogs, especially headaches. Bluish discoloration of wounds (Lach). Hydrophobia. Gagging, panic attacks at the sound or thought of water. Aggravated by shiny objects. Photophobia. Mania, delusions, hallucinations.

Hyperesthesia. Violent agitation and severe convulsions from air currents, approaching people, slightest touch, over hearing conversation. Convulsions from the thought of fluids, drinking, swallowing.

Convulsions from dazzling or reflected light from water or mirror (Stram.). Cannot bear heat of sun (Gels., Glon., Lach., Nat.).

Profuse salivation. Saliva tough, ropy, viscid, frothy in mouth and throat, with constant spitting (Hydr.). Sore throat, constant desire to swallow (Lac-c., Mer.). Difficulty in swallowing. Spasm of esophagus from swallowing liquids, gagging when swallowing water. Constant desire to urinate on seeing running water (Canth., Sulph.). Urine scanty, cloudy, contains sugar.

Prolapsed uterus, many cases of years standing have been cured. Leucorrhea, profuse, running down the legs (Alum., Syph., Tub.). Sensitiveness of vagina, rendering coition painful. Complaints resulting from abnormal sexual desire (from abstinence, Con.). Mental emotion or mortifying news always makes him worse (Gels).

RELATIONS - ***Compare:*** (1) Canth., Bell., Hyos. Stram., Lach., Nat-m. (2) Xanth. - said to be specific for hydrophobia and is recommended for chronic cystitis in women.

REFERENCES - Allen. Boericke. Clarke. Murphy. Phatak.

M

MACROTINUM

(Black Cohosh Resin)

PHARMACY - macrin. Macrotinum. Black cohosh resin. Macrotyn. Resinoid of Cimicifuga racemosa. N.O. Ranunculaceae. Trituration. ***Historical dose:*** Trituration and all potencies.

CLINICAL - Backache. Dysmenorrhea. Eye, disorders. Fears. Headaches. Irritable. Lumbago. Melancholy. Menses, disorders. Muscle, pain. Muscle, weakness. Neuralgic, pains. Rheumatism. Uterine, disorders.

HOMEOPATHIC - Muscular system exhausted after the least exertion. Muscular weakness. Excessive restlessness, better by moving about in spite of the weakness. Melancholic and irritable. Dullness of intellect.

Symptoms generally improved by onset of menses. Symptoms of the mind, eyes and breasts are worse before menses and better as soon as flow sets in (Cimic., mental symptoms worse during menses). Backache, better after menses.

MIND - Great restlessness. Fear of impending danger or having an incurable disease. Melancholic, irritable, better when menses come on. Dullness of mind. Sits for a long time thoughtless, moving hands and feet, frequent sighing.

COMMENTS - C. A. Howell noted the case of a woman, 63, who after an interval of eleven year began again to menstruate at 60, slightly but regularly.

Symptoms appeared suddenly at the time the flow was due, but failed to come on, including intense pain at the occiput, worse at every throb of heart. Retraction of head and neck. Neuralgic pains in limbs. Pulse 96, temperature 99.

Howell gave her Macrin. 2x, every two hours. The pain was relieved in a few hours and the menses came on.

REFERENCES - Clarke.

MAGNESIA CARBONICA

(Magnesium Carbonate)

PHARMACY - mag-c. Magnesia carbonica. Magnesium carbonate. Trituration. ***Historical dose:*** Trituration and all potencies.

CLINICAL - Acidity. Alcoholism. Antrum, disorders. Ascarides. ***Belching.*** Boils. Cataract. Catarrh. Constipation. ***Colic.*** Coma. Cornea, opacities. Cough. Deafness. Debility. ***Diarrhea. Dyspepsia.*** Emaciation. Epilepsy. Eyes, inflammation. ***Heartburn.*** Hernia. Hysteria. Indigestion. ***Insomnia. Leucorrhea. Malnutrition. Marasmus***. Menopausal, disorders. Menorrhagia. Menstruation, delayed. Metrorrhagia. Nausea. Nervousness. Neuralgia. Neurasthenia. Pregnancy, disorders. ***Prostration.*** Regurgitation. Spasms. Spleen, pain. ***Stomach, disorders.*** Taste, disordered. Tinnitus. Toothache. Tumors. Unconsciousness. Uterine, disorders. Vomiting.

HOMEOPATHIC - Nervous irritations and sleeplessness (Gels., Cham., Ars.), nerve exhaustion. Nervous systems that demand a permanently soothing and sustaining influence. Nerve prostration.

Numbness and distention in various parts. Intense neuralgic pains. Spasms. Epileptic attacks, while walking or standing he frequently falls down suddenly with consciousness. ***Sensitive to least touch***, noise or start.

Effects of shock, blows, mental distress. Ailments from excess of care and worry with constipation and heaviness. Broken-down, ***"worn-out"*** women with uterine and menopausal disorders.

Dryness of mucus membranes, skin. Tendency to boils, especially in children. Enlarged glands. Affections of the antrum of Highmore.

Malnutrition. Emaciation. ***Marasmus, children do not thrive*** in spite of feeding and medicines. ***Sour smell from the body*** (Rob.), especially in children, with vomiting, regurgitation, stools etc. Catarrhal condition of stomach and bowels with marked acidity. Tendency to constipation after nervous strain.

Walking fatigues, causes involuntary urination, prickings in rectum, smarting leucorrhea. Symptoms worse from cold winds or weather. Cannot bear hands covered, yet chilled by uncovering.

MIND - Mental exhaustion. Worse from mental exertion. Brain fag. Concentration difficult while writing. Absent-mindedness. Industrious, mania for work. Indolence, aversion to work.

Confusion of mind, as if intoxicated. Dazed feeling, packs and unpacks her clothes without consciousness of having done so. Automatic behavior. Aphasia. Slow learning to talk.

Trembling, anguish and fear as if some accident would happen, all day, better when going to bed. Anxious with perspiration all day. Anxiety on waking from frightful dreams. Anxiety about the future. Anticipation. Restlessness, nervousness in children.

Insecurity and fear with trembling and heat. Frightened easily. Fear of death, of misfortune, of robbers, of evil. ***Fear something bad will happen.*** Hypochondriasis. Least touch causes starting.

Moods changeable, variable. ***Capriciousness with toothaches.*** Sad mood with indisposition to talk. Morose, sulky, cross. Fretful, peevish. Ill-humor, in evening. Irritability during toothache. Censorious, critical. Abusive, insulting. Angry, violent. Discontented, disgust with everything.

Sensitive, oversensitive, mentally and physically. Startled, as from a fright. Shrieking, screaming, shouting in children, worse when touched (Cham.). Cannot bear to be looked at. Hysteria. ***Weeping, tearful mood during pregnancy.***

Despair with the pains. Despair of recovery. Moaning, groaning during sleep. Forsaken feeling. Feels unloved. Homesickness, nostalgia. Desire to travel Alcoholism, dipsomania. Loquacity during drunkenness. Unconsciousness, coma.

Abdomen - Great heaviness in bloated abdomen. Rumbling, gurgling. Dragging pain towards pelvis. ***Much flatus in bowels, with diarrhea.*** Cutting about navel better passing flatus. ***Very heavy***, contractive, pinching pain in right iliac region. ***Colic better bending double.*** Cutting, gripping, pressing colic, followed by thin green stools, which aggravates. ***Colic followed by leucorrhea.***

Back - Pain in back and small of back at night, as if broken. Violent bruised pain in back at night. Stiffness in neck. Tearing and pullings in nape of neck. Pain as if dislocated on raising arm. Shootings pain in loins. Sudden piercing in coccyx. Contusive pains in sacrum and back, at night.

Causations - Ailments from injuries, accidents. Ailments from emotional excitement, mental distress. Ailments from anger, fit of passion, vexation, fright or fear. Ailments from grief, sorrow, worry, care. Ailments from pregnancy. Ailments from dentition, cutting wisdom teeth. Poor nutrition, milk.

Chest - Oppression of chest, with sensation of constrictions. Constrictive pains in chest with dyspnea. Shooting pains in chest. Soreness in chest during motion.

Constitutions - Suited to ailing, worn out, nervous, flatulent and flabby persons, especially women, children, nurslings. Persons of lax tissue and sour smell. Hering noted it for "persons, especially children or irritable disposition, nervous temperament, lax tissue, sour smell." Cooper indicated it for "worn-out women and dark-haired, sensitive people, spare and thin."

Ears - Inflammation of the ears with external redness and sensation of great soreness. Numbness of outer ear. Feeling of distention of middle ear. Subdued tinnitus. Whizzing, buzzing, fluttering in right ear. Diminished hearing. Deafness, comes suddenly and varies, on taking cold, cutting wisdom tooth.

Eyes - Inflammation of eyes with redness, shooting pain. Sensation of burning and confused sight. Eyeballs sensitive to pressure. Eyeballs feel enlarged. Opacity of cornea. Cataract, lenticular. Dryness of eyes. Profuse lachrymation. Lids agglutinated in morning. Black motes before the eyes. Dimness of sight.

Face - Waxy pallor. Slovenly expression. Tension, as of white of an egg, dried on it. Tearing, digging, boring pain on one side, must move about. Swelling of malar bone with pulsating pain, worse exposure to cold wind, during rest and at night.

Female - Coryza and nasal stoppage before menses. ***Sore throat before menses appear***. Menses preceded by labor-like pains. Menses like thick dark molasses, tarry, viscid. ***Menses too late and scanty***, with dragging pains. Menses flow only in sleep, more profuse at night (Am-m.). Falls down in a faint at each menses. Mucus leucorrhea, white acrid, preceded by colic, regularly after the menses. Smarting pain when walking or sitting, with leucorrhea.

Food - Nibbling appetite. ***Aversion to vegetables,*** green food, green fruit. ***Craving for meat,*** fruits, acids, vegetables, bread and butter. Milk is refused, passes undigested in nursing children. ***Worse from milk***. Worse starchy food, potatoes, cabbages. Violent thirst for water, at night.

Head - Dullness of head from mental exertion. Brain heavy. Pulsation in forehead. Pressure, pain in forehead. Pain above margin of right orbit. Pain in the head, as if the hair were pulled, worse stooping. Sinking of occipital bone in marasmic children. Rush of blood to head when smoking. Hair falls out. Scalp is scaly, itching in wet weather.

Heart - Sharp pain from within outward in precordial region.

Kidneys - Involuntary urination while walking or rising from a seat. Frequent emission of urine, even at night. Sensation of burning and excoriation when urinating. Bladder and rectum become irritable. Urine, increased, pale, watery, or green. White sediment in urine.

Limbs - Heavy, tired and painful legs and feet. Swelling in bend of knee. Cannot put left foot on ground when walking. Tearing in shoulders as if dislocated. Right shoulder painful, cannot raise it (Sang.). Cannot bear hands covered, yet chilled by uncovering.

Liver - Hardness and sharp pains in liver region.

Lungs - Craves open air. ***Tickling cough with salty, bloody expectoration.*** Cough from tickling in the larynx, worse in evening till after midnight. Cramp-like cough at night. Expectoration of tubercles as big as a pea, very offensive in smell. Expectoration of blood.

Male - Inguinal and scrotal hernia. Discharge of prostatic fluid when passing flatus. Diminished sexual desire. Absence of erections. Frequent pollutions.

Modalities - ***Better motion. Better walking in open air.*** Better warm air. Cold water improves toothache for a short time, then aggravates. Worse rest, warmth of bed, uncovering. Worse every second day, every third week. ***Worse cold, wind. Worse change of weather.*** Worse drafts, night. Draft aggravates facial neuralgia. Pains are worse by rest insupportable, must get up and walk about.

Mouth - Bitter, sour taste. Dry, at night. Sticking pain in throat, hawking up fetid, pea-colored particles. Vesicular eruption, bloody saliva. Frequent, sudden stammering speech. Teeth feel too long. Toothache, especially during pregnancy, worse at night, cold and quiet, better cold drinks. Ailments from cutting wisdom teeth (Cheir.).

Nose - Vesicular eruption in nose with pressive pain. Chronic affections of nose. Dry coryza, breathes through mouth. Coryza and nasal stoppage, before menses. Nosebleed in morning.

Perspiration - Sour, greasy perspiration, difficult to wash off. Sweat stains yellow. Sweats with thirst after 12 p.m. until morning.

Rectum - Constipation after mental shock or nervous strain. Frequent ineffectual urging, with small stools or only flatus. Piercing pain in rectum, as from needles. Sharp pain in anus and rectum, with difficult stool. Stool preceded by griping, colicky pain. ***Sour stools with tenesmus*** (Rheum.). ***Stools, frothy, greenish like water like scum of frog pond.*** Stools, lienteric with gelatinous fatty masses, grass green or dry, hard, crumbling, white clay, putty like. Bloody mucus stools. Burning at anus after stool. ***Milk passes undigested*** in nursing children. Worms.

Sensations - As if everything was turning around. As if hair was pulled. As if white of egg had dried on face. As if teeth too long. As if rectum pricked with needles. Back as if broken.

Skin - Hair and nails unhealthy. Earthy, sallow and parchment-like, emaciation. Sore, dry, sensitive to cold. Violent itching and great dryness of skin. Itching vesicles on hands and fingers. Large nodosities between the skin and the flesh with shooting pains. Nettle-rash with much swelling. Small painless, red tetters, which exfoliate. Spreading blisters. Small blood boils. Corroding vesicles.

Sleep - Frequent and violent yawing. Inclination to go to sleep during day. Sleeplessness from flatus, from cutting wisdom-teeth, exhaustion. ***Many anxious dreams, with talking, cries, and starting from fright.*** Dreams of fire, flood, robbers, quarrels. Dreams of money, pleasures, misfortunes. Dreams of dead persons. Awakes at 2 a.m. or 3 a.m. and cannot fall to sleep. Unrefreshing sleep, more tired in the morning than on retiring.

Stomach - Sensation of emptiness in stomach. Constrictive pain in stomach. Pains, as from ulceration. Sour eructations and heartburn after cabbage, potatoes, greasy food, or milk. Acid risings. ***Sour belching and vomiting of bitter water***. Eructations tasting of rotten eggs during pregnancy. Nausea and vertigo during a meal, followed by retching, and vomiting of bitter or salty serum. Nausea and sour vomiting during pregnancy, during colic. Vomiting of undigested milk.

Temperature - Chilly in evening. Chilly, takes cold, before menses. Chill running down back. Chill, better out-door exercise. Fever at night, with night sweats and aversion to uncovering. Fever with dread of exposure, restlessness, sweat on head, redness and burning.

Throat - Sore throat with shooting pain when speaking and swallowing. ***Sore throat, worse before menses.*** Sticking pain in throat, worse talking and swallowing. Burning pain in throat and palate. Frequent rising of mucus in throat. Soft, fetid tubercles of color of peas are hawked up. Hawks up cheesy masses from throat.

Vertigo - Vertigo, worse when kneeling. Vertigo in evening with swooning. Continual giddiness, can hardly stand, with numbness of left arm. Vertigo, staggers in the street and fears to go out, lest people should strike against her.

COMMENTS - Cooper said that water containing magnesia, and that coming from magnesia limestone districts, is peculiarly soft feeling. It is often found that the physical characteristics of substances correspond with their dynamic influences, so there is reason for supposing that this softness has a soothing effect upon the nervous system when used in baths.

Mag-c. is to exhausted nerves what Chin. is to exhaustion from loss of fluids. Worn-out condition, often produced during pregnancy or menses as these are an additional tax on a women's strength.

Characteristic sensitiveness, mental and bodily, sensitivity to touch, to cold air. The least touch causes starting. Sensitiveness passes into neuralgic pains of the highest intensity. Lightening-like neuralgia, worse on the left side, insupportable during repose, must get up and walk about.

Tired and painful feeling, especially the legs and feet, aching, restless. Head injuries from shock, blows, mental distress. Unrefreshing sleep, more tired on waking than on going to bed.

Periodic symptoms, every second day, every three weeks, "all symptoms worse every third week." Worse from touch and pressure, but pressure in abdomen is better during the menstrual flow. Pain is worse on the side lain on. Smoking aggravates the headache.

Spasmodic disorders of stomach and intestines. Sour taste, breath, belchings, vomiting. Incarcerated gas causing severe abdominal pains. Colic with gas and bloating, cutting and stabbing pains in the abdomen (Cham.), with irritability. Diarrhea, green stools like the scum of a frog pond, jelly-like lumps, aphthae. Stool like chopped spinach, green flakes in stool (Cham.). Stool smells sour (Rheum.).

Puny and sickly children, who refuse their milk and get pain in the stomach if they take it. Food passes undigested in nursing children. Neonatal jaundice with gas, bloating and colic, light-colored stools and failure to thrive (Aeth.). Marasmus. Inordinate craving for meat in children of tubercular parentage, averse to vegetables.

Teething (Cham.), with colic. Cooper mentioned it as a possible remedy in pyorrhea alveolaris.

Menses preceded by labor-like pain, cutting colic, backache, weakness, chilliness. Menses late and scanty, flow only at night or when lying down, cease when walking. Flow acrid, dark, pitch-like, difficult to wash off. Vomiting and toothache during pregnancy.

Cooper gave the indication as a "worn-out women," that is, the state of nervousness induced by excess of cares and worries of life. Mag-c. 200c, repeated three or four times a day, has given untold relief to many a patient of this kind. When constipation and heaviness are present these will be removed at the same time.

Two cases of neuralgia, related by A. I. Harvey, are quoted in Amer. Hom. The first case is that of a carpenter, 50, who had a light complexion, spare. He had facial neuralgia for two years coming in attacks, lasting from three to seven days, at intervals of two or three weeks. Sharp pain, shooting from left side of face and head, worse at night, from pressure, from jar. Mag-c. cured promptly after the failure of Spig.

The second case was that of a blacksmith, 22, who had a light complexion, full figure. For several years he had attacks of facial neuralgia coming on after taking cold. Very severe pain in the left orbital region, shooting down into the eye and face and back to occipital region. Begins in morning, grows worse until noon, then subsides. No pain at night, rests well. Spig. and Kali-bi. failed. Mag-c., cured promptly.

RELATIONS - ***Antidoted by:*** Ars. and Cham. (neuralgia), Merc., Nux-v., Puls. and Rheum. (abdominal troubles). ***It antidotes:*** Acet-ac. ***Compare:*** (1) Cham., Rheum., Kreos., Aloe. (2) Cheir. - deafness, otorrhea, nose stopped up at night from *irritation of cutting wisdom-teeth.* (3) Mag-m., Mag-p., Aloe. (4) Ant-c. - headache from smoking. (5) Calc. and Rheum. - sour stools. Nux-v. - sour breath. (6) Cocc. and Sep. - worse from kneeling. (7) Ip. - nausea and grass-green stools. (8) Coloc. - griping pains with drawing up of legs, Coloc. has not the green slimy stools of Mag-c. (9) Cham. - neuralgia, better moving about, anxiety, restlessness, griping before stools, stools of Cham. more yellowish green like chopped eggs. (10) Calc. - sour stools, intolerance of milk, imperfect nourishment: Calc. has head-sweat, cold, damp feet, enlarged abdomen. (11) Lyc., Nit-ac., Sil., Lac-c., Lac-d. - intolerance of milk. ***Compatible:*** Caust., Phos., Puls., Sep., Sulph. ***Complementary:*** Cham. ***Planets:*** Jupiter, Saturn.

REFERENCES - Boericke. Clarke. Murphy. Phatak.

MAGNESIA FLUORIDE

(Magnesium Fluoride)

PHARMACY - mag-f. Magnesia fluoride. Magnesium fluoride. Remedy made from solution. Trituration. ***Historical dose:*** Trituration and all potencies.

CLINICAL - Auto-toxins. Goiter. Chronic suppurations. Fatigue. Hyperthyroidism. Infections. Influenza. Metabolic complaints. Neuralgia. Post-infectious conditions. Sinusitis. Staphylococcus. Streptococcus. Thrombosis. Tonsillitis.

HOMEOPATHIC - There is no homeopathic proving for Mag-f., but Mezger established symptomatology based on clinical usage and the characteristics of magnesium and fluorine.

Localized infections from bacteria. Streptococcus, enterococcus, staphylococcus. Nasal and pharyngeal infections of the maxillary sinus of the nose and tonsils. Post-infection conditions following influenza, sinusitis, tonsillitis, with fatigue, asthenia, nervous irritability, lack of appetite, muscular and neuralgic pains, pains in the ligaments and tendons and joint pains.

Metabolic complaints of senescence with cholesterol disorders. Action on the liver, pancreas, digestive passage. Capillary and venous stasis. Venous thrombosis. Goiter. Thyroid problems with the tendency to hyperthyroidism. Mag-f. is useful after the failure of Sulph. and Hep.

Modalities - Better from movement, in fresh air. Worse at 3 a.m., in the early morning, from sleep, especially after lunch. Worse a few days before menses.

RELATIONS - ***Compare:*** (1) Sulph. - Auto-intoxication with fatigue. Itching eruption, a alternating with other complaints, redness of the natural orifices, weakness at 11 a. m., sudden diarrhea. The need for fresh air. (2) Hep. - Tendency to suppuration. Hypersensitive, especially to the cold. Pain like that of a splinter. Skin unhealthy. Scrofulous lymphatic constitution. (3) Bar-c. - Hypertensive heart - vascular sclerosis. Glandular and ganglion hypertrophy. Cerebral slowness. (4) Stront. - Vascular and cerebral sclerosis. Pain in the bones. Muscular cramps. (5) Cresol. - Indifferent state with loquacity, tremors, trembling, paresis, oliguria, joint stiffness. Neuro-vascular sclerosis.

REFERENCES - Julian.

MAGNESIA MURIATICA

(Magnesium Chloride)

PHARMACY - mag-m. Magnesia muriatica. Magnesium chloride. Magnesia chloride. Solution. Trituration. ***Historical dose:*** Trituration, tincture and all potencies.

CLINICAL - ***Biliousness.*** Bladder, paresis. Cardialgia. Chronic, fatigue. ***Cirrhosis.*** Cold. Colic. ***Constipation.*** Coryza. Deafness. ***Diarrhea.*** Dysmenorrhea. Dyspepsia. Dyspnea. Fainting. ***Fatigue. Flatuence.*** Foot-sweat. Globus, hystericus. ***Headaches.*** Heart, disorders. Heartburn. Hemorrhoids. ***Hepatitis.*** Hernia. Homesickness. Hysteria. Influenza. Jaundice. Leucorrhea. ***Liver, disorders. Metrorrhagia.*** Milk, allergy. Nausea. ***Nerve, disorders.*** Nocturnal, emissions. Ozaena. ***Palpitations.*** Pregnancy, nausea. Rickets. Smell, disordered. Spleen, enlarged. Stomach, disorders. Taste, disordered. Tinea, ciliaris. Urine, straining. Uterus, pain. Water brash. Whooping cough.

HOMEOPATHIC - While Mag-c. and Mag-s. are recognized old-school remedies, there is no mention of Mag-m. or Mag-p. in allopathic text-books. Mag-m. first appeared in Hahnemann's book Chronic Diseases. The general features of Mag-c. appears in many Mag-m. symptoms, notably those of nervous disturbance and hysteria.

Guernsey noted that Mag-m. is found in many mineral waters and in seawater. It has a very bitter taste and in decomposed by heat. Mag-m. is similar to Nat-m. and Aq-mar. in their relation to seaside effects.

Constipation, ***"biliousness"*** and generally disordered health, when conditions appear as soon as the patient goes to the seaside. ***Ill effects of sea bathing.*** Excessive weakness after a sea bath.

General action on the ***liver and nerves,*** uterus and rectum. Cirrhosis. ***Chronic liver disorders*** with tenderness and pain, extending to spine and epigastrium, worse after food. Constipation. Fainting, fits, dyspnea, nausea and trembling occur after dinner, better by belchings.

Spasmodic, hysterical complaints. Globus. Soreness and sensitiveness to noises. Pains are boring, spasmodic, contractive, crampy, darting. Burnings. Shocks through the body like electric shocks when wide awake. Perversions of taste or smell.

Especially adapted to diseases of women with a long history of indigestion and uterine disease. Children who cannot digest milk.

MIND - Difficult concentration. Confusion of mind. Mental exertion aggravates. Aversion to conversation, prefers solitude. Reserved. ***Dislikes confrontations.***

Peevishness and chagrin. Obstinate, headstrong. Morose and sulky. Irritability, worse in morning. Moaning, groaning during sleep. Grief. ***Homesickness. Nostalgia.*** Forsaken feeling. Sadness and depression. Manic depression.

Capriciousness. Excited, unhappy, fitful, emotional. Restlessness, worse in evening. Uneasiness, nervous excitability with tendency to weep readily. Weeping, tearful moods with liver disease. Feels on the verge of a nervous breakdown.

Overwhelming anxiety. Anxiety and worrying at night. Anxiety during fever. Anxiousness in room, better in open air. Fears associated with liver disease. Fear of animals, spiders. Fear of robbers.

Abdomen - Cramps in abdomen. Distended abdomen with constipation. Flatulence with distension. ***Great flatulence, often incarcerated, causing numerous pains.*** Hysterical colic followed by leucorrhea. Colic, can't endure covering. Dragging sensation when lying on left side. Tearing, sharp pains in loins. Tingling, stinging in abdominal muscles.

Back - Bruised or burning pain in back after sex. Bruised pain in small of back and hips, during menses, better pressure. Cramps in back worse walking. Contractive, spasmodic pain in lumbar region. Sharp, tearing and burning pains in small of back. Throbbing below left scapula. Swelling of cervical glands.

Causations - Ill effects of sea bathing, especially weakness. Ailments from anger, vexation, sexual excesses.

Chest - Constrictive pain and tension in chest and scapulae. Congestion and soreness of chest, after sea bathing. Sudden heaviness of chest, with oppressed breathing, at dinner.

Constitutions - Suited to diseases of women, spasmodic and hysterical complaints complicated with uterine diseases. Women after suffering months or years from attacks of indigestion or biliousness. Puny, rickety children during dentition. Liver disorders in children who are puny and rickety and have eruptions about the eyes. Enlargement and congestion of liver. Men with disordered livers and sexual problems.

Cough - Cough, worse eating, fatty food, fruit. Spasmodic, dry cough at night, with tickling in throat, burning and sore chest. Spasmodic cough, worse rest, sitting, lying in bed, deep breathing, air of room, ascending steps, or speaking. Whooping cough.

Ears - Pulsations in ears. Itching of old herpes behind ears. Sensitive to noise. Deafness, as if something were lying before ear.

Eyes - Yellow sclera. Lachrymation and burning of the eyes when looking at anything in broad daylight. Nocturnal agglutination of eyelids. Tinea ciliaris with pimples on face.

Face - Pale, yellow. Eruptions on face, itching, burning vesicles. Pimples on the face and forehead itching worse night, warm room and before menses. Chapped lips. Blisters on lips. Prosopalgia. Facial neuralgia pains, dull, aching, worse damp weather, slightest draft, better pressure heat. Severe cramps in face.

Female - ***Menses, profuse, dark, lumpy like pitch, with cramps.*** Menses black, clotted, more copious when sitting than walking. Great excitement at every period. Dysmenorrhea, better by pressure on the back or lying on a hard pillow. Headache at menstrual period. ***Gushes of leucorrhea, after abdominal colic.*** Leucorrhea after exercise. Leucorrhea with stool. Leucorrhea followed by metrorrhagia. ***Metrorrhagia, worse at night.*** Uterine cramps, extending to thighs. Ovary enlarged and tender. Bearing down pain in right ovarian region. Pain in back and thighs. Labor pains interrupted by hysterical spasms. Tinea ciliaris, eruptions in face and forehead worse before menses.

Food - Appetite poor, bad taste in mouth. Ravenous hunger followed by nausea. Hunger but knows not for what. Inclination to nibble. Craves sweets, dainties. Better from lemons. Violent thirst. Worse from milk, salty food, fat food. ***Cannot digest milk*** (Nat-c.), especially children, causes pain in stomach and passes undigested during dentition.

Head - Bursting headache, worse motion, open air, better pressure and wrapping up warmly (Sil., Stront.). Sensitive to noise with headache. Squeezing pain in both temples in evening after lying down. ***Beating in forehead when pressing upon it.*** Tightness and pressure in forehead. Much sweating of head (Calc.,

Sil.). ***Thirst, belching during headache.*** Headache better lemons. As if boiling water on the side lain on. As if hair were pulled. Nodosities on occiput, tearing, painful to touch.

Heart - Sharp pain in heart, arresting breath. ***Palpitations, worse while sitting, lying on left side, better by moving about*** (Gels.). Pulse accelerated, with ebullitions while sitting. ***Heart disorders with liver enlargement***.

Kidneys - Numbness of urethra. In the dark one cannot tell whether one is passing urine or not. Urine can only be passed by bearing down with the abdominal muscles, straining and pressure. Stricture after dilatation. Urine passes in drops, some always seem to remain. Pale yellow urine, followed by burning in urethra.

Limbs - Rheumatic pains in limbs, better motion and pressure. Pain in back and hips, in arms and legs. Cramps in thighs, worse sitting. Thighs and calves tense, must move limbs. Ankles cold or nervous worse night. Cutting pain in heels. Feet sweaty. ***Arms "go to sleep"*** when waking in morning. Fingertips numb.

Liver - Jaundice. ***Hepatitis.*** Cirrhosis of the liver with a sluggish feeling. ***Liver sore, enlarged with bloating of abdomen, yellow tongue.*** Burning, tensive sticking in hepatic region. Pressing pain in liver, worse lying on right side. Hyperemia of liver with constipation. Liver affections with tendency to hemorrhage from various organs. Cramp in the gallbladder, better by eating. Pain from liver to spine or epigastrium, can only lie on back or affected side.

Lungs - Oppressed breathing, globus hystericus. Bloody sputum or congestion and soreness of chest after sea bathing. Purulent sputum, of fatty taste and offensive odor. Watery expectoration during day. Tough, yellowish mucus.

Male - Pain in testes and cords worse after sex. Itching on genitals and scrotum. Congenital hernia of scrotum. Scrotum relaxed and often covered with perspiration. Pain in testes and cords, worse after sex or after unrequited sexual excitement. Burning in back after sex. Frequent erections, early in morning, with burning in penis.

Modalities - Most symptoms, except headache, are better in cool, open air. ***Better from hard pressure.*** Better lying bent. Better hanging down affected part. Better gentle motion. Nausea and trembling better by belchings. ***Worse from sea bathing. Worse lying on right side***. Worse touch, noise. Worse at night, mental exertion. Worse immediately after eating. Worse salt, milk. Fainting worse at meals.

Mouth - Mouth dry, without thirst. Loss of taste. Bitter, sour taste at night. Continued rising of white froth into the mouth. Blisters on lips. Gums swollen, bleed easily. Toothache, worse if food touches the tooth.

Nose - Red, swollen. Nostrils ulcerated. Sore and burning, in nostrils, worse deep breathing, sneezing or touch. Acrid, crusty ozaena. ***Loss of smell and taste***, following catarrh. Sneezing with watery discharge. Discharge of yellow, fetid mucus. Coryza, with stoppage of nose, hoarseness. Nocturnal obstruction of nose, must breathe through the mouth. Cannot lie down.

Perspiration - Sweats on head or feet. Sweats from 12 p.m. until morning. Thirsty with sweats.

Rectum - ***Diarrhea after milk.*** Constipation of infants during dentition. Absence of desire for stools. Only passing small quantity. ***Stools are knotty*** like sheep's dung, gray. ***Stools crumbling at verge of anus***. Painful smarting hemorrhoids. Tape-worms.

Sensations - As if some one was running after her. As if boiling water was on side of head. As if hair pulled. As if tongue burnt, mouth scalded. Stools as if burnt.

Skin - Formication all over the body. Sweat on head and feet. Blood boils. Abscess with yellow, thin, foul pus. Jaundice.

Sleep - Sleepiness during day with yawning and sluggishness. Anxiety and restlessness of the body as soon as she closes the eyes. Restless at night on account of heat and shock. Sleeplessness from spasms. Anxious dreams with talking and crying out during sleep. Dreams of robbers in the house, on awaking will not believe to the contrary until a search is made. ***Sleep unrefreshing, tired in morning.***

Stomach - Coldness and weakness in stomach. Pressing pain in stomach, disappear while eating and reappear about an hour afterwards. ***Throbbing pain in stomach.*** Stomach pain as from ulceration, or from a bruise. Regurgitation while walking. Continued rising of white froth into mouth. Hiccough, during and after dinner, causes vomiting. Belchings like rotten eggs, like onions. Nausea and faintness, better eructations. Nausea in morning after rising, with salivation, faintness, weakness in stomach.

Temperature - Chill even near a stove, better open air. Chilliness, during and after loose stool, in morning. Sensitive to cold air, great disposition to take cold. Fever in evening, with aversion to uncovering.

Throat - Throat dry with hoarseness. As if a ball rising into the throat, better by eructation. Hawking of clammy, thick mucus, often mixed with blood.

Tongue - Tongue feels burnt, mouth feels scalded. Cracks in tongue with violent burning. Broad, yellow, scalloped tongue. Tongue large, flabby, white, tip and edges clean. Tongue coated white in early morning.

Vertigo - Vertigo during dinner, in morning on rising. Vertigo, better from open air.

COMMENTS - Liver conditions (Chel., Nat-s., Lyc., Ars., Nux-v., Phos.). Symptoms of liver deficiency or weakness. Liver disorders with enlargement and sensitiveness, worse from touch and lying on right side. Cirrhosis, with a sluggish feeling. Hepatitis with total exhaustion.

Liver rheumatism, arthritic symptoms associated with liver weakness. Severe chronic fatigue since hepatitis. Chronic neurasthenia (Sil., Phos.). Liver stasis, toxic feeling. Symptoms are worse in the morning, stiff, sore, achy, better with motion or as the day goes on (Rhus-t.).

Unrefreshed sleep. Generally sleeps on the left side, to avoid sleeping on the liver. Worse lying down, closing the eyes. Difficultly getting comfortable, desire to keep moving. May constantly wake in the night. Miserable in the morning, feel irritable and sluggish. Bitter taste in the mouth on waking.

Sluggishness comes from the liver, not from the joints (as in Rhus-t.). Drag themselves around, as if hung-over (Gels.). Heavy feeling, as if all their weight and energy are in the legs. Difficulty concentrating. Better open air and motion.

Anxious, restless, always better by mental exertion. Aversion to work, apathetic (Gels.), but a desire to move and keep busy. Bitter. Bilious, irritable temperament, dissatisfied look on their face. Passive, will avoid confrontation, complaining to others. Suffers when they see people arguing.

Influenza and mononucleosis with aching, malaise, sluggish, wiped out feeling, but also stiff, desire to move and stretch (Rhus-t. and Gels.). Viral infections with a sluggish, toxic feeling.

Palpitations, worse when quiet, better moving about. Boring and spasmodic contractive pains, dragging down. Marked hysterical symptoms, spasms, fainting, globus. Hysterical headaches.

Burning and heat. Numbness and heaviness of the extremities, with weakness. Burning in soles in the evening, must put feet out of bed. Chilly, but with warm feet. Sweaty feet. Aggravated by salt, salty foods, air or sea bathing. Can get headaches, red lips, and cracked corners of the mouth from salt.

Sweat about the head. Ozaena. Redness, swelling and scaliness of nose. Yellow tongue, imprinted with teeth. Tongue is large, coated and indurated. Perversions of taste and smell.

Weak digestion, exhaustion. Nausea and belchings during or after dinner. Trembling and faint spells are better by belching. Better from a light diet, generally vegetables, and fruits, aggravated from heavy, fried, fatty foods and meat. Aggravated from milk.

Intestinal atony. Constipation, stools break off or crumble at the anus. Stool is knotty, conglomerate. Painful urging before stool, burning in anus after. Tape worms. Bladder atony, urine can only be passed by bearing down with abdominal muscles.

Bearing down in uterine region, uterine spasms. Menses black or pitch-like, accompanied by pains in back when walking, pains in thighs when sitting. Leucorrhea after every stool or following uterine spasms.

Clarke frequently restored the loss of taste and smell after influenza with Mag-m.

Teste, who placed Mag-m. in his Ferrum group, noted that Mag-m. and Mag-c. "have been used for the cure of cachexia occasioned by long and painful diseases."

He said he saw Mag-m. produce great improvement in a case of "hydrarthrosis of left knee with emaciation of left thigh, consequent on a wandering neuralgia, which after having commenced in the form of cystitis with (non-venereal) discharge from urethra, had successively invaded the shoulder, left elbow, eyes and lastly, knees, where it had become seated."

R. M. Skinner reported a case in which a farmer had been treated allopathically for three months for chills, which were checked, but the man did not feel well. Spleen was very large, sensitive, felt heavy when he walked or rode.

He sought advice for his constipation, went three or four days without a stool. His abdomen was distended and hard, especially in ileo-cecal region. Cold on the left side and a crawling feeling like a cold snake. Beating in umbilical region as if his heart beat there.

Skinner gave him Mag-m. 200c, one dose on the tongue. At 8 p.m., the bowels began to act and went on acting with the exception of one hour until 3 a.m. He complained the next morning that the medicine had "almost killed him," and he looked thin and tired. No further medicine was given and in ten days he had no complaint, the spleen was normal in size and without tenderness.

RELATIONS - *Antidoted by:* Cham., Camph., Ars., Nux-v. *It antidotes:* Merc. (metrorrhagia). *Compare:* (1) Chel., Mag-c., Nat-m., Puls., Sep., Am-m. (2) Nast. (3) Hysteria, Mosch., Asaf., Valer., and Cast-eq. (4) Uterine spasms, Ign., Caust. and Sec. - both have continuous spasm. (5) Erections and burning in penis, Pic-ac., Nat-m. (6) Enlarged liver, worse by touch and lying on right side, Merc. (7) Foot-sweat and head-sweat, Sil. is offensive., scrofulous and rickety children, headache better wrapping, Sil. (8) Congestion of liver, enlargement, feeling of weight and pressure, Ptel. is better lying right side. (9) Enlarged liver of children, Calc-ar. (10) Sensitiveness to noise, Ign., Nux-v., Ther. *Compatible:* Bell., Sulph., Nat-m., Puls., Sep.

REFERENCES - Boericke. Clarke. Murphy. Phatak.

MAGNESIA PHOSPHORICA

(Magnesium Phosphate)

PHARMACY - mag-p. Magnesia phosphorica. Magnesium phosphate. Magnesia phosphate. Trituration. *Historical dose:* Trituration and all potencies.

CLINICAL - *Angina pectoris*. Catheterism. Chorea. *Colic.* Convulsions. Cough. Cracks. *Cramps.* Dentition. *Dysmenorrhea. Facial neuralgia.* Goiter. Headaches. Hiccoughs. *Intercostal, neuralgia.* Locomotor, ataxia. Membranous, dysmenorrhea. Meningitis. *Menses, painful. Neuralgias. Pains. Paralysis.* Parkinson's disease. Rectum, prolapsed. School, headache. *Sciatica.* Stomach, cancer. *Spasms.* Tic douloureux. *Toothaches.* Twitching. Vaginismus. *Whooping cough. Writer's cramp*.

HOMEOPATHIC - Mag-p. is one of the most important of Schüssler's additions to the Materia Medica. It has had a very fine proving in the potencies, conducted by H. C. Allen. Schüssler's picture of the remedy is confirmed in every point by Allen's proving and by the clinical use of Mag-p. in the highest potencies. Moreover, there is a very strong family resemblance between these features and those of Mag-c. and Mag-m.

But it is only right to say that Schüssler arrived at them by a way of his own, which shows that there are other means besides provings of finding the keynote symptoms of remedies.

Schüssler stated that Mag-p. is contained in the blood corpuscles, muscles, brain, spinal marrow, nerves, teeth. Disturbance of its molecules results in ***pains, cramps, and paralysis.***

Useful for cramps, convulsions, neuralgic pains and spasmodic effects, showing its influence on nerves and muscles.

Spasmodic effects. Cramping of muscles with radiating pains. The pains are shifting, better by rest, worse at night. Pains sometimes tense in paroxysms. ***Neuralgic pains relieved by warmth***. Parts are tender to pressure and numb. Allen noted that the pains rapidly change place, that cramping is the most characteristic type of pain.

Hiccough, yawning, chorea and hand cramps. Nervous, tense, sudden violent paroxysms of neuralgic pains. Sharp, shooting like lightning pains, that suddenly changing places. Radiating, boring, constricting pains, extorting cries, causing restlessness and prostration. Twitchings. Tics. Palsy. Parkinson's disease. Goiter.

Chorea better during sleep, worse at stool and emotions. General symptoms are worse by motion, cold air, draft of air, cold wind, ***cold washing, touch,*** uncovering, lying on the back stretched out, when eating. Dread of touching the affected part, of moving.

MIND - Very forgetful. Indisposition to study, to mental work. Mental dullness and inability to think clearly. Learning is difficult.. Ailments from mental work. Drowsiness on every attempt to study.

Capriciousness. Irritability. Ailments from suppressed anger, vexation. Mental depression and anxiety. Discontented, dissatisfied. Sadness, despondency. Weeping, tearful mood, during convulsions. Sobbing, crying.

Oversensitive to pain, noise, excitement. Restlessness and nervousness. Anxiety, depressed vitality. Fear of others approaching. Fear of being touched, motion. Excitable during convulsions.

Anxiety from the pains. Despair with the pains. ***Startled from the pains.*** Screaming, shouting from pains, cramps in abdomen. Hypersensitive to pain (Cham., Mag-s.). Complaining. Lamenting about pain in affected parts. Always talking about the pains.

Talks to himself constantly. Sits in moody silence. ***Carries things from one place to another and back again.*** Delusions, that he is about to die. Delusions, that another person is in the room. Illusions of the senses.

Abdomen - Abdomen contracted. ***Bloated, full sensation in abdomen,*** must loosen clothing, walk about and constantly pass flatus. Severe, griping colic, at times shooting up towards stomach, better by hot applications. ***Flatulent colic, forcing patient to bend double.*** Colic accompanied with belching of gas, which gives no relief. ***Colic relieved by rubbing, warmth, pressure. Colic in babies*** (Cham.). Cutting pain into thighs.

Back - Stiffness of neck and back. ***Cramps in back.*** One vertebra seems absent. Sore pain in neck and lower part of back. ***Very sharp, shooting, boring, shifting and remittent pains in nape.*** Aching pain in small of back. Dorsal spine, very painful and sensitive to touch.

Causations - Ailments from suppressed anger, vexation, mental work, study. Complaints of teething children (Cham.). Ill effects of overuse of muscles, standing in cold water, cold bathing, working in cold clay, catheterism.

Chest - Darting pains in chest, worse right side, which radiate from pain in bowels. ***Intercostal neuralgia, must sit upright.*** Oppression of chest, with desire to take deep breath, worse on first entering warm room, worse walking.

Constitutions - Hering thought it suited to young and very strong persons, teething children. Allen said that, though it is best adapted to emaciated persons, it acts promptly in stout, fleshy persons when well indicated. Suited to tired, languid, exhausted subjects.

Cough - Dry, tickling cough. Spasmodic cough, worse lying down, better cool air. Spasmodic cough during intervals of convulsions with contraction of fingers and staring, open eyes. ***Spasmodic, whooping cough*** (Dros., Cor-r.), better cool air.

Ears - Nervous otalgia, intermittent and spasmodic, better by heat. ***Severe neuralgic pain, worse washing face and***

neck with cold water. Neuralgic pain worse behind right ear, worse by going into cold air.

Eyes - Eyes, hot, aching, tired. Increased lachrymation. Twitching of eyelids. Photophobia. Nystagmus, strabismus, spasmodic, ptosis, worse right side. Itching and heat in lower eyelid. Supra-orbital pains, worse right side, relieved by the warmth.

Face - Cracks in corners of mouth. Face blue and swollen from violent spasmodic attacks of cough. Face distorted from pains and weakness. Lock-jaw, tetanus. Painful contraction of jaw joint with backward jerking. ***Spasmodic twitching of facial muscles.*** Trigeminal neuralgia worse slightest touch. ***Facial neuralgia,*** worse when body gets cold from washing or standing in cold water, ***better from warmth.*** Neuralgia on opening mouth to eat or drink. Neuralgia on right side of face alternating with toothache, rushing about like lightning.

Female - Menstrual colic, pain precedes flow. ***Menstrual cramps, better heat, bending over and by flow.*** Menses too early, dark, stringy, fibrinous, tarry. Menses flowing at night leaving a stain. ***Membranous dysmenorrhea.*** Swelling of labia, at times extremely painful. Vaginismus. ***Ovarian neuralgia, pain shooting and darting like lightning.*** Puerperal convulsions. Spasmodic labor pains, with cramps in legs.

Food - Appetite remains good. Thirst for very cold drinks. Food doesn't taste right. Acids taste stronger than usual. Aversion to coffee. Craves sugar.

Head - Headaches after mental labor with chilliness, better warmth (Sil.). Headaches of students. Sensation as if contents were liquid, as if parts of brain were changing places, as if a cap on head. ***Neuralgic or rheumatic pains, better external application of warmth.*** As if an electric shock in the head extending to all parts of the body. Boring pain over right eye, spreading over whole right side of head. Supraorbital pain worse right side, better external heat.

Heart - *Angina pectoris*. Constricting pains around heart. Pulse irritable. Nervous spasmodic palpitations.

Kidneys - ***Bladder neuralgic pains after use of catheter.*** Spasm of bladder of neck of bladder, spasmodic retention, tenesmus with constant and painful urging. Cutting pain in bladder before urinating. Nocturnal bedwetting from nervous irritation.

Limbs - General muscular weakness. Violent pains in acute rheumatism of joints. Pains in lower limbs, alternating sides. Sciatica with tender feet. Twitchings. Parkinson's disease. Involuntary shaking of hands. Chorea. Tetanic spasms. ***Spasmodic convulsions with stiffness of limbs, clenched fingers and thumbs drawn in. Cramps worse at night, in bed. Cramps from prolonged exertion.*** Cramps after prolonged use of tools. Crampy contraction of fingers. Skin of fingers tight. ***Writers' and players' cramps. Cramps in calves and feet.*** Runner's cramps. Cramps in limbs during pregnancy.

Lungs - Spasmodic nervous asthma. Asthmatic oppression of chest. Oppressed breathing, with desire to take deep breath, worse on entering warm room, worse walking. Difficult breathing with intercostal neuralgia.

Modalities - ***Better by heat, warmth***. Better hot water, bathing. ***Better from pressure.*** Better rubbing. ***Better bending double***. Better standing up. ***Worse from cold air.*** Worse drafts. Worse uncovering. Worse cold water. Worse periodicity. ***Worse night***. Worse exhaustion. Worse milk. Worse right side. Worse lying on right side. Worse touch.

Mouth - Bitter taste. Taste of bananas. Food does not taste right. ***Swelling of tongue.*** Tongue, clean with colic. Cracks in angles of lips. Painful contraction of jaw joint. Spasms without febrile symptoms. Spasmodic stammering.

Nose - Alternate stuffing and profuse gushing discharge. Discharge of a white, thin substance, worse from left nostril. Smarting and raw feeling in left nostril. Loss or perversion of sense of smell.

Rectum - Constipation in rheumatic subjects due to flatulence and indigestion. Constipation in infants. Torpid stool. Stool expelled with force. Dysentery with cramp-like pains, better by pressure or bending double. Dysentery with spasmodic retention of urine. ***Watery diarrhea with vomiting and cramps in calves.*** Stools loose, watery, with urging. Diarrhea ceases, spasms or other brain troubles set in. ***Cutting, darting, lightning-like pains in hemorrhoids.*** Itching and scratching feeling in anus.

Skin - Barber's itch. Herpetic eruptions with white scales. Rash on arms, legs and face, like insect bites. Rash red when scratched. Pricking sensation all over.

Sleep - Sleepy when attempting to study. Spasmodic yawning as if it would dislocate the jaw with tears. Sleepless on account of indigestion or toothache. ***Insomnia from exhaustion. Wakes at night with leg and foot cramps.*** Sleep disturbed by troublesome dreams. Drowsy in morning.

Stomach - ***Stomach cramps.*** Intense cutting, shooting, cramping pains in region of stomach. ***Colic, better eructation. Colic in babies*** (Cham.). Obstinate hiccough, causes long-lasting soreness. ***Hiccough with retching day and night.*** Burning pain, vomiting and hiccough, better hot drinks. Constant nausea. Persistent vomiting. Bilious vomiting, at times streaked with blood. Cancer of stomach.

Teeth - ***Toothache, better by heat and hot liquids***. Toothache, worse eating or drinking, cold things. Teeth sensitive to touch or cold air. Severe pain in decayed or filled teeth. Neuralgic pain in a filled tooth. Ulceration of teeth with swelling of glands of face, throat and neck. ***Complaints of teething children***, spasms during dentition without fever symptoms.

Temperature - ***Chilliness*** after dinner in evening. ***Chills run up and down the back.*** Chills with shivering, followed by a suffocating sensation.

Throat - ***Soreness and stiffness***, especially right side, parts seem puffy with chilliness and aching all over. Spasmodic constriction of throat on attempting to swallow liquids. Sensation of choking, of a corn-husk lodged in upper part of throat. Voice harsh, larynx sore and raw. Nervous angina.

Vertigo - Vertigo on moving. Vertigo falls forward on closing eyes, better walking in open air.

Vision - Vision blurred. Dark spots before eyes on attempting to read. Colored lights before eyes. Sees rainbow colors. Double vision during headache.

COMMENTS - Acute or chronic cramps and spasms. Writer's or musician's cramps, charley horses. Acute leg cramps in the elderly or in athletes. Lower leg cramps (Cupr., Calc-c.).

Paralysis, or cramping pains followed by paralysis. Cramps and spasms are better with heat, will often place a hot water bottle on the site (Cham. will want cold), better from pressure. Generally right sided (Coloc. is left sided).

Facial neuralgias (Kalm.) and sciatica, worse on the right side, better heat. Headache, better from applied heat. Chorea, respiratory spasms. Spasms of the glottis, whooping cough. Hiccoughs (Nux-v.).

Lockjaw, tetanus. For teething children or toothache, better drinking something warm or from warm applications. Useful for cracks at the corners of the lips. Allen's proving brought out canker sores in mouth, sore lips and cracked lips.

Stomach cramps. Abdominal cramps radiated from umbilical region, better by bending double, heat, sometimes with watery diarrhea. Colic in babies (Cham.), without irritability, better heat. Spasmodic retention of the urine. Inguinal hernia. Nondescript menstrual cramps. Labor pains.

Cramping, burning pain, better from heat (Ars.). Pains are shooting like lightning or boring, often combined with or alternating with a sense of constriction, at times wandering, better by warmth, pressure, worse by light touch.

Attacks of pain, often with great prostration or profuse sweat, leaving the patient "languid, tired, exhausted, unable to sit up."

More often called for in men than Mag-c, but the indication "worn-out women" applies to both. Disorders are often periodic.

Useful for complaints from standing in cold water, complaints of dentition, headaches of school children, professional neuroses, after effects of catheter.

Clarke cured a very severe attack of chorea in a girl of six with Mag-p. 6x. The spasms were general, but they affected the speech to such an extent that she could not make herself intelligible.

Rappaz of Montevideo cured with Mag-p. a young man, 17, of cerebral meningitis which began with violent pain and inflammation in his left eye with terrific pains in his head, delirium and intense fever. He was first treated allopathically, without success.

When Rappaz first saw him, he was hemiplegic with frequent and alarming convulsions, violent crying out, involuntary passage of feces and urine, dilated pupils, dropped jaw, escape of saliva, with difficult speech and comprehension. Under Mag-p. 6x in water, general improvement set in. Later the 12x was given and in two months he was well.

W. T. Ord cured Miss G., 48, of back pain extending down right sciatic nerve and up the back, following influenza with Mag-p. 3x, 5 grain doses.

Skinner has cured with Mag-p. a case of prolapsed of rectum with feeling as if rectum were torn, the symptoms being better by heat.

RELATIONS - ***Antidoted by:*** Bell., Gels., Lach. ***Compare:*** (1) Kali-p., Coloc., Sil., Zinc., Dios. (2) Cham. - vegetable analog, but Cham. has worse from heat. (3) Shifting pains, Puls., Lac-c. (4) Neuralgia recurring violently every night. (5) better warmth, Ars. (6) Dysmenorrhea, Caul., Cimic., Xan., Cact., Lil-t., Coloc. (7) Colic better bending double, Coloc. (8) better from hot drinks, Lyc. (9) Meteorism, Lyc., cracks on lips, Nat-m. (10) Headache from occiput to eye better warmth, Sil.

REFERENCES - Boericke. Clarke. Murphy. Phatak.

MAGNESIA SULPHURICA

(Magnesium Sulphate)

PHARMACY - mag-s. Magnesia sulphurica. Magnesium sulphate. Epsom salts. Magnesia sulphate. Trituration. ***Historical dose:*** Trituration and all potencies.

CLINICAL - Acidity. Acne. Allergies. Backache. Bedwetting. Boils. Constipation. Coughs, spasms. Diabetes. ***Diarrhea.*** Dropsy. Dysentery. Dysmenorrhea. ***Eczema.*** Epithelioma. Erysipelas. Eye, pain. ***Female, disorders.*** Gallbladder, pain. Gallstone, colic. Headache. Hernia. Intermenstrual, hemorrhage. Itching. ***Leucorrhea.*** Liver, complaints. Lumbago. Menorrhagia. Mental, problems. Migraines. Miliary, eruptions. Neuralgias. Pimples. ***Scabies. Skin, disorders.*** Tetany. ***Thyroid, weakness.*** Toothache. ***Urinary, disorders. Warts***.

HOMEOPATHIC - The ancient reputation of Mag-s. as a "refrigerant cathartic" under the familiar name of "Epsom Salts," or "salts" par excellence, has overshadowed its homeopathic uses.

Recently old-school authorities have discovered in this "cathartic" a remedy for dysentery. It is the chief ingredient in many laxative mineral waters and popular saline aperient mixtures.

Mag-s. is of diagnostic and therapeutic value in gallstone colic. The physiological dosage from 2 to 4 teaspoonfuls in glass hot water taken at onset of a colicky attack may abort or stop the colic.

Epsom salts is one of the most active saline cathartics, operating with little pain or nausea, especially if pure. Its action causing a rush of fluid into the intestine, which by producing a distention of the bowel produces evacuation.

It causes little or no irritation in the intestine. In common with the other salines, it is the classical evacuant to be employed in connection with mercurials and anthelmintics and in cases of poisoning.

It usually acts within from one to two hours, more quickly if taken in hot water and in the morning before breakfast.

The ordinary dose as a mild laxative is a heaping teaspoonful, as a cathartic, two to four teaspoonfuls. The taste may be improved, if necessary, by the addition of a little lemon juice and sugar. Use on compresses saturated with solution.

Besides Mag-s. chief use as a saline cathartic, magnesium sulphate is used to a considerable extent externally in saturated solution as an antiphlogistic and anti-itching in erysipleas, poison ivy poisoning, cellulitis and other local inflammations.

Percy Wilde noted that the purgative action of Mag-s. is not a quality of the drug, but a quality of its physical state, which renders its absorption impossible. The properties inherent in the substance itself can only be discovered by potency.

The ***skin, urinary and female symptoms*** are most marked. Greenish urine with red sediment. Profuse dark intermittent menses. Thick leucorrhea as profuse as menses. As of a lump between shoulders. Back feels broken. Left arm and foot numb. Crawling in fingertips. Small pimples all over the body which itch violently. Warts, large, soft.

Mag-s. has a depressive condition with hypersensitivity. Dysthyroidism. Tendency to spasms in the hollow organs. Liver weakness. Intermittent discomfort with prolonged periods of relief.

MIND - Apprehensive. Anxious, as though about to be struck by misfortune. Prostration from anxiety. Foreboding anxiety, as if some accident would happen. Irritable with a fear of dying. Hypersensitive to pain (Cham., Mag-p.).

Depression. Melancholy and disposition to weep and restlessness. Bad-tempered with nervous tension. Tendency to fly into a passion, every thing is taken in bad part. Misunderstands everything. Errors of imagination. Sees people who are absent.

Abdomen - Sharp pains in left hypochondrium. Tension, hardness and fullness of abdomen after a meal. Violent shooting pains in whole abdomen, around the navel. Painful drawing in abdomen. Rumbling in abdomen with emission of flatulence. Itching of left inguinal region, not removed by scratching.

Back - Pains in the lumbar region. Lumbago. Violent pain in the small of the back, as if bruised and as before menstruation. Bruised and ulcerative pain between the shoulders with a feeling as of a lump as large as the fist, on which account she could not lie upon her back or side, relieved by rubbing.

Constitutions - Allergic, tubercular types with nervous hyper-excitability.

Ears - Noises, tinkling in ears. Shooting pains in ears.

Eyes - Burning in eyes. Shooting pains in eyes. Pains in eyes, as if protruding from orbits. Lachrymation with photophobia. Dimness of eyes with frequent drowsiness. Supra-orbital neuralgia, left side.

Face - Face discolored, gray. Earthy color of face. Tearing in bones of face. Dryness and burning in lips, in evening.

Female - Premenstrual nausea. Menses too early or late, scanty or heavy. Blood thick and black. Discomfort during menses. ***Thick leucorrhea***, as profuse as the menses with weary pain in the small of the back and thighs, on moving about. Some blood from the vagina between the menses.

Food - Intense thirst, morning and evening. Want of appetite and repugnance to all food, even when thinking of it. Desire for fruits, green salad and refreshing dishes. Aversion to sausages, meat, fats and fatty foods.

Head - Headache with feeling of fullness in the head, blood in the head and a prickling, drawing, piercing sensation.

Heart - Pricking pain in the heart, ameliorated by sitting and resting and aggravated by heat. Palpitations and breathlessness from physical exercise. Wakes at night with palpitations, following sleep filled with nightmares.

Kidneys - Stream intermits and dribbles. The urine passed in the morning copious, bright yellow, soon becomes turbid and deposits a copious red sediment. The urine is greenish as passed is of a clear color and in a large quantity. Diabetes (Ph-ac., Lac-ac.). Stitches and burning in the orifice of the urethra after urinating.

Limbs - Sciatic pains, aggravated at night and during rest, ameliorated by walking. Chronic, non-inflammatory rheumatism of the hip. The left arm and foot fall asleep in bed in the morning after waking.

Liver - Pain in the liver region, especially on breathing. Painful sensitivity in the region of the gallbladder. Nightly attacks on the liver and gallbladder.

Lungs - Respiration panting after exercise. Laryngeal cough on waking, sometimes spasmodic and dry, sometimes with sputum. Dry and shaking cough after waking in morning, and which compels sitting up. Expectoration of sour mucus.

Male - Urethritis. Prostatitis. Frequent stinging about penis when sitting or walking. Erections without amorous fancies or sexual desire.

Modalities - Better from movement in the fresh air. Better from washing in cool water. Better from rubbing. Better walking. Worse morning. Worse on awaking. Worse from traveling on a train. Worse in a closed vehicle.

Mouth - Dryness and sweetish bitterness of the mouth, especially in the morning. Dryness of mouth with sensation of numbness. Roughness of tongue. Vesicles on edges of tongue with incisive pains. Toothache.

Nose - Congestive pain. Nasal discharge with painful ulceration inside the nose. Copious secretion of thick and yellow mucus in nose. Fluent coryza with loss of smell. Nosebleed, at night. Rough voice and frequent flow of water from nose.

Perspiration - Perspiration at night or in morning, accompanied by thirst. Hands moist from sweating.

Rectum - Neuralgia of rectum. Constipation. Feces at one time hard, at another soft. Liquid stools with tenesmus. Soft stools early after rising. Loose evacuations with violent thirst. Stools like diarrhea, grayish in color or constipation with gray stools covered with mucus. Diarrhea preceded by rumbling in abdomen. Diarrhea with diuresis. Diarrhea after eating pancakes. ***Acid diarrhea of children.*** Ejection of ascarides during every evacuation.

Skin - Generalized itching over the whole body, worse in bed. ***Eczema and vesicular eczemas.*** Miliary eruptions with burning and itching. Small pimples over the whole body, that itch violently. Boils. ***Suppressed scabies*** (Sulph.). Crawling in the tips of the fingers of the left hand, better on rubbing. ***Warts***. Erysipelas. Dropsy. Acne on the back. Epithelioma.

Sleep - Extreme sleepiness in the daytime. Sleepy, early in evening. Sleeplessness at night, caused by violent pains in head, abdomen and loins. Wakes at 3 a. m. with difficulty in falling asleep again. Many dreams at night, sometimes disagreeable and anxious. Sleep with worrying, with palpitations.

Stomach - Frequent belchings, tasting like bad eggs. Regurgitation of fluid, preceded by a quivering in stomach. Disgust and nausea with accumulation of water in mouth. Vomiting, first of food, then of mucus.

Temperature - Chill from 9 a.m. to 10 a.m. Chilliness with thirst, early in morning after waking. Shaking chill with violent headache in evening, succeeded by thirst. Shuddering in back, heat in one part and chill in another. Cold feet all day, although otherwise he feels hot. Heat of head with coldness of rest of body. Alternation of heat and shuddering, redness and paleness of face.

Throat - Deep, hollow, bass voice. Sore throat on swallowing and pricking pains spreading to the ear. Sore throat, with shooting pains at night, worse by swallowing. Dryness and sensation of numbness in throat. Accumulation of mucus in throat.

Vertigo - Vertigo, heaviness and numbness of the whole head. Vertigo during menses.

COMMENTS - Poisonings from Mag-s. have occurred from overdoses, death apparently occurring from collapse. The provings of the salts produced many symptoms of utter prostration.

The provings bring out effects common to the other magnesia. Tearfulness, restless uneasiness, pains in facial bones, sensitiveness to touch, better by walking. The diuretic action of the drug with great thirst has led to its successful use in diabetes.

Diarrhea, accompanied with great thirst. Toothache, worse coming into a room out of cold air, worse by contact with food, whether cold or warm, better in bed. Chill, accompanied or followed by thirst. Shuddering in back from below upward.

According to Med. Press in Sept. 9, 1891, eight cases of new growth having all the outward characters of epithelioma were cured by Graves with teaspoonful doses of a solution of three drachms to the pint.

Warts are allied to epithelioma, and H. T. Webster cured many cases in children, giving as much of the salts as would lie on a dime three times a day. One boy was literally covered with warts, his face being much disfigured. One girl of 16 was cured of large warts on her hands.

F. H. Pritchard gave his experience with Mag-s. (1/2 grains in a teaspoonful of water) in summer diarrhea with vomiting of food, copious yellowish, slimy and stinking stools and later merely watery serum. The first sign of improvement was that the stools became bile-tinged after which they soon became of thicker consistency. The copious stools seemed to be the cardinal indication.

RELATIONS - It is claimed that the addition of a small amount of Mag-s. to the usual hypodermic of morphine increases the value of the hypodermic from 50 to 100%. ***Compare:*** (1) Mag-c., Mag-m., Mag-p. (2) In diabetes, Nat-s. (3) Sadness, weeping, foreboding anxiety, Cimic., Puls. (4) Stinging in fauces between acts of deglutition, Ign. (5) Belchings, Hep. (6) Apprehension, Lyc.

REFERENCES - Boericke. Clarke. Julian. Phatak.

MAGNETIS POLI AMBO

(Magnet)

PHARMACY - m-ambo. (m-p-a.) Magnetis poli ambo. Magnet. Both poles of the magnet. Trituration of Sugar of Milk after exposure of the influence of the both poles of the magnet. Dilution of distilled water similarly exposed. ***Historical dose:*** All potencies.

CLINICAL - Colic. Coma. Constipation. Cough. Diarrhea. Dyspnea. Fainting. Flatulence. Headaches. Hemorrhage. Hemorrhoids. Orchitis. ***Pains.*** Paraphimosis. Prolapsed, anus. Rheumatism. Toothache. Ulcers. Vertigo. Wounds.

HOMEOPATHIC - General symptoms of the magnet produced by touching either magnetic pole indiscriminately while handling the magnet or by laying the whole of the magnetic surface upon the body.

Marked sensations of coldness. The eyeball feels cold, as if it were a lump of ice in the socket. Sensation as if the blood was rushing towards points. Burning sensation in the limbs and joints.

Burning lancinations across all parts of body in different directions. Pains as if broken in joints, when cartilages of two bones touch. Wrenching pain in the limbs.

Shooting and jerkings. Shuddering, which traverses the whole body. Shaking in the body with fright or shocks, which cause violent bending and straightening of the body, sometimes with the loss of consciousness.

Headaches as if a nail were driven in. Long-lasting swoons during which she feels her pains, but is not able to speak or move. Tendency of old wounds to bleed afresh.

MIND - Irresolution. Inadvertence. Hurried, heedless and forgetful. Busy precipitation. Absence of mind. Talks aloud to himself without being aware of it. Does things he doesn't intend to. Tendency to anger and rage.

Abdomen - Pressure and anxious fullness in abdomen, especially during mental exertion. Noisy, gas, grumbling and borborygmi in abdomen. Flatulent colic. Production of much flatus. Expulsion of flatulence with painful pressure.

Back - Jerking in the spine, as from something alive. Painful sensibility of the joint of the sacrum in morning in bed, when lying on side or by day, when stooping. Wrenching pain in shoulder joint or pain as from the starting of a tendon in wrist.

Chest - Burning insupportable lancinations in muscles of chest.

Ears - Humming in ears. Diminution of hearing.

Eyes - Itching in eyes, especially the lids. Pupils dilated. Scintillation of white light, beyond the range of vision in the twilight. Sparks before the eyes.

Face - Perspiration on face without heat in morning. Jerking, tearing in upper jaw. Small pimples with pain like that of a wound, on lips. Violent burning lancination in muscles of face in evening. Swelling of lips with salivation in evening.

Female - Menses premature, profuse and of too long duration.

Food - Fetid breath. Metallic taste in mouth. Insipid taste of tobacco and beer. Many things have a moldy taste. Speedy satiety. Good appetite in evening.

Head - Headache from over-strained memory and reflection. Digging, stupefying headache, which is immediately dispersed by movements of flatus. Head pain, as if a nail were driven into the head, as if caused by a wound, especially after a fit of anger. Jerking, tearing in head, appearing at intervals. Rushing or buzzing noises in whole head. Pain, as of a bruise in head, on waking in morning.

Limbs - Drawing pains in joints and muscles of arms, often from head to fingers. Tearing, jerking in muscles of arms after remaining some time in the cold. Red spots in palms like vesicles. Attacks of cramp in calves of legs and toes after waking in morning. Burning lancinations in heels and in corns on the feet.

Lungs - Paroxysms of dry cough at night. Spasmodic cough, especially after midnight, when awake or during reflection. Nocturnal dyspnea, excited by mucus in trachea, which is easily detached in morning.

Male - Burning sensation in region of spermatic vesicles, which excites sexual desire. Dullness of sexual feeling and aversion to sex. Erection without amorous thoughts. Retraction of prepuce behind the glans. Swelling of epididymis with pain during movement and when touched.

Modalities - Worse by motion and on waking. Toothache is worse from cold and on contact with anything cold. Touch aggravates pain in joints. Heat is better from uncovering.

Nose - Aberration of smell, a smoky or moldy scent is perceived.

Rectum - Constipation, as from contraction of rectum. Painless diarrhea with flatulence. Hemorrhoids, smarting pain in anus after evacuation with constriction in rectum. Blind hemorrhoids. Prolapsed rectum.

Skin - Tendency of old wounds to bleed afresh. Ulcers painful, like new wounds. Small furunculi. Small pustules with lancinating, drawing pain.

Sleep - Jerking of the body before going to sleep. Disturbed sleep with talking, snoring and continued tossing. Waking at 3 a.m. and falling into a drowsy lethargy towards sunrise. Lying on the back with the hand under the head, the legs wide apart and the mouth half open with snoring respiration. Amorous, lascivious dreams. After waking in morning, headache with pain, as of a fracture in all the joints, which forces constant change in position of limbs.

Stomach - Stomachache with cramp towards upper part, agitation, which allows no rest whatever, heaviness of tongue, paleness of face and coldness of body. Abortive risings. Risings with smell and taste of horn scrapings. Sour regurgitation, when stooping.

Teeth - Pressive, jerking toothache in isolated shocks. Toothache after drinking anything cold or from contact with cold air. Toothache in carious teeth with swelling of gums.

Temperature - Dry heat with need to be uncovered, at night and in morning in bed.

Vertigo - Vertigo, especially in evening after lying down, as if about to fall or as from concussion in head. Vertigo with staggering, when walking, objects seem to waver before eyes.

COMMENTS - The effect of the magnet as a whole and of each pole separately was tested by Hahnemann, and the symptoms are mainly from his pathogenesis.

He said he did not expect "ordinary mechanical, materialistic and atomistic heads" to be able to regard diseases as "immaterial alternations of the vitality or pure dynamic derangements of our state of health and medicinal powers as merely virtual, almost spiritual, forces."

Hahnemann asked how they can reconcile with their materialistic notions the fact that "a single imponderable spark from a Leyden jar gives a shock to the strongest man and yet to ascertainable ponderable substance is communicated to his body?"

Clarke's experience with magnetism is confined to M-ambo. 2,000c, but that is sufficient to give him confidence in prescribing potencies of these remedies when their indications arise, particularly burning lancinations throughout the body, pains as if broken in joints, where cartilages of two bones touch, shootings and jerkings, disturbed sleep, headache as if a nail were driven in.

Hahnemann said the symptoms "occurred from various powerful magnets brought in contact with various sensitive individuals without distinction of the poles.

"They were observed in experiments conducted for half a year for the purpose of ascertaining the proper and most efficacious mode of stroking the steel with magnets in which a horse-shoe magnet, capable of lifting a weight of twelve pounds, was held in the hands, which were held in contact with both poles for an hour at a time." Additional symptoms came from Andry, Thouret, Unzer and De Harsu.

Hahnemann noted that "Although each of the poles presents something peculiar in its power of altering the human health, yet each of them seems, when applied twice of oftener to produce alternating actions which resemble those of the opposite pole."

For curative purposes, Hahnemann recommended a much milder application of the magnet. The popular use of magnetic rings for rheumatism is analogous to this. The method of attenuating media saturated with emanations from the magnet does not seem to have occurred to Hahnemann.

RELATIONS - ***Antidoted by:*** Ign., Electr., Galv., Zinc. (imposition of Zinc plate). ***Compare:*** (1) M-arct., M-aust., Ferr-ma., Mang-o. (2) Burnt smell in nose, Anac. (3) Prolapsed anus, Podo., Caust., Ign. (4) Bell., Lyc., Nux-v., Petr., Puls., Stram., Sabin., Teucr.

REFERENCES - Clarke.

MAGNETIS POLUS ARCTICUS

(North Pole of Magnet)

PHARMACY - m-arct. Magnetis polus arcticus. North pole of the magnet. Potencies of saccharum lactis or water charged with the influence of this pole. ***Historical dose:*** All potencies.

CLINICAL - Amenorrhea. Clairvoyance. Coma. Constipation. Cough. Flatulence. Headache. Heartburn. Hernia. Menses, suppressed. Nosebleed. Panaritium. Salivation. Sleep, disturbed. Sleepwalking. Toothache. Vertebra, cracking. Vertigo.

HOMEOPATHIC - The symptoms of Mag-arct. were obtained by applying it in the region of the 4th to 6th thoracic vertebra, at a distance of four or five finger's breadth from the body.

Over-excitement with trembling, uneasy restlessness in limbs and great nervous weakness. Great lassitude and painful weariness of the whole body with dejection, especially in morning and in open air, as during sultry weather.

Sharp shocks, throbbing, trembling, coldness and sensation as if the blood were driven toward parts. Drawing sensation in periosteum of all bones, as at commencement of intermittent fever. Cracking in cervical vertebrae.

Marked affect in the teeth and jaws. Sensation of coldness with toothache. Increased flow of saliva. Swelling, heat and redness of one cheek. ***Coldness of eyes as if a piece of ice lay in orbit.*** Disturbed sleep, sleepwalking. Constipation, sopor, trembling. Abdominal flatulence.

MIND - Mildness, submission. Anxious hesitation and restlessness. Fickleness. Irresolution, followed by prompt execution after a resolution has been once formed. Indolence when seated, as if power of moving were lost.

Peevishness. ***Sensitive to noises.*** Weakness of memory. Tendency to make mistakes when writing. Loss of ideas. Loss of sense. Speaking loud while quite alone and engaged in business. Inclination to weep with shivering.

Abdomen - Inflation of abdomen. Shocks in abdomen, as if something in it were falling or blows proceeding from abdomen and passing upwards through chest, as far as the throat. Pressure and boring towards inguinal ring, as if preparatory to a rupture with relaxation of the inguinal ring. Production and incarceration of much flatus. Flatulent, pressive colic.

Back - Cracking in the cervical vertebra during movement. Pains in back, as if broken, on bending it backwards.

Ears - Murmuring in ears and internal heat, as from boiling water. Deafness, as if caused by a band over ears.

Eyes - Restless movements of eyes. Eyes prominent and fixed. Icy coldness of (weak) eye, as if a lump of ice lay in orbit instead of the eye. Lancinations, itching and jerking drawing in eyelids with lachrymation. Painful sensation of dryness in eyelids, on awaking in morning.

Face - Paleness in face. Tension in face. Painful squeezing in maxillary joint with sensation, while moving it, as if it were dislocated. Swelling of one cheek only. Trismus.

Female - Menses too feeble. Menses suppressed.

Food - Voracity in evening. Loss of taste. Acid taste in the mouth. Tobacco has a bitter taste.

Head - Headache is worse lifting or moving arm.

Kidneys - Increased secretion of urine. Deep-colored urine.

Limbs - Inflammation of back of hand with pulsative pain. Heaviness in arms, hands and fingers. Great lassitude in lower limbs, which feel as if they would break, when walking. Pains, as of a fracture in hip joints and lower limbs. Pain, as from excoriation in toes and corns on the feet.

Lungs - Dry, asthmatic, suffocating cough, worse by walking in open air. Constant want to cough in evening, which is removed only by restraining the cough. Spasmodic, shaking cough in evening, on going to sleep, which hinders sleep. Spasmodic, suffocating cough towards midnight, produced by irritation in bronchia. Cough shaking the head and whole body and exciting heat until a general perspiration ensues with cessation of the cough.

Male - Excitement of sexual desire. Immoderate erections with frequent pollutions.

Modalities - Better from uncovering, worse on waking. Toothache, worse breathing through the mouth.

Mouth - At night, collection of saliva in mouth, so profuse that every time he wakes the pillow is quite wet. Itching in point of tongue, compels him to scratch it.

Nose - Aberration of smell, smell of rotten eggs, fresh plaster or dust. Nosebleed. preceded by pressive head pain in forehead. Redness and heat in point of nose. followed by red spots, hot and plainly circumscribed, on cheeks.

Rectum - Obstinate constriction of abdomen and constipation. Hard feces of a large size, difficult to evacuate often preceded by drawing, dysenteric pains in the hypogastrium.

Skin - Tingling and lancination itching in skin. Burning sensation or burning tearing in tetters. Panaritium.

Sleep - Violent, spasmodic yawning, with wrenching pain in maxillary joint. Strong disposition to sleep by day. Coma. Profound sleep at night during which the patient generally ties on the back. Tossing during sleep, with troublesome heat and urgent inclination to be uncovered without thirst. Waking in the evening after sleep, in consequence of a violent shock in the head and muscles of the neck. Many vivid dreams, sometimes lascivious. Sings in her sleep, is wakened by it, falls asleep again, recommences to sing and again wakes up from it. Imperfect waking in morning (2 a.m.), with perfect inner consciousness, vivid memory, great concourse of ideas and reflections on some important subject.

Stomach - Frequent empty risings. Continued heartburn, especially after supper.

Teeth - Toothache in carious teeth, at intervals, as if they were being extracted. Pains in carious teeth with gums swollen and painful when touched, worse after a meal and by heat, better in open air and when walking. Toothache with red, hot, swollen cheeks. Toothache with shocks, which traverse the periosteum of the jaw or with drawing, pressive or else tearing, digging or burning sharp pains. Incisors set on edge, when breathing through the mouth. Numbness and insensibility of the gums, on the cessation of the toothache.

Temperature - Sensation of coldness or of coolness over whole body. Chilliness. Cool hands with cool perspiration upon them and over whole body. Cold sweat on hands and soles of feet. Shuddering, followed by transient heat and swelling of veins of hands. Sensation of heat over whole body with coldness of hands and lower limbs.

Vertigo - Vertigo, as from intoxication with staggering, when walking in open air and instability when standing.

COMMENTS - Swan reported a case cured by C. M. Conant in which Mrs. S., age 31, blonde, had pain in her left lower jaw as if out of joint, worse morning, on moving it. Sensation as if head of bone were squeezed and crowded into socket. Mag-arct. 1,000c cured.

One symptom of the proving, occurring in a half-waking state, suggests an approach to sleepwalking. He thinks out a "difficult subject in the best form in a foreign language," but when awake he cannot remember distinctly the subject.

Several provers complained of faintness. One had "sensation of dryness and lightness in the body with want of strength." Sensation as if scalp adhered to skull.

RELATIONS - ***Antidoted by:*** M-aust., Ign.; Zinc. ***Compare:*** (1) M-ambo. M-aust. (2) Sensation as if teeth being pulled out, Ip. (3) Worse raising arm, Bar-c., Con., Cupr., Ferr. (4) One cheek red, Cham. (5) Coff., Cham.

REFERENCES - Clarke.

MAGNETIS POLUS AUSTRALIS

(South Pole of Magnet)

PHARMACY - m-aust. Magnetis polus australis. South pole of the magnet. Potencies of alcohol saturated with emanations of the south pole. ***Historical dose:*** All potencies.

CLINICAL - Amblyopia. Borborygmi. Bulimia. Colds. Coryzas. Coughs. Dislocation, easy. Frostbite. Heart, palpitations. Hernia. ***Ingrown, toenails.*** Lachrymation. Levitation. Menorrhagia. ***Pains.*** Palpitations. ***Toothaches.*** Varicose, veins. Vertigo. Wisdom tooth.

HOMEOPATHIC - Hahnemann first noticed the symptoms that led to the use for ingrown toenails, including a sore pain on the inner side of the nail of the big toe when walking. As if the nail had grown into the flesh on the side, very painful on being slightly touched. The shoe presses on the toes and on the nail of the big toe when walking, as from corns.

The accurate response of M-aust. to these symptoms proved to Clarke the possibility of attenuating and so fixing this "energy" for use as an ordinary homeopathic remedy. Clarke cured so many cases of ingrown toenail with M-aust. 2,000c., that he invariably gave it in the first place when there were no symptoms plainly indicating another remedy.

Sharp, pulsative pains in roots of nails, as if about to suppurate. Easy dislocation of joints of foot, feet are painful when letting them hang down. Aching in patella, shooting in soles.

Drawings in fingers, feet and ankles. Pains with pinching or burning, lancinations in different parts of the body. Contusive pains in limbs and joints, as if the patient had been lying on flints.

Dryness of eyelids. Tendency of nose, ears, hands and feet to be frozen by a moderate degree of coldness. Liability to suffer from a chill. Sudden lassitude when walking with anxiety and heat or sudden inclination to sleep. Lightness of whole body.

MIND - Mood is changeable, variable. Capriciousness. Abrupt. Irritability. Instability of ideas. Inconstancy. Irresolution, indecision.

Confused, wandering thoughts. Absent-minded. Indifference, apathy. Indolence, aversion to work.

Anxiety with fear. Frightened easily. Fear of people, anthropophobia. Timidity. Aversion to anyone who comes near, even loved ones. Forsaken feeling. Weeping, tearful mood after anger, vexation. Guilt.

Morose and ill-humor, with aversion to conversation. Society is disagreeable, wants to be alone. Dislike to society and to laughing faces. Wants to say something hateful. Sulky. Ill-humor, peevish.

Asserts himself with vehemence and despises others. Anger at trifles. Anger with trembling. Harshness, rough. Abusive, insulting. Quarrelsome, scolding. Reproaches others. Violence, vehemence. Wild, hasty, harsh, violent in word and deed. Passion and rage.

Dreams of animals, fire. Nightmares. Amorous disposition. Stupefaction, as if intoxicated. Crawling around like a animal.

Abdomen - Noisy borborygmi and grumbling in abdomen. Pressive, flatulent colic with pinchings and inflation of abdomen. Sensation, as if inguinal ring were dilated, preparatory to the rupture with painful sensibility of that part, when coughing.

Back - Pressive, burning pain in loins during repose and movement. Pain, as of a fracture or wrenching pain in joint of sacrum and lumbar vertebra.

Causations - Ailments from anger, vexation, emotional excitement.

Chest - Oppression of the chest, as if the respiration were tremulous and produced an impression of coolness. Drawing pressure in both sides of sternum with anguish of conscience, which allows no rest.

Eyes - Dryness and smarting in eyelids, especially when moving them, worse morning and evening. Lachrymation. Amblyopia.

Female - Menses premature and profuse. Metrorrhagia.

Head - Great rush of blood to brain early in morning in bed. Heaviness, tingling and digging in head. Shocks in head, sometimes with tearing.

Heart - Violent palpitations of the heart with great heat in cardiac region. Palpitation of the heart during which it seems that it is not the heart that palpitates.

Kidneys - Involuntary emission of urine from paralysis of bladder sphincter, especially at night. Frequent emission of urine at night. Very feeble stream of urine. Emission of urine, drop by drop with torpor of urethra.

Lungs - Coughs and coryzas with expectoration of greenish mucus and shortness of breath. Paroxysms of fetid cough at night, when sleeping. Want to take full, sighing inspirations, with involuntary deglutition.

Male - Strong disposition to emission. Emissions in a hemiplegia patient, paralysis worse after the emission. Impotence with sudden cessation of all enjoyment in the moment of greatest excitement. Pain in penis, as if some tissues were torn or plucked away. Painful retraction of testes at night. Swelling of testes with tearing shocks and sensation of contraction.

Modalities - Worse when walking in open air, sitting, hanging limb down.

Mouth - Metallic taste, at one time sweetish, at another acidulous, on and under the tongue. Accumulation of watery saliva in the mouth. Speech embarrassed, as by a swelling of the tongue.

Rectum - Stools, soft, loose, preceded by gripings. Evacuation of liquid feces with a sensation as if flatus were about to be discharged. Contractions and painful constriction in rectum and anus, which hinder the expulsion of wind.

Sleep - Urgent inclination to sleep, evening and morning. Closing the eyes without power to sleep. Sleeplessness with over-excitement before midnight. Confused, frightful dreams. Prolonged dreams on the same subject with fatigue. Dreams of incendiary fires. Lying on the back during the night. Slow, noisy, snoring expiration. Congestion in head in morning, which compels lying with head high.

Stomach - All kinds of food appear insipid. Extreme indifference to food, drink and tobacco-smoke. Bulimia at noon and evening, sometimes during the febrile shiverings. Aching in scrobiculus during mental exertion.

Teeth - Tearing, jerking toothache, worse by hot things.

Temperature - Excessive dread of open air, which penetrates to the very marrow of the bones, even when the weather is hot, with ill-humor and inclination to weep. Shuddering with cloudiness before eyes. Trembling and tossing of limbs without shivering, followed by heat in head and face.

Throat - Burning sensation in gullet.

Vertigo - Vertigo, as from intoxication with staggering gait.

COMMENTS - Ingrown toenails, toothache, insomnia, and arthritis. Pinching, squeezing sensations and bruised pains. Faintness, comes on when walking, worse when sitting. Great rush of blood to the brain early in the morning in bed.

Berridge reported the case of Miss X, who had for three weeks aching in the middle of front of left lower leg, where she had varicose veins for eight months, when standing or when the leg is hanging down. Aching pain is removed by placing it horizontally.

Frequent feeling of hot water running down the affected part, but only when leg is down, at times throbbing when leg hangs down. She was given M-aust. 100,000c, one dose. The hot-water feeling never returned and the pain ceased in two days.

RELATIONS - ***Antidoted by:*** M-arct., Ign., Zinc. ***Compare:*** (1) M-ambo., Galv., Electr. in fetid cough, Caps. (2) Rush of blood to head, Aster. (3) Toenails, Graph., Sil., Nit-ac., Thuj.

REFERENCES - Clarke. Murphy. Phatak.

MAGNOLIA GLAUCA

(Sweet Magnolia)

PHARMACY - magn-gl. Magnolia glauca. Sweet magnolia. Sweet bay. Beaver-tree. N. O. Magnoliacee. Tincture of the flowers. ***Historical dose:*** Tincture and all potencies.

CLINICAL - Asthma. Fainting. Gout.

HERBAL - The Treasury of Botany said "M. glauca is a low-growing, deciduous tree, called in America Swamp Sassafras from the nature of the locality in which it grows and from the resemblance in its properties to Laurus sassafras. It is also called Beaver-tree, because the root is eaten by beavers, which the animals also make use of the wood in constructing their nests."

HOMEOPATHIC - S. A. Jones and T. F. Allen observed the effects of the flowers on three persons. Symptoms included a sense of great oppression about his chest, and a strong tendency to fainting.

A woman had oppression of chest, could not expand the lungs with a feeling as if she had swallowed food without chewing and it distressed her stomach. In a doctor, it increased the pain of inflammatory gout and evidently increased the paroxysm of a pain which came on every afternoon.

REFERENCES - Allen. Clarke.

MAGNOLIA GRANDIFLORA

PHARMACY - magn-gr. Magnolia grandiflora. Talauma mexicana. Magnolia yolotxochitl. N. O. Magnoliacee. Mexico. Tincture of the flowers. ***Historical dose:*** Tincture and all potencies.

CLINICAL - Aneurysm. Angina pectoris. Constipation. Dyspnea. Endocarditis. Flatulence. Headaches. Heart, disorders. Inter-menstrual flow. Leucorrhea. Migraines. Nausea. Pains. Pericarditis. Rheumatism. ***Stiffness.*** Vertigo.

HOMEOPATHIC - Allen, in his Handbook, gives a full pathogenesis of Magn-gr. Rheumatism and heart lesions are prominent features in the symptomatology of this drug.

Alternating pains between spleen and heart. Erratic shifting of pains. Pains rapidly change their place or alternate. Rheumatic action, particularly manifested in the chest and heart. ***Stiffness and soreness***. Bruised, constrictive and rheumatic pains in various parts, particularly the joints.

Patient tired and stiff. Tiredness impeding motion. Soreness when quiet. Marked action was developed in the female sexual sphere and an inter-menstrual flow was observed.

MIND - Confusion and dullness. Memory weak, lost. Repugnance to all occupation. Ill-humor with burning in hands. Sadness. Nervous, easily frightened. Uneasiness. Apprehensive, thinks she will die. Illusions and hallucinations of sight with sharp pains in eyes.

Abdomen - Rapid, pulsating pain with griping in intestines, extending to hypochondria, as from a blow. Burning in left side of abdomen, extending to chest. Contusive pain in liver and spleen, extending to the stomach. Flatulence. Lancinations in liver and spleen.

Back - Weight in neck with tiredness of spine. Stiffness, tiredness of neck and back. Contusive pain. Stitches in right side of back.

Chest - Oppression of chest with inability to expand the lungs. Constriction as from a band just beneath axilla. Tired feeling. Stiffness of sides of chest, as from exposure to a draft when over-heated. Stitches in sides of chest, in right side.

Ears - Lancinations in left ear, traveling to shoulder. Sharp pain in ears, in morning, traveling to throat.

Eyes - Sharp pain in eyes, from sunlight, with nervousness and visions. Vision weak, blurred. Lids heavy, sensation in lids as after weeping.

Face - Lancinations in jaw joints. Pain in right side in joints, worse pressure, also impeding opening of mouth. Sharp pain going to ear.

Female - Before menses, pain in small of back, hypogastrium and thighs with headache, flushes of heat to face, nausea and chill. Menses delayed, pale and scanty of coagulated blood for two days, then normal, painful. Bloody flow in interval between menses. Thick white or yellow leucorrhea, with constipation, straining when urinating. Congestion of left ovary with pain extending to left thigh.

Food - Appetite lost after vertigo, with lassitude.

Head - Migraines. Congestive, throbbing headache with griping in abdomen, flushes of heat. Pain in temples on bending forward, especially left temple. Pain in occiput and upper dorsal region. Pain in occiput as from a blow. Weight in occiput.

Heart - Endocarditis and pericarditis. Tendency to faint. Pulse weak and frequent. ***Sensation as if heart had stopped beating***. Alternating pains between spleen and heart. Crampy pain in heart. Angina pectoris. Stitches, which waking him frequently. Pain around heart accompanied by itching of the feet. Soreness after disappearance of pain.

Limbs - Stiffness and sharp erratic pains, worse in joints. Sprained pains in joints. Shooting in all limbs. Limbs tired, stiff. Stiffness of lower limbs. Sharp, erratic or rheumatic pains. Rheumatic pain in clavicles. Rheumatic pains in wrists. Numbness in left arm. Arms weak. ***Feet itch***.

Lungs - Dyspnea. Suffocation, with desire for stretching and uneasiness in paroxysms, when walking fast, when lying on left side after a meal. Hoarseness. Dry cough during the day, better at night.

Kidneys - Straining on passing water.

Modalities - Better dry weather, motion. Better inter-menstrual flow (Ham., Bov., Bell., Elaps.). Worse damp air, in morning, lying on left side.

Mouth - Pain in mouth, better by tepid water.

Rectum - Constipation.

Skin - Itching feet, sometimes with uneasiness of legs.

Sleep - Yawning during the day with sleepiness. Sleepless early in morning. Extravagant dreams.

Stomach - Sensation as from hunger with acidity. Emptiness with general lassitude, vertigo and nausea. Nausea in morning on rising, better by breakfast. Nausea as from tobacco. Feeling of a large bolus of food which distressed the stomach.

Teeth - Shooting in teeth. Soreness of teeth, impeding mastication.

Temperature - Erratic chill. Chill in afternoon, then fever lasting into night. Heat with burning in throat and headache, flushing with sweat of hands, hands and feet, upper limbs.

Throat - Red fauces. Burning and dryness with pain in pit of stomach and often extending to abdomen, preventing sleep. Difficult swallowing saliva. Sensation of mucus with fruitless attempts to remove it. Constriction, worse right side, worse bending forward. Pain in throat on turning head, waking him frequently at night.

Vertigo - Vertigo in evening, better going to bed with an emptiness at stomach with flushing of face. Vertigo with dislike for physical labor. Vertigo beginning with blurring of slight. Vertigo as from seasickness, causing loss of appetite.

COMMENTS - Allen gave indications including rheumatic pain in clavicles. Crampy pain in heart, alternating with lancinations. Pain in heart with suffocative constriction of throat. Aortic aneurysm. Nausea with vertigo and angina pectoris.

Dry cough. Rheumatic pains in back, especially when alternating with similar pains in different parts. Muscular rheumatism of left arm.

RELATIONS - ***Compare:*** (1) Rhus-t., Dulc., Aur. (2) Magn-gl., Anis. (3) In rheumatism, Kali-bi., Kalm. (4) Inter-menstrual hemorrhage, Ham., Bov., Bell., Cham., Elaps.

REFERENCES - Allen. Boericke. Clarke.

MALANDRINUM

(Grease of Horses)

PHARMACY - maland. Malandrinum. Grease of horses. Nosode of the disease in horses called "Grease." Trituration of Sugar of Milk saturated with the virus. Solution of the virus. ***Historical dose:*** All potencies.

CLINICAL - Acne. Boils. Eczema. Fistula. ***Impetigo.*** Knock-knee. Measles. Skin, unhealthy. ***Smallpox.*** Typhoid fever. ***Vaccination, effects.***

HOMEOPATHIC - According to Jenner, the origin of cow-pox is infection of the udders of cows by contact with grass on which a horse infected with "Grease" has trodden. This assertion is to some extent confirmed by the experience of homeopaths, who have found in Maland. a very effectual protection against infection with smallpox and against vaccination. Straube made provings of the 30c potency.

Clarke cured with it cases of unhealthy, dry, rough skin remaining for years after vaccination in smallpox, measles and impetigo. Burnett cured with it a case of knock-knee in a child who was constantly handling his penis.

Maland. has been used on inferential grounds with great success in ill effects of vaccination. Efficacious in clearing of the remnants of cancerous deposits. Bone-like protuberances. Toes feel scalded and itch terribly.

MIND - Dullness of mind. Dizziness. Confusion and lassitude of the mental faculties with a dread of any mental exertion. A lack of concentration.

Abdomen - Pains around umbilicus.

Back - Pain along back, as if beaten.

Causations - Ill effects of vaccinations (Thuj., Sil.).

Ears - Profuse, purulent, greenish-yellow discharge, mixed with blood.

Eyes - Red stripes under eyes.

Face - Scab on upper lip, with stinging pain when torn off.

Female - Vagina closed with crusts, yellowish-greenish-brown in color.

Head - Aching in forehead. Frontal and occipital headache. Impetigo covering head from crown to neck and extending behind ears. Thick, greenish crusts with pale, reddish scabs, itching worse in evening.

Limbs - Sore pains in limbs and joints. Pains, especially in left tibia with petechia-like patches on anterior aspect of left leg from knee to ankle. Petechia on both thighs, worse left. Knock-kneed. Impetiginous crusts on extensor sides of forearms. Run-around on nails of hands and feet.

Male - Child constantly handles his penis.

Mouth - Tongue is coated yellow with red streak down middle (typhoid). Tongue cracked and ulcerating down middle, swollen.

Skin - Smallpox. Measles, also as a preventive. Small, dusky red spots on legs, not disappearing on pressure. Petechial typhus. Impetigo covering back of head, extending over back to buttock and even into vagina, covering labia. Impetigo on extensors of forearms. Eczema. ***Dry, scaly,***

itching, cracks of hands and feet in cold weather and from washing. Boils. Malignant pustule. Bad effects of vaccination (dry, harsh skin).

Sleep - Dreams of troubles. Dreams of quarrels.

Stomach - Vomiting of bilious matter, nausea.

Stool - Dark, cadaverous-smelling stool. Yellowish, foul-smelling diarrhea.

COMMENTS - Burnett's indications are "Lower half of body, greasy skin and greasy eruption. Slow suppuration, never ending, as one heals another appears." Impetigo, ecthyma, fat, greasy-looking pustular eruptions are particularly acted on by this remedy.

A. L. Marcey related a striking experience with Maland. 30c. In the presence of a smallpox epidemic, he vaccinated himself, taking at the same time Maland. 30c night and morning. The vaccination did not take. It was twice repeated and still did not take, nor was smallpox contracted.

Called to vaccinate four children in a family whose parents were recovering from smallpox, he vaccinated all and gave Maland. 30c to three of them at the same time, the remaining child was the only one whose vaccination "took."

This was so severe that Maland. had to be given to modify its intensity, which it did effectively. The other three were re-vaccinated but none "took."

Of five children from six to seventeen years of age, only the eldest had been vaccinated and he had a good scar. All except the eldest were given Maland. and were vaccinated and none of the four "took." The eldest took smallpox. Maland. was then given and in a few days he was convalescent.

In another case of smallpox, Maland. was given and the disease only lasted a few days, the eruption drying up. In Straube's proving, the symptoms were worse in evening.

Burnett considers Maland. a very deeply acting remedy and one not to be repeated oftener than once a fortnight. Clears the remnants of cancerous deposits.

Heath cured with Maland. 30c fistula in a pony's neck, following strangles.

RELATIONS - ***Compare:*** (1) For the bad effects of vaccination, Vario., Vac., Thuj., Sabin., Ant-t., Apis, Sil. (2) In general, children handling genitals, Med. (but Maland. has deeper action). (3) In pustular eruptions, Hep., Merc. (4) Cast-eq., Hippoz., Hipp.

REFERENCES - Boericke. Clarke. Phatak.

MALARIA CO. NOSODE

(Malaria Nosodes)

PHARMACY - malar-co. Malaria co. nosode. Combination of the nosodes from all four types of malaria. (Plasmodium falciparum, Plasmodium malariae, Plasmodium vivax, and Plasmodium ovale). ***Historical dose:*** All potencies.

CLINICAL - Ague. Bilious, fever. ***Cachexia. Chills.*** Diarrhea. Emaciation. Fatigue. Fever. Headaches. Intermittent fever. Liver, disorders. ***Malaria.*** Nausea. Spleen, disorders. ***Sweats.*** Vomiting.

HOMEOPATHIC - The first episode of symptoms usually occurs about 8 to 30 days after the mosquito bite. Headache, fatigue, and nausea. Hard, shaking chills with fever for 12 to 24 hours. Rapid breathing. Heavy sweating, accompanied by a drop in temperature.

Episodes may recur every 2 or 3 days until the disease is treated. Without treatment, the disease can continue for years. Generally worse in crowded or unsanitary living conditions. Hot, humid climates. Malaria is endemic in Latin America, Asia and Africa.

COMMENTS - Malaria is an infection caused by a single-cell parasite, which is transmitted by the bite of an anopheles mosquito. Malaria affects the blood cells, blood vessels, liver, central nervous system.

There are four types of malarial parasites, they are transferred from person to person by a mosquito bite. The mosquito becomes infected with malaria after biting a person with the disease. The organism multiply in the mosquito, then enter the bloodstream of the next person the mosquito bites.

Once in a person's bloodstream, the parasites travel to the liver, where they thrive and multiply rapidly. After several days, thousands re-enter the bloodstream and destroy red-blood cells. Some parasites remain in the liver, continue to multiply and are released again at intervals into the bloodstream.

REFERENCES - Murphy.

MALARIA OFFICINALIS

(Decomposed Vegetable Matter)

PHARMACY - malar. Malaria officinalis. Decomposed vegetable matter. ***Historical dose:*** All potencies.

CLINICAL - Ague. Bilious, fever. ***Cachexia.*** Camp fever. Colic. Constipation. Cramps. Diarrhea. Emaciation. Fever. Gout. Hay fever. Headaches. Liver, disorders. ***Malaria.*** Nausea. Neuralgias. Rheumatism. Spleen, disorders. Tuberculosis. Typhoid. Vomiting.

HOMEOPATHIC - Malar. is made from vegetable matter decomposed in water in glass jars for one two and three weeks.

Malarial cachexia. Malaria and rheumatism. Rheumatic paralysis and emaciation. General sense of weariness. Sense of weariness from a very short walk. A kind of simmering all through the body.

Spleen disorders. Functional hepatic diseases. Typhoid, semi-paralytic condition. Right arm gets numb and has to be rubbed. Cold limbs, poor appetite but food does not distress her.

Fearful headache, nausea, aversion to food, distress through hypochondriac region, first in the spleen, then liver and stomach and chills. Bilious colic, nausea, cramps, diarrhea and headache. Urine red, scanty. Bowels sluggish but stools natural. Menses regular, rather scanty.

Dull headaches, dizzy and drowsy at all times, worse mornings. Eyes weak, blurring, reading difficult. Laryngeal irritation with cough and secretion of bloody mucus. Slow pulse.

MIND - Feels stupid and sleepy. Very forgetful. Dizzy and drowsy (Gels.).

COMMENTS - Yingling cured a Kansas volunteer with Malar. The volunteer, 28, after a week in camp in rainy, chilly weather had chill and fever, continuous nausea, vomiting bile, retching. Tongue white, thick coat. Mouth felt dry but was moist. Thirst for large quantities.

Symptoms were moderated by Ip. and later Bry., but not removed. Skin, eyes and face very yellow. Malar. 1m. Was given and improvement set in; in a week was in better health than usual.

Mrs. S. A. H., 63, had shooting pains all over muscles, bones ache. Diarrhea in morning, stools thin, yellow, foul. Bitter taste, parched mouth tongue white. Stretching and gaping. Malar. 1000c. cured quickly.

RELATIONS - Malar. belongs to the same order of remedies as Pyrog. (product of decaying animal tissues). Bowen found the best antidotes to Malar.: Nux-v., Bry., Ars., Rhus-t.. Eup-per. and Chin. gave negative results. ***Compare:*** (1) Spleen, Cean. (2) Liver, Bry., Lyc., Chol., Chel. (3) Pain under right scapula, Chel. (4) Effect of damp and wetting, Lem-m., Dulc. (5) Half machine-gun cough, Cor-r., Cocc-c. (6) better after urinating, Lith., Ambr. (7) Intermittents, Ip., Cedr., Nat-m., Meny.

REFERENCES - Anshutz. Boericke.

MALATHION

(Pesticide)

PHARMACY - malat. Malathion. Pesticide. Ovide. A pesticide and topical drug for lice, scabies. ***Historical dose:*** All potencies.

CLINICAL - Abdominal, cramps. Allergies. Aplastic, anemia. Asthma. Autoimmune, disorders. Birth, defects. Conjunctivitis. Convulsions. Diarrhea. Dyspnea. Eye, disorders. Immune, disorders. Impotency. Infertility. Intestinal, disorders. Kidney, failure. Learning disabilities. Leukemia. Miscarriages. Rash. Rheumatoid, arthritis. Stomach, cramps. Trembling. Twitching. Vertigo. Weakness.

HOMEOPATHIC - Malathion is an organophosphate parasympathomimetic which binds irreversibly to cholinesterase. Malathion is an insecticide of relatively high human toxicity. It weakens the immune system. Causes autoimmune disorders. Rheumatoid arthritis. Asthma and allergies. Leukemia. Aplastic anemia. Kidney failure.

Drowsiness. Unusual weakness. Slow heartbeat. Dizziness. Convulsions, seizures. Trembling. Clumsiness or unsteadiness. Difficult or labored breathing. Increased sweating. Increased watering of mouth or eyes.

Abdominal or stomach cramps. Diarrhea. Loss of bowel or bladder control. Intestinal disorders in children. Birth defects. Infertility or miscarriages. Lower sperm count. Slower sperm movement.

Muscle twitching of eyelids, face, and neck. Pinpoint pupils. Redness, pain, swelling of eye, eyelid, inner lining of eyelid. Burning, dry or itching eyes. Conjunctivitis. Eye discharges, excessive tearing. Skin rash. Stinging or irritation of scalp.

MIND - Anxiety and restlessness. Hyperactivity. Attention deficit disorder. Learning disabilities in math, reading, etc. Language or speech delays. Mental retardation. Memory weakness, confusion. Depression. Irritability. Aggressive behavior.

COMMENTS - Malathion breaks down into malaoxon, which is 60 times more toxic than malathion. For this reason, if malathion is used or somehow enters an indoor environment, as it breaks down into malaoxon, it can seriously and chronically poison the occupants living or working in this environment.

Malathion present in untreated water is converted to malaoxon during the chlorination phase of water treatment, so malathion should not be used in waters that may be used as a source for drinking water, or any upstream waters.

REFERENCES - Murphy.

MANCINELLA VENENATA

(Manganeel Apple)

PHARMACY - manc. Mancinella venenata. Manganeel apple. Hippomane mancinella. Manzanillo. N. O. Euphorbiacae. Caribbean. Tincture of fruit, fresh leaves and bark. ***Historical dose:*** All potencies.

CLINICAL - Asthma. ***Blindness. Blisters.*** Borborygmus. Chills. Cholera infantum. Colic. ***Dermatitis.*** Diphtheria. Erysipelas. Erythema. Esophagus, stricture. ***Eyes, disorders.*** Fever. Fungoid, growths. Hair, loss. Headache. Herpes. Melancholy. Menopause. Nausea. Nerve, disorders. ***Pemphigus***. Photophobia. Puberty. Scarlatina. ***Skin, disorders.*** Sore throat. Stomatitis. Tongue, patched. Typhoid fever. ***Vesicles***. Vomiting. Wounds.

HERBAL - The Treasury of Botany noted that "Mancinella is a species of the Euphorbiacae and has all the virulent properties of the family in a high degree. It is one of the trees around which the upas legends have clustered. It is certain that the juice, which resembles pure white milk, does possess a considerable amount of acridity and that some persons suffer great pain from incautiously handing it.

"Perhaps its most dangerous property is that of causing ***blindness***, if by chance the least drop of the milk or smoke of the burning wood, comes in contact with the eyes.

"Dr. Seeman states that at Veraguas some of the ship's carpenters were blinded for several days by the juice getting into their eyes while cutting down Manchineel trees, while he himself suffered from temporary loss of sight from merely gathering specimens. The same accident happened to a boat's crew from making a fire. Salt water is said to be an efficacious remedy."

HOMEOPATHIC - Marked skin symptoms. ***Dermatitis*** with excessive blistering, oozing of sticky serum, and formation of crusts. Acridity. Burning, smarting in various parts. Favors rapid healing of wounds. ***Loss of vision***. ***Pain in the thumb***.

Hering suggested it in mental depressed states at puberty and at menopause with an exalted sexuality.

MIND - Bashful and taciturn. Timid. Sympathetic. Weeps a great deal, especially when alone. Melancholy. Homesickness. Silent mood, sadness. Depression with sexual weakness.

Wandering thoughts. ***Sudden vanishing of thoughts.*** Forgets what she wishes to do next. Forgets her errands. Anger aggravates. Impatience during headache. Averse to work and answering questions.

Anxiety from becoming cold, during or after scarlatina, before menses.

Fear of becoming insane. Fear of evil spirits. Sometimes feels as light as if she could float or hover in the air. Delusions that he will be taken by the devil.

Abdomen - Rumbling in abdomen renewed by every motion and when taking a deep inspiration. Colic, worse cold drinks. Bowels sore and burn.

Back - Backache with nausea and tenesmus. Sharp pain in left scapula and left chest at intervals. Painful stiffness of small of back, neck, after sleep, could scarcely move neck.

Chest - Oppression of chest, better expectoration. Aching pain behind sternum. Severe pain in middle of sternum, worse pressure and breathing.

Ears - Ears feel as if closed. Redness and heat of ears.

Eyes - Lids, heavy and sore. Eyes smart or burn on closing them. Dull ache behind the eyes. Intense inflammation with loss of vision (for some days). Photophobia.

Face - Swollen, spotted. Herpes on lips.

Food - Craves cold water. Aversion to meat, bread, wine.

Head - Pain in vertex, worse lying. Heat in head, better from rest. Congestion of head before menses. Scalp itches. Hair falls out after acute sickness.

Heart - Pressure in region of heart. Needle like stitches at heart. Palpitations in evening, on turning in bed, as from eating. Palpitations with weakness. Pulse weak, very large and soft.

Limbs - Pain in thumb. Icy coldness of hands and feet. Biting vesicles on soles, desquamation and dryness of soles.

Lungs - Rattling in left lung during breathing. Violent cough and painful stitches in trachea from slightest exertion. Cough, worse cold drinks, at night.

Modalities - ***Worse from cold.*** Worse cold drinks. Worse cold feet. Worse dampness. Worse touch. Worse puberty, menopause. Worse anger. Worse after eating.

Mouth - Feels peppery. Burning and pricking in the mouth, not better by cold water. Burning of fauces. Dysphagia from constriction of throat and esophagus. Copious, offensive saliva. Profuse foul yellow saliva. Taste of blood.

Nose - Illusions of smell of gunpowder, dung, etc. Pressure at root of nose.

Perspiration - Cold sweats. Acrid, sticky foot sweat.

Rectum - Sensation of fullness in rectum with hollow feeling in stomach. Sudden desire to go to stool in morning. Profuse diarrhea with colic, vertigo, much discharge of flatus. Greenish stools. Burning pain during diarrhea. Pulsation in anus. Discharge of fetid blood from hemorrhoids.

Sensations - Head feels as if bruised or as if it had been exposed to the sun. Head as if hollow, as if lying on something hard. Ears as if closed. Electric thrusts in upper part of throat. As if flames rising from stomach. As if stomach drew together in a lump and then suddenly opened. As if something alive in stomach.

Skin - Intense erythema. ***Dermatitis with extensive blisters***, oozing of sticky serum and formation of crusts. Heavy, brown crusts and scabs. ***Large blisters, as from scalds***. Fungoid growths. ***Vesicles***. Erysipelas. ***Pemphigus***.

Stomach - Swollen epigastrium. Continual choking sensation rising from stomach. Vomiting of food, followed by severe colic and profuse diarrhea. Vomiting of ingesta, followed by griping and copious stools. Repeated green vomit. Burning pains and black vomit. As of flame rising from stomach.

Temperature - Chills with icy cold hands and feet. Burning heat, with inclination to cover himself in bed. Flushes of heat. Fever with tingling in skin, with thirst.

Throat - Cutting pains, worse cold drinks. Diphtheria. Tonsils swollen. Choking sensation rises in the throat when speaking, preventing drinking though thirsty.

Vertigo - Vertigo, head feels light, empty, while walking about.

COMMENTS - Manc. was introduced into homeopathy by Bute, who proved it. It was also proved by Mure and Ackermann. Marked affects on the head, eyes, throat, abdomen and rectum. The symptoms induced included burning in all parts, vesication and ulceration of the skin and mucus membranes.

Symptoms worse from drinking cold water, especially cough. Better from heat when lying down, but headache is worse from the warmth of a stove and there is an inclination to uncover. Cough is worse at night.

Med. Cent. quoted the case of a woman who for several years was possessed with the fixed idea that she would become insane. She had become a wife and mother, but still the ideas possessed her. Happening to see in Puhlmann's Therapeutics that Manc. has ***"fear of going crazy,"*** she took Manc. 12c and was permanently cured.

RELATIONS - ***Compare:*** (1) Crot., Jatr., Canth., Anac.

REFERENCES - Boericke. Clarke. Phatak.

MANDRAGORA OFFICINARUM

(Mandrake)

PHARMACY - mand. Mandragora officinarum. Mandrake. Atropa mandragora. Mandragora e radice. N. O. Solanaceae. Europe. Tincture of the whole plant. ***Historical dose:*** Tincture and all potencies.

CLINICAL - Allergic dermatitis. Backache. Blepharitis. Blisters. Boils. Chorea. Colitis. Congestive headache. Conjunctivitis. ***Constipation.*** Coryza. Digestive, weakness. Epilepsy. Erysipelas. Exanthemata. ***Eye, disorders.*** Gallbladder infections. Gallstones. Gastritis. Gout. Herpes. Hiccoughs. Hypersensitive. Hypertension. Iritis. Itching. Keratitis. Leucorrhea. Liver, migraines. Lupus erythematous. Motion sickness. Neuralgia. Night, sweats. Osteoporosis. Pancreatitis. Polyneuritis. Seasickness. Seborrhea. Shingles. Sterility. Styes. Ulcers. Uric, diathesis. Writer's cramp.

HERBAL - The mandrake does not derive its name from the shape of the human body which the root of the plant sometimes takes, but from the name by which it was known to the Greeks, Mandragora, and which signifies injurious to cattle. It was used by the ancient Egyptian physicians for many conditions.

The mandrake figures largely in legend and poetry. It is said to be the "insane root" spoken of by Macbeth and it is mentioned by name in Antony and Cleopatra and in Romeo and Juliet. Mandrake must not be confounded with Podophyllum or Bryonia dioica, which are also sometimes called "Mandrake" in this country.

HOMEOPATHIC - Dufresne experimented with Mand. on himself and another by repeatedly smelling, at short intervals, the expressed juice of the plant, ***"which has a nauseating odor like adder's flesh."*** W. B. Richardson also experimented with it.

There are two varieties of Mand., the vernal and the autumnal; Dufresne used the vernal. The symptoms were very similar to those of Belladonna, to which it is botanically closely related. Mand. is like a cooled or attenuated Bell.

Restless excitability and bodily weariness. Great desire for sleep. Striking tiredness, exhaustion, collapse. Depressive condition. Nervous, hypersensitive to noise and odors, ameliorated by urination. Exaggeration of sounds and enlarged vision.

Joint and muscular pains. The unpleasant symptoms go off at night in bed and are succeeded by a gentle perspiration. Lingering uneasiness and coldness after removal of other symptoms.

Congestive headache. Ocular complaints with mydriasis and dimming of the field of vision. Herpetic eruption on the face. ***Constipation. Inactive bowels with white, hard stools***. Liver, gallbladder and stomach complaints. Gout. Uric diathesis.

MIND - Alternating between good moods, euphoria, and depression, discontented. Depressive psychosis. Restless excitability, hysterical. Very nervous and irritable, hypersensitive to noise, ameliorated by urination. Poor powers of concentration.

Abdomen - Repletion and heaviness in the upper abdomen with dyspnea and palpitations, ameliorated by moving and getting up, and by belching and expelling gas. Gastric, duodenal, pyloric ulcers. Diaphragmatic hernia.

Back - Backache. Severe pain in the right shoulder and left wrist, worse with movement. Pain in the scapula and right hand.

Blood - Arteriosclerosis. Hypoglycemia. High level of urea in the blood.

Chest - Angina pectoris. Constriction of the heart, as if the chest were clamped in a vice, ameliorated by heat in bed and by rest. Anginal pain, lasting for an hour with cold sweat on the forehead.

Constitutions - Allergic and psoric constitutions. Arthritic tendencies. Uric diathesis.

Ears - Exaggeration of sounds. Persistent buzzing. Early otosclerosis.

Eyes - Red inflamed, tired, heavy. Pupils dilated. Conjunctivitis. Blepharitis. Keratitis. Iritis. Retinal infections. Painful, irritated with photophobia. Enlarged and confused vision. Eye movements painful, worse when reading. Eye neuralgia with spots before the eyes, dazzled and troubled vision. Stinging, smarting pains in the eyelids, which are red, swollen and itching, worse on the left side. Styes.

Face - Sudden pallor of the face, feeling that the fingers are dead. Herpetic blisters, boils on the face. Face dirty, seborrhea of the face and nape of the neck, clothes become dirty.

Female - Menses either a few days too early or late. Blood thick, sticky, dark. Brown leucorrhea with lumbar ache and pains in the low abdomen, ameliorated in bed and by resting. Sterility. Post-menopausal osteoporosis.

Food - Feeling of hunger quickly disappears after eating a little. Desire for spicy, piquant dishes, meat, cheese and sweets. Desire for sweets, which are not tolerated. Aggravated by coffee and fats. Aversion to and intolerance of alcoholic drinks.

Head - Head feels numb. Heaviness and confusion of head. Sense of fullness in vessels of brain. Headache resulting form an empty stomach, ameliorated by eating. Morning headache following bad digestion, accompanied by bad mood. Pulsating headache, as if in a fog and the skull seems enlarged.

Heart - Heaviness on the heart with paresis in the left shoulder and arm. Cardiac pains aggravated in the morning, before a storm, by exertion or movement, ameliorated in bed, by resting and in the fresh air. Arterial hypertension.

Kidneys - Kidney stones. Extreme atony of the bladder despite urgent pressing feeling. Urination difficult, must force the last drops. Thick urinary stream. Urine copious, pale, milky from phosphate deposits, brown. Urine with a strong odor, accompanied by conjunctiva jaundice. Nightly bedwetting. Amelioration of anger after urination.

Limbs - Cramping pains in all the joints with feeling of heaviness and numbing. Sciatic pain, worse in the morning on rising and letting the leg hang loose, better with heat. Muscular pains in the hips, thighs, legs. Legs heavy, cold, walking is painful. Numbness, heaviness and coldness in the arms. Needle-like pain in the upper part of the right arm, spreading to the hand with feeling of numbness. Cramps in the hands, causing great difficulty in writing.

Lungs - Slight cough with expectoration. Difficult breathing.

Male - Diminution of libido, aggravated after the proving. Sexual impotence. Prostatic adenoma.

Modalities - Better from discharges. Better menses, urine. Better after urination. Better from amelioration of anger. Better from heat. Better continuous movement, stretching backwards. Better resting in bed. Worse from the first movement. Worse dangling the legs, contact. Worse greasy food. Worse between 3 a.m. and 5 a.m. Worse changes in the weather, storms. Worse from the cold, except for head congestion which is better by the cold.

Mouth - Singular taste and sensation of acidity and dryness. Bad breath, which he notices himself. Lips, mouth, palate, dry and painful. Tongue dry, irritated, as if raw, as if scalded by hot water, benumbed. Tongue covered with a white coating. Aphthae on the tongue and inside of the cheeks. Ulceration of the gums and lips. Hemorrhaging of the gums. Inflammation of the roots of the teeth, painful to the touch.

Nose - Coryza. Irritation of the nasal mucus membranes with discharge and sneezing. Nasal crusts in the morning. Spasmodic rhinitis.

Rectum - Hemorrhaging recto-colitis. Spasmodic constipation. Bleeding hemorrhoids.

Skin - Skin itching. Allergic dermatitis. Erysipelas. Shingles. Lupus erythematous. Burning pain on the skin, resulting from exanthemata and boils. Sticky sweating on the palms, forehead, and at the hairline. Nocturnal sweating with strong odor. Exhausting, cold sweating from the trunk, around midnight, followed by feeling of improvement.

Sleep - Desire for sleep. Insomnia between 3 a.m. and 5 a.m. Sleep disturbed by unpleasant or horrible dreams, by muscular pains. Despite good sleep, feels tired, as if he had taken a sleeping pill.

Stomach - Cramping pains in the stomach, ameliorated by eating, drinking and lying down. Stomach painful like a wound, sensitive to pressure and movement, stinging pain, better by bending double and by resting. Hiccough with salivation, eructation and nausea. Travel sickness. Vomiting during pregnancy.

Stool - Inaction of bowels with white, hard feces when bowels are induced to act.

Temperature - Shivering in afternoon. Coldness remains after other symptoms. Febrile flush and pain in the bladder. Sensation of fever, with shivering in the back and persistent, sub-febrile condition.

Throat - Hoarseness. Husky voice. Throat insensitive, as if anesthetized. Swallowing painful. Cryptic tonsillitis, purulent with sore throat. Intense dryness of the larynx with irritating cough. Glairy secretion from the larynx and throat. Chronic laryngitis.

Vertigo - Frontal congestive headache with vertigo, dizziness of the head and extreme tiredness.

COMMENTS - The effects of the provings were removed by free indulgence in wine, coffee, and cigars. With regular dieting, the symptoms lasted much longer and were removed by Nux-v., Camph. and Bell.

RELATIONS - ***Antidotes:*** Nux-v., Camph. and Bell. ***Compare:*** (1) Bell. - Hypersensitivity and hyper excitability of all the senses, pupils dilated and fixed, photophobia. Dryness of the pharynx, pulse full and bounding, menses too early, blood hot, abdomen distended. (2) Dios. - Violent abdominal colic, ameliorated by leaning backwards, genital excitability, pains in the back and the right sciatic region, dryness of the mouth and flatulence. (3) Sulph. - Irritation of skin and mucus membranes, hepatic and portal intoxication, plethora in arthritis, sclerosis, fat or thin types.

REFERENCES - Clarke. Julian.

MANGANUM ACETICUM

(Manganese Acetate)

PHARMACY - mang. Manganum aceticum. Manganese acetate. Manganous acetate. Manganum carbonicum. Manganese carbonate. Triturations of the carbonate. Solutions of the acetate, according to Hahnemann. ***Historical dose:*** All potencies.

CLINICAL - Addison's disease. Albuminuria. Amenorrhea. Anemia. ***Ankles, weak.*** Arthritis. Asthenopia. Asthma. Bones, pain. Brain, concussion. ***Cellulitis***. Coughs. Deafness. Dysmenorrhea. Ear, infection. Gallstones. ***Growing, pains***. Gout. Headaches. Heel, pain. Hoarseness. Jaundice. Laryngitis. Lichen. Menopausal, flushings. Myopia. Nephritis. Palate, disorders. Paraplegia. ***Parkinson's, disease.*** Parotiditis. Periostitis. Pityriasis. Psoriasis. ***Reflexes, exaggerated***. Rheumatism. Scabies. Tongue disorders. Tuberculosis. Wilson's disease. Yawning.

HOMEOPATHIC - Manganese was isolated in 1774 and was introduced into the Materia Medica by Hahnemann, who made provings of the acetate and carbonate. The symptoms of the two have not been kept separate.

Manganese is a metal having a remarkable affinity for and in some respects a close resemblance to iron, of which it is an extremely frequent associate. Its medicinal as well as its physical relationship with iron is very close.

Symptoms of chronic manganese poisoning, according to Professor von Jaksch, were involuntary laughter, weeping and walking backwards. ***Exaggerated reflexes*** and physical disturbances, evidenced by men making fun of each other's gait. Paraplegia progressive, wasting, feeble and staggering gait. Anemia with destruction of red blood corpuscles.

Affinity for the ***inner ear,*** larynx, trachea, periosteum of shinbone, joints, ankles and lower limbs. Pain extends to ear from other parts. Everything affects the ear. Yellow-green lumpy or bloody discharges. Great accumulation of mucus. Asthmatic persons who ***cannot lie on a feather pillow.***

Bones are very sensitive, Painful, deep soreness of the whole body, every part of the body feels sore when touched, ears, joints, skin. Weak joints. Chronic arthritis with infiltrated, glistening joints. ***Growing pains.*** Diagonal pains. ***Wants to lie down in bed which improves all the troubles***.

Cellulitis, sub-acute stage, promotes suppuration and hastens regeneration. Suppuration of skin around joints. Necrosis and decay of bones. Malignant ulcers with blue border, following slight injury. Inflammation of bones or joints with nightly digging pains.

Progressive muscular atrophy. Motor paralysis, ascending paralysis. ***Parkinson's disease,*** paraplegia. Festinating, walks backwards.

Jaundice, nephritis with albuminuria. Fatty degeneration of liver. Gout. Typhoid fever, cases that are badly treated with prolonged convalescence.

Syphilitic and chlorotic patients with general anemia and paralytic symptoms. For speakers and singers. Valuable for boys and girls whose voices are changing.

MIND - ***Anxiety and fear.*** Anxiety as if something bad is going to happen, when moving in the room, better lying down. Fretful. Weak and nervous. Peevish. Irritability in morning, during music, while talking. Hatred of persons who had offended him.

Silent, reserved. Sad, weeping, silent. Depression, better sad music. Constant moaning or groaning. Confusion while sitting. Involuntary laughing and weeping. better open air. ***Mental conditions are better when lying down***.

Abdomen - Pressing in stomach and abdomen while eating, worse cold food. Rumbling in abdomen, from cold food. Abdominal colic, better eating. As if intestines were loose and shaking when walking about. Pain and constriction at the navel. Cutting in umbilical region worse on taking deep breath. Flatulence.

Back - Tearing pain in whole spinal column, from above downward. Pain in small of back on bending backward. Stiffness of nape. Red, swollen streak on left side of neck.

Chest - Heat, beating in chest. Sharp pains in chest and sternum running up and down. Bruised pain in upper chest when stooping, better raising head.

Cough - Dry cough, incessant, from irritation about middle of sternum. Cough with aphonia. ***Cough better lying down,*** worse evening, damp weather, loud reading, laughing, walking, or deep inspiration. Inclination to cough in morning.

Ears - Everything affects the ears. ***Pain extends to ear from other parts.*** Swelling of the parotid glands in fevers. Sharp pains in the ears from talking, laughing, swallowing. Feel stopped, cracking on blowing nose. Whistling tinnitus. ***Deafness in damp weather.*** Blowing the nose helps deafness.

Eyes - Burning in eyes during day. Pupils much dilated or contracted. Field of vision contracted. Dim vision during day. Eyestrain, with aching and pressure. Agglutination of eyes in morning. Eyelids swollen and painful to touch.

Face - Pale, sickly. Stolidly mask-like. Ulcerated at corners of mouth. Twitching, jerking pain from lower jaw to temples worse laughing. Cramp pain in upper and lower jaw after eating. Swelling of parotid glands, in fevers.

Female - Amenorrhea. First menses delayed. Menses, early, scanty, pale in anemic patients. Discharge of blood between periods with pressing in genitals. ***Flushes of heat at menopause.***

Food - Aversion to food from a feeling of satiety. Loss of appetite, in chlorosis. No thirst.

Head - Congestion to head, with throbbing, feels large and heavy, better open air. Frequent rush of blood to head, with thirst. Headache with stupefaction and confusion of senses while walking. Headaches worse, breathing, talking or laughing. Pains from above downwards, worse straining at stools, jarring, stepping. Sharp pains like needles, worse jarring or stepping. Cold feeling at a small spot on vertex.

Heart - Sudden shocks at heart and in left side of chest, from above downward. Palpitations of heart, strong, irregular, trembling. Pulse irregular, sometimes rapid, sometimes slow, but constantly weak and soft.

Kidneys - Darting in urethra on passing flatus. Cutting pain in middle of urethra between urination. Frequent desire to urinate during day. Urine profuse, sediment violet, earthy. Addison's disease.

Limbs - Muscular twitching. ***Parkinson's disease.*** Inflammation of bones and joints with nightly digging pains. Bones very sensitive. ***Every part of body feels sore when touched.*** Shiny red swelling of joints. Periosteal inflammation. Burning spots about joints. Suppuration of skin around joints. ***Knee pain*** and itching. Intolerable pain in skin of lower limbs. Legs feel numb. Stiffness in muscles of legs. Cramps in calves. Rheumatism of feet. Ankles painful. Children are unable to walk because of ankles are weak. Peculiar slapping gait, walks on metacarpo-phalangeal joint, walks backwards. ***Tending to fall forward, walks stooping forward***. Cannot walk backwards without falling.

Liver - Chronic enlargement of liver. Jaundice.

Lungs - ***Every cold becomes bronchitis*** (Dulc.). Mucus difficult to loosen after long hawking. Difficult expectoration of lumps of tough mucus in evening. Scanty mucus. Lumpy, yellow, adhesive mucus. Greenish masses. Expectoration of yellowish greenish lumps, even without coughing in morning. Bloody, reddish phlegm. Hemoptysis with stitching pains through right lung and dry cough. Asthmatic persons who ***cannot lie on a feather pillow.***

Modalities - Better from open air, sad music, eating, swallowing, ***lying down.*** Better or worse by change of weather. Worse cold, wet weather, damp, touching with cold things, touch. Worse at night, speaking, laughing, motion, bending backwards. Lying on the feather bed aggravates asthma.

Mouth - Dry, parched lips, with shriveling of skin, without thirst. Clear vesicles on upper lip. Nodes on palate and tongue. Tongue sore and irritable with ulcers or warts. Flow of saliva, while speaking with colic, paralysis etc. Oily taste. Toothache, worse anything cold, worse sucking, pain going up in the ears.

Nose - Crampy pain at the root of the nose. Dry, obstructed. Obstruction of nose and fluent coryza alternately. Chronic catarrh with bleeding, worse in ***cold damp weather***. Blowing is painful.

Rectum - Cramps in the anus while sitting, better lying down. Pain in rectum after dinner. Bowels are irregular, with constipation or diarrhea. Constipation with difficult, dry, knotty evacuations. Stool yellow, granular, with tenesmus and constriction of anus. Passes much flatus with stools.

Sensations - Head as if larger. Ears as if stopped. Throat as if excoriated. Trachea as if closed with a film. As if pit of stomach enlarged. As if bowels drawn together. As if tendons shortened.

Skin - Red, elevated spots. ***Itching***, better scratching. Itching of diabetes. ***Chronic eczema*** with amenorrhea, worse during menses or menopause. Psoriasis and pityriasis. Dry hard ulcers. Burning around ulcers. Suppuration of skin around joints. Rough, cracked (flexures), bluish. Deep cracks in bends of elbows, knees.

Sleep - Languor and sleepiness. Much yawning. Sleepy very early in evening. Many vivid dreams which are well remembered.

Temperature - Shaking chills in evening, with shooting pains in head, without thirst. Chills with icy cold hands and feet. Sudden flushes of heat in face in chest and over the back. Burning over whole body, in evening when rising from bed.

Throat - ***Chronic sore throat***, with cutting pain, as from excoriation, when not swallowing. Throat as if excoriated. Throat dry, scratching. Laryngitis. Larynx dry, rough, constricted. Tuberculosis of the larynx. Sharp pain in larynx when swallowing. Chronic disease of larynx, with Eustachian deafness. ***Chronic hoarseness***. Hemming and hawking all the time and annoying everybody. Low, monotonous voice. Rough voice better smoking.

Vertigo - Vertigo when sitting or standing, nearly falling forward.

COMMENTS - F. H. Pritchard, in an article on Mang., cited the action of the metal, noting that the mucus membranes are congested and secretions are increased or decreased. A powerful cholagogue, it induces inflammation and fatty degeneration of the liver.

Destroys red corpuscles and causes anemia. Sensitive bones and periosteum, with periostitis. Paralysis and progressive muscular atrophy of the cerebrospinal system. Fissures, excoriation, and suppuration of the skin.

Lippe noted the indication "Suppuration of skin round joints." Pritchard quoted observations of Grille that workmen in manganese mines do not get itch and those who come to the work with itch get cured of it. The manganese waters of Cransac cause "Ill-humor, weeping, despondency, sudden palpitation."

Guernsey noted that "The bones are very sensitive, red spots on the skin, which are elevated, owing to bone disorders. Ankles are particularly affected, children may have this trouble and be unable to walk.

"Typhus fever when the parotid gland is swollen and the bones are very sensitive to touch, disorders of the internal ear, upper part of chest. Hoarse voice, drawing sensation of the muscles."

Laryngeal tuberculosis, tuberculosis. Cough better by lying down. Deep cough, worse in damp weather. Single nodes on the palate. Chlorosis, if gastric symptoms and loss of appetite predominate.

Skin will not heal, slight scratches ulcerate. Anemia. Menses too frequent and too scanty in anemic girls. Boring, pressing headaches, proceed from above downwards. Headache like a concussion at every step or movement.

Inflammation of bones and joints with insupportable nightly digging pains. Every part of the body feels extremely sore when touched. Rheumatic patients cannot beat any weight on their heels. Rheumatic symptoms with dark, almost blue spots on skin.

Paralysis with inclination to run forward if he tried to walk. Paralysis which begins below, extending upward. Paraplegia. Paralysis from degeneration of anterior portion of cord.

Clarke has frequently verified the "cough better from lying down," and also this sensitiveness of the bones. Where these occur in connection with any other condition indicating Mang. it is sure to do good.

Clarke cured in an elderly woman a flat growth on the center of her palate with Mang. 30c. Bluish nodes on the skin, malignant ulcers with blue borders following slight injury.

Hansen cured with Mang. 6c a case of neuralgia of the tongue following the healing of a little ulcer on surface near left border after an application with lunar caustic. Shortly after the healing, the patient (a man, 60) had severe stinging burning at the left edge of his tongue and the inner side of his left cheek when touching the tongue.

In this state he came to Hansen after allopathic treatment. Several medicines were given without result, then Mang. was chosen and made a rapid and permanent cure.

A. W. Palmer reported a case of catarrhal deafness cured with Mang. 6c. Miss H., 38, had dull hearing, dry throat with hoarseness, itching in ears, loud rumbling, worse night, right ear, crackling on blowing nose, and deafness in damp weather. The last was the guiding symptom.

Cooper gave several ear-cases in which Mang. proved curative. The first concerned a nodule appearance of malleus handle, thickened irregularly, with history of bilious headaches and of previous discharges from the ears.

The ear drum membrane had a granular appearance. Purple glazed appearance of the malleus handles, which were thickened and very prominent, upper segment of membrane also purple and glazed.

The second concerned a case of chronic periostitis of the meatus and middle ear with otorrhea, left ear. Cooper also noted a case of otorrhea with earache, pain shot up from teeth to ear, the earache was worse after early dinner, up until 8 or 9 p.m. Pains extended to and concentrated in the ears from other parts.

The fourth case concerned sensitive ears, took cold and got a headache, history of gallstones and jaundice, sleepy and headache in afternoon, bitter taste in morning, lips glued together, whistling tinnitus worse in a cold. (explosions, Mag-carb., rasping, shrill tinnitus as well as cardiac tinnitus, pumping, Kali-i.).

The final case Cooper recorded was deafness in a woman, 36, which dated from when she was 14 from over-strain in singing, when she lost her voice and hearing for six months. Her left hearing returned, right remained deaf, worse after a cold or if over-excited or worried. Subject all life to bilious attacks which lasted twenty-four hours and left suddenly.

Head throbbed, couldn't put it down on a pillow. Headache came on in morning on awaking and reached a height at 3 or 4 p.m. and kept on until next morning. Bilious headaches went away and the hearing of right ear improved under Mang. 200c.

RELATIONS - ***Antidotes:*** Coff., Merc. ***Compare:*** (1) Mang-coll. - Boils and other staphylococcal infections. (2) Mang-m. - painful ankles, bone-pains. (3) Mang-s. - liver disorders, excess of bile, a powerful intestinal stimulant. (4) Arg-n., Rhus-t., Sulph.

REFERENCES - Boericke. Clarke. Phatak.

MANGANUM MURIATICUM

(Manganese Chloride)

PHARMACY - mang-m. Manganum muriaticum. Manganese chloride. Solution in water. ***Historical dose:*** All potencies.

CLINICAL - Ankles, painful. Ankles, weak. Belchings. Bone pains. Borborygmus. Constipation. Rheumatism.

HOMEOPATHIC - Mang-m. was proved by Lembke. The few symptoms obtained were manifested chiefly in the cranial bones, stomach, left shoulder, right knee and ankles. Violent pain in front part of left shoulder joint, worse by pressure and by any motion of arm. Violent drawing pain in inner side of the right knee.

Abdomen - Frequent rumbling.

Face - Pressive pain in right jaw joint.

Head - Boring in right cranial bones, tearing in right occipital bone.

Limbs - Pain in articulation of left thumb. Drawing pain with weary feeling in right thigh while sitting. Pressure in right knee extending into leg, a bruised sensation remains in ankles, afterwards same pain in left ankle. Pressure and drawing in ankle and ankle bones. Pressure in left foot.

Modalities - Stomach pains were worse by external pressure.

Rectum - Stool harder and scantier.

Stomach - Sour belchings of air. Pressure in stomach, worse by external pressure.

Vertigo - Vertigo and reeling when walking in open air, worse looking down, on descending or stooping.

REFERENCES - Clarke.

MANGANUM OXYDATUM NATIVUM

(Manganese Oxydatum)

PHARMACY - mang-o. Manganum oxydatum nativum. Manganese oxydatum. Pyrolusite. Native Black Oxide of Manganese. ***Historical dose:*** All potencies.

CLINICAL - Bulbar paralysis. Nervous disorders. Paralysis agitans. Parkinson's disease.

HOMEOPATHIC - Workers in Manganese binoxide are frequently affected with bulbar paralysis.

Mang-o. has some symptoms similar to Parkinson's disease, progressive lenticular degenerations and pseudo-sclerosis. Peculiar slapping gait. Muscular twitching, cramps in calves, stiff leg muscles.

Pain in tibia. Dysmenorrhea. Colic and diarrhea. Easily fatigued and heated, sleepy. Stolid, mask-like face. Low monotonous voice, ***"economical speech."*** Occasional uncontrollable laughter.

REFERENCES - Boericke.

MANGANUM SULPHURICUM

(Manganese Sulphate)

PHARMACY - mang-s. Manganum sulphuricum. Manganese sulphate. Solution. ***Historical dose:*** All potencies.

CLINICAL - Bile, excess. Gastritis. Liver, disorders. Toothaches.

HOMEOPATHIC - Cooper said, "This Salt of Manganese deserves more attention than seems to be at present given to it. It has been proved to cause vomiting, paralysis without convulsions and inflammation of the stomach and small intestines. As well as of the liver, spleen and heart."

C. G. Gmelin, who experimented with it, recorded its property of causing such an extraordinary secretion of bile that nearly all the intestines were colored yellow by it and the large intestines had a wax-yellow color communicated to them.

According to Rutherford, Mang-s. is a powerful intestinal, but a feeble hepatic stimulant. Toothache in a bad tooth, on right side, upper jaw. Shooting, darting extending up the whole side of face and head. Painful parts tender to touch.

Ure found Mang-s. to act on man as a purgative and cholagogue in doses of one to two drachms in half a pint of water. It has, however, caused vomiting and sweating as well as purgation and is uncertain in its action from an allopathic point of view.

Mang-s. 1x cured in one case of hepatic derangement where the stools were composed of large quantities of bile.

REFERENCES - Clarke.

MANGIFERA INDICA

(Mango Tree)

PHARMACY - mangi. Mangifera indica. Mango tree. N. O. Anacardiaceae. India. ***Historical dose:*** Tincture and all potencies.

CLINICAL - Chilly. Colds. Coryza. Dyspnea. Hay fever. ***Hemorrhages.*** Itching. Nausea. Pains. Pharyngitis. Rhinitis. Sneezing. Varicose veins. Vomiting.

HOMEOPATHIC - One of the best general remedies for ***passive hemorrhages,*** uterine, kidney, gastric, pulmonary and intestinal. Mangi. has atonic conditions, poor circulation and relaxed muscles. Rhinitis, sneezing, pharyngitis, and other acute throat troubles, suffocative sensation as if throat would close.

Hemorrhages of all kinds. Varicose veins. Drowsiness. Relaxation of mucus membrane of digestive tract. Chronic intestinal irritation. Catarrhal and serous discharges. Aching of left side of body. Chilly. Sticky mucus discharges. Tendency to suppurations.

Pains in spots. Pains shifting suddenly, or coming and going suddenly. Hay fever with whitish, sticky and stringy discharge. Dyspnea, starting with coryza. Skin as if sunburnt, swollen.

MIND - Ailments from anger. Easily offended. Feels like striking the person irritating her. Involuntary, sighing. Weeps easily. Melancholy. Feels bored. Worse being alone. Wants to remain busy.

Abdomen - ***Heaviness of abdomen after eating.***

Blood - Hemorrhage, venous blood with dark clots.

Face - Swelling of lips.

Female - Metrorrhagia, dark blood, painless, profuse.

Food - Better cold drinks. ***Desires mango.*** Desires sour. Desire for sweets. Worse sour, spicy foods.

Limbs - Itching of palms of hands.

Modalities - Better vomiting. Better open air. Better sitting bent forward or erect. Better cold drinks. Better continued motion. Worse sour food. Worse morning. Worse beginning of motion. Worse exertion, climbing. Worse 1 a.m. to 2 a.m.

Worse change of weather. Worse air-conditioned room. Worse closed room. Worse stooping. Worse bending forward.

Nose - Colds. Rhinitis with sneezing.

Skin - Skin as if sunburned and swollen. White spots intense itching. Itching of palms. Lobes of ears and lips swollen.

Stomach - ***Hyperacidity.*** Worse eructations. Better drinking cold water. Burning behind sternum at 2 a.m. to 3 a.m. Nausea and vomiting in morning.

Throat - Pharyngitis and other acute throat troubles. Suffocative sensation as if throat would close.

RELATIONS - ***Compare:*** (1) Erig., Epil.

REFERENCES - Boericke.

MANTIS RELIGIOSA

(European Praying Mantis)

PHARMACY - mant-r. Mantis religiosa. European praying mantis. N. O. Mantidae. Tinctures. ***Historical dose:*** All potencies.

CLINICAL - Backache. Belching. Coryza. Flatulence. ***Headaches.*** Heartburn. Herpes. Lumbago. Toothaches. ***Weariness.***

HOMEOPATHIC - Activity increased. Weariness with sleepiness. Lack of vital heat or heat sensation.

MIND - Hurry, haste. Anxiety alternating with cheerfulness. Anxiety about future. ***Fear bad something will happen. Fear with heart complaints.*** Delusions, that he is pursued. ***Ailments from domination by others.***

Contented. Cheerfulness, gaiety, happiness. Elated. Euphoria. Egotistic. Cheerfulness alternating with sadness. Mood changeable, variable. Morose, sulky, cross, fretful, ill-humor, peevish. Indifference, apathy. Unfeeling, hard-hearted. Sadness, despondency, depression, melancholy.

Concentration difficult while studying, reading, talking, when thinking. Memory weakness. Forgetful for what he was about to do. Loss of memory. Makes mistakes in localities, talking, writing. Stupefaction, as if intoxicated.

Abdomen - Bloating. Flatulence.

Back - Backache in dorsal, lumbar region. Lumbago. Stiffness, tension.

Breast - Itching in breast, nipples. Breast, nipple pain, stitching.

Dreams - Dreams lewd, lascivious, voluptuous, perverse. Dreams of anger, brutality, violence, mutilation, rape, war, escape. Dreams about children.

Ears - Noises in ears.

Eyes - Pain as from a foreign body. Burning, smarting, biting, pressing pain. Agglutinated inner canthi. Itching in inner canthi.

Face - Dryness, especially of the lips. Eruptions, pustules.

Female - Menses too late. Herpetic eruptions. Sexual desire diminished or increased.

Food - Desires juicy things. Aversion to alcoholic drinks, worse from coffee.

Head - Headache in the forehead. Headache, worse from changes of weather, ***draft of air***. Headache during fever. Pain in spots. Dull, pressing, stitching pain.

Heart - Palpitations. Stitching pain in heart.

Limbs - ***Weariness with heaviness of limbs.*** Numbness, insensibility. Trembling. Weakness in the lower limbs, especially in the right knee.

Modalities - Better open air. ***Worse draft of air***, or change of weather. Weariness better from lying.

Mouth - Dryness with thirstlessness, especially tongue. Sore, bruised gums on touch. Bleeding gums when brushing teeth. Scorbutic gums.

Neck - Pain in neck region. Stiffness, tension.

Nose - Coryza with fluent discharge. Watery discharge. Sneezing.

Rectum - Constipation.

Sleep - Falling asleep difficult or late. Bad sleep. Deep sleep. Position on right side, impossible to sleep on left side.

Skin - Itching.

Stomach - Heartburn. Acrid, sour belching. Pressing pain.

Teeth - Toothaches, pressing pain.

Throat - Rawness, roughness, scratching in throat. Sore, bruised pain. Throat pain during fever.

REFERENCES - Gluck.

MARRUBIUM ALBUM
(White Horehound)

PHARMACY - marr. Marrubium album. White horehound. Marrubium vulgare. N. O. Labiatae. Tincture of the whole plant. ***Historical dose:*** Infusions, tincture and all potencies.

CLINICAL - After, birth. Bites, snake. Bronchitis. Colds. Coughs. ***Dyspepsia.*** Fevers. Indigestion. Irregular, heartbeats. Itching. Liver, disorders. Lung, disorders. Malaria. Poisons. Rabies. Tetters. Throat, sore.

HERBAL - A valuable herbal remedy in coughs, colds and lung infections. Sold as "Horehound ale," a pleasant tasting beverage. An infusion of one ounce to one pint of boiling water, taken in hot wineglass doses as needed induces sweating. Horehound candies and cough drops are popular.

Marrubium is ***a bitter digestive tonic, expectorant and diuretic herb***. It has a bitter, aromatic taste and odor. Culpepper used it to repel the afterbirth, as an antidote to poisons, snakebites and to help indurated livers. It calms the nervous heart. Irregular heartbeats. Reduces fevers. Malaria.

RELATIONS - ***Compare:*** (1) Black Horehound - Stimulant, anti-spasmodic and vermifuge. Dioscorides said, "The leaves beaten with salt and applied the wound, cure the bite of mad dogs."

REFERENCES - Potter.

MATTHIOLA GRAECA
(Stock Gilliflower)

PHARMACY - matth. Matthiola graeca. Stock gilliflower. N. O. Crucifere. Tincture of fresh plant. ***Historical dose:*** Tincture and all potencies.

CLINICAL - Abscesses. Cancer. Neuralgia.

HOMEOPATHIC - Cooper studied Matth., and considered a leading indication for it ***"concentrated juices,"*** which should be compared with the action of its relative crucifere, Thlaspi., which has cured obstruction of bile duct from inspissated bile.

He cured with it abscesses in neck glands that had been discharging for twenty-five years, abscesses in hollow viscera, and one case of stomach cancer. Neuralgia of the left arm with numbness and paralysis.

COMMENTS - Cooper related a case which seems to indicate that morphine causes neuralgia and that Matth. antidotes morphine.

A man had neuralgia of his right arm from working in a damp house. Morphine was given. Then neuralgia of the left arm came on with numbness and paralysis. Lob. gave some relief. One dose of Matth. tincture completely cured. When the man came under Cooper's care, he was spending ten shillings a week on morphine.

RELATIONS - ***Compare:*** (1) Cheir., Thlaspi. and crucifere generally.

REFERENCES - Clarke. Cooper.

MDMA
(Ecstasy)

PHARMACY - ecst. MDMA. Ecstasy (3,4 methylenedioxymethamphetamine). A synthetic psychoactive drug similar to methamphetamine and mescaline. ***Historical dose:*** All potencies.

CLINICAL - Anorexia. Chills. Chronic fatigue. Attention Deficit ***Dehydration.*** Disorder. Drug, abuse. ***Empathy.*** Exhaustion. ***Fever.*** Headache. Insomnia. Paranoid, states. Malaise. Manic depression. Migraine. Narcolepsy. Nausea. Nystagmus. ***Restlessness.*** Tachycardia.

HOMEOPATHIC - MDMA produces ***intense activity***, physically, mentally, psychically. Restlessness, trembling. Exhaustion. Chronic fatigue. Chronic, influenza-like symptoms. Malaise. Analgesia.

Extreme sensitivity of the whole nervous system. Overstimulated mental states. All senses are enhanced, especially those of touch and sound. Heightened sense of balance and physical agility. ***Oversensitivity to environmental influences.***

Tranquility. Reduces physical and emotional stress. Release of "body armor." It has been used clinically, with much success, with patients undergoing periods of great psychic change.

MIND - ***Calmness.*** Pronounced feeling of personal well-being, at peace with the world. ***Acceptance.*** Deep sense of forgiveness and unconditional love. ***Feelings of bliss***, ecstasy, euphoria, fearlessness.

Empathy. Emotional warmth. Ease of communication. Desire to touch and be touched. Introversion or extroversion. Easy release of psychological trauma and deeply buried emotions.

Mood swings. Clarity of mind. Excessive loquacity. Inappropriate bonding. Racing thoughts. Difficulty in holding concentration. Nervous irritability. ***Restlessness.*** Low-grade anxiety without obvious cause. Paranoia. Fear of insanity, of losing control. Sudden depression. Chronic depression. Lethargy.

Abdomen - Bloating of abdomen.

Causation - Overstimulation. Over-work. Sexual abuse. Abuse of drugs, especially stimulants.

Chest - Warm full, sensation. Swelling.

Ears - Enhanced hearing. Sensitive to slightest sounds.

Eyes - ***Dilated pupils.*** Nystagmus. Increased clarity of vision. Colors look brighter, intense and painfully pleasurable.

Face - Flushed face. Tension in jaws.

Female - Dryness of vagina. Lack of clitoral response.

Food - Loss of appetite. Anorexia. ***Extreme thirstlessness.*** Intense thirst with dry mouth. Desire for cold, refreshing drinks, fruit juices.

Head - Headaches, pounding, explosive, occipital. Migraine.

Heart - Raised blood pressure. Tachycardia, fast, pounding heartbeats.

Limbs - Relaxation of muscular tension. Muscle cramping. Seizures. Tremors in upper and lower limbs, hands. Convulsive movements.

Male - Impotence with increased sensitivity. Orgasm impossible.

Modalities - Better fresh air, warmth, dancing. Better touch, stroking, massage. Worse alcohol. Worse sitting, standing still, overstimulation, suppression of emotions.

Mouth - Dryness of mouth. Continual desire to swallow. Intensely bitter taste. Enhanced sense of taste.

Perspiration - Copious, easy sweat.

Skin - ***Sensitivity to touch.*** Warm sensuality.

Sleep - Tired and drowsy but unable to sleep. Sleepless from excessive thoughts. Narcolepsy. Restless dreams, constantly changing.

Stomach - Nausea and cramping. Noisy eructations.

Teeth - Clenched jaws. Teeth grinding.

Temperature - Sudden chill, cannot get warm. Flu-like chills, alternating with flushes of heat. High fever.

Throat - Dry throat. Raw, scratching sensation. Constriction. Hoarseness, needs to keep clearing throat.

Vertigo - Dizziness on motion, with nausea.

COMMENTS - Ecstasy produces intensely pleasurable effects, including an enhanced sense of self-confidence and energy. Loss of inhibitions. Transfixion on sights and sounds. Feelings of closeness with others and a desire to touch others. Sense of peacefulness, acceptance and empathy.

Involuntary teeth clenching. Nausea, blurred vision, chills and sweating. Dehydration. Increases in heart rate and blood pressure. Seizures. Muscular breakdown. Kidney, liver and cardiovascular failure.

Sleep problems. Anxiety, depression. Memory loss or weakness. Disruption of serotonin levels, affecting mood, sense of pain, appetite, learning and memory.

RELATIONS - ***Compare:*** Agar., Anh. Hydrog., Nux-m., Salv-d., Sulph-ac., Tarent-h.

REFERENCES - Hammond. Murphy.

MEDORRHINUM

(Gonorrhea Nosode)

PHARMACY - med. Medorrhinum. Gonorrhea nosode. Glinicum. Potencies of the bacteria. ***Historical dose:*** All potencies.

CLINICAL - Abscess. ***Alcoholism.*** Allergies. ***Arthritis. Asthma.*** Backache. ***Bedwetting***. Bi-polar. ***Boils. Catarrh.*** Cellulitis. Clonic, spasms. ***Collapse. Condylomatas.*** Conjunctivitis. Corns. Coryza. ***Cystitis.*** Debility. Diabetes. Drug, abuse. Dysmenorrhea. Dyspnea. Epilepsy. Eyes, inflammation. Favus. Fibroids. Gleet. ***Gonorrhea. Gonorrhea, suppressed.*** Gonorrheal, rheumatism. Headaches. ***Impotence***. Incontinence. ***Infertility***. ***Insomnia. Itching.*** Joint, pain. Kidney, pain. ***Leucorrhea.*** Liver, abscess. Lumbago. ***Manic depression.*** Masturbation. Menstrual, colic. Metrorrhagia. ***Mucus, discharges.*** Nasal, congestion. Nephritis. Neuralgic pains. Ovaries, pains. Pains. Pelvic, problems. Polyps. Polyuria. Priapism. Psoriasis, palmaris. Ptosis. Rape, victims. ***Rheumatism.*** Sexual, abuse. ***Sexual, excesses.*** Schizophrenia. Sciatica. Shoulder, pains. ***Sinusitis.*** Stage-fright. Sterility. Stricture. ***Sycosis.*** Tenesmus. ***Trembling.*** Tuberculosis. ***Urethritis. Vaginitis. Venereal, diseases. Urethritis.*** Urticaria. Warts.

HOMEOPATHIC - Medorrhinum, one of the most important of the nosodes, is prepared from gonorrheal discharge. The nosodes may be used according to their indication in exactly the same way as other homeopathic remedies and also for manifestations of the disease from which they are derived. At the same time, a knowledge of the origin of obscure disorders, especially if hereditary, will often give the clue to the remedy required.

Medorrhinum is a powerful, deep acting medicine indicated for ***chronic ailments due to suppressed gonorrhea. History of gonorrhea,*** often restores a gonorrheal discharge. Poor reaction to remedies due to gonorrhea history.

It affects the mind, nerves, and mucus membranes. Great disturbance and irritability of nervous system. Intolerable pains, tensive, nerves quiver and tingle. Intensity of all the sensations. ***State of collapse and trembling all over***. Wants to be fanned all the time.

Arthritic, rheumatic pains. ***Chronic rheumatism***. Diseases of the spinal cord, even organic lesions ending in paralysis. Loss of power in the joints, joints feel loose. Many different kinds of pain, stiffness, aching, soreness, edema of limbs, dropsy of serous sacs.

Disseminated sclerosis. Numbness, internal formication. Burning. Small, very sore aphthae, blisters. Enlargement of the lymphatic glands all over the body with heat and soreness. Tumors, cancer, scirrhous etc. with history of sycosis.

Profuse acrid discharges, causing itching. Fishy odors of the secretions. Nose dirty, tonsils enlarged, thick yellow mucus from nostrils, lips thickened from mouth breathing. ***Chronic catarrhal conditions in children.*** Chronic pelvic disorders of women. Offensive, sour odor of the body especially children and women, cannot wash. Dwarfed and stunted children.

MIND - Sensitive, nervous, restless. Everything startles her. ***Hurried***, ***anxious*** and irritable. ***Wild feeling in head.*** Lack of self-control. Exhilaration at night. Cross through the day, merry at night.

Apprehensive, anticipates events. Anxiety if a time is set. Frighten, easily. ***Panic attacks.*** Stage-fright. Fears going insane (Calc., Manc.). ***Fear in the dark and of someone behind her,*** of being alone at night. Claustrophobia. Fear of animals. Fear of venereal diseases, cancer, misfortune, poverty.

Persistent ideas. Dwells on the past. Desperate. Sad, tearful and fearful. Melancholy with suicidal thoughts. Sad, dismal outlook, better after weeping. Cannot speak without weeping, tells it over and over again. ***Cries when telling her story.*** Great difficulty in stating her symptoms. ***Despair, hopeless of recovery.*** Suicidal thoughts, tendency.

Difficult concentration. ***Weakness of memory.*** Loses the thread of conversation. Forgets names, word, errands. Makes mistakes, reading, writings. Confusion of mind as to his identity.

Dread of saying wrong thing. Poor self confidence. ***Shuns responsibilities.*** Aversion to being touched. Stupefaction, as if intoxicated. ***Mentally retarded, children.***

Alternating or erratic states. Severe mood changes. Happiness alternating with gloominess. Contrasting extremes in one person. ***Manic depression***. Schizophrenia, paranoid. Abusive to others. ***Impulsive***, abrupt, rude, mean, cruel. Irritability, impatience over trifles. Censorious, critical. Jealousy.

Morbid impulses. ***Alcoholism and drug abuse.*** Fastidious. ***Bites nails.*** Cursing, swearing. Dictatorial, domineering, dogmatic, despotic. Cruelty, brutality, inhumanity to animals. Sexual excesses. Wild, strong, ***high sex drive***. Sexual perversions, ***fantasies and masturbation.*** Ailments from sexual abuse, rape.

Sensibility exalted. Sensitive to nature, animals, beauty, flowers. ***Feels life unreal, everything seems unreal like a dream.*** Things seem strange. ***Time passes too slowly*** (Cann-i., Arg-n.). Feels far off, as if things done today occurred a week ago. Sees faces peer at her from behind bed and furniture. Clairvoyance. Feeling of having committed the unpardonable sin and will be going to hell. Continually praying. Sensation of impending death.

Abdomen - Heaviness in lower abdomen. ***Rests more comfortably lying on abdomen.*** Grasping pain in liver and spleen. Burning in epigastrium. ***Agonizing pain in solar plexus***, applies his hands to stomach and to lumbar region. Left inguinal glands sensitive and slightly swollen. Grinding colic better bracing feet, lying on abdomen. Bilious colic with frequent vomiting and nausea. Flatulence with numbness.

Back - Spine sore and tender. Backache with burning heat in spine. Intense burning heat, commencing in neck and extending gradually down spine. Chills up and down back. Cutting, burning, crawling above left scapula. Drawing pain in cords of neck, causes desire to throw head back. Spasms of neck muscles, notably sterno-mastoid. Pain from left to right shoulder. ***Lumbar vertebrae sensitive to touch.*** Tenderness of spinal column when stretching. Pain in sacrum and coccyx. Lumbago from lifting.

Bladder - Cystitis with burning pains. ***Urethritis.*** Polyuria. Can't retain urine more than an hour. ***Nocturnal bedwetting***. Incontinence of urine on getting cold. Painful tenesmus when urinating. Urine flows very slowly. Debility after prolonged or complete urination.

Breasts - Breasts sore and swollen between periods. Breast sensitive, cold, icy, the rest of the body warm. ***Breasts and nipples sore and sensitive to touch.*** Sore, oozing or icy nipples during menses. Soreness of nipples, a gummy secretion drying on orifice, when picked off, nipple bleeds freely.

Causations - ***Ailments from suppressed gonorrhea.*** Ailments from verbal, sexual abuse. Ailments from anticipation, foreboding, bad news, rudeness of others.

Chest - Chest as if painfully contracted, when coughing. Sharp, along right edge of sternum. Pain and soreness through chest and breasts. Chest sore to touch. As if a cavity in chest. Coldness in chest. Pain, heat and soreness through chest.

Constitutions - Sycotic, rheumatoid and hydrogenoid constitution.

Coughs - Dry, hacking cough with weak, sinking sensation under sternum. Incessant, dry cough at night. Deep and hollow cough. ***Cough, better, lying on stomach***, worse from sweet things. Cough on entering warm room. Cough and retching, at night.

Ears - Opening of ear is sore and tight. Quick darting pains, in right ear. Pain passes up Eustachian tube. Aching in cartilage of ear. Aching or boring pain in left ear. Itching in left ear. Partial deafness, pulsation in ears. Hears voices. Frying and hissing noises in ears, mastoid.

Eyes - Eyeballs ache. Feels as if sticks in eyes. ***Neuralgic pain in eyeballs.*** Objects look double or small. Sees imaginary objects. ***Feels as if she stared at everything.*** Swelling under eyes. Lids irritated. Ptosis of lids. Upper lid hard as if it had cartilage. ***Swelling of upper lids.*** Eyelashes fall out.

Face - Freckles. Pallor. Grayish, greasy, greenish, yellow at the edges of hair. Flushes of heat in face and neck. Sweat on face. Blotches of red color. Acne, worse after menses. ***Small boils*** break out during menses. ***Red spiderlets on face.*** Risus sardonicus. Rigidity of muscles of face. Lips thickened from mouth breathing. Stiffness in jaws and tongue. Swelling of submaxillary glands. Warts.

Female - Dysmenorrhea. Intense menstrual colic, better pressing feet against support. Menstrual colic with drawing up of knees. ***Menses offensive***, profuse, dark, clotted. Menses stains difficult to wash out. Metrorrhagia. ***Vaginitis.*** Leucorrhea thick, acrid, excoriating, fishy odor. Intense itching, vagina better rubbing and by bathing with tepid water. ***Urethritis.*** Neuralgic pains. ***Sensitive spot near os uterus***. Os uterus, ulcerated. Ovarian pain, worse left side. Pain from ovary to ovary. Drawing in ovaries, better pressure. ***Infertility***, sterility. ***Sycotic infertility.*** Sycotic warts on genitals. ***Gonorrhea, suppressed.*** Passionate, wild, strong sex drive. Sexual perversions, ***fantasies and masturbation.*** Sexual excesses. Ailments from sexual abuse, rape.

Food - Ravenous hunger soon after eating. ***Craving for ice***, salt, sweets, sour things, refreshing things, ***green fruits***, ***oranges***. Desires ***fat, fish,*** tobacco, ale. Craving for liquors, which she used to dislike. ***Excessive thirst***, dreams of drinking water. Water tastes like perfume. Nausea after drinking water. Cough, worse sweet things.

Head - Head is heavy and drawn backward. ***Sensation as if tight band across forehead, worse bending head forward.*** Burning pain in brain, worse occiput. Weight and pressure in vertex. ***Tensive pains in head as if she would go crazy***, can't read or use mind. Sharp pains, comes and goes suddenly, worse light and coughing. Severe pain in back of head. Dull, aching pains. Aching, in base of brain with swelling of cords of neck. Burning in brain. ***Intense burning in cerebellum.*** Headache over eyes and in temples, on waking, worse sunlight. Headache from jarring, exhaustion or hard work. Headache during menses. Hair dry, crispy. Itching of scalp, dandruff.

Heart - Sensation of cavity where heart ought to be. Oppression of heart with difficult breathing. Heart as if hot and large. Heart with bursting sensation. Soreness in heart. Fluttering about heart. Heart beats very fast. Palpitations after slight exertion.

Kidneys - Nephritis. Deathly feeling in kidneys. Creeping chills in region of right kidney. ***Kidney colic*** (Berb., Oci., Pareir.). When stooping can't rise again without ***violent pain in region of kidneys.*** Pain in kidney region, better by profuse urination, with craving for ice. Bubbling in kidney region. Urine flows very slowly. Urine watery, colorless, intensely yellow, covered with a thick greasy pellicle. Scalding, ammoniacal urine. Urine stains clothes a dirty brown. Urinates frequently at time of menses. Passes an enormous quantity of high colored, strong smelling urine in bed every night.

Limbs - ***Stiffness*** throughout body and limbs. Gouty concretions. ***Rheumatism***. Edema of the limbs. Coldness of legs, hands, and forearms. Legs heavy, ache all night. ***Legs, cannot keep them still*** (Zinc.). Cramps in legs better stretching them. Ankles easily turn when walking. ***Heels and balls of feet tender*** (Thuj.), and itching, cannot walk on them, had to walk on knees. Edema of feet followed and better by diarrhea. ***Soreness of soles***. ***Burning of hands and feet wants them uncovered and fanned.*** Restless, better clutching hands. Finger joints enlarged, puffy. Fingertips cracked and burn. Bites nails. Nails depressed, as if they were bent.

Liver - Hepatitis. Abscess of liver. Violent, grasping pain in liver and spleen.

Lungs - Desire to breathe deep. ***Air hunger, cannot exhale.*** Dyspnea, cannot exhale (Samb.). Wakes gasping for breath. Much oppression of breathing. ***Asthma, only better lying on abdomen and protruding tongue.*** Asthma, sycotic infantile. Rattling, wheezing or whistling on coughing when lying on back or either side. Lungs feel stuffed up with cotton. Heat in lungs. Left lung very painful, feels drawn towards right side. Aching in left lung under scapula. As if left lung were collapsed and paralyzed, after talking. Darting pain through lung, causes startling. Painful shock at base of each lung on coughing. ***Bronchial catarrh.*** Ropy mucus, difficult to raise. Incipient tuberculosis.

Male - ***Urethritis.*** Whole urethra feels sore. Heaviness of prostate, painful. Prostate enlarged with frequent and painful urination. ***Gonorrhea infection.*** Gonorrheal flow thin, transparent, mixed with opaque, whitish mucus, stains linen yellow. ***Gonorrhea, suppressed.*** Gleet, persistent, yellow discharge. Heaviness in perineum. Sharp, cutting pains transversely across root of penis. ***High sex drive.*** Intense and frequent erections day and night. Amorous behavior. Sexual perversions, ***fantasies and masturbation.*** Sexual excesses. ***Impotence***. Prostration after seminal emission. Nocturnal emissions, followed by great weakness. Ailments from sexual abuse, rape.

Modalities - ***Better at the seashore***, damp weather (Caust.). Better being fanned, fresh air, at sunset. Better bending backward, stretching out, hard rubbing, ***lying on abdomen***. Chronic rheumatism of joints is worse inland, better near sea. ***Worse from damp, cold weather***, before storm, heat, covering, closed room, slight touch, after urinating. ***Worse 3 a.m. to 4 a.m.,*** during daytime, ***from sunrise to sunset,*** when thinking of ailments. Early morning aggravation. Salt-water bathing aggravates sore throat and colds in the head.

Mouth - Taste in mouth coppery, bad taste and foul breath in morning. Breath hot, feels so even when breathing through nose. Exhalation hot. Mouth feels burnt. Dryness of mouth. Water tastes like perfume. Copious salivation. Stringy mucus from mouth during sleep. Small very sore aphthae. Canker sores. Blisters on inner surface of the lips and cheeks.

Nose - Soreness and crawling in left nostril. Numbness. Burning pain in both nostrils when breathing through them. Coldness of tip. ***Intense itching of the tip.*** Obstruction at root of nose as if mucus membrane was hypertrophied. ***Hay fever and allergies.*** Coryza, better sea bathing, with loss of smell and taste. ***Nasal catarrh*** running down throat. Chronic nasal and pharyngeal catarrhs. ***Chronic sinusitis. Thick yellow-green discharges.*** Posterior nares obstructed. ***Post-nasal discharge, thick yellow.*** Snuffles in children. Nose dirty in children. Nosebleeds.

Perspiration - Great tendency to perspire on exertion. When asleep, day or night, no matter how short a time, profuse sweat on face and neck. Night-sweats and hectic fever. Sweat easy towards morning.

Rectum - Anus is red, moist. Fiery, red rash about anus in babies. ***Intense itching of anus***. Painful lump sensation on posterior surface of sphincter. Heaviness in perineum. Sharp, needle-like pains in rectum. Sensation of prolapsus of rectum. ***Dark fetid oozing moisture from anus of fish brine odor.*** Profuse bloody discharges from rectum. Inertia of bowels, with ball-like stools. White diarrhea. Stools tenacious, claylike, sluggish, can't be forced out. Can pass stools only by leaning very far back, then shivering. Cholera infantum with opisthotonus. Diarrhea, and headache, from motion of cars.

Sensations - As if sticks in eyes, lids and inner canthi, as if cold wind blowing in eyes, as if upper lid had a cartilage in it. As if something crawling in ear and nose. As if a lump in stomach. As if tumor in right side of abdomen. As if left lung collapsed or paralyzed. As if an abscess between left pectoralis major and minor muscles. As if the blood was boiling hot in veins. As if all bones were out of joint.

Skin - Pricking sensation all over body. ***Intense itching, sore, worse night and when thinking of it.*** Continuous itching. Skin cold, but feels as if the blood is hot, ***throws off covers.*** Yellow skin. Yellow, copper colored spots, remaining after eruptions. Sycotic red nodes. Deep red spots. Boils. Condylomatas and warts. Small, pedunculated warts. Tumors and growths.

Sleep - Dreads night to come. ***Insomnia.*** Sleepless from intolerable pains. Sleep prevented by aching in lower limbs. Spasmodic yawning, can't suppress it. ***Sleeplessness, falls asleep towards morning.*** Short sleep seems like a long one, which is better. Sleeps in knee-chest position. ***Sleeps more comfortably lying on abdomen.*** Can only sleep on back with hands over head. Asleep, but hears everything, answers questions as if she was awake. Dreams of drinking (Ars., Phos.), walking. Nightmares, of ghosts and dead people. Exhausting dreams. Wakes gasping for breath.

Stomach - Intense pain in stomach and upper abdomen, with sensation of tightness. Clawing pain in stomach worse drawing up knees. Cramps in stomach as from wind. Burning, trembling in pit. Throbbing in sides of stomach. Agonizing pains in solar plexus. Ravenous hunger soon after eating. Sick or gnawing feeling, not better eating or drinking. Coppery taste and belchings of sulphuretted hydrogen. Nausea in morning, before eating, during pregnancy. Vomiting of thick mucus and black bile, without nausea.

Teeth - Pale gums. Teeth yellow, easily decay. Teeth serrated, soft, crumbling. Eyeteeth sore, feel soft. Teeth sensitive while chewing.

Temperature - Creeping chills running down back and all over body in a zigzag course. Shivering chills with boring pains in chest. Chills after urinating, great coldness and shivering. Chilliness when bladder is too full, better urination. Cold skin but blood feels hot. Burning heat with sweat, wants to uncover, but is chilled. Flushes of heat, alternating with chills. Great internal heat after dinner and after slight exertion, as if blood was boiling hot in veins. Flashes of heat in face and neck. Wants to be fanned all the time (Carb-v.).

Throat - Great dryness of throat with swollen glands. Throat sore and swollen. Larynx feels sore as if ulcerated. Pains on swallowing. Swallowing of liquids and solids impossible. Choking. Spasm of glottis. ***Throat constantly filled with thick, gray or bloody mucus from posterior nares.*** Tenacious mucus in larynx. Sore throat and cold in head better salt water bathing. Hoarse while reading.

Tongue - Tongue coated brown and thick. Tongue white, with papillae showing through. Base of tongue white and foul. Tongue coated thickly in morning. Blistered tongue, canker sores. Skin peeling off in patches. Small, very sore aphthae. Bites tip of tongue in sleep.

Vertigo - Intense vertigo from sensation of tightening in head. Vertigo, worse in vertex and on stooping. Vertigo with sensation and fear of falling. Vertigo as if intoxicated, on waking. Walks zigzag.

Vision - Blurred vision. Objects look double or small. Many black, sometimes brown spots dancing over her book.

COMMENTS - An often prescribed polycrest remedy, especially if there is a history of a gonorrhea infection. Never well since suppressed gonorrhea. Symptoms are similar to Thuj. and Ars., but they work on different levels and can interrelate. Generally, Ars is a less serious Med., and where Med. is given for an acute, Thuj. would work for the chronic.

Confusion. Slow answering questions. Developmental problems. Difficulty concentrating. Restlessness. Hyperactivity, wildness. Temper tantrums and fits. Intense nervous sensibility, especially to touch of garment or a lock of hair by any one not en rapport. Sensibility is very exalted almost to clairvoyance.

Over excited. Starting at slightest sound. Spacey. Unpredictable, unstable, fitful and changeable. A disintegrated person, unharnessed. Lack of purpose or function in their life, concerned with fulfilling passions, particularly sexual passion.

Full of extremes. Can become obsessive, violent. Schizophrenia, manic-depression, depression with uncontrolled nature. Often violent, paranoid, can have persecution complexes.

Anticipation or panic attacks. Fear of losing control, about their mind not functioning correctly, of going insane (Cann-i., Calc-c.). Fear that something bad will happen, anticipates that something will go wrong, especially with their health. Think themselves incurable. Children can have severe nightmares and deep fears about monsters or people getting them. Delusion that someone is in their bedroom.

Exaggerated sexual development. Generally precocious children, may begin masturbating at an early age. Chronic masturbation. Preoccupation with sex, sexual fantasies.

History of sexual diseases such as vaginitis, bladder infections, herpes, gonorrhea. Often a history of promiscuity, history of gonorrhea. Attracted to the culture of sex, drugs, and wild behavior. Alcoholism. May be helpful for AIDS, stimulates the immune function and lessons recurring infections.

Tremor, spasms. State of collapse, with a desire to be fanned. The pains seem to tighten the whole body, especially the thighs. There is scarcely a spot on the body that is not full of pain. Acute arthritis with painful, swollen joints. Obstinate rheumatism. Sequela of acute rheumatism.

Insomnia from too much energy. Blood pressure or heart conditions. Chronic, recurring infections. Discharges, sensitivity. Conjunctivitis. Vaginitis, urethritis, uterine fibroids. Fishy odor to the vaginal discharge.

Multiple allergies, especially allergies with discharges since gonorrhea. Sore throats, earaches, sinus problems. Severe asthma. Great sensitiveness to draft of air, takes cold easily. Cough is better lying on face or stomach.

Generally worse motion, better rest. Worse stretching out, leaning head forward. Constipation is better leaning far back, can only pass stool so. Worse storms and damp weather. Better by the sea.

Worse from sunrise to sunset, always brighter in evening, worse in early morning hours (Syph. is worse from sunset to sunrise). Craves oranges and orange juice, particularly in children. Craves unripe fruit, alcohol and marijuana.

Craves tobacco (Staph, Thuj, Ars.), often as a nervous habit.

Many cases of stunted growth and arrested development in children are due to latent gonorrhea and syphilis. On this hypothesis, Clarke cured extremely offensive body odors in children with Med.

Negerath of New York and Angus Macdonald in England have pointed out a causal connection between post-partum pelvic cellulitis and latent gonorrhea in the husband. Macdonald published several fatal cases.

The effects of the poison, constitutional or acute, may be taken as data for homeopathic prescriptions, but the virus also has had an extensive proving in the potencies and symptoms have been largely verified in practice.

Burnett noted several cures with Med. 1,000c, including fits at every menstrual period, coming on in the early morning. Clonic spasms, the legs suddenly shoot up from the bed. Rheumatism of the right wrist.

Sycotic asthma, worse from 2 a.m. to 4 a.m. Psoriasis palmaris. Polyps having their origin in a chronic suppurating discharge. Albuminuria where the urine contains some mucus as well. Masturbation in children. Burnett regarded Med. as "a remedy of pus and catarrhs."

Clarke cured with Med. 200c a most aggravated case of constipation on learning that the patient was obliged to lean far back on the seat or he could not get rid of the stool. He was passing urine containing long white mucus shreds. He had gonorrhea many years before.

Deschere published a Med. case in which Miss S., 23, had chronic blepharitis since eleven. Her suffering was intense. Light, especially gaslight, was intolerable and this prevented her from going into society. She could not read in the evening, and in the morning the lids would be closed and she suffered much on getting them separated. There was much discharge.

Before coming under Deschere she had been under strict homeopathic treatment all the time. Deschere remembered treating her father for gonorrhea before his marriage and he suspected the taint had reappeared in this form. Med. was given in high potency, single doses repeated as the effect of each wore off and she was entirely cured.

Skinner traced a case of favus to the same hereditary cause. It had resisted all the external applications that allopaths could devise and which had such an appalling odor that the patient, a little boy, had to be isolated from the family. It was cured with Med. 1,000c.

McLaren related in Hahn. Advoc. a case in which a young French Canadian of delicate constitution, after working in a factory all winter, began coughing in spring and running down in health. He returned home and came under McLaren's care in May.

The cough persisted and prostration increased in spite of carefully selected remedies and the patient took to his bed. It was then observed by McLaren that the cough and general condition was better from lying on the face. This, coupled with a knowledge of there being a syphilitic taint in the boy's parentage, suggested Med., which was given.

The next day a profuse gonorrheal discharge appeared and the cough and all the threatening symptoms promptly disappeared. Exposure to contagion had occurred several weeks before, but from lack of vitality the disease could not find its usual expression and was endangering the patient's life.

Ernest Nyssens quoted some important observations by old-school authorities on constitutional gonorrhea. Wertheim, in a case of gonorrheal cystitis, watched the entrance of the gonococcus into the blood stream. With the gonococcus taken from the blood of this patient he made cultures to the fifth generation.

A youth who had never had a venereal disease volunteered for inoculation with this. The sub-acute urethritis which resulted was so grave and in spite of all, became complicated so cruelly with cystitis, epididymitis, prostatitis, synovitis and pleuro-pneumonia, that Wertheim asked whether the gonococcus did not redouble its virulence by passing into the blood.

Jullien and Sibut witnessed a case in Saint Lazare Hospital in which Louisa M., 17, entered the hospital June 8th with urethra-vaginitis and was treated with tampons of Ichtyhol dissolved in glycerine (1 to 5).

The urethritis ran a normal course until July 6, when the patient complained of sufferings in the abdomen. She had them for the previous week, but had made no complaint until the pain became so acute that an injection of morphine was needed.

Rectal temperature 100.2. Tongue coated. Right side abdominal pain. In spite of rigid contraction of the rectal muscles there seemed to be a swelling deep down, but the observers were not certain it was not a swelling of the muscles themselves. Intestinal functions were normal, rectum empty.

An eruption of roseola spots appeared on the body, abdomen and chest, so exactly like those of typhoid that the possibility of this was discussed. There was also acute pain in muscle of right calf. This pain persisted the following day when the abdominal pains had disappeared.

July 9, the right knee was painful, swollen. At the same time, synovitis of left wrist, dorsal aspect. Temperature normal. July 10, very few and slight traces of the eruption. Right arm the seat of acute sharp pain, especially at the level of the deltoid "V," deep down near the bone at the insertion of the tendon, (probably a hygroma).

On examining the Achilles tendon, there was pain at the level of the left ankle, nothing to the right at the same level, but the pain was, above all, acute along the inner border of the right tibia to five or six centimeters from the flat surface.

This part was edematous and painfully sensitive. Another painful spot in the abdomen was behind the right anterior superior iliac spine and beside the navel (probably muscular). The urethral discharge contained abundant bacilli beside only gonococci.

Treatment by daily injection of one centigram of Merc-c. was commenced. The next day there was sharp fever, coated tongue. The abdominal pains were muscular. Trace of albumen in the urine.

The next night there was delirium and nosebleed in the morning. This case went on to recover.

Another case, also in a girl of seventeen of tubercular history, complicated with syphilis, presented the same order of symptoms, along with the nosebleed, hemoptysis, albuminuria, endocarditis with suffocative attacks and violent palpitations, ending in permanent disablement.

These cases may be regarded as provings of Med. from the homeopathic standpoint. The rheumatic symptoms are of extreme intensity and Med. will cure many cases where the symptoms correspond. Following Burnett, there have been cures of many cases of dysmenorrhea using it.

Gilbert traced rickets to hereditary gonorrhea. In these cases, there are often glandular enlargements and the patient is better at seaside. In such cases he gave Med. When there was syphilitic paresis and the patient was better in the mountains, he gave Syph. In acute bowel troubles in rickety children he found Med. of great value.

Thomas Wildes considered that favus, scald-head and ophthalmia tarsi simplex (margins scaly, scurfy, often angry red, falling of lashes) were due to suppressed gonorrhea in one or both parents. The red, angry condition of skin may extend from face or scalp, down neck and back to perineum and genitals.

A girl, 11, had been treated by many physicians with salves and ointments to the general impairment of her health. Her face was mottled with a profusion of red scurfy sores, eyelids involved and nearly denuded of lashes.

Hairy scalp was one diffuse mass of thick yellow scabs from beneath which oozed a highly offensive mixture of ichor and sebum. Passing down neck, back, perineum and involving genitals and pubes was a fiery red band as broad as the child's hand, oozing a pale yellow serum that caused the clothing to stick to the body.

Wildes told the mother he could cure the case, but it would certainly get worse the first three months. This was not objected to.

Med. 100,000c was given, one dose on the tongue. The external appearance grew rapidly worse, but appetite, sleep and general health steadily improved and in nine months she was completely well.

In another case, a child, 6, was, since infancy, horribly disfigured with tinea capitis. The scalp was a mass of dense scabs exuding fetid ichor, the only semblance of hair being a few distorted stumps ending in withered roots.

One dose cured in a few months and, when Wildes was writing, the patient was a healthy and extremely talented young lady and the possessor of a luxuriant head of chestnut hair.

Wildes thinks that suppression of favus, when derived from gonorrhea in the father, leads to hydrocephalus, capillary bronchitis, severe teething diarrhea, cholera infantum, etc. If derived from the grandfather, suppression leads to tuberculosis and lingering diseases. A fiery red rash develops about the anus in babies a few days old, constipation with hard, dry stools. "Baby's water scalds it terribly."

Wildes regarded the latent gonorrheal miasm as the true explanation of many of the disease manifestations included by Hahnemann under Psora. Burnett, in a way, confirmed this, as he traced gout to a sycotic origin.

Wildes regarded Med. too strong a remedy to give in acute cases whether of gonorrhea, rheumatism or scarlatina, on account of the intensity of the aggravation it is liable to cause, though single doses are often useful when there is a tendency to sinking in dangerous cases of cholera infantum.

Wildes traced to the same source vascular meningitis in infants and cerebrospinal meningitis. In the former, the efficacy of Med. is doubtful, but in the latter it is very efficacious after Cimic. has allayed the first acute symptoms. In the convalescent stage, Lyc. was his chief remedy.

Wildes quoted from old-school authorities the following conditions traceable to latent gonorrhea communicated from husband to wife: ovarian tumors, endometritis, oophoritis, metritis, parametritis, salpingitis, and even peritonitis.

RELATIONS - ***Antidoted by:*** Ip. (dry cough), ***Compare:*** (1) Thuj., Nat-s., Puls. (2) Pic-ac. - inability to walk right, priapism. (3) Camph. and Sec. - collapse, skin cold yet throws off all covering. (4) Verat. - collapse with cold sweat. (5) Syph. - reverse aggravation, sunset to sunrise. (6) as if in a dream, Ambr., Anac., Calc., Cann-i., Con., Cupr., Rheum., Stram., Valer., Verat., Ziz. (7) better by leaning back, Lac-c. (8) Fish-brine odor, Sanic. (9) Breast-feeding - Galeg., Lact., Sulph., Zinc. ***Compatible:*** Sulph. (especially when stool drives out of bed).

REFERENCES - Boericke. Clarke. Murphy. Phatak.

MEDUSA

(Common Jelly-fish)

PHARMACY - medus. Medusa. Common jelly-fish. Arelia aurita. Sea-nettles. N. O. Radiata, class, Acalephe. Tincture of living animal taken in summer. ***Historical dose:*** All potencies.

CLINICAL - Breast-feeding, disorders. Desquamation. Edema. Leucorrhea. ***Nettle, rash.*** Urine, suppression. ***Urticaria.*** Vesicular, eruptions.

HOMEOPATHIC - The effects of encountering jelly-fish while bathing are well known and have been studied experimentally.

The effects of drinking two cupfuls of a decoction, warm, by a woman affected with stomach disease and leucorrhea was recorded. There was rapidly produced edema, anxiety and difficult speech. Secretion of urine, which had been suspended for days, returned.

Secretion of milk re-established in the woman's breasts three years after birth of her last child, she had twelve children and had not suckled any of them, having had no milk. Pricking heat and numbness of skin of face, arms, breasts and vesicular eruption, followed later by desquamation. Whole face puffed and edematous, eyes, nose, ears, lips.

MIND - Extreme anxiety, difficult speech. Aversion to change. Do not like a lot of changes and prefer pleasant routine. Easily offended. Taciturn. Coldness, hatred of others who are enjoying life. Difficult sexual relations. Love of music and dance (Sep.).

Breasts - ***Action on milk glands***. Lack of milk production in breasts.

Ears - Eczema of ear.

Eyes - Eyes puffed and edematous.

Face - Face, eyes, ears, nose are puffed and edematous.

Food - Very thin, doesn't like to eat very much. Craving for salt, fish. Intolerance of fish.

Kidneys - Retention of urine.

Modalities - Better from sleep, movement and food.

Skin - Numbness, burning, pricking heat. Pricking heat, numbness and burning of skin of face, arms, shoulders and breasts. Burning sensation very soon after contact. Burning more than itching. Vesicular eruption, especially on face, arms, shoulders and breasts. ***Nettle rash*** (Apis., Chlor., Dulc.). ***Urticaria and vesicles.*** Desquamation.

Sleep - Better after sleep. Need a lot of sleep otherwise they feel useless.

COMMENTS - Blackie wrote, "In looking at Medusa one must consider the two types of Sepia: [1] rather bright patients who go off at the deep end at the slightest provocation and are exceedingly irritable, and [2] rather stupid and tired out.

"Medusa is neither of these but fits somewhere in between. They can be silent and do not want to talk, they never finish their history in one go and do not want to answer questions. They always think of something else to add to their history."

RELATIONS - ***Compare:*** (1) Murx., Sep., Urt-u., Apis. (2) Pyrar., Physala-p. (urticaria), Hom. (3) Astac., Hom., Bomb-pr.

REFERENCES - Boericke. Clarke.

MEL

(Honey)

PHARMACY - mel. Mel. Honey. ***Historical dose:*** Topically and internally taken as a food or medicine. All potencies.

CLINICAL - Allergies. Athlete's foot. Asthma. Bites. ***Burns.*** Cough. Cuts. Diarrhea. Eczema. Fungal, infections. Hiccups. ***Mouth, ulcers.*** Nausea. Psoriasis. Rash. ***Skin, disorders.*** Stings. Sore throat. Stomach, ulcers. Sunburn. Surgery, effects. Ulcers. Vomiting. Worms. ***Wounds.***

HOMEOPATHIC - Honey is a by-product of bees concentrating plant nectars. The medicinal quality, taste, texture, color, aroma of honey differs according to the geographical area and the species of plants from which it has been collected. The characteristic flowery taste of raw honey comes from the pollen it contains.

It contains a variety of sugars and minerals and has been shown to be low in calories and useful as a sweetener for diabetics, people with heart disease or those who are overweight.

It was widely used in ancient Egypt as a food and as a remedy for many skin problems. Ancient Egyptians used honey as an application for emergencies including ***burns, bites, stings, cuts, sores and ulcers***. Useful for many ***acute and chronic skin disorders*** including eczema and psoriasis.

To heal wounds and treat infections, most commonly used as an anti-microbial agent for dressing wounds, burns and skin ulcers. A natural antiseptic, tonic and cleanser, it also is known for its antioxidant, antibiotic and antiviral capabilities.

Effective in the treatment of various ***wounds and infections*** because of its anti-microbial (antibacterial, antiviral and antifungal) properties. The use of honey reduces odors, reduces swelling, and reduces scarring, it also prevents the dressing from sticking to the healing wound. Postoperative wounds. Burns.

Modern research shows that honey blocks the growth of oral bacteria. Coats the throat and reduces throat irritation.

Effective when used in the treatment of gastric or peptic stomach ulcers. Allows the blood to circulate better and provide more oxygen to areas of the body such as the brain. Acts as a sedative and is very useful in bedwetting disorders. Itching of anus and worms. Allergies.

COMMENTS - Honey is used to cleanse wounds. It initiates growth of healthy granulation tissue. Helps in quick healing of deep wounds. Reduces the effects of poison. Honey is very good for the eyes and eyesight. Bronchial asthma, cough. Hiccoughs, nausea and vomiting. Urinary tract disorders, worm infestations, diarrhea.

RELATIONS - ***Compare:*** (1) Aloe-v., Calen., Mel-c-s. (2) Ric., castor oil, tea tree oil. (3) Urin.

REFERENCES - Murphy.

MEL CUM SALE

(Honey with Salt)

PHARMACY - mel-c-s. Mel cum sale. Honey with salt. ***Historical dose:*** Tincture and all potencies.

CLINICAL - Allergies. Itching. Metritis. Uterus, prolapsed. Worms.

HOMEOPATHIC - Mel-c-s. has been used for prolapsed uterus and chronic metritis, when associated with subinvolution and inflammation of the cervix. Uterine displacements and in the commencement of metritis. ***Soreness across the hypogastrium from ileum to ileum***. Sensation as if bladder were too full. Pain from sacrum towards pubes. Pain as if in ureters.

COMMENTS - Dr. Farrington wrote, "Now there is a combination of honey with salt, known as Mel cum sale. This was for years a popular remedy in Germany for bladder troubles and for diseases peculiar to women.

"I have used this remedy in prolapsus uteri and even in chronic metritis, especially when associated with subinvolution and inflammation of the cervix. The special symptom which leads to the selection of the remedy is a feeling of soreness across the hypogastrium from ilium to ilium."

Dr. Jeanes used a preparation of honey with salt, in the third or sixth potency, for a feeling of soreness in the uterus. Keynote feeling of soreness in the hypogastric region extending from ilium to ilium, especially in uterine displacements and in the commencement of metritis.

REFERENCES - Boericke. Farrington.

MELALEUCA ALTERNIFOLIA
(Tea Tree Oil)

PHARMACY - melal-o. Melaleuca alternifolia. Tea tree oil. New South Wales, Australia. (Do not store in plastic containers). The colorless to pale yellow oil. ***Historical dose:*** Tincture and all potencies.

CLINICAL - Abscess. Athlete's foot. Arthritis. Boils. Cervicitis. Cold, sores. Colds. Corns. Cradle, cap. Cuts. Dermatitis. ***Fungus.*** Gangrene. Hemorrhoids. Herpes zoster. Insect bites. ***Nail, fungus.*** Poison oak or ivy. Pyorrhea. Scabies. Sore, throat. Sprains. Sunburn. Thrush. Tinea versicolor. Trichomonal, infections. Ulcers. Vaginitis. Warts. Yeast, infections.

HERBAL - The tea tree grows in the swampy areas of New South Wales, Australia. The oil contains terpenes and terpineol which gives it a nutmeg-like odor. It contains viridflorene. Tea tree oil is has been used as an non-irritant anti-septic, fungicide and disinfectant of great repute.

When applied to pus filled infections, will clean and dissolve the pus without irritating the tissues. Dental treatment for pyorrhea and gingivitis. As a mouthwash or gargle for sore throats. In a vaporizer for congestions and colds. As a shampoo for head lice, ticks, scabies and cradle cap. Skin emollient. Creams for dry and cracked skin. Hand and body lotions.

HOMEOPATHIC - Skin fungus. ***Fungus of fingernails or toenails.*** Dermatitis. Poison oak or ivy. Tinea versicolor. Bad breath. Diabetic gangrene. Yeast infections and vaginitis. Sprains and muscle aches.

COMMENTS - Combine one part tea tree oil to ten parts olive oil (also almond or avocado oil). Add ten drops to an 8 oz. bottle of shampoo, to a bath, humidifier or vaporizer. Avoid eye contact.

RELATIONS - ***Compare:*** (1) Caj., Cajuput oil made from Melaleuca leucadendron, White Tea Tree. (2) Ric., castor oil use topically for many problems. Calen. (3) Echi., Plan.

REFERENCES - Olsen.

MELASTOMA ACKERMANI

PHARMACY - mela. Melastoma ackermani. N. O. Melastomacee. Tincture of leaves. ***Historical dose:*** Tincture and all potencies.

CLINICAL - Albuminuria. Chills. Colic. Diarrhea. Edema. Headache. Palpitations. Prostate, disorders. Prostration. Tenesmus. Vertigo.

HOMEOPATHIC - Mure described this plant and made a proving of the leaves. On the second day of the proving, the prover lost an inveterate diarrhea with colic. The most notable Mela. symptoms were a pain in the perineum and testicles and shuddering followed by heat without sweat. Prostration. Pains in perineum. Diarrhea. Prostatic disorders.

Abdomen - Borborygmi. Pain in the abdomen.

Chest - Pain in the sternal region, in the morning.

Ears - Roaring in the left ear.

Face - Pale face.

Head - Headache with sensitiveness of the scalp. Lancination and prickings at the vertex.

Heart - Palpitations of the heart.

Kidneys - Pricking in the urethra. Profuse light-colored and foaming urine. Urine more cloudy and less foaming. Urine deposits a white sediment. Red, odorless urine, with bloody clots. Fetid urine. Albuminuria.

Limbs - Edema of the legs. Pain in the loins. Weakness of the thighs.

Male - Hardness of the penis, without erection

Mouth - Looseness of the teeth. Digging pain in the teeth. White coated tongue. Copious flow of saliva. Bitter mouth.

Rectum - Pain at the perineum. Fearful pain and pulling from the perineum to the anus, when sitting, not ceasing in any position, lasting six hours. Lancinations in the perineum, urethra, and testicles. Heat and pricking at the anus. Tenesmus, with constriction of the sphincter. Inveterate diarrhea and colic.

Skin - Eruption on the lips, especially the upper. Itching and heat at night. Pricking over the feet, ankles, and wrists.

Sleep - Drowsiness in the daytime.

Stomach - Sour stomach.

Temperature - Chills, followed by sweat. Violent chills for four hours, followed by heat without sweat. General heat. Internal heat.

Vertigo - Vertigo and dizziness.

REFERENCES - Allen. Clarke.

MELATONIN

(Pineal Gland Hormone)

PHARMACY - melat. Melatonin. A pineal gland hormone. ***Historical dose:*** Tincture and all potencies.

CLINICAL - Amnesia. Breast, cancer. Cancer. Chronic, fatigue. Constipation. Depression. Drowsiness. Fatigue. Headaches. Hyperactivity. Infertility. ***Insomnia. Jet lag.*** Memory, weakness. ***Night, terrors. Nightmares.*** Night watching. ***Seasonal Affected Disorder. Sleep, disorders. Sleep, loss.***

HOMEOPATHIC - Melatonin is a hormone made by the pineal gland. Melatonin has been used as a treatment for a number of conditions, including jet-lag, seasonal affective disorder (SAD), depression and cancer.

Jet-lag, the desynchronization of the biological clock, drastic changes in the sleep-wake cycle. ***Night terrors***. Fatigue, early awakening or insomnia. Daytime drowsiness. Ailments from loss of sleep. Chronic fatigue.

Headache, fuzzy thinking, irritability. Dizziness. Mild depression. Low sex drive. Reduced immunity. Low blood pressure. Nausea. Vomiting. Abdominal cramps. Constipation.

Side effects from melatonin are not uncommon, even at doses that are significantly less than the recommended amount. When side effects from melatonin do occur, they may include an increase in blood pressure, fatigue, depression and problems with fertility.

MIND - Confusion. Dullness of mind. Memory weakness. Hyperactivity. Irritability. Depression. Seasonal Affected Disorder. Ailments from nursing loved ones.

Breasts - Breast cancer in women who sleep irregular hours, sleep with lights on, or work late hours, night shifts.

Causations - Sleep deprivation. Ailments from nursing loved ones.

Female - Infertility.

Head - Headaches.

Heart - High or low blood pressure. Stroke.

Modalities - ***Worse loss of sleep. Worse working night shifts.*** Worse irregular sleep patterns. Worse sleeping with lights on. Worse during winter.

Rectum - Constipation.

Sleep - Daytime drowsiness. ***Insomnia.*** Severe sleep disorders. Sleep deprivation. ***Altered sleep patterns.*** Sleep with lights on or work late hours, night shifts. Vivid dreams. Nightmares.

Stomach - Nausea. Vomiting.

RELATIONS - ***Compare:*** Cocc., Carc., Luna., Coff., Nux-v., Sep.

REFERENCES - Murphy.

MELILOTUS OFFICINALIS

(Sweet Clover)

PHARMACY - meli. Melilotus officinalis. Sweet clover. Yellow clover. Melilotus alba. White and yellow varieties. N. O. Leguminose. Papilionoideae. Tincture of whole fresh plant in flower. It would be well to include a specimen of both plants in the tincture. ***Historical dose:*** Tincture and all potencies.

CLINICAL - Blushing. ***Congestion.*** Coughs. ***Debility.*** Delusions. Dysmenorrhea. Epilepsy. Fears. Hemoptysis. Headaches. ***Hemorrhages.*** Insanity. Leucorrhea. ***Neuralgia. Nosebleeds.*** Ovaries, neuralgia. Pneumonia. Rheumatic pain. Shyness.

HOMEOPATHIC - Meli. was first proved by Bowen in 1851. A second proving was made by him fifteen years later. He used both the yellow and the white varieties.

H. C. Allen published a further proving of Meli. alba, using the entire plant. His proving entirely confirmed Bowen's and added many symptoms.

According to Allen the action of Meli. lasted about thirty days, the indolence and prostration being the first symptom to appear and the last to disappear. Congestions especially to the head, and profuse, bright red, hemorrhage which gives relief. ***Engorgements of any part or organ.*** Violent congestive and nervous headaches.

Pain and debility. Coldness, but also increase of temperature, tenderness and pain. Muscular system depressed. Spasms, eclampsia, convulsions. Epilepsy, from blow on head. Infantile spasms. Tired, bruised, listless, sleepy, chilly. Feeling of rawness. Dreams and emissions.

MIND - Irritable, impatient, discontented, fault-finding. Indolent. Unable to fix mind, stupid indifferent. Total inability to study, memory will not retain anything. Omits words and letters in writing.

Shyness and blushing. Attacks of weeping without much depression. Religious melancholy with intensely red face. Wants to kill himself or threatens to kill who approach. Furious, had to lock him in room. Loss of consciousness.

Panic and fear. Fear of talking loudly, she whispers. ***Fear of danger. Fear of being arrested.*** Wants to go home. Wants to run away and hide. Suspicious. Delusions, thinks everyone is looking at her, fears to talk loud.

Abdomen - Much distention, flatulent, worse during menses.

Back - Broken sensation in lumbo-sacral joint, on sitting and especially sitting upright. Constantly changes position to get relief, wants to strike the part or press it, better standing or walking.

Chest - Weight on chest causing difficult breathing, sensation of smothering, frequently examined clothes to see if they were not too tight.

Ears - Sensation of puffing of wind from ears. Each act of swallowing caused the wind to puff from both ears.

Eyes - Hot, heavy, blurred sight, wants to close them tightly for relief. As if they were too large. Eyes as if pressed outward. Eyelids very heavy. Vision dim, blurred, rubs eyes. Unable to focus. Floating bodies before eyes when studying.

Face - ***Intensely red and flushed with throbbing carotids*** and headache (Bell.). Very red before hemorrhages from nose, lungs, uterus. Face hot, flushed, all day, feverish.

Female - Leucorrhea, pain and soreness in back and pelvic region, excited by walking. ***Menses scanty, intermittent,*** with nausea and bearing down pains. Menses thin, watery, pale offensive. Dysmenorrhea. During menses, headache, bearing-down pain in pelvis. Recurring, sharp, darting pain in vagina and vulva at close of menses. Severe stitches or cutting pains through uterus. Ovarian neuralgia. Sticking pain in external parts.

Food - Ravenous about 10 a.m. with onset of frontal headache. Appetite capricious, especially in morning, impaired.

Head - Rushes of blood to head. ***Fullness all over head***. ***Violent, throbbing,*** nervous and periodical headaches. ***Congestive headaches.*** Headaches are better nosebleed, menstrual flow, application of vinegar. ***Sick headache***, ***relieved by nosebleed or menstrual flow.*** Headache with retching, vomiting, black spots before eyes. ***Neuralgia*** around and over right side of head and neck. Scalp sore and tender to touch. Headache alternating with backache.

Kidneys - Frequent and profuse urination. Urine profuse, watery and relieving the dull, congestive headache.

Limbs - Skin and limbs cold. Joints sore. Stiff and sore on rising, better by careful movement. Rheumatic pains in joints on approach of rain-storm or in rainy, changeable weather. Uneasy sensation in large joints. Numbness and aching in knee joints, right then left. Gnawing, throbbing in right knee joint, wants to stretch leg, but does not relieve. Arms heavy, too much prostrated to lift them without effort.

Lungs - Smothering sensations, cannot get air enough, from rapid walking. Cough harsh, dry, spasmodic, horribly distressing. Cough from fullness of chest better by nosebleed. Hemoptysis, blood bright red.

Modalities - Better from bleeding, profuse urination, vinegar application. Worse rainy, changeable weather, approach of storm. Worse motion, walking, 4 p.m., menopause.

Nose - ***Profuse and frequent nosebleeds***, bright red blood with general relief. Nosebleed with high fever and violent congestion of head and face. Stopped up, ***dry***, must breathe through mouth. Excessive dryness of nose, obstructed. Dry, hard clinkers in nose.

Rectum - Difficult, painful, constipated. Severe shooting cutting in rectum while walking, better sitting down. Anus feels constricted, full, throbs. No desire until there is a large accumulation (Bry., Alum.). Very difficult, painful stool with constriction in rectum. ***Discharge of stringy, glassy, milk-white mucus.*** Heavy throbbing and fullness in rectum from internal hemorrhoids.

Skin - Dry skin. Tendency to bruise and bleed easily.

Sleep - Drowsy, sleepy, stupid. Alternate sleep and wakefulness through night. Awakes regularly a few minutes before 3 a.m. Insomnia, cannot sleep after 3 a.m. Head seemed too high (although he had no pillow). Sleep prevented by unpleasant thoughts coursing through brain. Unpleasant dreams, of bickering.

Stomach - Gastric discomfort, flatulence, fullness and other symptoms appear when constipated. Acid belchings all day, causing burning and smarting.

Temperature - Chilly 10 a.m., begins in back, loins or occiput, passing in waves up to vertex. Chilly 12 p.m. to 1 p.m. with sharp pains in cardiac region of stomach and much flatulence. Chilly all forenoon. Uncomfortably chilly, feet and hands colds.

Throat - Throat sore, left side, swallowing difficult, painful. Tickling in throat with cough.

Vertigo - Vertigo worse on moving.

COMMENTS - Characteristic engorgement. Blood engorgement. Tending to hemorrhages, profuse, bright red, which give relief. Intensely red or even purple face attending any disorder.

Headaches with blushing and nosebleed. Headaches better by lying down, profuse urination, application of vinegar. Headaches more often in hot weather, worse after exposure or getting feet wet, on approach of storm, in rainy, changeable weather. Sensation of waving in the brain.

Alternation of pains, from right temple to right knee, pains in head alternating with pains in back. Marked periodicity. Generally better sitting, worse from walking, but pain in sacral region is opposite. Symptoms appear in the forenoon and wear off during the day. Relieved by discharges.

Bowen used Meli. successfully in all kinds of congestive or nervous headaches, nasal and pulmonary hemorrhages, congestion of spinal cord, pleura, lungs, ovaries, menstrual colic, palpitation and nervousness, cramps in stomach, spasms, convulsions and for relieving brain-pressure and irritation in insanity. He always gave it in pellets medicated with the 1c dilution.

In different cases, Bowen removed symptoms including a desire to run away, to hide, insists that everyone is looking at them. Mania to escape and kill himself, with insomnia. Nervous and timid. Dares not talk loudly, whispers. Vicious, threatens to kill those who approach. Thinks there is a devil in his stomach contradicting all he says.

H. C. Allen relieved with Meli. a fear of danger, fear of being arrested in mental cases.

In a schoolboy, Clarke cured with Meli. 30c a very distressing recurrent headache, accompanied by an intensely red face while the pain was on and with the same potency. Clarke gave great relief in a case of melancholia in a young woman.

C. F. Barker recorded the case of Miss X, 19, tall, blonde, for several years had severe, nervous and congestive headaches. The attacks recurred two to four times a month and were so severe that they compelled her to keep to her bed twenty-four hours.

The pain, mostly in temples and forehead, was a congested, full sensation with flushed face, drowsy, stupid feeling and sometimes much nausea.

Trivial things seemed to provoke the attacks. Spectacles had been supplied by oculists and teeth freshly stopped by dentists, diet, rest from study and outdoor exercise had all failed to relieve. Meli. 4x was given and she had only two attacks in six months and those very slight.

A writer in Hom. News tells of a Frenchman who came to him complaining of an incessant headache so bad that he thought he would die. A dose of Meli. was given on the spot and the doctor, thinking Nux-v. indicated, went into the next room to get it.

He returned in five minutes and found the patient on his hands and knees shaking his head. The doctor, thinking him crazy, asked what he was doing. He replied that the pain was entirely gone and he was only trying various attitudes and motions to make sure.

RELATIONS - ***Compare:*** (1) Meli-a., the white clover - has practically the same action. Hemorrhages, congestive headaches, engorged blood vessels. (2) spasms: Bell., Amyl, Glon. and Sang. in congestive headaches (but Bell. has worse lying down and worse from application of vinegar cloths). (3) In nosebleed after headache, Ant-c. (but with Ant-c. the nosebleed does not necessarily relieve). (4) Waving in brain, Cimic. (5) Rheumatic pains better moving, Rhus-t. (6) Hemoptysis, bright blood, Ip., Mill. (7) Discomfort from constipation, Op. (8) Congested head and nosebleed, Erig. (9) Red face with throbbing carotids, Bell. (10) Trif-r.

REFERENCES - Allen. Boericke. Bowen. Clarke. Phatak.

MELISSA OFFICINALIS

(Lemon Balm)

PHARMACY - melis. Melissa officinalis. Lemon balm. Bee balm. Sweet balm. N. O. Labiatae. North Africa. Europe. Tincture from fresh leaves picked just before flowering. ***Historical dose:*** Tincture and all potencies.

CLINICAL - Colds. Depression. Headaches. Herpes. Indigestion. Influenza. Insomnia. Nerves.

HERBAL - Avicenna recommended Melissa as a heart tonic, to make the heart merry and to lift the spirit. The volatile oil has a sedative effects in small doses that is soothing to the nerves. Melissa oil is has been used in aromatherapy for anxiety, nervousness, depression, insomnia and tension headaches. Infusions of lemon balm after meals eases the digestion.

Melissa oil helps with all kinds of allergies. Cold sores and herpes. Hot infusions have been used for treating colds and flus by inducing sweating. Depression, headaches and indigestion. Headaches and restlessness.

REFERENCES - Potter.

MELITAGRINUM

(Eczema Capitis Nosode)

PHARMACY - melit. Melitagrinum. Nosode of eczema capitis. ***Historical dose:*** All potencies.

CLINICAL - Crusta lactea. Eczema capitis.

HOMEOPATHIC - Dr. Skinner gave a brief account of this nosode introduced by him in Hom. World, xvii. 89. He prepared fluxional centesimal potencies from the lymph and blood of a case of eczema capitis.

Dr. Theobald treated cases with Melit. Very severe cases were cured with Melit. 100,000c potency, given in single doses at considerable intervals. In one case, there was an initial aggravation.

REFERENCES - Clarke.

MENISPERMUM CANADENSE

(Moonseed)

PHARMACY - menis. Menispermum canadense. Moonseed. Yellow parilla. N. O. Menispermacae. Tincture of root. Trituration of Menisperminum. ***Historical dose:*** Tincture, trituration and all potencies.

CLINICAL - Backache. Dryness. ***Headaches.*** Itching. Spine, pain. Tongue, swelling.

HOMEOPATHIC - Menis. is botanically related to Cocc. and the backache recalls the spinal action of the latter, but the Cocc. vertigo and intoxication were not elicited. Very considerable doses were taken in the proving of Menis.

The most notable symptom was an intense headache combined with aching all down the back. Megrim, associated with restlessness and dreams. Yawning and stretching were also a marked and frequent concomitant of headache and backache.

Dryness, itching all over (Cocc.). Dry mouth and throat. Pain in spine. Legs sore as if bruised with pain in bones. The pains were like those caused by large doses of quinine and were better by Chin. Restless, troubled and confused dreams, sudden starting from sleep.

MIND - Laziness, absent minded. Low-spirited, but attends to business rapidly. Quick-tempered.

Abdomen - Pain in umbilical region.

Back - Pain in whole length of back, with intense headache, yawning and stretching.

Eyes - Eyes feel dry and swollen during the night.

Face - Face hot. Pimples on face, bleed easily.

Head - ***Headaches.*** Sick headache, pain in forehead and temples, moving to occiput. ***Pressure from within outward, with stretching, yawning*** and pain down back.

Kidneys - Urine is high-colored and scanty, yellow, white thready clouds floating through.

Limbs - Pain in back, thighs, elbows, shoulders. Legs sore, as if bruised. Aching in thighs, elbows and shoulders in external muscles of thigh and upper arm, also under left scapula.

Lungs - Hurried respiration during the night. Morning expectoration less and of lighter color.

Modalities - Better walking in open air. Worse at night, warmth of bed.

Mouth - Tongue coated yellow, thicker at back with raised papilla, dry and parched, swollen, as if burnt. Much saliva. Mouth and throat dry during night.

Nose - Much sneezing. Discharge of nasal mucus, excoriating. Nostrils dry, especially the left, itch painfully, are sore.

Rectum - Tenesmus with regular stool.

Skin - Chilly. Skin cold and dry with some itching. Itching all over body, especially buttocks, worse warmth of bed.

Sleep - Yawning and stretching with backache and headache. Starting from sleep. Dreams of innumerable rats which creep under clothes, of cannonading. Sleeps late and heavy in morning, disinclined to rise.

Stomach - Appetite and thirst increased. Some nausea on waking.

Throat - Throat dry and parched without soreness.

RELATIONS - ***Antidoted by:*** Bry., Chin. ***Compare:*** (1) Cocc., Bry.

REFERENCES - Boericke. Clarke.

MENTHA PIPERITA

(Peppermint)

PHARMACY - menth. Mentha piperita. Peppermint. N. O. Labiate. Brandy mint. Curled mint. Balm mint. Tincture of whole plant. Dilutions of the essence. Essential oil. ***Historical dose:*** Tincture and all potencies.

CLINICAL - Aphonia. ***Colds. Coughs.*** Dyspepsia. ***Flatulence***. Headaches. Hoarseness. ***Indigestion. Influenza.*** Itching. ***Stomach, pains.*** Throat, sore. ***Voice, weakness.***

HERBAL - Demeures gave it to singers a short time before singing and it greatly helped them to hold the voice.

HOMEOPATHIC - A remarkable proving of Menth. was made by Demeures, who took a single drop of the tincture, the effects of which lasted into the third month. After the proving, Demeures found that he could rise earlier than usual and yet feel bright and fresh, whereas before it he could not.

Marked action on respiratory organs and skin. Stimulates the cold perceiving nerves so just after taking it a current of air at the ordinary temperature seems cold. Herpes zoster.

Broncho-tracheal catarrh and diseases of the skin. ***Dry cough,*** excited by air entering larynx, exposure to cold, reading aloud, shocks of any kind. Irritation in the suprasternal fossa. Dry, spasmodic cough which is worse in cold weather, and following the influenza.

Stomach pain, ***flatulence***, flatulent colic and hysteria, with nausea and vomiting. Deranged digestion. Vaginal pruritus.

MIND - Mental dullness, which follows early morning rising. Insensible. Confusion of mind. Eager for work, dispatches it quickly.

Back - Muscles around neck are painful to touch.

Ears - All day when walking, shooting from one ear to the other, as if abscesses were forming, worse left. When writing, sharp lancinations extend from left ear to left teeth.

Eyes - Flashes before eyes when writing.

Head - Headache with tension toward both ears, worse on rising, better returning to bed. Acute lancinations from ear to head, on stooping or turning head. Frontal headache from one temple to the other. Hair ceases to fall out.

Limbs - Sensation under right foot at extremity of metatarsus, as if shoe sole was too tight there.

Lungs - ***Frequent coughs and colds. Dry cough,*** excited by merely speaking, expectoration every morning of thick mucus like the core of a boil. Dry cough continues, not caused by titillation or mucus accumulations in the bronchi, but merely by the passage of air into the larynx. Cough excited from least feeling of cold, reading aloud, and smoke of all kinds.

Modalities - Better lying down in bed, while eating. Worse early rising, cold air, smoke. Worse stooping, turning head, reading aloud, writing.

Mouth - Very severe toothache in lower molars when chewing a bit of sugar.

Nose - Tip of nose sore to touch, swollen but not painful.

Skin - Every scratch becomes a sore. Pimples with much itching near left ear with heat in part. Frequent itching behind right ear. Formication in arm and hand when writing.

Sleep - Sleep good, refreshing. Waking early.

Stomach - Indigestion. In evening, two hours after dinner, weight in stomach which seems to extend to ears.

Throat - Entire trachea from larynx to pit of throat painful to touch. Throat dry and painful on swallowing, as if a pin stuck crosswise in pharynx. Momentary lancinations in parotids, better during breakfast and dinner. Throat externally painfully sensitive to touch. Husky voice from reading aloud.

COMMENTS - A case of fatal poisoning with the essence is on record. The patient, a boy of six took between 1 and 2 ounces and died in two hours. When seen, he was insensible, eyes fixed, pupils were fixed, stertorous breathing, cold skin and the lips were livid.

Demeures said he cured with Menth. every case of influenza that came under his care in the winter of 1847-8. "It is to dry cough, however caused, what Arn. is to injuries and Acon. to inflammatory complaints. It relieves even the cough of tuberculosis patients." A single globule of the 30c sufficed.

Gibson Miller related the case of a teacher, 43, who had a dry, spasmodic cough, worse in cold weather since whooping cough in boyhood. The inhalation of the smallest quantity of smoke, either of coal, wood or tobacco, at once induced a most distressing paroxysm.

Worse by the least breath of air or any fog. Scarcely any expectoration. Husky on attempting to sing.

Menth. 30c completely removed the cough and enabled him to sit in a room full of tobacco smoke and sing with clearness.

Hansen commended it in bilious colic with great accumulation of gas, severe pain of shingles and as an external remedy in itching of the vagina.

RELATIONS - ***Compare:*** (1) The labiates. (2) worse from smoke, Ign. (3) worse fog, Hyper. (4) worse rising, better lying down, Bry. (5) worse from cold air, Rumx.

REFERENCES - Boericke. Clarke.

MENTHA PULEGIUM

(English Pennyroyal)

PHARMACY - menth-pu. Mentha pulegium. English pennyroyal. European pennyroyal. N. O. Labiate. Tincture of plant. ***Historical dose:*** Tincture and all potencies.

CLINICAL - Faintness. Headaches. Itching. Rheumatic, pains. Salivation, nocturnal.

HERBAL - Pennyroyal is a common herbal remedy used for menstrual disorders. It is a popular herb for the uterus and acts painlessly and without much irritation or forcing down. Cooper noted that it often causes faintness.

HOMEOPATHIC - Berridge's provings with the 40th potency were all made on men, so its properties in the female sexual sphere remain untested. His proving brought out an affinity for the right side of the head, right eye and left kidney, shoulder and hand.

Jerkings of whole body directly after waking. Rheumatic pains flying about, chiefly on the right side. Sensation as of blood circulating quicker than usual. The symptoms were all worse when thinking of them.

Abdomen - Severe cutting pains in left groin and side while sitting. Sharp pains in the right hypochondrium, sometimes in middle of sternal region.

Back - Bruised, stiff feeling in small spot, upper part of right scapula with aching and empty feeling in right side of head. Sharp, cutting pains in region of left kidney, shooting up left side to left chest, better getting up.

Chest - Woke on right side and as soon as he had turned to left, sharp cutting pain in right chest for two minutes.

Female - Popular for the uterus, acts painlessly and without much irritation or forcing down.

Head - Aching in bones of forehead and sides of head, worse right after sunset. Headache in right forehead, forcing tears from right eye. Headache in right temple with pressing behind eyes, first right then both, worse towards evening and in night. Empty feeling in right side of head. Itching all around base of skull and roots of hair.

Limbs - Pinching pain in bones of legs and arms, chiefly right, better by a night's rest. Two sudden successive jerks upward of left shoulder and upper arm while lying on left side. Unable to hold a jug with left hand when pouring out water, hand trembles.

Mouth - Flow of saliva from left (side lain on) corner of mouth in night, waking him.

Sleep - Veins swollen at night, troublesome dreams.

Temperature - General creeping chilliness over back and half-way down front of left thigh.

Throat - Stitches down left eustachian tube into left side of throat, better pressing under left ear.

Vertigo - Faintness.

RELATIONS - ***Compare:*** (1) Hedeo., Menth. (2) In worse by thinking of symptoms, Pip-m., Ox-ac.

REFERENCES - Clarke.

MENTHA VIRIDIS

(Spearmint)

PHARMACY - menth-v. Mentha viridis. Spearmint. N. O. Labiate. Mackerel mint. Mentha spicata. Mentha crispa. Peamint. Yerba buena. Mint. Tincture of whole plant. Dilutions of the essence. Essential oil. ***Historical dose:*** Tincture and all potencies.

HERBAL - Spearmint is a simple but efficient diuretic and febrifuge. Stimulant, carminative, antispasmodic. Cases when the urine is scanty and there is a frequent desire to urinate. Use the infusion freely. This herb is added to many compounds on account of its carminative properties and its pleasant taste.

COMMENTS - Parkinson commended a decoction of spearmint to wash the hands of children when suffering from scabs and blotches.

RELATIONS - ***Compare:*** (1) The labiates. (2) Menth-p., Menth.

REFERENCES - Blackwood. Potter.

MENTHOLUM

(Menthol)

PHARMACY - menthol. Mentholum. Menthol. The stearopten from the essential oil of peppermint. ***Historical dose:*** Tincture and all potencies.

CLINICAL - Aphonia. Asthma. Cardialgia. Catarrh. Colic. Coryza. Coughs. Eustachian catarrh. Headaches. Itching. Laryngitis. Migraine. Neuralgias. Pharyngitis. ***Pruritus, vulvae***. Toothache. Vaginismus.

HERBAL - Menthol is anti-neuralgic, anti-spasmodic, sedative and a local anesthetic. Locally used for facial neuralgia and migraine. Cardialgia. Gastric and intestinal catarrh. Abdominal fermentation occurring in the stomach or intestines. Colicky pains and vomiting. Toothache. Pruritus vulvae. Vaginismus.

HOMEOPATHIC - Menthol. has proved curative in acute nasal catarrh, in acute Eustachian catarrh, pharyngitis, laryngitis and neuralgias. Affects the mucus membrane of the naso-pharynx and spinal nerve plexus. Neurotic pains and paresthesia. Itching, especially ***pruritus vulvae***.

MIND - Mental confusion.

Abdomen - Intestinal catarrh. Abdominal fermentation occurring in the intestines. Colicky pains and vomiting.

Back - Muscular pain in cervical region. Soreness of lumbar muscles.

Chest - Cardialgia. Stabbing pains in the precordia, radiating over entire chest.

Ears - Eustachian tubes feel blocked and some deafness.

Eyes - Pain in eyeballs. Supra orbital pain over left eye.

Face - Neuralgia. Pain in face above zygoma with numbness.

Female - ***Pruritus vulvae***. Vaginismus.

Head - Migraine. Headaches. Frontal headache, pain over frontal sinus, descends to eyeballs.

Lungs - Short, dry cough, worse smoking. Asthmatic breathing with congestive headache.

Mouth - Toothache.

Nose - Coryza with post-nasal dripping. Cold sensation in nose.

Stomach - Gastric catarrh. Fermentation occurring in the stomach. Colicky pains and vomiting.

Throat - Aphonia. Laryngitis. Tickling in the fauces. Pharyngitis.

COMMENTS - Externally for itching, use a 1 percent solution or ointment.

RELATIONS - ***Compare:*** (1) Kali-bi., Spig.

REFERENCES - Boericke.

MENYANTHES TRIFOLIATA

(Buckbean)

PHARMACY - meny. Menyanthes trifoliata. Buckbean. Bitterklee. Bog bean. N. O. Gentianacee. Tincture of whole plant. ***Historical dose:*** Tincture and all potencies.

CLINICAL - Amaurosis. Chest, disorders. Chilly. ***Cold.*** Cramps. Diabetes. Dyspnea. Fidgets. Headache. Heart, pains. Intermittent, fever. Jerkings. Malaria. Paralysis. Tinnitus.

HERBAL - The Buck-bean, or "Bog-bean" as it is also called in Ireland and Lincolnshire, is a water plant and abounds in the fen districts, where it is in great local repute as a remedy for malaria.

HOMEOPATHIC - Hahnemann proved it and well defined its sphere of action. The major features of Meny. are chill, sensations and pains of tension and compression, and spasmodic jerkings and visible twitchings, worse during rest and may be associated with neuralgia.

Tensive and compressive pains. Tension in skin, as if it was several sizes too small and he was crowded into it.

Shooting pains and pinching in limbs and joints, in arthritic disorders.

Jerking pain in outer parts, also pinching pain in outer parts. Spasmodic jerking and visible twitchings with neuralgia. Jumpy, fidgety women with urinary troubles. Diabetes.

Great general debility, on walking often accompanied by shivering. ***Icy coldness of single or affected parts***, nose, ears, fingers, knees, abdomen etc. Intermittent fever, coldness predominates, felt most acutely in abdomen and legs and tip of nose. Certain headaches.

MIND - Hurried. Anxiety and apprehension. Anxiety as if something evil were going to happen. Fear about the heart, driving him from place to place. Buffoonery and excessive gaiety.

Confusion, better open air. Dullness of mind. Indifference to everything, alternating with great joy. Aversion to amusement. Discontented with everything, with self. Dwells on past disagreeable occurrences. Taciturn and self-reflecting. Tearful sadness.

Abdomen - Distended and full, increased by smoking tobacco. Distention of abdomen by abundant flatus. Coldness, worse pressing upon it with hand. Pinchings in abdomen. Pain, as from excoriation in abdominal tissues.

Back - Rigidity and heaviness in muscles of neck, throat and nape. Extremely painful tearing between the scapula, extending downwards. Boring at scapula (left). Bruised pain in sacrum, worse stooping, walking.

Causations - Injuries to nerves (tooth broken in). Quinine.

Chest - Shooting compression on both sides of chest. Stitches in chest, worse during motion and when breathing. Aching in chest after dinner.

Ears - Tinnitus, when chewing. Tinkling in ears. Cracking in ear, when chewing. Shootings in ears. Feeling of coldness in ear. Discharge from ears (after exanthemata).

Eyes - Frequent spasmodic stiffness of eyelids. Pressing in eyes. Mist and flickerings before eyes. Cloudiness of eyes, when reading.

Face - Redness and heat of face during sleep. Heat in face with coldness of feet. Visible twitching of the facial muscles, worse rest. Pain and cracking in the articulation of jaw when chewing.

Food - Ravenous hunger, passing away after eating a little. Troublesome confusion in head after a meal. Desire for meat. Aversion to bread and butter. No thirst at any time.

Head - Bursting headache, pain ascends from nape, better stooping, sitting bent. Heavy, pressing pain in vertex, ***better hard pressure with hand***. Sensation as of weight in nape. Weight pressing on brain with every step on ascending. As if cold wind blowing on it.

Heart - Stitches in region of heart. Slightest exertion causes irregular action. Drawing pain in precordia, worse after eating. Anxiety about, as if some evil was going to happen.

Kidneys - Frequent desire to urinate with scanty urine.

Limbs - Cramp-like pains in limbs. Cramps in posterior thighs worse sitting. Cramps from ankles to calf (right). ***Legs jerk and twitch,*** worse lying down. Shocks and convulsive movements in thighs. Paralytic tearing and spasmodic drawings in arms, hands and fingers. ***Icy coldness of hands and feet***.

Lungs - Stitch in anterior regions of larynx, impeding swallowing. Dyspnea. Spasmodic contraction of larynx with excitation to cough, when drawing breath.

Male - Increase of sexual desire without excitement or erection. Both testicles drawn up, right more than left. Spermatic cord painful to touch.

Modalities - Better hard pressure on affected part, laying on hand, stooping, motion, twilight. Worse light, noise, during rest, walking, ascending, jar.

Mouth - Sweetish bitterness in mouth. Sensation of paralysis on left side of palate, when yawning and coughing.

Nose - Cold. Tension in root of nose. Nauseous smell before nose like that of rotten eggs.

Perspiration - Perspiration in evening as soon as he lies down, continuing all night.

Rectum - Constipation. Hard feces with pinchings in the abdomen. Bleeding, hemorrhoids.

Skin - Feels tight.

Sleep - Agitated sleep with vivid dreams. Doesn't remembered dreams.

Stomach - Sensation of coldness extending up esophagus with great nausea, following pressure in stomach. Heat in stomach, followed by excessive hunger. Contractive cramps in stomach. Continual rumbling in stomach, as if it were empty. Frequent empty belchings.

Temperature - Predominance of cold. Icy coldness of hands and feet. Shivering with yawning. Chill, which is better by heat of stove and only remains in back. Intermittent fever with coldness in abdomen. Pulse slow during cold stage and accelerated during fever. Heat in evening, mostly on head with cold feet. Quartan malaria.

Throat - Dryness of palate, stinging when swallowing. Dryness and roughness in throat, which impede swallowing of saliva, without thirst. When speaking hoarse and rough voice with obstruction of ears, as if something had been introduced into them.

COMMENTS - Teste, who also proved it, found it very similar to Dros. Both these drugs caused in him, as one of the first symptoms, obscuration of sight, a sort of white mist or vibrations, worse in open air or during a walk. This was so intense that he did not dare to cross a street.

The pains of Dros. and Meny. were the same in character, but those of Dros. were more intense. This analogy has not proved as close in other respects as Teste imagined it would.

"Jumps," "fidgets," and "urinary difficulties in women" are Burnett's leading indications. "

When sitting, the outstretched thigh and leg are four times spasmodically jerked up, but when standing or in drawing up the knees towards him, this is not perceptible."

Twitching in any part. Legs jerk and twitch, cannot rest when lying down. Stitches, numbness, tension. Tension sensation, as if the skin were several sizes too small. Cramp-like and paralyzing pains.

Severe pressure in the head. Pressing in vertex from above downwards, better during hard pressure with the hand, when ascending stairs, as of a heavy weight pressing on the head and brain at every step. Icy coldness of the hands and feet with the headache.

R. Farley reported the case of Miss D. W., long a sufferer from spinal irritation, had terrible attacks of bursting headache, a terrible tension in membranes of brain in paroxysms, which caused her to scream. Began in right side of nape, ascended to forehead and then spread over whole brain.

Terrible sensation of loneliness with the pain, begged her mother to stay with her. Worse from light, noise, jar, even if one walked lightly across the room. Better from sitting bent and by hard pressure on nape and vertex. Meny. 30c every ten minutes relieved immediately and completely removed everything in two hours.

RELATIONS - ***Antidoted by:*** Camph. ***It antidotes:*** Effects of quinine and Chin. ***Compare:*** (1) Caps., Puls., Calc., Ph-ac., Sang. (2) worse ascending, Calc. (3) Headache better hard pressure, Verat. (4) Weight on vertex at every step, Cact., Glon., Lach. (5) Intermittent fever with cold limbs, Lach. (but Lach. has livid skin, great prostration and filiform pulse). (6) Icy cold feet and legs, Calc., Gels. (7) Bursting headache pushing skull open, Sil. (Sil. better warmth, Meny. better pressure). (8) Pressive headache, Puls., Par., Mag-m. (9) Fidgets, Psor., Caust., Zinc. (10) the gentians. ***Compatible after:*** Cupr., Lach., Lyc., Puls., Rhus-t., Verat.

REFERENCES - Boericke. Clarke. Phatak.

MEPHITIS PUTORIUS

(Skunk Secretion)

PHARMACY - meph. Mephitis putorius. Skunk secretion. Mephitis mephitica. Mustela foetida. Mustelina. N. O. Mustelide. Alcoholic dilution of the liquid contained in the anal glands. ***Historical dose:*** Tincture and all potencies.

CLINICAL - Asthma. Blindness. ***Choking.*** Coldness. Convulsions. ***Coughs.*** Debility. Exhaustion. Eyes, disorders. Laryngismus. Otalgia. Rheumatic, pains. Spasms. Trembling. Vertigo. Vision, weak. ***Whooping cough.***

HOMEOPATHIC - The dilutions of this medicine are prepared from the liquid contained in the anal glands of skunk. Meph. was proved by Hering in the 30c. Should be given in the lower dilutions.

Meph. produced a suffocative feeling and spasmodic cough. Cough so violent, seems as if each spell would terminate life. ***Whooping cough.*** Child must be raised up, gets blue in face, cannot exhale. Mucus rales through upper part of chest. Asthmatic attacks.

Spasmodic effects. Trembling and choking with exophthalmos. Convulsions. Sensation of paralysis during the pains. Rheumatic pains. Shifting pains with want to urinate. Fine vibrations causing great uneasiness. Internal agitation of whole body with sensation of uneasiness.

Nervous exhaustion. Debility after severe illness. Great dejection and lassitude during which the muscles are painful when touched or exercised. Indolence with desire to stretch and stretching. Wants to bathe in ice cold water.

MIND - Excitement with heat in head. Talkative. Can neither sleep nor work. Unfit for intellectual labor, caused by too lively an imagination. Full of fancies. Excessive loquacity, as from drinking too much. Disinclination to work with inclination to stretch. Dejection with painful muscles. Ill-humor about trifles or imaginary troubles.

Abdomen - Pains in hypochondria. Aching and movements in abdomen, as if caused by a chill. Pains in abdomen in evening. Pains as from flatulency in left side. Aching in region of liver in with colic. Colic, as from diarrhea, but without evacuation.

Back - Pain and a sort of paralysis in back and in all limbs. Lancination in spine during motion. Pains in right side of neck. Tension in muscles of nape. Contusive pains in loins in morning.

Chest - Pains in chest when touching it. Chest pains when coughing and sneezing.

Cough - ***Spasmodic coughs or whooping cough.*** Cough, ***violent suffocative, spasmodic, nervous, worse at night,*** talking, loud reading, or drinking. Cough hollow, deep with rawness, hoarseness and pains through chest. Whooping or any kind of cough which is very violent, coming on spasmodically, and seeming as if each spell would terminate life. ***Cough with vomiting after eating.*** Loose cough, in morning, with some expectoration.

Ears - Otalgia. Itching heat, redness, blisters and erysipelas in the external part of the (right) ear. Tearing in the ears or in the jaw and teeth.

Eyes - Heat, burning and aching in eyes, morning and evening. As if fire in eyes. Conjunctiva red, eyes hot and painful. Injection of veins in sclerotica. Lancination in eyes like the pricking of needles. Pain from overexertion, blur, unable to distinguish letters. Inability to read fine print. Myopia. Nocturnal blindness.

Face - Bloated. Child gets blue in face and can't exhale with spasmodic cough.

Female - Burning leucorrhea. Excoriation of genital organs and swelling of labia majora. Soreness of genitals. Swelling of labia and uterus.

Food - Hunger, alternating with absence of appetite. Absence of appetite in morning and repugnance to tobacco-smoke. Painful weariness and desire to sleep after a meal. Desire for salted food.

Head - Violent pain in head as if a fullness were pressing upwards. Violent headache with sensation of fullness, as if caused by a weight or by pressure, especially in the occiput. Pain above eyes. Headache from motion of carriage.

Kidneys - Frequent want to make water, especially at night, with emission of clear urine. The urine becomes turbid in morning, and deposits a sediment in evening after an attack of fever.

Limbs - Drawing and rheumatic pains in thighs, hip and foot, but chiefly in leg. Contusive pains in knee. Rheumatic pains in arms with paralytic drawings, better by movement. Uneasiness in arm, as it were insensible. Trembling in arm on resting upon it. Jerking in hand.

Lungs - Dyspnea and cannot exhale. ***False croup and cannot exhale.*** Sudden contraction of glottis, when drinking or talking. Asthma, as if inhaling sulphur. Asthma, has to sit up in bed, worse ice water. Asthma of consumptives or alcoholics. Foul expectoration.

Male - Itching in scrotum. Heat in genital organs.

Modalities - Better from cold, icy, weather. Better bathing, sitting up, motion. Worse night, daybreak, morning, lying down , rest, touch, after menses, ice water.

Mouth - Metallic, coppery taste, as after eating onions. Foul breath. Painful jerks in root of teeth. Bloated face.

Nose - Dryness of the nose. Nosebleeds. Fluent coryza with pain, as from excoriation in the chest. Prolonged inclination to sneeze.

Rectum - Evacuations infrequent, but liquid. Diarrhea.

Skin - Pimples on thighs, forehead, face, neck and nates.

Sleep - Short nap, seems to refresh. Awakes at night with rush of blood to lower legs. Vivid dream of water, fire.

Stomach - Pressure in stomach, with colic. Belchings, better by discharge of flatus. Sensation of emptiness in stomach and nausea. Vomits food hours after eating.

Teeth - Drawing and tearing in teeth. Sudden shocks in roots of teeth. Pains in carious teeth, molars, in lower jaw.

Temperature - Coldness predominates. Less chilly in cold air, cold water is agreeable. Evening chilliness with desire to urinate. Increased heat in morning.

Throat - Tendency to choke when drinking and speaking. ***Food goes the wrong way***. Nausea with scraping in throat.

Vertigo - Violent vertigo, worse sitting, turning in bed. Vertigo on stooping suddenly, when moving the head, when seated.

COMMENTS - Rush of warmth to various parts. Enables patients to endure extreme cold, makes them less chilly in cold weather. Washing in ice water is pleasant. Awakens at night with congestion of legs. Legs uneasy, as if they would become insensible. Fidgety feet. Short sleep seems to refresh.

Choking while eating or drinking. Cough on reading aloud, while talking and after drinking, caused by choking. Lower ribs painful to touch or pressure, especially worse on coughing or sneezing.

Neidhard gave Meph. to "a young man affected with symptoms of tuberculosis," in whom it produced "a spasmodic cough with a crowing sound, lasting all night and returning several times."

This homeopathic aggravation suggested to Neidhard to use Meph. in whooping cough and his conclusion, quoted by Hering, notes that "If the facts collected since 1851, which are numerous, do not prove that Meph. will supersede all other remedies in whooping cough, it certainly may be considered a valuable specific. In order to ensure its full success, it should be exhibited in the lower dilutions from one to three, at least in severe cases."

Guernsey gave it as: "Whooping or any other kind of cough which is very violent, coming on spasmodically and seeming as though each spell would terminate life."

Farrington said the note of Meph. is nervous exhaustion. In whooping cough the catarrh is slight, whoop decided, worse at night and after lying down. Suffocative feeling, cannot exhale, vomits food sometimes hours after eating. Asthma of alcoholics of tuberculosis patients (after Dros.).

T. M. Stewart reported the case of a man, 47, who had a constant hacking cough coming on during conversation. For this the uvula was amputated.

When he recovered from the operation he had "Coughs after reading aloud or drinking any fluid, cough spasmodic, hollow, hoarse, worse at night and on lying down, loose in mornings." Amb., Cham., Kali-bi., Rumx., Phos., failed to relieve, Meph. 1,000c. cured promptly.

A. M. Cushing called attention to the possibilities of the remedy in weak sight and told of a friend of his who had a dose directly from the skunk injected into his eyes "It was as though fire had entered his eyes." For a time he was totally blind, but when his sight returned it was so keen that he could count the panes in a window said to be two miles distant.

In another case after getting the poison out of the eye, there was for weeks after a sensation on opening the lids as of breaking glass. On Farrington's advice it was antidoted by Crot-h.

RELATIONS - ***Antidoted by:*** Camph., but only temporarily. Crot-h. relieved eye symptoms. ***Compare:*** (1) Dros., Cor-r., Stict. (2) Whooping cough, Cor-r. has smothering before the cough and great exhaustion after. (3) Dros. has frequent spells of barking cough, worse after twelve midnight, holds sides, vomits if cannot raise sputa. (4) Cough worse from reading or writing, Aur., Nux-v., Plat. (5) Rumx. - cough at night, worse 2 a.m., Stict. with splitting headache. Aur. - awakes at night with congestion to legs. (6) Short sleep seems to refresh, Fl-ac., Menth. (7) Night blindness, Bell. (8) Aversion to tobacco smoke, Ign. (9) Easy choking, Lach. (10) Fidgety feet, Tarent., Meny., Zinc., Caust., Ars., Asaf., Asar., Cimic., Aur. (11) Loquacity, Agar., Lach. (12) Nervous symptoms generally, Cast-eq., Mosch. ***Follows well:*** Dros. (in cough of tuberculosis patients).

REFERENCES - Boericke. Clarke. Phatak.

MERCURIALIS PERENNIS

(Dog Mercury)

PHARMACY - merl. Mercurialis perennis. Dog mercury. N. O. Euphorbiacae. Tincture of whole fresh plant in flower. ***Historical dose:*** Tincture and all potencies.

CLINICAL - Amblyopia. Amenorrhea. Asthenopia. Belching. Breast disorders. Colic. Coma. Conjunctivitis. Diarrhea. Dysmenorrhea. Epiphora. Flatulence. Menses, late. Numbness. Palpitations. Pannus. Ptosis. Rheumatic disorders. Spleen disorders. ***Tension***. Tongue, paralysis. Trachoma. ***Vertigo.***

HERBAL - Dog's mercury is a common plant with poisonous properties, on account of which it is avoided by cattle.

HOMEOPATHIC - Merl. was proved by Hesse. Like other Euphorbians it has exceedingly acrid properties and many of its symptoms resemble closely those of the more corrosive salts of mercury.

Merl. has disorders of the muscular tissues, stomach, intestines, and bladder. Great exhaustion and drowsiness. Feeling of emptiness and weariness in the whole body. Persistent pains in muscles on motion. Prevalence of burning symptoms, irritation of eyes and nose, tenesmus after stool. Tumor at ensiform appendix, very sensitive.

Tension. Pain as if a band tied tightly across the forehead. Dragging, especially dragging down in small of back with rectal pains in groins and thigh as if a hernia might appear. Amenorrhea. Scanty and delayed menses. Dysmenorrhea, accompanied with orgasm, pains and swelling of breasts.

MIND - Hurry in movements. Excited mood like intoxication. Morose, quarrelsome. Fretful, ill-humored. Fear of insanity. Indifference to everything. Indifference to external things. Difficulty in collecting his senses. Coma.

Abdomen - Abdominal pulsation. Violent twanging in left hypochondrium. Warmth, gnawing, and pressure in spleen, worse lying down. Gnawing from pit of stomach to gallbladder. Rumbling, movings and workings in abdomen, emission of much flatus.

Back - Flushes of heat in back. Aching in nape. Drawing tearing along right scapula, extending into upper arm. Tensive dragging and dragging tearing in small of back, with anal symptoms.

Causations - Blow on the head.

Chest - Sticking in left, throbbing in right chest. Pressure and painfulness on chest in forepart and in stomach with dyspnea.

Eyes - Pain, burning, forcing-out sensation in eyes. Watery eyes. Dilated pupils with great sensitiveness of eyes to light. Asthenopia, as of a cloud, veil or cobweb before sight. Eyelids feel heavy and dry, difficult to move them. Weakness of upper lids. Trembling and twitching of upper lids. Blinking of eyes.

Face - Feeling of coldness, tension in face and head. Great redness of cheeks. Lips dry and parched with increased thirst.

Female - Amenorrhea. Menses scanty and delayed. Menses shorter with abdominal cramp too late. Menses profuse, violent orgasm of blood, great anxiety so that she nearly fainted, oppressed breathing, heat over whole body, especially head and face, anxious sweat. Dysmenorrhea, accompanied with orgasm, pains and swelling of breasts.

Food - Increased thirst with dry lips and mouth. Great dryness in mouth while eating. After eating, biting, burning on tongue, nausea, vomiting.

Head - Head confused as if inflated. Tension and heaviness of head with sensation of heat. Burning on vertex. Aching in forehead better by cold and pressure. Shooting in left forehead and temple, worse coming indoors. Numbness of occiput and vertex after a blow on head. Scalp feels tense and numb, is moved with difficulty.

Heart - Orgasm in the heart region. Constriction. Whirling and rushing, throbbing in heart, stomach and upper abdomen. Palpitations with oppression, as if chest would be constricted after stooping.

Kidneys - Burning, prickling, crawling in urethra and prepuce, with crawling in anus and tearing and dragging in small of back. Frequent urging with burning, urination somewhat increased.

Limbs - Tired and weary. Weakness of arms and legs as if she would fall to left without vertigo. Tearing, stitching, burning and smarting pains in limbs, almost in the skin, especially of hands and feet. Jerking, sticking, drawing tearings throughout upper limbs. Pressive tearing pain in tibia. Jerking tearing in left patella. Painful ache in knees.

Liver - Pressure in liver region extending to spleen. Sticking pain in liver.

Lungs - Breath hot, almost burning, lips almost made sore by it. stertorous, difficult breathing, especially right side.

Male - Dragging in inguinal region, at times sticking pain, worse walking, at times extending down into spermatic cord, sometimes one, sometimes both.

Modalities - Better by cold. Touch aggravates. Headache worse indoors. Sunlight aggravates the eyes. Open air causes blinking.

Mouth - Dryness of mouth, difficult to move tongue, impedes chewing. Burning in mouth and tongue.

Nose - Crawling and burning of nose. Sensation of heat rising from stomach into nose. The breath from nose is cold. Conscious of having a nose, nostrils feel sore. Feels as if she had two noses.

Rectum - Dragging, pressing in rectum, with pressure and tension in small of back. Dragging, burning, crawling, itching, smarting in anus. Diarrhea with constant colic. Thin stools. Profuse, soft stool followed by some straining.

Sensations - Heaviness in head as if pressed on pillow with a weight.

Skin - Pimples on chin with biting, itching. Burning, itching, tearing on skin.

Sleep - Frequent yawning and weariness. Dizzy sleepiness. Sleep unrefreshing, full of dreams, of animals.

Stomach - Chilly feeling or burning in stomach. Belching relieves. Vomits food as soon as eaten. Tumor inside pit of stomach size of hen's egg, worse pressure, cannot bear clothing.

Temperature - Cold over the whole body with hot flush in face. Goosebumps on the cold right arm, extending over whole body. Chill on going to bed in evening. Heat with intense thirst, perspiration in morning.

Throat - Burning dryness in throat. Ulcers on palate, tonsils and back of pharynx.

Tongue - Tongue feels heavy and dry, numb, insensible, with loss of taste. Burning blisters on tongue, inside of lips and cheeks, forming very painful spreading ulcers. Tongue painful if it touches palate as if there were blisters on it.

Vertigo - Giddiness. ***Vertigo by going downstairs.*** Whirling vertigo. Vertigo as if intoxicated, following headache. Feeling as if body would fall towards left side, when sitting, standing or even lying.

COMMENTS - Cooper said, "Compared with other Euphorbians, it dries up the mucus surfaces, causing burning locally and a general drowsiness, while the other Euphorbians set up violent irritation and diarrhea from the first. Moreover, its action is not expended on the skin so soon as that of the others."

Remarkable dryness of the mouth and throat, even sugar refuses to melt in the mouth. Eating aggravates the dryness. The breath from the mouth is hot and dries the lips. Hot or cold breath in the nose. Conscious of having a nose, "she feels as if she has two noses."

Head confused as if inflated. Numbness of head and dullness of mind. Vertigo as if intoxicated. Vertigo by going downstairs. Rolling, throbbing, trembling and orgasm in all the veins. The liver and spleen are influenced, warmth in spleen. Tension in rectum and back.

RELATIONS - ***Antidoted by:*** Acon., Bell. ***Compare:*** (1) Euph., Croto-t., Acal. (2) In worse descending stairs, Bor. (3) Straining after stool, Merc. (4) Dragging pains, Lil-t. (5) Numbness of head, Graph. (feels like wood). (6) Asaf., Caust., Kali-bi., Kreos., Lach., Led., Mag-m., Nat-m., Nat-ac., Nux-v., Nux-m., Rhod., Sulph., Thuj.

REFERENCES - Clarke.

MERCURIUS ACETICUS

(Mercury Acetate)

PHARMACY - merc-acet. Mercurius aceticus. Mercury acetate. Subacetate of Mercury. Trituration. ***Historical dose:*** All potencies.

CLINICAL - Chancre. Eyes, disorders. Dyspnea. Dysuria. Favus. Sternum, pressure. Syphilitic ulcer. Throat, sore. Tinea favosa. Ulcers.

HOMEOPATHIC - Hahnemann made a separate proving of Merc-a. which has furnished a few symptoms, not greatly differing from those of Merc. Hahnemann noted a symptom referring to the menses which came on at the new moon, four days before their proper time. The medicines whose action is influenced by the moon's phases are not numerous and thus worth remembering.

Congestion with stiffness, dryness and heat of parts affected. Lack of moisture. Throat dry, talking difficult. Throat lancinations, worse by coughing rather than by swallowing. Eyes inflamed, burn and itch.

Tinea capitis favosa, margin of ulcers painful. Chancre in urethra. Inflammation of the penis, worse cold water, better bathing with tepid water. Pressure in lower sternum and dyspnea on standing erect.

COMMENTS - Hansen said that burning in the urethra during urination and at other times has been confirmed in practice. He commended it in tinea favosa on a syphilitic base and for sharp pains in tabes syphilitica.

Donner of Stuttgart cured with Merc-a. a very painful syphilitic ulcer in the urethra.

RELATIONS - ***Compare:*** (1) Merc., Luna.

REFERENCES - Clarke. Hansen.

MERCURIUS CORROSIVUS

(Corrosive Sublimate)

PHARMACY - merc-c. Mercurius corrosivus. Corrosive sublimate. Mercuric chloride. Mercurius sublimatus. Triturations. Solution. ***Historical dose:*** All potencies.

CLINICAL - ***Albuminuria.*** Aphthae. Appendicitis. ***Bladder, disorders.*** Bones, disorders. Bright's disease. ***Burning, pains.*** Cancrum oris. Chancres. ***Cystitis.*** Delirium. Dermatitis. Diarrhea. ***Dysentery.*** Eczema. Edema. Esophagus, stricture. Eye, disorders. Fevers. ***Gonorrhea.*** Gums, disorders. Intestinal, fever. Intestines, ulcerated. Intussusception. ***Iritis.*** Jaundice. ***Kidney, disorders.*** Labor, pains. Leucorrhea. Measles. Miscarriage. Mouth, disorders. Mumps. ***Nephritis.*** Neuralgias. Paralysis. Paraphimosis. Pemphigus. Perimetritis. Peritonitis. Phagedenic, ulcers. Photophobia. Prosopalgia. Puerperal, fever. Pyorrhea. Retinitis. Rigg's disease. Syphilis. Tabes, mesenterica. Taste, disordered. ***Tenesmus.*** Throat, inflamed. Tongue, disorders. ***Ulcers. Urethritis.*** Uvula, elongated.

HOMEOPATHIC - Merc-c. is a powerful disinfectant and has a greater rapidity of action than Merc., causing violent effects. The chief effect of the chlorine element in this salt appears to be to intensify the mercurial action. The burning of Merc-c. is more intense than other mercury salts.

Inflammation with swelling and feelings of constriction. Internal burning in the throat, stomach rectum, neck of bladder and kidneys. Constriction of throat, rectum, bladder. ***Severe painful cystitis.*** Bright's disease. ***Albuminuria*** in early pregnancy, (Phos.). Destroys the secreting portions of the kidneys.

Dysentery. Severe ***tenesmus of the rectum,*** which is incessant and is not relieved by the stool. Tenesmus often involves the bladder as well. Dysenteric straining is excessive, for this reason Merc-c. is more generally prescribed in dysentery than Merc.

Syphilis. Gonorrhea, in the second stage with continuous tenesmus. Phagedenic ulcers. Chancres spread with great rapidity. Discharges acrid, tears, nasal discharge. Cracks on palms, soles, corners of mouth. Tibial pains. Lies on back with knees drawn up.

MIND - ***Restlessness at night.*** Anxious and restless, rocks back and forth. Anxiety during fever. ***Anxiety during sleep after menses.*** Fear arising from heart. Fear of misfortune. Anguish with pain in abdomen. Ill-humor. ***Irritability in daytime.***

Absent-mindedness. Confusion of mind. Difficult thinking. Disturbed speech. Wandering thoughts while talking. Stupid. Imbecility. ***Mind sluggish with torpid digestion.***

Coma vigil. Stupor. Stares at persons who talk to him and does not understand them. Delirium, springs up suddenly from bed and escapes. Shouting, brain cry.

Abdomen - Bloated, very painful to least touch. Bruised sensation, cecal region and transverse colon painful. Stitches in hepatic region. Pain in liver and right shoulder with frequent nausea and obstinate chronic constipation. Cutting colic, below navel. Painful flatulence. Appendicitis.

Back - Pott's disease, lies on back with knees drawn up. Cervical glands hard and swollen. Dorsal decubitus.

Bladder - ***Severe, painful cystitis. Tenesmus of bladder***. Intense burning in urethra. Stabbing pain up urethra into bladder. ***Urethritis.*** Burning and painful urination. Dribbling of urine, worse sitting. ***Albuminuria, during pregnancy,*** from abuse of alcohol. Urethra bleeds after urinating.

Breasts - Glandular swellings about the nipples. Nipples crack and bleed, pain worse when nursing.

Chest - Constriction of the chest. Stitches through side of chest. Frequent stitches shoot through thorax. All glands about thorax swollen.

Ears - Violent pulsation in ears. Stitches in ears with inflammation. Fetid pus.

Eyes - ***Burning, soreness of eyes.*** Pain severe at night, burning, shooting, tearing. Pain behind eyeballs, as if forced out. ***Iritis*** normal or syphilitic. ***Iris muddy in color, thick and neither contracts nor dilates***. Retinitis, albuminuria. Deep ulcers on cornea. ***Acrid lachrymation***. Ophthalmia neonatorum. Excessive photophobia. Objects appear smaller or double vision. ***Eyelids edematous*** red, excoriated.

Face - Red, puffy. Edematous swelling of the face. Yellow face. Face pale and anxious. Pale about mouth. Cracks in angles of the mouth. Lips, black, dark red, swollen, tender. Upper lip swollen and turned up. Jaws stiff. Necrosis of lower jaw. Darting pains along upper jaw, gums and roots of teeth. Swelling and tenderness of submaxillary glands. Facial neuralgia within the bones.

Female - Menses too early and too profuse. Burning heat and pain in genitals. ***Vaginitis. Urethritis.*** Mucus discharge as thin as water. Leucorrhea, pale yellow with sweetish nauseous smell. Fibroid tumors with profuse, muco-purulent, excoriating leucorrhea. Aching pain succeeding pressing or touching os uteri during sex.

Food - Attacks of violent hunger or no appetite. Great desire for cold food. Worse fat food. Unquenchable thirst, for cold drinks. Fluids return through nose.

Head - Heaviness of head. Frontal pain, congestion of head with burning in cheeks. Drawing pain in periosteum of skull. Pain in temples, worse looking sideways. Profuse sweat on forehead. Falling out of hair.

Heart - Tremulous undulating motion of heart, precordial anxiety. Pains in precordial region. Pulse rapid and intermittent, small, irregular. Palpitations during sleep.

Kidneys - Nephritis. Bleeding kidneys. Gonorrhea. Paraphimosis. Tenesmus of bladder, rectum. Frequent urine, pale, copious, dribbling, worse sitting. ***Urine hot, burning***, scanty or suppressed. ***Albuminous urine.*** Urine bloody, ***greenish discharge***. Urine brown, with brick dust sediment. Urine contains filaments, flecks or flesh-like pieces of mucus. Urine contains fibrin or fat globules. ***Urine passed drop by drop***. Urethra bleeds after urinating. Sweats after urination.

Limbs - Paralysis of limbs, trembling. Pains wandering from joint to joint, compelling him to stay in bed. Rheumatic pain after suppression of gonorrhea. Coldness in limbs, look purple. Feet icy cold. Cramps in calves in dysentery. Exostoses, on shin, sternum, ribs. As if legs had gone to sleep. Deltoid feels relaxed.

Lungs - Very difficult breathing. Slow, interrupted breathing. Sighing with palpitations. Burning and stinging in trachea. Breathes as through a metallic tube. Breathes through pectoral muscles. Cutting pain in larynx. Cough with bloody expectoration. Greenish mucus, worse at night. Asthmatic coughs, worse talking.

Male - Penis and testes enormously swollen. Chronic balanitis. Paraphimosis. Chordee, worse sleep. Painful stinging in left testicle. Hard, phagedenic chancres. Greasy, fatty, offensive smelling discharge. ***Gonorrhea,*** discharge thick, greenish. ***Urethritis.*** Urethra orifice red, swollen, glans sore and hot. Violent erections during sleep.

Modalities - Better while at rest. Pain in hip joints better from motion. ***Worse after urination and stool***, swallowing, acids, fat food. Worse from sex, motion. Worse night, cold, open air, autumn, hot days and cool nights. Dysentery and summer complaints from May to November.

Mouth - Salivation with salty taste. Metallic taste. Taste, astringent, salty, bitter. Discharge of albuminous mucus from mouth. Burning, scalding sensation in mouth. Aphthae, ulcers. Pyorrhea. Gums, purple, swollen, spongy with toothache. Teeth loose, nightly toothache. Necrosis of lower jaw.

Nose - Swollen, red nose. Rawness, smarting, burning and soreness of nostrils. Postnasal swelling, mucus membrane dry, red and covered with bloody mucus. Gluey nasal discharge. Stopped-up feeling with running of nose. Excessive coryza. Fluent, acrid coryza. Discharge excoriates upper lip. Ozaena with perforation of septum nasi (Kali-bi.). Frequent epistaxis.

Rectum - Violent burning in rectum. Burning in anus during stool. Continuous urging to stool and urine. Dysentery, tenesmus, not better stool. Most extreme tenesmus, with scanty evacuations of mucus and blood. Constipation, tenacious feces. ***Never get done feeling.*** Sweats before and after stool. Hemorrhoidal colic with congestion of liver and abdominal venous stasis. Spasms of rectum during sex.

Perspiration - Perspiration after urinating. Sweats from every motion, partial worse forehead and lower parts, foul, at night. Profuse sweat surfaces cold. Perspiration after urinating. Perspiration before and after stool. Foul sweats. Perspiration at night. Offensive sweats, towards morning. Cold sweats, often only on forehead, also general with anxiety.

Skin - Cold. Burning, stinging heat in skin. Burning and redness of skin with formation of small vesicles. Ulcers, perforating, spreading, serpiginous. Scorbutic spots over whole body, mingled with itch-like eruptions. Herpes and boils. Severe eczema from sweating parts of body. Condylomata. Nails gray colored.

Sleep - Frequent yawning and stretching. Sleepless at night. Starting from sleep. Sleeplessness from vertigo or anxiety. Wakeful after 3 a.m. Violent hiccough during sleep. Disturbed by toothache with anxious sensation. Frightful dreams.

Stomach - Burning gnawing, darting pains in stomach. Cramps in stomach and vomiting after eating rye bread. Cramp in epigastrium, worse least touch. Epigastrium very sensitive. Distention and soreness of the pit of stomach. Gastritis. Regurgitation, astringent. Spasmodic constriction of esophagus and stomach on attempting to swallow a drop of water. Spasmodic and very painful retching. Incessant, green, bilious vomiting. Vomiting of tenacious mucus with blood.

Stools - ***Stools, hot, bloody, slimy offensive,*** with cutting pains and shreds of mucus membranes. Stools yellow, green, bilious. Stools pasty, dark green, blackish, offensive. Oozing of corrosive ichor from anus, excoriating external parts. Passes pure blood or bloody water. Stools followed by slime and blood. Stools worse after midnight, worse autumn.

Teeth - Toothache at night. Teeth loose. Gums red and detached from teeth. Gums purple, swollen with toothache and spongy. Gums bleed easily. Pyorrhea,

Temperature - Chilly from slightest exposure, exertion. Chills when rising. Chilly after stools. Profuse perspiration, surfaces cold. Heat, fever when stooping and coldness when rising. Heat of skin causes great restlessness at night. Fever with anxiety. Fever often temporarily better drinking cold water. External heat with yellow skin.

Throat - ***Burning, sore, red, painful swelling,*** worse heat. Dark red color. Uvula, red, swollen, elongated. ***Tonsils swollen, covered with ulcers.*** Glands about throat swollen. ***Swallowing difficult and painful.*** Spasmodic constriction of glottis, on attempting to swallow a drop of liquid. Pricking in throat as from needles. ***Post-nasal discharge with sharp pains to ears***, worse pressure. Pain in larynx as cut with knife. Hoarseness quickly alternating with normal voice. Aphonia.

Tongue - Tongue coated and moist, with red edges. Tongue, patchy, swollen and inflamed. Papillae elevated, strawberry-like. Tongue very red, with blackish coat. Tongue covered with a grayish white crust. Tongue protruding from swollen lips. Tongue could not be protruded.

Vertigo - Vertigo with deafness when stooping. Vertigo with coldness, cold sweat.

COMMENTS - As with other ulcerating remedies, Merc-c. is a powerful antiseptic and disinfectant. Being much less irritating than carbolic acid, it took the place of the latter as the leading antiseptic. Before the proper degree of dilution had been ascertained many patients were poisoned by its external use.

In some of the poisoning cases, the bladder was found after death firmly contracted into a small hard lump. Keynote intense tenesmus of bladder with intense burning in urethra and discharge of mucus and blood with the urine or after it. Intussusception.

Tenesmus is worse or not relieved after the stool. Tenesmus with dysentery. Diarrhea with a "never-get-done feeling." Membranous threads in stool, blood, weakness, faintness, shuddering. Urine is albuminous, scanty, hot, bloody, may be retained or suppressed.

Gonorrhea. Greenish-yellow or bloody and watery discharge with violent burning, urging and painful erections, dark purplish swelling. Glans has a dark red or gangrenous appearance. Phimosis or paraphimosis.

Rapidly spreading chancres. Serpiginous ulcers, ulcers with ragged edges that will eat away half the penis in a few days. Skin disorders including syphilitic roseola, smallpox and condylomata.

Tibial pains, particularly when present in cases of enteric fever or after enteric fever, with symptoms of intestinal ulceration. Rheumatism and rheumatic fever (Merc.). Raging thirst for cold things. Desire for cold food and intolerance of hot things.

Sore throat characterized by the rapid spread of the infection and by the intensity of the burning pains. Constriction of the gullet, any attempt to swallow solids or liquids causes violent spasms and immediate ejection. Cutting pain, as from a knife in throat.

Thick and glue-like nasal catarrh, acrid excoriating. Tearing pains in bones and around eyes. Scrofulous, syphilitic ophthalmias. Burning, agonizing pains with excessive photophobia, causing excoriation of cheeks.

Clarke learned from Dr. McKechnie that long uvulas sometimes give rise to irritating coughs. If a low trituration of Merc-c. is applied to the uvula on a brush, it will in many cases immediately, and often permanently, relieve the trouble.

A patient of Clarke's who was treated under allopathic treatment with a solution of Merc-c. injected into his urethra for gonorrhea, not only suffered intensely in the urethra at the time, but for years afterwards had a painful spasm of the rectum every time he had sex.

Unna reported two cases of elderly women poisoned by sublimate lotion, lint and gauze after ablation of the breast. The dressings were removed on the second day in each case. The first symptoms were intense irritation of the skin and diffused redness of the part. The wounds failed to heal by first intention.

Widespread dermatitis followed and in the course of a few days a diffuse erythema spread over the whole body, creeping onwards like "water on blotting paper." Some fever, general malaise, nausea, restlessness.

In one case, the eruption lasted three weeks and changed its type, "scattered urticarial and erythematous itching spots on all parts of the body suggested that there was at that period a poisoning of the more central nervous system."

R. C. Markham recorded a cure with Merc-c. after the failure of Merc. in a case of dysentery. The symptoms were stool with bloody mucus, tenesmus after the stool, cutting colic below umbilicus, nausea, and perspiration before and after stool, most pronounced on lower part of body and thigh.

The symptoms of colic and perspiration were not found under Merc., but were under Merc-c. The patient felt better within ten minutes of receiving a dose of Merc-c. 1,000c.

RELATIONS - ***Antidote:*** Calc-s. is antidotal to bichloride poisoning. Use intravenous injection of 7 grains in 7 oz's. boiled water. ***Compare:*** (1) Ars., Lach. (2) Leon., Mons. - an African plant belonging to the Germaniacee used for dysentery in material doses.

REFERENCES - Boericke. Clarke. Murphy. Phatak.

MERCURIUS CYANATUS

(Mercury Cyanide)

PHARMACY - merc-cy. Mercurius cyanatus. Mercury cyanide. Bicyanide of Mercury. Solution. Trituration. ***Historical dose:*** All potencies.

CLINICAL - Albuminuria. Anorexia. Aphthae. Bilious. Coldness. Cyanosis. Diarrhea. ***Diphtheria.*** Dysentery. Edema. Enteric fever. Hoarseness. ***Hemorrhages.*** Keratitis syphilitica. Nausea. Nephritis. Phlebitis. Pneumonia. ***Prostration.*** Salivation. Throat, sore. Twitching. Typhoid. ***Ulcers.*** Varicosis. Vomiting.

HOMEOPATHIC - Merc-cy. is a valuable remedy for toxemia of acute infections, diseases, especially diphtheria, when there is early rapid and extreme prostration with cyanosis, coldness and tremors. Its action is similar to that of toxins in infectious diseases.

Acute infections. Great and rapid prostration. Livid states from great struggling, where suffocation is imminent and paralysis of lung threatening, great sweat. Rapid local destruction. Syphilitic ulcers when a perforation is threatening. Putridity. ***Hemorrhages of dark fluid blood.*** Twitching and jerking of muscles.

Affects most prominently the mouth, throat and larynx. Typhoid pneumonia. Cyanosis, rapid respiration and heart action. ***Malignant diphtheria with prostration.*** Efficient prophylactic in diphtheria. Coldness and nausea. Nephritis. Albuminuria.

MIND - Great excitement, fits of passion. Fury. Talkativeness. Frequent spells of unconsciousness.

Abdomen - Painful, tender to pressure.

Back - Constricting, between scapula.

Eyes - Eyes sunken, fixed. Injected and staring eyes, with barking cough at night.

Face - Face pale.

Food - Thought of food causes retching. Anorexia. Solids are swallowed better than liquids, which escape through nose. Milk relieves in general. Excessive ill-humor, after eating a little too much.

Head - Atrocious headaches, worse night.

Heart - Weak.

Kidneys - Nephritis with great debility and chilliness. Suppression of urine. Amber colored urine, very painful, albuminous, scanty.

Limbs - Varicose veins with great tenderness of leg (left). Cold limbs.

Lungs - Cutting pain in larynx. Croupy cough, causes suffocation. Hoarseness, talking painful.

Modalities - Better milk. Worse from speaking. Worse swallowing. Worse after eating.

Mouth - Astringent taste. Fetor of breath. Free salivation. Aphthae on tongue and lips, with a thick, yellowish white scab. Very painful, forming ulcers. ***Ulcerations of mouth*** with a gray membrane. Pain and swelling of salivary glands. Edema of soft palate. Gums swollen and covered with a white, adherent layer, under which is found a violet border.

Nose - Profuse nosebleed, dark blood, several times a day.

Perspiration - Moisture, sweat with icy coldness of skin. Profuse, sticky sweat on upper half of body. Cold sweat on forehead and cheek.

Rectum - Redness around anus. Intolerable pain. Frequent diarrhea preceded by severe colic. Stools are offensive, green, slimy, bloody and black. Discharge of fetid liquid with gangrenous odor. Frequent hemorrhage, stools with tenesmus.

Skin - Moist and cold skin.

Stomach - Early and complete anorexia. Incessant hiccough. Thought of food causes retching. Nausea. Bilious, bloody vomiting.

Throat - Intense redness of fauces. Feels raw and sore. Looks raw in spots, especially in public speakers. Hoarseness and talking is very painful. Swallowing very difficult, cutting pain on swallowing. Much thick grayish membrane in the throat. Mucus membranes broken down, ulcerated. ***Necrotic destruction of soft parts of palate and fauces.*** Septic diphtheria. Diphtheria of the larynx and nose (Kali-bi.). Tonsils enlarged. Dark blood from nose.

Tongue - Aphthae on tongue. Tongue pale with yellowish streak on base. Tongue swollen, edges red, tip dark red. Tongue dark red, almost black.

COMMENTS - When Dr. Alexander Villers was an infant, he had diphtheria. Known remedies had failed to arrest the disease. His father, Dr. Dominic von Villers, was in despair.

Taking counsel with his friend, Dr. Beck (of Monthly in Switzerland), the latter was struck with the likeness of the case to the effects of Merc-cy. in some poisoning cases, reports of which he had just been reading and he suggested the remedy.

A small quantity of the salt was procured and a potency was rapidly made and administered.

Improvement soon set in and recovered followed. Alexander Villers, saved by Merc-cy., lived to do brilliant work with the same remedy when practicing in St. Petersburg.

Merc-cy. has taken a sure place at the head of remedies for diphtheria, and as an efficient prophylactic in diphtheria cases. Villers had better results with the 30c than with any lower potency.

In the sensational New York poisoning case of February, 1899, Mr. Henry C. Barnett, the victim, was treated for diphtheria by his doctors before the cause of the illness was discovered.

Nash reported as particularly indicating it a chronic sore throat of public speakers with rawness in spots and a broken-down appearance, as if about to ulcerate and the feeling that "it hurts the patient to speak."

Diphtheria membrane in throat, mouth and at anus. Swallowing is impossible or causes severe cutting pains. Thought of food causes retching.

Beck noted the extreme feebleness, trembling, syncope. Profound prostration. Icy coldness, general coldness with nausea. Dark and persistent hemorrhage. Varicose veins with great tenderness on left leg. Cyanosis.

RELATIONS - ***Compare:*** (1) Arum-t., Caust., Hep., Kali-bi., Phyt., Echi., Lach., Gels.

REFERENCES - Boericke. Clarke. Phatak.

MERCURIUS DULCIS

(Calomel)

PHARMACY - merc-d. Mercurius dulcis. Calomel. Mercurous chloride. Subchloride of mercury. Trituration. ***Historical dose:*** All potencies.

CLINICAL - Aphthae. Blepharitis. Catarrh. Cirrhosis. Condylomata. Conjunctivitis. Constipation. Deafness. Diarrhea. Dysentery. ***Ear, disorders. Eustachian, catarrh.*** Gastromalachia. ***Glue ear.*** Jaundice. Meningitis. Nausea. ***Otitis media.*** Peritonitis. Pharyngitis. Pleurisy. ***Prostatitis. Swimmer's ear.*** Throat, sore. Ulcers. Vomiting.

HOMEOPATHIC - Merc-d. is responsible for a large amount of the mercury treatments of the past and for some of the present. As a comparatively mild and slow-aching form of mercurial, it has none of the corrosive effects Merc-c., but it has all the power of the metal in it, and it has had its own share of disasters.

It was at one time almost the only recognized remedy for constipation and any affection that could be ascribed to the liver. Some homeopaths adopted a modification of this by prescribing Merc-d. 1x in two-or three-grain doses as a direct purgative. As Merc-d. has caused both constipation and diarrhea, it is probable that the action is roughly homeopathic.

Keynote pallor, "pale as a corpse." A flabby, bloated appearance, ill nourished. Pale mucus membranes. Catarrhal inflammation of the ear. ***Eustachian catarrh*** and deafness (Kali-m.). ***Glue ear. Swimmer's ear infection.***

Diarrhea with soreness of anus. ***Prostatitis***. Inflammation with peritonitis, meningitis, pleurisy. ***Flabby, bloated*** and turgid flaccidity. Indicated in remittent bilious fevers in peritonitis and meningitis. Biliary stasis. For scrofulous children who are liable to remittent bilious attacks. Pale, scrofulous children who have swelling of cervical and other glands.

MIND - Bilious temperament. Moody, gloomy and irritable. Nervous, restlessness and agitated. Apprehensive. Anxiety about health. Hypochondriasis. Fear of impending disease. Whimpering. Desire to be silent, taciturn.

Abdomen - Violent pain in abdomen, griping, tenderness. Bloated, hot, painful abdomen.

Back - Swelling of cervical glands.

Chest - Great oppression in chest and heart.

Constitutions - Pale, scrofulous children, who have swelling of cervical and other glands.

Ears - ***Otitis media.*** Scrofulous otitis. Ear troubles of scrofulous children. Sudden fluttering. Itching in external meatus. ***Closure of eustachian tubes. Eustachian catarrh*** (Kali-m.). Eardrum retracted, thickened and immovable. ***Glue ear. Swimmer's ear infection.*** Deafness, occasioned by a swelling, which compresses eustachian tube. Deafness from every cold of old age. Deafness of old age.

Eyes - ***Irido-choroiditis.*** Scrofulous ophthalmia. Ciliary blepharitis. Eyes, red, dry. Gummy secretion on edges of lids, later, smarting and indistinct vision. Closure of lachrymal duct. Rapid winking. Symptoms worse after exercise and when heated from exercise.

Face - Face flushed, pale as a corpse. Swelling of cheeks. Exfoliation of lower jaw and death.

Female - Broad, moist and burning condylomata around external genitals, perineum and anus of exceedingly offensive smell.

Head - Painful scalp. Heaviness across forehead. Falling off of hair.

Limbs - Rheumatic stiffness and catching pain in muscles of legs and knee joints. Cramps in calves at night. Trembling of hands and feet.

Male - Acute inflammation of prostate after suppressed gonorrhea. Burning, pressing pains. Stinging and itching just back of corona glandis. Intense dysuria, urine scanty.

Modalities - Better from cold drinks, worse from acids.

Mouth - Offensive breath, salivation, sore gums. Constant flow of dark, fetid, putrid saliva, very offensive. Ulceration of throat with dysphagia. Granular pharyngitis. Aphthae on tongue. Tongue indented indurated, black. Ulcers in mouth, bleeding throughout night. Difficult to open mouth.

Nose - Blows lumps of mucus from nose. Dry, crusted nostrils. Sore right nostril. Violent nosebleed.

Rectum - Obstinate constipation. ***Anus is sore and burning***. Condylomata around anus. Tenesmus, constant disposition to stool. Dysentery, small stools of ***mucus and blood, covered with bile***. Diarrhea with vomiting.

Skin - ***Flabby and ill nourished***. Swollen glands. Desquamation of skin, especially of hands and feet. Copper-colored eruptions. Phagedenic ulcers with white bases and painful and inflamed margins in mouth, palate, face, genital and other parts.

Stomach - No appetite. Urgent thirst. Weight and pain at epigastrium. Nausea and vomiting. Cyclic vomiting of infants (Cupr-ar., Iris.).

Stool - Dysentery, small stools of mucus and blood, covered with bile. Black stools with great epigastric oppression, sinking. ***Stools scanty, bloody mucus, with bile, and constant desire***, without tenesmus. Stools coppery green, like chopped eggs. Dark green, watery stools, with griping. ***Acrid, grass-green diarrhea*** of infants, without tenesmus. Watery stools, colorless, or as if mixed with flocculent matter, or like washings of meat, occurring most often at night.

Teeth - Violent burning in teeth. Teeth become bare, shake and fall out. Gums swollen and bleeding when touched.

Temperature - Feverish heat, profuse nocturnal sweat, tearing pains in limbs, prostration of strength and trembling. Fever, sometimes hot, putrid.

Throat - Excessive ulceration of throat. Difficulty of swallowing.

COMMENTS - Blocked Eustachian tubes. Eustachian catarrh (Kali-m.) and deafness. Otitis media with closure of Eustachian tubes. Scrofulous inflammation in general, particularly of the eyes. Peritonitis. Soreness around the anus.

Hale noted its use in dropsies due to combined kidney and cardiac diseases, especially with jaundice. Cirrhosis of the liver, especially in the hypertrophic form.

Calomel in old-school practice rapidly resolved and cured a violent meningitis with wild delirium in a girl of five. In this case there was probably plastic exudation on the membranes. Inflammation with plastic exudation.

RELATIONS - ***Antidoted by:*** Hep. ***Compare:*** (1) Kali-m., Hydr. (2) In stringy stools, Sul-ac. (3) Catarrhal inflammation of middle ear, eustachian tube closed, deafness of old age, Kali-m.

REFERENCES - Boericke. Clarke. Murphy.

MERCURIUS IODATUS FLAVUS

(Mercury Iodide)

PHARMACY - merc-i-f. Mercurius iodatus flavus. Mercury iodide. Mercurius protoiodatus. Green iodide of mercury. Trituration. ***Historical dose:*** All potencies.

CLINICAL - Blepharitis. ***Breast, tumors.*** Catarrh. Chancre. Crusta lactea. Diphtheria. Eyes, disorders. Goiter. Intra-ocular disorders. Leucorrhea. Ozaena. Pregnancy, vomiting. Scabies. Syphilis. ***Throat, sore.*** Tonsillitis. Toothache. Writer's cramp.

HOMEOPATHIC - Merc-i-f. has had a valuable proving that developed a distinct individuality based on the general Merc. characteristics. Some symptoms of Merc-i-f. are very similar to Lyc, and Lyc. relieved some of the symptoms of the proving. The right-to-left direction was manifested in the throat and chest symptoms, but, unlike those of Lyc., the throat symptoms were worse by warm drinks.

Merc-i-f. has a strong affinity for glands of the throat, lymphatic and breasts. Throat disorders with greatly swollen glands and a characteristic coating of tongue. ***Sore throat, worse on the right side.*** Much accumulation of tenacious mucus in the throat. Characteristic thick yellow coat at the base of the tongue, anterior part clean and red.

Chancre induration remains a long time. Cervical and parotid glands enormously swollen. Goiter. Swollen inguinal glands, large and hard. ***Breasts tumors*** with tendency to much warm perspiration and gastric disturbances.

Pains in the eyes and orbits. Farrington mentioned "corneal ulcers looking as if they had been chipped out by finger-nail." Deep bone pains especially at night. Syphilis.

MIND - Capricious. Mood is changeable, variable. Moody and depressed. Anxiety. Full of cares and worries. Fear in narrow places, claustrophobia. Fear of suffocation. Confusion in warm room, better walking in open air. Confusion of mind, worse on waking.

Indolence, aversion to work. Irritability during pain. Destructiveness, can scarcely resist temptation to throw lamp through window. Lively, merry, talkative. Elated. Loquacity.

Abdomen - Pain in abdomen with pain in heart. Hardness of abdomen, as from flatulence. Faint sick feeling in hypogastrium before stools. Burning at umbilicus as from a hot coal, worse when inspiring. Indolent buboes.

Back - Sharp pain in back. Neck stiff. Bruised feeling over entire scapular region. Throbbing pain between scapula.

Breasts - Breast tumors with knots in axilla, blueness of the part, warm perspiration and gastric disturbances.

Causations - Cold draft when perspiring. Cold, damp weather, spring.

Constitutions - Suited to scrofulous and syphilitic patients, to mucus surfaces covered with squamous epithelium, to effects of drafts while perspiring.

Ears - Sudden, sharp pain in ears, worse touch. Throbbing, boring pains from within outward, deep in left ear.

Eyes - Dark circles around the eyes. Keratitis, cornea looks scratched or chipped out by fingernail. Photophobia. Throbbing, aching pains at night. Pannus. Ptosis, alternating with dimness of sight of left eye. Granular lids. Swelling below right eye.

Face - Dull aching and soreness in bones of face. Stinging pain in left cheek.

Female - Yellow leucorrhea of very young girls. Copious, muco-purulent discharge from vagina.

Food - Appetite variable, worse sweets. Excessive thirst for cold water, sour drinks.

Head - Catarrh of frontal sinuses, with offensive discharge. Dull frontal headache with pain at the root of nose. Throbbing, bursting sensation in temples. Shooting or sharp pains in temple. Soreness and stiffness in occiput. Headache better when mind and body actively engaged. Head pain follows heart pain. Itching of scalp, worse at night.

Heart - Pains in heart, preceded by headache. Suffocation about heart with nausea and dizziness. Palpitations with dyspnea, worse lying on back. Feeling as if heart had jumped out of its place. Pulse weak, irregular and labored.

Kidneys - Urine, copious, dark red, scanty.

Limbs - Excessive tired feeling of all limbs. Heaviness of limbs with indolence and drowsiness. Knees numb. Laming pain in right arm worse writing. Pain in right forearm with pain in left hip.

Male - Hard chancres, painless, with enlarged inguinal glands, not disposed to suppuration. Dreams of urination followed by seminal emission of which he knew nothing.

Modalities - Better from open air. Tired feeling in all limbs better lying on right side. Worse cold and damp weather, spring. Worse night, before 1 a.m., on waking, rest, lying on left side, warmth of bed, warm room. Worse raising up, touch, pressure, odors, warm drinks. Faint feeling worse at church.

Mouth - Bad taste in mouth. Coppery smell from mouth. Mouth, lips and tongue dry and sticky. Fine bright red eruption on roof of mouth. Stiffness of jaws, with inability to open mouth.

Nose - Mucus descends through posterior sinuses into the threat, causing hawking. Thick plugs of nasal secretion, with severe frontal headache. Chronic catarrh of posterior nares. Nostrils dilated with every inspiration. Shooting pain at root of nose, worse morning in waking.

Rectum - Diarrhea or discharge of fetid flatus, preceded by cutting, colicky pains. Frequent urging to stool. Black discharges with or without stools. Stools tough, almost like putty, with much straining. Stools thin, light-yellowish brown, frothy, soft, copious, dark.

Skin - Troublesome itching over whole body, worse at night. Persistent itching spots over whole body. Bright red, fine eruption on chest and abdomen. Flat warts.

Sleep - Sleeplessness without restlessness. Restless sleep from constant itching. Amorous dreams. Frightful dreams, nightmares. Dreams that he must urinate.

Stomach - Weak empty feeling in stomach. Burning at stomach with pain as from a blow. Sharp pain worse pressure. Cutting pain with nausea and inclination to vomit. Nausea at the sight or odor of food. Persistent nausea. Nausea with dizziness and suffocation about heart. Morning sickness.

Teeth - Desire to clench the teeth, jaw is stiff and tired from grinding, pain in teeth during sleep. Teeth sensitive, worse heat, cold and sweets. Teeth feel too long, cannot eat. Toothache after filling. Pyorrhea.

Throat - ***Sore throat, goes from right to left.*** Swelling begins on right side. Tonsillitis. Tonsils swollen, better cold drinks. When only the superficial part of the tonsils is involved. ***Constant inclination to swallow.*** Sensation of a lump. Small ulcers on posterior pharynx. Easily detached patches on inflamed pharynx and fauces, ***worse on right tonsil***, much tenacious mucus. Cheesy exudates with offensive breath. Goiter with suffocation.

Tongue - Tongue coated moist filmy. ***Tongue coated thickly, yellow at the base***. Tip and edges may be red and take imprint of teeth.

Vertigo - Faint or dizzy on rising from a chair or when reading.

Vision - Impaired vision with weakness of internal recti. Diplopia on holding eyes to left for some time. Distant objects look blurred. Black clouds float before eyes when lying on left side.

COMMENTS - Merc-i-f. a right-sided (Merc-i-r. is left-sided). Conditions can move from right to left. Characteristic concomitants including a heart pain immediately followed by a head pain, simultaneous pain in right forearm and left hip, and pain in heart with pain in abdomen.

Useful for abscessed tonsils, tonsillitis. Sore throats on one side with salivation and sweating (Merc-i-r.). Swollen glands and sores in the mouth (Phyt.). The teeth feel too long, worse by closing the jaws. Irresistible desire to clench the teeth. Jaw is stiff and muscles tired from clenching teeth in sleep.

Faint, sick feeling in hypogastrium. Nausea at the sight of food. Black stools. A cough worse by laughing. For conditions from the removal of mercury amalgams, particularly severe fatigue or recurring infections.

Kent mentioned the cure of "an ulcerated indurated lump in breast, as large as a goose's egg with knots in axilla, blueness of the part and no hope." Merc-i-f. 100c, given as often as the pains were severe, cured.

RELATIONS - ***Antidoted by:*** Hep., palpitations, Lyc. ***Compare:*** (1) Plb-i. - in breast tumors. (2) Right to left, Lyc. (Merc-i-r. to right). (3) Nausea in hypogastrium, Puls. (4) Black stools, Lept. (5) Cough worse laughing, Arg-n. (6) Pains all around orbit, Cinnb. (7) Worse warm drinks and empty swallowing, Lach. Thick yellow coating at base of tongue, Kali-bi. (Nat-p. golden yellow, Nat-s. dirty or greenish gray). (8) Worse lying left side, Phos., Arn., Spig. - opposite Merc., which has worse lying right side. ***Follows well:*** Lach. (scarlatina).

REFERENCES - Boericke. Clarke. Murphy. Phatak.

MERCURIUS IODATUS RUBER

(Mercury Bin-iodide)

PHARMACY - merc-i-r. Mercurius iodatus ruber. Mercury bin-iodide. Mercurius biniodatus. Trituration. ***Historical dose:*** All potencies, third trituration.

CLINICAL - Adenitis. Antrum, pain. Asthma. Buboes. Chancres. Coryza. Diphtheria. Eczema. Eye, inflammation. Hemorrhoids. Laryngitis. Liver, syphilis. Malaria. Nose, polyps, Nose, diseased bones. Parotiditis. Post-nasal catarrh. Quinsy. Rheumatism. Spleen, enlarged. Syphilis. Testicles, enlargement. ***Throat, sore.*** Tonsillitis. Typhus fever.

HOMEOPATHIC - Merc-i-r. acts on cellular tissue. Affects the lymphatic glands, throat, but more on the ***left side*** (Merc-i-f., right side). Wandering rheumatic pains with weariness. Much hard glandular swelling. Chronic suppurating buboes. Hard chancres. Old cases of syphilis in scrofulous patients.

Diphtheria and ulcerated sore throats, especially on left side with much glandular swelling. Early cases of cold, especially in children. Oppressed breathing.

Cases have been recorded in which small doses of Merc-i-r. 3x or 2x have cut short an attack of asthma or, if taken at bed-time, have prevented an expected attack from developing during the night.

MIND - Restlessness, nervousness. Better from occupation, diversion. Ill humor. Disposed to cry. Anxiety during sleep. Confusion of mind. Delirium during fever, scarlatina. Indifference, apathy.

Abdomen - Distended abdomen about navel, with pain on pressure. Heavy, painful feeling in region of liver, pancreas and spleen. Sudden cutting, in region of liver. Sore feeling all over bowels. Enlarged malarial spleens and livers. Inflammation of inguinal glands.

Back - Stiff neck. Cervical adenitis. Spine sore and painful.

Causations - Exposure to wet, weather changes.

Chest - Constriction across chest. Sharp cutting pain in chest. Sticking pain in muscles of ribs. Suppuration of axillary glands.

Ears - Itching in both ears. Pain in right ear. Increased earwax. ***Closure of eustachian tube***, opens with a pop. Dull hearing, better evening. Deafness, better after becoming warm on walking.

Eyes - Inflammation with burning. Stream of hot, acrid tears, mixed with yellowish flakes of fibrinous material. Bright light irritates. Granular eyelids. Trachoma. Blepharitis marginalis. Old cases of pannus.

Face - Slimy, sticky lips on waking. Eczema on chin. Scabs on right side of face. Pain in jaws and temples. ***Aching sore malar bones.*** Swelling of parotid glands.

Female - Profuse, acrid, green, yellowish leucorrhea. Stony hard fibroids.

Food - Desires food more salted.

Head - ***Heat and pulsation in vertex, worse evening.*** Painfully heavy occiput Frontal region as if bound by the cord. Small pustules on head. Syphilitic tumors in brain.

Kidneys - Ulcers in bladder. Urethra indurated. Frequent desire, can't retain urine for a moment. Increased flow of urine. Urine red, thick and dark when passing.

Limbs - Wandering rheumatic pains, especially muscular. Pain from calf up to sacrum. Middle humerus as if about to break.

Lungs - Catching pain under right breast, oppressing breathing. Asthma. Cough from elongated uvula with sore throat. Small quantity of loose, whitish, slimy sputum, with cough. Profuse, yellow mucus. Hoarseness on getting a little wet.

Male - Sharp shooting, in end of penis through glans. Nocturnal emissions. Sensitiveness of right testicle and cord. Sarcocele of testicles. Threatened gangrene of glans in paraphimosis. Stubborn suppurating buboes. Hard chancres.

Modalities - Open air ameliorates the head symptoms. Getting warm, walking ameliorates deafness. Worse empty swallowing, swallowing food, after dinner. Worse touch, pressure, after sleep, afternoon and evening. Worse weather changes, cold air, cold washing, getting wet, washing floor.

Mouth - Profuse saliva. Scalded feeling on tongue. Tongue, wrinkled stiff at base, pains when moving. Aphthae. Gums swollen. Toothache. Lips slimy and sticky on waking. Lips stick together during headache. Glands swollen.

Nose - Coryza with right side of nose hot and swollen. Hawks mucus from posterior sinuses. Boggy mucus membrane of nose and throat, closure of Eustachian tube, opening with a pop. Turbinated bones swollen.

Perspiration - Copious, hot sweat. Night sweats.

Skin - ***Syphilitic chancre and ulcers.*** Bubo. Hard papules. Pustules, with inflamed base, sore to touch. Freckles, liver spots. Lupus. Sarcocele. Small fissures and cracks. Moist cracks on palms. Chilblains.

Sleep - Sleeplessness from pain in ulcerated throat. Restless sleep from 12 p.m. until morning, with constriction in diaphragm. Lascivious, frightful dreams. Dreams of swimming, traveling.

Stomach - Pain in pit on pressure. Sinking at stomach and pit, with general sick feeling. Loud and bitter belching. Nausea while passing diarrheic stool.

Temperature - Intense shivering followed by fever. Chilly at bedtime. Chilliness, followed by flush over face. Flush of heat and feeling of being tickled.

Throat - ***Fauces dark red***, swallowing painful. Diphtheria. ***Sore throat, goes from left to right side.*** Tonsils greatly swollen, ***worse on left side***. Submaxillary glands painfully engorged. Parenchymatous tonsillitis. Cough with sore throat. Phlegm in nose and throat. Disposition to hawk with sensation of a lump in throat. Hawks much mucus from posterior sinuses. Laryngeal troubles with aphonia. Uvula elongated. ***Stiffness of muscles of throat and neck.***

Vertigo - Vertigo, things seem to reel around her. Vertigo during influenza.

COMMENTS - The liver, spleen and pancreas are affected and also the bladder and male sexual organs. Wandering rheumatism. Headaches, worse in open air. Eyes worse by bright light, psoric eye disorders. Right side of nose is inflamed. Troublesome dreams.

Will often abort peri-tonsillitis if given frequently. It acts well in old cases of syphilis, particularly in persons of lax tissue, scrofulous and those who have taken much mercury.

RELATIONS - ***Antidoted by:*** Hep. ***Compare:*** (1) In syphilitic eruptions, Bad., Carb-an., Nit-ac. (2) Ophthalmia, Jeqol. (3) Wandering rheumatism, Kali-bi. (4) worse after sleep, left to right, Lach. (5) Dreams of water, Merc-i-f.. (6) In disorders of antrum, Mag-c., Merc-c. ***Compatible after:*** Bell.

REFERENCES - Boericke. Clarke. Phatak.

MERCURIUS NITROSUS

(Mercury Nitrate)

PHARMACY - merc-ns. Mercurius nitrosus. Mercury nitrate. Mercurius nitricus oxydulatus. Liquor Hydrargyria. Nitratis acidus. Unguentum hydrargyria nitratis. Trituration. ***Historical dose:*** All potencies.

CLINICAL - Cachexia. Condylomata. Delirium. Eyes, disorders. Gonorrhea. Herpes. Impetigo. Leprosy. Malaria. Mucus, patches. Ophthalmia. Photophobia. Psoriasis. Ringworm. Stupor. Symptoms. Syphilis. Vegetations.

HOMEOPATHIC - The homeopathic authority for Merc-ns. is Hansen, who considered its special indication sticking pains and sticking itching. Hansen said Donner commended it in syphilis of the nerves and bones.

The symptoms are compiled from poisoning cases, including cachexia, tremors, frequent fainting, pains so intolerable he calls for a knife to kill himself. Coldness predominates, but there is the nitric acid flush of the face.

Merc-ns. has achieved a reputation as "a stimulating application" to indolent ulcers to the eyelids in ophthalmia and in a variety of skin diseases such as herpes, ringworm, impetigo, leprosy, psoriasis, and rupia. Vegetations.

Eye disorders with burning, sticking pains, photophobia and epiphora. Mucus patches with sticking pains. Gonorrhea with frequent burning, sticking itch on corona glandis and in the sulcus coronarius.

MIND - Memory poor. Extreme anxiety. Delirious. Rolled on the ground with excessive pain and called for a knife to kill himself. Stupor approaching a narcotic state.

RELATIONS - ***Compare:*** (1) Merc-d. in stinging and itching behind corona glandis.

REFERENCES - Clarke. Hansen.

MERCURIUS PRAECIPITATUS ALBUS

(White Precipitate of Mercury)

PHARMACY - merc-pr-a. Mercurius praecipitatus albus. White precipitate of mercury. Mercuric ammonium chloride. Trituration. ***Historical dose:*** All potencies.

CLINICAL - Blisters. Collapse. Dwarfism. Eczema, facial. Lachrymation. Nausea. Vesicles. Vomiting.

HOMEOPATHIC - The symptoms of Merc-pr-a. are taken entirely from poisonings. The most peculiar symptoms are a green tongue, bilious stools scalding anus. Slight subsultus. Collapse.

A child who was poisoned with 20 grains underwent a remarkable change one night. In the morning the child has changed to the appearance of an old man. During the night the child shrieked as from great pain.

Mossa related a case of chronic eczema of the face in an elderly man, a moistening eruption, worse in winter and from exposure to cold, vesicles on a reddened, swollen skin, dry into scales which exfoliate. Eyelids, especially the lower, edematous, the corners are reddened, lachrymation.

Ears involved, itching and burning on head preventing sleep. Merc-pr-a. 3 grains every third day was given. First the burning itching ceased. Then formation of blisters abated. Exfoliation continued a long time, but the skin finally became normal.

In another case, a girl, 2, had an eruption on face and large part of scalp, covered with thick yellow crust, matter exuding from cracks. Offensive odor, swollen cervical glands. Merc-pr-a. 3 grains once in three days cured in four weeks.

Abdomen - Pain in epigastrium, gradually spreading over whole abdomen. Great pain in abdomen, continuing after taking any, even liquid, food. Constant griping. Whole abdomen painful to pressure.

Face - Very flushed, greatly swollen.

Mouth - Tongue coated with thick greenish fur. Gums much swollen.

Perspiration - Cold, clammy skin, much congestion of cutaneous vessels. General perspiration.

Rectum - One copious stool with mucus shreds in some quantities, much dark blood. Numerous scanty stools with much blood. Almost pure bile causing great scalding of anus.

Sleep - Drowsy, semi-comatose.

Stomach - Urgent thirst. Much pain at stomach. Nausea and vomiting. Vomits deeply blood-stained fluid.

RELATIONS - ***Compare:*** (1) Dwarfish children, Bar-c., Carc. Syph. (2) Eczema, Mez., Aethi-a.

REFERENCES - Boericke. Clarke.

MERCURIUS PRAECIPITAT. RUBER

(Red Precipitate of Mercury)

PHARMACY - merc-pr-r. Mercurius praecipitatus ruber. Red precipitate of mercury. Red oxide of mercury. Mercurius oxydatus. Trituration. ***Historical dose:*** All potencies.

CLINICAL - Anus, burning. Barber's, itch. Blepharitis. Chancroid. Chemosis. Colic. Convulsions. Cramps. Diarrhea. Folliculitis. Gonorrhea. Mucus, patches. Otorrhea. Palpitations. Pemphigus, neonatorum. Phagedenic, ulcer. Salivation. Trembling. Ulcers.

HOMEOPATHIC - This intensely irritating mercurial was investigated by Hahnemann, all the usual mercurial symptoms were intensified.

Merc-pr-r. has produced suffocative attacks at night on lying down ***at the point of falling asleep.*** Patient is obliged to jump up suddenly, which relieves. Convulsions. Spasmodic contraction of limbs. Cramps of internal organs and in legs. General trembling.

Gonorrhea, ***urethra felt as a hard string.*** Chancroid, phagedenic ulcer and bubo. Pemphigus, mucus patches. Eczema with cracks and fissures. Barber's itch. Blepharitis internally and externally. Leaden heaviness in occiput with otorrhea.

MIND - Apprehension.

Abdomen - Abdomen distended and painful to contact. Occasional pain in left hypochondrium. Agonizing colic.

Eyes - Fierce intent look. Chemosis. Blepharitis.

Face - Dropsical condition of face. Remarkable redness of face and eyes. Cheeks and lips enormously swollen.

Heart - Violent palpitations that seemed as if it would burst the chest. Small, hard pulse.

Lungs - Larynx inflamed and swollen, even outside. Paroxysms of suffocation at night on lying down and while falling asleep, obliged to jump up suddenly, when it disappeared. Oppression of chest.

Mouth - Strong mercurial odor. Profuse salivation. Blood and saliva of the most fetid odor flowed constantly from mouth. Inside of mouth coated with a substance like decayed cheese. Mouth very sore, flakes of epithelium separate. Burning in mouth and throat, pains prevent sleep. Itching over whole mouth without salivation. Inflamed gums. Anterior portion of mucus membrane of cheeks, gums and under the tongue sloughed away and four teeth were lost in the process. As the parts healed the jaws became completely closed by contracting scars.

Rectum - Constant urging, gradually became worse and spread over whole intestinal canal, with constant sensation in anus as of a glowing hot iron moving up and down. Most excessive tenesmus with scanty discharge of blood with cutting and burning pains. Diarrhea excessively violent with violent cramps. Stools mainly blood involuntary, greenish and offensive.

Stomach - Unquenchable thirst. Pains in stomach and whole abdomen. Agonizing pain in stomach with burning heat and nausea. Nausea, vomiting. Vomiting, with cutting in abdomen, black blood, bloody mucus, followed by diarrhea.

Temperature - Cold, perspiring skin.

Throat - Throat inflamed. Burning like hot ashes on swallowing the powder.

Tongue - Tongue enormously swollen and protruding. Tongue was reduced and firmly adherent to floor of mouth and cheeks. Two holes in tongue.

COMMENTS - Hansen used Merc-pr-r. in practice and gave as indications gonorrhea when the urethra is felt as a hard string. Phagedenic ulcer and bubo. Indurated ulcer, deep with red, hard edges and especially when spreading. Syphilitic iritis when the pains have ceased. Pemphigus neonatorum and intertrigo syphilitica. Sensation "as of a hot iron in anus moving up and down."

Mucus patches on scrotum and by anus with or without fissures. Eczema, acute or chronic, much sero-purulent or purulent exudation, also externally (in ointment 1 to 40 of prepared lard). Tinea tonsurans, circinata and sycosis. Folliculitis.

RELATIONS - ***Compare:*** (1) Merc-pr-a.

REFERENCES - Boericke. Clarke. Hansen.

MERCURIUS SOLUBLIS

(Mercury Vivus)

PHARMACY - merc. Mercurius solublis hahnemanni. Mercurius vivus. Quicksilver. Argentum vivum. Mercurius oxydulatus niger. Hydrargyrum. Triturations. ***Historical dose:*** All potencies.

CLINICAL - Abscess. Anemia. ***Aphthae.*** Appendicitis. Balanitis. Bone, disorders. Brain inflammation. Breath offensive. Bronchitis. Bubo. Cancrum oris. Catarrh. Chancre. Chickpox. ***Colds***. Condylomata. Congestion. ***Coryza.*** Coughs. ***Dentition, abnormal.*** Deafness. Diarrhea. Dysentery. Dyspepsia. Ecthyma. ***Ear, infections.*** Eczema. Emaciation. Excoriation. Eyes, disorders. Fainting. Fevers. Fissures. ***Glandular, swellings.*** Gout. Gum-boil. ***Gum, disorders.*** Heart, disorders. Herpes. Hydrophobia. Jaundice. Joints, disorders. Leucorrhea. Liver, disorders. Lumbago. Mania. Measles. Melancholy. Meningitis. Mucous, patches. Mumps. Odors, offensive. Osteomalacia. ***Otitis, media.*** Ovaries, disorders. Pancreatitis. ***Parkinson's disease. Parotiditis.*** Peritonitis. ***Perspiration.*** Phimosis. Pregnancy, disorders. Prostate, disorders. Purpura. Pyemia. Ranula. Rheumatism. Rickets. Rigg's, disease. ***Salivation.*** Scurvy. ***Sinusitis.*** Smallpox. ***Sores.*** Stomatitis. Suppurations. Surgical, fever. ***Syphilis.*** Taste, disordered. Teeth, disorders. ***Throat, sore.*** Tongue, affections. ***Tongue, mapped. Toothache. Tremors.*** Typhus fever. ***Ulcers.*** Vaccination. Vomiting.

HOMEOPATHIC - There was a fitness in naming this metal after the mutable planet Mercury. It provides us with weatherglasses and thermometers and likewise it turns those who are under its influence into weatherglasses and thermometers.

Hahnemann invented Mercurius solublis in his pre-homeopathic days in response to a general desire for a mercurial preparation which should be at once soluble and non-corrosive and it at once took its place in the pharmacy, a place it has never lost.

The method of developing the medicinal power of metallic mercury by graduated trituration was a later discovery, through there was a suggestion of it in the well-known Hydrargyrum cum cretâ.

Although Hahnemann proved Mercurius solublis, he recommended the use of triturations of the pure metal in practice as being the simplest mercurial preparation and more easily obtained and equally available with Merc. The potencies are prepared from soluble black oxide of mercury, originally prepared by Hahnemann from pure metallic mercury.

There is no difference between the symptoms of these preparations, but it seems that when Merc. solublis fails, when indicated, Merc. vivus acts. Hahnemann recommended Merc. vivus as a superior preparation for homeopathic prescribing in his preface to the proving. No pains have been taken to keep distinct Merc. solublis and Merc. vivus.

Merc. is Hahnemann's typical anti-syphilitic remedy, as Sulph. is the typical anti-psoric and Thuj. the typical anti-sycotic.

Every organ and tissue of the body is more or less affected by this powerful drug.

It transforms healthy cells into decrepit, inflamed and necrotic wrecks, decomposes the blood, producing a profound anemia. Lesions, similar to those of syphilis. Hereditary syphilis manifestations. Often indicated in the ***secondary stage of syphilis*** when there is febrile anemia, rheumatoid pains and ulcerations. Ulcerations of the mucus membranes, especially of mouth and throat.

Lymphatic glands are enlarged, glandular activity increase, especially of salivary and mucus glands. Livid congestions. Destructive inflammations of bones, cellular tissues, and joints. Strictures after inflammation. Indurations. Rheumatism. Sycosis, scrofula, bullae.

Suppurations, tendency to formation of pus, which is thin, greening, putrid, streaked with blood. ***Breath, discharges smell foul. Secretions are watery,*** thin, slimy, acrid, burning, foul or thick greenish-yellow. Yellowness of eyes, teeth, nasal discharges. Biliousness, jaundice.

Tremors, convulsions. Tremblings, twitchings, disorderly motions of paralyzed parts. Cataleptic rigidity of the body. Parkinson's disease. Paraplegia. Contraction of joints. Burning, stinging pains. Painful exostoses. Softening of the bones.

Weakness with ebullitions and tremblings from least exertion. Exhausted and ready to sink down, worse after stools. Restless and sweaty, complaints increase with sweat and rest, and are associated with a great deal of weariness, prostration and trembling. Everything seems too short.

Redness. Swellings, edema, continued exudations. Parts are much swollen with raw, sore feeling. Profuse, oily perspiration does not relieve. Salt-lips, taste, expectoration etc. Stomatitis. Emaciation, marasmus.

A ***human thermometer***, extreme sensitivity to heat and cold. ***Worse from any change of temperature or weather.*** Catches colds easily. ***Hypersensitive to external impressions.*** Unstable and variable in mental and physical behavior, tremulous, weak and sweaty.

MIND - ***Changes their mind constantly.*** Instability of ideas, which constantly drive away each other. ***Irresolution.*** Precocious. ***Restlessness, is constantly changing from place to place, especially at night.*** Uncontrollable desire to travel far away.

Heedless. Weak memory, forgets everything. Hurried speech. Stammering, nervous with tremors. Slow in answering questions. Continuous moaning and groaning. Great anguish.

Apprehensive. Mistrustful, suspicious. Thinks he is losing his reason. Anxiety, anguish, trembling and sweat. Senses impending evil. Thinks he will die. Fear with desire to escape. Fear of robbers. Involuntary weeping. Ailments from fright, leaving one in a state of great anxiety, worse at night.

Moral dejection, with great listlessness, discouragement. Weary of life. Loss of will power. ***Poor self-confidence.*** Disgust. Dread of labor. Indifference to everything, does not even care to eat. Indifference to loved ones. Homesickness. Cheerful alternating with want of sympathy.

Ill-humor, disposition to be angry and to fly into a passion. Complaining of relations and surroundings. Agitation with excessive internal torment, as if conscious of having committed some crime. Quarrelsome, mistrustful, and suspicious. Raving.

Delirium, mental derangement of alcoholics. Confusion, loses his way in well-known streets. Weakness of memory for time. Time passes slowly. Delusions that he is a criminal, that everyone is an enemy. Confusion and vertigo in morning on waking. Loss of consciousness and of speech.

Fury, with dread of liquids. Filthy in mind and body, does foolish, mischievous, disgusting actions. Inclination to catch passing strangers by the nose. Violent, horrid impulses, homicidal, suicidal. Suicidal thoughts during menses, better weeping. Desire to kill the person that contradicts her. Postpartum mania, wants to throw child on fire.

Abdomen - Pressive pain in abdomen, as from a stone. Boring pain in right groin. External abdomen cold to touch. Stabbing pain with chilliness. Colic from cold.

Violent colic, with cutting and stinging pains, better recumbent position. Flatulent distention with pain. Shaking sensation of bowels when walking. Bowels feel weak, holds them. Intestines feel bruised when lying on right side. Intestines as if they fall to side on which one is lying. Appendicitis, better lying on back. Catarrh of pancreatic duct. Inguinal glands, pain on heavy pressure. Swelling of inguinal glands on taking cold. Inguinal glands swollen or suppurating. Buboes. Herpes zoster.

Back - Bruised pain in small of back, especially when sitting. Stinging pain in small of back with sensation of weakness. Violent pain in spine, worse motion and pressure. Burning pain in back, worse emission. Shooting pain in sacrum on breathing. Pain in sacrum, as if one had been lying on too hard a couch. Pricking itching in sacrum when walking. Tearing pain in coccyx, better pressing on abdomen. Pain forward from right scapula. Neck stiff, cervical glands enlarged. Cervical glands swollen and inflamed, with shooting pains. Psoriasis on nape. Herpes zoster.

Bladder - Great soreness in region of bladder when touching it. Frequent urging with copious or scanty urine. Must hurry, otherwise can't retain urine. Frequent urination at night, even involuntary. Sudden irresistible urging to urinate, passing large quantities. Burning in urethra on beginning to urinate, after urination, even when not urinating. Intolerable burning in forepart of urethra when passing last few drops. Cutting, during urination. Burning and stinging, with hemorrhage from urethra. Greenish discharge from urethra.

Breasts - Breasts swollen, become hard with ulcerative pain during menses. Swelling of nipples. Breast cancer. Palliative in breast cancer. Breasts painful and full of milk at menses. Milk in breast instead of menses. Milk spoiled. Milk in breast of boys.

Causations - Ill effects of fright, suppressed gonorrhea, foot sweat.

Chest - Burning or constriction in chest, worse night. Pain below breasts through to scapula, worse sneezing or coughing. Stitches from lower lobe of right lung to back. Feels as if everything in chest were dry. Sensations of bubbles or as of hot steam in chest. Sweating on chest with old people, from opium. Stabbing pain in left side under short ribs during every inspiration. Soreness from fauces to sternum. Cough with stitching pains in chest.

Constitutions - Suited to light-haired persons with lax skin and muscle, women and children. Scrofulous children. Merc. has relation to psora and sycosis as well as syphilis.

Cough - Whooping cough with nosebleed (Arn.). Cough causes pressing pains in head and chest. Cough in double bouts. Cough with hoarseness, salivation, vomiting, diarrhea. Cough with sensation as if head and chest would burst. Tickling cough before falling asleep. Dry cough at night, yellow-green sputum by day. Coughs only at night or only by day. Cough worse from tobacco smoke.

Ears - ***Otitis media. Chronic ears infections.*** Soreness and excoriation of inner ears. ***Otorrhea, thick yellow discharge.*** Fetid and bloody discharges. Watery discharge and hemorrhage from ears. Very offensive pus from ear, worse at night. ***Swimmer's ear infection. Glue ear.*** Red, hot swelling of external ear. ***Pains, worse warmth of bed***, at night. Sticking pains. Tearing and shooting pains. Pains extend to ear from teeth, throat etc. Sensation as if cold water running from the ear. Sensation of coldness in ears during pregnancy. Fungus excrescences. Polyps. Boils in external canal (Calc. pic.). Sounds vibrate in ears. Ringing and roaring. Whistling or running of trains. Deafness on becoming heated, better on swallowing and blowing nose.

Eyes - Conjunctivitis from taking cold. Scanty or profuse, ***burning acrid discharge.*** Iritis with hypopion. ***Keratitis*** of syphilitic origin with burning pain. Retinitis when worse by firelight and at night. Ophthalmia neonatorum. Arcus senilis. Optic nerve and eye disorders in those who work in foundries. Pupils dilated. Burning in eyes. Stitches in eyes. Cutting, stinging or aching pains when exerting eyes. Eyes draw together. Lids, red, thick, swollen, scurfy and swollen. Agglutinated lids in morning. Lids spasmodically closed. Styes on upper lids. Twitching of lids. Photophobia, worse heat and glare of fire of foundry men. Eyes sensitive to extreme heat or cold.

Face - Pale, ***earthy***, yellow, dirty looking. Puffy under eyes. Cheeks, swollen, red, hot. Syphilitic pustules on face. Mumps if suppuration threatens. Pimples on face. Corners of mouth ulcerated and painfully sore. Yellowish scabs around mouth. Swelling or cracking of upper lip. Lips, salty, dry, cracked in angles. Lips burn when touched. Swelling of cheeks during toothache. Aching in jaws. Spasms and immobility of jaws. Periostitis of jaw, progressing to necrosis. Masseter muscles contracted. Lockjaw from glandular swellings, with stinging pains. Aching in facial bones. Facial paralysis from cold. Trigeminal neuralgia from taking cold.

Female - Amenorrhea with congestions and ebullitions. Menses suppressed. Collapse and fainting at start of menses. Menses irregular, or every two weeks. Menses too late and scanty. Profuse menses with abdominal pains. Menses of short duration. Abscesses appear anywhere on body during menses and disappear after menses. Leucorrhea, thick, white with itching, worse urinating and washing with cold water. Leucorrhea excoriating, greenish and bloody. Leucorrhea in small girls, causing prostration. ***Sensation of rawness*** in parts. Genitals feel raw. ***Vaginitis.*** Itching of vulva. Burning, throbbing and itching of vagina. Swelling of labia. Pressure in genitals, obliging her to urinate often. ***Stinging pain in ovaries*** (Apis). Stitching, aching or boring pains in uterus. Prolapse of uterus with vagina, better from sex. Cancer of uterus and breasts. Bleeding excrescences on os uteri. Expels moles. Pregnant women with swelling of genitals. Edema, pruritus of vulva during pregnancy. Morning sickness with a profuse salivation. Tendency to miscarriage from uterine weakness. Infertility with too profuse menses.

Food - ***Intense thirst for cold drink and beer.*** Great thirst for ice water, though it aggravates cough. Much thirst day and night. Sweats when eating. Weak digestion with ***continuous hunger***. Craving for lemons. Appetite only for bread and butter. Bread tastes sweet. Aversion to meat, coffee, butter, oily things, sweets, salt, strong cheese. Sweet things and milk disagree, though he craves them. Wine, spirituous liquors, coffee and cold drinks aggravate.

Head - ***Catarrhal headaches***, much heat in head. Catarrhal affections of frontal and maxillary sinuses. Burning and pulsations in forehead. ***Tension about scalp, as if bandaged***. One-sided, tearing pains. Headache with ear and toothache. Headache alternating with foot sweat. Headache caused by suppression of foot sweat. Headache with suicidal tendency. Child turns head from side to side and moans. External head painful to touch. Stinging, burning, fetid eruptions on scalp. Scalp tense, fetid, sour smelling, oily sweat on head. Itching of scalp day and night. Falling of hair from sides and temples. Exostosis with soreness. Anterior fontanels open. Cerebrospinal meningitis from suppressed otorrhea. Hydrocephalus. Cephalhematoma.

Heart - Aching pain at apex and base of heart. Awakes with cardiac tremor. Weakness in heart as if dying. Palpitations on slight exertion. Palpitations with cough and bloody sputum. Palpitations with fear, worse at night. Pulse irregular, quick, strong and intermittent or soft and trembling. Pulse frequent at night, slower by day. Pulse irregular, generally full and fast. Pulse with violent beating in arteries. Pulse imperceptible, with warmth of body.

Kidneys - Dysuria. Greenish discharge from urethra, burning in urethra on beginning to urinate. Frequent urging to urinate day and night with copious or scanty urine. Urinates more than drinks. Stream of urine very small. Urine causes itching. Urine dark, scanty, bloody, albuminous. Hematuria, painless. Burning after urination.

Limbs - Weakness and weariness in all limbs. Pains in limbs, worse night. Bone pains, deep or near the surface, worse at night, must get up and walk about. Bones as if broken, joints as if sprained. Involuntary jerking in limbs. Convulsions in limbs. ***Trembling limbs, especially the hands. Parkinson's disease.*** Paralysis agitans. Stiffness and immobility of limbs. Osteoarthritis. Rheumatism of joints, with swelling and sensation of coldness. Lacerating pains in joints. Tendency to complete destruction of joints. Abscess in joints. Edematous swelling of hands, feet and face during menses, or with anemia. Phlegmasia alba dolens. Sensation as if knees were larger. Fingers numb. Icy cold hands after emission. Cold heels. Cold, clammy sweat on legs at night. Patient very sensitive to cold. Oily perspiration.

Liver - Liver enlarged, sore to touch, indurated. Jaundice from gallstones. Jaundice in newborn. Deficient bile secretion. Chronic atrophy of liver, with emaciation and desiccation of body.

Lungs - ***Dyspnea, when coughing or sneezing.*** Desire to take deep breath from anxious oppression. ***Shortness of breath on going upstairs or walking quickly.*** Breathing difficult, worse lying on left side, but cough worse lying on right side. Catarrh with chilliness, dread of air. Salty or bitter tenacious mucus. Easy expectoration. Yellow muco-purulent expectoration, with cough. Bloody expectoration on account of destroyed lung parenchyma. ***Asthma, worse change of weather,*** better tobacco smoke and cold air. Emphysema. Lungs as if heavy, in asthenic pneumonia. Pneumonia with cough and dyspnea. Pneumonia with jaundice. Suppuration of lungs after hemorrhages, or after pneumonia.

Male - Sweat on genitals with soreness between scrotum and thighs. Cold genitals. Swelling of lymphatic vessels along penis. Glans and prepuce inflamed and swollen, phimosis. Redness of meatus. Prepuce irritated, itches. Children or adults pull and scratch at the genitals from a kind of itching which makes them do so. Orchitis (Clem., Ham., Puls.). Testicles, swollen, hard with shiny, red scrotum. Dragging pain in testes and spermatic cords. Sensations of coldness in testicles. Gonorrhea. Gleet yellowish green and purulent. ***Syphilis. Vesicles on forepart and sides of glans of penis.*** Vesicles and ulcers, soft chancre. Herpes preputialis. Condylomata. Lascivious excitement with painful nightly erections. Nocturnal emissions, stained with blood. Emissions followed by burning pain in back and icy cold hands. Sexual power decreased, total loss of sexual power.

Modalities - Better from moderate temperature, in morning. Better from sex, rest, scratching. ***Worse drafts, taking cold***, touching anything cold, cloudy weather, damp, rainy weather, wet feet. ***Worse changing weather and temperature***, ***heat***, ***sweating***, warmth of bed, warm days with damp, cool nights, Fall. ***Worse at night, lying on right side***, bending forward, during and after urination, before stool.

Mouth - ***Great thirst with moist mouth. Saliva increased,*** flows during sleep. Saliva yellow, bloody, bad tasting offensive. Salivation, with nausea, waking her from sleep. ***Sweetish taste. Metallic taste.*** Offensive, ***putrid odor*** from mouth. Offensive breath during cough. Disagreeable, sweetish odor from mouth. Mucus membrane bluish-red and spongy. Sore pain on touch and from chewing. Itching palate. Ranula with salivation and sore gums. Confluent thrush. ***Aphthae.*** Stomatitis from chewing-gum. Painful ragged, swollen, bleeding gums. ***Gums spongy***, recede, bleed easily. ***Gumboils.*** Speech difficult from trembling of tongue. Stammering. Loss of speech, replies by signs and grimaces.

Nose - ***Sinusitis and colds. Colds*** travel to eyes, ears or throat. ***Coryza profuse, fluent.*** Coryza, acrid discharge, but too thick to run down the lip, worse warm room. Coryza with sneezing, sore, ***raw***, smarting sensation, worse damp weather. Copious discharge of corroding mucus. Yellow-green, fetid, pus-like discharge. Acrid nasal secretions having the odor of old cheese. ***Nostrils are raw, ulcerated***. Frequent sneezing without coryza. ***Sneezing in sunshine.*** Pain and ***swelling of nasal bones and decay with greenish fetid ulceration***. Nosebleed when coughing, blood hangs in dark coagulated strings. Nosebleed during sleep, at night.

Perspiration - General tendency to ***easy perspiration, but patient is not relieved from it***. Excessive odorous viscid perspiration, worse night. Oily sweat. Sweat, oily, foul, sour or with strong sweetish penetrating odor, on head, on chest, stains indelibly yellow. Stiffening linen. Foul, sour perspiration or with strong sweetish penetrating odor. Sweats immediately on drinking something warm. ***Profuse sweat without amelioration.*** Perspires while walking, eating. Day and night sweats, though more at night. Falls asleep while perspiring. Perspires easily during sleep, sweats through bedclothes. ***Profuse and very debilitating, at night.*** Sweats with pains. ***Clammy and cold sweats, driving out of bed*** with thirst and palpitation or nausea. Sweats on head, chest. Shriveling fingers.

Rectum - Rectal tenesmus with tenesmus of bladder. Great pressure at stool, as if bowels would be forced out. Ineffectual urging to stool with protruding hemorrhoids, which are painfully sore. Rectal discharge accompanied by chilliness, sick stomach, cutting colic and tenesmus. Constipation. ***Dysentery.*** Purulent diarrhea with chill between and hot flushes during stool. Long continued diarrhea. Diarrhea in children. Severe pain in anus, during stool. Never-get-done feeling. Rawness, burning and itching of anus and adjacent parts, after stool. Prolapse anus after stool. Constriction in rectum, causes faintness, after stool. Weakness after stool. Hemorrhage from rectum after urination. Discharge of ascarides and lumbrici.

Sensations - Vibration in forehead. Head as if in a vice, as if growing large. Crackling in head as from metal plates. As if weight on forehead, as if weight hanging on to nose. As of sparks being emitted from eyes, as of a body underneath lids, as if feathers came from corners of eyes. As if a wedge driven in ear, as if ice in it, as if cold water running out of it. As if teeth were loose, were fixed in a mass of pap. As if hot vapors rising into throat of worm rising into throat, must swallow it down of apple core sticking in throat. As if everything in chest was dry. As if breasts would ulcerate.

Skin - ***Constantly moist***. Insensible skin. ***Itching***, ***worse from warmth of bed***, perspiration. Itching as from fleabites. Jaundice with itching on abdomen. Yellow skin, tender, excoriated like raw meat. Scurfy eruptions. Vesicular and pustular eruptions. Moist vesicles surrounded by dry scales, easily bleeding. Red spots covered with small vesicles. Pimples around the main eruption. Phagedenic blisters. Moist eczema. Crusta lactea, with yellowish-brown crusts, considerable suppuration. Herpes, burning when touched. Herpes zoster, burning pains. Measles, tardy development. Nettle-rash. Buboes. Boils and abscesses form at the time of menses. ***Ulcers, bleeding with cutting pains and proud flesh.*** Ulcers, irregular in shape, edges undefined. Desquamation. Erysipelas of newborn children of syphilitic or scrofulous nature. Exanthemata spreading from pit over abdomen and chest. Varicella, chickenpox, water blotches turn yellow and maturate. Variola in stage of maturation.

Sleep - Excessive sleepiness day and night. Great sleepiness during day, not better long sleep. Sleeplessness from nervous excitability. Sleepless at night from ebullitions of blood to chest and head. Sleeplessness from pain or other troubles. ***Profuse perspiration without relief during sleep,*** with pains. Just after falling asleep, pains become more violent. Dreams of water, animals, thieves, misfortune.

Stomach - Stomach sensitive to touch. Feels constricted. Pit of stomach burns. Pressure in pit with deathly faintness. Heartburn all night. Heartburn during pregnancy. Frequent hiccoughs. Hiccough and regurgitation of water and food. Acrid, bitter, putrid or rancid eructations, worse at night.

Nausea when coughing. Water collects in mouth, causes nausea and vomiting of a bitter substance. Inclination to vomit while coughing. Nausea and vomiting during stool. Vomiting of bile and food. ***Morning sickness with profuse salivation.***

Stools - Stools with pain and tenesmus. Never get done feeling. Stools, painful, scanty. ***Greenish, bloody and slimy stools, worse at night.*** Stools ashen white, gray, acrid, then tenesmus or chill. Mucus stools preceded by chilliness, and followed by tenesmus. Stools like stirred eggs, pea green, slimy. Stools watery and colorless, with greenish scum floating on surface of water. Stools acrid and excoriating, purulent. Stools undigested, sour smelling. Stools pitch-like, tenacious or crumbling. Stools small, knotty masses, small like sheep dung. Stools form a narrow ribbon.

Teeth - Grinding of teeth. ***Looseness of teeth.*** Teeth feel tender and elongated. Alveolar abscess, worse at night. Inflammation of roots of teeth, which ulcerate and fall out. Toothache worse heat and cold, at night. Toothache at night, followed by general chilliness, with swelling of gums and salivary glands. Teeth, decayed, hollow, black. Crown of teeth decay. ***Gums spongy, recede, bleed easily.*** Gumboils. Large ulcers on protruding gums. Swelling of gums every night. Shooting pains into face and ears, better rubbing cheek.

Temperature - ***Patient very sensitive to cold.*** Easily chilled or overheated. ***Creeping chilliness***, worse in the evening and into night. Constant cold hands and feet. Sense of coldness with tremors. Chilly within abscesses. Debility, chilly and weakness. Cold, clammy sweat on legs at night. Chill alternating with flushes of heat in single parts. Heat and shuddering alternately. Easily chilled or overheated. Catarrhal, gastric, bilious fevers. Fever alternating with shuddering. Fever after midnight with violent thirst for cold drinks. Fever with aversion to uncover. Fever in bed, chill when out of bed.

Throat - Glands swell every time patient takes cold. Lymphatic glands of throat hard and large. ***Sore throats and colds.*** Sore, raw, smarting, burning throat. Putrid sore throat. Burning in throat, as from hot vapor ascending. Painful dryness of throat, with mouth full of saliva. Constant desire to swallow. Quinsy with difficult swallowing after pus has formed. ***Tonsillitis.*** Whitish, smeary concretions upon tonsils. ***Tonsils enlarged.*** Ulcers on tonsils, on pharynx. Bluish-red swelling. Stitches into ear on swallowing, fluids return through nose. Sensation as if a foreign object or something hanging in throat. Uvula elongated, enlarged, greatly swollen. ***Ulcers*** and inflammation appearing at every change in weather. Hawks large lumps from throat. Complete loss of voice, from straining voice. Hoarse, rough voice, worse least current of air. Chronic hoarseness with tendency to sweat and profuse salivation. Aphonia from nervous paralysis.

Tongue - Tongue thickly coated in morning. Tongue heavy, thick, moist coating. Tongue, broad, flabby, yellow, ***indented.*** Gray patches on edges of tongue, dirty-yellow coat on upper surface. Needle pricks at tip. Pricking pain in tongue with swelling. ***Furrow in upper surface of tongue lengthwise***, with pricking. Tongue feels as if burnt with ulcers. Ulcers behind the tongue. Severe pain on side of tongue from contact of teeth.

Urine - Urine flows in a thin stream or only drop by drop. Urine hot, acrid, dark, scanty, albuminous. Urine thick, white sediment as if flour had been stirred in. Urine yellowish, staining diaper, smells sour and pungent. Urine, flesh-like lumps of mucus, pus. Painless hematuria. Urine remaining on parts after urinating cause intense itching, has to be washed off.

Vertigo - Vertigo, worse lying on back, as if on a swing. Vertigo after stooping. Vertigo with headache and nausea. Vertigo with momentary loss of vision, everything turns black. Can't stand erect or even sit up in bed for fear of falling.

Vision - Dim vision, with involuntary closing of eyes. Foggy vision. Black spots, flames, sparks before the eyes. Sees green colors. Constant flickering and floating black specks. Letters seem to move. Object as if small. Periodical loss of sight. Scotoma of right eye after a fall.

COMMENTS - To the symptoms of Hahnemann's pathogenesis of Merc. solublis are added observed effects of mercury in those engaged in working with the metal, patients taking mercury, and the effects on those applying mercurial inunctions to patients.

Many people have been severely affected by absorbing it through their hands. An electrician, who at one time was required to work with his hands frequently in a trough filled with quicksilver, thereafter could not bear the slightest shock of electricity, though before he could stand very strong ones.

There is no difference between these effects and the symptoms of the proving so far as the general characteristics are concerned, but in the finer characteristics there must be differences. The symptoms of the proving are in general more particularly characterized than the effects of Merc. vivus.

The symptoms of nosebleed and the more finely characterized throat symptoms were produced by Merc. solublis, as were the majority of the symptoms in the male and female sexual organs. Stitches on tonsils, stitches into ear on swallowing, something hot rises into throat. This is not to say that Merc. vivus will not answer equally well or even better for curing them.

Hahnemann's typical anti-syphilitic remedy. Affects the bones, glands and skin. Inflammation leads to induration, then to ulceration. Merc. corresponds accurately to the true Hunterian chancre.

Pronounced tremors, usually commence in the finger. Tremor of weakness and paralysis. B. Cooper noted that it may attack the heart and cause sudden death on the smallest effort. Great tendency to fainting. The tremors may become jerkings and even convulsions. Parkinson's disease. Shaking and trembling with exertion.

Dissolves the living tissues by inducing emaciation. Offensive, rapidly decomposing ulcers. Ulcers, gray, ashy, lard or cheesy base, with burning or stinging pains. Obstinate varicose ulcers. Phagedenic ulcer that just gets bigger and spreads to other areas. General decomposition.

Bone ulcers, pains are deep and boring, aching. Deteriorating bones. The bones soften so that they will bend. Bone pains at night in the legs. Wounds and sores that are slow to heal. Bruise easily. Injuries may open up, ulcerate and discharge.

Scurfy, syphilitic, and pustular eruptions. Eruptions worse by warmth, at night, by cold. Moist, oozing, offensive eczema. Shingles. Suppurative stage of smallpox. Itching, voluptuous itching. Soreness and sensitiveness. Stabbing pains and stitches, burning, boring, digging, stinging and dragging pains.

Tendency to the formation of pus. Bloody pus, pus forms in cavities or abscesses that burn and sting. Discharges are yellow-green in color. Discharges are acrid, excoriating, irritating, except for vaginal discharges. Abscesses, boils, and ulcers with pus or pus with discharges that are yellow, green and acrid.

Chronic discharges from the lungs, nose and vagina, and colon. Gonorrhea. Vaginitis with yellow, green discharge, acrid over the whole vaginal area. Burning, itching, stinging, very offensive, the glands in the inguinal area can sweat.

Enlargement of glands with pricking pains, inflammation, suppuration. Chronic swollen glands. History of infections. Weakness and exhaustion, shortness of breath. Emaciation, shaky and fragile (Gels., Sil.). Immune weakness, AIDS. Allergies.

Suppressed measles or scarlet fever, causing acute problem with the brain, rolling the head back and forth, with severe head sweats. Profuse sweat accompanies nearly all complaints. Sweat does not relieve, may aggravate. Chronic night sweats. Nightmares and palpitations, wake up sweating.

Chronic colds (Psor.). Mono. Sensitive to every draft and yet worse by warmth, the nasal secretion is acrid and the nose red and excoriated. Old, catarrhal smell in the nose, smarting and burning inside nostrils.

Aching, tearing and pressing out in the bones. Recurring otitis media with foul, green discharge that is acrid and offensive.

Tendency to eardrum rupture. Sharp, stabbing pain in the ear. Fetid ear discharge.

Excessive saliva, bad taste in the mouth. Metallic taste in the mouth. Mercurial odor, offensive, breath excessively fetid, sweat offensive, mawkish, sweetish. Throat dry and forepart of tongue moist. Characteristic flabby, coated, teeth-indented tongue, foul breath and intense thirst. Mapped, cracked tongue.

Sore and raw feeling in the back of the mouth. Sores in mouth and nose. Abscesses. Canker sores, bleeding gums. Ulcers, white patches like thrush. Acute boils (Hep., Sil.). Children who get sores in their mouth while breastfeeding. Acute sore throats with stinging, raw feeling.

Aphthous stomatitis, severe pyorrhea. Teething with swollen gums, drooling. Loose teeth, receding gums, pockets of pus (Nit-ac., Hep.). Useful for the affects of dental work, especially if abscessed. Periodontal disease. Jaws crack and pop a lot (Ign., Rhus-t., Caust.).

Congested, enlarged, inflamed liver. Stitches in the liver. Sensitiveness in the liver and inability to lie on right side. Hepatitis. Disordered stomach. Thirsty, even with a moist mouth. Craves bread and butter. Aversion to meat, wine, brandy, beer, coffee, greasy food, butter. Aggravated from milk, sweets, lying on the right side. Food allergies.

Recurring bladder infections where indicated remedies don't work. During stool there is tenesmus, or tenesmus and no stool. Just before stool a sick, painful, faint feeling comes on. Slimy stools, acrid, knotty, containing pus, viscid. Diarrhea with slime.

Dysentery with much straining, never-get-done feeling when there is no more to come. Extreme exhaustion after a stool. Not well since dysentery, with diarrhea, sweating and dehydration.

Affects the generative organs of both sexes. Stinging, cutting pains in the ovaries (Apis.), cutting pains from left to right in lower abdomen. Burning and stinging in the ovaries with ovarian cysts. Breast cancer with ulceration and foul discharges (Ars.). Milk in the breast of non-pregnant women (Puls.).

Characteristic sensitivity to temperature changes, worse from both heat and cold. Sensitivity to draft. Creeping chills, shivering, shaking, and shuddering. Drowsiness during the day, sleepless at night. Symptoms are worse at night, particularly the bone pains. Aggravated by odors, noise, lights, changes of weather, exertion, cold. Ameliorated by lying down.

Extreme restlessness, overreacts, hurried (Med.). The mind is as weak and tremulous as the body, everything is done hastily. Lack of organized response. Speech and mind are slow. Slow comprehension. Time seems to pass slowly. Imbecility. Inefficient (Iod.), workaholics.

Desire to travel or change jobs because of instability. Homesick. Dreams of traveling, floods, delusions of water. Atrophy and deterioration of the brain. Memory loss. Problems with communication, stuttering, especially in children who have earaches (Caust.). Imbecility and senility in the elderly.

Difficulty adjusting to their environment. Tend to be closed, over protective. Anxiety, discontent. Can get anxious and worried about their illness (Ars.). Laughing and weeping spells, break downs. Can be impulsive. Impulses to kill, run away, fears people are after them. Murderous. Suicidal.

Guernsey noted it for "dirty-nosed children." Also that "Merc. is rarely indicated in these troubles where there is no slime."

Kent noted that "Kali-i. is better for the same bursting in the face, running coryza and worse from heat and warmth of the bed." Kent noted that it is useful "whenever cold settles in the eye in gouty and rheumatic patients."

Guided chiefly by the indications profuse sweat with no relief and worse at night, Clarke cured many cases of rheumatic fever with Merc. vivus 12c without any other remedy.

Hirsch of Prague related some striking experiences with a preparation of Merc. vivus that he learned from an old allopath. Quicksilver is boiled in water for half an hour, two teaspoonfuls being given every two hours.

Hirsch recorded cases of acute inflammation of the brain in which Bell. was indicated and in one of which Merc. had already been administered in vain.

Hirsch noted a case in which a black-haired girl, age 9, had a malignant scarlatina, which commenced six days before Hirsch (who came as consultant) saw the case. There were signs of brain inflammation that had set in on the third day.

Hirsch found her unconscious, sharply defined redness of cheeks, pulse 120, skin hot. Piercing screams were emitted from time to time, boring head in pillows, chewing motion of jaws, gnashing teeth.

Lips brown and dry, not much thirst, water not accepted readily, but milk seemed to be relished. Reddened patches here and there, especially along neck. Under the "decoction," which was given to the girl on Hirsch's suggestion, she slowly but steadily improved and in a week was convalescent.

RELATIONS - ***Antidote:*** Hep., Aur., Mez. ***Compare:*** (1) Bell. - very close analog, often complementary, commencing of abscess, difficult swallowing fluids, sharp pain through tonsils, pains come suddenly. (2) Hep. - chilliness, something sticking in fauces. (3) Meny. - coldness in ears. (4) Puls. - thick yellow nasal discharge, but that of Puls., is bland, otitis. (5) Nux-v. - coryza and sore throat, Nux-v. has scraped feeling, Merc. is always smarting, raw, or sore. Dysentery with Nux-v. tenesmus ceases after stool, with Merc. not, there is the never-get-done feeling. (6) Acon. - dysentery of hot days and cold nights. (7) Lept. - bilious troubles, horribly offensive stools, the griping of Lept. continues after stool but not tenesmus. (8) Ars. - Merc. worse by heat of, but better by rest in bed, Ars. better by heat of, but worse by rest in bed. (9) Ant-c. - dirty tongue, inflammation of eyes worse glare of fire or sunshine. (10) Kali-i. - stitching pains through lungs, Merc. right or left and shooting in different directions. (11) Bor. - sore mouth. (12) Cham. - diarrhea, dentition. (13) Syph. - syphilis, worse heat of stove or bed, worse night. (14) Apis - stinging pain, fetid breath, ovarian affections. (15) Psor. and Med. - foul body smell. (16) Mez. - decay of teeth, Merc. of crowns, Mez. of roots. (17) Chel. and Kali-c. - affect lower lobe right lung, stitches through to back. (18) Pic-ac. - boils in auditory meatus. ***Complementary:*** Bad.

REFERENCES - Boericke. Clarke. Murphy. Phatak.

MERCURIUS SULPHOCYANATUS

(Pharaoh's Serpents)

PHARMACY - merc-s-cy. Mercurius sulphocyanatus. Pharaoh's serpents. Sulphocyanide of mercury. ***Historical dose:*** All potencies.

CLINICAL - Diphtheria. Esophagus, stricture.

HOMEOPATHIC - The well-known scientific toy called *"Pharaoh's serpents"* is composed of the sulphocyanide of mercury. A boy ate one *"serpent,"* and a man took one in water. The symptoms were observed and included general prostration for some days. Heat and constriction in esophagus with difficulty in swallowing and burning in epigastric region and nausea.

MIND - Excessive anxiety.

Face - Pallor, great weakness. Cold skin and frequent shivering.

Limbs - Pain in shoulder joint.

Lungs - Voice rough and hoarse. Tenacious expectoration.

Mouth - Constant salivation. Disgusting, metallic taste.

Pulse - Pulse intermitting every three beats.

Rectum - Bloody stools.

Stomach - Vomiting. Epigastrium painful to pressure.

Throat - Extreme redness of throat with white membrane on tonsils. Violent burning in fauces.

Vertigo - Vertigo on attempting to rise.

REFERENCES - Clarke.

MERCURIUS SULPHURICUS

(Yellow Precipitate of Mercury)

PHARMACY - merc-s. Mercurius sulphuricus. Yellow precipitate of mercury. Hydrargyrum oxydatum sub-sulphuricum. Turpethum minerale. Turpeth mineral. Trituration. ***Historical dose:*** All potencies.

CLINICAL - Cardiac, pain. Debility. Diarrhea. Dropsy. ***Dyspnea***. Dysuria. Edema. ***Hydrothorax.*** Rheumatic pains. Sneezing. Ulcers.

HOMEOPATHIC - There is some confusion about the identity of this drug in books. Turpeth is correctly given by Allen. Hering, who proved and introduced it, calls it Turpethum and Turpeth mineral.

The Pharmacopeia of the American Institute of Homeopathy describes the white sulphate, $HgSO_4$, under the heading Mercurius sulphuricus, but says it is mentioned in Allen's Encyclopedia, vol. 6., p. 325, whereas it is Turpeth, the yellow precipitate, which is there spoken.

Merc-s. has ***intense dyspnea***, must sit up. Respiration rapid, short, burning in chest. Cardiac pain and weakness. ***Hydrothorax*** (Ars.). Debility with sleepiness. Rheumatic pains. Most pains feel as if a dull stick pressed on the parts and were moving in diverse curved lines, feels as if this pain were in the bones. Edema of legs.

Sneezing from direct rays of sun. Sore tip of tongue. Scanty, clear, scalding urine. Watery stools, burning in anus. Diarrhea early in the morning, stool bursts out in a hot stream of yellow matter. Intense evacuations like rice-water.

MIND - Morose. Low-spirited with chilliness and yawning. Ill-humor after eating.

Abdomen - Coldness or burning in abdomen. Wakes at 1 a.m. with severe pains along duodenum to umbilical region. Soreness in inguinal glands.

Chest - Pain in right side of chest, extending to scapula, can scarcely breathe, worse from 4 p.m. to 5 p.m. Pain in chest prevents him from breathing. Pressure on chest. Burning in chest. Hydrothorax from liver or heart disorders.

Ears - Burning in ears and in face after a chill.

Eyes - Oppression over eyes. Eyes worse from sunlight.

Face - Pale, anxious countenance. Swelling of parotid gland.

Head - Fullness in head with occasional stitches. Soreness and heaviness through head, after breakfast and when walking about. Sensation of giddiness while standing after headache. Violent itching of hairy scalp.

Kidneys - Diminished secretion of urine, does not urinate frequently, but has constant pressure. Increased secretion of urine without a sediment. Urine dark, becoming turbid with a scum on it. Urine scanty and scalding, but clear.

Limbs - Numbness in left forearm and hand, later numbness in right hand. Hands icy cold with blue nails. Stiffness in arms. Pain in knees and lameness, especially when walking. Foot-sweat with soreness at ends of the nails. Ulcers on ankles.

Lungs - Dyspnea in children. Sensation of heat in larynx. Increased expectoration of mucus from larynx and trachea.

Male - Gonorrhea and syphilitic diseases with great congestions to the parts. Swelling of testicles. Involuntary emission and lascivious dreams.

Mouth - Mouth clammy and full of mucus in morning. Salivation. Burning, smarting, stinging pain on tip of tongue, left side in evening. Lips, gums, fauces, mouth and tongue swollen, look dry and black. Gums and palate dark bluish (black), ulcerated margins.

Nose - Sneezing in sunshine with fluent coryza. Swelling and soreness of tip of nose. Itching of nose.

Rectum - After drinking coffee, pain in abdomen as if diarrhea would set in. Sudden and violent pressing to stool while walking compelling him to stand still, with anxious perspiration. Stools forcibly gush out in a hot, burning stream of yellow water, followed by great debility, hiccough and belching. Violent purging, rice-water motions, some yellow. Stools soft and earlier in morning than usual.

After stools, sensation of fullness as from congestion to legs, especially feet, feel numb when standing.

Skin - Induration of the glands. Psoriasis, leprosy.

Sleep - Frequent yawning and great sleepiness in afternoon. Sleeplessness after midnight. Awakens with headache in morning.

Stomach - Pain, weight in stomach, tenderness. Stomach so irritated nothing would stay on it an instant. Violent yellow vomiting, diarrhea.

Temperature - Chilliness running up back with yawning and depression of spirit, followed by dull pain in forehead, burning in face and ears and slight fever. Chilliness, restlessness and heaviness in upper part of abdomen, frequent yawning and diminished secretion of urine, in afternoon.

Throat - Heat and sensation of constriction in throat. Burning in mouth and throat. Dryness of tongue and throat. Roughness in the throat and hoarseness.

Tongue - Tongue, greenish yellow down middle, heavily coated white. Tongue yellowish at root. Enlarged papilla stand up like red points with flat taste in mouth and a reduced pulse.

COMMENTS - Lippe is the chief clinical authority for Merc-s. He considered it as important as Ars. in dropsies of the chest. The symptoms on which it has been prescribed are clinical and have been well confirmed. Among them is "Pain in right chest extending to scapula, he can scarcely breathe, worse 4 p.m. to 5 p.m."

When Merc-s. acts well, said Lippe, "it produces a profuse watery diarrhea with great relief to the patient." It is particularly suited to hydrothorax depending on liver or heart disorders.

Other confirmed symptoms include soreness of tip of tongue. Edema of legs. Scanty and scalding urine, but clear. Worse in afternoon, 4 p.m. to 5 p.m. Better by profuse diarrhea (dyspnea). After diarrhea stools, there is numbness of legs.

RELATIONS - ***Compare:*** (1) Merc-acet. - cutting in urethra when last drop is flowing out. (2) Cinnb., Aethi-a. and other mercuries. (3) Hydrothorax, Ars. (4) Worse afternoon, Lyc. (5) Dropsy, Dig.

REFERENCES - Boericke. Clarke. Lippe. Phatak.

_MERCURIUS VIVUS

(See Mercurius Solublis Hahnemanni)

METHYLENUM COERULEUM

(Methylene blue)

PHARMACY - meth-b. methyl. Methylenum coeruleum. Methylene blue. Teleamethylthionine chloride. One of the aniline dyes. A diphenyl amine compound, also classed as an aniline color. Trituration. Solution. ***Historical dose:*** All potencies.

CLINICAL - Albuminuria. Arthritis. Cancer. Chorea. Coma. ***Cystitis.*** Epilepsy. Epithelioma. ***Gonorrhea.*** Hemicrania. Kidneys, disorders. Malaria. Nephritis. ***Neuralgias.*** Neurasthenia. Pleurisy. Rheumatism. Spasms. Spinal irritation. Suppuration. Tremors. ***Typhoid fever.***

HOMEOPATHIC - Methylene blue consists of small, indigo-colored, scaly crystals with a bronze-like tinge, that are dark green in transverse fracture. Slightly soluble in water, forming a deep blue solution. It has been used in old-school practice in doses of about three grains in capsules or pills for rheumatism of joints and muscles and in rheumatoid arthritis.

The dyes are carcinogenic. Mosetig treated a man, 50, who suffered from cancer of the femur. Mosetig injected into the groin a 1 percent solution of "Trichlorate of Aniline," increasing the strength, until four grams were used at one injection. Almost an hour after the first injection the patient became dark blue, the next morning the discoloration was gone.

After the four-gram doses, poisoning symptoms appeared including unconsciousness, stertorous breathing, feeble pulse, the whole body becoming dark blue. Artificial breathing and stimulants brought the patient around in four hours. Smaller doses were used after that. In eight weeks he went home, cured to follow his ordinary work. Methyl-violet 1 to 500 and 1 to 1,000 produced equally good results.

Methyl. is a remedy for neuralgia, neurasthenia. Malaria. ***Typhoid fever***. delirium and fever.

Tendency to tremor, chorea and epilepsy. Later states of a stroke. Backache, sciatica. Gonorrheal rheumatism and cystitis. Pus infection.

Nephritis (acute parenchymatous), scarlatinal nephritis. Urine acquires a green color. Bladder irritation from its use is antidoted by a little nutmeg. Surgical kidney with large amount of pus in urine. Tympanites.

Cancerous ulcerations on the skin and mucus membrane and on internal organs such as uterus, lungs and the gastrointestinal tract. Hemorrhages are mostly bright red with few clots. Cough with blood-streaked expectoration and difficult breathing.

MIND - Neurasthenia. Unconsciousness.

Back - Backache with sciatica.

Bladder - Irritation of the bladder. Cystitis. Urine greenish. Gonorrhea.

Chest - Causes absorption of pleural effusion.

Head - Hemicrania. Habitual headache.

Limbs - Tremors. Spastic hysterical contractions.

Lungs - Stertorous breathing.

Skin - Turns the patient dark blue. Pus infection.

Temperature - Typhoid fever. Malarial fever. Fever from pus absorption.

COMMENTS - The kidneys have a distinct attraction for Methyl., as it appears in the urine within half an hour of the dose and, if the kidneys have their normal permeability, the whole is eliminated in thirty-six hours. If there is delay beyond this it indicates that the urea is not being perfectly eliminated and that a tendency to uremia exists. The aniline products have been used as remedies for malignant growths.

Mosetig of Moorhof published a case treated with Trichlorate of Aniline, "an aniline dye."

E. Thomson, stated that Methyl. in 1-5 grains doses, "with equal parts powdered nutmeg to prevent irritation of the bladder" (a useful item in view of the homeopathic employment) is valuable in habitual headache and hemicrania.

Cardamantes of Athens gave 10 to 12 grs. ten hours before an expected malarial attack. He said it is useful in combination with quinine or when quinine had failed. Immunity from malaria seems to follow its continued use.

Apt to cause cystitis. A gentleman who suffered excruciating pains from calculus in the kidney, giving rise to pyelitis and cystitis, derived no benefit from any treatment until his doctor gave him Methyl. with occasional doses of eucalyptus.

L'Art Medical gave an account of the use of Methyl. injection in pleurisy with serous effusion. C. H. Lewis of New York, first drew off by aspiration 100 cubic centimeters of the liquid, dissolved in this one grain of Methyl. and reinjected it into the pleural cavity.

The patient soon began to pass greenish urine and then the exudation quickly disappeared, partly from the diuretic effect of Methyl., partly from its stimulating action on the pleura. A watery solution is not borne, causing pain and irritation of the pleura.

The most homeopathic experience is that of Halbert. Utilizing the affinity of Methyl. for nerve tissues and nerve cells, Halbert gave it in 3x trituration with success in neuralgias of neurasthenia, tremor in neurasthenia, spasticity of hysterical contraction, trophic disturbances, the result of nerve-exhaustion, and spinal irritation.

Halbert confirmed its anti-malarial powers and commended it in typhoid as an intestinal anti-septic. An apparently hopeless case of typhoid was signally benefited by it, the tympanites disappearing as if by magic. Wherever there is pus infection it is indicated and it has "made a record" with him in gonorrhea and cystitis.

RELATIONS - ***Compare:*** (1) Anil., Pyrog..

REFERENCES - Boericke. Clarke. Grimmer.

MEZEREUM

(Spurge Olive)

PHARMACY - mez. Mezereum. Spurge olive. Daphne mezereum. Chameleons germanica. Mezereon. N. O. Thymelaceae. Hilly woods over nearly whole of Europe and Russian Asia. Tincture of fresh bark gathered just before the plant flowers in February and March. ***Historical dose:*** All potencies.

CLINICAL - Abscesses. Anus prolapsed. Bones disorders. ***Ciliary, neuralgia***. Coccyx, pain. Constipation. Contraction, tendons. Convulsions. Crusta lactea. Ear, affections. ***Eczema. Eruptions***. Erythema. Exostoses. Eyes, disorders. Glands, enlarged. Gleet. Gonorrhea. Hematuria. Hernia. Herpes, zoster. Impetigo. ***Itching.*** Leucorrhea. Lice. Mercury, effects. ***Neuralgias.*** Osteoma. Periostitis. Pityriasis. ***Pruritus, senilis.*** Rheumatism. Scrofula. ***Skin, disorders.*** Syphilis. Teeth, affection. ***Testicles, enlarged.*** Tinea, capitis. Tinea, versicolor. Tongue, disorders. Twitchings. ***Ulcers.*** Vaccination.

HERBAL - The plant flowers in very early spring, even when snow is on the ground. Suited to complaints that come on in the earliest months of the year.

HOMEOPATHIC - Hahnemann recorded the history of a robust man who took mezereum bark for some ailment and continued it after the ailment disappeared. Soon, unbearable itching set in all over his body, and he could not sleep a moment. Thirty-six hours after discontinuing it, the itching was still increasing. A few grains of camphor removed it.

Mez. is the vegetable analog of Merc., it and Mez. antidote one another. The mind, skin, eyes, mucus membranes and bones are affected in much the same way by both. They have the same sensitiveness to damp, cold and warmth and the same nightly aggravations.

Mez. affects skin, bones, nerves and mucus membranes of the mouth and stomach. Affinity for skin symptoms and disorders of bones and neuralgias, especially about the teeth and face.

Bruised, weary feeling in joints with drawing and stiffness. ***Pains of various kinds with chilliness and sensitiveness to cold air***. Sudden pains of various kinds followed by chilliness, numbness and soreness. Pains shoot upward and seem to draw the patient up out of bed.

Irritation, burning itching or burning smarting on the skin. Violent, burning, darting like fire in the muscles. Burning, darting sensation in the muscles, subsultus tendinum. Burning, boring pains in bones especially long bones, with neuralgia of the teeth and face or after shingles. Decay, exostosis of bones. Periostitis. Bones seem enlarged.

Internal burning with external violent itching in small areas or in single parts. Acrid secretions, pus, leucorrhea, etc. Ulcers. Eruptions after vaccination. Cystic osteoma. Abscesses of fibrous parts or tendons. Body feels light. Twitchings in the eyelids, on the right side of the face etc. Convulsions better by tight grasping.

Affected parts become cold or emaciate. One sided symptoms, whole or partial. Excessive sensitiveness to air, even of a fan. As if a cool breeze blowing on the part. Affections go from above downward, from within outward, and from right to left. Worse from cold, damp, cold winds, sudden changes of weather, heat, and warm food.

Nash mentioned an exception to the worse by warmth modality. In a man whom he cured with Mez. of obstinate facial neuralgia, the pains were brought on or greatly worsened by eating, and the only relief the man could get was by holding the painful side close to a hot stove. Only radiated heat was of any use, hot cloths, wet or dry, gave no relief whatever.

MIND - Forgetful. ***Vanishing of thoughts while speaking***, unable to repeat what has been learned by heart. Indifference to everything and everybody, looks through a window for hours without being conscious of objects around. Dullness of mind after sound sleep.

Apprehensive at the pit of the stomach when expecting some very unpleasant news or shock. ***Irresolution.***

Nervous, compelled to move and change positions. Aversion to talk, it seems to be hard work to utter a word.

Hypochondriac and despondent. Sadness about trifles, when alone. Religious or financial melancholy. Despair of eternal salvation. Anger alternating with quick repentance. Vexed and angry at trifles. ***Censorious.*** Reproaches or quarrels with others. Irritability during headache.

Abdomen - Burning and heat in abdomen. Swelling of glands with large abdomen in children. Contraction of diaphragm. Pressure in inguinal ring. Dull or severe pain in region of spleen. Stitches in left hypochondrium. Flatulent colic with shivering and difficult respiration.

Back - Pain in muscles of back. Pain in neck and back, worse motion and at night intolerant of all touch. Violent itching rash on nape. Stiff pain in nape and muscles of sides, worse motion. Rheumatic pain in right scapula, in morning after rising. Shuddering over back and limbs, when itching is most severe. Coccyx painful after a fall.

Causations - Ill effects of suppressed eczema capitis, vaccination and mercury.

Chest - Stitches in chest. Sore pain in right axilla. Soreness and burning in bones of thorax. Constriction across chest. Contraction of diaphragm. Painful tension in intercostal muscles. Chest feels too tight on stooping. Sensation as if ants were running over chest. Intercostal neuralgia following herpes zoster, worse at night and in warmth of bed. Red spots like fleabites on chest.

Constitutions - Suited to light-haired persons, phlegmatic temperament, irresolute. Gouty, rheumatic, syphilitic miasm.

Cough - Irritation in throat causes hacking cough. Dry tickling cough, into vomiting. Cough, worse eating, on taking a warm drink. Cough from beer. Must cough till food is vomited.

Ears - Thickening of tympanum. Ears feel too open, ***as if tympanum was exposed to the cold air and it blew into the ear***. Chronic diffuse otitis. Oozing eruption behind ear. Itching behind ears, scratching causes small elevations, when scratched off the spots feel sore. Desire to bore fingers into ears. Deafness after suppression of head eruptions.

Eyes - Eyes feel strained. Dryness of the eyes, they feel too large. Pains radiate and shoot downward with ***cold feeling and stiffness of bone.*** Pain outward along the brows. Smarting pain in eyes, with lachrymation. Lachrymation with any pains. ***Ciliary neuralgia after operations***, especially after removal of eyeball. Inclination to wink, jerking of eyelids. Obstinate twitching of muscles of left upper lid. Eczema of lids.

Face - Red. Facial muscles drawn tight. Face swollen, burning pains, confluent vesicles. Boils on face. Impetigo. Eruptions around the mouth with coryza. Cracks in corners of mouth. Scabs about mouth. Ulcers on upper lip. Lips swollen, dry, scaly externally, painful, sore and burning. Chin covered with elevated, white scabs. ***Violent neuralgia about face and teeth***, running towards ear, at night, ***worse eating***, better near hot stove. Neuralgic pains come and go quickly and leave part numb. Sudden pains, wakes from sleep. Left-sided prosopalgia. Twitching of muscles, right sided. Boring pains in bones of upper jaw. Violent itching of face and scalp.

Female - Menses scanty with face ache. Menses too frequent, too soon, too profuse. Leucorrhea like albumen, very corroding. Ulceration of vagina and cervix.

Food - Loss of appetite. Constant longing for food. Confusion after eating. Thirst during chill. Aversion to meat. Craving for bacon, ham, fat, coffee, wine. Desire for acid drinks. Beer tastes bitter and causes vomiting. Worse from wine. Itching temporarily better from wine and coffee.

Head - Violent headache on slightest touch, after vexation. Headache, worse from talking. Stupefying headache in right side. Numbness of one side of scalp or top of head. Pressing pains as if skull would split. Pains on slightest touch in temples and sides. Cranial bones painful. Boring pains in bones of occiput. Violent congestion to head during menopause. Affections of external head, scaly eruption, white scabs. Burning pain of scalp. Intolerable itching. ***Eczema capitis.*** Head covered with ***thick, leathery crusts, under which pus collects***. Milk crusts. Exostosis. Sore boils. White scabs or scales. Hair falls in handfuls. Dandruff, white, dry.

Heart - Pulse full, hard, accelerated evenings. Pulse at times intermittent. Pulse frequent mornings, slow evenings.

Kidneys - Red flakes float on top of urine. Hematuria, hot, preceded by cramps in bladder. After urinating, a few drops of blood are passed. Biting, burning in forepart of urethra at the close of urination.

Limbs - Trembling of limbs. Limbs feel cold, as if shortened. Joints feel bruised and weary, as if they would give way. Pain in hip and knee. Aching, itching in knee. Legs and feet go to sleep. Hands and feet cold, nails blue. One hand hot. Paralysis of flexors of fingers, cannot hold anything. ***Long bones inflamed*** and swollen, decay, exostosis. Pain, worse night touch, damp weather (Merc., Syph.). Burning in tibia and long bones.

Lungs - Dyspnea, as if from adhesions or contraction of lungs. Desire to take a long breath. Snoring in children. Yellow, viscid, salty expectoration. Expectoration during day or tasting like an old catarrh.

Male - ***Testicles enlarged.*** Painless swelling of the penis and scrotum. Heat and swelling of penis. Itching glans penis. Fine, pricking, stitches in penis and tip of glans. Urethra sore. Violent sexual desire. Gonorrhea with hematuria, discharge of watery mucus.

Modalities - Better open air, wrapping up, eating. Facial pains better radiated heat of stove. Head pains better wrapping up head. Headache better stooping. ***Worse at night***, evening until midnight, touch, motion. Worse warmth of bed, fire, warm food, cold, air, drafts, damp. Worse during menses, suppressions, vaccinations, mercury.

Mouth - Salivation. ***Mouth waters***. Taste bitter, sour, beer tastes bitter, which is vomited. Breath smells like rotten cheese. Burning in mouth and throat, sometimes better eating. Ranula, worse talking and chewing, ejects a watery fluid. Dry, dark red mouth. Flat, whitish ulcers on inner side of lips and corners of mouth.

Nose - Sneezing, coryza. Frequent sneezing with pain of excoriation in chest. Visible twitching at the root of nose. Interior of nose excoriated. Post nasal adenoids.

Perspiration - During sleep, following chill. Skin drips with cold sweat.

Rectum - Itching in anus. Biting, sore pain in anus on walking. Constriction of anus, stitches and prolapse of rectum. Burning in rectum. Much painless straining. Painful tenesmus. Constipation with hepatic and uterine inertia. Constipation after confinement. Summer diarrhea of children. Diarrhea with small, white glistening particles. ***Green discharges***. Constant passing of flatus, but in a short and interrupted manner.

Sensations - Head as if drunk, as if everything in the head would press asunder. As if skull would split, as if top of head gone, as if head bruised, as if head was in an ants' nest. Eyes as if too large, as if drawn back into head. Throat as if narrowing. As if food remained long time in stomach. Stools feel as if they would split anus. Limbs feel shortened. As if fire darting through muscles. Sensation of lightness of body. Bones are very sore and feel distended. Diseased parts wither.

Skin - Skin wrinkled and in folds. Eruptions ulcerate and form thick scabs under which purulent matter exudes (Chrys-ac.). ***Eruptions, ooze, acrid, gluey moisture, form thick crusts, scabs with pus beneath*** or chalky white. ***Intolerable, itching***, worse by warm bath, worse in bed. As if millions of insects were crawling on him. ***Crusty eruptions, white scabs***, bleeding when touched. Skin cold on places where itching is most intense. ***Pruritus senilis.*** Itching changes place on scratching, coldness after. Itching without eruption. Itch-like eruption, after vaccination, depriving child of sleep. ***Eczema.*** Psoriasis. ***Herpes zoster with burning pain.*** Liver spots on chest and arms become dark and desquamate. Ulcers itch and burn, surrounded by vesicles and shining, fiery-red areola. Deep, hard, painful ulcers worse touch and warmth. Old ulcers burn and sting. Ulcers form over bony protuberances. Desquamation over whole body. Scurf like fish scales on back, thighs, chest and scalp.

Sleep - Much yawning and stretching. Irresistible sleepiness during day. Sleepiness from debility. Sleeplessness from itching. Sleeplessness from cramps in calves. Sleep disturbed by violent pain in face. Nightmare at night, awakening after midnight.

Stomach - Chronic gastritis, burning, corroding pain. Constant, severe pain and pressure in stomach even after light foods. Induration of stomach. ***Stomach ulcer*** with much burning. ***Burning and corroding pain*** in stomach, better milk and eating. Constricting, pinching pain in stomach. Sensation of apprehension, fear, faintness and goneness at stomach as if something was going to happen. Sensation as if food remained for a long time undigested in stomach and caused pressure. Stomach pain culminates and ends with retching and vomiting of all food taken. Vomiting of chocolate colored substance with nausea. Vomit bitter, sour, slimy, oily or greasy. Water brash.

Stools - Stools preceded and followed by shivering. Stools, hard, large, as if they would split the anus. Stool soft, brown, sour, fermented, undigested, offensive.

Temperature - Chill of single parts as if dashed with cold water. Chill alternating with flushes of heat. General weakness. Great tendency to get remittent or typhoid fever. Ague.

Throat - Dark, red, burning, sore, worse winter. Burning in mouth and throat, sometimes better eating. Burning in pharynx and esophagus. Throat as if dry. Sensation as if posterior part of throat were full of mucus. Swallowing even of fluids difficult and painful, from severe burning and raw pain. Constriction of pharynx. Sensation of narrowing in throat. Nausea felt in throat, better eating.

Teeth - Teeth feel dull and elongated. Teeth feel cold. Teeth painful on biting on them and from cold air. Roughness from tartar on teeth. Roots of teeth decay. Rapid decay of hollow teeth. Toothache into temples, better with mouth open and from drawing in air. Toothache in gums from cold air. Toothache from congestion to head. Sensation as if tooth was being lifted out of socket.

Tongue - Burning in tongue with salivation. Tongue coated along one side only. Middle of the tongue fissured. Thick, white coating on tongue with large, red, elevated papillae.

Vertigo - Vertigo with contracted pupils, faintness. Vertigo and flickering before eyes, inclination to fall to left side.

COMMENTS - A case reported in Allen's Appendix recorded the history of a pale girl, 14, having been advised to use mezereum leaves to make her fat and rosy, went into the woods and used them freely on her cheeks and surrounding parts.

Burning soon set in, the whole face swelled enormously, especially the nose, eyelids and hairy scalp. Severe and painful sneezing, delirium, dull, unbearable, pressing pains in forehead, a nauseous dryness in throat and constant irritation to dry cough. The face soon showed the appearance of erysipelas bullosum, nostrils closed, she could only breathe through her mouth, febrile pulse, burning urine.

Oil and compresses were applied, and after the second day desquamation occurred in large areas. Health did not return. Debility followed, with loss of vitality, mental depression bordering on idiocy. Then typhoid fever, lasting fully for three months to which she finally succumbed.

Poisoning has also been observed from the effects of the berries, causing dryness and burning of throat and stomach, intense thirst, a narcotic state, coma, and convulsions of eyes and upper limbs.

In a child of four, poisoned with the berries, the lips swelled, the tongue was furred and swollen, protruding, with difficult swallowing. The tongue remained quite raw when other symptoms had passed away.

Mez. is one of Hahnemann's anti-psoric remedies. Ulcers, with thick, yellowish, white scabs. Vesicles, itch and burn. Lint dressings stick to them and when they are torn away, bleeding occurs. Burning vesicles on the sides of the fingers and ulcers on finger joints.

Canker sores with a scab, pus (Rhus-t., Nat-m.). Herpes zoster, shingles itch and burn and form scabs. Herpes zoster, during the eruption and for the neuralgia remaining after, especially if the pains are burning. Vaccination eczemas. Psoriasis and eczema, itching, worse in bed and from touch. Intolerable itching, migratory itching.

Skin is scabby looking, with an itch underneath the scab that aggravates. Pimples on ankles and backs of feet, horrid taste and clamminess of mouth in morning. Pimples better by hard scratching. Dry crust on the scalp and falling out of hair, accompanied with short sight.

Bone pains, particularly of the long bones. The least touch is intolerable. Affinity for the facial bones and teeth (Merc.). Decay attacks the roots or sides of the teeth, rather than the crowns (Merc.). Toothache is worse at night, from touch, even with the tongue. Better by holding the mouth open and drawing in air.

Neuralgia about the eyes, the pains radiate and shoot downward. Sensation in the eye as if a cold wind were blowing in it. Hypersensitiveness of the ear to air. Feeling as if air went through the ear to the throat.

Stitching, burning and itching in the rectum and anus. During stool, the rectum prolapsed and the sphincter closes upon the protruded part. Sluggish bowels. Constipation after confinement.

Constricting tendency in the throat, stomach and tendons. Enlarged testicles (Clem.). The leg is shortened with pain in the hip. Tension in muscles of the chest. Pain and stiffness in muscles of neck. Cramp-like contraction over chest and back and across front of chest.

Cooper noted that green discharges were particularly characteristic.

Carroll Dunham recorded a notable case of deafness, due to suppressed psora. A youth, age 17, deaf since four and incapacitated thereby, secluded himself and brooded over his trouble. Membranes thickened.

At the age of three, he had an eruption of thick, whitish scabs, hard, almost horny, covering the whole scalp. There were fissures through which exuded on pressure a thick, yellowish pus, often very offensive. There was much itching and disposition to tear off the scabs with the fingernails, worse at night.

The allopathic treatment was vigorous, a tar cap was placed on the head and when firmly adherent to the scabs was violently torn off, scabs and all, leaving the whole scalp raw. This was painted with a saturated solution of Arg-n. The eruption did not reappear, but from that time the child was deaf. The eruption was the very counterpart of an eruption observed in a proving by Wehle.

Mez. 30c, three globules in a powder of sugar of milk, was given on February 3, March 1, and September 28, 1857 and January 26, 1858. Improvement set in slowly after the first dose, which was only repeated when the effect of each preceding dose seemed to be exhausted. Finally, the hearing was for all practical purposes completely restored.

The action of Mez. in catarrhal cases is illustrated in the case of Miss M. R., 39, a brunette, who had chronic catarrh. The left ear had long been deaf and the right had begun to fail. There were noises in the ears. Drum membranes retracted and scarred.

The naso-pharynx mucus membrane was granular and irritable. There was excessive sensitiveness to the air, even of a fan and occasionally a sensation as if air went through to the throat. A dose of Mez. given before each meal entirely relieved the symptoms.

T. S. Hoyne collected many cases illustrating the action of the remedy including a case of a woman treated by W. E. Payne. She had no rest when alone, wanted company. Ideas vanished while talking, could not repeat what had been learned by heart. Looked through the window for hours without being conscious of objects around.

Did not know what she was doing, forgot what she was about to utter, looked ill-humored pale, wretched, fallen away. Apprehensiveness at pit of stomach, as when expecting some very unpleasant intelligence. All symptoms relieved in a single night by Mez. 20c.

S. R. Geiser noted the case of a man, 28, who had a violent neuralgia, boring pain in left lower jaw bone, extending to temple and ear. Pain was worse at night, better from pressure. Mez. 3c relieved in two hours.

J. W. Vance recorded the history of H. G., stout, healthy-looking, left supra-orbital neuralgia recurring daily at 9 a.m. increasing until noon, declining until 4 p.m., when it entirely departed leaving no soreness behind. Pain caused flow of tears. Mez. 1c cured permanently after other remedies had failed.

Hempel noted the case of a toothache in the incisor of a woman. Tooth felt elongated, loose, excessively sensitive with sensation as if being raised out of its socket. Upper part of tooth was excessively painful. Mez. 200c cured in a few hours.

Oehme noted the case of Mrs. X., who had pain in her right eye tooth, daily increasing. Felt too long. Pains much worse by pressure on crown and outside root. Mez. 2c cured.

Oehme also recorded a case in which the fastenings of a hammock broke and a woman on it fell, striking her sacrum and coccyx on the stump of a tree. She suffered excruciating pain. Arn. was applied locally. In a few weeks she came home and the coccyx was still so tender she could not sit, only lie or stand. Arn. internally and externally for two weeks had no influence. Mez. 2c cured in five days.

Cooper noted the case of a woman, 48, who had rheumatism which came on ten years before in her hands from wearing wet gloves and extended later to arms and knees. She had stiffness on walking with loss of muscular power, worse in hot weather, "pins and needles" in fingers on elevating arms. Could not grasp things, sometimes one hand burned when the other was cold, menopausal flushings. Great relief from Mez. tincture.

Cooper also noted that Daphne laureola, the British representative of the genus, cured scald-head when Mez. failed to work.

The symptoms in this case were worse by day, whereas Mez. has worse at night. The pains of D. laureola come on in the morning and affect the entire head or whole left side. Guai. pains are also worse by day and better by warmth.

H. B. Esmond cured with Mez. 3x a youth, 17, who had been afflicted with "salt rheum" as long as he could remember. It was absent in summer, but every autumn, as soon as cold weather came, his face, neck, hands and forearms would break out and continue sore until warm weather returned.

Mez. cured a girl, 18, getting thin with headache across forehead, temples and eyes, a throbbing with sickness of stomach and water brash, always worse by movement, bowels very confined, menses never appeared.

H. Noah Martin noted a patient that said "my stools are as hard as stone and as large a my arm. I feel as if they would split me open. They come in sections like mouthfuls and I becomes much exhausted and tremble with weakness. Every stool is immediately preceded by chills and followed by long stitches up rectum." Mez. 12c produced a natural stool in twelve hours.

RELATIONS - ***Antidotes:*** Kali-hp., Merc. ***Compare:*** (1) Merc., Phyt., Rhus-t., Guai., Syph.

REFERENCES - Boericke. Clarke. Murphy. Phatak.

MICROMERIA DOUGLASII

(Yerba Buena)

PHARMACY - micr. Micromeria douglasii. Yerba buena. California. ***Historical dose:*** Tincture and all potencies.

CLINICAL - Colic. Flatulence. Nausea.

HERBAL - A California mint-like plant acting on stomach and bowels. It is a pleasant beverage and febrifuge, blood purifier and tonic. Used as a tea for colic and to relieve flatulence. Nausea with pain in the stomach and bowels.

REFERENCES - Boericke.

MILLEFOLIUM ACHILLEA

(Yarrow)

PHARMACY - mill. Millefolium achillea. Yarrow. Achillea millefolium. N. O. Composite. Asteraceae. Tincture of whole fresh plant. ***Historical dose:*** Tincture and all potencies.

CLINICAL - Anemia. Ascites. Asthma. Bed-wetting. Bleeding. ***Blows. Bruises.*** Cancer. Chlorosis. Colic. Dentition. Diarrhea. Dysmenorrhea. Epilepsy. Fistula lachrymalis. Hematemesis. Hematuria. ***Hemoptysis. Hemorrhages.*** Hypochondriasis. Hysteria. Infertility. ***Injuries.*** Leucorrhea. Lochia, profuse. Lochia, suppressed. Milk, absence. Nipples, sore. ***Nosebleeds.*** Puerperal convulsions. Puerperal fever. Rodent ulcers. Sycosis. Tetanus. ***Trauma.*** Tuberculosis. ***Varicose, veins. Urine, bloody. Wounds.***

HERBAL - Yarrow was named Achillea by Linneus because the plant is mentioned in the Iliad as having been used by Achilles on the instruction of Chiron to heal the wounds of his soldiers.

Millefolium received its popular name, "nosebleed," because nosebleed comes on if the leaves are inserted into the nostrils. The other species of Achillea indigenous to Great Britain, Achillea ptarmic, is called "sneeze-wort" from its allergic properties.

HOMEOPATHIC - Mill. affects the ***capillaries of lungs,*** nose and uterus. Suited to all ***wounds which bleed profusely***, sprains and over-lifting. Profuse, painless, bright, red, fluid hemorrhages. ***Nosebleeds.*** Hemoptysis. Oozing of blood from the edges of closed wounds from over exertion.

Spasms or convulsions especially after the suppression of hemorrhages, menses, lochia, milk etc. ***Varicose veins in pregnancy.*** Bruised soreness and congestions. ***Sprains and over-lifting.*** Bad effects from fall from a height. Profuse mucus discharges. Piercing thrusts of pain. Incarcerated hernia. Smallpox with great pain in pit of stomach. ***Continued high temperature***.

MIND - Forgetfulness. Loss of memory. Difficulty thinking and comprehending. Confusion and dullness in evening. Confusion after coffee, wine. Desires nothing. Does not know what he is doing or wants to do. Aversion to mental work. Moaning, sighing and groaning of children.

Anxiety in chest, heart. Anxiety, excitement from pains. Anxiety better on rising from a seat. Very excited with pain in stomach. Sadness. Violent, irritable. Hysteria. Delusions, he has been poisoned. Hypochondriasis. Delirium. Knocking his head against wall.

Abdomen - Ascites. Abdomen distended. Pain in region of the liver. Congestions to portal system. Wind colic. Frequent emission of fetid flatulence. Colic during the menstruation. Violent colic with bloody diarrhea during pregnancy. Dysentery. Hemorrhage from bowels. Incarcerated hernia.

Back - Piercing, drawing pains, under left scapula. Fine piercing pains in left scapula, when standing.

Breasts - Sore nipples. Agalactorrhea. Suppressed secretion of milk.

Causations - Ill effects from operations for kidney stones, gallstones. ***Bad effects from a fall or sprain***, injuries, over-lifting, over-exertion. Suppressed lochia, menses, milk.

Chest - Oppression of chest with bloody expectoration or palpitations. Bubbles in chest as if warm blood was ascending.

Constitutions - Suited to the aged, atonic, anemic women and children.

Ears - Darting pain in left ear. Sense of cool air passing through the ears. Noise in left ear causes starting with fright. Sensation of stoppage in ears, after dinner.

Eyes - Glistening, brilliant eyes. Piercing pain from eyes to root of nose. Sensation of too much blood in eyes. Lachrymation and discharges from eyes. Fistula lachrymalis. Agglutination of eyes in morning. Spots on eyes.

Face - Sensation of heat, as if blood was rising to head. Redness of face without internal heat. Tearing pain in face to temples.

Female - Menses early, profuse, protracted. Menses suppressed, with colicky pain in abdomen. ***Convulsions and epilepsy from suppressed menses.*** Leucorrhea from atony of vaginal mucus membrane. Leucorrhea of children. Infertility with too profuse menstruation or tendency to miscarry. Cramps during pregnancy. ***Painful varicose veins during pregnancy.*** Uterine hemorrhages, bright red, fluid, after great exertion. ***Hemorrhage after labor, abortion or miscarriage.*** Prolonged bleeding during labor. Lochia too profuse. Suppressed lochia with violent fever. Curative of post-partum hemorrhage. Severe after-pains.

Food - Want of appetite. Sluggish appetite from stagnation in liver. Thirst during fever. Mouth dry, with thirst. Confusion after coffee, wine. Dullness after wine. Congestion to head from coffee. Symptoms worse coffee, better wine.

Head - Confused, dull headache, in evening, worse after coffee. Head seems full of blood. Fullness in head after siesta. Headache with twitching of eyelids and frontal muscles. ***Piercing thrusts*** of pain. Beats the head against the wall. Headache worse stooping. Throbbing in arteries of head and face.

Heart - Inflammation with tearing and piercing pains. Pains in heart with anxiety. Ebullitions from coughing blood. Violent palpitation with bloody sputum. Pulse accelerated and contracted.

Kidneys - Chilliness with pain in left kidney, followed by hematuria. Catarrh of bladder from atony. Stone in bladder with retention of urine. Pus-like discharge after surgery. ***Urine bloody*** (Senec.). Involuntary urination of children.

Limbs - ***Bad effects from falls and sprains.*** Convulsions, convulsive motion of all limbs and violent pain. Paralysis and contraction of limbs. Violent pains on a level with crest of left ilium. Pricking numbness. Left arm frequently feels as if going to sleep. Hot hands and feet. Right Achilles tendon pains as after a blow or sprain. ***Painful varicose veins during pregnancy.*** Painless or bleeding varices in pregnant women.

Lungs - Shortness of breath. Very difficult breathing, with tetanic spasms. Asthmatic affections. Inflammation of lungs. Excessive accumulation of mucus in bronchi. ***Hemoptysis with incipient tuberculosis.*** Hemoptysis after injury. Expectoration of bright red blood, without much coughing, sometimes in consequence of violent exertions. Cough with bloody sputum in suppressed menses or hemorrhoids. Lung disease with coughing blood.

Male - Wounds and injuries of penis. Swelling of the penis and testicles. Semen is not discharged during sex. Spermatorrhea. Gonorrhea, gleet. Sycotic excrescences.

Modalities - Better from bleeding, re-establishment of discharges. Better during the day, from wine, violent exercise. Violent exercise improves vertigo. ***Worse from violent exertion,.injury***, exertion, lifting, stooping, doubling the body, lying down. Worse evening and night, coffee, hemoptysis, suppression of discharges.

Mouth - Tongue swollen and coated. Thirst, mouth dry. Putrid sore mouth. Gumboils. Rheumatic pain with diseased gums. Toothache from eating things. Useful given before tooth extraction.

Nose - ***Nosebleed*** (Erech.), with congestions to head and chest. Piercing pain from eyes to root of nose. Stuffed nose.

Perspiration - Profuse sweats. Colliquative perspirations.

Rectum - Fetid flatus. Diarrhea, preceded by rattling of fluids in abdomen. Mucus diarrhea. Bloody dysentery. Bloody diarrhea during pregnancy. Hemorrhages from bowels after much exertion. Bleeding hemorrhoids. Pains from blind hemorrhoids. Profuse flow of blood from condylomata. Ascarides.

Sensations - As if he had forgotten something. As if all blood ascended to head. Right side of head as if screwed together. As if too much blood in eyes. As if cold air passing out of ear. As of a liquid moving from stomach to intestines. Pain as from a blow or sprain.

Skin - ***Bruises and bleeding from wounds.*** Wounds after operation for stone in the bladder. Painless varicose veins of pregnant women. Exanthemata and delirium. Suppressed itch, causing fever. Fistulous ulcers. Gangrenous ulcers. Ulceration of internal organs. Cancerous ulcers. Condylomata.

Sleep - Violent yawning without being tired. Goes to sleep late and does not feel refreshed in morning.

Stomach - Stomachache. Painful gnawing and digging in stomach as from hunger. Burning pain in stomach, extending to chest. Sensation of fullness in stomach. Pressure like a plug in stomach. Cramps in stomach with sensation as of a liquid flowing in intestines to anus. Eructations. Hiccough. Vomiting when coughing. Nausea with vertigo. Hematemesis.

Teeth - Toothache from eating things. Gumboil. Ulcers on gums. Rheumatic pain with diseased gums.

Temperature - Chilliness with pain in left kidney. Heat in hands and feet. Fever heat with thirst. Continuous high fever. Fever from suppressed itch or suppressed lochia. Hectic fever with hemoptysis. Malignant fever with tetanus. Intermittent fever. Quartan, tertian, irregular fever.

Throat - Rough feeling in throat. Rough voice. Elongation of palate. Uvula relaxed. Ulceration of throat, pain in left side when swallowing. Dull piercing pain, right then left. Throat catarrh.

Vertigo - Vertigo when moving slowly. Vertigo, falls to right side and backward. Vertigo with nausea when stooping, not when lying down. Violent exercise improves vertigo.

Vision - Vision nebulous with contortions of facial muscles. Clear, bright vision. Foggy vision, not near eyes, but at a distance.

COMMENTS - Hemorrhages and wounds (Arn.). Anti-convulsive. Convulsions occur, although not exclusively, as a result of suppressed hemorrhages, particularly the menses, or other discharges or secretions.

Trauma (Arn., Ham., and Phos.), with profuse bleeding. Hemorrhage with bright, red blood, florid hemorrhage. Tubercular hemorrhage. Bleeding hemorrhoids, bloody urine or stool. Useful for reabsorbing blood clots. Useful after surgeries (Phos.).

Copious mucus discharges, especially due to atony. Pronounced relation to pregnancy and the puerperal state.

Useful for varicose veins during pregnancy. Uterine tonic, particularly for profuse menses.

C. W. related an interesting case in which a man had severe diarrhea, with profuse dark, chocolate-colored stools, verging on black and slightly tinged with blood. A club doctor had failed to relieve, but an old woman cured the man with "yarrow tea."

C. W. had a collie dog that, when excited, would pull up grass or weeds and swallow them. When it happened to swallow Mill., this invariably caused a rattling of fluid in the bowels, followed by dark chocolate diarrhea, changing to black, very offensive, finally blood-tinged.

This lasted a day or two. It was found that Ars-i. 3x in solution was a complete antidote. Given every ten minutes, as soon as rattling came on, it effectually stopped it. The dog also had fissured pads. Ars-i. did nothing for these, but Ars. 30c cured.

RELATIONS - Ant-t. relieves the vertigo to Mill., Ars-i. the diarrhea. ***Antidotes:*** Ars-i., Arum-m. ***Compare:*** (1) Composite group generally, Arn., Bell-p., Calen. (2) Fic-v., Pakur. - hemorrhage from bowels and lungs. (3) Acal., Helix. - in hemoptysis, diseases of chest, tuberculosis. (4) Erech. - nosebleed and hemoptysis. (5) Senec. - hematuria. (6) Ham. and Ip. - hemorrhages. (7) Mill. red, clotted, Plat. dark, clotted. (8) Bry., Ust. and Ham. - hematemesis. (9) Acon. - hemorrhages, profuse flow of bright red blood. (10) Acon., anxiety, Mills., absence of anxiety. ***Incompatible:*** Coffee causes head congestion.

REFERENCES - Boericke. Clarke. Murphy. Phatak.

MIMOSA HUMILIS

(Sensitive Plant)

PHARMACY - mim-h. Mimosa humilis. Sensitive plant. N. O. Leguminose. Mimosoideae. Tincture of leaves. ***Historical dose:*** Tincture and all potencies.

CLINICAL - Ankle swelling. Borborygmi. Colic. Conjunctivitis. Coryza. Flatulence. Goosebumps. Numbness. Rheumatism. Sneezing. Trembling. Twitching.

HERBAL - Mimosa humilis is one of the remedies introduced and proved by Mure. The ***"sensitive plant"*** of the hothouses is M. pudica, but the leaves of M. humilis, said Mure, "close at the least contact."

HOMEOPATHIC - The most notable Mim-h. symptoms were lancinations in the back and limbs and ***swelling and redness of left ankle*** with tension and lancination. Smarting pain in legs with paralysis of knee. Stiffness of bends of knees. Pressure in nape and right temple. Prostration.

MIND - Indolent with indifference (Ph-ac.).

Abdomen - Borborygmi. Flatulent colic.

Back - Violent lancinations in back.

Ears - Whizzing in ears.

Eyes - Inflammation of eyes of left eye. Itching. Vision dim, halo around candle.

Head - Sensation of heat in head, as if enlarged.

Limbs - Lancinations in legs and hands, now in arm, now in leg. Swelling of left ankle with redness, tension and lancination. Trembling of legs. Twitching of arm, extending to chest. Numbness of arm and right hand, ceasing on movement. Inflammatory swelling of left hand.

Lungs - Dry cough in morning. Difficult breathing.

Male - Inflammatory swelling of scrotum.

Mouth - Bleeding of gums. Salivation.

Nose - Sneezing and coryza.

Rectum - Diarrhea. Frequent stools, colic.

Skin - Pimples and pimply excrescences about legs and arms. Goosebumps.

Sleep - Yawning. Drowsy in evening with frequent waking at night.

Stomach - Stomach aches and pains.

REFERENCES - Clarke.

MIMOSA PUDICA

PHARMACY - mim-p. Mimosa pudica. N. O. Leguminosae. Mimosoideae. Brazil and India. Tincture is prepared from the root and the flowers. ***Historical dose:*** Tincture and all potencies.

CLINICAL - Allergies. Backache. Blepharitis. Colic. Conjunctivitis. Coryza. Cough. Diarrhea. Enterocolitis. Fistulae. Headache. Hemorrhoids. Hydrocele. Hypersensitivity. Influenza. Otitis. Pains. Photophobia. Salivation. Scorpion, bites. Sinusitis.

HERBAL - Mimosa Pudica is ligneous with regular flowers in clusters with reduced corolla, meristenous androecium and albuminous seeds. It is a tropical plant originating from Brazil and in the warm parts of India. The root contains 10% tannin, and its common usage suggests that it is an aphrodisiac.

HOMEOPATHIC - The homeopathic proving is the work of Sankaran (Mumbai), who experimented with it on six young provers, for three weeks, using the potencies 3x and 6x in 1968-69.

Sensitiveness and headache above the eyes, aggravated by movement, ameliorated by closing the eyes. Irritation of the conjunctiva and nasal mucus membranes. Pains in the shoulders. Diarrhea with abdominal colic and irritating stools. Feeling that the body is too big.

MIND - General irritability. Annoyed by the thought of taking medicine. Easily angered, it takes a long time to forgive. Sensitivity, impression that the body is too large.

Abdomen - Pain in the epigastric region, worse when coughing.

Back - Backache. Dorsal pain. Sharp pain in both shoulders.

Chest - Thoracic pain, especially around the lower part of the large pectoral muscle. Better by a hot bath and by abduction movement of the arm, worse fresh air.

Constitutions - Allergic and psoric constitutions. Tubercular, nervous types, predominantly phosphoric.

Ears - Sudden, acute stinging pain, especially in the right ear. Pain coming in the evening, lasting through the night. Pain worse when lying on the right side with pressure and draft of air. Pain ameliorated by lightly covering the ear. Buzzing in the ears. Hears less well against a noisy background.

Eyes - Burning in the eyes, worse from a draft of air. Blepharitis. Conjunctivitis. Photophobia with headaches, aggravated by the sun. Vision slightly blurred. Eyelids secrete a yellowish pus, which forms in the corner of the corner of the eye.

Eyelids stuck together in the morning on waking.

Head - Headache above the eyes, especially at the left eyebrow. Headache aggravated by straining the eyes, or by quarreling. Headache, worse from movement, ameliorated by closing the eyes or by a tight bandage.

Lungs - Dry cough.

Male - Increase of sexual desire.

Modalities - Better by friction, tight bandage, hot bath. Worse from a draft, movement, bright light.

Mouth - Abundant ptyalism throughout the body. Nocturnal salivation when lying on the right side. Loss of sense of taste.

Nose - Irritation of the nasal mucus membranes. Coryza. Constant discharge of a watery secretion.

Rectum - Irritating stools with abdominal colic. Stools frequent, as often as ten times a day. Better after evacuation. Ameliorated by rubbing the abdomen.

Throat - Pain and tickling in the throat, ameliorated by a hot drink, aggravated by speaking and by coughing.

COMMENTS - Mim-p. has been used as a decoction of the root (1:10), to be prescribed for gravel and all urinary complaints. The infusion of the leaves has been used as a blood cleanser. Powder of the leaves and root is for fistulae and hemorrhoids. The juice can be used as an application for insect and scorpion bites, hemorrhoids and fistulae. A paste made from the leaves is an effective application for hydrocele. The leaves can be used in the bath for cases of lumbar and hip pains.

RELATIONS - ***Compare:*** (1) Euphr. - Inflammation of the nose and eyes. Aggravated by light and air, ameliorated in darkness when lying down. (2) Sabad. - Senses: irritation of the mucus membranes in the nose and the throat. Ameliorated by hot drinks. (3) Psor. - Periodic migraines, worse from the slightest draft, hypersensitive to the cold, sudden nocturnal diarrhea with a fetid odor.

REFERENCES - Julian.

MIMULUS

(Bach Flower Essence)

PHARMACY - mimul-b. Mimulus. Mimulus guttatus. Flowers are picked, placed in a bowl of water and left to the sun's action for several hours. The water imbued with healing power is then prepared as medicine. ***Historical dose:*** Take two drops from the stock bottle into a one ounce dropper bottle, (add brandy or alcohol, if this bottle will be used for days or weeks). This is the dosage bottle, take a few drops straight into the mouth or as needed in a little water or juice.

HOMEOPATHIC - Mimulus belongs to Bach's group ***"For Those who have Fear,"*** along with the remedies of Rck-r-b., Cher-p-b., Asp-b. and Rd-ch-b. Anxiety disorders and phobias when there are concrete objects, persons, or situations of fear (Rck-r-b.).

Nervousness, lowered stamina and decrease in vitality. Dread with internal agony or a slumping of vitality. Hypochondriacal. Obsessive anxieties, intensifying minor symptoms. Excessive self-observation. Fear of being rejected.

Frequent loose bowels and intestinal griping pains during acute states of anxiety. Chronic diarrhea. Heart neurosis, with duodenal ulcers in the passive-dependent patient, emotional diarrhea, urticaria and atopic dermatitis.

Useful during physical rehabilitation after accidents or surgery, or during sickness or old-age infirmities, when every move frightens and small pains intimidate.

MIND - Constant fear. Dreaded things, persons, or events are seen as a hurdle, or as a dangerous deterrence. Shyness and nervousness. Desire to hide shyness.

Anticipatory fears. Chronic phobias. Fixations or obsessions. Fear of death, accidents, poverty, loneliness, misfortunes. Hypochondriasis (Chic-b., Heath-b.) and excessive self-observation (Cer-b., Lar-b.).

REFERENCES - Bach.

MITCHELLA REPENS

(Partridge Berry)

PHARMACY - mit. Mitchella repens. Partridge berry. Partridge-beans. N. O. Rubiacae. Tincture of whole plant. ***Historical dose:*** Tincture and all potencies.

CLINICAL - Amenorrhea. Belchings. Bladder, irritation. Catarrh. Constipation. Depression. Dysmenorrhea. Dysuria. Hemorrhages. Kidneys, pain. Menorrhagia. Menses delayed. Metritis. Uterine, hemorrhage.

HERBAL - Mitchella is a small, trailing evergreen bearing a scarlet bean and is common throughout the United States. It belongs to the same order as Chin., Coff. and Ip. and shows its affinity with these in its power over hemorrhages.

Indian women drink a decoction of it before confinements to make labor safe and easy. Herbalists use a concentrated decoction as an application to sore nipple.

HOMEOPATHIC - Duncan induced pains and burning in the kidneys in his proving and Hale, who observed the effect on a woman, recorded some characteristic symptoms in the urinary and uterine sphere.

Congestion of the uterus with bladder irritation. Irritation at neck of bladder with urging to urinate (Eup-pur., Apis.). Engorged uterus, hemorrhage, bright with dysuria. Lassitude. All muscles feel sore. Whole digestive tract feels cold, transverse colon tender to pressure.

MIND - Inability to concentrate mind. Depression, followed by buoyant spirits.

Abdomen - Griping. Distention with flatus. Rumbling.

Back - Aching pains running down back. Dull pain between shoulders in kidney region.

Bladder - Uneasiness in neck of bladder, urging to urinate, burning, 11 a.m. Catarrh of bladder. Urethra and neck of bladder swollen and irritated, especially in females).

Ears - Burning in left pinna. Dull aching in right ear.

Eyes - Eyes dull and heavy.

Female - Amenorrhea. Menses delayed. Menorrhagia. Dysmenorrhea and uterine hemorrhage, blood bright red. Uterus irritated, severe pain in it. Cervix engorged, dark red, swollen. False pains in last mouth of pregnancy. Slow, feeble ineffective labor pains.

Food - Appetite impaired.

Head - Severe frontal headache on waking. Burning in vertex. Throbbing in occiput. Scalp sensitive to touch.

Heart - Burning pains, uneasy feeling as if its action was being interfered with. Beats irregular.

Kidneys - Heat in kidneys with dull pain. Dysuria, accompanying the uterine complaints. Increased quantity of urine, acid. Urine high-colored, white sediment.

Limbs - Aching and burning sensation in right upper limbs. Walk unsteady, inclines to fall to right. Aching in lower limbs in knee joint.

Lungs - Much mucus in bronchi. Dry, backing cough in morning. Breathing difficult, 11 a.m.

Male - Pain, drawing in right testicle.

Mouth - Burring and prickling on tongue.

Rectum - Tenesmus, urging. Constipation, feces small, thin, difficult.

Sleep - Yawning, drowsy. Woke in a fright, frightful dreams.

Stomach - Burning in stomach extending whole length of esophagus. Acid belchings.

Temperature - Chill over whole body with flushes of heat, very sensitive to cold air.

Throat - Fauces dry. Pharynx feels constricted, impeding swallowing. Tonsils enlarged, painless, especially the left. Some enlargement of left submaxillary gland.

RELATIONS - ***Compare:*** (1) Chim., Senec., Uva., Ger., Goss. (2) In congested cervix associated with irritation of neck of bladder, Sep. - Mitch has no general resemblance to Sep., (3) Eup-pur. - bladder irritation in women. (4) Hydrc. has in addition heat and itching in vagina. (5) Apis, Vesp. - has ulcer around os. (6) Caul., Chim., Cimic., Helon., Puls., Senec.

REFERENCES - Boericke. Clarke.

MOMORDICA BALSAMICA

(Balsam Apple)

PHARMACY - mom-b. Momordica balsamica. Balsam apple. Momordica balsamina. N.O. Cucurbitaceae. Momordica. Tincture of fresh ripe fruit. ***Historical dose:*** Tincture and all potencies, externally used as a liniment and poultice for burns, chapped hands, etc.

CLINICAL - Colic. Dropsy. Dysmenorrhea. Flatus. Leucorrhea. Menorrhagia.

HOMEOPATHIC - Mom-b. was introduced by Dr. Mercer, whose wife made the proving with twenty-four drops of the tincture, producing some very well characterized symptoms.

Griping and colic (Coloc. and Elat.). Accumulation of flatus in splenic flexure of colon. Dropsy. Severe pains in back and hypogastrium with painful and excessive menses. Sensation as if the whole contents of the head had greatly diminished in weight.

Abdomen - Rumbling, griping, colicky pains, starting from back, spreading over abdomen.

Eyes - Mist before eyes.

Female - Painful and profuse menses, labor-like pains, followed by gushes of blood, pain at small of back coming towards front of pelvis.

Vertigo - Dizzy, contents of head feel lighter.

COMMENTS - Farrington gave as a keynote "distention and rumbling in splenic flexure of colon," which he compared with the effects of Lyc.

RELATIONS - ***Compare:*** (1) Mom-ch., Lyc.

REFERENCES - Boericke. Clarke.

MOMORDICA CHARANTIA

PHARMACY - mom-ch. Momordica charantia. Indian variety. N. O. Cucurbitaceae. Momordica. ***Historical dose:*** Tincture and all potencies.

HOMEOPATHIC - This remedy has more severe symptoms than Mom-b. Mom-ch. has gallbladder symptoms. The intestines full of yellow watery fluid, ***discharged explosively,*** cramps, thirst and prostration.

RELATIONS - ***Compare:*** (1) Similar to Crot-t., Elat.

REFERENCES - Boericke.

MONOSODIUM GLUTAMATE

(MSG)

PHARMACY - mono-s-g. Monosodium glutamate. MSG. Sodium salt of glutamic acid.

CLINICAL - Allergies. Anaphylactic, shock. Asthma. Cramps. Flushings. Headaches. Hives. Insomnia. Migraine. Nausea. Numbness. Palpitations. Rash.

HOMEOPATHIC - MSG is made by either a bacterial fermenting process, protein hydrolysis (a breaking of protein into its constituent amino acids), or by synthesis. When a product is 99% pure MSG, the product is called "monosodium glutamate" by the FDA and must be labeled as such. However, when a hydrolyzed protein contains less than 99% MSG, the FDA does not require that the MSG be identified.

Many food products manufacturers advertise "No MSG" on their food packages, but MSG may be disguised as "hydrolyzed vegetable protein," "glutamic acid," "enzyme modified," "natural flavor," "yeast extract," "maltodextrin," or "autolyzed yeast."

There have been reports of allergies and/or sensitivities to MSG, sometimes attributed to the free glutamic acid component. It has been blamed for causing a wide variety of physical symptoms including migraines, nausea, stomach cramps, bloating, irritable bowel syndrome. Extreme dryness of the mouth, mouth lesions. Hives or rash.

Numbness to the tongue and face, burning sensation in the neck, facial pressure or tightness. Drowsiness, insomnia, anxiety, panic attacks, mental confusion. Asthma, runny nose, sneezing. Flushing, heart palpitations, and anaphylactic shock. "Chinese restaurant syndrome" is often used as an example of the symptoms purported to be caused by MSG.

MSG has been shown to cause lesions on the brain, especially in children. These lesions cause cognitive, endocrinological and emotional abnormalities.

In children, excess glutamate affects the growth cones on neurons. Growth cones are vital in laying down chemical pathways in the brain to enable the brain to operate effectively. MSG could affect human children's cognitive skills and cause learning difficulties.

REFERENCES - Murphy.

MONOTROPA UNIFLORA

(Indian Pipe)

PHARMACY - mono. Monotropa uniflora. Indian pipe. Ghost flower. Corpse plant. Convulsion weed. Fit root. N. O. Monotropaceae. ***Historical dose:*** Tincture and all potencies.

CLINICAL - Bunions. Colds. Convulsions. Epilepsy. Eye, disorders. Eye, inflammation. Fainting. Fevers. Gonorrhea. Sores. Toothache. Ulcers. Warts.

HERBAL - The plant was used by some North American Indian tribes to treat eye problems, the stem was bruised and the clear fluid of the stems applied to the eyes. An infusion of the root is antispasmodic, hypnotic, nervine, sedative, tonic.

The flowers have been chewed in order to bring relief from toothache. Water extracts of the plant are bactericidal. The crushed plant has been rubbed on bunions and warts in order to destroy them. A poultice of the plant has been applied to sores that are difficult to heal.

The juice of the plant used alone or combined with water helps ophthalmic inflammation, ulcers, gonorrhea, and inflammation and ulceration of the bladder. The juice from the stems has also been used to treat nervous irritability, including fits and spasms.

It is a good remedy for spasms, fainting spells and various nervous conditions. It has been given to children who suffer from fits, epilepsy and convulsions.

Because of the salicylic acid, the base of asprin, Monotropa unifora is considered a pain reliever. It has been suggested in the past as a possible asprin or opium substitute.

An infusion of the leaves has been used to treat colds and fevers.

An infusion has been used for sore, tired swollen eyes. A tea is made from equal parts juice of Indian pipe and fennel seed.

The infusion of Indian pipe to douche to help ease vaginal irritations. Safety is undetermined and it is possibly toxic at high doses as it contains several glycosides.

REFERENCES - Murphy.

MORBILLINUM

(Measles Nosode)

PHARMACY - morbill. Morbillinum. Measles nosode. ***Historical dose:*** All potencies.

CLINICAL - Adenitis. Catarrh. Conjunctivitis. Coryza. Coughs. Ear, disorders. Erythematous, lupus. Exanthema. Eye, disorders. Lachrymation. Laryngitis. ***Measles.*** Optic neuritis. Otitis. Photophobia. Rash. Skin, disorders. Splenomegaly. Spontaneous, abortion. Tachycardia.

HOMEOPATHIC - The well-known symptoms which characterize an attack of measles may all be taken as guides for its homeopathic use. Its chief use has been as a prophylactic against infection and to clear up after-effects of an attack.

Morbillinum is extremely useful for cases of debility, weak eyes, blepharitis, conjunctivitis, etc., left after severe measles. Treated in fever hospitals, children who simply will not put on weight, are anemic, weary, and often with some bronchitis, morbillinium will help to remove all these symptoms, prevent lung complications and help them to assimilate their food well and to put on weight rapidly.

Affinity for the mucus passages, eyes, ears and the respiratory mucus membranes. Diffused bronchial rales. Nasal voice, rough cough, lachrymation. Fevers, nasal and eye catarrh.

Koplik spots. Macular exanthema, begining on the face and behind the ears. Fine scaly desquamation. Aggravation of a first infection of measles. Troubles of the perception. General convulsions. Grumbling children.

Mind - Mental dullness, sluggishness. Difficulty of thinking and comprehending. Moaning, groaning in children. ***Fear of the sea.***

Abdomen - Abdominal pain, localized at the appendix region. Acute mesenteric adenitis. Splenomegaly. Swollen lymph glands.

Ears - Acute otitis.

Eyes - Optic neuritis. Lachrymation. Photophobia.

Female - Spontaneous abortion.

Heart - Tachycardia.

Lungs - Cough. Paroxysmal respiratory dyspnea. Purulent pleurisy.

Mouth - Koplik spots. Small white patches, surrounded by a red areola, slightly raised seen on the internal walls of the cheeks and on the mucosa of the gums.

Nose - Flapping of the nasal wings, snoring. Catarrh of the nose.

Skin - Rosy maculae, round and oval, of different shapes separated by healthy skin disappearing by pressure. Papulous eruption. Miliary, confluent, scarlatina-like eruptions. Ecchymotic spots.

Throat - Hypertrophy of the superficial glands of the neck. Throat red, irritated. Striduous laryngitis.

COMMENTS - This nosode was prepared by Gross, a contemporary of Hering. Gross used to soak some globules in the blood of the patient suffering from measles, dynamised and used via olfaction.

According to another version, Gross gave some natural globules to the patient suffering from measles, who kept them in his hands firmly closed, and afterwards Gross made dilutions from these globules.

Clarke would prescribe a dose of the Morbill. 30c 2 or 3 times daily as a prophylactic given to those who are or may be exposed to infection. For an attack of the disease, he found nothing better than Morbill. 30c, eight or ten globules in six ounces of water, a dessert spoonful every two hours.

Clarke noted that the effect of this is heightened by alternately giving Bell. 30c in the same way. These two medicines will be sufficient to carry through any uncomplicated case and in his experience do even better than Puls.

Dr. D. Sheppard case: Baby Jean, aged 13 months, who had done well on repeated doses of Silica, so that she weighed 22 lb. and had 7 teeth without any disturbance, developed measles at the beginning of June, 1941. When seen again on June 19th, she was not her usual bright self, very quiet and miserable, had lost about a pound in weight.

Morbillinum 100 given at once. The next week she was extremely lively and happy as always, and had gained 6 oz. Morbillinum was repeated weekly until July 10th, when she weighed 22 lb. 3 oz., a gain of nearly 20 oz. in three weeks, plus the eruption of another tooth and four more nearly through; always cheerful and bright now.

Dr. D. Sheppard writes: "Let me repeat once more: remember the measles serum, Morbillinum, in potency during the convalescence period after measles. There will be no need to send the child to the seaside or give innumerable doses of the nauseating cod - liver oil and malt mixture. This treatment is much simpler, less costly and more efficacious."

"And if in an older child or even an adult you find that the individual had one or more attacks of measles, and has not been doing too well since, interpose a dose or two of Morbillinum 30 or higher, and then go back to the other constitutional remedies as may be necessary; and you will be surprised how quickly various states of ill-health will clear up."

RELATIONS - ***Compare:*** (1) Puls., Hep., Merc., Sulph. ***Complementary:*** Bell.

REFERENCES - Clarke. Julian.

MORGAN BACILLUS

(Bowel Nosode)

PHARMACY - morg. Morgan bacillus. Morgan pure. Proteus morgani. A bowel nosode. ***Historical dose:*** All potencies.

CLINICAL - Alopecia. Anal, fissures. Arthritis. ***Asthma. Bartholinitis.*** Boils. ***Bronchitis.*** Callosities. ***Catarrh.*** Chilblains. Cholecystitis. ***Congestions***. Conjunctivitis. Constipation. ***Cystitis.*** Dysmenorrhea. Eczema. Edema. Emphysema. ***Fibrositis.*** Flatus. Foot sweat. Gallbladder, disorders. Growing, pains. Headaches. Hemorrhoids. Herpes zoster. Hiatal, hernia. High blood pressure. Hot, flashes. Insomnia. ***Jaundice.*** Laryngitis. ***Leucorrhea***. Liver, disorders. Lumbago. Meniere's disease. Menopause. Menorrhagia. Metrorrhagia. Migraines. Neuritis. Nodules. Numbness. Osteoporosis. ***Otorrhea.*** Pes, planus. Pharyngitis. ***Phlebitis.*** Pneumonia. Rheumatic fever. Rheumatic, pains. Salivation. Styes. Thrombosis. Thyroid, enlarged. Tonsillitis. Tracheitis. Ulcers. ***Varicose veins.***

HOMEOPATHIC - There are two sub-types of the nosode Morgan Pure, which is closest to Sulph. and particularly good in skin conditions, and Morgan Gaertner, which is like Lyc. and is helpful in cholecystitis, adrenal colic. It is often useful in hiatal hernia and diverticular disease.

Keynote ***congestion***. Broncho-pneumonia, where the indicated remedy fails to act even in the acute state or to clear up a residual infection. Selective on skin and liver in headaches with flushed face, aggravation from heat and raised blood pressure.

Congestion of the stomach lining and the liver with dirty mouth, indigestion, and bilious vomiting. Gallbladder conditions, constipation and hemorrhoids.

Pelvic congestion and dysmenorrhea. Hot flashes during menopause. Circulatory disturbances of the limbs, blueness, chilblains, varicose veins, edema and hot feet, etc. Congestion around the joints in arthritis. History of rheumatic fever.

Hyperemia of the surface circulation (Sulph.), deep internal venous stasis (Ham., Graph., Petr. and Psor.). Skin ailments with heat and itching. Eczema, red raw with exudate, itching and bleeding.

Giving the nosode in 30c potency, followed by Sulph. in 3x or 6x tablets twice daily, can help the acute itching in bad eczema or dermatitis.

MIND - ***Tense, active.*** Excitable. Introspective and anxious. Apprehensive about state of health, fear of impending disease. Agoraphobia. Fears crowds but often shows mental anxiety if left alone. Fear of the unknown, of the dark, that something bad will happen. Claustrophobia.

Irritable with a tendency to depression. Weeping, tearful mood. Sadness, despondency. Idiocy. Suicidal disposition. Mental depression often with suicidal tendency by jumping.

Abdomen - Epigastric pain or discomfort. Tenderness in epigastrium. Pain right and left hypochondrium. Pain right and left iliac fossae. Flatus. Redness and moisture at umbilicus, bad odor.

Back - Lumbago, acute or chronic. Arthritis spine, sacro-iliac joints. Pain generally better moving, worse on beginning to move, heat.

Blood - High blood pressure. ***Varicose veins. Varicose ulcer.*** Cerebral thrombosis. ***Phlebitis.*** Sluggish circulation. Easy bruising. Tendency to hemorrhoids.

Chest - Pleurodynia. ***Fibrositis of chest wall.*** Angina. Pain since shingles.

Constitutions - Red, coarse, blotchy appearance. Introspective, anxious about their health.

Ears - ***Otorrhea.*** Boils on meatus. Noises in ears. Meniere's disease. ***Catarrhal deafness.***

Eyes - Conjunctivitis. Iritis, keratitis. Tarsal cysts. Styes. ***Lids granular.*** Spots before eyes.

Face - Acne rosacea. Eczema on chin and forehead, in ear passages. ***Cracks and eruption behind ears.*** Eruption ***pustular, weeping, scalding and very itchy.*** Eruption on margins of scalp, pustular, itchy and scaling. Erysipelas. Hot, red, dry and fissured.

Female - ***Pruritus vulvae and vagina.*** Boils vulva. Menorrhagia and metrorrhagia. Fibroids of uterus. ***Leucorrhea, corrosive,*** offensive, brown, green, yellow. Urethral caruncle. ***Bartholinitis.*** Pain on sexual intercourse.

Food - ***Desires fats, sweets, eggs and butter***. Worse from fats and eggs, or avoids fats and eggs.

Head - Congestive headache with flushed face. Frontal, occipital headache, on vertex. Migraines. Weekly sick headache. Headaches worse from hot atmosphere, thunderstorm weather, excitement, traveling in bus or train. Scalp sensitive. Hair falling out. Complete alopecia.

Kidneys - *Cystitis* with frequency and pain. Urine of strong smell, corrosive, containing sugar.

Limbs - Osteoporosis. Rheumatic shoulders. Neuritis arms. Numbness and tingling arms. Rheumatoid arthritis of wrists, thumb. Hands puffy, stiff and grip poor. Nodules on fingers. ***Finger joints swollen and painful.*** Fingers stiff in morning. Lack of power in legs. Tingling legs. Growing pains in legs. Knee joints are large and stiff. Pain in soles, heels. Thick skin soles of feet with ***cracked heels.*** Pes planus. Feet too hot, offensive foot sweat. Chilblains.

Liver - Pain in liver and gallbladder. ***Gallstones.*** Congestion of liver. Attacks of jaundice. ***Bilious attacks*** with severe headache, relieved by vomiting large quantities of bile-stained mucus.

Lungs - Suffocative attacks. Shortness of breath. Morning cough, dry tickling cough, loose or sticky. Emphysema. ***Asthma.*** Congestion of nasal and bronchial membrane, especially in children, bronchi and lobar pneumonia. Infantile asthma. ***Bronchitis, each winter.*** History of pneumonia or bronchopneumonia and never well since.

Mouth - Salivation. Bad taste in the mouth, taste deficient or lost. Mouth and lips dry, lips stiff in the morning. Angles of mouth cracked, lips very red. Ulcers. Jaw bones ache. Periostitis jaw.

Neck - Adenitis neck. Fibrositis neck and shoulders.

Nose - Catarrh. ***Post-nasal catarrh.*** Sinus and antrum infection. Dry mucus membrane. Cracks angle nose. Sense of smell lost. Nosebleeds.

Perspiration - Profuse in axilla.

Rectum - Constipation. Bowel motion without help, loose, urgent in the morning. Bowel motion immediately after food. Stool may be pasty, foul and contain blood and mucus. Hemorrhoids, bleeding itching or painful. Itching of anus. Anal fissures.

Skin - ***Eruptions dry, cracked, fissured, weepy, itchy*** and burning. Tremendous thickening and congestions of skin with deep cracks. Itching eruption, worse from heat. Raw, red eczema, exuding freely with itch and heat, bleeding from scratching. Callosities. Herpes zoster. Skin sensitive to sun, prickly heat. Cannot wear wool next to skin.

Sleep - Insomnia, light and restless.

Stomach - Burning in throat and stomach. Pain and acid, worse with food. Duodenal and peptic ulcer. Bilious attacks. Water brash, heartburn. Sour, acid, bitter, mouthfuls. Belching and heartburn. Nausea, vomiting, hematemesia.

Throat - Throat dry and burning. Throat parched, raw and granular. Apple core sensation, easy choking. Pharyngitis, laryngitis, tracheitis. Recurring tonsillitis, cheesy pieces come out. Thyroid enlarged.

Tongue - Burning in tongue. Tongue raw and dry, coated, slimly, swollen. Tongue stiff in the morning. Warts on tongue. Pain in the root of tongue.

Vertigo - Vertigo from high blood pressure.

COMMENTS - Congestion of gastric mucosa and liver. Heartburn. Dirty tongue, bitter taste in mouth in the morning with accumulation of mucus causing gagging as soon as rises from bed.

Appetite absent in the morning but, by 11 a.m., a sinking feeling relieved by eating. Recurrent bouts of indigestion, with vomiting of mucus and occasionally blood without ulceration. History of bilious attacks, especially occurring at menopause.

A history of repeated attacks of congestion of the lungs or bronchi pneumonia in children is indicative for the use of the nosode Morg. or one of the subtypes: Morgan-Pure or Morgan-Gaertner.

Dr. Sargunar, who used this nosode in 5300 cases, reported that Morg. relieved the attacks of bronchial asthma as quickly as Adren. Chest infection where the indicated remedy fails to act or in cleaning up residual infection after a bronchi pneumonia, especially in cases following Sulph. or Nat-s.

Dr. William B. Griggs said that he used Morg. from 200c to the 100,000c in cases of asthmatic children where Nat-s., Ars. and various asthmatic remedies failed completely.

Dr. Griggs said, "Morgan Bacillus has been one of my most successful remedies in eczema of young children. You take the moist type of eczema where the child scratches and has the exudate on its face and bleeds. Clarke has seen Morgan clear that up after failure of Graph., Psor. and Med."

RELATIONS - Miasmatic relation: Morgan has deep range of action covering the field of a number of anti-psoric remedies. ***Compare:*** (1) Sulph., Calc. and Lyc. and also many carbonates.

REFERENCES - Bach. Paterson.

MORGAN GAERTNER

(Bowel Nosode)

PHARMACY - morg-g. Morgan gaertner. A bowel nosode. ***Historical dose:*** All potencies.

CLINICAL - Alopecia aerata. Anal fissure. Anal pruritus. Angina pectoris. Asthma. Bedwetting. Bladder pain. Blepharitis. Catarrhal, rhinitis. Chalazions. Constipation. Dysmenorrhea. Dyspnea. Eczema. Furuncles. Gallbladder, pain. Hemorrhoids. Herpes. Intercostal neuralgia. Kidney, stones. Leucorrhea. Mastoiditis. Myocarditis. Nasal polyps. Nephritis. Nosebleeds. Otitis. Palpitations. Pleurodynia. Polyuria. Psoriasis. Pustules. Pyelo-nephritis. Rectal, prolapsed. Rheumatic, pains. Sinusitis. Styes. Urticaria. Vomiting. Warts.

HOMEOPATHIC - Pale, impatient, claustrophobic persons. Subjects with fine brown hair. Polyarticular rheumatic pains of upper extremities specially of the right side. Vesiculous, squamous, papulo-squamous eruptions. Pyelo-vesical burning congestion. Dysmenorrhea.

MIND - Impatient. Tense, with strong reaction. Full of apprehensions, gets excited in company. Chews nails. Irritable. Jealousy. Claustrophobia. Nocturnal fears cries out in sleep. Manic depressive psychoses.

Abdomen - Gallbladder painful. Intestinal lethargy. Flatulent dyspepsia. Flatulence of the left and right hypochondrial region.

Back - Cervical rigidity.

Breasts - Warts on the breasts, nipples.

Chest - Intercostal neuralgia. Thoracic pain. Angina pectoris. Constriction in the chest, painful irradiation to the left hand. Sensation of coldness in the chest.

Ears - Otitis. Mastoiditis. Furuncles in the auditive conduit. Buzzing in the ears.

Eyes - Chronic inflammation of the eyelids. Blepharitis. Styes. Chalazions. Ulcer of the cornea. Vitral opacity.

Face - Facial neuralgia, dominating left side. Sudden edema of the face. Herpetiform eruption on the left side of the face.

Female - Irritation at the approach of menstruation. Painful menses. Dysmenorrhea. Thick, brown, corrosive, bad smelling leucorrhea. Vulvar pruritus.

Food - Desire for sweets, salted things, fatty foods, eggs, meat. Sometimes aversion to fat, eggs, meat.

Heart - Myocarditis. Precordial uneasiness. Angina pectoris. Nocturnal palpitations, wakes up the patient. Palpitations, better by eructations, better by emission of gas, better by movement.

Kidneys - Pain in the kidney region. Nephritis. Pyelo-nephritis. Pyelo-vesical pain, congestion. Kidney stones. Bladder pain with frequent urination. Polyuria. Burning urine. Bedwetting.

Limbs - Nocturnal pains of the arms. Rheumatoid pains in shoulders, arms, elbows, wrists, deltoid muscles (right).

Painful swelling of the thumbs. Knees, numb and painful. Excessive heat of the feet at night.

Lungs - Dyspnea. Shortness of breath. Pleurodynia. Asthma. Tickling cough morning and evening, while walking up, while lying down.

Modalities - Better by movement, passing flatus, eructation. Worse in company, after meals, before menses, at night, heat of bed, right side.

Mouth - Bad mouth, bitter taste. Thick saliva. Tongue burning, as if pricked by needles. Inflamed gums, pyorrhea. Cracks in corner of lips.

Nose - Sinusitis. Hypersecretion of nasal fossa and of maxillary sinus. Crusty coryza with ulceration in the nose. Catarrhal rhinitis. Nasal polyps. Nasal herpes. Nosebleed.

Rectum - Constipation. Hard, dry stools with mucus. Spontaneous expulsion of mucus through rectum even when the patient is not constipated. Rectal prolapsed. Anal fissure. Anal pruritus. Painful hemorrhoids, bleeding, pruriginous.

Skin - Skin sensitive. Sudden edema of the face. Herpetiform eruption on the left side of the face. Psoriasis. Eczema. Urticaria. Pustulous eruption on face, on brows, knees. Skin, oozing, crusty, desquamating with fissures. Giant urticaria on arms. Warts on hands, big flat or lacerated. Erythematous squamous eruptions in round plaques on elbows, knees, integument, sacral region, nails and heels. Herpetic eruption on soles. Alopecia aerata. Loss of hairs in bunches.

Stomach - Fullness of the epigastrium without eating. Noisy eructations with bad smell. Vomiting of foods after meals, afternoon or night.

Throat - Inflammatory congestion of tonsils. Edema of the uvula. Sensation of burning in the base of the throat as if from acid.

RELATIONS - *Compare:* Lyc., Puls., Sil., Kali-bi., Nat-m., Nux-v., Sulph., Sep., Graph., Calc.

REFERENCES - Julian. Paterson.

MORPHINUM ACETICUM
(Morphine)

PHARMACY - morph. Morphinum aceticum. Morphine. Opium alkaloid. Morphinum muriaticum. Morphinum sulphuricum. Morphia. N. O. Papaveraceae. Trituration. Solutions. ***Historical dose:*** All potencies.

CLINICAL - Albuminuria. Amenorrhea. ***Bradycardia***. Chorea. Colic. ***Coma.*** Constipation. Convulsions. ***Delirium***. Delirium tremens. Delusions. ***Depression***. Diabetes. ***Drug, addictions. Drug, overdose.*** Electric shock. Eyes, disorders. Headache. Herpes zoster. Hysteria. Impotency. Infertility. ***Itching.*** Jaws, clenched. Lightning-stroke. ***Nausea***. Neuralgias. ***Neuritis***. ***Numbness***. ***Pains.*** Palpitations. ***Paralysis. Ptosis. Shock***. Sleep, disordered. Strabismus, divergent. ***Strangury. Tachycardia.*** Trismus. ***Tympanitis***. ***Uremia***. Urticaria. Vertigo. Vision, illusions. ***Vomiting.***

HOMEOPATHIC - Morphine is the alkaloid of opium, which contains the most characteristic properties of the drug. The alkaloid, the acetate, the muriate and the sulphate have all been used as painkillers and sleep inducers.

Morphine bears a similar relation to opium as atropine is to belladonna, that is, it represents its nervous side. It is less stimulating, less convulsive and more decidedly hypnotic. Constipates less and affects contractility of the bladder more. It is less diaphoretic and more itching.

Restlessness, hyperesthesia, trembling, twitching, jerking, convulsions. Violent and sudden neuralgic pains and sudden fainting. ***Multiple neuritis***. Neuralgias after herpes zoster (Mez.). ***Extremely susceptible to pain***. Pain causes twitching and jerking of limbs. Sore feeling all over. ***Bed feels too hard***.

MIND - Mental exhaustion. Incapable of thinking or fixing mind. Concentration difficult. Memory weakness. ***Forgetfulness, hunting for words while speaking.*** Makes mistakes in writing. Makes gestures. ***Indifference, apathy.***

Great anxiety, thought she was going to die. Anxious, restless, ran about the room.

Ailments from fright or fear. Frightened easily. ***Shock induced by terror.*** Terror, cried out in great alarm. Suspicious, mistrustful.

Emotions very easily excited. Hysteria. Excitable during childbirth. Flow of ideas rapid and pleasant, but without control of the will. Lies, never speaks the truth, does not know what she is saying.

Ill-humor. Irritable, wants to be alone. Censorious, critical. Fault-finding. Anger at trifles. Intolerant of contradiction. Deceitful, sly. Want of moral feelings.

Delirium, melancholic in character. Delirium during fever, sleep. Delirium, springs up suddenly from bed and escapes. Howling. Delusions, sees faces, hears voices, perceives various odors. Sensation of death. Delirium tremens. ***Drug addictions, overdose***.

Profound depression. Sad, melancholy, despair. Despair with the pains. Could not describe symptoms because tears and sobs. Suicidal disposition. Stupefaction, as if intoxicated. ***Dream-like state.*** Confusion of mind. Unconsciousness, coma. Uremic coma.

Abdomen - Distended. Acute pain in abdomen and along spinal column. ***Tympanitis***. Pain in umbilical region. Colic better turning on back in morning.

Back - Great pain in back. Pain extending along spine. Pain and twitchings all down spine. Aching across lumbo-sacral region, cannot walk erect (Cimic.). Weakness of the loins. Stiff-neck.

Causations - Ailments from fright or fear. Drug addiction, overdose. Electric shock, lightning-stoke. Thunderstorms. Ailments from apoplexy, stroke.

Chest - Chest tight. Pain in middle of sternum. Ill with an indescribable sensation, worse then any pain, behind lower half of sternum. Neuralgia after herpes zoster (Mez.).

Constitutions - Nervous constitutions.

Ears - Left ear throbs painfully, better heat. Severe pain in left ear with pain at side of left eye all day. ***Seems to hear circulation all over body.*** Ringing, surfing, roaring, tinnitus.

Eyes - ***Itching*** of eyes. Pupils unequally contracted. ***Paresis of recti internal.*** Staring, injected, diverging strabismus. ***Look unsteady.*** Double vision with disturbed accommodation. Sight blurred, obscured by fogs. Delusion of vision on closing eyes. Eyes feel too small for sockets. Eyeballs protrude. Bluish, drooping eyelids. ***Ptosis.*** Nystagmus.

Face - Heavy, confused, wild, haggard expression. Intensely flushed face, puffed, livid, cyanotic. ***Dusky red or pale face, lips tongue, mouth or throat.*** Trismus, teeth clenched.

Female - Amenorrhea. Menses too profuse, and too early. Infertility. Sexual desire at first increased, afterwards abrogated.

Food - Loss of appetite. ***Aversion to meat***, pastry. ***Thirst***, burning.

Head - Head dull, heavy as lead, hot. Bursting pain, head drawn back. Brain feels tense as though wound up tightly. Headache with drowsiness. Congestions of head, palpitations of heart, starts in fright if approached, touch causes cramp and twitchings.

Heart - Cardiac muscular tissue is intact, even if severely exhausted. Violent throbbing in heart and carotids. ***Alternation of tachycardia and bradycardia***. Palpitations. Pulse small, weak, dicrotic.

Kidneys - Suppression of stool and urine. Paresis of bladder. Prostate enlarged. ***Strangury. Uremia***, acute and chronic. ***Slow and difficult urination.*** Urine is turbid and slimy. Albuminuria. Diabetes.

Limbs - Tremors, twitchings, contractions, stiffness of limbs. ***Numbness***. Cramps in several muscles. Violent pain in joints. Staggering gait. Legs swollen. Wandering, sharp pains in legs and feet. Stiffness and pain in arms after sleep. Icy coldness of left sole as if standing on oil-cloth.

Lungs - Faint and struggling for breath. Breathing is stertorous, difficult, slow. ***Diaphragmatic paralysis***, hiccough, dyspnea, paroxysmal, on first falling asleep (Lach., Grind.). Cheyne-Stokes respiration. Dry, hard, ***teasing***, exhausting cough, worse at night. Strangling cough with viscid mucus sputum, thin, scanty, but sounds loose and abundant.

Male - Pain in right spermatic cord (Ox-ac.). Impotency. The sexual excitement, voluptuous sensations and erections are incomplete or do not occur. Diminished desire.

Modalities - Better by coffee. Worse by eating, vinegar. Worse after sleep, in morning, slightest movement, especially of the head.

Mouth - ***Very dry mouth***, with thirst, nausea, bitter, sticky vomiting. Discharge of watery saliva from mouth. Palate scarlet. Speech is hasty, stammering, embarrassed and feeble.

Nose - Sneezing in paroxysms, coryza. Tickling in nose and larynx as before a sneeze. ***Intense itching***, tingling, numb feeling on end of nose, rubs it constantly.

Perspiration - Profuse sweat. Cold, clammy sweat. Viscid, colliquative sweat.

Rectum - Stool retained. Constipation for a long time. Constipation, stools large, dry, knotty with tendency to bruise and fissure. Diarrhea watery, brown or black with horrible tenesmus.

Sensations - Tight sensations in head, as if skull too small for the brain. As if brain wound up. Something shot to head like lightning the instant the injection look place. Sight as if obscured by a fog. Ticking of nose and tip of nose. Tongue as if thick. Teeth as if clenched. As if worms in legs.

Skin - Skin lost its elasticity. Skin deathly pale. ***Livid, purple spots.*** Eruption like herpes zoster, but without pain. ***Itching is constant***, violent, all over, nose, neck, loins, inside thighs. Urticaria appearing at the menopause.

Sleep - Heaviness, drowsiness. Sleepy, but cannot sleep. Sleepless, restless sleep with frequent startings. Yawning, ***drowsy***, prolonged, deep sleep. Muttering in sleep. Dreams are pleasant, frightful. Half waking, half stupid condition. Aggravation after sleep (Lach.).

Stomach - Pain in stomach, worse by eating. Constriction, pressure, cramps. Colic, crawling in stomach. Belchings, violent, with much acid mucus. ***Nausea incessant and deathly***, faintness, constant retching. ***Nausea and vomiting on rising up.*** Nausea with drowsiness. Vomiting of green matter, sour, bright green fluid, bitter, greenish water.

Temperature - Icy coldness. Chills and rigors. Burning heat, profuse sweat. Heat, burning, itching, cheeks hot and flushed.

Throat - Dry and constricted. Burning back of fauces. Hoarseness. Pharynx paralyzed, swallowing almost impossible, better hot drinks, worse solids. Jugular veins swollen, carotid arteries pulsating.

Tongue - Tongue is dry, brown, red tip and margins. Tongue violet in middle, at times trembles on putting in out.

Vertigo - Vertigo from the ***least movement of the head.*** Giddiness and drowsiness, everything turns around.

COMMENTS - Extreme susceptibility to pain. Cannot describe symptoms for tears and sobs. Neuralgia where the pains are so violent as to threaten convulsions, pain causing twitching or jerking of limbs. Nervous spasms brought on by lightning-strike, worse by any exposure to heat, better by cold.

Tremblings, twitching, jerking and convulsions, even tetanus. Marked clenching of the jaws. Restlessness and hyperesthesia. Restlessness of legs, wants them held, feels as if worms in them.

Heavy and hot head. Intense drowsiness. Deep sleep, but also sleeplessness and restless sleep with starting up. Half sleeping state, "a half-waking, half-stupid state, but with perfect ability to think of different things, though at the same time he was busy with confused fantasies, limbs stiff."

Green vomit is a constant effect. Nausea during pregnancy (Lac-d., Ip.). Sudden fainting. Useful for the after affects of morphine, or morphine withdrawal.

Both the muriate and the sulphate are able to cure symptoms produced by Morph. In Clarke's experience, the acetate has produced much more violent gastric symptoms than the muriate, but not different in kind.

Rufus Thurston recorded a short but very important proving of Morph. on a patient who took a grain for sleeplessness.

Among the symptoms he emphasized "vertigo from least movement of the head."

Not long after, Skinner had a case of vertigo with the tendency to fall forward and become unconscious. Symptoms were worse from movement of any kind, especially of the head, and by eating and drinking. Morph-m. 500c cured the case.

Boger cured with Morph-s. 100,000c the case of Miss M., 22, who was dark and spare. She had a headache with the sensation of being wound up tight. Sleepiness and numbness of lower limbs. Intense vertigo on least motion of head.

Thurston also had a case with the "wound-up" headache. That case also had sudden faintness.

That same symptom was produced by one-eight of a grain of the sulphate in a case reported by E. V. Ross. Spells of feeling faint came on suddenly with great anxiety, as though he was going to die. Visual delusions on closing eyes, "sees a man standing at foot of bed. The room seems full of white and colored babies."

RELATIONS - ***Compare:*** Apom., Herin., Op., Nux-v.

REFERENCES - Boericke. Clarke. Murphy.

MOSCHUS MOSCHIFEROUS

(Deer Musk)

PHARMACY - mosch. Moschus moschiferous. Deer musk. Musk. N. O. Mammalia. Ruminantia. Trituration of inspissated secretion contained in preputial follicles. ***Historical dose:*** All potencies.

CLINICAL - Alcoholism. Angina pectoris. ***Awkwardness.*** Backache. Catalepsy. Choking. ***Coldness***. Coma. Convulsions. ***Coughs.*** Croup. Deafness. Diabetes. Dysmenorrhea. Dyspnea. Epilepsy. ***Fainting.*** Flatulence. Globus, hystericus. Headache. Heart, failure. Herpes. ***Hiccoughs.*** Hypochondriasis. ***Hysteria.*** Impotence. Laryngismus. Lungs, paralysis. Nymphomania. Palpitations. Pregnancy, complaints. Rage. Somnambulism. Stings. Twitching. Typhoid. Vertigo. Whooping cough.

HOMEOPATHIC - Musk is a well-known perfume, which can produce fainting in some by smelling it. Useful for all complaints that have easy fainting as a chief indication. Faints easily, faints dead away from the least excitement. Faints while eating, during menses, from heart disease. Scolds and rages until she falls unconscious.

Hysteria and nervous paroxysms, ***Fainting fits*** and convulsions, catalepsy. Globus hystericus ending in unconsciousness. Spasmodic, nervous effects with a feeling of coldness. Twitching, choking. Epilepsy with shuddering as from a rigor or chilliness.

Much nervous trembling and frequent fainting. Nervous, shuddering, laughter, hiccough etc. Tension in muscles, skin, mind. Great flatulence. Parts lain on feel dislocated or sprained. Buzzing, squeezing, plug like sensation.

Aggravation by cold, great sensitiveness to air. ***Coldness*** in general or of single parts. As of a cool wind blowing on part. Wants to uncover. Poor reaction, diseases do not follow the normal course. Complains without knowing what ails him. Imaginary diseases.

MIND - Absent-mindedness. Sudden loss of memory. Confusion of mind. Mental activity with weakness, so that everything falls from the hands. ***Awkwardness.*** Hurried, tremulous. Talks to himself and gesticulates.

Frightened easily. Anxiety with palpitations. Fear of noises, going crazy, something bad will happen. Fear of dying, suffocation. Afraid to lie down, as they might die. Talks of death. ***Imaginary sufferings.*** Sexual hypochondriasis. Nymphomania.

Censorious, critical. Abusive, insulting. Violent anger. Desire to break things. Deceitful, sly. Aversion to being asked questions. Talks excitedly, raves, scolds, until mouth becomes dry, lips blue, eyes staring and she falls unconscious.

Hysteria. Uncontrollable laughter. Weeping, tearful mood alternating with laughter. One feels as if being rapidly turned around. Delirium during convulsions. ***Sensitive to odors, to musk.*** Somnambulism. Coma vigil. Alcoholism, dipsomania.

Ailments from domination by others.

Abdomen - Greatly distended. Tension in abdomen as if clothes were too tight. Incarceration of flatus.

Back - Backache. Tension in back, before menses.

Causations - Chills. Ailments from anticipation, deceived ambition, reproaches, domination by others.

Chest - Chest oppressed, hysterical spasms of the chest. Tightness of chest is obliged to take a deeper breath.

Constitutions - Suited to spoiled, sensitive natures and hysterical women and men. Girls who are selfish, obstinate, self-willed and pampered, they resort to all kinds of cunning to have their whims gratified.

Ears - Sounds as from report of a cannon. Rushing, fleeting sound. Nervous deafness.

Eyes - Turned upwards, fixed and glistening.

Face - One cheek red but cold, other pale and hot. Lips blue. Chewing motion of the lower jaw.

Female - Menses too early, too profuse, with disposition to faint (Nux-m., Verat.). Dysmenorrhea with fainting. Drawing and pushing in the direction of the genitals, sensation as if menses appear. Sexual desire with intolerable titillation in parts.

Food - Desire for black coffee, beer and brandy, stimulants. Aversion to food, everything tastes flat. Faints while eating.

Head - Compressive pain over root of nose. Pressure on top of head. Headache with coldness, fainting, involuntary stools, and polyuria. Shivering in scalp. Scalp sensitive.

Heart - Trembling around heart. Weak pulse and fainting. Anxious palpitation with fear of death. Hysterical palpitations.

Kidneys - Diabetes. Copious, watery urine. Urine normal during day, but dark red, offensive at night.

Limbs - Painful, restless. Limbs, tense, feel too short. Coldness in tibia. One hand hot and pale, the other cold and red.

Lungs - Sudden nervous suffocation, wants to take deep breath, worse from becoming cold, better after belching. ***Difficult respiration, chest oppressed.*** Spasm of glottis. Impending paralysis of lungs. Asthma with intense anxiety, fear and smothering sensation. Hysterical asthma. Globus hystericus. ***Cough ceases, and mucus cannot be expectorated***. Cough with pain under left breast.

Male - ***Sexual desire increased*** with insupportable tickling in the parts and tensive pain in penis. Involuntary emissions without erections. Erection with desire to urinate. Nausea and vomiting after sex. Impotence with diabetes (Coca.). Premature senility.

Modalities - Better in open air. Better rubbing. Better smell of musk. Worse cold, open air, which is felt very cold. ***Worse from excitement.*** Worse suppressions. Worse after and during a meal. Worse menses. Worse from pressure. Worse motion, must lie down and lie still, but worse on side lain on. Vomiting worse after sex.

Nose - Bleeding with spasmodic jerking of muscles.

Rectum - Stools of sweetish odor. Stools are passed involuntarily in sleep.

Sensations - As if falling from a height. As of being turned about so rapidly he perceived the current of air produced by the motion. As if cold air blowing on him. As if cold, wet poultices on head. Headache as if from a heavy weight. As if larynx closed on breath.

Sleep - Sleepy by day, sleepless at night, awakes frequently. Somnambulism.

Stomach - Distended. Faints when eating. ***Spasmodic, nervous hiccough*** (Hydr-ac., Sul-ac., Ign., Caj.). Violent belchings. Nausea, on seeing or thought of food. Anxiety in chest with stomach symptoms.

Temperature - Sensitive to cold air, which makes him shudder. Skin cold. Burning heat with restlessness. Sweat smelling like musk.

Throat - Sudden constriction of larynx and trachea.

Vertigo - Vertigo with fainting, as if falling from a height, worse stooping, better rising. Vertigo on least motion.

COMMENTS - Tendency to faint often. Fainting spells (Am-c.). Spasms and twitches. Spasm of chest of heart, general convulsions. Laryngeal spasm. Subsultus tendinum of fever. Tension in muscles in skin, in mind. Tension in back before menses, tension in limbs, they feel too short. Pressure outward in heart.

Characteristic coldness in general, or it may affect single parts. Coldness with pallor. Sensation as if cool wind blowing on parts. Coldness in tibia. Hysteria, laughing and crying fits. Sexual desire is much excited in both sexes, even in the aged. Diabetes with impotence, with excessive thirst.

H. N. G. noted that it is useful "in nervous or spasmodic complaints where the patient feels very cold: in epileptic fits where there is rigor or chilliness or shuddering as though the patient was very cold."

RELATIONS - ***Antidotes:*** Camph., Coff. ***Compare:*** (1) Nux-m., Asaf., Valer., Sumb., Ign., Cast-eq. ***Planets:*** Moon. ***Compatible:*** Ambr.

REFERENCES - Boericke. Clarke. Murphy.

MUCUNA URENS

(Horse-Eye)

PHARMACY - muc-u. Mucuna urens. Horse-eye. N. O. Leguminose. Papilionoideae. Venezuela. The pulverized bean is macerated five times its weight of alcohol. ***Historical dose:*** Tincture and all potencies.

CLINICAL - Hemorrhoidal discharges. Hemorrhoids.

HERBAL - In New, Old and Forgotten Remedies is a letter by Delgado Palacios of Venezuela, pointing out that the name Dolichos, given to Cowhage of Cow-itch in homeopathic literature is not in accordance with botanical terminology.

Cowhage is really a Mucuna, Mucuna and Dolichos being separate genera of the Leguminose. Allen gave Linneus as the authority for the name Dolichos pruriens. There is no pathogenesis.

HOMEOPATHIC - Muc-u. is used for hemorrhoids and problems arising from the hemorrhoidal diathesis. The keynote symptom is burning. There may or may not be bleeding. Affections of liver, uterus, bladder and the testicles, when accompanied by hemorrhoids.

COMMENTS - Palacios said modern botanists consider Cowhage identical to Muc-u., but he does not name his plant M. pruriens, an alternative name of Cowhage. He said, further, that M. urens is a "special plant which grows in the calid regions of Venezuela," and that the beans are "very difficult to obtain."

Palacios used the pulverized bean for making his tincture. He gave one drop daily of the tincture and sometimes made an ointment of it as well, He placed more reliance in it than in Ham. and Aesc. In Dol. the entire pod is used, the stinging hairs being the most important part of it.

REFERENCES - Clarke.

MUREX PURPUREA

(Purple Fish)

PHARMACY - murx. Murex purpurea. Purple fish. Murex purpureus. N. O. Gasteropoda. Trituration of desiccated juice. Trituration or tincture of fresh juice. The fresh preparation is to be preferred, though the dried is the usual one. ***Historical dose:*** All potencies.

CLINICAL - Breasts, pains. Cervix, disorders. Diabetes. Dysmenorrhea. Endometritis. Leucorrhea. Menopausal sufferings. Menorrhagia. Metrorrhagia. Miscarriage. ***Nymphomania***. Pregnancy disorders. Uterus, disorders. Uterus, prolapse.

HOMEOPATHIC - Petroz first proved Murx., which like Sep. produces the chief intensity of its action in the female generative sphere. They are chiefly distinguished in that Murx. produces frantic sexual desire and tends to have excessive hemorrhage with large clots, Sep. having in general a scanty flow.

Murx. is for sensitive, nervous, lively, affectionate women. Those who are very tired, weak and run down, must lie down, which aggravates. Walking is difficult, all the joints are weak during pregnancy. Pains are diagonal, ovary to opposite breast. Menopausal sufferings.

MIND - Great depression of spirits, a sort of deep hypochondriacal state. Great sadness, anxiety, and dread. Imagines herself sick. Seemed to her she was hopelessly ill. Impatient. Memory weak, cannot find correct words to express himself.

Conscious of uterus. Anxious, apprehensive, better leucorrhea. Sadness before menses. ***Unconsciousness before menses.*** Wants to die, from intense abdominal pain during menses. ***Nymphomania from suppressed menses.*** Nymphomania during metrorrhagia.

Abdomen - Painful weariness of loins. As if a weight in hypogastrium.

Back - Lumbago, sometimes burning and with pain like excoriation. On extending the body, pain in hips and lumbar region. Pains in pelvic region. Sensation as if bones of pelvis getting loose.

Breasts - Benign tumors in breasts. Pain in breasts during menstrual period. ***Pain from right side of womb to right or left breast.***

Chest - Wheezing in chest. Pain in chest, as if it had been bruised. Sharp and burning pains below false ribs on left side. Sensation as of a snake creeping over entire region of short ribs.

Constitutions - Suited to the melancholic or sanguine, lymphatic temperament. Especially adapted to nervous, lively, affectionate women. Menopausal sufferings.

Ears - Cramp-like squeezing behind ears. Noise in ears with aggravation of heaviness of head.

Face - Burning sensation of one cheek, right in evening, left in morning.

Female - Conscious of a womb (Helon.). Pulsation in neck of womb. Feeling of protrusion. Prolapsed, enlargement of uterus with pelvic tenesmus and sharp pains. ***Must keep legs tightly crossed***. Sore pain in uterus. Feeling as if something was pressing on a sore spot in the pelvis, worse sitting. Least contact of parts causes ***violent sexual excitement. Desire easily excited, nymphomania***. Menses irregular, profuse, frequent, large clots. Dysmenorrhea and chronic endometritis. Leucorrhea green or bloody, alternate with mental symptoms and aching in sacrum.

Food - Hunger, sometimes in morning only and unfelt during a meal. Awful hunger and emptiness, even after a meal.

Head - Squeezing at the back of head, better putting hand on it or by throwing head backwards.

Heart - Palpitations of heart and throbbing of arteries.

Kidneys - Constant urging (Kreos.). Slight discharge of blood while urinating. Urine frequent at night, smells like valerian.

Lungs - Cough in morning while fasting, dry, hard with oppression of chest.

Modalities - Better before menses, pressure support, putting head back, eating. Worse in sun, exertion, least touch, sitting, lying down, night, after sleep.

Nose - Distressing coldness of the nose all day.

Rectum - Pressure in anus like painful lancinations. Sensation of heavy weight pressing on rectum. Swelling of hemorrhoids. Difficult evacuations, constipation. During stool, bloody leucorrhea, discharge of pure blood by vulva.

Skin - Dry, as if about to crack. Hives.

Sleep - Urgent inclination to sleep. Drowsiness, sometimes with sadness. Sleep interrupted by pains. Distressing dreams. Awakening with fright.

Stomach - Sinking, all-gone sensation in stomach (Sep.). Hungry, must eat. Violent hunger even after eating.

Throat - Voice changed, hoarse.

COMMENTS - Consciousness of the womb, sore pain in uterus. Cutting pains confined to the cervix and os. Sensation of dryness and constriction in the womb. Feeling of bearing down and prolapse (Sep.).

General sensitiveness to touch. Feeling as if something were pressing on a sore spot in the pelvis. Pains are frequently diagonal and shoot from ovary to opposite breast. Must lie down from weakness, but lying down aggravates all symptoms.

The least contact with the parts causes violent sexual excitement. Cervix is sensitive to the examining finger. The slightest touch causes bleeding of excoriation on cervix. Cauliflower excrescences.

Hungry, sinking, all-gone sensation (Sep.).Diabetes. Excessive secretion of urine and frequent necessity to rise at night to urinate. Great depression of spirits, a sort of deep hypochondriacal state, better when leucorrhea is worse and vice versa.

RELATIONS - ***Compare:*** (1) Plat., Lil-t., Sep. the latter lacks sexual weakness of Murx. (2) Uterine congestion, cervix affected, Sep. is passive, Murx. feels disgust and despair at her sexual desires. (3) Shooting pains in uterus, prolapse, melancholy, Aur. has induration. (4) Nocturnal polyuria, Kreos. (5) Sexual weakness, Lil-t., Plat. Orig. (6) Dragging down, Bell. (7) Prolapsed uterus, Sec., Plat., Bell., Lil-t., Nux-v., Nux-m., Podo., Puls., Sep. (8) Consciousness of womb, Helon., Lyss. (9) Menopausal, Lach., Sep., Sulph. (10) Better throwing the head back, Seneg.

REFERENCES - Boericke. Clarke. Phatak.

MURIATICUM ACIDUM

(Hydrochloric Acid)

PHARMACY - mur-ac. Muriaticum acidum. Hydrochloric acid. Muriatic acid. First dilutions with distilled water. ***Historical dose:*** Tincture and all potencies.

CLINICAL - Achilles tendon, disorders. ***Acidity.*** Alcoholism. Aphthae. Ascites. Anus, prolapse. Backache. ***Bedsores.*** Belching. Carbuncles. Chilblains. Chorea. Cirrhosis. Deafness. Delirium. Diarrhea. Diphtheria. Drug addiction. Dysentery. Feet, pains. Fevers. Flatulence. Hemiopia. Hemorrhages. ***Hemorrhoids.*** Hernia. Impotence. ***Intestinal, fever.*** Measles. Mercurial, ulceration. Morphinism. Mouth, ulcers. Muscular, exhaustion. ***Nosebleeds.*** Palpitations. ***Prostration. Septic fever.*** Scarlatina. Scurvy. ***Soreness.*** Stomach, disorders. ***Stomach ulcers.*** Tongue, disorders. ***Typhoid, fever. Typhus. Ulcers.*** Varicose veins. Vomiting. Whooping cough.

HOMEOPATHIC - The alchemist's name of hydrochloric acid is the "Spirit of Salt," which describes at once its nature and origin. It is a colorless gas with a pungent, suffocating odor and acid taste, manufactured from salt (Nat-m.) by the action of sulphuric acid. It is freely soluble in water and the saturated solution contains 43 percent of the hydrochloric gas.

Mur-ac. is a constituent of the gastric fluids and must therefore be considered as allied to the sarcodes and proximate principles of the tissues, e.g., Chol. Teste, who helped define the powers, groups it with Agn. and Hyos. He considered its action to correspond perfectly to a typical case of typhus.

Mur-ac has an affinity for blood, producing ***septic conditions*** similar to that found in low fevers with high temperatures and great prostration. Scorbutic states. Muscular exhaustion. Paresis of muscles, including the heart, bladder, tongue, and, in particular, the mouth and anus.

Burnings and tearing pains. Dropsical swelling. Decomposition of fluids. Violent hemorrhages. Pulse rapid and feeble. Pulsations in single parts. ***Soreness of the body causing restlessness.*** Frequently changes position, but soon grows weak and very debilitated. Wants to lie down, slides down in bed, eyes fall shut, lower jaw drops.

Mucus membranes of the mouth and digestive tract are dry, bleeding, cracked and deeply ulcerated. Bloody mucus membranes. Bluish tongue, hemorrhoids, ulcers. Involuntary discharges. Involuntary stools while passing urine. Itching of anus and scrotum, not better by scratching.

MIND - Irritable and peevish, fretful. Sad and taciturn. Introverted. ***Suffers in silence***. Loquacity. ***Muttering. Loud moaning***. Conscientious about trifles. Obstinate, headstrong. Great restlessness.

Indifference, apathy to pleasure. Discontented in open air. Delirium with fever, sleeplessness. Weary of life. Absorbed in thought during menses. Anxiety during fever. Anxiety about future. Want of self confidence. Cowardice.

Memory weakness. Absent-mindedness. Confusion of mind. Irresolution, indecision. Thoughts intrude and crowd upon each other while at work. Stupefaction, as if intoxicated. Ailments from anger. Morphinism. Drug addiction. Alcoholism, dipsomania.

Abdomen - Fullness and distention in abdomen from small quantity of food. Pressing pain and tension in hypochondria. Liver enlarged, sore. Ascites from cirrhosis of liver. Cramp in abdomen, with griping in umbilical region. Empty sensation in abdomen, after stool, in morning. Rumbling. Flatulence with distension. Hernia.

Back - Backache. Aching pain in back, as from having been having bent double for a long time or from a strain. Shootings in shoulder blades. Furunculi in back.

Chest - Deep respiration with groans. Oppression across chest. Tensive pain in sternum. Incisive shocks in chest. Sharp pains in chest.

Constitutions - Suited to persons of black hair and dark eyes.

Ears - Cuffing from mastoid to nape. Tingling, creeping, cold pain running up to vertex. Distant voice, talking causes headache. Deafness.

Eyes - Eyes close on sitting from exhaustion. Vertical hemiopia.

Face - Dark or glowing red face with cold hands, but no thirst. Lips sore, cracked and scabby. Lower jaw fallen. Pimples and freckles. Freckles due to exposure to sun.

Female - Leucorrhea with backache. Leucorrhea during menses, soreness of anus. Menses appear too soon. Ulcer in genitals. Pricking in vagina. Genitals very sensitive, cannot bear least touch.

Food - At times, ravenous appetite and constant desire to drink. Cannot bear sight or thought of meat.

Head - Occipital pains, leaden heaviness, worse looking intently at any object. Pain as if brain were crushed. Periodical pain over left eye with numbness down right arm and aphasia. Sound of voice is intolerable. Hair as if standing on head.

Heart - Shootings in region of heart. Shock in heart at night. Large full and soft pulse. ***Pulse, drops every third beat.*** Pulse rapid. ***Pulse feeble and small.*** Palpitations felt in face.

Kidneys - Atony of bladder, must wait a long time, before urine will pass or has to press so hard that anus protrudes. Cannot urinate without having bowels move at same time. Urine, red, violet, milky, copious, night and day, escapes from passing wind.

Limbs - Heavy, painful and weak. Tottering gait. Staggers when walking from weakness of thighs and knees. Pain in achilles tendon. Red, swollen burning fingers and toes. Eczema of dorsum of hands. Cramps in the ball of thumb (right) when writing, goes off when moving it. Forearms heavy.

Liver - Liver enlarged, sore. Ascites from cirrhosis of liver.

Modalities - Better from motion. Better warmth. Better uncovering during fever. Better lying on left side. Better after drinking. Worse from touch. Worse human voice. Worse walking, sitting. Worse before midnight. Worse rest. Worse after sleep. Worse cold, drinks, bathing. Worse damp weather. Worse sun. Diarrhea worse after eating.

Mouth - Dry. Fetid breath. Everything tastes sweet. Beer tastes like honey. Tongue, pale, bluish, swollen, dry, leathery, shrunken or burnt looking. Tongue, heavy, stiff, hinders talking, paralyzed. Hard lumps in tongue. Deep ulcers on tongue. Cancer of tongue, epithelioma, edges bluish-red (Carb-ac.). Aphthous mouth. Gums are swollen, bleeding, ulcerating. ***Sordes on teeth***. Teeth, worse acids and sweets. Lips, burn, heavy, bloated. Glands swollen.

Nose - Nose stopped up. Coryza thin, acrid, excoriating, with itching, tickling and sneezing. Stinging pain in sore nostrils. ***Nosebleed*** with much sneezing. Dark and putrid blood from nose.

Perspiration - Cold sweats, on feet, evening in bed. Sweats during first sleep, until 12 p.m., worse head and back. Sweats at night and in morning. Aggravated when sweating, wants to uncover.

Rectum - Smarting and burning in anus. Anal itching and prolapsed anus while urinating. Involuntary stools or prolapse of rectum, on urinating or passing flatus. ***Stools very difficult, as from inactivity of bowels.*** Diarrhea with much flatus. Diarrhea with intolerable anal itching, not better scratching. Dysentery, blood and slime separated. Stools too thin, but round. Stools greenish in typhoid. Burning in anus after stool. Anus sore during menses. Hemorrhoids bluish, hot with violent stitches. Very sore hemorrhoids, better heat. Hemorrhoids protruding like a bunch of grapes. ***Hemorrhoids most sensitive to all touch,*** even sheet of toilet paper is painful. ***Hemorrhoids during pregnancy.***

Sensations - Hair, as if drawn upwards, as if standing on end. Brain as if loose, beaten or torn to pieces, brain clasped by a hand and bruised and torn. Occiput as if filled with lead. Deadness and numbness in forehead, in fingers. Mouth as if glued up with mucus. As if some obstruction must be pulled out of throat. Burning as if under skin of coccyx. As if place was jammed in Achilles tendon.

Skin - Papular and vesicular eruptions with great itching (Rhus-t.). Eczema on back of hands. Scarlet fever, livid with petechia, scanty eruption. ***Bedsores.*** Carbuncles. Foul-smelling ulcers on lower limbs. Ulcers throb on walking.

Sleep - Great drowsiness during day, which disappears with exercise. Sleeplessness before midnight. Before midnight, continued snoring, groaning tossing, talking and tendency to slide downwards in bed. Anxious dreams. Frequent and early waking, caused by a coldness that is felt in bed.

Stomach - Achlorhydria. Lack of stomach acids and fermentation of food. ***Stomach will neither tolerate nor digest food.*** Sensation of emptiness in stomach and esophagus, not better eating. Weak feeling in stomach from 10 a.m. until evening. Acid reflux. Bitter, putrid eructations. ***Stomach ulcers.*** Burning pains. Vomiting with belching, coughing. Gulping up of contents of stomach into esophagus, sometimes going down again.

Temperature - Cold in bed in early morning. Cold limbs. Intense burning heat with aversion to covers. Heat without thirst. ***Typhoid types of fever, septic fevers***.

Throat - Dry with burning in chest. Edematous, dark, raw. Ulcers and false membrane. Uvula swollen. Involuntary swallowing. Attempt to swallow produces spasms and choking.

Vertigo - ***Vertigo, worse lying on right side***. Vertigo, occiput heavy as if filled with lead. Vertigo worse moving eyes, slightly. Vertigo lying on right side or on back.

COMMENTS - Mur-ac. is a powerful antidote to Merc. (as is Nit-ac.), and it meets conditions caused by Merc. as well as similar conditions. Like other disinfectants, it causes as well as remedies rapid decomposition of tissues and dynamically cures low, putrid conditions met with in disease. Characteristic muscular prostration from blood poisoning progressing to paralysis, finally of brain or heart.

Teste gave common features of the group in which he classified Mur-ac as a stupefying headache, obscuration of sight and optical illusions, whizzing noises in the ears and hardness of hearing, nosebleed and loss of smell. Rough, cracked lips and foul breath, scurvy of mouth, paralysis of tongue, loss of taste. Distended, sensitive abdomen, pricking, bruised pain in abdominal walls.

Mucus membranes are very dry, bleeding, cracked and ulcerated. Burning, particularly burning eruptions on lips. Ulcers. Eruptions and hemorrhoids. Varicose veins. Black pocks. Blind boils, frothy when touched. The skin is sensitive to the sun, eczema solare and freckles.

Low, febrile states. Puerperal, diphtheria, exanthematous, and typhoid fevers. Fever with stinging heat, frequent, small intermittent pulse, earthy or livid skin. Stitches about the heart. Excited sexual desires. Impotence. Hahnemann noted a tendency "to slide down to the foot of the bed."

Offensive, sour, acrid excretions. Offensive breath and body smell. Deafness, otitis and glandular swellings about the ears. Sordes on teeth. Shrunken and paralyzed tongue, parched. Throat pains. Hoarseness, spasmodic cough.

Serous, fetid diarrhea, not very painful. Involuntary stool. Paralysis of bladder. Prolapse of rectum, while straining to pass water. Involuntary or difficult urination. There is straining and dribbling, and the straining can cause a prolapsed rectum or involuntary stool.

Hemorrhoids like a bunch of grapes that look purple and burn when touched.

Cooper cured the case of a man, 52, whose sister had died of cancer, who had a hard, deep, warty ulcer, size of a small bean on under surface of tongue, on the left side, with much surrounding hardness and little discharge. Swollen tongue made his speech thick. It was ulcerated, especially on the right side that was hard with swelling. This was followed by a lupoid ulcer on the corresponding side of nose, and had been going on ten months.

RELATIONS - ***Antidoted by:*** Carbonates of alkalis and earths in poisoning cases, to small doses: Camph., Bry. Teste said the surest antidote is Ip. ***It antidotes:*** Merc., Op. It cures the muscular weakness following the excessive use of opium (Hering). ***Compare:*** (1) Ph-ac., Ars., Bapt. (2) In typhoid state Bry. has worse motion. (3) Rhus-t. - restlessness, better by motion, Rhus-t. has less debility. (4) Ph-ac. has less prostration is apathetic indifferent. (5) Mur-ac. taciturn. (6) Apis has blisters on tongue and it catches teeth when attempt is made to protrude it. (7) Ars. has scanty evacuations. (8) Bapt. has besotted look tongue red on edges. (9) Bell. more active, hyperemia. (10) Kali-perm. - throat symptoms, edematous uvula. ***Follows well after:*** Bry., Rhus-t., Merc.

REFERENCES - Boericke. Clarke. Murphy. Phatak.

MUSCA DOMESTICA

(House Fly)

PHARMACY - musc-d. Musca domestica. House fly. ***Historical dose:*** All potencies.

CLINICAL - Arthritis. Awkwardness. Backache. Boils. Catarrh. Delusions. Dysmenorrhea. Eczema. Headache. Herpes. High, fever. Masturbation. Memory, weak. Mumps. Rashes. Rheumatism. Salivation. Stupefaction. Styes. Toothaches. ***Weakness.***

HOMEOPATHIC - Lassitude. Heaviness, sensation externally and internally. Heaviness, internally, alternating with lightness. Lack of vital heat. Heat alternates with a chill. Sensation of paralysis. Weakness, with restlessness. Worse during a storm.

MIND - Fastidious. Conscientious, about trifles. Restlessness with pain. Restlessness, driving from place to place. Desire for exercise and physical activity. Industrious. Elation. Extravagance. Irresolution. Impatience, with children. Easily angered. Cursing.

Anxiety, with congestion, when alone. Fear of abandonment, sensation of isolation. Anxiety about health. Anxiety about time. Fear of accident, sexual assault, men. Aversion to company, to certain people.

Memory, weakness. Forgetfulness, feels as if he had forgotten something. Confusion of mind. Rapid thoughts. Confounds objects and ideas. Awkwardness. Mistakes in talking, words, localities, names. Confusion of mind, identity. Stupefaction, as if intoxicated. Indolence.

Causeless crying. Tendency to weep. Sadness, before menses. Pities herself. Self loathing. Despair, hopeless. Dwells on past disagreeable circumstances. Reproaches others. Desires sympathy. Worries for others. Forsaken. Suicidal thoughts.

Delusion, that he died, and is alive again. That body and mind are separated. That he is being watched. That fingers are scratching his body. Everything is dirty, foul. Visions of dead animals. Sees maggots, vermin, insects.

Abdomen - Dull, knotting pain, sharp over bowel.

Back - Backache. Dull, throbbing pain. Pain in nape, neck. Neck pulling to left. Tension in neck, shoulders. Pain in coccyx. Sensation of gap in mid-back. As if back were separated.

Breasts - Pain and swelling in breasts, before menses. Pain in nipples, in men.

Chest - Radiating pain, gas in center of chest. Aching pain, constriction.

Dreams - Dreams of sexual violence, abortion, sick babies, dying from cholera.

Ears - Cutting, aching pain. Oozing eruption on the earlobe. Sensitive to high pitched noise. Ringing noises.

Eyes - Dryness. Discharge in right eye. Stye, in right eye. Eyelid opens and shuts involuntarily.

Face - Eruptions, painful to touch, on forehead, eyebrows, over left eye. Herpetic eruption on lower lip, corners of mouth. Inflammation of parotid gland.

Female - Painful menses, dysmenorrhea. Menses, profuse, brown discharge, spotting, intermittent. Pain in lower vaginal region. Sharp pain in cervix, in left ovary. Herpetic eruptions. Boils on labia. Sexual desire increased. Masturbation.

Food - Aversion to water. Desires chocolate, cheese. Desires bacon. Desires vinegar, sour food. Desires coffee. Desires beer in the morning. Worse from cheese.

Head - Headache, frontal pressure. Pressure in temples, worse lying down. Dull aching in occiput. Dull, gripping like too much caffeine. Throbbing head and above eyes. Head pain before menses. Dry, flaking, scalp.

Kidney - Musty smelling urine.

Limbs - Insensibility, limbs. Stiffness of limbs. Joint pain. Numbness in arms on waking. Aching pain, in upper limbs, shoulders, upper arms, at night. Pinching, throbbing pain in wrist. Awkwardness, lower limbs, hands. Throbbing pain in hip. Cracking pain in groin, worse walking. Lancinating pain in knee. Cold, numb feet. Soreness in feet, soles.

Lungs - Greenish yellow expectoration. Shortness of breath.

Male - Pinching pain in testes. Sexual desire increased. Penis, flaccid. Impotency.

Modalities - Worse lying down. Worse from cheese.

Mouth - Profuse saliva, in gushes. Frothy mucus on waking. Salivation with mumps. Taste of lemons in mouth. Breath, fetid odor. Bleeding, spongy gums. Lower gum line feels thin and stings. Chancre sore on tongue, lip. Lip, split, cracked.

Nose - Obstruction. Catarrh. Acute sense of smell. Odors, imagined and real, fruit, peaches, sulphur.

Perspiration - Night sweats.

Rectum - Constipation, must strain. Urging absent. Incomplete, unsatisfactory bowel movements. Excessive flatulence, smelly. Stools are dry, pasty, soft, light brown, loose.

Sensations - Heaviness sensation. Alternating heaviness with lightness sensation. Paralytic sensation.

Skin - Greasy skin. Herpetic eruptions. Boils on right upper back. Flat, pink, scaly rash on chest. Eruption in cervical area. Red rash above left axilla, after bathing. Eczema on hand. Raised red bumps on upper thigh.

Sleep - Snoring during nap. Overwhelming desire to sleep. Sleeping early. Sleeps in fetal position, right side. Deep, soporific sleep. Recurring vivid dreams, of houses, fire, water, falling into water. Deep, unrefreshing sleep. Restless. Waking groggy, late.

Stomach - Appetite wanting for dinner. Upset stomach, worse drinking cold water. Sharp pain, with belching, gas. Sour eructations. Spikes or flashes of nausea.

Teeth - Toothache while eating chocolate. Pain in right lower teeth.

Throat - Sore throat, with tickling in the ears, worse tea. Mucus stuck in throat.

Vertigo - Light-headed. Drifts or falls, to the left, worse in morning.

Vision - Difficulty focusing. Blurry when reading. As if a bug was flying in peripheral sight.

REFERENCES - Sonz, Stewart.

MUSA SAPIENTUM

(Banana)

PHARMACY - musa. Musa sapientum. Banana. N. O. Palmacee. Araceae. Tincture of the dried flowers. ***Historical dose:*** Tincture and all potencies.

CLINICAL - Anemia. Blood pressure. Brain, fatigue. Bronchitis. Constipation. Cystitis. Depression. Dyspnea. Hangovers. Headache. Heartburn. Hemorrhoids. Morning, sickness. Mosquito, bites. Overweight. Premenstrual syndrome. Seasonal Affective Disorder. Strokes. Tobacco, smoking. Ulcers. Warts.

HERBAL - C. Campbell commended bananas baked in their skins as an ideal food or even a "cure" for brain workers, nervous persons and the anemic. A syrup made with the juice of bananas extracted by heat is commended as a remedy in chronic bronchitis with insufficient expectoration and marked dyspnea.

Clarke had a case of profusely bleeding hemorrhoids, which had resisted every kind of treatment, showed improvement and an ultimate cure.

HOMEOPATHIC - Jenner proved the tincture of banana flowers, producing costiveness and a sensation of fullness about the anus in a person of regular habits. He cured a bad case of bleeding hemorrhoids with it. Musa also produced pain in the bladder and passage of mucus with urine.

MIND - Brain fatigue. Depression.

Abdomen - Rumbling in stomach and bowels with expulsion of flatus.

Head - Dull, heavy, frontal headache.

Kidneys - Discharge of large quantities of mucus with the urine, with dull, aching pain in bladder region.

Mouth - Dry, rough and extremely astringent taste and feeling in mouth, tongue, and fauces, but afterwards an increase of saliva.

Rectum - Constipation with feeling of fullness about anus.

COMMENTS - Bananas contain three natural sugars, sucrose, fructose and glucose, combined with fiber. They also contain tryptophan, a protein that is converted into serotonin. Vitamin B6, which regulates blood glucose levels and affect mood. High in iron, bananas can stimulate the production of hemoglobin. They also contain potassium and are natural antacids.

Can be useful for depression, seasonal affective disorder and stress. Anemia. High blood pressure, strokes. Premenstrual syndrome. Morning sickness. Hangovers. Constipation. Heartburn, ulcers. Neutralizes over-acidity and reduces irritation by coating the lining of the stomach.

REFERENCES - Clarke. Murphy.

MUSCARINUM

(Muscarine)

PHARMACY - muscin. Muscarinum. Muscarine. Muscarineis the alkaloid of Agaricus muscarius. ***Historical dose:*** All potencies.

CLINICAL - Lachrymation. Perspiration. Salivation.

HOMEOPATHIC - Muscin. increases the lachrymal, salivary, hepatic secretions etc., but diminishes kidney secretions. ***Salivation, lachrymation and excessive perspiration.***

REFERENCES - Boericke.

MUSTARD

(Bach Flower Essence)

PHARMACY - must-b. Mustard. Sinapis arvensis. The flower heads are picked above any seed pods and boiled for half an hour. The water is strained and prepared as medicine. ***Historical dose:*** Take two drops from the stock bottle into a one ounce dropper bottle, (add brandy or alcohol, if this bottle will be used for days or weeks). This is the dosage bottle, take a few drops straight into the mouth or as needed in a little water or juice.

HOMEOPATHIC - Must-b. belongs to Bach's group ***"Lack of Interest in Present Circumstances,"*** along with Clem-b., Honey-b., Wld-r-b., Oliv-b., Wh-ch-b., and Ch-bd-b. Affects of head injury, nerve damage or misalignment of the skull plates along fissures. Dampened consciousness (Horn-b., Scler-b., Wld-o-b.).

Depression and gloom. Lowered vitality, lethargy. Chronic fatigue and appetite disturbances (Chic-b, Crb-a-b.). Solace found in eating and constipation (Chic-b., Will-b.), resulting in weight loss or gain. Sleep disturbances (Pine-b., Wh-ch-b.). Disinterest in physical recreation and general decline in healthful interests and habits (see Wld-o-b.).

MIND - Depression and gloom, with sensation of a weight or downward pull, better in the sun. Desires light. Sadness, regret, weepy. Introverted. Absent-minded, disinterested in present circumstances. Lack of appeal for life. Boredom, sense of meaningless. Morose and ill-tempered. Sense of desolation, loneliness. Self-pity. Withdrawal and joylessness in retardation (Horn-b., Wld-o-b.).

REFERENCES - Bach.

MUTABILE BACILLUS

(Bowel Nosode)

PHARMACY - mut. Mutabile bacillus. Bacillus coli. A bowel nosode. ***Historical dose:*** All potencies.

CLINICAL - Asthma. Cystitis. Eruptions. Malnutrition.

HOMEOPATHIC - Mutabile bacillus is so named because it mutates almost as soon as it is sub-cultured from a non-lactose to a lactose fermenter, and is of interest mainly from a bacteriological point of view as it is an intermediary form between the B. Coli and the true non-lactose fermenting type.

This nosode is likely to be of value in treatment where there is alternation of symptoms. Associated with Puls. Skin eruptions alternate with asthmatic symptoms (Calad.). Skin has a sallow color. Cystitis. Malnutrition.

RELATIONS - ***Compare:*** (1) Puls., Calad.

REFERENCES - Bach. Paterson.

MYGALE LASIODORA

(Black Cuban Spider)

PHARMACY - mygal. Mygale lasiodora. Black Cuban spider. Bird spider. Mygale avicularia. Aranea avicularia. N. O. Arachnida. Latin America. Tincture of whole spider. ***Historical dose:*** All potencies.

CLINICAL - Chill. Chordee. ***Chorea.*** Convulsions. Dyspnea. Fever. Gonorrhea. Nausea. Palpitations. Syphilis. ***Trembling***. Twitching.

HOMEOPATHIC - The pathogenic data of Mygale consist of a proving by a young woman and the effect of a bite on a man. In the latter case, inflammation ensued which spread along the lymphatics, violet and afterwards green discoloration, chill followed by fever, dry mouth and great thirst, trembling, dyspnea, despondency and fear of death.

The prover developed sadness, dry mouth, nausea with great palpitation, trembling, dim sight and great general weakness increased flow of urine, hot, scalding with stinging in urethra. This last symptom led to the successful use of Mygal. in gonorrhea, chordee and syphilis.

The ***"trembling"*** observed in the man suggests its use in nervous cases, but the sphere of Mygal. in chorea has been developed from the clinical side. In the cases cured with it, twitching and contractions of facial muscles have been very prominent, convulsive movements of head to right side, twitching of one side of body, mostly right. The twitchings may be so violent as to prevent walking.

Chorea, especially of the upper parts. Constant motion of whole body. Convulsive, uncontrollable movements of arms and legs. Twitchings and contraction of facial muscles and head, which is jerked to the right side. Limbs are quiet during sleep, movements worse in morning.

Unsteady gait, limbs drag while walking. Mouth and eyes open in rapid succession. Words are jerked out in the effort to talk. Nausea with palpitations and dim vision. Intense red streaks along lymphatics. Sexual symptoms, violent erections, chordee. Weakness, nervousness, fear.

MIND - Sad, despondent with anxious expression. Fear of death. Delirious, talking about his business, restless all night.

Back - Pain in back, extending around to front.

Ears - Acute aching in right ear.

Eyes - Nausea with dimness of sight, weakness, palpitation.

Face - ***Twitching of facial muscles***. Mouth and eyes open in rapid succession. ***Hot and flushed***.

Food - Excessive thirst. Aversion to food, no appetite. Better after eating.

Head - Head jerked to one side.

Heart - Strong palpitations, with nausea, dimness of sight and general weakness. Pulse frequent.

Limbs - ***Constant motion of whole body***. Twitching of limbs. Tremulous. ***Convulsive, uncontrollable movements of arms and legs.*** Restless hands. Limbs drag while walking. Unsteady gait. Intense redness in streaks, following course of lymphatics.

Lungs - Difficult breathing. Words jerked out when effort is made to talk.

Male - Violent erections. Chordee (Kali-br., Camph.). Protracted gonorrhea. Syphilis.

Modalities - Better during sleep. Worse in morning, eating. Legs in constant motion, worse sitting.

Mouth - Tongue dry and parched, put out with difficulty. Grating of teeth at night.

Sleep - Restless all night, with ridiculous dreams.

Stomach - Nausea with strong palpitations, dim sight.

Temperature - Severe chill lasting thirty minutes, then fever with excessive thirst and trembling of limbs.

Urine - Urine is increased, stinging in urethra, burning hot, scalding.

RELATIONS - ***Compare:*** (1) Agar., Tarent., Cupr., Ziz. (2) in chorea, Agar., Cimic., Ign., Stram., Ziz. Tarent., Ant-c.

REFERENCES - Boericke. Clarke.

MYOSOTIS SYMPHYTIFOLIA

(Forget-me-not)

PHARMACY - myos-s. Myosotis symphytifolia. Forget-me-not. Black-root. N. O. Boraginaceae. Marshy places in Indiana. Tincture of fresh plant. ***Historical dose:*** Tincture and all potencies.

CLINICAL - Bronchitis, chronic. Bronchorrhea. Coughs. Emaciation. Lung, disorders. ***Night-sweats.*** Tuberculosis. Vomiting.

HERBAL - Hale collected some clinical experiences with Myosotis symphytifolia, which differs from Myosotis palustris in having large symphytum-like leaves, showing it to have a strong affinity for the respiratory organs.

HOMEOPATHIC - Myos-s. affects the left lower lung. Chronic bronchitis and tuberculosis. Bronchorrhea. Cough with profuse muco-purulent expectoration, gagging and vomiting during cough, worse during or after eating. Pain in left lung (lower), painful while coughing and sensitive to percussion. Copious expectoration, emaciation, ***night-sweats***. Profuse sweat day and night.

RELATIONS - ***Compare:*** (1) Symph., Stann. - lung disease.

REFERENCES - Boericke. Clarke.

MYRICA CERIFERA

(Bayberry)

PHARMACY - myric. Myrica cerifera. Bayberry. Wax myrtle. Candleberry. N. O. Myricacee. Tincture of fresh bark of root. ***Historical dose:*** Tincture and all potencies.

CLINICAL - Achilles tendon, pain. Cancer. Catarrh. Conjunctivitis. Diphtheria. Headaches. Heart, disorders. ***Insomnia. Jaundice.*** Leucorrhea. Liver, disorders. Pharynx, disorders. Stomatitis. Throat, sore, Urticaria.

HERBAL - According to Hale, though Myrica was known to old herbalists, it was Samuel Thomson, of lobelia fame, who established its reputation. Thomson had a crude pathology of his own which served him to some extent.

Myrica formed the chief ingredient in Thomson's once famous "Composition powder." One of his ideas was that the digestive tract was liable to become fouled with a copious mucus lining. This he called "canker" and he stated of Myrica that it "has the power of disengaging the thick, viscid secretions of the mucus membrane of the stomach."

HOMEOPATHIC - The provings of Myric. confirmed Thomson's observation, that it produced a characteristic abundant, offensive secretion of tenacious mucus in the throat, difficult to detach. Liver disorders with ***jaundice*** and mucus membranes. Combined liver and heart disorders. Persistent ***insomnia***.

MIND - ***Gloomy, despondent*** and dejected. ***Irritable***, indifferent. Cannot concentrate mind on any subject. Dull and drowsy state. Exhilaration, then excitement or depression, preventing sleep, with restlessness.

Abdomen - Dull pain in the liver with pain under either scapulae. Fullness and burning in gallbladder. Fullness in the stomach and abdomen. Flatus is passed continuously while walking.

Back - Pain under scapulae with liver complaints.

Eyes - Yellow sclerotica. Very red eyelids.

Face - Yellow, jaundiced. Itching and stinging. Creeping sensation.

Female - Acrid, fetid, thick, yellow, long lasting leucorrhea.

Food - Desire for sour things. Strong desire for acids. Imagines he cannot eat, the taste is so foul. Loss of appetite, loathing of food.

Head - Pain and stiffness in nape of neck. Headache with drowsiness, yellow sclerotica, aching in eyeballs. Pressure in vertex and forehead. ***Dull, heavy aching in temples and forehead on waking in the morning***. Scalp feels tight.

Heart - Pulse, slow, feeble, irregular

Kidneys - Dark, frothy, scanty, high-colored, biliary urine.

Limbs - Pain under shoulder blades and back of neck, in all muscles, in hollow of right foot. Staggering gait.

Liver - Liver disorders with heart complaints, with urticaria with jaundice. ***Jaundice*** of infants. Liver cancer, with bronze-yellow skin.

Modalities - Better from open air, eating, breakfast. Worse from warmth of bed, after sleep, morning, after breakfast, motion.

Mouth - Dry, water relieves only partially. ***Tenacious, thick, nauseous mucus*** in mouth and throat. Taste bitter and nauseous with offensive breath. Tongue, thick yellowish, dark, furred. Tender, spongy and bleeding gums (Merc.).

Rectum - Urging to stools but passes only great amount of flatus. Constant discharge of flatus when walking. Stools, foul, pasty, of gray color. Loose, light-colored stool, ash-colored and destitute of bile. Adhesive mucus in stools.

Skin - Yellow and itching. ***Jaundice***. Creeping sensation, as of insects.

Sleep - Drowsiness. ***Insomnia.*** Disturbed, bad dreams and frequent waking.

Stomach - Complete loss of appetite, but with a feeling of fullness in the stomach after a hearty meal. Weak, sinking feeling in the epigastrium, approaching nausea increased after eating, relieved by rapid walking.

Throat - Constricted and rough feeling with a constant desire to swallow. Diphtheria. Stringy mucus, detached with difficulty.

COMMENTS - Long-lasting, profuse catarrhal discharges, offensive, tenacious and difficult to detach. Leucorrhea, bronchorrhea intestinal catarrh, pharyngeal catarrh, stomatitis. Nasal obstruction, post-nasal catarrh which often accompanies disordered liver.

Drowsiness, despondency. Weakness. Muscular soreness, aching in limbs. Sharp pains about the heart with increased, audible pulsations, but slow pulse, worse lying on left side (Dig.). Pains in left chest and under scapula (especially left) and pain in middle lobe of right lung.

Aching pain in liver, fullness. Jaundice. Itching of jaundice. Dull, heavy headache, worse in morning. Dirty, yellow tongue. Yellowish white of eyes. Dirty, lids abnormally red. Ash-colored stools.

Douglass noted the case of Miss O., 18, who complained of itching and stinging on face, neck, right forearm and leg. Sensation as if insects crawling on face, must brush them away. Skin yellowish tongue, thickly coated yellow. Felt sick all over and rather irritable. Myric. 6x every two hours improved at once and cured in ten days.

Hale said it rivals Guai. as a local application in diphtheria. Burnett used Myric. with excellent effect with jaundice, given in material doses. It has generally been given in the lower potencies.

RELATIONS - ***Antidote:*** Dig. - jaundice. ***Compare:*** (1) Ptel., Corn., Chel., Lept., Fago. (2) in tenacious secretions, Kali-bi., Hydr. (3) Jaundice, light-colored stools, slow pulse, Dig. (Dig. has pulse irregular as well as slow, the tongue of Dig. has not the thick, tenacious coat of Myric.). (4) Liver, Berb., Chel., Chim., Podo., Hep., Merc., Chol., Hydr. (5) Urticaria and liver disorder, Astac. (6) Sore all over, Arn., Bapt. (7) Leucorrhea, Hydr. (8) Pain through left chest to scapula, Ther., Anis., Pix.

REFERENCES - Boericke. Clarke. Phatak.

MYRISTICA SEBIFERA

(Brazilian Ucuba)

PHARMACY - myris. Myristica sebifera. Brazilian ucuba. N. O. Myristicacee. Brazil. Trituration of red, acrid, very poisonous gum obtained by incising bark. ***Historical dose:*** Tincture and all potencies.

CLINICAL - Abscesses. Arthritis. Boils. Carbuncles. Elephantiasis arabum. Erysipelas. Fistulas. Headache. ***Injuries.*** Joints, disorders. ***Panaritium***. Parotiditis. ***Suppurations.*** Traumatic, infections. Ulcers. ***Whitlow.*** Wounds.

HOMEOPATHIC - Mure proved and introduced Myris., which belongs to the same order as the nutmeg tree, Nux-m. In the proving there was ***"pain in the fingernails with swelling of the phalanges."*** This, apparently, led to its use in ***whitlow*** in which many successes have been reported, including some from Chancerel Pere.

Spanish homeopaths used Myris. extensively. Olive of Gros reported cures of scrofulous osteitis, callous ulcers, and phlegmonous erysipelas.

Works as an antiseptic. Inflammation of skin, cellular tissue and periosteum. Hastens suppuration and shortens its duration. Traumatic infections. ***Panaritium***. Parotiditis. Fistulas. Carbuncles.

Phlegmonous inflammations. Inflammation of middle ear, suppurative stage. Coppery taste and burning in the throat. Tongue is white and cracked. Fistula in ano. Hands are stiff, as if from squeezing something a long time.

MIND - Heedless and careless. Indifference, apathy to business affairs. Stupefaction, as if intoxicated. Concentration is difficult. Persistent thoughts. Vexed by a song which keeps running in his head. ***Excitable, alternating with chilliness.*** Dreams of neglected business, quarrels, strife. Startled during sleep.

Abdomen - Sensation as if a foreign body, as large as a walnut, has lodged in left inguinal region, all forenoon.

Back - Pinching, right side of neck.

Chest - Hard pressure during night on both sides of chest, not affecting breathing.

Ears - Inflammation of middle ear, tympanum, myringitis. Suppuration of middle ear, tympanum. Abscess of external meatus. Ringing noises.

Eyes - Redness of eyes and eyelids.

Face - Very red face.

Food - Thirst.

Head - Head heavy. Pain with pressure outwards. Headache in frontal eminence, at noon, better in open air.

Kidneys - Less frequent urination, scanty although he drinks much. Urine reddish yellow.

Limbs - Hands stiff as if from squeezing something for long time. Pain in left hand. Pain in hands worse when they touch each other. Formication on left thumb joint. Pain in fingernails with swelling of phalanges. Pinching pain in right calf.

Mouth - Tongue white and cracked. Whole mouth with tonsils and upper pharynx painful and sensitive to contact, every mouthful seems to wound the parts when chewed or swallowed. Taste bitter of copper, which excites spitting of blood. Palate insensible with loss of taste.

Rectum - Stools mixed with yellow mucus.

Skin - Malignant pustules. Abscesses. Carbuncles. Two pimples on left cheek, quickly disappearing.

Sleep - Cannot get to sleep. Restless sleep with unconnected dreams, about business, disputes, houses being built commencing with top stories. Violent starting in sleep.

Throat - Burning at bottom of throat. Constriction at isthmus of pharynx, pain increases progressively. Difficulty in swallowing saliva.

Urine - Red color.

Vertigo - Dizziness in morning. Vertigo, right to left on waking in morning. Vertigo, swaying toward left.

COMMENTS - Myris. is useful for abscesses from splinters and foreign objects, especially splinters under the nails causing infection, pus and pain (Sil.). Suppuration of the joints. Kippax, according to Hansen, noted that it is the principal remedy in elephantiasis arabum.

Cartier noted two cases in which he used Myris. The first was a young girl who had had her leg in a splint for inflammation of the knee and doughy swelling of the entire limb for three months. Cartier came to the conclusion that there was pus in the joint.

Myris. 3c, five drops three times a day, was given for three months.

Five months later, the swelling and inflammation were all gone, walking gave no pain, but the joint was anchylosed.

The second case was an old man, 87, who was seized with sudden arthritis of the shoulder with intense fever. Cartier was sent for and found the shoulder quite full of pus with a particularly painful spot on the scapula, at a point where the bone was said by one authority to be attacked.

Myris. 3c, five drops three times a day, was given. In ten days there was no longer suppuration, the size of the joint has become normal and the tender spot was gone.

RELATIONS - ***Compare:*** (1) Sil., Nux-m., Calc-s., Sulph., Pyrog.

REFERENCES - Boericke. Clarke. Murphy.

MYRRH

(Gum Myrrh)

PHARMACY - myrrh. Myrrh. Gum myrrh. Commiphora myrrha. Commiphora molmol. Balsamodendron myrrha. N.O. Burseraceae. Middle East and Africa. Tincture from bush or small tree. ***Historical dose:*** Tincture and all potencies, third potency.

CLINICAL - ***Abscess.*** Amenorrhea. Anemia. Asthma. Bronchitis. Colds. Constipation. Coughs. Debility. Dyspepsia. Flatus. Gastritis. ***Gum, diseases. Mouth, disorders.*** Pharygitis. ***Pyorrhea. Sores.*** Stomach, disorders. Throat, sore. Thrush. Tonsillitis. Ulcers.

HERBAL - The Myrrh plant is a shrub or small tree. Myrrh is highly prized for its bitter, cleansing perfume. The aromatic pale yellow, gum resin seeps out from fissures in the bark. It was part of the embalming mixtures of the ancient Egyptians.

It is a stimulant, tonic and antiseptic. The tincture is used for sore throats, ulcers and thrush. Mouthwash for infected gums or ulcerated tongue. The dry, powdered resin is often added to tooth formulas.

Myrrh is an excellent antiseptic, a slow and mild stimulant, possessed of moderate astringency, and acting as a stimulating tonic. Its use occasions an agreeable sense of warmth in the stomach, large quantities causing decided gastric excitement. It slowly increases the fullness and force of the pulse, and exerts a well-marked influence on the capillary circulation.

It diminishes mucus discharges, leaves a sense of warmth in the respiratory passages, arrests decomposition, and removes foul odors from sores. It is also a very good styptic in passive hemorrhages. Emmenagogue properties have been attributed to it.

HOMEOPATHIC - Large doses of Myrrh quicken the pulse, raise the temperature, cause gastric burning, great sweating, and prostration, vomiting and purgation may follow. Myrrh is a remedy for enfeebled states with excessive mucus discharges.

Muscular debility. Respiratory weakness with difficult expectoration. Tonsillitis with large and infected glands. Chronic gastritis and dyspepsia. Gas and frequent mucus stools.

Female - Dragging and weight sensation in the female pelvis. Leucorrhea. Suppressed menses in anemic young girls.

Mouth - Pale tongue. Salivation. Abscesses. Sores in the mouth. Inflamed and sore gums. ***Pyorrhea.*** Spongy and bleeding gums.

Throat - Sore throats. Pharyngitis. Infected and enlarged tonsils. Abscessed glands.

COMMENTS - As a local application in degenerate ulcers, it is of great value. Especially in phagedaenic, malignant and fetid sores. Carbuncles, malignant scarlatina, putrid sore throat and diphtheria. After an indolent bubo has been opened. In all such local cases it may be used in powder, tincture, or watery solution. It is a favorite appliance in aphthous sores, and bleeding or spongy gums.

REFERENCES - Clarke.

MYRTUS CHEKAN

PHARMACY - myrt-ch. Myrtus cheken. Eugenia cheken. N. O. Myrtacae. South America. ***Historical dose:*** Tincture and all potencies.

HERBAL - The constituents and properties of chekan correspond with those which generally characterize the family myrtacea. To this family belong cloves, allspice, eucalyptus and jambul, all possessing, in the part used, stores of aromatic oil to which, at least, in great part, is due their valuable properties.

Dessauer considers it to possess tonic, expectorant, diuretic and antiseptic properties; he states that he has used it with great success in bronchitis, vesical catarrh and other affections of the mucous membrane, also that digestion is improved.

HOMEOPATHIC - Dr. Dessauer, physician-in-chief to the German hospitals in Valparaiso, and Dr. Murrell, of London, both were instrumental in introducing this remedy to the profession. Dr. Dessauer first had his attention called to the plant by the successful self-treatment by one of his patients in a case of purulent bronchitis. He then tried the chekan on members of his own family with equal success.

Myrt-ch. has chronic bronchitis with dense, yellowish sputum, difficult to detach. Copious expectoration keeps patient distressed and coughing. Dr. John B. Garrison writes: "Myrtus chekan, should prove a valuable remedy in bronchial catarrh.

The chief indications for its use are severe paroxysmal cough with dense yellow expectoration which is difficult to 'bring up. ' Sometimes the secretion is so abundant that it rattles in the deeper bronchial tubes, but, owing to its tenacious character, only small amounts are expectorated. Shortness of breath is also a marked feature, but the cough is the more important of the two symptoms.

This remedy is not a 'cure-all' for all forms of bronchitis, but only in those cases which present, at least, the symptoms, 'thick, yellow, sticky sputum, difficult to expectorate. ' Good results may be anticipated from its use. In all elderly people who suffer from weakened power in expectoration and inability to thoroughly clear the bronchial tubes, Myrtus chekan is most reliable."

COMMENTS - Chekan has done its best work in cases of chronic bronchitis associated with emphysema, particularly in elderly persons suffering from 'winter cough. ' As an example of this reference is made to Murrell's report of fifteen cases of chronic bronchitis which were treated at the Royal Hospital for Diseases of the Chest, London. All of the patients, with one exception, were men. The age of the woman was 51 years; the ages of the men ranged from 36 to 58 years. They were all bad cases, many of them of many years' duration.

Most of them had been attended at the hospital for some considerable time, and, almost without exception, they had in former years undergone much medical treatment without much benefit. Their occupations exposed them to cold, wet and draught, and in some cases they had the additional disadvantage of working in a dusty atmosphere.

They complained chiefly of a paroxysmal cough with thin, yellow expectoration, and much shortness of breath on exertion. On physical examination of the chest emphysema was detected, with, or without, a little bronchus of the bases behind. They were, in fact, ordinary cases of winter cough.

REFERENCES - Boericke.

MYRTUS COMMUNIS

(Myrtle)

PHARMACY - myrt-c. Myrtus communis. Myrtle. Closely allied to Granatum, the pomegranate tree. N. O. Myrtacae. Tincture of fresh shoots and leaves. Tincture of fresh flowering shoots and leaves. ***Historical dose:*** Tincture and all potencies.

CLINICAL - Bronchitis. Catarrhal, fevers. Chest, pain. Coryza. Coughs. Cystitis. Hemoptysis. Pyelitis. Syphilis. Tuberculosis.

HERBAL - The leaves contain Myrtol and an active antiseptic.

HOMEOPATHIC - Myrt-c. is an unproved remedy, the symptoms are entirely clinical, of which Hering gives an account.

Powerful action on the left lung, especially the upper part (Ox-ac., lower). Chest pains, as found in tuberculosis patients. Incipient tuberculosis. Nerve sedative and stimulant to mucus membranes, bronchitis, cystitis and pyelitis.

Breasts - ***Stitching pain in left breast, running through to scapula*** (Anis., Ther., Pix.).

Chest - Acute pressing pain in chest. Pain in upper part of left chest, through to shoulder, worse taking a deep breath and making a strong motion. Stitching in left apex straight through to scapula, worse breathing, yawning, coughing. Burning in left chest with throbbing, aching, tickling. Hepatization of lungs. Tuberculosis from maltreated syphilis. Cough with tightness. Hemoptysis.

Lungs - Dry, hollow cough from tickling in upper anterior lobes of lungs, worse morning, better evening, great lassitude in afternoon. Cough, coryza and catarrhal fever setting in with every atmospheric change.

Modalities - Worse from changes of atmosphere.

Nose - Coryza with cough.

Temperature - Catarrhal fevers with pain in elbow and knee joints, with dry, hollow cough, caused by tickling in upper and front part of lungs, especially in morning, better evening, accompanied by lassitude in afternoon.

Throat - Dryness in throat, pains in throat and chest with expectoration of blood.

COMMENTS - Dr. John B. Garrison writes: “Myrtus communis, the common myrtle, was though highly of by Hering, who made clinical tests with it, and found it to be useful in pain in the upper left lung, going right through, from front to back, under the left scapula.

‘Great lassitude in the afternoon' he considered a very important symptom.”

Pain in upper left lung going right through from the front to the left scapula. The pain is mostly stitching, but may be throbbing, aching or burning. It is worse in morning, better evening, worse by breathing, yawning, coughing.

Cough is dry, hollow, excited by tickling in upper anterior lobes. Hemoptysis, Tuberculosis, lung syphilis, hepatization. Cough and tickling in afternoon is better in evening. Every atmospheric change causes cough, coryza and catarrhal fever.

Hering cured catarrhal fever with tickling cough worse morning and better evening with great lassitude in afternoon.

RELATIONS - ***Compare:*** (1) Myrt-ch. (2) pains through left chest to scapula, Ther., Anis., Pix., Sulph. (3) pain through lower lobe of left lung, Ox-ac. (4) Phos., Bry.

REFERENCES - Boericke. Clarke.

N

NABALUS SERPENTARIA

(White Lettuce)

PHARMACY - nabal. Nabalus serpentaria. White lettuce. Prenanthes serpentaria. Rattlesnake root. N. O. Composite, suborder Chicoracee. Tincture of whole fresh plant. ***Historical dose:*** Tincture and all potencies.

CLINICAL - Constipation. Diarrhea. Dysentery. Dyspepsia. Emaciation. Headaches. Leucorrhea. Ophthalmia.

HERBAL - Nabalus is a Native American plant used in domestic practice for diarrhea and dysentery.

HOMEOPATHIC - There is only one proving with 1c and 3c dilutions by a married woman, age 19. The symptoms somewhat resemble those of its botanical relative, Lact-s., especially in constipation and somnolence. Susceptibility to magnetic contact and to the personal aura of others.

Pain in the abdomen and rectum, with emaciation. Dyspepsia with acid burning eructation. ***Craving for acid food.*** Constipation and chronic diarrhea (Lact.), worse after eating, at nights and toward morning.

Leucorrhea with throbbing in uterus. Heaviness, as if blood vessels filled with lead, body heavy, she leans about. Dull pains in joints and numbness on waking. Irritability of temper and occipital pain, worse in the evening. Ophthalmia.

MIND - Continued melancholy. Depression followed by unusual buoyancy. Irritability of temper and occipital pain.

Eyes - Great and lasting irritation of eyelids and margins, the margins sting and smart and are slightly swollen. Sight weak.

Female - Sharp throbbing in uterus. Menses delayed. White, jelly-like discharge from vagina with weakness.

Food - Appetite and thirst diminished. ***Craving for acid food,*** lemons.

Head - Deep-seated frontal pains behind right eyeball and over eye. Occipital pains with stiffness in neck, worse evenings. Headache with irritability and irritation of eyes, throat and skin. Tipsy sensation.

Kidneys - Sharp, transient pain in right kidney. Diminished urine.

Nose - Right nostril sore. Smell and taste slightly impaired.

Rectum - Constipation, only three stools in twelve days, hard, painful, followed by prostration.

Skin - Subcutaneous glands irritated and swollen, especially behind right ear and in neck. Prickling as from suppressed perspiration, general itching.

Sleep - Somnolence. Sleep prolonged, afterwards lighter and more broken.

Stomach - Burning belchings.

Temperature - Chilliness, not better by heat of fire. No febrile reaction except occasional flushes over head and face.

Throat - Throat sore, tickling and scraping (left), worse lying down and swallowing saliva, then both eyes, worse left.

RELATIONS - ***Compare:*** Lact-s.

REFERENCES - Clarke.

NAJA TRIPUDIANS

(Cobra Venom)

PHARMACY - naja. Naja tripudians. Cobra venom. Cobra di capello. N. O. Elapide. India. The hooded snake of Hindustan. Tincture of the fresh venom. Trituration of saturated with fresh venom. ***Historical dose:*** All potencies.

CLINICAL - Angina pectoris. Asthma. Collapse. Dysmenorrhea. Edema. Esophagus, stricture. Hay fever. Headache. ***Heart disorders.*** Ovaries disorders. Plague. Sepsis. Spinal irritation. Throat, sore.

HOMEOPATHIC - P. C. Majumdar noted that cobra poison had been used by Indian practitioners from ancient times in many nervous and blood diseases. Naja. is not a hemorrhagic or septic medicine like Lach. and Crot-h.

Naja. produces a typical bulbar paralysis. Causes no hemorrhage but only edema, hence the victims of this reptile frequently bear very little sign of external injury, the only indication is often a small scratch or puncture.

The tissue lying beneath the wound is colored dark purple and a large quantity of viscid, blood-like fluid collects in the vicinity of the wound. The first symptom is an intense burning pain at the bite. There is an interval, usually an hour, before other symptoms develop, after which they develop rapidly.

A feeling of intoxication is produced, followed by a loss of power over the limbs. Loss of speech, swallowing and the control over the movement of the lips. Saliva is ejected in large quantities. The respiration gradually becomes slower and slower and at length ceases. Victim remains conscious throughout.

The action of Naja. settles around the ***heart, hypertrophy and valvular diseases***. Affects medulla and cerebellum, respiration, throat, ovary. Diseases primarily depending upon degeneration of motor cells. Sepsis.

Nervous, excited and tremulous with heart disorders, often reflex. Marked surging of blood upwards. Heart is enlarged. Affections of heart with paucity of symptoms. ***Organs seem to be drawn together***. Constrictions in chest, throat. Concomitant with the heart symptoms are pain in forehead and temples. Collapse. Swooning fits.

Feeling of intoxication. Loss of power over limbs and sphincters, unable to speak. Marked dyspnea, inability to lie on left side. Insensible right side. Left sided symptoms. Very susceptible to cold. Sensation of wasting away. Burnings as of hot irons. Screwed up sensation.

MIND - Absent-mindedness. Very forgetful. Stupid and confused feeling. Irresolution, indecision. Wandering of the mind. ***Brooding, over imaginary troubles and disease.*** Blurred speech. Insensible and speechless. Aphasia. Aversion to talking. Affected easily by wine or alcoholic drinks.

Nervous, excited and tremulous. Want of self confidence. Anxiety from pain in heart region. Forebodings. Hypochondria. ***Fear of death,*** disease, being incurable, ***rain,*** accidents, misfortune. Dreads to be left alone. ***Feels anguish for others.*** Anguish from pain in abdomen.

Melancholy. Sorrow felt in the heart. Depressed, as if everything were done wrong and could not be rectified. Depressed with distress about sexual organs, better in evening. Despair with the pains. Loathing of life. Suicidal disposition (Aur.). Ailments from grief.

Insanity. Antagonism with self. Confusion as to his identity. Sensation of duality. Delirium during fevers, with meningitis, typhus, typhoid fever. Sees images, phantoms. Delusion that he is a failure, that he has neglected his duty, that he is being injured. Consciousness almost lost. Comatose.

Abdomen - Aching in loins. Cutting, twisting, griping pains. Much flatulence with rumbling and colicky pains. Flatulence during day, at night with pain. Frequent cutting in umbilical region and small of back in afternoon, then profuse and sudden leucorrhea.

Back - Rheumatic pains in neck and back. Cutting, aching in nape. Tired feeling in thoracic vertebra all day with burning and exhaustion. Shooting from inner and upper angle of left scapula to front of chest. Pain between the shoulders as if in spine afterwards involving scapula in morning on waking, worse moving arms. Dragging sensation in spine between shoulders. Acute pain in small of back, gnawing pain.

Breasts - Milk decreased, next day returned freely, afterwards scanty. Occasional pain at top of both breasts.

Causations - Ailments from anticipation, grief, sorrow.

Chest - Constriction in chest, in evening. Oppressive weight on chest, as if a hot iron had been run in. Uneasiness and dull, heavy pain in chest. ***Sharp pains, worse on deep inspiration.*** Ribs feel broken. Heavy pain over lower half of right chest with stabbing on deep inspiration, cannot cough for the stabbing, worse lying left side, better lying on affected side. Tenderness over sternum and in throat.

Cough - ***Irritating, dry cough.*** Cough from sticky mucus and saliva. Cough with tightness and fullness in larynx. Cardiac cough. Dry, hacking cough with blood-spitting. Hoarseness, short, hoarse cough.

Ears - Burning heat of ear. Otalgia. Chronic otorrhea, black discharges, smells like herring brine. Noises in ears. Whizzing in left ear with insipid, almost nauseous taste in mouth. Noise as of a mill, waking him in morning. Illusions of hearing.

Eyes - Fixed and staring, wide open and insensible to light. Pupils dilated. Loss of vision. Hot pains at back of eyeballs. Ptosis of both lids. Heaviness in eyelids. Lids swollen in morning.

Female - Pain in left groin, especially in post-operative cases, ***seems to be drawn to heart.*** Neuralgia of left ovary. Crampy pains in left ovary. ***Aching in left ovary with pains in heart,*** come on a week before menses, grow worse until menses appear, then easier until next month.

Food - Loss of appetite. Thirsty. Craving for stimulants, which aggravate.

Head - Pain in forehead and temples with heart symptoms. ***Pain in left temple and in left orbital region,*** extending to occiput with nausea and vomiting. Severe throbbing and aching in temples. Constriction across forehead. ***Severe headache with intense depression.*** Headache supervening on cessation of menses. Neuralgic headache extending backwards from orbital region. Shooting up occiput. Vertex sensitive to cold. Aching in vertex with cold feet. ***Feeling as of a blow from behind on head and neck.*** Sensation as if brain was loose. Entire head feels hollow. Confusion and dullness in head in morning. Sensitiveness of scalp. Hair falls off the vertex

Heart - ***Acute and chronic septic endocarditis. Damaged heart after infectious diseases.*** Hypertrophy, weakness. ***Valvular heart disorders. Heart lesions*** (Spong., Laur.). ***Low blood pressure*** (Elaps., Vip.). Visible palpitations. Palpitations prevent speech because of choking. Chronic nervous palpitations, worse after preaching. Threatened paralysis of heart, body cold. Sharp pain in region of heart. Angina pains extending to nape of neck, left shoulder and arm with anxiety and fear of death. Heart symptoms with pain in forehead and temples. Dragging and anxiety in precordia. Feeling of weight on heart. ***Irregular in force***. Pulse slow, irregular, weak, tremulous.

Kidneys - Uneasiness and pressure in bladder. Urine of deep straw color. Urine deposits red sediment, mixed with mucus, loaded with gravel and mucus.

Limbs - Sudden loss of strength in limbs. Rheumatic pains in limbs. Drawing, lacerating, worse motion. Cramps in shoulders, nape or thighs. Aching in ankles, lower part of thighs, wrists and shoulder joints, on waking. Violent racking in marrow of thighs. Numb left arm. Puffy or sweating hands and feet with cough. Acute pain under the left thumb nail running up the arm.

Lungs - Labored and difficult breathing. Gasping for breath. Puffing breathing. Breathing very slow, shallow and scarcely perceptible. Suffocative spells after sleeping. (Lach.). Dry or empty feeling in left lung. Asthmatic constriction of chest, cannot expand lungs, followed by mucus expectoration. Asthma preceded by coryza, worse lying, better sitting up. Cardiac asthma. Expectoration of whitish viscid mucus in morning on waking. Spitting of blood, which had no tendency to coagulate.

Male - Stinging, somewhat burning pain along right side of penis, immediately under skin, at night in bed and in morning after rising. Increased sexual desire. Desire on going to bed with frequent waking, vivid imaginations. Nocturnal emissions. Involuntary emissions, then prostration and distress. Peculiar distress, great desire, but no physical power, with depression.

Modalities - Great relief of pain and breathing by lying on right side. ***Better from walking or riding in open air,*** sneezing, smoking. Worse from stimulants, alcohol, cold air, drafts, riding in carriage, touch, pressure of clothes. ***Worse lying on left side***, after sleep, after menses. Headache worse at 3 p.m.

Mouth - Great dryness of the mouth. Wide open, flow of saliva. Foaming at mouth. Taste insipid, bitter, sour, metallic. Tongue cold, coated thick yellow, white, dry, no thirst. Ulcers on frenum. Loss of speech.

Nose - Hay fever with dry larynx. Hay asthma. Flow of water from nose, then intense sneezing which betters the breathing.

Rectum - Urging always sudden, whether followed by diarrhea or not. Sudden urging, then small, bilious stool. Constipation, feeling of a large stool which when voided was small. Diarrhea with pain in abdomen, profuse, sudden, slimy, white or green, bilious. Heat in anal region with itching, smarting at anus.

Sensations - ***Screwed-up sensations*** and crampy pains. As if head screwed together. As if heart and ovary were drawn up together. Pains in temple and ovarian regions. Pain from heart to scapula. Sensation as if a hair in larynx. Pain as from needles in tonsil. The left side is predominantly affected.

Skin - Itching scars. Creeping, itching and tingling sensation in skin. Skin swollen, mottled and of dark purple, livid color. Gangrene. Small, white itching blisters on inflamed base, on neck, nose and body in afternoon. Large pimples on inflamed base. Pimple on upper lip, on left ala nasi, on tip of nose, sore in consequence, painful on brow. Boil-like swelling on back of middle phalanx of right little finger. Painful chilblains on feet.

Sleep - Yawning, great sleepiness. Dozing and moaning. Sleepiness in evening and weakness. Deep, profound, comatose with stertorous breathing. Restless, disturbed sleep. Long and vivid dreams, little recollection of the subjects, affairs of the day recalled with additions and new plans for the morrow. Dreams of murders, suicides, fires, etc.

Stomach - Uneasy, disagreeable feeling in stomach, as from indigestion, pressure as from stones after a meal. Acidity in stomach. Heartburn, belchings tasting like barley water or hot and foul. Nausea with faint feeling, vomiting.

Temperature - Body cold and collapsed. Limbs very cold, icy coldness of feet. ***Very sensitive to cold.*** General sweat, cold, clammy. Free perspiration. Flushes of heat in face at different times of day, worse left side. Head hot and full of blood and much sweat in palms. Feels very uncomfortable, hot and feverish. Heat, but he refused water, heat with prostration with discomfort, dry lips and tender, hot mouth.

Throat - Roughness and scraping in throat. Soreness and pricking in left side of throat. Dryness and constriction of throat and fauces. Dark red color of the fauces. Redness of left side in morning with pain on swallowing. Irritation and tickling in larynx and trachea. Stricture of esophagus, swallowing difficult or impossible. Grasping at throat with sense of choking. As a lump in throat. Much mucus in throat. Shooting in left tonsil.

Vertigo - Vertigo, lasting a short time, followed by ***astounding pain*** in right side of head.

COMMENTS - Naja. was introduced into homeopathy by Russell and Stokes, who made the first provings along with some forty other provers including Gillow, Pope and Drysdale. Provings were made with low potencies.

Majumdar had no success with Naja. until he obtained fresh venom from snake charmers and made potencies. Previously the Naja. used by Indian homeopaths had been re-imported into India from England in the form of potencies.

Deane, in his experience in the plague epidemic of 1899-1900, found Naja. prepared from the fresh venom more efficacious than Lach.

Naja. has an affinity for the medulla oblongata and cerebellum. Heart failure and distress. Weak valves with regurgitations, stenosis, prolapse. Acute and chronic endocarditis. Heart damage after infectious diseases.

Low blood pressure. Fluttering palpitation sensations outside the chest. Depression and weakness about the heart. Inability to speak with choking, nervous chronic palpitations. Pulse is slow, irregular.

Severe pains in left temple, cardiac and ovarian region. Diphtheria with impending paralysis of heart. Sensation of weight, of a hot iron, on the chest. Sensation as if heart and ovary were drawn together.

Pains about heart extending to nape of neck, left shoulder and arm with anxiety and fear of death.

Neuralgic pain in head, preceded or followed by nausea or vomiting. Severe throbbing in left orbital region drawing back to occiput, from over-eating, mental or physical exertion. Headache after cessation of menses. Dull, heavy constriction in forehead on waking.

Characteristic grasping at the throat with choking sensations. Esophageal spasms. Worse at night, patient wakes gasping, surface blue. Worse by lying on left side. Useful for snake bites (Lach.).

According to Hering, nervous phenomena predominate in Naja. over other serpent poisons. It acts primarily upon the nervous system, especially on respiratory nerves, pneumogastric and glossopharyngeal.

Majumdar related the case of a young woman suffering from a heart affection who had oppression of the chest amounting almost to suffocation, feeble, irregular, almost imperceptible pulse, anemic appearance, inability to speak.

One dose of Naja. was given, followed four hours later by a second. These sufficed for the cure. The next day, when the doctor called, his patient addressed him in a loud voice, "Doctor, you gave me a poison last night." When asked to explain, she said that after the first dose she "felt awful heat in her system."

Majumdar saved a number of apparently hopeless cases of cholera with Naja. in the collapse stage with lack of pulse and difficulty of breathing.

In a case cured by Russell there was dragging and anxiety in the precordia occurring in great grief.

Andrew M. Neatby related a cure with Naja. 6c that had nervous palpitations and faintness, frequent sensation of swelling, of "choking" in the throat, with dyspnea and occasionally of anesthesia down the right side.

Mahlon Preston cured himself with Naja. 30c of asthma with difficult breathing, worse lying down, better sitting up. He cured many cases of hay fever and autumnal catarrh that had a flow of water from the nose for a few minutes, then intense sneezing, which relieved the breathing. After recurring for a few days, there is dryness in the lungs with great difficulty of breathing, worse on lying down.

Bunn cured the case of Miss S., 22, who had dysmenorrhea since her menses were established. Dilatation, galvanism., etc., had been tried in vain. She had shooting pain in the region of the left ovary and faintness. Hypogastrium revealed nothing abnormal except sensitiveness of the ovarian region.

Extreme restlessness with the pain. During the menses the pains suddenly became very severe. The flow stopped when the pain was at its worst and returned the next day with relief from pain. Naja. 30c was given and the next period passed absolutely free from discomfort.

RELATIONS - ***Antidoted by:*** Ammonia, stimulants (effects of bite), tobacco (to potencies). ***Compare:*** (1) Snake venoms. (2) Bung-f.- this venom produces a condition like an acute polioencephalitis and myelitis. (3) Lach., Crot-h., Spig., Spong. (4) Depression and suicidal tendency, Aur. (5) Ulcer of frenum lingue, Nat-c. Agar. (6) Headache from before backwards, Anac., Bry., Nux-v. (7) from behind forwards, Gels., Lac-c., Sang., Sil., Spig. (8) Diphtheria, Arum-t. (9) Heart, Ars., Cact., Iber., Lach., Spig., Dig. (10) Collapse, Carb-v., Camph., Tab. (11) Mouth wide open tongue cold, Camph. (12) Loss of speech, Dulc., Gels., Caust., Hy., Laur. (13) Dark red color of fauces, Ail., Bapt., Phyt.

REFERENCES - Boericke. Clarke. Murphy. Phatak.

NAPHTHALINUM

(Tar Camphor)

PHARMACY - naphtin. Naphthalinum. Tar camphor. Naphthalene. A chemical compound from coal tar. Trituration. ***Historical dose:*** All potencies.

CLINICAL - Albuminuria. Amblyopia. Asthma. Bronchitis. Cataract. Diarrhea. Eczema. Flatulence. Gleet. Gonorrhea. Hay asthma. Psoriasis. Retina, detached. Tuberculosis.

Typhoid fever. Whooping cough. Worms.

HOMEOPATHIC - Naphthalene is a hydrocarbon obtained by distillation from coal tar. It consists of colorless, transparent, lustrous scales or, when crystallized, of rhombic tables or prisms.

Naphtin. is an unproved remedy, though it has been used in old-school practice as an intestinal antiseptic and vermifuge, as an expectorant, as a remedy for eczema and psoriasis, and as an antiseptic application to wounds.

Naphtin. is for the expulsion of thread worms after the bowels have been freely opened by a cathartic, given in doses of grains 1/4 to grains 1/2 four times a day for two days. The dose should not be given after a meal and all fats and oils should be abstained from during the treatment, which may be repeated once or twice after leaving a week's interval.

Affinity for the eyes. Detachment of the retina, deposits an exudation in the retina. Opacity of cornea, cataract, amblyopia. Long and continued attacks of coughing, unable to get a breath, sometimes so violent as to cause perspiration. Whooping cough.

Abdomen - Incarcerated flatus in the transverse colon causing cardiac distress.

Eyes - Eyes inflamed, painful, bloodshot, in hay fever. Cataract. Amblyopia. Detached retina. Shiny bodies in vitreous. White patches on retina of oxalate, sulphate and carbonate of calcium.

Face - Lips and face cyanotic. Face pale, yellow. Twitching of facial muscles.

Food - Loss of appetite.

Head - Headache with fever, drowsiness and loss of appetite.

Head - Saliva flows from the mouth.

Kidneys - Sudden, violent desire to urinate, urethra meatus red and swollen, prepuce edematous. Urine is dark brown, becoming black after standing, albuminous. Incontinence of urine. Gonorrhea. Gleet.

Lungs - Breathing is labored and irregular, asthmatic. Cough in violent, incessant paroxysms almost arresting breath, compelling the patient to hold his head for the pain. Cough with blue or purple face. Expectoration free, thick, tenacious, almost absent. Night cough preventing sleep.

Male - Edema of prepuce.

Nose - Coryza, thin, excoriating discharge, much sneezing. Hay fever. Attacks of sneezing. Irritation of nose. Rubs his nose to remove the irritation.

Rectum - Incontinence of urine and feces. Thin, offensive diarrhea of tuberculosis.

Skin - Eczema. Psoriasis.

Sleep - Very great drowsiness lasting some days.

Temperature - Sudden onset of a fever, with headache and loss of appetite. Temperature reduced in typhoid.

COMMENTS - Some cases of Naphtin. poisoning have been reported. Evers recorded chronic illness, loss of appetite, headache and eczema over both legs as due to Naphtin. which was used as a moth powder and sprinkled on bedding.

In another case, a boy, 12, came home one evening apparently drunk, semi-conscious, staggering, unable to answer questions. He had eaten two candies which were really moth-destroyers, each tablet containing two grams of pure naphthalin. An emetic was promptly administered and the next day the boy was still drowsy but quite conscious. The drowsiness lasted four days.

Attacks of sneezing from nasal irritation, frequently attempting to remove the irritation by rubbing his nose. In two hours incoordination had increased. Twitching of facial muscles. Saliva flowed freely from the mouth.

Lippincott was the first to use Naphtin. in cases of hay fever, having heard that hay fever sufferers who went into factories where Naphtha was much used were always cured. His experience of its value was speedily confirmed by other observers. Naphtin. 1x and 2x were used in the first trials.

W. Louis Hartmann of Syracuse is the chief homeopathic authority for this remedy. His leading indications for it are acute coryza with fluent excoriating discharge and much sneezing. Paroxysms of coughing, following each other in rapid succession so that the patient is unable to take his breath (as in asthma and whooping cough). He found it more often indicated than any other drug in whooping cough.

The spasmodic action and the cyanosis of the drug are good indications here, though it is not necessary to wait until the child is blue before prescribing Naphtin. Followed well by Dros.

In a case of tuberculosis of the left lung, Naphtin. removed an inability to sleep for cough. Exhausting night-sweats and offensive, thin diarrhea during the day.

In three cases in which Naphtin. had been applied to wounds there was sudden onset of fever, headache, loss of appetite. In one of them, there was temporary mania with incontinence of urine and feces. In two of them, albuminuria. All symptoms rapidly disappeared when Naphtin. was discontinued.

J. Meredith cured with the Naphtin. 6x incarcerated flatus in transverse colon causing cardiac distress.

Hartmann used the 1x trituration, having been disappointed with higher potencies.

RELATIONS - ***Compare:*** (1) Salol., Carb-ac., Anil., Methyl-b. and coal-tar products generally. (2) In coughs, Dros. which follows Naphtin. well. (3) Coc-c., Arn., Bell., Cor-r. Ip. (4) In tuberculosis, Petr., Basil. In eye affections, Chol. (5) In gonorrhea, Thuj., Petros., Salol. (6) In hay fever, Psor., Sabad., Ars., All-c., Kali-i. (7) In worms. Cina, Teucr.

REFERENCES - Anshutz. Clarke.

NARCISSUS POETICUS
(Daffodil)

PHARMACY - narc-po. Narcissus poeticus. Daffodil. N. O. Amaryllidaceae. Tincture of unexpended blossom-buds, stem, leaf and flower. The young buds, stems and leaves are macerated in two times their weight of alcohol. ***Historical dose:*** Tincture and all potencies.

CLINICAL - Bronchitis. Coryza. Cough. Diarrhea. Whooping cough.

HERBAL - The name of the plant, Narcissus, is not from that of the fabled youth who fell in love with his own image reflected in the water, but is from the Greek Narkao, *"to be numb,"* on account of the narcotic properties of the drug. The classic Asphodel and the Narcissus are the same, from which it may be seen that the plant dates back as far as man's records go.

Dr. Charge's work, Maladies de la Respiration, quoted the great Laennec as an authority in regards Narcissus.

Fernie, in his excellent Herbal simples, also said "An extract of the bulbs applied to open wounds has produced staggering numbness of the whole nervous system and paralysis of the heart. Socrates called this plant the 'Chaplet of the Infernal Gods,' because of its narcotic effects."

He also noted that a decoction of the dried flowers is emetic and when sweetened will, as an emetic, serve most usefully for relieving the congestive bronchial catarrh of children.

On the other hand, the alkaloid from the bulbs after flowering produces copious salivation, increases cutaneous secretion, contracts the pupil of the eye, produces slight relaxation of the pulse and slight faintness and nausea.

Daffodil bulbs contain an alkaloid the action of which, according to authorities, varies as to whether the alkaloid is extracted from the flowering bulb or from the bulb after flowering.

The National Dispensatory noted that "The emetic action of Narcissus has been used to break up intermittent fever and relieve bronchial catarrh with congestion or obstruction of the air tubes. Like Ipecacuanha, it has also been prescribed in dysentery, especially of the epidemic form. Its influence upon the nervous system is attested by the vogue it has enjoyed in hysteria, chorea, whooping cough and even epilepsy."

HOMEOPATHIC - The concluding paragraph in Fernie's section on the Narcissus states: "The medicinal influence of the daffodil on the nervous system has led to giving its flowers and its bulb for hysterical states and even epilepsy with benefit."

Narc-po. is peculiarly homeopathic to long-continued coughs, especially of nervous origin. Bronchitis. Convulsive stage of whooping cough. Coryza, frontal headache. Faintness and drowsiness. Symptoms of nausea followed by violent vomiting and diarrhea.

Eyes - Running at eyes. Pupils contracted at first, dilated later.

Head - Frontal headache.

Heart - Pulse increased.

Mouth - Increased flow of saliva. Free salivation of very ropy saliva.

Nose - Severe coryza.

Rectum - Diarrhea with severe aching below left free ribs. Stools are watery, relaxed, loose, some solid.

Skin - Erythema of a papular, vesicular and pustular types, aggravation in wet weather.

Stomach - Sinking, sick sensation. Rumbling. Heartburn. Hiccough. Vomiting.

Temperature - Hand which was quite wet with perspiration became dry in twelve minutes.

Throat - Dryness in throat.

COMMENTS - A patient of Clarke's once had a very severe cough set up by daffodils used in some profusion as a decoration of a dinner table.

A fatal case of poisoning from eating the flowers is on record. A salad of onions in which were mixed some bulbs of Narcissus poeticus, caused burning, copious stools with dreadful griping, obtuse senses, fainting, cold hands, and cold sweat. Symptoms were not distinguishable from the usual effects of Colch. and similar to those of Narc-ps.

J. Meredith made a conserve of flowers, buds and stems by mashing them with six to ten times their weight of sugar in a Wedgwood mortar with a wooden pestle. Counting this as 1x, he made sugar potencies to 4x, and with these he cured a case of bronchitis with continuous cough which had resisted many of the standard remedies.

In Ringer's experiments, the bulb preparation produced the greater number of effects including salivation, sinking, vomiting and diarrhea. The flower preparation acted on the head and eyes and dried up a profuse perspiration of the hands.

RELATIONS - ***Compare:*** (1) All-c., Colch., Lil-t. Narc-ps.

REFERENCES - Anshutz. Boericke. Clarke.

NARCOTINUM

(Opium Alkaloid)

PHARMACY - narcot. Narcotinum. Opium alkaloid. Noscapinum pura. Papaveraceae. Trituration. ***Historical dose:*** All potencies.

CLINICAL - Bladder, paralysis. Vertigo.

HOMEOPATHIC - Narcot. has been rather extensively proved, but very few distinctive symptoms were elicited. The most notable were dry, clammy mouth, thick indistinct speech and paralysis of bladder. The vertigo symptoms were like those of Morph., and the general symptoms those of Op. and its other alkaloids.

REFERENCES - Clarke.

NASTURTIUM AQUATICUM

(Water-cress)

PHARMACY - nast. Nasturtium aquaticum. Water-cress. Nasturtium officinale. Roripa nasturtium. Roripa aquaticum. N. O. Cruciferae. Tincture of the whole plant. ***Historical dose:*** Tincture and all potencies.

CLINICAL - Cirrhosis. Hysteria. Neurasthenia. ***Tobacco, poisoning.***

HERBAL - Nasturtium is useful in scorbutic disorders and constipation, related to strictures of urinary apparatus. Supposed to be an aphrodisiac.

HOMEOPATHIC - Nast. is antidotal to ***tobacco poisoning***. Sedative in neurotic affections, neurasthenia, hysteria. Cirrhosis of liver and dropsy.

REFERENCES - Clarke.

NATRUM ARSENICUM

(Sodium Arsenate)

PHARMACY - nat-ar. Natrum arsenicum. Sodium arsenate. Atoxyl. Hydric di-sodic arsenate. Solution. Trituration. ***Historical dose:*** All potencies.

CLINICAL - Anemia. ***Asthma.*** Blepharitis. Conjunctivitis. Coryza. Cough. Diphtheria. Edema. Emaciation. Esophagus, constriction. Eyes, inflammation. Granular, eyelids. Hemoptysis. Interscapular pain. ***Leukemia. Miner's asthma.*** Nose, disorders. Pityriasis rubra. Post-nasal catarrh. Testicles, neuralgia. Tuberculosis.

HOMEOPATHIC - Nat-ar. has been very extensively proved, notably by Imbert Gourbeyre. The principal clinical use of Nat-ar. has been in diphtheria, when it presents with a dark purple throat, great swelling, much prostration, and not much pain.

Useful in disorders of the eyes and nose. Generally irritating effects. ***Miner's asthma from coal dust.*** Lungs feel as if smoke had been inhaled. Racking cough with profuse greenish expectoration. Oppression of chest and about the heart. Nasal catarrh with headache, pain at root of nose, dry and painful eyes. Bronchitis of children, chronic.

Feels tired all over. Psoriasis (Ars., Thyr.). ***Leukemia*** (Ars.). Emaciation. Edema. As if the thyroid gland were compressed by a thumb and finger. Cartier noted that it facilitates the termination of a cold and conserves strength and appetite.

MIND - Mental dullness, listless. Concentration difficult while studying, reading. Forgetfulness. Imbecility. Timidity. Depressed, as if something bad impending. Lamenting, bemoaning, wailing. Hysteria. Ailments from anger, vexation. Quarrelsomeness, scolding. Reproaches himself and others.

Conscientious about trifles. Fastidious. ***Nervous restlessness at night.*** Anxiety with palpitations. ***Anxiety about the future. Frightened easily.*** Fear of impending disease, that something bad will happen, of evil. Fear of people, in a crowd, anthropophobia. Aversion to company. ***Suspicious.***

Abdomen - Pain from abdomen at times, shifting through bowels, better by passage of flatus or stool. Gas forms rapidly, better when bowels move, colic from flatus and before stool. Pain in groin.

Back - Pain and soreness in back. Neck stiff and sore. Soreness at lower cervical vertebra down to joints of scapula and under both scapula. Severe pain between scapula, better moving forward, worse from inspiration. Pain in lumbar region.

Chest - Oppression of chest and about heart, worse exertion and full inspiration. Roughness and irritation in bronchi mornings, with slight cough. Eruption on chest, dark brown scaly spots on a red base, no itching.

Coughs - Teasing, dry cough, during day. ***Dry cough, with feeling of tightness and oppression in chest.*** Dry, hacking cough, from an uneasy feeling and soreness beneath ribs, worse any exertion. Racking cough with profuse, greenish expectoration. Hemoptysis.

Ears - Ears feels heavy and drooped.

Eyes - Catarrhal conjunctivitis and blepharitis marginalis. Dry, painful, burning, stinging. Eyes feel weak, soon tire. Stiffness of eyeballs, feel too large. Smarting and lachrymation on going into open air. Agglutination in morning. Tendency of lids to close, cannot open them as wide as usual. Edema of orbital region. Supraorbital pain.

Face - Feels puffed, bloated. Swollen face. Hot and flushed. Malar bone feels large, as if swollen. Masseter muscles stiff, painful to move jaw. Eruptions around mouth. Corners of mouth fissured.

Female - Menses protracted, scanty. Leucorrhea, thick, offensive, yellow.

Head - Heat and fullness in head. Floating sensation on turning head quickly. Aching pain in frontal region, root of nose, and over orbits. Boring pain in temples. Headache, worse pressure. ***Headache from tobacco smoke.*** Periodical headaches, worse noise.

Heart - Oppression about heart on least exertion. Can feel heartbeat through chest distinctly. Sounds heard through nearly every part of chest. Pulse irregular, variable in volume. Pulse slower than usual.

Kidneys - Dull, aching pain in kidneys, with profuse urine. Sore feeling in region of bladder, worse urinating. Urine copious, frequent, clear. Urine contains some epithelial scales, casts and fat globules.

Limbs - Neuralgic pain, recurring frequently. Pain in anterior crural nerves. Pains erratic, worse in joints and on left side. Feels tired all over. Joints stiff. Knee joints crack. Aching in arms, worse in shoulder.

Lungs - ***Oppression of chest and about heart*** and also larynx. Pneumonia and tuberculosis. Lungs feel as if smoke had been inhaled. Asthma, worse dust and smoke. ***Miner's asthma*** produced by inhalation of coal dust.

Male - Dull, cutting pain along inguinal ligament, followed by sickening sensation in left testicle as from a blow, testicle very sensitive while pain lasts.

Modalities - ***Worse on moving***, jarring, least exertion, pressure, during the day.

Nose - ***Feels stopped up, pain at root. Nasal catarrh, with pain at root of nose.*** Coryza, worse open air, fluent alternating with dry. Watery discharge, drops into throat. Post-nasal dropping of thick, bland, yellowish mucus. ***Crusts in nose.*** Dry crusts, on removal, leave mucus membrane raw. Smell defective or lost.

Perspiration - Surface cool, covered with cold, clammy sweat.

Rectum - Diarrhea, alternating with constipation. Stool thin, dark, soft, followed by burning at anus. Yellowish, watery, copious, painless, hurries out of bed in morning. Diarrhea worse at night. Diarrhea from milk.

Sensations - Some of the peculiar symptoms are wavering, floating sensation on turning head. Eyeballs feel stiff, feel too large for lids to close over. Scratching beneath lids on rolling eyeballs. Pain at root of nose. Feeling of lump in throat of blow on testicle, as if smoke inhaled into lungs. Feeling as if the body were compressed by thumb and finger.

Skin - Squamous eruption, scales thin, white, and when removed leave skin slightly reddened. Scales cause itching, worse getting warm from exercise.

Sleep - Drowsy, heavy sleep. Restless sleep, when aroused awakes nervously as from a fright.

Stomach - Stomach tender. Sensation of fullness. Sinking sensation, with dull feeling in supraorbital and frontal region. Hematemesis. Belching and sour eructations.

Throat - ***Dark, purplish, swollen, edematous***, red and glassy. Roughness causes hemming, with spasmodic cough. Hawking of tough, gelatinous, greyish yellow mucus from throat and posterior nares. Dark slate-colored, scanty mucus in larynx, detached with difficulty. Elongation of uvula. Sensation as if thyroid were compressed by a thumb and finger.

Tongue - Tongue coated yellow, deep red, corrugated, anterior part fissured. Tongue large, moist, fissured, flabby.

Vertigo - Floating sensation on turning head quickly.

Vision - Vision weakened, objects blur when he looks at them for a short time, eyes sensitive to light.

COMMENTS - Leukemia (Ars., Nat-m.), especially in children. Pain between scapula, better bending forward. Headache, worse from heat. Restlessness, thirst, chilliness with a hot head (Ars.). Nasal obstruction and chilliness, worse at night.

Sensitive to cold air. Itching is worse when heated, by exercise. Warm things cause burning in stomach, cold drinks aggravate nausea. Wind causes conjunctivitis. Right side of head, left testicle and left leg are most affected.

RELATIONS - ***Compare:*** (1) Ars., Kali-c. - edema about eyes and face. (2) Apis - diphtheria with sac-like swelling of uvula, but Apis has much pain, Nat-a. has not. (3) Arum-t. - diphtheria, Arum-t. has less swelling and more pain. (4) Kali-bi. - tenacious mucus. (5) Nat-m. - throat. (6) Lyc. - stopped catarrh.

REFERENCES - Boericke. Clarke. Murphy.

NATRUM CACODYLICUM

(Sodium Cacodylate)

PHARMACY - nat-cac. Natrum cacodylicum. Sodium cacodylate. Trituration. Solution. ***Historical dose:*** All potencies.

CLINICAL - Dermatitis. Neuritis. Paralysis. Tuberculosis. Wrist-drop.

HOMEOPATHIC - This acid (and more particularly its sodium salt) has been used on the recommendation of Armand Gautier, Professor of Chemistry at the Faculty of Medicine of Paris, as a "cure" for tuberculosis. The non-poisonous nature of this salt enables the patients to take it in large doses, but it is not always harmless.

Cacodyl, which signifies evil-smelling, is like Cyanogen, a compound radical. It was first obtained by Bunsenis 1873 as di-cacodyl. It is a clear liquid that refracts light strongly, heavier than water, of insupportably offensive smell, its vapor being highly poisonous.

Cacodylic acid is a crystalline arsenic compound, soluble in water, odorless and, though containing 54.4 percent of metallic arsenic, not an active poison.

Useful for malignant diseases and growths. Tuberculosis. Foul breath and mouth with bad odor. Dry dermatitis of the skin of abdomen.

COMMENTS - Murrell gave Nat-cac. in pills of one grain, three times a day, to a young woman, 21. Poisoning symptoms set in suddenly after the eleventh dose, including constant vomiting, tongue like a piece of raw beef, inflamed conjunctive, eyelids edematous. Breath of gangrenous odor, peripheral neuritis, wrist-drop, paralysis of left leg. The odor was noticed on second day, the other symptoms came suddenly.

REFERENCES - Clarke.

NATRUM CARBONICUM

(Sodium Carbonate)

PHARMACY - nat-c. Natrum carbonicum. Sodium carbonate. The common "Soda" of the shops, purified, not the Bicarbonate of Soda. Trituration. Solution. ***Historical dose:*** Trituration and all potencies.

CLINICAL - Acidity. Albuminuria. Anemia. Anidrosis. ***Ankles, weak***. Backache. ***Belching.*** Burns. Candida. Chills. Colic. Constipation. Cornea, ulcers. Corns. Coryza. Coughs. Deafness. ***Debility. Diarrhea***. Dysmenorrhea. ***Dyspepsia***. Eczema. Elephantiasis. Emaciation. Fever. ***Flatulence. Food, allergies.*** Glands, disorders. Goiter. Hands, chapped. ***Headaches.*** Heartburn. Heat, flushes. ***Heatstroke.*** Heels, blisters. Herpes. Hiccough. Hoarseness. Hypochondriasis. Hysteria. Ichthyosis. ***Indigestion***. Infertility. Keratitis. ***Leucorrhea.*** Lisping. ***Malassimilation.*** Malnutrition. ***Milk, allergies.*** Moles. Nausea. Nose, eruptions. Nose, swollen. Nosebleed. Ozaena. Palpitations. Photophobia. Post-nasal, catarrh. Presbyopia. Priapism. Rheumatism. Ringworm. School, headaches. Scrofula. Stammering. Sterility. ***Sunstroke.*** Throat, mucus. Toothache. Ulcers. Vertigo. Vomiting. Warts. Waterbrash.

HOMEOPATHIC - Nat-c. was proved by Hahnemann and is one of the anti-psoric remedies. All the natrums stimulate cellular activity and increase oxidation and metabolism. It had been used in old-school practice as an external application in solution to burns and eczema, and as a douche in nasal or vaginal catarrh.

The common practice of taking sodium bicarbonate for indigestion and heartburn is founded on a true relationship (though Nat-c. is the carbonate and not the bicarbonate), but the indiscriminate and excessive use of it only intensifies the trouble.

Nat-c. forms the alkaline basis in most soaps, excess alkali almost burns off the superficial layers of the epidermis and leaves the skin dry and cracked. The provings confirm this irritating action. Nat-c. is particularly useful for chapped hands and faces, rough, dry skin, eczema, herpes, warts and scrofulous conditions of the skin.

Swelling and induration of glands. Exhaustion. Emaciation, anemia. Milky, watery skin. ***Very weak ankles***. Puffiness. Relaxation, easy dislocation. Twitching in the muscles and limbs. Contraction of muscles, tendons. Pains cause tremors, cold sweat, anxiety etc.

Irritation of the mucus membranes. Irritation, vesicles, ulcers and catarrh in the digestive tract from the mouth to anus. Keratitis and ulceration of the cornea. The nose is swollen and ulcerated with a thick yellow or green offensive discharge. Thick, yellow, putrid leucorrhea (Sep.).

Oversensitive to open air, music, noise and dietetic errors. Worse from any physical or mental exertion, strain, from the least effort, from sun and gaslight. ***Debility from heat of summer***, every spell of warm weather causes headache. ***Chronic effects of sunstroke***. ***Headache from sun*** or working under lights.

Children when asleep, jump, cry, grasp the mother. Startled, nervous children. ***Children cannot tolerate milk*** but thrive better on cereals.

MIND - Mental weakness. Weak memory. Difficulty thinking or concentrating. Slow comprehension. Mental work is impossible. Transposes words. Spacey. Stupefaction in morning on waking.

Impatience while reading. Restlessness better mental labor. Conscientious about trifles. Sympathetic. ***Mild and kind.*** Pathologically cheerful. Tendency to sacrifice for others. Refined sensibility. Dislikes intruding on people, bothering people (Staph., Sil.). Selective friendships, air of detachment.

Elusive nature. Strong sense of integrity. Humane, empathetic. Very self-conscious. Closed, controlled emotions. Avoidance of stress. Meditative. Difficulty dealing with suffering and pain in the world.

Profound sadness, depression and melancholy. Constantly occupied with sad thoughts, though there is also the opposite, great gaiety and talkative. Philosophical about grief, resigned. Internal sorrow, melancholy. ***Suffers grief with dignity.*** Unassimilated emotions. ***Sadness from errors of diet.*** Thoughts of suicide, overwhelmed with suffering.

Cross, irritable. ***Irritability during fever.*** Aversion to society, even that of their own family or spouse. ***Sensitive to the presence of certain persons.*** Indifferent. Anxious and fearful. Anxiety, trembling and sweat during pains. Delusions of being deserted, forsaken.

Very sensitive to noise, cold, change of weather. Worse thunderstorms, electric changes in the atmosphere. ***Very nervous during thunderstorm, hides in cellar.*** Anxious and restless during thunderstorms. Desires to be magnetized.

Starting from noise. Sensitive to music (Ambr.). Music causes tendency to suicide, sadness, religious insanity. ***Playing on piano*** causes anxiety and trembling. Sensitive to sensual impressions.

Abdomen - Griping colic just after a meal. Abdominal colic somewhat better eating. ***Indigestion, gas and bloating.*** Accumulation, incarceration, and painful movements of flatus in abdomen. Flatus changes places, abdomen bloated here and there. ***Hard, bloated, swollen abdomen.*** Epigastrium painful to touch and talking. Colic with retraction of naval and hardness of skin. Colic somewhat better eating and warmth. Pressure in lower abdomen, as if everything in abdomen would fall out. ***Violent sharp pain*** in right hypochondriac region, followed by griping in lower abdomen. Swelling of glands of groin and axilla. Itch-like eruption on lower part of abdomen.

Back - Backache, violent pain in lumbar region after walking. Burning pain and distress along spine. Tingling in back. Cervical glands swollen. Cracking in cervical vertebrae, when moving the neck. Boring pain at tip of left scapula. Coldness between scapulae. Stiffness and drawing between scapulae. Pustules on lumbar region.

Causations - Sun, gaslight, heat, changes in temperature. Ill effects of sunstroke (chronic). Suppression of sweat. Cold drink when over-heated. Extreme sensitivity to electrical changes, like thunderstorms. Over-study, strains, grief. Errors in diet, milk.

Chest - Chilliness in one side of chest. Pressing, sharp pains in chest. Burning soreness in right mid chest.

Constitutions - Suited to light-haired people and persons of leuco-phlegmatic constitution with aversion to open air and mental or physical exercise.

Ears - Dryness and heat. Sharp stitching pain in ears. As if something moved in ear on swallowing. As if a bubble bursting in ears. Oversensitive hearing. ***Sensitive to noise, music.*** Stopped sensation. Deafness with recurring earache, with amenorrhea. Loss of hearing of right ear, sounds seem to come from left side when they really come from right. Hardness of hearing and roaring in left ear, worse before menses.

Eyes - Burning pain in eyes, worse reading and writing, with dryness. Shooting pain from within outward. Needle-like stitches in both eyes, after dinner. Ulcers on cornea, with shooting pains. Dim eyes, has to wipe them constantly. ***Photophobia.*** Lachrymation during forenoon. Agglutination of eyes in morning. Eyes close involuntary. Heaviness of upper lids. Lids swollen. Inflammation of eyelids with photophobia.

Face - Pale, withered, bloated face. Pale face, with dark streaks under eyes. Blue rings around eyes, swollen lids. ***Freckles, yellow spots, pimples***. Yellow blotches on forehead and upper lip. Burning crack in lower lip. Lips swollen, particularly upper lip. Swelling of both cheeks, with glowing redness. Swelling of submaxillary glands. Pains in bones of face, with chronic naso-pharyngeal catarrh.

Female - Soreness. Deficient menses in adult females. Menses too early, late, scanty, like meat-washings (Nit-ac.). Menses with pain in lumbar region and abdomen. Dysmenorrhea. Leucorrheal discharge, offensive, irritating. ***Leucorrhea thick, yellow, ropy.*** Leucorrhea better after urination. Profuse leucorrhea, after frequent attacks of colic. Induration of cervix. ***Bearing down sensation*** (Sep., Murx). Motion, as if fetus in uterus. Sterility. Infertility from non-retention of semen. Promotes conception. Labor pains weak, or with anguish, sweat and desire to be rubbed. Prevents false conception. Expels moles.

Food - Hungry at 5 a.m. Greedy, always nibbling. ***Very weak digestion***. Food tastes bitter. ***Food allergies. Oversensitive to errors in diet.*** Craving for sweets. Must drink in order to swallow solids. Aversion to milk. ***Worse from milk***, causes flatulence, diarrhea. ***Children who can't tolerate milk*** but thrive better on cereals. Drowsiness after meals. Heartburn after fats. Diarrhea from starch. Indigestion is worse from vegetables and starchy foods. Ill effects of drinking cold water when overheated.

Head - Head pains out through eyes, head bent backwards. Stupefying pain in forehead, with nausea, eructations and dimness of sight. Headache alternating with digestive troubles. Headaches from slightest mental exertion. ***Headaches from exposure to sunlight*** (Glon.), gaslight. Dullness of head when at rest or when in sun. ***Headaches in hot weather.*** Head feels too large. Pulsating, in vertex every morning. Almost painless boil on occiput. Falling out of hair.

Heart - Painful cracking in region of heart. Palpitations from noise, on going upstairs, when attention is directed to something, when lying on left side. Palpitations, a general accompaniment of indigestion. Pulse excited at night, with ebullitions.

Kidneys - Pressure in region of bladder. Burning in urethra during and after urination. Frequent need to urinate, with copious or scanty discharge. Bright or dark yellow urine. Urine smells like horse's urine, from vegetable or milk diet. Involuntary urination at night.

Limbs - Great weakness of limbs, especially in morning. Locomotor ataxia, fulgurating pains better eating. Heaviness of legs and feet with tension in them. Unsteady walk, small obstruction on pavement causes him to fall, or falls without apparent cause.

Hollow of the knee is painful on motion. Popliteal, painful on motion. Legs are icy cold up to knees. ***Weak ankles.*** Cramps from ankles to toes. ***Easy dislocation and spraining of ankles. Foot bends under*** (Caust.). ***Old sprains.*** Heel and Achilles tendon affected. Tender soles, needle-like pain, burning while walking. Soles of feet raw and sore. Burning wrists and ankles. Jerking of hand on going to sleep. Contractions of fingers. Folds of fingers and toes sore. Chapped hands. Vesicles on tips of all fingers and toes.

Lungs - Dyspnea and shortness of breathing, from tension of chest. Short cough with rattling in chest. Cough with rawness in chest, worse morning. Cough, dry, tickling, worse at 9 to 11 a.m. Cough with coldness of left side of breast. Violent and dry cough on passing from cold to hot temperature. Cough with rumbling, incarcerated flatus. Loose, hollow cough, with salty, purulent, greenish sputum. Bloody expectoration.

Male - Straining and tenesmus, with voluptuous sensation in genitals. Glans penis becomes sore easily. Inflammation, swelling and easy excoriation of prepuce and glans penis. Prostatic affections, discharge of prostatic fluid at stool and when urinating. Bruised pain in testicles. Heaviness and drawing in testicles. Soreness between scrotum and thighs. Increased sexual desire with priapism and painful pollutions. Incomplete sex, erection weak, emissions speedy. Nightly emissions. Sweats after sex.

Modalities - Better from eating, sweating. Better wiping with hand. Better boring into nose or ears with fingers. Better rubbing, motion, pressure. Aversion to cold air. ***Worse from heat of sun***. Worse drafts, damp weather. Worse getting wet, change of weather. Worse extremes of temperature. Worse before a storm or during a storm. Worse drinking cold water, cold drinks when over heated. Worse from vegetable diet, starchy food. ***Worse milk, dietetic errors. Worse from music, noise.*** Worse mental or bodily exertion. Worse at 5 a.m. Worse alternate days. Worse the full moon. Worse sun exposure.

Mouth - Constant dryness of mouth and lips, which she was constantly obliged to lick. Saliva increased. Bitter taste in the mouth, food tastes bitter. Taste perverted, too sensitive. Taste sour, metallic. Redness and soreness of mouth, with flat, painful blisters. Vesicles and smooth ulcers in mouth with burning, mouth open. Sensitiveness of lower teeth. Toothache, in lower jaw, worse eating fruits, sweets, better smoking. Nightly pressing toothache with swelling of lower lip and of gums.

Nose - Swollen or peeling. Pimples and puffiness. Red nose with white pimples on it. Many troubles of external nose (Caust.). Humid herpetic eruptions and ulcers on nose, around mouth and on lips. Ulceration high up in nostrils. Nosebleed. Stoppage at night. ***Catarrh, post-nasal catarrh.*** Catarrh, foul, thick, yellow or green discharge. ***Hawking mucus from throat,*** worse slight draft. Constant coryza, obstruction of nose. Coryza, worse least draft, alternate days. Coryza, with burning in eyes. ***Bad odor of nasal secretions***. Musty smelling discharge. Violent sneezing. Squeaking sensation at root of nose.

Perspiration - Profuse sweat from the least physical exertion. Perspiration while eating, in morning. Patient breaks into a cold sweat. Burning sweat on forehead where hat presses. Anxious sweat during pain, with dreams. Perspiration all over, during fever. Night sweat alternating with dryness of skin. Perspiration in morning.

Rectum - Sudden call to stool without result. Emission of much sour-smelling or fetid flatus. Stools escape with haste and noise. Constipation, insufficient stool, with tenesmus. Constipation alternating with soft and liquid stools. Gushing diarrhea, preceded by cutting pain in upper abdomen. Discharge of tinea during evacuation. Diarrhea with cutting pain. ***Diarrhea from starches, milk***, taking cold. Burning and cutting pain in anus and rectum during stool. Burning pain in rectum after stool. Lancinations in perineum. Itching and tingling in anus.

Sensations - As if head too large, as if forehead would burst, as if head would be drawn back. As if ears were closed up, as of a bubble bursting in ear. As if tip of tongue were cracked. Dryness of mouth as if caused by heat of breath. As if veins of right leg were bruised. Blisters on points of toes as if scalded. Motion as from a fetus in uterus.

Skin - Dry, rough, milky, watery. Inclination to perspire easily or dry, rough, cracked skin. Full veins. Formication. Itching as from fleas over whole body. Pustular eruptions. Blisters on small joints, tips of toes or fingers. Red vesicles filled with fluid. Vesicles with shooting pains and itching. Vesicular eruption in patches and circles. Yellow rings like remains of herpes. Herpetic eruptions, sometimes suppurating. Ulcers, burning, pricking and pulsating. Ulcers, pus corroding, acrid, putrid and yellow. Ulcers, with swelling and inflamed redness. Warts, ulcerate, sensitive to touch. Elephantiasis.

Sleep - Drowsy during day after meals. Falls asleep late at night. Sleeps with mouth open. Jerking and shocks during sleep. Restless sleep with ebullitions, palpitations and nightmares. Pleasant, amorous dreams. Anxious, frightful dreams. Dreams of traveling, floods, quarrels, robbers, devils, thieves, death. Wakes too early in the morning. Sleepiness in morning.

Stomach - Stomach feels swollen and sensitive. Heaviness and pressure in stomach. ***Weak digestion***, worse from slightest errors in diet. ***Dyspepsia relieved by soda biscuits. Old dyspeptics, always belching, have sour stomach and rheumatism.*** Gastric pains, better eating. ***Indigestion.*** Cramp in stomach, pressing, drawing, cutting pain. Depressed after eating. Bitter taste. Acidity. Waterbrash. Heartburn after fats. ***Sour eructations.*** Frequent hiccough. Nausea and retching, with pain and soreness in stomach. Violent retching in morning, without actual vomiting. Vomiting of bile, bitter. ***Food allergies.*** Ill effects of drinking cold water when overheated.

Stool - Stools, black, hard, smooth, crumbly. Watery stool. ***Yellow substance like pulp of orange*** in stool in menopausal women. Discharge of ball of mucus like peas. Stool spotted with blood, discharge of blood during stool.

Temperature - Sudden chilliness. Chill, without thirst. Shivering fits induced by over fatigue and anxiety. Chill with cold hands and hot cheeks, or the reverse. Cold hands and feet, with hot forehead. Coldness of lower limbs. Heat with great debility and sleep. Heat with perspiration over whole body. Febrile shuddering, with cold hands and hot cheeks. Heat flushes, with aversion to uncovering.

Throat - Hoarseness with coryza, chilliness and scraping, painful cough. Throat painful when yawning and swallowing. Must drink to swallow solids from roughness, dryness of esophagus and throat. Hawks much mucus from the throat. Taste of blood, pus in throat. Glandular swellings in throat. Resistant swelling of middle lobe of thyroid gland. Hard goiter, with pressing pain.

Tongue - Tongue coated, dry. Burning about tip of tongue, as if it was cracked. Pimples on tip of tongue, which burns as if full of cracks. Affections of under-surface of tongue. Tongue heavy, immovable, with difficult speech. Stammering on account of heaviness of tongue.

Vertigo - Vertigo from wine, mental exertion, exposure to sun, better from exercise in open air.

Vision - Dim vision, has to wipe eyes constantly. Can't read small print. Sensation as if feathers before eyes. Flashes and streaks of light before closed eyes at night. Dazzling flashes or stars before eyes, on waking. Black spots before eyes when writing.

COMMENTS - Sensitive digestion (Nat-s.). Chronic dyspepsia, stomachaches. Very weak digestion, burning, gas and bloating. Belching, ulcers, and indigestion. Heartburn with acid regurgitations and esophageal problems.

Malassimilation, food allergies. Difficulty swallowing foods. Emaciation, anemia, and bloating. May get bloated from starchy foods. Ill effects of drinking cold water. Worse from milk, especially in children (Aeth.), causing diarrhea. Worse from wine.

Stomach problems will often alternate with headaches. Depression and irritability is worse after a meal, the aggravation diminishing as digestion advances, "as the food passes through the duodenum."

Characteristic blue ring around the eyes of children with allergies. Ptosis of the eyelids. Photophobia. Chronic nasal congestion.

Women can have a "discharge of mucus after an embrace" causing infertility. Candida. Bearing down pain, dragging feeling in the stomach (Sep.). Worse after sex, exhaustion. Emotional detachment.

Symptoms of hysteria. Contractions of muscles and tendons, relaxation of tissues. Twitching in muscles and limbs. Paralysis of the left leg. Conditions resulting from malabsorption. Swelling and induration of glands. Bone problems, curved spine. Stooping forward. Ankle joints are weak and burn.

Stitches go from within out. Right upper and left lower are particularly effected. Great debility from any exertion, unsteady walk, any little obstruction on pavement causes falling, or he falls without any apparent cause. Aversion to exercise. Symptoms are worse from mental or bodily exertion.

Generally chilly. Worse extremes of temperature. Sensitivity to changes in atmosphere. Worse before a storm or during a storm. Restless before a storm or with a storm. May get migraine headaches or stomach problems before a storm. Conditions resulting from exposure in the sun. Heat exhaustion. Headache from mental exertion, sun exposure.

Sensitivity to music, worse from loud music. Sensitive to particular things, not a general sensitivity (as is Phos.), certain foods, people, sounds, light conditions. Pet peeves. Aggravations cause headaches, stomachaches, heartburn, indigestion, depression. Aware of limitations and sensitivities.

RELATIONS - ***Antidoted by:*** Ars., Camph.. ***It antidotes:*** Chin. ***Compare:*** (1) Sodium bicarbonate - in vomiting of pregnancy with acetonuria. (2) Nat-s. is preferable for yeast-like vomiting, with pallid, dirty, livid tongue. (3) Nat-m. - hypochondriasis. That of Nat-c. keeps pace with indigestion, that of Nat-m. with degree of constipation, head and face better uncovering, leucorrhea. (4) Caust., Nat-cac. (5) Sep. - Indifferent to family, melancholy, apprehensive, worse by music, backache worse by sitting, bearing down, boring through from tip of left scapula. (6) Pic-ac. - priapism, towards morning, emission and no desire. (7) Nux-v. - hypochondriasis, morning retching, Nux-v., of pregnancy, or after debauch. (8) Phos., Rhod., Sil., Petr., worse from thunder storm. (9) Lyc. - better uncovering, ulcer on heel. Lyc. on instep, right upper, left lower. (10) Debility from heat of summer, Ant-c. (11) Headache from sun or gaslight, Glon., Lach. (12) Bearing down as if everything would come out, Sep., Agar., Lil-t., Murx. (13) Easily sprained ankles, Stront., Led. ***Complementary:*** Sep., Kali salts. ***Compatible:*** Calc., Nux-v., Puls., Sep., Sul.

REFERENCES - Boericke. Clarke. Murphy. Phatak.

NATRUM FLUORATUM

(Sodium Flouride)

PHARMACY - nat-f. Natrum fluoratum. Sodium flouride. Triturations from the salts. ***Historical dose:*** All potencies.

CLINICAL - Constipation. Cramps. Diarrhea. Muscle, pains. Mydriasis. Proteinuria. Stomachache. Tetany. Writer's cramp.

HOMEOPATHIC - Nat-f., molecular weight 42, appears in the form of colorless crystals, cubic or tetragonal in shape. The triturations were prepared from the salt. The work was completed in 1956 by Gutman New York, on twenty-one provers. The proving lasted fifty days using a 6c in tablet form.

Due to the fluorine, the action of the remedy is myoneurotrophic. Sudden muscular contracture. Sudden muscular pains, coming and going in the muscles and joints. Pains while resting or from lack of distraction, reduced by pressure. Pains in the region of the left scapula.

MIND - Agitation and depression. State of stupor. Loss of ability to speak.

Abdomen - Gastric and intestinal cramps.

Back - Muscular, cramping, sudden pains. Pain in the shoulders.

Eyes - Mydriasis. Cramping pains in the eyelids.

Food - Lack of appetite.

Heart - Weak heart. Irregular pulse, rapid, weak, jumping.

Kidneys - Oliguria. Urine retention. Proteinuria.

Limbs - Sudden pains, coming and going in the muscles and joints. Hardening of the bones. Cramps in the calves and cyanosed, bluish coloring of the legs.

Modalities - Better from pressure, distraction. Worse from resting.

Mouth - Pain in the mouth with salty or soapy-tasting saliva.

Rectum - Constipation or diarrhea with expulsion of wind.

Skin - Itching of the skin without eruption. Itching eruption in the left axilla. Passing eruption on the legs. Copious, cold perspiration.

Stomach - Cramping pain in the stomach. Digestive heaviness and discomfort, nausea. Stomachache, painful hungry feeling, not eased by nourishment. Blood-streaked vomit.

RELATIONS - ***Compare:*** (1) Cupr. - Violent intermittent, cramping pains of the eyelids, stomach, calves and feet, aggravated by the cold.

REFERENCES - Julian.

NATRUM HYPOCHLOROSUM

(Labarraque's Solution)

PHARMACY - nat-hchls. Natrum hypochlorosum. Labarraque's solution. Natrum chloratum. Liquor soda chlorate. It comes from hypochlorite of soda or potassium-chloride water. Potencies of the solution. ***Historical dose:*** All potencies. Fifteen to twenty drops of Labarraque's solution in water.

CLINICAL - Albuminuria. Allergies. Anaphylaxis. ***Ankles, weak.*** Aphonia. Backache. Breast pain. Bronchitis. Chlorosis. Cough. Diarrhea. Dyspnea. ***Eczema.*** Edema. Emaciation. Fainting. Flatus. Globus. Gravel. Headache. Hematuria. Hemorrhoids. Hysteria. Kidney stones. Leucocytosis. Leucorrhea. Liver, disorders. Metrorrhagia. Nephritis. Nosebleed. Ovaries disorders. Priapism. Proctitis. Scurvy. Smarting eruptions. Sub-involution. Tongue, shriveled, swollen. Toothache. Uterus, water-logged. Vertigo. Vomiting.

HOMEOPATHIC - Nat-hchls., the well-known disinfecting fluid, is one of Cooper's additions to the Materia Medica. His proving brought out some very characteristic features, although there is a close general resemblance to Nat-m. The chlorine radical determines irritation of the skin and mucus membranes, the sodium induces extreme sensitivity to humidity.

The indications are not the result of a Homeopathic proving, but the result of the information given by the toxicology and the clinical usage of the remedy.

Nat-hchls. affects profoundly the entire organism and causes rapid emaciation, fainting, weakness with a flabbiness most pronounced along the mucus tracts with a diffused hydrogenoid condition and a tendency to leucocytosis.

Eczema and itching, more particularly localized on the upper limbs and the face. Anaphylaxis caused by cutaneous intolerance of a product. Chronic catarrhal diseases of the middle ear. Phlegmatic. Congested and atonic states of the uterus and its ligaments with hepatic disorders. Both hands swollen in morning. Depressed, faint.

Abdomen - Swelling low in abdomen going up to chest and causing dyspnea, worse after eating with much flatus. Bloated, tight feeling across upper abdomen.

Back - Much pain across small of back, worse morning on rising.

Constitutions - Phlegmatic, flabby, debilitated constitutions.

Coughs - Cough with aphonia.

Ears - Pain under right ear when swallowing with much tenderness and swelling up side of head.

Eyes - Eyes red, weeping, eyelids puffy, red and itching. Amelioration by cold compresses.

Face - Edema of the face.

Female - Violent metrorrhagia. Leucorrhea and backache. Womb is feels heavy, sodden with tendency to prolapse. Feeling as if the uterus were pushed up on sitting down (Ferr-i.). Feels as if it opened and shut. Passive, bearing-down pains from heavy condition of uterus. Subinvolution. Itching of the vulva, perineum, and anus.

Head - Headaches. Swimming feeling, as if top of head would float off.

Kidneys - Much pain across small of back. Diffuse nephritis. Dark urine with albumen and casts.

Limbs - Extreme ***weakness in ankles*** and knees. Hands swollen every morning.

Lungs - Pulmonary edema, capillary bronchitis. Dyspnea, aggravated by the coughing. Dry, irritating, painful cough in fits and then frothy, pink sputum. Cough with aphonia.

Modalities - Better after stool, from cold applications. Worse from eating or drinking, drinking least drop of cold water, warm drinks. Worse by washing, damp, warmth, lying on either side. Worse before each menstrual period, before stool.

Mouth - Putrid taste. Furred tongue, large, flabby indented. Flat ulcer on tongue far back towards root. Sore, irritable spots along sides of tongue and throat. Gums sore, tongue swollen, aphthous ulceration. Stomatitis, aphthosis.

Nose - Nosebleed, clots of blood.

Rectum - Anal and rectal burning, burning diarrhea. Proctitis. Hemorrhoids, anal fissure.

Skin - Generalized or localized itching, better by scratching. Recurring erythema with appearance of vesicles filled with a whitish, oozing liquid. Weeping eczema. Dry eczema in nursing children.

Sleep - Drowsiness after meals. Drowsy by day, wakeful by night. Cannot sit down without falling asleep. Disinclined to rise in morning. Child looks ghastly, as if dead, when asleep, his sleep is quiet.

Stomach - Drowsy after meals. Burning in epigastrium, with acrid vomiting, hematemesis.

Throat - Throat red and sore, with difficult swallowing. Burning in the pharynx with redness, choking cough.

Vertigo - Vertigo with aching across forehead. Swimming feeling, as if top of head would float off.

COMMENTS - Drowsiness, cannot sit down without falling asleep. A weight seems to fall from pit of chest to pit of abdomen with aching, dull sensation on vertex. Vertigo causing falling. Paralyzed feeling in brain. Sensation as if top of skull were about to float off, as though cranial bones were being crossed over each other.

Swelling, neuralgic pains and suppuration about jaws. Tongue swollen or shriveled at sides. Swelling low down in abdomen, going up to chest and causing dyspnea. Swelling of both hands in morning on waking. Gatherings on fingers. Swelling on both hands in morning on waking. Pain in hip joint reflected from ovary.

Dr. Robert Cooper's grand characteristic indication for Nat-hchls. is a water-logged uterus. The womb is sodden, heavy, low down in pelvis, bearing down in pelvis with tendency to prolapse.

The state of subinvolution after confinement corresponds very closely to this and Clarke frequently saw Nat-hchls. do good work in such cases.

RELATIONS - ***Antidoted by:*** Puls. - rheumatic and myalgic symptoms, Guai., also, probably, the antidotes to Nat-m. ***Compare:*** (1) Aur-m. Nat-m., Calc., Sep., (2) Helio. - has uterine displacement with active bearing-down sensation and loss of voice, membranous dysmenorrhea. (3) Nat-c., Nat-m., Kali-chl., Chlor. (4) In uterine bearing down, Helio., Sep. (5) Womb feels as if it opened and shut Sep. has clutching and relaxing. (6) Feels as if uterus were pushed up when ever she sits down. Ferr-i. (7) Uterine engorgement and induration, Aur-m-n. (8) Bloated feeling after meals, worse by warm drinks, Lyc. (9) Easily overpowered with heat, Sep., Nat-m., Nat-c. ***Complementary:*** Sep.

REFERENCES - Boericke. Clarke.

NATRUM IODATUM

(Sodium Iodide)

PHARMACY - nat-i. Natrum iodatum. Sodium iodide. ***Historical dose:*** All potencies.

CLINICAL - ***Angina pectoris.*** Arteriosclerosis. Catarrh. Dyspnea. Endocarditis. Heart, disorders. Rheumatism. Vertigo.

HOMEOPATHIC - Nat-i. has various symptoms, such as ***angina pectoris*** and vertigo. Dyspnea become less marked after continued use. Chronic catarrhal affections, arteriosclerosis and rheumatism. Incipient rheumatic endocarditis. Chronic bronchitis and tertiary syphilis.

Nat-i. will be found to give most excellent results where there is organic disease of the heart, associated with the angina pectoris. There is an oppression in the region of the heart that is attended with a fear of death and a feeling as if something dreadful was about to happen. Angina pectoris and dyspnea.

REFERENCES - Blackwood. Boericke.

NATRUM LACTICUM

(Sodium Lactate)

PHARMACY - nat-l. Natrum lacticum. Sodium lactate. Solution. ***Historical dose:*** All potencies.

CLINICAL - Fatigue. Gout. Rheumatism. Vomiting.

HOMEOPATHIC - Allen collected a few observation on the effects of large doses. Skinner removed with it in potencies gouty or rheumatic concretions, ***"chalk stones"*** in fingers. Gout, rheumatism. Rheumatic pains. Abnormal sense of fatigue, yawning and sleepiness.

Food - Unusual hunger and thirst.

Limbs - Great weakness of lower limbs after great physical exertion.

Sleep - Yawning and sleepiness. Sleep more prolonged and sounder.

Stomach - Vomiting from very large doses.

RELATIONS - ***Compare:*** (1) The lacs, Lac-ac. (2) In "chalk stones," Lyc., Calc.

REFERENCES - Clarke.

NATRUM MURIATICUM

(Sodium Chloride)

PHARMACY - nat-m. Natrum muriaticum. Sodium chloride. Common Rock Salt. Trituration. Solution. ***Historical dose:*** All potencies.

CLINICAL - Acne. Addison's disease. ***Allergies.*** Alopecia. Amenorrhea. Anemia. Anorexia nervosa. Aphthae. ***Asthenopia.*** Asthma. Atrophy. ***Autism.*** Backache. Bee, stings. Blepharitis. Brain-fag. ***Canker, sores.*** Cataract. Catarrh. Chlorosis. Chorea. ***Cold, sores. Colds.*** Colic. ***Constipation.*** Convulsions. ***Coryza.*** Coughs. Cracks, skin. Deafness. Debility. ***Depression.*** Diabetes. Diarrhea. Disparunia. Dropsy. Dysmenorrhea. Dyspepsia. Eczema. Edema. Emaciation. Epilepsy. Erysipelas. Eye, disorders. ***Eyestrain. Fever, blisters.*** Gleet. Glossopharyngeal, paralysis. Goiter. Gonorrhea. Gout. ***Grief.*** Hair, loss. ***Hay fever. Headaches. Heart, disorders.*** Hemiopia. Hemorrhages. Hernia. ***Herpes.*** Hiccough. Hodgkin's disease. ***Housemaid's knee.*** Hydremia. Hydroa. Hydrocele. ***Hypertension.*** Hyperthyroidism. Impetigo. ***Impotency. Infertility.*** Intermittent fevers. Jaundice. Lachrymation. Leucocythemia. Leucocytosis. ***Leucorrhea.*** Lice. Lips, sores. Lungs, edema. ***Malaria.*** Menstruation, disorders. ***Migraines.*** Mouth, sores. Multiple sclerosis. Mumps. Nettle rash. Neuralgia. Nosebleeds. Orchitis. ***Otitis.*** Otorrhea. ***Palpitations.*** Paralysis. Phimosis. ***Photophobia.*** Psoriasis. Ptosis. Ranula. Ringworm. Self-abuse. ***Sinusitis.*** Skin, unhealthy. Sleepwalking. Sneezing. ***Sore throat.*** Speech, embarrassed. Spermatorrhea. Spinal, irritation. Spleen, enlarged. Sterility. Stomatitis. Strabismus. Styes. ***Sunstroke.*** Taste, disordered. Tongue, blistered. ***Toothache.*** Tri-facial-nerve, paralysis. Ulcers. Uterine, cramps. Varicose veins. ***Vaginismus.*** Vertigo. Vesicles. Warts. ***Whooping cough.*** Worms. Yawning.

HOMEOPATHIC - Nat-m. is one of the remedies Schussler adopted from homeopathy. His indications are, for the most part, identical with Hahnemann's. In old-school practice, Nat-m. was used chiefly in solution as a douche or spray in nasal and other catarrhs, and in the mixture of "Brandy and Salt," in which large quantities of salt are given for pulmonary hemorrhages.

Affects the emotions, heart, kidney, and spleen. Suited to thin patients who are thirsty, poorly nourished on account of digestive disturbances. Craves salt. The skin, may be corrosive (salt-rheum). Clear vesicles on skin or conjunctiva. Lachrymation. Salty taste in the mouth. Salivation, toothache with salivation. Constipation. Lack of mucus. Catarrh of stomach with vomiting of mucus. Water brash. Watery, mucus diarrhea.

Tendency to catch colds, coryzas or ***hay fever. Dry mucus membranes***. Mucus membranes and skin may be dry or may produce thick, white or clear, watery, acrid discharges. Dryness of mouth, throat, rectum, vagina etc. Disturbances of the digestive tract and skin.

Emaciation, most notable in the neck. Emaciation from malaria. Anemia. Hyperthyroidism. Goiter. Addison's disease. Diabetes. Gouty or rheumatic gout. Chlorosis. Bloating. Hydremia. Leucocytosis. Intermittent fever

Contraction of muscles and tendons. Twitching in muscles. Frequent starts in upper part of body. Chorea, jumping after fright. Neuralgic pains with tears. Numbness of one side, parts lain on with paralysis. Fingers, parts seem too short. Constrictive sensation throughout the body. Trembling of the whole body from smoking tobacco.

Great weakness and weariness. Weakness felt in the morning in bed. Easy exhaustion. Tired, sleepy. Inclination to weep. Oversensitive to all sorts of influences. ***Coldness***. Cold limbs, cold sensation along the spine. Likes to be covered but does not relieve. Children talk late, are cross, irritable, cry from slightest cause.

MIND - ***Reserved and introverted.*** Depression, with spells of irritableness and crossness. ***Severe depression and feelings of isolation.*** Depression after death of loved ones, divorce, broken relationships, broken hearts. ***Acute and chronic grief.*** Suicidal after grief. Emotionally shut down and closed off since grief.

Dwells on past unpleasant memories. ***Holds grudges for years.*** Offended easily. Revengeful. ***Cannot cry in front of others.*** Company distresses. ***Consolation aggravates***. Thinks he is pitied for his misfortunes and weeps. Laughter with tears. ***Ailments from grief, disappointed love,*** fright, anger.

Mental behavior and physical symptoms are hopeless or awkward in nature. Chronic affects of ***grief, disappointed love,*** fright, anger. ***Depressed and introverted***. Dwells on past unpleasant memories. Cannot cry or express grief. Averse to consolation. Depression or paralysis from hurt emotions. ***Young girls fall in love with married men.***

Very sensitive, romantic, sentimental, intellectual. Sympathetic. Fear of hurting others emotionally. Need for unconditional love. Inability to receive and give affection. ***Sulking, sighing*** (Ign.). Despair about future.

Afraid of close relationships, feels too vulnerable and shy. Poor confidence in relationships. Difficulty trusting, believing in people. Difficulty communicating emotions. ***Tendency to fall in love with unattainable people, particularly married people***. Lovesick with one of her own sex.

Appears to bid for sympathy, yet angry when consoled. Cannot cry or urinate in public. Aversion to presence of strangers during urination. Aversion to men in women. ***Aversion to sex.*** Low sex drive. Lack of enjoyment during sex. ***Sadness before menses.*** Sadness in pregnancy.

Inclination to weep and be excited. ***Cries from music.*** Weeps bitterly, involuntary, whenever alone. Tears with laughter. Hysterical laughter, laughs at serious things. Child irritable and cross when spoken to, crying from slightest cause. Excitement followed by melancholy. Hypochondriasis and hysteria with constipation.

Hurriedness with anxiety and fluttering at heart. Anxiety and fear. ***Fear of intimacy, rejection, betrayal,*** of losing control, of relationships. Fear of being ridiculed, embarrassed, being late. Claustrophobia. Fear of robbers, the dark, heights. Fear of insects, especially bumblebees, spiders. Fear of insanity.

Alternating mental conditions. Irritable, gets into a passion about trifles. Abrupt. Absent minded. Extremely forgetful. Scattered thoughts. Mistakes in speaking, what he doesn't intend to. Awkward speech. Awkward, hasty, drops things from nervous weakness. Shy and timid. Mental retardation. ***Children late learning to talk and walk.*** Autism.

Abdomen - Anxiety in abdomen. Cutting pain in abdomen. Much pain and soreness in left hypochondrium. Pressure in upper abdomen. Pain in abdominal ring on coughing. Epigastric pulsation. Epigastrium swollen and painful. Tightness of skin across abdomen from hip to hip, must loosen clothes. Tension groins. Rigidity of the left side. Sudden distention. Abdomen swollen, rumbling and incarceration of flatus. Great fermentation, loud gurgling. Colic with nausea, better flatus. Bilious colic. Burning in intestines. Abdominal viscera loose and dragging as if when walking. Jaundice with drowsiness. Yellowish discharge from navel.

Back - ***Backache with desire for firm support*** (Rhus-t., Sep.). Backache is better lying on back, on something hard or from pressure. Can stoop readily, but hurts to straighten. Bruised pain, early in morning, worse coughing and after sex. ***Spine oversensitive to touch or pressure.*** Sensitiveness between vertebrae. Spinal irritation from grief, anger, sexual excesses, etc. Paralytic feeling in lumbar region. Violent pulsations in lumbar region. Sacral region as if beaten. Painful stiffness of neck. Cervical glands enlarged, sore when coughing. Impetigo or itching tetter on margin of hair at nape.

Breasts - Breasts emaciate. Stitches beneath nipples. Loss of hair during breast-feeding. Child refuses breast, from sore mouth.

Causations - Ill effects of ***grief, guilt, betrayal, disappointment***. Fright, fit of passion. Loss of fluids, masturbation. Injury to head. Silver salts, eating salt. Sunlight.

Chest - Sore pain or bruised feeling in chest. Oppression of chest. Sensation as if constricted or if lungs were too tight, with burning hands, while at work. Sensation and pain in chest as from tension. Sharp pains all over chest, on deep inspiration and when coughing. Tearing, sharp pain, from left upper region of chest to shoulder joint, after suppressed facial neuralgia. Single stitches along sternum. Pain like a cutting cramp through left chest to scapula. Severe pain in right side.

Constitutions - Suited to sensitive, anemic, chlorotic people with catarrhal troubles. Cachectic persons, old people, teething children. Tuberculous, scrofulous, dropsical, emaciated persons.

Cough - Spasmodic, suffocative cough at night in bed. ***Whooping cough with flows of tears with cough.*** Dry cough with rattling in chest. Cough with hawking of mucus. Cough from tickling in the pit of stomach, with asthma, or with stitches in liver and spurting of urine (Caust., Squil.). Cough with palpitations. Cough with bursting pain in head. Sticking in liver while coughing. Cough in the morning, evening after lying down in bed. Cough worse in winter. Chronic cough of tuberculous subjects.

Ears - ***Chronic catarrhal otitis with acrid discharges.*** Purulent discharge from ears. Catarrh of tympanitic cavity and eustachian tube, non-suppurating. Throbbing and beating in ears, ears red from congestion, otorrhea. Swelling and heat of outer ear. Itching behind ears. Painful cracking in the ear when chewing. ***Noises, buzzing, humming, ringing, and roaring.*** Roaring and buzzing in ears and head, with inability to work, read or think. Difficult hearing. Deafness from swelling of tympanitic cavity. Deafness with watery conditions of tongue.

Eyes - Sensation as if eyes were filled with salt. Burning pain in eyes. Eyes itch and burn, must wipe them and pull at lashes. ***Photophobia, worse bright light, sunlight.*** Lachrymation with redness, burning, acrid from affected side from sneezing, coughing, laughing etc. Eyes appear wet with tears. ***Tears stream down face on coughing*** (Euphr.). Stricture of lachrymal duct with suppuration. Cataract incipient.

Ptosis on lying down. Blepharitis with marked photophobia and spasmodic closure of lids. Divergent strabismus, coming on from fatigue, more marked in hot weather and worse in winter. ***Asthenopia*** due to the insufficiency of internal recti muscles. ***Muscles weak and stiff. Eyestrain.*** Eyes give out in reading and writing. Cannot read by artificial light. ***Pain in eyes when looking down***. Feel bruised with ***headache in school children***. Eyes feel drawn together. Protruding eyes, due to goiter. Styes. Lids swollen. Eyelids heavy.

Face - Dry skin. Oily, shiny skin, as if greased. Earthy complexion. Acne. Pimples on face. Eruptions and ulcers on chin. ***Fever blisters and cold sores. Herpes about the lips***. Lips and corners of mouth dry, ulcerated, and cracked. Lips tingle, feel numb. ***Crack in the middle of the lower lip.*** Swollen upper lip. Throbbing in lower jaw, worse biting, heat and cold. Down on the face in hysteria, passes away as the patient improves. Falling out of whiskers and beard. Prosopalgia. Neuralgia. Cheekbones as if bruised, when chewing. Mumps with profuse flow of saliva. Submaxillary glands swollen.

Female - Delayed first menses. Amenorrhea. ***Suppressed menses from grief,*** from putting feet in cold water. Menses irregular, usually profuse. Hot during menses. Menses painful from getting feet wet. Dysmenorrhea with convulsions. Menses preceded and followed by headache. Sore burning in vagina before menses. White leucorrhea turns green gradually. ***Leucorrhea acrid, watery.*** Debilitating, white, thick leucorrhea, instead of menses. ***Genital herpes, eruptions worse from stress, emotional upsets.*** Uterine cramps with burning and cutting in groins. Ineffectual labor-pains. Prolapse of uterus with aching in lumbar region. Bearing down pains, worse in morning (Sep.), with aching in lumbar region. Burning and soreness of vagina after urinating. Dryness and soreness of vagina, with itching. Burning, smarting in vagina during sex. ***Aversion to sex,*** which is painful from dryness of vagina. ***Low sex drive since grief.*** Sterility, with too early and too profuse menses. ***Infertility***. Labor progresses slowly, pains feeble, seemingly from sad feelings and forebodings. Loss of hair in childbed or during period of lactation.

Food - ***Hungry, yet loses weight*** (Iod.), ***with depression.*** Anorexia nervosa. Hunger without relish. Hunger without appetite during pregnancy. Unquenchable thirst. Thirsty, drinks large quantity of water. ***Craving for salt and salty foods,*** especially during pregnancy. Eats more salt since a grief. Desires sour things, lemons. Desires bitter things, beer. Desires chocolate, farinaceous food, oysters, fish, milk. ***Averse to anything slimy like oysters, fats***. Averse to meat, coffee, tobacco. Averse to bread, acidic foods. Aversion to rich food, chicken, salt, milk. Worse from bread, fat. Worse salt, acid food. ***Bad effects from eating salt and salty foods.***

Head - ***Migraine headaches,*** bursting, maddening, heavy. ***Blinding headache.*** Aches as if a thousand little hammers were knocking on the brain, throbs. Headaches over eyes, on vertex, with partial numbness or disturbed vision. Headaches from eyestrain. ***Headaches from sunrise to sunset***. Headaches during, before or after menses. Burning on vertex during menses. Headaches on coughing. ***Headaches from sunlight.*** Sunstroke. ***Headaches with photophobia.*** Pains, aggravated by motion, even of eyes, worse frowning, reading. ***Anemic headaches of schoolgirls,*** nervous, discouraged, broken down. Headaches are better sleep, pressure on eyes, lying with head high, and sitting still. Headaches worse on waking. Headaches with constipation. ***Headaches from grief.*** Nodding motions of the head. Rush of blood to head. Throbbing and heat in head, with red face, nausea and vomiting. Hemicrania with sour vomiting and eructations. Falling out of hair. Chronic effects after injury to head. White scurf on scalp, dandruff, alternating with catarrh and loss of smell.

Heart - Tachycardia. ***Fluttering of the heart*** with a weak, faint feeling, worse lying down. Chronic forms of valvular disease, with weak, faint feeling, must lie down. ***Hypertrophy of heart. Palpitations***, shaking the body or alternating with beating in head. Palpitations, anxious, worse exertion, emotions, lying on left side. Palpitations before menses. Palpitations on falling asleep and on awaking. Palpitations with sensation of weakness, exhaustion and heaviness. ***Heart feels weak and vulnerable, worse after grief.*** Sensation of coldness or emptiness about heart. Heart and chest feel constricted. Painful stitches in region of heart, after reading aloud. ***High blood pressure from excess salt eating.*** Fluttering, palpitating, intermittent every third beat, worse lying down. Pulse, full and slow, weak and rapid.

Kidneys - ***Difficulty urinating in the presence of others.*** Has to wait a long time for it to pass if others are present (Hep., Mur-ac.). Must wait before the urine will start. Polyuria, thirst for large quantities of water. Frequent or sudden desire to urinate, can't retain urine, copious flow. Urination every hour at night. Tension and heat in renal region. Clear urine with red sediment. Hematuria. Urine dark, like coffee. Milky urine after menses. Involuntary urination on coughing, laughing, sneezing, walking, sitting. ***Pain just after urinating*** (Sars.).

Limbs - Multiple sclerosis. Paralysis after grief, intermittent fevers. Convulsive jerking of the limbs on falling asleep. Every motion accelerates the circulation. Cracking in joints on motion. Urticaria about joints. ***Coldness of legs*** with congestion to head, chest and stomach. Hamstrings seem short, painful, drawing in (Caust.). Arms and legs, but especially knees, feel weak. ***Housemaid's knee.*** Ankles weak and turn easily. Soreness of toes or between toes. ***Numbness and tingling*** in fingers and lower limbs. Buttocks emaciated in infants. ***Children do not learn to walk or late learning to walk.*** Icy coldness of hands and feet. ***Palms hot and perspiring. Hangnails***. Dryness and cracking about fingernails. Hands tremble when writing.

Lungs - Acute edema of lungs. Attacks of suffocation. Difficult breathing after menses. ***Sighing from emotional states.*** Shortness of breath, especially on going upstairs (Calc.). Breathing better from exertion of arms, and better in open air. Lungs feel raw and sore from continual coughing. Spasmodic cough, face blue. Pneumonia, with much rattling, mucus clear, serous and frothy, coughed up with difficulty. Pleuritis when serous exudation has taken place. Respiratory catarrh after suppressed sweats. Yellow or blood-streaked mucus, in morning. White, salty mucus. Bloody expectoration, with cough. Profuse, frothy or watery expectoration, with asthma. Expectoration in clots, most in morning.

Male - Genital organs smell strongly and badly. Violent itching on and under scrotum. Itching and crawling sensation at corona glandis. Scrotum relaxed, flabby. Edema of scrotum. Hydrocele. Phimosis. Loss of hair from pubes. ***Genital herpes, eruptions worse from stress, emotional upsets.*** Gonorrhea, when chronic, discharge usually clear, sometimes yellowish, cutting in urethra after urinating. Suppressed gonorrhea. Aching in testes, orchitis, after suppression of gonorrhea or mumps. ***Discharge of thin fluid from urethra, causes itching and burning.*** Loss of prostatic fluid during stool. Emission of prostatic fluid without erection when thinking of sexual things. Erections in morning, without sexual excitement. Emission, even after sex. ***Impotency, with retarded emission.*** Sexual desire with physical weakness. Backache, weak legs and depression after sex. Weakness, even paralysis after sexual excess. ***Aversion to sex, since grief.***

Modalities - Better from open air, deep breathing. Better cool bathing, sweating. Better talking long. Better from tight clothing, rubbing, rest. Better lying on right side, sitting up. Better before breakfast, going without regular meals. ***Worse from***

sunlight, heat of sun. Worse summer, seashore. Worse dampness. Worse talking, reading, writing. Worse exertion of the eyes, mental exertion. ***Worse from strong emotions, consolation, sympathy.*** Worse puberty, sex. Worse alternated days after menses. Worse the moon. Worse from 9 a.m. to 11 a.m. Worse noise, music. Worse touch, pressure. Worse chronic sprains. Worse quinine, bread, fat, sour foods.

Mouth - Breath, hot offensive. Bitter taste. ***Loss of taste and smell.*** Salivation with thrush, obstinate. Saliva, profuse, watery, salty, bloody. Constant spitting. Salivation in morning. Sense of dryness of mouth. Vesicles and ulcers in mouth and on tongue, smart and burn when touched by food. Blood-blisters on inside of upper lip. Scorbutic gums. Dental fistula. Epulis or small tumor on the gums. ***Numbness, tingling of lips and mouth.*** Aphthae in mouth, on gums and cheeks, with great burning and impeded speech. ***Canker sores, herpes, fever blisters.*** Eruptions around mouth and vesicles like pearls on lips. ***Dry and chapped lips.*** Lips and corners of mouth dry, ulcerated and cracked. ***Deep crack in middle of lower lip.***

Nose - Allergies and colds. ***Colds begin with sneezing. Hay fever, watery discharge from eyes and nose.*** Alternate fluent and dry coryza. ***Fluent coryza***, lasting from one to three days, then changing into stoppage of nose, making breathing difficult. ***Discharge thin and watery like raw egg white***. Violent sneezing. Sneezing early in the morning. ***Sinusitis.*** Frontal sinus inflammation. Internal soreness of nose. Dryness. Exfoliation of skin on dorsum of nose. Little ulcers in nose. ***Fever blisters*** on wings of nose and on lips. One side numb. Burning pain in nasal bones. Nosebleeds, on stooping or when coughing, at night. ***Loss of smell and taste.***

Perspiration - Sweats on every exertion. ***Sweats while eating,*** on face. Sweats at edge of hair. Sweats on nose, face while eating. Sweats in axilla and on soles of feet. Sweats with aversion to uncover. Scanty sweats. Much better during sweat. Sweats relieving headache and other pains, though it weakens. Sour sweat, weakening. Profuse, and offensive sweats, at night.

Rectum - Ineffectual urging. Constipation from inactivity, grief. ***Constipation on alternate days,*** alternating with diarrhea. Chronic, painless, watery diarrhea, in the morning. Diarrhea preceded by pinching pain in abdomen. Diarrhea on moving about. Diarrhea after menses. Diarrhea from abuse of opium. Constriction of rectum. Stools tear the anus or cause burning. Burning, tearing, itching about anus after stool. Stinging pain in hemorrhoids and soreness at anus after stool. ***Anus contracted torn, bleeding***. Ripping up sensation in anus after stool. Anal fissures with bleeding and smarting. Soreness at and around anus when walking. ***Herpes about anus.*** Disposition to get worms. Seat worms.

Sensations - As if head too heavy and would fall forward. As if some displacement in head had taken place, as if cold wind blowing though head. As though forehead would burst on coughing, as if head in a vice, pain like a rope around head drawing tighter and tighter, as if nail driven in left side of head. As if foreign body in eyes, as if eye being torn open. As if eyeballs too large. As if a small worm squirming in nose. As if hair on tongue.

Skin - ***Dry and chapped skin.*** Greasy, oily skin, especially on hairy parts. Herpetic eruptions, worse flexures. ***Fever blisters, cold sores.*** Vesicles, with watery contents, burst and leave a thin scurf. Pemphigus, blisters starting up on burning spots, with clear, watery contents. Small boils, blood boils. Eruption like ringworm, with itching, worse warmth. Hives, itching and burning after exertion. Nettle-rash over whole body, large red blotches, with violent itching. Itching, better from sweating. Eczema, dry, raw, red, and inflamed, worse eating salt, at seashore. Herpes zoster. Crusty, dry eruptions in ***bends of limbs, margin of scalp***. Dry eruptions behind ears (Caust., Graph.). Urticaria. Corns. Comedones. Fungus hematodes. ***Insect bites, stings of bees, mosquitoes.*** Painful scars, redness of old scars. ***Sunburns eas-***

ily. Affects hair follicles. Alopecia. Warts on palms of hands.

Sleep - Sleepy in forenoon. Sleepiness during day, with frequent yawning. Sleepy, but can't sleep at night, and in morning feels unrefreshed. ***Sleeplessness after gnawing grief, from depressing events, dwelling on past events.*** An idea clings to mind, preventing sleep. Prostration from loss of sleep. Twitching and electric shocks through whole body on falling asleep. Nervous jerking during sleep. Starts and talks in sleep. ***Sobs during sleep.*** Sleep-walking, rises and sits about room. Dreams during siesta. Vivid dreams like a living reality. ***Dreams about grief, past events.*** Dreams about work, which she is busy with a long time after waking. Dreams of burning thirst. Dreams of robbers, waking from fright, thought there were robbers in house. Very anxious dreams with weeping in sleep. Awakes feeling weak and unrefreshed.

Stomach - Anxiety in stomach rises into head. Feels better on an empty stomach. ***Great weakness in stomach, comes in spells.*** Faint, weak, gone sensation in stomach during pregnancy. Heartburn during pregnancy. Heartburn with palpitations. Violent hiccough. Burning pain and belchings after eating. Sweetish eructations in morning, before or during menses. Throbbing in pit. Sticking sensation in cardiac orifice. Pressure as from a stone in stomach, with nausea. Vomiting of white, slimy mucus. Vomiting first of food, then bile. Continuous nausea with thirst and profuse water brash. ***Morning sickness with vomiting of frothy, watery phlegm.***

Stools - Hard, difficult and painful stool, followed by liquid stool. Involuntary stools. Irregular stools, sometimes two or three a day, then constipation. Stools, dry, hard, crumbling (Am-m., Mag-m.), or coated with glassy mucus. Stools, black, watery, corrosive. Green, bloody, watery or brownish stools, mostly during day. Stools transparent, glassy, slimy. Stools like white of an egg. Stools without feces.

Teeth - Dentition with dribbling of saliva. Teeth sensitive to air or touch, pain worse on chewing. ***Toothache with lachrymation or salivation.*** Drawing, tearing pains, extending to ears and throat. Toothache after eating and at night. Toothache worse drawing in air, touch, pressure, after chewing. Toothache before menses, beginning of menses. Scorbutic gums. Spongy and bleeding easily. Epulis or small tumor on gums. Dental fistula. Cheek swollen.

Temperature - ***Coldness of the body***. Morning chill with thirst, between 9 a.m. and 11 a.m. Chilly, but worse in sun. Chills beginning in feet or lumbar region. Chills predominates, mostly internal, hands and feet cold. Chills with yawning, chattering of teeth. Chill alternating with fever, at various times of day, without sweat. Heat, violent thirst increases with fever. Intermittent fever. Malaria. Hydremia in chronic malarial states with weakness, constipation, loss of appetite. ***Fever blisters.*** Sunstroke.

Throat - Dry, sore spot in the throat, tickles and causes cough etc. Soreness and feeling of dryness in larynx and trachea. Sore throat with sensation as if she has to swallow over a lump. As if a plug in throat. Sensation of a splinter sticking in throat. ***Tobacco smoker's sore throat.*** Uvula hangs to one side. Sore throat, with transparent mucus covering tonsils. ***Throat glistens.*** Hawks much mucus, bitter, salty. Only fluids can be swallowed. Solids reach a certain point and then are violently ejected. Food goes down the wrong way in post diphtheria paralysis. Swelling of cervical glands. ***Hypertrophy of tonsils.*** Exophthalmic goiter. Goiter with chronic sore throat. Hoarseness in morning. Weakness of organs of speech. Voice weak, faint, exhausting from talking. Bad effects of long speaking.

Tongue - Sense of dryness on tongue. ***Tongue mapped*** (Ars., Rhus-t., Tarax.). ***Numbness, tingling of tongue.*** Tongue broad, pale, puffy, with pasty coat. Frothy coating on tongue with bubbles on side. Tongue, beaded or striped along edges. Burning at tip of tongue. Aphthae on tongue. Herpes on tongue from sea-bathing. Tongue, heavy, difficult speech. Sensation of a hair on the tongue.

Vertigo - Vertigo, as if falling, worse standing near a window. Vertigo on closing eyes, better lying with head high. ***Vertigo during pregnancy***. Vertigo from straining eyes or close study. Vertigo with jerking in head, with tendency to fall forward or to left. Vertigo in morning on rising. Vertigo after stool.

Vision - ***Eyes give out on reading or writing.*** Frequent obscuration of vision, when stooping, walking, reading, writing. Amaurosis, from debilitating weakness. Weakness of vision after debilitating illness. Diplopia or vertical hemiopia. Hemiopia, followed by headache. Retinal images are retained too long. Vision blurred, wavering. Letters run together. Sees sparks, fiery, zigzag appearance around all objects. Sparks, black spots. Dim vision, as if looking through gauze or feathers. Objects seem covered with a thin veil. Dark veil passes before eyes.

COMMENTS - Can antidote the effects of the crude salt, allows patients to cut down intake. Antidotes the effects of Arg-n. Scrofulous ophthalmia which has been treated locally in vain with Arg-n., sore throats that have been cauterized, the effects local and remote of uterine injections of Arg-n. or cauterizing of the os uterus.

Symptoms are worse at the seaside or cannot stay by the sea. Constipation at seaside. Can also be better at seaside. Great desire for open air and washing in cold water. Sensitivity to the sun.

Fluttering palpitations with faint feeling, worse lying down. Characteristic sense of coldness at the heart of precordia, with trembling of the heart. In one case of hypertrophy with degeneration of most of the valves, the patient told Clarke that nothing gave her so much relief as Nat-m.

Periodic, intermittent fevers. Chilliness predominates. Chill from 10 to 11 a.m. with thirst, drinks after a meal, fever blisters around mouth. Fever with violent headache, great thirst, nausea, vomiting, blueness, faint, averse to uncover. Fever may come on without chill 10 to 11 a.m. Fevers and chills from malaria (Ars.). Antidotes quinine.

Headaches from over study. Headache with partial blindness. Throbbing, beating as with little hammers, pain as if the head would burst. The throbbing headache has its analog in palpitation of the heart. Headache much worse by coughing. Migraines, worse during the day and better at night. Worse from the sun or light.

Lambert recorded several cases of headache associated with errors of refraction and consequent eyestrain cured with Nat-m. 30c. The headache was noticed on walking. In one case it was like a cloud over the brain with intense depression and lasted ten years. It disappeared before the vision was corrected.

Indicated in some cases of multiple sclerosis and lupus. Psoriasis. Hydroa. Eczema on hair margins, especially at back of head. Warts on palms of hands. Corns. Painful scars. Greasy skin, an excess of sebaceous secretion. Disorders due to loss of fluids. Copious lachrymation. Burnett noted the characteristic "flow of tears with cough" in whooping cough.

Schussler noted the specific relation to catarrh. Excessively fluent coryza with much sneezing, sore nose, especially the left wing. Tendency to loss of smell and taste. Allergies.

Dry skin and lips. The lower lip has a crack down the middle. Cold sores on lips and nose. Herpes infection. Cold sores, canker sores, fever blisters and genital herpes that are worse from emotional stress or fatigue.

Mapped tongue with red islands, or a clean, shining tongue with froth along each side. Sensation as if there is a hair on the tongue. Numbness and stiffness of one side, heavy, embarrassing speech. The tongue is blistered, sticks to roof of mouth. Dryness of mouth and throat.

Sinking sensation. Hypoglycemia. Great hunger with no appetite. Eats heartily, ravenous appetite, but emaciates, especially about the neck. Feels better when stomach is empty. Strong aversion to fats and slimy foods. Craves chocolate, sweets, fish.

Craves salt. One patient, who said she could "eat the brine out of a mackerel kit," was cured with a single dose of Nat-m.

Unquenchable thirst. After eating there are empty belchings, nausea, acidity, sleepiness, heartburn, palpitation, epigastric pressure and heat radiating up to chest. Indigestion. Violent hiccough. Nausea. Vomiting. Constipation and diarrhea. Constipation often associated with anemia, chilliness, cold feet and chills down the back.

Women can have an aversion to sex, an aversion to men. Delayed first menses. Menses may be early and profuse or scanty and delayed. Bearing down pain (Sep.). Leucorrhea, with backache that is better pressure of from lying down on something hard. Characteristic dryness of the vagina with painful sex. Morning sickness during pregnancy. Infertility or amenorrhea from grief.

Useful for children who are late in talking. Autism. Learning or speech disabilities.

RELATIONS - ***Antidoted by:*** Smelling Nit-s-d., Phos. - especially abuse of salt in food. Ars. - bad effects of sea-bathing. Nux-v. will relieve headache after Nat-m. ***Antidote to:*** Arg-n. - abuse of, as cautery. Quinine - in diseases continue intermittent and patients suffer from headache, constipation, disturbed sleep. Apis - bee stings. ***Compare:*** (1) Bry., Apis, Ign., Sep., Thuj., Graph., Alum. (2) Bor., Nat-c., Nat-h., Kali-chl. (3) In mapped tongue, Ars., Rhus-t., Kali-bi., Tarax., Ran-s. (acidity). (4) Hypochondriasis with indigestion, Nat-s. (5) Lachrymose, Puls. - better consolation. (6) schoolgirls' headache, Calc., Calc-p. (7) Headache coming and going with sun, Spig., Gels., Glon., Sang. (8) Headache with partial blindness, Kali-bi., Iris-v. (9) Half sight, Aur., Lith., Lyc., Titan. (9) Headache with cough, Caps., Bry., (Sulph. occiput, Nat-m. forehead). (10) Ravenous yet wastes, Iod. (11) Ringworm, Sep., Bar-c. Tell. (12) Paralyzed by emotion, Gels., Staph. (13) Intermittents, chill beginning in small of back, Eup-per., Rhus-t. - chill begins in one leg, or thigh, or between shoulders, Gels. - runs up spine. (14) Sadness during menses, Lyc., Nit-ac., Sep. (15) Laughs at serious things, Anac., Phos., Lyc., Plat. (16) Aq-mar. ***Complementary:*** Apis, Sep., Caps. Nat-m. is the chronic of Ign., Bry., Apis and Caps. ***Compatible:*** Before - Sep., Thuj., after - Ign., Kali-m., Kali-p., Con., Nat-s., Calc-p., Ferr-p.

REFERENCES - Boericke. Clarke. Murphy. Phatak.

NATRUM NITRICUM

(Sodium Nitrate)

PHARMACY - nat-n. Natrum nitricum. Sodium nitrate. Cubic nitre. Chili saltpetre. Trituration. Solution. ***Historical dose:*** All potencies.

CLINICAL - Anemia. Asthma. Belching. Constipation. Croup. Distention. Exhaustion. Exophthalmic goiter. Flatulence. Headaches. Hematuria. Hemoglobinuria. Hemoptysis. ***Hemorrhages***. Hydremia. ***Influenza***. Laryngitis. ***Nosebleeds***. Pneumonia. Purpura hemorrhagica. Otalgia. Otitis. Rheumatism. Tracheitis. Variola. Weakness.

HOMEOPATHIC - According to Hansen, Nat-n. was called Rademacher's Aconite; he used it in inflammations of all kinds, especially laryngitis, tracheitis, croup, and acute pneumonia. Acute rheumatism and heart affections. Exophthalmic goiter. Purpura, hemorrhages inflammations of the eye.

Inflammations and hemorrhages. Hemorrhages from the mucus membranes, particularly the nasal tissues. ***Influenza***. Pressing-inward pains in temple and forehead, in malar bones.

Anemia and hydremia. Exhaustion, must rest frequently when walking. Drowsiness. Pains of tabes. Heat spreading left to right. Heat in left ear, coldness in right. Coldness streaming through upper part of body. Coldness of left foot.

Asthma with urine supersaturated with solids. Flatulent troubles with weight in lower abdomen. Painful retraction of abdominal muscles. Painful constipation.

MIND - Great ill-humor. Mental indolence. Indisposed to mental and bodily exertion.

Abdomen - Abdominal muscles painfully contracted towards the spine. Distended.

Constitutions - Uric acid diathesis.

Ears - Otalgia.

Head - Dull pain. Pressing inward pain. Inward pressing in malar bones. ***Nose-bleeds***. Headaches.

Heart - Pain in region of heart. Pulse slower and softer.

Modalities - Worse by deep inspiration. Worse exertion, ascending stairs. Worse sitting bent over.

Rectum - Difficult stool, feels as if more remained to pass.

Stomach - Sour risings. Aversions to coffee. Flatulence with pressure in pit of stomach and pain in chest, worse motion, better eructation.

RELATIONS - ***Compare:*** (1) Kali-n. (2) Abdomen mostly contracted, constipation, Plb.

REFERENCES - Boericke. Clarke. Rademacher.

NATRUM NITROSUM

(Sodium Nitrite)

PHARMACY - nat-ns. Natrum nitrosum. Sodium nitrite. Trituration. Solution. ***Historical dose:*** All potencies.

CLINICAL - Angina pectoris. Collapse. Cyanosis. Diarrhea. Fainting. Gastro-enteritis. Roseola. Strokes.

HOMEOPATHIC - Ringer and Murrell gave ten grains of Nat-ns., dissolved in one ounce of water to fourteen men and four women. It was given in five grain doses to twelve men and four women.

In almost all it produced alarming symptoms of the apoplectic attack. The concomitance of fainting with other disorders may prove a keynote. Copious liquid stools at night with faintness. Better lying down, worse motion.

COMMENTS - Collischorm related two cases of accidental poisoning with Nat-ns. The first patient was affected with diarrhea and fainting, heavily coated tongue, bitter belchings, and an eruption like syphilitic roseola on the chest. Traces of albumen in urine. During the night, copious alvine discharges with faintness.

The following day, there was intense cyanosis. Urine dark yellow, containing copious urates. The next day, he took 2.5 grain, cyanosis diminished and the measly eruption spread all over the body except the face.

The second patient had the cyanosis, diarrhea and faintings in an aggravated form so that collapse threatened. Strong coffee and omission of the drug removed the symptoms.

RELATIONS - ***Antidoted by:*** Coffee. ***Compare:*** (1) Amyl-n., Glon. (2) worse by motion, Bry.

REFERENCES - Clarke.

NATRUM PHOSPHORICUM

(Sodium Phosphate)

PHARMACY - nat-p. Natrum phosphoricum. Sodium phosphate. Hydric disodic phosphate. Trituration. Solution. ***Historical dose:*** All potencies.

CLINICAL - ***Acidity***. Allergies. Arthritis. Belching. ***Blisters***. Boils. Colic. Conjunctivitis. ***Cystitis.*** Diabetes. ***Diarrhea.*** Dyspepsia. ***Dysphagia***. Enteralgia. Erysipelas. ***Flatulence.*** Glands, swelling. Goiter. Gonorrhea. Gout. ***Heartburn. Hives***. Indigestion. Infertility. Intertrigo. ***Jaundice.*** Leucocytosis. ***Leucorrhea. Marasmus***. Morning, sickness. Morphine addiction. Oxaluria. ***Peptic ulcer.*** Post-nasal catarrh. Rheumatism. Scrofula. Sighing. Stomach pain. Thread, worms. Tuberculosis. Urticaria. ***Vaginitis.*** Vertigo. Vomiting. ***Worms.***

HOMEOPATHIC - Schussler, who introduced it, noted that Nat-p. is contained in the blood-corpuscles, in the cells of the muscles, of the nerves, and of the brain, as well as in the intercellular fluids. Nat-p. breaks down lactic acid into carbonic acid and water. It then binds to the carbonic acid, allowing it to be exhaled and exchanged for oxygen.

Affinity for diseases caused by an ***excess of lactic acid***. In oxaluria, Nat-p. 1x four times daily prevents formation of stones, keeps the oxalate of lime in solution. Ailments with ***excess of acidity***.

Affects duodenum, bile ducts, mesenteric glands and genitals. Leucocytosis. Bladder infections, vaginitis and gout. Oxaluria.

Diabetes. ***Jaundice.*** Swelling of lymphatic glands.

Sourness, belchings, vomiting, stomach, stools, leucorrhea, expectoration, sweats. Flatulence with sour risings. ***Yellow, creamy coating at the back of the roof of mouth and tongue.*** Inflammation of the throat with sensation of a lump.

Debility. Nervousness, tired feeling. Cracking in joints. Pricking sensation. Tightness of muscles and tendons. Trembling and palpitation from thunderstorms. Ill effects of mental exertion or sexual vices, or both.

Marasmus of bottle-fed babies. Infants who have been fed to excess with milk and sugar. ***Worms.*** Colic with symptoms of worms.

MIND - Mental weakness. ***Confusion from mental exertion.*** Nervous, forgetful, after sexual excesses. ***Easily frightened.*** Fear that something would happen, especially at night. ***Starting from noise.*** Imagines that he hears footsteps in the next room. Imagines that pieces of furniture are people.

Sensitive and offended easily. Irritability before breakfast. Vexed at trifles. Sighing (Ign.). Grief with a craving for cold drinks. Sadness from music, from masturbation. Indifferent to everything. ***Indifference to loved ones.*** Sits still for a long time.

Abdomen - Fullness in abdomen, worse standing or eating a little. Gastro-duodenal catarrh. ***Noisy flatulence.*** While at stool, sensation as if a marble dropped down descending colon.

Back - Heavy dragging in the back. Rheumatic arthritis. ***Synovial crepitation***. Swelling of glands of neck extending to chest. Weakness after sex.

Causations - Acids, citrus fruits, alcohol, milk, sugar. Fat or bitter foods. Thunderstorms.

Chest - Chest feels empty after eating, or pain through chest after dinner. Pain in chest, worse deep breathing and pressure. Burning deep in chest, worse right side. Sudden feeling of fullness. Weight above ensiform cartilage with empty feeling.

Constitutions - Acid diathesis.

Ears - One ear red, hot, itching, scratches until it bleeds, with gastric disorders and acidity. As if water falling in from a height.

Eyes - One pupil dilated. Whites of eyes are dirty yellow. Discharge of ***golden-yellow, creamy matter*** from the eyes. Eyes weak, worse gaslight. Squinting with worms.

Face - Paleness of bluish, florid appearance of face. Pale or red on alternate sides. Face burns. Itching about mouth.

Female - Menses too early, pale, thin, watery. During menses, feet icy cold during day, burn at night in bed. ***Leucorrhea***, sour, ***creamy,*** honey-colored, or acid and watery. Sour-smelling discharges from uterus. Infertility with acid secretions from vagina. Morning sickness with sour vomiting.

Food - Canine hunger with gone feeling in stomach. Desires strong tasting things, eggs, fried fish, beer, which ameliorate. Aversion to bread and butter. ***Worse acids, citrus fruits.*** Worse alcohol, milk, sugar. Worse fat or bitter foods.

Head - Feels dull in the morning, full feeling and throbbing. Cutting pain in temples (right) while studying. Pressure and heat on top of head as if it would open.

Heart - Heart pains alternating with rheumatic pains. Heart pains are better when big toe pains. Anxious palpitations after a thunderstorm. Trembling about heart, worse going upstairs, after menses. Feeling as if a bubble started from heart was forced through arteries.

Kidneys - Frequent urination. Must wait for urine to start. Bladder semi-paralyzed, flow soon stops and requires straining. Increased urine, pale, scanty, dark. Urine too acid. Burning during urination. Diabetes, hepatic form. Urging to urinate, burning and itching at meatus after sex.

Limbs - Aching in wrists and finger joints. Cramps in hands while writing. Rheumatism, particularly of the knee joint. Legs give way while walking. Feet icy cold during day, burn at night. Synovial crepitation. Trembling of limbs after sex.

Liver - Jaundice. Sclerosis of liver and hepatic form of diabetes especially when there is a succession of boils.

Lungs - Difficult respiration. Constant cough and hawking, pain in chest in mammary region. Cough, worse sitting. Cough from drinking water, from tickling in throat.

Male - Emissions without dreams, with ***weakness in back and trembling in limbs***. Desire without erection. Thin, watery semen, smells like stale urine. Itching of scrotum, prepuce. Gonorrhea.

Modalities - Better from cold. Worse from sugar, milk. Worse bitter or fatty foods. ***Worse acids, citrus fruits.*** Worse from sex. Worse walking upstairs. Worse mental exertion, gaslight. Worse thunderstorms.

Mouth - Canker sores of lip and cheeks, worse acid foods. Pricking, numbness of whole mouth. ***Blisters on tip of tongue*** with stinging in evening. Thin, moist coating on the tongue. ***Yellow creamy coating at the base of tongue,*** on tonsils or roof of mouth. Sensation as of a hair on tongue. Teeth grinding in children.

Nose - Offensive odor. Naso-pharyngeal catarrh. Thick, yellow offensive mucus. Itching of nose. Prickling with lachrymation. Child picks nose.

Rectum - Urging to stool and urination after sex (men). Afraid to pass flatus lest the stool escape. ***Greenish diarrhea.*** Stools hacked. Itching at anus. Round or thread worms.

Skin - Yellow. Smooth, red, shining. Erysipelas. ***Hives***. Itching in various parts, ***especially of ankles.*** Feet icy cold in daytime, burn at night. Swelling of lymphatic glands.

Sleep - Cannot get to sleep feels so hot, thoughts crowd in mind. Very drowsy, falls asleep while sitting. Sleepy in the forenoon, but sleepless before midnight. Anxious, amorous dreams, of dead people.

Stomach - Emptiness in stomach and abdomen, even in chest, worse after eating. Heaviness and pressure in epigastrium. ***Peptic ulcer. Heartburn, acidity, water brash.*** Acid dyspepsia. ***Sour belchings***. Belchings after eating. Spits mouthfuls of food. ***Vomiting of sour,*** cheesy masses. Attacks of gastralgia and enteralgia, with vomiting of fluid sour as vinegar. Morning sickness, with sour vomiting.

Temperature - Feet icy cold in day, burn at night. Chilly during menses, mostly on chest, followed by hot flushes around body. Flashes of heat and sweat. Exceedingly sour-smelling sweats. Intermittent fever with vomiting of sour masses.

Throat - Hoarseness. ***Dysphagia***. Thick, yellow, creamy membrane over tonsils and soft palate. As of a lump, preventing speech. Swallowing difficult. Goiter with feeling of pressure.

Vertigo - Vertigo from stomach problems. Dizzy, as if he would fall, objects turn around on rising or moving.

COMMENTS - Nat-p. was proved under Farrington's direction. Charles Mohr, who was one of the provers, related the effect it had on him and the use he made of it. After being under the influence of the drug for some time, without knowing what it was, he had much itching at the ankle joints with an eczematous eruption. Headache, some nausea, vision problems, one pupil dilated. Fear, especially at night, that something would happen. The symptoms had to be antidoted with Sep.

Two years after, Mohr had a patient with visual disturbance and headache. When symptoms were at their worst, the patient had a sense of fear, worse at night, and an eruption about the ankles that began with itching, Nat-p. 6x cured promptly.

Acid diathesis. Gout. Spasms with acidity. Sour belchings, vomiting of sour, cheesy masses, yellowish-green. Heartburn and indigestion. Stomachaches with burning and acidic indigestion, particularly in children. Colic.

Candida symptoms, diarrhea, sores in the mouth after eating acidic foods. Low blood sugar causes frequent urination or diarrhea. Atony of bladder. Kidney infections or achiness in the kidneys. Hacked diarrheas. Diarrhea since antibiotics (Nit-ac.). Allergies to sugar and milk.

Recurring cases of worms in children with nasal irritation and itching of the anus. The back of the tongue is coated creamy yellow. Sensation of a hair on the tongue. Tightness of muscles and tendons.

Seminal emissions. Vaginitis, cystitis. Creamy, yellow discharge. Itching of the vulva and labia after sweets and acids. Herpes outbreaks from eating sugar, acids or alcohol.

Symptoms are worse walking, especially up stairs, worse from sex, during thunderstorms. The warmth of bed causes itching at anus from worms. Worse pains, causes trembling and palpitations. When big toe pains, heart pains are better. Periodic action. Sighing (Ign.). Grief with a craving for cold drinks.

M. J. Luys successfully overcame the morphine habit by subcutaneous injections of Nat-p. with glycerine and water.

RELATIONS - ***Compare:*** (1) Acidity and scrofula, Calc., Rheum. Gout, Benz-ac., Guai., Lyc., Urt-u., Sulph. (2) Gastric catarrh, Calc., Carb-v., Kali-c., Nux-v., Rob., Carb-ac. (3) Speech impeded, Nat-m. (4) Hair sensation. Nat-m., Kali-bi., Sil. (5) Worse from sex. Kali-c., Caust. (6) Worms, Abrot, Cina, Teucr. (7) Drinking water causes cough, Sil., Caust. better cough. (8) Emissions causing weak back and knees, Nat-m. (9) Nat-lac. - rheumatism and gout, gouty concretions, rheumatism with diabetes. (10) Nat-ns. - angina pectoris. Cyanosis, fainting, copious liquid stools at night, throbbing and fullness, faintness, nervous pain in head, nausea, belchings, blue lips. (11) Nat-sil-f. - a cancer remedy, tumors, bone affection, decay, lupus, ethmoiditis. Must be used carefully. (12) Nat-sel. - chronic laryngitis and laryngeal tuberculosis, hoarseness of singers, expectorate small lumps of mucus with frequent clearing of throat. (13) Nat-sulo. - diarrhea with yeasty stools.

REFERENCES - Boericke. Clarke. Murphy. Phatak.

NATRUM SALICYLICUM

(Sodium Salicylate)

PHARMACY - nat-sal. Natrum salicylicum. Sodium salicylate. Trituration. Solution. ***Historical dose:*** All potencies.

CLINICAL - Abscess. Amblyopia. ***Arthritis.*** Boils. Debility. Depression. Diarrhea. Dyspnea. Ears, noises. Edema. Fever. Fibrositis. Head, noises. ***Headaches. Influenza.*** Iritis. ***Joint, pain. Meniere's disease.*** Nosebleed. Periostitis. ***Prostration. Rheumatism.*** Stammering. Strabismus divergens. ***Tinnitus.*** Tonsillitis. Unconsciousness. Vertigo. Vomiting.

HOMEOPATHIC - The introduction of Salicylic acid and Nat-sal. into general practice as remedies in rheumatism which led to much overdosing. Affinity for the joints. Affects the head, ear, throat, kidneys, liver and metabolism. Increases the quantity of bile.

Vertigo when objects seem to move to the right, worse on rising from lying. Giddiness, worse on rising from lying. Marked effect upon the internal ear with vertigo, deafness, noises in the ears with loss of bone conduction. ***Meniere's disease***. Intense tinnitus aurium with deafness.

Hemorrhages, especially nosebleed. Follicular tonsillitis. ***Prostration after influenza.*** Temperature subnormal with slow pulse. Lassitude, drowsiness, listlessness, tremor. Periosteal rheumatism. ***Pains of gout and rheumatism*** in the joints.

MIND - Severe mental prostration, worse since influenza. Weariness and depression. Listlessness. Apathetic. Highly nervous dread. Perfectly rational periods, alternate with manifestations of insanity of a somber character. Incipient dementia.

Abdomen - Inguinal glands swollen, sensitive.

Chest - Dyspnea, breathing noisy, shallow, panting, irregular pulse. Complete loss of voice.

Ears - Auditory vertigo. Giddiness, deafness, noises in ears. ***Tinnitus*** of a low tone. Deafness.

Eyes - Pupils dilated, very slightly sensitive to light marked divergent strabismus. Eyes have a peculiar sparkle. Retinal hemorrhage. Iritis due to trauma. Amblyopia. Does not see distant objects, mydriasis.

Face - Anxious expression, red face. Left face red, both eyelids, upper lip edematous. Burning pains on skin of forehead.

Food - Great thirst. Appetite lost.

Head - Severe headache as though head would burst. Dull headaches and confusion. Fibrositis of the scalp.

Limbs - Axillary abscess. Strong itching on back of right hand. Feet swollen, soles tender, veins of dorsa much congested.

Lungs - Dyspnea with great heat. Breathing so noisy it was heard in street, gasps for air. Breathing is shallow. Panting respiration, like that of a hunting-dog.

Mouth - Speech hoarse, indistinct, stammering, some words she cannot pronounce. Dryness in mouth and throat with great thirst.

Pulse - Pulse stronger, arterial pressure increased. Pulse irregular, small, weak, compressible.

Rectum - Diarrhea, great thirst.

Skin - Tingling and itching. Edema and urticaria, red in circumscribed patches. Pemphigoid eruption.

Stomach - Vomiting, unconsciousness.

Temperature - Wild delirium, with great heat, dyspnea. High fever with intense thirst. Fever and rash come only with disappearance of rheumatic pains.

Vertigo - Vertigo, giddiness, worse raising head or sitting up, better lying down. All objects seem to move to the right.

COMMENTS - Nat-sal. has been used freely in the manufacture of beer to prevent fermentation and this has caused poisoning symptoms, notably sweating and tenderness of the feet with dark colored and enlarged veins.

In some of the overdoses, high fever with delirium was produced. Divergent strabismus and stammering were marked pathogenic effects in one case. Irritation of inguinal glands, abscess in axilla.

Clarke gave Nat-sal. 3c to a patient recovering from influenza who had symptoms of vertigo with noises in the head, the patient was so much relieved by the medicine of her weakness and depression that she named the remedy her "tonic."

W. R. Rice published a case in which he gave a woman 10 grain doses of Nat-sal. every four hours. After the third dose "most alarming prostration, mental and bodily" set in. Pulse became weak and compressible and the temperature became subnormal. On stopping Nat-sal., the symptoms rapidly passed off.

Ebstein claimed for Nat-sal. in ordinary dosage a controlling power over glycosuria and R. T. Williamson confirmed this in some cases.

RELATIONS - ***Compare:*** (1) Gaul., Chin. (2) Lob-p. - drowsiness, dizzy headache between eyebrows, cannot keep eyes open tongue white-feels paralyzed as also do the heart and lungs intense prostration of all vital forces, deadly chill without shivering, useful for the low, nervous prostration of influenza. (3) Pyrus-m., Crab apple tree – Labyr., vertigo (Cooper). (4) Salx-m., Salx-n., Sal-ac., Salol. (5) In Meniere's disease, Chin., Kali-i., Carb-s.

REFERENCES - Boericke. Clarke. Phatak.

NATRUM SELENICUM

(Sodium Selenate)

PHARMACY - nat-sel. Natrum selenicum. Sodium selenate. Trituration. ***Historical dose:*** All potencies.

CLINICAL - Laryngitis. Tuberculosis.

HOMEOPATHIC - This is an unproved remedy, but it has a decided affinity for the larynx. According to Hansen, its use in homeopathy was first suggested by Meyhoffer, who gave the indication in laryngeal tuberculosis.

Expectoration of small lumps of bloody mucus with slight hoarseness. It is best suited to the early stage of the disease. Laryngeal tuberculosis. Chronic laryngitis.

REFERENCES - Clarke. Hansen.

NATRUM SILICICUM

(Sodium Silicate)

PHARMACY - nat-sil. Natrum silicicum. Sodium silicate. Natrium silicatum. Trituration. ***Historical dose:*** All potencies.

CLINICAL - Abscess. Ankles, weak. Bone, diseases. Chilly. Diarrhea. Gout. Headaches. Hemophilia. Nasal, discharge. Osteomalacia. Tuberculosis.

HOMEOPATHIC - Nat-sil. is useful in hemophilia, pulmonary tubercle, chronic gout, osteomalacia and scrofulous diseases of bone. Marked lack of vital heat. Chilly. Marked lassitude and desire to lie down.

Headache from mental exertion. Headache worse evening, noise and uncovering the head, better pressure and warm application. Pain in occiput. Nasal discharge offensive, thick and purulent. Swelling of submaxillary glands.

Breathing deep, difficult and short. Dryness of mouth and throat. Sputum offensive and purulent, often with a salty taste. Cold feet. Weakness of ankles. Abscess, relieves the pain and hastens the flow of pus. Restrains progress of cancer of cervix.

Diarrhea from milk. Sweats on the least exertion. Aversion to open air. ***Worse from exertion***. Worse motion, forenoon, evening and night. Better lying down, pressure, warm applications.

MIND - Weakness of mind and nerves. Can't stand mental exertion. Headache from mental exertion. Sadness and weeping during menses. Easily frightened and starting from noise. Anxious and vivid dreams.

REFERENCES - Clarke. Pulmann.

NATRUM SILICOFLUORICUM

PHARMACY - nat-sil-f. Natrum silicofluoricum. Salufer. Solution. ***Historical dose:*** All potencies.

CLINICAL - Bone disorders. Bone caries. Ethmoiditis. Lupus. Tumors.

HOMEOPATHIC - Cooper is the chief authority for this remedy. Nat-sil-f. must be used carefully, as it has an extraordinary penetrating power. Particularly useful for bone disorders.

Cooper called it the medicinal ***"bone scraper"*** in cases of caries. With a lotion of three grains to a tumbler of water he healed a case of lupus. Cooper saw ethmoiditis set up by it. Burnett cured tumors with Nat-sil-f. given internally.

REFERENCES - Clarke. Cooper.

NATRUM SULPHURICUM

(Sodium Sulphate)

PHARMACY - nat-s. Natrum sulphuricum. Sodium sulphate. Glauber's salt. Sal Mirabile. Soda vitriolata. Trituration. Solution. ***Historical dose:*** All potencies.

CLINICAL - Abscess. Alcoholism. ***Asthma.*** Bedwetting. Biliousness. ***Blindness***. Brain, injuries. Chills. Colic. Coma. ***Concussions.*** Condylomata. Conjunctivitis. ***Convulsions. Cough.*** Debility. ***Depression.*** Diabetes. Dropsy. Dyspepsia. ***Epilepsy.*** Fever. Fistula. ***Flatulence.*** Gallbladder, disorders. ***Gonorrhea.*** Gout. ***Head, injuries. Headaches.*** Heartburn. Heatstroke. ***Hepatitis.*** Hydremia. Influenza. Jaundice. Leucorrhea. Leukemia. ***Liver, disorders.*** Malaria. Meningitis. ***Migraines.*** Morning sickness. Nausea. Nephritis. Nosebleeds. Ophthalmia. Opisthotonos. Panaritium. Phlegmasia alba. ***Photophobia.*** Rheumatism. Sciatica. Scrofulous, glands. Sinusitis. Spinal, injuries. ***Spinal, meningitis***. Spleen, disorders. ***Suicidal***. Sunstroke. ***Sycosis.*** Tuberculosis. Typhlitis. Vertigo. Vomiting. Warts.

HOMEOPATHIC - Nat-s., named Sal Mirabile, was discovered by the alchemist Glauber in 1658. It has since been named after him, Sal Glauberi. Nat-s. was proved by Schreter, Hartlaub, Trinks and others.

Nat-s. was studied by Grauvogl, who found in it the typical remedy for his "hydrogenoid constitution," and it forms one of the tissue remedies of Schussler. It corresponds to Hahnemann's sycosis miasm. The indications from these studies are generally agreed upon by all, although homeopaths have the widest field.

Grauvogl described the hydrogenoid constitution as the state in which there is extreme sensitiveness to damp wetting, bathing, watery foods and residence near fresh water, especially standing water. Periodicity is also another feature of this state. He considered this constitution as providing the soil for gonorrheal infection.

Schussler wrote, "The action of the Sodium sulphate is contrary to that of the Sodium chloride. Both indeed, have the faculty of attracting water, but the end is a contrary one, Nat-m. attracts the water destined to be put to use in the organism, but Nat-sulph. attracts the water formed during the retrogressive metamorphosis of the cells and secures its elimination from the organism."

Especially affects the occiput, liver, and pancreas. Head symptoms from ***injuries to head***. Mental troubles arising from a fall or other injuries to head. ***Epilepsy or depression after head injuries***. ***Spinal meningitis***. Sudden violent effects in ailing patients. Pains worse from thinking of them.

Sycosis. Tendency to warts. Suppressed gonorrhea. Yellow, watery, secretions, stools, skin, vesicles etc. Thick yellow-green pus. Sour, bilious and lithemic. Fistulous abscesses. Dropsy. Chronic gout (Lyc.). Trembling. Fingers and toes affected.

Skin disorders return every spring. Worse in rainy weather, water in any form, cannot eat plants growing near water, or fish. ***Feels every change from dry to wet***. Always feels best in warm, dry air.

MIND - Inability to think. Mental exertion aggravates. Industrious. Periodical attacks of mania. Sensitive and suspicious. Fear of crowds, evil. Fear from noise, from noise at night. ***Mental troubles arising from injury to head. Mental effects of falls, blows.*** Cheerful after stools. ***Confusion better after stools.***

Depression, worse music or mellow light. Sadness sitting near a stained glass window. Moved to tears by music and soft light. Sadness in morning. Very irritable, ill-humored, worse morning. Dislikes to speak or to be spoken to. Weeping, better in open air.

Aversion to life, with photophobia. Estranged from her family, from his wife. ***Suicidal impulses,*** has to use self-control to prevent shooting himself (Aur.). ***Wants to commit suicide by shooting, or by hanging.***

Abdomen - Burning pain in abdomen and anus. Duodenal catarrh. Cramps at umbilicus. Cramps with flatulence, before breakfast, better eating. ***Incarcerated flatulence,*** painful, pushes here and there, right abdomen. Flatulency, wind colic in ascending colon, worse before breakfast. Colic better rubbing or kneading abdomen, lying on sides. Lead colic. Bruised pain with urging to stool. Abdominal flatulence after confinement. Tension in right hypochondrium as if it would burst. Inflammation of right groin, typhlitis. Tympanites in bilious fevers. Tuberculosis abdominalis.

Back - Violent pain in back of neck and at base of brain. Soreness up and down spine and neck. Piercing pain between scapulae. Sharp cutting pain in back spreading upwards like a fan. Bruised pain in lumbar region. Lumbar region pains if one attempts to retain the urine. Contusive pains in sacrum. Chronic swelling of cervical glands. Spinal meningitis. Opisthotonos. Itching when undressing.

Breasts - Nipples retracted (Sars.).

Chest - Chest feels all gone, empty. Oppression in chest. Pressure on chest, as of a heavy load. Soreness of chest when coughing, better pressure. ***Pain through lower left chest.*** Stitches in left side of chest. Swelling of ribs, near sternum. Spasmodic motions of muscles, worse left side. Swelling and induration of axillary glands. Furuncles near axilla. Foul axillary sweat.

Constitutions - Hydrogenoid constitutions where complaints are such as due to living in damp houses, basements, and cellars. Patients cannot eat even plants growing near water, or fish.

Cough - ***Cough*** with thick, ropy, greenish, copious expectoration. Cough with purulent sputum and pain about last ribs, left side. ***Must hold chest when coughing***. Springs up in the bed the cough hurts so, holds painful side (Bry.). Loose cough from tickling in throat, better sitting. Dry cough with roughness in throat, worse morning after rising, worse night.

Ears - Heat in right ear, evening. Piercing, stitches, sticking pains in ears, worse in damp weather. Piercing pain in right ear inward. Lancinations in ears. Irritable mucus membrane of ears and nose. Pressing in ears as if tympanum was pressed out. Earache as if something was forcing its way out. Ringing, tinkling in ears, as of bells.

Eyes - Yellow conjunctiva. Conjunctivitis with granular lids, green pus, terrible photophobia. ***Photophobia,*** on waking in morning. ***Sensitive to sunlight.*** Crawling or burning in eyes. As if eyeballs were hot. Granular lids. Itching on edges of lids mornings. Heaviness of eyelids. Aching in eyes in evening, when reading by candlelight. ***Blindness from head injury.*** Dimness of sight from weakness of eyes. Confused sight. Sparks before eyes after blowing nose.

Face - Yellow complexion, pale, sickly. Itching of face. Tearing in face and in cheekbones. Vesicles and pimples on face. Pimples on chin that burn when touched. Vesicles on lower lip. Lips burn like pepper. Dryness on upper lip.

Female - Scanty menses, too late, with knotty stools. Acrid and profuse menses, with nosebleed. Burning in pharynx during menstruation. Leucorrhea acrid, corrosive, parts inflamed. Yellow-green leucorrhea following gonorrhea, with hoarseness. Leucorrhea with hoarseness. Herpetic vulvitis.

Food - Want of appetite and repugnance to food. Desire for ice and ice-cold water. Thirst at the start of fever only. Desire for salty fish, beer and cold drinks. Desire for or aversion to yogurt. Aversion to meat and bread. Starchy food, milk and potatoes disagree. Beer is distasteful. Vegetables, fruit, pastry, cold food or drink and farinaceous food causes diarrhea.

Head - ***Ill effects of falls and injuries to the head***. Mental or physical troubles after injury. ***Headaches since head injury.*** Gnawing pain in occiput. Base of brain as if crushed in a vise. Boring in right temple, preceded by burning in stomach. Headaches, worse by noise, stooping, during menses, light, eating, better in dark room, vomiting. Salivation with headache. Head jerks to side (right). Brain feels loose when stooping. Bursting feeling on coughing. Pressure and heat in vertex during menses. Pulsating, from congestion of blood to head. ***Spinal meningitis***. Head jerks to right side. Creeping in scalp of vertex. Scalp sensitive, combing hair painful.

Kidneys - Frequent urination. Polyuria. Diabetes. Urging to urinate, with piercing in both groins. Burning pain in urethra. Urine loaded with bile. Urine with sediment of a yellow color or like brick-dust. Scanty, dark urine, had to get up several times at night.

Limbs - Rheumatism, worse in damp, cold weather. Rheumatic pains with gastric symptoms. Gout. Pain in limbs, compels frequent change in position. Sciatica on rising from sitting or turning in bed, no relief in any position. Pain in hip joint worse rising or sitting down. Stiffness of knees, cracking of joints. Edema of feet. Throbbing, piercing in heels. Burning in soles. Vesicles on soles. Itching between toes. Trembling of hands on waking and also when writing. Twitching of hands and feet during sleep, more after midnight. Inflammation around root of nails. Hangnail. Swelling of axillary glands.

Liver - Sore and tender liver, worse deep breathing, stepping, jar. Liver sore to touch. Region of liver sensitive when walking in open air, stitching pain. As of a lump below liver. Irritable liver sometimes after excessive study or mental work. Jaundice after anger. ***Hepatitis, icterus and vomiting of bile.*** Gallbladder disorders. Clawing pain in gallbladder.

Lungs - Dyspnea during damp weather. Constant desire to take deep, long breath. ***Humid asthma,*** rattling in chest, at 4 a.m. and 5 a.m. ***Asthma worse damp weather.*** Asthma, with early morning diarrhea. ***Asthma, sycotic in children***. Every fresh cold or any unusual exertion, brings on an attack of asthma. Attacks of hay asthma. Bronchial catarrh, with glairy sputum, worse damp weather. Delayed resolution in pneumonia. Hemoptysis, in hydrogenoid constitutions. Copious expectoration, thick, ropy, greenish. Chest feels all gone with cough.

Male - Edema of prepuce and scrotum. Sweat on scrotum in evening. Itching of glans, of scrotum with burning after scratching. Violent itching of glans of penis or scrotum. Enlarged prostate, with pus and mucus in urine. Condylomata, soft, fleshy excrescences, greenish discharges. Warts. Chronic gonorrhea, thick, greenish discharge, little pain. Increased sexual desire. Voluptuous feeling during stool.

Modalities - Better from open air, warm, dry air. Better change of position, lying on back, pressure. Better after dinner, breakfast. ***Worse from damp weather*, *dampness of cellars***, night air, late evenings, wind. Worse subdued light, music, lifting, lying long in one position, touch, pressure. Worse cold food and drinks, vegetables, fruits. ***Worse from head injuries***.

Mouth - Offensive breath with malarial symptoms. ***Bitter taste.*** Taste unpleasant, slimy. Slimy, thick, tenacious, white mucus. Salivation during headache. Mouth as if rough and numb. Blisters on palate. Burning in mouth as from pepper. Burning of palate as if sore and raw during menses. Gums burn like fire.

Neck - Violent pains in back of neck and at ***base of brain***. Stitches in nape of neck at night. Jerking, tearings and tension in muscles, on left side of neck.

Nose - Nose stopped up, great dryness and burning. Root of nose feels stopped up. ***Nasal catarrh with thick, yellow discharge*** and salty mucus. Coryza with obstruction of nose. Sneezing with fluent coryza. Yellowish-green nasal discharge becomes green on exposure to light. Watery discharge at night. Ethmoiditis. Nosebleed, before and during menses, stops and returns often.

Perspiration - Sweats without thirst. Sweats at night, in morning. Sweats on face, on scrotum.

Rectum - Bruised pain and urging to stool. Involuntary stools, when passing flatus. Rumbling, gurgling in bowels, then sudden noisy spluttering stools in the morning, can drive from bed. ***Loose morning stools***, worse after spell of wet weather. ***Great size of the fecal mass.*** Diarrhea, yellow, watery stools. Foamy or yellow diarrhea, mixed with green slime. Burning pain in anus after stool. Itching of perineum and mons veneris. Itching of anus, as from worms. Knotty, wart-like eruption on anus and between thighs.

Sensations - As if forehead would burst, as if a screw being driven in, as if top of head would split. As if brain was loose and fell to left temple, as if brain crushed in a vice or something gnawing there. Creeping in scalp to vertex. Crawling in eyes. As if bells ringing in ears. As if tympanum was pressed out, as if something forcing its way out of ears. Lump or ball in throat. Weight on chest. Burning on top of head, right eye, edges of lids, gums, palate, anus, abdomen, soles to knees.

Skin - Jaundiced skin, after anger. Chronic skin eruptions. Eczema, moist and oozing profusely. Erysipelas, smooth, red, shiny, tingling or painful swelling of skin. Wheals containing a yellow, watery, not glutinous secretion. ***Watery, yellow blisters.*** Yellow scales after breaking of vesicles. Sycotic excrescences, wart-like red lumps all over body. Itching pimples. Itching while undressing. Chafing of skin in children with bilious symptoms.

Sleep - Great sleepiness during day. Drowsiness in forenoon when reading or writing. Sleeplessness caused by great agitation. Jerking of limbs during sleep. Awakes from the pain of flatulence. Uneasy sleep with anxious and disagreeable dreams. Dreams of running water, of flying. Dreams of being insulted or fighting. Frequent waking from unpleasant, fantastic dreams.

Stomach - Stomach feels distended and heavy. Squeamishness in stomach before meals. Slow digestion. Acid dyspepsia with heartburn and flatulence. Water brash in evening. Frequent hiccough after eating bread and butter. Hiccough in evening. Nausea with pain in eyes. Sour vomit or regurgitation. Green bilious vomiting. Green, bilious vomit. Morning sickness, vomiting with bitter taste in mouth.

Teeth - Drawing pains in teeth. Throbbing toothache with restlessness, worse warm, but intolerable to hot drink. Tearing in carious teeth, on getting out of bed, at night. Toothache better by holding cold water in mouth. Gums burn like fire.

Temperature - Chills up back, with icy coldness, gooseflesh, shaking and chattering of teeth, with anguish and thirst. Cannot get warm even in bed. Internal chills with stretching and yawning. Sudden flashes of heat towards evening. Increased warmth of body, with restlessness. Fever with aversion to uncover. Foul axillary sweat, profuse at night. Perspiration in morning.

Throat - Dry throat. Sore throat. Tearing pain down throat. Burning in pharynx during menses. Impeded swallowing. Feeling of a lump on swallowing. Frequent constriction of throat. Inflammation, with profuse, tenacious mucus. Thick, yellow mucus drops from posterior sinuses. Hawking of salt mucus, worse morning. Tonsils and uvula inflamed and swollen. Ulcers on tonsils. Goiter.

Tongue - ***Brown, bitter coating on tongue.*** Dirty brown or greenish yellow, thick, pasty tongue, especially at base. Tongue covered with mucus, slimy taste in mouth. Burning blisters, vesicles on tongue. Tip of tongue feels burnt. Root of tongue coated a dirty greenish gray or greenish brown.

Vertigo - Vertigo, relieved by sweat on head. Vertigo after dinner, from gastric derangements. Vertigo at 6 p.m., followed by vomiting of sour mucus.

COMMENTS - Grauvogl and Schussler used Nat-s. in the lower trituration. It was Schüssler's specific for epidemic influenza, but homeopaths need not confine themselves. When the correspondence is exact, the highest potencies will act better than the lower; when the likeness is more general, the lower will give the best results.

Headache, with drowsiness. Basal headache, as if the bones at the base of the brain were crushed, pressure on both sides or on right side of occiput. Sun headaches. Severe migraine, especially after a head injury or after grief. Nausea, vomiting, bursting and splitting migraines. Worse mental effort.

Spinal meningitis with violent, crushing pain in the occiput. Traumatic epilepsy from injury to the head. Blindness after head injury, cortical blindness. Personality change after head injury. Injuries to the spine, although more specifically for the head.

Mental troubles arising from injury to the head. Nervous exhaustion brought on by debilitating diseases. Chronic fatigue. Overly concerned with the future. Tend to project and plan a lot. Irritability, worse morning. The mind clears as the day goes on. Mental symptoms worse from music.

Sentimental. Worse from nursing loved ones, never been well since nursing a loved one. Overwhelming sense of being overburdened. Very independent. Angry, verbally violent. Resentment about life, regretful. Holds grudges.

Difficulty expressing emotions after a grief. Low spirits, even to suicidal impulse. Suicidal depression typified by a great conflict about whether to do it or not (Aurum has conflict over when they will do it). May act impulsively. Tendency to hanging or shooting themselves.

Postpartum depression, especially if the birth was traumatic (Sep. first). Feeling overwhelmed and overworked with new baby. Depression worse in the morning. Despair over recovery.

Hydremia, worse in humid weather, near the water and in moist, damp, underground dwellings. Ailments arise or are worse from dwelling in damp houses, from damp weather, damp soil, weather changing to damp, getting wet. Chest eruptions every spring. Warm-blooded, worse heat. Better from warm, dry weather, and being in the open air.

Asthma, particularly found in malarial districts. Humid asthma. Asthma after a cold. Attacks frequently occur in the early morning hours. Skin symptoms during or after asthma. Asthma in children, with restless legs.

Catarrhs with yellowish green or green secretions. Discharges are thick, green, yellow and painless (Med., pain and inflammation with the discharge). Bronchitis and coughs with a lot of mucus. Gonorrhea, sinusitis, and chronic urethritis.

Scrofulous ophthalmia. Granular lids. Photophobia (Nat-c., Nat-m.). Sensitivity in the eyes. Nosebleed before and during menses (not vicarious like Bry). Toothache is worse by warm things, intolerable by hot things, and better by holding cold water in the mouth.

Edema, edematous erysipelas. Vesicles on the skin containing yellowish water, moist herpes, ringworm, sycotic excrescences. Burning of the feet (Sulph.) and stiffness of the joints (Rhus-t.). Limbs feel bruised and weary, especially with migraines. Drowsy, weak, weary and heavy feeling.

Functional disturbances in the secretion of bile. Chills and fever, bilious fever, influenza, diabetes, bilious vomiting, bilious diarrhea. History of hepatitis. Gallstones with severe right-sided pain and cramps. Bad taste in the mouth in morning. Tongue is coated yellow or white.

Diarrhea in the morning (Sulph.), especially after eating fruits, pastries or ice cream. Diarrhea driving one out of bed. "Cheerfulness after loose stools." Craves yogurt. Likes dairy and cheese, but not as strong. Desires sweets, but aggravate. Worse from fruits or pastries.

Generally right-sided (Thuj., left sided). Hydrogenoid and sycotic miasm (Thuj.). Pain in the right colon, the right shoulder. Headaches over the right eye. Warts on the right foot and right hand (Thuj.).

H. C. Allen said that with the possible exception of Graph., no remedy has "such terrible sensitiveness to light."

Hermann of Paris cured a young woman, a patient whose sleep was disturbed by dreams of fighting.

Leonard cured a case of violent asthma induced by unusual exertion with Nat-s. 200x.

W. J. Guernsey recorded a similar case. Mrs. S., 36. had violent attacks of asthma, with greenish, purulent sputa, and a loose evacuation immediately after rising the last two days. Nat-s. 500c was given in water, every two hours. She was able to lie down the same night and all her symptoms rapidly cleared up.

Guernsey also had the case of Mrs. C., 42. who had been subject to attacks for years. Copious expectoration of greenish mucus. She was given Nat-s. in water every three hours. Improvement began after a few doses, expectoration became paler and less abundant. She felt better than she had for years previously.

Mahlon Preston cured many cases of threatened tuberculosis having "pains flying from the chest beginning with a dry cough."

Gregg gave the symptoms "all-gone, empty feeling in chest, a sense of weakness in chest, must hold chest with both hands when coughing for support to relieve the weakness." "Must hold chest because of pain and soreness, feels as if it would fly to pieces" (Bry., Phos.).

RELATIONS - ***Compare:*** (1) Nat-suc. - catarrhal jaundice. (2) Malar. (3) Nat-ch., Fel. (4) Mom-b. - colic, dysmenorrhea with gushes of blood. (5) Pulm-v. (6) Peumus boldus. (7) Nat-i., Nat. hydrosulph. - liver-spots, locally and internally. (8) Sulph., Thuj., Merc., Still. ***Complementary:*** Ars., Thuj.

REFERENCES - Boericke. Clarke. Murphy. Phatak.

NATRUM SULPHUROSUM

(Sodium Sulphite)

PHARMACY - nat-sulo. Natrum sulphurosum. Sodium sulphite. Sulphite of Sodium. Trituration. Solution. ***Historical dose:*** All potencies.

HOMEOPATHIC - Clarence Bartlett related a case of chronic diarrhea in which "the stools were watery and looked very much like yeast." The patient had pain in right scapula as if bathed in hot water, was much debilitated, taking food provoked a stool. The face was whitish waxy, except the cheeks, which were a "light freckle color."

Farrington, on the indication "yeasty stools," suggested Nat-sulo. 3x, which cured after the failure of many other remedies.

REFERENCES - Clarke.

NECTRIANINUM

PHARMACY - nectrin. Nectrianinum. Nosode of tree cancer. Nectria ditissima. Dilution. Trituration of the parasite. ***Historical dose:*** All potencies.

CLINICAL - Cancer. Epithelioma. Hemorrhages. Neoplasm.

HOMEOPATHIC - Nectrianinum is a clear liquid of a yellowish-brown hue which was prepared by Bra and Chaussé. Two month old nectria cultures on grape broth were evaporated on a water bath until reduced to one-third of their original volume.

They were filtered through paper, and again through porcelain. The liquid was then taken to the autoclave at a temperature of 120 degrees centigrade. This assured that all spores are killed.

Observers said that Nectrin. caused "An arrest or diminution of hemorrhages. Suppression of fetid discharges. A tendency at times to epidermization of the neoplasm with a corresponding well-defined arrest in its evolution."

The patients were worse when treatment was discontinued and better when it was resumed. In very advanced cancer, reaction may not occur.

RELATIONS - ***Compare:*** (1) Carc., Cadm-s., Scirr.

REFERENCES - Clarke.

NEGUNDIUM AMERICANUM
(Box Elder)

PHARMACY - neg. Negundium americanum. Box elder. Acer negundo. Ash leaved maple. Negundo aceroides. Negundo fraxinifolium. N. O. Sapindaceae. The bark of the root is macerated in twice its weight of alcohol. ***Historical dose:*** All potencies.

HERBAL - Dr. O. S. Laws of Los Angeles, California, wrote of a new "pile" remedy, Negundo. "In botanical language it is known as Negundium americanum.

The common name is 'box elder.' It is a native of Kansas. It is a distant relative of the Acer family. The bark of the root in the yearling plants is preferred."

HOMEOPATHIC - Neg. has writhing with an engorged rectum. Engorgements of rectum and hemorrhoids with great pain. Recent cases of hemorrhoids can be completely cured with five to ten drop dose of tincture every two hours, and the old hard cases temporarily relieved.

REFERENCES - Anshutz. Boericke.

NEON

PHARMACY - neon. Neon. ***Historical dose:*** All potencies.

CLINICAL - Asthma. Colds. Cough. Down's syndrome. Headache. Urticaria. ***Yawning.***

HOMEOPATHIC - Down's syndrome. Headache, in temples, amel. hot bath. Eyes dry, tired, desire closing them. Heaviness and numbness of eyelids, as if they have been in chlorine. Hot face. Colds, much mucus, itching, blocked nose.

Sore throat, scraping, amel. water and tea, rasping, as if something stuck in it. Low voice, deep voice. Respiration asthmatic, cough agg. morning. Wart on first joint of right index finger. Urticaria.

Walking upright and gracefully. Worse right side. Weather, cold, as if freezing or very hot. Worse 5 p.m. Worse 5 a.m. Desires nothing. Desires oranges. Aversion to cold drinks, bread. ***Yawning.*** Worse from neon lights.

REFERENCES - Sherr.

NEPENTHES DISTILLATORIA

PHARMACY - nep. Nepenthes distillatoria. Nepenthaceae family, related to the Aristolochiaceae. The mother tincture is prepared from the entire plant. ***Historical dose:*** Tincture and all potencies.

CLINICAL - Amenorrhea. Diabetes insipidus. Dyspepsia. Endometriosis. Fatigue. Headaches. Hyperthyroidism. Menorrhagia. Migraines. Narcolepsy. Neurasthenia. Ovaritis. Torticollis. Ulcers. Vertigo.

HOMEOPATHIC - The Nep. symptomatology was established by Julian with a group of twenty-one people, five men and sixteen women, using the 15x, 6x, and 3x potencies and placebo in 1960-61.

Julian stated, "It is possible to confirm without being misleading, that is digestive and genital infections, for which we have described the clinical indication above, Nepenthe is a sure and faithful remedy of great value."

Feeling of general, cerebral and physical tension. General fatigue with complete exhaustion around 3 p.m. Weariness and prostration, followed by a general improvement. Extreme tiredness with shivering.

Feverish, irritated, restless, hasty in actions. Over activity. General internal trembling, ameliorated by resting. Diminution of nervous tension. Pain in the 'nerves,' unfamiliar, new depressive sensation.

Painful sensitivity of the scalp. Dryness of the skin. Dyspepsia with dryness in the mouth, hunger-pangs, feeling of bruising in the epigastrium. Abdominal distention. Menstrual disorders with female frigidity. Hyperthyroidism.

MIND - Optimism, everything seems easier, less wasting. Hasty in actions. Irritation. Impatience, nerves jangle and feeling of anguish. Anguish, accompanied by sadness and depression. Neurosis from anguish. Depressive state with prostration, sadness and fatigue. Fatigue, prostration, sadness. Neurasthenia. Apathy. No desire to smoke. Narcolepsy. Hypochondria.

Abdomen - Dull aching in the liver. Feeling of a hard ball in epigastric region. Distention. Flatulent dyspepsia. Gastric and duodenal ulcers. Diaphragmatic hernia.

Back - Pains in the lumbar region when bending down. Lumbar area is fatigued. Chronic lumbar rheumatism. Torticollis.

Chest - Retro-sternal discomfort after meals.

Constitutions - Pre-senility. Carbo-flouric constitution. Thyroid conditions with cancerous tendency. Syphilitic poisoning.

Eyes - Pricking of eyelids. Conjunctivitis.

Female - Hypogastric heaviness. Congestion of the pelvis. Feeling of swelling of whole body 10 days before menses. Menses repeat after a period of amenorrhea lasting 6 months. Menses early by 5 days and copious. Secondary amenorrhea. Metrorrhagia and menorrhagia. Endometriosis. Stinging, needle-like, flashing pains around the right ovary in the morning. Left ovarian pain, spreading to the left kidney. Cystic ovaritis. Frigidity. Diminution of sexual desire. Infertility.

Food - Appetite wanting. Hunger with feeling of weakness. Hunger-pangs at 6 a.m. and around 11 a.m. Feeling of thirst. No desire to smoke.

Head - Migraines. Head heavy.

Heart - Feeling of a lump in the precordial region and in the arms, fairly violent, but not spreading and disappearing gradually after half an hour, not aggravated by movement. Habitual hot flushes. Cardiac neurosis. Digestive cardiac pains.

Kidneys - Increased urinary excretion. Polyuria in the morning.

Limbs - Cramps in the left leg, soothed by bending the leg. Arthrosis of the hip. Pains in the left hip.

Lungs - Reflex cough, related to the thyroid area.

Modalities - Better in the fresh air. Worse at night. Worse towards the end of the day. Worse on the left side.

Mouth - Peculiar indefinable taste in the mouth. Insipid taste. Persistent taste of pimentos in the mouth. Taste like iron in the mouth during the morning. Burning flavor with feeling of dryness in the mouth. Dryness in the mouth, especially the pharynx with expulsion of mucus. Palate rough. Gingivitis.

Nose - Head cold. Atrophic rhinitis. Dryness of the nasal mucus membranes. Dry cough.

Rectum - Nausea. Heartburn. Stools easy, but can be painful to expel. Stools easy with bleeding hemorrhoids. Stools more difficult to expel.

Skin - Dryness of the skin and mucus membranes. Dry skin on the face with small eczematous eruptions. Ichthyosis. Pityriasis-type eczema. Herpes on the upper lip, on the right side. Rapid, clear regression of malleolar edema. Violent itching, situated at the fold of the left elbow. Labial herpes. Painful sensitivity of the scalp. Hair is more alive and is easier to arrange.

Sleep - Yawning, after eating, sleepiness. Sleep light and disturbed. Insomnia at first, then deep sleep. Wakes early.

Stomach - Gastric pains. Gastric dyspepsia. Swelling, heaviness in the stomach with the need to take deep breaths, ameliorated by alkalis, by walking in the open air. Feeling of bruising in the stomach. Stomach cancer.

Throat - Larynx, sensation of hardness, sensitive on palpation. Laryngitis.

Tongue - Glossitis. Tongue dry, thick. Feeling like parchment at the tip of the tongue and below the roof of the mouth. Tingling at the tip of the tongue. The median line of the tongue stands out from the tip to the root. Tobacco aggravates the tongue complaints.

RELATIONS - ***Compare:*** (1) Arg-n. - Phobic, asthenic conditions, irritation of the mucus membranes. Anxious agitation, weakness of the legs with trembling. Feeling of a splinter of wood lodged in the pharynx. (2) Merc-v. - Mental slowness, weakness and trembling at the slightest exertion. Fetid odor in the mouth with metallic taste, nocturnal sweating, diarrhea, copious menses and burning, itching leucorrhea.

REFERENCES - Julian.

NEPETA CATARIA

(Catnip)

PHARMACY - nepet. (catar.) Nepeta cataria. Catnip. Catmint. Cataria nepeta. Cataria vulgaris. N. O. Labiatae. Europe and North America. Tincture of the whole plant. ***Historical dose:*** Tincture and all potencies.

CLINICAL - Abdominal, pain. Amenorrhea. Bronchitis. Catarrh. Colds. ***Colic.*** Coryza. Cramps. Diarrhea. Dysmenorrhea. Dyspepsia. Exanthemata. Fever. ***Flatulence.*** Headaches. Hiccoughs. Hyperactivity. Hysteria. Indigestion. Influenza. Menstrual, cramps. Nausea. Nightmares. Sleeplessness. Stomach, cramps. Vomiting.

HERBAL - Nepeta cataria is diaphoretic, tonic, antispasmodic, diuretic, refrigerant and carminative. As it produces free perspiration it is very useful in colds, etc.

C. D. Collins, M.D., in the Electic Medical Journal, noted, "The infusion of the fresh plant certainly has something in it or about it that produces excellent results, and is soul satisfying when given to the crying baby. The infusion of the dried plant does not do so well.

"In fact, the tincture is preferable to the use of the dried article. Catnip relieves pain and produces sleep. We give it to the colicky baby. Its persistent crying and kicking and writhing soon ceases, and balmy sleep causes baby to forget its troubles.

"Catnip is not necessarily a baby remedy. many think of it only in this field. It is a woman's remedy, and produces just as certain and pleasant effects in nervous headache, nervous irritation, hysteria, amenorrhea, dysmenorrhea.

"It is an excellent remedy to bring about the relaxation necessary to the appearance of the exanthemata. In acute coryza or catarrh, bad colds, or la grippe, no remedy surpasses full doses, say ten to twenty drops, in hot water every hour or oftener."

The infusion of 1 oz to 1 part boiling water may be taken by adults in doses of 2 tablespoonfuls, by children in 2 or 3 teaspoonfuls frequently, to relieve pain and flatulence.

Ten to thirty drops of the tincture, added to five teaspoonfuls of hot, sweetened water, and given freely, constitutes a good treatment for colicky and fretful infants.

Culpeper stated, "The green herb, bruised and applied to the part for two or three hours, easeth the pain arising from piles. The juice also, being made up into an ointment, is effectual for the same purpose. Washing the head with a decoction thereof taketh away scabs, and may be used to the like effect on other parts of the body."

Some of the herbalists recommend the use of the herb against barrenness. Avoid catnip during pregnancy.

HOMEOPATHIC - Nepet. is a children's

remedy for ***colic and indigestion*** (Cham. and Mag-p.). Colic and sleeplessness in babies (Cham.). Abdominal complaints, with pain, flexing of thighs, twisting of body, crying. ***Fretful and irritable children from indigestion.*** Nervous headache and hysteria. Nervous irritability and insomnia in adults.

COMMENTS - Catnip is so named because of the general fondness of cats for this plant. It is said that when the plant starts to wither cats will roll themselves in it and chew it. There is an old belief that it makes cats "frolicsome, amorous and full of battle."

There is also an ancient belief that "if the root be chewed it will make the most quiet person fierce and quarrelsome."

RELATIONS - ***Compare:*** (1) Cham., Coloc., Mag-p.

REFERENCES - Boericke. Collins. Murphy.

NEUROLAENA LOBATA

(Jackass Bitters)

PHARMACY - neuro-l. Neurolaena lobata. Jackass bitters. Golden bitters. Alligator's foot. Kayabim. N. O. Asteraceae. ***Historical dose:*** Tincture and all potencies.

CLINICAL - Amoebas. Candida. ***Diabetes.*** Giardia. Fungus. Hypoglycemia. Lice. Malaria. ***Parasites.*** Ringworm. Wounds

HERBAL - Neurolaena lobata is a member of the Asteraceae family and a common Central American plant. It has yellow flowers and bitter-tasting leaves which contain a potent anti-parasitic agent (sesquiterpene dialdehyde), that is active against amoebas, candida, giardia and intestinal parasites.

A tea made from the root is used to cleanse the blood, and a leaf tea is used to treat intestinal parasites, malaria, fungus and ringworm. It is also topically to bate wounds to prevent infection, and to use as a hair wash for ridding the hair of head lice. Boiled and strained leaves have been used as an insecticide for house and garden plants.

There is some preliminary research that indicates N. lobata helps ***regulate blood sugar levels***, which can ultimately help diabetics manage their condition. A subsequent animal study showed that a tincture of this plant lowered blood glucose levels in animals.

RELATIONS - ***Compare:*** Chin.

REFERENCES - Buttimer. Murphy.

NICCOLUM CARBONICUM

(Nickel Metal)

PHARMACY - nicc. Niccolum carbonicum. Nickel metal. Niccolum metallicum. Nickel carbonate (Ni, At. Wt. 58.6). Trituration. ***Historical dose:*** Trituration and all potencies.

CLINICAL - Asthenopia. Clavus. Coryza. Cough. Dysmenorrhea. Face, chapped. ***Headaches.*** Hoarseness. ***Hiccough. Migraines.*** Nasal, catarrh. Neck, cracking. Ophthalmia. Sneezing. Speech, impeded. Throat, sore. Tongue, stiff. Toothache. Vertigo. Vision, impaired. Whooping cough.

HOMEOPATHIC - Nickel is found associated with cobalt. It is said to have received its name, the devil, from miners who considered it "false ore" as they were mining for copper. Cobalt (Kobold) possibly has a similar derivation as nickel forms the chief ingredient in the alloy known as "German silver."

Nickel was proved by Nenning and the pathogenesis contains some striking symptoms, many of which have been confirmed.

Sir James Y. Simpson used the sulphate of nickel in ***"periodic headaches of a very severe character,"*** and the provings show that the metal and the carbonate are equally appropriate in this connection.

Periodic nervous headaches with asthenopia, weak digestion, constipation of debilitated literary persons. Cracking in cervical vertebra on moving the head. Catarrh. Violent hiccough with thirst.

Hoarseness. "Must sit up and hold head with both hands with the cough." The child must be held up when coughing or it will go into convulsions. Must sit up and hold the head with hands or has to put the arms on thighs when coughing, worse night.

Great debility in evening. Restlessness, worse at night, from agitation. Tearing and shooting in the limbs and other parts. Compelled to change position continually with vomiting and colic after suppressed menstruation. Dysmenorrhea.

MIND - Dullness of mind, does not comprehend the conversation and is unable to relate properly in conversation. Dislike to conversation. Taciturn, fretful. Low-spirited. ***Disposition to contradict***. Vexed and very angry from least contradiction. ***Irritability during headache.*** Quarrelsome in evening.

Anxious moroseness and inquietude. Anxiety on moving as if sweat would break out. Fears something evil will happen. Trembling and fright with desire for solitude. Restlessness, after midnight. Confusion, as after intoxication, in morning.

Abdomen - Abdominal pains go from left to right. Violent stitches, as with knives in hypochondria. Pinching around navel. Painless rumbling in abdomen. Tension of abdomen and discharge of flatulence.

Back - Cracking in cervical vertebrae when moving the head. Pain in neck, as from a sprain. Stitches in small of back, in afternoons. Pain in the small of back during a soft stool.

Chest - Pressure and heaviness on chest. When coughing, dyspnea and pressure on chest. Stitches in chest when breathing. Shootings in chest, especially when laughing. Pain, as from excoriation in chest.

Constitutions - Hering said it is suited to literary people who suffer from periodical nervous headaches, weak, asthenopic, weak digestion, constipation, worse morning on awaking.

Ears - Stinging in ears. Shootings in ears. Sudden deafness with roaring and humming in ears, in evening.

Eyes - Heat and redness of eyes with pressing in them. Violent twitching in eyes, with lachrymation and difficulty of vision. Agglutination of eyes in morning. Vision very much impaired, especially in the evening. Objects appear too large.

Face - Skin of face chapped. Right side of face red and hot. Redness of face with burning and itching like erysipelas. Swelling of right side of face with sore throat. Painful sensitiveness and cramp in maxillary joint, which hinders mouth from being easily opened. Twitching of upper lip. Itching tetters on cheeks. Eruption on lips.

Female - Menses premature, scanty and of too short duration. Menses late, scanty with great debility and burning in eyes. During menses, bloated abdomen, colic, pain in small of back, great debility, burning of eyes. Profuse leucorrhea, worse after menses, after urinating (Mag-m., Plat.), watery after urination.

Food - Farinaceous taste in mouth on rising in morning. Risings with taste of roasted meat. Aversion to meat. Want of appetite. Thirst in evening. Violent thirst day and night.

Head - Migraines, first on left side. Periodical headaches, every two weeks. Headache all day in forenoon with vomiting of bile. Pain on top as from a nail. Pressure on vertex in morning, worse until noon and in warm room. Stitches.

Kidneys - Increased secretion of urine, also at night. Burning at orifice of urethra during urination. Burning urine. After urination, discharge of thin leucorrhea.

Limbs - Headache feels heavy, tremble, feel bruised. Pain in shoulders as if sprained. Rheumatic pains in elbows, extending to hands in fingers. Heaviness in the hands and feet, better by motion. Feet feel heavy, tremble and are weak. Stitches in left heel.

Lungs - Hoarseness. Dry, hacking, regular cough with stitches in chest. ***Obliged to sit up and hold head, must put arms on thighs***. Violent cough at night. Dry, scraping cough with sleeplessness. Cough from tickling in trachea. Expectoration of white mucus.

Male - Itching on a small spot of scrotum, scratching does not relieve. Erections, worse after dinner.

Modalities - Better in open air, evening, after eating. Cold helps pain in face. Coughing helps roughness of throat. Worse periodically, every two weeks, yearly, forenoon. Worse from motion, pressure, after midnight. Talking and yawning aggravates sore throat.

Mouth - Breath is offensive, of which he himself is not aware. Bitter taste in mouth in morning. Abundant accumulation of sweetish saliva in mouth. Stiffness of the tongue, it is difficult to talk.

Nose - ***Violent sneezing.*** Obstruction of nose, nose stopped up at night. Coryza, fluent during day and dry during night. Nasal catarrh with redness and swelling at tip of nose. Acute pain at root of nose, extending to vertex and through temples. Stinging, tearing and soreness at root of nose. Eruption on nose. Dryness of nose.

Rectum - Constipation, ineffectual urging to go to stool. Stool very hard and only discharged with great effort, has to press hard to discharge the stool. Diarrhea with yellow mucus, expulsion with great force and much flatulence. Diarrhea after drinking milk with tenesmus, preceded by cuttings or burning in anus. During stool, burning and stitches in rectum and anus. After stool, anal itching, burning and stitches.

Sensations - As if sweat would break out. As if brain were cut to pieces. As if she had not slept enough. As if a nail was sticking in head. As if neck sprained.

Skin - Itching over the whole body, but mostly on the neck, as from fleas, not better by scratching, but followed by small vesicles. Itching and pimples in small of back. Itching on shoulders, scratching does not relieve. Itching tetters.

Sleep - ***Sleeplessness*** from midnight until 4 a.m. Wakefulness. Frequent awakening at night from agitation. Pain in swollen face wakens him at night, it is better by cold. Awakens after midnight with colic. Feels as if she had not slept sufficiently.

Stomach - ***Gone, empty feeling in epigastrium without desire for food.*** Acute stomach pains, extending to shoulder. Painful sensation of constriction of stomach. Fullness in stomach after eating. Thirst and ***intense hiccough***, especially in evening. Bitter and sour belchings. Nausea. Diarrhea and tenesmus after milk.

Teeth - Swelling of gums. All teeth feel loose and elongated. Gnawing toothache in evening. Toothache with tearing in ears toothache with tearing in right ear. Sour, fetid secretions ooze from decayed molar teeth.

Temperature - Chill is preceded or begins with yawning and sleepiness. Chill with chattering and shaking, followed by profuse general perspiration. Continuous chill with moist palms of hands. Heat with perspiration and thirst, followed by chill. Anxious heat with violent thirst. Fever, restlessness and vomiting at night. Morning sweat.

Throat - Hoarseness, every year at same time. Sore, right side with great tenderness, ***Soreness to touch externally***. Sore throat, worse when speaking or yawning. Throat feels sore as if ulcerated on swallowing. Stitches in throat on swallowing. Spasmodic contractions and sensation of strangulation in throat. Roughness in throat better by coughing. Accumulation of thick mucus in throat with stinging pain. Swelling of tonsils on right side, as well as of face and neck, which are painful when touched.

Vertigo - Vertigo with nausea and desire to vomit. Vertigo with dizziness and staggering, as from weakness, worse on getting in up in the morning. Vertigo in the morning, when rising after stooping in evening.

COMMENTS - W. A. Clausen noted that, in the sore throat, the right side had exquisite tenderness, soreness to touch externally on affected side. Must sit up and hold the head with both hands when coughing, or has to put arms on thighs when coughing.

Mahony cured with Nicc. 200c a middle-aged woman who had "loose hacking cough day and evening and at 9 a.m., has to put arms on thighs when coughing."

H. Moser cured cases when the pain was worse at 10 a.m. to 11 a.m. and could be so intense as to cause the patient to cry out, appeared first left side, could jump to right, disappeared in evening.

RELATIONS - ***Compare:*** (1) Cob., Plat. (2) In "objects appear large," Hyos., Nat-m., Phos. (3) objects appear small, Hyos., Plat, Stram. (4) objects appear blue, Lyc., Stram., Zinc. (5) Diplopia, rainbow colors around light, Phos.,

Gels. (6) Coryza, Nux-v., Sulph. (7) Red face, Ferr. (8) Chapped face Nat-c. (9) Toothache with tearing in ear, Mang. (10) Periodical headache, Gels. Sil., Sulph. (11) Emptiness in stomach, Carb-an., Ign., Sep. - Nicc. has it without desire for food. (12) Cracking in neck and stiff jaw, Petr. (13) Headache, menses, chilliness, Puls. (14) Feels refreshed in morning without having slept, Fl-ac., Cob. (15) Annual hoarseness, Ars. (16) Literary men, Nux-v. (17) Sore throats, Lyc.

REFERENCES - Boericke. Clarke.

NICCOLUM SULPHURICUM

(Nickel Sulphate)

PHARMACY - nicc-s. Niccolum sulphuricum. Nickel sulphate. Trituration. ***Historical dose:*** Trituration and all potencies.

CLINICAL - Headaches. ***Hot flashes.*** Menopause. Migraines. Neuralgia, periodic. Spinal, pains.

HOMEOPATHIC - Nicc-s. is for weak, asthenopic literary persons with weak digestion and constipation, who are worse in morning and suffer from periodic headaches and hoarseness.

Urine and saliva increased. Coppery taste in mouth. Periodic neuralgias of malarial origin. Menopausal disturbances.

MIND - Nervous, uneasy. Restlessness, cannot settle down to any occupation. Desire to recline, tired.

Back - Stiff, numb sensation, worse in neck. Spine sore. Spinal pains, legs and arms heavy and weak, cannot lie on back.

Female - Dull aching in ovaries with sensation as if menses appear. ***Hot flashes***, followed by perspiration on parts touching each other, when separated become dry.

Head - Periodic headaches, occipital pain, extending down to spine, worse lying on back, sore pain in eyes.

Limbs - Awakened in morning with burning soles.

COMMENTS - J. Y. Simpson cured with Nicc-s. periodical headaches of very severe character. Hale used with success the Nicc-s. 2x trituration in periodic neuralgias of malarial origin.

REFLRENCES - Boericke. Clarke.

NICOTIANA RUSTICA

(Tobacco)

PHARMACY - nicot-r. Nicotiana rustica. Tobacco. Nelson's horsenettle. N. O. Solanaceae. Tincture of whole fresh plant. ***Historical dose:*** Tincture and all potencies.

CLINICAL - Abdomen, pain. Absent-minded. Allergies. Asthma. Backache. Belching. Brain-fag. Bronchitis. Cancer. Canker, sores. Chills. Collapse. Convulsions. Coryza. Coughing. Delirium. Distension. ***Dyspnea.*** Emaciation. Epilepsy. Fainting. Flatuence. Hay fever. Headaches. Insomnia. Itching. Lachrymation. Lung, disorders. ***Nausea.*** Palpitations. Photophobia. Rumbling. Salivation. ***Seasickness.*** Sinusitis. Spasms. Tetanus. ***Tobacco, effects.*** Ulcers. Unconsciousness. ***Vertigo.*** Vesicles. Vomiting. Weakness.

HERBAL - Tobacco refers to a genus of broad-leafed plants of the nightshade family indigenous to North and South America, or to the dried and cured leaves of such plants. Tobacco leaves are often smoked (see tobacco smoking) in the form of a cigar or cigarette, or in a smoking pipe, or in a water pipe or a hookah. This could damage the lungs and could also potentially cause lung disorders such as asthma. Tobacco is also chewed, "dipped" (placed between the cheek and gum), and sniffed into the nose as finely powdered snuff.

Nicotiana rustica is a very potent variety of tobacco. The high concentration of nicotine in its leaves makes it useful for creating organic pesticides. It is also used for religious purposes by South American shamans. Growing in the rainforest it contains up to twenty times more nicotine than common North American varieties such as Nicotiana tabacum.

HOMEOPATHIC - Richard Pitt conducted a recent proving of Nicotiana rustica which was written up in his book called Tobacco. Tobacco contains the nicotine, a powerful neurotoxin that is particularly harmful to insects. All means of consuming tobacco result in the absorption of nicotine in varying amounts into the user's bloodstream, and over time the development of tolerance and dependence.

Nicotine is the key alkaloid found in tobacco. Extremely addictive and poisonous, one or two drops of pure nicotine can be lethal. In some varieties of Nicotiana rustica, the nicotine content of the leaves can be as high as 20 percent.

Toxic effects of tobacco include perspiration, light-headedness, general weakness, tremors, convulsions and respiratory paralysis.

Interestingly, one of the keynote symptoms of Tabacum is a sinking feeling, usually associated with nausea. This was confirmed in the Nicotiana rustica proving, but the ***feeling of sinking was also seen in its psychological sensations***, making it a theme of the remedy. The sinking was explained in different ways, from a falling from a high place into the earth, a falling through space, a general sinking feeling in the body. The sinking feeling was confirmed in the stomach and abdomen region.

The ***vertigo*** symptoms were confirmed and also elaborated on with Nicotiana rustica. This falling, sinking feeling was consistent throughout the remedy picture, and more modalities were confirmed than are currently found with Tabacum. Physically, there were strong vertigo symptoms, one prover experienced debilitating vertigo for over 4 weeks.

There were characteristic headache symptoms, often described as being neuralgic in nature, and also eye and face symptoms which were neuralgic in nature. In the ear and nose symptoms, there was a particular feeling of "openness", which could parallel some of the mental experiences, a sense of opening to other dimensions, or like the earth opening up, creating an abyss or chasm.

The nose also had some itching and tickling and a delusion of smelling smoke or a herb. The mouth had symptoms of tingling, and also a feeling of numbness, showing the alternating state of the remedy.

Deathly nausea is one of the well-known characteristics of Tabacum. The stomach and abdomen showed similarities to that of tabacum, with a sinking feeling, an emptiness and hollowness, along with the characteristic nausea. Along with the sinking feeling, there was a rising feeling, and feeling like a wave, revealing a similar state to the mental experiences of rising and sinking.

In the respiratory system, there were some cough symptoms, often of a tickling nature, worse by any cold, air or water and in the chest some sharp, stitching pains, similar to heart symptoms.

There were some characteristic symptoms in the back and limbs with aching, burning and stitching sensations. Also in the limbs, there were sensations of weakness, heaviness, fatigue, a sprained feeling, and jerking spasms. All the joints were affected, including the feet and hands. The shoulder and arm symptoms and general aching should be compared with Lycopersicum (tomato), another solanaceae remedy.

There were some interesting sleep symptoms, especially waking suddenly from sleep, as if from a jolt or a feeling of being half awake and asleep. There was extreme tiredness, even a feeling of complete collapse. Similar to Tabaccum, there was an extreme feeling of chill, going through the whole body, including the bones. The coldness was felt both externally and internally.

In general, there was a feeling of weariness, heaviness and exhaustion and also the opposite, a feeling of energy circulating the body, a feeling as if to take off, to fly, along with an up and down feeling, a rocking sensation and vibrations throughout the body, a nervous excitation and pulsating in the body. There was a desire for salty food, sweets and ice cream and an increased thirst. Faintness. Emaciation.

MIND - The mental image of the proving also revealed a heightened sense of awareness, clarity and lightness. Full of ideas. Anxiety from smoking tobacco. Mental excitement. Joy and cheerful feelings.

Increased mental dullness. Absent-minded. Confusion of mind. Difficult concentration. Sadness. Depression about being away from loved ones. Hurried feelings. Nervousness and restless. Impulsive. Fear of heights. Fear of falling. Fear to go to sleep. Awkwardness. Aversion to exertion.

Delusion to be sinking. Delusion of being possessed. Mind and body are separated. Delusion of floating in air. Delusion that air is flowing through him. As if in a dream. Delusion of once being in an earthquake.

The clarity and light seemed psychedelic in nature and was connected to the feelings of being between sleep and waking. The connections between life and death were also seen in the dreams, with themes of birth and death and also dreams of the past. Both the dreams and waking state revealed a sense of being in between both states.

Abdomen - Coldness. Distension. Rumbling. Flatuence after eating. Flatuence from emotions. Fullness sensation. Itching. Abdomen pain, better from belching, passing flatus. Cramping pain in morning on waking. Cutting pain umbilicus region. Sinking sensation. Swelling of abdomen in morning on waking.

Back - Bubbling sensation in spine. Buzzing sensation in lumbar region. Backache. Neck, sore, aching pains. Back pain between the scapulae. Aching pain. Burning pain in spine. Sharp pains dorsal region. Lumbar spasms. Stiffness of back, neck.

Breasts - Aching pains. Burning pains above nipples. Nipple pains. Sharp pains in breasts, nipples.

Chest - Anxiety in chest. Chest pain. Constriction. Burning pains axilla.

Coughing - Asthmatic coughs. Dry cough. ***Coughing with gagging.*** Painful, irritable coughs. Tickling cough. Sudden coughs. Paroxysmal coughs. Violent coughs with jerking of body. Coughing from eating, cold drinks.

Ears - Fullness sensation. Redness. Itching. Heat sensation in left ear. Pulsation of eardrum. Ear pains, in morning, on waking. Burning, pressing pains. Crackling noises in ears. Sensitive hearing to high pitched noises.

Eyes - Itching of eyes. Dryness. Lachrymation. Eye pains. Burning pain. Stinging and stitching pains. Photophobia. Sensitive to sunlight, must close the eyes. Tired sensation, better from closing eyes. Eye tension and strain. Swelling.

Face - Eruptions. Red face, cheeks. Rash on chin, forehead, cheeks. Pimples, tingling, painful to touch. Numbness. Jaw pains. Pressing, stitching pains. Clenched, stiff jaws. Crunching noise when closing jaws.

Female - Menses bright red, copious. Menses, scanty. Itching of vagina. Increased sexual desire. Irregular menses, returns after having been ceased.

Food - Thirst. Desires ice cream, sweets and salt.

Head - Itching of head. Congestion. Constriction sensation. Heaviness sensation, in morning, on waking. Headache from tobacco smoke. Headache from strong odors. Dull pain in forehead and temples. Fullness sensation. Pressing, pulsating pains. Pain on sides of head. Tingling, vibrations, wavelike sensations. Sinus headache. Opening sensation in frontal sinuses, in the morning, on waking.

Heart - Anxiety in heart region, worse when thinking of it. Palpitations. Sensation of pulse reverberating throughout the body.

Limbs - Icy cold foot. Burning pains. Convulsion on side not lain on. Dryness of hands. Eruptions, red spots. Itching of hands and feet. Heaviness sensation of lower limbs while walking. Paralysis sensation. Sensation as if shoulder is dislocated. Stiffness of lower limbs. Tinglings. Pulsations in wrist and shoulders. Trembling and weakness. Sensation as if ankle is sprained.

Lungs - Catching respiration. Bronchitis. Shortness of breath. Expectoration difficult. Tingling. Sensation as if lungs are expanding.

Modalities - Better open air. ***Worse in mornings, on waking.***

Mouth - Dryness of mouth, lips. Tingling of lips, mouth. Itching of the corners of mouth. Salivation. Vesicles, gums. Taste wanting. Canker sores. Ulcers.

Nose - Nasal congestion, obstruction. Allergies. Hay fever. Coryza. Nasal discharge clear, watery or yellow. ***Nasal discharge*** in morning on waking. Sinusitis. ***Sensitive to odors*** of flowers, food, mothballs, smoke. Burning in nostrils. Sneezing. Sensation of air flowing through bridge of nose.

Rectum - Constipation. Ineffectual urging and straining. Flatus. Inactivity of rectum. Soft stool. Dark stool. Hard stool.

Sensations - Pulsations. Rocking sensation and vibrations. ***Wavelike sensation***. Sinking, emptiness, sensation. ***Hollow sensation***. Sensation of air flowing.

Skin - Cold skin. Eruptions, itching. Sensation of air flowing in and out of skin. Pimples. Stinging pain.

Sleep - Insomnia, protracted. Sleeplessness after waking. Wakes after midnight. Wakes 2:30 a.m. to 3:30 a.m. Wakes unrefreshed in the morning. Half awake while dreaming. Dreams of childbirth. Dreams of falling. Dreams of high places. Amorous dreams. Dreams of mortification, grief. Dreams of old friends, children. Dreams of animals, pets.

Stomach - Acidity. Burning pain. Cramping pain. Churning sensation. Indigestion. Belching, bending forward, agg. Stomach distension after eating. Flatus. Rumbling. ***Nausea.*** Nausea in morning. ***Deathly nausea.*** Nausea, better drinking. Nausea from smoking tobacco. Nausea, better urination. ***Wavelike sensation***. Sinking, emptiness, sensation. ***Hollow sensation*** in stomach.

Temperature - Chilliness. Icy coldness of body. Bones cold. Chill, morning, forenoon. Chills beginning in the feet, moving upward. Fever alternating with chills. Cold feeling upper body.

Throat - Constriction. Dryness of throat. Itching. Sore throat, worse on swallowing. Burning pain. Sore throat on waking in morning. Scraping sensation, better cold drinks. Disposition to hawk. Swallowing difficult. Tickling in throat, better coughing. Larynx, cold sensation.

Tongue - Tingling of tongue. Sensation as if tongue is enlarged, swollen. Tongue numbness.

Vertigo - Vertigo with disorientation and weakness. ***Vertigo as if in an earthquake.*** Vertigo with nausea. Vertigo with wavelike sensations. Vertigo as if floating. Vertigo worse exertion, morning. Vertigo better from sitting. Vertigo on rising.

Vision - Blurred vision. Acute vision. Objects seem to approach then recede. Sensation that their vision was lost. Weakness of vision.

COMMENTS - Tobacco smoking carries significant risks including the potential to develop various cancers as well as strokes, and severe cardiovascular and respiratory diseases.

Significantly shorter life expectancies have been associated with tobacco smoking. Many jurisdictions have enacted smoking bans in an effort to minimize possible damage to public health caused by tobacco smoking. The substantially increased risk of developing cancer as a result of tobacco usage seems to be due to the plethora of nitrosamines and other carcinogenic compounds found in tobacco and its residue as a result of anaerobic heating, either due to smoking or to flue-curing or fire-curing.

The word death is interesting in relation to this substance. The above facts of the use of tobacco are testament to the toxicity of tobacco and its impact on societies throughout the world. It is the most widely used drug known to man, having spread originally from the Americas to the rest of the world. Nicotiana plants were frequently seen in cemeteries, reinforcing the connection between tobacco and the other world.

RELATIONS - ***Compare:*** Tab., Nicot.

REFERENCES - Pitt.

NICOTINUM

(Nicotine)

PHARMACY - nicot. Nicotinum. Nicotine. An alkaloid from Nicotiana tabacum. N. O. Solanaceae. Solutions in distilled water or alcohol. ***Historical dose:*** All potencies.

CLINICAL - Aura of epilepsy. Brain-fag. Collapse. Delirium. ***Dyspnea.*** Epilepsy. Fainting. Headache. Lachrymation. Lung, disorders. Nausea. Seasickness. Spasms. Tetanus. ***Tobacco, effects.*** Unconsciousness. Vertigo. Vomiting. Weakness.

HOMEOPATHIC - Nicot. had a very heroic proving by Flak, Wochenfeld, Wertheim, Schroff and Reil. Very violent tonic and clonic spasms were produced. Dullness of senses. Loss of consciousness.

Alternate tonic and clonic spasms, followed by general relaxation and trembling, nausea, cold sweat and speedy collapse. Coldness extends from fingertips and toes over trunk.

Jerking respiration. Breathing difficult and impeded, every respiratory effort consisting of a series of short jerks in quick succession. So weak could scarcely hold up head. Paroxysms of faintness beginning with a vanishing of senses and ending with loss of consciousness.

Great aversion to tobacco and tobacco smoking. One prover, a smoker was unable to smoke more than a few whiffs, the other, a non-smoker, could not approach any one who was smoking.

MIND - Excitement. Inability to think or fix attention on any subject. Delirium with frightful vision. Uneasiness. Brain-fag. Loss of consciousness.

Abdomen - Distended. Disagreeable sensation through whole intestinal canal.

Chest - Oppression, compelling deep breathing. Sensation of foreign body behind sternum.

Ears - Indistinct hearing, sensation as if ears filled with cotton.

Eyes - Pupils dilated. Indistinct vision with sensitiveness of eyes to light. Lachrymation. The eyelids feel too heavy.

Face - Face pale, features drawn. Sensation of an aura in upper jaw.

Head - Dullness of head, heaviness, dizziness, stupefaction. Head drawn back with rigidity of muscles of neck and back.

Heart - Pulse and respiration very irregular, sometimes becoming very rapid, sometimes sinking. Constant sinking of pulse. Pulse increased in frequency in direct proportion to dose.

Kidneys - Urgent desire, urine copious, increased.

Limbs - Formication, beginning in fingertips, extending to the wrists and afterwards to elbows. Weakness of lower limbs, on going up stairs,

Lungs - Breathing, very rapid and difficult.

Mouth - Increased saliva. Scraping, burning taste, especially low down in throat, causing hiccough and hawking. Sharp, burning sensation in tongue.

Nose - Expired air had odor of alcohol.

Rectum - Excessive desire for stool, better by emission of flatus and urine. Stool retarded.

Sensations - Great sensitiveness of eye to light, along with indistinct vision. Aura in upper jaw. As though a sharp brush had been drawn through esophagus to stomach,

Skin - Dryness of skin.

Sleep - Sleepy. Restless night, sleepless, hot and excited.

Stomach - Loss of appetite. Emptiness and faintness in stomach and intestines. Disagreeable sensation extending from stomach upwards and downwards. Hiccough. Eructation with some vomiting which relieves.

Temperature - Shaking chill. Limbs icy cold. Coldness beginning in fingertips and toes and extending to trunk. Cold sweat. Sensation of warmth commencing in stomach, rapidly extending over chest and to head and like a streaming into fingertips and toes, not followed by sweat.

Throat - Dryness and scraping in throat. Sensation as though a sharp brush drawn through esophagus to stomach. Sensation of dysphagia.

Vertigo - Vertigo and headache.

COMMENTS - Increasing clonic spasms, trembling limbs, extending over whole body, which violently shakes. Head drawn back, contraction of eyelids and masseter muscles, muscles of neck and back rigid, hissing respiration from spasm of laryngeal and bronchial muscles.

RELATIONS - ***Antidotes:*** See under Tab. ***Compare:*** (1) Tab., Dig., Lob., Absinth.

REFERENCES - Clarke.

NIGELLA SATIVA

(Black Cumin)

PHARMACY - nig-s. Nigella sativa. Black cumin. Common Fennel flower. Blessed seed. N. O. Ranunculaceae. Tincture from rectangular black seeds. ***Historical dose:*** Tincture and all potencies.

CLINICAL - Allergies. Amenorrhea. Asthma. Belching. Bites. Bronchitis. Colic. Coughs. Dysmenorrhea. Gallstones. Gout. Fevers. Flatulence. Hemorrhoids. Indigestion. Jaundice. Leucoderma. Paralysis. Parasites. Ringworm. Salivation. Whooping cough. Worms.

HERBAL - Nigella sativa is the fennel flower of the buttercup family. It is sometimes confused with the fennel plant (Foeniculum vulgare). It has blue flowers and black seeds, which have been used in Egyptian and Arabic medicine.

Avicenna maintained that it is an expectorant and tonic for low energy and apathy. Affects the digestive tract and the respiratory tract. It acts as a tonic for weak digestion, colic, gas and belching. Dry coughs, asthma, bronchitis and whooping cough. Leucoderma, skin allergies, periodic fevers, hemorrhoids.

A special oil is extracted from Nigella which was used in herbal formulas as a digestive tonic and stimulant. Undiluted Nigella oil causes irritation to the stomach and intestines, increases the flow of breast milk, stimulates the menstrual flow and causes excessive salivation. It helps prevent gout if added to the diet.

COMMENTS - Placing the powdered seeds in a cloth and inhaling them helps reduce the common cold. A decoction of the black seeds helps amenorrhea, dysmenorrhea, intestinal worms, fevers, paralysis and hemorrhoids.

Adding the seeds to the diet will help prevent gout. Drinking a tea made from the crushed seeds with honey can help dissolve gallstones and kidney stones. The tea also increases the flow of the breast milk, the menses and urine.

An ointment was used to stimulate the growth of the beard and helps prevents hair graying. Used externally for ringworm. Dog bites and spider bites. The smoke of black seeds drives insects away.

RELATIONS - ***Compare:*** (1) Lyc.

REFERENCES - Al-Akili. Murphy.

NITRI SPIRITUS DULCIS

(Sweet Spirits of Nitre)

PHARMACY - nit-s-d. Nitri spiritus dulcis. Sweet spirits of nitre. Aethylium nitrosum. Spiritus etheris nitrois. Nitrous ether. A mixture of alcohol, water and ethyl nitrite: it contains no "nitre" (Kali-nit.). Dilution. ***Historical dose:*** Tincture and all potencies.

CLINICAL - Backache. Canker, sores. Chills. Colds. Colic. Constipation. Cough. Diarrhea. Dropsy. Dysentery. Dyspnea. Fever. Gallstones. Headaches. Mouth, sore. Nausea. Nephritis. Paralysis. Photophobia. Prosopalgia. ***Salt, abuse.*** Scarlet fever. Scurvy. Tibia, pains. ***Typhoid fever.*** Vertigo. ***Vomiting***. Warts.

HOMEOPATHIC - Nit-s-d. was proved by Lembke. Poisonings give a perfect picture of the typhoid state. Hahnemann recommended it for hospital typhoid with apathy In fevers, Hahnemann advised that Nit-s-d. should be given a few drops dissolved in an ounce of water, a teaspoonful every three hours.

Typhoid fevers with symptoms of cerebral paralysis. ***Sensorial apathy*** in low fevers when there is stupor, difficulty of arousing patient is met by this remedy. Great fatigue, a recumbent position can alone mitigate and tranquilize it. Excessive emaciation. Swelling of veins. Very sensitive to cold. Catching cold in stormy weather causes prosopalgia.

Ill effects of excessive salt intake (Phos.). ***Sore mouth of salt eaters.*** Salty taste. Dry skin, nausea, flatulence. Dropsy. Excellent diuretic. Acute nephritis following scarlet fever. Urine very scanty. Bloody diarrhea. Scurvy. Hands covered with warts.

It has been used as a remedy for incarcerated gallstones, given beaten up with an egg yolk and applied outwardly in the same form.

The symptoms of Nit-s-d. go from below upward, worse on passive motion, riding in carriage. Worse from cheese. Nit-s-d. has been found to be an antidote to several medicines. It increases the action of Digitalis.

MIND - Excessive ill-humor. Irascibility, passion and quarrelsome disposition with tendency to weep. Complete apathy, without desire for anything. ***Lies indolently without sleeping or speaking.*** Dislike to labor and conversation.

Delirious and incoherent in manner. ***Hears and desires nothing, unconscious.*** Dizzy as if intoxicated, when roused could answer questions, complained of headache and said he found it difficult to walk straight.

Abdomen - Shootings, cutting and burning pains in abdomen. Cutting in umbilical region. Stitches in left side below navel. Rumbling in abdomen. Colic. Incarcerated gallstones.

Back - Backache. Violent pressure in nape and cervical vertebra. Pressure and stitches in region of spine. Drawing in scapulae. Sensation as hot water creeping through back from below upward.

Causations - Salt, cheese. Stormy weather.

Chest - Painful constriction behind sternum. Pressure and stitches in chest. Stitching in skin of left axilla.

Eyes - Black spots and rings float before eyes. Pupils contracted. Pupils somewhat dilated, acting feebly. Stitches in eyes and lids, burning on margins. Twitching of eyelids.

Face - Prosopalgia with photophobia. Burning in cheeks. Very sensitive to cold. Boring in facial bones in angles of lower jaw. Twitching in middle of left upper lip. Chronic soreness in corners of mouth, patient eats much salt.

Food - Want of appetite. Worse after eating, from cheese. ***Ill effects of excess salt*** (Nat-m., Phos.).

Head - Confusion, fullness, heaviness in forehead. Violent boring pain in forehead. Drawing, tearing pain, pressure and heaviness in head. Boring or pressure in temple. Pressure, heaviness and heat in occiput. Stitches in vertex. Drawing pain on scalp.

Heart - Feeling of pressure in heart. Violent beating of heart.

Kidneys - Frequent desire. Increased urination, clear urine.

Limbs - Wandering pain in limbs. Pressure, boring and stitches in muscles and joints.

Lungs - Short, dry cough. Dyspnea. Shortness of breath and wheezing, while eating, before attack of prosopalgia. Inhalations intermit. Very rapid breathing by going only a short walk.

Male - Violent cutting pain in tip of urethra.

Modalities - Worse from mental disturbance. Worse when cold, during winter and spring, afternoon. Walking aggravates breathing and heat.

Mouth - Heat in mouth, sour taste. Salivation. Accumulation of water, mucus in mouth. Taste, salty on tip of tongue. Tongue dry. Cutting, burning and stitches in tongue. Tearing drawing pain in teeth. Canker sores after eating cheese.

Rectum - Bloody diarrhea after purging from salt. Bloody diarrhea after purpura, caused by excessive use of salt. Epidemic dysentery with lethargy. Marked constipation.

Perspiration - Inclination to perspire during fever.

Skin - Crawling in skin. Skin and tongue dry. Warts from having used too much salt. Shiverings and acute drawing pains in the bones.

Sleep - Lies in bed motionless.

Stomach - Empty eructations. Paroxysmal cutting deep in stomach, with flushes of heat and hot sweat. Contractive pain and aching in stomach with sensation of fullness, immediately after a meal, from eating too much salt. Continued nausea and loathing. After a meal, vomiting of sour matter and mucus, followed by headache. ***Vomiting, followed by lassitude.*** Vomiting and purging.

Temperature - Internal chills with cold hands. Creeping chills under skin. Typhoid fever with sensorial apathy and semi-paralysis of brain, wild, staring eyes. Adynamic fevers with nervous symptoms such as shootings, jerkings, etc.

Throat - Increased mucus, dryness in throat. Sensation of contraction in throat with pain. Stitches in larynx, constriction. Sensation as if a plug in gullet. Cramp from below upward in esophagus.

Vertigo - Vertigo with dullness. Vertigo while sitting, upper part of body sways to and fro.

RELATIONS - ***Antidoted by:*** Calc., Carb., v., Caust., Con., Kali-c., Nat-c., Nat-m., Kali-nit., Op., Sep. ***Antidote to:*** Nat-m. (crude or in potencies), Nat-c., Phyt. ***Compare:*** (1) Ph-ac., Lyc. - worse afternoon, fullness after meals. (2) Coloc. - worse from cheese. (3) Hell., Ph-ac. - typhoid, sensorial apathy, stupor, Ph-ac. has apathy more pronounced than Nit-s-d., Hell. most of all. ***Incompatible with:*** Dig., Ran-b.

REFERENCES - Boericke. Clarke.

NITRICUM ACIDUM

(Nitric Acid)

PHARMACY - nit-ac. Nitricum acidum. Nitric acid. Aqua fortis. Solution. ***Historical dose:*** All potencies.

CLINICAL - Actinomycosis. Allergies. ***Antibiotics. Anus, fissures.*** Arthritis. Axilla, perspiration. Blisters. Bladder, catarrh. Breath, offensive. Bright's disease. Bronchitis. Bubo. ***Cachexia.*** Chancre. Chilblains. Choking, easy. Colds, easily taken. Condylomata. Constipation. Corns. Coughs. ***Diarrhea.*** Dysentery, Dyspepsia. Ear, disorders. Epilepsy. Esophagitis. Eyes, disorders. Feet, perspiring. Fistula. Freckles. Frostbite. Glandular, swellings. Gleet. Gonorrhea. Gums, sore. Hay fever. Hematuria. ***Hemorrhages. Hemorrhoids*** Hernia. Herpes. Herpes. Ingrown toenail. Iritis, syphilitic. Irritation. Jaundice. Jaw, joint. Keloids. Leucorrhea. ***Mastoiditis***. Menopause. Menses, profuse. Metrorrhagia. Mouth, sore, Mucous, patches, Muscae volitantes. Myopia. Nails, disorders. Ozaena. Palpitations. Paralysis. Perspiration, abnormal. Phimosis. Polyps. ***Proctitis.*** Prolapsed, anus. Prostate, suppuration. Ranula. Rectum. Rickets. ***Ringworm.*** Salivation. ***Spinal, injury. Syphilis.*** Taste, disordered. Tongue, ulceration. ***Tuberculosis***. ***Ulcers.*** Vaginitis. Vertigo. ***Warts.*** Wens. Whooping cough.

HOMEOPATHIC - The Aqua Fortis of the alchemists. Used in old-schools practice as an escharotic for warts and warty tumors, for phagedenic ulcers, chancres, poisoned bites. Had been used internally in fevers to quench thirst in bronchitis and tuberculosis to diminish the excessive secretions in some cases of syphilis in phosphaturia. Brunton noted that it has been injected into the bladder in a dilute form to dissolve stones.

When strong nitric acid comes in contact with the skin it destroys the upper layers and turns them yellow, but as it coagulates their albumen it forms a barrier against its own further action, its action therein differing from that of Sulphuric acid.

When swallowed it acts as an irritant poison. When its fumes are inhaled, it may cause suffocating spasms of the glottis or intense bronchitis.

In the store of Mr. Harold Woolley, in Manchester, a two-gallon bottle of nitric acid fractured. Water was thrown upon the bottle and whiting placed about it to neutralize the fumes which issued from the fracture.

Mr. Woolley supervised the process and was in contact with the fumes for two hours. This happened in the afternoon. The next day, Mr. Woolley complained of being unwell and although medical aid was promptly summoned, he died at 5 o'clock in the afternoon. Death was attributed to rapid congestion and inflammation of the lungs in consequence of inhaling the fumes.

Nitric acid belongs almost equally to all three of Hahnemann's miasms: psora, syphilis and sycosis. It is one of the chief antidotes of Merc., and is useful in cases of syphilis that have been overdosed with Merc. As the nitric acid patient begins to improve, skin symptoms may appear for a time, a favorable indication.

Marked affinity for the ***margins of the outlets*** especially of the throat, anus and mouth. Orifices are red, swollen and cracked. Mucus membranes are dark, smooth. It affects glands, particularly the liver, prostate and salivary. Patients are greatly debilitated, trembling, shivery, sensitive and sore. Excessive physical irritability.

Pains as from splinters. Sticking pains. Ulcerative grating. Pains as if flesh is torn from the bones. Slight pain affects him violently. Pains appear and disappear quickly (Bell.). Bones painfully sore.

All discharges are very offensive, especially urine, feces and perspiration. Discharges are ***acrid,*** thin, dirty or brown, they cause redness or destroy hair. Stubborn suppuration. Malignancy. Decay and exostoses of bones. Ozaena, foot or night sweats on parts lain on.

Hemorrhages, easy, bright or bloody water. Capillary bleeding after currettage. Blisters and ulcers in mouth tongue, genitals, bleed easily. Fissures with pain during stool, as if rectum were torn.

Cachexia, due to syphilis, scrofula intermittent fever with liver involvement and anemia, etc. Phagedena. Fistula. Syphilis. Gravel. Arthritis. Sycosis. Cancer. Convulsions, epileptiform, at night and going to bed. Frequent vertigo during the day.

Marked improvement of all symptoms while riding in a carriage. Sensitive to medicines given in high potency.

MIND - Mind is weak. Weakness of memory. Confusion. Indifference. Thoughts vanish after mental exertion. No disposition to work to perform any serious business. Mind easily affected, inclined to weep. Weeps from discontent of himself. Sensitive to noise, pain touch, jar. Impetuous during daytime.

Anxiety from thinking about it. ***Anxiety about health.*** Fear of cholera, ***death***. Easily frightened. ***Anxiety from night watching, loss of sleep.*** Anxiety during a thunderstorm. Anxiety on ascending steps. Restlessness after midnight.

Discontented, with everything, with himself. ***Pessimism***. Sadness. Taciturn. Despondency. Hopeless despair. Refuses consolation on one's misfortune. Sadness before menses. Suicidal disposition with fear of death.

Sympathetic. ***Holds grudges.*** Constantly thinks about past troubles. ***Unmoved by apologies***. Estranged from family. ***Hatred of persons who had offended.*** Inveterate ill-will. Anger, over his mistakes. ***Irritable, hateful, vindictive, headstrong.*** Irritability when spoken to.

Excitability, peevishness, quarrelsome. ***Violent anger.*** Fits of rage and cursing. Trembling from anger while quarrelling. Profane, cursing, using vulgar language. Quarrelsome delirium, talks to spirits in other tongue. Delusions, thought he was about to die, yet is not physically ill.

Abdomen - As of a dry, hot cloth on abdomen. Colic relieved from tightening clothes. Inguinal hernia of children.

Back - Stitching pain in lumbar back when coughing. Pain in back at night, better lying on abdomen. Stitches in and between scapulae. Stiff neck.

Breasts - Hard nodes or atrophy of breasts.

Causations - Ill effects of loss of sleep from nursing the sick. Injury to spine. Antibiotics drugs, penicillin, mercury.

Chest - Congestion in the chest with palpitations and fear. Sensation as if bound by an iron band. Catching at every attempt to breathe. Stitches in sides of chest. Soreness at lower end of sternum. Offensive sweat in axillae at night.

Constitutions - Hydrogenoid constitution. Sycotic remedy. Persons who have chronic diseases and take cold easily, disposed to diarrhea. Acts best on the dark complexioned, middle age or older. Persons of dark, swarthy complexion with black hair and eyes, lean persons of rigid tissue. Brunette rather than blonde. Nervous temperament. Old people with great weakness.

Ears - ***Very sensitive to noise*** (Coff., Nux-v.). Cracking in ears when chewing. Decay of mastoid. One's speech echoes in ears. Deafness from enlarged and indurated tonsils after measles, better noise in trains or riding in a carriage. Swelling of glands behind and beneath ears. Cystic tumors on lobes of ears.

Eyes - ***Sharp, sticking pains***. Gonorrheal ophthalmia, photophobia, constant lachrymation. Syphilitic iritis. Ulceration of cornea. Fistula lachrymalis. Double vision. Eyelashes, stiff, all point towards nose (right). Paralysis of upper eyelids.

Face - Yellow, sickly. Dark freckles. Pimples on face. Blood boils on chin. ***Comedones.*** Peeling of lips. Angles of lips raw, cracked or scabby. Corners of mouth raw, cracked or scabby. Stitches as from splinters in upper lip when touched. Submaxillary glands swollen and painful. Cracking in jaws when chewing.

Female - Menses early, profuse like muddy water with pain in back, hips and thighs. Leucorrhea, brown, flesh-colored, watery or stringy, stains yellow or leaves spots with black border. Bloody water from vagina or hemorrhages from overexertion. ***Uterine hemorrhages*** after childbirth or curetting. Vaginitis. Stitches through vagina. Voluptuous itching of vagina after sex. External parts sore with ulcers (Hep., Merc., Thuj.). Hair on genitals falls out (Nat-m., Zinc.).

Food - Appetite variable or absent. Great hunger with sweetish taste. Great thirst. Aversion to cheese, bread, sight and smell of meat. Dislikes meat, things sweetened with sugar, bread. Longing for indigestible things, chalk, earth. ***Loves fat, herring and salt*** (Sulph.). Craving for cheese, fish, carbonated drinks, sweets. Worse milk and fatty food. Worse after eating. Bitter taste after eating.

Head - Head feels hot. ***Sensation of a band around head***. Crushing head pains. Headaches from pressure of hat, full feeling, worse from street noises. ***Painful tension*** within head with nausea. Headaches as if head were in a vice. Piercing pain in temples. ***Pulsating headache.*** Violent throbbing, hammering pains. Headaches, worse motion and jar, better riding in a carriage. Skull sore. ***Decay of mastoid bone.*** Scalp sensitive. Puffy swelling on scalp. Moist scabby, itching eruption on scalp. Falling of hair from vertex.

Heart - Nervous palpitation caused by slightest mental excitement. Palpitations and anguish on going upstairs. Palpitation with heat, anxiety and trembling, during menses. Pulse rapid and small beats. Pulse intermits at fourth beat, irregular.

Kidneys - Infective nephritis. Contracted kidney. Cramps from kidney to bladder. Burning and stinging. Dyspepsia with excess of oxalic acid, uric acid and phosphates in urine and great mental depression. As of a hot tire in urethra. Painless retention or incontinence of urine. Stream thin, as from stricture. ***Urine, smells strong as horse's or offensive.*** Urine feels ***cold*** when it passes, alternately profuse and scanty. ***Scanty, dark offensive urine***. Urine bloody and albuminous. Alternation of cloudy, phosphatic urine with profuse urinary secretion in old prostatic cases. Hematuria with shuddering along the spine.

Limbs - Offensive foot sweat, causing soreness of toes with sticking pain, chilblains on toes. Offensive sweat in axilla at night. Sweating of palms, hands, cold. Warts on back of hands. Finger joints swollen. Herpes between fingers. Blue nails. Nails, distorted, discolored, yellow, curved. Ingrown nails with ulceration and a feeling of splinter, worse touch. White spots on nails. Tibia painfully sore. Pain in patella, impeding walking. Weak ankles, cracking when walking.

Liver - Jaundice, aching in liver.

Lungs - ***Shortness of breath*** on going up stairs (Sil., Calc.). Panting breathing when reading or stooping. Short breath from uterine displacements. Cough in sleep without waking. Cough shattering from a dry spot in larynx, with stitching pain in lumbar region, worse cold, winter. Empyema. Expectoration, muco-purulent, yellow, bitter offensive, smeary, accompanied with sweat. Hemoptysis. Cavernous tuberculosis.

Male - Itching, burning foreskin. Edema of prepuce. Phimosis. Strictures from gonorrhea or syphilis. Soreness and burning in glans and beneath prepuce. Ulcers, burn and sting, exude offensive matter. Red, scurfy spots on prepuce or on corona glandis. Phagedenic chancres.

Modalities - Better from gliding motion, riding in a carriage. Better steady pressure and mild weather. ***Worse from touch, jarring***, rattling, motion, mental exertion or shock, noise. ***Worse cold air,*** cold climate, dampness, evening and night, changing weather, ***hot weather***, heat of bed. Worse mercury, loss of sleep.

Mouth - Putrid breath. Salivation. ***Bloody saliva*** with green coating on tongue. Sore palate. ***Ulcers in soft palate with sharp, splinter-like pains***. Ranula. Bites the tongue and cheek. Gums, swollen, sore, flabby. Gums bleeding inner side. Margin of mouth covered with sores and blisters.

Nose - ***Nosebleeds,*** dark, clotted with chest affections, worse crying. Allergies, hay fever. Nasal diphtheria with watery and excoriating discharge. Frequent sneezing, without coryza during sleep. Coryza with shortness of breath. Coryza with sore and bleeding nostrils. Chronic nasal catarrh with yellow offensive, ***corrosive*** discharge. Ozaena. Green casts from nose every morning. Stitches, as of a splinter in nose. Cutting pain in the nose, decay of bones. Red, scurfy tip.

Perspiration - Sweats easily, then takes cold. Exhausting profuse sweats in morning. Sweats in axillae, on feet and hands (in spinal injuries). Night sweats on part lain on.

Rectum - Bowels constipated with fissures in rectum. Great straining, but little passes. Tearing pains during stools. Stools tear the anus, even though soft. Diarrhea, slimy and offensive. ***Diarrhea from antibiotics drugs, penicillin.*** After stools, irritable and exhausted. ***Violent cutting pains after stools,*** walks in agony (Rat.). Ulcerations after dysentery. Hemorrhages from bowels, profuse, bright. Hemorrhages from rectum after removal of hemorrhoids. ***Hemorrhoids bleed easily.*** Anus, itching, eczematous or oozes moisture. Burning in rectum after urination. Prolapsed anus.

Sensations - As if a mouse running up and down left side. ***Pain as from splinters in eruption. As if splinters in great toe, in carbuncles, etc.*** As if a band about or weight hanging to the part. As if head in a vice from ear to ear over vertex. As if someone were forcibly pressing head, head tightly bound, constricted by tape, contused. As if a gathering in left temple. As if warm water were flowing from and over eyes (first right, then left). As if teeth soft and spongy. As if abdomen would burst, as if a boiler working in bowels. As if a band around bones. As if dogs were gnawing flesh and bones and as if sinews were being pulled up. As if ball of great toe had been frozen.

Skin - Actinomycosis. Warts, large, jagged, bleed on touch or washing. Condylomata. ***Ulcers bleed easily, sensitive. Ulcers with splinter-like pains.*** Ulcers zigzag, irregular edges, base looks like raw flesh. Stubborn suppuration. Burrowing pus. Exuberant granulations. Crusts form and fall. Black pores on face, papules worse on forehead. Coppery spots, on shinbones. Dry skin, eroded, cracked in every angle. Skin itches on undressing. Old scars become painful in cold weather.

Sleep - Sleepiness during day. Drowsy all day from debility with vertigo. Shocks on going to sleep. Pains come during sleep. Starts in fright on falling asleep. Frequent waking and inability to fall asleep again after a long time. Sleeplessness after 2 a.m. Sleeps badly latter part of night. Sobbing during sleep, with anxious dreams. Anxious, unrefreshing sleep with frightful dreams. Wakes too early in morning, or difficult waking.

Stomach - Dyspepsia with excess of oxalic acid, uric acid and phosphates in urine and great mental depression. ***Dyspepsia from abuse of salt.*** Esophagitis. Pain in cardiac orifice. Eructations sour, empty. Eructations during menses. ***Indigestion and nausea.*** Nausea with sour belchings, cannot take food. Nausea with occasional vomiting, better riding in a carriage. Bitter and sour vomiting with much eructation. Vomiting of tenacious or bloody mucus. Vomiting of mucus and food, from cough.

Teeth - Yellow teeth. Teeth feel elongated. Coldness in teeth. Teeth as if soft and spongy. As if teeth would fall out. Decay of teeth. Teeth become loose, gums soft and spongy. Toothache on taking anything cold or hot into mouth. Toothache and swelling of gums during menses. Pulsating, stinging in evening in bed and all night. Gums red and enlarged between teeth. Gums white, swollen. Itching on gums. Bleeding of gums.

Temperature - Icy coldness of soles. Chilly, continuous. Chills after lying down. Chills from least exposure. Chills in room or at fire. Chills in waves up each side of spine and over chest. Chills with aversion to heat. Chills with internal heat. Dry heat, at night, with violent thirst. Heat flushes with sweat on hands. Heat flushes of single parts, or over entire body. Dry heat, internal, at night, wants to uncover. Blood seems hot at night, causes sleeplessness.

Throat - Dryness and heat in throat. Sharp, stinging pains, with rawness as if sore and ulcerated. Throat pain goes into ears. ***Sharp pains, as from splinters, on swallowing.*** Difficult swallowing. Cutting in the larynx. Diphtheritic patches on tonsils and fauces. Uvula and tonsils edematous. ***Tonsils, red, swollen, uneven with small ulcers.*** Hypertrophy of tonsils, after angina. Hawks out mucus from posterior sinuses. White patches. Hoarseness. Aphonia with dry, hacking cough from tickling in larynx and pit of stomach.

Tongue - Tongue, clean, red with center furrow. Moist fissured or mapped tongue. Painful pimples on the sides of the tongue. Tongue sensitive, even to soft food, causes smarting.

Vertigo - Vertigo with obscuration of sight. Vertigo with nausea followed by eructations. Vertigo with weakness, must sit down. Vertigo with pulsation in head and pressure in middle of brain. Vertigo when raising head after stooping. Vertigo in evening, after lying down. Vertigo in morning on rising. Vertigo during menopause.

COMMENTS - Affinity for the mucocutaneous orifices and adjoining parts, particularly the intestines, throat, and mouth.

The mouth, especially in the angles, and anus are prominent seats of syphilitic action and also of the action of the other miasms, the condylomata and fissures of sycosis, the fissures, fistula, hemorrhoids and sore mouth of psora. Salivation, sores in the mouth, sore throats. Mouth symptoms are often confused with Merc.

Characteristic offensive discharges, thin, excoriating. If purulent, they are a dirty yellowish green, not laudable pus. Ulcers on the skin and in the mouth. Ulcers have profuse exuberant granulations and bleed easily. Suppuration. Painful scars.

Characteristic sticking pain, as if from splinter, in any part of the body. Pain comes after touch or movement. Pains, even slight ones, affect him violently. Cramp-like pains, stinging, shooting, burning, pressure and soreness. Twitchings in various parts, frequent starts in upper part of body. Left-sided paralysis.

Sensitiveness to touch runs through the entire symptomatology including the symptoms of the mind. The head is sensitive to the slightest jar, to the rattle of wagons in the street, or even to the step of one walking across the floor, to the pressure of a hat, sensitive to combing and on part lain on.

Eruptions and ulcers bleed easily when touched. Eyes are sensitive to light. Sensitiveness of the head while out driving, stopping suddenly. The tongue is sensitive even to soft food. Chilly. Easily catches colds. Hyperallergic, multiple allergies.

Excessive physical irritability, hysteria. Anxiety (Ars.), obsession about their health. Fixed ideas that they have a disease. Extremely pessimistic. Negative attitude, irritable, complaining. Arrogant. Hateful and vindictive.

Prostration, sick feeling, faints from least motion. Deafness, epilepsy, better riding in carriage. Emaciated. Ailments from nursing loved ones (Cocc., Caust., Nux-v.). Night watching (Caust., Cocc., Nux-v., Carc., Phos.).

Exhausting sweats towards morning, chilly. Profuse, fetid sweats on feet, hands or in axilla. Flashes of heat in hands and feet.

Sudden rush of blood to the chest. Hectic, frequent hemorrhages, bright, red, profuse. Hemorrhages occurring in cachectic women after confinement or abortion. Sharp stitches through right chest to scapula. Tuberculosis when the chest walls are extremely sore to touch.

Great dyspnea, cannot talk for getting out of breath. Morning hoarseness. Tickling cough, seems to annoy all night, at times loose and rattling. Loud rales through chest, offensive sputa, bloody.

Strong smelling urine, very offensive. Typhus when pneumonia supervenes, also when the bowels hemorrhage. Stools are green, slimy offensive, may be purulent, exhausting. Slimy stools from excess of mucus passed with much straining.

Stools may be pale, pasty, sour, and offensive, especially in scrofulous children. The stool is putrid in children, may contain lumps of casein. Dysentery and colitis. Tendency to acute or chronic diarrhea. Diarrhea with every cold (Ars.). Diarrhea from diet, or since antibiotics.

Rawness and soreness of the anus with diarrhea. Pain after stools, whether loose or constipated. As if anus and rectum were torn and pierced, violent pains after stool lasting for hours. Anal fissures with bloody stools and mucus. Anal warts.

Burnett made a cure of actinomycosis with Nit-ac. 3x in a patient who had seen many London consultants and had doubtless taken much Kali-i. The localities in which the disease manifested itself, the region of the mouth and anus, gave Burnett his indication.

H. N. Coons recorded the case of an anemic woman who, four weeks after miscarriage, had constant pelvic hemorrhages, at times coming with a gush, a constant heavy feeling, much worse standing or walking. Nit-ac. 2x, 20 drops in three ounces of water, a teaspoonful every two hours, quickly arrested bleeding and cured.

W. M. James cured a case in which a girl had frequent attacks of petit mal, sometimes as many as fifty a day, between the periods. At the beginning of menses she had spasms so violent that they dislocated both humeri. Giving Nit-ac. 200c persistently gradually put an end to the attacks. The first few times after beginning treatment, there were spasms but no dislocation.

D. C. Perkins related the case of a woman who said she was very ill, but could only describe her illness by saying that she "felt like a pulp-mill." Nit-ac. has "borborygmus as if a boiler was working in the bowels," and proved to be the remedy.

Mohr gave Nit-ac. 3x to a man who suffered from liver cancer with bloody diarrhea, followed by constipation, and violent pains in the stomach and liver. He was unable to sleep or to take any food without much pain, vomiting. Nit-ac. removed the pain and relieved the constipation entirely, and the patient died without an hour's suffering from the time he received treatment.

J. H. Fulton cured M., 28, with one dose of Nit-ac. 200c. M. had bleeding hemorrhoids for eighteen mouths. He had frequent bloody and slimy stools, and bright red blood after stools ranging in quantity from a dessert spoonful to half a tea cupful. When the stools were hard there was much pain in passing them. Burning in the anus after stools.

RELATIONS - ***Antidoted by:*** Calc., Hep., Merc., Mez., Sulph. ***It antidotes:*** Calc., Dig., Merc. ***Compare:*** (1) Merc., Kali-c., Thuj., Hep., Calc. (2) Calad. (3) Ars. - morbid fear of cholera. (4) Med., Syph., Mur-ac., Nit-m-ac., Merc. (5) better riding in carriage, Graph. (6) Spinal injuries, Arn., Rhus-t., Hyper., Calc. (7) Punctured wounds, Hyper., Led. (8) Worse on awaking, Lach., Nat-m. Sulph. (9) Ingrown toenail. Mag-aust. (10) Stringy leucorrhea, Kali-bi. (11) Pains appear and disappear suddenly, Lyc., Bell. (12) Pains affect violently, Acon., Cham., Hep. (13) Strong odor of urine, Benz-ac. (14) Splinter pains, Arg-n., Hep., Sul. (15) Sore, excoriated anus, Merc., Sul., Cham., Ars., Puls., Syph., Chin. (16) Ulcers threatening to perforate cornea, Sil., Calc. (17) Condylomata, enlarged tonsils, fissures, balanorrhea, greenish leucorrhea, Thuj. (18) Ulcers, Merc. ***Compatible before:*** Calc., Puls., Sulph., Arn. - collapse in dysentery, Kreos. - diphtheria dysentery, Sec. - gangrene of mucus membrane, Sulph. (scrofulous ophthalmia). ***Compatible after:*** Calc., Nat-c., Puls., Sulph., Thuj., Carb-an. - bubo, Kali-c.- tuberculosis, etc., Aur. - abuse of Merc., Mez. - secondary syphilis, Hep. - throat, etc. ***Incompatible:*** Lach.

REFERENCES - Boericke. Clarke. Murphy. Phatak.

NITROGENIUM OXYGENATUM

(Nitrous Oxide Gas)

PHARMACY - nitro-o. Nitrogenium oxygenatum. Nitrous oxide gas. Laughing gas. Solution. ***Historical dose:*** All potencies.

CLINICAL - Anesthesia. Bedwetting. Convulsions. Drowsiness. Epilepsy. Faintness. Headache. Hemoptysis. Hemorrhoids. Hysteria. Lungs, congestion. Muscular, weakness. Opisthotonos. Unconsciousness. Vertigo. Weakness.

HOMEOPATHIC - This well-known anesthetic was introduced by Sir Humphrey Davy. Nitrous oxide has given rise to some pathological symptoms including epileptic convulsions during the anesthesia, pain in forehead where the aura commenced. Increased muscular rigor. Muscular weakness. Muscular pains in revived joints.

Some of the symptoms were observed by Clarke on a girl of twelve who had congestion of the right lung setting in within a few hours of the anesthesia.

A man, 30, who had blisters around and inside his mouth on two occasions after being under gas was troubled with drowsiness for weeks after and had acne-like spots on his face.

Other symptoms are from the observation of Mr. Silk and from provings recorded by Allen. Silk observed that females were very much more liable to ill effects than males. One of his patients, an epileptic girl, otherwise healthy, when he removed the face-piece, struggled to get her hands up and afterwards described her feelings as "pain in the forehead where the aura commenced."

In a patient suffering form valvular disease of the heart there was a more than usual degree of lividity during anesthesia and a tendency to syncope afterwards.

In one epileptic patient a fit actually did occur. Rhythmic movement of the arms or legs is a common occurrence. Opisthōtonos, most common in females, much struggling. One prover had his hemorrhoids cured as an incidental result of his experiments.

MIND - Unusual exaltation of the mind, most agreeable sensations and fancies. No command over himself. Mind extremely susceptible to suggestion. ***Involuntary desire to laugh.*** After the giddiness, rapid rush of thoughts afterwards unconsciousness. Mental torture beyond endurance.

Back - Tension in sides of neck in region of carotids. Drawing in neck, as though skin were contracted or cords shortened. Sensation of drawing in muscles, especially the lumbar muscles.

Chest - As if something which was obstructing the chest dropped down into stomach. Sharp pain in front of chest, worse lying on right side. Right chest congested and dull on percussion. Great pain at chest, cough with hemoptysis, better hot applications to chest.

Ears - On waking from unconsciousness, voices of others seemed to come form a great distance or to be in a whisper.

Eyes - Widely dilated pupils. Pupils first dilated, later contracted. Protruding eyeballs.

Face - Face swollen. Acne. Jaws firmly clenched. Blue lips, ears, face, afterwards face dusky. Face livid with unconsciousness.

Female - Erotic movements and sexual illusions. Bilious attacks in a nursing woman, making the infant ill.

Fever - Fever every afternoon from 3 to 6 p.m. Face covered with perspiration after return of consciousness. Coldness of feet and legs to knee between the paroxysms of consciousness. Delirium in evening.

Head - On going into open air, vertigo and staggering to left. A kind of waving of the head. Aching in head and along spine as if they were asleep. Giddiness after palpitations. Numb feeling on head, spreading over body, before the paroxysms. Headache after return of consciousness.

Heart - Great lividity and tendency to faint. Palpitation of heart, afterwards felt and heard in head.

Kidneys - Involuntary urination.

Lungs - Breathing is quick, thick and stertorous. Suffocative feeling. Cough with hemoptysis. Cough early morning.

Mouth - Eruption of blisters around mouth inside. Point of tongue thrust between teeth. Mouth and head feel numb, as though asleep.

Rectum - Hemorrhoidal pains.

Sleep - Sleepy. Drowsiness continued for weeks after the gas. Screamed whenever she fell asleep.

Stomach - Pressure in epigastrium. Nausea and vomiting on return of consciousness, next day a bilious attack.

Throat - Weakness and feeling of construction in throat, dysphagia.

RELATIONS - ***Antidoted by:*** Bell. ***Compare:*** (1) Nit-ac. (2) In congestion, Verat-v.

REFERENCES - Clarke.

NITROMURIATIC ACIDUM

(Aqua Regia)

PHARMACY - nit-m-ac. Nitromuriatic acidum. Aqua regia. A mixture of chloro nitric acid, chloronitrous acid, chlorine and water. Prepared by mixing 18 parts of nitric acid with 82 parts of muriatic acid. Dilutions. ***Historical dose:*** All potencies.

CLINICAL - Anus, constricted. Bilious. Canker, sores. Catarrh. Cirrhosis. Constipation. Depression. Digestion, slow. Dysphagia. Gravel. Headache. Hepatitis. Mouth, sore. ***Oxaluria.*** Palpitations. Ptyalism. Salivation. Scurvy. Vertigo. Weakness.

HOMEOPATHIC - Aqua Regia, the royal water of the Alchemists, has been proved in the lower dilutions, in the 30c.

Some experiments were made by Dr. Scott, who acidulated his bath with the acid and sponged his body with acidulated water. Sponging and bathing had the same effect. Scott noticed that the symptoms were more marked as the proportion of muriatic acid was increased.

Salivation and sore mouth and throat with dysphagia were produced in Scott and the provers. Scott noticed that the salivation was intermittent. Weakness. Headache with drowsiness. Slow digestion. Pricking pains.

Clinical reputation in ***oxaluria*** and gravel. Removes the distressing skin symptoms resembling psoriasis. Weak, physically and mentally depressed. Constricted anus. Gravel. Bilious conditions torpid liver, hepatitis and early cirrhosis of liver.

Hale noted that it is more adapted to liver torpor and gastric catarrh common in hot and damp climates and ***aggravated by meat eating and alcohol***.

MIND - Nervous irritation and restlessness. Low spirits, depression.

Abdomen - On rising, sensation from left hypochondrium to rectum as of desire for stool. Slight colic in lower abdomen.

Back - Catching pain in back muscles while taking a cold bath.

Food - Aggravated by meat and alcohol.

Head - Headache and great sleepiness, worse 3 p.m. Sensation in temples as if brain distended. Sudden sticking ache in left temple while leaning to left side, preceded by twitching of anterior tissues of temporal muscle.

Heart - Palpitations. Fluttering at heart, while eating or moving.

Kidneys - Urging in penis and bladder, aching in hips, thighs and small of back, after a short delay some pale urine passed. Burning in urethra. ***Oxaluria***. Cloudy.

Limbs - Heavy pain in loins. Sticking in various parts of limbs successively, while walking. Languid aching through hips and front of thighs and small of back.

Liver - Bilious conditions, torpid liver, hepatitis and early cirrhosis of liver. More adapted to liver torpor and gastric catarrh common in hot and damp climates. Sudden increase of secretion of bile.

Lungs - Inflammation of larynx and bronchi. Breathing easier than usual.

Modalities - Worse after eating and from exercise.

Mouth - Metallic taste (Cupr.). Ptyalism. Extreme salivation, could not spit it out fast enough. ***Constant drooling at night*** (Merc.). Salivation intermittent, no fetor. Pain in palate or mouth. Small superficial ulceration over inside of mouth and tongue, excoriation. Cankers. Large blister inside lower lip. Gums bleed easily.

Rectum - Sphincter constricted. Constipated with ineffectual urging. Constipation, desire for stool, but unable to pass anything owing to constriction of anal sphincter. Anus moist and sore. Loose, yellowish, pappy stool after breakfast.

Sleep - Sleepy with headache. Slept unusually well and felt better for it.

Stomach - ***Salivation, worse at night.*** Food takes longer to digest than usual. Sour belchings with empty hungry feeling in stomach, not relieved by eating. Evacuation of flatus and belchings.

Temperature - Chill passing upward, while sitting near stove. Mild fever. Perspiration increased, often to a great extent.

Throat - Pain on swallowing all down esophagus with burning there and in roof of mouth. Spasmodic, tremulous contractions in pharynx near levator palati muscles, while writing at a very low table.

Vertigo - Frontal headache with dizziness. Sensation on rising from bed as if brain was all in occiput, making it feel heavy.

REFERENCES - Boericke. Clarke. Phatak

NUPHAR LUTEUM

(Yellow Pond-lily)

PHARMACY - nuph. Nuphar luteum. Yellow pondlily. Nymphaea lutea. N. O. Nympheacee. Tincture of fresh root. ***Historical dose:*** Tincture and all potencies.

CLINICAL - Cholerine. Colitis. Diarrhea. Dyspepsia. Entero-colitis. Exhaustion. Headaches. Impotence. Psoriasis. Pityriasis, capitis. Rhus poisoning. Seminal emissions. Sexual, weakness. Typhoid fever.

HOMEOPATHIC - Nuph. was proved by Pitet, and many of his symptoms have been clinically confirmed. Yellow diarrhea coming on in the early hours of the morning, with great exhaustion. Typhoid fever.

Produces nervous weakness with marked symptoms in the sexual sphere. Sexual weakness and pollutions. Pityriasis capitis very much aggravated, with much itching and falling out of the hair.

MIND - Impatient of slightest contradiction. Excessive moral sensibility. Sympathetic. Acute pain in witnessing sufferings of animals.

Abdomen - Colitis. Entero-colitis. Colicky pains all around waist, worse 5 a.m. to 7 a.m.

Back - Dull pain in left lower lumbar region. Sensitive in kidney region. When walking, painful stitch to flank, better from pressure.

Chest - Pain behind sternum, when running, as though subjacent organs violently shaken.

Eyes - Sparks filled field of vision, converging from circumference to center, when standing.

Head - Heaviness of head. Bruised shaking in brain. Dull pains in front part of base of brain on level of orbits. Lancination in right and left anterior lobes of brain. Headaches attending depressed states of generative organs.

Limbs - Weakness and loss of power in limbs, worse evening.

Male - Pain in testicles and penis. Spermatorrhea. Weakening nocturnal omissions while convalescing from typhoid. Impotency with involuntary emissions during stool, when urinating. Complete absence of sexual desire, parts relaxed, penis retracted.

Modalities - Diarrhea worse 4 a.m. to 6 a.m., worse after the least excess of any kind. Weakness and itching worse evening. Walking causes painful shocks in hams and pain in flank, better by pressure. Worse the day after sex.

Mouth - Sweetish taste. Tongue white, mouth pasty.

Rectum - Stitches as from needles in rectum, above. Smarting and burning at anus after every stool. Much exhaustion with stools, sense of exhaustion in epigastric region.

Skin - Violent itching. Red blotches, regular in outline, ovoid or circular, prominent and covered with little silvery white scales. As eruption disappeared, scales ceased to be reproduced and the skin at place of each blotch became pale red or yellowish.

Stomach - Painful sensation of weariness in stomach. Exhaustion in epigastrium. Digestion slow, wind colic with liquid, sour-smelling stools.

Stool - Diarrhea during typhoid. Soft stools preceded by some colic for several days, or painless diarrhea. Yellow diarrhea, worse in the morning. Stools liquid, yellow, fetid.

Urine - Urine deposits copious reddish sand, hard, adheres to the vessel.

COMMENTS - A marked feature of the proving was the excessive depression of the male generative system. Nuph. has done good work in analogous conditions and headaches associated therewith.

RELATIONS - ***Compare:*** (1) in sexual weakness, Agn., Kali-br., Lyc., Sel., Yohim., Nym. (2) In diarrhea: Chel., Gamb., Sulph., (3) Early morning diarrhea: Sulph., Nat-s., Rumx., Podo. (4) Sexual debility, Gels., Con., Dig., Nat-m., Chin.

REFERENCES - Boericke. Clarke.

NUX MOSCHATA

(Nutmeg)

PHARMACY - nux-m. Nux moschata. Nutmeg. Myristica fragrans. Myristica officinalis. Myristica moschata. N. O. Myristicacee. Tincture of powdered seeds deprived of the Mace. A fresh nut and fresh plant tincture should be prepared and tested. ***Historical dose:*** All potencies.

CLINICAL - Acne. Asthma. Backache. Belchings. Brain, softening. Catalepsy. Chilblains. Clairaudience. Clairvoyance. Colic. Convulsion. Cough. Debility. ***Drowsiness. Dryness.*** Dysmenorrhea. ***Dyspepsia.*** Eyes, disorders. ***Fainting.*** Fevers. ***Flatus.*** Freckles. Frostbite. Gastralgia. Hemorrhage. Headaches. Head, movements. Hemorrhages. Hiccoughs. Hoarseness. ***Hysteria.*** Intermittent fever. Locomotor ataxia. Lumbago. Mania. Marasmus. Menopausal disorders. Menorrhagia. Metrorrhagia. Miscarriage. ***Narcolepsy.*** Pelvis, congestion. Perspiration, bloody, hysterical. Pregnancy, complaints. Ptosis. Puerperal convulsions. Kidney colic. Rheumatism. ***Sleep, overpowering.*** Speech, defective. Stammering. Strangury. Strokes. Toothache. Turpentine, effects. Typhoid, hemorrhage. Uterus, prolapse. Vertigo. Worms.

HERBAL - Nux-m. is one of the many examples of poisonous and medicinal substances commonly used as food. The use of nutmeg as a condiment doubtless originated because Nux-m. is specifically related to weak digestion.

Ground nutmeg is popularly used in conditions of excessive flatulence and when the smallest excess in eating or drinking sets up indigestion. Used for diarrhea and boils. Nutmeg has a reputation for putting off the menstrual period or else for bringing it on.

Using nutmeg for these purposes has led to many cases of poisoning, supplying a large number of the homeopathic symptoms.

HOMEOPATHIC - There is a characteristic ***"irregularity"*** in the remedy. It produces states of exaltation resembling hysteria, as well as the mesmeric state with exalted senses and consciousness of double personality. Profoundly disturbs the sensorium, mind and nerves.

Characteristic ***drowsiness***, conditions accompanied by drowsiness, especially if there is also chilliness, coldness or ***thirstlessness.*** General inclination to become unconscious during acute attacks.

Marked tendency to ***fainting fits*** with heart failure, worse at stools, at menses, with slight pain, from sight of blood, while standing (when dressing). Epilepsy with consciousness. Paralysis with spasms and trembling of tongue, eyelids, esophagus. Catalepsy. Automatism. Mania. Hysteria. Mental depression from grief.

Feels as if drunk, staggers on trying to walk. Cold limbs. Humming, buzzing, funny feeling in body. Hard parts feel soft. Fleeting pains. Parts lain on feel sore. Heaviness of eyes tongue etc. Sensation as of a hard lump in stomach, liver, throat. Puffiness.

Extreme dryness of the mucus membranes and skin. Female organs are affected. Bearing-down pain, dark blood. Dark hemorrhages. Uterine prolapse and displacements. Useful for threatened miscarriage. Affinity for pregnancy, labor, and the puerperal state.

Disturbed digestion. Indicanuria. Spasms of children with diarrhea. Marasmus of children. Useful to scrawny, delicate, hysterical women who have small breasts and who laugh or cry by turns. Clairvoyant.

MIND - Confused mind and impaired memory. Memory weakness, loss associated with dryness in the brain (Alum., Anac., doesn't have dry skin). Senile dementia (Alum.), Alzheimer's disease. Entire loss of memory of his past life.

Thoughts suddenly vanish while talking, reading or writing. Weak memory with headache. ***Uses wrong words during headaches.*** Slow ideation. Slow learning to talk. Ailments from overtaxing mental powers.

Changeable moods, laughing and crying. Fickle and wavering in his undertakings. Listless, indifferent. ***Dreamy and bewildered, as in a dream.*** Does things automatically, does not recollect what she has done.

Staggering state, helpless as if drunk. Unconsciousness, after mental excitement, worse just before menses. Stupefaction during menses. ***Confusion during pregnancy.*** Ailments from disappointed love. Depression with grief.

Strange feelings with irresistible drowsiness. Fears to go to sleep. ***Starting, as if electric shocks though body during sleep; wakening her. Starting on recovering consciousness.*** Fright causes trembling of heart, fear and sadness. Aware of danger, but no apprehension.

Mental disturbances. Hysteria and mania. Hysterical fainting. Loss of emotional control. Mania with odd speeches and ridiculous gestures. Incoherence. Talks loudly to herself. Answers irrelevantly. Mockery. Everything seems ludicrous. Laughing, in open air, before menses. Loud talking and bewildered manner, with pelvic congestion. Jesting.

Clairvoyant states. ***Sense of duality,*** thinks she has two heads, seems to be two persons (Plat.). Sense of impending dissolution. Surrounding seems changed, does not know the well-known streets. Short time seems very long. Objects seem changed or grow larger. Sense of levitation.

Abdomen - ***Enormously distended***. As of a board across the hypogastrium. Paralytic weakness of the intestines. Abdominal colic from cold drinks. Colic immediately after eating. Flatulent colic. Navel is sore, even ulcerated, festering.

Back - Neck so weak, head drops forward on chest. Pain in back, moves to sacrum or lumbar region. Pain along spine. Lumbago. Backache and neuralgia of sacrum and coccyx worse riding in a carriage. As if a piece of wood stretched across sacrum, worse before menses.

Breasts - Nipples retracted. Breasts too small.

Causations - Ill effects of fright, mental exertion, suppressed eruptions, suppressed menses. Bathing. Over-eating, milk, bad beer, alcohol.

Chest - Oppression of chest, generally coming from epigastrium. Fullness and distressing sensation of a load on chest. Burning in chest, peculiar dead feeling and swelling. Stitches in chest, tightness, spitting of blood.

Constitutions - Suited to children, women and pregnant women. Persons with cool, dry skin, who do not easily perspire. Weakness of old age. Dyspepsia of old people. Constitutions with stiff, straight hair rather than crisp and curly. Delicate constitutions. Hydrogenoid constitution.

Cough - Dry cough, with sudden loss of breath. Cough with great soreness in larynx or chest. Cough excited by scratching in throat, crawling in upper part of trachea. Cough from getting overheated, getting warm in bed. Cough during pregnancy.

Ears - Pain in Eustachian tube as from a foreign body. Tearing or sharp pains in ears. Sharp pain in left ear, worse moving jaw. Oversensitive hearing, distant sounds increased. Buzzing and ringing in ears, as if stopped up.

Eyes - Eyes seems dry, which impedes the movement of the eyelids. Pterygium over cornea. Mydriasis. Blindness, then fainting. Motes before eyes. Objects look larger or too small, very distant, oblique, too close together, vanish, or are red.

Face - Deathly pale, worse in damp air. ***Sleepy, stupid, debauched look.*** Foolish, childish expression, diabolic grin. Distorted face during headache. Blue rings around eyes. Cheeks sometimes red and hot. Eruptions spreading from face to neck. Pustules with broad red borders on chin. Chapped lips. Lips, swollen, stick together, retracted. Jaws as if paralyzed, cannot close them.

Female - Suppressed menses with persistent fainting attacks and sleepiness (Kali-c.). Menses scanty or suppressed from fright, debility, getting cold, overexertion. ***Variableness of menses, irregularity in time and quantity.*** Menses too long, dark, thick. During menses great pressure in back from within outward. Leucorrhea, muddy, bloody. Leucorrhea replaces menses. Continuous and obstinate flooding. Flatus from vagina. Pain of uterus from pessary. Prolapse of uterus and vagina. Uterine hemorrhage. Sterility. Puerperal convulsions. ***Threatened abortion, in hysterical females disposed to fainting.*** Deficient labor pains. Labor pains weak, irregular. Uterus remains uncontracted after delivery.

Food - Hunger or loss of appetite after a few mouthfuls. ***Thirstlessness.*** Loathing when eating or thinking of food. Food tastes like sawdust. Craving for highly seasoned food. Worse cold food, milk, ***alcohol, wine.*** Brandy has a kind of electrifying effect from roof of mouth downward in a straight line to feet.

Head - Head feels full. As if head expanding with ***sleepiness***. Cerebral congestion. Brain feels loose, striking the sides, on motion. Painless pulsating in head, in small spot. Cracking sensation in head. Convulsive movements of the head, could not talk or swallow. Head drops forward while sitting. Raising head from pillow causes deathly sickness. Headaches, bursting in temples. ***Headaches better hard pressure.*** Headaches from eating a little too much. Headache from wine. Headache of alcoholics.

Heart - Trembling, fluttering, as from fright, fear, or sadness. Palpitations, better walking about, drinking warm water. Sensation as if something grasped the heart. As if beating in a vacuum. Pulse intermits at long interval, exciting fear of death. Pulse, weak, irregular. Pulse frequent, trembling, accelerated after wine.

Kidneys - Renal colic. Pain from stone in bladder or gravel. Dysuria from exertion of body. Dysuria with dysmenorrhea or from uterine complaints. Dysuria after eating, from beer or wine. Tenesmus of bladder. Urging at night, with scanty emission. Frequent urination, sometimes involuntary. Burning, cutting in urethra, during urination. Urine smells like violets.

Limbs - Fatigue on slight exertion. Hysterical paralysis. Limbs as if floating in the air. Rheumatism, drawing, wandering pains, worse cold, damp air, wet clothes, better from warmth, dry clothes. Rheumatism from getting feet wet, from exposure to drafts. Pain in right hip to knee, worse motion, especially going up stairs. Feels as if treading on hard peas when walking. Feet cold with appearance of menses. Soles always moist. Dry palms.

Lungs - Paroxysms of suffocation. Dyspnea with feeling of weight in chest. Dyspnea, with upward pressure, during pregnancy. Oppressed breathing. Difficult breathing from fullness in stomach. Loss of breath when standing in water. Hysterical asthma, difficult inhalation. Wheezing, snoring, rattling in chest. ***Hysterical cough,*** worse when getting warm in bed. Cough when getting warm in bed.

Modalities - Better from moist heat, warm room, dry weather. Worse from exertion, motion, shaking head, jarring, lying on painful side, bruises. Worse from mental exertion, ***shock, emotions, excitement. Worse menstruation***, pregnancy. ***Worse from alcohol.*** Worse damp, wind, drafts, fog, cold bath, cold feet. Worse changes of season, summer, hot weather, overheating.

Mouth - Chalky taste in morning, when fasting. Thick saliva like cotton (Berb.). ***Dry mouth without thirst, worse sleep.*** Tongue numb, paralyzed, speech difficult. Tongue adheres to the roof of the mouth. Teeth seem pulled, loose. Teeth painful while eating. Toothache of pregnant women, better warmth.

Nose - Dry nose, stopped up, must breathe through mouth. Catarrh worse cold, damp weather. Nosebleed of dark blood.

Oversensitive sense of smell, followed by loss of smell.

Perspiration - Sweat is red, bloody or absent. ***Lack of perspiration***. Sweats with aversion to be uncovered.

Rectum - Inactive rectum. Constipation in women who are disposed to faint or who bolt their food. Difficult stool during pregnancy. Hard alternating with soft stools. ***Stool is soft and yet is unable to expel it***, even with long straining (Alum.). Summer diarrhea from cold drinks. Epidemic diarrhea in autumn, with want of appetite, but frequent thirst. Diarrhea during dentition, pregnancy, from boiled milk. Stool, soft, putrid, bright yellow and lienteric, worse at night. Slimy stools with slimy taste in mouth. Sharp pain in anus during stool. ***Faintness during or after stool***. Acrid feeling in rectum and anus during and after stool. Passing fetid flatus. Protruding hemorrhoids. Worm affections in children.

Sensations - Forehead as if pushed out, as if brain struck against side of head or loose. Objects appear much too large. As if drunk. Pain as of a rough body in Eustachian tube. Pricking as of electric sparks on cheek. As if wind incarcerated in stomach, as if a piece of bacon were in throat. Limbs as if floating in the air. As if left shoulder contained lead. As if a string were tied around arms. As of a grasping hand in upper arm.

Skin - ***Cold, dry skin.*** Dryness of inner parts. Bluish spots on the skin. Skin sensitive to cold, damp air. Anasarca, dropsy of external parts. Freckles. Acne. Chilblains. Irregular red scaling patches on face and neck during congestions, at time of menses. Ulcerations of skin. Complaints after suppressed eruptions.

Sleep - Narcolepsy. Attacks of sleepiness, with vertigo. ***Great drowsiness*** (Indol.). ***Complaints cause sleepiness***. Great sleepiness with great inclination to laughter. Starting in sleep, but doesn't always awake. Starts with shocks as if electricity were passing through body. Dreams of falling from high place, of being pursued. Coma.

Stomach - ***Excessively bloated.*** Retrocession of gout to stomach. Eating a little too much causes headache. Digestion weak, all food turns to gas. ***Flatulent dyspepsia.*** Hiccoughs and craving for highly-seasoned food. Deathly sickness on raising head from pillow. Nausea when riding in a carriage. Nausea and vomiting, with sleepiness. Nausea and vomiting, from irritation of uterine pessary, during pregnancy.

Temperature - Chill with stupor, pale face. Chill begins in left hand (Carb-v.). Desire to sleep between chills, if left alone. Chill alternating with heat, without thirst.

Throat - ***Great dryness of throat, without thirst.*** Difficult swallowing from paralysis of muscles. Scraping in throat. Contraction on throat like strangulation. Globus hystericus. Hoarse voice when walking against the wind (Hep.).

Vertigo - Vertigo as if drunk, staggering. Vertigo when walking in open air. Vertigo with headache and nausea, with lightness and emptiness of head. Vertigo feels as if floating in air.

COMMENTS - Stonham reported a case in which a dark-haired young man ate two nutmegs one morning. In the afternoon, he was exhilarated, able to do more than usual, to argue on any subject. At dinner, his mouth was dry, he had great thirst, felt he could not drink enough to quench it.

After dinner, his head felt strange, as if in a dream, but he jointed a small musical party as he had intended. He seemed to be two people. His real, conscious self seemed to be watching his other self playing. He could not play well and had to stop. He seemed lost and when spoken to would come to himself with a start. He could hear distant sounds much more acutely than usual.

A woman who ate several nutmegs in an attempt to bring on a miscarriage hallucinated that she had two heads.

A. P. Williamson recorded one case of a woman who took grated nutmeg for diarrhea. After the second dose of half a nutmeg, her head felt queer and dizzy, then her head felt large.

She could not reply to questions, although her eyes were open and she seemed to understand.

Her pupils dilated, eyes starting, face pale, respiration was labored. She was semi-conscious and had to be shouted at, but relapsed into semi-consciousness. Pulse was at first small or rapid, but during the unconscious period it was irregular, fuller and weak.

When consciousness first returned, she kept her hands to her head "to prevent it falling off, was obliged to move her head with her hands, it being too large and heavy for her body." Her chest felt as if in a vice. For some days she was unable to use words properly, frequently obliged to stop in the middle of a sentence and change it entirely from not being able to use the appropriate words.

General exaltation of the senses. One hypersensitive patient given a single dose of Nux-m. 30c, said it seemed to put a coat of cotton wool over her. Clairvoyant state, answers questions accurately quite out of her sphere and on returning to consciousness knows nothing about it.

Pains as if bruised, sprained, wrenched. As if the bones smashed. As if electrified. Pressure, throbbing, drawing, burning. Parts lain on are sore. Puffiness, swellings, dropsy of outer parts. Buzzing sensation with numbness of hands and feet.

Spasms and convulsions. Jactitation of muscles, chorea. Locomotor ataxia excited by cold and wet. Jerks in inner parts, in muscles, recovers with a start. Paralysis with spasms and trembling of tongue, eyelids, and esophagus. Catalepsy.

Characteristic drowsiness (Op.), particularly if accompanied by chilliness and thirstlessness. Irresistible tendency to fall asleep, narcolepsy. For any disease with the concomitant overpowering sleep. Tendency to faint. Persons who easily faint from the sight of blood or from standing. Dark hemorrhages.

Dryness, either actual dryness or the sensation of it. Dry skin, lack of perspiration. Dryness of the mouth and tongue (Nat-m., Alum., Bry.), usually without thirst.

The tongue is so dry it adheres to the roof of the mouth. Eyes dry, too dry to close the lids. Neurotic patients who always awaken with a very dry mouth and tongue. Dryness during pregnancy.

Severe constipation, inactive bowels with dry skin. Constipation with drowsiness (Op.). Faintness during or after stool. Hemorrhage of typhus, fetid flatus. Protruding hemorrhoids. Incontinence of urine.

Diarrhea from milk. Eating a little too much causes a headache. Worse from alcohol. Drinking causes dry cough, colic. Drinking beer causes strangury. Brandy causes an electrifying effect.

Generally worse by cold and damp, better by warmth. Aggravated by wet weather. Cough when warm in bed, or worse in bed.

Clarke cured with Nux-m. 30c a very bad cause of indigestion with acne in a youth who had the symptom "the saliva seems thick like cotton."

P. P. Wells said that "in brain disorders of infants in the stupor with insensibility and unconquerable desire to sleep. Whether in idiopathic disorders of the brain or in those occurring during cholera infantum, Nux-m. is one of the most precious remedies in the Materia Medica."

J. White gave a striking instance of a Nux-m. headache, better by hard pressure, in a man convalescing from a severe gunshot wound to the head. He wanted the nurse to "bear her whole weight on it."

With the headache was rapid, anxious breathing, as if he could not get air enough and the "wind would be shut off." Nux-m. always relieved. The 3x was first given, then a higher potency.

RELATIONS - ***Antidoted by:*** Camph., Laur., Gels., Nux-v., Op., Zinc, Valer. ***It antidotes:*** Ars., Laur., Rhod., lead colic, turpentine, alcohol, bad yeasty beer. ***Compare:*** (1) Ol-myr., oil of Nutmeg - as a remedy for boils, felons, poisonous ulcers, it has been used in the 2x potency. (2) Orni. (3) Myris. - Ulcerative tendency in all tissues. Inflammation, hastens suppuration, powerful anti-septic. Said to act more powerfully than Hep. and Sil. (4) Nux-v.,

Puls., Rhus-t., Ign., Asaf. ***Compatible:*** Lyc., Nux-v., Puls., Rhus-t., Stram., Ant-t.

REFERENCES - Boericke. Clarke. Murphy. Phatak.

NUX VOMICA

(Poison Nut)

PHARMACY - nux-v. Nux vomica. Poison nut. Strychnos nux vomica. N. O. Loganiacae. Tincture and trituration of imported seeds. ***Historical dose:*** All potencies.

CLINICAL - Acne rosacea. Addictions. ***Alcoholism.*** Amaurosis. Amblyopia. Anger, effects. Asthma. Belching. ***Biliousness.*** Bladder, disorders. Bone, nodes. Brain, disorders. Breath, sour. Catarrh. Clavus. Colds. ***Colic.*** Constipation. Convulsions. Coughs. Cramp. Cystitis. Delirium. ***Delirium tremens.*** Diarrhea. ***Drug, abuse. Drug addictions.*** Dysentery. ***Dyspepsia.*** Epilepsy. Eye, affections. Gallstones, pain. Gastrodynia. Gout. ***Hangovers. Headaches.*** Heart, disorders. Heartburn. ***Hemorrhoids.*** Hepatitis. ***Hernias.*** Hydroceles. Hypochondriasis. Impotence. ***Indigestion.*** Intermittent fever. ***Insomnia.*** Intussusception. Jaundice. ***Liver, disorders.*** Locomotor ataxia. Lumbago. Masturbation. Migraines. Morning, sickness. Motion, sickness. Musca volitantes. Myelitis. ***Nausea.*** Night-blindness. Nightmares. Nymphomania. Paralysis. Paraphimosis. ***Photophobia.*** Pregnancy, affections. Pylorus, disease. Kidney, stones. Seasickness. Sexual, mania. Sexual, weakness. ***Sleep, disorders.*** Spermatorrhea. ***Stomach, disorders.*** Strabismus. Strokes. Taste, disordered. Tea, effects. Tenesmus. Tobacco, habit. Tongue, disorders. Trachea disorders. Umbilical, hernia. Urethra, spasm. Urination, frequent. Uterus, prolapse. Vagina, prolapse. Vertigo. ***Vomiting.*** Water brash. Worms. Yawning.

HOMEOPATHIC - Strychnos nux vomica is a moderate-sized tree, native to the Coromandel Coast and Cochin China. The fruit is like an orange in appearance and contains numerous seeds of flattened circular outline, about the size of a half penny, ash-gray in color, covered with fine silky hairs.

The seeds are intensely bitter owing to the presence of strychnia and brucea that exist together with certain peculiar acids, but the pulp is innocuous and is said to be eaten by birds. If nitric acid is added to the seeds a deep orange-yellow color is produced. The wood of the tree is very bitter.

Nux-v. is used in India in cases of intermittent fever and snakebites. The Treasury of Botany noted that a decoction of the leaves is used externally in rheumatism.

The difference in the character of Ign. and Nux-v. proves the wisdom of Hahnemann's simple methods of studying medicines. If there was nothing more than the chemistry of the drugs to go by Ign. and Nux-v might be used indifferently, but with the knowledge of their characteristic features, they are seldom even thought of in connection with the same case.

Nux-v. is useful to those who lead a sedentary life doing much mental work, or to those who remain under stress and strain of prolonged office work, business cares and worries. Generally thin, spare, quick, active, nervous and irritable.

Pre-eminently for men. Firm-tissued brunettes. Debauchees, much drugged patients. Useful for the ill effects of wine, women, rich food, tobacco and sedative drugs. Indulgences result in a thick head, dyspepsia and irritable temper.

Irritable nervous system, hypersensitive and over-impressionable. Digestive disturbances, portal congestion and hypochondriacal states. Dyspepsia. ***Zealous fiery temperament.*** Easily chilled, avoids open air.

Lightning-like pains. Neuralgia, prodromal. Internal scrapy sensation or rawness in throat, larynx. Bruised soreness of abdomen, brain etc. Reflexes increased.

Twisting and jerks. Convulsions. Spasms, tetanic with consciousness, worse by slightest touch, but better by grasping tightly or when elbow was stretched. Tense, contracted feeling. Fainting. Trembling. Paralysis from a stroke in high livers, partial with vertigo and nausea, with sticking pains.

Hemorrhages. Varicose veins without tortuosity, black hard cords from standing or from sedentary habits. Reversed peristalsis. ***Biliousness.*** Fainting after stools. Epilepsy during stool. Vomiting after labor pains.

MIND - Overactive mind. ***Very irritable***, sensitive to all impressions. ***Cannot bear noises, odors, light***, touch, music. Sensitive to singing. Every harmless word offends, every little noise frightens, anxious and beside himself. Cannot stand pain, so mad, he cries.

Loses connection of ideas, thinks she will lose her reason. ***Concentration difficult while calculating.*** Easily makes mistakes. Confusion of mind after vexation. Stupefaction worse in sun. Wants to be quiet, desires repose and tranquility. Despondency alternating with buoyancy. Averse to work. Time passes too slowly.

Headstrong, self-willed. Zealous, fiery temperament. ***Angry and impatient.*** Offended easily. Obstinately resists wishes of others. Can't bear conversation or reading. Quarrelsome if disturbed. Quarrels, reproaches, scolds, insults, from jealousy.

Angry when consoled. Faultfinding. Reproaches others. Can't endure slightest contradiction. ***Impatient when spoken to, gets angry and violent without any provocation.*** Spiteful. Cursing. Ugly, malicious. Violent and abusive. Disposition to slander.

Nervous and excitable. ***Workaholics.*** Anxiety about business affairs. ***Ambitious and competitive.*** Obsessive and compulsive behavior. ***Fastidious.*** Anxiety in morning on waking. Melancholy. Pessimistic. Sullen. Nagging.

Alcoholism. Delirium tremens. Drug addictions. Frightened easily, wakes in fright from least noise. Frightfully apprehensive about getting married. Fears poverty. Hypochondriasis. Even the least ailment affects them. Talks about one's condition. Fear of knives, lest she should kill herself or others. Suicidal, homicidal impulses.

Abdomen - Contraction of abdominal muscles. ***Bruised soreness of abdominal walls*** (Apis., Sulph.). ***Weakness of abdominal ring region***. Bowels gripe here and there. ***Sore bowels, worse coughing and stepping.*** As of a hand about waist, clothes oppress it. Forcing in lower abdomen towards genitals. Intussusception, crampy, remittent pain in bowels. Gastroduodenal catarrh. Sense of goneness in the groins. ***Loud rumbling and gurgling in abdomen, in morning. Incarcerated flatus.*** Flatulent distention with spasmodic colic. Colic with upward pressure, causing short breath and desire for stool. Colic with cold hands and feet. Colic of brandy and coffee drinkers. ***Colic in nursing infants*** from stimulating food eaten by the mother (Cham.). Colic from suppressed hemorrhoidal flow, from uncovering. Strangulated hernia (Op.). Umbilical hernia of infants from constipation or crying.

Back - ***Sudden sharp pains in back when turning, with dull pain while sitting.*** Spinal irritation with sudden loss of power in legs. Lateral spinal sclerosis. Spinal anemia. Myelitis and early stages of locomotor ataxia. Crawling sensation along spine. Burning in spine, worse 3 a.m. to 4 a.m. Acute lumbago. ***Lumbar region feels bruised and lame.*** Lumbar ache, as if breaking, must sit up in order to turn in bed. Sacral region as if lame after childbirth. Bruised pain below scapulae. Sharp pains between scapulae. Cervical-brachial neuralgia, painfully stiff neck, pains down shoulder (right), worse touch. Drawing pain in muscles of neck. Torticollis from cold or nervous shock, fright.

Bladder - Catarrhal cystitis. Cystitis after suppression of menses or hemorrhoidal flow. Pressure on bladder before urinating. Itching burning in region of neck of bladder in morning in bed. ***Irritable bladder from spasmodic sphincter***. Ineffectual urging, spasmodic and strangury. ***Paralysis of bladder***. Spasms of bladder from undue use of stimulants. Spasms of bladder, especially if caused by sexual excesses. Burning and tearing pain in neck of bladder, itching in urethra, during urination. Frequent scanty urination when becoming warm from working, can't empty bladder. Involuntary urination when laughing, coughing, sneezing. Nocturnal and diurnal bedwetting. Vesical calculi.

Breasts - Nipples, sore, white spot in center. Tensive pain when nursing. Nipples painful during suckling with little or no soreness or rawness. Painless gathering of milk in breast from not nursing the child.

Causations - Ill effects of alcohol, drugs, spices, stimulants, sexual excess.

Chest - Spasmodic constriction. Chest as if drawn together, at night in bed. Tightness across chest during coryza or chill. Intercostal neuralgia, worse lying on painful side. Spasms of chest from vapors of copper or arsenic. Itching and scraping under middle of sternum, causes cough. Sensation as if something were torn loose in chest during cough.

Constitutions - Very particular, zealous persons inclined to get angry and excited or of a spiteful, malicious disposition. Ardent persons or disposed to anger, spite or deception, always irritable or impatient. Nervous, melancholic people, with indigestion, venous constitution with tendency to hemorrhoids. Thin, irritable, choleric persons with dark hair, who make great mental exertion or lead a sedentary life. Bilious temperament. Vigorous persons of tense tissue, ardent and irascible temperament disposition. Persons addicted to wine, coffee or pepper and condiments, who lead a sedentary life with much mental exertion. Debauches, thin, irritable, venous.

Cough - Cough of nervous or gastric origin. Cough at night, preventing sleep. Dry cough, after midnight, violent in morning before rising. Dry cough with rattling of mucus. Cough after motion or mental effort. Cough with sensation as if something torn loose in the chest. Tight, dry, hacking cough, at times with bloody expectoration. ***Cough brings on bursting headache*** and bruised pain in epigastric region. Cough with sensation as if something were torn loose in chest. Cough with vomiting or bleeding from nose or mouth. Cough after yawning. Desire to eat during cough.

Ears - Auditory canal dry and sensitive. External meatus dry and sensitive. Itching in ear through the Eustachian tube. Sharp pain, when swallowing. Otalgia, worse in bed. Hyperesthesia of auditory nerves, ***loud sounds are painful and anger him.*** Ringing, roaring and hissing in ears. Strong reverberation of sounds in ear.

Eyes - Bloodshot eyes. Lower eyeballs yellow. Eye affections with liver disease. Burning and smarting pain as from salt, with lachrymation. Sensation of hot water in eye. Burning pain when looking at a light. ***Photophobia, much worse in morning.*** Loss of vision due to alcohol and tobacco. ***Twitching and blinking.*** Orbital twitching radiating towards the occiput. Paresis of ocular muscles. Optic neuritis. ***Optic nerve atrophy from habitual use of tobacco or intoxicants.*** Strabismus. Trachoma and follicular conjunctivitis. Conjunctivitis in spring. Smarting, dry sensation in inner canthi. Lachrymation from affected side. Exudation of blood from eyes.

Face - Red, turgid or yellowish. Face yellow with a red flush. Yellow around mouth and nose. ***Twitching and spasmodic distortion.*** Distortion of face. Trigeminal neuralgia with numbness of face. Submaxillary glands swollen. Erysipelas. Itching pimples on chin. Acne from eating cheese, from excessive use of liquors. Infra-orbital neuralgia with swelling of cheek intermittent, better when lying in bed. Drawing and stiffness in masseter muscles. Drawing tearing, in jaws. Jaws snap shut, stiff. Lower jaw hangs down. Left angle of the mouth drops. Child passes hand constantly over face (brain disease).

Female - Menses interrupted and beginning again. ***Menses irregular***. ***Menses too early***, too long, prolonged. ***Menses with black blood*** with fainting spells. ***Dysmenorrhea*** with pain in sacrum and constant urging to stool. ***Prolapse of uterus*** from straining or lifting. Cramping, in uterine region, causing her to double up and cry, must stay in bed. Contractive uterine spasms with discharge of clots. ***Metrorrhagia with sensation as if bowels wanted to move***. Metrorrhagia at menopause. Metrorrhagia from high living. Irritation and inflammation of ovaries, caused by rich living, highly seasoned food, stimulating drinks. Uterine fibroid. Leucorrhea, fetid, staining yellow. Itching and tingling of vulva, causes masturbation. Sexual desire too strong with burning in vulva. Soreness across pubes. Threatened miscarriage. Profuse bleeding after miscarriage. Inefficient, weak labor pains. Retained placenta. Scanty, offensive lochia.

Food - Hunger, yet aversion to food. Ravenous appetite after drinking beer. ***Craving stimulants***, coffee, tobacco, drugs. ***Craves alcohol, beer, brandy. Craves pungent, bitter things and tonics.*** Craves meat, milk, gravy and spicy food. ***Loves fats*** and tolerates them well (Puls., opposite.). Aversion to bread, coffee, tobacco, meat. Bread has a bitter taste. Worse cold food, cold water. ***Worse from coffee. Worse alcohol, liquor, beer, wine.*** Worse over eating, condiments, stimulants, narcotics, drugs. Worse coffee, tobacco, purgatives. Intoxicated feeling, worse tobacco, alcohol, coffee. Artificial food disagrees and causes vomiting and purging. Coffee, milk, beer, water, don't taste right. Thirst during chill, thirstless during heat.

Head - Migraines. Headache in occiput or over eyes. Frontal headache with desire to press the head against something. Bruised sensation of the brain. Pressing pain on vertex, as if a nail driven in. Pressive and throbbing, at vertex from fixed attention of mind. ***Headache in the sunshine*** (Glon., Nat-c.). ***Toxic headaches from drugs, alcohol.*** Headache after drugging. ***Hangover headaches with irritability.*** Headache from constipation. Congestive headache, associated with hemorrhoids. Head feels distended and sore after a debauch. Supraorbital neuralgia with great restlessness. Scalp sensitive to slight touch.

Heart - Angina pectoris, patient lies on knee with body leaning backwards, worse at night. Angina pectoris with loss of appetite and accumulation of gas in bowels. ***Angina pectoris from using coffee, tobacco or alcohol to excess.*** Heart feels tired. Distension, aching pains and anguish in region of heart and hypochondria. Dilatation of heart with nervous palpitations. Palpitations after stimulants, after eating, after wine, from mental emotions. Palpitations on lying down. Pulse rapid and irregular, at times intermitting.

Kidneys - Pressure, burning and heat in region of kidneys, in nephritis. Nephritis from abuse of liquors. Severe sharp pains in region of left kidney, worse rising from seat and motion. Kidney colic (right), extending to genitals and legs with dribbling urine. Spasmodic strangury, after beer. ***Painful ineffectual urging to urinate.*** Frequent calls, urinates little and often. Tenacious mucus passes with the urine, without pain. Urine pale, later thick, whitish, purulent, reddish, with brick-dust sediment. Hematuria from suppressed hemorrhoidal flow or menses (Ip., Ter.). Urine dribbles in old men with enlarged prostate or gonorrhea.

Limbs - Chorea. ***Convulsions from abuse of alcohol.*** Progressive locomotor ataxia from alcoholism. ***Cramps and spasms of limbs.*** Cramps in calves and soles. Paresis of arms with shocks. Automatic motions of hand towards mouth. Partial paralysis from overexertion of getting soaked (Rhus-t.). Crawling and formication in paralyzed parts. Legs numb, feel paralyzed. ***Sudden loss of power of arms and legs in the morning.*** Aching, drawing or bruised pains in limbs, worse motion and at night. Limbs heavy as lead. Rheumatism attacking mostly muscles of trunk and large joints. Legs stiff. Knee joints as if dry, cracking during motion. Drags his feet while walking, legs tremble, unsteady gait. Shooting from toes to thighs, worse after stool. Heat of hands, feet, yet they must be covered. Arms go to sleep, numb, stiff feeling. Varicose veins attributable to high living.

Liver - Great soreness and tenderness in region of liver, with pain in right shoulder. Liver sore, enlarged, sticking pain. Sharp pain in region of liver, worse from contact or motion. Pressure and stinging pains. ***Weak liver from bad diet, meat, fats, spices, alcohol, etc.*** Gallstone colic. Throbbing pain as from hepatic abscess. ***Hepatitis from bad food or water.*** Jaundice from anger. Jaundice from habitual use of alcohol. Cirrhosis from alcohol abuse. Enlarged liver of alcoholics. ***Toxic liver from drugs, chemicals and alcohol.***

Lungs - ***Shallow and oppressed breathing.*** Awakened every night by ***intolerable sense of suffocation***. Dyspnea in morning and evening. Loud, snoring, during sleep. Difficult breathing, from accumulation of gas. Dyspnea during pregnancy. Asthma from disordered stomach. ***Asthma with fullness in stomach,*** worse in mornings or after eating. Asthma with feeling as if clothing were too tight, better belching. Asthma from spasmodic constriction. Yellow, grey, cold mucus. Sour or sweetish expectoration. Bright red blood. Hemoptysis from anger, suppressed hemorrhoidal flow. Pneumonia with catarrhal irritation. Pneumonia, after suppression of hemorrhoidal flow, when hepatization occurs, from becoming chilled. Pneumonia of the elderly, also of children. Pneumonia in sick people compelled to lie upon back.

Male - Drawing pain in testicles and spermatic cords. Testes hard and retracted. Constricting pain in testes. Orchitis (Ham., Puls.). Sharp pain in testes. Heat in testicles. Hydrocele. Chronic prostatitis. Increase of smegma. Gonorrhea, thin discharge, with burning on urinating and frequent urging to stool. Spermatorrhea with dreams, backache, burning in spine, weakness and irritability. High sex drive. Cannot be in female society without having emission. ***Premature ejaculation.*** Bad effects of onanism, sexual excess. Emissions from high living. ***Impotency.*** Penis becomes relaxed during sex.

Modalities - Better from a nap, if allowed to finish it in evening. Better moist air, damp, wet weather (Caust.). ***Better from free discharges***. Better strong pressure, wrapping head, lying on sides, resting, frequent stretching. Better hot drinks, milk, fats. ***Worse from overeating, coffee, condiments, liquor, stimulants.*** Worse from high living, debauched, sedentary habits. ***Worse narcotics, drugs tobacco, purgatives.*** Worse anger, mental exertion, vexation, mental shock, wounded honor, disappointment of ambitions. ***Worse cold, open air***, dry air, drafts, wind. ***Worse disturbed sleep, early morning.*** Worse noise, music, odors, after eating, yawning. ***Worse pressure of clothes*** at waist, touch, ***uncovering.***

Mouth - Dry mouth. Foul, sour breath. Offensive breath in morning. ***Sour, bitter, bad taste in morning.*** Internal mouth, tongue and palate slimy, and feel raw and sore. Small aphthous ulcers in mouth and throat. ***Bloody saliva*** runs out at night. Itching of palate, Eustachian tube. Gums, swollen, white and bleeding. Teeth chatter. Toothache, worse cold, better warm drinks. Jaws contracted. Articulation and speech difficult.

Nose - ***Stuffy colds, snuffles*** after exposure to dry, cold atmosphere, worse in warm room. Snuffles in a newborn. ***Stuffed up at night and outdoors*** or alternates between nostrils. Sudden fluent coryza after rising. Coryza, fluent in daytime, worse warm room, better open air. Coryza with lachrymation. Acrid discharge, but ***with stuffed-up feeling***. Violent sneezing, abortive, from intense crawling in nostrils (left). Bloody mucus in nose. Nosebleeds in morning (Bry.). Nosebleeds during sleep, from suppressed flow of hemorrhoids, from coughing. Oversensitive to strong odors, even fainting. Smell before nose like old cheese, burning sulphur. Nose looks sharp and pointed. Picking at nose, worms.

Perspiration - Sour perspiration, on one side of body. Rather light sweat. Cold, clammy sweat on face. Odor of sweat, musty straw. Sweats during sleep, disappears on waking. Sweats after midnight and in morning.

Rectum - Constriction of rectum. ***Constant uneasiness in rectum***. Irregular, peristaltic action. ***Constipation with frequent ineffectual urging or passing but small quantities at each attempt.*** Urging to stool felt throughout abdomen. Constipation, the harder he strains the harder it is to pass stool. ***Feeling as if part of***

stool remained. Sharp pain in rectum after stool. Frequent small evacuations. ***Dysentery, stools relieve pains for a time.*** Alternate constipation and diarrhea after abuse of purgatives. Diarrhea after a debauch, worse morning. Diarrhea after night watching, after overexertion of mind, after anger, after ginger or brandy. Diarrhea with jaundice (Dig.). ***Itching, blind hemorrhoids*** with ineffectual urging to stool. Burning pain in hemorrhoids, intolerable to least touch. Hemorrhoids very painful after drastic drugs. Hemorrhoids during pregnancy or after childbirth. Dragging pain at anus when not at stool. Prolapsed rectum.

Sensations - As if something heavy fell into head. As if his head were immensely larger than his body. As if pressing a nail into brain into vertex, as if skull pressed asunder. Chest as if drawn together, as if something torn loose in chest. As if blood would be jerked out of veins. Navel as if drawn in. As if hernia would occur, as if everything in region of umbilicus were being shattered and torn. As of a band above knees, around body.

Skin - Pale or yellowish color of skin. Jaundice. Blue mottled skin. Skin red and blotchy. Skin as if numb. Ecchymosis, blue spots. Goose bumps. Eruptions with burning, pricking, itching. Burning, pricking like fleabites. Miliary and pimpled eruptions. White miliary eruption. Acne. Furunculi. Urticaria with gastric derangement. Ulcers with elevated margins of a pale red color. Chilblains, burning itching. Tendency to boils. Abscesses.

Sleep - ***Better after a nap***, unless aroused. Yawning. Drowsy after meals and in early evening. ***Sleeplessness from abuse of coffee, wine, liquor, opium or tobacco.*** Sleepless from rush of ideas. ***Sleeplessness from mental strain.*** Awakens in fright from least noise, as if someone were in room. Awakens at 3 a.m., lies awake for hours, with a rush of thoughts. ***Cannot sleep after 3 a.m. until towards morning.*** Weeping and talking during sleep. Amorous dreams. Dreams about exerting the mind. Anxious dreams. Dreams full of bustle and hurry, anxious. Dreams of being pursued by animals, dogs and cats. Dreams of quarrelling, of mutilations, of fatal accidents. Nightmare after a heavy supper or alcoholic beverages. Wakes feeling wretchedly.

Stomach - ***Weight and pain in stomach,*** worse eating. Severe pain in stomach from injury, worse least food. Ravenous hunger, especially about a day before an attack of dyspepsia. ***Region of stomach very sensitive to pressure*** (Bry., Ars.). ***Indigestion from alcohol.*** Disordered stomach from debauchery, from high living, from drugs, from sedentary habits. Indigestion, after business anxiety, from sedentary habits, night watching. Dyspepsia from drinking strong coffee. Cramps in stomach in morning and after eating. ***Sour taste and nausea in the morning***. Food lies like a heavy knot in stomach. Epigastrium bloated with pressure as of a stone several hours after eating. ***Hiccough from overeating***, from cold or hot drinks. Flatulence and heartburn. Sour, bitter belchings. Difficult belching of gas. ***Nausea and vomiting every morning***, with depression of spirits. ***Nausea and vomiting with much retching.*** Nausea, better if he can vomit. Wants to vomit, but cannot. Vomiting of sour mucus, oily, greasy or black substances. Vomiting of greenish matter, undigested food, blood. Vomiting of bile with thirst, after anger. ***Motion sickness from riding in cars or seasickness.***

Stool - ***Stool is incomplete and unsatisfactory.*** First part of stool soft, last part hard. ***Scanty stool with much urging.*** Black, dark or brown stool. Hard and knotty stool, consisting of little balls. Stool often mixed with mucus and blood. Black, hard stool, often streaked with blood.

Teeth - Teeth seem too long. Sensation as if tooth were wrenched out. Tearing pain in teeth and jaws, worse cold drinks, better warmth. Stinging pain in decayed teeth. Pain in hollow tooth. Sharp pain in teeth on drawing in air or just after eating. Toothache, worse mental exertion, when reading or thinking. Toothache worse from exercise, better external warmth. Toothache with swollen face. Chattering of teeth. Gums swollen, white, and bleeding. Gumboils, which seem about to burst.

Temperature - Chilliness alternating with heat. Cold stage predominates. Chills with backache on slightest motion. Chills on being uncovered, ***must be covered*** in every stage of fever. Chill with thirst, and heat without thirst. Fever with internal chilliness. Fever with anxiety and restlessness. ***Body burning hot,*** especially the face, ***yet cannot move or uncover without feeling chilly.*** Warm on upper most side, on lying down. Dry heat of the body. Paroxysms in morning. Excessive rigor with ***blueness of fingernails***. Aching in limbs and back, and gastric symptoms.

Throat - Sensation of ***roughness,*** tightness and tension. ***Stitches into ear.*** Pharynx constricted. Acute catarrhal laryngitis. Spasmodic constriction of larynx with suffocating spells. ***Tickling*** in throat after waking in morning. Sore rawness in throat. Catarrhal hoarseness with scraping in throat. Tenacious mucus in upper part of trachea. Putrid taste in throat on coughing. Dark gray patches on right tonsil. Small ulcers in the throat, pain worse during empty swallowing. Diphtheria. Elongation and swelling of uvula.

Tongue - First half of tongue clean, posterior covered with deep fur, white, yellow, cracked edges. Tongue black and dark red, cracked on edges. Tongue red, sore and yellow at base. Needle-like stitches at edges of tongue. Painful vesicles on tongue. Tongue seems heavy when talking.

Vertigo - Vertigo in morning, on empty stomach, after dinner. ***Intoxicated feeling, worse morning, mental exertion, tobacco, alcohol, coffee, open air.*** Vertigo, brain and other objects turn in circle. Vertigo with black spell. ***Vertigo with momentary loss of consciousness.*** Dizzy and faint in a crowd or where many lights are burning. Vertigo from night watching and mental overexertion. Vertigo from opium, smell of flowers, gas, etheric oils, etc.

Vision - Weakened power of accommodation from overexerting eyes. Diplopia from muscular asthenopia. Diplopia from paralytic strabismus. ***Blurred vision from overeating.*** Dim vision, can see better on cloudy day. Obscuration of vision in morning. ***Printed matter is seen with difficulty.*** Sees flashes from external canthi towards pupils, like a circle of fire, before headache. Sees streaks like lightning. Glittering appearance just outside of distinct field of vision. Floating black and grey points.

COMMENTS - Clarke stated, under Brucea antidysenterica, how the bark of the tree was imported into Europe in mistake for Angustura. The tree from which the ignatia "beans" are obtained is unknown, but it is not doubted to be a strychnos, the seeds actually contain a larger proportion of strychnia than those of Nux-v.

In poisoning cases, the most marked feature is the spasms and convulsions which cause death by arresting the respiratory movements. The general effect of the spasms was to cause opisthotonos and throwing the head back. In some, the body was spasmodically drawn sideways.

Tetanus, differing from traumatic or idiopathic tetanus in that the spasms of the former are less continuous, do not invariably begin with the muscles of the jaws, but preferably in the lower limbs and are not accompanied by rise of temperature.

Characteristic spasms. Spasms affect all the muscles, including the esophagus, stomach, intestines, uterus, bladder, rectum. Intestinal spasms after eating unripe fruit. Tetanic seizures with a drawn facial expression.

Respiratory spasms. Asthmatic states. Asthma, coryza from drafts or air conditioning. A dry, persistent fatiguing cough that causes headache as if the skull would split. Cough, worse at night, after midnight. Clarke cured with Nux-v. many cases of bronchitis with copious moist rales and expectoration. Acute flus. Flu with muscle aches, toxic feeling. Gastric flus with cramps, spasms, irritability and nausea.

High blood pressures, heart attacks, often from severe exhaustion. Hepatitis, cirrhosis of the liver with irritability.

Kidney conditions, liver weakness. Crave fats (Nit-ac.), sweets, salt, spicy foods, coffee, tobacco, stimulants. Desires alcoholic drinks, but they aggravate.

Pressure two or three hours after eating (Nux-m. and Kali-bi., have it immediately after). Severe cramps and spasms in the stomach and colon. Severe peristalsis. Colitis, ulcers, gas and bloating with irritability, depression, and frustration. Colic with alternating diarrhea with mucus in the stool and constipation with severe cramps and spasms.

Irritability of the bladder and rectum. Constant urging and desire, very little passed. Tenesmus. Incontinence of urine or feces. Constipation with ineffectual urge. Alternate constipation and diarrhea. Sudden diarrhea, drives the patient out of bed. Involuntary diarrhea, can come on after a meal. Straining ceases as soon as the stool passes. Improvement for a short time after a stool.

Portal stasis. Prolapse of rectum with constipation. Lack of bowel tone. Itching and burning hemorrhoids (Sulph.), worse from alcohol. Hernias in infants, or from lifting things. Incipient hernia. Inguinal and umbilical hernias. Clarke saw a case of strangulated hernia resolved by Nux-v. while preparations for an operation were in progress.

Tendency to faint after diarrhea stools or after vomiting. Fainting from odors in a warm room after eating, after every labor pain. Epilepsy attacks during stool. Headaches with nondescript achiness, irritability, often associated with dietary errors.

Hemorrhage. Metrorrhagia, menorrhagia. Uterine bearing down and prolapse, cramps at menstrual periods and pressure on bladder and rectum. Menses too early and profuse, dark flow, faints easily, irregular, cease flowing at nighttime. Cramping pains, cause nausea and fainting, twisting, moving about in abdomen, soreness across pubes, cramps in bladder.

Nash gave a characteristic of the menses of Nux-v., "Menses a few days before the time and rather too copious or keeping on several days longer with complaints at the onset which remain until it is over." Menses return at full moon.

Pregnancy with irritability, hiccough, morning sickness, varicose veins, hemorrhoids. False labor pains. Irritability with labor pains (Cham.), with nausea or indigestion or vomiting (Sep.). Labor pains are violent and causes fainting. Lochia scanty offensive. Nipples sore, with a white spot in center. Tensive pains when nursing.

Strong sexual desire in both sexes, even the slightest provocation excites sexual passion. May be impotent from overuse of drugs or excessive sexual activity.

Keynote over sensitiveness. Morbid sensitiveness. Severe irritability. Languor, great nervous debility (as from sexual or other excesses). Over stimulation, particularly in sedentary people. Trembling, excitement with trembling. Locomotor ataxia. Hemiplegia. Paralysis, after a stroke, parts cold, numb, emaciated.

Sleeplessness, from excitement, anger or resentment. Wakes at 3 a.m. and lies awake for hours. Falls asleep when it is time to rise and feels heavy and unrefreshed. Sleep is unattainable except from a stimulant. Symptoms are better after undisturbed sleep, worse when sleep is disturbed.

Chilliness. Cannot get warm in bed at night. Coldness of the whole body with blue hands and skin. Cold, moist hands with cold tip of nose. Repugnance to cold or cold air. Chilly on least movement, from being uncovered, must be covered in every stage of fever, chill, heat or sweat.

H. C. Allen noted that in the fever there is great heat, whole body burning hot, face red and hot, yet patient cannot move or uncover without being chilly.

Boenninghausen's keynote is "Feels worse in morning, soon after walking, also after mental exertion after eating and in cold air." Worse cold, dry weather. Worse from music.

General toxicity, usually from addictions to drugs, stimulants, and strong foods. Bilious affects, ailments due to high living. Alcoholism. Rage when drunk. Drug withdrawal (with Aven.). Hangovers (Ran-b., Coff.). Toxic drugged feeling, particularly in the morning.

Ambitious personality, impatient, irritable. Craves stimulants. Very competitive from a young age, aggressive. Hyper or over active children, but purposeful (unlike Med.). Robust, energetic, passion behind a quick intellect. Often from an early sibling comparison (Lyc.).

Career and work oriented, can be workaholics. Not sentimental. Stress and tension lead to over sensitivity, weakness. Anxious, overreact, never satisfied. Fear of failure, of not being successful. Worry. Suicidal depression. Homicidal, suicidal impulse, insanity.

RELATIONS - ***Antidoted by:*** Wine, coffee, Acon., Bell., Camph., Cham., Cocc., Op., Pal., Plat., Stram., Thuj. (ineffectual desire to pass water). ***It antidotes:*** Narcotic, drastic and vegetable remedies. Bad effects of anomalies on foods, e.g., ginger, nutmeg, pepper and so-called *"hot"* medicines, alcohol, Merc. (tremors), Mez. (neuralgia), ether, Thuj. (urination). ***Compare:*** (1) In tetanus, Picro., Verin., Thebin., Cic., Hy-ac., Bell., Acon., Phys., Phyt., Cur., Camph. (2) Cerebrospinal affections, Pic-ac. (3) Fainting in nervous women, Ign., Nux-m., Mosch. (4) Gastric troubles, Bism., Ars., Kreos., Lyc., Puls., Carb-v. (Carb., v. often follows Nux-v. in ill effects of debauchery). (5) Asthma, Zing., Carb-v., Lyc., Nat-s. (6) Paralysis of sphincters, Sep., Bell., Sulph. (6) Bad temper before and during menses, Cham., Mag-m., Sep. (Lyc., before menses). (7) Wakes 3 a.m. and cannot get to sleep, Kali-c., Ars., Calc., Sep. (8) Night watching effects, sensitiveness, effects of noise, traveling by land or sea, umbilical hernia, Cocc. (9) Fear of losing senses, Calc., Lyc., Sulph. (10) Desire to kill love ones, Hep., Ars. (11) Fainting or faints after every evacuation, Dig., Nux-m. (12) Hemorrhoids, Aesc., Ham. (13) Leucorrhea staining yellow, Agn., Carb-an., Chel. (14) Impotence from abuse, Agn., Calc., Sulph. (15) Stricture of rectum, Nat-m., Op. ***Compatible after:*** Carb-v., Ars., Ip., Mag-m., Phos., Sep., Sulph. ***Compatible before:*** Bry., Puls., Sulph. ***Incompatible:*** Zinc.

REFERENCES - Boericke. Clarke. Murphy. Phatak.

NYCTANTHES ARBOR TRISTIS

(Sad Tree)

PHARMACY - nyct. Nyctanthes arbor tristis. Sad tree. Arbor tristis. Paghala tree. Sephalika. Harsinghar. Night-Jasmine of India. N. O. Jasminacee. Verbenaceae. Forests of Central India. Tincture of fresh leaves, collected March to April. ***Historical dose:*** Tincture and all potencies.

CLINICAL - Chills. Constipation. Fevers, bilious. Fevers, remittent. Rheumatism. Sciatica. Vomiting.

HERBAL - Nyctanthes is a small tree of the Jasmine family, having brilliant, highly fragrant flowers, white and yellow, which do not expand until evening and which fall off about sunrise. During the day the tree lose all its brightness and hence is called "The Sad Tree." "Nyctanthes" means "Night-flowering."

S. C. Ghose gave an account of the medicinal properties of this plant. He used it extensively in cases of bilious and remittent fevers, rheumatism and sciatica and the constipation of children.

Nyctanthes is "a bitter tonic and expectorant and a mild purgative." In the fever there is thirst before and during chills, and bitter vomiting at close of chill. Not much sweat.

HOMEOPATHIC - Ghose, who made a short proving of it, compared Nyct. with Eup-per. Bilious and obstinate remittent fevers, sciatica, rheumatism. Constipation of children.

MIND - Anxious and restless. Depression.

Food - Insatiable thirst, before and during chill and fever.

Head - Dull headache.

Kidneys - High-colored urine.

Liver - Tenderness of liver. Stitches in liver region, which is very sensitive to touch.

Mouth - Tongue coated.

Rectum - Constipation. Profuse, bilious stool with nausea.

Stomach - Burning sensation, better cold application. Constant nausea may or may not be present. Bilious vomiting occurs every time he takes a drink.

Temperature - Thirst, before and during chill and heat. Bitter vomiting at close of chill. Sweat not generally marked.

COMMENTS - Dr. Sarat Chandra Ghose of Calcutta, India recorded his observations of clinical experiences and provings made about the years 1898-1903.

The first case noted a woman at the house of Babu I. C. Chakrabarti, B. A., Head Master. Town School, Midnapore, was suffering from a complicated attack of intermittent fever. No medicine could give her any relief.

In another case, a boy, aged 7, was suffering from intermittent fever for some time. The fever came on every evening at 7 p.m. Violent thirst during chill and fever. Bilious vomiting. Constipated bowels. Ghose prescribed Nyct. tincture in five drop doses thrice daily. The boy was cured within three days.

The third case, a woman, aged 68, was suffering from remittent fever for ten days. Ghose took her under treatment on the eleventh day.

The son of Babu Sarada Kanta Chatterjee was suffering from a malignant type of ague with great constipation. He was treated by some allopaths and native Kabirajes for nearly five months, but no perceptible improvement was wrought by the administration of their remedies. He was eventually placed under Ghose's treatment.

The son of Mr. M. M. Ray, Deputy Magistrate and Collector of Midnapore, was suffering from remittent fever, associated with bilious symptoms for five days. On the sixth day the boy was placed under Ghose's treatment.

The son of Mr. G. C. Dutt, Deputy Magistrate of Midnapore, was suffering from an attack of intermittent fever for some time. The fever came on every morning at about 7 a.m. Violent thirst was present during all the stages. Bilious vomiting came on in the hot stage. Constipated bowels. Ghose prescribed Nyct. tincture in three-drops doses. The boy was all right within three days.

Nyct. proved an excellent remedy for the symptoms and Ghose treated nearly 120 cases with this medicine alone and an overwhelming majority of them were cured.

REFERENCES - Anshutz. Boericke. Clarke.

NYMPHAEA ODORATA

(Sweet Water Lily)

PHARMACY - nym. Nymphaea odorata. Sweet water lily. N. O. Nympheacee. Tincture of the root. ***Historical dose:*** Tincture and all potencies.

CLINICAL - Back, pain. Bronchorrhea. Coryza. Diarrhea. Leucorrhea. Throat, sore. Ulcers.

HERBAL - Hale mentioned this emblem of purity and its traditional reputation as a dissipater of venereal desires. Like Nuph., it has early morning looseness of bowels.

HOMEOPATHIC - Nymph. has early morning diarrhea, and backache. Acrid leucorrhea. Offensive ulcers. Bronchorrhea. Ulcerative sore throat.

REFERENCES - Boericke. Clarke.

NYSTATIN

(Antibiotic Drug)

PHARMACY - nyst. Nystatin. Antibiotic drug. ***Historical dose:*** All potencies.

CLINICAL - Acne. Blisters. Dermatitis. Hair, disorders. ***Skin, disorders.*** Stretch marks.

HOMEOPATHIC - Blistering, burning, dryness of skin. Eruptions resembling acne. Excessive discoloring of the skin. Skin irritation, itching, peeling, prickly heat. Reddish purple lines on skin. Secondary infections.

Severe inflammation of the skin. Softening of the skin. Stretch marks, stretching or thinning of the skin. Excessive hair growth, especially on the face. Hair loss, especially on the scalp. Inflammation around the mouth. Inflammation of hair follicles.

REFERENCES - Murphy.

O

OAK

(Bach Flower Essence)

PHARMACY - oak-b. Oak. Quercus robur. Red female flowers are gathered and put in a bowl of sunlit water for several hours. The water is strained and prepared as medicine. ***Historical dose:*** Take two drops from the stock bottle into a one ounce dropper bottle (add brandy or alcohol, if this bottle will be used for days or weeks). This is the dosage bottle, take a few drops straight into the mouth or as needed in a little water or juice.

HOMEOPATHIC - The remedy Oak-b. belongs to Bach's group of ***Despondency and Despair***, along with Crb-a-b., Will-b, Star-b-b., Sw-ch-b., Elm-b., Pine-b. and Lar-b. States of stoic perseverance and willpower in the face of hardship.

Mental/emotional and physical weariness. Over-work and strength of will may lead to physical strain and undue stress. Older people may become bent from over-exertion and one-sided activity.

Great determination to not succumb to invalidity. Avoids necessary rest and restful recreation, even though both may be of vital need. Psychosomatic diseases from the continued rule of willpower over the need for healthful diversion and renewal (Cent-b.).

MIND - Self-discipline, seriousness of intention. Tendency to over-work. Loyalty. Focused on completing tasks. Perseverance in duties, even though strength and vitality may be failing. Unceasing disappointments or lack of rewards despite efforts made will increase resolve to struggle on with great strength of will and ever renewed hope. Inner weariness and lack of motivation.

REFERENCES - Bach.

OCIMUM CANUM

(Brazilian Alfavaca)

PHARMACY - oci. Ocimum canum. Brazilian alfavaca. Hoary basil. Ocimum incanescens. Ocimum fluminense. N. O. Labiate. Portuguese. Tincture of fresh leaves. ***Historical dose:*** Tincture and all potencies.

CLINICAL - Albuminuria. Allergies. Arthritis. Belching. Breasts, painful. Bubo. Diarrhea. Edema. Gravel, urinary. Headaches. Herpes. Hiccoughs. ***Kidney, diseases. Kidney, pain. Kidney, stones.*** Nausea. Pyelonephritis. Salpingitis. Urine, abnormal. Vagina, prolapse. Vulvitis.

HERBAL - All the members of the Ocimum genus are aromatic. The Sweet or Common Basil, Ocimum basilicum, is one of the best known. Mure reported that it is used in Brazil as a specific for diseases of the kidneys, bladder and urethra.

P. C. Majumdar added that Ocimum sanctum is the sacred tulsi of India and that the Kabirajes use it in diseases of the liver and bilious remittent fevers.

HOMEOPATHIC - Oci. is useful in diseases of kidneys, uterus, bladder and urethra. ***Kidney pain with violent vomiting*** every fifteen minutes. Wrings one's hands and moans and cries all the time. Kidney colic, especially on the right side. Pronounced symptoms of ***kidney stones***.

Uric acid diathesis. Red sand in the urine. Red urine with brick-dust sediment after the attack. The urine may be saffron color or thick, purulent with an intolerable smell of musk.

Febrile condition, shivering, sweating and with congestive headache. Vomiting, cries tossing about and wringing hands. Arthritis. Allergies.

Pain in the left testicle. Prolapsed vagina. Vulvar congestion. Breast congestion. Swelling of inguinal glands and breasts. Excessive sensitiveness of the breasts and pain on nursing.

MIND - Difficulty concentrating. Confused state. Anxiety.

Abdomen - Abdomen distended, painful on the right side during menses. Glands in the groin swollen. Edema on the right side of the testes or labia.

Breasts - Constrictive tension in the breasts. Breasts feel full and tense, itching. Neuralgic pains in the breast. Nipples painful and sensitive to the touch. Congestive pains in the breasts as after nursing. Puerperal mastitis.

Chest - Chest painful on right side. Dry cough in the evening and early morning. Copious sputum.

Constitutions - Allergic constitutions. Psoric constitutions. Neuro-arthritic temperament.

Ears - Boil on the meatus of the right ear. Noise heard painfully in the ears.

Eyes - Blurred vision.

Female - Menses late, short or abundant. Whitish-yellow leucorrhea. Vulvitis. Vulva swollen, darting pain in labia majora. Vaginal prolapse. Salpingitis.

Food - Lack of appetite. Desire for cold drinks during fever.

Head - Stinging pain in the head. Pain in the head, as if a nail were being driven in, ameliorated by pressure. Pulsating, throbbing headache. Headaches followed by shivering.

Kidneys - Pyelonephritis. Cramps in kidneys. ***Kidney colic on the right side*** with vomiting ever quarter of an hour with calling out. Restlessness and groaning. Pronounced symptoms of ***kidney stones,*** especially of right side. Stones in the bladder. Tenesmus of the bladder. ***Sore pain in ureters***. Burning pain in the urethra during urination. Urine abundant, burning.

Male - Pain in the testes. Tenderness, heat and swelling of the left testicle. Increase, then diminution of sexual desire. Absence of erection.

Modalities - Better in a room, in rainy, humid weather. Worse in the morning, from cold, right side.

Mouth - Lips dry, face red. Tongue furred, yellow, yellowish-white with a brown spot in the center. Toothache on the right, ameliorated by pressing the teeth together.

Nose - Nasal congestion.

Rectum - Constipation with dry, hard, evil-smelling, yellow or greenish stools. Diarrhea several times a day.

Skin - Herpes. Eczematous eruptions.

Stomach - Belching, hiccoughs. Nausea.

Temperature - Shivers, fever and lack of thirst. Profuse sweating with strong odor. Fever of the tertian or quartan type.

Urine - High acidity, formation of spike crystals of uric acid. ***Brick-dust red or yellow sediment.*** Red sand in saffron colored urine. Urine ***foul-smelling with odor of musk.*** Turbid, thick, purulent, bloody urine. Urinary complaints with proteinuria. Scanty urine, which aggravates.

Vertigo - Vertigo on rising and on sitting down.

COMMENTS - Majumdar related the case of a medical man, 45. Majumdar was sent for at 4 a.m. one morning and found the patient in great agony, pain in upper part of region of right kidney, extending downwards and forwards to pubes.

Constant vomiting, bilious, acid tossing about without any relief. After Calc., Lyc., Sep., Sars. and Berb. had been given in vain, Oci. 3x gave immediate relief and no other remedy was required.

Majumdar also noted the case of a man, 50, with excruciating pain in his left kidney, for which he had received opium under allopathic treatment without relief. Majumdar saw the patient on the sixth day of the attack. The suffering was extreme, vomiting of bile, constant nausea, bowels constipated.

Oci. 3x, one drop every three hours, speedily gave relief, and two days later two small uric acid stones were passed. There was no recurrence.

Clarke published two cases. The first concerned a man, 27, who was seized with violent pains of a leaden character in the right side of the abdomen, every three or four weeks. The pains commenced in morning, lasted twelve to fifteen hours. For four hours from commencement of attack the pain steadily increased, culminating in vomiting, first of sour fluid, then slime, then a fluid like coffee.

After the vomiting there was some relief of pain. Urine contained no sediment. The attacks had lasted seven years. At first they began in the evening. There was a history of epilepsy in the family, and as a child the patient had three fits.

Oci. 200c, one dose, was given and there were no more attacks for about two years. On their recurrence Oci. failed to control them, but Dios. tincture succeeded.

In the second case, a woman, 24, had severe pain in her right flank shooting around to her back. Frequent urination, sometimes depositing clots. Terebe. 3c gave some relief, but it was not permanent. Oci. 200c, a few globules in water, a teaspoonful every two days, rapidly relieved the symptoms and cleared up the case.

RELATIONS - ***Compare:*** (1) In kidney colic, Berb., Dios., Coloc., Calc., Lyc. (2) Berb., Hedeo., Lyc., Urt-u. (3) Pareir., Coloc., Tab. (4) In painful breasts, Lac-c., Bor. (5) Crot-h., Phel. (6) Prolapsed vagina, Staph. ***Followed well by:*** Dios.

REFERENCES - Boericke. Clarke. Julian. Phatak.

OCIMUM SANCTUM

(Holy Basil)

PHARMACY - oci-s. Ocimum sanctum. Holy Basil. Tulsi. N. O. Labiate. Brazil. ***Historical dose:*** Tincture and all potencies.

CLINICAL - Aphthae. Asthma. Bites. Bronchitis. Broncho-pneumonia. Catarrh. Colds. Constipation. Cough. Delirium. Diarrhea. Headache. Hiccoughs. Influenza. Intermittent fevers. Leucorrhea. Memory, weak. Ophthalmia. Ozaena. Pneumonia. Ringworm. Ulcers. ***Urethritis.***

HERBAL - Ayurvedic physicians like Charaka, Harita, Chakradatta, Bangasena, and others have found Ocimum sanctum very efficacious in cough, cold, catarrh, nose affections, ozaena, scorpion bites, remittent and intermittent fevers and constipation.

The medicated oil is used as drops, in the ears in earache and purulent discharges, and into the nose in ozaena. The leaves, with lime juice, are rubbed over ringworm. The seeds are mucilaginous and used as a diuretic in scanty urine and cough. The leaves are expectorant, and given, sweetened with honey, in chronic cough, especially in children.

The expressed juice of the herb has traditionally been administered to children who are attacked with catarrh, cough with fever and constipation, with very gratifying and beneficial results.

HOMEOPATHIC - Ocimum canum is a species of this shrub which grows abundantly in Brazil. Dr. Mure, who proved and introduced it, noted that it is largely used in Brazil ***"as a specific for diseases of the kidneys, bladder, and urethra."*** He gave a short list of nineteen symptoms which are partly clinical and partly pathogenetic.

Dr. Mure's experience was several times verified by several noted homeopaths. Drs. Pramada Prasanna Biswas of Pabna, Bengal, N. Sinha and N. C. Ghosh have made provings of this drug.

MIND - Memory weak. ***Forgetfulness***. Mistakes in talking. Difficulty concentrating. Prostration and drowsiness. Patient falls asleep while answering questions. Child is peevish and cries, does not like to lie in bed. Irregular delirium, disturbed.

Abdomen - Abdomen distended. Heaviness in abdomen. Griping pain in the abdomen. Pain is felt over the region of liver and spleen. Pain in the right iliac region. Hepatic pain. Gurgling sound can be felt on pressure.

Chest - Pains are felt on both sides of the chest, worse while coughing or sneezing. Pleuritic pains in the chest. Pain is felt in the middle of sternum. Patient cannot lie quiet in bed.

Ears - Watery secretion from the ear. Offensive pus from the ears. Ears painful due to nasal catarrh. Hot flushes come out from the ears. Noises in the ears, loud sound appears to be very painful. Shortness of hearing.

Eyes - Eyes red. Pain in the eyes, lachrymation, eye complaints due to nasal catarrh. Ophthalmia. Foggy vision. Mist before eyes, especially when fixing them on something.

Face - Face red or pale with reddish hue. Flushed and hot.

Female - ***Menses too late.*** Metrorrhagia. Leucorrhea alternating with bloody discharge. Leucorrhea offensive, profuse, white, yellow. Metritis after childbirth. Profuse bloody discharges after delivery. Lochia offensive, profuse, fetid, lasts for a long period. Sexual desire diminished or increased.

Head - ***Headache as from a nail.*** Heavy, throbbing pain as if thousand nails were being driven into it, relieved by pressure. Giddiness of head, worse while walking, likes to keep quiet, relieved by wrapping up the head. Heat on the vertex, relieved by pouring cold water on the head or by fanning.

Kidneys - Kidney colic. ***Urethritis.*** Desire to urinate off and on. Burning in the urethra while urinating. Yellow like saffron, urine. Discharge of mucus with urine. Involuntary urination of the children.

Limbs - ***Aching pains, better from pressure.***

Lungs - Asthmatic attack, wheezing and rattling sound felt in the chest. Asthma better from bending head forward, rocking. Asthma of infants and children. Croupy cough. Hacking cough, profuse expectoration.

Male - Troublesome erections. Sexual desire increased or decreased. Impotency.

Mouth - Lips bright red. Lips dry and black as if burnt. Watery salivation or spitting from the mouth. Putrid and bitter taste in mouth. Ulcer, aphthae in mouth. Ulcer in mouth and tongue of children. The tongue is bright red or its edges and sides are red and the middle portion is deeply coated. ***Toothache, better pressing the gums together,*** warmth, pressure.

Nose - Nasal obstruction. Nasal catarrh associated with frequent sneezing, white or yellow secretions. Coryza. Watery discharge from the nose. Nostrils ulcerated. Nosebleeds.

Perspiration - Offensive sweats.

Rectum - Constipation. Incomplete stools. ***Diarrhea with high fever.*** Diarrhea during rainy season and autumn. Stools liquid, copious, watery, very offensive. Yellowish or greenish liquid stools. Mucus or bloody or streaked with blood. Involuntary stools during high fever.

Skin - Skin disease.

Stomach - Want of appetite. ***Thirstlessness during chill.*** Eructations, Hiccough.

Temperature - Chills and fever. Influenza. Remittent and intermittent fevers. Bilious, continued fever. Quartan fever, tertian fevers. Typhus, typhoid fever.

Throat - Pain in the throat while walking or during cough. Pain and difficulty in swallowing. Redness, ulceration of throat. Glairy phlegm. Enlargement of tonsils. Hoarseness. Voice gets changed.

Vertigo - Vertigo on rising.

COMMENTS - Oci-s. has an assured place in the treatment of influenza and in common nasal catarrh. Remittent fever associated with cough, cold or diarrhea, pneumonia, broncho-pneumonia, bronchitis and asthma.

Typhoid fever or fever associated with delirium, comatose condition, prostration, and falls into slumber or drowsiness while answering questions (Bapt.). Fever in influenza, associated with cough, acute pains in the body, bone pains, soreness of the muscles, and terrible headache (Eup-per.).

Fevers associated with cough, cold and diarrhea, especially in children. Fevers prevalent in rainy season, winter or spring. Intermittent fever. Fever with thirst or absence of thirst.

Fever comes on in the afternoon with extreme chilliness, with shivering. Chilliness, even when exposed to the sun. Hands and the feet become cold and do not become warm easily. Numbness and tingling in hands and feet.

Extreme heat and flushes of heat felt over the face and eyes during hot stage. Burning sensation in the palms of hands and soles of feet, relieved by cold breeze or placing cold water on the head.

Sweat with heat. Heat, sweat, and chilliness may appear alternately. Sweat, delirium, drowsiness or comatose condition.

Remittent fevers of children, fever during dentition period, diarrhea and worm affections (Cina.). Worm complaints of children, fretful and peevish, start from sleep, and do not allow the physician to examine them. The children become awfully peevish, always cry, become quiet while they are being carried (Cham.).

Aching pains, in the feet and legs. Pains are felt all over the body. Offensive and filthy odor. Putrefaction. Contagious and infectious diseases caused by bacteria or bacilli.

Terrible headache. Headache due to congestion, common cold, influenza or fever. Headache relieved by application of cold water on the head or by fanning the head. Better from keeping quiet or wrapping the head with a cloth, worse while walking or by motion.

Face is flushed and hot, lips are red and parched, eyes are drowsy. Pain in the throat, felt while swallowing, coughing or sneezing. Redness inside the throat, both tonsils are enlarged.

Offensive smell comes out of the mouth, offensive salivation. Tongue is red or reddish and shining at the edges with yellow or brown coating in the middle (Bapt.). Aphthae. Putrid ulcer in the mouth and teeth. Toothache, with terrible pains, worse at night, from touch or cold.

Eyes congested, red, with lachrymation, especially in cases of the common cold. Watery discharges and sticky discharges. Ophthalmia, ophthalmia neonatorum. Earache and purulent discharges from the ear. Shortness of hearing.

Difficult respiration. Asthma, the patient cannot lie on the back. Bends forward and supports the head with the hands, the elbows resting on the knees or leans forward and puts the head on the hands lain flat on such support (Aral., Lob., Blatta.). Asthma of children.

Gastric and intestinal catarrh, with inflammation of the intestinal mucous membrane, fever and diarrhea. Pain in the region of liver and spleen. Abdomen distended, distension does not abate in spite of stools passed.

After gurgling in the stomach, copious watery and offensive stools appear. Diarrhea with fever and cold, cough, pneumonia, broncho-pneumonia and bronchitis. Involuntary stools.

Irregular, long lasting menses. Leucorrhea. Uterine complications after delivery. Terribly offensive lochia, of unnatural color, long lasting. Discharge mixed with mucus, is pus-like and like washing of fish.

Ocimum sanctum is supposed to drive away mosquitoes; it may prevent malarial fevers if cultivated near a house.

REFERENCES - Ghose.

OENANTHE CROCATA

(Water Dropwart)

PHARMACY - oena. Oenanthe crocata. Water dropwort. Hemlock drop-wort. N. O. Umbelliferae. Marshy places. Tincture of fresh root at time of flowering. ***Historical dose:*** Tincture and all potencies.

CLINICAL - Albuminuria. Amenorrhea. Breast, pain. Coma. ***Convulsions.*** Cough. Delirium tremens. Diaphragm, spasm. ***Epilepsy.*** Esophagus, stricture. Gastroenteritis. ***Hysterical, epilepsy.*** Ichthyosis. Insanity. Leprosy. ***Menstrual, convulsions.*** Nausea. Priapism. Puerperal, convulsions. Sciatica. Speech, lost. ***Status, epilepticus.*** Stomatitis. Strokes. Tetanus. Tongue, swollen. Tongue, ulcerated. Tympanites. Vertigo. Vomiting.

HOMEOPATHIC - Oenanthe crocata is one of the most poisonous of the Umbelliferae, and many accidents have occurred from the use of the root in mistake for parsnips and of the leaves in salads and soups. These have furnished many of the symptoms of the pathogenesis.

Epileptic convulsions, worse during menstruation and pregnancy. Epilepsy, utters a loud cry before falling backward. ***Status epilepticus.*** Face swollen, convulsive twitching of facial muscles, foaming at mouth, lockjaw. Cold as if dead during convulsions, noise in throat as if being choked. Burning heat. Numbness. Legs stretches straight out.

Skin affections, especially leprosy and ichthyosis. Rosy red blotches on face and chest, arms, abdomen. Profuse, offensive sweat. Burning in throat and stomach, nausea and vomiting. Obstinate vomiting for days, not relieved by anything.

MIND - Epileptic condition at periods when menses are due, in amenorrhea. Epileptic insanity. Coma after convulsions. Sudden and complete loss of consciousness. Insanity, hallucinations. Delirium tremens. Furious delirium. Tendency to cry over little things. Averse to be questioned.

Abdomen - Great tenderness, slightest touch on any part of abdomen causes great pain. Distended with colic pains. Gastroenteritis with violent pain and vomiting. Tympanites with the convulsions.

Back - Pain along spinal column. Intense action of dorsal and lumbar muscles, opisthotonos.

Breasts - Swollen breasts. Pain in breast. Nipples painful to least contact.

Causations - Menstrual disturbances. Injuries.

Chest - Pain in right side under the ribs. Chest firmly fixed. Pleuritic exudation. Lungs hyperemic, hepatized in spots.

Eyes - Sunken, full and projecting, inflamed. Redness. Pupils first contracted, then dilated. Eyes turned upward and inward, firmly fixed. Vision disturbed, obscured.

Face - Countenance livid, rose-colored spots on face. Lips blue. Eyes fixed, pupils dilated. ***Rapid, convulsive twitching of facial muscles***. Trismus, foaming at mouth, locked jaws. Risus sardonicus.

Food - Total loss of appetite with debility. Thirst, craves cold drinks, evening. Cannot bear to drink anything hot.

Head - Hyperemia of brain, extravasation and serous exudation. Pains all over head, dizzy. Headache and giddiness. Violent pain in head. Apoplectic conditions. Suddenly falls down backward. Hair fell off.

Heart - Pain in region of heart. Pulse is small, feeble, irregular and scarcely perceptible, accelerated before the fit.

Kidneys - Painful urination. Urine copious, dark, turbid, reddish, with thick yellow sediment.

Limbs - Numbness and feebleness of limbs. Pain along crural and sciatic nerves, commencing in back. Cold hands and feet. Numbness of hand and foot. Cramps in calves. Arms flexed at elbow in a right angle. Hands clenched during tetanus. Convulsions, opisthotonos.

Lungs - Spasms of the diaphragm. Heavy, spasmodic, stertorous breathing. Tickling cough with rattling in the lower part of the chest. Cough, worse at night, excited by tickling at top of throat. Rattling in the chest, sputa thick, heavy, white and yellow. Thick, frothy expectoration, reddish, bloody, white.

Male - Priapism.

Modalities - Worse from water, injury, sexual and menstrual disturbances. Pressure aggravates pain in throat, but ameliorates deep pain in thorax. Swallowing causes soreness of throat.

Mouth - Mouth dry and parched. Foaming at mouth, bloody mucus. Excoriation inflammation, blisters. Convulsive movement of teeth. Loss of speech.

Nose - Nosebleeds.

Rectum - Involuntary stool, diarrhea.

Sensations - As if a bug creeping under the skin about the waist, worse touch of clothes.

Skin - Rose colored rash on face, chest, arms and abdomen. Loss of nails and hair.

Sleep - Much yawning. Drowsy. In a deep sleep, snoring loudly and moaning. Roused with difficulty.

Stomach - Tender stomach. Burning heat in stomach. Esophagitis. Distressing hiccough. Nausea, better if vomiting occurs. Vomit is clear water liquid, blood. Vomiting and diarrhea.

Temperature - Extreme coldness, loss of animal heat. Deadly cold and pale. Face and limbs cold and blue. Burning heat that mounted to head. Slight fever with pain at pit of stomach. Profuse, offensive sweat, accompanies symptoms.

Throat - Burning and constriction in larynx. Pharyngitis. Violent constriction and burning in the throat. Pressure on throat gives pain, sore when swallowing. Power of swallowing lost.

Tongue - Tongue sore, swollen and protruded. Tongue slightly furred, raw at tip, ulcerated at edges. Tongue clean, moist, trembling. Tongue half bitten through.

Vertigo - Vertigo with falling. Vertigo with nausea, vomiting, syncope and convulsions.

COMMENTS - Oena. is a valuable convulsive remedy, useful in epileptiform, puerperal and uremia convulsions. Hormonal epilepsy, since or during pregnancy, in childbirth, abortion, miscarriage, menstrual period, amenorrhea, and menopause. Epileptic symptoms since birth control pills. Epilepsy after vaccinations. Epilepsy after errors in diet.

Severe, violent epileptic attacks. Sudden attacks (Bell.). Grand mal, petit mal, and particularly status epilepticus attacks. Risus sardonicus, a fixed smile. Feeling of dread and anxiety before attacks. Can hear bells ringing before. Followed by deep sleep or coma. Vomiting after epilepsy.

Vertigo during the menstrual period. Toxemia during pregnancy with convulsions and protein in the urine. All symptoms are worse from water and drinking.

D. A. Baldwin of Englewood, N. J., entirely controlled the convulsions in a young man of 16 with Oena. Dr. Ord reported a case of petit mal cured with Oean. 3x. In a South American homeopathic journal a Dr. Rappaz reported the cure of a case of three years' standing with increasing seizures with the remedy in doses ranging from the 6c to 12c.

Henderson reported the cure of an epilepsy case of 9 years standing, where the patient was almost idiotic, the convulsions were relieved and the mental condition was greatly relieved and improved. In two other cases equally satisfactory results were had.

S. H. Talcott, in the report of the Middletown Asylum, 1893, noted that Oena. possesses a marked power in epilepsy. He stated that it makes the attacks less frequent, less violent and improves the mental state of the patient. Talcott prescribed it in the tincture, 1 to 6 drops daily.

F. H. Fisk reported the cure of a case that had lasted two years with the tincture. This patient was having 6 to 10 attacks daily during the last month before Fisk took the case.

Dr. Garrison of Easton, Penn. reported a case of reflex uterine of hystero-epilepsy in which the Oena. 2x acted promptly. J. S. Cooper of Chillicothe, Ohio, reported the cure of a case of 25 years standing with Oena. 4x.

J. Ritchie Horner reported that the Oena. 3x greatly modified the attacks in a woman who had the disease over 20 years and who, for the two months previous, had a convulsion daily.

W. A. Dunn reported a cure of a young woman of 16 who had been epileptic for 7 years, having as many as 4 or 5 attacks during a night. The remedy caused these attacks to disappear entirely. The girl commenced menstruating at age 12, so the establishment of the menses had nothing to do with the cure.

Charles A. Wilson of San Antonio, Texas, reported a number of cases cured with Oean. 3x, and the same potency greatly lessened the number of seizures in others. Dr. Purdon of the University of Dublin, related a case of epilepsy cured with this remedy in 1 to 6 drop doses several times a day.

F. E. Howard, in a case that had 3 or 4 attacks a week, gave 5 drops of the tincture every two hours, which caused violent pains in the head, but complete recovery followed on reducing the dose.

McClellan of New Jersey told of a case of his in which a young woman, 19, of a very healthy family, who had never menstruated and had become almost idiotic in consequence. At the periods when the menses should have come on there were epileptiform seizures of minor intensity. The state of mind was such that after taking the best advice in Paris and the States without avail, the patient was about to be put away.

Oean. was given and the next period passed without any epileptic symptoms. But there was no sign of the flow. Bell. was given and at the next period, the flow came on and the patient's mind was entirely restored.

J. S. Cooper related the case of a clergyman in attendance on one of the Federal generals at the battle of Gettysburg, who was wounded in the forehead by a fragment of shell, taken prisoner and kept in prison twenty months.

On his release he was quite a wreck and soon began to have light epileptic seizures, which gradually got worse. When seen by J. S. Cooper, twenty-five years later, he was having four or five fits a day, could write his name and at time would take to his heels and run four or five miles into the country before he could be caught.

Oean. 4c, five drops every four hours, was prescribed. After the first dose he had a very bad fit. The dose was then diminished. He began to improve and in less than a year was in perfect health. Oean., was not taken continuously, but when he "felt nervous" he would take a few doses.

F. H. Fish cured a girl, 16, sanguine, well grown, who at eight began to have fits of absentmindedness at irregular intervals. At 12, menstruation commenced; at 14, epileptic seizures occurred, having no relation to the menstrual periods. The fits were so severe that sixty to one hundred grains of potassium bromide were required to keep them under control.

Oean. tincture was given, five drops in six ounces of water, a teaspoonful every three hours, and later less often. She had not another spasm, lost her absentmindedness and became cheerful and active.

W. K. Fowler reported a case of a teamster, 60, who had gotten into a fight nineteen years before from which he had three ribs broken and was struck in stomach with the butt of a gun.

Two weeks later, he had pneumonia on the injured side, and after that, epileptic seizures. Before the attacks he had a pain in the stomach going through to the spine and pain in the second cervical vertebra. Attacks were induced by worry and by becoming very tired. He had severe attacks when the day's work was finished.

Oean. was given on discs, four discs every three hours for a month. After this there was only one slight attack after a hard day's work during the four months he was under observation.

Several cured cases of epilepsy have been reported in which Oena. alternated with Sil. or some other drug, but they need not be given as it was unclear which remedy cured.

RELATIONS - ***Compare:*** (1) Cic., Kali-br. (2) Phel., Con. (3) In epilepsy, Bufo. (4) In priapism, Pic-ac.

REFERENCES - Boericke. Clarke. Murphy. Phatak.

OENOTHERA BIENNIS

(Large Evening Primrose)

PHARMACY - oeno. Oenothera biennis. Large evening primrose. Tree primrose. N. O. Onagracee. North America. Tincture of fresh plant. ***Historical dose:*** Tincture and all potencies.

CLINICAL - Cholera infantum. Diarrhea. Hydrocephalous. Nervous exhaustion. Paralysis.

HOMEOPATHIC - T. Riker Nuted recorded a proving on a woman who took Oeno. twice, the first, a teaspoonful, the second, 30 drops of the liquid extract for the relief of a wearisome feeling of mental and physical oppression. On each occasion, notably the first, distinct poisoning symptoms were developed.

General paralysis of mental and bodily forces, with copious and easy evacuations of bowels and bladder, followed by relief of the general symptoms. General numbness, general warm sweat with urgent desire to urinate, better after evacuation of bowels and bladder. Effortless diarrhea.

Farrington gave the indication exhausting, watery diarrhea without effort with nervous exhaustion, even incipient hydrocephalous. Hurd cured a man, 65, who had "severe pains in his stomach after meals for over two years" with 25 drop doses of the tincture.

RELATIONS - ***Compare:*** (1) In diarrhea, Ip., Gnaph., Nuphar. (2) In better from copious urination, Ign., Gels. (3) In better after stool, Bry., Colch., Coloc., Crot., Oxyt., Rhus-t., Spig., Sulph. (4) Paralytic symptoms, Gels.

REFERENCES - Boericke. Clarke.

OLEANDER

(Rose Laurel)

PHARMACY - olnd. Oleander. Rose laurel. Nerium oleander. N. O. Apocynaceae. South Europe, North Africa, West Asia. Thrives best in moist ground. Tincture of the leaves. ***Historical dose:*** Tincture and all potencies.

CLINICAL - Brain, disorders. Eczema. Fainting. Headaches. Hyperesthesia. Lienteria. Memory, weakened. Numbness. Nursing, disorders. Palpitations. Paralysis. Perichondritis. Rheumatism. Scalp, eruptions. Spasms. Spine, disorders. Strabismus. Tongue, coated. Vertigo.

HERBAL - In the Cap de Verde Islands, the petals of oleander blossoms are used with dried orange-peel in all kinds of fevers to promote perspiration and drive out the rash.

HOMEOPATHIC - Olnd., which is one of the remedies proved by Hahnemann, has been recognized as a powerful poison from antiquity. In animals poisoned by it, the heart becomes paralyzed, first the auricles, then the entire heart.

Goullon referred to poisoning cases in which "anguish inflammation of the stomach, diarrhea, swoons," and even death had occurred. "Palpitations of the heart, anxiety insomnia and unconsciousness," were observed by Petrus de Alvano, and Morgagni noted "vomiting, thirst, slumbering, speechlessness and death." Goullon also quoted instances of suffering from exhalations of the flowers and even from the plants when not in flower.

Marked action on the skin, heart and nervous system. Paralytic conditions with cramp like contractions of upper limbs. Hemiplegia. Paralytic rigidity. Paresis after infantile paralysis.

General crampings. Numbness. Sopor. Weakness with trembling in nursing women. Sense of vibrations. Difficult articulation, or unable to speak. Emptiness in stomach and chest after eating, better brandy. Involuntary discharges.

MIND - Memory weak, slow perception. Morose. Peevish. Sadness with lack of confidence and power. Melancholy with obstinate constipation.

Abdomen - Borborygmus with profuse, fetid flatus. Gnawing around navel.

Chest - Oppression as from a weight, asthmatic when lying down. Obtuse stitches in chest.

Eyes - ***Sensation as if eyes were drawn back into the head.*** Lachrymation, when reading. Double vision. Can see objects only when looking at them sideways.

Face - Pale, sunken, with blue rings around eyes (Ph-ac.). Numb upper lip. Lower jaw trembles when yawning.

Female - Tremors after nursing, so weak she can scarcely walk across the room.

Food - Desires cold water. Aversion to cheese.

Head - Numb feeling. Dull, unable to think. Indolence. Pain in brain, as if head would burst. Headache better by looking crossways, sideways or squinting. ***Corrosive itching on forehead and edge of hair***, worse heat. ***Eruption on scalp***. Humid, fetid spots ***behind ears*** (Graph., Petr.) and occiput, with red, rough, herpetic spots in front.

Heart - ***Palpitations*** with weakness and empty feeling in chest, better brandy. Pains on stooping.

Kidneys - Involuntary urination.

Limbs - Limbs stiff and cold. Crampy contraction of upper limbs in paralysis. Stiffness of joints. ***Weakness of lower limbs***. Painless paralysis. Paralysis of legs and feet. Trembling knees when standing. Edema. Swelling, burning stiffness of fingers. Veins on hands swollen. Constant cold feet.

Lungs - Dyspnea.

Modalities - Better from looking sideways, brandy. Squinting helps headache. Worse in open air, draft, undressing after nursing. Worse rubbing, scratching, friction of clothes. Worse rest, looking sideways. Rising up aggravates headache, vertigo. Stooping causes pain over heart.

Mouth - Toothache only when masticating. Tongue numb. Loss of speech.

Rectum - Ineffectual urging. Burning pain in anus. ***Passes food undigested*** in the morning. ***Stools, pass when emitting flatus***, thin involuntary.

Sensations - Peculiar sensations suggestive of paralysis. Numb or painless paralyzed feeling as if inner parts were distended. Buzzing and humming. Pulsations in outer parts. Gnawing, itching, biting or pungent pain after scratching. Numbness of skin or itching numbness.

Skin - ***Very sensitive skin***, slightest friction causes soreness and chapping. Nocturnal burning. ***Violent itching eruption, bleeding, oozing,*** want of perspiration. Itching, especially of scalp, which is sensitive. Itching, scurfy pimples, herpes, sensitive and numb. Eruptions with itching, biting as of lice. Skin numb.

Sleep - Sopor. Yawning with trembling of lower jaw.

Stomach - ***Canine hunger with hurried eating*** without appetite. Thirst. Empty feeling even after eating, better brandy. Extreme debility of digestive power. Throbbing in pit. Empty belching. Vomiting of food, greenish water.

Temperature - Heat from mental exertion.

Throat - As if a cool wind blowing on throat (left).

Vertigo - Vertigo for a long time before paralysis. Vertigo, worse looking fixedly at an object or looking down, turning to either side in bed with diplopia.

COMMENTS - A young man, 18, fell sick, had attacks of vertigo, suffered from great weakness of the muscles, headache better in evening, worse every morning after waking, which was a difficult process.

He had a pale face, white-coated tongue, slow pulse. On leaving for change of air he soon got quite well, but ill again as soon as he returned. Some oleanders in his bedroom were then suspected by his doctor, and on their removal all the trouble vanished.

The doctor recalled that when he was a student he had some oleanders before his windows and in autumn, when the nights were cold, he took them into his bedroom. On waking in the morning, he had a heavy head and sensation of weariness, could only leave his bed by great exertion.

As soon as be put his foot to the ground, he was seized with vertigo and reeled. Having traced this to the oleanders, he purposely repeated the experiment, always with the same result.

Weak memory and slow perception. Pressive and stupefying headache. Pressure as if a hundredweight were pressing brain forward and as if everything would come out at forehead. Headaches better by looking cross-eyed or looking sideways.

Cloudiness of vision, worse by looking sideways. Momentary loss of sight. Eyes distorted. Strabismus.

Functional paralysis. The left side is most affected, violent contraction of muscles, worse left side. Numbness of upper and lower limbs.

Digestion is paralyzed, the food passes completely undigested. Gastro-enteritis. Involuntary evacuation of feces and urine. Infants soil their diapers every time they pass flatus. "Trembling after nursing" in nursing women.

The skin is very sensitive and easily chafed and chapped. Olean. is in the front rank of remedies affecting the scalp, more particularly the back part of the scalp or commencing there.

Clarke confirmed the symptoms "desquamation of the epidermis of the scalp," and "violent gnawing itching on the scalp, as from lice after scratching, a smarting as if scratched raw."

Cooper reported a case of a schoolboy whose head was very sore and irritable, covered with crusts, sore to the touch. Glands in his neck were swollen and sore to the touch. Olean. was given, two drops in a powder at bedtime on November 14th.

On November 27th an aggravation was reported and the eruption had spread from the head to the back. From this time rapid improvement set in. Cooper noted that a single dose of the tincture may give the best possible results in such cases.

RELATIONS - ***Antidoted by:*** Camph. - acute effects, Sulph. - the chronic effects. ***Compare:*** (1) Con., Nat-m., Rhus-t., Caust., Lath. (2) Oleander contains Oleandrin and also Nerein which is said to be closely related, if not identical with Digitalin. (3) In irritability, Staph., Hyos., Nux-v. (4) In fits of passion followed by quick repentance, Croc. (5) disorders of nursing women, Carb-an. (7) In lienteria, Ferr., Ars. has diarrhea from chilling stomach indigestion of cold things, stool yellow with stool great pain, burning, worse after midnight, great thirst. (8) Arg-n. - bowels act as soon as patient drinks. (9) Chin. - watery stool containing undigested food, very debilitating, stools may escape involuntarily after a meal, caused or worse by eating fruits. (10) Apis, Phos. and Ph-ac. - wide-open anus. ***Compatible:*** Con., Lyc., Nat-m., Puls., Rhus-t., Sep., Spig.

REFERENCES - Boericke. Clarke. Phatak.

OLEUM ANIMALE

(Dippel's Animal Oil)

PHARMACY - ol-an. Oleum animale. Dippel's animal oil. Aethereum dippeli. Oleum cornu cervi. Bone-naphtha. Dilutions in alcohol. This volatile oil is prepared by Dippel first by distillation of stags' horn. ***Historical dose:*** Tincture and all potencies.

CLINICAL - Asthma. Breast, disorders. Cancer. Colds. Constipation. Coryza. Facial, paralysis. Faint. Gonorrhea. Headaches. Migraines. Neurasthenia. Polyuria. Prostate disorders. Spermatic cord, neuralgia. Testes, neuralgia. Testes, retraction.

HOMEOPATHIC - Ol-an. is an oil obtained from the preparation of bone-black and further distilled and rectified for medicinal use. It was discovered in 1711 by Johann Conrad Dippel, the alchemist, who was the discoverer of Prussian blue.

Dippel obtained it in the first instance by a distillation of stags' horns, the deciduous horns of the stag partaking more of the nature of bone than the permanent horns of cattle. This lead to the name Oleum cornu cervi, with which the Ol-an. is at present prepared is considered identical.

Sircar noted that though it is not the panacea which Dippel imagined it to be when he discovered it, Ol-an. in a very powerful medicinal substance and since it has been well proved by Nenning, Schreter and Trinks, it has a definite place in the Homeopathic Materia Medica.

Grimmer indicated it in cases of breast cancer with burning or sticking and pressure radiating in all directions, relieved by rubbing and in the open air. A uterine tumor cured with several doses of Ol-an. 1000c potency given at long intervals shows its relationship to new growths.

Pain in spots. Stitches, burning pains, as with red hot needles. ***"Pulled upward"*** and ***"from behind forward"*** pains in malar bones, testicles, breasts. Flesh feels torn from bones. Affected part feels sore. Symptoms appear here and there or in single parts.

Affects the nerves, especially pneumogastric nerve, digestive organs. Neurasthenia. Migraine, neuralgia of spermatic cord. Tremulous weakness of hands, knees, feet etc. Shuffling gait.

Icy coldness from tips of teeth in throat, stomach etc. Chilliness (and coryza) are worse in a warm room and better in open air. Sensation as if stomach were full of churning water. Urinous odor with belchings, leucorrhea etc.

MIND - Ill-tempered. Nervous irritability. Sad introverted, absorbed in self, speaks in whispers. Indolent, inclined to sit, taciturn. Vanishing thoughts. Faintness from gastric origin.

Abdomen - Flatulence and rumbling. Bruised pain in abdomen after stool.

Back - Cracking in cervical vertebrae on raising the head. Aching in right scapula, better pressure. Sprained feeling in sacrum. Unsteady gait.

Breasts - ***Stitches in breast*** from behind forward.

Causations - Ill effects of suppressions, especially of foot sweat.

Chest - Stitches at clavicle. Chest feels constricted. Oppression.

Eyes - Smarting in eyes, misty vision. Lachrymation when eating. Short-sighted. Glistening bodies before the eyes. Twitching of lids (Agar.). A skin seems to overhang the eyes.

Face - Cramp-like pains. Feels drawn. White of an egg seems dried on lips. ***Twitching of lips***. Malar bone feels pulled upward. Swelling beneath right lower jaw. ***Toothache, better from pressing teeth together.***

Female - Stitches in breast from behind forwards. Sore breasts before menses, outward stitches in nipples in scirrhus. ***Menses, early, scanty,*** black flow. Urinous leucorrhea.

Food - Drinking cold water causes pressure in stomach, worse from hot drinks. Desires bread. Worse eating (sweat, lachrymation, headache). Especially worse after dinner.

Head - Migraine with polyuria. Pain in spots. Tearing pain with sadness and irritability, worse after dinner, relieved by rubbing. Itching, burning vesicles, better friction. Malar bones feel pulled forcibly upward.

Heart - Anxious palpitations. Pulse slow.

Kidneys - ***Polyuria***. Frequent and urgent want to urinate with tenesmus and scanty emission. Small stream of urine. Profuse, pale urine of fish brine odor, worse hysteria, migraine. Greenish urine. Itching in urethra.

Limbs - Sprained feeling in small of back. Cracking of vertebrae on raising head (Aloe, Nat-c., Thuj.). Rheumatic pain in shoulders. Restlessness. Fish-brine odor of sweat of heels.

Lungs - Asthma from suppressed foot-sweat.

Male - Desire increased, ejaculation too soon. Pain along spermatic cord to testicles. ***Testicles feel seized and pulled forcibly upward,*** worse right. ***Pressure in the perineum***. Prostate hypertrophy. Seminal losses, on straining at stool.

Modalities - Better from rubbing, pressure. Better stretching, changing position. Better in open air. Better eructation. Worse from cold. Worse in warm room, hot drinks. Worse eating. Worse suppressions, noise. Worse from 2 p.m. to 9 p.m. Worse before, during and commencement of menses.

Mouth - Bites cheek while eating (Caust.). Snow-white cottony saliva. Greasy feeling in mouth. Tongue sore as if scalded. Toothache, better pressing teeth together with sensation of coldness coming out from tips.

Nose - Watery, excoriating discharge, worse in open air.

Rectum - Ineffectual urging to stool, with burning in anus.

Sensations - Sensation in scalp as if skin had been cut and reunited. As if blood were rushing to head to occiput on entering a warm room. As if red-hot needles in chest. As if testicles were seized and pulled forcibly upward. As if thumb (and toe) would ulcerate.

Skin - Excoriation in bends of joints.

Stomach - ***Sensations as if water were in stomach,*** of coldness, constriction, and burning, better belchings. Urinous belchings. Water brash, better chewing tobacco.

Temperature - Alternate chill and heat. Cold, foul foot-sweat, fishy smell on heels.

Throat - Sore, dry, constricted, empty swallowing difficult, though food and drink pass easily. As if cold air penetrates the throat. Acrid vapor or raw streak in throat, worse cough. Hawks out gluey, brown lumps.

Vertigo - Vertigo from gastric origin, better bending head backwards.

COMMENTS - Dippel's Animal Oil is "a colorless or slightly yellow, thin, oily liquid with a penetrating but not disagreeable odor and an acrid, burning taste, which changes to a cool and bitter one. It darkens and thickens on exposure to air and light and is extremely volatile. A drop on paper evaporates without leaving a greasy stain."Its composition is extremely complex, but it may be regarded as belonging to the group of volatile carbons.

Burning pains and burning sensations in almost all parts, stitching pains, "stitches as with red-hot needles" (Kali-c., other carbons). Stitches and pressure in all directions, particularly from behind forward.

Cramp-like pains in different parts. Sensation of part being pulled upward. The left side is predominantly affected, when direction is noted it is from before backward and from behind upward. Cracking in vertebra of neck on raising head.

Twitching of lips and swelling beneath right lower jaw. Malar bone feels as if pulled forcibly upward. Greasy feeling in mouth and accumulation of quantities of saliva white as snow. Relaxation of buccal mucus membrane, patient cannot avoid biting cheek when he eats.

Sensation as of white of egg dried on lips. Soreness of tongue as if scalded. Sensation as if cold air penetrated throat although the air is warm, better eating and drinking, worse empty swallowing. Desire for soft-boiled eggs or for bread, with aversion to meat. Sensation as if water were in stomach, as if a lump of ice there. Belchings taste like urine and burn.

Both testicles are drawn up and very painful. "Stitches from behind forward in breasts, pressure from both sides of the back extends forward." Menses too early and too scanty.

Clarke gave great relief in a case of cancer of right breast in which the patient complained of pains darting forward out of the nipple.

Dr. Leggett related the case of a very stout Dutch woman, 56, who had been under constitutional treatment for uterine tumor, engorged liver and cerebral congestion. She fancied the tumor had increased to the size it was years ago. She had the sensation as if water rushing back and forth in stomach. She had been walking, standing and shopping and had eaten many sweets.

Of the remedies having "stomach as if full of water," Ol-an. was chosen as more similar to the case than Mill. or Phell. and was given in 1000c potency, a single dose. A month later she was better in every way and a second dose brought still further improvement.

A case of long-standing neuralgia of the spermatic cord was cured. There were excruciating attacks three or four times every year, pains as if testicles were seized by a hand and pulled very severely. Ol-an. 18c gave almost instant and permanent relief.

Dever cured a toothache in an extremely irritable patient, pain better by pressing the teeth together. The provings had "stitches in right upper molar removed by pressure after dinner."

The cure of a case of migraine is quoted in H. M., July, 1895. Zwingenberg, after failing with Sang., gave Ol-an. 2x, five drops in warm water, morning and evening to a woman who always suffered from migraine the day after a party, at which she usually wore a heavy diadem on her head.

Polyuria of clear urine accompanied the migraine and suggested the remedy. This accompaniment may indicate Ol-an. in any nervous disorder. Zwingenberg also cured a case of nervous asthma following repelled foot-sweat.

RELATIONS - ***Antidoted by:*** Camph., Nux-v., Op. ***Compare:*** (1) Puls., Ars., Sil., Sep. (2) in headache with concomitant polyuria, Ign., Gels. (3) Twitching eyelids, Agar. (4) Gastric symptoms after drinking cold water, Ars., Phos., Carb-v. (5) Pains in testicles, Puls. (6) worse by noise, Graph. better by noise. (7) better by rubbing, Phos., Nat-c., Carb-ac., Canth. (8) Coryza worse in open air, All-c. (9) Numb head, Graph. Cracking in nape on moving head, Nicc. (10) Dried white of egg sensation, Alum., Bar-c., Mag-c., Ph-ac., Sul-ac. (11) better eating and drinking, worse empty swallowing, Lach. (12) Belchings taste like urine, Agn., smell like old urine. (13) Sad, despondent, Puls. - unlike Puls., bad tempered. ***Follows well:*** Bry. ***Followed well by:*** Sep.

REFERENCES - Boericke. Clarke. Phatak.

OLEUM JECORIS ASELLI

(Cod-liver Oil)

PHARMACY - ol-j. Oleum jecoris aselli. Cod liver oil. Oleum jecoris morrhue. Oil obtained from the livers of Gadus morrhua and some other allied fishes. N. O. Gadide. Tincture. Trituration. ***Historical dose:*** Tincture and all potencies.

CLINICAL - Addison's, disease. Alopecia. Amenorrhea. Anemia. Asthma. Bones, disorders. Bright's, disease. Cold, abscess. Constipation. Coryza. Coughs. Diarrhea. ***Dwarfishness. Emaciation.*** Fever. Fistula. Goiter. Hair, abnormal. Headaches. ***Indigestion.*** Intermittent, fever. Joints, stiffness. ***Liver, diseases.*** Lumbago. ***Malnutrition. Marasmus.*** Palpitations. Pneumonia. Rheumatism. Ringworm. Sacrum pains. Sciatica. Scrofulous ophthalmia. Sleeplessness. Spinal irritation. Tuberculosis. Vision disorders.

HOMEOPATHIC - The number of people who "cannot take cod-liver oil" is very great, which means that Ol-j. is a pathogenic as well as a curative agent.

Neidhard proved it and elicited some very definite symptoms and to these have been added curative and pathogenic effects observed on patients. The oil contains a large number of proximate principles of great complexity to which its specific medicinal properties are due.

Decided pains in the liver and liver region with great soreness were noted in Neidhard's provings and these symptoms give one of the keynotes of the remedy as ***soreness***. Not only the liver, but the throat, chest, abdomen, kidneys, ovaries, joints and back are all sore. The spine is sore as in spinal irritation.

Sore pains. Burning in spots. Rheumatic disorders. ***Pains in liver region***. Yellow discharges. Scrofulous diseases. ***Faulty nutrition.*** Emaciation. Anemia, weakness. Deficiency of vital heat. Always taking cold. Lassitude. Hot hands and head. Frontal headaches, over right eye, bursting after coughing. Palpitations of the heart, with cough, short breath.

The nutrition of the skin is improved and the medicinal properties of the oil are absorbed without any tax being put on the organs of digestion. Burnett said that olive oil and almond oil acts as well.

Atrophy of infants, emaciation with hot handle and head, restless and feverish at night. ***Emaciated, dwarfish***, chilly babies and children, a nightly rubbing with cod liver oil soon revolutionizes their condition. Children who cannot tolerate milk.

Abdomen - Soreness and heaviness in the region of liver, worse exercise.

Back - Chilly or fluttering from sacrum up back to occiput.

Causations - ***Malnutrition.***

Chest - Sharp, stitching pains. Burning spots. ***Soreness through chest.*** Coughing causes soreness of chest, headache.

Face - Growth of short, thick hair on chin and upper lip in women.

Female - Establishes menses. Yellow leucorrhea with weak back.

Food - Children who cannot take milk.

Heart - ***Palpitations***, accompany other symptoms.

Limbs - Chronic rheumatism with rigid muscles and tendons. Aching in elbows and knees, in ***sacrum***. ***Burning in palms.*** Palms hot toward evening.

Lungs - ***Dry, hacking, tickling cough***, especially at night. Cough with palpitation. Soreness or stitches in chest. Yellow sputum. Hemoptysis (Acal., Mill.). Early tuberculosis. Whooping cough in miserable, scrofulous children. Dahlke indicated giving give drop doses increasing daily, one drop up to twelve, then descend in the same way for whooping cough.

Modalities - Worse from milk. Worse from exposure to cold, draft of air. Worse living in cold. Worse damp localities. Worse touch, motion. Worse raising arm, bending side inwards. Worse stooping, walking. Worse riding, falling. Laughing aggravates cough. Lying down causes oppressed feeling.

Mouth - Tongue yellow. Fetid breath.

Skin - ***Yellowness***. Cold abscesses. Milk crusts. Ringworm (local application).

Temperature - Constantly chilly towards evening. ***Hectic fever.*** Night-sweats.

Throat - Hoarseness.

COMMENTS - Ol-j. is a liver remedy, an ally of Chol., confirmed by the provings. Burnett noted that cod liver oil is a nutrient and affects the chest, liver, pancreas and tendons. Internally, a nutrient and a hepatic and pancreatic remedy.

Burnett showed that ringworm generally has its constitutional basis in a tuberculosis miasm. In recent ringworm, the application of the plain oil at bedtime is at once the most innocent and most effectual of known local measures. Before the application, the part should be washed well with soft soap.

"Dry, hacking cough, night-cough, cough with tough expectoration, yellow or white, soreness of chest, especially on coughing, sharp stitches here and there, through chest, burning through to back, burning in spots."

Tuberculosis, in the beginning stages. Scrofulous diathesis. Cough is worse from exposure to cold, worse in damp weather. Cough relieved by onset of fever.

Marked fever symptom, both hectic and intermittent. "Fever worse towards evening with burning in palms." Chilly, sensitive to drafts, feels as if continually taking cold. Chills running down the back. Feet constantly cold. Sensitive to chill and damp. Thirst before and during the chill.

Affection of the spleen. Yellow discharges, particularly expectoration, coating of the tongue, yellow mucus from sore throat.

Increases the menstrual flow, and restores it when in abeyance. Abnormal growth of hair on the face of a woman. Yellow leucorrhea. Passage of mucus from urethra with burning during stool.

RELATIONS - ***Antidoted by:*** Iris v. (chill with sick stomach and diarrhea). ***Compare:*** (1) Chol., Tub., Phos., Iod. (2) One liter of Ol. Jecoris contains 0.4 gram of iodine. (3) Gad., Cod, - frequent breathing with flapping of ala nasi, rush of blood to chest, pain in lungs and cough, dry heat in palms. (4) Fel. and sarcodes generally. (5) In tuberculosis, ringworm, emaciation, Bac., Phos. (6) Emaciation and ravenous appetite, Iod. (7) Intolerance of milk, Aeth., Calc., Lac-v., Mag-c. (8) Pains in head with cough, Caps., Bry., Nat-m. (9) Chilly, effects of damp localities, Nat-sulph., Aran. (10) Heavy eyelids, Gels., Op.

REFERENCES - Boericke. Clarke. Phatak.

OLEUM OLEA EUROPEA

(Olive Oil)

PHARMACY - ol-o-e. Oleum olea europea. Olive oil. N. O. Oleaceae. ***Historical dose:*** Tincture, oil and all potencies.

CLINICAL - Constipation. Dehydration. Heart, disease. Malnutrition. Skin, disorders.

HERBAL - Olive oil is obtained from the fruit of the olive tree, now common to the shores of the Mediterranean. It is used in cooking, cosmetics, soaps and as a fuel for traditional oil lamps.

Olive oil is pleasant and bland, very nutritious, and mildly laxative. It is regarded as a healthful dietary oil because of its high content of monounsaturated fat (mainly oleic acid) and polyphenols.

Very well tolerated by the stomach. It's protective function has a beneficial effect on ulcers and gastritis. Activates the secretion of bile and pancreatic hormones, lowering the incidence of gallstone formation.

For infants it is especially serviceable as a cathartic, being easily taken and of mild action. Suitable for adults in irritated or inflamed conditions of the bowel or stomach, and may be given after acrid poisons. As a laxative enema, one to two fluid ounces should be taken, two teaspoonfuls or less for a child one year old.

Externally, it is a lubricant and is valuable for shielding irritated surfaces, relax contracted tendons, and promote healing. Olive oil massage is helpful in preventing dehydration from fever. Daily breast massage with the oil is helpful in preventing breast cancer and tumors. Olive oil foot massages are good for relaxation and will promote sleep.

Olive oil is often the basis in which to incorporate other medicaments, or is compounded with dense fatty or resinous substances to give them pliancy in the formation of ointments, cerates, or plasters.

RELATIONS - ***Compare:*** Alf., Mel., Aloe-v., Calen., castor oil.

REFERENCES - Murphy.

OLEUM SANTALI

(Sandalwood Oil)

PHARMACY - ol-sant. Oleum santali. Sandalwood oil. Oleum santalum. ***Historical dose:*** Tincture and all potencies.

CLINICAL - Acne. Bronchitis. Colds. Colic. Coughs. Cystitis. Diarrhea. ***Gonorrhea. Kidney, pain.*** Laryngitis. Nausea. Skin, dry. Sore throats. Wrinkles. Wounds.

HERBAL - Ol-sant. is a stimulating, disinfectant expectorant and antispasmodic. Antiseptic, anti-inflammatory, and a mild pain reliever. Acne, wounds, dry skin and wrinkles.

Two or three drops on sugar will frequently relieve the hacking cough, when only little sputum is expectorated. Bronchitis when the cough is dry and hacking. Coughs, sore throats and laryngitis.

Affects the urinary and sexual spheres. ***Gonorrhea,*** discharge is thick and yellow. Swelling of the prepuce, painful erections. Urine is passed slowly and causes burning and smarting of the urethra. Gonorrhea where the prostate gland is implicated and there is pain deep in the perineum.

Nausea, diarrhea and colic. Aids in digestion, relaxes the muscles of the digestive tract. Stimulates the production of urine, restores hormonal balance.

MIND - Aggression and irritability. Stress, anxiety, nervous tension and depression. Difficult concentration.

Bladder - Chronic cystitis. Frequent, burning, smarting, swelling and redness of meatus. Sensation of a ball pressing against the urethra, worse standing.

Kidneys - ***Aching in kidney region***. Gleet with profuse, thick discharge. Stream small and slow.

Lungs - Bronchitis when the cough is dry and hacking.

Male - ***Gonorrhea.*** Thick, yellowish, muco-purulent discharge. Deep pain in perineum. Swelling of the prepuce. Painful erections.

RELATIONS - ***Compare:*** Cann-s., Buchu, Cop.

REFERENCES - Boericke. Blackwood. Clarke.

OLIVE

(Bach Flower Essence)

PHARMACY - oliv-b. Olive. Olea europea. The flowering clusters are placed in sunlit water for several hours. The remedy is prepared from the strained water. ***Historical dose:*** Take two drops from the stock bottle into a one ounce dropper bottle (add brandy or alcohol, if this bottle will be used for days or weeks). This is the dosage bottle, take a few drops straight into the mouth or as needed in a little water or juice.

HOMEOPATHIC - Olive, together with the remedies Clem-b., Honey-b., Wld-r-b., Wh-ch-b., Must-b. and Ch-bd-b., belongs to Bach's group ***Lack of Interest in Present Circumstances***.

States of exhaustion in mind/emotions, body and spirit. Weariness and exhaustion. Emotional weariness. Sadness, depression, discouragement. Sense of meaninglessness and apathy with exhaustion.

MIND - Weary. Intense exhaustion: Cannot complete tasks. Absent-minded, disinterested, lethargic. Especially after prolonged sickness or for those in social service.

REFERENCES - Bach.

ONISCUS ASELLUS

(Wood-louse)

PHARMACY - onis. Oniscus asellus. Wood louse. Oniscus armadillo. Armadillo officinalis. Sow-bug. Sow-louse. Cellar-worm. Millipedes. N. O. Isopoda, class Crustacea of the Articulate. Tincture of whole animal. ***Historical dose:*** Tincture and all potencies.

CLINICAL - Asthma. Bladder, disorders. ***Colic.*** Epilepsy. Hemoptysis. Rectum, disorders. Strangury. ***Tenesmus***. Toothache.

HOMEOPATHIC - In Germany, Onis. has a popular reputation as a remedy for epilepsy. Hering proved a tincture and Wolf recorded the effect of swallowing three cellar-worms in a glass of brandy before an attack of fever. This experience provided the most characteristic symptoms of the remedy, showing it to be related to Canth., Apis and their cognates.

The symptoms of Hering's proving showed pains in the head, over the eyes and down the nose. Constriction of gullet and stomach. Hawking up of blood-streaked mucus. Burning in anus. Many erections with disinclination to work (Canth.). Frequent yawning and desire to stretch.

Asthmatic conditions with bronchial catarrh. Pale face, wild expression, constant vomiting. Very severe colic with meteorism and tension of abdomen. Tenesmus of bladder and rectum. Cutting burning in urethra. Dropsy.

Abdomen - Distended, ***meteorism, very severe colic.*** Very severe colic with meteorism and tension of abdomen.

Bladder - Cutting burning in urethra. ***Tenesmus of bladder and rectum*** with absence of stool and urine.

Face - Pale face, wild expression.

Head - Boring pain behind right ear in the mastoid bone (Caps.). Violent pulsation of arteries (Poth., Glon.). Painful pressure above the root of nose.

Kidneys - Cutting, burning in urethra.

Lungs - Hawking up of blood-streaked mucus. Asthmatic conditions with bronchial catarrh.

Male - Many erections with disinclination to work (Canth.).

Rectum - Burning in anus. ***Tenesmus of rectum*** with absence of stool and urine.

Stomach - Persistent pressure in cardiac orifice. Constant vomiting.

RELATIONS - ***Compare:*** (1) Poth., Canth., Glon.

REFERENCES - Boericke. Clarke.

ONONIS SPINOSA

(Rest-harrow)

PHARMACY - onon. Ononis spinosa. Rest-harrow. Ononis arvensis. Cammock. N. O. Leguminose. Papilionoideae. Tincture of fresh plant. ***Historical dose:*** Tincture and all potencies.

CLINICAL - Epilepsy. Headaches. Nephritis. Nosebleeds.

HERBAL - The Treasury of Botany notes that ononis arvensis is indigenous to Britain, growing on barren pastures and on the borders of ill-cultivated fields. It owes its name, "Rest-harrow," to its tough underground roots, which cause stoppages to harrow and plough.

In some parts it is called "Cammock," and the country people, having the idea that it communicates its nauseous, goat-like odor to cheese made from the milk of cows who have eaten it, call the cheese so tainted "Cammocky."

HOMEOPATHIC - Nosebleed three or four times in one day, worse when washing his face. Hansen gave "chronic nephritis" as having been cured by Onon.

COMMENTS - Cooper recorded the case of a brick field laborer, 45, who at 13 was prostrated for a week, apparently with sunstroke, something seemed to catch the back of his head. At 25, had similar attacks. In March, 1900, he began to have daily attacks.

An aura seemed to spread over his head from the occiput, he made frightful grimaces, but did not scream out, became unconscious, turned deathlike and blue in face and fell down.

After the attacks he had a violent headache, giddiness and wakeful nights. Onon. tincture in single doses at rare intervals produced improvement at once and cured in nine months.

REFERENCES - Clarke.

ONOPORDON ACANTHIUM

(Cotton Thistle)

PHARMACY - onop. Onopordon acanthium. Cotton thistle. Scotch thistle. N.O. Compositae.

CLINICAL - Chilliness. Headache. Heart, disorders.

HOMEOPATHIC - Constriction in left side of chest. Sensation as of a stone in the chest. Characteristic heart rhythm disorders. Excessive depressive tendency. Headache better change of weather, to warm and dry weather. Stuffed sensation in ears and nose. Pain in right maxillary sinus.

Increased sensory perceptions. Chilliness. Sensitiveness to cold and to drafts of air. Worse cold, damp weather. Better warmth and rest. Pains in back and limbs, better motion, and worse sitting and after sleep.

Sensation of cold and the dryness of the mucous membranes of nose and throat. Dryness of mouth, lips. Better eating. Desire for sweets. Swelling and redness of the part of the abdomen where a belt is worn. Cold feeling in lower abdomen during scanty menses. As if icicles in rectum.

MIND - Difficult concentration. Sensitiveness to external impressions. Euphoria, alternating with sadness.

Food - Desires sweets.

Head - Headache better change of weather to warm and dry weather.

Heart - Dull pain in region of heart, extending to left arm.

Limbs - Fleeting pains in small joints. Limbs heavy like lead. While walking, feet turn frequently.

Modalities - Better warmth and rest. Better eating. Worse cold, damp weather.

Nose - Smell more acute.

REFERENCES - Murphy.

ONOSMODIUM VIRGINIANUM

(False Cromwell)

PHARMACY - onos. Onosmodium virginianum. False cromwell. Lithospermum virginicum. N. O. Boraginacee. Tincture of entire fresh plant including root. ***Historical dose:*** Tincture and all potencies.

CLINICAL - Amblyopia. Aphasia. Bladder, irritation. Breasts, disorders. Colic. Color-blindness. Debility. Diarrhea. Diplopia. ***Eye, disorders. Eyestrain. Headaches.*** Locomotor ataxia. Meniere's disease. ***Migraines***. Neurasthenia. Nose, dryness. Paralysis. Pregnancy, sickness. Presbyopia. Seminal emissions. ***Sexual, weakness.*** Spine, congestion. Throat, sore. Tinnitus. Urethra, irritation. Uterus, prolapse.

HOMEOPATHIC - Onos. is a member of an American branch of the borage family closely resembling the British Onosma. Its common name is False Cromwell, the real Cromwell being another borage, Lithospermum.

It was proved in material doses by W. E. Green of Arkansas. The most remarkable feature of the proving was the want of power of concentration or coordination produced by the drug. This appears in an inability to concentrate thought, to focus eyes, to coordinate muscles, or to judge the height of impediments on stepping.

General prostration, weariness. Acts and feels as if born tired. Seems to tread on cotton. Staggering. Vertigo, numbness with muscular prostration. Neuralgic pains. Aching, soreness and stiffness of muscles after a pain.

Marked association of head and eye symptoms with muscular tiredness and weariness. Disturbance in the sense of proportion. ***Migraine headaches***. Onos. has probably cured more cases of ***headache associated with eye-strain*** (Ruta). than any other remedy since it was proved.

Headaches from sexual weakness. Diminution of sexual desire in both sexes, similar to ***sexual neurasthenia***. Depressed or lost sexual life in women.

MIND - Loss of concentration and coordination. Confused mind, slow thinking. Irresolution. Aphasia. Forgetful, loss of memory. Fear of falling on going up or down stairs.

Abdomen - Distended feeling, better removing clothing, with griping and grumbling. Colic is better bending backward.

Back - Tired feeling in lower part of the back. Pain in dorsal and lumbar regions. Numbness and tingling in feet and legs.

Breasts - Sore, aching in breasts, feel swollen and sore. Nipples itch.

Causations - Eyestrain. Sexual excess.

Ears - Fullness in ears. Hearing impaired, ringing as from quinine.

Eyes - Eyes heavy and dull. ***Eyestrain, strained feeling in eyes,*** worse using eyes. Muscular asthenopia. ***Ocular muscles tense***. Internal eye muscles paretic. ***Pain in eyeballs*** between orbit and ball, extending to left temple. Eye symptoms with ovarian symptoms.

Female - ***Sexual desire completely loss***. Feels as if menses would appear. Menses too early and too prolonged. Leucorrhea, acrid, yellow offensive, profuse, running down the legs. Severe uterine pains, bearing down pains, old pains return. Soreness in uterine region. Pains alternate between ovaries. Soreness of ovaries with rectum.

Food - Craving for ice water and cold drinks, wants to drink often. Distaste for water. Appetite and thirst diminished. Appetite increased. Hunger after siesta, nervous, all day.

Head - ***Migraine headache from eyestrain*** or sexual weakness. Dull, heavy, dizzy, pressing upward in occiput. Occipital headache as if screwed, worse eyestrain and lying down. Occipital-frontal pain in morning on waking, ***Chiefly on the left side***. Pain up and down from occiput (left) to shoulder worse exertion. Pain in temples and mastoid (Caps.).

Heart - Pain in heart causing fear of death. Pain in region of apex. Oppression of heart. Depressed feeling in heart, as if it would stop beating. Pulse rapid, irregular and weak, and slow. With every third or fourth beat the diastole is prolonged.

Kidneys - Pain in prostatic urethra before and after urination. Seldom any desire to urinate. Urination frequent, scanty. Urine is high-colored, very acid, aromatic, of balsamic odor and heavily loaded with urea.

Limbs - Great muscular weakness and weariness. Pain in back. Pain in left scapular region. ***Tired and numb*** feeling in legs, popliteal spaces and below knees. ***Staggering gait***. Sidewalk seems too high.

Lungs - Hacking cough with sticky, white sputum, better drinking cold water.

Male - Burning in urethra with itching. Sexual excitement. Constant, severe erections. Speedy emissions. ***Psychological impotence***. Loss of sexual desire. Deficient erections.

Modalities - Better from cold drinks, eating, undressing. Better lying on back, rest, sleep. ***Worse eyestrain***, sprains, jarring, motion, tight clothing. Worse sexual excess, darkness, warm, humid air.

Mouth - Dryness of mouth, and of lips, without thirst, better cold water, with scanty saliva. Clammy, sticky, feeling in mouth. Bitter taste.

Nose - Dryness of nose, with feeling as from taking cold. Pain in nasal bones. Stuffed feeling or discharge in posterior sinuses. Sneezing in morning, left side of nose and left eye seem affected.

Rectum - Stools with tenesmus, yellow, mushy, hurrying him out of bed in morning. Stool is shining, bloody and stringy.

Skin - Formication in calves.

Sleep - Sleeplessness. Sleep is uneasy and interrupted, restless and waking early. Many, varied dreams.

Temperature - As if would have a chill every day about twelve or one o' clock. Flushed feeling over body. No perspiration in very warm weather.

Throat - Severe dryness and tightness, all symptoms are better by cold drinks and eating. Raw, scraping. Laryngeal cough, better from drinking cold water, with expectoration of whitish, sticky phlegm. Husky voice.

Vertigo - Vertigo, numbness and muscular prostration. Vertigo with headache, worse lying on left side, raising the hands above the head.

Vision - Vision blurred, optic disc hyperemic and retinal vessels enlarged. Misjudges distances. Color blindness for red and green.

COMMENTS - Vertigo and sensations of numbness and general muscular prostration. Neuralgic pains, dull, heavy aching, affecting the cervical and spinal nerves, pelvic organs, eyes, occiput and sacrum. These are the chief centers of pain along with the throat, bowels, breasts, heart and limbs. The left side of the body is more affected than the right.

Characteristic paralyzing effects on the internal eye muscles. "Feeling of tension in the eyes, as from straining them to read small print," and "desires to have things far off to look at them." The eyeball aches, aggravated by reading small print. Glaucoma. Blurred or double vision. Eyestrain headaches (Ruta.).

Marked "soreness and stiffness." In the occiput there is pressure upward and the pains may go from the eye backward. Gluey expectoration with laryngeal cough. Catarrh of the Eustachian tube (Kali-m., Merc-d.). Meniere's disease.

Characteristic dryness of the nose, mouth and throat. Ameliorated by a great thirst for cold water. Strictures of the urethra where there's painful urination and there are adhesions or blockages in the urethra.

Great loss of sexual desire. Fibroids. History of enlarging breasts when given in tincture (Sabad.). Equalizes the size of unequal breasts.

E. S. Norton published several illustrative cases including the case of Miss C., 23, who suffered three years from a headache. Pain especially in occiput, which felt "sore and stiff," often extending down spine, which was somewhat sensitive to touch.

There was a dull, aching pain on the left side of head, with occasional darting pain through the eyes. Aching in eyes, stiff, strained feeling in them if she read a lot, worse on the left. Headache worse in the morning with some dizziness. The patient had some astigmatism that was corrected with glasses and Onos. 1x at once relieved all the symptoms.

Norton also noted the case of Mrs. D., who had excessive myopia and a severe headache with a constant dull, stupid ache in right occiput and right eye, worse when tired, from coughing or from any sudden motion. There was a little vertigo and a strained feeling in right eye. Onos. 3x cured.

Norton suggested that neurasthenia and neurasthenic headache may be met with Onos. when connected with strains of other kinds besides eye strains. He pointed to the case of Mrs. B., who was deaf for nine years.

For four years she had a constant roaring, hissing noise in both ears with constant dull, pressing pain in occiput, worse in the evening. She had some pain in the ear and sharp shooting pain in front of auricle, with slight vertigo. Chronic catarrh of both middle ears, membranes thickened. Onos. 1x immediately relieved all the pains, though it did not alter the hearing or noises.

H. F. Ivens cured a case of headache of ten years duration, with the modality worse in the dark. The pain was in the left temple and over the left eye, not worse by noises, light or use of eyes, but worse in the dark and on lying down. Pellets of Onos. tincture were given every twelve hours.

W. A. Yingling found that the depressing action of Onos. extends to the generative sphere, desire being abolished in both men and women. He quoted S. A. Jones as suggesting that this is the primary action of the drug, thereby distinguishing it from Pic-ac. in which excitement precedes debility.

Onos. will correspond to the developed consequences of sexual abuse and Pic-ac. to the initial step of sexual debility manifested in weakness. Yingling many times verified "complete loss of desire" as a leading indication.

Yingling had an interesting experience in the case of a woman to whom he gave Onos. for dryness of the nose and throat.

Not only did it cure this, but it also restored the breasts, which were diminutive and almost absent to their normal size. Yingling's results were from the tincture, and not marked from 30c.

W. J. Guernsey greatly relieved with Onos. a man, 38, who suffered from seminal emissions, the result of masturbation. The pains were better by undressing and lying on the back.

Green published some very striking cases with some pathogenic symptoms as well as cures, and also gives an interesting comparative experience with potencies.

RELATIONS - ***Compare:*** (1) Nat-m., Lil-t, Gels., Ruta. (2) Myos., Helio., Symph. (3) In uterine misplacement, Helio., Helon., Lil-t., Sep., Nat-m., etc. (4) Disorder of vision, Lil-t. - astigmatism, Pic-ac. - myopia, Nat-s. - Myopia. (5) Ocular headache, Gels. more right, Onos. more left, Lil-t., Spig., Bapt. (6) Eyestrain - Ruta.

REFERENCES - Boericke. Clarke. Murphy. Phatak.

OPERCULINA TURPETHUM

(Nishope)

PHARMACY - oper. Operculina turpethum. Nishope. N. O. Convolvulaceae. ***Historical dose:*** All potencies.

HOMEOPATHIC - Fevers. Delirium associated with restlessness, loquacity. Tendency to escape from bed, ravings, pains cause fainting.

Bubonic plague. Lymphatic glands are enlarged and indurated. Boils and slowly suppurating abscesses. Hemorrhoids. Cholera morbus. Watery diarrhea, profuse with sinking sensation.

REFERENCES - Boericke.

OPIUM

(Poppy)

PHARMACY - op. Opium. Poppy. Papaver officinale. Papaver somniferum. Thebaicum. N. O. Papaveracee. Opium is the gummy exudation of the unripe capsule of the poppy, contains morphine. Tincture. ***Historical dose:*** Tincture and all potencies.

CLINICAL - After-pains. Bladder, paralysis. Brain disorders. Cancer. Catalepsy. Chilblains. Colic. ***Coma.*** Constipation. Delirium. ***Delirium, tremens***. Diabetes mellitus. Dreams. Dysmenorrhea. Epilepsy. ***Fear, effects.*** Fetus, movements. Hernia. Hystero-epilepsy. Ileus. Intestines, obstruction. Labor pains, abnormal. Lead, colic. Marasmus. Measles. Melancholia. Meningitis. Opisthotonos. ***Paralysis.*** Puerperal convulsions. ***Shock.*** Sighing. ***Sleep, abnormal.*** Snoring. Starting. ***Strokes.*** Sunstroke. ***Trauma.*** Tympanitis. Uremia. Urine, suppression. Uterus, inertia. Veins, fullness. Whooping cough.

HOMEOPATHIC - Opium is one of the most complicated substances in the Materia Medica. Opium contains about eighteen alkaloids of which the apomorphine, morphine, heroin and codeine are well known. Brunton noted that besides mucilage, albumen, fat, sugar and salts of ammonia, calcium and magnesia, it contains "seventeen or eighteen alkaloids and two neutral substances, as well as a meconic acid."

Opium played a very prominent part in old-school therapeutics due to its painkilling properties, often with the end result of addiction. The pathogenesis is made up of provings, clinical observations and, in large part, the effects observed in opium-smokers and in those poisoned with massive doses.

The effects of a poisonous dose of opium are scarcely to be distinguished from a fully developed attack of a stroke. There is absolute unconsciousness, complete muscular relaxation, pupils are contracted to a pinpoint aperture, turgid, bloated. Very red or bluish face, stertorous breathing, pulse slow and full. Death takes place by asphyxia, the heart continuing to beat after breathing has ceased.

Smaller doses produce a deep sleep, pleasant, fantastic or frightful dreams, and delirium like delirium tremens. On waking there is a severe headache, nausea, furred tongue, and a loss of appetite.

Want of susceptibility to remedies even though indicated. Insensibility of the nerves, ***painlessness,*** depression, drowsy stupor, torpidity and general sluggishness of function and lack of vital reaction, a kind of negative state. All complaints are characterized by a ***stupor***.

Lessens voluntary movements and contracts the pupils. Painless paralysis of brain, tongue, bowels etc. Depresses higher intellectual powers, lessens the self-control and power of concentration, judgment. Stimulates the imagination. Useful for diseases that originate from fright. Idiocy from masturbation.

Tremors, twitchings, jerking during sleep. Convulsions, worse heat of room or bath. Epilepsy in sleep, from the approach of strangers (children), from fright, worse glare of light, from anger, insult. Throws limbs or stretches arms at right angle to the body, stupor between spasms.

Strokes. Venous, passive congestion. Faints every fifteen minutes. Stupid sleep, accompanies all complaints during spasms, violent chill etc. Complaints are ***painless*** and are accompanied by ***heavy, deep sleep, and stertorous breathing.*** Sensation of bodily well-being, great happiness. Painless ulcers. Suppuration.

Checks all secretions except that of the skin. ***Sweaty skin.*** Hot sweat, hand. Complaints appear with sweat. Reappearance and aggravation from becoming heated. Bed seems hot, hunts a cold place. Internal dryness. Dropsical swelling of the whole body. Dark, mahogany-brown face.

MIND - ***Apoplectic (stroke) state. Coma from drug overdose, fright, stroke or injury. Loss of consciousness.*** Dreamy. Sluggish. Dull. Stupid. No will power. ***Placid.*** Wants nothing, says nothing ails him.

Unable to understand or appreciate his sufferings. Indifferent to pain or pleasure. Nervous, irritable, tendency to start.

Frightful fancies, visions of mice, scorpions. ***Fears after fright,*** which remains. ***Delirium tremens*** with terror.

Delirious talking with wide-open eyes. Exaltation of the mind, vivid imaginations. Gaiety. Talkative. Rash. Bold, increased courage. Tendency to lie. Deceptive, vision, taste touch, perversion of all senses. Imagines parts of his body are very large. Thinks he is not at home. Carphology.

Abdomen - Hard, bloated, tympanitic. As if a weight in the abdomen. ***Lead colic.*** Colic with urging to stool and discharge of hard feces. Intestinal spasms, child cries day and night. Incarcerated umbilical or inguinal hernia. Difficult emission of flatus. Bowels feel completely obstructed. Paralytic atony of bowels after laparotomy.

Back - Pulsating arteries and swollen veins on neck. Opisthotonos.

Causations - Ill effects of fear, fright, anger, shame, rape, sudden joy. Charcoal fumes, alcohol, lead, drug overdose, sun.

Chest - Heat in chest, burning about heart. Tension and constriction in chest. Compression of diaphragm. Aching in chest with shootings in sides.

Constitutions - Suited to persons of light hair, lax muscles and want of bodily irritability. Children and the elderly. Persons insensitive to well-chosen remedies. Alcoholics.

Ears - Acuteness of hearing, clocks striking at a great distance keep her awake. Tinnitus like sea roaring. Buzzing, tinkling in ears.

Eyes - Red, bulging eyes. Staring, glassy. ***Pupils fixed,*** contracted, dilated, ***nonreactive to light.*** Embolism of central artery of retina. Visual hallucinations. Cloudiness of sight. Sensation as if eyeballs were too large, or of dust in eyes. Quivering of eyes and lids. Eyes half open and are turned upwards. Eyelids hanging, as if paralyzed. Ptosis (Gels., Caust.). Swelling of lower lids.

Face - Red, bloated, ***swollen, dark suffused, hot***. Looks intoxicated, besotted (Bapt., Lach.). Distorted. Trembling, spasmodic facial twitching, especially corners of mouth. Veins of face distended. Lips swollen, protruding. ***Lower jaw hangs down.*** Lockjaw. Old look after cholera infantum.

Female - Dysmenorrhea, forcing her to bend double with urging to stool. ***Suppressed menses from fright.*** Prolapse from fright. Softness of uterus. Horrible labor-like pains in uterus. Hiccough during pregnancy. Lively or violent fetal motion. ***Threatened miscarriage*** from fright with sopor. Puerperal convulsions, drowsiness or coma between paroxysms. Convulsions from stoppage of labor pains. Suppression of lochia from fright.

Food - Hungry, but no desire to eat. Attacks of bulimia with want of appetite and repugnance to all food. Slowness and weakness of digestion. Burning thirst, especially for beer.

Head - Heavy occiput. Pain in back of head, great weight there (Gels.). Bursting feeling. Head hot with hot sweat. Paralysis of brain. Confusion in head. Dull, heavy, stupid. Complete insensibility, no mental grasp for anything.

Heart - Weakness. Burning about the heart. Pain in heart with great anxiety, trembling, sleeplessness, talkative delirium. ***Palpitations after stressful events***, fright, grief, sorrow, etc. Full, slow pulse.

Kidneys - Kidney colic, pain radiates to bladder and testicles. Loss of power or sensibility of bladder. Paralytic atony of bladder after laparotomy. ***Retained or involuntary urination after a fright.*** Retention of urine in nursing children from spasms of neck of bladder. Slow to start, feeble stream.

Limbs - Trembling of the limbs after fright. ***Twitching of limbs***. Jerks as if flexors were overacting. Convulsions, worse from glare of light, coldness of limbs. One or other arm moves convulsively to and fro. Shuffling and trembling gait. Feels as if lower limbs were severed and belong to someone else. Numbness, weakness. Painless paralysis (Olean.). Veins of hands distended.

Lungs - ***Stertorous breathing***. Difficult, intermittent, deep. Hoarse. Sighing. ***Deep snoring with rattling,*** unequal breathing. Breathing stops on going to sleep, must be shaken to start it again (Grind.). Cough, tickling with blue face or profuse sweat on whole body, better drinking water. Cough with dyspnea and blue face with bloody expectoration. Hemoptysis. Yawning after cough.

Male - Increased sexual desire with frequent erections and pollutions. Diminished sexual desire and impotence. Spasmodic stricture from drinking poorly fermented liquor and in alcoholics.

Modalities - Better from cold, uncovering, constant walking. Worse heat, ***sunstroke***. Worse odors, stimulants, ***alcohol***, ***suppressed discharges*** and receding eruptions. ***Worse emotions, fear,*** anxiety, reproaches, shame, joy. Worse during and after sleep (Apis, Lach.).

Mouth - Dry. Intense thirst. Copious salivation. Bloody froth. Hemoptysis. Ulcers in mouth and on tongue. Difficult speech and swallowing. Blubbering of lips. Looseness of teeth.

Nose - Loss of smell.

Pulse - Pulse is full, slow, quick, hard, irregular, imperceptible.

Rectum - ***Involuntary stools after fright***, black offensive, frothy. Obstinate constipation, no desire to go to stool. ***Round, hard, black balls***. Feces protrude and recede (Thuj., Sil.). Spasmodic retention of feces in small intestines, from ileus. Violent pain in rectum as if pressed asunder. Bloody mucus oozes from open anus.

Sensations - As if from smoke on the brain. As if flying or hovering in air. As if drunk. As if eyes too large for orbits, as if sand or dust in eyes. As if eyelids paralyzed. As of a band around chest. As if something was forced through a narrow space in abdomen. Rolling, as of a hard body in right hypochondrium. As if intestines would be cut to pieces, as of a stone in abdomen. As though anus closed. As if lower limbs severed from body.

Skin - Dry. Rough and dirty. Whole body looks red. Skin blush with blue spots. ***Hot perspiration over whole body,*** except lower limbs. Constant desire to uncover. Dropsical swelling of whole body. General itching. Crawling here and there. Erythema, scarlatina-like eruptions. Painless indolent ulcers. Desquamation of epidermis. Chilblains.

Sleep - ***Great drowsiness*** (Gels., Nux-m.). Falls into a heavy, deep sleep. ***Profound coma.*** Suffocates on falling asleep (Grind.). Sleepy, but cannot go to sleep. ***Sleeplessness*** from acuteness of hearing, distant noises keep him awake. Bed feels so hot cannot lie on it. Picking at bedclothes. Dreams of cats, dogs, black forms. Pleasant, fantastic, amorous dreams. Coma vigil.

Stomach - Painful sensitiveness and inflation of stomach and epigastrium. Heaviness and pressure in stomach. Incarcerated hernia. Nausea with vomiting and retching. Retching from emotions. Vomiting with colic and convulsions. Vomiting of blood or of greenish matter. Vomiting in peritonitis of fecal matter, of urine.

Temperature - General low temperature with inclination to stupor. Hot, sweaty and drowsy with cold limbs. Heat extending over body. ***Hot perspiration.*** Sweats without relief. Pulse ***full and slow***. Fever characterized by stupor, ***snoring respiration,*** twitching of limbs intense thirst and sleepiness.

Throat - Dryness of throat. Inability to swallow. On swallowing food either goes the wrong way or returns through the nose. Bitter or sour taste in throat. Aphonia from fright. Voice weak with inability to speak loudly without great exertion.

Tongue - Tongue purple, white, black. Tongue protrudes to right side, dry. Paralysis of tongue and difficult speech.

Vertigo - Vertigo after fright. ***Lightness of the head in the elderly*** from injuries to head.

COMMENTS - Complaints brought on by fear, fright, anger, shame, shock. Ailments from excessive joy (Acon., Coff.). Also from alcohol, lead, charcoal fumes. For fright where the image reoccurs. Fright leading to an excited state, hypersensitive, sleepless.

Mentals similar to those of drug addicts. May lie and steal, lack of conscience. Pathologically courageous people. State of confusion or delirium. May go in and out of a stupor. Time seems to move too slowly. Frightened terror (Acon.). Fear of being murdered, of impending death.

Visions and nightmares, wakes in a panic. Visions of fire and ghosts. Visions of great beauty and misery, similar to manic-depression. Astral visions. Exhilaration. Ecstasy (Acon., Phos.).

Shock, total painlessness (Arn., Resc-b.), improbable lack of pain. More rarely, shock with unbearable headaches. Deception in their symptoms and behavior, their senses can be deceptive. State of desirelessness. Stupor. Pinpoint, frozen pupils, irregular pupils.

Polarizing narcosis. In crude doses it causes insensibility, numbness. Total relaxation, calmness, tranquility. Can also cause hypersensitivity, insomnia, heightened senses. Sensitivity to light and noises (Coff.). Hyperacute hearing (Lach.).

Grimmer noted that "this is a remedy of many phases and opposite extremes and alternating states, and of symptoms such as diarrhea with burning pains and violent tenesmus, and involuntary stools. Or there may be an inveterate constipation, often ending in complete bowel obstruction and paralysis of the bowels, cancers and gangrenous ulcerations are most often painless."

Hahnemann described a "deathly paleness, coldness of the limbs and whole body, cold perspiration, timorous anxiety, trembling and despair, mucus stools, transient vomiting and short cough and very rarely certain kinds of pain." He noted that it was a rare and transient effect in excitable subjects, occurring as a reflection of the secondary state.

Keynote abnormal painlessness, but there are also acute pains. Hahnemann recorded one example, "horrible labor-like pains in uterus, which compelled her to bend the abdomen double with anxious, almost ineffectual urging to stool."

Characteristic drowsiness. Inertia, torpor. Absence of sensation, absence of reaction. Great stupor, painlessness, complains of nothing, wants nothing. "Want of susceptibility, trembling." Lack of vital reaction.

Exalted sensitiveness and timidity, sensitiveness to fright and other emotions. Sleepy but cannot sleep, sleepless with acuteness of hearing disturbed by sounds ordinarily not heard at all. Nervous and irritable, tendency to start. Twitching, trembling of head, hands and arms.

Spasms in children at the approach of strangers, from nursing after the mother has had a fright, from crying, eyes half open and upturned. Screaming before and during a spasm. Tetanus, the spasms are ushered in with a loud shriek.

Epileptic attacks occur during sleep. Epilepsy after a fright. Deep sleep after attacks. Deep, rapid breathing, stertorous breathing while sleeping. Children sleep deeply and snore, as if in a coma. Coma, near death-like states (Carb-v., Ant-t.). Coma from uremia, kidney failure. Comatose-like states with high fevers.

Fever, the skin is hot and damp. Secretions are generally checked except that of the skin. Sweat is a characteristic concomitant. "Very hot, sweltering perspiration." Guernsey noted that the "patient may not feel cold all day, but may have only a little chill and at night, when in bed, complain that the sheets feel so very hot."

T. F. Allen remarked that the Op. fever may be closely allied to that of Acon. because the Ranunculaceae are not far removed from the Papaveracee. May have a high temperature without a distinct inflammatory process. Intense thirst and great sleepiness, without the anguish, fear and restlessness of the Acon. fever.

Fever is similar to Gels., but with thirst. May be periodic, intermittent or remittent. Happy with a high fever. Brain damage from high fevers, lack of oxygen or drugs, particularly in children (Hell.).

Delirium with great loquacity, visions of animals starting out of various parts of the room. Feels well in delirium.

Delirium tremens, very little drink is sufficient to bring on an attack. The bed feels too hot. Better cool, fresh air, worse warmth (Apis.).

Besotted face, dusky, mottled (Bapt.). Can be bloated, purplish with dark blue color. Emaciation, wrinkled skin, sunken eyes. Dry skin. Wasting infants who look aged, jerking and twisting of the body. Constant expression of fright.

Pinpoint pupils, unequal, fixed. Glassy eyed children, especially with an arched back and high fever. Childhood meningitis, arched backs, high fever, may have convulsions. Dreamy, sleepy state in meningitis (Gels.).

Stroke with dizziness and paralysis (Arn., Plb.). Deep red face. Strokes with labored breathing, a dusky, dark color on the face, fixed pupils. Stroke, with insensibility and partial or complete paralysis, resulting from charcoal vapor, inhaling gas, alcohol, fright, the fear still remaining. After a stroke, dropped jaw, paralyzed bowels, and dry skin. Multiple sclerosis with paralysis.

Paralysis of sphincters. Severe constipation (Plb.), painless, after a shock or fright. Impacted bowels, particularly in babies. Complete constipation with no desire for stool (Alum.). Lack of sensation, cannot strain. Retention of urine due to lack of sensation. Constipation with round stool, hard, black balls that look like sheep dung.

Involuntary and unconscious passage of urine and feces. Reversed peristalsis and fecal vomiting. Ileus and strangulated hernia. Inertia of the intestines results in constipation of the bladder, retention of the uterus, suspension of the menses.

Threatened abortion or miscarriage from fear. Uterine inertia during labor. Excessive fetal movements. Birth trauma. Asphyxia of the newborn (Acon.), the child is unaware. Puerperal convulsions.

Drug overdoses. Stupor and slurred speech from overdose (Gels.). Nausea or constipation from drugs. Antidotes the effects of morphine (Nux-v.). Side effects of chemotherapy (Ip.). Antidote for lead poisoning, especially where there is constipation, colic, cramps in the colon.

J. P. Willard repeatedly gave permanent relief in cases of suffering with Op. 2x without producing any narcotic effect.

J. B. S. King noticed that in seven opium eaters, there was marked arching of the back, especially of the upper part of the back. In as many morphine takers he had not met with a single case of arched back.

Villers cured with Op. 200c a case of hystero-epilepsy in which the attack was preceded by a sensation of swelling of body. Veins protruded, face bluish red. Complete unconsciousness.

In one of the worst cases of painful menstruation Clarke ever treated, Op. 30c gave greater and more lasting relief than any other remedy. In one patient he gave Op. 30c for constipation. With the onset of the next period, Op. caused a "sharp pain which caused vomiting and a desire to sit doubled up and keep warm."

C. N. Payne related the case of a little girl, aged two, who had never slept properly since birth. She went to sleep at the usual time and slept until 10 p.m., when she woke moaning, crying and tossing about. Seemed frightened, almost fell asleep again but woke with a start. She screamed and kept one arm and one leg in motion after waking. Seemed sleepy but could not sleep. Usually napped during the day.

Nux-v., Bell., Cham. were given in succession in vain. It then transpired that before the baby was twelve hours old it had four different medicines put into its stomach. One of them was paregoric, and had been given since, as well as a "quieting medicine."

During the early months the baby had colic with constipation, stools in dark, hard, round balls. Clearly, it was a proving of opium. Op. 200c was given. The first night she slept much better, rapid improvement and cure followed.

RELATIONS - ***Antidoted by:*** Strong coffee, Atropine, Kali-perm. solution, oxygen inhalations, Camph., Bell., Ip., Nux-v., Chronic opium poisoning. Ip., Nux-v., Passi., Aven. is useful to counteract opium, morphine or heroin habit. ***Antidote to:*** Bell., Dig., Lach., Merc., Nux-v., Stry., Plb., Stram., Ant-t. ***Compare:*** (1) The alkaloids, Apom., Cod., Morph., Chel., Sang. (2) Apis, Bell., Gels., Nux-m. (3) Morphine - an extreme susceptibility to all pain, twitching, tympanites, much itching, (4) Codeine - dry, teasing incessant cough, twitching of muscles, especially those of eyelids. (5) Esch. - California Poppy - a harmless soporific. (6) Stroke of alcoholics, Bar-c. (7) Lack of vital reaction, Psor. (8) Spasms after fright - Hyos., from anger, Cham., Nux-v., Effects of fright, the fear still remaining, Acon., Hyos. (9) Diarrhea from fright, Gels., Puls., Verat. (10) Effects of sudden joy, Coff. (11) Violent movements of fetus, Arn., Sil., Thuj., Sulph., Croc. (12) Uterine inertia, Morph., Chloral., Sec. ***Followed well by:*** Acon., Bell., Bry., Hyos., Nux-v., Nux-m., Ant-t.

REFERENCES - Boericke. Clarke. Murphy. Phatak.

OPUNTIA VULGARIS

(Prickly Pear)

PHARMACY - Opun-v. Opuntia vulgaris. Prickly pear. Cactus opuntia. Opuntia alba spina. Opuntia italica. Opuntia pumila. N. O. Cactaceae. Opuntiae. Tincture of flowers. Tincture of the juice, stems and leaves. ***Historical dose:*** Tincture and all potencies.

CLINICAL - Diarrhea. Enteroptosis. Nausea. Priapism. Spleen, pains.

HOMEOPATHIC - Two kinds of "Prickly pear" have been proved, Opun. vulg. and Opun. alba spina. Burdick took one or two deep inhalations of the tincture of the flowers of the former. J. Fitch, who proved many of the Cactaceae took ten drops of the tincture of the second potency.

Opun-v. has a sick feeling in the lower third of the abdomen. ***Feels as if bowels were settled down in lower abdomen***. Diarrhea with nausea. Enteroptosis with loose and frequent evacuations.

COMMENTS - The bulk of the symptoms of the proving are Fitch's, but the most peculiar symptom (which has also been verified) is Burdick's, "Nausea extending from stomach down into bowels with sensation as if diarrhea would set in." Also "feeling as if bowels had settled down into lower abdomen." Fitch had actual diarrhea.

All the urinary and genital symptoms were his except "bloody urine," which is an effect of Opun-v., but not Burdick's. Coldness was observed by both provers. The peculiar mental symptoms recalling the swearing tendency of Anac., are Fitch's. Sticking and pricking pains predominate, also numbness and tension.

RELATIONS - ***Compare:*** (1) Chap. - which Mexican physicians laud as a specific in chronic diarrhea. (2) Ric. - diarrhea, dysentery, obstinate chronic diarrhea. (3) Cact., Cer-b., Anh. (4) In nausea and sinking-down sensation in stomach and abdomen, Ip. (5) Blasphemy, Anac.

REFERENCES - Boericke. Clarke.

ORCHITINUM

(Testes extract)

PHARMACY - orch. Orchitinum. Testicular extract. Sperminum. A sarcode. Trituration. ***Historical dose:*** Tincture and all potencies.

CLINICAL - Debility. Hot flashes. Impotency. Menopause. Senility. Sexual, weakness.

HOMEOPATHIC - The use of a testicular extract in cases of senile decay and nervous breakdown was first proposed by Brown-Sequard, and formed one of the examples by which he illustrated his doctrine of "inner secretions."

He maintained that the various glands of the organism had, in addition to their obvious secretion or excretion, an additional secretion which was not obvious, but which materially contributed to the welfare of the organism.

The doctrine is now generally accepted and the use of the sarcodes in general is based upon it. Homeopathy can use these remedies in both ways.

Orch. has been used with success in the triturations in menopausal sufferings and in old-school practice in the sequelae of ovariotomy in cases of debility, sexual weakness and premature senile decay.

COMMENTS - Generally a remedy for men. Impotency (Sel.) and sexual debility. Weakness in the testes, particularly before puberty. Hot flashes. Senility.

REFERENCES - Clarke. Murphy.

OREODAPHNE CALIFORNICA

(California Laurel)

PHARMACY - oreo. Oreodaphne californica. California laurel. Mountain laurel. Spice-bush. Balm of Heaven. N. O. Lauracae. Tincture of the leaves. ***Historical dose:*** Tincture and all potencies.

CLINICAL - Backache. Colic. Diarrhea. Headaches. Meningitis. Vertigo.

HOMEOPATHIC - Oreodaphne is a tree which grows to a hundred feet in height. When bruised, it emits a strong, spicy odor which may cause sneezing.

J. Murray Moore proved on himself and friends a tincture of the leaves and produced well-marked fronto-occipital headache, worse by movement, better by rest. The symptoms were more violent when the tincture was smelled than when taken internally.

Neuralgic headaches, cervical-occipital pain, cerebro-spinal meningitis. "Dull ache in occipital and cervical regions, extending down to scapula, great heaviness of the head with a constant desire to move the head, which, however, gives no relief." Atonic diarrhea and intestinal colic.

Back - Constant, dull ache in ***cervical and occipital region***, extending to scapula down spine.

Eyes - Drooping eyelids. Eyelids heavy,

Head - Head heavy, twitching. Intense aching with ***pressure at inner angle of either orbit***. Headaches, worse light, noise, better closing eyes and perfect quiet. Pains, worse left side, extending through brain and across scalp to the base of the occiput. Pain extending to ears.

Rectum - Atonic diarrhea.

Vertigo - Dizziness, worse on stooping or moving.

REFERENCES - Boericke. Clarke.

ORGANOPHOSPHATE

PHARMACY - org-p. Organophosphate. *Historical dose:* All potencies.

CLINICAL - ***Allergies.*** Ataxia. ***Chronic fatigue.*** Chemical, sensitivity. Colic. Coma. Convulsions. Cramps. Dementia. Dystonia. Food, allergies. Heart disease. Incoordination. Multiple sclerosis. ***Muscle weakness.*** Nausea. Neuropathy. Palpitations. Paralysis. Parkinson's disease. Osteoporosis. Twitching. Vertigo. Vomiting. ***Weakness.***

HOMEOPATHIC - Organophosphate compounds are a diverse group of chemicals used in both domestic and industrial settings. Examples include insecticides (malathion, parathion, diazinon, fenthion, dichlorvos, chlorpyrifos), nerve gases (soman, sarin, tabun, VX), ophthalmic agents (echothiophate, isoflurophate), and antihelmintics (trichlorfon). Herbicides (tribufos [DEF], merphos) are tricresyl phosphate–containing industrial chemicals.

Severe anxiety. Restlessness. Confusion. Impairment of concentration and memory. Confusion, irritability, lethargy. Tearfulness. Depression, with suicidal tendencies. Hallucinations. Psychosis.

Muscular contractions. Ataxia. Seizures. Convulsions. Dysarthria, tremors. Polyneuropathy. Paralysis. Insomnia. Cancer. Coma.

Respiratory distress. Bronchospasm and laryngeal spasm, can lead to airway obstruction. Weakness and paralysis of respiratory muscles. Chest pain. Cerebral ischemia.

Chronic fatigue syndrome. Malaise. General sick feeling. Severe, debilitating fatigue which is physical and mental. Loss of muscular strength. Muscle aching, flitting from one group of muscles or joints to another. Degeneration of handwriting. Episodic blurred vision.

Immune weakness, tendency to acquire infections and difficulty getting rid of infections, autoimmunity. Multiple chemical sensitivity. Drug intolerance (such as alcohol, antidepressants). Food intolerances. Birth defects.

MIND - Poor short term memory. Unable to learn new things. Poor concentration. Speech difficulty with poor word finding. Irritability and aggression. Severe anxiety. Nervousness and apprehension. Impairment of concentration and memory.

Destabilization of mood. Mood swings. Increased tearfulness. Depression and psychosis. Impulsive suicidal thoughts. Dementia. Rage. Hallucinations.

Abdomen - Abdominal pain and bloating. Colic. Irritable bowel syndrome.

Chest - Chest pain.

Eyes - Optic neuropathy. Retinal degeneration. Myopia, and miosis. Pupils dilated. Excess lachrymation. Blurred vision.

Female -

Food - Loss of appetite. Hypoglycemia or hyperglycemia. ***Food allergies.***

Head - Headache. Cerebral ischemia.

Heart - Heart disease. Cardiac arrhythmias. Palpitations. Bradycardia. Hypotension, hypertension.

Kidneys - Frequent urination. Urinary incontinence.

Limbs - ***Muscle weakness.*** Muscle aching. Muscle twitching or cramps. Clumsiness. Incoordination. Dystonia, cogwheel rigidity. Paralysis. Osteoporosis.

Lungs - Shortness of breath. Pulmonary edema.

Modalities - Worse from diesel fumes, perfumes, cigarette smoke, alcohol.

Mouth - Salivation.

Nose - Allergies. ***Acute sense of smell.***

Perspiration - Increased sweating.

Rectum - Bowel incontinence. Diarrhea and constipation.

Skin - Numb patches.

Sleep - Sleep disturbance. Insomnia.

Stomach - Nausea and vomiting.

Temperature - Hypothermia. Heat flushes.

Vertigo - Vertigo, with poor balance and dizzy spells.

RELATIONS - ***Compare:*** Mal., Phos., Ph-ac., Phys.

REFERENCES - Murphy.

ORIGANUM MAJORANA

(Sweet Marjoram)

PHARMACY - orig. Origanum majorana. Sweet marjoram. N. O. Labiate. Tincture of whole fresh plant. The whole plant, without the root, gathered when in flower, is macerated in two times its weight of alcohol. ***Historical dose:*** Tincture and all potencies.

CLINICAL - Breasts, disorders. Headaches. Hysteria. Leucorrhea. ***Masturbation.*** Nipples, irritation. ***Nymphomania.*** Restlessness. Seminal, emissions. ***Sexual, mania.***

HERBAL - The "Wild Marjoram" of this country is Origanum vulgare, grows on limestone or chalky soil and yields an oil called Oil of Thyme.

HOMEOPATHIC - Orig., the "Sweet Marjoram" which is used for seasoning in cookery, was proved by Dr. Cessoles, on himself and two young women. The symptoms of the proving showed a distinct relation to the sexual organs, which clinical experience verified and expanded.

Orig. strongly affects the ***female sexual organs***. Acts on the nervous system generally and is effective in masturbation and excessively aroused sexual impulses. Increases the desire for sex.

Sexual excitement driving her to masturbation. Lascivious ideas, impulses, dreams. Affections of the breasts (Bufo.). Great physical prostration. Desire for active exercise ***impelling her to run.***

MIND - ***Lascivious ideas, impulses and dreams,*** with sexual irritation. Great sexual excitement driving her to masturbation. Eroticmania with inclination to commit suicide.

Sadness the whole day, followed by lively mood and excessive joyfulness. Thoughts of marriage, which dispel sadness. Fearful, silent, sad, discontented, despairing and weary of life. Irritable. Uneasiness. Restless with great anxiety and full of ideas. Need for active exercise of running in open air. Impulses to run.

Abdomen - Violent pain in abdomen wakes her from sleep at night.

Back - Pains beneath the scapula.

Breasts - Swelling and itching of nipples and pains in breast.

Female - Great sexual irritation, deep moroseness, believes herself lost or despised. Great sexual excitement driving her to onanism, daily indulgence. Nearly idiotic from masturbation. ***Sexual mania***, powerful lascivious impulses. Sexual mania with inclination to suicide in a young girls. Hysteria. Sexual irritation with leucorrhea and irritation of pudenda. ***"Flatulence of uterus."*** Infertility.

Food - Loss of appetite. Excessive thirst at night

Head - Headache in temples. Heat of head, as heat increased, head was involuntarily turned from side to side.

Kidneys - Frequent desire to urinate, waking him from sleep as many as four times in one night.

Limbs - Cramp in sole of right foot, in left leg, in fingers and shoulders. Pains in right hand. Rheumatic pains in right foot frequently recurring and disappearing. Pains in the toes.

Male - Nocturnal emissions.

Nose - Tickling and sensation of constriction in tip of nose. Nosebleeds.

Skin - Pale red spots on legs, thighs and abdomen. Painful red pimples on outer portion of both legs.

Sleep - Frequent waking from sleep in fright, with trembling. Vivid, anxious, lascivious, exciting dreams.

Stomach - Hiccough.

Temperature - Heat of head, as the heat, as the heat increased the head was involuntarily turned from side to side.

Vertigo - Vertigo on lying down in evening.

COMMENTS - A treatise on the "Sexual Passion," by Dr. Gallavardin, Lyons, France, reported that a clergyman of Mississippi, the founder of an orphan asylum, discovered that Origanum majorana, or common marjoram, in a certain sense may be considered as a specific against sexual passion. It proved effective in masturbation and excessively aroused impulses.

Gallavardin used it in the 4c dilution as he has not found the higher potencies effective. He dissolved five or six globules of this dilution in four teaspoonfuls of fresh water and the young masturbator takes of this every two days, a quarter of an hour before the meal, one teaspoonful.

If the cure is not accomplished eight days after this solution is used up, the same dose is repeated in the same way.

When desired, this remedy can be used according to Gallavardin without the knowledge of the patient, by pouring a teaspoonful into the soup, milk or chocolate. The effect frequently appears very rapidly, but sometimes it does not appear.

Clarke verified the power of Orig. in morbid sexual excitement in both sexes.

The sexual symptoms were developed chiefly in the female provers and included sadness followed by joyfulness and thoughts of marriage. Lascivious dreams. Increased desire for sex. Swelling and itching of nipples and pains in breasts.

"Impulse to run." "Heat of head, as the heat increased the head was involuntarily turned from side to side." Symptoms were worse evening on lying down (vertigo) and worse at night (excessive thirst).

RELATIONS - ***Compare:*** (1) Ferul. - in violent sexual excitement in women, icy coldness in occiput. (2) Plat., Valer., Canth., Hyos. (3) In masturbation in girls, Grat. (4) In masturbation, desire to run, heat to head and movements of head, disorders of breasts, Bufo. (5) In impulse to run, Iod. (6) Canth., Cann-i., Coll., Hedeo., Helon., Plat., Valer.

REFERENCES - Anshutz. Boericke. Clarke. Phatak.

ORIGANUM VULGARE

(Wild Oregano)

PHARMACY - orig-v. Origanum vulgare. Wild oregano. Wild marjorum. Greek oregano. N. O. Lamiaceae. ***Historical dose:*** Tincture and all potencies.

CLINICAL - Acne. Arthritis. Asthma. Athlete's foot. Bad, breath. Bed-sores. Bites. Boils. Bronchitis. Bruises. Burns. Bursitis. Candida. Canker, sores. Cellulitis. Cold, sores. ***Colds.*** Coughs. Cystitis. Dandruff. Diaper rash. Diarrhea. Ear, infections. Eczema. Fleas. Food, poisoning. Frostbite. Fungus. Giariasis. Gum, disease. Headaches. Hepatitis. Hives. Impetigo. Leg, cramps. Lice. Nail, fungus. Peptic, ulcer. Pneumonia. Poison, ivy. Poison, oak. Psoriasis. Prostate, disorders. Radiation, burns. Ringworm. Rosacea. Scabies. Shingles. Sinusitis. Sore, throat. Thrush. Toothaches. Tuberculosis. Varicose, veins. Vertigo. Warts. Wounds.

HERBAL - Oregano grows wild in the mountains of the Mediterranean region. The name is derived from a Greek word meaning "joy of the mountains."

It was used by Greek physicians for trauma, wounds, headaches, lung disorders and venomous bites and was the traditional cure for hemlock poisoning. Over the centuries it gained widespread use for lung conditions, asthma, pneumonia, bronchitis, sinusitis, allergies, and cough.

Britain's Gerard, in his 17th century manuscript, explained the use of oregano as a top remedy for ***head colds.*** The 19th Century eclectic physicians used oregano as a general tonic and a promoter of menstruation (which is why it should not be used during pregnancy).

REFERENCES - Murphy.

ORNITHOGALUM UMBELLATUM

(Star of Bethlehem)

PHARMACY - orni. Ornithogalum umbellatum. Star of Bethlehem. N. O. Liliaceae. Hyacinthaceae. A plant of which there are many varieties, nearly allied to garlic, Allium sativum. Tincture of fresh plant. ***Historical dose:*** Tincture and all potencies.

CLINICAL - ***Cancer***. Constipation. Depression. ***Flatulence.*** Gastric, ulcer. Prostration. Restlessness. ***Stomach, cancer.*** Stomach, ulcers. ***Vomiting.***

HOMEOPATHIC - Orni. is to be considered in chronic gastric and other abdominal indurations, like cancer of intestinal tract, especially of stomach and cecum.

Pains in stomach with sickness, vomiting two or three times a day. Swollen feeling across lower chest. ***Flatulence***. Heartburn and rising of food. Gastric ulcer and cancer. Painful contraction in the pylorus with duodenal distention. Feels ***as if a bag of water turns*** when she turns over in bed.

Complete prostration. Cold before the pains. Feels a pressure in every nerve of the body, sometimes in one part or another with pain across chest, sometimes after food or at night and sometimes on an empty stomach.

Restlessness on account of creepy feeling in feet, cannot sit still, cannot read without walking about. Painful sinking across pit of chest and a feeling of sickness that kept her awake the greater part of the night. Writhing in agony, unable to keep anything long on stomach, better by warm food, worse by cold drinks.

MIND - Hateful. Depression and desire for suicide.

Abdomen - Hardness and distention of abdomen, with frequent belching of mouthfuls of offensive flatus. Wind rolling in balls from side to side. Obliged to loosen clothing.

Limbs - Legs and feet go to sleep on sitting. Legs and feet swollen, preventing walking. Legs swollen, great red streaks and patches coursing along them. Right leg felt bruised and sore, later, angry and red. Creepy feeling in legs keeps him awake at night.

Mouth - Tongue red, coated towards back. Nasty taste in morning.

Rectum - Constipation. Diarrhea, which ameliorates.

Sleep - Great difficulty in going to sleep because of a creepy feeling in limbs. Sleep disturbed by pains. Waking in perspiration at night. Wandering dreams.

Stomach - Loss of appetite. Painful sinking across epigastrium. Agonizing feeling in chest and stomach, starting from pylorus with flatus that rolls in balls from one side to the other. ***Pains increased when food passes pyloric outlet***. Frequent belching of offensive flatus. Phlegm retchings and loss of weight. ***Vomiting of coffee-ground looking matter***. Gastric ulceration with hemorrhage.

COMMENTS - For stomach cancer (Hydr., Cad-s.), stomach ulcers, or a history of ulcers followed by stomach cancer. Stomach cancer after a vaccination. The abdomen is distended and hardened. Writhing in agony from stomach pain. Keynote belching. Emaciation (Hydr.). Used in the Bach Flower system for shock.

In his "Cancer and Cancer Symptoms" Dr. Cooper published several cases of cancer helped by Orni. Cooper particularly insisted on his method being followed: a dose of a single drop being allowed to act until all trace of its action has disappeared.

Cooper noted the case of a man named George, 40, who suffered from stomach cancer. His father had died of a stomach ulcer at 73. He was sent to the cancer hospital in London. They began to operate, but abandoned the operation because of overwhelming numbers of adhesions.

Cooper first saw him July 22, 1898. The patient was writhing in agony on his bed, unable to keep anything down. He was better by some warm foods, worse by cold drinks. The pains were worse at night.

Cooper gave one drop of Orni. tincture on July 23 at 6:00, this was followed by an aggravation of great pains and the patient was frantic until 3:00 a.m. At 1:00 p.m. the next day he had a bowel movement.

Then he developed flatulence and pain, and was given Carb-v. 3x as an acute, which cured those symptoms. Three days later, Cooper saw the patient and the pain that was in his stomach had begun spreading out to the rest of his body.

A second dose of Orni. was given on the evening of July 28. Immediately after taking that dose, he vomited a black, jelly-like substance that greatly relieved the pains and generally improved his energy and appetite. From that time on there was steady progress.

On August 29th, the patient reported that he was getting some pain in the lower abdomen. He had difficulty getting to sleep and he had started getting creeping sensations in his legs.

He repeated a dose on September 9. On September 18, he reported that he was sleeping better, there was more pain in the legs, but it was not so bad, and there were slight pains in the stomach. His appetite and energy were improved. On September 23, his right leg felt bruised and began to swell. He started choking on food. He was given another dose.

Some flatulence returned. In a few days, the man came to Cooper's office in a great fright. Both his legs were swollen with red streaks. Believing these were to do with the rapid elimination of the cancer, Dr. Cooper thought he was being too aggressive in the case, so he gave no medicine. The man was astonished.

The legs became swollen and inflamed, then returned to normal. In July 1901, Cooper visited his patient to find him in good health without any signs of cancer or pain.

In the same volume, Cooper reproduced from H. W. (April, 1898) cases of ulceration of the stomach in elderly women cured with the same remedy.

Miss J., 50, was a thin, drawn-featured woman. Her sister died of stomach cancer. She had vomited blood fifteen years ago and had been subject to gastric pains since. Pains in stomach with sickness. Vomited two or three times a day. Felt a pressure in every nerve of body, sometimes in one part, sometimes in another, with pain across the chest. Pain at night, or after food and sometimes on an empty stomach.

She had a great deal of wind and sometimes a swollen feeling across the lower chest. Occasional heartburn with rising of food. Nasty canker taste in the morning. Could not sleep from the pains, had wandering dreams. Bowels were confined.

Orni. tincture was given, one dose, on November 6. On November 13, the patient was seen again. Symptoms had moderated, vomiting ceased. A new symptom appeared, "wakes in perspiration at night." That diminished by November 27. Pains better, "gets cold before the pains." No heartburn, still a nasty taste and confined bowel. The dose was repeated.

The day after this dose, the bowels loosened with general relief. This went on, increasing under more doses of the remedy, until the patient regained almost perfect health and was quite changed in appearance.

Mrs. K., 62, had been seized with profuse vomiting of blood eighteen months before. Since then she lived on slops and Quaker oats. Lately, she spat up clots. Whenever she turns in bed she "feels as if a bag of water turns also." Feet and legs swollen, unable to walk with ease. A brother is said to have died of cancer.

On January 12, 1898, one dose of Orni. in tincture was given. On January 23, she was so much better that she could hardly believe the effect. The oppression of the stomach was gone. The "fluid sack" that rolled about in her seemed to go down and she felt nothing of it. She felt cheery and light. On February 10, there was a threatened return of the symptoms, but another dose permanently removed them.

Cooper added the account of how he was led to think of Orni. in cancer. "My acquaintance with it in cancer cases was due to the very distinctive disturbance it produced in a woman very sensitive to all alliaceous flavoring substances in food. The dose was taken at midday and the same evening distention of the stomach and duodenum came on.

"Also frequent belching of mouthfuls of offensive flatus obliging her to loosen her clothes. This was accompanied by the most hateful depression of spirits and desire for suicide. A feeling of complete prostration and painful sinking across the pit of the chest. A feeling of sickness that kept her awake the greater part of the night and that did not pass off for several days.

"The subject of this disturbance was about fifty-four years of age of quite a sanguine temperament inclined to the enfeebled digestion and with a history of pleuritic seizures and a possible tubercular tendency, but otherwise not subject to any settled form of disease. Since the medicinal thrill above recorded, her general strength, digestion and capacity for the enjoyment of life have manifestly improved.

"The Ornith. in those sensitive to it goes at once to the pylorus, causes painful spasmodic contraction of it and distends the duodenum with flatus, its pains being invariably increased when the food attempts to pass the pyloric outlet of the stomach."

Clarke had several opportunities to confirm Cooper's observations on the action of Orni. for cancer the stomach, including the case of Mr. W., 44, who came to him in August, 1899. Both parents had died of cancer. He had a weak stomach for two or three years and was wasting. He had to get up in the night to vomit, bringing up green and yellow liquid.

He had much flatus, "swells up in balls of wind." His abdomen was large and hard, with a rather large spleen. Venous zigzag. Stools were loose, watery, slate-colored. Urine was scanty, dark. He had been vaccinated three or four times.

He made good progress under Thuj. 30c once a week, the vomiting ceased and he began to put on flesh. He developed an offensive body odor, which disappeared under Sulph. 30c, but on October 13, symptoms were rather worse. He had some distention, wind did not pass freely. Rumbling before stool. Balls of wind rolled about, but not as badly as at first. Frothy, acid vomiting, which relieved.

Clarke then gave Orni. tincture, one dose, repeated three weeks later with manifest improvement in the symptoms. His body was much less hard and distended. Sleep and appetite were good, cessation of vomiting and gain of three pounds in weight. When he returned, the symptoms were different and another remedy was required and then he considered himself cured.

RELATIONS - ***Compare:*** (1) All-s., in flatulent indigestion. (2) Abies-n., Cham., Chin., Carb-v., Lyc.

REFERENCES - Boericke. Clarke. Murphy.

OSCILLOCOCCINUM

PHARMACY - oscilloc. Oscillococcinum. Lysate from Oscillococcus. Virus. ***Historical dose:*** All potencies.

CLINICAL - Aches. Anxiety. Bronchitis. Conjunctivitis. Ear pain. ***Epidemic, influenza***. Fears. Headaches. ***Influenza.*** Gastro-intestinal disorders. Mastoiditis. Otitis. Rhinitis. Sinusitis. Varicose ulcer.

HOMEOPATHIC - In the year 1925, Joseph Roy is believed to have observed in some conditions of a culture the existence of a germ animated by an oscillating movement. He named the nosode Oscillococcinum because of this fact. These researches helped him to describe a remedy of which the clinical experiments in the infections of influenza were carried out in particular by Paul Chavanon.

Oscilloc. was developed by Boiron Laboratory in France. Pierre Schmidt said Oscilloc. is for "influenza at the beginning as a preventive, as well as during convalescence"

Influenza of all types, especially in the earlier stages. ***Epidemic influenza***. Bursting headaches and muscle aching. Gastro-intestinal troubles with the influenza. ***Beginning of influenza***, rhinitis and otitis. Tendency to get influenza.

Given early it is very efficacious. To obtain good results in a case which begins and to cut short the manifestations of influenza, it is necessary to use one dose of Oscillococcinum 200c every 2 to 3 hours or repeat only if necessary.

Anxiety, paleness, chill. Sensitiveness to barometric weather changes. Tuberculous patients sensitive to cold. Asthenia, hyperthermia. Eye and nasal catarrh. Bronchial congestion. Painful congestion of the ear drum. Schmidt noted it for "Mastoiditis, at the beginning of a disease which does not develop."

MIND - Subjects with fixed ideas, obsessions. Obstinate. Agony, anxious without any motive. A busy body. Maniac, cannot bear disorder. Fear of dirt, of being polluted. Has the need to wash his hands very often and is afraid of giving his hand to others for the fear of pollution, contagion.

Abdomen - Abdominal cramping pains followed by fetid diarrhea. Pains in the appendix region.

Ears - Pains sometimes as if from needles in one or both ears. Tympanum red and swollen. Mastoiditis. Diminution of hearing acuity.

Eyes - Yellow conjunctiva. Conjunctivitis of influenza. Eye catarrh.

Face - Pain in the frontal and maxillary region.

Food - Can digest neither milk nor eggs.

Head - Bursting headaches. Headache with considerable throbbing.

Kidneys - Turbid urine, less abundant, deep color. Painful urination.

Lungs - Muco-purulent expectoration with humid cough.

Modalities - Better by heat, rest. Worse by milk, eggs.

Mouth - Tongue white.

Nose - Nasal voice. Nasal catarrh. Stuffed nose, nasal obstruction, sneezing. Serous discharge from the nose, then muco-purulent.

Rectum - Constipation.

Skin - Varicose type of ulcers of the legs.

Stomach - Swelling of the stomach. Putrid regurgitations. Vomiting of water or food.

Temperature - Bruised sensation, chill, hyperthermia.

Throat - Aphonia, dry painful cough.

RELATIONS - Eup-per. is to be associated with it. ***Compare:*** (1) Eup-per., Gels., Pyrog., Bapt., Ars., Influ. (2) Gaulphimia glauca - Hypersecretion of the nasal and ocular mucous, sneezing, hypersensitivity to change of weather. (3) Gelinsoga purviflora - Morning headache, makes mistakes when writing numbers and letters, stuffed nose, augmentation of diuresis, joint pains, lassitude, feels as if bruised. (4) Gink. - Pale face, drawn traits, numbness and chill. Laryngeal irritation with cough, frontal and left supra - orbita pain. (4) Luf-op. - Frontal-occipital headache, acute or chronic inflammation of the mucus membrane of the nasal fossa, lassitude and bodily fatigue.

REFERENCES - Julian.

OSMIUM METALLICUM

(Osmium Metal)

PHARMACY - osm. Osmium metallicum. Osmium metal. Osmium tetroxide. The element (At. Wt. 190.3). Trituration of the precipitated metal. Osmium acidum. Dilutions with absolutely pure water. ***Historical dose:*** Trituration and all potencies.

CLINICAL - Asthma. Bronchitis. Colds. Coryza. Cough, spasmodic. Eczema. Erections. ***Glaucoma.*** Headache. Hernia. Herpes iris. Larynx, pain. Penis, sores. Pollutions. Post-nasal bleeding. Post-nasal, growths. Spermatic cords, pains. Sternum, pain. Syphilis. Syphilitic eruptions. Testicles, pains. Tongue, sore. Trachea, pain.

HOMEOPATHIC - Osmium is a metal of the platinum group in association with which it is always found. It is the heaviest of them all and the most refractory, having never been fused. It derives its name from the pungent odor of the fumes of osmic acid, which are evolved in the process of separating platinum from its ore.

The odor of Osmium closely resembles that of chlorine, as also do its irritating effect on the respiration mucus membrane. The odor imparted to the secretions is various, it makes the urine smell like violets, the belchings like radishes, the axillary sweat like garlic.

Triturations of the pure metal have been proved. The symptoms of the metal and of the acid are taken together.

Osm. affects the respiratory tract, especially the trachea. Irritation and catarrh of respiratory organs. ***Pain in trachea***.

Pains go up and down. Crawling on back and shoulders. Increases and gives odor to local perspiration. Albuminuria. Eczema. Causes ***adhesion of the nail fold.***

MIND - Morose, irritable, impatient. Weeping mood, screaming with cough. Weak, gives up. Consciousness of mental weakness, misplaces words. Thoughts of accidents having happened to others. Disinclination for work.

Abdomen - Distention of stomach and abdomen in evening, with difficult passage of flatus. Rumblings. Pain in groins, on coughing the pain extended into testicles. Weakness in groins towards spermatic cords. Pressure on inguinal rings. Constriction in epigastrium before dinner.

Back - Crawling on back and shoulders. Pressive pain in back and loins. Pain in sacral region. Peculiar pain extending from scapula to sacral region, worse motion and cough.

Chest - Oppression, better deep inspiration. Tightness. Dryness in chest. Sticking near left lower rib. Pain beneath sternum on coughing, extending to sides of chest. Sternum is sore, painful to touch, independent of cough. Shooting up and down in sternum. Wandering pneumonia.

Ears - Earache evenings, first right then left ear. Perforations with irritation of meatus. Itching in the ears, profuse nasal catarrh. Tingling and pain in right ear. Ringing in right ear. Deafness, ears pain when nose is blown, mouth open, sleep noisy.

Eyes - Increase in intra-ocular tension, dim sight, photophobia. Conjunctivitis. ***Glaucoma*** with iridescent vision. ***Green colors surround candlelight.*** Greenish or rainbow colors around the light. Violent supra and infra-orbital neuralgia, violent pains and lachrymation.

Food - Aversion to cocoa, coffee and tobacco, disgust at their odor.

Head - Feels as if a band around head. Dull, heavy headache. Violent headache above and under the eyes. Sharp bewildering pain in center of forehead. Aching in base of brain and jaws at night. Pain in vertex and occiput, worse throwing head backward. Falling off of hair (Kali-c., Fl-ac.).

Heart - Anxious palpitations. Pulse rapid.

Kidneys - Bright's disease. Diminution or suppression of the urinary secretions. Urine is albuminous, strong-scented, smelling of violets. Urine is high-colored, full of bile, dark brown and scanty. Deposits bright-red sediment.

Limbs - Heaviness and weariness of limbs, worse knees. Twitching of fingers with spasmodic cough. Fold of skin remains attached to growing nail. Axillary sweat smells like garlic.

Lungs - Sensitive air passages. Dread of breathing, sore pain when air enters lungs. Moist rales on breathing and in larynx. Convulsive cough, feels as though membrane were torn from larynx. Noisy, ***dry, hard, cough*** in violent short bursts, coming from low down, shaking the whole body. Spasmodic cough, sounds as if coughing in an empty tube with torn loose feeling and sticky sputum. Twitching of fingers with spasmodic cough.

Male - Steady aching in glans penis. Violent pain on the point of penis and prepuce. Pain in testes and spermatic cord. Pain in testicles, preventing sleep. Erections every morning, earlier and harder.

Modalities - Open air helps the smarting in eyes. Worse coughing, talking, riding, touch. Worse in evening. Cough worse until midnight. Open air aggravates coryza, cough.

Mouth - Aching in jaws, pain in muscles of mastication. Mouth sticky and pasty. Copious salivation. Taste of blood, metallic, cigars cannot be smoked, because they provoke cough and worse the rawness in larynx, taste blunted.

Nose - Nose and larynx sensitive to air. Full feeling in nose. Coryza, fluent with a feeling of stoppage. Snuffling. Small lumps of phlegm from posterior sinuses.

Rectum - Constipated. Stool hard, then soft, mushy, frequent. Bilious stools with burning at anus. Burning in anus during and after stool. Tendency to hemorrhoids.

Sensations - As of a band around head. As if he had swallowed broken stones. Cough as if caused by resonance of contiguous parts. As if insects crawling on back and shoulders. Legs and feet as if too full.

Skin - Irritated skin. Eczema. Itching pimples. Bromidrosis, sweat in axilla smelling of garlic, worse evening and night. Fold remains attached to growing nail.

Sleep - Sleepless. Restless sleep, with painful dreams. Sleepiness is overpowering. Sleep heavy, interrupted by nightmare. Dreams of fire, confused, but not frightful. Dreams of activity and of serious events. Dreams not remembered.

Stomach - Feels full of broken stones or lumps. Qualmishness and extreme discomfort with dull pain and heaviness in pit of stomach. Belchings smelling like radishes. Nausea in morning. Vomiting of watery mucus of the odor and taste of the acid. Chronic vomiting, with pressure in stomach.

Temperature - Shivering, worse back. Fever, with difficult respiration, fever, with hot and dry skin. Sweat in axilla, smelling of garlic, worse evening and night.

Throat - Acute laryngitis, cough and expectoration of tough, stringy mucus. Talking causes pain in the larynx. Hoarseness, sore sternum.

Tongue - Tongue coated, red stripe in middle, fissured, one spot denuded. Tongue edges rough and covered with pimples. Tongue sensitive to touch when eating and drinking. Bad taste to coffee.

COMMENTS - The respiratory tract is irritated and pained from beginning to end. The nostrils and larynx are sensitive to cold air. Pain in larynx, trachea and in and under sternum on coughing. Talking causes pain in larynx.

Cough convulsive in paroxysms, hollow sounding as if one coughed into an empty tube, caused by irritation in larynx or low down in chest. Violent headaches, affecting the base of the brain.

Skin irritation, irritating eruptions, eczematous and herpetic. In the provings, the erections were severe almost to priapism and the ejaculations were longer-lasting and more copious than normal.

A woman, 62 to whom Clarke once gave Osm. 2x for a spasmodic cough with pain in the head had a severe aggravation, the headache taking this form: "Sharp pain in center of forehead going through to back, better by hard pressure on forehead." She discontinued Osm. and in two or three days that pain went away, leaving only an ordinary headache. The cough was not relieved.

G. S. Norton suggested that Osm. may be a remedy in many cases of glaucoma.

Cooper had a case of a girl of 14 with post-nasal growths who improved rapidly under Osm., 3x, but was seized with exhaustion, then under Hydr-ac., got quite well.

In one of Blackley's cases, a child born during the time that his father was under the influence of Osm. developed eczema, though none of the previously born children were eczematous. The kidneys were affected in another of Blackley's cases, incipient nephritis being set up.

C. M. Boger cured a case in which there was pain in both directions, "Stitching pain upward in left spermatic cord. Creeping sensation downwards in left spermatic cord. Weakness in calves, they give out while walking." Shootings in the sternum are up and down.

In another case of a man, 44, syphilitic was cured of "dull, steady pain in hypogastrium, sore to pressure. Steady aching in glans penis."

RELATIONS - ***Antidoted by:*** Sulfuretted hydrogen, Phos-ac., Sil. - swollen gums, Hep. and Psor. - pain in larynx, Bell. and Merc. - laryngeal catarrh. ***Compare:*** (1) Arg-n., Sel., Mang. (2) Irid., Tell., Thal., Plat., Pall. (3) In eyes and lungs, Chlor., Brom. (4) Skin of nails, Fl-ac. (5) Itch, Sulph. (6) Coryza, cough with pain in larynx, All-c. but it has better in open air. (7) Eruptions, Ars., Rhus-t.

REFERENCES - Boericke. Clarke. Phatak.

OSTEO-ARTHRITIC-NOSODE

PHARMACY - o-a-n. Osteo-arthritic-nosode. Made from the synovial liquid of arthritic joints. ***Historical dose:*** All potencies.

CLINICAL - Arthritis. Joint, pains. Osteo-arthritis. Rheumatism.

HOMEOPATHIC - A proving of the Osteo-arthritic-nosode of hip was read in the 18th All India Homeopathic conference at Madras on 10 Oct., 1970. The O-A-N. that originated from Dr. Foubister, comes from the knee of a patient suffering from an osteo-arthritic affection, and the other stock from the hip of a similar case.

State of stupor, indifference to others. Extreme weakness with somnolence in the afternoon and profound sleep. Weakness, worse in the morning when waking up. Great desire for sleep, with deep sleep at night.

MIND - Apathy. State of indifference. Nonchalance. Idleness, no desire to work. Indecision, needs relaxing. Irritability, worse towards evening.

Eyes - Styes of upper eyelid of the left eye.

Kidneys - Highly colored urine and less abundant, worse at noon.

Limbs - Pain in the right shoulder. Temporary redness and swelling of the right shoulder. Redness and swelling of the right forearm and right wrist. Muscular pain of the right hip. Pain of the Achilles tendon. Pain aggravated by the first movement, ameliorated by continued movement.

Male - Increase of sexual desire in men. Furuncle on the scrotum.

Modalities - Aggravation by the first movement, at night. Better by prolonged movement. Worse right side.

Skin - Furuncles.

RELATIONS - ***Compare:*** (1) Calc., Calc-p.

REFERENCES - Julian.

OSTRYA VIRGINIANA

(Ironwood)

PHARMACY - ost. Ostrya virginiana. Ironwood. Hop-hornbeam. Lever-wood. N. O. Cupulifere. Betulaceae. Tincture of heart wood. ***Historical dose:*** Tincture and all potencies.

CLINICAL - Anemia. Headache, dull. Head, numb. Intermittent fever. Liver disorders. Lumbago. Malaria. ***Nausea.***

HOMEOPATHIC - Ost. is sometimes regarded as a variety of the common Hornbeam naturalized in America, though native to southern Europe. The chief difference between them is that Ost. vulg. has pendulous catkins, and Ost. virg., upright. The wood is exceedingly hard and heavy.

The preparations of which the provings by Burt and others were made were from the wood. Marked action on the liver with the usual dull headache and pain in back and shoulders, cutting, sinking pains in abdomen. Nervous, languid, weak, uneasy. Very nervous with dull headache.

Increased appetite, hunger wakes the patient at 4 a.m. Sinking at the epigastrium. Sickening pains. Black stools. Bilious conditions and intermittent fever. Anemia from malaria.

Abdomen - Dull pains in right lobe of liver with sour belchings. Retraction of umbilicus. Rumbling, flatus, pain waking him in night.

Back - Back so painful, can hardly turn in bed, cannot sit up (better from Macro., Bry., Nux-v). Dull pain in whole dorsal region, extending to left hypochondrium. Constant lumbar and sacral pain, worse stooping or walking.

Ears - Drawing pain deep in left ear.

Face - Moist freckles in face, head and hands.

Food - Appetite greatly increased, woke with hunger at 4 a.m. Loss of appetite.

Head - Dull headache with numb, prickly feeling in head, face and hands, worse head. Dull, frontal headache with nausea. Right side headache, morning.

Limbs - Aching, dull pains in arms and legs. Fine drawing rheumatic pains in left fingers, morning. Drawing pains in right ankle.

Modalities - Worse moving, walking, stooping. Worse 6 a.m., 4 a.m., 3 p.m.

Mouth - ***Tongue yellow, coated at the root***. Taste is coppery, slimy, sweet, slimy, bitter, rough. Boring and sharp pain in right lower molars.

Rectum - Rectum feels sore, protruded feeling after stool.

Stomach - Sour stomach. Nausea and distress after riding in cold air. Burning distress in epigastrium. Hard sickening pains in epigastric and umbilical region, awaking him at night. Sinking in epigastrium. ***Frequent nausea*** with dull, frontal headache. Sickening pains.

Stool - Loose stools, bilious with tenesmus and straining, loose without tenesmus. Tenesmus followed by diarrhea stool. Mushy stool with burning at anus and tenesmus. Black stools, dry lumps.

COMMENTS - Allen mentioned "***Tongue coated yellow at root.*** Loss of appetite for breakfast and dinner. Frequent nausea with the dull frontal headache."

RELATIONS - ***Antidoted by:*** Macro., Bry., Nux-v. (lumbago). ***Compare:*** (1) Waking in night hungry, Ign., Lyc. (2) Black stools, Lept.

REFERENCES - Boericke. Clarke.

OVARY GLAND

(Oophorinum)

PHARMACY - ov. ovar. Ovary gland. Oophorinum. Ovininum. Ovarian extract. A sarcode. Trituration of expressed juice of ovary gland of sheep or cow. ***Historical dose:*** Trituration and all potencies.

CLINICAL - Acne, rosacea. Hormonal, imbalance. ***Hot flushings.*** Infantile, genitalis. Infertility. ***Menopause.*** Menstrual, disorders. Nervousness. Oophorectomy. Ovaries, disorders. Ovaries, cysts. Ovaries, tumors. Prurigo. Seborrhea. Sexual, weakness.

HOMEOPATHIC - Ov. has been used with much success in cases of suffering following excision of the ovaries (Sep.) and for the menopausal sufferings of women. Clarke had good results with it in such cases in the lower triturations.

Ov. has been suggested as a remedy in ovarian cysts. ***Menopausal disturbances*** in general. Cutaneous disorders and acne rosacea. Prurigo.

Female - Menses are frequent. too early. Menses are clotted, coagulated, copious. Menses of short duration. Infertility. Hot flashes. Menopause. Infantile genitalis.

COMMENTS - Characteristic amelioration from the menses, all symptoms better during menses (Lach., Zinc.). Generally associated with ovarian conditions, often after removal of ovaries (Staph., Phos.). Ovarian cysts (Thuj., Sil.), when nothing else works. Useful for menopausal symptoms, particularly hot flashes (Sep., Puls., Thuj.).

Severe hormonal acne (Sep., Puls., Thuj.). Spacey. Indecision, difficulty deciding who they are, about changing careers, about health.

E. Saalfeld, in view of Landau's observations on the effect of Ov. on the nervous sufferings of women at menopause, gave Ov. to women suffering from acne rosacea and other skin disorders of menopause.

A woman, 20, after a double oophorectomy, had lichen-like eczema. This was relieved by Ov. as well as the accompanying nervous symptoms and adiposity.

Saalfeld also obtained good results in some non-menopausal cases, including acne and seborrhea in chlorotic women. He had a case of prurigo that had lasted from childhood in a woman of 26. In this case, the itching was better for a short time after the period.

RELATIONS - ***Compare:*** (1) Orchitinum, Testicular extract - after ovariotomy, sexual weakness, senile decay.

REFERENCES - Boericke. Clarke. Murphy.

OVI GALLINAE PELLICULA

(Egg-shell Membrane)

PHARMACY - ovi-g-p. Ovi gallinae pellicula. Egg shell membrane. Membrane of the shell of a hen's egg. The fresh membrane is triturated in 95% alcohol, allowed to digest several days and then potentized (Swan). ***Historical dose:*** Trituration and all potencies.

CLINICAL - Amenorrhea. Backache. Catarrh. Coryza. Debility. Heart, oppression. Hip, pain. Leucorrhea. Menstruation, irregular. Ovaries, pains. Post-nasal catarrh. Pruritus vulvae. Throat, sore. Uterus, displacements, retroverted. Vertebra, pain. Vulva, soreness.

HOMEOPATHIC - Historically, egg shells were used powdered, fresh, or roasted, in the treatment of oxyuris vermicularis. Swan prepared the membrane. As an ovarian product, it might be expected that all parts of the egg should have an action on the ovaries, and that eggs would have a stimulating effect on the sexual functions. The provings confirmed this relation.

Sudden onset and ceasing. Sudden pains. Bearing-down sensation. Pushing and rushing feeling in womb, as if blood might rush out in torrents. Sensation as if something turned over inside.

Debility. Heat in sacrum, the rest of the body being cool. Pain in heart and left ovary. Backache and pain in left hip. Intolerance of bands on wrists, arms, waist, etc. Jerkings on going to sleep and in sleep.

Causations - Over-exertion. Strain.

Modalities - Dyspnea better bending backward, jarring or beating breast. Worse by movement, reaching, lifting arms, descending stairs, over-exerting. Worse pressure and touch, pressure of clothing, at full moon. Worse before, during and after menses, though some symptoms were better when flow appeared.

COMMENTS - This preparation was made by Swan. He noted that it has an ancient reputation for "immoderate flux of the menses" (Calc.) and for nocturnal bedwetting.

The first prover was a young woman, a patient of J. C. Boardman, who was known to be unable to bear any extra exertion, but the details of this were not known until after she had taken the first dose of the Ovi-g-p. 100,000c sent by Swan.

Some years before, she had felt something "give way" in the groin while shoveling snow, bringing on a left ovarian pain, extending down the left limb. The trouble was suddenly removed after the dose. The sensitiveness to exertion never returned, though the dose created much disturbance of the generative functions before it had finished its action.

The symptoms of a second prover, a married woman who took the Ovi-g-p. 30c, confirmed the symptoms experienced by the first. This prover had also hemorrhage from the rectum, incontinence of urine while sneezing or coughing, and post-nasal catarrh.

Yingling contributed the case of H. E., 42, blonde, who had a dull, hard, heavy aching in region of heart, generally about apex, extending at times to left ovarian region.

Occasionally a cutting which extended to base of heart and prevented breathing, after the cutting a sensation as if something went "thud," after which pain seemed to recommence at apex. At times, heavy aching in base of heart, which made breathing very difficult. Only bending backward alleviated respiration.

Ovi-g-p. (a preparation of Fincke's) was given, one dose, dry on the tongue. In a very few minutes the pain was all gone. "Feels splendidly since taking the remedy." Without knowing what it was, said she had "a taste of fresh eggs in the mouth since taking the powder."

RELATIONS - ***Compare:*** (1) Calc., Naja. (2) Ova tosta - Tosta preparata, Roasted egg-shells. Calc-o-t. - has leucorrhea and backache. A feeling as if the spine were broken and wired or tied together with a string. Pain of cancer. Warts. (3) Egg vaccine for asthma. Much interest is shown in Dr. Fritz Talbot's method to cure one form of asthma in children by the use of egg vaccine. Asthma due to susceptibility of the protein substance in eggs can be cured by immunizing against egg poisons by repeated doses of egg white. After the skin has been cleansed with soap and alcohol the egg-white is rubbed into a slight scratch.

REFERENCES - Boericke. Clarke.

OXALICUM ACIDUM

(Oxalic Acid)

PHARMACY - ox-ac. Oxalicum acidum. Oxalic acid. Sorrel acid. Hydrogen oxalate. Trituration. Tincture. ***Historical dose:*** All potencies.

CLINICAL - ***Allergies.*** Angina, pectoris. ***Aphonia***. ***Backaches***. Bedwetting. Chest, disorders. Cholera, infantum. Convulsion. Deltoid, rheumatism. ***Dyspnea***. Eyes, disorders. Gastrodynia. Gout. Gravel. Hernias. ***Hives.*** Indigestion. ***Kidney, stones.*** Meningitis. Myelitis. Nails, blue. ***Neuralgias. Neurasthenia***. Nose, disorders. Numbness. ***Oxaluria. Pains, severe.*** Paralysis. Pregnancy, sickness. Side, pain. Spasms. ***Spermatic cord, pain.*** Stomach, disorders. Tetanus. Testes, pains. Tongue, disorders. Tuberculosis. Urine, abnormal. Voice, altered.

HOMEOPATHIC - Although certain oxalates are constant constituents of vegetable food and of the human body, the acid itself is a violent poison when taken internally, producing gastro-enteritis, motor paralysis, collapse, stupor and death.

If Op. is the painless remedy, Ox-ac. may be considered its antithesis. It causes the ***most excruciating pains*** beyond description, which are all worse when the patient thinks of them.

Thinking of pains and conditions will bring them on when they are not actually present. Symptoms are worse by touch (small spots on head), slightest touch causes excruciating pain. Worse motion and ***thinking of pains.***

Neuralgias. Excruciating pains like lightning in streaks, burning in spots. ***Violent pains in spots*** (Kali-bi.). ***Rheumatism of left side.*** Periodical disorders. ***Periodical remissions***.

Neurasthenia. Weak, cold, livid and numb all over, worse lower limbs. Influences the spinal cord and produces motor paralysis. Paralysis of the left side from spinal meningitis.

Spasmodic symptoms of throat and chest. ***Angina pectoris, sharp, sharp pain in left lung coming on suddenly,*** depriving of breath. Tuberculosis. ***Severe back and kidney pains. Kidney stones.***

After eating pains at navel, colic, rumbling in abdomen, urging to stool, weakness. Pain in stomach, better from eating. Gnawing in stomach better from soup. ***Cannot eat strawberries, severe allergies.*** Sugar, coffee and wine disagree. Worse from shaving.

MIND - Exhilarated, quicker thought and action. Nervous and sleepless. ***Symptoms worse by thinking of them***, thinking of the conditions will bring them on when they are not actually present.

Abdomen - Stitching pains in the liver, better deep breathing. Burning in small spots in abdomen. Pain in upper part of abdomen after eating, with much flatulence. Chronic inflammation of bowels. Colic about the navel or involuntary muddy brown stools better lying. Flatus passes with difficulty. Fainting and vomiting during stool.

Back - Numb pricking in back. ***Backaches***, feels numb. Back feels too weak to hold the body. Cold creeps up spine.

Chest - Chest fixed. Sharp pain through lower region of left lung, extending down to epigastrium. Left lung painful.

Eyes - Severe pain in eyes, feel expanded. ***Hyperesthesia of retina***. Small, and especially linear objects, appear larger and more distant than they are. Sight vanishes with the nosebleed.

Face - Pale, cold, livid. Feeling of heat.

Food - ***Cannot eat strawberries, severe allergies.*** Sugar, coffee and wine disagree.

Head - Headache, before and during stool. Band like sensation about the head, as of a screw behind each ear, better after stool. Sense of heat. Numb pricking in occiput. Sore tender spot on scalp.

Heart - Precordial pains which dart to the left shoulder. ***Angina pectoris, sharp, sharp pain in left lung coming on suddenly,*** depriving of breath. Palpitations and dyspnea in organic heart disease, worse when thinking of it. Palpitations worse lying down. Pulse feeble. Beats of heart intermit when thinking of it. Aortic insufficiency. Fluttering in heart. Heart symptoms alternate with aphonia.

Kidneys - ***Severe kidney pains. Kidney stones.*** Must urinate when thinking of it. Frequent and copious urination. Oxaluria. Burning in urethra and pain in glans when urinating.

Limbs - Multiple sclerosis. Myelitis. Muscular prostration. Numb, tingling. Numbness extends from shoulders to fingertips. Lower limbs blue, cold insensible. Weak trembling, hands and feet. Hands cold as if dead. Drawing and ***sharp pains*** shooting down limbs. Pains start from spine and extend through limbs. Sharp pains in various parts, jerking pains. Wrist painful, as if sprained (Ulm.). Pain in fleshy part of thumb (right).

Liver - Stitches in liver.

Lungs - Spasmodic breathing with constriction of larynx and chest. ***Dyspnea, short, jerking inspirations***. Burning sensation from throat down. ***Left lung painful. Hoarseness.*** Paralysis of the tensors of vocal cord. ***Aphonia***.

Male - Seminal vesiculitis. ***Neuralgic pains in spermatic cord,*** worse from slightest motion. Testes, throb or feel crushed. Testicles feel contused and heavy.

Modalities - Better after stools. Change of position helps pain in back. ***Worse thinking of symptoms***. Worse from light, mental exertion, motion, ***left side,*** slightest touch, shaving, cold. ***Worse from strawberries,*** sour fruits, grapes. Worse evening, night and early morning. Worse from being aroused about 3 a.m. with gastric and abdominal pain. Lying down causes swimming sensation.

Mouth - Sour taste. Belchings, with difficult swallowing.

Rectum - Diarrhea from coffee.

Sensations - Sensation as if all blood had left the brain. As if blood in head was coursing upward and outward. As from a screw behind each ear. Hypogastrium as if bound. Back as if broken or bruised. Wrist as if sprained. Hands as if dead. Jerking pains like short stitches, confined to small spots, lasting only a few seconds. Sensation as from chafing during shaving.

Skin - Sensitive, soreness, smarting, worse shaving. Mottled, marbled in circular patches. Perspires easily.

Stomach - Emptiness with gnawing, compelling one to eat. Burning pain goes upwards, worse slightest touch, sugar. ***Cannot eat strawberries.*** Violent pain in epigastrium, discharge of flatus relieves. Gastralgia, heartburn, sensation of coldness below epigastrium. Bitter and sour eructation, worse at night.

Throat - Hoarseness with cardiac derangements. Voice altered. Low voice. Nervous aphonia (Coca, Hydr-ac.). Aphonia from paralysis of vocal cords.

Vertigo - Confusion and vertigo. Vertigo, swimming sensation on lying down, while looking out of window.

COMMENTS - Ox-ac., the chief constituent of Sorrel (Rumx-a.) and Wood Sorrel (Oxal.), exists in plants that are ordinarily deemed anti-scorbutic and are remarkable for the grateful acidity of their herbage.

Ox-ac. is said to enter largely into the inspissated juice of the Clover (Trif-p.) which formed Thomson's "Cancer plaster," and which is strongly escharotic.

Inspissated solutions of sorrel have been used successfully as local applications for epithelioma and with a solution of Ox-ac. and of Tannic acid, applied locally. With a solution of 5 grains to 3 ounces of water, Cooper removed troublesome small nevi in infants upon the face and elsewhere, using it for weeks or even months.

Cooper removed a large patch of erythematous lupus on the cheek. From this it would appear, taking into account that Ox-ac. produces wart-like growths, it may have a beneficial influence, locally and probably internally as well, upon epithelial proliferations of the cuticle.

In an interesting study of Ox-ac., J. W. Ellis cited a fatal case of poisoning recorded by Boericke through exposure of the hands to a saturated solution used for chemical purposes.

The symptoms were intense pains in head, hyperesthesia, especially to light. Spasms of pain down limbs, along throat muscles and through spermatic cord. Sensitive spots on spine.

Excruciating pain in lower back and loss of power in the lower limbs shows an unmistakable action on the spinal cord and its meninges. These symptoms are better seen in less severe cases of poisoning. In animals poisoned with Ox-ac. the first symptom is stiffness of hind limbs.

Farrington summed up the indications of Ox-ac. in spinal affections, including weak loins, hips, legs, numb back, numb limbs. Limbs blue and cold, weak and numb, worse going up stairs. Limbs stiff, paroxysm of dyspnea (as in spinal meningitis). Pains in small spots, especially linear spots. Pains worse when thinking of them. Erections with dullness in occiput. Left-side rheumatism.

Sharp shooting pain in left lung and heart, extending down to epigastrium. In afternoon, stitches several times in left lung. Sharp, sharp pain in lower lobe of left lung, coming on so suddenly that it deprives him of breath for a few seconds. Sore sticking in chest extending back to between scapula.

Pleurisy, pneumonia, tuberculosis. The heart may be paralyzed, becomes flaccid or distended with blood. Angina pectoris. Coldness of surface, numbness. Mottled skin, blue nails. Generally left sided.

Sugar aggravates the stomach pain. Wine causes headache. Oxaluria, with backache, numbness. Frequent ineffectual urging to stool, preceded by a sick, distressing feeling from navel downwards, worse when thinking of it, worse from drinking coffee. Faintness and vomiting during stool. Pain in back better after stool.

John Moore reportd the case of a sea captain who suffered from indigestion. Two years before Moore saw him he had to undergo an operation for strangulated hernia. Ever since he had been subject to pain in region of navel coming on two hours after eating, accompanied by much flatulence and bitter and sour belchings.

Pain worse in night, arousing the patient 3 a.m. and keeping him awake. Burning sensation from throat downwards to the region of the pain. The patient had always has a weak digestion and had met with many severe accidents at sea.

He was given Ox-ac. 3c, two drops, an hour after meals. He was a little better the first night and after that slept the night through and said he had not had so much comfort for years.

Bedwetting has been cured with Ox-ac. 6c in a blonde boy of six. The guiding symptom was "Sharp shooting pain in left chest, close to sternum and parallel to it."

D. Walker told Clarke of a case of his in which the patient, an elderly, gouty man, was suddenly seized with congestion of spinal meninges with great coldness, blueness and numbness with complete prostration of strength. Ox-ac. 6c rapidly cured.

A patient of Clarke who used Ox-ac. in his work suffered from "Rheumatism of left side. Starting on falling asleep. When actually at work, acidity."

W. M. Butler gave great relief with Ox-ac. 3c. in a case of paraplegia, affecting first the right then the left leg of a year's duration in an American woman, mother of four children.

In a few weeks the motor symptoms were better then the sensory. Sensation to heat and cold was restored, general tactile sensibility was improved. Some control was gained over bladder and rectum.

Hale cured a case of palpitation with action of heart irregular in force and rhythm, alternating with aphonia with Ox-ac. 6c. It was a favorite remedy with S. A. Jones in cardiac trouble, occurring in highly "nervous" patients. Ellis suggested that Ox-ac. corresponds to many cases of neurasthenia.

RELATIONS - ***Antidoted by:*** Carbonates of lime and magnesia. Lime water, antidote to poisoning of Ox-ac. ***Compare:*** (1) Ars., Colch., Arg-n., Pic-ac. (2) Cice., Chickpea - Lithiasis, jaundice, liver affections, diuretic. (3) Scol. - terrible pains in back and loins, extending down limbs, return periodically, commencing in head to toes. Angina pectoris. Inflammation, pain and gangrene. Pustules and abscesses. (4) Caes. - Pain in lumbar region and testicle. Headache, darting through temples. Diarrhea and colic. Languor. (5) Kali-ox. (6) In cholera infantum, Ars., Ip., Verat. (7) In gastralgia, Colch. (8) In spinal disease, Pic-ac., Arg-m., Ph-ac. (9) Induration of testicles, Puls. (10) Headache worse from wine, Zinc.

REFERENCES - Boericke. Clarke. Phatak.

OXALIS ACETOSELLA

(Wood Sorrel)

PHARMACY - oxal. Oxalis acetosella. Wood sorrel. N. O. Geraniaceae. Great Britain. ***Historical dose:*** Tincture and all potencies.

HERBAL - Diuretic, refrigerant. Reputed of value in febrile diseases, urinary affections, catarrh, and hemorrhages. The herb may be infused with water or boiled in milk and administered freely, although excess should be guarded against.

Joseph Miller said, "The juice, when clarified is a fine red color and makes a very agreeable syrup."

RELATIONS - ***Compare:*** Ox-ac. Rumx-a.

REFERENCES - Potter.

OXYDENDRON ARBOREUM

(Sorrel-tree)

PHARMACY - oxyd. Oxydendron arboreum. Sorrel-tree. Sour-wood. Elk-tree. Andromeda arborea. N. O. Ericacee, tribe Andromedee. Rich woods of the Alleghenies. Tincture of leaves. ***Historical dose:*** Tincture and all potencies.

CLINICAL - Ascites. Bladder stones. Dropsy. Prostatic enlargement.

HOMEOPATHIC - Oxyd. is the only species of its genus. It is an unproved remedy for dropsy, ascites and anasarca. Deranged portal circulation. Prostatic enlargement. Suppressed urine. Bladder stones. Irritation of neck of bladder.

COMMENTS - M. E. Douglass treated Mrs. H. for general dropsy, ascites and anasarca, which dated from an attack of measles treated with ice-drinks and ice-applications seven months before.

When Douglass saw her, the urine was nearly suppressed, but contained very little albumen. Great difficulty of breathing even when sitting, lying down impossible. Had to sit in one chair with feet in another. Menses suppressed.

After the failure of Apoc. and several carefully chosen medicines, the legs having burst in several places, Douglass was about to tap the abdomen, but before doing so put Oxyd. 3x in a tumbler of water and gave three teaspoonfuls every three hours.

In forty eight hours the breathing was better and urine increased. Oxyd. was continued (with the exception of three days during which Rhus-t. was given to combat erysipelas which had set in on left leg).

On the tenth day, the patient lay down on the bed and slept for three hours. Appetite increased, and in two months she was quite free from dropsy and felt perfectly well though much emaciated.

RELATIONS - ***Compare:*** (1) Ceref. - dropsy, Bright's disease, cystitis.

REFERENCES - Boericke. Clarke. Phatak.

OXYGENIUM

(Oxygen)

PHARMACY - oxyg. Oxygenium. Oxygen. Ozonum. Nascent Oxygen. Oxygen including ozone, which is nascent oxygen. Oxygen (At. Wt. 16). Dilutions of distilled water charged with the gas. Dilutions. ***Historical dose:*** Tincture and all potencies.

CLINICAL - Anemia. Cancer. Canker, sores. Coryza. Cough. Diabetes. Influenza. Morphine, poisoning. Mouth, sores. Strychnine, poisoning. Whooping cough.

HOMEOPATHIC - Oxyg. is said to liberate oxygen in nascent state in the tissues when it is taken internally, diluted with five or six parts of water. Undiluted, its taste is disagreeably metallic, though it can be used as a gargle without inconvenience. Diluted, it has no taste at all.

When taken as directed in doses of a tablespoonful with six of water it sometimes causes relaxation of the bowels followed by constipation.

Clarke said it set up all the symptoms of a common cold. Clarke found it of great value as an anti-septic lotion and application, and as a gargle in cases of sore throat. It has been known to stop the irritation of a raw throat, when ushering in a cold, from going further either up or down.

In cases of gonorrhea, Oxyg. renders the urine anti-septic, supplying an anti-septic lotion from within without interfering with the action of a specific homeopathic remedy.

Clarke gave it in a number of cases of cancer, and obtained favorable temporary results in some. Inhalations of oxygen have palliated some late cases of cancer, producing profuse discharges from the ulcerating mass of tumor with reduction of its growth, but no cure followed and death supervened.

Abdomen - Great flatulence, passing large quantities at stool.

Back - Excessive pains in whole sacral region, apparently in articulations, especially a sensation of tiredness all through pelvic viscera, even in perineum.

Causations - Morphine. Strychnine.

Chest - Bursting sensation in chest. Suffocating feeling in chest, tendency to breathe slowly. Tightness under sternum, worse bringing shoulders forward.

Eyes - Lancinating, paroxysmal pain in right eyeball, a little to left of pupil. Occasional rush of pain, filling whole right eyeball and extending into right temple, which then became hot. Tingling of conjunctive and skin of face.

Face - Tingling of skin of face. Rawness in throat.

Head - Dull frontal headache, worse in spot over left eye. Headache in outer half of right eyebrow, pain still in frontal region. Pain in left temple, which feels cold to touch. Continued sweat on scalp.

Limbs - Thighs and legs as if overworked, excessively fatigued. Eruption of pimples in the fold of right side of buttocks, near anus, becoming very sore and seemingly like blisters, as skin rubbed off it was left very sore. Itching of skin of metacarpal end of first phalanx of left index finger, no redness of eruption.

Lungs - Irritation of respiratory tract as when recovering from attack of influenza. Violent irritating cough and sneezing, followed by rawness in throat and air passages. Hoarseness and hard, shaking, tearing cough from tickling under sternum in night, worse lying either side, better lying on back with profuse, lumpy, tasteless whitish sputa. The sputa occasionally yellow, purulent. Dry, hacking cough, 2 to 5 a.m. Cough causes hawking, blowing nose, and a bursting sensation in chest.

Male - Fine stinging rash on right side of scrotum, lasting one day.

Mouth - Canker sores in mouth and cheeks.

Nose - Much indurated mucus in nose, necessitating frequent picking in morning, blowing out of lumps, generally tough, opaque, whitish yellow. Sneezes with the cough.

Perspiration - Sweat all over and headache between eyes. Sweat on scalp and slight moisture over body.

Rectum - Flatus seems to accumulate in rectum, causes desire for stool and fears to pass flatus lest stool should also pass.

Skin - Tingling of skin of face and conjunctive.

Throat - Rawness in throat. Irritation of fauces and glottis. Slight hoarseness, dryness of throat towards evening dryness increased around rim of glottis, at midnight woke with choking, burning dryness of glottis and upper larynx, no thirst. Aphonia with difficulty of controlling voice.

COMMENTS - Oxyg. is not chemically distinguishable from hydrogen peroxide, but it has none of the disagreeable features of that substance; it does not bleach articles it may touch or cause effervescence.

A cure of diabetes with large doses of Oxyg. is on record and many cases of whooping cough have been cured with inhalations of ozone. Dilute Oxydol is a useful preparation as a mouth wash in canker sores.

D. T. Playfair cured a desperate cases of morphine poisoning (30 grains Morph. had been taken) in a young woman of 37 with inhalation of oxygen kept up for ten hours. All the usual antidotes had been given before without avail. The patient was entirely well in twenty-four hours.

In one case, an elderly working class woman had a large fungating cancer of the left breast. Oxyg. was given internally and applied externally. It caused excessive discharge with corresponding reduction of the tumor.

After several, weeks the patient's legs suddenly swelled, rapidly increasing, and she sank, the tumor had at least three-quarters disappeared. The effect of the Oxyg. was probably to liberate the disease elements too rapidly for the organism to eliminate them, as Dr. Cooper suggested in his account of Orni.

Oxyg. 1,000c cured a case of cough from dryness in upper larynx and constant tickling in throat-pit. Hard, shaking cough causing soreness in epigastric region. Expectoration with every cough, thick, lumpy, tasteless.

Oxyg. 100,000c cured a cough excited by tickling in throat and causing soreness of chest, 2 to 3 a.m., better lying on back. In another case, Oxyg. 100,000c cured a case in which the patient was passing quantities of uric acid like ruby sand.

RELATIONS - ***Antidote to:*** Morphine and strychnine poisoning. Antidotes, Camph. ***Compare:*** Ozone. Chr-ac., Kali-bi., Kali-chl., Kali-perm., Osm., and oxidizing agents generally, Chlor., Electr.

REFERENCES - Clarke. Grimmer. Murphy.

OXYTROPIS LAMBERTI

(Loco-weed)

PHARMACY - oxyt. Oxytropis lamberti. Loco-weed. Oxytropis campestris. Rattle-weed. Astragalus campestris. N. O. Leguminose. Papilionoideae. Tincture of fresh plant without the root. ***Historical dose:*** Tincture and all potencies.

CLINICAL - Amblyopia. Apathy. Belchings. Bladder, irritability. Coughs. Delirium. ***Depression.*** Fevers. Impotence. Locomotor ataxia. Mania. Ovary, pain. Paralysis. Rheumatism. Spermatic cord. Sphincters, relaxation. ***Staggering, gait.*** Testicles, pain. Vertigo.

HOMEOPATHIC - The "Crazy-weed" or "Loco-weed" is of Spanish origin and has been variously identified by Gray as Astragalus legum, by others as Astragalus mollisimus, and by W. S. Gee, who made the proving, as Oxytropis Lamberti.

In Gee's proving, the tincture and potencies from 1x to 30x were used. A number of mind and brain symptoms were produced including despondency, forgetfulness, a feeling as if consciousness would be lost, fullness in the head and instability standing. There were pains both in testes and ovaries, and one male prover, naturally passionate, became impotent.

W. D. Gentry in June, 1895, sent Boericke & Tafel specimens of Oxyt. and as this firm is extremely careful about the botany of the plants they make their tinctures from, Gentry made these remarks concerning the plants he sent:

"My attention was first called to this plant last winter during January. Soon after my arrival on the territory, as it was almost the only green thing showing itself above the snow. Which covered the ground at that time for two or three days.

"Some cattle had been eating the weed and as I approached them they tried to move away, but in spite of their efforts they backed towards me and in their efforts to escape made some ludicrous maneuvers. I observed them closely for more than an hour and was reminded most forcibly by their actions of the symptoms of locomotor ataxia."

Gentry's observation of loco-disease in winter bears out what is said by other writers, namely, that it is only in winter, when food is scanty, that animals can be induced to commence eating the weed and then they cannot leave off.

Gentry made provings of the tincture of the whole plant and seeds on three persons. Two provers had "symptoms worse when thinking of them." They had "pleasant intoxicated feelings."

Both Gentry's and Gee's provers had well-marked pains in the eyes and disturbance of vision and Gentry's had "numb, pithy or woody feeling about and on the spine," and "loss of power to control movements of limbs."

Marked action on the nervous system producing uncertain, staggering or backward gait. Staggering gait. Reflexes lost. Trembling, sensation of emptiness. Vertigo. Congestion of spine and paralysis. Pains come and go quickly. Sphincters relaxed. Urging to urinate when thinking of it. ***Great mental depression.***

MIND - ***All symptoms worse when thinking of them*** (Ox-ac.).Stimulation of mind, pleasant, intoxicated feeling (Gent.). Mono-maniac tendency. Cannot think or concentrate his thoughts. Very forgetful of familiar words and names. Indifference to all interests. ***Depression***. Feeling as if he would lose consciousness. Disinclination to talk or study. Desires to be alone.

Abdomen - Full feeling in abdomen, causing short breathing after lying down in bed. Sharp, sharp pains all through abdomen. Sharp pain, running from right to left across bowels. Slight griping pain in region of umbilicus. Tenderness in epigastric region.

Back - Pain and stiffness of muscles of back of neck. Numb, pithy or woody feeling about and in the spine (Gent.).

Chest - A warm tingling sensation over left chest, just under skin. Oppression in lungs at 9 p.m.

Ears - Roaring sound in ears.

Eyes - Sight obscured, pupils contracted, do not respond to light. Paralysis of nerves and muscles of eyes.

Female - Pain in left ovary like something grasping or holding tightly.

Food - Loss of appetite. Appetite gradually increasing. Symptoms worse after eating, better after an hour.

Head - Full, warm feeling about head. Feeling of intoxication with loss of vision. Pain in maxillary bones and masseter muscles. Pressure on head, better after sleep.

Kidneys - Pain in kidneys, worse in right, with some tenderness (Berb.). Awoke with a heavy pain in kidneys. Urging to urinate when thinking of it. ***Profuse flow of urine***.

Limbs - Pain along ulnar nerve. Pains come and go quickly, but muscles remain sore and stiff. Numb feeling about spine. ***Staggering gait***. Patellar tendon reflex lost. Loss of coordination.

Lungs - Short and quick breathing from the full feeling in abdomen. Hard breathing, as though lungs and bronchials were closing. Short cough with tightness across chest. A dry cough, from any little exercise.

Male - No desire or ability. Pain in testicles and along spermatic cord and down thighs.

Modalities - Better after sleep, on side lain on. Pains better when moving about, better in cool air. Worse thinking of symptoms, every other day. Worse immediately after eating, better an hour after.

Mouth - Mouth very dry, especially in morning. Metallic taste in mouth. Gumboil on left lower jaw, profuse saliva. Pain in left lower jaw.

Nose - Frequent, violent sneezing with fluent coryza. Fluent coryza, somewhat bloody. Nose very dry, scabs form in it. Nose feels as if sunburned, red and shining, especially on ale. Feeling of pressure over bridge of nose.

Rectum - Sphincter seems relaxed. Looseness of bowels. Stools slip from anus like ***lumps of jelly***, mushy.

Sleep - Twitching of muscles on falling asleep. Wakes often. Restless, dreams of quarrel. Dreamed of spiders, bugs, of swimming in water. Dreams of a pleasant or lascivious nature. On rising feels sad, weary, despondent.

Stomach - Belchings with colicky pains. Belchings, as after taking soda-water with colicky pains. Stomach cold during the chill.

Temperature - Chill lasted until 2 p-m., then disappeared. As chill passes off a smarting in throat and a feeling as though lungs and bronchials would close up, making breathing very difficult. No thirst in either stage.

Throat - Throat dry and sore. Slight inflammation of pharynx, a "husky" feeling. Slight accumulation of mucus in larynx, hard to cough it up.

COMMENTS - The botanical articles in the Century Dictionary noted that Loco-weed is "any one of the several Leguminous plants producing the loco-disease in animals. Among them are Astragalus mollisimus and A. Hornii with several other species of the genus and Oxytropis Lamberti."

Henry's Botany reported that the foliage of "Oxytropis Lamberti is said to be injurious to cattle," so Dr. Gee was quite justified in taking this plant for the proving. The Astragali are very closely related to the Oxyt.

RELATIONS - ***Compare:*** (1) Astrag., Lath., Ox-ac., Bar-c. Loco plant is rich in Baryta. Lol. (2) Lath., Astra-me., Phys. and other Leguminose. (3) In symptoms worse when thinking of them, Ox-ac. (better, Camph.). (4) Pain in cord and tests, Ox-ac. (5) Pains right to left, Lyc. (6) better moving about, Rhus-t.

REFERENCES - Boericke. Clarke. Gentry.

OZONUM

(Ozone)

PHARMACY - ozone. Ozonum. Ozone. ***Historical dose:*** Tincture and all potencies.

CLINICAL - Aphonia. Backaches. Belching. Cancer. Heartburn. Hoarseness. Keloids. Nausea. Night-sweats. Photophobia. Sinusitis. Vertigo. Vitiligo. Vomiting.

HOMEOPATHIC - The name ozone derives from the Greek, which means "to smell," "to spread an odor."

Back - Backache in lumbar region. Lancinating and cutting pains.

Eyes - Tired eyes. Burning and twitching. Photophobia.

Nose - Sinusitis. Thick nasal discharges. Sensitive to smell.

Perspiration - Night-sweats.

Skin - Dry skin. Darker coloration of different parts of skin. Vitiligo. Itching. Scars that itch. Keloids.

Sleep - Falling asleep difficult despite tiredness, with tension. Sleep unrefreshing, troubled, wakes up often, tosses and turns. Frequent yawning and tired eyes, better after nap.

Stomach - Heartburn. Sour belching. Nausea and vomiting.

Throat - Dry throat in heated rooms, better fresh air with open window. Feeling as if a lump of mucus in throat, worse swallowing. Tries to get the lump out by coughing and clearing my throat, but this doesn't help. Shrill voice. Hoarseness. Husky voice when singing. Aphonia.

Vertigo - Vertigo, tottering, staggering on rising from crouching, with nausea. Sensation of falling, worse bending down, better lying down.

RELATIONS - ***Compare:*** (1) Oxyg., Carb-v.

REFERENCES - Murphy. Schadde.

P

PAEONIA OFFICINALIS

(Peony)

PHARMACY - paeon. Paeonia officinalis. Peony. N. O. Ranunculaceae. Tincture of the fresh root dug in spring; in autumn the root is said to be inert. ***Historical dose:*** Tincture and all potencies.

CLINICAL - ***Abscess. Anal, disorders.*** Bedsores. Breast, ulcerations. Ciliary, neuralgia. Coccyx, ulcer. Colic. ***Fissure. Fistula.*** Headaches. ***Hemorrhoids.*** Nausea. ***Nightmares.*** Perineum, ulcer. Sternum, pain. ***Ulcers.*** Varicose, veins. Vertigo. Vomiting.

HERBAL - Paeon. belongs to the great order of Ranunculaceae, which includes the aconites, acteas and hellebores.

HOMEOPATHIC - Chronic ulcers on lower parts of body, leg, foot toes, also breast, rectum. Skin is very sensitive, ulcerations from pressure of tight boots, bed sores etc. Shooting or splinter like pains. Rolls on floor from pain.

Congestion. Rush of blood to head, face, chest, burning heat and redness of eyes and face, burning, itching and swelling of anus, heat in throat in skin. Varicose veins.

Anal varicose veins. Anal disorders such as ***fissure, fistula, abscess and hemorrhoids***. Biting, itching, swelling, burning. Intolerable during and after stool. Oozing of moisture.

Both Dioscorides and Pliny cured ***nightmares*** with Paeon., the former with the seeds, the latter with the root. The dreams experienced by the provers were of a terrifying nature.

MIND - Ill-humor. Depression with irritability. Much affected by bad news. Excitement. Nervous. Apprehension in evening with anxiety. Anxious, afraid to talk with any one. Delirium.

Abdomen - Griping pain. Pinching in muscles. Cutting in umbilical region. Sensitiveness, worse along transverse colon and epigastric region. Crawling in abdomen. Colic with diarrhea, transversely across upper abdomen. Borborygmi.

Back - Sticking in last cervical vertebra. Pinching or griping. Boring in left scapula, better motion. Ulcers over sacrum, bedsores.

Breasts - Ulcer on lower part of left breast, consequent on abscess.

Chest - Heat in chest. Dull shooting from chest to back through the heart. Sticking pain in left chest. Cutting in left side when sitting bent over. Sharp pain in ribs above hepatic region in morning.

Ears - Jerking in cartilages. Sticking outward in right ear. Pinching behind right ear. One ear cold, the other hot. Itching in concha. Ringing, roaring in ears.

Eyes - Eyes red and watery. Dry and smarting, not easy to open. Burning, itching and dryness of eyes and lids. Conjunctivitis with lachrymation and contracted pupils. Inflammation of left ball with pain as if a grain of sand were under upper lid. Sticking in right upper lid towards inner canthus.

Face - Face red and puffy. Burning heat in face. Crawling in upper lip.

Female - External genitals swollen and painful.

Food - Appetite lost. Thirst.

Head - Rush of blood to head and face. Pain and confusion of head. Dullness, heaviness, vertigo and feeling of heat in head. Gnawing headache. Boring outward in right temple. Pain in occiput and in nape. Heaviness in occiput.

Heart - Pain beneath the heart as from anxiety. Dull shooting from front to back through heart. Pulse contracted.

Kidneys - Frequent and copious urination, disturbing sleep at night. Constriction in region of neck of bladder, so that urine passed only in droplets. Burning and scanty urine.

Limbs - Pain in wrist and fingers, knees and toes. Cramp in ulna at wrist. Weakness of legs, inhibiting walking. Jerking and tearing in limbs, then numbness. Weary pain in ankles when sitting. Pain in corns.

Modalities - Drinking water helps vertigo with nausea. Worse from touch or pressure, motion. Worse coming into warm room, night, ***during stool***.

Mouth - Tongue red.

Nose - Stoppage of nose, in evening in morning in bed with dryness. Crawling in tip of nose.

Rectum - Diarrhea with burning and internal chilliness. Sudden, pasty diarrhea with faintness in abdomen. Excruciating pain at anus, continues long after stools, must rise and walk about. Biting, ***itching in anus,*** orifice swollen. Burning in anus, then internal chilliness. ***Ulceration of anus and perineum, purple, covered with crusts.*** Painful ulcer, oozing offensive moisture on perineum. ***Anal fissures. Anal fistula. Hemorrhoids,*** large and ulcerated.

Skin - Sensitive, painful. Sensitive ulcers on lower part of body. ***Ulcers*** from pressure, bedsores. Painful ulcer, oozing offensive moisture on perineum, near anus. Ulcers below coccyx, around sacrum, varicose veins. Itching, burning, as from nettles.

Sleep - Sleepiness all afternoon. Sleep is restless. Sleep unrefreshing, disturbed by many dreams. ***Terrifying dreams, nightmares,*** of the death of relatives.

Stomach - Anxious aching in epigastrium. Periodical sticking upward from middle of epigastric region. Burning in epigastric region at night. Nausea. Vomiting and painful diarrhea.

Temperature - Shivering. Coldness of limbs with (burning) heat in face, back and chest. Rush of blood to head and face with sweat. Hot skin. Heat at night, disturbing sleep.

Throat - Biting posteriorly in palate in evening. Swallowing difficult. Scraping in throat. Sensation as if an acrid, burning vapor ascended throat. Heat extending to pharynx in throat and esophagus, worse hawking. Hawking caused by tenacious mucus in throat.

Vertigo - Vertigo when moving. Vertigo on every motion in a warm room. Vertigo with constant reeling and staggering.

COMMENTS - "Small ulcers on perineum near anus that constantly oozes very offensive moisture, painful for eight days." This symptom has been expanded by clinical observation, principally Ozanam's, into ulceration in general, ulcers from pressure, as bedsores and from ill-fitting boots.

"Sensation of splinter sticking in skin of right great toe when touched and violent pain as from pressure in left little toe." Ulcers are the seat of severe shooting pains. Tissues sensitive to pressure and injury, sensitive mind (Hell.).

"Griping pain in the abdomen, preceded and especially followed, by anxiety, trembling of legs and arms as though he were frightened, he became apprehensive if any one spoke to him and unpleasant news affected him exceedingly."

Fainting with diarrhea, stools are followed by intense chilliness, occurring generally a few hours after he felt the worst. Bad pain in anus compelling him to walk the floor all night or to roll on the floor. Symptoms worse by motion, walking. The right side is more affected than the left.

RELATIONS - ***Antidoted by:*** Aloe., Rat.

Compare: (1) Glech. - rectal symptom. (2) Ham., Sil., Aesc. (3) Rat. - great constriction of anus, stools forced with great effort. (4) in varicose veins, Ham. (5) In splinter sensation, anal fissures and abscess in ulcer, Nit-ac. (6) In splinter sensation and ulcers, Arg-n., Hep. (7) In ulcers, Hell., Hell-v., Sil. (8) In ulcers about the toes, M-aust. (9) In diarrhea, Sulph. (10) In effects of bad news, Gels.

REFERENCES - Boericke. Clarke. Phatak.

PALLADIUM METALLICUM

(Palladium Metal)

PHARMACY - pall. Palladium metallicum. Palladium metal. (Pd, At. Wt. 1065). Trituration. ***Historical dose:*** Tincture and all potencies.

CLINICAL - Constipation. Egotism. Eyelids, blisters. Flatulency. Headaches. Hysteria. Leucorrhea. Oophoritis. ***Ovaries, disorders. Ovarian, tumors.*** Sciatica. Sexual weakness. ***Tumors.*** Uterus, disorders. ***Uterine, prolapse***. Warts.

HOMEOPATHIC - Palladium, one of the rare metals, was first separated from native platinum by Wollaston in 1803 and was named after the planet Pallas, which had been discovered just before that time by Olbers. The metal is closely associated with platinum and gold.

Hering, who made the first provings in 1850, said that platinum and palladium, both proved in dust form, showed such similarity in their effects that the question arose whether corresponding differences might be found. Subsequent clinical experience has done much to distinguish between these two remedies.

F. Aguilar noted that Pall. is indicated in gynecological conditions where the disease had its inception in the right ovary, the uterine prolapse and retroversion, sub-acute pelvic peritonitis and concomitant symptoms being secondary.

Pall. affects the ovaries, especially the right, the uterus and the mind. ***Disorders of the right ovary,*** attended with pains that are better from pressure. Chronic oophoritis.

Bruised soreness. Stitches, rheumatic pains, suddenly changing and often lasting but a short time. Pains fleeting, transient. Every step causes pain in groin. Motor weakness, averse to exercise. Undressing causes itching all over body.

MIND - ***Love of approbation.*** Seeks the good opinion of others and attaches great importance to them. Desires flattery. Haughty. Pride, easily offended. ***Wounded pride*** and fancied neglect. Effected profoundly by slight offensives, real or imaginary.

Irresolution in morning. Irritability, takes everything in bad part. Irritability and impatience from headache. Very impertinent. Tries to appear as amiable as possible, but is obstinate. Anger with trembling. Inclined to use violent language. Curses and swears (Anac.).

Weeping mood. ***Keeps up brightly when in company***, much exhausted afterwards and pains aggravated. Excitement in company. Conversation aggravates. Desire for company, worse when alone.

Averse to mental exertion. Apprehension that something horrible will happen. Depressing news aggravates all symptoms. Ailments from bad news. Feels as if she were going crazy. Time passes too slowly. ***Delusion that he is neglected***, that she is not appreciated, that he has been insulted. Delusion had grown taller while walking.

Abdomen - Soreness of abdomen, swelling in right groin. Hollowness in groins. Shooting pain from navel into breasts or pelvis, better after stools. Intestines feel strangulated. Sensation as if intestines were bitten off. Flatulency. Abdomen feels sore after menses. Pain in abdomen worse coughing and sneezing.

Back - Tired feeling in small of back. Frequent, painful spasm in muscles of right side of neck, especially morning. Painful drawing in neck, shoulders and down left arm. Pain in back and hips with coldness of limbs.

Breasts - Sharp, stitching pain in right breast near nipple, worse from deep inspiration.

Causations - Ailments from bad news.

Chest - Stitches in right side of chest, through to the back. Worse from taking a long breath, better when walking in the open air.

Eyes - Blue half-circles under eyes. Dryness and itching of eyes in evening, which is not better by rubbing. Sensation of dryness on the edges of the lids. Small watery blisters on edges of lower lids. Dull, heavy pain in and behind left eye. Pain around left eye, extending beyond right eyebrow. Pain in right eye, temple and ear. Pustule under right eyelids, worse touch.

Face - Sallow complexion, blue. Soreness and painfulness of the right corner of the mouth. Pain in right and left lower jaw. Itching pimples on the face, the nose, behind the ears, in facial hair. Slower growth of facial hair.

Female - Menses come on at full moon. Menstrual discharge while nursing. Glairy, yellow leucorrhea before and after menses. ***Pain and swelling in region of right ovary***. ***Ovarian tumors.*** Ovarian pains, better pressure. ***Uterine prolapse with retroversion.*** Cutting pains in uterus, relieved after stool. Sub-acute pelvic peritonitis with the right-sided pain and backache, menorrhagia. Pelvis leaden heavy, worse standing. Shooting or burning pain in pelvis. Bearing-down pains, relieved by rubbing. Soreness and shooting pain from navel to breast.

Food - No desire for beer. Headache at dinner and after coffee.

Head - Headache, causing irritability and impatience. Headache, better fixing attention on it. Morning headache with weakness in back. ***Pain across top of head from ear to ear***, worse after an evening's entertainment with irritability and sour belchings. Temporo-parietal neuralgia with pain in shoulder. Sensation as if head were swung from behind forward, as if brain were being shaken. Itching on sides of head.

Heart - Pain in region of heart. Heart pain with paralysis of left arm. Pressing deep in the left side of the chest periodical, as if in the heart.

Kidneys - Cutting pain in bladder, better stool. Pressure in bladder, as if very full, but little urine is passed. Dark urine with brick-dust sediment or coloring the vessel red. Muddy (not dark) urine, urine like water mixed with blood.

Limbs - Fleeting neuralgic pains in various parts of the body. Sciatica. Rheumatic pain in right shoulder, in right hip. Heavy and tired limbs. Tired feeling in small of back. Darting pains from toes to hips. Itching.

Lungs - Stitches in chest on taking a deep breath. Frequent hawking of small solid lumps that he must swallow. When expectorating, sensation as if something were pushed into head. Abdominal pain is worse coughing and sneezing.

Male - Single stitches in urethra, extending down to corona glandis. Sensation as if testicles were bruised with pain in abdomen. In evening and at night no proper erection could be obtained.

Modalities - Better from diversion, touch, pressure, rubbing, after sleep, rest and stools. Sciatica, and colic are better from warmth (hot cloths). Worse from lively emotions, chagrin, social excitement, social functions. Worse standing, exertion.

Mouth - Tongue red in the middle (morning). Burning sensation on surface of tongue near tip. Tough mucus in mouth, slimy taste. Sensation as if upper incisors projecting. Left upper and outer incisor sensitive and feels like a foreign body.

Nose - Burning in nose with coryza, in evening. Painful pustule on point of nose, bleeds long after being squeezed. Blood pustule on right cheek, near wing of nose. Abdominal pain worse when sneezing or coughing.

Rectum - Constipation, stools are hard, frequently whitish like chalk. Dull pains in rectum, as from too long retained stool without urging. Frequent soft stool. Diarrhea with very little pain, night and day.

Sensations - As if he had grown taller. As if she could not touch anything. As if head were swung from behind forward. As if brain were being shaken. As if neck becoming stiff. As if bladder was filled. As if uterus would prolapse. As if parts of groins would tear. As if testicles were bruised. As if heads of femurs were forced out of their sockets and expanded. As if hand shattered.

Skin - Itching all over after undressing. Itching and crawling as from fleas on different spots, back, arms, abdomen, thighs, ankles. Redness of knuckles, warts on knuckles.

Sleep - Great sleepiness in afternoon (3 p.m.) and early evening. Wakeful until 2 a.m. Starting in afternoon sleep. Dreams every night of buildings, wide stairs, many rooms. Symptoms better by sleep.

Stomach - Nausea. Tasteless belchings, which do not relieve.

Temperature - Chilliness with cold hands and feet, with colic. Coldness of the limbs with pain in the back.

Throat - Tough mucus in throat, slimy taste. Glairy mucus from throat. Frequent hawking of small solid lumps, which he must swallow. Tickling (or sticking) as if a crumb of bread had lodged in throat. Sensation when swallowing as if something hanging near hyoid bone. Dryness in throat and on tongue without thirst.

Vertigo - Reels on coming into a room from exhaustion.

COMMENTS - Right-sided ovarian tumors (Thuj. for the left side). Uterine and ovarian disorders. Bearing down feeling, achiness. Uterine prolapse. "Headache across top of head from one ear to the other." Hering noted that the pains are fleeting, transient and hard to describe. Pressure relieves pains.

"Love of approbation." Easily hurt from slights, real or imaginary. "Wounded pride and fancied neglect." Depressed, weep easily (Puls.). Irritability, leading to violent expressions. Can curse and swear (Anac.). Better in society and worse after the party or entertainment.

Skinner cured a young woman who had excessive pain in the right ovary during the menses with Pall. The only relief she could get was by inducing her sister to sit on that region. This "better by pressure" distinguishes the pain of Pall. from the similar ovarian of Plat.

RELATIONS - ***Antidoted by:*** Chin. (diarrhea), Glon. and Bell. (headache). ***Compare:*** (1) Irid., Osm., Plat. (2) Right ovary, Apis, Graph., Podo., Plat. (3) Left ovary, Arg-m. - feeling as if left ovary growing enormously large. Lach. - worse pressure. Lil-t., Cimic., Sulph. (4) Tired backache, Helon. (5) Hysteria introverted state of mind, Tarent. (6) Crumb in throat, Hep. (7) Pain in spleen, Cean. (Pall. at menses). ***Complementary:*** Arg-n., Helon., Lil-t., Apis, Plat.

REFERENCES - Boericke. Clarke. Murphy. Phatak.

PALOONDO

(Gobernadora)

PHARMACY - palo. Paloondo. Gobernadora. Zygophyllum tridentatum. Larrea mexicana. Creosote-bush. N. O. Zygophyllaceae. Northern Mexico, California and Texas. The tincture is prepared from the leaves and young branches. ***Historical dose:*** Tincture and all potencies.

CLINICAL - Allergies. Anorexia. Bone, disorders. Colds. Influenza. Migraines. Nausea. Neuralgia. Osteoporosis. Rheumatism. Sinusitis.

HERBAL - Paloondo is a Mexican plant already familiar to the Aztecs. It grows in the dry territories of Northern Mexico, in California and in Texas. Dr. Willmar Schwabe introduced it into Europe.

Paloondo has been used for different illnesses affecting the locomotor system, especially for arthritic and rheumatic afflictions.

HOMEOPATHIC - Schutt proved the remedy in 1960 on two groups of provers, producing few symptoms of rheumatism. A clinical proving was first undertaken using 3x and 4x, for cases of muscle pain and polyarthritis with favorable results.

Palo. has allergic complaints, sneezing, face puffy on waking. Nasal allergic syndrome. Neurotic pains. At times, the pains are accompanied by vertigo. The pains are aggravated in the evening, on waking and after mental exertion. Nerve and rheumatic pains in the lower limbs and vertebral column. Growth dystrophy of the bones and cartilages. Bone dislocations, fractures and inflammations.

MIND - Irritable, extreme sensitivity to noise. Tired, stunned. Depressive or euphoric condition with excitability. Bad-tempered, but more often, euphoric to the point of hyper-excitability.

Female - Menses early and painful.

Food - Anorexia.

Head - Acute pains in the head. Drawing pains coming from the occiput and spreading across the top of the head to the eyes. Occipital neuritis.

Heart - Heartbeat irregular with extra systole.

Limbs - Feeling of lead weight in the legs. Sensation of cracking. Pricking sensation in the limbs. On waking, pains in the limbs and the back, better by moving. Iliac and sacral pain, worse by being seated or lying down, ameliorated by walking.

Modalities - Better from walking. Worse in the evening, after mental exertion, on waking.

Rectum - Foul smelling, constipation or diarrhea.

Skin - Redness with sensation of heat. Dryness of the skin with itching. Dry eczema.

Sleep - Dreams lively, especially in people who do not usually dream at all. Anguished dreams.

Stomach - Distention. Nausea, especially in morning. Cramping abdominal pains.

Temperature - All the provers experienced a febrile influenza-type condition. Shivering, as at the onset of influenza.

RELATIONS - ***Compare:*** (1) Rhus-t. - Generalized stiffness with physical and cerebral restlessness. (2) Eup-per. - Generalized stiffness and sensation of cracking with pains between the bones. (3) Asar. (4) Ther. - Intolerance of the slightest noise.

REFERENCES - Julian.

PANCREATINUM

(Pancreas Extract)

PHARMACY - pancreat. Pancreatinum. Pancreas extract. Pancreatic glands of ox or sheep. Sarcode. Trituration. ***Historical dose:*** All potencies.

CLINICAL - Diabetes. Diarrhea. ***Gout.*** Hypoglycemia. Mumps. Pancreas, disease.

HOMEOPATHIC - Pancreat. has been used with success in conditions due to disease or faulty action of the pancreas on the analogy of thyroid and the other sarcodes. Pancreat. is a combination of several digestive enzymes.

Pancreas disease. Pancreatic diabetes. Hypoglycemia. ***Atonic dyspepsia***, due to impaired secretion or defective composition of the digestive enzymes secreted. ***Dyspepsia, when the power of digesting fatty and starchy food is deficient.*** Acid dyspepsia, resulting from abnormal digestion of food.

Intestinal indigestion, pain an hour or more after eating. Indigestion of fats and starches. Indigestion of children who are fed chiefly upon milk and sweets, and starches. Lienteric diarrhea. Mumps.

COMMENTS - Burnett noted that Pancreat. is often of great service in gout.

RELATIONS - ***Compare:*** (1) In action on pancreas and salivary glands, Iris, Nux-v., Puls., Merc., Iod., Jab., Piloc.

REFERENCES - Boericke. Clarke.

PANDANUS CONOIDEUS LAM

(Buah Merah)

PHARMACY - pand-c. Pandanus conoideus lam. Buah merah. Red fruit. Blood fruit. ***Historical dose:*** Tincture and all potencies.

CLINICAL - AIDS. Asthma. Baldness. Bone, cancer. Brain, cancer. Breast, cancer. Cachexia. Cancer. Cirrhosis. Cough. Cysts. Dengue fever. Diabetes mellitus. Fatigue. Gout. Heart, disease. Hepatitis. Hypertension. ***Immune, problems.*** Leukemia. Lymph, cancer. Osteoporosis. Parkinson's disease. Rheumatism. Sinusitis. Stamina. Stroke. Toxoplasmosis. Tumors. Uterine, cancer.

HERBAL - Buah Merah is grown only at the eastern portion of the Indonesian Islands, Papua, (east of Borneo and Bali). It is reported to be an effective tonic for the blood and immune system. The active substances are high in antioxidant and antivirus effects, proven to support the body's natural defenses in illness.

Useful to assist the healing process of multifarious diseases including cancer and tumors. Leukemia. Lymph, bone cancer, brain, liver, breast, uterine, and ovarian cancer, cysts. Lung spots in infants.

Hypertension. Heart disease. Lung weakness. Stroke. Parkinson's disease. Epilepsy. Rheumatism and osteoporosis. Hepatitis and cirrhosis. Diabetes mellitus. Eye irritation, blindness. Sinusitis. Lack of stamina, emaciation. HIV, AIDS. Dengue fever. Toxoplasmosis. Baldness.

COMMENTS - People who took Buah merah were found to have much less incidences of HIV/AIDS, hepatitis, cancer, heart and hypertension diseases.

REFERENCES - Buttimer. Murphy.

PAPAYA VULGARIS

(Papaya Tree)

PHARMACY - papay. Papaya vulgaris. Carica Papaya. Papaw. N. O. Cucurbitaceae. A tincture is made of the milky juice of the green fruit of the "Papaw." ***Historical dose:*** Tincture and all potencies.

CLINICAL - Colds. Constipation. Cough. Dyspepsia. Eczema. Epithelioma. Headache. Itching. Nausea. Neuralgia. Numbness. Pimples. Toothache. Tumors. Vertigo. Warts.

HERBAL - The ripe fruit is refreshing and palatable, it is sometimes used as a sauce, the seeds are very similar to capers, it is sometimes preserved in sugar or boiled like turnips. The juice is used to remove freckles and is also a strong vermifuge. The leaves are used as a substitute for soap.

Papain is the dried, white, powdered, unripe juice of Papaw, a ferment, and strongly suggests pepsin in odor, taste and appearance. When the unripe fruit is pierced with a knife, a milky juice exudes which is collected in a basin and allowed to coagulate. This is dried in the sun and contains a propeolytic enzyme which acts as a neutral or alkaline solution, and is given for impaired digestion.

It is said to dissolve the fibrinous membrane in croup and diphtheria when a solution over the pharynx painted every five minutes. When injected into the circulation in large doses, it paralyses the heart. Glossal fissures and ulcerations, and particularly syphilitic ulcerations of the throat, mouth and tongue, are asserted to have yielded to alkaline solutions of papain.

Applied to the skin, it renders it softer and smoother, and appears to destroy the projections formed at certain points by a greater thickening of the epidermis. Hardened tissues, produces by irritation, etc. Warts, corns, chronic forms of scaly eczema. Cutaneous tubercules, epithelioma. Injected into indolent glandular tumors to promote their absorption.

It is not caustic or astringent, but has the virtue of dissolving muscular and connective tissue. The seeds possess an identical property, and will probably be found preferable for administration. It is likewise said to cause the destruction and expulsion of the tapeworm.

Catarrh of the stomach. Atonic and fermentative dyspepsia, with painful acid eructations, flatulence, and constipation. Digestive failure accompanying continued fevers. Stimulates the stomach in the beginning of convalescence, and in some cases increases the appetite and promotes absorption of the digested pabulum.

HOMEOPATHIC - Muscular debility. Languor and drowsiness. Dull feeling in morning on rising. Pains worse towards evening, better by rubbing. Loses flesh. Catches colds easily when riding, during menses. Nervous before and during menses.

MIND - Impatient. Unusually active, can study longer without weariness, likes to read. Unable to think quickly. Stupid, confused feeling. Could hardly trust herself to do anything during menses for fear of making mistakes. Forgetful. Listless, lacking in ambition. Wants to be alone. Dislikes to be talked to or to answer.

Back - Sore pain in point under left scapula. Bruised pain in left side. Pain in region of kidney region, of left kidney, running around ilium.

Bladder - Tearing in bladder, with desire to urinate. Frequent desire to urinate. Irresistible desire at sound of running water, even in horse's throat when drinking. Straining with the first urinary effort in morning, with burning as if an obstruction were being overcome, which being removed, the urine passes easily. Burning in urethra during and after urination, with continuous desire. Urine increased, scanty. Less sediment than formerly.

Ears - Itching behind left ear.

Eyes - Prickling in eyes. Pain in eyeballs. Dry feeling in eyeballs. Inflammation of right lid, feeling as if a foreign substance were in it, preventing much reading by artificial light. Vision not as good as usual.

Face - Neuralgia on left side of face.

Female - Itching on mons veneris.

Food - Appetite diminished in morning. Thirst, but inability to drink cold water on account of toothache. Drinks much water.

Head - Headache towards evening. Headache after eating popcorn and candy. Headache worse bright light, warm air and motion, better cold air, rubbing, sleep. Pain involving eyeball, passing backward to occiput and nape, drawing head backward. Frontal pain. Piercing pain traveling like lightning from right side of head to right side of foot. Bruised feeling in left side. Soreness of parietal region with throbbing. Dullness. Fullness in evening. Itching greater, but dandruff less than usual.

Heart - Shooting pain in heart. Pulse slow and weak. Pulse 100, temperature 102.

Limbs - Numbness, pricking and sleepiness. Limbs go to sleep easily. Numbness, better walking. Trembling of lower limbs, with weakness of them. Prickling in lower limbs, but not in foot, with tingling. Right leg went to sleep when writing. Pain on ball of right foot under little toe, with swelling and with heat extending to toes. Itching on right ankle on going to bed. Itching forearms and anterior part of thighs, with diffused redness, worse warmth of bed. Rheumatic pain in left shoulder, left arm helpless. Numbness of right hand and fingers while asleep, especially little finger. Numbness of right ring finger, worse on outer side.

Lungs - Cough keeping him awake at night. Violent, sudden, spasmodic cough with easy expectoration and soreness of left lung. Shooting in lungs and around heart. Pain in left lung. Deep pain in upper lobe of left lung. Pain from left chest to left thigh and knee. Heavy pain, in left lung, extending through to back and becoming stabbing. Lungs feel tired and hot.

Male - Pain running from perineum to middle of penis as if a rough, jagged body forced its way out. Pain in left testicle, waking him at night. Instinct abnormally aroused. Erections towards morning. Erections, but no emissions, not long-lasting and not due to sexual thoughts. Emissions without lascivious dreams. Flaccid and lifeless. Functions depressed.

Mouth - Toothache in lower molars, with soreness, worse cold water. Tongue dry at night. Food tastes flat.

Nose - Nose stopped, worse left side. Thick discharge from nose watery, colorless, bland coryza.

Rectum - Irregular bowel movements. Constipation. First part large and hard, breaking into balls, later part mushy, with wind. Soft stool.

Skin - Itching all over body. Red, itching elevations, worse evening and warmth to bed, better scratching. Itching eruption over right eye. Eruption in groins, bends of knees and right elbow, extending along flexor surface, and on right forearm and abdomen. Pimples on face and body. Red, sore, elevated points, like acne, on thighs. Pinkish erysipelatous swelling on dorsum of left great toe, with itching, better scratching or rubbing. Eruption like nettle-rash after scratching.

Sleep - Yawning and stretching. Drowsy, but cannot sleep. Disturbed. frequent waking. Heavy sleep. Horrible, vivid dreams, of shipwreck, drowning, being shot, fire.

Stomach - Faint for want of food, but food distresses stomach. Pain around waist. Tasteless eructations. Nausea after dinner.

Temperature - Chilly at night, in open air. Cold hands and feet, forefingers, with deadness, stoppage of circulation.

Throat - Pain in larynx. Hoarse in evening.

Vertigo - Vertigo and throbbing frontal headache with nausea.

COMMENTS - Psoric conditions, particularly when caused by suppression of an itch.

Digestive disorders causing great pain when food is taken. Digestive disorders of pregnancy, stimulating appropriation and assimilation, particularly when the digestion is seriously interfered with during the last three months of pregnancy.

REFERENCES - Allen. Ellingwood. King. Murphy.

PARAFFINUM

(Purified Paraffin)

PHARMACY - paraf. Paraffinum. Purified paraffin. Obtained by distillation of wood peat bituminous coal petroleum and others. Trituration. ***Historical dose:*** Tincture and all potencies.

CLINICAL - Abdomen, swelling. Breasts, disorders. ***Constipation.*** Diaphragmitis. Indigestion. Leucorrhea. Menorrhagia. Musca, volitantes. Spinal, pain. Spleen, pain. Umbilicus, pain. Uterus, disorders. Vertebrae, disorders. Vision, disorders.

HOMEOPATHIC - Paraffin as a generic term includes all those substances which have no affinity for sulphuric acid and cannot be destroyed by it, including petroleum.

Specifically, Paraffin is a tasteless, inodorous, fatty matter, which resists the action of acids and alkalis, obtained by the dry distillation of wood, peat, bituminous coal, petroleum, etc. In the distillation of petroleum, naphthalin is the first substance that comes off, paraffin the next.

The homeopaths of Rome found it serviceable in uterine and other troubles, particularly constipation.

Pains in the groins, stabbing in mons veneries, cutting pain from one iliac crest to the other. Leucorrhea, pruritus vulvae and other disturbances of the female generative system with pains. Uterine disorders.

Knife-like pains. Pains extend from one part to another and alternate. Pain in stomach alternates with pain in throat and spine. Aversion to tobacco, smoking causes pain in stomach. Stomach pain with palpitations. Constipation.

Abdomen - Pain in lower abdomen, extending to genitals, rectum and coccyx, better sitting.

Back - Pains in spine, extending into lumbar vertebra. Pains in spine as if it had been injured, as bad during rest as when in motion. Back pains are worse by bending. Drawing and stinging between the shoulders. Pains as if from fatigue in both loins.

Breasts - The nipple is painful on touching them, as if sore inside.

Chest - Chest pains as if compressed. Stinging in chest. Diaphragm, as if it was inflamed.

Ears - Roaring in right ear like rumbling of a mill wheel, afternoon. Gurgling in left ear like beating of pulse. Ringing in both ear, morning. Stinging and twisting in left ear.

Eyes - Vision dim, with black specks. Sensation as if there were fat on the eyes. Lids red.

Face - Itching in face as from urticaria, smooth red spots appear.

Female - Menses too late, black, abundant. Milky leucorrhea. Nipples pain when touched, as if sore inside. Stabbing pain in mons veneris. Very hot urine with burning pains in vulva.

Head - Left side of head and face suffer most, pains stinging and twisting. Pain as if a nail were driven in left side of vertex. Twisting in left ear.

Heart - Pulse weak, thready, increased in frequency.

Limbs - Pain in spine extending to inguinal region and in both loins, when ascending the stairs. Feeling of electric shocks in all joints. Wrenching pain in calves, extending into toes in joints. Feet swollen with tearing in ankles and soles.

Modalities - Better after sleep, rest. Better by supporting the part. The pains are worse bending over. Worse standing or walking (soon bring back the symptoms).

Mouth - Tearing, twisting pain in teeth down to lower jaw. Full of saliva, feels sticky, bitter taste.

Nose - Odor of cordials in nose. Nose moist, frequent desire to blow it, but without sneezing. Nosebleed, dark red.

Rectum - Frequent desire for stool. Chronic constipation with hemorrhoids and continual urging to stool without result. ***Obstinate constipation in children*** (Alum., Nyct.).

Skin - Frost bite. Burns, even of third degree with sloughing and sepsis; wash with sterile water and dry and spray with paraffin and cover with thin layer of cotton.

Sleep - Continued yawning, although the joints of the jaw are painful. Frequent gaping with great somnolence. Cannot keep awake and goes to sleep in her chair, her feet go to sleep. Sensual, lascivious dreams.

Stomach - Hungry all the time. Pain across stomach. Pain in stomach alternates with pain in throat and spine, extends to chest with belching. Fixed pain in left hypochondrium, as if parts were being twisted. Stomach pains with palpitations.

Teeth - Tearing in teeth. Stabbing pain in one of the left lower molars. Twisting in teeth with stinging in ear. Twisting pain in left lower teeth and left temple, sleep impossible.

Temperature - Chill, heat, and sweat, frequently alternating. Chill, followed by dry heat with thirst, which is soon followed by sweat. Face and hands hot and red, hot sweat on upper part of body, especially forehead.

Throat - Dryness of throat, fauces as if dried up, but without thirst. Sense of suffocation in pharynx.

COMMENTS - Knife-like stabs, twisting, wrenching pains, stinging and twisting, electric pains. Pains extend from one part to another and alternate. Pain in the stomach alternates with pains in throat and spine.

Clarke recorded the case of Mrs. W., 37, mother of three children, who suffered since her last confinement, five years before, with bearing-down pains, excessive menses, and leucorrhea. Constant and violent indigestion with morning retching or vomiting.

Pain in back, shoulders and abdomen after, any food, however light. The pains, which "double her up" were worse on standing. Much thirst. Constipation with hemorrhoids. Constant desire to pass water.

After Murx., and Alstonia constricta had given some relief, the indigestion returned in full force. A few globules of Paraf. 30c were dissolved in water and a teaspoonful taken every two or three hours.

In a few days, all symptoms of indigestion were gone and did not return. Other symptoms were ameliorated. The menses, instead of recurring too soon, were delayed much beyond the normal time.

Paraf. also has a remarkable action in joints with nodules. Cooper saw swollen joints lessen considerably from its use as a liniment.

RELATIONS - ***Compare:*** (1) Napht., Petr., Eupi. (2) Desire to walk fast, Buff., Iod. (3) Uterine symptoms, Sep., Murx., Nat-m., Nat-s. (4) Intolerance of tight clothing, Lach.

REFERENCES - Boericke. Clarke.

PARAQUAT

(Nitrogen Herbicide)

PHARMACY - paraq. Paraquat. Nitrogen herbicide (1,1'-dimethyl-4,4'-bipyridinium). ***Historical dose:*** All potencies.

CLINICAL - Abdominal pain. Coma. Convulsions. Diarrhea. Dyspnea. Eye, problems. Incoordination. Kidney, failure. Liver, problems. Lung, problems. Lung, scarring. ***Nail, problems.*** Nausea. Pulmonary, edema. Respiratory, failure. ***Skin, problems.*** Tachycardia. Vomiting.

HOMEOPATHIC - Paraquat is a quaternary nitrogen herbicide widely used for broadleaf weed control. It is a quick-acting, nonselective compound, that destroys green plant tissue on contact and by translocation within the plant. It is also used as a crop desiccant and defoliant, and as an aquatic herbicide.

Paraquat affects the lungs, heart, liver, kidneys, cornea, adrenal glands, skin, and digestive system. It causes skin and eye irritation and also has caused skin sensitization. Paraquat splashed in the eye can irritate, burn, and cause corneal damage and scarring of the eyes.

Direct contact with paraquat solutions or aerosol mists may cause skin burns, dermatitis, and damage to fingernails. After prolonged skin exposure, workers get damaged fingernails as indicated by discoloration, nail deformities, or loss of nails.

Effects due to high acute exposure to paraquat may include excitability and lung congestion, which in some cases leads to convulsions, incoordination, and death by respiratory failure.

If swallowed, burning of the mouth and throat often occurs, followed by gastrointestinal tract irritation, resulting in abdominal pain, loss of appetite, nausea, vomiting, and diarrhea. After a person ingests a large amount of paraquat, he or she is likely to immediately have pain and swelling of the mouth and throat.

The next signs of illness following ingestion are gastrointestinal symptoms, such as nausea, vomiting, abdominal pain, and diarrhea (which may become bloody). Severe gastrointestinal symptoms may result in dehydration, electrolyte abnormalities (not enough sodium and potassium in the body), and low blood pressure.

Ingestion of small to medium amounts of paraquat may lead to development of liver, kidney or heart failure, or lung scarring, within several days to several weeks. Ingestion of large amounts leads to pulmonary edema, lung scarring, respiratory failure, leading to possible death, heart injury, increased heart rate, confusion, seizures, or coma, within a few hours to a few days.

Other toxic effects include thirst, shortness of breath, rapid heart rate, kidney failure, lung sores, and liver damage. Some symptoms may not occur until days after exposure. Persons with lung problems may be at increased risk from exposure. Many cases of illness and/or death have been reported in humans.

REFERENCES - Murphy.

PARATHYROIDINUM

(Parathyroid Hormone)

PHARMACY - parathyr. Parathyroidinum. Parathyroid hormone. Sarcode. ***Historical dose:*** All potencies.

CLINICAL - Arthritis. ***Bone, disorders. Calcium, deposits.*** Chilblains. Emaciation. Fibrocystic, osteitis. Hematuria. Kidney, stones. Multiple, myeloma. Muscular, hypotonia. Myasthenia. Osteogenesis, imperfecta. ***Osteoporosis. Paget's disease.*** Pancreatitis. Polyuria. Rheumatism. Tabes. Varicose, ulcer.

HOMEOPATHIC - Parathyroid secretion plays an important part in phosphorus and in the regulation of calcium in the blood. The hypercalcemic parathyroid hormone was first isolated in 1925 by Hansen. It increases the level of calcium in the blood, reduces the level of calcium in the urine and increases the amount of phosphorus in the urine.

General weakness. Asthenia. Fatigue. Depression. Pallor. Emaciation. Tabes. Dry skin, eczema. Hair loss. Grave's disease. Hypersensitivity. Nervous irritability. Hypomania.

Paralysis agitans. Puerperal convulsions and epilepsy. Tetany, when there is a disturbance of the calcium metabolism and it is associated with muscular irritation and hyperexcitability. Chronic rheumatism. Pains in the thorax, lumbar region and lower limbs.

Arthritis of the wrists, ankles, knees, hips. ***Demineralization of the bones. Osteoporosis.*** Diffuse pain in the bones, especially in the long bones. Paresis of the limbs. Walking painful, difficult, dragging. Myasthenia gravis. Muscular hypotonia. Paget's disease.

Belated gastric attacks. Polyuria. Hematuria. Increased level of calcium and reduction of phosphorus in the blood, increased alkaline phosphate liberating enzymes. Great calcium loss.

MIND - Depression. Mental confusion. Agitation. Hypomania.

Abdomen - Slow digestion, eructation of gas. Chronic pancreatitis. Gastric and duodenal ulcer.

Back - Weakness and curved spine. Strong pain in the lumbar region, spreading towards the bladder and thigh, tenesmus of the bladder with occasional vomiting.

Blood - Increase in the level of calcium in the blood. Reduction in the level of phosphorus in the blood. Increase in the alkaline phosphate-liberating enzymes.

Constitutions - Syphilitic condition in a phospho-fluoric type.

Eyes - Scleritis.

Face - Pale face.

Female - Dysmenorrhea and rare menses. Uterine fibromyoma.

Food - Anorexia, loss of appetite.

Heart - Palpitations and tachycardia. Infarction of the myocardium. Precordial pains. Inflammation of the coronary arteries.

Kidneys - Increase in the level of calcium in the urine with or without an increase of calcium in the blood. Calcium deposits in the kidney parenchyma. Calcium kidney stones. Polyuria and hematuria. Disorder of glomerular clearance and urea clearance.

Limbs - Diffuse pains in the bones, especially the long bones, aggravated by standing and walking. Deformity of the fingers. Bones sensitive to pressure. Paget's disease. ***Demineralization of the bones.*** Painful post-traumatic osteoporosis. ***Osteoporosis.*** Osteogenesis imperfecta. Fibrocystic osteitis. Painful non-inflammatory lesion of the bones. Chilblains.

Mouth - Caries and arthritis of the tooth sockets.

Rectum - Atonic constipation or frequent stools, abundant, whitish and fetid.

Skin - Strumous edema of the legs. Varicose ulcer.

Stomach - Gastric acidity. Painful after-meals gastric attack. Stomach and duodenal ulcers. Vomiting of blood. Sickness of pregnancy.

COMMENTS - Experimental results have indicated the existence of a parathyroid secretion whose action diminishes the level of calcium in the blood. It was the clinical syndrome of the primitive hyperparathyroid hormone which drew Fouche's attention to establishing a homeopathic symptomatology.

Primary hyperparathyroidism is explained by an osseous syndrome whose clinical manifestation is expressed by pain in the bones, aggravated by standing or walking and also expressed by spontaneous fractures, swelling in the bones and bone deformities.

In radiology, one can observe abnormal transparency of the skeleton, the cortex of the long bones is decalcified, the medullary canal is enlarged and these signs are especially present in the hands and jaws. Cavities can also be seen, again, primarily in the hands and jaws, as well as tumors, which enlarge the bones by pushing back the periosteum.

The extra-osseous syndrome occurs in 40% of the cases. It is characterized by its effects on the urinary organs, polyuria, kidney stones and nephrocalcinosis. Effects on the digestive system with anorexia, post-prandial epigastric pains and constipation. Gastric atony and ulcers in the low duodenum.

Effects on the heart muscles with palpitations, tachycardia and shortening of the Q. T. interval on the electrocardiogram. Effects on the muscles with asthenia and muscular hypotonia. Psychological effects with depressive tendency and mental confusion.

The syndrome is characterized by an increase of calcium and reduction of phosphorus in the blood, as well as an increase of phosphates in the urine and an increase of the alkaline phosphate-liberating enzymes. Fouche noticed that the removal of the parathyroid gland improved the condition of patients with chronic ankylosing rheumatism, but only temporarily.

Secondary hyperparathyroidism can occur as a defense reaction by the organism, which aims to maintain the normal level of calcium in the blood.

The level can become reduced as a result of a diminution in the calcium deposits in the bone or disorders of alimentary deposits or because of absorption complaints.

It can also be reduced from destruction of the skeleton following osseous carcinoma or myelomas, or from kidney infections, kidney malfunctioning, glomerulonephritis, tubular nephritis, idiopathic increase in the level of calcium in the urine.

RELATIONS - ***Compare:*** (1) Calc., Calc-p., Calc-f. (2) Syph. - Nightly linear pains in the bones, loss of memory, especially of proper nouns, obsessions. (3) Astra-e. - Confused state, paretic weakness of the limbs. (4) Mez. - Periosteal pains at night, worse in cold, damp weather.

REFERENCES - Blackwood. Julian.

PAREIRA BRAVA

(Virgin Vine)

PHARMACY - pareir. Pareira brava. Virgin vine. Cessampelos pareira. Velvet leaf. Chondrodendron tomentosum. N. O. Menispermacae. Tincture of fresh root. Tincture of dried root. ***Historical dose:*** Tincture and all potencies.

CLINICAL - Bladder, catarrh. Calculus. ***Dysuria.*** Gonorrhea. Kidney, disorders. Leucorrhea. Prostate, enlargement. Kidney, colic. Urethritis. Urine, slimy.

HERBAL - Pareira is a climbing plant, a native of the West Indies, Central America and India. The root has a traditional use in diseases of the bladder and urinary organs.

HOMEOPATHIC - Pareir. affects the genitourinary organs and the left side. It is useful in kidney colic, prostatic disorders and catarrh of bladder. Cartilaginous induration of mucus membranes of the urethra and bladder. Sensation as if bladder were distended with pain.

Kidney colic, enlarged prostate with retention of urine and catarrh of the bladder. ***Dysuria.*** Constant urging to urinate, violent pain in the glans penis and ***down the thighs*** during efforts of urination, must get on knees and hands pressing head firmly to the floor to urinate. Urine contains thick, stringy, white mucus or red sand.

Back - Excruciating pains in the left lumbar region, pain radiates from left kidney to groin, following course of ureter.

Bladder - Feeling of the bladder being distended. Almost cartilaginous induration of mucus membrane of bladder. Itching along urethra. Can emit urine only when he goes on his knees, pressing head firmly against the floor.

Kidneys - Bruised pains in region of kidneys. ***Constant urging, great straining,*** pain down thighs during efforts to urinate. ***Dysuria. Painful urination*** since confinement cannot urinate in any position except on hands and knees. Dribbling after urination (Sel.).Urethritis with prostatic trouble.

Limbs - Dropsical swelling of feet and legs.

Lungs - Viscous matter lodged in and obstructing bronchi.

Male - Urethritis with prostatic disorders. Enlargement of prostate glands with retention of urine, pains extending down thighs. Severe pain when urinating and discharge of mucus from urethra. ***Violent pain in glans penis***. Gonorrhea.

Urine - Urine smells strongly of ammonia and contains a large quantity of viscid, thick, white mucus. Black, bloody, foaming urine, depositing a brick-dust sediment of uric acid, deep red and mucus urine.

COMMENTS - A short proving by C. M. Fox of Denver, Colorado, brought out some characteristic symptoms which have been clinically confirmed.

Violent pains with strangury, must go on "all-fours and press head against floor to pass water at all. Urethritis with severe pain when passing water and discharge of mucus from urethra. Pains down thighs and even to feet when attempting to pass water. Violent pain in glans penis" with the straining.

Fox related two cases of prostatic enlargement with dysuria in which Par. gave complete relief. The first concerned a man, 68, who had an old prostatic affection, constant urging with entire inability.

Feet and legs much swollen, had to be put in a warm bath before catheter could be passed. Only on hands and knees with forehead pressed on the floor, could he pass a few drops of scalding urine.

Pareir. 1x gave rapid relief. Swelling disappeared from legs and he was able to resume his business and continue at it for ears.

Fox's second case recorded a man with an enlarged prostate with retention, severe attacks two or three times a years, when he would have to have the urine drawn off for a week or two.

After using Pareir., the catheter was not required more than twice in two years. When he felt the symptoms coming on, a few drops of Pareir. would relieve him at once. Many other remedies had been used in vain before Pareir. was prescribed.

RELATIONS - ***Compare:*** (1) Pariet. (2) Chim. - chronic catarrhal congestion following cystitis, acute prostatitis, feeling of a ball in perineum when sitting. (3) Fab. - dysuria, post-gonorrheal complications, gravel, bladder catarrh. (4) Uva., Hydrang., Berb., Oci., Hedeo. (5) Cocc. (6) Spasm and burning in bladder, ropy urine, Chim., Uva. (7) Prostatic affections, Hydrang., Sabal. (8) Kidney colic, Oci., Berb. (9) Dysuria - Berb. has pain in back extending to hips, Pareir. has pain extending to thighs and even toes. Berb. urine lacks the ammoniacal smell of Pareir. (10) Dribbling urine after urination, Sel.

REFERENCES - Boericke. Clarke. Phatak.

PARIETARIA OFFICINALIS

(Pellitory-of-the-Wall)

PHARMACY - pariet. Parietaria officinalis. Pellitory-of-the-wall. N. O. Urticaceae. Tincture of fresh plant. ***Historical dose:*** Tincture and all potencies.

CLINICAL - Kidney stones. Nightmares.

HOMEOPATHIC - Pariet. belongs to the nettles, it grows on old walls and its ashes contain a lot of nitre (Kali-n.). Cooper used it with success in a case of kidney stones, and in one case it produced nightmare, the patient dreaming of being buried alive in the midst of ruins.

RELATIONS - ***Compare:*** (1) Urt-u., Kali-n.

REFERENCES - Boericke. Clarke.

PARIS QUADRIFOLIA

(One Berry)

PHARMACY - par. Paris quadrifolia. One berry. True Love. Herb Paris. N. O. Trilliaceae. Sometimes considered a sub-order of Smilacee or of Liliaceae. Europe. Moist, shady woods in Great Britain. Tincture of whole plant when in fruit. ***Historical dose:*** Tincture and all potencies.

CLINICAL - Acidity. After-pains. Brachial neuralgia. Ciliary neuralgia. Ciliary paralysis. Digestion, weak. Gonorrhea. Headache. Hiccough. ***Hoarseness***. Hysteria. Mania. Neuralgia. Panaritium. Paralysis. Saliva, sour. Spine, affection. Touch, sense, disordered.

HERBAL - The Treasury of Botany said of Paris that the leaves and stems were "formerly used in medicine, the juice of the berry, though considered poisonous, has been employed in curing inflammation of the eyes."

Paris betrays its relation to the lilies and arums in the symptoms of irritation which it causes in mucus membranes and the skin with burning sensations and cramps.

HOMEOPATHIC - The provings made by Hahnemann, Stapf and others, brought out a very marked and characteristic action on the eyes and developed some of the keynote symptoms of the drug.

Affects the head, spine, eyes and one side. Sensation of expansion and consequent tension. Sensation of heaviness, numbness, parts feel too big or drawn together. Whole body painful especially when touched. Broken feeling of joints.

Generally a left side remedy, but it has coldness of the right side, while the left side is natural or hot. Catarrhal complaints, stuffed feeling at root of nose. Disorder of sense of touch, objects feel rough. The scalp is very sensitive to touch. Pressure on a sore spot on head causes cries.

Mucus secretions are green and tenacious. The eyes give out of fetid, ulcer-like smell. Great sensitiveness to offensive odors, also imaginary bad smells, milk and bread smell like putrid meat. Diarrhea stool smells like putrid meat.

"Hunger soon after a meal," the ***"sinking"*** of the anti-psorics, hellebores, and veratrums.

MIND - Loquacious mania. ***Garrulous***, prattling, vivacious. Inclination to treat others with rudeness and contempt. Silly conduct. Feels too large. Imaginary foul smells.

Abdomen - Tensive pain throughout abdomen. Hard pressure in abdomen. Rumbling and rolling in abdomen, cutting, griping pains. Incisive drawing and boring in one side of abdomen.

Back - Weight and weariness in nape of neck. Violent pain on both sides of neck extending down to fingers worse mental exertion. Stitches in coccyx on sitting.

Causations - Ill effects of injury, suppressions.

Chest - Shootings in chest and sides of chest. Aching in the right side of chest.

Ears - Pain as if the ears were pressed out or forced apart by a wedge, worse swallowing.

Eyes - Eyes feel too large and heavy for their sockets. ***Sensation of a string through eyeballs***, drawing them tightly backward to the middle of the brain. Eyes as if they were projected. Expanded, as though eyelids did not cover. Affections of the eyebrows.

Face - Neuralgia, hot stitches in left malar bone, which is very sore. Seems drawn into root of nose. Inflammation of the antrum, where eye symptoms coexist.

Female - Premature menses. Increased sexual desire. Intense after-pains. Suppressed lochia with ineffectual urging to stool.

Food - Voracious appetite. Hunger very soon after a meal.

Head - Chronic headaches. Headache worse by thinking. ***Headaches as from pulling a string from eyes to occiput.*** Occipital headache with a feeling of weight. Head feels very large, expanded. Numb feeling on left side of head. Head feels as if distended and the scalp too tight. Sensation as if scalp were contracted and bones scraped. Soreness of top of head, scalp sensitive, cannot brush hair.

Limbs - Numbness of upper limbs. ***Sense of weight and weariness in nape of neck*** and across shoulders. Neuralgia, beginning in left intercostal region and extending into left arm. Neuralgia of coccyx, pulsating, sticking, when sitting. Joints feel broken, swollen or dislocated at every motion. Arm becomes stiff, fingers clenched. ***Fingers feel numb***. Everything feels rough.

Lungs - Stuffed condition and fullness at root of nose. Periodical, ***painless hoarseness***. Cough as from vapor of sulphur in trachea. Constant hawking, on account of viscid, green mucus in larynx and trachea.

Modalities - Better from rest, pressure, belching. Worse touch, hiccough, eating. Worse from thinking of problems, mental exertion, thinking, eyestrain. Smoking tobacco causes headache.

Mouth - Tongue feels too large. ***Tongue dry when awaking***, Coated white ***without thirst*** with bitter or diminished taste.

Nose - Imaginary foul smells. Bread, fish, and milk smell putrid.

Rectum - Frequent but scanty evacuations of the consistency of pap. Loose, fetid evacuations, which smell like putrid flesh.

Sensations - Sensation of expansion and consequent tension. As if scalp were contracted and bones scraped sores. Heavy load on nape. As if a thread were drawn tightly through eye to middle of head. Ear as if forced apart by a wedge, as if pressed out or torn out, as if a burning heat was rushing out of ears. Tongue feels too large. Ball in throat. Throat constricted. Stone in stomach. As if internal parts contracted. Fingers as if asleep, dead. All joints as if broken, swollen or dislocated at every motion.

Skin - Painfully sensitive.

Stomach - Heavy as from a stone, better by eructation. Weak digestion. Red curved streak above navel.

Temperature - Unilateral coldness or heat. Heat descending the back from the neck.

Throat - Burning, when eating and drinking. As of a ball in the throat. Hawks up tough, green mucus. Periodical painless hoarseness.

Vertigo - Vertigo on reading aloud.

COMMENTS - Par. is one of the drugs which are credited with producing garrulity, vivacity, with love of prattling, like tea.

B. Nath Banerjee recorded a case of loquacious insanity cured with Par. 3c. Mrs. B., 45, suddenly become loquacious and insane. After a mouth of Kavirajee treatment without benefit she came under his care, October 3, 1893.

A year before, the last of her five children, a grown-up son, died and she could not be consoled and gradually became morose and dull. She ceased to menstruate in February, 1893, but had no uterine troubles or any other illness previous to the present. Loquacity, but not continuous. Every three or four days, if interfered with, maniacal attacks lasting about half an hour. At times foolish behavior.

With difficulty Banerjee obtained the following symptoms from the patient: vertigo and whenever she thinks of her lost son, severe headache, the vertex being sensitive to touch. When telling these symptoms, suddenly her looks became wandering and her eyes appeared as if protruding from their sockets.

She could not relish her food because everything, especially fish, smelt putrid. Whole body painful, especially when touched. She complained of a ball lodging in the throat and giving her trouble with burning. Acidity and badly smelling diarrhea. A peculiar feeling of coldness of right side of the body while the left side was hot.

All symptoms worse in evening and on motion. Ign. 30c and later 200c, was given without any effect. Par. acted promptly, and on the third day the patient assured the doctor that she was quite well. The remedy was not repeated and the cure held.

Clarke cured with Par. a "numb feeling of left side of head." Numbness affects the upper limbs. The left arm is paralyzed, and it feels stiff with fingers contracted.

"Numbness and prickling in left hand" was removed in a case of spinal affection.

"Fingers often feel as if asleep, objects seem rough to touch." Disorder of the sense of touch, with great sensitiveness of the surface. Hot stitches in left malar bones. Acidity, sour saliva.

RELATIONS - ***Antidoted by:*** Coff. ***Compare:*** (1) Past., Sil., Calc., Nux-v, Rhus-t. (2) In spinal headache rising from nape, Sil. (3) Wild look in eyes, Bell. (4) As if eyes drawn back by thread, Croto-t. (5) Eyeballs feel too large, Sil. (6) Garrulity, Lach., Meph., Stram., Cimic., right, Agar. (7) Laryngeal affections, Arg-n. (Par. has expectoration noticed mostly in morning and it is green and tenacious). (8) String-like pain, All-c. (9) Heart, Lil-t., Conv. (10) Panaritium, Bor-ac. (11) Imaginary foul smells, Anac. (12) worse from motion, Bry. ***Compatible:*** Calc., Led., Lyc., Nux-v., Phos., Rhus-t., Sep., Sulph. ***Incompatible:*** Ferr-p.

REFERENCES - Boericke. Clarke. Phatak.

PARONICHIA ILLECEBRUM

PHARMACY - paro-i. Paronichia illecebrum. Tiangius pepetla. Alternanthera sessilis. Sanguinaria of Cuba. Illebraceae or Paronychiaceae family. Cuba. The tincture is prepared from the whole fresh plant. ***Historical dose:*** Tincture and all potencies.

CLINICAL - Angio-hematic typhus. Appendicitis. Blepharitis. Bronchial pneumonia. Cancer. Conjunctivitis. Encephalitis. Endometritis. High fever. Infectious diseases. Mastoiditis. Menorrhagia. Metrorrhagia. Pleurisy. Pneumonia. Rhinitis. Septicemia. Sinusitis. Typhoid fever. Typhus.

HERBAL - This plant is a very close relation to the Caryophyllaceae, which gives the saponarias to the Materia Medica. Paronichia illecebrum is a grass whose trailing stem has branches, oblong pale green leaves and capitate flowers.

HOMEOPATHIC - The proving was established by Manuel M. De Legarreta. Paro-i. has fever, dry, oppressive heat and symptoms of catarrh. The patient wants to uncover himself all the time. When lying on his side, he can no longer move, feels weary, weak and sleepy.

Acute congestion of the nerves, lungs and blood vessels. Feeling of emptiness in the brain and doubling of personality. High fever. Encephalitis in eruptive juvenile diseases. Involuntary passing of stools and urine. Poisoning of the nursing child.

MIND - Calm, tranquil state of mind. Sleepy and in a semi-awake state. Nervous weakness. Doubling of personality. Feeling that there are two different people inside him, who contradict each other and argue about their illness (Anac.).

Abdomen - Rumbling in the right iliac cavity. Gas difficult to expel. Acute inflammation of the gallbladder and biliary passages. Sub-phrenic abscess. Chronic appendicitis.

Chest - Chest painful. Dyspnea with intercostal pains. Shooting pains in the left intercostal region. Thoracic pains when changing position.

Ears - Outer ear hot and painful. Auditory canal dry. Discharge of a hot, excoriating serum from the left ear, forming crusts which, when scratched, bleed easily. Acute congestive otitis. Suppurating inflammation of the ear-drum (Sil.). Mastoiditis. Hears well.

Eyes - Eyes look sad. Eyes bloodshot, red, tearful. Conjunctivitis. Blepharitis. Eyelids heavy, burning with need to refresh them.

Female - Hemorrhaging endometritis. Menorrhagia or metrorrhagia during the menopause with violent headaches. Uterine cancer.

Food - Thirsty for water, which is vomited as soon as it is absorbed. Thirsty for ice-cold water with stomach, as if burning.

Head - Acute pain in the temples, as if compressed by an iron helmet. Scalp very painful, cannot tolerate combing. If he moves his head, he hears a rush of water.

Heart - Pulse violent, full and bounding, resounds in the ear and is annoying. Myocarditis. Pericarditis.

Kidneys - Acute glomerulonephritis. Involuntary urination. Urine dark, but copious. Hematuria. Dysuria with tenesmus, with involuntary passing of stools.

Lungs - Painful cough with great difficulty in expectorating and desire to vomit. Bronchial crepitant rales, abundant expectoration, sputum frothy, rusty or blood-streaked. Pleurisy. Bronchial pneumonia. Pneumonia. Abscess on the lung. Pulmonary gangrene.

Male - Prostatic congestion with tenesmus and burning during urination. Prostatic adenoma.

Modalities - Worse from movement or the slightest effort. Worse left side, but not exclusively.

Mouth - Tongue pasty, covered with a yellow-white coating. Mouth dry, tongue coated, rough. Breath fetid, putrid, nauseating. Taste of copper in the mouth. Saliva thick and dark yellow. Teeth covered with thick, yellow tartar. Cracks at the corners of the lips. Lips chapped.

Nose - Ozaena. Rhinitis. Sinusitis. Nostrils blocked by crusts. Light nosebleeds. Loss of sense of smell.

Rectum - Involuntary intestinal evacuation and fetid odor. Diarrhea with greenish stools, smelling of sour milk. Perianal burning with anal excoriation and anal trickling. Rectal hemorrhaging.

Skin - Petechial exanthema on the backs of the hands. Rheumatoid purpura. Hyperglobulinemic purpura. Infectious purpura. Pressure sores. Copious sweating, especially from the groin and armpits. Sweating with excoriation of the skin which forms wounds.

Sleep - Sleepy and in a semi-awake state.

Stomach - Acute gastritis. Acridity, bringing up of air and food. Nausea.

Temperature - Temperature between 39.5°C and 41°C. Copious sweating, smelling of curdled milk.

RELATIONS - ***Compare:*** (1) Anac. - Clouded mental state, feels as if he had two opposed wills, headaches, nausea, vomiting, amelioration by eating. (2) Bapt. - Prostration with putrid odor of all discharges. Feeling of painful cracking in the muscles. Putrid smell of breath. Diarrhea is fetid, sometimes involuntary. (3) Anthr. - Septic infections, burning pains, prostration, bleeding from the orifices or black blood, which decomposes rapidly. (4) Ars. - Prostration, agitation, anxiety about death. Burning pains, with burning diarrhea, peri-anal excoriation, oppression, palpitations, worse between midnight and 3 a.m.

REFERENCES - Julian.

PAROTIDINUM

(Mumps Nosode)

PHARMACY - parot. Parotidinum. Mumps nosode. Nosodes. ***Historical dose:*** All potencies.

CLINICAL - Cholera. Cryptorchism. Eustachian, catarrh. Fibroma. Gland, disorders. Lymphangioma. Meningitis. ***Mumps.*** Myoma. Orchitis. Otalgia. Parotitis. Salivation. Sterility. Stomatitis. Tonsillitis. Tumors.

HOMEOPATHIC - This nosode is prepared from inactivated mumps viruses, which belong to the paramyxovirus group and can cause mumps. Parot. has been used as a prophylactic against infection by mumps.

The well-known complications which sometimes occur with mumps, cerebral inflammation and orchitis, suggest its possible use in these conditions.

The main indications are painful swellings of the parotid gland, fever, otalgia, difficulty hearing, and sometimes pancreatic involvement. Pancreatic affections. Diseases of the oral mucosa such as stomatitis, tonsillitis. Eustachian catarrh and hearing problems of catarrhal origin.

Cryptorchism, benign or malignant tumors of the testes. Fibroma, myoma, lymphangioma, adenomatoid tumors. Teratoma and dermoid cysts.

COMMENTS - Mumps is to be distinguished from the parotitis which is seen in scarlet fever, cholera and other infectious diseases, and also from the secondary parotitis, arising from throat infections and diseases of the oral mucosa.

Parot. is generally given in the 30c two or three times a day to those exposed to the infection. In cases of mumps, it may be given every four hours, either by itself or alternated with other indicated remedies.

RELATIONS - ***Compare:*** (1) Merc., Jab., Piloc.

REFERENCES - Clarke. Reckeweg.

PARTHENIUM HYSTEROPHORUS

(Bitter-broom)

PHARMACY - parth. Parthenium hysterophorus. Bitter-broom. Congress grass. Escoba amargo. N. O. Composite, Synanthereae, tribe Helianthee. The dry plant is macerated in five parts by weight of alcohol. Trituration of solution of the alkaloid Parthenia. ***Historical dose:*** Tincture and all potencies.

CLINICAL - Amenorrhea. Cheyne-Stokes breathing. Debility. Dyspepsia. Ear disorders. Fainting. Fevers. Headaches. Liver, pain. Milk increased. Miscarriage. Neuralgia, periodic. Salivation. Spleen, disorders. Toothache. Vision, disordered.

HOMEOPATHIC - A Cuban remedy for fevers, especially malarial. An alkaloid, Parthenia, was isolated by C. J. Ulrice of Havana; and Dr. J. L. Duenas published experiments with this on humans and animals.

In the proving, the pains were sudden, congestive, out-pushing. Pains in the head and ears. Singing and fullness in the ears. Heaviness and dullness of head. Tendency to vertigo. Malaise, apathy, lassitude. Stupor, desire to be quiet. Indifference.

Profuse and very fluid salivation. Sensation of heat and weight in the stomach. Increased appetite, or refusal of food. Gastric intolerance, nausea and vomiting. Increased flow of milk. Amenorrhea and general debility. Cheyne-Stokes breathing. After-effects of quinine. Antidotal action to quinine.

MIND - Feels dull and stupid. Difficult to fix attention. Malaise, apathy, lassitude. Indifference.

Abdomen - Spleen disorders. Spleen painful to pressure, pain in right side, worse in some parts than in others, with shiverings. Severe pains in the left hypochondrium with tertian fever. Loud rumbling in bowels, about navel. Slight colicky pains at navel. Colic deep in pelvis, pains run down backs of thighs to knees.

Breasts - Great increase of milk in breasts of nursing women.

Ears - Sharp pain in ears. Stabbing pain in left ear. Dullness and aching in ears, coming suddenly. Stitching at lobe of left ear, deep in and above external auditory meatus. Tinnitus, ringing in ears, worse left.

Eyes - Eyes heavy, drowsy. Aching in eyeballs. Aching over eyes, wants to close them. Disordered vision. Must look intently to see the words, when writing the letters seem pale and eye ache.

Face - Seems as if bloods would burst through face. Bursting pain in right malar bone. Aching pains run up from above left eye-tooth to eye and over face, occurs by starts and stops.

Female - Given to pregnant women for fevers, it has caused miscarriages and premature deliveries. In a case of subacute tuberculosis, it restored the menses, which had been absent since the illness commenced.

Head - Headaches, extending to nose, pain in frontal eminence. Stitching pain in left temple of short duration. Aching pain at left supra-orbital foramen. Pain at root of nose, feels swollen. Heaviness and dullness of head. Full feeling in vertex, pressing from within.

Heart - Excited heartbeat. Progressive slowness of pulse, followed by syncope, cardiac paralysis and death. Pulse slow, soft compressible.

Kidneys - Kidneys enlarged and congested. Increased urine.

Limbs - Pains run from pelvis down backs of thighs to knees. Marked diminution of reflex in hips and extinction of voluntary movements.

Lungs - Slow, irregular, breathing. Cheyne-Stokes.

Modalities - Better after rising and walking about. Worse after sleep, from sudden motion.

Mouth - Tingling in tip of tongue. Profuse, very fluid salivation.

Nose - Pain at root of nose, in nose, in bones of nose, worse left. Stuffed feeling at root of nose, as with dry coryza. Nose feels swollen and tender to touch. Aching in bridge of nose (worse left side) and of upper left molars. Aching at end of nose, which feels full of blood.

Rectum - Stabbing pain runs up rectum after passing flatus. No desire at usual time, 10:30 p.m., mushy stool.

Sleep - Restless night, wakes at 3 and 4 a.m., then dozes and dreams until 7:30. Increased stupor, desire to be quiet.

Stomach - Emptiness sensation in epigastrium, hunger. Heat and weight in stomach. Irrepressible, tasteless belchings. Belchings tasting of the drug.

Teeth - ***Teeth feel on edge,*** too long. Aching in teeth. Upper teeth, pricking pains in sockets. Sharp aching twinges in upper molars. Upper incisors tender at sockets when biting.

Temperature - Rise and fall of temperature, shivering, diminished perspiration.

Vertigo - Vertigo, while sitting with heat of face and blurred vision.

COMMENTS - Dr. B. H. B. Sleight proved increasing doses of the tincture and, later on, of 6x, which reproduced most of the symptoms of the first proving.

Fornias reported the case of his niece, 5, living in Havana, who had been suffering from a continued fever with periodical midday exacerbations, which later on assumed an intermittent form. She had been saturated with quinine and complained at the time of malaise, lassitude, headache, gastric intolerance, etc.

Dr. Govantes prescribed an extract of Parth., three doses a day, each the size of a pea. In four or five days she was free from fever and made a quick recovery.

Dr. Ramirez Tovar reported several cures by Parth. The first was a woman living in the lower part of the city, where the rain left channels of infection, who had daily attacks of intermittent, more intense each day.

One grain of the alkaloid was divided into six powders, one every hour after the attack. No further attacks. The patient was nursing at the time and she noticed a marked increase of milk in the breasts. Half a grain divided into five doses completed the cure.

In the second case, a tailor, 30, moved to a lower part of the city and contracted tertian intermittent, the fourth seizure being attended with much pain in the left hypochondrium.

One grain in five doses cured, though the conditions were unchanged. (The removal of this left hypochondriac pain is important in connection with Burnett's experience with Helia.)

The third case was a girl, 6, lymphatic, who lived near the harbor, ill for seventeen days with malaise, loss of appetite, sleepiness and fever. She had quinine internally and externally, and was wasting visibly. The alkaloid, aided by a tonic wine prepared from the extract of the plant, cured

In his fourth case, Tovar noted a man, 45 of delicate constitution, poorly nourished, straw-yellow face, yellow sclerotics, enlarged liver and spleen, spleen painful to pressure. He had a fever in Panama, had taken quinine, complained of a pain in right side, which commenced 1 p.m. with shiverings, disappeared in two hours and returned at precisely the same hour the next day.

Five doses of ten centigrams each removed the pain. About six weeks later there was a relapse, the pain this time being located in the stomach. One grain in five doses, one dose every two hours, removed the pain, but it returned the third day. The same treatment then removed it permanently.

The fifth case concerned a young woman, 18, who had periodical facial neuralgia, cured by the same treatment.

RELATIONS - It antidotes quinine. ***Compare:*** (1) In spleen affections, Helia., Cean. (2) In malaise and periodic neuralgia, Malar. Off., Chin., Cedr.

REFERENCES - Anshutz. Boericke. Clarke.

PASSIFLORA INCARNATA

(Passion Flower)

PHARMACY - passi. Passiflora incarnata. Passion flower. N. O. Passifloracee of the Violal alliance. Tincture of fresh or dried leaves gathered in May. Fluid hydro-alcoholic extract. Powdered inspissated juice. ***Historical dose:*** Tincture and all potencies.

CLINICAL - Addictions. ***Alcoholism. Asthma.*** Burns. Chancre. Cholera infantum. Convulsions. Delirium. ***Delirium tremens.*** Dentition. Diarrhea. Drug addictions. Dysmenorrhea. Epilepsy. Erysipelas. Exophthalmos. Headaches. Hemorrhoids. Hysteria. ***Insomnia.*** Levitation. ***Morphine, habit.*** Nerve, disorders. Nervousness. Neuralgia. Opisthotonos. Puerperal, convulsions. Sciatica. ***Sleeplessness.*** Spasms. ***Tetanus***. Ulcers. Whooping cough.

HERBAL - Passion flower is a climbing plant, leaves cordate, ovate and palmately three lobed. The plant bears solitary, large, and very beautiful flowers, white with a purple center. The edible fruit is a large berry.

Passion flower is a safe and Used as a herbal remedy in nervous, irritative, and neuralgic pains with debility. harmless soporific herb that will allay irritation of the brain and central nervous system. It is a nerve sedative, narcotic, antispasmodic.

Used in derangements of the nervous system such as insomnia, chorea, convulsions and headache. Nervous headache. Hysteria spasms. Convulsions, especially in those of childhood when it should be given in large doses before the approach of the convulsion.

Insomnia from exhaustion and excitement. Wakefulness of infants and elderly people. Produces a restful sleep, the patient awakens refreshed. Hypnotic. Should not be given in insomnia with flushed face and determination of blood to the head.

HOMEOPATHIC - Passi. has not been proved. Hale introduced it to homeopathy, citing a paper by Phares in the New Remedies. Its curative action appears to be a direct kind.

Quieting effect on the nervous system, hence an efficient nervine and anti-spasmodic remedy. Excitement with spasms. Hysteria, puerperal convulsions. Convulsions in children with neuralgia. Convulsions of children during teething.

Tetanic convulsions affecting mainly the muscles of the trunk, with predominant opisthotonos. Violent ***tetanus***, with opisthotonos, trismus, and convulsions. Tetanus infantum. Neuralgias, internal and of the limbs.

Worm fever, teething and spasms. ***Insomnia of infants and the aged***. Sleeplessness, with great restlessness and suicidal mania. Restlessness of fevers. Nervous disorders.

General atonic condition. Mentally worried and over-worked persons.

Asthma. Whooping cough. Painful diarrhea. Cholera infantum with restlessness. Tedious labor pains when the patient becomes nervous and excitable. Delirium tremens. ***Alcoholism.*** Abuse of narcotics. Drug addictions. ***Breaks off morphine habit*** (Aven.).

MIND - Mentally worried and over-worked. ***Insomnia of infants and the aged***. Sleeplessness, with great restlessness and suicidal mania. Nervous and excitable. Restlessness. Hysteria. Acute mania. Excitement and spasms. Neurosis of children. Alcoholism. Delirium tremens. Drug addictions. Abuse of narcotics. ***Breaks off morphine habit*** (Aven.).

Back - Pain in coccyx.

Eyes - Sensation that the eyes are being pushed out.

Female - Painful menses, dysmenorrhea.

Head - Violent ache as if top of head would come off. Top of head seemed to lift off.

Limbs - Sensation that her heels are up in the air.

Lungs - Nocturnal cough.

Rectum - Severe attack of hemorrhoids. Irritable hemorrhoids.

Skin - Chancre. Erysipelas.

Sleep - Restless and wakeful, resulting from exhaustion. Insomnia with tendency to convulsions. ***Insomnia in screaming children***, of infants, the aged, the mentally worried and overworked. ***Sleeplessness in alcoholics.*** Sleeplessness with delirium.

Stomach - Leaden, dead feeling after or between meals, flatulence and sour belchings.

COMMENTS - Phares learned its action from W. B. Lindsay, who used it with extraordinary success in tetanus of the newborn. Lindsay commended an aqueous extract of the root as an application for chancre, erysipelas, irritable hemorrhoids and new burns.

Phares confirmed the efficacy of Passi. in erysipelas, ulcers, neuralgia and tetanus. He cited the case of an old woman who was seized with convulsions of a tetanic nature as well as the case of his hors, cured by himself and his son, J. H. Phares.

One of his own horses was seized with tetanus and all hope of saving him was given up, when Phares gathered some Passi. stems, leaves and flowers. They were pounded, moistened with water, expressed ten or twelve ounces and poured it down the animal's throat through a tube introduced at the side of his mouth. Though not expected to live half an hour, the horse was found grazing the next morning.

J. W. Covert reported the case of Mrs. X., 28, who had epileptic convulsions for years from one to twenty fits in a week. The aura was a tight feeling in the chest. By homeopathic treatment, Covert succeeded in diminishing the frequency of the attacks, but they would invariably return at the menstrual period.

Passi. tincture 6 drops, six times a day, was given. The next period passed without a convulsion, but the patient had a violent headache as if the top of the head would come off. This was rapidly controlled by Glon. 6c. The three following period passed without any attack.

Farrington considered Passi. suited especially to tetanus of hot countries and referred to two cures by Archibald Bayne of Barbados with the tincture and 1x. It has also been used in convulsions of children and other complaints of dentition, and even in epilepsy.

E. S. Prindle related a case of delirium tremens. A German, driver of a beer wagon, was laid up with a broken arm when he was seized with delirium tremens of a most ferocious type, which the usual remedies entirely failed to control.

Passi. succuss was then given, two drachms every half-hour. After the third dose the patient quieted down and slept three hours. On waking, he again began to rave, but not as badly as before. Another teaspoonful of Passi. put him to sleep and the next morning he was quite sane and allowed his arm to be reset.

G. C. Buchanan observed some curious effects in a patient, Mrs. V., to whom he gave teaspoonful doses for neuralgia, sleeplessness and nervousness.

"Her eyes seemed to push out of her head and lie on the quilt, her heels seemed to be up in air top of her head seemed to lift off."

To the observer, the eyes seemed to protrude. Later a severe attack of hemorrhoids developed. The dose was reduced to half-teaspoonfuls, which produced sleep and caused no ill effects.

RELATIONS - ***Compare:*** (1) Valer., Cypr. (2) In tetanus and epilepsy, Oena., Nux-v. (2) Heels seem to go up, Ph-ac.

REFERENCES - Boericke. Clarke.

PASTINACA SATIVA

(Parsnip)

PHARMACY - past. Pastinaca sativa. Parsnip. Pastinaca urens. N. O. Umbelliferae. Tincture of roots of second year. ***Historical dose:*** Tincture and all potencies.

HERBAL - Roots used as a food, cooked in water, as broth, or as salad, for tuberculosis patients and kidney stones.

HOMEOPATHIC - After the first year, the root is very poisonous and some cases of poisoning have been observed. A state of perfect ***"delirium tremens"*** was observed in several persons, illusions of vision, catching at imaginary objects, fighting with one another. Loquacity. Intolerance of milk. A peculiar effect was produced on the stomach, the irritability was depressed and emetics would not act.

RELATIONS - ***Compare:*** (1) Aeth., Ziz.

REFERENCES - Boericke. Clarke.

PEARL

(Oyster Pearl)

PHARMACY - pear. Pearl. Oyster Pearl. Aragonite, about 82-86%; conchiolin, 10-14%; and water, 2%. Pearls are calcified objects made by oysters and are usually pale white or cream colored, though darker blue, gray, and even black variations exist. Layers of aragonite, known as nacre, are secreted around the irritant and gradually build up to form the solid pearl. ***Historical dose:*** Tincture and all potencies.

CLINICAL - Arthritis. Breasts, disorders. Coughs. Headaches. Hypertension. Infertility. Tuberculosis.

HOMEOPATHIC - Soothing influence. Enhances curative powers. Promotes body fluids and the blood, nourishing the body tissues and the nerves.

Said to lessen stress and related maladies (hypertension, headaches, and exhaustion), which may help prevent heart attacks and strokes. Pearls supposedly aid in digestion and may reduce the chance of developing ulcers. Strengthens the female reproductive system, improves fertility, and calms the emotions.

A good pearl (not pierced) triturated in rose or kewra water, made into paste, dried and taken orally, is very beneficial for diseases caused by calcium deficiency. The ashes provide relief to body heat, are good for the eyes. Cures tuberculosis, chronic fevers, cough, breathing problems, palpitations, high blood pressure, heart ailments, exhaustion and weaknesses.

MIND - Pearl increases emotional stability, mental strength, friendliness and contentment. Weakness or afflictions are shown by anxiety, mental and emotional swings, worry, isolation or the inability to cope with relationships and people.

COMMENTS - The Arabs called pearls "tears of the gods," and said they were formed by drops of rain falling into oyster shells. The Chinese, regard pearls as the hidden soul of the oyster. "Margarithe," another name for this gem, means "child of light." It has become a symbol of purity and virtue.

Pearls were essential toiletry articles, used to clean face and teeth. Applying the oyster shell containing a pearl to the affected area was said to heal leprosy and other skin diseases.

The gem was considered beneficial for easing indigestion, curing hemorrhoids, and counteracting poison. Taken in milk, they were used to cure ulcers. Nursing women took pearl concoctions to make their milk healthy and plentiful.

6 grains in water sweetened with manna (ash tree sap) was said to ward off the plague. Burnt pearl powder drunk in water stopped hemorrhages; inhaled, it cured headache. Oil of pearls was believed to fortify the nerves.

A pearl tonic can be made to increase vitality, relieve eye strain, and soothe burning urination; place several small pearls in water overnight and drink the water following day. The tonic is a natural antacid and anti-inflammatory.

RELATIONS - ***Compare:*** (1) Calc., Luna, Arg-n.

REFERENCES - Murphy.

PECTEN JACOBAEUS

(Scallop)

PHARMACY - pect. Pecten jacobaeus. Scallop. N. O. Pectinide. Trituration or tincture of whole animal. ***Historical dose:*** All potencies.

CLINICAL - ***Asthma, humid.*** Coryza. Cough. Dyspnea.

HOMEOPATHIC - Swan learned from a gentleman that every time he entered a room where scallops were being opened he had such a severe attack of asthma that he had to leave or suffocate. Swan potentized the scallop and used the preparation with success in similar cases.

Asthma preceded by coryza, sneezing and burning in throat and chest. Attack ends with copious expectoration of tough, stringy, frothy mucus, worse at night. ***Humid asthma.*** Quick and labored breathing. Constriction of chest, especially right side. Pulse very quick and wiry. Fullness of the head. Cough worse after 6 p.m., at night.

COMMENTS - T. Franklin Smith reported a case of humid asthma, with quick, labored breathing, cannot lie flat or on left side. Constriction of chest, especially right side. Cured quickly and permanently with Pect. 1,000c and 100,000c potencies.

REFERENCES - Boericke. Clarke.

PEDICULUS CAPITIS

(Head Lice)

PHARMACY - ped. Pediculus capitis. Head lice. Head louse. N. O. Hemiptera. Tincture of the insects. Pediculus belongs to the same class of remedies as Cimx. and Trom. ***Historical dose:*** All potencies.

CLINICAL - Children, diseases. Colic. Diarrhea. Edema. Ganglion, foot. Hair, loss. Irritation. Lice. Psora, hereditary. Skin, disorders. Stammering.

HOMEOPATHIC - Ped. was proved by Mure, who said that he thought that nature pointed to the louse as a specific for hereditary psora, which was strengthened by the fact that Psor. develops pediculosis in healthy persons. He added that he found Ped. to be one of the most useful agents in diseases of children.

Five people took part in the proving, but no particulars were given as to the doses they took. All developed symptoms, including eagerness and aptitude for study and work. One prover, a stammerer, had unusual fluency of words.

Constriction of pharynx. Jerks and starts in evening when sitting or lying. Miliary eruptions, itching and formication almost all over. Symptoms were worse by contact, in evening, after eating, standing, stooping, or walking.

RELATIONS - ***Antidoted by:*** Chin. (anasarca). ***Compare:*** (1) Colic and diarrhea after eating, Trom. (2) Skin, Psor., Sulph.

REFERENCES - Clarke.

PEGANUM HARMALA

(Syrian Rue)

PHARMACY - peg-h. Peganum harmala. Syrian rue. African rue. N. O. Zygophyleaceae. Russia. Tincture of the seeds. ***Historical dose:*** Tincture and all potencies.

CLINICAL - Acne, vulgaris. ***Alcoholism.*** Amenorrhea. Asthma. Baldness. Breast, disease. Colic. Delusions. Diabetes. Endometriosis. Epilepsy. Fever. Hemorrhoids. Hirsutism. Hysteria. Lice. Malaria. Menstrual, problems. Myoma, uterus. Neuralgia. Parkinson's disease. Rheumatism. Sexual, disorders. Stomach, disorders. Syphilis. Tapeworms. Urinary, disorders. Uterus, prolapse. Worms.

HERBAL - The seeds of this Middle-Eastern shrub have a long history of medical and psychoactive use. Widely known and used in its native areas, the seeds yield a dye ("Turkish" or "Syrian" red) long used in "Persian" carpets. The seeds and roots contain b-carboline alkaloids, mostly harmine, as well as harmaline, harmalol, etc.

Egyptian studies found the extract to be markedly fungicidal and bactericidal, mostly due to harmine. It is reported to be used as an incense and spice, and as an abortificant, narcotic, aphrodisiac, stimulant, sedative, emmenagogue, emetic, vermifuge, or soporific.

Consumption of the seed in quantity induces a sense of euphoria and releases inhibitions. It has been used in the past as a "truth drug." The seed has also been used as an anthelmintic in order to rid the body of tapeworms.

Harmine, which is being used in research into mental disease, encephalitis and inflammation of the brain. Small quantities stimulate the brain and are said to be therapeutic, but in excess, harmine depresses the central nervous system. A crude preparation of the seed is more effective than an extract because of the presence of related indoles.

The seed is used externally in the treatment of hemorrhoids and baldness. The oil obtained from the seed is said to be aphrodisiac, and to have galactagogue, ophthalmic, soporific and vermifuge properties.

The root has been used as a parasiticide in order to kill body lice, and used internally in the treatment of rheumatism and nervous conditions. A decoction of the leaves is used in the treatment of rheumatism.

This remedy should be used with caution, and preferably under the guidance of a qualified practitioner, since excessive doses cause vomiting and hallucinations.

HOMEOPATHIC - Peg-h. has been reported to be used in India for syphilis, fever in North Africa, and elsewhere for fever, hysteria, malaria, neuralgia, parkinsonism, prolapse of the womb, rheumatism, colic, asthma, and eye complaints.

The fruit and seed are digestive, diuretic, hallucinogenic, narcotic and uterine stimulants. They are taken internally in the treatment of stomach complaints, urinary and sexual disorders, epilepsy, menstrual problems, mental and nervous illnesses.

MIND - Excitement. Euphoria. Indifference. Sadness. Ailments from grief. ***Irritability. Anger.*** Desire to curse, fight, to strike others, to break things, to kill, to die. Hatred of close relatives, parents.

Delusion of belonging to the opposite sex. Confusion as to their sexual identity. ***Delusion of being surrounded by vampires***. Delusion that he is a vampire. Delusion that he follows or belongs to the devil. ***Delusion that he has been cursed by the evil eye.***

Abdomen - Pain in right hypochondria. Sharp, cutting pains.

Face - Acne vulgaris. Pimples on chin.

Female - Amenorrhea. Suppression of menses. Sexual desire decreased or increased.

Food - ***Desires alcohol,*** drugs, smoking.

Head - Occiput pain, worse lying down, moving the head.

Limbs - Convulsions. Cramps, twitching.

Male - Sexual desire increased.

Mouth - Swelling of gums.

Nose - Pimples. Red blister on surface of top.

Rectum - Constipation. Painless diarrhea.

Skin - Acne vulgaris. Pimples. Red blisters.

Sleep - Insomnia. Sleepiness. Nightmares. Dreams of talking with the devil, of vampires, or murder, ***of death of his relatives***, of talking with dead relatives. Dreams that he is a woman.

Stomach - Sharp, cutting pains. Nausea.

REFERENCES - Timofeeva. Tiraspolski.

PELARGONIUM RENIFORME

PHARMACY - pelarg. Pelargonium reniforme. Rabassum Dutch. Umckaloabo. N. O. Geraniaceae. Tincture of fresh root. ***Historical dose:*** Tincture and all potencies.

HERBAL - Pelarg. is a Kafir remedy for dysentery. The root is cut up finely or bruised, and then boiled in milk for a considerable time. Many British soldiers were cured of dysentery with it in the Boer War.

Pelarg. was also used for purging in horses. When a horse was attacked during a journey the root (which is very thick) was wrapped up and tied to the bit. The juice mingled with the saliva and was swallowed.

REFERENCES - Clarke.

PENICILLINUM

(Penicillin)

PHARMACY - penic. Penicillinum. Penicillin. The antibiotic drug. The sodium salt of Benzyl-penicillin of Penicillin G is used. Crystalline powder, white, odorless, soluble in water with a slightly bitter taste. ***Historical dose:*** All potencies.

CLINICAL - ***Allergies.*** Angina. Asthenia. Asthma. Boils. Chills. Chronic, fatigue. Colds. Colitis. Collagen, diseases. Conjunctivitis. Constipation. Coryza. ***Diarrhea.*** Ecchymosis. Eczema. Fever. Headache. Lumbago. Neuralgia. Proctitis. Reticular, endotheliosis. Toothache. Tubercular, conditions. Sinusitis. Styes. Sycosis. Vaginitis. Vertigo.

HOMEOPATHIC - The antibiotic penicillin has been used homeopathically to antidote the affects of penicillin when it has been over prescribed to patients.

Indicated in those who have never been well since taking this drug. Chronic fatigue syndrome. Nervous trembling. Limbs cold with paresthesia. Intermittent neuralgic pains. Asthenia, shivering, sub-febrile condition.

Fever continues for a very long time, worse in the evening. Hot or cold perspiration with a stale odor. Changeable sycotic condition with boils, skin diseases, warts and muco-purulent weeping. Ecchymosis. Recurring angina. Chronic diarrhea.

MIND - Increased cerebral activity, quickly followed by considerable asthenia. Mental cloudiness. Everything seems sad. Indisposition to talk. Feels very lax and tired. Fidgety.

Abdomen - Epigastric and peri-umbilical cramping pains with flatulence.

Back - Lumbago, worse morning, better motion. Rheumatic pains in the muscles and small of the back. Aching in side of neck. Painful swelling in glands of the neck below the ear.

Chest - Pain in right side of chest wall.

Ears - Buzzing in the ears. Boil or eczema in the auditory canal.

Eyes - Tearful. Conjunctivitis with eyelids stuck together and puffy in the morning, especially the lower lid. Eczema on the lids. Styes, which appear slowly. Neuralgia above and behind the right eye.

Female - Menses late and scanty. Yellow or white leucorrhea, non-irritating.

Food - Great thirst. Desires sweets.

Head - Head heavy with nausea, worse on movement, better when lying down and resting and by eating. Sharp pain in forehead over the left side. Pain in the occipital region and just below, worse on awakening and in the evening. Right frontal headache with sinusitis.

Heart - Pain in the precordial region, worse on waking. Extra systole, rapid, irregular pulse.

Kidneys - Bilateral kidney pains, spreading towards the lumbar and sacral regions. Urine scanty, albuminous, edema. Deposit of lithates in the urine.

Limbs - Shooting, wandering pains in various parts of upper and lower extremities, worse night. Lightning pains, aggravated by movement, accompanied by prickling beneath the skin. Intermittent pains in the legs. Numbness of hands, arms, and legs in bed at night. Violent cramp in right leg at night. Joint pains with muscular edema, aggravated by movement. Pain on ball of right shoulder worse night, and light motion. Pain in right shoulder and interior of right upper arm and forearm. Pain left shoulder and arm. Aching in fingers and finger tips.

Lungs - Dry, raucous cough, sometimes fitful, making the patient bend double, better by resting. Thick, yellow or whitish-yellow sputum. Sternal and supra-sternal pains. Asthmatic dyspnea at 4 a.m.

Modalities - Better by rest, pressure, warmth, dry sunny weather. Worse from cold and damp, movement, 4 a.m. The pains are worse at night and in damp, stormy weather.

Mouth - Dryness of mouth. Mucus membranes of the mouth red with whitish spots and slight bleeding from the gums. Root of tongue yellowish-brown and imprint of the teeth stays marked on the tongue.

Nose - Coryza with thick, yellow, trailing discharge. Yellow mucus discharges. Right frontal sinusitis.

Perspiration - Sour smelling sweat.

Rectum - Constipation with empty urging. Chronic diarrhea. ***Loose stools.*** Stabbing pain up rectum. Proctitis.

Skin - Changeable sycotic condition with boils, skin diseases, warts and muco-purulent weeping. Boils, especially on the face, with edema. Eczema, oozing out a pale liquid. Herpes-type eruption on the face. Weeping, macerated impetigo mycosis of the epidermis. Warts. Acne.

Sleep - Heavy or light sleep, waking in the early morning, at 4 a.m., accompanied by feeling of discomfort.

Teeth - Teeth feel too long. Incisors feel on edge. Teeth painful, especially the upper right incisors and canines, spreading towards the right maxilla. Toothache, aching, upper right side, changing from place to place, worse hot or cold drinks.

Temperature - Chilliness, feeling of icy-coldness in different parts of the body, especially the thorax and loins. Sub febrile condition with slight rise in temperature in the evening, which does not go above 38°C.

Vertigo - Vertigo, aggravated by movement with nausea. Dizzy, worse towards evening.

RELATIONS - ***Compare:*** (1) Bry. - Joint pains, aggravated by movement, edema. (2) Nat-s. - clammy, puffy, hydrogenoid type, aggravated by humidity. (3) Thuj. - clammy, sycotic type with dirty, warty skin. (4) Ars. - aggravation from midnight to 3 a.m., chilly, diarrhea, anxious, restless. (5) Puls. - muco-purulent, catarrhal condition, moody, yearning for consolation.

REFERENCES - Julian.

PENTHORUM SEDOIDES

(Virginia Stonecrop)

PHARMACY - pen. Penthorum sedoides. Virginia stonecrop. N. O. Crassulaceae. Penthoraceae. Tincture of fresh plant. ***Historical dose:*** Tincture and all potencies.

CLINICAL - Aphonia. Coryza. Diarrhea. Headache. Hemorrhoids. Hoarseness. ***Post-nasal catarrh***. Sacrum, pain. Sinusitis. Varicocele.

HOMEOPATHIC - Hale said Pen. is reputed to be curative in catarrh and in diarrhea. A scalded sensation in the tongue is one of the symptoms. A sense of levitation was also produced. The symptoms proceed from above downward.

Chronic disorders of mucus membranes with irritability. Chronic post-nasal catarrh, chronic pharyngitis, mucus membrane purple and relaxed. Coryza with rawness and wet feeling in nose. Hypersecretion of mucus membranes.

Posterior sinuses feel moist and raw, nose and ears feel full. Throat feels raw. Aphonia, hoarseness, relaxed vocal cords. Trouble in pharyngeal vault and Eustachian tube. Itching of anus and burning in rectum. General malaise, headache, weakness of limbs inability to attend to business.

MIND - Dull, discouraged and despondent. Mind is dull, study impossible. Inability to attend to business.

Abdomen - A clawing, uneasy sensation about umbilicus, which gradually passed to lower bowel. Twitching in muscles of abdomen. Parietes of abdomen felt thickened. Borborygmus.

Back - Aching through basilar region from back to front. Aching in sacrum and sacroiliac joint. Heat in sacrum with headache.

Ears - Ringing and singing in both ears.

Eyes - Inner, upper tarsal borders itch and burn. Full sensation in supra-orbital region. On closing eyes, felt like floating, vertigo.

Food - Appetite increased.

Head - Dull, heavy headache with heat and soreness in sacrum. Catarrhal aching in forehead. Weight in sinciput. Itching of hairy scalp.

Kidneys - Dull aching in kidneys. Bladder sore to pressure. Urine increased, alkaline, burning along urethra when urinating.

Limbs - Arm numb. Hand felt swollen. Trembling feeling of legs for several days with soreness of knees.

Lungs - In morning a cough from deep in chest with soreness throughout chest.

Male - Sexual orgasm. Weakness, almost satyriasis, followed by long-continued depression, approaching impotence. Varicocele.

Mouth - Prickling, burning sensation on tongue as though scalded. Increased flow of saliva (bloody).

Nose - ***Constant wet feeling in nose***, which no amount of blowing will relieve. Discharge thick, pus-like, streaked with blood. Posterior sinuses feel raw as if denuded of epithelium. ***Post-nasal catarrh*** of puberty.

Rectum - Constipation, an atonic condition of bowels and rectum. After being constipated, semi-fluid evacuation next morning. Burning in rectum at stool, continuing after. Itching of anus, hemorrhoids with aching in sacrum and sacroiliac joint. Crawling in lower rectum as though a worm tried to escape.

Stomach - Disgust and nausea. Forcible eructation and ejection of small quantities of odorless flatus.

COMMENTS - Pen. was proved by Dr. D. B. Morrow (twice), Dr. Scudder and a young man, who all took substantial doses. The majority of the symptoms are Morrow's, including the catarrhal symptoms, which have been verified in practice.

"A peculiar wet feeling in sinuses as though a violent coryza would set in," but it did not, the secretion became thickened and pus-like but not increased.

The same "wet feeling" was experienced at the same time in trachea and bronchi, which passed from above down as if coryza would set in, followed by a slight feeling of constriction in the chest, which also passed from above down.

The next day the nose felt stuffed. The third day the first symptoms were repeated and the discharge became thick, pus-like and streaked with blood and there was an odor in the nose as if from an open sore.

Scudder had "fullness in nose and ears." Morrow experienced itching at anus, hemorrhoids and pains and sensations in rectum, sacrum and sacroiliac joints, his first proving cured "heat and soreness in sacrum with a dull, heavy headache."

Morrow reported two cures, the first, Miss P., 17, blonde, had severe cough of several weeks' duration. Worse by talking or singing. Frothy, greenish sputa. Puls. and Phos. failed, Pen. soon cured.

The second concerned a decrepit old woman, 75, suffered from eczema for twelve years. Previous winter cured of asthma (probably from suppressed eczema) with Sulph. 100,000c. Now paretic right side, for which Phos. was given.

But Phos. did not relieve a loose, continual, rattling cough, caused by tickling at bifurcation of bronchi with raising much thick, frothy, greenish sputa. Pen. pellets quickly cured.

RELATIONS - ***Compare:*** (1) Pen. often follows Puls., Sang., Hydr. (2) Sedum acre., Hydrang. (3) In scalded sensation on tongue and in catarrh, Sang. (4) Catarrh, Puls. (5) Levitation, Cann-i., Cocc., Ph-ac., Stict., Sulph., Thuj. (6) Jerking of limbs, Meny., Psor.

PEPSINUM

(Pepsin)

PHARMACY - pep. Pepsinum. Pepsin. Digestive enzyme from the mucus membrane of the stomach of pigs sheep or cow. ***Historical dose:*** All potencies, first to thirtieth potency.

HOMEOPATHIC - Imperfect digestion with pain in gastric region. Diarrhea due to indigestion. Marasmus of children who are fed on artificial foods. Diabetes. Gout. Diseases of pancreas.

REFERENCES - Boericke.

PERSEA AMERICANA

(Avocado)

PHARMACY - pers. Persea americana. Avocado. Alligator pear. N. O. Lauraceae. ***Historical dose:*** Tincture and all potencies.

CLINICAL - Arthritis. Coughs. Diarrhea. Emaciation. Gout. Hair, loss. Impotence. Infertility. Malnutrition. Skin, disorders. Worms. Wounds. Wrinkles.

HERBAL - Throughout the Aztec empire, avocado was used as both a food and medicine. All parts of the tree was used for medicinal purposes. Native Guatemalans have long used the avocado to stimulate hair growth, repel worms, and treat diarrhea.

The fruit is highly nutritious, containing calcium, phosphorus, iron, and vitamins. Avocado is rich in potassium and vitamins B6 and E, which can help in relieving stress and sexual problems, such as infertility and impotence.

Although many believe that avocados are fattening, they contain a high amount of mono-unsaturated fats, particularly oleic acid, making it a powerful antioxidant foot. The oleic acid offers protection against heart disease, strokes, and cancer. There is some evidence to suggest the fruit can help lower cholesterol.

The fats are also easily digestible and contain anti-fungal and antibacterial actions that, when pureed, make an excellent food for invalids, convalescents and sick children. In some parts of Africa, the fruit pulp is used as a baby food.

Externally, the fruit soothes the skin, helps heal wounds, and stimulates hair growth. Avocado oil nourishes and softens rough, dry, or flaking skin. Stimulates the production of collagen, helping reduce the appearance of wrinkles.

Avocado leaves have anti-tussive properties and increase biliary secretions. The leaves and bark are used to treat diarrhea, gas, and bloating, as well as to relieve coughs, liver obstructions, and clearing out uric acid. They can also stimulate menstruation and induce abortion.

The rind can expel worms. The seed is rich in tannins, and used as a cloth dye or to treat diarrhea. The oil has been used to help reduce gout pain. A decoction reduces arthritis pains.

REFERENCES – Murphy.

PERTUSSINUM

(Whooping Cough Nosode)

PHARMACY - per. Pertussinum. Whooping cough nosode. Pertussin. Coqueluchinum. ***Historical dose:*** All potencies.

CLINICAL - Anorexia. Asthenia. Bronchitis. Chemosis. ***Choking***. Convulsions. ***Coughs***. Cyanosis. Mastoiditis. Myelitis. Nosebleed. Paralysis. Polyneuritis. Tachycardia. Vomiting. ***Whooping cough.***

HOMEOPATHIC - Per. is taken from the glairy and stringy mucus containing the virus of whooping cough. Introduced by Clarke for the treatment of whooping cough and other spasmodic coughs.

In Clarke's experience, it agrees well with all other whooping cough remedies and when their specific indications appear he gave them in alternation or alone. Per. is an unproved remedy, except in the sense that every case of the disease is a proving. Can be used a preventive in ***whooping cough*** or to treat the disease.

Spasmodic coughing attacks. Dry cough, spasmodic of different intensity, comes suddenly. Repeated coughing fits which end in vomiting. Increasing jerking cough with cyanosis, with a phase of apnea followed by the taking of respiration. Predisposition to tuberculosis.

Asthenia. Convulsions. Muscular jerkings. Neuro-motor deficit. Polyneuritis. Paresis. Paralysis. Myelitis. Hemorrhage from the meninges. Anorexia. Sleepy and in a state of confusion. Troubles of conscience.

MIND - Psycho-motor or sensorial troubles. State of confusion. Restlessness. Troubles of conscience. Cries, tears.

Chest - Stinging pain in or on the chest with cough.

Ears - Mastoiditis.

Eyes - Chemosis. Tears. Coryza with hacking cough.

Face - Intense flushing with cough.

Heart - Cyanosis, sweats, weakness. Tachycardia.

Lungs - Bronchitis. Dyspnea with cough. ***Whooping cough.*** Strangling sensation with cough on waking. ***Spasmodic choking cough.*** Spasmodic cough with intense flushing of face. Hacking cough with coryza. Deep-sounding croupy cough. ***Coughing in frequently repeated attacks***. Cough provoked by intense tickling in throat, fauces or trachea. Sobbing or sighing at end of cough.

Modalities - Worse by laughing, emotion, effort, rest or nervous shock.

Mouth - Itching of the palate on lying down at night. Ulceration of the tongue.

Nose - Nosebleed.

Stomach - Vomiting or nausea at end of cough.

Throat - Laryngo-spasms. Spasm of the glottis. Intense tickling in throat causing cough.

COMMENTS - Clarke gave the 30c every four hours in all cases of whooping cough, suspected or defined, as a matter of routine, and as a rule it quickly assumed control of the case and did all that was necessary.

Dr. Sheppard wrote about giving Per. for whooping cough prophylaxis. "Pertussin 30c acts well as a protective against whooping cough. 364 cases were given daily doses of pertussin for two weeks after contact.

"Many of these cases were seen in the day nurseries under my care and not one of these children developed the disease. As two of the nurseries took in children from two weeks old, it was most essential that they should not be exposed to the infection, and it was gratifying to find that Pertussin was a means of preventing the spread of the disease.

"In another private school, a child came back after the holidays with a fully developed whooping cough, in spite of carrying a doctor's certificate as being free from any infectious disease. All the twelve children in her class were infected.

"The headmistress, on my advice, gave Pertussin 30 four doses hourly, and the children had the mildest attack of whooping cough she had ever seen. She was grateful to Homoeopathy, and to the nosode Pertussin for turning so serious a disease into a mild one."

RELATIONS - ***Compare:*** (1) Dros., Bell., Cor-r., Cupr., Napht., Meph., Passi., Coc-c., Mang-p.

REFERENCES - Boericke. Clarke. Julian.

PESTINUM

(Plague Nosode)

PHARMACY - pest. Pestinum. Plague nosode. Plaguinum. Trituration of the micro-organism. ***Historical dose:*** All potencies.

CLINICAL - Bubo. Plague. Typhus.

HOMEOPATHIC - The prophylaxis and treatment of plague with injections of a more or less modified virus of plague by old-school practitioners affords evidence that the nosode of plague is available, like other nosodes, for the treatment of cases of the disease from which it is derived.

REFERENCES - Clarke.

PETIVERIA TETRANDRA

PHARMACY - peti. Petiveria tetrandra. Erva de pipi. N. O. Phytolaccaceae. Trituration of fresh root. ***Historical dose:*** Trituration and all potencies.

CLINICAL - Conjunctivitis. Paralysis. Paraplegia.

HERBAL - Allen said that P. tetrandra is probably identical with the Mexican and West Indian species, P. alliacea.

Mure's figure corresponds to this and he said the roots, which are branching and fibrous, ***"smell strongly of garlic."***

P. alliacea, according to the Treasury of Botany is called "Guinea-hen Weed" in West Indies and "Raiz de Guine" in Brazil. In Brazil it is put into warm baths to restore motion to paralyzed limbs. Mure did not mention these names or this use, but his proving brought out some strongly confirmative symptoms.

HOMEOPATHIC - Mure's proving showed some strongly confirmative symptoms in numbness and paralytic sensations, weariness and weight of eyelids. Cold saliva internal coldness, coldness inside bones were experienced.

Modalities - Worse by movement, bending backwards, during and after dinner. Worse in the morning, on waking and on rising, after breakfast.

RELATIONS - ***Compare:*** (1) Phyt. (2) Rhus-t. - In paralysis. (3) Cist. - Cold saliva.

REFERENCES - Clarke.

PETROLEUM OLEUM

(Crude Rock-oil)

PHARMACY - petr. Petroleum. Crude rock oil. Oleum petrae album. Kerosene. Coal oil. Trituration and tincture of the rectified oil. ***Historical dose:*** Trituration, tincture and all potencies.

CLINICAL - Allergies. Addison's disease. Albuminuria. Anemia. Angina pectoris. Anus, fissure. Bedsores. Breath, offensive. Burns. Chilblains. Chlorosis. Constipation. Cracks in skin. Deafness. Diarrhea. Dysmenorrhea. Dyspepsia. Ear disorders. ***Eczema.*** Face, rough. Facial paralysis. Feet, painful. Fester, tendency. Fistula. Frostbite. Gastric ulcer. Gonorrhea. Hands, chapped. Headache. Hemorrhoids. ***Herpes.*** Herpes. Irritation. Jaw, dislocated. ***Motion, sickness.*** Myopia. Nose, sore. Otorrhea. Perspiration strong. Pregnancy. Presbyopia. Prostatitis. ***Psoriasis.*** Rheumatism. ***Seasickness. Skin disorders.*** Sprains. Syphilis. Tabes mesenterica. Tinnitus. Toothache. Urethra, stricture. Varicose veins. ***Vertigo.*** Vomiting. Warts.

HOMEOPATHIC - Petrolatum (vaseline) consists of hydrocarbons of the paraffin series, obtained from residues after distillation of lighter oils from crude petroleum, or deposited from crude petroleum on standing.

Petroleum is made by agitating the liquid commercial petroleum with sulphuric acid and then rectifying the portion which this acid does not act upon. It is "a light oily fluid, colorless or of a pale straw color and strong characteristic naphthalic smell. Dropped on white paper it evaporates completely, leaving no greasy stain."

Petr. was proved by Hahnemann and is one of his leading anti-psorics, closely related to Graph. It is suited to long lasting, deep-seated, wasting diseases, lingering gastric and intestinal troubles with or without ulceration. In Clarke's experience, no remedy corresponds to more cases of chlorosis in young girls, with or without ulceration of the stomach.

The disorders met with in petroleum extractors and refiners are diseases of the skin and subcutaneous tissue, depressed nutrition, anemia, dyspepsia, nerve troubles, irritability insomnia, respiratory disorders. In addition to these is a kind of intoxication.

Petr. chiefly acts on the skin, especially folds, scalp, face and genitals, sweat and oil glands. Cracked skin. Unhealthy granulations after severe burns. Discharges are thick, purulent, yellowish green.

Car, train or seasickness. Ailments from riding in cars, carriages or ships. ***Long-lasting complaints*** follow mental states-fright, vexation, etc. Ailments are ***worse during the winter***. Dread of open air with shivering when exposed to it.

Great weakness, fainting, tremor, twitching of limbs, catalepsy tonic spasms, left-sided paralysis. Tremulous weakness. Wooden feeling. Bruised soreness, worse in joints. Internal itching. Coldness in spots, in abdomen, in heart, after scratching.

Dryness in ear, nose, etc. Catarrhal condition of the mucus membranes, of stomach and bowels. Lingering gastric and lung troubles, chronic diarrhea.

Strumous diathesis, especially the dark type, who suffer from catarrhal conditions of the mucus membranes, gastric acidity and cutaneous eruptions.

Enlarged glands. Emaciation, especially of chest. Feels sick internally. Hemorrhages, blood light red, worse lifting or riding. Dropsy. Burnings.

MIND - Mental weakness and forgetfulness, with deep-seated disease. Very forgetful, disinclined to think. Loss of memory. Irresolution. Confusion while walking in open air.

Presence of strangers aggravates. Anxiety in a crowd. Worries but does not know why. Anxiety and apprehension about his family. Anxiety with fear. ***Fear,*** long lasting. Anxiety increases until he becomes inconsolable.

Feeling of helplessness. ***Low-spirited with dimness of sight.*** Sadness during menses, with weeping. Melancholy. ***Feels that death is near and must hurry to settle affairs***.

Irritable, easily offended, vexed at everything. Excited, irritable after sex with inclination to be angry and to scold. Cursing. Intolerant of contradiction. Anger with fright. Quarrelsome in morning.

Sense of duality, thinks he is double of someone else lying alongside or one limb is double. ***Delusion there are two babies in the bed.*** Delusion that she has a third leg which would not remain quiet.

Abdomen - Inflated abdomen. Sensation of coldness inside. Pinching colic, better bending double. Navel ulcerated in infants.

Back - Neck, stiff and painful, cracks when moved. Weakness in small of back. Pain in spine and all over the body with sciatica. Coccyx painful on sitting. Pain in sacrum, worse standing erect. Sharp pains shooting up dorsal spine into occiput, in confinement.

Breasts - Itching and mealy coating of nipple.

Causations - Ailments from riding in cars, carriages or ships (Nit-ac has deafness). Vexation. Ill effects of sprains or suppressed eruptions. Cabbage.

Chest - Oppression of chest, worse cold air.

Constitutions - Suited to persons with light hair and skin. For lean, slender persons.

Ears - Ears sore to touch. Dryness in ears. Eczema in and behind ears with intense itching. Moist spots behind the ears. Fissures in meatus. Discharge of pus and blood from the ears. Itching deep in ears in Eustachian tubes. Chronic Eustachian catarrh. Dry catarrh with deafness and noises. Ringing and cracking in ears. Diminished hearing. Deafness with noises in ears in the elderly. Noise from several people talking is unbearable.

Eyes - Inflamed tarsi. Fistula lachrymalis (of recent origin). Blenorrhea of lachrymal sac. ***Marginal blepharitis***. Canthi fissured. Skin around eyes dry and scurfy. Loss of eyelashes. Dim sight, far-sighted, cannot read fine print without glasses.

Face - Dry, as if covered with albumin. Pale or yellow, hot after eating. Easy dislocation of jaw.

Female - Dry, obstinate eruptions. Genitals sore and moist. Aversion to sex. Before menses, throbbing in head (Kreos.). Menstrual flow causes itching. Leucorrhea, profuse, albuminous (Alum., Calc-p.), with lascivious dreams. Prolapsed uterus from constant diarrhea.

Food - ***Hunger***, causing nausea, wakes at night. Hunger immediately after stool. Desire for dainties, aversion to meat, fats, cooked or hot foods. Worse eating cabbage. Thirst for beer.

Head - Headache, worse shaking, while coughing, must hold temples for relief. Occiput, aching, heavy (Op.). Head feels numb as if made of wood. Scalp, sore to touch, followed by numbness. Sensitive scalp, ***as if a cold breeze blowing on it. Moist eruption on scalp***, worse back and ears. ***Falling of the hair.***

Heart - Cold feeling about heart (Carb-an., Nat-m.). Fainting with ebullitions, heat and palpitations.

Kidneys - Cystitis, urethritis. Stricture from chronic urethritis. Acute sudden urging, if not attended to immediately, will cause severe pain. Involuntary urine on rising.

Bedwetting at night. Dribbling of urine after urination.

Limbs - Limbs go to sleep. Chronic sprains. Cracking in joints. Joints stiff, particularly knees. Scalding sensation in knee. Stitches, blisters, cracks in heels. ***Fingertips rough, cracked, fissured every winter***. Ragged, chapped hands and fingers, bleeding in housemaids. Psoriasis of the palms. Offensive sweat in axilla.

Lungs - Dry cough at night, coming deep from chest, waking the patient (in young girls and boys). Cough at night or worse at night. Shatters the head, better pressing. Cough produces headache.

Male - Sweaty genitals. Herpetic eruption on perineum. Itching in urethra. Prostate inflamed and swollen.

Modalities - Better warm air, dry weather, lying with head high. ***Worse from motion of cars, trains, carriage, boat. Worse from dampness,*** cold weather, ***winter***, changing weather, before and during a thunderstorm. Worse from mental states, vexation, sex, touch. Worse eating, cabbage.

Mouth - Dry. Offensive smell like garlic. Ulcers on the inner cheek, painful when closing the teeth. Soreness, while chewing. Tongue, white in center, dark streak along edges.

Nose - Dry. Tip of nose itches. ***Nostrils ulcerated, cracked, burn***. Ozaena with scabs and muco-purulent discharge. Nosebleed.

Rectum - ***Diarrhea***, watery, gushing. Diarrhea or dysentery during the day, worse cabbage, then empty feeling. ***Itching of anus*** after stools. Hemorrhoids and fissures of anus with great itching. Herpes on perineum.

Sensations - Brain as if wrapped in a fog. As if everything in head were alive. As if head made of wood or as if bruised. As if a cold breeze were blowing on head. As if head would burst. Veil before eyes, sand in eyes. Jaw as if distended. As if something were tearing off from pit of stomach. As if a cold stone at heart. Upper and lower limbs as if stiff without joints. Splinter in heel.

Skin - Eczema with cracks in skin, worse in winter. ***Psoriasis***, especially of hands. ***Deep cracks*** in skin folds, nipples, fingertips. ***Cracks bleed easily***, worse in winter. ***Dirty, hard, rough, thickened*** like parchment. Skin gets raw, festers or ***won't heal,*** worse in folds. Slight injuries suppurate (Hep.). ***Thick, greenish crusts, burning and itching, redness, bleeding.*** Itching at night. Itching orifices with burning. Herpes. Chilblains, moist, itch, burn and turn purple. Brown spots. Bedsores. Skin is extremely sensitive, all clothing is painful.

Sleep - Restless with frightful dreams.

Stomach - Feeling of emptiness. Stomach pain when stomach is empty, relieved by constant eating (Anac., Sep.). Ravenous hunger. Must rise at night and eat (Psor.). Smells of garlic. Distention. Heartburn, hot, sharp, sour eructation. Pungent, acrid belchings. ***Nausea*** with accumulation of water in mouth. Vomits bitter green substance. ***Seasickness and motion sickness.*** Nausea during pregnancy, must stoop.

Temperature - Chilly with dry mouth. Chilliness, followed by sweat. Flushes of heat, particularly of the face and head, worse at night. Flushes of heat all over in frequent attacks during day. Palms and soles hot. Perspiration, foul on feet and axilla. Sweat in spots.

Throat - Dry. Hoarseness (Carb-v, Caust., Phos.). Foul mucus in throat, hawks out in the morning. Croup and laryngeal diphtheria.

Vertigo - ***Vertigo on rising***, felt in occiput. Vertigo, as if intoxicated or as if seasick. Vertigo like that produced by swinging motion.

COMMENTS - Kent suggested Petr. for low conditions in which there is an inability to throw out eruptions on the skin or conditions in which an eruption has disappeared without improvement in health. Mucus membranes have catarrh. Ozaena, intestinal catarrh. Soreness and cracks about mucocutaneous orifices.

Severe irritability of the skin. Affinity for the scalp, behind the ears, skin folds, scrotum, and genitals.

Eczema (Sil., Graph.), especially of the hands and toes. Psoriasis (Nat-m., Graph.). Severely chapped skin. Chapped, rough hands.

Induration with cracks. Deep cracks that bleed. Painful cracks of the heels of palms of the hands. Fissures that ooze clear or yellow fluid. Skin feels tight, like wrapped leather. Thickened skin, hard, splitting.

Fingertips crack and bleed. Nails split and turn dark. Cracked nostrils. A slight wound or injury can suppurate easily. History of suppressed eruptions with unhealthy looking skin that doesn't heal well.

Marked burning sensations. Feet and palms burn (Sulph.). Severe itching, will scratch until the skin is raw and bleeding (Sulph.). Itching without eruptions. Feet feel frozen, tingling, numbness. Diabetic neuropathies (Agar.). Stinging and red. Very sensitive to clothing.

Scalp eruptions, moist and sensitive to touch. Athletes foot (Thuj., Sil., Graph., Psor., Sanic.), with offensive foot sweats, deep cracks between the toes, burning and itching of the skin. Offensive, smelly feet (Sil.).

Genital herpes (Nat-m., Rhus-t., Apis.). Vesicles with yellow fluid. Crusty appearance. Vesicles with yellow thick crusts that become moist, ulcerating, rawness. Sores pop, leaving a painful ulcer. Groin is itching and red. Groin eczema, fungal infections.

Chilblains. Frostbite (Agar., Zinc.). Intermittent claudication, painful cramps and spasms, burning in hands and feet from poor circulation. Pain on touching something cold.

Skin symptoms are worse in winter. This modality gave Nash the key to several cases of eczema, chapped hands, chilblains and one case of chronic diarrhea, as soon as he discovered that the patient had eczema of the hands in winter. Petr. 200c was given.

A man, a patient of Clarke's who suffered from inveterate eczema and who had formerly been employed in a factory where much petroleum was used, noticed that his eczema was much better while working with petroleum.

He told Clarke that the vapor had the singular effect of making some of the workmen insane, causing desire to kill, hallucinations, they will see things not actually visible, for instance, "they will see the rails in a station when a train is on them."

"Falling out of the hair." Cooper clarified that Petr. "probably acts on the sebaceous rather than the sudoriferous secretions of the skin and its local action is on parts where the sebum is abundant."

Vertigo and heaviness, often associated with nausea and bilious vomiting. Useful for motion sickness or seasickness (Tab., Cocc.). Carsickness, feels as if intoxicated. Faint and weak. Pale, cold, cold sweat, sinking nausea. Worse motion, better fresh air and cold water on face, closing eyes.

Headache in the occiput region with sickness. Heaviness like lead, pressure, sticking, pulsating, worse on shaking head or any jar. Pain travels from occiput to eyes and is associated with temporary loss of sight and fainting. Blocked Eustachian tubes and itching in the ears (Kali-m., Cham.). Dizziness, ringing in the ears.

"Oppression of the chest, worse in cold air." Cough coming from deep down in the chest and frequently waking the patient up at night, usually in children. Thick, purulent and yellowish green discharges.

Kent remarked on the awful ravenous hunger. Empty feeling, gnawing hunger, must eat small amounts. Hunger immediately after a stool in diarrhea, nervous affections, spinal disease, etc.

Irritability of the mind. Excitable, angry at trifles. Characteristic illusion that there is another person or another baby in bed has led to cures in cases of typhoid and puerperal fever with Petr.

RELATIONS - ***Antidoted by:*** Cocc., Nux-v., Phos. ***Antidote to:*** Nit-ac., Lead poisoning - one of the best remedies. ***Compare:*** (1) Carb-v, Graph., Sulph., Phos. ***Complementary:*** before Sep. ***Compatible:*** Bry., Calc., Lyc., Nit-ac., Nux-v., Puls., Sep., Sil., Sulph.

REFERENCES - Boericke. Clarke. Kent. Murphy. Phatak.

PETROSELINUM SATIVUM

(Parsley)

PHARMACY - petros. Petroselinum sativum. Parsley. Carum petroselinum. Apium petroselinum. N. O. Umbelliferae. Tincture of whole fresh plant when coming into bloom. ***Historical dose:*** Tincture and all potencies.

CLINICAL - Blindness. Catheter, fever. Chills. ***Cystitis.*** Dyspepsia. ***Dysuria.*** Fevers. Flatulence. Gleet. ***Gonorrhea. Gravel. Hemorrhoids***. Intermittent fever. Night-blindness. ***Polyuria.*** Priapism. Prostate, enlargement. Urethritis. Urinary, difficulties. Urticaria.

HERBAL - Parsley tea is a recognized domestic remedy for gonorrhea. Parsley eaten after meals, with or without salad oil, is reputed to act as a solvent on uric acid if there is a tendency to its formation in the urine. Fresh butter and parsley applied warm is an old remedy for bruises.

Cooper noted that an infusion is given to all children recovering from scarlatina by the matron of a suburban infectious hospital. An old gleet has been known to disappear from parsley infusion, and an Edinburgh surgeon used to given it in all nephritic and bladder diseases that were chronic. Parsley is said to be poisonous to ferrets.

HOMEOPATHIC - Hahnemann noted the usefulness of Petros. as a gonorrheal remedy when there is a frequent desire to urinate. Affinity for the genito-urinary sphere. The leading indication is ***sudden urging to urinate*** and drawing, tingling, crawling or itching in navicular fossa. During urination, burning and tingling from perineum through whole urethra. After urination, cutting and biting in fossa navicularis. Very ***painful urination*** causing him to shiver, dance around the room in agony.

Gonorrhea with a milky or yellow discharge. ***Dysuria*** with prostatic enlargement. Urinary difficulties of babies. ***Hemorrhoids with much itching***.

Back - Jerking or bubbling sensation in muscles of back and arms.

Ears - Shrill singing in ears like a bell ringing out of tune, which affects the whole organism.

Eyes - Blindness at night with swelling of eyes.

Food - Thirsty and hungry, yet as soon as they begin to eat or drink they lose all desire.

Kidneys - ***Tingling***, lancinating, pressure and drawing in urethra. Burning, tingling from perineum throughout whole urethra. ***Dysuria and polyuria.*** Frequent and almost fruitless desire to urinate, every half-hour. ***Sudden urging to urinate***, voluptuous tickling in fossa navicularis. Child suddenly seized with desire to urinate, if not gratified immediately, jumps up and down with pain. Urethritis. ***Gonorrhea with intense biting, itching, deep in urethra***. Milky fluid, albuminous yellow discharge from urethra. Orifice of urethra agglutinated with mucus.

Male - Priapism, without curvature of penis. Urethritis. Pollutions, profuse emission toward morning.

Rectum - Whitish evacuations like clay, chronic diarrhea. ***Hemorrhoids with much itching***. Burning at anus.

Skin - Urticaria.

Sleep - Sleep late, with many anxious dreams.

Stomach - Twitching, jerking pains in epigastrium. Flatulent belchings, colic, nausea and vomiting.

Temperature - Ague, especially quotidian, marked periodicity, regular stages. Acute fevers from defective assimilation or perverted innervation, accompanied by flatulent dyspepsia. Intermittent fevers with abdominal disorders. Fevers with traumatic or chronic inflammation of urethra or even stricture.

COMMENTS - Petros. was proved by Bethmann. He obtained only thirty-six symptoms, all in the genito-urinary sphere, but these were very characteristic and have given the remedy a definite place in homeopathic medicine, especially in gonorrhea and gleet.

Farrington said Petros. is a great "baby medicine" for urinary difficulties. Hering collected symptoms from other observers. It has cured many cases of intermittent fever and traumatic or other urethral fevers.

Acute cystitis, urethritis. Burning and tingling in the urethra. Irresistible desire to urinate, frequent urination. Children will scream and yell with the urge to urinate, anticipating the pain. Bladder infections in children. Gonorrhea. Trauma to the urethra from catheters.

Clarke confirmed its efficiency in gonorrhea and gleet, giving ten-drop doses of the tincture. In a case of dysuria from prostatic enlargement there was frequent urging to urinate every half to three-quarters of an hour with burning pains in bladder and urethra.

Petros. 4x, three drops every hour took away all the pains and relieved the tenesmus in a few days. The prostate gland itself was not influenced.

RELATIONS - ***Compare:*** (1) In gonorrhea with sudden and frequent urging, Cann-s., Canth., Merc. (2) Screams before urinating from irritation of mucus membrane, Acon., Caust., Bor. (3) Sars., Lyc. and Benz-ac. have screaming before urinating when due to gravel. (4) Gonorrhea, strangury, frequent urging to urinate, white stools, Dig. (5) Dig. has slow pulse often puffed prepuce, Sulph. indurated prepuce. (6) Cystitis, Con. - has intermittent urination, Petros. has inflammation that has traveled back, sudden, irresistible desire. (7) Bubbling in back, urinary disorders, Berb. (8) Uric acid tendency intermittent fevers, Urt-u.

REFERENCES - Boericke. Clarke. Murphy. Phatak.

PHALLUS IMPUDICUS

(Stinkhorn Fungus)

PHARMACY - phal. Phallus impudicus. Stinkhorn fungus. N. O. Fungi. Tincture or infusion of whole fungus. ***Historical dose:*** Tincture and all potencies.

CLINICAL - Gastro-enteralgia. Sweat, viscid. Vertigo. Vomiting.

HOMEOPATHIC - Kalieniczensko took five or six teaspoonfuls of an infusion of Phal. in twenty-four hours and observed the effects, which included vertigo, dullness, vision disordered, gastro-enteric disturbance and viscid sweat.

There is a general resemblance to the effect of Agar.

REFERENCES - Clarke.

PHASEOLUS NANUS

(Dwarf-bean)

PHARMACY - phase. Phaseolus nanus. Dwarf-bean. Phaseolus vulgaris. Kidney-bean. N. O. Leguminosae. Papilionoideae. Trituration of the dried bean. Decoction of dried beans and pods. ***Historical dose:*** Trituration and all potencies.

CLINICAL - Albuminuria. Breast, tumors. Diabetes. ***Dropsy.*** Hematuria. Headache. ***Heart, disorders.*** Hernia. Hydrothorax. Impotency. ***Palpitations.*** Pericarditis. Pleurisy. Prostate, diseases. Wounds, punctured.

HERBAL - Clarke included under Phaseolus both Phaseolus nanus and Phaseolus vulgaris. The New Eng. Med. Gaz. published a translation of a pamphlet by Dr. Heinrich Ramm on the uses of ***"Bean tea."***

A woman whom Ramm had treated in vain for mitral valve disease with liver and kidney complications and dropsy, presented herself one day apparently cured by drinking "Bean tea."

This led Ramm to try it in other cases and he found that kidney and cardiac dropsies were speedily relieved, urine largely increased in quantity and in cases of albuminuria, where the albumen quickly disappeared.

HOMEOPATHIC - Some effects of eating mildewed beans in a child were recorded by W. Dale. A. M. Cushing and Demeures both proved Phaseolus nanus, but Cushing only published the symptoms observed on the heart.

Demeures, in his proving, experience severe headache from fullness in the brain. Breathing slow, pulse slow or extinct. "Irregular, weak pulse and heart failure." Soreness to touch in eyeballs, right rib, epigastrium, and right humerus. Diabetes.

Cooper noted that the inside of the pod rubbed on warts is said to cure them. A decoction of the shells has been used as a drink for diabetes, but can cause severe headaches.

Ramm noted it for dropsical effusion into pleural cavity, pericardium and peritoneum. Chronic disorders of the urinary tract from kidneys to urethra, pyelitis, bladder catarrh, gravel, stones, uric acid.

Ramm considered Phase. an important remedy in gout and diabetes. He used a decoction of the whole dried ripe pod "of the taller variety," Phaseolus vulgaris.

MIND - Could only be roused by speaking loudly. Frightened by irregular action of heart. Feeling that she would die with palpitations.

Abdomen - Pressure on abdomen gave pain, child shrank from it and drew up legs. Dropsy. Pain like hernia in right inguinal ring, lasting all day.

Chest - Breathing slow and sighing. Sick feeling about heart with weak pulse. Pulse rapid. ***Palpitations.*** Right ribs sore. Dropsical effusion into pleura or pericardium.

Eyes - Pupils dilated, insensible to light. Eyeballs (especially right) painful to touch as from a blow. Scalding pain in right orbit. Very smart itching in inner canthi. Pain over right orbit worse from mental exertion.

Face - Features expressed suffering.

Head - Aches chiefly in forehead or orbits from fullness of brain, worse any movement or mental exertion.

Heart - ***Fearful palpitations*** and feeling that death is approaching.

Kidneys - Diabetic urine. Bloody urine. Uric acid gravel.

Limbs - Pain to touch in extremity of head, of right humerus.

Lungs - Breathing slow and sighing.

Male - Complete impotence. Prostate enlargement.

Modalities - Headache was worse by movement of the head or any mental exertion, reading or writing. Pressure aggravates.

Stomach - Pain in epigastrium when touched, especially in region of pylorus. Severe, dull pain in epigastrium, vomiting.

Temperature - Cold perspiration.

COMMENTS - Cushing's proving recorded disturbance of the nervous system, genital organs, impotence, stomach, bowels and kidneys and this symptom, which brought the proving to an abrupt close:

"I suddenly felt a curious sensation in the region of the heart. It was so sudden and strange I immediately felt my pulse and found it very irregular and feeble, so much so I think I was frightened, at least, I did not take any more of the medicine."

Cushing used this in his case of a female doctor, 30, married, no children, never ill except with children's diseases, had much mental trouble two years before and had done much cycling. Since then her heart had given trouble. About five times in a minute the heart would give one hard, unpleasant throb, then omit one beat. During the night it was much worse and prevented sleep. Phase. 10c was given.

Thirty-six hours later the heart would beat a hundred beats without varying and improvement continued, but the patient had to give up the remedy on account of the headache it caused, "as if something were pressing hard against each temple", much worse after each dose of the medicine. The patient was never subject to headaches.

He had another case, in which a man, 45, had dropsy, heart and other complications. Bean pod decoction enabled him to lie down on a couch and markedly diminished the dropsy.

A clergyman, 69, many years invalid on account of heart disease after unusual exertion was greatly exhausted and became entirely pulseless and so remained four days in spite of treatment until Phase. 9x was given. In a few hours pulse returned. In thirty-six hours it was regular and strong and so remained until his death, which occurred two weeks later.

In another case, Cushing observed a woman, 50, weak, tired, badly acting heart for some years. Phase. 9x was given and in forty-eight hours "her heart wheeled into line all right and remains so."

Another woman, 87, heart acted badly, every third beat omitted. After taking Phase. two days pulse quite right.

A nurse, 50, "had fearful time with her heart palpitating and feeling as if she should die," Phase. 15x cured. The patient "never took anything in her life that did her so much good."

In a confinement case, with primipara, urine loaded with albumen, frightful convulsions, forceps delivery. Two hours later the heart failed and no stimulants would start it.

Phase. 9x was given and in ten minutes the heart was all right. Twice in the night the dose had to be repeated, but that was all. The albumen rapidly disappeared and a quick recovery was made.

S. R. Stone reported the case of Mr. T., 69, whom he found semi-conscious, yet suffering severely, having been seized with distress in heart region, respiration labored, pulse 51. He had attacks previously, but lighter and the pulse in them had always been slow.

Phase. 6x was given, at first every half-hour, then every hour. The next day the patient was nearly well and said he "could feel every dose working."

RELATIONS - ***Compare:*** (1) The Leguminosae. (2) In heart, Dig., Crat., Spig., Lach., Thyr., (3) Punctured wounds, Hyper., Led. (4) Diabetes, Syzyg., Nat-s., Uran-n.

REFERENCES - Boericke. Clarke.

PHELLANDRIUM AQUATICUM

(Water Dropwort)

PHARMACY - phel. Phellandrium aquaticum. Water dropwort. Oenanthe phellandrium. Fine-leaved water-hemlock. Horse-bane. N. O. Umbelliferae. ***Historical dose:*** Tincture and all potencies.

CLINICAL - Bronchitis. Emphysema. Tuberculosis.

HOMEOPATHIC - Phel. acts on lungs and nerves. The respiratory symptoms are most important and have been frequently verified clinically.

Catarrhal conditions of the respiratory tract. Bronchitis and emphysema. ***Offensive expectoration and cough in tuberculosis***. Hemoptysis. Tuberculosis, affecting generally the middle lobes.

Everything tastes sweet. Hectic and colliquative diarrhea. As if all the blood vessels were in vibratory motion. Feeling of tiredness while walking.

MIND - Peevish arrogance.

Breasts - Pain in nipples. ***Pain in milk ducts,*** intolerable between nursing.

Eyes - Only half open and look as if one has been crying for a week. Burning in eyes. Lachrymation. Ciliary neuralgia, worse any attempt to use eyes. Intolerance of light.

Face - Livid red in the evening.

Head - Headache involving nerves going to eye. Clang like striking on metal in brain, waking him. ***Weight on vertex, aching and burning in temples and above eyes***. Crushing feeling in vertex.

Lungs - Expectoration, horribly offensive (like bedbugs), loose, profuse, smeary, causing dyspnea. Cough compels him to sit up. Sticking pain through from left border of right breasts to between shoulders. Pains going backwards through chest.

Modalities - Better while nursing. Worse air, cold, open. Worse from using eyes.

Sleep - So sleepy, would fall asleep while standing at work.

Stomach - Everything tastes sweet. Desires sour things, milk or beer. Aversion to water. Belchings smelling of bed bugs.

Vertigo - Vertigo, dizzy when lying down.

COMMENTS - This remedy, proved by Nenning, has a few striking symptoms, although it is rarely used and very little known. Generally right-sided.

Continuous cough for hours in the morning accompanied by dyspnea and prostration. Coarse rales, compelling the patient to remain in a sitting posture. Bronchitis and tuberculosis. Last stage of tuberculosis when a cavity has formed in the lungs and there is edema of the limbs. Diarrhea, difficult respiration and profuse sweat.

Affinity for the female breasts, specially the right one. The nipples pain each time the child is put to the breast. The pain shoots inward and backward to the shoulder and to the sacrum.

Intolerable pain in the right breast along the course of the lactiferous tubes immediately after nursing, causing physical and mental distress, loss of strength, and hysterical weeping. Removes abnormal sleepiness in women after childbirth.

Usher reported a cure with Phel. in a woman, who would go off to sleep standing over her wash-tub.

REFERENCES - Boericke. Clarke.

PHENACETINUM

PHARMACY - phenac. Phenacetinum. Para-acetphenatidine. Derivate of anilinum. ***Historical dose:*** All potencies.

CLINICAL - Cyanosis. Face, eruptions. Fevers. Headache. Perspiration, excessive. Typhoid fever. Uremia.

HOMEOPATHIC - Phenac. belongs to the Aniline group and was introduced into old-school practice as a remedy in febrile states and neuralgias.

Clarke added a symptom observed on a young woman who had taken Phenac. for headaches. She had a circumscribed rash on both cheeks which came out red, lasted four days and then peeled and as soon as it was clear the process was repeated.

Clarke tried many remedies with varying success, but it finally disappeared under Alum. 30c, one powder at bedtime.

REFERENCES - Boericke. Clarke.

PHENOBARBITALUM

(Phenobarbital)

PHARMACY - phenob. Phenobarbitalum. Phenobarbital. Gardenalum. Allopathic drug. ***Historical dose:*** All potencies.

CLINICAL - Acetonemia. Allergies. Asthma. ***Convulsions.*** Coryza. Digestive, disorders. Eczema. Edema. ***Epilepsy.*** Erythema. Food, allergies. Headaches. Liver, deficiency. Phenobarbital, poisoning. Urticaria. Vesicles.

HOMEOPATHIC - Phenobarbital is derived from phenylethylmalonylurea or gardenal.

Chronic poisoning from phenobarbital and the other barbiturates, especially in cases of digestive or skin intolerance. Eczema, especially weeping eczema. Food, allergies. Digestive complaints from intolerance to foods (fish, crustacea, cream). Physical and psychological depression, tiredness and sleepiness.

Liver deficiency. Alternation of classical allergic phenomena including asthma, eczema, and spasmodic coryza. Nasal and pharyngeal itching. In the child, prurigo coexists or alternates with acetonemia.

Urticaria, either in patches, confluent or isolated. Vesicles dry or weeping when scratched with a syrupy liquid, which is usually cloudy. Itching edema. Itching and often vesicular erythema.

MIND - Mental depression alternating with hyper-excitability. Hypersensitive. Acrimonious. Memory weak.

Abdomen - Abdominal heaviness. Intestinal sluggishness. Chronic or occasional hepatic deficiency.

Blood - Acetonemia in the child.

Constitutions - Phospho-fluoric or flouric, normal or with hypo-laxity with irregular teeth and marked clinical manifestations.

Eyes - Eyes tearful, eyelids heavy, puffy, itching. Sight tires easily, especially after prolonged reading.

Face - Edema of the face. Impression of peripheral congestion of the face and hands.

Female - Menses ameliorate the complaints.

Food - Food, allergies. Worse from eating fish, crustacea or cream.

Head - Headaches with heaviness in the head, at any time.

Modalities - Better from diet, rest, calm and menses. Worse from rest, heat, heat of the bed, at night, from air. Worse from eating fish, crustacea or cream. Worse from being contradicted.

Mouth - Bitter taste in mouth.

Nose - Nasal and pharyngeal itching.

Skin - Hot feeling in the fine areas of skin. Itching with stinging and burning, changed little by heat or cold, attended by excessive scratching to the point of smarting and discharge. Urticaria. Erythema, more or less intense, locality varies. Scarlet fever type erythema. Vesicular eczema, usually oozing with syrupy or oily liquid.

Sleep - Easily tired, sleepy during the day, needs sleep.

Stomach - Nausea in the morning. Epigastric discomfort.

COMMENTS - The proving was carried out by Vannier on four people, using potencies from 30c to 1c, two doses a day, for one week, decreasing the doses from potency to potency, over a period of ninety weeks. All the symptoms appeared with 4c, also with 3c, 2c and 1c.

RELATIONS - ***Compare:*** (1) Urt-u. - Urticaria appears, especially after too much shell-fish and often is more marked on knees and elbows. (2) Apis - Rosy edema, burning and red of the eyelids. Always improved by the cold. With phenobarbital, it is somewhat whiter and unaffected by the cold. (3) Kali-c. - Swelling of the inner corner of the upper eyelids. He wants to be alone. (4) Bell. - Erythema without edema, general symptoms more violent with intense redness, but no real itching. (5) Rhus-t. - Edema with herpetic vesicular eruptions, burning discharge from the eyelids. Need for movement and cold very marked. (6) Ran-b. - Blisters and itching, but no edema. (7) Sulph. - Pruriginous redness with or without blisters with or without edema and frequent alternation with other allergic complaints or complaints caused by self-intoxication.

REFERENCES - Julian.

PHLORIZINUM

PHARMACY - phlor. Phlorizinum. Phlorizin. A substance discovered in the fresh bark of the apple, pear, cherry and Plb. solution. Trituration. ***Historical dose:*** All potencies.

CLINICAL - Diabetes. Glycosuria. Herpes. Intermittent fever.

HOMEOPATHIC - Phlor. exists in fine, silky, four-sided, colorless needles, soluble in water. It has a bitter and slightly astringent taste and has been used in old-school practice as a remedy for intermittent fever.

While being administered for this it has produced glycosuria. This observation led to its successful use by homeopaths in cases of diabetes.

Successes with the 3x and 6c have been reported.

A patient to whom it was given by Burnett accused him of having given him a preparation of apples. The man discovered it because it produced herpes along the dorsum of the penis, an effect which invariably occurred whenever he ventured to eat apples.

V. Mering produced glycosuria in dogs with Phlor., but if Syzyg. was given simultaneously with Phlor., no glycosuria appeared.

REFERENCES - Clarke.

PHOSPHORICUM ACIDUM

(Phosphoric Acid)

PHARMACY - ph-ac. Phosphoricum acidum. Phosphoric acid. Dilution. The dilute acid forms the homeopathic 1x. The first solution is made of glacial phosphoric acid. ***Historical dose:*** Tincture and all potencies.

CLINICAL - Amblyopia. Anemia. ***Apathetic***. Asthma. Bedwetting. Boils. Brain-fag. Breast-feeding, disorders. Bronchitis, capillary. Chancre. Chilblains. Cholera. Coccyx, pain. Condylomata. Corns. Coughs. ***Debility. Diabetes. Diarrhea.*** Dyspepsia. Eclampsia. ***Emaciation.*** Emissions. Enteric fever. ***Fatigue, chronic.*** Feet, sore. Flatulence. Ganglion. Gout. Gravel. ***Grief. Hair, loss.*** Headache, school children. Hectic. Herpes. Hip joint disease. ***Homesickness.*** Impotence. Levitation. Lienteria. Locomotor, ataxia. ***Love, disappointed.*** Masturbation. Menopausal flushes. ***Mental, weakness.*** Navel, pains. ***Neurasthenia.*** Nymphomania. Osteomyelitis. Perspiration, profuse. Phosphaturia. Physometra. Pimples. Polyuria. Pregnancy, nausea. Psoas abscess. Purpura. Rheumatism. Rickets. Sciatica. Scurvy. ***Self-abuse. Spermatorrhea.*** Spinal decay. Sycosis. Syphilis. Tetters. Typhus fever. Ulcers. Urine, phosphates. Uterus, prolapsed. Varicose veins. Vertigo. Warts. ***Weakness.*** Wens. Worms.

HOMEOPATHIC - Ph-ac. is less poisonous than Phos. Proved by Hahnemann, there is a marked action on the emotional and sensorial faculties, a drowsy, depressed, apathetic state is produced, such as is met with in typhoid fevers.

Ph-ac. affects the mind, especially its emotional side. It influences sensory nerves, the sexual system and bones. The debility commonly found in acids is very marked in this remedy, producing a nervous exhaustion.

Conditions from a weakened immune system caused by ***acute disease, sexual excesses, grief, loss of vital fluids. Weakness and debility*** with free secretion, profuse urination, loss of fluids, sweatings etc. except with diarrhea. Heartburn, flatulence. Diarrhea, diabetes, rickets and periosteal inflammation.

Characteristic stupor on which the patient is easily arouse, then is fully conscious. Indifference. The mind is confused, thoughts cannot be connected, thinking makes him dizzy. Neurasthenia.

Hemorrhages with dark blood. Hemorrhages in typhoid. Formation of abscesses after fever. Decay. External parts become black, senile gangrene. Bone diseases. Osteitis. Gnawing pain in bones. Neurosis in stump after amputation, better from deep breathing.

Loose joints. Bruised soreness like growing pains. ***Cancer pain***. Pains go to part lain on. Sense of pressure, as of causing weight in forehead in sternum in vertex in eyes, navel, breasts etc. Formication, at root of hair, along the spine, limbs. Coldness of parts. Sensitive to light, sound and odors, which takes away her breath.

Particularly suitable for young people who grow rapidly and who are mentally or physically overtaxed.

MIND - ***Mental debility, followed by physical.*** Difficult comprehension. Slowness of mind and special senses. Impaired memory (Anac.). Prostrated and stupefied with ***grief, effects of disappointed love. Homesickness.*** Brain fag. Cannot collect his thoughts or find the right word. Forgetfulness of old people. Vanishing of thoughts on reading. Reflects long, then answers correctly, but slowly.

Mild, yielding disposition. ***Apathetic. Indifferent to everything.*** Listless and dullness. Answers reluctantly and slowly, or short and incorrectly. Aversion to talking. Wants to be left alone. ***Wants nothing and cares for nothing.*** Indifferent to those things that used to interest her the most.

Mental ailments with drowsiness, night-sweats toward morning, emaciation. Silent ill-humor. Sadness only while walking, the longer he walks the worse he gets. Sadness from masturbation. Effects of ***grief and mental shock.*** Ailments from disappointed love, with silent grief.

Anxiety and doubt concerning recovery. Despair. Hopelessness. Dread of future, broods over one's condition. Discouraged in open air. ***Pining with emaciation. Homesickness*** with inclination to weep.

Hysteria at menopause. Hysterical affections of young women, with excessive sensibility and irritability. Wildness from vexation. Mild delirium, easily aroused. Delirium with great stupefaction. Unconscious after strong emotions.

Abdomen - ***Aching in umbilical region***. Enlarged spleen (Cean.). Coldness. Distention and fermentation in bowels. Loud rumbling. Offensive, garlicky flatus.

Back - Pain in back and limbs, as if beaten. Lumbar region heavy, increases pain in legs. Boring pain between scapulae. Paralytic weakness along spine. Formication or burning along spine. Spondylitis of cervical vertebrae. Fine stitches in coccyx and sternum. Boils on buttock.

Breasts - Sharp pressure in left breast. Milk scanty, health deteriorated from nursing. Infants vomit milk constantly.

Causations - Ill effects of bad news, disappointed love, grief, chagrin, shock. Separation from home. Loss of fluids, sexual excesses. Over-lifting, over-study. Injuries, operations.

Chest - Takes cold from drafts on chest. Chest troubles after brain-fag. Pressure or twisting behind the sternum, rendering breathing difficult. ***Weak feeling in chest from talking*** (Stann.). Dry cough from tickling in chest. Salty expectoration.

Constitutions - Suited to persons of originally strong constitution weakened by loss of fluids, excesses, violent, acute diseases, chagrin or a long succession of moral emotions. Children and young people who have grown too rapidly, tall, slender and slim with pains in back and limbs as if beaten, growing pains. Persons of mild disposition.

Ears - Earache after blowing the nose. Shrill sound in ears on blowing the nose. Intolerance of noise, especially music, which causes stitches, even while singing himself. Illusions of hearing, hears bell pealing. Every sound re-echoes loudly in the ear. Roaring with difficult hearing. Nervous deafness after typhoid-like fevers.

Eyes - ***Blue rings around eyes***. Lusterless, glassy, staring, sunken, dull appearance. Yellow spots on conjunctiva. Pupils dilated. Eyeballs feel large. ***Pain as if eyeballs were forcibly pressed together and into head.*** Optic nerves seem torpid. Photophobia, averse to sunlight. Sees colors as if a rainbow. Loss of vision from masturbation. Lids inflamed and cold.

Face - Pale, earthy, sickly. Tense as if egg white had dried on it. Sensation of coldness of one side of face. Acne from onanism. Hairs of beard fall out.

Female - Menses too early and profuse, with pain in liver. Itching, yellow leucorrhea after menses. Uterus bloated, as if filled with wind. Dysuria during pregnancy.

Food - Loss of appetite. Craves juicy things. Thirst for cold milk, ***sodas, carbonated drinks,*** mineral water, ice water. Sour food and drinks disagree.

Head - Crushing weight on vertex, pain as if temples were crushed, worse shaking or noise. ***Pressure on top***. Dull headache after sex, from eyestrain (Nat-m.). ***School girl's headache*** from over use of eyes (Ruta). Hair thins, turns gray early, falls out. Hair loss after grief or loss of fluids.

Heart - Irregular, intermittent pulse. Palpitations after grief, after masturbation, in children and young persons who grow too fast.

Kidneys - Burning in kidney region. ***Diabetes***. ***Frequent urination at night***. Bedwetting during first sleep. Urination preceded by anxiety and followed by burning. Urine is profuse, watery, ***milky***. Phosphaturia. Whey-like urine shortly before menses.

Limbs - Weak. ***Great debility***. Pains at night ***as if bones were scraped.*** Tearing pains in joints, bones and periosteum. Numbness along radial nerve. Stumbles easily and makes missteps. Formication in limbs. Burning below the waist. Cramps in upper arms and wrists. Heavy forearms. Wens on hands between metacarpal bones. Itching, between fingers or in folds of joints.

Liver - Liver, seems to be too heavy, painful during menses.

Lungs - Spasmodic tickling cough. Salty expectoration.

Male - Sexual power deficient. Weak, relaxed genitals during sex, preventing emission (Nux-v.). Weakness and pollutions after sex. Nightly emissions with lascivious dreams. Seminal vesiculitis (Ox-ac.). Prostatorrhea, even when passing a soft stool. Tender and swollen testes. Edema of prepuce and swollen glans penis. Sycotic excrescences (Thuj.). Herpes. Eczema of scrotum.

Modalities - Better from warmth, after short sleep, stool. ***Worse from loss of vital fluids,*** sexual excess, fatigue, surgery, convalescence from fevers. ***Worse from emotions, grief, chagrin, mental shock,*** homesickness, unhappy love. Worse chronic fright (Carc.). Worse from being talked to, talking, sitting, standing, lifting. Worse cold drafts, music.

Mouth - Lips dry, cracked. Mouth dry. Taste of rotten eggs. Tongue swollen, dry with viscid, frothy mucus, slimy. Red streak in middle of tongue. Bleeding, swollen gums, retract from teeth. Painful nodosities on the gums. Teeth become yellow and feel dull. Teeth feel cold. At night, bites tongue involuntarily.

Nose - Bleeding. Nose swollen with red patches or pimples on tip of nose. ***Itching***. Bores fingers into nose.

Rectum - Stools involuntary, escape with flatus. ***Profuse, painless, dirty white, watery or lienteric stools***, odorless, with ***little debility.*** Diarrhea in weakly, delicate children with rickets.

Sensations - As if intoxicated, as if head would burst. As if weight in head, as if brain crushed. Bones as if scraped with a knife. As if eyeballs too large. As if egg white had dried on face. As if lower jaw were going to break. Nausea as if in soft palate in throat. Heavy load in stomach. Uterus as if filled with wind. Tickling in chest as with a feather, as with down in larynx. Red-hot coal on arm and shoulder. As if ants crawling over body. As if feet going up.

Skin - Clammy, wrinkled. Pimples, acne, blood boils. Burning red rash. Tendency to abscess after fevers. Painless ulcers with stinking pus. Formication in various parts. ***Falling out of the hair*** (Nat-m., Sel.).

Sleep - Weakness is better from short sleep. ***Sleepy by day,*** hot and wakeful at night. Deep sleep, but when aroused, fully conscious, during fevers. Lascivious dreams with emissions.

Stomach - ***Symptoms following sour food and drink.*** Pressure as from a weight, with sleepiness after eating (Fel.). Acidity. Sour risings. Nausea.

Temperature - Low types of fever with dull comprehension and stupor. Sluggish, painless fevers. Fever with sweat. ***Profuse sweat*** during night and morning. Chilliness. Cold parts, one side of face, abdomen.

Throat - Dry palate. Hoarseness. Hawks up tough mucus.

Vertigo - ***Vertigo toward evening,*** when standing or walking. Vertigo, as if floating in the air, while lying in bed with ringing in the ears and glassy eyes.

COMMENTS - Convalescent remedy. Chronic fatigue since a debilitating acute. Heavy limbs, droopy eyelids, drained feeling, chills and fever (Gels.). Mononucleosis and flu with extreme weakness. Draining, debilitating chronic illness. Emaciation with dark circles around their eyes, sunken faces and apathy. Spacey and empty eyes.

Chronic fatigue with weight loss, especially after grief, emotional loss, loss of fluids, or fevers. Debilitated and tired since grief (Gels., Sil.). Grief, leading to falling of hair, premature senility and depression. The hair may turn gray or fall out in patches.

Homesickness (Caps.), with weight loss, insomnia, and pining. Chronic mental exertion or worry. Lack of emotions (Aur., Sep.). Apathetic (Gels.). Aversion to loved ones (Sep.), with weakness. Feels indifferent about future. Listless. Decreased mental function. Lack of direction, empty (Ign.). Blank mind, spacey, cannot concentrate.

May have a history of excessive sexual activity and loss of sexual fluids. Chronic seminal discharge, prostatorrhea. Weakness and apathy from masturbation or excessive sexual activity (Sel., Agn.). Effects of chronic masturbation. Severe impotence with a history of masturbation or too much sex. Lack of sexual desire or function. Used in some countries as a tonic for sexual debility. May have a history of drug use.

Vertigo with the sensation as if the feet were rising until he stood on his head. This symptom occurred in a patient of Skinner's suffering from smallpox. The disease had been cut short by Vario., when the patient, a woman, complained that her feet were rising to the ceiling and begged her nurses to keep them down. Ph-ac. speedily put her straight.

Illusions of the senses as well as of the sensorium, bells are heard, ciphers, sparks, etc., are seen. Exalted sensitiveness to light, sound and odors, "odors take away his breath."

Becher, one of Hahnemann's provers, noted that his right pupil became widely dilated while the left remained normal. The more he strained the eye, the wider the pupil became until the iris had almost disappeared.

Great weakness, better by short sleep (Phos.). Legs tremble when walking, limbs are difficult to control. "Weak feeling in chest from talking, coughing or sitting too long, better by walking." Hoarseness and nasal voice. Dyspnea, capillary bronchitis.

Cough, as if a feather tickling from middle of chest to larynx, low down in chest. The cough is worse in evening, after lying down. Muco-purulent, salty, bloody, offensive expectoration. Cough causes headache, nausea and vomiting of food, spurting of urine. Every draft of air causes fresh cold.

Dry mouth and throat. Involuntary biting of tongue in sleep. Thirsty for ice cold drinks, bubbly drinks and mineral waters, fresh fruit juice with ice, sparkling fruit juices. Diabetes, when there is a history of sexual excess or of severe mental or emotional over-strain. Emaciation with diabetes.

Copious discharges appear in the sweat and urine. Polyuria. White, milky urine and also white stools. The urine may be clear as it is passed, but turns milky at once and is very offensive. Bedwetting, the child passes a great quantity of urine.

Excessive flatulence. Distention and passing of flatus in large quantities, sometimes with the odor of garlic. Weakened sphincters, involuntary escape of feces and urine, especially on coughing or movement.

Keynote "persistent, painless, watery diarrhea often containing undigested particles of food and which does not debilitate." Diarrhea in children who are emaciated and dehydrated. Weight loss from severe diarrhea. Children feel better when they're having diarrhea (Calc., better constipated).

Bloating of the uterus with gas. Menses are excessive and premature. Debility from breast-feeding. Dark, profuse, passive hemorrhages.

H. Maandblad offered the case of a married woman, 36, mother of eight children, who had for some time been so melancholy and depressed as to be unable to fulfill her household duties. There was no discoverable mental cause, though her condition had been made worse by a sudden death in the family.

The beginning of the illness was apparently a weakness of the stomach, small appetite, always pain and distention after eating, the food seemed to lie long in the stomach undigested. Ph-ac. 6x, ten drops three times a day, soon restored the patient.

RELATIONS - ***Antidoted by:*** Camph., Coff., Staph. ***Compare:*** (1) Carc., Chin., Nux-v., Mur-ac., Pic-ac., Lac-ac., Phos. (2) Oeno., Evening primrose - effortless diarrhea with nervous exhaustion. Incipient hydrocephaloid. Whooping cough and spasmodic asthma. (3) Nect. - watery diarrhea, dry tongue, colic, bluish ring around sunken eyes, restless sleep. ***Compatible:*** Chin., before or after in colliquative sweats, diarrhea and debility after Nux-v. in fainting after a meal after Rhus-t. in typhoid. ***Followed well by:*** Ars., Bell., Caust., Lyc., Nux-v., Puls., Sep., Sulph., Calc-p., Ferr-p., Kali-p., Nat-p.

REFERENCES - Boericke. Clarke. Murphy. Phatak.

PHOSPHORUS

PHARMACY - phos. Phosphorus. The element (P., At. Wt. 30.96). Saturated solution in absolute alcohol. Trituration of red amorphous Phosphorus. ***Historical dose:*** All potencies.

CLINICAL - Alopecia areata. Amaurosis. Amblyopia. Anemia, pernicious. Anus, fissure. Arteries, disease. Asthma. Bone, diseases. Brain, disorders. Breast, abscess. Breast-feeding, disorders. ***Bronchitis.*** Bruises. Cancer. Catalepsy. Cataracts. Catarrh intestinal, nasal. Chilblains. Chlorosis. Chorea. Ciliary neuralgia. Coccyx, pain. ***Colds.*** Constipation. Corpulency. ***Coughs.*** Croup. Dandruff. ***Diabetes.*** Diarrhea. Dropsy. Epilepsy. Esophagus, pain. Exophthalmos. Exostosis. Eye disorders. Fainting. ***Fatty, degeneration.*** Fistula. Flatulence. Fungus hematodes. Gastric, fevers. Gastritis. Glaucoma. Gleet. Gums, ulceration. Hemoglobinuria. ***Hemophilia. Hemorrhages.*** Headaches. Heart, degeneration. ***Hepatitis.*** Hydrocele. Hydrocephalus. ***Hypoglycemia.*** Hysteria. Impotence. Infertility. Injuries. Intussusception. ***Jaundice.*** Keratitis. Laryngitis. ***Lightning, effects. Liver, disorders.*** Locomotor ataxia. ***Lung, disorders.*** Marasmus. Menorrhagia. Menstruation, disorders. Morphinism. Musca volitantes. Muscular, atrophy. Nevus. Nails, disorders. Neuralgias. ***Nightmares. Nosebleeds.*** Osteomalacia. Osteomyelitis. Osteoporosis. ***Pancreas, disorders. Paralysis.*** Periostitis. Petit mal. Plague. ***Pneumonia.*** Polyps. Pregnancy, vomiting. Proctitis. Pruritus, ani. Psoriasis. Puerperal, convulsion. ***Purpura, hemorrhagia***. Pylorus, thickened. ***Retinitis.*** Rheumatism, paralytic. ***Rickets. Scurvy***. Sexual mania. Shiverings. Sleep, disorders. Sleepwalking. Spine, curvature. Spleen disorders. Sprains. Stammering. Syphilis. Syringomyelia. ***Throat, sore.*** Tobacco, effects. Trachea, tickling. ***Tuberculosis.*** Tumors, cancerous. Typhus fever. Ulcers. Urethra, stricture. Vaccinosis. Variola. Voice, loss. Whitlow. ***Wounds.*** Yellow fever.

HOMEOPATHIC - Phosphorus was discovered in 1673 by Brandt, an alchemist of Hamburgh, and shortly afterwards by Kunkel in Saxony. According to Teste, attempts were made to use it in medicine immediately after discovery. Kunkel made it into his "luminous pills," and Kramer claimed to have cured with it diarrhea, epilepsy and malignant fevers.

Teste offered a list of old-school cures, which included continuous, bilious and intermittent fevers, general edema, measles, two cases of pneumonia of the left lung with ataxic symptoms, chronic rheumatism of the legs, strokes, hydrocephalus, periodic headaches, catalepsy, epilepsy, and chronic lead poisoning.

Hahnemann's provings have been added to by later provings, by numerous cases of poisoning and by the effects on workers in match factories, most notably, necrosis of the lower jaw.

The vapor given off by unignited phosphorus is phosphorus oxide. The jaw affection, called "the phossy-jaw" by the workers, is accompanied by profound adynamia and frequently ends in death.

The form of the disease differs according to whether the upper or lower jaw is attacked. In the former case, it generally pursues a chronic and mild course, ending in exfoliation, scars and cure. In the latter, the necrosis may be either acute or chronic, but is always severe and the patients usually die of "tuberculosis" fever.

Phos. irritates, inflames and degenerates the mucus membranes. It inflames the serous membranes, the spinal cord and nerves. It causes paralysis and destroys bone, especially in the lower jaw and tibia. It disorganizes the blood, causing fatty degeneration of blood vessels and every tissue and organ of the body. It gives rise to hemorrhages and hematogenous jaundice.

Phos. produces a picture of destructive metabolism. It causes yellow atrophy of the liver and sub-acute hepatitis.

Ill effects of iodine and excessive use of salt. Great sensitivity to external impressions to light, sound, odors touch, electrical changes, thunderstorms. ***Human barometer*** (Merc.). Great susceptibility to external impressions, light, sound, odor touch, electrical changes, etc.

Insidious onset, gradually increasing debility, ending in severe or rapid disease. Sudden symptoms, sudden prostration, faints, sweats, shooting pains, etc. Sudden prostration from a profound shock. The left side is more affected than the right, the venous more than the arterial system.

Polycythemia. Blood extravasations. Hemophilia. ***Hemorrhages,*** recurrent, vicarious, small wounds bleed much. Blood streaked discharges. Purpura hemorrhagica. Easily bleeding polyps. Healed wounds break out again and bleed. Pyemia. Jaundice, as a concomitant, hematogenous.

Internal, itching, tickling, throbbings here and there. Numbness. Burnings. Jerking, localized, subsultus. Joints, stiff with little pain, sprains, easily dislocated, weak spells in joints, worse exertion. Pain or soreness in spots.

Decay of the bones, spine, upper jaw. Hard swelling here and there. Osteomyelitis. Bone fragility (Calc-p.). Exostoses. ***Fatty degenerations.*** Lipoma. Cancer. Erectile tumors. Tertiary syphilis, skin lesions and nervous debility.

Muscular pseudo-hypertrophy, neuritis. General paralysis of the insane with mania of grandeur, in a stroke. Duchenne's ***pseudo-hypertrophic paralysis*** in locomotor ataxia and other paralyzes. Ataxia and adynamia. Uncertain, involuntary acts. Spasms on the paralyzed side. Epilepsy with consciousness. Petit mal.

Symptoms due to heart and lung disorders. Inflammation of the respiratory system. Recurrent effects colds, croups etc. (Ferr-p.). ***Tightness in chest***, cough etc. Emptiness or heaviness in the chest, stomach etc. ***Craves ice cold drinks and food.***

Acidosis (Nat-p.). Cirrhosis. ***Scurvy***. Emaciation. Flabby muscles. Totters while walking.

Ailments from losses of fluids, over-work of brain, sexual excesses and abuse. ***Worse lying on left side***.

MIND - Mentally and emotionally sensitive. ***Over-sensitive to external impressions***, noise, odors and lights. ***Excitable, impressionable.*** Quickly prostrated by unpleasant impressions. Great tendency to be startled from noises. Can't endure sound of piano, from great weakness of head. Sensitive to bad news, horror stories. ***Sympathetic to others***. Sensitive to others pain and sufferings. Nervous and restless in crowds.

Anxious, restless, fidgety, can't sit still or stand for a moment, better while standing. Anxiety for others, about friends at home. ***Anxiety, when lying on left side, during thunderstorm.*** Anxiety as if he had committed murder.

Frightened easily, better weeping. Fear arising from stomach. Fear of being alone, of death when alone. Fear at twilight, ***of the dark***, of ghosts, monsters, of imaginary things. ***Fear of thunderstorms***. ***Fear something bad will happen***, when thinking of disagreeable things. Fear about future, of insanity.

Timid and irresolute. Lacks willpower to undertake anything. Loss of memory. Brain feels tired. ***Spacey can't keep mind on any subject.*** Stupor, is aroused with difficulty and immediately relapses. Apathy is unwilling to talk and answers slowly. Indifferent even towards her own children (Sep.). Retarded development of speech in children.

Melancholy, disinclined to work, study, converse. Sadness during headache. Sadness in darkness. Great lowness of spirits. Depression arising from belief that he has an incurable disease of heart. Weary of life. Prostration of mind from trifles.

Suicidal disposition, better weeping. Weeps before menses. Weeping during palpitations. ***Wants sympathy.*** Better from company and consolation. Weeping alternating with attacks of involuntary laughter. Laughs at serious things. Laughing when sad.

Irritable and spacey when misses a meal. Offended and hurt easily. Easily angered and vehement, beside himself with anger and suffers physically from it. Rage when aroused. Hypocrisy.

Insanity with exaggerated idea of one's own importance. Monomania in chronic alcoholism. ***Clairvoyant.*** Ecstasy. ***Desires to be magnetized.*** Confusion, better washing face. Paralysis of the insane.

Amorous, will uncover his body and expose his genitals. Sexual thoughts intrude and crowd upon each other. Shamelessness. Accuses herself of obscene actions of which she had not been guilty.

Delirium, loquacious, with difficult respiration. Delirium that he was in several pieces and could not collect them. Fearfulness, as if something were creeping out of every corner. Imagines he sees faces grinning at him from the corners of the room. Destroys everything, spits at nurse, kisses those who comes near her.

Abdomen - Feels cold (Caps.). Abdomen distended and painful to touch. Rubs abdomen for relief. Sharp, cutting pains. ***Very weak, empty, gone sensation*** felt in whole abdominal cavity. Weakness in abdomen, before menses. Sore spot in pit of stomach. Pressure above epigastrium. Painful pulsation in right hypochondrium. Varicose veins all over abdomen. Boils. Large, yellow spots on abdomen. ***Pancreatic disease and diabetes.*** Pancreatic disease with fatty stools. Loud borborygmi. Incarcerated flatus. Flatulent colic, worse hot drinks. Frequent pinching pain in bowels as if diarrhea were about to come on. Inguinal hernia with relaxed abdomen.

Back - Back pains as if broken, impeding all motion, especially during menses. Weak spine. Spinal irritation, worse heat. Burning in spots along spine. Spondylarthrocace. Weakness and paralytic feeling at junction of lumbar and sacral vertebrae. Spinous processes of dorsal vertebrae painful on pressure. Stiff neck. Lipoma on neck with hectic fever. Cramps, burning, between scapula. ***Heat between the shoulder blades***. Pain forward from left scapula. Burning spot in lumbar region, better rubbing. Stitching pain from coccyx up the spine to occiput, worse during stool. Coccyx pain as if ulcerated. Sacrum pain as if broken, on coughing. Pain in sacrum after confinement.

Bladder - Tension over region of bladder. Bladder is full without urging. Burning and twitching in urethra, with frequent desire to urinate. Frequent urination at night, with scanty discharge. Involuntary urination in children who grow too rapidly.

Breasts - Stitching pain in breasts. Left infra-mammary pains. Nipples, hot and sore. Enlargement of mammary gland. ***Suppuration of breasts***, burning, offensive watery discharge. Fistulous tracks after breast abscess. Breast cancer with sharp lancinating pains or bleeding easily. Amenorrhea with milk in breast. Increased secretion of milk, with great debility. Metrorrhagia in nursing women.

Causations - Ill effects of anger, fear, grief, worry. Ill effects of exposure to drenching rains, washing clothes, having hair cut. Tobacco. Iodine. Excessive use of salt or sugar. Electrocution.

Chest - Sharp stitches in chest, ***breathing quickened, oppressed.*** Stitches in left upper chest, rattling worse cold drinks. Full, heavy chest, pains into throat, right arm, or alternating sides. ***Oppression, as if a great weight on chest***. Great pressure on middle of sternum, impossible to lie on back. ***Tightness across chest.*** Burning pains. ***Heat in the chest***. Intense heat behind sternum. Dry, hot feeling in chest with cough, dry, then loose. Yellow spots on chest. Swelling of axillary glands. Violent itching in right axilla. Boils in left axilla.

Constitutions - Suited to tall, slender persons of sanguine temperament, fair skin, blonde or red hair, quick, lively perceptions and sensitive nature. Young people who grow too rapidly and are inclined to stoop, chlorotic, anemic. Persons of waxy, translucent skin, half anemic, half jaundiced. Tall, slender, narrow-chested, tubercular patients, delicate eyelashes, soft hair. Tall, slim, dark-haired persons, especially women, disposed to stoop. Nervous, weak persons who like to be magnetized. Hemorrhagic patients, slight wounds bleed profusely.

Cough - Cough with burning dryness in throat. Dry cough, with pain in head as if it would burst. Dry cough, waking from sleep. Hollow cough, mostly in morning in bed, also at night, prevents falling asleep. Cough in morning after rising with expectoration of transparent mucus. Cough from tickling in throat, worse ***cold air***, reading, laughing, ***talking*** from going from warm room into cold air. Cough before thunderstorm. Nervous cough, provoked by strong odors. Whole body trembles during cough. Must sit up when coughing.

Ears - Otitis media. Mastoiditis (Caps.). Polyps in the ear. Tickling and itching in ears. As if foreign bodies were lodged. Something seems constantly in front of ears. Echoes and reverberations of sounds, especially music (Caust.). Ringing noises, with palpitations. Roaring, from rush of blood. Constant buzzing. ***Hearing difficult***, especially human voice. Dull hearing after typhoid.

Eyes - Glaucoma. Cataract (Calc-f.). Vitreous opacities. ***Atrophy of optic nerve.*** Degenerative changes in retina. Thrombosis of retinal vessels. ***Retinal bleeding.*** Choroiditis. Yellow eyes. Frequent itching in eyes. Sensation of sand in left eye, better rubbing. Burning in eyes, with profuse lachrymation in wind. Photophobia. Aversion to light. Symptoms after an iridectomy. Eyes turned outwards. Eyeballs feel large, stiff. Fatigue of eyes and head even without much use of eyes. Paresis of extrinsic muscles. Edema of lids and about eyes. Pain in orbital bones. Hollow, with blue rings around eyes.

Face - Pale, sickly complexion, blue rings under eyes. Puffiness under eyes. Color of face very changeable. Hippocratic countenance. Skin as if too tight. Skin burns on shaving. Burning heat and redness of one or both cheeks. Lips, blue, dry, cracked, sooty, scabby. Crack in middle of lower lip. Ulcerated corners of mouth. Facial neuralgia. Prosopalgia, worse opening mouth. Mouth drawn to left. Tearing pain in facial bones. ***Swelling and necrosis of lower jaw*** (Amph., Hecla.).

Female - Chlorosis. Amenorrhea with vicarious menstruation, with blood spitting, bleeding from the anus or hematuria, or with milk in breast. Before menses, bearing down pains, nymphomania, weeping. Menses too early and scanty, not profuse. Menses too late but very copious. ***Menses last too long***. Leucorrhea, profuse, smarting, corrosive instead of menses. Milky leucorrhea early in morning, when walking. Slight hemorrhage from uterus between periods. Frequent and profuse or short uterine bleeding in between the periods in nursing women. Metritis. Uterine polyps. Condylomata. Cauliflower cancers bleeding profusely. Cancer of the uterus with metrorrhagia. Edema of labia. Phlebitis. Aversion to sex. Vagina numb during sex in spite of sexual excitement. Violent sexual desire during pregnancy and breast-feeding. Infertility from excessive voluptuousness or with profuse or too late menses. Labor pains distressing, ineffectual.

Food - ***Ravenous hunger during fever***, nightly, before the attack of sickness. Hunger soon after eating. Hypoglycemia, low blood sugar. Loss of appetite alternating with bulimia. Headache from fasting. ***Craving for cold, iced drinks.*** Craves ice during chill. ***Craving for ice cream***, cold milk, carbonated drinks, refreshing things. ***Desires salt,*** acids, spicy foods. ***Desires chocolate,*** candies, cheese, cucumbers, chicken, fish, wine. ***Aversion to warm drinks, warm food.*** Aversion to coffee, tea, boiled milk, puddings, sweets. Aversion to fruit, garlic, onions, tomatoes, meat, salt fish, beer. ***Bad effects of eating too much salt***. Unable to drink water during pregnancy, the sight of water makes her vomit, has to close her eyes when taking a bath.

Head - Headaches, heavy, over one eye, with hunger. Sick headache, with pulsations and burning. Headaches with weakness and strained feeling of eyes. Pains preceded by dimness of sight. ***Headaches with increased sensitiveness to odors.*** Headaches before thunderstorm. Chronic congestion of head. ***Heat comes up from spine***. Burning pains in temples. Shooting pains from one temple to other. Pulsating, pressing, boring and burning, in one or the other temple. Stupefying headache, in vertex. Vertex throbs, hot after grief. Chronic meningitis. Neuralgia, parts must be kept warm. Burning pains. Brain-fatigue with ***coldness of occiput***. Softening of the brain with formication, numbness of limbs. Tendency to atrophy of brain in old age. Periostitis of skull. Feels as if pulled by hair. Skin of forehead feels too tight. Clammy sweat on head. Copious dandruff. Itching of scalp. Falling of hair in large bunches, in spots.

Heart - Anxiety about heart with nausea and peculiar sensation of hunger, somewhat better eating. Pressure in middle of sternum and about heart. Pains go into right arm. Congestion of blood to heart, excited by sensual impressions. Dilatation of the heart from fatty degeneration or endocarditis. Endocarditis or myocarditis during course of acute inflammatory rheumatism or during pneumonia. ***Palpitations with anxiety while lying on left side.*** Palpitations from least excitement. Palpitations during menses. Palpitations with numbness, stiffness and coldness of left arm. Weak heart, pulse rapid, small and ***soft***. Blowing sounds in heart. Feeling of warmth in heart.

Kidneys - Fatty or amyloid degeneration of kidneys. Dull pain in renal region. Burning pain in kidneys, can't lie on back. Bright's disease. Nephritis with hydrops and diarrhea. Hematuria in acute nephritis (Canth.). Hematuria with jaundice. Periodical albuminuria.

Limbs - Limbs heavy as lead. Tingling and formication in limbs, better rubbing. Muscular rheumatism. Weakness and trembling from every exertion, can scarcely hold anything with his hands. ***Joints suddenly give way.*** Ascending sensory and motor paralysis from ends of fingers and toes. Post-diphtheria paralysis with formication of hands and feet. Hands and arms cold during diarrhea. ***Arms and hands become numb***. Stitches in elbow and shoulder joints. Tearing left shoulder at night. Paralyzing stitches in hips, then up back. Pains in tibias, periostitis. Ankles, as if to break, easy dislocation. Burning of feet. Icy cold feet. Toes cramp. Suppressed foot sweat. Cold feet and hands during menses. Can lie only on right side.

Liver - ***Acute and chronic hepatitis.*** Congested liver. Acute yellow atrophy of liver. Fatty degeneration of liver (Carb-tcl., Ars., Chlor.). Cirrhosis. Jaundice with pneumonia or brain disease. Jaundice during pregnancy. Jaundice from nervous excitement, malignant, hematogenous. Liver weakness and sensitivity. Disordered liver in men from tropical climates.

Lungs - Oppressive breathing, worse least motion. Tight suffocative breathing, worse cough. Congestion of lungs. Bronchitis. ***Pneumonia*** of left lower lung, with oppression, ***worse lying on left side***. Pleuro-pneumonia. Lobular pneumonia. Threatened paralysis of lungs at an early stage of pneumonia in old people. Whole body ***trembles*** with cough. Hard, dry, tight, racking cough. ***Sputa rusty, blood-colored or purulent.*** Repeated hemoptysis (Acal.). Easy sputum, frothy, rusty bluish, salty, sour, sweetish or cold. Nervous coughs provoked by strong odors, entrance of a stranger, worse in the presence of strangers, worse lying upon left side. Asthma after cough. Congestive asthma, worse lying on back or on falling asleep. ***Tuberculosis*** in tall, rapidly-growing young people (Calc-p.). Pulmonary edema. Typhoid pneumonia, with sensitiveness and gurgling in ileocaecal region and diarrhea.

Male - Constant discharge of thin, slimy, colorless fluid from urethra. Discharge of prostatic fluid during hard stool. Ulcers on prepuce. Testes sore, swollen, painful. Hydrocele after gonorrheal orchitis, with sexual weakness. ***Irresistible desire,*** but impotent. Erections feeble or none at all. Erection ineffectual during sex. Impotence from or preceded by overexcitement of sexual organs. Premature ejaculation. Involuntary emissions with lascivious dreams. Lascivious, strips himself, sexual mania.

Modalities - Better in dark, sleep, lying on right side, sitting. Better rubbing, massage, magnetism. Better eating, cold food, washing with cold water, cold, open air. Worse from the change of weather, windy, cold, ***thunderstorms, lightning.*** Worse putting hands in cold water, getting wet in hot weather. ***Worse twilight, evening,*** light. Worse from warm food or drink, salt. ***Worse lying on left side*** or painful side, on back. Worse from touch, physical exertion, ascending stairs, shaving, odors. Worse mental exertion, emotions, talking, puberty, sexual excess, loss of fluids.

Mouth - Much watery saliva. Salty or sweetish salivation. Taste bitter of rotten eggs in morning. Sour taste after milk, bitter, sweetish, when coughing. Aphthous patches on roof of mouth and tongue. Itching of palate. Abscess of hard palate. Gums bleed easily, sore behind central incisors. ***Persistent bleeding after tooth extraction.*** Mouth drawn to the left. Speech difficult, stutters. Sore mouth from nursing.

Nose - Nose swollen, red, shiny, painful to touch. Ulcers in the nose. Decay. Periostitis of nasal bones. Nervous fan-like motions of alae nasi (Lyc.). ***Polyps, bleeding easily*** (Calc., Sang.). Nosebleed instead of menses. ***Nosebleeds in children, youths.*** Nosebleed, then pneumonia with cough during stool. Chronic catarrh with ***hemorrhages***, handkerchief is always bloody. Acute coryza, with dull headache. Coryza, alternately fluent and dry, on alternate sides. Sneezing, worse odors, smoke with dyspnea, causes pain in the throat. Sneezing and coryza on putting hands in water. Nose obstructed in morning. ***Oversensitive smell*** (Carb-ac., Nux-v.). Faints from smell of flowers. Foul imaginary odors (Aur.). Loss of smell and taste.

Perspiration - Cold, clammy sweats. Profuse sweat at night during sleep. Profuse sweat in morning. Early morning, sticky sweats, without relief. Perspires on slight exertion. Sweat smells of sulphur. Exhausting sweats. Perspires on head and hands, frequently alternating with coldness. Mostly sweats on head, hands and feet, with increased urine. Perspires only on forepart of body.

Rectum - Urging for stool, on lying on left side. Stool difficult to expel. Stricture of rectum, stools flattened. ***Great weakness after stool***. Dysentery. ***Exhausting diarrhea.*** Diarrhea during pregnancy or confinement. Morning diarrhea of old people. Alternating diarrhea and constipation in old people. Nervous, involuntary stool after fright. Anus open, prolapsed. Painful cramps in rectum. Needlelike stitches in rectum. Tearing in anus, better warm cloth. Fissure of anus. Burning in rectum. Discharge of blood from rectum during stool. Bleeding hemorrhoids. Hemorrhoids burn like fire. Polyps with proctitis.

Sensations - As if about to die. As if immersed in hot water. As if chair were rising. As if he had been lying at night with head too low. As if everything had stopped in head. As if eyes would be pressed out or pressed down by weight about them. As if painful nodes under scalp. Anxiety as if below left breast. As if great weight lying on middle of sternum. Back as if broken. As if quicksilver moved up and down spinal cord. Coccyx as if ulcerated. Soles as if he had walked too much. Feet as if asleep. Ankles as if sprained.

Skin - Anesthesia of skin. Burning in skin with restlessness. ***Scurvy***. Jaundice. Petechia. ***Purpura hemorrhagia***. Ecchymosis. ***Wounds bleed very much, even if small***. Wounds which appear to have healed break out again and bleed. Little ulcer outside of large ones. Ulcers bleed during menses. Thin foul, bloody pus. Brownish or blood red spots. Red streaks after scratching. Psoriasis on knees, elbows, legs and eyebrows. Blood-boils. Fatty cysts. Fungus hematodes and excrescences. Chilblains. Skin burns on shaving.

Sleep - Great drowsiness, especially after meals. ***Short naps ameliorates***, frequently waking. Sleepiness during coryza. Sleepy by day, sleepless before midnight. Sleepless, cannot close the eyes from internal heat. Difficulty falling asleep on account of excitement. Sleeplessness in elderly people. ***Vivid dreams*** of fire, of hemorrhage, of biting animals. Dreams of restless work and business which he could not finish. Lascivious dreams. Sleepwalking. Goes to sleep late and awakens weak. Feels in the morning as if he had not slept enough. Coma vigil.

Stomach - Tremors, fluttering or something rolling over in stomach. Sore spot in pit. Stomach cold as if frozen. Empty, hollow feeling in stomach, as if hanging down, worse emotions. Gnawing pain. Pain in stomach, better cold drinks. Burning in stomach, worse eating. Burning in esophagus. Gastritis with heartburn. Water brash. Hiccough. Sour taste and sour belchings after every meal. Bitter, tasteless eructations. Nausea on putting hands in warm water. Constant nausea with confusion of head. Regurgitates ingesta. ***Throws up food by the mouthfuls***. Water is thrown up ***as soon as it gets warm in the stomach.*** Vomiting of bile, blood, coffee grounds. ***Post-operative vomiting, after chloroform.*** Stomach ulcer.

Stool - ***Very fetid stools and flatus***. Long, narrow, hard stool, like a dog's. ***White***, hard stools. Green mucus with grains like sago. Stools hot, sour-smelling, corrosive. Painless stool, copious, gray, bluish, watery, pouring out. Stools scanty, semi-fluid. Stools green, yellow, watery, with flakes of mucus and clots of blood. Discharge of blood from rectum, during stool.

Teeth - Numb teeth. Rapid decay of teeth. Tearing and shooting pains in teeth, worse open air and warm food. Toothache in morning when chewing. Toothache from washing clothes, from having hands in cold or warm water. ***Persistent bleeding after tooth extraction.*** Inflammation of gums and gumboils in lower jaw. Gums sore behind central incisors. Boring pain sometimes passing into numbness, worse cold, heat and chewing, with soreness and swelling of gums. Swollen and easily bleeding gums. Gums ulcerated. Irregular formation of teeth of lower jaw of scrofulous children with mesenteric disease.

Temperature - Chilly every evening in warm room. Cold knees at night. Craves ice water during the chill. Chill alternating with heat, at night. Chill descends, heat ascends (up back). Burning heat, up back. Internal heat, with sensation of hot water in stomach. Flushes all over, beginning in hands. Profuse perspiration. Hectic fever with small, quick pulse, viscid night-sweats. Fever in warm room, heat down back. Fever with anxiety, burning in face and hands, flushed cheeks. Painless fevers. Fever on falling asleep. Fever at night, without thirst. Stupid delirium.

Throat - Dryness in pharynx and fauces. Dry, glistening. Rawness, roughness and scraping in throat, worse toward evening. ***Tendency to get sore throats that go into the lungs. Larynx very painful***, sore, painful on speaking. Feeling of rawness in larynx from passage of inspired air. Larynx feels as if lined with fur. Violent tickling in larynx while speaking. Burning in esophagus. Stricture of esophagus. Tonsils and uvula swollen. Uvula elongated. As of cotton or something hanging in throat. Pain in throat on coughing. Sweetish taste while coughing. Low, hoarse voice, worse morning and evening. Hoarseness, worse evenings. Can't talk on account of pain in larynx. Croupy voice, followed by bronchitis. Sudden aphonia. Aphonia, worse evenings, with rawness.

Tongue - ***Tongue dry, smooth***, red or white, not thickly coated. Tongue coated white, yellow, grey, with brown center. Tongue coated only in middle. Tongue dry in middle, cracked, parched or glossy, with stinging in tip. Burning pain on tongue. Tip of tongue somewhat swollen, with enlargement of its papillae and feeling as if it had been burnt.

Urine - Constant discharge of thin, slimy, colorless fluid from urethra. ***Diabetes, sugar in urine.*** Turbid urine, brown, with red sediment. Profuse pale, watery urine, then weakness. Urine acrid, smelling offensive. Urine turbid, whitish, like curdled milk, with brick-dust sediment and variegated cuticle on surface. Pellicle on urine. Albuminuria, periodical. Sediment white, sandy or flocculent, albuminous, containing fatty casts. ***Urinates pure blood.***

Vertigo - Vertigo with faintness, nausea and headache. Vertigo, floating sensation, on waking. ***Vertigo after rising*** (Bry.), with weakness of legs. ***Vertigo on exertion of vision.*** Vertigo, worse looking up or down. Vertigo from smell of flowers, gas, ethereal oils, turpentine, with fainting. Vertigo of the elderly.

Vision - Narrow field of vision. Partial loss of vision from abuse of tobacco, sexual excess, lightning. Diplopia. Amaurosis from sexual excess. Misty vision, with attacks of vanishing of sight. Retinal trouble with the lights and hallucination of vision. Colors before eyes followed by migraine. ***Green halo about the candlelight*** (Osm.). Muscae volitantes. Black points seem to float before the eyes. ***Letters appear red.*** Patient sees better by shading eyes with hand. Sensation as if everything were covered with a mist or veil or something pulled tightly over eyes. ***Blindness after lightning-stroke.***

COMMENTS - Profoundly affects the nutrition and function of all tissues, notably the hardest (bone) and the softest (nerve and blood). Causes irritation, weakness, exaltation of all the senses, and later a typhoid state and fatty degeneration.

Pareira observed in phosphorus workers "a peculiar sallow, bloated complexion with dull expression of eye and gastric derangement," when there was no affection of the jaws. Wagner found Phos. symptoms long before local disease appeared, e.g., cardialgia, anorexia, eructation of gas smelling of Phos., also dizziness, faintness and cachectic appearance.

The first symptoms in the jaws are tearing pains, the teeth being sound, swelling and suppuration of the gums and lessening of the teeth follow, and the bone becomes denuded. Langenbeck objects to the term "necrosis," stating that it is a periostatics in which bony deposit occurs, enclosing the jaws more or less as in a sheath. There is no exfoliation. This osteo-periostitis may arise from rheumatism.

Painful burns and burning sensations. "Glowing sensation throughout the epigastrium and chest." "A flame seemed passing through me." "Warming sensation right side of heart and below left clavicle.

This heat spread to apex of left scapula and to acromion, when it left the heart." "From 11 a. m. until 4 p.m. remarkable numb feeling in left leg from knee to toes, sometimes sensation as if hot blood flowed into it."

Burning pains with inflammation. Burning between the scapula, burning in spots along the spine, feeling of intense heat running up the back. Flashes of heat beginning in hands and spreading to face. Burning palms, cannot bear to have the hands covered.

Nervous or hectic fever. Low delirium, muttering, stupid or violent or there may be a state of ecstasy or odd ideas. In intermittents when there is heat at night beginning in the stomach, faint and hungry in night, heat in hands.

Chilliness towards evening, icy coldness of hands, knees and feet, even in bed. Sweat is anxious, profuse, exhausting on slightest exertion, profuse at night, cold and clammy, smelling of sulphur or of garlic.

Fibrillary twitching of individual bundles of tissues in muscles. Numbness and formication in paralyzed limbs. Spasms on paralyzed side. Uncertain gait, neuralgic pain and fuzzy feeling of the feet. Locomotor ataxia. Epilepsy from masturbation. Petit mal, epilepsy with consciousness.

Sudden prostration from shock or malignant types of disease, either acute or chronic. Overly sensitive, impressionable. Excitable condition, exaltation of mental faculties, and the condition that follows over-exertion. Overextended feeling. Tendency to overreact in situations.

Sense of immediacy, living in the present. Anxiety. Lack of focus, spaciness. Can have a lack of direction. Fears of death, solitude, darkness, thunderstorms. Better from company, extroverted. Sympathetic, tends to nurse others.

Sensitive to effects of storms, especially thunderstorms. Headache with a thunderstorm. Blindness from lightning stroke. Sleep relieves most symptoms. Refreshed from naps. Exertion, physical or mental, aggravates complaints. Better from open air, warm wraps.

Heart palpitations and irregularities of the heart. Palpitations aggravated by lying on the left side. Peripheral numbness, circulatory problems, Raynaud's disease. Stroke. Transient ischemic attacks. Panic attacks associated with blood sugar and the heart.

Pulmonary hemorrhage and congestion. Nosebleeds, hemophiliacs. Hemorrhagic diathesis. Small wounds bleed profusely. Bright red blood. Blood-streaked discharges. Blood-streaked or rusty sputa, tasting salty. Acute pernicious anemia and bone cancer. Cancers that bleed profusely and persistently, bright-colored blood. Tendency to bruising.

Ulcers, bleed easily at the slightest touch. Open cancers or fungus hematodes. "Large ulcers surrounded by smaller ones." Ulcers affecting the nails. Ulcers, psoriasis, lichen, eczema, blood boils, purpura. Eruptions. Exanthema with pustules like smallpox.

Inflammation and eruptions around joints, particularly the hip and knee. Fistulae with callous edges from glands. The left side of the lower jaw is more affected than the right. Decay and exostoses of spine (Calc-f.).

Rheumatism with great stiffness of the joints, more stiffness than pain. Paralytic rheumatism from exposure to rain. Stiffness of old people. A drawing, tearing, tight feeling, in the girdle, pain of spinal affections, tightness of skin of face and forehead.

"Splitting headache caused by cough." Headache and other sufferings from grief. Hot vertex after grief. Shocks in occiput, coldness in cerebellum, congestion of brain seeming to rise from spine into head. Neuralgic pain. Impending paralysis. Attacks induced by mental exertion, worry, washing clothes and are worse by music, noises, strong odors.

Cataract and glaucoma. Pustule on cornea. Burning pains. Retinal hemorrhage. Retinitis albuminuria from suppressed menses. Halo around candle. Colors appear black before the eyes. Sees green. Letters appear red while reading. As if a gray veil is over everything. Blindness after typhoid, sexual excess, loss of fluids, or lightning. Twitching of eyelids.

Suffocative pains in upper part of chest with constriction of larynx and engorgement of lungs. Bronchial catarrh. Cough causes tearing pain under sternum as if something was being torn loose. Mucus rales, panting and labored breathing. Emphysema. Asthma after the cough.

Pneumonias. Indicated when the morbid action becomes localized in the right lung, particularly the lower lobe. Hard, dry cough, rusty sputa, worse at twilight and until midnight. Worse lying on left side, better lying on right side.

Tendency to colds and sore throats. Tuberculosis florida. "Stomach" or "liver" cough. Cough comes on after eating and starts from a tickling in pit of stomach. Cough worse when strangers enter the room, or from strong odors.

Sinking, faint feeling in the abdominal cavity, head, chest and stomach. Violent tearing pains in esophagus, chest, stomach. Bloating of abdomen, distended, sore, sensitive to touch. Hemorrhages from all offices. Stomach ulceration with severe burning pains, hemorrhage, and persistent vomiting.

Tenderness of the liver. Disorganization of the liver and blood with jaundice, hemorrhages. Hepatitis. Acute fatty degeneration of the liver and fatty degeneration of pancreas with gastric symptoms and oily stools. Fatty and amyloid degeneration of the kidneys. Degeneration with engorgement of the lungs, particularly the right lung.

Hunger with great weakness and faintness. Hungry soon after a meal, hungry during the night. Hypoglycemia. Ice cream ameliorates the gastric pains. Desires cold milk, which agrees. Wants to suck ice (Med.). Longing for acids and spicy things, desires salt things (Nat-m.). Antidotes the effects from excess of salt in diet.

Desire for cold foods and preference for cold meat, may be vomited as soon as it becomes warm. Burning thirst for cold water, which relieves, but as soon as it becomes warm in the stomach it is vomited.

Regurgitation of ingesta in mouthfuls. The sight of water causes vomiting during pregnancy. Nausea on putting hands into warm water. Sneezing and coryza from putting hands in water. Vomiting and diarrhea. Typhoid. Diabetes. Diabetic peripheral neuropathies.

Rectal, bladder, and uterine tenesmus. Stool voided with great difficulty and straining. Stools are long, tough and hard, like a dog's. Stools offensive, involuntary, the anus appearing to remain open. Bloody stool, blood-streaked stool, stool like shreddy membranes.

Diarrhea as soon as anything enters the rectum. Profuse diarrhea pouring away as from a hydrant. Watery diarrhea with sago-like particles. Painless, involuntary stool during cholera, in the morning, of old people. Burning in the anus, notably stitches shooting up rectum. Hemorrhoids.

Menses are profuse and long lasting. Vicarious menstruation in the form of hemoptysis, nosebleed or hematuria. Leucorrhea which causes blisters. Left ovarian pain (Thuj., Coloc.).

Burning, shooting, and cramping pains in the breasts. Breast abscess and fistula. Erysipelatous appearance, red streaks starting from opening, thin, ichorous discharge. Morning sickness with nausea and burning. Aversion to sex. Nymphomania.

Frequent erections in men and sexual thoughts entirely beyond the patient's control. Strong sexual desire, constant wish for sex. Erections in spite of efforts to control passion in young men. Impotence from over-indulgence or from celibacy.

A man, 48 inhaled the vapor of burning Phos. Among his symptoms was a sensation as if something twitched under his skin or was creeping between skin and flesh. Twitching of single bundles of tissues at different times like playing on a piano. Tongue often refused to move when speaking so that he stammered.

E. R. Heath had some decidedly "phosphorescent" symptoms. Darting, cutting pains, causing much distress, starting from different points and flashing over the whole abdomen. He imagined an aurora borealis and seemed to distinctly hear voices shouting "Beautiful, oh! was not that splendid?" as the pains became more severe and lasting.

He sprang from the bed and tried to collect his thoughts, had numbness all over with sensation of myriads of needles slightly pricking him. Throat dry and parched, a flame seemed to pass through him. Feet seemed glued to the floor.

With great difficulty he reached the vessel and as soon as the bowels began to act the pains changed to cramps. Stools were like scrapings of intestines. They were almost constant, with tenesmus, for over two hours. He lay down in bed after, weak, sore, and almost helpless.

Clarke reported a case of spinal decay with paralytic symptoms in a woman aged 67. She had a history of a strained back thirty-five years before, and of lumbago and sciatica five years before he saw her. Pains in the scapula and chest, she could not walk unless supported about the waist. She was cured with Phos. 1,000c, the curvature remained, although the decay and paralysis were removed. The Phos. caused dryness of her mouth, lips and throat.

W. A. Nicholas reported the case of T. B., 51, whom he saw after a four months' illness. The case began with congestion of the brain on the sudden death of his wife and was followed by bronchitis. During all this time he was heavily drugged. A rather long walk brought on a severe attack of angina pectoris. Bell. 1x gave much relief. Nicholas noticed the patient at times put his hand to the back of his neck. Phos. 1c relieved entirely.

Hansen cured a case of purpura in a girl of 10. The disease began with loss of appetite and pains in the stomach, but as soon as the purpura spots appeared, the pains ceased and the appetite returned. The inner thighs were affected. Phos. 2c cured.

Walker cured with Phos. 6c a large exostosis of the femur which had been pronounced as osteosarcoma by old-school authorities.

In a case of rheumatism in an old woman who had a waxy pallor, Cooper gave Phos. and set free all the joints.

Dr. Mills related a typical case of thunderstorm effect. Mrs. F., tall, thin, dark of mild and gentle disposition, was seen by the doctor during a thunderstorm. He found her sitting on the stairs, trembling, cold, and bathed in cold, clammy sweat, full of nervous dread and almost beside herself. One dose of Phos. 100,000c cured. Some weeks later she witnessed a storm with complete unconcern.

RELATIONS - ***Antidote to:*** Phos. poisoning: Turpentine with which it forms an insoluble mass. Kali-perm. ***Compare:*** (1) Tub. follows Phos. well and complements its action. (2) Phos-h. - crumbling of teeth, hyperesthesia, locomotor ataxia. (3) Amph. - right jaw swollen and painful. (4) Thymol - typical sexual neurasthenia, irritable stomach, aching throughout lumbar region, worse mental and physical exertion. (5) Calc., Chin., Ant-t., Sep., Lyc., Sulph. (6) For pneumonia, Pneu. Pneumonia and paralytic phenomena, pleuritic pain and pain in ilio-cecal region (Cartier). ***Complementary:*** Ars., All-c., Lyc., Sil., Nux-v. Phos. antidotes the nausea and vomiting of chloroform and ether. Sanguis. 30c - Leech - persistent hemorrhages, effects of use of leeches. Phos-pchl. - great soreness of mucus membrane of eyes and nose, throat and chest sore. ***Incompatible:*** Caust.

REFERENCES - Boericke. Clarke. Murphy. Phatak.

PHOSPHORUS HYDROGENATUS

(Phosphoretted Hydrogen)

PHARMACY - phos-h. Phosphorus hydrogenatus. Phosphoretted hydrogen. Phosphine. Solution. ***Historical dose:*** All potencies.

CLINICAL - Amblyopia. Anus, weak. Diarrhea. Hyperesthesia. Locomotor ataxia. Paralysis. Stammering. Teeth, crumbling.

HOMEOPATHIC - Breunar related the effects of inhaling this gas, given off in the preparation of ***"hypophosphites."*** The symptoms began to appear after three months including vision disturbances, diarrhea, paralysis and a complete state of locomotor ataxia, worse on closing eyes.

The teeth crumbled without pain. Speech and swallowing were difficult. Diarrhea, accompanied by weakness of the anus.

RELATIONS - Electricity antidoted the effects. ***Compare:*** (1) Locomotor ataxia, Arg-n., Alum., Helo. (2) Vision defects, Benz-d., Carb-s.

REFERENCES - Clarke.

PHOSPHORUS MURIATICUS

(Phosphorus Pentachloride)

PHARMACY - phos-pchl. Phosphorus muriaticus. Phosphorus pentachloride. Solution. ***Historical dose:*** All potencies.

CLINICAL - Asthma. Coryza, Ophthalmia.

HOMEOPATHIC - J. Meredith recorded the effects observed on a science student from grinding up this salt and inhaling the fumes. The main symptoms were eye soreness, coryza, sore throat and chest with difficult breathing. The symptoms lasted fourteen days from the exposure and were cured by Bell. 3x internally and a one percent iodine lotion locally as a compress.

REFERENCES - Clarke.

PHYSALIA PHYSALIS

(Portuguese Man-of-war)

PHARMACY - physala-p. Physalia physalis. Portuguese man-of-war. Physalia pelagica. N. O. Physophoridae. Hydrozoa. Radiata. ***Historical dose:*** All potencies.

CLINICAL - Blisters. Hives. Nettle, rash. Numbness. Stings. Urticaria.

HOMEOPATHIC - G. Bennett was stung by the animal on his second and ring fingers. The sensation was as if stung by a nettle, succeeded in a few minutes by violent aching, affecting the finger joints and spreading up the arm, involving the elbow joint.

The pain spread to the shoulder joint and pectoral muscles causing oppression of breathing. After half an hour the symptoms began to abate, leaving a numbness of the limb and a blister at the spot which was stung. The pain was aggravated by application of water, worse by motion and worse when joints became affected.

RELATIONS - ***Compare:*** (1) Apis, Medus., Urt-u.

REFERENCES - Clarke.

PHYSOSTIGMA VENENOSUM

(Calabar Bean)

PHARMACY - phys. Physostigma venenosum. Calabar bean. Ordeal-bean. Esere. N. O. Leguminosae. Papilionoideae. Trituration of the bean. ***Historical dose:*** All potencies.

CLINICAL - ***Astigmatism.*** Backache. Bathing, effects. Blepharospasm. Chorea. Ciliary spasm. Constipation. Coccyx, pain. Dentition. Diarrhea. Dyspepsia. Epilepsy. ***Eyes, disorders.*** Glaucoma. Headaches. Heart, disorders. ***Hemiplegia.*** Hemorrhoids. Herpes. Hiccough. Hysteria. Iris, prolapsed. Leucorrhea. Locomotor ataxia. Meningeal, irritation. Menopausal. Muscular atrophy. ***Myopia.*** Navel, inflammation. Palpitations. Paralysis. Paraplegia. Parkinson's disease. Polymyelitis. Prostration. Sleeplessness. ***Spinal, irritation.*** Spinal sclerosis. Stiff neck. Tremors. ***Tetanus.*** Throat, sore, fish-bone sensation. Water, effects. Wounds.

HERBAL - Calabar is the type of a genus of Leguminosae of the tribe Phaseoleae. It has flowers very like Phaseolus except that its bearded style is terminated by a great oblique hood, covering the blunt stigma. It is this hood that distinguishes the genus and gives it its name. It is a great twining climber and has purplish flowers.

Physostigma is the "ordeal-bean" of old. The seeds are very poisonous and are used by the Calabari to determine guilt and innocence. When ingested, the person either vomits or dies, if they die they are considered guilty, if they vomit, they are innocent.

Observed cases showed twitchings, especially in the back, and death in thirty minutes. In poisoning cases, the most notable feature was complete muscular prostration.

A group of children in Liverpool ate beans that they found among the sweepings of a ship from Africa. Forty-six were admitted to a hospital with loss of muscular power, prostration, feeble, slow pulse.

Cold, perspiring skin, cold limbs, vomiting in nearly all cases, diarrhea in one-third of them. At first there was colic, but later on remarkable freedom from pain.

Pupils contracted in many, in one they contracted during sleep, dilated when aroused.

· Only one (a tubercular boy) succumbed. He staggered as he walked, then fell, kicking and rolling as if in pain, but afterwards became quiet, much purged, pulse hardly perceptible, skin cold, face livid, quite conscious and able to swallow water.

Directly after drinking he died without a struggle, some froth issuing from nose and mouth. After death the blood was found to be fluid, the heart distended with it and its muscular substance very flaccid.

HOMEOPATHIC - Physostigma and its active principle, eserine, form a valuable addition to the Materia Medica. Stimulates heart, raises blood pressure and increases peristalsis. Causes contraction of the pupil and of the ciliary muscles. Induces a condition of near-sightedness. Eserine is used locally to produce contraction of pupil.

Spinal irritation, loss of motility, prostration with very sensitive vertebrae. Depresses the motor and reflex activity of the cord and causes loss of sensibility to pain, muscular weakness. This is followed by complete paralysis, although muscular contractility is not impaired. Meningeal irritation with rigidity of muscles. Paralysis and tremors. Chorea.

Fluttering tremors in the muscles, they do not respond to the will, or draw into knots, even the intestines are seen twisted in knots. Fibrillary tremors. Ataxic gait, shooting pains down the limbs. ***Tetanus***. Trismus. Tremors. Polymyelitis anterior. Progressive muscular paralysis. General paralysis of the insane.

Horror of cold water, drinks or bathing. Cold water feels too cold. Shuddering worse every draft. Floating sensation. Darting pain here and there. Flushes of heat, worse palms. Pain, beginning at any hour, continues to 12 o'clock following, either noon or midnight.

MIND - The mind is active even during sleep. Nothing was right. Too many things in the room, continually counting them. Paralytic state of mind and body from grief.

Abdomen - Navel, sore, bloated, red. Hypogastrium sore, bloated worse standing. Gripe in right hypochondrium. Groins pain alternately. Colicky pains, worse diarrhea, better extending legs.

Back - Sensitive spine. Cramp-like stitches up and down the spine. Drawing on turning head. Creeping numbness from occiput down spine. Chilly, creeping sensations up back. Dull pain in back. Backache in kidney region. Back very weak, unable to stand erect.

Breasts - Stitches in left breast, unable to draw in breath.

Causations - Ill effects of emotions, grief. Injuries, falls, blows, and bathing.

Chest - Stitches in the chest. Stitches under inferior angles of scapulae during expiration. Heavy weight at chest. Twitches across pectoral muscles.

Ears - Sharp, shooting pains in the ears. Sudden pain from throat to middle ear, worse eructation. Pain in the ear when writing. Painful pressure on tympani. Crawling in left ear. Sensitive to every sound. Hissing, buzzing, ringing in the ears. Fullness. Stopped feeling. Partial deafness.

Eyes - Bloodshot eyes with burning. Muscae volitantes, flashes of light. Glaucoma, especially after injury. ***Contraction of pupils.*** Vision trembling. ***Increasing myopia***. Accommodation affected, ***astigmatism.*** Night-blindness, photophobia. Profuse lachrymation. Exophthalmus. ***Spasm of ciliary muscle with irritability after using eyes.*** Post-diphtheria paralysis of eye and accommodation muscles. Twitching of eye muscles. Pain over orbits, cannot bear to raise eyelids. Eyelids tense, cannot close or open them.

Face - Face pale, flushings of the face, heat. Lips numb, licks them. Lockjaw. Neuralgic pain in right side of face. Spastic conditions of the face muscles. Sensation of cramps or spasms in face.

Female - Pain as if menses were coming on. Menses are irregular with palpitations. Leucorrhea worse during the day, when exercising. Sighing, worse when leucorrhea is worse. Metrorrhagia. Rigid muscles. Numbness of womb with pain in back.

Food - Hunger but can find nothing to satisfy it. Food has a flat taste. No appetite, disgust for food, tobacco and coffee, and especially for cold drinks.

Head - Headache unbearable, worse at night. Constant pain on vertex. Pain over orbits. ***Headache, cannot bear to raise eyelids***. Pain from forehead down nose. As of a band about the head, as of a tight cap on head. Heartbeats felt in head on lying down. Cerebro-spinal meningitis, general tetanic rigidity. Brain, falls to side lain on, wavering in. Tremors in head.

Heart - Fatty degeneration of heart (Phos., Cupr-acet.). ***Fluttering of heart felt in throat.*** Heartbeats distinctly perceptible in chest and head. Feeble pulse. Palpitations, spasmodic action with feeling of pulsation through the whole body.

Kidneys - Bruised, sore feeling in region of kidneys. Bladder feels distended. Frequent desire to urinate, often ineffectual. Urine is yellow, high colored, strong-smelling, clear, muddy, pale and copious.

Limbs - Limbs feel weary, as after great fatigue. Sudden jerking of limbs on going to sleep. Tetanic convulsions. Locomotor ataxia. Numbness in paralyzed parts, crampy pains in limbs. Pain in deltoid (right) better violent motion. ***Pain in right popliteal space***. Burning and tingling in spine. Hands and feet numb. Flushes of heat in palms. Offensive odor from hands.

Lungs - Labored, sighing respiration, yawning. Cannot fill left lung as inspiration causes dull pain at left apex, better by pressure. Cough from tickling in throat. Slight constant inclination to cough from filling lungs.

Male - Frequent erections with but slight desire. Emissions without dreams or excitement. Strong-smelling sweat about genitals.

Modalities - Better in cool open air, exerting the will. Better closing eyes, sleep, warmth to feet, lying on right side, lying on abdomen or with head low. Hiccough better by sleep. Worse lying on left side, on waking, in church. Worse motion, stepping, descending, misstep, jar, falls, blows. Worse pressure, bathing, heat and cold, cold water, cold bath, change of temperature at 4 p.m. (Lyc.).

Mouth - Bad taste in mouth. Profuse salivation, thick, leathery saliva. ***Tongue feels sore on tip***. Tongue feels oily, scalded, swollen in chorea. Feeling of loose skin on roof of mouth. Teeth feel rough. Dentition stressful in nervous children.

Neck - Pain at base of brain. Inclination to stretch out neck. Stiffness in neck. Rheumatic pains in left neck.

Nose - Fluent coryza, burning and tingling of nostrils, nose stuffed and hot. Fever blisters around nostrils. Small boil inside right nostril. Nosebleed while at supper. Smarting at end of nose. Twitching of muscles of nose. Tension in skin of nose and forehead.

Perspiration - Easy sweat with excitement. Copious, cold sweat in drops over whole body. Strong-smelling sweat around genitals.

Sleep - Irresistible desire to sleep, soporific sleep. Restless sleep with dreams. During sleep, mind so active was unaware he had been asleep.

Stools - Copious stools, soft, thin, watery. Yellowish stools, bilious, part natural, part black like tar. Stools lumpy, mixed with watery discharge, dark and offensive.

Rectum - Constipation from atony. Tenesmus and burning with diarrhea. Stools are irregular and loose. Sphincter swollen and rigid, evacuation painful. Anus sore and inclined to protrude. Severe hemorrhoids, following childbirth.

Sensations - Sensations of contraction and tension. Wavering in brain. As if she will lose her mind. Tongue as if burnt, swollen and paralyzed. As if a ball were coming up throat. As if stomach were full. Weak feeling in stomach. Back as if paralyzed. Lower limbs as if asleep.

Sleep - Attacks of overpowering sleepiness with feeling as if to lose consciousness.

Stomach - Great pain immediately after eating. Sensitive to pressure in epigastric region. Pain extends into chest and down arms. Gastralgia, chronic constipation. Hiccough with short break, better from sleep.

Temperature - Cold, clammy skin. Hands and feet cold. Every movement and draft causes shuddering. Creeping, chilly sensation in back. Heat in head and face, flushed and hot. Dry burning in hands. Perspires very easily.

Throat - Tonsils enlarged, swollen. Elongated uvula. Feeling as if a ball came up throat. Strong heartbeats felt in throat.

Vertigo - Vertigo, stumbles on ascending or descending steps. Vertigo with constrictive feeling of head.

COMMENTS - According to Brunton, the tetanus properties of the bean belong to the alkaloid calabarine. The paralysis, to eserine, or as it is now called, physostigmine.

In cases of poisoning, people experience a speedy general paralysis. Death occurs from failure of respiration, although the heart may be poisoned both directly and through its nerves.

The paralysis is seated in the spinal cord. The muscles are affected by fluttering tremors. Involuntary muscles are excited to active movements and expulsive efforts. The intestines are often twisted up in knots. All the secretions are somewhat increased.

Many provings have been made with Phys., among which a proving made by Christison on himself is remarkable. Simpson and Douglas MacLagan were sent for to attend to him in his collapsed state. Simpson could only compare it to the state produced by severe flooding, though Christison's only sensation was one of "extreme but not unpleasant faintness." MacLagan thought it a lot like aconite poisoning. Christison could not get his will into his muscles except by a tremendous effort.

Warmth to Christison's feet and a mustard plaster to his whole abdomen gave great relief and he was then able to turn on his left side, but only remained there a very short time on account of the tumultuous action of the heart it caused.

He became drowsy and slept, but his mind was so active in sleep that on awaking he did not know that he had slept. The tumultuous action of the heart continued on waking, but strong coffee quickly restored the whole condition and made the heart regular.

Indigestion was observed by Christison and many other provers, "as if large pieces of food had been suddenly swallowed." It began under the upper sternum, descending and increasing in intensity until it reached the epigastrium.

Belchings then occurred and a reversal of direction followed, the sensation ending where it began. With other provers, there was a sensation of weight and hardness. Christison also experienced giddiness and dimness of vision.

Phys., and its alkaloid eserine, are best known in old school practice for its action on the eye, especially of contracting the pupil. The effects are more definite when the drug (tincture, extract or solution of alkaloid) is applied to the eye directly, but one myopic prover had his myopia much diminished.

Dudgeon related the case of A. E., 26, struck by the cork of a soda-water bottle on the inferior and outer part of the left eyeball. Intense burning pain and effusion into the eyeball followed.

Under Arn., prescribed by Mr. Engall, the effusion disappeared and later the pain and inflammation subsided under Acon. and Merc-c. The pupil was now egg-shaped, the long diameter perpendicular, smaller end downwards, vision extremely myopic.

Bell. dilated the pupil, but it had no effect on the vision. Engall sent the patient to Dudgeon, who found the pupil was sluggish and a book had to be held within four inches of the eye to be read. Phys. 3x, every three hours, was given.

After the first dose, objects could be seen at a considerable distance and the next day sight was nearly as good as ever. Dudgeon believed that the lens was tilted by the blow and that Phys. restored the over-stretched or paralyzed portion of the ciliary muscle.

Woodyatt stated that Phys. produced corneal astigmatism in a young woman who found any attempt at close work caused redness of tarsal edges and a hot, sandy feeling in conjunctiva. Lil-t. 30c cured.

For ocular tension, especially when glaucoma has been the result of injury. Eye injuries (Calen., Hyper.). Conjunctivitis with sharp, shooting pains. Pinpoint pupils (Op.). Paralysis of certain eye muscles.

Astigmatism. Double vision, severe blurry vision, worse in the right eye. Holes in the field of vision. The eye feels full of fluid. Eye problems associated with extreme insomnia. Muscae volitantes.

Paralysis and tremors predominate, but also cramps, twitchings, stiffness and tension. Tetanus. Paralysis and numbness is more apparent on the left side, especially in left arm. Nervous disease with extreme tremors or trembling. Paralysis of the spinal cord and respiratory failure. Parkinson's. Guillain-Barre syndrome.

Muscular prostration. Polio, diaphragm paralysis (Con.). Labored respiration. Paralysis with an inability to get the will into the muscles. Paralytic state of mind and body from grief.

Ataxic gait, shooting pains down limbs. Locomotor ataxia. Spinal, sacral and coccygeal pains, with numbness of the womb. One prover noted a feeling of levitation on stepping.

Dread of cold water, aversion to bathing. Weakness on change of weather and on cold, bracing days. Sleeplessness.

Nash cured with Phys. 12c and 30c persistent sleeplessness in a patient who had been in an insane asylum and feared she would have to go again. Her symptoms were "If we chanced to get a nap she awoke suddenly as if in a fright and felt no better from what she had slept."

H. L. Chase, another prover, had a "very severe pain in the right popliteal space," and he afterwards cured a patient who came to him with pain in the same region two years later.

REFERENCES - Boericke. Clarke. Murphy. Phatak.

PHYTOLACCA DECANDRA

(Poke Root)

PHARMACY - phyt. Phytolacca decandra. Poke root. Poke weed. Virginian Poke. Pole-root. Red ink plant. Garget weed. N. O. Phytolaccaceae. Tincture of fresh root dug in winter. Tincture of the ripe berries. Tincture of fresh leaves. Solution of the resinous extract, Phytolaccin. ***Historical dose:*** Tincture and all potencies.

CLINICAL - Adenitis. Albuminuria. Angina pectoris. Anus, fissure. Asthma. Barber's itch. ***Boils.*** Bone, diseases. ***Breasts, disorders. Breast-feeding. Breasts, tumors. Cancer.*** Cholera. Ciliary, neuralgia. Colic. Conjunctivitis. Constipation. Cough. Dentition, difficult. Diarrhea. Diphtheria. Diplopia. Dysentery. Dysmenorrhea. Ears, disorders. Erythema nodosum. Eustachian tubes disorders. Galactorrhea. ***Gland, disorders. Glands, enlarged.*** Glossitis. Gonorrhea. Gout. Headaches. Hearing, disorders. Heart, disorders. Hepatitis. Hemorrhoids. Impotence. Influenza. Laryngismus. Leucorrhea. Lichen. Liver, disorders. Lumbago. Lupus. ***Mastitis.*** Mercury, effects. Miscarriage, threatened. Mouth, ulcerated. ***Mumps.*** Nephritis. Neuralgia. ***Nipples, painful.*** Nursing, painful. Obesity. Orchitis. Ozaena. Paralysis, diphtheria. Parotiditis. Prostate, disorders. Rectum, cancer. Respiration, abnormal. ***Rheumatism.*** Ringworm. Rodent, ulcer. Salivation. Scabies. Scar. Sciatica. Sewer-gas poisoning. Spinal, irritation. Spleen, pain. Stiff-neck. Syphilis. Tetanus. Throat, sore. Tinea capitis. ***Tonsillitis.*** Toothaches. ***Tumors.*** Ulcers. Uterus disorders. ***Venereal buboes***. Warts. Wens.

HERBAL - Phytolacca is a branching herbaceous plant with a thick, perennial root, sometimes larger than a man's leg in diameter. The plant is common throughout North America, the Azores, North Africa and China. It grows in damp places.

The young shoots, though extremely acrid, are rendered harmless by boiling and are eaten like asparagus in the United States. The berries have a popular repute as a remedy for cancer and rheumatism.

The berries of Phytolacca octandra are used in Mexico and the West Indies as a soap.

According to Raffinesque, the ash of the plant is 45 percent caustic potash, and the plant contains an acid, phytolactic acid, which is closely allied to malic acid. Phytolacca has been used as an escharotic in cancers, ulcers, etc.

HOMEOPATHIC - Phyt. is pre-eminently a ***glandular and rheumatic remedy***. It powerfully affects the fibrous and osseous tissues, and the sheathes and fascias of muscles. Hence it becomes an admirable remedy in rheumatic affections.

It has a special affinity for the muscles of the shoulders and arms. Acts on the muscles of the neck and back, tendons and joints, periosteum, throat, digestive tract and the right side.

General soreness over the whole body, the patient moans and groans every time he moves. Lameness, soreness and a bruised feeling are felt all over the body. It combines with the pain, intense prostration and great exhaustion.

Rheumatic pain, tendency to affect the outer aspect of limbs. ***Sudden achiness.*** Pains come and go suddenly, change places. ***Sore, hard aching pains.*** The pain occurs in such quick succession that it renders the leg powerless numb and heavy. Each movement elicits groans. Spreading pains.

Rheumatism after tonsillitis. Lassitude with rheumatism, makes him lie down every now and then. Sciatica and hip joint disease, with pain shooting from sacrum down the outer aspect of thighs to knees and toes. Syphilitic bone pains, chronic rheumatism.

Glandular swellings with heat and inflammation, particularly ***breasts and tonsils***. Hard and painful nodes. Acts on scar tissue. Hastens suppuration. Pus is watery, fetid, ichorous. Discharges are shreddy, stringy, stools, menses etc.

Affinity for the breasts and glands of women, which are prone to become cancerous in those of a cancer constitution.

Breast cancer, as well as cancers of the uterus and rectum. ***Mastitis, breast disorders***. Pressure with hand ameliorates pain in breasts. Great sensitivity in breasts.

Sore throat, quinsy and diphtheria. ***Sore throats, right-sided***, relieved by swallowing cold drinks, worse from warm drinks and empty swallowing. Enlarged and painful cervical glands accompany the inflamed sore throats. Bluish-red parts, throat glands. Burning pains in cancerous ulcerations and in inflamed throats.

Restlessness and prostration. Tetanus, general muscular rigidity, alternate spasms and relaxation of muscles. Opisthotonos. Decrease of weight. Obesity. Retarded dentition.

MIND - Irritable and nervous. Restlessness. Indisposition to mental exertion. Disgust for business. Feels faint on rising. Stupefaction with vertigo and dimness of vision. Refuses food in spite of continuous insistence. Irresistible compulsion to clench the teeth.

Melancholy, gloom, indifference to life. Depression of spirits with headache. Weeping at night during menses. Great fear, sure she will die. Predicts death, with mastitis. Desires death in morning on waking.

Confusion while sitting, better open air. Delirium. Loss of personal delicacy, complete shamelessness and indifference to exposure of her person. Oversensitiveness to pain. Cannot endure pain, it is intolerable. Unconsciousness from pain.

Abdomen - Great rumbling in abdomen and pain in umbilicus. Heavy aching pain in the hypochondrium, worse lying on affected side. Sore spot in right hypochondrium. Soreness and pain in right hypochondrium during pregnancy. Rheumatism of abdominal muscles. Bruised feeling through the epigastrium and abdomen. Colic at navel, with burning griping pains. Bearing down pains. Intense vomiting and purging with griping pains and cramps in abdomen. Ulceration of mucus membrane of upper part of digestive tract.

Back - Pains streaking up and down the spine. Back stiff, especially in morning on rising and during damp weather. Aching pain in lumbar and sacral region. Shooting pain in sacrum. Weakness and dull pain in region of kidneys. Hardness of glands in right side of neck. Neck stiff in morning on waking. Pale red spots on neck and arms. Both scapulae ache continually.

Breasts - ***Heavy, stony, hard swollen or tender breasts.*** Severe stinging pains, throughout breasts, with oozing out of milk, better pressure with hands. ***Swollen breast.*** Irritable breasts, before and during menses. Tender and sore breasts, before and during menses. ***Mastitis,*** with breasts hard and very sensitive. Mastitis from taking cold. Mastitis during pregnancy. Galactorrhea (Calc.), causes great exhaustion. When child nurses, ***pain goes from nipple all over body***. Milk thick, scanty and unhealthy, dries up too soon. Breast hard as a stone, after weaning. Cracks and small ulcers about nipples. Nipples, cracked, very sensitive inverted. Tumors or hard nodes of the breasts with enlarged axillary glands. Breast is hard, painful and of purple hue. ***Breast cancer***, with shooting, lancinating pains, great exhaustion and prostration. Breast abscess. Bloody, watery discharge from breasts. Affection of old scars in breasts.

Causations - Emotions, grief, injuries, blows, bathing, and exposure to cold, damp weather.

Chest - Aching pains in chest, through mid-sternum with cough. Rheumatism of lower intercostals, from exposure to cold and dampness. Tenderness and lameness of muscles of chest, as if bruised. Swelling of axillary glands.

Constitutions - Suited to rheumatic or syphilitic subjects, sensitive to damp weather. Cancer constitution.

Ears - Shooting pains in both the ears, worse swallowing. Obstruction in left Eustachian tube. Irritation in one Eustachian tube. Increased sense of hearing with pain in forehead.

Eyes - Dull aching in eyes, worse motion, light or exercise. Orbital cellulitis. ***Burning, smarting, tingling in eyes.*** Feeling of sand under lids. ***Profuse hot lachrymation.*** Fistula lachrymalis (Fl-ac.). Lids agglutinated and edematous. Lids as if on fire. Tarsal edges feel hot. Photophobia. Green vision. Eyeballs ache on reading and writing. Diplopia. Motion of one eye only, independent of the other.

Face - Face very pale, hippocratic. Yellowish, sickly. Blotches in face, worse evening, after washing and eating. Blueness around eyes. Chin drawn closely to sternum. Glands swollen at the angle of jaw. Jaws ache, as in mumps. Aching malar bones. ***Mumps.*** Tension and pressure in parotid gland.

Female - Amenorrhea, with ovarian irritation or disease. Menses too copious and frequent, followed by leucorrhea. Menses with salivation and lachrymation. Dysmenorrhea in barren women with erosion of cervix membranous. Leucorrhea, thick, tenacious and irritating. Leucorrhea profuse, thick, tenacious. Ovarian neuralgia of right side. Ovaritis with rheumatic complications. ***Venereal buboes***. Swollen nabothian cysts. Glandular swellings and abscesses. Suppression of lochia.

Food - Intense thirst. Hunger, soon after eating. Loss of appetite. Can't swallow any hot food or drinks (Lach.), causes choking. Diarrhea after lemonade. Vomiting of food and milk, in teething children.

Glands - Swelling and induration of glands. Swollen glands and burning pains, worse at night. Glands swollen at the angle of jaw. Glandular abscesses. ***Venereal buboes***. Hardness of glands in right side of neck. Swelling of axillary glands.

Head - Pain from frontal region backwards. Pressure in temples and over eyes. Brain feels sore, head as if beaten. Violent headache, with stupid expression of face and enlarged pupils. Headache with vertigo and dim vision. Nausea and headache better eating, but returns soon with vomiting. Rheumatism of scalp, pains come on every time it rains. Cold sweat on forehead. Scaly eruption on scalp. Tinea capitis.

Heart - Feeling as if heart leaped into throat (Podo.). Pains in region of heart, worse walking. Shock of pain in cardiac region alternating with pain in right arm. Fatty heart. Small, irregular pulse with great excitement in cardiac region.

Kidneys - Dull and sore pains in kidneys. Pains in kidney region, with scanty, suppressed urine. ***Hard aching pain in kidney*** with scanty urine. Nephritis. Urine coffee-colored. Dark red urine, chalky sediment. Urine stains the clothes yellow. Albuminuria after diphtheria, scarlatina. Copious nocturnal urination.

Limbs - Rheumatic pains, worse in morning. Syphilitic sciatica. ***Pains fly like electric shocks***, shooting, lancinating, shifting rapidly (Puls., Kali-bi.). ***Wandering pains*** passing from one joint and place to another, with swelling and redness. ***Muscular soreness all over.*** Shooting pain in right shoulder with stiffness and inability to raise arm. Painful, hard, shiny swelling of finger joints. Pain in hips and thighs on change of weather. Sharp cutting, drawing pains in the hip, legs drawn up, cannot touch floor. Pain in legs, patient dreads to get up. ***Aching of heels***, relieved by elevating feet. Feet puffed, pain in ankles and feet. Neuralgia in toes. Cold hands and feet.

Liver - Chronic hepatitis (Chin., Phos.), with enlargement and induration of liver.

Lungs - Difficult breathing. Pains and suffocating feeling in throat and lungs. Panting breathing. Hoarseness. Paroxysmal cough and very profuse and exhausting expectoration of thick starch-like mucus. Dry hacking, tickling cough, worse at night (Menth., Bell.). Cough with burning in trachea. Cough as soon as he lies down. Cough with pain in chest and side. Croupy cough, with burning in larynx and trachea, worse night and in cold, damp weather. Chronic cough, generally hard and dry. Thick, tough expectoration. Thick expectoration, starch-like mucus, profuse and exhausting. Copious, yellow mucus.

Male - ***Shooting along perineum to penis.*** Painful induration of the testicles. Orchitis, acute and chronic, with suppuration and fistulous ulcer. Spermatic cord sore. Gonorrhea and gleet. ***Venereal buboes***. Ulcers on genitals. Impotency.

Modalities - Better warmth, dry weather. Better from lying on abdomen or left side, lying on stomach, rest. Rubbing ameliorates pain in hip. Pressure on trachea facilitates expectoration. Sensitive to electric changes. ***Worse exposure to damp, cold weather, rain, cold night,*** changes of weather, washing, heat. Worse ***movement***, raising up, stepping down from high step, right side, from touch, during menses. Worse from swallowing, particularly hot drinks. Pressure aggravates pain in joints and ulcers. Riding aggravates nose and breathing.

Mouth - Dry sensation in mouth, from cough. Metallic taste in mouth. Much stringy saliva. Profuse saliva, sometimes yellowish, often thick, ropy, tenacious. Bleeding from mouth. Very painful small ulcers on side of cheek, cannot chew on that side. Jaws firmly set, chin drawn down on sternum. Ulcers on lips. Upper lip excoriated. Lower lip drawn down. Lips everted and firm.

Nose - Coryza with lachrymation and photophobia. Acrid coryza. Coryza, ***flow of mucus from one nostril and from posterior sinuses.*** Thin watery discharge from nose. Feels congested and heavy. Pain at root of nose, with stoppage. Obstruction of nose while riding. Mucus hangs down in strings from posterior nares, hawked with difficulty. Cancerous affection of nose, lupus.

Rectum - Continuous urging to stools, even in sleep. Constipation of the aged and those with weak heart. Diarrhea after lemonade. Dysentery, passage only of mucus and blood or like scraping from the intestines. Stools thin, dark brown. Bloody discharges with heat in rectum. Bleeding from rectum. Bleeding hemorrhoids. Fissures of anus. Cancer of rectum.

Sensations - Brain as if bruised. Right side of head as if pressed firmly. As if sand in eyes. As if eyes too large. As if lids granulated. As if tarsal edges raw. As if lids on fire. As if lump in throat. As if apple core in throat. Throat so full it felt choked. Pharynx feels like a cavern, chest as if it were a big empty cask. Body as if bruised, pounded all over. As if joint were being chopped with an ax.

Skin - Dry, harsh, shriveled. Skin becomes dry, shrunken, pale. Itching. Papular and pustular lesions. Erythematous blotches, irregular, slightly raised, pale red, ending in dark red or purple spots. ***Disposition to boils*** and carbuncles, with swollen glands and burning pains, worse at night. Painful boils on back and behind ears. Squamous eruptions. Syphilitic eruptions. Swelling and induration of glands. Scarlatina-like rash. Warts and moles. Lipoma. Corns. Barber's itch. Lipoma. Pityriasis. Ringworm. Ulcer, chronic, surrounded by boils. Cancerous ulcers.

Sleep - Frequent yawning and drowsiness. Restlessness at night. Pains drive him out of bed. On awaking, feels wretched.

Stomach - Hunger soon after eating. Heat in stomach. Stomach cramps and coldness. Pain in region of pylorus. Pains, worse deep breathing. Nausea, eructations of flatus and sour fluids, with severe pain in umbilical region. Easy vomiting without nausea. ***Violent vomiting with retching, desires death to relieve vomiting.*** Vomiting of clotted blood and mucus. Vomiting and diarrhea, with griping pains and cramps in abdomen.

Teeth - Difficult dentition, better biting on something hard. Teething children with ***irresistible desire to bite the teeth together***. Teeth and jaws clenched. Teeth feel sore and elongated. Inflamed gums and teeth, with mercurial ptyalism.

Temperature - Chills at night and every morning. Cold hands and feet. High fever, alternating with chilliness and great prostration. ***Mastitis. Mumps.***

Throat - Aphonia. ***Dark red or bluish red***. Much pain at root of tongue, soft palate and tonsils swollen. Sensation of a lump in throat (Bell., Lach.). ***Throat feels rough, narrow, hot.*** Ulcerated sore throat and diphtheria, ***throat feels very hot, pain at root of tongue extending to ear***. Pseudo-membranous exudation, grayish-white, thick, tenacious yellowish mucus. ***Shooting pain into ears on swallowing***. ***Cannot swallow anything hot*** (Lach.). Tension and pressure in parotid gland. ***Tonsils swollen***, especially right, dark-red appearance. ***Tonsillitis with fauces swollen*** with burning pain, cannot swallow even water. Uvula large, dropsical. Follicular pharyngitis.

Tongue - Tongue thickly coated, yellow at base, ***fiery red at tip.*** Tongue mapped, indented, fissured, with yellow patch down center. Tongue feels rough and scalded, burnt on back of tongue. Pains at root. Tongue protruded.

Vertigo - Vertigo on rising, feels faint. Vertigo, staggering with danger of falling. Vertigo with dim vision.

COMMENTS - Closely related to Merc. and Kali-i., especially in syphilitic rheumatism. General action of tissue absorption, especially new growths. Tumors and indurations of the glands. Muscles, joints, bones, brain and spinal cord, as well as the special senses, were all more or less disordered.

In cases of poisoning, the most common symptoms were vomiting, diarrhea, frontal headache and a sore throat. Irritation of the eyes, nose and throat, a severe headache and diarrhea have occurred after inhaling the dust of the powdered dried root, or from the odor of the fresh root when it is sliced.

Phyt. has caused convulsive symptoms, vomiting and vomiting of worms when given to animals. Wild pigeons and other birds that eat the berries acquire a red color and lose fat. This observation has led to the use of a tincture of Phyt. berries as an anti-fat remedy, and successful results have been reported.

Hale tells us that among American dairymen the root is used to regulate any abnormality in cows' milk, whether it is scanty, thick, watery, curdy, or containing blood or pus. Its chief repute is for caked udders.

One boy, who drank two or three drachms of a tincture of the root, developed complete tetanus in which his limbs were stiff, hands firmly shut, feet extended toes flexed, lower lids drawn down, teeth clenched, lips everted and firm, general opisthotonos. Respiration was difficult, rales were heard all over the room.

For an hour muscular rigidity increased with convulsive action of muscles of face and neck, chin drawn close on sternum.

This condition lasted five or ten minutes, followed by perfect relaxation and return in twenty minutes more with the same violence.

After cold-water infusion, cupping, and mustard plasters, the boy slept about twenty-five minutes. On waking he had some twitchings, especially of lower limbs, pain in back of head and stomach. The next day he was quite recovered.

A boy, 8, who ate a quantity of the berries, was found in great agony, complaining that his stomach was "inched together." He had nausea, violent vomiting, his throat was sore and dry, fauces dark red, tonsils swollen.

After his vomiting ceased, purging set in, stools dark brown and thin, severe pain in stomach on pressure, extorting a cry. Later he had burning griping in umbilical region, dim vision, tongue coated white, and spasmodic jerkings in his arms and legs.

In a woman, 45, who took Phyt. as a "blood purifier," a general rash in appearance not unlike the rash of secondary syphilis was set up.

A family of four was poisoned by eating the root with their food by mistake. They had a dread of movement. Seemed stupid, fell asleep after a paroxysm of cramping pain had ceased. Pain in the forehead, worse after eating.

Vomited clotted blood and slime. Copious discharge of blood and mucus that looked like scrapings of the intestines. Involuntary stools from straining, which occurred even in sleep.

In the mother of the family, who was seven months pregnant, it nearly produced miscarriage. The uterus could be felt contracting under the hand, and there was involuntary straining and hemorrhage from the vagina. Intense griping pain in small of back and cramps in legs coming and going suddenly. Coldness and withered appearance of limbs, the whole body cold.

Phyt., used externally, produces good results in cases of ulceration. Clarke found that a gargle of a few drops of the tincture in a tumbler of water was useful in many throat cases.

Hundall successfully used a preparation of the leaves as an external application for cancerous growths in dogs. An ointment prepared with a strong tincture of the leave, as well as the juice of the leaves, has been used for malignant ulcers in humans.

A case of cancer of the rectum was cured with Phyt. 3x. Nash removed many breast tumors by giving a single dose of Phyt. 100,000c during the wane of the moon. The tincture may take away nondescript lumps in the breast when there are few symptoms.

Breast cancer, especially with axillary involvement, especially right sided. Breast cancer that suppurates with horrible burning pains in the breasts. Advanced cases of cancer or tumors. Hard nodules with a bluish appearance and enlarged axillary glands. Scirrhus tumors, hard like cement (Con.). Scars of the breast, cicatrix (Graph., Sil.).

Sharp pain from the breast. Breast neuralgias, painful nerve irritation. Swollen glands, indurated (Brom.). Paget's disease of the breast. Breast induration and abscesses in nursing women.

Mastitis with a hot, painful, congested and sensitive breast, worse cold and damp. Breasts are hard and lumpy, heavy with mastitis (Bry.). Cracks and fissures in the nipples. Blocked ducts in the breast. Problems with nursing, if the milk dries up, bad milk, thick or lumpy milk. Painful, sore nipples in nursing women. Pain radiates all over the body when the child is put to the breast.

Rheumatic swellings are hard, tender and intensely hot. Arthritis, particularly of the shoulder (Rhus-t.), the joints swell before a storm or when damp. Worse at night, change of weather. Wandering pains, migratory arthritis.

Sciatica with sharp, cutting pains in the hip and down the thigh. Stiff neck. Generally swollen, stiff and sore, worse on the right side. Electric shocks, sharp pain in the joints with the stiffness (Ruta.). Very restless, but worse from motion. The tendons feel too short (Ruta.).

When pain in intestines disappears, pain in limbs comes on. Pain leaves heart and appears in right arm. Pains in head and chest go from before backward.

Pains run down spine from nape, from sacrum down outer aspect of thighs to toes. The outer aspects of the limbs are chiefly affected.

Frontal headaches, pressive, involving the eyes, worse right side. Headache associated with increased sense of hearing. Apathetic, gloomy. Restless with a fear of dying (Ars.). Generally self-centered (Ars.). Nervous irritability.

Disorders of dentition. Teething, better pressure. Teething with bad breath and sores in the mouth. Irresistible inclination to bite the teeth or gums together. Toothache with digging in pain, shooting pain. Sensation as if the teeth are too long. Jaw problems, with or without swollen glands. The tongue feels burnt and rough, may be blistered, with a red tip (Rhus-t.).

Influenza with general body ache, back pain and wandering joint pains. Swollen, tender glands with throat symptoms. Stiffness. Bone ache. Fevers with pain and vertigo (Gels.). Apathetic, internal shivering (Gels.). Feels sore and bruised (Bapt., Eup., Arn.). Delirium.

Diphtheria (Lac-c.). Sore throat, strep throat, tonsillitis. Burning in the throat with a stiff neck (Rhus-t.), worse from warmth. Dry, raw, rough sore throats. Throat appears dark and purplish. Very swollen and tender glands, particularly on right side of the throat. Great pain at root of tongue when swallowing, pains shooting from throat into ears on swallowing, worse on right side.

Hot feeling as if a red-hot ball in throat, burning worse by hot drinks. As if a red-hot iron in the throat (Kali-c., in the rectum; Alum., in the spine). Throat feels plugged (Caust.). Dark redness of fauces. White or gray patches on the tonsils, with offensive breath. Tonsils may appear ulcerated, with crypts. Tenacious, thick mucus in the throat, especially in the morning. Burning of the tongue. Ulcers of the mouth.

The Eclectics gave the expressed juice of the berries in "spasmodic or membranous croup or diphtheria." Clarke used Phyt. 30c for the so-called "diphtheria sore throat."

With the throat symptoms there are generally headache, backache, wandering rheumatic pains and fever. Nash relieved chronic follicular pharyngitis in public speakers when there was much burning, as if a hot substance in throat.

Rapid and profound prostration. Diphtheria paralysis. Faint and dizzy when standing. Soreness of the muscles. Restlessness, but he fears to move because motion worse the pains. Stiff neck, especially right side.

Angina. Sense of constriction in the chest. Radiating pains down the right arm (Lil-t.). Heart palpitations followed by severe aching down the right arm. Sensation of the heart beating in the throat.

The right side is most affected. Many symptoms were experienced in the liver and the spleen. Liver pains were worse lying on right (painful) side. The spleen pain was better lying on left (painful) side. Hepatitis with an enlarged, indurated liver.

Sensation in the stomach as if something is being pinched with violent vomiting attacks and pains in the pit of the stomach. Colic during teething, clenching their teeth with severe stomach or abdominal cramps, diarrhea.

One characteristic pain, noted in a case of constipation, is a shooting pain from anus to lower part of rectum, along perineum to middle of penis.

"Gurgling sensation in the prostate gland, repeatedly in the afternoon," was noted by one prover along with pains in spermatic cords. Suspension of sexual appetite with relaxation of the genitals. Syphilis, with bone pains, ulcers on the genitals and sore throats, worse at night.

Discharges are tough, stringy, difficult to detach. Generally offensive and acrid. Clinkers. Shreddy discharge in certain forms of intestinal catarrh and dysmenorrhea. Hemorrhagic and hemorrhoidal, acting strongly on rectum and anus, curing tenesmus, bloody discharges and heat.

Psoriasis, ringworm and barber's itch. Chronic eczematous eruptions of the face. Old scars that never heal, and when the weather changes the scars flare up and become painful (Graph.).

RELATIONS - ***Antidotes:*** Milk and salt, Bell., Mez. ***Compare:*** (1) Tincture of Phyt. berry - sore throats and in the treatment of obesity. (2) Bry., Rhus-t., Kali-hp., Merc., Sang., Arum-t. ***Inimical:*** Merc.

REFERENCES - Boericke. Clarke. Murphy. Phatak.

PICRICUM ACIDUM

(Picric Acid)

PHARMACY - pic-ac. Picricum acidum. Picric acid. Picronitricum acidum. Trinitrophenolum. Carbazotic acid. Tri-nitro-carbolic acid. Trituration. Solution in rectified spirit. ***Historical dose:*** All potencies.

CLINICAL - Acne. Anemia. Backaches. Bedwetting. ***Boils.*** Brain, pain. ***Brain-fag. Burns.*** Cachexia. Cancer. Condylomata. Conjunctivitis. Deafness. ***Debility.*** Dementia. Diabetes. ***Ears, boils.*** Emissions. Erythema. Hands, sweat. ***Headaches.*** Hemiplegia. Hemoglobinuria. Jaundice. Leucorrhea. Leukocythemia. Liver, congestion. Locomotor, ataxia. Masturbation. ***Memory, weakness.*** Myelitis. ***Neurasthenia.*** Nosebleeds. Otitis. Ovary, pain. Paralysis. Paraplegia. Pernicious, anemia. ***Priapism.*** Pruritus, vulvae. Sexual, mania. Spinal, exhaustion. Spinal, irritation. Spinal, sclerosis. Styes. Sycosis. ***Uremia***. Urine, bloody. Writer's cramp.

HOMEOPATHIC - Pic-ac. was discovered by Hausman in 1788. It is formed by the action of nitric acid on carbolic acid, salicin, silk and many other substances. Pic-ac. and its compounds are among the most powerful explosives known, lydite being an example.

Picric acid crystallizes in bright yellow needles or scales of very bitter taste, sparingly soluble in water. The yellow color is imparted to the eyes and skins of patients who take it in the crude, and it not only produces a semblance of jaundice, but actually disorganizes the liver if pushed.

Acts upon the brain, spinal cord, lumbar region, occiput, kidneys and sexual organs. Weakness, heavy, tired feeling in body and mind. It causes degeneration of the spinal cord with paralysis. It acts upon the generative organs probably through the lumbar centers of the spinal cord.

Occipital and bursting headaches (Glon.). The headache, frontal or occipital is worse on any attempt to use the mind and it may extend down the spine. Headache extending from the top of the spine up over the head to the eyes.

Neurasthenia (Ox-ac.). ***Worn out persons, mentally and physically.*** Cachexia. Progressive, pernicious anemia. Prostration, weakness and pain of back. Muscular debility. Heavy tired feeling. Numbness. Formication. Pins and needle sensation in limbs. Burning in many parts, along spine in legs.

Sallow complexion. ***Uremia*** with complete anuria. Brain-fatigue and sexual excitement. Degeneration of the spinal cord with paralysis. Myelitis with spasms and prostration. Acute ascending paralysis. Typist's or writer's palsy.

Thery of Paris accidentally discovered in Pic-ac. solution a remedy for burns. He twice dropped burning matter on his hands while working with a Pic-ac. disinfectant and was astonished at the absence of pain or injury.

From that date Pic-ac. became his principal remedy for burns and though others have complained that it caused violent pains, Thery has only once in some thousands of cases had to abandon its use on that account. A one percent solution applied on lint is the best application for burns until granulations begin to form.

MIND - Anxiety. ***Dread of failure at examination.*** Mental weakness after prolonged strain and anxiety. ***Memory, weakness.*** Forgetfulness. ***Mental exertion aggravates.*** Mental prostration after reading a little, worse after writing a little. Inability to collect thoughts or to study. ***Brain-fag.*** Inability to exert the mind, talk or think. Lack of willpower, disinclined to work.

Aversion to talking or movement, during headache. Sits still and listless, does not take interest in surroundings. Cerebral softening. Dementia with prostration, sits still and listens. In women, although enjoying the society of men, idea of marriage unendurable. Lascivious thoughts in presence of any woman. Lewdness.

Delusion that parts of body enlarged. As if stairs or ground coming up to meet him.

Abdomen - Fullness of the abdomen. Sharp pain in left side of umbilicus. Shooting, wandering pain. Crawling, stinging. Rumbling in small intestines with colic. Crampy pain and flatus. Emission of flatus during the day in evening.

Back - Burning along spine. Painful boils on nape of neck. Backache with languor, patient is unable to sit straight and burning along spine, worse study. Keeps legs wide apart when standing. Aching, tired legs. Writer's cramps or palsy. Back seems as if bandaged, also limbs. Anesthesia of legs as if one has on elastic stockings. Legs weak, heavy like lead, lifts with difficulty.

Chest - Tightness of chest, as if encircled by a band. Numbness in lower part of sternum.

Constitutions - Suited to dark complexioned persons with a dirty appearance from bile pigments, anemic and cachectic persons. Worn-out person, overtaxed mentally and bodily.

Ears - Boils within ears and back of neck. ***Painful boils*** in meatus. Puffy and burning sensation in ears. Buzzing and hissing in ears. Noises in ears with vertigo and headache at the base of brain. Chronic deafness.

Eyes - Pupils dilated. Eyes yellow. Catarrhal conjunctivitis with copious, thick yellow discharge. Lachrymation. Styes with a sore pain.

Female - Pain in left ovary and leucorrhea before menstruation. Extreme exhaustion at menstrual periods. Pruritus vulvae.

Food - Appetite increased, then lost for breakfast. Aversion to food, at noon. Great thirst with bitter taste, unquenchable. Thirst for cold water.

Head - ***Headaches, relieved by bandaging tightly.*** Headache, worse mental exertion, better nosebleed. Headache, worse with sexual excitement and violent erections. Headache during daytime better in sleep. Headache of businessmen, teachers and students from grief and other depressing emotions. ***Brain-fag. Occipital pain***, worse slightest mental exertion. Heavy occiput, down spine and lower limbs.

Kidneys - Inflammation of kidneys with profound weakness, dark, bloody, scanty urine. Dribbling urine. Albuminuria. Ammoniacal. Urine contains much indican, granular cylinders and fatty degenerated epithelium. Uremia with ***complete anuria.*** Diabetes. Nightly urging.

Limbs - ***Great weakness, tired, heavy feeling all over body, especially limbs. Worse exertion***. Acute ascending paralysis. Feet cold. Cannot get warm.

Liver - Liver full of fat granules. Sticking through hepatic region, worse in muscles. Tendency to jaundice. Jaundice with itching.

Male - Enlargement of the prostate gland. Hard erections with pain in testicles up spermatic cord. ***Priapism,*** penis distended. Lascivious thoughts in presence of any woman. Extreme prostration from frequent seminal emissions. Impotency with tendency to boils and carbuncles.

Modalities - Better from cold air, cold water, sun. Better tight pressure, bandaging, rest. Worse least exertion, especially mental, fatigue, study, mental shock. Worse after sleep, seminal losses. Worse wet weather, hot weather.

Mouth - Bitter taste with thirst. White, frothy saliva hang in strings to the floor.

Nose - Boil in left nostril. Stinging on right side of nose. Acne. Nose full of mucus, can breathe only through mouth, better open air.

Rectum - Diarrhea from mental exertion. Stools thin, yellow, oily. Burning in rectum while passing stools.

Sensations - As if sand or sticks in eyes. As if throat would split. As of a lump back of thyroid cartilage. As if chest encircled in a tight band. As if legs enclosed in elastic stockings. Pricking as from needles in legs. As if stairs or ground coming up to meet him. As of ants crawling over surface.

Skin - Jaundice. Small, painful, sore boils, especially on neck.

Sleep - Sleepy during day and sleepless during night. Sleepiness. Sleep sound but unrefreshing.

Stomach - Vomits suddenly, without warning. Vomit bright yellow, bitter.

Throat - Redness of throat with raw, scraped, stiff and hot feeling. Soreness back of and above soft palate with debility. Dry and husky.

Vertigo - Vertigo and noises in ear.

COMMENTS - Grimmer said this remedy's sphere of action centers in the brain, spinal cord and the bloodstream. It produce in the provings a marked cachexia and pernicious anemia and these conditions in the sick have many times been cured.

In some experiments by Parisel, symptoms were observed including buzzing and whistling in ears, sparks, whirling around of objects, heaviness of head alternately with sense of emptiness. Copious, oily-looking, yellowish stool with amelioration of cerebral symptoms.

Pulse slow, small, very feeble. Great weakness, compelling to lie down, limbs hardly able to stir themselves, no anxiety, profound calm. Vivid coloration of sclerotics and tissues, urine colored blood-red. These were effects of 0.5 grains doses. Slow poisoning set up an intermittent fever of quotidian type and "anorexia, thirst often sweat, cancerous tint about skin, tendency to cachexia."

These observations give the chief features of the remedy's action: fatigue, mental and bodily, symptoms worse by least exertion, fatigue going into actual paralysis, brain fatigue, nerve fatigue, at the same time absence of anxiety indifference. The right upper part of the body is more affected than the left, the left leg more than the right.

Cachectic tint to skin, suggestion of malignancy, skin merging into a jaundice as the disease advances. Cachexia and cancerous tints. "Tired-out, washed-out feeling must give in." Jaundice, with itching. Small, painful furuncles, particularly in the auditory meatus. Fig warts. Erythema and itching of abdomen and feet.

Heat and congestion of the head, with nosebleeds. Heaviness of head alternates with emptiness. Frequent severe headache. Pain in eyes, worse from lamp light, strong light, moving the eye. Spinal congestion. Colds. Chilliness predominates.

Amorous fancies. Lascivious thoughts in the presence of any women. Great sexual desire with emissions. Terrible erections, disturbing sleep. Long-continued erections at night with emissions, followed by more erections and lewd dreams, priapism day and night. Priapism, penis distended almost to bursting. Gonorrhea. Burning during and after urination.

Exhaustion and complete prostration of mind and body from sexual excesses, mental and physical fatigue. Over-excitement of sexual system is associated with spinal or cerebral disorders in either sex.

A. C. Blackwood detailed the uses of Pic-ac. for burns of the first and second degree. He used a saturated solution diluted with one quart of water. The clothing was removed and the burnt surface cleansed with the solution and absorbent cotton. Blisters were opened but he carefully preserved the epithelial covering.

If extensive, the whole surface might be bathed with the solution and strips of sterilized gauze soaked and applied to entirely cover it, a layer of absorbent cotton held with a light bandage over all.

After three or four days the dressing was removed carefully after thorough moistening, as it adhered closely. The second dressing was applied as at first and allowed to remain a week. The staining of the hands and linen caused by the dressing can be removed by boric acid.

Blackwood found it painless, anodyne, antiseptic, preventing inflammation, suppuration and septic poisoning. It coagulates the albuminous exudation and healing takes place under the coagulum.

Gaucher removed acute vesicular eczema by the same treatment. He noted that the skin and kidneys are intimately related and Pic-ac. has a powerful action on the latter. Among other disorders, it has cured diabetes.

Kent said Pic-ac. cures fig-warts and gonorrhea, he was led to infer its relation by its power over pernicious anemia, which he had often traced to a gonorrheal base.

In a case of spinal irritation, Clarke relieved with Pic-ac. 30c a pain which shot up from the spine into the head. The pains referable to the spinal cord are strongly marked. Any attempt to study causes burning along spine with great weakness of back and legs, soreness of muscles and joints.

Halbert reported a case illustrating the power of Pic-ac. over the effects of fatigue in professional neuroses. A stenographer and typewriter, after using her right index finger continuously for six years, noticed weakness of her thumb and index.

Then, she noticed the inability to hold a pen or pencil. Next there was difficulty in striking correctly the keys of the typewriter and some wrist-drop. The finger, when Halbert first saw her, was quite rigid and straight, showing extreme spasticity.

Massage, electricity, etc., had failed to give any relief. Pic-ac. 3x six times daily cured the case and made great improvement in the patient's general health.

Halbert reported the case of Mrs., C., 49, who had "nervous prostration" since the shock of the loss of a child three years before. Wasting with great appetite. Intense thirst and copious urination, especially at night.

Great perspiration and some jaundice. Heart flabby, mitral bruit, Dyspnea, emaciation, anemia, exhaustion. Urine 1040, 7 1/2 percent of sugar and some albumen. Pic-ac. 6x six times daily was given, rapid and continuous improvement followed.

Nash cured an old man who have been failing for a year with Pic-ac. 6c trituration. The man complained of heaviness in the occiput, inability to exert the mind, talk or think and general "played-out" feeling. Nash had feared brain softening.

Evans found it curative in girls and young women who, under the strain of many studies, show signs of breaking down. They lose appetite, sleep lightly and lie awake, exhaustion after the day's studies, fatigued even from a short walk, twitchings of muscles when asleep or awake, hysterical state, loss of will power, constant headache, irregular menses. Such patients are usually given iron, which does little or no good.

RELATIONS - ***Compare:*** (1) Ox-ac., Gels., Phos., Sil., Arg-n. (2) Zinc-pic. - facial palsy and Parkinson's disease. (3) Ferr-pic. - buzzing in ears, deafness, chronic gout, nosebleed, prostatic troubles. (4) Calc-pic. - boils in and around ears.

REFERENCES - Boericke. Clarke. Phatak.

PICROTOXINUM

(Picrotoxin)

PHARMACY - picro. Picrotoxinum. Picrotoxin. Alkaloid obtained from the fruit of Cocculus indicus. Menispermaceae. Trituration. ***Historical dose:*** All potencies.

CLINICAL - Dysentery. Dyspepsia. Hernia. Locomotor ataxia. Night-sweats. Urine, excess.

HOMEOPATHIC - Falk noted that Cocc. is used to stupefy fishes and when Picro. is added to water in which fishes are swimming "they make winding and boring movements of the body. Alternating with quiet swimming, open their mouths and gill caverns frequently, fall on their side and rapidly die of asphyxia."

J. H. Henry proved Picro. on himself. The symptoms were so severe that he was alarmed and took Op. and Camph. to antidote them.

Nausea with tendency to faint, violent intestinal pain and purging, dysenteric diarrhea and excessive secretion of urine, cramps and paralytic sensations were experienced. The symptom which gave the most concern was the pain in the bowels and sensation as if the bowels would protrude at left inguinal ring.

COMMENTS - Brunton said the local application of Picro. as an ointment to the head for tinea capitis and to destroy lice has been followed by convulsions and death.

Hansen mentioned that it has been given at bedtime to relieve the night-sweats of tuberculosis. With Pictx-ac 3x, Dorr cured in a few weeks a case of advanced locomotor ataxia with amaurotic amblyopia.

RELATIONS - ***Compare:*** (1) Cocc. (2) In tetaniform convulsions, Nux-v. with Picro. respiration is accelerated more from spasm of glottis then of respiration and there is less susceptibility to slight touch, more chorea symptoms.

REFERENCES - Clarke.

PILOCARPINUM

(Pilocarpine)

PHARMACY - piloc. Pilocarpinum hydrochloricum. Pilocarpine. Jaborandi alkaloid. Pilocarpinum muriaticum nitricum purum. Rutaceae. Solution in distilled water. Trituration. ***Historical dose:*** All potencies.

CLINICAL - Albuminuria. Alopecia. Convulsions, uremia, Deafness. Exhaustion. ***Eye, disorders.*** Faintness. ***Hair, loss.*** Meniere's disease. ***Mumps.*** Myopia. Paralysis. ***Perspiration, excessive.*** Pregnancy, nausea. Salivation. ***Tinnitus.*** Vertigo, aural.

HOMEOPATHIC - Piloc. is one of the most characteristic of several alkaloids which have been isolated from jaborandi (Pilocarpus pinnatus). It has been used like Jab. to produce and cure profuse sweating, and by oculists to produce contraction of the pupil, which it does whether it is injected subcutaneously or applied directly to the eye. It has also an action on the ear.

The hair as well as the skin is affected by Piloc., which is an ingredient in many "hair restorers." Schmitz of Cologne treated two bald men with injections of Piloc. mur. to produce absorption of inflammatory residue within the eye.

In both a secondary effect occurred, the growth of young downy hairs on the bald parts of the scalp. One, age 60 in four months and his head covered "partly with gray and partly with black hairs" of considerable growth, so as to entirely obliterate his previous baldness. Piloc. has also been known to turn white hair black.

In a case of lead paralysis, it produced profuse salivation and sweat with sensation of great coldness and excessive tremors of limbs. Salivation and sweating speedily occur.

Dilatation of blood vessels, temporal artery becomes a thick, pulsating cord, veins of forehead stand out blue. Exhaustion (after the perspiration) during which most of the patients fell asleep. Faintness.

Ears - Aural vertigo. Tinnitus of left ear. Deafness with tinnitus. Labyrinthine deafness, worse when tired. Increased secretion of wax.

Eyes - Profuse lachrymation. Pupils contracted to pin-head. Sight for distance improved.

Face - Forehead and face red, veins stand out. Perspiration begins on face.

Female - Menses two days early.

Food - Intense thirst following the sweating.

Head - Throbbing in temples with acceleration of pulse. Turns white hair black.

Heart - Weakness of the heart. Pulse accelerated, blood pressure diminished. After the perspiration the pulse sinks to normal.

Lungs - Increased bronchial mucus, much cough and expectoration. Constantly taking cold and in fear of bronchitis.

Mouth - Saliva thick, stringy, exceedingly tenacious. Sudden salivation, maximum reached in fifteen minutes, continues two hours, one and a half pints of thin saliva being secreted in that time.

Nose - Nasal secretion increased.

Rectum - Urging to stool.

Skin - Irritable skin.

Sleep - Patients fall asleep under its influence.

Stomach - Nausea, only occurring when salivation is complete (does not go on to vomiting as that of Jab. does). Nausea and retching.

Temperature - Sensation of coldness and shaking chill without fall of temperature. Increase of temperature with feeling of intense cold. Sweat profuse, may lose from tow to four pounds in the sweating. After sweat, thirst, feeling of relief and sense of increased vigor.

COMMENTS - G. P. Field gave it with good effect in labyrinthine deafness, tinnitus and auditory nerve vertigo.

The cases least amenable to its influence were those in which the hearing was better in a noise as of a train, etc. and those in which the hearing is worse after a cold. Subjects of syphilis, hereditary or acquired and patients who are more deaf when tired, are the most suitable.

Wood went to see a woman three months pregnant. She was a picture of distress and despair. For eight weeks she had saturated from six to ten handkerchiefs daily with tenacious saliva. Nausea and vomiting were constant, emaciation extreme. Nausea worse by slightest movement.

Alternate redness and paleness of face, flushes of heat and perspiration. Urine scanty, high colored, depositing much uric acid. Very chilly, obstinate constipation. Piloc. was given, a teaspoonful every two hours.

The next day Wood found his patient sitting up, cheerful and free from nausea and salivation. The improvemen,t with some fluctuations, continued. Merc., Ip., Nit-ac., Kali-bi., Hydr., Cimic. had all previously failed.

A woman who had Piloc. injections complained to Cooper that thereafter she had been constantly catching colds and had fears of getting bronchitis. Her skin too, became irritable. Piloc. 3x is Burnett's chief remedy in mumps. He regarded it (and Jab.) as an organ remedy of the sweat glands, parotid and pancreas.

Frohling related a case showing the power of Piloc. over debilitating sweats left after acute diseases. With Merc. 12c he cured a case of rheumatic fever so far as the joint affection was concerned, but the sweats persisted and strength declined in spite of remedies until Piloc. was given, when the sweating stopped after the first dose.

RELATIONS - ***Antidoted by:*** Atro., Am-c. (sal volatile), brandy. ***Compare:*** (1) Jab., Myos., Esin., Phys. ***Follows well:*** Merc. (in sweating of rheumatic fever).

REFERENCES - Clarke.

PIMENTA OFFICINALIS

(Allspice)

PHARMACY - pime. Pimenta officinalis. Allspice. Pimento. Eugenia pimenta. Eugenia acris. Myrtus pimenta. Jamaica Pepper. N. O. Myrtacae. West Indies. Pimento consists of the dried berries. Tincture of the fruit. ***Historical dose:*** Tincture and all potencies.

CLINICAL - Chills. Neuralgia.

HERBAL - "Allspice" is so named because its odor is said to resemble a combination of cinnamon, nutmeg and cloves. A tincture was proved by Becket, and developed one-sided neuralgias and disturbed sensations of heat and cold.

HOMEOPATHIC - Pime. has helped disturbances in the body's temperature and sensitivity. Parts of body burning hot, other cold. Peculiar cold sensation as if sponge filled with cold water passed here and there over the surface, succeeded by sensation of heat, as in the reaction after a cold bath. Very imperious desire to eat. Semi-lateral neuralgic lesions.

RELATIONS - ***Compare:*** (1) Eucal., Eug.

REFERENCES - Clarke.

PIMPINELLA SAXIFRAGA

(Bibernell)

PHARMACY - pimp. Pimpinella saxifraga. Bibernell. Pimpinella alba. Burnt saxifraga. N. O. Umbelliferae. Saxifrage. Tincture of the fresh root. ***Historical dose:*** Tincture and all potencies.

CLINICAL - Chilliness. Corns. Nosebleed. Fever. Headache. Lumbago. Stiff neck. Tinnitus.

HOMEOPATHIC - The majority of the symptoms were obtained by Shelling from chewing the fresh root. The rest were contributed by Berridge, who proved the 1x on a man.

Marked chilliness, chilly in the back even in a warm room and much worse if a window was opened. Sensitive to drafts. Sensation of coldness in occiput as from a cutting wind behind.

Cold stream from hip and into right leg. the pains and sensations extended from one part to another, principally from above downward and from before backward (temples to nape, forehead to eyes, nape to shoulders) from within outward or alternated between different parts.

Rush of blood to head, followed by nosebleed, whizzing in head, roaring in ears. Sinking sensation in intestines. Weariness and falling asleep of parts rested on. Frequent yawning and desire to take a long breath, which was difficult. Great drowsiness.

Modalities - Vertigo and sweat worse morning. Heat and rush of blood to the head, worse afternoon. Weary pain in limbs worse from rest. Worse reading, writing, reflecting. Worse by chewing, standing, stooping, walking. Worse by opening window in warm room.

RELATIONS - ***Compare:*** (1) Rush of blood preceding nosebleed, Graph. (2) Occipital pains, Hell., Nat-s., Glon.

REFERENCES - Clarke.

PINE

(Bach Flower Essence)

PHARMACY - pine-b. Pine. Pinus sylvestris. N. O. Pinaceae. Twigs with male and female flowers are picked and boiled for half an hour. The boiled water is strained and prepared as medicine.

Historical dose: Take two drops from the stock bottle into a one ounce dropper bottle, (add brandy or alcohol, if this bottle will be used for days or weeks). This is the dosage bottle, take a few drops straight into the mouth or as needed in a little water or juice.

HOMEOPATHIC - Pine-b. belongs to Bach's group of ***Despondency and Despair,*** with the remedies of Crb-a-b., Oak-b., Will-b., Star-b-b., Sw-ch-b., Elm-b. and Lar-b.

States of guilt, regret and self-reproach. Obsessive-compulsive states and too much over-conscientiousness. The body may show signs of becoming burdened, depressive, or rigid, due to excessive introversion and self-blame. Deep-seated conflict and obsessive guilt.

Gastric and duodenal ulcers, irritable colon, nervous breathing syndrome and insomnia (Must-b., Wh-ch-b.). Skin disorders with itching.

MIND - Introverted, subdued by the burdens of guilt and regret. Preoccupied or obsessed with guilt and self-reproach. Deep sense of unworthiness. Internal sense of failure. Over-conscientiousness.

Feelings of shame, regret and self-blame at not having fulfilled one's high ideals. Despondency and despair. Unable to forgive self. May assume responsibility and blame for failure caused by others. Frustration, anger, rigidity and alienation from oneself and others.

Obsessive-compulsive, self-punitive and perfectionist or ritualistic behavior and thinking, as in obsessive-compulsive personality disorder (Crb-a-b., Rck-w-b., Verv-b.). Delusions and paranoid personality disorders. Fear of being punished or persecuted (Asp-b.).

REFERENCES - Bach.

PINUS LAMBERTIANA

(Sugar Pine)

PHARMACY - pin-l. Pinus lambertiana. Sugar Pine. N. O. Confierae. Pinaceae. North America. Trituration of inspissated sap. ***Historical dose:*** Trituration, all potencies.

CLINICAL - Abortion. Amenorrhea. Constipation.

HERBAL - The inspissated sap of Pinus lambertiana makes a sugary substance like manna. A small quantity from a bit the size of a pea to a teaspoonful, has a decided but gentle laxative action, and in larger quantities emphatically so.

HOMEOPATHIC - Pin-l. has also an action on the menstrual function, restoring menses when suppressed and producing abortion in pregnant women. It was used by Indian women to restore the menstrual flow and remove painful sensations resulting from the suppression. It has a gentle cathartic action.

RELATIONS - ***Compare:*** (1) Sabin., Juni., Pin-s. and other coniferae.

REFERENCES - Clarke.

PINUS SYLVESTRIS

(Scotch Pine)

PHARMACY - pin-s. Pinus sylvestris. Scotch pine. Scotch fir. Red Norway. Riga Pine. Baltic Pine. N. O. Coniferae. Pinaceae. The typical pine of Europe. Tincture of leaves and young twigs. ***Historical dose:*** Tincture and all potencies.

CLINICAL - ***Ankles, weak.*** Anus, itching. Bronchitis. Constipation. Diarrhea. Dysuria. Emaciation, lower limbs. Glands, swollen. Gout. ***Headaches.*** Hemorrhoids. Joints, stiff. Kidneys, pains. Liver, enlargement. Lumbrici. Palpitations. Rheumatism. Scrofula. ***Squint.*** Tinnitus. Urine increased, strong. Vertigo. Walking, late. Worms.

HERBAL - Pine baths may also be made by adding Oleum pinus sylvestris to an ordinary bath in the proportion of one minim to the gallon. These baths have a reputation in the treatment of rheumatism, gout, paralysis, scrofula and skin diseases.

HOMEOPATHIC - Pin-s. was proved by Demeures in the tincture, and Patzack observed the effect of bathing in an infusion of the leaves.

Rheumatic, bronchial and urticaria symptoms. Rheumatic, gouty and paralytic pains in limbs, bones and joints. Stiffness. Glandular swellings. Enlarged and painful liver and spleen. Sensitiveness to touch. Scalp sensitive. Chest walls sensitive with a feeling of thinness, as if they would give way at a touch.

Chilliness alternating with flushing, the face is alternately red and pale. Itching in general. Emaciation of lower limbs. ***Weak ankles.*** Late walking in scrofulous and rickety children.

Bronchial mucus was increased. The kidneys were stimulated, burning on urination, flow increased, urine strong. Itching of the nose and discharge of round worms was noted. The menstrual function was deranged.

MIND - Anxiety. Despondency. Mind dull, unable to think, caused by any exertion. Wants to do many things, undertakes all and finishes none.

Abdomen - Distention of hypochondrium with pressive and burning pains. Enlargement of liver. Pressure and fullness in liver and spleen. Colic with incarcerated flatus. Pain in inguinal glands with swelling.

Back - Drawing and stiffness in nape extending into occiput. Pressive, tensive drawing pain between shoulders and small of back, motion difficult.

Chest - Oppression. Anterior portion of chest painful to touch. Burning in sides of chest. In middle of sternum sensation as if a cupping-glass had been applied inside.

Ears - Sticking in ears. Roaring in ears.

Eyes - Eyes inflamed. Margins of lids red. Vision dim, veiled. Squint.

Face - Face alternately pale and red. Tearing in face.

Female - Menses, earlier, delayed. Menses, usually scanty, became more profuse.

Food - Appetite at first decreased, afterwards increased.

Head - Dullness, fullness, heaviness of head. Tearing in temples. Pressive headache. Headache worse by any movement of eyes. Scalp sensitive.

Heart - Palpitations.

Kidneys - Violent boring-burning pains in kidneys, extending along ureters. Burning pains when urinating. Spasms of bladder. Urination is difficult. Very greatly increased secretion of urine. Urine of strong odor.

Limbs - Stiffness, gouty pain in all joints, especially finger joints. Cramps in calves.

Lungs - Hoarseness. Breath tight, especially when walking. Increased bronchial mucus. Short, dry cough. Expectoration greater when coughing.

Modalities - Worse by exertion, walking, touch. Worse in morning, evening.

Mouth - Pain in teeth with heat of face and pain in head. Dry mouth with increased thirst.

Nose - Violent nosebleed several days in succession. Mucus discharge from nose. Sensation of coryza. Itching of nose.

Rectum - Constipation. Stool thin, pasty with colic and great excitement, bilious. Bloody, slimy, hemorrhoidal discharge. Troublesome itching at anus. Discharge of round worms.

Skin - Nettle-rash. Itching all over, especially about joints and on abdomen. Nose itches.

Sleep - Great sleepiness, especially forenoon with restless sleep in evening. Sleepless. Dreams which seem when remembered like real occurrences.

Stomach - Pressure in pit of stomach after eating with great distention.

Temperature - Chilliness, especially towards evening, alternating with flushes of heat. Perspiration general, easy.

Throat - Uneasiness in throat as if something in the way. Painful swelling of submaxillary glands.

Vertigo - Vertigo, even to falling down.

COMMENTS - In a patient of Cooper's, Pin-s. caused a "headache worse by any movement of the eyes" and it cured a case of squint.

Hansen gave "emaciation of lower limbs" and "weak ankles in children" as indications for it and mentioned that the tinctures may be used externally, while the potencies are given internally.

RELATIONS - ***Compare:*** (1) Pin-l. - constipation, amenorrhea, miscarriage. Pinus lambertina sap is a decided cathartic. Delayed and painful menstruation. (2) Abies-c., Abies-n. (3) Terebe., Sabin., Juni., Thuj., Aloe., Pix. (4) Strong urine, Benz-ac. (5) Red margin of eyes, Sulph., Bac.

REFERENCES - Boericke. Clarke.

PIPER AUGUSTIFOLIA

(Matico)

PHARMACY - pip-a. (mati.). Piper augustifolia. Matico. Artanthe. N. O. Piperaceae. Tincture of the leaves. ***Historical dose:*** Topically a hemostatic. Tincture and all potencies.

HOMEOPATHIC - Pip-a. is an aromatic, stimulant and urinary tonic. Has been used in gonorrhea, hemorrhage from lungs, catarrhal condition of genitor-urinary organs and gastro-intestinal tract. Chronic mucus discharges, such as leucorrhea, gleet and catarrh. Difficult, dry, deep, winter cough. Hemorrhages. Locally used for cuts, wounds and indolent ulcers.

REFERENCES - Boericke.

PIPER METHYSTICUM

(Kava-kava)

PHARMACY - pip-m. Piper methysticum. Kava-kava. Kawa. Macropiper methysticum. N. O. Piperaceae. Tincture of fresh root. ***Historical dose:*** Tincture and all potencies.

CLINICAL - Albuminuria. Anus, prolapsed. ***Arthritis deformans***. Brachialgia. Brain-fag. Catalepsy. ***Chordee***. Colic. Cystitis. Dysuria. Eczema. Emaciation. Gonorrhea. Headache. Ichthyosis. ***Insomnia.*** Intoxication. ***Leprosy.*** Liver, disorders. Neuralgias. Neurasthenia. Orchitis. Paraplegia. Prostate, disorders. Rheumatism. Skin, disorders. Toothaches. Urethritis. Uric acid, excess.

HERBAL - Piper methysticum furnishes the root called Kava in Polynesia. The natives use it as a stimulant, either chewing the root or drinking a beverage made of it before undertaking any important business or religious rites.

Kava causes exaltation of the mind, lively and inclined to work. Faculties sharpened, capable of working more without fatigue or brain-fag. From increased doses, there is intoxication of a sorrowful, silent and sleepy character, different from that produced by alcohol.

Excessive indulgence in it produces a skin disease like leprosy, called Tahiti Arevareva. Lutz described the disease as observed amongst natives of the Sandwich Islands,

"The skin, par marked ichthyosis, associated with a certain degree of atrophy, such as is observed in senile skin. There is an absence of inflammatory symptoms."

HOMEOPATHIC - Kava-Kava is an intoxicant which produces liveliness and inclination to do more work without fatigue. Silent and drowsy intoxication, with incoherent dreams, loss of muscular power.

Nervous system strung up to its highest tension. Trembling. Uneasiness and weakness during day with timidity and apprehension. Weakness in morning, better rising and moving around. Want of tone and life in all functions towards night.

Dizziness and vertigo, better on closing eyes. Full forehead, ***"solid with pain,"*** shifting to occiput and cervical spine, where it became a compression, extending as a constricting sensation to stomach and chest. Marked and persistent sensation of enlargement of head.

All the symptoms, especially pains are temporarily better by diverting attention, changing position or topic. ***Arthritis deformans***. Emaciation and decrepitude. Colic with flatulence. Urinary and skin symptoms have been verified.

MIND - Mental symptoms, excitement or depression, and the headache, better by diversion of mind. ***Amelioration of pains by diverting the attention.*** Restless desire to change position. Intoxication with fantastic ideas and desire to skip about, although he cannot for a moment hold himself on his legs.

Exaltation of mind. Very sensitive. Mental tension. Lively and inclined to work. Faculties sharpened, capable of working more without fatigue or brain-fag. Lazy and drowsy. Want of vigor, timid, apprehensive.

Back - Pain in back only felt on pressure. Soreness about second dorsal vertebra.

Chest - Constriction of chest and stomach, extending from base of brain. Heaviness behind upper part of sternum, as from wind that cannot be belched out.

Ears - Singular pressure in lobules of pinna of left ear.

Eyes - Conjunctivae red. Pain along right optic nerve when reading. Pain deep in left eye as if ball would be pressed out. Dizzy blindness when dressing

Face - Pressure outward in face at 7 p.m.

Food - Appetite is formidable, but not able to eat much.

Head - Brain tired in morning on waking, better getting on feet. Heaviness of head. Feeling as though the head were enlarged even to bursting. Headache with pressure in upper part of orbits with sleepiness.

Kidneys - ***Chordee***. Cystitis. Burning in urethra during urination, gonorrhea and gleet. Urine increased, scanty in morning. Urine nearly neutral, hot and over-acid at night.

Limbs - Numbness of the lower limbs. Weakness, as if unable to stand. Heaviness of legs when walking. Sticking in left knee at 4 p.m. when walking. Pain in right arm. Numbness of right elbow. Pain in right wrist, worse writing. Weakness of left hand. Hands feel paralyzed. Pain in the thumb joint.

Male - Shooting in penis. Pain in right testicle. Erection in afternoon, at night after an emission. Emission early in morning without dreams. Amorousness.

Modalities - Better moving, open air. Better by turning mind to another topic, changing position. Vertigo better closing eyes. Worse reading and thinking. Worse in open air, motion, walking. Going down stairs causes symptoms to rush up. Sour belchings worse before meals. Burning in urethra worse urinating.

Mouth - Burning in whole mouth followed by numbness. Dryness of mouth on waking from afternoon nap with sweat (on a hot day). Salivation. Taste is nauseous, sweet, then piquant and sharp, pappy, everything tasteless, lost to food, but ravenous haste in eating. Taste and relish to food not as usual, at noon, but appetite usually good.

Rectum - Urging all day, every evening. Continuous desire, next day forced a large stool, which caused prolapsed anus. Constipation, hard, large, light-colored. Stool difficult, large, soft. Pain after first stool. Burning in rectum.

Skin - Dryness, especially where it is thick, as on hands and feet with scales, cracks and ulcers. Ichthyosis. ***Leprosy***. Scaly. Fall of scales leaves ***white spots***, which often ulcerate.

Sleep - Difficult falling asleep. Sleepless. Sleepiness at 10 p.m., soon afterwards irresistible liveliness and wakefulness. Restless sleep last part of night. Stupid sleep. Heavy sleep with disturbing but unremembered dreams. Dreams are curious, nonsensical, wild, amorous of traveling by rail, active, vivid, last part of night of a fire, heard the engines and firemen.

Stomach - Warmth in stomach. Crampy pain, better pressure against edge of table. Sour belchings, worse an hour before meals.

Teeth - Teeth deep yellow. Teeth sensitive to cold water, cold air, brushing,

Tongue - Tongue feels as if covered with velvet or fur at night. Burning on tongue.

Vertigo - From 5 to 9 p.m. very dizzy, swimming sensation and faintness. Vertigo in morning in bed with frontal pressure.

COMMENTS - W. N. Griswold proved the third and second dilutions and developed a large number of nervous, mental and brain symptoms, among which are some which have proved to be keynotes. The mental symptoms of Pip-m. or the "Intoxicating Pepper" are the most interesting feature of the drug's action.

Feeling of buoyancy, as if every nerve was strung up to the highest pitch, feels he can work without fatigue, quickly followed by a feeling of tired brain and over-sensitiveness to all external impression.

Griswold cured a case having burning in chest, better by diverting mind, and three cases having "Agonizing pain with tossing, twisting and writhing, patient driven irresistibly to change position, which generally gives little or no better." These cures were with the 1x or tinctures.

Skinner gave fractional doses of tincture in water to a highly excitable young girl. She had severe toothache and earache and had worn out her family by the incessant day and night attendance she required.

The pains were dragging, heavy, worse at night in bed and after or when eating, "forgets all about her pains if amused with anything, but directly she is tired of it she exclaims 'Oh, my tooth or ear!' "

She had "Agonizing pain with tossing, twisting and writhing, irresistibly driven to change position." The patient slept well that night the first time for a fortnight and had no more pain. The remaining swelling was removed by Puls. 200c.

Skinner also reported the case of Miss R., 20, who had a toothache in a decayed molar, better if attention is diverted by anything, is diverted by anything sufficiently exciting. When pain is at all violent she has no rest in any position, must keep continually changing it. Pip-m. 500c (F. C.) was given and there was relief very soon after the first dose. A few doses completely removed the pain.

Farrington said convulsions simulating catalepsy are produced. Cerna, as a result of his investigations, found Pip-m. a general and local anesthetic. It diminishes reflex action by its action on the cord and kills by paralyzing respiration.

Cerna illustrated its relationship to Cub. by citing cases of gonorrhea, acute and chronic cystitis, gleet, prostatorrhea, vaginitis, cured with it.

RELATIONS - ***Antidoted by:*** Puls. and Rhus-t. (partially). ***Compare:*** (1) Cub., Pip-n., Mati. (2) Is better by diverting mind, Ox-ac. (3) better by motion, Rhus-t. (4) Feeling of buoyancy, Coff. (but with Coff. the reverse condition of brain-fatigue does not quickly follow). (5) Neurasthenia, Pic-ac., Arg-n., Aven. (6) Unbearable pains, Coff., Acon., Cham. (7) Chaul. (8) Bix.

REFERENCES - Boericke. Clarke. Phatak

PIPER NIGRUM

(Black Pepper)

PHARMACY - pip-n. Piper nigrum. Black pepper. N. O. Piperaceae. Trituration or tincture of dried fruits, peppercorns. ***Historical dose:*** Tincture and all potencies.

CLINICAL - Anus, fissure. Blenorrhagia. Breasts, swelling, eruption. Constipation. Cough. ***Diarrhea.*** Dysuria. Flatulence. Headache. Hemorrhoids. Menses, irregular, scanty. Milk, excessive flow. Neuralgia. Obesity. Priapism. Speech, difficult. Teeth, decay. Tongue, eruption, heavy. Toothache. Tympanites. Uterus, cramps. ***Worms.***

HERBAL - The Treasury of Botany noted that the peppers are tropical climbing shrubs. Pip. nigrum. yields the pepper of commerce. When ripe, the fruit is red. Black pepper is gathered before it is fully ripe and spread on mats in the sun, when it loses it red color and becomes black and shriveled. White pepper is the same fruit freed from its outer skin by maceration in water and subsequent rubbing.

HOMEOPATHIC - The symptoms of the Pip-n. proving are Houat's. The only additional symptom is one recorded by Berridge as having occurred in a woman on two occasions from taking a large quantity of pepper: "Feeling as if temples and malar bones were pressed in, worse on left side." Sensation of burning and pressure everywhere.

Clarke can confirm the full, heavy headache of Houat's provings by personal experience. He gets the headache whenever he takes food highly peppered and he knows of others who do the same.

MIND - Sad, apprehensive. Unable to concentrate, starts at any noise. Hot-headed, irascible and often gay. Amorousness with hypochondriasis. Fear of being poisoned.

Abdomen - Disposition of abdomen to obesity. Abdomen swollen, hard, burning. Inflammation of intestines with great thirst. Tympanites. Borborygmi. Colic and cramps, sensation as intestines would burst. Flatulence.

Back - Burning in loins and kidneys with contractive movements.

Breasts - Great flow of milk.

Chest - Dyspnea, cough with pain in chest in spots, feels as if spitting blood.

Ears - Crusty ulcers in concha of ears.

Eyes - Bursting aching in eyeballs. Eyes inflamed and burning. Lachrymation and photophobia. Lids ulcerated and bleared. Dim sight and vertigo with headache, nausea and vomiting.

Face - Red burning face. Lips dry and cracked.

Female - Menses difficult, retarded, capricious, irregular. Menses with colic and black blood. Ovaries and uterus congested with pricking and sharp pains. Burning and distending pains in uterus.

Food - Desire for coarse and extravagant food. Constant, unquenchable thirst.

Head - Heavy headache, as if temples were pressed in, pressure in nasal and facial bones.

Heart - Palpitations, cardiac pain, slow, intermittent pulse.

Kidneys - Bladder feels full, swollen, frequent inclination without success. Burning in bladder and urethra. Difficult urination. Priapism.

Male - Inflammation and swelling of penis with priapism and burning pains. Burning, pricking, excoriating pains in glans.

Modalities - Worse from change of temperature, damp weather, evening. Worse by motion.

Mouth - Burning dryness of mouth and throat. Heat and dryness of palate and tongue, as if burned.

Limbs - Inflammation and swelling of joints.

Lungs - Dyspnea and attacks of suffocation. Severe coughing, especially in evening and when going to sleep. Cough is violent, occasionally spitting of blood, croupy, hollow.

Nose - Nose itches, sneezing, nosebleed.

Rectum - Inflammation of rectum, anus swollen and burning. ***Diarrhea.*** Fear to go to stool on account of the difficulty and pain. Fissures in the anus. Long-lasting constipation, then involuntary, thin stools. ***Worms.*** Large flowing hemorrhoids.

Sensations - Burning sensation. Pressure in nasal bones in temples and facial bones. Sensation of a foreign, round body rising to stomach. Contraction of uterus and sensation as if something about to enter it.

Skin - Large pustules on face, leaving scars. Very tender skin. Itching, by scratching, heat and motion. Eczema on lips. Crusty ulcers in ears.

Sleep - Irresistible drowsiness. Lethargic sleep. Nightmares. Wakens at night without being able to sleep again.

Stomach - Full feeling. Gastric discomfort. Sensation of heat and dryness in stomach. Cramps and drawing in stomach. Vomiting with great exertion, it seemed as if stomach itself would be vomited.

Teeth - Tooth decays. Violent toothache, worse in warmth and evening.

Temperature - Dryness and coldness of skin, heat with biting dryness. Heat in forehead with heaviness of head and vertigo. Cold sweat with great heat through whole body. Sweat which seems to corrode the skin.

Throat - Sore, feels raw, burns. Burning pain in tonsils. Constant accumulation of mucus in throat and expectoration. Paralysis of muscles of throat, can cry but not articulate intelligibly.

Tongue - Eruption of little vesicles on margin of tongue. Painful, heavy tongue, impeded speech. Whitish coating on middle of tongue.

RELATIONS - ***Compare:*** (1) Piper-m. (2) Cub., also mental, genito-urinary, skin and general symptoms.

REFERENCES - Boericke. Clarke.

PIPERAZINUM

(Piperazidine)

PHARMACY - pipe. Piperazinum. Piperazidine. Diethylen-diamine. Trituration. Solution. ***Historical dose:*** All potencies.

CLINICAL - Glaucoma. Gout. Lead paralysis. Kidney, colic.

HOMEOPATHIC - Pipe. is a synthetic product which was intended to replace Spermin and was named Dispermine. It was found, however to be a different body both in chemical and physiological properties.

It occurs in well-defined, colorless, acicular crystals (Helbing) or in lustrous tables (J. Gordon), is deliquescent and mostly soluble in water.

It readily unites with uric acid, forming a very soluble compound (urate of piperazine). When taken by the mouth it is not entirely oxidized, as part is discoverable unchanged in the urine.

John Gordon experimented with Pipe. and found that a 1 percent solution in normal urine at body temperature dissolved to a large extent a fragment of uric acid calculus and converted undissolved portions to a granular and pulpy condition. The amount of urea is increased in the urine of those taking it.

J. R. Hamilton of Hawick reported success in treating kidney colic with Pipe. and Walter of Odessa, cleared up two cases of glaucoma, giving one grain daily in carbonated water, all the symptoms disappearing within three weeks.

According to Cooper, a patient, after a teaspoonful dose of an effervescing preparation of Pipe., complained that he was seized with a bad attack of acute gout, that was quite unexpected.

Helbing said it has been used with success in mental diseases and in a case of lead paralysis with "very remarkable results."

RELATIONS - ***Compare:*** Phlor., Hydrang., Urt-u.

REFERENCES - Clarke.

PISCIDIA ERYTHRINA

(Jamaica Dog-wood)

PHARMACY - pisc. Piscidia erythrina. Jamaica dogwood. White dogwood. N. O. Leguminosae. Papilionoideae. Tincture of root bark obtained when the plant is in flower, before leaf. ***Historical dose:*** Tincture and all potencies.

CLINICAL - Asthma. Bronchitis. Coughs. Fever. ***Insomnia.*** Neuralgias. Pains. Spasm. Sweat, profuse. ***Teeth, decay. Toothaches.*** Tuberculosis.

HERBAL - This small tree has unequally pinnate leaves and entire, oval leaflets. The flowers are in lateral clusters, and appear in profusion before the leaves. The bark of the tree is very astringent, and acts as a narcotic poison. When Pisc. is chewed, there is an unpleasant acrimony in mouth like that of Mez.

Locally the tincture is used for ***toothaches in decayed teeth.*** Piscidia is sedative, hypnotic and narcotic. A good nerve sedative and pain killer. The pounded leaves and young branches of Piscidia and some allied species are used like cocculus, for poisoning fish hence the name Piscidia (Piscis-caedere).

HOMEOPATHIC - Excessive restlessness and insomnia. ***Insomnia due to pain, worry*** or nervous excitement, it usually produces a quiet, deep sleep. Dysmenorrhea pains. Pains of irregular menstruation, regulates the flow. Neuralgias, ovarian or uterine. Neuralgic and spasmodic affections. Tetanus.

Toothaches in decayed teeth. Spasmodic coughs, especially cough of phthisis. Bronchial catarrhs, bronchitis. Asthma, nervous cough.

Fevers with a violent sensation of heat generally increasing in intensity, the sensation of burning gradually extended to the surface and a profuse diaphoresis burst out from every pore.

COMMENTS - The experiment recorded in Allen is by W. Hamilton, who took a drachm of the Pisc. tincture in water for toothache and went off to sleep with great suddenness. Profound sleep, he remained motionless the whole night, when he awoke, twelve hours later, he was still holding the glass and uncorked vial from which he had taken the dose.

When he returned to consciousness, he was free from every pain or ache and without any of the unpleasant sensations which invariably succeed an overdose of opium.

RELATIONS - ***Compare:*** Coff. and Op.

REFERENCES - Allen. Boericke. Clarke.

PITUITARIA GLANDULA

(Pituitary Gland)

PHARMACY - pitu-gl. Pituitaria glandula. Pituitary gland. Hypophysis. The tincture comes from the gland. Sarcode. Prepared by maceration in a mixture of water and alcohol-glycerine from the whole pituitary gland. ***Historical dose:*** All potencies.

CLINICAL - Amenorrhea. Angina pectoris. Anuria. Asthma. Backache. Bedwetting. Blood, clots. Breast, disorders. Cardiac, neurosis. Colitis. Coryza. ***Delayed, growth.*** Dyspnea. Enterocolitis. Hair, loss. Headache. Hypertension. Incontinence. Nephritis. Pharyngitis. Prostatitis. Recto-colitis. Septicemia. Stroke. Tachycardia. Tonsillitis. Valvular disease. Vertigo. Vitiligo.

HOMEOPATHIC - The proving was established by the Hering Proving Committee in 1935 on five provers, using the potency 12x.

George Fuller noted that Pitu-gl. exercises a superior control over the growth and development of the sexual organs, stimulates muscular activity and overcomes uterine inertia. Uterine inertia in second stage of labor where os is fully dilated.

Affects the female glands. Painful menses with disturbed cycle. Cervical pains. A vasoconstrictor and parturient, used chiefly for its action on the uterus either to aid in childbirth or to check bleeding after delivery.

Cerebral hemorrhage. It will check hemorrhage and aid absorption of clots. High blood pressure. Chronic nephritis, prostatitis. Bedwetting. Incontinence when the patient loses a few drops.

The action of this remedy has a clear antispasmodic tendency, especially affecting the vessels in the head. Vertigo, difficult mental concentration, confusion and fullness deep in frontal region. Congestive headaches. Pigmentation disorders and loss of hair.

MIND - Mental weakness. Difficult concentration. Nocturnal anxiety and anguish. Anxiety, aggravated at nightfall. Weeping, the patient cries involuntarily and even without noticing.

Obsessive ideas linked to the uro-genital area; fear of impotence, of passing urine. Obsession of ideas, especially of depressive, or of erotic, of impotence.

Abdomen - Enterocolitis. Recto-colitis. Spasmodic colon infection. Inflammation of the gallbladder.

Back - Pains in the nape of the neck, spreading to the occiput and shoulders. Neck ache. Backache.

Breasts - Breasts hypertrophy or atrophy. Amenorrhea with breast atrophy.

Chest - Growth of hair on chest.

Constitutions - Phosphoric, flouric types, tubercular poisoning or syphilitic, with obsessions or depressive complaints.

Ears - Earache. Buzzing. Deafness in the left ear.

Eyes - Mydriasis. Pupils very dilated. Weeping, the patient cries involuntarily and even without noticing. Styes, especially on the left. Conjunctivitis. Blepharitis.

Female - Amenorrhea with breast atrophy. Menses late, cycle longer than 30 days. Menses scanty. Menses with pain during the day. Menses very painful, especially the day before and the day after the start. Dysmenorrhea. Uterine pains from muscular contraction. Painful uterine contractions during childbirth. Difficult childbirth.

Food - Desires cold drinks.

Head - Congestive headache. Pulsating, throbbing headaches, related to hypertension. Headaches, starting at the occiput and spreading towards the base, cervical column and shoulders. Headaches, aggravated by heat, confined space, at the end of the day. Alopecia of the scalp, which is very dry.

Heart - Feeling of heaviness in the precordial region, aggravated by the slightest movement. The patient can "feel his heart." Sensation of heart constriction, aggravated by the slightest exertion. Arterial hypertension with the feeling of pounding arteries in the temples and carotid arteries. Coronary arthritis. Angina pectoris. Valvular disease. Cardiac neurosis. Arrhythmia. Tachycardia. Hypertension. Septicemia.

Kidneys - Nephritis. Anuria. Incontinence of urine, worse in the evening. Incontinence of urine in women with fibromatous uterus, the patient loses a few drops of urine on rising. Presence of albumin in the urine.

Lungs - Asthma. Asthmatic dyspnea, accompanied by intestinal and rectal spasms. Dyspnea from anguish. Dyspnea with abundant, watery, salty-tasting sputum, sensation of constriction in the thoracic cage. Laryngitis. Tracheitis and bronchitis.

Modalities - Better from fresh air, open air. Worse from the heat, in a closed room, at the end of the day.

Mouth - Excessive salivation. Saliva tastes salty.

Nose - Coryza.

Rectum - Rectal tenesmus, the patient wants to pass stools, but cannot. Diarrhea with painful intestinal spasms. Hemorrhaging recto-colitis. Proctitis.

Skin - Skin cold, discolored or strongly pigmented. Alternating white and dark patches. Vitiligo. Skin is swollen, edematous, itching. Eruptions of a urticaria type. Skin very dry, scaly.

Stomach - Nausea and post-prandial distention, worse after the evening meal.

Throat - Tonsillitis. Pharyngitis.

Vertigo - Vertigo when not moving body or head.

RELATIONS - ***Compare:*** (1) Ign. - Cortical and visceral rhythm disorders, characterized by mobility instability and paradoxical, contradictory state of symptoms. (2) Syph. - Changing moods, forgets proper nouns, obsessions, all aggravated at night. (3) Thuj. - Fixed ideas, sad, varicosities in the nostrils, skin sticky.

REFERENCES - Boericke.

PITUITARIA GLAND ANTERIOR

(Anterior lobe of Pituitary Gland)

PHARMACY - pitu-a. Pituitaria glandula anterior. Anterior lobe of pituitary gland. Hypophysinum anterioris. Adenohypophysis. Remedy made from the pituitary glands of sheep. Sarcode. ***Historical dose:*** All potencies.

CLINICAL - Acne. Backache. Breast, nodules. ***Constipation.*** Coryza. Dermatitis. Diarrhea. Dyspnea. Headache. Hemorrhoids. ***Hormonal, disorders.*** Insomnia. Nausea. Obesity. Ovarian, pain. Photophobia. ***Premenstrual syndrome.*** Sinusitis. Tonsillitis. Vertigo. Vitiligo. Vomiting. Warts.

HOMEOPATHIC - The homeopathic indications are based upon 5 years of clinical observations by Dr. David Flores Toledo of Mexico, who named the remedy Hypophysinum anterioris.

He wrote, in The Journal of the American Institute of Homeopathy, September, 1987, "Hypophysinum anterioris may well become one of the great polychrests, but it needs a careful proving. Numerous cases of acne, obesity, one of sterility, headaches related to menses, asthma, hemorrhoids, breast nodules, fungal infections of the nails, recurrent tonsillitis, vitiligo, and warts have been resolved with this medicine."

Hormonal, disorders. Sexual desire diminished, enjoyment absent (Sep.). Premenstrual syndrome. Flushes of heat in young girls. Weakness and cold perspiration on rising. Obesity. Allergy, metal dermatitis (Morg-g.).

Worse before menses, headache, coryza, pallor of face, nausea, vomiting, distended abdomen, yellow leucorrhea, pain in ovaries, pain in uterus, difficult respiration, painful swollen breasts, low backache, sleeplessness. Better after menses (Zinc-p.).

MIND - Aversion to everything, to friends, husband. Dislike of oneself. Easily depressed and avoids her friends. Fear to be alone. Anticipatory diarrhea before a date or engagement (Arg-n.).

Emotionally, worse before menses, fearfulness, irritability, sadness. Discouraged during menses. Causeless weeping. Weeping at trifles. Desire to weep, but finds it difficult. Ailments from disappointed love. Sexual desire diminished, enjoyment absent (Sep.).

Irritability before and during menses. Irritability at trifles. Anger during ovulation. Anger in morning on waking. Anger from contradiction.

Desire to strike. Screaming and crying from anger.

Abdomen - Distension, causing to bend double. Rumbling after eating, after milk. Flatulence, all food seems to turn to gas. Flatulence from fruit, vegetables. Pain after eating, after milk. Pain before and during menses.

Back - Acne, on back and cervical region. Low backache before menses. Pain in sacral region, coccyx, during menses.

Bladder - Involuntary urination when rising from a seat.

Breasts - Painful, swollen breasts before menses. Painful nodules in breasts.

Chest - Palpitations while lying on back. Eruptions, confluent acne. Perspiration in axilla during menses.

Eyes - Redness of eyes. Photophobia. Nausea preceded or attended by visual disturbances.

Face - ***Brown spots on face.*** Pale discoloration about eyes (Ptel.). Sensation as if face were burnt. Acne before menses. Acne on forehead during menses. Cold perspiration on face before or at beginning of menses.

Female - Hormonal disorders. Premenstrual syndrome. ***Worse before menses,*** headache, coryza, pallor of face, nausea, vomiting, distended abdomen, yellow leucorrhea, pain in ovaries, pain in uterus, difficult respiration, painful swollen breasts, low backache, sleeplessness. Pain in ovaries before menses, worse stepping. Menses brown at onset, clotted. Menses coagulated during first day and last days. Menses irregular, protracted with clots. Lack of vital heat during menses. Offensive leucorrhea like fish brine. Metrorrhagia between menses. Sexual desire diminished, enjoyment absent (Sep.). Sterility.

Food - Diminished appetite during menses (Mag-c.). Thirst for large quantities. Craving for cakes, sweets and chocolate. Desires fried potatoes, fruit, solid food. Indigestion from eggs. Worse from milk, seafood, fruit, vegetables. Worse from fats and rich food (Puls.).

Head - Headache before or at beginning of menses. Headache in temples at beginning of menses. Headache worse light, noise, sun, warm room. Headache due to contact lenses. Perspiration on scalp at night.

Limbs - Discoloration, white, depigmentated burning spots on upper limbs, worse sun. Itching eruptions on upper limbs, worse summer. Nails do not grow (Ant-c.). Swelling of thighs before menses.

Lungs - Asthmatic respiration in morning on waking. Asthma after anger. Asthma better copious expectoration. Asthma sudden attacks, from change of weather. Difficult respiration and headache. Difficult respiration before menses (Zinc.).

Mouth - Mapped tongue (Tarax.). Bad taste in mouth before menses.

Nose - Susceptible to sinusitis and obstruction to nose. Obstruction in evening, alternates with pain in root of nose. Discharge watery with sneezing (Cob-n.). Pain as if nose were extremely dry. Nosebleed during sleep.

Perspiration - Perspiration of hands and feet during menses. Weakness and cold perspiration on rising.

Rectum - Hemorrhoids. ***Constipation.*** Bowel movement every two or three days. Stool large, dry and hard. Stool like sheep dung. Anticipatory diarrhea before a date or engagement. Diarrhea from seafood, milk and milk products.

Skin - Eruptions, confluent acne. Moist eruptions. Brown spots. Discoloration, itching white spots worse menses. Vitiligo. Warts pedunculated, soft and small.

Stomach - Empty feeling in stomach without hunger. Nausea preceded or attended by visual disturbances. Nausea on looking at or smell of fatty food. Nausea better after eating. Pains better after eating a little, eructations, worse rich food (Puls.).

Throat - Susceptible to tonsillitis. Sore throat. Voice, hoarseness in hot weather. Hoarseness from talking.

Vertigo - Vertigo with tendency to fall, worse before and during menses. Vertigo with trembling. Vertigo as if intoxicated. Vertigo worse entering dark room from a lighter place, lying on back, moving head, rising from stooping, better when sitting. Perception of colors (pink, red, yellow, green).

RELATIONS - ***Compare:*** Sep., Puls., Calc., Nat-m.

REFERENCES - Toledo.

PITUITARIA GLAND POSTERIOR

(Posterior lobe of Pituitary Gland)

PHARMACY - pitu-p. Pituitaria glandula posterior. Posterior lobe of pituitary gland. Hypophysis posterium. Pituitarum posterium. Neurohypophysis. Sarcode. From the pituitary glands of sheep. ***Historical dose:*** All potencies.

CLINICAL - Angina, pectoris. Arterial, spasms. Diabetes, insipidus. Diarrhea. Eclampsia. Edema. Heart, attacks. Hemorrhage. Hypertension. Lactation. Moles. Salivation. Urticaria. Uterine, atony.

HOMEOPATHIC - The posterior lobe of pituitary gland releases the oxytocin and antidiuretic hormones. Removal or injury to the posterior lobe will lead to the symptoms of diabetes insipidus. It acts upon the parasympathetc center in the hypothalamus. Rate of secretion is controlled from the hypothalamic nucleri.

Antidiuretic hormone, or vasopressin, promotes the reabsorption of water in the kidneys. It raises the blood pressure and plays a role in the water balance. Also affects the production of breast milk.

It constricts the arteries of the abdominal organs, therefore it use to stop hemorrhage involving abdominal blood vessels. It may produce cerebral or coronary arterial spasms in large doses.

Oxytocin causes uterine contractions at term. Allopaths used it for the induction or stimulation of the labor. It has been given to relieve painful breast engorgement. Promotes breast milk release during lactation. Also for postpartum hemorrhage and uterine atony.

Its action is controlled in pregnancy by progesterone, which diminishes its action, and estrogen, which increases it.

An enzyme in the blood plasma of pregnant women appears to mediate this control.

Mind, anxiety, Head, pain. Dropsy. Basal metabolism rate increased. Blood pressure elevated. Blood sugar increased, Blood vessels constricted. Pulse, slow. Weakness.

Abdomen - Distention.

Bladder - Frequent or diminished urination.

Breast - Milk increased.

Chest - Bronchi constriction.

Ears - Noises in ears.

Eyes - Dilated pupils. Lachrymation. Vision loss.

Face - Dark discoloration, during pregnancy.

Female - Contracted uterus. Eclampsia. Weak labor pains.

Head - Headache in occiput, extending downwards. Hair falling out.

Kidney - Suppression of urine.

Lungs - Respiration difficult.

Mouth - Salivation.

Perspiration - Profuse perspiration.

Rectum - Diarrhea.

Skin - Dry and red. Dark discoloration. Coldness of skin. Moles. Urticaria. Angioneurotic edema.

Stomach - Nausea.

Urine - Copious urine, with albumin, sugar, increased levels of chloride, potassium and sodium.

COMMENTS - On the basis of these observations, Ghose made use of this sarcode in its 30th potency in anginal attacks with coronary spasms.

Ghose's first case was that of a middle aged man of 45, suffering from diabetes for two years. He developed mild anginal attacks after slight exertion and an occasional sense of heaviness in the precordium.

His cardiograph showed coronary disorder and was advised perfect rest. Blood pressure was more or less normal, pulse was 72 bpm. He was apparently a well-built man and was on a restricted diet for a long time due to diabetes.

Pitu-p. 30, three times a week, brought great relief of the precordial pain and heaviness; within a fortnight he could walk about in plain ground without any discomfort.

Ghose also used it in a case of old man, 70, with dyspepsia who used to get severe attacks of pain in the heart when walking, and particularly when getting up at night to attend calls for urination.

He was relieved with the very first dose of Pitu-p. 30 and could move about freely without any discomfort and could also attend to his nature's calls at night without feeling any pain.

In a third case, Ghose treated an old man, 65, suffering from coronary thrombosis for about a year and a half. He had W. R. 10/10 which was treated homeopathically.

He was living without any heart symptom for any other trouble for about a year, when suddenly he felt agonizing pain in the heart at 11 o'clock at night, with severe dyspnea and moist sounds all over the chest. All these symptoms pointed to edema of lungs. Pulse was soft and slow. Blood pressure was rather low.

Pitu-p. 30, repeated every half an hour, relieved the pain completely and made the dyspnea tolerable. A sanguinous expectoration followed for which he was given one dose of Merc-s. 200 and later on a few doses of Thyr. 200 which stopped the dyspnea completely.

RELATIONS - ***Compare:*** Pitu-a., Bell., Nat-m., Phos., Sec., Thyr.

REFERENCES - Ghose.

PIX LIQUIDA

(Pine-tar)

PHARMACY - pix. Pix liquida. Pine tar. Liquid tar. N. O. Confierae. Pinaceae. A product of dry distillation of various coniferous woods. Tincture. ***Historical dose:*** All potencies.

CLINICAL - Acne. Alopecia. Ardor urine. Bed-wetting. Bronchitis. ***Chest, pain.*** Desquamation. Diarrhea. Eczema. Eruptions. Hair, loss. Hands, eruptions. ***Itching.*** Psoriasis. ***Stomach, pain.*** Tuberculosis. ***Vomiting.***

HOMEOPATHIC - In old-school practice, tar is known as a "stimulant expectorant" in chronic bronchitis and tuberculosis, and a stimulant to the skin in psoriasis and scaly eczema.

Tar and its constituents act on various mucus membranes.

Cough. Bronchial irritation after influenza (Kreos., Kali-bi.). Tuberculosis and chronic bronchitis. Pain at the third left costal cartilage, where it joins the rib, pain of the left bronchus, with an offensive muco-purulent expectoration the indications for Pix are complete.

Scaly eruptions. Much itching. Alopecia (Fl-ac.). ***Constant vomiting of black fluid with pain in stomach***.

Abdomen - Excessive pain in bowels and loins.

Chest - Suppuration of left lung with pain at third rib. ***Pain at a spot about the third left costal cartilage,*** where it joins the rib. Rales through the lungs and chest.

Kidneys - Ardor urine. Dark-colored urine.

Lungs - Chronic bronchitis. Cough chronic, worse night, expectoration purulent, fever at night. ***Muco-purulent sputum,*** offensive odor and taste.

Rectum - Dark-colored stools.

Skin - Acute eczema. Acne. Desquamation. Skin cracked, ***itches intolerably***, bleeds on scratching, with sleeplessness. ***Eruptions on back of hands***.

COMMENTS - Buckley recorded severe constitutional effects following the local application of preparations of tar in skin disorders, including a high fever, black vomit, black stools, dark-colored urine, acute eczema, and acne.

In the Hom. News., Raynaud noted a case of chronic bronchitis in a merchant, 55. The cough was worse nights, breath short, copious expectoration, some fever and night-sweats. He had been ill three years and was growing worse.

Raynaud prescribed wood tar, a teaspoonful four times a day after meals and at bedtime, which cleared up most of the symptoms.

Pix. often cures the bedwetting of children.

RELATIONS - ***Compare:*** (1) Terebe., Pin-s., Kreos., Eupi., Petr. (2) In chest pains, Anis, has pain at third right costal cartilage, occasionally also left, Myric., Ther. (3) Desquamation, Chin-s. (4) Ter., Carb-ac.

REFERENCES - Boericke. Clarke. Phatak.

PLACENTA HUMANA

(Human Placenta)

PHARMACY - plac. Placenta humana. Human placenta. Sarcode. ***Historical dose:*** All potencies.

CLINICAL - ***Abdominal, pain.*** Backache. Belching. Constipation. Depression. Diarrhea. Earache. Eyestrain. ***Flatulence. Headaches.*** Night-sweats. ***Nightmares***. Nosebleeds. Palpitations. Photophobia. Sciatica. Styes. Toothache. Vertigo.

HOMEOPATHIC - ***Loss of energy.*** Weariness. Weakness and trembling. Restlessness, worse on waking. Poor co-ordination with extreme tiredness. Lack of vital heat, sensation of coolness. Averse to warm stuffy rooms. Worse on right side.

MIND - Apathetic and emotionless. No emotions, very little reaction to things going on. Calmness, almost to the point of no reaction. Completely passive. Confused, dazed and distant. Confusion of identity. ***Feel isolated, lonely, vulnerable and weepy.***

Weak memory, forgetful. Concentration difficult with an inability for mental work. Sadness, depressed and despondent. Nostalgia with flashbacks to past events. Feeling unappreciated, cross and sorry for self.

Irritability and anxiety. Anxiety, as if forgotten something important. Nervous anxiety about being on time. Anxiety about family, finances, work, the future. Anxiety about health and heart disease. Ailments from bad news.

Fear, as if something would go wrong. Fear of failure. Fear of closed places, sensation of claustrophobia. fear of crowds. Fear of rats. Sexual thoughts increased.

Abdomen - Bloated and uncomfortable after eating. ***Bloated and tender.*** Lower abdomen sore and bloated, better from sitting with legs wide apart. ***Abdominal***

pain associated with distension. Rumbling. Painful ***flatulence***, with abdominal tension. Flatulence with short, cramping, twisting pains making one double up. Shooting pain right to left, as if in labor when the head is low, better for lying on abdomen. As if needed to pass stool. Stabbing pain to right of groin.

Arms - Heavy weight sensation in arms with numbness. Lancinating pain in right elbow.

Back - Lower backache. Back pain, worse from sitting and relieved when lying down, worse during menses. Cervical and lumbar spine stiff. Right sided pains. Dull ache behind and between shoulder blades with twitching muscles. Sensation of inflammation in back.

Bladder - Pain during urination. Offensive, strong smelling urine.

Breasts - Breasts swollen and tender, before period. Nipples sensitive and tingling, as if milk coming in. Left nipple itchy with hard cheesy discharge. Shooting pains in right breast going through to back. Stitching pain, left breast.

Breathing - Difficulty breathing, like old asthma. Accelerated breathing. Breathless on talking. Difficult breathing on walking up the hill. Hyperventilation.

Chest - Constriction. Tight, suffocative feeling in chest, worse from emotions. Sensation of tight band around chest, worse at night, extending into throat. Chest feels tight and wheezy. Sensation of a lump in chest, extending to throat and back, worse swallowing, and pressure, better movement. Chest raw with a feeling of warmth. Eruptions on the chest.

Cough - Dry cough with nasal discharge.

Ears - Earache, hot, painful, itchy. Aching, throbbing ear pain. Popping of ears with crusty discharge. Ears feel hot inside with a low pitched hum and bloody discharge. Fleeting, sharp pains in right ear. As if ears had been in the wind. Sensitive to vibrations.

Eyes - Heavy and aching. Soreness. Stabbing pain, better sleep. As if eyes strained. Must keep blinking. Hard to open eyes. Puffy on waking. Dark eyelids as if punched, worse right. Swelling of the eyelids. Styes. Photophobia during the day.

Face - Anxiety felt in face with a mild ache in cheekbones. Pain in right cheekbone. Aching. Dry, sore patch right side of nose. dry and flaky. Worse left side, after exposure to wind and rain. Left temple, dry skin erupted, lumpy. Numb patch. Tingly, numb sensation, below left eye. Right side of face numb. Red spots on the face.

Feet - Cold feet. Numbness, loss of sensation in feet. Pins and needles in feet.

Female - Menses delayed. Period heavy. Menstrual pain in back and abdomen. Cramps in uterus. Uterus aching and uncomfortable. Dragging period pains, better warmth and pressure. Painless period. Blood bright red. Shooting pain in ovaries and fallopian tubes(left side morning, right side evening) during ovulation, with increased mucus. Right ovarian pain during ovulation. Streaks of blood at ovulation. Herpetic eruptions and cysts on the labia. Itching. Less vaginal discharge than normal. Small amount of dark purple, sticky mucus. ***Libido, strong. High sexual energy.*** Urge to have sex and reproduce. Strong feeling of pregnancy, as if baby moving around in belly and sensation of breasts filling up with milk. Sexual when premenstrual.

Food - ***Lack of thirst.*** Appetite changeable. Appetite lost but better for eating. ***Appetite decreased.*** Reduced appetite, increased after 6 p.m. When eats, feels sick. Easy satiety with difficulty eating. Snacks rather than a meal. Snacking with weight loss. Obsession for the amount of food eaten. Increased appetite. Appetite increased for breakfast and then reduced with weight loss. ***Desires spicy food,*** curry, delicate hot foods. ***Desires sweets and chocolate.*** Intolerant to milk. Thirst increased for cold drinks, beer, carbonated drinks and tea. Strong aversion to nuts. Strong disinterest in vegetables.

Hands - Itchy, flaky, dry, cracking and sore. Heels of palms of both hands hot, itchy, burning. Fingers as if numb with cold. Pins and needles sensations. Right hand stiff and slightly painful, especially fingers.

Head - ***Headache, worse in the forehead,*** as if the head were in a vise. Headaches, worse noise, and on right side. Dull, pressing head pain. Tightness. Pain in right temple. Bursting, stabbing pains. Sensation of coldness on vertex. Head cold, body hot, better if head is wrapped. Hair greasy.

Hearing - Ears with pulsating blood flow. Noise, as if under water, with distortion of hearing. Sounds distinct, more able to hear high pitched sounds. Sensitive hearing, particularly to the noise of children. Averse to loud noises. Competing, conflicting noises irritates.

Heart - Sensation of heart on right side. Heart rushing. Accelerated heartbeat. Heart racing and palpitations on going to sleep. Palpitations and breathlessness, feeling unable to breathe. Panic and palpitations with a sensation as if heart would be crushed on sitting.

Hips - Muscular stiffness in left hip. Aching pain in bed.

Knees - Stiff knees, worse in one position too long, worse rising.

Legs - Shaking, weak legs. Legs heavy and uncoordinated. Pain in back of left thigh. Achy legs with pins and needles in right leg. Muscle spasm in right leg muscles with twitching and jerking. Numbness in right calf.

Limbs - Sciatica. Trembling of limbs, worse sitting. Coldness and itching of the extremities. Burning pain in the legs.

Lungs - Tightness of lungs in waves. Cough, worse deep breathing. Tickly cough, high pitched with a sensation of hollowness in right lung. Slightly throaty, croupy cough when chest feels tight. Expectoration thick, stringy and green.

Mouth - Tingling of the lips. Lips, redness and swelling, peeling and dry. Ulcerated lips with yellow crusts and scabs, burning, cracking, sensitive to hot food and bleeding. Worse from eating, talking. Lips sensations, tingling, pins and needles. Crack in top lip. Vesicles on the lips and aphthae in the mouth, on the tongue. Sore lumps on roof of mouth with numbness. Gum ulceration, gums as though hardened after a burn. Gums sore, not bleeding.

Neck - Neck feels knotted. Stiffness. Achy and sore, neck aches in waves.

Nose - Sneezing. Clear, watery discharge from right nostril. Clear catarrh. Copious discharge. Right nostril runny, with clear discharge, while left nostril is blocked. Discharge that drips down the back of the throat. Thick and green discharge. Lots of green, yellow, sticky mucus, worse at 3 p.m. Nosebleed on washing face. Pain on bridge of nose, left nostril sore inside, as if scratched. Sensitive smell, worse perfume, people, body odor, car fumes and dogs.

Perspiration - Night sweats.

Rectum - Sharp shooting pains, worse sitting, as if sword up inside. Sudden urging for stool. Constipated, better from standing to pass stool. Constipation alternating with diarrhea. ***Soft and watery stools,*** alternating with hard and dry stools. Diarrhea is gushing, watery, urgent, loud and explosive with abdominal pain. Bowel movements increased to three a day. Burning and sensation of heat during and after stools.

Shoulder - Lancinating pain in right shoulder. Pain at base of left shoulder blade, worse breathing deeply. Right shoulder blade aches.

Skin - Dry skin. Itching with and without eruptions. Painful warts. Wounds slow to heal.

Sleep - Disturbed and difficult to get to sleep. Deep sleep. Offensive perspiration during sleep. Vivid dreams, ***nightmares***, frightful and anxious dreams. Dreams of falling, of being pursued, of being raped, of dead people. Waking after midnight. Restlessness, worse on waking.

Speech - Voice croaky, hoarse. Loss of speech.

Stomach - Nervous trapped energy in stomach. Stomach cramps, worse eating, at night. Cramping pain. Pain top of stomach, connected to back. Burning stomach pain extending upward into the esophagus. Gas and acidity in stomach, worse wine. Heartburn associated with nausea. Belching. Deep, long, loud belching. A lot of wind. Hiccoughs on and off throughout day. Nausea on eating. Nausea, pill tasted bitter. Nausea with sudden vomiting around midnight.

Stool - Large painful, dry stool. Loose and windy. Loose, fast stool, smelling of onions or garlic, 8 a.m. and 9 a.m.

Taste - Mouth dry, with a bad taste, and breath smells. Dry, metallic taste on front of tongue. Foul taste. As if soaking up chemicals, smells and pollution. As if been licking metal.

Teeth - Teeth sensitive. Feel loose, difficult to bite. Bottom right side molar section loose, fell out. Toothaches. Gums receding.

Throat - Hoarseness. Throat dry and tickly. ***Sore throat,*** dryness and rawness, worse on swallowing. Sore throat with numbness, particularly on left side, worse morning, 3 p.m. Sore throat, on waking, better hot and cold drinks. Sore, swollen and hot, better cold food. Sensitive to pressure. Stinging throat pain extending down to the esophagus. Stinging from smoking. Pressing, choking sensation in throat, worse right side with a need to clear it. ***Need to clear mucus from the throat.*** Mucus in back of throat. Loose phlegm at back of throat, coughs to clear it, worse 10 p.m.

Tongue - Tongue is slightly red, but not sore, with ulcer under the right side. Tongue yellow and furry, big and rough sensation.

Vertigo - Light headed. Vertigo on motion of head, worse sitting, worse on closing eyes and lying down. Vertigo with fear of brain tumor.

Vision - Blurred vision. Lack of focus, has to keep blinking. Fuzzy, as if drunk. Heightened vision, more sensitive.

RELATIONS - ***Compare:*** Carc., Lyc., Puls., Sep.

REFERENCES - Biggs. Gwillim.

PLANTAGO MAJOR

(Plantain)

PHARMACY - plan. Plantago major. Plantain. Ribwort. N. O. Plantaginaceae. Plan. must not to be confounded with Musa, sometimes called "Plantain," which belongs to a different class. Tincture of whole fresh plant. Tincture of the root. ***Historical dose:*** Tincture and all potencies.

CLINICAL - Ague. ***Bedwetting.*** Bites. Breast inflammation. Burns. Ciliary neuralgia. Chilblains. Depression. Diabetes. Diarrhea. Dysentery. Earache. Ears inflammation. Emissions. Erysipelas. Erythema. Frostbite. ***Gumboils. Hemorrhoids.*** Herpes. ***Injuries.*** Impotency. Insomnia. Mastitis. Neuralgias. Otorrhea. Polyuria. ***Pyorrhea.*** Rhus poisoning. ***Snakebites.*** Spleen, pain. ***Tetanus.*** Tobacco, habit. ***Toothaches.*** Urination, delayed. Urticaria. Vaccinations. Worms. ***Wounds.***

HERBAL - Plantago has a reputation in herbal medicine from remote antiquity, including for use in intermittent fevers. In 1558 the Herbal of Dodoens commended the juice of leaves or roots for ***"toothache and bleeding of gums."*** External use in toothache in hollow teeth, otorrhea, itching and poison oak. Incised wounds.

John Parkinson, in his Theater of Plants (1640), said that "the root taken fresh out of the ground, washed and gently scraped with a knife, then put into the ear, cures the toothache like a charm."

Reutlinger noted that in Switzerland the leaf tissues were frayed out and put into the ear for the same purpose. If they relieve the pain they "turn black" and have to be removed, if there is no relief the leaves remain green.

Hale summed up the ancient and modern history of Plantago Maj., the weed that furnishes food for cage-birds. In herbal practice, it is constantly resorted to as an application in all disorders of the skin with irritation, pain and heat, the bruised leaves being applied to the part.

HOMEOPATHIC - Hale noted that erysipelas, rhus poisoning, erythema, burns, inflammation of the glands, bruises, incised wounds, animal bites, chilblains, and frostbite had all been relieved by its use.

Plan. has a considerable clinical reputation in the treatment of earache, ***toothache and bedwetting***. Pyorrhea alveolaris. Gums bleed easily. Sharp pain in the eyes, reflex from decayed teeth or inflammation of middle ear. Eyeball is very tender to touch.

Affects the nerves, causing neuralgia of ears, teeth, face, of shingles. Pains are sharp, shifting, play between ear and teeth. Can be applied locally for neuralgia. Inflammation of the breasts. Soreness. Sensation as of a foreign body between ears in the groins, etc. Inflamed and painful hemorrhoids.

MIND - Great mental prostration, worse by mental exertion, which causes rapid breathing and anxiety. Mind inactive with dullness. Confusion of thought. Irritable, morose, impatient. Restless mood with dull, stupid feeling in brain. Despondency. Depression and insomnia of chronic nicotinism. Disgust for tobacco in chewers and smokers.

Abdomen - Gone sensation. Severe pains in the hypochondrium. Violent griping in upper abdomen. Bowels seem cold. Distention with passage of fetid flatus. Colic, flatulent, better by eating.

Back - Cold sweat on sacrum. Pain in sacrum. Throbbing, pulsative pain between scapulae. Neck stiff and sore. Stiffness of sternocleidomastoid mastoid.

Breasts - Inflammation the breasts. Erysipelas of breasts. Mastitis. Neuralgia of nipples.

Causations - Ill effects of bites, bruises, burns, cuts, punctured wounds, snakebites, stings.

Chest - Oppression, worse reading or talking. Sharp stitches. Orgasms of blood. Muscular drawing.

Ears - Sticking pain in ears. Otalgia with toothache. Neuralgic earache, ***pain goes from one ear to the other***. Pain in right ear with pains in teeth and face. Pains sharp, twinging. As of a foreign body between ears. Hearing acute, noise painful. Loud noises go through body. Ringing in ears.

Eyes - Sharp pains in the eyes, reflex from decayed teeth. Dull, heavy ache in left eye. Eyes red, dim, inflamed, sore. Aching deep in orbit. Lids sore, swollen. As of a hair before eye.

Face - Neuralgia of left side of face, pains shooting and tearing, extending from jaw to ear. Violent bruised, aching pain, right face. Pain radiating to temples and lower jaw. Drawing in right malar bone. Lips livid, dark, sickly, rough. Dry, scaly eruption on lower lip. Eruption on forehead.

Food - Appetite poor. Thirst. Causes disgust for tobacco in chewers.

Head - Dull headache. Headache with toothache. Sense of something lying in the head, through one ear to the other. As if brain turned over. Itching of scalp.

Heart - Heat in precordia when walking in open air. Violent palpitations on ascending stairs. Pulse strong, full, intermittent.

Kidneys - Tenderness over region of kidneys on pressure. Irritable bladder with frequent urination. Urethra tingling with unpleasant itching in meatus. Delayed, dribbling urine. Frequent passage of large quantity of pale urine, worse night, with thirst. Diabetes. Profuse flow of urine. ***Nocturnal bedwetting*** from laxity of sphincter (Rhus-a., Caust., Bell.).

Limbs - Disposition to stretch. Stinging, dull pains here and there. Numbness and trembling legs. Great pain and stiffness in left leg and knee, worse stooping. Hard, white, flattened, papules on inside of thighs.

Lungs - Hoarseness. Cough in cold air. Panting breathing, inclined to sigh.

Male - Sexual debility. Unconscious emission in sleep.

Modalities - Better from sleep. Colic is better by eating. Worse at night, heat of room, heat and cold, cold air, sharp wind. Worse contact, motion, mental exertion.

Mouth - Profuse flow of saliva. Saliva flows with pains. Dirty taste. Breath putrid. Tongue coated white, with dirty, putrid, clammy taste. Food tasteless. ***Gumboils***. Gums bleed easily. Aphthae in children. Swelling of cheeks.

Nose - Red papules around nose. Sensation

at bridge as if nasal bones being pressed together. Frequent sneezing, with sudden attacks of profuse, watery, bland coryza. Sudden discharge of yellow colored water from the nose.

Rectum - Wants to defecate, goes often, but cannot. Chronic diarrhea. Stools are brown, frothy, watery, fermented, papescent, excoriating. Cholera infantum. Dysentery. Worms. Painful hemorrhoids, bloody, can hardly stand (used locally).

Skin - Sensitive skin. Burns. Violent itching, worse night. Burning, pricking, stinging pains. Burning after rubbing where scratched. Redness, swelling, and vesicles on hands and face. Papules which exude yellowish humor and form a crust. Erythema. Urticaria, chilblains (Agar., Tam.). ***Rhus poisoning*** (external use).

Sleep - Excessive and continued yawning. Insomnia from abdominal trouble. Grinding teeth during sleep. Sleep restless, disturbed by dreams. Gloomy dreams exciting tears.

Stomach - Belchings, frequent, empty, tasting like sulphur, of carbonic acid gas. Nausea with drowsiness or faint, tremulous feeling. Sinking sensation. Heaviness of stomach as from a stone, even after a light meal.

Teeth - Teeth feel too long. Teeth are sensitive and sore to touch. Rapid tooth decay. ***Toothache in decayed teeth*** or shooting up left side of face. Toothache, better while eating. Toothache with reflex neuralgia of eyelids. Sharp stabbing pains. Grinds teeth at night.

Temperature - Chilliness with erratic pains. Chilliness on moving about, cold hands in a warm room. Chill without thirst, with goose bumps. Coldness of body with shivering. Heat with thirst, and great excitability, mental agony, restlessness. Sweat is cold over lumbar and the sacral region, heat of room unbearable, producing perspiration.

Throat - Dry, parched throat. Scraping in throat. Profuse secretion of thick sticky, mucus with much hawking. Soreness and swelling of submaxillary glands on both sides.

COMMENTS - The tincture has been extensively proved by F. Humphreys (who wrote a monograph upon it), Heath and others. Neuralgic pains of teeth, ears and face were especially pronounced. Shingles, neuralgia.

Great surface sensitiveness. Tearing, boring, bruised pains. Pains come suddenly and are apt to be erratic. Unendurable pains. The left side is most affected. Snake bites, bee stings, animal bites. Burns. Frostbite. Loud noises go through body. Sudden discharge of yellowish or saffron-colored water from the nose.

Toothaches, especially in cavities (Hyp. tincture, Hecla.). "Toothache with earache," particularly if with salivation. Toothache with boring and digging pains. A deep aching in hollow or rotten teeth. Neuralgic pains shooting up the face, from the tooth area. Gumboils. Grinds teeth at night (Cina., Tub.).

Produces disgust for tobacco in chewers and cures neuralgia resulting from tobacco. Foul breath. Sinking and weight in stomach. Offensive flatulence. Darting up and down the urethra. Bedwetting in children. Lax sphincters. Very copious urine, with thirst. Diabetes. Diarrhea, dysentery. Worms. Painful hemorrhoids.

Clarke used it with success in numberless cases of toothache and earache. It has given relief in the painful neuralgia of shingles and in pleurodynia.

F. P. Stiles related three cases of its use. Mrs. S., 39, had terrible neuralgic pain in the right side of her face, shooting into temporal, superior, maxillary and orbital regions for 10 days. Plan. was applied locally to the gums, temple and cheek removed the pain in a few minutes. Some days later a slight return was promptly relieved in the same way.

Mr. R. had neuralgia in left superior maxillary and lower orbital region of long standing. Promptly relieved in the same way.

Mrs. N. had neuralgia of the right upper jaw, unbearable pain, radiating to ear, temple and cheek. A tooth had been extracted without relief. Plan. removed all the pain.

There is a case of one man who allowed himself to be bitten by a rattlesnake. He cured himself by frequently drinking the juice.

RELATIONS - ***Antidote to:*** Apis, Rhus-t., Tab. ***Antidoted by:*** Merc. (toothache). ***Compare:*** (1) Punctured wounds, Led., Hyper. (2) Wounds and bruises, fetid breath and flatus, Arn. (3) Earache with toothache intolerance of warm room, Puls. (4) In neuralgias, Cham., Merc., Spig., Kalm., Coloc. (5) Wounds, Calen. (6) Kalm., Cham., Puls. (7) Hemorrhoids, external and internal, Ham. (8) Equis., Bell., Caust. - bedwetting. (9) Unendurable pains, Acon., Cham., Hep.

REFERENCES - Boericke. Clarke. Murphy. Phatak.

PLATANUS OCCIDENTALIS

(Sycamore Buttonwood)

PHARMACY - platan. Platanus occidentalis. Sycamore buttonwood. Platanus acerifolia. Platanus vulgaris. London plane tree. N. O. Platanaceae of the Urtica alliance. Tincture of young shoots. ***Historical dose:*** Tincture and all potencies.

CLINICAL - Cataract. Ichthyosis. ***Tarsal tumors.***

HERBAL - Burnett named the remedy Plat. occidentalis, but his tincture was made from Platanus acerifolia. It sheds its bark annually, which was the signature of its skin action.

HOMEOPATHIC - The tincture, applied topically, has been used for ***tarsal tumors***, both acute and old, neglected cases. It restored to practically normal conditions areas where destruction of tissue occurred and scar tissue caused marked deformity. Ichthyosis. Must be used for some time; acts best in children.

COMMENTS - Burnett recorded a case of ichthyosis in an elderly woman in which Platan. caused considerable improvement in the condition of the skin.

Another case of Burnett's was that of a girl, 5 1/2, "of the coal-black variety of the strumous, her forehead low and projecting," who was blind from double cataract due to the shock of a fall in the first instance, the lenses having gradually silted up.

In this case Platan. was given, five drops night and morning, for a number of months, "with very evident improvement in the nutrition of the child's lenses."

REFERENCES - Boericke. Burnett. Clarke.

PLATINUM METALLICUM

(Platina Metal)

PHARMACY - plat. Platinum metallicum. Platina metal. The element (Pt. At. Wt. 195.08) Trituration. ***Historical dose:*** All potencies.

CLINICAL - Amenorrhea. Chlorosis. ***Colic. Constipation.*** Convulsions. Delusions. Dentition. Depression. Dysmenorrhea. Fears. Gout. Hemorrhage. Hemorrhoids. Hysteria. Insanity. Lead, poisoning. ***Masturbation.*** Melancholia. Menorrhagia. Menses, suppressed. ***Multiple personalities.*** Neuralgias. Neurasthenia. ***Numbness. Nymphomania.*** Ovarian, disorders. ***Painter's colic.*** Pruritus, vulvae. Rape. Rheumatism. ***Sexual, abuse. Sexual, mania.*** Spasms. Tapeworms. Uterus, disorders. ***Vaginismus.*** Vaginitis. Vertigo. Yawning, spasmodic.

HOMEOPATHIC - The original name of platinum was "Platina," a Spanish word meaning "like silver." The metal was introduced into Europe from South America in the middle of the eighteenth century. It is always found in association with other metals, chiefly rhodium, osmium, iridium, and palladium.

Hahnemann was the first to think of it as a medicine and his proving in the Chronic Diseases is the basis of the knowledge of its action.

Strong tendency to paralysis, anesthesia, localized ***numbness and coldness*** are shown. Hysterical spasms, pains increase and decrease gradually (Stann.). Tremulousness. ***Alternation of mental and physical symptoms***, as physical symptoms disappear mental symptoms appear and vice versa. Oversensitive mind, emotions and nerves.

Plat. is pre-eminently a woman's remedy. Many and various symptoms reflex from ovaries and uterus or sexual organs. Sticky discharges, tears, stools, menses, etc. Catalepsy during menses.

Hemorrhages with black clots with fluid. Irregular spasms, congestion of blood.

Violent cramping, squeezing, thrusting or numbing pains, then spasms. Hysterical spasms. Spasms alternate with dyspnea. Tonic and clonic spasms with laughter. Violent shocks, as from pain. Contortions of limbs. Epilepsy, catalepsy.

Painful tremors. Pains increase and decrease gradually. Bandaged feeling. Sensation of pricking. Localized, coldness of single parts, eyes, ears etc. or numbness of scalp, face, coccyx, calves etc.

MIND - ***Alternate mental and physical symptoms.*** Physical symptoms disappear as mental symptoms develop. Mental troubles better at twilight. Mental troubles with suppressed menses.

Changing moods. Cheerfulness alternating with depression. Weeps and laughs alternately. Whistles, sings, dances. Laughs at wrong time. Irritability alternating with tenderness. Irritable about trifling things.

Morose and discontented mood, worse being spoken to. ***Sadness better open air.*** Sits in a corner, broods and says nothing. Bad humor, yet weeps. Inconsolable weeping, worse when spoken to. Weeps with pains.

Unkind, abrupt and quarrelsome. ***Contempt for others***. Faultfinding. Proud and erotic. Self-exaltation. Feels tall and stately. Haughty, looks with disdain upon everyone and everything. ***Arrogant***. ***Wounded pride.***

Absent-minded and forgetful. Any serious thought is terrifying. Weary of everything. Alone, deserted feeling. Indifference while in company. Past events trouble her. Everything seems changed or different. ***Feels she does not belong to her own family***. Thinks she has no place in the world. Forsaken, deserted feeling. Feels everything seems changed. Disordered sense of proportion, ***objects seem smaller,*** strange, frightful.

Anxiety when speaking in company. Sensation of dread and horrors. Fears of death. Fear of imaginary forms, ghosts. Thinks her husband will never return, something will happen to him. Screams for help.

Impulse to kill her own child, her husband. Aversion to children.

Delusion of superiority. Delusions she is alone in the world. Delusions she is not appreciated. Delusions she is disgraced. Delusions everyone is an enemy. ***Delusion that all persons are devils.***

Mental symptoms alternating with sexual symptoms. Sexual excitement brings on mental symptoms. Religious affections alternating with sexual excitement. Inclination to embrace everybody. Perverted sexual desire. Unchaste talk. Hysteria before menses. ***Nymphomania,*** worse during menses. Sexual mania.

Abdomen - Pressing and bearing down in abdomen, extending into pelvis. Constriction. Pinchings in umbilical region. Pain in umbilical region extending through into the back, turns and twists in all possible positions. Fermentation, much flatulence. Flatulent soreness towards hypogastrium. ***Colic from lead poisoning.***

Back - Pains in back and small of back as if broken, after a walk. Bruised backache, worse pressure, worse on bending backwards. Contusive pain in loins and in back. Sensation of numbness in coccyx, as after a blow. Weakness and sensation of tensive numbness in nape of neck. Rigidity of nape of neck.

Causations - Ill effects of fright, vexation, bereavement, fit of passion. Ill effects of sexual excess, prolonged hemorrhages and masturbation.

Chest - Sensation of weakness. Anxious oppression of chest with sensation of heat, which ascends from epigastrium. Pain in chest, as if a weight were pressing upon it with desire to take a full inspiration. Tension, pressure and shootings in sides of chest, which do not permit lying down on either side. Aching and dull blows in the chest. Increasing to a certain intensity and gradually diminishing in same way. Dull lancinations in sides of chest during an inspiration.

Constitutions - Suited to women with dark hair, thin, sanguine, bilious with too frequent and too profuse menses, sexual organs exceedingly sensitive. Hysterical and hemorrhoidal patients.

Ears - Cramp-like twinges. Shocks in ears. Sensation of numbness and of coldness in ears, extending to cheeks and lips. Gnawing tingling in ears. Roaring, whizzing and ringing in ears. Dull thundering, rumbling in ears.

Eyes - Eyes feel cold. Cramp-like pain in orbits. Aching in eyes with sleep. Pain in eyes after fatiguing the sight by looking attentively at an object. ***Objects look smaller than they are***. Quivering and sparkling before sight. Confused sight, as if directed through a veil, often with painless twitchings around the eye. Twitching of the eyelids (Agar.).

Face - Distortion of muscles of face. Grimaces. ***Coldness, creeping and numbness*** in whole right side of face. Facial pain with numb feeling in malar bones, as if the parts were between screws. Pain at root of nose, as if squeezed in a vise. Pains increase and decrease gradually (Stann.). Boring, cramps in the jaws. Lockjaw. Smarting and sharp vesicles on lips. ***Numbness of lips,*** dry and cracked.

Female - ***Painfully sensitive genitals*** with itching, tickling or crawling. Tingling internally and externally (Kali-br.). Pruritus vulvae with voluptuous angling. ***Excessive sexual desire*** that leads to masturbation. ***Nymphomania,*** worse in puerperal state. Sexual mania. Frequent sensation as if menses would appear. Menses with chilliness, sensitive genitals. Menses too early, too profuse. ***Menses dark, clotted,*** with spasms and painful bearing-down. Dysmenorrhea with shrieks and jerks. Amenorrhea in emigrants. Leucorrhea like white of an egg. ***Vaginismus from excessive sensitiveness of sexual organs, sex is impossible*** (Staph.). Prolapse of uterus. Induration, uterine cancer. Fibroids. Ovaries sensitive and burn. Infertility from ovaritis or excessive sexual excitement.

Food - ***Ravenous hunger,*** persistent nausea with anxiety and weakness. Hasty eating, eats everything around her or detests it. Loss of appetite after first mouthful. Repugnance to food from sadness. Worse from fasting.

Head - Constriction about forehead and right temples. ***Cramp-like, squeezing pain***. Tensive confusion in forehead, as if head were compressed in a vice. Tense, pressing pain, confined to a small spot. Pain in sides of head, as if caused by a plug. Tense scalp. Constrictive headache, as if a tape were tightly drawn around it with sensation of numbness in brain. ***Numbness with headache.*** Attack of headache with nausea and vomiting. Headache with leucorrhea. Headache commences on waking. As of water in forehead.

Heart - Burning and sticking low down by heart. A dull pressure in region of apex of heart. Anxious palpitation of heart.

Kidneys - Slow but frequent emission of urine. Red urine with a white cloud, or turbid and deposits a red sediment.

Limbs - Limbs feel weary, numb, paralyzed. Tingling restlessness, sensation of weakness and trembling in limbs. Paralytic weakness. Attack of spasmodic rigidity in limbs. Cramp-like jerking and drawing pains in limbs and joints. Cramp in calves. Tightness of thighs, as if too tightly wrapped. Distorted fingers. Numbness of little finger or fingers.

Lungs - Inclination to draw a long breath, prevented by a sensation of weakness in chest. Shortness of breath with a constrictive oppression of chest. Short, difficult and anxious respiration. Short, nervous, dry cough with palpitations and dyspnea. Walking against wind causes sudden arrest of breathing.

Male - Ill effects of masturbation before puberty. Perverted sexual desires. Unnatural ***increase of sexual desire*** with frequent erections, especially at night (with amorous dream). Sex, short duration with little enjoyment. Flow of prostatic fluid. Burning pain and gnawing in scrotum. ***Voluptuous tickling, itching with excessive sexual desire.*** Voluptuous crawling in genital organs and abdomen with anxious oppression and palpitations, then painless pressure downwards in genitals with sticking in sinciput and exhaustion.

Modalities - Better from walking in open air, sunshine, stretching and motion. Obliged to stretch, which ameliorates. ***Worse from emotions***, chagrin, nerve exhaustion. Worse sex, during menses. Worse touch, pressure, sitting, standing and bending backwards. Worse evening and night, in a warm room.

Mouth - Mouth feels cold. Sensation as if palate or uvula were elongated. As if tongue were scalded. Sweet taste on tip of the tongue. Numb pain in left lower teeth. Cramp-like drawing in teeth. Toothache with pulsative and digging pain. Fissures in gums.

Nose - Cramp-like pain with sensation of numbness in nose and at root of nose. Ineffectual want to sneeze and tingling in nose. Dry coryza often semi-lateral. Corrosive sensation on nose, as of something acrid.

Rectum - Constipation after lead poisoning, sometimes very obstinate. Constipation of pregnancy. ***Constipation of travelers,*** who are constantly changing food and water. Frequent want of stool, retarded, feces scanty, evacuated with difficulty in pieces. Stool seems to stick to anus and rectum like putty. Crawling, itching anus in evening. Voluptuous crawling in rectum. Violent and dull lancinations in rectum.

Sensations - As if her senses would vanish. As if everything about her were very small. As if she were constantly growing longer and longer. As if she did not belong to her own family. As if head were enlarged. As if parts of malar bones were between screws. As if throat constricted, palate elongated tongue scalded. As if abdomen, chest, nape, limbs, thing, great toe, tightly wrapped or constricted. Back and small of back as if broken. Crawling, tingling, numb sensations.

Skin - Tingling, gnawing with pain as of excoriation and itching or burning, pricking and shooting pain on various parts of skin, which provokes scratching. Ulcers, on fingers and toes.

Sleep - Convulsive and spasmodic yawning, especially in afternoon. Great disposition to sleep in evening. Sleeps with legs far apart. Sleeps on back with knees drawn up and spread apart, wants to uncover entirely. Waking at night with frightful dreams, want of consciousness or with anxious, sad and distressing thoughts. Anxious dreams of wars and bloodshed. Lascivious dreams. Prolonged sleep in morning.

Stool - Stool as if burnt. Stools hard, black passed in small portions with great straining, Stools adhere to rectum like soft clay. ***Sticky stool***. Tinea and ascarides are discharged from rectum. Worms.

Stomach - Aching, pressure in stomach, especially after a meal. ***Sensation of constriction*** in pit of stomach, extending into abdomen. Fermentations in epigastric region. Ineffectual effort to belch. Empty, noisy belchings. Continued nausea with lassitude, trembling and anxiety.

Temperature - Pulse small, feeble, frequently tremulous. Constant shivering and shuddering over whole body, especially in open air. Chilliness predominates with low spirits, which ceases during heat. Heat with sensation of burning in face without any visible change in color of face. Flushes of heat interrupted by chilliness. Gradually increasing and decreasing heat. Perspiration only during sleep, ceasing as soon as one wakens.

Throat - Cramp-like drawing in throat like a constriction. Scraping and accumulation of phlegm in throat. Hawking up of phlegm. Aphonia.

Vertigo - Transient attacks of vertigo in evening with loss of consciousness. Vertigo on sitting down or ascending stairs. Vertigo as if torn and pulled with threads.

COMMENTS - Plat. has a lost sense of proportion in both ocular and mental vision. Objects look small or the patient thinks they are small. Distortions of distance and size (Cann.).

Pride and hauteur, the patient (generally a woman) looks down on everything and everybody. Delusion of grandeur.

Megalomania (Cann., Hyos.), but seen as arrogance, not insanity. Arrogant, proud, particularly after grief, fright, rape or sexual abuse. Deep hatred for men.

Alternating between one mental state and another. Changing moods, sad and gay, laughs and cries by turns. Laughs immoderately, but in the wrong place, laughs at serious things. Homicidal. Manic depression. Multiple personality disorders (Anac.). Identity crisis, they forget who they are.

Jahr cured with Plat. a woman who had an inspiration to kill her child.

Jule Gaudy recorded the case of a woman who was tormented with an almost irresistible impulse to kill her husband, whom she loved passionately and with whom she was perfectly happy. The sight of a knife had an irresistible fascination for her and she was often obliged to leave the table to free herself from the impulse.

A few months before, she had lost a child a short time after confinement, which had been followed by profuse and persistent hemorrhage. Recovering from this she became restless, irritable and her whole existence was ruled by this terrible impulse. Plat. 6x and 30x relieved and finally cured her.

Kent recorded the case of a middle-aged woman, the mother of several grown-up daughters, who complained of a fear in the absence of her husband, that he would never return, that he would die or be run over. She wept all the time he was away.

Kent discovered that she had been treated for uterine displacement and was then wearing a pessary. This was removed. Menstrual flow was copious, black, clotted. The external genitals were so sensitive that the usual napkin was intolerable. Plat. cured the whole case including the displacement.

Nash cured a case of insanity of some duration with Plat., being led to the remedy by an alternation of the mental symptoms with a pain the whole length of the spine.

Keynote occurrence of cramps, cramping pains and spasms, developing into convulsions. Cramping pains causes numbness and tingling in the parts affected. Pains as if nipped, squeezed in a vice and these pains increase gradually to a climax and then, as gradually, decline.

Cramping tendency, antidotal to lead poisoning. Tenesmus. Constipation, stools are tenacious and sticky, adhere to the rectum and anus like putty or they may be hard as if burnt. Constipation comes on while traveling, in emigrants, during pregnancy.

Spasms alternate between convulsions and opisthotonos, full consciousness. Spasms alternate with dyspnea. Spasmodic yawning. Pains go from right to left. The right side is somewhat more affected than the left. The symptoms are periodic and paroxysmal, as well as alternating.

Severe, painful menstrual cramps. Catalepsy during menstruation. With the menses, uterine spasms, convulsions. Convulsions of puerperal state. Excessive itching in uterus, pruritus vulvae. Vaginismus. Severe stitches in right ovary. Ovarian tumors.

Generally centers in and radiates from the sexual organs, male and female. The sensitiveness of the external genitals is often so great as to make sex impossible (Staph., Cact.). Digital examining of such a patient causes great pain. Prostate problems (Pall.).

Masturbation before puberty and also to the effects of masturbation. Premature and excessive development of sexual instinct and organs, before puberty. Severe vaginal irritation that leads to vaginal discharge and masturbation in young girls (Med.).

Excessive desire, especially in virgins. Nymphomania, worse in puerperal state. Characteristic tendency to uncover completely in sleep. It was one of Gallavardin's remedies for the impulse to pederasty and sodomy.

RELATIONS - ***Antidote:*** Puls. Plat. antidotes the bad effects of lead. ***Antidoted by:*** Puls., Teste, who classes Plat. with Thuj., Brom. and Cast., says Colch. is the best antidote to all four. ***Compare:*** (1) Rhodi., Stann., Valer., Sep. (2) Plat-m. (3) Sed-ac - sexual irritability, relieves irritation of nerve centers and gives rest. (4) Self-pride, Pall., Plat. egotistical, despises others, Pall. easily wounded, attaches importance to others, Lyc. - imperious. (5) Spasms, emaciation from pre-puberty masturbation, Staph. (6) Uterine affections, nymphomania, Aur., Sep. (the nymphomania of Plat. is more intense. Plat. is intermediate between Aur. and Sep. in weariness of life, the uterine cramps of Plat. are followed by numbness, those of Sep. are a clutching as if suddenly seized then suddenly relaxed. (7) Hysteria indurated ulcers, Tarent. (8) Sees ghosts spirits and demons, Hyos., Kali-br. (9) Shamelessness, uncovers, Phos., Hyos. - sees things larger, Plat. smaller. (10) Thinks death near and fears it, Acon., Ars. (11) Dark, stringy hemorrhage, Cham., Croc. has sensation of something alive. ***Complementary:*** Plat. and Pall. both affect right ovary, but Pall. has better from pressure. ***Compatible:*** Bell., Ign., Lyc., Puls., Rhus-t., Sep., Verat.

REFERENCES - Boericke. Clarke. Murphy. Phatak.

PLATINUM MURIATICUM

(Platina Chloride)

PHARMACY - plat-m. Platinum muriaticum. Platina chloride. ***Historical dose:*** All potencies.

CLINICAL - Acne. Bone, disorders. Cancer. Caries. Condylomàta. Gonorrhea. Fever. Headaches. Laryngismus. Syphilis.

HOMEOPATHIC - Plat-m. was experimented with by Hofer of Pau, who applied a saturated solution locally and administered solutions internally.

There is only a fragmentary proving, the mental symptom ***"thinks she has been poisoned"*** might be helpful as a guide in certain cases. The local application produced acute irritation of the skin and glans penis with an eruption on the latter like commencing chancre.

Decay and caries of the nasal and tarsus bones. Syphilitic caries and syphilitic rheumatism. Laryngismus. Stricture of esophagus and cancer of the stomach. Canker, condylomata. Acne. Mercury abuse. Chronic gonorrhea.

Involuntary movement of tissues of muscles of nape, back and limbs for several hours. Fever, headaches, constricting sensations and fibrillary twitchings were induced by internal doses.

Plat-m. has achieved beneficial results after Kali-i. failed to cure in syphilitic affection, violent occipital headaches, dysphagia and syphilitic throat and bone affections, decay of bones of feet.

MIND - ***Thinks she has been poisoned*** (Ars., Lach.).

Head - Some headache with slight acidity of stomach. Severe headache, especially in occiput with fever.

Kidneys - Acute inflammation of urethra, pain on urinating, slight dysuria.

Male - Violent itching on glans and prepuce with sensation of warmth. Eruption about glans penis, somewhat livid, raised, size of pin head, looks like commencing syphilitic sore, but disappears in twelve hours.

Mouth - Metallic taste.

Skin - Discolored yellow. Skin becoming covered with rosy red eruption that disappears after a few minutes from local application.

Stomach - Acidity of stomach with headache. Warmth and heaviness in epigastrium. Nausea and vomiting.

Temperature - Slight shuddering, pulse accelerated, warmth in epigastrium.

Throat - Violent constriction of larynx, so that speech and swallowing were impeded.

REFERENCES - Boericke. Clarke.

PLATINUM MUR. NATRONATUM

(Sodium Chloroplatinate)

PHARMACY - plat-m-n. Platinum muriaticum natronatum. Sodium chloroplatinate. Solution. ***Historical dose:*** All potencies.

CLINICAL - Eructation. Flatus. Nausea. Polyuria. Salivation. Vomiting.

HOMEOPATHIC - Hofer experimented with Plat-m-n. on the same man who took Plat-mur. The chief additional symptom was decided increased secretion of urine and saliva.

Slight headache. Feeling of warmth and heaviness in stomach. Rumbling in abdomen. Transient colic. Emission of flatus. Eructation of gas. Nausea and inclination to vomit.

REFERENCES - Clarke.

PLECTRANTHUS FRUTICOSUS

PHARMACY - plect. Plectranthus fruticosus. N. O. Labiatae. Tincture of fresh plant. ***Historical dose:*** Tincture and all potencies.

CLINICAL - Abdomen, coldness. Cholera. Cramps. Dentition. Diarrhea. Dysphagia. Fever. Intermittent, fever. Lumbrici. Neuralgia. Rheumatism. Shoulder, pains. Spastic, paralysis. Stiff neck. Sweat, local. Throat, sore. Toothache. Wrists, pains.

HOMEOPATHIC - Plect. was proved by the Austrian Provers' Association. Severe symptoms were induced in the head, throat, intestines and rectum, limbs and joints. Hansen mentioned spastic paralysis as having been remedied by it.

Toothaches with swelling of face and difficulty of opening mouth. "Pain near right jaw joint as if a tooth were coming through" suggests a use for the remedy in difficult cutting of wisdom teeth.

Burning sensation throughout the digestive tract. Coldness of abdomen, better in open air. Pressure on rectum and bladder. Discharge of white mucus from anus, causing scratching. Whites of eyes yellow, worse left. Sweat of right foot, left foot dry of right foot and both hands and no other part of scalp.

Pains and other symptoms come and go suddenly. Exhaustion, bruised sensation, general discomfort. Cramps and paralytic pains in joints. Pains of many kinds in right shoulder. Pains about the navel. Affects the right side more than the left.

Modalities - Better by application of ice, belchings. Burning in mouth worse from all food and drink. Chewing causes pain in temples. Worse by motion, moving head, turning body, swallowing. Worse while urinating, better after urinating. Worse by warmth of stove. Pressure in stomach, pain in umbilical region, worse after eating.

Sensations - Cool sensation followed by burning at root of tongue and palate. As if a morsel stuck in the throat after swallowing. Pressure as from a heavy weight in stomach. As through air were piercing the marrow of the bones.

RELATIONS - ***Compare:*** (1) Urinary symptoms, Oci. (2) Black stools, Lept. (3) Stitches in chest, Kali-c. (4) Pains come and go suddenly, Lyc., Bell. (5) Crumb in throat, Hep., Nit-ac., Arg-n.

REFERENCES - Clarke.

PLUMBAGO LITTORALIS

PHARMACY - plumbg. Plumbago littoralis. Plumbago scandens. Bay of Rio Janeiro. N. O. Plumbaginaceae. Tincture of leaves. ***Historical dose:*** Tincture and all potencies.

CLINICAL - ***Blisters.*** Eyes, inflammation. Fever. Kidneys, pain. Saliva, milky. ***Ulcerations.*** Vertigo.

HERBAL - Mure says Plumbg. is a creeper inhabiting the shores in the bay of Rio de Janeiro. Many of the plants of this genus are acrid and caustic in the highest degree.

The Treasury of Botany noted that the root of Plumbago scandens, the Herbe du Diable of San Domingo, is a blistering agent when fresh, so also is that of Plumbago rosea. The beggars employ Plumbago europea to raise ulcers on their body to excite pity, and used internally it is said to be as good an emetic as ipecac.

HOMEOPATHIC - Mure proved Plumbg. The most peculiar symptoms were profuse, milky saliva. ***Ulceration of commissures of lips***, which is an evidence of its acridity. Costiveness with red urine. Pain in humerus on lifting anything. Hot arms with cold hands. Vertigo after eating. ***Aversion to everything***.

RELATIONS - ***Compare:*** (1) Costiveness with red urine, Lyc. (2) The Plumbaginaneae are allied to the Primulaceae. (3) Plantaginaceae - the root of Plumbg-eu. is used dried as a remedy for toothache.

REFERENCES - Clarke.

PLUMBUM ACETICUM

(Lead Acetate)

PHARMACY - plb-acet. Plumbum aceticum. Lead acetate. Trituration. ***Historical dose:*** All potencies.

HOMEOPATHIC - Care must be used, as sufficient lead can be absorbed to produce lead poisoning, one to two drams of the Liquor plumbi sub-acetatis to the ounce of water. Also in pruritus pudendi, equal parts of the Liquor plumbi and glycerin.

Plb-acet. has painful cramps in paralyzed limbs, severe pain and muscular cramps in gastric ulcer, locally, as a non-homeopathic application in moist eczema and to dry up secretions from mucus surfaces.

REFERENCES - Boericke.

PLUMBUM CHROMICUM

(Lead Chromate)

PHARMACY - plb-chr. Plumbum chromicum. Lead chromate. Chrome yellow. Trituration. ***Historical dose:*** All potencies.

CLINICAL - Colic. Convulsions. Cramps. Diarrhea. Dysphagia. Erythema. Paralysis. Screaming. Tenesmus.

HOMEOPATHIC - Several cases of poisoning by Plb-chr. have been observed. The symptoms present the cardinal features of lead poisoning. Cramps. Convulsions with terrible pains. Pupils enormously dilated. The face was red and hot and there was heat of the body generally.

Erythematous redness of chest and abdomen. Retracted abdomen. ***Violent diarrhea of yellow color***. Yellow stools with constipation. The symptoms were worse towards evening. Better by drinking warm milk.

REFERENCES - Clarke.

PLUMBUM IODATUM

(Lead Iodide)

PHARMACY - plb-i. Plumbum iodatum. Lead iodide. Plumbic iodide. ***Historical dose:*** All potencies.

CLINICAL - Arteriosclerosis. Breast infections, indurations. Paralysis. Pellagra.

HOMEOPATHIC - Plb-i. has been used empirically in various forms of paralysis, sclerotic degenerations, especially of spinal cord. Atrophies, arteriosclerosis, pellagra.

Associated with very dry skin. Indurations of great hardness. ***Indurations of breasts,*** especially when a tendency to become inflamed appears, sore and painful. Sharp pains of ***tabes.***

REFERENCES - Clarke.

PLUMBUM METALLICUM

(Lead Metal)

PHARMACY - plb. Plumbum metallicum. Lead metal. The element (Pb. At. Wt. 206.39). Plumbum aceticum. Lead acetate. Sugar of Lead. Plumbum carbonicum. Lead carbonate. Pure White Lead. Trituration. ***Historical dose:*** All potencies.

CLINICAL - Amaurosis. Anus, prolapsed. ***Anemia.*** Anesthesia. Aneurysm. Anidrosis. Appendicitis. Arteriosclerosis. Asthma. ***Atrophy.*** Bone, tumors. Brain, disorders. Bright's disease. ***Colic. Constipation.*** Convulsions. ***Cramps.*** Cystitis. Depression. Diplopia. Dropsy. Dysuria. ***Emaciation.*** Epilepsy. Epulis. Esophagus, stricture. Eyes disorders. Ganglion. ***Glaucoma***. Gout. Hemoptysis. Headaches. Hemorrhoids. Hernia, strangulated. Hyperesthesia. Hypertension. Hypopion. Ichthyosis. Intermittent fever. Intestines, obstruction. Intussusception. Jaundice. Jaw, tumor. Kidneys, disorders. ***Lead, poisoning.*** Liver disorders. Lockjaw. Locomotor ataxia. ***Marasmus***. Metrorrhagia. Multiple sclerosis. Myelitis. ***Nephritis.*** Neuritis. Numbness. ***Painter's colic. Paralysis. Parkinson's disease.*** Perichondritis. ***Progressive muscular atrophy.*** Rectal pain. Sciatica. ***Spasms. Spine, diseases.*** Spleen, disorders. Stricture. ***Strokes.*** Tabes mesenterica. Tobacco habit. Tongue, paralysis. Typhlitis. Umbilicus, disorders. Uric acid. ***Vaginismus.*** Varicose veins. ***Wrist drop.***

HOMEOPATHIC - Plb., the Saturn of the Alchemists, has been proved by Hartlaub, Trinks, Hering and Nenning. To those symptoms have been added those of numberless cases of poisoning among workers with lead and painters, symptoms from drinking lead-contaminated waters, from the use of lead in cosmetics, and from cases of suicide.

Teste noted that metallic lead was seldom used in old school practice as it was considered inert, but Boerhaave gave it internally, reduced to an impalpable powder, for leucorrhea, dysentery, syphilis and gout.

The salts of lead, in the form of plaster and "Foulard water," have been largely used as external applications in skin diseases, vaginal and urethral injections. Injury has frequently resulted, especially from repelled eruptions.

Among painters and lead manufacturers, the best-known symptoms are ***colic and wrist drop***. Kidney irritation with albuminuria, ending in granular degeneration with attendant heart hypertrophy, optic neuritis and blindness.

There is an excess of uric acid in the blood of persons under the influence of lead and actual gouty deposits and gouty attacks have been observed. In one case of lead poisoning, there was an enlargement of the knees and contraction of the lower limbs, completely crippling the patient.

Useful for general sclerotic conditions. It affects the muscles, nerves, spinal cord, abdomen, navel, kidneys, blood vessels and blood. Particularly affects the blood, alimentary and nervous systems.

Lead paralysis is chiefly of extensors, forearm or upper limb from center to periphery with partial anesthesia or excessive hyperesthesia, preceded by pain. Localized neuralgic pains, neuritis.

Progressive muscular atrophy. Infantile paralysis. Locomotor ataxia. Bulbar paralysis. Peripheral disorders. ***Paralysis of single parts, wrist drop,*** flaccid with hyperesthesia, worse touch. Tremors, followed by paralysis.

Attacks of the neural axons and the anterior horns. Multiple sclerosis, posterior spinal sclerosis. Contractions and boring pain. Retraction, sense of a string pulling back or in. Constrictive sensation in internal organs. ***Violent contractions.***

Convulsive trembling and jerking of the limbs. Convulsions, chronic epilepsy with marked aura with hemorrhages. Boring, cramps. Lightning pains that extort cries. Small aneurysms all over the body. Dropsical swelling. Arthralgia.

Symptoms appear slowly, insidiously, progressively, often with violent side effects of very changeable and incoherent character, coming in single parts, etc. Anesthesia is as marked as excessive hyperesthesia. Exaggerates her condition. Perception slow, comprehension is difficult. Delirium, coma and convulsions.

Hematosis is interfered with, rapid reduction in number of red corpuscles, causing pallor, jaundice, and anemia. Hypertension and arteriosclerosis. ***Gout***. Acute nephritis with amaurosis and cerebral symptoms.

Impulse to stretch with abdominal distress. Retraction of abdomen, anus, testes, navel etc. Excessive and rapid emaciation. Emaciation of limbs with plump body, of paralyzed parts, of single parts after neuralgias. ***Marasmus of infants*** in apparently hopeless cases, abdomen large and hard and constipation extreme.

MIND - Mental exhaustion from physical labor. Confusion of mind while standing. Weakness or loss of memory (Anac., Bar-c.). Deficiency of ideas. Increasing slowness and apathy. Slow perception. Stupid, imbecile. Timid, restless and anxious. Unable to find proper word while talking. Amnesia aphasia.

Mental depression. Quiet and melancholy. Gloom alternating with excitement. Censorious. Taciturn. Aversion to company. Timidity about appearing in public. Restlessness at night, wants to go from one bed to another.

Anxiety with restlessness and yawning. Hysteria, only while being watched. Screams from time to time. Fright without cause. Frantic, bites, strikes. Fears of poisoning, ***of being assassinated***. Thinks every one about her is a murderer. Delusion of dead persons. Paretic dementia.

Feigns sickness or exaggerates her condition. Inclined to cheat and deceive. Plays antics. Foolish behavior. Cursing. ***Wild delirium with distorted face.***

Delirium, nocturnal, alternating with colic or pain in the limbs. Delirium from hearing music. Delirium after epilepsy. Disposition to suicide or do himself some bodily injury. Time passes too slowly.

Abdomen - ***Colic***, accompanies many symptoms. Colic alternates with delirium and pain in atrophied limbs. Obstructed flatus with intense colic. Abdominal wall feels ***drawn by a string to spine***. ***Navel feels retracted.*** Abdomen is drawn into uneven lumps. Radiating abdominal pains to all parts of the body. Hernia, navel. Intussusception, strangulated hernia. Boring or as if forced through a narrow place. Pain causes desire to stretch.

Back - Spinal cord sclerosis. Lightning-like pains, temporarily better by pressure.

Breasts - Stitches and burning pains in breasts (Apis, Con., Carb-an., Sil.). ***Induration of breasts***. Breasts become momentarily harder or smaller with colic.

Causations - Ill effects of repelled eruptions. Sexual excess. Lead, cadmium or aluminum poisoning.

Chest - Oppression of chest, appearing periodically. Pressure on chest, especially when breathing deeply or laughing. Shootings in chest and sides, sometimes with obstructed respiration. Apices of lungs affected. Small red papules on chest, desquamation.

Constitutions - Particularly adapted to adults, males more than females, particularly to persons of a dry, bilious constitution with somewhat jaundiced, irascible, hypochondriac or disposed to religious monomania.

Ears - ***Tinnitus*** (Chin., Nat-sal., Carb-s.). Hears music with frightful delirium. Occasional sudden deafness.

Eyes - Pupils contracted. Yellow or deep bluish red sclerotics. Optic neuritis, central scotoma. Intra-ocular, suppurative inflammation. ***Glaucoma*** from spinal disorders. Sudden loss of sight after fainting. Paralysis of upper lid. Profuse hot lachrymation.

Face - Yellow, corpse-like, cheeks sunken. Skin, greasy, shiny. ***Pale and emaciated***. Swelling of face, one side. Twitching of side of face (right). Tremor of naso-labial muscles.

Female - ***Vaginismus*** with emaciation and constipation. Vulva and the vagina hypersensitive. Ovarian pain, better stretching legs. Menorrhagia with sensation of string pulling from abdomen to back. Cannot pass urine in pregnancy from lack of sensation or paralysis. Tendency to abortion from undeveloped uterus. Feeling of lack of room for fetus in uterus.

Head - Headache, as if a ball was rising from the throat into the head. Delirium alternating with colic. Hair very dry, falls from beard.

Heart - Cardiac weakness. Pulse soft and small, dicrotic. Pulse wiry, slow sinks even to 40. Painful constriction of peripheral arteries.

Kidneys - ***Chronic interstitial nephritis*** with great pain in abdomen. Contracted kidney. Paralysis of bladder, difficult urination or retention, suppression. Frequent ineffectual tenesmus. Scanty urine. Urine profuse, but flows slowly, drop by drop. Albuminous, low specific gravity. Diabetes mellitus. Uremia.

Limbs - ***Paralysis of lower limbs.*** Paralysis of ***single muscles.*** Pain in ***atrophied limbs,*** alternating with colic. Sciatica and muscular atrophy. Lightning like pains better by pressure. Stinging and tearing in limbs, also twitching and tingling, numbness, pain or tremor. Weakness and painful lameness of arms and hands. Extension is difficult. Paralysis from overexertion of the extensor muscles in piano players (Cur.). Arms shaky when attempting to use them. ***Wrist drop***. Paralysis of lower limbs after childbirth. Pains in muscles of thighs, ***come in paroxysms.*** Cramps in calves. ***Loss of patellar reflex.*** Hands and feet cold. Feet swollen. As if feet were made of wood. ***Pain in right big toe,*** very sensitive to touch.

Male - Testicles drawn up, feel constricted. Frequent pollutions. ***Loss of sexual power.***

Modalities - Bending back ameliorates pressure in stomach, pain in epigastrium, pain in back. Bending double ameliorates colic. Better by hard pressure, rubbing, physical exertion, stretching limbs. Better at rest, lying down. Worse from motion, grasping smooth objects, touch. Worse mental exertion, company. Worse at night, open air, clear weather, foggy weather. Damp weather causes profuse salivation. Swelling in abdomen and cough are worse lying on right side.

Mouth - Sweet taste. Sticky saliva, blue. Yellow inside the mouth. Aphthae, fetid ulcers. Gums swollen, pale. Hard tubercles on gums. ***Distinct blue lines along margins of gums.*** Tongue tremulous, red on margin. Cannot put it out, seems paralyzed. Loud motion of lower jaw and frightful grinding of teeth.

Nose - Coldness of the nose. Erysipelatous inflammation of nose. Obstruction of nose. Accumulation of tenacious mucus in nostrils. Fluent coryza with discharge of serous mucus. Fetid smell in nose. Loss of smell with epilepsy.

Rectum - Anus feels drawn up or painfully contracted. Neuralgia of rectum. Prolapsed anus with paralysis. Constipation. Stools, ***hard, lumpy, black with urging and spasm of anus***. Stools, granular, hard black balls like sheep dung, passed with an urging cramp in anus. Obstructed evacuation from impaction of feces (Plat.). Stubborn constipation or colics of infants.

Sensations - As if everything were weighed down. As if something were working at top of head with a sense of screwing from throat into brain. As if a wheat hull in throat. As if abdomen and back were too close together, abdomen drawn to spine with a string. Bowels as if twisted, constricted, distended with gas. As if abscess forming near umbilicus. Anal sphincter as if drawn in. As if a bag not quite filled with fluid lay in bowels. As if fluid rolled from one side to other of abdomen. As if thighs pierced with needles. As if feet made of wood.

Skin - Oversensitive to open air. Dry, wrinkled, shriveled and drawn over the bones. Jaundice. Yellow, dark-brown liver spots. Bluish, red spots. Dilated veins of forearms and legs. Small wounds easily inflamed and suppurate. Dry, burning ulcers. Bed sores. Blisters, corns, bunions. Gangrene.

Sleep - Falls asleep while speaking, talking during sleep. Nocturnal sleeplessness with abdominal spasms. Jerks during sleep. Odd position during sleep. Must stretch in every direction. Many dreams, sometimes lascivious with erections. Coma and lethargy, sometimes with dizziness.

Stomach - Contraction in esophagus and stomach, pressure and tightness. ***Gastralgia,*** better hard pressure, bending backwards. Foul or fecal belchings. Periodical or persistent vomiting of food. Vomiting of brown-black liquid or of green mucus. Vomiting of fecal matter with colic and constipation.

Temperature - Coldness from exertion. General cold sweat during stools. Feet cold, only when walking.

Throat - Solids cannot be swallowed. Dysphagia, fluids can be swallowed. Paralysis of gullet with inability to swallow. Globus hystericus. Stricture of esophagus from spasms.

Vertigo - Fainting in a room full of people or on going from one room to another.

COMMENTS - Tunzelmann reported a number of cases of acute poisoning from drinking water containing lead.

In one such case, a cook was ill for three weeks. Unable to retain any food in the stomach, constant nausea and, even when no food was taken, frequent vomiting of greenish watery fluid, worse at night.

Skin was yellowish, conjunctiva decidedly yellow. Tongue was furred, coated at back, very yellow, horrible taste, fetor of breath, bowels confined. Extreme debility. Hydr. 3c gave great relief, but three months later the hands became paralyzed, which led to the testing of the drinking water and the discovery of lead.

A boy, age 12, had bronchial catarrh with a loose cough and consolidation of left apex. As soon as the poisoned water was stopped, he rapidly recovered.

An elder brother had hemoptysis, and coughed up half a pint of blood. Nothing was found wrong with the lungs beyond a slight feebleness of respiration at the apices. Three months later, after a day's rowing, the hematemesis returned with a nosebleed. Now distinct dullness was found at right apex. Rapid recovery followed stopping the water.

Women who work with lead frequently abort. Women who do not work with lead but whose husbands do, abort in even greater proportion. Children born under these conditions are frequently idiotic or epileptic.

Characteristic retraction and sense of retraction. Sensation of or actual drawing in of abdominal wall, were drawn back by a string to the spine. The cheeks are retracted, sunken. Excessive and rapid emaciation. Emaciation of certain parts (Caust.). Anemia. Memory loss.

Progressive muscular atrophy. Parkinson's disease. Paralysis of single muscles. Paralyzed parts lose flesh. Progressive locomotor ataxia. Stroke, with spastic paralysis. Epilepsy preceded by vertigo, sometimes sighing, followed by a stupid feeling.

Cramps, spasms, convulsions, paralyzes, tremors. Clonic or tonic convulsive movements of limbs from cerebral sclerosis or tumor. Cramps in the fingers. Wrist drop, weak wrist from overuse. Lead palsy.

Spasm of bladder of esophagus. Violent colic. Strangulated hernia. Colon spasms. Painful impacted bowels (Alum. and Op. are painless). Vaginismus, spasm of uterus and expulsion of its contents. Useful for vaginismus resulting in paralytic symptoms. Sensation as if there was not room enough for fetus.

Anesthesia and hyperesthesia. Restlessness, lassitude, faintness. Sensation in abdomen at night that causes patient to stretch violently for hours, must stretch in every direction. Assumes strange positions in bed at night.

Pains are wandering or radiating, vague, paroxysmal. Ailments develop slowly and can intermit for a time. Alternations are common, delirium with colic, diarrhea and constipation, jerks of flexors and extensors, paralysis and colic. Right side is most affected, symptoms go from left to right (throat). Symptoms worse 8 a.m. to 9 a.m.

Frohling related the case of N., a farmer, 46, who was taken ill in November 1893 with attacks of colic with vomiting and extreme constipation, action only obtained by large enemata. Had been constipated in former years, but without illness. Op. had given only temporary relief.

After December 1983, vomiting was rare, but colic increased in intensity up to February 1894, when Frohling saw him first and found him wasted to a skeleton, abdomen drawn in, appetite bad, feeling ill.

His mind was somewhat affected, unable to give sensible answers to questions. Constant urgent call to stool, but only small, hard, black balls were passed. Liver dullness only heard from upper border of sixth to upper border of seventh rib.

Lead poisoning was suspected, but as no evidence of it could be found, Plb. 6c three times a day was prescribed. In six days the colic attacks were less frequent and less severe, two stools passed without enema, his mind clearer.

Improvement continued in all respects, and in fourteen days N. was able to leave his bed to which he had been confined since November. By the middle of March he made an hour's journey to see Frohling and was hardly recognizable, he had gained so much flesh and his liver was of normal size.

Wingfield reported two characteristic cases. The first concerned Mrs. D., 50, no children, sparely built, very nervous, constipated fifteen years, took a teaspoonful of Cascara extract every other night. Tongue coated with yellowish white fur. Had constant headaches and after each motion was thoroughly exhausted and had to lie down the rest of the day.

Plb. 6x was given, three grains twice a day. In two days, bowels began acting naturally.

In three weeks the headaches were gone, tongue clean, much less nervous.

Wingfield's second case was Miss M., 25, florid, had boils appear on face and arms and chronic constipation. The constipation had been a trouble since she was twelve years old. Slight spinal curvature. Tongue furred, occasional headaches. Suffered much during menstrual periods. Plb. 6x twice daily at once relieved the constipation and soon the boils disappeared. Patient soon felt quite well.

Arriage, of Mexico City, reported the case of a woman, 73, seized with symptoms of intestinal occlusion, violent colic, nausea, constipation, meteorism, complete anorexia and no fever. Nux-v. relieved the colic, and then Plb. 12c and later 13c, gradually brought about recovery in four days.

Nash cured a severe case of post-diphtheria paralysis in a middle-aged man. The leading symptom was excessive hyperesthesia, he could not bear to be touched anywhere due to the pain. A single dose of Plb. 40,000c cured.

Nash told of a man, 70, attacked with severe pain in his abdomen and finally a large, hard swelling developed in the ileo-cecal region, very sensitive to contact or least motion. It began to assume a bluish tint and, on account of his age and weakness, the man's life was despaired. But his daughter, the wife of a medical man, found the symptoms in Raue under Plb. in the chapter on Typh., and Plb. 200c cured.

Theuerkauf cured a case of hypopion with great pain in six weeks using Plb. 6c.

Skinner cured a case of epilepsy in which the head turned to the right after a fit.

W. H. Woodyatt reported a case of "vasomotor neurosis" affecting the left eye. Mrs. D., 29, had been ill for two weeks and supposed she had caught cold in the eye. She had a drooping upper lid, intense photophobia, very profuse lachrymation of hot tears, peri-corneal injection, deep bluish redness of sclerotica, most marked at corneal margin. Cornea was very faintly hazy. Pupil contracted. Sight misty.

Ars. 6x and Plant. 6x failed to relieve. Plb. 6x was then given with immediate improvement, which went on to cure in seven days.

Plb. cured a case of right-sided sciatica that had been greatly benefited by Gnaph. 1c, but which had returned. The symptoms included stiffness, soreness from great trochanter and point of exit of nerve to knee, weakness in thigh, worse by stooping, walking causes sensation as if pushing a knife in thigh.

Plb. 6c was given four times day. Up to the twelfth day there was no change, on that day, the pain suddenly disappeared. The case had lasted nine months.

RELATIONS - ***Antidotes:*** Plat., Alum., Petr. ***Compare:*** (1) Plb-acet. (2) Plb-i. Alum., Plat., Op., Podo., Merc., Thal. (3) Plect. - paralysis, spastic, spinal form, (4) Plb-chr. (5) Plb-p. - loss of sexual power, locomotor ataxia.

REFERENCES - Boericke. Clarke. Murphy. Phatak.

PLUTONIUM NITRICUM

(Plutonium)

PHARMACY - plut-n. Plutonium nitricum. Plutonium. ***Historical dose:*** All potencies.

CLINICAL - AIDS. Bone, cancer. Bone marrow, affections. Brain, tumors. Cancer. Diarrhea. ***Fatigue.*** Fibrosis. Hodgkin's diseases. Leukemia. Lung, cancer. Lung, complaints. Radiation, poisoning. Thyroid, enlarged. Virus infections. Vomiting.

HOMEOPATHIC - Very serious pathologies. Cancers, leukemia. ***Periodical fatigue.*** Paralyzing fatigue. Chilliness and shivering, yet great feeling of heat in head and face.

Desire to lie down from feeling of extreme heaviness. Body seems to be heavy like lead. Head very heavy, like an enormous weight, difficult to keep head up. Feels the pull of gravity. Desire to lie down on one's back and on the floor.

Sensation of dryness in throat, as if swallowing of food would be impossible. Paralyzing pain in sacral region. Pain as if broken or twisted. Great restlessness at night. Weakness of lower limbs. Cannot walk upright, must crawl on all fours.

MIND - Serious, no smile on the face, as if carrying burden of world on their shoulders. Extremely conscientious. Delusion of having too many responsibilities. Fastidious, impulse to put things in order. Deep religious feelings or philosophical thoughts. Feels alone and empty.

Aggressive, reckless impulses. Irritability and aggression. Resentment, controlled anger. Reproachful, reproaches his wife. Outbursts of violence. Aggressive fantasies. Dominant behavior.

Anxiety about health. Fear of falling ill, of catastrophes. Fear of narrow places, claustrophobia. Fear of one's own impulses, of being too aggressive. Panic-stricken. Persistent feeling of existential threat. Delusion of being threatened. Delusion of decaying and disintegrating.

Depressed, dark gloomy mood. Weeping on account of physical pain. Sadness better company. Restlessness, cannot find a place or position to relax. Delusion of changing one's identity. Clairvoyant. Severe mental illnesses.

Abdomen - Cutting pain, better bending double.

Back - Paralyzing pain in sacral region. Back pain extending to posterior part of thigh and popliteal region.

Breasts - Sensation of heaviness and fullness in breasts. Sensation of tension in breasts, desire to wear a bra.

Eyes - Burning sensation.

Food - ***Desires bacon, raw meat,*** lamb, pork, ham, fat.

Head - Shattering headache, in forehead. Pain as if vertex comes up, as if it would explode. Pressing pain in forehead. Sensation of enormous heaviness. Sensation of great heat in head and face.

Limbs - Sensation of leaden heaviness. Sensation as if left leg were shorter. Pain in soles of feet on account of vesicles on toes.

Modalities - Better warmth, sitting in the sun, ***hot applications, hot bathing.*** Better massage, strong pressure, after long sleep. Worse from walking. Worse 3 p.m., sunset, evening, night. Worse overcast weather, first ray of sun.

Rectum - Anal warts. Sensation of insecurity in rectum when passing flatus.

Sleep - Short sleep improves. Sleeplessness and restlessness from pain in sacral region, tossing about to relieve pain; sleeplessness from feeling of heat. Dream of falling. Dream of killing or murders, of dead people, of bodies.

RELATIONS - ***Compare:*** Androc., Aur., Carc., Hydrog., Med., Rad-br., Stram., Syph., Tarent., Uran-n., X-ray.

REFERENCES - Sherr.

PNEUMOCOCCINUM

(Pneumococcus Nosode)

PHARMACY - pneu. Pneumococcinum venenosum. Pneumococcus nosode. Bacteria of the Diplococcus genus, Micrococcales. Non-pathologic bacteria of the mucus membranes. Nosodes. ***Historical dose:*** All potencies.

CLINICAL - Hemicrania. Hypochondria. Memory, loss. Neuralgia of the skull. Pneumonia.

HOMEOPATHIC - Pneumococcus is a gram positive bacteria of the Diplococcus genus and of the Micrococcaceae family. Pneumococcus is a saprophyte host of the mucus membranes. It is found in the saliva, nasal and pharyngeal mucus, or the conjunctiva of 50% of healthy subjects. Sevaus conducted a clinical symptomatological study, but there is no homeopathic proving.

Respiratory complaints localized in the bronchial region. Cardiac palpitations. Dysmenorrhea with late menses and premenstrual syndrome. Intoxication.

Depressive condition associated with pains situated all over the cervical and dorsal regions. Acute pains, which come suddenly of the stinging (Nit-ac.) or cramping type (Cupr.), lasting only a short while. Constricting pains, as if in a vice (Cact.).

MIND - Loss of memory. Depressive condition with anguish, anxiety. Desire to stay at home, horror of going out (Sep.). Lack of taste for life. Impression that the patient is going to collapse, that he cannot walk. Very afraid of being ill, of dying.

Abdomen - Bad digestion. Hepatic deficiency. Air in the stomach and colon. Distention and pain in the left hypochondrium, eased by expulsion of wind. Gas with alternation of constipation and fetid stools.

Back - Dorsal and lumbar arthrosis. Dorsal pains, preventing standing.

Constitutions - Bilious and nervous, depressive, anxious. Allergic, psoric constitutions. sycotic, cancerous, and tubercular constitutions.

Ears - Otitis media.

Eyes - Fatigue from neon light. Frontal pains above the eyes.

Female - Premenstrual aggravation. Menstrual cycle short, every 22 or 24 days. Menses stopping on the 2nd day. Menses late, scanty, legs heavy and swollen before menses. Menstrual migraines and vertigo. Bearing down pain and crosses legs (Sep.). Burning sensation during intercourse in cases of fatigue. Frigidity. Lack of orgasm.

Food - Ameliorated by eating (Anac.).

Head - Pains in left frontal sinus. Headaches lasting for 3 to 4 consecutive days. Headache on coughing or bending the head. Frequent headaches, localized at the nape of the neck, worse by noise. Right or left hemicrania, worse by walking, which causes throbbing in the head. Feeling of liquid in the head on stooping.

Heart - Aching in the precordial region with pains. Cardiac neurosis. Basedow's heart. Rhythmic anomalies. Emotive palpitations. Frequent palpitations at any time of the day. Palpitations forcing him to stop when walking rapidly or climbing stairs. Frequent redness of the face when going into a hot room.

Kidneys - Weakness of the bladder. Passes urine when coughing (Caust.).

Limbs - Pains in the arms. Pains in the legs. Legs restless, especially before menses (Zinc., Lach.). Legs heavy in the morning on waking. Trembling in the legs. Cramps in the feet. Poly-arthrosis.

Lungs - Sinusitis. Tracheitis. Chronic bronchitis. Emphysema. Incessant cough with no expectoration, especially at night with nausea. Feeling of having a feather in the throat (Kali-bi.). Dry cough in the cold or heat. Coughs in the heat, particularly when entering a hot room and clears the throat (Rhus-t.). Sickening cough in the morning after breakfast. Does not cough any more after 9 a.m. Coughs a great deal as a result of frequent bronchitis during childhood. Has to stoop to cough.

Modalities - Better from the open air, in the country. Better from movement, a hot foot-bath, a short nap after meals (Nux-v.). Worse on entering a warm room, from damp before menses. Worse from inactivity (Rhus-t.), sitting for a long time, especially when remaining motionless, rest at night. Pains aggravated by rest, at night, better by movement (Rhus-t.).

Mouth - Aphthae in the mouth.

Neck - Neck pains with frontal aching. Cervical pains with back aching. Chronic degenerative rheumatism of the cervical column.

Rectum - Gas with the alternation of constipation and very fetid stools. Constipation with empty urging (Nux-v.). Constipation when traveling (Ign.).

Skin - Itching with eruptions spread over the neck and forehead. Small eruptions on the face. Hands clammy.

Sleep - Sleepiness around 3 p.m.

Stomach - Acrid dyspepsia. Frequent nausea after eating. Gastric pains, especially when hungry. Stomach cramps with burning sensations.

RELATIONS - *Compare:* (1) Med. - amnesia for recent facts. Hasty with restless legs and burning in the heels. Burning pains in the joints and vertebral column. Improvement at the seaside and in the knee-chest position. (2) Thuj, - hydrogenoid condition, melancholy, worse from changing weather or after a trauma. Flatulence, diarrhea, periodic skin complaints.

REFERENCES - Julian.

PODOPHYLLUM PELTATUM

(May-apple)

PHARMACY - podo. Podophyllum peltatum. May-apple. American mandrake. N. O. Berberidaceae by some placed in Ranunculaceae. Closely related to both. Tincture of root gathered after fruit has ripened of whole fresh plant of ripe fruit. Solution of resinous extract, podophyllin. ***Historical dose:*** Tincture and all potencies.

CLINICAL - Acidity. Amenorrhea. Anus, prolapsed. Asthma, bronchial. Bedwetting. ***Bilious, attack.*** Bronchitis. Cataract. Cholera. Cornea, ulcer. ***Dentition.*** Deafness. Depression. Diabetes. ***Diarrhea.*** Duodenum, catarrh. Dysentery. Dysmenorrhea. Dyspepsia. Fevers. Flatus. Gagging. Gallstones. Gastric, disorders. Goiter. Headaches. Heart, pain. Hemorrhoids. Jaundice. Liver, disorders. Ovary, disorders. Ovarian, tumor. Palpitations. Pneumonia. Proctitis. ***Prolapsed, uterus. Prolapsed, rectum.*** Prostatitis. Pustules. Sciatica. Stomatitis. Strabismus. Taste, disorders. Tenesmus. Tongue, burning. Urticaria. Uterus, prolapsed. Vomiting. Whooping cough. ***Worms. Yellow, diarrhea.***

HERBAL - Podophyllum grows throughout the United States in damp, shady places, usually in woods. It has five to nine-lobed leaves, large white nodding flowers, and yellowish, egg-shaped fruits. The fruits are not unlike a small lemon, hence the plant is sometimes called "wild lemon." It flowers in May and June, and the fruit ripens in October.

Indian tribes used the root to expel worms, and dropped the juice of the root into the ear to cure deafness. "All the tribes are fond of the fruit," said Raffinesque, quoted by Hale, who gave an account of the medicine.

The herbal practitioners adopted the remedy and used it as the "vegetable mercury." The first homeopathic proving was made by Williamson.

HOMEOPATHIC - Podo. is a remedy for bilious constitution. It affects chiefly the ***duodenum***, small intestines, liver, rectum, ovary, scapula and throat. It generally affects the right side.

Torpidity of the liver. Jaundice. Hypogastric pain. Gastro-enteritis with colicky pain and bilious vomiting. Painless cholera morbus. ***Profuse diarrhea***. Stool is watery with jelly-like mucus, painless, gushing and offensive. Diarrhea, while being bathed or washed, of dirty water soaking through napkin, with gagging.

Portal engorgement with a tendency to hemorrhoid. Fullness of superficial veins. Relaxed sphincters. Prolapsed uterus. Pendulous abdomen after confinement. Troubles during pregnancy.

Alternating conditions, diarrhea alternating with constipation, headache alternating with diarrhea. Sudden shocks from jerking pains. Constantly shaking and rubbing region of liver with hands.

Much drowsiness and desire to stretch. Great loquacity during chill and heat. Thirst for large quantities of cold water. Viscid mucus in mouth, coating teeth. Intense ***desire to press the gums together***.

MIND - Fidgety and restless, cannot sit still. Whining. Child wants to be carried. Depression of spirits. Disgust for life, during headaches. Imagines he is going to die or be very ill. Delirium from eating acid fruits.

Fatigue of mind from business. Aphasia. Want of power of expression even of simplest ideas. Absurd words being chosen in place of right ones. Stupid during paroxysm of fever patient.

Loquacity during chill and fever, afterwards forgets what has passed. Inclined to talk, but would drop a sentence before half finished. Great desire to talk during chill, but can't because he forgets words.

Abdomen - Distended abdomen, heat and emptiness. ***Sensation of weakness or sinking***. Can lie comfortably only on stomach. Fullness in right hypochondrium, with flatulence, pain and soreness. Rumbling and shifting of flatus in ascending colon. Rubs for relief. Weight in hypogastric region. Pain in right inguinal region, shoots down inner thigh to knees. Colic, in abdomen, with cramp-like knots, better flexing limbs. Colic continues after stool. Abdominal viscera are sore, worse during vomiting, diarrhea, before and during menses. Abdominal pains and stool excited by eating and drinking. Sick, empty feeling after stools.

Back - Nape of neck stiff, muscles sore. Pain under right scapula. Pain between shoulders. Pain in small of back. Pain in lumbar and sacral regions, worse during stool, and still worse after stool. Pain in loins, worse walking on uneven ground or from misstep.

Chest - Oppression in chest. Pains in chest worse by deep inspiration. Catarrh of chest during dentition.

Constitutions - Suited to persons of bilious temperament, especially after mercury poisoning.

Ears - Aching pain in right ear, with rough feeling extending along right Eustachian tube.

Eyes - Jaundiced. Eyes sunken. Eyes glazed and motionless. Cataract. Smarting, inflammation of lids. Lids half closed. Pain in eyeballs and temples.

Face - Hot. Cheeks flushed during diarrhea. Jaundiced.

Female - Suppressed menses with pelvic tenesmus. Menorrhagia from straining. Sensation as if the genitals would come out during stool. Pain in the region of the ovaries (right), down the crural nerve worse stretching the legs. Ovarian tumor with pain extending to shoulder. ***Pain in uterus and right ovary with shifting noises along ascending colon***. Can lie comfortably only on the abdomen during early months of pregnancy. Swelling of labia during pregnancy. Hemorrhoids with prolapsed anus during pregnancy. ***Prolapsed uterus*** on straining or overlifting after childbirth.

Food - Thirst for large quantities of cold water (Phos., Bry.). Appetite variable, at times voracious. Indifference to food. Loss of appetite. Smell of food causes loathing. Satiety from small quantity of food, followed by nausea and vomiting. Craves acids, which disagree. Worse after eating and drinking, especially acid fruit and milk. Diarrhea after sour milk, canned fruits, acid fruit and milk.

Head - Headache, dull pressure, worse morning, with heated face and bitter taste. ***Headache alternating with diarrhea***, or better by diarrhea. Darting pain in forehead, must close the eyes. Rolling of head from side to side with moaning, during dentition, from business worry. Child perspires on head during sleep.

Heart - Palpitations with a clucking sensation, rising up to the throat, from emotions.

Kidneys - Frequent urination, at night, during pregnancy. Urinates immediately after drinking. Bedwetting. Diabetes mellitus and insipidus.

Limbs - Paralytic weakness on left side. Pain between shoulders, under right scapula, in loins and lumbar region. Pain along ulnar nerve of both arms. Pain in right inguinal region, shoots down inner thigh to knees. Cramps in calves with stools.

Liver - Sore and painful liver, better rubbing. Stitches in liver region, worse while eating. Liver and whole abdominal viscera are sore. Jaundice with gallstones.

Lungs - Inclination to breathe deep, sighing. Sensation of suffocation. Pneumonia. Chronic bronchitis. Bronchial asthma, worse after catching cold. Loose, dry, hacking cough, with remittent fever. Whooping cough with constipation and loss of appetite.

Male - Diseases of prostate gland associated with rectal troubles.

Modalities - External heat ameliorates pain in bowels. ***Better by pressure, rubbing or stroking liver.*** Better lying down, lying on abdomen, stretching in bed. Hot weather, summer, aggravates diarrhea. ***Worse in early morning***, 2 a.m. to 4 a.m., night. Worse open air, washing. Worse eating, swallowing, drinking, acid fruits, milk. Worse before, during and after stool, ***dentition***, mercury. Worse from motion, walking, ascending stairs, exertion.

Mouth - Offensive odor. Bitter, foul, putrid taste. Everything tastes sour or putrid. Loss of taste, could not tell sweet from sour. ***Tongue, broad, large, moist.*** Tongue coated as of mustard spread on it. ***Burning,*** rough or flabby indented tongue. Grinding the teeth at night. ***Difficult dentition***

with intense desire to press the gums together (Phyt.).

Rectum - Fetid flatus. Long standing diarrhea. Diarrhea alternating with other symptoms. ***Diarrhea early in morning, during teething, with hot, glowing cheeks.*** Diarrhea while being bathed or washed, in hot weather, after acid fruits. Morning, painless diarrhea when not due to venous stasis or intestinal ulceration. ***Gurgling through the bowels, then yellow profuse putrid stools gush out painlessly***. Cholera infantum and morbus. Constipation alternating with diarrhea (Ant-c.). Constipation, clay-colored, hard, dry, difficult. ***Prolapse of rectum*** before or with stool. Internal and external hemorrhoids. Sensation of weakness in rectum. Severe burning, deep in rectum, after stool. Anus feels very sore, sensitive and swollen.

Perspiration - Profuse, offensive sweat with sleep. Warm sweat on head and legs. Sweats on head with coldness of skin.

Sensations - As if strabismus would occur. Pain in head as from ice on occipital protuberance. As if tongue, throat and palate had been burned. Ball in upper esophagus. As if heart ascending to throat. As if a thousand live things moving about in abdomen or of fish turning over. As if everything would drop through pelvis.

Skin - Moist, warm, jaundiced. Cold, clammy skin. Sallow skin, jaundice, also in children. Rawness and itching of genitals. Erysipelas. Intolerable itching of body and arms. Urticaria. Pustules, slow in healing. Scabs on arms and legs.

Sleep - Sleepy after paroxysms of malaria. Heavy sleep, fatigue on waking. Moaning and whining during sleep. Rising up in sleep without waking. Sleep disturbed, full of confused dreams.

Stomach - Stomach so weak that rice wouldn't digest. Heartburn, gagging or empty retching. Hot, sour belching, nausea and vomiting. Belchings smelling like rotten eggs. Constant gagging. Vomiting of a hot, frothy mucus. Vomiting of milk in infants.

Stool - ***Stools yellow with undigested food.*** Stools green, watery, at times mixed with mucus, gushing. ***Yellow, fetid profuse diarrhea***. Stools, white like water. Pale, hard, chalky stools. Stools foaming with meal-like sediment. Stools run right through the diaper, followed by weakness. Muco-gelatinous stools after miscarriage. Stools involuntary during sleep, when passing flatus.

Temperature - Chills at 7 a.m. with pain in hypochondria and knees, ankles, wrists. ***Great loquacity during fever.***

Throat - Gagging in infantile diarrhea. As of a lump in esophagus. Sore throat, pain extends to ears. Dryness, swallowing painful. Sore throat right extends to left. Rattling of mucus in throat. Goiter.

Vertigo - Vertigo, tendency to fall forward. Vertigo with sensation of fullness above eyes. Vertigo while standing in open air. Vertigo from gastric or bilious disorders.

COMMENTS - An unintentional Podo. proving recorded by E. V. Rose brought out the chief characteristics and showed that its reputation as a "vegetable mercury" is well deserved.

At 11 a.m., Mr. J., 26 took grains x of Podo. 1x to "stir up his liver." At 6 p.m. he was taken with an indescribable sick feeling all over and a persistent, dry, rough feeling in pharynx and esophagus, extending along right Eustachian tube with dull, aching pain in right ear, feeling as though a ball or lump in upper esophagus.

At 8 p.m., he had a dull and stupefying headache, chiefly frontal, worse lying down. Fullness in stomach, belching of gas, sour belchings, marked salivation and an offensive odor from the mouth. Sleep was disturbed, full of confused dreams, rolled and tossed about, bed felt too hard and a feeling as though head and shoulders were lying too low.

At 3 a.m., urge to stool, which was profuse, watery, and dark green. Frequent urging. Before stool there was a peculiar weak, dull, griping pain below umbilicus, fullness in rectum. During stool there was a weak feeling in the stomach. After stool, tenesmus and faint feeling.

These symptoms passed off in two or three days, the diarrhea was followed by constipation, which was quickly removed by Nux-v.

External irritant. Produces a rawness like intertrigo when applied on the skin. The dust of the powdered root sets up intense inflammation, ulceration and leucoma if it gets into the eyes. Useful in potency for eye disorders.

Irritation of the brain, generally reflected to the abdominal viscera (cholera infantum), or the teeth (dentition). Moaning and whining during sleep, the head is thrown back and rolls from side to side, the child grates its teeth. Great desire to press gums or teeth together. Salivation, foul breath and moist, tooth-indented tongue (Merc.). Burning sensation on the tongue. Thirst.

Bilious, remittent, and intermittent fevers. Loquacity during chill and heat. Prone to sweat. Delirium, apt to be loquacious. Much drowsiness and desire to stretch. Congested, sensitive liver with excess or absence of bile.

Generally for diarrhea with any other symptoms, painful or painless. Children's diarrhea (Ars., Nit-ac.). Yellow, profuse, offensive and excoriated diarrhea in infants with a raw and burning anus. Profuse stools, yellow or white. Early morning diarrhea. Dysentery, colitis. Cholera. Hepatitis concomitant with severe diarrhea. Severe cases of jaundice, gallstone attacks, and worms.

The stools may be painless or may be preceded, accompanied, and followed by colic, tenesmus and other symptoms. Pains in sacrum in lumbar region with rectal and uterine symptoms, cramps in calves with stools.

Fullness and tenderness of the rectum. Proctitis, inflammation of the rectum and anus. Tendency to prolapse in the rectum and genital organs. "Symptoms of prolapse uterus with pain in sacrum with mucogelatinous stools," and "sensation at stool as if the genital organs would fall out."

Pains in the ovaries, especially the right, extending down the anterior and inner side of thighs. Vomiting during pregnancy. Swelling of labia during pregnancy. "Can lie comfortably only on stomach" during the early months of pregnancy. Severe afterpains with strong bearing-down sensation, hemorrhoids and prolapsed rectum after confinement.

Alternating conditions. Diarrhea alternating with constipation, headache alternating with diarrhea, headache in winter, diarrhea in summer, inflammation of scrotum or of the eyes, not of both. Antidotal to mercury. Worse hot weather.

Nash cured an obstinate case of intermittent fever with violent chills, followed by intense fever with great loquacity. When the fever was past, the patient fell asleep and, on waking, remembered nothing of his loquacious delirium.

W. A. Burr related a case of a young man who had for some weeks a burning sensation along the left edge of his tongue, occasionally shooting to tip or through to opposite edge. He had been in poor health, "bilious," for years. With catarrh of stomach, duodenum and bile ducts, extreme discomfort followed even the blandest foods. Podo. 3x improved in two days and the tongue was well in a week.

Clarke often cured prolapsed anus in children with Podo. 6c. With Podo. 1x, Mr. Knox Shaw relieved "continual urging and straining" in a case of rectal cancer too far gone for operation.

L. M. Barnes noted the case of a stout woman, 60, who complained of burning, aching, cutting pain in rectum. She was obliged to be on her feet all day. Nervous, cross, irritable. Podo. cured.

Barnes also reported the case of a woman who, for four months after a miscarriage, had ovarian pain, worse at night. She was sleepless, nervous, restless. Bearing down in abdomen and back. She was a large, stout woman with a pendulous abdomen. Podo. cured after Puls. and Cimic. had only partially relieved.

Guernsey mentioned that it is often called for in complaints of pregnant and parturient women with the sensation as if intestines were falling down. He mentioned also whooping cough with costiveness and loss of appetite.

RELATIONS - ***Compare:*** (1) Mand. - Great

desire for sleep, exaggeration of sounds and enlarged vision. Bowels inactive, stools large, white and hard. (2) Aloe, Chel., Merc., Nux-v., Sulph. (3) Prune. - colitis.

REFERENCES - Boericke. Clarke. Murphy. Phatak.

POLYGONATUM MULTIFLORUM

(Solomon's Seal)

PHARMACY - polygo-m. Polygonatum multiflorum. Solomon's Seal. Lady's Seals. St. Mary's Seal. Sigillum Sanctae Mariae. N.O. Liliaceae. Tincture of the root. ***Historical dose:*** Tincture and all potencies.

CLINICAL - Abscess. Alopecia. Back, pain. Bone, disorders. ***Bone, injuries.*** Bone, spurs. Bruises. Bunions. Calcifications. Carbuncles. Constipation. Dysentery. Erysipelas. Hair, loss. Hemorrhoids. Hyperlipidemia. Injuries. Joint, pains. ***Joint, weakness.*** Leucorrhea. Malaria. Metrorrhagia. Muscle, weakness. Pyorrhea. Sores. Sprains. ***Tendon, disorders.*** Tinnitus. Tumors. Vertigo. Wounds.

HERBAL - Polyg-m., in material doses of tincture or low potencies, has been found useful in treating all kinds of musculoskeletal disorders.

Astringent, demulcent and tonic. Combined with otherremedies, Solomon's Seal is given in pulmonary consumption and bleeding of the lungs. It is useful also in female complaints.

It is used mainly in the form of a poultice and is believed to prevent excessive bruising and to stimulate tissue repair.

The infusion of 1 oz. to a pint of boiling water is taken in wineglassful doses and is also used as an injection. It is a mucilaginous tonic, very healing and restorative, and is good in inflammations of the stomach and bowels, piles, and chronic dysentery.

A distilled water made from the whole plant has been used as a skin tonic and is an ingredient of expensive cosmetics.

Young shoots can be cooked, boiled and used as an asparagus substitute, they make an excellent vegetable and are widely used in Turkey. Root - cooked. Rich in starch. The root should be macerated for some time in water in order to remove bitter substances. Normally only used in times of famine, the root was powdered and then made into a bread by the North American Indians.

COMMENTS - According to the English-Chinese Rare Chinese Materia Medica, raw ho-shou-wu, that is, the dried root that has not been prepared with soybeans, is used to treat toxicosis (infections yielding abscess, swellings beneath the skin, sores, carbuncles, and eruptive diseases like rubella), inflammation, constipation, and hyperlipidemia.

The soybean-prepared ho-shou-wu is used as a tonic for yin and blood, nourishing the hair, strengthening the bones and muscles, and used to treat pale complexion, dizziness, tinnitus, premature graying of hair, weakness of loins and knees, numbness of extremities, metrorrhagia, profuse leucorrhea, weakness due to lingering diseases (e.g., malaria), and hyperlipemia.

According to evaluations done with raw and processed ho-shou-wu, the processed version does have different properties, and is the one with the most dramatic effects on preserving the immune system functions.

Processed ho-shou-wu is currently the only one that is regularly exported from China. During the past thousand years in China, processed ho-shou-wu has been used to nourish the liver and kidney, promote the growth of hair, treat alopecia, and premature graying of hair.

RELATIONS - ***Compare:*** Bell-p., Ruta, Calc., Symphytum.

REFERENCES - Murphy.

POLYGONUM AVICULARE

(Knot-grass)

PHARMACY - polyg-a. Polygonum aviculare. Knot-grass. Knotweed. Doorweed. Crawlgrass. N. O. Polygonaceae. Tincture of the whole plant. ***Historical dose:*** Tincture and all potencies.

HERBAL - Polyg-a., in material doses of tincture or 1c potency, was found useful in lung tuberculosis and intermittent fever and especially in arteriosclerosis. Erythema.

REFERENCES - Boericke.

POLYGONUM PUNCTATUM
(Smartweed)

PHARMACY - polyg. Polygonum punctatum. Smartweed. Polygonum hydropiper. Polygonum acre. Persicaria urens. Water pepper. Pursh. N. O. Polygonacae. Britain, North America. Tincture of whole fresh plant. ***Historical dose:*** Tincture and all potencies.

CLINICAL - Amenorrhea. Antrum, pain. Blepharitis. Colic, flatulent. Cough. Diarrhea. Dysentery. Dysmenorrhea. Dysuria. Eczema. Epilepsy. Gonorrhea. Gravel. Heart, disorders. Hemorrhoids. Hysteria. Laryngitis. Nephritis. Neuralgia. Orchitis. Prostatitis. Sciatica. Spermatic cord, pain. Spleen disorders. Strangury. Ulcers.

HERBAL - The Polygonum are named by Gerarde "Arse-smarts." Burnett regarded it as a splenic and as useful in old cases of syphilis. As a splenic, he found it was often required in cases of gout and in gouty eczema with much irritation; he used it with much benefit in the 6c, 12c and 30c.

Hale stated, "Smart Weed is a popular domestic remedy throughout U.S.A. Applied externally it has the effect of a mustard plaster and the leaves saturated with hot water are applied to relieve cramps and colic. Also as an emollient in inflammation and sprains."

HOMEOPATHIC - Polyg. was proved by W. E. Payne and others. The provers were all men, but clinical experience has shown a definite action in the female generative sphere, as amenorrhea, aversion to sex and congestion of the ovaries have been cured by it.

Acts upon the genito-urinary organs and the intestines, causing ***cutting pains,*** along the ureters, along ovarian ducts, up spine with bearing down. Pulsating, flashing, wandering pains in prostate. Coldness alternating or coincides with heat in the same or other part, burning in chest with cold feeling in pit of stomach. Smarting discharges.

Leading symptoms include aching pains in hips and loins with weight and tension in pelvis and tearing in groin, worse right. Metrorrhagia, also amenorrhea in young girls. ***Varicose veins***, hemorrhoids and rectal pockets. Burning in stomach followed by feeling of coldness in the pit of the stomach.

Abdomen - Cold feeling in stomach with burning in chest. Cutting pains with great rumbling, as if whole intestinal contents were in a fluid state. Griping pain with great rumbling, nausea and liquid feces. ***Flatulent colic***. Nausea..

Breasts - Shooting pains through the breasts.

Ears - Acute pain, on bending head down, better bending backwards.

Eyes - Puffiness under right eye. Lids twitch when closed and when lying down.

Face - Coldness in right face, when pain is most severe in left.

Female - Metrorrhagia, amenorrhea in young girls. Cutting pain along the fallopian tubes with bearing down. Aching pains in hips and loins. ***Sensation as if hips were being drawn together***. Sensation of weight and tension within pelvis.

Head - Acute pulsative pains in temples.

Kidneys - Nephritic colic with grinding, griping, cutting ***bellyache.*** Suppurative nephritis. Cystitis. Painful constriction at neck of bladder. Cutting pain along ureters. Urine scanty, dribbling, dark or calcareous, adherent sediment.

Limbs - Aching in lower limbs. Feet alternately hot and cold. Sore pains in heels.

Male - Scrotum excoriated. Pulsating, burning pain in prostate on urinating. Pain in testes, spermatic cord on urinating.

Modalities - Better from warmth. Worse pressure of clothes. Worse by cold, damp, change of temperature. Lying down causes pressure in occiput, dizziness and wavering of sight. Rising causes sudden pain in occiput.

Mouth - Itching, burning palate, wants to scratch it. Tongue feels swollen.

Rectum - ***Hemorrhoids with itching.*** Interior of anus studded with itching eminence. Liquid feces.

Sensations - As of sudden rising of scalp. As if whole intestinal contents were fluid. As if hips drawn together. As of galvanic shock through lower limbs.

Skin - ***Superficial ulcers and sores on lower limbs***, especially in females at menopause. Urticaria.

COMMENTS - Lancinating, cutting, pulsating, shooting, wandering and flashing pains. One prover described them as like aurora borealis, and a case of sciatica with pains of this description was cured with Polyg. The left temple was markedly affected, left side generally more so than right.

Epilepsy and hysteria. Marked diarrhea (Rheum. and Rumx.) and dysuria. Excessive weakness, trembling and sensitiveness to cold.

Cold sensations, alternating or coinciding with heat in the same or other parts. Coldness of right side of face when pain in left side was most severe. Burning in chest with cold feeling at pit of stomach. Feet burning, then suddenly cold.

RELATIONS - ***Compare:*** (1) Card-m. - ulcers. (2) Ham., Senec. (3) Polyg-pe. - kidney colic, stones, gangrene. (4) Polyg-s. (5) Polyg-a.

REFERENCES - Boericke. Clarke.

POLYGONUM SAGITTATUM

(Arrow-leaved)

PHARMACY - polyg-s. Polygonum Sagittatum. Arrow-leaved. N. O. Polygonaceae. ***Historical dose:*** Tincture and all potencies.

HOMEOPATHIC - Boger used Polyg-s. 2x for pains of nephritic colic, suppurative nephritis. Sharp pains along spine, burning inner side of right foot and ankle, itching of hard palate.

REFERENCES - Boericke.

POLYPORUS PINICOLA

(Pine Agaric)

PHARMACY - polyp-p. Polyporus pinicola. Pine agaric. N. O. Fungi. Tincture of fresh fungus. ***Historical dose:*** Tincture and all potencies.

CLINICAL - Anus, prolapse. Constipation. Hemorrhoids. ***Intermittent, fever.*** Liver, disorders. Malar bone, pain. Neuralgias. Prolapse, anus. Rheumatism. Spleen, disorders. Tonsils, enlarged.

HOMEOPATHIC - The pine agaric, Polyp-p., like the larch agaric, Polyporus officinalis, or Bol., was proved by Dr. Burt. The symptoms of the two have a very close resemblance and many are common to both.

Hale said it is a remedy for ague in the middle and southern states, taken during the intermission macerated in whisky. Quotidian fevers are most suited to it. Intermittent, remittent and bilious fevers with headache, yellow tongue, constant nausea, faintness at epigastrium and constipation.

Despondency, aching distress in many parts. Stiffness of back of fingers, enlarged tonsils with dysphagia and constant inclination to swallow. Neuralgic pains in head, face and temples, pain in liver and spleen with diarrhea or constipation and hemorrhoids these are the chief features of the proving.

Modalities - Better by rest. Worse in damp air. Worse after stool, motion, walking.

COMMENTS - Great lassitude. Congestion of head with vertigo, face hot and flushed, prickling sensation all over. Headache about 10 a.m. with pain in back, ankles and legs increasing until 3 p.m., then gradually better. Restless at night from pain in wrists and knee, rheumatic pains. Profuse perspiration.

RELATIONS - ***Compare:*** (1) Similar to its botanical relative, Polyporus officinalis or Bol. Deep dull, severe pain in shin bones, preventing sleep. (2) Bol-lu., Agar.

REFERENCES - Boericke. Clarke.

POPULUS CANDICANS

(Balm of Gilead)

PHARMACY - pop-c. Populus candicans. Balm of Gilead. Populus balsamifera. N. O. Salicaceae. The name Balm of Gilead tree is given to the Black Italian Poplar. Tincture of the resinous buds. ***Historical dose:*** Tincture and all potencies.

CLINICAL - Aphonia. Asthma. Brain, congested. Bullae. ***Colds.*** Constipation. Dysmenorrhea. Dyspepsia. Dysphagia. Ecthyma. Heart disorders. Liver, disorders. Phosphaturia. Sinusitis. Sunstroke. Throat, sore. Vagina, burning.

HERBAL - The name Populus balsamifera applies especially to the variety Populus candicans, but also to all P. balsamiferae. In England, the name "Balm of Gilead tree" is given to the Black Italian Poplar, which abounds in Italy, but the origin of which is not known.

C. F. Nichols gave an account of Pop-c., the effects of which he observed. "The resinous gum exuding from buds and stalks, deliciously aromatic in perfume is widely used to heal wounds, open sores and eruptions and often suppresses these latter to the harm of the patient."

As an application, Nichols said, it is like Arn., dangerous, though most people are not susceptible to its poisonous effect. He never saw blisters of the size of those of Pop-c. produced by any other drug. Blisters hung down like bags of water the size of walnuts. Burning was a common symptom in the eyes, nose, throat, bowels, vagina.

HOMEOPATHIC - Pop-c. seems to have a remarkable power over ***acute colds***, especially when accompanied by a deep, hoarse voice or even aphonia. Instantaneous voice-producer (Coca).

General insensibility of surface, worse back and abdomen, rubbing and pounding borne without pain and is grateful on account of warmth produced. Fingertips thickened, horny insensible to pinching and prickling.

MIND - Loquacity. Discusses her symptoms with everyone. Hopeless foreboding, worse after sleep. Fear and anguish. Expectation of death. Feels as if the will were paralyzed. Vanishing of thought. Forgets to finish a sentence. Voices sound distant and words just spoken seem as if uttered long ago, objects seem multiplied.

Abdomen - Flatulent colic, doubling the body forward. Pain in right hypochondrium with enlargement. Wears her clothes loose.

Back - Numbness in back radiating from spine. Burning weariness in lower back.

Chest - Rawness, soreness of chest, throat.

Eyes - Sensation as if left eye were twisted during the headache. Burning irritation in eyes, nose, mouth, throat, and air passages.

Face - Face yellow. Burning, prickling on face.

Female - Menses scanty, usually delaying, afterwards absent, then abundant, early, with dysmenorrhea, better hot cloths. Vagina burns as if scalded.

Food - Appetite lost, loathes meat. Nothing relished. Hungry but dares not eat for fear of choking.

Head - Weight on vertex. Hot head with cold limbs. Cold-sores on lips (Nat-m.). Burning irritation of eyes, nose, mouth, throat and air passages.

Heart - Pain in heart, stitches. Palpitations when rising or lying on left side with vertigo. Heart's sound irregular, usually muffled, worse before menses.

Kidneys - Urine strong, high colored, hot, scanty, increased, variously colored, red, dark, light, phosphates abundant. Urine dark, straw color, smoky.

Limbs - Fingertips thickened, horny, insensible to pinching and pricking. Nails blue as in ague (not thickened).

Lungs - Suffocation. Breathing dry, asthmatic with dyspnea. Sits bent forward with dry cough, worse lifting arms. Dry cough when tired. Cough caused by "cobwebs" in his throat. Cough of children caused by naso-pharyngeal catarrh, mucus drops from posterior sinuses.

Modalities - Better hot applications. Worse on moving, lifting arms, contact of clothes. Worse after sleep, before menses. Worse after food and drink.

Mouth - Speech thick. Taste bitter, sweet in morning.

Rectum - Stools small, round, preceded by cramps in abdomen, lack of expulsive power. Constipation, bowels feel hot and dry. Stools watery, green, alternating with constipation.

Sensations - Whole body feels swollen, bruised, lame, sore and painful, exhausted as in dry, sultry weather. Eye feels twisted with the headache.

Skin - Skin harsh, dry and cold with burning-stinging. Burning, prickling on face, chest, and hands. Blisters hanging down like bags of water.

Sleep - Sleepless after midnight with restlessness. Dreams frightful, vivid, fearful after fitful sleep.

Stomach - Belching of gas, feeling like hot steam. Nausea with a sinking in epigastrium. Vomits bile.

Temperature - Fever and unrest. Fever with congestion of brain, fullness, heaviness, dullness, soreness. Dry heat. Sweat on head and neck. Sudden coldness of limbs with numbness of them and heat of head.

Throat - Rawness and soreness of throat. Throat is red, dry. Throat and nostrils burn. Burning and paralysis in throat. Pharynx and larynx feel dry and the voice weak and toneless. ***Acute hoarseness***.

Tongue - Tongue white, dry, feels thick and numb. Tongue and mouth feel burnt and dry, but are moist, worse after food and drink.

Vertigo - Vertigo from lifting head. Vertigo and heat of head as if scorched by sun.

COMMENTS - W. C. Stilson related a case of poisoning in a man who one evening drank rum in which Balm of Gilead buds had been placed for making a liniment. A few hours later his wife heard him breathing heavily and on waking him found he could not speak.

Stilson found him only able to speak in hoarse whispers and he would forget in the middle of a sentence what he was going to say. Face ashy pale, wild look. Tongue and mouth dry. Throat dry, burning, constricted, felt as if spiders had spun webs on it. It was some days before he recovered.

Since this occasion, Stilson cured several cases of catarrhal hoarseness and aphonia with Pop-c. and one case of nervous aphonia. Mrs. S. had nervous prostration and, during the attack, aphonia. The aphonia remained after the patient got well otherwise.

Among the peculiar symptoms observed by Nichols is surface anesthesia with or without numbness. The fingertips are thickened, horny, insensible to pinching and pricking. Skin is harsh, generally dry and cold with a stinging burning behind the surface as if an eruption would appear or as if sweat would break out.

Numbness in back radiating from spine. Constipation, bowels feel hot and dry. The menses were at first scanty, later abundant and early, with dysmenorrhea pain, better by application of hot cloths.

RELATIONS - ***Antidoted by:*** Rhus-t. ***Compare:*** (1) Salx-a., Pop. (2) Salicylates. (3) worse contact of clothes, Lach.

REFERENCES - Boericke. Clarke.

POPULUS TREMULOIDES

(American Aspen)

PHARMACY - pop. Populus tremuloides. American aspen. Aspen. Poplar. N. O. Salicaceae. The American Aspen; the British Aspen is Populus tremula. Tincture of inner bark. Solution of Poplin. ***Historical dose:*** Tincture and all potencies.

CLINICAL - ***Acidity. Ague***. Ardor urine. Bladder, catarrh. ***Flatulence***. Gleet, chronic. ***Indigestion. Malaria.*** Nausea. ***Night-sweats.*** Prostate, enlarged. Vomiting.

HOMEOPATHIC - Pop. is a good remedy in bladder troubles after operations and in pregnancy. Dyspepsia and catarrh of the bladder, especially in elderly people. Cystitis. Fullness of head. Sensation of heat of the surfaces of the body. ***Night-sweats. Ague***.

Bladder - Severe tenesmus, painful scalding. Urine contains mucus and pus. Pain behind pubis, at end of urination.

Male - Prostate enlarged.

Stomach - ***Indigestion with flatulence and acidity***. Nausea and vomiting.

COMMENTS - The symptoms were provided by Pane (an eclectic), whom Hale quoted. Pane used Populus tremuloides in disorders of the bladder, urethra and prostate. Hale confirmed its action in bladder tenesmus and inflammation of the neck of the bladder.

Hale gave the case of a woman who had metritis, vaginismus and cystitis and was apparently cured. A ride on the cars brought back weight, pressure and aching in pelvis and bladder tenesmus with frequent desire to urinate. Pop. 3x removed all these symptoms in three days.

Hale noted that in the cases he cured there was little pain during urination, but as soon as the last drops were voided or a little before, there was a severe cramp-like pain just behind pubes, lasting ten to fifteen minutes.

RELATIONS - ***Compare:*** (1) Pop-c., Salx-n., Gaul. (2) Salin. and Salicylates. (3) Nux-v., Chin., Corn-f., Cann-i., Canth. ***Follows well:*** Cann-s., Canth. (succeeded after they had only partially helped).

REFERENCES - Boericke. Clarke.

PREDNISONE

(Corticosteroid)

PHARMACY - predn. Prednisone. A synthetic corticosteroid drug. ***Historical dose:*** All potencies.

CLINICAL - Acne. Adrenal glands. Allergies. Arthritis. Asthma. Blood, disorders. Bone, fractures. Bruises. Cancers. Cataracts. Colitis. Connective tissue. Crohn's disease. Cushing's syndrome. Enteritis. Eye, diseases. Facial, swelling. Fluid retention. Glaucoma. Growth, stunted. Headache. High blood pressure. Hives. Lung, diseases. Lupus erythematosus. Meningitis. Menses, irregular. Multiple sclerosis. Muscle, weakness. Nephrotic syndrome. Osteoporosis. Poison ivy. Rheumatism. Skin, diseases. Stomach, ulcer. Thyroiditis. Trichinosis. Tuberculosis. Ulcerative colitis. Urticaria. Vertigo. Wounds.

HOMEOPATHIC - Prednisone is a synthetic corticosteroid drug. Abnormal adrenal gland development. Cushing's syndrome. Thyroid gland inflammation. Certain cancers. Blood disorders. High blood pressure. Congestive heart failure.

Increased appetite. Weight gain, "moon-faced" appearance. Stunted growth in children. Sweating. Distended abdomen. Inflamed esophagus or pancreas. Fluid retention due to nephrotic syndrome. Peptic ulcer. Irregular menses.

Muscle weakness. Brittle bones, bone fractures. Osteoporosis. Painful hips of shoulders. Convulsions. Vertigo. Nervousness. Insomnia. Hyperactivity. Depression, mania or other psychiatric symptoms. Unusual fatigue or weakness.

Diseases of the connective tissue, including systemic lupus erythematosus. Flare-ups of multiple sclerosis. Rheumatoid arthritis and related disorders. Severe flare-ups of ulcerative colitis or enteritis. Lung diseases, including tuberculosis. Prevention of organ rejection. Trichinosis.

Skin diseases. Severe allergic conditions. Hives. Acne, rash. Thin, fragile skin. Purplish stripe marks on the skin. Bruising. Poor healing of wounds. Infections. Eye diseases of various kinds, including eye infection, cataracts and glaucoma. Bulging eyes. Blurred vision. Increased pressure in the eyes or skull. Headache. Meningitis.

MIND - Euphoria, severe depression. Insomnia. Mood changes, personality changes, psychotic behavior. May worsen any existing emotional instability.

RELATIONS - ***Compare:*** Cortico., Ars.

REFERENCES - Murphy.

PREMARIN

(Conjugated Estrogens)

PHARMACY - prem. Premarin. Conjugated estrogens. ***Historical dose:*** All potencies.

CLINICAL - Allergies. Backache. Breast, disorders. Constipation. Cough. Cramps. Depression. Diarrhea. Dysmenorrhea. Edema. Eye, disorders. Fatigue. Fever. Flatus. Hair, growth. Hair, loss. Headache. Hemorrhages. Hot, flushes. Indigestion. Joint, pain. Leucorrhea. Migraine. Nausea. Nervousness. Rash. Skin, disorders. Sleep, disorders. Sore, throat. Tumors. Vaginitis. Vomiting. Weakness.

HOMEOPATHIC - Nervousness. Depression. Sleep disturbances. Fatigue. Weakness. Dizziness. Fever. Changes in blood pressure. Blood clots. Increased heartbeat. Twitching. Increased muscle tone. Muscle pain. Backache. Leg cramps. Joint pain.

Migraine headache. Hair loss from the scalp, increased body hair. Eye disorders. Intolerance to contact lenses. Runny nose. Sore throat. Cough. Infection. Allergic reactions. Skin darkening, especially on the face. Skin rash or redness.

Skin tingling. Swelling of wrists and ankles. Yellow eyes and skin.

Appetite changes. Weight gain or loss. Bloating, fluid retention. Indigestion. Abdominal cramps, gas. Nausea, vomiting. Diarrhea, constipation. Gallbladder disease. Inflammation of the pancreas.

Abnormal vaginal bleeding. Painful menstruation. Heavy bleeding during menstruation. Vaginal yeast infection. Enlargement of benign tumors in the uterus. Breast swelling and tenderness. Excessive flow of breast milk. Sex-drive changes.

RELATIONS - ***Compare:*** Sep., Foll., Estro., Lach., Puls.

REFERENCES - Murphy.

PRIMULA OBCONICA

(Primrose)

PHARMACY - prim-o. Primula obconica. Primrose. Tibetan Primrose. N. O. Primulaceae. Primulae. Tincture of whole fresh plant. ***Historical dose:*** Tincture and all potencies.

CLINICAL - Blisters. Chapped, hands. Eczema. Eyes, inflammation. Itching. Liver, pain. Skin, disorders. Spleen, pains. ***Weakness***.

HERBAL - Prim-o. is an ornamented variety of primrose. Gardeners, amateur and professional, have discovered after much suffering that in some people it has a powerful action on the skin, taking place chiefly by contact but partly by effluvia.

HOMEOPATHIC - The poison of the Primrose is in its *glandular hairs*, which break easily and discharge an irritating fluid which is absorbed into the skin. But skin symptoms of poisoning appear in sensitive patients even without coming in direct contact with the plant, mere nearness begin sufficient, like poison ivy.

Prim-o. has deep infiltration and tension of tissues. ***Paralyzed sensation. Weakness***. Pain in liver and spleen. Pharyngeal soreness alternates with diminished facial irritation. Blisters. Intermittent symptoms, worse right side.

Abdomen - Pain in region of liver, and a less severe pain in spleen, worse by bending from side to side.

Eyes - Burning irritation of eyeballs and eyelids, nostrils, and mouth. Lids greatly swollen, covered with large bullae. Lids half closed, stiff and immovable.

Face - Moist eczema. Papular eruption on chin. Burns at night. Urticaria-like eruption. Eyelids swollen.

Limbs - Eczema on arms, wrists, forearms, hands, papular and excoriated. Purple blotches on back of hands, palmar surface stiff. Blisters on fingers. Palms dry and hot. Cracking over joints and fingers. Rheumatic pain around shoulder.

Skin - Eruption between fingers. ***Great itching***, worse at night, red and swollen like erysipelas. Tumefied. ***Small papules on a raised base.*** Skin symptoms accompanied by febrile symptoms.

Temperature - At night feverish, hands and face would burn, then intolerable itching.

COMMENTS - The Rev. F. H. Brett, who was one of the first to notice its poisonous properties, undertook to prove it. He had handled the plants freely up to that time without experiencing any ill effect. He cut up some young plants and added some vigorous fresh leaves of an old one and made a tincture.

This he allowed to stand for a week and then took three or four drops, three times a day for four days. Two days after ceasing to take it symptoms began to develop in the right little finger and two days afterwards in the right thumb. These became very intense and ran a chronic course.

He could not go near a plant of Prim-o. without worsening the symptoms. They were also worse at night, and by rubbing or scratching. At the same time, Brett noted that the pains in the liver and spleen to which he had been subject now troubled him no more. The right hand was much more affected than the left.

Clarke cured a chronic psoric dry eruption on the leg of a woman with Prim-o. 3c. Cooper relieved a case of severe eczema on the leg with bleeding.

RELATIONS - ***Compare:*** (1) Rhus-t., Fago. (antidotal). (2) Hume., similar skin symptoms. (3) Anag., Prim-v., Verat.

REFERENCES - Boericke. Clarke.

PRIMULA VERIS

(Cowslip)

PHARMACY - prim-v. Primula veris. Cowslip. Primula vulgaris. Primula officinalis. N. O. Primulaceae. Primulae. Tincture of entire fresh plant. ***Historical dose:*** Tincture and all potencies.

CLINICAL - Dropsy. Eczema. Fevers. Gouty, pains. Migraine. Neuralgia. Rheumatic pains. Strokes, threatened. Vertigo. Voice disorders.

HERBAL - According to The Treasury of Botany, the flowers of Prim-v. are said to be narcotic. "Cowslip wine" is a favorite remedy in the country for many small disorders.

HOMEOPATHIC - Schier, of Mentz, proved a tincture of the fresh plant including the root. The duration of action is only a few days in healthy persons.

Prim-v. has threatened strokes, arising from depression. Cerebral congestion with neuralgia. Migraine. ***"Pressure at heart."*** Wandering dropsy. Rheumatic and gouty pains. Chronic eczema.

Ears - Buzzing in ears, better in open air.

Head - Sensation of a band around head, cannot keep hat on (Carb-ac.). Skin of forehead tense.

Kidneys - Urine smells strongly of violets.

Limbs - Weight and lassitude in limbs, especially the ***shoulders***. Right axillary muscles painful. Burning in hollow of right hand. Drawing pain in thumb and big toe.

Lungs - Cough with burning and prickling in respiratory tracts. Weak voice.

Modalities - Worse by bent position, stooping, movement. Worse in a room, in a closed carriage, traveling by rail. Worse in open air.

Vertigo - Violent vertigo, as if everything turned around. Fear of falling when standing up.

COMMENTS - Schier commended it as an external application when there is no skin lesion, "as this remedy has a certain relation with the skin. Prudence is necessary here, especially for persons with sensitive and easily vulnerable skin."

Cooper cured with Prim-v. a case of eczema of the hands after Prim-o. had failed. He also cured with it eczema palmaris of years' duration in a man, aged 70.

Cooper also cured a case of wandering dropsy with Prim-v. In a cancer case, one dose caused the disappearance of dropsy from the leg and led to oppression at the heart. Cooper thought this a characteristic aggravation.

RELATIONS - ***Compare:*** (1) Cycl., Ran-b. (2) Evening Primrose - exhausting, watery diarrhea, cholera infantum, hydrocephalus. (3) Prim-f. - the wild primrose - dermatitis, especially on index fingers and thumbs.

REFERENCES - Boericke. Clarke.

PRINOS VERTICILLATUS

(Black Alder)

PHARMACY - prin. Prinos verticillatus. Black alder. N. O. Aquifoliaceae. Tincture of the berries. Tincture of fresh bark. ***Historical dose:*** Tincture and all potencies.

CLINICAL - Diarrhea. Fever.

HERBAL - The genus Prinos is very closely allied to the hollies. The Treasury of Botany reported that "The bark of Prin. is bitter and has been used in the treatment of fever and in the form of a lotion as an application in cases of gangrene. The berries are tonic and emetic."

HOMEOPATHIC - The only recorded experiment with Prin., swallowing twenty berries, showed the effect to be vomiting, plus an extremely profuse greenish diarrhea. Prin. increased the appetite and produced a feeling of well-being in spite of great loss of weight.

REFERENCES - Clarke.

PROGESTERONE

PHARMACY - prog. Progesterone. ***Historical dose:*** All potencies.

CLINICAL - Acne. Amenorrhea. ***Bloating.*** Breast, disorders. Constipation. Cramps. ***Depression.*** Edema. Endometriosis. Epilepsy. ***Fatigue.*** Hair, growth. Hair, loss. Headache. Hemorrhages. Hormonal, disorders. Hot flashes. Infertility. Insomnia. Menopausal, disorders. Menstrual, disorders. Migraine. Miscarriage. Nausea. Obesity. Osteoporosis. ***Premenstrual syndrome.*** Vaginal, dryness.

HOMEOPATHIC - Progesterone is a hormone secreted by the ovary in the second two weeks of the menstrual cycle in reproductive age ovulating women. Progesterone, or progesterone-like substances called progestogens or progestins, are ingested by women in birth control pills and menopausal hormone replacement therapy.

Progesterone acts to stabilize the tissue lining of the uterus (endometrium) so if it is absent, such as with ovarian anovulation, irregular and heavy menstrual bleeding often occurs after a period without any menstrual bleeding. Thus progesterone is used to prevent this irregularity of bleeding if it is given continuously.

If, on the other hand, a onetime bolus of progesterone is given such as with a shot or with only 5 days of oral pills, then the falling progesterone levels will actually cause an estrogen-primed endometrium to slough and therefore start a menses.

It is sometimes used to induce a menstrual period or regulate abnormal bleeding problems if menses are skipping or bleeding is irregular or prolonged. Progesterone has been used as therapy for premenstrual syndrome and for women with infertility or frequent miscarriages.

Too much progesterone often causes tiredness and even sedation. This side effect can be beneficial in a women who has epilepsy or even uterine irritability causing preterm labor because progesterone in high doses can decrease seizure activity and uterine contractions.

Progesterone tends to promote vaginal dryness by counteracting the effect on lubrication of estrogens, and it can also decrease the amount of menstruation or block it entirely by reversing estrogen effect on the growth of the uterine lining.

Progestegens can cause some medical conditions to worsen, examples are asthma, heart failure, epilepsy and migraine headache. Natural progesterone tends to have fewer side effects.

Progesterone can cause blood clots, particularly in the legs. Irregular vaginal bleeding. Breast tenderness. Liver disease. Painful swelling of the abdomen. Bloating. Nausea. Constipation. Increased appetite. Weight gain.

Headache. Insomnia. Hot flashes. Profuse sweat. Acne. Unwanted hair growth. Tiredness, irritability. Loss of concentration. Depression, anxiety. Moodiness. Overly emotional.

MIND - Loss of concentration. Foggy thinking. Inability to make decisions. Inability to handle even the smallest amount of stress. Anxiety, irritability. Anger. Anti-social. Panic attacks. Very emotional, feeling overwhelmed. ***Mood changes.***

Severe depression. Feeling of despair and hopelessness. Uncontrollable crying, immense sadness. Suicidal depression. Psychotic. Delusion, feel like they are in another's body.

Abdomen - ***Bloating in abdomen,*** cramps, worse before menses.

Back - Back pain.

Breasts - Breasts tender and sore.

Face - Puffiness in face. Whole face broke out in acne.

Female - Premenstrual syndrome. Amenorrhea. Menses skipping, bleeding is irregular or prolonged. Infertility or frequent miscarriages. Vaginal dryness. Menopausal disorders.

Food - Increased appetite. Craving for sweets.

Head - Sick headaches.

Limbs - Puffiness in hands. Joint pains.

Lungs - Shortness of breath.

Modalities - Worse heat, before menses, before menopause.

Perspiration - Profuse sweating.

Rectum - Constipation.

Skin - Greasy skin. Unwanted hair growth.

Sleep - Sleeplessness. Strange dreams.

Stomach - Sick feeling. Bloating. Nausea.

Temperature - Hot flashes.

RELATIONS - ***Compare:*** Sep., Foll., Estro., Lach., Puls., Aur.

REFERENCES - Murphy.

PROPOLIS

PHARMACY - propo. Propolis. Red or brown resinous substance collected by bees from buds for use in constructing hives. ***Historical dose:*** All potencies.

CLINICAL - Acne. Allergies. Bruises. Burns. Cancer. Chilly. Colds. Coughs. Earache. Fatigue. Fungus. Herpes. Herpes zoster. Immune system. Influenza. Lung, ailments. Lung, infections. Nasal congestion. Polyuria. Shingles. Skin, disorders. Sore, throats. Sunburns. Ulcers. ***Weariness.*** Wounds.

HOMEOPATHIC - Depending upon its precise composition, propolis may show powerful local antibiotic and anti-fungal properties. Generally efficient in treating skin burns. Allergies.

Great weariness. More tired in the morning than usual, even after sleeping longer. Symptoms appear and disappear suddenly. The action of the remedy is quick and violent. It can be compared with Acon., Bell. and Cham.

It may stimulate the immune system, but some warn that it should not be taken if the user is likely to have severe allergic reaction to bees. Old beekeepers recommend a piece of propolis kept in the mouth as a remedy for a sore throat.

Ears - Earache.

Face - Herpes labialis. Red blotches and spots on face.

Food - ***Increased appetite.*** Desire for every kind of food, especially fruit, bread. On waking strong desire for sweets. Increased thirst.

Head - Headache. Various pains of the head, similar to sinus troubles.

Kidneys - Frequent urination at night in spite of normal intake of fluids.

Modalities - Weariness, cough, worse morning on waking.

Mouth - Bad smell from mouth. Tongue coated grayish, except for the tip of the tongue.

Nose - Watery discharge from nose, preceded by fleeting pain in frontal sinuses. Tingling in nose.

Sleep - Anxious dreams. Dreams of traveling. Dreams of quarrels. Awakes with anger.

Temperature - Chilly. Icy-cold hands. Coldness of fingers between 10 a.m. and noon. Freezing sensation over whole body. Transitory chilliness at 4 p.m.

Throat - Dry sensation in throat and posterior nares.

RELATIONS - ***Compare:*** Alf.

REFERENCES - Murphy.

PROPYLAMINUM

PHARMACY - prop. Propylaminum. Trimethylaminum. Found in many plants and in herring-brine. Solution. ***Historical dose:*** All potencies.

CLINICAL - Ankles, pains. Diarrhea. Fever. Joint, pains. ***Numbness.*** Prosopalgia. Rheumatic fever. Rheumatism. Wrists, pains.

HOMEOPATHIC - Prop. is found in many plants (Chen-v., Crat., Phal., Pyrus-c., Arn., Cot., Fagu., etc.) and in the Trimethylaminum, which is, among other sources, prepared from herring-brine, and has a very unpleasant and penetrating fish-like odor.

At one time it was regarded as a panacea in cases of acute rheumatism. Dissipates fever and pain in a day or two in acute rheumatism. Rheumatic prosopalgia and rheumatic metastases, especially heart lesions. Rheumatism, needle held in fingers gets too heavy.

Pain in wrists and ankles, worse slightest motion (Bry.), unable to stand. ***Tingling and numbness of fingers***. Great restlessness and thirst. Experiments show that Prop. diminishes the amount of urea excreted.

COMMENTS - Hansen indicated great pains in the wrist joints, also great restlessness. Pains in ankle joints from standing, worse slight movement.

Dr. C. Smith noted "Rheumatism, when the needle held in the fingers gets so heavy she cannot sew." "Copious diarrhea with pains in ankle joints but not in wrists, thirst for large quantities of cold water like Bry." Weakness in lumbar and lower dorsal region.

REFERENCES - Boericke. Clarke.

PROTEUS BACILLUS

(Bowel Nosode)

PHARMACY - prot. Proteus bacillus. Bowel nosode. Proteus bacteria. Intestinal bacteria. Bacillus proteus mirabilis reltgeri. Nosodes. ***Historical dose:*** All potencies.

CLINICAL - Acne. Aerophagy. Agoraphobia. ***Allergies.*** Alopecia. Angina pectoris. Backaches. Blood, clots. ***Boils.*** Convulsions. Coronary, disease. Cystitis. Diarrhea. Duodenal, ulcers. ***Dyspepsia. Food, allergies.*** Eczema. Edema. Gastric, ulcers. Headache. Hematemesis. Herpes. Hysteria. ***Indigestion.*** Intermittent, claudication. Leucorrhea. Meibomian cyst. Melancholy. Ménière's disease. Meningitis. ***Migraines.*** Neuralgia. Neurasthenia. Otitis. Phlebitis. Premature, senility. Pyelitis. Pyelonephritis. Raynaud's syndrome. Rhinitis. Sciatica. Senility. Spinal, neurasthenia. Ulcers. Vaginitis. Vertigo. Worms. Writer's cramp.

HOMEOPATHIC - Culture of a bacteria of the Proteus genus: Proteus vulgaris, mirabilis, morganii, reltgeri. Proteus, a bacterium frequently found in the intestinal region, is a nosode whose range of action concerns essentially phenomena of digestive problems. G. Sevaus conducted a detailed clinical study, but there is no homeopathic proving.

Digestive allergies. Sudden nervous symptoms. Extreme feeling of intra-cranial tension. Meningitis with attacks of fever. Premature senility.

Convulsion, epileptiform fits. Cramps leg, calf. Neuro-arthritic diathesis. After-attack of phlebitis. Long, drawn-out convalescence. Pain aggravated by effort. Intermittent claudication. Icy cold feet.

Morbid alternations (Psor., Sulph.).

MIND - Prostration of mind, mental exhaustion. Brain fag. Confusion of mind. Memory weakness. Forgetfulness of words while speaking. Vanishing of thoughts. Premature senility.

Restlessness, nervousness. Feeling of extreme nervous tension and over-exertion. ***Cannot handle things anymore, overwhelmed by stress.*** Anxiety in stomach. Anguish during discomfort. Ailments from excitement.

Melancholy. Sadness, despondency, depression. Suicidal disposition. Thinks about suicide without really wanting to die. Weeping, tearful mood when telling about her illness.

Sensitive. Horrible things, sad stories affect her profoundly. Frightened easily. Fear of being alone, of the dark. Agoraphobia. Fear something will bad happen. Fear of losing his reason. Hysteria.

Timidity. Want of self confidence. Offended easily. Fear of opinion of others. Aversion to company. Intolerant of contradiction. Anger from contradiction. Tense, irritable. Quarrelsomeness, scolding.

Brainstorm, outbursts of anger. Anger, throws things away, ***impulse to kill. Temper tantrums.*** Destructiveness. Hurls objects held in the hand, kicks out. Children rolling about on the floor when angry.

Abdomen - Hematemesis and melaena. Aerophagy. Acrid dyspepsia. Gastric and duodenal ulcers. Spasmodic colon infections. Oxyuric diseases.

Back - Backaches. Spinal neurasthenia. Hernia.

Chest - Eruptions, boils in axilla.

Constitutions - Allergic and psoric constitutions. Carbonic, flouric, and phosphoric constitutions.

Ears - Acute or burning pains like otitis, but without fever. Noises during vertigo. Ménière's disease.

Eyes - Burning pains. Acute pains, stitching. Pains ameliorated by pressure. Eyes red, tired by light. Intermittent failing of sight. Meibomian cyst.

Face - Dryness of lips. Corners of mouth cracked. Itching of upper lip. Herpes about lips. Acne on chin.

Female - Blood-streaked, brownish discharge before menses. Menses regular, with blood clots for seven days. Menses clotted, protracted. Fibrous blood clots at the end of menses. Leucorrhea before menses, between menses. Leucorrhea, acrid, brown, copious. Leucorrhea offensive, thick. Copious white discharge, worse during ovulation. Vaginitis. Metritis of the cervix. Vulvar pruritus. Anal and vulvar boils.

Food - ***Food allergies.*** Desires fats, butter, eggs, rich food. Desires sweets, sugar, salt. Aversion to butter, pork, beef. ***Aversion to eggs, especially hard-boiled eggs.*** Aversion to cranberries, raw food, salads, green beans, cucumber, onions, garlic. Aversion to chocolate, which he cannot digest. Worse fats, rich food, eggs, garlic, cranberries, cucumber and chocolate.

Head - ***Digestive migraine.*** Frontal headache with feeling of heaviness, aggravated during the week preceding menses. Headache in the morning. Headache with diarrhea and furred tongue. Pressing pains. Beats head against the bed. Knocks head against things. Hair falls out. Alopecia.

Heart - Coronary disease. Angina pectoris. Feeling of weight in the precordial region. Palpitations after excitement. Palpitations from the slightest emotion, when lying down.

Kidneys - Pyelitis. Pyelonephritis. Pain in the loin. Cystitis, after eating pork. Violent, burning pains in the urethra. Urine cloudy and fetid. Whitish tissues in the urine.

Limbs - Arthritic diathesis. Sciatic pain. Intermittent claudication. Legs look bruised. Pain in the calf, pain forcing him to walk with a stick, cramps in the legs. Pain in calves of legs after walking. ***Muscular cramps.*** Functional or professional contracture. Writer's cramp, pianist's cramp, dancer's cramp. Spasms of the hands. Flexor contraction of the little finger. Cannot close the hand. Awkwardness of hands, drops things. Moist eruptions, eczema, on backs of hands. Coldness and blueness of hands. Feet numb, as if frozen, aggravated by cold weather. Hammer-toes.

Lungs - Cough with sputum.

Modalities - Better resting, lying down, one hour after rising. Better from stretching, eating, drinking whisky. Better from mild temperature, in the mountains. Aggravation in the morning on waking, from exertion, from climbing stairs. Worse from drinking wine. Worse in stormy weather, cold, winter, heat, exposure to sun. Worse from lying down, at night.

Mouth - Aphthae and mouth ulcers. Taste of salt in the mouth. Gums sensitive. Cracking at the corners of the lips, resistant to treatment.

Nose - Impression of greasy discharge at the back of the nose. Hypertrophic chronic rhinitis. Nasal blockage. Nasal obstruction in warm room.

Rectum - ***Diarrhea from excitement.*** Diarrhea with headache and furred tongue. Alternation of diarrhea and constipation. Constipation with empty urging. Sensation of a lump. Hematemesis and melaena. Presence of oxyuris in stools. Stools yellow, soft, in the morning after breakfast.

Skin - Eczema. Itching vesicles. ***Boils maturing slowly.*** Herpes. ***Herpetic eruptions at muco-cutaneous margins.*** Papular, pustular eruption, erythematous, dry, peeling. Severe pruritus. Nails split. Hair falls out. Alopecia.

Sleep - Dreams of dead people, of death or dying.

Stomach - Stomach pain while fasting. Empty sensation in stomach, not better eating. Acidity, heartburn, sourness. Acrid dyspepsia. Aerophagy. Gastric and duodenal ulcers.

Temperature - Copious perspiration from the axilla, falling in large drops, clammy hands.

Throat - Acute pharyngitis with difficulty speaking. Dryness during excitement.

Vertigo - Vertigo when looking at moving objects, while riding in a carriage, during railroad travel. Vertigo with feeling that the ground is coming up to meet him. Vertigo, accompanied by colored lights.

COMMENTS - Keynote ***suddenness and***

violence with nervous symptoms and spasm. Slow build up of stress with a sudden catastrophe. Emotional hysteria (Ign., Nat-m.). Violent temper in a child with kicking.

Spasm in peripheral vessels, Raynaud's Syndrome (Sec.). Migraines headaches with blurred vision and Meniere's syndrome. Petit mal attacks of epilepsy.

Herpetic eruptions with pain out of proportion to the lesion. Angioneurotic edema. Hemorrhage or perforation without any previous stomach symptoms but with a history of nervous strain.

RELATIONS - ***Related:*** Ign., Nat-m., Apis, Cupr. ***Compare:*** (1) Psor. - Inhibition, chilliness, sadness, periodic migraine, nocturnal need to eat, morning diarrhea, weakness in the back and joints, evil-smelling eruptions, appearing in winter, disappearing in summer. (2) Sulph. - Allergic, psoric conditions, burning skin with eruptions and itching. Impatient, quarrelsome, asthenic. (3) Tub. - Unstable, emotional, aggravated by physical or mental effort, emaciation, sweating, morning diarrhea. Aggravated by damp and cold and weather changes.

REFERENCES - Bach. Julian.

PROZAC

(Fluoxetine Hydrochloride)

PHARMACY - proz. Prozac. Fluoxetine hydrochloride. An allopathic anti-depressant drug. ***Historical dose:*** All potencies.

CLINICAL - Acne. ***Allergies.*** Amenorrhea. Amnesia. Anemia. Angina, pectoris. Arthritis. Asthma. Belching. Bi-polar, disorder. Blood, clots. Bronchitis. Bruising. ***Bulimia.*** Bursitis. Chronic, fatigue. Colitis. Coma. Conjunctivitis. Convulsions. Cough. Depression. Dehydration. Diabetes. Diarrhea. Duodenal, ulcer. ***Eating, disorders.*** Eczema. Edema. Gallstones. Gout. Hair, loss. Headaches. Heart, attack. Heart, failure. Hemorrhages. Hepatitis. Hirsutism. ***Hives.*** Hypertension. Hypotension. ***Impotency.*** Indigestion. Influenza. ***Insomnia.*** Itching. Kidney, disorders. Menstrual, disorders. Migraines. Miscarriage. Nausea. Nervousness. ***Obsessive compulsive disorder.*** Premenstrual, syndrome. Psoriasis. ***Rashes.*** Salpingitis. Seborrhea. Shingles. Skin, disorders. Spasms. Stomach, ulcer. Strokes. Tooth, problems. Tremors. Twitching. Urticaria. Vomiting. Weakness.

HOMEOPATHIC - Changes in sleep habits. Increased fatigue. Difficulty concentrating. Slowed thinking. Feelings of guilt or worthlessness. Suicidal thoughts. Decreased sex drive.

Involuntary movements. Lack of muscle coordination. Twitching. Tremors. Weakness. Vague feeling of bodily discomfort. Nervousness. Drowsiness and fatigue. Headache. Flu symptoms. Sweating. Chills. Fever. Skin inflammation. Hemorrhage. High blood pressure.

Enlargement of or increased activity of thyroid gland. Inflammation of the esophagus. Tooth problems. Changes in appetite. Weight gain or loss. Fluid retention. Dehydration. Kidney disorders. Diabetes. Flatus. Diarrhea.

Pelvic pain. Premenstrual syndrome, with anxiety, depression, irritability or persistent anger, mood swings, and tension. Physical problems that accompany premenstrual, syndrome include bloating, breast tenderness, headache, and joint and muscle pain.

MIND - Changeable moods and emotions. Anxiety. Irrational ideas. Agitation. Paranoid reaction. Hostility. Antisocial behavior. Nervousness. ***Obsessive-compulsive disorder. Bulimia, binge-eating*** followed by deliberate vomiting.

Euphoria. Exaggerated feeling of well-being. Apathy. Confusion. Difficulty concentrating. Slowed thinking. Amnesia. Depersonalization. Hallucinations. Delusions. Feelings of guilt or worthlessness. ***Suicidal thoughts.*** Loss of consciousness. Coma.

Abdomen - Bloating and gas. Colitis. Duodenal ulcer. Hemorrhage from intestines.

Bladder - Urinary tract disorders. Frequent urination. Hematuria, albuminuria, polyuria.

Blood - Anemia. High blood sugar. Leukocytosis. Leukopenia. Blood clots. Thrombophlebitis. Stroke.

Breast - Enlargement. Breast pain and swelling. Breast tenderness. Fibrocystic breast.

Chest - Angina pectoris. Severe chest pain.

Ear - Ear pain. Ringing in the ears. Deafness.

Eyes - Dry eyes. Dilated pupils. Conjunctivitis (pinkeye). Glaucoma. Bleeding. Amblyopia. Sensitivity to light. Photophobia. Vision problems. Double vision. Nystagmus.

Face - Facial swelling due to fluid retention. Excess growth of coarse hair on face.

Female - Amenorrhea. Abnormal stoppage of menstrual flow. Premenstrual syndrome. Menstrual disorders. Painful menstruation. Excess uterine or vaginal bleeding. Miscarriage. Salpingitis. Decreased sex drive.

Food - Increased appetite. Lack or loss of appetite. Thirst.

General - Chronic fatigue.

Head - Headaches. Migraines. Hydrocephalus. Hair loss.

Heart - Angina pectoris. Low blood pressure upon standing. High blood pressure. Slowing of heart rate. Irregular heartbeat. Rapid or throbbing heartbeat. Heart attack. Heart failure.

Kidney - Pyelonephritis. Kidney calculus.

Limbs - Abnormal gait. Gout. Arthritis. Rheumatoid arthritis. Bursitis. Bone pain. Tremors. Muscle spasm. Leg cramps.

Liver - Gallstones. Liver enlargement. Hepatitis.

Lung - Bronchitis. Cough. Asthma. Rapid breathing. Temporary cessation of breathing. Lung fibrosis.

Male - Abnormal ejaculation. Impotence. Decreased sex drive.

Mouth - Sores. Tingling sensation around the mouth. Dry mouth. Increased salivation. Bleeding gums. Gingivitis. Inflammation. Stomatitis. Slurred speech.

Nerves - Neuralgia. Convulsions. Uncoordinated movements. Decreased reflexes.

Nose - Sinus or nasal inflammation. Nosebleeds.

Rectum - Inability to control bowel movements. Diarrhea. Dark, tarry stool. Bloody diarrhea.

Skin - Itching. Sweating. Skin discoloration. Acne. Eczema. Psoriasis. Hives. Shingles. Urticaria. Rashes. Reddish or purplish spots on the skin. Bruising. Seborrhea.

Sleep - Drowsiness and fatigue. Yawning. Insomnia. Inability to fall or stay asleep. Strange dreams.

Stomach - Esophagitis. Gastritis. Indigestion. Hiccups. Belching. Nausea. Vomiting. Inflammation of the stomach lining. Stomach ulcer. Vomiting blood. Hemorrhage.

Temperature - Reduction of body temperature. Chills and fever. Flu symptoms. Infection.

Throat - Sore throat. Difficulty in swallowing.

Tongue - Taste altered, lost. Inflammation, swelling of the tongue.

Vertigo - Dizziness.

COMMENTS - Muscle spasms and weakness. Muscle inflammation. Tissue inflammation, below skin. Skin inflammation and disorders. Inflammation of eyes and eyelids. Fluid buildup in larynx and lungs. Spitting blood, stomach and intestinal. Colitis. Female milk production. Stupor.

RELATIONS - ***Compare:*** Aur., Carc., Staph., Anac.

REFERENCES - Murphy.

PRUNELLA VULGARIS

(Self Heal)

PHARMACY - prune. Prunella vulgaris. Self Heal. N. O. Labiatae. ***Historical dose:*** Tincture and all potencies.

CLINICAL - Headache. Leucorrhea. Sore, throat. Wounds.

HERBAL - Prunella vulgaris is useful in sore and relaxed throat. Astringent. Internal bleeding, leucorrhea, etc. The infusion of 1 oz to 1 pt of boiling water is taken internally in doses of a wineglassful. Externally it is used as a gargle and injection.

Culpeper wrote, "Here is another herb of Venus, Self-heal whereby when you are hurt you may heal yourself; it is a special herb for inward and outward wounds. Take it inwardly in syrups for inward wounds, outwardly in unguents and plasters for outward. The juice thereof used with oil of roses to annoint the temples and forehead is very effectual to remove headache."

COMMENTS - There is an old German saying that "He needs neither physician nor surgeon that hath Self-heal and to help himself. "

REFERENCES - Murphy. Potter.

PRUNUS PADUSRHEUM

(Bird Cherry)

PHARMACY - prun-p. Prunus padusrheum. Bird cherry. Cerasus padus. Padus racemosa. Padus vulgaris. N. O. Rosaceae. Tincture of leaves and bark of small twigs collected when in blossom. ***Historical dose:*** Tincture and all potencies.

CLINICAL - Headache. Heart, disorders. Rectum, pains.

HERBAL - The fruit is small, black and nauseous to the taste. In Scotland it is known as the Hayberry. The Treasury of Botany noted that in the north of Europe it is made into a liqueur. The juices can also be expressed and drunk with milk, while the residue of the fruit can be kneaded into cakes. The plant is now classed with the cherries, but Clarke retained it under its old name.

HOMEOPATHIC - Lembke's proving of Prun-p. brought out marked symptoms in the head, rectum, chest and heart. Pains were pressive in head and beneath sternum, sticking in rectum. Tumultuous heartbeats. The symptoms were worse by pressure, sitting, standing, stooping and walking.

RELATIONS - ***Compare:*** (1) Heart, Crat., Prun., Prun-v., Laur.

REFERENCES - Clarke.

PRUNUS SPINOSA

(Blackthorn)

PHARMACY - prun. Prunus spinosa. Blackthorn. Sloe. N. O. Rosaceae. Tincture of buds just before flowering. ***Historical dose:*** Tincture and all potencies.

CLINICAL - Angina pectoris. Appetite, lost. Ascites. Breast, pain. Cardiac, dropsy. Choroiditis. ***Ciliary, neuralgia.*** Cystitis. Dropsy. Dyspnea. Dysuria. Earache. Eyes, choroiditis. Flatulent. Glaucoma. Heart, affection. ***Headaches.*** Hernia. Herpes zoster. Leucorrhea. Menorrhagia. Metrorrhagia. ***Neuralgias.*** Sprains. Strangury. Stricture. ***Toothache.*** Vitreous, opacities.

HOMEOPATHIC - Prun. was proved by Wahle. The symptoms resemble those of Prun-p. in general, but some very strongly characterized ones were produced. Acts especially on the nerves, respiratory orbital and on urinary organs. Special action on the urinary organs and the head.

Shooting from within out, from before backward. The pains were pressive, and out pressing and out-shooting. Lightning like pains, wandering, causing ***shortness of breath.*** Spraining pains and pains which take away the breath.

Pains are felt in the skull, eye, root of the nose and ears. The teeth feel raised out of their sockets. Glaucoma, choroido-retinitis, irido-choroiditis, irido-cyclitis. ***Ciliary neuralgia*** (Spig.). Neuralgias. Nerve paralysis. Anasarca and edema. Dropsy caused by defective heart. Ankle and foot feel sprained. Pains after shingles. Cramps. Compensatory effects.

MIND - Restlessness, walks about constantly, cannot remain in one place.

Abdomen - Ascites. Cramp-like pain in bladder region, worse from walking.

Back - As of a lump below the left scapula.

Causations - Ill effects of sun, sprains, over-lifting.

Chest - Angina pectoris.

Eyes - Ciliary neuralgia. Shooting like lightning through the brain to occiput. ***Sudden pain in eyeball as if it would burst,*** better by lachrymation. Irido-choroiditis. Opacity of vitreous humor.

Female - Menses, thin, watery, too early, too copious, with sacral pain. Leucorrhea, acrid, watery purulent, staining yellow.

Head - Pressing, tearing pain beneath skull. ***Shooting from right frontal bone through brain to occiput.*** Headache from heat of sun. Piercing toothache, as if teeth were pulled out, worse taking anything warm.

Heart - Hypertrophied. Cardiac dropsy. Angina pectoris. Throbbing of carotid arteries. Knocking at heart with labored breathing, worse least motion. Furious beating of heart, worse slightest motion.

Kidneys - Neuralgic dysuria. Tenesmus of bladder. Ineffectual effort to urinate. Urgent desire to urinate, urine reaches glans penis and then ***returns with violent pain and spasms*** and tenesmus in rectum. Cramp in bladder from pressure of flatus, must double up to urinate. Glans pains on urinating. Must press a long time before urine appears. Pulsating pudendum. Stream of urine thin like a thread or forked.

Limbs - Edema of feet. Itching at the fingertips as if frozen. Thumb as if sprained, hindering writing.

Lungs - Oppression of chest, anxious, short respiration. Wheezing when walking. Short breath with pains. Feeling as if air inhaled did not reach the pit of stomach, has to yawn and try to take a deep inspiration. Air hunger.

Male - Pulsation in glans from jar of walking.

Modalities - Better from rest, doubling up. Biting the teeth together helps toothache. Worse stooping, ascending, motion, jarring, must walk carefully. Worse by touch, pressure, night. Toothache worse from warm food.

Mouth - Teeth feel pulled out. Toothache better by biting teeth together.

Rectum - Hard, nodular stool with rectal pain, as if angular body were pressed inward. Burning in anus after slimy diarrhea.

Sensations - As if a sharp corner pressing against top of head. As is skull would be pressed outward by a sharp plug. Headache as if from sun. As if inner portion of eye would be torn out. Eyeball as if crushed or pressed asunder. Sighing as if climbing a steep mountain. As if small of back had been injured. As if right thumb sprained, as if left ankle sprained, as if first joint of big toe pulled out.

Skin - Herpes zoster. Dropsy. Itching on fingertips, as if frozen.

Temperature - Night sweat.

COMMENTS - "Breath always seems to remain sticking in pit of stomach." This symptom, with "pain as if sprained in left ankle," led Lippe to make a remarkable cure in the case of a young woman, 16, who jumped from a carriage while the horse was running away and sprained her ankle. Left ankle and foot much swollen.

As swelling abated, breathing became rapid, great oppression with constantly recurring desire to take a long breath, felt as if air inhaled did not reach pit of stomach and until she could force air so far down had to yawn and try to take a deep inspiration. The tightness, stitches and sticking pains in chest have marked Prun. as a remedy in many cases of neuralgic pains with or following herpes zoster.

"Flatulence presses on bladder and causes cramps in bladder so that he is obliged to double up." Strangury. Hurriedly compelled to pass urine, which seems to pass forward into glans penis and then return and cause most violent pain in urethra.

Menses are too early, too profuse, last too long, and are thin and watery. There is lectureship, which weakens and stains yellow. The right side is much more affected than the left.

C. M. Boger gave the case of a man, 60 with enlarged prostate, had frequent urging to urinate, day and night. Shooting pains in neck of bladder unless desire to urinate is at once gratified.

Urination delayed if any great amount has accumulated.

Spasmodic tenesmus of bladder and rectum at close of urination with pains in glans. Pulsation in glans from jar of walking. Prun. 1,000c. (Fincke) removed the symptoms.

RELATIONS - ***Compare:*** (1) Laur. (2) Prun-p., bird-cherry - sore throat, pressure behind sternum and sticking pain in rectum. (3) Pyrus., mountain ash - irritation of eyes, constriction around waist, spasmodic pains in uterus, bladder, heart, cold-water sensation in stomach, coldness extends up esophagus, neuralgic and gouty pains.

REFERENCES - Boericke. Clarke.

PRUNUS VIRGINIANA

(Choke-cherry)

PHARMACY - prun-v. Prunus virginiana. Choke-cherry. Wild cherry. Cerasus virginiana. N. O. Rosaceae. Tincture of fresh inner bark. Solution of concentrated resinous extract, Prunin. ***Historical dose:*** Tincture and all potencies.

CLINICAL - Acidity. Anorexia. Bronchitis. ***Coughs***. Dyspepsia. Heart, hypertrophy. ***Heart, weakness.*** Heartburn.

HERBAL - Hale said the cold infusion of Prunus virginiana has been used from time immemorial for irregular intermittent action of the heart with deficient impulse.

HOMEOPATHIC - Prun-v. is a ***heart tonic.*** It relieves the flagging and distended ventricle, irritable heart, dilatation of right heart. ***Cough, worse at night on lying down.*** Chronic bronchitis. Weak digestion, especially in elderly people. Increases muscular tone.

Hale noted it for cough, sympathetic with heart troubles, dyspepsia with tendency to acidity, slow digestion, loss of appetite and heartburn. Excessive doses have caused a "dull, heavy feeling in head" like that of the other Pruneae.

COMMENTS - Seymour Taylor said it is especially useful in dilatation of right heart, whether as a result of chronic bronchitis or of mitral stenosis.

Burnett used it for weak digestion especially of elderly people. He regarded it as a mild form of Hydr-ac.

Laidlaw gave as a particular indication persistent coughs acquired in winter, worse at night on lying down. Spasmodic and asthmatic coughs. Attacks of wheezing and whistling in trachea and large bronchi and cough left behind after an attack of influenza.

Laidlaw's first case was a delicate girl, 20, who took cold, which began with coryza and in a few days passed into a cough with scanty expectoration and soreness under the sternum. Cough was persistent and annoying at all times, but worse at night.

After many other remedies had failed, Prun., one grain every two hours, relieved in two days and cured in a week. A recurrence some months later was rapidly cured by the same remedy.

REFERENCES - Boericke. Clarke.

PSILOCYBE CAERULESCENS

(Psilocybe Mushroom)

PHARMACY - psil. Psilocybe caerulescens. Psilocybe mushroom. N. O. Strophariaceae. (Agaricaceae). ***Historical dose:*** All potencies.

CLINICAL - Aphthae. Coryza. Delusions. ***Fatigue.*** Headache. Heat, flushes. Nausea. Palpitations. Salivation. Sneezing. Tonsillitis. Vertigo. Weakness.

HOMEOPATHIC - ***Extreme weakness and tiredness.*** Weakness and nausea. Great weakness after eating, desire to take a nap, better motion. Flushes of heat at night. Increased sexual desire at night.

Voracious appetite, gets up at midnight to eat. Sour eructations after spicy and fatty food. Sensation of heaviness in stomach and indigestion, better drinking water. "Slow digestion with sensation of suffocation at night, better cold drinks." Thirst, not better drinking.

Dryness. Watery, mucus nasal discharge with sneezing. ***Throbbing headache, especially on the right side***. Great pain in right shoulder, as if covered with ice.

Sexual desire increased, especially in females.

Pains appear and disappear suddenly. Pains pricking and stinging. Fleeting and erratic pains. Pain worse by small movements rather than by big movements. Painlessness of complaints usually painful. Sensation of strength.

MIND - Mental weakness. Absent-minded when conversing. Abstraction of mind and fixed eyes. Distraction. Loses the thread of his conversation. Listens with interest but only some minutes later it occurs to him what was said. Forgets everything, from lack of involvement, yet without feeling worried about it.

Sadness. "Great depression, recalling the past as if something was left undone, recalling occurrences with great detail, making one melancholic." Vindictiveness, "without knowing why or against whom." "Want of ethical and religious principles." Indifference to everything around him.

Idea that one can be in several places at the same time and think differently in each place. Sensation of being two or three personalities at the same time that cannot fuse, as if looking into several mirrors.

Telepathic speaking with superior spirits. Sensation of being in visual touch with God. Alternatively attracted to God and the devil. Sensation of being possessed by a divine force.

Involuntary laughing. Feels that someone is spying on him from behind and to the right, which makes him turn over in an summersault. Sensation of being in the moon. Sensation of being able to resolve whatever problem of mathematics or being able to understand any language. Thinks he is well.

An old and badly dressed woman looks young and beautiful. Vivid hallucinations of luminous colors. Time appears shorter, passes too quickly.

Suddenly changing delusions (Cann-i.). Delusion of having creative power. Delusion of being in communication with God. Delusion of being under a powerful, superhuman influence, alternately by God and the devil. Delusion that he is hovering in the air like a spirit.

Abdomen - Pain in liver after cold food (Mang.).

Back - Coldness as from ice.

Chest - Sudden, paroxysmal palpitations.

Eyes - Sensation of enlargement of left eye (Arg-n.). Burning pain in eyelids on winking.

Food - Thirst, vanishing at sight of water. Worse cold food.

Head - Heaviness in forehead when stooping. Pain, headache, on head getting cold. Headache increasing gradually. Headache simultaneous with other pains. Pain in forehead from sunlight (Ign.). Pain in temples while chewing. Pressing pain as if by a band.

Limbs - Desquamating eruption of palms of hands, soles of feet. Itching of soles of feet. Wrinkling of fingertips, as if dehydrated.

Modalities - Better from cold. Worse cold, wet weather. Worse in the morning on waking, right side.

Mouth - Aphthae, bleeding easily. Salivation and dryness of tongue. Metallic taste, at tip of tongue, seemingly originating from the teeth, with sensation as if esophagus were knotted up.

Nose - Violent attacks of coryza. Coryza in warm room. Obstruction and watery discharge. Sneezing in morning, after rising.

Sensations - Sensation of flying. Sensation of obstruction of nose and watery discharge. Sensation of dryness of mouth and salivation. Sensation of dryness of throat, not better drinking. Sensation of sweating around the mouth, but the skin is dry.

Sleep - Falling asleep from weakness. Short sleep refreshes. Sleepiness during pain. ***Unrefreshing sleep***. Difficult waking in morning. Waking from hunger. Dreams of being robbed and attacked in his own house and being incapable of defending oneself. Dreams of being chased by a vampire in a big house. Dreams of eating frogs with thorns and waking up with epigastric pain.

Stomach - Emptiness, weak feeling, better

pressure. Nausea, in morning on waking, from odors, while smoking.

Throat - Sensation of mucus. Mucus in morning on waking. Pain when touched. Dryness of throat, worse emotions, not better drinking. Inflammation of tonsils from smoking or from tobacco smoke. Constant disposition to swallow from lump in throat. Weakness of voice after talking.

Vertigo - Vertigo and trembling, better sitting. Vertigo and momentary loss of consciousness. Sensation as if the earth were slipping away under one's feet. Vertigo with weakness and trembling of legs, tendency to fall to the right side.

Vision - Colors, black spots during headache (Meli.).

RELATIONS - ***Compare:*** Anh., Cann-i., Sulph., Lach., Agar.

REFERENCES - Murphy. Toledo.

PSORINUM

(Scabies Nosode)

PHARMACY - psor. Psorinum. Scabies nosode. The product of *"Psora sicca"* epidermoid efflorescence of pityriasis by Gross. The salt from a product of psora by Hering. Nosodes. Triturations. ***Historical dose:*** All potencies.

CLINICAL - Acne rosacea. Adenoids. ***Allergies.*** Anus, itching. ***Anxiety.*** Asthma. Backaches. Bedwetting. Blepharitis. Boils. Cancer. Cholera infantum. Colds. Cough. Constipation. Cornea, ulcers. Crusta lactea. Crusta serpiginosa. ***Debility.*** Depression. ***Despair***. Diarrhea. Diphtheria. Dyspepsia. ***Eczema.*** Emaciation. ***Eruptions, itching.*** Gleet. Gonorrhea. Gouty. ***Hay fever. Headaches.*** Hemorrhages. Hemorrhoid. Hernia. Hydrocele. Hypoglycemia. Impotency. Influenza. Injuries. ***Itching. Leucorrhea. Lice.*** Lienteria. Liver, disorders. ***Malnutrition.*** Melancholy. Nose, redness. Odor, fetid. Ophthalmia. Otorrhea, fetid. Ozaena. Pericarditis. Peritonitis. Plica polonica. Polyps. Psoriasis. Quinsy. ***Scabies.*** Sciatica. Scurvy. ***Skin, disorders.*** Spina bifida. Spleen, disorders. Sprains. Syphilis. Throat, mucus. Tinea, capitis. Tonsils, concretions. Ulcers.

HOMEOPATHIC - Dr. Hering prepared this nosode from the sero-purulent matter of scabies vesicles. The therapeutic field of action is found in the psoric manifestations, when there is a lack of reaction in chronic diseases, and when well related remedies fail to relieve or to permanently improve.

Psor. chiefly affects the folds of the skin, sebaceous glands, ears, bowels, respiration system and the right side. ***Allergies and hay fever.*** Syphilis, inherited and tertiary. Cardiac weakness. Looseness of joints, teeth.

Prominent ***skin symptoms***. Unhealthy skin. Severe itching, worse at night, heat of bed, worse from ***wool clothing***. ***Itching leads to despair.*** Eczema and psoriasis. Eruptions and rashes disappear in summer, appear in winter.

Offensive discharges. Thick secretions. ***Secretions have a filthy smell***. ***Foul discharges,*** odor of the body, stools, eruptions, sweat, stubborn foot sweat. Profuse sweating. Easy perspiration when walking. Night-sweats.

Otorrhea is horribly offensive. Emaciation. Cholera infantum. Diarrhea is profuse, watery, dark brown and even black and is putrid smelling like carrion.

Debility independent of any organic disease. ***Prostration after acute disease*** or after loss of fluids. Feels good and bad by turns. Feels sick all over. Recurrences of diseases. Hopelessness, despair of recovery. ***Lack of reaction,*** when well-chosen remedies fail to act (Op.).

A cold medicine, wants the head kept warm, ***wants warm clothing*** even in summer. ***Extreme sensitiveness to cold***. ***Dread of least cold air or draft.*** Weak, tender and thin. Clothing seems large or he feels pushed down when walking in the sun. ***Hungry or unusually well before an attack.*** Wants to wash parts constantly, especially hands and feet.

Scrofulous patients. Nervous, restless persons who are easily startled. Adapted to dirty people with a filthy smelling body, even after bathing. Pale, sickly, delicate, unhealthy looking children, who have a disagreeable smell around them.

Sick babies will not sleep day and night but worry, fret and cry or good and play all day, troublesome screaming all night. Difficulty in breathing when standing in open air, wants to go home and lie down. Enlarged glands. Often gives immunity from catching colds.

MIND - Dull, beclouded mind. Confusion, better open air. Difficult thinking. Stupefaction. Aversion to work. Inability for calculating, due to confusion of senses. Vanishing of thoughts after over-lifting. Memory weak, can't remember, doesn't even know his room.

Anxiety and restlessness. Gestures, wringing hands. Anxiety while riding downhill. Anxiety about salvation. Foreboding. Fears the business will fail. Fear of fire. Fear of being alone, of becoming insane. Restless during a thunderstorm. Thought pains would drive him crazy.

Pessimism, thinks he is very ill when he is not. ***Despair of recovery. Despair from itching of skin.*** Constant thoughts of dying. Religious melancholy. Horrid thoughts, ***suicidal tendency***. Weeping at night.

Great depression during menopause. ***Hopelessness.*** Great despondency, makes one's own life and those about him intolerable. ***Forsaken feeling.*** Sentimental. Melancholy and gloomy. Seeks solitude. Desires to remain in bed.

Severe ailments from even slight emotions. Thoughts which he can't get rid of constantly reappear in his dreams. Feels himself poor. Feels his business is going to be a failure, though it is prosperous.

Children very fretful, day and night. Children intolerably self-willed, annoying those about them. Peevish, irritable, noisy. Easily startled. Irritability on waking at night. Irritability while talking.

Abdomen - Constant feeling of emptiness and looseness in abdomen. Pain in abdomen after eating. Abdominal affections during menopause, with high degree of ill-humor. Chronic indurations of spleen. Stitches in spleen better standing, worse moving, and continuing when again at rest. Stinging, sharp, in inguinal glands. Inguinal hernia. Lumps in right groin, preventing stooping. Pain through right groin when walking. Griping in abdomen and desire for stool while riding. Painful bearing down with painful, burning micturition. Sensations as if intestines were hanging down. Colic better eating and passing fetid flatus. Flatus like bad eggs. Flatulent symptoms with distension.

Back - ***Backache and debility***. Severe backache, as if bruised, can't straighten out. Backaches after suppressed eruption. Spina bifida. Boring in vertebrae in morning with colic, as from rheumatism. Bruised feeling in evening, cannot straighten it. Lumbar ache worse standing or walking. Pain in lumbar region, like weakness, worse motion. Pressing pain in lumbar region, worse motion. Sticking in back. Drawing pain extending to shoulder. Tearing and sharp pains between scapulae. Painful stiffness of neck, soreness and tearing pain on bending backward. Swelling of glands of nape, with bruised pain.

Breasts - Breasts swollen and painful, nipples red. Burning and itching pimples around nipples. Eruptions on breasts causing excoriation. Breast cancer.

Causations - Poor hygiene and diet. Ill effects of infectious diseases lasting for years. Over-lifting injuries, blows, sprains, dislocations. Slight emotions cause severe ailments.

Chest - Hot sensation in chest. Pain in chest, better lying down. ***Feeling of ulceration under sternum***. Knife-like cutting pain in chest. Burning, pressing pain in chest. Dull pressure in right side of chest. Chest expands with great difficulty. Soreness as if everything were torn in chest. Chest pain extends to shoulder, worse cold drinks. Anxious oppression in chest every morning. Paroxysmal, in chest, with great anxiety. Eruption in axilla.

Constitutions - Suited to scrofulous, nervous, restless persons who are easily startled. Psoric constitutions, lack of reaction after severe diseases. Complaints of psoric origin, patients emit a disagreeable odor. Pale, sickly, delicate children. Peevish, unhealthy-looking children, who have a disagreeable odor about them. Dirty people in whom the body has a filthy smell which no amount of washing can remove. Those subject to diseases of the glands and skin and who have had eruptions suppressed.

Cough - Dry, hard cough with great weakness in chest. Severe, dry cough with pain as if everything in chest were raw and scratched. Cough from tickling in larynx, with soreness under sternum and heaviness on chest. Coughs a long time before expectorating. Cough from suppressed eruption, talking. Cough worse mornings, evenings, lying down, drinking. Cough returns every winter.

Ears - Putrid otorrhea, with headache, with offensive watery diarrhea. ***Moist fetid pus*** from ears, brownish, offensive. Ulceration of tympanum. Reddish wax. ***Raw, red, oozing scabs around ears***. Eczema, humid sores, behind the ears. ***Offensive discharge*** from eczema around ears. ***Intolerable itching***. Itching in ears, child can hardly be kept from picking or boring at meatus. Herpes from temples over ears to cheeks. Severe pains. Sore pain behind ears. Illusory noises, as if he heard with ears not his own. Impaired hearing with singing, cracking, humming, buzzing and ringing in ears.

Eyes - ***Recurring chronic ophthalmia.*** Acrid secretion. Profuse flow of hot tears. Sharp pains in eyes. Soreness of eyes and burning, must close them frequently. Lachrymation. Agglutinated. Gummy. Edges of eyelids red. Pterygium. Everted eyelids. Blepharitis. Tendency to styes. Objects tremble, then get dark. Darkness before eyes. Sensation as if something were moving or one were playing with his fingers before eyes. Aversion to light. Photophobia when walking in open air, walks with eyes bent upon ground.

Face - Pale, delicate, sickly, dirty, fuzzy or puffy. Broad blue rings around eyes. Down on the face. Burning heat and redness of face. Acne rosacea, red, small pimples, on nose, chin and middle of cheeks. Pimples on forehead. Coppery eruption on face. ***Humid eruptions on face***. Lips dry, brown, black. Swelling of the upper lip. Cheekbones pain as if ulcerated. Soreness of jaw, right side, could not open mouth. Painful tension and pressure in right zygoma. Submaxillary and sublingual glands swollen, sore to touch.

Female - Amenorrhea. Menses, early and profuse. Menses delayed and scanty. Dysmenorrhea, near menopause. Menstrual disorders during menopause. Leucorrhea and debility. ***Fetid leucorrhea***, gushing, lumpy, with violent pain in sacrum, with ***backache and debility***. Pimples oozing an acrid fluid that burns and excoriates the glands. Ulcers on labia. Pinching pain in pubic region. Obstinate vomiting during pregnancy. Fetus moves too violently. Flow starts anew when the woman gets on her feet after a miscarriage.

Food - Canine hunger preceding attacks. Very hungry always, must have something to eat in middle of night. Ravenous appetite, but grows thin. Hypoglycemia. Hungry during attacks of headache. Loss of appetite after illness with great thirst. Anemia with aversion to food. Generally worse fasting. Desires beer, acids. Aversion to pork. Dinner tastes oily. Thirst during dinner. Drinking causes cough.

Head - Migraines. Headache as from a heavy blow, follows visual disturbances, better nosebleed. ***Headaches from suppressed eruptions***, suppressed menses. Chronic headaches, hungry during attacks of vertigo. Hammering pain. Awakens at night with pain as from blow on head. Dull, pressive pain in occiput. Pain alternates with other complaints. Brain feels too large, worse change of weather. Head feels separated from the body. Sensitive to drafts about head, wants it covered in hot weather. Twitching in temples. Whole head burns. Viscid sweat about head. ***Humid eruption on scalp, hair matted.*** Pustules, boils on head. Spots of white skin with white lock of hair. Dry, lusterless, rough hair. Tangled hair. ***Head lice.*** Scurfy eruption of children.

Heart - Heart murmurs and mitral regurgitation. Gurgling in the heart, worse lying down. Purring in region of apex, cyanotic lips. Pericarditis. Heart pains, better lying down. Thinks the sharp pains will kill him if they continue. Stitches in cardiac region, for a moment breathing is impossible. Palpitations with anxiety. Palpitations in those suffering from hepatic disorders. Pulse weak, feeble, irritable. Weak, irregular pulse.

Kidneys - Has to pass urine several times from weakness of bladder. Burning and cutting pain in urethra. Frequent, scanty urine. Urine thick, whitish, turbid, red deposit, cuticle forms on surface. Escape of urine when coughing. Obstinate bed-wetting, worse full moon.

Limbs - Caries, rachitis. Chronic forms of rheumatism. Tearing pains. Joints feel loose, weak, as if they would not hold together. Eruptions around joints, makes walking difficult. ***Eruptions around fingernails***. Hot itching soles. ***Fetid foot sweat*** (Sil.). Hands and feet feel as if broken early in morning and after a little work. Heat in hands and feet.

Liver - Deep, heavy pain in region of liver, worse pressure or lying on right side, worse sneezing. Stinging, sharp pain in region of liver and spleen. Flatulence with disorders of liver. Chronic hepatitis.

Lungs - Difficult breathing, when standing in open air. Dyspnea wants to go home and lie down. Shortness of breath on walking in open air. Anxious dyspnea with palpitations and pain in cardiac region. ***Asthma with dyspnea***, worse sitting up, better lying down and keeping arms spread wide apart. Asthma, feels as if he would die. Asthmatic attacks with hydrothorax. Hydrothorax. Tedious recovery in pneumonia. ***Allergies. Hay fever*** returning irregularly every year. Bloody expectoration with hot sensation in chest. Green mucus sputa, worse mornings when awaking and evenings on lying down. Tenacious mucus, difficult to expel. Green and yellow, salty taste. Small lumps of mucus.

Male - Offensive genitals. Hydrocele. Inflamed ulcer on glans. Discharge of prostatic fluid before urination. Chronic, painless discharge from urethra, staining yellow. Griping pain in testes. Drawing pain, in testes and spermatic cords. Chronic gonorrhea, painless discharge from urethra staining yellow. Aversion to sex. Impotency. Absence of erections, parts flabby, torpid. Want of enjoyment of emission during sex. Excessive, uncontrollable sexual desire.

Modalities - Better heat, warm clothing, even in summer. Better washing, hard pressure, rest, being in a room. Better from coffee, profuse sweating, nosebleed. ***Better from lying with head low or quietly***. Better when eating, but rush of blood to head is worse immediately after. ***Worse from cold, open air.*** Worse changing weather, storms, before thunderstorms. Worse evening, before midnight, night, morning on waking. Worse from heat of bed, wool clothes. Worse exertion in hot sunshine, walking, moving, washing. Worse pressure, rubbing, scratching, touch, contact of own limbs, bandage. ***Worse from suppressions***. Liver is worse lying on right side. Over-lifting causes thoughts to vanish. Winter causes cough. Summer causes diarrhea, itching eruptions. Bedwetting is worse periodically, yearly, at the full moon.

Mouth - Mouth inflamed, sore, worse warm food, not annoyed by cold food. Mouth dry, burning. Bad taste in mouth, better open air. Bitter taste, better eating or drinking. Filthy taste. Tough mucus of foul taste adheres to soft palate. Gums, bleed, spongy, settled away from the teeth. Pyorrhea. Cyanotic lips. Burning, painful vesicles inside lower lip. Obstinate cracks in corners of mouth.

Neck - Glands of neck swollen, bruised pain extending to head on touch. Sticking in neck with pustules. Herpetic eruption on side of neck extending from cheek. Nape excoriated by discharge from eczema capitis.

Nose - Recurring colds. Allergies. ***Hay fever,*** regularly returning every year. Hay fever coming on in August. Watery acrid discharges. Dry, coryza with stoppage of nose. Coryza with loss of smell. Chronic catarrh, dropping from posterior sinuses. Tough mucus in nose. Burning pain followed by thin nasal discharge, which relieves. Nose sensitive when inhaling air. Bloody, purulent discharge. Smell of blood. Septum inflamed, white, suppurating pustules. Small, red pimples. Acne rosacea.

Perspiration - Profuse sweats, improves all complaints. Colliquative sweats. Sour, clammy sweats. Easy, profuse sweat, worse night. ***Profuse, offensive at night.*** Sudden outbreaks of sweat on slight exertion, which is offensive, followed by debility and easily taking cold. Sweats easily on limbs. Sweats if he turns in bed. Heat with steaming sweat. Sweats on face, palms of hands and perineum when moving about. Cold sweat, on palms. Lack of perspiration and dry skin.

Rectum - Constipation with pain in lumbar region. Obstinate constipation with coryza and obstruction of nose. ***Constipation of infants*** in pale, sickly scrofulous children. Cholera infantum. Chronic diarrhea, early morning, urgent. Involuntary stools with sleep. Soft, difficult stools, has to go several times to pass normal stools. Hard, difficult stool with blood from rectum. Desire for stool when riding. Soreness in rectum and anus when riding. Burning in rectum. Burning hemorrhoids. Hemorrhages from rectum in old women.

Sensations - As if frightened. As if he would lose his senses. As if stupid in left half of head. As if brain had not room enough in forehead. As from heavy blow on forehead. As if brain would protrude. As if sand in eyes. Eyes as if pressed outward. As if he heard with ears not his own. Cheekbones as if ulcerated. Condyle of jaw as if lame. Tongue as if burnt. Teeth as if glued together. Plug in throat. Throat as if narrowing. As if intestines hanging down.

Skin - ***Unhealthy skin.*** Abnormal tendency to skin diseases. Sebaceous glands secrete excessively, oily skin. Urticaria, worse exertion. Crusty eruptions all over. Herpetic eruptions, especially on scalp and bends of joints, with itching. Eruptions bleed easily and constantly tend to suppurate. Dirty, rough, scabby, greasy, breaks out in folds. ***Eczema behind ears.*** Pemphigus. Psoriasis. ***Intolerable itching,*** worse heat of bed. Scratches raw or until it bleeds. Rubbing skin causes small vesicles to arise. Condylomata on edges of skin. Pustules near fingernails. Indolent ulcers, slow to heal. ***Suppressed eruptions.*** Enlarged glands. ***Scabies. Recurring body lice.*** Burning itching pustule after vaccination. Skin troubles disappear in summer, only to occur again in winter.

Sleep - Easily started. Sleepy by day. Sleepless from anxiety and despair, ***from intolerable itching,*** from congestion to head. Sleepless after 12 p.m. In morning lies in same position as when he fell asleep. On waking, can't get rid of the one persistent thoughts from dreams. Vivid dreams, continue after waking. Dreams of robbers, danger, traveling.

Stomach - Hypoglycemia. ***Very hungry always, must have something to eat in the middle of the night***. Weakness of stomach. Cramps in stomach. Sharp stinging pain in pit. Water brash when lying down, better getting up. Sour, rancid belchings, tasting and smelling like rotten eggs. Eructations, sour, rancid, room is filled with an offensive odor. Nausea after suppressed itch. Nausea all day, in morning, with pain in lumbar region. Vomiting first of blood, then of sour, slimy fluid. Vomiting of sweet mucus every morning at 10 a.m. and in evening. Nausea, vomiting of pregnancy.

Stool - Hot flatus, smelling like rotten eggs. Stools like rotten eggs or carrion, worse at night. Mucus stools. ***Stools bloody, excessively fetid, dark fluid, brown, horribly putrid, gushing***. Stools have a penetrating odor, going through the whole house. Involuntary stools during sleep. Diarrhea after severe acute disease. Fetid diarrhea during dentition.

Teeth - Teeth stick together as if glued, from tough mucus in mouth. Looseness of teeth, fears they may fall out, worse touch. Sensations of soreness of teeth. Stitching pain in teeth from one side to other. Toothache worse at night and from cold, better warmth. Gums bleed, spongy, settled away from teeth. Pyorrhea.

Temperature - Internal shivering, creeping chills and icy cold feet. Chilliness in evening, on upper arms and thighs, with thirst. Sudden heat over whole body, with trickling sweat all over face. Fever with steaming sweat. Fever at night, with dryness of mouth. Fever when riding in a carriage. Thirst during chill and heat.

Throat - Throat burns, feels scalded. Tension and swollen feeling in throat. Dryness of throat in morning. Recurring quinsy. ***Eradicates tendency to quinsy***. Tonsils greatly swollen, painful swallowing with pain in ears. Tonsillitis with swelling of submaxillary glands and fetid otorrhea. Profuse, offensive saliva, tough mucus in throat. Hawking up of cheesy, pea-like balls of disgusting smell and taste (Agar.). Sensation as if a plug in throat impeding hawking. Sensations of suffocation, with paroxysmal, dry, hacking cough. Tickling, throat as if narrowing, must cough to better it. Hoarseness when talking, phlegm sticks in larynx. Voice weak, trembling, talking very fatiguing. Herpetic eruption on side of neck extending from cheek.

Tongue - Tip of tongue feels scalded. Tongue thickly covered with whitish-yellow slime. Tongue, gums ulcerated. Tough mucus of foul taste adheres to soft palate.

Vertigo - Vertigo in morning. Vertigo, objects seem to go around with him. Vertigo with headache, eyes feel pressed outwards. Vertigo with confusion and drawing in forehead, and roaring in ears.

Vision - Sensation as if something were moving or one were playing with his fingers before eyes. Objects seem to tremble for a few moments, then get dark. Obscuration, with ringing in ears. Fiery sparks. Misty, after anxiety. Black spots or rings, flickering, dancing about of objects, before headache. Blurs and blue stars, during headache.

COMMENTS - Psoric manifestations. Similar symptoms to Sulph., particularly for psora conditions, itch and itch-like eruptions. Exceedingly chilly, likes to have a fur cap on in summer (Sulph. is hot).

H. C. Allen noted that Psor. is indicated in chronic cases when well-selected remedies fail to relieve or to permanently improve (in acute diseases, Sulph.), and when Sulph. seems indicated but fails to relieve. Clears up confused cases. Useful as an intercurrent, when indicated remedies palliate or fail to act.

Feeble reactions, lack of reaction. Weakness from loss of fluids, after acute disease, with or without organic lesion. Debilitated, worse exertion. Weak since loss of fluid. Emaciation. Feels unusually well before attacks, sense of well being. Lies with arms out, as if crucified (Puls.). Whole body painful, easily sprained and inured.

Unhealthy skin. Skin is dirty looking, scurfy. Sores refuse to heal. Severe eczema, psoriasis, dermatitis. Scabies. Lice, worms, parasites. Bruises and scars easily (Sulph.). Rough skin, cracks and sores (Petr.). Scaly skin. Skin will ooze and crust. Sallow and greasy face, several pustules on chin and neck that itch intensely and bleed when scratched.

Constant irritation. Formication. Itch and scratch until they bleed (Alum.). Wandering itching. Tormenting, despairing itching, drives a person crazy, especially at night and in bed. Can pick at skin. Can't stand clothes or the covers. Skin problems along the hairline with inflammation and itching. Dry, lusterless hair, plica polonica. Scabs, pus, seborrheic dermatitis (Graph., Mez.).

Extreme dullness. Fears inflammation of brain, better by nosebleed. Dull, heavy pain in the base of brain, in the afternoon. Headache better by eating, nosebleed, suppressed menses. Very hungry during headaches. Headache following darkness before eyes. Black spots before eyes.

Chronic colds from little drafts and getting chilled easily. Chronic bronchitis with severe shortness of breath. Quinsy, throat burns, feels scalded. Tendency to quinsy. Cutting, tearing, intense pain on swallowing. Profuse, offensive saliva, tough mucus in throat, must hawk continually. Hay fever. Allergies. Allergic to wool (Sulph.).

Sudden gnawing hunger. Wakes up in the middle of the night hungry. Large appetite, but loses weight. Malnutrition. Starvation (Sil., Calc-p., Calc.). Low blood sugar. Aversion to pork (Puls.). Desires acids. Thirst for beer. Chronic headaches with hunger (Anac.). Worms that irritate the colon (Cina.).

Sensation as though skin of abdomen was greatly relaxed and drawn down. Decomposition. Belching like rotten eggs (Arn., Chin., Carb-v.). Flatus with pungent, carrion-like odor. Smell penetrates the room. Horribly offensive, nearly painless, almost involuntary, dark and watery stool, only in night and most towards morning. Cracking and bleeding anal fissures.

Vertigo with poor circulation. Dizzy after exertion. Great sensitiveness to cold air, change, storms, sun. Lack of vital heat. Steaming perspiration. Restless for days before a thunderstorm. Symptoms are worse during menses from fats, sugar, coffee, meat. Dislikes bathing.

Depression, mental anguish. Very insecure. Possessive. Sense of depletion. Anxious about health. Despair about survival. Fear of poverty, of the future, of being forsaken. Ailments from illness, malnourishment, nutritional weakness, lack of hygiene.

Sick babies will not sleep day or night, but worry, fret, cry or good and play all day, restless, troublesome, screaming all night.

Clarke frequently saw Psor. develop its own symptoms in patients whom it has benefited in other ways. A man who complained of "cloudiness of mind and difficult thinking," and who had, among other symptoms, his "left foot colder than right," received Psor. 30c. It removed these symptoms, but while under its influence new symptoms appeared, including a heavy headache across the [illegible]brows, and greasiness of face and [illegible].

Hahnemann noted the symptom "spasmodically contracting headache." A woman to whom Clarke gave Psor. 30c complained that after each dose she had a feeling "as if something in the head were being screwed up and drawn."

A patient who took Psor. 500c complained that it had a "filthy taste." Psor. 20,000c. has produced an eruption of boil-like indurations in both axillae, first in the left then in right. The general symptoms were relieved at the same time.

Clarke noted that Psor. cured more cases of hay fever than any other single remedy in his practice. Many cases have a psoric basis and when the basic taint is corrected, the irritating agents have no effect. Nasal polyps have also been cured with Psor. when the general symptoms indicate the remedy.

Hawley reported a case of cholera infantum that seemed to defy every remedy. Stools were very thin and watery, dirty greenish, smelled like carrion. Child was very fretful and had no sleep for two days and nights. Hawley gave Psor. 42,000c (Fincke), one dose in water. In two hours the child went to sleep, in four days it was well without repetition of the dose.

Hawley also had the case of Miss N., 20, who had an eruption in the bends of elbows and knees. It was dry, scaly, with little pointed vesicles around the reddened edges. It disappeared entirely in summer and reappeared when cold weather set in. Violent itching, worse by warmth of bed or by scratching. Psor. 42,000c, two doses at six weeks interval, cured, it did not return the following winter.

Wesselhoeft observed that headaches and eruptions were worse during changeable weather.

Miss C., when convalescing from typhoid fever, reported that she was "stationary, no appetite." Psor. 400c produced immediate change and ravenous appetite.

Mr. P., age 50, complained of nothing but weakness, no appetite, least exertion put him into a perspiration. Psor. 40c cured rapidly.

Mr. X., age 21, was obliged one day to run until nearly exhausted. Though strong and well before, he now became weak, perspiring easily, severe pains on right side, worse by coughing, laughing and motion. Psor. 40c cured rapidly.

Mr. C., age 43, was spare, dark. Hypochondriacal. "Nervous" nine months, had to give up business, took quinine and other drugs. Complained of a very disagreeable feeling about the head and manifested mental depression, thought he would never recover, lost all hope.

Could not apply his mind to business. Seemed confused, could not reckon. Numbness of legs and arms, worse left side, worse going to bed, formication and crawling with prickling and smarting on scalp and on limbs. Tongue coated white.

After three months, treatment was stationary. It was then ascertained that he sweated very easily on least exertion and somewhat at night, and had loss of memory. Psor. 400c soon caused improvement and enabled "the patient to return to business."

G. A. Whippy cured with Psor. 200c, a dose every third night, the case of a carpenter, 40, with a long-standing discharge of reddish cerumen from left ear, worse at night. There was a sensation of a valve opening and shutting in left ear, worse afternoon. Buzzing in ear, which stopped suddenly and was followed by violent itching.

RELATIONS - ***Compare:*** (1) Ped. - psoric manifestations in children. Eruption on dorsum of hands, feet, neck. Prurigo, pellagra. Unusual aptitude for study and work. (2) Ped. - transmit typhus and trench fever. (3) In lack of reaction compare Op., Calc. and Nat-ar. (4) Gaert. ***Complementary:*** Sulph.

REFERENCES - Boericke. Clarke. Murphy. Phatak.

PTELEA TRIFOLIATA

(Hop Tree)

PHARMACY - ptel. Ptelea trifoliata. Hop tree. Shrubby trefoil. Water ash. Wafer ash. N. O. Xanthoxylaceae of the Rutaceae. Tincture of bark of root. ***Historical dose:*** Tincture and all potencies.

CLINICAL - Asthma. ***Ascarides.*** Bilious, headaches. Constipation. Dysentery. Dyspepsia. Erysipelas. Gallstones. Gastric, headaches. Headaches. Intermittent, fever. Jaundice. ***Liver, disorders.*** Nightmares. Phosphaturia. Rheumatism. Spleen, disorders. Stomach, pain. Urticaria. ***Worms.***

HERBAL - Ptelea is the Greek name for the Elm and was applied by Linnaeus to a genus of shrubs and small trees, natives of North America and Asia and included in Xanthoxylaceae. The Treasury of Botany noted that the fronds are bitter and aromatic, and have been used as a substitute for hops.

In Canada, the young green shoots of Ptelea are used as an anthelmintic in the form of an infusion. One of the provers of Ptelea confirmed its anthelmintic powers by "a very copious expulsion of ascarides."

HOMEOPATHIC - The proving was very thorough and extensive, and T. Nichol, Burt and Cowperthwaite were among the provers. Marked action on the liver and in those erysipelatous and urticaria eruptions that are so often concomitant with disorders of the liver.

Ptel. is a remarkable remedy in stomach and liver disorders. ***Atonic states of stomach***. The aching and heaviness in the region of the liver is ***greatly aggravated by lying*** down on the left side. Stomach and liver symptoms associated with pain in limbs. ***Worms.*** Ravenous hunger, empty sensation in esophagus and stomach.

Taste bitter and belchings either bitter or like rotten eggs. Aching and heaviness in the region of liver worse lying on left side. Headache with hunger, especially on awaking, may prove a keynote. Right (liver) side most affected.

Asthma. Difficult breathing coming on as gastric symptoms improve. Alternating symptoms. Nervous pains alternated from left arm to left eye and temple. Liveliness alternates with sadness. Sensitive to light, sound, open air. Enlarged feelings, head feels large, fingers feel numb and large and clumsy.

Abdomen - Much weight and pain in right side, heavy, aching feeling, relieved by lying on right side. Retraction of abdomen.

Ears - Swelling of gland under right ear, sharp pain behind ear. Shooting pains from left ear down spine. Intolerance of loud talking. Roaring and singing in ears.

Eyes - Eyes heavy. Pressure over eyes, worse lifting eyebrows. Pains over eyes. Sensitiveness to light.

Face - Face pale, especially around eyes, sickly, yellow. Burning in face.

Food - Appetite voracious. Tired before finishing eating. Desire for acid food. Aversion to meat, butter and rich food. Thirsty, drank much water. Absence of thirst with bitter taste.

Head - Feels dull and stupid. ***Pain from forehead to root of nose, pressing-outward pain. Frontal headache***, worse noise, motion, night, rubbing eyes with acidity. Temples as if pressed together. Headache better after stool.

Limbs - ***Edema of feet*** and legs with liver disorders. Stomach and liver symptoms associated with ***pain in limbs***.

Liver - ***Liver congestion.*** Liver sore, swollen, sensitive to pressure. Weakness of liver.

Lungs - Feeling of pressure on lungs and of suffocation, when lying on back. ***Asthma***, dyspnea, cramp-like pain in cardiac region.

Modalities - Better eating sour, acid things. Better in cold air, morning and evening. Worse lying down, lying on left side, after sleep, on waking, early morning, afternoon. Worse in hot room, walking, speaking, mental exertion, moving eyes, raising eyebrows. Worse after eating, cheese, butter, meat, puddings. Worse before, during, and after stool.

Mouth - ***Excess of saliva with dry, bitter taste***. Tongue coated white or yellow, feels rough, swollen. ***Papillae red and prominent*** (Arg-n.). Coating may be brownish-yellow. Breath, hot, burns the nostrils.

Nose - Sneezing. Nose stopped, sore, breath burns and irritates nostrils. Influenza.

Rectum - Pressure in rectum, urging to stool. Stool followed by tenesmus and succeeded by itching and smarting at anus. Smarting in anus after hard stool, with diarrhea stool.

Sleep - Restlessness with frightful dreams, nightmares. Awakes languid and unrefreshed.

Stomach - Stomach feels empty after eating. Weight and fullness. Heat, dryness and distressing feeling of emptiness in esophagus. Constant sensation of corrosion, heat and burning in stomach. Belching, nausea and vomiting.

Throat - Dryness, roughness, heat, constriction in throat. Throat sore, ulcerated, worse right side. Burning and pricking pains, especially in tonsils.

COMMENTS - Hale said Ptel. has not the violent action of Podo. or Iris-v., but "a slow, pervading" action and causes chronic ailments. He found it useful in "bilious headache, dyspepsia, gastralgia, congestion of the liver, chronic hepatitis and chronic erysipelas." Others used it in chronic rheumatism, dysentery and constipation.

Hale said the oily constituent of Ptel. resembles turpentine and one of the most marked symptoms of the proving is: "Pressure as from a stone in pit of stomach," recalling Abies-n. and the conifers. In the proving, the liver was swollen and tender, but it was better lying on right side and worse lying on left

H. K. Leonard cured a seemingly hopeless case with Ptel. 1x on the symptom weight, aching distress, dull pain in hepatic region, better lying on right side, turning on left causes a dragging as if liver pulling on its ligaments. The dull, muddled headed feeling is another liver symptom.

J. Preston cured with Ptel. a case of jaundice following gallstones with great emaciation. Aching distress, general aching and soreness, malaise.

RELATIONS - ***Compare:*** (1) Merc., Mag-m., Nux-v., Chel.

REFERENCES - Boericke. Clarke. Phatak.

PUERARIA LOBATA

(Kudzu Vine)

PHARMACY - puer. Pueraria lobata. Kudzu Vine. Kuzu. ***Historical dose:*** Tincture and all potencies.

CLINICAL - ***Alcoholism.*** Anemia. Asthma. Bronchitis. Constipation. Diabetes. Diarrhea. Dysentery. Edema. Enteritis. Fevers. Hangovers. Headaches. Hypoglycemia. Impotence. Infertility. Influenza. Insect, bites. Measles. Migraines. Pneumonia. Sinus, problems. Snake, bites. Tonsillitis.

HERBAL - Traditional Asian herbalists have long valued kudzu's root and flowers for treating colds, flu, high blood pressure, chest pain, allergies, and a host of other ailments. Research indicates that a compound in the root (an isoflavone called puerarin) may also increase blood flow to the heart and brain which may explain certain traditional uses.

In traditional Chinese medicine, kudzu has been used to relieve muscle pain. Animal studies and some human case reports suggest that kudzu may have some anti-inflammatory effects.

Chemicals in kudzu may also lower the heart rate and regulate its rhythm, as well as widen the blood vessels near the heart and the brain. This may support its uses in heart conditions and for the treatment of migraine headaches.

HOMEOPATHIC - Other medicinal uses for kudzu include influenza, cough, colds, tonsillitis, measles, and fevers. Bronchitis, pneumonia. Asthma. Sinus problems.

Lack of energy. Sexual apathy, impotence, infertility. Muscle shrinking. Dizziness. Headaches, migraines. Hangovers. Diaphoretic. Removal of excess fluids from the body. Anemia, internal bleeding. Snake and insect bites.

Thirst, hunger. Bad breath. Diarrhea, dysentery, intestinal ailments, enteritis, constipation, and digestive disorders. Diabetes. Can reduce blood sugar levels and result in hypoglycemia when taken in large amounts.

Strengthens the spleen, stomach and intestines, as well as the entire immune system.

RELATIONS - ***Compare:*** Nux-v., Sul-ac., Lach.

REFERENCES - Murphy. Yui.

PULEX IRRITANS

(Common Flea)

PHARMACY - pulx. Pulex irritans. Common flea. Insecta. ***Historical dose:*** All potencies.

CLINICAL - Abdomen, bloated. ***Headache.*** Leucorrhea. Salivation.

HOMEOPATHIC - Pulx. has marked urinary and female symptoms. Cannot retain urine, must attend the call immediately. Stains of menses and leucorrhea are very hard to wash out. As if cotton ball inside the vagina.

MIND - Very impatient. Restlessness. Cross and irritable, does not want to be looked at or spoken to. Memory confused. Cannot think. When walking has a sensation of lightness. Glad feeling, as though she had heard good news. Felt a dread of going to bed.

Back - Backache (Ox-ac.). Back weakness. Drawing of muscles below scapula.

Eyes - Eyes feel as if enlarged.

Face - ***Face wrinkled and old-looking***.

Female - Menses delayed. Increased flow of saliva during menses. Leucorrhea, profuse, foul, staining a greenish yellow, stains of menses and leucorrhea very hard to wash out. Intense burning in vagina.

Food - Thirst, especially during headache.

Head - Frontal ***headache with enlarged feeling of eyes.*** Very impatient, cross and irritable.

Kidneys - Urine scanty with frequent urging with pressure in bladder and tenesmus in urethra. Cannot retain urine, must attend to the call without delay. Irritable bladder before menses. Urine foul. Flow of urine stops suddenly, followed by pain.

Modalities - Better sitting or lying down. Worse left side, moving about.

Mouth - Metallic taste. Sensation of a thread in throat. Thirsty, especially during headache.

Skin - Sore spots all over. Prickly itching. Skin emits foul odor.

Stomach - Breath and taste foul. Intense nausea with vomiting, purging and faintness. Stool very offensive.

Temperature - Feels a glow all over, like being over steam. ***Chilly***, sitting near by fire.

Throat - As if a thread hanging in throat.

REFERENCES - Boericke. Clarke. Phatak.

PULMO VULPIS

(Fox's Lung)

PHARMACY - pulm-v. Pulmo vulpis. Fox's lung. Sarcode. Trituration. ***Historical dose:*** All potencies.

CLINICAL - Asthma. Bronchitis. ***Dyspnea.*** Catarrh. Heart, disease. Lungs, catarrh. Lungs, edema. ***Shortness of breath.***

HOMEOPATHIC - The uses of tissues and organs as remedies have thrown light on many curiosities of ancient medicine. As the fox is probably the longest-winded of all animals, the doctrine of signatures pointed to his lungs as a likely remedy for short breath.

Pulm-v. has ***persistent shortness of breath,*** causing a attack of asthma on the slightest motion. Strong, sonorous bubbling rales.

COMMENTS - Grauvogl put on record his case of a women, 65, much reduced in flesh by a persistent condition of humid asthma. It commenced with chronic catarrh and symptoms of edema of the lungs.

Strong, sonorous bubbling, rattling, whistling sounds over whole chest and at some distance away, perceptible also to hand laid on chest. Accelerated short breath amounting to suffocation, even without corresponding heaving of the chest, frequently with cough and inability to expectorate.

Sometimes in light cases, there is no catarrh present and only persistent shortness of breath, becoming a paroxysm of asthma on the least bodily exertion. The patient could only live sitting up, bent forward, constant lividity of face, lips and limbs and dropsy of legs.

Heart's pulsations irregular and death seemed imminent. Pulm-v. 1x grains right was given and repeated in an hour. Visible improvement set in but without increased expectoration. After a third powder the patient was able to lie down and fell into a refreshing sleep lasting several hours. In eight days she engaged in her domestic duties.

REFERENCES - Clarke.

PULMONARIA OFFICINALIS

(Lungwort)

PHARMACY - pul-o. Pulmonaria officinalis. Lungwort. Pulmonaria maculosa. Jerusalem sage. N. O. Boraginaceae. ***Historical dose:*** Tincture and all potencies.

CLINICAL - Asthma. Bronchitis. Coughs. Hemoptysis. Hemorrhoids. Lung, disorders. Urinary, incontinence. Tuberculosis.

HERBAL - Pulmonaria officinalis is an evergreen perennial species of lungwort, native to locations throughout Europe. A rhizome, P. officinalis produces small bunches of pink flowers which turn to blue-purple in spring.

The plant has been cultivated for centuries as a medicinal herb, the ovate spotted leaves were thought to be symbolic of diseased lungs. The appearance of the plant makes it easy to see why the lungwort was used for diseases of the lung (putrid bronchitis, hemoptysis), and also for hematuria, and urinary incontinence (see also under Myos.).

The medicines are prepared from the fresh, flowering herb. It is an astringent, demulcent, diaphoretic, diuretic, emollient, expectorant, ophthalmic, and resolvent.

The leaves and flowering shoots are often used for their healing effect in pulmonary complaints. The leaves can also be used externally to stop bleeding. They are harvested in the spring and dried for later use. A distilled water made from the plant is an effective eyewash for tired eyes.

The tannins in lungwort have a slight astringent effect when applied to the skin, thereby reducing secretions, relieving irritation, and improving tissue firmness.

It has been used as a wash, poultice, or soak for hemorrhoids and minor skin injuries such as scrapes and sunburn.

Lungwort has a high mucilage content and this makes it useful in the treatment of chest conditions, being of particular benefit in cases of chronic bronchitis. The herb is very mucilaginous and contains silica, tannins and saponins. It combines well with other herbs such as coltsfoot (Tus-fa.) in the treatment of chronic coughs including whooping cough and can also be taken to treat asthma.

Lungwort is good for coughs, hoarseness, and mild lung problems. It acts as a good expectorant, which breaks up chest congestion. Soothes throat irritation. It can also be used for diarrhea, which makes it useful for a stomach virus accompanied by a cough.

HOMEOPATHIC - Pul-o. is used in the treatment of bronchitis, coughs and diarrhea. Bronchial catarrhs, colds. In the past, lungwort was given for the coughing up of blood arising from tubercular infection.

REFERENCES - Murphy.

PULSATILLA NIGRICANS

(Wind Flower)

PHARMACY - puls. Pulsatilla nigricans. Wind flower. Pasque flower. Pulsatilla pratensis. Anemone pratensis. N. O. Ranunculaceae. Pastures in Central and Northern Europe, parts of South of England. Tincture of entire fresh plant when in flower (it flowers in spring and again in autumn). ***Historical dose:*** Tincture and all potencies.

CLINICAL - Acne. Allergies. Amaurosis. ***Amenorrhea. Anemia.*** Bladder, catarrh. Blepharospasm. Breast-feeding, disorders. Breasts, pain. Bronchitis. Cataract. Catarrh. Chest, pains. ***Chickenpox.*** Chilblains. Clavus. ***Colds. Conjunctivitis.*** Coughs. Diarrhea. Distention. Dysmenorrhea. Earache. Epilepsy. ***Ear, disorders. Eye, disorders.*** Fears. Feet, painful. ***Fetus, mal-position***. Freckles. Gonorrhea. Gout. Hands, painful. Heart, palpitations. Heartburn. Hemorrhoids. Hydrocele, congenital. Hysteria. Intermittent, fever. Faints. Labor, pains. ***Leucorrhea. Measles. Menstruation, abnormal.*** Moles. ***Mumps.*** Neuralgias. Nosebleed. Nymphomania. Ophthalmia. ***Otitis, media.*** Ovaries, inflammation. Phlegmasia alba dolens. Pregnancy, troubles. Priapism. Prostatitis. Prostatorrhea. Puerperal convulsions. Puerperal fever. Puerperal, mania. Retained, placenta. Rheumatism, gonorrheal. ***Sinusitis. Smell, loss.*** Spine, curvature. Styes. Synovitis. Tapeworm. Taste, lost. Tongue, coated. Toothaches. Urinary, incontinence. Uterus, prolapse. ***Vaginitis.*** Varicose veins. Whitlow.

HERBAL - Pasque flower is in bloom at Easter, its flowers have been used for coloring Easter eggs. It is a medicine of ancient times, and its affinity for the eyes seems to have been noted from the beginning. Perhaps its tearful propensities gave rise to the legend that it sprang from the tears of Venus. Dioscorides mentions it as a remedy for headache and ophthalmia.

HOMEOPATHIC - Stoerck was the forerunner of Hahnemann in the modern use of Puls.; he employed it especially in chronic disorders of the eyes (catarrh, amaurosis, spots on cornea). Pulsatilla affects the emotions, veins, mucus membranes, respiration and one side. It is pre-eminently a female remedy, especially for mild, gentle, yielding disposition.

Useful in acute as well as chronic diseases. Most suitable when not only the physical symptoms correspond but also when the mental and emotional disorders peculiar to the remedy encounter similar states in the disease to be cured, or at least in the temperament of the patient.

The disposition and mental state are the chief guiding symptoms. Sad, crying readily, weeps when talking. ***Moody***, contradictory. ***Changing, shifting symptoms,*** known as a weather cock remedy. Alternations. Symptoms rise to a certain pitch, then suddenly cease.

Changeable nature. Erratic temperatures in fevers. Alternate pallor and redness of face. Wandering pains shift rapidly from one part to another, also with swelling and redness of the joints. Hemorrhages apparently stop and in a few hours return. Stools constantly changing color, no two stools alike.

When one set of symptoms comes on another vanishes. Symptoms appear on one side or go to side lain on.

The patient seeks the open air, always feels better there, even though he is chilly. ***Thirstless, chilliness and shortness of breath*** with digestive or menstrual disorders. Chilliness with pains but burning with stitching pains with numbness.

Mucus membranes are all affected. Mucus ***discharges are profuse, bland, thick, yellowish-green***. Metastasis. Hemorrhages, passive, vicarious, blood dark, easily coagulating. Varicose veins. Anemia. Emaciation of suffering parts. Symptoms in distant parts of the body cause dyspnea.

Epilepsy with absent or irregular menses. ***Never well since puberty.*** Chorea from amenorrhea or dysmenorrhea.

Peevish. Great sensitiveness. Scraping, jerking, tearing, ulcerative pains, wandering pains. Numbness, partial, hands, feet etc. of the part lain on of suffering parts. Heaviness. Pulsation through whole body. Wants the head high. Feels uncomfortable with only one pillow. Lies with hands above head. The longer he lies in the morning, the longer he wishes to lie. ***Child wants to be carried slowly.***

Sensation of distention in size, as if one part or every part were growing too large during pain. Bandaged sensation. Wearing of flannels or woolen clothes cause itching and eruptions. Great inclination to stretch feet. Often indicated after abuse of iron tonics and after badly managed measles.

MIND - ***Changeable moods.*** Timid, irresolute. ***Mild, emotional and tearful.*** Highly emotional, easily moved to tears and laughter. ***Craves affection and sympathy.*** Desires company. Capricious. Easily discouraged. Whining. Wandering thoughts.

Forsaken feeling. Sadness from disagreeable news. Sadness from injuries of head. ***History of abandonment or grief.*** Silent grief with submissiveness. Remorse in evening.

Weeps easily. Can hardly give her symptoms without weeping. ***Better being held and hugged. Weeps at everything, whether it is joyful or sorrowful.*** Weeping when disturbed at work. ***Weeps easily before menses.***

Over-sensitiveness to pain. Given to extremes of pleasure and pain. ***Consolation improves all symptoms.*** Children like to be carried slowly and held. Children like affection and caresses. Children are extremely affectionate, which they manifest by kissing and caressing.

Very irritable, touchy, feels slighted or fears slight. Sensitive to reprimand. Easily offended. Answers yes or no by nodding head. Selfishness. Miserly. Jealousy. Envy. Delusion she is alone in the world, that she is always alone.

Suspicious. Disgusted at everything. Fastidious. Fixed ideas about food, sex, religion. Imagines that certain articles of food are not good for the human race. Fixed ideas about marriage. Thinks that sex is a sinful act. Religious melancholy. Religious mania. Mania from suppressed menses. Despair of salvation, seeks aid in constant prayer. Weary of life, thinks of drowning.

Full of cares about domestic affairs. Anxiety better open air, better motion. Anxiety and uneasiness in bed, must uncover. Fear, wants to hide or run. ***Fear of abandonment, of being unlovable.*** Fear of marriage. Morbid dread of opposite sex. Fear of being alone, of dark, of ghosts in the evening. Fear of high places. ***Fear of insanity.***

Abdomen - Great soreness of epigastrium. Cutting, pulsation in epigastrium. Abdominal walls sensitive and swollen, tender to touch. Feeling of numbness. Chilliness from abdomen. Tense distension in upper abdomen. Pressure as from a stone. ***Painful, distended abdomen loud rumbling. Abdominal colic from ices, fruits, pastries, fat or greasy things.*** Colic, with chilliness in evening. Colic and rumbling of wind in upper abdomen. Colic from getting feet wet. Incarcerated flatus. ***Flatulence***. Cholera morbus from drinking ice-water. Pains extend into groins. Hard painful lumps in both groins.

Back - Curvature of the upper part of the spine. Pain in back and small of back as from prolonged stooping. Back painfully stiff, like a board. Backache worse lying on back, better lying on sides or changes of position, especially during pregnancy. Back feels bandaged. As if cold water was poured down the back. Chilliness and pain in sacral region during menses. Chilliness in lumbar region after stool. Lumbago, must move, yet motion gives no better. Shooting pain in the nape and back, between shoulders, in sacrum, after sitting. Swelling of cervical glands. Stiffness of neck after stool.

Bladder - Region of bladder painful to touch. Sensation as if a stone rolling in bladder. Sharp pain, pressure on neck of bladder. Burning in orifice of urethra during and after urination. Pain and tenesmus in urinating. Constrictive pain in region of bladder with urinary tenesmus and involuntary emissions of a little urine. Spasmodic pain in bladder, after urinating. Urination more frequent during attack of headache. Hematuria with burning at orifice of urethra. Retention of urine after childbirth. Involuntary urination at night, on coughing or passing flatus. Involuntary urination on laughing, sneezing. Dribbling of urine from anger. ***Nocturnal bedwetting*** after measles, worse in autumn, especially little girls.

Breasts - Lumps occurring in breasts of young girls, painful and affecting arm of corresponding side. Thin, milky fluid escapes from breasts before puberty. Aching, sore breasts. Secretion of milk during menses. Milk suppressed or very scanty. Weeps when the child is put to breast. Child refuses breast. Galactorrhea, in women who are not nursing their children. After weaning, breasts swell, feel stretched, tense, intensely sore, milk continues to be secreted.

Causations - Ill effects of suppressions, otorrhea, menses, lochia, milk etc. Abandonment. Grief. Eating ice cream, pork, fats, pastry, desserts, mixed rich diet, tea. Chill. Wetting feet.

Chest - Smothering sensation on lying down. ***Pressure and soreness upon the chest.*** Chest oppressed, as by a load. Soreness beneath clavicles. Tension in chest, worse drawing a long breath. Pain as from ulcer in middle of chest. Paroxysms of burning in chest. Hard, painful, throbbing glandular swelling in right axilla. Congestion to chest and heart at night with anxious dreams. Chest symptoms, worse lying on painful side.

Constitutions - For females of mild, gentle, plethoric, yielding disposition, who cry readily and weep when talking. Pale, chilly blondes.

Cough - Dry cough in evening and at night, must sit up in bed to get relief. Loose cough in morning, with copious mucus sputum. Dry, hacking cough from tickling in epigastrium. Short, dry cough, worse becoming warm and after sleeping. Cough from dryness in larynx and trachea, worse eating and evening. Dry cough, often with palpitations, nausea, retching, headache, backache. Loose cough by day, dry after every sleep. Cough with retching and desire to vomit. Loose cough, with vomiting of mucus. Cough with diarrhea. Cough after measles.

Ears - External ear swollen and red. Lobes of ear swollen. ***Catarrhal otitis media. Ear infections, worse at night.*** Otorrhea, discharge of pus, blood, thick yellow humor, offensive after exanthemata. Threatened ulceration and perforation of tympanum. Itching deep in ears. ***Severe earache, not better warm applications.*** Earaches, worse night. Sensation as if something were being forced outward. Hearing difficult, deafness, as if ears were stopped up. Can hear better in car and in a warm room. ***Deafness after suppressed measles.*** Impaired hearing, worse cold, damp weather, better in warm room. Sounds of wind or rushing water.

Eyes - Pupils dilated or contracted. Ophthalmia neonatorum. Ophthalmia after suppressed gonorrhea. Ophthalmia with amenorrhea. Spots on cornea. Superficial ulcers on cornea. Incipient cataract. ***Catarrhal conjunctivitis.*** Sub-acute conjunctivitis with dyspepsia, worse in warm room. Conjunctivitis from colds. ***Thick, profuse, yellow, bland discharges***. Burning, itching in eyes, must rub. Child frequently rubs eyes. Profuse, acrid lachrymation and secretion of mucus. Pressure, as from sand in eyes, when reading. Weeping eyes. Fistula lachrymalis, discharging pus on pressure. ***Lids inflamed, agglutinated.*** Veins of fundus oculi greatly enlarged. ***Styes,*** recurrent, upper lids. Blepharitis with acne of face. Oversensitive to light. Allergies.

Face - Face puffed, blue, red. Flushes. ***One cheek red, the other pale, during fever.*** Paleness of face during vertigo. Painful sensitiveness of skin of face. Facial erysipelas with stinging, pricking pains, skin peels off. Acne of young, growing girls. Prosopalgia towards evening until midnight, chilly with pain. Facial neuralgia. Right-sided neuralgia, with profuse lachrymation. ***Mumps, especially metastatic to the breast or testes.*** Tension of face and fingers, as if parts would become swollen. Boring pain in left malar bone. Frequently licks dry lips. Swelling of lower lip. Licks lips, crack in center of lower lip. Sweat on one side of face.

Female - ***Amenorrhea*** (Ign., Cimic., Polyg., Senec.), from wet feet, nervous debility, anemia or chlorosis. ***Menses delayed at puberty.*** Suppressed menses. Dark, thick menses. ***Menses too late, scanty*** after bathing. Menses clotted, changeable. Flow more during day while walking about. Menses intermittent, irregular, or vicarious. Tardy menses. Bearing down pain, worse lying. Dysmenorrhea beginning in puberty. Dysmenorrhea, with chilliness, paleness of face, stretching and yawning. Metrorrhagia after abuse of quinine and iron. Leucorrhea worse lying down. ***Acrid, milky leucorrhea, thick like cream***, with swollen vulva. Leucorrhea with pain in the back and exhaustion. Leucorrhea after masturbation. Vaginismus. Serous cysts, indurations or polyps in vagina. Promotes expulsion of moles. Nymphomania. Threatened miscarriage after fright. ***Malposition of fetus, breach position.*** Labor pains causes palpitations. Labor pains too weak or ceasing, with somnolence. ***Weak labor pains.*** Bearing down pain, worse lying. After-pains too long and too violent. Post-partum hemorrhages from retained placenta.

Food - ***Hunger, but doesn't know for what.*** Changeable appetite. Sudden loathing, worse eating. Food tastes too salty. ***Thirstlessness with nearly all complaints.*** Aversion to butter, pork, meat, fats, milk, bread, buckwheat. Aversion to warm food and drink. Aversion to smoking. Craving for what disagrees, pungent food, cheese, sweets, ice cream, peanut butter, soft-boiled eggs, herring. Craves or dislikes butter. Desire for tonics, acids, sour, lemonade, refreshing things, beer or alcoholic drinks. ***Worse from rich foods, fats, pork. Worse pastries, desserts, ice cream***. Bad effects from onions.

Head - Confusion of head as after intoxication. Headaches from overwork, suppressed sexual desire, indigestion. ***Headache from overloaded stomach, from pastry, fats, ice cream. Headache from abuse of coffee, spirits or chamomile tea.*** One-sided headaches, pulsating, bursting, with scalding. ***One-sided headaches, lachrymation of the affected side.*** Headaches of schoolgirls at puberty. ***Headaches, better walking in open air.*** Occipital pain, worse coughing. Numbness of head during headache. Occipital headache worse coughing. Shooting pains in temples. Wandering stitches about head, pains extend to face and teeth. Frontal and supra-orbital pains. Neuralgic ***scalding*** pains, beginning in ***right temporal side***. Pressure on vertex. Head seems heavy, cannot hold upright, cannot raise it. Sensations of emptiness in head. Humming in head. Tumors on scalp, suppurating. Profuse sweat on hairy scalp.

Heart - Burning in region of heart. Catching pain with short breath, better by pressure of a hand and walking. Murmur in jugular veins. Anxious palpitations with amenorrhea, from emotions, after dinner. Nervous palpitations in young girls during puberty, or from amenorrhea. Palpitations, worse lying on left side. Pulse with distended blood vessels. Beat of pulse is felt in pit of stomach. Pulse frequent in evening. Pulse slower in morning. Heart symptoms reflex from indigestion.

Kidneys - Cystitis with weeping. Urging to urinate when lying on back. Sensation as of a stone rolling in the bladder. Stricture, urine passed only in drops and stream interrupted (Clem.). Urine dribbles when angry. Spasmodic pain in bladder after urinating. Burning in orifice of urethra during and after urination. Hematuria after urination. Heavy pressure or cramp in bladder after urination. Involuntary urination at night during sleep, while coughing, sneezing or passing flatus. Involuntary on lying down, laughing, hearing sudden noise after surprise, shock.

Limbs - Swollen, red joints. Pains down lower limbs, alternating sides. ***Pains, worse from letting the affected limb hang down*** (Vip.). ***Tensive pain, letting up with a crack***. Drawing, tensive pain in thighs and legs with restlessness, sleeplessness and chilliness. ***Pain in limbs, shifting rapidly***. Rheumatism caused by getting wet. Rheumatism from protracted wet weather. Legs feel heavy and weary. Numbness in legs when after long standing. Painful hip joint. Knees swollen with tearing drawing pains. Sticking in tibia worse lying better cool air and walking. Milk leg. Periostitis. Inclination to stretch the feet. Feet red inflamed, swollen, edematous. Boring pain in heels toward evening. Cold sweat on legs. Foul foot sweat. Arms feel broken and dislocated. Elbows numb. Veins in forearms and hands swollen. Veins full, varicose, painful.

Lungs - ***Craves open fresh air, must open the window. Shortness of breath,*** anxiety and palpitations worse lying on left side (Phos.). Smothering sensation on lying down, ***worse in warm, stuffy rooms.*** Asthma in evening after a meal. Asthma from suppressions. Dry, hacking cough, from tickling in epigastrium. Dry cough in evening and at night. ***Cough must sit up in bed to get relief.*** Loose cough in the morning with copious mucus expectoration. Urine emitted with cough (Caust.). Cough after measles. Expectoration, thick, purulent, slimy, sweet, salty, bitter as it loosens up. ***Bland, yellow, greenish expectoration***. Large quantities of yellow, thick, lumpy mucus, worse mornings. Groaning or rattling breathing. Broncho-pneumonia in chlorotic or anemic women. Acute suppuration of lungs. Pneumonia from hepatic troubles or during measles.

Male - Orchitis, pain from abdomen to testicles. Orchitis, gonorrheal or from sitting on cold stones. Testicles hang low down. Soreness of testes. Burning and aching of testes, with or without swelling. Burning down left spermatic cord. Epididymitis. ***Acute prostatitis*** with pressure and great heat in perineum. Enlarged prostate. Hydrocele, varicocele, sarcocele. ***Thick, yellow discharge from urethra, late stage of gonorrhea.*** Bloody emissions. Pain and tenesmus while urinating, ***worse lying on back.*** Venous congestion of penis. Sexual desire in morning on waking, long-lasting morning erections. Nocturnal emissions, without dreams. Sexual excesses resulting in headache, backache, limbs heavy.

Modalities - ***Better from cool, fresh, open air.*** Better uncovering, cold applications, cold food and drinks, though not thirsty. Better from erect posture, lying with head high. ***Better continued, gentle motion***, pressure, rubbing, massage. ***Worse from warmth of air, stuffy rooms,*** clothes, bed, sun. Worse getting feet wet, before and during thunderstorms. ***Worse at twilight, sunset,*** evening and night. Worse rest, beginning motion. Worse lying on one side, hanging down limbs. ***Worse puberty, before menses, pregnancy***. Worse from eating, long after. ***Worse from rich foods, pastry, fats, ice cream,*** pork, eggs, tea. Worse hot food, is vomited immediately, aggravates toothache. Worse from iron, quinine. Never been well since puberty (anemia, bronchitis, phthisis).

Mouth - ***Crack in middle of lower lip.*** Frequently licks dry lips. Offensive breath. Offensive odor from mouth (Aur., Merc.). Copious salivation during pain in stomach. Much ***sweet saliva.*** Tenacious saliva, like frothy cotton. Watery saliva like water brash. ***Dry mouth without thirst***, wants it rinsed frequently. ***Yellow or white tongue, covered with a tenacious mucous***. Diminished taste and smell to all foods. Loss of taste with nasal catarrh. ***Alterations of taste***, bitter, bilious, greasy, salty. ***Foul taste***. Greasy taste. Food, especially bread, tastes bitter. Food leaves an aftertaste. Taste as of bad meat.

Nose - Foul discharge or odor before the nose. Bad smells, as of old catarrh. Imaginary smells. Stoppage of nose with loss of smell, taste and appetite. Coryza, stoppage of right nostril, pressing pain at root of nose, better going out in the open air. ***Chronic bland yellow discharge. Yellow mucus,*** abundant in morning. ***Sinusitis with thick yellow, green nasal discharge. Yellowish-green discharge, worse indoors, better open air.*** Nose stopped up in house, fluent in open air. Nose swollen and itching in evening. Frequent sneezing. Sneezing in sleep. Large green fetid scales in nose. Sore nasal bones. Nosebleed, before, during menses. Nosebleed from suppressed menses.

Perspiration - One-sided pains during sweat. Sweats only on face and scalp. Sweats at night, with stupid slumber. Profuse sweat in morning. Sweats during cough. Sour, musty sweat. Sweetish acid odor sweat. Sweat like musk.

Rectum - ***Changeable stools.*** No two stools alike after fruit (Ars., Chin.). Rumbling, watery, worse at night. Obstinate constipation. Constipation with headache, irregular menses. ***Constipation alternating with diarrhea.*** Frequent urging, as if diarrhea would occur. Dysentery, mucus and blood with chilliness (Merc., Rheum.). Diarrhea in jaundice with sensation of heat. Diarrhea after fright. Diarrhea during or after menses. Discharge of blood from rectum even when not at stool. Pressure in rectum after stool. Burning and cutting pains in rectum during stool. Smarting of anus after stool. Blind hemorrhoids with itching and sticking pains, worse menses, lying down.

Sensations - As if beside himself. As if death were near. As if looking through a sieve. As if one had turned in a circle a long time, as if he would fall, as if he were dancing. As if in a hot atmosphere. Chill as if drenched with cold water. As if brain would burst and eyes fall out of head, on coughing. Limbs as if bruised, as if asleep. Tongue as if burnt. Pain as from subcutaneous ulceration. As of a hot coal above ulcer.

Skin - Skin itches on being heated. Itching as from numerous fleas. Herpes zoster. Erysipelas. Moles or freckles in young girls. ***Urticaria after rich food, with diarrhea.*** Urticaria from delayed menses, worse undressing. Urticaria in summer. Acne at puberty. Ulcers with hard, red, glistening areola. Wounds suppurate. Pus thick, yellow, bland, too profuse. Swollen glands. ***Measles with catarrhal symptoms.*** Varicose veins.

Sleep - Sleeps late in morning. Wakes unrefreshed, confused. Great sleepiness during day. Irresistible sleepiness in afternoon. Frequent yawning. Yawning during cough. Sleeplessness on account of an anxious sensation of heat. Sleeplessness from ideas crowding on mind. ***Wide awake in the evening***, restless first sleep. Talks, whines or screams during sleep. Chattering in sleep. ***Lies upon back, with hands over head***, or with arms crossed on abdomen and feet drawn up. Dreams, frightful, disgusting, voluptuous, confused. Anxious dreams when lying on left side. Dreams of cats, of black beasts, of men, of falling. Sad dreams with weeping.

Stomach - Pain as from subcutaneous ulceration. Visible pulsations in the pit of stomach (Asaf.). All-gone sensation, especially in tea drinkers. Weight as from a stone, especially in morning on awakening. Gnawing, hungry feeling (Abies-c.). ***Bitter taste***, diminished taste of all food. ***Stomach disordered, feels heavy.*** Pain in stomach an hour after eating (Nux-v.). ***Indigestion from rich, greasy, fatty foods.*** Worse after ices, fruits, pastry. Dyspepsia with great tightness after a meal, must loosen clothing. ***Flatulence***. Heartburn. Water brash with foul taste in the morning. ***Belchings, taste of food remains a long time.*** Hiccough when smoking tobacco. Persistent nausea. Nausea, with colic, better after vomiting. ***Vomiting after fruits, fats, pastry, ices.*** Vomiting with pale face and chilliness. Vomiting of food eaten long before. Morning sickness.

Stools - ***Changeable stools.*** No two stools alike after fruit (Ars., Chin.). Green, bilious, stools. Stools resembling stirred eggs, perfectly white, yellowish white. Discharge of acrid, mucus stools, with sensation of weakness in loins, during urination. Mucus, blood, mixed with stool.

Teeth - Sensation as if teeth would be forced out. Sharp, shooting pains in teeth. Looseness of painful teeth. Toothache, better holding cold water in mouth (Coff.). Toothache from picking teeth. Toothache from abuse of quinine. Toothache better outdoors, returns on coming into room. Sore gums, with gnawing pain.

Temperature - Body hot, limbs cold. Childhood fevers, ***chickenpox, earaches, measles and mumps.*** Prophylactic for measles. Erratic temperature in fevers. Feverish, hot, body temperature normal. ***Moaning during fever.*** Attacks of flushes of heat. Fever just at sunset. ***External heat is intolerable***. Intolerable burning heat at night with ***distended veins***. Heat in parts of body, coldness in other. Partial sweat. During apyrexia, headache, diarrhea, loss of appetite, nausea. Chilly, yet averse to heat in ***warm, stuffy rooms*** with pain, on lying down at night. ***Chilliness without thirst***. Chilly with pains in spots, worse evening. Chill about 4 p.m. One-sided coldness with numbness. One hand cold.

Throat - Great dryness of throat, in morning. Dry, sore throat with sense of dysphagia. Food lodges in throat. Constricted feeling about throat. Rawness and scraping. Stinging, sharp pain worse swallowing saliva or after food. As if a lump in it, when swallowing. Tough mucus in throat, worse night and morning. Hoarseness, comes and goes. Hoarseness and roughness of throat, can't speak a loud word. Nervous aphonia. Sensation of a worm wriggling up. Dilated or varicose veins in throat. As of a sulphur vapor when coughing.

Tongue - Dryness of tongue in morning. Edges of tongue feel sore as if scalded, middle of tongue feels as if burnt. Tongue feels too broad, too large. Yellow or white tongue, covered with tenacious mucus. Tongue bright red and covered with a network of dilated and congested veins. Blisters on sides and tip of tongue. Biting pain on tip of tongue. As if tongue would be torn out.

Vertigo - ***Vertigo caused by indigestion.*** Vertigo with nausea and gastric disturbances. Vertigo on stooping, with nausea. Vertigo as if intoxicated, with whirling. Vertigo with loss of sight. ***Vertigo, better in open air***, worse sitting up, looking up. Vertigo before, during menses, after suppressed menses.

Vision - Diplopia. Amblyopia, with diminished hearing. Obscured vision in morning on rising, and on going into a warm room. Dim vision, as from accumulation of mucus. Dim vision, after getting warm from exercise, before menses. As if veil before eyes, worse in bright light. Loss of vision at night, as if eyes were tightly bound by a cloth, with menstrual disturbances. Day blindness with amenorrhea. Fiery circles. Bright streaks and rainbow colors.

COMMENTS - Hahnemann gave in the picture of Puls. "a timid, weeping disposition with a tendency to inward grief and silent peevishness or at all events a mild and yielding disposition. Especially when the patient in his normal health was good-tempered and mild or even frivolus and good-humored.

"It is therefore especially adapted for slow, phlegmatic temperaments, on the other hand, it is but little suitable for persons who form their resolutions with rapidity and are quick in their movements, even though they may appear to be good-tempered.

"Puls. acts best where there is a disposition to chilliness and thirstlessness. It is suitable for females when their menses come on some days after the proper time. Especially when the patient must lie long in bed at night before he can get to sleep and when the patient is worse in the evening. It is useful for the ill effects caused by eating pork."

Rapid, changeable moods and desires. Capricious. Changeable and soft. Generally healthy, affectionate, loving, humble, particularly as children. Very sociable, needs attention, desires company. Exaggerated mothering instincts (opposite of Sep.). Better from consolation. Babies better from picking up, gentle rocking.

Strong fear of loneliness, often an etiology. Fear of abandonment, grief over abandonment, "forsaken feeling." Helpless feeling. Depression, insomnia, stemming from loneliness. Fear of being alone, the dark, more often in children. Fear of being unlovable.

Weeps easily, poor confidence, jealous. Self pity. Dependent, strong desire to please. Inability to make decisions. Fixed ideas, from parents, about diet, relationships, religion. Seeks stability. Can smother people in relationships, drive them away because of their neediness. Likes sex because of closeness, company.

Generally soft and fleshy. Great desire for fatty, creamy, buttery foods. Worse from fatty foods, rich foods, pastries, pork, sweets. Can have digestive problems, even nightmares, from overly rich foods. Dependency on food, eats when depressed. Emotional addiction to food, bulimia. Obliged to exercise to lose weight and to rationalize food choices.

Food cravings, but doesn't know what for. May eat too late in the evening, leading to nightmares, headaches and stomachaches. All-gone sensation in stomach, especially in tea-drinkers. Thirstless. Great dryness of mouth without thirst.

Chilly or warm blooded, but susceptible to cold, wet weather, worse sinus and menstrual symptoms. Craves fresh, open air. Will cover themselves with many blankets, then open a window to feel a cool breeze.

Loves to walk slowly outdoors, improves symptoms. Likes the seashore, walking by the ocean. Better slow, passive motion in the open air. Worse from warm, stuffy rooms. Dislike the confines of clothing. Fear of suffocating, drowning. Feels closed in.

Better lying with the head higher than the rest of the body. Worse at twilight, sad at twilight (Rhus-t., Phos.).

Measles, mumps, typhoid fevers, bilious, catarrhal intermittent, or rheumatic. In fevers, "chilly, worse by warmth, thirstless." Chilliness may be one-sided and associated with numbness. Chilliness flitting in spots, now here, now there. Heat with distended veins and burning hands that seek cool places, without thirst. Profuse sweat, may be one-sided, sour, sweetish sour or musty in odor.

"Mousey" odor, similar to measles, as well as a cough, catarrhal symptoms and rash. Ear trouble as a sequelae or complication of measles or other fever. Effects of suppressed rashes and metastases, as of mumps to testes or breasts. Prophylactic against measles (Bell.). For scarlatina, give 3c three times a day.

Pains appear suddenly and leave gradually, or tension increases until very acute, then "lets up with a snap." Characteristic wandering pains. When lying down, pain is in side on which patient is not lying, but when changing position, pain goes to the side that had been lain on before change of position. Rheumatoid arthritis. Rheumatic pains shift from joint to joint. Suffering parts emaciate. Vascular engorgement.

Congestion in respiratory system. "Pressure upon the chest and soreness." Coughing with a copious expectoration. Sinusitis. Secretions are generally thick, bland and yellowish green. Earaches (Cham.), sore throats, particularly with clinging and changeable moods. Colic, in babies. Can have a history of many acute infections and drug treatment.

Can almost be regarded as an organ remedy for the generative organs of both sexes. Gonorrhea with thick, purulent secretion. Effects of suppressed gonorrhea orchitis and cystitis, prostatitis, sarcocele, varicocele, and hydrocele. Metastasis of mumps to testes or breasts.

Useful for the sexual period from puberty to menopause, including menstruation, pregnancy, the puerperium and breast-feeding.

First serious impairment of health is referred to age of puberty, "never been well since," anemia, bronchitis, tuberculosis.

Premenstrual syndrome. Irritable before menses, weeps easily. Delay of menses in spite of evident symptoms of a flow of blood towards the uterus. Menstrual blood is black, coagulated, impoverished if menses either too early or too late. Menstrual cramps with chills and weeping. Epilepsy with absence or irregularity of menses.

Vaginitis with thick yellow or yellow green discharge, or without specific symptoms (Thuj., Nat-p.), may or may not have itching. Menopause with heat and flushing, desire for fresh air.

Weeping during pregnancy. Fears during pregnancy, that they are unloved, that no one will help with the baby. Feelings of helplessness, lead to weeping. Fear that they will not be a good mother, that something is wrong with the baby. Morning sickness with headaches, vomiting and nausea, and a large appetite. Labor pains. Ineffectual and weak labor (Caul.).

Bojanus related two cases, the first in which a girl, 18, of good constitution with no hereditary predisposition, had amenorrhea for six months and a fit occurred at the time each period was due. In the epileptic aura, she looked sad, pale as death, had chewing movements. Puls. 6c one dose a day was given. The next month, menses returned and there were no more fits.

The second case was of a robust girl, 14, with no hereditary predisposition. She had fits for twelve months. The exciting cause was the non-appearance of menses. She had one great fit per month, small fits daily. In the epileptic aura she was self willed, angry, stood on one spot, stared into vacancy, stamped her foot. In the fit she cried, had deathly paleness, bit her tongue, urine flowed. She continued the occupation she was engaged with at the beginning of the fit. Puls. 30c one dose a day was given.

Some weeks after, she had a slight fit. A month later, menses came on for first time, she had no great fits, and small ones were rare. She was given Puls. 30c one dose a week. A month later, she had a great fit. Puls. was then given once a day. She had no more great fits, only a few small ones. The cure was permanent.

Teste noted a case of Stoerck's, in which a young girl who had amaurosis of both eyes since infancy. Stoerck cured in two months, administering an extract internally and externally a dry powder. The latter caused at first an acute pain and profuse flow of tears after which the pains, which had existed previous to the lachrymation, diminished as soon as it commenced and finally disappeared with it.

RELATIONS - ***Antidoted by:*** Cham. and Puls. antidote each other and follow each other well. If either one has over-acted the other will probably neutralize the ill effect and carry on the good. Coff., Ign., Nux-v. When the improper use of Puls. has affected the air passages, Calc-p. has proved the best antidote. ***Antidote to:*** Chin., Chin-s., Ferr. (in chlorotic girls who have been damaged by iron, Puls. has excellent effect). ***Compare:*** (1) Puls., similar effects. Cycl., Kali-bi., Kali-s., Sulph. (2) Tearfulness, Sep., Nat-m., Ign. (3) Varicose veins, varicocele, orchitis, milk leg, Ham. (4) Ophthalmia, Arg-n. (5) All-c., both have worse in room, better open air, but All-c. discharge is thin and excoriating, Puls. thick and bland. (6) Stinging pains in throat worse swallowing saliva and after eating, Apis. (7) Feeling as if food lying in esophagus, Chin., Abies-n. (8) Effect of fat food, Ip. Thuj., Carb-v. (9) Effect of ice cream, Ars., Carb-v., Ip., Bell-p. (10) Mixed diet, Nux-v., Ip., Chin. (11) Desire for lemonade, Cycl., Sabin., Bell. (12) Gastric ailments from pork, (13) Retained placenta, Canth. after-pains, Cham., Xan., Cupr. (14) Non-appearance of milk, Urt-u., Ric., Agn. (15) Uterine affections, Caul., Helon., Alet., Cycl., Hydr., Lil-t. (16) Measles, Morbill., Kali-bi. (17) Earache, Bor. ***Compatible:*** Ars., Bry., Bell., Ign., Kali-bi., Lyc., Nux-v., Phos., Rhus-t., Sep., Sulph. ***Complementary:*** Coff., Cham., Nux-v., Pen. often indicated after Puls. in later colds.

REFERENCES - Boericke. Clarke. Murphy. Phatak.

PULSATILLA NUTTALIANA

(American Pulsatilla)

PHARMACY - puls-n. Pulsatilla nuttalliana. American pulsatilla. American Pasque Flower. Anemone Ludoviciana. Anemone nuttaliana. N. O. Ranunculaceae. Tincture of whole plant. ***Historical dose:*** Tincture and all potencies.

CLINICAL - Amenorrhea. Clavus. Cold, liability to. Deafness. Diarrhea. Dyspepsia. Feet, fidgety. Homesickness. Knees, rheumatism. Liver, pains. Measles, prophylaxis. Menses, retarded. Ptosis. Rheumatism. Sciatica. Shoulder, pain. Tinnitus. Uterus, pains.

HERBAL - The American pulsatilla is more similar to Puls. vulgaris than to Puls. nig. in its botanical characters. It flourishes especially in the dry and sandy bluffs which form the bed of the Mississippi.

Hale wrote "The flower is pale purplish. The odor of the dried plant is rather faint, being slightly camphor-like, the taste of the dried flowers simply sweetish and herbaceous, that of the leaves more astringent with very slight acrimony. The taste and to some extent the odor of the fresh plant are both acrid and irritating."

A. W. Miller, a pharmacist, analyzed Puls-n. The extracted substances had an acrid, almost caustic taste and well-marked camphor-like odor. When volatilized, they produced an irritating, pungent vapor, affecting the eyes and causing sneezing.

His analysis revealed constituents including organic grape-sugar, gum, resin, an alkaloid and anemonic acid. Inorganic sulphate of potash, carbonate of potash, chlorate of potassium, carbonate of lime, magnesia and "a proto-salt of iron."

HOMEOPATHIC - Dr. W. H. Miller, an allopath, claimed to have used Puls-n. with success in many chronic eye affections, particularly catarrh, amaurosis and corneal opacities, skin eruptions and secondary syphilis.

Homesick feeling. Trembling weakness, weariness, heaviness. Great debility, on rising in evening. Languid, feverish, depressed. Snapping noise in ears. Hands constantly hot and dry. Stiffness of fingers. Fidgety feet. Colic before and after stool. Colic after eating a pear.

MIND - Sad, gloomy, with frequent belchings. Homesick, despondent. Anxiety, at night. Irritable, quick, nervous motions. Dull, disinclined for work.

Abdomen - Dull pains in the right hypochondrium. Aching in one spot worse by moving. Aching in left groin, above left iliac crest on moving or bending. Dull pains in the abdomen, by spells in hypogastrium. Severe pain in umbilicus, 6 a.m., with desire for stool, stool dark, covered with mucus, severe pains for half an hour after. Rumbling after dinner of wind in distended abdomen moving from epigastrium to hypogastrium. Colicky pains after eating a ripe pear.

Back - Stiffness right side of neck, in the morning. Backache. Woke frequently with backache. Lameness in back, especially loins. Weakness of loins, feeling as if menses coming on.

Chest - Sharp, stabbing pain in pectoralis major muscle, followed by burning distress. During evening, severe pain under left arm nearer back. Aching pain in chest all forenoon. Itching blotches on right breast, right side chest.

Ears - With the pains in head and eyes, frequent drawing pains in ears from within out. Hard, drawing pains along right Eustachian tube. Sharp pains in right ear and temples. Left ear feels closed, later both. Snapping noises in ears, fluttering in right. Deafness with edema of left upper eyelid.

Eyes - Neuralgic pains in eyeballs, while walking, worse right side. Dull pain deep in eyes with smarting. Dryness, smarting, profuse flow of tears. Profuse secretion of mucus from eyes. Profuse lachrymation with dull pains in eyeball extending to malar bone. Tarsal edges red, dry, irritable. Eyelids agglutinated, profuse secretion of soft, yellow or white matter. Paralysis of lids. Edema of left upper lid. Twitching of left brow and upper lid for half an hour after going to bed, right lids worse reading.

Face - Face red, hot, flushed. After eating, flushed, pressure of blood in face. Complexion at first rough, later very clear after disappearance of rash. Painful drawing in left cheekbone and jaw. Lips dry.

Female - Feeling as if menses coming on. Menses, weak, too soon (discharge, which had been formerly too dark and with pain, was this time natural in color and painless). Menses, always copious, increased to flooding and lasted three days. In morning on awaking found menses had returned first time since weaning babe (two months). Painless leucorrhea. Leucorrhea, bland but so profuse and with so great depression that the prover refused to take more of the drug although it removed a pleuritic pain. Stinging, darting pains passing through uterus from side to side.

Food - Great hunger, rapidly returned after eating. Loss of appetite. More thirst than usual, cold water extremely grateful.

Head - Dull heavy headache, in the mornings, better by active exercise before breakfast. Dull, oppressive, frontal headache, on waking. Hard pains in upper forehead pass in wave to occiput involving whole brain. Flying pains in head and feet. With headache cutting pains in the epigastrium. Hard pain over left eye, as if a nail being pressed into forehead. Pain over right eye afternoon, better walking in open air, worse in warm room with sense of heat, fullness in head and dryness of eyes. Sharp, shooting pains through both temples in right temple. Dull pain in right temple in vertex. Severe throbbing on vertex. Full, hot feeling at cerebellum. Headache arising from nape of neck and upwards.

Heart - Audible pulsation of heart. Pulse accelerated.

Kidneys - Frequent urination. Tenesmus, extending up ureters, uneasiness in kidneys. Pain on urinating, at end of urethra. Urine pale, albuminous, excess of water, skunk-like odor.

Limbs - Muscles stiff. Cramp. Nervous sensation, irresistible fidgets, worse night, with desire to urinate afternoon and at night. Legs heavy while walking, trembling weakness, nervous pains. Aching in limbs and loins wakes him frequently. Sharp neuralgic pains along sciatic nerve from hip joint to middle of thigh. Pain in both knees, rheumatic. Dull pain in ankles, flying pains. Very cold feet, evening. Frequent flying pains in hands, feet, toes. Rheumatism of right shoulder. Lameness in muscles of right upper arm. Frequent momentary pains in wrists and fingers. Hands dry and hot all day. Fingers stiff.

Lungs - Constant inclination to cough. Small sore spot in upper trachea.

Male - Distressing erection, soon subsiding. Emission. Pain in penis on waking, worse on urinating. Hard, sticking pains in left spermatic cord and testes. Dull pains in testes, worse right.

Modalities - Better walking in open air. Better from rubbing with brush, scratching. Worse coming in from open air, warmth, at night. Worse from reading, walking, urinating, after eating, eating a pear.

Mouth - Tongue coated white, covered with tough slime, red, rather dry and swollen, yellowish coat along center, unusually red after eating. Teeth indented on tongue. Breath offensive to self and others after eating. Mouth filling with saliva. Mouth and lips dry. Smarting of velum palati. On waking, dry, flat, pappy taste in mouth, as if tongue thickly coated (which it was not). Flat, bitter, rough, sweetish, bad taste. Wakes with vinegar-like acidity in mouth and dull, pressing pain in stomach.

Nose - Dryness and heat in nose.

Rectum - Feeling as if must go to stool immediately, with constant distress in lower epigastrium and umbilicus. Constipation. Sudden attack of diarrhea while riding on horseback. Stools dark, thin, pap-like, watery, light yellow, painless, mushy, dark, slightly covered with mucus, dry, hard, lumpy.

Skin - Red rash on body, face, neck, back, chest, abdomen, limbs, worse chest and abdomen. Itching, scattered pimples, right side of chest, light red, rash-like blotches on right breast, itching severely at night, worse when heated. Slight rash on back and shoulders. Elevated, blotchy eruption on legs and back. Erythema, nodules, turn white after scratching. Intense itching all over, worse night before bedtime, better rubbing, worse riding in cold air, returned repeatedly throughout the winter.

Sleep - Sleepy, sleep not refreshing. Sleepless for an hour at 4 a.m., for several hours from over-eating. Restless with frontal headache. Many confused dreams.

Stomach - Gnawing, empty sensation. Painful emptiness, pressure, then rising towards esophagus like heartburn. Emptiness after action of bowels, after eating. Fullness in stomach preventing eating in spite of appetite. Weight and pressure in stomach after eating with faintness. Distress with severe cutting pains in epigastrium. Heartburn. Belchings, of food, hot, tasteless wind, sour air. Thick gulping. Nausea and dull headache, then faintness at stomach, on entering house.

Temperature - Chilly, with a full, uncomfortable feeling in stomach, with inclination to yawn, with papescent stool, shaking. Heat, feverish with debility, skin hot, flaccid, better cool, blustering wind. Hot face, cold feet, hands hot and feverish.

Throat - Scratchy, husky feeling in throat. Sensation of plug in lower throat. Frequent inclination to clear throat. Throat dry, smarts on waking, contains much tough mucus that is hard to dislodge. After eating, slight irritation in throat with easy expectoration of white, tough mucus.

Vertigo - Dizziness on entering house from open air, sudden in afternoon, with fullness of head.

COMMENTS - Hale instituted the first homeopathic research and Burt was the first prover. The symptoms have a strong resemblance to those of Puls. and cases cured with Puls-n. are mostly such as would be amenable to Puls.

The Puls. flying pains were very noticeable in the proving. Feeling as if needles being pressed through stomach. Heat in stomach gradually increasing to pain, worse in spots under sternum, burning, pricking burning.

The proving showed a powerful effect on the menstrual function and Hale reported many cures of amenorrhea, including the case of a young woman, formerly subject to retardation of menses.

She had constant chilliness, cold hands and feet, loss of appetite, sour belchings, nausea after meals, hemicrania, toothache, melancholy, and general malaria. Menses were two weeks late, took a chill at the time they were due, when she had precursory symptoms, no symptoms of menses now.

Hale gave Puls-n. 1x in water every two hours. After the first dose, the menses came on and the constitutional symptoms cleared off.

Hale also noted the case of a plethoric, usually healthy young woman, who had menses delay two weeks. Continual severe headache, a heaviness and fullness, worse moving or stooping. Sight dim, complete blindness on stooping or rising suddenly, weight in uterine region severe aching extending to back, worse evening. Hands and feet cold, weakness in lower limbs. Act. failed to relieve.

Puls-n. 1x, 5 drops every three hours, brought speedy improvement. The next day menses came on profusely but without pain, two days before the expiration of the eighth week.

Hale reported the case of a strong, healthy looking man who had wandering rheumatic pains chiefly in dorsum of right foot, loins, thighs, chest, arms, head. The head pain was a dull, heavy pressure in vertex, nearly constant with occasional sharp pains.

Some fever but no local inflammation of joints or muscles. Urine scanty, depositing gravel. Acidity of stomach. Appetite good. Bowels normal. Puls-n. 1x cured in three days.

A patient of Clarke's was incidentally cured of a tendency to catch colds by taking Puls-n. for some weeks as a prophylactic against measles.

Burnett cured with Puls-n. a case of deafness and edema of left upper eyelid.

RELATIONS - ***Antidoted by:*** Ant-c. ***Compare:*** (1) Puls. (2) In fidgety feet, Zinc, Caust.

REFERENCES - Clarke.

PYRARARA

(Amazon Fish Lard)

PHARMACY - pyrar. Pyrarara. Amazon fish lard. The lard of the Pyrarara fish of the Amazon river. ***Historical dose:*** All potencies.

CLINICAL - Chloasma. Dermatitis. Elephantiasis. Gangrene. Leprosy. Nodules. Scleroderma. Syphilis. Tuberculosis. ***Ulcers. Varicose veins.*** Vitiligo. Wounds.

HOMEOPATHIC - Pyrar. has been used clinically for various skin affections, leprosy, tuberculosis, syphilis, varicosities, etc.

COMMENTS - Dr. Frederick M. Dearborn, New York, 1915, who brought some of the "lard" from South America and turned it over to Boericke and Tafel wrote, "I had curiosity enough to inquire of my homeopathic friends, while visiting Rio recently, if they knew of any 'new' remedies.

"While a number were suggested that I had never heard of, Pyrarara appealed to me because of its manifest dermal indications and because I was able to procure, through the endeavors of Dr. Theodore Gomes, a small supply of the extract, and by the courtesy of Dr. Marques de Oliveira, a genuine clinical record."

"Before proceeding to the recital of the clinical case, it might be well to mention that the use of Pyrarara is not limited to the treatment of leprosy, but has been used to relieve a number of dermatoses."

"The exact diagnoses of these conditions were hard to determine, but their descriptions would lead me to think of the tuberculosis, the syphilis, scleroderma, vitiligo, chloasma, elephantiasis, varicosed vessels and the attendant dermatitis, gangosa, jaws and the varieties of gangrene. I received some positive assurances as regards its use in varicosities."

"Pyrarara is not listed in any group of Brazilian or South American remedies that I can discover and has not been scientifically proven, but I hope the following translation of Dr. Oliveira's notes may be of interest:

"The lard of the Pyrarara, a fish of the Amazon river, was brought from Acre by Major Carpenter of the Engineers, who offered it as a curiosity to Mr. Liberato dos Santos. The Major said that he had heard from the inhabitants of the Amazon valley that the lard has the property of changing the color of the plumage of parrots fed upon it, and that a person abusing the use of the fish, as a food, would develop leprosy or symptoms similar to that disease. After a talk with Mr. dos Santos, he gave me some of the lard for homeopathic experimentation on people affected with leprosy."

"The following is the result: Maria Theresa, 36 years old, has suffered from leprosy since she was 19 years old. The first appearance of the disease was on the extremities of her fingers and on her face after suppression of menstruation. She was treated by Dr. Gabizo for three years without any result and by many other doctors, using various medicines and electricity, but still no result was attained."

"The disease had reached the highest state of development; her anatomic structure had become deformed and her facial changes took away from her the appearance of a human being. Her body was covered with nodules and ulcers in constant suppuration; her ears were inflamed and deformed; her nose was ulcerated and corroded; her lips were tumefacted and ulcerated; her throat was so affected that her voice was completely lost; her arms looked like a piece of raw flesh; and the phalanges of all her fingers were destroyed. Certain areas of the skin were anesthetic and there was a general coppery discoloration."

"It was at this period that she came to me. I proposed experimenting upon her with the new medicine, which she reluctantly accepted, after many days of insisting. In June, 1905, we began our treatment, at first using the 3x trituration with a dose of three tablets every three hours applying, externally, vaseline with calendula. The first month there was no apparent dermal improvement, but her appetite increased.

I then began to use the 5x potency and during the first two weeks there was a great transformation."

"Through the open lesions came an abundant discharge of a whitish color tinted with blood and very thick, and the body was covered with bullae, where there were no ulcers before, but always the same kind of discharge. Her appetite became very good and digestion regular, but she became prostrated and suffered from neuralgic pains in the head, face, and feet. During the month of August the inflammation of the lips was disappearing and the wounds of the lips healing. She was very cheerful with the result. As her sight was getting feeble, Asafoetida was given to her and the eye symptoms improved to a great extent."

"At the beginning of September the ulcers had ceased suppurating, the bullae did not appear any more and her general state was very good. As the menstrual periods came, she felt great pain in the lumbar and ovarian regions and Pulsatilla 30th was given to her and the menses appeared, although very feeble. I then gave Pyrarara in the 30x potency for a few days and she continued to improve. The nodules diminished in size and the ulcers became almost dry, with scant discharge, while the tumefaction disappeared."

"About this time Aurum met. 5th potency and afterward Apis 5x potency and Cuprum met. 5x potency were used as the symptom called for. On the following month the menses came freely. In November I returned to the use of Pyrarara 30x potency. The healing of the wounds continued and only three ulcers were to be found on the whole body, one on the forearm, on the foot, and one on the middle finger. The tumefaction gradually disappeared, except on the ears. General condition was very good. By the 25th of December one could hardly detect her sickness."

"The intense redness of her face was gone; the forehead was white, the natural color having returned; the lips, mouth and throat were normal; while the ears were still tumefacted, the nodules had disappeared; the body was free from ulcers and nodules; the forearm completely well. Only one ulcer on the middle finger was to be found. Her organic functions were re-established, sensibility had almost returned and she could move the deformed fingers, but the sense of touch was not complete. By January, 1906, after seven months of treatment, she disappeared."

"This medication has been tried since on different people with splendid results, but lack of persistency has prevented complete cures. On the other patients the Pyrarara has been used, employing the centesimal scale of potencies."

REFERENCES - Anshutz.

PYRETHRUM PARTHENIUM
(Feverfew)

PHARMACY - pyre-p. Pyrethrum parthenium. Feverfew. Chrysanthemum parthenium. Anacyclus officinarum. Leucanthemum parthenium. N. O. Compositae. Tincture of fresh plant. Tincture of dried roots. ***Historical dose:*** Tincture, all potencies.

CLINICAL - Convulsions. Delirium. Diarrhea. Dysentery. Fevers. Loquacity. Rheumatism.

HERBAL - Pyrethrum has bitter tonic properties like those of chamomile (Anthemis nobilis) and is a popular remedy in slight fevers, hence the name "feverfew."

The Treasury of Botany noted that the smell of the whole herb is said to be particularly offensive to bees. Some popular insect powders were made of the dried flowers of Pyrethrum roseum.

Radix pyrethri, or Pellitory of Spain, which is used as an irritant and as a toothache cure is the root of Anachycles pyrethrum. The roots of the genus have a hot taste, the source of the name pyrethrum (fire).

HOMEOPATHIC - One observation was recorded with pyrethrum; a boy, 3 1/2 took 50 minims of the tincture. It nearly proved fatal, causing diarrhea, convulsions of a tetanic nature, twitchings, loquacious delirium, restless, rapid and weak pulse and profuse sweat at night.

Twitching of muscles, of limbs, subsided by morning of third day.

Violent convulsions lasting an hour and leaving the child apparently moribund, but he gradually recovered.

Feet, legs and body, which were swollen, were decidedly reduced and the next menstrual period was dark and deficient in a gouty woman, age 50. She also had convulsive movements like tetanus. Restlessness. Stupor.

Cooper cured cases of sub-acute rheumatism with Pyrethrum roseum.

MIND - Very excited, talks incessantly for hours. Lying in state of stupor, easily roused but quickly relapsing.

Limbs - Old sub-acute rheumatism of hands and small bones.

Mouth - Soreness of tongue.

Pulse - Pulse very rapid (120 to 130) and feeble.

Rectum - Tenesmus followed by involuntary evacuations of mucus, slightly tinged with blood, better next morning. Diarrhea, 5 a.m. with pain, at first profuse and exhausting.

Temperature - Profuse perspiration and restlessness at night.

RELATIONS - ***Compare:*** (1) Cham., Cina, Absin., Art-v. (2) other Compositae.

REFERENCES - Clarke.

PYROGENIUM

(Rotten Meat Pus)

PHARMACY - pyrog. Pyrogenium. Rotten meat pus. Pyrogen. Pyrexin. Sepsin. A product of the decomposition of chopped lean beef in water, allowed to stand in the sun for two or three weeks. Nosodes. Dilutions. ***Historical dose:*** All potencies.

CLINICAL - ***Abscesses.*** Appendicitis. ***Bedsores. Bites. Blood, poisoning.*** Boils. Bright's disease. Boils. Bones, pain. Constipation. Debility. Diarrhea. Dysentery. Eczema. ***Enteric, fever. Fevers, high.*** Fistula. ***Food poisoning.*** Headache. Heart, disorders. ***Hectic, fever.*** Hepatitis. ***Influenza.*** Injuries. Intestines, ulceration. ***Lymphangitis.*** Malaria. Miscarriage. ***Offensive, discharges. Ovary, abscess. Palpitations. Peritonitis.*** Plague. Ptomaine, poisoning. ***Puerperal, fever.*** Pyemia. Tabes mesenterica. Tuberculosis, lungs. Typhoid. ***Restlessness. Septic, fever. Septicemia. Sores.*** Syphilitic. Ulcers. Varicose veins. ***Wounds.***

HOMEOPATHIC - John Drysdale, in 1880, was the first to suggest the use of this substance as a medicine. This nosode is prepared from decomposed lean beef allowed to stand in the sun for two weeks, or from septic pu.

Pyrog. is the great remedy for ***septic states with intense restlessness.*** H. C. Allen indicated that it is an anti-septic, useful in septic fevers, especially puerperal. Chronic complaints that date back to septic conditions.

For all types of ***septic states when blood is disorganized.*** The heart becomes weak and muscles prostrated. Hectic, typhoid, typhus, ptomaine poisoning, and diphtheria states. Dissecting wounds. Sewer-gas poisoning.

Characteristic carrion-like odor of bodily emaciation, secretions and excretions. ***Horribly offensive discharges,*** foul, menstrual, lochia, diarrhea, vomit, sweat, breath, taste, body odor. Constipation from impacted feces in fevers, stool large, black, carrion-like. Great pain and violent burning in abscesses.

Septic fevers. Temperature rises rapidly. Quickly oscillating temperature. Fever commencing with pains in the limbs. ***High fevers with sore limbs and delirium.*** Threatening heart failure in zymotic and septic fevers. Influenza, typhoid symptoms. Cerebrospinal meningitis. Chronic malaria. ***Rosy red streaks, lymphangitis.*** After-effects of miscarriage. ***Food poisoning.***

Great heat with profuse sweat, but ***sweating does not cause a fall in temperature***. Sweats without relief. Shivers and begins to move about restlessly. Cold and chilly all day. No fire will warm, sits by fire and chilly whenever he leaves it. Chill begins in back, between scapulae. Severe general chill of bones and limbs.

Aching, bruised, sore pains and prostration, yet restless. Bones pain. ***Restless, must move to ameliorate the soreness of parts.*** Cannot lie more than few minutes in one position, better change. ***Bed feels too hard*** (Bapt., Arn.), aching all over. Great muscular debility, rapid recovery in few hours. Debility in morning, staggered on trying to walk.

MIND - Sensitive, anxious, confused. Confusion of mind. Active mind, making speeches and writing articles at night. Loquacious, thinks and talks faster than ever before. Prostration of mind, mental exhaustion, brain fag.

Weeping, tearful mood. Morose, sulky, cross, fretful, ill-humor, peevish. Anxiety in morning. Full of anxiety and insane notions. ***Desires to be rocked.*** Talks or whispers to herself in sleep. Cannot tell whether dreaming while awake or asleep. ***Semi-conscious and muttering.*** Stupor.

Bed feels too hard (Bapt., Arn.). ***Restlessness, tossing about in bed. Restlessness and delirium with fever***. Delirium on closing the eyes. ***Delirium, anxious and confused.*** Delirium from sepsis.

Delusions, sees images, phantoms. Delusion that he is very wealthy. Delusions, he is enlarged, body parts were scattered about bed. Sensation as if she covered the whole bed. Feels if crowded with arms and legs. Confusion as to his identity. Sensation of duality. Feels when lying on one side, one person, and another person, when turning, on the other side. Disgust at his own body odor.

Abdomen - Distension. Full feeling of abdomen. Bloated, sore, cutting pain. Soreness of abdomen can hardly breathe or bear any pressure over right side. Sore, bruised pain and tenderness. Cutting pain. Cramping, griping pain in hypochondria. Severe cutting pains right side going through back, worse by every motion. Bubbling or gurgling sensation in hypochondria, extending back to left of spine. Rumbling, gurgling noises. Colitis. Peritonitis, enteritis. Tabes mesenterica. Pain in umbilical region with passage of sticky, yellow stool. Ileus, obstruction of bowels, impaction. Appendicitis. Hepatitis. Cholecystitis. Buboes.

Back - Weakness, tired feeling in back. Weak feeling in back, stitching pain on coughing. Coldness, chill. Sharp, shooting pain. Caries, necrosis of spine. Lumbago. Pulsation, cervical region. Throbbing of vessels of neck running up in waves from clavicles.

Breasts - Sore, bruised pain. Pains in the region of left nipple.

Causations - Chronic complaints since septic conditions. After-effects of miscarriage. Remote effects of hepatitis, diphtheria, chronic malaria. Typhoid fever, puerperal fever. Bites, cuts, dissecting wounds, blood poisoning. Ptomaine poisoning, sewer-gas poisoning.

Chest - Pain in right lung and shoulder, worse talking or coughing. Aching pain behind sternum. Chest sore, with purple spots. Oppression of chest. Severe contracting pain within lower sternum, sometimes extending to rib joints and up to throat, as if esophagus was cramped.

Cough - Cough with large masses of phlegm from larynx, worse by motion, in warm room. Coughs up yellow sputa at night. Cough, with night-sweats, frequent pulse. Cough causes burning in larynx and bronchi. Cough better sitting up, worse lying down.

Ears - Burning pains. Discharges, offensive. Ears red, as if blood would burst out of them. Ears feel cold. Pulsation, synchronous with pulse. Noises like steam escaping. Loud ringing like a bell.

Eyes - Cornea, keratitis. Sore, bruised pain. Eyeballs sore, worse looking up and moving eyes, particularly left eyeball. Swelling of eyes. Projecting eyes. Photophobia. Roughness of margins, edges of lids. Styes.

Face - Face, burning, yellow, very red, pale, greenish, chlorotic, sunken and bathed in cold sweat. Hippocratic. Bluish around eyes. Circumscribed redness of cheeks. Hectic flush 3 p.m. to 4 p.m., lasting until midnight, then covered with large drops of cold perspiration.

Female - Fever at each menstrual period. Menses, bright red, clotted. ***Menses horribly offensive, carrion-like.*** Menses too short, last but one day, then a horribly offensive, bloody leucorrhea. Genitals severely swollen (Bright's disease). Pelvic peritonitis or cellulitis. Abscess in ovaries. Abscess of left ovary, acute throbbing pain, great distress with fever and rigors. Ovaritis. Pulsating pain in ovaries. Salpingitis. ***Prolapse uterus***, better holding the head and straining. Uterine hemorrhage of bright red blood with dark clots. Metrorrhagia, bright red, clotted, coagulated. Puerperal peritonitis with extreme fetor. Septicemia following a miscarriage with the ***fetus or placenta retained and decomposed.*** Retained placenta. ***Septic infections after childbirth***. Lochia thin, watery. Lochia, acrid, offensive, bloody, intermittent. Lochia suppressed, followed by fever, chills and profuse fetid sweat. Post-operative cases with overwhelming sepsis.

Food - No appetite or thirst. Great thirst for small quantities of cold drinks, but the least liquid is instantly rejected. Better by drinking very hot water. Nausea, better very hot drinks.

Head - Excruciating, violent, throbbing headache, better bandaging. ***Bursting pain with restlessness.*** Great throbbing of arteries of temples and head. Painless throbbing all though front of head, sounds like escaping steam. Dull throbbing in mastoid region. Rolls head from side to side. Skull-cap sensation. Forehead bathed in cold sweat. ***Erysipelas.***

Heart - Anxiety in region of heart. Consciousness of the heart. Sensation as if heart enlarged, too full of blood. As if the heart were pumping cold water. Purring at region of heart. Cardiac weakness from septic conditions. ***Threatened heart failure in zymotic and septic states.*** Fluttering sensation. Heart tired, as after a long run, increased action worse least motion. ***Palpitations,*** worse by motion. Palpitations are increased without corresponding increase of temperature. ***Pulse quick, out of all proportion to temperature or the reverse.*** Loud heartbeats, audible to herself and others. Throbbing felt in head and in ears, preventing sleep.

Kidneys - ***Bright's disease.*** Intolerable tenesmus of both bladder and rectum. Urging to urinate before fever. Frequent calls to urinate as fever comes on. Urination twice a day, scanty. Urine clear like water, adhesive, red, slimy, sediment, deposits like red pepper. ***Putrid smelling urine, horribly offensive, carrion-like odor.*** Urine scanty, yellow after standing, cloudy with substance looking like orange peel. Urine, containing casts. Red sediment in urine hard to wash off. Albuminous urine during and after delivery, parturition. Suppression of urine, anuria.

Limbs - Soreness, better from motion (Rhus-t.). Aching in bones, all over body as from a severe cold with soreness. ***Bed feels too hard*** (Bapt., Arn.). ***Rapid bedsores of septic origin.*** Great debility in the morning. Chilliness. Cold limbs. Numbness of hands, arms and feet, extending over whole body. Cramps. Pain in right shoulder, worse coughing, talking. Automatic movement of right arm and right leg, in cerebrospinal meningitis. Tingling in right little toe as if frostbitten. Feet and legs swollen (Bright's disease). Milk leg, phlegmasia alba dolens, phlebitis. Perspiration on limbs. Ulcers. Varicose ulcers on lower limbs. Panaritium. Exfoliation of nails. Nails threaten to fall off or feel loose.

Lungs - Pain in right lung, worse coughing, talking. Neglected pneumonia. Pleuritis. Empyema. Tuberculosis, last stage. Difficult breathing during sleep. Dyspnea, better open air. Wheezing when expiring. ***Horribly offensive expectoration***, rusty mucus. Bloody expectoration, spitting of blood. Rusty sputum. Rattling expectoration. Thick, offensive, purulent, viscid expectoration. Abscess opens, discharging pus.

Male - Testes hang down, relaxed. Relaxed scrotum. Scrotum looks and feels thin. Prostatitis.

Modalities - Better from heat, hot bathing, hot drinks. Better from pressure, stretching, motion, changing position, hard rocking and walking. Worse cold, damp. Worse sitting, motion, moving eyes, passing flatus.

Mouth - Dryness of mouth. Horribly offensive, cadaverous, putrid breath. Taste sweetish, terribly fetid. Excoriation of mucus membrane. Sordes. Abscess of teeth, roots.

Nose - Cold feeling in nose. Obstruction, alternating sides. Fan-like motion of the alae nasi. Sneezing from uncovering. One-sided coryza. ***Nosebleed with sepsis.*** Nosebleed during fever. Nosebleeds, awakened by dreaming it and found it was so. Disgust at his own body odor.

Perspiration - Clammy sweats. Shivering with sweats. Great heat with profuse hot sweat. ***Sweating does not cause a fall in temperature***. Sweats without relief. Profuse sweats at night. ***Perspiration horribly offensive, carrion-like.*** Sour smelling sweats. Disgust, up to nausea, about any effluvia arising from her own body.

Rectum - Inactivity of rectum. Constipation with complete inertia (Op.). Obstinate constipation from impaction. Constipation, stool remains long in rectum with no urging. Intolerable tenesmus of both bladder and rectum. Involuntary stool during urination. ***Diarrhea with fever.*** Diarrhea from excitement, emotions. ***Diarrhea from septic conditions.*** Painless diarrhea. Hemorrhage from anus. Sore, bruised pain. Fistula. Perspiration about the anus and perineum.

Skin - Pale, cold, dry. Dryness and burning. Unhealthy skin, every scratch festers or heals with difficulty. Small cut or injury becomes very swollen and inflamed, discolored. ***Septic cuts, bites, wounds.*** Abscess. Ulcers offensive, putrid, purulent, fetid, sloughing. Ulcers with bloody discharges. Varicose ulcers. ***Offensive ulcers of old persons.*** Bedsores during fever. ***Lymphangitis, red streaks on skin.*** Boils. Blood boils. Carbuncles. Scarlatina. Smallpox. Purpura hemorrhagica. Obstinate varicose veins. Erysipelas. Ecchymosis. Actinomycosis.

Sleep - ***Restlessness.*** Unable to sleep for brain activity and crowding of ideas. Sleepless from fevers. ***Sleeplessness, bed feels too hard.*** Sleeplessness from thoughts. Kept awake by purring of heart. Seems to be in semi-sleep. ***Position changed frequently.*** Slept awhile, wakes to roll and tumble. ***Whispering in sleep.*** Cries out in sleep that a weight is lying on her. ***Restless sleep from dreams.*** Vivid dreams all night, of various things, of business. Frightful, anxious dreams.

Stomach - Coldness, chilliness in stomach. Stomach feels too full. Eructations sour. Belching of sour water after breakfast. ***Nausea, vomiting and purging.*** Urging to vomit with cold feet. Nausea, better very hot drinks and vomiting. Vomits water when it becomes warm in stomach. Persistent, brownish vomiting, offensive smelling. Bile or bloody vomit, or like coffee-grounds. Vomiting, fecal with impacted or obstructed bowels. Vomiting with constipation.

Stool - Hard, dry stools, like small black balls, sheep dung. Knotty, nodular, lumpy stools. ***Offensive, putrid, carrion-like stools***. Bloody streaks in stools. Mucus, slimy bloody stools. Long, narrow stools. ***Horribly offensive, brown-black diarrhea.*** Painless, involuntary stools. Insufficient, incomplete, unsatisfactory stools.

Temperature - Chilliness with perspiration. Cold sweat over body. ***Violent chill,*** begins in back between scapula, felt in bones with sweat, at night. ***Shivers and begins to move about restlessly.*** Cold and chilly all day, no fi Temperature rises rapidly. Quickly oscillating temperature. Great heat with profuse sweat. ***Sweating does not cause a fall in temperature***. re would warm, sits by fire and chilly whenever he leaves it. Cold, then hot. Quotidian fever. ***Septic fevers***. Latent pyrogenic condition. Cerebrospinal meningitis. Fever commencing with pains in the limbs. ***High fevers with sore limbs and delirium.*** Slowly advancing hectic fever. ***Fever and pulse don't match, high fever, slow pulse.*** Frequent calls to urinate as soon as fever came on, urine clear as water.

Throat - Septic sore throats. Abscessed tonsils. Diphtheria with extreme fetor. Membrane, exudation, malignant diphtheria. Dry throat, difficult articulation. Hoarseness. Voice husky, weak.

Tongue - Tongue ***red and dry***, clean, cracked, smooth, as if varnished. ***Brown streak down center.*** Red stripe down center. Cracked, fissured tongue. Excoriation of tongue. Fiery-red, glistening, tongue. Yellow tongue. Smooth, shining, glazed, glistening, glossy tongue. Large, flabby tongue, with imprints of teeth. Clean, clear tongue. Protruding the tongue is difficult.

Vertigo - Staggers as if drunk on rising in morning. Dizziness on rising up in bed.

COMMENTS - Drysdale prepared a tincture of Pyrog., which he preferred to call Pyrexin since it is not a mere fever-producer. Others have called it Sepsin, but this is too close to Septicemia, a name given to a related and perhaps identical nosode.

The provings and most of the clinical experience have been obtained from this preparation. Subsequently, Dr. Swan potentized some septic pus, which has also been proved and clinically applied. There does not seem to be any marked difference in their effects.

As Drysdale put it, "The most summary indication for Pyrog. would be to term it the Aconite of the typhus or typhoid quality of pyrexia," and it is likely useful wherever there is poisoning by bacterial products (e.g. in the hectic of tuberculosis). Sepsis is the essence of its action.

H. C. Allen, who published the proving and most of the cases in Med. Adv., rightly describes Pyrog. as a "Product of Sepsis." He gave the indication for its use in septic state, "When the best selected remedies fail to relieve or permanently improve," analogous to the action of Psor. and Sulph. in other conditions.

Drysdale's original cases include a number in which threatened typhoid was averted, a case of tabes mesenterica cured, and one of ulceration of the colon greatly benefited. Drysdale's success was encouraging, but as he continued to use the tincture and the lowest potencies it was difficult to keep the preparation.

The remedy did not come into extensive use until Burnett published his pamphlet on Pyrogenium in Fevers and Blood-poisoning in 1888. Burnett used chiefly the 6c dilution, which is perfectly harmless and which will keep indefinitely. Heath, who made one of the preparations used by Burnett, gave some of it to Swan of New York, who ran it up into the high infinitesimal.

Much of the American experience is with Swan's potencies, including a proving by Sherbino. Yingling collected symptoms from many reported cases and arranged them with the symptoms of the proving.

In Sherbino's proving, he was cured incidentally of a consciousness of the heart, and its working and palpitation from least excitement or anxiety, worse beginning to move, congestion to head as if a stroke would ensue. Cact. had done no good.

Sherbino cured a case of puerperal fever with Pyrog., being led to its selection by the very high pulse rate. He also had a case of relapsed typhoid, with pulse 140, temperature 102 F., both were normal in twenty-four hours.

He had a third case of a young woman, 17, with a fever and aching bones where the bed felt very hard. She had a numb, paralytic feeling. As the fever left, the pulse kept mounting up. Sherbino used Swan's potency, Pyrog. 100,000c, repeated as often as effect ceased.

Clarke had ample opportunity to observe the power of Pyrog. over typhoid fever, typhoid, and hectic states, including one of discharging abscess connected with Pott's disease of the spine.

Burnett had cases of fully developed typhoid cut short at the height by Pyrog. 6c given every two hours. In his pamphlet he included Dr. Shouldham's successful experience with Pyrog. 6c in two cases of diphtheria sore throat.

Burnett also recorded that Pyrog. 5c, five drops in water night and morning, assisted in the cure of a case of anal fistula. Under its action a sweating at the seat, which the man had for many years, disappeared. The skin of his hands, which were subject to dry eczema, assumed a much cleaner aspect.

J. S. Hunt reported five cases of varicose ulcers, all of which healed quickly under Pyrog.

Bellairs gave Pyrog. 200c to an elderly woman who suffered for years with an ulcerated leg, which was riddled with deep, burrowing wounds, extremely painful and discharging freely. Hep., Sil., Ars., and Ham. did no good. Under Pyrog. once or twice a day, "a large boil" formed on the calf of the leg and discharged its contents after which the various ulcers healed up directly.

Septicemia (Bapt., Merc., Rhus-t., Lach., Ars., Echi.), after surgery. Septic bites, cuts, wounds, and snakebites (Led., Hyper.). Blood poisoning, from dissecting wounds. Gangrene (Sec.).

Abscesses with violent, burning pain. Abscesses in the muscles and major organs. Abscesses of the ovaries. Ruptured abscess of the lung, pus in the lungs. Ruptured organs, blood filled with pus. Septic organs, rotting away.

Septic kidney with offensive urine. Ulceration of the colon with blood and pus in the stool. Severe, acute, abdominal infections; acute appendicitis, peritonitis. Septic varicose veins. Large boils with accompanying fever.

Septic fever with pus, decomposed tissue, abscesses (Acon. and Bell., are clean, inflammatory). Sudden, septic onset (Bapt.). Infected bite, cute or wound that lead to an infected fever. High fevers, 105-106 F.

Fever and pulse don't match, high fever, slow pulse. Throbbing pains, sudden chills, rigors. Chill felt in the bones. Cold, clammy hands. Never well since septic fever (Bapt.). Typhoid, diphtheria. Toxic flu (Ars., Nux-v.).

Delirium. Loquacity. Confusion about the body, delusion of too many limbs. Feel as if their body fills the whole bed. Cannot find their body. Delusion of a man at the foot of the bed. Staggers as if drunk, vertigo. Confused, muttering, talking in a whisper.

Toxic state. All discharges and odors are offensive and fetid, diarrhea, sweat, breath, menses.

Putrid, fetid, offensiveness. Stench-like odors; cadaver-like (Kreos., Bapt.). Offensive perspiration (Merc.).

Bitter, offensive taste. Tongue is brown, yellow at the back. The tip of the tongue can be red (Rhus-t.). Constipation with black, putrid balls. Infected anal fissures with abscesses and offensive pus. Vomit of bile, blood and water, coffee grounds (Ars., Cadm-s.).

Rapid, irregular heartbeats, high pulse. Feels as if the heart is pumping cold water. Hemorrhage of dark, offensive blood with high fever, especially with pelvic infections and abscesses. Nosebleeds with offensive blood.

Uterine hemorrhage. Horribly offensive menses (Kreos.). Bloody, vaginal discharges that are offensive, no matter the cause. Septicemia after a miscarriage. For expelling a dead fetus (Sec.), beginning to decompose in the womb, with a fever. Decomposing placenta after labor.

Severe muscle aches and soreness. Restless in bed. The bed feels hard (Arn., Bapt.). Difficulty getting comfortable. Flesh feels tender and sore. Bone aches, bruised feeling (Arn.). Pains better motion. Cannot lie in the same place very long, must move (Ars.).

RELATIONS - ***Compare:*** (1) Echi., Carb-an., Ars., Lach., Rhus-t., Bapt. (2) Sepin. - a toxin of Proteus vulgaris, prepared by Dr. Shedd, same symptoms as Pyrogen of which it is the main constituent. (3) Malar., Lach. (4) In typhoid with soreness, bed feels hard, Bapt., (5) Arn., Rhus-t., better motion and stretching limbs, Rhus-t. (6) Cough worse by motion and in warm room, Bry. (7) Uterine hemorrhage, Ip. (8) Offensive diarrhea, Psor. (9) Black stools, Lept. (10) Constipation, Op., Sanic., Plb. (11) Lochia thin, fetid, Nit-ac. (12) Vomits water as soon as warm in stomach, Phos. ***Complementary:*** Ars., Bapt., Bry.

REFERENCES - Boericke. Clarke. Murphy. Phatak.

PYRUS AMERICANUS

(Mountain Ash)

PHARMACY - pyrus. Pyrus americanus. Mountain ash. N. O. Rosaceae. The British is Pyrus aucuparia. Swamps and mountain woods from Maine to Pennsylvania. Tincture of fresh bark. ***Historical dose:*** Tincture and all potencies.

CLINICAL - Bladder, irritation, prolapse. Chills. Clairvoyance. Dyspepsia. Gout. Heart, disorders. Hysteria. Rectum, constriction. Rheumatism. Sciatica. Tongue, paralysis. Uterus, prolapse.

HOMEOPATHIC - Pyrus Americanus, the Mountain Ash, was proved by Gatchell on himself, a married woman and two boys. Gatchell's only symptom was "irritation of the eyes." Another prover had a similar symptom.

By far the greatest number were induced in the woman, though hers were largely confirmed by those of the boys, and included severe neuralgic pains, and rheumatic and gouty symptoms. Labor-like or spasmodic pains were frequent in uterus, in bladder, like prolapse. Constrictive at base of lungs and around waist, like spasm of heart.

Aches in every joint, acute intense pains like inflammatory rheumatism. Pains seem to move in lines. Worse motion, dreads to move on account of joints. Feels as if full of cold water. Worse cold, sensitive to cold and air.

MIND - Brain active, intellect clear, thoughts vivid, whole being intensified. Indolent, indifferent, no inclination to read. Full of gloomy determination. Feels gloomy and discouraged but cannot cry. Sad, weeping mood, tears will come.

Hypochondriac, not nervous, lazy, would like to lie in bed and be waited on. Feels weak as if about to die, moans, groans, calls for help. Cries and feels apprehension, fears something terrible going to happen. Seems to her that fundus of stomach is depressed in abdomen and pyloric end of fire, a red spot like raw beef there as if stomach burnt up with raw whiskey.

Thinks she is clairvoyant, can read character and understand motions, see into herself. Seems to be able to go out of herself for a short distance to walk around and return into her body.

Abdomen - Feels constricted around waist, obliged to loosen clothes at once.

Back - Sick feeling under right scapula.

Chest - Feels as if lungs congested, especially at base and constricted.

Eyes - Irritation of eyes. Eyes feel as if they had been crying a long time, smart.

Female - Bearing down and pressing out as if swollen and burning all over. Sense of prolapse of womb.

Food - Craves hot tea. Wants soft food, feels as if meat would not digest.

Head - Headache begins over eyes, pains knife-like, left side of headaches terribly like a toothache. Headache extends to right side. Head feels as if it would burst. Great weight at vertex. Shooting pains in forehead. Headache penetrating in temples.

Heart - Oppression about heart as if it had stopped beating, as if going into convulsions. Sense of spasm at heart, as if blood too thick to circulate (better by Camph.). Heart aches as if from some great sorrow.

Kidneys - Irritation of bladder and urethra. Sensation as if bladder prolapsed.

Limbs - Twinging pains in arms, legs and toes. Drawing, cutting pain. Joints feel constricted and sore. Some pain in finger joints. Pains drawn, rending along backs of thighs to toes, worse left. Feels as if left leg drawn up and would never straighten again. Tight feeling of patella. Pain in knees is followed by pain in tendons and along calves. Knees and toes feel as if immensely swollen and ache. Left great toe feels as if torn from its socket. Toes burn. Unendurable aching of bones of toes.

Lungs - Can hardly breathe, as if cold water in stomach. Spasmodic breathing as of nervous women. Dry cough, as if pharynx stuffed with cotton. Hoarseness. Can't talk loudly, voice gone.

Mouth - Tongue partially paralyzed, cannot direct it.

Rectum - Sensation as if rectum were shrunken and dried up.

Sensations - As if she were outside of herself and could see into herself. As if stomach full of cold water, coldness extends up esophagus under sternum. As if rectum were shrunken and dried up. As if left leg drawn up and would never straighten again.

Skin - Clammy feeling of skin.

Stomach - Stomach feels weak as if nothing would digest, it feels dry and wrinkled. Feels as if stomach full of cold water. Thinks mucus accumulated in cold stomach. Feeling of coldness extends up sternum and esophagus.

Temperature - Chilly when air strikes him. Chilly down back and both legs. Very cold, shivering internally, thinks she must look blue. Cold creeping all over. Chilly and with a very tranquil feeling, especially of consciousness. Glow all over, hands sweat.

Throat - Throat feels obstinate.

RELATIONS - Antidoted by: Camph. ***Compare:*** (1) Neuralgic and gouty pains, Prun. (2) Heart, Crat. (3) Chilliness, Camph.

REFERENCES - Clarke.

Q

QUASSIA AMARA

(Quassia Wood)

PHARMACY - quas. Quassia amara. Quassia wood. Picrena excelsa, (Jamaica) and Quassia amara (Surinam). N. O. Simarubacee. Tincture or cold infusion of the wood. ***Historical dose:*** Tincture and all potencies.

CLINICAL - Amblyopia. Ascites. Cataract. Cirrhosis. Dyspepsia. Dysentery. Headaches. Heartburn. Indigestion. Intermittent fever. Threadworms. Worms.

HERBAL - The Quassia now found in the shops in the form of "Quassia chips" is the wood of Picrena, the Jamaica Quassia. The name "Quassia" was given by Linneus to Quassia excelsa of Surinam from the name of a healer, Quassi or Coissi, who employed its bark as a remedy for fever.

The wood of this tree was formerly employed under the name of Surinam Quassia. The wood is very bitter and yields its properties best to cold, distilled water. In the old school the infusion is used as a bitter tonic in dyspepsia, and in enemas for clearing the rectum of threadworms.

HOMEOPATHIC - Quas. acts on digestive organs as a tonic (Gent., Hydr.). Pressure and stitches in liver and sympathetically in spleen. Pain in right intercostal muscles above the liver. Seems to possess a marked action on eyes, producing amblyopia and cataract.

Abdomen - Sticking pains between umbilicus and stomach. Abdomen feels empty and retracted. Abdomen hard and distended.

Back - Sensation of coldness running over back with constant inclination to yawn and stretch out the feet.

Head - Constant dullness of head.

Kidneys - Excessive desire, impossible to retain urine. Secretion of urine increased, solid constituents diminished. Copious urination day and night. As soon as the child wakes up the bed is drenched.

Limbs - Prostration, with hunger. Inclination to yawn and stretch (Rhus-t.). Sensation of coldness over back. Cold limbs with sensation of internal coldness (Helo.). Drawing pain in calves.

Liver - Very acute sticking in hepatic region, followed by dull pain. Cirrhosis of liver with ascites.

Neck - Severe drawing pains in cervical muscles.

Rectum - Stools at first hard with great effort, afterwards pasty, once very thin.

Stomach - Dyspepsia after infectious diseases, especially influenza, dysentery. Atonic dyspepsia with flatus and acidity. Heartburn and gastralgia. Regurgitation of food.

Tongue - Tongue dry or with brown sticky coating.

COMMENTS - There is a short homeopathic proving. J. O. Muller took a single dose of the tincture, Eidherr four doses of Quas. 30x. Lembke took the extract.

The most peculiar characteristic symptoms were drawing in hypochondria and sensation as if abdomen were empty and retracted, with sensation as if he would have a stool. Stool at first hard with effort, later pasty. Sticking in liver and abdomen. Peculiar beating through abdomen, extending into limbs.

Eidherr had "coldness running over back with constant inclination to yawn and desire to stretch out the feet," which gives a clue to its action in fevers.

RELATIONS - ***Compare:*** (1) Fevers - Cedr. (2) Worms - Cina.

REFERENCES - Boericke. Clarke.

QUEBRACHO ASPIDOSPERMA

(White Quebracho)

PHARMACY - queb. Quebracho aspidosperma. White quebracho. Aspidosperma quebracho. N. O. Apocynaceae. Tincture and trituration of the bark. Trituration and solutions of the alkaloid aspidospermine and its salts. ***Historical dose:*** Tincture and all potencies.

CLINICAL - Asthma. Cardiac, asthma. Cyanosis. ***Dyspnea.*** Emphysema. Fever. Heart, disorders. Paralysis. Pulmonary stenosis.

HERBAL - Quebracho is a Brazilian herbal remedy from which the alkaloid aspidospermine has been isolated. The alkaloid takes the form of small, very brilliant, white crystals, sparingly soluble in water, readily soluble in alcohol and ether.

Queb. removes obstruction to the oxidation of the blood by stimulating respiratory centers. Increases oxidation and excretion of carbonic acid.

HOMEOPATHIC - ***Shortness of breath*** during exertion. ***Dyspnea***, respiratory paralysis, slowed heart and paralysis of limbs. Dyspnea with cyanosis. Dyspnea in tuberculosis and pleurisy. Uremic dyspnea. Asthma, cardiac asthma. Emphysema. Pulmonary stenosis. Thrombosis of pulmonary artery.

COMMENTS - Dr. Hale reported that Aspin. or Queb. is derived from the Chilean "White Quebracho" (Aspidospermine Quebracho). At Santiago de Chile, the bark is used as a substitute for chinchona as a febrifuge. The alkaloid forms salts with citric, hydrochloric and sulphuric acids.

Hale said Queb. produces in animals dyspnea, respiratory paralysis, slowed heart and paralysis of limbs. It relieves dyspnea in tuberculosis and pleurisy, but without influencing the fever.

The 1x relieved asthma with livid face, and dyspnea with cyanosis is frequently relieved by it. Following this were signs of emphysema and severe attacks of asthma. Rales were heard and "pearls" of rounded gelatinous masses were expectorated. Aspin. 3x gave more relief than any other remedy.

Hale noted two cases relieved by it, one of mitral incompetence and stenosis with severe nocturnal dyspnea, the other of fatty heart (Queb. had no influence on the edema, which was removed by Dig.).

Jos. P. Cobb recorded a case of heart affection of some duration in a man, age 24. There was some heart enlargement, especially of right side. Much dyspnea and a slight mitral murmur.

REFERENCES - Boericke. Clarke. Hale.

QUERCUS GLANDIUM SPIRITUS

(Acorn Kernels)

PHARMACY - querc. Quercus glandium spiritus. Acorn kernels. Aqua glandium quercus. Quercus robur var. English oak. Quercus pedunculata. Quercus sessilifera. N. O. Corylacee or Cupulifere. Fagaceae. Tincture of acorns are peeled and crushed or shredded. Water extract of acorns with addition of alcohol for Aqua glandium quercus. ***Historical dose:*** Tincture and all potencies.

CLINICAL - ***Alcoholism.*** Breath, offensive. Constipation. Diarrhea. Dropsy. Fistula. Giddiness. Gout. Intermitting, fever. Leucocythemia, splenica. ***Liver, disorders.*** Spleen, disorders. ***Spleen, dropsy***.

HERBAL - Rademacher gave the tincture of acorns to an old brandy drunkard who had long suffered from the spleen, which was at times very painful and who was at that time ***"sick unto death"*** with ascites and dropsy of the legs. The urine at once increased, but the patient complained that each dose of the medicine caused constriction of the chest.

This led Rademacher to prepare the Distilled Spirit and finally the Aqua, as milder preparations, which they proved to be, for the remedy completely cured the patient without causing further constriction of the chest.

In the course of cures of spleen cases Rademacher noticed that not only was the flow of urine increased, there was also, especially in old spleen engorgements, an eliminative diarrhea with amelioration of the symptoms generally. A passing diarrhea often appears for a time when using it.

HOMEOPATHIC - Querc. is one of Rademacher's splenic remedies. It was introduced to homeopathic practice by Burnett, who published a translation of Rademacher's account of the remedy.

Chronic spleen disorders and ***spleen dropsy***. Dropsy and liver disorders. Useful in gout, old malarial cases with flatulence. Flushed state. Vertigo, deafness with noises in head. Exceedingly nervous.

Antidotes effects of alcohol. ***Desire for alcoholic drinks***. Burnett does not find Querc. a remedy for the liquor habit, it stops short at that, but it diminishes the craving and antidotes the alcoholic state.

Clarke noted that Querc. acts well in trituration of the Acorn 3x in splenic cases, flatulence, old malaria and alcoholic history. Missionaries who used Querc. on Burnett's indications in spleen disorders found it no less effective in the intermittent fevers which gave rise to the enlarged spleens.

Powdered oak bark is an excellent dry dressing for ulcers and discharging wounds.

MIND - Nervous, depressed, glum, taciturn. Easily moved to tears, not quite capable of stating his own case.

Abdomen - ***Pain in spleen region***. Pain in hypochondria, worse left, much worse by stooping. Ascites.

Chest - Constriction of chest in precordia.

Ears - Deafness and noises in the head.

Eyes - Eyes yellow, puffy underneath.

Face - Flushed.

Head - Peculiar sensation in head, feel as when drunk, sensation lasts a minute or two. Gouty eczema of scalp, poll and backs of hands.

Heart - Fluttering, irregular heart.

Kidneys - Increased flow of urine.

Limbs - Gouty eczema of backs of hands. Hands tremble. Dropsy tottering gait. Varicose veins.

Liver - Enlarged liver and spleen.

Mouth - Foul breath, stercoraceous. Tongue foul.

Rectum - Diarrhea. "It keeps his bowels open. " Fistula in alcoholics.

Stomach - Gnawing at pit of stomach. Flatulent dyspepsia. Removes craving for alcohol.

Vertigo - Wheeling vertigo. Vertigo with disorders of spleen and left side. Afraid to move for fear having a stroke or giddiness would come on.

COMMENTS - Burnett noted the symptom "Certain few people feel, as soon as they have taken it, a peculiar sensation in the head, lasting barely a minute or two, which they say is like being drunk." This led him to use it in the treatment of alcoholism and its effects, which he elaborated in his Gout and its Cure.

The first case Burnett noted was that of a military man, 64, broken down with gout and alcoholism and pretty severe chronic bronchitis. Heart irregular. Liver and spleen enlarged. Complained bitterly of gnawing at pit of stomach. Gait tottering, hands quivered.

He had lost his wife and had to keep himself up with nips of spirits, for which he had a constant craving. Querc., ten drops in water, three times a day, completely revolutionized his state and took away his abnormal craving for spirits.

In a merchant of 57, given to nips of sherry, Querc. threw out a gouty eczema on scalp, poll and backs of hands, which took three months to cure after which Querc. was again given and completed the cure.

An officer who drank too much had foul breath, eyes yellow, puffy underneath. Querc. cured.

A hunting man, 40, free liver, gouty, had varicose veins of legs originating apparently in enlarged spleen, left by typhoid fever. Querc. cured. The patient said it kept his "bowels very regular."

A country squire, 60, bachelor, appeared in a hopeless condition. Was unable to state his own case. Flushed, much pain over the eyes and in both rib regions. Stooping caused great pain, worse left hypochondrium. Liver and spleen much enlarged. Nervous, depressed, glum, taciturn, easily moved to tears. Could not walk without support on account of his great giddiness.

Breath in highest degree disgustingly stercoraceous, nearly caused Burnett to vomit when examining him. That smell of breath, said Burnett is an unmistakable sign of the chronic tippler indicating undigested alcohol. Burnett subsequently ascertained that he was quite a sober man, but took frequent nips, particularly when confined to the house by wet weather.

The pain in left side, giddiness, and flushed state indicated Querc., which was given. In a week the breath was normal, giddiness a little better, tenderness of rib region much diminished. In six weeks he was quite well.

Clarke, noting that giddiness with spleen trouble is met by it, gave Querc. to a young woman for extreme whirling vertigo, an affect of influenza. The patient was greatly relieved when she took it in a severe attack, but if she took it when the giddiness was only slight it caused severe aggravation.

Patients to whom Cooper gave Querc. complained that they "felt as if in a vice, dared not move for fear of having a stroke or an attack of giddiness." "Deafness with noises in the head" is another effect observed by Cooper.

RELATIONS - ***Compare:*** (1) Ange., Nux-v. (2) Lach., Nat-m. (3) Helia., Cean. - spleen enlarged and painful.

REFERENCES - Boericke. Clarke.

QUILLAYA SAPONARIA

(Chile Soap Bark Tree)

PHARMACY - quill. Quillaya saponaria. Chile soap bark tree. N. O. Rosaceae. Soap bark contains saponine. Tincture of the dried bark. ***Historical dose:*** Tincture and all potencies.

CLINICAL - Bronchitis. Catarrh. ***Colds. Coryza.*** Coughs. Lung, disorders. Sneezing. Sore, throats.

HOMEOPATHIC - Quill. is most effective in the ***beginning of colds, coryza,*** often checking its further development. Colds with sore throat, heat and dryness of throat. Acute catarrh, sneezing and sore throat. Coughs with difficult expectoration. Squamous skin.

COMMENTS – Quill. is used herbally to loosen cough in chronic bronchitis and pulmonary complaints. The infusion of 1/2 oz of bark in 1 pint of boiling water is taken in tablespoonful doses or more as required. It is also used externally as a cleansing application to cutaneous ulcers and eruptions.

RELATIONS - ***Compare:*** (1) Kali-hp., Gels., All-c., Squil. (2) Sapo. - sore throat involuntary urination. Seneg.

REFERENCES - Boericke. Murphy.

R

RADIUM BROMATUM

(Radium Bromide)

PHARMACY - rad-br. Radium bromatum. Radium bromide. Triturations. Radium brom. of 1,800,000 radio-activity was employed (At. Wt. 226). ***Historical dose:*** All potencies.

CLINICAL - Acne. Albuminuria. Appendicitis. Arteritis. ***Arthritis.*** Atheroma. ***Backaches.*** Bones, disorders. ***Burns.*** Callosities. Cancer. Carbuncle, urethra. Corns. Dermatitis. Diarrhea. Duodenal, ulcer. Eczema. Epithelioma. Erythema. Eyes, disorders. Gout. Hemorrhage. Headaches. ***Itching.*** Leucocytosis. ***Lumbago.*** Lupus. Menopausal, flushes. Moles. Nephritis. Neuralgia. Neurasthenia. Nevus. Nose, disorders. Nosebleeds. Ophthalmia. Phimosis. Prurigo. Pruritus, anus. Pruritus, vulvae. Psoriasis. ***Radiation, burns. Radiation, ulcers.*** Rheumatism. ***Rodent ulcer.*** Sclerotitis. Skin disorders. Tic douloureux. Trachoma. ***Ulcers.*** Warts. ***X-ray dermatitis.***

HOMEOPATHIC - Pure radium is a white metal which "oxidizes in water, burns paper, turns black on exposure to air and has the property of adhering firmly to iron." This last quality is not without significance and shows a close affinity with ferrum. It is found in ore pitchblende.

The discovery of radium and its properties in 1898 by Pierre and Marie Curie set many persons thinking and among them, naturally, those who are engaged in the healing of the sick. Curie himself made the first "proving."

He put a tiny bit of radium salt in an India rubber capsule and fastened it to his arm, leaving it there for ten hours. When he took it off the skin was red, the place turned into a wound, which took four months to heal, leaving a white scar the size of a shilling surrounded by discolored, puckered skin.

On another occasion he left it for half an hour. A wound appeared at the end of a fortnight and took another fortnight to heal. On a third occasion, it was left for eight minutes only, two months later the skin became red and a bit sore, but it soon passed off.

Skin and nerves are affected. Acne rosacea, nevi, moles. Cancer. Lymphoid tissue. ***Ulcers due to radium burns,*** that take a long time to heal. Effects of ***x-ray burns***. Effective for rheumatism and gout. Chronic rheumatic arthritis.

Severe aching pains all over with restlessness, better moving about. Nerves are affected causing suddenly shifting or electric pains, must lie down. Electric shocks through the body during sleep.

Dull, hard aching pains all over, deep in joints, very restless. Numbness, worse stretching the part. Dry burning heat, as if on fire, through the entire body, craves cool air.

Constriction of the chest, heart etc., with air hunger. Lowered blood pressure. Necrotic changes. Marked increase in the white blood cells. Lateness in appearance of symptoms. Weakness, lassitude, tiredness. Great weakness.

MIND - Apprehensive, depressed. Tired and irritable. Cross. Easily vexed. Torpid, apathetic. Great desire to be with people, wants to have someone near. Fear of being alone, of the dark.

Abdomen - Alternating with chest or ear symptoms. Pain over McBurney's point and at location of sigmoid flexure. Colic better bending double and passing stools. Pain, violent cramps, rumbling, full of gas. Much flatulence.

Back - Aching in back of neck. Pain and lameness in cervical vertebrae, worse dropping head forward, better standing or sitting erect. Weakness between scapulae. Backache between shoulders and lumbar-sacral region, better after walking. ***Lumbar and sacral aches***, pain appears to be in bone, continued motion relieves, better hot bath, worse going upstairs.

Breasts - Right breast sore, better hard rubbing.

Causations - Ill effects of x-ray, radiation burns.

Chest - Tightness of chest. Chest pain alternating with indigestion and stuffed up feeling.

Ears - Sound of rushing water, better lying on face.

Eyes - Red, smarting, worse reading. Sensation as if pieces of cotton in eyes, better rubbing.

Face - Flushed. Acne rosacea. Aching pain in angle of right lower jaw. Violent trifacial neuralgia.

Female - Itching genitals, pruritus vulvae. Aching over pubes during menses. Delayed and irregular menstruation and backache. Menses last one day, then bloody leucorrhea. Leucorrhea, white and scanty, curdy and cheesy. Uterine hemorrhage (Ip.). Lochia putrid, scanty or suppressed.

Food - Nausea, better eating. Usual food not relished, sour things taste good. Craves pork. Aversion to sweets, ice creams, of which she is usually very fond.

Head - Both eyes ache. Severe pain over right eye, spreading back to occiput and to vertex, better in open air. Occipital and vertex pain, accompanying severe lumbar aching. Frontal headache. Head feels heavy. Aching pain of right lower jaw. Violent trifacial neuralgia.

Heart - Constriction. Wakes with palpitations. Pulse, rapid, irregular, fluttering. Low blood pressure.

Kidneys - Nephritis with rheumatism. Kidney irritation, albuminuria, granular and hyaline casts. Increased elimination of sediment. Bedwetting.

Limbs - *Arthritis*, aching pains, worse at night. Deep pain in joints, knees and ankles. Muscles of legs and hips sore. *Pain in toes*, calves, hip joint, popliteal spaces. Legs, arms and neck feel hard and brittle, as though they would break on moving. Cracking in shoulder. Sharp pains in shoulders, arms, hands and fingers. Arms feel heavy. Rheumatism of the hands. Dermatitis of the fingers. Trophic changes in the fingernails.

Lungs - Tightness of chest, feels as if she could not get enough air. Spasmodic cough. Persistent cough from tickling in throat pit. Cough, worse lying, smoking, better eating and open air, sitting up, exercise.

Male - Eczema of penis and inner surface of thighs. Itching. Dysuria, then erection.

Modalities - Better lying down, after sleep. Better continued motion, pressure, hot bath, open air. Better eating, cold drinks. Worse from smoking, shaving, washing. Worse getting up, warmth of the bed. Worse at night, noon, 3 a.m., 4 a.m., 7 a.m., and 11 a.m.

Mouth - Dry mouth. Breath seems hot. Metallic taste. Prickling sensation on end of tongue.

Nose - Burning in nose. Itching and dryness of nasal cavities, better in open air.

Rectum - Alternating constipation and loose movements. Stools, soft, dark or offensive, slate colored. Rectum sore, prolapsed. Itching of anus and hemorrhoids.

Sensations - As if skull too small, as if foreign body in eye, as if something dropped into trachea. Knees feel as if the bones would protrude. Intolerance of tobacco can be produced.

Skin - ***Itching all over body***, burning of skin, as if on fire. Irritable, thick, moist if scratched, worse face and genitals. Erythema and dermatitis with itching, burning, swelling and redness. Eczema. Psoriasis. Small pimples. Branny scabs. Scabby on ears. Scleroderma. Callosities. Cancer. Necrosis and ulceration. Epithelioma.

Sleep - Restless. Sleepiness with lethargy. Wakes panting with palpitations. Dreams vivid, busy, of fire, which seems true.

Stomach - Empty feeling in stomach. Warm sensation in stomach. Nausea and sinking sensation, belching of gas.

Temperature - Cold sensation internally, with chattering of teeth. Internal chilliness followed by heat of the skin, associated with bowel movements and flatulence.

Throat - Dry, sore, raw with earache. Feeling in throat as from eating pepper.

Vertigo - Vertigo with pain in back of head, left when in bed.

COMMENTS - After investigating radium for ten years, Dieffenbach reported that when the provings commenced, one prover's hands had eczematous eruptions, cracks, scaly excrescences and wart-like growths as a result of X-ray and radium-ray experiments. These gradually disappeared after his proving with 6x.

This is confirmed by a case reported by Mr. E. S. Pierrepont. A girl employed in the X-ray department of the hospital with which he was connected developed dermatitis of the right hand and fingers. An ointment was prescribed without benefit, and cracks appeared on the skin. Two doses of Rad-br. 30c were given, on Mr. Pierrepont's suggestion, one in the morning and one in the evening.

The following day the patient came out in a rash, which the matron mistook for measles. Her eyes watered, fingers very sore and she felt very ill. By the following day, the rash had disappeared and she felt well. The fingers were now better and they got quite well, except that a sore feeling was left after washing.

A feature of Dieffenbach's proving was the disappearance of small nevi, which is significant as the rays are used for the destruction of nevi.

Useful for indolent and phagedenic ulcers. Sores that refuse to heal. Skin cancers, especially cancerous ulcers. Severe psoriasis. There is some history of moles and birthmarks disappearing.

Dermatitis and eczema after radiation exposure. Radium burns. Ulcers due to radiation treatment (Fl-ac.). After affects of radiation exposure, weakness, tendency to infections, where nothing else seems to work (Stront.).

Rad-br has been used in cases of lupus, epithelioma, carcinoma of the cervix uterus and urethral caruncle. There are numerous cases of skin cancers cured with Rad-br. in potencies.

T. Simpson recorded one such case. A retired officer had an intractable eruption on his genitals and the inner surface of thighs and legs that had prevented him from getting any refreshing sleep for three years. One tablet of Rad-br. 30c each morning was prescribed for a month. All conditions were vastly improved and the patient got well without further medication.

Clarke reported the case of a young, unmarried woman who, after the application of a belladonna plaster to the back for lumbago, developed an edematous rash involving the whole face and neck. It was extremely irritating, worse at night, preventing sleep.

At the back of the neck was a sore, oozing patch. After temporary relief from some remedies, there still remained an irritating, oozing rash, sore eyes, first right, then left, lids swollen, oozing from corners, lips hard, swollen.

One dose of Rad-br. 30c was given. The result was dramatic. The first night she was able to sleep, waking only once. Two days later, the rash had nearly gone and the eyes had ceased to water. In a few days all had vanished and the patient could enjoy open air.

Dr. S. L. Guild-Leggett recorded the case of a girl, 2.5 years, who had shifting rheumatism from her left foot to right knee, then to left knee, hands and toes. She had also a peculiarity about her stools, they were slate-colored, very offensive, urgent and came at noon during a meal.

Guild-Leggett used symptoms from Dieffenbach's proving: "defecation at noon, stool soft, dark or offensive, slate-color, clay-color, pains in limbs, wakes 4 a.m., pains in all joints knees, ankles, feet, could not walk, had to lie down." Rad-br. was given and cured entirely.

RELATIONS - ***Antidotes:*** Rhus-v., Tell. ***Compare:*** (1) Anac. - the ulceration produced by it is like radium. It may appear elsewhere than on place of contact and appear late. (2) X-ray, Rhus-t., Sep., Uran-n., Ars., Puls., Caust.

REFERENCES - Boericke. Clarke. Murphy. Phatak.

RADON

(Radioactive Gas)

PHARMACY - rado. Radon. Radioactive gas. ***Historical dose:*** All potencies.

CLINICAL - Adenocarcinoma. Emphysema. ***Lung cancer. Lung, disorders.*** Pneumonia, interstitial. Pulmonary fibrosis. Respiratory lesions. Silicosis.

HOMEOPATHIC - Radon is a toxic radioactive gas, formed by the natural radioactive decay of uranium in rock, soil, and water. It is colorless, odorless, tasteless, and chemically inert.

Radon gas decays into radioactive particles that can get trapped in the lungs when breathed in. The primary adverse health effect associated with chronic exposure to radon is ***lung cancer***. Squamous cell carcinoma. Small cell carcinoma. Large cell carcinoma. Adenocarcinoma.

Other harmful respiratory effects associated with chronic exposure to radon include emphysema, pulmonary fibrosis, respiratory lesions. Chronic interstitial pneumonia. Silicosis.

COMMENTS - Uranium changes to different elements as it decays down to its final element of lead. All of the elements it changes into are solids except one, radon, which floats freely in the soil and is easily drawn into the lower level of homes by the natural flow of air.

Radon's primary hazard is caused from inhalation of the gas and its highly radioactive heavy metallic decay products (polonium, lead, and bismuth) which tend to collect on dust in the air.

REFERENCES - Murphy.

RAJANIA SUBSAMARATA

PHARMACY - raja-s. Rajania subsamarata. Amphypterygium adstringes. N. O. Anacardiaceae or Dioscoreaceae family. Tincture from the triturated and macerated bark in 80% alcohol. ***Historical dose:*** Tincture and all potencies.

CLINICAL - Abscesses. Anthrax. Bacillary, dysentery. Blepharitis. Boils. Colitis. Diphtheria. Encephalitis. Fevers. Mastoiditis. Measles. Meningitis. Myelitis. Typhoid. Vaccination, reactions.

HERBAL - Rajania subsamarata is a shrub 1.50m high, which grows in the Michoacan in the warm territories of Morelos and Guerrero. It has dioecious leaves, a trilocular herbaceous stem and the limb is cut near the top. It has six fibrous stamens, an ovary linked to the perigon tube with two to three seeds in the receptacle.

HOMEOPATHIC - De Legarreta proved the remedy, reporting symptoms of high fevers, general exhaustion. Stares, stunned, closes eyes as if to think more easily. Jaw hangs, muscles relaxed, slips into bed. No longer has the strength to speak.

Swelling of the neck and parotid region. Measles, diphtheria or whooping-cough. Epidemic, spinal and cerebral meningitis. Acute post infectious encephalitis in the child. Post-vaccination encephalitis.

Circumscribed inflammation of the skin with swelling or ulceration. Congestion of the nerves and blood vessels. The diarrhea is muco-purulent and blood-streaked. Metrorrhagia of black, putrid blood.

MIND - Indifferent towards everything around him, bewildered. Loss of sense of identity. Mumbles in his delirium, weeps and sighs and speaks incoherently. Sings bawdy or religious songs. Fits of exaltation, fury and lasciviousness.

Abdomen - Hypogastric region painful, especially when speaking. Abdomen retracted into a boat shape. Rumbling and abdominal wind. Gurgling in the right iliac cavity and pain at McBurney's point. Cholera-like enteritis. Enteritis. Ileitis. Bacillary dysentery. Hemorrhaging recto-colitis.

Ears - Mastoiditis. Catarrhal discharge. Suppurating inflammation of the eardrum. Sensitive to sharp sounds. Buzzing. Sensation of blocked ear, as if full of earth. Sounds seem far off like distant rain. Later total deafness.

Eyes - Eyes bloodshot. Eyes bright at first, then lusterless, as if covered with a film of gum or tears, which are burning and corrosive. The pupil is contracted and insensitive to light. Conjunctivitis. Eyelids are heavy, eyelashes stuck together. Blepharitis.

Face - Face dull, serious at first, then aspect becomes hippocratic, cadaverous. Earthy, dirty, moist.

Female - Menses ameliorate the general condition. Menses with evil-smelling blood, black and irritating. Menses with a bitter odor. Metritis. Profuse, sticky leucorrhea, causing vaginal insensitivity. Labia majora excoriated. Puerperal fever. Venereal granuloma. Ulcerous vulvar elephantiasis.

Head - Acute headache, like a nail being driven into the head. Pain in the head persisting for a long time, accompanied by anguished lamentation.

Heart - Fall in arterial tension. Sub-acute myocarditis. Pericarditis. Palpitations and diffuse pains in the precordial region. Pulse thready, weak. Heartbeat irregular, moderate tachycardia. Hears the heart heat when lying down, as if the heart were on the pillow.

Limbs - Limbs trembling and slack with convulsions. Limbs are cold, purple. Continual involuntary movements of the hands, as if seizing particles in the air.

Lungs - Chest swollen, panting and anguish. Respiration weak, becoming imperceptible. Pulmonary gangrene. Pulmonary abscess. Breath fetid.

Male - Soft canker. Ulcers. Epithelioma of the glans. Penis limp, scrotum slack. Fetid sweating, smelling of rancid cheese.

Modalities - Better from coolness, discharges. Worse from moving, speaking.

Mouth - Breath fetid, putrid, repulsive. Sticky saliva, nicotine-colored like that of a tobacco chewer. Aphthae and ulcerations which bleed at times, on the tip of the tongue. Tongue fissured with black stripe in the middle and red, excoriated edges. Teeth tarnished with yellow, then brown, deposit, despite frequent brushing. Lips swollen. Mouth open, lower jaw dropping. Slight trismus at times.

Nose - Rhinitis. Sinusitis. Ozaena. Nose dry. Hairs inside the nose bristling, as if dusty. Attacks of nosebleed, which ameliorate. If abundant, they are exhausting.

Rectum - Constipation for the first few days, then diarrhea. Diarrhea, mucopurulent, blood-streaked, loosely bound, very fetid.

Skin - Skin rough, sticky sweat. Earthy appearance with petechiae on the chest, abdomen and on the inside of the arms. Erysipelas. Pimples, boils, suppurating abscesses. Bedsores. Varicose ulcers. Painful, purulent anthrax. Soft canker with fetid, blood-streaked discharge. Gangrenous patches. Septic gangrene. Cancerous tumors and ulcerations with blue-black edges, painful and bleeding.

Stomach - Paresis of the esophagus with difficulty in swallowing. Hiccoughs, nausea, vomiting.

Temperature - Fever high, general exhaustion. Temperature between 39.5°C and 41°C.

Throat - Throat dry with need for liquid in order to swallow. Cold foods go down better than warm foods. External swelling of the throat and parotid region.

COMMENTS - Rajania has been used in compress form for ulcerations, diluted in water with 1% or 2% of the mother tincture.

RELATIONS - ***Compare:*** (1) Mur-ac. - Adynamic conditions, prostration, hyperthermia, deep, bleeding ulcerations. The patient is so exhausted that he falls into bed. (2) Lach. - Acute infections, adynamic condition with tendency to hemorrhage and decomposition of the blood. Loquacity, burning pains, cannot bear anything tight, cardiac failure, ameliorated by drainage, spontaneous ecchymosis. (3) Anthr. - Septic infections, burning pains, extreme prostration. (4) Bapt., Hyos., Bell., Stram. and Crot-h.

REFERENCES - Julian.

RANUNCULUS ACRIS

(Goldcup)

PHARMACY - ran-a. Ranunculus acris. Goldcup. Crowfoot. Ranunculus acer. N. O. Ranunculacee. Tincture of whole plant. ***Historical dose:*** All potencies.

CLINICAL - Erysipelas. Fever. Gangrene. Lumbago. Neuralgia. Rheumatism. Ulcers.

HERBAL - Ran-a. is distinguished from Ran-b. by its slender cylindrical flower-stalk, that of Ran-b. being furrowed. Both are common buttercups, and have acrid and poisonous properties.

HOMEOPATHIC - Ran-a. was proved by Franz and Lembke. The chief skin symptoms were observed in a woman of seventy who applied a handful of the herb to her limbs with the result of setting up violent constitutional symptoms, fever and intense inflammation, going on to gangrene of the skin of the legs.

Rheumatic pain in the muscles and joints, especially ankles and wrists. Pains when walking and at rest. Lumbar pains, worse on bending or turning the body. Heat, faintness and fever.

RELATIONS - ***Compare:*** (1) Ran-b.

REFERENCES - Clarke.

RANUNCULUS BULBOSUS

(Buttercup)

PHARMACY - ran-b. Ranunculus bulbosus. Buttercup. Bulbous crowfoot. North America. N. O. Ranunculacee. Tincture of whole plant. ***Historical dose:*** All potencies.

CLINICAL - Adhesions. ***Alcoholism.*** Breast, pain. Cachexia. Chest, pains. Chilblains. Corns. ***Delirium tremens.*** Depression. Diarrhea. Dropsy. Dyspnea. Eczema. Epilepsy. Feet, pains. Gastralgia. ***Hangovers.*** Hay fever. ***Herpes zoster.*** Hiccoughs. Hydrocele. Hydrothorax. ***Intercostal, pain.*** Jaundice. Liver, pain. ***Neuralgias.*** Nyctalopia. Ovaries, neuralgia. Pemphigus. Pleurodynia. Rheumatism. Sciatica. Spinal, irritation. Warts. Writer's cramp.

HOMEOPATHIC - Ran-b. was proved by Franz and some effects of its external application have been observed and results of inhaling the fumes while preparing the plant or when it has been burned. The last caused headache and in one instance epilepsy, followed by cachexia, gout, headache and death.

One prover, who expressed the juice with the fingers, reported a long-lasting and recurrent eruption of vesicles on the fingers, with blue vesicles and horny scabs.

"Small, deep, transparent, dark blue little elevated blisters of the size of an ordinary pin's head. Crowded together in oval-shaped groups of the size of a coin with intolerable burning itching, emitting when opened a dark yellow lymph afterwards becoming covered with a herpetic, horny scurf."

Symptoms rising from the acrid vapor while the juice of the plant was being prepared included "Smarting from eyes as from smoke in evening. Smarting in eyes, nose and fauces, the eyes run and are very painful. He has to stop using them for half an hour because he cannot see anything, whites slightly inflamed, mucus runs in torrents from nose."

Ran-b. is a painful remedy, affecting nerves, muscles, eyes, serous membranes, chest, skin, fingers toes and left side. Its most characteristic effects are upon the chest walls like pleurodynia. Hydrothorax. Fauces painful as if sore during an inspiration, less during deglutition. Hay fever.

Pains are stitching, stabbing, shooting, extort tears with shuddering, cannot rest in any position. Burning, biting, bruised soreness or as of deep ulceration. Sore, spots. Burning in small spots from sedentary living. Neuralgia. Herpes.

Bad effects of alcohol, including hiccough, epileptiform attacks, and ***delirium tremens***. Spasmodic hiccough. Epilepsy of alcoholics. Weak and tottering patients, from the prolonged use of whisky, brandy or other alcoholic stimulants.

Sudden weakness and fainting. Trembling from anger. Distended feeling. Shocks throughout the whole body. Sensitive to air and touch. As of a cold wet cloth, especially on chest, worse on going into cold air.

Caustic and pain producing properties. Ran-b. forms a constituent of some arsenical plasters used to disperse cancers.

M. Jousset noted it for chronic sciatica, he applied the tincture to the heel of affected leg.

MIND - Quarrelsome, angry mood. Irritability, with pains. Anxious. Worse thinking of complaints. Restlessness at night. Obtuse intellect. Vanishing of thoughts on reflection. Stares at one point. Cowardice. Weeping in evening. Depression of spirit and desire to die.

Great fear of ghosts in evening, dares not be alone. Ailments from fright, vexation or anger. ***Delirium tremens***, with hiccough. Delirium tremens, with talkative mania, unusual exertions and powerful efforts to escape from bed. ***Bad mental effects of alcohol.***

Abdomen - Hypochondria bruised. ***Tenderness of abdomen to pressure.*** Pinching colic, alternating with chest pains.

Back - ***Muscular pain along lower margin of the shoulder blade***. Pain extending through lower half of left chest. Burning in small spots from needlework, type writing, piano playing. Scapula adherent. Muscles of neck rigidly contracted, can speak only by moving shoulders up and down.

Causations - Bad effects of alcohol injury, fright, vexation. Cold air brings on all sorts of ailments.

Chest - Various kinds of pains and ***soreness, as if bruised in sternum,*** ribs intercostal spaces and both hypochondria. ***Intercostal rheumatism.*** Rheumatic pain in chest. ***Sharp, cutting, stitching*** in chest, bilateral. Stitches in chest, worse when inspiring, moving. Small sore spot as from subcutaneous ulceration in chest. ***Herpes zoster.*** Pleurodynia. Pleurisy, adhesions after intercostal neuralgia. ***Chilliness in chest when walking in open air***.

Ears - Shootings in ears, especially in evening. Cramp-like sensation in and on ears.

Eyes - Herpes vesicles on cornea with intense pain, photophobia and lachrymation. Eyeballs sore on moving them. Hemiopia during pregnancy. Day-blindness, mist before eyes, pressure and smarting in eyes, as from smoke. Night-blindness. Lids burn. Pain over right eye, better standing and walking.

Female - Acrid and gnawing leucorrhea. Ovarian neuralgia always excited by atmospheric changes.

Food - Thirst augmented in afternoon. Feeling of hunger and rumbling in stomach early in morning. Butter tastes too sweet. Bitter, empyreumatic taste while eating or after having eaten dry food.

Head - Irritable with pains in forehead and eyeballs. Aching in forehead and vertex as if pressed asunder with nausea and sleepiness. Pressing pain in forehead from within outward. As if too large and distended. Creeping sensation in scalp.

Limbs - Crawling and tingling in fingers. Itching palms. Sudden jerking, stitching pain in forearm (right) while writing. Pain in heels as if pinched by boots.

Liver - Jaundice with itching of body, especially palms.

Lungs - Anxious, oppressed breathing with desire to draw deep breath. Dyspnea from anger.

Modalities - Better from standing, sitting bent forward. Worse from open air, drafts, change of temperature, atmospheric changes. Worse damp, cold, rainy and stormy weather. Worse from change of position, motion of arms, standing, breathing, touch. Worse evening and morning. Worse after eating, alcohol. Worse from fright, vexation, anger.

Mouth - Increased saliva. Butter tastes too sweet. Crawling on palate, wants to scratch it. Cramp, spasms of lips.

Nose - Crawling and tingling in nostrils, in posterior sinuses, Tries to relieve it by hawking and blowing the nose.

Sensations - Confusion of head as if intoxicated. As if head would be enlarged. As if head pressed asunder. Hypochondria in lowest ribs painful as if bruised. Burning in left side of chest in region of short ribs. As if a full breath could not be drawn. As of a knife thrust through side and into back. As if something tearing in chest. As if cold wet cloths applied.

Skin - ***Herpetic eruptions*** with great itching. Vesicular and pustular eruptions. ***Shingles, bluish vesicles. Burning and intense itching, worse contact***. Flat, burning, stinging ulcers. Pemphigus. Blister-like eruption in palms, itching. Fingertips and palms chapped. Horny scabs. Hard excrescences. Corns, smart or burn worse touch.

Stomach - Pains in stomach. Pressure on scrobiculus. Frequent risings. Nausea in afternoon or evening, sometimes with headache. Spasmodic hiccoughs of alcoholics.

Temperature - Chilliness, worse open air. Shivering in evening with heat in face. Heat in head with coldness in hands.

Throat - Inflammatory burning pains. Scraping, burning down the throat. Accumulation of much tough mucus in throat. Spasmodic sensation of something which ascends esophagus and passes into throat.

COMMENTS - Pains in nerves, serous membranes, muscles, tendons, joints, eyes and internal organs. The pains are lancinating, pressing and outpressing, jerking and sticking, as if bruised with external sensitiveness. Pains are sharp, stitching, shooting, come in paroxysms.

Pains are induced by atmospheric changes, sudden exposure to cold or heat, worse in wet, stormy weather, from touch, motion or turning the body. General sensitiveness to cold air and change. "Worse during inspiration." Sensitiveness to touch with a sore, bruised sensation, soreness of parts affected.

Pains particularly in the chest. Muscular pains about the margins of shoulder blades in women of sedentary employment. H. C. Allen noted burning pains in small spots from close work.

"Jerks and shocks and sudden tearings in right forearm and between thumb and index finger while writing." Writer's cramp and professional neuroses. "Pressure and smarting in eyeballs." Day-or night-blindness. Herpes. Spinal neuralgia.

White-coated tongue. Bitter, sour or sweetish taste with accumulation of saliva. Scraping, burning in throat. Spasmodic hiccough, spasmodic feeling in esophagus and pharynx, ascending. Painful indigestion. Belchings, nausea.

Pressure on sternum with labored breathing. Violent burning in cardiac end of stomach, hunger early in morning, thirst in evening. Pains in liver and spleen region, worse by touch. In pleurisy, pleurodynia intercostal neuralgia.

Hering mentioned "hemeralopia" as having been cured with Ran-b. in a woman during pregnancy and in her three-year old son. The word "hemeralopia" has been used to denote both day-blindness and night-blindness. Hering used it in the latter (rarer) sense, for he says of the woman, she "can see well during the day."

The concomitant symptoms were "heat, biting and pressure in eyes, redness of conjunctiva and lids, especially inner surface of lower lids, lachrymation, pus in canthi, pustules on eyes. Eyes look weak, pupils dilated, candlelight appears as a bright circle, can see well during day."

In a child who was cured of ague with subsequent dropsy and hydrocele by applying Ran-b. to the wrist, ulcers of the fingers penetrating down to the flexor tendons were produced.

The "cold-water feeling" occurred in a patient of Burnett's. A woman, 30, had a fall two years before Burnett saw her and ever since had the peculiar sensation that whenever she goes out of doors she feels as if wet cloths were applied to three different parts of the anterior walls of thorax-both infra-clavicular fossae and under left breast. Never felt indoors, but constant as long as she is out.

Guided by this symptom, "Unusual chilliness of outer parts of chest when walking in open air, with the worse in open air and worse walking in open air," Burnett gave Ran-b. In two days, the patient was better; in three weeks, the sensation had completely gone and the general health very much improved.

Dudgeon reported the case of a woman, 27, who went for a drive three weeks after confinement.

The day was cold and an accident occurred to the carriage which frightened her.

In the evening she had a slight rigor and complained of pain in her left side about sixth and seventh ribs. Worse slightest movement, better sitting rather bent forward and leaning a little to the left. Pulse 120, no heat of skin. No signs of lung or pleural involvement.

Bry., and later Arn., gave no relief and for two days the symptoms grew worse. The patient had to be propped up with pillows, leaning forward and to the left. Her head rested on her breast, not daring to breathe at all deeply.

Ran-b. 1c relieved her in ten minutes, when she "felt a wrench in her side and the pain was gone." She was able to lie down, slept all night and made a rapid recovery. There were some slight returns of pain, now on one side, now on the other. But Ran-b. soon removed them.

RELATIONS - ***Antidoted by:*** Bry., Camph., Puls., Rhus-v. ***Compare:*** (1) Rad-a. - pain in lumbar muscles and joints by bending and turning body. (2) Rad-g. (3) Rad-r. - crawling sensation in forehead and scalp in evening in bed. (4) Rad-fl. (5) Bry., Crot-t., Mez., Euph. ***Incompatible:*** Sulph., Staph., Nit-s-d., alcohol, wine, vinegar.

REFERENCES - Boericke. Clarke. Phatak.

RANUNCULUS FICARIA

(Lesser Celandine)

PHARMACY - ran-fi. Ranunculus ficaria. Lesser celandine. Pilewort. Ficaria ranunculoides. Ficaria verna. Scrophularia minor. N. O. Ranunculacee. Tincture of whole fresh plant. ***Historical dose:*** All potencies.

CLINICAL - Hemorrhoids.

HERBAL - The "lesser celandine" is not botanically related to the true celandine, Chelidonium majus, or to the Figwort tribe (Scrophularia) although it is named Scrophularia minor in old books.

Ran-fi. is in all respects a true crowfoot except that it has three deciduous instead of five persistent sepals and nine petals instead of five. Gerarde noted that "It growth in meadows, by ditches and trenches and it is common everywhere in moist and dark places.

It comes forth about the Calends of March and flower a little after: it beginneth to fade away in April, it is quite gone in May afterwards it is hard to be found, yea scarcely the root."

Gerarde wrote that the idea of its use in hemorrhoids was derived from the cluster of small tubers growing around the crown of the root, which bear a striking resemblance to a bunch of hemorrhoids.

REFERENCES - Clarke.

RANUNCULUS FLAMMULA

PHARMACY - ran-fl. Ranunculus flammula. N. O. Ranunculacee. Tincture of whole plant. ***Historical dose:*** All potencies.

CLINICAL - Gangrene. Ulceration.

HOMEOPATHIC - Ran-fl. produces abdominal distention and inflammation and gangrene of abdominal organs in horse who eat large amounts of it, but it is only hurtful if eaten in excess.

It promotes digestion when eaten in moderation. In a woman who applied the plant to her wrist, it produced gangrene of the arm down to the tendons and bone. Ulceration.

REFERENCES - Clarke.

RANUNCULUS GLACIALIS

(Reindeer Flower)

PHARMACY - ran-g. Ranunculus glacialis. Reindeer flower. N. O. Ranunculacee. Tincture of whole plant. ***Historical dose:*** All potencies.

CLINICAL - Cerebellum, pain. Dyspnea. Headaches. Night-sweats. Strokes. Thighs, sweat.

HOMEOPATHIC - Dr. Codde of Spoleto proved the tincture and the 3rd and 9th dilutions of this plant. It produced an enormous weight in the head with vertigo and feeling as if a stroke were impending, better from coffee.

Pulmonary affections, broncho-pneumonia. Dyspnea, worse when lying down and compression of chest. Intolerance of weight of coverlet.

Influenza with an enormous weight in head with vertigo and sensation as of impending stroke. Right-sided early morning headache, better by rising. General copious night-sweat, especially abundant on thighs. Coldness of thighs.

REFERENCES - Clarke.

RANUNCULUS REPENS

(Creeping Buttercup)

PHARMACY - ran-r. Ranunculus repens. Creeping buttercup. N. O. Ranunculacee. Tincture of whole plant. ***Historical dose:*** All potencies.

CLINICAL - Back, pulsation. Coma. Eyes, disorders. Feet, weakness.

HOMEOPATHIC - Ran-r. has furrowed flower-stalks like Ran-b., but it has a spreading calyx and creeping scions.

Franz reported a number of symptoms experienced from preparing the juice of this plant, including phantasmagoria.

Jahr quoted an account of the effects of eating Ran-r. observed in a flock of sheep. Several fell down as if struck by lightning, eyes rolled, breathing hurried. Some reeled and died with heads bent towards left groin.

Great weakness in feet remained behind. Sleep, short but refreshing. Mucus membranes of eyes injected, mouth dry. Abdomen slightly distended, ruminations ceased. Bleeding worse. Some raised themselves, reeled, fell down again, bleated piteously, most were in profound coma. Ether in milk gave much relief.

REFERENCES - Clarke.

RANUNCULUS SCELERATUS

(Marsh Buttercup)

PHARMACY - ran-s. Ranunculus sceleratus. Marsh buttercup. Marsh crowfoot. Celery-leafed crowfoot. N. O. Ranunculacee. Europe, North Asia and North America. Tincture of whole plant. ***Historical dose:*** All potencies..

CLINICAL - Aneurysm. Anus, itching. ***Blisters.*** Chest, sternum, pain behind. Corns. Coryza. Diphtheria. Earache. Glossitis. Gout. Hemorrhoids. Herpes, zoster. Liver, pain. Neuralgia. Nose, ulceration. ***Pemphigus***. Quinsy. Sternum, pains. Stomatitis. Toes disorders. Tongue, peeling, mapped. Varicose veins.

HOMEOPATHIC - Ran-s. has the most acridity of all the Ranunculi, causing burning in mouth, throat, stomach, chest, urethra and other parts. It causes blisters on the skin which leave a raw surface with acrid discharge.

The effects of Ran-s., which German shepherds call "cold fire," on horned cattle is loss of appetite, trembling and shivering, and distention of abdominal veins. A dog poisoned with it became anxious, howled, tossed about, bent double, and was very restless at night.

Affinities for the chest, skin, vertex and right side. ***Rawness, burning, smarting, gnawing or boring pains.*** Overall sore feeling. Convulsive twitchings. Periodical complaints. Shortness of breath. Fainting with pain in stomach.

Burning in the mouth, throat, stomach, chest, urethra. Sensation as of a plug. Characteristic "***mapped or peeled tongue***," with smarting, burning and rawness. ***Pemphigus***.

Ran-s. cured pemphigus in a three-months old infant with continual thirst, weak intermitting pulse, trembling with anxious features. After Ars. 4c had caused improvement, Ran-s. 3c healed up the resulting ulcers.

MIND - Indolence and aversion to mental work. Sadness and melancholy in the evening.

Abdomen - Sensation of a plug behind umbilicus. Pressure as of a plug behind right false ribs, worse deep inspiration.

Chest - Integument sensitive. Bruised pain and weakness in the chest every evening.

Sore burning behind xiphoid cartilage.

Face - As if covered with cobwebs.

Head - Fluent coryza with sneezing and burning urination. Gnawing pain in small spot on vertex or either temples. Biting, itching on the scalp. Frightful dreams about corpses, serpents, battles, etc.

Heart - Sensation as if a plug in heart.

Limbs - ***Boring pain***. Gnawing in knee, left palm. Gout of fingers and toes. Sudden burning, ***sticking pain in right toe***. Sudden stitches in big toes, passing into burning. Corns with burning and soreness, especially when feet hang down.

Liver - ***Pain over region of liver with sensation as if diarrhea would set in***.

Lungs - Stitches in chest muscles, chest and sternum are sensitive to touch. Sore burning behind sternum. As of a plug forced between ribs, worse deep breathing.

Modalities - Pains better after midnight. Worse from motion, walking, letting limb hang down. Worse by touch, pressure, blows. Worse deep breathing, open air. Worse evening, after midnight, morning. Worse after a meal.

Mouth - ***Burning and rawness of tongue***. Tongue cracks and peels off, denuded patches. ***Tongue mapped***. Mouth sore and raw. Teeth and gums sensitive. Blunt teeth with toothache.

Nose - Fluent coryza, with sneezing, with burning urination.

Skin - Vesicular eruption with ***tendency to form large blisters. Acrid exudation,*** which makes surrounding parts sore.

Sensations - As if head were too full and too large. As if a plug were lodged in umbilicus. Pressure as from a dull instrument. As if diarrhea would set in. As of a needle thrust deep into big toe. With pains in stomach there is fainting. Convulsive twitches of limbs. Gnawing and boring sensations.

Skin - Yellow vesicles. Bullae with acrid contents. Pemphigus.

Sleep - Dreadful dreams of dead bodies, snakes and fights.

Stomach - Nausea worse after midnight. Pain with fainting.

Throat - Burning scraping in throat.

COMMENTS - External sensitiveness, especially of chest and sternum. Chest disorders, including aneurysm. Arrest of breathing. Pains in liver, spleen, chest or heart, worse on deep inspiration and associated with external soreness.

Most of the symptoms are right-sided, but there is one left-side symptom that is peculiar: continual gnawing in left palm. The right toes, especially the right big toe, are the seat of many acute pains, giving the remedy a high place in acute attacks of gout and painful corns.

Mahoney cured with Ran-s. 3c an aged woman subject to gout aching in dorsum of feet, especially the right, with wakefulness at night. Kali-c. 30c had previously removed pain passing downward over the glutei.

RELATIONS - ***Antidoted by:*** Puls. Wine and coffee antidote only partially. The ulcers were somewhat relieved by Peruvian Balsam. ***Compare:*** (1) Ran-b. - Ran-s. more irritative. (2) Headache, gnawing in small spot at vertex, Puls. (3) Mapped tongue, Nat-m., Ars., Rhus-t., Tarax. (4) Ran-s. has more burning and rawness than any. (5) Cobweb sensation, Am-c., Bor., Brom., Bry., Calc., Con, Graph., Mag-c. ***Follows well:*** Ars. in pemphigus. ***Followed well by:*** Lach. in diphtheria with denuded tongue.

REFERENCES - Boericke. Clarke. Phatak.

RAPHANUS SATIVUS

(Black Garden Radish)

PHARMACY - raph. Raphanus sativus. Black garden radish. Wild radish. Raphanus raphanistrum. N. O. Cruciferae. Tincture of fresh root immediately before flowering in spring. Tincture of whole fresh plant. ***Historical dose:*** Tincture and all potencies.

CLINICAL - Abscess. Alcoholism. Amblyopia. Axilla, inflamed. Breast pains. Catalepsy. Coughs. Diarrhea. Emaciation. Esophagus. Faintness. Fevers. Flatulence. Flushings. ***Gas, pains***. Headaches. Heart, disorders. Heel, pain. Hernia. Hysteria. Insomnia. Intoxication. Lienteria. Liver, affections. Menorrhagia. Metrorrhagia. Myopia. Nosebleeds. Nymphomania. Palpitation. Pemphigus. Seborrhea. Tonsillitis. Toothache. ***Tympanitis***. Vomiting.

Yawning.

HOMEOPATHIC - Nusser proved both the garden radish and the wild radish (the former probably only a cultivated variety of the latter). He took tinctures of the long, round and black (the favorite in Germany) varieties of garden radish, and ate the different radishes themselves.

Raph. affords a marked example of a common article of diet being at the same time a poison and a medicine. The symptoms are from effects of eating radishes and provings by Curie made on a woman with 15c and 30c dilutions. The symptoms will not appear if salt is used with the Radish.

Cooper wrote "A man, has these symptoms whenever he eats even a single radish: "Burning sensation in epigastrium, followed by hot belchings, lasting a whole day and ending in a headache." Turnips (Brassica rapa) produce in him a similar effect, but in less degree.

Raph. produces in provers hysterical, mental and uterine symptoms. Numbness, changing places. Coldness of one foot. Can only lie on back. Seborrhea with greasy skin. Pemphigus. Stopped sensation in ears. Teeth feel as if made of paper.

Produces pain and stitches in liver and spleen. Increases of bile and salivary secretion. Globus, as of hot ball from uterus goes up to the throat. Appetite without hunger 4 a.m. in bed. Drinks more than one urinates. Urine thick like milk.

Great accumulation and incarceration of flatulence. Retained flatulence, cannot be passed up and down. ***Post-operative gas pains***. Loss of vision and hearing just before vomiting. Vomiting of fecal matter.

Hysteria, chilliness in back and arms. Epilepsy, reflex from removal of an adherent prepuce, the healing being delayed by furious priapism. Sexual insomnia. (Kali-br.) Nymphomania.

The leaves of Raph. are said to antidote its roots, and the arum root is said to antidote the effects of radish leaves.

MIND - Forgetful during menses. Hysteria during first day of menses. Brain excitement. Extreme anxiety with feeling of impending death. Fear of becoming a burden. Anguish with fear of death, which is supposed to be near.

Capricious, stupefaction, sadness, tears. Hopefulness alternating with sadness. Weeping on waking. Sadness with aversion to children. Aversion to her own sex and children especially girls. Dread of men. Nymphomania. Sexual insomnia.

Delusion she has an unrecognized disease. Fancies herself talking. Delusion of being in different places. Sense of intoxication. Alcoholism.

Abdomen - Distended. ***Tympanitis, no flatus emitted upward or downward***. Griping about navel. Retching and vomiting, loss of appetite.

Back - Weak back. Burning, itching on the back. Acute pains in coccyx, as if an abscess forming. Cracking in nape of neck. Numbness of muscles of neck near left ear, coldness in left eye.

Chest - Pain in chest extends to back and throat. Heavy lump and coldness in center of chest.

Ears - Tearings and shootings in left ear. Lancinations in right ear. Itching in concha of left ear, which is painful to the touch. Loss of sight and hearing just before vomiting.

Eyes - Eyes filled with blood, sight lost. Edema of lower eyelids. When she turns her eyes in the direction of the ear she feels a pain in the ear, temple and parietal bone.

Face - Face, red, somber. Cheeks burn, are red, whole head and face red. Face disfigured.

Female - Menses very profuse and long-lasting. Nervous irritation of genitals. ***Nymphomania,*** with aversion to her own sex and to children, and sexual insomnia.

Head - Headache, brain feels tender and sore. Headache after dinner. Severe headache in temple, eyes and root of nose. Aching above root of nose. Dull pain in occiput, better by throwing head back. Gnawing in occiput followed by numbness. Sharp pains in vertex. Tightness in skin of vertex. Sweat on head after rising.

Kidneys - Urine scanty or else more in quantity than the drink swallowed. Urine more copious, thick like milk. Turbid urine with yeast-like sediment. Pale urine of a dirty yellow.

Limbs - Weakness and bruised feeling in limbs. Trembling of limbs. Sticking pains in left shoulder. Gland in right armpit, swollen and tender to touch. Numbness of soles and buttocks. Cramp in calf, at night in bed.

Modalities - Better walking in open air. Throwing back head ameliorates pain in occiput. Worse at night, morning on waking, 3 a.m. to 4 a.m. Worse eating or drinking. Worse from touch, jarring. Motion aggravates pain in belly. Laughing causes a cough. Cough causes painful shock in brain, efforts to vomit, pain in chest. Riding in carriage causes pain in heart. Pain in heart worse after breakfast.

Nose - Nose pointed. Dull pain in root of nose extending to occiput. Pressure, as from a weight, on back of nose. Breath feels burning hot in nose. Stoppage of nose. Mucus in posterior sinuses. Frequent sneezing or at least frequent want to sneeze. Nosebleed of deep red blood. Smell of horseradish.

Rectum - Stool liquid, frothy, profuse, brown, with colic and pad-like swelling of intestines. Vomiting of fecal matter.

Sensations - Sensation of stiffness. Sensation of an iron band around waist. Swelling of abdomen. Hot breath, hot belchings. Sensation of a number of balls rising from abdomen to throat. Sensation of a hot foreign body like a ball going up from uterus to throat. Numbness in hands in soles of feet and buttocks of the parts near the painful bones. Sensation of swelling of bones of hands, arms, eyes, yet feet feel small.

Skin - Skin greasy. Painless pemphigus. Itching and heat of skin, fever, pimples under skin. Itching of whole body, scratching causes burning.

Sleep - Nervous yawning. Inclination to sleep. Sleep with dreamy reveries, lascivious dreams.

Stomach - Pains in stomach, which urge continual eating. Burning in epigastrium, followed by hot eructation. Putrid belchings. Black vomit. Vomiting of fecal matter.

Throat - Hot-ball feeling from uterus to throat, stopping there. Heat and burning in throat.

Vertigo - Vertigo with loss of vision. Vertigo with dim sight in evening, head feels tightly bandaged.

COMMENTS - The hysterical, mental and uterine symptoms of Curie's prover were very well marked, including a state approaching catalepsy: "On returning a little to herself she was unable to speak or stir."

"Globus" symptoms. Sensation of a number of balls ascending from abdomen to throat. Sensation of a morsel, too large to be swallowed, sensation of something hard to digest, leaving an empty sensation with hunger.

Constant, violent thirst. "Drinks more than he urinates." "Pains more severe when he drinks liquid." Pressure in hypogastrium as if a hernia would protrude. Flatulence. Accumulation of gas almost stops the breathing, cannot be passed either up or down.

Hot, foreign body goes up like a ball from uterus and stops at the beginning of the throat. Nymphomania. Aversion to her own sex and to children, especially girls.

Cough, causing jarring of head and chest, seems to come from epigastrium. Low cough to loosen phlegm. Expectoration of a large amount of tenacious white mucus from pharynx and esophagus, with sensation of stricture in throat.

Pain in vertebral column as if a foreign body passed through it from top to bottom and was stopped at certain points by obstacles causing pain. Pains in the back on swallowing. On breathing, pain under breasts and in back. Heavy lump and coldness in center of chest between breasts, preventing sleep.

Acute pains in coccyx, sensation as if an abscess forming. Sensation as of an abscess in liver. Throbbings in the body that became lancinations. Chilliness along the back and posterior surfaces of arms. Icy cold knees. Sensation as if she had put her cold feet into very hot water. Fever sensation, as if a cold coming on.

E. T. Blake reported two cases of sexual insomnia cured with Raph., one of which shows that Raph. has an influence on the male sexual sphere analogous to that it has on the female.

A young man suffering from reflex epilepsy had a generally adherent prepuce removed. Healing was delayed by furious priapism, which caused dragging at the sutures. Raph. 1x given each night cured.

Blake's second case was in a woman of 40 with old pelvic troubles. Orig. had failed and Plat. had helped only slightly. Raph. cured.

RELATIONS - ***Antidoted by:*** Copious draft of cold water (Milk and water worsen the pains in abdomen). ***Compare:*** (1) Mom-b. - Worse near splenic flexure. (2) Carb-v, Anac., Arg-n., Brass. ***Follows well:*** Lyc., Coch., Brass., Cheir., Thlaspi., Matth., Sin a.

REFERENCES - Boericke. Clarke. Phatak.

RATANHIA PERUVIANA

(Rhatany Root)

PHARMACY - rat. Ratanhia peruviana. Rhatany root. Mapato. Krameria triandra. Pumacuchu. N. O. Polygalacee or Leguminosae according to some. Tincture of the dried root. ***Historical dose:*** Tincture and all potencies. Locally, the Cerate has proved invaluable in many rectal complaints.

CLINICAL - ***Anus, fissures. Breast, fissures.*** Breast pain. Breath offensive. Constipation. Diabetes. Dysentery. Dyspepsia, atonic. ***Fissures***. Gonorrhea. Hemoptysis. Hemorrhages. ***Hemorrhoids***. Hemoptysis. ***Hiccoughs.*** Hydrothorax. Itching. Metrorrhagia. Miscarriage. Metrorrhagia. ***Nipples, fissures.*** Nosebleed. Pimples. ***Pinworms***. Pleurisy. Pterygium. Scurvy. Snoring. Speech, arrested. Stomach, disorders. Throat, contraction. Tinnitus. ***Worms.***

HERBAL - Ratanhia is remarkable for its entire, ovate, acuminate leaves, covered on both sides with silky hair; it is one of the species most known as yielding the Rhatany root of commerce. All the species of Krameria, as far as known, are intensely astringent. The root of several species of Krameria, especially Krameria triandra, is used to make the remedy.

The Treasury of Botany noted that the infusion of the root is blood-red, and has a history of being used to adulterate port wine. The infusion has been used as a gargle and wash, and the powder, mixed with charcoal, forms an excellent tooth-powder.

In Peru, an extract is made that is a mild, easily assimilated astringent medicine, useful for passive, bloody or mucus discharges. As a tonic, it is used for the weakness of digestive organs and muscular debility, and restores tone to relaxed parts.

Ratanhia is useful for delicate and nervous women, and to prevent miscarriage in those with a history of it. Can arrest passive hemorrhages. Styptic action, astringent. Used in intermittent and putrid fevers.

HOMEOPATHIC - Teste put Rat. in his Sulph. group. He wrote, of its pre-homeopathic use, "There is perhaps no plant the properties of which have been so well indicated by chance as this."

Anal and rectal symptoms have received a great deal of clinical confirmation. ***Pinworms***. Various forms of incontinence of urine. Mucus discharges, such as chronic catarrh of the bronchia, vagina, large intestines, etc. ***Violent hiccoughs***.

Hemorrhages, passive. Nosebleed, hemoptysis and metrorrhagia. Cracks, fissures. ***Cracked nipples*** (Graph., Sil.). Chronic edema of the skin. Scurvy. Pterygium.

Weakness and prostration with anxiety and sweat over whole body. Pains are here and there. Shooting pains, as from excoriation. Jerking in different parts. Sense of constriction. Dark thin scrawny persons.

MIND - Irritable, peevish and quarrelsome humor. Changeable mind. Depression when alone, better in company. Desire for company. Fear something will happen when alone, better conversation. Anxiety at night on waking. Starting from sleep. Desire to die during pains.

Abdomen - Griping in lower abdomen, externally violent itching. Heat and burning sensation in epigastrium. Repeated violent sticking in hypochondrium. Pinchings in abdomen and sides of abdomen, sometimes with a burning sensation. Pullings and a sensation of coldness in umbilical region. As if abdomen had been cut to pieces, worse deep breathing. Movements in sides of abdomen as of something alive.

Back - Tearing in nape of neck with heaviness of head. Stiffness in nape on turning head, better on violent motion. Drawing tension from nape of neck to the bottom of spine. Bruised pain in whole spine. Bruised pain in loins and hips, morning rising, better on motion.

Breasts - Fissure of the breasts. ***Cracks in nipples*** in nursing women.

Chest - Painful constriction in both sides of chest. Sticking, burning, cutting pains. Burning stitch in last ribs near back, on stepping. Rush of blood and heat to chest with difficult breathing. Violent pressure in chest as from a stone, with short breath on slight exertion. Ulcerative pain in chest during and after coughing.

Ears - Tearing, itching and shooting in ears. Violent stitch in right ear. Crawling as if insect in right ear. Chirping in right ear. Nocturnal tinkling and ringing in ears.

Eyes - Pains in eyes as if compressed in a vice and could not be moved. Inflammation of sclera. Contractions and burning sensations in eyes, especially in evening. Agglutination of eyes at night and lachrymation in morning. Jerks and quivering of eyes and eyelids. Very rapid twitching of eyelids. Stiffness of upper lids with soreness of upper tarsal edges. Pterygium. White spot before eye, which obstructs the sight with constant urging to wipe the eyes. Vision dim for distant objects. Myopia.

Face - Heat in face. Burning vesicles on the red part of upper lip. Tearing pain in face and jawbones. Violent tearing in left malar bone, evenings. Tearing in left side of lower jaw and corresponding teeth. Tearing in inner surface of lips in a small spot. Sensation of cobwebs above right side of mouth.

Female - Menses suppressed with swelling of abdomen and breasts, simulating a pregnancy of several months with profuse leucorrhea and kidney pain. Menses delayed. Menses too early and of too long duration and too copious, with pains in abdomen and loins. Metrorrhagia. Pressure in groin, as of a general bearing-down pain towards genital organs, followed by leucorrhea. Leucorrhea with itching in rectum and discharge of bloody mucus. Miscarriage. Compelled to get up at night and walk about during pregnancy, with toothache.

Food - Thirst in evening. Constant desire to eat. Anorexia with dislike of food and drink.

Head - Bursting headache when straining at stool or after stools. Bursting in head when sitting with head bent forward. Pain in middle of forehead, as if brain would fall out, while straining at stool. Long-lasting headache, as if screwed in a vice. Dullness of head, as if intoxicated. Sensation as if scalp from nose to vertex were stretched. Itching of scalp, not better by scratching.

Heart - Sharp sticking in precordial region, rather external. Full pulse.

Kidneys - Frequent and urgent want to urinate with scanty emission. More frequent and more abundant emission of urine, even at night. Pale urine. Urine more scanty, deposits a cloud and becomes turbid. Burning in urethra and root of penis when urinating.

Limbs - Tearing in limbs. Tearing in shoulder, arms, forearms and wrists. Contraction of flexor muscles. Spasmodic and painful contractions in elbows and fingers. Pain in bend of elbow when flexed, better extended. Jerking, tearing and stitches in thumbs. Drawing and tearing in thighs, knees, legs, feet and toes. Tension and burning sensation in thighs. Tearing from left Achilles tendon, up the leg. Sticking and burning tearing in left big toe. Tickling on heels on soles. Voluptuous itching in left sole.

Lungs - Malaise with frequent yawning, repeated and labored attempts to draw a long breath and distressing constriction across chest. Dry cough with tickling in larynx and pain of ulceration in chest. Some tight mucus evacuated with great difficulty.

Male - Chronic gonorrhea. Burning in root of penis while urinating. Itching in scrotum, not better by scratching.

Modalities - Better from hot water applications, hot bath, cool bathing. Better walking in open air, exercise. Pressure ameliorates pain in chest. Worse from anxiety, uneasiness of mind, at night. Worse exertion, touch, sitting bent over, stooping, straining at stool. Eating aggravates, better emission of flatus.

Mouth - Offensive breath. Dryness of mouth at night. Tasteless water collects in mouth. Acid blood from gums on sucking them. Tension and burning sensation at tip of tongue. As if cool air came from teeth. As of a cobweb about the right side of the mouth.

Nose - Itching in nose. Violent itching on tip of nose, better by rubbing. Nostrils inflamed and scabby with burning sensations. Dryness of nose with frequent sneezing. Dry coryza with complete stoppage of nose. Violent nosebleed, three times a day, for five days in succession.

Rectum - Constriction or as of sharp splinters of broken glass in rectum. Dry heat at anus with sudden knife-like stitches. ***Fissure of anus with great constriction, burning like a fire.*** Hemorrhoids burn like fire, temporarily relieved by cold water, protrude with straining. Stool is forced with great straining and followed by prolonged aching and burning, better hot water. Fetid, thin diarrhea, stools burn, burning pains before and after stools. Discharge of blood from rectum with or without stools. Oozing at anus. Dry, itching anus. ***Pinworms*** (Sant., Teucr., Cina.). Ascarides.

Sensations - As if intoxicated. As if head in a vice. As of a white speck before eyes, skin before eyes. Eyelids feel stiff. As if coldness rushed out of molars. As of cobwebs about right side of mouth. As if abdomen or chest cut to pieces. Movement as if something alive in abdomen. As if rectum and anus were all twisted up. As if splinters of glass in rectum and anus. As if rectum protruded and then suddenly went back with a jerk. Jerkings and quivering. Right side is most affected.

Skin - Sickly looking skin. Small red and white pimples that do not suppurate, especially between shoulders and on loins. Pimples, itching and burning after scratching. Formication and itching eruption on back. Itching in nape and between scapula, on scrotum, front of thigh, bends of knees.

Sleep - Disposition to sleep, especially after dinner. Violent yawning. Retarded sleep. Snoring. Frequent waking and prolonged wakefulness. Waking with a start, with trembling inquietude and fear. Dreams of battles, sick people, quarrels, anger, vexation, funerals, death of friends, and earthquakes.

Stomach - Stomach feels too full. Sudden painful bursting in pit of stomach. Pains as from ulceration in stomach. Heat and burning sensation in stomach. Cutting like knives or griping pain better belching. Empty belching with taste of food. ***Violent hiccough,*** which causes pain in stomach. Long-continued hiccough after dinner. Nausea and disgust with retching and vomiting of food, worse in open air. Vomiting of water, of mucus streaked with blood.

Teeth - Toothache in evening, especially after lying down, compelling one to rise and walk about. Toothache with tearing or jerking. Digging pains. Pulsative pain in teeth. Bleeding of teeth. Painful sensation of coldness and elongation in the molars and as if coldness rushed out of them. Violent pain in incisors, painful to the touch.

Temperature - Predominance of coldness and shivering, especially in evening. General chill 8 or 9 p.m. Chilly even in warm room. Heat of whole head with heaviness. Heat and puffiness of face. Dry heat in anus with cuttings. Nocturnal perspiration. Wakes 1 a.m. with sweat, thirst and dry mouth.

Throat - Sore throat, generally felt during empty swallowing. Painful spasmodic contraction in throat, which stops the voice. Unable to speak a loud word.

COMMENTS - Teste quoted from Trousseau and Pidoux a case in which Bretonneau cured a fissure of the rectum. In the case, a woman suffered from constipation and fissure of the rectum that caused her horrible pains and had damaged her health. Bretonneau ordered a daily injection mixed with one-fourth of Rat. and in a short time the constipation and fissure were cured.

Other similar cases were also cured and the treatment was shown to be successful in cases of fissure without constipation. One patient of fissure, cured by Rat., was better by an application of hot water, he sat in a sitz-bath as hot as he could endure, the relief only lasted while in the bath.

The provings of Hartlaub and Trinks bring out the keynotes of Rat. in rectal cases: "straining, stool so hard she cried out with great protrusion of hemorrhoids, followed for a long time by burning in anus."

Burning in the anus, persists for a long time after the stool and it occurs when the stool is diarrhea as well as hard. Burning also precedes and accompanies the stool. Dry heat with sudden stitching, like knife-stabs.

Oozing at anus. Dropping of blood from anus. Anal fissures (Graph., Nit-ac., Sil.). The anus and rectum feel as if they're sitting on glass. Hemorrhoids with severe bleeding and burning pains. Worms with severe itching.

Bursting headache that accompanies and follows a straining at stool. "Pains in middle of forehead, as if brain would fall out," and a similar pain after stool. Head pains are worse on bending forward. Violent nosebleed.

Burning, smarting of the eyes. Obscured vision. Inflammation of the whole eye, a membrane seemed to extend to central point of eye, which burned. Pterygium. Twitching of lids.

Bleeding gums, toothache, worse lying down. Aching molars with a sensation as if coldness rushed out of them. Toothache during pregnancy, compelling the patient to get up at night and walk about. Tasteless water collects in mouth.

Contractive sensations in stomach, groin, anus, eyes, neck, muscles, throat, "painful spasmodic contraction of throat during which she could not speak a loud word." Causes and prevents miscarriage, metrorrhagia and leucorrhea. Fissure of the breasts or nipples in nursing women.

Dr. Tournel, who, no doubt, did not suspect that Ratan. produced abortion, had the idea of prescribing it as a tonic in cases of incipient miscarriage and thus preventing that accident in delicate and nervous females who had never yet been able to go their full time.

Rummel related the case of a servant girl who had rapid twitching of the lids of right eye to such an extent as to hinder her seeing. There seemed to be also a rotary motion of the ball. Bell. and Calc. failed to relieve. Rat. 12c relieved quickly.

Cushing, who made a proving of Rat., said it caused great itching in the rectum and he has cured with it since nearly every case of pin-worms in his practice. Cushing considered that, next to Sang-n., Rat. meets more rectal cases than any other remedy.

In an old and feeble woman, he cured with Rat. 3x internally and a Rhatany rectal suppository each night. There were frequent discharges of mucus, blood and pus from the bowels night and day with great pain and burning in rectum almost wholly preventing sleep.

RELATIONS - ***Compare:*** (1) Pleurisy, Seneg. (2) Fissure of anus, Nit-ac. (3) Anal symptoms, Sulph., Iris-v., Canth., Peon. (4) Graph. is similar, but has not the constriction of Rat. (5) Splinters of glass in rectum, Thuj. (Sticks, Aesc.). (6) Pain in head from straining at stool Ind., Puls., Sil. (7) Hiccough, Cycl. (8) Burning on tongue, Raph., Ran-s., Sang. (9) Toothache of pregnancy, Raph., Mag-c., Cham. (10) Alive sensation, Croc., Thuj. (11) Cobweb sensation, Ran-s., Bar-c. ***Follows well:*** Sulph., Bov., Sep. in uterine affections (Teste).

REFERENCES - Boericke. Clarke. Murphy. Phatak.

RAUWOLFIA SERPENTINA

PHARMACY - rauw. Rauwolfia serpentina. N. O. Apocynaceae family. Java and India. Containing, among others, the alkaloid reserpine. The tincture is prepared from the root. *Historical dose:* Tincture and all potencies.

CLINICAL - Addison's disease. Angina pectoris. Basedow's disease. Colitis. Dystonia. Hypotension. Pancreatitis. Parkinson's disease. Thyroid, disorders. Vasomotor complaints.

HERBAL - Rauwolfia serpentina, found in Java and India, belongs to the Apocynaceae family. A very old drug in Ayurvedic medicine, the roots and rhizomes contain hypotensive and neuro-depressive alkaloids.

In 1952, the Russian chemist Muller isolated the specialized reserpine under the name of "serpasil." Most of the alkaloids are built on the base of reserpine, a harmonic group linked with a second isoquinoleic group.

HOMEOPATHIC - The homeopathic proving was conducted in 1954 by Leeser and Schrenk at the Robert Bosch Hospital in Stuttgart. The proving was carried out on twenty-four doctors, using the 1x and 3x potencies, for a period of fourteen to twenty-eight days.

W. Lee Templeton also conducted a proving at the Faculty of Homeopathy in London in 1954-55 on six provers, using the 3x, 6x, 12c, and 30c potencies, depending on the subject, for a period of six months.

Beja of Orléans began a self-proving in July-August 1956 using the 3x potency, for one month, at the rate of 10 drops four times a day. Finally, Julian undertook detailed clinical studies to determine the range of action of Rauw. in a homeopathic potency.

Rauw. has a general and cerebral hypotonia. Lack of tone in the nerves and circulatory system. Congestive vascular condition. Pallor, alternating with redness and hot flushes. Insomnia after midnight.

Chronic allergic condition progressing to cancer. Chronic neurotic conditions with development of arthrosis or depression. Rapid, widespread trembling. General stiffness. Heaviness in the legs. Libido disorders. Dripping after urination.

MIND - Uneasiness with irritability and apprehension. Aversion to company, better when alone. Abrupt. Face expressionless and he avoids any effort. Dullness from alcohol.

Diminution of the memory and powers of concentration. Phases of increased ability to work and well being, alternating with phases of fatigue and exhaustion. Alternating excitability and depression. Maniacal depressive psychosis. Psychosis in elderly people.

Restlessness at night in bed. Neurosis from anguish. Psychological complaints during the menopause. Melancholic conditions. Hyper-emotiveness. Unstable personality. Delusions, everything seems unreal. Sudden impulse to kill.

Abdomen - Abdominal plethora and dropsy. Chronic pancreatitis. Feeling of gastric and abdominal repletion. Heartburn, nausea, malodorous flatulence. Aerophagy, air in the colon. Colitis from fermentation, enterocolitis.

Blood - Circulatory dystonia. Hypotension, faintness. Temporary rise and then fall in arterial tension. Vasomotor complaints. Vascular or febrile congestion.

Chest - Angina pectoris.

Constitutions - Carbo-phosphoric types with nervous or sanguine temperament.

Face - Congestion of the face and possible nosebleed. Neuralgia of the upper maxilla, ameliorated by heat. Numbness sensation in the right half of the face, followed by shooting pains.

Female - Heaviness in the small pelvis with frequent need to urinate. Amenorrhea. Menses too early, accompanied by cramping pains. Too frequent menses. Endometriosis. Fibroma. Menopausal complaints. Frigidity.

Head - Congestive headache with arterial palpitations in the temples and forehead. Frontal headache, spreading towards the occiput, ameliorated in fresh air, accompanied by hot flushes, dizziness.

Heart - Hypotonia with diarrhea. Constriction, angina pectoris and rhythmic anomalies. Bradycardia, aortitis. Aortic aneurysm. Palpitations, prickling and irregular heartbeat. Palpitations and irregularity of the heart when lying down, ameliorated by standing and walking. Cardio-renal edema.

Kidneys - Difficulty in urinating with need to squeeze to push. Dysuria. Cystitis. Urine reddish-brown. At the end of urination, a little urine is passed, drop by drop. Bedwetting from compression (fibromas, prostate).

Limbs - Chronic rheumatism. General stiffness and pain in all the limbs. Legs heavy, black and blue, as if shattered. Joint pains in the left hip and big toes, which are hot and swollen. Arthrosis of the knee. Painful flat feet in adolescents. Gout. Soft edema, puckered, located in the malleolar region, at times connected to a generalized edematous infiltration including the upper limbs and the face.

Liver - Cirrhosis of the liver. Pigmentary cirrhosis or glandular pigmentation or hypertrophic pigmentary cirrhosis in sugar diabetes. Biliary sycosis.

Lungs - Dyspnea from exertion with lack of air. Tracheal bronchitis. Fitful cough with expectoration of sticky, sometimes blood streaked, mucus.

Male - Clear diminution in libido, sometimes with a temporary phase of excitement. Impotence. Sterility. Prostatitis.

Modalities - Better in the open air, fresh air. Better from violent exercise, prolonged movement, strong pressure. Better from the emission of gas or stools. Worse from heat, confined air. Worse on waking, after meals, from 6 p.m. to 8 p.m.

Mouth - Excessive salivation. Impression of a rotten taste in the mouth.

Nose - Dryness of the nasal mucus membranes. Nosebleed with ulcerations on the nasal wall. Sinusitis. Spasmodic rhinitis.

Rectum - Morning attacks of colic with evil-smelling black diarrhea-type stools. Sudden urging, followed by pallor of the face with sweating, thirst and faintness. Anal fissure. Congestive hemorrhoids, bleeding at times.

Skin - Clammy, odorous sweating from the axilla, hands and feet. Dyshidrosis. Lymphaedema. Elephantiasis-type edematous dystrophy. Sweating. Fissures. Cracks. Ulceration of the heel.

Sleep - Insomnia. Slow in going to sleep and stays awake for hours after midnight. Erotic dreams. Dreams of wasps, drowning, death, dying.

Stomach - Excessive hydrochloric gastritis. Alcoholic gastritis.

Temperature - Sensation of heat on the whole body with or without sweating and accompanied by congestive headache and general uneasiness.

Throat - Dryness of mucus membranes of the nose and throat. Tickling in the throat with need to cough, aggravated by lying down. Laryngitis.

Vertigo - Vertigo and precordial heaviness, cramping pains spreading towards the neck, discomforts, tendency to faintness with sticky sweating from the hands and feet. Amelioration from movement in the open air.

RELATIONS - *Compare:* (1) Lach. - Circulatory dystonia with localized congestion, amelioration by discharges, occurring predominantly on the left side. (2) Phos. - Agitation with uneasiness, worse at dusk, vertigo on waking, burning sensation at the hands and between the shoulders. (3) Ars. - Anxious, especially between 1 a.m. and 3 a.m., edema of the lower eyelids, thirst for small quantities of iced water, diarrhea with vomiting, physical and mental agitation. (4) Nux-v. - Nervous irritability. Sleepy after meals, ameliorated by a short nap. Heaviness in the stomach, constipation and hemorrhoids. (5) Aur. - Congestions, disgust for life, obsession with suicide, palpitations. Pains in the bones and right testicle, worse at night and from contact.

REFERENCES - Julian.

RED CHESTNUT

(Bach Flower Essence)

PHARMACY - rd-ch-b. Red chestnut. Aesculus carnea. The flowering clusters are boiled for half an hour. The boiled water is strained and used as medicine. ***Historical dose:*** Take two drops from the stock bottle into a one ounce dropper bottle (add brandy or alcohol, if this bottle will be used for days or weeks). This is the dosage bottle, take a few drops straight into the mouth or as needed in a little water or juice.

HOMEOPATHIC - Rd-ch-b. belongs to Bach's group ***For Those who Have Fear,*** with Rck-r-b., Mimul-b., Cher-p-b. and Asp-b. Fear for the welfare of others. Extreme physical nervousness and anxious weakness, with tightening in the stomach and abdominal region from fear.

MIND - Fearful worries about loved ones' welfare. Nervous energy. Grief and worry. Sense of danger. Fears for life and limb. Helplessness, self-blame.

REFERENCES - Bach.

RESCUE REMEDY

(Bach Flower Essence)

PHARMACY - resc-b. Rescue Remedy. Rescue Remedy is made up of a combination of five Bach flower remedies. Add two drops from stock bottles of each of the five remedies listed below to a one ounce (30cc) bottle filled with brandy or alcohol. ***Historical dose:*** Add three drops of the Rescue Remedy to a glass of water. The patient should sip this frequently and as he or she grows calmer, at intervals of fifteen minutes, and then every half hour according to the progress made.

HOMEOPATHIC - Bach discovered this unique combination of five remedies which aim at restoring balance and calm to a person in acute emergency situations.

Cher-p-b. - for desperation, to balance intense tension and the fear that events and one's own life, including one's mental power, is out of control. ***Clem-b.*** - for that faraway, out-of-the-body state that precedes fainting or loss of consciousness. Can reduce faintness or coma.

Imp-b. - to counteract inner turmoil, tension and impatience. ***Rck-r-b.*** - to counteract terror and panic. ***Star-b-b.*** - to reduce shock, trauma, sadness and prevent the trauma's possible long-lasting effects on mind, emotions and body from imprinting.

Rescue remedy is of great value immediately after accidents or similar moments of shock and panic when there is faintness, trembling, or other failing of normal physical functioning. Useful as the first medicine administered on arrival at the accident. After accidents, shocks, traumas or during severe illness, mental or physical.

Can be given before stressful events to help calm the anticipation or fear. Anxiety, panic attacks and sudden fear. Speechless and trembling. Can also be used as a daily remedy in chronic situations of intense nervousness and tension when the vital force needs to recharge and recuperate. Can prevent or give a peaceful death if given at the right moment.

MIND - Rescue Remedy helps to bring balance, calm and synchronicity of functioning within the levels of the human being, these being the mind, emotions and body.

REFERENCES - Bach. Murphy.

RESERPINUM

(Reserpine)

PHARMACY - reser. Reserpinum. Reserpine. Alkaloid of Rauwolfia serpentina. ***Historical dose:*** All potencies.

CLINICAL - Allergies. Cancer. Catalepsy. Diarrhea. Duodenal, ulcer. Dyspepsia. Headache. Hemorrhoids. Hypotension. Hypothermia. Jaundice. Migraines. Melancholy. Nasal polyps. Parkinson's disease. Pharyngitis. Rhinitis.

HOMEOPATHIC - It is one of the alkaloids of Rauwolfia serpentina and was found commercially under the name of serpasil ciba. The proving was carried out by Julian on a group of thirteen provers during the winter of 1964-65, using the 3x, 5c, 7c, 9c, 15c and 30c potencies.

Sleepiness. Sleeping after meals. Slowing down of the mind and body. Asthenia, particularly accentuated between 3 p.m. and 4 p.m. General condition of weakness. Habitual trembling. General excitability. Anxiety. Suicidal tendencies.

Muscular hypertonia and a total lack of movement. Hard trophic edema. Intermittent stomach pains. Hypotension. Bradycardia. Vertigo. Allergies. Cancer.

MIND - Slowing down of the mind and body. Lassitude and aversion to work in the evening. Catalepsy. Nervous depression. Melancholy. Anxiety and suicidal tendencies. Difficulty working. Very hyperactive and aggressive. Feeling that the nerves are at skin level in the evening. Premature senility.

Abdomen - Spasmodic attacks of pain in the colon.

Breasts - Excessive milk in the mother.

Constitutions - Allergic and psoric constitutions. Syphilitic, asthenic types with tendency to inhibition of nervous reactions.

Eyes - Myosis.

Head - Headache on waking, better by breakfast and worse again at the end of the morning.

Heart - Hypotension. Tension instability. Bradycardia, with vertigo. Permanently slow pulse.

Limbs - Fidgets in the legs.

Lungs - Laryngitis and tracheitis.

Mouth - Tongue covered with a yellowish coating. Excessive salivation.

Nose - Nasal obstruction. Congestive rhinitis. Nasal polyps.

Rectum - Jaundice. Constipation followed by diarrhea. Diarrhea. Hemorrhoids.

Skin - Dry, ligneous scabs. Hard, trophic edema. Lymphaedema. Dull and damp hair.

Sleep - Sleepiness. Sleeping after meals.

Stomach - Acrid dyspepsia. Slight nausea. Gastric pain coming late after meals in painful bursts. Gastric and duodenal ulcer. Cancer of the stomach.

Temperature - Hypothermia, at 31°c, adynamic condition, hypertonia total indifference.

Throat - Pharyngitis. Throat sensitive.

Vertigo - Violent attack of vertigo with feeling of a black hole in front of the eyes and leaving an empty feeling for a few minutes, then return to former condition.

RELATIONS - ***Compare:*** (1) Rauw. (2) Aur. - Depressive suicidal condition. (3) Lach. - Emotional instability. (4) Ars. - Anguish and fear of dying. (5) Nux-v. - Complaints of the nervous and digestive systems.

REFERENCES - Julian.

RHAMNUS CALIFORNICA

(California Coffee-tree)

PHARMACY - rham-cal. Rhamnus californica. California coffee tree. ***Historical dose:*** Tincture and all potencies.

CLINICAL - Bladder, tenesmus. ***Constipation***. ***Dizzy***. ***Dysmenorrhea***. Gastralgia. Heart, disorders. Lumbago. Muscular pains. Pleurodynia. Rheumatism.

HOMEOPATHIC - Provings were done using the 2x potency.

Rumbling, griping and cutting pains in ileocecal region. Bladder tenesmus. Pleurodynia. Gastralgia. ***Dysmenorrhea*** of muscle origin, pain in head, neck and face. Rheumatism and muscular pains. ***Inflammatory rheumatism***, joints swollen, painful. Lumbago. Rheumatic heart. Tendency to metastasis. Profuse sweat.

MIND - Nervous, restless, irritable. Lassitude, mentally dull and dazed, unable to concentrate mind on studies.

Chest - Sub-sternal oppression. Tenderness on pressure of right intercostal muscles.

Ears - ***Dullness of hearing***. Soreness, deep under right tragus, on swallowing.

Face - Flushed, hot and glowing. Outward pressure from malar processes.

Head - ***Dizzy*** full feeling. Heavy bruised sensation, better from pressure. ***Bursting feeling*** with every step. Soreness, especially in occiput and vertex, worse bending over. Dull pain in left temple. Dull aching in frontal region (left), extending backwards and over forehead. Deep, right-sided frontal headache. Twitching eyelids.

Heart - Variation of pulse. Slow pulse.

Kidneys - Increased urination. Tickling in anterior urethra, small morning drop (no previous gonorrhea). Sexual desire increased.

Limbs - Legs sore. Unable to control muscular action. Walked like a drunken man.

Modalities - Worse in evening.

Mouth - Canker sore between gums and lips. Tongue coated, with clean, pink, central patch.

Rectum - ***Constipation*** with some flatus. Tenesmus and dry stool. Flatulent diarrhea.

Throat - Dry, rough. Soreness on right side and tonsil.

RELATIONS - ***Compare:*** (1) Rham-cath. or Rham-f., European Buckthorn - a rheumatic remedy, abdominal symptoms, colic, diarrhea, hemorrhoids, especially chronic. (2) Rham-p. (3) Cas-s. - palliative in constipation, as an intestinal tonic and dyspepsia dependent thereon. 10-15 drops of tincture.

REFERENCES - Boericke. Clarke.

RHAMNUS CATHARTICA

(Purging Buckthorn)

PHARMACY - rham-cath. Rhamnus cathartica. Purging buckthorn. Buckthorn. N. O. Rhamnacae. Tincture of fluid extract of ripe berries. ***Historical dose:*** Tincture and all potencies.

CLINICAL - Appendicitis. Canker, sores. Colic. Constipation. Diarrhea. Tympanites. Typhlitis.

HOMEOPATHIC - The common buckthorn produces black, shiny, four-sided berries with an acrid taste. A syrup is made from these berries, and forms the Rhamni succus of the old school. Symptoms were observed in a boy poisoned by eating the berries.

Copious watery stools. Nausea and severe vomiting. Rham-cath., in doses of a few drops, is a useful palliative in cases of constipation. The ileo-cecal symptoms seem to indicate it as a possible remedy in cases of appendicitis. Milne noted that it was formerly given in dropsy.

Abdomen - Abdomen hard, tympanitis. Colic. Violent rumbling and griping. Cutting pains in ileo-cecal region and in transverse colon.

Eyes - Eyes glistening and injected.

Face - Trembling of lips. Commencing trismus.

Food - Complete loss of appetite.

Head - Unable to rise, seemed to desire to press his head against the wall.

Kidneys - Urine highly colored.

Limbs - Weakness and prostration in all limbs.

Lungs - Respiration short, anxious.

Mouth - Coated tongue. Extremely bitter taste.

Pulse - Pulse variable.

Rectum - Diarrhea. Liquid stools.

Temperature - Violent chilliness. Skin at one time warm, at another cold.

Throat - Scraping in throat.

RELATIONS - ***Compare:*** (1) Cas-s. (2) Cean. in appendicitis, Iris-t.

REFERENCES - Clarke.

RHAMNUS FRANGULA

(Alder Buckthorn)

PHARMACY - rham-f. Rhamnus frangula. Alder buckthorn. N. O. Rhamnacae. Tincture and trituration of the bark gathered in spring from the younger branches. Tincture of bark of root. Tincture of ripe berries. ***Historical dose:*** Tincture and all potencies.

CLINICAL - Anus, itching. Appendicitis. Ardor urine. Cecum, gurgling. Diarrhea. Flatulence. Urethritis. Vomiting.

HOMEOPATHIC - All parts of Rham-f. appear to produce irritant and cathartic properties. The majority of the symptoms were the result of the root bark, but the leaves were no less active.

There was more vomiting with Rham-f. than with Rham-cath., and the former was abandoned as a cathartic because it so frequently produced vomiting instead.

Burning in urethra while urinating and frequent urination may prove an indication in gonorrhea. Stools of a dark-green color, copious, thin or pasty. Much rumbling in the ileo-cecal region and along the transverse colon with weakness after stool.

RELATIONS - ***Compare:*** (1) Rham-cath., Cean. and Cas-s.

REFERENCES - Clarke.

RHAMNUS PURSHIANA

(Cascara Sagrada)

PHARMACY - rham-p. (cas-s.). Rhamnus purshiana. Cascara sagrada. Sacred bark. N. O. Rhamnacae. California. Extract of bark. ***Historical dose:*** Tincture and all potencies.

CLINICAL - Cholera. Cirrhosis. ***Constipation.*** Headache. Hemorrhages. Hemorrhoids. Indigestion. Jaundice. ***Rheumatism.*** Vomiting.

HERBAL - Cas-s. is a palliative for constipation, fifteen drops of fluid extract restores normal function by its tonic effects. Only material doses have been used.

HOMEOPATHIC - Pathogenic effects on patients taking it for constipation have been recorded, including vomiting, severe griping, and hemorrhage. In one case, temporary insanity was produced from a homemade decoction of the bark. In two cases, cholera symptoms were produced.

This is a well-known purgative as it has been found curative in cases of acute and ***chronic rheumatism with constipation.*** Chronic indigestion, cirrhosis and jaundice. Hemorrhoids and constipation. Gastric headache. Broad, flabby tongue. Foul breath.

Kidneys - Must wait before flow starts, then comes in drops at first.

Limbs - ***Rheumatism of muscles and joints with obstinate constipation***.

Liver - Cirrhosis and jaundice.

Rectum - Hemorrhoids. ***Severe constipation***.

Stomach - Chronic indigestion. Gastric headache. Vomiting.

RELATIONS - ***Compare:*** (1) Hydr., Nux-v. (2) Rham-cal - tincture for constipation, tympanites and appendicitis and especially rheumatism.

REFERENCES - Boericke. Clarke.

RHEUM PALMATUM

(Turkey Rhubarb)

PHARMACY - rheum. Rheum palmatum. Turkey rhubarb. Rheum officinale. Rhabarbarum. N. O. Polygonacae. China. Tincture and trituration of the dried root. A tincture of the fresh leaves and young stalks should be investigated. ***Historical dose:*** Tincture and all potencies.

CLINICAL - Ardor urine. Breath offensive. Constipation. Deafness. Dentition, difficult. ***Diarrhea.*** Duodenum, catarrh. Dysentery. Ears, thickening. Esophagus, constriction. Headaches. Jaundice. Kidneys, disorders. Meniere's disease. Milk, abnormal. Mouth, mucus. Nipples, pain. Nose, pain. ***Nursing disorders.*** Rheumatism. Salivation. Screaming, children. Snoring. ***Stomach, disordered. Sour smell.*** Taste, bad. Tongue, numbness. Urination, difficult. Urine, red.

HERBAL - Rhubarb, called "Turkey rhubarb," comes from China, but the exact species is unknown.

Milne summarized its action from the traditional point of view as being "tonic, cathartic and a feeble astringent, the latter property being overborne by the cathartic and only coming into play afterwards," i.e., the constipation which follows rhubarb purgation.

"In small doses, it improves digestion and appetite and renders the kidney secretions more healthy. In larger doses it is an excellent cathartic, acting on the whole bowel and especially the duodenum and increasing the peristaltic action." It affects the liver, duodenum, bile ducts and intestines.

HOMEOPATHIC - Hahnemann's proving of Rheum confirmed many of its traditional uses. Rheum is a remedy for nursing infants and children especially during dentition, and suited to pregnant and nursing women.

The whole child smells sour, washing does not remove it. Colicky children who are always screaming and crying. ***Sour diarrhea***, taste, vomits, stools, sweat etc. Difficult dentition. Requires very little sleep and not much food. Sensation of crepitation.

MIND - Impatient and vehement, desires many things and cries (Cina.). Impetuous desire for particular objects. Temper of child is as acrid as are the stools. Child dislikes even its favorite things. Child cries and tosses all night.

Full of fear. Fear of death, and restlessness, in first days after confinement, with diarrhea. Anxiety from motion, when stooping. Indolent. Taciturn. Asks for nothing. Morose. Delirious talking. Quarrelsome in sleep. Restless with weeping.

Abdomen - Wind seems to rise up to chest. Colicky pain about navel. Colic with screaming, better doubling up, worse uncovering any part, then diarrhea.

Back - Stiffness in sacrum and hips, cannot walk straight. Cutting pain in lumbar region, worse after stools.

Causations - Eating prunes, unripe fruit. Dentition. Spasms, dislocations.

Chest - Lancinations in chest. Rush of blood to chest. Crackling bubbling (even audible) in right then left pectoral muscles.

Constitutions - For nursing children, especially during dentition, and for pregnant and nursing women.

Ears - Otalgia with itching in ear. Pressure and throbbing in ears. Dullness of hearing.

Eyes - Weak when looking steadily at any object. Convulsive twitching of eyelids.

Face - ***Cool sweat on face,*** especially about mouth and nose, on upper lip. Tendency to frown. Forehead wrinkled. Twitching.

Female - Urinary complaints after abortion. Diarrhea after childbirth. Yellow and bitter milk in nursing women, infant refuses breast.

Food - Loss of appetite. Requires little food. Loathing after first bite. Food tastes bitter, even sweet things. Desire for various things, but cannot eat them. Plums and prunes disagree.

Head - Sweat on hairy scalp. Wet, sopping hair.

Kidneys - Burning in bladder and kidney, before and during urination. Unsuccessful urging to urinate before stool.

Limbs - Limb on which he lies falls asleep. Twitching in arms, hands and fingers. Bubbling sensation in elbow joint from bend of knee to heels. Lameness of wrist and knee after sprains and dislocations.

Liver - Jaundice from eating unripe fruits, with white diarrhea.

Lungs - Snoring inspiration during sleep. The cough is dry in evening, with expectoration of mucus.

Modalities - Better from warmth, wrapping up. Better lying bent, lying doubled up, takes the queerest positions in order to rest awhile. Worse uncovering, summer, night, after sleep, and morning. Worse motion, dentition. Worse after eating, plums. Worse before, after and during stools. Worse in nursing women.

Mouth - Salivation with colic or diarrhea. Offensive mucus in the mouth after sleep. Breath smells sour (Cham.). Food tastes bitter, even sweet things. Teeth feel cold. Difficult teething, restless and irritable.

Nose - Stupefying drawing from root of nose to tip, where it tingles. Heat in nose.

Perspiration - ***Child smells sour, even if washed or bathed***. Sweat on scalp, about mouth, nose, and on upper lip. Easy perspiration, on forehead and scalp. Stains yellow.

Rectum - Frequent, ineffectual urging to stool, worse motion and walking. Tenesmus. Before stool, unsuccessful urging to urinate. Renewed urging after stool, when moving. Colicky, even ineffectual urging to evacuate altered fecal stools. Severe constipation. Diarrhea only when walking. White diarrhea from eating unripe fruits with jaundice. Sour diarrhea during dentition. Diarrhea in first days after confinement, with colic. Loose, sour-smelling stool with colic, immediately after nursing child.

Sensations - Sensation as if brain moved when standing. Heaviness as on waking from a heavy sleep. Coldness in teeth. Blunt feeling in teeth. Tongue numb, numbness of part of limb lain on. Constriction of stomach of gullet. Crackling, crepitation or bubbling in muscles and any part of body.

Skin - Sweat stains yellow. Pemphigus on face, scalp and hands, face, lips and tongue swollen, face livid. Itching rash on forehead and arms.

Sleep - Restless with whining and crying. Twitching of face and fingers. Requires very little sleep and not much food.

Stomach - Throbbing and shootings pain in pit of stomach. Contractions in stomach. Fullness in stomach with pressure, as if overloaded. Nausea during colic.

Stool - ***Stools smell sour***, with shivering and tenesmus, and burning in anus. Sour diarrhea during dentition. Diarrhea of varying color and consistency, usually frothy and of a sour odor. Diarrhea only when walking. Stools pasty, pappy, brown, green, fermented, slimy or acrid. ***Yellow stool, turning green on standing.*** Stools with shivering, tenesmus and burning in anus. ***Thin, pasty, sour-smelling stools***, with straining before, and colicky, constrictive cutting in abdomen after. Stools worse from eating unripe fruit, or in the evening.

Temperature - Chilliness alternating with heat. Internal, with external heat. Heat all over, mostly on hands and feet, with cold face, no thirst.

Throat - Contraction of gullet.

COMMENTS - Characteristic sourness and acidity. The stools are sour, the taste is sour, the whole body has a sour smell. No amount of washing will wash the sourness out. The breath, stools, and sweat smell sour (Mag-c., Nat-p., Calc.). Sopping-wet hair.

Often indicated in nursing babies when they get sores in their mouth and sour-smelling diarrhea. Dentition with sour stools. Colic with night screaming. "Screaming of children with urging and sour stools." Sour disposition (Cham.). Peevish, impatient, screams for things, dislikes even his favorite playthings.

Stomach disorders with a sour, flat, slimy, insipid or nauseous taste. Food tastes bitter, even sweet things. The mouth is covered with offensive mucus after sleeping, with a bad taste and offensive breath.

Hunger for various kinds of food, but the first few mouthfuls nauseate. Bad effects of eating plums or unripe fruit. Nausea. Severe colic, compelling one to bend double, worse standing, worse just before stool, not better after, worse at once by uncovering an arm or leg. Evacuations accompanied by shivering and renewed urging. "Shivering with stool."

Symptoms are mostly left-sided or go from above down or from right to left. Generally affects the left loin, brain, upper part of body (sweat).

With a few drops of Rheum, Clarke relieved severe constipation in an acid child who was intolerant of almost all remedies in the potencies.

On the indication "diarrhea only during active exercise," Hundall cured a horse of a diarrhea that only came on when he was at work.

Cooper noted that "Rheum has the property of setting up pains in old disease, in the old cellulitis and old psoriasis patches. Hot burning pains therein as well as in the unaffected veins of the thighs and other parts. Its good effect in old middle and internal ear thickenings seems due to the creation of tissue-activity in dormant structures."

Cooper offered two cases, the first was that of a woman who suffered from characteristic symptoms of Meniere's disease, feeling of things spinning around with extreme giddiness and noises in the head. She was cured by a chemist giving her 10 grains of powdered rhubarb based on the idea that it was due to the liver. Before this, great suffering had been endured without any relief.

The second case concerned vertiginous symptoms due to brain exhaustion with flushings followed by perspiration and awful muffled and discordant tinnitus. Great relief followed the sniffing of 3x trituration of Rheum.

RELATIONS - ***Antidotes:*** Camph., Cham. ***Compare:*** (1) Mag-c., Mag-p., Hep., Podo., Cham., Cina, Ip. ***Complementary:*** Mag-c.

REFERENCES - Boericke. Clarke. Murphy. Phatak.

RHODIUM METALLICUM

PHARMACY - rhodi. Rhodium metallicum. Rhodium metal and element, (Rh. At. wt. 103). ***Historical dose:*** All potencies.

CLINICAL - Cough. Headache. Nausea. Rheumatism.

HOMEOPATHIC - Proved by MacFarlan with the 200c potency. Nervous and tearful. Frontal headache, shocks through head. Fleeting neuralgic pains in head, over eyes in ear, both sides of nose, teeth. Dull headache. Loose cold in head. Feels weak, dizzy and a tired feeling.

Stiff neck and rheumatic pain down left shoulder and arm. Cough scratchy, wheezy. Thick, yellow mucus from chest. Lips dry. Itching in arms, palms and face. Hyperactive peristalsis, tenesmus after stool. Loose stools with gripings in abdomen. More urine passed. Nausea, especially from sweets.

REFERENCES - Boericke.

RHODIUM OXYDATUM NITRICUM

PHARMACY - rhodi-o-n. Rhodium oxydatum nitricum. Nitrate oxide of rhodium. Solution. ***Historical dose:*** All potencies.

CLINICAL - Anus, itching, burning. Constipation. Ears, pains. Hemorrhoids. Headache. Hearing, illusions. Impotence.

HOMEOPATHIC - Rhodium is often found in association with platinum. Hering's preparation was obtained from exposing a small quantity of rhodium sponge, hydrate of potash and nitre to the action of a blowpipe until oxidized.

After having the oxide well washed and boiled in nitric acid for a few minutes and exposed to a gentle heat for an hour, the nitrate was obtained from the oxide, producing a fluid of a golden color of the consistency of syrup.

Dilutions of this were made and the 4th was proved for Hering by Dr. Person, the 2nd and 3rd by Dr. Negendank. The bowels were affected in both, constipation with hemorrhoids being relieved in one and constipation with itching of the anus being caused in the other.

Headache on being woken in the night. Headache alternating with faintness. Faintness better by passage of stool. Heat preceding chill and alternating with it. Sensation as if teeth blunt, as if sand between them. A scraping or harsh noise causes disagreeable sensation in teeth. The hearing is more acute, illusion that he hears whispering.

REFERENCES - Clarke.

RHODODENDRON CHRYSANTHUM

(Yellow Snow Rose)

PHARMACY - rhod. Rhododendron chrysanthum. Yellow snow rose. Rhododendron aureum. Siberian rhododendron. Gout rose. N. O. Ericacee. Tincture of fresh leaves. ***Historical dose:*** Tincture and all potencies.

CLINICAL - Amenorrhea. ***Arthritis.*** Asthenopia. Bone, pains. Bunions. Chorea. ***Ciliary, neuralgia***. Colic. Coryza. Delirium. Diarrhea. Diphtheria. Dysmenorrhea. Earache. Eye, disorders. Fever. Flatulence, incarcerated. ***Fibrositis.*** Gout. Gums, itching. Headaches. ***Hydrocele.*** Lienteria. Lumbago. Memory, weak. Meniere's, disease. Neuralgias. Nightmares. Nosebleeds. ***Orchitis.*** Ovary, cyst. Periostitis. ***Rheumatism.*** Spleen, pain. Sprains. Stiff-neck. ***Testes, disorders.*** Tinnitus. Toothaches. Vagina, cysts. Wrists, pains.

HERBAL - The golden flowered rhododendron grows among the fog and storms of the Siberian mountains. It is not well known in general medicine, but the Treasury of Botany said that "it is narcotic in its properties and is used medicinally."

Gmelin, during his travels in Siberia, noted that the Cossacks and Mongolians used it for rheumatism and gout. The hunters and mountain rangers would drink an infusion of it to remove the weariness and pains from their limbs after fatiguing expeditions.

Gmelin was the first to recommend rhododendron in Europe as a remedy for gout and rheumatism. The first publication on the subject was by Professor Kolpin, of Stettin, in 1779. It was used with greater or less success, and recommended accordingly by many German physicians.

HOMEOPATHIC - Rhod. is a gouty, rheumatic remedy, affecting the ***fibrous tissues***, forearm, lower legs, small joints, bones, genitals, nerves, and single parts. ***Fibrositis. Arthritis.*** Great weakness after slight exertion. Formication with sweat. Undulating sensation. Tearing, zigzag, boring, rapidly changing, descending, paralytic pains.

Rhod. produces delirium, fever, headache, neuralgias, rheumatism and inflammations. ***Symptoms come on or are worse on the approach of a storm, worse during a storm or in wet weather.*** Sensitiveness to electric changes, lightning (Phos.). Weather vane, can predict an upcoming change (Calc., Rhus-t., Dulc.).

Arthritis cases are especially sensitive to barometric changes. Aggravated symptoms before a storm, usually arthritis, headaches, neuralgias, toothaches and earaches. Increased warmth of hands even in cold weather.

Sensitive to windy or stormy wet weather, even if he is in the house. For nervous persons who are afraid of thunder, dread of storms. Chorea before storm. Disorders which come on in the spring and autumn. Rheumatism in the hot season. Symptoms alternate.

MIND - Dread of a storms. ***Fear of thunderstorms*** in nervous persons (Phos.). Nervous before storms. Fits of anxiety. Confused and stupid. Impatience. Irritability. Peevish, without any apparent cause. Phlegmatic mood, he is affected by neither pleasant or unpleasant impressions. Gloomy mood. Sadness, being alone aggravates.

Indifferent. Aversion to everything, especially to occupations. Aversion to his business. Stupefaction. Obscuration or loss of senses. ***Forgets what he is talking about, leaves out whole words while writing.*** Does not recollect what he had been talking about until he has thought a while. Vanishing of thoughts. Easily affected by wine.

Mental derangement. Frightful visions. Delirium, he staggers, tosses his head about and reels. After a short time, falls asleep upon his knees. In vain he attempts to rise, but is overcome with sleep for an hour and a quarter, during which he starts continually and appears terrified, but awakes cheerful.

Abdomen - Colic at navel. Flatus felt in back. Undulating sensation arising from abdomen. Sickening pain in spleen on walking fast. Pain from rectum to genitals. Paroxysmal pain, lying on abdomen impossible. Pain in left hypogastrium. Umbilical pain.

Back - Stiff neck. Sacrum pains, w rse sitting. Pain between scapulae. Backache, lumbar region. Stitching pain, extending to pit of stomach.

Bladder - Frequent desire to urinate. Burning in the urethra before and during urination. Copious urine.

Causations - Catching cold. Stormy weather, thunder, getting wet. Sprains. Eating fruit.

Chest - Violent pleuritic pains running down the left anterior chest. Crampy pain under short ribs. Stitches in spleen from fast walking. Breathless and speechless from pain.

Constitutions - Suited to nervous persons who dread a storm and are particularly afraid of thunder.

Cough - Choking. Suffocative coughs, worse motion. Cough from tickling in trachea. Paroxysmal coughs with retching, choking. Morning coughs, from 6 a.m. to 9 a.m.

Dreams - Erotic dreams. Exhausting, frightful dreams. Nightmares.

Ears - Earache. Sensation as of a worm in the ear. As if hot air was flowing from throat to ears. Tinnitus with vertigo. Difficult hearing with whizzing and ringing in ears. Hearing better in the morning, noises come on after patient has been up a few hours. Deafness, long after rising.

Eyes - Muscular asthenopia. ***Ciliary neuralgia*** involving orbit, eyeball and head, worse before storm. Heat in eyes when using them. Darting pains, red-hot needles darting from within out. Contractive pain behind the eyes, with pain in forehead. Pain in eyes before a storm.

Face - Prosopalgia, violent jerking pain involving dental nerves from temple to lower jaw and chin. ***Pains better warmth and eating***. Painful pimples, better pressure.

Female - Suppressed menses. Painful menses. Dysmenorrhea. Fever with headache, with each menstrual period. Serous cysts in vagina. Burning in uterine region after childbirth, alternating with pain in limbs, fingers spasmodically flexed. Sexual desire increased.

Food - Desires sweets. Dullness of taste, food has no flavor. Gnawing, hungry sensation before a meal. Speedy satiety with good appetite, followed by uneasiness. Augmented thirst.

Generals - Burning, stitching pain. Pressure on certain points ameliorates. Trembling. Weakness. Weariness, worse afternoon. Lack of vital heat. Sensation of heat. Desires open air.

Head - Headaches, worse wine, wind, cold and wet weather, early in the morning, better eating. Aching in temples. Throbbing in right side. Bursting pains, better pressure and rubbing forehead. Tearing pain in bones. Drawing, tearing under scalp. Hair stands up as if electrified. Heat in afternoon, evening. Pressure in temples, as if compressed. Contracting, as if scalp stretched tight.

Heart - Warm undulation at heart. Strong heartbeat.

Kidneys - Frequent urging to urinate with drawing in the bladder region. Pain in the urethra as from subcutaneous ulceration. Profuse, foul, greenish urine.

Larynx - Dryness. Hoarse voice. Trachea irritation, mucus. Sensation of mucus that he is not able to eject. Burning pains, like splinters.

Limbs - Swollen joints. ***Rheumatic and tearing pains*** in all the limbs, especially right side. ***Rheumatic pains worse at rest and in stormy weather.*** Rheumatism in hot weather. Numbness. Numbness as if limbs have gone to sleep, must move about. Stitching pain. Pain, better motion. Drawing, tearing in periosteum of long bones. Pain in bones, in spots, and reappear by change of weather. Coldness of limbs. Sensation like a cool draft of air over limbs. Gout. Gouty inflammation of great toe joint. ***Cannot sleep unless legs are crossed.*** Lower legs, cold, skin wrinkled, feel as if asleep. As of a weight hanging to feet. Feet cold even in warm room, even in bed. Pain in Achilles tendon on stepping. Shoulder pain, better firm pressure and warmth on certain points. Pain in shoulders, arms, wrists, worse when at rest. Bruised, sprained feeling in wrist. Hands feel warm in cold weather.

Lungs - Bruised, sprained feeling in chest. Breathless and speechless from violent pleuritic pains, running down anterior chest. Expectoration in mornings, 6 a.m. to 9 a.m. Crumbly expectoration, left-over food, like leaves in the mouth.

Male - ***Hydrocele*** of boys from birth (Sil.). Drawing from spermatic cord into abdomen and thighs. Orchitis. Itching, wrinkled, sweaty, scrotum. ***Testes, especially the epididymis, are intensely painful to the touch swollen***, drawn up, worse left. Contusive pain in the testes. Induration and swelling of testes after gonorrhea. Glans feels crushed. Burning, sore pain between the genital organs and thighs, especially when walking.

Modalities - Better after the storm breaks, when the sun shines. Better heat, warmth, wrapping up, wrapping head. Better motion and eating. ***Worse before a storm, rough weather***. Worse during windy, cold, damp, cloudy weather. Worse when the seasons change, midsummer. Worse getting wet, catching cold. Worse at night, towards morning, from rest. Worse wine, eating fruit.

Mouth - Salivation with nausea and intermittent pain in stomach. Insipid, bitter taste. Dryness in the mouth, palate, and tongue. Speech impossible due to numbness of cheeks, and lips, in morning after waking.

Nose - Dryness, soreness inside nose. One sided nasal obstruction. Nostrils obstructed, alternately with fluent coryza, better in open air. Nasal discharge, viscid like gravel on dry mucus membranes. Paroxysmal sneezing. Nosebleed. Diminished smell.

Perspiration - Offensive smell in the axillary sweat, but the general sweat may be aromatic in odor and not unpleasant.

Formication with sweat.

Rectum - Diarrhea worse fruits, does not weaken. Difficult evacuation, even of soft feces. Feces of pap consistency. Mucus evacuations.

Sensations - Brain as if in a fog. Scalp as if bruised. As if a worm in ear. As if water rushing into ear. As if throat lined with mucus. As from tension under short ribs. As if a fist pressed forcibly against stomach. Undulating sensation arising from abdomen. Warm undulations in heart. Testicle as if violently contused or crushed. As if blood ceased to circulate in arms. As if arms asleep. As if feet and legs asleep. As if heavy weights hanging to feet. As of subcutaneous ulceration. Bruised pains. Pains flying about. Crawling sensations.

Skin - Eruptions. Burning and tearing with erysipelas. Itching, burning and creeping.

Sleep - Cannot sleep unless legs are crossed. Wakes, as if called.

Stomach - Empty feeling in morning. Weak feeling, better eating. Feels full after a little food. Paroxysmal pain. Heartburn. Belching, after eating eggs. Heavy pressure from cold drinks. Nausea, better fresh air. Green, bitter vomiting after drinking cold water.

Teeth - Swollen gums. Stumps of teeth are loosened. Toothache in damp weather and before a storm. Toothache, better eating and warmth. Toothache ceases suddenly, worse again in two or three hours.

Temperature - Formication and itching of skin with sweat. Chilliness, 11 a.m. to 11:30 a.m. Shaking, shivering rigors. Cold feet, even in warm room or bed. Hands warm in cold weather.

Throat - Dryness. Burning pain. Swelling of throat. Chocking, constriction and burning sensation in throat. Scratching, scraping in throat, sensation as if lined with mucus. Mucus tough, gluey, green, difficult to detach with cough and retching. Sensation of foreign object. Heat, as if hot air were to gush out from throat to ears.

Vertigo - Vertigo, when lying in bed, better when moving about. Tinnitus with vertigo.

COMMENTS - Characteristic loss of memory. Words are omitted while writing, thoughts suddenly disappear, forgets what they are talking about, has to think a while before they can recall it. Narcotic symptoms. Intoxication, and sensitivity to wine. One pupil dilated, the other contracted.

Vertigo and confusion, "brain feels as if surrounded by fog." Vertigo while lying in bed, better by moving about. Tinnitus aurium, associated with the vertigo. Meniere's disease. "Loud sounds re-echo long in ears."

Symptoms frequently alternate, left and right nostril, burning in uterus and pains in limbs, chilliness and heat. Pains go from within outward. Both sides are affected.

Arthritis, worse rest and better motion (Rhus-t.). Better from warmth and wrapping the area up. Chorea of left leg, arm and face, worse on approach of a storm. Splenic stitch on walking fast.

Offensive smell in the axillary sweat, but the general sweat may be aromatic in odor and not unpleasant. Formication with sweat.

Like the other Ericacee, Rhod. has a strong effect on the kidneys, producing increased urine with offensive smell, clear, brown red or of greenish tinge and, whatever color it may be, of offensive smell.

Diarrhea. Paralytic condition of the rectum, effort is required to expel a soft stool. "Flatus felt in the back," in cases of flatulent indigestion.

Pains in rectum extend to genitals. The scrotum shrinks, testes are retracted or else they swell (especially at night) and are the seat of a bruised pain, as if they had been crushed violently. Pains are worse by touch, worse sitting, better moving about. Pains may be so violent as to arrest breathing.

The menses are too early and too profuse. Menses are accompanied by fever and headache. Menses reappear soon after they have ceased. In one prover,

Rhod. restored the menses after six months' absence. Vaginal cysts, has caused the rupture of ovarian cysts.

The paralyzing effect of Rhod. was exemplified by the poisoning of a flock of sheep from eating the leaves. A number of them died and the autopsy showed that cause of death was paralysis of the swallowing muscles.

Cooper cited a parallel case of death from post-diphtheria paralysis affecting the throat muscles, occurring a few minutes after drinking tea. In both instances, the fluid entered the trachea instead of the gullet and caused suffocation.

H. S. Budd related the case of Mrs. X., 44, who was married ten years and had three children. She had neuralgia for three years. Attacks usually occurred on Friday or Saturday and would last until Monday or Tuesday, but were induced any time by high winds, damp weather or an approaching storm. Passi. only partly relieved, sometimes enabling the patient to get sleep.

The pain was worse after hard work, during any movement, in very cold weather or from hot applications. She had intense soreness all over the right half of her head, she could not rest on a pillow or endure even the lightest hairpins when pain was worst. Worse at night.

She was intensely nervous and hysterical at being touched, even by accident. During the pain, she had increased activity of the kidneys, that ceased when pain ceased. Pain was greatest in her right lower jaw. Sometimes better for an hour by chewing gum or eating. Afraid of thunder. Omitted words when writing.

Rhod. 16x every hour was given on May 12. Each dose caused an immediate worsening of symptoms. The next morning, pains stopped suddenly and did not return. On June 7th there was a premonitory twinge and a powder of Rhod. 1,000c was given, after which there was complete immunity.

E. V. Moffat treated a girl, 10, for neuralgia, which had existed for several years. The patient was of a marked gouty heredity and had been treated by leading old-school doctors in New York. She was well during the summer, but suffered intensely during winter.

Pains were general and shifting, sometimes intercostal, sometimes sciatic in bad weather, never absent. The last form was a prostrating headache incapacitating her for schoolwork.

Her eyes were normal. While the sun shone, she was comfortable. If it stormed or threatened, she was miserable. If she had a headache on a stormy day and the sun came out in ten minutes she was relieved, and it returned at once if snow or rain came on. A cold day, especially if damp, was almost as bad as a storm.

Rhod. in repeated and increasing doses, cured in three weeks. Color, spirits, strength returned and she no longer minded the weather or missed her school.

RELATIONS - ***Compare:*** (1) Ampe-qu. - hydrocele and kidney dropsy. (2) Med., Dulc., Rhus-t., Nat-s. (3) It is analogous to and follows as regards the testes, Puls., Aur., Spong., as regards hydrocele, Clem., Graph.

REFERENCES - Boericke. Clarke. Murphy. Phatak.

RHUS AROMATICA

(Fragrant Sumac)

PHARMACY - rhus-a. Rhus aromatica. Fragrant sumac. Rhus canadensis. Rhus suaveolens. Betula triphylla. Lobadium aromaticum. Turpinia glabra. N. O. Anacardiacae. Tincture of fresh root bark. ***Historical dose:*** Tincture and all potencies.

CLINICAL - Atony. Bedwetting. Bladder, hemorrhage. Cystitis. Diabetes. Diarrhea. Dysentery. ***Hematuria. Hemorrhages.*** Kidneys, hemorrhage. Uterus, hemorrhage, atony.

HERBAL - J. T. McClanahan's account of Rhus-a.: "It is a shrub, growing from two to six feet high, on high, rocky soil, stems straight, branching near the top. The flowers are yellow, fruit clustered, red, seedy and acid. When the bush is fractured it emits a strong odor. The bark of the root is the proper medicinal part."

HOMEOPATHIC - Rhus-a. has kidney and urinary disorders. ***Diabetes***, large quantities of urine of low specific gravity (Ph-ac., Acet-ac.). Bedwetting due to bladder atony, senile incontinence. Hematuria and cystitis. The urine is ***pale***, albuminous. ***Incontinence of urine. Severe pain at beginning or before urination***, causing great agony in children. Constant dribbling.

COMMENTS - McClanahan mentioned hemorrhage from kidneys, bladder and uterus, menorrhagia and other discharges accompanied by a relaxed condition of the uterus as indicating the remedy, also atonic conditions generally.

These experiences have been confirmed by others. McClanahan's grandfather, Dr. John Gray, used Rhus-a. as a remedy in diabetes, and his father, Dr. F. McClanahan, in other genito-urinary diseases.

J. T. McClanahan recorded several cases, including the case of Mr. A., 27, cadaverous, emaciated, haggard, had diabetes insipidus. Rhus-a., teaspoonful doses of the powdered root bark in sweet milk, three times a day, completely cured in four months.

Mrs. B., 37, had diabetes mellitus. First noticed increase of urine ten months before, became so weak she had to abandon house-work. Pain in back, thirst, appetite, now ravenous, now deficient. Skin sallow, doughy. Cough and night-sweats occasionally. Diarrhea at times.

Rhus-a., half-teaspoonful doses every four hours, was given. Quantity of urine diminished next day and as this diminution progressed the doses of Rhus-a. were given at increasing intervals, and in three months it was discontinued. Proper diet had been observed in the meantime.

Mr. C. had incontinence of urine more than a year, constant dribbling. Rhus-a. tincture 10 drops, three times a day, improved at once and cured completely in eight weeks.

A girl had bedwetting during the day and night for two years. Rhus-a. tincture, one part to glycerine three parts, a teaspoonful three times a day, cured.

A boy, early in summer had diarrhea, stools pale and thin, running from him like water, no particular pain or fever. Pale, emaciated, limbs trembling, scarcely able to stand. Abdomen flabby. Rhus-a. tincture 3 drops in water after each stool, cured rapidly.

A laborer had "chronic dysentery" for two months. On the average, had five stools a day, sometimes copious and painless, sometimes scanty and with pain. Stools consisted largely of blood and mucus or clear blood. Patient was thin, anxious, bowels (abdomen) flabby. Skin sallow. Rhus-a. tincture in ten-drop doses with boiled milk diet, cured.

J. A. McKay related the case of Mrs. S., 45, who had severe, profuse uterine hemorrhage for eight days, which three old-school doctors failed to arrest. The condition was becoming desperate, large clots passing away and the patient fainting from the loss.

Rhus-a. tincture 10 drops, every six hours, was given. The first dose checked the flow, which ceased entirely after the second.

REFERENCES - Boericke. Clarke.

RHUS DIVERSILOBA

(California Poison Oak)

PHARMACY - rhus-d. Rhus diversiloba. California poison oak. N. O. Anacardiacae. Tincture of fresh leaves. ***Historical dose:*** All potencies.

CLINICAL - Chickenpox. Eczema. Erysipelas. Fatigue. Skin, sensitive. Sprains.

HOMEOPATHIC - Rhus-d. is an antidote to Rhus-t. Affects the skin with violent skin symptoms with frightful itching. Much swelling of the face, hands and genitals. The skin is very sensitive with eczema and erysipelas. Tired from least effort, goes to sleep from sheer exhaustion. Great nervous weakness.

Causations - Ailments from overexertion, lifting, physical labor. Strains. Sprains.

COMMENTS - Murray Moore observed the effect of Rhus-d. on three persons. The first was Miss M., 25 of brown hair and fair complexion. She walked up a hill one warm morning and, while perspiring, gathered ferns which grew among the Rhus-d. trees, the leaves of which she must have touched, though she did not pull any. The result was a very severe poisoning.

J. W., a light-haired, robust Englishman, 23, lay down while sweating among the bushes and was smartly poisoned. Ver-v. tincture internally and a lotion of magnesia sulph. externally checked the spread of the disease.

A boy, 10, pure blond type with thin, freckled skin, plucked some of the leaves and in eighteen hours the poisoning symptoms came on, facial erysipelas with extreme edema, closing both eyes, itching and burning. The symptoms became general.

M. Moore also related the case of a man who was poisoned in California in September, returned to the eastern states, and suffered from an annual eruption for six successive years. During the seventh attack he was carried off with pneumonia, which Moore thought would not have been the case but for the Rhus-d. complication.

RELATIONS - Rhus-d. is an antidote to Rhus-t. *Compare:* Rhus-t.

REFERENCES - Clarke.

RHUS GLABRA

(Smooth Sumac)

PHARMACY - rhus-g. Rhus glabra. Smooth sumac. Rhus carolinas. Rhus elegans. Rhus virginica. Pennsylvania sumac. Upland sumac. N. O. Anacardiacae. Rocky or barren soils in North America. Tincture of fresh bark of root. Tincture of berries. ***Historical dose:*** Tincture and all potencies.

CLINICAL - Aphthae. Debility. Diarrhea. Dreams, annoying. Dysentery. Hemorrhages. Headache. Mouth ulcers. Nosebleed. Pharyngitis.

HERBAL - Rhus trypanosomiasis, Rhus glabra and Rhus coriaria have acid fruit and astringent bark, which is used in tanning. Rhus-g. is a deciduous shrub with a stem 2 to 12 feet high and has terminal flowers and fruit clothed with acid crimson hairs like the other non-poisonous Rhus.

A tincture made of the whole pannicle, *"Sumac-bobs"* cured a patient who had every spring an attack of laryngeal cough with dyspnea and almost complete loss of voice. Farmers place *"bobs"* in the mangers of hoses who have *"heaves."*

HOMEOPATHIC - The tincture of the bark was proved by Dr. A. V. Marshall on himself with very substantial doses. The symptoms are his and they bear out the traditional uses of the remedy.

One of these is ***"profuse perspiration arising from debility."*** Marshall had "profuse sweat during sleep" and such a degree of debility that he was obliged to leave off the proving.

Hale mentioned that an infusion of the root had a popular repute in diarrhea and dysentery, especially when the discharges are fetid, and that the berries were used for chronic cough, wheezing cough and laryngeal asthma.

It was claimed that this remedy will so disinfect the bowels that the flatus and stools will be free from odor. It acts well in putrescence conditions with tendency to ulceration. ***Fetid flatus.***

Used locally on soft, spongy gums, aphthae, pharyngitis, etc. Ulceration of mouth. Nosebleeds and ***occipital headaches. Dreams of flying through the air*** (Stict.). Exhaustion and painful fatigue. Loss of weight.

MIND - Stupid, forgetful, indifferent to surrounding objects. Distaste for society.

Abdomen - Sharp cutting in umbilical region and abdomen. Umbilical region tender to pressure.

Back - Pain in small of back.

Food - Loss of appetite. Hunger at breakfast, could eat but little though feeling as if he had fasted many days.

Head - Dull, heavy headache on waking, better by exercise. Dull heavy pain in front and top of head.

Kidneys - Scanty, high-colored urine.

Limbs - Aching and fatigue of lower limbs, can hardly stand.

Modalities - Better by movement. Worse after sleep. Abdomen, ulcers in mouth, worse from touch.

Mouth - Taste flat, alkaline. Taste of drug remains long. Tongue furred white. Bleeding from mouth. Aphthous stomatitis. Several small, very sensitive ulcers on mucus membrane opposite the bicuspids. Scurvy, nursing sore mouth (Vero-o.).

Nose - Bleeding from left nostril and mouth. Bloody scabs in left nostril. Left nostril hot and dry.

Perspiration - ***Profuse perspiration arising from debility*** (Chin.). Sweat, profuse during sleep.

Rectum - Diarrhea in afternoon, worse towards evening. Dry, hard stool, later moist, then natural, and again diarrhea.

Sleep - Sleep disturbed by annoying dreams, very restless. Dreams of flying through the air.

Stomach - Distress in stomach, disturbed, very restless. Pain in stomach, much worse by all food or drink.

Temperature - Sense of coldness while there is actual increase of heat in the skin. Skin hot, dry with thirst.

Throat - Expelled two clots of blood from throat soon after waking.

COMMENTS - Cooper observed an aggravation in a case of psoriasis in which the patient felt irritable and despondent and the skin became irritable. Aggravation of stomach symptoms by either food or drink.

In the proving there were dull, heavy headaches, better by exercise. Hale said Rhus-g. has cured occipital headaches.

RELATIONS - Said to be antidotal to the action of Merc. and has been employed in the treatment of secondary syphilis after mercury. ***Compare:*** (1) Rhus-t. Anac. and other Anacardiace, and the Xanthoxylaces, which are an allied order.

REFERENCES - Boericke. Clarke.

RHUS LAURINA

(Laurel Sumac)

PHARMACY - rhus-l. Rhus laurina. Laurel sumac. N. O. Anacardiaceae. ***Historical dose:*** All potencies.

CLINICAL - Edema. Itching. Skin, eruptions. Swelling. Urticaria. Vesicles.

HERBAL - This variety grows abundantly in the Sacramento and San Joaquin valleys, as well as in the mountains and is found in all parts of California. It differs from Rhus-t. principally in the shape of the leaves, and in the entire absence of the slightest pubescence, both on their superior and inferior surfaces.

The sap of the plant is a thin milky fluid, but when allowed to touch the skin, it produces a dark purple stain, and for three or four days afterwards, whenever the part is washed, it looks as if it had been recently touched with silver nitrate.

HOMEOPATHIC - M. J. Rhees, M.D. wrote, "Some persons are much more readily and severely affected by this plant than others, while a very few are entirely exempt from its influence. The great majority are more or less susceptible to its action. I have seen very many cases of poisoning by it.

"Some have presented the same symptoms and the same kind of eruption as were present in my own case, but in more severe form. I have seen eyes completely closed for 24 hours by the swelling, and the scrotum and prepuce have been so badly swollen in a few cases as to render it necessary to support them with a suspensory bandage.

"In other instances, the vesicles are much longer than in my case, and become confluent, forming a dark scab of an inch or more in diameter. I have not seen any case in which the tongue or pulse were materially disordered. I have been informed by a gentleman in this city, that two persons with whom he was acquainted, died from the effects of the poison, but I have been unable to learn anything concerning their symptoms.

"Dr. Lewis Post, of San Jose, California, informs me that if he rides within ten feet to leeward of the plant, he is speedily affected by it, particularly and almost exclusively on the scrotum and prepuce. It seems to have a great affinity for this part of the body, as almost all the cases I have seen have complained of the intense voluptuous itching of the external genital organs and the inside of the thighs."

COMMENTS - Recorded in proceedings of the American Institute of Homeopathy on rhus-l., M. J. Rhees, M.D. wrote, "On the 4th of the present month, at 10 o'clock a.m., I procured several branches of both sexual varieties of Rhus laur., and cut the leaves tenshoots, and clusters of flowers into small fragments, and put them into a vial, with the intention of making a tincture.

"While doing so, I was troubled with a smarting and burning in the eyes. My hands were protected at the time by kid gloves, and I washed them carefully with strong soap before I touched any part of my body. In the evening I began to experience slight itching and burning in the face, particularly about the eyes and forehead; and voluptuous itching on the scrotum and prepuce. At night, felt a sense of oppression as if the air was too heavy.

"April 5th. Last night the sleep was disturbed and full of dreams, which were lascivious, and of venereal pleasure; felt heavy and unrefreshed in the morning; during the day the itching in the face has increased and spread over the nose, the edges of the nostrils, the upper and lower lips, the external ears, and the inferior portion of the neck immediately above the sternum and clavicles; the skin on these parts feels rough, and is covered with a minute eruption of lenticular vesicles, filled with transparent serum.

"Itching on the back of the hands, particularly between the fingers. The itching on the scrotum and prepuce has become more troublesome, and is much increased by scratching; scratching, or rubbing of the parts is followed by intense burning; the prepuce is slightly swollen. In the evening the nose is quite red and shining; the redness is not removed by pressure.

"April 6th. This morning I felt weak and languid. Dull, aching pain, and weakness across the loins. Redness, and swelling of the skin of the forehead, eyelids, nose, cheeks, lips, and ears, behind the ears, and on the front of the neck.

"The skin on these parts is covered with the minute lenticular vesicles spoken of yesterday, which are more filled with serum. These vesicles seem to be situated in the rete mucosum; at least they involve a deeper tissue than the cuticle. During the day some of them find their way to the surface, and are ruptured while being scratched.

"The itching is so intolerable that it is impossible to resist the inclination to scratch. After scratching, the parts burn and sting, become more swollen, and feel stiff and dry; the prepuce is much swollen and very red, and the itching is unbearable about once in five or six hours on this part and the scrotum; the scrotum is red, swollen, and much corrugated.

"After scratching for a few minutes, the itching is entirely relieved for several hours; eruption of pimples and minute vesicles with excessive itching on the backs of the hands and between the fingers; itching on the inside of the thighs.

"April 7th. The same symptoms continue as were noted yesterday, but with increased violence. The eyes were nearly closed in the morning, by the swelling of the lids. Chilly sensation during the day, through the whole body, while sitting in a warm room.

"April 8th. The itching and swelling on the face, between the fingers, and on the scrotum and prepuce, became so intolerable, that, fearing it would incapacitate me for business, I took Rhus tox. 6th, every four hours, and bathed the parts with cream. This treatment alleviated the symptoms somewhat. At night itching and redness on the inside of the thighs, from the perineum to the knees.

"April 9th. The itching and swelling in the face is very much abated, as well as that on the scrotum and prepuce. The itching on the hands and between the fingers is very harassing, and is much increased by rubbing and scratching.

"The itching comes on at intervals of 5 or 6 hours, but it may be produced at any time by rubbing or scratching.

Scratching is followed by excessive burning, and between the fingers by a dull, aching pain, the skin becoming more swollen, hard, and white, as in urticaria.

"This evening took a hot bath, as hot as it could be borne, using Castile soap and the flesh-brush freely. This was followed by immediate and complete relief for several hours. Continued the Rhus tox. as yesterday, and the cream externally.

"April 10th. The itching in the neck returned at bed time, last night, and was somewhat troublesome through the night. This morning the itching returned with great severity in the hands, and was again relieved by bathing them in hot water, which was repeated this evening.

"The face is very dry and rough, and has a scurfy appearance, and the skin seems to be thickened and indurated; all other parts have been comfortable through the day, with the exception of the thighs and the skin covering the lower portion of the abdomen, which has at long intervals itched considerably.

"April 11th. Bathed the hands in hot water this morning, and they have not been at all troublesome through the day. There has been some itching on the thighs and scrotum, but not nearly so much as formerly.

"April 12th. The hands have been very troublesome at intervals of 12 hours during the day. This morning vesicles made their appearance in the palm of the left hand wherever the sap of the plant had touched the skin, in gathering it.

"April 19th. Up to the present time, the itching and burning in the palm of the left hand, and between the fingers of both hands, have been very annoying, almost painful, at intervals of 10 or 12 hours. Wishing, however, to know how long the effect of the plant would continue, I have made use of no remedies since the 11th. It is now evidently abating."

RELATIONS - ***Compare:*** Rhus-t. Anac. and other Anacardiace, and the Xanthoxylaces, which are an allied order.

REFERENCES - Rhees.

RHUS RADICANS

(Climbing Poison Ivy)

PHARMACY - rhus-r. Rhus radicans. Climbing poison ivy. Poison vine. Toxicodendron radicans. N. O. Anacardiaceae. Tincture of fresh leaves gathered at sunset just before flowering time. ***Historical dose:*** All potencies.

CLINICAL - ***Arthritis. Backaches.*** Boils. Chills. Colic. Constipation. Cough. Debility. Dermatitis. Diabetes. ***Dislocated, joints.*** Dyspnea. Eczema. ***Erysipelas.*** Faintness. ***Fever, blisters.*** Fevers. ***Fibrositis.*** Glossitis. Headaches. ***Herpes zoster.*** Hives. Housemaid's knee. ***Influenza. Injuries.*** Intermittent fever. ***Joint, pains. Lumbago.*** Muscular, pains. Nausea. Neuralgia. Nosebleeds. Palpitations. Palsy. Paralysis. Periosteum, pains. ***Poison ivy, oak.*** Rashes. ***Rheumatism. Sciatica.*** Spine, diseases. ***Sprains. Stiffness. Strains. Tendonitis.*** Typhoid fever. Typhus. Ulcers. ***Urticaria.*** Vesicles. Vertigo. ***Whiplash.***

HERBAL - Dispute whether Rhus radicans differs from Rhus toxicondendron continues. Botanists agree in recognizing little distinction other than that of habit between the two.

Millspaugh, in his book "American Medicinal Plants," tells in his account of the plant that he had seen the two varieties springing from the same root-stock. He advises that the tincture should be made from specimens of both.

Rhus-t. is a dwarf, erect, shrub, while Rhus-r. is a climber, with stem five to forty feet long, furnished with numerous radicles by which it adheres to trees and climbs up them like ivy. The leaves of Rhus-r. are almost entire and glabrous. The leaves are smoother at the margins than Rhus-t.

HOMEOPATHIC - Under the name "Rhus," Hahnemann published his proving of "Rhus radicans, also called Toxicodendron." The two forms have been proved independently. The American provings were made with Rhus-r. and the majority of the poisonings have occurred from this plant.

It acts on the brain, mucus membrane, skin, muscles, joints, and tendons. Inflammation of fibrous tissues. Neuralgias. Palsy of the limbs.

Rheumatism of the chest, neck, and back. ***Wandering, rheumatic pains***, first one joint, then another. ***Pains and stiffness*** are often semi-lateral and in various parts, often remote and successive.

Traumatic inflammation of the joints. Sprains. The pains are worse when first beginning to move in the morning, relieved during the day, when occupied, and when walking in the open air.

Ailments from straining a single part, muscle or tendon, over-lifting, particularly from stretching high up to reach things. ***Whiplash. Dislocated, joints.*** Injuries and traumas to the joints. ***Tendonitis.*** Sprained joints.

Severe backaches, chronic, low back pain. Burning in the spine. ***Stiffness in the sacrum,*** better with cracking and adjustments. Coldness in left tibia. Old injuries that never healed, stiffen with weather changes.

Headache in occiput, even pain in nape, and from there pains draw over the head forwards. Jaws are tight and stiff, can crack and pop. Inflammation of the tongue Burning in tongue, tip feels sore (Rhus-t.).

Erysipelas, red, itching, phlegmonous swelling, with vesicular eruption extending like a band around right ankle. Large open ulcer on ankle, pain worse after, not during motion (Rhus-r. cured after failure of Rhus-t.).

Intermittent fever. Fever with debility. Excessive debility. General languor. Inclination to lie down. Faintness and dyspnea. Typhoid. Typhus conditions. Diabetes.

Symptoms better after a storm has thoroughly set in, especially after an electric storm. Pronounced yearly aggravation (Lach.). Symptoms increased after drinking cold water.

MIND - Unfit for any mental labor. Confusion at night on lying down. Irresolution in projects. Mistakes in speaking. Jesting. Melancholy. Mental depression. Great discouragement and apprehension about the future. Delusion that she is criticized. Unconsciousness while standing.

Abdomen - Distention and flatus. Constriction and pain in left hypochondria. Dull pains. Lancinations in right hypochondria during inspiration. Sharp pains. Shooting pain after drinking cold water. Griping colic. Colic that compels him to flex the trunk.

Back - ***Backaches and stiffness.*** Severe backaches, chronic, low back pain. ***Stiffness of back in the morning.*** Aching in the back and in the renal region. Aching in the lumbar spine and ileum when lying down at night. ***Lumbago.*** Pain across the back, loins and quadratus lumborum. ***Stiffness in the sacrum*** that's better with cracking and adjustments. Weakness in the whole spine. Burning in the spine. Pains in and between the scapulae. ***Rigidity of the neck. Stiff neck.*** Pain in the cervical muscles on motion, feel tender.

Chest - Chest sensitive to pressure. Chest pains that seem to proceed from the stomach. Pain in chest, near the nipple. Dull pain. Pains worse on inspiration.

Ears - Pain in one ear. Small boil. Sensation as if the beating of the heart and arteries were heard. Sound of rushing water.

Eyes - Pain in the eyes when opening them. Burning, smarting in the eyeballs. Lachrymation. Itching at the inner canthus. Swelling and redness of the lids, with itching and burning. Edema of the lids. Confusion of sight. Vision obscured. Dimness at candlelight.

Face - Neuralgia. Pain in the left side of the face and lower jaw. ***Erysipelas***, burning, smarting, heat, and redness. Boils. Pustules. Vesicles. Pimples on the face and forehead. Large red pimple on the cheek. Eruptions at the angle of the mouth.

Food - Appetite deficient or lost.

Head - Head feels as if it were swelling, and had become too large. Heaviness, fullness. Sensation as if the crown of the head were rising up. Heat, pain, and throbbing in the head. Continual dull pain in forehead. Semi-lateral pain in the temple. Pain over the eye. Headache, with nausea worse when lying down, better after rising. Pain in vertex and nape of neck. Scalp tender. Small elevations. Eruptions. Itching.

Heart - Palpitations of the heart with fullness in the head. Pulse frequent and small.

Kidneys - Pressure on the bladder. Increased secretion and flow of urine. Milky urine. Deep red urine, with pink deposit.

Limbs - ***Rheumatism.*** Inflammation of the joints with heat, redness, and swelling. ***Wandering pains from joint to joint. Traumatic inflammation of the joints.*** Instability. ***Stiffness of joints.*** Weakness, and feeling of heaviness in the limbs, when walking. ***Sprains. Dislocated joints. Pain as though the muscles or tendons were strained.*** Pain and stiffness in hip. Soreness and excoriation about the nates. ***Swelling, stiffness and lameness of the knee, ankle.*** Pain in knee, near the patella, worse on moving the joint. Pains in calf when walking. Cramps in the calf when lying in bed, or extending the limb. Pains at the ankles. Sharp pains in the feet. Pains in the sole of the right foot. Coldness of the feet. Coldness, with numbness. Severe pain in shoulder and the acromion process. Aching in the wrists, especially during exertion of the fingers. Numbness of the arms, hands and fingers. Erysipelatous inflammation of the hands and fingers. Vesicles between the fingers. Scratches and injuries tend to inflame and suppurate. Itching, red eruption on the legs, and about the ankles. Vesicles.

Lungs - Dry cough. Hacking cough, excited by tickling. Cough on movement or lying down.

Male - Penis swollen, bloated. Scrotum, inflamed and irritated by walking. Rash in genital area. Vesicles.

Mouth - Increased saliva. Disagreeable bitter or metallic taste. Air feels unusually cold in the mouth. Sore pain, as if the mouth had been scalded. Ulcers. Vesicles inside the mouth. Gums inflamed, tender. Transient throbbing in the teeth. Pains in carious teeth. Toothache, with flow of saliva.

Nose - Frequent sneezing. Nostrils excoriated and encrusted. Fluent coryza, with copious secretion of mucus. Nosebleed.

Rectum - Anus, sore, excoriated, especially after walking. Constipation with headache. Diarrhea, with slimy, yellow stools. Pale evacuations. Evacuations streaked with blood. Bright blood after a stool.

Skin - Itching, pricking, stinging. Dermatitis. ***Poison ivy and poison oak rashes.*** Hard, red eruptions. Inflamed tubercles, elevations, hard pimples. Pustules, blisters, watery pimples. ***Vesicular eruption***, some disappear without rupture of the cuticle, others burst. Yellow, acrid fluid from eruptions. Erysipelas, especially in hot weather. Small boils. Ulcers. Swelling of the lymphatic glands.

Sleep - Sleepy by day, and early in the evening. Imperfect sleep at night, disturbed by frequent waking. Dreams of danger and horses. Fear on waking.

Stomach - Stomach sensitive to pressure. Severe pain in stomach with dizziness. Shooting, sharp pain. Pain after food. Pressure and fullness in epigastrium. Empty eructations. Nausea. Vomiting of tasteless water.

Temperature - Chills, general or partial, generally in the back. Coldness of the extremities. General body heat with dry skin. Intermittent fever, every day, at 1 p.m. Fever, with pain in the legs. Typhoid fever with brown tongue, red tip.

Throat - Rawness, excoriation. Pricking, smarting, stinging, irritation. Red, hot, burning, and swollen, constriction. Painful deglutition.

Tongue - Tongue feels dry, sore. Burning, pricking. Scalded feeling, tip of the tongue feels sore or burnt. Vesicles at tip. Rough tongue. Yellow coated tongue.

Vertigo - Vertigo, and pains in the limbs. Vertigo with confusion and momentary loss of consciousness.

COMMENTS - Rhus-r. has almost identical action as Rhus-t.; characteristic burning in the tongue, tip feels sore. Pains are often one-sided and in various parts, often remote and successive. Pronounced yearly aggravation (Lach.).

H. C. Allen noted a periodicity in Rhus-r. that marks it as a great anti-psoric. It is, he said, on deeply psoric or tubercular constitutions that its toxic effects are most felt and longest lasting, and these constitutional effects "seem incurable without the anti-psoric."

Guernsey considered Rhus-r. deeper acting than Rhus-t., being indicated in phlegmonous erysipelas, especially where it begins in ankles and moves gradually up the leg, moving in the deeper tissues, with no fever, and for axillary glands when the swelling is very deep and hard.

Millspaugh summarized the effects of Rhus poisoning: the majority of poisonings have been caused by Rhus-r., as first redness and swelling of the affected part with intolerable itching and burning, flowed by vertigo, weariness and a sort of intoxication.

Farrington gave, as distinctive indications for Rhus-r., an occipital headache with rheumatic stiffness of the nape. Drawing, tearing pains in legs. Pleurodynia when the pains shoot into the shoulders.

Mahony reported a case of eczema on the perineum and scrotum with sweat in cleft of buttocks, both relieved in a week with Rhus-r., 12c, twice daily.

RELATIONS - Rhus-r. is said to be antidotal to the action of Rhus-t. and has been employed in the treatment of cases where Rhus-t. had failed. ***Compare:*** Rhus-t. Anac. and other Anacardiace, and the Xanthoxylaces, which are an allied order.

REFERENCES - Buck. Clarke.

RHUS TOXICODENDRON

(Poison Oak)

PHARMACY - rhus-t. Rhus toxicodendron. Poison oak. N. O. Anacardiaceae. Tincture of fresh leaves gathered at sunset just before flowering time. ***Historical dose:*** All potencies.

CLINICAL - Abortion. Acne, rosacea. After-pains. Allergies. Amenorrhea. ***Ankle injuries.*** Anus, fissure. Appendicitis. Appetite, lost. ***Arthritis.*** Beriberi. ***Back, injuries.*** Bones, pain. Cecum, inflammation. Chilblains. Circulation, poor. Cyanosis. Dengue fever. Dermatitis. Diarrhea. Diphtheria. ***Dislocated, joints.*** Dysentery. Dysmenorrhea. Dyspepsia. Ear, eczema. Ecthyma. Enteric fever. Erysipelas. Erythema nodosum. Exostosis. Eyes, disorders. ***Fever, blisters. Fevers.*** Gastro-enteritis. Glandular, disorders. Gout. Hemorrhages. Hemorrhoids. Hernia. ***Herpes. Herpes zoster.*** Hives. ***Hoarseness.*** Housemaid's knee. Hydrocele. ***Influenza. Injuries.*** Intermittent fever. ***Joint, injuries.*** Liver, abscess. ***Lumbago.*** Measles. Menorrhagia. Metrorrhagia. Muscular, pains. Neuralgias. Ovary, tumor. Paralysis. Paraphimosis. Pemphigus. Periosteum, pains. Pleurisy. Pleurodynia. Pneumonia. ***Poison ivy. Poison oak.*** Ptosis. Pyemia. ***Rashes.*** Relapsing fever. ***Rheumatism. Rhus, poisoning.*** Scarlatina. ***Sciatica.*** Sleep, restless. Smallpox. Spine, diseases. ***Sprains. Strains.*** Strictures. ***Tendonitis.*** Throat, sore. Tongue, disorders. Typhoid fever. Typhus. ***Urticaria.*** Vesicles. Warts. ***Whiplash.*** Wens. Yawning.

HERBAL - Poison ivy grows in thickets and low grounds in North America, flowering in June. It was introduced into England as a plant in 1640. In 1798, Dufresnoy of Valenciennes first used it as a medicine.

It was brought to his notice by the cure of a young man of a herpetic eruption (darter) of six years duration, through his being accidentally poisoned with the plant. Dufresnoy used it successfully in eruptive diseases, paralysis, rheumatism and amaurosis.

A peculiarity of the plant is that it is more poisonous during the night, and when bursting into leaf, or at any time in June or July when the sun is not shining upon it. The absence of sunlight together with dampness, seems to favor the exhalation of toxicodendric acid.

"An acrimonious vapor, combined with carburetted hydrogen, exhales from a growing plant of the Poison Oak during the night. It can be collected in a jar and is capable of inflaming and blistering the skin of persons of excitable constitution who plunge their arms into it."

Though it is not certain that Hahnemann used Rhus-t. at all or exclusively, Jahr gave a separate presentation of the Rhus radicans symptoms. Under the name of Rhus, Hahnemann published his proving of "Rhus radicans, also called Toxicodendron."

Botanists agree in recognizing no distinction other than that of habit between the two.

The milky juice, which turns black on exposure, is used as a marking ink (like Anac.), and as an ingredient in varnishes for finishing boots.

HOMEOPATHIC - Rhus-t. affects the fibrous tissue, joints, tendons, sheaths, etc., producing pains and stiffness. Irritating agent to the skin, especially of the face, scalp, genitals and mucus membranes.

Rheumatism in cold damp season. Stiffness of muscles and joints. Motion ***"limbers up"*** the Rhus-t. patient, hence he feels better for a time from a change of position. Inclination to stretch. ***Dislocated joints.*** Stretching causes cracking in knees, soreness in abdomen. Sciatica, better by warmth from exercise.

Ailments from straining a single part, muscle or tendon, over-lifting, particularly from stretching high up to reach things. Injuries and traumas to the joints. ***Tendonitis.*** Sprained ankles. ***Whiplash.*** Old injuries that never healed, stiffen with weather changes.

Pains are tearing, shooting, stitching, worse at night, ***cannot rest in any position. Tearing asunder pains***. Parts feel sore, bruised and ***stiff.*** Pains as if the flesh was torn loose from the bones. Dislocated joints sensation. Soreness of prominent projection of bones. Muscles twitch. Crawling, trembling. turning, swelling and lividity.

Severe backaches, chronic, low back pain. Burning in the spine. ***Stiffness in the sacrum*** that's better with cracking and adjustments. Affections of ***nerves and spinal cord*** give rise to ***paretic effects.*** Numbness of parts paralyzed.

Unwanted exercise causes paralysis. Hemiplegia, right sided, sensation as if gone to sleep. Infantile paralysis from exposure to cold damp. Paralysis after unwonted exertion, after childbirth. Over-exertion causes palpitations, aggravates coxalgia. Limbs lain on fall asleep, no sweat on them. Ailments from getting wet, while perspiring.

Septic conditions. Cellulitis and infections, carbuncles in early stages (Echi.). ***Septicemia***.

Inflammation and swelling of the long bones, scraping, gnawing, tearing loose in periosteum. Strictures after inflammation. Mucus discharges are acrid, rusty red like meat water, musty, causing eruptions. Post-operative complications.

Influenza. Smallpox. ***Glands are swollen,*** hot and painful indurated, suppurating. Boils, abscesses. ***Typhoid-like fevers. Headache in occiput,*** even pain in nape of neck, and from there pains draw over the head forwards. Jaws are tight and stiff, can crack and pop. Coldness in left tibia.

Symptoms appear on the left side or go from left to right. Characteristic modalities, particularly worse at night and from damp. "The more he moves the better he is," (opposite of Bry.). Worse during rest, and after rest.

Nausea, worse after eating. Craves cold water, which is vomited immediately. Many symptoms are better after a storm, especially after an electric storm.

MIND - Confusion. ***Mind and senses becomes cloudy.*** Low, mild delirium, incoherent talk, answers correctly but slowly, or hastily, or reluctantly. Forgetful and cannot remember the most recent events. Recalls with difficulty things and names. Vanishing of thoughts while standing. Can't hold mind on one subject long enough to answer. Stupefaction, with tingling in head and pains in limbs, better motion.

Anxious, sadness, helplessness and profound despondency. ***Causeless weeping, without knowing why.*** Inclination to cry, worse in evening without knowing why, with desire for solitude. Forsaken feeling.

Inexpressible anxiety with pressure at heart. Anxiety about one's children. Anxiety, worse twilight, with restless change of place. ***Great apprehension at night, cannot remain in bed***. Mental and physical restlessness at night. ***Extreme restlessness with continued change of position***. Restlessness during menses.

Anguish as if she had committed a crime or as if some terrible calamity impended, driving her from one place to another. Superstitious fears. Fears, with sighing, worse at night. Fear and despair on account of sad thoughts. Delirium with fear of being poisoned (Hyos.). Complaints from fright.

Fretful, impatient, ill-humored, easily vexed. ***Irritability at night, better walking in open air.*** Discouragement and dissatisfaction. Satiety of life. ***Dwells on past disagreeable occurrences after midnight.*** Talking of business in sleep.

Aversion to company alternating with bursts of pleasantry and sarcasm. Delusion he is roaming over fields, or hard at work. Delusion of being watched. Suicidal disposition in twilight. Thoughts of suicide, wants to drown himself.

Abdomen - Ileo-cecal symptoms, appendicitis. Swelling of inguinal glands. Incarcerated hernia. Hourglass contraction. Excessive distention after eating. Mucus colitis. Colic after getting wet. Colic, compelling to walk bent. Violent pains, relieved by lying on abdomen. Pain in region of ascending colon. Rumbling of flatus on first rising, but disappears with continued motion. Soreness of navel. Sensation as if water swashing in abdomen. Sensation as if a lump in abdomen.

Back - ***Back strain or injury. Pains from over-lifting or overuse.*** Backache, as if back would break, better hard pressure. ***Backache, compelling him to move constantly in bed.*** Contractive or breaking backache, better hard pressure, lying on something hard, walking about or bending backwards. ***Pain and stiffness in small of back, better motion or lying on something hard***, worse while sitting. Pain between shoulders on swallowing. Aching and stiffness in lumbar region as after long stooping or bending. Burning in lumbar region. Lumbago, coccyx aches into thighs. Curvature of dorsal vertebrae. Acute spinal paralysis of infants. Spinal membranes inflamed, from getting wet or sleeping on damp ground. Myelitis. Stiffness and lameness in sacrum, worse resting.

Breasts - Great soreness of nipples after confinement. Breast pain with itching, burning papular eruption about nipples.

Causations - Effects of drinking cold water (Bell-p.), beer (headache). Cold, getting wet, especially after being heated, cold bathing, sea bathing (Mag-m.). Wetting head, damp sheets, bathing. Slightest anger. ***Strains***, over-exertion, ***over-lifting***. Raising arms high to lift things.

Chest - Oppression of the chest, cannot get breath, with sticking pains. Tickling behind upper sternum, causing dry, hoarse, tearing, tormenting cough. Tingling in chest with tension in intercostal muscles, worse rest. Numb sensation in chest. Chest pains worse using arms. Pleurodynia, chest pains shoot into shoulders. Pain as if sternum were pressed inward. Stitches in chest and sides of chest. Herpes axillaris. Axillary abscess after delivery.

Constitutions - Suited for the psoric or tubercular constitutions. Rheumatic constitutions.

Cough - Bronchial coughs in old people, worse on awaking and with expectoration of small plugs of mucus. Dry teasing coughs. Dry coughs from midnight until morning. Coughing and sneezing worse uncovering body (Rumx.). Coughing during chill, or when putting hands out of bed. Coughing prevents sleep at night. Cough with profuse sweat and pain in stomach. Frequent hacking cough with bitter taste in throat.

Ears - Lobes swollen. Swelling of ears. Otalgia. Pain in ear with a feeling as if something were inside. Painful throbbing in ear at night. Discharge of bloody pus, with deafness.

Eyes - ***Orbital cellulitis***. Suppurative iritis. Iritis after exposure to cold, dampness. Iritis of rheumatic origin. Corneal injection with intensive ulceration. Suppuration of cornea. Ulceration of cornea. Glaucoma. ***Pustular inflammations***. Saccular conjunctiva. Acute retro-bulbar neuritis. Swollen, red, edematous. Profuse flow of yellow pus. Lachrymation when yawning. Profuse gush of hot, scalding tears upon opening lids. Photophobia. Eye painful on turning it or pressing. Paralysis of the eyeball muscles. Eyelids, stiff agglutinated, dry, firmly closed. Edema of lids.

Ptosis. Styes or abscesses, on lower lids. Old eye injuries.

Face - Pale, sickly look, with sunken eyes. Blue rings about eyes. Cyanosis of face and hands. ***Swollen face***. Erysipelas, shining redness with formation of vesicles. Moist eruptions and thick scabs on face. Suppurating eruptions on face. Acne rosacea. ***Crusta lactea*** (Calc., Viol-t.). Corners of mouth ulcerated. ***Fever blisters around mouth and chin*** (Nat-m.). Red spots on left cheek. Parotiditis (left) with fever. Joints painful. Pains in maxillary joint. Painful cheekbones, sensitive to touch. Facial neuralgia with chilliness, worse evening.

Female - Amenorrhea, from getting wet with milk in breast. Menses early, profuse and prolonged, acrid. Menstrual flow light-colored and acrid, causes biting pain in vulva. Dysmenorrhea, cramping, with backache, worse lying on back. Membranous dysmenorrhea in rheumatic women. Violent pain in vulva during menses. Soreness in vagina shortly after sex, or preventing coition. Swelling with intense itching of vulva. Bearing down pain when standing or walking, with backache. Pelvic joints stiff when beginning to move. Consciousness of uterus. Prolapse uterus from lifting or overstraining. Uterine infection, septic. Polyps of uterus after getting chilled from sea-bathing. Metrorrhagia, clotted blood, with labor-like pains. Miscarriage from a strain. ***Lochia thin, protracted offensive diminished*** (Puls., Sec.). ***Lochia with shooting pain upwards in vagina*** (Sep.). Frequent after pains.

Food - No appetite for any kind of food. ***Drowsy after eating***. Food tastes bitter, especially bread. Desire for sweets, oysters, tonics, beer, acids. ***Desires cold milk, yogurt and cheese.*** Dairy relaxes. Nausea worse from ice cream. Aversion to meat and bread. Great thirst with dry mouth and throat. Drinks little and often during fever. Craves cold drinks, though they aggravate cough, chill. Worse after ice-water. Sweats from warm drinks. Pulse affected by beer, coffee or alcohol. Aversion to spirituous liquors, beer.

Head - Headache in occiput (Rad-br.), painful to touch. Stupefying headache, must lie down, worse least chagrin. Headache after taking a cold bath, from beer, immediately after a meal. ***Heavy feeling*** in head. Pain in forehead, proceeding backward. Feels as if a board were strapped on the forehead. Brain feels loose and as if struck against skull on walking or rising. Burning in forehead when walking. Aching in occipital protuberances. Painful tingling in head, occiput. Vesicular erysipelas of scalp, going from left to right. Dry herpes on hairy scalp. Scalp sensitive, worse on side lain on. Humid eruptions on scalp, itching greatly.

Heart - Hypertrophy from overexertion. Weak and tremulous feeling about heart, after walking. Acute, stabbing pains in cardiac region on deep inspiration or raising left arm suddenly. Heart feels tired, pains go down left arm. Left arm aches with heart disease. Anxious palpitations in morning on awaking. Palpitations after overexertion. Severe palpitation and pain in heart when lying on left side. ***Trembling and palpitations when sitting still***, better from walking. Pulse quick, weak, irregular. Pulse intermittent with numbness of left arm.

Limbs - Arthritis and rheumatism. ***Stiffness of all the joints, better warmth, motion and massage.*** Hot, painful swelling of joints. ***Cracking of joints when stretching.*** Synovitis. Rheumatic pains spread over a large surface at nape of neck, loins and limbs, better motion (Agar.). ***Pains tearing in tendons, ligaments and tissues***. ***Sciatica***, worse cold, damp weather, at night. Sciatica better warmth, exercise. ***Limbs stiff, paralyzed.*** the cold fresh air is not tolerated, it makes the skin painful. ***Numbness and prickling in limbs after over-work and exposure to damp.*** Paralysis, trembling after exertion. Paraplegia after childbirth, sexual excess, fever. Pain along ulnar nerve. Soreness of condyles of bones. Tension as from shortening of muscles. Legs feel dead, wooden. Involuntary limping. Tearing pains down thighs. Tenderness about knee. Cramps in calves.

Ankles or knees are swollen, stiff after sprain or injured. Tingling in feet. Sensation as if walking on needles. Itching of legs and feet. Gangrenous ulcers on legs, runs bloody water, on dropsical legs. Cold hands and feet. Arms nervous and shaky (left). Paralytic pains in elbows. Loss of power in forearm and fingers, crawling sensation in the fingertips. Cracks on back of hands. Palms, dry, hot, cracked and sore, washing causes burning.

Lungs - Oppressed breathing, as if breath were stopped at pit of stomach. Anxious breathing, as if not able to draw a long breath. Hurried and very short breathing at night. Dyspnea from pressure and painfulness in pit of stomach. Hot air from trachea. Shortness of breath during stool. ***Asthma alternating with skin eruptions.*** Hemoptysis from overexertion or from blowing wind instruments. Hemoptysis bright blood. Sudden hypostasis or edema of lungs. Pale, clotted or brown blood. Rust colored sputum. Expectoration, acrid pus. Gray-green cold mucus of putrid smell. Pneumonia with typhoid symptoms, often after reabsorption of pus.

Male - Painful, persistent erections, better lying on back. Erections at night with desire to urinate. ***Intense itching*** of genitals. Dark-red, erysipelatous. Humid vesicles on glans. Humid eruptions on genitals and between scrotum and thighs. Swelling of glands and prepuce. Paraphimosis. Hydrocele from over-lifting. Scrotum, swollen, ***edematous.*** Scrotum thick and hard, with intolerable itching. Edema of scrotum and penis after scarlatina, with recurrence of fever. Metastasis of mumps to testes.

Modalities - ***Better from heat,*** hot bath, warm wrapping, warm applications. Better warm dry, weather. ***Better stretching limbs, continued motion***, change of position, walking. Better rubbing, holding affected part, abdomen, head. Better from nosebleed. ***Worse from cold, dampness, wet rainy weather. Worse before storms***, after rain. ***Worse exposure to wet, cold***, air, draft. Worse being chilled, when hot or sweaty, ice cold drinks. Worse uncovering parts. ***Worse beginning of motion, rest, sprains***, blows, jar. ***Worse overexertion, lifting***, after exertion. Worse prolonged sitting, rising from bed or a seat, riding. Worse at night, after midnight, during sleep, lying on back or right side. Worse on side lain on.

Mouth - General dryness of the mouth, with thirst. Coppery, herby, or ***bitter taste*** (Cupr.). Salivation, must spit frequently. Much tough mucus in mouth and throat. Bloody saliva runs during sleep. Gums sore. ***Mouth filled with herpes sores.*** Herpes on lips. ***Fever blisters around mouth and chin*** (Nat-m.). Lips dry and parched, covered with reddish-brown crusts. Lips, dry, brownish, cracked, at corners, crusty. Corners of mouth cracked, ulcerated. ***Jaws crack when chewing***. Cramp-like pain in joint of jaw, when yawning. ***Pain in maxillary joint***. Easy dislocation of jaw (Ign., Petr.).

Neck - Carbuncle on nape. Neck strain or injury with stiffness. ***Neck stiff after injuries. Whiplash.*** Stiff neck with painful tension, when moving. Stiff neck from a draft, or dampness, better heat and massage.

Nose - Swelling of nose. Violent aching in bones of the nose. Red, sore, ulcerated tip of nose, drips water. Soreness in nostrils. Hot breath burns nostrils. Dryness and stoppage of nose. Sneezing with fluent coryza, from getting wet. Spasmodic sneezing after sudden cessation of cough. Sneezing and coughing worse uncovering body. Nasal discharge thick, yellow mucus, green, offensive pus. Nosebleed, worse at night, stooping, at stool, gives relief in fevers. Loss of smell.

Perspiration - Sudden outbreak of sweat while sitting, often with violent trembling. Sweats with violent itching of eruptions. Perspires with pains, often with trembling. Sour, musty, putrid sweat. Perspires all over, except on head. Profuse sweat on exterior parts of body, but not on parts on which she lay. Sweat, worse during pain, with sleepiness. Night sweat with miliary itching eruption. Profuse sweat in morning.

Rectum - Constriction in rectum. Shooting pain up rectum. Painful tenesmus without stools. Colitis mucosa. Dysentery with tearing pains down thighs. Diarrhea alternating with constipation. Diarrhea of blood, slime and reddish mucus. Diarrhea after walking through moist ground with bare feet. Remission of pains and urging after stools. Fissure of anus, with periodical profuse bleeding. May abort a beginning suppurative process near the rectum. Hemorrhoids, worse lifting. Hemorrhoids protruding after stool, with pressing in rectum, as if everything would come out.

Sensations - As if intoxicated. As if asleep. As of a band strapped across forehead. As if head were swelling out. Brain, as if loaded, as if torn, as if loose, as if fluctuating, as if a quantity of blood shot into it when stooping. As of a weight behind right orbit. Legs as if made of wood. As if hamstrings and tendons of limbs too short. As if walking on needles. Joints as if bruised. As if bones ached. As if sinking through bed. As if whole body was burning. As if cold water poured over him. As if blood ran cold through veins.

Skin - Skin sensitive to cold air. Dry, hot, burning. Red, swollen, ***intense itching***. ***Cellulitis***. ***Dermatitis.*** Eczema. Burning eczematous eruptions with tendency to scale formation. ***Poison ivy, oak. Shingles, herpes zoster.*** Burning and neuralgic pains after herpes zoster. Herpetic eruptions alternating with dysentery and pains in chest. Boils and abscesses. Vesicles, herpes, pemphigus, erysipelas, vesicular suppurative conditions. Vesicles over abscess. Hives. ***Urticaria*** from getting wet with rheumatism. Urticaria during chills and fever. Bluish, gangrenous carbuncles. Smallpox. Swollen glands. Milk crusts. Baker's itch. Warts on hands and fingers. Pus erodes the hair. ***Itching better hot water.*** Itching with burning and smarting, feeling as if pierced with hot needles. Itching all over, worse on hairy parts. Itching worse sweating. Burning after scratching. Rubbing affected part aggravates eruptions. Eruptions, alternating with dysentery.

Sleep - Drowsy after eating. Yawning, frequent, violent, spasmodic. Yawning without inclination to sleep. Yawning with stretching. Sleepy during day, sleepless at night, with inability to remain in bed. Sleepless before midnight. Sleeplessness at night with burning of whole body. ***Restless sleep tossing about can't get comfortable.*** Sleep prevented by cough. Heavy sleep, as from stupor. Sleeps with mouth open. Somnolence with snoring, muttering and grasping at objects. Laborious dreams. ***Dreams of great exertion***, rowing, swimming, working hard at his daily occupation. Dreams that the world was on fire, with palpitations on awaking. ***Awakens, stiff and sore must stretch.*** Awakes tired or nervous.

Stomach - Hunger and emptiness in stomach, without appetite. Fullness as if overloaded. Pressure as from a stone (Bry., Ars.). Pressure in pit, as if swollen or as if drawn together. ***Pain in stomach after ice water.*** Ulcerative pain in stomach. Violent throbbing in epigastric region. Eructations with tingling in stomach, worse rising from lying. Nausea, vertigo and bloated abdomen after eating. Nausea, worse from ice cream, at night. Vomiting while lying on back. Vomiting from coughing.

Stools - ***Involuntary stools with great exhaustion.*** Stools involuntary during sleep, or with tenesmus, worse drinking. Stools, lumps of transparent mucus. Stools, frothy, watery, slimy, gelatinous, painless, bloody. Black blood from bowels. Stools of cadaverous odor.

Teeth - Teeth feel as if asleep. Teeth feel loose and long. Sensation as if teeth were being torn out. Shooting pain, in evening and night, better external heat. Teeth painful with stinging at root of nose. Toothache at night, better application of cold hand. Toothache worse at night, cold, vexation. Sordes on teeth. Gums sore.

Temperature - Easily chilled, worse least uncovering with pain in limbs. Chills, as if cold water were poured over him, followed by heat and inclination to stretch the limbs. Chills as if cold water in the veins, preceded by cough, alternating with heat. Chill in single parts. Wants to yawn and stretch during chill. ***Intermittent fever,*** chill with dry cough and restlessness. Rapid alternations of burning heat and shivering. Sudden flushes of heat follow or alternating with chills. Fever after chill, with sweat which better. General heat, as from hot water or hot blood running through veins. ***Influenza fever, restlessness, stiff and sore,*** with aching in all bones (Eup-per.). ***Typhoid fever,*** tongue dry and brown, sordes, bowels loose, great restlessness. Fever with busy delirium. Urticaria during fever. Hydroa.

Throat - ***Sore, stiff feeling in throat after straining throat.*** Sore throat with bruised pain. ***Soreness,*** better warm drinks with swollen glands. ***Hoarseness from overstraining the voice*** (Arn.). Hoarseness, better after talking a while. Hoarseness with roughness and soreness in chest. Hoarseness, worse evening and change of weather. Red, puffy itching fauces. Sensations of dryness of throat. Sore throat with swollen glands. Esophagitis from swallowing corrosive matter. Tonsils covered with yellow membrane. Larynx cold when breathing. Sticking or stinging pain in tonsils, worse beginning to swallow. Difficult swallowing of solids as from contraction of saliva.

Tongue - Tongue, red and cracked, dry and red at edges. Tongue shows imprint of teeth. ***Tongue coated, except red triangular space at the tip***. Tongue coated diagonally or on one side only. Yellowish-white coating at root of tongue. Tongue coated with brown mucus, except on edges, in morning on rising. Feeling as if tongue covered with skin.

Urinary - Nephritis. Tearing pain in region of kidneys with edema, worse after exposure to wet. Dysuria with loss of blood. Retention of urine, with restlessness and backache. Tenesmus of bladder, with discharge of a few drops of blood-red urine. Dark, high colored, white sediment, scanty urine. Urine turbid when passed. Urine passes in a divided stream. Frequent, profuse urination day and night. Frequent and painful urination from prolapsed uterus. Incontinence or urine, worse lying at night, or sitting in boys. Dribbling of urine in cold air or from becoming cold.

Vertigo - Vertigo with heaviness in limbs. Vertigo when rising, as if she were going to fall forward or backward. Vertigo while walking. Vertigo with staggering, as if intoxicated. Vertigo in the aged, whirling, then headache. Nausea, vertigo and bloated abdomen after eating.

COMMENTS - The worst poisonings with Rhus divers. happened to persons who were moist and heated. One prover of Rhus-t. was not influenced by contact with the leaves when his skin was dry, but only when perspiring.

Millspaugh noted several instances of rhus poisoning. In one poisoning case, ten men were employed to clear a piece of land of shrubs, among which the poison vine predominated; only four escaped without symptoms. "Most of the men soon began to show signs of being tired and at the end of the fourth day six of them were flat on their backs too sick for anything."

Actual contact with the plant is not necessary in order to produce its effect. One such instance occurred on a sultry day in June. A young woman drove a croquet ball across a lawn to a clump of poison ivy that grew beside it. Knowing her susceptibility, she reached under the plant and drew out the ball without touching a leaf.

In the evening of the same day her face began to itch and burn. That night her face swelled so badly that the eyes were not merely closed, but the lashes even disappeared in the swelling. It took nearly two weeks for her to recover.

Generally, there is infiltration of the face and eyes, and agglutination of the lids after sleep. Great restlessness, pain, thirst and fever. The surface of the skin becomes studded with confluent bullae where the cellular tissue is loose.

Then a dermatitis follows, resembling erysipelas; this may spread rapidly and finally be communicated to the mucus membranes.

This is followed by swelling of the mouth and throat, cough, nausea and vomiting.

Rheumatoid pains develop about the joints and a painful stiffness asserts itself in the lumbar region while the legs and arms become numb. Confusion of mind and delirium may then set in, during which the patient may become so ill-humored, restless and anxious that he will jump out of bed.

Concomitants include inflammation of the eyes, dilation of the pupils, weak vision, and sometimes diplopia. Nosebleed, brown-coated tongue with triangular red tip. Swelling of parotids, difficult swallowing. Griping, diarrhea, profuse urination. Oppression, rapid pulse, prostration, soreness of muscles, worse by exercise, bleariness, chilliness followed by fever and copious sweat.

Neidhard added a note which brought out a modification of "worse by rest," which is of the greatest practical importance. Neidhard said that the disease in which he had made the most use of Rhus-t. is a form of rheumatism common in North America and characterized by the following symptoms:

"Rigidity, paralytic weakness of the joints with stinging pain along the tendons and muscles. Swelling and redness on or near the joints. Rheumatism of the hip joint and wrist seem to be most effectually controlled by its action. The greatest rigidity and pain is experienced on first moving the joints after rest and on waking up in the morning. After the joints are moved for a while the pain is lessened."

Nash noted that the restlessness of Rhus-t. will be found to qualify the symptoms in a large proportion of the cases in which it will be called for. It is as restless as Acon. and Ars., but in a different way from either. With Rhus-t. it is due to the pain and soreness, temporarily better by movement or a nervous internal uneasiness which makes the patient want to be on the move when there is no particular pain present.

Conditions can often change from Rhus-t. to Bry., as well as the reverse. Hahnemann wrote about "these two antagonistic sister remedies."

Each in its place successfully met with typhus which prevailed in the countries desolated by the war which raged from the summer of 1813 and onwards. Of 183 cases treated by Hahnemann in Leipzig, not one died.

Hahnemann perceived the keynote of the Rhus-t. symptoms: "We observe," he said in his preface to the proving, "this curious action, the severest symptoms and sufferings are excited when the body or the limb is at rest and kept as much as possible without movement.

"The opposite of this, namely, an increase of the symptoms by movement in much more rarely observed." He contrasted Rhus-t. with Bry., which has almost the same rheumatic pains but with opposite modalities.

Hahnemann pointed out another keynote of Rhus-t.: "Multiplied experience has taught me that Rhus-t. is the most efficacious and the specific remedy for the frequently fatal effects of over-lifting inordinate exertions of the muscles and contusions." He might have been led to this inference by the "bruised and sprain-like pains" and "stiffness" of the provings. Rhus-t. is in the front rank of vulneraries.

Restlessness in fevers, typhoid and other. Clouded sensorium, stupefaction, muttering delirium. Characteristic stiffness, better heat, manipulation. Worse remaining in one place and sitting. Worse damp weather, causes stiffness. Worse in the morning, better from hot shower. Worse twilight (Puls., Phos.).

Demands exertion, better from exertion, exercise. Tendency to overwork physically. Stiff personality. Worrisome. Tendency to dwell on things. Projects into the future. Difficulty relaxing. Can turn to exercise as a cure for tension, may become an addiction.

Irritable, bored without a physical outlet. Can have fixed ideas, superstitions. Fear of not functioning, of injury. May have a history of auto accidents, fear of accidents, of fast motion in a car (Calc.). Fear of infection.

Rheumatoid arthritis. Rheumatic paraplegia from getting wet, lying on damp ground, sleeping in damp sheets after exertion, after childbirth, sexual excess or fevers. Paralysis of single limbs.

Numbness of parts paralyzed. Facial neuralgia, lumbago and sciatica (left side) with restlessness, coming on after a wetting or after a bath. Ptosis. Neuralgic pains.

Burning pains, better heat, particularly in blistering skin rashes or allergic reactions. Skin can feel tight, like its wrapped. Dermatitis. Chickenpox (Puls., Sulph., Ant-t., Ant-c.). Scalp sensitive, worse turning hair back. Herpes zoster. Herpes alternating with asthma and dysentery. Fever blisters around mouth, herpes in the mouth. Yellow blisters in herpes. Shingles. Inflamed and burning blisters.

Rheumatic fever. Flu. Chronic sinusitis, colds and sore throats. Sore throat with hoarseness. Straining, rheumatic coughs. In intermittents, "cough during the chill." Taste of blood with cough (no blood being raised). Chokes easily on swallowing. Swallowing causes pain in middle of back.

Tongue is dry or dark, coated with a triangular red tip. Craving for cold drinks, milk, yogurt and cheese. Dairy relaxes. Likes sweets. Aversion to meat and bread. Anorexia. Nausea in chest. Hour-glass contraction of abdomen.

Threatened miscarriage from a sprain. Prolonged after pains and other effects of the strain of a severe labor. Axillary abscess from severe labor.

RELATIONS - ***Antidotes:*** Bathing with milk and Grindelia lotion very effective. Aloe vera gel topically. Desensitizing against Poison Ivy by use of ascending doses of the low potencies by mouth is recommended. Especially for acute reactions: Rhus-t. 30c and 200c and Anac., Crot-t., Grind., Mez., Cypr., Plumbg. - eczema of vulva., Graph. ***Compare:*** (1) Rhus-r. (2) Rhus-d. - California Poison-oak, antidote to Rhus-t., violent skin symptoms with frightful itching, much swelling of face, hands and genitals, skin very sensitive, eczema and erysipelas, great nervous weakness, tired from least effort, goes to sleep exhausted. (3) Xero. - dysmenorrhea and skin symptoms. (4) Arn., Bapt., Lach., Ars., Hyos. (4) Op. - stupefactions more profound. (5) Mim-h. - Sensitive Plant - rheumatism, knee stiff, sharp pains in back and limbs. Swelling of ankles. Legs tremble. (6) Ampe-tr. - Toxic dermatitis due to vegetable poisons. Very similar to Rhus poisoning. ***Complementary:*** Bry., Calc-f. Phyt. (Rheumatism). In urticaria follow with Bov. ***Inimical:*** Apis.

REFERENCES - Boericke. Clarke. Murphy. Phatak.

RHUS VENENATA

(Poison elder)

PHARMACY - rhus-v. Rhus venenata. Poison elder. Poison sumac. Swamp sumac. N. O. Anacardiacae. North America in swampy ground. Tincture of fresh leaves and stem. ***Historical dose:*** All potencies.

CLINICAL - Boils. Chilblains. Diarrhea. Dyspepsia. Dysphagia. Eczema. Eruptions. Erysipelas. Erythema nodosum. Glands, cervical, ulceration. Hemorrhoids. Herpes. Hydroa. Impetigo. Irritation. Lips, swollen, sore. Lumbago. Measles. Menorrhagia. Ophthalmia. Paraplegia. Prurigo. Purpura. Scabies. Sore throat. Stiff neck. Tongue, cracked. Urticaria.

HERBAL - Named "Rhus Vernix," the name belongs properly to the allied Varnish-tree of Japan. Rhus-v. in one of the most actively poisonous of the Rhus.; the skin symptoms of this species are most severe.

HOMEOPATHIC - P. B. Hoyt, who first drew attention to it and made the first provings, said it is more poisonous than Rhus-t., which he could handle with impunity, while he was violently affected by Rhus-v. in spite of extreme caution. Further, he considered it more actively curative in a case of Rhus sore throat, when Rhus-t. failed, Rhus-v. acted with excellent effect.

Persons poisoned by Rhus-t. are more liable to be poisoned by Rhus-v. Children are more readily poisoned than adults. Rhus-v. in the potency is credited with the cure of Rhus-t. poisoning.

Butman observed that blondes are more susceptible to Rhus-v. poisoning than brunettes. When once affected, persons are liable to a renewal of the affection (without further poisoning) each year at the same time.

Rhus-v. has many symptoms referring to the bones and, according to Hering, it affects those parts where the bones are directly covered with skin, especially the forehead, backs of fingers, etc.

Pain as if sprained. "Pain half way down the esophagus" which is probably a variant of the Rhus-t. "Pain between the shoulders on swallowing food." Eating raw things aggravates burning of lips. Diarrhea 4 a.m. Washing with cold water or snow improves itching on back. Chills in warm room.

Clarke found Rhus-v. an excellent remedy for arsenical overdosing. A minor use of Rhus-v. is as a topical remedy in itching, burning chilblains. The tincture painted on relieves almost instantly and practically cures the chilblains in a large number of cases.

MIND - Great melancholy. Gloomy and depressed. No desire to live.

Abdomen - Pain in hypogastrium before every stool. Stools with colicky pains, expelled with force. Profuse, watery, white stools in morning, 4 a.m.

Back - Back very stiff. Sharp pain under left scapula, extending through to ribs. Rheumatic pains between scapulae. Lumbago from a strain or a cold.

Breasts - Burning in left breast and left side of body. Breast must be supported, it aches when it hangs down,

Chest - Violent stitches through chest with great suddenness.

Ears - Transient stitches in right concha. Jerk-like tearing in bone behind right ear. Earache, hammering-throbbing deep in ear after dark. Jerk-like cutting stitches in ear. Vesicular inflammation of ears.

Eyes - Eyes nearly closed with great swelling, red. Eyes ache as though pressed on. Eyes feel as if sand in them.

Face - Heaviness in swollen face. Boring in right upper jaw. Itching of upper lip and chin. Lips sore, swollen, blistered, cracked. Sensation as if sand on lips.

Female - Menses with very large clots like pieces of meat. Soreness of vagina during menses.

Head - Heavy, frontal headache, worse walking or stooping.

Limbs - Paralytic drawing in right arm, especially wrist and extending to fingers.

Modalities - Better moderate exercise or open air. Better hot bath, gently rubbing and scratching. Worse before stools. Worse damp days, hot weather. Worse rest, after waking, morning. Worse mental exertion, touch and pressure. Motion aggravates pain in elbow. Walking aggravates frontal headache.

Neck - Stiff neck or crick in neck. Ulceration of cervical glands.

Nose - Nose red and shiny, redness not removed by pressure. Nose dry, sore. Erysipelas. Both nostrils filled with tenacious mucus. Loss of smell.

Rectum - Neuralgic pains in anus. Intolerable burning and itching in anus. Bleeding hemorrhoids with extensive itchings and burning. Discharge of blood from rectum after a stool.

Sensations - As if mouth and throat had been scalded. As if sand on lips in mouth. Sensation in arm as if the bone would break. Pains wander about, upward and downward along the periosteum, come and go suddenly, chill runs up back.

Skin - ***Vesicles. Erysipelas, skin dark red.*** Itching, relieved by hot water. Erythema nodosum with nightly itching and pains in long bones.

Temperature - Chills over whole body, run up back even when warm and in a warm room. Feeling of coldness when moving.

Throat - Irritation and acridity about throat and eyes. Tonsils red, congested, dull aching distress in them. Soreness left side throat. Frequent desire to swallow. Swallowing difficult.

Tongue - Red at tip. Fissured in middle. Vesicles on under side.

COMMENTS - Hoyt, wishing to prepare a tincture, went to a swamp and procured a sample. He wore a pair of buckskin gloves and kept carefully to the windward side of the plant.

Nevertheless, in an hour and a half a most intense itching and burning (more burning) set in scrotum and penis. The glans was very painful, slight friction better for a moment the itching but nor the burning.

The symptoms continued through the next day. At 11 a.m. he made the tincture, using great caution in manipulating the plant. At 3 p.m. itching and burning began on back of right hand. A restless night followed.

He awoke in the morning with itching, especially on palmar surface of wrists. This spread all over his body, symptoms steadily advancing. Dizziness, eyes and ears became affected, fever set in. When the symptoms passed off it was found that some chronic dyspeptic symptoms and inflammation of the eyes had been much benefited.

Clarke frequently used Rhus-v. with good effect in skin diseases. Bayes told him of a case of universal eczema with intense in an old man which he cured in a fortnight with Rhus-v.

A case of pemphigus in a young man of 27 came after years of treatment under allopathic specialists who had given him arsenic until they could give no more, telling him at the same time that nothing but arsenic could do him any good. Rhus-v. 3x and 30c completely cured in a few month and the cure enabled the patient to marry.

Hale had a case showing the comparative action of Rhus-v. with Rhus-r and Rhus-t. A woman had several times every year a sore mouth with intense redness of mucus membrane of tongue, cheeks and fauces, in small vesicular points intense burning and feeling as if mouth and throat had been scalded.

If unchecked, every mucus membrane, including those of rectum and vagina, became involved. No remedy helped until Rhus was tried. Rhus-r. and Rhus-t. only slightly relieved, but Rhus- v. 3c always removed the affection quickly.

RELATIONS - ***Antidote:*** Clem. The California Poison-oak (Rhus-d.) is identical with it. ***It antidotes:*** Rad. and follows it well. ***Compare:*** (1) Skin - Anac., Com., Rhus-t. (2) Stitching pains, Kali-c. (3) Wandering pains, Puls. (4) Pains come and go suddenly, Lyc. (5) Pain at root of tongue, Kali-i.

REFERENCES - Boericke. Clarke.

RIBES NIGRUM

(Black Currant)

PHARMACY - ribs-n. Ribes nigrum. Black currant. Leaves, fruit. ***Historical dose:*** Tincture and all potencies.

CLINICAL - Arteriosclerosis. Arthritis. Colic. Gout. Gums, bleeding. Hoarseness. Kidney, problems. Rheumatism. Sore, throat.

HERBAL - Ribes nigra is a diaphotic, diuretic, sudorific, refrigerant, detergent, and has been used as a substitute for tea as it also contains tannins. The leaf tea stimulates the kidneys and is good for gouty and rheumatic problems, as well as for arteriosclerosis. Drunk cold, it is also useful for hoarseness and other throat ailments.

Both the leaf tea and the expressed juice of the berries can be used for whooping cough in children. The berries or their juice is beneficial for kidney problems and colic pains. An infusion of the dried berries can be used as a gargle for inflammation in the mouth and throat and as a mouthwash for bleeding gums.

REFERENCES - Murphy.

RIBONUCLEINICUM ACIDUM

(RNA)

PHARMACY - rib-ac. Ribonucleinicum acidum. RNA. Ribo nucleinic acid. ***Historical dose:*** All potencies.

CLINICAL - Allergies. Cancer. Eczema. Epilepsy. Herpes. Hypoglycemia. Hypotension. Hypothyroidism. Insomnia. Leukemia. Urticaria. Varicose ulcer. Weight, unstable.

HOMEOPATHIC - The proving of RNA was conducted in 1971 and 1972, by O. A. Julian. Twenty-two people, two females, took part in the experiment, taking the 3x, 7c, and 30c potencies, plus a placebo, in a single-blind trial.

Symptoms are the result of provings incorporated with the clinical research of several Belgian homeopaths, including Dr. Guiot of Wavre who gave a report on a self-proving. Recommended by Jenaer for treatment for cancer and leukemia.

Lively feeling, optimistic, dynamic. General lassitude. Lessened physical strength. Feels depressed, ill at ease in his skin. Wants to run, to disappear. Tiredness, vertigo, stiffness. Tired in the morning to the point of not hearing the alarm bell ring. Sleepiness.

Extreme chilliness. Cortical and medullary hyposthenia. Endocrine glands produce a mucus which is too viscous. Slight edema of the feet and hands.

Desire to sleep, to eat, to make love. ***Hunger with need to nibble throughout the day, especially sugar***. Unstable weight, sudden increase in weight, then sudden loss of weight two days later.

MIND - Psychological and physical slowness. Mental over-exertion. Cannot concentrate on intellectual work. Dullness of mind. Slowness at schoolwork. Personality disorders in children.

Ugly character. Aggressiveness. Wants everything and nothing. Cannot bear anything, cries at anything. Clings on to everything, breaks everything and becomes even more annoyed. Feels as if he is living on his nerves. Desire to go away, to escape. Feels weary and leaves everybody.

Abdomen - Distention, especially at the end of the afternoon. Cramps in the transverse colon at 4 p.m. Biliary sycosis. Entero-pancreatic syndrome.

Back - Joint pains in the shoulders and feet. Pain all along the vertebral column.

Blood - Circulatory discomfort. Hypotension. Leucopenia. Leukemia.

Constitutions - Allergic, psoric, tubercular constitutions. Cancerous conditions.

Female - Increase in libido. Sexual weakness. Frigidity. Fetid leucorrhea. Mycosis vaginitis.

Food - Extreme hunger. Must eat often. ***Strong desire and need to eat sugar.*** Hypoglycemia. Hungry sensations. Desires vinegar and cold, spicy food, which goes down more easily. Aversion to fats and hot food. Loss of appetite.

Limbs - Lymphaedema. Arthralgia in the back and lumbar regions. Swelling of the lower limbs, more marked in the morning and the evening. Hands and feet slightly swollen. Infection around the nails, especially of the index, second and third fingers of the right hand.

Male - Increase in libido. Impotence.

Modalities - Better from lying on the stomach (Med.), worse from lying on the back. Worse from the cold.

Mouth - Fever sores on the middle of the lower lip.

Nose - Small pimples in the nostrils.

Rectum - Tendency to constipation. Watery diarrhea with colic.

Skin - Recurring herpes. Tendency to eczema. Chronic recurring eczema. Small red patches on the forehead, disappearing rapidly. Urticaria. Varicose ulcer. Fissures on the heels and the skin of the heels flakes off in long strips. Tendency to reopening of old healed ulcerations.

Sleep - Sleepiness around noon, beginning of the afternoon. Persistent insomnia, between 2 a.m. and 4 a.m. Sleeps badly, wakes up excited and tired.

Stomach - Acrid dyspepsia. Nausea.

RELATIONS - ***Compare:*** (1) DNA, Sil., Cortiso., Tub. (2) Alf. - increase appetite, weight gain. (3) Cann-s. - appetite increased, desire for sweets.

REFERENCES - Julian.

RICINUS COMMUNIS

(Castor Oil Bean)

PHARMACY - ric. Ricinus communis. Castor oil bean. Palma christi. N. O. Euphorbiaceae. Tincture made with hot alcohol and water. Trituration of fresh seeds. Tincture of fresh plant. ***Historical dose:*** All potencies.

CLINICAL - Albuminuria. Aphthae. Arthritis. ***Breast, disorders. Breast-feeding. Cholera.*** Cholera infantum. Constipation. ***Diarrhea.*** Duodenum, catarrh. Dysentery. Eruptions. Gangrene. ***Gastro-enteritis.*** Jaundice. Muscle pain. Peritonitis. Sprains.

HERBAL - The castor oil plant is a native of Egypt and India. In the tropics, it is a small tree growing to the height of eight or ten feet. It can be cultivated as an annual, its stems reaching from three to five feet.

Castor oil, obtained from the seeds, can be rubbed into muscles and joints. Castor oil packs, warm oil-soaked flannel, can be applied to inflamed tissues or organs. Leaves can be applied topically.

The blandest form in common use is "cold drawn," i.e., expressed without the aid of heat and contains the smallest amount of the acrid principle. A decoction of the seeds, used in the East and West Indies, contains a much larger proportion.

Ric. has great power over breast-feeding. O. McWilliams observed in the Cape Verde Islands that the leaves of the plant were applied to the breasts to increase the flow of milk if it were delayed and even to produce it in women who had never borne children or who had not suckled for years.

In increasing the flow of milk in nursing women, the breasts were fomented with a decoction of the leaves of the plant, the boiled leaves being afterwards thinly spread on the breasts.

For producing milk in others more vigorous measures were resorted to. The women had to sit over a boiling decoction of the leaves, care being taken to prevent the escape of steam. When the decoction was sufficiently cool the parts were bathed with it, and also the breasts to which the leaves were applied as in the other case.

Women with well-developed breasts were more easily influenced. When the breasts were small and shriveled this treatment acted more on the uterine system, bringing on the menses long before their time or causing immediate flow if the time is near.

HOMEOPATHIC - Hale made the first collection of the pathogenetic effects of Ric. and pointed out its analogy to cholera, which Salzer confirmed.

Cases of poisoning, some of them fatal, have been recorded from the ordinary oil, but the greater number of the pathogenetic effects have resulted from eating the seeds. Fatal effects have followed eating three seeds, and one seed has caused violent effects. After twenty seeds, gastroenteritis and death preceded by general convulsions and collapse occurred.

Ric. has marked action on gastro-intestinal tract. Vomiting and purging. Very painful cramps in trunk and limbs. Collapse. Convulsions. Muscular contractions. Languor and weakness. Pale and listless. Anemia. Profound adynamia.

The leaves have an especially powerful action on the breasts and female generative organs. ***Increases the quantity of milk*** in nursing women.

Abdomen - Rumbling. The different parts of the abdominal muscles can be seen successively and individually contracting under the skin. Feels as if all the intestines violently drawn together. Violent colic and yellowish green vomiting. Cramps with the diarrhea. Pain over abdomen, worse by pressure.

Back - Pains in back like after-pains.

Breasts - Breasts thick, swollen with swelling of axillary glands and pains running down arms. Thin discharge from breasts, becomes milky. Brings milk in breasts of virgins and women who have not nursed for years.

Ears - Buzzing and humming in ears.

Eyes - Conjunctiva is injected. Copious lachrymation, pupils only moderately dilated. Eyes convulsed and turned up.

Face - Face slightly congested. Face pale, features strongly contracted. Twitchings of mouth.

Female - Menses too early, excessive. Leucorrhea.

Food - Anorexia. Thirst, great, burning.

Head - Brain seems exhausted and easily overpowered, in open air. Severe headache. Sudden pain as if seized by something in occiput extending around to backs of ears, eyes and forehead with rush of blood to head and shocks which come and go as from electricity, thirty times in five days.

Heart - Pulse is extremely small, scarcely perceptible, though normal in frequency.

Kidneys - Complete anuria. Passes a little dark, thick, highly albuminous urine.

Limbs - Prurigo on wrists and bends of knees. Gangrene of one foot necessitates amputation.

Mouth - Tongue, coated white and dry, furred. Salivation.

Rectum - Incessant diarrhea with cramps and chilliness, colliquative like cholera. Diarrhea without pain. Violent purging with the diarrhea. Rice-water stools. Stools serous liquid mixed with mucus. Bloody diarrhea. Complete confinement of bowels for five days, causing headache.

Skin - Pronounced jaundice, skin saffron yellow. Pruriginous eruptions or redness and itching, at wrists and bends of knees.

Sleep - Great desire for sleep.

Stomach - Pit of stomach very sensitive, pains radiate from this center, shooting to umbilicus and hypochondria. A kind of bar across stomach, which caused profound anguish. Cramps, burning in stomach. Heartburn. Nausea and vomiting persistent, vomited mattery liquid, slightly colored by a little bile, contains only a few mucus threads in suspension. Vomiting and purging. Painless vomiting. Vomiting profuse with burning in gullet and all the symptoms of Asiatic cholera.

Temperature - Chilliness with the diarrhea. Skin moist and cool, especially lower limbs. Forehead covered with cold sweat. Perspiring freely.

Throat - Burning pain in the gullet accompanied the vomiting. Voice altered, veiled.

COMMENTS - Salzer gave to Ric. the same importance in cholera with diarrhea that Camph. occupies in relation to spasmodic cholera. The stools of Ric. correspond exactly to the rice-water stools in cholera, while those of Ver-a. do not.

Ric. also has painless evacuations which are met with in many cases of cholera. Ric. therefore corresponds to the diarrhea stage of cholera and also to the collapse stage if vomiting and purging continue.

Salzer quoted B. L. Bhaduri as having observed "rice-water stools, cramps and suppression of urine brought on by eating the seeds."

Hale said that before he had learned to used Ric. as a homeopathic remedy he has often been discomfited by seeing aphthous diarrhea cured with small (half-teaspoonful) doses of castor oil, repeated three or four times a day, by old nurses or impatient mothers.

Such diarrhea often arises in improperly-fed children. It begins with sickness, frequent and griping evacuations, greenish yellow to dark green, becoming more liquid and more or less mixed with slimy or gelatinous mucus or blood.

Each stool is accompanied with pain and tenesmus, mouth dry and aphthous. The anus is inflamed, belly tumid and painful, child becoming more and more feverish and somnolent.

Hale later gave a Ric. 1x trituration of the oil with sugar. In acute and chronic dysentery and in those cases in which there is impaction of feces, Hale saw the oil promptly curative.

Hering remarked that puerperal fever had become much less common in Philadelphia (where it used to be very common) since homeopaths interdicted the use of castor oil in confinements.

Tyler Smith experimented with the leaves, in his cases the application produced swelling of the breasts, throbbing and other pains in them, swelling of the axillary glands with pains running down the arms.

Pains in the back like after-pains were caused in every case. Leucorrhea was increased. Discharges from the breasts became milky and menses came on too soon. The radiating pains, bar sensation, constricting and cramping pains are the most peculiar.

RELATIONS - ***Compare:*** (1) Tea tree oil. Olive oil. (2) Crot-t., Jatr. and Euphorbiaceae. (3) In cholera, rice-water stools, Agar. Phos., Jatr. (4) Galactagogues, Alf., Agn-c. Asaf., Lec., Puls. (5) Duodenal catarrh, Berb., Chin., Hydr., Lyc., Merc., Podo.

REFERENCES - Boericke. Clarke.

RITALIN

(Methylphenidate Hydrochloride)

PHARMACY - rital. Ritalin. Methylphenidate hydrochloride. An allopathic stimulant drug. ***Historical dose:*** All potencies.

CLINICAL - Angina pectoris. ***Attention deficit disorder.*** Bi-polar. Coma. Convulsions. Delirium. Depression. Dermatitis. Dizziness. Drowsiness. Dyslexia. Fever. Glaucoma. Hair, loss. Hallucinations. Headaches. Hives. ***Hyperactivity. Insomnia. Learning, disability.*** Narcolepsy. Nausea. ***Nervousness.*** Palpitations. Schizophrenia. Tremors. Tourette's syndrome. ***Twitchings.*** Urticaria. Vomiting. Weight, loss.

HOMEOPATHIC - Methylphenidate is a central nervous system stimulant. Excessive doses of Ritalin over a long period of time can produce addiction; it is also possible to develop tolerance to the drug, so that larger doses are needed to produce the original effect.

Common side effects may include an inability to fall or stay asleep, nervousness. In children, loss of appetite, abdominal pain, weight loss during long-term therapy, inability to fall or stay asleep, and abnormally fast heartbeat.

Chest pain. Abnormal heartbeat. Palpitations. Fluttery or throbbing heartbeat. Pulse changes. Rapid heartbeat. Blood pressure changes. Dizziness. Abnormal muscular movements. Jerking. Joint pain. ***Severe twitching.***

Reddish or purplish skin spots. Hives. Skin reddening. Skin inflammation with peeling. Skin rash. Hair loss. Headache. Fever. Drowsiness. Abdominal pain. Loss of appetite. Nausea. Retardation of growth in children.

MIND - ***Attention deficit disorder.*** Distracted. Short attention span. ***Learning disability.*** Dyslexia. ***Hyperactivity.*** Agitation. Confusion. Emotional impulsivity. Feeling of elation. ***Nervousness and restlessness.*** Depression.

Delirium. Hallucinations. Psychotic episodes. Paranoia. Bipolar disorder. Schizophrenia. Minimal brain damage. Tourette's syndrome.

Abdomen - Abdominal pain.

Chest - Angina pectoris. Chest pain.

Blood - Increased blood pressure. Leukopenia, and anemia. Necrotizing vasculitis. Thrombocytopenic purpura. Increased blood sugar.

Eyes - Dilated pupils. Glaucoma. Blurred vision. Difficulty with accommodation.

Food - Loss of appetite. Weight loss.

Head - Headaches. Alopecia. Hair loss.

Heart - Angina pectoris. Blood pressure changes. High blood pressure. Cardiac arrhythmias. Abnormally fast heartbeat. Palpitations and irregular heartbeats.

Limbs - Arthralgia. Joint pain. Muscle cramps. ***Hyper reactive reflexes.*** Abnormal muscular movements. Jerking. Convulsions. Tremors and tics. ***Twitchings.*** Tourette's syndrome (severe twitching).

Skin - Reddish or purplish skin spots. Pruritus. Urticaria. Hives. Skin reddening. Skin inflammation with peeling. Exfoliative dermatitis, erythema multiforme. Dryness of mucus membranes.

Sleep - ***Insomnia.*** Inability to fall or stay asleep. Drowsiness. Narcolepsy.

Stomach - Loss of appetite. Nausea, vomiting.

Temperature - Extremely elevated body temperature. Heat, flushing.

Vertigo - Dizziness.

COMMENTS - Exaggerated feeling of elation. Hyperactivity. Agitation, confusion. Transient depressed moods. Nervousness and insomnia. Delirium. Psychotic episodes including hallucinations.

Dry mucus membranes. Dilated pupils. Extremely elevated body temperature, flushing. Fever. Sweating. Vomiting. Dizziness, drowsiness, headache, and dyskinesia. Headaches. High blood pressure. Irregular or rapid heartbeat.

Rash, pruritus, urticaria. Exfoliative dermatitis, erythema multiforme with histopathological findings of necrotizing vasculitis, and thrombocytopenic purpura. Alopecia.

Arthralgia. Muscle twitching. Tremors. Convulsions, muscle cramps, choreoathetoid movements, tics, or exacerbation of pre-existing tics, Tourette's syndrome.

REFERENCES - Murphy.

ROBINIA PSEUDACACIA

(Yellow Locust)

PHARMACY - rob. Robinia pseudacacia. Yellow locust. Common acacia. False acacia. North American locust. N. O. Leguminosae. Papilionoideae. Tincture of fresh bark of young twigs. Trituration of the beans. ***Historical dose:*** All potencies.

CLINICAL - ***Acidity. Belchings***. Coryza. ***Dyspepsia.*** Flatulence. Headaches. ***Heartburn.*** Hyperchlorhydria. ***Indigestion.*** Intermittents. Neuralgia. ***Stomach, disorders.*** Urticaria.

HERBAL - The Treasury of Botany stated "The roots of Robinia have the taste and smell of liquorice, but are a dangerous poison and accidents have occurred from their being mistaken for liquorice roots."

HOMEOPATHIC - The recorded poisonings were due to eating the beans or chewing the bark. Of thirty-two boys so poisoned, in the mildest cases there was vomiting of ropy mucus, dilatation of pupils, dry throat, flushed face.

In the severest, the vomit was more copious and mixed with blood with retching, epigastric pains, debility, stupor, cold limbs, dusky pallor, heart's action feeble intermittent, limbs pulseless. Recovery took place in two days.

Acidity of children. Child cries when its arms were laid hold. ***Sour infants with sour smell of the body, sour stools and vomiting of sour milk.***

Hyperchlorhydria, when the belchings and taste is sour and vomiting is so sour that it sets the teeth on edge or dulls them. The gastric symptoms with the most ***pronounced acidity*** are well authenticated and are the guiding symptoms. Acid dyspepsia. Burning in stomach and between scapulae. Squeezing in stomach. Heartburn and acidity worse lying down especially at night. Water brash.

Albuminoid digestion is too rapid and starch digestion is perverted. ***Intensely acrid belchings***. Acrid and greenish vomiting, colic and flatulence, nightly burning pains in stomach and constipation with urgent desire.

Stools and perspiration sour. Incarcerated flatus. Acidity accompanied by frontal headache. Constant dull frontal headache worse motion and reading. Sick headache with acid vomiting.

MIND - Excessively irritable. Very low-spirited. Tried to write but could not. Can hardly tell what she is doing.

Abdomen - Constant dullness in epigastric region with cutting pains in stomach and bowels and a good deal of rumbling. Burning distress in stomach and region of gallbladder. Bowels greatly distended with flatulence, seemed to fill up whole abdomen, tympanites, better passing flatus. Soreness in bowels when moving or from pressure.

Causations - Ill effects from fat, gravies, flatulent food, cabbages, turnips, new bread, ice cream, raw fruit, etc.

Eyes - Eyes sunken. Eyes sore, watery with rough throat. Pupils contracted (in poisoning cases, dilated).

Face - Neuralgic face ache, spreading to eyes, forehead, ears and teeth, changing the whole features. Spasmodic pains in jaws, feels as if they would be broken or dislocated, intensely sour taste in mouth. Face flushed (in mild poisoning cases), dusky, pale (in severe cases).

Female - Menses too late, black. Bleeding between the periods, accompanied by purulent leucorrhea. Leucorrhea, acrid, fetid, whitish, greenish, yellowish, thick and purulent. Ulcerative pains in vagina with acrid, yellowish leucorrhea of most fetid smell. Cramps in uterus. Tumefaction and bruised feeling in neck of womb and general prostration. Hard swelling of uterus. Herpes on vagina and vulva. Nymphomania.

Food - Worse from eating, fats, cabbages, turnips, raw fruit, ice creams. Thirst.

Head - Constant dull, heavy, frontal headache, much worse by motion and reading. Dull headache, with profuse nasal discharge and frequent sneezing, with sharp stitches in temples. Stinging pain in temples, changing from right to left side. Gastric headache with acid vomiting. Sick headache with sour stomach from fat meat, gravies, flatulent food, cabbage, turnips, warm bread, pastry, ice creams, raw fruits. Steady headache with sensation as if head full of boiling water. As if brain struck against skull when moving. Unable to hold his head upright.

Heart - Almost pulseless. Heart's action is very feeble, embarrassed when moved from horizontal position.

Kidneys - Urine scanty, painful or profuse, turbid.

Limbs - Could not move in slightest degree fingers, hands, arms or legs, later could move fingers of right hand a little, later could stir legs, but not draw them up, tickling feet caused much distress.

Lungs - Voice reduced to a whisper and efforts to cry exceedingly feeble, suddenly ceasing with a slight sigh, as if from exhaustion. Feeble respiration.

Modalities - Worse at night, by motion. Neuralgia from contact of food, worse by touch. Headache worse by reading. Heartburn and acidity worse lying down. Nausea and vomiting worse being raised from the horizontal.

Mouth - Burning, sharp pains, especially in carious teeth, spreading to cheeks, eyes and temples, worse at night or on contact of food, especially if cold or spiced. Teeth become loosened from the spongy and easily bleeding gums. White coating on tongue with red tip. Tongue covered with whitish-brown fur, smooth and slimy. Mucus membrane of mouth pale.

Nose - Profuse continual discharge from nostrils with sneezing and dull headache. Wax-like tumor on nose.

Rectum - Heat and pressure in epigastrium, cramps. Bowels costive with frequent ineffectual desire for stool. Desire for stool, but only flatus passes, finally constipated stool. Sudden attacks of purging and vomiting. Stools are loose, black, fetid with great tenesmus, watery, whitish, excessively frequent and generally involuntary. ***Sour stools of infants with sour smell from body and vomiting of sour milk.*** Diarrhea stools, yellow, green, burning with nervous agitation, weakness, cold sweat, dyspnea. Sensation as if whole body would pass away with stool. The daily motion has a slimy look and bilious tinge.

Sensations - As if head were full of boiling water. As if brain revolved. As if brain struck against skull. Jawbone as if dislocated. Stomach as if scalded. As if whole body would pass away with stool. The left side was most affected. A sleepy, dull feeling in head and limbs changed from right to left.

Skin - Covered from head to foot with urticaria.

Sleep - Sleepiness and dullness in limbs and head. Restless sleep all night on account of frequent sneezing from indigestion.

Stomach - Everything turns to acid. ***Sour stomach.*** Regurgitation of acid and bitter substances. Heartburn and acidity of stomach at night on lying down. Heavy, aching dullness in stomach. Very severe, sharp pains in stomach all day and night. Great distention of stomach and bowels. Flatulent colic (Cham., Dios.). Nausea with ***sour belchings.*** Profuse ***vomiting of an intensely sour fluid*** (Sul-ac.). Vomiting of ropy mucus, tinged with blood, retching and epigastric pains. Vomiting with slight convulsions.

Temperature - Hands and feet cold. Hectic fever with night-sweats. Paroxysms of pain late in afternoon, lasting until 3 to 4 a.m., face hippocratic, much flatulence.

Throat - Dry scratching in throat, with flushing of face. Rough soreness, with sore eyes.

Vertigo - Faintness, worse when raised from horizontal position. Vertigo and dullness of head in whatever position it is placed. Sensation as if brain revolved, worse lying on right side. Vertigo with unsteadiness and nausea.

COMMENTS - The provings of Burt and Spranger developed the symptoms which have led to the chief clinical uses, but some of Houatt's symptoms have also been confirmed. Clinical experience has added to the symptoms.

Among Houatt's symptoms was a facial neuralgia spreading to eyes, forehead with contraction of the jaw and features and also a sensation as if the jaws would be dislocated or fractured. Hering gave a case of neuralgia as having been cured with Rob. "Jawbone feels as if dislocated intensely sour taste and vomiting."

The paralytic symptoms were very marked in one of the poisoning cases. Flatulence and diarrhea were produced and also constipation with constant ineffectual urging.

The chief keynote of Rob. is acidity, especially at night. Cooper observed improvement under Rob. cease at night-time.

Sour stomach, heartburn and acidity coming on when lying down at night and preventing sleep. Vomiting of intensely sour fluid which set the teeth on edge. Belchings of a very sour fluid. Sour stools of infants with sour smell of body and vomiting of sour milk.

Halbert related a case of hyperchlorhydria treated with Rob. Mrs. S., 40, had stomach troubles for many years, for which she had bitter tonics, stomach douching, and electric massage. She had acid belchings and vomitings of intensely sour food.

Extreme appetite, but gastric pains an hour or two after meals. Stomach and bowels distended with gas almost constantly, and extremely irritating flatulence. Craved meats, but could not tolerate vegetables. Craved solid food, but did not dare take it. Emaciated and cachectic.

Lavage was performed every alternate day and after it the patient was directed to eat a full meal. Rob. 3x was given every two hours and steady improvement occurred in ally particulars, until health was practically restored.

Burt had a severe neuralgia in left temple, preventing sleep from midnight to daylight. He had also a "dull, heavy aching in stomach," and a "constant dull, heavy frontal headache, much worse by motion and reading." The combination of gastric and head symptoms has placed Rob. among the chief remedies in migraine and sick headaches.

A. L. Fisher relieved with Rob., when everything else failed, the intensely acid vomiting in four cases of gastric cancer.

RELATIONS - ***Compare:*** (1) Cyt-l. (2) In acidity, Rheum, Calc., Aeth., Mag-c., Puls. (3) In neuralgia, Ars., Chin., Flatulence, Chin., Carb-v., Lyc. (4) Ineffectual urging to stool, Nux-v. (5) Gastric headaches, Iris-v. (6) Jawbone as if dislocated, Rhus-t. (7) Changing sides, Lac-c. (Rob. Right to left). (8) Heart, Phase. (9) Dilated pupils, dry throat and flushed face, Bell.

REFERENCES - Boericke. Clarke. Phatak.

ROCK ROSE

(Bach Flower Essence)

PHARMACY - rck-r-b. Rock rose. Helianthemum nummularium. Rock Rose flowers are gathered and put in a sunlit bowl of water for several hours. The water imbued with healing power is strained and prepared as medicine. ***Historical dose:*** Take two drops from the stock bottle into a one ounce dropper bottle (add brandy or alcohol, if this bottle will be used for days or weeks). This is the dosage bottle, take a few drops straight into the mouth or as needed in a little water or juice.

HOMEOPATHIC - This remedy belongs to Bach's group ***"For Those who Have Fear,"*** with Mimul-b., Cher-p-b., Asp-b. and Rd-ch-b. Rck-r-b. treats states of intense fear and panic, plus a chronically weakened nervous system.

Acute anxiety states cause accelerated heartbeat and breathing, shortness of breath, choking sensation, dry mouth, indigestion with possible nausea, vomiting and diarrhea, dizziness and fainting and internal and external trembling.

Chronic, advanced nervousness, characterized by nervous weakness, insomnia, lack of physical and mental/emotional endurance, shakiness, digestive problems including lack of appetite, heightened sensitivity to noise and touch, first signs of a nervous breakdown and other typical symptoms of an exhausted nervous system.

Restores equilibrium after a nervous breakdown (Cher-p-b., Verv-b.).

MIND - Fright and heightened anxiety. Extreme agitation and nervousness. Chronic state of nervousness, frequent starting and inner trembling. Anxiety disorders. Prolonged fearful worry, chronic loss of sleep. Exhaustion of nerve power.

Anger, hatred, irrational resentment. Impatience, aggressiveness. Feelings of helplessness, despair. Easily aroused weeping. Longing for help. Desire for peace and rest.

Frequent nightmares, fixations and obsessions of a fearful nature, as in phobias or panic disorders. Fright from near death or the near death of a loved one. Post-traumatic stress disorder and adjustment disorder, trauma was related to fear or terror (Star-b-b.).

Repeated fearful experiences or one-time traumas of fright have become linked with a certain person, object, or circumstance which will trigger renewed fear on contact even when the real danger has passed.

REFERENCES - Bach.

ROCK WATER

(Bach Flower Essence)

PHARMACY - rck-w-b. Rock water. Aqua petra. Water from any special well known to carry healing power is placed in a sunlit bowl for only one hour and used as medicine. ***Historical dose:*** Take two drops from the stock bottle into a one ounce dropper bottle (add brandy or alcohol, if this bottle will be used for days or weeks). This is the dosage bottle, take a few drops straight into the mouth or as needed in a little water or juice.

HOMEOPATHIC - This remedy belongs to Bach's group ***"Over-Care for Others' Welfare,"*** along with Beech-b., Vine-b., Verv-b. and Chic-b. These remedies heal the tendency to overly influence and control others. Rigidity and hardening of physical structures. Excessive willpower resulting in inner tension and strain.

MIND - Disappointment or despair, leading to a sacrifice or loss of pleasure.

Inner conflict. Intense self-control, leading to personal pride and the desire to inspire others to be equally strong. Rigidity and self-centered toughness, with frustration, sadness, depression, or anger. Hardened. Sense of loss.

Ritualistic, perfectionist, obsessive-compulsive behavior (Cher-pl-b., Crb-a-b., Pine-b., Verv-b.). Tendency to adhere to routines and one-sided acceptance of limitations. Self denial and habitual patterns in the rehabilitation of addictive drugs or behavioral patterns.

REFERENCES - Bach.

ROSA CANINA

(Dog Rose)

PHARMACY - ros-ca. Rosa canina. Dog-rose. Cynorrhodon. N. O. Rosacea. Europe. Tincture of ripe fruits. ***Historical dose:*** Tincture and all potencies.

CLINICAL - Bladder, disorders. Dysuria.

HERBAL - Rose hips are used for making the very pleasant "Confection of Roses" used in general medicine as a basis for pills and electuaries. Rosa canina has been used in ancient times as a remedy in urinary difficulties.

HOMEOPATHIC - A proving only evoked a somewhat increased flow of urine and a little heat in the urethra. Burnett confirmed this to some extent.

REFERENCES - Clarke.

ROSA DAMASCENA

(Damascus Rose)

PHARMACY - ros-d. Rosa damascena. Damascus rose. Damask rose. N. O. Rosacea. Tinctures of the flowers. ***Historical dose:*** Tincture and all potencies.

CLINICAL - Allergies. Coryza. Deafness. ***Eustachian, catarrh***. Hay fever. Hearing, problems. Rose-colds. Tinnitus.

HOMEOPATHIC - Hay fever and allergies. Hardness of hearing, tinnitus. Rose-colds. ***Eustachian catarrh*** (Kali-m., Merc-d.), Eustachian tube swollen.

Farrington mentioned that Ros-d. was introduced by Jeanes as a remedy at the beginning of rose-cold when the Eustachian tube is involved with some degree of deafness and tinnitus.

RELATIONS - ***Compare:*** (1) In hay fever: Phle., (Timothy grass) - Hay fever with asthma, watery coryza, itching of nose and eyes, frequent sneezing, dyspnea. Use 6c to 30ç potency. (2) Eustachian tube catarrh: Kali-m., Merc-d. (3) Succ-ac, Sabad., Euph., Psor., Kali-hp., Napht.

REFERENCES - Boericke. Clarke.

ROSMARINUS OFFICINALIS

(Rosemary)

PHARMACY - rosm. Rosmarinus officinalis. Rosemary. N. O. Labiatx. Tincture of whole plant. ***Historical dose:*** Tincture and all potencies.

CLINICAL - Baldness. Dandruff. Dizziness. Headache. Lice. Menses, too early. Memory, weak. Miscarriage. Sleeplessness.

HERBAL - Rosemary oil has an ancient reputation as a remedy for baldness, headache and flagging mental powers. It has been called the "Herb of Memory," which Shakespeare alludes to when he has Ophelia say, "There's Rosemary, that's for remembrance."

HOMEOPATHIC - ***Memory deficient.*** Head heavy, ***drowsy.*** Menses too early, violent pains followed by uterine hemorrhage. Chilly with icy coldness of lower limbs without thirst, followed by heat.

MIND - Anxiety. Memory weak. Dullness.

Female - Violent pains followed by uterine hemorrhage and miscarriage, succeeded by faintness, spasms of chest, cold hands and feet, small, rapid, irregular pulse. Menses four days too early.

Head - Headache. Heaviness and dullness of head. Weight and tension around head. Baldness.

Lungs - Oppression of breathing. Spasms in chest.

Skin - Hair loss. Dandruff. Lice.

Sleep - Overpowering sleepiness with yawning. Sleeplessness.

Temperature - Coldness so that she could not leave the bed. Chill over whole, legs icy cold, no thirst and no subsequent heat.

Vertigo - Dizziness.

COMMENTS - The most violent of the symptoms of Rosm. were observed on a woman who took a strong infusion for eight days resulting in a miscarriage. In another woman, it brought on the menses four days too soon. Chilliness predominated, the chill not being followed by heat.

RELATIONS - ***Compare:*** (1) Hedeo., Menth., Puls.

REFERENCES - Clarke.

RUBIA TINCTORUM

(Madder)

PHARMACY - rub-t. Rubia tinctorum. Madder. N. O. Rubiaceae. Tincture of the root. ***Historical dose:*** Tincture and all potencies.

HOMEOPATHIC - Burnett found Rub-t. an excellent remedy for anemia and under-nourished conditions, especially in splenic anemia. Useful for the spleen (Cean.) Anemia with undernourished conditions. Chlorosis amenorrhea and tuberculosis. Bone disorders.

RELATIONS - ***Compare:*** (1) Chin., Coff., Gali. (bot.). (2) In anemia, Ferr.

REFERENCES - Clarke.

RUBUS FRUTICOSUS

(Blackberry)

PHARMACY - rubu-f. Rubus fruticosus. Blackberry. Brambleberry. Dewberry. Cloudberry. Tincture of the leaves. N. O. Rosaceae. ***Historical dose:*** Tincture and all potencies.

CLINICAL - Anemia. Appendicitis. Coughs. Cystitis. Diarrhea. Dropsy. Dysentery. Eczema. Gingivitis. Gums, bleeding. Hemorrhoids. Insect, bites. Laryngitis. Leucorrhea. Menorrhagia. Mouth, sores. Pharyngitis. Sore, throat. Tonsillitis. Toothache. Ulcerations. Whooping cough. Wounds.

HERBAL - Blackberry is also known by the common names brambleberry, dewberry, and cloudberry. The berry grows on small, bushy vines, each berry being a cluster of tiny black knobs. In England, they are often referred to as brambleberries because of the prickly thorns, or brambles.

It is astringent, tonic, mild diuretic, and hemostatic. The fruit and juice is considered a refrigerant and tonic. The root-bark and the leaves are strongly astringent, depurative, diuretic, tonic and vulnerary. Blackberry leaf is more specific to the stomach and intestines. The fruit is more specific to liver and kidneys.

The root is the most astringent part. It has been used as a preventative for dropsy. It makes an excellent remedy for diarrhea, hemorrhoids, and cystitis. The root-bark as well as the dried and powdered fruit have been used for dysentery. Extract of the root has been used for stomach problems as well as an antidote to poison.

In American folk medicine the root was also used for tonsillitis. It has been used as an anti-inflammatory for conditions such as laryngitis and pharyngitis. The root decoction was once used during the spasmodic phase of whooping cough. A decoction of the root has been used for lung problems in general, as well as amenorrhea.

Medicinally, the leaf of the Blackberry is most often used. The white underside of the leaves was said to "draw" while the smooth green upper side was said to "soothe."

The leaves, root, and root bark have been used for inflammation of the throat, mouth and gums (also bleeding gums), as well as hemorrhoids and leucorrhea. The leaves were used in England for burns and scalds. Blackberry leaves were also used as a poultice for wounds and insect bites, and as a wash for oily skin.

Blackberry leaves have been made into a tea to ease the discomfort of sore throat. It has also been used internally to loosen phlegm. The leaves were chewed to treat bleeding gums and mouth sores. Blackberry leaf tea was used as a gargle to treat sore throats, mouth ulcers and gum inflammations.

A strong tea of the leaves has been used externally for eczema. Another method was to soak leaves in hot wine to make an infusion, then placing a cloth dipped in the liquid on the ulcerations morning and evening. A decoction of the leaves was once used as a fomentation for ulcerations.

Blackberry leaves have also been used to inhibit excessive menstrual bleeding. Blackberry tea made from the roots was a remedy for pregnant woman who were in danger of miscarrying due to overwork. The leaves have been used as a uterine tonic.

Blackberry tea, made of the scrapings of the bark of the branches, was used for bronchial infections. As a poultice, it was used to treat pneumonia. Boiled vines, roots, and berries for a drink for those vomiting and spitting blood. Boiled the cane to use as a diuretic and used a root tea for diarrhea.

The fruit and juice have been used for anemia and to regulate menses. The flowers and fruit were once used for venomous bites and the young shoots eaten to tighten loose teeth. The ancient Greeks used blackberries to treat gout, mouth inflammation, and bowel inflammation.

Blackberry was believed useful for appendicitis. Steeped berries in water was drunk as a vermifuge. European settlers to North America used blackberry jam to remedy diarrhea.

Blackberry jelly was an English folk remedy for swelling of the limbs (especially those associated with heart problems). The jelly was added to apple cider vinegar and used as a compress. Blackberry glycerite was also used as a compress on swollen joints.

COMMENTS - The common name blackberry also includes the species Rubus villosus, Rubis lacinniatus, Rubus procerus, and other Rubus species, which are used interchangeably with Rubus fructicosus.

The primary constituents of this herb include tannins, gallic acid, villosin, and iron. The fruit portion contains vitamin C, niacin, pectin, sugars, anthocyanins, and flavonoids (kaempferol, quercitin).

The tannin content of blackberry leaves makes it an effective astringent. It also has diuretic properties. The tannins in blackberries also contribute to the plant's ability to treat diarrhea and dysentery, as well as to constrict blood vessels, which inhibits bleeding.

REFERENCES - Murphy.

RUBY

(Gemstone)

PHARMACY - ruby. Ruby. Gemstone. ***Historical dose:*** All potencies.

CLINICAL - Allergies. Anemia. Anger. Angina. Belching. Blood, disorders. Circulation, weak. Constipation. Cough. Debility. Diarrhea. Earache. Flatulence. ***Heart, disorders.*** Heartburn. Hemorrhages. Hemorrhoids. Hepatitis. High blood pressure. Immune, disorders. Infections. Leucorrhea. Migraine. Nausea. Nosebleed. Palpitations. Vomiting. Wounds.

HOMEOPATHIC - Ruby has an affinity for the blood, immune system, heart and circulation. It is a blood cleanser, blood tonic. Wounds, stab or lacerations. Hemorrhages. Encourages speedy coagulation. Anti-septic properties. For the after-effects of bacterial and viral infections.

Chronic fatigue and all states of debility. Poor vitality due to liver dysfunction. Chilliness, affecting one side of the body, generally the right. Patches of cold, especially if they are felt to move around the body.

Affinity for children and adolescents and for those from the Indian sub-continent and Southeast Asia.

MIND - Clear mind, sensation of energy breaking free all over body. Mental and physical clutter. Mental blankness with an inability to focus one's ideas or thoughts. Forgetful. Cannot remember details. Fastidious.

Feels isolated. Helps to restore a sense of self-worth (Aur.). Feeling of unworthiness due to the recognition of how much worse off are others, while feeling that there is nothing that can be done to redress the balance.

Sense of being consumed by worldly events or by family emotions. Inability to let go of emotions. Guilt and shame. Resentment. Confused and distressing thoughts. Escapist daydreaming.

Anger comes up in outbursts. Anger that is expressed inappropriately. ***Suppressed anger*** (Staph.). Anger associated with sexual frustration. Vehemence and intolerance. Impatience with slowness and poor articulation of expression. Teenage anger.

Anticipation. Shaking or trembling with fear. Fear of new situations. Fear of the dark. Fear of one's own dark side, of being in someone else's power. Fear of death, of being sacrificed.

Abdomen - Ache in epigastrium. Epigastrial discomfort, as though the lateral edges of the muscles contract in towards each other, better with massage. Ache in left hypochondrium. Pain in right hypochondrium. Fullness and heaviness in lower abdomen. Sharp tweaks in lower abdomen, right side (psoas muscle), constant heaviness like pressing down. Mild cramping in lower abdomen, comes straight up midline. Bloating more than usual. Foul gas, rumbly (not painful), very bloated lower abdomen. Loud, painless gurgling in stomach. Reduction in abdominal gas.

Back - Pain in lower sacral, right side.

Bladder - Frequent urination.

Blood - Anemia. Blood disorders. Immune disorders.

Chest - Heat in chest and pressure in the morning, around esophagus, centrally located. Heavy constricted chest, all day belching and heartburn, need to burp feeling, know it will taste bad. Dull pain in heart region, lasted several minutes. Circulation feels dull.

Ears - Aching pain in left ear, with fullness like earache. Ears feel full. Hearing not registering. Heightened sense of hearing, all sounds are so clear.

Eyes - Pupils dilated, eyes were very wild and maniacal looking. Bloodshot and glassy, red and dry. Eyes tired and burning, itching. Pain in the corner of the right eye as if stabbed by a finger. Heavy eyelids, burning sensation.

Face - Face puffy. Tingly cheeks. Face grayish with blemishes, irritated.

Female - Labia feels swollen and itchy. Vaginal discharge yellow and curdsy. Leucorrhea, yellow, lumpy, and not itchy. Early sexual awareness. Increased desire. High sexual energy. Uses sex as a way of avoiding hidden emotions. Decreased or absent sexual desire.

Food - Appetite diminished, not hungry. Appetite increased, very hungry, wakes hungry. Thirsty. More thirstless than usual. Craving meat, salty food, fatty foods, bread.

Head - Head pain started at left front and moved to the back of my head. Migraines with nausea and vomiting, especially when the liver is involved. Pain from the cervical area and up and over the head to the forehead. Compression down the back from the head and neck. Sensation of pushing down on the vertex or of pushing inwards. Head feels split. Hair fuller, thicker, healthier and stronger. Hair feels dry. Cannot detangle hair at nape of neck.

Heart - Heart disorders. High blood pressure. Compression of the cardiac area. Pain in heart, seized up, sharp constriction for five minutes. Pain behind the sternum as if a heart attack would come on. Angina. Palpitations.

Limbs - Right side feels alive while the left side feels dead. Tingling in the legs. Fidgety and restless. Pins and needles in the right leg. Itching and aching in the right leg. Tweak in right hip. Feet and legs are cold. Goosebumps on upper arms and thighs. Poison oak like rash between wrist and elbow, itching and oozing. Mark on right arm (the underside in the middle of forearm which itches on occasion). Backs of the hands feel itchy. Nails healthier and stronger.

Liver - Useful after hepatitis when the body is weakened and cannot restore itself to full strength.

Lungs - Cough in the middle of the night. Dry, gagging cough, with thick phlegm. Wakes with choking cough.

Male - Anger associated with sexual frustration. High sexual energy. Not interested in sex.

Mouth - Taste somewhat enhanced. Food tastes funny. Burning, dryness on sides of tongue. Pain under left side of tongue, at the root, could be felt even exteriorly. Sore under tongue, behind teeth, very painful. Sores on inside of lip, on lower gums. Swollen gums.

Nose - Middle separation of nostrils is sore to touch. Rawness in nose and throat came and went, itchy and dry. Nose very wet and damp in the morning. Pain at the root of the nose as if it is blocked. Nose plugged, crusted, hard. Nose mucousy, tight without discharge. Intermittent sneezing, relieves. Sneezing, nose is running, like allergies or hay fever. Profuse nosebleeds. Sensitivity to smells, especially vinegar and beer. Everything smells different.

Perspiration - Body sweaty, unusual. Sweating at peak of anxiety attack. Sweats all night long. Hot and sweaty had to take covers off. Apple-like smell coming off body.

Rectum - No bowel activity. Constipation. Diarrhea, explosive, loose, watery, painless. Gassy diarrhea, gassy expulsion. Bouts of loose stool with sudden urge (9 a.m. to noon). Small stool with urination. Foul gas, rumbly, painless. Blood from the hemorrhoids with each stool. Prolapsed old hemorrhoids.

Skin - Flushed, mottled skin. Itching rash, especially on buttocks. Itchy all over, better with scratching.

Sleep - ***Deep sleep.*** Sleep interrupted, woke often beginning at 2 a.m. then 3 a.m., 4 a.m. Awoke unrefreshed, feeling almost drugged, hard to open eyes. Groggy in morning. Sleepy in the morning. Difficult getting up. Nap in the afternoon, did not feel good from nap. Can't get enough sleep.

Stomach - Digestion sluggish. Sensation of a stone in the stomach. Heaviness in the upper abdomen. Empty pit feeling. Bloating, both flatulence and flatus. Constant heartburn. Belching to the point of interrupting conversation. Burping loudly, involuntary, repeatedly. Foamy belching. Constant nausea. Empty, nauseous feeling. Nausea, not from stomach but umbilicus.

Morning sickness. Cancer.

Stool - Diarrhea, explosive, loose, watery, painless. Defecate with expulsion, gassy diarrhea, gassy expulsion. Five bouts of loose stool with sudden urge. Small, dry stools with blood.

Teeth - Grinding teeth. Hard to floss, teeth are tight.

Throat - Heat around esophagus, in morning, with heat in chest and pressure. Burning esophagus. Closing up. Rawness in throat and nose, came and went, itchy, dry. Instantly dry throat. Throbbing sore throat. Sore throat, tight and dry, mild headache, sneezy, running nose. Wakes with slight dryness in back of throat, full ears.

Urine - Smells acidic, like acidosis.

Vertigo - Some vertigo and weakness in the sun. Dizzy feeling when stands up, like wavering in a clockwise motion.

COMMENTS - Ruby is one variant of the simple mineral corundum, the other is sapphire. Corundum is a compound of aluminum and oxygen, AL2 O3 (aluminum oxide). Chromium is responsible for the color of ruby, while iron, titanium and other elements cause the coloration of sapphires.

The name "corundum" is derived from the Sanskrit word "kuruvinda" via the Tamil name for ruby, "kuruntam." The name "ruby" comes from the Latin word for red, "ruber."

Sluggish system with low energy. Circulation feels dull and weak. Heavy feeling, body heavy like lead, heaviness, hard to exercise. All over tiredness. Felt need to lie down, fighting gravity. Very tired in the evening, barely made it to bed. Hungover or fluish feeling. No desire to exercise. Better as day goes on. Weight gain.

Body warm all over. Cooler temperature. Goosebumps on upper arms and thighs. Tingling all over body. Sensation as if air were passing through certain areas of the body. All senses acute. Left ear painful with dull ache, ear fullness.

RELATIONS - ***Compare:*** Amber, Staph., Ferr.

REFERENCES - Murphy.

RUMEX ACETOSA

(Sorrel)

PHARMACY - rumx-a. Rumex acetosa. Sorrel. N. O. Polygonacae. Tincture of the leaves. ***Historical dose:*** Tincture and all potencies.

CLINICAL - Convulsions. Esophagus inflammation. Gastritis. Paralysis. Throat, sore. Uvula, elongated.

HERBAL - Sorrel was at one time cultivated as a salad. The Buckler-shaped or French Sorrel is cultivated in France, where it is considered a powerful anti-scorbutic. The leaves contain a large quantity of Bin oxalate of Potash (Kali-ox.).

HOMEOPATHIC - The Rumx-a. symptoms were observed on three men who ate largely of the leaves. In one, very violent convulsions were induced of a peculiar kind, the limbs being thrown reciprocally backwards and forwards and the head from side to side. The hands being alternately clenched and unclenched, the eyes prominent.

Other remarkable symptoms included swelling of the lower eyelid. Elongated uvula. Pain all down esophagus worse by swallowing. Persistent short, dry cough. Complete paralysis of bodily powers, copious green vomit, constipation.

RELATIONS - ***Compare:*** (1) Kali-ox., Lapa. (2) In persistent cough, Rumx.

REFERENCES - Clarke.

RUMEX CRISPUS

(Yellow Dock)

PHARMACY - rumx. Rumex crispus. Yellow dock. Curly dock. Sour dock. Narrow dock. N. O. Polygonaceae. Tincture of fresh root. ***Historical dose:*** Tincture and all potencies.

CLINICAL - Abortion. Acne. ***Anemia.*** Aphonia. Asthma. Borborygmi. ***Bronchitis.*** Catarrh. Corns. Coryza. ***Coughs.*** Diarrhea. Dyspepsia. Dyspnea. Feet, tender. ***Flatulence***. Gastralgia. Headache. Heart, disorders. Heartburn. Hiccough. Indigestion. Irritation. Jaundice. Lichen. Miscarriage. Mouth, ulceration. Nausea. Nosebleeds. Phimosis. Prurigo. Rheumatism. Throat, sore. ***Trachea, disorders.*** Tuberculosis. Urticaria.

HERBAL - Rumex is an old Latin word for "lance," referring to the shape of the leaves. Crispus means "curly," also in reference to the leaf shape. The yellow dock or curly dock is a common British weed, a member of the buckwheat family. It grows abundantly throughout North America.

The common yellow dock includes the species Rumex occidentalis, Rumex venosus, Rumex obtusifolius and Rumex sangineus, which are used interchangeably with Rumex crispus.

The common dock of fields and roadsides, Rumex obtusifolia has a well deserved reputation among children as the best antidote to the nettle's sting. Rumex crispus, according to Joslin, was used by herbalists internally and externally for the cure of scabies.

Yellow dock has been used for hundreds of years for its astringent properties, treating a variety of skin problems, including boils, rashes, blemishes and burns. Topically, the crushed leaf of yellow dock can soothe the stings from nettle plants.

It can also be added to a tooth powder for spongy gums, and to a gargle for laryngitis. Salves, poultices or compresses of this herb have been used for eczema, hives, itchy skin, scabies and ringworm.

The properties of this herb are alterative, laxative, purgative, cholagogue, and astringent. It has been used for nutritional support of the blood, lungs, and urinary system. Yellow dock is valued today as one of the ***best available sources of iron***. Its high iron content makes it beneficial for treating anemia and pregnant women.

Yellow dock has also been known to help improve bladder and liver functions, and reduce bowel inflammation and glandular swelling. This herb can be used to treat some cases of jaundice, and skin eruptions associated with the toxicity of the intestines.

HOMEOPATHIC - Hale noted that among the constituents and salts of Rumx. are Sulph. and Calc-p., and Sulph., Calc. and Phos. are strongly represented in its action. Rumx. is a close ally of Rheum and has analogous purgative and other properties.

The provings were made by Houghton, Joslin, Paine, Bayard, Rhees and Co., both with the tincture and potencies, and its characteristics were well defined.

Dry, hacking, tickling cough (Bry.). Constant tickling in the pit of the throat, runs into bronchi. Trachea sore to external pressure, feels excoriated, as do the fauces. Lump sensation in the throat that descends and comes back up after they swallow.

Cough is excited by pressure on throat. Touching the throat brings on the cough. Violent cough with a scanty difficult expectoration. Rattling cough. Coughing as if a piece of phlegm is stuck in chest.

Cough caused by an incessant tickling in the throat, tickling runs down to the bifurcation of the bronchial tubes. ***Cough, worse from the least cold air or uncovering.*** Cough ceases by covering the body and head with bedclothes.

Marked action on the skin, producing an ***intense itching.*** Numerous and varied pains, neither fixed nor constant. Sharp pains, neuralgias. Acts on joints, especially ankles, the skin, left side, chest. Cold affects the joints. Obesity.

Rumx. diminishes the secretions of mucus membranes and at the same time exalts sensibility of the mucus membranes of the larynx and trachea. Dry and sensitive mucus membranes. Mucus secretions decrease causing stickiness with burning. ***Lymphatics are enlarged*** and secretions perverted.

MIND - Disinclination to mental exertion. Indifferent about his surroundings. Restlessness in evening. Patient refuses to speak or even listen to conversation, lest his attention should be withdrawn from the supervision of his respiratory acts. Low spirited with serious expression of the face. Suicidal mood. Feels like killing herself in despair.

Abdomen - Annoying rumbling flatulence in women. ***Flatulence***. Flatulent abdominal colic soon after a meal. Creeping near navel better by discharge of offensive flatus.

Back - Pain under scapulae, right.

Breasts - Pain in the left breast after meals.

Chest - Pain under sternum, under right nipple. Pain in left side of chest after meals with flatulence. Burning, sticking pain in left chest near the heart, worse deep breathing. ***Rawness or burning*** under clavicle as if the air penetrated there, worse hawking. Clavicular pain, worse hawking. Soreness behind sternum, especially left side in region of left shoulder.

Constitutions - Tubercular or nervous constitutions.

Cough - Suffocative choking coughs. ***Tickling in throat*** causes cough. ***Dry, tickling cough, preventing sleep.*** Barking cough. Cough worse by pressure, talking, lying on left side, ***inspiring cool air and at night***. Cough provoked by changing rooms. Cough by change from cold to warm and warm to cold. ***Cough from uncovering, drafts.*** Cough comes regularly at 11 p.m., 2 a.m. and 5 a.m., in children. ***Continuous coughing.*** Cough in the daytime only. Cough worse during early pregnancy, may cause miscarriage.

Ears - Ringing in ears. Itching deep in ears. Pain, throbbing, stopped sensation in ears.

Eyes - Burning indoors, puffed up in morning. Pain in eyes as from dryness, lids inflamed, worse evening. Sore feeling in eyes without inflammation. Deep-seated pain in right eye. Sharp, shooting pain in left eye. Lachrymation when yawning.

Face - Sodden complexion. Pale, while standing. Pain in right jaw, morning.

Female - Pain from right ovary to back. Tendency to miscarriages, in early stage of pregnancy (Sep.). Miscarriage with dry, shaking, spasmodic cough, in paroxysms of great violence.

Food - Ravenous appetite. Worse when eating and after meals. Worse after excessive use of alcohol. Gastric disturbances, from tea drinking. Can't eat meat, it causes eructations, pruritus. Worse from apples.

Head - Headache after waking in morning. Headache and nausea after eating. Catarrhal headache with great irritation of larynx and trachea. Darting or sharp piercing pains, in left side. Bruised feeling in forehead. Dull feeling in head during cough.

Heart - Feels as if suddenly stopped, followed by heavy throbbing through the chest.

Kidneys - Sudden urging, involuntary with cough. Copious, colorless urine in afternoon. Urine less copious, flocculent deposit, oily surface, marked brick-dust sediment.

Limbs - Pain in left shoulder on coughing, on raising arms. Hands cold when coughing. Spasmodic cramps in ankles and feet.

Liver - Jaundice after excessive use of alcohol.

Lungs - Dyspnea on retiring. Better closing the mouth or covering the head. Breathing worse in wind. Asthma. ***Copious mucus discharge*** from nose and trachea. Profuse, frothy, thin expectoration, stringy and tough, by the mouthful.

Male - Tendency to phimosis. In evening, feeling of soreness and excoriation with redness of end of prepuce. Itching of prepuce. Sexual desire diminished, lost.

Modalities - Better from covering mouth. Better wrapping up, lying on right side. Better from discharge of offensive flatus. Worse weather change, warm to cold, cold to warm. ***Worse from cool air, inhaling,*** open air. Worse deep or irregular breathing. Worse uncovering. Worse motion, riding, lying on left side. Worse from pressure on trachea, talking. Worse eating, after meals. Worse evening and night, morning, on waking. Worse 3:30 p.m., 11 p.m., 2 a.m. to 5 a.m.

Mouth - Bitter taste in morning. Dry tongue and mouth. Tongue sore at edges, coated. Tongue feels as if burned. Tongue coated yellowish-brown or reddish-brown. Toothache, entirely better after dinner, rinsing mouth with cold water. Toothache with acute colds. Ulceration of mouth and throat.

Nose - Nose obstructed, dry sensation in posterior sinuses. Copious mucus discharge from nose and trachea. Yellow mucus from posterior nares. Sneezing attacks, fluent coryza. Violent sneezing and painful irritation of nostrils. Itching that extends from the end of the nose to pharynx. Desire to pick nose. Nosebleed.

Rectum - Brown, watery ***diarrhea, early in morning*** with cough, driving him out of bed. Sudden, profuse, foul, painless, brown, black or thin, watery stools. Itching of anus with sensation as of a stick in rectum. Hemorrhoids. Valuable in late stage tuberculosis (Seneg., Puls., Lyc., Ars.).

Sensations - Eyes pain as if from dryness. Tongue as if burned. As if cough did not reach low enough to raise phlegm. Lump in throat, it descends on deglutition, but immediately returns. Hands cold when coughing. As if head would fly to pieces with cough. As if he might raise blood any minute. Hard substance in pit of stomach. As if heart suddenly stopped. Pressure of a stick in rectum.

Skin - Acne vulgaris on back. Intense itching of skin, especially of lower limbs, ***worse exposure to cold air or when undressing***. Urticaria, contagious prurigo. Jaundice after excessive use of alcohol.

Sleep - Sudden sleepiness. Sleep disturbed, wakeful, restless, short naps and unpleasant fancies, even when awake. Unpleasant dreams of danger and trouble.

Stomach - Tight, suffocative, heavy ache in epigastrium to back, clothes feel tight. Chronic gastritis, aching pain in pit of stomach and shooting in the chest, extends towards the throat, worse any motion or talking. Hiccough, heartburn. Nausea, better by belchings. ***Eating meat causes belching and itching.***

Teeth - Pain in teeth of both sides, morning. Toothache better after eating dinner, better by rinsing with cold water.

Temperature - Sweat on waking from a sound sleep.

Throat - Throat feels hollow. Rawness of larynx and trachea. Hawks much tenacious mucus. Lump, not better by hawking, descends and rises again after swallowing. Irritation in larynx when eating, causes cough.

COMMENTS - Guernsey described the cough of Rumex as a "cough caused by an incessant tickling in throat-pit, which tickling runs down to the bifurcation of the bronchial tubes touching the throat brings on the cough, by covering up all the body and head with the bed-clothes there is no cough."

Shakes head as if it would fly to pieces and chest so that he feels he might raise blood any minute. Exhausting paroxysms, rapid coughing spells (Coc-c., Cor-r.). Coughing if the hands get cold. Headache during cough. Cough causes expulsion of urine and it may even cause expulsion of the fetus in pregnant women. Palliates late stage tuberculosis (Phos., Ph-ac., Stann.).

Cold air and drafts bring on coughing spells, as well as itching and skin aggravations. Characteristic sensitivity to cold air. The cough and skin symptoms are worse by uncovering or exposure to air. Wants to be covered (Hep.).

Worse from change of weather, temperature, talking with cough, eating. Worse motion, lying on the left (Phos.). Worse touching the throat. Irritated by irregular or deep breathing. Coughing worse at night around 11 p.m., and from 2-4 a.m.

Flu with a dry, hacking cough. Dryness of the nose and throat. Tendency to colds easily, with cough. Asthmatic cough, allergic asthma with constriction and a hacking, tickling cough.

Allergies with more coughing than sneezing, with a runny nose. Irritation of the nose. Burning, smarting, rawness in nasal passages (Caust.). Rapid sneezing. Severe sinus headaches, especially when the discharge dries up.

Thick, white discharges deep in the lungs or in the sinuses. Mucus or dryness alternating with total obstruction of thick mucus. Catarrh of the nose, eyes and chest that is gluey, thick, white, gelatinous, ropy and lumpy (Ant-t.). Nosebleeds from hawking.

Lachrymation of the eyes. Aphonia, aphasia. Hoarseness and change of voice (Spong.). Toothache, worse from inhaling cold air, may be better from cold drinks. Raw, burning sensation on inhaling.

Disturbed circulation. Violent palpitations of the heart and throbbing throughout the whole body.

Itching with burning, worse scratching, after bathing (Sulph.). Skin is worse being uncovered (Hep.). Scabies with severe itching. Eczema with small, red pimples. Itching without eruptions (Spong., Alum., Sulph.).

Sensation of weight in stomach. Borborygmi, particularly on the left. Flatulence and rumbling. Diarrhea in the early morning, driving the patient out of bed. Morning diarrhea, brown, watery, offensive. Diarrhea after catarrh, often associated with a cough.

Sadness and aversion to work, with irritability. Restless, sleep with vivid dreams, especially when the cough wakes them. Dreams of danger and robbers. Can wake up coughing or with diarrhea.

Paine noted a particular symptoms that led to many cures of skin cases where exposure to air is the exciting cause, "while undressing and for some time after, considerable inching of surface of lower limbs."

P. P. Wells related the case of Mrs. X., who had eight miscarriages all in the early months of pregnancy. Each miscarriage was attended with a severe dry, shaking, spasmodic cough in violent attacks. This was regarded as the cause of the miscarriages.

At the beginning of the ninth pregnancy she came under homeopathic treatment. The cough came on very dry, harsh, loud, shaking, worse at night, preventing sleep, excited instantly by pressure on the trachea. Rumx. 30c promptly relieved.

Wells also cured with Rumx. 200c a cough in a man that began with tickling behind top of sternum, sometimes in paroxysms lasting for five to ten minutes.

Joslin pointed out the left chest had more verified symptoms than any other region. Conditions are worse lying on left side, better lying on right side. Worse at 11 p.m. and 4 a.m.

RELATIONS - ***Antidoted by:*** Camph., Bell., Hyos., Con., Lach., Phos. ***Compare:*** (1) Caust., Sulph., Bell., (2) Rumx. contains chrysophanic acid to which the skin stitches correspond. (3) Rumx-a. - Sheep sorrel - Gathered in June and dried, used locally for Epithelioma of face. Dry, unremitting short cough and violent pains in bowels, uvula elongated inflammation of esophagus, also cancer. (4) Rumex obtusifolius - Broadleaf dock - nosebleed and headache following, pain in kidneys, leucorrhea.

REFERENCES - Boericke. Clarke. Murphy. Phatak.

RUSSULA FOETENS

PHARMACY - russ. Russula foetens. N. O. Fungi. Tincture of the fresh mushrooms. ***Historical dose:*** Tincture and all potencies.

CLINICAL - Bedwetting. Blindness. Chorea. Coma. Convulsions. Cyanosis. Dyspnea. Spasms. Tremors.

HERBAL - Some species of Russula are edible and are much esteemed as a food.

HOMEOPATHIC - Alphonse Barrelet observed the effects of eating cooked Russula foetens, which produced a very severe poisoning. Russ. has produced hallucinations, muscular tremors and clonic spasms recall the effects of Agar.

The eye symptoms were even more pronounced, complete blindness lasting many days occurred with this peculiarity of the pupil, that it was sometimes normal, sometimes dilated and sometimes contracted.

Constant trembling of muscles, at times interrupted by tonic contractions increasing to general clonic spasms with complete loss of consciousness. Muscular spasms, deathly anxiety, dyspnea. Patient recovered after two or three weeks.

MIND - Hallucinations constant for three days after spasms ceased. Unconsciousness. Deathly anxiety.

Abdomen - Nausea, colic, vomiting, diarrhea, with cold limbs.

Eyes - Pupils at one time normal, at another time dilated, at another contracted. Consciousness returned on third day, patient could hear but was completely blind.

Face - Cyanosis.

Kidneys - Involuntary urination.

Lungs - Dyspnea.

Pulse - Pulse small and contracted.

Skin - The attack was followed by pseudo-erysipelas on elbows and painless furuncles over whole body, especially on scapulae and small of back.

REFERENCES - Clarke.

RUTA GRAVEOLENS

(Garden Rue)

PHARMACY - ruta. Ruta graveolens. Garden rue. Bitterwort. N. O. Rutaceae. Tincture of whole fresh plant. ***Historical dose:*** Tincture and all potencies.

CLINICAL - Amblyopia. Anus, prolapse. Arthritis. Asthenopia. ***Backache.*** Bedwetting. ***Bone, bruised.*** Bruises. Bursitis. Cancer. ***Carpal tunnel.*** Cartilages, bruises, pains. Chest, pains. Constipation. ***Dislocated, joints.*** Dyspepsia. Exostosis. ***Eye-strain.*** Facial paralysis. Fevers. Fractures. ***Ganglions.*** Hemorrhages. Hands, pains. ***Injuries. Joint, injuries. Lameness.*** Nosebleeds. Paralysis. Perichondritis. Periostitis. Rectum, cancer. Rectum, prolapsed. Restlessness. ***Rheumatism.*** Sciatica. Spleen, disorders. ***Sprains.*** Stammering. ***Strains. Tendonitis.*** Tongue, swelling. Urination, difficulty. Varicocele. Veins, swollen, varicose. Vision, weak. Warts.

HERBAL - The common rue is a native of southern Europe. Teste noted that it was formerly in great repute in medicine for epilepsy, hysteria, hydrophobia and weakness of sight from excessive reading. Ozaena, nosebleed, foul gumboils, flatulent colic, and inertia of the bowels have been cured with it empirically.

Teste added that Ruta graveolens was supposed to be a kind of universal antidote, "Even in our own time the Roman ladies imagine that the most odoriferous flowers may be left in their rooms without the least danger provided a bush of garden rue be amongst them."

Practitioners have perhaps been deterred from employing it by the symptoms of acrid-narcotic poisoning induced by an overdose. It is noted, in The Treasury of Botany, that locally applied rue is a powerful irritant and one species, Ruta montana, is dangerous to handle even with gloves

Green's Herbal mentioned that Ruta is "useful in feverish complaints, promotes perspiration and removes noxious material in headache, nervous and hysteric complaints, weakness of the stomach and pains in the bowels, suppressed menses and if taken for a long time it benefits epilepsy. The expressed juice benefits nightmare."

M. Helie indicated that, in large doses, it causes violent gastric pains, excessive and sometimes bloody vomiting, profuse salivation and swelling of the tongue. Great prostration and confusion of the mind. Convulsive twitchings and, in pregnant women, miscarriage.

HOMEOPATHIC - Hahnemann's proving showed how largely the old uses were founded on a homeopathic relationship. The vulnerary remedies indicate in symptoms of their provings the peculiar form of injuries for which they are adapted.

Like the sprained pains of Rhus-t. and the bruised pains (in skin and muscles) of Arn., Ruta also has bruised pains, but these are more particularly manifested in bones. Historically, it was used to ward off plague.

Affinity for fibrous tissue, flexor tendons, joints, ankles, wrists, cartilages, periosteum, uterus and skin. Acts upon the eyes and uterus. ***Eyestrain.*** Overstrain of ocular muscles. Jaundice.

For ***injured joints***, tendons, bones and especially ***bruised bones***. Rheumatism. ***Tendonitis.*** Formation of deposits or nodes in the periosteum, tendons and about the joints especially wrists. Brittle bones. Lain on parts become sore, even in bed.

The pains are bruised, ***sore, aching with restlessness***, a feeling of intense, painful weariness. ***Lameness after sprains. Sprains with weakness in joint*** (Arn.). Complaints from straining ***flexor tendons*** especially. All parts of the body are painful, ***as if bruised***.

Heaviness, as of a weight in forehead or hanging to feet or lower limbs. As of a rough blunt plug in part, head, nose etc. Paralytic rigidity. Distortions. Grating, burning pains, neuralgia.

MIND - Stupefaction. Thought and comprehension slow. ***Feeling of intense lassitude, weakness and despair***. Indifference. Disinclined to work. Quarrels and contradicts. Inclined to anger and vexation. Morose, peevish, fretful. Disposed to weep.

Frequent anxiety, with despondent thoughts and fear. ***Fear of death during fever.*** Anxious restlessness. Anxious all day, as though he had done something wrong. Fear that someone will come to arrest him.

Melancholy, dissatisfied with life, and sad. Dissatisfied with himself and others. Mistrustful. Suspicious, imagines that he is always being deceived. Delusion someone is behind him. Starting from sleep from slightest touch. Desire for light.

Abdomen - Painful swelling of the spleen. Gnawing ache in region of liver. Gnawing and eating pain about navel. Sick feeling in abdomen followed by soft stools. Pinching pain in abdomen after bread and butter. Cancer of lower bowel. Colic in children, from worms.

Back - ***Backache from injury or strain,*** better pressure and lying on back. Bruised pain in coccyx, sacrum. Spine and limbs feel bruised. ***Vertebrae slip out of place easily.*** Coldness of spine, downwards. Drawing in nape of neck and in the shoulder blades. Tension and pressure in nape and shoulders. Pain in small of back, groin and nape. Weak, bruised feeling in lower back. Lumbago worse morning before rising. Stitches in lumbar region.

Bladder - Constant urging to urinate, can hardly retain urine. If urine forcibly retained, could not pass afterwards, with severe pain. Urging with scanty urination. Sensations as if bladder were still full, after urinating. Pressure in neck of bladder after urinating, painful closure (Apis). Sensations as if bladder is moving up and down at every step. Scanty, green urine. Frequent urination at night. Incontinence at night, or even during day when walking.

Causations - Ill effects of bruises, fractures, carrying heavy weights. Bone or joint injuries. Overuse of tendons. Sprains. Going up and down stairs causes hamstrings to feel shortened and weak. Dyspepsia from straining stomach by carrying heavy weights. Over-exertion of eyes.

Chest - Short breath with tightness of chest. Painful spot on sternum. Sensation of coldness or heat in chest. Gnawing, biting and burning pains in chest. Tuberculosis after mechanical injuries to chest. Ill effects of mechanical injury to chest.

Constitutions - Suited to robust, bloody persons and corresponds to hemorrhages from nose (with pressure at root), gums, and rectum.

Ears - Earache with scraping pressure. Itching lancinations in ear. Cartilages of ears as if bruised. Pain in ear and under mastoid process as from a bruise. Pain as from a blunt piece of wood.

Eyes - Amblyopia. Asthenopia. Weakness of ciliary muscles. Spots on cornea. Eyes burn like fire. Lachrymation in open air, not indoors. Pressure deep in orbits. ***Eyestrain with headaches.*** Weary pain while reading. Red, hot and painful from reading fine print, sewing (Nat-m., Arg-n.). Itching inner canthi. Tarsal cartilage feels bruised. Spasm in lower eyelids, when it ceases, lachrymation starts. Pressure over eyebrow.

Face - Acne. Acne rosacea. Eruption of pimples on lips. Lips dry and sticky. Pain as if bruised in periosteum of facial bones. Spasmodic tearing in cheekbone. Itching and gnawing at face and on cheeks. Coldness beneath left eye. Erysipelas in forehead with swelling. Facial paralysis after catching cold.

Female - Menses very irregular. Menses scanty, lasting but two days, preceded and followed by leucorrhea. Corrosive leucorrhea after irregular or suppressed menses. Symptoms worse at menstrual period. Vaginal pruritus. Bearing-down pains. ***Prolapsed uterus.*** Metrorrhagia as a forerunner of miscarriage. Miscarriage, at seven months. Lameness and soreness all over with feeble contractions during labor. Sterility.

Food - Appetite normal, but aversion to everything as soon as he begins to eat. Disgust at first mouthful with a sensation of fullness and satiety in abdomen. Great thirst during chill. Violent thirst for ice cold water. Headache from abuse of alcohol. Worse after eating bread, butter, eating meat, grapes, raw or indigestible food.

Head - Heat in head, with anxious restlessness. ***Headache from eye-strain.*** Stitches, worse reading. Aches as if a nail is driven into it. Pain as from a nail after excessive intoxicating drinks. Pressure over eyebrow. Pulsative, pressive, in forehead. Head externally painful, as if bruised or beaten. Periosteum sore. Erysipelas and swelling of forehead. Erysipelas of scalp, arising from wounds. Corrosive itching on scalp. Humid scabs on head.

Heart - Anxious palpitations. Pulse somewhat accelerated only during fever.

Limbs - Bursitis. Cracking in joints, worse walking in open air. Paralytic weakness of legs after spraining of the back. Sciatica, worse lying down at night, pain from back down hips and thighs. ***Hamstrings feel shortened (Graph.).*** Great restlessness. ***Thighs feel broken,*** worse when stretching the legs. Legs give out on rising from a chair (Phos., Con.). ***Knees give way,*** while ascending and descending stairs. Pains as if deep in long bones, must walk about. ***Tendons sore***. Aching pain in Achilles tendon. Pain in bones of feet and ankles. Ankles swollen from strain or injury. Contraction of fingers. Pain and stiffness in wrists and hands. ***Ganglion of wrist*** (Benz-ac., Calc-f.). Nodes in palms.

Lungs - Cough with copious, thick, yellow expectoration, chest feels weak after. Waking from cough, about midnight. Violent cough, with expectoration of tough mucus and nausea. Shortness of breath from tightness of chest.

Male - Varicocele following a strain. Injury to genitals, testes. Hematocele in which the effusion is small and firmly coagulated.

Modalities - Better from lying on back. Better warmth, motion, rubbing, scratching. ***Worse from overexertion, lifting, injury, sprains.*** Worse exertion, ascending or descending stairs. Worse lying down, sitting, stooping. ***Worse eyestrain,*** reading. Worse pressure on an edge. Worse from cold air, damp, wind, wet. Worse during menses. Worse from uncooked or indigestible food. Warm stove causes chilliness.

Mouth - Woody taste. Dryness in mouth and throat. Mouth dry and glutinous. Profuse salivation and swelling of tongue. Cramp in tongue, causing embarrassment of speech. Boring pains in lower teeth. Gums bleed easily.

Nose - Pressive, hard aching at the root of nose, with nosebleed. Perspiration on back of nose.

Perspiration - Cold sweat on face. Perspires in morning in bed. Sweats after walking in open air.

Rectum - Constipation from impaction of feces following mechanical injuries. Constipation, alternating with mucous, frothy stools, discharge of blood with stool. ***Difficult stool***, evacuated only with straining. Feces often escape when stooping. Protrusion of rectum when stooping. When sitting, tearing stitches in rectum. Urging to stool, causing rectum prolapses. ***Rectal prolapse.*** Sudden prolapsus recti, with tenesmus, after eating grapes. Anal prolapse on stooping. Anal prolapse after delivery, during hard or soft stools. Stricture of rectum. ***Cancer affecting lower bowel.*** Nausea felt in rectum.

Sensations - As if a nail were driven into head. Head as if bruised or beaten. Eyes, as if strained, as if a shadow flitting before them, as after looking too long and intently at an object, as if eyes were balls of fire. As if one were digging about in the ear with a blunt piece of wood. As of a lump in throat. Bladder as if constantly full. Spine as if beaten and lame. Pain as if from a fall in periosteum. As if pain were in marrow of bone or as if bone were broken. ***Wrists as if sprained.*** Thighs as if beaten, as if weak. As if there were an ulcer on ankle. All parts of body bruised at night, feeling as if it were time to rise.

Skin - Easily chaffed from walking, riding, also in children. Flat, smooth, painful warts, on palms. Warts with sore pains. Corrosive itching over whole body, better scratching. Itching of skin from every attempt to eat meat. Erysipelas after mechanical injuries of hands. Skin becomes easily chafed, from walking and riding.

Sleep - Sleepiness during day, with stretching. Yawns, stretches and extends hands. Yawning and stretching, after eating. Frequent waking at night, as if it were time to rise. Vivid, confused dreams.

Stomach - Epigastric region sensitive. Aching, gnawing pains in stomach. Tension in stomach, better drinking milk. Pains in stomach after eating bread or crude and indigestible food. Burning, gnawing pain. Dyspepsia caused by straining stomach when carrying heavy weight. Frequent odorless eructations. Hiccough, with depression. Sudden nausea when eating, with vomiting of food. Nausea felt in rectum.

Temperature - Coldness and shivering, with great thirst. Cold shivers run over back. Coldness running over one side of head. Chills mostly left-sided, worse up and down back, shakes even near a warm stove. Heat of face and dull head. Frequent attacks of quick flushes of heat. Glowing heat on face, skin etc.

Throat - Sensation as if a lump in throat on empty swallowing. Larynx as if bruised.

Vertigo - Whirling vertigo, which causes falling when rising in morning. Vertigo when seated, when walking in open air.

Vision - Amblyopia dependent upon anomalies of refraction. Amblyopia from writing by artificial light. ***Disturbances of accommodation***. Obscuration of vision as if one had looked too long and intently at an object. Blurred vision with burning, aching in eyes and strained feeling. Blurred vision from fine sewing, reading too much, worse using eyes in evening. Letters seem to run together. Dim vision, as if a shadow were flitting before objects. Green circle around light in evening.

COMMENTS - The vulnerary power of Ruta does not appear to have been known before the provings were made, but an old use of the remedy for impaired sight due to eyestrain, corresponded to symptoms from the provings.

"His eyes feel as if he had strained the sight too much by reading," "weak, pressive-like pain in right eye with dimness of surrounding objects, as if from having looked too long at an objects that was fatiguing to the eyes," "a feeling of heat and burning in the eyes and pain in them when he reads (in the evening and by candle-light)."

Eyestrain, with burning and itching in the eyes. Eyestrain headaches (Onos.). Blurry vision. Contracted pupil. Eyeballs ache. Paralysis of the eye muscles and neuralgias. Facial paralysis from catching cold in robust, sanguine persons.

Rheumatic paralysis of wrists and ankles. Affinity for the joints, especially the tendons and ligaments. Joints feel weak and bruised. Chronic weakness and inflammation. Structural abnormalities. Torn or overstretched ligaments. Often a history of injury, remaining weakness in injured spot. Often follows or is complementary to Rhus-t.

Twisting injuries to the spine (Arn., Hyper., Rhus-t.). Wrenching injuries. Injuries to the shin and face. Injuries that are close to the bone. Bone injuries with torn ligaments, muscles or nerves (Arn., Calc-p., Symph.). Hard lump after injury (Arn.).

Overuse of joints, particularly the wrists. Dislocated joints, or the tendency to dislocate. Weak ligaments or joints. Carpal tunnel syndrome (Caust.). Shooting pain in wrist (Rhus-t., Hyper.). Chronic shortening of tendon due to overuse. Fibrositis. Bursitis, tendonitis, from overuse. Chronic knee complaints. Frozen shoulder. Thickening of the periosteum or nodules after injury (Bellis).

Stiff and aching (Arn., Rhus-t.). Sharp pains (Hyper.). Deep, grinding pain. Sharp, tearing nerve pain. Drawing pain, as if area is being pulled shorter. Feeling of lameness ever since injury. Worse sitting or lying down. Chronic weakness after an injury.

Gnawing, grinding pains, especially in the shoulder. Pain worse in cold, damp weather. Stiffness, worse in the morning, better from motion and heat (Rhus-t.). Coldness down the spine, leg or sciatic nerve. Tearing pain down the sciatic nerve.

Great weakness, pain in limbs after a short walk. Limbs feel bruised, pain in small of back and loins. Tottering as if thighs were weak. Uneasiness and heaviness in legs, difficultly finding a comfortable position. All parts of the body on which he lies, even in bed, are painful as if bruised. Restlessness.

Sore spot on sternum. Pain below right scapula and stitches in small of back. Backache. Lying on back ameliorates many conditions, has led to relief in cases of malignant disease of kidneys and bladder.

Cramp in the tongue with embarrassed speech. Swollen tongue. Toothache with digging pain. Dry sockets, with achy pain. Slow pulse. Hangovers. Rhus poisoning, itching, inflammation, and rashes. Skin is red, swollen with watery vesicles.

Rectal polyps. Constipation, since trauma to the area (Bell-p.), since childbirth (Sep.). Constipation from inactivity of rectum or impaction of feces following mechanical injuries. Hemorrhoids and impacted feces after an injury.

Prolapse of the rectum after confinement. Prolapse is worse by stooping and crouching, comes on immediately on attempting a passage. Tearing stitches in rectum when sitting. Tearing in rectum and urethra while urinating. Sensation of nausea located in the rectum.

Rushmore cured with one dose of Ruta 900c (Fincke) a case of prolapse preceding a very difficult stool.

A prolonged use of Ruta 3x has cured ganglion in front of left wrist.

Cooper said, "It certainly acts strongly on deposits of scirrhus material in both the breasts and in the vagina and sometimes lessens the size of these." He used Ruta ointment, prepared by extracting the plant in warm Vaseline, as an application in broken cancer of the breast.

RELATIONS - ***Antidoted by:*** Camph. ***Antidote to:*** Merc. ***Compare:*** (1) Arn., Bell-p., Rhus-t., Hyper., Calc., Calc-f. (2) Restlessness, effects of cold and damp, Rhus-t. (3) Eye-strain, Nat-m., Onos., Seneg. (4) Prolapsed rectum, Aesc. Bell., Chin-s., Nit-ac., Podo. (5) Pain in back, worse in morning before rising, Pet. (6) Sore as if bruised in parts lain on, Arn., Bapt., Pyrog. (6) Constipation after injuries, Arn. (7) Warts on palms, Nat-c., Nat-m. - on backs of hands, Dulc. chafing. (8) Arg-n., Con., Euphr., Lyc., Cham., Sep. (9) In diseases of bone, Ang., Conch. ***Compatible:*** after Arn. in joint injuries, after Symph. in bone injuries, Calc., Caust., Lyc., Ph-ac., Puls., Sulph., Sul-ac. - diseases of bone. ***Complementary:*** Calc-p. in joint disorders.

REFERENCES - Boericke. Clarke. Murphy. Phatak.

S

SABADILLA OFFICINALIS

(Cevadilla Seed)

PHARMACY - sabad. Sabadilla officinalis. Cevadilla seed. Cebadilla. Asagraea officinalis. Scoenocaulon officinale. Veratrum officinale. N. O. Melanthaceae of the Liliaceae. Tincture of seeds. ***Historical dose:*** Tincture and all potencies.

CLINICAL - ***Allergies.*** Ascarides. ***Chilliness***. Colds. ***Coryza.*** Coughs. Debility. Diarrhea. Diphtheria. Dyspepsia, pregnancy. Earache. Esophagus, stricture. ***Hay fever.*** Headaches. Imaginary diseases. Influenza. Intermittents. ***Lice.*** Mania. Melancholia. Neuralgia. Nosebleeds. ***Pinworms.*** Rheumatism. Tapeworm. Throat, sore. Toothache. Uvula, elongated. Vertigo. ***Worms.***

HERBAL - Asagraea is a Mexican genus belonging to the Colchicum family, Melanthaceae. It has only one species, Asagraea officinalis, furnishing the cebadilla seeds from which Veratrine is prepared. According to the Treasury of Botany, the seeds were formerly used to destroy vermin.

HOMEOPATHIC - Sabadilla first appears in homeopathic literature as one of Stapf's additions; Hahnemann was one of the provers. Stapf's additions form a kind of appendix to the Materia Medica Pura. Stapf said that the plant was first described by Monades around the year 1572. At first, it was almost exclusively used for destroying lice and worms in putrid ulcers and the intestines.

Sabadilla has affinities for the ***mucus membranes of the nose,*** lachrymal glands, anus, digestive tract, and the nerves. Coryza and symptoms like ***hay fever***. Allergies. ***Chilliness***, sensitive to cold.

Nerves are affected, producing weakness. Alternate nervous and bodily symptoms. Cutting pains in bones. Formication. Worms. Reflex nervous symptoms with twitching, convulsive trembling or catalepsy. Children's diarrhea with constant cutting pains.

MIND - Nervous, timid and easily startled. Mental exertion aggravates. ***Thinking produces headaches and sleeplessness.*** Feels miserable. Fright causes hysterical paroxysms. Unresponsive to questions. Loss of consciousness, then he jumps up and runs recklessly through the room. Rage. Mania better washing head in cold water. Delirium during intermittents.

Erroneous, fixed ideas about himself. Imagines he is very sick. Imagines that she is pregnant or that she has cancer. Imaginary diseases. Imagines that parts are sunken, limbs are crooked, chin is elongated. That one side is longer than the other.

Abdomen - Bowels feel knotted. As of a lump or thread moving rapidly in abdomen.

Back - Contusive pain in back and loins, especially when seated. Burning, tingling, stinging sensation between scapulae. Stitches in rapid succession in right side of back.

Causations - Ill effects of fright, mental exertion, thinking. Worms, causing convulsions, nymphomania.

Chest - Burning sensation on chest. Pressure on the chest. Breathing obstructed, as if there were a stone in the chest. Shootings in sides of chest. Inflammation of pleura. Red spots and points on chest.

Constitutions - Suited to sensitive persons of light hair, fair complexion with a weakened, relaxed, muscular system. Children and old people.

Ears - Otalgia with troublesome pressure, with snapping as of electric sparks before ears. Tickling in ears. Itching in ear, alternately with itching at anus. Burning, itching and shootings in tips of ears. Humming, gurgling, and detonation in ears. Deafness as if there were a band over ears. Boring in parotids.

Eyes - ***Red, burning eyelids.*** Redness of margins of eyelids. Lachrymation, worse during pain, sneezing, coughing, yawning. Pressure on eyeballs, especially when looking up. Weakness of sight.

Face - Lips hot, burn as if scalded. Heat of face with fiery redness, especially after drinking wine. Blue circles around the eyes. Boring in lower jaw and submaxillary glands. Cracking of the articulation of the jaw on opening mouth wide.

Female - Menses too late, come by fits and starts, intermit, sometimes stronger, sometimes weaker (Kreos., Puls.). Nymphomania from worms.

Food - ***Thirstless.*** Canine hunger for sweets and farinaceous food. ***Desires hot things***, milk. Loathing for strong food. Aversion to all food, meat, sour things, coffee, garlic. During pregnancy, no relish for food until she takes first mouthful, then she makes a good meal.

Head - Dullness and oppression. Unilateral head pains or alternating sides, worse thinking, better eating. Burning, itching, crawling on hair and scalp, better scratching. Headache in schoolgirls.

Heart - Palpitations with pulsations through whole body.

Kidneys - Urgent want to urinate, especially in evening, with tenesmus and scanty emission. Increased secretion of urine. Turbid, thick urine, like clay-water. Burning in urethra when urinating.

Limbs - Upward jerking of arms. Cutting pains in bones. Red spots on arms and hands. Yellow spots on fingers. Swelling of feet with painful soles. Cracking of skin under and beneath toes. Inflammation under toenails. ***Thickened,*** deformed horny nails (Ant-c.).

Lungs - Wheezing respiration. Short, difficult breathing. Breathing obstructed, as if there were a stone in the chest. Asthmatic breathing with itching of skin, nose and anus. Violent coughing attacks, muffled, worse anger with lachrymation. Hawking up of bright red blood, which comes from the nose. Cough dry with perspiration and water in the eyes. Cough immediately on lying down. Pleurisy with great paralytic debility.

Male - Digging and pressive pain in testes. Tensive and painful erections, without desire for sex. Pollutions with flaccidity of penis. Diminished sexual desire.

Modalities - Better from heat, warm food and drink, swallowing. Better being wrapped up, open air. Better quick motion of affected part. Warm stove ameliorates chilliness. ***Worse from cold air***. Worse forenoon, new and full moon. Worse periodically, every week, two weeks, four weeks, same hour. Worse odors, wine. Worse undeveloped rash. Worse mental exertion. Worse forenoon.

Mouth - Itching of the soft palate. Dryness of the mouth without thirst. ***Sweetish taste.*** Copious saliva, jelly-like saliva. Cannot bear anything hot or cold in mouth. Lips as if scalded. Tongue as if burnt, as if full of blisters. Pricking, soreness in tip of tongue. Cannot protrude tongue with sore throat.

Nose - Influenza. Hay fever. ***Spasmodic sneezing with running nose.*** Copious, watery, nasal discharge. Coryza with severe frontal pains and redness of eyes and lachrymation. ***Fluent coryza,*** worse from the ***odor of flowers,*** even thinking of flowers increases the discharge. ***Oversensitive to odors***, cannot tolerate the smell of garlic. Dry, ***itching,*** tickling in nose, rubs or picks at it. Tickling in nose spreads over the whole body, then dyspnea. One or the other nostril stuffed up. Hawks bright red blood from naso-pharynx.

Rectum - Constipation. Stools burning, frothy, loose, brown, floating. Broken, hard, scanty stools. Itching, crawling in rectum and anus, as from ascarides, alternating with itching in nose or ears. ***Pinworms***, lumbrici, tapeworm.

Sensations - As if things were turning around each other. As if she would fall if she did not hold on to something. As if eyes went around with the whirling sensation. As if uvula were down. As if esophagus would be closed. As of a lump in abdomen. As if a ball of thread were moving and turning rapidly through abdomen. As if knives were cutting abdomen. As if abdomen were shrunken, were empty. Croaking as of frogs in abdomen. As of something alive in abdomen. As if stomach were gnawed.

Skin - Parchment-like dryness of skin. Hot burning, creeping and crawling sensation. Itching with asthmatic breathing. Tingling and burnings shooting under skin.

Red bands, spots, and points in different parts of skin.

Sleep - Great inclination to sleep during day. Sleep comes on when thinking, meditating or reading. Agitated and unrefreshing sleep at night, with anxious dreams. Sleep retarded by a multitude of thoughts. Starts up as from a fright in the morning.

Stomach - Spasmodic pain in stomach with dry cough and difficult breathing. Heartburn, copious salivation. Cold, empty feeling in stomach.

Teeth - Toothache with drawing and pulsative pain. Shooting pains in molars. Tooth decay. Pricking in gums. Bluish gums.

Temperature - ***Chill predominates*** from below upwards. Heat in head and face, hands and feet icy cold with chill. Thirstless, thirst after chill only. Lachrymation with chill. Shivering as a concomitant.

Throat - Chronic sore throat, worse from cold air. Sore throat, ***left to right,*** worse empty swallowing, better hot drinks. Tonsillitis after coryza. Much tough phlegm. Sensation of a skin hanging loosely, must swallow it. ***Warm food and drink relieve***. Painful empty swallowing. Dry fauces and throat. Sensation of a lump in throat with constant need to swallow.

Vertigo - Vertigo with sensation as though all things were turning around each other. Vertigo accompanied by blackness before eyes and sensation of fainting. Vertigo, sudden on waking at night or rising from stooping, better resting head on table.

COMMENTS - Stapf pointed out that the provings reveal strong febrile symptoms. Sabad. may be as clock-like as Cedr., and is a leading remedy in intermittent fevers and neuralgias. Sabad. is a chilly remedy, the symptoms, especially the coryza, are generally worse in the open air.

Intolerant of mental exertion, thinking causes a headache. Tendency to be startled. Erroneous impressions as to the state of his body. Imaginary diseases, imagines parts shrunken. Imagines she is pregnant if there is distention from flatus.

Giddiness, may cause staggering and even fainting. Objects seem to whirl around or to whirl around each other. Sitting aggravates vertigo. Rising from seat causes vertigo. Lying perfectly still ameliorates vertigo.

Severe catarrhal symptoms. Hay asthma. Allergies. Hay fever with itching and tingling in the nose (All-c., Ars.). Tingling and numbness in the nose (Petros. in the urethra.). Itching in the roof of the mouth, rubbed raw by the tongue (Wye.). Spasmodic sneezing. Coryza, sneezing and runny nose (All-c.). Thick, yellow discharge, worse stuff rooms, better fresh air (Puls.), alternates with watery discharge.

Sore throats characterized by a sensation of a lump or foreign body in the throat and a constant need to swallow. Pressure on larynx causes sore throat. Lying down causes cough immediately, worse expectoration.

Kent said it is suited to "old, chronic sore throats that are worse from cold air. The patient is sensitive to cold air. Every time he takes cold it settles in his nose and throat. Tonsillitis going from left to right."

Desires hot drink (opposite of Lach.). Overly sensitive to the smell of garlic (Thuj.). Opening mouth wide causes cracking of jaw joints.Disordered digestion and loaded tongue. Sinking at stomach and gnawing hunger. Indigestion, during pregnancy.

"Violent itching of hairy scalp, compelling her to scratch until blood comes." "Itching of the vertex as if a quantity of vermin had collected there, obliging him to scratch incessantly." "Itching of anus and rectum as from ascarides." "Itching of anus alternating with itching of alae nasi and meatus auditorius." Scratching ameliorates itching of scalp, causes burning of anus.

Kent gave Sabad. to a pet dog which had great irritation of anus and soon afterwards the dog passed a very large number of worms.

RELATIONS - ***Antidoted by:*** Camph., Lach., Lyc., Puls., Con. ***Compare:*** (1) Colch., Nux-v., Bry., Arund. and Poll. (2) Veratrina is alkaloid of Sabad., not of Verat., locally in neuralgias and for removal of dropsy. Five grains to two drams. Lanolin, rubbed on inside of thighs, causes diuresis. (3) Phle. - Timothy-Hay - Potentized to 12c a specific to many cases and evidently acts in a desensitizing manner.

(4) Cumin. - hay fever. ***Follows well:*** Bry. (Pleurisy). ***Followed well by:*** Ars. Bell., Merc., Nux-v. ***Complementary:*** Sep.

REFERENCES - Boericke. Clarke. Murphy. Phatak.

SABAL SERRULATA

(Saw Palmetto)

PHARMACY - sabal. Sabal serrulata. Saw palmetto. Serenoa serrulata. N. O. Palmaceae. South Carolina to Florida. The tincture must be prepared from the fresh berries to be effective. ***Historical dose:*** Tincture and all potencies.

CLINICAL - Appendicitis. Asthma. Atrophy. Backaches. ***Bedwetting.*** Breast, disorders. Bronchitis. Catarrh. ***Cystitis.*** Debility. Dysmenorrhea. Dysuria. ***Epididymitis***. Gland disorders. Gleet. ***Gonorrhea.*** Headache. Hoarseness. ***Impotency.*** Infertility. Iritis. Laryngitis. Lumbago. Malnutrition. Menses, delayed. Neuralgia. Neurasthenia. Obesity. Ovaries disorders. Peritonitis. Pharyngitis. Proctitis. ***Prostate, disorders. Prostate, enlarged. Prostatitis.*** Puerperal fever. Rhinitis. ***Sexual, debility.*** School, headache. Strangury. Testes, atrophy. Throat, sore. Tuberculosis. ***Urine incontinence.*** Uterus, disorders. Whooping cough.

HERBAL - Sabal serrulata was introduced into medicine by J. B. Read and A. A. Solomon, both of Savannah, Georgia. Dr. Read gave a "Saccharated oil," of which he said, "By its peculiar soothing power over the mucus membranes it produces sleep and relieves the most troublesome coughs, promotes expectoration, improves digestion and increases fat, flesh and strength.

"It has been used with benefit in cardiac asthma, tuberculosis, especially laryngeal, chronic bronchitis and dilatation of the bronchial tubes. Sabal's action in catarrhal disorders in rapid and permanent. A cold in the head may be checked with two or three doses (of the saccharated oil) mixed with boiling water and used by inhalation it has been found beneficial in chronic ozaena."

HOMEOPATHIC - In the provings, the tincture or fluid extract were used, from 5 to 10 drop doses, repeated two or three times a day. A similar dosage has been adopted in the clinical use of the remedy.

Sabal is an organ remedy of great power, selecting the uterus and prostatic gland (which is the male analog of the uterus), ovaries and testes and bladder. For irritability of the genito-urinary organs, especially the prostate, ovaries, breasts, bladder and urethra. It is soothing to the mucus membranes and is tonic, nutritive and stimulating to the overworked brain.

Prostate enlargement and weakness. Prostatitis. Epididymitis and urinary difficulties. Iritis with prostatic trouble. Homeopathic catheter for retention of urine due to enlarged prostate.

General and sexual debility. Nervous irritability with loss of sexual desire in both sexes. Sexual neurotics. ***Valuable for undeveloped breast glands.*** Small and undeveloped genitals.

Sharp, stinging and wandering pains. Languor, apathy and indifference. ***Fear of going to sleep.*** Promotes nutrition and tissue building.

MIND - Difficult thinking, cannot grasp or remember what is read. Confused. Impatience, fretfulness. Irritability and depression, particularly before menses. Irritability from loss of sexual desire. ***Dislikes sympathy, makes them angry***. Self-concentrated on their own sufferings, wants to be left alone. Apathy. Wants to go away and die alone. Indifference to wants of others. Fears to fall asleep lest something should happen. Starts up with fear as he is dozing.

Abdomen - Sudden, intense, cramp-like pain through abdomen. Sharp, stinging pains running up and down front of abdomen, and also right side. Pain extending to thighs.

Back - Aching across lower part of back. Deep pains in lower back. Fearful backache, pain in sacral region, before and at commencement of menses. Backache after sex.

Bladder - Feeling as if bladder too full. Heavy, aching pain and sense of coldness in bladder, extending to external genitals. Painful starting the flow, as if forced through very narrow meatus. Feeling as of a stricture about two inches down urethra. Urethra sensation of narrowness (Arg-n.). Difficult urination, smarting, burning in urethra. Paresis of bladder sphincter. ***Cystitis from prostate enlargement.*** Painful urination, connected with ovarian pain. Urinary sediment. Incontinence from any exertion, lifting, laughing. Constant desire to pass urine at night. ***Bedwetting***. Chronic gonorrhea.

Breasts - One breast smaller than other. ***Breasts shrink in size*** (Iod., Kali-i.), or increase rapidly. Breasts, sore, tender and full feeling, itching. Stinging in breasts, soreness worse after cold bath. Sharp pains in mammary glands. Pain in breasts, worse coldness, pressure. Defective lactation.

Chest - Sharp pain in left side of chest, running through left breast.

Constitutions - Sycotic constitutions.

Ears - Chronic inflammation of middle ear. Fullness in nose and ears. Frequent sharp, stitch-like pains inward from ears. Hearing diminished, voices seem far off.

Eyes - Iritis when prostate gland is involved. Dim vision during headache.

Face - Papular eruption on left temple and about mouth. Slight neuralgia in right temple and right jaw. Pallor.

Female - Amenorrhea. Ovaries tender and enlarged. Stinging pain in ovary, pains running down the thighs. Stinging pain in uterus. Uterine tumor. Heavy feeling over womb. Vulva feels open. Sensation of coldness in genitals. Awakened by a most distressing itching of labia majora. Furious sexual passion. Loss of sex drive. Sexual neurotics with suppressed or perverted sexual inclination.

Food - Appetite poor and capricious. Malnutrition and great emaciation. Better from bread, milk. Constant desire for buttermilk, milk (Rhus-t., Tub.), which is usually disliked. Aversion to mother's milk. Worse meat, pudding, vegetables.

Head - Severe headache with giddiness and dim vision. Headache of weak persons. Neuralgia in feeble patients. Sharp, darting pains here and there, coming and going suddenly. Pain runs up from nose and centers in forehead. Dull, aching pain in right temple and on vertex. Pain and irritation at base of brain and upper third of cervical spine (Gels.). Sensation as if something tightening in brain.

Kidneys - Pain or irritation in region of kidneys. Excruciating pain and fainting on being raised up to urinate.

Limbs - Pains into thighs, radiating in different directions, settling in ovaries. Sharp pain running down thigh. Aching in knee and calf. Annoying eczema of hands.

Lungs - Chronic bronchitis (Stann., Hep.). Copious expectoration with catarrh of nose. Wheezing cough, worse lying down, until 6 a.m.

Male - Coldness of genitals. Drawing pains in spermatic cords. Slight twisting chordee as if stretched from the root. Atrophy of testes. Testes drawn up, painfully. Epididymitis. Gonorrhea. ***Impotency, loss of sexual power***. Hard erections. Semen thick, causes hot feeling along the cord. Sex is painful at the time of emission. Loss of sex drive. ***Sexual neurotics*** with suppressed or perverted sexual inclination.

Modalities - Better after sleep, from milk. Worse from cold, damp, cloudy weather. Worse in early morning, from rising, at bedtime. Worse from sympathy. Worse before menses. Worse from motion. Backache worse after sex. Catarrhal symptoms are worse in cold, damp weather. Cough worse on lying down at night. Depression worse before menses.

Mouth - Pungent, burning sensation in mouth and fauces, causing sneezing, coughing, and gagging. As if mouth coated with fat. Burning on tongue as if scalded.

Nose - Pain at root of nose. Pain running up from nose and centering in forehead. Fullness in nostrils, compelling him to pick them. Catarrhal symptoms, worse cold, damp weather. Sneezing and lachrymation, coughing and gagging.

Prostate - ***Prostatitis.*** Emission of prostatic fluid during stool, on straining at stool, during urination. ***Prostatic weakness*** with discharge of prostatic fluid. ***Enlarged prostate.*** Dull aching in prostate extending into abdomen. ***Cystitis from prostate***

enlargement. Dribbling of urine from prostate enlargement.

Rectum - Constipation and enlarged prostate. Hemorrhoids with dryness of stool and pressure from within out. Stools dark, almost black. Stools unusually easy, free from hemorrhoidal troubles.

Skin - Papular eruption on face. Eczema of hands.

Sleep - Fears to fall asleep lest something should happen, starts up with this fear when he is dozing. Wakes from coldness. Awakened by stinging pains in ovaries, or by a distressing itching of labia majora.

Stomach - Sharp pain running through stomach. Severe pain in left side of stomach. Irritation of stomach. Belching and acidity. Acute gastritis, fearful burning as from sulphuric acid. Could not take meat, vegetable, or pudding, only bread and milk.

Throat - Voice changed, throat feels husky. Sharp pain in left side of throat. Pungent, burning sensation in fauces, followed by smooth sensation, as if coated with oil.

Vertigo - Vertigo with headache from fumes of oil.

COMMENTS - In his book, Saw Palmetto, Hale put together most of the available knowledge regarding this plant. It is a dwarf palm with a creeping (or leaning), branching stem, the edges of leaf and petioles serrate, roots fibrous, large, half exposed.

The fruit, so-called "berry," is a one-seeded dupe about the size of an olive, dark purple when ripe, and ripening in October and November. The fruit is richer in sugar than sugar cane and contains two oils, one volatile and one fixed. The volatile oil is considered to possess the most characteristic properties of the medicine.

Hale described it as "yellow," but he quoted John Uri Lloyd of Cincinnati, as writing to him, "The principal constituent is a volatile oil. This oil possesses a deep green color." And he goes on to say that the color is not due to chlorophyll nor to the copper of the form used in condensing it.

This agrees with Estep's contention that the preparation of Sabal should be dark-green or grass-green. The preparation Estep used was a fluid extract prepared by Burrough Brothers of Baltimore from the "fresh green berries." Hale directs that the fresh ripe berries should be used.

Hale's tincture was of fresh ripe berries and seeds, all crushed and macerated in 90 percent alcohol for fourteen days and decanted. He noted that the fluid extract was "probably four times stronger than the tincture."

C. S. Estep used a dark-green fluid extract that was made from the fresh green berries and as "almost as green as grass and has an oily surface." He made his dilutions from this. Other preparations disappointed him.

Oil can be prepared from the expressed juice of the fruit by allowing it to stand a few days. Saccharated oil is one part of the oil to seven parts of cane sugar. Malted Sabal is one part of the oil to seven of Maltine. Aqua Olei Sabal, for use as a spray, is a preparation suggested by Hale made by triturating 15 drops of the oil with Mag-c. 3j., gradually adding a pint of distilled water and decanting.

The preparation used by Dr. Mullin's prover was made by Boericke and Tafel. All are agreed that preparations of the dried fruit and of the root-bark do not possess the curative powers of the remedy.

While on a trip through the wilds of Florida, Hale observed the great fattening properties of the berries on animals. During summer, food is scanty and the wild animals become very thin, but as soon as the palmetto fruit ripens they improve rapidly. In a few weeks have put on so much fat that they become easy prey. This fat, said Hale, "consists principally of olein and will not make lard."

Dr. Langton said that she gave 5 drop doses four times daily in cases of overworked brain and school-headache for the "tonic, nutritive and stimulating" effect of the remedy. She gives the 1x as soon as relief has been obtained and she finds that the dilution often gives greater relief than the larger doses for the headaches.

Mullins said "I now found the use of the drug in the 3c and 6c potency curative in nearly all of the diseases of the uterus and appendages. Also in headache from reflexes uterine troubles in breast abscess, mental irritations and nervous debility." He thought that it well deserved the name of "The Homeopathic Catheter," but he added that it must be given on its individual indications.

W. E. Rely published three cases illustrating the prostatic action of Sabal. The first, Mr. J., 56, was very despondent, irritable. Sympathy seemed to anger him. Great tenesmus in neck of bladder with heavy, aching pains with sense of coldness extending into external genitals. Occasional sharp pains extending up into abdomen and down into thighs. Capricious appetite. Chronic constipation. Urination too frequent, disturbing sleep.

Sabal tincture was given, five drops, night and morning. Steady improvement followed, and in eight weeks all the symptoms had gone and with them an annoying eczema of the hands.

The second case was Mr. M., 45, who had increasing frequency of urination for a year. Despondent, distressed. Capricious appetite. Vertex headache and gastric catarrh. Little sexual desire. Sex followed by digging pain in back and tenesmus of bladder with difficulty in commencing to urinate.

Genitals were cold, dull aching in region of prostate, extending to abdomen and thighs. Sabal tincture gradually relieved and cured in three weeks.

The third case concerned Mr. E., 35. He had frequent urination for one and a half years. Heavy, dragging pains, extending into back and thighs, back pains much after sex. Considerable loss of prostatic fluid at times. Sexual desire much impeded. Severe headache on vertex and gastric catarrh. All symptoms were removed by Sabal tincture.

Hale said that E. S. Evans of Columbus, Ohio, considered Sabal "almost specific in iritis when the prostate gland in involved. I have cured cases with the 3x which could not be relieved in any other way."

A. L. Davidson related a case of impotence in a man, 51, who had difficult urination, tenderness of prostatic portion of urethra, loss of power. His testicles shrunk, penis shrunk and cold.

Sabal tincture, 15 drops, four times a day, was prescribed. At the end of the first week he complained of drawing pains in spermatic cords, there was freer flow of urine, he slept better and felt better. At the end of the second week the testes gradually increased in size. The urethral tenderness had nearly disappeared and erections were established. In two weeks more the cure was complete, the testes were even larger and firmer than normal.

J. Martin Kershaw of St. Louis, treated a young woman, 23, who had great difficulty in controlling her urine all her life. Undue exertion, lifting, straining, or laughing caused it to dribble away. Unless she rose several times in the night, she was sure to wet the bed. Sabal tincture, one drop, four times a day, was given. In one month she was much improved and under the same remedy she gradually got quite well.

Elias C. Price reported three cases. The first was a case of a very nervous, sensitive woman with chronic inflammation of the bladder, frequent, painful urination, ten to twelve times in the night and every fifteen to thirty minutes during the day. Spells of pressing pain on rectum, better by warm water enemas, which generally brought away hardened feces.

Lil-t. 3x removed this temporarily. Rectal examination disclosed a hard, fleshy tumor the size of half a hen's egg on the posterior aspect of the uterus. Sabal fluid extract 5 drops, thrice daily, diminished the tumor by half in two months and removed it entirely in three more.

Prices' next case was of Mrs. X. who, five days after confinement after her first child, had irritation of kidneys and a week later symptoms of pelvic peritonitis. Her uterus was much enlarged, very tender. She did not urinate very often, but when she did the pain was so excruciating that she fainted away and sometimes did not come to for an hour.

For three days no remedy did any good. Then she had a violent pain on the right side of her head above and behind the ear, and paralysis of her left arm and leg. She became unconscious and could not be aroused, at times would talk of things that had occurred before her illness, insensible to external impressions.

She remained so for ten days. Sabal fluid extract, 20 drops, every two hours, relieved the pain on being raised to urinate after the second dose. Recovery from the other condition was very gradual.

The third case was of Miss X., 22, who had irregular menses for years, having once gone nine months without a period. When she came to Price she was three months past her time, one breast was much smaller than the other.

Sabal fluid extract was given, 5 drops, thrice daily. In about a month the menses came on freely, lasting four days instead of the usual two. Breasts began to increase in size. In three months one was as large as the other. The following year she again missed her time and Sabal brought it right in a week.

Using Sabal, Price has cured cases of pelvic cellulitis, peritonitis, puerperal fever inflammation of uterus, tubes, ovaries and even appendicitis and proctitis, especially if the prostatic gland is involved. Enlarged prostates. Acute prostatitis. Prostate conditions relating to impotence. Prostate cancer (Con.). Frequent urination. Chronic bladder inflammation. Benign prostatic hypertrophy.

Characteristic stinging pains. Wandering, radiating and cramping pains were also prominent. Sabal has several groups of associated regions of pain: pains affecting head and ovary, ovaries and breasts, lower back and right temple, prostate and eye. Mainly used in tincture.

RELATIONS - ***Antidoted by:*** Sil. - Sabal grows on the sandy shore. Puls. delayed menses, Puls. also grows on sandy soils. Sabal. is most fruitful nearest the sea, compare Sil-mar. ***Compare:*** (1) Stinging pains in ovaries, Apis, Merc. (2) Pain in right ovary and thigh, Apis. (3) Breasts painful, Con., Calc. (4) School-headaches, worse by sympathy, Nat-m. (5) Prostatic affections, Ferr-pic., Cham., Arg-n., Dig., Solid. (6) Prostate and eye, Solid. (7) Worse from sex, Kali-c. (8) Wandering pains, Kali-bi. the roots of Sabal. are very rich in potash salts. (9) Over-worked women, Mag-c.

REFERENCES - Boericke. Clarke. Hale. Murphy. Phatak.

SABINA OFFICINALIS

(Savine)

PHARMACY - sabin. Sabina officinalis. Savine. Juniperus sabina. N. O. Coniferae. Cupressaceae. Tincture of the young, fresh tops of the branches. Tincture of the oil. ***Historical dose:*** Tincture and all potencies. Locally, tincture for warts.

CLINICAL - Abortion, effects. After-pains. Boils. Condylomata. Cystitis. ***Dysmenorrhea.*** Fibroids. Gonorrhea. ***Hemorrhages.*** Inter-menstrual, flow. Leucorrhea. ***Menstruation, excessive. Miscarriages.*** Moles. Nephritis. Nymphomania. Ovary, disorders. Penis, swelling. Phimosis. Retained, placenta. Rheumatic, gout. Strangury. Sycosis. Toothache. ***Uterus, bleeding***. ***Warts***.

HOMEOPATHIC - Stapf made the first collection of the symptoms of Sabin., and Hahnemann and his son were among the provers. A number of observations on women who had taken the drug to bring on menses or procure miscarriage have also been added, and some cases of fatal poisoning are recorded.

A close botanical ally of Thuj., Sabin. is not too close to be complementary to that great anti-sycotic. Broad condylomata, fig-warts with much itching and exuberant granulations are characteristic. Like Thuj., it removes wart-like growths from the mucocutaneous surfaces.

Cooper noted that Sabin. acts as a widespread irritant, inflaming the pyloric end of the duodenum and causing patches of inflammation in other portions of the intestines, especially the upper intestines, the omentum and the peritoneum. In addition, it affects the fibrous tissue of small joints, serous membranes and heels.

Pronounced action on the generative organs of both sexes. It produces fig-warts with itching and burning of the external genitals, phimosis of the male, swelling of the dorsum of the penis, and gonorrhea. Uterine hemorrhages, abortion.

Hemorrhages, where blood is fluid and clots together. Hemorrhage is partly pale red and partly clotted, worse from the least motion, but may be better by walking. The flow is in paroxysms and is accompanied by labor-like pains.

Tendency to miscarriage especially at the third month. Warmth ameliorates pain of dysmenorrhea. The dysmenorrhea pains were better lying on flat of back with limbs extended out. Walking ameliorates the metrorrhagia.

Pain from ***the sacrum to the pubis.*** Pain increases suddenly and decreases slowly. Cold applications ameliorates wandering pains in joints. Red, shiny, swelling of affected parts. Acutely inflamed arthritic nodes.

Violent pulsations, wants windows open. Heaviness and indolence of body, wants to lie down. Sense of fullness. Lies on left side during sleep. Sleepless and restless after midnight.

MIND - Dejection, discouragement and sadness. Feeling of deep-seated trouble, which makes him melancholy and sad. Sadness with great tiredness and laziness. Melancholy. Moroseness with dislike to conversation, especially when exercising in open air. Weeping aloud. Desires repose and tranquility. Reserved while walking in open air. Taciturn while waking in morning.

Nervous and hysterical. Great anxiety, fear and apprehension. Irritable nerves. Much irritability of temper. Irascibility with tears and sobs. Listlessness. Weakness of memory. Hypochondriacal mood. Sensitive to slightest noise. Starting from noise. Music goes through bone and marrow. ***Music is intolerable***, it produces nervousness. Distraction from sound of piano.

Abdomen - Tympanitic distention. Congested. Quivering as if something were alive, resembling fetal movements. Bearing-down, constrictive pain. Colic, mostly in hypogastric region.

Back - Paralytic pain in small of back. ***Pain between sacrum and pubis***.

Breasts - Crawling, voluptuous itching in nipples. Stitches in left nipple.

Chest - Pressure on chest. Pressive, spasmodic tension in chest in middle of sternum. Trembling in the lungs with dull rattling and crackling. Lancinations.

Constitutions - Suited to hot-blooded women with gouty or rheumatic diathesis, arthritic pains. For the chronic ailments of women, tendency to miscarriage, hemorrhagic tendency, nosebleeds and hematuria. Farrington said it is suited to "plethoric women who suffer from what they call rheumatic inflammation" of the heels.

Ears - Pinching in ears. Hardness of hearing. Gets deaf when tired, in foggy weather, or at any change of weather.

Eyes - Tensive pain in eyes, as if muscles too short. Heat in eyes. Eyes dull and downcast. Clouds before eyes. Smarting tears. Jerking quivering of lids.

Face - Pale with blue circles around eyes. Black pores in cheeks and around nose. Paralytic pain and pressure in zygomatic process.

Female - Menses, too profuse too early, gushing of hot, watery, ***bright, blood, mixed with dark clots.*** Dysmenorrhea, better lying flat on the back with limbs extended. Bleeding between periods with sexual excitement. Increased desire for sex. Vaginitis. Leucorrhea from suppressed menses or copious menses. Leucorrhea, foul, acrid, thick, yellow. Leucorrhea after menses, corrosive, offensive. Atony of uterus. Uterine pains extend into thighs. ***Pain from sacrum to pubis*** and from below upwards. ***Shooting pain up the vagina***. Uterine hemorrhage, partly clotted, ***worse from least motion***. Bleeding fibroids (Thalspi). Promotes expulsion of moles from uterus (Canth.).Tendency to miscarriage, especially at the third month. Menorrhagia in women who abort readily. Itching of pudenda during pregnancy. ***Retained placenta, intense after-pains.*** Inflammation of ovaries and uterus after childbirth.

Food - Poor appetite. Bitter taste of food, especially milk and coffee. Desire for acids, especially lemonade.

Head - Rush of blood to head and face. Bursting headache, coming suddenly and going slowly. Splitting sensation in forehead and temples. Pulsative headache with heaviness and stupefaction. Drawing pains in masseter muscles.

Heart - Violent pulsation in blood vessels through whole body. Augmented and extended beating of the heart. Pulse unequal, generally quick, strong and hard.

Kidneys - Burning and throbbing in region of kidneys. Bladder inflamed, throbbing. Bladder irritability with gouty diathesis. Inflammation of urethra. Bloody urine with much urging.

Limbs - ***Arthritic pain in joints***. Red, shining swelling. Gouty nodosities (Am-p.). Gout, worse in heated room. Knots and enlargements in varicose veins. Bruised pains in anterior portion of thighs. Shooting in metatarsal bones. Shooting, intermittent aching in the heels. Swelling, redness and stitches in right big toe.

Lungs - Dry, hacking cough and tickling in the trachea. Hemoptysis. Expectoration of mucus streaked with blood.

Male - Burning, sore pain in glans. Prepuce painful with difficulty in retracting it. Sexual desire increased with violent continuous erections. Hard swelling on dorsum of penis. Sycotic warts, growths. Gonorrhea with pus-like discharge.

Modalities - Better from cold, cool open air. Better exhalation. Worse from foggy weather, night. Worse heat, warm air. ***Worse heat of bed*** or room. Worse exertion, stooping, least motion, taking a deep breath. Worse letting limbs hang down. Worse pregnancy, menopause. Worse music. Worse by touch, though better pressure.

Mouth - Drawing pain in the muscles of jaws. Toothache, worse only when chewing. ***Bitter taste*** to food especially milk or coffee.

Nose - Dry coryza.

Rectum - Sense of fullness. ***Pain from back to pubis***. Constipation. Hemorrhoids with bright, red blood, bleed copiously. Hemorrhoids alternate with pain in limbs.

Sensations - As if she would fall. As if parts of temporal eminence were pressed asunder. As if skin had grown fast in forehead. As if eyes would be pressed out. As if tooth would burst. As if he had to swallow over a foreign body. As of a lump in throat. As if vomiting would come on. As if something alive in abdomen. Right shoulder joint as if sprained.

Skin - Black pores in skin, especially face. Foul, itching, burning. Exuberant granulations (Thuj., Nit-ac.). ***Warts***. Fig-warts, moist with intolerable itching and burning.

Sleep - Sleeplessness and restlessness after midnight. Disturbed sleep with frequent waking. Talking and loud snoring during sleep. Tendency to lie on left side when sleeping. Anxious, continued dreams, full of fanciful images and intellectual efforts.

Stomach - Fullness and inflation of region of stomach. Pain from epigastrium to back. Stomachache. Acidity in stomach after a meal. Empty risings and heartburn. Nausea with fullness in stomach. Vomiting of bile or of food eaten the previous day.

Temperature - Intolerable burning heat of whole body, with great restlessness. Great chilliness through the day. Chill in the evening with attacks of chilliness. Fever in evening, first shivering, then heat and lastly perspiration.

Throat - Sore throat during deglutition, as from a foreign body or an internal swelling in gullet, with pressure and choking. Dull lancinations in throat. Dryness in throat with drawing pain.

Vertigo - Vertigo with suppressed menses. Stupefying vertigo, leading to falling, with cloudiness of sight. Giddiness with congestions to and heat in head.

COMMENTS - Characteristic pain from sacrum to pubis. Pains are paroxysmal and labor-like. Pain suddenly increases and then slowly disappears. Wandering pains (Puls.). Numbness, goes through bone and marrow. Inflamed sacrum, or severe aching pains in the sacrum. "Intermittent aching" in the heels.

Tendency to bleed (Phos.). Nosebleed (Phos., Ferr-p.). Tendency to warts, genital warts, venereal warts, and anal warts. Bleeding warts (Nit-ac.). Gonorrhea, or a history of gonorrhea, with genital warts (Thuj.). History of vaginitis with genital warts.

Hemorrhage of bright red blood, with clots (Bell.), comes in gushes. Heavy menstrual bleeding, with swelling, fatigue and headaches, worse motion. Menses too early, too abundant, may last too long. Painful dysmenorrhea with heavy bleeding, pains from the pubic bone back to the sacrum, better lying on the back, limbs extended. Pains can be sharp and stabbing. Bearing down pains. Drawing pains.

Endometriosis (Med.). Pelvic inflammatory disease, with a throbbing uterus. Discharge of blood between the periods with sexual excitement. Bleeding fibroids. Blood streaked leucorrhea. Vaginitis with offensive, irritating, profuse discharge.

Severe morning sickness, spasmodic vomiting. Miscarriages due to spasmodic vomiting. Tendency to miscarriage (Caul., Sep.), usually in the third month (Bell.), with bleeding, passing clots and membranes. Retained placenta (Sec., Caul.). Hemorrhage after an abortion. Postpartum hemorrhage. Severe after-pains.

Hemorrhage during menopause. Pulsating sensation and hot flashes during menopause. Throbbing with hot flashes. Turmoil in the circulation. Hot flashes, worse clothing, wants to take off clothing and fan themselves. Desires fresh air. Irritable and ill humored during menopause. History of being worn out, overworked, with many children. Menopause brought on by a weakened uterus. Varicose veins.

Obscure abdominal pains due to inflammatory states of the peritoneum. Sensation of something alive in the abdomen (Thuj.). Rumbling with indigestion and uterine problems, as if something is kicking or moving. Bleeding hemorrhoids, especially with a history of constipation and uterine problems. Bloody urine.

Irritability, hysteria and hypochondriasis. Discouraged and adverse to conversation. Music is intolerable. Overheats easily, dislikes stuffy rooms. Desires juicy, sour things. Can complain that food tastes too bitter. Generally left sided. Worse at night and from physical contact.

RELATIONS - ***Antidoted by:*** Puls. ***Compare:*** (1) Croc., Calc., Tril., Ip., Mill., Erig. (2) Hir. - the leech. (3) Rosm. (4) Worse by music - Ambr., Thuj., Sep. (5) Inter-menstrual flow, Ham., Ambr. (6) Condylomata, Thuj., Nit-ac. (7) Hemorrhage, worse from least motion, Sec. (8) Menses partly fluid, partly clotted, Ferr. (9) Retained placenta, Caul., Sec. Promotes expulsion of moles or foreign bodies from uterus, Canth. (10) Better in fresh air, desires lemonade, Puls. (11) Clotted hemorrhage, Mill., Plat. is dark, Sabin. bright red. ***Compatible:*** Ars., Bell., Rhus-t., Spong. ***Complementary to:*** Thuj., Nit-ac.

REFERENCES - Boericke. Clarke. Murphy. Phatak.

SACHARINUM

(Sacharin)

PHARMACY - sacchin. Sacharinum. Sacharin. Benzoic sulphinide. Saccharine. Artificial sweetener. ***Historical dose:*** All potencies.

CLINICAL - Allergies. Bladder, cancer. Bladder, tumors. Hypoglycemia. Insomnia.

HOMEOPATHIC - This substance is a derivative of benzoic acid, and is made synthetically from coal-tar. It is a white powder, readily soluble in warm water, but to only a slight extent in cold water.

Saccharin is the foundation for many low-calorie and sugar-free products and is used in table top sweeteners, baked goods, jams, chewing gum, canned fruit, candy, dessert toppings and salad dressings.

Saccharin is about 300 times as sweet as sucrose, but has an unpleasant bitter or metallic aftertaste, especially at high concentrations. Saccharin goes directly through the human digestive system without being digested. It does not affect blood insulin levels, and has effectively no food value.

Saccharin is not recommend for children with "sulfa" allergies, and has been linked to short-term problems with infant muscle tone, "lazy" eye, irritability, and insomnia.

Saccharin has been implicated in the development of photosensitive skin eruptions in humans, and as a hypoglycemic agent in animals. Increased incidences of bladder cancer and tumors have been found in toxicity studies.

RELATIONS - ***Compare:*** (1) Aspart., Sac-alb.

REFERENCES - Murphy.

SACHARUM ALBUM
(Cane Sugar)

PHARMACY - sac-alb. Sacharum album. Cane sugar. Sucrose. Sacharum officinale. White sugar. Sugar cane. N. O. Gramineae. Trituration. Solution. ***Historical dose:*** Tincture and all potencies.

CLINICAL - ***Acidity. Anal, itching***. Anorexia. Aphthae. Ascites. Bilious. ***Blood, sugar.*** Bulimia. ***Cachexia.*** Cataract. Chills. Chlorosis. Constipation. Cornea, opacity. Cramps. Coughs. ***Diabetes.*** Diarrhea. Dropsy. Dyspepsia. Edema. Emaciation. Epilepsy. Fainting. Fatigue. Fever. Gangrene. Gout. Hair, growth. Headache, periodic. Heartburn. Hemorrhoids. Hoarseness. ***Homesickness. Hyperactivity. Hypoglycemia.*** Hysteria. Intermittent, fever. Insomnia. Leg, ulcers. Liver, disorders. ***Malnutrition.*** Migraine. Myocardial, degeneration. Nausea. Neurasthenia. Ophthalmia. Pancreas, disorders. Panaritium. Poisoning. Quinine, effects. Ranula. ***Restlessness.*** Rheumatism. Rickets. Scurvy. Sleeplessness. Spleen, disorders. ***Sugar, effects.*** Tabes mesenterica. Teeth, decay. Ulcers. Vertigo. Vomiting. ***Worms.***

HOMEOPATHIC - According to Hering, a large proportion of chronic diseases of women and children are developed by using too much sugar. Like so many other articles of diet, Sugar may be a poison and a medicine as well as a food. Sugar preserves food, as salt does, and both sugar and salt have produced scurvy.

Cases of scurvy, rickets in bottle-fed children have been traced to excess of sugar in their food and the exclusion of sugar from the dietary of the gouty, rheumatic and the diabetic, shows the pathogenetic power it is credited. Acidity of the stomach and itching at the anus are common effects of taking too much sugar.

Sugar is an antiseptic. Combats infection and putrefaction. It has a solvent action on fibrin and stimulates secretion by the intense osmotic changes induced, thus rinsing out the wound with serum from within outward, favoring healing. Leg ulcers.

Sensitive to pain or ***not sensitive to pain at all. Fainting from pain.*** Fainting on seeing blood. Fainting from a blood puncture. Fainting spells. Plethora. ***Weakness,*** lack of energy. Sudden weakness, ameliorated by eating. Weakness after sweets. ***Physical tension. Waking very early in the morning.***

Extreme ***dryness***, dryness of skin, hair, nails, hands, feet, inside of nose, eyes, mouth, throat, vagina, stool. Tingling in the limbs. Pains in bones from head to foot. Edema of feet.

Cold expectoration. Opacity of cornea. Dim sight. Myocardial degeneration. Headache every seven days. ***Emaciation with great appetite.*** Obesity with compulsive eating, especially sweets, cakes and pastries, potato chips, anything. ***Acidity and anal itching***.

Children who are ***cross, peevish***, whining, capricious. Very aggressive children, often emaciated. Children who want dainty things, tidbits and refuse substantial food. Scurvy, rickets in children. Fat, bloated, large limbed children. Family history of diabetes and cancer.

MIND - ***Discontented*** with himself and with everything. Hard to please. Lack of joy in life, feeling that life is not worth living. Want of childish cheerfulness. ***Sadness, worse after sweets. Loneliness.*** No real feelings of relationship with other people and with life in general. ***Longing and melancholy, as if homesick.***

Lack of love. Possessive love. ***Jealousy, from fear of losing the loved one.*** Fundamental frustration in affection in the past, mostly in early childhood. ***Very uncertain about the love of partner or parents.***

Fear of failure. Sensitive to criticism.

Great need of approbation. ***Ailments from lack of affection***, lack of physical contact in early childhood. Lack of attention. ***Loquacity,*** mostly to have attention. ***Plays antics*** to have attention. ***Forsaken feeling.*** Desire to be held in the mother's arms. Desire to be carried.

Great need to be caressed and touched, or difficulty in admitting this need and refusing every contact. Often a lack of contact with the mother. ***Sucking the fingers or thumb.*** Sucking thumb almost the whole day and during the night, or never sucking the thumb at all. Sucking the thumb until an advanced age. ***Biting nails,*** up to the quick. Biting toenails. ***Touches everything.***

Alternating moods, gentleness alternating with aggression. Peevishness. Melancholic mood with chilliness. ***Capriciousness.*** Low spirited, hypochondriacal mood. ***Restlessness, aggravated after eating sweets.***

Indifference. Disinclined to talk, want of interest. ***Antisocial.*** Thinks he is neglected and placed at a disadvantage. Feels despised. Envious. ***Jealous. Lack of self-confidence. Timidity.*** Increased modesty of women. ***Great modesty.*** Stupidity. ***Irresolution.*** Dainty, cross and whining, indolent.

Anxious. Worries about all sorts of things at night. Fear of fainting, of seeing blood. Fear of falling. Felt afraid to go to bed, ***of the dark***. ***Fear of failure*** (Carc.). Fear of losing beloved persons and parents. Hypochondriacal mood. ***Intense nervousness.*** Jumps from her seat at the least unusual noise. Seems as if she would fly out of her skin.

Irritable, in morning, until breakfast. ***Irritable when hungry, better by eating.*** Offended easily. Cross and fault-finding. Censorious and sarcastic. Bilious sanguineous temperament.

Quarrelsomeness. Violent temper. ***Extremely aggressive***, quarrelsome, violent, malicious and defiant, especially after eating chocolate or sweets. ***Fits of anger, unapproachable.*** Kicks and hits. Ailments from anger. Bad effects from violent anger. Ailments from excitement, stress. ***Fainting from pain.***

Delusion of being persecuted. ***Delusion that her parents don't love her or that she is less loved than her siblings.*** Imagined that her mother wanted to kill her. Imagines that some one is behind her. Feeling that everybody in the world is against him.

Abdomen - Abdomen swollen and enlarged. Abdomen as hard as a stone. Painful hardness of the abdomen. Hard swollen abdomen after scarlet fever. Swelling and induration of the mesenteric glands. Tabes mesenterica. Abdomen shows the presence of water on percussion. Dropsy. Flatulency. ***Pain in the spleen*** (from a blow received a long time ago) and liver. Swelling of the spleen.

Breasts - Atrophy of breasts. Fullness and swelling of breasts before menses. Pain in breasts before menses.

Causations - Sugar. Anger.

Chest - Sharp pains in the left side of the chest. Rheumatic pain in the region of the heart. Fullness in the chest, in the morning and relieved by expectoration of mucus. Swelling of the lower part of the sternum. Emaciation of the chest, the muscles dwindle away.

Constitutions - Bilious, sanguine temperament. Plethoric constitution.

Ears - Discharge of pus from the ears.

Eyes - Dullness of eyes. Dryness. Eyes closed by swelling and inflammation of lids. Varicose distention of vessels of eyes. Ophthalmia. Cataract, opacity of lens. Opacity of cornea. Dimness of the cornea. Dimness of sight. Obscuration of sight. Inflammation of the eyelids. Edematous swelling of the eyelids.

Face - Changed expression of the countenance. Face pale, deathlike. Face bloated, edematous. ***Healthy fresh color of the face.*** Twitching of muscles of right cheek, over malar bone.

Female - Amenorrhea. Menses diminished, scanty. Menses painful, dysmenorrhea. Menstrual pale blood, watery. Painful ovulation and menses. Brown leucorrhea. Suppressed leucorrhea. Complaints before menses including sadness, irritability, swelling and painful breasts (Sep., Carc.). Brown bloody discharge preceding menses. ***Leucorrhea, bloody before menses.*** Dryness of vagina. Increased sexual desire. Swelling of the genitals.

Food - ***Compulsive eating.*** Bulimia with obesity. Ravenous appetite soon after eating with feeling of emptiness in stomach and general weakness. ***Insatiable appetite not ameliorated by eating.*** Morbid hunger with the fever. Anorexia, no feeling of hunger at all at any time, no desire to eat. Little or no appetite in the morning, but insatiable appetite in the evening, especially for sweets. ***Hypoglycemia.*** Has to eat at the normal times, otherwise weak, dizzy, trembling, headache. Tendency to eat frequently between meals. ***Better after eating,*** after breakfast, from sweets. ***Desires sugar, sweets, chocolate,*** pastries and cakes. Desires sweets after dinner and before menses. Desires bread, butter, fat, salt, sour, lemons, mustard. Desires raw vegetables. ***Worse from chocolate, sweets.*** Aversion to sweets, butter, fat, warm milk, warm food, cooked vegetables. Aversion to anything except sweets. ***Thirst for large quantities.*** Thirstlessness. ***Desires licorice.*** Desires cold drinks, especially water, tea, warm milk. ***Desires alcohol.*** Bad effects from spirituous liquors.

Head - Giddiness from indigestion. Migraine. One-sided headache. Headache every week the same day. Severe headache with the chill. Cold in the head. Hair grows rapidly. Perspiration only on the head.

Heart - Myocardial degeneration. Endocarditis. Rheumatic pain in heart region. Weakness of heart. Pulse weak and irregular.

Kidneys - Great pains in kidneys. Sharp burning pains run from kidneys to shoulders, passing under scapulae. Increased urination, strong odor, white sediment. ***Diabetes mellitus. Sugar in urine.*** Urine diminished. Scanty urine.

Limbs - Stiffness. Legs swollen and as hard as a stone. Emaciation, especially of lower limbs. ***Heat of lower limbs, must uncover feet.*** Gouty pains, wandering. Sharp pains. ***Weakness of the legs.*** Tingling in limbs. ***Restlessness of legs.*** Cramps in the calves of the legs. ***Caries on the feet.*** Ulcers on legs. Edematous swelling of the legs, water oozes out from them. Sensation as if water, oozing from legs. Swelling around the ankles. Panaritium. Felon. Nail disorders. ***Edematous swelling of the right arm with stinging***, less painful when uncovering the arm, more painful in the evening and during damp weather. ***Fistulous ulceration of the right forearm with tingling and stitches***, discharge of yellowish thin pus (Bute-j.).

Liver - Pain in liver and spleen. Liver is swollen, indurated. Increased secretion of bile. Hypoglycemia.

Lungs - Breathing oppressed with cold expectoration. Suffocative attacks, must be bolstered up. Can only breathe in an erect position. Respiration difficult, oppressed in the morning, relieved by expectoration. Accumulation of mucus in the lungs. Expectoration with the cough is very offensive. ***Suppressed expectoration is restored.*** Expectoration very fetid, offensive odor. Expectoration white, yellow. Expectoration tastes salty. Expectoration thin, watery, while walking in open air. Dry, loose cough. Cough with children. Pneumonia.

Male - Enormous swelling of scrotum, right genitals. Swelling of the penis. Increased sexual desire. Frequent involuntary emissions.

Modalities - ***Better after eating***, in evening. Dyspnea better in erect position. Worse in early morning, difficulty starting the day. Worse from warm weather. Worse from anger (Staph., Coloc., Cham.). ***Worse sugar, sweets,*** chocolate. Bad effects from spirituous liquors.

Mouth - Dryness of mouth. ***Salivation.*** Inflammation of salivary glands. Inflammation of lining membrane of mouth. ***White coating on tongue, so thick as to cause stiffness in it.*** Cracked, fissured mouth, tongue. Ranula. ***Thrush.*** Aphthae of children. Scorbutic gums. Teeth feel as if on edge. Dullness of teeth with sour vomiting. Scurvy. ***Sucking the fingers or thumb.*** Children put fingers in the mouth. ***Biting nails.***

Nose - Dryness inside nose. Coryza, dry without discharge. Sneezing.

Perspiration - ***Perspiration day and night.*** Profuse sweat at night, especially on head. Sweats on head, neck and shoulders. All perspiration is suppressed.

Rectum - Lump sensation. Dragging and heaviness sensation in rectum. Constipation alternating with mucus diarrhea. Constipation, stools difficult, dry. Diarrhea, stools watery and debilitating. Stools of mucus and blood, bilious. ***Itching at the anus.*** Congested and painful hemorrhoids. ***Hemorrhoids bleed.*** Painful hemorrhoidal tumors. ***Worm affections of children.***

Skin - ***Dryness of skin.*** Chlorosis, after anger, with dropsy. Eruptions, red blotches. Pale red blotches over the body. ***Anasarca after scarlet fever.*** Scurvy. Panaritium. Ulcers. Excessive granulation in the ulcers. Proud flesh in the ulcers. Gangrenous ulcers, cold dry gangrene. Old herpes.

Sleep - Sleeplessness. Starts in sleep. Dreams of dead persons, of falling. Slow to wake up and revive after rising in the morning.

Stomach - ***Acidity of the stomach.*** Disordered stomach. Slow digestion. ***Indigestion, weak with acidity.*** Burning at pit of stomach. Stomach bloated, overloaded with sour mucus. ***Empty, weak, hungry feeling in stomach.*** Painful constriction of stomach. Painful sensitiveness of the pit of the stomach. Coldness or heat in the stomach. ***Gurgling and rumbling noises in stomach.*** Pressure in the stomach in the morning when fasting. Stomach pain with hypochondriacal persons. Nausea early in morning. ***Violent retching and gagging.*** Vomiting of white, viscid tough mucus. Vomiting of blood. Vomiting acid, making teeth dull. Vomiting, occasional with the chill. Periodical vomiting. Vomiting of alcoholics. ***Malnutrition.***

Temperature - Instability of body temperature. Extreme chilliness alternating with heat, especially at night. Chilliness from 10 a.m. until evening with melancholic mood. Chills beginning in lower back, spreading up and down. Chilliness alternates with perspiration. Chill followed by profuse sweat. Intermittent fever every one, two or three days, irregular in its type. Evening fever. Rheumatic fevers. Malignant plague fevers. Suppressed fevers from quinine sulphate. Hot feet, sticks them out of bed, often only one foot. Sticks one or two arms out of bed or sleeps with the upper half of body uncovered.

Throat - Dryness of throat. Dry, rawness in the larynx. Irritation of larynx, causing a slight hacking cough with yellow, salty sputa, which floats on water. ***Ulceration of the larynx.*** Ulcers in throat. Hoarse, catarrhal voice. Hoarseness from reading but a short time.

Vertigo - Fainting attacks. ***Giddiness from indigestion. Harassing giddiness with gout.*** Vertigo with low blood sugar, weakness. Vertigo better after eating. Vertigo while lying down. Vertigo as if sinking down through the bed.

COMMENTS - ***Restlessness, aggravated after eating sweets.*** Running, moving all the time. Restless while sitting. Difficult concentrating, particularly when eating sweets. Very uncertain. Fear of unknown situations (Lyc., Stram.). Sensitive to reprimand, or not sensitive to reprimand at all (Tub.). Impossible to correct.

Alternating moods, gentleness alternating with aggression. Extremely ***aggressive,*** quarrelsome, violent, malicious, and defiant, especially after eating chocolate or sweets. Kicks and hits. ***Fits of anger.*** Insolence. Disobedience. Unapproachable.

Waking early in the morning. Aphthae. Profuse salivation.

To these symptoms have been added others observed by Swan from a patient who accidentally discovered after twenty-five years of suffering, that the cause of his trouble was sugar. All the symptoms disappeared when he abstained from sugar in food or drink and only reappeared when he took it again by way of experiment.

Then from two to four days after taking sugar, the same train of symptoms invariably occurred. Burning at pit of stomach. A white coat on tongue, so thick as to cause stiffness of it. Sharp burning pains run up from head to foot, causing a rigidity of the muscles so that it was impossible to rise from bed until he had been rubbed.

Chill commencing in small of back and spreading up and down. Severe headache and occasional vomiting with the chill. Fever followed with headache, morbid hunger and a hectic flush.

Increased urine, strong odor, white sediment. Great pain in kidneys. Constipation. Sleeplessness. Edema of feet and ankles. Weakness of legs, as if paralyzed, causing staggering. Painful jactitation of feet and legs during the burning in the stomach. Oppression of chest with a cough. Profuse cream-like expectoration, that was very offensive and cold.

Sac-alb. 10,000c and 5,000c cured him of some remaining symptoms and the 41,000c enabled him to eat sugar with impunity.

Swan also reported the case of a woman who was continually eating candies of which she was very fond, until her digestive organs were affected. A few doses of Sac-alb. 30,000c changed her taste so that she ate no more and could not even bear the sight of them.

Farrington traced a great similarity between Sac-alb. and Calc. Sac-alb. is indicated, he said in children who are large-limbed, fat and bloated with a tendency to dropsy.

Sac-alb. has produced opacity of the cornea and ought to cure it. The children are dainty and capricious, care nothing for substantial food, but want little "knick-knacks," always cross and whining and, if old enough, are insolent and do not care to occupy themselves in any way. Everything is too much trouble.

H. C. Allen related a case of opacity of cornea cured with Sac-alb. and with the same remedy in 2,000c potency he cured swelling around the ankles following rheumatism.

According to Lippe, black-and-tan terrier dogs that eat sugar go blind. The cataract and amblyopia of diabetics are well known. Here, again, salt and sugar meet as Burnett has shown in his super salinity of the blood that excess of salt in food has been an important factor in the production of cataract.

Sugar must be considered a sustainer and developer of the musculature of the heart and hence useful in failure of compensation and a variety of cardio-vascular troubles. It acts as a nutrient and tonic in wasting disorders, anemia, neurasthenia, etc. increasing weight and power.

One ounce of lump sugar morning and evening valuable adjunct in the treatment of obstinate cases of heart failure due to deficient heart muscle without valvular lesion. Epilepsy, blood with reduced sugar content irritates the nervous system with tending to convulsions.

Sugar as an oxytocic has its most suitable application toward the end of labor when there is no mechanical obstruction and delay is due to uterine inertia. 25 grams dissolved in water, several times every half hour.

RELATIONS - ***Compare:*** (1) Sac-l., (2) Sacchin - hinders both the salivary and peptic ferment actions with consequent dyspepsia. Prof. Lewin believes its action to be on the secretory cells themselves and it has caused pain, (right hypogastrium), loss of appetite, diarrhea and wasting. (3) Arg-n., Lyc., Sulph. - craving for sweets. (4) Sil. - rickets. (5) Arg-n. - diabetes, swollen ankles, (6) Santa. - Kidney ache.

REFERENCES - Boericke. Clarke. Lippe. Smits. Swan.

SACHARUM LACTIS

(Milk Sugar)

PHARMACY - sac-l. Sacharum lactis. Milk sugar. Lactose. ***Historical dose:*** All potencies.

CLINICAL - Amblyopia. Angina pectoris. Body, odor. Diabetes. Dyspepsia. Earache. Gout. Headache. Hysteria. Labia, soreness. Nervousness. Neuralgia. Ovaries disorders. Over-exertion. Ptosis. Sciatica. Sighing. Styes. Umbilicus inflammation.

HOMEOPATHIC - Hahnemann chose globules of Sacharum lactis as the chief vehicle of his remedies because he considered it the most inert substance he could find. But his method of attenuating remedies had shown that no substance is inert in potencies and experience shows that no substance is absolutely inert in any form.

Sac-l. in large doses develops the bacillus acidophilus to correct putrefactive intestinal conditions and also constipation. Diuresis. Amblyopia.

Sensitive in every part of body. Small shooting pains all over in morning. Throbbing in parts of body. ***Cold pains,*** as if produced by fine, icy cold needle with tingling, as if frost bitten. ***Great physical exhaustion and weakness, caused by overwork.*** Prostration from mental excitement.

MIND - Extremely nervous, jumps from her seat at least unusual noise. Sudden fear and trembling of whole body, as from fright. Sarcastic and fault-finding, could not speak a pleasant word to any one. Laziness.

Longing and melancholy as if homesick, with oppressed breathing. Her heart aches as if it would burst, yet she cannot weep. Fear of death during pain in heart. Hysteria in evening, laughing and crying, jumping up and lying down.

Sensation as if she were kept together by a great effort. Loses her way in well-known streets. Imagines that there is a large hole in her back just above sacrum, that her mother wants to kill her, that some one is behind her.

Abdomen - Sore to touch, painful from the jar caused by walking. Severe pain passing through abdomen during stool. Sharp pain passing across bowels just above navel and all around body. Pain in left hypochondrium passing under left breast. Pain above left hip, which would come when leaning back, followed by severe pain in forehead.

Back - Dull ache all over back and in right arm. Backaches the whole length of spine. Pain passing up and down along right side of neck. Hot flashes all over back of neck and shoulders. Pain with soreness at upper right scapula. Pain in sacral region, worse when taking a breath. Pain passing up back from sacrum. Pain in lumbar region, worse by leaning backward.

Breasts - Sharp pain into right breast, very sore to touch. Constant pain under left breast, worse when bending forward. Severe pains under left breast at every inspiration.

Causations - Mental excitement. Over-fatigue.

Chest - Feeling as if ulcerated over right short ribs, worse from touch and when stooping. Pain in axilla.

Ears - Pain in right ear and underneath it. Painfulness of right external ear with burning like an ulcer, also when touched. Pain passing from right ear to shoulder. Pain from right ear to lower part of inferior maxillary bone. Pain in left ear and sensation as if there were a gathering. Shooting pains in and behind ears and all over face. Pains in external ears and behind them. Reverberation of voice when speaking. Buzzing sound in right ear. Sensation as if she could not hear, but she could.

Eyes - Pain through right eye inwards. Sensation as if needles were sticking in eyes. Dryness of eyeball so that the lid would stick to it. Looking at bright light dazzles and makes her close eyes, no pain. Sight fails, eyes tire very easily. Styes. Swelling of right upper lid. Can only elevate upper lids half way.

Face - Sad expression of face, eyes look as from weeping, though she has not wept. Wretched appearance. Great pallor of face with dark places under eyes. Burning in cheekbones towards temples and lower jaw. Pain passing from corner of mouth of forepart of right axilla. Pain all over face, then centering in right ear. Corners of mouth, chin smart and burn.

Female - Menses commenced too early, no pain. Menses very dark. Profuse greenish-yellow leucorrhea. Bloody leucorrhea. Soreness and rawness of labia with profuse greenish-yellow leucorrhea. Itching of labia. Lobulated growths on each side of vagina, extremely sore and sensitive to touch. Pain in region of right ovary. Ovarian region very weak and painful when walking. Dragging-down sensation in pelvic region.

Food - Hungry all the time. When first getting out of bed feels faint for something to eat. Desire for dainties. Feeling of distention after eating. Great thirst, wanted large quantities of very cold water.

Head - Sharp pains behind right ear. Pain in left eyebrow. Left temple sore to touch. Burning like fire, extending from right frontal eminence to vertex. Sensation as of pressure on frontal bone at inner canthi of left eye, felt very sore. Sharp darting pain on left side of head from temple to occiput. Forehead feels very heavy with a tendency to fall forward. Sharp pain in forehead from one temple to the other. Head feels large and as though all the blood in the body had gone into the head. Head feels confused and as if it were tossing on a rough sea.

Heart - Sensation as if a fire in heart. Feeling as if heart would burst. Awoke at midnight with severe numb pains about heart, great fear of death, when the pains passed off they left great soreness around heart. Pulse intermittent.

Kidneys - Constant pain in region of left kidney. Soreness of urethra during urination. Constant, urgent desire to urinate with cutting pain up urethra. Sound of running water produced urination, no power to restrain it. Involuntary urination during night. Urinates large quantities very frequently. Urine causes intense pain when coming in contact with the labia, which are very sensitive. Urination followed by a thick yellow discharge. Urine stains a dark yellow.

Limbs - Pain from right shoulder passing down to waist. Pain from right shoulder to left breast. Pain in forepart of right upper arm. Pain in right wrist. Pain, itching in palm of right hand. Grasping anything with right hand causes pains to pass from all the fingers into palm. Sharp pain in all right fingers except little finger. Skin under nails looks dirty. Awful pain extending down the right sciatic nerve. Pains in thighs and hips. Hot flashes in lower limbs. Pain in right instep when bending foot. Pain like gout in right toe. Balls of feet covered with little corns, which are very painful when walking.

Modalities - Worse by a coming storm, the approach of which was felt some twelve hours previously. Pains, worse in damp room or basement, but better if there was a fire. All symptoms better after 4 p.m. Worse by blue and yellow colors, better by red.

Mouth - Burning in whole mouth. Sensation of coolness as of ice in mouth and throat. Roof of mouth sore. Soreness like blisters in mouth and on tongue. Sore on left side of tongue. Tongue, coated white, yellow. Taste, putrid in mouth after eating or fine spicy taste like fresh nuts. Thick bitter mucus in mouth during morning. Lips feel very sore, raw and dry with great thirst.

Nose - Pain in sides, end of nose. Ridge of nose extremely sore, it feels sore to touch or from the least movement of facial muscles, the left side is the worst and somewhat swollen.

Rectum - Stool preceded by shooting pains across abdomen, which are better by stool. Before stool, pains in breasts and upper abdomen. Urgent inclination to stool, felt as though there were a great ball in rectum, much straining and some flatulence, but no stool and not better from the flatulence. Stools smell like rotten eggs. Soreness around anus, extending up rectum. Creeping, itching and crawling around anus, extending inside rectum. Shooting pains in rectum.

Skin - Very restless at night from itching all over body as soon as she is covered in bed. Itching of both shoulders.

Sleep - Yawning all day. Sleeplessness after midnight. Cannot sleep on right side. Cannot go to sleep without putting arms over head. Impossible to lie straight in bed, finds herself continually lying diagonally across bed. Has to lie on left side. Fatiguing dreams all night. Awoke with the impression that she had dreamed of dreadful pains in chest, does not know whether it was a dream or a reality.

Stomach - Pressure in stomach as if she had eaten something indigestible. Dyspepsia after eating hot pie-crust. Heartburn with sweet taste coming from stomach without water brash. Violent sickness, going on all day. Nausea does not affect appetite. Nausea like seasickness.

Temperature - Great coldness as if a chill were coming on. Fingers, feet toes, icy cold, could not keep warm in bed covered with clothes. Hot flashes inside body pressing from below upward. Feeling of heat all over, the body is covered with a light sweat, enough to feel uncomfortable. Strange restlessness at night.

Throat - Spasmodic stricture in esophagus. Globus hystericus after lunch at noon with dull, sick headache. Throat very sensitive to external pressure, the least pressure causes a feeling as if she were choking. Sensation when swallowing as of a fish-bone in throat.

COMMENTS - Swan is the authority for Sac-l. as a homeopathic remedy. He published a full pathogenesis of Sac-l., proved in the potencies from 30c upward, together with confirmed and cured symptoms.

One of Swan's provers had the symptom "Sight fails, eyes tire very easily." Another patient, when taking pilules of Sac-l. three times a day complained that they made his "eyes ache and feel weak."

Sensations of both coldness and heat. One of the cold sensations is "Sensation of extreme cold passing in a fine line from center of pubes to a point two or three inches above."

Swan regarded cold pains as a keynote and recorded the case of Mr. S., who had an excessively cold neuralgic pain in the cartilage of both ears, the right being the worst with tingling as if frost-bitten, rubbing with difficulty restored the warmth.

Lancinating, neuralgic pains in forehead in occiput, extending from region above ears down through ears into muscles of neck in both eyes, worse by least breath of air, skin sensitive to touch as in inflammatory rheumatism.

These pains were icy cold, as if produced by an extremely fine ice-cold needle. As Sac-l. has "fine cold pains" and pains passing in all directions, Sac-l. 1,000c was given and relieved all the pains within an hour.

H. A. Hare said of Sac-l., "Scientific and clinical studies have shown it to be possessed of very great diuretic powers when given in full doses."

He said further, that its direct action on the kidneys and its slight action elsewhere indicate it in kidney dropsy and kidney inactivity, that it acts best in cases where albuminuria is absent and that it causes profuse diuresis in infants fed on it.

RELATIONS - Camph. aggravates the effects of Sac-1. ***Compare:*** (1) Sac-alb. in rickets, acidity, fat children, Calc., the Lacs. (2) Right cheekbone, Mag-c. (3) Roof of mouth, Mang. (4) Ball sensation in rectum pains, Kali-bi. (5) Kidney ache, Santa, Sacchin. (6) Fatigue, Pic-ac., Mag-c. (7) Heat in heart, Lachn. (8) better lying on left side, Lil-t. (9) worse from damp, Dulc. (10) Sensitiveness, Kali-i. Mag-c.

REFERENCES - Boericke. Clarke.

SALICYLICUM ACIDUM

(Salicylic Acid)

PHARMACY - sal-ac. Salicylicum acidum. Salicylic acid. Acetylsalicylicum acidum. Found in spiraea blossoms, Gaultheria. Prepared from Phenol. Trituration. ***Historical dose:*** Trituration and all potencies.

CLINICAL - ***Arthritis. Belching.*** Bone, decay. ***Canker sores.*** Colds. Colitis. Coryza. Deafness. Diarrhea. Diphtheria. Dyspepsia. ***Flatulence.*** Foot-sweat, suppression. Gastritis. Hematuria. Hot flashes. Influenza. Intestine ulceration. Iritis. Melancholy. ***Meniere's disease.*** Menopausal. Necrosis. Pharyngitis, herpetic. Puerperal fever. Purpura. ***Rheumatism. Rheumatoid arthritis.*** Scarlatina. Sciatica. Septicemia. Stomatitis. Tapeworm. Throat, sore. ***Tinnitus.*** Ulcers. Urticaria. Vertigo.

HOMEOPATHIC - Salicylic acid is found in nature in the leaves and barks of willows and in wintergreen oil (Gaultheria), which is one of the chief sources of its supply, and is obtained synthetically from carbolic acid. Like Carb-ac. it has been largely used as a disinfectant, and, as it is supposed to be non-poisonous, it is used for mixing with and so preserving foods.

MacLagan of London and Senator of Berlin, introduced it into medicine as a remedy for rheumatism. It has a specific relation to rheumatism, but the massive doses given in allopathic practice have been attended with so many unpleasant symptoms of vital depression, fainting, flatulent dyspepsia and delirium.

Overdoses led to the discovery of its power to set up Meniere's disease, auditory nerve vertigo, gastric disturbances and delirium. Roaring and ringing in the ears. Deafness with vertigo. Prostration after influenza, also tinnitus aurium and deafness. Hematuria. Effects of suppressed foot sweats.

MIND - Melancholy, wants to be quiet, feels faint. Anxiety, worrying, restless. Excited mood. Maniacal exaltation. Talked incessantly and disconnected. Mistakes in speaking and writing. Awkwardness, drops things, bumps into things. Delirium, stupid, can hardly collect his ideas, then laughed without cause.

Abdomen - Abdominal distention. Violent, constant pressure in abdomen with feeling of incarcerated flatus. Ulceration of bowels.

Chest - Spasmodic, flatulent asthma, fetid bronchitis, gangrene of lungs. Firmly seated pressure at side of sternum as large as the hand, with feeling as if the bone was sore.

Causations - Suppression of foot-sweat. Aspirin overdose.

Ears - Meniere's disease. ***Tinnitus,*** dependent on hyperemia. ***Roaring and ringing in ears***, hears music, swarm of bees or buzzing of flies. Auditory nerve vertigo with a troublesome nausea accompanying the head symptoms. Hearing diminished. Nervous deafness. Deafness with noises in ears, with vertigo.

Eyes - Retinal hemorrhage. Retinitis after influenza, also albuminuric. Plastic iritis following acute rheumatism. Diminished acuteness of vision.

Face - Dull, heavy aspect, face flushes quickly on slight excitement.

Female - Leuco-phlegmatic woman, frequent hot flashes with irritability, forgetfulness, dull, heavy pain in cerebellum. Septic puerperal fever.

Head - Piercing pain in temples. Headache commencing on top or back of head, running down neck, which is tender to touch. Headache, confusion in head on rising suddenly. Dullness of head, stupefaction. Rush of blood to head. Buzzing sensation in the brain as if blood were forced violently through a contracted vessel.

Kidneys - Diabetes mellitus. Albuminuria, rheumatic diathesis. Urine scanty, clear, brown.

Limbs - ***Arthritis and rheumatism.*** Acute joint rheumatism, worse touch and motion, profuse sweat. Pain shifts. Sciatica, burning pain, worse at night. Knees are swollen and painful. Copious foot-sweat and ill effects if sweat is suppressed.

Lungs - Respiration hurried. Spasmodic, flatulent asthma, fetid bronchitis, gangrene of lungs. Dry cough of a hard, racking, spasmodic character, worse at night, in old people.

Modalities - Better by hot applications, especially by dry heat. Worse by motion. Worse at night, cold air, touch of anything cold.

Mouth - Taste extremely disgusting, as of something burnt, bitter. Burning, scalded feeling. Burning and scraping in mouth and throat. Redness of mouth and fauces. Mouth dotted with white patches. ***Canker sores*** with burning soreness and fetid breath. Tongue purplish, leaden-colored, foul breath. Ulcers on tip of tongue. Stomatitis, mouth hot and dry, tongue covered with burning vesicles.

Nose - Sneezing. Coryza. Incipient catarrh, patients, especially children, sneeze all day.

Rectum - Putrid diarrhea, gastro-intestinal derangements, especially in children, stools like green frog's spawn (Mag-c.). Stools green, flushes easily as in hectic, acid, sour, or putrid smelling. Cholera infantum with peculiarly putrid belchings. Worms. Pruritus ani.

Skin - Hot and burning skin. Itching vesicles and pustules, better by scratching. Skin red and sensitive, points like flea-bites. Urticaria. Herpes zoster. Purpura. Necrosis and softening of bones.

Sleep - Yawning. Dreams of being pregnant. Frequently awakens from sleep thinking he heard music.

Stomach - Weak, nervous sensation in stomach. Burning in epigastric region. Erosions and ulcers in stomach and bowels. ***Putrid fermentation and dyspepsia***. Water brash. ***Flatulence, hot, sour belching***. Gagging, frequent vomiting.

Temperature - Slight chill, crawling in spine, yawning, chill in fingertips. Fever continuous, burning, then sweat with relief, fever again till exacerbation of symptoms. Weak, faint after fever and sweat. Flushes easily as in hectic. Profuse sweat, as sweat increased strength declined.

Throat - Burning in throat. Sore, red and swollen. Tonsils red, swollen, studded white. Scraping in throat causing cough. Hemorrhagic pharyngitis with difficulty of swallowing.

Vertigo - Vertigo, tendency to fall to left side. Deafness with vertigo. Meniere's disease.

COMMENTS - Sal-ac. has been notably used for corns and warts, as well as to hasten the peeling of palms and soles after scarlet fever.

Brunton noted that "A mixture of 2 parts with 100 of tallow, applied directly to the feet, not to the stockings, has been found most useful in preventing sweating and soreness of the feet in soldiers after a long march."

Sal-ac. has had an accidental proving which has led to some homeopathic uses, including blood-poisoning conditions, such as puerperal fever and septicemia. Like carbolic acid and other disinfectants, Sal-ac. produces fermentative dyspepsia and diarrhea with putrid-smelling stools. Disorders following suppressions of foot sweat.

RELATIONS - ***Compare:*** (1) Nat-sal., Salol. (2) in rheumatism and subsequent weakness, Colch. (3) Piercing in temples, throat, diarrhea, ulcers, anti-septic properties, Kreos. (4) In anti-septic properties, dyspepsia, fever, urine, Carb-ac. (5) Tinnitus, Nat-sal., Chin., Chin-s., Carb-s. (6) Bones, Phos. (and throat), Lac-ac. (7) As if blood forced through contracted vessel, Coc-c. (8) Foot-sweat and suppressed foot-sweat, Sulph. Sil. (9) Loquacity, Lach.

REFERENCES - Boericke. Clarke. Phatak.

SALIX MOLLISSIMA

PHARMACY - salx-m. Salix mollissima. N. O. Salicaceae. Tincture of fresh leaves and young shoots. ***Historical dose:*** Tincture and all potencies.

CLINICAL - Neuritis. Rheumatism. Sciatica.

HOMEOPATHIC - Cooper used Salx-m. with success in rheumatic affections, especially in sciatic neuritis in nervous subjects in whom the capillary cutaneous circulation showed up visibly and there was some tenderness and swelling of the limb.

REFERENCES - Clarke.

SALIX NIGRA

(Black Willow Bark)

PHARMACY - salx-n. Salix nigra. Black willow bark. Pussy willow. N. O. Salicaceae. Tincture of fresh tree bark. ***Historical dose:*** Tincture and all potencies.

CLINICAL - Diarrhea. Emissions. Fevers. Gonorrhea. Impotence. Masturbation. Night-sweats. ***Nymphomania.*** Prostatitis. Satyriasis. Sexual mania. Spermatorrhea.

HERBAL - The black willow of North America has a reputation as a purgative and febrifuge. Salx-n. has been largely used by herbalists in a great variety of disorders of the genito-urinary system.

HOMEOPATHIC - A proving by E. D. Wright, who took half an ounce of the tincture in a day, is given in Allen's Appendix. He developed soreness of muscles, a tired, sleepy state, loose bowels, sore gums and fever.

Salx-n. has a positive action on the generative organs of both sexes. It reduces the irritability of sexual organs, moderates sexual passion, and controls genital irritability. It has been used after a history of masturbation or spermatorrhea.

Acute gonorrhea with much erotic trouble, chordee. Satyriasis and sexual mania. Libidinous thoughts and lascivious dreams. Seminal emissions in presence of woman or when talking with her. Hysteria and nervousness.

Back - Pain across sacral and lumbar region. Unable to step out quickly.

Face - Red, swollen, especially the end of nose. Nosebleed. Eyes blood-shot, sore to touch and on motion. Roots of hair hurt.

Female - Before and during menses much nervous disturbance, pain in ovaries, difficult menstruation. Menorrhagia. Bleeding with uterine fibroid. Ovarian congestion and neuralgia. Nymphomania.

Head - Skin on temples sore to touch.

Male - Painful movement of the testicles.

Mouth - Gums sore.

Rectum - Looseness of bowels.

Sleep - Disposition to lie down and sleep.

COMMENTS - Dr. John Fearns wrote of the tonic and anti-septic properties of this species of Salix, but also of its usefulness as a sedative to the generative system. As a sedative on these lines he had very goods results from its use.

Fearns gave Salx-n. in doses of thirty to sixty drops on retiring and repeated at midnight or towards morning, if needed. He found it particularly useful in cases of acute gonorrhea with much erotic trouble, chordee with great irritation, and excessive sexual desire, amounting to satyriasis.

Salx-n. seems to control the venereal appetite in a very satisfactory manner. It can be given in cases where the bromides have always been considered appropriate and it can be given where the bromides would be very inappropriate and there is no reflex effect on the brain or nervous system.

W. B. McCoy related a number of cases illustrating this action. The first concerned a man, 35, who lost control of his sexual appetite. The more he indulged the worse the craving became, and indulgence made him a physical wreck. Salx-n. tincture in teaspoonful doses thrice daily, cured in five weeks.

The second case concerned a youth, 23, who had masturbated since he was a boy. Salx-n. tincture, 20 drops, four times a day, was given for a fortnight, the quantity being gradually diminished, until in a few weeks the young man was quite cured.

A teacher, 21, five years before had a spell of fever which left him with a tendency to seminal emissions which had become very frequent and had reduced him to a very low condition. Extremely thin, sallow, nervous. Cold hands and feet even in heat of summer. Extremely cross and irritable.

Salx-n. tincture, 1c one drop four times a day, was given with speedy improvement. Later on the dose was reduced to thirty drops. The losses ceased and in three months the patient had gained 41 pounds in weight.

A man, 53, had sexual desire but without ability, yet during the night he would have emissions without erections. Salx-n. tincture, 15 drops, four times a day, cured in three weeks.

McCoy also used Salx-n. successfully in gonorrhea, but other remedies were given as well.

RELATIONS - ***Compare:*** (1) Dam., Yohim., Canth., Con., Agn., Pic-ac. (2) In gonorrhea, Salol, Petros. (3) Aven., Sabal.

REFERENCES - Anshutz. Boericke. Clarke. Phatak.

SALIX PURPUREA

(Purple Willow)

PHARMACY - salx-p. Salix purpurea. Purple willow. Red willow. N. O. Salicaceae. Tincture or infusion of fresh bark. ***Historical dose:*** Tincture and all potencies.

CLINICAL - Diarrhea. Fever. Parotiditis. Vertigo.

HOMEOPATHIC – T. C. Duncan and his wife proved Salx-p., taking drachm doses of the infusion of the bark. The chief symptoms were giddiness, loose stools, swelling of the right parotid gland. Fever, marked by heat preceding chill and perspiration.

Duncan chewed the bark on one occasion and this caused the astringent effect on the mucus membrane of the mouth. The only rheumatic symptom was aching in right acetabulum.

MIND - Very nervous, irritable and despondent all day. Dullness of intellect.

Abdomen - Pain in abdomen. Flatulence.

Face - Swelling of right parotid gland.

Head - In a few minutes dizzy feeling commencing just in front of ears and passing up to vertex like a wave, compelled to sit down.

Heart - Pulse feeble, circulation torpid.

Kidneys - Urine slightly acid, excess of phosphates and epithelium, less uric acid crystals.

Limbs - Aching in right acetabulum.

Mouth - Peculiar astringent taste, puckering mucus membrane and closing Steno's duct. Taste of undigested food.

Rectum - Bowels loose, two stools in one day with griping.

Sleep - Rested poorly, woke often, first too hot, then too chilly.

Temperature - First too hot, then chilly and at last towards morning in a profuse perspiration.

REFERENCES - Clarke.

SALMONELLA TYPHI

(Salmonella Nosode)

PHARMACY - salm-t. Salmonella typhi. Salmonella nosode. Bacteria. ***Historical dose:*** All potencies.

CLINICAL – Cholecystitis. Dehydration. Diarrhea. Enteritis. Fever. ***Food poisoning. Gastroenteritis.*** Heartburn. Nausea. Pancreatitis. Salmonellosis. Typhoid fever. Ulcers. Vomiting.

HOMEOPATHIC – The attenuations of this bacteria nosode are prepared from washings of a culture of Salmonella typhi. Disease-causing salmonellae have recently been re-classified into a single species, Salmonella enterica, which has numerous strains. Salmonella typhi is a well-known strain that causes typhoid fever.

Other salmonellae are frequent causes of food-borne illness, especially in poultry and raw eggs, and more generally from food that has been cooked or frozen, and not eaten straight away.

The acute symptoms of salmonella gastroenteritis include the sudden onset of nausea, abdominal cramping, and bloody diarrhea with mucus. The onset of symptoms usually occurs within 6 to 72 hours after the ingestion of the bacteria.

Salmonella infections usually resolve in five to seven days, and often require no treatment, unless the patient becomes severely dehydrated or the infection spreads from the intestines. Persons with severe diarrhea may require rehydration, often with intravenous fluids.

Some salmonella bacteria have become resistant to antibiotics, however, and this has occurred possibly as a result of the use of antibiotics to promote the growth of feed animals.

Confusion and mental vagueness, e.g. in cerebral degeneration. Highly febrile illnesses. Enteritis. History of intestinal infections or acute inflammatory fever. Chronic cholangitis and cholecystitis. Cholelithiasis. Duodenal and gastric ulcer. Chronic pancreatitis.

RELATIONS – ***Compare:*** Ars., Echi., Pyrog.

REFERENCES – Murphy. Reckeweg.

SALOL

(Phenol Salicylate)

PHARMACY - salol. Salol. Phenol salicylate. Salolum. Trituration. ***Historical dose:*** All potencies.

CLINICAL - Arthritis. Diarrhea. Dysentery. Fever. Gonorrhea. Headaches. Influenza. Neuralgia. Rheumatism. Smallpox.

HOMEOPATHIC - Salol. was primarily used as an anti-rheumatic, especially in the treatment of acute cases. It was given as an antipyretic in 30 to 45 grain doses in powders or tablets. It is soluble in ether and petroleum spirit, very sparingly, if at all in water.

It does not disturb digestion because it passes through the stomach unaltered, being decomposed in the duodenum, by the ferments of the pancreas into salicylic acid and phenol (it contains 38 percent phenol).

These are excreted by the kidneys and the condition of intestinal digestion has been estimated by the length of time required after the ingestion of Salol., for them to appear in the urine.

Helbing reported that it has been used in acute diarrhea, dysentery, cholera and other diseases where intestinal asepsis in indicated and also in disorders of the bladder and urethra as a substitute for ordinary mechanical irrigations and injections.

Its internal use in gonorrhea (in 5-grain doses three times a day) has met with much success.

Dull aching in head and all over body. Can hardly go up stairs, and it is dreadfully painful to sit on a hard stool. The hands shrink when cold, cannot straighten the little fingers without much pain.

Head - Dreadful headache, especially over eyes. Dull aching in head and all over body.

Kidneys - Urine smelled strongly of violets.

Limbs - Rheumatic pains. Feeling of stiffness in joints. Limbs sensitive to touch. Pain in shoulder. Pain in right arm in evening. Pain in wrists. Cramp in hand on writing. Hurts even to carry a book in hand. Buttocks sore. Pain in left buttock, especially on walking.

Modalities - Worse walking, raising eyes, ascending stairs. Pain in buttocks worse sitting on hard stool. Worse by touch, in evening.

Skin - Burning and itching eruption. Smallpox.

COMMENTS - The only proving of Salol. was made incidentally on a chemist from making up powders of the remedy. He experienced very severe symptoms from inhaling the odor, and possible also some of the powder. Rheumatic pains in joints with soreness and stiffness were marked, especially pain and soreness in the buttocks, knees, and wrists.

The prover was subject to headaches, but he never had so violent a headache as that produced by Salol. and conversely after the proving, Salol. 12c immediately relieved him when threatened with one of his usual headaches.

The first symptom he noted was that his urine smelled of violets and it was only when this passed off that the other symptoms came on. The joints felt stiff, "as if they wanted oiling."

C. Beg referred to the use of Salol. in smallpox and other skin disorders attended with burning and itching. The relief of itching in smallpox was a constant and most satisfactory result. When administered early it prevented maturation of pustules.

RELATIONS - ***Antidoted by:*** Bry. ***Compare:*** (1) Sal-ac., Salin.., Nat-sal., Carb-ac. (2) Wrist rheumatism, Act-sp., Led., Viol-o. (3) Urine smells of violets, Terebe. (4) Gonorrhea, Napht., Petros. (5) Smallpox, Carb-ac., Sarr., Vario.

REFERENCES - Clarke.

SALVIA DIVINORUM

(Shepherdess's Herb)

PHARMACY - salv-d. Salvia divinorum. Shepherdess's herb. Ska pastora. Shka pastora. Maria pastora. Mexican mint. Yerba de Maria. N. O. Lamiaceae. Tincture of fresh leaves and blossom-tips. ***Historical dose:*** Tincture and all potencies.

CLINICAL - Amnesia. Ascites. Debility. ***Delusions.*** Depression. Diarrhea. Drug, addictions. Edema. Headache. Intoxication. ***Memory, loss.*** Nightmares. Panic attacks. Personality, disorders. Rheumatism. Visions.

HERBAL - The Latin name Salvia divinorum literally translates to "sage of the seers." The genus name Salvia is derived from the Latin salvare, meaning "to heal" or "to save." The words salvation and savior also come from this root.

Salvia divinorum is a sprawling perennial herb which grows wild only in the Sierra Mazatec region of Mexico. Its leaves contain the extremely potent salvinorin-A. It has a history of use as a divinatory psychedelic for oral use and has been widely available since the 1990's primarily as a smoked herb.

Salvia divinorum is traditionally used by chewing pairs of leaves. Modern use includes both smoking and chewing the leaves. When the leaves are chewed, the quid and bitter juice are held in the mouth to increase absorption.

Strong effects can be difficult to attain from smoking dried leaf, but extracts and potency-bred leaves can cause dramatic, sometimes frightening deep mind-states. Many people who try S. divinorum do not find the effects at all pleasant and choose not to repeat the experience.

Historical uses include headache, diarrhea, rheumatism, debilitation and ascites. Intense shaking of body. Inability to control muscles and maintain balance. Tendency to stagger, fall. Depression. May prove to be useful for those troubled with addictions.

MIND - Altered perceptions. Clarity of thought. Introspection. Insights into life and existence. Trances and visionary states of intoxication. Dreamlike experiences. Powerful visions with open or closed eyes. Visions of past lives and times. Feels the presence of entities. ***Delusions and visions.***

States of tranquility and ecstasy. Great relaxation and bliss. Uncontrollable hysterical laughter. ***Restlessness.*** Panic attacks. ***Intense experiences of fear, terror and panic.*** Speechless. Complete loss of memory.

Overlapping realities. The perception that one is in several locations at once. Feel detached from reality with a heightened senses of space, sight smell and sound. ***Loss of the body and personal identity.***

Sensation of dying. Near death experiences. ***Out of body experiences.*** Sensation of entering or perceiving other dimensions, alternate realities. Revisiting places from the past, especially childhood.

Back - Prickling and tingling up and down the spine.

Perspiration - Increased perspiration.

Sensations - Sensation of pins and needles all over my body. Prickling and tingling. ***Sensation that the body becomes suddenly very heavy***. Sensations of physical push, pressure, or wind. Various sensations of motion, or being pulled or twisted by forces of some kind.

Temperature - Change in body temperature, flushing.

COMMENTS - One person wrote, "For the next two hours I felt light headed and restless. I couldn't sit still. Whenever I sat down I felt compelled to get up. I tried to eat something and drink a little wine in order to get grounded and relaxed, but I couldn't seem to swallow anything. I had been shaken to the soul."

RELATIONS - ***Compare:*** (1) Anh., Bani-c., Cann-i., Op.

REFERENCES - Murphy.

SALVIA OFFICINALIS

(Common Sage)

PHARMACY - salv. Salvia officinalis. Common Sage. N. O. Lamiaceae. Tincture of fresh leaves and blossom-tips. ***Historical dose:*** Tincture and all potencies.

CLINICAL - Cough, tickling. Fever. Gums, bleeds. Mouth, sores. ***Night-sweats. Perspiration, excessive.*** Tuberculosis.

HERBAL - Gerard wrote, "Sage is singularly good for the head and brain, it quickened the senses and memory. Sage strengthen the sinews, restore health to those that have palsy and take away shaky trembling of the members."

French doctors called attention to sage for gargling in cases of inflammation of the throat and for washing the mouth in disorders of the gums.

HOMEOPATHIC - Salv. exerts a tonic influence on the skin. Controls excessive sweating when circulation is enfeebled. ***Night-sweats*** in persons suffering from disorders of the respiratory organs, especially tuberculosis. ***Colliquative perspiration.*** Soft skin, relaxed with enfeebled circulation and cold limbs. Suffocating, tickling cough. Galactorrhea.

COMMENTS - Salv. should be given in doses of 20, 30 or 40 drops in a tablespoonful of water. The effects manifest themselves very quickly, two hours after taking a dose, and these effects persist for two to six days. The tickling cough of tuberculosis and the night-sweats are entirely relieved by doses of 20 to 40 drops in a tablespoonful of water.

In the numerous experiments made with it, there were never any disagreeable concomitant effects. Salv. acts even more favorably on the tickling coughs in tuberculosis patients than Bell., Rumx., so that preparations of morphine and codeine could be dispensed with.

In one case, Ms. Smith had for three weeks an irritating cough following an attack of pneumonia. The irritation being particularly great, she was given, fresh from the garden, some sage to chew, and the irritation was instantly relieved.

RELATIONS - ***Compare:*** (1) Phel., Merc., Tub. (2) Chrysan. (3) Salv-sc - tonic influence on nervous system, dose, teaspoonful to one pint hot water, as inhalant for sponging. (4) Rub-t.

REFERENCES - Boericke. Clarke.

SAMBUCUS CANADENSIS

(Elder-bush)

PHARMACY - samb-c. Sambucus canadensis. Elder-bush. Marsh elder-bush. Sambucus humilis. Sambucus glauca. N. O. Caprifliaceae. Tincture of buds, flowers, tender shoots and leaves. ***Historical dose:*** Tincture and all potencies.

CLINICAL - Albuminuria. Angina pectoris. Asthma. Blotches. Cuts. Larynx, dry. Lumbago. Wounds.

HERBAL - The indigenous North American elder grows in rich alluvial soils, flowers in July and fruits in September.

The species, said Millspaugh is not sufficiently distinct from the European elder (Samb. nigra), differing only in being less woody and having more loose cymes, larger flowers and more compound leaves.

Millspaugh said of Samb-c. that a decoction or ointment of the flowers and leaves was used as an application to large wounds.

HOMEOPATHIC - The severe chest symptoms and blotched face recall symptoms of Samb. with which it is probably identical in action. Uneasiness, and unrest. Exhaustion. Recurrence of symptoms.

MIND - Depression and dread of undefined danger.

Back - Back felt sprained. Pressing pain in lumbar region.

Chest - Palpitations. Heaviness and constriction in chest, as from a heavy load. Aroused from sleep by a terrible constriction of chest and heart, cannot lie down for fear of choking.

Face - Face flushed and broken out in blotches, looks ill.

Head - Severe drawing in head with fullness, motion causes sensation as if water were undulating in it. Head heavy, confused with drawing and darting pains.

Heart - Constriction of chest and heart, lying down causes choking. Sharp pain in heart (region of valves), with palpitations, at times visible through the clothes. Heart labors heavily. Pulse rose to 100, but became normal at end of perspiration.

Kidneys - Pressure in kidney region, followed by profuse flow of clear urine. Frequent urination. Urine albuminous.

Limbs - Sharp, darting rheumatic pains hands and feet.

Lungs - Breathing labored, asthmatic, wheezing. Has to sit up in bed to get breath.

Modalities - Better by sweat, getting out of bed. Worse from lying down.

Mouth - Mouth parched, dry, desire for drink.

Temperature - Sweat, soon becoming profuse, which gradually ameliorates all other symptoms (except exhaustion). Head perspired less than rest of body.

Throat - Pharynx and larynx felt dry and swollen, impeding free respiration.

REFERENCES - Clarke.

SAMBUCUS NIGRA

(Elder)

PHARMACY - samb. Sambucus nigra. Elder. N. O. Caprifliaceae. Tincture of fresh leaves and flowers. ***Historical dose:*** Tincture and all potencies.

CLINICAL - Angina pectoris. Asthma. Chest, oppression. Choking. Colic. Contusions. Coryza, dry. ***Coughs. Croup.*** Cyanosis. Edema. Emaciation. Headaches, catarrhal. Hoarseness. Hydrocele. Ileus. Laryngismus. ***Spasms. Snuffles. Suffocation. Tuberculosis.*** Whooping cough.

HOMEOPATHIC - Samb. was proved by Hahnemann and appears in his Materia Medica Pura. It acts especially on the respiratory organs, kidneys and the skin.

Spasm, mainly affecting the respiratory system, larynx, chest and nasal passages. ***Shortness of breath. Snuffles in infants*** preventing breathing and nursing. Dry coryza. When it occurs lower down in the tract, it causes dyspnea.

The child awakens suddenly nearly suffocated, face livid, blue. Sits up in bed, turns blue, gasps for breath, which it finally gets. The attack passes off but is again repeated. Child inspires but cannot expire. Sleeps into the attack. The breathing is rattling. Croup, whooping cough, asthma.

Profuse sweat during waking hours, dry heat when asleep, particularly in tubercular or febrile conditions. A deep, dry cough precedes the fever paroxysm. Fever without thirst. Dreads uncovering.

Edema, dropsical swellings in various parts of the body, especially legs, instep and feet. When edema affects the nose it may give rise to obstruction. Contusions cause dark red swelling.

MIND - General trembling with anxiety. ***Constant state of fretfulness.*** Very easily frightened. Fright followed by suffocative attacks. Worse from fright or strong emotions. Sees images when shutting eyes.

Abdomen - Pressive pain in abdomen with nausea. Spasmodic tearings, shootings and pinchings in abdominal muscles, with expulsion of flatus. Colic with nausea and flatulence. Frequent, watery, slimy stools.

Back - Aching in middle of spine during repose and movement. Lancinations in scapulae.

Causations - Ill effects of fright, grief, anxiety, excessive sexual indulgence. Fright causes suffocative attack.

Chest - Oppression of chest with pressure in stomach, nausea and weakness. Pressure on sternum. Sudden sensation of contraction in sides of chest.

Constitutions - Suited to diseases of scrofulous children that affect the air passages especially. Suited to persons previously robust and fleshy who suddenly become emaciated.

Ears - Sharp stitches in right inner ear, with cramp pain in it. Itching, creeping in ears and in throat.

Eyes - Pupils at first contracted, then greatly dilated. Photophobia. Half open in sleep.

Face - Pale, bluish, puffy. Turns blue with cough. Blotches on face. Red, burning spots on cheeks. Heat and perspiration of face. Hot face with icy cold feet.

Female - Menses too profuse, like metrorrhagia. Debilitating sweats after childbirth.

Food - Thirst without relishing the drinks.

Head - Headache as from intoxication. Motion of head causes tension and dizziness. Pressure and expansion in head. Sudden shocks in the brain. Digging pain in vertex. Scurf on head with intolerable itching.

Heart - Orgasm in whole body. Occasional omission of heartbeat. Pulse generally very frequent and small, sometimes slow, full. Intermitting. Angina pectoris where pressure proceeds from spine.

Kidneys - Dropsical symptoms with vomiting of bile and distress in stomach after eating. Acute nephritis. Profuse urination with a sensation of heat in the body, dry heat of skin. Urine frequent and scanty.

Limbs - Tension in hamstrings as if they were too short. Tearing in legs and ankles. Edematous swelling in legs, insteps and feet. Icy-cold feet with a warm body. Hands and feet bloated and blue. Drawing in forearms and bones of hands. Paralytic heaviness in elbow joint. Lancinations in wrists. Trembling of hands (when writing).

Lungs - Spasmodic croup. Asthma. Cyanosis. ***Sudden suffocation*** or strangling on falling to sleep, or waking him at midnight with violent sweat. ***Child awakes suddenly, nearly suffocating, sits up, turns blue.*** Paroxysmal, ***suffocative cough, coming on about midnight*** with crying and dyspnea. Loose choking cough. Spells of coughing, before fever. Dry coryza. ***Sniffles of infants***, nose dry and obstructed. ***Cannot expire*** (Meph.). When nursing child must let go of nipple, nose blocked up, cannot breathe. Whistling breathing.

Male - Hydrocele from injury. Swelling of scrotum.

Modalities - Better sitting up in bed, motion, from pressure over a sharp edge, and wrapping up. Worse from dry, cold air, uncovering. Worse cold drink while over heated, eating fruits. Worse motion. Worse sleep, rest, lying down in bed, on left side. Worse about midnight, after midnight, 2 to 3 a.m., wakes with sense of stoppage of air tubes. Head low aggravates, must sit up to regain breath.

Mouth - Dryness of the mouth and throat without thirst. Half open in sleep. Toothache with tearing and lancinations in all the teeth and with a sensation as if cheeks were swollen.

Neck - Pressive heaviness in nape. Deep incisive lancinations in muscles of neck. Sweat on throat and neck with children.

Nose - Dry coryza with snuffles in infants. Sensation of numbness in nose with itching on bridge. Obstruction of nose with accumulation of thick and viscid mucus in nostrils. Dry coryza of children.

Pelvis - Pains in loins with drawing pressure. Incisive blows in loins.

Perspiration - Very debilitating sweats. ***Profuse sweat over entire body during waking hours***. Continued perspiration while awake, changing into dry heat as soon as one goes to sleep. Night sweats, except on head, worse towards morning.

Rectum - Irritable anus with hemorrhoids. Frequent, watery, slimy stools.

Sensations - As if head were filled with water. Skull as if stretched. As if suffocating.

Skin - Dry heat during sleep. Tingling, itching of skin. Sudden painful drawing in all points over surface while sitting. Edema, anasarca. Bloated and swollen, general dropsy, ***profuse sweat on waking***.

Sleep - Frequent waking with a start, with obstructed respiration. Child starts up suddenly as if suffocating. Incomplete sleep with mouth and eyes half open. Sleeps with arms above head. Dry heat during sleep, profuse perspiration after waking. Lascivious dreams.

Stomach - Pressure in stomach. Acute lancinations under the stomach, worse by pressing upon it. Vomiting in morning, first of mucus and milk (or food) that had been taken, followed by bile.

Temperature - Shuddering with shivering. Icy coldness of hands and feet. Pricking, tingling in skin. Intermittent fever. Dry, burning fever while asleep, copious sweating on waking. Fever with excessive perspiration, especially at night. Debilitating night sweats (Salv., Acet-ac.). ***Dreads uncovering.*** Dry, deep cough precedes the fever paroxysm. Sweats with cough.

Throat - Hoarseness with tenacious mucus in larynx. Screeching voice. Spasms of glottis. Itching, tingling in throat.

Vertigo - Dizziness and confusion in the head, during movement, on rising.

COMMENTS - The leaves of Sambucus nigra have an unpleasant odor when bruised, which is supposed to be offensive to most insects. A decoction of the leaves is sometimes used by gardeners to keep caterpillars off delicate plants.

Green noted that sheep that have the rot can be cured by letting them eat the bark and young leaves of Samb. Herbalists use the inner bark, as well as the leaves, to make an ointment. The flowers serve for fomentations or are made into a medicinal tea. According to the Treasury of Botany, the berries are the principal ingredient in elderberry wine.

Millspaugh said that the bark contains viburnic acid, which is identical with valerianic acid. This no doubt accounts for the odor and suggests a relationship in action between sambucus, valerian and the viburnum.

Nash once relieved with Samb. 200c a very bad case of asthma in an old woman, who had suffocative attacks. The relief was accompanied by a profuse flow of urine, which carried off a large amount of dropsical effusion in her legs and abdomen.

Severe croup, whooping cough, bronchitis, and asthma. Infants with chronic snuffles (Thuj., after vaccinations). Suffocating attacks (Ip.). Tendency for attacks to recur. Croupy attack "passes off but is again repeated." Spasms in the throat. Severe coughing with mucus. Thick, white, upper respiratory mucus that suffocates and gags the person (Ant-t.)

Patient can wake up in the middle of the night, grab at their throat, face turns blue. Waking with a spasm where the oxygen gets cut off (Cup.). Worse about midnight or after midnight, worse 2:00 to 3:00 in the morning. Worse dry, cold air.

RELATIONS - Samb-c. may be regarded as practically identical with Samb-n. ***Antidoted by:*** Ars., Camph. ***Antidote to:*** Ars. - relieves ailments from abuse of Ars. ***Compare:*** (1) Ip., Meph., Op. (2) Samb-c. - great value in dropsies. (3) In Miller's asthma, Arum-d. (4) Dyspnea, inspires, cannot expire, Chlor., Meph. (5) Sleeps into the attack, Lach. (6) Peculiarities of sweating, Chin., Con., Thuj., Puls. (7) Dreads uncovering, Nux-v. (8) Fat people emaciate suddenly, Iod., Tub. (9) Tenacious mucus in larynx, Kali-bi. (10) Effects of cold drink when over-heated, Bell-p. (11) Effects of dry cold, Acon. Snuffles, Am-c., Nux-v. ***Compatible:*** Bell., Con., Nux-v., Phos., Rhus-t., Sep. ***Follows well:*** Op. (effects of fright).

REFERENCES - Boericke. Clarke. Murphy. Phatak.

SANGUINARIA CANADENSIS

(Blood-root)

PHARMACY - sang. Sanguinaria canadensis. Blood-root. Puccoon. N. O. Papaveraceae. Tincture of fresh root. The resin, leaves, seeds, seed-vessels, powdered root and expressed juice have also been used. ***Historical dose:*** Tincture and all potencies.

CLINICAL - Alcoholism. Anemia. Aphonia. Arthritis. Asthma. ***Bilious, disorders. Blood, disorders.*** Breast, tumor. Bronchitis. Cancer. Catarrh. Chest, pains. Cold. Croup. Deafness. Diphtheria. Dysmenorrhea. Dyspepsia. Ear, polyps. Gleet. Granular, lids. ***Headaches.*** Heartburn. Hemoptysis. Hot, flashes. Influenza. Keratitis. Liver, disorders. Menopause. Menstruation, painful. Migraines. Nails, ulceration. Neuralgias. Edema, glottidis. Ophthalmia. Pharyngitis. Tuberculosis. Physometra. Pneumonia, acute. ***Polyps.*** Pregnancy, disorders. Quinsy. ***Rheumatism.*** Rhus poisoning. ***Shoulder, rheumatism. Sinusitis.*** Smell, loss. Stomach, neurosis. Syphilis. Tinnitus. Tumors. Vomiting. Whitlow. Whooping cough.

HERBAL - The bloodroot is commonly found throughout the United States and Canada, and is the sole representative of the genus Sanguinaria of the Papaveraceae. It is herbaceous, has a thick, branching root stock, which creeps along underground.

In early spring, it sends up from the ends of the little side branches a single long-stalked leaf and another stalk bearing a solitary flower. The leaf is wrapped around the flower bud when it rises from the ground and is bluntly five to nine-lobed, roundish at first, but later kidney-shaped.

The Treasury of Botany noted that Native Americans used the orange-colored juice of the root for smearing their bodies and for staining various domestic articles. The plant had also been successfully used by American and French dyers.

HOMEOPATHIC - Sang. is a ***right-sided remedy,*** affecting the head, liver, chest and deltoid. Affects chiefly the mucus membranes, especially of the respiratory tract. Suited to pulmonary disorders with liver involvement.

Marked vaso-motor disturbances, as seen in the circumscribed redness of the cheeks, flashes of heat, determination of blood to head and chest, general pulsations and distention of temporal veins.

Burning heat and ebullitions. Burning in various parts. ***Burning sensations*** like from hot water. Burning in palms and soles. Burning in throat, under sternum, spots or stitches in chest, palms and soles. Burnt feeling in tongue. Applicable to menopausal disorders.

Influenza coughs. ***Sudden stopping of catarrh of respiratory tract followed by diarrhea.*** Tuberculosis. Mucus membranes become dry. Acrid, blood-streaked or foul discharge. ***Sick and faint from odor of flowers.***

Polyps, nasal, uterine. Fungus excrescences. Pains in places where bones are least covered. Internal rawness. Lies on back with head elevated. Bilious. Pains increase and decrease with the sun. Symptoms ascend or end in bilious vomiting.

MIND - Hopefulness, confident of recovery. Mind confused, better by belchings. Anxiety and dread preceded vomiting and delirium. Borrows trouble. Grumbling. Angry, irritability, moroseness. Rage after insults. Disgusting thoughts and ideas. Sensitive to noise.

Mental torpor, stupor, heaviness, sleepiness. Lassitude, indisposed to move or make any mental effort. Indolence. Dreamy state with eyes open. Sensation as if paralyzed and unable to move while lying on her back. Recognizes everything but can't move.

Abdomen - Throbbing in abdomen. Tension in epigastrium. Awoke with severe pain in region of spleen. Violent stitches in spleen. Sensation as if hot water poured itself from breast into abdomen, followed by diarrhea. Flatulent distention with escape of flatus from vagina. Colic with torpor of liver.

Back - Soreness down muscles of back. Pain in inner border of right shoulder blade. Pain in sacrum from lifting.

Breasts - Sore and enlarged breasts, at menopause. Pain in right breast to shoulder. Severe soreness under right nipple. Hot streaming from breast towards liver. Pain in breast with periodic cough.

Chest - Pain, burning soreness, in right chest to shoulder. Burning in chest, as of a hot steam extending to abdomen with cough. Tickling behind sternum, causes a constant hacking cough, worse at night on lying down. Hemoptysis. Hydrothorax. Pneumonia.

Ears - Burning of ears with redness of cheeks. Cracking in right ear while stroking cheek. Earache with headache. Polyps. Humming and roaring in the ear, painfully sensitive to sounds, at menopause. Throat disorders causing deafness and earache.

Eyes - Acute conjunctivitis. Yellow sclera, jaundice. Retinal congestion. Catarrhal ophthalmia, granular lids. Redness of eyes in morning. Burning dryness in eyes, followed by copious lachrymation. Lachrymation with coryza, tears hot. Vapor or cloud before eyes. Eyeballs painful on moving them. Swelling over eyebrows. Blepharitis.

Face - ***Hectic flush, redness and burning of cheeks.*** Neuralgia, pain extends in all directions from upper jaw. Fullness and tenderness behind angle of jaws.

Female - Amenorrhea. Before menses, itching of axilla. Menstruation too early with a discharge of black blood. Menses offensive, profuse. Leucorrhea fetid, corrosive. Uterine polyps. Menopausal disorders, especially flushes of heat. Burning of palms and soles at menopause.

Food - Loss of appetite with great weakness of digestion. Unquenchable thirst. Craves, knows not for what. Craving for spicy things. Aversion to butter, leaves a sweetish taste. Sweet things aggravate, taste bitter, cause burning. Bilious headaches if he goes without food.

Head - ***Periodical sick headache,*** pain begins in occiput, spreads upwards or ***ascending from occiput to over right eye.*** Pain in the occiput like a ***flash of lightning***. Pain in small spot over upper left parietal bone. ***Veins and temples are distended***. Headaches if he goes without food. Headaches, better sleep, vomiting and passing copious flow of urine. Headaches return at menopausal, every seventh day (Sulph., Sabad.). Sun headache. Hemicrania increases and decreases with the sun.

Heart - Weak feeling, irregular action. Palpitations. Valvular disease with lung development, phosphates in urine and loss of flesh. Metastasis of rheumatism (or gout) to heart from outward applications.

Kidneys - Dull, heavy pain across kidneys. Urine dark yellow with jaundice. Copious and frequent, clear, worse at night. Urine high-colored, red sediment. Ardor urine.

Limbs - ***Rheumatism of right shoulder.*** Pain in shoulder, worse night. Cutting pain or stiffness in right deltoid, worse raising or turning arm. Pain in arm better swinging arm to and fro. Itching in axilla, worse before menses. Aching and swelling of ball of thumb (right). Palms wrinkled. ***Burning of palms and soles***, worse covers, at menopause. Rheumatism of left hip joint and nape of neck. Pain in bones near surface. Neuritis better by touching the part.

Liver - Pain over region of liver. Jaundice. Liver-cough.

Lungs - ***Severe dyspnea*** and constriction of chest. Asthma with stomach disorders (Nux-v.). ***Pneumonia***, catarrhal, right side, better lying on back. Sudden stoppage of catarrh of air passages brings on diarrhea. Tuberculosis. Hemoptysis from suppressed menses. ***Cough of gastric origin***, relieved by eructation. Cough with burning pain in chest, worse right side. Tough, ***rust-colored***, purulent, offensive sputum, almost impossible to raise. Spasmodic cough after influenza and ***after whooping cough***. Cough returns with every fresh cold.

Male - Burning in glans. Cheesy secretions from glans (syphilis). Gleet, old cases. Emissions two nights in succession, after which he felt very well.

Modalities - Better acids, sour things. Better vomiting, passing flatus. Better cool air. Better darkness, sleep, lying on back or on left side. Worse from motion, raising arms, looking up. Worse touch, ***right side***. Worse light, sun, odors, and sweets. Worse 3 a.m., weekly, nightly, periodically. Worse menopause.

Mouth - Ulceration of mouth and fauces with dry, burning sensation. Palate feels scalded. Tongue white, feels burnt. Anterior tongue looks red, like raw beef. Offensive breath. Sweet things taste bitter.

Neck - Soreness of nape on being touched. Rheumatic pain in nape, shoulders and arms. Pain in right side of neck as if strained in left side.

Nose - ***Nasal polyps***. Chronic rhinitis, membrane dry and congested. Hay fever. Ozaena with profuse, offensive, yellowish discharges. Coryza, followed by diarrhea. Pain at the root of nose. Rose-cold with subsequent asthma. Sensitive to odors. Loss or perverted sense of smell, smell in nose like roasted onion.

Rectum - Alternate diarrhea and constipation. Colic followed by diarrhea. Diarrhea as coryza improves. Dysentery. Urging to stool, but only discharges of flatus. Ineffectual urging to stool, then vomiting. Bilious, liquid, gushing diarrhea (Nat-s., Lyc.). Copious apple-green stools with flatus. Hemorrhoids. Cancer of rectum.

Sensations - As if forehead would burst. As of a band across forehead. As if head were drawn forward. As if electric current shooting through head. As if temples and scalp were alive with irrepressible pulsation. As if eyes would be pressed out. As if hairs were in eyes. As if paralyzed. As if she was in a railway car that was moving and jarring her and as if all about her moved rapidly and confusedly.

Skin - Heat and dryness of skin. Prickling heat spreading over body. Burning and itching, worse by heat. Circumscribed red spots. Red, blotchy eruptions, worse in spring. Acne with scanty menses. Scaly eruptions, carbuncles. Itching and nettle-rash before the nausea. Old indolent ulcers with callous borders and ichorous discharge. Fungus excrescences. ***Antidotes rhus poisoning***. Jaundice.

Sleep - Drowsiness causing mental and bodily indolence. Sleeplessness at night, awakens in a fright as if he would fall. Can't sleep without brandy. Slightest noise disturbs, yet is sleepy and dreamy. Dreams of sea voyages with sensation of being rocked. Dreams of frightful business matters.

Stomach - Sinking, faint, all-gone feeling (Phos., Sep.). Stomach pains to right shoulder. Burning in stomach with headache, and vomiting. Hiccough while smoking. Nausea with salivation, not better by vomiting. Vomiting of bitter water, sour, acrid fluids, of ingesta, of worms. Spitting of bile, gastro-duodenal catarrh.

Teeth - Looseness of teeth, with salivation. Toothache from picking teeth. Pain in hollow teeth, especially when touched by food. Pain in decayed teeth after cold drinks. Bleeding, spongy, fungoid gums.

Temperature - Fever, heat and delirium. Intermittent fevers, marsh fevers, nervous fever. Fever from pulmonary, hepatic or gastric inflammation. Flushes of heat, rising into face and head with headache. Burning, scanty sweat. Copious sweat, cold sweat. Heat flying from head to stomach. Chill with nausea, headache. Chill and shivering in back. Shaking chill.

Throat - Dry cough, tickling in throat. Tonsillitis. Ulcerated sore throat, as if raw and denuded. Sore, swollen (right), pains to ear and chest. Burning, worse eating sweet things. Dry and constricted. Sensation in pharynx as if scalded by hot drink. Edema of larynx. Larynx, full and dry in singers. Aphonia.

Tongue - Burnt, sore feeling. Tip of tongue burns as if scalded. Crawling, pricking on tip of tongue. Stitches in left side of tongue. White coated tongue with slimy, fatty taste. Red streak through middle of tongue.

Vertigo - Vertigo, worse looking up and moving head rapidly, with nausea, fainting and headache.

COMMENTS - Acts powerfully on the outer chest, sternum and breasts. Reputed to cure cancer, polyps and new growths (Chel.). Clarke saw breast tumors diminish under its action.

Grimmer stated that this remedy has cured breast cancer with severe burning pains and inflammatory symptoms of the mucus membranes, the respiratory and gastrointestinal tracts, and the skin. Pronounced heat, flushing and redness of the skin. Characteristic burning pains (wherever pain exists).

S. L. Mitchell recorded the fatal poisoning of workmen who drank the tincture in mistake for brandy. They were all soon seized with severe racking and burning pains in the stomach and bowels with intense thirst. "Burning" is one of the leading notes of the remedy and is found in many different parts.

Winterburn published a case illustrating this indication in the region of the stomach. Mr. F., 48, of sanguino-bilious temperament, energetic and refined, had been ill with pains in the stomach for several months. A clairvoyant had recommended "a decoction of blood-root and bone-set in tablespoonful doses." Each dose produced "intense burning pains in the stomach lasting for hours," and it had to be discontinued.

Weeks later, Winterburn was consulted and found Mr. F with burning in his epigastrium with pressure, worse at night, but coming on soon after lying down and compelling the patient to rise. Belching gave no relief. Great appetite, torpid bowels, an unsatisfactory relief each morning, leaving a sense of discomfort.

There was a peculiar drawing pain in the shoulders and arms during sleep, so that when he woke his fists were tightly clenched and flexed on the sternal end of his clavicle, lameness and weariness of the muscles followed.

Sang. 200c, was chosen after careful comparison with Nux-v., Graph. and others. It was given every night at bedtime. After the first dose, the symptoms disappeared "like magic," and the patient was soon well.

Leonard said "a circumscribed burning in the chest, commonly followed by heat through abdomen and diarrhea," is a strong indication for Sang. in pneumonic conditions.

Sang. also has the circumscribed hectic flush on the cheeks, as in tuberculosis in which it is frequently indicated. Flushed face, at times dark red or livid (Op.). It has the "hopefulness" of tubercular patients.

Severe headaches. Migraine, starting at the back of the head and moving to above the right eye (Sil.). Headaches begin at occiput, spreading upwards and forwards, settling over the right eye. Pains like a flash of lightning in occiput. Bursting headaches, as if the eyes would be pressed out. Better by sleep. Symptoms begin in the morning, increase to noon, then diminish. Headaches return at menopause. Right-sided headaches with the flu. Bilious or gastric headaches.

Hering described the headache as the "American sick-headache." There is a rush of blood causing faintness and nausea, pains are sharp or throbbing. Patients cannot bear light, odors, or the least jar, as that of anyone stepping across the floor. There can be vomiting of food and bile. Pain so violent the patient goes out of her mind or seeks relief by pressing head against pillow or pressing with the hands.

Cooper gave as a keynote, "If he goes without food, gets bilious headaches." Violent, throbbing headache with extreme nausea and vomiting, frequent, fetid belchings and great salivation.

Severe burning in stomach, vomits bitter water and sour, acrid fluids. Nausea may not be relieved by vomiting. Sweets taste bitter, aggravate the burning. Vomiting of worms. Tormenting thirst. Offensive breath and flatus.

Irritation of the nasal mucus membrane. Polyps. Coryza with pain at root of the nose. Influenza, hay fever and ozaena. Sinusitis, more on the right side. Lost or perverted sense of smell, sensitive to the odor of flowers.

Laryngitis and membranous croup. Tracheal and bronchial coughs in epidemic influenza. Cough after influenza or whooping cough, particularly in children. Cough returns with every fresh cold. Violent, dry cough, wheezing, whistling, metallic. Offensive and acrid discharges. Sputa is almost impossible to raise.

Clarke recorded several cases in which Sang. relieved patients who had thick plugs of suffocating mucus which the patients were too weak to dislodge.

Offensive menses, bright red flow, later blood darker and less offensive. Itching of axillae before menses. Eruptions on the face of young women, during scanty menses. Menopausal disorders, flashes of heat, leucorrhea, and painful enlargement of breasts.

Neuralgia of the face, ameliorated by kneeling down and pressing head firmly against the floor. Pain extends in all directions from the upper jaw.

Rheumatism. Rheumatic pain in right arm and shoulder, worse at night. Cannot raise the arm, but can swing it to and fro. Frozen shoulder. Great affinity for the right shoulder. Right side generally more affected. Symptoms go from right to left. Marked periodicity. Pains in places where the bones are least covered.

Cooper gave the case of a woman, 19, who had a condition of her throat from scarlatina three years previously, and lately increasing deafness. There were noises all over her head and vertigo. Sudden flushings in daytime, menses too frequent, and profuse leucorrhea. Backache, paining her to walk, forcing her to give up teaching from the pain.

Poor appetite from the headaches and tinnitus, she often had pain behind the angles of lower jaw and swollen glands. All symptoms disappeared after a single dose of Sang. tincture, although at first the leucorrhea was increased.

F. Nichol, in giving Hale his experience with Sang. in croup, said he used a solution of Sanguinarine in vinegar, and he found that the most effective preparation.

RELATIONS - ***Compare:*** (1) Just. - bronchial catarrh, coryza, hoarseness, oversensitive. (2) Dig. (migraine). (3) Bell., Iris, Meli., Lach., Ferr., Op. (4) Chel., Op. In rheumatism of right deltoid, Mag-c. (5) Headache extending forward from occiput and settling over right eye, Spig. (6) Headache better by hard pressure, Chin., Indg., Mag-m. (7) Paroxysms of headache ending in profuse urination, Ign., Gels., Verat. (8) Menstrual headache, Sep. scanty flow, Sang. profuse. (9) Right side, throbbing, congestive headache, worse light and noise, Bell. (10) Periodic sick headaches, Iris-v. (11) Pneumonia, Phos., Ant-t. ***Compatible:*** Bell. - in scarlatina rashes. ***It antidotes:*** Op. ***Complementary:*** Ant-t.

REFERENCES - Boericke. Clarke. Murphy. Phatak.

SANGUINARINUM NITRICUM

(Sanguinarine Nitrate)

PHARMACY - sanguin-n. Sanguinarinum nitricum. Sanguinarine nitrate. Trituration. ***Historical dose:*** All potencies.

CLINICAL - Adenoids. Allergies. Asthma. Borborygmus. Bronchitis. Catarrh. Colic. Colds. Coryza. ***Coughs.*** Deafness. Eustachian catarrh. Hay fever. Headaches. ***Influenza***. Laryngitis. Pharyngitis. Polyps. Post-nasal catarrh. Quinsy. Stiff-neck. Throat, sore. Tinnitus.

HOMEOPATHIC - Sanguin-n. is a very fine brownish-red powder, pungent, acid, bitter and inodorous. It is soluble in alcohol, ether, water and oils, but not in the same proportion in all. Pure sanguinarine is a pearly-white substance, but when combined with any of the acids the result is a salt of some shade of red, crimson or scarlet. The color of the blood-root may be due to the presence of some native salt of Sanguinarine.

Sang-n. was proved in 3x trituration by Professor Owens of Pulte Medical College. Nasal polyps. Acute and chronic catarrh. Acute pharyngitis (Wye.). Smarting and burning in throat and chest especially under sternum. ***Influenza***. Chronic follicular pharyngitis. Lachrymation, pains in eyes and head, sore scalp, ***sense of obstruction***.

Abdomen - Borborygmus and pains in abdomen, as if diarrhea would set in, with sharp, cutting pains.

Back - Stiffness in muscles of left neck and shoulder.

Causations - Driving in cold wind, winter weather, exposure.

Chest - ***Pressure behind center of sternum***. Tightness in the chest. Tension in chest, burning and accumulation of mucus behind center of sternum. Short, hacking cough arising from sensation of tightness in chest.

Ears - Obstruction of Eustachian tube. Roaring in right ear. Difficulty in distinguishing sounds.

Eyes - Sore, aching pain in eyeballs. Burning, pressing aching, and sore pains in eyes. Profuse lachrymation, tears gush out. Redness and soreness of inner canthi. Redness of lids and conjunctiva. Sight dim, as if looking through gauze.

Food - Little appetite. Everything tastes dry like chips. Coffee did not taste natural, wanted something succulent, not pungent, but soothing to mouth and throat.

Head - Pain in supra-orbital region. Burning pain in forehead and root of nose. Sensation of obstruction and fullness in head, ameliorated by discharge of a large quantity of thick, yellow, sweet-tasting mucus.

Kidneys - Passed urine every hour during the night. Urine had bright yellow or white sediment.

Limbs - Stiffness in muscles of left shoulder and neck.

Lungs - ***Strong desire for fresh air.*** Sense of suffocation. Dryness and burning in throat and bronchials. Feeling as if air passages lined with thick, stiff mucus or pus. Chronic nasal, laryngeal and bronchial catarrh. Raises thin, frothy mucus, which is very tenacious. ***Tickling cough***. Short, hacking cough with expectoration of thick, yellow, sweetish mucus. Cough is deep and rattling.

Modalities - Worse touch, at night. Pressure aggravates soreness of eyes. Bathing with warm water ameliorates heat in forehead. Headache is ameliorates by discharge of much mucus from nose.

Mouth - Acrid, burning sensation on tongue. ***Ulceration on the side of the tongue.*** Roughness and dryness in mouth and throat. Heat in mouth as if pepper had been taken. Increased flow of mucus and saliva with sneezing and burning in forehead. Bitter taste extending back to root of tongue.

Nose - Dry and burning nostrils. ***Feels obstructed.*** Enlarged turbinates at beginning of hypertrophic process. ***Profuse, watery mucus with burning pain,*** with pressure over root of nose. ***Sneezing***. Secretion scant, tendency to dryness. Nostrils plugged with thick, yellow, bloody mucus. Small crusts which bleed when removed. Post-nasal secretions stuck to naso-pharynx, dislodged with difficulty. Rawness and soreness in posterior sinuses.

Sleep - Sleep poor, restless from feverish and irritable condition.

Stomach - Sensation of burning in stomach and esophagus. Belching up of putrid-smelling gas though she had eaten nothing since morning.

Throat - Voice altered, deep, hoarse. Rough, dry, ***constricted, burning***. Right tonsil sore, swallowing difficult.

COMMENTS - The catarrhal symptoms of Sanguin-n. appear in great intensity, the nose, eyes, throat and bronchi being affected. Sensation of obstruction and fullness in the head, accumulation of mucus obstructing nose, awakes frequently with dry mouth, the nose being obstructed.

Accumulation of mucus behind center of sternum, sense of suffocation, feeling as if air-passages lined with thick, stiff mucus or pus. Heat and tension behind sternum is characteristic and so is expectoration of quantities of sweet-tasting mucus. Expectoration of thin, frothy, very tenacious mucus.

Lachrymation, pains in eyes and head, sore scalp, obstructed nose and burning pains throughout all regions were experienced. Symptoms of influenza, even to the loss or perversion of taste. "Sensation arising to nostrils as if he had eaten strong horse-radish."

Hale reported the case of Mr. B., 40, dark, had for eight years in spite of continuous old-school treatment, chronic post-nasal catarrh, bronchitis and laryngitis. Voice altered, deep, hoarse, speech with effort, as if from chest. Severe pressure from behind sternum. Mucus membrane dry, raised only a few balls of gray mucus.

He spent two winters on St. John's River, Florida, and was better there, but worse again on his return north. Sanguin-n. 6c trituration. was given every two hours. In one week he was better, there was more moisture in his throat than three had been for two years. Voice markedly better.

Sanguin-n. was given every four hours. In ten weeks he regained six pounds of his lost weight and strength in proportion. The voice not having improved in the same degree, Caust. 6c and afterwards Dros. 3c, were given and in sixteen weeks he was perfectly well.

Mrs. S., city missionary, 49, had constant hacking cough, raw, sore feeling in throat, sore aching and pressing behind sternum. She was much exposed to cold winds of winter, which set up coryza and irritation. Sanguin-n. 6c. every two hours, enabled her to follow her occupation without suffering and in ten weeks she was completely cured.

O. W., 55, subject to frequent attacks of cold in head, throat and chest. After a long drive in open trap contracted a severe cold in head, throat, lungs. Sore and lame all over, frequent sneezing, lachrymation.

Next day sore throat very marked, constant tickling in throat-pit, exciting cough, at first short and hacking, but in two days it became violent and convulsive. Bell. and Dros. did little good. Pressure behind sternum became very severe.

Sanguin-n. 6c was given every two hours. In four hours copious perspiration came on with frequent sneezing. Next day, sore throat appeared after waking from a troubled and restless sleep, constriction of throat with difficult swallowing, tension across chest radiating from behind sternum.

Sanguin-n. was given every hour. In one hour, free discharge from nose set in; three hours, moisture and relaxation of constriction across chest. The discharge was yellow and sweetish-tasting, continued all day. Slept well and woke next morning feeling quite free. But little cough or coryza during the day. The following morning he was quite well.

C. Wesselhoeft regarded Sanguin-n. as the simillimum for "New England colds." Adenoids and polyps have been cured with it. There is great craving for air.

RELATIONS - ***Compare:*** (1) Sanguin-t. - exophthalmos. (2) Mydriasis, dim vision. Arum-t., Psor., Kali-bi., Sang. (3) Burning in nostrils, Arum-t. (4) Tenacious mucus, Kali-bi. (5) Hay fever, Psor. (6) Sweet expectoration, Stann.

REFERENCES - Boericke. Clarke.

SANGUINARINUM PURA

PHARMACY - sanguin. Sanguinarinum pura. N. O. Papaveraceae. Trituration. Solution in vinegar. ***Historical dose:*** All potencies.

HOMEOPATHIC - Sanguin. is a pearly white substance. Thomas noted that in smallest physiological doses it acts as ***"expectorant,"*** in large, it causes nausea and still larger vomiting. In repeated doses, it lowers the pulse rate.

Useful for croup. Pseudo-membranous croup. Great dyspnea. Hoarse, muffled cough, with complete aphonia. Grasped his throat in agony. Nausea and vomiting.

COMMENTS - T. Nichol gave his experience with a solution of one grain of Sanguin. in two ounces of vinegar in cases of pseudo-membranous croup. He related the case of W. G., age 5, who had been ill some days.

Nichol found him with a hoarse, muffled cough, complete aphonia, pulse 132. Soft palate and fauces covered with pearly, fibrinous exudation, a hissing sound was heard on auscultating larynx.

Great dyspnea. The child stretched back his head and grasped his throat in agony. Features swollen and dark. Sangn. acet. was given and in fifteen hours there was notable improvement. In forty-eight hours the boy was out of danger.

REFERENCES - Clarke.

SANGUINARINUM TARTARICUM

(Sanguinarine Tartrate)

PHARMACY - sang-t. Sanguinarinum tartaricum. Sanguinarine tartrate. Papaveraceae. Trituration. ***Historical dose:*** All potencies.

CLINICAL - Exophthalmos. Mydriasis. Stool, bilious. Vision, dim.

HOMEOPATHIC - Tully and Terry experimented with Sang-t. in considerable doses. Tully said he repeatedly witnessed all the effects of sanguinaria root, save the neuralgic pains and the convulsive disorders, from the use of Sang-t.

The most peculiar of the symptoms are starting and protrusion of the eyes, extreme mydriasis, haggard expression and cold surface and cold sweats.

REFERENCES - Clarke.

SANICULA AQUA

(Mineral Springs)

PHARMACY - sanic. Sanicula aqua. Mineral Springs of Ottawa, Ill., USA. Containing, approximately in grains per gallon, Nat-m. 93, Calc-m. 23.5, Mag-m. 23.25, Calc. bi-carb. 14.25, Calc-s. 9.5, Kali-s. 5, Nat-bic. 1, Nat-br. 3, Fe. bi-carb. 1, Nat-i. 12, Sil. 5, Alum. 01 and traces of Lith. bi-carb., Nat-p., Bor. Dilutions of the spring water. Triturations of the evaporated salt. ***Historical dose:*** Tincture and all potencies.

CLINICAL - Amenorrhea. Anterior crural, neuralgia. Asthma. Bedwetting. Bee stings. Boils, blind. Borborygmus. Coccyx, soreness. Condylomata. Conjunctivitis. Constipation, children. Cornea, ulceration. Coryza. Cough. Dandruff. Debility. Diabetes. Diarrhea. Digestion slow. Dropsy, during pregnancy. Eczema. ***Emaciation.*** Excoriations. Foot sweat. Gastritis. Gumboil. Headaches. Indigestion. Influenza. Intermittents. Itch, suppressed. Itching. Leucorrhea. Liver, soreness. Lumbago. ***Marasmus.*** Melancholy. Milk, thin. Morning, sickness. Motion sickness. Mouth, sore. Neuralgia. Neurasthenia. Night-terrors. Nose, crusts. Ophthalmia, tarsi. Os uterus, dilated. Ossification, early. Ozaena. Perspiration, excessive. ***Pot-bellied children.*** Rectum, cramp. Rheumatism. ***Rickets.*** Ringworm. Scurvy. Seasickness. Shoulder, rheumatism. Throat, sore. Tongue, burning. Toothaches. Uterus, prolapsed. Uterus, tumor. Vomiting, milk, water. Wrist, boils.

HOMEOPATHIC - Sanic. has sometimes been confused with the plant Sanicula marylandica, or black snake-root. The water is odorless and colorless, and has an agreeable and slightly alkaline taste.

Sherbino proved Sanic. in the potencies and a large number of the symptoms of the provings have been confirmed. It's a polycrest and anti-psoric of wide range. Guernsey considered Sanic. the chronic of Cham.

Sanic. affects the nutrition, female organs, rectum, neck and skin. Useful for bedwetting, seasickness, motion sickness, constipation, etc. ***Rickets. Marasmus.*** Thick, acrid, yellow pus. Body smells like old cheese.

Bursting in perineum, bowels, bladder, vertex, chest. Shifting pains. Cannot bear to have one part touch another or cannot lie near another person. Enlarged feeling in throat, vagina etc. Child kicks off covers at night, wants to lie on something hard though thin. Clothes feel cold, damp.

MIND - Irritable, least word or action would upset her. Misconstrues everything. Crossness quickly alternating with playfulness in children. Headstrong, obstinate, touchy children. Restless desire to go from place to place. Instability of purpose. Does not want to be touched. Constant desire to look behind. Dread of downward motion. Fear of the dark.

Abdomen - Bowels bloated as if they would burst. Sore pains in groin. Loud gurgling, pot-bellied children.

Back - Neck weak and emaciated, child cannot hold its head. Stiff backache, worse least turning, raising arms or putting hands behind him. Must turn whole body to look around. Sits, head forward, to ease the pain. Cold lumbar spine. Lumbago, better lying on right side. Lumbar vertebras as if dislocated or were gliding past each other. As if back is broken in two pieces. As if a damp cloth on sacrum.

Causations - Poor diet, strains.

Chest - Tickling under sternum. Great soreness of upper chest, must hold it with hands when coughing.

Constitutions - Patients are thin and look old, especially children.

Ears - Eustachian catarrh. Soreness behind ears with discharge of white, gluey, sticky substance. Stuffed feeling in left ear.

Eyes - Lids agglutinated in morning. Lachrymation in cold, open air or cold application. Eyes burn, exuding a sticky fluid. Ulcerated cornea. Dim sight. Photophobia. Dandruff of the eyebrows.

Face - Acne about eye and cheek. Itching eruptions in beard, especially under chin, worse when warm. Excoriation of upper lip.

Female - Leucorrhea with strong odor of fish-brine, worse stools. Bearing down as if contents of pelvis would escape, worse jar, walking. Supports the relaxed parts by placing the hand against vulva, better rest. Vagina feels large, cannot stop menstruation. Os cervix open and dilated.

Food - Child wants to nurse all the time, yet loses flesh. Craves, salt, bacon or ice cold milk. Eating causes urging for stool, must leave the table. Feels better after eating. Great longing for the spring water. Thirst little and often.

Head - Bursting in vertex. As if a cold cloth around brain. Cannot bear cold air on occiput and neck. Profuse sweat on occiput and neck, worse during sleep. Electric crackling in hair when combed. Profuse scab dandruff, falling of hair. Small boils on head that do not mature.

Kidneys - Bursting in bladder with urgent call to pass urine. Frequent, profuse, sudden urination, urging ceases if desire is resisted. Briny urine, stains diaper red. Child cries before urinating, strains to urinate while at stools.

Limbs - Pain in shoulders, worse raising arms or putting them behind back. Hands become sweaty when putting them together. Cold, clammy hands and feet. Burning of palms and soles. Feet as if in cold water. Cramps in feet. Foul foot sweat, chafes toes, destroys shoes or stiffens the hose.

Liver - Soreness through hepatic region. Enlargement of liver, sensitive to pressure and jar.

Lungs - Asthmatic breathing, worse after supper. Wheezing, rattling under sternum, worse during or after eating. Deep, hollow cough with loud rattling, caused by tickling under sternum. Tickling on lying down at night and on waking. Rattling cough, child gags and vomits a mouthful of tough, stringy matter. Expectoration of large, yellow, cheesy masses.

Male - Increased sexual desire at first, then much decreased. Discharge of semen too early, with little sensation. Scrotum relaxed, clammy sweat about parts. Briny odor of the genitals, a few hours after sex. Child's parts smell of fish brine even after bathing.

Modalities - Better from open air, warmth. Better vomiting. Worse from strain, jarring. Worse motion, raising arm, putting hands behind, descending. Worse cold wind on occiput or neck.

Mouth - Offensive breath. Mouth and palate covered with ulcers, white aphthae. Profuse flow of white, clear, transparent, stringy saliva when teething. Teeth sensitive to cold air, as if they were very thin. Teeth feel too long. Gums sore and painful, worse from eating. Gumboils.

Nose - Sneezing and itching of nose. Nose sore and stuffed with yellow scabs. Fluent coryza, worse eating. Water smells like old, musty rainwater.

Rectum - Constipation with ineffectual urging. Pain, bursting in the perineum during stool. Even soft stool requires great effort to expel. Stool of one large heavy mass, foul like rotten cheese, or dry, small balls. Stools, misshapen, changeable, involuntary. Stools must be removed or crumbles at the verge of anus.

Skin - Eczema exuding sticky fluid, behind ears, on wrists, fingers and toes. Itching, worse by scratching. Skin is dry, brownish, flabby. Skin about neck wrinkled and hangs in folds. Copper-colored syphilitic sores. Fissured hands and fingers. Cracks on fingers. Tendency to small boils that do not mature.

Sleep - Falls asleep after vomiting. Frequent waking at night. Dreams of robbers and cannot sleep until the whole house is searched. Dreams of murder and remorse, lascivious dreams. On waking, child rubs eyes and nose with its fist.

Stomach - Bloating of stomach on beginning to eat. Sensation of a lump in stomach. Thirst little and often, water is vomited as soon as it reaches the stomach. Sour, rancid, burning belchings. Nausea after eating with sick feeling, better from smoking. Vomiting of milk soon after nursing.

Temperature - The cold air chills him. Chill every day at same time. Whole body feels too hot at night. Begins to sweat as soon as covered. Sticky sweat, particularly on side lain on. High fever every night with sleeplessness.

Throat - Dry throat. Hoarseness following sore throat, must clear throat before speaking. Cold, icy sensation, like peppermint. Throat feels too large. Can swallow solids better than fluids. Ulcers with yellowish base on tonsils.

Tongue - Sides of tongue turn up. Tongue adheres to roof of mouth. Tongue, large, flabby, burning, must protrude to keep it cool, ringworm on tongue. Thick yellow coating on back of tongue.

Vertigo - Vertigo on rising from stooping. Vertigo while sitting at table or desk. Vertigo after eating with nausea. Faint, smothering sensation with great desire for open air. Seasick sensation.

COMMENTS - Itching skin, eczema, worse bathing (Sil.). Sweaty, smelly feet, particularly in children (Sil.). Fear of the dark, sensitivity to storms (Phos.). Children are very obstinate, stubborn, hard to please.

Offensive vaginal discharges that smell like fish brine or dead fish (Hep.). Strong fishy odor in hemophilis, gardnerella and trichomonas. Discharge can also smell like rotten cheese.

RELATIONS - W. J. Guernsey considers Sanic. the chronic of Cham. ***Compare:*** (1) Sil., Phos., (2) The constituents of the Sanic. water, especially Nat-m. and Calc. (3) Dread of downward motion, Bor. (4) Head sweat, Calc., Sil. (5) Soreness behind ears, viscid discharge, Graph., Psor. (6) Ringworm on tongue, Nat-m., Ran-s., Tarax. (7) Drinks little and often, vomits as soon as it reaches stomach, Ars. (8) Symptoms change constantly, Carc., Lac-c., Puls. (9) Sphincter not under control, Aloe soc. (10) Stool recedes, Sil., Thuj., must be removed mechanically, Sel.

REFERENCES - Boericke. Clarke. Murphy. Phatak.

SANTALUM ALBUM

(Sandalwood)

PHARMACY - santa. Santalum album. Sandalwood. Santalum freycinetianum. Santalum paniculatum. N. O. Santalaceae. India, Sandwich Islands. The oil distilled from the wood. Dilutions with alcohol. ***Historical dose:*** Tincture and all potencies.

CLINICAL - Cystitis. Gonorrhea. Kidney pain.

HERBAL - The word "Santalum" is of Persian origin. Sandalwood oil is obtained from several species of Santalum, S. album being the chief. Its chief use in old-school practice is in gonorrhea.

HOMEOPATHIC - Shirtliff observed in a man taking the oil for gonorrhea, soon after each dose, an acute aching pain felt in the kidney region, so severe that if he was standing he was obliged to sit, which slightly relieved.

Shirtliff gave the same indication in his case of an elderly man, who looked worn and haggard, complained of pain in region of left kidney from ribs to iliac crest, brought on by walking, better leaning forward, completely better by lying down. Better pressing clenched fist into back.

The pain lasted six months and was very acute; Sulph., Berb. and Bry. gave no relief.

Santal. (oil), one drop every four hours, soon gave great relief and entirely removed the pain in two months.

REFERENCES - Boericke. Clarke.

SANTONINUM

(Santonin)

PHARMACY - sant. Santoninum. Santonin. A neutral active principle obtained from Cina. N. O. Compositae. Trituration. ***Historical dose:*** All potencies.

CLINICAL - Amblyopia. ***Bedwetting. Blindness.*** Cataract. ***Color blindness***. Convulsions. Cough. ***Cystitis.*** Delirium. Diarrhea. ***Dysuria.*** Eyes, paralysis. Enteralgia. Enteritis. Epilepsy. Gastroenteritis. ***Hallucinations.*** Hemoglobinuria. Hemiplegia. Hysterical. ***Incontinence.*** Nephritis. Infantile remittents. Melancholy. ***Night, cough.*** Nosebleed. Photophobia. Strangury. Tetanus. Urination, frequent. Urticaria. ***Vision, yellow.*** Vomiting. ***Worms.***

HOMEOPATHIC - Sant. is the active principle of Santonica, the unexpanded flower heads of Cina Artemisia Maritima.

Sant. is the favorite anthelmintic of the old school and it has been chiefly given against lumbrici. Fatal poisonings have caused convulsions, left side paralysis, delirium, vomiting and purging.

Worm affections, corresponding to the ***"pain in shocks"*** (Cina.). Gastro-intestinal irritation, ***itching of nose***, restless sleep, twitching of muscles. Ascaria lumbricoides and thread worms, but not tapeworms.

Color blindness and yellow vision. Visual illusions, ***yellow sight***, violent light not recognized, colors not distinguishable. ***Chronic cystitis***. Urine deep saffron color. Chronic gastric and intestinal troubles. ***Night cough*** of children. Laryngeal crises and lightning pains of tabes.

Spasms and twitchings. Violent convulsions, unconscious, head hot, face flushed, purplish. Spasm begins in face and spreads to limbs. Partial paralysis of one (left) side. Restlessness and prostration.

MIND - Delirium. Excited, laughs and sings. Hysterical. Restless and irritable. Wants everything, but satisfied with nothing. Profound and unusual depression with irresolution and want of confidence, unfitting him for work of any kind. Melancholy like that produced by jaundice. Coma.

Abdomen - Rumbling, very sensitive abdomen. Bruised but soft, hot, full. Severe abdominal pains with vomiting and purging. Every night pain in intestines before stool.

Chest - Paralysis of lungs, needs artificial respiration.

Eyes - Dark, blue rings around eyes. Eyes rolled convulsively, distorted, staring. Pupils dilated and insensible. Pressure in eyes. Photophobia with lachrymation. Sudden dimness of sight. Flickering before eyes. Objects seem to totter and dance, visions of figures, cherries, animals. ***Color blindness***, xanthopsia. Yellow soup looks red, blue evening sky looks green, objects look green, white looks yellow, violet. ***Yellow vision,*** objects as if in yellow haze or yellow light. Strabismus due to worms.

Face - Red, hot face, staring eyes. Face pale. Pale around mouth, worse afternoon. One cheek white, the other one is red. Lips swollen, glistening with the distention. Swelling under chin, left side of face. Face pinched, drawing in of lips over teeth with pinched expression of mouth and nose. Convulsive movements of muscles of face, especially lips and lids.

Food - Deficient appetite. Thirst intense, continual for ice cold water.

Head - Occipital headache with ***chronic hallucinations.*** Head turning and twisting, restless. Dullness of head. Pain in forehead.

Heart - Pulse is quick and full, rapid, lowered, left absent, right soft and steady.

Kidneys - Nephritis. Feeling of fullness of bladder. ***Incontinence and dysuria. Bedwetting***. Frequent efforts to urinate, only passes a few drops at a time, that color linen yellow. Urine greenish if acid and reddish purple if alkaline. Urine deep saffron yellow, thick, sulphur yellow, greenish. Hemoglobinuria.

Limbs - Spasms of limbs. Convulsive jerking of upper limbs. Twitching of hands and feet. Gait unsteady and tottering, staggered.

Lungs - Coughed incessantly all night from tickling in larynx and trachea. Breath is rapid, sighing, quick and catchy, rattling.

Mouth - Frothing from mouth. Tongue deep red, dry. Burning pains apparently torment her, as she forces everything into her mouth. Hallucinations of taste.

Nose - Nosebleeds. Hallucinations of smell. Things smell peculiar.

Rectum - Well-marked tenesmus. Purging of watery, flaky, foul-smelling stools, followed by vomiting. Stools copious, grayish, putrid-smelling.

Skin - Urticaria, with edema of nose, lips, and eyelids, over almost entire lids, with vomiting.

Sleep - Sleepy, tired. Sleep restless, disturbed, woke unrefreshed with sickness, frontal headache, and deficient appetite.

Stomach - Dull pain in pit of stomach. Frequent belchings. Nausea and vomiting. Nausea, better after eating. Vomiting and purging of yellowish, slimy mucus with severe abdominal pains.

Teeth - Grating teeth during sleep. Teeth clenched.

Temperature - Whole body icy cold, lips and ears blue, face white as snow. Limbs cold, very clammy coldness. Cold sweats. Hot sweat in occiput, more clammy in front. Violent fever, rapid pulse, burning heat of skin, face puffy, eyes brilliant, fixed.

Throat - The glands of neck, parotid and submaxillary are swollen.

Vertigo - Giddiness and intense headaches, every object looks bright green.

COMMENTS - A case recorded by Demme was quoted in Brit. Med. Jour., 1892. A boy, 3, was given fifteen tablets over three days by his mother. Each tablet contained 1/3 grain of Sant.

The symptoms produced were vomiting, dilatation of the pupils, collapse, cyanosis, dyspnea and finally convulsions. Dilatation of the pupils, collapse, cyanosis, dyspnea, and finally convulsions.

After a warm bath with cold applications to the head and spine, consciousness returned. The temperature was 103.5, nosebleed and hemoglobinuria occurred and a scarlatina-like eruption was noticed.

The child ultimately recovered. After a dose of 7 centigrams, a child, 2, was seized with prostration, convulsions, cramps and jaundice, followed on the third day by salivation and ulceration of the gum.

Less serious but very characteristic are the effects on the senses, especially the sense of sight. Visions of figures have been produced and colored vision is a frequent phenomenon, even when the lower triturations have been used.

Yellow is the predominant color, but green and violet vision are also marked. The urine also is yellow colored and stains yellow and is passed with much urging and painful burning. A kind of giant urticaria occurred in one case.

Hale recorded that Sant. cured cases of ***"nervous blindness."*** It was given to an old man, quite blind, for worms and his sight partially returned. This led to further trials in which it was given in nine cases of cataract and, according to Hale, four were cured, the rest not benefited.

Hale also mentioned bedwetting, strangury, chronic cystitis, as having been cured by it. Chronic catarrh of the bladder. Infantile remittents with or without worms,. In one prover there was ***"sensitiveness of the abdomen."***

RELATIONS - ***Compare:*** (1) Cina, Teucr., Napht., Nat-m. Phos., Spig. (2) Amaurosis, Benz-d., Carbn-s. (3) Colored vision, Cycl.

REFERENCES - Boericke. Clarke. Phatak.

SAPONARIA OFFICINALIS

(Soap Root)

PHARMACY - sapo. Saponaria officinalis. Soap root. Soapwort. Hedge pink. N. O. Caryophyllaceae. Tincture of the roots. ***Historical dose:*** Tincture and all potencies.

CLINICAL - Ciliary, neuralgia. Colds. ***Coryza***. Exophthalmos. Glaucoma. Sore throat. Trigeminal, neuralgia.

HOMEOPATHIC - Acute colds, coryza, sore throat, etc. Will often ***"break up"*** a cold. Worse at night, mental exertion, left side.

MIND - ***Depressed with sleepiness***. Apathetic. Utter indifference to pain or possible death.

Eyes - Violent eye pains. Hot stitches deep in eyeball. Ciliary neuralgia, worse left side. Exophthalmos, worse reading and writing. Increased intra-ocular pressure. Glaucoma. Photophobia.

Face - Left-sided trigeminal neuralgia, especially supra-orbital.

Head - Stitching pain, ***supra-orbital***, worse left side, evening, motion. Throbbing over orbits. Congestions to head, tired feeling in nape.

Heart - Impulse weak, pulse less frequent. Palpitations with anxiety.

Nose - ***Coryza***. Stopped up feeling in nose, also itching and sneezing.

Stomach - Difficult swallowing. Nausea, heartburn, full feeling not relieved by eructation.

Vertigo - Sensation of drunkenness with constant endeavor to go left-wards.

RELATIONS - ***Compare:*** (1) Sapin. (2) Verb., Cocc. - both containing Sapin. (3) Quill., Anag., Helon., Sars., Par., Agrostema, Cycl. and others contain Saponin.

REFERENCES - Boericke.

SAPONINUM

(Saponin)

PHARMACY - sapin. Saponinum. Saponin. A glucoside obtained from Saponaria officinalis. Trituration. Solution. Watery solution speedily decompose. ***Historical dose:*** All potencies.

CLINICAL - Acne. Bedwetting. Boils. Colic. Constipation. Diarrhea. Dysmenorrhea. Fevers. Headaches. Leucorrhea. Migraines. Menstrual disorders. Nausea. Photophobia. Rheumatism. Sleeplessness. Spleen, pain. Strabismus. Tongue, strawberry. Tonsillitis Vomiting.

HOMEOPATHIC - Sapin., a glucoside found in Quillaya, Yucca, Senega, Dioscorea and other plants, has had a somewhat extensive proving in potencies ranging from 1x to 30c, conducted by A. J. Hills.

One prover, who took the 30c, was for many years a sufferer from joint rheumatism, but had none of his usual pains during the proving and a great enlargement of the left knee was entirely removed.

Tired, indifferent. Migraine. ***Pain in left temple, eye,*** photophobia, hot stitches deep in eye. Fifth nerve disorders. Much pain before the menstrual flow, severe sore throat, worse right side tonsils swollen, worse in warm room. Sharp burning taste and violent sneezing.

Modalities - Better by stool, onset of menses. Better by cold, cold bathing. Better while sitting. Worse by moving, even motion of the eyes. Worse mental labor. Worse by warmth. Worse swallowing. Desire to vomit and defecate, worse when quiet.

COMMENTS - Two female provers had marked disturbance of the menstrual functions, especially pain and sufferings before the flow. Miliary eruption, colic and leucorrhea before the menses, pain better but not removed when the flow was established.

Severe sore throat, worse right side, was experienced by several provers, and Hills had so much swelling of the tonsils that he was obliged to abandon the proving. Bodily and mental depression. Exophthalmos and strabismus.

Roughness of mouth mucus membrane, raised papillae on palate and tongue. Strawberry tongue. Involuntary emission of urine when walking. Nausea and vomiting, colic and diarrhea, "nausea more in esophagus and throat, worse in a warm room."

This worse by warmth was met with in relation to many symptoms and is probably a keynote. At the same time there was much chilliness and lowered temperature is a characteristic feature.

RELATIONS - ***Compare:*** (1) Tough mucus, Kali-bi. (2) Onset of menses ameliorates, Lach. (3) Spleen pain, Cean. (4) Kidney pain, Santa. (5) Worse by movement, moving eyes, Bry. (6) Sleepy but cannot sleep, Bell. (7) Early waking, Bell., Nux-v. (8) Worse in warm room, Puls. (9) As if damp stockings on, Calc., Sanic. (10) Strawberry tongue, Frag., Bac. (11)

Involuntary emission of urine when walking, Ferr., Caust. (12) Seneg.

REFERENCES - Clarke.

SARCOLACTICUM ACIDUM

(Sarcolactic Acid)

PHARMACY - sarcol-ac. Sarcolacticum acidum. Sarcolactic acid. Dextrum lacticum acidum. Isomer of lactic acid. ***Historical dose:*** All potencies.

CLINICAL - Addison's disease. ***Chronic fatigue. Diabetes.*** Dyspnea. Headache. ***Influenza.*** Lichen planus. Myasthenia. Myasthenia. Myotonia. Neurasthenia. Polyuria. ***Prostration.*** Psoriasis. ***Rheumatism.*** Raynaud's syndrome. ***Rhinitis.*** Tumors.

HOMEOPATHIC - Sarcol-ac. is formed in muscle tissue during muscle exhaustion. It differs from ordinary lactic acid in its relation to polarized light. It represents a much broader and more profoundly acting drug and its pathogenesis is quite dissimilar from the normal acid.

The proving was the work of W. Griggs of the Hering Laboratory, Philadelphia. The experimentation was carried out in 1940 on eleven people (nine men and two women), using the 4x, 6x, 15x, and 30x potencies.

Wm. B. Griggs found Sarcol-ac. of great value in the most violent form of ***epidemic influenza, especially with violent and retching and greatest prostration***, when Ars. had failed. ***Influenza with rhinitis.*** Locally in the tuberculous ulceration of vocal cords.

Intra-muscular lactic acid, following prolonged exercise, which generates fatigue. This ***chronic fatigue***, when pushed to an advanced stage, results in an almost paralyzing weakness with prostration. Spinal neurasthenia, muscular weakness, dyspnea with myocardial weakness.

Extreme fatigue, anxiety, prostration. Muscular cramping pains, aggravated by movement. Digestive intolerance. Dryness and itching of the skin. Morning sickness, ***diabetes and rheumatism*** offer a field for this remedy. Troubles in the breasts.

MIND - Feeling of laziness, weakness. Dejection. Irritability, becomes easily annoyed by the smallest thing.

Abdomen - Sedative, palliative for gastro-intestinal tumors.

Back - Tired feeling in back and neck and shoulders. Paralytic weakness. Cramping pains in the back and lumbar region, aggravated when standing.

Chest - Aortic pain and rapid pulse after exertion.

Head - Headache and vomiting, pain situated on the forehead and above the eyes, ameliorated by going to stool.

Heart - Cardiac rheumatism. Raynaud's syndrome.

Kidneys - Polyuria. Profuse nocturnal urination. Urine clear with traces of proteinuria.

Limbs - Psoric rheumatism. Rheumatoid arthritis. Fibrous rheumatism. Paresthesia, joint numbness and pains. Extreme weakness from climbing stairs. Stiffness of thigh and calves. Cramp in the calves. Arms feel as if no strength in them. Wrist tires easily from writing. Writer's cramp. Difficulty in brushing hair.

Lungs - Dyspnea, feeling of cardiac weakness, croupy cough, especially at night. Bronchitis. Dry, painful pleurisy.

Modalities - Worse at night. Worse from movement, from standing upright.

Nose - Coryza, throat dry and painful, swallowing impeded, alleviated by day, aggravated at night.

Rectum - Burning hemorrhoids. Stools acrid and expulsion of gases in profuse, easing the condition.

Skin - Intense general itching, improved by the cold. Keratotic eczema. Lichen planus. Psoriasis. Scleroderma (Graph.).

Sleep - Difficulty in going to sleep, sleep light when it comes. Wakes aching and exhausted.

Stomach - Heavy, painful feeling in the pit of the stomach. Digestive intolerance, especially of cold water. Acrid dyspepsia. Nausea. Uncontrollable vomiting even of water followed by extreme weakness.

Temperature - General chilliness with coldness of the limbs. Extreme chilliness in bed. The right hand does not become warm by external heat.

Throat - Constriction in pharynx. Sore throat with tightness in naso-pharynx. Tickling in throat.

COMMENTS - According to Dr. Kuhl, lactic acid has an anti-cancerous preventive action and he recommended a special diet with additional lacto-fermented products.

RELATIONS - ***Compare:*** (1) Eup-per. - cracking sensation with acute pains in the bones. (2) Bry. - aggravation by movement. (3) Arn. - muscular bruises.

REFERENCES - Boericke. Julian.

SAROTHAMNUS SCOPARIUS

(Scotch Broom)

PHARMACY - saroth. Sarothamnus scoparius. Scotch broom. Spartium scoparium. Cystisus scoparius. Genista scoparia. N. O. Leguminosae. Papilionoideae. Europe. The tincture is prepared from the flowers. ***Historical dose:*** Tincture and all potencies.

CLINICAL - Acne rosacea. Albuminuria. Alopecia. Angina pectoris. Bacillary, dysentery. Cheyne-Stokes. Choroiditis. Collagen diseases. Diabetes insipidus. Emaciation. Glaucoma. Hay fever. ***Heart, disorders.*** Hodgkin's disease. ***Hypertension.*** Hypotension. Impetigo. Insomnia. Iritis. ***Kidneys, disorders.*** Leukemia. Nephritis. Ozaena. Palpitations. Parasites. Pityriasis. Sinusitis. Tobacco, heart. Worms.

HERBAL - Sarothamnus scoparium is a shrubby tree, widespread throughout Europe. The twigs are used for the extraction of the official spartein, the flowers are rich in flavonoids, and the plant contains aromatic amines.

Sparteine sulphate, an alkaloid found in scotch broom, causes a lowering of the systolic and diastolic pressures of the provers. It also lowers blood-pressure.

Depresses the heart by its poisonous action on the myocardium, and this, with the stimulating action of the drug upon the vagus, accounts for the lowered blood pressure and reduced pulse rate. It weakens the cardiac contraction. The total amount of urine is increased, diuretic properties, useful in dropsy.

HOMEOPATHIC - Hinsdale attempted the first homeopathic proving in 1918, on three students. In 1897, Schier conducted a proving on six people, using the tincture and the infusion of the winter root, as well as the tincture and infusion of the fresh flowers.

Mezger undertook a true proving on twenty-seven provers of whom seven were women, at the Robert Bosch Hospital in 1951-52. He used the 4x, and 2x potencies as well as the mother tincture.

Saroth. is a ***heart tonic***, affects the kidneys, cord, muscles and left side. Sparteine sulphate increases the strength of the heart, slows it and reduces the blood pressure. Hinsdale reported that it continues the good effects of Verat. and Dig. without any of the undesirable effects of either.

Irregular heart action from influenza or other infectious diseases. Arterial hypertension, arteriosclerosis. Relieves the congestion of kidneys enabling them to eliminate and relieve the distress upon the heart. Heavy aching.

Cheyne-Stokes respiration. Irregular heart following grip and various infections. Hypotension. Very useful in sustaining heart after stopping habit of morphine. Indicated when primarily the muscles of the heart and especially the nervous apparatus is affected. Acts rapidly and lasts three to four days. Does not disturb digestion.

Specific action on the kidneys, enabling them to eliminate and relieve the stress on the heart. Nephritis. Albuminuria.

Congestion of the thyroid gland, hands clammy, sleep disturbed, hot flushes, emaciation. Increase in the size of the thyroid. Extreme tiredness. Leukemia with eosinophil.

MIND - Irritable, loses his temper at the slightest thing. Irritability from trifles. Inner agitation, ideas escape him. Easily irritated and likely to explode. Excitement at night. Melancholic disposition is upset easily.

Apathetic without spirit, distracted. Absent-minded. Everything is too much for him, difficulty in concentrating. Weakness of the senses and body. General inhibition, but especially erotic. Obsession with erotic thoughts. Sexual thoughts intrude and crowd around each other.

Abdomen - Stomach and bowels seem to be filled with stones or as a firm mass. Spasmodic entero-colitis. Flatulency with much mental depression. Sensation of abdominal repletion and stomach feels hollow. Passage through intestines accelerated with three to six evacuations a day. Bacillary dysentery. Intestinal tuberculosis. Intestinal parasites.

Back - Pain in the lumbar region.

Blood - Leukemia. Eosinophilia. Attacks of vasodilation at the limbs in the big toe and foot.

Breasts - Nodular congestion of the right breast (especially in men).

Chest - Angina pectoris. Constriction in the precordial region with sensation of tightness and anguish.

Constitutions - Tubercular, thyroidism or nervous. Allergic, psoric constitutions.

Ears - Monotonous rumbling and crackling in both ears, particularly intense between 7 p.m. and 8 p.m. Buzzing and other noises.

Eyes - Chronic glaucoma. Choroiditis. Iritis. Burning and stinging pains, especially behind the left eyeball. Pain on moving the eyes. When looking at an area of light, the brightness of the light and the rainbow colors of the halo seem more intense.

Face - Barber's itch.

Female - Excessive menses and long intervals between menses. Menses late and prolonged. Sex drive increased. Loss of libido, genital deficiency and evil-smelling sweating from the genital region.

Food - Appetite increases, constant need to eat. Persistent feeling of hunger, despite constant feeling of nausea. Loss of appetite with aversion to food and strangling feeling. Aversion to eggs and meat.

Head - Pulsating headaches, as if the skull would burst. Headache, as if wearing a helmet, going from the eyes towards the occiput (glaucoma). Congestion in the head. Flashes of heat in head.

Heart - Anxious oppression, radiating to left shoulder and neck. Hypotension. Tobacco heart. Angina pectoris. Irregular action, disturbed rhythm due to gas, feeble in nervous hysterical patients. Myocardial degeneration, failing compensation. Palpitations with congestion to head.

Kidneys - Drawing pains in the kidneys with colic pains. Increased urination. Very profuse, bright foaming urine, then burning in the pudendum. Hydronephrosis. Albuminuria. Diabetes insipidus. Frequent need to urinate at night, especially around 5 a.m. Bedwetting.

Limbs - All the muscles are painful, as if stiff. Shooting pains. Sudden pains, regularly in the sciatic nerve. Sciatica. Neuralgic pains, beginning on the right side, moving towards the left and diminishing on the right. Drawing joint pains. Chronic inflammation of the hip. Nocturnal pain in the hips and sacrum, left shoulder, left elbow and fingers of the right hand. Fidgets in the legs, which prevent him from falling asleep. Strumous edema of the legs. Deadness of right arm and fingers. Chilblains. Acrocyanosis.

Lungs - Asthma.

Male - Loss of libido, genital deficiency and evil-smelling sweating from the genital region.

Modalities - Better from cool air, rapid motion, passing flatus. Worse turning on left side.

Mouth - Vesicles on the lips and mouth.

Nose - Hay fever. Ozaena. Maxillary sinusitis. One-sided obstruction. Nostrils blocked alternately. Nasal secretions, streaked with blood and abrasion of the nasal orifices. Tickling in the nose with frequent sneezing. Small new growths on the nasal wall.

Rectum - Tenesmus, ameliorated by emission of wind. Colic, then bright acrid foaming stools followed by burning in anus. Stools yellow, glairy with tenesmus. Stools hard like balls, covered with mucus and mixed with a frothy diarrhea. Alternating diarrhea and constipation. Hemorrhoids with splinter-like pain.

Skin - Allergic eruptions. Urticaria. Folliculitis. Boils. Pityriasis. Dysidrosis. Adenitis of the sweat glands. Impetigo. Acne rosacea. Small vesicles, extremely irritating. Eczematous eruption, both damp and dry.

Infiltration and bluish coloring in the joints of the toes. Copious nocturnal sweating with a strong odor. Hair stiff, dandruff. Loss of hair in patches. Alopecia.

Sleep - Insomnia. Sleep long in coming with abundant ideas. Sleep light, easily woken by noise. Waking between 3 a.m. and 5 a.m. Dreams are pleasant and colorful. Dreams at times, about disappearances, murders, deaths. Unrefreshing sleep. On waking, feels tired and has the impression of not having slept enough. Great need for sleep, spends a large part of the day in bed.

Stomach - Ptosis of the stomach and intestines. Dyspepsia. Aggravation of stomachache by food.

Temperature - Sensitive to the cold, worse in the evening, feeling of head, sweating, numbness.

Throat - Irritation of the larynx with dry cough, coming from the throat. Tickling in the throat. Acute and chronic laryngitis.

COMMENTS - Weakness of the senses and body. Sensation of uneasiness and cold, which is worrying, only the head needs fresh air. Sensation of coldness, except for the head, which is better in fresh air.

Pain in the cardiac region and rhythmic anomalies. Pains and cardiac palpitations with tingling and feeling of soreness, especially when lying on the left side. Palpitations, especially at night and when resting, but also from slight exertion. Violent cardiac pulsations, which shake the whole body.

Pulse accelerated. Extra systole, notices the irregularity of the contractions. Left ventricular cardiac deficiency. Angina pectoris. Rhythmic anomaly. Basedow's heart. Aortitis.

Bubbling sensation in the head. Precordial constriction with anguish. Rheumatic pain, moving from right to left. Sudden pain in the left sciatic nerve around 10 p.m. Hollow sensation in the stomach and abdominal repletion. Sleep long in coming.

RELATIONS - ***Compare:*** (1) Kalm. - Pains along the nerves from the center to the periphery and from top to bottom. Sudden pain, which moves around. Palpitations, worse when lying on the left side. Pulse slow. (2) Spig. - Violent palpitations with oppression and anxiety. Must lie on the right side with the head high. (3) Iber. - Violent palpitations at the least exertion. Pulse full, irregular. Aggravated in a warm room and when lying on the left side.

REFERENCES - Boericke. Julian.

SARRACENIA PURPUREA

(Pitcher Plant)

PHARMACY - sarr. Sarracenia purpurea. Pitcher plant. N. O. Sarraceniaceae. Grows in boggy places from Canada southward. Contains a very active proteolytic enzyme. Tincture of fresh plant. Tincture of root. ***Historical dose:*** Tincture and all potencies.

CLINICAL - Back, pains. Bones, pains. Borborygmus. Constipation. Coxalgia. Diarrhea. Eruptions, scrofulous. Femur, pains. Herpes. Influenza. Lumbago. Psoriasis. Smallpox. Vision, disordered.

HERBAL - The use of the pitcher plant in smallpox is a discovery of the Native Americans of North America, the spotted appearance of the plant probably suggesting a resemblance to the disease.

HOMEOPATHIC - A proving by T. C. Duncan, Thomas and others brought out symptoms of fever, backache, headache and gastric disturbance. Hale collected much confirmatory evidence of its power to antidote the smallpox poison.

Sarr. is a remedy for variola. Congestion to head with irregular heart action. Sick headache, throbbing in various parts, especially in neck, shoulders and head, which feels full to bursting. Visual disorders. Chlorosis.

Feels dull and heavy, sweats freely. Insensibility of right side, paralysis of hearing and smell. Debility, heavy, languid. Dull, heavy, sore feeling in all bones. Phlegmonous swelling with a rosy tint on various parts. Unrefreshed though slept soundly.

MIND - Melancholy. Great depression of spirits with frontal headache. Dullness of mind. Forgetful. Loss of memory with the headache. Difficult to concentration. Alternate apathy and intellectual activity. Anxious about everything.

Abdomen - Transient pains in bowels. Bloated about navel. Borborygmi and some pain in bowels with constipation, dry throat.

Back - Deep-seated pain in back. ***Pains shooting in zigzag*** course from lumbar region to middle of scapula. ***Weakness between the shoulders***. Warm sensation passed up back into head. Back weak, wants to lean on something. Pain and soreness in sacrum.

Chest - Pains in third and fourth ribs, with great apprehension of heart disease. Pain in angle of ribs. Soreness of pectoralis major.

Ears - Ringing in ears. Sticking pains deep in right ear, transient but recurring often, same in left ear. Intense earache, fears he will lose his senses. Swelling of parotids.

Eyes - Eyes feel swollen and sore. Pain in orbits. Photophobia. Black objects move with the eye.

Face - Face flushed. Heat and redness of face. Face pale with heat and chill alternating. Erysipelatous swelling of face. Miliary eruption. Scaly herpes on face. Intense neuralgic pains from temples to jaws.

Female - Bloody discharge at other times menstrual period, as during menopause. Watery or milky leucorrhea, foul-smelling, with spasmodic pains in uterus. Pulsative pains in womb with swelling as if from a tumor or dropsy. Uterus swollen as if full of cysts. Cervix swollen, hot. Miliary eruption and heat in vulva.

Food - Hungry all the time, even after a meal. Appetite unusually active. Little appetite, but what is eaten agrees. Great desire to sleep during eating.

Head - Light feeling in head. Sensation as if he had received a knock on the head, drowsiness and staggering gait. Sensation as if head were split.

Heart - Congestion to chest, heavy feeling about heart. Feeling of congestion about head, with irregularity of heart's action.

Kidneys - Urine phosphatic, scanty, limpid.

Limbs - Limbs cold when still, as from poor circulation. Weakness of limbs with paralytic debility. Limbs weak, bruised pain in knees and hip joints. Pains and soreness in diaphyses of all long bones. Bones in arm pain.

Lungs - Paroxysms of suffocation and nosebleed. Tuberculosis and bronchial disorders. Cough with desire to vomit, and vomiting. Hemoptysis, thick cough, continual tickling in larynx and bronchi. Hard cough, shaking chest and bowels. Expectoration of mucus, tenacious, filamentary, with a bitter, putrid, oily taste.

Modalities - Better in fresh air, out of bed. Worse about midnight, in the morning, at 3 p.m. Worse rising from lying, trying to walk. Worse in stormy weather. Open air causes chilliness, hands and feet cold, causes head to be hot, sore and feel full. Cold air causes to chilliness and aggravates bone pains.

Mouth - Tongue is dry, coated brownish white. Mouth dry, lips and mouth parched. Toothache at night in bed, from least contact, and cold air.

Nose - Nosebleed nearly producing fainting. Nose swollen, red, with pressure and pulsation at root. Fluent coryza with cold chills and loss of smell. Foul-smelling, green, yellowish, or bloody discharges. Fetid smell.

Rectum - Rectum and anus swollen and inflamed. Much flatus. Much tenesmus, dysenteric diarrhea. Stool copious, dark, fetid, evacuated with great straining, morning. Stools very hard, covered with mucus, and dark. First part of stool natural, last diarrhea. Morning diarrhea, faint after stool.

Sensations - Heat in face as if on fire. Left eye as if congested. Swelling in uterus as if from a tumor or dropsy, as if full of cysts. As if bones of leg were too thick.

Skin - Eruptions similar to crusta lactea. Herpes. Psoriasis. Scrofulous eruptions. Smallpox, aborts the disease, arrests pustules.

Sleep - Sleepy in daytime, sleep disturbed by strange and frightful dreams. Awakes early in a fright with urging to urinate.

Stomach - Sleepy during meals. Empty, hungry feeling, can keep nothing in his stomach. Burning pains in stomach with palpitations and contraction. Pinching pain in stomach, it feels distended and torn. Copious, painful vomiting.

Temperature - Feverish and shaking chills, worse morning. General chills between shoulder blades. Chills, heat, and sweat, 5 p.m. Skin hot and dry. Hands hot, warm all over. Head and body warm. Perspires freely.

Throat - Throat dry, not better by tea or water.

Vertigo - Vertigo with cramps in neck, worse at night.

COMMENTS - Hering quoted several instances of Sarr. action. The first was a woman far advanced in pregnancy who was cured of smallpox with Sarr. 3c, 6c and 9c, delivery as accomplished during her convalescence, the infant bearing on its body numerous red blotches indicating that it had been affected with the disease.

A second case concerned an infant a few months old who was attacked with a grave form of smallpox with variolous angina so severe that it was with difficulty it could take the breast, the mother took Sarr. 3c, 6c and 9c and continued to nurse the infant, which promptly recovered, the mother not taking the disease.

In an epidemic occurring in the environs of Wavre, Sarr. was given to two thousand people living in the very middle of the disease and coming in constant intercourse with it, but all who took Sarr. escaped. During the same epidemic, two hundred cases were treated with Sarr. without a death.

Bilden, who used the 1x tincture in an epidemic with success, concluded that Sarr. is to smallpox what Gels. is to bilious fever.

Hale quoted Surgeon-Major C. G. Logie's (an allopath) account of his experience with Sarr. (decoction probably) in smallpox: "Four of the cases in my hospital have been severe confluent cases. They have throughout the disease all been perfectly sensible, have had excellent appetites, been free from pain and have never felt weak.

"The effects of this medicine, which I have carefully watched, seemed to arrest the development of the pustules, killing, as it were, the virus from within, thereby changing the character of the disease and doing away with pitting."

A number of eye symptoms appeared in the provings and Sarr. has cured disordered vision. A case of "phlyctenoid herpes" has also been reported cured by it. Extreme lassitude and pains in the bones were prominent in the provings. Week feeling in the arms. Very sensitive to cold air.

Sarr. has the empty, hungry, sinking sensation of the anti-psorics. Dryness of mouth and throat. Faint after stool. Bladder and rectal tenesmus. Stool smells of musk. The right side was more affected than the left.

RELATIONS - ***Antidoted by:*** Podo. ***Compare:*** (1) In smallpox, Ant-t., Merc., Vac., Vario., Maland. (2) In bone pains, Eup-per.

REFERENCES - Boericke. Clarke.

SARSAPARILLA OFFICINALIS

(Wild Licorice)

PHARMACY - sars. Sarsaparilla officinalis. Wild licorice. Smilax officinalis. The root of several species of Smilax. N. O. Smilaceae, by some classed as a sub-order of the Liliaceae. Triturations and tincture of the dried rhizome. ***Historical dose:*** Tincture and all potencies.

CLINICAL - Asthma. Bedwetting. Bladder, disorders. ***Blood, disorders.*** Bones, disorders. Breast, scirrhous. Bright's disease. Constipation. ***Cystitis.*** Cracks, skin. Dysmenorrhea. Dyspepsia. ***Dysuria. Emaciation.*** Eruptions. Eyes, disorders. Faintness. Glands, enlarged. Gonorrhea. Gout. Gravel. Hands, chapped. Headaches. Hernia. Herpes. Hiccoughs. Intermittent fever. ***Kidney, colic.*** Kidney, disorders. Marasmus. Masturbation, effects. Melancholy. Menopause. Mercury, abuse. Mycosis. Nephritis. ***Nipples, retracted.*** Plica polonica. Rheumatism. Seborrhea. Spermatic cords, swelling. Spermatorrhea. ***Stones.*** Strangury. ***Syphilis.*** Ulcers. Warts.

HERBAL - The dried root or rhizome of sarsaparilla, as imported, is of the thickness of a goose quill, many feet in length, reddish brown, odorless, mucilaginous in taste, feebly bitter, and faintly acrid.

It was historically reputed, according to Mile, to be a diaphoretic tonic, alterative. It was given in scrofula and secondary syphilis and the concomitants of these diseases such as ulcers, cutaneous eruptions, nodes indurated glands, decay, and necroses. Joint swellings and rheumatism often improve under a protracted course of it. Some think it a kind of restorative after an exhausting course of mercury.

HOMEOPATHIC - Hahnemann proved Sars., confirming many of the historical uses. Sars. is *"restorative"* after over-dosing with Merc., because it is a homeopathic antidote to Merc. It covers the syphilitic, sycotic and psoric constitutions.

Affinity for the genito-urinary organs, skin, bones, and lower right extremity. Marasmus, emaciation. Kidney colic. Marked urinary symptoms. Moist eruptions about the genitals or between the scrotum and thighs. Periosteal pains due to venereal disease. Retraction of nipples in those of cancerous inheritance or constitution.

Clears the complexion. Eruptions following hot weather and vaccinations, boils and eczema. Fig warts. Scratching causes itching to begin in another place, causes eruption on forehead to become humid.

Parts feel screwed together. Nightly bone pains. Pains shoot in different directions and are accompanied by depression and anxiety. As if salt were put upon the wound. Very sore, gouty nodes. Rheumatism.

MIND - Depression and anxiety from pain. Despondent, gloomy without any cause. Ill humored and taciturn. Sensitive, easily offended.

Abdomen - Rumbling with sensation of emptiness. Much flatus, rumbling and fermentation. Colic and backache at the same time, with diarrhea. Cholera infantum.

Back - Emaciation of neck. Backache with colic. Pain from small of back down the spermatic cord after emission.

Bladder - Bladder distended and tender. Tenesmus of bladder. Urging to urinate before menses. Pain at meatus, in urethra going back to abdomen. Jerking along the urethra. Can pass urine only when standing, ***urine dribbles while sitting***. Urine passes in thin, feeble stream. Urine scanty, slimy, flaky, sandy, pus, ***bloody***. Air passes from bladder during urination. Crusty urinary sediment. Sand on diaper. ***Severe pain at conclusion of urination.***

Breasts - Sore, shriveled breasts. ***Nipples retracted or cracked, small and shriveled.*** Nipples retracted before menses.

Constitutions - Anti-syphilitic and anti-sycotic. Suited to children with faces like old people and enlarged abdomens, to thin, frail, shriveled, old looking persons. To dark-haired persons, and to lithic or sycotic diathesis.

Ears - Words reverberate in ear to the root of nose.

Eyes - Foggy vision, worse seminal emission. Itch like eruptions on eyelids.

Face - Yellow, wrinkled, old looking. ***Eruptions on face and upper lip***, worse during menses.

Female - Moist eruption and soreness in right groin before menses. Menses late and scanty. Dysmenorrhea, with retracted nipples or sore breast.

Head - ***Itching and humid eruption of forehead***. Moist eruption on scalp. Scalp sensitive. Crusta lactea beginning in face. Shooting pain from above right temporal region. ***Pains from occiput to eyes*** or to root of nose. As of a painful tight band around the head. Periosteal pains due to venereal disease. ***Pains cause depression***.

Kidneys - ***Pain from right kidney downward***. Kidney colic and painful urination, in infants. ***Child screams before and while passing urine***. Gravel.

Limbs - Rheumatism, bone pains, worse at night. Rheumatic pains after gonorrhea (Thuj.). Paralytic, tearing pains. Affections of any kind in general in right lower limb. Trembling of hands and feet. Burning on sides of fingers and toes, under nails. Deep cracks on fingers and toes, worse sides. Cutting sensation under nails (Petr.). Tetter on hands, ulceration around ends of fingers (Psor.).

Male - Genitals moist and offensive. Itching on scrotum and perineum. Herpetic eruption on genitals. Syphilis, squamous eruption and bone pains. Intolerable stench on genitals. Bloody semen. Spermatic cord painful after emission, swollen after unrequited sexual excitement. Jerking along urethra.

Modalities - Better from uncovering neck and chest, warmth. Standing improves difficult urination. ***Worse at the close of urination***. Worse from cold, wet, dampness, spring, at night. Worse from touch, pressure, tight clothes. Worse motion, sitting, going up and down stairs. Worse scratching, yawning. Worse after urinating, before menses, from suppressed gonorrhea.

Mouth - ***Aphthae***, ***salivation***. Offensive breath. Metallic taste, no thirst. White tongue. Pain in jaw, worse bending head back.

Nose - Stoppage for years. Swelling at the root of nose.

Rectum - Cholera infantum. Obstinate constipation with frequent want to urinate. Sand in stools.

Sensations - As if in a dream. Buzzing as if a large bell had been struck in head. As if he had been hit with a hammer on top of head. As of a great weight in head. As if breath were stopped by a spasm. Breastbone as if bruised. As if chest were too short. Limbs as if paralyzed. As if fingertips ulcerated or as if salt were put on a wound.

Skin - ***Emaciated, shriveled, skin lies in folds*** (Abrot., Sanic.). Dry, flabby skin. Skin hard, indurated. Cracks on hands and feet. New skin cracks and burns. Itching, scaly spots. Dry, itching rash from exposure to open air, ***comes on in spring,*** becomes crusty. Summer cutaneous disorders. Herpetic eruptions, ulcers. Irritating pus. Copper-colored eruptions. Ecchymoses in old age. Edema.

Sleep - Yawning. Complaints concomitant to yawning. Worse when yawning. Sleep early in evening. Nocturnal sleeplessness and frequent waking. Frightful dreams.

Stomach - Sensation of emptiness after a meal as while fasting, or else nausea or disgust when thinking of what has been eaten. Drinking water causes vomiting.

Temperature - Chill starts from region of bladder to back. Influenza.

COMMENTS - Sars. chiefly affects the urinary organs, genitals, rectum, skin and bones, right lower extremity, right lower side inner, and one-sided head. General "sinking" sensation of the great anti-psorics. General sensitiveness.

Acute and chronic bladder infections. Kidney stones, and the tendency to form kidney stones. Acute kidney stone colic (Berb.). Cystitis. Bladder infections in children, the child screams when they feel the urge because they anticipate the pain (Petros.).

Cannot pass urine freely except when standing, dribbles when sitting. Excessive pain in urethra that runs back into abdomen. Great pain and burning at end of urination (Equis.). Tenesmus. Urine is turbid, full of flakes and mucus or gravel, red or gray sand, or particulate matter. Urine with mucus or blood.

Gonorrhea, and the effect of suppressed gonorrhea. Herpes. Moist eruptions on scrotum and thighs. Spermatorrhea with swollen cords. The semen may be bloody. Offensive odor about genitals in both sexes.

"Moist eruption in right groin before menses." Painful and disordered menstruation. Nipples are soft, unexcitable, retracted, inverted. Cracked nipples (Cast-eq.), associated with cancer (Aster., Phyt.). Breast abscesses (Phyt.), with inverted nipples. Scirrhus of the breast. Helpful in patients of cancerous history with retracted nipples.

Herpetic eruptions in all parts. Moist and dry tettery eruptions. Cracks. Itch-like eruptions, prone to appear in spring. Itching eruption on forehead during menses. Emaciation, causing the skin to be shriveled and lie in folds.

Pains shoot in different directions. Anxiety accompanies the pains, and can cause depression. Warmth generally relieves. Warm diet aggravates, cold diet relieves. Warm room aggravates vertigo. Washing, bread and yawning aggravates.

Grimmer wrote, "Ulcers, cutaneous eruptions, nodes indurated glands, decay, necroses, joint swellings and rheumatism often improve under a persistent course of this remedy."

One of Sars. popular uses was for "clearing the complexion." When it succeeds it is by virtue of its similarity, for Clarke saw a very extensive crop of blotches it produced in a young woman.

Farrington offered several indications for Sars., including sycotic eruptions with little spots scarcely raised above the skin, often scaling a little, but looking like the roseola of syphilis and itching intolerably, worse in spring.

Moist eruption on scalp, the pus from which causes the inflammation of any part it touches. Sycotic headache, beginning at back of head, coming forward and settling at root of nose with swelling of nose. Moist eruption about genitals or between the scrotum and thighs.

With Sars., Skinner cured many cases of retraction or flattening of the nipple in nursing women. On two occasions with high potencies of Sars. he enabled a woman to nurse her child when it was utterly hopeless.

ELATIONS - ***Antidoted by:*** Bell., Merc. ***It antidotes:*** Merc. ***Compare:*** (1) Berb., Lyc., Nat-m., Petr., Sass. (2) Saur. - Lizard's tail - irritation of kidneys, bladder, prostate and urinary passages. Painful and difficult urination, cystitis with strangury. (3) Cuc-c. - Watermelon, infusion of the seed acts promptly in painful urination with constriction and backache, relieves pain and stimulates flow. ***Compatible:*** Hep., All-c., Phos., Rhus-t., Sulph., Sep. ***Complementary:*** Merc., Sep.

REFERENCES - Boericke. Clarke. Grimmer. Murphy. Phatak.

SASSAFRAS OFFICINALIS

PHARMACY - sass. Sassafras officinalis. N.O. Lauraceae. ***Historical dose:*** Tincture and all potencies.

HERBAL - Sassafras is a warm, aromatic stimulant, alterative, diaphoretic, and diuretic. Also used in diseases of the kidneys and bladder.

The oil is said to relieve the pain caused by menstrual obstructions, and pain following parturition, in doses of 5 to 10 drops on sugar, the same dose having been found useful in gleet and gonorrhea.

Dr. Shelby of Huntsville stated that it would both prevent and remove the injurious effects of tobacco. The mucilage of the pith (2 drachms to 1 pint of water) is used as a local application in acute ophthalmia, and is a demulcent drink in disorders of the chest, bowels, kidneys, and bladder.

Externally, as a rubefacient, in painful swellings, sprains, bruises, rheumatism, etc., and is said to check the progress of gangrene. A lotion of rose-water or distilled water, with sassafras pith, filtered after standing for four hours, is recommended for the eyes.

An infusion of the bark administered internally and applied externally is reputed an excellent treatment for rhus poisoning. Dr. King has also derived some benefit from its internal use in gonorrhea and obstinate gleet, 5 to 10 drops on sugar, 3 times a day.

REFERENCES - King. Murphy.

SAURURUS CERNUUS

(Lizard's tail)

PHARMACY - saur. Saururus cernuus. Lizard's tail. N. O. Piperaceae. The entire plant including the root is macerated in twice its weight of alcohol. ***Historical dose:*** All potencies.

CLINICAL - Cystitis. Kidneys, disorders. Prostate, disorders.

HOMEOPATHIC - The Saur. plant is an indigenous perennial found in swampy localities in some parts of the United States. It has been and is still used in domestic practice for those conditions for which Dr. Phares commended it, including irritation and inflammation of the kidneys, bladder, prostate and urinary passages.

Phares considered it peculiarly adapted to all such cases if they were attended by strangury or painful difficult urination. He used the remedy both externally and internally and he found that the stomach was very tolerant of the rather heroic doses he prescribed.

RELATIONS - ***Compare:*** (1) Canth., Berb.

REFERENCES - Anshutz.

SCAMMONIUM

(Scammony)

PHARMACY - scam. Scammonium. Scammony. Convolvulus scammonia. N. O. Convolvulacae. Triturations of the dried milky juice of the root. ***Historical dose:*** Tincture and all potencies.

CLINICAL - Diarrhea. Gastro-enteritis. ***Vomiting.***

HOMEOPATHIC - Scam. is a drastic cathartic, producing copious watery evacuations and griping. Scam. must be compared with Jalap., another purging convolvulus. Sprengel recorded a case of fatal poisoning in an infant whose mother took a large quantity of Scam. and herself suffered no effects. Symptoms included ***sudden vomiting and copious green stools,*** distention and sensitiveness of the abdomen, and finally death.

Abdomen - Distention and sensitiveness of abdomen. Violent pain and rapid succession of stools, leaving inactivity of lower intestines for several days.

Rectum - Copious green stools. Loose evacuation of feces with slight pain in stomach. Rapid succession of stools.

Stomach - Sudden vomiting. Pain in stomach with the bowel movements. Inflammation of mucus membrane attended with loss of appetite and headache.

REFERENCES - Clarke.

SCARLATININUM

(Scarlet Fever Nosode)

PHARMACY - scarl. Scarlatininum. Scarlet fever nosode. Nosodes. ***Historical dose:*** All potencies.

CLINICAL - Albuminuria. Nephritis. ***Scarlet, fever.*** Skin disorders. Throat, sore.

HOMEOPATHIC - Scarl. has been used, like other nosodes, for the prevention and cure of the disease from which it takes origin. Its well-known affinity for the skin, throat and kidneys suggests its applicability for disorders of those organs.

COMMENTS - Zinke reported a case in which a patient suffered from angina with hyperthemia. Profound asthenia and infectious look. Grave hyperthemia of tonsils swollen, pillars, the uvula dark red, the submaxillary glands swollen, painful. The patient had suffered from scarlatina treated by penicillin. Since that time the general condition was bad.

Zinke prescribed Scarl. 12x, twice 2 globules the first day. Immediate amelioration which the patient had not had till then. Repeated once 12 and 14 days after one dose of Scarl. 30x. The patient was cured.

RELATIONS - Bell. is the nearest analog and should be its antidote and the various Mercuries come next. ***Compare:*** (1) Apis, Ars., Rhus-t., Morbill., Diph.

REFERENCES - Clarke.

SCHINUS MOLLE

PHARMACY - schin. Schinus molle. N. O. Anacardiacae. Tincture of leaves and berries. ***Historical dose:*** Tincture and all potencies.

CLINICAL - Diarrhea. Esophagus, dryness. Flatulence. Heartburn. Liver, pain. Spinal cord, drawing. Vomiting.

HOMEOPATHIC - Allen reported that schinus is an evergreen shrub, native of Mexico and South America and frequently cultivated in Southern California under the names "Pepper tree" and "Chili pepper."

The Schin. symptoms were observed by Dr. P. W. Poulson on a young woman who ate a few berries after dinner, as well as on himself. He ate the leaves as well as the berries and experienced heartburn, griping in liver and "a kind of drawing sensation a in the spinal cord and cerebellum."

Abdomen - Rolling and flatulence in the bowels. Griping sensation in the liver.

Back - Drawing sensation as in the spinal cord and cerebellum.

Rectum - Painless diarrhea following painful vomiting. Profuse diarrhea continuing all night.

Stomach - Long continued vomiting, ***"as if all the bowels would be emptied out."*** Vomiting very painful, as the vomiting subsided diarrhea came on, the diarrhea being painless. Heartburn, dryness of esophagus.

RELATIONS - ***Compare:*** Anac., Rhus, Com.

REFERENCES - Clarke.

SCIRRHINUM

(Cancer Nosode)

PHARMACY - scirr. Scirrhinum. Cancer nosode. Durum. Carcinominum. The nosode of scirrhus cancer. Trituration. ***Historical dose:*** All potencies.

CLINICAL - Breast, cancer. ***Cancer.*** Glands, enlarged. Hemorrhages. Tumors. Varicose veins. ***Worms.***

HOMEOPATHIC - Burnett is the authority for this nosode. He proved it on himself and produced "a tremendous sinking at the navel," which he regarded as a keynote for its use. Burnett particularly noted its usefulness on cases of breast tumors.

This cancer nosode corresponds to cancerous diathesis, cancer of the breast with enlarged glands. A valuable intercurrent remedy to be given during the course of the broad constitutional treatment, enhancing and complementing the action of the other indicated remedies.

Constitutions - Cancerous diathesis.

Modalities - Worse 5 p.m. to 6 p.m. Worse irregularly on through the night.

COMMENTS - A patient to whom Burnett had given Scirr. mentioned to him that it had caused the passage of an enormous number of thread worms. On this hint, Burnett gave it with great success in many cases of this troublesome complaint. In inveterate cases where Cina and Teucr. have given little relief, Scirr. has wrought a great change for the better.

With Scirr., Burnett cured a man of hard glands which appeared on the left side of the neck after other glands had been removed by the patient's brother, a surgeon. Hemorrhages and varicose veins of legs and feet with purple points, have also been cured by Scirr.

RELATIONS - ***Compare:*** (1) Con., Carc. (2) Worms, Cina, Teucr., Sulph., Sabal. (3) Sinking sensation, Sulph., Sep., Hell., Hydr. (4) Cancer, Con., Hydr., Phyt., Sang., Carc., Cund., Ars.

REFERENCES - Clarke. Grimmer.

SCLERANTHUS

(Bach Flower Essence)

PHARMACY - scler-b. Scleranthus. Scleranthus annuus. The flowering sprigs are placed in a bowl of water and left in the sun for several hours. The water is strained subsequently and used as medicine. ***Historical dose:*** Take two drops from the stock bottle into a one ounce dropper bottle (add brandy or alcohol, if this bottle will be used for days or weeks). This is the dosage bottle, take a few drops straight into the mouth or as needed in a little water or juice.

HOMEOPATHIC - Scler-b belongs to Bach's group ***For Those who Suffer Uncertainty,*** with Cer-b., Gent-b., Gors-b., Horn-b. and Wld-o-b.

States of indecisiveness and vacillation between options. The body is marked by a changeability of symptoms as well. Symptoms may alternate between mental, emotional and physical states.

Vacillating between feeling loved and rejected. Bipolar disorders, manic-depressive states, dissociative personality disorders, such as multiple personality disorder and in conversion disorder (Chic-b., Heath-b.). Hysterical neurosis when symptoms vacillate between extremes.

Quick changes in weight. Travel sickness due to disturbance in equilibrium. After head injuries (Horn-b., Must-b., Wld-o-b.), when the mind is imbalanced or over-stimulated, with a sense of chaos. Susceptibility to lung tuberculosis, other lung conditions.

Gives mental calm and restores the mind's ability to be in charge, to regain an overview (Elm-b.). State of prolonged indecisiveness, usually in regard to a vital decision, has been found to precede the onset of illness.

MIND - Inner uncertainty. Unable to come to a satisfying decision. Changes mind frequently. Preoccupied, over stimulated with internal arguments, disoriented and exasperated. Dread about possibly making the wrong choice paralyzes the mind.

Over stimulated by details and cares. Confusion. Inability to calm the mind. Feels overwhelmed, inadequate. Emotional instability, Capriciousness, mood swings. Too easily impressed, overreacts. Sudden interest and disinterest.

REFERENCES - Bach.

SCOLOPENRDA MORSITANS

(Centipede)

PHARMACY - scol. Scolopendra morsitans. Centipede. Centipeda. The insect is triturated with sugar of milk in the usual way. Tincture of whole animals. ***Historical dose:*** All potencies.

CLINICAL - Angina pectoris. Backache. Constipation. Convulsions. Deafness. Dysmenorrhea. Gangrene. Headache. Hyperacidity. Leucorrhea. Malignant pustule. Nausea. Vertigo. Vomiting.

HOMEOPATHIC - When the centipede bites, it secretes a very active venom which contains cyanhydric acid and sulphuric acid. Swelling, pain inflammation and gangrene of the bitten part, often with appearance like malignant pustule. Vomiting and precordial anxiety.

In one fatal case the paroxysms of vomiting increased in intensity until the child, in a convulsive struggle, ceased to breathe. In the case of a man bitten in the arm by a centipede, reported in the Nashville Journal of Medicine, 1870, among the striking symptoms was no perspiration in the arm for three months.

Dr. Sherman of California reported the following symptoms as prominent in a woman bitten by a centipede: vertigo with blindness, worse in the morning, nausea and vomiting, unable to retain either food or liquid.

Terrible pain in back and loins, spasmodic and irregular, at times extending down the limbs. Pains returned every few days for three weeks, commencing in the head and going out at the toes. "Resembled labor pains as nearly as anything I ever saw."

MIND - Severe headache that makes him think that he has some brain tumor. Fear he is going to lose his mind. Delusion that he has been bewitched. Awakes with fear and a start. Loss of memory.

Abdomen - Tympanitis. Weakness in the epigastrium.

Chest - Pain in the chest on the right side.

Ears - Severe pain in the ears. Itching in the ear. Abundant wax. Buzzing noise. Deafness.

Eyes - Burning in the eyes. Pupil is red. Inflammation of the cornea. Sensation of gravel. Sensation as if the eye would burst. Sensation of pressure over the eyes. Weakness of vision.

Female - Irregular menstruation. Menses, the blood is black and coagulated. Dysmenorrhea. Leucorrhea, purulent discharge. Inflammation of the uterus and the vagina. Itching in the nipples.

Food - Anorexia.

Head - Headaches in forehead. Sensation as if the head would split open. Burning pain. Piercing sensation. Vertigo.

Heart - Precordial anxiety.

Limbs - Feet cold and aching. Cramps from the feet up to the calf. Arm greatly swollen. Erysipelatous blush extending half over arm. No perspiration on right arm.

Lungs - Respiration short. Dry cough. Mucus rales. Expectoration purulent.

Mouth - Burning of the tongue with diminution of the taste. Tongue is coated. Bad breath. Severe toothache, especially on the left side.

Nose - Sinusitis with severe pain in the forehead. Acute rhinitis. Itching and sneezing. Greenish discharge.

Rectum - Severe constipation. Stool is hard. Stool of a strong odor.

Skin - A large red spot, becoming black in the middle. Malignant pustules, associated with swelling of lymphatic glands. Violent itching, followed by violent pain in bitten part.

Stomach - Hyperacidity. Burning in the stomach. Sensation of fullness. Nausea. Vomiting of a pale yellow, glairy matter, continued at short intervals with increasing violence.

REFERENCES - Anshutz. Clarke.

SCROPHULARIA NODOSA

(Knotted Figwort)

PHARMACY - scroph-n. Scrophularia nodosa. Knotted figwort. Scrophularia marylandica. American variety introduced from Europe and Asia. N. O. Scrophulariaceae. Tincture of whole fresh plant. Apply locally to cancerous glands (Semp.). ***Historical dose:*** Tincture and all potencies.

CLINICAL - Adenoma. Appendicitis. Bedwetting. Breast, disorders. Breast, tumors. ***Cancer.*** Colic. Crusta lactea. Deafness. Dyspepsia. ***Eczema***. Eyes, disorders. ***Glands, enlarged. Hemorrhoids***. Hodgkin's disease. Liver, pains. ***Lymphoma.*** Nodosities. Palms, cramp. Pemphigus. Peritonitis. Rheumatism. Sigmoid flexure. Sleepiness. Stiff-neck. Ureter, pain.

HERBAL - The plants of the genus Scrophularia generally have an unpleasant smell. The generic name is derived from the supposed property of the roots to cure scrofula. The Treasury of Botany noted that a decoction of one of the common British species, S. nodosa, is sometimes used by farmers to cure the scab in swine.

HOMEOPATHIC - Scroph-n., according to Dr. Cooper of London, has an especial affinity for breast tissue. ***Adenoma and cancer*** come within its curative range. ***Enlarged glands***. Hodgkin's disease. Epithelioma. Nodosities in the breasts (Scirr.). Breast tumors. ***Scrofulous swellings*** (Cist.). Threatened abscesses that show no sign of disappearing. Lupoid ulceration. Tubercular testis. ***Eczema of the ear***. Vaginal itching. ***Painful hemorrhoids***.

Pain in all flexor muscles. Cutting pains in the joints (Rhus-t.), but more intense and longer-lasting, worse by rest and in open air, better in warm room. Darting pain from knee to ankle joints, which feel stiff. Weakness, languor, wants to lie down.

MIND - Despondency, much troubled about the past and very apprehensive about the future. Miserable and sluggish feeling in mind when moving about.

Abdomen - Eczema around the navel. Peritonitis. Pain in sigmoid flexure. Pain in right hypochondrium, worse deep inspiration or lying right side. Twisting-pinching pain in umbilicus (left side). Dull, heavy, periodic pain worse when abdomen compressed, legs extended. Colic just below navel. Griping below naval, in the side in afternoon, 7 a.m., after a slight vexation. As a local remedy for appendicitis.

Back - Pain in spinal column with slight opisthotonos. Stiff neck with pain and contraction of right sternomastoid muscle.

Chest - Oppression with tremulous movement as from much weeping. Constricted feeling, which causes uneasiness. Cramp-like pain transversely across lower chest. Stitches in right chest, about 6th rib with shivering. Violent pinching stitches near right last true ribs, while walking during rest, seeming to be in liver.

Ears - Inflammation about auricle. Deep ulcerated auricle. Eczema around ear, behind right ear. Ringing in ears and sudden loss of hearing. Deafness in bull-necked boys. Deafness before and after menses, improving during the flow.

Eyes - Scrofulous keratitis. Sore eyeballs. Severe cutting pains in eyes, unable to move them, passed off with profuse sweat. Distressing photophobia (Con.). Black spots before eyes. On closing the eyes visions of objects. Pulsating stitches in right eyebrow. Blepharospasm.

Face - Pleasant warmth in cheeks. Recurrent periostitis of lower jaw in a syphilitic.

Female - Recurring metritis with painful hemorrhoids. Irritation, soreness and burning in vagina and anus.

Head - On rising, indescribable pain and fullness in head, especially occiput and vertex, causing congestion of conjunctive with puffiness, followed by nosebleed. Heaviness and distress in head, as after eating too much. Pain at exit of right facial nerve from hypo-mastoid foramen, darting to right eye. Headaches above the eyebrows while walking. Severe headache through temples, appearing every morning, extending to vertex and occiput. Severe, sharp pain in vertex, forehead and temples, dull and throbbing, returning periodically, worse resting, worse in open air, worse leaning forward, worse by study. Eczema behind ear.

Heart - Anguish in precordia, worse after food. Indescribable sensation in heart, with severe audible palpitations. Pulse full, regular.

Kidneys - Pinching and tearing as if in ureter, extending from anterior superior spine of ilium down to pubis. Increased secretion of urine with burning in urethra. Frequent, scanty emission of urine in afternoon. Bedwetting.

Limbs - Drawing rheumatic pain in all flexors of arms and legs. Tingling in limbs as from a blow on a nerve. Deep-seated cutting pain in all muscles of arms. Tingling or buzzing in arms and hands. Sticking and drawing in right palm from joints of fingers to middle of hand as far as carpal bones, muscular cramp of palms.

Liver - Cutting, ***pains in liver*** on pressure.

Lungs - Violent dyspnea, oppression of chest with trembling. On turning on either side, violent dyspnea, worse on right, with cutting in liver on pressure. Asthma in scrofulous patients. Pain about bifurcation of trachea. Pain in right lung, on taking a deep inspiration, which causes cough without expectoration. Cutting in upper left lung, worse breathing cold air.

Modalities - Better in warm room. Worse lying on right side, in morning. Worse pressure, rest, after food. Worse deep breathing, breathing cold air and studying in cold air.

Mouth - Bitter taste. Accumulation of sweetish water in several parts of tongue. Sick, sticking taste just above pit of throat, frequently lasting an hour with sensation as if a soft substance (a plug of mucus) were lodged there. Increased saliva, then dry mouth. Teeth feel loose. Pain in carious teeth, worse upper jaw. Gums bleed freely.

Nose - Dry coryza.

Rectum - ***Rectal pain***. Several stools daily with tenesmus. ***Painful, bleeding, protruding hemorrhoids***.

Skin - Sallow. Surface burns when rubbed. Prickling, itching, worse back of hand, inside wrists and between fingers. Pemphigus gangrenous. Falling off of hair stopped by lotion of Scroph-n.

Skin - Irritating vesicles on inside of lip, loaded with spindle-celled epithelium.

Sleep - ***Great drowsiness*** in morning, with weariness and fullness in whole body. Sleep irresistible before and after a meal. Prolonged afternoon sleep.

Stomach - Appetite greatly increased at first, later nausea with weakness and oppression at epigastrium. Feeling as if he had missed his regular meal. Dyspepsia.

Temperature - Chilliness for several hours on moving about in cool air, after rising in morning, passing off with profuse sweat, followed by stupor and absence of all symptoms. Body feels dry and hot with burning sensation, followed by profuse sweat.

Throat - Thick, tenacious, offensive mucus in throat in forenoon. Rancid taste in throat with great weakness and stiffness in hollows of knees. Irritation of esophagus.

Vertigo - Dizziness, fullness and pressure in vertex. Vertigo in top of head when standing, even with severe aching in supra-orbital region.

COMMENTS - Scroph-n. was proved by Franz, and later in America by W. H. Blakeley, who took from 10 to 60 drops of the tincture several times a day. Blakeley's proving showed pain in sigmoid flexure. Both Franz and Blakely noted pains in the liver.

The most remarkable of Franz's Scroph-n. symptoms included excessive drowsiness in forenoon, in afternoon, and before and after eating. Sensation of a soft body in the gullet. Constriction of the chest. Oppression of chest with trembling as after much weeping.

A sickly, giddy feeling with a sense of weakness and sinking at pit of chest, too weak to speak, along with pain from forehead to back of head. Most of these symptoms were confirmed by Blakeley.

Gerard mentioned "hard kernels" and painful, swollen hemorrhoids as its indications.

Cooper saw Scroph-n., in the form of a poultice, relieve peritonitis affecting the lower abdomen. Colic from slight vexation occurred in Franz's proving.

Cooper gave Scroph-n. to a patient who had been poisoned by an Indian arrow-poison which produced inflammation and suppuration of the glands. Scorph-n. relieved a most painful condition of the rectum and purulent discharge that had kept up for years afterwards.

Cooper reduced strumous glands with it, cured deafness in a "bull-necked" patient, and cured a case of sycosis using Scroph-n. externally as well as giving it internally. "Nodosities in the breast" is another indication of Cooper's.

RELATIONS - ***Antidoted by:*** Bry. - chest symptoms. ***Compare:*** (1) Dig., Euphr., Grat. (2) Pains in joints worse by rest, better in warm room, Rhus-t. (3) Sleepiness, Nux-m., Op., Lup. Lob-e., Ruta, Carc., Con., Aster. ***Followed well by:*** Dig. in enlarged glands.

REFERENCES - Boericke. Clarke. Cooper. Murphy.

SCUTELLARIA LATERIFOLIA
(Skullcap)

PHARMACY - scut. Scutellaria laterifolia. Skullcap. Mad-dog. N. O. Labiatae. Tincture of fresh plant. ***Historical dose:*** Tincture and all potencies.

CLINICAL - Ardor, urine. Brain, irritation. Chorea. Delirium tremens. Dentition. ***Diarrhea***. Exophthalmos. Flatulence. ***Headache.*** Hiccoughs. Hydrophobia. Hysteria. ***Insomnia.*** Nervousness. Night-terrors. Sleeplessness. Tobacco-heart.

HERBAL – Hale, who introduced scutellaria into homeopathy, noted that it is in the domestic practice of North America with the equivalent usage of valerian in Europe. "Its calming effects on the nervous system have been known ever since the settlement of New England."

HOMEOPATHIC - Scut. is a nervous sedative. ***Nervous fear*** or excitement predominates. ***Chorea, twitching of muscles. Restlessness.*** Chronic fatigue. Tired weak feeling. Uneasiness. Languor. Nervous weakness after influenza. Nervous irritation and spasms of children during dentition.

Cardiac irritability. Tobacco-heart. Like its relation, Lycopus, it caused weak and irregular action of the heart and protrusion of the eyes.

Hale used Scut. with success in sleeplessness, night-terrors, hysteria, nervous agitation from pain or exciting emotions, cerebral irritation of children from dentition or intestinal irritation.

MIND - Confusion of mind. ***Fear of some calamity***. Apathy. Irritability. ***Inability to study or fix the attention on one's work*** (Aeth.).

Abdomen - Gas, fullness and distention, colicky pain and uneasiness.

Constitutions - Suited to persons of a nervo-bilious temperaments.

Eyes - ***Aching in eyeballs***. Eyeballs painful to touch. Eyeballs feel too large, pressed outwards.

Face - Flushed face.

Head - ***Dull, frontal headache***. Migraine, worse over right eye. Nervous sick headaches, worse noise, odor light, better night, rest. Explosive headaches of school teachers with frequent urination, headaches in front and base of brain.

Kidneys - Frequent urination but quantity small. ***Quantity of urine diminished. Biliary salts increased***.

Limbs - Chorea. Twitchings of muscles, must be moving. Tremors. Sharp, stinging pains in upper limbs. Nightly restlessness. Weakness and aching.

Male - Seminal emissions and impotency, with fear of never being better.

Modalities - Better by sleep. The hemicrania is better moving about in open air. Headache worse from motion. Worse by overwork or over-exertion. Worse by work or excitement.

Mouth - Bad taste, sour, bitter.

Rectum - *Diarrhea*. Light colored. Stools preceded by colicky pain in abdomen.

Sleep - ***Restless, must move about***. Disturbed sleep and frightful dreams. Night terrors. Sleep is ***unrefreshing***.

Stomach - Poor appetite. ***Sour belchings***. ***Nausea.*** Vomiting of sour ingesta, hiccough, pain and distress in stomach.

Throat - Sensation of lump in throat which could not be swallowed.

COMMENTS - Provings by G. W. Gordon and G. H. Royal gave the homeopathic data. Royal's provers took 3x and 30x. Gordon took repeated doses of 10 to 50 drops. Royal had this indication for Scut. given to him by a friend: "Nervo-bilious headache with the nervous symptoms uppermost and nothing the matter with her."

He related the case of Miss M., 32, who was the head of a large school, complained of being used up, unable to sleep or think. Pain in head almost constant, sometimes frontal, mostly at base of brain.

Whenever called upon to overdo herself, she could not sleep that night and then there is either a nervous explosion the following day or a nervous sick headache, either being followed by complete collapse.

This was in May. Pic-ac. and later Phos-ac., gave relief and in September the patient resumed work. Late in December there was another breakdown, and Stych-p. was given.

A week later after a very long and fatiguing day's work, Royal was summoned at 2 a.m. He found the patient screaming. Every few minutes she had to urinate and passed only a few drops. Stools frequent, loose, watery. Pulse irregular.

Scut. was given, ten drops every half-hour. Patient was better after the second dose, slept after the fourth. Since then she kept the medicine by her, but only took it when overworked. She never had another nerve explosion or headache. In this case there was "nothing the matter with her" i.e., no organic defect to which the sufferings could be attributed.

Hale quoted many eclectic writers who give various indications King mentioned depression of nervous and vital powers after long sickness, over-exercise, over-study, long-continued and exhausting labors. It controls nervous agitation. It was Burnett's chief remedy in the nervous debility after influenza.

Scudder mentioned chorea, delirium tremens and hydrophobia, as its popular name "Mad dog" suggests. Rafinesque cited cases of prevention of hydrophobia and Hale observed it produce in a patient taking it "Spasmodic or constrictive closing of jaws and a tightness of the muscles of the face."

A writer, quoted in the N. Y. Med. Times, said Scut. has the remarkable effect of calming fear in delirium tremens.

Paine added the indications subsultus tendinum following fevers in delirium tremens, epilepsy, catalepsy, and hysteria. Coe, who used Scutellarin, the concentrated preparation, mentioned sunstroke, tenesmus, tetanus, cramps.

Churton gave 60 drops of the tincture every two hours in a case of "severe and rapid hiccough" which chloroform, morphine and pilocarpine had failed to relieve permanently. After the eighth dose, the patient slept and the spasms gradually diminished and stopped for good by the fourth day.

RELATIONS - ***Compare:*** (1) Heart, Grave's disease, Lycps. (2) Nervous exhaustion, Cypr. according to Hale, acts more on brain, Scut. on spinal cord. (3) Trismus, Nux-v. Hydrophobia, Agar., Fagus, Lach., Bell. (4) Overworked women, Mag-c.

REFERENCES - Boericke. Clarke.

SECALE CORNUTUM
(Ergot of Rye)

PHARMACY - sec. Secale cornutum. Ergot of Rye. Spurred Rye. Claviceps purpurea. N. O. Fungi. Pyrenomycetae. The black, hornlike spur into which the grains of rye cereal are changed by the fungus Claviceps purpurea. Tincture of the fresh spurs collected just before harvest. ***Historical dose:*** Tincture and all potencies.

CLINICAL - After-pains. Blindness. Cataracts. Childbirth. Collapse. ***Debility***. Delirium. Diarrhea. Emaciation. ***Ergotism. Gangrene. Hemorrhages.*** Labor, pains. ***Leucorrhea. Locomotor, ataxia.*** Lymphoid, tumors. Mania. Menstrual, colic. Metritis. ***Miscarriage.*** Myelitis. ***Nosebleed***. Numbness. Nymphomania. Paraplegia. Petechia. Prostration. Puerperal, fever. Puerperal, mania. Raynaud's disease. Tetanus. Thrombosis. Varicose, veins. Varicose, ulcers.

HOMEOPATHIC - Rye and grasses are apt to be affected with the ergot disease in damp seasons and when grown on damp, ill-drained lands. If breeding cows are turned on pastures where infected grasses grow, they are very liable to drop their calves. Ergot has been known to hasten childbirth from remote times.

Secale's other actions have been, for the most part, learned from the terrible epidemics of ***"ergotism"*** which have occasionally devastated districts in which rye infected with ergot has been ground into flour and eaten by the population.

Death takes places in convulsions, from gangrene and consequent exhaustion, or from exhausting hemorrhages or discharges, as diarrhea. Many who escape immediate death are reduced to a cachectic state from which they never recover, are paralyzed, have limbs distorted and senses impaired. In general, the sufferer retains a clear intellect and a good, even abnormally good appetite to the last.

Sec. contracts the muscles of ***blood vessels and the uterus.*** It also decomposes the blood, producing hemorrhage which is thin, fetid, watery, black, oozing continuously. Small wounds bleed much. Mortification, ***gangrene. Traumatic gangrene,*** from application of leeches or mustard, better from cold. Lymphoid tumors.

Useful for old people with shriveled skin or for thin, scrawny, old women. Produces contraction of the unstriped muscular fibers, hence a tight feeling throughout the body. Produces an anemic condition, with coldness, numbness, petechiae.

Restlessness, anxiety, extreme debility and prostration. Collapse. ***Emaciation, though appetite and thirst may be excessive.*** Discharges are dark, thin, foul and exhausting. Varicose veins. Thrombosis. Hinsdale noted that Sec. decreases the flow of pancreatic juice by raising the blood pressure.

Chronic, sharp, stinging neuralgic pains, which burn like fire, better application of heat. Tetanic spasms with full consciousness. Facial and abdominal muscles twitch. Twitchings, spasms with fingers spread apart. Gnawing and cramps with stiffness. Numbness. Insufferable tingling, crawling, better rubbing. Sensation of burning in the whole body or as of sparks falling on them or here and there like fire. Loss of power of voluntary motion.

Coldness, but does not want to be covered up. Symptoms are ***better from cold***, the whole body is pervaded by a sense of great heat. Sensation of deadness in any part. Everything feels loose and open. Walking causes giddiness. The right side is predominantly affected.

MIND - Mania fear or depressed by fear. Anxiety with fear of death, restlessness and difficult breathing. Fear of death before menses. ***Suspicious***. Unconsciousness during pregnancy or childbirth. Unconsciousness, with heavy sleep.

Excessive sadness, gradually changes to cheerfulness. Seems besides herself after miscarriage. Forgetful after sex. Weakness of mind after spasms or exhausting sex. Indifference to exposure of person.

Impotence. Nymphomania during menses. Grasping at genitals during spasms.

Puerperal mania, exposes the body, tears at the genitals, inserts her finger into the vagina and scratches until it bleeds, all ideas of modesty lost. Sardonic laughing. Madness, inclination to bite or drown himself. Laughs, claps her hand over head, seems besides herself.

Delirium, abandons her relatives. Mocking at his relatives. Treats his relations contemptuously and sarcastically. Wants to fight. Rage, followed by continuous deep sleep.

Wandering talk and hallucinations. Raving delirium. Delusion that two sick people were in bed, one of whom got well and the other did not. Foolish behavior during spasms. Impulse to jump into river.

Abdomen - Excessively inflated and tight, wants uncovered. Empty feeling in hypogastrium or bearing down, must lie doubled up in bed. Twitching of abdominal muscles. Formation of large lumps and swelling in abdomen.

Back - Spinal irritation, tingling of lower limbs, can bear only slightest covering. Tingling in back, extending to fingers and toes. Formication and numbness. ***Locomotor ataxia***. Myelitis. Pressure on affected portion causes pain there as well as through the chest.

Breasts - Suppression of milk with stinging in breasts. Breasts do not fill with milk properly.

Causations - Abortion, ***miscarriage***, childbirth. Hemorrhages, wounds. Suppressions of tears, lochia, milk, or sweat.

Chest - Dyspnea and oppression with cramp in diaphragm. Boring pain in chest. Angina pectoris. Pains through chest, on pressing spine. Burning in lungs.

Constitutions - Hemorrhagic diathesis. Suited to irritable, plethoric subjects or to thin, scrawny, feeble emaciated women. To very old, decrepit persons. Women of very lax muscular tissue, everything seems loose and open, no action, flabby vessels.

Ears - Great difficulty in hearing, with roaring, humming in ears. Confused hearing or lost, after chorea. Sensitiveness of hearing, so that even the slightest sound re-echoed in her head.

Eyes - Dilated pupils, distortion and strabismus. Incipient cataract, senile, especially in women. Pustulous conjunctivitis. Suppuration of cornea. Diabetic retinitis. Ptosis. Catarrh. Suppressed tears. Sparks before the eyes. Double or triple vision. Blindness. ***Eyes sunken and surrounded by blue rings.*** Paralysis of upper lid from coal gas.

Face - ***Spasmodic distortion***, or sunken. ***Pale, pinched***. Wild look. Livid spots on face. Tingling, twitching, or cramps in face, which spread over the body. Lockjaw.

Female - Menstrual colic with coldness and intolerance of heat. Menses irregular, copious, dark, ***continuous oozing of watery blood*** until next period. ***Passive hemorrhages*** in feeble, cachetic women. ***Brownish offensive leucorrhea***. Burning pains in uterus. ***Threatened miscarriage*** about the third month (Sabin.). Never well since miscarriage or abortion. During labor no expulsive action, though everything is relaxed. Bearing down pain with coldness. Puerperal fever and putrid discharges. Contracted uterus, hourglass labor contractions. Septic placenta. ***Severe after-pains.*** Dark offensive, green lochia. Prolapsed uterus after forceps delivery. Tympanitis, coldness, suppressed urine. Vagina hot or cool. Weak uterus. Metritis. Gangrene of female organs.

Food - Unquenchable thirst. Thirst with dry mouth or burning. Unnatural, ravenous appetite. ***Craves acids*** and sour things. Averse to fat and meat.

Head - Passive, congestive headache, rises from back of head. Twisting of head to and fro. Head drawn back. Feels light or heavy, with tingling in legs. Falling of hair. Hair is dry and gray.

Heart - Precordial tenderness. Palpitations with contracted and intermittent pulse. Palpitations after sexual excess in males.

Kidneys - Paralysis of bladder. Retention with unsuccessful urging. Suppressed urine, pale, watery. Bloody urine, white, cheesy deposit. Discharge of black blood from bladder. Bedwetting in the elderly.

Limbs - Paralysis with distorted limbs, of lower limbs, of one side of one arm or one leg, with tingling, numbness and prickling. Paralysis after spasms. Paraplegia. Locomotor ataxia. Formication, pain and spasmodic movements. ***Violent cramps,*** in hands, legs, feet and cramps. ***Icy coldness of limbs***. Numbness. Fingers and feet bluish, shriveled, ***spread apart or bent backwards***. Cold, dry hands and feet in heavy smokers, with feeling of fuzziness in the fingers. ***Varicose ulcers***, foul indolent. Trembling, staggering or shuffling gait, as if feet were dragged along. Violent pain in fingertips, tingling in toes. Toes drawn up.

Lungs - Heavy, anxious, obstructed breathing with moaning, sighs, sobs. Spitting of blood, with or without cough. Expectoration of blood during violent efforts to breathe.

Modalities - Better lying doubled up in bed, rocking, forcible stretching. Better cold applications, cold bathing. Better open air, uncovering, fanning. Better after vomiting. ***Worse from heat, warmth, warm cover***. Worse touch, motion, exertion. Worse eating, smoking. Worse loss of fluids, sexual excess. Worse just before or during menses. Worse pregnancy and after miscarriage.

Mouth - Salivation, with fetid breath. Much acid fluid in mouth. Spitting of blood. Bloody or yellowish green foam at mouth. Dryness of mouth. Stuttering, indistinct speech. Speech difficult, slow and weak.

Nose - ***Nosebleed***, oozing, dark blood, with great prostration in old people, alcoholics or young women.

Rectum - Cholera-like stools with coldness and cramps. Gushing offensive, painless, watery stools with collapse and great exhaustion. ***Olive-green, thin, putrid, bloody stools with icy coldness*** and intolerance of being covered. ***Involuntary stools***, no sensation of passing feces. Anus feels loose and wide open.

Sensations - As if intoxicated while undressing. As of a solid plug in nose. Uterus as if burnt. As if contents of uterus would fall forward. As if soft air were creeping through back. As if sacrum would be forced out. As if something alive creeping under skin. As if limbs had been a long time in hot water. As if sparks of fire falling on different parts. As if mice creeping under skin. Fuzzy feeling in limbs.

Skin - ***Shriveled skin***, numb, mottled, dusky-blue tinge. Skin cold, dry, wrinkled or bluish, worse over affected part. Raynaud's disease. Edema neonatorum. Twitchings or quivering in the skin. ***Formication*** under skin. ***Burning sensation***, better by cold, ***wants parts uncovered***, though cold to touch. ***Aversion to heat***. Petechiae. ***Dry gangrene***, developing slowly. Slight wounds continue to bleed. Bloody blisters. Livid spots. Boils with green pus, matures slowly.

Sleep - Deep, lethargic, profound and long sleep. Insomnia with restlessness, fever, anxious dreams. ***Insomnia of drug and liquor habits.***

Stomach - Burning in stomach and abdomen. Tympanites. Hiccough. Belchings of bad odor. Empty retchings. Nausea, easy vomiting of blood and coffee-grounds fluid. Hematemesis.

Temperature - ***Coldness***. Cold, dry skin, clammy sweat, excessive thirst. ***Internal burning with icy coldness externally, yet averse to being covered,*** worse abdomen. Heat as of sparks. Puerperal fever. Erysipelas. Cold or foul sweat destroys shoes.

Throat - Painful tingling, burning. Post diphtheria paralysis. Feeble voice inaudible, stammering. Voice hoarse and hollow. Painless aphonia in morning, as the day goes on he gets hoarse.

Tongue - Tongue dry, ***cracked, blood like ink exudes***. Tongue coated thick, viscid, yellowish. Cold, livid. ***Tingling of tip of tongue, which is stiff***. Tongue swollen, feels paralyzed. Stuttering as if tongue were paralyzed. Tongue clean, with dry, red tip.

Vertigo - Vertigo with stupefaction and heaviness of head. Reeling, inability to stand erect. Vertigo as from intoxication. Vertigo on slightest motion. Vertigo while sitting.

COMMENTS - Convulsive nervous symptoms. The body is at times rigid, at times alternating with relaxation. This is especially seen in the hands, which are either clenched or have the fingers spread widely apart (a keynote symptom).

The muscles of the face and abdomen twitch. Spasmodic twitchings of muscles in various parts (especially spreading of fingers), eyes sunk, features pinched, shriveled, dry, as though no moisture were left in the body. Anesthesia.

Cold to the touch, but cannot bear to be covered. Characteristic burning sensations, burning in all parts of the body as if sparks were falling on the patient. Worse from warmth and external heat. Characteristic numbness, tingling as if ants were crawling all over, better from rubbing.

Contraction and then dilatation of blood vessels. Vascular headaches, constriction. Migraines. The fingers turn bluish black. Hemorrhagic diathesis, persistent offensive bleeding. Hemorrhages with tingling.

Small wounds bleed persistently. Purpura. Hollow viscera and violent palpitations. Dry gangrene. Threatened amputation. Gangrene aggravated by heat, affected part feels cold. Shriveled, dry skin. Harsh and sallow complexion. Small and painful boils with green contents, mature very slowly, heal slowly and are very weakening. Exophthalmic goiter.

Spasmodic retching, the stomach is violently contracted. Incontinence or retention of urine. Involuntary diarrhea with wide-open anus. In cholera where the patient is cold, almost pulseless. Exhausting and offensive discharges. Loss of fluids, debility.

Threatened miscarriage, especially at the third month. Tendency to miscarriage. Prolonged, forcing pains, bearing-down, bearing down forwards (Sep. is bearing down downward). Irregular, too weak, feeble or ceasing labor pains (Puls., Caul.).

Everything seems loose and open, but no expulsive action. Used to hasten and promote delivery. Fainting. Hourglass contraction of the uterus. Too long, excessive after-pains. Postpartum hemorrhage of dark, oozing blood. Retained placenta. Suppression or non-appearance of the milk.

Menses are irregular, copious, dark, fluid, accompanied by labor-like pains in abdomen. There may be a continuous watery discharge of blood during the whole time between the periods.

Teste recorded the case of a woman, 50, fat, very soft flesh, who had flooding which nothing could stop. After several useless attempts, Teste gave large doses of Sec. with scarcely any effect. The patient asked for infinitesimal doses. At that time, Teste had no faith at all in infintesimals, but he yielded to the patient's request and gave one drop of the 6c. Then the bleeding ceased immediately and permanently.

RELATIONS - ***Antidoted by:*** Camph., Op. ***Compare:*** (1) Ergot. (2) Pedi-can. - symptoms of locomotor ataxia, spinal irritation. (3) Brass. - dropsical swellings, scorbutic mouth, voracious appetite, tympanitis, dropping of nails, gangrene. (4) Cinnam., Colch., Ars., Aur-m. 2x - locomotor ataxia. (5) Agro. (6) vertigo, headache, difficult locomotion, burning sensation, Ust., Carb-v. (7) Pituin. - dilated os, little pain, no progress. ***Compatible:*** Chin., Ars., Acon., Bell., Merc., Puls. Teste classes Sec. with Chin. in his Ferr. group.

REFERENCES - Boericke. Clarke. Murphy. Phatak.

SEDUM ACRE

(Small Houseleek)

PHARMACY - sed-ac. Sedum acre. Small houseleek. Wall pepper. Crassulaceae. Tincture of the whole plant. ***Historical dose:*** Tincture and all potencies.

CLINICAL - Anal, fissures. ***Fissures***. Hemorrhoids.

HOMEOPATHIC - Hemorrhoids. ***Fissures***. Pains like those of anal fissures. Constricting pains, worse a few hours after stool.

RELATIONS - ***Compare:*** (1) Muc-u. - for the hemorrhoid diathesis. (2) Sed-t. - uterine hemorrhages, also for bowels and rectum, menorrhagia, at menopausal. (3) Sed-r. - Cancer, specific action on abdominal organs, pain, loss of strength.

REFERENCES - Boericke.

SELENIUM

PHARMACY - sel. Selenium. The Element (Se, At. Wt. 79.5). Trituration. ***Historical dose:*** All potencies.

CLINICAL - Alcoholism. Bedwetting. Comedones. Constipation. Debility. Diabetes insipidus. Eczema, scalp. ***Hair, loss.*** Headache. Hoarseness. ***Impotency.*** Laryngitis, tubercular. Liver, disorders. Masturbation. Myasthenia. Prostatitis. ***Prostatorrhea.*** Psoriasis. Scabies. Skin, disorders. ***Spermatorrhea.*** Stammering. Sun, effects. Syphilis. Tea, effects.

HOMEOPATHIC - Selenium was discovered in 1818 by Berzelius and was named by him after the moon, because it is found associated with tellurium (Tellus, the earth). It is also found associated with sulphur. All three belong to the same group of elements. Selenium is found either in its natural state or, more often, as a metallic selenide.

Colloidal selenium has been used as an injection for inoperable cancer. Pain, sleeplessness, ulceration and discharge are markedly diminished.

Marked effects on the ***genito-urinary organs***. The larynx and liver are also affected. Often indicated in elderly men, especially for ***prostration and sexual atony***. Bedwetting. Chronic urethritis. Diabetes insipidus.

Irritability after sex. ***Sexual weakness.*** Lascivious, but impotent. ***Loss of sexual power*** with sexual thoughts. ***Prostate weakness*** with dribbling of urine. Escape of semen especially when straining at stool. Chronic gleet.

Great debility, worse heat. Debility after exhausting diseases, fevers. Patient becomes easily debilitated by heat or hot weather, a little mental or physical exertion makes him sleepy. Easy exhaustion, mental and physical in old age. Early senility.

Hemicrania. Neuritis and neuralgia of the head. Marked effects on the supra orbital nerves (left). Myasthenia. Chronic diseases of the bone-marrow. Emaciation of single parts, face, hands, thighs etc. ***Pulsation in the whole body*** especially in abdomen, worse eating. Cramps, then stiffness. Biting, here and there. Aversion to draft of air, warm cold or damp.

MIND - Dullness of mind. Difficult comprehension, concentration. Mental labor fatigues. Total unfitness for any kind of work. Forgetful in work, but dreams of what he has forgotten.

Great forgetfulness when awake with distinct recollection during half sleep. Fails to understand what he hears or reads. Lack of enthusiasm and of interest, indifference. Apathy. Talkative, when excited, stammers, pronounces some words incorrectly. Stutters.

Extreme sadness. Depression in the morning, aggravated in the evening. Despair, melancholy. Aversion to company of intimate friends. Dread of society. Reveries of a religious and melancholy character.

Easily irritated by noise, people and conversation. Easily antagonized. Irritability after sex. Confusion after emissions. ***Dipsomania before menses.*** Erotic thoughts with impotence. Lascivious thoughts. Becomes drunk easily.

Abdomen - Sensation of abdominal distention on the left side, ameliorated by pressure, aggravated by going to stool or by coughing. Left abdominal hyperesthesia, spreading towards the left kidney area. Violent shootings in spleen when walking. Pulsation all over the body especially in abdomen after eating which hinders sleep.

Back - The back becomes almost paralytic after a temporary illness. Paralytic pain in small of back, better lying on abdomen. Sensation of paralysis in loins. Pain as from lameness in small of back in morning. Hard swelling on back. Severe pain in the coccyx, aggravated when sitting, ameliorated by walking. Pain through left side of neck and down back of left leg.

Bones - Osteoporosis during menopause. Inflammation of the bones and cartilages in the young adult, attacking the knee, then the elbow and the hip. Bones fragile.

Breasts - More or less acute pain, prickling or dull aching in the left or right breast.

Causations - Bad effects from excess of tobacco or tea. Ill effects of debauchery, alcohol, sugar, salt, lemonade, loss of vital fluids, masturbation, sexual excess, over-study. Walking, exertion.

Chest - Constrictive or stinging pain behind the sternum and in the upper left thoracic region. Pains in right side, around under last ribs, especially on inspiration, extending to region of kidneys.

Constitutions - Suited to blondes and persons of light complexion.

Ears - Deafness from hardened wax. Ear stopped.

Eyes - Blurred vision, with difficult accommodation. Myopia. Pains deep in orbits. Discharge of a thick, yellow secretion, especially in the morning. Heavy, painful, burning, blood-shot with red marks on the eyelids. Spasmodic twitching of left eyeball. Itching vesicles on eyebrows and margins of lids. Styes. Blepharitis. Dacyrocystitis. Falling off of eyebrows.

Face - Great emaciation of face and hands. Twitching in muscles of face. Greasy, shining skin of face. Upper lip cracked. Comedones.

Female - Rare menses. Menses early, scanty, painful. Menses painful on the first day. Awakened by pain of menses. Menses copious and dark. Menses delayed about eight days. Throbbing in abdomen during pregnancy, worse eating.

Food - Thirstless. Anorexia in morning with white-coated tongue. Hunger at night. Craves stimulants, brandy, tea etc. Desire for alcoholic drinks. Aversion to salty food. Worse from tea, sugar, salt, lemonade, wine. Sweetish, disagreeable taste after smoking.

Head - ***Pain over left eye, worse walking in sun, strong odors and tea***. Nervous headaches. Headache from intellectual labor. Headache every afternoon. Headache after drinking lemonade, wine or tea. Headache of alcoholics, headache after debauchery. Pain in the scalp as if hair were pulled out. Scalp feels tense. Does not want hair touched. Hair falls out from eyebrows, whiskers and genitals.

Heart - Pulse very accelerated. Arterial pulsation, especially in the abdominal aorta, preventing him from sleeping. Pain in the heart region. Rhythmic anomalies. Syphilitic aortitis.

Kidneys - Frequent urination with urgent need to urinate. Sensation in the tip of urethra, as if a biting drop were forcing its way out. Red, itching irritation at the tip of the penis. Urine dark red, thick, scanty, gritty with deposits. ***Dribbling of urine*** after urination and after stool. Involuntary dribbling, when walking. Urination predominantly at night. Nocturnal bedwetting.

Limbs - Pains in all the limbs, as if caused by a chill. Legs feel weak, with fear of paralysis after typhus. Sudden left sciatic pain leaves soreness behind. Itching pimples on buttocks and thighs, near the scrotum. The knees crack when they are bent. Cramps in calves and soles. Flat ulcers on lower legs. Itching in feet, especially around ankles in evening. Blisters on toes. Emaciation of hands, of legs. Dry, scaly eruption on palms with itching, having syphilitic base. Psoriasis of palms. Painful hang-nails. Scabies-like pimples on hand. Tearing in hands at night with cracking in wrists. Itching at wrist in palms, itching vesicles on and between fingers. Miliaria in forearm.

Liver - Chronic liver affections. Pain in the liver, especially on taking an inspiration, extending to the kidney region with sensibility to external pressure. ***Enlarged with fine rash over liver region.***

Lungs - Weak feeling in the chest. Frequent efforts to breathe deeply like sighing. Difficulty breathing when walking in open air. Respiration obstructed at night, when lying down, by pains. Dry hacking cough, worse in the morning. Hawking up of mucus and of small clots of blood. Hawks up clear mucus in the morning. Frequent necessity to clear the throat in singers. Tubercular laryngitis.

Male - Irritability after sex. ***Loss of sexual power*** with lascivious fancies. Lascivious but impotent. ***Increases desire, decreases ability***. Sexual weakness. On attempting sex, penis relaxes. Easy loss of semen during sex with feeble erection, but long continued voluptuous thrill during stools. Semen watery, odorless. Dribbling of semen during sleep. ***Prostatitis,*** prostatic adenoma. Oozing of prostatic fluid during sleep, while sitting, walking and at stool. ***Hydrocele***. Chronic gleet. Bedwetting, chronic urethritis. Papillomas on the penis.

Modalities - Better after sunset. Better inhaling cool air, taking cold air or cold water into mouth. Worse loss of sleep, night watching, after sleep, rest. Worse in open air, draft, even if warm. Worse hot weather, sun and with the sun's increase. Headaches worse every afternoon. Worse singing, mental exertion. Worse by touch, pressure, motion. Worse after seminal losses, after stools. Worse wine, cinchona.

Mouth - Sweetish taste. Bitter taste in the mouth. Extreme dryness of the mouth. Tongue loaded with a thick white coating in morning. Burning at the tip of the tongue. Pain under root of tongue. Pain in the left molars, which spreads to all the teeth. Bleeding gums and ulcerations in the mouth. Stammering speech, articulates with great difficulty.

Neck - Glands of neck large and hard. Cramp in neck. Rigidity of muscles of neck and nape, which hinders head being turned.

Nose - Sinusitis. Atrophic rhinitis. Coryza, ending in diarrhea. Fluent coryza in evening. Yellow, thick, gelatinous mucus in nose. Full of thick glairy mucous. Complete chronic obstruction of nose. Nasal itching with the need to scratch the inside of the nose. Inclination to bore fingers in the nose. Sense of smell diminished at times. Smells a repulsive odor like garlic.

Rectum - Anal and rectal itching, especially towards evening. Constipation from rectal weakness with flatulence. Hard evacuations, followed by a discharge of mucus or of blood when passing the last portion of it. Stools large, hard, requiring a great effort, even a mechanical aid to expel them. Stools exceedingly difficult and threaten to tear anus from their immense size. Somewhat liquid feces with tenesmus. Filament like hair in feces.

Skin - Seborrhea, ***comedones with an oily surface of the skin.*** Oily. Frequent tingling in circumscribed parts of skin with great provocation to scratch. Red rash on region of liver. Miliary eruption. Vesicular eruption between fingers (Rhus-t., Anac.). Dry, scaly eruption in palms with itching. ***Itching about the ankles*** and folds of skin, between fingers. ***Acne***. Prolonged oozing from parts which have been scratched. Flat ulcers. ***Loss of hair*** from the head, armpits, pubic region and eyebrows. Hair falls off head, whiskers and other parts. Alopecia.

Sleep - ***Sleep prevented by pulsation in all vessels,*** worse abdomen. Sleepless until midnight, awakens early and always same hour. Insomnia, following alcoholism, infectious diseases, heart diseases. Disposition to sleep early in evening with imperfect sleep and frequent waking during night. Jerks in body when going to sleep. Erotic dreams. Dreams of fire, murders, robbers, quarrels and unnatural cruelty. Waking early in morning and always at same hour.

Stomach - After eating, pulsation all over, especially abdomen. Pressure in stomach as if cramp would occur. Cramp in stomach. Belching. Hiccough and belchings after smoking. Inclination to vomit. Feels very sick after sleep. Nausea, vertigo, thirsty for cold water, general weakness one hour after eating.

Teeth - Teeth covered with mucus. Toothache from tea. Toothache with feeling of coldness, better taking cold water and cold air into mouth. Toothache which compels use of toothpick until the blood comes. Boring in molars. The teeth become free of mucus, hard and smooth and crack when rubbed.

Temperature - Chilliness, followed by hot flushes. Constant alternation of heat and cold. Sweating from the armpits and genital region. Burning heat, extending over the skin. Perspiration from least exertion. Perspiration as soon as he sleeps, day or night. Tendency to profuse perspiration when walking or during an afternoon sleep. Perspiration on chest, genitals and under axilla, which leaves yellow or white spots on linen and stiffens it. External heat with burning in skin and only in single spots.

Throat - Chronic laryngitis. ***Voice hoarse*** and husky, as soon as he begins to sing, talk or read, affected by even cold. Voice rattles. Nodes on vocal cords. Incipient tubercular laryngitis. Throat dry, painful on waking, especially on the left side with extreme thirst. Cough in the morning, expectoration of a bloody mucus. Much clear, starchy mucus (Stann.). Laryngeal cough. Hawking and raising transparent lumps of mucus every morning.

Vertigo - Vertigo on lifting head, rising from a seat, raising himself in bed, moving about with nausea, vomiting. Faintness, worse for an hour after breakfast and dinner.

COMMENTS - The Sel. proving was conducted by Hering. In London, Raeside repeated a complete proving on sixteen provers and six controls in 1959-60, using the 6c, 12c, and 30c potencies.

A leading feature of Sel. is the weakness it causes, a weakness involving all parts of the body, easy fatigue from any labor, night watching, mental exertion and especially from hot weather. The hotter his body the weaker he is; strength rises as the sun sinks.

Irresistible desire to lie down and sleep, strength leaves him suddenly, especially in hot weather. Sluggishness, wants to sleep from sheer exhaustion and is worse after. Cannot bear any nervous drain, hence worse after sex or seminal emissions. Impotence. Debility after fevers, infectious diseases.

Great emaciation of face, hands, legs, feet, affected parts and single parts. Pulsation in whole body, especially in abdomen after eating. Very great aversion to a draft of air, either warm, cold or damp.

Irritability, headaches and other troubles following or worse by seminal emissions. Headaches are accompanied by profound melancholy and may be caused by indulgence in alcoholics or in tea, by hot weather, by over-study, and they are worse by strong odors. Headaches may be periodical and are frequently located above the left eye.

Chronic liver disorders. Sensitiveness of liver. Enlargement of liver with loss of appetite. In the morning, sharp stitching pain worse on any movement or pressure. "Fine rash over liver region."

Coryza ending in diarrhea. Hungry at night, longing for spirituous liquors, an almost irresistible maniacal desire. Aversion to salted food. Sensation as if a biting drop were forcing its way out of the urethra.

Constipation from weakness with impacted feces. Dribbling of semen after stool and after urination. Sufferings after seminal emissions mental confusion, headache, almost paralytic weakness of spine, involuntary escape of prostatic fluid.

Itching in folds of skin, as between fingers and about joints, especially the ankle-joint (Sulph.). The itching may occur in small spots and be accompanied by tingling (showing involvement of the nervous system).

Clarke frequently relieved "psoriasis palmaris" with Sel., which shows that it has a relation to syphilis. The scalp is affected with an eczematous eruption which oozes thin fluid after scratching. Hair falls off scalp and all parts of body.

Clarke cured with Sel. many cases of hoarseness, the special indications being hoarseness of singers, appearing as soon as they begin to sing or after long use of the voice with frequent necessity to clear the throat from accumulation of clear, starchy mucus. Scrofulous and incipient tubercular laryngitis have been cured with Sel.

RELATIONS - ***Antidoted by:*** Ign., Puls., Mur-ac. ***Compare:*** (1) Agn., Calad., Sulph., Tell., Ph-ac. (2) Arg-n. - Nervous imbalance with weakness, trembling, vertigo, ataxia. (3) Alum. - Paretic weakness, especially of the rectum and bladder. (4) Stann. - Nervous exhaustion and extreme weakness of the respiratory organs. (5) Calad. - Depressive state as a result of excess of tobacco and sexual over-indulgence. (6) Rauw. ***Compatible after:*** Calad., Nat-c., Staph., Ph-ac. (in sexual weakness). Itch checked by Merc. or Sulph. often requires Sel. ***Incompatible:*** Chin., wine.

REFERENCES - Boericke. Clarke. Phatak.

SEMPERVIVUM TECTORUM

(Houseleek)

PHARMACY - semp. Sempervivum tectorum. Houseleek. N. O. Crassulaceae. Tincture of fresh leaves. ***Historical dose:*** Tincture and all potencies.

CLINICAL - Bites, insects. Breast, cancer. ***Cancer.*** Hemorrhoids. Herpes zoster, Menopause. Menses, suppressed. Ringworm. Scirrhus. Tongue, indurations. ***Tumors. Warts.*** Wounds, poisoned.

HERBAL - In Hufeland's Journal, said Kallenbach, the fresh juice of Sempervivum tectorum is recommended in chronic aphthae in grown persons in causal relation to hemorrhoids, as well as in scirrhus indurations of the tongue.

In many countries, it has a popular reputation for indurations and sores on the tongue. Reichel of Staben, considered it curative in spasms of the uterus and in menstrual disturbances of all kinds. Cases of too exalted vascular activity in the sexual sphere. Also in ear troubles consequent on hardened earwax and in inflammatory exudations of the ear.

It is externally used for bites of insects, stings of bees and poisoned wounds, ***warts***. Herpes zoster and ***cancerous tumors***. Breast cancer. Ringworm. Hemorrhoids.

HOMEOPATHIC - Grimmer stated, "Sempervivum tectorum has cured many cases of induration and sores on the tongue, it also has definite action on the uterus and menstrual function in cancer constitutions, it could be thought of in cases of tongue cancer."

COMMENTS - Kallenbach was consulted by Mrs. S., 44, childless of sickly looks, for an affection of the tongue. For the previous six months menses had appeared only every eight to ten weeks and were accompanied with pains darting from small of back to uterus and vulva.

During the six months, she had stitching pain on the right rim of her tongue about 3/4 inch from the point, at which place after a few weeks, a swelling formed, the size of a small bean.

The swelling bled at times, and at night caused a burning sensation as of a small coal, disturbing sleep. Sour food caused pain. The swelling was not hard on the surface, but contained two hard nodules the size of lentils, one of which was denuded and bled on touch.

Three enlarged veins crossed the swelling and entered the tongue muscle behind it. She had been treated for over a month with Aur., Ars., Carb-v. in vain.

Kallenbach moistened the swelling with the fresh juice of Semp. thrice a day. Within three days it was smaller and folds appeared, the enlarged veins were contracted, formed thin, tense vessels crossing the swelling and seemingly tying it.

During the next three days, the patient applied the juice too energetically and Kallenbach found the surroundings in inflammatory irritation and very sensitive.

The applications was stopped and Semp. 2x was given internally. After a week's use the swelling had shriveled to one-third the size, and ten days later the menses, which had ceased altogether, reappeared and continued very profusely for five days.

The swelling shriveled to the size of a small pea, was firmer, harder, devoid of sensation and gave no further trouble. The menses continued regularly.

In another instance, Mrs. X., 27, a mother of a six month old healthy boy, formerly frequently afflicted with swelling of the glands, very sensitive to homeopathic remedies, complained of a pain under her tongue of ten days' duration, interfering with eating and speaking.

There was a bluish red elevation on under side of tongue the size of a split bean. It was hard, and along both sides there were enlarged veins. On the side a denuded spot exuded a whitish albuminous matter which could easily be wiped off.

Semp. 6c was given, one powder every forty-eight hours. On the second day, the swelling was less sensitive, and in a week, much smaller. Then the menses reappeared (first time since confinement) and in three weeks the whole swelling was gone, leaving only in its place a somewhat engorged vein.

Kallenbach treated with applications of 1x General V. B. who had nodules on the left rim of his tongue with swollen veins, the nodules disappeared and the sensitiveness was removed and the patient was so well that he refused to stay for the completion of the cure and failed to report.

Clarke's experience with Semp. was in domestic practice. For some child affections of the eyes he used rags moistened with "house leek and cream" (about equal parts of the juice and fresh cream) were applied and his recollection of it is that the application was exceedingly pleasant.

REFERENCES - Boericke. Clarke. Grimmer.

SENECIO AUREUS

(Golden Ragwort)

PHARMACY - senec. Senecio aureus. Golden ragwort. Senecio gracilis. Squaw-weed. N. O. Compositae. North America, found in swamps. Tincture of fresh plant in flower. ***Historical dose:*** Tincture and all potencies.

CLINICAL - ***Amenorrhea.*** Ascites. Cirrhosis. Coryza. Cough. Dropsy. Dysmenorrhea. Dysuria. Fainting. Gleet. Gonorrhea. Hemorrhages. Homesickness. Hysteria. Kidney, colic. ***Kidney, inflammation.*** Leucorrhea. Lumbago. Mania. Menorrhagia. ***Menstruation, disorders.*** Nails, brittle. Nervousness. Neurasthenia. Nosebleeds. ***Prostate, enlarged.*** Prostatitis. Puerperal, mania. Sciatica. Spermatic cord, pain. Tuberculosis. Wounds.

HERBAL - The golden ragwort had a reputation in domestic and eclectic practice as a regulator of menstrual functions when Hale introduced it into homeopathic practice. Its action on the female organism was clinically verified.

Lyman Watkins said, "Females taking Senec. generally improve in health and strength, accumulate flesh, become light-headed and cheerful. This may be due to some tonic influence."

HOMEOPATHIC - A. E. Small and others proved it and clinical additions have filled out the picture. Like many other Compositae, the Ragworts or Groundsels, have power over hemorrhagic conditions, whether arising from disease or from wounds.

Marked action on ***female and urinary organs,*** especially bladder. Lack of reaction in genito-urinary tract. Hemorrhagic tendency from other organs especially with suppressed or delayed menses. Dropsy after hemorrhage.

Debilitating or vicarious discharges. Backaches of congested kidneys. Early cirrhosis of liver. Tightness in nose, throat etc. Muscles draw into a knot. Nervous, pale, weak and sleepless hysterical women. Globus. Very sensitive to open air, tendency to catarrhs.

MIND - Despondent. Nervous and irritable, whining. Self centered. Elated and sad alternately. Inability to fix mind upon any one subject.

Abdomen - Pain about umbilical region, spreading in all directions better stools, bending double. Ascites from suppressed menses.

Back - Lumbar backache, as if to break with amenorrhea. Kidney disease.

Breasts - Burning in left nipple. Pains from ovaries to breasts.

Causations - Ill effects of suppressed or delayed menses, wounds, venesection.

Chest - Chest sore and raw.

Constitutions - Suited to women and little girls of nervous temperament.

Ears - Itching in Eustachian tube.

Eyes - Tears are irritating, causing itching.

Face - ***Sharp, cutting pain*** in left side. ***Dryness*** of fauces, throat and mouth.

Female - Before menses, inflammatory conditions of throat, chest and bladder after menstruation commences, these improve. Feels like the menses would come. ***Menses, retarded,*** suppressed with concomitant symptoms, dropsy, cough, backache. ***Amenorrhea of young girls***

with backache. Premature and too profuse menses (Calc., Erig.). Menorrhagia, a copious flow which continues until they become anemic. Anemic dysmenorrhea with urinary disturbances. Dysmenorrhea after abortion. Leucorrhea, thick, yellow, profuse, flows down thighs. Profuse flow of mucus from vagina from sexual excitation. Sexual irritation causing, itching, burning and swelling of labia. Pains from ovaries to breasts.

Food - Aversion to all food, especially sweets and coffee which she was very fond.

Head - *Wave-like dizziness* from occiput to sinciput. ***Sharp pains over left eye and through the left temple***. Dull, stupefying headache. Headache precedes leucorrhea and irritation in bladder.

Kidneys - Kidney colic (Pareir., Oci., Berb.). Nephritis. ***Great heat and constant urging***, with kidney pain. Irritable bladder of children with headache. Dysuria in women with dysmenorrhea or uterine displacements and in children with headache. Scanty, high-colored, ***bloody*** with much mucus sediment and ***tenesmus***.

Limbs - Wandering rheumatic pains, periodical. Feet cold in bed. Brittle nails (Sil., Thuj.).

Lungs - Dyspnea on ascending (Calc.) Acute inflammatory conditions of upper respiratory tract. ***Loose cough*** with copious mucus expectoration and labored breathing. Cough tickling with blood-streaked sputum with suppressed menses. Dry teasing cough, stitching chest pains. Hoarseness.

Male - Lascivious dreams with involuntary emissions. ***Prostate enlarged,*** feels hard and swollen to touch. Dull, heavy pain in spermatic cord, extending to testicles.

Modalities - Colic is better bending forward and better by stool. Better at onset of menses, from menstruation. Worse puberty, sexual excitement. Worse dampness, cold open air. Worse at night, in afternoon. Worse sitting, must keep moving about.

Mouth - Twitching about mouth. Teeth very sensitive.

Nose - Burning in nostrils. Fullness of nasal passages, burning, ***sneezing***, profuse flow. Tightness in nasal passage. Nosebleed or nasal catarrh take the place of menses when suppressed from any cause. Coryza with nosebleed.

Rectum - Thin, watery stool intermingled with hard lumps of feces (Ant-c.). ***Straining at stool, thin, dark, bloody with tenesmus***. Stools, thin, watery, mingled with hard lumps of feces or thin, dark, bloody.

Sensations - As of a wave from occiput to sinciput. As if he would pitch forward. As of a ball rising from stomach to throat.

Skin - Dry.

Sleep - Nervousness and sleeplessness. Sleepless women with uterine troubles and amenorrhea. Drowsy during day. Great drowsiness with unpleasant dreams. Many dreams, erotic.

Stomach - Sensation of a ball rising from stomach to throat. Sour belchings. Nausea and vomiting of kidney origin.

Temperature - Hectic fever with anorexia.

Throat - Dry mouth, throat and fauces. Burning in pharynx, raw feeling in nasopharynx, must swallow, though painful.

Vertigo - Wave-like sensation of dizziness from occiput to sinciput.

COMMENTS - Hale noted that the country people call Senec. "Wild Valerian," and use it for nervousness, hysteria and low spirits, sleeplessness, especially in women.

He referred to this "globus" symptom of the pathogenesis: about the middle of the afternoon, sensation as if a ball was in the stomach. Rising up into the throat, lasting for about an hour. Sensation of tightness in the throat with a disposition to attempt to relieve it by swallowing.

Respiration as if greatly fatigued. Coughs and tuberculosis. "It is especially serviceable in mucus coughs." "In chronic coughs, catarrhal affections, hemoptysis incipient tuberculosis attended with troublesome cough, the result of obstructed menstruation."

Pains are radiating, shifting, lancinating. Symptoms alternate.

"Dull, heavy pain in left spermatic cord, moving along cord to testicle. Prostatic gland enlarged, feels hard and swollen to touch. Lascivious dreams with pollutions."

Hemorrhagic function of menstruation. Menses, profuse and early, retarded or absent. Ailments from non-appearing menses. Nosebleed or nasal catarrh when menses are suppressed.

C. M. Foss reported the case of Miss L., 18, who had seen no period for fifteen months. She was chlorotic, had a dry, hacking cough with frequent pulse, made still more frequent by any excitement, headache, poor sleep, constipation. The abdomen had been gradually enlarging for six months and tapping had been decided upon when Senec. 1x was given. All symptoms rapidly cleared up and the menses returned within a short time.

Senec. 1x also cured a girl, 21, who had suppression of urine in addition to chlorosis, ascites and suppressed menses.

S. H. Talcott reported an important case bearing on the same point. Mrs. X., 26, a mother of two children. Before confinement, the patient was haunted with the idea that her child would be stillborn.

Nine days after its birth, strong and healthy, she was admitted to hospital in a state of violent acute mania, which continued with high temperature, for three months. with great physical activity.

The mental state was that of a wild, violent and almost uncontrollable person. There was severe pain in the head, great nervous irritability and sleeplessness and hysterical weakness.

These symptoms, coupled with the fact (now first ascertained) that the lochia had ceased suddenly after confinement and the menses had not come on, led to the choice of Senec., which was given in drop doses of the 3x every two hours.

Steady improvement resulted and after a few weeks the patient was allowed out on parole. A relapse followed and Bell. did no good. Senec. was again given with good effect and complete recovery took place.

Talcott remarked that recovery from puerperal mania seldom occurs unless menstruation is re-established. Talcott's case becomes more significant in the light of Cooper's observation of the brain action of Senec-j.

Hale reported the following case of dysmenorrhea: Mrs. X., mother of one child, had an miscarriage three years before and another (at the second month of pregnancy) four months before Hale saw her.

Since the last miscarriage she had suffered from painful menstruation, which had not been the case previously. Menses every three weeks, profuse, lasting eight or nine days, accompanied by much cutting pain in sacrum, hypogastrium and groins. Pale, weak, nervous, slight cough, generally at night.

Senec., 5 drops, was given three times a day until the next period, which came on at the twenty-ninth day and was perfectly normal in quantity and without pain.

Hale said he also found Senec. useful in advanced stages of gonorrhea and in prostatic disorders.

Small, who proved Senec., recorded the case of a woman, 30, who had been ill six weeks, the symptoms steadily increasing until the following picture was presented: face bloated, abdomen enlarged, feet edematous, urine alternately profuse and watery or dark and scanty, frequent desire to urinate day and night. Senec., 10 drops, three times a day, cured quickly.

Small remarked that he has found Senec. useful in the dysuria of women and children when evidently of catarrhal origin and in dysuria with uterine displacement. Mucus sediment in the urine is an indication. But the benefits of Senec. are not confined to the female sex.

Small related the case of a man, 50, nervo-sanguine, subject of kidney inflammation affecting right kidney generally, causing intense pain, fever, prostration. On one occasion the pain was particularly intense and the bladder seemed implicated.

Every time he passed water he cried out in agony. Urine reddish, very hot and acrid. Bowels constipated. Dull headache, mouth and throat dry, chilly, fever and perspiration.

Senec., 20 drops in half a tumbler of water, a dessert spoonful every hour. There was relief from the first dose and the pain soon subsided entirely, leaving the patient freed from recurrence of the attacks.

RELATIONS - ***Compare:*** (1) Senec-j. - cerebrospinal irritation, rigid muscles, chiefly of neck and shoulders, also in cancer. (2) Alet., Caul., Sep. (3) Arn., Calen., Bell-p. (4) Uterine, chest and bladder symptoms, Puls., Helon. (5) Vicarious menstruation, Bry. Senec. has bloody expectoration. (6) Homesickness, Caps., Ph-ac. (7) Worse 4 p.m., Lyc. (8) Prostatitis and gonorrhea, Sabal., Solid., Puls., Pip-n., Cop., Thuj. (9) Nervousness, Coff., Cham., Valer., Ambr. (10) Fidgety feet, Caust., Zinc.

REFERENCES - Boericke. Clarke. Phatak.

SENECIO JACOBOEA

(St. James Wort)

PHARMACY - senec-j. Senecio jacoboea. St. James' wort. Staggerwort. Ragwort. N. O. Compositae. Tincture of fresh plant. ***Historical dose:*** Tincture and all potencies.

CLINICAL - Arthritis. Brain, disorders. Cerebrospinal, irritation. Depression. Bedwetting. Headaches. Twitchings. Ulcers.

HERBAL - This is the common ragwort, which, with its yellow flowers, is such a conspicuous feature of English roadsides and commons throughout the summer months. Gerarde mentioned "green wounds and old filthy ulcers" as benefited by it, also "old aches and pains in the arms, hips and legs."

HOMEOPATHIC - Cooper published several observations with Senec-j.

MIND - Depressed in body and mind, it seemed as if brain would not work. Talks incoherently.

Back - Constant rigidity of muscles, chiefly of neck and shoulders, especially at night, seems like a habit, but finds it most difficult to relax them, it seems to return involuntarily, so that the weight of the head is somehow held in this way and though touching the pillow does not rest on it.

Head - Exhaustion felt in back of head, after this felt lighter and better.

Kidneys - The bladder, which had been rather weak, became more so, the bed-wetting continuing day and night for several days.

Limbs - Sometimes in the day the upper part of the legs gets a sort of ague fit of shaking.

Rectum - Bowels (before fairly regular) began acting in gushes, large stools occasionally, but in no way regular.

COMMENTS - Cooper gave a woman, 57 who had slight otorrhea of left ear with deafness on that side, a single dose of Senec-j. Immediately after, she began to feel depressed in mind and body, it seemed as if her brain would not work, for she talked incoherently. The bowels began acting in gushes and a bladder weakness was aggravated, so that there was bedwetting night and day for three days.

Another woman from a single dose of the same had "exhaustion in the back of the head."

Yet another woman, 51, had depression all her life, coming in fits. "Memory and everything goes," could not talk coherently to herself and dislikes conversation in others.

On July 1, 1900, she wrote, "Have suffered agony from awful feeling of torpor of brain, which has made it an effort to put words together, memory seemed to go, felt altogether insensible, bowels have been confined."

One dose of Senec-j. was given and removed the depression and relieved all the other symptoms. It also produced constant rigidity of muscles, chiefly of neck and shoulders, worse at night, it seems like a habit.

"And I try to relax them but find it most difficult, it to run back involuntarily, so that the weight of the head is somehow held in this way and though touching the pillow does not rest on it. Sometimes in the day the upper part of the legs gets a sort of ague fit of shaking."

On this Cooper remarked, "The exhaustion felt after a dose of Senec-j. in the back of the head in case 2 and the cropping up as a new symptom of this strange-looking rigidity of the muscles of the neck, at night chiefly together with the shaking of the legs in the daytime, points to incoordinated muscular action due to deranged cerebral control."

Cooper added the case of a man, 68, many years apoplectically inclined, who had constant twitchings at night with cascular deafness of right ear, loss of memory, pressure and heat of head. After a dose of Senec-j., he remained comfortable for three months and hearing improved.

Senec-j. has been used like Senec. in cases of menstrual irregularity.

REFERENCES - Clarke. Cooper.

SENEGA OFFICINALIS

(Snake-wort)

PHARMACY - seneg. Senega officinalis. Snake-wort. Snake-root. Polygala senega. N. O. Polygalaceae. Tincture of powdered dried root. ***Historical dose:*** Tincture and all potencies.

CLINICAL - Allergies. Amblyopia. Ascites. Asthma. Bedwetting. Bladder, irritable. Blepharitis. Bronchitis. Chest disorders. Constipation. Cornea, opacity. Coughs. Esophagus, stricture. Facial paralysis. Hay fever. Headaches. Hydrothorax. Hypopion. Influenza. Iritis. Lungs disorders. Pleurisy. Pneumonia. ***Snakebites.*** Sneezing. Sprains. Styes. Throat, sore. Tuberculosis. Whooping cough.

HERBAL - Senega is one of the sources of Saponin. It has a nauseous taste and leaves a scraping sensation in the throat. It is in disorders of the chest, eyes and bladder that homeopaths have found it of most service and the extensive provings have supplied excellent data for prescribing.

Teste reported that Seneg. was introduced to medical practice by Dr. Tennant of Virginia, who was led to test its properties through hearing that the Native Americans used it as an antidote to snakebites as it relieved the symptoms of snakes' venom.

Tennant concluded that it might also relieve dyspnea, cough and hemoptysis arising from other causes and gave it with success in cases of pneumonia, pleurisy and hydrothorax.

Other old-school practitioners used it as an expectorant in chronic respiratory catarrh, acute tuberculosis, rheumatic fever, dropsies incipient cataract, croup. It is regarded as "a stimulant, diaphoretic and expectorant in chronic bronchitis."

HOMEOPATHIC - Seneg. affects the ***mucus membranes*** causing catarrhal symptoms especially of the respiratory tract and bladder. Eyes, serous membranes of chest, muscles and left side are also affected. Distinct eye symptoms of a paralytic type.

Great soreness of walls of chest. Pressure on chest as though lungs were forced back to spine. Pleurodynia. Lying on right side causes pain in chest. Motion causes pain under sternum. Motion of arms causes soreness of walls of chest. Circumscribed spots in chest left after inflammations.

Hoarseness. The throat is so dry and sensitive it hurts the patient to talk. Cough often ends in sneezing. Lying down causes tickling in larynx. Great accumulation of clear albuminous mucus, which is difficult to expel. Whooping cough in fat, chubby children, clear mucus like white of egg, difficult to raise, cough worse towards evening.

MIND - Anxiety with hasty respiration. Fear of suffocation. Inclined to quarrel. Readily takes offense. Suddenly remembers unimportant regions which he saw long ago.

Abdomen - Boring and digging pains in abdomen. Flatulent disorders with a sensation of a general bearing down towards hypogastrium.

Back - Bursting, distending pain in kidney region.

Causations - Ill effects of poisonous bites, sprains.

Chest - Chest feels oppressed on ascending. Pressure on chest as though lungs were forced back to spine. Pain in spots, as if bruised shifting pains on stooping. As of a crushing weight or weakness starts in chest. Sore from coughing, pressure, sneezing or moving arms. Burning in chest before or after coughing. Dry scraping in chest worse talking. Thorax feels too narrow. Exudation in pleura. Hydrothorax. Circumscribed spots in chest left after inflammations.

Constitutions - Suited to plethoric, phlegmatic persons, persons tending to obesity, fat persons of lax tissue, fat, chubby children and old persons. Suited to females of slender and tall, but having retained a good deal of sprightliness and moral power.

Ears - Aching in the ear when chewing.

Eyes - Oculomotor paralysis. Muscular asthenopia (Caust.). Opacities of the vitreous humor. Promotes the absorption of fragments. Staring. Lachrymation. Dryness with ***sensation as if too large for orbits***. Eyeballs feel distended or like balls of ice. Sensation of trembling without visible trembling. Flickering, must wipe eyes frequently. Objects look shaded. Double vision, better only by bending head backward. Ptosis. Blepharitis, lids dry and crusty (Graph.).

Head - Dullness with pressure and weakness of eyes. Pain in temples. ***Bursting pain*** in forehead into eyes, better cool open air.

Kidneys - Bursting, distending pain in kidney region. Scalding before and after urinating. Increased or decreased in amount. Greatly diminished urine, loaded with shreds and mucus. Urine, foamy, acrid with mucus shreds.

Lungs - Bronchial catarrh with ***sore chest walls,*** much mucus, sensation of oppression and weight of chest. Bursting pain in back on coughing. Hacking cough. ***Cough often ends in a sneeze. Rattling in chest*** (Ant-t.). Albuminous or blood-streaked sputum. ***Exudations in pleura***. Pleuro-pneumonia. Hydrothorax (Merc-s.) ***Difficult raising of tough, profuse mucus*** in the aged. Asthenic bronchitis of old people with chronic interstitial nephritis or chronic emphysema. Old asthmatics with congestive attacks.

Modalities - Better walking in open air, sweat, ***bending head backwards***, walking in open air. Rest helps dry cough. Worse from inhaling air, open air, cold, wind, walking in open air. Worse in warm air, warm room. Worse going up stairs, stooping, bending forward. Worse by touch and pressure, rubbing. Worse rest, morning and night. Worse looking intently at an object.

Mouth - Dry scraping in mouth, worse talking. Taste, metallic like urine.

Nose - Dry. Coryza, much watery mucus and sneezing. Sneezes, so often and so violently that the head grows dizzy and heavy. Nostrils feel peppery.

Sensations - Eyes, as if they were pressed out, as if eyeballs were being expanded, as if soap in eyes. As if red pepper throughout nostrils and air passages. Dyspnea as from stagnation in lungs. As if lungs pushed back to spine. As if chest would burst. As if chest too narrow. Wrist as if sprained. Joints as if lame.

Stomach - Loathing and nausea with inclination to vomit.

Throat - Catarrhal inflammation of throat and fauces with scraping hoarseness. Catarrh of larynx. Hawks viscid mucus in detached small clots. Burning and rawness. Sensation as if membrane had been abraded. Dry scraping, worse talking. Loss of voice. Voice unsteady, vocal cords partially paralyzed. Hurts to talk.

COMMENTS - The prover took from 40 to 6 drops of the tincture. Extreme tenderness. Worse bending head forward and worse from stooping. Generally left-sided.

Disordered digestive organs. Gnawing hunger and empty feeling. Irritability and catarrh of the urinary organs. Frequent urging, scalding in urethra before or after urination. Urine is loaded with mucus threads. Seneg. has been used as an emetic.

Pressure, dullness, heaviness in the head. Painful sensitiveness of hearing. Eye symptoms as an accompaniment of head symptoms. "Violent rush of blood to head when stooping, especially to eyeballs, where a painful pressure is experienced."

Pains, inflammation both of the exterior and interior of the eye and lids, and much disorder of vision. The eye troubles are worse when looking intently at an object and better bending head backwards.

The symptom in which it was first noticed was "When walking towards the setting sun he seemed to see another smaller sun hover below the other, assuming a somewhat oval shape when looking down, disappearing on bending head backwards and on closing the eyes."

Guernsey outlined its action, "Where there is a great burning in the chest, either before or after coughing, profuse secretion of mucus. Dryness of inner parts which are usually moist, dry skin. General disorders of the windpipe, left side of chest particularly, right eye, lower eyelids."

Nash, who had only obtained success with low potencies of Seneg., cured many cases of "cough with great accumulation of mucus, which seems to fill the chest with much rattling, wheezing and difficult breathing."

A very stout elderly woman of tubercular family history had pneumonia of both bases, especially right. She had a very violent paroxysmal cough with ropy, difficult expectoration tinged with blood. Seneg. 30c quickly relieved a very dangerous condition when other remedies had failed.

Clinton Enos related a case of a very fat girl, age 10, with cold, damp feet and hands and sweating about the head, had spells of sneezing for two years, even since whooping cough.

Several sneezing spells a day lasting about half an hour. Sharp pains in chest and temples during the attacks. In nose a large quantity of mucus with stuffed-up feeling. One dose of Seneg. 200c removed the whole trouble in a week.

RELATIONS - ***Antidoted by:*** Bry., Arn., Bell., Camph. ***Compare:*** (1) Sapin. - a derivative of Senega root. (2) In bronchial affections, Am-c. (3) Fat, plethoric people disposed to catarrhs, Calc. (4) Muscular asthenopia, loss of voice, paralysis (facial, etc.), Caust. (5) Laryngeal and pulmonary catarrh, Phos. (6) Bronchial catarrh, Spong. (7) Whooping cough, Coc-c., Kali-bi. (Seneg. clear phlegm, cough worse towards evening, Coc-c. clear phlegm worse morning, Kali-bi. yellow phlegm in morning). ***Follows well:*** Calc., Phos., Lyc., Sulph.

REFERENCES - Boericke. Clarke. Phatak.

SENNA

(Cassia Acutifolia)

PHARMACY - senn. Senna. Cassia acutifolia. Alexandrian senna. Cassia angustifolia. Cassia obovata. N. O. Leguminosae. Caesalpinioideae. The leaflets of several species of Cassia. Trituration or tincture of the dried leaves. ***Historical dose:*** Tincture and all potencies.

CLINICAL - ***Acetonemia. Colic. Constipation.*** Exhaustion. Fainting. ***Flatulence.*** Liver, disorders. Nitrogenous, waste. Oxaluria. Sleeplessness. Sneezing with heat.

HOMEOPATHIC - The symptoms are mostly derived from overdosings. Senn. is used as a laxative in ordinary practice.

Senn. has proved an excellent remedy in the colic of infants with incarcerated flatulence and sleeplessness. ***Infantile colic,*** when the child seems to be ***full of wind. Constipation*** with colic and flatulence. Oxaluria with excess of urea increased specific gravity. Liver enlarged and tender.

Exhaustion. General swelling. Ebullitions of blood at night. "Repeated sneezing, which caused heat (especially of hands), exhaustion and panting breathing." ***Acetonemia***, prostration, fainting. Unclean body swell.

Abdomen - Sensation of coldness in the abdomen with emptiness and uneasiness in the stomach. Accumulation of flatus with grumbling and fermentation in the abdomen and discharge of fetid flatus. Painful colic from incarcerated flatulence. ***Colic,*** especially in children, infants.

Face - Livid lips. Commissure of lips covered with small burning blisters.

Food - Anorexia. Thirst.

Head - Heaviness of the head when stooping, as if it were pressed down.

Kidneys - Specific gravity and density increased. Hyperazoturia, oxaluria, phosphaturia and acetonuria.

Limbs - Heat in limbs, especially of hands.

Liver - Liver enlarged and tender.

Nose - Repeated sneezing, which caused heat, especially of hands, exhaustion and panting breathing.

Rectum - Burning in rectum with strangury of bladder. ***Constipation*** with colic and flatulence. Stools hard and dark with loss of appetite, coated tongue, bad taste and weakness. Diarrhea with straining and prolapsed rectum and sore anus in children. Liquid stools with griping pains. Loose evacuation with tenesmus and followed by a burning sensation in the anus. Yellowish fluid, with pinching pains before. Greenish mucus, never-get-done sensation (Merc.).

Sleep - Ebullition of blood, especially at night, disturbing the sleep. Sleeplessness with cries and tossing, especially in the case of infants.

Stomach - Empty or watery and fetid, risings. Loathing and nausea with inclination to vomit. Sinking immediately after meals.

COMMENTS - Farrington said it is one of the best remedies in the Materia Medica for "simple exhaustion with excess of nitrogenous waste." The exhaustion is exemplified in the sinking immediately after meals.

The pods caused an unclean smell from the body of a woman taking them for constipation. Acts as a tonic where the system is broken down, bowels constipated, muscular weakness and waste of nitrogenous materials.

RELATIONS - ***Antidotes:*** Nux-v., Cham. ***Compare:*** (1) Cassi-s., Kali-c., Jal.

REFERENCES - Boericke. Clarke.

SEPIA SUCCUS

(Cuttlefish Ink)

PHARMACY - sep. Sepia succus. Cuttlefish ink. Sepia officinalis. N. O. Cephalopoda. Trituration of dried liquid contained in the ink-bag. ***Historical dose:*** All potencies.

CLINICAL - Abortion. Addison's disease. Alcohol, effects. ***Amenorrhea.*** Anal, problems. Appetite, depraved. Ascarides. Baldness. ***Bedwetting. Bladder, weak.*** Birth control pills. Cancer. ***Childbirth.*** Chloasma. Chorea. Condylomata. ***Constipation***. Cortisone, effects. Cushing's disease. Cystitis. Depression. ***Dysmenorrhea.*** Dyspepsia. Eczema. Estrogen, effects. Eyes, disorders. Face, yellow. Freckles. Gleet. Gonorrhea. Gravel. Hair, loss. Hemorrhoids. Herpes. ***Hormonal, disorders.*** Hormonal, drugs. ***Hot, flushes.*** Hysterectomy. Hysteria. ***Infertility.*** Jaundice. Labor, pains. Leucorrhea. ***Libido, low.*** Liver, spots. Liver, torpid. ***Menopause. Menstruation, disorders.*** Mental, disorders. ***Miscarriages. Morning sickness.*** Neuralgias. Nose, inflamed. Nosebleed. Ovarian, disorders. Ozaena. Phimosis. Pityriasis, versicolor. Pleurisy. ***Pregnancy, disorders. Premenstrual, syndrome.*** Pruritus. Psoriasis. Ptosis. ***Puberty, disorders.*** Pylorus, induration. Quinsy. Rectal, disorders. Ringworm. Sacrum, pain. Sciatica. Seborrhea. ***Sexual, disorders.*** Smell, disorders. Spermatorrhea. Strokes. Styes. Toothache. Urinary, incontinence. ***Uterus, disorders. Uterus, prolapsed. Vaginitis.*** Varicose, veins. ***Venous stasis***. Warts. Whooping cough.

HOMEOPATHIC - The inky juice of cuttlefish, known as Indian ink, is one of the remedies of the Chronic Diseases, and was proved by Goullon, Von Gersdorff, Gross, Hartlaub and Wahle.

It is preeminently a woman's remedy, although the first symptoms were found by Hahnemann accidentally proved by a male artist. It affects the generative organs of both sexes and a large number of the symptoms occurring in other organs have some relation thereto.

Sep. affects the venous circulation, especially of the ***female pelvic organs*** and of the digestive tract. It acts especially on the portal system with venous congestion. ***Venous stasis,*** ptosis of viscera. Violent ebullitions of blood with pulsation throughout the body. Pulsating headache in cerebellum. Bleedings.

Hormonal disorders. Affections in pregnant women. ***Tendency to miscarriages***. ***Bearing down in pelvic region. Uterus prolapsed.*** Hot flashes at menopause with weakness and perspiration. Excess of sexual indulgence. Loss of vital fluids. Milky secretions.

Upward tendency of its symptoms. Symptoms settle in back, in ileo-cecal region, ovaries. Pains extend down to back, chills easily. Shuddering from pain. Burning pains in different parts of the body. Rheumatism, chronic cases. Fits of uneasiness and hysterical spasms. Spasms, clonic, tonic, cataleptic. Jerking in muscles. Fidgety.

Sudden prostration. Easy fainting. ***Feels cold,*** even in warm room. Short walk fatigues much. Weariness and misery. Weakness, yellow complexion. Weak, empty, hollow feeling in epigastrium, chest, muscles, lumbar back, hips, knees etc. or sensation of fullness. As of a lump or something rolling over internally. ***"Ball"*** sensation in inner parts.

Females dragged down by overwork. Tubercular patient with chronic hepatic troubles and uterine reflexes. Children who take cold easily when the weather changes. Relaxed, plethoric females. Weak, pot-bellied mothers with yellow complexion. Diseased conditions which drag on, linger. Atrophy of children, their face like an old man. Warty growths. Big belly, dry flabby skin.

MIND - ***Mentally and physically worn-out patients.*** Industrious. Indisposed to mental labor. Repugnance to customary business, disgust of life. Makes mistakes while writing or reading. Poor memory. Confused, wants to run away. Confusion of mind when spoken to. Irresolution.

Anxious fear, over trifles. Anxiety during heat flushes. Constantly worries, frets and cries about her real or imaginary illness. Despair about recovery. ***Cries when telling her symptoms.*** Fear of poverty. Fear of thunderstorms. Nervous, so that she wants to hold on to something or she should scream.

Sense of helplessness. Feels unfortunate without cause. ***Weeping, worse from consolation.*** Breaks down in spells of weeping. Miserly. Dwells on past disagreeable occurrences.

Self-pity. Complaints and grievances. Sad and gloomy moods. Sad over her health and domestic affairs. Tendency to burst into tears. They have too much work to do. People are not kind to them. No one realizes how much suffering they have or with what difficulties they have to contend.

Depression, suicidal. Depression on awaking in morning. Depression related to pregnancy, menses or menopause. ***Unhappy married life.*** Great sadness during pregnancy or lactation. ***Post-partum depression.*** Emotional stillness.

Sexually shut down, no libido. Low sex drive since childbirth, hysterectomy, menopause. Aversion to the opposite sex. Women who dislike men and men who dislike women. ***Loss of sex drive and sexual disorders.*** Nausea, disgust at the thought of sex. Anxiety after sex. Dullness of mind after sex.

Aversion to those loved best, to family. Aversion to sympathy and company, yet dreads to be alone. Averse to occupation, house work. Indolent. Desires solitude, lies with closed eyes. Sits quietly and answers either with yes or no.

Irritable and easily offended. ***Irritability***, alternating with indifference or sulks. Bad-tempered. Resents criticism of any kind. Spiteful. Lack of sympathy. ***Angry, sensitive,*** easily offended and miserable. Anger about past events. ***Anger from contradiction.*** Anger related to pregnancy, menses or menopause. Anger in morning.

Censorious. Takes pleasure in teasing others. Never seems happy unless annoying someone. Says and does strange things. Mania before menses. Sensitive to least noise, odors. ***Excited during thunderstorms.*** Cheerful when it thunders and with lightning. ***Loves to dance.***

Abdomen - Brown spots on abdomen. Coldness in abdomen. Lax feeling in abdomen. Falling out or heavy, bearing down feeling in hypogastrium, better by holding it or crossing legs. Burning and shooting pains. Violent pain in umbilical region. Bloated abdomen after eating. Loud rumbling in abdomen after eating. ***Flatulence*** with headache. Colic and faintness before menses. Soreness and pain as if menses would appear. Pot-belly of mothers.

Back - Backache, causes nausea and faint feeling while standing. Sudden pain in back, as if struck by a hammer, worse stooping, kneeling. Back pain, better belching, by pressing back against something hard. Heaviness in back in morning on waking. Burning pressure in spine. Spine tender to touch or pressure. Aching and dull pain in lumbar and sacral regions. Aching in inter-scapular or lumbar region, paralytic, wants to be pressed. ***Weakness in small of back,*** when walking, from uterine disease. ***Weakness in lumbar region.*** Lumbar region as if sprained. Throbbing in lumbar region. Cramps in buttocks when stretching out legs. Coldness between scapula, as from an icy hand. Collar feels tight.

Bladder - Chronic cystitis. ***Prolapsed bladder***, must cross limbs to prevent protrusion or press against vulva. ***Bladder weak.*** Sensation as if bladder falls to side lain on. Cutting pain in bladder before urination. Involuntary urination, worse coughing, sneezing, laughing, hearing sudden noise, fright or inattention, especially in women. Slow urination with bearing down sensation above pubis. ***Bedwetting*** during first part of sleep.

Breasts - Swollen, sensitive breasts before menses. Sensation as if breasts were enlarged. Stitches, tender, burning pains. Induration of breasts. Scirrhus breasts. Burning pain in a fixed spot under right nipple. Nipples cracked across the crown. Nipples bleeding and sore, preceded by itching.

Causations - Ill effects of overwork, anger and vexation. Ill effects of blows, injury, over-lifting, falls. Ill effects of getting wet, laundry work, boiled milk, fat, pork, tobacco, alcohol. Snowy air. Puberty, hormone treatment, birth control pills, hysterectomy, pregnancy, childbirth, menopause. Sexual abuse.

Chest - Oppression of chest, morning and evening. Oppression when walking or from slightest exertion. Pain in sides of chest, when inspiring or coughing. Sensation of emptiness in chest. Chest symptoms better by pressure of hand. Stitches in chest when coughing. Fungus hematodes in clavicular region, bleeding profusely. Boils in axilla. Swelling and suppuration of axillary glands. Humid tetter in axilla. Brown spots on chest.

Constitutions - Hering said it was suited to young persons of both sexes of nervous and delicate constitution, who are disposed to sexual excitement or worn out by sexual excess. Women during pregnancy, in childbed, and while nursing. Children who take cold readily when the weather changes. Scrofulous persons. Men who have been addicted to drinking and sexual excesses. Pot-bellied mothers, yellow saddle across nose, irritable, faint from least exertion, leuco-phlegmatic constitutions. Bahr indicated it for sanguine, excitable temperaments inclined to congestions.

Coughs - Cough in morning with profuse expectoration, tasting salty (Phos., Ambr.). Rotten-egg taste with coughing. Cough excited by tickling in larynx or chest. Cough better eating. Cough with nausea and bitter vomiting. Dry, fatiguing cough with foul sputum, as if coming from stomach, worse rapid change of temperature. Spasmodic cough, evening and at night in bed, preventing sleep. Child cries each time it coughs at night. Whooping cough that drags on.

Ears - Chronic otalgia. Discharge, thick yellow pus offensive. Discharge of thin matter. Itching in affected ear. Pain as if from sub-cutaneous ulceration. Dragging or stitching pain in ears. Swelling of and eruptions on external ear. Herpes, behind ears, on lobe of ears, on nape of neck. Tetter on lobes of ear and behind ears. ***Oversensitive to noise,*** especially music. Loud sounds and humming in ears. Sudden deafness, as if caused by the plug in ears.

Eyes - Eyes feel tired and look injected. Conjunctivitis. Muscular asthenopia. Asthenic inflammations with uterine trouble. Burning in eyes with lachrymation. Aching at back of eyeballs. Eyes feel sore as if bruised. Falling out feeling in eyes during headache. Pressure as from sand in eyes. Arrests cataract in women. Photophobia. Cannot tolerate reflected light. Aggravation of eye troubles morning and evening. Agglutination of eyelids. Epithelioma of eyelids. Eyelids red, itching. Styes.

Ptosis. Drooping eyelids. Eyelids as if too heavy to open. Venous congestion of the fundus. Tarsal tumors. Tarsi, red, itching cancer.

Face - Old, wrinkled skin with spots. Black pores. Face changes color. ***Chloasma.*** Dark circles under eyes. ***Yellowish-brown saddle across nose.*** Yellow-brownish discoloration on nose and cheeks. Yellow blotches, pale or sallow, yellow about mouth. Rosacea. Acne, worse before menses. Warts. Swollen, cracked lower lip. Cancer of the lips, epithelioma. Swelling of submaxillary glands. Numbness of malar bones. Jerking of facial muscles while talking. Facial neuralgia during pregnancy.

Female - Hormonal disorders. ***Never well since puberty, childbirth, after weaning or hormone pills.*** Amenorrhea. ***Menses irregular, early and profuse***. ***Menses too late and scanty***. Menses cause faintness, chilliness and shuddering. Mania from profuse menses. Dysmenorrhea in women with scanty menses. Dryness of vagina and vulva after menses. Leucorrhea, yellow, greenish, milky in large lumps, with much itching, instead of menses. Leucorrhea, foul, gonorrheal with stitches up in vagina from uterus to navel. Leucorrhea in little girls. Pelvic organs relaxed. Weak uterus. Dragging or ***bearing down sensation as if everything would escape through the vagina*** (Bell., Lil-t., Nat-c.), must cross limbs to prevent protrusion or press against vulva. ***Prolapsed uterus or vagina***. Sub-involution. Violent stitches upward in the vagina from uterus to umbilicus. Griping, burning or sticking in uterus. Sharp clutching pains. Labia swollen, abscessed. Severe itching in vulva causing abortion. ***Tendency to miscarriage*** from the fifth to the seventh month. Labor-like, during seventh month of pregnancy. ***Morning sickness.*** Motion of fetus is intolerable. Retained placenta after abortion. Offensive, excoriating lochia. ***Infertility.*** Sterility. ***Aversion to sex,*** worse since childbirth. ***Low sex drive.*** Nausea and irritability on thought of sex. Sexual parts tender to touch. Sex painful from dryness of vagina. Bleeding after sex. Exhaustion after sex. ***Sudden flushes of heat*** with weakness and sweat during menopause. Metrorrhagia at the time of menopause.

Food - Voracious appetite or no appetite. Sudden cravings and sudden satiety. Everything tastes too salty (Carb-v., Chin.). ***Desires chocolate,*** sweets, wine, ***vinegar***, acids and pickles. Great sensitiveness to smell of cooking food. ***Nausea at thought or smell of food.*** Aversion to all food during headache, to bread and milk during pregnancy. Aversion to fat, meat, milk. Aggravated from acids and fats, loathes fats. ***Worse from boiled milk.*** Great nervous irritability from coffee. Water brash after eating or drinking. Thirst during headache.

Head - Headache alternating sides of occiput. Headache worse lying on painful side, indoors. Headache better after meals. Headache with ***terrible shocks*** at menstrual time, with scanty flow, or before menses. Weekly or monthly headaches. Headache worse from shopping, mental labor, better after meals. Headache with nausea and vomiting. Smell of food repulsive during headache. Jaundice with headache. Hair falls out after chronic headache. Shooting pains. Screams with pain. Stinging pain within out or upwards. Stinging pain over left eye. Heavy feeling on vertex. Cold sensation on vertex. Involuntary jerking of head backwards and forwards, with open fontanelles in children. Prodromal symptoms of a stroke. Hemicrania. ***Hair falls out at menopause***. Root of hair sensitive to combing. Pimples on forehead along the margins of hair.

Heart - Irregular circulation, seems to stagnate. ***Venous stasis.*** Congestion of blood vessels. Dropsy in consequence of valvular insufficiency. General pulsations. Ebullitions at night. Tremulous feeling with flushes. Beating in all arteries. Violent, intermittent palpitations. Palpitations with anxiety. Nervous palpitations, better walking fast, worse lying on left side. Visible palpitations, ascends to occiput. Palpitations before scanty menses. Wakes up with violent beating of heart. An occasional hard thump of the heart. Sensation as if heart stood still. Pulse full and quick during night and then intermitting. Pulse slow during day. Pulse accelerated by motion or being angry.

Kidneys - Weak kidneys. Kidney pain and backache. Nephritis. Feeble stream, urine is ***thick, foul,*** white, milky, bloody. Gritty, red, ***adhesive***, ***sandy sediment*** in urine.

Limbs - ***Poor circulation.*** Venous stasis. Heaviness and a bruised feeling. ***Restlessness in all limbs***, twitching and jerkings night and day. Sensation of running, as from a mouse in lower limbs. Tension in limbs as if they were too short. Lower limbs lame and stiff. Short walk fatigues. ***Limbs go to sleep easily.*** Coldness of legs, knees, feet, and heels. ***Coldness of limbs during fever.*** Hot hands with cold feet or vice versa. Cold hands in warm room. Rheumatic pains. Stiffness of joints. Weakness of joints, especially the knees. Swelling of veins of affected limbs. Sciatica, better during pregnancy, chronic, localizing in heels. Ulcers on small joints, fingers, toes. Thick crusts on elbows. Hands sweaty, purple. Skin of palms peels off. Crippled nails.

Liver - Aching, throbbing, shooting, stitching, pressing in hepatic region. ***Liver sore and painful, relieved by lying on right side***. Pain in the region of liver or gallbladder, worse stooping.

Lungs - Dyspnea, worse after sleep, better rapid motion. Dyspnea better dancing or walking rapidly. Dyspnea in dry air, fog, east and north wind. Loss of breath, with palpitation, after mental emotions. Suffocation in stormy weather. Asthma, wheezing expiration. Spasmodic asthma. Suddenly aroused from a deep sleep by asthma. Neglected pneumonia. Pleuritis. Copious, very offensive expectoration. Expectoration of blood, after lying down. Yellow, green or grey pus. Expectoration milk-white, tenacious mucus, generally of salty taste, in morning. Can raise sputum if he turns from left to right side.

Male - Offensive perspiration on scrotum. Itching and dry eruption on genitals. Herpes. Prepuce ulcerates and itches. Cracks on foreskin. Condylomata surrounding head of penis. Swelling of scrotum. Cutting pains in testes. Weak prostate gland. Weakness of genitals. Genitals cold. Impotency. Insufficient erections. Sexual desire increased or decreased. Nightly emissions with sexual dreams. Watery semen. Complaints after sex. Gonorrhea. Gleet, discharge from urethra only during night, no pain.

Modalities - Better sitting with legs crossed, crossing or drawing limbs up. ***Better from exercise, running, dancing, vigorous motion***. Better pressure, warmth of bed, hot applications. Better after sleep. Better cold drinks, cold bathing, open air. ***Worse from cold, air,*** dampness, north wind, snowy air, snowfall. Worse before thunderstorms. Worse washing clothes, laundry-work. Worse morning and evening. Worse after first sleep, falling to sleep. ***Worse left side.*** Worse after sweat. Worse sitting, standing, kneeling, jarring, stooping. Worse ascending, lifting. Worse from touch, rubbing, scratching. Worse after sex, sexual excess. Worse before menses, after pregnancy, miscarriage.

Mouth - Swelling and cracking of lower lip. Mouth and tongue feel as if scalded. Offensive or sour smell from mouth. Profuse flow of salty saliva. Taste of rotten eggs on coughing. Taste salty, putrid, cheesy, fishy. Taste bitter, sour, putrid, offensive. Everything tastes too salty. Hawks foul or cheesy grains in the morning.

Nose - ***Yellowish-brown saddle across nose.*** Dry feeling in nose. Pressive pain in root of nose. Tip of nose inflamed and swollen. Nostrils ulcerated. Chronic nasal catarrh. Post-nasal catarrh, dripping of heavy, lumpy discharge, must be hawked through the mouth. ***Thick greenish discharge***, foul, plugs and crusts. Ozaena. Ascending throat colds. Frequent sneezing without coryza. Fluent coryza. Nosebleed, when the nose has been struck by anything, even lightly, during menses or pregnancy, with hemorrhoids. Great sensitiveness to odors. Odors are ***repulsive to the smell of cooking food***. Fetid smell before nose.

Perspiration - Hot sweats, worse menopause. Easy, offensive sweat, with orgasms, on genitals, in axilla or back, between menses. Hands sweaty, purple. Sweats from least motion. Sweat on feet, worse on toes, intolerable odor. Cold sweats at night, on chest, back and thighs. Continuous, debilitating sweats. Sweet-smelling sweat.

Rectum - ***Sensation of weight or ball in anus,*** not better by stool. ***Shooting pains*** up rectum and vagina. ***Prolapsed anus*** (Podo.), ***rectum,*** worse from smoking. Rectum is constricted and powerless, almost constant oozing from anus. Bleeding at stool and fullness of rectum. Weak feeling in rectum. Obstinate constipation, no urging for days. ***Constipation***, large, hard stools, cannot strain, with great tenesmus. ***Constipation during pregnancy.*** Infantile diarrhea, ***worse from boiled milk*** and rapid exhaustion. Heat, burning and swelling of anus. Itching in rectum and anus. ***Hemorrhoids during pregnancy.*** Hemorrhoids prolapsing with sticking pain. Hemorrhoids bleed while walking. Soreness between buttocks. Cancer of rectum. Anus encircled by ring of condylomata.

Sensations - As if something twisting in stomach and rising to throat. As if viscera turning inside out. As if bladder full and contents would fall out over pubes. As if drops came out of bladder. As if bladder and urinary organs would be pressed out. ***As of everything would fall out through vulva***. As if everything would fall out of uterus. Uterus as if clutched. As if vulva enlarged. As if something heavy would force itself from vagina. As if heart stood still. As of a ball in inner parts. As of hot water poured over body. As if roots of hair were sore, as if cut short near roots.

Skin - ***Chloasma***. Spots on skin. Yellowish-brown spots. Blotched, raw, rough, hard or cracked, worse flexures. Wine colored skin. Delicate skin, least injury tends to ulceration. Ulcers, on small joints. Herpetic eruption on lips, about mouth and nose. ***Ringworm*** in isolated spots. Ringworm-like eruption every spring. Itching, not relieved by scratching, worse in bends of elbows and knees. Itching vesicles. Urticaria, worse open air better warm room. Boils in axilla. Hyperidrosis and bromidrosis. Lentigo in young women. Ichthyosis with offensive odor of skin. Ichthyosis with offensive odor of skin. Skin pinkish after scratching. Indurations from constant pressure with purple color. Large, hard, seed warts. Small, itching, flat warts on hands and face. Epithelioma, on eyelids, lips.

Sleep - Sleeplessness from excitement. Insomnia from rush of thoughts. Talks loudly during sleep. Wakes frequently as if he has been called. Frequent starts with fright, screaming. Waking at night from frightful dreams, with screaming out. Dreams of rape, being pursued, chased with a knife. Dreams of urinating and finds on waking an urgent desire to do so. Dreams, worse if he lies on left side. No desire to rise in morning. Very sleepy during day, falls asleep as soon as she sits down.

Stomach - Gnawing in stomach, better eating. Sinking down feeling and weakness. ***Faint sinking feeling at epigastrium,*** not better by eating. Severe cramping pains. Hardness in pyloric region. Burning in pit of stomach. Heartburn. Sensation of a lump in stomach (Carb-an.). Sensation of something twisting about in stomach and rising into the throat. Disordered stomach after bread, milk, fat food or acids. Stomach pain and vomiting of mucus after simplest food. Acid dyspepsia with bloated abdomen, sour belchings. Dyspepsia from over-lifting, from smoking. Belchings, milky, sour, bitter, rancid of tough, foamy mucus. Eructations like rotten eggs. ***Nausea at thought or smell of food***. ***Nausea in morning before eating***. Nausea worse lying on side. ***Morning sickness,*** motion sickness. Disposition to vomit after eating. Vomiting of milky fluid during pregnancy. Vomiting of bile and food.

Stool - Stools passed after prolonged straining, followed by cupful of jelly like yellow-white, very offensive mucus. Insufficient stool, mixed or covered with mucus. Dark-brown, round balls glued together with mucus. Large, hard stools, constipated. Soft stool, difficult. Narrow stools, sometimes triangular. Greenish loose stool. Stool has a putrid, sourish, fetid smell, expelled suddenly. Almost constant oozing from anus.

Teeth - Bleeding of gums. Gums painful, as if burned. Grinding teeth. Teeth decay. Teeth feel dull. Hollow molar pains as if elongated and swollen. Toothache from hot or cold things. Toothache better cold water, returning as soon as water gets warm. Toothache better inhaling cold air. Toothache after sweets and from tea-drinking. Toothache when biting teeth together. Toothache during pregnancy. Toothache and throbbing in gums during menses.

Temperature - ***Poor circulation.*** General lack of warmth of body. Cold in spots, on vertex, between scapula. Easily chilled. Chilly in warm room, during day. Chilly with air hunger. Chilliness during stool. Feet cold and wet in bed. Very sensitive to cold air. Shivering with thirst, worse toward evening. Irregular fevers. ***Hot flashes.*** Heat ascending or as if hot water were poured over her. ***Frequent flushes of heat***. Anxious hot flushes preceded by sudden weakness.

Throat - Dryness and soreness. Roughness and soreness of larynx and throat. Roughness and burning in fauces, worse hawking. Raw pain when swallowing. Pressure in the throat, feels neck cloth tight. Sensation of dryness in larynx. Sensation of a plug. Sore throat with swelling of cervical glands. Ascending throat colds. Hawks foul or cheesy lumps in morning. Hoarseness. Aphonia.

Tongue - Tip of tongue as if scalded. Tongue white and feels burnt. Tongue coated with mucus, dirty yellow, brown with red edges. Tongue pale, flabby and indented. Tongue stiff. Vesicles on tongue. Tongue dirty, becomes clear during menses.

Vertigo - Fits of vertigo, worse walking in open air, least movement of arms. Vertigo with a sensation as if something rolling around the head. Vertigo as if intoxicated. Vertigo as if every object were in motion. Vertigo as if suspended in air.

Vision - Black spots, points, before the eyes. Amaurosis, with contracted pupils. Hemiopia. Vision was dimmed from sexual excess, masturbation or uterine diseases. Vanishing of sight during menses, better lying. Flashes of light when closing eyes. Sparks, veil, streaks before the eyes. Intolerance of reflected light from bright objects.

COMMENTS - Historically, physicians used the flesh, the eggs or even the only bone that constitutes the skeleton of this animal, for "leucorrhea, gonorrhea, catarrh of the bladder, gravel, spasms of the bladder, baldness, freckles and certain kinds of tetters which is sufficiently remarkable in the light of the provings."

Sep. acts on the vital forces as well as on organic tissues. The sphincters and all non-striated muscles are weakened. Sep. disturbs the circulation, causing flushes and other irregularities, throbbings all over, hot hands and cold feet or vice versa. The flushes run upward and end in sweat with a faint, weak feeling. Nosebleed may occur from a blow, from being in a warm room, or from suppressed menses. Low thyroid with hormonal components.

Grimmer stated "This remedy has cured cancer of rectum and uterus, it acts strongly on the sexual organs of both sexes and a great many symptoms and conditions are manifested in this sphere. Young people of both sexes frequently have ailments calling for this medicine, women during the pregnant state after childbirth, men who have been addicted to drinking and sexual excesses are often helped by this remedy. Sex aggravates it in both sexes."

Difficulty with hormonal changes, associated with headaches, constipation, hemorrhoids and irritability. Never well since puberty (Puls.), childbirth, miscarriage, abortion, menopause. Ailments from the birth control pill, hormonal creams or patches.

Premenstrual syndrome, with irritability, headache, generally fastidious before menses. Irregular menses, painful, may have a heavy flow. Low energy, bloating, irritability and sensitivity before period.

May crave chocolate. Somewhat offensive, yellowish-green leucorrhea.

Prolapse or induration of uterus and cervix. Engorgement of the uterus going on to induration. Prolapse or retroversion. Bearing-down pains of great intensity, in the abdomen, back, extending into thighs, and sometimes even seem to interfere with breathing. Bearing down worse standing or walking.

Constant sense of pressing into vagina, compelling the patient to cross the limbs to prevent prolapse. Uterine symptoms with hysteria, weakness, palpitation, orgasm of blood, faintness.

Loss of sex drive. Aversion to sex, to affection, or being touched and held since hormonal change. Aversion to the smells of their partner. Aloofness, disgust for sex. May fake orgasms, have sex out of a feeling of duty, obligation. Anorgasmic or may take a long time to orgasm. Ailments from rape, with emotional and sexual shutdown (Staph. has anger). Drained of love and affection for all loved ones. Empty, sinking feeling.

Morning sickness with aversion to sight, smell, thought of foods. Vomiting of food, bile and milky fluid, in the morning. Strains so that blood comes up. "The thought of food sickens her with sense of a great weight in anus." Hypersensitive to odors, delusions of odors. Disgusted feeling. May want to back out of pregnancy.

May have a history of many childbirths or miscarriages. Miscarriage from sex, causes contractions. Tendency to miscarriage. Hering is reported to have said "All women prone to miscarriage should take Sep. or Zinc." Physical affects from abortions (Nat-m. for emotional trauma).

Difficulty making decisions, confusion, anger during pregnancy. Sinking sensation in pregnancy. Premature delivery or false labor pains associated with low energy or depression. Traumatic, loss of blood and energy. Long and exhausting labor.

Postpartum depression. Emotionally shutdown after childbirth. Loss of mothering instincts. Aversion to breastfeeding. Ill effects of breastfeeding. Weight gain since pregnancy (Calc.). Depression with menopause. Hot flashes, low sex drive, depression after a hysterectomy.

Indifference to loved ones. Aloof and detached, insensitive. Critical, cold hearted, tendency to nag and complain, especially with hormonal changes. Easily upset, frustrated (Ign.), from hormonal imbalance. Ailments from grief (Nat-m.). Impulse to do violence.

Fits of weeping, without knowing why. Fear of not understanding their emotions. Worse from consolation, desires to be left alone. Lack of mental thought, of emotional feeling. Mind becomes dull, struggle to thing. Weak, dragged feeling.

Venous stasis, weak veins. Slowed circulation, better from vigorous exercise. Raynaud's disease. Tendency to bruise easily. Cold hands and feet. Varicose veins (Phos.), during or since pregnancy. Weakened uterine tissues, bearing down feeling. Lack of tone and weakness leading to congestion, then to bearing down pain. Hemorrhoids, ever since childbirth. Hemorrhoids with menses. Prolapsed rectum in cases of hemorrhoids.

Sensation of emptiness, sometimes connected with the pelvic bearing down. Empty sensation in the epigastrium and throughout the abdomen. Lump sensation in the throat and rectum. "Ball" sensation in inner parts, most notably in rectum, not relieved by stool. Clarke has cured both constipation and diarrhea when that symptom was present. Upward stitches in rectum and vagina.

Portal stasis. Fullness, soreness and stitches in liver region, as well as stitches in left hypochondrium. Diabetes with a hormonal component. Low blood sugar. Dyspepsia, from injury, by over-lifting. Severe constipation (Alum., Calc.), or constipation during pregnancy. Craves chocolate, bitter, sour and tart foods, particularly during pregnancy. Tendency to stimulate their taste buds. Strong aversion to fat.

Irritation of the urinary tract. Catarrh of bladder and urethra. Frequent strong urging to urinate. Stitches along the urethra. Relaxed sphincters. Bedwetting, "The bed is wet almost as soon as the child goes to sleep, always during the first sleep." Discharge of urine may be difficult even with urgent desire. Gonorrhea after the acute stage has subsided. Gleet and gonorrheal warts.

Delicate skin, the least injury tends to ulceration. Itching, which often changes to burning when scratched. Soreness of skin, humid places on bends of knees. Painful eruption on tip of nose. Herpetic eruption on lips and about mouth.

Skin condition relating to hormonal changes. Tendency to dry skin from low estrogen. Severe dryness of the vagina (Nat-m.). Chloasma. Liver spots, brown spots. Hair falls out after childbirth or with menopause. Acne, mole growth, freckles related to hormonal change, including puberty, childbirth, or birth control pills. Brittle nails. Addison's disease.

Psoriasis, skin funguses (Thuj.), ringworm (Thuj., Bac., Tell.). Ringworm-like eruptions, pityriasis, every spring on different parts of body. Herpes circinatus. Round, yellow spots. Nettle rash, appears on going into open air, better in warm room. Desperate itching, especially when it affects the genitals and anus.

Bursitis from kneeling and scrubbing the floors, overwork. Patient is worn out from domestic duties. Arthritis, worse cold, wet (Calc.). Backache (Bry., Nat-m.). Stiffness of limbs worse after sleep. Stiffness of uterine region. "Involuntary jerking of head backward and forward, especially at forenoon when sitting." Jerking in hysteria. Open fontanelles in children.

Vertigo with sensation of something "rolling round" in the head. "Faints easily," after getting wet, from extremes of heat and cold, riding in a carriage, kneeling at church.

Chronic nasal catarrh. Inflamed tonsils from colds, tending to suppuration. Nash had a case in which the discharge was thick, bland and copious. Puls. relieved the catarrh but increased the menstrual flow too much. Sep. cured both.

Whooping cough when it has lasted eight weeks or longer and the paroxysms, though reduced in number and virulence, do not disappear and occur especially before midnight. The patients are reduced in strength, dyspeptic, irritable, tearful, easily angered or apathetic.

Symptoms are generally left-sided. Worse standing, kneeling, on the left. Very chilly, sensitive to cold. Better deep pressure but worse light touch. Irritable in the mornings from toxicity in the liver (Nux-v.). Need movement, but worse from exertion. Cheerful with thunderstorms.

Kunkel reported a case of pulmonary affection in a boy, 14, who had been under treatment five weeks for cough and hoarseness. Hoarseness was worse evening, cough with purulent sputa during the day. Slept well but dreamed when he lay on left side. Emaciated. Phos. 10x produced little change.

There was remarkable tightness of the chest on breathing with inclination to take a deep breath, this was better in open air, on motion, while at work, worse while in the house and at rest. Though the weather was bad he had a constant desire to be out of doors. Sep. 10x made a rapid cure.

Boenninghausen recommended Sep. in cases of cough, either with or without expectoration with blood-streaked, purulent, yellow greenish or stinking sputa, and especially in tuberculosis.

Nash mentioned a case of cholera infantum that he cured with Sep. on the indication "always worse after taking milk." He compared it with Ant-c. for moisture oozing from the anus, which has the first place.

Bahr said Sep. afforded considerable help in a certain condition of the system that had only been noticed in females. After the exacerbation of a chronic gastric catarrh has lasted a few days with intolerable burning pains, the kidney region becomes painful, more particularly the left side.

Violent burning pain in the kidney region and a quantity of saturated, highly-colored urine is discharged. Urine deposits copious quantities of urates, or else a clear urine with copious sandy sediment, coated with uric acid. After the discharge, the pains generally abate and only return if the stomach has not been restored to its normal condition.

Hering noted its usefulness for "condylomata completely surrounding head of penis."

Clarke cured a crop of small, velvety warts completely encircling the mouth of the prepuce. Thuja had failed. Clarke also cured with Sep. 3x a large horn-like wart on the abdomen of a woman. It was as large as a crown-piece but shaped like a bean and raised a quarter of an inch from the surface.

Clarke confirmed the experience of Dr. Swallow, who found the fresh preparation of Sep. to possess a wider range than the ordinary preparation and to act as an "organ remedy" in a great variety of uterine disorders not definitely indicated by the pathogenesis. Clarke used it in potencies from the 5c to 30c.

RELATIONS - ***Antidoted by:*** Smelling Nit-s-d., by vegetable acids, Acon., Ant-c., Ant-t., Rhus-t. ***It antidotes:*** Calc., Chin., Merc., Nat-m., Nat-p., Phos., Sars., Sulph. ***Compare:*** (1) Nat-m., Bell-p., Lil-t., Murx., Sil., Sulph. (2) Vesicular eruptions and ulcers about joints, Bor., Mez. (3) Indifferent to his occupation, Fl-ac., Ph-ac. (4) Sensation of ball in inner parts, Lach. (5) Ringworm in isolated spots, Bac., Calc., Tell. (6) Psoriasis, Ars., Ars-i. (7) Chloasma, Lyc., Nux-v., Sulph., Cur. (8) Constipation during pregnancy, Alum. (9) Pain in rectum long after stool, Nit-ac., Sulph. (10) Empty feeling better eating, Chel., Lyc., Phos. (11) Bedwetting almost as soon as child goes to sleep, Kreos. (12) Bearing down as if everything would protrude from pelvis, Agar., Bell. Lil-t., Murx., Sanic. (13) Sight or thought of food sickens, Nux-v. Smell of cooking food nauseates, Ars., Colch. ***Complementary:*** Nat-m., Phos. Nux-v. intensifies action. Guaiacum is often beneficial after Sep. ***Followed well by:*** Nit-ac. ***Inimical:*** Lach., Puls.

REFERENCES - Boericke. Clarke. Murphy. Phatak.

SEQUOIA SEMPERVIRENS

(Redwood Tree)

PHARMACY - seq-s. Sequoia sempervirens. Redwood. N. O. Taxodiaceae. ***Historical dose:*** All potencies.

CLINICAL - Asthma. ***Constipation.*** Edema. Flatulence. Headache. Lungs, collapsed. ***Nausea.*** Pneumonia. Polyuria. Rheumatism. Salivation. ***Sneezing.***

HOMEOPATHIC - Birch and Rockwell, wrote, in A Homoeopathic Proving of Sequoia sempervirens, 1994, "The tree grows in the fog where it is damp and wet, it also grows near the ocean.

"The source of the remedy is the burl, a growth on the tree from which new life sprouts. If one were to study the logging industry, one would find that in man's greed and desire for more, bigger and better, he shows no restraint from destroying the last few virginal growths of these incredible giants.

"It seems to affect some people in one way, while in others the effects are opposite. In the lungs there is ease of breath or there is difficulty of breath. In the heart we find pressure, shooting pains and symptoms from grief, or absence of symptoms and complete happiness. Blurry vision or clarity of vision."

Seq-s. is a sycotic remedy. Hydrogenoid propensity, overproduction of mucus, voracious appetite, rheumatic complaints. Wandering pains. Pains gripping, constrictive, aching. Stiff and tight feeling in body (Guai.).

Feeling of well-being. Great exhaustion. Voracious appetite. Strong desire for whatever is available. Increased salivation. Fluid retention Absence of fluid being collected. Vision extremely clear. Blurred vision, worse wind. Worse lying, sitting, continued motion.

MIND - ***Clarity of thought***, as if a fog or haze had lifted in the mind. Feeling of well-being. Feels new and rejuvenated. Relaxed, in tense situations. Difficult concentration. Confusion. Confused by simple tasks.

Overwhelming feeling of being old

(Gink.). Feels cut down. Desires solitude. Aversion to company, desire to go somewhere where no one will bother. Sadness, hard to raise oneself to get up and go in the day. Sympathetic, takes on other peoples sufferings, only feels good while rescuing someone.

Irritability, about trifles, about noises. Desire to scream that gets suppressed. Delusion of being fragile, as if she would emotionally fall apart. Delusion of being unappreciated. Delusion as if she is falling in love, of having a broken heart, as if his wife of many years never loves him. Time appeared to be slowed down.

Abdomen - Burning pain in abdomen. Gripping pain in abdomen, worse after eating, motion, better after sleep.

Back - Pain extending down to hips and knees.

Bladder - Pressing pain in bladder. Polyuria. Desire to urinate even after having just done so.

Chest - Limp feeling in chest. Short sharp pain in right side of chest. Shooting pain in heart from being heart broken. Band of tightness in diaphragm, desire to stretch, which causes soreness.

Ears - Outward pressing pain.

Face - Looks much older. Sensation of fullness, as if more fluid were under the skin. Obstruction of facial sinuses. Pressing pain in maxillary area.

Female - Menses starts and stops; copious.

Head - Headache between the eyes.

Heart - Feeling as if he would die from a broken heart. Sensation of a wall of bricks and stones fall away from the heart and a yellow and white light encompass the heart.

Limbs - Sharp pain in elbows, shoulders and feet. Sensation of tightness in hands and feet.

Lungs - History of collapsed lungs, pneumonia. Feeling as though one couldn't get enough air into lungs, breathing deeper and deeper yet still wanted more. Asthmatic respiration, worse night, better steam and fresh air. Sore pain in lungs. Coughing up thick mucus. Feeling as if lungs are hyper-clear, as if more air can move in and out of the lungs.

Male - Sexual desire diminished.

Mouth - Salivation increased. Bitter taste. Sensation of stiffness in jaws. Hard to articulate words that require more motion of the jaw.

Nose - ***Burning pain in nasal passages. Sneezing.***

Rectum - ***Constipation during menses.*** Flatulence, frequent, like rotten eggs. Loose and putrid stool.

Skin - Eruptions, raised circular or oval bumps of a light brown discoloration. Itching, worse night.

Sleep - Sleepiness in the afternoon. ***Deep sleep,*** refreshing. Dreams, of being happy and finding someone who really loves them. Dreams of responsibility, of rescuing some children by the side of the road. Wakes unrefreshed; wakes in a sweat.

Stomach - ***Nausea.*** Thirst diminished.

Teeth - Desire to clench teeth, to scratch teeth.

Throat - Nausea felt in pit of throat.

Vision - Objects have a haze to them. Edges of objects seem to swim. Vision, as if on a hallucinogenic drug.

RELATIONS - ***Compare:*** (1) Lyc.

REFERENCES - Birch. Rockwell.

SEROTONIN

PHARMACY - serot. Serotonin. A brain neurotransmitter. ***Historical dose:*** All potencies.

CLINICAL - ***Alcoholism.*** Alzheimer's disease. Anxiety. Autism. Bipolar disorder. Bulimia. Clumsiness. ***Compulsive disorders. Depression.*** Drowsiness. Edema. Insomnia. ***Learning, disorders.*** Migraine. Nightmares. Palpitations. Restlessness. Schizophrenia. Suicidal. Twitching. Vertigo.

HOMEOPATHIC - Serotonin is a neurotransmitter produced in the brain known to influence the functioning of the cardiovascular, renal, immune, and gastrointestinal systems. In the nervous system, serotonin is believed to play an important role in the regulation of mood, sleep, vomiting, sexuality and appetite.

Serotonin has been thought to play a part in many disorders, notably as part of the biochemistry of depression, migraine, bipolar disorder and anxiety. Recent research suggests that serotonin also plays an important role in liver regeneration.

It is well known that abnormal serotonin levels can cause various types of sexual dysfunction such as anorgasmia, erectile dysfunction, and diminished libido. Serotonin also causes problems such as insomnia, depression, obesity, eating disorders, premenstrual syndrome, panic attacks, alcoholism, anxiety disorders, and bulimia.

Serotonin, at increasing levels, stimulates nervous tension, drowsiness, heart palpitations, water retention and inability to concentrate and perform.

Any disruption in the synthesis, metabolism or uptake of this neurotransmitter has been found to be responsible for certain manifestations of ***schizophrenia, depression, compulsive disorders and learning problems.*** Increase in brain levels of either of neurotransmitter, serotonin, produces a ***craving for alcohol, anger, or anxiety,*** especially for those who have a history of alcoholism.

Drowsiness. Tiredness. Sustained rapid eye movement. Overreaction of the reflexes. Rapid muscle contraction and relaxation in the ankle causing abnormal movements of the foot. Clumsiness. Muscle contraction and relaxation in the jaw. Twitching of the muscles. Rigidity. High body temperature. Sweating.

MIND - Euphoric feelings. Feelings of intoxication. Substance abuse. Impulsive behavior, recklessness, exhibitionism. Restlessness. Hostility, argumentative behavior. Violence, violent nightmares. Insomnia.

Depression, anxiety, suicidal tendency. Psychosis. Schizophrenia, mood disorders. Organic brain disease, mental retardation, autism and Alzheimer's.

RELATIONS - ***Compare:*** Melat.

REFERENCES - Murphy.

SERUM ANGUILLAE

(Eel Serum)

PHARMACY - ser-ang. Serum anguillae. Eel serum. Freshwater Eel Serum. Anguilla anguillae. Ichthyotoxinum. Potencies are made with glycerine or distilled water. ***Historical dose:*** All potencies.

CLINICAL - ***Albuminuria.*** Anuria. Dyspnea. Edema. Elephantiasis. Heart, disorders. Hemoglobinuria. Hematuria. ***Hypertension.*** Kidney, disorders. ***Kidney, failure. Lymphaedema.*** Mitral, insufficiency. ***Nephritis. Oliguria***. Uremia.

HOMEOPATHIC - Jousset considered Ser-ang. a specific in disorders of the heart and kidneys without much edema. Ser-ang. affects the kidneys, which becomes acutely affected, either from cold, infection or intoxication. The attack is characterized by ***oliguria, anuria and albuminuria***.

Jousset's experiments have demonstrated the rapid hematuria, albuminuria and oliguria caused by it. But its really specific indication seems to be for sub-acute and ***acute nephritis***. Repressed kidney function and sexuality. Acute nephritis with threatening uremia. Diuresis. Albuminuria. ***Kidney failure.***

Cardiac uremia. ***Hypertension and oliguria without edema***. Heart diseases in cases of failure of compensation and impending asystole. Functional heart diseases. Mitral insufficiency. Asystole with or without edema, dyspnea and difficult urinary secretion.

Warm-blooded. Chilliness when tired. Desire for warm room. ***Lymphaedema*** after operation on breast tumor. Elephantiasis. Faintness and nausea.

MIND - Indifference and lack of will power. Irresolution. Every effort is too much. Aversion to change. Irritability and dissatisfaction with oneself. Nervousness. Restlessness. Sensitive to noises and odors. Anger from noise. Mental dullness. Difficult concentration. Memory weakness. Brain fatigue. Mental and physical symptoms better from appearance of menses.

Abdomen - Pain in abdomen when retaining urine.

Eyes - Sudden sparks before the eyes.

Food - Appetite increased or decreased. Ravenous appetite in evening. Appetite decreased, thirst increased or vice versa. Desire for salty and pungent foods. Desire for coffee.

Head - Congestive headaches, often one-sided. Pressing sensation in head. Sensation as if head enlarged. Sudden heat in face and head.

Heart - Consciousness of heart. Oppression. Constriction. Stitches in heart. Palpitations. ***Cardiac uremia***. Heart diseases with failure of compensation and impending asystole. Mitral insufficiency. ***Hypertension and oliguria without edema***.

Kidneys - ***Kidney failure.*** Repressed kidney function. Acute nephritis. Uremia. Hematuria, albuminuria and oliguria.

Limbs - Wandering joints pains. Pains wander from fingers to elbows and shoulders. Pains wander from toes to knees and hips. Restless legs, impossible to remain seated, must move.

Modalities - Aversion to warm room. Worse deep inspiration, swallowing, bending head backward. Worse from noises and odors.

Perspiration - Sweat smells sweetish.

Sleep - Dreams of traveling, of black snakes. Erotic dreams of naked women.

Stomach - Eructations better after eating. Nausea concomitant with heart or kidney diseases.

Throat - Dry feeling in pharynx.

Vertigo - Dizziness on rising. Faintness and nausea.

COMMENTS - The serum of the eel has a toxic action on the blood, rapidly destroying its globules. The presence of albumin and kidney elements in the urine, the hemoglobinuria, the prolonged anuria (24 and 26 hours), together with the results of the autopsy, plainly demonstrate its elective action on the kidneys. Secondarily, the liver and the heart are affected and the alteration observed are those usually present in infectious diseases.

Boericke wrote, "When during the course of heart disease, the kidney, previously working well, should suddenly become affected and its function inhibited and when besides we observe cardia irregularities and a marked state of asystole, we may yet expect good results from this serum. But to determine here the choice of this remedy is not an easy matter."

RELATIONS - Vip. ***Compare:*** (1) Dig., Lach., Apis.

REFERENCES - Boericke. Rohrer.

SILICA MARINA

(Sea Sand)

PHARMACY - sil-mar. Silica marina. Sea sand. Silica maritima. Trituration. ***Historical dose:*** All potencies.

CLINICAL - Abscess. Constipation. Glands, enlargement. Glands, suppuration. Gonorrhea. Tartar.

HOMEOPATHIC - W. B. Clarke of Indianapolis told of the use of Sil-mar. as a remedy for constipation. He used it in patients of all ages with excellent results, giving it in crude doses.

W. B. Clarke's preparation was taken from the beach, just as it was left by the tide, on a part of the coast many miles distant from a river estuary or a drained town. He preferred the rather coarse sand taken from a river sand-bar. He thought a finer variety may be better for younger patients.

This was thoroughly washed and baked in an oven. The sand is taken plain or enclosed in capsules or made into pills. In either case it is washed down with water and water is to be drunk freely during the treatment.

Sil-mar. has Sil. and Nat-m. symptoms. ***Inflamed glands*** and suppuration. Constipation.

W. B. Clarke mentioned this case as the hardest he had encountered: a man, 60, had suffered for thirty years with severe constipation often sitting at stool for an hour and nearly fainting. He took a teaspoonful after dinner daily for a week without particular effect.

Then he took it three times a day for a week. After this he was able to return to the one dose a day and soon required it but once a week.

"The peculiarity of this treatment is the ease with which evacuation is accomplished after the first impression is made, the discharges being soft, mushy and yellow and the regular habit then seems established, for the treatment can then be discontinued."

If there is any return of the trouble, a dose or two more will be sufficient to put it right. This experience is of great value and interest as Sil. in the potencies (as well as Nat-m.) is a great constipation remedy. W. B. Clarke never observed any ill effects of the treatment.

In the case of a child, age 4 to whom Cooper gave Sil-mar. 6x "a thick mass of tartar which had accumulated behind the front teeth came away in flakes.

COMMENTS - Clarke had a specimen triturated and run up to the 30c potency. He had not long to wait for an opportunity of testing it. A tall, fair young man of 24, a violinist, presented himself with a mass of scrofulous glands on the right side of the neck softening at one point.

Clarke gave him Sil-mar. 3c, three or four times a day and warned him not to poultice. The mass of glands soon began to diminish. The abscess matured and discharged itself through a minute opening and eventually healed without leaving a perceptible scar. The rest of the glands, in the meantime, disappeared.

Sil-mar. 3c, three times a day, rapidly cured a case of gonorrhea in a patient who had many previous attacks, as well as stricture which had been treated with cauterizations and strong silver nitrate.

It was this history which partly led Clarke to give the remedy on account of the Nat-m. element contained in it. The discharge was creamy and there was tenderness in the middle of the urethra.

For three days after commencing the Sil-mar. there was a sharp aggravation, the discharge became very profuse, was worse at night and accompanied by painful erections.

Burnett told an interesting experience of his in which he was consulted about a boy who persisted in spite of punishment in eating sand when playing on the beach. Burnett advised the parents to let the boy eat as much as he liked. He kept it up for a fortnight, at the end of which time he was vastly improved in health and he neither wanted nor ate any more sand from that day.

REFERENCES - Boericke. Clarke.

SILICA TERRA
(Pure Flint)

PHARMACY - sil. Silica terra. Pure Flint. Silex. Silicic anhydride. Silicon dioxide. Trituration of pure, precipitated silica. ***Historical dose:*** All potencies.

CLINICAL -***Abscess.*** Acne. Anemia. Ankles, weak. Anus, fissures, fistula. Appetite, depraved. Back, weakness. Bedwetting. ***Boils.*** Bones, necrosis. Brain, concussion. Brain-fag. Breast, abscess. Breast-feeding, disorders. ***Bunions. Cachexia.*** Cancer. Carbuncle. Cataract. Cellulitis. ***Cephalohematoma.*** Chin, eruptions. Circulation, poor. Coccyx, pains. Conjunctivitis. ***Constipation.*** Convulsions. Coryza. Cough. ***Cysts.*** Debility. Diabetes. Ear, disorders. Elephantiasis. ***Emaciation. Emphysema.*** Enchondroma. Epilepsy. Eruptions. Excrescences. Eyes, disorders. Feet, burning. Fester. Fibroma. Fistula. ***Foot sweat, suppressed. Foreign bodies.*** Fractures. Ganglion. Gastric, catarrh. Glandular, swellings. Headaches. Hernia. Hip joint, disease. Homesickness. Housemaid's, knee. Hydrocele. Hypopion. Iritis. Jaw, bone, decay. ***Keloids.*** Keratitis. Kyphosis. Lachrymal, fistula. Locomotor ataxia. ***Malnutrition.*** Mania. Ménière's disease. Meningitis. Metritis. Metrorrhagia. Migraines. Miner's, disease. Miscarriage. Molluscum, contagiosum. Morphinism. Morvan's disease. ***Nails, problems.*** Nails, splitting. Necrosis. Neuralgias. Nodes. Panaritium. ***Perspiration, offensive.*** Phimosis. Pleurisy. Potts' disease. Psoas, abscess. Pyorrhea. Rheumatism, chronic. Rickets. ***Scars.*** Sinuses. Sleepwalking. Spermatorrhea. Spina bifida. ***Spinal, curvature.*** Spinal, irritation. Strains. Strangury. ***Styes. Suppurations.*** Synovitis. Teeth, decay. Tenesmus. ***Tumors.*** Ulcers. Urethra, stricture. Urethritis. Urine, incontinence. ***Vaccination, effects.*** Vagina, spasms. Vertigo.

Walking, late. Whitlow. Worms. Writer's cramp. Wounds.

HOMEOPATHIC - Outside homeopathy, flint is practically unknown as an internal remedy. Hahnemann introduced it into medicine and it was his method of attenuating insoluble substances that enabled him to discover its powers. Sil. forms one of the most important remedies for chronic diseases.

Want of grit, moral or physical. Proud flesh. Prostration of mind and body. ***Tendency to easy exhaustion*** and abnormal sweats. ***Defective nutrition*** due to imperfect assimilation, especially in children. ***Emaciation. Arrested development.***

Enlarged glands. Slow, incomplete inflammation of glands, cellular tissue and skin, then induration. Edema in morning. Cancer. Contracted sphincters. Cerebral softening. Diseases of bones and cartilages, decay and necrosis, softening of bones. Exostosis.

Skin is unhealthy, every injury festers. ***Suppurative processes***, stubborn, fistulous openings, abscesses. Pustulous burrowings. Ripens abscesses, promotes suppuration. Ailments attended with ***pus formation***. Discharges offensive, pus, sweat, stools etc.

Sil. can stimulate the organism to reabsorb fibrotic conditions and scar-tissue. Scars indurated, hard, nodular, shiny, glassy, tender with shooting pain. ***Keloid*** growth. J. Weir noted that it must be used with care in cases of tuberculosis as it may cause the absorption of scar tissue and liberate the disease. ***Removes foreign bodies.***

Neurasthenic states with increased susceptibility to nervous stimuli and exaggerated reflexes. Epilepsy, aura in the solar plexus creeping into the chest and stomach. Convulsions begin in the solar plexus, after vaccination. Feeling of coldness before spasms or epileptic attacks.

Spinal curvature. Nervous disorders after spinal injury, especially when pressure on spine causes pain in remote parts. Hysteria, paralysis and obstinate neuralgias caused by dissipation, hard work with close confinement. Progressive locomotor ataxia.

Organic changes, it is deep and slow in action. Periodical states. Ascending effects. Pains are violent and sticking, localized in ears, throat, ulcers etc. Parts lain on to go to sleep. Sensation as if she were divided into halves and left side does not belong to her. Sensation of a hair on tongue, in trachea.

Generally cold, chilly, hugs the fire, wants plenty warm clothing, hates drafts, hands and feet cold, worse in winter. ***Want of vital heat*** even when exercising. ***Intolerance of alcoholic stimulants***. Sensitive to pain, noise, starts at least noise. Restless, fidgety.

Ill effects of vaccination. Scrofulous, rickety children with large heads, open fontanelles and sutures, distended hot and hard abdomen, slow in walking and wasted in body, especially legs. Children crawl nervously or are dragged in on their mother's arms, on running they become pale. Cachectic and senile patients, persons of fair, clear complexion.

MIND - Complaints from anticipation. ***Faint hearted, anxious***. Nervous and excitable. ***Loss of self-confidence.*** Anticipates failure. Performance anxiety. Fear of speaking in front of a group (Arg-n., Gel., Lyc., Nat-m.). ***Timidity about appearing in public.*** Irresolution. ***Bashful.*** Worries about their mind and its ability to perform. Undertakes nothing lest he fail.

Mental acuteness with physical weakness and torpidity. Cannot express himself correctly. Mental confusion. Abstracted. ***Conscience about trifles.*** Fastidious for details. Inconstancy. Forgetfulness better after eating. Restlessness while sitting, on waking.

Procrastinates, dread at any mental effort. Intellect lacks stability and clarity. Poor concentration, inability to focus, poor memory. Brain-fag of businessmen, lawyers, preachers and students. Brain exhaustion (Sulph., Cann., Arg-n., Lyc., Pic-ac.). Fear of literary work. Prostration of mind after writing.

Can overexert their minds. Avoid things that take away their energy. Tendency to monitor energy function. Afraid of draining activities. Anxiety about health, worse during menopause.

Fear of injury. Fear of becoming weak. Fear of being incapable.

Sensitive to all impressions. Starts from slight noise. ***Timidity.*** Fidgety. Sensitive weeping mood. Cries when spoken to kindly. ***Yielding disposition.*** Lacks courage. Homesickness. Longing for his relations and home. Obstinate, stubborn, headstrong, in children. Mental dullness in children.

Hopeless. Sad. Sullen. Disgust for life, wishes to drown herself. Melancholy and weariness of life during menses. Worse from mental exertion, talking, nervous excitement.

Mild and yielding when calm but irritable and irascible when aroused. Intolerant of contradiction. Indisposed to talk loud. Screaming violently, groaning, in epilepsy. Fixed ideas. ***Fear of needles, pins and sharp objects.*** Thinks only of pins, searches for them, and counts them. Somnambulism during increase of moon.

Abdomen - Hard, bloated. Distended, hard and hot, with thin legs, especially in children. Abdomen feels thick and heavy like a weight. Clothing across abdomen feels too tight, after eating. Tightness transversely across abdomen. Pain or painful cold feeling in abdomen, better external heat. Soreness of abdominal walls. Cracks on abdominal wall. Much rumbling in bowels. Flatulence with much rumbling. Ascites with great effusion, with frequent attacks of watery diarrhea. Flatulence incarcerated with constipation. Colic, cutting pain with constipation. Colic from worms. Inguinal glands swollen and painful. Inguinal hernia.

Back - Constant aching in center of spine. Spinal irritation after injuries to spine. Spine, weak, very sensitive to drafts on back. Spina bifida. ***Spinal curvature.*** Painful kyphosis. Pott's disease. Decay of vertebrae. Diseases of bones of spine. Backache as from riding in carriages for a long time. Burning in back, when body is being heated, after walking in open air. Rheumatism. Aching, beating, throbbing, in lumbosacral region. Coccyx hurts after riding. Painful coccyx. Lameness in region of sacrum. Stiff neck with headache. Hard, cold swelling of cervical glands. Boils or carbuncles.

Bladder - Pressure in bladder during urination. Burning and soreness in urethra during urination. Frequent urination with tenesmus. Chronic urethritis, foul discharge from urethra, thick, curdy, purulent, bloody. Chronic urethritis with twisting pain. Continuous urging with scanty discharge, or without emission. Renal and vesical calculi. Involuntary urination. Nocturnal bedwetting in children with worms.

Breasts - Milk suppressed. Sharp pain in breasts and uterus. Breasts swollen, hard and painful. Great itching of swollen breasts. Scirrhus with itching. Darting, burning, in left nipple. Nipples very sore, ulcerated easily. Nipples drawn in like a funnel. Fistula in breasts. Fistulous ulcers of breast (Phos.). Threatened abscess of breast. Hard lumps in breast (Con.). Breast cancer.

Causations - Ill effects of ***suppressed sweat, especially of feet***. Stone-cutting. Loss of fluids. Injury, strains. ***Vaccinations***. Splinters, foreign objects in tissue. Overwork, mental or physical.

Chest - General sensation of weakness in chest, can hardly speak (Stann.). Can't breathe deeply without chest pain. Sticking pain in chest on inspiration. Bruised pain in chest on coughing. Stitches in chest, through the back. Painless throbbing in sternum. Tight feeling around chest, as if tied in with tape. Pressure at lower sternum as from a stone. Eruption like varicella, covering chest and itching violently. Axillary glands swollen, enlarged. Offensive axillary sweat.

Constitutions - Demineralized constitution. Constitutions that suffer from deficient nutrition due to lack of assimilating power, oversensitive physically and mentally. Children with large heads, open fontanelles and sutures, much sweating about the head, which must be kept warm. Distended abdomen, weak ankles, slow in learning to walk. Nervous, irritable persons with dry skin, profuse saliva, diarrhea, and night sweats. Weakly persons, fine skin, pale face, light complexion, lax muscles. Scrofulous children who have worm diseases during dentition. Stonecutters' ailments, chest disorders and total loss of strength.

Cough - Cough and sore throat. Cough with expectoration in day, bloody or purulent. Loose cough day and night. ***Violent cough when lying down with a thick, yellow lumpy expectoration***, suppurative stage of expectoration (Bals-p.). Cough gagging, shaking, retching, worse cold drinks, talking, lying and after waking. Dry cough at night, waking patient from sleep. Dry, hacking cough with hoarseness.

Ears - Earaches. Abscess. Boils. ***Otorrhea, fetid discharge.*** Crusty formations in ears. ***Perforated eardrum.*** Itching in ears when swallowing. Itching of outer ears. Shooting pain in left ear. Feeling of stoppage in the ear, better when yawning or swallowing. Decay of mastoid process. Child bores into its ears with fingers when asleep, causing a discharge of pus and blood. Sensitive to noise. Ménière's disease. ***Hissing, roaring in ears***. Hissing in perforated ear. Ringing in the ears or loss of hearing. Loud pistol-like report. Deafness, hears again with a loud report or on blowing the nose and coughing, worse full moon.

Eyes - Eyestrain and headaches. Keratitis, pustular, perforating. Iritis and iridochoroiditis with pus in anterior chamber. ***Perforating or sloughing ulcer of cornea.*** Abscess in cornea after traumatic injury. Opacities of the cornea after smallpox. Cataracts and weak vision, from over use. Cataract in office workers after suppressed foot sweat. Inflammation of eyes. Sharp pain through eyes. Eyes tender to touch, worse when closed. ***Swelling of lachrymal duct***. Stricture of lachrymal duct. Hypopyon. Angles of eyes affected. Affections of canthi, tear-ducts. ***Styes***. Encysted tumors of lids. Aversion to light, especially daylight, it produces dazzling. Amblyopia from abuse of stimulants.

Face - Pale, cachectic, waxy. Red spots on cheeks with burning heat. Lupus. Burning about mouth. Skin of face cracks. Cracks in lips, on skin of face. Indurated fissures at the corners of lips. Cancer of lower lip. Comedones. Eruptions on chin. Herpes on chin. Rheumatic pain in jaw and decayed teeth. Swelling of jaw. Swelling of maxillary glands. ***Parotid glands swollen*** (Bell., Rhus-t., Calc.), enlarged. Facial neuralgia, throbbing, tearing, face red, worse cold damp. Boring, tearing pains.

Female - Amenorrhea. Watery discharge instead of menses. Early, scanty menses. Increased menses with paroxysms of ***icy coldness over whole body***. Menses strong-smelling, acrid. Discharge of blood between menstrual periods. Discharge of blood from vagina every time child is nursed. Leucorrhea milky (Calc., Puls., Sep.). Leucorrhea acrid gushing, worse during urination. Burning and soreness about vulva. Cutting pain around the navel with leucorrhea. Cutting upward in vagina, worse urinating. ***Vaginal cysts*** (Lyc., Puls., Rhod.). Abscess of labia. Itching of vulva and vagina, very sensitive. Pressing-down feeling in vagina. Prolapsus uteri in consequence of myelitis. Salpingitis with accumulation of pus or serum that escapes from uterus from time to time. Nausea during sex. Nymphomania. Sterility. Miscarriage or no conception due to weakness. Too violent motion of fetus. After-pains felt in hips. Promotes expulsion of moles.

Food - Want of appetite, thirst excessive. Loss of appetite and of taste. Voracious appetite, but disappears on attempting to eat or loathing of food. ***Desires only cold things,*** ice cream, ice water, feels comfortable when it is in stomach. Aversion to cooked or warm food and meat. ***Disgust for meat and warm food, milk.*** Pain in head better while eating. Worse after eating. Aversion to mother's milk, child vomits as soon as it nurses. Milk, aggravates, causes diarrhea and vomiting. Drinking cold water causes dry cough. Warm drinks improves cough, causes sweat about head and face. Water tastes badly. Intolerance of alcoholic stimulants.

Head - Chronic, periodical headaches since some severe disease. Migraines. ***Headaches located over one eye***. Headache as if vertex will burst. Vertex throbs. ***Sick headaches*** as if coming from spine or occiput. Headache, then blindness. Headache while fasting or when not eating at proper time. Headache worse by exertion, study noise, motion, jar, light, cold air, talking and straining at stools. Headache better by wrapping warmly, binding and pressure. Profuse urination, relieves the headache. Swelling filled with grumous fluid between scalp and bone. ***Must keep head covered or catches a cold.*** Lumps on scalp. ***Profuse sweats on head.*** Moist crusty eruptions on the scalp. ***Premature falling of hair, baldness.*** Swelling of glabella. ***Cephalohematoma.*** Fontanelles open with distended abdomen.

Heart - Circulation easily agitated. Heart troubles from nervous exhaustion. Throbbing all over the body, when sitting or while in motion. Palpitations while sitting, with trembling of hand. Violent hammering palpitation, after every quick or violent motion. Orgasm of blood at night, throbbing in all vessels. Pulse small, hard, rapid. Pulse irregular and then slow. Pulse imperceptible.

Kidneys - Chronic urethritis, foul discharge from urethra, thick, curdy, purulent, bloody. Frequent urination with tenesmus. Profuse urination, better headache. Urine is bloody, with red or yellow sediment. Pus in urine. Kidney and bladder stones. Nightly incontinence after a blow upon the head. Nocturnal bedwetting in children from worms.

Limbs - Pott's disease. Psoas abscess. Felons, deep-seated pain. Axillary glands swollen, enlarged. Ulcers around the joints. Sciatica, pains through the hips, legs and feet. ***The parts lain on go to sleep.*** Limbs distorted during convulsion. Slovenly gait. Legs feel paralyzed, trembling while walking. Loss of power in legs. Pain in knee, as if tightly bound. Calves tense and contacted. Cramp in calves and soles. Weak ankles and feet. ***Icy cold and sweaty feet.*** Voluptuous tingling in soles. ***Soreness in feet from instep through to the sole*** (Ruta.). Pain beneath toes. Bunions. Soft corns in between toes. Distorted ingrown, yellow nails. ***Affections of fingernails***, especially if white spots on nails. Nails, splitting. Nails, rough, yellow, crippled, brittle, white spots, blue in fever. Fingertips, as if suppurating, painful, dry, at night. Tremulous hands when using them. Paralytic weakness of forearm. Panaritium. Arms (left) shake before epilepsy.

Liver - Throbbing ulcerative pain in the region of liver. Abscess of liver. Beating soreness in liver, worse motion, walking, lying on right side.

Lungs - Weak lungs. ***Shortness of breath***, from manual labor, walking fast. Deep sighing. Dyspnea when lying on back, when stooping, running, coughing. Dyspnea from draft on neck. Breathing so difficult that eyes seemed to protrude. Neglected pneumonia. Pneumonia resulting in suppuration. Slow recovery after pneumonia. ***Emphysema.*** Emphysema after pleurisy. Stone-cutter's disorders. ***Miner's disease.*** Sycotic asthma worse lying down. Asthma with spasm of larynx. Hay asthma coming on about the last of August. Asthma, can't bear a draft of air on back of neck. Chronic colds that settle in chest and bring on asthmatic attacks after being overheated or exertion. Colds fail to yield, sputum persistently muco-purulent and profuse. Rattling in chest. Profuse foul, yellow, lumpy sputum, granular, offensive when broken.

Male - Burning and soreness of genitals. Squeezing pain in testes. Sharp pricking pain in penis. Itching moist spots on scrotum. Elephantiasis of scrotum. Hydrocele. Painful eruptions in pubic region. Chronic urethritis with twisting pain. Prostate gland enlarged. Discharge of prostatic fluid when straining at stool. Burning in prepuce after stool. Sexual desire increases or decreases. Sexual weakness, nocturnal emissions. ***Extreme exhaustion after sex,*** takes 8 to 10 days to recover. ***Worse after sex***, sensation on right side of head as if paralyzed. Chronic gonorrhea with thick, foul, urethral discharge.

Modalities - ***Better warmth***, warm room, warm wraps, especially around head. Better summer, wet or humid weather. Better from profuse urination. Better magnetism and electricity. Worse from change of weather. ***Worse cold, air, drafts,*** damp. Worse lying down, lying on left side. Worse uncovering, bathing, washing during menses. Worse jarring of spine, touch, pressure. Worse combing hair. Worse mental exertion, talking, nervous excitement. Worse light, noise. Worse alcohol. ***Worse suppressed perspiration, especially of feet.*** Worse from moon changes, new moon, increasing moon and full moon. Worse night, in morning. ***Worse from vaccinations.***

Mouth - Saliva runs out of mouth. Inflammation and suppuration of salivary glands. Offensive odor from mouth in morning. Water tastes badly, vomits after drinking. Dryness of mouth. ***Sores in mouth.*** Sore mouth, gangrenous with perforating ulcer of palate. Abscess at the root of the teeth. Pyorrhea. ***Boils on gums*** (Merc-c.). Gums sensitive to cold air. Sensitive to cold water.

Nose - Obstinate colds, with ear affections. Sinusitis. Chronic catarrh and coryza. Coryza with nosebleed. Frothy nasal discharge. Acrid, excoriating discharge. Sneezing in morning. Obstructed and loss of smell. Burning, shooting pain. Drawing pain in root of nose and right malar bone. Nose, dry, cold. Sore, sensitive nasal bones. Itching at tip of nose. Herpetic eruption around nostrils and lips. Ulcers high up in nose. Cracks in nostrils. Perforation of septum. Dry, hard crusts form, ***bleeding when loosened***. Nosebleed in infants. Dryness and stoppage after suppressed foot sweat.

Perspiration - Debilitating at night. Profuse sweats at night, worse towards morning. Foul, acrid sweat, as soon as he falls asleep. Sweats on upper part of the body, head or affected parts. Wetting pillow. ***Offensive sweat,*** hand and axilla. ***Profuse sweat of head*** offensive and extends to neck. ***Offensive sweat on feet***, itching, acrid, destroying shoes, suppressed. Warm sweat after epilepsy. Sweats from least exertion. Sour and offensive sweats.

Rectum - Feels as if rectum is paralyzed. Constant but ineffectual desire for stool. Straining with soft stools, with exhaustion. Great straining, rectum stings, closes upon stool. Feces remain a long time in rectum. Itching in rectum and anus during stool. Moist anus, foul flatus. Chronic diarrhea. Diarrhea after milk. Diarrhea of cadaverous odor. ***Constipation always before and during menses***. Burning, smarting and pressing in anus, after stool. Pain in anus as if constricted during stool. Painful spasms of sphincter. Cutting, cramping pain in rectum extending to testes, worse sex. ***Fistula in anus*** (Berb., Lach.), alternating with chest symptoms. ***Painful hemorrhoids***, protrude during stool. Sensation as of a heavy lump in anus during menses. Tapeworm.

Sensations - As if she would die. As if beaten all over. As if he had lain in an uncomfortable position. As if gradually losing senses. As if feeling for pins. Sensation as if she were divided into halves and that the left side does not belong to her. As if head would burst with throbbing in it internal and external at same time. As if forehead would be torn asunder, as from a heavy weight over eyes. As if head were forced asunder. As of a splinter in finger. As if a panaritium would form in index finger. As if fingertips were suppurating. As if finger were thick and bone enlarged. As if joints of fingers were being pulled out of sockets. Nails as if decayed.

Skin - Delicate, pale, waxy skin. ***Unhealthy skin, every injury suppurates.*** Rose-colored blotches. Coppery spots. Acne, eruption itches and burns. Acne rosacea. Carbuncles. ***Felons, abscesses, old scars, ulcers.*** Boils and pustules everywhere. Boils come in crops. Long lasting suppuration and fistulous tracts. ***Impetigo.*** Psoriasis inveterata. Herpes zoster. ***Promotes expulsion of foreign bodies from tissues***. Abscesses after vaccination. Acuminate eruptions. Eruptions itch only in daytime and evening. Proud flesh forms in ulcers.

Ulcers, painfully sensitive, foul, spongy, on feet, toes, and nails, better heat. Sensation of coldness in ulcers. Offensive pus. Bursitis. Elephantiasis. Leprous nodes. Indurated tumors. Painless swelling of glands. Large fleshy warts. Warty growths. Gooseflesh. ***Crippled and brittle nails***. Dry, cracked fingertips. ***Keloids.*** Scars suddenly become painful.

Sleep - Sleepiness all day. Great sleepiness after eating, and in evening. Excessive yawning. Sleepy but cannot sleep. Sleeplessness with great orgasm of blood and heat in head. Restless, unrefreshing sleep. Unrefreshed sleep, wishes to remain in bed. Talks in sleep loudly, whines or laughs. Whining and laughing during sleep, loud talking. ***Sleepwalking*** at new and full moon. Frequent starts in sleep. Lascivious dreams. Dreams of his youth, past events. Anxious, frightful dreams, wakes with trembling of the whole body. Nightmares of murders, horrid things, corpses and dead persons. Dreams of some one choking her.

Stomach - Anguish in pit of stomach, with attacks of melancholy. Pit of stomach painful to pressure. Gnawing, twisting pain in epigastrium, worse by pressure. Sensation as if a cold stone were in stomach. Sensation of emptiness in stomach, with nausea. Induration of pylorus. Slow and painful digestion. Griping in stomach after eating. Screwing, pressing, twisting pain in stomach after drinking. Swallowing food easily gets into posterior sinuses. Burning or throbbing in pit. Intense heartburn. Sour belchings after eating (Sep., Calc.). Nausea, with good appetite. Nausea during sex in females. Nausea and vomiting during pregnancy. Vomiting after drinking (Ars., Bism., Verat.). Sour vomiting. Vomiting of food at night. Water brash with chilliness.

Stool - Stools comes out with difficulty ***when partly expelled, recedes again.*** Stools retained for fear of pain. Stools offensive, painless, lienteric, of cadaverous odor. Stool composed of hard lumps, light-colored and very hard.

Teeth - Teeth feel too large and too long for the mouth. Tearing pain at night. Constant aching in all teeth. Teeth break down, lose their enamel, become rough, carious. Stinging toothache, preventing sleep. Toothache during menses. ***Abscess at root of teeth.*** Swelling on gums and roof of mouth after extraction of teeth. ***Pyorrhea*** (Merc-c.). ***Boils on gums*** (Merc-c.). Cold feeling in upper gums. Gums sensitive to cold air and to cold water. Difficult dentition, teething delayed.

Temperature - Chilly, worse lying in bed, exertion. ***Chilliness***, very sensitive to cold air. ***Always chilly,*** even when exercising. Shuddering all over body whole day, before menses. Icy chills. Creeping, shivering over the whole body. ***Suffering parts feel cold.*** Cold limbs, feet, even in a warm room. Hectic fever in debilitated persons, worse after meals. Hectic fever during long suppurative processes. Intermittent fever heat predominating. Spotted fever. Typhoid fever with desire to be magnetized. Fever during dentition.

Throat - Sore throat. Burning in throat. Chronic pharyngitis. Periodical quinsy. Colds settle in throat. Tonsillitis. Tonsils swollen, suppurating. ***Pricking as of a pin in tonsil***. Enlarged thyroid gland. Right lobe of thyroid gland swollen, having the appearance of an elastic cyst. Swallowing is painful, stinging, difficult, hysterical. Sticking pain on swallowing or on touch. Food is ejected through nose, when swallowing. Swelling of larynx. Roughness and soreness in larynx. Tickling in larynx causes slight cough and hoarseness. Foreign bodies in larynx. Hawks foul lumps. Bitter taste. Husky voice, worse mornings with chronic coryza. Hoarseness.

Tongue - ***Sensation of a hair on tongue***. Tongue feels sore. One sided swelling of tongue. Tongue coated with brownish mucus. Indurations in tongue.

Vertigo - Vertigo when closing eyes. Vertigo from excessive use of eyes. Vertigo as if drunk. Vertigo with nausea, sleepiness. Vertigo from looking up, ***when lying on left side*** (Mag-m., Stront.). Vertigo with tendency to fall backward. Vertigo ***better wrapping up warmly,*** must sit down.

Vertigo in neurasthenia and epilepsy. Ménière's disease.

Vision - Vision is confused, letters run together on reading. Spotted vision. Objects appear pale. Objects as if in a fog. Black spots. Day blindness, with sudden appearance of furuncles. Momentary loss of sight. Foggy vision, better wiping eyes. Lightning-like flashes during headache. Dim vision and flickering, worse after headache. Dim vision after suppressed foot sweat.

COMMENTS - Sea sand (Sil-mar.) is mainly composed of silica. The spicules of many sponges are made up of silica. Silicates are taken up by plants and silica is often deposited on the surface or in the interior of their stems. The strength of straw is due to silica. Equisetum generally contains as much as 18 percent silica. Flint supplies the "grit" of the earth's crust, of plant life and to a large extent of animal life also.

Schussler, who was a homeopath before he was a biochemist, noted that silicic acid, from the tissue remedy point of view, is a constituent of the cells of the connective tissue or the epidermis, the hair and the nails.

It may be used if a suppurative center is formed either in the connective tissue or in a portion of the skin. These cells are thereby enabled to throw off inimical substances (the pus). In consequences, the pus is either absorbed by the lymphatics or it is cast out. In the latter case there is a breaking open of the suppurative center. Sil. may also cause an effusion of blood in any tissue to be absorbed through the lymphatics.

Teste put Sil. in his Puls. group of remedies, the other members of it being Calc., Hep., Graph., and Phos. According to Teste, Sil. is the "chronic" of Puls. Sil. corresponds to the chronic form of such diseases as Puls. cures when acute, including rush of blood to the head, especially to the right temple and vertex, headache every day, photophobia, lachrymation, loss of taste, and aversion to fat food with rancid or oily taste in the mouth.

The symptoms of Sil. differ from those of Puls., being more constant, more deep-seated and lasting longer. For instance, the mucus secretions of Puls. easily become purulent under the action of Sil.

Sil. is useful for chronic arthritic or rheumatic affections as it forms a soluble combination (sodium silicate) with the soda of the urate of soda, this combination is then absorbed and removed through the lymphatics. For the same reason it may also be used in kidney gravel.

"Sensitive to noise and anxiety therefrom. Sensitive, weeping mood. Yielding, faint-hearted. Children become obstinate, headstrong, cry when kindly spoken to." "Fixed ideas: the patient thinks only of pins, fears them, searches for them and counts them carefully."

Nice, sensitive, timid and shy (Sil., Phos., Nat-m.). Obstinate, strong will power but lack of energy. Poor confidence (Lyc.), due to lack of strength. Afraid of falling apart. Feeling of fragility. Yielding and mild. Arguing drains them. Irresolution. Lack firmness. Aristocratic, sophisticated. Aggravated by a coarse environment or people. Well behaved because they lack stamina, energy. Overwhelmed and drained from conflicts and confrontations. Startled and upset easily.

Poor stamina, poor endurance, easily exhausted. Brain fag, worse mental or physical exertion. Chronic fatigue. Aversion to exerting themselves. Mental, emotional and physical weakness.

Premature babies with a failure to thrive (Calc-p.). Fontanelles that have slow closures. Slow learning to walk. Delayed development. Weak and malnourished children. Malnutrition. Protein deficiency, mineral imbalances, poor assimilation and poor deposition of minerals. Difficulty breast-feeding, tendency to regurgitate milk and have colic and diarrhea from breast milk (Calc-p.).

Weak muscles and bone structures. Easily injured, weak joints and ligaments, especially when tired. Shin splints, bones don't heal well. Curvature of the spine. Stooped shoulders, generally weak. Brittle nails with white spots. Fragile, brittle hair and nails. Crippled nails, produces inflammation around and under them. "Sensation as if the finger-tips were suppurating."

Unhealthy skin, every little injury ulcerates. Inflammation, swelling and suppuration of all the lymphatic glands and the glands of the skin. Tendency to form scars and keloids. Boils or cysts. Deep scars with unhealthy skin. Matures abscesses and reduces excessive suppuration. For indurations after suppuration, particularly in tonsils which refuse to heal after the pus has been evacuated and in abscesses which leave sinuses and fistula.

Useful to expel foreign objects, especially in the eyes. For splinters under the nails (Hyper.). In the provings, Sil. produced a sensation of a "splinter in the finger," of "a pin in the throat." For foreign bodies embedded in the tissues. Sil. will cause suppuration and expulsion of necrosed tissues caused from embedded objects. Sil. should be used with caution as the expulsion of harmless, encysted objects might risk the patient's life.

For restoring the perspiration of the feet when this has been suppressed, thus it is an indirect remedy in diseases arising in consequence of such suppression (e.g., amblyopia, cataract, paralysis, etc.). In such a case, the meatus is dry and enlarged.

Athlete's foot from suppression of sweat. Heavy foot sweats, foul odor, sweat eats away at their socks. Pungent, penetrating odor, sour, carrion-like. Sweat on hands and feet. The feet may give off an intolerable odor without any sweat. Offensive head sweat. Symptoms are better from sweat.

Keynote sensitiveness. Over-susceptibility to nervous stimuli. The senses are hypersensitive. The surface is tender and the least touch is painful. Brain and spine cannot bear even ordinary vibrations. This condition may be caused by losses of fluids as in spermatorrhea, or by over-worked brain.

Tendency to paralysis. Paralytic weakness from defective nutrition of nerves, brain, and spinal cord. Constipation with paralytic weakness. Epileptic convulsions, starting from the solar plexus, worse at full and new moon, and worse from any overstrain of mind or emotions.

Locomotor ataxia when the fingers feel stiff, with loss of power in them. Spinal irritation. The neck is stiff, causing headache. The small of the back aches as if beaten. The part of the body lain on goes to sleep. Sciatica, numbness and tingling around the legs. Worse lifting and straining. Arthritis, worse cold, damp.

Chronic headaches, which may owe their origin to some severe disease of youth. Headaches ascend from the nape of the neck to the vertex, as if coming from the spine and locate in one eye, especially the right. Headaches worse from draft of air or uncovering head, better pressure and wrapping head up warmly, better profuse urination. Headaches from over study (Calc., Nat-m., Phos., Ign.). Head injuries that lead to exhaustion and convulsions.

Vertigo, ascends from the back of the neck, as if one would fall forward (sometimes backward), worse looking up, closing eyes, lying on left side. Sleepwalking (Puls.).

Asthma, worse change of weather with yellow mucus. Asthma from exertion. Asthma is worse physical exertion, worse change of weather and worse cold, damp. Sinusitis, allergies, from low resistance. Shortness of breath, particularly in the elderly. Emphysema, particularly in those who inhale particulate matter. Problems with changes in altitude.

"Discharge of blood from the vagina every time the child takes the breast." "Nipple is drawn in like a funnel." Cysts and nodules in the breast. Constipation before and during menses. Prostration after sex.

Constipation, difficult stool. As from inactivity of rectum with great straining, as if rectum was paralyzed. Bashful stool, when partly expelled, recedes again. Feces remain a long time in rectum. Cracking and dryness around the anus. Hemorrhoids. Fistulas and fissures, particularly in the anus, rectum and breasts.

Sensitivity to food. Aversion to milk, meat, fatty foods, sometimes sweets. Thirsty for cold drinks but not for ice (Phos. would want ice). Desires eggs, cold food. Aggravated by coffee, alcohol.

Weakness after vaccinations. Worse

since vaccination (Thuj.) or never well since vaccinations. Epilepsy, asthma, headaches, chronic infections, abscesses, lack of stamina, loss of weight, excessive sleep, after vaccinations.

Worse from excessive stress, from pregnancy or surgery. Exhaustion and stress lead to physical ailments. Worse thinking about problems. Sensitive to noise and pain. Want of vital heat, even exercise will not get up any warmth. Heated and chilled easily. Chilly, but worse heat and stuffy rooms. Sensitive to cold, damp and changes of weather. Aggravated from drafts, from getting wet. Sensitive to the moon (Calc.).

Rushmore verified a peculiar symptom of Sil. in a woman suffering from scirrhous of her left breast. She had a feeling of dryness in her fingertips, as if made of paper, at night. Ant-t. and Sil. have this symptom, but only Sil. in afternoon. Sil. removed this and took away sharp, stinging pains in the tumor as well.

Clarke recorded a case of recurrent keloids, "Eleanor W., 14, had a growth on left temple. Five months previous she was an inmate in St. Bartholomew's Hospital and had a tumor removed from the spot, the tumor having existed for two years.

"A month after the operation a new growth appeared on the scar. Two months later this was removed. But it rapidly recurred and when I saw her there was a linear elevation an inch long, three lines wide and raised about two lines. It was red, shiny and slightly modulated, was tender to touch and the seat of shooting pain. Before the first operation there had been no pain and no discoloration of the skin.

"Hahnemann gives this symptom in the proving of Sil. "Stitching, aching pain in the spot where an ulcer had been formerly on the leg." Sil. 3c, night and morning, was prescribed.

"There was no further increase in the size of the growth, though it was still painful, the pain being apparently somewhat increased. In three months there was evident diminution in size and from that time the pain began to diminish. In seven months the growth had entirely disappeared."

RELATIONS - ***Antidoted by:*** Camph., Hell., Fl-ac. ***It antidotes:*** Merc-c., Sulph. ***Compare:*** (1) Gunpowder - abscesses, boils, carbuncles, limb purple. Wounds that refuse to heal, ailments from bad food or water. (2) Hep., Kali-p., Pic-ac., Calc., Phos. (3) Nat-sil. - tumors, hemophilia, arthritis, dose, three drops three times daily in milk. (4) Ferr-cy. - epilepsy, neuroses with irritable weakness and hyper-sensitiveness, especially of a periodical character. (5) Sil-mar. (6) Head-sweat and open fontanelles, Calc. (7) Head must be kept warm, Sanic., Mag-m. (8) Ailments from suppressed foot-sweat, Cup., Graph., Psor. (8) Want of vital heat, Led., Sep. (9) Vertigo as if one would fall forward from looking up, Puls. (10) Chronic sick-headaches since some severe disease of youth, Psor. Headache better pressure and wrapping up warmly, Mag-m., (11) Fistula in ano alternates with chest complaints, Berb., Calc-p. (12) Somnambulism, Luna, Kali-br. (13) Vaccination ill effects, erysipelas, convulsions, diarrhea, Thuj. Apis, Sulph., Maland. (14) Scars, fissure of anus, Graph. ***Complementary:*** Thuj., Sanic., Puls., Fl-ac. Sil. is the chronic of Puls. ***Follows well:*** Bell., Bry., Calc., Calc-p., Cina, Graph., Hep., Ign., Nit-ac., Phos. ***Followed well by:*** Hep., Fl-ac., Lach., Lyc., Sep. ***Incompatible:*** Merc. and Sil. do not follow each other well.

REFERENCES - Boericke. Clarke. Murphy. Phatak.

SILICONE

PHARMACY - silic. Silicone. ***Historical dose:*** All potencies.

CLINICAL - Anemia. Arthritis. Autoimmune, disease. Fatigue. Fibromyalgia. Headaches. Lupus. Lymphadenopathy. Neuropathy. Pericarditis. Pleurisy. Rheumatism. Scleroderma. Sleep disturbance.

HOMEOPATHIC - Autoimmune disease. Chronic rheumatism, producing a painful thickening and contraction of the fibrous structures, interfering with motion and causing deformity. Neuropathy. Diseases involving the cranial or spinal nerves.

Connective tissue diseases. Systemic lupus erythmetosus, polyarteritis, scleroderma. Dermatosclerosis, hide-bound or skin-bound disease. Thickening of the skin caused by swelling and thickening of fibrous tissue, with eventual atrophy of the epidermis.

Rheumatoid arthritis. Inflammation or degeneration of connective tissue, accompanied by deposition of fibrinous material. Collagen disease. Fibromyalgia, aching, soreness, stiffness, with fatigue, sleep disturbance, headaches. Muscular rheumatism.

Diffuse erythematous skin lesions on the face, neck, or upper extremities, with liquefaction degeneration of the basal layer and epidermal atrophy. Lymphadenopathy (enlarged lymph nodes). Pleurisy or pericarditis. Glomerular lesions of the capillaries. Anemia, hyperglobulenemia.

RELATIONS - ***Compare:*** Calc-f., Sep., Sil.

REFERENCES - Murphy.

SILPHIUM LACINIATUM

(Rosin-weed)

PHARMACY - silphu. Silphium laciniatum. Rosin-weed. Rosin-wood. Compass plant. Pilot weed. Polar plant. Turpentine-weed. N. O. Compositae. Tincture of fresh plant. ***Historical dose:*** Tincture and all potencies.

CLINICAL - Asthma. Bladder, catarrh. Bronchitis. Cachexia. Cancer. Dysentery. Influenza. Nausea. Tuberculosis.

HOMEOPATHIC - The leaves of this plant, when they first come up, present their faces uniformly north and south, later on, when the leaves become heavy, the winds carry them in different directions and the polarity is not to be observed. The stem of the plant exudes an abundance of resin, as some of its names indicate.

Cooper used Silphu. in single doses of tincture with notable effect in cases of cancer of the throat and mouth. The great "sensation of emptiness" of the proving shows a relation to the cancer cachexia.

Hale mentioned that Silphu. has been used in all forms of asthma and in chronic bronchitis with large quantities of stringy, frothy, light-colored mucus and in catarrh of the bladder. Catarrhal influenza. Dysentery, attack preceded by constipated stools covered with white mucus.

Chest - Constriction and tightness of chest. Hacking, spasmodic cough.

Kidneys - Frequent urination with sense of heat or burning at meatus during urination. Urine, high-colored, scanty.

Lungs - Constriction of lungs. Catarrh with copious, stringy, mucus discharges. Irritation of posterior sinuses involving mucus membranes of nasal passages with constriction of supra-orbital region. Cough with expectoration, ***profuse***, stringy, frothy, light-colored. Excited by sense of mucus rattling in chest and worse by drafts of air.

Mouth - Tongue, whitish slimy coat, with dry sensation as if burned with hot soup.

Nose - Irritation extends from throat up posterior sinuses to nose causing sneezing, followed by discharge of limpid, acrid mucus. Constriction and pressure in supra-orbital region.

Rectum - Stool natural, but covered with slimy mucus.

Stomach - Nausea, sick, faint feeling and a sense of emptiness in epigastrium.

Throat - Scraping, tickling and irritation of fauces and throat. Desire to hawk and scrape throat and throw off a thin viscid mucus. Engorgement and thickening of mucus membrane of throat extending down.

COMMENTS - Hale gave the case of Mr. H., 55, who had tuberculosis for twenty years. On the slightest exposure or cold he would have congestion of mucus surfaces, followed by copious expectoration of stringy, frothy, light-colored mucus (from one to three pints in twenty-four hours). Rapid exhaustion, at times keeping him in bed for weeks. Silphu. 2x trituration was used, 2 grains every two hours.

During the next night, less than a tea cupful of mucus was raised and its sudden decrease alarmed the patient so much that he left off the remedy until his doctor assured him that he was very much better and that the remedy had been more successful than he himself had expected.

RELATIONS - ***Compare:*** (1) Aral., Cop., Just., Tereb., Cub., Samb. (2) Silpho. - tuberculosis pulmonum with incessant cough, profuse night-sweats, emaciation. (3) Polyg-a. has been found useful in tuberculosis, when given in material doses of the mother tincture, salvia tickling cough. (4) Arum-d. - loose cough at night on lying down. (5) Just. - bronchial catarrh, hoarseness, oversensitive.

REFERENCES - Boericke. Clarke.

SIMARUBA AMARA

(Mountain Damson)

PHARMACY - sima. Simaruba amara. Mountain damson. Simaruba officinalis. Simaruba glauca. N. O. Simarubacae. West Indies and tropical America. Tincture of the dried root-bark. ***Historical dose:*** Tincture and all potencies.

CLINICAL - Diarrhea. Dysentery. Snakebite. Worms.

HERBAL - Simaruba bark is used as a bitter tonic and as a local remedy for dysentery and diarrhea. The part used is the bark, which is really the rind of the root of which, domestically, a decoction is made. "In large doses," said the Treasury of Botany, "it is said to act as an emetic, purgative and diaphoretic."

Simaruba versicolor, a Brazilian species, has similar properties. The fruits and bark are used as anthelmintics, an infusion of the latter is employed in cases of snakebite. The plant is so bitter that insects will not attack it, on which account the powdered root has been used to kill vermin.

Simaruba glauca, a native of Cuba, furnishes a glutinous juice which is employed in certain cases of skin-disease. And it is well to remember that Cedron, which is "Simaba Cedron," belongs to the same order.

COMMENTS - Clarke's first practical acquaintance with Sima. as a homeopathic remedy was in the case of a traveling patient who suffered from a chronic tendency to looseness of the bowels. He had stools like yellow ochre, for which Gamb. had been very helpful.

When in the south of France, he consulted a homeopath who prescribed Sima. with excellent effect. Since then, Clarke used it in similar cases.

H. H. Beamish said that for dysentery the simaruba bark is boiled and, by way of strengthening the astringent effect, Alum is added to the decoction. But Simaruba is the specific agent.

RELATIONS - ***Compare:*** (1) Cedr., Ail., Chap., Quas. (2) Vac., Chin., Rheum. Gamb.

REFERENCES - Clarke.

SINAPIS ALBA

(White Mustard)

PHARMACY - sin-a. Sinapis alba. White mustard. Brassica alba. Senescent. N. O. Cruciferae. Trituration and tincture of the seeds. ***Historical dose:*** Tincture and all potencies.

CLINICAL - Anus, disorders. Backaches. Breast-feeding, disorders. Chills. Colic. Dyspepsia. Esophagus. Flatus. Gastric ulcers. Gastritis. Headaches. Heartburn. Mouth, inflammation. Pregnancy, problems. Salivation. ***Threadworms.*** Vomiting. Worms.

HERBAL - Sin-a., like Sin-n., is indigenous to Great Britain. The Treasury of Botany reported that "Its seeds are larger than those of Black Mustard and of a yellow color externally. Chemically they differ in containing a crystalline substance known as sulpho-sinapisin.

Moreover, its myrosine yields with water a pungent oil of a different character from the Volatile Oil of Mustard. The seed-leaves or cotyledons of Sin-a. furnish the "mustard" of "mustard and cress," the "cress" being Lepidium sativum.

HOMEOPATHIC - Bojanus proved Sin-a., taking substantial doses of the triturated seeds and of a tincture made therefrom.

Under Sin-a. the prover, who had no sign of threadworms since his thirteenth year, passed many both living and dead and had all the usual rectal symptoms which accompany their presence. The urine too, was turbid, as is often the case in helminthiasis.

Marked throat symptoms, especially ***pressure and burning with obstruction in esophagus,*** sensation of a lump in esophagus behind the sternum and with eructations, similar symptoms in rectum.

The well-known emetic effects of mustard were produced by it and also its ***"burning"*** sensations in many parts, notably anus, stomach and esophagus. Flatulence. Headache, (better walking in open air, worse in warm room). Salivation.

MIND - Distracted in mind, while reading must make great efforts to keep thoughts from wandering.

Abdomen - Movements in abdomen. Heaviness as of a weight, fullness and distention in abdomen. Rumbling and gurgling with emission of odorless flatus. Emission of offensive flatus. Griping colic.

Back - Pains in small of back and coccyx, as if sprained and bruised with urging to stool.

Chest - Oppression of chest, compelling frequent deep breathing. Burning beneath sternum.

Eyes - Sudden sensation of warmth with stitching in left eye compelling winking, eye fills with tears, after which the sensation disappears.

Food - Thirst.

Head - Sensation as if head hollow. Rush of blood to head. Headache better in open air worse in warm room. Heaviness in the forehead, as from intoxication or too great warmth of room. Pain in left frontal eminence, paroxysmal, pressive in the evening. Pressive pain in right frontal eminence worse moving head back and forth. Dullness with obscured vision, especially of forehead over eyes, worse walking.

Kidneys - Urine dark yellow, soon forming transparent cloud, bright golden yellow, dark brown like beer. Many grains of red sand deposited and iridescent film on surface. Thick, fatty pellicle. Cloud remains suspended in urine. Sediment white, like chalk and containing grains of white sand.

Limbs - Heaviness in lower limbs.

Male - Emissions without lascivious dreams.

Modalities - Better rest, open air. Worse by touch, pressure, motion, warm room. Crawling in anus worse swallowing. Sensation of hard substance in stomach worse after eating.

Mouth - Root of tongue thickly coated yellow, on rising in morning, later extends along sides, especially left. Profuse salivation with nausea, nausea better at rest, worse walking about. Saliva frothy, salt.

Pulse - Pulse full and hard.

Rectum - Burning, itching in anus, obliging to scratch. Crawling biting in anus. Violent, sudden pain in anus. Spasmodic griping in anus, worse after swallowing anything. Sensation as though a hard substance were lying in anus and could not be evacuated, not better by stool. Stools, black, hard, covered with mucus. Stools, small, thin, soft, greenish, copious, pasty, partly hard partly soft, sour, fermented, yellowish gray. Stools with dead threadworms.

Sensations - As if head hollow. As of a plug in throat of hard substance high up in esophagus under sternum, something hard lying in stomach after a moderate meal, hard substance in rectum not better by stool.

Sleep - Sleeps in afternoon with vivid dreams, after eating. Vivid dreams of dead people and of death. Dreams confused and unremembered of foreign countries and dangerous expeditions.

Stomach - Burning, pressure, fullness and distention in pit of stomach. Thirst without heartburn, drinking water causes sensation of heaviness and fullness in abdomen as after eating. Belchings are tasteless and odorless. Belchings of acid liquid with griping scalding in pharynx, tasting of food. Nausea, qualmishness inclination to vomit, salivation. Nausea better at rest, worse by movement. Retching and vomiting of water. Vomits flakes of mucus with black streaks, yellow, odorless, tasteless matter with much tenacious, jelly-like mucus. After vomiting, scraping in throat and burning rising from stomach.

Temperature - Creeping chills on moving about, over whole body after vomiting with coldness of hands and feet and frequent belchings of gas. Inclined to perspire.

Throat - Scraping in fauces, provoking frequent hawking. Burning in pharynx in esophagus rising up from stomach like heartburn and pressure in esophagus. Sensation of hard body high up in esophagus, worse swallowing hard food and on empty swallowing in afternoon seems as if a plug sticking in pharynx (this sensation alternated with biting and crawling in anus). Sensation of constriction on swallowing hard food. Sensation as if a large morsel of food had been swallowed.

COMMENTS - A. L. Fisher said that for twenty years Sin-a. has had a prominent place in his armamentarium. He used it on the indications of the proving and he found that the states of pregnancy and breast-feeding seem to favor development of the conditions calling for it.

He verified "Excessive accumulation of watery saliva or mucus." "Acute bruised pain, even on slight pressure, just beneath ensiform cartilage." "Vomiting, ejecta consisting of flakes of mucus with black veins like clots of blood." "Crawling and burning in anus with griping in abdomen." "Spasmodic griping in anus, appearing at intervals and especially noticed after swallowing anything."

He cured with Sin-a. "Sore mouth with intensely red mucus membrane, dotted with minute white ulcers, the least food, even of blandest character increasing the burning that is present all the time and also in the throat."

Bojanus noticed an alternation between the symptoms of the anus and those of the pharynx.

Clarke cured with Sin-a. "Sharp, shooting pain in right frontal eminence, worse in warm room, better moving about and in open air."

RELATIONS - An overdose of table mustard, which contains both Sin-a. and Sin-n. with starch is immediately antidoted by smelling bread. ***Compare:*** (1) Sin-n. - plug sensation. (2) Anac. - ball in anus, Sep. lump in stomach. (3) Bry., Abies-n., Nux-v., Puls. (4) Cina, Sant., Teucr., Napht., Scirr., - worms, helminthiasis.

REFERENCES - Clarke.

SINAPIS NIGRA

(Black Mustard)

PHARMACY - sin-n. Sinapis nigra. Black mustard. Brassica nigra. N. O. Cruciferae. Trituration and tincture of seeds. ***Historical dose:*** Tincture and all potencies.

CLINICAL - ***Allergies.*** Amenorrhea. Asthma. Catarrh. Chlorosis. Chordee. Chorea. Colds. Constipation. ***Coryza.*** Coughs. Diarrhea. ***Hay fever.*** Headache. Heartburn. Hemorrhoids. Hiccoughs. Intermittents. Menses, premature. Mucous, fever. ***Pharyngitis***. Post-nasal catarrh. Priapism. Scurvy. Strokes. Variola.

HERBAL - Sin-n. yields the greater part of the condiment so generally used in England. The plant is indigenous, but is nevertheless largely cultivated in Yorkshire and Durham.

Like many other Crucifers, Sin-n. has antiscorbutic properties and it has cured cases of ague, mucus fever, catarrh of bladder of stomach and of air passages. It has been most used in the treatment of hay fever.

Cooper suggested the use of Sin-n. as an aperient. He considered that the chief agent in effecting dislodgement of feces in constipated states is flatus. His method of producing this is as follows:

A tumblerful of hot water is to be taken in sips in the early morning, the same at breakfast time with some plain brown bread or with no solid food at all. At 11 a.m. one or two capsules of pure mustard, each containing about five grains of the powder to be taken, followed by half a tumbler of hot water.

"This last is most important, as the water drives on the capsule and prevents its staying about the cardiac orifice of the stomach and consequent distress to the patient. It also causes contraction of the walls of the stomach and consequent expulsion of flatus into the duodenum."

HOMEOPATHIC - Sin-n. is of use in ***hay fever, coryza and pharyngitis***. Mucus membrane dry and hot, no discharge, worse afternoon and evening, either nostril may be affected alone or they may be affected alternately. Dry sinuses and pharynx with thick, lumpy secretion.

Mucus hawked or coughed from posterior sinuses felt cold. "Sweat on upper lip and forehead." Smallpox.

During the proving, symptoms were noted including "It seemed to double him up, could hardly stand, tears ran from eyes intense pain across epigastric region. Rose late, feeling sore and stiff all over. Weakness in all muscles."

MIND - Mind worked rapidly. Better by study or mental diversion. Irritable, difficult to think and study. Unreasonably cross.

Abdomen - Dull pain in left hypochondriac region. Heavy, dull pain as from weight below umbilical region. Severe twisting in umbilical region. Pain from left of umbilical region to left iliac region, later to right side, ascending colon. Accumulation of flatus with twinges of pain about umbilicus. Rumbling. Left inguinal gland swollen and painful. Sharp pain in right inguinal gland. Dull pain in right inguinal region better by pressure.

Back - Rheumatic pain in intercostal and lumbar muscles, sleeplessness from pain in back and hips. Severe, dull, pulsating pain under inferior angle of left scapula. Slight backache, becoming intolerable towards bedtime, better motion.

Bladder - Pain in bladder. Frequent ***copious*** urine flow day and night. Desire frequent, flow increased. Urine, pale, straw colored without sediment.

Causations - Damp weather, summer.

Chest - Wandering pains in chest. Pain in left side of chest in region of heart. Sensation in right chest as if heart were on right side. Respiration at base of left lung roughened.

Eyes - Eyes feel weak, pressure causes pricking in them. Pressing feeling in eyes.

Face - Shrunken features. Burning prickling in face. ***Sweat on upper lip and forehead***. Lips dry and feel as if tissues were stiff. Red around mouth with smarting of lips. Sensation as if cheek were bulged outward by bubble of air, just below malar bone in afternoon.

Female - Menses appear long before the proper time. Amenorrhea and chlorosis.

Food - Appetite good. All food tastes of horseradish, later tasteless. Aversion to sweets.

Head - Headache over right eye worse stooping. Head dull, heavy, better when mind occupied by study, shutting eyes, in open air, worse in warm room, when thinking of it. Frontal headache, most over bridge of nose and around edge of orbits. Forehead hot and dry. Sensation as if scalp were adherent to bones. Scalp hot and itches.

Heart - Dull, continual pain in heart toward apex in evening, seemingly in heart substance. Heart pains return daily. Sensation as if heart were on right side. Pulse accelerated, full.

Limbs - Dull, heavy ache in legs. Weariness in limbs, with cramps in calves. Weakness in calf-muscles. Constant pain in ankles and calves. Occasional dull pain in left shoulder joint.

Lungs - Allergies. Asphyxia. Pituitous asthma. Asthmatic breathing. Loud coughing-spells with barking expiration. Cough is relieved by lying down. Cough mostly dry or with expectoration of lumps of mucus worse in cold air, better lying down. Expectoration from posterior sinuses much mucus, which felt cold, white in tenacious masses.

Male - Violent erections during day and night, obstinate, painful and continued. Awakening him at night with lascivious thoughts, dreams and emissions at night.

Modalities - Better by study or mental diversion. Better sitting erect, shutting eyes. Better hearty meal. Better lying down at night, except dreams. Worse by touch and pressure. Worse motion, leaning forward, stooping. Worse thinking of symptoms. Worse warm room, July, August, damp weather. Worse evening, 4 p.m. to 6 p.m., 7 p.m. to 9 p.m. Laughing causes cough.

Mouth - ***Offensive breath***, smelling like onions (Asaf., Coch.). Taste of garlic, causing nausea of horseradish. Profuse saliva. Dry, burning, extending to stomach. Tongue feels blistered. Black tongue. Tongue fissured in middle, dirty white coat, sore, raw. Teeth sensitive to warm drinks and cold air, especially stopped teeth. Swollen bleeding gums.

Nose - *Severe colds. Allergies. Hay fever.* Mucus from posterior sinuses. Scanty, *acrid* discharges, making skin smart. ***Stoppage of left nostril all day*** or in afternoon and evening. ***Nostrils alternately stopped.*** Dry, hot with lachrymation, sneezing, hacking cough, better lying down. Dryness in both nostrils. Scurvy with copious and frequent nosebleed.

Rectum - Before stool uneasy feeling in rectum after stool, smarting cutting low down in rectum and anus. Desire for a stool without passage. Constipated, stools hard like balls. Diarrhea. First stool normal, second loose. Stools offensive. Smarting, cutting pain low down in anus after a stool.

Sensations - Vertex as if empty. As if she had taken cold. As if scalp was adherent to bones. As of pins sticking in eyeballs. Eyeballs as if pressed on from above. As if nostrils stopped up. As if movements impeded all around the chest. As if something heavy oppressed her on all sides from neck to diaphragm. As if cheeks were bulged out by a bubble of air below malar bone. Skin of lips as if stiff. As if blisters on tip of tongue. As if a load on stomach. Pain as if heart were on right side. As of hot water in blood vessels.

Skin - Burning heat and stitches in skin. Skin turns red. Ecchymosis. Chronic eczema. Smallpox. Ulcers on legs. Frightful suppuration and gangrenous inflammation reaching down to sternum (fatal effects of mustard applied to swollen glands of neck).

Sleep - Sleepiness during day, sleepless at night. Sleeps little at night, but does not feel loss of sleep. Restless sleep from pains in back and hips. Vivid or lascivious dreams.

Stomach - Burning in stomach, extending up esophagus, throat and mouth, which is full of canker sores. Ulceration of stomach and intestines. Pressure in epigastric region. Pain in region of stomach with sensation of faintness compelling to bend forward, which relieves. Hiccough. Heartburn and belching. Hot sour belchings. ***Colic, pains come on while bent forward, better sitting up straight.*** Sweat relieves when nausea comes on.

Temperature - Severe chills, chattering of teeth, sensation of general coldness with shrunken feeling (from mustard bath). Heat through whole body, especially down spine. Quartan ague and inflammatory fever. Sweat and feeling of hot water in all blood vessels, better when menses came on. Sweat general, especially on forehead and upper lip. Sweat free from mental or physical exertion, from external heat.

Throat - Hoarseness, evening from 4 p.m. Feels scalded, hot inflamed. Dry sensation back of nose and throat. Throat sore, left side, on swallowing saliva. Whole throat behind uvula injected light red. Sore throat right side extending to left.

Vertigo - Vertigo of old people, violent attacks with hard hearing after eating heavy food, fat.

COMMENTS - Hansen added "Acute coryza with thin, watery, excoriating discharge, lachrymation, sneezing. Hacking coughs, better from lying down. Acute pharyngitis, throat feels scalded, hot inflamed. Loud coughing spells with barking expiration, heard at a great distance."

RELATIONS - ***Antidoted by:*** Smelling bread (immediate effects of taking excess of condiment): Nux-v., Rhus-t., or when blistering has been produced by a mustard poultice, soap is the remedy. ***Compare:*** (1) Sin-a., Thiosin., Coch. (2) Scalded sensation on tongue, Sang. (3) Cough worse laughing, Arg-n., Phos. (4) Cough, better lying down, Ferr., Mang. (5) Worse from 4 p.m. to 6 p.m., Lyc. (6) Amenorrhea, Sulph., Puls. (7) As if hot water in blood vessels (Rhus-t. as if blood running cold). (8) Sulph., Caps., Coloc. (9) Sin-a.. (10) Mustard oil by inhalation - acts on the sensory nerve endings of the trigeminal. Relieves pain in middle ear disease and in painful conditions of nose, nasal cavities and tonsils.

REFERENCES - Boericke. Clarke.

SIUM LATIFOLIUM

(Water Parsnip)

PHARMACY - sium. Sium latifolium. Water parsnip. N. O. Umbelliferae. Tincture of root. ***Historical dose:*** Tincture and all potencies.

CLINICAL - Convulsions. Dizziness. Opisthotonos. Spasms. Tetanus.

HOMEOPATHIC - Knowledge of water parsnip is derived from cases of poisoning through eating the root. The Sium. symptoms bear a strong resemblance to those of the other poisonous Umbelliferae.

The most pronounced features of the convulsions were the drawing of the arms to the middle of the body, flexure of the fingers and the preponderance of the contractions on the left side.

Opisthotonos. Spasms, at first violently clonic, diminishing with each succeeding convulsion until they became little more than tremors. Loss of voluntary motion. Lack of mental energy (Aeth.).

MIND - Mentally excited. Lack of mental activity. Fear of death.

Abdomen - Sense of swelling and flatulence about bowels.

Eyes - Pupils dilated, responded steadily to bright light.

Head - Dizziness, headache.

Lungs - Breathing slow and stertorous.

Stomach - Nausea and vomiting, followed by a convulsion.

Temperature - Skin cold and clammy. Head hot, rest of body cold. Wet with perspiration.

Throat - Burning along digestive tract, especially esophagus.

REFERENCES - Clarke.

SISYRINCHIUM GLAXOIDES

(Blue-eyed Grass)

PHARMACY - sisy. Sisyrinchium glaxoides. Blue-eyed grass. N. O. Iridaceae. The fresh root is macerated in twice its weight of alcohol. ***Historical dose:*** Tincture and all potencies.

CLINICAL - Coma. Delirium. Snakebites. Wounds.

HERBAL - Sisyrinchium was one of the old "Thompsonian remedies." Dr. W. U. Reed of Indiana contributed the following in 1892 to the Hom. Recorder, concerning this little known remedy.

"The roots of Sisyrinchium are used in the treatment of snake bites. A tincture is made from the roots, it is said to have been used by the Indians in treating snake bites, by bruising and moistening the roots and applying to the wound."

The symptoms of the snake bites cured with Sisy. are bluish black colored skin, as if dreadfully bruised. The whole body becomes very red, hot and dry, face dark red. The leg and foot are enormously swollen and of the same general appearance. The foot, calf of the leg and thigh turn black. Patient delirious but would cry out if touched. Wild delirium all night. Unconscious. Pulse quick and hard.

COMMENTS - Dr. W. U. Reed stated "We have growing in our woods and fields a small plant, which I believe to be a specific for the treatment of persons or animals bitten by the rattlesnake. From my own experience and observation in the use of this remedy, I believe it to be a positive cure in all cases if exhibited in any reasonable time.

"I have never known it to fail in a single instance, even where the alcoholic treatment and many other kinds had failed. I am not aware of its ever having been used as a medicine by the profession and, so far as I know, I am the first to prepare and use it in the form of a tincture."

Dr. Reed gave these cases: "(1) Bessie A., aged six years, while playing in the yard on a farm, some twelve miles in the country, was bitten in the hand by a rattlesnake which was killed a moment after by the mother of the little girl who was attracted by the screams of the child.

"Sixteen hours after I arrived, everything having been done in the meantime that had ever been heard of by the parents, even to applying a poultice the wound with entrails of a black chicken.

"The little sufferer was indeed, an object of pity. The hand and arm were swollen almost to bursting, the swelling extending to the shoulder and spine, being of a blush black color as if dreadfully bruised. This discoloration extended over the back to the hips. Skin hot and dry, face flushed, pulse quick and hard. Child unconscious.

"I felt that the case was hopeless. But, through the earnest entreaties of the mother, I proceeded to do what I could. Saturating a piece of cotton with the tincture I had prepared, I bound it on the wound, then dropping twelve drops in a glass of water I directed that a teaspoonful be given every hour, the compress to be renewed every hour also, until my return.

"I confess I had little hope of seeing my little patient alive again but on my return the following day I was much rejoiced to find a decided change for the better in the condition of the little sufferer. The swelling was not nearly so tense, the fever had subsided, the delirium gone and the danger seemed past. The treatment was continued and a speedy and permanent recovery followed.

"(2) Burt Whitten, aged ten, while out in a marsh with a number of older boys gathering huckleberries, was bitten in the right ankle by a rattler. He was so frightened when he saw the snake, as it bit him, that he ran all the way home, a distance of nearly a mile, although the day was very hot.

"This patient came to my hands after the usual alcoholic treatment for twenty four hours by an allopathic physician with the patient growing worse all the time. I found this patient in about the same condition as the first.

"The leg and foot were enormously swollen and of the same general appearance, the foot, calf of the leg and thigh were black, the whole body was very red, hot and dry, face dark red, pulse quick and hard, patient delirious but would cry out if touched.

"Fifteen drops in a glass of water. Teaspoonful every hour with cotton saturated with the tincture applied to the wound. In this case the change, I was informed by the father, was quite noticeable in two hours.

"The boy had been in a wild delirium all night and up to the time he received the first dose of Sisy. After the second dose he became quiet and in two hours the delirium had passed away. Under this treatment the patient was able to be out on the streets again in four days, though the discoloration did not disappear for some time after.

"Many more cases might be given where this remedy has been given to both man and beast with the same results."

REFERENCES - Anshutz.

SKATOLUM

(Skatol)

PHARMACY - skat. Skatolum. Skatol. Methyl-indol. Minerals, carbon compounds. ***Historical dose:*** All potencies.

CLINICAL - Acne. ***Belching.*** Dyspepsia. Headaches.

HOMEOPATHIC - Skatol represents the ultimate end of protein decomposition and is a constituent of human feces. Sluggishness with no ambition. Acne with auto-intoxication dependent upon intestinal decomposition. Stomach, abdominal symptoms and frontal headache.

MIND - Lack of concentration, impossible to study, ***despondent***. Lack of ambition. Desire to be with people. Irritable. Felt mean towards everyone. Desire to curse and swear.

Food - Appetite increased.

Head - Frontal headache, worse over left eye in the evening, ***better by short step***.

Kidneys - Frequent, scanty, burning, difficult.

Mouth - Tongue coated. ***Foul taste***. Salty taste to all cereals.

Sleep - Increased desire to sleep, wakes unrefreshed, half doped feeling.

Stomach - ***Belching***.

Stool - Light, yellow, narrow, ***very offensive stool***. Intestinal dyspepsia.

RELATIONS - ***Compare:*** (1) Indol., Bapt., Sulph.

REFERENCES - Boericke.

SKOOKUM CHUCK AQUA

(Mineral Springs)

PHARMACY - skook. Skookum chuck aqua. Mineral springs. Skookum limechen chuck. Medical lake. Strong Medicine Water. Salts of water from Medical Lake near Spokane, Wash. A lake in Western USA containing in grains per gallon: sodic carbonate 63.54, sodic chloride 16.37, sodic silicate 10.63, potassic chloride 9.24, ferrous carbonate. 526, Mag-c. 237, Calc. 186, aluminic oxide. 175 with traces of lithic carbonate, Bor. and potassic sulphate. Trituration of the dried salt. ***Historical dose:*** Tincture and all potencies, third trituration.

CLINICAL - Allergies. Breast, tumor. ***Catarrh.*** Coryza. ***Eczema. Hay fever***. Lithemia. Otitis media. Ozaena. Rheumatism. ***Skin, disorders.*** Urticaria. Vaccination, effects.

HOMEOPATHIC - The medical and curative properties of this remarkable lake were known to the Native Americans of the northwest; they have many legends and tribal history concerning the lake, and it was held in much reverence by them.

The country around this lake was called "Sahala Lyee Illihe," or "Sacred Grounds," and no matter how hostile the tribes were to each other no members journeying to or from the "Skookum Limechen Chuck," or "strong medicine water," were ever molested.

"In the Skookum Chuck we have a remedy for all our ailments. We only have to bathe in and drink its water and we are made well. If we sign the treaty we will forever offend the Great Spirit, we will sign away our mother and she will cry. Her tears will dry up these lakes and we will be hungry and sick. We will go the Skookum Chuck only to find that its water have disappeared."

It is an anti-psoric remedy. Affinity for the skin and mucus membranes. ***Skin disorders. Eczema.*** Urticaria. Lithemia. Vaccinal eczema. ***Dry skin. Hay fever***. Profuse coryza and constant sneezing. ***Catarrh***. Profuse, ichorous, cadaverously smelling discharge. Otitis media.

Back - Heaviness in sacrum.

Food - Appetite increased.

Limbs - Severe rheumatic pains in limbs.

Nose - Profuse coryza with constant sneezing as in hay fever.

Skin - ***Eczema.*** Urticaria. ***Dry skin.***

COMMENTS - In the U. S. Med. Investigator, 1889, Dr. W. D. Gentry told the story of a Frenchman passing by the lake, before the properties of the water became known to the white men, with a drove of sheep afflicted with a skin disease called "the scab."

As soon as the sheep saw the water they ran to it, but would not drink. They stood in the water for some time, and in a few days they were well of the "scab." The Frenchman was suffering with rheumatism and decided to try the water for his disease. He was steadily cured.

Stories of marvelous cures were reported by the Native Americans and by seeing those who had been taken there on litter, appearing at the point of death, return in health and vigor.

The cure of many cases of inveterate skin disease is on record, the external use of Skook. soap or ointment has been employed as well as the internal administration.

W. D. Ingalls reported the case of Mrs. D., 48, who had eczema of her feet. Fissured skin, exuding an acrid secretion. So excessively sore that the patient had not been able to wear shoes or walk any distance for two years.

Skook. 2x was given internally, an ointment of a drachm to the ounce of vaseline applied and Skookum soap used for washing. In two months the patient was able to wear shoes and in three months the feet were well.

Mrs. H., 23, had a benign growth in left breast, noticed eight months. No history of tuberculosis or cancer in family. Skook. was given for the first week, one grain of 1x every four hours, for the second week, two grains of Skook. 2x every four hours, for the next seven weeks, five-grain powders of Skook. 3x, when the patient was cured.

Mr. J., had chronic nasal catarrh, discharge greenish yellow having odor of ozaena, was greatly relieved and apparently on the way to cure.

B. F. Bailey reported the cure of Mrs.

X., 40 of lithemic diathesis, never free from eczematic trouble for years. At times much rheumatism. Not infrequently the rheumatism disappears and is immediately followed by styes on the eyelids.

Formerly treated allopathically and also homeopathically. Skook. 3x every four hours. Improvement soon showed itself and the patient was well in three months and remained so.

Mrs. Y., 26, lithemic with flushed face and yellowish background. Urine, 1030 and with marked uric acid deposits. Much difficulty of digestion. Great dryness of skin, especially of scalp. Hair falling out to such an extent that baldness was feared.

Skook. 3x was given every four hours. Hair ceased to fall out. The heated, congested feeling of head and face disappeared and the patient became well.

RELATIONS - ***Antidoted by:*** Tab. ***Compare:*** (1) Nat-c., Nat-m. (2) Skin disorders, Graph., Med., Maland., Vac. (3) Saxon. - appears has remarkable cleansing, deodorizing and soothing properties for the skin. Eczema, scalds, burns, sores and hemorrhoids.

REFERENCES - Anshutz. Boericke. Clarke. Phatak.

SLAG

(Pulverized Slag)

PHARMACY - slag. Slag. Pulverized slag. Blast-iron-furnace cinder. Slag silica. Silico-sulphocalcite of alumina. Slag was analyzed and found to contain the following: Silica, Alumina, Calcium, Sulphur, part of these occur as Calc-s., Ferrum, Phosphorus, Magnesium, Manganum. ***Historical dose:*** Tincture and all potencies.

CLINICAL - Constipation. Debility. Diarrhea. Flatulence. Headache. Hemorrhoids. Housemaid's knee. Lumbago. Spleen, disorders. Tuberculosis.

HOMEOPATHIC - Slag was introduced into medicine by J. Meredith who gave the 6x trituration to a patient suffering from housemaid's knee and in addition to relieving this it took away "a dreadful anal itching, hemorrhoids and constipation as if by magic."

Meredith confirmed the rectal power of Slag by experiments on his own person. Acting on Meredith's suggestion, George Herring instituted a proving with the 3x on himself and others.

Herring's only symptom was a creeping irritation of the skin or under the skin in the umbilical region, sufficiently severe to keep him awake.

Drowsiness in evening. Digestive weakness and flatulence. ***Soreness of the anus***. Constipation and diarrhea. Hemorrhoids with anal itching and soreness. Tuberculosis.

Housemaid's knee. Lumbago. Spleen disorders. Spleen pain and stitches in heart. A pain (dull, heavy sensation) alternated between inter-scapular region and spleen. Stiffness at back of head, neck and pain between shoulders. Dull, stupefying frontal headache.

COMMENTS - One prover, in which Slag produced no symptoms, was cured of flatulent distention in the evening and an oppressive feeling over the heart. Another prover had constipation relieved, but Slag produced "soreness of anus."

In a delicate woman of tubercular history, took Slag 3x twice a day, and experienced diarrhea, debility, quick pulse, lumbago with pain in back, distention of stomach, so that she had to loosen her dress, profuse night-sweat, cough and expectoration. Phos., Ph-ac., Carb. v. were given to this patient in succession and all helped.

Another proving of Slag was made by F. C. B. The prover was age 33, rather dark, nervo-bilious, had chronically enlarged tonsils and tendency to colds in the head. He took Slag by way of experiment, hoping to cure his tonsils.

RELATIONS - Effects were relieved by: Phos., Ph-ac., Carb-v. ***Compare:*** (1) Constipation, flatulence, Lyc., Carb-v., Sulph. (2) Anal symptoms, Graph., Nit-ac. (3) Intolerance of tight clothing, Lach. (4) Housemaid's knee, Stict., Apis., Sep.

REFERENCES - Clarke.

SOL

(Sunlight)

PHARMACY - sol. Sol. Sunlight. Lactose is exposed to concentrated sun's rays and stirred with a glass rod until saturated. Potencies made by Fincke. ***Historical dose:*** All potencies.

CLINICAL - Allergies. Backache. Burns. Cancer. Cataracts. ***Chills.*** Constipation. Dermatitis. Faintness. Freckles. ***Headaches.*** Heat, stroke. Lupus. Menses, premature. Paralysis. Photophobia. Radiation, sickness. ***Skin, cancers***. Skin, disorders. Snow-blindness. ***Sunburns.*** Sunstroke.

HOMEOPATHIC - Dr. Finsen, of Copenhagen, revived and confirmed much of the ancient light-therapy. O. V. Thayer published, in 1893, a series of cases in which he had used concentrated rays of sunlight (solar cautery) including cases of skin cancer, rodent ulcer, parasitic diseases, moles, small wens, and birthmarks.

H. T. Webster gave details of a case of epithelioma in which the growth was removed by solar cautery and a scarcely perceptible scar left. Sunlight has cured ***skin cancers*** and lupus in the hands of Finsen.

Potentized sunlight has been used for sun dermatitis, heat stroke, cancer and radiation. Chronic sun headaches (Verat., Glon., Nat-c, Nat-m.). Violent headache from vertex down to forehead with hot sensation in face. Keynote photophobia. Very sensitive to sunshine.

Sunburns easily. ***Never well since severe sunburn.*** Sunlight damage of the eyes, from over-exposure, snow-blindness, sun-blindness. Cataracts. Radiation exposure with nausea, vomiting, hair loss, emaciation (Cadm-s., X-ray.).

Mental excitement and anxiousness, at first with trembling of the heart, finally remaining in the stomach pit. Faintness, prostration and general stiffening up of the whole system, the body strength seems more equalized. Spasm coming with sunrise and ceasing with sunset. Some spasms appearing at sunset.

MIND - ***Decisiveness*** and assertive. Impatient to make decisions. Cheerful. Urge to be healthy, to eat fruit. ***Mental restlessness***. In control, then out of control. Irresolution. Light headed and mentally disorientated. Loses his way in well-known streets.

Depression, tearful. Sensitive. Suspicious. Irritable, impatient and frustrated. Irritability over trifles. Fastidious. Argumentative and angry. Nasty. Desire to bang head and scream. Escapism.

Excitement. Anxiety with trembling in heart. Anxiety in solar plexus. Anxiety if somebody comes towards her. Nervous, as if all the nerves were trembling. Very sensitive and easily frightened. Frightened on the approach of anyone coming toward them. Delusion of being pursued.

Abdomen - Anxiety in solar plexus. Swollen sensation on right side. Distention and hardness. Abdominal cramps with menses. Cramping pain on right side, better bending double. Griping pain, like diarrhea. Foul flatulence. Sensation as after childbirth or at conception (with great excitement).

Back - Backaches. Pain in left side of back, hip joint area. Heat rash, red blobs, on back. Spots on back during menses. Itchiness, worse evening and in bed, better scratching.

Breasts - Tender, swollen breasts, before menses. Sharp pain in left breast.

Chest - Sensation as if a weight on chest. Chest very tight with wheezing. Armpits perspired without exertion. Sharp pain, top of rib cage.

Ears - Sharp shooting pain from left ear to nose, continued at intervals for some time. Partial deafness.

Eyes - ***Painful eyes from glare of sunlight.*** Photophobia. Light offends eyes. Snow-blindness. Diminished sensitivity of eyes, odd-blindness. Blurry vision with headaches. Suffusion of veins, of sclerotica. Cataracts. ***Stinging pains.*** Sensation of swelling, as if eyes would force themselves out of sockets. Puffiness around the eyes.

Face - Jaws rigidly set as in trismus. Painful large spot on cheek. Pressing pain with sensation of heat in face. Perspiration on face, warm and tingly. Hot sweat on face, cold to touch. Dripping perspiration.

Female - Achy and bloated before menses. Diarrhea before menses, on going to bed. Menses six to seven days too soon. Menses, bright red blood. Menses slow, spotting. Very heavy menses, bright red blood, occasional clots, abdominal cramps. Sharp pain in uterus which turned to cramp, worse bending forward. Spots on back during menses. Green leucorrhea at night, with yellow-brown diarrhea. Itching genitalia, some discharge.

Food - Diminished appetite and thirst. Loss of appetite first thing in the morning. Desire for hot chocolate. Desire for juicy, refreshing things, oranges and grapefruit. Desire for cheese and salty foods. Desire for meat, prawns. Thirst, desires cold sweet drinks, lime juice. Thirstless, sips lemon squash, which relieves the throat.

Head - Light headed and mentally disorientated. Violent headache from vertex down to forehead. Headache with the excitement and anxiousness at stomach pit. Left sided headache. Pain in forehead, as if forehead would crush itself down upon the eyes. ***Headache from sunshine on bare head***, better by laying a glass of water on solar plexus. ***Very sensitive to sunshine on the vertex.*** Extreme painfulness if the sunshine strikes the bare head. Violent stitches in brain. Stitching pain if she does not gain the shade, stomachache and nausea follow. Sensation of undulating or floating in head after mental excitement. Instantaneous shock to brain, followed by prostration and a scalding sensation on top of head. Excessive perspiration of head and neck.

Heart - Anxiety with trembling in heart. Weakness about heart.

Kidneys - Increased urine though drinking less, night as well as day. Polyuria, urinates five times in night. Nocturia. Urine and stool invariably suspended.

Limbs - Drawing through all his limbs after rising. Right side, arm and foot, weak as from partial paralysis. Pain in left elbow. ***Hands and feet cold.*** The back of hand exposed to sunshine feels warm, while at same time a coolness appears in palm and runs up whole arm into temple. Cool, refreshed sensations. Pains as if bruised. Pain like toothache deep inside left hip, better as day progressed, better walking. Fingers numb with cold, chilled to bone.

Lungs - Wheezing, difficulty in breathing, before bedtime. Wheezing on exhalation and inhalation. Coughs on talking. Coughed up green catarrh and blood, worse evening.

Male - Loss of libido. Increased libido.

Modalities - Ameliorated by cloudy weather. ***Better hot bath***, when chilled to bone. ***Better short naps***, sleep. Better bending double, sitting down. Eyes better hot flannel. Throat better cold sweet drinks. Headaches better pressure, cold application, orange juice. Worse sunlight (Nat-m.), from sunrise to sunset. Spasms coming with sunrise and ceasing with sunset. Worse from standing. Eyes are worse from wind.

Mouth - Offensive breath. Brown tongue, unpleasant taste on tongue. Food tastes like something she cannot tell. Food is more palatable if put in the sunshine. Dry mouth in morning. Sore gum, right side, top of mouth. Nail biting. Stupid, cannot articulate a word. Articulates with difficulty.

Nose - Sneezing with a little sore throat, as if she had taken cold. Stopped up, right nostril blocked completely.

Perspiration - Perspiration streaming out of stomach pit over whole body. Perspiration under armpits with no exertion.

Rectum - Constipation. Pale colored stool. Diarrhea at night in bed, yellow/brown, painless with green leucorrhea. Diarrhea on going to bed just before menses. Loose stools. Pains better stool. Hemorrhoids.

Skin - Freckles. Itching, red skin. Red blotches from sunlight. ***Skin sensitive to sunlight.*** Sunburns easily. ***Never well since severe sunburn. Skin cancer.*** Dermatitis, often with cold limbs, degenerates into megrim. Nevi. Painful spot on cheek. Spots on back during menses. Peeling of skin on left hand.

Sleep - Sleeplessness until 3 a.m. to 4 a.m. Head very much excited, could not sleep for hours. Great sleepiness all through the head and not merely in the eyes, heavy, sound sleep all through night. Sound sleep, oversleeping. Dreams of being lost, of travel. Tired on waking. Tired all day with irritability, worse early evening, better sleeping. Sleepiness, better short naps.

Stomach - Anxiety in solar plexus. Heat in pit of stomach. Empty feeling in stomach, as if she had not eaten anything substantial yesterday and today. Sensation of faintness and vacuity in stomach pit. Nausea, no hunger, desires cold drinks. Nausea on waking, worse as morning progressed. Nausea after lunch. Slight inclination to vomit, or actual vomiting. Desire to vomit but unable to.

Teeth - Grinding of teeth as in helminthic spasms.

Temperature - Cold shivers with aching neck glands. ***Chilled to bone, very cold.*** An agreeable coolness extends over whole body. ***Chills.*** Running chills of increasing sensation of cold in all limbs from holding wires partially exposed to the sun. ***Shivering.*** Felt cold in night, drew up more cover and perspired. Congestive chill from exposure to sun right after drinking cold water freely.

Throat - Swollen glands. Yellow ulcer on right side of throat, no pain. Swollen throat, white pus on left side. Sore, achy throat, on waking, desire for cold drinks. Sore throat better eating, worse after dinner. Catch in throat after sudden dry mouth in morning. Sensation of loose skin flopping on back of throat on swallowing. Catarrh.

Vertigo - Vertigo on waking at 6 am, better lying, worse closing eyes. Dizziness with nausea, worse standing, sitting. Dizziness with nausea, much better lying, sleeping.

COMMENTS - In 1880, Swan published a pathogenesis which contained information obtained from four provers and from Reichenbach's experiences from hypersensitives. The common effects of strong sunlight, such as sneezing, freckling and sunstroke, may be added to the list.

Dr. Thayer, in 1893 in southern California, wrote a paper on sunlight for a homeopathic journal. He described how to "Concentrate the sun rays to a diseased part until slightly burned or charred and then wait until it heals and then repeat the procedure."

He claimed to have cured all kinds of cancers, removed birthmarks, tattoos, warts, sebaceous cysts, ulcers, varicose veins and all other types of benign growths. "Unlike other caustics, it can be applied upon the most delicate of tissues and it causes only slight irritation and most heal with only the slightest scar."

Dr. Thayer coined the term "solar cauterization." A magnifying glass was used and the sunbeam was focused right on the skin cancer, until a burning sensation was felt, then stopped. This would be repeated once or twice a day. After a week or ten days the melanoma would fall off and it would heal without a scar.

Thayer had a whole practice based on the magnifying glass and focusing the sunlight in 1893 and very few homeopaths used his methods.

Dr. Foubister revived interest in Sol in its potentized form as an antidote for radiation poisoning from radiation therapy with cancer patients.

RELATIONS - ***Antidoted by:*** Acon., Bell., Glon., Gels. and other sunstroke remedies. ***Compare:*** (1) Luna, Elect., M-aust., X-ray. (2) Cadm-s., radiation poisoning. (2) Dislike of sun, Lach., Nat-c., Nat-m., Glon.

REFERENCES - Clarke. Daws. Foubister. Murphy. Scriven.

SOLANINUM ACETICUM

PHARMACY - solin. Solaninum aceticum. Solanium aceticum aut purum. An alkaloid obtained from various Solanums, especially dulcamara and nigrum, also from the potatō plant. Trituration. Solution. ***Historical dose:*** Tincture and all potencies.

CLINICAL - Lungs, paralysis. Tetanus. Ticklishness.

HOMEOPATHIC - Solin. is obtained from many of the Solanaceae. and especially from Dulc. It exists in potatoes, and under certain conditions of germination, potatoes may contain a poisonous amount.

An accident of that kind occurred in soldiers at Pfuhl who were supplied with potatoes containing about 24 percent Solin. Sixty-six soldiers had marked poisoning symptom including shivering, fever, vomiting, syncope and in one case convulsions. Skin and conjunctiva were tinged yellow.

Clarke's first acquaintance with Solin. was through seeing the effect of Solin. 2c in solution given by Dr. Hughes to a diabetic and semi-paralytic man of 60 who had frequent threat of respiratory paralysis with accumulations of mucus which he was unable to expel. Solin., more than any other remedy, rescued him from danger and prolonged his life.

Solin. was proved by Clarus and Schroff, among others. Slowed and oppressed respiration was a marked feature. Respiration was slowed in inverse proportion to the increase in the pulse rate.

Cerebrospinal irritation, hyperesthesia and convulsions, worse by touch. Fainting. Weakness. Sensitiveness to light, noise and touch. Skin more easily tickled than usual. In animals, the hind limbs were rigid and paralyzed and in the provers the lower limbs were weakened.

MIND - Stupefaction without previous excitement. Fainting.

Abdomen - Rumbling in abdomen.

Chest - Convulsions of thorax, which were associated tonic spasms of limbs.

Eyes - Pupils slightly contracted.

Head - Vertigo. Cerebrospinal meningitis. Head hot, heavy, dull, painful. Pain in occiput.

Heart - Pulse increased in rapidity, weak, thready. Pulse and respiration slowed. Increased pulse rate with slowed respiration.

Kidneys - Albumen in urine.

Limbs - Weakness of lower limbs. Slight tonic spasms of lower limbs.

Lungs - Hoarseness. Breathing is slow, superficial, difficult and oppressed, distressed, especially on inspiration. Moist rattle during inspiration. Frequent violent outcry. Masses of mucus in larger air-passages. Paralysis of respiration.

Mouth - Salivation. Bitter taste. The pure alkaloid has a cooling, acid and salt taste and when chewed causes a glutinous sensation in pharynx and throat with scraping which extends to stomach, where it becomes a peculiar sticking pain.

Skin - Yellow discoloration of skin. Skin dry. Hyperesthesia, creeping along spine when touching the skin, more easily tickled than natural. Itching.

Sleep - Frequent yawning. Great sleepiness with inability to sleep. Sleep restless, frequently disturbed by frightful dreams. Sleep frequently interrupted, without dreams.

Stomach - Constant belchings. Nausea and diarrhea and vomiting. Nausea, violent ineffectual efforts to vomit. About 5 p.m., vomiting three times without previous nausea or pain or any intestinal symptoms.

Temperature - Limbs cold. Shivering, fever, vomiting and syncope. Profuse perspiration without weakness.

Throat - Scraping in throat.

RELATIONS - ***Compare:*** (1) Dulc., Bell., Sol-c., Sol-nig., Sol-tub. or Sol-t-ae. (2) In respiratory paralysis, Dulc., Bell. (3) Sleepy but cannot sleep, Bell. (4) Hyperesthesia, Nux-v, Tetox.

REFERENCES - Clarke.

SOLANUM ARREBENTA

PHARMACY - sol-a. Solanum arrebenta. Solanum acleatissimum. Solanum rebenta. Arrebenta cevallos, the Brazilian name. Tincture of the leaves. ***Historical dose:*** Tincture and all potencies.

HOMEOPATHIC - Mure, who proved Sol-a., said of it, "The bush grows spontaneously in the provinces of Rio Janeiro, along roads and in cultivated places. It is from ten to sixteen inches high."

Sol-a. has been used for strokes, boils. "Redness of face and rush of blood to brain" (Bell.). Swelling of the glands. Swelling and pains in breasts (Bell.). Urticaria and vertigo.

REFERENCES - Clarke.

SOLANUM CAROLINENSE

(Horse-nettle)

PHARMACY - sol-c. Solanum carolinense. Horse-nettle. N. O. Solanaceae. The fresh, ripe berries are macerated in twice their weight of alcohol. ***Historical dose:*** Tincture and all potencies.

HERBAL - In 1889 Dr. Napier called attention to Solanum carolinense as a remedy for the treatment of epilepsy, stating that it was used as a domestic remedy in for convulsions and "that he had successfully prescribed it in his practice."

HOMEOPATHIC - Sol-c. has ***convulsions and epilepsy***, twenty to forty-drop doses is of great value in grand mal of ***idiopathic epilepsy***, where the disease has begun beyond age of childhood, hystero-epilepsy, also in whooping cough.

COMMENTS - Dr. Charles S. Potts of the University of Pennsylvania, contributed a paper to The Gazette, Dec., 1895, on the remedy, giving several cases.

H. T., male, aged thirteen years. Idiopathic epilepsy, had his first spell five years ago, averaged one paroxysm daily. Sol-c. was first given in 10 drops doses without effect. When increased to 25 drops, the spells were lighter in severity, but occurred about as often.

The dose was finally increased to a teaspoonful four times daily. After being put upon this dose he was under observation six weeks during which time he had six seizures much lighter in severity.

T. H., male, aged twenty-eight years. He had epileptic seizures for three years, following an injury to the head which rendered him unconscious, but produced no other visible injury. Since this, however, had almost constant headache. The first spell was six months after the injury and have been frequent after, averaging three to four weekly, of an ordinary type.

Sol-c. in 40-drops doses three times daily was given, the spells at once decreased in frequency and severity. During the last six weeks he was under observation he only had three spells, very mild in type.

A. N., male, aged thirty years. First spell one year ago, have since occurred every two weeks, good deal of headache. Sol-c. 30c drops three times a day. No spells for one month and headache ceased. He then stopped attendance.

J. D., female, aged eighteen years. First spell when thirteen years old, had one spell a month at the time of her menstrual period. About a week before her next period, she was given Sol-c. 40 drops three times a day and escaped the usual spell. The following month however, she had one.

I. K., female, aged twenty-five years. Nocturnal epilepsy for past three years, about one spell a month. While using Sol-c. 40 drops three times a day, went three weeks longer than usual without a spell. The dose was then increased to 1 fluid drachm, she then ceased her visit.

F. S., female, aged twelve years. First spell five weeks before her visit, had been having them daily since. Sol-c. 30 drops ordered, this dose was gradually increased to 1 fluid drachm. During the three months that she was under observation her spells averaged in number about one a week.

H. B., male, aged eighteen years. First convulsion at age of ten years, then had none until three months before visit, had general convulsions about once daily since. Sol-c. 40 drops ordered. He was only under observation nine days, having during that time four spells, much milder in character.

A. C., female, aged fifteen years. First convulsion one year before, they had been increasing in frequency, up to one about every three days. During the three weeks she was taking Sol-c. 30 drops three times a day she had one spell, occurring during the third week.

H. K., male, aged eighteen years. First spell when fourteen years old. Every three or four days had several attacks in succession, an average of about one daily. While taking Sol-c. 40 drops, afterwards increased to teaspoonful-doses, he had twelve in thirty-eight days, an average of a little less than one in three days, going six without having any.

REFERENCES - Anshutz. Boericke.

SOLANUM MAMMOSUM

(Apple of Sodom)

PHARMACY - sol-m. Solanum mammosum. Apple of sodom. N. O. Solanaceae. Tincture of fresh ripe fruit. ***Historical dose:*** Tincture and all potencies.

CLINICAL - Coxalgia. Coughing. Hemoptysis. Irritability. Sleep, abnormal. Thought, difficult. Tobacco, effects. Twitching.

HOMEOPATHIC - Hering is the authority for Sol-m. The chief symptoms are irritability and inability to think. Uneasiness and inability to keep quiet. Sleepiness without being able to sleep, a kind a stupor worse at time of flood tide, at the full moon, better with ebb tide. Hawking, of blood-streaked mucus. Sensitiveness to tobacco (Ign.).

MIND - Irritability. Becomes exasperated at what he thinks may happen. Mental confusion. Inability for continuous thought. Difficulty expressing ideas.

Back - Twitching of large muscle below right scapula, as if the flesh were pinched up by the hand and shaken back and forth.

Limbs - Sticking pain in left hip joint that made him quite lame, frequently during and after walking, disappearing after standing and sitting down.

Lungs - Mucus hawked from the larynx contains streaks of bright blood.

Rectum - No stool, stool occurred later than usual and after much pressure.

Skin - Causes blotches over whole body from poisoning.

Sleep - Great weariness and desire to sleep without ability to sleep, followed by slumbering without real sleep. Deep sleep, from which he awoke and could not collect his senses for a long time and remained long in an irresolute condition. Sleepy in evening and sleeps well all night, even after afternoon sleeping. Dreams of death with violent weeping.

REFERENCES - Clarke.

SOLANUM NIGRUM

(Black Nightshade)

PHARMACY - sol-n. Solanum nigrum. Black nightshade. N. O. Solanaceae. Tincture of fresh plant. ***Historical dose:*** Tincture and all potencies.

CLINICAL - Amaurosis. Blindness. Chorea. Convulsion. ***Coryza.*** Delirium. ***Headaches.*** Heartburn. Hydrocephalus. Mania. ***Meningitis.*** Night-terrors. Parotiditis. Peritonitis. Psoriasis. Puerperal convulsions. Scarlatina. Skin, disorders. Smallpox. Stammering speech. Tetanus. Trismus. Tympanitis. Typhoid fever. Ulcers. Varicose veins. Vertigo.

HERBAL - Sol-n. is a common weed found in waste places. It has white flowers and black berries.

Green's Herbal recorded that "The leaves applied externally ease the pain and abate inflammation. Too large a quantity occasions violent sickness and headaches, giddiness, drowsiness and other dangerous symptoms. The Arabs apply the leaves to burns and ulcers, skin diseases and scrofulous and cancerous affections, they are diaphoretic, diuretic and purgative."

HOMEOPATHIC - Hale said some country practitioners used Sol-n. with much success under the impression that it was "an indigenous Belladonna," having been misled by the name "nightshade."

Hale verified its use in meningitis and headache. Also in scarlatina when the eruption is blotchy. He justly pointed out the close affinity of Sol-n. with Bell.: Delirium, headache, flushed face, sparkling eyes, pains coming and going suddenly, fiery rashes, burning skin and sweat.

"Frightful" headaches. Splitting, throbbing, bursting, piercing headaches, worse by least movement of head, least movement after sitting, light, noise, stooping. Headache is worse in a warm room and better in open air. Great sensitiveness to cold air.

Marked action on head and eyes. Brain irritation during dentition. Restlessness of a violent and convulsive nature. Formication with contraction of limbs.

Ergotism with tetanic spasms and stiffness of whole body with mania. Black appearance, bruised feeling all over the body. Chronic intestinal toxemia.

MIND - Mania. Furious delirium, characterized by the cephalic cry, efforts to escape and stammering speech. Night-terrors. Complete cessation of the mental faculties due to headaches.

Chest - ***Pain in left side***, sore to touch.

Eyes - Pain over both eyes. Alternate dilatation and contraction of pupils, weak sight, floating spots.

Head - ***Terrible headaches*** and complete cessation of the mental faculties. ***Congestive headaches*** (Bell.). Splitting, throbbing, bursting, piercing pains. Headaches at 10 a.m. Headache causes him to close eyes. Headaches, worse by least movement of head, light, noise, stooping.

Lungs - Constrictive feeling in chest with difficult breathing, cough with tickling in throat. ***Expectoration thick, yellow***.

Modalities - Better closing eyes. Worse by touch, motion. Worse moving head, beginning to move after sitting. Worse walking (inclines to left), misstep. Worse swallowing. Worse morning on waking, light. Worse bright sunshine (eyes).

Nose - ***Acute coryza, profuse, watery discharge*** from right nostril, left stopped up with chilly sensation, alternating with heat.

Sensations - Brain as if swimming. As if things moving in a circle, when stooping. As if brain shaking about in skull, on moving head. As if head would split. As from a blow on forehead. As if sand in eyes. As if splinter in right tonsil. Tongue as if scalded. Pains come and go suddenly. Symptoms extend upward. Right upper, left lower. Alternate coldness and heat.

Sleep - Night terrors.

Temperature - Alternation of coldness and heat. Scarlet fever, eruption in spots, large and vivid.

Vertigo - Vertigo with a terrible headache and complete cessation of the mental faculties. The vertigo is worse on moving the head. Sensation as if the bed was being rapidly turned in a circle. Inclines to left on walking.

COMMENTS - The provings and symptoms of poisoning cases are unusually distinctive. Tendency to blackness of the skin. Painful swelling, it enlarges, becomes shiny, hard and deep red and in several places, quite black.

Marked dilatation of the pupils (Bell.). Dryness of mouth and throat. Spasms, convulsions and tetanic rigidity of the whole body. "In the midst of these convulsions the children frequently stretch out their little hands, then carry them eagerly to their mouths and go through the motions of chewing and swallowing."

A patient of Cooper's, after one dose of the tincture, patches of psoriasis on the knees, elbows and forehead, scaly with red irritating spots at roots of hair disappeared. The day after taking a single dose of tincture, another patient of Cooper's had, "Head feels full across forehead, eyes heavy and forehead burns, could not apply himself to work."

RELATIONS - ***Compare:*** (1) Bell. (2) Sol-m. - pain in left hip joint. (3) Sol-t. - cramps in calves and contraction of fingers, spitting through closed teeth. (4) Sol-v. recommended in facial paralysis. (5) Sol-a. - threatening paralysis of the lungs in the course of bronchitis in the aged and children must cough a long time before able to raise expectoration. (6) Sol-ps. - acute pains in lower abdomen, Sol-t. (7) Aegrotans - diseased potato. (8) Sol-t. Potato berries - cramps in the calves of the legs and fingers.

REFERENCES - Boericke. Clarke.

SOLANUM OLERACEUM

(Juquerioba)

PHARMACY - sol-o. Solanum oleraceum. Juquerioba. N. O. Solanaceae. Tincture of flowers. ***Historical dose:*** Tincture and all potencies.

CLINICAL - Breast-milk, profuse. Breasts, swelling. Catarrh. Glands, swelling. Herpes Leucorrhea. Pustules. Sleep excessive. Styes. Urticaria.

HOMEOPATHIC - Mure reported that this plant is herbaceous, stem somewhat woody, the upper branches being covered with short and crooked thorns. It grows on the shores around Rio Janeiro in damp and shady places.

The most remarkable symptom of the proving was ***"swelling of the breasts with profuse effusion of milk"*** occurring in a woman of 60. "Pain and swelling of face and throat with inflammation." "Cold feeling in left chest after drinking." Drowsiness with headache. The generally deranged sleep of the other Solanaceae.

REFERENCES - Boericke. Clarke.

SOLANUM TUBEROSUM

(Potato)

PHARMACY - sol-t. Solanum tuberosum. Potato. N. O. Solanaceae. Tincture of the berries. Tincture of green potatoes. Tincture of fresh plant. ***Historical dose:*** Tincture and all potencies.

CLINICAL - Amaurosis. Colic. Cramps. Diarrhea. Faintness. Headache. Iritis, rheumatic. Stammering. Trismus. Tumors. Vomiting.

HOMEOPATHIC - The poisonous properties of the berries and leaves of the potato plant are well known, and the tubers are popularly believed to have anti-scorbutic properties when eaten as food. Under some conditions the tubers have been known to contain poisonous quantities of Solanin.

The symptoms are the result of eating new potatoes, green potatoes, an extract and the berries. The last proved fatal in a number of instances. Sickness and diarrhea with tenesmus, giddiness, dilated pupils and indistinct vision. Tossing to and fro in bed. A paralytic condition of the tongue, cramps and tetanic spasms. General rigidity. Patient is exceedingly weak. Faintness.

MIND - Almost lost consciousness.

Abdomen - Violent colic and vomiting. Pain in bowels. Tumors.

Eyes - Eyes deep in sockets. Pupils dilated. Staring look. Vision indistinct.

Face - Hippocratic face. Anxious expression.

Female - Tumors around cervix, uterus.

Limbs - Cramps, especially in calves with spasmodic contractions of fingers and thumbs.

Lungs - Difficult breathing. Respiration is hurried, irregular, at times suppressed, usually short and incomplete, only seldom slow and sighing.

Mouth - Constantly spitting through the closed teeth, viscid, frothy phlegm. Tongue covered with brown, moist fur. Tongue is heavy and difficult to move, hardly able to articulate. Speech thick. Speechless.

Pulse - Pulse small, rapid, scarcely perceptible.

Rectum - Diarrhea with tenesmus. Tends to relax bowels.

Skin - Skin livid.

Stomach - Epigastric region sensitive to pressure. Felt sick, a darkness over her eyes, skin cold, cramped all over. Violent retching followed by vomiting and diarrhea.

Temperature - Skin cold. Face, chest and limbs cold. Skin beaded with cold, clammy sweat.

Vertigo - Vertigo, headache, stupor.

COMMENTS - Cooper relieved with a single dose of Sol-t. tincture a case of rheumatic iritis.

Burnett cured a case of tumors feeling like masses of potatoes in the abdomen with Sol-t. It also assisted him in the cure of a case of tumors all around the cervix uterus. Urt-u. finished this cure.

RELATIONS - ***Compare:*** (1) Solin. (2) In paralysis of tongue, Caust., Dulc. (3) Iritis, Bell. (4) Stammering speech, Merc., Stram.

REFERENCES - Clarke.

SOLANUM TUBEROSUM AEGROTANS

(Rotten Potato)

PHARMACY - sol-t-ae. Solanum tuberosum aegrotans. Rotten potato. Diseased potato due to several fungi. Tincture of the affected tubers. ***Historical dose:*** All potencies.

CLINICAL - *Anal, prolapse.* Breasts, painful. Constipation. Nosebleed. Headache. Ileus. Menses interrupted. Noma. Pruritus vulva. ***Rectal, prolapse.*** Scalp, painful. Sciatica. Scurvy. Tenesmus. Tongue, cracked. Vertebra, pain, pulsation.

HOMEOPATHIC - According to the Treasury of Botany, the "potato murrain" is characterized by "the rapid putrescence of the leaves and haulm, which is first indicated by the presence of a little mold, Peronospora infestans, which preys upon the tissues, spreading rapidly in every direction. The tubers also exhibit brown spots on their surface and within their tissues and according to circumstances decay with greater or less rapidity."

In 1846, the sudden inroad of this disease led to the famine in Ireland, resulting in the death of thousands.

Mure made the first proving of Sol-t-ae., using a potato "in an entire state of decomposition without, however, being completely rotten." Effects of eating diseased potatoes, some of them fatal, have been observed and these have been added to Mure's.

Dark skin. Breath and odor of body are offensive. Excruciating muscular pains. Cold water causes shock. The urine has an oily pellicle. ***Prolapse of the rectum and anus***. Tumors of rectum look like decayed potato. Dreams of pools of blood. Irritability.

MIND - Quarrelsome, irritable mood. Bad temper. Dread of work. Hypochondriac mood. Fancies she is miserable, and dwells much on the future. Wants to enjoy a change of scenery. Crowd of ideas. Attention is easily disturbed by other things. Confusion of mind.

Abdomen - Painfulness of abdomen to contact along the median line. Belly hard, swollen, dropsical. Pain after eating, spasmodic pains, as though the bowels became twisted together, rumbling. Pain, as if sprained, in right groin. Stitch in right groin near inguinal ring. Flatulence.

Back - Violent beating in spine, early, when lying. Prickling sensation in spine. Stinging pain. Sensation of weariness in whole back. Stiffness in muscles of back. Tingling in sacrum. Prickling in psoas muscles. Pain in lumbar vertebra, impeding walking. Swelling of muscles of neck.

Breasts - Breasts are painful, especially when raising arm.

Chest - Oppression in chest. Congestions to chest. Tearing in chest. Prickling as from a thousand pins on the inner surface of sternum. Violent stitching pain above right breast. Acute pain in the sides like a stitch.

Ears - Ringing in the left ear.

Eyes - Congestion of the conjunctiva. Prickling and burning in eyes. Profuse lachrymation, on waking. Burning in lids. Prickling about the lids, the surface of which is red. Spasmodic contraction and twitching of left upper lid.

Face - Face pale, bloodless. Swollen, especially about eyelids, nearly closing them. Face hot and red. Red pimples on cheeks. Desquamation of face. Bluish-black, fetid ulcer of left cheek. Upper lip is bleeding, cracked.

Female - Suppression of the menses. Menstrual blood rose-colored. Menses smelling of foul fish. Small pimples and intolerable itching of labia. Burning and itching in vagina. Flatulence presses on uterus. Spasmodic pains in uterus. Twisting pains through uterus. Feeling of dislocation in hip joint with pain in womb after a slight exertion.

Food - Canine hunger. Salt taste. Taste of raw potatoes. Food tastes as bitter as gall. Great desire for spirits and oranges. Burning thirst.

Head - Heat in head, evening. Heaviness of head. Catarrhal dullness. Lancinations, as if brain would burst open. Headache at noon, worse by the smell of spirits. Sensation of water splashing in head. Painful sensitiveness of scalp and roots of hair, cannot bear combing.

Heart - Weight and pain in heart region. Lancinations in heart. Palpitations of heart. Pulse is irregular, sometimes weak, hard and tense.

Kidneys - Region of bladder distended. Difficult urination. Urine reddish, mingled with mucus. Urine is very thick, soapy, turbid, of a dingy yellow with copious white sediment. Constant urination while at stool. Heat and pain in urethra after urinating.

Limbs - Sense of weariness in all the limbs. Inclination to stretch. Joints swollen and very painful. Acute pains in hip joint caused by least motion. Feeling of dislocation of hip joint. Legs edematous. Shuddering in right leg. Heat in hands.

Lungs - Constriction and difficulty breathing. Constant involuntary sighing. In trachea, tearing, prickling with cough. Cough with expectoration of yellow mucus, at night. Dry cough, day and night. Expectoration of lumps of black blood, early in the morning. After eating choking and difficult breathing caused by dryness of mouth. Hoarseness on walking.

Male - Weight in right testicle all day.

Modalities - Worse by touch, pressure, walking. Worse from smell of alcohol. Worse at 5 p.m., sleeping. Headache is worse on waking, from working.

Mouth - Dry mouth. Breath horribly fetid. Tongue pale, coated white or yellowish white. Tongue yellowish along the median line. Tongue swollen, cracked, early in the morning. Prickling in right half of tongue.

Nose - Repeated sneezing, followed by feeble cough. Pressure at root of nose. Nosebleeds. Smell of blood.

Rectum - Alternate protrusion and retraction of rectum during stool. Contraction of anal sphincter. ***Prolapsed rectum and anus.*** Acute pain in anus. Great heat in anus. Frequent urging to stool. Has to strain until tears come. Hard, large, lumpy stool, with violent burning in anus and rectum. Constipation. Copious greenish-yellow diarrhea. Violent colic previous to stool.

Sensations - Of water splashing on head, as if brain were leaping in skull (on stooping). As of something sticking in throat. As if there were a fleshy growth in throat. As if a spring unrolled in left hypochondrium. As if a hollow body were turning rapidly in chest. Of stoppage in trachea. Of something becoming detached from sacrum.

Skin - Skin is tender. Rose-colored patches appear and as suddenly vanish. Small red pimples cause violent itching.

Sleep - Irresistible drowsiness. Sleepless. Restless sleep. Starting from sleep, as in a fright. Amorous dreams. Dreams about men who become transformed to talking animals. Confused dreams, about fires, revolution, corpses, thieves.

Stomach - Pain in stomach, with red face, after breakfast. Spasmodic pains, griping-tearing at night. Acidity, bitterness, and gulping-up, after eating. Belchings followed by rumbling in stomach. Sour belchings causing a cough.

Teeth - Teeth covered with white mucus. Swelling of mucus membrane of the inner margin of the two incisors. Teeth loose and very painful. Gums, especially lower, spongy, oozing blood.

Temperature - Chilliness and sensation of internal coldness. Alternate burning heat and chilliness, at night. Sweat all over, early is morning, in bed, cold night-sweat. The sweat makes the bed smell of potatoes. Heat all over with sweat. Fever, afterwards dropsical appearance. Violent paroxysms of heat.

Throat - Feeling as of a fleshy growth in throat. Feeling as if something sticking in throat. Mucus accumulates in throat. Fauces and mouth inflamed, ulcerated in patches. Inflamed fauces, unable to swallow saliva.

COMMENTS - The symptoms of the Sol-t-ae. proving were severe, and one of the most important, prolapse of the rectum, has been confirmed by the poisoning cases.

A man and three children ate boiled diseased potatoes and among their symptoms were "Pain of an acute character was referred to the region of the anus, which on examination was found perfectly patulous and exquisitely tender to the touch.

Two of the four patients had prolapsed anus, which was probably caused by the violent and ineffectual efforts to discharge the contents of the rectum.

There had not been an evacuation of the bowels, nor had they passed water, except in drops and with extreme suffering, for six days. On introducing the finger into the rectum, which caused acute pain, it was found that the intestine was completely filled to within an inch of the orifice with a solid substance."

The foul odor of the diseased potato is reproduced in the breath and body odor of the patients. Lips cracked and raw, gums bleeding tongue coated, thick, cracked, throat inflamed and ulcerated with sensation of something sticking in it or a fleshy growth.

In one poisoning case a condition of noma of left cheek was induced.

RELATIONS - ***Compare:*** (1) Bry., Ars., Plb., Nux-v., Sep., Stron., Viol-t., Squil., Puls., Graph., Alum., Merc., Nat-m., Ign., Calc. (2) Sensation of machinery inside, Nit-ac. (3) Constipation, black balls, Op. (4) Prolapsus anus, Podo., Ruta. (5) Patulous anus, Apis., Phos.

REFERENCES - Clarke.

SOLANUM XANTHOCARPUS

(Kantikari)

PHARMACY - sol-x. Solanum xanthocarpus. Kantikari. N. O. Solanaceae. Root, bark, fruit and flower. ***Historical dose:*** Tincture and all potencies.

CLINICAL - Abscesses. Asthma. Boils. Bronchitis. Buboes. Cough. Cystitis. Dropsy. Dysuria. Hemorrhoids. Hoarseness. Kidney, disorders. Kidney, stones. Lung, disorders. Ophthalmia. Pneumonia. Smallpox. Teeth, decay. Urinary, stricture. Vomiting.

HERBAL - Ayurvedic physicians prized Sol-x. as an excellent remedy for cough, respiratory troubles, cough associated with hoarseness, ophthalmia, stone or calculus, stricture, and retention or suppression of urine.

Sol-x. is an aperient, carminative, expectorant, and diuretic. It is given in asthma, cough, catarrhal affections of the lungs, fever, flatulent and pain in the chest. As a diuretic, the decoction is given in dysuria, cystitis, calculi and dropsy, also given in costiveness.

A paste of the seeds is locally applied to promote suppuration of boils, buboes, and other indolent chronic abscesses. Fumigation of the fruit is largely used by natives as sialogogue and applied for the relief of pain in carious teeth.

Charaka recommended Sol-x. in hemorrhoids, cough, delirium tremens, urinary difficulties, stone and calculus. Shushruta found it efficacious in ophthalmia, respiratory troubles, cough, urinary difficulties and troubles and stricture.

Chakradatta said that Sol-x. is useful in cough, stricture, and urinary troubles. Bangasena has recommended it in the cough of children.

Sol-x. is used by them separately or as a principal ingredient in their compound medicines for the above mentioned complaints.

HOMEOPATHIC - Hoarseness (Caust., Phos., Sel.), associated with cough. Bronchitis, pneumonia, or bronco-pneumonia associated with voice loss. Asthma.

Fevers associated with thirst, vomiting, aversion to food, burning sensation felt over the body and pains felt over the collective body of the ribs. Stricture, suppression or retention of urine and kidney stone.

Preventive against smallpox. The Ayurvedic physicians also used it against smallpox, dose being 1/8 tola of its root (white variety) to be given in the morning in empty stomach.

RELATIONS - ***Compare:*** In the cure of kidney maladies it can be compared with Berb., Canth., Sars. and Lyc.

REFERENCES - Ghose.

SOLIDAGO VIRGAUREA

(Goldenrod)

PHARMACY - solid. Solidago virgaurea. Goldenrod. N. O. Compositae, Tribe, Corymbifere. Tincture of whole fresh plant. Tincture of flowers. The fresh blossoms are macerated in twice their weight of alcohol. Infusion of dry leaves and flowers. ***Historical dose:*** Tincture and all potencies.

CLINICAL - Albuminuria. Allergies. Asthma. Backache. Bright's disease. Bronchitis. Calculus. ***Colds.*** Conjunctivitis. Coughs. Croup. Cystitis. Deafness. Dysentery. Dysuria. Eczema. Edema. Eruptions. Gangrene. Gout. Hay fever. Hemorrhages. ***Kidney,***

disorders. Leucorrhea. ***Nephritis.*** Ophthalmia, scrofulous. Phosphaturia. Prostate, enlarged. Prostate, weak. Rheumatic fever. Rheumatism. Sciatica. Scrofula. Tuberculosis. ***Urine, suppressed.***

HERBAL - The common golden rod is the only British species of Solidago. It is common in woods and healthy thickets. "This herb," said Rademacher, "is a very old and good kidney medicine. It is a specific for kidneys and brings the patients back to the normal condition."

HOMEOPATHIC - Solid. has helped diseases arising from or complicated with defective functions of kidneys. It affects the digestive tract, lower limbs and blood. Hemorrhages. ***Feeling of weakness,*** chilliness alternating with heat.

Homeopathic replacement for the catheter. Pain in region of kidneys with dysuria. ***Kidneys sensitive to pressure***. Bright's disease. Chronic nephritis. Uremic asthma. "Clear, stinking urine" is an indication of Cooper's.

Hay fever when golden rod is the exciting cause. ***Takes cold easily.*** Inhalation of the pollen has caused hemorrhage from the lungs in tuberculosis. ***Repeated colds of tuberculosis***. Naso-pharyngeal catarrh, burning in throat, pains in limbs and thoracic oppression.

Abdomen - Costiveness, sensation of pain in the abdomen on both sides of the navel, upon deep pressure, gas. Severe pricking in both hypochondria to the region of the kidneys, reaching to the lower limbs.

Back - Backache. Lumbar ache, makes her sick all over.

Bladder - Cystitis. Catarrh of the bladder. Obstructed flow of urine. Scanty urine. Nightly dysuria. Catheterizing of bladder.

Chest - Rheumatism of the inter-costal muscles.

Constitutions - Especially suited to scrofulous subjects.

Ears - Sudden deafness with ringing in the ears and albuminous urine.

Eyes - Conjunctivitis. Scrofulous, herpetic inflammation. Red with enlarged prostate gland.

Female - Uterine enlargement organ pressed down upon the bladder. Fibroid tumors. Hemorrhage. Chronic leucorrhea in connection with copious, watery urine and sediments of mucus particles and uriniferous tubules, epithelium.

Kidneys - Kidneys, sore and tender, ache, feel distended. Pain in kidneys extends forward to abdomen, bladder, down the thighs. ***Chronic nephritis.*** Urine, voided with difficulty.

Limbs - Chronic pains in the loins. Rheumatic pains in the leg. Pains in the thighs, the leg can be moved horizontally. When limbs are moved perpendicularly they feel lame. Limping, dragging gait.

Lungs - Oppressed breathing. Continuous dyspnea. Allergies. Asthma. Periodical asthma with nightly dysuria. Bronchitis. Chronic catarrh of the lungs. Cough with much purulent expectoration blood-streaked. Heavy expectoration in coughing, croup and diminished urine.

Male - Enlarged prostate gland, obstructing flow of urine or inflammation. Weak prostate gland.

Modalities - Better from profuse urination. Worse from pressure, at night.

Mouth - Continuous bitter taste. Tongue heavily coated, clears when urine becomes normal. Flat ulcers in the mouth and throat.

Nose - Allergies and hay fever. Dry, inner surface of the nose covered with blood crust, scalding and very scanty urine. Paroxysms of sneezing with abundant mucus discharge.

Rectum - Chronic catarrh of the bowels. Dysentery, diarrhea. Profuse involuntary mucus stools.

Skin - Petechiae, on lower limbs with edema and itching, Gangrene, diabetic. Eczema worse from suppressed urine. Scrofulous rash, little blotches on hands and feet. Very obstinate, itching exanthemas. Exanthema of the lower limbs without swelling of the inguinal glands, but with disturbance in urinating.

Sleep - Insomnia.

Temperature - Rheumatic fever, very frequent pulse, high fever.

Urine - Dark urine, especially at night with very scanty brown and sour urine. Scalding and very scanty urine. Urine, dark and scanty or clear, stinking. Urine, voided with difficulty. Urine, albuminous, mucous, phosphatic.

COMMENTS - Anshutz wrote, "A lady, by administering, morning and evening, an infusion of the dry leaves and flowers of Golden Rod (Solidago virgaurea) tells me that she cured her husband of an affection of the bladder which had compelled him to use a catheter for a year or more.

"A friend of homeopathy desired to test the energetics of this plant. He had the first dilution of its tincture to be taken three times a day by seven patients. From forty-two to seventy-fours years of age. They had been obliged to catheterize themselves for weeks, months and years.

"Homeopathy cured them so thoroughly that they had no relapses. Surgeons who spend much time in catheterizing such patients for months and years could often cure them much more rapidly by prescribing for them the remedy just mentioned."

Gallavardin told of a woman who cured her husband, who had been compelled to use the catheter for more than a year, by administering an infusion of the dried leaves and flowers of Solid. morning and evening.

Dr. White said "I have used it in several other cases where it seemed indicated by the tenderness in kidney region and the inability to control the water from whatever cause, always the perfect satisfaction to patient and myself."

Gucken confirmed Rademacher's clinical observations and quoted further confirmations and cures by Dr. Buck of Wurtemburg.

The grand keynote of this remedy lies in the condition and the action of the kidneys and the quality of their secretions. Diseases arising from or complicated with defective action of the kidneys are very likely to be benefited by Solid.

Pain and tenderness in kidney region, pains extending from kidneys to abdomen, bladder and down limbs, urine dark, red-brown, scanty, thick, voided with difficulty, albuminous, mucus and phosphatic urine. Affections of any other parts or organs complicated with these symptoms will probably find their remedy in Solid.

Buck mentioned scrofulous inflammation of the eyes. Clarke saw very sharp attack of conjunctivitis produced in a patient who was taking Solid. Also for prostatic troubles.

Buck noted several cases, including that of a boy, age 8, who had severe membranous diphtheria with scarlet rash, which was removed by Merc-cy. and Bell., but a fever of the typhoid type remained. The urine was albuminous and scanty, pulse weak and intermittent, feet swollen. Kali-ar. 4c was given, but the symptoms grew worse.

A thorough examination of the patient showed great sensitiveness of the kidneys to pressure in spite of the otherwise apathetic condition. Solid. 3x was given and in one day the urine became more profuse with corresponding improvement in the general condition. The body peeled and recovered completely.

A clerk, 45, had sleeplessness and pain in the back. He casually mentioned that it took him a long time to urinate for want of the necessary pressure. This he attributed to gonorrhea, which he had years before. No sleep until 3 a.m. when he got some sleep, which was not refreshing.

On rising, tired, especially upper part of thighs, then would begin the pain in the back, which extended to the loins and lasted until bedtime. Nux-v. did not relieve. The urine was found dark, slimy, reddish, slightly acid, not albuminous. Kidneys sensitive to pressure.

Solid. 3x, taken steadily for three months, cured. A year afterwards there was a relapse, but this time it took the form of sciatica and Solid. again proved to be the remedy.

Mrs. F., 53, wife of a farmer, stout, fresh-looking, had her present trouble twenty-six years. After her confinement, which was difficult and followed by prolapse uterus, still existing. Her legs began to swell and an itching rash broke out by degrees.

Menstruation had always come on at

the proper time, but suddenly stopped six months before Buck saw her. Since then the itching had been almost intolerable, the legs more swollen and always cold.

Appetite very poor, constant bitter taste in mouth tongue thickly coated, at the same time a rising from the stomach as if she would suffocate and at the least exertion she lost her breath. Urinated very little and mostly at night.

No pains in the back, but the kidneys were sensitive to pressure. "The appearance of the lower limbs of this patient," said Buck, "frightened me. From knee to heel they formed a bluish-red mass in the shape of a stove-pipe and were covered with little blotches and crusts."

The prolonged use of Solid. 3x, though it did not effect a cure, produced a mitigation of the whole body, so that the woman induced her eldest son to consult the doctor.

This man had also trouble in his lower limbs not unlike his mother's. A year before he had some severe throat trouble after which his lower limbs began to swell and itch. They were also tinted blue-red and covered with vesicles, his urine was scanty and his kidneys sensitive to pressure. Solid. 3x cured him in a few months.

RELATIONS - ***Compare:*** (1) In prostatic and urinary affections, Sabal., Santa., Hydrang., Tritic. (2) Kidney-ache, Santa. (3) Gonorrhea and its effects, sciatica, Med.

REFERENCES - Boericke. Clarke. Phatak.

SPHINGURUS MARTINI

(Porcupine Tree)

PHARMACY - sphing. Sphingurus martini. Porcupine tree. Spiggurus martini. Hystrix prehensis. N. O. Sphingurinae. Trituration of prickles taken from one of the sides. ***Historical dose:*** Trituration and all potencies.

CLINICAL - Hair, loss. Jaw, pains. Stammering. Zygoma, pain.

HOMEOPATHIC - The old world porcupines have the name Histricinae, those of the new world, Sphingurinae. Mure proved the 3x trituration of the prickles.

The most noteworthy symptoms were falling out of the hair, especially of whiskers. Itching of the pubes after taking tea. Pain in the jaw-joint and right zygoma. Embarrassed speech. Nausea at sight of food.

Modalities - Better walking on open air, after dinner. Worse lying down, after tea.

REFERENCES - Clarke.

SPIGELIA ANTHELMINTICA

(Pinkroot)

PHARMACY - spig. Spigelia anthelmintica. Pinkroot. Demerara. N. O. Loganiaceae. Middle and South America. Tincture of dried herb. ***Historical dose:*** Tincture and all potencies.

CLINICAL - Adenoids. Amaurosis. ***Angina pectoris.*** Anorexia. ***Anxiety.*** Ascarides. Bulimia. ***Ciliary, neuralgia.*** Colds. Colic. Concussions. Constipation. Depression. Diaphragm, stitches. ***Dyspnea.*** Exophthalmic, goiter. ***Eyes, pains. Face, pains.*** Gastric, catarrh. Glaucoma. Headaches. ***Heart, disorders.*** Hernia, inguinal. Iritis. Jaw, pain. ***Migraines.*** Nausea. ***Neuralgias.*** Otalgia. ***Palpitations.*** Pericarditis. Photophobia. Post-nasal, catarrh. ***Prosopalgia.*** Prostatorrhea. Pterygium. Rectum, cancer. Rheumatism. Scarlatina. Sigmoid flexure, cancer. Stammering, speech. Strabismus. Tinnitus. Tobacco habit. Toothache. Vertigo. ***Worms.***

HERBAL - Spigelia anthelmia is a common weed in South America. Spigelia Marylandica, *"Pink-root"* or *"Worm-grass,"* is a native of the southern states of North America. Spig. was known in Europe in Hahnemann's time as an anthelmintic, the drug properties were learned from the natives of the Antilles.

HOMEOPATHIC - Spig. markedly affects the nerves, trifacial, heart, eyes, teeth, fibrous tissue and left side. Useful for pericarditis and other diseases of the heart. ***Heart disorders and neuralgias.*** It produces combined heart and eye symptoms, or the latter as an accompaniment.

Affected by the sun. Headache beginning at sunrise, at its height at noon, declining to sunset.

Pains of neuralgias and headaches increases and declines with sun. Sun pains.

Neuralgia of the fifth nerve. Stabbing pains. ***Pains are violent, burning like hot needles or wires,*** jerking, tearing, stitching, radiating to other parts. ***Very sensitive to touch. Parts feel chilly, send shudder through frame.*** Body feels light while walking, heavy and sore when rising from a seat. Moves very carefully.

A remedy for stitches due to the presence of worms. ***Child refers to the navel as the most painful part*** (Gran., Nux-v., Plb., Mosch.).

MIND - Mental exertion difficult. Weakness of memory. Absence of ideas. Difficulty of thinking. Unfit for intellectual labor. Confusion on stooping. Sadness and discouragement. Stammering, repeats first syllable three or four times. Sits as if lost in thought, stares at a single object.

Agitation and anxiety, with restlessness. Anxiety about future. Restless and anxious. So nervous he can't control himself. feels as if he must run. Anxiety on seeing any one move quickly, on breathing deeply. ***Afraid of sharp, pointed things, pins, needles*** (Sil., Apis.). ***Delusions about pins.*** Excitement after sadness. Irritability during chill.

Mental irritability. Easily offended. Very restless and anxious. ***Cannot tolerate thinking of pain.*** Can become suicidal because the pain is too severe. Gloomy, suicidal mood. Desires death during chill. Great dejection in evening, he could have killed himself. Timidity.

Abdomen - Abdomen hard and painfully tight. Contact and pressure of clothes is unbearable. Colic with pinching pains in the umbilical region. Expulsion of fetid flatus.

Back - Neck stiff, pains into right temple or pain from left shoulder to neck. Cutting about the left scapula.

Causations - Concussions. Worms, ascarides and lumbrici. Sunlight. Tobacco.

Chest - Aching at the chest with painful oppression. ***Angina pectoris.*** Contraction of chest with anguish and obstructed respiration. Stitches in diaphragm with dyspnea. Craving for hot water which relieves chest pain.

Constitutions - Adapted to anemic, debilitated, rheumatic and scrofulous subjects. Suited to persons with light hair, pale, thin, bloated, weak with wrinkled, yellow, earthy skin. Children afflicted with worms, ascarides and lumbrici.

Ears - Roaring, buzzing and pulsation in ears. Stoppage of ears. Periodical deafness, ears feel as if stuffed.

Eyes - Pupils dilated. Rheumatic ophthalmia. Feel too large, ***pressive pain on turning the eyes. Severe pain in and around the eyes,*** extending deep into socket, worse thinking of them. ***Ciliary neuralgia,*** neuritis. As if needles were thrust in. Profuse lachrymation, from affected side, tears acrid. Eyes, red, sore, drawing ache. Yellow rings about the eyes. Difficulty in raising the eyelids with painful sensation of stiffness. Everted eyelids. Inclination to wink. Difficult to fit glasses, no settled focus, no fixed vision, latent errors of vision. Pricking in lids. Squints with worms. Photophobia.

Face - ***Prosopalgia*** involving eye, zygoma, cheek, teeth, temples. Worse from touch, stooping, from morning until sunset, drinking tea, suddenly going and coming.

Food - Ravenous hunger. Anorexia with violent thirst. Bulimia, sometimes with nausea and thirst. Putrid, fetid taste. Aversion to coffee, tobacco smoke and snuff. Craving for hot water which relieves chest pain.

Head - Feels too large. Migraines. ***Pain from beneath frontal eminence and temples, extending to eyes*** (Onos.). Semi-lateral involving left eye, pain violent, throbbing, worse making a false step. Pain as if a band around head (Carb-ac., Cact., Gels.). Pain from left occiput to over left eye, worse stooping, making a false step, opening mouth. Supra-orbital neuralgia.

Heart - ***Violent sticking or compressive pains,*** radiating to throat, arms, scapula, worse least motion or bending double. Soreness, purring, cracking in the region of heart. ***Angina pectoris.*** Neuralgia extending to arm or both arms. Craving for hot water which relieves. ***Violent palpitations,*** audible, attending other symptoms. Frequent attacks of palpitations, especially with foul odor from mouth. Throbbing of carotids and subclavian arteries. Precordial pain and great aggravation from movement. Pericarditis. Rheumatic carditis, trembling pulse, whole left side sore. Pulse intermittent with palpitations, weak tremulous irregular.

Kidneys - Frequent want to urinate with profuse emission, even at night. Sudden and involuntary dribbling of urine with burning sensation in anterior part of urethra. Urine with whitish sediment.

Limbs - Fatigue. Drawing, tearing, twitching pains in limbs and joints. Left arm numb. Pulsation in patellae. The limbs are affected mostly when walking.

Lungs - ***Dyspnea, must lie on right side with head high***, worse moving in bed, raising arms. Hydrothorax. Trembling in chest. Stitches in chest worse least motion or when breathing.

Male - Discharge of prostatic fluid from the urethra.

Modalities - Better from rest, lying on right side with head high. Better inspiring, steady pressure, warmth. Pressure helps the neuralgia, cold application helps temporarily. Better while eating, worse immediately after. Worse light touch but better firm pressure. Worse motion, jar. Worse turning, rising, raising arms, stooping, bending forward. Worse from sex. Worse slightest draft, cold, damp, rainy, stormy weather, cold air, cold washing. Worse with the sun (Nat-m.). Worse morning, on waking. Worse blowing nose, expiration, tobacco. Worse noise. Worse thinking of problems.

Mouth - ***Foul odor from mouth.*** Offensive taste. Tongue, coated yellow or white, cracked, with burning or stitching pain. Tongue fissured, painful. Opening mouth aggravates headache.

Nose - Tickling and itching of nose. Forepart of nose always dry. ***Chronic catarrh*** with post-nasal drip of bland mucus. ***Discharge through posterior sinuses.*** Flow of water during prosopalgia.

Rectum - Constipation and diarrhea. Frequent, ineffectual urging to stool. Faints at stool. Stools of large lumps of mucous. Itching, tickling and crawling in anus and rectum. ***Worms,*** ascarides.

Sensations - As if he would fall. As if intoxicated. As if head would burst. As of a band around head, as if head tightly bound. As if electric sparks in temples. Brain as if loose. As if eye would be pushed out of head. As if hairs or feathers on lashes. Face feels as if it had been scorched. As if heart compressed or squeezed with a hand. As if everything in chest were too short, loose and wobbling about. As if something tearing in chest.

Skin - Pale, wrinkled skin of body. Painful sensibility when touched. Painful glandular swellings. Red pimples with pain when touched, as from excoriation.

Stomach - Pressure in stomach. Accumulation of mucus in the stomach. Sour risings. Nausea with sensation of a worm rising in throat. Nausea when fasting.

Teeth - Tearing pains, worse after eating, cold, and when thinking of it. Toothache with facial pain, better by warmth or the warmth of the bed. Nerve toothache. Toothache, worse cold drinks (Mag-p., better warm drinks.), better by smoking tobacco.

Temperature - Chilliness on the slightest motion. Cold, offensive sweat on upper part of the body, on hands. Heat, flushes at night in back.

Throat - Sore throat with lancinations and swelling in palate. Discharge of mucus from fauces all day, most from posterior sinuses. Swollen cervical glands.

Vertigo - Vertigo on stooping with heat of head. Vertigo as if they are drunk. Vertigo, the feet as if higher than head. Vertigo worse looking down, must look straight ahead, worse standing, walking. Vertigo, hearing exalted.

COMMENTS - Hahnemann said Spig. has the peculiarity that the primary action of a single unrepeated dose usually increases somewhat daily during the first seven to ten days. Experiments should be conducted with caution, seeing that 60, 80 to 100 drops of the tincture produce violent effects even in robust persons.

Keynote violence. More left-sided than right, but by no means exclusively left-sided. Primarily affects the head, eyes, face, teeth and heart. Sensitivity to cold, wet and stormy weather.

Produces intense pains in all parts. Hypersensitive to all pain. Burning, jerking, tearing, pressing and stitching pains, radiate and extend to other parts. Pains are largely out-pressing and proceed from within outward and below upward. Pains are worse by noise, jar, movement, change of weather, especially stormy weather. The pains were worse night and morning and in damp weather. Sensitive to pain remedies (Cham., Nux-v., Ign., Hep.).

Darting and aching pains in head, nose and eyes and similar pains about the heart with slow, irregular action, but no murmur. Sudden pains at bottom of back. The body is painfully sensitive to touch. Pain feels like shiver in the body, eye or face. The part touched feels chilly. Touch sends a shudder through the whole frame. Pain radiates from a spot, not in a straight line. Darting pain. Pain will transfix (Bry.).

Neuralgia, especially facial neuralgias. Pains over the left eye or the left side of the face, trigeminal neuralgias. Neuralgias with burning sensations or electric-like sensations. Intercostal neuralgias (Ran-b.). Often with neuralgia, their whole left face consists of tearing pain as if someone is cutting their face or tearing the skin off their face.

Neuralgias and inflammation of the eye, amaurotic conditions, and glaucoma. Exophthalmic goiter. Intolerable pressive pains, worse on motion. Stabbing pains through eye backwards into brain. Uveitis. Ciliary neuralgia or affection to the optic nerve with cutting, stabbing pain, the eye becomes inflamed and watery. Sensation as if eye would burst. Deep pain in eye socket.

Dilated pupils, can see sparks and rays of light. Severe photophobia, especially with headache, they want to be in the dark with a hand covering their left side and making no noise and staying from noise.

Migraine, from occiput, settling in or over left eye (Sang. starts at the occiput and settles in the right eye; Sil. and Gels. are from occiput to forehead.). Occiput feels numb and stiff.

Heart attack, aching pain. Acute heart attacks with sharp, stabbing, burning pains down the left arm (Lat-m.), or it feels as if a hot, red, burning knife is stuck into the heart and turned. The heart feels as if squeezed or compressed, sense of suffocation. Palpitation as if the whole chest will shake. Violent palpitation, can hear or see the heart beating. Irregular heartbeat. Left-sided angina.

Suffocative attacks, can become anguished, think they are going to die. Chest pain, worse during deep breathing (Bry.). The movement of the rib cage aggravates. Stitching pains synchronous with the pulse. Heart disorders from rheumatism. Rheumatism.

Abdominal ailments with worms. Masses of lumbrici have been expelled and also threadworms. Itching of anus and nose, colic and borborygmus. Fetid breath and fetid flatus.

In one prover, the accustomed evening smoke caused violent toothache. Clarke cured a case of cardiac neuralgia caused by tobacco. He saw cardiac murmurs appearing in acute rheumatism disappear under Spig.

Hochecker related the case of Miss O., 27, who was blonde, tall, and robust, and had neuralgia for several weeks without traceable cause. Pains came suddenly, twitching and tearing of left side of face, now in ear, then in lower jaw, particularly worse by mastication. Whenever the pains were about to commence a diarrhea set in. A single powder of Spig. 6c cured.

Hochecker also cured with Spig. 3c, 6c, 10c and 20c a case of tic douloureux of the right side that had lasted fifteen months. In this case, each lower potency, after first relieving, caused an aggravation. So the potencies were successively raised. Spig. 20c completed the cure. This patient had dark hair and dark complexion. She attributed her trouble to taking cold in a draft when heated by dancing.

A patient Clarke successfully treated for a serious heart affection with Spig. 3c said that under the treatment he had lost a pain in the right knee that he had for eighteen months and which he had not mentioned at first. The pain was as if dislocated, unable to rise from kneeling, could not find an easy position often for hours at night.

Clarke found it especially useful in heart cases where constipation has been a troublesome complication.

Hering gave this case, "Helminthiasis: dilated pupils, strabismus, putrid smell from mouth, itching of nose, griping pain in belly, throat inflamed, swallows often, pale redness in throat and swelling of mucus membrane, palpitation."

Meninger had a severe case of nausea during pregnancy that he cured with Spig. The only leading symptom in the case was that she was afraid of pointed things and asked her husband to take away a fork, crochet-needle, etc. Sil. has a somewhat similar symptom, but the Sil. patient hunts for pins although afraid of them.

RELATIONS - ***Antidoted by:*** Camph., Aur. (restlessness in limbs), Cocc., Puls. ***Antidote to:*** Merc., Colch. (heart). ***Compare:*** (1) Spig-m., Nux-v., Ign., Cur. (2) Acon., Cact., Cimic., (3) Arn., Spig. is a chronic Arn. (4) Cinnb. - supra-orbital pain. (5) Naja, Spong. - heart. (6) Sabad., Teucr., Cina - worm symptoms. (7) Pains, left eye, Acon. (8) Neuralgia in left eye, Ther. (9) Headaches, coming and going with sun, Nat-m., Sang., Tab. (10) Eye pains, Bell., Ciliary neuralgia, Cedr., Mez. (11) Heart pains, white stools, Dig. (12) Stitches in heart, Hep., Nat-m., Kali-c., Ars., Caust. (13) Headache begins occiput and goes to left eye, (Sang. to right, Sil. to both). (14) Tic douloureux, Thuj., Cocci-s. (15) Neuralgia with pallor (with redness, Bell.). (16) Worms, Sabad., Cina, Teucr., Scirr. (17) Worse tight clothing, Lach., sensitiveness to touch, Kali-c. ***Compatible:*** Acon. (endocarditis), Ars., Dig., Kali-c., Zinc. (heart), Iris (prosopalgia), Arn. (Carbuncle).

REFERENCES - Boericke. Clarke. Murphy. Phatak.

SPIGELIA MARYLANDICA

(Worm Grass)

PHARMACY - spig-m. Spigelia marylandica. Worm grass. N. O. Loganiaceae. Tincture of dried root. ***Historical dose:*** Tincture and all potencies.

CLINICAL - Mania. Strabismus. Vertigo.

HOMEOPATHIC - The symptoms of Spig-m. are mainly from overdosing. A state of mania was induced in a boy from large and frequent doses of a decoction of the root. Strabismus of right eye was noted in one case. On attempting to assume erect position, seized with general tremor lasting a few seconds and leaving her exhausted.

Maniacal excitement, paroxysmal laughing and crying, loud, disconnected talking, vertigo, dilated pupils, congestions. On attempting to assume erect position, seized with general tremor lasting a few seconds and leaving her exhausted.

MIND - Suddenly affected with complete mental derangement (Stram.). Countenance distorted, running and skipping. Fits of laughing and crying. Wild and incoherent talking.

Eyes - Pupils greatly dilated. Irregular movement of adductors and abductors of eyes. Strabismus of right eye. Pain in and about the eyes. Sensation of stiffness of eyelids.

Face - Wild, staring, ludicrous expression. Swelling of face and about eyes. Face flushed.

Heart - Pulse is accelerated, irregular.

Mouth - Tongue pointed and tremulous.

Skin - Hot and dry.

Sleep - Drowsiness.

Vertigo - Dizziness.

REFERENCES - Clarke.

SPILANTHES ACMELLA

(Toothache Plant)

PHARMACY - spil. Spilanthes acmella. Toothache plant. Paracress. N. O. Asteraceae. Paraguay cress. Brazil. Tincture of fresh leaves, root and flower heads. ***Historical dose:*** Tincture and all potencies.

CLINICAL - Allergies. Bacteria, infections. Candida. Colds. Dysentery. Fungal, infections. Glands, swollen. Gum, disease. Herpes. Influenza. Lyme disease. Malaria. Parasites. Ringworm. Salivation. Sore throats. Toothaches. Viral, infections. Wounds.

HERBAL - Also known as "Toothache Plant" or "Paracress," Spilanthes acmella is a flowering herb in the Asteraceae family. Its leaves and flower heads contain an analgesic agent that may be used to numb toothaches. It is native to the tropics of Brazil, though it is grown as an ornamental (and occasionally as a medicinal) in various parts of the world.

Chewing on one of the flower buds will numb your mouth and make you salivate. The leaves may be used topically to treat bacterial and fungal skin diseases such as ringworm. Leaf decoction is used as diuretic and lithotriptic. Root decoction is used as purgative. The whole plant is used in treatment of dysentery.

Useful for enhancing the immune system's resistance to infections. It stimulates wound healing, protects the individual from colds and flu. Decreases allergic symptoms. Antibacterial. Inhibits the yeast/fungal organism Candida albicans.

Indicated for swollen glands, gum disease and all manner of acute bacterial, viral and fungal infections. Herpes. Sore throats. Useful against blood parasites, particularly malarial spirochetes, either as a prophylactic or as a treatment for malarial paroxysms. Lyme disease.

Because of their high isobutylamide content, both Spilanthes and Prickly Ash have similar stimulating and therapeutic actions.

REFERENCES - Murphy.

SPIRAEA ULMARIA

(Meadow-sweet)

PHARMACY - spirae. Spiraea ulmaria. Meadow-sweet. Hardhack. Queen of the Meadows. N. O. Rosacea. Tincture of fresh root. ***Historical dose:*** Tincture and all potencies.

CLINICAL - Bites. Conscientiousness, morbid. Convulsions. Eclampsia. Epilepsy. Esophagus, stricture. Eyelids, disorders. Gleet. Hydrophobia. Prostatorrhea. Ptosis. Rabies. Urine, deposits.

HOMEOPATHIC - Bojanus proved Spiraea ulmaria, taking substantial doses. A leading symptom was the production of general and local heat. Heat in throat in esophagus, under sternum, under ensiform cartilage.

Bojanus was seized with remorse, a kind of morbid conscientiousness. Fullness and heaviness of head. Washing with cold water was very unpleasant and caused a feeling as if the head were too large.

A scurfy condition of eyelids and heaviness of lids after afternoon sleep were noted. The urine was turbid as if mixed with clay and deposited red sand, had an oily film on the surface.

The burning in esophagus was better by eating and drinking but not by empty swallowing. Burning and pressure in esophagus, feels contracted but not made worse by swallowing.

Relieves irritation of the urinary passages influences the prostate gland. Checks gleet and prostatorrhea. Bites of mad animals. Heat in various parts.

Hansen mentioned that Spirae. was recommended in hydrophobia, epilepsy and eclampsia.

MIND - Restlessness, obliged to rise and walk about. ***Morbid conscientiousness***. Remorse over a long-past slight indiscretion. Fearful qualms of conscience. Loathing of himself. Hydrophobia.

Abdomen - Sensation of heaviness in the lower part of the abdomen. Very offensive flatus. Odorless flatus.

Bladder - Burning in the urethra while urinating.

Eyes - Sclera is bright red. Sensation as if something hot in the eyes. Eyes filled with mucus. Lachrymation with smarting and increased sensation of warmth. Indistinct vision, as through a mist, relieved by blinking and rubbing the eyes. Heaviness of the eyelids with headache.

Face - Redness of the face. Sensation of heat in the face and eyes.

Head - Headache on shaking the head. Pulsations. Dullness and heaviness in the head. Pain as if a ring were tightened about the head. Sensation as if the brain wobbled to and fro.

Food - Hunger disappeared. No relish for smoking.

Limbs - Heaviness in all the limbs.

Lungs - Dry cough. Cold feeling in lungs on inspiration.

Male - In the morning, in bed, violent erections, with great sexual desire.

Modalities - Better moving about. Better in open air. ***Worse left side.*** Worse indoors. Worse moving head, sneezing.

Mouth - Drawing pain. Toothache in back teeth.

Rectum - Sensation as if drawn rectum inward. Sensation as if the anus would not open sufficiently. Prickling constrictive sensation in the anus. Crawling and prickling in the rectum. Frequent desire for stool, that suddenly disappeared. Hard stool. Feces lumpy, like balls of rabbit's dung, without being hard.

Sleep - Overpowering sleepiness. Restless sleep, frequent waking and tossing about. Sleep full of vivid dreams. Lascivious dreams and emission.

Stomach - Cold sensation in the esophagus. Burning pressure in the esophagus, better belching. Heartburn. Frequent eructations of odorless gas.

Throat - Sensation of increased warmth in the pharynx.

Urine - Urine turbid. Bright lemon yellow urine, almost straw-colored. Cloudy urine with an iridescent film. Looks like red sand, brick-dust powder.

RELATIONS - ***Compare:*** (1) Salicylic acid is in Spirae. (2) Bell.

REFERENCES - Allen. Boericke. Clarke.

SPIRANTHES AUTUMNALIS

(Lady's Tresses)

PHARMACY - spira. Spiranthes autumnalis. Lady's tresses. N. O. Orchidaceae. Tincture of the root. ***Historical dose:*** Tincture and all potencies.

CLINICAL - Acidity. Belching. Breasts, painful. Breath, putrid. Burns. Colic. Coryza. Dyspareunia. Eczema. Hysteria. Jaundice. Kidneys, pain. Lumbago. Milk, excessive. Nausea. Nosebleed. Rash. Rheumatism. Skin, disorders. Toothache. Vision, dimness. Vomiting.

HERBAL - The Treasury of Botany reported that the genus to which this orchid belongs received its name from the spiral arrangement of flowers. Spiranthes is an anti-phlogistic remedy akin to Acon. Its symptoms showing congestion and inflammation. The tuberous roots of Spira. were formerly esteemed as an aphrodisiac.

HOMEOPATHIC - Spira. has been used for milk-flow in nursing women, lumbago and rheumatism. Pulsations in arteries over whole body. Acidity and burning in esophagus with eructation. Colic with drowsiness and spasmodic yawning. Appears intoxicated. Lies on left side rather than right.

MIND - Melancholy. Complaining and sobbing. Ill-humor. Confusion of ideas. Indolence and boredom. Worse from mental effort. The least emotion or excitement causes palpitations.

Abdomen - Intermittent pressure in umbilical region. Pain, weakness, tympanites after a meal. Borborygmi. Desire to tighten clothes. Piercing, sharp insupportable pain in colon, on becoming erect. Laughing heat in lower abdomen. Eruption in groin.

Back - Cramp-like pain in neck at night compelling change of position. Lumbago preventing walking. Pain in center of scapula. Pain in scapula, when standing, worse walking.

Bladder - Bladder, pain on urinating, pain and burning after waking. Urine, abundant, scanty, decomposes rapidly. Urine, deposits a gelatinous red sediment.

Breasts - Pain in breast on raising it. Burning on tips of breasts, especially the left. Milk abundant, more in left breast.

Chest - Sensation of weakness of lungs. Sensation of dilatation of left lung. Pleuritic and intercostal pains, worse left side.

Ears - Pain in left auditory canal. Itching in ear, externally and internally.

Eyes - Eyes brilliant, fixed. Pain in eyes on looking up. Burning in eyes with lachrymation. Eyes hot inflamed. Vision dim, obscured with sleepiness instantaneously lost, objects at a distance seem to move, on closing lids, sees wheels of fire. Lids swollen. Heaviness of brows.

Face - Swollen, red and hot, black, pale. Fixed, meditative expression. Burning in upper lip. Chin is red with pain. Burning itching in left cheek near mouth.

Female - Pressing pain in uterus. Dryness of vagina. Itching, red vulva and burning in vagina. Burning pain in vagina during sex. Bloody discharge from vagina. Yellowish leucorrhea.

Food - Loss of appetite. Desire for acid, sour foods. Constant thirst.

Head - Brain troubles, worse bending or raising arm. Heaviness and heat in brain. Sensation of band tied about head. Weight on forehead. Pain in forehead and nasal bone. Pain in roots of hair. Hair falls out.

Heart - Pain in heart. Palpitations with difficult respiration from least emotional excitement. Pulse full and hard at beginning of proving afterwards small and quiet.

Kidneys - Cramp-like pain at night in kidneys, obliging change of position. Burning pain preventing stooping, worse going up stairs, better lying on back, coldness and heat.

Limbs - Trembling in limbs, weakness. Sciatic pain, especially right side. Pain in shoulders. Swelling of veins of hands. Pain in all articulation of hands. Coldness of feet and toes.

Liver - Pain in liver and spleen, on pressure.

Lungs - Breathing difficult, short, panting on walking. Hacking cough, caused by tickling in larynx. Dry cough at night with burning in throat.

Male - Constant erections, on waking. Great desire for or repugnance to sex. Pricking pain in cords.

Modalities - Better lying on left side, on back. Worse by touch, stooping. Worse bending or raising arm, raising breast. Rheumatism of shoulders worse when bending over. Laughing causes heat in lower abdomen.

Mouth - Putrid odor from mouth. Taste acid, sweetish like nitre, bitter in morning. Salivation with dryness of mouth. Irritation of sublingual glands. Numerous small excresences on palate, which was bloody. Gums red and burning. Sensation of coldness in teeth. Pain and elongation of teeth. Toothache only at night.

Nose - Pain in right nasal bones. Burning, itching at root of nose. Itching of right nostril. Dry coryza. Dripping of water from nose. Nosebleed in clots. Smell very acute.

Rectum - Burning and itching in anus, worse during evacuation. Stool preceded and followed by prickling and itching in anus. Diarrhea or constipation, stools sour in children.

Sensations - Sensation of a band tied around head. Sensation of a foreign body in throat. Coldness of teeth. Coldness of the affected part. Pulsation in arteries over whole body. Preference for lying on left side or else on back. Pain followed by numbness.

Skin - Dryness of skin. Jaundice. Yellow spots. Whole skin red, red in spots. Miliary rash. Eruption of red points on buttocks with itching and heat. Blisters as from a burn with purulent secretion. Pricking over whole body. Itching in axilla in pubes, scrotum, forearms at night, backs of hands.

Sleep - Incomplete yawning. Sleeping during day. Late falling to sleep in evening. Sleeplessness in infants. Starting up during sleep. Lascivious dreams with emissions.

Stomach - Epigastrium distended, intolerant of touch, painful after a meal, the pain corresponding to the pain in loins. Heat rising from stomach to head. Regurgitations. Belchings preceded by heat in lower abdomen and lancinations in colon, acid, bitter, difficult, empty. Nausea after eating. Vomiting of food right after eating.

Temperature - Alternations of cold and heat. Hands alternately hot and cold. Coldness, evening, especially of hands. Affected part colder than rest of body. Coldness of feet and toes. Heat of whole skin, flushes of heat in head, followed by sensation of cold. Flushes of heat. Fever, followed by thirst. Fever at night, sweat in morning. Hands very hot. Sweat of palms.

Throat - Globus rising from lower abdomen to esophagus. Burning in larynx. Sensation of foreign body in throat. Incessant desire to clear throat, caused by a thick mucus. Burning in pit of throat. Irritation of tonsils. Tickling in throat, provoking cough. Sensation of acidity and burning in esophagus. Incarceration of air in esophagus. Pain on swallowing.

Vertigo - Vertigo, obliged to lean head against wall, on rising from bed, worse sitting or lying.

COMMENTS - The tincture of the root was proved by Dr. Patti Chagon, Duc de Sorentino, who said of it, "The action of this drug begins with decided symptoms of inflammation of the eyes, chin, chest, which become red and hot, the whole skin is dry and hot, the hands are burning, the limbs of the feet are cold most of the time, there is a sensation of oppression and heat with palpitation and a desire to uncover.

"This condition lasted two hours and gave place to others including desire to meditate and complain, vertigo, pains in shoulders, boredom, loss of appetite.

"The last symptoms to appear are: pains in scalp, on vertex, distress in kidneys and intestinal troubles after eating. The secretions of urine and milk were first diminished afterwards increased.

"The aphrodisiac property of Spira. was shown in some of the symptoms of the proving and this bears on the increased secretion of milk. A number of symptoms appear in the lower abdomen. The globus hystericus rises from thence to esophagus. Heat in lower abdomen, preceding belchings, caused by laughing."

RELATIONS - ***Compare:*** (1) Cypr. (2) Skin and mucus membranes, Arum-t. (3) Desire for tight clothing, dryness of vagina, Nat-m. (4) Pain followed by numbness, Gnaph.

REFERENCES - Boericke. Clarke.

SPONGIA TOSTA

(Roasted Sponge)

PHARMACY - spong. Spongia tosta. Roasted sponge. Common Sponge. Porifera. Radiata. N. O. Coelenterata. Tincture of the powdered sponge after toasting. ***Historical dose:*** Tincture and all potencies.

CLINICAL - Amenorrhea. Aneurysm. Angina, pectoris. Asthma. Bronchitis. Catalepsy. Chin, disorders. Clumsiness. Colds. Constipation. ***Coughs. Croup.*** Diphtheria. Diplopia. Dyspnea. Endocarditis. Epididymitis. ***Exhaustion***. Exophthalmos. Fainting. Gland, disorders. ***Goiter, exophthalmic.*** Headache. ***Heart, hypertrophy.*** Hernia. Hyperthyroid. Jaw joint, pain. Laryngismus. Laryngitis. Lung, disorders. Myopia. ***Orchitis***. Rheumatic, fever. Rheumatism. Somnambulism. Testicles, disorders. ***Thyroid, disorders.*** Tuberculosis. Varicose, veins. ***Whooping cough.*** Worms.

HOMEOPATHIC - According to Hahnemann, toasted sponge was first mentioned as a specific for goiter by the alchemist Arnold Von Villanova in the thirteenth century, but it was generally given mixed with other substances and had fallen into disuse when Hahnemann proved it.

The virtues of Spong. have been attributed to the iodine contained in it and partially liberated by the presence of roasting. But Spong. contains many other elements besides iodine and has a distinctive action of its own.

Affects the ***heart valves***, larynx, trachea and glands, especially ductless. Useful for the symptoms of the respiratory organs, cough, croup, heart disorders and tubercular diathesis.

Keynote ***dryness of mucus membranes,*** of tongue, pharynx, larynx, and trachea. Cough is caused by dryness, hacking, crowing, ***"dry as a bone,"*** sounding like a saw being driven through a pine board. Cough is excited by talking, by ***dry, cold winds***, better by eating or drinking, swallowing, especially from warm food.

Dry, chronic, sympathetic cough of organic heart disease. Anxiety with pain in the region of heart or dyspnea. ***Hypertrophy of the heart***. The right heart is affected, with asthmatic symptoms.

Anxiety and difficult breathing, terrible sinking sensation. Dry asthma. In laryngismus, croup and asthma the patient rouses up generally after midnight with ***fear of suffocation and death***. Contraction of larynx as if suddenly grasped. The larynx is sensitive, but has not the hyperesthesia of Lach. The sputa cannot be raised, must be swallowed, swallowing relieves.

Exhaustion and heaviness of the body with slight exertion, he must lie down with orgasms of blood to chest, face etc. Feels stuffed up. Hard swelling of glands, thyroid. As if everything were shaking and moving about in goiter.

Clothes feel uncomfortable. Numbness of lower half of the body. Stiff without ability to move. Faint, when losing her breath, on raising hands above head. Worse after sleep (Lach.). Rises up in sleep as if in a great fright.

MIND - Timidity. ***Anxiety and difficult breathing.*** Fear of future. Terror. Anxiety with pain in the region of heart or dyspnea. Aggravated from excitement and thinking of symptoms. Every excitement increases the cough. ***Starting from sleep.*** Starting from trifles.

Fear of death from suffocation (Puls., Acon, Phos., Stram.), wakes frightened and anxious. Fear of dying. Anxiety about his heart, fear of heart disease. Attacks of anguish and pain with fear. Anxiety during flushes of heat.

Obstinate and improper behavior. Abusive. Quarrelsome. Tired of life. Despair during fever. Apprehension of a fatal termination of his disease. Inconsolable. Despondent about loss of sexual power. Suicidal disposition during perspiration. Weeps with dreams, whooping cough, fever, sweat.

Ill humor, crying, indifference to everything, during croup. Taciturn and discontented mood, not disposed to talk. Indifference to everything. Cheerful alternating with aversion to work. Irresistible desire to sing with excessive mirth, followed by sadness. Singing alternating with distraction.

Abdomen - Violent action of abdominal muscles during inspiration. Viscera drawn up against diaphragm. Pain in abdomen instead of menses.

Back - Neck as if a cord about. Pain in sacrum instead of menses. Cramps in the muscles of neck. Coldness in back, not better by warmth of stove.

Chest - Oppression and heat of chest with sudden weakness. Chest weak, can scarcely talk, choking on falling to sleep. Fullness and obstruction in chest. A fixed, sharp and pressive pain. Spasmodic, constrictive pains. Shootings in chest. Burning, rawness, soreness in chest.

Constitutions - Suited to blue-eyed, fair-haired patients (Iod. acts best on brunettes). Children with a fair complexion, lax fiber, swollen glands. Suited to scrofulous disorders.

Cough - ***Dry, barking, croupy*** cough, larynx sensitive to touch. Deep, resonating coughs. Foghorn coughs. ***Croup, worse during inspiration and before midnight***. Asthmatic cough. ***Cough abates after eating or drinking***, especially warm drinks. Irrepressible cough from a spot deep in chest, as if raw and sore. ***Dry, chronic, sympathetic cough of organic heart disease.*** Cough is caused by dryness, hacking, crowing, ***"dry as a bone,"*** sounding like a saw being driven through a pine board. Cough is excited by talking. Cough worse by ***dry, cold winds***, better by eating or drinking, swallowing, especially from warm food. ***Whooping cough.***

Ears - Otalgia with contractive pain. Ulceration of external ear. Boils on left ear painful to touch. Inflamed nodule in left concha. Heat, pressure in ears. Hard of hearing. Dull ringing in ears.

Eyes - Protrude, staring. Red with lachrymation and burning. Watering, gummy or mucus discharge. Diplopia, better lying down.

Face - Terrified, anxious expression. Blue lips. Pale from exercise instead of ruddy glow. Cold sweat on chin. Chin numb.

Female - Hunger and palpitations of heart before menses. Pain in sacrum before menses or instead of menses. Awakes with suffocative spells during menses (Cupr., Iod., Lach.). Amenorrhea with asthma (Puls.).

Food - Excessive thirst, ***great hunger.*** Desire for dainties, sweets aggravate.

Glands - Glands painful on pressure. ***Swelling and induration of glands***. Cervical glands swollen with tensive pain on turning head. ***Thyroid disorders.*** Hyperthyroid. Thyroid gland swollen, even with the chin. Exophthalmic goiter. Goiter with suffocative spells, worse touching neck or pressure or pains with heart.

Head - Rush of blood, bursting headache, worse forehead. Throbbing, pulsation, heaviness and fullness of head. Headache with lachrymation. Pressing headache. Sensation as if hair were standing on end, on vertex. Violent itching in scalp.

Heart - Angina pectoris, faintness and anxious sweat. ***Surging of heart into chest, as if it would force out upward***. Blood surging up to neck, head and face with closure of eyelids and tears. ***Hypertrophy of heart***, especially right, with asthmatic symptoms. Valvular insufficiency. Aneurysm of the aorta. Rheumatic endocarditis. Pulse frequent, hard, full or feeble. Rapid and violent palpitations with dyspnea, cannot lie down, feels best resting in horizontal position. ***Awakened suddenly after midnight with pain and suffocation,*** flushed, hot and frightened to death (Acon.). Dry, chronic sympathetic cough of organic heart disease (Naja.).

Limbs - Fingers numb. Numbness of lower half of the body. Thighs, numb and cold. Pain in the knees, when rising from kneeling. Thickening of joints after rheumatic fever.

Lungs - ***Great dryness of all air-passages.*** Noisy, whistling inspiration on falling to sleep. ***Suffocation,*** as from a plug, valve or leaf. Anxious, gasping breathing. As if breathing through a dry sponge. Respiration short, panting, difficult. Asthma, must throw head back, worse full moon. ***Croup, worse during inspiration and before midnight***. Bronchial catarrh with wheezing, asthmatic cough, worse cold air with profuse expectoration and suffocation.

Male - Screwing, squeezing or stitches up into cord and testes. ***Orchitis***. Testes hard and swollen. ***Swelling of spermatic cord and testicles*** with pain and tenderness. Epididymitis. Fistulous opening in scrotum with little, thick, white discharge. Genitals hot.

Modalities - Better descending. Better lying with head low, resting in horizontal position. Better eating or drinking warm food or drink. Frosty weather helps the cough. ***Worse from dry, cold, wind***. Worse warm room. Worse from sweets. Worse from exertion, motion, walking, stooping, rising, raising arms, ascending. Worse talking, singing. Worse touch, pressure. Worse lying on the right side. Worse at night, before midnight, full moon, after sleep.

Mouth - Sweetish taste. Salivation. Tongue dry and brown. Mouth and edge of tongue covered with vesicles. Burning pain. Speech difficult.

Nose - Nose pinched, cold. Chronic dryness. Dry, nasal catarrh. Dry coryza, nose feels stuffed up. Fluent coryza, alternating with stoppage. Nostrils wide open, fan like motion.

Rectum - Hard and retarded evacuations. Loose, whitish evacuations. Tenesmus in the anus during the evacuation. Itching, smarting and pain as from excoriation in anus. Passage of ascarides from rectum and tingling in rectum. Diarrhea with ascarides.

Sensations - As if head would fall to one side. As if tipsy. As if skull would burst. As if hair were standing on end. Eyes as if twisted around. As if a battery of guns were discharged in ears. Stitches as if passing through tympanum. As if skin of neck were compressed between fingers. As if air were passing up and down thyroid and cervical glands.

Skin - Sensitive to touch. Biting, itching of the whole body. Red, itching blotches. Herpes. Ringworm. Ulcers with scanty discharge. Erysipelas, erythema. Pricking, itching during fever. Measles. Itching in swollen glands.

Sleep - Sleeplessness with fantastic dreams and delirium on going to sleep. Generally worse after sleep or sleeps into an aggravation (Lach.). ***Awakes in a fright and feels as if suffocating*** with terror and fear. ***Starting from sleep.*** Sad, anxious, frightful dreams. Somnambulism.

Stomach - Cannot bear tight clothing. Stomach feels flaccid as if standing open. Chill in pit of stomach. Sour regurgitations. Frequent hiccough. Nausea with acidity in mouth. Vomiting after having partaken of milk.

Temperature - ***Attacks of heat with anxiety***. Heat, redness of face, perspiration. Heat in flushes with anxiety, cardiac pain, would rather die, with cold moist thighs, worse thinking of it. Heat and sudden weakness after walking in open air, must lie down.

Throat - Burning and stinging. Stitches and dryness. Bitter taste. ***Sensation as if plug in larynx***. Diphtheria. Larynx, painful, dry, constricted worse touch, singing, talking or swallowing, he grasps it. Laryngeal tuberculosis. Sore throat, worse eating sweet things. Clears throat constantly. Throat symptoms better lying on back. Swallows water in small quantity and with difficulty. Numb externally. ***Hoarseness*** with many complaints, cough, coryza. Voice gives way when singing or talking.

Vertigo - Vertigo with giddiness to such an extent as to fall. Vertigo with a sensation as if head were about to fall on one side. Vertigo with nausea, on waking at night.

COMMENTS - The action of Spong. on the respiratory organs is closely connected with its action on the glandular system, the lymphatics. The thyroid and testes are indurated. The blood, heart and veins are also involved and, with the protruding eyes, a perfect picture of exophthalmic goiter is produced.

Tuberculosis of the larynx. Tuberculosis of apices, with commencing solidification, tubercles spreading downwards. Tuberculosis of the lungs with weakness of the voice and a chronic, dry, hacking cough. Congestion of chest coming on when the patient is moving about, with sudden weakness as if he would fall. Croup (Acon., Hep., Samb., Brom., and Iod.), of the larynx. Croupy deposits on the valves of the heart.

Chronic bronchitis with a deep, resonating cough, especially in the elderly, worse excitement or exertion, with constant dryness, hacking. Must sit up and lean forward. Respiratory symptoms in excited children. Dry asthma with asthmatic cough, wheezing and whistling. Laryngitis with change of voice, the throat feels plugged up, like the larynx was grabbed.

Rapid and suffocative breathing with a deep, resonating cough. Slow and deep breathing. Paralyzed with dryness and constriction, must breathe slowly. Sensation of a sponge in the throat, as though they had to breathe through a sponge. Wakes up at night suffocating (Acon., Lach.), with dryness. Fear of suffocation.

General dryness of the mucus membranes (Bry., Alum., Nux-m.). Suffocating, constricting dryness. Dry nasal passages with dry cough, worse in a cold, dry wind (Acon.). Chronic sore throat, especially with swollen glands and cough. Dry, hacking coughs (Bry., Rumx.). Deep, resonating coughs. Foghorn coughs with a shrill at the end, peaks at the end. Burning and rawness in the chest with the coughing. As though the chest would burst because of all the coughing.

Cough is worse in cold, dry weather, wind, warm and stuffy rooms. Cough worse from exertion. Tobacco aggravates the cough. Worse lying down and with head lowered. Talking aggravates, can't talk during attacks. Desires warm fluids.

Hypertrophy of the heart with asthma. Sensation as though the heart will burst.

In a heart attack the heart feels bigger and bigger (Cact. feels smaller and smaller.). Constriction of the chest and the heart (Cact.). Stinging, pressing pain in the heart with violent gasping.

Excitement of the nerves, tendency to start, twitching of muscles with fever. Stiff, without ability to move. "Conscious but unable to act on her limbs" as in a cataleptic state. Clumsiness of the body. Faint when losing breath. Feeling of numbness of lower half of body.

Thyroid problems (Calc-i., Fuc., Sep., Nat-m., Thyr.). Hyperthyroid. Goiter. Exophthalmic goiter, protruding eyes, staring, headaches and enlarged thyroid. Keynote sensation of something alive in the goiter, as if something moving there. Swollen and hard glands, causes difficulty in breathing, suffocative dryness. There may be tingling or shooting pain in the thyroid.

Testicular problems. Metastasis of mumps to the testes (Puls., Carb-v.), or to the breast. Hard, swollen, indurated testicles. Pressing, squeezing or sharp pains in the testicles. The testicles are swollen and very painful (Clem., Aur., and Puls.). Orchitis, with heaviness and screw-like squeezing pain in cord and testicles. Orchitis from suppressed gonorrhea (Thuj.).

Chill usually commences across the back, cannot be warmed. Chill, followed by heat, extendiung over the whole body except the thighs, which remain numb and chilly. Frequent flashes of heat. Skin is hot and dry. Etiology of exposure to cold, dry wind (Acon.), but takes a day or so to come out.

Worse after sleep, or sleeps into the aggravation (Lach.). Worse when thinking of the symptoms (Ox-ac.). Aversion to tobacco and aggravated from it. Problems may start on the right and go to the left.

Kent gave the indication "Rheumatic fever after having been over-heated with arising heart complications."

Nash gave the keynote of Spong. in valvular diseases, "Awakes out of sleep from a sense of suffocation with violent, loud cough, great alarm, agitation, anxiety and difficult respiration." Nash said it is better than Lach., and relieves the "dry, chronic, sympathetic cough of organic heart disease" more frequently and more permanently than Naja. Psor. also meets thickening of joints after rheumatic fever.

Boenninghausen's croup powders consisted of a sequence of Acon., Spong., and Hep., given in that order. Spong. is dry, Hep. rattling, Spong. worse before midnight, Hep. worse after midnight.

RELATIONS - ***Antidoted by:*** Camph. ***Compare:*** (1) Acon., Hep., Brom. (2) Iod. - goiter. Hep. (3) Lach., Merc., Prot. (4) Laryngitis, Samb., Lach. (5) Cough better by eating, Anac. (6) Dry tongue, Nux-m. (7) Better warm drinks, Ars., Alum., Lyc., Nux-v. (8) Heart, Naja, Sep., Kalm., Lach. (9) Orchitis, Gels., Puls., Ham. (10) Jaw-joint as if dislocated, Rhus-t. (11) Worse thinking of symptoms, Ox-ac., Pip-m. (12) Tubercular diathesis, Bac., Tub., Dros. ***Follows well:*** Acon., Hep. ***Followed well by:*** Brom., Carb-v.

REFERENCES - Boericke. Clarke. Murphy. Phatak.

SQUILLA MARITIMA

(Sea Onion)

PHARMACY - squil. Squilla maritima. Sea onion. Squill. N. O. Liliaceae. Red variety. Hyacinthaceae. Tincture of fresh bulb. ***Historical dose:*** Tincture and all potencies.

CLINICAL - Angina, pectoris. Ascites. Asthma. Bright's, disease. ***Bronchitis. Broncho-pneumonia.*** Conjunctivitis, phlyctenular. Coryza. ***Cough, catarrhal.*** Diabetes, insipidus. Dropsy, splenic. ***Dyspnea***. Eyes, disorders. Fidgets. Heart, palpitations. Hydrothorax. ***Lungs, disorders.*** Measles. ***Pleurisy. Pneumonia.*** Spleen, disorders. Toothaches. Urine, excessive. Whooping cough. Worms.

HERBAL - Squilla maritima grows on the shores of the Mediterranean Sea and has had a place in medicine from the most ancient time. The genus Squilla is distinguished from Allium by having the flowers inserted one above the other on the scape, and from Ornithogalum by having the petals deciduous.

Green's Herbal noted that Squil. promotes expectoration and urine in large doses, vomiting and purging. "Its cardiac action is exactly the same as that of Digitalis." An old rule runs "Put squills in every cough-mixture."

Mile recorded "Diuretic, expectorant, emetic, cathartic and a narcotic-acrid poison in large doses it produces inflammation of the alimentary and urinary canals and a dose of 24 grains has proved fatal."

According to Hamilton, Avicenna employed Squil. "in complaints of the gums in inveterate coughs in diseases of the spleen in dropsy and jaundice and forbids its use in ulceration of the viscera," the last caution also being mentioned by Celsus.

HOMEOPATHIC - Cooper noted that Squil., if much handled, irritates the skin, and in large doses excites nausea, strangury, bloody urine and hemorrhoids. Fatal inflammation, gangrene of stomach and bowels in small doses. The continuous use of squills seems to cause teeth and gums to ache.

The reputation of Squil. as a splenic was revived by Rademacher, whom Burnett quoted, "I have found it quickly and surely helpful in painful spleen diseases disorders painful and beyond any doubt in and of the spleen. In those dull pains on the border of the left hypochondriac and epigastric regions, there being no signs of any liver affection, I have used Squil. as a remedy with advantage."

Rademacher also mentioned as cured by Squil. those so-called ***"stomach pains"*** that are made much better by lying on the left side and probably in reality splenic, one case of asthma from a splenic affection with nocturnal exacerbation, and possibly splenic dropsy.

Burnett improved on Rademacher's teachings and applied Squil. successfully in cases of spleen-cough. Hahnemann's proving brought out many symptoms, apparently arising from the spleen, notably stitches under the free ribs of the left side.

Squil. affects the serous and mucus membranes of the respiratory and digestive tract and acts also on the kidneys, heart and spleen. Slow acting, useful for those condition which require several days to reach their maximum. Persistent, dull, rheumatic pains throughout the body.

A ***spleen remedy***, stitches under left free ribs. Heart and kidney ailments. ***Broncho-pneumonia.*** Valuable in chronic bronchitis of old people with mucus rales, dyspnea and scanty urine.

Exudations and profuse secretions. Dropsy with profuse urine. Gurglings. Cardio-urinary effects. Action is like Dig.; follows Dig. when it fails to relieve dropsical conditions.

MIND - Great anxiety of the mind. Angry about trifles. Malicious. Haughty. Aversion to mental and bodily labor. Inclination to sit, aversion to bed. Confusion after sleeping, on walking. Delirium after hemorrhage. Fear of death.

Abdomen - Painful diseases of the spleen. Aching in hypochondria. Cutting pain in abdomen. Rumbling and gurgling in paroxysms above pubic region, better eating. Bubbling sensation in muscles of right side. Frequent discharge of fetid flatulence. Ascites with scanty urine.

Back - Stiffness of nape of neck. Bubbling beneath scapula. Painful jerking above left scapula. Drawing in left scapula.

Chest - Stitches in chest. Perspiration in armpit.

Ears - Tearing behind left ear. Tearing pains in both ears.

Eyes - Left eye looks much smaller than right. Child rubs eyes and face much, as if to relieve itching in brain affectations, measles. As if swimming in cold water. Tears with cough. Staring look, eyes wide open.

Face - Changeable expression and color of face. Distorted countenance. Child rubs the face with fist during cough. Lips twitch and are covered with yellow crusts. Humid, spreading eruption on upper lip. Black, cracked lips and black teeth.

Female - Atony of the cervix, uterus. Hemorrhage from uterus.

Food - Insatiable appetite. Longing for acids. The food tastes bitter, especially bread. Tastes sweet, especially soup and meat.

Tastelessness of tobacco when smoked. Thirst for cold drinks. Drinks in sips during dyspnea.

Head - Stinging headache. Headache in morning on waking, with pressing pains. Painful sensitiveness of vertex every morning. Pulsation in head when raising it.

Heart - A cardiac stimulant affecting the peripheral vessels and coronary arteries. Pulse small and slow, slightly hard.

Kidneys - Great urging, ***much watery urine*. *involuntary*** spurting of urine when coughing (Caust., Puls.). Frequent calls to urinate at night, passing large quantities (Ph-ac.). Bloody urine. Feces escape when urinating.

Limbs - Hands and feet cold, body hot (Meny.). Feet get sore from standing. Nails become brittle and split.

Lungs - Wheezing. Splenic asthma. ***Dyspnea and stitches in chest*** and painful contraction of abdominal muscles. Sneezing, throat irritated, short, dry cough, must take a deep breath. Pleurisy. Bronchopneumonia. Fluent coryza, margins of nostrils feel sore. ***Sneezing with coughing.*** Cough, stubborn, dry, rattling, disturbs sleep. ***Child rubs face with fist during cough*** (Caust., Puls.). ***Violent***, exhausting cough with much mucus, with ***involuntary spurting of urine and sneezing.*** Expectoration, easy, heavy, difficult in small round balls of sweetish taste, white or reddish offensive. Profuse, salty, and a slimy expectoration. Cough provoked by taking a deep breath or cold drinks from exertion. Cough changes from warm to cold air. Cough of measles.

Male - Erotic pollutions. Dull stitches in glans causing anxiety. Compressive pain in testicles.

Modalities - Better from rest, lying down in bed, sitting up, wrapping warmly. Better expectoration even a small quantity. Worse early morning. Worse motion, exertion, ascending. Worse inspiration, coughing, cold air, uncovering. Drinking cold water causes cough.

Mouth - Taste, sweet of food, especially soup and meat. Bitter taste to bread. Increased saliva. Open, dry mouth. Scraping, burning on palate. Vesicles on tongue. Black spots on teeth.

Nose - Violent sneezing with fluent acrid coryza. Sneezing during cough. Copious running worse in morning. Coryza with ulcerated nostrils. Humid eruptions under nose with itching.

Rectum - Stitches in anus when walking. Itching in anus. Painless constipation. Stools dark, brown, frothy, very offensive. Diarrhea, stool very offensive, watery. Passes thread worms and white tissues with tenesmus.

Sensations - Prominent stitches, in teeth, in chest, in head. Eyes as if swimming in cold water. Nostrils as if sore. As if chest too tight. Tickling creeping in chest. As if intestines would burst through abdomen. As if diarrhea would set in.

Skin - Handling the fresh squills caused blisters. Eruptions like itch, with burning-itching. Small red spots all over the body with pricking pain. Soreness in the bends of the joints. Hard swellings. Gangrene.

Sleep - Frequent yawning without sleepiness. Restless sleep, with much tossing about. Dreamed that his body was excessively swollen.

Stomach - Pressure in stomach as from a stone. Stomach pains are better lying on left side. Constant nausea in pit of stomach. Nausea during the morning cough.

Temperature - Chill internally at night with external heat. Heat with aversion to uncover. Heat, dry, burning, internally predominates. Whenever he uncovers himself during the fever he suffers from chilliness and pain. Perspiration wanting, even during the violent burning heat.

Throat - Dryness in throat. Burning in mouth and throat. Irritation in throat causing constant cough. Pain in submaxillary glands.

Vertigo - Vertigo in the morning with nausea. Vertigo as if he would fall sideways on rising from bed. Cloudy dizziness.

COMMENTS - Burnett used the Acetum Squil. and Clarke gave this (five drops of in water three times a day) with excellent effect in the case of an elderly woman, very gouty, who had a distressing paroxysmal cough with a pain extending from splenic region into the throat. The cough caused sneezing, flow of tears, spurting of urine and even involuntary stools.

The kidneys are acted on by Squil. and many of the traditional uses of the drug have been with the idea of eliminating dropsical effusions by reproducing a great flow of urine. Hahnemann pointed out that the excessive flow of urine accompanying dropsy and other complaints was one of the best indications for its use.

Boger added the heart to the organs primarily affected by Squil. He gave three cases. Mr. B. suffered from angina pectoris, forcible cardiac contractions, profuse urine, much loose mucus in throat and trachea, heart pain indefinite but very severe. Squil. 30c relieved in a few hours and kept him free from an attack for three months.

Miss L., pleuro-pneumonia, pulse 132, temperature 103 F, respiration 30, must sit erect in bed. Stitching pains in left chest, constant hacking cough. Frequent, hot, scanty urine, great weakness and anorexia. Squil. 100,000c cured.

A boy, 7, hay fever for third year in succession. Teeth show black marks, constantly rubs eyes and sneezes, bloated about eyes and face, loose cough. Under Squil. there was complete relief in two days and no further trouble that season.

Boger mentioned that Lippe noted "black teeth" as a symptom of Squil. Boger added that the nails become brittle and split and that veterinarians use Squil. for cracked hoof in horses.

The use of Squil. as an "expectorant" depends on its power of producing free secretion from the respiratory mucus membranes; in homeopathy this free secretion is one of the leading indications.

Hering said Squil. is suited to the pleurisy and pneumonia that follow blood-letting.

RELATIONS - ***Antidoted by:*** Camph. ***Compare:*** (1) Headache, worse motion, chest symptoms, Bry. (2) Bry. cough is worse change to warm, Squil. cough worse change to cold air. (3) Stitches, swollen upper eyelids, Kali-c. (4) Cold drink causes or worse cough, Lyc., Sil. (better by cough, Caust.). (5) Expectoration sweetish and offensive, Calc., Stann. (6) Spurting of urine when coughing, Caust., Alum., Con., Nat-m., Puls. (7) Dig., Stroph., Apoc., Bry., Kali-c. ***Compatible after:*** Bry. Squil. follows Dig., if this fails to relieve water-logged cases.

REFERENCES - Boericke. Clarke. Phatak.

STACHYS BETONICA

(Wood Betony)

PHARMACY - stach. Stachys betonica. Wood betony. N. O. Labiate. Tincture of whole fresh plant. ***Historical dose:*** Tincture and all potencies.

CLINICAL - Belching. Colds. Diaphragm, paralysis. Headaches. Vertigo.

HOMEOPATHIC - Berridge published the proving of Stach. made by Croker and himself with some others. Pains in various parts, dizziness, fullness in head and eyes with disposition to take cold.

Tired, especially in legs. Great sensitiveness to take cold. A feeling of oppressed breathing as from paralysis of diaphragm. Stach. has been used in eye-waters and as a remedy for headaches.

MIND - Inability to concentrate mind. Distracted easily. Mental dullness.

Abdomen - Pains in abdomen, hepatic region and of transverse colon, also in gallbladder and right inguinal region and spermatic cords.

Ears - Slight earache.

Eyes - Heavy, sleepy feeling in eyes. Pain in eyeballs as if too tense, worse looking at light, reading, thinking, bending head down.

Head - Stitches in right temple. Fullness over and in eyes as if they would burst. Dull, heavy action in frontal region better walking about in room.

Kidneys - Woke with desire to urinate in night. Urine high-colored, ammoniacal.

Limbs - Shooting pain in back of both wrist joints. Wrist drops. Pain in right popliteal space down leg, which feels paralyzed.

Liver - Pains in hepatic region and gallbladder.

Lungs - Breathing oppressed as from paralysis of diaphragm, constriction just behind ensiform cartilage, on walking up hill must keep mouth open.

Nose - Frequent sneezing, increased nasal mucus on going indoors from open air.

Stomach - Warmth in stomach increasing to sharp cutting pain. Weight in stomach with feeling of sickness. Belchings, tasting of drug.

Temperature - Free perspiration. In night profuse sweat, limited to head, neck and chest.

Vertigo - Dizziness better open air, worse closing eyes or moving head.

RELATIONS - ***Compare:*** (6) Lycps. and the Labiate.

REFERENCES - Boericke. Clarke.

STANNUM IODATUM

(Tin Iodide)

PHARMACY - stann-i. Stannum iodatum. Tin iodide. Trituration. ***Historical dose:*** All potencies.

CLINICAL - ***Coughs.*** Lung, disorders. ***Tuberculosis.***

HOMEOPATHIC - Stann-i. is valuable in chronic chest diseases characterized by tissue changes, with persistent inclination to cough. It is indicated in cases that ***'hang fire'*** and need an alternative.

Stann-i. has been used in preference to Stann. in some tubercular cases in which the general features of Stann. were present.

Persistent inclination to cough, excited by tickling dry spot in the throat, apparently at root of tongue. Dryness of throat. Tracheal and bronchial irritation of smokers. Pulmonary symptoms, cough, loud, hollow, ending with expectoration (Phel.). Purulent infiltration.

Stonham noted that in ***advanced tuberculosis*** when Stann-i. has not taken effect, an additional dose of iodine in milk caused the drug to have its usual beneficial effect.

Chest - Feeling of dryness, weakness in chest and throat and increased oppression.

Lungs - Persistent cough, excited by tickling, dry spot in the throat. Cough beginning with a weak sounding cough with short breath, soon gathers strength and sound. Coughs up a copious, pale yellowish expectoration. Consolidation in middle of right lung.

COMMENTS - O. S. Haines considered Stann-i. especially indicated where the patient "has a clear complexion and long eyelashes and where the progress of the disease is rapid." He used the 2x trituration.

M. D. Youngman found it a deeply acting drug, chiefly of value in chronic chest diseases characterized by plastic tissue changes. Stann-i. is indicated in cases that "hang fire" and need an "alterative."

Youngman gave the keynote, "A persistent inclination to cough. Cough excited by a tickling dry spot in the throat, sometimes in one place, sometimes in another often apparently at root of tongue."

This cough, which begins as a weak-sounding cough, accompanied by shortness of breath. The cough soon gathers strength and sound and induces raising of a free, copious, pale yellowish expectoration, which at first aggravates. But is soon followed by a feeling of dryness, weakness in throat and chest and increased oppression.

An inveterate smoker, who had a cough of this kind, said it came from his throat and ascribed it to his smoking. Youngman found consolidation areas in the middle of the right lung. There was weak feeling in chest after coughing.

Stann-i. 3x trituration. greatly relieved. The man was sent to a high altitude, where he enjoyed perfect health and was freed from his smoking habit.

REFERENCES - Clarke.

STANNUM METALLICUM

(Tin Metal)

PHARMACY - stann. Stannum metallicum. Tin metal. (Sn, At. Wt. 118.102). Trituration of the pure metal. ***Historical dose:*** All potencies.

CLINICAL - Anemia. Asthma. ***Bronchitis***. ***Chest, weakness.*** Chilblains. Colic. Convulsions. Cramps. ***Debility.*** Dentition. Diaphragm, pains. Dyspepsia. Ears, ulceration. Epilepsy. Gastralgia. Hematemesis. Hemoptysis. Headaches. Hectic, fever. Hemiplegia. Hypochondriasis. Hysteria. Lachrymal fistula. ***Lungs, weak.*** Milk, altered, Nails, splitting. Neuralgias. Neurasthenia. Nosebleeds. Opisthotonos. Paralysis. Ptosis. Sleeplessness. ***Sore, throat.*** Styes. Tapeworms. Trachitis. ***Tuberculosis***. Uterus, prolapsed. Vagina, prolapse. ***Voice, weak***. ***Weakness.*** Worms.

HOMEOPATHIC - Stannum is the Jupiter of the alchemists. "The ancients have recorded wonderful cures of the most serious diseases with Tin," said Hahnemann, but in his day, until he proved it, its main use was as a vermifuge. The chief action centers on the nervous system, respiratory organs, and liver.

Marked ***debility***. Debility in chronic bronchial and pulmonary conditions, characterized by profuse muco-purulent discharges upon tuberculosis basis. ***Talking causes a very weak feeling in the throat and chest.***

Extreme weakness in the chest, throat, stomach, upper arms and thighs. The patient is unable even to talk, drops into a chair instead of sitting down, trembles on moving. Weakness is felt much more on going downstairs than going up. ***Paralytic heaviness or weakness***. Paralysis from worms after spasms, emotions, onanism. Hemiplegia, part constantly moist.

Pains increase gradually and gradually subside. Pressive drawing pains. Spasms with pain in abdomen and diaphragm. Epileptic spasms with tossing of limbs, clenching of thumbs, opisthotonos, unconsciousness and sexual complications.

Cramps, hysteria. Neuralgia, diaphragmatic, suppressed.

Affections of mucus membranes produces yellow, muco-purulent secretions. Bland secretions. Emaciation. Girdle sensation with yawning. Trembling more from slow motion or exercise. Child wants to be carried across shoulders.

MIND - Depressed and hopeless with lung problems. Low spirited, despondent and without hope, feels like crying all the time, but crying aggravates. ***Anxious,*** nervous, sad, worse before menses. Miserable. ***Sad and discouraged***.

Discontented with everything. Uneasy, knows not what to do with himself. Forgetful and absent-minded. Forgetful on waking in morning. Thinking makes her feel wretched. Cannot get rid of an idea once fixed in her mind.

Taciturn and dislike to society. Dread of seeing people. Fear in a crowd. Fear of men, during pregnancy. Suspicious. Aversion to certain persons (Nat-c.). Child wants to be carried across shoulders. Very sensitive as to what others say about her. Changeable mood. Sudden fits of passion. Can't answer questions from weakness.

Abdomen - Abdomen painfully distended and sensitive to touch. Incarceration of flatus. Cutting, pinching, cramp-like colic, around navel. Colic with hunger, diarrhea and a feeling of emptiness, exhausting, ***relieved by hard pressure.*** Colic in children, better by carrying them on shoulder. Spasmodic pain in abdomen, hysterical.

Back - Stitches in back, small of back, and into limbs. Opisthotonos. Weakness of the muscles of the nape of the neck.

Breasts - A child leaves the breast of its mother and will not nurse (Sil.).

Causations - Ill effects of emotions, fright, masturbation, dentition, using voice.

Chest - Oppression of chest when coughing, with emptiness in pit of stomach. Oppression as if chest were internally constricted. Tension across upper part of chest with emptiness in lower. Weak, empty sensation in chest, is constantly obliged to stop and take a breath. ***Chest***

feels weak, can hardly talk. Chest feels raw or hollow. Aching in chest from reading aloud. Diaphragmatic neuralgia, hysterical. Soreness. Stitches in left side of chest, when breathing or lying on that side. Knife-like pains, below left axilla. Itching, tickling in chest. Sharp pains in chest and sides hinder respiration. Sharp, cutting stitches in left side of chest, worse stooping. Gnawing pain at middle of sternum.

Constitutions - Tubercular constitutions.

Cough - Cannot walk, cannot do anything without coughing. Short breath from every effort, must loosen clothes. Hemoptysis with copious expectoration. Concussive, in paroxysms of three coughs. Violent, dry cough in evening until midnight. ***Cough excited by laughing***, singing, talking. Cough worse lying on right side. Influenza cough from noon to midnight with scanty expectoration. Hoarse, mucus expelled by forcible cough. Cough during day, with copious green, sweetish expectoration, most profuse in morning. Retching with coughing.

Ears - Cracking, shrieking noise in ear when blowing nose. Tinkling, ringing in ears, particularly the left. Earache with drawing tearings. Ulceration of holes pierced for earrings.

Eyes - Sunken, dull, clouded eyes. Pupils contracted. Eyes sore. Itching, smarting and burning sensation in eyes. Great sensitiveness to light during headache. Jerking and quivering of eyes. Burning lancinations in lids. Agglutination of eyelids at night. Pustular swelling of left inner canthus. Blenorrhea. Ptosis. Styes.

Face - Face pale, sickly-looking, flushing easily on exertion. One cheek hot and red. Painful swelling of submaxillary glands. Swelling of cheeks and upper jaw. Spasm in jaw. Prosopalgia, pains increase and decrease gradually. Drawing pains in malar bones. Malar neuralgia, at menses.

Female - Strong body odor during menses. ***Menses early and profuse. Bearing-down sensation***. Gushing leucorrhea, yellow-white or transparent mucus, with much debility. Prolapse uterus and vagina, worse stools. Prolapse with ***weak, sinking feeling in stomach*** (Sep.). Uterine symptoms with a weak, drawn sensation in the chest. Pain in vagina upward and back to spine. Scratching of distant parts (of arms) produce an intolerable sensation of pleasure in genital organs producing orgasm. Increased sexual desire, early orgasm.

Food - Increased hunger, which cannot be satisfied. Increased thirst. Bitter taste of all food. Bitter, herbaceous taste of beer. ***Smell of cooking causes vomiting.*** Excessive weakness of digestion. Nausea and vomiting after a meal.

Head - Severe, painful constriction in forehead and temples. Pressive and stupefying headache. Migraine of cerebral origin, better by vomiting. Aching in temples and forehead. Pains worse motion, ***gradually increasing and decreasing***. Violent, glowing, beating pains, as if the head would burst with inward blows. Jarring of walking resounds painfully in head. Drawing pains in malar bones and orbits. Ulceration of hole in lobe of ear. Obstinate acute coryza and influenza with cough.

Heart - Pain in precordial region and hiccough. Pulse frequent and small.

Kidneys - Dull stitches inward in kidney region. Insensibility of the bladder, only the sense of fullness indicates the necessity to urinate. Atony of bladder. Retention of urine. Blister on margin of meatus.

Limbs - Paralytic weakness, drops things. Limbs suddenly ***give out when attempting to sit down***. Tremulous knees. Swelling of the hands and ankles. Spasmodic twitching of muscles of forearm and hand. Cramps in hands, cannot let go the broom. Fingers jerk when holding pen. Typist's paralysis. Contraction of fingers, retraction of thumbs. Neuritis. Aching in deltoid from reading.

Liver - Pressure and burning sensation in hepatic region. Weak liver, poor digestion. Bitter and sour taste.

Lungs - Asthma. Emphysema. Pneumonia. Bronchiectasis. Takes deep breaths. Shortness of breath on exertion. Short, oppressive respiration, stitches in left side when breathing and lying on same side. ***Lungs***

feels weak, can hardly talk. Sharp pains in lungs which hinder respiration. Much mucus in trachea. ***Copious green, sweetish*** expectoration. Easy expectoration, quantities of sweet, salty, sour, putrid or bright yellow pus or ball of mucus. ***Catarrhal tuberculosis.*** Last-stage tuberculosis remedy, used for tuberculosis epidemics. Last stages of respiratory illnesses heading toward lung failure.

Male - Increased sexual desire. Voluptuous feeling in genitals ending in emission, which exhausts. Frequent pollutions with excessive prostration.

Modalities - Pains are better walking, but must soon rest. Better by pressure, lying across something hard, bending double. Better rapid motion. Better coughing, expectorating and open air. ***Worse using voice,*** laughing, talking, singing. Worse going down stairs, ascending. Worse lying, gentle motion, touch. Worse from weakness of chest. Worse from cold, warm drinks. Worse during stool. Worse at 10 a.m.

Mouth - Sweet, sour, ***bitter taste***, for all food except water. Fetid exhalation from mouth. Flow of acid saliva. Tickling at the root of the tongue. Tongue coated with a yellowish mucus. Tongue red or yellow. Difficult, weak speech, occasioned by weakness.

Nose - Oversensitive to smells. Heaviness and sensation of obstruction. Stuffed feeling and heaviness high up in nostrils. Burning sensation in nose. Dry coryza on one side only. Obstinate coryza and influenza with cough. Nosebleed on moving, on rising from bed.

Perspiration - Heat in evening, ***exhausting night sweats***, towards the morning. Perspiration at 4 a.m. Debilitating perspiration, principally on forehead and nape of neck. Sweat smelling musty or offensive.

Rectum - Burning in anus, constant itching. Constipation. Monday constipation, occurring after working days. Frequent ineffectual want to evacuate. Hard, dry, knotty feces or else scanty and greenish. Stools are green, curdy with colic. Passes worms.

Sensations - As if all objects were too far off. As if she would faint. As if forehead were shattered. As if forehead would be pressed inward. Tickling as from soreness in trachea. Inclination to hawk as if mucus were in chest. Chest, as if eviscerated, as if internally constricted. As of a heavy load in affected arm and side of chest. Epigastric region as if beaten. As if limbs beaten. As if sweat would break out.

Skin - Itching, burning, shootings over skin of whole body. Itching pimples on face, sore to touch or on washing. Chilblains. Flaws in nails. Painful hangnails.

Sleep - Nocturnal agitation and many vivid dreams, anxious or lascivious. Moaning, weeping and plaintive lamentations while sleeping. Sleeps with one leg drawn up, the other stretched out.

Stomach - Pain better pressure, but sore to touch. Sensation of ***emptiness in stomach***. Uneasy feeling. Smell of cooking causes nausea and vomiting. Bitter taste. Vomiting, violent of blood of bile, early in the morning with odor of ingesta.

Teeth - Sensation of elongation and looseness in teeth. Toothache after a meal with jerking pain and heat in the face. Ulcer on gums with swelling of cheeks.

Temperature - Chill 10 a.m. with numb fingertips. Hectic fever. Burning palms and soles. Heat in evening, ***exhausting night sweats***, towards the morning.

Throat - Throat dry and stings. Sore throat, as from an internal swelling. Rawness in larynx. Cutting in pharynx and esophagus on swallowing. Nausea in throat. Adhesive mucus, difficult to detach, efforts to detach cause nausea. Voice deep, hollow, hoarse, better hawking mucus. ***Hoarseness with weakness of voice.*** Laryngitis.

Vertigo - Dizziness and weakness when ***descending***. Vertigo, all objects seem too far off. Vertigo on sitting down, with loss of ideas.

COMMENTS - Hahnemann's Stann. proving appears in his Materia Medica Pura and in his Chronic Diseases. A number of worm symptoms appeared, including a sinking, empty, all-gone feeling, and diaphragmatic and abdominal pains. Tendency to excessive mucus secretions. Pale, sunken, sickly countenance with dark rings around the eyes. Convulsions. Hectic fever.

Compressive and cramp-like pains. Cramps and spasms. Opisthotonic convulsions, thumbs are drawn in, particularly in teething children, in children who masturbate, or who have worms.

Pains associated with the hypochondriac or hysterical mental state. Pains begin lightly, increase gradually to the highest point and then gradually decline, particularly in headaches, facial and dental neuralgias, abdominal and other pains. Diaphragmatic neuralgia.

Characteristic weakness, exhaustion of mind and body. Nervous weakness with trembling. Neurasthenia. Depressed and hopeless with lung problems. Low spirited, despondent and without hope. Trembling of arms and legs, limbs as heavy as lead. Palpitations and anxiety occur from slightest exertion.

The chest is so weak as to make talking impossible. Weakness in the throat in singers and speakers. Weakness and aching of the deltoid and arm, felt when using the voice. The patient will drop into a chair instead of sitting down. Must sit down several times to rest while dressing in the morning. Weakness felt more going down stairs than on going up. Weak, empty, sinking sensation felt at the epigastrium.

Characteristic respiratory or lung weakness. Last-stage tuberculosis remedy, used historically tuberculosis epidemics. Last stages of respiratory illnesses heading toward lung failure. Emphysema. Pneumonia. Hoarseness, laryngitis, hollow voice.

Keynote weakness in the lungs and breathing. Patient talks extremely weakly, must put ear to patient's mouth to hear. Weak, empty feeling in the chest, in tubercular conditions. Stitches in the chest. Shortness of breath on exertion.

Deep, hollow, shattering cough (Spong.). Deep, husky, hollow voice, better by hawking or expectorating mucus. Profuse expectoration, like an egg white (Nat-m.), sweetish, salty, sour, putrid, musty, yellow-green pus. Thick globs of green sputum. Coughs up green pus and globs of green mucus (Kali-b.). Yellow secretions, including sputa, leucorrhea and coating on the tongue.

Dyspepsia, with nausea and vomiting from the smell of cooking. Stomach pain compels the patient to walk about for relief, yet the weakness is so great that he is soon compelled to rest. Colic, better by hard pressure, as by laying the child with its abdomen across the knee or on the point of the shoulder.

Menses are early and profuse. Uterine and vaginal prolapse, worse during stool, especially during pressure. Labor pains are spasmodic and put the patient out of breath. The milk of nursing woman is changed and the child rejects it.

Sexual excitement in both sexes. Emissions with excessive prostration. Orgasm is easily produced, "Scratching arm produces an intolerable sensation of pleasure in genital organs which extends to uterus and produces orgasm."

Clinique quoted a typical case of a neuralgia cured by Stann. A man, 30, suffered for eight years off and on and for some months continuously with neuralgic headache. Pain centered over one or the other eye (usually the right) and extended over whole or part of head and was at times unbearable.

It began in the early morning (4 to 5 a.m.), increased gradually to noon, when it gradually declined to sunset, reappearing again the following morning. Two doses of Stann. cured in a fortnight.

Hering gave as cured by Stann. "Monday constipation," that is, constipation occurring on days following rest-days. Stann. has marked periodicity.

T. H. Urquhart cured an affection of the nails characterized by breaking and splitting, and a sequel of scurvy, with an application of Stannum oleate on a narrow flannel bandage. All symptoms were cured in two months.

Alston obtained indirectly from "a woman of Leith in Scotland" this prescription of which he had witnessed the efficacy in a case of tapeworm:

"Take an ounce and a half of Tin, (pewter metal) and grind it small to powder, mix it with sugar syrup and take, on a Friday before the change of the moon, one-half of it, the following day the half of the remainder and the Sunday following the rest, but on the Monday a purgative."

Alston also noted in his Materia Medica that he had seen hematemesis cured by this remedy.

RELATIONS - ***Antidoted by:*** Puls., Phos. ***Compare:*** (1) Stann-i., Phos., Caust., Calc., Sil., Tub., Bac., Helon. (2) Myrt-ch. - chronic bronchitis, cough of tuberculosis, emphysema with gastric catarrh and thick, yellow difficult sputum. Old persons with weakened power of expectoration. (3) Sour sensation in stomach, Chel., Phos., Sep. (4) Weeps all the time, but crying aggravates. (5) Worse descending, can go up well enough, Bor. (6) Pain increases and decreases gradually, Plat., Stront. (7) Nausea from smell of cooking food, Ars., Colch. (8) Weak from talking, Cocc., Verat., Sulph., Calc. (9) Catarrhal tuberculosis, Sil. (10) Paralysis by emotions, Staph., Nat-m. ***Complementary:*** Puls. ***Follows well:*** Caust., Cina. ***Followed well by:*** Calc., Phos., Sel., Sulph., Bac.

REFERENCES - Boericke. Clarke. Murphy. Phatak.

STAPHYLOCOCCINUM

(Staphylococcus Nosode)

PHARMACY - staphycoc. Staphylococcinum. Staphylococcus bacteria. Nosodes. ***Historical dose:*** All potencies.

CLINICAL - ***Abscesses.*** Acne. Adenitis. Allergies. Anthrax. Aortitis. Blepharitis. ***Boils.*** Carbuncle. Cellulitis. Conjunctivitis. Dacrocystitis. Edema. Endocarditis. Empyema. Fever. Folliculitis. Furuncle. ***Impetigo.*** Kidney, disorders. Lymphadenitis. Mastitis. Mastoiditis. Meibomian cysts. Meningitis. Myelitis. Osteomyelitis. Parotiditis. Pemphigus. Phlebitis. Prostatitis. Pyelonephritis. Pyemia. Radiculitis. ***Septicemia.*** Staphylococcal, infections. Styes. Sycosis. Thrombophlebitis. Whitlow.

HOMEOPATHIC - Staphycoc. is used for diseases where the staphylococcus bacteria is the chief bacterial factor, such as acne, abscess, furuncle, empyema, impetigo, and endocarditis. Morbid conditions where the staphylococcus pyogenes aureus or albus or citreus is notably symbiotic or is the direct and chief bacterial factor.

Julian wrote that the main indications for Staphycoc. are chronic illnesses in which staphylococci are present, e.g. in boils, impetigo, blepharitis, styes, Meibomian cysts, osteomyelitis, whitlow, but possibly also in perinephritic abscess, malignant staphylococcal infections of the face, acne vulgaris, cystic acne, thrombophlebitis, and possibly also in anthrax.

Psoric and sycotic. Allergic conditions. Pre-diabetic conditions. Syndrome of acute ***septicemia.*** Oscillating fever with great chill, general condition is weakened, an enlarged spleen. Radiculitis. Myelitis. Meningitis. Abscess of the brain.

Heart - Endorcarditis. Pericarditis.

Kidneys - Pyelonephritis. Prostatitis. Acute prostatic abscess.

Limbs - Spondylitis. Osteitis. Ostemyelitis.

Lungs - Pulmonary abscesses.

Skin - Abscess. Purpura vesicles, pustular. Follicular pustule. Follicultis of the integument. Sycosis of the mustache. Adenitis of the armpits. Anthrax. Ecthyma. Panaris. Onyxis. Perionyxis.

COMMENTS - Dr. P. W. Shedd of New York noted that Staphycoc. is made from the Staph. alb. aur. citreus, a species whose variations in color are dependent upon what the plant gets as nourishment.

The attenuations of this nosode are prepared from the washings of cultures of staphylococci. While preparing this particular remedy, the maker was compelled to get out of the room several times because of a decided, though indefinite, malaise.

The odor, aroma or effluvium was ambrosia compared to the atmosphere of the dissecting room with its lumps of putrefaction, but it had much greater expulsive power, not nauseating, but sickening and chemically probably due to some of the fatty acids.

Anshutz wrote, "In the human economy the staphylococcus does best where weakness of the protective mechanism or debility due to other than bacterial agencies, e.g., overwork, worry, lack of proper food, heredity, excess, etc., is prominent."

Staphycoc. may be of value in conditions due to damage from staphylococcal toxins. Auto-immune diseases of all kinds, in which staphylococci were involved. Myocardial lesions, nephritis, hepatic lesions, connective tissue lesions and thyroid illnesses.

RELATIONS - ***Compare:*** Strept., Ars., Bapt., Sil., Pyrog.

REFERENCES - Anshutz. Boericke. Clarke.

STAPHYSAGRIA

(Stavesacre)

PHARMACY - staph. Staphysagria. Stavesacre. Delphinium staphysagria. N. O. Ranunculaceae. Southern Europe. Tincture of the dried seeds. ***Historical dose:*** All potencies.

CLINICAL - Adenoids. ***Anger, suppressed.*** Anus, itching. Backaches. Blepharitis. Bones, diseases. Cauliflower, excrescences. ***Chalazion. Colic. Colitis.*** Condylomata. Cough. ***Cystitis. Cystocele.*** Cysts. Dentition. Dysentery. ***Dyspareunia.*** Eczema. Eyes, tumors. Fistula, dentalis. Gastralgia. Glands, disorders. Hip joint, disease. ***Humiliation.*** Hypochondriasis. Impotency. Iritis. Jaw, dislocation. ***Lice.*** Lumbar, abscess. Mania. Masturbation, effects. Nausea. Neuralgias. Night-sweats. Nymphomania. Ovaries, disorders. Perspiration, offensive. Prostate, disorders. Psoas, abscess, Ranula. ***Rape.*** Rheumatism. Sciatica. Scurvy. Seasickness. Seborrhea. ***Self-abuse.*** Sexual, abuse. ***Sexual, excesses.*** Spermatic cords, disorders. Spermatorrhea. Steatoma. Stiff, neck. ***Styes. Surgery.*** Swallowing, constantly. Teeth, decay. Testicles, disorders. Tibia, pains. Tobacco, effects. Toenail, ingrown. Tonsillitis. Toothaches. Tumors. Warts. Wounds.

HERBAL - Dioscorides used the seed of Stavesacre to producing vomiting and salivation and to cure a toothache, "the origin of which application," said Hahnemann, "was evidently domestic practice."

HOMEOPATHIC - Diseases of the genito-urinary tract and skin. Acts on teeth, urinary organs, fibrous tissue of lids, tarsi, skin, glands and right deltoid.

Sphincters, lacerated and stretched. ***Lacerated tissue,*** perineum (Calen., Hyper.). ***Pains, remaining after surgery.*** Squeezing or stinging smarting pains, as if cut. Whole body painful with feeling of weakness. Compressive pains. Sensation of squeezing between stones or in a vice in intestines, testes, head. Pains that move into teeth. Pain and nervousness after extraction of teeth.

Painful swelling of glands. Exostosis. Swelling and suppuration of bones of periosteum. Hemiplegia after anger. Arthritic nodosities on joints. Stiffness and sensation of fatigue in all joints. Warts. Condylomata.

Marked nervous disorders with trembling, irritability. Ill effects of ***anger and humiliation.*** Physical and moral sexual disturbances. Provokes excesses and irregular sexual appetites. High or low sex drive. Suppressed sexual desire, tendency to fear sex because it makes them feel out of control. Deep, sexual fears.

Sexual excesses. Insomnia due to sexual fantasies. Vivid sexual fantasies at night. Headaches after sex. Guilt and depression with the headaches. A tendency to masturbation and ailments from masturbation. ***Rape or a history of sexual abuse.***

MIND - Great indignation about the things done by others or by himself, grieves about the consequences. ***Humiliation, deep guilt and shame.*** Believes he will lose his fortune, his wife will leave him. Sadness without any cause with irritability. Want of self-control. Hypochondriacal. Poor memory.

Violent ***outbursts of passion.*** Always angry. Gloomy and petulant, throws things. Peevish. Child cries for many things and refuses them when offered. ***Rape or sexual abuse.*** Dwells on sexual matters, prefers solitude. Unsatisfied sexual urge in widows. Irritable, nervous, excitable and violent.

Morbidly sensitive, the least word that seems wrong, hurts her very much. Very sensitive as to what others say about her.

Imagines insults. Special senses become irritable, cannot tolerate touch. Sensitive to odor, noise, taste. Everything is painfully sensitive. Fear of his shadow.

History of verbal, sexual or physical abuse, mortification, humiliation (Lyc., Anac., Nat-m.). History of being put down by someone, verbally or physically abusive (Lyc.). ***Ailments from shame, punishment, vexation and suppressed anger.*** Effects of reserved or ***suppressed anger***. Ill effects after scolding or punishment in children. Fears of being punished, abandoned, hurt, failing, of not being good enough, of being unlovable.

Overly nice, timid. Passive, pathological desire to please (Puls.), but anger underneath. Fears the person, but still loves them, turns them passive. Difficulty resisting others, defenseless. Feels guilty, reproach themselves. Feels trapped. ***Self-pity, resignation.***

Hurt easily. Very poor confidence, low self-esteem. Deep feelings of worthlessness (Aur.), severe depression. Manic depression. Easily offended, take things to heart (Nat-m.). Cries easily (Puls.), and worse consolation (Ign.).

Acute anger. ***Speechless when angry.*** They act out their anger in a dream or fantasy. Afraid of their anger. Tendency to suppress anger, with periodic rages, tendency to throw or break things. Grief with anger (Caust.), sense of an injustice done to them. Acute and chronic griefs, particularly over broken relationships.

Abdomen - ***Severe pain following abdominal operations*** (Calen.). Feeling of weakness in abdomen, as if it would drop, wants to hold it up. Spasmodic cutting in abdomen after eating and drinking. Swollen abdomen in children with much flatus. Incarcerated flatus, hot, smells like rotten eggs. Colic with pelvic tenesmus. Colic, pain after anger. Colic of pot-bellied children. Colic with urging to stool or urging to urinate. Dysentery in weak, ailing, pot-bellied children.

Back - ***Backache, worse in morning, before rising.*** Pain in small of the back, as after over lifting. Backache worse sex and rising from a seat. Back feels broken. Rheumatic drawing pains. Violent stitches move upward in back. Stiffness. Itching pimples on nape.

Bladder - Honeymoon cystitis, worse after sex. ***Irritable bladder in young married women***. Cystitis after too much sex. Cystitis in lying-in patients. ***Cystocele***. Pain after use of catheter. Frequent urging to urinate with scanty or profuse discharge of watery urine. Urinates in thin stream or drop by drop. ***Sensation as if a drop of urine were rolling continuously along the channel***. Burning in urethra during urination. ***Burning pain when not urinating*** (Thuj., Sabal, Ferr-pic.). ***Pain after urinating.*** Pressure upon bladder, feels as if it did not empty.

Causations - ***Ailments from shame, punishment, vexation and suppressed anger.*** Effects of suppressed or reserved anger. ***Humiliation***. ***Rape***, sexual abuse. Ailments after sex, sex excesses, masturbation. ***Surgery***, cutting wounds, injury, falls. Tobacco, mercury, dentition.

Chest - Soreness and rawness in chest on coughing. Muscles of chest as if bruised. Sticking pain in lower part of chest and diaphragm. Sticking pain, itching between costal cartilages. Tightly adherent mucus in chest. Itching, sharp pain in axilla.

Ears - Shootings in ears. Tensive stitches in left ear. Eruption behind ears. Tinkling in ears. Sensations as if wind blew into ears. Roaring in ears during headache. Ringing in ears on moving head. Impaired hearing in children from enlarged tonsils or from adenoids.

Eyes - Eyes sunken with blue rings. Dryness and pressure in eyeballs and eyelids. Lacerated or incised wounds of cornea. Bursting, burning pain in eyeballs of syphilitic iritis. Heat in eyeballs, dims spectacles. Pupils dilated. Dry eyes with lachrymation. Hot tears run from eyes on looking at sun. Margin of eyelids itch. Affections of angles of eye, particularly the inner. Blepharitis. Steatoma of upper lid. ***Chalazion*** (Platan.). Nodes on eyelids. ***Recurrent styes***. Stye doesn't suppurate and break, but remains a hard nodule.

Face - Brown and blue color of face when getting angry. Sickly, peaked, nose. Easy dislocation of jaw. Neuralgia from tooth decay, pains go into the eyes. Painful submaxillary glands, with or without swelling, abscess. Prosopalgia, pain starts from lips over face, worse mastication. Sharp, burning stitches in left cheek, which provoke scratching. Submaxillary glands painful with or without swelling.

Female - Menses irregular, late and profuse. Menses first of pale blood, then dark and clotted. Menses, regular with loss of power in limbs. Amenorrhea from indignation. Leucorrhea. ***Painful sensitiveness*** of genital organs, worse sitting down (Berb., Kreos.). Itching or sensitive vulva. Granular growths of vagina. Salpingitis. Prolapse with sinking in the abdomen, aching around the hips. Ovarian pains, going into thighs, worse pressure, sex. First sex is very painful, causing acute mental and bodily suffering. Nymphomania. Sexual desire increased, mind dwells too much on sexual subjects. Unsatisfied sexual urge in widows. ***History of rape, sexual abuse victims.***

Food - Canine hunger, even when stomach is full. Hunger before and after chill. Sleepy after eating. Thirstlessness. Food tastes bitter. Desire for bread and milk. ***Craving for tobacco,*** stimulants, wine, brandy. Desire for soup, sweets, meat. Aversion to ***milk,*** cheese, solid food. Worse meat, bread, smoking. Worse from drinking cold water. Cold drinks aggravates pain in roots and in hollow teeth.

Head - Compressive, stupefying headache, better much yawning or leaning head against something. Burning in left temple. Pressing, stinging and tearing pains. Brain feels squeezed or torn. Dullness in middle of forehead. As of a heavy load or of a round ball in forehead. Brain feels numb and occiput feels hollow. As if back of brain were made of wood and couldn't think. Dandruff. ***Head lice.*** Hair falls off from occiput and around ears. Moist, foul, eroding milk crusts, worse occiput. Itching eruption above and behind ears (Olean.). Neuralgia of scalp.

Heart - Heart feels weak. Stitching pains in heart. Trembling beating of heart. Visible palpitation, shaking the whole body. Palpitations from emotional excitement. Palpitations when listening to music.

Kidneys - Itching, needle-like stitches in region of kidneys. Constant darting pains in region of left kidney, worse cold, lying in cold bed, better heat, becoming warm in bed. Weak kidneys from sexual excesses. Nephritis. Urging and pain after urinating. Pain after lithotomy.

Limbs - Limbs feel beaten and painful. Muscles, especially of calves, feel bruised. Joints stiff. ***Crural neuralgia.*** Fine tearing or numb fingertips. Bones of fingers imperfectly developed, osteitis of fingers. Arthritic nodes on finger joints. Buttocks ache while sitting. Knees weak. Shuffling gait. Suppurating swelling in psoas muscles.

Lungs - Dyspnea with constriction. Dyspnea at close of sex or after seminal emission. Dyspnea, with oppression of chest and fear of suffocation, after becoming angry. Cough, worse cleaning teeth, eating meat or alternating with sciatica. Cough worse tobacco smoking.

Male - ***Persistent dwelling on sexual subjects, especially after self-abuse.*** Masturbation. Priapism. Seminal emissions followed by great prostration. Impotence with irritability of bladder and urethra, brought on by sexual excess. Sexual neurasthenia. Spermatorrhea with sunken features, guilty look, emissions with backache and weakness. Dyspnea, worse during or after sex. Prostate troubles. ***Prostatitis***, pain extends from anus to urethra. Chronic prostatitis in old men. Enlarged prostate and hemorrhoids. Soft humid excrescences behind corona glandis. Orchitis from mumps. Atrophy of testicles. Voluptuous itching of scrotum.

Modalities - Better at night, from rest, after breakfast. Better warmth, sex. Worse from anger, indignation, grief, mortification. Worse night, new moon, before full moon. Worse loss of fluids, onanism, sexual excesses. Worse touch, least touch on affected parts. Worse stretching parts.

Worse from lacerations. Worse cold drinks, tobacco. Worse after urinating, when not urinating.

Mouth - Salivation with pale, spongy, bleeding gums (Merc., Kreos.). Pyorrhea (Plant.). Musty taste. Thrush. Swollen submaxillary glands. Stomatitis. Canker sores with a bluish-red or yellowish bottom.

Nose - Coryza now thick, now thin, with ulcerations. Violent coryza, one nostril is stuffed up. Coryza with much sneezing and lachrymation. Coryza with nasal voice. Nasal voice from stoppage of posterior nares. Frequent sneezing without coryza. Scratching in choanae. Nose ulcerated with scabs, deep in interior.

Perspiration - Profuse, cold sweats. Perspiration smelling like rotten eggs. Perspiration with a desire to uncover. Sweats easily during day, even when sitting. Cold sweat on forehead and feet. Fetid sweat at night. Inability to sweat.

Rectum - Itching in anus, while sitting. Discharge of hot flatus during stool. Flatus hot, smells like rotten eggs. ***Constipation***. Stool hard, round, dry. Diarrhea after drinking cold water, with tenesmus. Dysentery in weak, ailing, pot-bellied children. Dysenteric stools, worse after the least food or drink. Griping and dysenteric stools after least food or drink. Stool yellowish, slimy. Stool hot, excoriating. Stool smelling like rotten eggs. Hemorrhoids with enlarged prostate, very sensitive worse by touch. Worms.

Sensations - As if stupefied. As of a round ball in forehead. As if head would burst. As if brain were compressed. As if something were loose in pit of stomach. As if chest were bruised. As if small of back were broken to pieces. As if bones would be pressed out. As if legs would go under him. As if done up after much hard work.

Skin - Skin unhealthy, doesn't heal. Biting pain and itching. Dry herpes, with scabs on joints. Dry, scurfy eruption in joints. Frequent boils. Ulcers, new growths extremely sensitive to touch, may bring on convulsions. Eczema of head, ears, face and body. Eczema with yellow, acrid moisture oozing from under the crusts. Itching eruptions, burning after scratching. ***Scratching changes location of itching***. Dry, thick scabs, itch violently. Fig-warts pedunculated (Thuj.). Arthritic nodes. Inflammation of phalanges. Night sweats. Pain that precedes shingles. Skin symptoms alternating with joint pains.

Sleep - Violent yawning and stretching bring tears to the eyes. Yawning, as if he had not slept enough. Body aches all over. Sleepy all day, awake all night. Goes to sleep late from activity of mind. Amorous dreams with emissions. Unpleasant dreams. Child wakes as from frightful dreams. Child wakes, pushes everything away and wants everybody to go out, calls for mother often.

Stomach - Canine hunger, even when stomach is full. Stomach pains after becoming angry. Sensation as if stomach were hanging down relaxed. Flabby and weak. Heartburn after indignation. Heartburn after eating, with frequent nausea and constipation. Bread causes heartburn. Bitter eructations after sour food. Bitter or salty eructations after eating meat. Frequent hiccoughs. Hiccough while smoking. Nausea and salty-bitter eructations after becoming angry. Nausea, especially after operations. Nausea from vertigo, as in seasickness.

Teeth - Teeth loose, show black streaks, better hard pressure and heat. ***Teeth black and crumbling.*** Decayed teeth exceedingly tender. Fistula dentalis. ***Teeth decay*** as soon as they erupt. Tearing pain in gums of lower incisors, and their roots when eating. ***Toothache*** if slightest food remains in cavities of hollow teeth. Violent pain goes into roots. Toothache during menses. Decay of teeth during pregnancy. Cold drinks seem to penetrate teeth, as if they were hollow. Gum painfully sore. Pyorrhea [Plan.]. Gums white, swollen, ulcerating. Gums receding. Gums bleed when pressed upon and on cleaning teeth. Caries of lower jaw, following osteitis, latter being brought about after extraction of decayed tooth. ***Dentition***, child very sensitive to mental or physical impressions.

Temperature - Predominating chilliness

and coldness, without thirst. Exercising in open air improves chills. Chills in evening, with heat in face. Ascending chills from neck over head. Chills running down back. More chills in a warm room. Intermittent fever paroxysm, consisting mostly of coldness, preceded by unnatural hunger. Tertian fever with symptoms of scurvy, constipation

Throat - Swallows continuously while talking. Constriction and pressure in throat-pit after anger, worse swallowing. ***Sharp pains flying to the ear on swallowing, especially left***. Roughness and painful soreness on talking and on swallowing. Induration and hypertrophy of tonsils, with nasal voice. Chronic tonsillitis. Scratching in throat from belching, followed by cough.

Vertigo - Vertigo when sitting, better by walking about in a circle. Vertigo turning rapidly on heels. Vertigo on stooping and turning head rapidly.

COMMENTS - J. H. Schultze, when suffering from toothache, took some of the Staphysagria seed in his mouth, but it gave him such a violent exacerbation that he thought he should go mad.

Brunton noted that the seed was called "an exterminator of vermin" by the Greeks and as such it enters into the composition of an ointment (unguentum pediculosum). This last is the only use of Staph. known to orthodox medicine.

Teste remarked that Staph., like Cocc., is used in some countries for the purpose of stupefying fish. Teste found Staph. 6c, like Cocc., useful as a remedy for seasickness. To be successful, Staph. had to be taken at the moment when dizziness and nausea commenced, before vomiting set in and it always helped "nervous persons, not over fat and disposed to sadness."

Staph. produced in Teste a "long lasting vertigo, accompanied by continued nausea as in sea-sickness" and "vertigo, which ceases on rapidly turning round on one's heel."

This corresponds with one of Hahnemann's symptoms, "wheeling vertigo, especially while sitting, better by walking about in a circle."

It is noteworthy that Staph. and Cocc. are both head remedies and both effective against head lice. Both also affect the genitals, Staph. more so, and are remedies for crab lice.

An application of one part a dilution of the tincture to four parts water will destroy the parasites, although concurrent internal treatment (probably with a dilution of the same remedy) increases success.

In Teste's experience, Staph. was no less effective in nausea during pregnancy than nausea caused by seasickness. Tab. is another remedy for sickness and Teste cured with Staph. effects of tobacco smoking (excoriated tongue, stomach pain) and the habit of "swallowing the tobacco smoke."

For anger and for the effects of anger, especially if the indignation cannot have its natural expression. "Was insulted, being too dignified to fight, swallowed his wrath and went home sick, trembling and exhausted."

Great sensitiveness to the least impression, "the least word that seems wrong, hurts her very much." Sensitive to criticism. Irritated by trifles. Sudden, violent outbreaks provoked by mere trivial causes. Want of self-control and self-confidence. Fears, afraid of his shadow.

"Apathy, weak memory, caused by sexual excesses or constantly dwelling on sexual subjects." Weak memory after multiple abortions. Inability to make decisions, spaciness.

Sycotic and syphilitic condylomata. Seed warts. Keynote styes (Puls., Thuj.), tendency to get styes. Ulcers are generally very painful and sensitive. Pressing, stinging, tearing pains in periosteum. Exostoses and gouty nodes on fingers and toes. Dry, scaly eruptions over the ends of bones. Eruptions are foul smelling when moist. "Inability to perspire." Sweat smells of rotten eggs. Chilly. Shortness of breath.

Effects of "wounds made by clean-cutting instruments." Ailments from surgery and scars (Calen.). Stab wounds.

"Teeth turn black and have dark streaks through them, cannot be kept clean, crumble: decay on edges, scorbutic cachexia." Toothache during menses, affects sound as well as decayed teeth, worse from touch of food or drink, but not from biting or chewing. Toothache worse drawing cold air into mouth, worse from cold drinks and after eating.

Extreme "sinking" sensation. The stomach and abdomen feel as if hanging down relaxed. There is extreme hunger even when the stomach is full. Ravenous hunger for days before an attack of fever.

Feels guilty and depressed, turns to food, then feels guilty about food (Puls., Ign.). Bulimia. Tendency to binge on sweets, custards, creamy things. Thirstless, worse warm stuffy rooms. Craving for tobacco, cough excited by tobacco smoke. They may like milk or be aggravated by milk.

Colic from anger. "Colic of screaming, ugly, pot-bellied children, especially if they suffer much from their teeth, which turn black with tender, spongy gums, sensitive and painful." Colitis cases, Crohn's disease, inflammations of the colon from anger. Colic, vomiting, or dysentery, all worse from least food or drink. Colic after an operation on the ovaries or intestines.

Cystitis from anger. Burning in the urethra when not urinating. Urinary difficulties after severe labors. Prolapse of bladder. Prostatitis with pain running from the anus along urethra, inflamed testicles with shooting and drawing in the cords, stitching towards groin and testicles.

Vaginismus. Vaginitis. Fibroids, ovarian cysts or tumors. In one female prover, Staph. brought on the menses a year after they had ceased, at the new moon. The symptom did not recur the following month, which led Hahnemann to conclude that this "was only the primary action of the drug."

A tendency to masturbation, ailments from masturbation. Staph. is one of Gallavardin's chief remedies for removing the habit of masturbation in children and for removing improper appetites in adults.

Worse from sex. Dyspnea occurring during or after sex, dyspnea and prostration after an emission. Genitals are sensitive, itching, stinging, stitching, shooting pain, worse by touch. In women, sex is painful because the external parts are excessively sensitive. Impotence. Acute for rape. Ailments after rape, anger after rape. Fear from sexual abuse or rape, images may come back during sex (Op.).

Clarke had known Staph. to have an impulse to throw things at persons who had caused a trifling or imaginary irritation.

P. C. Majumdar gives two cases in which loss of memory following masturbation and seminal emissions was cured with Staph. 30c. The first case was a student, naturally robust and intelligent, who lost his memory when he contracted the habit of masturbation. His symptoms included a vacant countenance, with no aptitude or inclination for mental work. Despair of the future, great languor and weakness. Occasional nocturnal emissions, or constipation.

When he read anything he forgot it the next moment. Heaviness, headache and vertigo after the least mental exertion. Staph. 30c was given morning and evening. Improvement began at once and the cure was complete in a month.

The second case involved another student who had constant involuntary emissions, weak memory, languor, headache every morning on rising, no appetite, constipation. Staph. 30c, once a day, cured.

Clarke saw Staph. 30c give relief to complaints in newly married women. "Constant urging to urinate in young married women." Honeymoon cystitis. Clarke saw cystocele relieved by Staph.

Bibby used Staph. tincture with much success, three drops in two ounces of water, a teaspoonful every two hours in cases of night sweat in patients bordering on tuberculosis.

RELATIONS - ***Antidote:*** Camph. ***Compare:*** (1) Coloc., Cham., Caust., Ign. (2) Ph-ac., Calad. (3) Ferr-py. - tarsal cysts. (4) Nux-v., Calc-p. ***Complementary:*** Caust., Coloc. ***Inimical:*** Ran-b.

REFERENCES - Boericke. Clarke. Murphy. Phatak.

STAR OF BETHLEHEM

(Bach Flower Essence)

PHARMACY - star-b-b. Star of Bethlehem. Ornithogalum umbellatum. The flower heads are boiled for half an hour. Subsequently, the water is strained and used as medicine. ***Historical dose:*** Take two drops from the stock bottle into a one ounce dropper bottle (add brandy or alcohol, if this bottle will be used for days or weeks). This is the dosage bottle, take a few drops straight into the mouth or as needed in a little water or juice.

HOMEOPATHIC - Star-b-b. is listed in Bach's group of ***Despondency and Despair,*** with Crb-a-b., Oak-b., Will-b., Sw-ch-b., Elm-b., Pine-b. and Lar-b. States of grief and shock. Post-traumatic stress disorder (Rck-r-b.). Ailments after accidents.

Lack of appetite, digestive problems, shock and collapse. Ulcerative colitis and Crohn's disease. The diaphragm is known to tighten during grief and impair breathing, leading to frequent sighing.

MIND - Shock and grief. Sadness, heart wrenching impact, deepest pain and despair. Despondency and hopelessness. Fear, shame, frustration, and guilt. Anger and prolonged outrage (Holly-b.).

Thoughts of nihilism and meaninglessness (Sw-ch-b.). Internal numbing or taking lightly those things that cannot be changed. Hidden internal agony (Agri-b.). Hides inner feelings from others (Must-b.).

REFERENCES - Bach.

STELLARIA MEDIA

(Chickweed)

PHARMACY - stel. Stellaria media. Chickweed. N. O. Caryophyllaceae. Tincture of whole fresh plant in bloom. ***Historical dose:*** Tincture and all potencies.

CLINICAL - Constipation. Gout. Liver, inflammation. ***Rheumatism.*** Psoriasis. ***Synovitis***. Vomiting.

HOMEOPATHIC - The first mention of Stel. by F. H. Brett recounted an experience in the case of his wife in which the tincture was applied externally to enlarged, inflamed gouty fingers-joints, and in his own case to painful, aching great toes.

In each case a few applications removed the trouble. Brett was led to this use by having heard a rumor that "chickweed poultices" were good for gouty joints.

F. Kopp published a proving of the tincture on himself. Kopp took frequently repeated doses of the tincture and also chewed some of the weed. The pains induced were of a rheumatic character and were so severe that they had to be antidoted with Nux-v. and Bry.

Kopp confirmed Brett's observations in the value of external applications of Stel. Internally, he gave Stel. 2x.

Stasis, congestion and sluggishness of all functions. Pain, swelling and soreness of the liver, better by motion and accompanied by soreness. ***Rheumatism***, darting pains in almost every part, stiffness of joints, parts sore to touch, worse motion. ***Chronic rheumatism. Shifting pains*** (Puls., Kali-s.). Psoriasis. Enlarged and inflamed gouty finger joints. Morning aggravation.

MIND - General irritability. Lassitude, indisposition to work.

Abdomen - Bowels sore, worse by touch. Burning pressure in region of liver. Bilious feeling. Pains in right groin.

Back - Dull pain under right scapula. Rheumatic pains across small of back, worse bending. Loins stiff and sore.

Chest - Constriction, oppression, heat. Tickling in upper part.

Eyes - Right eyeball sore to touch. Darting pain in right eye. Smarting and burning in eyes, feel protruded. Flushes of heat below right lid. Vision dim.

Face - Neuralgic pains in right side of face. Burning on lower lips.

Head - Dull, frontal headache, worse in morning and left side with sleepiness. Neck muscles stiff and sore. Eyes feel protruded.

Kidneys - Kidney region sore to touch.

Limbs - Rheumatoid pains in different parts of the body. Bruised feeling. Joints stiff. ***Synovitis***. Sharp pain in small of back, over kidneys in gluteal region, extending down thigh. Rheumatic pains in calves of legs. Pain in shoulders and arms.

Liver - Hepatic torpor. Burning pains all over liver. ***Liver engorged, swollen with stitching pain and sensitive to pressure***. Sensation as if liver too large for body.

Lungs - Short cough from tickling on upper chest, worse deep inspiration. Hawking of viscid, salty mucus.

Modalities - Better evenings, cold air. Better motion. Worse mornings, warmth, tobacco.

Mouth - Persistent taste of the drug with slight acrid feeling. Heat and dryness of mouth, numbness of lower gums and tip of tongue. Sensation as if incisors set on edge.

Nose - Dryness of nostrils.

Rectum - Constipation or alternating constipation and diarrhea. Stools loose, dark brown, attended with slight pain. Clay-colored stools.

Sleep - Sleeps well but unrefreshed on waking.

Stomach - Slight nausea with frequent belchings, tasting of the drug. Sharp pains in stomach.

Throat - Numbness and dryness in throat. followed by sharp stitches in left tonsil.

COMMENTS - Bellairs published the case of E. B., 18, who had rheumatic fever which had left him in a hopeless state of chronic "shifting" rheumatism, pains now in ankle, now in knee, now in arm, wrist or fingers.

Stel. 2x, was taken three times a day, completely cured in a month. Bellairs suggested that "shifting-pains" may be a keynote and Kopp confirmed this.

Brett cured himself with Stel. 1c of a violent attack of sickness with sharp pains in stomach increasing in violence and culminating in an explosive vomit. The liver was much enlarged, hard to the touch. The pain began in the region of the gallbladder. Vomiting ceased after the first dose and the liver enlargement quickly subsided.

Cooper gave much relief with a single dose of in the case of a woman, 55, who had psoriasis, dating from twenty-one years back with irritation in the spots, chiefly on flexures of joints with much irritation of scalp and soreness of eyeballs.

RELATIONS - ***Compare:*** (1) Puls. - similar in rheumatism, pains shifting, worse rest, warmth, better cold air.

REFERENCES - Boericke. Clarke.

STICTA PULMONARIA

(Lung-wort)

PHARMACY - stict. Sticta pulmonaria. Lungwort. Lobaria pulmonaria. N. O. Lichenes. Tincture of dried lichen. ***Historical dose:*** Tincture and all potencies.

CLINICAL - Allergies. Angina pectoris. Anus, pain. Asthma. ***Bronchitis.*** Catarrh. Chorea. Clergyman's sore throat. Colds. Conjunctivitis. Coryza. ***Coughs.*** Diabetes. Diarrhea. Glands, swollen. ***Hay fever.*** Headaches. Hemoptysis. ***Housemaid's knee***. Hysteria. Influenza. Laryngitis. ***Lung, disorders.*** Measles, cough. Migraine. Milk, scanty. Neuralgias. Ozaena. Post-nasal catarrh. Pott's disease. ***Rheumatism.*** Rhinitis. Seminal, emissions. Sick, headache. Sleeplessness. Syphilis. ***Tracheitis.*** Tuberculosis.

HERBAL - Sticta pulmonaria received its name, lungwort, from the likeness of the plant to lung tissue. It was a popular remedy of great repute in catarrhs and coughs when Hale introduced it to homeopathy.

HOMEOPATHIC - S. P. Burdock, C. H. Lutes and S. Lilienthal proved it and elicited some very remarkable and valuable symptoms. Hering added many clinical symptoms.

Stict. is a remedy for coryza, bronchial catarrh, nervous and rheumatic disturbances. Influenza, better in open air. Painful dry mucus membranes. ***Coughing aggravates*** cough, the more he coughs, the more he wants to. Cough worse nights, comparatively free from it during day.

Rheumatic stiffness of neck. Diagonal pains (Lac-c.). ***Nervous and rheumatic disturbances***. Nervous, sense of levitation of different parts. General feeling of dullness and malaise, as when a cold is coming on, dull, heavy pressure in forehead, catarrhal conjunctivitis, etc. Hysteria, chorea after loss of blood.

MIND - Confusion of ideas. Inability to concentrate. ***Patient must talk.*** Lively, kicks her heels up. ***Feels as if floating in air*** (Dat-a., Lac-c.). Horror of night, when he suffers the most.

Abdomen - Dull pains in the right hypochondrium. Feeling of fullness in left hypochondriac region. Rumbling as if full of yeast.

Back - Rheumatism. Red spots on affected joints. Chorea like spasms. Cold moist limbs. Sore stiff neck, pains to shoulder. Legs as if floating in the air. Bursitis, especially about the knee. Profuse sweat on hands. Restless hands and feet.

Breasts - Absence of milk after delivery. Scanty flow of milk.

Causations - Ill effects of falls or hemorrhages.

Chest - ***Pulsation from right side of sternum down to abdomen.*** Oppression of chest and feeling a hard mass there. Pain from sternum to spine, worse motion. Pain through chest from sternum to spinal column.

Constitutions - Suited to neuralgic, rheumatic, gouty individuals.

Coughs - Barking cough, worse night and morning, when tired. ***Dry, hacking cough during night, worse inspiration***, prevents sleep. Loose cough in morning. Cough from cold, damp weather. Cough after measles (Sang.), after influenza, after whooping cough.

Ears - Acute neuralgic pains in mastoid apophysis, rather deep in.

Eyes - Burning in eyes and soreness of eyeballs. Burning of eyelids on closing lids or turning eyes.

Face - Darting pains in side of face and in lower jaw.

Female - Uneasiness in the pelvis. Menses more abundant and paler than usual.

Head - Heaviness in the forehead. Dull headache with dull heavy pressure in forehead and ***root of nose. Catarrhal headache before discharge appears***. Sensation as if scalp were too small.

Heart - Attacks of anxiety about heart. Dull, oppressive pain in cardiac region.

Kidneys - Profuse urination with sore painful bladder.

Limbs - Swelling, heat, redness of joints. ***Spot of inflammation and redness over affected joint***. Pain severe and drawing. Chorea-like spasms, legs feel floating in air. ***Housemaid's knee*** (Sep., Rhus-t., Kali-hp., Slag.). Shooting pains in knees. Joints and neighboring muscles red, swollen, painful. Rheumatic pain in right shoulder joint, deltoid and biceps. Rheumatic pains precede catarrhal symptoms.

Lungs - Bronchitis. Tracheitis, facilitates expectoration. Tickling high up in pharynx. Air passages numb. Expectoration, scanty, whitish or frothy. Expectoration, entirely absent.

Modalities - Better from free discharges. Better open air, pressure. Worse as day advances, lasting all day. Worse at night, lying down. Worse sudden changes of temperature. Worse by touch, motion.

Nose - ***Fullness at the root of the nose*** (Nux-v.). Obstruction of nose, worse at night, preventing sleep, better open air. Tingling in right side of nose. Painful ***dryness*** of mucus membranes. Atrophic rhinitis (Calc-f.). ***Hay fever,*** incessant sneezing (Sabad.). Coryza from slightest cold. Coryza which dries up soon, forming scabs, difficult to dislodge, particularly at night. ***Constant need to blow the nose, but no discharge***. Loss of smell.

Rectum - Diarrhea, stools profuse, frothy. Diarrhea worse in morning.

Sensations - As if she cannot keep her tongue still. Throat and mouth burn as if scalded. As if hard mass collected in lungs. As if stomach full of yeast. As if floating in air. The right side is more prominently affected.

Sleep - Sleepless from nervousness from cough after surgical operations.

Throat - Dryness. Clergyman's sore throat with great dryness of mucus membranes. Tracheitis. Tickling in throat causes cough. Raw throat, dripping of mucus posteriorly.

COMMENTS - Hale said, "It was first used for severe harassing cough," and such good results accrued that provings were made to ascertain its full value. Dewey conducted a proving on several persons which further enriched the pathogenesis.

Severe coryza with violent sneezing intense headache and conjunctivitis. Attacks preceded or followed by rheumatic pains and swelling of the small joints.

Dry cough, worse evening and night, can neither sleep nor lie down, must sit up. Coughs left by measles, whooping cough, or influenza. Hard, dry barking coughs following colds. Obstructive catarrh. Discharge dries quickly and forms crusts or scurf. Constant need to blow the nose, but no discharge comes on account of dryness.

"Dull, heavy pressure or stuffed feeling in root of nose" in catarrh and headaches. "A deep-in headache" (Bac.). Rheumatism, related to catarrh. Tuberculosis and hemoptysis. "Oppression at chest, sensation as if a hard mass on it. Sudden pain from sternum to spine, constant, worse on movement."

Sleeplessness, due to nervousness or cough. Hysterical chorea coming on after profuse hemorrhage. Sensation of levitation, the legs feel as if floating in the air, head as if floating off, as if the body and limbs did not touch the bed.

P. C. Majumdar cured two cases of whooping cough with Stict. 6x. The cough began just after sunset and went on until vomiting occurred and all the contents of the stomach were thrown off.

M. D. Youngman related a number of cases of catarrhal and pulmonary disorders cured with Stic., with harsh coughing, racking incessant, "unprofitable" cough of spasmodic type. Youngman considered it especially suited to neuralgic, rheumatic, gouty individuals.

Youngman noted the case of Mrs. H., 42, who had an attack of bronchitis in January and when seen, on March 20th, she had a harsh, racking cough with pain all through chest on coughing. Spongy state of mucus membrane of pharynx, which bled easily.

She had several attacks of asthma, hay fever every August, paroxysms of cough often ended in convulsive sneezing, which she dreaded because it was followed by asthmatic symptoms.

"She takes cold in her head, which in a day or so goes down in her throat and thence into her chest." Every cold she got did this. Stict., 1x gave relief in five days.

Hale said Stict. is indispensable in February, March and April in the American climate.

O. Rogers prescribed Stict. for a patient with the cough of the remedy, at the time she was nursing her seventh child. She had always been annoyed because of a lack of milk, it had been occasionally suppressed. While taking Stict. the flow became ample and remained so as long as an occasional dose was being taken. Rogers subsequently verified this effect in a number of cases.

Elias C. Price related the case of a boy, 8, who had acute rheumatism with inflammation and redness of one knee, ankle toes, wrist and fingers, valvular heart disease from a previous attack. Acon. and Sulph. failed to relieve.

Stict. 1x was given every hour. The next day, there was a considerable quantity of fluid in the knee joint, apparently an aggravation by Stict., but otherwise the boy was better. Stict. was continued. The next day, half the fluid was gone, and the third day it was all gone. The boy was cured in nine days.

Price remarked that he had noticed one symptom so frequently present in the cases he cured with Stict. that he began to regard it as a characteristic although it was not in the provings: a spot of inflammation and redness on the affected joint like the hectic flush on the cheeks in tuberculosis. In housemaid's knee, Stict. comes as near being a specific as a remedy ever can.

RELATIONS - ***Compare:*** (1) Lung affections, headache, Pul-o., Bac. (2) Catarrhs and coughs, Dros., Nux-v., Rumx., Samb., Meph. (3) Rheumatism, Cimic., Stel. (4) Nerve symptoms, Asar., Tarent. (5) Asthma of tuberculosis patients associated with splitting headache, Rumx., Meph. (6) Levitation symptoms, Calc.,

Sil., Cann-i. (7) Sensation of lightness of body, Cocc., Gels. (8) The more he coughs, the more he wants to, Ign. (9) Heaviness from front to back, Naja. (10) headache, as if skull being raised and lowered, Cann-i.

REFERENCES - Boericke. Clarke.

STIGMATA MAYDIS

(Corn-silk)

PHARMACY - stigm. Stigmata maydis. Corn-silk. Zea mays. Maize. Indian Corn. N. O. Gramineae, Tribe, Phalarideae. (1) Stigmata maydis. Green pistils. Tincture: One part, by weight, of the corn silk to two parts of alcohol. Fluid Extract. (2) Shucks. Decoction or tincture of the husks of maize after the removal of the grain. ***Historical dose:*** Tincture and all potencies.

CLINICAL - Albuminuria. Bladder, disorders. Cystitis. Dropsy. Dysuria. Edema. Gonorrhea, chronic. Heart, disorders. Heart, failure. Malaria. Kidney, colic. Kidney, stones. Pyelitis. Urine, retained. Urine, suppressed.

HERBAL - The grain in bulk appears to be capable of generating a poisonous gas, as four men were suffocated, one fatally, on opening a cargo of maize for the purpose of discharging it in the London docks.

Generally, two parts of maize have been used in medicine, the pistils and the husks, but Clarke thought it best to take them together. Dr. E. C. Lowe, of England, used a decoction of corn shucks for chronic malaria, teaspoonful doses freely.

Irritable conditions of the urinary tract, ureters, bladder, urethra. A powerful diuretic in kidney disorders unconnected with cardiac involvement. Heart and urinary conditions combined.

HOMEOPATHIC - Marked urinary symptoms. Organic heart disease with much edema of lower limbs and scanty urination. Enlarged prostate and retention of urine. Uric and phosphatic. Gonorrhea. Cystitis.

Hansen confirmed the value of Stigm. in 20 drop doses of the fluid extract in organic heart disease with dropsy, much edema of lower limbs and scanty urination. He mentioned also as suitable cases kidney stones with nephritic ulcer and discharge of small stones, red sand and blood.

Chronic pyelitis from catarrh. Chronic retention of urine with great tenesmus after urinating. Suppression of urine with lack of solids and low specific gravity. Bladder catarrh, tenesmus of neck of bladder, ammoniacal urine, much mucus. Chronic gonorrhea, prostate involved, painful urination.

Bladder - Cystitis. Tenesmus after urinating. Bladder catarrh. Gonorrhea.

Kidneys - Kidney stones, nephritic colic. Suppression and ***retention of urine***. Dysuria. Blood and red sand in urine.

COMMENTS - J. H. Cook gave an account of Stigm. in the Med. Cent. He quoted the results of Dumont's investigation of its action on the heart: "It makes the heart's action slower and stronger. Regulates its rhythm. Its diuretic action is manifested first. Its action is more powerful and evident in cardiac disorders with dropsy. With the disappearance of the dropsy arterial tension increases and venous tension diminishes."

Cook gave the case of Mr. X., 63, florid, robust, temperature, had been many months under treatment with intense prostration, intermittent pulse, and dyspnea, traced originally to cooling off too rapidly when perspiring.

The urine contained much albumen, mucus and some blood, specific gravity 1010. Great tenderness over entire abdomen, especially in region of ureters. Under remedies he would improve for a few days, when a slight chill would be followed by fever and the symptoms would come back in full force.

The microscope revealed pus cells and granular epithelial cells in abundance. Stigm. was then given, a teaspoonful of the fluid extract every four hours. In less than a week there was visible improvement. The constant calls to urinate ceased and the patient could go through the night without being disturbed more than once or twice.

The specific gravity of the urine increased and pus, blood and albumen disappeared. Only a little abdominal tenderness remained, which did not prevent the patient from attending to his business and enjoying life.

Another use of Stigm. was communicated to the profession by Dr. J. W. Pruitt. Pruitt's son took a chill in the Arkansas river bottom. The chills were stopped with the usual remedies, Chin., Ferr., Pipe., but every fourteen days would come back with increased severity.

Presently gastric symptoms set in with anemia and other symptoms of chronicity. "Shuck tea" was recommended by a lay friend and was taken for one day only. There was never a chill after. Pruitt thence forward used Stigm. largely and he found it was only in the chronic cases that it was beneficial.

RELATIONS - ***Compare:*** (1) In bladder affections, Equis., Tritic., Sabal. (2) Kidney colic - Oci., Berb. (3) Heart - Dig., Crat., Stroph.

REFERENCES - Clarke.

STILLINGIA SYLVATICA

(Queen's Root)

PHARMACY - still. Stillingia sylvatica. Queen's root. Queen's delight. Pine barrens. N. O. Euphorbiacae. Pine barrens grows from Virginia to Florida. Tincture of the root after flowering. ***Historical dose:*** Tincture and all potencies.

CLINICAL - Bones, diseases. Clergyman's, sore throat. Elephantiasis. Headaches, catarrhal. Headaches, syphilitic. Hemorrhoids. Hip joint, disease. Influenza. Larynx, disorders. Liver, disorders. Nodes. Periostitis. Psoriasis. Rheumatism. Scrofula. Sore throat. Syphilis.

HERBAL - Stillingia has long been a popular remedy for syphilis in the southern states of North America. T. Y. Simons introduced it into medicine and Hale to homeopathy.

HOMEOPATHIC - H. R. Frost, A. B. Nichols, J. M. Cunningham and others proved it, chewing the root or taking the tincture. One prover chewed the bark.

The Still. proving shows an action closely parallel with that of syphilis, attacking the genito-urinary organs, throat, pharynx, larynx and trachea, mouth, head and bones. It has a popular repute in scrofula, skin affections, liver diseases and rheumatism, confirmed in the provings.

One prover was cured of a pustular eruption. In chronic rheumatism, Hale classed it with Phyt. and Kali-i. Chronic periosteal rheumatism, syphilitic and scrofulous disorders. Well marked respiratory symptoms. Torpor of lymphatics torpid liver with jaundice and constipation.

MIND - ***Gloomy forebodings,*** depressed. Fear that something bad will happen.

Abdomen - Heavy pain in hypogastric region. Severe cramps in both hypochondria. Sharp darting in left hypochondrium, followed by passage of flatus. Borborygmi. Colic, periodical.

Back - Aching in back and down thighs and legs. While sitting, pain in left lumbar region, darting forwards.

Bones - Bones, diseases. Nodes.

Chest - Oppression of chest. Darting pain in thorax. Raw feeling in chest, whole length of sternum.

Constitutions - Hydrogenoid constitution.

Ears - Burning in left ear in evening, next morning a vesicular eruption.

Eyes - Eyes inflamed and watery. Sharp, darting pain over left eye. Lachrymation of both eyes after reading.

Face - Stinging, darting pains in face with frontal headache. Periostitis of facial bones.

Female - Both ovaries pained very severely. Copious muco-purulent leucorrhea with rheumatic pains.

Food - Appetite increased, then lost.

Head - Persistent dull headache in vertex. Sharp darting pains in right occipital protuberance. Bone swellings in head and forehead in latter size of hen's eggs.

Heart - Boring pains about region of heart with irregular pulse. Pulse weak and very irregular.

Kidneys - Dull pain in region of kidneys. Incontinence of urine. ***Deposits white sediment***. Urine colorless, milky and thick.

Limbs - Aching pains in bones of limbs and back.

Liver - Torpidity of liver with jaundice, great depression, constipation.

Lungs - Dry, spasmodic cough. Larynx constricted with stinging in fauces. Trachea feels sore when pressed. Croup. Cough deep and loose.

Male - Slight drawing up in right testes. Dull tearing pain in left testes. Gonorrhea.

Modalities - Better in morning, dry air. Warmth helps itching of legs. Worse in afternoon. Worse by movement, walking. Worse exposure to cold or to air, damp air.

Mouth - Heat in mouth and fauces. Taste salty, bitter in morning. Increased flow of saliva. Tongue coated heavily yellowish white. Tongue feels rough and sore. Scalded sensation on tongue with soreness in region of larynx. Paroxysms of neuralgic toothache.

Nose - Catarrhal discharge, first watery then muco-purulent. Influenza. Necrosis of bones of nose.

Rectum - Severe attack of hemorrhoids. Burning and tenesmus. Constipation, stools delayed. Bowels loose and irregular. Stools copious, acid, frothy, bilious, papescent, white like curds, dysenteric.

Sensations - As of a heavy substance pressing on brain. Tongue as if scalded. As if room were too warm.

Skin - Ulcers, chronic eruptions on hands and fingers. Ulcers with unhealthy skin. Leprosy. Itching and burning. Exostosis. Vesicular eruption on ears. Scrofulous, venereal and other skin diseases. ***Enlarged cervical glands***. Elephantiasis.

Sleep - Unusual drowsiness all day with general malaise and headache. Very sleepy after eating.

Stomach - Faint, empty sensation in stomach. Distress, griping, cramps in stomach. Sickness and salivation. Regurgitation and vomiting of ingesta. Nausea with constipation.

Throat - Laryngitis. ***Hoarseness*** and chronic laryngeal disorders of public speakers. Smarting, stinging, dryness and rawness of fauces. Intense burning in fauces and throat. Constriction of throat.

COMMENTS - Clarke cured with Still. syphilitic cough of the hoarse, barking type. In one case of secondary syphilis the patient, who was taking Still. 1c, complained that the medicine made his legs and feet feel tired and his feet feel sore.

Still. attacks the periosteum and produces pain in the bone. Nodes on the forehead, tibia and elsewhere. Decay of the nasal bones. Pain in the cranial bones and the headaches of syphilis, though it is not confined to syphilitic cases. Pains are sharp, shooting, darting. The cartilages of larynx and trachea are sore and feel bruised. Dryness.

Hale quoted a case of secondary syphilis treated by Preston, one of the provers. The patient, a man, suffered extreme torture from bone pains. After receiving Still. he slept well.

The immense nodes disappeared from head and legs and "from the most deplorable, down-hearted, sometimes almost raving from derangement, miserable, thin-looking object, he changed into a buoyant, joking, rotund-looking fellow."

RELATIONS - ***Antidote to:*** Merc. ***Antidoted by:*** Ip. - nausea from the fumes. ***Compare:*** (1) In syphilis, Syph., Med., Merc., Kali-i. (2) Chronic rheumatism, Guai., Phyt. (3) Nodes, Mang., Corydalis, Staph. (4) Hip disease, Nat-s. (5) Still. secondary or inherited syphilis, pains in and through hip, worse night, worse wet weather, Nat-s. (6) the hydrogenoid constitution, pains Worse night rouse patient from sleep, better turning over in bed.

REFERENCES - Boericke. Clarke.

STRAMONIUM

(Jimson Weed)

PHARMACY - stram. Stramonium. Jimson weed. Thornapple. Datura stramonium. Jamestown-weed. Stink-weed. N. O. Solanaceae. Grows in vicinity of cultivation on rank soil where refuse is deposited in all parts of the world. Tincture of fresh plant in flower and fruit. ***Historical dose:*** All potencies.

CLINICAL - Alcoholism. Anasarca. Aphasia. Bedwetting. Burns. Catalepsy. Chordee. ***Chorea. Delirium. Delirium tremens. Delusions.*** Ecstasy. Epilepsy. Esophagus, spasms. Eyes disorders. ***Fevers.*** Headache, sun. Hiccoughs. Hysteria. Injuries. ***Insanity.*** Lochia offensive. Locomotor ataxia. ***Mania.*** Meningitis. Nymphomania. Parkinson's disease. ***Rabies.*** Sexual mania. Scarlatina. Schizophrenia. Stammering speech. Starting. Strabismus. Strokes. Sunstroke. Tetanus. Thirst. Tremors. Trismus. Typhus.

HOMEOPATHIC - According to Teste, Stoerck, one of Hahnemann's predecessors, was the first to use Stram. in modern times. Stoerck first tried it in mental alienation, because it was supposed to produce "a marked and persistent disorder of the mental faculties."

Hahnemann proved it and introduced it into the Homeopathic Materia Medica. In his introduction to the remedy he pointed out that, although it produces many symptoms, it does not in its primary effects cause actual pain.

Hahnemann attached a good deal of importance to this. Hahnemann said "Stram. allays some spasmodic movements and restores suppressed excretions in several cases in which absence of pain is a prominent symptom."

Teste specifically mentioned its usefulness in some kinds of mania, particularly in nymphomania of lying-in women.

Marked and persistent disorder of the mental faculty. Hysteria, weeping, laughing with sexual excitement. Certain forms of religious mania in exaggerated and ridiculous scruple of conscience. Fixed notion that some unpardonable sin has been committed which the patient is unable to remember. Notion that he is possessed of the devil.

Hallucinations. Delusions as to size and distance. Sensation as if limbs were separated from the body. Delirium tremens. Suppressed secretions and excretions, including urine and stool.

Absence of pain and muscular mobility especially of muscles of expression and of locomotion. Gyratory and graceful motions. Increases the mobility of the muscles of expression and of locomotion, the motions may be graceful, rhythmic or disorderly of head and arms.

Parkinson's disease. Trembling of limbs. Nervous tremors. Convulsions, spasms worse at night after masturbation. Tonic and clonic spasms alternately. Paralysis of one side, convulsions of the other side or unilateral paralysis with twitching. General paralysis of the insane. Chorea, epilepsy from fright. Catalepsy, limbs can be moved by others. Traumatic neuritis.

MIND - Hallucinations, fixed notions, terrifying delirium etc. Active variable delirium, delirium tremens. ***Delirium with desire to escape*** (Bell., Bry., Rhus-t.). ***Raving mania*** with cold sweat. Maniac, curses, tears ones clothes with teeth. ***Devout, earnest, beseeching and ceaseless talking***. Violent and lewd speech.

Paranoid. Schizophrenia. Manic-depression. Religious insanity. Wants to kill people or himself. Exposes himself. Rapid changes from joy to sadness. Wife thinks husband neglecting her. Man thinks his wife faithless. Stupid, imbecile.

Fearful hallucinations that terrify the patient, sees ghosts, vividly brilliant or hideous phantoms, animals, jumping sideways out of ground or running to him. Wildly excited, as in night terrors. Hears voices, talks with spirits. Delusions about his identity, thinks himself tall, double, a part missing.

Terrors, cannot bear solitude or darkness, ***must have light and company***. ***Dread of darkness*** and has a horror of shining objects. Fear and anxiety on hearing water run. Sight of water or anything glittering brings on spasms. ***Anxiety when going***

through a tunnel.

Abdomen - Abdomen inflated, hard, distended. Contusive pain in abdomen during movement. Violent pains in abdomen, as if navel were being torn out. Hysterical spasms in abdomen. Borborygmi with fermentation in abdomen. Expulsion of much flatus. Swelling of inguinal glands.

Back - Neck stiff, cannot bend it backwards. Drawing pain in the back. Spine sensitive, slightest pressure causes outcries and ravings. Opisthotonos.

Causations - Ill effects of shock, fright, sun, childbirth. Dog bites. High fever. Head injury. Hydrophobia.

Chest - Constrictive oppression on chest with dyspnea. Pressure on chest, worse by speaking. Spasm in pectoral muscles. Red rash on chest.

Constitutions - Suited to ailments of young, plethoric persons, especially of children (chorea, mania, fever, delirium).

Ears - Sensation as if air rushing out of ear. Deafness. Hallucinations of hearing.

Eyes - Fixed, sparkling, ***staring wide open***. Half open in sleep. Pupils dilated. Lachrymation with headache, fever, otalgia. Diplopia. Night-blindness. Green vision. Hallucinations in which everything looks jumbled. An objects look black, crooked, small, large. Parts of the body seem enormously swollen. ***Small objects look large.*** Loss of vision, complains that it is dark and ***calls for more light.*** All objects look black. Squint in brain disorders during convulsions, worse terror, fear. Strabismus.

Face - Pale face. Red, bloated, hot, circumscribed redness of cheeks. Blood rushes to face, distorted. ***Expression of terror.*** Expression rapidly changing, now flushed, now pale, a sardonic grin, then expression of terror. Thinks face elongated. Forehead wrinkled, frowning in brain diseases. Lips, dry, glued together. Chewing motion. Lockjaw.

Female - Excessive menstrual flow, preceded by sexual excitement. Menses have strong smell as of semen. Loquacity and singing during menses. Sobs and moans after menses. ***Uterine bleeding with loquacity***. Hands constantly kept on genitals. Nymphomania, lewd talking, sings obscene songs. Puerperal, convulsions, mania with mental symptoms and profuse sweating. Convulsions after childbirth.

Food - Food tastes bitter, like straw. ***Aversion to all fluids.*** Violent thirst. Great desire for acids, citric acid better. Lemon juice ameliorates.

Head - Headache with tendency to speak incoherently. Pain in forehead and over eyebrows, beginning at 9 a.m., worse until noon. Boring pain, preceded by obscure vision. ***Headache from sun.*** Rush of blood to head, staggers with tendency to fall forward and to the left. ***Meningitis*** from suppressed ear discharge. ***Raises head frequently from the pillow*** and drops it again during unconsciousness, delirium, puerperal fever.

Heart - Pressure about heart. Heart disorders with constrictions of the chest and mental symptoms. Angina pectoris. Palpitations. Feeble, pulse irregular.

Kidneys - Suppression of urine, especially during typhoid, bladder empty. Loss of power of bladder in the aged, stream flows slowly, cannot make haste. Rigor during urination. Bladder empty.

Limbs - ***Chorea***, spasms partial, constantly changing. Convulsions of upper limbs and of isolated groups of muscles. ***Graceful and rhythmic motions.*** Clasps hands over head. Hands open and shut. Wringing of hands. Staggering gait. Misses step of stairs while descending. Heels numb, sometimes painful. ***Violent pain in left hip***. Abscess of left hip joint with violent pain. Trembling of limbs. Inside of right thigh red and swollen. Hemiplegia with convulsions in unparalyzed parts.

Lungs - Inspiration slow, expiration quick. Nervous asthma. Cough with jerking of lower limbs, when sitting. Cough worse looking at light, fire or bright objects. The spasmodic cough of alcoholics, whooping.

Male - ***Sexual passion exalted*** with indecent speech and action. Hands constantly kept on genitals.

Modalities - ***Better from bright light,***

company, warmth. Worse from shining objects, mirror, surface of water. Worse from fright, when alone. Worse sun, cloudy days, in dark room. Worse suppressions, intemperance, after sleep. Worse by touch, pressure, swallowing.

Mouth - Dry, dribbling of viscid saliva. Constantly spits saliva. Cannot swallow on account of spasm. Chewing motion. Grinding of the teeth. Fine red dots on tongue. Tongue, dry, parched, swollen, hangs out of the mouth. ***Stammering***. Aphasia. Risus sardonicus.

Nose - Alae nasi white with a red face. Obstruction of the nose. Nasal discharge yellow, bad-smelling. Nose feels obstructed and dry, though she is able to breathe through it.

Rectum - Putrid, dark, painless involuntary diarrhea with a squint and pale face. Cholera infantum. Stools suppressed.

Sensations - As if spinning or weaving. As if objects were smaller than they really are. As if dizzy. As if drunk. As if he was seeking something. As if he had no limbs. As if bones were sawed through. Head as if drawn backward. As if pins and needles were in forehead. As if nose were shifted. As if front teeth would fall out. Teeth as if pressed together.

Skin - Fiery red patches on skin. Shining red flush. Burns and scalds. Crawling as of many bugs. Chronic abscesses, fistulae. Abscesses and tumors with severe pain. Non-appearance of exanthemata. ***Effects of suppressed eruption in scarlatina*** with delirium.

Sleep - Sleepy, but cannot sleep (Bell.). Sleepless in darkness. Deep snoring sleep. Lies on back with thighs and knees flexed. ***Frightful dreams.*** Weeping in dreams. Laughs, screams, starts during sleep. Awakes terrified, knows no one, screams with fright, clings to those near him (child). Comatose.

Stomach - Hiccough obstinate. Nausea. Vomiting of mucus and ***green bile.*** Watery vomiting with colic and diarrhea.

Temperature - Profuse sweat which does not relieve. Cold sweat during spasms. Violent fever. Heat over whole body with red face and perspiration. Heat with anxiety and redness of cheeks or else with thirst and vomiting. Retention of urine in any fever.

Throat - Dry with great thirst, yet dreads water, it chokes him. Spasms, twitching of larynx. Up and down movement of larynx as in swallowing. Swallowing, difficult, hasty. As if boiling water rising in throat. Voice hoarse and croaking, suddenly fails in higher tones.

Vertigo - Vertigo, worse walking in dark or with eyes closed. Head bent backwards in vertigo, supports head with hands while bending or rising after sunstroke.

COMMENTS - J. Emmons Briggs recorded a case of poisoning. Briggs had an urgent call to see James M., 4, in "convulsions." He found him lying on the bed in a state of wild delirium, requiring the constant combined efforts of two people to keep him in bed.

Face was exceedingly flushed, expression rapidly alternated between pleasant and anxious. Pupils widely dilated, iris scarcely visible, giving the eye a very brilliant appearance.

Marked convergent strabismus, skin hot and dry, resembling scarlatina eruption. Abdomen tense. The most alarming symptom was rapidly recurring convulsions with twitching of the arms and lower limbs. Clonic spasms and contractions.

Grasped at imaginary objects before the eyes, when expression frequently became anxious, as if the patient was trying to ward off imaginary foes. At times the mind was very active and the patient talked rapidly and incoherently. Between the spasms, laughter and crying frequently occurred.

The boy, it transpired, had been chewing a thorn apple. When he came home he seemed rather dazed, and vomited. He then threw himself on the sofa and slept very soundly until he awoke in the convulsions. The boy recovered under Kali-br. in five-grain doses, though it was with great difficulty that he was made to swallow.

Schizophrenia (Lach., Anac.). Paranoid schizophrenia. Religious mania. Insanity, mania, and dementia. Violent mania (Lach., Hyos. has a passive mania), rages, and wild violence. Loquacious (Lach.).

Characteristic wild, animal-like look in the eyes. Clinical possession, they talk in other languages, other voices, violent speech, rages and ravings. Primitive instincts and fears. Vithoulkas described it as an "uncontrolled eruption of the unconsciousness."

May have a history of frights, strokes, head injuries or meningitis leading to mania. Fear of dogs and wolves, often hallucinate that they see dogs attacking them. Visions of animals. Claustrophobia. Fear of the dark, of tunnels. Fears of mirrors and crosses. Afraid of shiny objects, fire. Hydrophobia, rabies (Bell., Lyss.). Cries as if from sight of hideous objects.

Terrifying delirium. Delirium tremens. Delirium with high fever, hallucinations. High fevers with sudden onset, flushed face, dilated pupils, rashes, hallucinations (Bell.). Scarlet like scarlatina, petechiae, vesications, and spots on the arms like flea bites. Burns and scalds. Mania after exposure to the sun (Bell.).

Absence of pain. Epilepsy and convulsions. Extreme muscular mobility. Movements are generally gyratory and graceful when they occur in the arms. Continually jerks head up from pillow, head bent back, boring head into pillow. Twitchings of single muscles, squint. Chorea. Moving fingers as if searching for something. Coxalgia and morbus coax, with severe pain.

Characteristic difficulty swallowing, with intense thirst, delirium and hallucinations. Suppressed secretions, menses, lochia, sweat, or eruptions. Discharges are foul, even cadaverous.

Congestions without actual inflammation, but with high mental exaltation and furious delirium and little or no fever without pain but with some coma. Constriction of the chest, asthmatic symptoms and cough of the whooping cough type. The common practice of smoking stramonium leaves for asthma is roughly homeopathic.

Clarke had a case of severe pleuro-pneumonia of right side, supervening on scarlatina, in which the patient, a young man, said he saw a large black dog about the room. This led Clarke to give Stram., which rapidly altered the whole case for the better including the pneumonia, and resolved the situation.

Nash reported a case or a woman, 30, with acute mania after being overheated in the sun. She called Nash for 6 days straight to come watch her die. She imagined herself eternally lost and begged everyone to pray for her. Talked day and night. Thought her head was as big as a bushel, her legs as large as a church. Nash cured with Stram. 6c after Glon., Lach., and Nat-c. failed. All symptoms and any traces of mania were gone after 24 hours.

S. A. Jones related the case of a little girl with brain symptoms for whom he had prescribed a remedy. The report was brought late at night that the patient was much worse. "She vomits," said the father, "if she even raises her head from the pillow."

The vomit was green. Jones found this under Stram., which he gave, and the next morning the case was entirely changed for the better. Acting on this analog, Jones also cured a "vomiting of green stuff always induced by bright light."

RELATIONS - ***Antidotes:*** Bell., Tab., Nux-v. ***Antidoted by:*** Lemon juice, Vinegar tobacco injections, Senn. for cerebral symptoms, Bell., Hyos., Nux-v. and *"Particularly Camphor"* (Teste). ***Antidote to:*** Merc., Plb. ***Compare:*** (1) Hyos. and Bell. It has less fever than Bell., but more than Hyos. It causes more functional excitement of the brain, but never approaches the true inflammatory condition of Bell. (1) Metrorrhagia, from retained placenta with characteristic delirium, Sec. (2) Pyrog. with fever and septic tendency. (3) Delirium, Bell., Lach., Agar., Cupr., Zinc. (4) Illusions of shape, Bapt., Petr., Thuj. (5) Erysipelas, Bell., Rhus-t. (6) Stuttering, unable to combine consonants with vowels, Bov. Bright light causes convulsions, Kali-br. (7) Better light, Stront. (8) Hears voices from far off talking to him, behind him, Anac. (9) Loquacity, Cupr., Hyos., Lach., Op., Verat. (10) Laughs and weeps by turns, Aur., Puls., Alum., Lyc., Caps., Graph., Phos., Sep., Sulph., Verat. (11) Tetanic convulsions worse touch and light, Nux-v. (12) Desire to escape in delirium, Bell., Bry., Op., Rhus-t. (13) Rabies, Lyss. ***Follows well:*** Cupr., Bell. ***Incompatible:*** Coff.

REFERENCES - Boericke. Clarke. Murphy. Phatak.

STREPTOCOCCINUM

(Streptococcus Nosode)

PHARMACY - strept. Streptococcinum. Streptococcinum bacteria. Nosodes. Made from streptococcus pyogenes and marcy. ***Historical dose:*** All potencies.

CLINICAL - Adenitis. ***Arthritis.*** Bronchitis. Cellulitis. Chorea. ***Colds. Debility.*** Ear, pain. Epilepsy. Fevers. Fibrositis. Infections. Mastoiditis. Otalgia. Otitis media. Psoriasis. Rheumatism. Scarlatina. Sinusitis. ***Sore, throats.*** Tonsillitis.

HOMEOPATHIC - Strept. should be considered in chronic disease where there is a history of acute streptococcal infection, including severe infection in the mother during pregnancy. Especially when the streptococcal infection immediately precedes chronic illness or when it is an outstanding event in the history of the patient.

Rapid action, especially in its effect on temperature. Anti-febrile action. Chilliness. Oversensitive. Intolerance to the least current of air caused by the moving of a person. Intolerance to noise, light.

Chronic sore throats and streptococcal infections. Severe or repeated tonsillitis or quinsy. ***Susceptible to catching colds and sore throats***. Acute sinusitis. Severe influenza, pneumonia, bronchitis, pleurisy.

Debility after streptococcal infections. Septic symptoms in infectious diseases. Puerperal sepsis. Epileptiform attacks. Chorea-like movements. Acute rheumatism. Retarded growth in delicate children.

Erysipelas. Otitis media. Meningitis. Dental caries. Acute parenchymatous nephritis. Peritonitis and cholecystitis. Intestinal toxemia, sometimes with amebic dysentery or other intestinal infection.

Scarlet fever has its own nosode, but Stept. is often effective when Scarl. fails.

MIND - Depressed. Weeping without reason, ***weeps on being given sympathy.*** Despair of recovery. Oversensitive. Highly strung, emotional, apprehensive. Exaggerated obsequiousness. Tormenting thoughts and anxiety. Obsessions. Thinks that he will become mad. Auditory hallucinations, hears cry for help.

Abdomen - While lying down cannot bear the weight of hand on the abdomen. Pain in the appendix.

Back - Pain of the backbone. Acute pain on the clavicles. Sensation of vibrations in the vertebral column and in the limbs.

Causations - Streptococcal infections. Ailments after tonsillectomy.

Ears - Otitis and mastoiditis. Otalgia specially if the person is lying down on the left. Intermittent puffs of wind in the ear. Auditory hallucinations, hears cry for help.

Eyes - Troubles of vision with ocular hypertension. Eye fatigue with the need of wearing glasses. Visual hallucination, sees the room full of flies.

Head - Tenacious migraine with vomiting of bile. Pain of the whole head as if it is going to burst.

Heart - Sensation of weakness of the heart. Pain of the point of the heart. Cramping pain in the precordial region.

Limbs - Muscular pain. Rheumatism of small articulations of the wrist, of the hand, with local redness, sometimes with hydro-arthrosis. Parethesia of lower limbs. Cold feet.

Modalities - Better from movement, in open air. ***Worse by consolation.*** Worse by humid weather, wet weather. Worse on beginning to move, better from subsequent movement.

Mouth - Feeling of having salty lips. White tongue with the tip red, without papilla in the front and in the back part. Gums painful when chewing.

Nose - Serous nasal discharge, mucopurulent with nasal crusts. Sinusitis with headache.

Skin - Vesicular and pustulous eruptions. Cellulitis. Exanthema. Erysipeltoid patches of the limbs. Fibrinous dermatitis, edema of the face. Scarlatina. Recurrent suppuration. Abortive pus formation. Loss of hair.

Sleep - Agitated sleep. Dreams of violence, scuffles.

Stomach - Sudden pains in the esophagus after meals. Dull, deep pain in the epigastric region. Nausea with vertigo and vomiting of bile.

Throat - Persistent pain and redness of the throat. Acute and chronic laryngitis. Red angina. Adenopathy of the neck. Big, infected, purulent tonsils.

Vertigo - Vertigo while rising and while lying down.

COMMENTS - When there has been a number of severe acute illnesses, Dr. Gordon, of Edinburgh, maintained that the best results can be obtained by antidoting the most recent infection first by its appropriate nosode, proceeding backwards and thus "curing in layers."

Another view is that, other things being equal, the first lapse from health is of greatest importance and that this should be antidoted first to undermine the superstructure and then deal with the case according to the remaining symptoms.

Ghose wrote, "I have used Streptococcin with very remarkable results in acute Bacillary dysentery with excessive hemorrhage and high rise of temperature with toxemia. The more the blood the more it is indicated like Mercurius, but there is no tenesmus or urinary complications of Mercurius in Streptococcin.

"In very bad cases of bacillary dysentery, very bad complications will follow and take a very long time to cure if it cannot be checked in the very beginning. In chronic cases of Dysentery where blood with mucopurulent discharge does not respond to indicated remedies or recurs and prolongs unduly. I have seen it to stop the bloody and mucopurulent discharge within a very short time with a dose of Streptococcin 200c."

RELATIONS - ***Compare:*** (1) Bell., Pyrog, Rhus-t. (2) Staphycoc., Scarl.

REFERENCES - Boericke. Foubister. Ghose. Julian.

STRONTIUM BROMATUM

(Strontium Bromide)

PHARMACY - stront-br. Strontium bromatum. Strontium bromide. Trituration. Solution. ***Historical dose:*** All potencies.

CLINICAL - Cellulitis. Dyspepsia. Gravel. Indigestion. Legs, swollen. Phlebitis. Varicose veins. Urine, offensive. Vomiting.

HOMEOPATHIC - Stront-br. often gives excellent results where a bromide is indicated. Anti-fermentative and neutralizes excessive acidity. Nervous dyspepsia. Vomiting of pregnancy.

COMMENTS - Cooper gave several experiences with Stront-br., including the case of a woman, 40, who had tenderness of her limbs and veins of legs showed up and were inclined to inflame. Chronic cellulitis, left ankle inclined to swell, vertigo, at times darkness comes over sight, appetite not good, bowels regular, menses every three weeks, cannot keep awake in evening.

Great relief came from Stront-br. 3x, but after taking it for ten days, severe ardor urine with constant bedwetting day and night set in, which yielded to Ferr-p. 6x. after failure with other remedies.

Woman, 60, had left leg and left foot swollen, hard and tender, red and pitting. The right also but less in degree. Indigestion with pain after food and sickness after food. For seven or eight years has been rheumatic and has had sciatica off and on. For two years, bowels confined, sleep very restless generally.

Stront-br. 3x was given and in two weeks the legs had gone down very much and she felt altogether better. Urine had become clear, but though ravenous for food had to stop eating and felt more sick and the bowels were more confined. After this, the patient got quite well without further medicine.

Stront-br. 30 gave great relief to a woman broken down by sorrow who could not digest food. Stront-br. 6x produced in a woman, 70, thick and offensive urine, dark-looking with grains of red sand.

REFERENCES - Boericke. Clarke.

STRONTIUM CARBONICUM

(Strontium Carbonate)

PHARMACY - stront-c. Strontium carbonicum. Strontium carbonate. Strontianite. Trituration. ***Historical dose:*** All potencies.

CLINICAL - Angina pectoris. ***Ankle, sprains.*** Anus, burning. Arteriosclerosis. Bedwetting. ***Bones, diseases.*** Cardialgia. Constipation. Cramp. Diarrhea. Emaciation. Feet, cold. Femur, decay. Headaches. Heart, disorders. Hemorrhoids. Hiccoughs. Hoarseness. Leucorrhea. Menses, disorders. ***Neuritis***. Phlebitis. ***Photophobia***. Sciatica. ***Shock. Sprains.*** Sternum, pains. Strokes. Sycotic, eruptions. Varicose, veins. Vision disorders.

HOMEOPATHIC - Strontianite was first discovered in the lead mines of Strontain in Argyllshire, from which it received its name. It occurs in massive, fibrous, stellated, rarely ortho-rhombic, crystals. The metal stronlium is dark yellow. Strontium carbonate varies in color from white to yellow and pale green.

Stront-c. was proved by Nenning, Schreter, Seidel, Trincks and Woost. It affects the circulation, causing a congestive feeling of tension. The heart, kidneys, marrow, ankles and right side are also affected.

Rheumatic pains, chronic sprains and stenosis of esophagus. Pains make patient faint or sick all over. Pain and itching alternate. Pains are fleeting, can hardly tell where they are, seemingly felt in marrow of bones. Pains increase and decrease gradually or make the patient faint and sick all over. Burning, gnawing. Right side most affected.

For the shock after surgical operations. Chronic ***sequelae of hemorrhages,*** after operations with much oozing of blood and coldness and prostration.

Arteriosclerosis. High blood pressure, with flushed face pulsating arteries, threatened strokes. Edema, especially about the ankles as a concomitant. Numbness. Soreness. Restlessness at night, smothering feeling. Affections of bones, especially femur.

Violent involuntary starts. Immobility of one side. Sense of paralytic weakness. Formication in limbs. ***Neuritis***, worse cold. Coldness in spots, on calves. Pressure in stomach is better by eating and worse after a meal. Emaciation.

MIND - Depression of spirits. Excessive forgetfulness. Inquietude and anguish. Apprehension as from bad conscience. Irritable, suddenly becomes angry, beats anything that comes in his way. Peevishness with tendency to fly into a rage.

Abdomen - Sticking in the abdominal ring. Uncomfortable fullness and swelling of abdomen. Colic in umbilical region.

Back - Pain, as of a fracture in loins and back. Drawing pain in back and lumbar region.

Causations - Hemorrhages, chronic sequelae. Injuries, sprains. Shock. ***Surgical shock after blood loss.*** Great exhaustion after surgery.

Chest - Pressure at chest in sternum. Constriction, pressive pain, worse walking. Drawing pain in muscles of chest. Angina pectoris.

Constitutions - Suited to bone disorders of scrofulous children when associated with diarrhea.

Ears - Tearing in front of right ear as if in the bone. Sticking in front of left ear in frequent paroxysms. Humming in the ears.

Eyes - Burning and redness of eyes. Pain and lachrymation on using eyes, with dancing and alternation of colors of objects looked at. ***Photophobia,*** remaining after operation, especially when objects appear covered with blood. Green spots before the eyes in the dark.

Face - Flushed face, worse from exertion. Violent, pulsating flushes in face. Red with burning heat or very pale, every time the patient walks. Red face, burns, itches.

Female - Flushes of heat, worse during menopause. Profuse perspiration at night, menopausal.

Food - Loss of appetite, food tasteless. Craving for bread, beer. Aversion to meat.

Head - Aches into upper jaw with vertigo and nausea. Headaches from nape of neck, spreading upwards, better wrapping head up warmly (Sil.). Distensive pressure on head. Aching eyebrows. Supra-orbital neuralgia, pains increase and decrease slowly (Stann.).

Heart - Heart feels smothered. Heart block. Dull, intermitting pressure in precordial region. Violent beating of arteries and of heart.

Kidneys - Pale urine with strong smell of ammonia. Increased secretion of a yellow, deep-colored urine. Diminished secretion of urine. Nocturnal emission of urine.

Limbs - Rheumatic pain, in joints, in right shoulder. Rheumatism with diarrhea. Sciatica with edema of ankle. Immobility of the limbs of one side only, like paralysis. Gnawing as if in marrow of the bones. Chronic sprained joints. ***Ankles sprained or swollen***. Swelling of ankle remaining after a sprain. ***Weakness of ankles.*** Chronic spasms, especially of ankle joints. Cramps in calves and soles. Icy-cold feet. Veins of hands engorged. Hands numb.

Lungs - Pressure, as of a load on chest. Pain in the left breast, with oppression, worse after meals. Dry cough, excited by irritation in trachea, worse at night. Dyspnea, when walking with heat and redness of face.

Modalities - Aversion to darkness. Better from light, heat, and sun. ***Better immersing in hot water***. Better wraps, hot bath, covering, warm stove. Worse change of weather. ***Worse cold***, uncovering, drafts. Worse evening, night and early morning. Worse 2 a.m. or 3 a.m., from being quiet. Worse when beginning to move, ***walking***, stooping Worse sprains, bleeding. Worse touch, rubbing, scratching.

Mouth - Feels numb and dry on waking. Bad odor from mouth. Teeth as screwed together.

Nose - Itching, redness and burning of nose. Bloody crusts in nose. Blowing of dark scabs from nose. Quivering on one side of nose. Twitching of left side of nose.

Rectum - Exhausting diarrhea with ***constant urging*** of yellow water with gripping, worse at night, better towards morning. Periodical diarrhea. Burning in anus lasts a long time after stool (Rat.). Hard, knotty stools, evacuated slowly with much effort, then burning in anus lasting for a long time.

Sensations - As if head were expanded from within. As if scalp were too tight. As if tendons of neck were drawn up. As if a load on chest. As if all power had left right arm. As if bruised in back and sacrum. Gnawing as if in marrow of bones. Symptoms as if in marrow of bones. Symptoms like phantoms, difficult to locate.

Skin - ***Sprains of ankle joint with edema***. Moist, itching, burning eruption, better in open air, especially warm sunshine. Violent perspiration at night.

Sleep - Retarded sleep. Jerking in body and starts when sleeping. Frequent waking at night, principally caused by a dry cough. Many fantastic dreams.

Stomach - Pressure in stomach during digestion. Heartburn. Belchings after eating. Violent hiccough causes chest pains, cardialgia. Nausea, with burning heat in face.

Temperature - Flushes of heat in face, with aversion to uncovering. Profuse perspiration at night, menopausal.

Throat - Hoarseness and roughness in throat, which excites a cough.

Vertigo - Vertigo with ***headache and nausea***.

COMMENTS - Congested state. Flushing in the face and violent pulsation of the arteries, congestion to heart, lungs and head. Symptoms better by warmth and wrapping up and worse by cold. All complaints are worse walking, particularly headache, leucorrhea, dyspnea and pressure in the sternum.

Headaches are boring, pressive and tensive. Tension from vertex to upper jaw, as if head were expanded from within and as if scalp were too tight, worse in evening, when lying with head low, slowly increasing and decreasing, better from heat. Tension in the nape, as if the tendons were drawn up. Tensive drawing in dorsal and lumbar muscles. External soreness, numbness.

Venous tension in the arms. "The veins of the arms and hands are injected and tense with great prostration and ill-humor." Phlebitis, varicose veins. Angina pectoris.

Predisposition toward strokes and high blood pressure. Surgical shock after blood loss. Great exhaustion after surgery.

Pressure in the stomach, better by eating and worse by walking. Pressure after eating. Diarrhea and constipation. Stools are accompanied and followed by burning in the rectum. Diarrhea is worse at night, urgent, with yellow stools. Emaciation.

Calcification, osteoporosis. Weak and brittle bones that break easily. Bony growths and enlargements. Bone pains, especially the femur, the thighbone. Bone disorders, particularly the femur. Bone disorders in scrofulous children when associated with diarrhea.

Characteristic weak ankles (Nat-c.). Chronic sprains of the ankle with edema. Sciatica associated with weak ankles. Ice cold feet. Leg and foot cramps (Calc.).

C. M. Boger cured a sciatica accompanied by edema of left ankle with Stront-c. after other remedies had failed.

A. P. Bowie cured a case occurring after a tedious labor. The stools were large and hard, expelled with great effort, followed by great pain in anus, burning, lasting a long time and compelling patient to lie down. Anus violently contracted after stool. Complained of coldness in spots on calves of legs. Stront-c. 6c entirely relieved.

RELATIONS - ***Antidoted by:*** Camph. ***Compare:*** (1) Arn., Ruta, Sil., Bar-c., Chin. (2) Stront-br., Stront-n., Stront-i. - Arteriosclerosis.

REFERENCES - Boericke. Clarke. Murphy. Phatak.

STRONTIUM NITRICUM

(Strontium Nitrate)

PHARMACY - stront-n. Strontium nitricum. Strontium nitrate. Solution. ***Historical dose:*** All potencies.

HOMEOPATHIC - C. M. Boger had a case in a menopausal woman of passive congestion of the kidneys completely relieved by Stront-n. The menses, which were usually exceedingly scanty, became profuse.

Morbid cravings. Eczema behind ears. Headaches. Kidney congestion. Menses scanty.

COMMENTS - Boger recorded the following case of Miss D., 18, brunette, who had dull pains over eyes worse by sunlight, motion, loss of sleep, sewing, reading. Pains were better after stool, with headache, swelling of upper lids, worse in morning. Bad taste in mouth.

Menses irregular, profuse, dark. Felt tired and weak. Addicted to eating cloves. In hot weather, sweats profusely and easily about head and chest, staining yellow. Very susceptible to cold. Cough provoked by oppression of breathing and talking.

Formerly had catarrh, followed by right-sided deafness. She had typhoid fever two years before and during the fever was allowed unlimited quantities of ice. Preceding the fever she had a post auricular eczema suppressed by salves, now is anemic and bloated. Urine contained epithelium, excess of chlorides, calcium oxalate and a trace of albumen (due probably to the clove habit).

Glon. helped the case, but for a time only. Stront-n. was chosen because Stront. irritates the kidneys and Nit-ac. corresponds to the vasomotor disturbance besides having cravings for odd things.

Stront-n. 6x was given and in a few days the headache vanished. At the end of a month the post-auricular eruption had reappeared. Five months later there had been no return of headache or palpebral edema, the craving for cloves had gone, the patient had taken on good flesh and color. The eruption had not all gone.

REFERENCES - Boericke. Clarke.

STROPHANTHUS HISPIDUS

(Kombe Seed)

PHARMACY - stroph. Strophanthus hispidus. Kombe seed. Strophanthus gratus. Inee. Onaye. Onage. Poison of Pahonias. N. O. Apocynaceae. Tincture of the seeds. ***Historical dose:*** Tincture and all potencies.

CLINICAL - ***Alcoholism.*** Anasarca. Anemia. Arteriosclerosis. Colitis. Cough. Cystitis. Diplopia. Dropsy, cardiac. Edema. Exophthalmia goiter. Faintness. ***Heart, disorders.*** Hemoptysis. ***Hives***. Levitation. Nausea. obesity. Pneumonia. Urticaria.

HOMEOPATHIC - Strophantus is an ornamental, evergreen and a climbing shrub, native of tropical Africa and Asia. The mother tincture comes from the seeds of the plant. It is used as an arrow-poison by natives of Africa. Among the alkaloids is strophanthin.

Stroph. occasions no gastric distress, diuretic. It has no cumulative action, safe for corpulent, aged persons with rigid arteries, as it does not affect the vaso-motors. Restores tone to a ***weak tissue***, especially of the heart muscle and valves.

Stroph. increases the contractile power of all striped muscles, especially the heart, increasing the systole and diminishing the rapidity. Acts on the heart ***increasing the systole and diminishes the rapidity***. Tones the heart and run off dropsical effusions.

Especially useful in failing compensation dependent upon fatty heart. After the long use of stimulants. Arteriosclerosis, rigid arteries of aged. Precordial anxiety. Retrosternal pain. Functional disturbances of heart from alcohol, tobacco, tea.

In small doses for weak heart, that feels enlarged. In mitral regurgitation, where edema and dropsy have supervened (Dig.). Severe prostration from hemorrhage after operations and acute diseases.

Anemia with palpitations and loss of breath. Faintness. Pneumonia. Rapid alternations of symptoms with slow pulse. Undulating sensation in whole body. Throbbings. Stitching pains. Twitchings of the muscles.

Obesity. Increased secretions. Nausea with special disgust for alcohol. ***Alcoholism***, with drop doses of Stroph-h. tincture. ***Hives***. Exophthalmia goiter.

MIND - Worse from strong emotions. Irritable. Anxiety and fear. Fear of ordeals. Feels lifted up during sleep. Precociously talkative children.

Abdomen - Abdomen distended, painful, especially in the umbilical and inguinal regions. Rumbling and pinching at navel. Shooting pains in right hypochondrium. Stitches in region of sigmoid flexure. Acute entero-colitis. Colic.

Back - Joint and muscular pains in the limbs, back and lumbar region with stiffness, muscular weakness, coldness at the limbs.

Causations - Alcohol, tea, tobacco.

Chest - Pressive pain in middle of right third rib on anterior half, worse by pressure. Thoracic pain on left side. Constrictive, cramping pain behind the sternum, crushed, gnawing, needle-like sensation.

Eyes - Pupils quivering, dilating and contracting alternately. Eyes brilliant. Glimmering in vision. Impaired sight of left eye with nausea and faintness. Double vision.

Face - Flushed, red spots. Lips scarlet.

Female - Uterine hemorrhage. Uterus heavily congested.

Food - ***Craving for alcohol,*** tea, coffee, stimulants. Nausea with special disgust for alcohol. Loss of appetite. Loathing of food, followed by choking and vomiting after eating.

Head - Temporal pains with double vision, impaired sight, brilliant eyes, flushed face. Violent, pulsating headache, aggravated by movement.

Heart - Weak heart with aching or anguish. Heart's action weak, rapid, irregular, due to muscular ***debility and insufficiency***. Cardiac pain and dyspnea. Chronic, nervous palpitations and arrest of breathing. Violent palpitations, worse by emotion and exercise. Sense of lively action. Mitral regurgitation. Stitches and twitches at apex beat. Pulse, rapid, alternating with slow, weak, small irregular.

Kidneys - Kidneys become hyperemic. Cystitis. Urinary tract infections. No urine passed for hours. Frequent urination. Urine increased secretion or scanty albuminous. Urine strong, odor is fruity or like horse urine, pale.

Limbs - Swollen, dropsical. Anasarca. Swelling of legs. Itching and stitching in both feet. Dorsum of foot painful and tense. Muscular and joint pains with stiffness and coldness of the limbs. The pains are aggravated by movement. Heaviness and pain in forearms and the fingers.

Liver - Pressure in liver region.

Lungs - Edema of lungs. Bronchial and cardiac asthma. Breathing deep, difficult, thirsty for air, feeling of dryness in the mucus membranes, aggravated by movement. Cough worse by lying down. Expectoration of bright red blood.

Modalities - Better from rest, lying down. Worse from exertion, exercise, standing. Worse tobacco, tea, alcohol. Worse from emotions.

Mouth - Dryness of tongue and fauces.

Rectum - Stool with burning and tenesmus in anus. Diarrhea with burning and tenesmus in anus. Frequent diarrhea with violent colic but good appetite. Infectious or toxic diarrhea.

Skin - Hives, chronic, receding. Urticaria, especially more chronic forms.

Stomach - Bulky feeling in the stomach. Twitching in stomach. Burning in esophagus and stomach with loss of appetite and extreme gastric distress. Cramping, acrid stomachache with belching and nausea. Eructation and hiccough. Nausea with special disgust for alcohol.

Temperature - Coldness of limbs. Temperature raised, skin dry. Profuse sweat.

Throat - Seems dry, constricted. Burning in throat and esophagus to stomach, compelling empty swallowing.

Vertigo - Vertigo with swimming vision. Senile vertigo. Undulations in head.

COMMENTS - The homeopathic proving was conducted by Templeton on five provers, using 2x, 3x, 6c, 12c, 30c and by O'Hanlon on twelve provers, using 6c, 12c and 30c.

Piedvache proved the tincture, but only with reference to the pulse. Gisevius proved Stroph-h. tincture, beginning with 5 drops increasing to 80 drops during the five days of his proving. Matthes proved Stroph-h. tincture in 10 drops doses.

Some well-marked symptoms were produced on two chemists from preparing the tincture. Other effects curative and pathogenetic have been observed on patients taking the drug. Stroph-h. disorders the digestion, causes burning in the esophagus and stomach, nausea, vomiting and diarrhea.

A. P. Skworzow gave an infusion of Stroph. to an alcoholic, 63, for weak heart and intermittent pulse, 7 drop doses three times a day. The first dose caused nausea and a repugnance to alcohol which proved to be permanent. The man entirely discontinued the habit.

On this hint, Stroph. was given to two other alcoholics with the same result of abolishing the taste for alcohol. It caused nausea and profuse sweating and the sudden withdrawal of alcohol was not attended with delirium.

A case of Clarke's illustrates the gastric and cardiac action of the remedy. W. G., 16, a delicate-looking boy, was admitted to a hospital. He had rheumatic pains for three months and an attack of rheumatic fever two years previously. He had been laid up a month before admission and a week before was taken with cough, shivering and occasional vomiting.

When admitted, he had a frequent, short, dry cough, worse lying down, had to be propped up in bed, had edema of feet, especially left. Tongue white, unable to retain any food for three days, no pain after food, but much flatulence, belchings giving much relief.

Heart greatly dilated, pulsation diffused, double mitral bruit. Dullness at bases of both lungs, moist rales, halfway up right lung. Expectoration of bright blood for seven days.

Stroph. tincture, one drop every four hours, was given. Improvement in all the symptoms was immediate, sickness, cough, hemoptysis and dropsy all disappeared and the heart sounds had cleared up to a large extent when the boy went home, less than three weeks after admission.

Hamer mentioned that Stroph. cured "functional disturbance of the heart from alcohol tobacco and tea." This agrees with the relation of Stroph. to alcoholism and symptoms of indigestion.

A writer gave his experience with Stroph.: a woman had constant outbursts of urticarial rash dating from exposure to an offensive effluvium from a dead whale cast on the sands. The attacks would recur after drinking a glass of table beer. Stroph-h. cured.

Any accompanying cardiac weakness would be an additional indication. The same writer considered Stroph. of great service in the anemia of young girls when palpitation and breathlessness are marked features.

An accidental proving on a girl of five was made through the mother giving twenty drops of the tincture by mistake. Some half an hour later her face was flushed, lips scarlet, eyes brilliant, temperature raised, skin dry, tongue normal. Pupils quivering, dilating and contracting every few seconds. Pulse 140, arteries distended.

Heart sounds vigorous, slight regurgitant mitral murmur. Intellect clear, precociously loquacious during the five hours the poisonous symptoms lasted. An ipecac emetic was administered. No urine passed for ten hours after the dose.

RELATIONS - ***Compare:*** (1) Heart, dropsy, Apoc. (2) Heart, Dig. is cumulative, Stroph-h. is not. (3) Crat., Phase., Cact. (4) Anemia, Ferr. (5) Alcoholism, Chin., Nux-v., Aven., Querc. (6) Kali-c. - heart weakness, fatigue, chill, acute stinging pains, aggravated by the cold and at 2 a.m. (7) Acon. - Sharp intolerable pains, much more agitated with fear of death. (8) Lach. - worse left-side, aggravated on waking, hyperesthesia of the skin, tendency to hemorrhage. (9) Sarcol-ac.- Pains and muscular weakness, extreme asthenia, aggravated by the slightest movement. (10) movement, feeling of fullness in the epigastrium, constipation. ***Compatible:*** Ferr. in anemia.

REFERENCES - Boericke. Clarke. Phatak.

STRYCHNIA PHOSPHORICUM

(Strychnine Phosphate)

PHARMACY - stry-p. Strychnia phosphoricum. Strychnine phosphate. Alkaloid obtained from several species of Strychnos. Solution. Trituration. ***Historical dose:*** All potencies.

CLINICAL - Atelectasis. Heart, disorders. Headache. Paralysis. Pulse, irregular. Spinal cord, disorders. Tachycardia.

HOMEOPATHIC - Stry-p. is useful in chorea, hysteria, acute asthenia after acute fevers. ***Hands and axilla covered with clammy perspiration***. Cold and clammy feet. Better rest and in open air, worse from motion.

Acts through the cerebro-spinal system upon muscles, causing twitching, stiffness, weakness and loss of power. Anemia of spinal cord, paralysis, burning, aching and weakness of spine, pain extends to front of chest, tenderness on pressure in mid-dorsal region.

Atelectasis and break in the compensation of a hypertrophied heart, the beginning of fatty degeneration of the heart muscle. Tachycardia. Irregular pulse. Rapid and weak pulse.

MIND - Affects upon the mind, producing lack of control, ***uncontrollable desire to laugh*** and disinclination to use the brain.

COMMENTS - A woman to whom Clarke gave Stry-p. 3x in five-drop doses twenty minutes before meals, felt at once constriction of the throat and after each meal violent headache in forehead over the eyes. The choking sensations were a constant feature in provings and poisonings.

REFERENCES - Boericke. Clarke. Royal.

STRYCHNINUM

(Strychnine)

PHARMACY - stry. Strychninum. Strychnine. Alkaloid obtained from several species of Nux vomica, Loganiaceae. Trituration. Solution. ***Historical dose:*** All potencies.

CLINICAL - Amaurosis. Aorta, pain. Aphonia. Asthma. Athetosis. Bedwetting. Bladder, paralysis, pains. Breasts, pains. Coughs. Cramps. Diaphragm, spasms. Emphysema. Exophthalmos. Eye, disorders. Headaches. Hemiplegia. Influenza. Joints, stiffness. Laryngeal, crises. Locomotor, ataxia. Malar, bones, pains. Neurasthenia. Night-blindness. Paraplegia. Proctalgia. Rheumatism. Scrotum, abscess. Spinal irritation. ***Tetanus***.

HOMEOPATHIC - Liquor Strychnie is responsible for many of the poisonings, the powdered crystals, either pure or mixed in pills or rat-poison, for others. Strychnia itself is very sparingly soluble in cold water (1 in 5760). A homeopathic proving of Stry. was made by Henry Robinson on two provers, a man and a woman.

The man took 900 drops in twenty-three days, the woman 445 drops in fifty-three days. These have furnished the most distinctive symptoms. Extreme nervous excitability. Visions of an ugly face. Fits of laughing with light. Idiotic-like chuckle. Confusion of ideas, stupor and weariness were some of the mental symptoms. Swimming sensation in the head and giddiness involuntary.

Stimulates the motor centers and the reflex action of the spinal cord. Stimulates the central nervous system, mental activities, special senses rendered more acute. All reflexes are made more active.

Spasmodic rigidity. Spasms of muscles, cramps from an undue reflex excitability of the cord, spasms of the bladder, etc. Stiffness in muscles and face and neck. Athetosis. Tetanus with violent jerking, twitching and trembling.

Tetanic convulsions with opisthotonos. The muscles relax between paroxysms, worse slightest touch, sound, odor. Influences more directly the spinal cord and is less appropriate in visceral derangements than Nux-v.

Explosive nervousness. The ***pains and sensations come suddenly*** and return at ***intervals***. Darting, pinching lancinating, fulgurating, electric pains. Spine is cold. Gushing sweat from head and chest.

Drowsiness, with headache. Frontal headaches, momentary dartings like electric shocks. Respiration increased. Inability to take deep breath, fixation of chest walls. Sudden palpitations.

The direct "tonic" action of Stry. was shown in one of Robinson's provers, who had "unusually good appetite, she enjoys her food amazingly."

Stry. is an antidote to chloral, used in asphyxia from gas and chloroform and early stages of opium poisoning.

Abdomen - Sharp pain in abdominal muscles, griping pain in bowels.

Back - ***Rigidity of cervical muscles***. Sharp pain in nape and down spine. ***Back stiff***, violent jerks in spinal column. ***Icy sensation down spine***.

Ears - Hearing very acute, burning, itching and roaring in ears.

Eyes - Hot, painful, protruding, staring. Pupils dilated. Spasmodic contraction of ocular muscles, twitching and trembling of lids. Sparks before eyes.

Face - Pale, anxious, livid. Jaws stiffened, lower jaw spasmodically closed.

Female - Desire for sex increased (Plat.). Any touch on body excites a voluptuous sensation.

Head - ***Over irritability***. Restless. Full and bursting headache with heat in eyes. Vertigo with roaring in ears. Jerking of head forwards. Scalp sore. Itching of scalp and nape.

Limbs - ***Cramp-like pains***. Rheumatism with stiff joints. Limbs stiff. ***Violent jerking, twitching and trembling.*** Tetanic convulsions and opisthotonos, spasms provoked by slightest touch and attempt to move. Shocks in the muscles.

Lungs - ***Spasm of muscles*** about larynx. Sharp, contractive pains in muscles of chest. Excessive dyspnea. Persistent cough, recurring after influenza.

Modalities - Better from lying on back. Worse morning, after meals. Worse touch, noise, motion, exertion, walking.

Rectum - Very obstinate constipation. Feces discharged involuntarily during spasms.

Sensations - Feeling as if head and face were enlarged, after affects of debauches (Nux-v.). As if an iron cap were on head. Paralyzed feeling in left half of head and face. Scalp sore, as if hair had been pulled. As if nerves suddenly pulled out of teeth. As of a lump in throat. As if water dripped off right elbow, at intervals and off right shoulder. As if chopped in half at waist, at night.

Skin - Itching of whole body, especially nose. Icy sensation down the spine.

Stomach - Constant retching. Violent vomiting. Nausea of pregnancy.

Temperature - Cold chills down spine. Perspiration in a stream down head and chest. Lower limbs cold.

Throat - Dry, contracted, feeling of a lump. Swallowing impossible. Burning along and spasms of esophagus. Violent itching in roof of mouth.

COMMENTS - Innumerable poisonings with strychnine are on record, the symptoms being convulsions of a tetanic nature, in the fatal cases ending in asphyxia. The spasms are intermittent and the least touch or movement is sufficient to induce an attack. Lying on the back is the only tolerable position.

"Lying on her back, body rigid, jaws set, arms and hands flexed, the thumbs nearly touching across the chest and the whole muscular system convulsed with short, jerky spasms. Which would continue for about a minute and then remit, the muscles remaining contracted and as hard as wood during the intervals between the paroxysms."

The convulsions generally take the form of opisthotonos, cries, terror, hippocratic countenance and frothing at the mouth are common occurrences.

Meyhoffer experimented with Stry. on himself and two other persons, one of whom was a woman of lymphatic temperament.

"It always brought on electric shocks, occurring whenever the prover was touched or whenever any one lightly shook the bed on which he or she was lying. This happened to all, only the woman (lymphatic and feeble) needed a stronger dose." Any touch on any part of the body caused a voluptuous sensation.

Gamper of St. Petersburg experimented with Stry-n. on healthy young hospital assistants and found that it increased the amount of gastric juice secreted, the general acidity and the quantity of free acid in the secretion. It hastened the absorption from the stomach and strengthened mechanical movements. The effects continued some time after the administration was stopped.

Marked action on the rectum and genito-urinary organs (Ign. and Nux-v.). The male prover had his left testicle and cord swollen and an abscess of the scrotum developed and discharged.

"Gurgling noise in rectum with electric darts" is a symptom of one prover. Many pains center about the lips and eyes. Pains and chills occur in the occiput and nape and run down whole length of spine. Stiffness is a leading note of Stry. and Cooper gave "rheumatism with stiff joints" as an indication.

Itching of the whole body and "violent itching in roof of mouth." Jerkings, twitchings and shocks in all parts. Increased activity of the spinal senses. Dread of touch, shrinks from drafts.

Clarke found Cooper's suggestion that many cases of persistent cough recurring after influenza are met by Stry. to be correct. The influenza cough has in it a strong spasmodic and asthmatic element, whether dry or not, and this seems to give one point of correspondence.

C. W. Lawson related the case of a medical man who took continuously for two years, Stry. hydrochlor., 5 to 10 minims, thrice daily with a little sal volatile. He was at first benefited, but afterwards experienced a desire to take deep inspirations. "He felt that to do so would overcome the inhibitory power over the lung, probably the action of the diaphragm."

One morning after a dose of Stry., he was taking such an inspiration and from that moment experienced the sensations complained of an inability to take a deep breath. Fixation of chest walls compelled him to stoop, weakness on exertion, great confusion of thought and memory, occasional clay-colored feces, usually greater in amount than ordinary.

After six months, the apex beat descended to the 6th interspace and headache and drowsiness became marked. He traveled for six months without benefit. All attempts to act on the heart with drugs increased the headache. Lawson then found the heart dilated, wide sub-costal angle, chest emphysematous, moving en mass.

After a full year of treatment with Hyos. tincture at bedtime, which proved strikingly beneficial, drowsiness ceased entirely and improvement in all other respects followed.

Hale mentioned the following uses of Stry. and its salts as observed by him and others. Stry. 6c. in the tetanic spasms of cerebro-spinal meningitis. Amaurosis from atony of retina. Diplopia and night-blindness. Stry-s., and in one case when all other Stry. preparations had failed, Stry-val. cured facial neuralgia and neuralgic headache.

Spasms of esophagus in an hysterical woman. Stry-val. 2x. cured brain exhaustion of women in whom high nervous weakness exists. Stry. 12c or 30c for chorea, when the convulsions do not cease during sleep.

RELATIONS - ***Compare:*** (1) Eucal. - neutralizes ill effects of strychnine. (2) Cic., Arn. (tetanus). (3) Stry. ars. - Paresis in the aged, relaxed musculature. Prostration. Psoriasis, chronic diarrhea with paralytic symptoms. Compensatory hypertrophy of heart with beginning fatty degeneration. Stry-ar. - Marked dyspnea when lying down, edema of lower limbs, urine scanty, high specific gravity, heavily loaded with glucose. Diabetes. use the 6x trituration. (4) Stry-f-c. - chlorotic and paralytic conditions, dyspepsia with vomiting of ingesta, 2x and 3x trituration. (5) Stry-n. - 2x and 3x. Said to remove craving for alcohol. Use for two weeks. (6) Stry-s. - Gastric atony. (7) Stry-val. - exhaustion of brain-power, women of high nervous weakness, 2x trituration.

REFERENCES - Boericke. Clarke. Phatak.

STRYCHNOS GAULTHERIANA

(Hoang Nan)

PHARMACY - stryeh-g. Strychnos gaultheriana. Hoang nan. Tropical Bind-weed. N. O. Loganiacee. Tincture of dried bark. ***Historical dose:*** Tincture and all potencies.

CLINICAL - Albuminuria. Boils. Cancer. Carbuncles. Colic. Convulsions. Diarrhea. Eczema. Fatigue. Hydrophobia. Leprosy. Paralysis. Prurigo. Pustules. Rabies. Snakebites. Syphilis. Ulcers. Vertigo.

HERBAL - The Strych-g. plant is indigenous to Tonquin, where it has a great reputation as a remedy for leprosy, hydrophobia, snakebites and diseases of the skin. The red dust of the bark contains the most active properties.

HOMEOPATHIC - The native method of preparing the medicine is by moistening the mixture of the three powders with a little vinegar and forming the paste into pills of about a centimeter in diameter.

When taken by a healthy person these pills cause fatigue, general indisposition, vertigo, tingling of the hands and feet involuntary movements of jaw. When a person is bitten by a poisonous animal, a dose of three or four grams is administered in vinegar.

If none of these symptoms appear it is understood that the medicine is antagonized and the dose is increased until some of the symptoms manifest themselves, when the poison is considered to be destroyed. The use of alcohol is forbidden while a patient is taking this medicine. Vinegar appears to modify its virulence.

In animals poisoned with it, tetanic convulsions always begin in the hind legs and spread all over the body. Brain, liver, kidneys and lungs were found congested post mortem.

Generally improves nutrition, especially in constitutional syphilis. Exhaustion with vertigo, numbness and tingling in hands and feet involuntary action of lower jaw. Tetanic convulsions beginning in legs and spreading over body.

Eczema, prurigo. Pustules and boils. Old ulcers. Leprosy. Snakebites. Tertiary syphilis and paralysis. Glandular disorders. Cancer of glandular structures. Removes fetor and hemorrhage in cancer, revives the healing process.

MIND - Apathy. Lassitude, indisposition to make mental effort.

Abdomen - Colic and diarrhea.

Head - Vertigo, headache.

Kidneys - Albuminuria. Mucus casts.

Skin - Malignant ulcers, pustular eczema, boils, carbuncles, leprosy.

COMMENTS - In 1883 a proving of Strych-g. was made by seven people, producing a few symptoms. According to Hansen, there is prurigo, pustular eczema in parts well supplied with sebaceous glands (face, neck, genitals).

General malnutrition. Glandular cancer. Boils, carbuncles, constitutional syphilis. The dose of which is 5 to 30 drops of the tincture three times a day.

RELATIONS - *Compare:* Nux-v., Cur., Ang., Bruc., Hydrc. Follows well after Ars.

REFERENCES - Boericke. Clarke.

SUCCINUM ACIDUM

(Succinic Acid)

PHARMACY - succ-ac.Succinum acidum. Succinic acid. Amber oil. A mineralized fossil resin not to be confounded with Ambergris, Ambra. Trituration. Solution of the non-rectified oil prepared by dry distillation of Amber. Solution of Succinic acid. ***Historical dose:*** All potencies. Drop doses of the oil.

CLINICAL - Asthma. Fears. Globus. Hay fever. Hiccough. Hysteria. Leucocythemia splenica. Spleen disorders.

HOMEOPATHIC - Dr. Morris Weiner tested Succ-ac., which he prepared himself from amber by dry distillation. The fumes of the crude acid, he said, are inflammable and produce asthma, cough, sneezing, weeping, dropping of watery mucus from nostrils, pain in chest and headache.

On this indication, he treated thirty people suffering from hay fever and cured them all, saving them the necessity of making an annual exodus. He gave one or two grains of the 3x trituration of Succ. diluted in twelve teaspoonfuls of water, a teaspoonful every two hours.

Burnett wrote in Diseases of Spleen, that the non-rectified oil is used as an organ remedy in spleen affections, especially when accompanied by nervous and hysterical phenomena. The crude oil is a thick brown liquid having a strong empyreumatic odor. It is a powerful local irritant and has been used with success as such in lumbago, rheumatism and sciatica.

Succ-ac. enters into the composition of "Roche's Embrocation," and "Haarlem Oil," and has a popular reputation as a remedy for whooping cough, the directions being for it to be rubbed into the spine night and morning.

Succ-ac. produces many nervous and hysterical symptoms. Asthma. Fear of trains and closed places. Affections of spleen. Burnett noted it for hysterical convulsions in women.

MIND - Fear of trains and closed places.

Eyes - Lachrymation.

Head - Headaches.

Lungs - Pains in chest. Asthma. Incipient tuberculosis. Chronic bronchitis. Whooping cough.

Nose - Sneezing, dropping of watery mucus from nostrils.

Stomach - Persistent hiccough. Violent vomiting.

Throat - Globus.

COMMENTS - A tablespoonful dose, said Murrell, has caused persistent vomiting, diarrhea and symptoms of collapse and the patient aborted. He gave the oil, six ounces of acorn-water added half a scruple of the oil. They do not mix chemically, but by shaking each time a dose is taken the required division and potency is attained.

Burnett's keynote was "Painful spleen disorders where there are convulsive attacks such as the hysterical and hypochondriacal often have."

Burnett related in his book a most remarkable case of "chronic enlargement of the spleen with hyperesthesia, head pain, Dyspnea orthopnea, convulsions" in a young woman "towards the end of her teens."

After years of treatment, Burnett concluded from Rademacher's account of Succ-ac. that it might provide the remedy. It was given in five-drop doses three times a day. In forty-eight hours the convulsive attacks ceased and all the phenomena slowly disappeared.

A keynote of Burnett's is "Fear of trains and close places." His dose is five drops of the oil three times a day.

RELATIONS - *Compare:* (1) Amber gemstone. Succinum purum. (2) Ars-i. - Hay fever. Paroxysmal sneezing, dropping of watery mucus from nostrils, asthma. Inflammation through respiratory tract, causing asthma, chest pains, etc., itching of eyelids and canthi and nose worse drafts. (3) Arund., Wye., Sabad, Sinapis nigra.

REFERENCES - Boericke. Clarke. Phatak.

SULFANILAMIDE

PHARMACY - sulfa. Sulfanilamide. Para-amino-phenylsulfamide. Allopathic drug. ***Historical dose:*** All potencies.

CLINICAL - Addison's disease. Anemia. Audio-visual, disorders. Boils. Cataract. Coma. Cyanosis. Delirium. Dermatitis. Goiter. Hypoglycemia. Jaundice. Ménière's disease. Muscular, atrophy. Myxedema. Nephritis. Schizophrenia. Thyroid, deficiency.

HOMEOPATHIC - In medicine, Sulfanilamide is known in one form as Exoseptoplix. It was the active part in the decomposition of prontosil which was used in experiments by Domagk in 1935. The homeopathic proving of sulfanilamide was conducted by Sutherland, who used the 3x, 6x and the 200th potency.

Sulfa. has a slowing down of all physical and mental functions. Halt in development and puberty comes late in the child. Myxedema. Fatigue, general weariness. Indefinable discomfort with giddiness or vertigo, with apathy.

Febrile condition with rash, aching, conjunctivitis, which may be accompanied by fever with shivering, pain in the joints increase in leucocytes with granulocytosis. Paresis and muscular atrophy of the feet and hands. Cramping pains in the hypogastric region. Oliguria and kidney colic. Hypoglycemic conditions.

Heart rhythmic anomaly, cyanosis and comatose condition. Cyanosis with violet or livid coloring of the lips, nose, ears, fingertips. Vesicular eruptions. Goiter. Thyroid deficiency and congestion of the thyroid gland.

MIND - Mental backwardness. Clouded mental state. Idea association complaints. Concentration complaints. Difficulty in determining contrasts and shapes. Loss of memory for graphic movements and for sounds and words. Loss of memory with diminution in auditory acuity. Physical and mental apraxia.

Alternating psychological condition. Cyclical moods. At times happy, joyful, then sad and dejected. Indolence, apathy, state of confusion. Attacks of delirium. Schizophrenia.

Abdomen - Sensation of fullness. Pain in the hypogastric region. Cramping abdominal pains. Congestion of the liver with alternate constipation and diarrhea. Gastric and duodenal ulcer. Jaundice.

Blood - Anemia. Aplastic anemia. Hemolytic anemia. Chronic leukemia. Thrombopenia. Acetone elimination in the urine or excessive nitrogen in the blood. Agranulocytosis syndrome with fever, leucopenia, necrotic angina and light hemorrhaging of the skin and mucus membranes.

Chest - Pain and heat in the chest.

Ears - Pustules and papules on the outer ear. Buzzing in the ears, as if produced by a bell. Bilateral diminution in auditory acuity. Deafness through atrophy of the auditory nerve. Ménière's disease. Boils in the auditory canal.

Eyes - Chemosis of the left eye. Cloudiness of the crystalline lens or capsule. Cataract. Hemorrhaging of the retina. Optic neuritis. Stye on the lower left eyelid. Eruption of yellow pustules on the edge of the eyelids.

Face - Acne of the chin.

Food - Hypoglycemic syndrome with condition of weakness, sweating, hunger pangs and tendency to faint with or without convulsions. Loss of appetite.

Head - Frontal or occipital headache increasing towards evening.

Heart - Rhythmic anomaly, especially in elderly people.

Kidneys - Chronic interstitial nephritis. Kidney colic. Kidney stones. Paresis of the bladder with retention of urine. Slow urination, urinary stream weak. Urine cloudy. Oliguria. Presence of porphyrin in the urine. Hematuria. Uremia.

Limbs - Severe muscular pains. Acute rheumatism. Sciatica. Neuritic, especially sciatic pains. Progressive symmetrical muscular atrophy, beginning in the hands. Paresis or paralysis of the feet with muscular atrophy and absence of the Achilles' reflex. Acrocyanosis with formication and numbing of the limbs of the legs. Pain in the right leg. Pain and weakness in the small muscles of the feet and hands.

Lungs - Dyspnea, difficulty in breathing deeply. Bronchial asthma.

Male - Inhibition of the production of spermatozoa. Sterility.

Modalities - Better from hot compresses, discharges.

Nose - Pustules in the left nasal fold. Sneezing. Boils.

Rectum - Alternate constipation and diarrhea.

Skin - Burns. Acne of the chin. Burning papular and pustular eruptions. Dermatitis. Sycosis of the beard. Chronic eczema. Pityriasis rubra. Erythema. Pigmentation disorders of the skin. Vesicular eruptions on uncovered areas exposed to the sun. Dermatitis from photosensitization. Measles-type, urticarial eruptions. Eruptions ameliorated by hot compresses and by discharges.

Stomach - Nausea, vomiting.

Temperature - Basal metabolism reduced.

Vertigo - Vertigo with nausea, ameliorated in the open air and by leaning forwards.

RELATIONS - ***Compare:*** (1) Ars. - Anxiety and agitation, especially between 1 a.m. and 3 a.m. Burning pains. Edema of the lower eyelids. Thirsty for small amounts of iced water. Vomiting and diarrhea with severe prostration. Oppression. Scaly, burning eruptions and itching, worse between 1 a.m. and 3 a.m. (2) Cresol. - Asthenia with euphoria. Loquacious mood, talks non-stop. Paresis of the lower legs with ataxia. Hypertrophy of the muscles in the hands. Hypertension and oliguria. Hardening of the cartilages. Thickening and hardening of the skin. Itching, pigmented erythema of the skin. (3) Cic. - Convulsions, contraction of the muscles of the entire body. Pupils dilated. Pustular eruptions with thick, yellow scabs.

REFERENCES - Julian.

SULFONALUM

(Sulfonal)

PHARMACY - sulfon. Sulfonalum. Sulfonal. Diethylsulphone dimethyl methane. Coal tar product. Trituration. ***Historical dose:*** All potencies.

CLINICAL - Albuminuria. Chorea. Constipation. Cramps. Cyanosis. Diarrhea. Epilepsy. Headaches. Heart failure. Hematoporphyrinuria. Insomnia. Locomotor ataxia. Nausea. Paralysis, ascending. Ptosis. Reflexes, abolished. Tinnitus. Twitching. Vertigo. Vomiting. ***Weakness.***

HOMEOPATHIC - Sulfonal was at first regarded as one of the safest of hypnotics, but many cases of poisoning by medicinal doses have occurred and the schema is made up of reported effects produced on patients.

Sulfon. is a coal tar product which produces ataxic symptoms, staggering gait, anesthesia of legs with absence of knee jerks. Chorea. Cerebellar disease. Vertigo of cerebral origin. The symptoms disappear slowly.

Reflexes abolished. Epilepsy, with over-excitability of the cortical substance. Twitching of muscles, especially of face and flexors, worse by voluntary movement, but always present in sleep. Muscular incoordination. Paralysis of body, better by cold water, and cold douches. Great prostration. Paralysis progressive sometimes with hyperesthesia and abnormal sensation, affecting first legs, then arms.

Profound weakness, faint feeling and despondency. Fainted and vomited. Loss of control of sphincter. Livid, especially the face. Cyanosis. Death by respiratory failure preceded by unconsciousness.

MIND - Mental confusion, incoherence, illusions, apathetic. ***Alternation of happy, hopeful states with depression and weakness***. Extreme irritability. Stupidity. Unconscious with dilated and fixed pupils, profuse sweat.

Abdomen - Spleen enlarged, hyperemic.

Back - Chronic leptomeningitis.

Ears - Tinnitus.

Eyes - Pupils dilated and fixed. ***Eyes bloodshot and restless***. Ptosis, heavy look about eyes. Double vision.

Face - Livid.

Head - Headache and tinnitus aurium. Pain on attempting to raise head.

Heart - Heart failure and edema of lungs. Heart's action feeble, occasionally intermittent.

Kidneys - Constant desire to urinate. Retention of urine, had to be drawn off, dark-colored. Urine very scanty, albuminous, almost solid when cooled, with casts. Pink color. Urine cherry-color, later like dark port wine. Hematoporphyrinuria, urine oscillated between deep claret and light claret color. Dark brown urine.

Limbs - Restlessness, muscular twitchings. Ataxic movements, ***staggering gait***, cold, weak, trembling, legs seem too heavy. Knee-jerks. Plantar reflex deficient. Cramps of legs and single muscles. Stiffness and paralysis of both legs. Anesthesia of legs.

Lungs - Congestion of lungs, stertorous breathing. Sighing dyspnea. Edema of lungs. Signs of bronchopneumonia.

Male - Erythema on prepuce.

Mouth - Breath smells of onions. ***Tongue as if paralyzed.***

Rectum - Diarrhea and vomiting. Great constipation.

Skin - Itching, bluish purpura. Discolored patches like purpura on skin. Erythematous measles-like eruption.

Sleep - Insomnia. Fidgety, wakeful, drowsy. Sleepiness and weariness with unsteady gait. Stupor. Heaviness and drowsiness.

Stomach - Constant retching, vomiting and soreness over epigastrium. Vomiting, diarrhea and violent chills. Great disturbance of digestion with scanty urine.

Temperature - Violent chills.

Throat - Aphasia, dysphagia, difficult speech.

Vertigo - Vertigo of cerebral origin, unable to rise from seat.

COMMENTS - Ataxic gait and diminished or abolished reflexes. Locomotor ataxia. Ascending paralysis. Stupor. Headache with noises in ears. Rashes on the skin, purpura, erythematous, etc. Vomiting and diarrhea. Urine retained or secretion arrested, claret-colored, containing albumen, porphyrin. Weak heart, fainting occurs and death takes place by heart failure.

One man observed uniform skin effects every time he took Sulfon., more intense the larger the dose. This occurred from 5 grains: patches of erythema appeared first on inner side of first phalanx of right little finger, next over proximal ends of metacarpal bones of left thumb and index, on posterior surface of left forearm a little below elbow, fourth on prepuce. The symptoms were better by cold douches.

RELATIONS - ***Compare:*** (1) Trion. - insomnia associated with physical excitement, vertigo, loss of equilibrium, ataxia, nausea, vomiting, Diarrhea, stertorous breathing, cyanosis, tinnitus, hallucination.

REFERENCES - Boericke. Clarke. Phatak.

SULPHUR

(Brimstone)

PHARMACY - sulph. Sulphur. Brimstone. Sulphur lotum. Sulphur sublimatum. Sulphur (At. Wt. 31.98). Trituration of Flowers of Sulphur. A saturated solution of Sulphur in absolute alcohol constitutes the tincture. A trituration of amorphous Sulphur has also been used. Sulphur prepared by precipitation from a solution of Calc-s. with hydrochloric acid, are included. ***Historical dose:*** All potencies.

CLINICAL - Acne. Adenoids. ***Alcoholism***. Allergies. Amaurosis. Amenorrhea. Anemia. Anus, prolapsed. Asthma. Atelectasis. Backache. Bedsore. Belching. Biliousness. ***Boils.*** Brain, congestion. Bright's disease. Bronchitis. Cataract. Catarrh. Chancre. Chest, pains. Chilblains. Chloasma. Colds. Constipation. Corns. Cough. Crusta, serpiginosa. Dental fistula. Diabetes. ***Diarrhea. Eczema.*** Epilepsy. ***Eruptions.*** Esophagus, constriction. Eyes, disorders. ***Faintness. Feet, burning.*** Fever. Freckles. Ganglion. Glands, disorders. Gleet. Globus hystericus. Gonorrhea. Gout. Headache. Head, congestion. ***Hemorrhoids.*** Herpes. Hydrocele. Hydrocephalus. Hydrothorax. Hypochondriasis. Impotence. Influenza. Intermittents. Irritation. ***Itching***. Jaundice. Keloids. Laryngitis. Leucorrhea. Lichen.

Liver, disorders. ***Lumbago.*** Lungs disorders. Mania. Masturbation. Measles. ***Memory, weak***. Meningitis. Menstruation, disorders. Miscarriage. Molluscum. ***Nettle rash.*** Neuralgia. Nipples, sore. Nosebleed. Ophthalmia. Phimosis. Phlegmasia dolens. Peritonitis. Pleurisy. ***Pneumonia.*** Pregnancy, disorders. Prostatorrhea. ***Psoriasis. Rectal disorders.*** Rheumatic fever. Rheumatism. Ringworm. ***Scabies.*** Sciatica. ***Senile, dementia. Skin, disorders.*** Sleep, disorders. Smell, illusions. Spinal curvature. Spleen, pain. Stomatitis. Taste, illusions. Tenesmus. Tonsillitis. Toothache. Trachea. Tuberculosis. Ulcers. ***Urticaria.*** Uterus, prolapsed. Vaccination. Varicocele. Varicose veins. ***Vertigo.*** Warts. Worms.

HOMEOPATHIC - Sulphur is an elementary substance, occurring in nature as a brittle crystalline solid, burning in the air with a blue flame, being oxidized to Sulphur dioxide (Sulphurous acid).

Sulphur is a product of volcanic eruptions, found free in nature and was used from ancient times to remove skin disorders. The reputation of Sulphur as a remedy is perhaps as old as medicine. "As early as 2,000 years ago," said Hahnemann, "Sulph. had been used as the most powerful specific against the scabies.

"The itch with which the workers in wool are so much affected, causes an intolerably agreeable, tingling, itching, gnawing as of vermin. Some designate it as an intolerably voluptuous titillating itching, ceasing as soon as the parts are scratched and commencing to burn, which burning continues after the scratching.

"Sulph. frequently produces in healthy persons burning-itching pimples and vesicles resembling the itch vesicles and especially itching in the joints and in the night."

The domestic use of Sulph. as a "Spring medicine" is based on its anti-psoric properties. "It is one of the most popular diaphoretics of the day," said Milne, "few old women failing to use it when any eruption is supposed to be struggling through the skin."

The specific power of Sulph. to cure itch can be abused if applied externally as baths and ointments. Instead of being cured, the skin affection can be repelled and a host of secondary disorders will appear in its place.

Sulph. is a major anti-psoric. A great reabsorbent and is frequently needed after acute illnesses which do not entirely clear up. ***Complaints that relapse. When carefully selected remedies fail to act, especially in acute diseases***. It is often of great use in beginning the treatment of chronic diseases and in finishing acute ones or when the ***reaction is deficient***.

Irregular distribution of circulation, causing ***local burning, throbbing or congestion,*** flushes of heat, rush of blood to head, chest, heart. Its action is centrifugal from within outward. ***Ascending effects***.

Affinity for the skin, where it produces heat and ***burning*** with itching, made worse by heat of the bed. ***Dry, unhealthy hair and skin.*** Very red lips and face, flushing easily. ***Redness of orifices*** or of single parts is another prominent feature due to irregular circulation, ***lips,*** ears, nose, eyelids, ***anus,*** vulva.

Weak faint spells, frequently during the day after nursing or night watching with great sleepiness. Empty, sinking feeling, in stomach. Sensation of fullness, roughness or numbness. Inertia and relaxation of fiber, characteristic feebleness of tone.

Chorea, chronic after suppressed eruptions. Epilepsy with a feeling that mouse is running up arms to back, before the fit. Child jumps, starts and screams fearfully. As if swinging or standing on wavering ground.

Nutrition is affected on account of defective assimilation in spite of voracious appetite, the patient emaciates (especially children). Thin and weak, even with good appetite. Hungry and always tired. Cat-nap sleep.

Glandular swelling indurated and suppurating. Mucus discharges and exhalations are acrid, blood streaked offensive and cause itching. Serous effusions or deposits are absorbed slowly.

General offensive character of discharge and exhalations. Body offensive in spite of washing. Aversion to being washed, always worse after the bath. Aversion to water.

Child looks dried, a little old man, big head, big belly with emaciated limbs. Dirty, filthy people, prone to skin disorders. Patient is unable to walk erect, ***stoop shouldered, unwashed, tall and lean, untidy***. Coal miner's disorders. Ragged philosopher.

MIND - ***Absent-minded.*** Dullness of mind. Brain fatigue. Difficult thinking. Very forgetful. Weak memory, especially for names. Misplaces things, words, cannot find proper words when talking or writing. Scatter-brained, burnt out brains (Sil., Ph-ac., Med., Cann.). Repeats everything said to him on account of difficult comprehension.

Awkwardness at his work. Aversion to do mental or physical work. ***Bored easily.*** Lazy, cannot arouse himself. Lazy, hungry and always tired. Averse to business, or busy all the time. Workaholics, ambitious, aggressive (Nux-v.).

Often irritable, depressed. Irritated greatly by least advice. Dislikes having anyone near him. Quarrelsome and impatient nothing pleases. Impatience about trifles. Censorious, critical. Despises literary people and education. Anger over his mistakes. ***Alcoholism***.

Melancholy. Sadness from injuries of head. Sadness during labor. Tired of life. Strong impulsive tendency to suicide by drowning or leaping from a window. Imagines giving wrong things to people, causing their death.

Worried by trifles. Anxiety about others, imagination leads them to worry. Anxiety from pressure on chest. Anxiety about friends at home. Fear of failure, or poverty, of starving. Fear of ghosts at night, of robbers. Childish peevishness in adults. Moaning and complaining day and night, with wringing of hands.

Anxiety with an overactive mind, preventing sleep. Restlessness at night. ***Persistent thoughts***, expressions and words heard recur to his mind. Absorbed in thoughts in evening. Obsessive, curious. Intellectuals.

Haughty. Egotistical and obstinate. ***Very selfish,*** no regard for others. Indifference to the welfare of others. Megalomania. Delusions of grandeur. Foolish happiness and pride. ***Imagines himself a great person***. Fear of not being recognized. Insecurity, poor self-confidence. ***Indifference to personal appearance.***

Monomania. Strong tendency to ***philosophical or religious reveries*** with fixed ideas. Makes many plans and theories. ***Philosophical mania,*** wants to know who made this or that and how. Racks his brain about metaphysical subtleties. ***Ragged philosophers.*** Religious melancholy. Religious aversion to opposite sex. Indisposition to play in children. Religious affections in children.

Laughing over serious matters. Thinks himself in possession of beautiful things, everything looks pretty. Senility. ***Senile dementia.***

Abdomen - Sore, very sensitive to pressure, internal feeling of rawness and soreness. Abdomen heavy, as of a lump. Movements as of something alive (Croc., Thuj.), as of the fist of a child. Stitches in region of spleen, worse coughing or deep inspiration. Intestines feel as if strung in knots, worse bending forward. Bearing down against rectum. Colic after eating or drinking, obliging one to bend double, worse sweet things. Colic after drinking. Colicky babies. Big belly, emaciated limbs in children. Eczema about navel.

Back - Curvature of spine. Drawing pain between shoulders. Neck stiff. Muscles of neck weak, child cannot hold head. Boils on neck. Sensation as if the vertebrae glide over each other or crack on bending backwards. Aching between scapulae. Lumbar pains to stomach, walks bent from pain in the back, can only straighten up after moving. Supports weight on hands when sitting. Coccyx pains during stools. Aching in small of back, worse when urinating.

Breasts - Sharp burning in breasts. Nipples, cracked, around the base, smart, burn, bleed after nursing, pain extends to back. Cancer of breast or uterus. Breast and uterus develops imperfectly.

Causations - Suppressions. Alcohol. Sun. Chills. Sprains, over-exertion, reaching high. Falls, blows. Bedsores.

Chest - Burning sensation in chest. ***Oppression, as of a load on chest.*** Shooting pains in chest extending to back worse coughing, lying on back and deep breathing. Pain backward from left nipple. As of a band or load on chest. Red, brown spots all over chest. Heat, throughout chest. Sensation of burning or coldness in chest, extending to face. Feeling of weakness in chest, while talking.

Constitutions - Suited to lean, stoop-shouldered persons, who walk and sit stooped, standing is the most uncomfortable position. Persons of psoric temperament, nervous, quick-motioned, quick-tempered, plethoric, skin excessively sensitive to atmospheric changes. Dirty, filthy people with greasy skin and long, straight, matted hair, prone to skin disorders. Children who cannot bear to be washed or bathed, emaciated, big-bellied, restless, hot, kick off clothes at night, have worms. Persons of scrofulous diathesis, subject to congestions, especially of portal system. Lymphatic temperaments, nervous constitutions disposed to hemorrhoids with constipation or morning diarrhea, diseases caused especially by suppressed eruptions. Emaciated children, old-looking faces, big bellies, dry, flabby skin. Full-blooded persons with great irritability, restlessness and hastiness. Old people. People with hot, sweaty hands. ***"Ragged philosophers,"*** dirty-looking persons who are always speculating on religious or philosophical subjects.

Ears - Purulent, offensive otorrhea, catarrhal discharge even on the eighth day. Bad effects from the suppression of an otorrhea. Very red ears in children. Sensation as if sounds do not come through the ear but through forehead. Whizzing in ears. Swashing as of water. Deafness preceded by exceedingly sensitive hearing, catarrhal deafness.

Eyes - Painful inflammation of eye from presence of foreign body. Cutting as from sand. Heat and ***burning in eyes*** (Ars., Bell.). Bursting pain in eyeballs. Trembling of eyes, quivering of eyelids. Chronic ophthalmia with much burning and itching. First stage of ulceration of cornea. Photophobia. Parenchymatous keratitis. Keratitis, cornea like ground glass. Retinitis caused by overuse of eyes. Oily tears. ***Burning*** ulceration of margin of lids. Agglutination of lids. Styes and tarsal tumors. Eczema of lids. Trachoma. Opacities of vitreous. Obscuration of vision like black gauze or motes before eyes. Halo around lamplight. Objects seem more distant than they are.

Face - Pale, sickly and ***old looking.*** Circumscribed redness of cheeks. Lips, bright red, swollen (upper), dry, rough, cracked, burning, twitching or trembling. Freckled, spotted. Acne. Mumps. Swollen veins on forehead.

Female - Amenorrhea. Suppression of menses from excitement. Menses preceded by headache. Menses too late, short, scanty and difficult, thick, black, ***acrid, making parts sore***. Leucorrhea of yellow mucous, burning, excoriating. Weak feeling in genitals. Offensive genitals with offensive sweat on thighs. Pudenda ***itches. Vagina and vulva burn***, itch and sore, worse sitting is scarcely able to keep still. Sore feeling in vagina during sex. Bearing down in pelvis towards genitals, worse standing. Puerperal sepsis with high fever, profuse sweat of whole body, tenderness of abdomen and drowsiness. Prolapse of uterus from reaching high. Cancer of uterus. Uterus develops imperfectly.

Food - Complete loss of appetite or ravenous appetite. Feels hungry, but when comes to the table, he loathes the food, turns away from it. Eats anything and everything. Headache or feels tired if he does not eat often. Food tastes too salty. Aversion to meat. Desire for sweets (Arg-n.), for raw food. Sweets, ***milk disagrees***. Water fills the patient up. Drinks much, eats little.

Head - Hot head with cold feet. Constant ***heat on top of head*** (Cupr., Graph.). Hot.

throbbing, heavy, sore vertex. Heaviness and fullness, pressure in temples. As of a band about or pain deep in brain. Beating headache, worse stooping and with vertigo. Sick headaches recurring periodically, on every Sunday, preceded by photopsia. Head bent forward when walking. Fontanelles remain open too long. Hydrocephalus with convulsions, red face and pupils dilated. Tinea capitis, dry form. ***Itching, scratching causes burning. Scalp dry***. Sweaty scalp. Hair, dry, cold, hard, falling off, worse washing.

Heart - Heart feels too large. Pericarditis with effusion. Sharp pains go through chest to between shoulders. Palpitations, worse lying at night in bed, going up an ascent. ***Pulse more rapid in morning*** than in evening.

Kidneys - Painful, ineffectual efforts to urinate, retention. Itching, burning in urethra during urination, lasting long after. ***Parts sore over which it passes.*** Thin stream, intermits. ***Great quantities of colorless urine***, greasy particles, mucus and pus in it. Sudden call to urinate, must hurry. Urination involuntary while passing flatus or on coughing. Frequent urination, especially at night. ***Bedwetting,*** especially in scrofulous, untidy children. Every cold settles in the bladder.

Limbs - Heaviness, paretic feeling in limbs. Jerks one limb on dropping to sleep. Rheumatic gout with itching. Swelling of the joints with hydro-arthrosis. Joints stiff, especially knees and ankles. Tense hamstring (left). Cramp in calf (left). ***Soles, burn, wants them uncovered,*** at night, cold in bed, dry. Poplitiae tight on stooping. Tuberculosis of the knee and hip joints. Unsteady gait. Ganglion. Cannot walk erect, ***stoop-shouldered***. Heavy shoulders. Rheumatic pain in left shoulder. Left arm numb, worse lying. Numb fingers. Tremulous sensation in hands, when writing. Palms, dry, bum, crack, peel, eczema on, warts on. Ulcers around the nails. Whitlow with rapid swelling of the finger, redness, stiffness and excessive burning stitching. Involuntary contraction of hands as if about to grasp something. ***Hot, sweaty hands.*** Sweat in armpits, smelling like garlic.

Liver - Pain and soreness of liver. Stitches in region of liver. Gallbladder colic and chronic jaundice. Relapsing jaundice.

Lungs - ***Difficult respiration, wants windows open,*** nightly suffocative air hunger. ***Dyspnea*** in middle of night, relieved by sitting up. Irregular breathing. Asthma preceded by colds. Loose cough, worse from talking, morning, greenish, purulent, sweetish expectoration. ***Much rattling of mucus*** and heat in chest, worse 11 a.m. ***Pleuritic exudations***. Cough, violent in two or three incomplete bouts, tickling as from down in larynx. Greenish, sweetish and purulent expectoration. Violent cough with headache worse lying on back. As of rivet through upper third of left lung. Neglected pneumonia.

Male - Hydrocele. Testes hang low. Induration of testes. Discharge of prostatic fluid after urination and stool. Stitches in penis. Penis cold. Prepuce stiff, hard like leather with copious smegma, causes itches. Fetid sweat on genitals. Itching of genitals when going to bed. Organs cold, relaxed and powerless. Involuntary emissions. Seminal emission on touching a woman. Seminal emission with burning in urethra. Semen, odorless, watery. Sexual power weak, impotence. Exhaustion in the morning after seminal emission. Backache and weakness of the limbs after sex, with sadness and irritability.

Modalities - ***Better dry, warm weather***, dry heat. Better open air, motion. Better sweating, walking. Better lying on right side, drawing up affected limbs. ***Standing*** is the most uncomfortable position. Worse at rest, stooping, reaching high. Worse talking, looking down. Worse crossing running water, washing, bathing. Worse in morning, 11 a.m., at night. Worse full moon, atmospheric changes. Worse from alcoholic stimulants. Worse periodically. ***Worse from suppressions, milk,*** sweets. ***Worse warmth, over-exertion in bed.*** Worse woolens. Worse vaccinations. Worse suppressed hemorrhoids. Worse menopause.

Mouth - Bitter taste in morning. Sour, sweetish, foul taste. Food tastes like straw or too salty. Profuse saliva, with nauseous taste. Nursing sore mouth. Aphthae, thrush. Tongue white with red tip and borders. Dry, tremulous tongue. Sensitive, tender teeth. Jerking, shooting, throbbing pains in teeth. Grinding of the teeth. Gums bleeding. Swelling of gums, throbbing pain. Lips dry, ***bright red***, burning.

Nose - ***Pale, red and scabby.*** Fluent burning coryza, worse outdoors, stopped indoors. Frequent sneezing. Obstructed on alternate sides. ***Chronic dry catarrh, dry scabs and readily bleeding***. Nosebleeds, worse at night, on lying on right side. Polyps and adenoids. Herpes across the nose. Freckles and black pores on nose. Tip of nose or alae nasi red, swollen, worse cold. Sensitive to smell. Imaginary odors.

Rectum - ***Redness around the anus*** with itching. Pain, urging and burning in rectum. Involuntary stools on sneezing or laughing with emission of flatus. ***Morning diarrhea, drives out of bed*** with prolapsed rectum. ***Painless diarrhea,*** changing, mushy, foul, painless, watery, grayish, frothy worse milk. Stools flat and thin. Diarrhea of infants with profuse sweating, drowsiness, suppression of urine and the child wakes up screaming. Children afraid, hold stools back on account of pain. Diarrhea alternating with constipation. Habitual constipation. Frequent, unsuccessful desire, hard, knotty, insufficient. Odor of stool follows him as if he had soiled himself. Hemorrhoids, oozing and belching. External and internal hemorrhoids, great bunches that are sore, tender, raw, burn, bleed and smart. Hemorrhoids during pregnancy.

Sensations - As if a band were tied tightly around forehead or cranium. Vertigo as if swinging. As if one stood on wavering ground. As if hair on vertex stood on end. As if hernia would form. As if lungs came in contact with back. Heart as if enlarged. Like a weight on shoulder. As if something heavy hanging on upper arm. Arms as if beaten. As of a mouse running up arms and back. Thigh as if broken. As if too short in popliteal space. As if bed were not large enough to hold him.

Skin - Skin as if denuded and sore. ***Unhealthy skin, breaks out,*** dry, scaly. Skin festers and would not heal, ***every little injury suppurates***. Excoriation, especially in folds (Lyc.). Voluptuous, violent ***itching***, worse at night, heat of bed, scratching and washing. ***Burning when scratched,*** painfully sensitive to air, wind, washing. ***Itching***, ***especially from warmth*** in evening, often recurs in spring, in damp weather. Pimply eruption, pustules, cracks, hangnails. Freckles. Crops of boils. ***Scabies.*** Cracks. Eczema. Ulcers. Creeping erysipelas. Suppuration with air bubbles. Varicose veins, ulcerate, rupture and bleed. Eruptions, can alternate with other complaints, asthma etc. Skin disorders after local medication. Feeling of a band around bones.

Sleep - Drowsy, then migraine. Sleeps in ***catnaps***, slightest noise awakens. Drowsy by day, wakeful at night. Heavy, unrefreshing. Talks, jerks and twitches during sleep. Awakes with starts or screams. Sings during sleep or wakes up singing. Vivid dreams, remain impressed on the memory. Wakes frequently and becomes wide awake suddenly. Cannot sleep between 2 and 5 a.m.

Stomach - Burning, painful, weight-like pressure. Heaviness in stomach. ***Very weak and faint about 11 a.m.,*** must have something to eat. ***Great acidity***, sour eructation. Belchings on pressing on stomach. Putrid belchings tasting like bad eggs, worse eating or at night. Milk causes sour taste and sour belchings. Vomiting of undigested food or sour vomiting. Nausea during pregnancy.

Temperature - Dry skin and great thirst. Chill spreading up back. Flushes of heat. Feels too hot. ***Frequent flashes of heat. violent ebullitions of heat throughout entire body***. Heat with general throbbing, between scapulae. Sweat on single parts in axilla, hands and feet. Profuse sweat at night with sulphur odor. Night sweat, on nape and occiput. Sweat without relief. Sweat may occur on one side of the body only or on neck only. Remittent fever. Septic, puerperal fever.

Throat - Burning, redness and dryness. External redness. Sensation, as of a lump, hair or splinter or as of a vapor rising in. Ball seems to rise and close the pharynx. As if swollen. Dry, exciting cough. Deep, hoarse voice. Aphonia.

Vertigo - Vertigo in forehead, worse when crossing a river, stooping with headache.

COMMENTS - Sulph. is used in various countries for allaying pain in a variety of forms. A piece of stick Sulph. carried in the pocket is commonly used in England to ward off rheumatism. Natives of South America apply Sulph. in solid form to painful parts and allow it to act for an hour before result is effected. For lumbago and chronic rheumatic pains a bag filled with Flowers of Sulphur, heated and applied to the part, immediately relieves the pain.

An experienced sea captain testified to the extreme frequency of rheumatism among his sailors, but, he added, when carrying cargoes of Sulph., he had never had a case of acute rheumatism on board.

Dr. Laugardiere of Toulouse, reported to the Academy of Medicine that he had discovered a cure for croup: a tablespoonful of Flowers of Sulphur dissolved in a tumbler of water. After three days of this treatment his patients were rescued from imminent death and fully recovered. Many practitioners spoke highly of a local application of Sulph. to the fauces in the treatment of croup and diphtheria.

Nettle rash is often relieved by a little Flowers of Sulphur, water and Sulph. mixed with sea sand and rubbed over itch vesicles destroys the acarus at once. In the early days of vaccination it was found that the action of Sulph. was adverse to the receptivity of vaccine. According to Dr. Tierney, Dr. Jenner failed in vaccinating thirty soldiers, all under treatment by Sulph.

Cooper noted that operatives in sulphur mines enjoy an immunity against ague when prevalent in surrounding districts, and that, before going on hunting expeditions in malarious districts, men in Ethiopia submit themselves to fumigations with Sulph. and find it an efficient prevention of ague. Cooper thought there was a great probability of Sulph. having a power of destroying the organisms in the blood of ague patients.

Hahnemann found in Sulph. the homeopathic counterpart of the peculiar constitutional weakness which tends to manifest in itch-like eruptions and which he named Psora. Sulph. is the chief of the anti-psoric remedies. It is this property of Sulph. to divert to the surface constitutional irritants which renders it the chief of Hahnemann's anti-psorics.

Sulph. has also an anti-psoric action independently of its power of "bringing out" rashes. The psoric poison may be present and active in a case of disease and "apparently well-indicated remedies may fail to act" in consequence.

In such cases, one or two doses of Sulph. will frequently antidote the psora and either clear up the case or open the way for the action of other remedies. In such cases there will almost certainly be some Sulph. indications present.

Sulph. is a potent antiseptic and is one of the most certain destroyers of scabies. The exact relation of acarus itch to psora and other itching eruptions need not be considered, but as Sulph. has the power of repressing constitutional eruptions when locally applied, as well as the power of destroying the acarus, it is best to use other means (e.g., oil of lavender) for the latter purpose and give Sulph. or other indicated remedies internally.

The symptoms of latent psora are detailed in Hahnemann's Chronic Diseases. They are, for the most part, almost exact reproductions of the symptoms of Sulph. But while Sulph. is the chief of anti-psorics, it is only one of many and Sulph. is in no way limited in its uses to cases of latent or declared psora.

When well-selected remedies fail to act or act too short a time because of the patient's feeble reactive powers, Sulph. will often build up the vital powers of the patient to effect the cure. It will clear the way by removing the psoric miasm to permit other similar remedies on their indications to cure the patient.

Useful for complaints that are always relapsing (menses, leucorrhea, etc.), patient seems to get almost well when the disease returns again and again.

Irregular distribution of the circulation, flushes of heat, rush of blood to the head, chest, and heart. Plethora from suddenly suppressed eruptions, hemorrhoids, discharges. Heat and burning sensation of all parts or coldness, and sweating of many parts.

Hot flushes during the day with weak, faint spells, passing off with a little moisture. Sensation of burning on vertex, of vesicles in mouth, and dryness of throat. Smarting in eyes, cutting, stabbing pain in right eye. Congestions to single parts, eye, nose, chest, abdomen, ovaries, arms, legs or any organ of the body, marking the onset of tumors or malignant growths, at menopause.

First right, then left in stomach, in rectum, in anus and itching. Heat in chest rising to face and skin, with hot flushes in spots below scapulae. Burning soles, must find a cool place for them at night. Hot head with cold feet. Lutze found that Sulph. 1,000c will make feet that have been cold for years comfortably warm.

Irregularities may go on to actual inflammation with effusions and to fever of intermittent or other types. Will cause absorption of effusions from pleuritis, hydrocephalus or synovial.

Periodical headaches, headaches occurring every week, every month. Sick headaches. Headaches are accompanied by red face and hot head, are better in warm room, at rest, worse in open air, worse from stooping. Headache on coughing. Clarke cured a severe occipital headache worse on coughing with Sulph. 30c.

Stopped catarrh, nose obstructed indoors, better outdoors. Nasal catarrh where the nose is stopped indoors and free out of doors. White, frothy expectoration. Asthma. Alternation between skin irritation and asthma.

Tuberculosis with marasmus, with hunger at 11 a.m., sore, red orifices, flushes of heat. Tuberculosis of the lungs when the "body feels too hot." Must have windows open.

Rheumatism and sciatica, better morning and worse at night in bed. Rheumatism, begins below and spreads upwards.

Unhealthy skin, tendencies to eczema, psoriasis. Burning and heat. Voluptuous itching, worse scratching, scratching causes burning, worse from heat of bed, soreness in folds. Red blotches. Sores that don't heal well. Boils, coming in crops in various parts or a single boil is succeeded by another as soon as the first is healed.

Offensive odor of body despite frequent washing. Aversion to bathing. Aggravated by water (Petrol.), with itching and burning. Poor hygiene or poverty (Psor.). Unkempt appearance. Allergic to wool. Skin disorders that have been treated by medicated soaps or creams, hemorrhoids that have been treated by ointments.

Redness of orifices and parts near orifices. Red ears, eyelids and borders around eyelids. Brilliant red lips, bright red anus in children, red meatus of urethra, red vulva. Red nose, worse by cold, the colder the redder. Orifices are red, congested, sore and hypersensitive. The passage of all discharges or excretions is painful.

Feeling of emptiness. "Faint, sinking, all-gone sensation at 11 a.m." Empty sensation in head, heart, stomach, abdomen. "Must have something between breakfast and dinner-time." Low blood sugar. Ravenous hunger. Defective assimilation, hungry yet emaciated. Poor breakfast eaters.

Poor dietary habits. Toxicity. Ulcers and burning in the stomach. Dyspepsia from suppressed eruptions, from farinaceous food. After eating, dyspeptic patients feel puffed up, heavy, sluggish, and low-spirited.

Cannot take milk, vomits it at once. Sour vomit with undigested food. Crave sweets, fats, spicy foods, wine, beer and marijuana. Alcoholism (Nux-v.). They crave beer, and marijuana. Aversion to eggs.

Dyspepsia of alcoholics. Craving for alcohol. Chronic alcoholism, dropsy and other ailments in alcoholics, they reform but are continually relapsing. Gallavardin cured many apparently hopeless alcoholics with Sulph. 1,000c.

Scalding urine like fire. Portal congestion. Constipation with ineffectual urging, constipation alternating with diarrhea. Stools are hard, dry, knotty, as if burnt, large, painful.

Child is afraid to have stool on account of pain, or pain compels child to desist on first effort, alternating with diarrhea. Diarrhea, after midnight, painless, driving out of bed early in morning, as if bowels were too weak to contain their contents. Hemorrhoids with burning and itching.

Drowsy in afternoon, after sunset, wakeful the whole night. Chronic insomnia from an overactive mind. Nightly suffocative attacks, wants doors and windows open. Becomes suddenly wide awake at night. Happy dreams, wakes up singing. Cramp in calves and soles at night. Will stick their feet out from the covers to cool down the body at night in bed.

"Worse by heat," by warmth of the bed, humidity. Worse at night, 11 a.m. Aversion to being washed, always worse after a bath. Not well since vaccinations, especially skin problems. Ailments from the abuse of metals.

Taken altogether there are more symptoms on the left side than the right. It acts strongly on the left side of the chest. "Sharp stitching pains through left lung to back, worse lying on back, worse by least motion."

The child looks dried up, a little old man, skin hanging in folds, yellowish, wrinkled, flabby. Head large in proportion to body. Lymphatic glands enlarged.

Clarke frequently cured ganglion of the wrist with Sulph. given on general indications. Sulph. 30c rescued a patient from a condition that seemed desperate in a case of left pleuro-pneumonia following a violent hemoptysis.

Lippe cured a case of menorrhagia with "a single dose of Sulph. at new moon," the patient had not been well since her last miscarriage.

Skinner gave a single dose of Sulph. 100,000c with instructions to take it on a certain date (when the moon was full) to a man who had paresis of the lower limbs. The man recovered suddenly.

Cooper used it to keep his regiment of sepoys in India healthy when many others were in the hospital with fever.

One writer treated nine cases with the pilules and arrested the fever in twenty-four hours. One of the cases was a particularly obstinate one and had been pronounced by the doctors to be complicated with liver affection. Quinine had been tried before to Sulph. cured.

Cooper, in a case of "Charges fever" of West Indies, which had lasted three months, ordered a Sulphur bath as well as the Sulph. pilules. That single bath seemed to alter the whole condition and the patient, an unhealthy, anemic, bilious-looking man, rapidly became the picture of health.

RELATIONS - ***Antidoted by:*** Acon., Camph., Cham., Chin., Merc., Puls., Rhus, Sep., Thuj. ***Antidote to:*** Acon., Aloe., Chi., Iod., Merc., Nit-ac., Olean., Rhus, Sep., Thu., ailments from abuse of metals generally. ***Compare:*** (1) Acon., Ars. - Sulph. often follows in acute diseases. (2) Merc. and Calc., Lyc., Sep., Sars., Puls. (3) Tann-ac. - nasal hemorrhage, elongated uvula, gargle, constipation. (4) Pyrar. - a fish caught in the Amazon, clinically used for various skin affections, leprosy, tuberculosis, syphilis, varicosities, etc. (5) Meningitis, Apis. (6) Early-morning diarrhea, Bry. (as soon as he moves), Nat-s. (with much flatus), Podo. (stools changeable, go on all day, though worse at noon, Sul. raw, sore anus), (7) Defective reaction, Psor., Op., Carc. (8) Hot flashes at menopause, Lach., Sul-ac., Amyl-n., Kali-bi. (9) Intermittent fever and neuralgia, Chin., Ars., Bapt. (10) Ravenous hunger with heat at vertex, Calc., Phos. (11) Tuberculosis, Bac., Calc., Tub., Phos. (12) Itch, Merc., Sep., Caust. (13) Dyspepsia, Lyc., Nux-v., Sep. (14) Pneumonia, restoration imperfect, Sang. ***Complementary:*** Aloe, Psor., Acon., Ars. Nux-v., Lyc., Sars., Sep., Puls., Thuj. ***Follows well:*** Merc-s. complements Rhus-t. in paralysis.

REFERENCES - Boericke. Clarke. Murphy. Phatak.

SULPHUR HYDROGENISATUM

(Sulfuretted Hydrogen)

PHARMACY - sul-h. Sulphur hydrogenisatum. Sulfuretted hydrogen. Solution of the gas. ***Historical dose:*** All potencies.

CLINICAL - Asphyxia. Asthma. ***Blood, poisoning.*** Convulsions. Delirium. Fever. Headache. Mania. Prostration. Tetanus. Typhoid fever.

HOMEOPATHIC - Sul-h. is a colorless inflammable gas, having a sweetish taste and an exceedingly fetid smell resembling rotten eggs. It is extremely poisonous when inhaled. It is evolved when animal or vegetable tissues containing sulphur decay. It also occurs in mineral springs, being liberated by the reduction of gypsum or other sulphates through the action of a microbe.

Sulph-h. is one of the remedies which help ***"blood poisoning"*** especially when bad smells are encountered. Asphyxia, tetanus, delirium, low continued fever have been observed as resulting from the gas.

COMMENTS - J. Wiglesworth recorded two cases of insanity, one certainly and both probably, due to inhaling the gas. The first concerned R. H., 32, an engine man at chemical works, who had been kept at home with an attack of bronchitis for ten days. A few days after his return to work he became "gassed" (i.e., accidentally inhaled Sul-h.).

This caused headache, stupor, prostration, compelling him to stay at home for a few days, when he became wildly delirious. He passed into a very excited state, shouting and gesticulating, said he was Jesus Christ.

He tried to bury his head in the floor and to raise his feet above his head. Three days later he was admitted to Rainhill Asylum and there was still very violent and excited, gesticulating and talking incoherently, chiefly on religious subjects. At the end of a month there was some improvement and he was discharged, he recovered five months after admission.

In the other case, that of a laborer at chemical works, Wiglesworth is not quite certain that Sul-h. was the poison inhaled. This patient was greatly excited, threw his arms about, shouted and laughed by turns, was excited and talkative. He remained permanently insane.

REFERENCES - Clarke.

SULPHUR IODATUM

(Sulphur Iodide)

PHARMACY - sul-i. Sulphur iodatum. Sulphur iodide. Trituration. ***Historical dose:*** All potencies, third trituration.

CLINICAL - ***Acne.*** Allergies. Asthma. ***Barber's itch.*** Coryza. Ears, noises. Eczema, weeping. Gonorrhea. Hay fever. Influenza. Kidneys, pain. Lichen planus. Lips, eruption. Parotid glands, hypertrophy. prostate disorders. Scalp, soreness. Spine, weakness. Stricture, urethral. Tongue, thickening. Tonsils, chronic hypertrophy.

HOMEOPATHIC - Sul-i. was proved by Kelsall on himself and some others. Hale used it in "obstinate skin diseases, notably barber's itch, for which it is almost a specific." The provings indicate this in "pustular eruption on upper lip" and "erythema on chin."

Hale also noted it for large and painful suppurating acne. Weeping eczema. He used the 3x trituration. internally and applied a cerate of one or two grains of Sul-i. to an ounce of Cosmoline.

Useful for psoric, allergic constitutions. Obstinate skin affections. Suppuration. Acrid discharges. Painless enlargement of glands and infiltration of tissues with thickening and induration after inflammation.

Weakness, as from the influenza. Prostration, sensitive to everything. Faint and sick. Raw burning heat internally with external coldness. Single parts, fingers etc. turn white and insensible.

MIND - Doubtful. Dread of exertion. Incapacity for business. Feverish excitement. Hurried, impatient, sad. Restlessness at night. Starting, frightened on waking.

Abdomen - Mesenteric disease.

Eyes - Zigzag before vision.

Face - Acne. Suppurating pimples. Parotid hypertrophy after mumps.

Female - Irregular menses. Copious thick, burning, leucorrhea worse before and after menses.

Food - Anorexia. Appetite increased in marasmus of children. Desire for acids.

Head - Headache better sundown. Hair seems erect.

Kidneys - Urine, scanty, purulent, with brown sand. Urine smells like raspberries. Stricture after gonorrhea, painful urination, stream twisted. Burning at the end of penis, dull pain in prostate.

Limbs - Aching soreness below knees. Soles of feet ache, bum and sore, when standing.

Lungs - Chest constricted, dropsy of pleura and eruptions on chest. Breathing asthmatic, irregular, rattling and suffocative. Cough worse a.m., spasmodic. Expectoration greenish, purulent, copious, viscid and yellow.

Male - Testes soft. Prepuce cracked. Hydrocele of small boys. Deficient erections.

Modalities - Better by expectoration. Better from cool air, winter. Better standing. Worse from exertion, even slight. Worse lying on right side, leaning forward, stooping, ascending stairs, rising. Worse before storms. Worse night, in morning.

Mouth - Raw, dry, wants to moisten it. Cold sores on lips. Tongue is glazed, thickened after inflammation. Teeth feel soft. Parotid hypertrophied.

Rectum - Stubborn constipation. Bright yellow stools. Foul anal discharge.

Sensations - Hair feels as if erect. As if a band across forehead. As if heat in heart.

Skin - Moist eczema. ***Suppurating acne.*** Barber's itch. Lichen planus. Papular eruption on face. Itching. Ulcers. Itching on ears, nose and in urethra. Arms covered with itching rash. Boils on neck. Hair feels as if erect.

Stomach - Tremors in epigastrium on exertion.

Throat - Raw, dry, painful in swallowing. Uvula and tonsils enlarged and red. Swollen.

Vertigo - Vertigo worse stooping, binding of the hair, fasting, before and during menses.

COMMENTS - Dr. Berlin treated with Sul-i. two cases of "weeping eczema" associated with varicose veins of the leg and pronounced itching. Also a child with eczema of arms. The keynote was "dark red, swollen and sweeping eczematous surface which itches terribly." Sul-i. 3x trituration. was given.

Hansen mentioned, among the therapeutic uses of Sul-i., thickness of tongue remaining after glossitis. Hypertrophy of parotids after parotiditis. Chronic hypertrophy of tonsils. Lichen planus, chronic and simple.

Bradford reported a case of burning at the end of penis, dull pain in prostatic region, weakness across kidneys. Frequent desire to urinate with slight flow, eats very little, does not go out of doors is much discouraged about himself. Sul-i. 3x cured.

Violent attack of pain in kidney region with shootings down ureters, pain and weakness about kidneys, constant desire to urinate, urine thick and whitish with creamy sediment. Sul-i. 3x and 6x cured.

Stricture after gonorrhea, chordee, very painful urination, twisted stream. Yellow discharge. Sul-i. cured.

RELATIONS - ***Compare:*** (1) Band across forehead, Manc. (2) Difficult expectoration, Kali-bi. (3) Heat in heart, Lachn., Rhod. (4) Sleepy by day, restless at night, Staph. (5) Acne, Bell-p., Kali-br.

REFERENCES - Boericke. Clarke. Phatak.

SULPHUR TEREBINTHINATUM

(Terebinthinated Sulphur)

PHARMACY - sul-ter. Sulphur terebinthinatum. Terebinthinated sulphur. One part of purified Sulphur is dissolved by heating in one hundred parts of Turpentine. Dilutions. ***Historical dose:*** All potencies.

CLINICAL - Chorea. Rheumatoid, arthritis. St. Vitus's dance.

HOMEOPATHIC - Sul-ter. is referred to in the Hon. Robert Boyle's works. A Sul-ter. 1x dilution cured a most obstinate case of St. Vitus's dance and has often relieved pain in chronic rheumatic arthritis.

REFERENCES - Clarke. Cooper.

SULPHURICUM ACIDUM

(Sulphuric Acid)

PHARMACY - sul-ac. Sulphuricum acidum. Sulphuric acid. Vitriol. Dilution. ***Historical dose:*** All potencies.

CLINICAL - Acidity. ***Alcoholism.*** Alopecia. ***Aphthae.*** Backaches. Back, pain. Bedsores. Brain, concussions. Breath, offensive. ***Bruises. Burns.*** Cachexia. Cancer. Cancrum, oris. Chafing. Chilblains. Constipation. Corns. ***Debility.*** Diabetes. Diarrhea. Diphtheria. Dyspepsia. Erythema nodosum. Esophagitis. ***Gangrene.*** Gastritis. Glossitis. Hair, loss. ***Heartburn.*** Hemorrhoids. Hernia, inguinal. Hiccoughs. ***Hot, flushes***. Impotence. Infertility. Injuries. Intermittent fever. Irritation. Lead, poisoning. Liver disorders. Menopausal. Menorrhagia. Metrorrhagia. Myopia. Nephritis. Nightmares. Paralysis. Perspiration, great. Pneumonia. Pregnancy, sickness. ***Purpura hemorrhagica***. Pyorrhea. Rheumatism. Scurvy. Spleen, disorders. ***Thrush.*** Tuberculosis. ***Ulcers.*** Uterus, prolapse. Vagina, prolapsed. Varicose, veins. Warts. ***Weakness.*** Wounds. Writer's cramp.

HOMEOPATHIC - Known as vitriol to the Alchemists., Sul-ac. was a favorite remedy of the Middle Ages. It was used extensively in dilution for scrofulous, phagedenic, cancerous and venereal ulcers, as a gargle and mouthwash for aphthae, ulceration of the gums and diphtheria. It was given as "Mineral Lemonade" in cases of lead poisoning. Clarke verified this last use by giving water acidulated with the 3x.

The "Acid Soap" of Achard was prescribed as a dissolvent in scirrhous of the breast and nephritis, obstinate intermittent fevers, visceral obstructions, dropsy, jaundice, cachexia and "certain tumors of the feet."

Elixir of vitriol is a mixture of the sulphuric acid, alcohol and water. It was a popular remedy for nervous weakness in women. Dippel, Haller and others each had an "Elixir," differing only in the proportions of the chief ingredients.

The elixirs were used in intermittent, putrid, malignant, contagious, comatose and petechial fevers, scarlatina, confluent and malignant variola, dysentery, plague, leprosy, itch and other skin diseases, nocturnal emissions, suppression of menses and hemorrhoids, nephritis and gout, tuberculosis, and chorea.

Grimmer stated that patients needing this remedy are weak and exhausted, yet mentally impatient and hurried. Prone to suffer from ulcerations, both externally and internally, that readily tend to become gangrenous or cancerous. Ulcers become red, blue and painful. Gangrene following mechanical injuries. Profuse, acrid or stringy discharges.

Hemorrhages of dark blood, from lungs, stomach, uterus and rectum. Violent hemorrhages of thin, black blood from all the orifices. Veins (of feet) distended. Purpura hemorrhagia. Removes long lasting black and blue spots with soreness and stiffness of the part after trauma (follows Arn.).

Weakness or debility, especially in the ***digestive tract,*** giving a very relaxed feeling in the stomach. ***Tremor and weakness***, everything must be done in a hurry. ***Trembling internal,*** wants to be held. Weakness is out of proportion to the disease, from some deep seated dyscrasia. ***Hot flushes***, followed by perspiration with trembling.

Stomach pain and hypochlorhydria. Sour stomach. ***Craving for alcoholic stimulants.*** Inflammatory ulcerations and malignancy of the stomach occur in those who are chronic users of alcohol to excess.

Parts feel stiff and tight. Pains increase gradually and end abruptly. As of a blunt plug being driven in. Great painfulness. Pains felt during sleep. Disappear on waking. Gnawing pains. Burning, darting pains. Shocks as from pain. Writer's cramp. Lead poisoning.

MIND - Irritable, impatience about trifles. Fretful, impatient. ***Hurried feeling.*** Must do everything in great hurry. ***Hurried while walking, movements,*** eating, in writing, occupation. Sullen, impatient, angry because things move so slowly. Nervous fatigue and tendency to take fright.

Changeable mood during perspiration. Vacillating and morose. Disheartened. Constant crying or weeping. Unwilling to answer questions, says yes or no with difficulty. Speech monosyllabic. Extreme mental dejection, unfit for work, would sit and weep whole day long.

Abdomen - Colic with sensation ***as if hernia would protrude***, especially left side. Spleen enlarged, hard, painful, on coughing. Sinking sense in abdomen after stools.

Back - Weak feeling with dragging into the hips and small of back. Weakness of spine, cannot sit or stand. Large abscess on right side of neck.

Causations - Burns. Mechanical injuries. Falls, bruises, concussion of brain. Chafing. Surgical operations. Sprains, wounds.

Chest - Great weakness in the chest with difficult speech.

Constitutions - Suited to topers, old persons, especially women in menopausal years, weak children with no other complaint. Light-haired people. Sour babies. When some deep-seated dyscrasia prevails. Cases where the weakness is out of proportion to the disease.

Ears - Feeling as of a leaf lying before the ear. Tearing and shaking in right ear. Violent tickling. Rhythmical roaring in ears. Ringing of bells before ears. Humming in ears in evening.

Eyes - Intra-ocular hemorrhage, following trauma. Great chemosis of conjunctiva with aching and sharp pain. Eyes, smart, burn and lachrymation, while reading. Feeling as of a lump in outer canthi, moves to inner canthi on closing eye and returns to outer on opening. Eyelids difficult to open.

Face - Deathly pale or wrinkled. Feels as if the white of an egg had dried on it.

Female - Distressing nightmares before menses or after menses. Menses too early and too profuse. Acrid, burning leucorrhea often of bloody mucus. Prolapse of vagina and uterus from weakness. Gangrene of vagina after prolapse. Erosion of cervix in the aged, easily bleeding. ***Hot flushes.*** Flushes of heat, followed by sweat and a feeling of tremors all over the body during menopausal.

Food - Averse to smell of coffee. ***Craves alcohol***, brandy. Desires fruits, fresh food. Wine aggravates. Worse drinking cold water. Sweats after eating, especially warm food.

Head - Concussion of brain where skin is cold, body bathed in cold sweat. Sensation as if brain was loose in forehead and falling from side to side (Bell., Rhus-t.). Compressive pain in occiput, ***better by holding the hand near head***. Electric like shocks in forehead, temples. Right-sided neuralgia, painful shocks, skin feels pinched. ***Thrust in right temple as if plug were pressed in.*** Pain of outer parts, as if there were subcutaneous ulceration, painful to touch. Hair falls out, turns gray.

Kidneys - Pain in the bladder if urging for urinating is not attended to. Diminished secretion of urine. Slimy sediment in the urine. Hematuria. Diabetes with lassitude, debility, despondency.

Limbs - Cramp-like paralytic contraction in arms, hands. Jerking of the tendons. Fingers jerk while writing, sleeping. Writers' cramp. Knees, ankles weak, cannot walk.

Lungs - Rapid respiration. Bronchitis in children with short, teasing cough. Cough, then belchings or vomiting. Larynx moves up and down violently, rapid motion of alae nasi during dyspnea, better hanging down legs. Bloody expectoration during menopause.

Modalities - Better from warmth, moderate temperature, hot drinks. Better lying on affected side, hands near head, rest. Worse from excessive heat, open air. Worse cold, drinking cold water. ***Worse alcohol, odor of coffee***. Worse towards evening. Worse from touch, pressure. Worse lifting arms. Worse injuries, sprains, surgical operations. Worse concussion of brain. Worse during menopausal period.

Mouth - Offensive breath. Bloody saliva from mouth. Aphthae during protracted disease, especially in children with marasmus. Ulcers spread rapidly. Gums bleed easily. Pyorrhea. Destruction of teeth in diabetes mellitus.

Nose - Dry coryza with loss of smell and taste. Coryza with thin, lemon-colored discharge. Flow of water from nose. Nosebleed in evening. Oozing of dark, thin blood, worse odor of coffee, of old people. Pimples on side of nose

Rectum - Diarrhea with sour odor of body and empty, faint feeling in abdomen. Diarrhea, very foul, green, black or of hacked stools orange yellow, from unripe fruit and oysters, from least indigestion. Hemorrhoids, with oozing moisture. Hemorrhoids prevent stools. Rectum feels as if it has a big ball.

Sensations - As if brain were loose and falling from side to side. As if one side of head filled with smoke. As if a plug were thrust quickly into head. As from subcutaneous ulceration in scalp. As if white of egg had dried on face. As if skin of cheek and chin were pinched. As of want of elasticity of vocal organs. As if there were a lump in throat. As if rectum were torn to pieces during stool. As if hernia would protrude. As if menses would come on.

Skin - Bad effects from mechanical injuries, with bruises and livid skin. Petechia. Livid, red, itching blotches. ***Purpura hemorrhagica***. Hemorrhage of black blood from all outlets. Ecchymosis. Nodular urticaria. Carbuncles, boils and other staphylococcic and streptococcic infections. Itching all over the body. Scars turn red and blue, become painful. Chilblains with gangrenous tendency. Bed sores, abscesses.

Sleep - Sleeplessness from mental excitement. Sleepiness. Retarded sleep and early waking. Jerkings during sleep. Anxious dreams, nightmares before menses.

Stomach - ***Weak, relaxed feeling at stomach***, worse after stools. Coldness of stomach relieved by applied heat. Heartburn, ***sour belchings, sets teeth on edge*** (Rob.). Drinks chill the stomach and rejected unless mixed with liquor. Nausea with chilliness. Sour vomiting, ***hiccough of alcoholics***, nausea with shivering. Vomits mucus instead of food. Coughs before vomiting during pregnancy.

Temperature - ***Hot flushes***, then trembling or cold sweat, worse after warm ingesta, worse upper parts, better motion. Drenching sweats. Disproportionate weakness during fevers like typhoid.

Throat - Sore. Liquids regurgitate, on swallowing. ***Larynx moves up and down violently.*** Throat looks whitewashed. Stringy lemon-yellow mucus hangs from posterior sinuses in diphtheria.

Vertigo - Vertigo when sitting down, disappearing in the open air. Vertigo in room, better open air. Vertigo, must lie down, as soon as he raises himself dizziness returns.

COMMENTS - Hahnemann noted that Sul-ac. is useful for disorders characterized by "tension in the eyelids in the morning, shortsightedness, hardness of hearing inguinal hernia, chronic looseness of the bowels, roughness in the throat, asthma, profuse menses, metrorrhagia, swelling of the feet, coldness of the feet." Hahnemann's proving with homeopathic experience confirmed many of the ancient uses of Sul-ac.

Characteristic weakness and prostration. Suited to cases where the weakness is out of proportion to the disease. Weakness that seems to come from deep-seated dyscrasia. General internal trembling, as if trembling from head to foot, but without visible trembling.

Symptoms often appear on right side, but the left cheek and left parotid are most affected. Pain travels from left to right around hypochondria. Pains felt during sleep and disappearing on waking. Jerking on falling asleep.

Neuralgic pains increase gradually and end abruptly. Dull pain, pressure as of a plug thrust in. External soreness and sensitiveness. Severe pain over the whole left side of the head, face and neck, coming on from exposure to draft.

Agues and periodic neuralgias. Concussion, with cold sweats and great fatigue after the head injury. Easy sweating, mostly on upper body. Sour body odor, cannot be washed off, particularly in children. Severe hot flashes with profuse perspiration.

Trauma. Hemorrhage. Keynote of black blood (Croc.). Easily bleeding ulcers. Easily bruised. Extensive bruising (Arn., Ham.), when bruises turn black or very dark blue. Purpura hemorrhagica. Bruises of soft parts (Arn.), glands (Con.), and bones (Ruta.). Bruising pains. Long-lasting black and blue spots with soreness and stiffness of the parts. Scars turn black or dark blue. Gangrene after injury. Boils, bedsores. Blotches.

Menses are too early, too profuse, may cause infertility. Menses with oozing of dark thin blood. Prolapse of vagina and uterus, weakness. Flushing, with sweat, particularly during menopause. Cervicitis where the cervix has been eroding and bleeding. Cervix bleeds when touched, friable.

Bloody saliva. Throat is filled with ulcers. Aphthous ulcer with pinpoint bleeding. Thrush in nursing infants.

Heartburn, burning in the stomach, with sour belchings that set the teeth on edge. "Vomiting in morning, acidity in stomach, burning is esophagus and stomach, sour, acrid or foul belchings."

Pain in bladder unless call to pass water is immediately attended to. Cholera, diarrhea. Diarrhea in emaciated children. External hemorrhoids, sensitive to touch, accompanied by itching.

Thirsty, but water is not tolerated. Water chills the stomach unless qualified with alcohol. Uncontrollable craving for alcohol (Lach.). Cirrhosis of the liver in alcoholics. Vomiting after alcohol.

For inebriates who are "on their last legs," long after Nux-v. had ceased to help. Hering said the craving for liquor has been subdued by taking for two or four weeks, thrice daily, ten to fifteen drops of a mixture of one part of Sul-ac. with three parts of alcohol.

Cooper contended that many ague cases, supposed to have been cured with Chin-s., were really cured by the sulphuric acid used in dissolving it. "Moreover," said Cooper, "in all epidemic diseases influenza, cholera, small-pox, etc."

With Sul-ac. 30c, a dose every night, Clarke gave great help to a delicate woman who had nightmare, waking in a fright, before each menstrual period.

A chemist in Covent Garden used a lotion of Sulphuric acid, well diluted, for all the cases of itch that came before him.

RELATIONS - ***Antidoted by:*** Puls. ***Antidote to:*** Lead poisoning. ***Compare:*** (1) Arn., Calen., Led., Sep., Calc. ***Complementary:*** Puls. ***Follows well:*** In injuries, Arn., Con., Ruta.

REFERENCES - Boericke. Clarke. Murphy. Phatak.

SULPHUROSUM ACIDUM

(Sulphur Dioxide)

PHARMACY - sulo-ac. Sulphurosum acidum. Sulphur dioxide. Sulphurous acid. Sulphurous anhydride. The remedy is obtained by dissolving sulphur dioxide in water. ***Historical dose:*** All potencies.

CLINICAL - Acne rosacea. Allergies. Colds. Constipation. Croup. Diphtheria. Eczema. Epidemics. Favus. Hands, chapped. Heartburn. ***Infections.*** Influenza. Nipples, sore. Pityriasis versicolor. Stomatitis, ulcerative. Tuberculosis.

HOMEOPATHIC - Sulo-aç. is soluble in water, it produces an acid solution containing sulphurous acid. In this way, relatively weak solutions are obtained.

Gutman carried out a clinical study, and taking as a base the results obtained, he drew up a clinical symptomatology in 1968. Julian completed Gutman's description with reference to the symptom data which resulted from acute and chronic poisoning cases.

Sulo-ac. irritates any mucus membrane with which it comes into contact and by becoming oxidized, it is transformed into sulphurous acid and then into sulfuric acid. Acting on the upper respiratory tract, it is known even to create retro-sternal constriction and phenomena such as anoxia ischemia and myocarditis.

Predisposition to pulmonary tuberculosis. Chronic, purulent hyper secretion of bronchial mucus in the young without dilatation of the bronchi. Need for fresh air, vertigo. Irritation of the nose, pharynx and larynx.

Dyspnea, wheezing, coughing and retro-sternal constriction. Pulmonary tumors. Cold in the head, influenza. Asthma, bronchitis, croup. Chronic tuberculosis. Clergyman's sore throat.

Dyspepsia with ptyalism and gastric acidity. Keratitis and conjunctivitis. Chilblains, chapped hands. Diphtheria. Scarlatina malign. Typhoid fever. Sensitivity to infections.

Chest - Angina pectoris. Constriction behind the sternum.

Eyes - Irritation of both conjunctivae and cornea. Tension of the artery of the retina. Change in the reaction of the pupil. Conjunctivitis. Superficial epidemic spotted keratitis. Herpes of the cornea. Chronic glaucoma. Choroiditis. Dacryocystitis. Blepharitis. Edema of the eyelids.

Heart - Rapid pulse, cold sweating. Accentuation of the second pulmonary sound. Systolic pulsation in the pit of the stomach. Inflammation of the coronary arteries.

Limbs - Chilliness at the limbs.

Lungs - Feeling of suffocation and cyanosed face. Wheezing and rhonchi widespread in the chest. Bronchiectasis. Emphysema, asthma. Chronic pulmonary tuberculosis. Chronic bronchitis. Oppression, sneezing and spasmodic coughing. Expectoration of dirty-gray or bloodstained mucous.

Mouth - Brownish stains on the teeth, especially on the incisors. Dental caries. Ptyalism, gingivitis. Ptyalism in pregnant women.

Nose - Burning sensation in the nose and discharge of a viscous liquid. Mucopurulent rhinitis. Nasal polyps.

Skin - Eruption of vesicles and edema. Brownish coloring of the skin. Eczematic eruption, very sensitive. Leucoderma. Urticaria.

Stomach - Acrid dyspepsia. Dyspepsia and hyperchlorhydria.

Temperature - Septic fevers of all kinds. Epidemic influenza. Typhoid fever. Tuberculosis. Smallpox. Plague.

Throat - Burning sensation in the throat. Feeling of tightness around the throat. Lingering huskiness of voice. Scratching in the throat and chest.

COMMENTS - Some forty years ago, when the germ theory of disease in its present form was in its infancy, Dewar of Fite, conceived the idea that sulphurous acid was an innocent and at the same time universal germ destroyer and consequently universal remedy. His views met with cordial acceptance and inhalations of sulphurous acid given off from burning sulphur became the fashion.

Dewar's method was simple. A few red cinders were put in a kitchen shovel, this was placed in the center of a room and flowers of sulphur sprinkled thereon. In a very short time every person in the room was sneezing violently, coughing and wheezing and running at the eyes and nose.

Dewar also used the ordinary solution and a spray. Wounds, sore nipples, bruises were also amenable to its local use. For erysipelas, a local application of equal parts of the acid and glycerine.

Sulo-ac. doubtless shares the anti-septic properties of Sulph. The symptoms are from observations of the effects on workmen in mines from air contaminated with Sulo-ac.

Milne summed up its virtues, "Anti-septic, disinfectant, a powerful deoxidizer and destroyer of vegetable life." As a gargle it is used in the strength of one to six. In parasitic skin disorders the B. P. solution is used and is effective.

Ringer said that ten to fifteen minims taken ten minutes before each meal will remedy heartburn in most instances. It prevents flatulence and fermentations and that "the solution, either strong or diluted in varying proportions, speedily removes thrush." In potencies, it has cured ulcerative inflammation of the mouth. Headache, better by vomiting.

C. Wootton tasted the acid with this result it at once stopped the mucus secretion of the bowels. The constipation was so severe that he was in misery for nine months, until he took Hydr., which cured. The use of Sulo-ac. as a hair-wash at a later time produced the same result.

RELATIONS - ***Antidoted by:*** Hydr. (constipation). ***Compare:*** (1) Sulph. in ulcerated sore mouth, Nat-m., Caps., Sul-ac. (2) The effects on the back recorded by Hahnemann as from the fumes of burning Sulph. were antidoted by electricity. (3) Brom. - Persistent, excoriating cold in the head, huskiness worse in the evening, dry cough and attacks of suffocation. (4) Kali-i. - Streaming, burning, excoriating, cold in the head, with violent cough and soapy, salty, greenish expectoration. (5) Tub. - Emaciation, varying pains, chronic swelling of the tonsils, palpitations, perspiration, very sensitive to the cold, coughing hoarseness.

REFERENCES - Clarke. Julian.

SUMBULUM MOSCHATUS

(Musk Root)

PHARMACY - sumb. Sumbulus moschatus. Musk root. Sumbul. Ferula sumbul. N. O. Umbelliferae. Tincture of the powdered root. ***Historical dose:*** Tincture and all potencies.

CLINICAL - Acne. Ascarides. Asthma. Breasts, pains. Chorea. Diarrhea. Epilepsy. Fainting. Heart, disorders. Pneumonia. Hysteria. ***Insomnia.*** Neuralgias. ***Numbness. Palpitations.*** Spermatorrhea. Throat, catarrh. Throat, spasms. Typhoid fever. Worms.

HOMEOPATHIC - Sumbul, as its name, "Musk-root," implies, has an odor resembling that of musk. The resemblance is so close that Sumbul is used to adulterate musk. Sumb. was proved by Lembke, Cattell and others.

The symptoms are as like to those of Mosch. as the physical resemblance would imply. Hysterical and nervous disorders. Easy fainting, nervous palpitations. Nervous, irritable and sleepless.

Anomalous, functional, cardiac disorders. Sclerosed arteries. Menopausal flushings. Asthma. Yellow tenacious discharges. The left side was more affected than the right.

Neuralgia. Chorea, constant jerking of the head and limbs with protrusion of the tongue. ***Numbness on becoming cold***, on left side. ***Insomnia*** of delirium tremens (fifteen drops of tincture). Sensation as if water dropped down spine. As of a hot water flowing through part. Early senility.

MIND - Emotional and fidgety. Mistakes in writing and adding. Weeps and laughs by turns. Fear of becoming insane. Faintness from hearing music.

Abdomen - ***Abdomen full, distended and painful.***

Back - Trickling along spine.

Breasts - Pulling like a string in right breast. Neuralgia around left breast and left hypochondriac region.

Face - Neuralgia. As of a hair or cobweb on face. Idiotic expression.

Female - Ovarian neuralgia. Screwing pain in left side of uterus. Sexual excitability. Menopausal flushes.

Head - Dull in morning, clear in evening.

Heart - ***Nervous palpitations*** in hysterical subjects or at menopause, worse least exertion and thinking of it. As if heart beating in water. Neuralgia around left breast simulating angina pectoris. High blood pressure due to arteriosclerosis. ***Cardiac asthma***. Aching in left arm, heavy, numb and weary. Pulse irregular.

Kidneys - ***Oily pellicle on surface of urine.***

Limbs - Left arm aching, heavy, numb, weary.

Lungs - Asthma, cardiac, hysterical. Oppressed tightness in left chest, as if clogged. Loses breath on any exertion.

Modalities - Better from gentle motion, warmth. Worse from cold, inspiration. Worse menopausal. Worse motion, active exercise. Worse left side, after sitting. Worse thinking of symptoms. Worse in morning. Music causes faintness.

Mouth - Tongue feels rough as if scraped.

Nose - Comedones. Tenacious yellow mucus from nose.

Sensations - Tongue as if scraped. Clogged sensation in left chest. As if heart beating in water. Like a string pulling in right breast. Corkscrew pains in (left) uterus and appendages.

Skin - Pale, cold. Internal itching.

Sleep - Dreams of falling, of sex, followed by profuse, sudden emission.

Stomach - Burning water brash. Belching of gas from stomach.

Throat - Choking constriction, with constant swallowing. Hysterical. Spasm of pharyngeal muscles. Tenacious mucus in throat.

COMMENTS - Hale gave indications for Sumb. including nasal and pharyngeal catarrh with nervousness, sleeplessness and tendency to spasms (especially in children), discharge of tenacious, yellow mucus.

Catarrhal, spasmodic or cardiac asthma. Ascarides with bloated, drum-like abdomen and constipation, picking nose cured with Sumb. 15c. Oily pellicle in urine. Pain in left uterine region. Menopausal flushings.

Neuralgia, facial or ovarian in women of quick and lively nervous constitutions. Neuralgia of the left hypochondrium, simulating angina pectoris with palpitation in nervous women. Insomnia of chronic alcoholism.

RELATIONS - ***Compare:*** (1) Asaf., Mosch. (2) Mosch., Asaf., Melit., Med., Mez. (3) Oily pellicle on urine, Sulph., Puls., Petr. (4) Tenacious, yellow mucus, Hydr. (5) Infra-breast pain, Cimic., Puls., Lil-t. (6) Worse thinking of symptoms, Ox-ac., Pip-m.

REFERENCES - Boericke. Clarke. Phatak.

SWEET CHESTNUT

(Bach Flower Essence)

PHARMACY - sw-ch-b. Sweet chestnut. Castanea sativa. Flowering sprigs with both male and female flowers are boiled for half an hour. The water is strained and used as medicine. ***Historical dose:*** Take two drops from the stock bottle into a one ounce dropper bottle, (add brandy or alcohol, if this bottle will be used for days or weeks). This is the dosage bottle, take a few drops straight into the mouth or as needed in a little water or juice.

HOMEOPATHIC - Sw-ch-b. belongs to Bach's group of ***Despondency and Despair*** with Crb-a-b., Oak-b., Will-b., Star-b-b., Elm-b., Pine-b. and Lar-b. States of apathy and anguish.

Severe and prolonged physical suffering, leading to anguish. Suffering seems to be unbearable. Physical side effects of deep depression. Morbid preoccupation and depression (Must-b.). Existential doubt, despair. Suicidal.

MIND - Anguish. Apathy, faithlessness, nihilism and despair. Religious despair with loss of faith. The "dark night of the soul." Depressive disorders (Must-b.), especially when suicide is threatened with deep-seated despair Morbid preoccupation with death.

Void of emotional life. Despair and despondent. Sense of meaninglessness of life may lead to carelessness of attitude. Lack of aspirations and meaningful purpose.

REFERENCES - Bach.

SWERTIA CHIRATA

PHARMACY - swer-ch. Swertia chirata. N. O. Gentianaceae. Tincture from the flowers and leaves. ***Historical dose:*** Tincture and all potencies.

CLINICAL - Acidity. Bilious. Boils. Cough. Dropsy. Dyspepsia. ***Fevers.*** Flatulence. Indigestion. Intermittent fever. Leprosy. Malaria. Typhoid fever. Worms.

HERBAL - Charaka recommended Swertia in hematemesis and dropsy. Habita found it efficacious in vomiting of pregnancy.

Ayurvedic physicians extolled its therapeutic virtues in typhoid and intermittent fevers, malarial fever, respiratory troubles, bilious troubles, impurities of blood, burning, cough, dropsy, thirst, leprosy, boils and worms.

Swertia is a well-known and well-tried febrifuge among these practitioners and they very often use it in all sorts of fevers. It has been in constant demand among the Kavirajas of India.

Like cinchona and other bitter tonics, it is bitter, stomachiec, laxative, anthelmintic and febrifuge. It excites the appetite, strengthens digestion, but does not constipate. It diminishes flatulence and hyperacidity. Removes biliousness in atonic dyspepsia, liver troubles. Removes acidity of the stomach and flatulence, gout, intermittent and other fevers.

HOMEOPATHIC - Dr. Kali Kumar Bhattacharjea, of Gouripore, Assam, made a short proving of Swer-ch. An account of the proving and the symptoms developed therein were published in the Hahnemann of Falgoon. Dr. Bhattacharjea prepared a tincture from the flowers and leaves of the plant.

MIND - Dullness of mind, laziness, desire to lie down always.

Abdomen - Accumulation of wind in the abdomen.

Ears - Hissing sound in the ears.

Eyes - Severe burning sensation in the eyes.

Food - Desire for bitter substances and meat.

Head - Dull pain over both the temples, gradually extending to the whole of the head. Coldness is felt over the head.

Kidneys - Dull pain in the kidney, especially on the right side. Urine is of high red color. Burning while urinating.

Limbs - Aching pains in the hands and feet. Weakness of the legs, difficulty in walking.

Liver - Enlargement of both liver and spleen associated with pain.

Lungs - Hurried respiration during fever. Dry mucus, dry hacking cough. Dry cough in the bronchial region.

Male - Weakness of the male sexual organ, slight discharge of semen.

Mouth - Bad taste in the morning, offensive odor.

Nose - Flushes of heat come out of the nostrils.

Temperature - Stage of coldness lasts long, but there is no desire for drinking. Cold with nausea, bilious vomiting. Desire for hot water. Hot stage generally lasts for three hours, and afterwards sweating stage appears. Sweat only on chest, axilla and thighs. Slight thirst with heat. No fixity of the appearance of fever. Burning sensation in the eyes during fever.

Throat - In the morning and evening, pain is felt in the throat, not relieved by hot drinks.

Tongue - The middle of the tongue is enveloped with a thick yellowish coating. Heaviness of the tongue. Difficult speech.

COMMENTS - A noted febrifuge. Acute and chronic malarial fevers. Chronic fevers. Liver troubles after fever has stopped. Debility after fevers. Long-lasting malarial fever, turns into Kala-azar associated with enlarged spleen and liver.

The fever may come on at any time of the day and night; in chronic cases the fever appears usually in the afternoon. In the morning attacks, cold stage lasts for a long time, there is no appreciable thirst in this stage and if there be any, it is generally relieved by hot drinks.

Before the appearance of hot stage, nausea and bilious vomiting trouble the patient. The hot stage lasts for 3 to 4 hours and there is slight thirst. Severe burning sensation in the eyes, continues as long as the fever is present.

Indigestion, atonic dyspepsia. Flatulence. Loss of appetite. Troubles arising out of worms. Catarrhs, leprosy and some skin diseases.

RELATIONS - ***Compare:*** Chin., Ars.

REFERENCES - Ghose.

SYCOTIC CO. BACILLUS

(Bowel Nosode)

PHARMACY - syc-co. Sycotic co. bacillus. Sycotic bacillus. Bowel nosode. Bacillus streptococcus faecalis. Sycotic co. from non-lactose fermenting cocci of intestinal tract. ***Historical dose:*** All potencies.

CLINICAL - Albuminuria. Allergies, food. Alopecia. Amenorrhea. Anemia. Arthritis. Asthma. Backaches. Bedwetting. ***Conjunctivitis.*** Cough. Cystitis. Deafness. Dysmenorrhea. Enteroptosis. ***Fibrositis.*** Food, poisoning. Gastroenteritis. Headaches. Indigestion. Leucorrhea. ***Lumbo-sacral pain.*** Menorrhagia. Metrorrhagia. Neuritis. ***Otorrhea***. Photophobia. Polyps. Rheumatism. Sebaceous, cysts. Vaginitis. Warts.

HOMEOPATHIC - Characteristic ***irritation***, particularly in relation to the mucus membranes. Catarrhal states of the respiratory tract, the bladder and the vagina. Asthma, sinusitis. Cough about 2 a.m., worse from change of atmosphere.

Irritation of synovial linings in rheumatism. Enlarged lymphoid tissue of tonsils and adenoids, glands. Meningeal irritation. Convulsions. Cold and sensitive to dampness. Warty growths. Ailments from vaccinations.

Vulvo-vaginitis, leucorrhea. Gastroenteritis. Bedwetting, cystitis. Albuminuria. Stools are excoriating, loose and offensive with urgent call to stool on rising.

MIND - ***Nervous and tense.*** Ailments from anticipation. Bites the fingernails. Nervous irritability. ***Cross, irritable and restless***. Quick tempered, outbursts of temper from resentment. Oversensitive. Shy, sensitive and fussy. Exhausted. Timidity. Weepy and depressed. Fears of dark, of being left alone, of animals and dogs.

Abdomen - Distended abdomen, colon. Enteroptosis. Chronic irritation of whole digestive tract. Acute or chronic gastroenteritis in the child.

Back - Severe backache. Pain in morning on rising. Backache from damp weather. Stiff all over. ***Fibrositis,*** myositis. Neuritis of head and neck. Sebaceous cyst back. ***Lumbo-sacral pain.*** Pain in sacral-iliac joints. Hips stiff.

Blood - Anemia and hydremia.

Chest - Pleurisy. Pleurodynia. Fibrositis of chest wall. Sudden pain at the base of right lung. Intercostal neuralgia. Pain in left shoulder blade.

Constitutions - Pale, sallow, flabby and soft with long eyelashes (Tub.), and sweat of the head.

Ears - ***Otorrhea.*** Excessive formation of wax. Deafness. Itching of meatus. Cracks under ears.

Eyes - Conjunctivitis. Vitreous opacities. Pain in eyeballs. Photophobia, hemiopia. Blinking. Tarsal cysts. Cystic tumors on eyelids. Swelling of upper eyelids.

Face - Puffy in morning, especially under eyes. Acne rosacea. Eruptions, herpes about mouth. Erythema. Vesicular eruption on cheeks. Malignant growth on right cheek. Hair on face and upper lip. Facial neuralgia. Twitching facial muscles.

Female - Amenorrhea. Pain left ovary at menstrual period. Menorrhagia. Metrorrhagia. Dysmenorrhea. Leucorrhea acrid, excoriating. Leucorrhea copious, yellow. Leucorrhea profuse, bland. Vaginal discharge, offensive, fishy. Pruritus vulvae, vulvo-vaginitis, balanitis. Tumors, ovarian cysts. Uterine polyps. Genital warts, herpes.

Food - Desires butter, fat, cheese. Desires sweets, milk and salt. Averse to breakfast. Aversion to egg, fat, cheese, milk, milk pudding, cream. Aversion to salt, vinegar, sugar, tea. Aversion to bread, potato, tomato, vegetables, meat. Aggravated by egg, causing nausea, vomiting, bilious attack and hay fever. Worse from fat, eggs, onion and oranges.

Head - Irritation of meninges, sub-acute or chronic. Headache from infection of sinuses. Aching pain deep in brain. Headache on left side. Frontal congestive headache which lasts for many days. Sick headache, worse at menstrual period. Throbbing, better heat and rest, worse noise. Sweating of head at night. Painful dry scaly spots. Premature gray hair. Alopecia. Baldness.

Kidneys - Irritation of mucus membranes from kidney to urethra. Kidney pain. Nephritis, pyelitis, nephrosis, cystitis. Frequency and urgency. Urine corrosive. Albuminuria. Urinary tantrums.

Limbs - Fibrositis, shoulders. Muscular rheumatism of arms. Arthritis fingers, pain generally better dry day and hot water. Fingers deformed, nodules on fingers. Fingertips cracked. Fingers go dead, numb, with spasm of the fingers. Prickly feeling in hands. Nails brittle. Feet and legs painful when walking as if walking on loose cobble stones. Feet and legs painful at night. Pes planus. Rheumatism of knees. Ankles swollen and stiff. Feet swollen at night. Fidgety feet at night in bed. Soles of feet painful. Big toe joint painful.

Lungs - Dyspnea in morning on waking. Asthma and bronchitis, worse with damp and frost and better at the sea side. Frequent bronchial colds. Bronchitis in winter. Tracheitis. Wheeze and coughing at 2 to 3 a.m. Irritable cough of croupy nature at night, wakes from sleep. Coughs until sick. Chronic spasmodic persisting cough. Cough with tough sputum.

Male - Impotency. Genital warts and herpes.

Modalities - Worse from change of atmosphere, damp.

Mouth - Salivation increased. Bad taste, sense of taste lost. Pins and needle sensation on tongue. Pain like a splinter in tongue. Tongue sore, scalded, dry, fissured, furred. Tongue dry, sticks to roof of mouth. Warts on tongue. Deep ulcers on tongue. Ulcers in mouth. Lips dry and cracked. Cracks in angles of mouth. Herpes of mouth.

Neck - Fibrositis in neck, shoulders and back.

Nose - Nasal, post nasal catarrh. Catarrh extending to frontal sinuses. Turbinates congested, sinus infection. Vasomotor rhinorrhea. Hay fever. Coryza after eating eggs. Polyps. Nose dry, crusting and burning. Cracks at corners of nostrils. Nosebleed. Sense of smell lost.

Perspiration - Profuse perspiration at night during sleep.

Rectum - Condylomata around anus. Anal warts. Splinter pain. Distended feeling in rectum. Prolapse. Constipation or looseness. Stool pale, crumbly, bad odor. Loose, offensive stool, excoriating (Med.). Diarrhea from excitement of emotions. Diarrhea after eating, fatty food. Liquid motion after every meal. Urgent call to stool as soon as rising out of bed.

Skin - Sallow and oily skin. Impetigo. Warts large, flat and rugged. Herpes on face, neck and chest. Herpes groin. Varicellar eruption of limbs since immunization. Intertrigo breasts. Eczema of face in infants. Eczema on back of hands. Palmar dermatitis. Cracks on fingertips. Paronychia. Nails and toenails brittle and painful. Cracks on heals. Varicose eczema of ankles. Chilblains on feet.

Sleep - Insomnia. Restless sleep. Perspiration of head and body during sleep. Wheeze or cough. Can't sleep until 3 a.m. Wakes 2 to 3 a.m. Night terrors. Nightmares, of dead bodies.

Stomach - Anorexia. Burning pain in stomach. Pain and distention in the epigastrium. Flatulence. Acidosis attacks. Eructation acid, bilious attacks. Nausea from the smell of cooking. Nausea or sickness after eating eggs (Ferr.). Nocturnal vomiting, must empty stomach.

Throat - Fibrositis of neck and throat. Goiter. Glands enlarged. Enlargement of tonsils and adenoids. Tonsillitis, cheesy masses from tonsil. Quinsy. Throat feels raw, scorched, dry. Profuse mucus from throat in morning. Swallowing difficult, chokes easily.

COMMENTS - This organism of the intestinal tract is related morphologically and clinically to the gonococcus bacteria. Hahnemann related what he called "the Sycotic Miasm" to the disease, gonorrhea, but this disease is only one form of catarrhal infection of the mucus membrane of the urinary tract.

There are many non gonorrheal organisms associated with the symptom picture of "Catarrh" and according to Dr. John Paterson the miasm "Sycosis" may be considered synonymous with "Catarrh." Gonorrhea is an infection of mucus membrane, but catarrhal manifestations (sycotic) are not at all due to gonorrheal infection.

Characteristic warty growths. Exanthema of chickenpox. Chronic and recurring cystitis, often treated several times with antibiotics. Usually additional remedies are required, particularly a constitutional prescription, but intercurrent doses of Syc-co. can be of great help.

Griggs noted it for human "flu," cat "flu," foul pest, foot and mouth disease and canine distemper are all the signs of Syc-co. Convulsions, meningitis or epileptic forms of seizures are to be found in the clinical picture and also chorea, though less frequently than in Dysentery Co.

Syc-co. 200c in nosebleeds of long standing in a girl without any apparent reasons, cured completely with a few doses at long intervals.

RELATIONS - ***Compare:*** (1) The related sycotic remedies are Thuj, Nit-ac., Nat-s. and Bac. (2) Vesicular type of rash related to Ant-t., Rhus-t., Bac., and Thuj. ***Complementary:*** Lyc., is often complementary to this nosode.

REFERENCES - Bach. Paterson.

SYMPHORICARPUS RACEMOSUS

(Snowberry)

PHARMACY - sym-r. Symphoricarpus racemosus. Snowberry. N. O. Caprifliaceae. Tincture of fresh ripe berries. ***Historical dose:*** Tincture and all potencies.

CLINICAL - ***Constipation***. Hematemesis. Indigestion. ***Morning sickness.*** Nausea. ***Vomiting.*** Water brash.

HOMEOPATHIC - Prof. S. Burdick investigated the medicinal properties of many plants hitherto unused by the profession, including Symphoricarpus racemosa.

Useful for persistent ***vomiting of pregnancy.*** Nausea during menstruation. Nausea, ***worse from any motion. Averse to all food***, better when lying on the back. Gastric disturbances, fickle appetite, nausea, water brash, bitter taste. Smell and thought of food repugnant. ***Constipation***.

COMMENTS - When Burdick gave some of the Sym-r. to the first prover, a woman, she felt the marked nausea, and exclaimed, as soon as it was produced, "Doctor, this is precisely like the morning sickness I always experienced during pregnancy."

Dr. Burdick became more interested, repeated the experiment with other provers, and obtained almost uniform results, viz., a feeling varying from qualmishness to intense vomiting. It was given to female provers only and merely tested far enough to verify that symptom.

Upon this clue, Dr. Burdick gave Sym-r. in the higher potencies to patients suffering from the vomiting of pregnancy with the most satisfactory results. After a trial of many years, he found it so far superior to other remedies that he relied on it altogether with rarely any but entirely satisfactory results.

Burdick mentioned the drug in his course of lectures, so Moaffat bore it in mind waiting for a test case. Soon that came in the person of a young woman three months advanced in her first pregnancy.

She was suffering from a deathly nausea with vomiting and retching so prolonged and violent as to produce hematemesis. The smell or thought of food was repugnant in the extreme.

An examination disclosed no malposition or apparent cause for the trouble, so he procured some Sym-r. 200c from Dr. Burdick and gave her one dose in the midst of a violent paroxysm.

In a few minutes she stopped vomiting and said she felt soothed and quieted all over. In half an hour the nausea began again, but a few pellets checked it promptly and she fell asleep. Once during the night she awoke distressed and took a dose, but slept again quite soon.

For a month or so she felt very well until after over-exerting herself she became nauseated once more, but it was promptly checked, nor did it return during her pregnancy. The indications have been observed in cases of pregnancy with a feeling of qualmishness, with indifference to food.

In more severe cases, there is a deathly nausea, the vomiting is continuous, violent retching. Sym-r. does not seem to be confined to any particular morning aggravation, a prominent symptom is the disgust at the sight, smell or thought of food.

In one case, the patient was comparatively comfortable while lying on the back, but would be nauseated by the slightest motion of the arms, particularly raising them. The case was completely relieved by a few doses of Sym-r.

REFERENCES - Anshutz. Boericke. Clarke. Phatak.

SYMPHYTUM OFFICINALE

(Comfrey)

PHARMACY - symph. Symphytum officinale. Comfrey. Knit-bone. Healing herb. N. O. Boraginaceae. Tincture of fresh root-stock collected before flowering and in autumn. Tincture of fresh plant. ***Historical dose:*** Tincture and all potencies. Tincture, externally as a dressing for sores and ulcers and itching of anus.

CLINICAL - Abscess. Amputation. Backache. Bone, cancer. ***Bone, fractures***. ***Bone, injuries.*** Breasts, sore. ***Eyes, injuries.*** Fractures. Gingivitis. Glands, enlarged. ***Gunshot wounds.*** Hernia. Menses, suppressed. Osteoporosis. Periosteum, painful. Periostitis. Psoas, abscess. Sexual excess. Sprains. ***Stump, pain.*** Tennis elbow. Wounds.

HERBAL - Symphytum is also called consolida, and the word comfrey is derived from confirnare. The common name, knit-bone or bone-set, gives the indication for this remedy. The root contains a crystalline solid that stimulates the growth of bone cells and epithelium on ulcerated surfaces.

The glutinous juice of the root seems, according to Gerarde, to have given the key to its action as a vulnerary. Symphytum may be considered the orthopedic specific of herbal medicine.

HOMEOPATHIC - Symph. is a bone remedy. It may be administered internally in the treatment of gastric and duodenal ulcers, and in stomach pain, and externally for anal itching. External application disposes the swelling, due to injury or other growths.

Wounds penetrating to perineum and bones. ***Injuries to bones***, cartilages, ligaments, joints, tendons and the periosteum, with excessive pain. ***Pricking pain*** and soreness of periosteum. Pricking, sticking, jagging pains.

Fractures, broken bones. Painful bone at point of fracture. Pricking, stitching pains, remaining after wound is healed, worse touch. ***Non-union of fractures.*** Painful, irritable stump after amputation. Painful old injuries.

Bruises, sprains and inflammation of bones, diseased spinous processes. Deficient callus. Acts on joints generally. Neuralgia or arthralgia of the knee. Sore breasts. Psoas abscess. Sarcoma.

Abdomen - Pain about navel, worse sitting. Pains across epigastrium from one side to the other, when sitting. Griping pain.

Back - Backaches from excessive sexual indulgence, or from violent motion. Low back pain from injury, overexertion, or excess sexual activity. Spinal injury. ***Pain in back from a fall.*** Pott's disease from a fall. Decay of vertebrae. Caries of spinal and other bones.

Breasts - Sore breasts.

Causations - ***Broken bones.*** Injures to eye, bone, periosteum. Falls. Blows from blunt instruments. Sexual excess.

Ears - Cannot hear well, feels as if ears were stopped up. Inflamed ears.

Eyes - ***Injuries to the eyes*** from blunt instruments, blows, knocks, to the eyeball, eye socket, or sclera. Black eyes (Arn., Led.). Bleeding inside the eye after injury. Retinal bleeding. Traumatic conjunctivitis. Long-lasting pain or soreness in the eye after injury. Eyelids spasmodically closed.

Face - Facial injuries. Inflammation of inferior maxillary bone, hard, red swelling. Cancer, tumor of antrum. Cancer of jaw bone.

Female - Menses stopped. Leucorrhea.

Head - Headache in occiput, in top of head, in forehead, changing places. Pain comes down bone of nose. Inflammation of inferior maxillary bone, hard, red, swelling. Skull fracture or head injury (Hyper., Nat-s.).

Kidneys - Stricture of urethra.

Limbs - Bone fractures. Comminuted fracture. ***Non-union of bones.*** Accelerates the formation of callus. Reduces healing. Prickling, stitching pains. Bruises. Injuries from blunt instruments. Pain in area of bony protuberances, elbow, epicondyles, ankles. ***Injury to periosteum.*** Injury to hard tissue, shins. Bone inflammation, periostitis with pain and soreness. Osteoporosis. Brittle bones. Knee arthralgia. Tennis elbow. Psoas abscess. Bone cancers. Pain at the site of old wounds or fractures, past injury to cartilage or bone. Post-surgical pain at the site of amputation or bone puncture.

Male - Testicles become painful and tender, prevent walking. Backache from excessive sexual indulgence, with spermatorrhea.

Modalities - Better gentle motion, warmth. Worse from ***injuries.*** Worse sexual excess. Worse touch, motion, pressure. Stooping causes weight in forehead. Sitting causes pain about navel. Walking causes pain opposite spleen.

Nose - Pain comes down bone of nose and sometimes down both sides of nose.

Rectum - Dysentery. Inflamed and bleeding hemorrhoids.

Sensations - As if upper lid passed over an elevation on closing eye. As if ears were stopped up.

Skin - Cold.

Stomach - Ulcers of the stomach.

Teeth - Periodontal disease. Toothache after injury. Jaw swollen and painful after dental work. Pain worse after tooth extraction.

COMMENTS - Grimmer noted that, though the proving was meager, there was a rich clinical history.

According to Gerarde, "The roots of Comfrey stamped and the juice drunk with wine, help those that spit blood and heal all inward wounds and bursting. The same bruised and laid to in manner of a plaster, do heal all fresh and green wounds and are so glutinous, that it will solder and glue together meat that is chopped in pieces, seething in a pot and make it in one lump."

Gerarde added that it eases pains in the back from violent motion such as wrestling or from excessive sexual indulgence (Arn.), even when spermatorrhea has been induced thereby.

Peter Squire gave, as the medicinal properties of Symph., "Astringent, mucilaginous, glutinous, useful to form cases for injured limbs. The black rind of the root is scraped off and the mucilaginous root is then scraped carefully into a nice even pulp. This spread upon cambric or old muslin in wrapped round the limb and bandaged over, it shortly stiffens and forms a casing superior to starch, giving support and strength to the part."

Squire knew a bonesetter who rendered himself famous for setting compound fractures with this root, which he kept secret. He never removed the bandage after the first dressing until the limb was well.

Sir Wm. Thomson of Dublin related a case of malignant tumor of the face that had extended to the nose. Microscopic examination proved it to be round-celled sarcoma. The patient, a man, refused advice at the time, and was examined by Felix Semon, who saw the man later. After still further delay, Thomson performed the operation in the month of May, 1896.

A month later the growth began to show again, increased rapidly, closed the right eye, was blue, tense, firm, lobulated, but did not break. Thomson declined to operate again. Early in October, the man walked into Thomson's study well. "The tumor had completely disappeared from the face and I could not identify any trace of it in the mouth." The man had applied poultices of comfrey root and the swelling disappeared.

Comfrey's therapeutic history is rich with clinical cures of round-cell sarcoma of the antrum and many cases of bone cancer. It seems to have special curative action on the periosteum and bony structures, facilitating the formation of callus in fractures, bringing about union, even in compound fractures, and in cases of slow or delayed union.

Curative in injuries to the eyeball by blows etc. It follows Arn. in such cases, as well as in injuries to and bruising of the testicles. Backaches after strains and from sexual excesses. Pott's disease, psoriasis and abscesses from a fall. One case of inguinal hernia has been cured with the topical application of the tincture of the root.

H. C. Allen referred to the following indications for Symph. given by Lippe: when the bone or periosteum has been injured and the soft parts have recovered from the bruised soreness under Arn., the remaining pain and soreness of periosteum may be promptly relieved by Symph.

Symph. was the only remedy Lippe had seen which was efficient in traumatic injuries of bone or periosteum. He cured many cases after others had used Arn. and failed.

H. C. Allen gave the following cure, reported by Fowler. Mrs. J. stepped on the edge of a scantling, which rolled and she turned her ankle. In a few minutes the ankle began to swell and become painful, pain increased rapidly, so that in hour or two the patient was in great agony.

She declared that her leg was broken, she "could feel the rough ends of the broken bones jagging into the flesh." She could not bear any one to approach her for fear of being hurt. No discoloration whatever. Symph. promptly relieved, so that she went about her usual duties in forty-eight hours.

Allen regarded pricking pain as a guiding symptom. He noted its usefulness, next to bone injuries, for injuries to the eyeball. "I have long since ceased to use Arn. in injuries of the globe of the eye, Symph. having given such prompt and permanent relief."

Croserio was one of the first to use Symph. in the potencies for fractures. "Injuries of the bones are healed most promptly with Symph. 30c internally, once a day."

Wells gave cases of his own, including the case of a boy, 14, who broke the bone of his forearm at the junction of middle and lower thirds, two years before. He had twice repeated the fracture by slight falls. The ends were now slightly movable on each other, and the arm was of little use. Three doses of Symph. 30c made a perfect cure and the boy became robust and much better in health than he had ever been before.

Wells also recorded the case of a boy, 8, with a fractured humerus near the junction of condyles and shaft. Arn. 30c immediately arrested the spasmodic jerks of muscles of the injured arm. Arn. was continued three days, by which time all traumatic fever had subsided. Symph. 3c was given, one drop in half a tumbler of water, a teaspoonful morning and evening. The splints were removed the ninth day and the bone was found to be consolidated. The cure was entirely without pain.

F. H. Brett cured himself of inguinal rupture by rubbing the part with tincture of the root. On another occasion, a blow on the lower part of the back from a fall resulted in a secondary affection of the spine in the mid-dorsal region, a protuberance as if from a light dislocation appearing at the spot. Again Symph. was applied. The tenderness at the point subsided after three applications, and in a few days the protuberance disappeared.

Brett mentioned a case he had heard of a diseased arm that had begun to mortify. It was dressed with a poultice of comfrey root and this "drew off the mortified substance. The arm became sound again."

Cooper noted that one patient, just before her marriage, had a dangerous attack of scarlatina, leaving abscesses on both sides of the neck and great internal swelling, so that she could swallow only liquids and those with great difficulty.

The external swelling extended from ear to chin and was hard and very painful. Poultices of comfrey root were applied. The pain was immediately relieved and her abscesses decreased rapidly until they were entirely absorbed without external opening so far as the patient could remark.

For bone tumors, osteomyelitis, bone ulcers. Sarcomas. Bone cancers of the jaw or bones (Hecla.). Bone cancer, even if there is no bone injury (Calc-p., Hecla.). Non-union of fractures. Broken bones that don't heal well. Acutely for osteoporosis, or osteogenesis imperfecta (Calc., or Calc-p. chronically). Stump pain after amputation of a limb (Hyper., All-c., Coff., Calen.), strong aching pains.

Spinal diseases after trauma and injury. Injuries that result in a lump or tumor. For swellings, nodules and tumors in bones and limbs after an injury (Bell-p. and Con. after injury to soft tissue). Tailbone injuries (Arn., Hyper.), with an aching pains.

Blows to the eyes (Led., Arn.). Corneal abrasions. Hernias (Nux-v., Calc., Lyc.). As a compress for mastitis. In tincture for stomach ulcers.

RELATIONS - ***Antidote to:*** Canth. ***Compare:*** (1) Arn., Bry., Calc-p. - fractures. (2) injuries, Arn., soft parts, Symph., hard, Arn., sore, bruised lame, Symph., pricking, stitching, jagging pains. (3) Calen., Fl-ac., Hep., Sil., Staph., Led., Rhus-t., Hyper. (4) Effects of sexual excess, Arn. (5) Calc., Calc-f. ***Follows well:*** Arn. - for pricking pains and after the bruising of the soft parts is healed.

REFERENCES - Boericke. Clarke. Murphy. Phatak.

SYPHILINUM

(Syphilis Nosode)

PHARMACY - syph. Syphilinum. Syphilis nosode. Luesinum. Lueticum. ***Historical dose:*** All potencies.

CLINICAL - ***Abscesses. Alcoholism.*** Anus, fissures. Aphasia. Asthma. Baldness. ***Bone, disorders.*** Breasts, sensitive. Bubo. Cachexia. Cancer, Chancres. Constipation. Deafness. ***Debility.*** Deltoid rheumatism. Dentition. Diplopia. Dysmenorrhea. Epilepsy. ***Hair, loss.*** Headache, syphilitic. Hoarseness. Hodgkin's disease. ***Insomnia.*** Iritis. ***Leucorrhea.*** Mouth, ulcers. Myopia. ***Nerve, disorders.*** Neuralgia. Night-sweats. Ophthalmia. Otorrhea. Ovaries, disorders. Ozaena. ***Pains, severe.*** Paralysis. Pemphigus. ***Prostration.*** Psoas, abscess. Ptosis. Rectum, stricture. Rheumatism. Sciatic pain. ***Sleeplessness.*** Spine, decay. Strabismus. Strictures. Sunstroke. ***Syphilis. Teeth, decay.*** Throat, ulcerated. Tibia, pains. Tongue, cracked. Tongue, ulcerated. Tuberculosis. Ulcers. Whitlow.

HOMEOPATHIC - The syphilis nosode is mainly used on the general symptomatology with the family and personal history of the patient. Its ***nightly aggravation*** of complaints, with extreme mental and physical restlessness, together with its intense irritability, are striking indications for its use.

It's frequently used to great advantage as an intercurrent remedy in the course of treatment in chronic disease, prior to or following the apparently indicated remedy when the patient's response to that remedy is feebly or nil.

Syph. has been used in cancer, tuberculosis, severe types of neuro-arthritis, mental disturbances or various forms of paralysis. Syphilitic disorders. Especially useful when there is hereditary tendency to ***alcoholism*** or a ***syphilitic miasm.***

Affects the nerves, mucus membranes and bones. Utter ***prostration and debility in the morning.*** Great weakness with very few symptoms.

Shifting rheumatic pains. Chronic eruptions and rheumatism. Persistent pains in any part of the body. Cold pains. ***Pains from darkness to daylight***, decrease and increase gradually. Violent or linear pains. Knots in muscles. Pains in bones. Bones, sore, decay, curvature. Exostoses.

Ulceration of mouth, nose, genitals, skin. Stubborn ***ulcerations. Succession of abscesses.*** Fetid discharges, foul or green pus. Foul odor of the body. Ichthyosis Slowly advancing hemiplegia. Glands enlarged. Hodgkin's disease. Epilepsy, worse after menses. As of hot water in blood vessels.

Crying infants, who begin crying immediately after birth. Dwarfed, shriveled up, old looking babies and children, bald head, pouting lips and big belly.

MIND - Loss of memory, but remembers everything previous to his disease. Difficulty in making arithmetical calculations.

Apathetic. Severe insomnia and suicidal depression (Aur.), especially during extreme attacks of pain. Sad and lamenting. Antisocial, aversion to company. Cross, irritable, peevish. Does not want to be soothed.

Anxiety about health. Great restlessness and paces the floor at night. ***Hopelessness. Despair of recovery.*** Fear of suffering and pains. Desperate, can't take the pain or suffering anymore. Fear of dying. ***Fears the night.*** Fears from exhaustion.

Very nervous. Fastidious. Fear of germs, of catching an infection. ***Always washing or wringing the hands.*** Causeless weeping. Laughs or weeps without cause. Nightly delirium. Senile dementia. ***Feels as if going insane or being paralyzed. Insanity***, syphilitic insanity.

Abdomen - Pain or distress deep in abdomen as if in omentum. Feeling of heat internally in hypogastric region. Pain in right groin followed by swelling of glands. Large, painless bubo in right groin, opened and discharged freely.

Back - Neck feels short. Pain at coccyx with sensation as if it is swollen, worse sitting. Pain in the back in the region of kidney, worse after urinating.

Breasts - Sensitive to touch, feel sore during menses and other times.

Causations - Sun. Syphilis. Damp weather, thunderstorms.

Chest - Soreness of chest. Rattling in chest and throat. Oppression of chest to such an extent as almost to arrest breathing. Sensation of pressure under upper part of sternum.

Constitutions - Syphilitic.

Ears - Deafness without any obvious cause, nervous with cachexia. Abscess of the middle ear. Calcareous deposit on tympanum. Decay of ossicles in ear, of syphilitic origin.

Eyes - Ophthalmia, neonatorum. Tubercular iritis. Amaurosis, atrophy of optic nerve. Spots on cornea. ***Chronic, recurrent, inflammation of cornea.*** Successive crops of phyctenules and abrasions of epithelial layer of cornea. ***Intense pain at night.*** Feeling of cold air blowing on eye (Fl-ac.). Photophobia and profuse lachrymation. Glimmering vision. Diplopia. Vertical diplopia. Squints. Ptosis. Lids swollen, especially upper eyelids. Eyelids glued together.

Face - ***Pale, wrinkled, old looking.*** Pain over eyes (right) worse protruding tongue. Paralysis of one side with difficult speech, mastication and twitching of eyes, lids. Twitching of muscles.

Female - Menses, with putrid meat-like odor. ***Leucorrhea profuse, thin, watery, acrid*** with sharp, knife-like pain in ovaries. Yellow, offensive, acrid leucorrhea, so profuse it soaks through napkins and runs to the heels, with itching of the genitals. Ulcers on labia. Ulcers on the vulva with ovarian pain, sensitive to touch. Cutting pain in ovary during sex, at the moment of orgasm. Habitual abortion.

Food - Capricious appetite. No food agrees or satisfies him. Total loss of appetite for months. ***Craves alcoholic drinks.*** Aversion to meat.

Head - Stupefying headaches. Pain in bones of head. ***Deep, crushing head pains across the base of temples.*** Linear pains from temples across, or from eyes backward, cause sleeplessness and delirium at night. Beats head against the wall. Feels pulled back. Top of head feels as if coming off. Cerebral softening. ***Falling of the hair.*** Tubercles all over the scalp.

Heart - Large, soft pulse. Valvular disease of heart. Sharp pains in heart from base to apex (Med. has reverse), at night. As if hot water flowing in the veins.

Kidneys - Urine frothy, scanty, yellow. Urinates only once a day, but profuse. Passes urine better while standing. Nocturnal bedwetting.

Limbs - Muscles contracted in hard knots. Indolent ulcers. Sciatica, worse at night, better about daybreak. Bones pain as if sawed. Bilateral exostoses sore and painful. Osteo-sarcoma in center of tibia. Cold pain in legs. Shin bones painful, better pouring cold water on them. Soles painful with feeling of contraction, worse standing on them. Cannot sit on low chair or squat. Redness and rawness between toes (Sil.). Rheumatism of shoulder joint, at insertion of deltoid, worse from raising arm laterally or in front. Itching eruptions about elbows. Affections of middle fingers. ***Always washing the hands.***

Lungs - Asthma with wheezing and rattling (Ant-t.). Chronic asthma, worse in summer, during thunderstorms, at night, humid weather. Dry cough, worse lying on right side, worse at night, windpipe sensitive to touch (Lach.). Sharp pains from base of heart to apex at night.

Male - Nodular formation in testes, spermatic cord and scrotum. Chancres. Aching of genitals, cannot sit still.

Modalities - Better inland, mountains, high altitude. Better during day, from applied heat. Better continued or slow motion. Better changing positions. ***Worse at night, from sundown to sunrise.*** Worse full moon. Worse damp, thunderstorms. Worse extreme heat or cold, winter, summer. Worse at the seashore. Worse in any position, squatting. Worse motion, raising arms laterally. Worse protruding tongue.

Mouth - ***Excessive flow of saliva, it runs out of mouth when sleeping.*** Putrid taste, before epileptic fit. Ulcers, smart and burn. Tongue, coated, indented, deep longitudinal cracks along center. Paralysis of tongue. Aphasia.

Nose - Decay of nasal bones, hard palate and septum with perforation. Ozaena offensive, thick yellow-green discharge. Attacks of fluent coryza. Snuffles. Green lumps from posterior sinuses. Sinuses, painful, from inhaled air. Saddle across the bridge of the nose (Sep.). Itching nostrils.

Perspiration - Perspires at night, with exhaustion. Sweats at night, most marked between scapulae and down to waist. Peculiar disagreeable odor from body.

Rectum - Fissures in anus and rectum, prolapsed. Feels tied up with strictures. Obstinate constipation. Diarrhea, bilious, painless worse seashore, drives her out of bed about 5 a.m. Water from enema escapes, with pain.

Sensations - A seething feeling as if hot water or hot oil running through all veins of the body, all night long. A far-away feeling with apathy. As if going insane or about to be paralyzed. As if top of head were coming off. As if teeth were loose. Tongue feels as if paralyzed. Fluttering as of something alive in teeth. As if throat tearing to pieces. As of a nervous chill commencing in anus and running down legs. Palms and soles as if pricked by needles. As if bitten by bugs.

Skin - Extreme emaciation. Reddish-brown eruption with a disagreeable odor. Swollen and blotched. Biting as from bugs. Wandering erysipelas. Conical crusts. Bullae. White or pockmark scars. Coppery spots. Distorted nails.

Sleep - ***Sleeplessness.*** Great restlessness at night, impossible to keep leg in one position. Wakes soon after midnight and cannot sleep again until 6 a.m.

Stomach - Nausea. Vomiting for weeks or months due to erosion from superficial ulceration of lining of viscous. Heartburn with pain and rawness from stomach to throat pit, often with cough.

Temperature - Chilly. Nervous chills preceded by pains in head. Fever dry, hot, shortly after going to bed, parted lips, great thirst. Sweats at night with exhaustion.

Throat - Aphonia before the menses. Continuous pain in the larynx, worse touch. Sore, right to left, worse cold drinks. Chronic hypertrophy of tonsils with syphilitic taint.

Teeth - Teeth feel sticky, as of a worm in. Feeling as if teeth had all got out of place. Teeth decay at the edge of gums. Toothache better pressing them together, worse hot or cold things. Teeth cupped in children.

Vertigo - Vertigo on looking up, seems to be caused by heat.

COMMENTS - Syph. is useful for ailments since syphilis, or a history of syphilis in the family. Pains get worse or better gradually, are shifting and require frequent change of position. Unbearable pains (Aur.). Linear pain. Ulcers and bone pains (Merc.).

Characteristic aggravated by night, pains from darkness to daylight, begin with twilight and end with daylight. All symptoms are worse at night. Terrible dread of night, because of mental and physical exhaustion on waking. Neuralgia and headache, asthma, coughs worse from sunset to sunrise, whether syphilitic or not. Sleeplessness (Sulph.).

Epilepsy. Parkinson's disease. Facial paralysis. Hemiplegia, "persistent pains in any part of the body." Neurotic behavior, especially wringing and washing of the hands. AIDS, dementia, sleeplessness, anxiety, fear of infection, and neurotic behavior.

Ulceration, affecting the mouth, nose, genitals or skin. Ulcers have grayish bases. Abscesses with foul secretions. Fetid pus formations. Succession of abscesses. Eruptions with copper-colored spots. Pemphigus.

Ozaena with discharge of fetid clinkers. Catarrhal and nerve deafness. Itching of nostrils. Fetid discharges from the ear. Alopecia universalis. Dark purple lines between alae nasi and cheeks. Itching, scabby eruptions on face or breast, singly or in clusters, looking like herpes. Pain and pressure behind sternum.

Ophthalmia neonatorum, the lids adhere during sleep, pains worse 2 to 5 a.m., profuse pus, better cold bathing. Iritis, syphilitic or rheumatic. Diplopia, one image seen below the other. Ptosis, sleepy look from drooping lids.

Teeth decay at the edge of the gums and break off. Cupped teeth, serrated edges, dwarfed in size and converge at their tips. Deformities of the teeth. The teeth come in rotten and deformed (Calc-f., Kreos.). Paralysis of tongue. Aphasia.

Craving for alcohol in any form. Hereditary tendency to alcoholism. Impaired nutrition, emaciation. Burnett recorded many instances of Syph. helping stunted children. Progeria. Babies that never stop crying and screaming ever since they were born (Jal., Acon.).

Leucorrhea, profuse, soaking through napkins and running to heels. Rectal pain. "Obstinate constipation for years, rectum seems tied up with strictures, when enema was used the agony of passage was like labor."

H. C. Allen said "Syphilitics or patients who have had chancre treated by local means and as a result have suffered from throat and skin troubles for years, are nearly benefited by this remedy at commencement of treatment unless some other remedy is clearly indicated."

Thomas Wildes noted that, in his experience with Syph., the chancre increases for the first two weeks and then gradually fades away, not being followed by secondaries.

Wildes cured a bookkeeper who, for many months, had a piercing, pressing, excruciating headache over his right eye extending deep into his brain. It was so severe, he was losing continuity of thought and memory.

Under Syph. 1,000c every night, the headache disappeared entirely in ten days and his mental faculties were fully restored. But in six weeks the whole eyebrow on that side broke out into a sickly, yellow, syphilitic eczema with a red, angry and oozing base extending under the arch to the lid, from canthus to canthus, up into forehead and down the side of the nose.

The cure of this was tedious; Wildes attributed it to his change of remedy instead of continuing with Syph. This man had syphilis a few years before.

In 1879 a woman, 26, extremely bright and intelligent, came to Wildes with a dreadful ozaena. She also had a spinal curvature and congestion of right ovary. She had always been delicate.

Syph. cured the ozaena and improved her health, but it "drove out a saddle to which the Sepia saddle is but a shadow." A furious inflammatory mass of syphilitic sores, scabs and eczema, red and angry with a fiery base extending from one malar prominence to the other, across nose up to eyes and forehead. This took eighteen months to cure. The ozaena never returned.

A boy, age 4, had an obstinate rash, a combination of prurigo and herpes, on his chin, lips, cheekbone, forehead and hairy scalp, on arms, chest, back, bends of joints and on the joints and on fingers and hands, nowhere profuse. In spite of authorities to the contrary, Wildes maintained that syphilitic rashes may itch and that prurigo is infectious and is one of the initial stages of leprosy.

This boy had a spot of eruption on the left thigh the size of the top joint of a man's thumb. This was distinctly a leper spot. Syph. 1,000c caused the rash to come out strongly all over the body in patches, the face was one-third covered with a thick, yellow, scabby eruption. The remedy was continued and the boy got well, wonderfully improved in health, was no longer nervous, grew well, slept well, with good appetite.

A girl, 16, had measles a year before which did not come out properly. A year and a half prior she was subject to neuralgic headaches. She had been ailing about two years, very despondent, wanted to die, headaches growing more violent.

During the headaches, the temple veins stood out, had pains all over the body, was very irritable, restless, walked about much of the time, did not wish to be soothed, violent on being opposed, had tremors and seemed on the verge of convulsions, dazed, absent-minded and almost insane. Always washed her hands. She was formerly constipated, but now subject to "a kind of diarrhea."

Menses never came on properly and for the past year had been very irregular, much delayed, scanty and always extremely painful.

Often feverish. Anxious sleep, distressed and often wakeful and violently restless. The symptoms indicated Syph. and under this she steadily recovered.

A young woman contracted "leprosy-syphilis" from vaccination. She had a blood-boil on her arm that would not heal. Face broken out with a fiery rash. With Syph. 1,000c at bedtime she recovered rapidly. The arm healed quickly and her face became free from eruption.

A boy, 3, had a cluster of yellow blotches on his fingers and roots of nails, distorting the nails. The boy's father was epileptic. The boy was helped with Fl-ac. and cured with Syph., the nails became straight.

G. H. Carr related the case of an old man who had been troubled for two or three winters with an intense cold pain in both legs. It came on every night on lying down and lasted all night, the only relief was from getting up and walking.

Magnetic leggings had given the most relief. Syph. 1,000c, one dose daily, was given. He lost the pain for six weeks, when it returned in milder form. Syph. 100,000C was given and he had no more pains all the winter. The medicine, he said "made his genitals ache so that he couldn't sit still." This lasted over a month.

Syph. 100,000c cured a woman of "asthma" that she had for twenty-five years, the attack coming on only at night after lying down or during a thunderstorm.

Swan said he gave crying infants one dose of Syph. 100,000c, when they developed the propensity immediately after birth and did not cease, and it was difficult to make them cry after that.

Yingling reported the case of Rev. D., 30, who was dark and free from venereal disease. Haggard look. He had a constant dull, heavy ache above inner angle of right eye, very distressing with an occasional thrust as of an iron rod from the same spot through to lower part of occiput. This thrust was excruciating.

He was due to preach the next day, but the pain quite incapacitated him, which led him to appeal for help. Syph. 100,000c, one dose, was given. He was free from pain before he reached home, and was perfectly well the next morning.

RELATIONS - ***Compare:*** (1) Merc., Kali-hp., Nit-ac., Aur., Alum.

REFERENCES - Boericke. Clarke. Murphy. Phatak.

SYRINGA VULGARIS

(Lilac)

PHARMACY - Syringa vulgaris. Lilac. N. O. Oleaceae. ***Historical dose:*** All potencies.

CLINICAL - Fever. Malaria. Worms.

HERBAL - The leaves and the fruit are anti-periodic, febrifuge, tonic and vermifuge. The bark or leaves have been chewed by children as a treatment for sore mouth.

REFERENCES - Murphy.

SYZYGIUM AROMATICUM

(Clove Oil)

PHARMACY - eug-c. Syzygium aromaticum. Clove oil. Eugenia caryophallata. ***Historical dose:*** Tincture and all potencies.

CLINICAL - Arthritis. Asthma. Bronchitis. Rheumatism. Sprains. Strains. ***Toothache.***

HERBAL - The clove plant originated in the lowlands, valleys, and hillsides of the southern Philippine islands. The essential clove oil, the most popular clove product, is extracted from the flower of the clove.

Clove oil constituents include eugenol, eugenyl acetate, caryophyllene and io-caryophyllene.

Clove oil is used in connection with respiratory ailments such as asthma and bronchitis, muscle aches, sprains and strains, arthritis and rheumatism. Many individuals use clove oil for its analgesic effects for body pain.

Clove oil is considered by many to be an effective antibiotic, antiseptic, antiviral, analgesic, antioxidant, carminative, expectorant, antifungal, anti-parasitic, spasmodic, and stimulant.

REFERENCES - Murphy.

SYZYGIUM JAMBOLANUM

(Jambol Seeds)

PHARMACY - syzyg. Syzygium jambolanum. Jambol seeds. Syzygium cumini. Eugenia jambolana. Jumbul. N. O. Myrtacae. India. Trituration of the seeds. Tincture of the powdered fruit-stones. ***Historical dose:*** Tincture and all potencies.

CLINICAL - ***Diabetes.*** Glycosuria. Pimples. Prickly heat. Ulcers.

HERBAL - Syzygium jambolanum is a native of India. It has an edible fruit, the powdered stones of which have a popular use in India as a remedy for diabetes. Syzyg. has an immediate effect of increasing the blood sugar, glycosuria results. The dose is five to ten grains of the powdered stones three times a day, also, the tincture.

HOMEOPATHIC - Syzyg. is a most useful remedy in diabetes mellitus. Dudgeon used Syzyg. in the lower homeopathic potencies with marked success, which has been repeated by many others.

Diminution and disappearance of sugar in the urine. Great thirst, weakness, emaciation. Very large amounts of urine, specific gravity high. ***Prickly heat in upper part of the body***, small red pimples itch violently.

Hansen mentioned "old ulcers of skin, probably of a diabetic foundation" as having been cured with Syzyg.

COMMENTS - Dudgeon related the case of a scientific man, 56, who complained of "prickly heat" all over upper part of body and arms. The skin was covered with small, red papules, which itched so intensely he could get no rest.

There was much thirst and great flow of urine, which he was obliged to pass every two hours, night and day, mouth very dry. Urine 1036, very saccharine.

Syzyg. tincture, mixed with three times the quantity of alcohol, was given of this two drops every three hours. The specific gravity of the urine steadily declined, sugar disappeared and all the symptoms passed off. This in spite of the fact that the dietetic rules were relaxed.

RELATIONS - ***Compare:*** (1) Insulin. - an aqueous solution of an active principle from pancreas which affects sugar metabolism. If administered at suitable intervals in diabetes mellitus, the blood sugar is maintained at a normal level and the urine remains free of sugar. Overdosage is followed by weakness and fatigue and tremulousness and profuse sweating.

REFERENCES - Boericke. Clarke.

T

TABACUM FUMUS

(Tobacco Smoke)

PHARMACY - tab-fum. Tabacum fumus. Tobacco smoke. ***Historical dose:*** Tincture and all potencies.

CLINICAL - Allergies. Asthma. Bronchitis. Coughs. Lung, disorders. Tobacco, addiction.

HOMEOPATHIC - Tab-fum. is made by blowing cigarette smoke into a bottle of water, which is then mixed and potentized. A homeopathic proving of Tab-fum. was done by Chachanidze. It has been used to reduce the cravings for smoking of cigarettes. Allergies to cigarette smoke, headaches and irritability from smell of tobacco. Asthma in cigarette smokers.

MIND - Concentration difficult during study. Anxiety, which comes from the heart. Anticipation as if something bad will happen. Irritability in the crowd, desire to escape. Dullness. Indifference to habitual deeds. Sensation as if one has a disease of throat (fixed idea).

Eyes - Burning, itching and lachrymation, worse in the right eye.

Face - Aching of the left upper jaw-bone in the morning after awaking, as if it is toothache. It is extending to the left eye-socket and left side of the nose bone, lasts whole day. Pain goes to the forehead and nose in the evening.

Head - Sensation of emptiness in the right half of the head with the nausea. Dull pain in the head. Headache, aggravation from the sun. Heaviness in the occiput, more in the left side, began in the morning awaking after. Heaviness of the whole head. Sensation as if head is bursting. As if all bones of the scull are aching, especially along the sutures. Nausea and emptiness in the head. Amelioration from the stool.

Lungs - Shortness of breath even after slight physical exertion, worse ascending stairs. Hoarseness, burning of throat and weakness of voice. Dry cough, as if would choke.

Mouth - Tickling. Heat in the mouth, as if hot air go out from mouth. Sensation that mouth is dirty. Desire to clean teeth. Sensation of loosening of teeth with bitter saliva. Salivation. Pressure of parotid glands as if after sour lemon. Desire to make massage with tongue of gums. As if toothache in upper incisors. Ache in the root of the tooth of upper jaw-bone. Sensation as if teeth are unnecessary. Desire to rub gums and teeth. Pain like from little nail. Stretching pain in the right submaxillary region. Sensation of swelling of the inner cheek. Little white ulcer on inner cheek.

Nose - Sensation of smell of smoke. Stuffed-up nose, amelioration in open air. Discharge of mucus to the postnasal region.

Sensations - Sensation as if faint, as if body is like cotton wool.

Sleep - Drowsy from 7 to 8 p.m. Dreams of heavy shower, rain, flood, dirty water. Dreams of being dirty, desire to take a shower.

Stomach - Hunger, burning in stomach as if hot water is pouring, in the morning. Increased appetite with impatience. Hunger after eating. Desire chocolate.

Tongue - Sensation of coating at the root of the tongue. Tickling and itching of tongue. Pricking in tip of tongue. As if beating of electricity to the tip op of tongue. Dryness, burning of tongue. Shooting pain in the root of tongue extending to the right Eustachian tube and to the right ear.

Throat - Sensation of coating at the throat and at the postnasal region. Numbness of posterior part of gullet and of throat and hoarseness. Sensation feel like tissues are hanging from the gullet. Sensation as if ulcers on gullet.

Vertigo - Sensation of vertigo, as if falling to the right. Vertigo with palpitations during walking.

REFERENCES - Chachanidze. Murphy.

TABACUM NICOTIANA

(Tobacco)

PHARMACY - tab. Tabacum nicotiana. Tobacco. Nicotiana tabacum. N. O. Solanaceae. Tincture of the fresh leaves collected before the flowers are developed. ***Historical dose:*** Tincture and all potencies.

CLINICAL - ***Amaurosis.*** Anemia. Angina, pectoris. Anus, prolapse. Asthma. Backaches. Brain, anemia. Brain-fag. Catalepsy. Cholera. Cholera, infantum. Color-blindness. Constipation. Diarrhea. Epilepsy. Esophagus, stricture. ***Fainting.*** Freckles. ***Giddiness***. Glands, enlarged. Heartbeats, disorders. Heartburn. Hernia. Hiccough. Idiocy. Itching. Leg, jerking. Lip, cancer. Lung, disorders. ***Masturbation, effects.*** Ménière's disease. Morning sickness. ***Motion, sickness. Nausea.*** Optic, neuritis. Pregnancy, disorders. Prostatorrhea. Rectum, paralysis. ***Seasickness.*** Speech, disorders. Strabismus. Strokes. Tetanus. Toothache. Varicocele. ***Vertigo. Vomiting.***

HERBAL - When Columbus and his followers landed in Cuba in 1492, the practice of smoking tobacco was in common use among the natives throughout the island and also throughout the continent of America. On their return to Spain, the practice rapidly spread throughout the Peninsula.

Nicotiana tabacum received its specific name from Jean Nicot, the French ambassador to Portugal, who was the means of introducing the tobacco plant into France about 1560.

Sir Walter Raleigh and his companions introduced the practice into England in 1586. From that time, the cultivation, manufacture and use of tobacco, either by smoking, snuffing or chewing, rapidly became popular.

HOMEOPATHIC - Tab. has ***nausea, giddiness, deathly sinking***, vomiting, icy coldness and sweat, with intermittent pulse. Complete prostration of the entire muscular system. Collapse. ***Seasickness***.

Marked anti-septic qualities, antidotal to cholera germs. Cholera infantum, cold, but ***wants abdomen uncovered***. Vigorous peristaltic activity. Diarrhea.

Produces high tension and arteriosclerosis of the coronary arteries. Angina pectoris with coronary sclerosis and high tension. Constriction of throat, chest, bladder and rectum. Pallor, breathlessness, hard cord-like pulse. Vagus, sympathetic, cerebro-spinal nerves and heart are prominently affected.

Complete prostration and relaxation of the entire muscular system with free secretions, vomiting, profuse sweat, lachrymation, salivation etc. Constriction of the muscles of hollow organs, throat, bladder, rectum, chest etc. Cramps, then paralysis of bowels, heart etc. Convulsions, head firmly drawn back. Jerking throughout the body. Trembling.

Pains are worse from heat. Excessive emaciation, especially of the muscles of back and cheeks. Gait slow and shuffling, unsteady, difficulty in ascending stairs. Faintness. Tetanus. Paralysis of sphincters. Slides in bed. Coughing causes hiccough, stitches in pit of stomach. Symptoms come in paroxysms, are periodical. Gastralgia, enteralgia.

MIND - Mental confusion and fatigue. Confusion from motion. Brain fag. Idiotic, epileptic idiocy. Slow perception. Forgetful. Indifferent. Desire for company in evening and at night.

Morose, sensation of extreme wretchedness. Feels wretched during menopause period and menses. ***Feels very despondent***. Discontented. Apathetic, indifferent. Sadness is better after complaining. Sadness with impeded respiration. Weeping ameliorates symptoms. Suicidal disposition but lacks courage.

Nervous and restlessness. Anguish when walking in open air. Sudden anxiety, with angina pectoris or oppression of chest, driving him from place to place. Anxiety from thinking about it. Anxiety better after crying. Anxiety at night. Fear after eating food. Fear from noises.

Cheerful, merry and talkative. Sings all day. Silly talk. Talks nonsense. Talks to himself. Delusions, preventing sleep. Feels as if someone were coming to arrest him or murder him. Doesn't recognize his relatives. Unconsciousness, as in a trance, better when cold water poured over head.

Abdomen - Coldness in abdomen. ***Wants abdomen uncovered***, it lessens the nausea and vomiting. Sinking feeling in epigastrium with dreadful faint sense. Retraction of navel, abdominal muscles contracted. Violent burning in abdomen, extorting cries. Painful distentions. Intestinal obstruction. Incarcerated hernia. Strangulated hernia. Gurgling in bowels. Horrible colic, must shriek, with weakness. Colic during stool.

Back - Emaciation of the muscles of back. Pain in the small of back worse lying, better while walking. Heat down spine. Throbbing in sacral region. Red eruption on back. Pustules on nape and upper limbs. Violent pain, in lumbar region. Neck stiff. Neuralgia of neck, with tightness of throat. Head drawn back in convulsions.

Causations - Effects of sunstroke. Bee-sings and mosquito bites.

Chest - Angina pectoris. Tightness of chest, better inspiration. Violent constriction of chest. Oppression of the chest with anguish. Pain radiates from the center of sternum. Sticking under sternum with inability to take a deep breath. Nocturnal attacks of tightness across chest. Tuberculosis is said to make less rapid progress among tobacco workers.

Cough - Cough dry, teasing, must take a swallow of cold water (Caust., Phos.). Cough followed by hiccough. Cough and hiccough at the same time. Suffocative cough from irritation in throat and larynx, worse at night. Dry cough, cardiac in origin. Coughing causes stitches in pit of stomach.

Ears - Burning heat and redness of the ears. Hyperesthesia to music and loud talking. Hearing music causes pain in the ears. Ménière's disease with feeling of seasickness. Sensation as if ears were closed. Nerve deafness.

Eyes - Sunken eyes, blue around them. Heat and burning in eyes. Pupils dilated. Retina retains the image too long. Eyeballs injected, cornea covered with mucus, must wipe it off. Contraction of eyelids. Strabismus.

Face - Emaciation of face. Deathly pale, blue, pinched, sunken, collapsed, covered with cold sweat (Ars., Verat.). One cheek hot and glowing, other pale. Freckles. Miliary rash on cheeks. Violent tearing in facial bones and teeth, worse evening. Pain in maxillary joint, worse laughing. Spasms of the lower jaw.

Female - Retarded and profuse menses. Leucorrhea of serous fluid, worse after menses. During menopause and menses, subjective coldness, epigastric sinking, palpitation, slight diarrhea, muscular relaxation. Excessive sense of wretchedness during menopausal period and menses. ***Morning sickness*** of pregnancy, nausea and vomiting, patient dreads least movement. Severe itching of the whole body during pregnancy.

Food -. Thirstlessness. Great thirst, worse at night, in cholera infantum. Complete loss of appetite. Constant hunger, nausea if stomach is not satisfied. Incessant nausea, worse smell of tobacco smoke. Desires sweets, ice cream, salt. Immoderate smoking of cigars causes vertigo.

Head - Head drawn back in convulsions. ***Sick headache with deathly nausea.*** Periodical headache from fatigue or excitement. Headache better in the open air. ***Headache with nausea and vertigo.*** Tight feeling as from a band. Heaviness sensation with heat of head, better open air. Sensation as if head would burst, or as if brain were being bored out. Sudden pain as if struck by a hammer, worse while passing urine. Hair falls out. Secretion from eyes, nose and mouth increased.

Heart - Angina pectoris, pain in precordial region. Angina pectoris with nausea, cold sweat and collapse. Shooting pain from heart down left arm or up into neck. Pain radiates from center of sternum. Bradycardia. Tachycardia. ***Acute dilatation*** of heart caused by shock or violent physical exertion. Twisting about the heart. Unsteady heartbeat. Precordial oppression with palpitations and pain between shoulders. Violent beating of heart and carotids. Violent palpitations, worse lying on left side (Phos.). Palpitations due to tobacco. Pulse rapid and small. Pulse thready, intermittent, hard, cord like, imperceptible.

Kidneys - Kidney pain with cold sweat, deathly nausea. Kidney colic, violent pain along ureter, left side. Renal region sensitive to pressure. Paralysis of sphincters, urine dribbles. Enuresis. Urine increased, or scanty high-colored urine. Urine yellowish-red with increased secretion. Inflammation of the orifice of the urethra. Bedwetting.

Limbs - Formication. Feebleness of arms. Fingertips fuzzy. Cramps in single fingers, worse washing. Legs and hands icy cold, limbs tremble. Paralysis following a stroke (Plb.). Cramps in legs. Gait shuffling, unsteady. Can't walk with angina pectoris. Tremor and disabling weakness of feet.

Liver - Stitches in liver. Pressure in liver region as from a heavy body. Hepatic region sensitive to pressure.

Lungs - Difficult, violent constriction of chest. Dyspnea with tingling down left arm when lying on left side. Difficult breathing, worse ascending, with distress in heart and palpitations. Paroxysms of suffocation. Hurried, anxious, irregular breathing. Inability to take a deep breath, from sticking under sternum. Periodical attacks of asthma, sits up in bed, suffering with extreme dyspnea. Asthma with blueness of face and swelling of jugular veins.

Male - Frequent erections. Nocturnal emissions. Impotency. Genital organs flabby, no erections or little sexual desire. Masturbation and its consequences. Discharge of prostatic fluid. Hyperesthesia and neuralgia of penis. Varicocele.

Modalities - Better when uncovering abdomen. Better cold, open fresh air, cold applications. Better walking. Better weeping, vomiting. ***Worse from motion of boat,*** riding in cars. Worse extremes of heat and cold, being indoors. Worse stimulants. Worse motion, pressure. Worse in evening, rising up, opening eyes. Worse lying on left side, causes palpitations. Music causes pains in ears.

Mouth - Profuse salivation. Salivation with burning in mouth and throat, tickling, dryness, rawness. Spits much with other complaints. Frothing from the mouth. Mouth full of white tenacious mucus. Dryness of the mouth and tongue with violent thirst. Tongue feels swollen. Swelling of glands under tongue. Drawling, monotonous style of reading. Lips retracted. Lips cracked, swollen, covered with a brown crust. Speech difficult. Weak, interrupted speech.

Nose - Burning sensation and tingling in the nose. Paroxysms of sneezing. Secretion increased. Dryness and obstruction of nose. Nasal catarrh with crawling sensation in nostrils. Naso-pharyngitis and tracheitis.

Perspiration - ***Cold sweats.*** Sudden cold sweats with chill, angina pectoris, kidney colic etc. Perspiration at night. Cold, clammy sweats at night on hands, forehead and face.

Rectum - Habitual constipation. Constipation with rectum paralyzed, prolapsed. Rectal tenesmus. Involuntary stool, watery or thick curdled stools like sour milk. Sudden diarrhea, watery with nausea and vomiting, prostration and cold sweat. Cholera infantum, warmth of body with icy-cold hands. Watery diarrhea, urgent, painless in morning. Evacuations like cholera, with deathly faintness, cold skin, irregular pulse. Sudden, papescent, yellow-green or greenish, slimy stools.

Sensations - As if struck by a hammer on right side of head. As if a band around head. As if brains were being bored out. As if black dots filled visual field. As if ears were closed. As of a plug in esophagus. As if throat influenced by a hand. As if chest too tight. As if a crowbar were twisted around the heart. As if seasick. As if stomach were relaxed.

Skin - Skin swollen, yellow, hot and dry. Itching over the whole body, as from flea or insect bites. Eruption of itching pimples or vesicles with yellow serum and red areola. Red spots on face and on right shoulder, burning when touched. Violent itching of whole surface. Dark, color of skin. Vesicles containing yellow serum and surrounded by red areola. Cold skin in cholera, livid, with angina pectoris. Jaundice.

Sleep - Drowsiness, better in open air. Urgent inclination to sleep, especially after a meal and towards evening with frequent yawnings. Insomnia with dilated heart with cold, clammy skin and anxiety. Disturbed sleep at night with fright. Nightmares. Stupefying sleep at night.

Smell - Diminished power of smell. Sensitive to smell of wine. ***Smell of tobacco, aggravates*** (Ign.). Patient tormented by smell of tobacco.

Stomach - Coldness in stomach, with nausea. Shocks in stomach, at night while sleeping. Gastralgia, pain from cardiac end extending to left arm. Frequent fluttering sensation in pit, with heartburn. Acidity. Burning in stomach. Eructations, sour, hot, of small amounts of food, loud, noisy. Sense of relaxation of stomach with nausea (Ip.). ***Terrible faint, sinking feeling in pit of stomach***. Incessant nausea, worse smell of tobacco smoke (Phos.). Deathly nausea and violent vomiting, worse least motion, better uncovering abdomen. ***Seasickness, motion sickness.*** Morning sickness. ***Nausea during pregnancy, with much spitting.*** Retching. Vomiting of fecal matter.

Temperature - Icy cold skin. ***Chills with cold sweat***. Coldness and shivering, sometimes with chattering of teeth. Chilliness after eating and drinking. Heat down spine, of one cheek, internal. Body warm, with icy coldness of hands and legs.

Throat - Throat dry, can hardly swallow. Much viscid mucus in throat. Nasopharyngitis and tracheitis. ***Hemming cough***. Morning cough, sometimes with vomiting. Hoarseness of public speakers. Violent constriction of throat in angina pectoris. Swallowing difficult on account of spasms of pharynx. Scraping in larynx causes frequent hawking and coughing. Laryngismus stridulus.

Vertigo - ***Vertigo with seasickness***. Excessive vertigo, with copious cold sweat, worse opening eyes. ***Vertigo on opening eyes***, in sick headache with deathly nausea, periodical. ***Vertigo on rising or looking upward.*** Vertigo with nausea, worse indoors, better open air. ***Vertigo and fainting, loss of consciousness.*** Vertigo followed by vomiting of food and tremulous weakness. Ménière's disease with feeling of seasickness.

Vision - ***Amaurosis***. Muscae volitantes. Central scotoma. Retina retains image too long. Diplopia. Dim and confused, as if black dots filled visual field. Sudden loss of vision without lesion, followed by atrophy of optic nerve. Loss of sight on looking steadily at any white object. Strabismus.

COMMENTS - M. E. Douglass, in the Homeopathic News of 1897, wrote about the "medicinal uses" of tobacco and it seems that it was regarded as a perfect panacea by the Virginians for diseases of men and cattle.

Douglass mentioned its palliative use for bee stings and mosquito bites. A portion of a leaf was moistened with vinegar and applied to the part. Ip., one of the antidotes of Tab., has a similar reputation. Strong tobacco-juice is the most effectual destroyer of the burrowing-flea, Chigoe.

Leaves of tobacco are moistened with vinegar or camphor solution and applied to the forehead and nape for headaches. The pain is allayed and sleep induced. The local application over the pit of the stomach relieves nausea.

Douglass used small doses of vinegar for the acute symptoms of nicotine poisoning, either chewing or smoking, with excellent results. Nothing, he said, relieves the sensation of constriction of the esophagus as quickly as vinegar. There is violent rectal tenesmus, paralysis, and prolapsed anus. The bladder sphincter is paralyzed, debility of urine, and bedwetting. Cholera.

The power of Tab. to paralyze sphincters and morbid constrictions accounts for its traditional use in cases of strangulated hernia and obstruction of the bowels. Kidney colic comes under the same heading. Impotency in males, prostate discharges (Calad.), and constant dribbling of the urine.

The same pair of opposites, relaxation and constriction are seen in the weakness, paralysis, and convulsions. All shades of nervous tremors, faintings, cramps, jerkings and restlessness. Tab. holds its place in society by its power of antidoting such conditions. Intermittent heartbeats and arrhythmias, especially in elderly people.

Central nervous action that can lead to degeneration of nerve tissue, as seen in tobacco blindness. Amaurosis, optic nerve degeneration following blindness (Phos.). Tab. also produces a condition like brain-fag, an inability to concentrate thoughts that may even go on to a state of idiocy. Silly talking in boys.

Profoundly influences nutrition, retards growth in children. Characteristic deathly, sinking nausea. It is no doubt by virtue of this, acting homeopathically, that Tab. enables persons who cannot have proper meals endure starvation better than they otherwise would.

Terrible faint, sinking feeling at pit of stomach. Pallor, coldness, icy cold surface, covered with cold sweat. Motion sickness (Cocc.). Morning sickness with cold sweats, sinking nausea and dizziness. Violent vomiting, as soon as he began to move, better on deck and in fresh air.

Keynote better by uncovering abdomen. Child wants abdomen uncovered, it helps the nausea and vomiting. There may be a coldness of the abdomen at the same time. Skin affections with itching.

Teste cured with it several cases of freckles, he repeated the remedy and gave it for weeks at a time: "A country girl had her face and hands covered with freckles, two-thirds of which disappeared completely [under Tab.] in summer, the season in which they are most frequent and obstinate."

Terry cured a case of seasickness, with heat along the spine from the nape down, cold sweat, then vomit. He also cured a case of Ménière's disease with a feeling as if seasick.

Boger cured, with Tab. 100,000c, a persistent backache, worse lying down, better walking, with a history of angina-like attacks.

Burnett noted that an infusion of tobacco is a popular German remedy for scrofulous glands. Cooper gives as an indication, "intermittent heart in old people."

C. W. was troubled with spasm of lower jaw, worse outdoors. No remedy worked until he remained one evening with two friends who were smoking and saturated himself with the smoke. That cured him. Slight subsequent returns were always removed by Tab.

J. W. Scott observed a case of epileptiform convulsions brought on by tobacco. For five months the patient had two attacks weekly and they grew worse in spite of treatment until the tobacco habit was discontinued.

RELATIONS - ***Antidote:*** Vinegar, sour apples. Camphor in the physiological antagonist. ***Compare:*** (1) Calad., Daph., Lob. and Plan. - cause aversion to tobacco. (2) Nicot. (3) Ars. - chewing tobacco. (4) Ign. - aversion to tobacco smoke. (5) Sep. - neuralgia and dyspepsia), Lyc. impotency. (6) Nux-v. - bad taste due to tobacco. (7) Phos. - tobacco heart, sexual weakness. (8) Hydrobr-ac., Camph., Verat., Ars.

REFERENCES - Boericke. Clarke. Murphy. Phatak.

TABERNANTHE IBOGA

(Iboga Bark)

PHARMACY - tab-ib. Tabernanthe iboga. Iboga bark. Black bugbane. Bitter grass. N. O. Apocynacae. Bark and root. ***Historical dose:*** Tincture and all potencies.

CLINICAL - Addictions. Alcoholism. Delirium tremens. Drug, abuse. Fatigue. Heroin, habit. Tobacco, habit.

HERBAL - Tabernanthe iboga, also known as black bugbane, is a perennial rainforest shrub and hallucinogen, native to western Africa. Iboga stimulates the central nervous system when taken in small doses and induces visions in larger doses.

Ibogaine is the active chemical in the African root. It is a strong, long-lasting psychedelic used traditionally in a coming of age ritual, but also known for its modern use in treating heroin addiction.

The drug's story as an anti-addictive began in 1962, when college dropout and heroin addict Howard Lotsof obtained a dose from a chemist friend. Iboga relieved him of all cravings for heroin.

In 1986, Lotsof began to supply ibogaine to a clinic for addicts in Holland. The clinic found that ibogaine works in three stages. First the addict has about four hours of waking dreams in which he seems to confront inner demons.

This is followed by an eight- to 10-hour "cognitive evaluation period," during which the user analyzes the waking dream. Then comes a sleepless day or two, which Lotsof calls the "residual stimulation phase."

Lotsof said ibogaine allows addicts, especially heroin users, to put aside their fears of withdrawal and begin the process of detoxification.

One methadone patient said that in just four days he reached a state that normally would have taken him three months, but without the agony.

The heroin addiction therapy may last several days and upon completion the subject is generally no longer physically dependent. Research suggests that ibogaine may also help to treat addictions to alcohol and nicotine.

Ibogaine breaks down in the liver into a metabolite called nor-ibogaine. This metabolite has been shown in clinical research to prevent cravings for several weeks after a single dose in some individuals.

Others have observed Iboga having some undesirable side effects regarding blood pressure and heartbeat.

COMMENTS - The Iboga was brought back from Gabon in 1864 by Dr. Griffon du Bellay, a navy surgeon. He wrote, "The root of this plant is the part that the Gabonese eat. They say that it is inebriating, aphrodisiac, and, with it, they claim that they feel no need for sleep."

However, as early as 1885, Father Henri Neu had written in a manuscript entitled "Le Gabon" (Neu 1885), "The natives use an infusion of iboga root scrapings as a potent philter that enables one to discover hidden things and to tell the future. The one who drinks it falls into a deep sleep during which he is obsessed by uninterrupted dreams which, until the time that he awakens, he takes to be actual events."

REFERENCES - Lotsof. Murphy.

TAMARINDUS INDICA
(Tamarind)

PHARMACY - tama. Tamarindus indica. Tamarind. N.O. Leguminosae. Tamaricaceae. Africa. India. Tincture of the fruit. ***Historical dose:*** Tincture and all potencies.

CLINICAL - Acidity. Asthma. Boils. Constipation. Rheumatism. Spleen, disorders. ***Tobacco, habit.***

HERBAL - People in India use tamarind as a souring agent like vinegar. It is used in common preparations like chutneys. It is also eaten as a fruit by those who have a craving for sour things. Tamarind flavored beverages are popular in Italy and Latin America.

Patients suffering from rheumatic problems are said to be aggravated from tamarind.

MIND - Indifference, apathy. Indolence. Lethargy, no desire to work, even if it is important and requires immediate attention. Mental dullness, sluggishness. Difficulty thinking and comprehending. Forgetfulness.

Restlessness, nervousness. Starting easily. Fear of his own shadow. Fear of passing stool, on account of pain. Irritability from trifles. Tolerance in persons normally easily annoyed and irritated. Quiet disposition. Involuntary sighing. Weeping, tearful mood. Dreams of talking to deceased grandfather.

Back - Pain in one spot under right scapula, worse lying on back.

Eyes - Lachrymation, especially in left eye.

Food - Increase thirst. Desires ice-cold water, cold drinks, ice cream, tamarind, sour foods, spicy foods. ***Craves tobacco.*** Worse from spicy foods and tobacco.

Head - Heaviness of head.

Modalities - Better drinking cold water, worse from spicy foods and tobacco.

Worse morning. Worse from the sun.

Mouth - Dryness of mouth, lips and throat. Stringy salvia.

Nose - Obstruction of nose.

Rectum - Ineffectual urging with unsatisfactory stools. Constipation. Rectal pain worse passing stools, walking, sitting, squatting.

COMMENTS - Vakil stated, "People consuming tobacco in any form, chewing or smoking, are especially affected. Tamarindus may be useful to give up the habit of tobacco chewing or smoking. Provers addicted to tobacco developed some unbearable symptoms of tobacco, e.g. vertigo. One prover who had stopped smoking one year back, developed increased desire for smoking again and now he is not able to give it up."

Joseph Miller, in Potter's Cyclopedia, wrote about Tamarindus, "They are accounted specific for all disorders of the Spleen, as being believed to lessen it much; nay they used to drink out of cups made of this wood to cure those illnesses."

RELATIONS - ***Compare:*** Phos., Ph-ac., Mangi, Sulph.

REFERENCES - Murphy. Vakil.

TAMUS COMMUNIS

(Ladies Seal)

PHARMACY - tam. Tamus communis. Ladies seal. Black bryony. Black bryonia. Blackeye root. Tamus cretica. N. O. Dioscoreaceae. Tincture of fresh root. Tincture of the berries. ***Historical dose:*** Tincture and all potencies.

CLINICAL - Broken, bones. Bruises. Chilblains. Splinters.

HERBAL - The Greeks used the young suckers like asparagus, which they resemble.

Tamus is a popular remedy for removing discoloration caused by bruises. The fresh root is scraped and the pulp rubbed into parts affected by gout, rheumatism, or paralysis. It is also reputed as a diuretic. The fruits steeped in gin are a popular remedy for chilblains. The tincture also has a reputation for curing chilblains when applied externally.

The root-plaster of Tamus has been used to removed scars and deformities and it softens harden tissues (Thiosin.). It draws forth splinters and heals broken bones, dissolves congealed blood. If laid on hip or knuckles or any other part where there is great pain, it takes away the pain speedily.

COMMENTS - Gerarde reported, "The root is very great and thick oftentimes as big as a man's leg, black without and very clammy or slimy within, which having been scraped with a knife, it seems to be a matter fit to be spread upon cloth or leather in manner of a plaster of sear-cloth."

Dioscorides, according to Gerarde, said the fruit or berries take away sun-burns and other blemishes of the skin, and Gerarde added that these, "very quickly waste and consume away black and blue marks that come of bruises and dry beatings: which thing also the roots perform being laid upon them."

Joseph Miller stated, "A cataplasm of the root with vinegar and cow-dung, helps the gout" and he added significantly, "It is but rarely used."

REFERENCES - Boericke. Clarke.

TANACETUM VULGARE

(Tansy)

PHARMACY - tanac. Tanacetum vulgare. Tansy. Chrysanthemum vulgare. N. O. Compositae. Tincture of the fresh plant in flower. Potencies of the oil. ***Historical dose:*** Tincture and all potencies.

CLINICAL - Abortion. Abscess. Amenorrhea. Chorea. Convulsions. ***Dysentery***. Dysmenorrhea. Epilepsy. Eyes, inflamed. Eyes, sclerotica. Hallucinations. Hydrophobia. Labia, abscess. Menorrhagia. Paralysis. Poison ivy. Strabismus. ***Worms.***

HERBAL - The word "tansy" is derived from immortality with its deep-yellow button-like flowers, a close companion of the Ragwort (Senecio facobea). In olden times puddings were made containing tansy leaves and these puddings were called "tansies" also.

Gerarde also said that the seeds kill and ***expel worms*** of every sort, the root is good in gout, and being drunk with wine relieves pain in the bladder and dysuria when a man is only able to urinate by drops.

HOMEOPATHIC - Hale noted it for amenorrhea, dysmenorrhea, menorrhagia, uterine cramps and metritis. In one instance it caused a large abscess of the labia majora. Hale said a crystalline acid identical with Santonin has been isolated from it.

Abnormal lassitude, a nervous and tired feeling. "Half dead, half alive feeling" all over. It is of use in chorea and reflex spasms due to worms. Tanac. is said to be a specific against effects of poison ivy.

Tanac. induces all the cardinal features of rabies, including abundant salivation, excitability, tendency to bite. Hoarse cry. Hallucinations. Diminished sensibility and mobility, momentary paralysis. Frothy, bloody mucus in the air passages. Convulsions, without loss of consciousness. Opisthotonos. Spasms of pharynx, larynx and the thorax.

MIND - Mental fatigue, nausea and vertigo, worse in a closed room. Inability to think coherently. Confusion of thought. Dullness of all the senses. Fatigue of the mind after the least exertion. Ambitious. Wants to stand on his head, stretches and draws up his feet, and says, "it does me good."

Sadness, with desire to be let entirely alone. Irritable, sensitive to noise. Irritable and lazy. Very nervous and low spirited, annoyed by trifles; noise of the children almost unbearable. Extremely sensitive to noise. Coma and violent convulsions.

Abdomen - Dull pains in the right hypochondrium, sharp in left. Sharp, sticking pains in whole umbilical region.

Back - Severe attack of lumbago. Constant dull ache in loins.

Ears - Stitches in internal ear. ***Ears seem to close up suddenly.*** Roaring, ringing in ears. Her own voice sounds strange in her ears.

Eyes - Eyes open, very brilliant, pupils equal, widely dilated, immovable. Pupils contracted. Sclerotic congested, dark purple, glassy-looking. Dull aching in eyeballs. Slight inward squint, right eye. Lids agglutinated in morning.

Face - Features seemed fixed, giving an expression of deep solemnity. Face dusky, flushed, cheeks bright red. Fullness of head and face.

Female - Menses suppressed, later, profuse. Dysmenorrhea with bearing-down pains, tenderness, drawing in groins. Miscarriage in the early months of pregnancy.

Head - Weariness in head. Heavy, dull, confused. Dull, frontal headache with cutting in temples. Headache with least exertion.

Heart - Feeble heart-action and all signs of impending dissolution. Pulse increased in force and frequency, feeble.

Kidneys - Constant desire. First suppression, then profuse flow. Marked diuresis, must rise in night to urinate. Urine is very fetid, high-colored increased. Urine caused slight scalding.

Limbs - Numbness and sensation as though arms and legs were suddenly swelling. Prickling, coming and going, over limbs and along spine with flashes of heat. Cold numbness over limbs, going on to paralysis.

Lungs - Breathing laborious. Hurried, stertorous respiration. Frothy mucus obstructs the air-passages.

Modalities - Worse at night, at 4 a.m. Suddenness is a characteristic of a number of the symptoms.

Mouth - Flat insipid taste. Tongue white coated, feels rough. Mouth, blood-stained, frothy.

Nose - Profuse secretion of mucus in nose with fluent coryza. Dryness of nostrils.

Rectum - Pain in bowels, relieved by stool. ***Dysentery***. Desire for stool immediately after eating.

Sensations - As if something closed the ears very suddenly. His own voice sounds strange in his ears. Sensation like a thrill all through body. As though arms and legs suddenly swollen.

Stomach - Thirst. Drawing, cutting pains in epigastrium. Faint and sick at stomach. Constant belchings, tasting of the oil. Belchings of sour air at night. Nausea and vomiting.

Temperature - Surface cool and moist. Cold, clammy sweat. Feeling of warmth diffused over whole abdomen.

Throat - Roughness of throat. Feeling in throat as if one could cough all the time. Unable to swallow.

COMMENTS - Like Senec., Tanac. has an action on the female generative organs and a large proportion of the observations with it have been on women who have taken it to procure abortion. Other effects are from its use as a vermifuge, and in addition to these are provings by Burt and others.

In Russia, Tanac. has a reputation as a remedy for hydrophobia. M. Peyraud even used Tanac. as a substitute for Pasteurian "vaccinations," and reported success.

W. H. Pierson observed a woman who took two drachms of the oil to procure abortion. The attempt failed, but throughout her pregnancy she suffered from mixed tonic and clonic convulsions. Frothing at the mouth, clenched hands, thumbs turned in, followed by exhaustion and a short coma. Since then, Pierson treated every case of epilepsy which came to him with drop doses of the fluid extract of Tanac. four times a day, with marked success.

RELATIONS - ***Compare:*** (1) In uterine symptoms, Sabin., Tereb., Hedeo., Ruta. (2) In convulsions, Stram., Cic., Cupr. (3) Worm symptoms, convulsions, paralysis, Sant., Cina, Chen-a. (4) Abscess on labium majus, Stry., abscess of scrotum. ***Follows well:*** Cimic., Cina, Absin., Nux-v.

REFERENCES - Boericke. Clarke. Hale.

TANGHINIA VENENIFERA

PHARMACY - tang. Tanghinia venenifera. N. O. Apocynaceae. Trituration of the seed. ***Historical dose:*** All potencies.

CLINICAL - Anxiety. Debility. Delirium. Numbness. Paralysis. Stupor. Vomiting. Weakness.

HERBAL - Tanghinia, the Tanghin or Tanquen of Madagascar is the only representative of its genus of Apocynaceae. The fruit of the tree is ellipsoid, between two and three inches long, having a smooth, purplish skin tinged with green, containing a hard stone surrounded by a thick fibrous flesh.

HOMEOPATHIC - Intense and distressing vomiting, accompanied by anxiety and weakness. Great debility and anxiety with the vomiting. General weakness. Numbness, over whole body, especially of the hands.

Staggers if attempts to walk, is unable to support his own weight and falls down helpless and paralyzed. Complete paralysis. Death, preceded by spasmodic movements of fingers and toes.

MIND - Anxiety, with the vomiting. Stupor. Lies as if asleep and when roused answers like a drowsy man and then relapses into former condition. Delirium.

Limbs - Hands numb. Spasmodic movements of the fingers and toes.

Mouth - Numbness, tingling in mouth and fauces.

Rectum - Purging and urination.

Stomach - Vomiting intense, distressing and repeated, first of contents of stomach, then of bile and mucus.

Vertigo - Giddy, staggers.

COMMENTS - The seed has been used as an "ordeal" test for those thought to have committed a crime. The seed is pounded and a small piece is swallowed by the person to be tried. Those in whom it causes vomiting escape punishment. Those whose stomachs retain it are thought to have been proven guilty, and are quickly killed.

REFERENCES - Clarke.

TANNICUM ACIDUM

(Tannic Acid)

PHARMACY - tann-ac. Tannicum acidum. Tannic acid. Tanninum. There are two forms of tannic acid, Gallo-tannic acid, derived from nut-galls. Also querc-tannic acid, derived from healthy leaves and bark of the oak. The former is the most used. Trituration. Solution in rectified spirit. One-half percent solution. ***Historical dose:*** All potencies.

CLINICAL - Colic. Conjunctivitis. Constipation. Hematuria. Ileus. Nosebleed. Ophthalmia. Palpitations. Vomiting. Weakness.

HOMEOPATHIC - Tannin, or tannic acid, of which gallic acid is a derivative, has produced effects on healthy persons and on those taking it for diarrhea. Mostly used locally against excessive secretion of mucus membranes to contract tissue and check hemorrhage.

Leathery dryness of mouth and intestinal canal, a condition like ileus and a very aggravated state of constipation. Obstinate constipation. Typhoid fever and dysentery. Intestines can be felt like cylindrical enlargements. Pain in abdomen, sensitive to pressure. Diabetes. Hematuria. Ulcerated tissues. Fetor of the perspiration. Weakness. Chronic nervous coughs.

Abdomen - Abdomen is sensitive to pressure but not distended. Irritable bowel. Intestines could be felt like cylindrical enlargements through walls of abdomen. Ileus. Colic. Ulceration of bowels. Hemorrhage.

Eyes - Acute and chronic conjunctivitis. Granular lids and vascular cornea. Chemosis and pannus. Ophthalmia. Purulent ophthalmia of infants.

Female - Sore breasts and nipples. Uterine bleeding. Syphilitic ulceration of the cervix.

Food - Loss of appetite. Thirst.

Heart - Palpitations.

Kidneys - Dysuria. Urine scanty, dark-colored. Albuminuria. Hematuria.

Lungs - Tuberculosis. Bronchial catarrh. Nervous coughs. Whooping cough.

Mouth - Leathery dryness of mucus membrane of mouth and intestinal canal. Hemorrhage and sponginess of the gums. Mercurial salivation. Toothache.

Nose - Nosebleeds. Chronic catarrh and coryza.

Rectum - Obstinate constipation. Chronic diarrhea. Painless and bloody discharge from bowels. Foul stools. Prolapsed rectum. Hemorrhoids.

Skin - Ulcers with copious discharges.

Stomach - Painful sensation in epigastric region and abdomen. Violent pains in stomach. Dyspepsia. Obstinate vomiting of bilious substances.

Tongue - Tongue white, dry.

RELATIONS - ***Compare:*** (1) Querc., Gall-ac., Op., Plb.

REFERENCES - Boericke. Clarke.

TARAXACUM OFFICINALE

(Dandelion)

PHARMACY - tarax. Taraxacum officinale. Dandelion. Leontodum taraxacum. Taraxacum dens-leonis. N. O. Compositae. The tincture from the whole plant when in flower. ***Historical dose:*** Tincture and all potencies.

CLINICAL - Ague. ***Bilious.*** Cancerous, conditions. Debility. Diabetes. Flatulence. ***Gallstones. Headaches.*** Hepatitis. Jaundice. ***Liver, disorders.*** Liver, weakness. Neuralgias. ***Night, sweats.*** Rheumatism. ***Tongue, mapped.*** Typhoid fever.

HERBAL - Taraxacum's chief traditional uses are as a remedy for jaundice, liver obstruction in dysentery, involuntary emissions and in difficulties in passing water.

The young leaves of the dandelion are sometimes eaten in salads. They have a bitter chicory like taste, as does the root. Children may eat the flowers, although they are supposed to cause bedwetting.

HOMEOPATHIC - The first provings were done by Hahnemann and his pupils. Hahnemann's provings brought out the leading symptoms "painless urging to urinate," and "frequent urging to urinate with copious discharge of urine."

Hahnemann pointed out that the urging to urinate with thirst may indicate Tarax. in some cases of diabetes. Hahnemann's dosage was a single drop of the tincture.

Langhammer noted the ***"mapped tongue."*** The tongue is coated white and clears off in patches, leaving dark red, very sensitive spots.

Affinity for the liver and bladder. A ***bilious*** remedy. Pains in both splenic and liver regions. Heaviness in the liver region. Gastric headaches, bilious attacks with mapped tongue and jaundiced skin. Jaundice with enlarged, indurated liver. Disorders of the liver, sour taste, darting pains in outer parts. ***Hysterical tympanites***. Flatulence. Cancer of bladder.

Hands and nose cold at 8 p.m. ***Cold fingertips***. Feeling of sickness and exhaustion, inclined to sit or lie down. Muscular pains with shuddering and muscular prickling.

Stitching pains. Affections in left upper side, right lower side, back of foot, sole of foot. Almost all symptoms appear while the patient is seated and are dissipated by walking.

MIND - Depressive, morose, sad condition. Memory weak. Apathy, lack of reactions. Dislike for labor, but after beginning works well. ***Impatient and irritable.*** Anxiety while sitting. Restlessness on waking. Irresolution. Constant muttering to himself. Inclined to talk, laugh and be merry. Loquacity during perspiration. Unconsciousness.

Abdomen - Stinging abdominal pains. Sharp stitches in left side. Grumbling and movements in abdomen. Sensation of bubbles bursting in bowels. Hysterical tympanites. Pinching in abdomen. Pressive shootings in abdomen and sides of abdomen, in left side of the hypogastrium.

Back - Tearing pain from ear down to neck. ***Sternomastoid muscle*** very painful to touch. Pressive jerkings and shootings in muscles of neck, throat and nape. Pressive and tensive shootings in back and loins, when lying down with obstructed respiration. Pressing, stinging in spine and sacrum with dyspnea. Vibration and quivering in right scapula.

Chest - Pressure at chest. Shootings in chest and sides of chest. Jerkings in muscles.

Ears - Shootings in ears. Drawing pain in external ear. Stinging, rending pains in the ears.

Eyes - Pain in eyes, as if a grain of sand were in internal canthus. Burning and stinging pains in the eyes. Inflammation of eyes. Lachrymation and photophobia. Nocturnal agglutination of lids. Aversion to light.

Face - Hot and red face. Sensation of heat and redness in face. Shootings and pressure in cheeks. Upper lip cracked. Pustule in right corner of lips. Purulent pimples on face, cheeks, alae nasi and lips.

Female - Suppressed menses.

Food - Loss of appetite. ***Food tastes sour.*** Salt or acid taste of food. Butter and meat taste salty. Bitter taste after eating. Tobacco smoke is very disagreeable, causes heartburn and interrupts respiration. Great chilliness after drinking or eating. No thirst during fever. Thirst during sweat.

Head - Heavy and numbing headache. Stinging pains in the head and face. Neuralgic headaches. ***Headaches due to liver disturbances.*** Headaches, as from contraction or expansion of brain. Violent headache, felt only when standing or walking. Sensation of great heat in vertex. Drawing pain in left temple while sitting, ceasing when walking or standing. Tearing pain in occiput. Lancinations in forehead and temples. Tension of scalp.

Kidneys - Bladder weakness. ***Frequent desire to urinate*** with copious urine. Urination with painless urging. Bedwetting during sleep.

Limbs - Muscular pains with shuddering and prickling in the muscles. Restless limbs. Limbs painful, tenderness of all limbs when touched. Tearing pains in limbs. Dull, joint pains. ***Fingertips cold.*** Pressive pains in loins. Heaviness of the legs, ameliorated by walking. ***Neuralgia of knee,*** better pressure. Jerking pain in calf (right) better on touch. Toes burning.

Liver - Pain in the region of liver and spleen. Liver enlarged and indurated. Sensation of heaviness in the liver region. ***Deficiency of the liver***. Liver weakness. Chronic cholecystitis. ***Gallstones.*** Jaundice. Hepatitis with jaundice.

Lungs - Cough after eating.

Male - Pain in testes. Permanent erections. Frequent pollutions, on alternate nights.

Modalities - Better from touch. Better moving, walking, open air. Burning in throat is better by drinking. Worse while lying down, resting, at night. Worse from fat food.

Mouth - ***Sour, bitter taste.*** Acid saliva in mouth. Salivation with sensation as if larynx was pressed shut. Bitter taste, rising from pharynx into mouth. Smarting, burning and rawness in mouth and fauces. Accumulation of sour water in mouth. Tough, ropy, sour-tasting saliva.

Nose - Cold nose. Nosebleeds.

Perspiration - Very debilitating perspiration, causing biting on the skin. Sweat on falling asleep. ***Profuse night sweats,***

mostly before midnight, when just going to sleep.

Rectum - Stools white. Inefficient urging to go to stool. Evacuations often, but accomplished with difficulty, even if stool is soft. Feces of the consistence of pap, followed by tenesmus. Bilious diarrhea. Constipation following an abundant expulsion of feces. Voluptuous itching in perineum.

Sensations - As if brain was constricted. As if teeth were set on edge. As if larynx were compressed. As if bubbles were forming and bursting in abdomen. As of rolling and gurgling in right scapula. As if limbs were bound or powerless.

Skin - Stinging on skin. Unhealthy, pimply, sycotic skin. Eruptions over body and limbs, itching severely and appears to be a mixture of lichen and urticaria. ***Profuse night sweats***, biting in skin with sweat.

Sleep - Irresistible drowsiness after meals. Sleepiness in daytime and yawning while sitting. Sleepiness and going to sleep while listening to a scientific discourse. Vivid, unremembered dreams, frequent waking and tossing.

Stomach - Gastric bilious attacks. Bitter taste, risings, belchings and hiccough. Empty belching after drinking. Nausea, as after an excess of greasy food. Nausea with inclination to vomit or vomiting from very fat food, with anxiety and pressive headache, better in open air. Nausea, with headache, anxiety, after fat food.

Teeth - Toothache with drawing pain in carious teeth, extending to eyebrows. Pressive pains in teeth. Teeth set on edge as from acids. Flow of acid blood from decayed teeth. Blunt teeth. Hawking up of sour mucus, causing teeth to feel dull.

Temperature - Chill in open air. Chilliness after eating and drinking. Chilliness, shiverings, all over with pressive headache. ***Fingertips cold.*** Heat at night on waking, especially on face and hands. Heat without thirst, in face or ***toes***.

Throat - Hawking up of acid mucus. Sore throat with pressive pain, as from internal swelling. Dryness, shootings and bitter mucus in the throat. Burning in throat from smoking, better drinking.

Tongue - ***Tongue, coated, mapped.*** Tongue covered with a white film. Tongue feels raw, comes off in patches, leaving ***red. sensitive spots***. Tongue dry, loaded with a brown coating on waking in morning.

Vertigo - Vertigo with giddiness and staggering when walking in the open air. Vertigo with unsteady gait, falls to either side.

COMMENTS - The Treasury of Botany noted that "the bright-yellow flowers of Taraxacum open in the morning between 5 a.m. and 6 a.m. and close in the evening between 8 p.m. and 9 p.m. Hence this was one of the plants selected by Linneus to form his floral clock."

Cooper noted the case of an old Indian officer who, when in India, suffered from gallstones and was advised to take dandelion infusion every day. He did so and soon the symptoms left him and he remained free from them for over twenty years.

Gastric and bilious attacks, especially gastric headaches. The headaches are generally pressive. Pains in both splenic and liver regions. Jaundice with enlarged, indurated liver.

Pressure in lower occiput after lying down. Debility, loss of appetite, profuse night sweats, especially when convalescing from bilious or typhoid fever. Restlessness of limbs in typhoid. Sweat between toes.

RELATIONS - ***Compare:*** (1) In gastric and bilious affections, Card-m., Bry., Chel., Hydr., Lyc., Nux-v. (2) Mapped tongue, Ars., Nat-m., Merc., Ran-s. (3) Restlessness of limbs with tearing pains, Rhus-t. (4) Chel.- Tongue dry, yellowish with red edges, retains the imprint of the teeth. Epigastric pain, spreading to the lower corner of the right shoulder blade. Pressing sensation in the hepatic region. (5) Bry. - Dryness of the mucus membranes, acute, stinging pains, aggravated by movement. Intense thirst, stubborn constipation. (6) Nux-v. - Impatient, sleepy after meals, sensation of a weight in the stomach, constipation with empty urging. ***Compatible:*** Ars. - Night-sweats.

REFERENCES - Boericke. Clarke. Murphy. Phatak.

TARENTULA CUBENSIS

(Cuban Tarentula)

PHARMACY - tarent-c. Tarentula cubensis. Cuban tarantula. Mygale cubensis. Aranea peluda. N. O. Araneideae. Tincture of whole decomposed spider. Tincture of whole spider. ***Historical dose:*** All potencies.

CLINICAL -***Abscesses***. Anthrax. Bites, insect. Boils. ***Bubonic plague. Carbuncles***. Chills. Chorea. Convulsions. Delirium. Diarrhea. Diphtheria. Felon. Fever. Gangrene. Headaches. Intermittent, fever. ***Itching.*** Meningitis. Paralysis. Pruritus, vulvae. Scirrhus. ***Senile, ulcers.***

HOMEOPATHIC - Tarent-c. affects the cellular tissues. It is useful in septic conditions, when incubation is slow, but further progress is rapid with alarming prostration, atrocious burning or sharp stinging pains, board like ***hardness of affected part*** and copious sweat.

Intermittent septic chills. Severe types of inflammation and pain. Purplish hue and burning, stinging pains. ***Itching, especially about genitals.*** Diphtheria with intense fever and numb aching pains.

Various forms of malignant suppuration. Gangrene. ***Bluish abscesses, painful.*** Felon. ***Carbuncles.*** Bubo. ***Bubonic plague,*** as a curative and preventive remedy especially during the period of invasion.

Early and persistent prostration. Restless feet. Paralysis then convulsions. Tarent-c. is a ***remedy for the pain of death, soothes the last agony.***

MIND - Nervous restlessness. Sensitive to others. Anxiety. Excessive hyperesthesia. ***Hysteria.*** Lacks emotional control. Delirium due to pains. Agony of pains, compels the patient to walk on the floor for nights Keeps hands busy, picks fingers.

Back - Itches across kidney region.

Female - Pruritus vulvae.

Head - Dull ache on top of head. Fullness in head. Headaches. Shooting pain through left eye across frontal region. Meningitis.

Kidneys - Retention of urine. Urine hot, thick. Cannot hold urine on coughing.

Limbs - Hands tremble, turgid with blood. Fidgety feet. Unsteady gait.

Lungs - Spasmodic difficulty of breathing. Shattering cough, whooping cough.

Modalities - Better from tobacco smoking. Worse from cold drinks. Worse exertion. Worse at night.

Rectum - Diarrhea.

Skin - Feels puffed all over. Pungent burning, stinging pains. Red spots and pimples. Purple discoloration. ***Carbuncles***. Abscesses, where pain and inflammation predominate. ***"Senile ulcers."*** Gangrene. Anthrax. Scirrhous of breasts.

Sleep - Drowsiness. Sleep restless, prevented by harsh cough.

Stomach - Feels hard, sore. Loss of appetite, except for breakfast. Tendency to vomit.

Temperature - Pungent heat of surface.

Vertigo - Dizziness after heat and hot perspiration.

COMMENTS - Hering stated "The Mygale Cubensis, which may be called the Cuban Tarentula, also found in South Carolina and Texas is a larger spider of a dark brown color, less poisonous and covered with more hairs than the Tarentula Hispanica."

Tarent-c. seems to be a toxemic remedy, acting directly on the blood, and is in this way an analogue of Crot-h., Apis, Ars., etc.

The bite is painless. The person is not sensible of it until next day. Then an inflamed pimple is found surrounded by a scarlet areola. From the pimple to some other part of the body a red erysipelatous line is seen, which marks the line followed by the spider over the skin after biting.

The pimple swells, the inflamed areola spreads, chills and fever set in with copious sweat and retention of urine, the pimple becomes a hard, large. Exceedingly painful abscess, ending by mortification of the tissues over it and having several small openings.

Discharging a thick, bloody matter containing pieces of tissue, fascia and tendons. The openings grow, run into one another, forming a large cavity. At this period the fever takes the intermittent type with evening exacerbations.

In two cases in delicate children, the bite proved fatal, but the majority recover in from three to six weeks.

A case of chorea in a girl of twelve was reported cured with Tarent-c. 6c. The movements were confined to the left side and occurred chiefly at night, when Tarent-c. was prescribed.

Dr. Burt related the case of Don M. B. Aet. 72, good constitution, with an abscess in the back of his neck, whose burning, excruciating pain had completely banished sleep for six or seven nights.

Fever, with great thirst and prostration. On examination, it was found to be anthrax, with all the accompanying train of symptoms. Burt gave Tarent-c., 6c one dose every two hours; after the second dose, the pain was greatly relieved, and that very night the patient was able to sleep through the whole night. Under the use of this remedy, the patient recovered without using any other, except Sil. to aid cicatrization.

Carbuncle, even to sloughing with great prostration and diarrhea. Intermittent fever with evening exacerbation. Atrocious pains.

RELATIONS - ***Compare:*** (1) Ars., Pyrog., Crot-h., Echi., Anthr., Bell., Apis. (2) in intermittents, Aran-d. (3) Carbuncle, Anthr., Lach., Sil.

REFERENCES - Boericke. Clarke.

TARENTULA HISPANICA

(Spanish Tarentula)

PHARMACY - tarent. Tarentula hispanica. Spanish tarantula. Wolf spider. Lycosa tarentula. Lycosa fasciiventris. N. O. Araneideae. Italy and Spain. Tincture of the whole spiders. ***Historical dose:*** All potencies.

CLINICAL - Angina, pectoris. Bites, spider. Boils. Callosities. Cancer. ***Chorea***. Coccyx, pain. Cornea, opacity. Cystitis. Depression. Diabetes mellitus. Diphtheria. Dysmenorrhea. Dyspnea. Fibroids. Headaches. Hiccough. ***Hysteria. Insanity.*** Intermittent fevers. Kleptomania. Leucorrhea. Levitation. Locomotor, ataxia. Mania. Ménière's disease. Migraine. Multiple sclerosis. ***Nervous, disorders.*** Noma. Nosebleeds. Numbness. Onanism. Ovaries, enlarged. Parkinson's disease. Photophobia. Physometra. Proctalgia. Pruritus, pudendi. ***Pruritus, vulvae.*** Quinsy. Septic, fever. Sexual, mania. Spinal, irritation. Spinal, sclerosis. ***Suffocation.*** Tonsillitis. Tumors. ***Twitching***. Uterus, cancer. Uterus, neuralgia. Vertebrae, tumors. Vertigo. ***Violent, pains.***

HOMEOPATHIC - The name tarantula covers a number of poisonous spiders, but in homeopathy, unless distinguished, it refers to Tarentula hispanica. Nunez instigated the proving and collected much outside information bearing on the action of the poison.

"Tarantella" is a dance named from the city of Tarentum. "Tarantism" is a dancing mania, set up in persons bitten by the tarantula or in those who imagine themselves bitten. The cure is music and dancing. These symptoms give a keynote indication to this remedy.

Affects the nerves, which are highly strung, producing remarkable ***nervous symptoms, hysteria*** with chlorosis, ***chorea***, often reflexive from generative sphere. The heart, spine, respiration and right side are also prominently affected.

Extreme restlessness, fidgety, hurried, must keep in constant motion even though walking aggravates. ***Music causes excitement***. Rolls on ground from side to side or strikes vehemently with his feet or rolls the head and rubs it to relieve her distress. Chorea with arm symptoms. Irregular movements. Can run better than walk.

Symptoms appear suddenly, with violence. Quivering, jerking, trembling, twitchings. ***Violent pains,*** neuralgias, as if thousands of needles were pricking. Joint pains. Headache with pain in uterus, throat with eye pains, face pain with stomach pain, pain in the ear with hiccough. Tickling, burning, scorching and numbness with prickling. Palliates the ***death pains and agony of dying process.***

Nervous phenomena, dysmenorrhea, spinal irritability. Bladder tenesmus. ***Constriction sensation***. Deep septic conditions, abscess, evacuates pus rapidly. Noma. Emaciation, as if the flesh fairly fell off the bones, worse in the face. Cancer, fibrous tumors. Hysterical epilepsy.

Intense sexual excitement, causing pain. Formication. Diabetes mellitus with great prostration and pain as if whole body were bruised.

MIND - Adroit. Crafty, sly, cunning. Instability of intelligence. ***Obstinacy.*** Selfish and demanding. Very impatient and irritable with others. Hateful. ***Destructive impulses.*** Throws things away. Kleptomania. Desire to strike herself or others. Angry with despair. Discontented. Melancholy.

Intolerant to any criticism. Averse to company, but wants someone present. Ungrateful. Conceited and deceptive behavior. ***Feigns fainting, insensibility.*** When there are no observers, there is no hysteria, when attention is directed to her, she begins to twitch.

Suddenly changing moods, fancies or strength. ***Lacks emotional control. Erratic. Impulsive.*** Fits of nervous laughter then screaming. Moral depravity. ***Restlessness and compelled to walk. Tormenting and intense behavior.*** Anxious and full of fears.

Erratic moods. Sometimes a sweet cheerfulness and gaiety, while at other times, anger, irritability. Quarrelsome, excitable, exhilarated or sad. Self-indulgence. Hysterical emotions. Intense sexual excitements, lasciviousness. ***Mania***, very excitable.

Sensitive to music. Dances up and down. Laughs, mocks, runs, dances, makes gestures and jokes. Cries and sings until hoarse or exhausted. Aversion to colors, black, red, yellow, green. Mental symptoms better in evening after eating. Refuses to eat.

Delirium, mania, shrieking, singing, erotic mania. Stupefaction. Indisposed to talk. Sensation of being small (contrast to Aur., Plat., Stram.). Weeping, causeless, during sleep. Palliates the ***agony and pains of the dying process.***

Abdomen - Violent burning in abdomen. Burning in hypogastrium with great weight, interferes with walking. Hepatic region painful to touch. Pain in hepatic region, with nausea and vomiting, worse before paroxysm of malaria. Sharp pain in umbilical region.

Back - Painfully sensitive spine, touch excites pains in chest, heart etc. Coccygodynia, better standing, worse slightest movement, touch. Tumors around vertebral column. Painfully sensitive spine.

Bladder - Bladder seems swollen and hard, during cystitis. Pains in region of bladder. Very painful, frequent urination, worse at night. Incontinence when coughing, laughing, or making any effort whatever. Urine foul, with sandy sediment.

Causations - Ill effects of unrequited love, bad news, scolding, punishment, falls, sepsis.

Chest - Panting with oppression of the chest. Sensations of oppression of chest when raising arms or lying on left side. Rheumatic pains in chest. Angina pectoris.

Constitutions - Suited to nervous, hysterical patients subject to chorea disorders; to persons of foxy, mischievous and destructive tendency. Suited to chorea disorders when whole body or right arm and left leg are involved.

Ears - Snapping, cracking in ears (right), with pain and hiccough. Noises, ringing as of bells, worse on waking in the morning. Singing, like a tea-kettle, in left ear.

Eyes - Itching of the eyes with thick tears. Stitching in eyes as sand or thorn. One pupil dilated, other contracted. Eyes are wide open spasmodically and staring. Photophobia. Squinting of eyes which remain open during epileptic attack.

Face - Acne in face since menopause. Fiery red, bloated. Expression of terror. Wrinkled. Pains in angles of lower jaw.

Female - Menses early. Profuse menstruation with frequent erotic spasms. Dysmenorrhea with very sensitive ovaries. Dysmenorrhea better during warm weather, when outdoors, worse during cold weather. ***Pruritus vulvae*** after menses. Leucorrhea alternating with bloody discharge. Leucorrhea of clear acrid, sticky lumps. Dry, hot raw, itching vulva and vagina, worse scratching. Great sexual desire. ***Violent nymphomania***, worse sex. Sensation of motion in uterus like a fetus. Sensation of burning. Expulsion of gas from vagina. Strong bearing-down pelvic pains. Displacement of uterus. Neuralgia of uterus, with sadness and despair. Violent tearing pains in uterus. Fibroid tumors of uterus with bearing-down pains. Ovaries, sensitive to pressure. Cancer of cervix.

Food - Loss of appetite. ***Refuses to eat.*** Food tastes sour. Mental symptoms better evening, after eating. Craving for sand or raw food. Craving for raw food during pregnancy. Desires highly seasoned food, salty things. Desires ashes, cuttlefish, smoking. Aversion to meat, bread. Thirst for cold water. Thirst often and for large quantities.

Head - Intense pain, as if thousands of needles were pricking into brain. Heavy pain in temples, extending to face and neck with nausea and impatience. Violent crushing headaches. Migraine, can't open eyes, with tendency of head to incline backward. Fullness in head with throbbing carotids, better nosebleed. Burning heat in occiput with pricking and itching over whole body. Neuralgia in temples. Meningitis. Wants hair, brushed, pulled or head rubbed. As if cold water were poured on head and body.

Heart - Diseases of heart, worse by wetting hands in cold water. Angina pectoris. Palpitations, precordial anguish. Trembling and thumping of heart as from bad news or fright. Sensations as if heart twisted and turned around. Heart takes sudden jumps. Pulse, hard infrequent, irregular. Heart suddenly ceases to beat, patient fears to die. Heart as if squeezed or compressed.

Kidneys - Foul urine with sandy sediment. Incontinence on laughing, coughing etc. Diabetes mellitus. Polyuria with violent pains in lumbar region and paralysis of lower limbs.

Limbs - Multiple sclerosis with trembling. ***Chorea movements. Twitching and jerking.*** Extraordinary contractions and movements. Legs restless, impulse to walk. Can run better than walk. Numbness of legs. Weak legs, cannot plant them firmly, do not obey. Yawning with uneasiness of legs, must move them constantly. Festination. Kneeling difficult. Soles itching. Cold, moist feet and hands. Restless arms, keeps hands busy, picks fingers.

Lungs - ***Attacks of suffocation,*** with crying, screaming and restlessness, must have fresh air, worse coughing. Panting with oppression of the chest. Cough when expectorating, gagging, fatiguing. Cough worse after sex, noise, better smoking.

Male - Sensitive genitals. ***Extreme sexual excitement.*** Lasciviousness almost to insanity, worse sex. Prostatic ailments after masturbation. Seminal emission hot, bloody. Indolent tumors of testicles.

Modalities - Better open air, sun. Better bright colors. ***Better from music***. Better pressure, rubbing affected parts. Better relaxation. Better warm water, sweating, smoking. Better riding in a carriage. Motion improves headache but aggravates uterine pains and pains in coccyx. Worse from rest, touch, contact, motion. Worse noises. Worse seeing others in trouble. Worse damp, cold, washing head or putting hands in cold water. Worse after menses. Worse at night, evening. Worse periodically, yearly, at the same hour. ***Worse after sex***: sadness, difficult respiration, cough, and general weakness specifically increased by sexual excitement.

Mouth - Dry mouth and teeth. Tongue drawn backward, preventing speech. Pain in lower jaw, as if teeth would fall out. Grinding of teeth.

Nose - Catarrh, dryness, burning, sneezing and bleeding, worse right side. Nosebleed better throbbing carotids and fullness in head.

Perspiration - Profuse excoriating sweat. Copious perspiration, worse after excitement.

Rectum - Weakness of anal sphincter. Violent burning in abdomen and rectum. Burning pain with profuse, dark, fetid, bloody stools and violent urging. Severe constipation, not relieved by purgatives or enema. Constipation with involuntary passing of urine on coughing or any effort.

Sensations - As if thousands of needles were pricking into brain. As of needles sticking into muscle of neck when touched. As of insects creeping and crawling. As if occiput were struck with a hammer. As of a hair in eye. As if lower teeth were going to fall out. As if heart turned and twisted around.

Skin - Purplish skin. Ecchymosed spots. Cold spots or as of a cold matter flowing or dropping on part. ***Boils, burning and painful.*** Carbuncle. Deep abscesses. Helps evacuation of pus. Dry eczema (Ars., Sulph.). Miliary eruptions and furuncles, with diabetes. Itching, as of insects creeping and crawling.

Sleep - Sleepless before midnight from excitement. Sad dreams, with weeping.

Stomach - Gastric symptoms, worse at onset of fever. Gastric disturbances, accompanied by pains in head, face, teeth etc. Bitter belchings, hysterical. Vomits all food eaten. Vomiting during pregnancy.

Stools - Stools oily, black offensive, worse by washing head. Very dark, fetid, partly formed stools, containing much mucus, expelled with difficulty. Stools followed by smarting and burning in anus, but no tenesmus.

Temperature - Alternate chill and heat. General heat with cold feet. Septic fever. Sweat profuse, excoriating. Intense chill all over before convulsions.

Throat - Tonsils greatly swollen, with offensive odor. Diphtheria both tonsils covered by a firm membrane, color of pearl.

Vertigo - Vertigo after breakfast, with bad taste in mouth. Vertigo when fixing sight on any object. Vertigo at night, when descending stairs. Vertigo before or following epileptic attack. Vertigo, worse carrying burden on head, then spasms.

Vision - Sees ghosts, faces, flashes. As if a cloud before left eye, before epileptiform fits.

COMMENTS - Clarke recorded two cases of poisoning. The first was the case of a girl, three months old, who was bitten by a tarantula. She appeared at first uneasy, then exhibited dyspnea and complained. Showed signs of suffocation, vomited. She was agitated and convulsed. Music was played, movements of the limbs were set up, resulting in a profuse sweat, followed by sleep and complete recovery.

Clarke also noted the case of Francis Mustel, a peasant, who was bitten by a tarantula on the left hand about the middle of July as he was gathering corn. He went home with his companions but on the way fell as if struck by a stroke. Dyspnea followed and his face, hands and feet became dark. Knowing the remedy, his companions fetched musicians.

When the patient heard their playing he began to revive, to sigh, to move first his feet, then his hands and then the whole body. At last getting on his feet he took to dancing violently with sighing so labored that the bystanders were almost frightened.

At times he rolled himself on the ground and struck it vehemently with his feet. Two hours after the music began the blackness of his face and hands went off, he perspired freely and regained perfect health.

Every succeeding year at the same season the pain and attending symptoms returned, but less violently and they could always be averted by music. But if the imminent paroxysm was not averted in time, he was found by his friends struck down as at first and was restored in the same way.

Hysterical hyperesthesia. The least excitement irritates, followed by languid sadness. Great excitability of nerve endings. Fingertips are extremely sensitive. Sore and bruised feeling all over, worse moving about. Spinal irritation, slightest touch along spine causes spasmodic pain in chest and heart regions. Hypersensitive to the least touch.

Neuralgias, particularly in the head, "as if thousands of needles were pricking to the brain." Worse by noise touch, strong light. Better by rubbing head against pillow. Keynote better by rubbing. "Ends of nerves become so irritated. That some kind of friction is necessary in order to obtain relief."

Chorea (Ign., Staph.), most marked on right side. Characteristic unceasing movements, twitching, jerking, and dancing. Restlessness, particularly in the lower limbs, with desire to cry. Must keep moving about though all symptoms are worse walking.

Farrington noted that "When there are no observers there is no hysteria, when attention is directed to her she begins to twitch," and "cunning attempts to feign paroxysms of wild dancing."

Mental symptoms in connection with sexual disorders. Sighing, yawning, laughing and crying. Joking and profound melancholy. Insanity. Better by music. Music at first excites then it subsequently relieves.

Dark red or purplish coloration and swelling of skin and tissue. Septic boils that turn really blue and painful. Spider bites in general (Hyper., Led.). Periodicity, deep action returning annually on the date of the bite.

Diphtheria tonsillitis, threatening suffocation. Apparent imminent choking. Cystitis. Septic and intermittent fevers. Constrictive headache with pain in uterus.

P. C. Majumdar reported the case of a woman, 18, who had oppression of the chest, with a suffocating sensation. She had continuous jerking and movement of her hands. Foam at mouth. Complete insensibility. Profuse and delaying menses. Very sleepy. Hysterical epilepsy was diagnosed. Ign. 30c did nothing. Tarent., 200c, brought her out of the fit and restored her completely in a few minutes.

C. M. Boger cured a case of irritative cough with Tarent. 30c. Mr. B., 41, was sore all over, throat felt dry. Coughed when lying down at night and in morning after rising. Dry with tearing pain in chest. Excited by pressure of phlegm in chest. Felt short of breath for at least an hour after each coughing attack. Only better from smoking. Bad taste in the evening. Three doses cured.

In Med. Ad., a case of hyperesthesia of the fingertips was mentioned. The patient, a woman, 33, could not dress herself without gloves. The irritation caused a sensation in the teeth as if set on edge by a strong acid. The pain was not in the fingers. Tarent. gave relief after Asar., Gels. and Sul-ac. had failed.

Farrington related a case of typhoid in a child cured by Tarent. The child rolled its head and bit its nightgown. Apis. and Agn. improved. Tarent. slightly aggravated at first, then rapidly improved.

RELATIONS - Tarent.'s action is similar to Ars. in many symptoms, therefore when Ars. seems indicated but fails, it is better to give Tarent. ***Antidote to:*** Lach. ***Antidotes:*** Puls., Mag-c., Mosch., Cupr., Chel., Gels., Bov., Carb-v. ***Compare:*** (1) Agar., Ars., Cupr., Mag. phos. (2) Kali-br. - Irritation of periphery of nerves better exercising and rubbing. (3) Chorea, Mygal., Cimic., Agar., Stram. (4) Desire to jump, Stram., Croc., Nat-m., Stict., Asar., Agar., Hyos., Cic. (5) Bores head in pillow, Bell. (Tarent. is more rubbing). (6) Croc. (7) As if occiput struck with a hammer, Naja. (8) Deep-in headache, Bac. (9) Extreme joy, Coff. (10) Unfortunate love, Ph-ac. (11) Ménière's disease, ague, Chin-s. (12) Sees faces, Sulph.

REFERENCES - Boericke. Clarke. Murphy. Phatak.

TARTARICUM ACIDUM

(Tartaric Acid)

PHARMACY - tart-ac. Tartaricum acidum. Tartaric acid. Trituration. Solution. ***Historical dose:*** All potencies.

CLINICAL - Convulsions. Debility. Gastritis. Heels, pain. Paralysis.

HOMEOPATHIC - Found in grapes, pineapple, sorrel and other fruits. Tart-ac. is an anti-scorbutic anti-septic, stimulating the mucus and salivary secretions.

Extreme weakness. In evening feels very tired, can scarcely drag himself along. General bruised sensation, especially of lower limbs. Convulsions just before death.

Abdomen - Pain around umbilicus and region of loins. Pinching below navel with emission of flatulence, cold feeling in abdomen.

Face - Face instantly became red as fire and having exclaimed that he was poisoned, became speechless, died on tenth day (drank 2 oz. in solution). Lips, turn brown and black on their inner edges. Constant dryness of lips, must moisten them continually. Burning of lips.

Food - Excessive, very urgent thirst.

Heart - Very weak action of the heart. Feeble pulse.

Limbs - Sharp pain in region of loins. Paralysis of thighs and legs. Tearing pains at soles, near the heel, which prevents him setting his foot on the ground after luncheon.

Lungs - Breathing accelerated, then laborious and slow.

Modalities - Better in open air. Pasty taste is better after eating.

Mouth - Teeth set on edge. Brown and dry tongue. Taste, pasty in morning, ceases on eating.

Rectum - Many stools during night. Stools like color of coffee grounds.

Sleep - Frequent yawning and stretching.

Stomach - Dyspepsia with copious secretion of mucus. Belchings. Nausea. Vomiting is repeated and almost continuous. Continued vomiting with burning in throat and stomach. Vomited deep green matter.

Temperature - General cold feeling, evening in bed.

Throat - Hoarseness and scraping in larynx. Burning sensation in throat and stomach as if on fire.

Vertigo - Confusion in head, dizziness.

COMMENTS - A proving by Nenning and some poisonings have furnished the pathogenesis of Tart-ac. One of the most marked symptoms was intense burning in throat and stomach, feeling "as if on fire." Tongue brown and dry. Almost constant vomiting, vomited matter of deep green color. Feces coffee-ground color.

Dullness and lassitude. Paralytic debility. "Weakness in the evening, can scarcely drag himself along." Difficult respiration. Great weakness with diarrhea with dry and brown tongue. "Tearing pain on the soles of the feet, near the heel, which prevents him putting his foot on the ground after luncheon" (Phyt.).

REFERENCES - Boericke. Clarke.

TAXOL

(Alkaloid of Pacific Yew Tree)

PHARMACY - taxol. Taxol. Alkaloid of Pacific Yew Tree, (Taxus brevifolia). Taxol is an anti-cancer chemotherapy drug. N. O. Taxaceae. ***Historical dose:*** All potencies.

CLINICAL - Allergic reactions. Anemia. Arthritis. Breast, cancer. ***Cancer.*** Chemotherapy, effects. Chills. Diarrhea. Dyspnea. Edema. ***Fatigue.*** Fever. Hair loss. Hypersensitivity. Hypotension. Hives. Kaposi's sarcoma. Liver problems. Lung, cancer. Lung, disorders. ***Mouth, sores.*** Nail, discoloration. Nausea. Ovarian, cancer. ***Peripheral neuropathy.*** Radiation, effects. Rheumatism. Stomach, disorders. Skin, disorders. Tumors. Ulcers. Vertigo. Vomiting. Weight, gain.

HERBAL - The Taxol compound belongs to a family of compounds called Taxanes that are unique to the Yew species. During the Taxol studies, several yew taxanes in addition to the Taxol tanane were found to exert anti-cancer properties. Other Pacific Yew taxanes (also called diterpenes) are known by various names such as baccatin 111, brevitaxin, brevifoliol and cephalomannine, as well as variations of taxol compounds. Taxol is only one of hundreds of organic compounds in Taxus brevifolia.

Taxol was originally approved for use as a treatment for ovarian cancer, ongoing research was showing its efficacy in other arenas such as cancers of the lung, breast, bladder, prostate, testes, esophagus, head and neck, cervix, and endometrium. Also used to treat Kaposi's sarcoma and melanoma.

HOMEOPATHIC - The homeopathic indications for prescribing Taxol can be determined from the side effects of Taxol cancer therapy. Homeopathic potencies of Taxol maybe given to lessen the toxic side effects of the treatment.

The following Taxol side effects are common for patients taking Taxol: Low blood counts. White and red blood cells and platelets may become decreased. Hair loss. Pain in the joints and muscles. Peripheral neuropathy, numbness and tingling of the hands and feet. Nausea and vomiting. Diarrhea. Mouth sores. Hypersensitivity reaction with fever, facial flushing, chills, shortness of breath, or hives after Taxol is given.

The following are less common side effects for patients receiving Taxol: Swelling of the feet or ankles (edema). Liver problems. Low blood pressure. Darkening of the skin where previous radiation treatment has been given. Nail changes, discoloration of nail beds.

Fever, chills. Shortness of breath, wheezing, difficulty breathing, closing up of the throat, swelling of facial features, hives. Allergic reaction. Redness or pain at the site of injection. Nausea. Vomiting. Diarrhea. Unusual bleeding or bruising. Black or tarry stools. Blood in stools or urine

Extreme fatigue. Mouth sores, painful redness, swelling or ulcers. Yellowing of the skin or eyes. Swelling of the feet or ankles. Sudden weight gain. Signs of infection such as redness or swelling, pain on swallowing, coughing up mucus, or painful urination.

RELATIONS - ***Compare:*** Taxus brevifolia (Pacific Yew) belongs to the botanical family Taxaceae, which is a small family with one main genus - Taxus. Species include Taxus baccata (European Yew), Taxus cuspidate (Japanese Yew), Taxus globosa (Mexican Yew) and Taxus canadensis (Canadian Yew).

REFERENCES - Murphy..

TAXUS BACCATA

(Yew Bark)

PHARMACY - tax. Taxus baccata. Yew bark. N. O. Coniferae. Tincture of the fresh young shoots. Tincture of the berries. ***Historical dose:*** All potencies.

CLINICAL - Abscess. ***Cancer.*** Chemotherapy, effects. Ciliary, neuralgia. Collapse. Convulsions. Cystitis. Delirium. Digestion, quick. Dysuria. Ear, polyps. Eruptions. Fainting. Gout. Hair, loss. Headaches. Heart, disorders. Kidneys, disorders. Knees, abscess. Lachrymation. Nose, eruptions. Rheumatism. Purpura. Spermatorrhea. Strangury. Stupor. Trembling. Uterine, tumors. Vision, dim.

HERBAL - The poisonous properties of the yew have been recognized and disputed from ancient times. Gerarde said that in his school days he and his companions ate their fill of yew berries and slept not only under its shade, but on its branches without any ill effect, but there is plenty of evidence on the other side.

In the Med. Press, May 29, 1901, a patient of Mullingar Asylum died suddenly from eating the leaves. Some years ago a correspondence in the Times brought to light instances of the lethal effects of yew leaves on cattle.

One correspondent, Mr. James Simmons of Haslemere, mentioned an observation made by himself and others, that yew leaves are more poisonous some time after they have been cut than when fresh.

"Yew cropped green from the tree has no fatal effect," and animals do not eat it fresh, they prefer grass, but if Yew has been cut and allowed to wither cattle will eat it in large quantities and in that state it is deadly poison." "My people," said Mr. Simmons, "once buried some Yew cuttings deep in the dung of a farmyard, a number of large hogs dug it up, ate it and all died."

HOMEOPATHIC - Tax. is for pustular diseases of skin and night-sweats. Gout and chronic rheumatism. Pains in the knees, elbows and back. Slight tremor over whole frame. Trembling. Convulsions. Fainting and collapse. Relaxation of muscles. ***Cancer,*** chemotherapy effects.

MIND - Impatience, which unfits the patient for mental application. Delirium. Stupor.

Abdomen - Tension in abdomen, as if the stomach were overloaded. Squeezing and tension across abdomen. Aching in umbilical region. Borborygmi.

Back - Drawing pain in muscles of neck (left). Constant pain in back. Sacral pains, which allow no rest either in a standing or sitting posture and which compel the patient to remain in bed. Incisive pain in sacrum. Pain in shoulder blade, which subsequently removes to loins.

Chest - Oppression, when stomach is either too full or too empty or else with pain below xiphoid cartilage. Sharp pain in left side. Chest full and hot. Lungs engorged.

Ears - Polyps in the ears.

Eyes - Pupils widely dilated. Drawing with lachrymation and pressure. Lachrymation of left eye. Itching of external angle of left eye. Burning itching in eyelids. Vision dim.

Head - Supra-orbital and temporal pain on right side with lachrymation.

Heart - Irregular action of heart. Pulse rapid, slow, feeble, small, wiry, almost imperceptible.

Face - Puffy and pale. Looks ill. Face livid, convulsed. Lips are purplish, livid, black brown, especially upper. Frothing at mouth.

Female - Uterine cancer and tumors.

Food - Violent hunger. Frequent want to eat with activity of digestive functions.

Kidneys - Cutting pain at base of kidneys which allows him neither to sit still nor stand up and even prevents turning in bed. Urinary tenesmus. Frequent want to urinate with difficult emission in a fine stream. Strangury, urine red.

Limbs - Numbness of limbs and paralysis after several sweats. Sharp, transient, wandering pains. Contusive and incisive pain, which hinders walking. Abscess at right knee. Violent pinching in left calf. Tingling crawling sensation in whole left foot. Lancinations in hand. Burning dryness of palms of hands. Dull pain in joints of fingers. Rheumatic pain in fingers.

Lungs - Violent and fatiguing cough. Short cough after every meal, excited by full inspirations with oppression.

Male - Flow of semen without erection or sexual pleasure for several successive nights. Great excitement during sex. After sex, weakness and great oppression.

Modalities - Worse by pressure, by application of liquids. Worse before and after each meal. Worse after sex. Coughing causes headache. Deep breathing causes cough. Rubbing improves the itching of eyelids.

Mouth - Sensation of coldness in teeth. Mouth dry. Burning pricking on tongue. Tongue excoriated, moist, tremulous. ***Saliva hot***, acrid. Saliva increased, extremely viscid, acrid. Bitter taste like that of Cinchona.

Nose - A round spot of a reddish-brown color, on the end of the nose with desquamation of skin.

Rectum - Hard, difficult, dry evacuations. Occasionally a stool which is soft or of a natural consistence. Diarrhea with insupportable tenesmus and burning at every evacuation.

Skin - Large, flat, itching pustules. Badly smelling and offensive night-sweats. Peculiarly offensive sweat with eruption of vesicles. Podagra. Erysipelas. All hairy parts become denuded. Black jaundice. Skin red. Body covered with pustules. Miliary eruption. Eruption of large pimples. Dry tetter causing much itching.

Sleep - Sleeplessness during whole night, yawning without inclination to sleep.

Stomach - ***Feeling of emptiness***, must eat frequently. Violent hunger, soon after breakfast with general uneasiness and weakness in region of stomach. Aching, burning and pinching in region of stomach. Pain in pit of stomach and region of navel. After eating, cough. Feeling of pins and needles at pit of stomach. Nausea with accumulation of saliva. Retching. Vomiting ending in death. Vomit, tenacious, containing bile.

Temperature - Perspiration from least exertion with great prostration of strength. Profuse night-sweats. Commencing with shivering followed by dry heat of hands and feet. Offensive viscid sweats with itching and redness.

COMMENTS - The symptoms of the Tax. pathogenesis are made up of poisonings by leaves and berries and also of provings by Gastier. Fainting is a very prominent feature with Tax. And, in the fatal cases there are convulsions, collapse and syncope.

Death from yew poisoning, said Cooper, is remarkably painless. "Empty feeling" in the stomach was prominent and it was noted that the digestion was very rapid. "Must eat frequently." Gastric catarrh is set up with vomiting of tenacious mucus. Increased saliva, viscid.

Pustular skin affection. Large, flat, strongly itching pustules. Viscid sweat. Shooting pains in the toes. Gout. Irritation in the kidneys and bladder. Disturbed heart. Tax. has been recommended as a substitute for Dig., being considered superior to the latter in having no cumulative effect.

On the suggestion of Cooper, Clarke once gave a single dose of Tax. tincture in a case of ear polyps (bright red) with catarrh in a youth with the result that the polyps shriveled up to one-third of its former size.

RELATIONS - ***Antidoted by:*** Staph - prostration with oppression after an embrace. ***Compare:*** (1) Ars., Bell., Nux-v., Colch., Dulc., Kali phos., Lyc. (2) The Coniferae. (3) Load at stomach, Abies-n. (4) Rapid digestion, Sulph. (5) Podagra, Urt-u.

REFERENCES - Boericke. Clarke.

TELA ARANEAE

(Cobweb)

PHARMACY - tela. Tela araneae. Cobweb. Araneae tela. Spider's web. Aranearum tela. N. O. Arachnida. The cobweb of the black spider found in barns, cellars, dark places. Tincture or trituration. ***Historical dose:*** Tincture and all potencies.

CLINICAL - Aphthae. Asthma. Chills. Chorea. Coryza. Coughs. Delirium. Eczema. Fatigue. Headaches. Hectic fevers. Hiccoughs. Hydrothorax. Insomnia. Intermittent fever. Leucorrhea. Nervous, weakness. Numbness. Sleeplessness. Tuberculosis. Urticaria.

HOMEOPATHIC - The spider's web has been used as a remedy since ancient times. Tela. has been experimented with on healthy persons; t very rapidly lowers the frequency of the pulse rate.

In some it produced "a calm and delightful state of feeling, followed by a disposition to sleep. The most delicious tranquility, resembling the action of opium and followed by no bad effects."

Twenty grains given to an old and infirm asthmatic produced "slight but pleasant delirium." Muscular energy is increased, could not be kept in bed, but danced and jumped about the room all night.

In cases of febrile depression, deficient animation or indifference to surrounding objects, the exhibition of eight or ten grains of cobwebs was often followed by exhilaration, the eyes sparkled.

The countenance assumed a temporary life and, though the course of the disease might not be changed or the danger averted, more respite was obtained than is gotten from wine, opium or anything else within my knowledge.

"In spasmodic disorders of various kinds in asthma in periodic headaches in general restlessness and muscular irritability, its good effects are often signal. The cobweb gives sleep, but not by narcotic power, tranquility and sleep here appear to be the simple consequence of release from pain and irritation."

Tela. acts on arterial system. The pulse is full, strong, and compressible. Lowers pulse rate frequency. Cardiac sleeplessness increased muscular energy. Excitement and nervous agitation in febrile states.

Dry asthma, harassing coughs, periodic headaches with extreme nervous weakness. Obstinate intermittents. Masked periodical diseases, hectic, broken down patients. Symptoms come on suddenly with cool, clammy skin. Numbness of hands and legs when at rest. Continued chilliness.

MIND - Absent-mindedness. Mental dullness, brain as if enveloped in a fog. Makes mistakes in spelling, time. Disoriented feeling. Spaced-out feeling. Thoughts, disconnected. Prostration of mind. Tranquility and a sense of well-being.

Sadness, despondency, depression with heaviness of body. Pities herself. Sighing. Offended easily by jokes. Censorious, critical. Cursing. Irritability. Aversion to being touched. Kleptomania. Anxiety with chest constriction. Anxiety about health. Fear of disease. Fear of being bitten. Bites himself.

Abdomen - Distension. Sensation of fullness, heaviness. Abdomen sensitive to clothing. Stabbing pain in left hypochondria. Spasms and twisting in the bowels

Back - Heat flushes. Heaviness sensation. Pain in dorsal region, left scapulae. Stabbing, sensation of a knife in the back. Pulling sensation. Burning pain in cervical region. Stiffness in cervical region. Stiffness of spine. Desire to stretch, neck region. Sensation as if stretched backwards.

Chest - Anxiety with chest constriction. Heaviness feeling. Stabbing pain. Stinging pain in sternum. Wave sensation, behind sternum. Pain in axilla. Perspiration in right axilla. Hydrothorax.

Ears - Boring pains. Heaviness sensation in ears. Heat sensation. Noises while eating. Sounds seem far away.

Eyes - Dryness of eyes. Heaviness sensation. Aching pain, better cold application. Eye inflammation, better from cold. Discharges are green. Pains, burning and sore. Injected, inner canthus. Lachrymation, in the wind.

Face - Fullness, heat sensations. Numbness, heaviness of jaw. Heat flushes. Aphthae on lips. Twitching of lips. Facial paralysis.

Female - Leucorrhea, offensive smell. Sexual desire decreased or increased.

Food - Appetite increased. Desires beets, chocolate, ginger, ice, warm soup. Fruit aggravates.

Head - Headaches with flushes of heat. Boring and pressing pains. Tingling pains in scalp.

Heart - Anxiety with constriction. Cardiac sleeplessness. Piercing pain, heart, region. Pulsation in heart region. Pulse is full, strong, and compressible. Lowers pulse rate frequency.

Kidneys - Pain at close of urination.

Limbs - Awkwardness. Chilliness. Heaviness sensation in limbs, hip. Numbness. Aching pains. Stitching pain in knee, patella. Eczema in the hollow of the knee. Urticaria on the leg, calf. Heat with alternating cold in feet. Weakness of legs during stool. Sharp pain in shoulders. Trembling of hand, right.

Lungs - Difficult breathing with palpitations, stabbing pains. Dry, irritating coughs.

Male - Stitching pains in penis.

Modalities - Aversion to air, drafts. Cold, better applications. Better when it rains.

Mouth - Metallic taste. Aphthae on the tongue. Biting sensation on tongue. Itching inside cheek. Mucus on teeth.

Nose - Coryza, as if about to get a cold or flu, with anxiety. Coryza with fever. Nosebleed during exercise. Twitching of nose.

Perspiration - Clammy, offensive sweat. Perspiration of hands, feet. Perspiration with fever.

Sleep - Sleeplessness with heat in feet. Cardiac sleeplessness.

Skin - Clammy skin. Eczema. Urticaria.

Stomach - Appetite increased. Indigestion. Hiccoughs. Vomiting, with spasms and twisting.

Temperature - Fever alternating with chills. Obstinate intermittents. Perspiration with fever, shivering, at night. Hectic fevers.

Throat - Constriction of throat. Dryness, sore pain, on waking. Congested. Sensation of a lump. Unsteady speech and voice .

Vertigo - Vertigo after exertion, exercising.

Vision - Focusing difficult. Vision is blurred, worse after eating chocolate.

COMMENTS - Dr. Chapman wrote of Tela., "I have cured some obstinate intermittents, suspended the paroxysm of hectic fevers. Overcome morbid vigilance from excessive nervous mobility and quieted irritation of the system from other causes and particularly as connected with protracted coughs and other chronic pectoral disorders."

Dr. Gillespie of Edinburgh reported, "I cured an obstinate intermittent with cobweb after other means had failed."

Dr. Jackson wrote, "I think I may venture to say that it prevents the recurrence of febrile paroxysms more abruptly and more effectively, than quinine bark or arsenic or any other remedy employed for that purpose with which I am acquainted: that like all other remedies of the kind, it is only effectual as applied under a certain conditions of habit, but that the condition of susceptibility for cobweb is at the same time of more latitude than for any other of the known remedies."

"If the cobweb," said Dr. Jackson, "was given in the time of perfect intermission, the return of paroxysm was prevented, if given under the first symptoms of a commencing paroxysm, the symptoms were suppressed and the course of the paroxysm was so much interrupted that the disease, for the most part, lost its characteristic symptoms.

"If it was not given until the paroxysm was advanced in progress the symptoms of irritation, viz., tremors, startings spasms and delirium, if such existed as forms of febrile action, were usually reduced in violence, sometimes entirely removed. In this case sleep. calm and refreshing, usually followed the sudden and perfect removal of pain and irritation.

"Vomiting, spasms and twisting in the bowels, appearing as modes of febrile irritation, were also usually allayed by it, there was no effect from it where the vomiting or pain was connected with real inflammation."

Jackson noted particular changes induced on the existing state of the system, and characterized it as powerfully stimulant base on its affects.

Where the pulses of the arteries were quick, irregular and irritated, they became calm, regular and slow after the cobweb had passed into the stomach. The effect was accompanied, for the most part, with perspiration and perfect relaxation of the surface.

When the pulses were slow, regular and nearly natural, they usually became frequent small, irregular, sometimes intermitting.

Languor and depression characterize the disease, sensation of warmth and comfort are diffused about the stomach and increased animation is conspicuous in the appearance of the eye and countenance.

Dr. Jackson likewise effected perfect cures with it in some troublesome spasmodic disorders and gave it with the most marked benefit in dry, irritating coughs, usually termed nervous. In the advanced stage of tuberculosis it procured a respite beyond his expectation.

He also found it useful in restraining a troublesome hiccough. Remembering the fame of Mygale avicularia in chorea, this other spider to be of use "in some troublesome spasmodic affections."

Dr. Thatcher cited the following case from a paper of Dr. Jackson's: "W. Sands has been afflicted for many years a distressing asthma, which has proved fatal to his father and two sisters. The complaint being hereditary and aggravated by malformation of the thorax, no remedy gave any permanent relief, nor did change of climate procure any alleviation of symptoms.

"For a considerable time back he has never been able to lie down in bed on account of a sense of suffocation, but is obliged to be supported half sitting by pillows and is seldom able to sleep.

"He swallowed nearly a scruple of the spider's web, he swallowed it at bed time and to his utter astonishment enjoyed sound and uninterrupted sleep all night, a blessing to which he had been an entire stranger above six years.

"Since he began with the cobweb thinks his health is improved, the cough has entirely abated, but whenever the remedy is omitted the complaint returns."

Dr. Oliver found that by the use of this remedy a patient laboring under organic disease of the heart and hydrothorax obtained great relief and refreshing sleep, who had not before slept for three nights.

Another, under similar affection, experienced uncommon relief from the same prescription. To one suffering much pain from cancer, it afforded ease and comfortable sleep.

A patient in tuberculosis pulmonalis being affected with distressing agitation of mind and nervous irritation, it answered like a charm and soon induced great sleep like a moderate dose of opium.

REFERENCES - Anshutz. Boericke. Clarke.

TELLURIUM METALLICUM

(Tellurium Metal)

PHARMACY - tell. Tellurium metallicum. Tellurium metal. An element (Te, At. Wt. 125). Trituration of the precipitated element. ***Historical dose:*** All potencies.

CLINICAL - Axilla, sweat. Backache. ***Barber's itch.*** Boils. Cataract. Cholecystitis. Conjunctivitis. Coryza. ***Coughs.*** Eczema. Entropion. Eruptions. Eye, inflammation. Deafness. Emphysema. Foot, sweat. Gastritis. Gleet. Gonorrhea. Heartburn. Hepatitis. ***Herniated, disks***. Herpes. Hoarseness. ***Injuries.*** Insomnia. Levitation. Mastoiditis. Migraines. Numbness. ***Offensive, sweat.*** Otitis. Pityriasis, versicolor. Post-nasal, catarrh. Psoriasis. ***Ringworm.*** Scarlet fever. ***Sacro-iliac, pain.*** Sciatica. ***Spinal, irritation.*** Threadworms. Vertigo. Worms. Yawning.

HOMEOPATHIC - Tellurium occurs in the native state and in combination with gold, silver, lead and antimony. It resembles sulphur and selenium in its chemical reactions. Tellurium is an element situated between antimony and iodine; it was discovered in a gold mineral by the Austrian Muller in 1782.

The proving was conducted by Hering in about 1850 on fourteen provers, using the low potencies. A new proving was established by Raeside in London. He conducted a proving on seventeen provers, eleven women and six men. The provers took the remedy night and morning for fourteen days. The potencies 6x and 6c produced the maximum symptoms.

The most notable feature of the provings was the irritation of the skin, including the skin of the eyelids and ears, of the spinal column and of some nerves. Dryness of the skin and mucus membranes. Herpes circinatus, ***ringworm***, especially of the face and body. Vesicular, burning, itching eruptions. Itching, urticarial or macular eruption.

Offensive discharges. Chronic fetid suppuration from the ear. Persistent fetid body odor. Heavy perspiration from the feet, extremely foul-smelling.

Restlessness and pains all over body. ***Very sensitive back***. Pain in the cervical, right lumbar and sciatic regions. Sacral and sciatic pains. Slight amnesia with frontal headache. Lassitude. Afraid, cannot bear to be touched on sensitive areas. Slow development of symptoms (Rad-br.).

MIND - Rough and angular disposition. Excitable, disposed to fly into a passion. Afraid of any movement and of anyone approaching them. ***Fear of being touched in sensitive places.***

Lassitude. Quiet disposition. Absent-minded. Neglectful and forgetful, when engaged in doing one thing, forgets and neglects others. Incapable of mental activity. Amnesia, inability to fix the memory on immediate events. Depressed. Depressive psychosis. Serene and cheerful, then impatient and irritable.

Abdomen - Fullness and oppression in hypogastrium, clothing must be loosened. Pressing first left, then right side, as from wind. When lying on left side, throbbing under right ribs, and vice versa. Pinching in abdomen. Frequent spasmodic pains in bowels as from incarcerated wind, mostly from 5 to 9 p.m.

Back - Weak feeling in back. ***Vertebral pain from last cervical to fifth dorsal vertebra,*** very sensitive to pressure and touch (Chin-s., Phos.). ***Herniated disks*** (Aesc, Agar.). Sensitive spinal column with ***coughing, straining***. Pressing ache in scapula. Numbness in nape and occiput. Pain in sacrum. Neck pain, spreading to the shoulder and between the scapulae. Lumbar pain spreading to the right thigh, ameliorated by walking. Afraid of any movement and of anyone approaching.

Breasts - Cutting around and in left nipple, through to scapula. Eruption about nipple.

Causations - ***Falls, injuries.*** Eating rice causes vomiting. Eating and drinking improves sore throat.

Chest - Pain in the sternum, aggravated by deep breaths and by bending. Pressure in middle of chest under sternum, better in open air. Shooting in left chest, fifth rib. Feeling as if some fluid is pressing downward in, from right lung.

Ears - ***Catarrh of middle ear.*** Chronic suppurating otitis. Otitis after scarlet fever. ***Fetid, irritating discharge, smells of brine*** from the ear, especially the left ear. Chronic mastoiditis. Itching, swelling, throbbing in meatus. Dull, throbbing pain in ears, day and night, thin, watery, excoriating discharge. Ache in the left ear. Vesicular eruption on the eardrum, suppurating and perforating. Eczema behind ears with formation of thick crusts. Deafness. Buzzing, ringing in the ears.

Eyes - Pustular conjunctivitis, with eczema on lids and much purulent discharge from eyes. Deposit of chalky-looking white mass on anterior surface of lens. Cataract, following ocular lesions. Aids the absorption of infiltrations in iris and choroid. Herpes conjunctivae, phlyctenules near edge of cornea, worse from crying. The eyelids are ***thickened and inflamed,*** with pustules, pale red, edematous and oozing. Feeling as if lashes of lower lid were turned in.

Face - Heat in face. Sudden flushes of redness over face. Distortion and twitching in left facial muscles, left corner of mouth drawn up when talking. ***Ringworm on face. Barber's itch.*** Pimples on face. Burning in lips.

Female - Shooting deep in pelvis across to left. Premenstrual colic in lower abdomen. Menses painful and late. Menses too early in menopausal years. Long intervals between menses.

Food - Craving for apples, fatty bacon, salt, bread during the evening, cold drinks, beer. Hungry at night. After meals, great drowsiness. Vomits after eating rice.

Head - Feeling of heat in the head. Heaviness and fullness of head in morning. Pain in left side of head and in forehead above left eye. Periodic headaches. Migraines. Sudden rush of blood to head. Congestion to head and nape of neck, followed by weakness and faintness in stomach. Brain feels as if beaten on slightest movement. Violent linear pain in small spot over left eye. Itching of scalp, red spots. Numbness of nape and occiput.

Heart - Dull pain in region of heart when lying on left side, better lying on back. Heart irregular when lying on the back or right side. Palpitations with throbbing through whole body and full pulse, followed by sweat. Palpitation with sensation of thoracic constriction and pain. Rapid pulse rate.

Kidneys - Painful soreness in kidneys, extending downward like a weight, worse morning, making her irritable. Increased, high-colored, acid urine.

Limbs - Aching all over, mostly in limbs, worse right side and in walking. Sciatica, right side, worse lying on affected side. Sciatica with sensitiveness of vertebral column. Weakness of the legs in the morning. Bruised pain in hip joints after walking. ***Contraction of tendons in bends of knees.*** Sharp, quick pains in elbows, ankles and other parts. Fetid sweat on feet, mostly on toes. Fingertips feel dead on stretching hand. Rheumatism of right little finger, worse moving it.

Liver - Hepatitis and gastritis. Chronic cholecystitis.

Lungs - Coughing on laughing, worse aching in small of back. Wakened by cough. Cough towards morning, looser after a few days. Wheezing, scraping cough with mucus. Emphysema.

Male - Herpes on scrotum and perineum. Secondary gonorrhea. A drop of viscid fluid in meatus. Increased sexual desire, followed by long-lasting indifference. Erections all night.

Modalities - Better lying on back. Worse while at rest, at night, lying on painful side. Worse in morning, on waking. Worse cold weather. Worse coughing, laughter. ***Worse from touch***, friction. Spine sensitive to touch. Eating causes drowsiness.

Mouth - Dryness of the lips and mouth with raw, irritated areas. Ulcerations on the gums tongue, mouth, palate. Gums bleed easily and profusely. Tongue somewhat swollen, furred white, shows print of teeth. ***Breath has odor of garlic.*** Copious saliva. Tenacious mucus runs from mouth. Taste earthy, metallic. Coldness of mouth and pharynx on drawing in air.

Nose - Hawks dried yellowish-red phlegm from posterior sinuses, salty tasting, in mornings. Coryza, lachrymation and hoarseness, better in open air (All-c.). Nose obstructed, must breathe through mouth. Head cold with running of a blood-streaked liquid accompanied by tears and hoarseness, ameliorated in the open air. Nostrils itch. Boils.

Perspiration - ***Offensive foot-sweat.*** Heavy perspiration from the feet, extremely foul-smelling. Offensive sweat of armpits, smelling of garlic. Sweat on face, on spots.

Rectum - Very offensive flatus. Spasmodic pains with urging to stool. Stools soft at first, then hard. Copious stool with feeling of flatulence in bowels. Costive. Itching anus, rectum and perineum after stool. Tetter on perineum, itching. Passes many threadworms with stool.

Sensations - As if in air on going to sleep. Brain as if beaten. As if lashes were turned in. As if air whistled through left Eustachian tube. As if strapped together in epigastric region. As if fluid wanted to discharge in lobe of right lung.

Skin - Skin dry, hot. Stinging in skin. Barber's itch. Herpetic spots, ***ringworm*** (Tub.), worse lower limbs, on single parts. ***Ring-shape lesions.*** Circular patches of eczema. Small red pimples, very bright red and very sharply defined with minute vesicles upon them. Psoriasis. Scrofulous eczematous eruption. Eczema, back of ears and occiput. Itching of hands and feet. Itching worse in cool air. Offensive odors from affected parts. ***Fetid exhalations*** (Sulph.).

Sleep - Drowsy after a meal. Yawning and belching. Insomnia with unpleasant dreams. Sleepless, restless turning from weariness and bruised feeling. At night, pains all over. On going to sleep, feels as if in air, quick drawing towards feet wakens him. Wakes with a start during the night.

Stomach - Empty and weak feeling. Sensation of weakness, like faintness in the stomach after local congestion of blood to head and nape, also with chest symptoms. Heartburn with warmth in stomach as from alcohol. Belching with taste of food eaten. Fullness in pit of stomach, must lie down after dinner. Constrictive feeling in stomach as if strapped together.

Temperature - Inner shivering and fever, fetid, repulsive sweating, forcing him to be alone. Chilly with pains. Sweat on face, on spots, with increased itching of these places, often throbbing through whole body, generally warm, while sitting in a cool breeze. Skin hot and dry, sensation as if overstrained, as if bruised, as if he had taken cold after severe exertion.

Throat - Hoarseness in morning with fluent coryza, a rough, pressing, tickling sensation in larynx. In morning, hawks pieces of salty, yellowish-reddish phlegm. Painful dryness of fauces. Rough, scratching sensation in throat, worse towards evening. Throat feels sore with a prickly, rough sensation evening and morning. Throat sore on swallowing, better after eating or drinking. Pain in throat extends into ear.

Vertigo - Vertigo, when going to sleep, morning after rising. Vertigo worse walking, sitting up or turning head. Vertigo better lying perfectly quiet and still.

COMMENTS - Ringworm, herpes. Offensive, garlic-like odor of the body and sweat. Fishy odors and discharges (Hep., Sanic). Offensive foot sweats (Sil.). Vesicating effect on the skin, hair-roots, breasts, perineum and anus. Acrid discharge, blisters any part of the skin it touches.

Otorrhea. Discharge of the ear smells of fish brine. Nash cured several cases of post-scarlatina otorrhea using Tell. 6c, higher potencies had failed. Eyelids are inflamed. Phlyctenular conjunctivitis. Itching in the rectum after stool. Threadworms.

Great sensitiveness to touch. Neuralgic hypersensitive state of the spine. Painful spots along the spinal cord (Agar.). Injuries to the spine and pelvic bones. Radiating pain down both thighs from an injury to the sacroiliac area. Pains are sharp and radiating, or electric-like. Contractures. Pressing pain in the scapula. Neuralgic symptoms, especially on the right side.

Sciatica. Sciatic pain deep in the leg, behind the knee. Herniated disks (Aesc, Agar.). Sacro-iliac problems with radiating pains (Aesc, Hyper.). Worse lying on the affected part, from touch, worse in C7 to T5 and in the Sacro-iliac joint.

Many of the pains and symptoms come and go suddenly. The ears are suddenly stopped. Sudden rushes of blood to the head. Drowsiness. Yawning after retching, drowsy after eating.

Clarke once gave Tell. to a child for an eruption and cured it incidentally of constant yawning with which it had been troubled. The eruption improved at the same time.

Clarke also cured with Tell. an Indian officer home on furlough whose body was covered over with a ringworm-like eruption.

Kent had a case in which a boy, 4, slid down banisters and struck his head on a tiled floor. He became unconscious and a surgeon was summoned, who found him unconscious with a clear, watery discharge from the ear, which the surgeon pronounced to be cerebrospinal fluid.

This condition lasted three days and the case had been pronounced hopeless when Kent first saw the boy. Kent noticed that the discharge was acrid and reddened whatever part it came in contact with. One dose of Tell. was given. In two hours the child vomited, a sign of reaction, and in two weeks was well.

Shelton related three cases using Tell. The first concerned a widow, 50, who had pain and soreness in the upper part of her back for a long time. She shrank from the slightest touch on the part. The sensitiveness was so acute that, when touched, the pain extended into the occiput and all over the upper region of the back. Tell. 6c cured in eighteen days.

The second case concerned Miss X., 45, who had a fall, striking a severe blow on the sacrum. She suffered for some weeks from concussion with one point of great soreness in the sacral region, just above the spot where the blow was received. She was kept in bed for some weeks and improved generally, but the painful spot remained and sensitiveness appeared over the back, especially its upper third. Tell. 6c cured all completely.

The third case concerned Miss Y., 29, who had severe spinal meningitis ten years before, and consulted Shelton for a burning, pressing pain at base of brain. He diagnosed the condition as meningitis. The patient grew worse and gradually ptosis, and then right and then left hemiplegia set in.

Finally hyperesthesia of the back became so distressing that it was a question of finding any support that did not intensify the pain. She could not bear the slightest touch, complaining that it not only hurt her at the point of contact, but that she felt it in the head and in remote parts of the body. Tell. cleared up the case.

RELATIONS - ***Antidoted by:*** Nux-v. (epigastric oppression). ***Compare:*** (1) Rad-br., Berb., Hyper., Sel. (2) Tet. - coccygodynia, ulceration of nails, pains in hands in small spots, ankles, heels and Achilles tendon, (3) Sep., Ars., Rhus-t. (4) Restlessness, garlicky odor, Ars. (5) Coryza, All-c. (6) Otitis, Puls., Bell., Ter. (7) Ringworm, Bac., Sep., Nat-m. (8) Ringworm in clusters Sep., Calc. (9) Threadworms, Teucr. (10) Pains come and go suddenly, Bell., Lyc. (11) Worse laughing, Phos. (12) Worse straining at stool ind. (13) Cough and skin, Osm.

REFERENCES - Boericke. Clarke. Murphy. Phatak.

TEPLITZ AQUA

(Teplitz Mineral Springs)

PHARMACY - tep. Teplitz aqua. Teplitz Mineral Springs of Teplitz in Bohemia. Teplitz aqua, contains: Natrum carbonicum, Natrum muriaticum, Natrum fluorica, Natrum silicata, Kali sulphuricum, Kali muriaticum, Calcarea carbonica, Silica, etc. Dilutions. ***Historical dose:*** Tincture and all potencies.

CLINICAL - Amenorrhea. Bones disorders. Breast, tumors. Eruptions. Erysipelas. Flatulence. Gout. Hemorrhoids. Irritability. Leucorrhea. Metrorrhagia. Nosebleed. Paralysis. Rheumatism. Sciatica. Scurvy. Speech, difficult. Spine, pains. Tongue, paralysis. Toothache. Ulcers. Vertigo.

HOMEOPATHIC - The waters of Teplitz are chiefly in repute for the treatment of gouty patients, especially those suffering from atonic gout. The springs are alkaline and hot, and the temperature forms a leading feature in their action.

The symptoms of Tep. are from Perutz, who experimented on himself and several healthy individuals, together with symptoms by Hromada. Symptoms of Nat-c. and Nat-m. appear throughout. Tearfulness, low spirits and irritability were noted and giddiness of much intensity. "Giddiness, when she walks all the houses seem to move too."

Modalities - Better by friction. Better drinking cold water. The symptoms are worse at night, especially bone pains. Worse from motion.

COMMENTS - On moving head it seems as if something fell from one side to the other. Cold feelings in upper arm in foot. Increased sensitiveness to cold. Paralysis of tongue of limbs.

Vesicles in mouth and on tongue. Vesicular erysipelas. Burning sensation in many parts. Burning in stomach, better drinking cold water. Hemorrhage, nosebleed, hemorrhoids with stool, metrorrhagia. Better from hemorrhoid bleeding.

RELATIONS - ***Compare:*** (1) Nat-c., Nat-m., Kali-s., Mang., Lith., Sil., Alum.

REFERENCES - Clarke.

TEREBINTHINIAE OLEUM

(Oil of Turpentine)

PHARMACY - ter. Terebinthiniae oleum. Oil of Turpentine. Turpentine. Oleum terebinthine. Pinaceae. The oil distilled from the oleo-resin (turpentine) obtained from various species of Pinus, purified by repeated rectification with water. Solution in rectified spirit. Ozonized oil of Turpentine (prepared by exposure of the common oil to sun and air in a half-filled bottle and shaking from time to time). ***Historical dose:*** All potencies.

CLINICAL - Albuminuria. Amblyopia. Ascites. Asthma. Backache. ***Bladder, irritable.*** Brachial neuralgia. Bronchitis. ***Chilblains.*** Chordee. Chorea. Ciliary neuralgia. Coma. ***Cystitis.*** Dentition. Dropsy. Dysentery. Dysmenorrhea. Enteric, fever. Epilepsy. Erysipelas. Erythema. Fibroma. Gallstone, colic. Glands, swelling. Gleet. Gonorrhea. Headaches. ***Hematuria. Hemorrhage***. Hemorrhoids. Hernia. Herpes. Hypochondriasis. Injuries. Insanity. Intestines, ulceration. Iritis. Jaundice. ***Kidneys, disorders.*** Lumbago. ***Nephritis.*** Neuralgias. Ovaries, dropsy. Ovaries, pains. Peritonitis. Pityriasis. Purpura hemorrhagica. Rabies. Scabies. Scarlatina. Sciatica. Spermatorrhea. ***Strangury.*** Stricture. Tetanus. Tympanites. ***Uremia.*** Urethritis. ***Urine, retention.*** Worms.

HOMEOPATHIC - Ter. was introduced to homeopathy by Hartlaub. The symptoms have been added to from poisonings and overdosings in allopathic practice. According to Dr. Taylor, children are particularly sensitive to its action. Illness caused by sleeping in newly painted rooms is due in great part to the turpentine.

Milnes noted that Ter., as an internal remedy, is "A stimulant and tonic to the mucus membranes, especially of the bladder and urethra: it proves useful in leucorrhea and gleet."

Selective affinity for the mucus membranes of ***kidneys,*** bladder, respiration, bronchi, heart and blood. ***Bleeding mucus surfaces***, oozing hemorrhage of a passive, black offensive fluid. Purpura hemorrhagica.

Marked tympanites and urinary symptoms. ***Inflammation of kidneys*** with dark, passive, fetid hemorrhages. Affections of kidneys with rheumatism. Goullon indicated it for Bright's disease preceded by dropsy.

Aching, soreness and stiffness of the muscles. Even minor bumps cause bruises. ***Unbroken chilblains***. Burning in various parts, tip of tongue, epigastrium, small of back, kidney, uterus etc. Exhausted, sensitive and tired. Disturbed sense of equilibrium. Drowsiness and strangury. Coma.

MIND - Anxiety on going to bed. Confusion of mind, better when urinating freely. Tired and difficult concentration of thoughts. Intense irritability, children fly into temper during dentition. Muttering delirium. Hydrophobia.

Despondent during nervous headache. Fear of apoplexy during fullness and pressure in head. Loathing of life. Suicidal disposition, by hanging. Comatose, can be roused only by shaking out of apparent stupor, but falls immediately into it again. Unconsciousness after stool.

Abdomen - Bruised soreness. Dropsy, pelvic peritonitis. ***Enormous distention***. Tympanites. Ascites. Flatulence. Enterocolitis, hemorrhage and ulceration of bowels. Bowels were drawn towards spine. Bleeding ulcers in the intestine.

Back - Backache and soreness in kidney disorders. ***Burning pain in region of kidneys***. Drawing in right kidney, extending to hip.

Causations - Ill effects of alcohol, falls, strains, tooth extraction, damp cellars.

Chest - Burning and tightness across chest.

Constitutions - Suited to children, dentition, nosebleed, worms. Complaints of elderly people, people of sedentary habits. Chronic rheumatism and gouty complaints. Bleeders. Nervous women with headaches, amenorrhea and dysmenorrhea. Hydrogenoid.

Ears - Disturbed sense of equilibrium. Own voice sounds unnatural, humming as of a seashell. Loud talking is very painful. Otalgia. Sensation in ears as of striking of a clock.

Eyes - Opens eyes when swallowing in coma. Eyes dark red, face red on affected side. Intense pain in eye and side of head. Ciliary neuralgia over right eye. Amblyopia from alcohol.

Face - Pale, earthly, sunken. Hot flushes followed by sweat.

Female - Intense ***burning in uterine region***. Metritis and puerperal peritonitis. Metrorrhagia with burning in uterus. Uterine diseases after wearing pessaries.

Food - Hunger and thirst with debility. Diminished appetite, loss of appetite, great thirst. Desire to eat more after a satisfying meal. Aversion to animal food.

Head - Dull pain like from a band around the head (Carb-ac.).

Heart - Warmth in heart while sitting in evening, obliged to yawn a great deal. Frightful oppression in precordial region. Palpitations. Rapid, small, thready, intermittent pulse.

Kidneys - Nephritis after exanthemata with violent bronchitis. Burning, drawing pain in region of kidney, along ureters. Cystitis. Urethritis with painful excretions (Canth.). Bleeding bladder. Constant tenesmus. ***Strangury with bloody urine.*** Scanty, suppressed urine, ***odor of violets.*** Urine, smoky with coffee grounds or thick, yellow, slimy, muddy sediment. Pains alternate between navel and bladder, better walking.

Limbs - Brachial or sub-scapular neuralgia. Intense pain along the larger nerves, worse damp weather. Stiff muscles. Hands feel swollen. Cramps in knees. Stands with feet apart, has no power of balancing the body. As if pitched forward while walking. Walks bent like an old man.

Lungs - Dyspnea. Difficult breathing, the lungs feel distended, hemoptysis. Bronchitis of children with drowsiness and retention of urine. Bronchial asthma or catarrh with profuse expectoration. Bloody expectoration.

Modalities - Better from motion, stooping. Better belching and passing flatus. Loose stool better nausea. Burning in anus better cold water. Worse from dampness, cold. Worse at night, 1 a.m. to 3 a.m. Worse walking in open air. Worse lying, sitting. Worse pressure, touch. Worse by pressure in region of bladder it causes convulsions. Worse lying on left side, better turning to right. Pain in crest of ilium worse from motion and least jar. Damp dwellings aggravates. Damp cellar causes diarrhea. Damp weather causes neuralgia in legs.

Mouth - Foul, cold breath. ***Dry, red, sore, shining***, smooth and glossy tongue, burning in tips with prominent papillae (Arg-n., Bell., Kali-b., Nux-m.). Choking sensation in throat. Aphthae from mouth to anus. Dentition.

Nose - Discharge of serum without coryza. Cold in head with sore nostrils, with disposition to bleed. Passive nosebleed in children.

Perspiration - Suddenly checked sweat causes neuralgia. Suppressed foot sweat causes rheumatic iritis. Cold sweat on legs. Cold, clammy, all over with prostration. Profuse sweat on legs in evenings in bed.

Rectum - Pain before flatus with and relief after stool. Fainting after every stool. Diarrhea with watery, greenish, fetid stool. Diarrhea with tetanic spasms. Bloody stools. Hemorrhage from bowels. Worms, lumbrici.

Sensations - As of a band around head. As if sand thrown violently in eye. As of a seashell sounding in left ear. Sound in ear as of a clock striking. As from hasty swallowing in epigastrium. As if he had swallowed a bullet, which had lodged in stomach. As if he would pitch forward on walking.

Skin - General sensibility increased. Acne. Erythema, itching pustular, vesicular eruption, urticaria. Purpura hemorrhagica, advancing. Ecchymosis, dropsies. Scarlatina. Chilblains with excessive itching and pulsative pains. Aching soreness of the muscles.

Sleep - Drowsiness with urine retention. Lethargy. Retarded sleep. Agitated sleep at night with tossing and frequent waking. Many dreams, nightmares. Wakes frightened at night, looks ghastly and shrieks.

Stomach - Rancid, flatulent, acrid belchings. Burning in epigastric region. Nausea and vomiting with intense burning. Nausea, better loose stool. Aversion to meat.

Temperature - Heat under the skin. Heat with violent thirst, dry tongue, profuse cold, clammy sweat. Cold sweat on legs. Typhoid fever with tympanites, hemorrhages, stupor, delirium. Prostration.

Vertigo - Vertigo with vanishing of vision, nausea. Disturbed sense of equilibrium. Vertigo as if intoxicated, as if he would fall forward, when walking.

COMMENTS - Brunton noted that Ter., when applied to the skin, acts as an irritant and rubefacient, causing vesicles and a sensation of burning if applied for any length of time. Inhaled, it causes sneezing, tightness across the eyes and dyspnea.

Given internally, it causes burning in the mouth and salivation in stomach, sensation of heat or cold, gastro-enteritis with vomiting and diarrhea, and ulceration of the intestines. The pulse is sometimes slowed, sometimes quickened.

Respiration is quickened and spasmodic, the chemical is partly excreted by the lungs and acts on the mucus membrane, lessening its secretion. The temperature sometimes rises, or falls. Voluntary movement is diminished, reflex action lowered, blood pressure lowered and vessels dilated.

Acute and chronic nephritis. Kidney infections. Protein or blood in the urine. Albuminuria and hematuria after scarlatina and also to the consequent dropsy. Effects of chemical inhalation of exposure, particularly if there is kidney damage.

Diminished quantity of urine. Urine has an odor of violets. Lumbar pain, burning in urethra, painful urination. Hematuria with smoky, turbid urine depositing a sediment like coffee-grounds. Dull pain or burning pain in region of kidneys. Burning during urination.

Brunton mentioned its usefulness in treating gallstone colic, given in ether in the proportion of one part of the oil of turpentine to three of ether. Homeopaths have confirmed the value of this treatment.

Characteristic burning. Burning in gums, tongue, tip of tongue, mouth, throat, stomach, rectum and anus, kidneys, bladder and urethra, uterus, air passages, and chest. Burning in the sternum, particularly after warm drinks, the pain running along the sternum with the drink and spreading in the chest. Burning extends from kidneys along ureters.

"Burning in uterus." Peritonitis, metritis, metrorrhagia with burning. Passive, dark and fetid hemorrhages. Hemorrhages from any orifice. Purpura hemorrhagica with fresh ecchymoses in great numbers from day to day. Smooth, glossy, red tongue, as if deprived of papillae.

Drowsiness. Drowsiness with capillary bronchitis, in child. Stupor and great weakness, particularly in cases of typhus, typhoid, and uremic poisoning. "Drowsy with retention of urine."

Excessive tympanites, with extreme sensitiveness to touch. Sensitivity of the hypogastrium and pains in symphysis pubis with cystitis. Urogenital and rectal troubles. Pains go from left to right across bowels and then shoot upward.

Sense of anxiety and utter prostration about epigastrium. Umbilical region feels as if covered with a round, cold plate. Sprained pains, contusive pains and rheumatic pains appear, notably pressure and drawing pains.

Irritation of the meninges and often ascarides or other intestinal worms. Maniacal fury. Cooper found Ter. indicated in children (especially teething children) when they fly into passions.

Lippe observed that this irritability manifests itself in some cases of spasms and convulsions. He had a case of a woman who had made her feet sore by walking and applied turpentine to them. This was followed by a state like hydrophobia, she had spasms whenever she saw water, heard it poured, or saw a bright object and also whenever she attempted to urinate.

Cooper noted the case of a woman, 35, who, from being exposed to the odor of turpentine, got pain as from pinchings in the throat with lifeless feeling in the tongue and dryness of the mouth, followed by pain in her right eyeball, which extended back to the same side of occiput.

S. H. Roberts maintained that Ter. had a specific effect in tonsillitis when applied externally.

Marc Jousset gave Ter. 1x with marked benefit in two cases of bronchial asthma. He was led to give it in the first case by coincident hematuria, but this was not present in the second.

A young man who was badly poisoned by a low potency of Phos. got more relief from Ter. 3x than from any other remedy.

Brunton argued that it is only ozonized Ter. that is effective in such cases. Dr. Hering says the ozonized oil is recommended as a prophylactic in malarial and African fevers, a few drops being given daily on a lump of sugar.

George Royal gave three cases illustrating the action of Ter. The first concerned a man, 24, with typhoid in the third week. He had extreme distention, with a rapid, small and compressible pulse. Cold sweat in lower limbs.

Ter. 6x was given, two drops in water every half-hour. Oil of Ter. was applied locally to the abdomen, mixed with lard. Later in the evening, when there was already slight improvement, an injection containing turpentine was administrated. This relieved the patient of a large quantity of flatus and he began to recover the next morning.

The second case concerned pyemia after miscarriage at the third month, brought on by the patient herself. Enormous distention, lower limbs covered with cold sweat, lochia thin, scanty offensive.

Ter. given in another case brought about slow improvement for three days, when Chin. 30c was indicated and finished the cure.

The third case from Royal concerned a teamster, 36, who had severe nephritis after being out in cold rain. He had a constant desire to urinate, severe pain in back, down ureter to bladder, urine scanty, very high-colored. Temperature 102. Pulse weak, 130. Ter. 6x was given every half-hour and hot fomentations on kidneys greatly relieved. After three days he was able to leave his bed.

Royal considered cold sweat of lower limbs and rapid pulse with the distention, as leading indications. A keynote of Burnett's for Ter. is "Pains in the bowels which causes frequent urination."

RELATIONS - ***Antidoted by:*** Phos. ***Antidote to:*** Phos., Merc. ***Compare:*** (1) Alumn., Sec., Canth., Nit-ac. (2) Terebe. 1x - chronic bronchitis and winter coughs, sub-acute stages of inflammation of respiratory tract. Loosens secretion, relieves tightened feeling, makes expectoration easy. Neurotic coughs. Huskiness of public speakers and singers. (3) Cystitis when urine is alkaline and offensive. (4) Onon. - Diuretic. Chronic nephritis, diuretic effects like Juniper, calculus, nosebleed, worse washing face. ***Followed well by:*** Merc-c.

REFERENCES - Boericke. Clarke. Murphy. Phatak.

TERMINALIA ARJUNA

PHARMACY - term-a. Terminalia arjuna. N. O. Combretaceae. Bark. ***Historical dose:*** Tincture and all potencies.

CLINICAL - Angina pectoris. Boils. Contusions. Diarrhea. Dysentery. Ecchymosis. Fractures. Gonorrhea. Heart, diseases. Hemorrhages. Palpitations. Spermatorrhea. Tuberculosis. Ulcers. Wounds.

HERBAL - Terminalia arjuna is a large, deciduous tree measuring a height of 60 to 80 feet. Sanskrit writers found the bark to be a cardiac tonic. Bagbhata was the first to prescribe the bark in heart diseases.

The ayurvedic physicians of India have been using this herb independently or as one of the ingredients in all sorts of heart diseases with marked success for a long time. They use it in both functional and organic diseases of the heart. Angina pectoris, palpitations of the heart, pain in the heart, weakness of the heart.

Fractures. Pains all over the body owing to a fall. Ecchymosis. Hemorrhages. Spermatorrhea and gonorrhea.

Charaka used it in hematemesis. He prescribed equal quantities of the bark, pulverized red sandalwood, sugar and rice water. Its leaves are also used for boils.

Sushruta used a decoction of the bark with equal quantity of white sandalwood in spermatorrhea. Harita found it useful in gonorrhea.

Bangasena has recommended it in chronic diarrhea and dysentery. Bagbhata recommended its decoction for suppression and retention of urine. He also recommended an ointment prepared of the bark and honey in acne.

Chakradatta found it useful in bloody dysentery and in cardiac affections. He also recommended it in fractures. Bhavaprakasha recommended it for tuberculosis of the lungs and for suppression and retention of urine.

COMMENTS - R. N. Khory in his Materia Medica of India, vol. II, wrote, "Astringent ad tonic given in heart disease. Locally used as a wash for wounds, ulcers, contusions and specially used in promoting union of fractures and dispersion of ecchymosis. Internally, largely used by the natives in hemorrhagic and other fluxes and as a lithontriptic."

REFERENCES - Ghose.

TERMINALIA CHEBULA
(Myrobalans)

PHARMACY - term-c. Terminalia chebula. Myrobalans. ***Historical dose:*** Tincture and all potencies.

CLINICAL - Catarrh. Colds. Colic. Constipation. Cough. Delirium tremens. Diarrhea. Dropsy. Dysentery. Elephantiasis. Glands, enlarged. Hemorrhages. Hemorrhoids. Hiccoughs. Jaundice. Rheumatism. Salivation. Scorpion, sting. Spleen, enlarged. Stomach, disorders. Typhoid fever. Vomiting. Whitlow.

HERBAL - R. N. Khory, Materia Medica of India, vol. II, p. 260, said, "Purgative, astringent and alternative. The ripe fruits are generally purgative and the unripe ones astringent and aperient."

Lt. Col. R. N. Chopra, I. M.S., wrote in his book Indigenous Drugs of India, p. 532, "It is astringent, laxative, alternative; used in scorpion sting."

Charaka found it useful in bleeding piles, diseases of the stomach, chronic dysentery, jaundice due to cough, cold and catarrhs, and vomiting.

Sushruta recommended it in rheumatism, blind piles, elephantiasis, chronic enlargement of the spleen and glandular enlargement of the abdomen and hiccough.

Bagbhata prized it is an excellent remedy for piles, stone and calculus and throat affections ad as a tonic. Harita recommended it in hemorrhages of the stomach and lungs, and delirium tremens.

Chakradatta found it useful in rheumatism, dropsy and in several affections of the eye. Bhavaprakasha recommended it in typhoid fever, chronic diarrhea and dysentery and biliary colic.

Bangasena said that it is an excellent remedy in diarrhea associated with colicky pains and also in whitlow.

HOMEOPATHIC - Term-c. is an indigenous remedy, very much used in ayurvedic medicine. The symptoms for homeopathic use are ineffectual desire, hard stools, distended abdomen, and bleeding hemorrhoids.

Therapeutic action to clear the bowels. Constipation, chronic dysentery, dropsy, chronic diarrhea. Frequent in effectual desire to pass stools, but the patient passes only small quantity of feces with great force. Sweat breaks out during stool. For piles, some skin diseases.

Vertigo, relieved by cold bathing. Profuse salivation with great thirst which accompanies all affections. Offensive odor comes out of the mouth. Tongue is flabby, dry, and covered with a brown coating on tip of the tongue.

MIND - Mind indifferent. Single mindedness. Easily indisposed to yawn, constant yawning.

Abdomen - Rumbling and gurgling sounds in abdomen. Flatulence. Pain in right lower abdomen.

Back - Intense pain in back (right lumbar region and lower spinal column). Sitting is painful due to pain, often at intervals. Pain increased while sitting straight, and decreased altogether while lying on bed and during sleep. Pain in back of neck.

Chest - Intense pressive pain in right chest.

Food - Thirst for drinking cold water.

Head - Headache in occiput and right cranium with intense vertigo. Stitching pain in right temporal region and occipital suture.

Heart - Pressive pain in region of heart. Pulse is accelerated and quick in motion, irregular. Pulse for some moments is rapid, hard and for some moments is weak simultaneously. Some heartbeats are feeble or of low sound, some normal and some of loud sound, everything in successive order.

Limbs - Muscular pain in right upper hand. Pain in the region of deltoid muscle. Itching pains relieved by scratching.

Liver - Slight pain in the region of liver (large lobe). Pain better temporarily by external pressure.

Lungs - Hot deep breathing.

Modalities - Every complaint is better by cold bathing. Better dry, cold air. Better while eating. Better closing the eyes, sleeping, evening. Better during complete rest of mind and body.

Mouth - Fetid odor in mouth. Profuse salivation with intense thirst. Sensation of dryness in upper jaw. Gums of teeth swollen and hard.

Rectum - Sweats while passing stool. Pressive itching and full sensation in rectum. Constipation, stool hard, of small quantity, and slightly yellowish. Diarrhea, stools is liquid, and small in quantity. Feces mixed with some mucus, flatulence associated with burning sensation in the stomach.

Stomach - Sensation of fullness in stomach. Distension of stomach. Downward pain in stomach and epigastrium. Rumbling and gurgling sounds in stomach. Fetid eructation. In the morning constant acid, empty eructation.

Stool - Frequent ineffectual desire for passing stool, but passes very small quantity of feces with great force or sometimes with ineffectual action to pass stool. After much trying a little quantity of feces comes out with great force.

Tongue - Flabby, dry, tongue. Brown coating on tip of tongue. Sore and raw tongue.

Urine - Quantity of urine is slightly diminished. Frequency of urination is increased at night.

Vertigo - Vertigo remains all the day and night for hours. Vertigo is worse by hot sun's rays, hard pressure and motion. Vertigo is better by cold bathing, evening dry cold air and during sleep and eating. Intense vertigo begins in occiput and spreads to the whole right side of the head (right temporal region to right frontal region).

RELATIONS - ***Compare:*** Chin., Nux-v., Lyc.

REFERENCES - Ghose.

TESTOSTERONE

PHARMACY - test. Testosterone. Male hormone. ***Historical dose:*** All potencies.

CLINICAL - Acne. Baldness. Bleeding. Cancer. Emaciation. Fatigue. Hepatitis. Impotency. Jaundice. Menstrual, disorders.

HOMEOPATHIC - Low levels of Testosterone can cause symptoms of fatigue, malaise, loss of sex drive, and loss of muscle tissue.

Anabolic steroids are compounds related to testosterone. The most common side effects of using Testosterone in both men and women include increased facial and body hair, oily skin or acne, male pattern baldness, water retention, joint stiffness, and soreness at the injection site. Lab tests may show increased levels of liver enzymes.

A deepened or hoarsened voice, growth of the clitoris, and menstrual irregularities have been reported in women. The masculinizing side effects may be irreversible in women, even with short term use.

At higher doses over longer periods, increased or decreased sex drive, mood swings, aggressive behavior, persistent painful erections, shrinking testicles, and breast growth have been reported in men. Long term use of high dose anabolics can damage the liver, causing jaundice, hepatitis, bleeding, or, possibly, cancer.

RELATIONS - ***Compare:*** Orch., Sep.

REFERENCES - Murphy.

TETRACYCLINE

(Antibiotic)

PHARMACY - tetra. Tetracycline. Antibiotic. The attenuations are prepared from the antibiotic, Tetracycline hydrochloride. Potentized allopathic drug. ***Historical dose:*** All potencies.

CLINICAL - Agranulocytosis. Allergies. Anemia. Blood, disorders. Convalescence. ***Diarrhea.*** Dystonia. Headache. Hives. Nausea. Photophobia. Rash. Skin, disorders. Sores. Tinnitus. Vomiting.

HOMEOPATHIC - Protracted convalescence. Post-infectious anemia. Agranulocytosis. Blood disorders. Dizziness, light headedness. Headache, bulging soft spot on head (in infants). Blurred vision. Ringing in the ears. Muscle weakness.

Extreme allergic reactions. Rash. Skin peeling. Skin eruptions. Inflammation of the tongue, of the upper digestive tract. Hives. inflammation of large bowel. Genital or anal sores or rash. Inflammation of the penis.

Sore throat and inflammation. Sore mouth and perineal itching due to overgrowth of yeasts. Difficult or painful swallowing. Indigestion. Irritation of the gastrointestinal mucosa. Autonomic dystonia. Diarrhea or loose stools. Cramps or burning of the stomach. Abdominal pain, nausea and vomiting. Loss of appetite.

Bone deformation. Discoloration of teeth. Swelling due to fluid accumulation. Liver poisoning. Photosensitivity. Prone to sunburns. Exaggerated sunburn.

RELATIONS - ***Compare:*** Ars., Fl-ac., Nit-ac.

REFERENCES - Murphy. Reckeweg.

TETRADYMITUM

(Tetradymite)

PHARMACY - tet. Tetradymitum. Tetradymite. Rare Tetradymite crystals from North Carolina and Georgia, contain about 60 parts of bismuth, 33 of tellurium, 6 of sulphur and traces of selenium and iron. Triturations. ***Historical dose:*** All potencies.

CLINICAL - Achilles tendon, pain. Coccyx, pain. Nails, ulceration ingrown. Urticaria.

HOMEOPATHIC - Hering proved Tet., taking about five grains of the first trituration. The most prominent symptoms were pains occurring in small spots, ulcerative pains about the nails and a sharp attack of urticaria from eating shell-fish. Pains in ankles, heels and Achilles tendons were also severe, worse rising from a seat.

REFERENCES - Clarke.

TEUCRIUM MARUM VERUM

(Cat thyme)

PHARMACY - teucr. Teucrium marum verum. Cat-thyme. Marum verum. N. O. Labiatae. Tincture of whole fresh plant. ***Historical dose:*** Tincture and all potencies. Locally for polyps, dry powder.

CLINICAL - Anorexia. Anus, itching. ***Ascarides***. Cachexia. Colic. Concussion. Eyelids, tumor. Fibroma. Hiccoughs. Ingrown, toenail. Nasal, catarrh. Otalgia. ***Ozaena. Polyps.*** Psoriasis. Rheumatism. ***Threadworms***. Urethra, excrescences. Uterine, fibroids. Worms.

HERBAL - The Germander group of the Labiatae, to which the Teucriums belong, had an important place in old herbal medicine, and homeopathy has placed Teucr. on a firm foundation. Stapf and others proved it.

HOMEOPATHIC - Worm infestations, irritation of anus and nose. ***Threadworms***. Worms and polyps suggest a tubercular taint and Clarke has used both Teucr. and Teucr. scorod. in tubercular cases.

Nasal polyps. Guernsey noted "Polyps with stoppage of nose on side lain on, large red pimples under right nostril near septum, sore and smarting to touch."

Chronic nasal catarrh with atrophy, large offensive crusts and clinkers. ***Ozaena. Loss of sense of smell***. Fibrous tumor of the eyelid.

Affections of children. Suitable after too much medicine has been taken. Over sensitiveness. ***Desire to stretch***. Urethral granulations following gonorrhea and also uterine fibroids.

Abdomen - Pressure in abdomen. Expulsion of much flatus, having the smell of rotten eggs. Incarceration of flatus. Colic with tearing drawings. Cutting pain after drinking beer or water.

Back - Burning in left scapula. Rheumatic drawing and tension in back.

Causations - Concussion (brain). Injuries likely to set up tetanus.

Chest - Chest loaded, with sensation of dryness in trachea. Squeezing pressure in lower part of chest, with anxious uneasiness, without affecting the breathing.

Constitutions - Suited to elderly persons and children. When too much medicine has produced an over-sensitive condition and remedies fail to act.

Ears - Otalgia. Shootings and tearings in ears. Hissing and ringing.

Eyes - Eyes red, inflamed. Smarting in canthi, lids red and puffy, tarsal tumor (Staph.).

Female - Smooth pedunculate, pear-shaped polypus of vagina, protruding three inches beyond hymen.

Food - Hunger in morning and evening. Appetite increased. Sensation of hunger, as if the food were unsatisfying and which hinders sleep. Bitter taste in gullet after dinner. Cuttings or nausea with inclination to vomit after drinking water.

Head - Excited, tremulous feeling. Frontal pain, worse stooping. Strengthens brain after delirium tremens.

Limbs - Tearing pains in arms and legs. Affection of fingertips and joints of toes. ***Pain in toenails***, as if they had grown into flesh.

Lungs - Dry cough, excited by a tickling in trachea, as if dust had been inspired, worse by coughing. ***Moldy taste in throat*** when hawking up mucus, expectoration profuse.

Male - Sexual desire decreased. Drawing pain behind left side of root of penis, extending to left side of scrotum, became sore to touch. Pressive, drawing sensation from abdomen into cords and testes. Burning, pressing, biting in fore part of urethra when not urinating. Excrescences in urethra following gonorrhea.

Modalities - Desires exercise in open air, which does not fatigue. Moving improves. Worse by touch. Worse sitting, stooping, on side lain on. Disinclined for exertion. Worse warmth, warmth of bed, wet weather. Worse evening and at night.

Mouth - Foul breath. Mouth clammy. Much mucus in mouth. Smarting as from pepper, first on left, later also on right side. Smarting in root of the tongue.

Nose - Catarrhal condition of both anterior and posterior nostrils. ***Mucus polyps***.

Chronic catarrh, ***Discharge of large, irregular clinkers. Crawling in nostrils*** with lachrymation and sneezing. Coryza with stoppage of nostrils.

Rectum - ***Itching of anus and constant irritation*** in the evening in bed. Crawling in the rectum after stool. ***Ascarides*** with nightly restlessness. Swelling, itching, and creeping at anus as from ascarides. Frequent itching and tingling in anus, often after the evacuations. Copious fetid evacuations of the consistence of pap.

Sensations - As if air forced through mucus in ear. As if right nostril were partly stopped. Chill as from abdomen. Sensation as from flea bites. As if nail had grown into flesh of right great toe.

Skin - Very dry skin. Itching causes tossing about all night. Suppurating grooves in the nails.

Sleep - Sleep retarded in evening. Restless with twitching, choking and starting up frightened. Unrefreshing sleep and difficulty in waking in morning. Agitated sleep at night, from excessive excitement. Vivid dreams and frequent starts.

Stomach - Vomiting of large quantities of dark-green masses. Constant hiccough, attended with pain in back. Hiccough on eating after nursing.

Temperature - Shivering and shaking, often with icy coldness in hands, and frequent yawning. Chilliness after eating, and when talking about unpleasant things. Heat worse in evening, with exaltation and great loquacity. Frequent feeling of flushing in face, without external redness.

Throat - Sore throat with shooting pain and impeded deglutition. Pressure or drawing and tearing in throat. Frequent necessity to hawk. Hawking up of much mucus of a moldy taste.

COMMENTS - Clarke gave Teucr. tincture in five-drop doses three times a day to a man of 44 who had tuberculosis affecting the right lung with severe recurrent hemorrhages. Teucr. helped him, and with other remedies he got quite well. While taking Teucr. he noticed that he passed a large quantity of threadworms to which he was not at all subject.

C. M. Boger related a case of cough in which his patient had with the cough a moldy taste in the throat when hawking up mucus. Expectoration profuse. Rapid loss of weight and strength. Anorexia. A brother had died of tuberculosis four years before with very similar symptoms. Teucr. 3x helped and 20x finished the cure.

Teucr. has the craving hunger of the antipsorics and worm remedies, it prevents sleep at night. Nervous, irritable, sensitive. Rheumatic and gouty symptoms and scapular pains, both in the bones and joints. Limbs go to sleep with tingling when sitting.

RELATIONS - ***Antidoted by:*** Camph. ***Compare:*** (1) Teucr-s. (2) Cina, Ign., Sang., Sil. ***Compatible:*** Chin., Puls., Sil.

REFERENCES - Boericke. Clarke.

TEUCRIUM SCORODONIA

(Wood Sage)

PHARMACY - teucr-s. Teucrium scorodonia. Wood sage. Wood germander. N. O. Labiatae. Tincture of whole fresh plant. ***Historical dose:*** Tincture and all potencies.

CLINICAL - Asthma. Bronchorrhea. ***Catarrhs***. Coryza. Coughs. ***Epidymitis***. Nasal, catarrh. Testicle, tuberculosis. Tuberculosis.

HERBAL - Teucrium scorodonia is an extremely bitter plant with the smell and taste of hops, for which it has been substituted. Some have observed an alliaceous smell and Cazin said that it gives a garlicky taste to the milk of cows, goats and sheep which eat it.

HOMEOPATHIC - Teucr-s. has been used in tuberculosis with muco-purulent expectoration. Dropsy orchitis and ***tuberculous epidymitis, especially in young,*** thin individuals with tuberculosis of lungs, glands, bones and uro-genitals.

It is used as an adjuvant in severe afflictions of the lungs. Remarkable results have been observed in ***chronic catarrhs*** of the lungs and bronchi, in nasal catarrhs, coryza, cough and asthma bronchiale.

COMMENTS - Dr. Criquelion told how Dr. Martiny one day in the Ardennes, had occasion to examine a man of thirty who was apparently in the last stage of consumption and had a cavity in one apex. Martiny gave his opinion that he had not long to live.

A year later, being in the same district, he called at the house and inquired of a man whom he saw there, apparently in perfect health, what had become of the invalid. "I am he," was the reply. It was the fact, though it took some time to convince Martiny of it.

An old woman had recommended him to make a tisane of the wood germander which grew abundantly about there. He had taken it daily and got well. "A similar case," said Cooper, "was told me by a distinguished scientist.

Martiny introduced Teucr-s. into his practice and used a tisane of it with much success in bronchorrhea and consumptive disorders with tuberculous elements and muco-purulent expectoration. Clarke confirmed this, using the tincture in five or ten-drop doses two or three times a day.

Criquelion pointed out that Teucrine has been used as a subcutaneous injection in tubercular cases as a substitute for Koch's Tub. Criquelion had a patient, a farmer of scrofulous habit, high color, thick neck, who had for ten years an enlarged testicle the size of a quince, which he diagnosed to be tuberculous.

Teucr-s. 6c was given, one drop in four spoonfuls of water, a spoonful three-quarters of an hour before each meal. After three months the testicle was softer in six months it had almost returned to its proper size.

RELATIONS - Teucr-s. is allied to Marrubium vulgare (Common or White Horehound), a well-known cough remedy. Also to Nepeta glechoma (Ground Ivy), which was formerly much used with snail-jelly for chest affections."

Compare: (1) Bac., Tub., Teucr., Helix.

REFERENCES - Clarke.

THALAMUS

PHARMACY - thala. Thalamus. Gray nuclei around the encephalon. Nerve-hormonal tissue from brain. Sarcode. ***Historical dose:*** All potencies.

CLINICAL - Angina pectoris. Catatonia. Contractures. Cyanosis. Hebephrenia. Hyperthyroidism. Menopausal, complaints. Neuralgias. Pains. Parkinson's disease. Raynaud's syndrome. Sciatica. Vasomotor, complaints.

HOMEOPATHIC - Thala. belongs to the group of gray nuclei around the encephalon. It is a large ganglion, even and symmetrical. Situated in front of and outside the quadrigeminal bodies inside the striped bodies. Laterally bordering the third ventricle, surrounded on its convexity by the caudate nucleus. It is egg-shaped and the distal end is large.

Hardy conducted a clinical proving, but there is no homeopathic proving. Complaints of the psychological system, including spasmodic laughter and crying, consciousness disorders inner sensitivity disorders. Patient misinterprets his illnesses.

Pseudo-bulbar paralysis. Neuralgias, cervical and brachial, sciatica. Tabes. Painful stumps. Vasomotor disorders. Parkinson's disease. Pre-cancerous conditions, predominantly painful.

Paresthesia in the female during the menopause. Formication, painful numbness situated particularly in the arms and which keeps the patient awake. Tingling, which is always distal and which appears with no apparent cause. Neuralgia of the left cervical region and arm with formication.

Pains accompanied by phenomena of anguish, ill-defined feeling of uneasiness, painful discomfort. Spontaneous pains, appear suddenly and then immediately reach their peak intensity. The painful sensation is much greater than the stimulus. Exaggerated pain. Violent attacks of paroxysm. Pains reside in one half of the body, predominantly of the limbs. Pain accompanied by sweating.

MIND - Catatonic conditions. State of inertia, desire for solitude and peace, loss of initiative. The patient does not want to do anything. He sits in a corner, immobile. Condition of psychological strain, which causes the feeling of being ill at ease in his body. Hebephrenia.

Spasmodic laughing and crying without any real cause, expressed by involuntary, automatic contracture of the muscles in the face and by mimicry, which is either ill-times or irrelevant or exaggerated.

Abdomen - Epigastric pain in a continuous

transverse bar, not changed by eating, but aggravated by emotion. Pain is diffuse, badly localized. Accompanied by discomfort. Abdominal meteorism ameliorated by emission of wind. Abdominal pains with emission of soft stools.

Chest - He feels as though his thoracic cage were trapped inside an iron corset.

Constitutions - Psoric, syphilitic or tubercular disposition. Nervous, biliary and lymphatic temperament.

Ears - Hallucinations of hearing with feeling of strangeness and fright. Buzzing in the ears, sound of a bell in the fog or of a foghorn. Noises in the ears. Feeling of confusion in the ears.

Eyes - Sight becomes weaker on one side of the field of vision. Objects seem lost in a halo of light. Diminution of sight on one half of the field of vision.

Female - Frigidity. Libido disturbed, impotence, frigidity, sexual asthenia. Menopausal complaints with hot flashes, aggravated at night. Hyperthyroidism during the menopause with swelling at the base of the neck.

Head - Occipital headaches, worse on the left side, spreading to the entire left side of the body.

Heart - Vasomotor complaints. Vascular disorders, accompanied by pain. Pain in the left side of the thorax, which may spread to the arm, aggravated by physical exercise and capable of stimulating an attack of angina pectoris.

Limbs - Raynaud's syndrome. Cyanosis of the limbs with tingling and burning sensation. Movements badly coordinated for the upper as well as the lower limbs. Often drops things. Hands in a contracted state without total paralysis. Numbness of the hands with cyanosis and trembling. Numbness of the feet with cyanosis, formication, swelling and edema of the ankles. Copious perspiration from the feet. Spastic gait.

Lungs - Asthmatic dyspnea, the patient has difficulty in exhaling.

Male - Impotence with dwindling or libido and lack of orgasm. Sex painful with premature ejaculation.

Modalities - Better by fresh air and movement. The pains are better at night. Worse by the cold, heat. Worse from emotions, especially unhappy emotions.

Nose - Ozaena. Reduction in the olfactory sensitivity. Sensation of evil-smelling, unpleasant whiffs like sulphur. Smells are badly tolerated.

Skin - Dermographia. Burning sensation on the skin, aggravated by heat and cold. Excessive sweating, predominantly on one half of the body. Lesion caused by parasites, on the nails. Deformity of the nails, which are concave, ridged, breaking. Nails extremely fragile. Inflammation beneath the nails.

Stomach - Pains with nausea, worse after ingestion of food. Cramping stomachache, accompanied by nausea and meteorism.

Temperature - Vascular complaints, the skin is either very red or very pale, but always cold. Cyanosis and edema at the limbs, accompanied either by an increase in the local heat or, the opposite, by decrease in the heat.

RELATIONS - ***Compare:*** (1) Agar., Op., Hyos., (2) Hypoth., Pitu-gl.

REFERENCES - Julian.

THALLIUM METALLICUM

(Thallium Metal)

PHARMACY - thal. Thallium metallicum. Thallium metal. Thallium aceticum. A Rare Metal. Trituration. Solution of the Sulphate. ***Historical dose:*** All potencies.

CLINICAL - Acne. ***Alopecia***. Amenorrhea. Atherosclerosis. ***Baldness.*** Cachexia. Conjunctivitis. Cyanosis. Dysuria. Emaciation. Emphysema. Folliculitis. Glomerulonephritis. ***Hair, loss.*** Hematuria. Hyperthyroidism. Insomnia. Locomotor ataxia. Malaria. Muscular, atrophy. Myelitis. Neuritis. Night-sweats. Paraplegia. ***Paralysis.*** Pleurisy. Pneumoconiosis. Polyneuritis. Rheumatism. Sciatic pains. ***Trembling***. Tremors. Tuberculosis.

HOMEOPATHIC - Thallium is a rare metal discovered by Crookes in 1861. He found it in the residue left from the distillation of selenium and named it thallium (a green shoot) from the green it gives in the spectrum. Thallium and its derivatives are toxic.

Thallium has been experimented with by Lamy and Marme. The symptoms picture of Thallium were established in 1965-66 by Panos, Rogers and Stephenson, on seven male and nine female provers.

Combermale of Lille, used Thal. with success in the night-sweats of tuberculosis, but this treatment had the effect of causing profuse falling of the hair, so serious as to contraindicate its use. Huchard had patients become quite bald in several days. Hansen said Thal. relieves the violent pains of tabes dorsalis.

Horrible, neuralgic, spasmodic shooting pains. Pains like electric shocks. Muscular atrophy. Tremors. ***Trembling***. Chorea-like movements. Locomotor ataxia with pain. ***Paralysis of lower limbs.*** Paraplegia. Polyneuritis. Neuritis. Trigeminal neuralgia. Spinal neurasthenia. Pseudo-bulbar paralysis. Intermittent paralysis.

Muscular pains. Muscular atrophy. Numbness or formication starting in the fingers and toes, extending up to lower limbs and down to feet and involving lower abdomen and perineum. General emaciation with a lack of strength.

Hyperemia, swelling and excessive secretion. Night-sweats of tuberculosis. Dermatrophic lesions. ***Alopecia, hair loss*** following acute, exhausting diseases. Loss of body hair and hair of the head.

Influences the endocrine glands, especially the thyroid and adrenalin. Hyperthyroidism symptoms. Emaciation, hypotonia, chilliness.

Pains in the legs, aggravated when lying on the affected side. Unable to find a position in the bed which eases the pain. Pain in the right knee on bending or stretching it. Pain in the sciatic nerve.

Discomforts are of a periodic nature, recurring in strength, at the same hour and then disappearing again. Permanent state of jangled nerves. Trophic conditions of the nails.

MIND - Growing impatience. Extreme irritability and violence, uneasiness with insomnia. Extreme anxiety for no reason. Hysterical symptoms with hyperesthesia and then hypoesthesia.

State of jangled nerves of excitability and bewailing with weeping and shouting. Attacks of weeping, excitement. Bursts into tears for the least thing, only to blow up soon after. Stubborn. Indifferent resignation. Apathy. Depression.

Abdomen - Retraction or depression of abdomen. Distention of the abdomen. Heavy flatulence, even after a light meal. Spasmodic pain in the stomach and intestines with abdominal pains. Pain in intestinal canal.

Back - Formication on the back. Lumbar aching.

Blood - Attacks of hypertension with hyperthyroid phenomena. Bleeding from the capillary vessels. Atherosclerosis. Cyanosis. Increase of carbon dioxide in the blood plasma.

Chest - Painful, heavy feeling on the sternum. Retro-sternal pain in the esophagus. Neuralgia after herpes zoster.

Eyes - Dacryocystitis. Iritis. Blepharitis. Purulent conjunctivitis. Frequent conjunctivitis with abundant production of mucus. Muco-purulent discharge from the right eye, worse in the morning. Glittering spots in front of the eyes with formication on the face. Visual complaints with feeling of heaviness behind the eye. Scotoma. Eyebrows fall out.

Face - Facial neuralgia. Hair loss from beard.

Female - Menses prolonged with black blood. Amenorrhea. Loss of pubic hair.

Food - Thirst. Voracious appetite. Loss of appetite.

Head - Headaches. Pain in occiput in morning. ***Alopecia.*** Hair falls off with great rapidity. Falling out of hair after diseases. Hair falls off in handfuls. Hair loss in spots

Heart - Diminished frequency of pulse. Pulse rapid with precordial constriction.

Kidneys - Involuntary passing of urine. Casts in urine. Acute glomerulonephritis. Dysuria. Proteinuria. Hematuria.

Limbs - Sharp pains like electric shocks. Very tired. Disorders of movement coordination. Chorea-like movements and rapid movements like convulsions. Exaggerated reflexes and muscular atrophy. ***Trembling***. ***Paralytic feeling***. Chronic myelitis. Numbness in fingers and toes with extension up lower limbs involving lower abdomen and perineum. ***Paralysis of lower limbs***. Cyanosis of limbs. Formication, beginning in fingers and extending through pelvis. Emaciation of fingertips. Deformed nails.

Liver - Gallbladder distended. Coating of liver white and granular-looking.

Lungs - Slow and difficult breathing. Dyspnea. Respiration difficult with pain all over the thoracic cage. Emphysema. Pleurisy. Pneumoconiosis. Cyanosis.

Male - Impotence. Loss of pubic hair.

Modalities - Better from walking. Worse at night. Worse from contact, pressure.

Mouth - Lips dry with thirsty feeling. Bad breath, irritation of the mucus membranes in the mouth with excessive salivation. Stomatitis. Aphthae. Gingivitis. Dental caries. Toothache. Numbness.

Rectum - Spasmodic, stubborn constipation, alternating with attacks of diarrhea and anal and rectal pains. Diarrhea, bloody stools.

Skin - Dryness of the skin. Red stripes after scratching. Acne. Folliculitis. Skin pigmentation disorders. ***Loss of hair on the body*** (axillary and pubic). Skin sensitive in particular areas, especially on the soles of the feet. Pustular formations. Trophic complaints of the nails, which are deformed. Inflammation beneath the nails. Deformed nails.

Sleep - Sleep is light, wakes often. Great difficulty in falling asleep again.

Stomach - Acrid dyspepsia. Bitter belchings and bitter taste in the mouth. Feels nauseated but cannot vomit. Nausea and vomiting. Pain in stomach and bowels, terribly severe lancinations, following each other with the rapidity of electric shocks.

Temperature - Profuse sweating in cases of severe illness. Night-sweats of tuberculosis.

Throat - Goiter. Swollen thyroid gland.

RELATIONS - Thal. belongs to the Lead group of metals and approaches Plb. closest in its symptoms. ***Compare:*** (1) Thal-s. Plb., Lath., Caust., Arg-n. (2) Baldness, Jab., Pilo., Petr. (3) Baldness and tuberculosis, Phos. (4) Aran. - Feeling of constant coldness. Periodic return of symptoms. Severe pain in the heels. (5) Cedr. - Periodicity of symptoms, supra-orbital neuralgia, periodic migraines. (6) Aran-ix.

REFERENCES - Boericke. Clarke. Julian. Phatak.

THALLIUM SULPHURICUM

(Thallium Sulphate)

PHARMACY - thal-s. Thallium sulphuricum. Thallium sulphate. The attenuations are prepared from Thallium sulphate (Tl2SO4). ***Historical dose:*** All potencies.

HOMEOPATHIC - The main indications are falling of hair. Emaciation. Tremors. Paralytic states. Night-sweats in pulmonary tuberculosis.

RELATIONS - ***Compare:*** Thal.

REFERENCES - Reckeweg.

THEA SINENSIS

(Chinese Tea)

PHARMACY - thea. Thea sinensis. Chinese tea. Camellia thea. N. O. Ternstromiaceae, Theaceae. Tincture or infusion of dried leaves and flowers. Trituration of Theine. ***Historical dose:*** Tincture and all potencies.

CLINICAL - Delirium, tremens. Mania. Homicidal. Insanity. ***Insomnia.*** Kidney, disorders. Mania. Megrim. Nervousness. ***Neuralgias.*** Paralysis. Sleeplessness. Suicidal.

HERBAL - Tea contains an alkaloid, Thein, which is considered by some identical with caffeine, and both tea and coffee are used to stimulate the jaded faculties. The stimulation will enable persons to endure fatigue and get more enjoyment out of themselves than they could obtain by mere food.

Coffee and tea are different in their effects though they may be alike in their chemistry. The after-effect of all stimulation is reaction, unless it is kept off by a repetition of the stimulant as the effect of the last dose wears off.

The sign that the first dose of tea is wearing off is a nervous, restless, depressed, ill-tempered state, which is visible in persons who rely on tea, at about 5 p.m.

HOMEOPATHIC - ***Neuralgia and insomnia.*** All-gone, sinking sensation at the epigastrium. Nervous sleeplessness, heart troubles, palpitations and dyspepsia of old tea-drinkers. ***Sensitive kidneys***. Sick headaches. Allen noted it was antidotal to Tab.

MIND - Nervousness and want of confidence. Great nervous excitability with exaltation of intellectual faculties. Ill-humored. Peevish. Disposition to quarrel at the most harmless speech.

Nocturnal fright, suicidal thoughts. Temporary mental exaltation. Delirium with ecstasy, laughed incessantly, talked in rhyme. Delirium tremens. Mania. Suicidal and homicidal. Impulses to kill. Impulse to jump out of the window.

Abdomen - Borborygmi. After lunch, stitch below ribs in paroxysms. Intestines relaxed. Liability to hernia.

Chest - Oppressed and constricted. Fluttering in left side and feeling of suffocation.

Ears - Neuralgic pains in cartilage of ears. Roaring in ears. Hallucinations of hearing.

Eyes - Eyes are unusually bright. Dilated pupils. Neuralgia of eyes. Sight is dim, dark before eyes, fiery lines, sparks.

Face - Wild, distressed expression. Face is pale, with congested redness, flushed.

Female - Soreness and tenderness in ovaries. Menses delayed, scanty with severe cramp-like pains. Uterine bearing down from beginning to end of period.

Food - Very hungry, but little satisfies. Thirst, but every mouthful of cold water affects the head like a shock. Craves acids, lemons.

Head - Rush of blood to head. Sick headache radiating from one point. Sleepless and restless. Hallucinations of hearing. Cold damp feeling at back of head. Scalp tender can scarcely comb hair.

Heart - Anxious oppression. Precordial distress. Palpitation, unable to lie on left side. Fluttering. Pulse rapid, irregular intermittent.

Kidneys - Very marked increase of urine. Must pass water immediately after drinking tea.

Limbs - Paralyzed numbness of limbs. Joints of hands and feet tender. Nervous excitability in wrists, hands, and feet. Hand trembled violently. Restlessness of feet. Neuralgic pains in outer hamstrings. Sensation as if the weight of a sheet even would crush toes.

Lungs - Edema of respiratory tract. Breathing increased in frequency and amplitude. Breathlessness on least exertion. Paroxysm of asphyxia. Cough is dry, severe and bloody expectoration.

Male - Erections. Unnatural excitement.

Modalities - Better warmth, warm bath, applying hand or warm clothes to occiput. Worse at night, from cold water, walking in open air. Worse after meals.

Mouth - Bitter taste in mouth. Much viscid saliva. Whole mouth cavity dry and sensitive. Tongue clean and pale. Tongue red, blistered, painful as if scalded. Teeth frequently decayed.

Nose - Dryness, soreness of nose. Sensation at root of nose as if nosebleed would occur. Nosebleed before menses.

Rectum - Swelling of lower end of rectum, with slight itching. Chronic relaxed bowels. worse by beer, better by port wine. Constipation.

Sensations - As if on the verge of fainting. As if a foreign body in throat. As if the stomach hung down relaxed in the body like an empty bag. As if the weight of a sheet on the feet would crush the toes. Cold sensations are prominent, cold, damp feeling at back of head with pain spreading thence to eyes, also dryness and swelling of mucus membrane.

Skin - Skin dry as if pores obstructed. Skin of fingertips peels from excessive dryness. Eruption of red, indolent pimples. Itching, crawling, prickling in different parts.

Sleep - Sleepy in daytime, sleepiness at night with vascular excitement and restlessness and dry skin. Horrible dreams cause no horror.

Stomach - A sinking sensation at the epigastrium. ***Faint, gone feeling*** (Sep., Hydr., Olean.). Weakness about stomach. Sudden production of wind in large quantities. Nausea, and vomiting after eating. Vomits bile, when pain at its height.

Temperature - Intense coldness passing over whole head. Lowered temperature. Hands and face cold as marble. Beaded with chilly moisture. Excessive internal heat with flushes of heat on the surface, coming and going quickly. Disposition to perspire.

Throat - Scraping in larynx. Hoarseness. Diphtheria sore throat. Painless swelling of mucus membrane. Uneasy feeling in pharynx, as if obstructed by a foreign body.

Vertigo - Vertigo with darkness before eyes, sudden in open air.

COMMENTS - The symptoms are made up of observed effects of overdosing and some direct provings. A woman who was addicted to drinking tea showed very pronounced delirium tremens indistinguishable from that caused by alcohol, though there was no alcoholism in the case.

Another woman, who kept a pot of tea boiling on the stove and drank several bowls every day, developed both suicidal and homicidal mania, impulse to jump out of the window, to cut her baby's throat or throw it downstairs. Thea 100,000c, Fincke, cured.

A man who had been many years in the East and was used to one-story houses, on his return to the West had a curious impulse to jump out of the window, which he traced to tea-drinking and which disappeared when he left it off.

Teste noted that the homicidal impulse appeared in the dreams of one prover, who was so far from being horrified by his dream-murders that he even took pleasure in them after awaking. The talkativeness of Thea. is one of its chief allurements.

Among tea-tasters, who do not drink the tea they taste, but only hold it in the mouth a short time, yet long enough for the mouth to absorb some, there is sometimes developed what is known as tea-tasters' paralysis, affecting mostly the lower limbs with loss of sensation of both upper and lower.

A man, after drinking tea, had pain in his epigastrium going through to his back with a feeling as if he wanted to be sick and could not, better sitting down and stretching out. Thuj. 30c cured.

Guernsey gave these as indications for Thea, "Nervous sleeplessness, heart troubles. of old tea-drinkers, palpitations of the heart, can't lie down."

RELATIONS - ***Antidote:*** Thuj., Ferr., Kali-hp. - Material doses for tea-taster's cough. ***Antidoted by:*** Beer. ***Compare:*** (1) Gone, faint feeling, sick-headache radiating from one point and pain in left ovary, Sep. (2) Averse to work, especially writing, Hydr. (3) Relaxed feeling in stomach, Ip. (4) Desire for acids, Verat., Sulph., Ant-c., Phos., Sabin.

REFERENCES - Boericke. Clarke.

THERIDION CURASSAVICUM

(Orange Spider)

PHARMACY - ther. Theridion curassavicum. Orange spider. Latrodectus curassavicus. N. O. Arachnida. West-Indies. Tincture of the whole spider. ***Historical dose:*** All potencies.

CLINICAL - Angina pectoris. Anthrax, sheep. Bone, disorders. Decay. Menopause. Coughs. Dysmenorrhea. Eye-teeth, pains. Fainting. Headaches. Hysteria. Liver, disorder, abscess. Marasmus. Ménière's disease. Nausea. Necrosis. Nose, catarrh. Ozaena. Photophobia. Pregnancy, sickness. Rickets. Scrofulosis. Seasickness. Spinal, irritation. Tetanus. Toothache. ***Tuberculosis.*** Vertigo.

HOMEOPATHIC - Ther. was introduced and proved by Hering in 1832. The spider is found in the West Indies, chiefly in the island of Curacao. It is about the size of a cherry-stone and is found on orange-trees. It is velvety black when young with antero-posterior lines composed of white dots, on the posterior of the body there are three orange-red spots and on the belly a large square yellow spot.

The spider is very poisonous. It produces a highly sensitive, nervous condition with weakness, trembling, coldness, anxiety, faintness and easily excited cold sweat. Venom produces hypersensitiveness of the nerves. ***Sensitive to noise, which penetrates the body.***

It affects the teeth, causes nausea, chills and pains all over, strikes the painful parts etc. Nervous hyperesthesia. Noises seem to strike on painful spots over the body.

Affinity for the ***tubercular diathesis***. Tuberculosis, stitch high up in left apex (Anthr.). Where the indicated remedy does not hold long. Rickets, decay, necrosis. Vertigo, sick headache, peculiar pain around heart region, tuberculosis florida, and scrofula.

Spinal irritation. Decay and necrosis of the bones. Bones feel broken. Rickets. Burning pains. Water feels too cold. Bounding internally, as of a child. Sense of duality. Effects of sunstroke. Hysteria during puberty and at menopause. Infantile atrophy, glands enlarged with marasmus. Nodes on various parts especially buttocks. Seasickness. Left side most affected.

MIND - Restless, finds pleasure in nothing. Time passes too quickly. ***Sensitive to slightest noise.*** Startled by least thing. Confusion of mind, worse laughing. Insanity during menopause. Hysteria. Talkativeness and hilarity.

Want of self confidence. Aversion to work. Joyful during headache. Depression during headache. Weeping from toothache. Feels and looks as if dying, but hears and understands all that is said.

Abdomen - Violent burning in liver region. Abscess of liver. Pain in the groins after sex, motion and drawing up the limbs. Stinging pain on left side over anterior aspect of spleen.

Back - Stinging pains. Spine is sensitive to pressure and jar, sits sideways in a chair to avoid pressure. Sensitiveness between vertebra.

Causations - Seasickness. Washing clothes. Riding.

Chest - Stitches high up in chest, back through apex of left lung. Pain in upper left chest (Myrt., Pix., Anis.). ***Pain in left floating ribs.*** Pinching in left pectoral muscle.

Constitutions - Tubercular diathesis.

Ears - Least noise, even sound penetrates her whole body, especially teeth. Rushing in both ears like a waterfall.

Eyes - Glittering vision, on stooping. Luminous vibrations before eyes. Blurred vision. Sensitive to light. Pressure behind eyeballs. Throbbing over left eye.

Face - Pale. Jaws immovable in the morning.

Female - Hysteria during puberty, at menopause. Menses suppressed.

Food - Constant desire to eat and drink but knows not for what. Craves oranges and bananas, acid fruits and drinks, wine, tobacco smoke.

Head - Head internally hot, oppressed and heavy. Head feels thick, thinks it belongs to another, that she can lift it off or she would like to remove it. Migraine. Headache, felt during sleep, worse jarring, with nausea and vomiting, at menopause. Headache worse after stool. Cannot lie down with headache. Pain worse anyone walking over floor.

Heart - ***Cardiac anxiety and pain***. Anxiety about the heart, sharp pain radiates to arm and left shoulder. Pulse slow with vertigo.

Kidneys - Increased urination, at night, does not pass much during day.

Limbs - Burning in upper arm. Restless feeling in hands, wrings them. Stinging from elbow to shoulder. Lies or sits with feet crossed, cannot uncross them.

Lungs - Cough, jerks body together, head forward and knees upward. Too much air seems to enter the chest. Breathing difficult going up and down stairs, hysteria. Tuberculosis.

Male - Gonorrhea. Prostate enlarged, sense of a lump and heaviness in perineum, worse at even step. Seminal emission during afternoon sleep.

Modalities - Better from rest in horizontal position. Warm water improves nausea and retching. Warmth improves. ***Worse touch, pressure***, jar, left side. Worse least motion, exertion, stooping, rising, walking, going up or down stairs. Worse sex, particularly groin pain. Worse on shipboard, riding in carriage. ***Worse from noise.*** Worse from cold, washing clothes, sunstroke. ***Worse closing eyes***.

Mouth - Mouth feels furred, benumbed.

Froth before the mouth with shaking chill. Teeth feel as if cold water is too cold. Bites tip of tongue during sleep. Lockjaw, morning on waking. Remains open involuntarily, cannot close.

Nose - Pain over root of nose. Ozaena. Chronic catarrh, yellow-green, thick offensive, discharge. Discharge is yellowish and offensive. Post-nasal catarrh (Puls., Thuj.).

Sensations - As if her head was another strange head. As if vertex did not belong to her. Like a pressing pain in root of nose and about ears. As of a veil before eyes. As if something in esophagus were slipping towards epigastrium. Like labor pains in lower abdomen. As if a child were bounding in body. As if bones were broken and would fall asunder. As if dying.

Skin - ***Stinging, stabs everywhere***. Itching sensations. Sensitive skin on the thighs.

Stomach - Seasickness. Nausea and vomiting when closing eyes and on motion (Tab.). Nausea worse least motion, looking steadily at one object from noise. Nausea and retching better drinking warm water.

Temperature - Shaking chill with foam at mouth. Internal coldness. Cold sweat easily excited.

Vertigo - Faints after washing clothes. Vertigo with nausea, worse stooping, kneeling. ***Vertigo with nausea and vomiting on least motion***, worse when closing eyes.

COMMENTS - Grimmer stated, "The orange spider poison can cure when indicated on the totality of its symptoms. Decay of bones, abscesses and cancer of the liver and lungs. It acts profoundly on the nervous system, producing extreme sensitivity to noise the vibration penetrating to the teeth."

Keynotes extreme sensitiveness to noise, worse by least noise, "sounds penetrate the teeth." The sensitiveness extends to vibrations of any kind, jar of a step, riding in a carriage or in a boat.

"Worse closing eyes," especially in vertigo and symptoms of the head and stomach. Seasickness or sickness of pregnancy. Severe headaches, affecting the eyes, especially the left. The ears are highly sensitive. Intolerance of light.

Frequent cough, convulsive, head spasmodically jerked forward, knees jerked up to abdomen. Hallucinations of sight and hearing, luminous vibrations and rushing sounds. A kind of intoxication is induced, hilarity, talkativeness. "Time passes too slowly."

Burning pains and itching are common and a stitch high up in apex of left chest has proved a guiding symptom for Ther. in the cure of cases of tuberculosis. "Burning in liver region" led to the cure of abscess and even cancer of that organ.

H. C. Allen noted it for spinal irritation and disease of the spine and other bones. Decay, necrosis and scrofulous disease of bones have all been cured with it. "In scrofulosis when the best remedies fail to relieve."

Chackravarti related a case of headache cured with Ther. Mr. B., 35, well built of bilious temperament, had for three months severe headache with nausea and vomiting like seasickness and shaking chills. Dullness and fullness in the head with throbbing beginning in occiput, preceded by flickering before the eyes.

Head felt large and heavy. The pains began in the morning increase during the day and last until evening. Excessive irritation with loss of sustaining power. Worse from least overwork and motion, better by keeping quiet in horizontal position. Constipation, stools hard, small, dry.

Ther. 3x was given, one drop in water twice daily. The pain was much better the next day and was gone in less than a week.

RELATIONS - ***Antidoted by:*** Acon. (sensitiveness to noises), Mosch. (nausea), Graph. (more chronic effects). Follows well: Sulph., Calc., Lyc. (scrofula). ***Compare:*** (1) Aran-d. and Spiders generally. (2) Hemicrania worse closing eyes, worse noise, Sep. (But Sep. worse from noise is less intense). (3) Vertigo and faintness on closing eyes, Lach. (4) Headache, nervousness, hysteria, Tarent. (5) Stooping down, violent stitch high up in left chest, thence to back, Myrt-c. through to left scapula. (6) Time passes too quickly (too slowly Cann-i., Arg-n., Nux-m.). (7) Vertigo on closing eyes, Lach., Thuj. (on opening them, Tab., on looking up, Puls. Sil.). (8) Headache, worse lying down, Lach.

REFERENCES - Boericke. Clarke. Grimmer. Phatak.

THEVETIA NERIFOLIA

(Ahovai Tree)

PHARMACY - thev. Thevetia nerifolia. Ahovai tree. Cerbera thevetia. Ahovai tree of the Antilles. N. O. Apocynaceae. Tincture or trituration of the seeds. ***Historical dose:*** All potencies.

CLINICAL - Diarrhea. Somnolence. Throat, disorders. Vomiting.

HOMEOPATHIC - J. Balfour observed the effect of eating the seeds on two boys, age 7 and 8 years old. He noted "A tendency to sleep, disturbed every three to four minutes by irritation in the throat and the discharge of a mouthful of frothy mucus with a sort of gulp, then the child would lie down and close his eyes until again disturbed."

RELATIONS - ***Compare:*** (1) Apoc. Stroph. Upa.

REFERENCES - Clarke.

THIOSINAMINUM

(Mustard Seed Oil)

PHARMACY - thiosin. Thiosinaminum. Mustard seed oil. Rhodallinum. Rhodallin. Cruciferae. Allyl sulphocarbamide, derived from Mustard seed oil. Trituration of the crystals. Solution in alcohol. ***Historical dose:*** Tincture and all potencies.

CLINICAL - Adenitis. Adhesions. Allergies. Alzheimer's disease. Ankylosis. Arteriosclerosis. Arthritis. Carpal tunnel syndrome. Cataract. Cicatrices. Contractures. Cornea, opacities. ***Deafness.*** Dupuytren's, contracture. Ectropion. Emphysema. Fibroids. Frozen, shoulder. Glands, enlarged. Glands, indurated. Indigestion. Indurations. ***Keloids.*** Lupus. Lymphatic glands, enlarged. Ménière's disease. Old, age. Otitis, media. ***Otosclerosis.*** Painful, adhesions. Premature, aging. Rectum, stricture. ***Scar, tissue.*** Scleroderma. Senile, dementia. Stiffness. Strictures. Tabes dorsalis. Tennis, elbow. ***Tinnitus.*** Tumors. Urticaria. Uterine, tumors. Wounds.

HERBAL - Thiosinaminum belongs to the same chemical group as Urea. The colorless, bitter crystals are soluble in water, alcohol and ether.

HOMEOPATHIC - Thiosin. has been effective in curing adhesions, scars, lupus and enlarged lymphatic glands. It's a dissolvent, externally and internally, for ***dissolving scar tissue, keloids***. It has been used for tumors, enlarged glands, lupus, strictures, adhesions. Inflamed, swollen glands, adenitis.

Ectropion, opacities of cornea, cataract, ankylosis, fibroids, scleroderma. Noises in ear. ***Tinnitus aurium***, deafness. Gastric, vesicle and rectal crises. Strictures of rectum. Tumors of the uterus appendages.

For tabes dorsalis, improving the lightning pains. Sensation of heat and burning in affected parts. Increases body weight and reduces glandular swellings. Dr. A. S. Hard suggested Thiosin. for retarding old age.

MIND - Depression of spirits. Aversion to consolation. Moody, alternating moods. Alzheimer's disease. Senile dementia.

Abdomen - Flatulence. Internal adhesions after surgery, after hysterectomy, etc. Intestinal strictures.

Back - Torn ligaments in the shoulder. Frozen shoulder.

Ears - Ménière's syndrome, vertigo. Noises in ear. ***Tinnitus*** caused by fibrous bands. Formation of fibrous bands impeding free movement of the ossicles. ***Otosclerosis.*** Suppurative otitis media. ***Thickened eardrum.*** Catarrhal deafness with scar thickenings. Deafness due to some fibrous change in the nerve. Adhesions of the Eustachian tube. Eustachian tube catarrh.

Eyes - Cataract of the lens or cornea. Stricture of the lachrymal duct.

Female - Painful uterine adhesions, pelvic inflammation. Uterine tumors. Infertility.

Food - Increased appetite.

Kidneys - Strictures of the urethra and painful urination. Urine increased in quantity, no albumen or formed elements. Increased urination at night.

Limbs - Locomotor ataxia. Stiffness of joints.

Lungs - Accelerated respiration. Emphysema.

Nose - Allergies.

Rectum - Stricture of rectum.

Skin - Wounds that are slow to heal. Wounds that form a lot of scar tissue. ***Scar tissues.*** Granulations, scars, keloids after burns, wounds. Inelasticity of the skin. Indurations. Urticaria. Lupus.

Stomach - Indigestion, flatulence of stomach and bowels, worse after eating. Pyloric stenosis. Stricture of esophagus.

Vertigo - Arteriosclerotic vertigo. Ménière's syndrome, vertigo.

COMMENTS - The mustard seeds of Sin-n. are of a reddish-brown color. Mixed with those of Sin-a., they are crushed between rollers and subsequently powdered and sifted at least twice. A fixed oil is obtained by pressure from the residue left on the sieve. The powdered mustard is mixed with a considerable quantity of wheaten flour and a small quantity of turmeric powder.

The Treasury of Botany noted that "The term 'flour of mustard' is not quite accurate, as the mustard seeds themselves contain little or no starchy material. The chemical ingredients are somewhat complex. Among them are a peculiar acid called Myronic acid, noticeable as containing a large proportion of Sulphur. When mixed with water and a peculiar substance called Myrosine, (analogous to albumen), also found in mustard seeds, yields a volatile Oil of Mustard.

"This has no separate existence in the seeds, but is formed artificially in the manner just stated. This oil is very acrid and has been used as a rubefacient. The fixed oil before mentioned as existing in the seed itself has little or no acridity and has been used as a purgative and vermifuge."

Scar tissue and adhesions. Ringing in the ears. Tinnitus or deafness in elderly people from otosclerosis. The bones of the ears get calcium deposits. Scarred eardrums or eardrums that thicken and cause hearing difficulties. Chronic ruptured eardrums in children (Calen. acutely). Ménière's disease (Chin-s.). Vertigo. Opacities of the cornea, cataracts.

Torn ligaments, especially in the shoulder. Painful adhesions affecting mobility of a joint. Internal adhesions of the uterus, adhesions after surgery. Strictures of the urethra and painful urination.

Dr. McCullogh found that it exerts a marked beneficial action on ear diseases accompanied by the formation of new connective tissue. He believed that this beneficial action was due to an increased pliability of this tissue. Its administration should always be accompanied by mechanical measures; better and more prompt results may be obtained in recent cases.

McCullogh also noted a beneficial action on vertigo and better results may be obtained with it in the relief of tinnitus aurium than with any drug used previously.

C. H. Pennoyer related the case of Mrs. C., 69, who had been ill for several years with gastric distress, sciatica, pains in hips down to knees, worse by motion. She had indigestion, flatulence of stomach and bowels, worse after eating. Pain in back. Inability to walk, much perspiration, depression of spirits and subnormal temperature. Her father had died at 69 of stomach trouble, mother at 58 of stricture of the bowel.

Examination showed stricture of the rectum two inches above the anus, there being a tense fibrous band forming a ring opening, which would not admit the index finger. Bougies and mechanical measures failed to relieve. Weakness was so great, the patient would faint at stool. Nutrition improved under general treatment, but the local condition was unchanged.

A year later the stricture was slightly increased. Thiosin. was then given, 2 grains. twice daily. The following year the patient was found to be much improved. Examination showed that the scar band had gone, the speculum could be introduced and the mucus membrane was normal in appearance, though not as elastic as a normal rectum should be.

W. Spencer applied this property of

resolving scar tissues in cases of tinnitus aurium "where the ossicles are bound down and the function of the tympanic cavity so much impaired by fibrous bands or adhesions." In such cases he had encouraging success. Enlarged lymphatic glands have been reduced in the same way.

RELATIONS - ***Compare:*** (1) Sil., Calen., Sinapis and Cruciferae. (2) Uterine tumors, Thlaspi. (3) Diuresis - also chemical. (4) Urea. Lup., Tub. (5) Scars. Sil., Graph., Fl-ac. (6) Affections of rectum, Nit-ac., Graph., Scirr.

REFERENCES - Anshutz. Boericke. Clarke. Grimmer. Murphy. Phatak.

THLASPI BURSA PASTORIS

(Shepherd's Purse)

PHARMACY - thlaspi. Thlaspi bursa pastoris. Shepherd's purse. Bursa pastoris. Capsella bursa pastoris. N. O. Cruciferae. Tincture of fresh flowering plant. ***Historical dose:*** Tincture and all potencies.

CLINICAL - Albuminuria. Colic. ***Cystitis.*** Dropsy. Dysentery. Dysuria. Fibroma. Fibroids, uterine. Flatulence. Gallstones. Gonorrhea. Hematuria. ***Hemorrhages.*** Kidney, stones. Leucorrhea. Liver, disorders. Metrorrhagia. Miscarriage. Nausea. Nosebleed. Ranula. Strangury. Urethritis. ***Uric acid, diathesis. Uterine, bleeding***. Uterus, cancer. Whitlow.

HERBAL - The Treasury of Botany noted that Thlaspi is "A native of Europe, it has accompanied Europeans in all their migrations and established itself wherever they have settled to until the soil." It does not refuse to grow in the poorest soils, but it luxuriates in the richest.

Burnett noticed that it flourished best in the neighborhood of dunghills and the odor of the tincture is much suggestive thereof. Some have seen in the seed-vessel the signature of the shape of the uterus.

Burnett found in it an organ remedy of vast importance. He said the tincture is the best thing to give for menses that have been checked, for uterine hemorrhages he preferred the potencies.

HOMEOPATHIC - Hemorrhagic and ***uric acid diathesis.*** Hemorrhages are profuse, periodic, blood dark, clotted. Uterine hemorrhage with cramps and expulsion of clots. Hemorrhage from uterine fibroid with aching in back or general bruised soreness. Bleeding fibroids.

Bleeding between the menses. Tendencies to miscarriage. Bleeding at ovulation or postpartum hemorrhage of dark, red, oozing blood (Ham.). Passive bleeding. Hemorrhage with burning or a mild bladder problem.

Uterine hemorrhages concomitant with bladder infections. Albuminuria during pregnancy. Kidney and bladder irritation. Kidney stone formation (Sars., Lyc.). ***Chronic cystitis.*** Craves buttermilk. The toes are affected along with cramping pain in stomach. Chronic neuralgia. Aching between scapulae.

MIND - Impulse to walk far. Restless, goes from room to room. Agony because of pains. Spells of causeless weeping. Stupefied and dull, as if she had not slept enough.

Abdomen - Flatulence. Pain between end of sternum and umbilicus like needles or an electric shock. Cramping pain, better bending over. Bloated after eating, with loud emissions of flatus; bowels feel as if drawn down and out.

Back - Continued pain in small of back. Morning backache. Wakes with violent pain between the shoulders. Weakness between scapula. Weakness between shoulders on rising.

Breasts - Milky water from right nipple. Shooting pains in right breast.

Causations - Suppression of hemorrhages or vaginal discharges.

Chest - Pulsative pain in left chest. Pain, uneasiness, and pressure behind the sternum.

Ears - Deafness and pain in left ear. Sensation as if something pushing in right ear. Spasmodic drawing from right ear to right lower jaw. Dry eruptions behind the ears. Small vesicles, with yellow points, above right ear. Scaly eruptions behind ears, with fissures in the fold. Sensation as of an insect entering the left ear, making buzzing noise, relieved by boring in ear with fingers.

Eyes - Eyes puffy. Dusky eyes, shiny and with dilated pupils. Dull ache behind eyes on awaking in the morning with aching in nape. Blurred vision. Sensation as if eyes are swollen, as if the ball was pressed inward. Sensation as of dust in eyes, worse after sewing or using eyes.

Face - Eyes and face puffy. Face feels parched and dry. Miserable countenance.

Female - Menses bright red and profuse. Menses too frequent and copious. Every alternate period very profuse. Menstrual blood stains indelibly. Leucorrhea before and after menses, bloody, dark offensive. ***Leucorrhea stains indelibly,*** smells foul, excites itching. Scarcely recovers from one period before another begins. Metrorrhagia. Cutting pain from side to side across pubes, worse by standing. ***Sore pain in uterus on rising. Uterine bleeding with violent uterine colic.*** Uterine fibroids with cramps and expulsion of clots. Sexual excitement.

Food - Aversion to the sight of food. Aversion to potatoes. Craves buttermilk, juicy fruits. Oat cakes are eaten with a relish. Desire for bread and butter, which does not taste good. Nausea better after strawberries.

Head - Headache, with great fullness. Frontal pain, worse toward evening. Pain from above eyes up over head to nape. Scaly eruption behind ears. Sharp pain over right eye, drawing eye upwards, behind right eye. Heaviness over eyes. Pressing pain in forehead. Stupefying pressing pain in forehead. Violent headache, lasting all night.

Heart - Feels large and sore, then throbbings go up into back of neck. Stitching pains at the apex. Palpitations worse in the morning in bed. Palpitation ending with cough. Pain left side of apex.

Kidneys - ***Chronic cystitis.*** Kidney colic and stones. Urethritis, urine runs away in little jets. Frequent desire. ***Urine heavy***, phosphatic. Accumulation of gravel, ***brick-dust sediment***. Hematuria. Albuminuria during pregnancy. Dysuria and spasmodic retention, after forceps delivery. Dysuria in the elderly, with dribbling. Often replaces the use of the catheter.

Limbs - Weariness in lower limbs, can hardly stand. Drawing pain in left thigh like gout. Severe pain and stiffness in right knee cap. Tearing, gouty pains left leg, worse in forenoon. Strained pain in right shoulder. Gouty pain in arm. Tearing, gnawing pain from elbow to throat. Rheumatic pain in left arm and shoulder blade, extending to throat. Hands tremble when holding anything. Swelling of veins of hand and arm. Tearing, wrenching pain in left wrist. Redness around root of nails. Lame feeling in right forefinger. Pain in the periosteum.

Liver - Gallstone colic, liver affection being secondary to uterine condition.

Lungs - Accumulation of phlegm in lungs. Convulsive cough, relieved as soon as phlegm is loosened. Hemoptysis. Dry cough on lying down with aching under left breast. Cough with irritation behind sternum. Fits of coughing as if the sternum pressed inward.

Male - Spermatic cord sensitive to concussion of walking or riding. Stitching in penis, running through to anus. Soreness of prepuce with intense itching or cold sensation (Agar.).

Modalities - Better bending over. Better cold bathing, dampness, Better open air, rapid motion. Worse every other month. Worse toward night. Worse suppression of hemorrhages or vaginal discharges.

Mouth - Bitter, slimy taste with dryness of mouth. Taste like bad eggs. Scratchy feeling in the palate. Mouth feels raw, as if from smoking strong tobacco. Mouth cracked in right corner and sore. Upper lip cracked. Teeth sore on closing jaws. Gums sore, neuralgic feeling in teeth.

Nose - Dull pain at root of nose. Gnawing pain in nasal bones. Soreness in nose, with tenderness on touch. Dryness of nose, preceded by sensations of bleeding. Bruised feeling each side of bridge, with bleeding from nose. Frequent nosebleeds. Nosebleed after nasal operations. Especially passive hemorrhage. Free discharge of blood and mucus from left nostril.

Perspiration - Sweat profuse at night.

Rectum - Passage of blood. Diarrhea mushy, brown, dark, urgent, and sometimes with nausea. Diarrhea yellowish color. Constipation. Slow and difficult stool. Obstinate slow stool with severe pressure and urging without effect. Hard, difficult, dry stool, leaving anus sore. Bleeding after hard stool. Troublesome itching and protrusion of hemorrhoids.

Sensations - Sensation as of needles or shocks between end of sternum and umbilicus. As if neck and left shoulder would break with pain.

Skin - Skin dry, hot, even to burning.

Sleep - Restless tossing about. Frequent wakening. Sleeplessness. Sleepy after eating or falls asleep while eating. Confused and unpleasant dreams when asleep.

Stomach - Sick, faint feeling in stomach. Emptiness feeling in stomach. Cramping pain in stomach, toes hurt as well as stomach. Flatulence. Sour rising like heartburn. Attacks of nausea. Nausea so severe, could hardly raise head from pillow. Tobacco smoke, of which she was fond, now nauseates her. Nausea in the forenoon. Nausea with loathing of food. Vomited brown, sourish blood in the afternoon. Vomiting and purging, with great debility.

Temperature - Alternate chill and sweat during headache. All night chills, with wakefulness and slight diarrhea with swelling of tonsils. Chill at 9 a.m. or from 7 p.m. to 9 p.m. Chilly when uncovering during fever. Chill worse from going into warm room during fever. Continued fever with quick pulse.

Throat - Hoarse in morning with slight sore throat. Soreness of upper part of throat. Swelling of throat and face, worse left side. Tonsils swollen. Dry throat on swallowing. Dryness of fauces, with sensation of constriction of the throat. Dry sensation and scraping. Violent sore throat. Sensation as if the throat was laced together.

Tongue - Tongue and palate feel as if scalded. Ranula, caused enlargement of submaxillary duct. Tongue white, coated. Taste like bad eggs.

Vertigo - Vertigo with sensation as if drunk. Dizziness in the forehead, like seasickness. Vertigo, worse rising.

COMMENTS - "Shepherd's purse," said Gerarde, "stayeth bleeding in any part of the body, whether the juice or the decoction thereof be drunk or whether it be used poultice-wise or in both or any way else. In a clyster it cureth the bloody flux, it healeth green and bleeding wounds, it is marvelous good for inflammations new beginning and for all diseases which must be checked back and cooled."

Gerarde added that the decoction will stop diarrhea, blood-spitting, hematuria and all other fluxes of blood. Burnett noted it for the effects of suppressed uterine disease.

Burnett observed it cause sexual excitement like Canth. It aided him in the cure of an inveterate case of gallstones, the origin of which he traced to the uterus.

Dudgeon reported the case of a woman who had recovered from jaundice. She then had a peculiar discharge after the menses flux of a brownish-green blood which was attended with obscure abdominal pains. The cervix uterus was swollen and soft but not ulcerated.

Dudgeon failed to cure this, but Rafinesque of Paris, after trying other remedies, succeeded with Thlaspi. 6c, which had an immediate positive effect. Rafinesque then gave the tincture, and then again the 6c, and in a few weeks the cure was complete.

Dudgeon, in an article on Thlaspi., quoted a case of Rademacher's showing the action of Thlaspi. on uric acid excretion.

A woman whom Rademacher had relieved ten years before of a large quantity of urinary sand, again presented herself; her abdominal cavity was full of water, extremely swollen and she was passing urine of a light red color with bloody sediment. Thlaspi. tincture, 30 drops five times a day, was given solely with the idea of stopping the hematuria. The result was a more copious discharge of urinary sand than ever before, the urine increased, the dropsy disappeared and the woman was cured.

Dudgeon's own cases are no less striking. One such case concerned a woman, 76, who had rheumatic muscular pains in various parts and an abundant secretion of uric acid, which passed away with every discharge of urine.

Sometimes small stones formed and there was much pain in their passage along the ureter, but generally it passed in the form of coarse sand, which formed a thick layer at the bottom of the utensil. This sand continued to pass after the cessation of the rheumatic pains, which lasted six or seven weeks. Puls., Pic-ac., and Lyc. had no effect. Thlaspi. 1c diminished the sand to an insignificant amount.

Dudgeon also noted the case of a man, 57, who, in addition to other dyspeptic symptoms, had unusually large discharges of coarse uric acid, coming away in masses as large as a big pin's head but without pain. Thlaspi 1x stopped this.

He also recorded the case of a woman, nearly 80, who suffered from the presence of a calculus in left ureter. She had previously passed much sand. Thlaspi. 1x caused a great discharge of sand and a speedy relief of her pain.

Dudgeon referred to a case of Harper's illustrating the action of Thlaspi. on the bowels. An elderly woman had suffered for years from a copious discharge of mucus, pus, sometimes mixed with blood, sometimes nearly all blood, which passed from the bowels after each evacuation. She had been under high homeopathy, oxygen treatment and for a long time under Harper's care, all without effect. He then gave Thlaspi. tincture in 5 drop doses and cured the case in a few days.

Clarke, with Thlaspi. 1x, saved a woman who had been curetted several times with little success from a further curetting, which was advised as being essential to the cure. Thlaspi. stopped the hemorrhages, restored the periods to their proper term and the patient immediately began to recover her strength, which had been drained to the last degree. There was no return of the trouble.

RELATIONS - ***Compare:*** (1) Urt-u., Croc., Trill., Mill. (2) Cruciferae, especially Sinapis. (3) Thiosin. - fibroma, uterine tumors. (4) Matth. - inspissated secretions, grows near sewage stream. (5) Kidney stones, Oci. (6) Uric acid, pain in shoulder, Urt-u. (7) Uterine hemorrhages, Trill., Vib., Ust., Senec. (8) Hemorrhages from bowel, Merc., Nit-ac., Sulph., Caps., Merc-c., Phos.

REFERENCES - Boericke. Clarke. Murphy.

THUJA LOBBI

(Red Cedar of Alaska)

PHARMACY - thuj-l. Thuja lobbi. Red cedar of Alaska. Thuja menziessi. Thuja plicata. N. O. Coniferae. The tincture is prepared with the fresh leaves. ***Historical dose:*** Tincture and all potencies.

HOMEOPATHIC - Thuja lobbi or Red Cedar is a tree which is almost 50 meters high and which originates from Alaska. From the heart-wood are separated out the Thuja plicines with antibiotic, as well as anti-fungal properties. These substances also exist in Thuja occidentalis.

There is no homeopathic proving for this remedy, but Dano conducted a clinical proving with it in 1934. Thuj-l. has emaciation and constipation. Chilly and the limbs are cold.

MIND - Anxious melancholy. Weeps and moans easily. Indifferent to everything except for his obsessions with his own suicide. Depressive neurotic condition. Psychosis from anguish. Lack of will-power. Personality problems with those around him. Hebephrenia.

COMMENTS - If the development within the compass of homeopathic remedies is followed, according to Roy, Thuja lobbi can be situated on the line: Aur., Sep., Thuja lobbi.

The tendency to suicide, which is characteristic of Aur. and the indifferent psychological disposition which characterizes Sep., can be anticipated in the development of a symptomatological picture for this remedy.

RELATIONS - ***Compare:*** (1) Tendency to suicide (Aur.) and indifferent disposition (Sep., Ph-ac.).

REFERENCES - Julian.

THUJA OCCIDENTALIS

(Arbor Vitae)

PHARMACY - thuj. Thuja occidentalis. Arbor vitae. N. O. Coniferae, Tribe, Cupresineae. Tincture of the fresh green twigs. ***Historical dose:*** Tincture and all potencies. Locally, for warts and excrescences, tincture or cerate.

CLINICAL - Abdomen, distended. ***Anal, warts.*** Angina pectoris. Anus, fissure. ***Asthma.*** Balanitis. Bedwetting. Cancer. Catalepsy. Chorea. Clavus. Colic. ***Condylomata.*** Constipation. Convulsions. ***Cysts.*** Diarrhea. Dyspareunia. Dysmenorrhea. Ear, polyps. ***Emaciation***. Epilepsy. Epulis. Eyes, inflammation. Eyes, tumors. Fatty, tumors. Feet, fetid. ***Flatulence.*** Fibroids. ***Fig, warts***. Ganglion. ***Gleet. Gonorrhea.*** Hemorrhage. Hair, disorders. Headaches. Hemorrhoids. Hernia. Herpes zoster. Ichthyosis. Intussusception. Joints, cracking. ***Leucorrhea.*** Miscarriage. ***Moles.*** Morvan's, disease. Mucous, patches. Muscae, volitantes. Myopia. ***Nevus. Nasal, catarrh.*** Neck, stiff. Onanism. ***Ovarian, cysts.*** Ovary, pain. Ozaena. Neuralgias. Nose, catarrh, polyps. Paralysis. Pemphigus. ***Polyps. Post-nasal, catarrh.*** Pregnancy, imaginary. Prostate, disease. Ptosis. Ranula. Rheumatism. Rickets. Sciatica. Seminal, emissions. ***Sinusitis.*** Smallpox. ***Sycosis.*** Syphilis. Tea, effects. Teeth, decay. Tongue, ulcers. Toothache. Tumors. ***Vaccination, effects. Vaccinosis***. Vaginismus. ***Vaginitis.*** Variola. ***Venereal, warts. Warts.*** Whooping cough.

HERBAL - Thuja was introduced to France from Canada during the reign of Francis I, and it now has an honored place in many gardens and shrubbery. The native habitat of Thuja is not without its importance in relation to therapeutics. It loves swamps, it is Hahnemann's typical anti-sycotic and Grauvogl's hydrogenoid.

HOMEOPATHIC - Thuj. is one of Hahnemann's discoveries. Most of the remedies of his Materia Medica had been known in a fashion before his time, but practically nothing was known of the therapeutic properties of Thuj. until Hahnemann proved it. Old-school observers found in Thuj. an efficient hemostatic, locally applied, especially after tooth extraction.

Hahnemann found Thuj. to be an antidote to the sycotic miasm, meaning the constitutional disease resulting from suppressed gonorrhea and having ***warty growths*** as its characteristic manifestation. Soft, spongy warts, emitting a fetid fluid with a sweetish odor something like herring brine. Warts that bleed readily and having the coxcomb or cauliflower form.

Thuj. acts chiefly on the mucus membranes of genito-urinary tract intestines, skin, mind, nerves, glands, occiput and left side. Acts on skin, blood, gastro-intestinal tract, kidneys and brain.

Wart-like growths on mucus and skin surfaces. Soft, exuberant, fungoid tissue, ***polyps, condylomata, warts,*** pediculated, black, suppressed. Spongy tumors, ***fig warts***, bleeding fungus growths. Birthmarks. Moist mucus tubercles.

Antibacterial action, as in gonorrhea and vaccination. ***Vaccinosis, never well since vaccination,*** neuralgia, skin troubles etc. Variola, aborts the pustule and prevents the suppurating fever. ***Suppressed gonorrhea.*** Crying babies with a sycotic taint from the parents. Complaints from moonlight.

Burning, sticking, numbing, drawing or wandering pains worse warmth. Sycotic pains, tearing in muscles and joints, worse at rest, better in dry weather, worse damp humid atmosphere, lameness. Left-sided and chilly medicine.

Great prostration. ***Rapid exhaustion and emaciation***. Neurasthenia, prostatic weakness. The patient is exhausted and soft, body feels thin and delicate, frail. Deadness of the affected part. Sensation of lightness of body when walking.

Flesh feels as if beaten off the bones. Edema about the joints. Pains keep extending from original site. Stitching, tearing pains in the glands as if they were being torn to pieces. Rheumatism. Paralysis. Jerking of the upper part of the body of spinal origin, chorea.

Discharges are foul, acrid, musty, rancid or of sweetish odor. Oily, stools, skin, sweat. Trickling in urethra. Congenital inguinal hernia. Venous stasis. Aneurysm by anastomosis, swelling of the blood vessels.

MIND - Introverted and private. ***Dullness of mind.*** Cannot concentrate. Speech slow, hunts for words. Hurried with ill humor, talks hastily, swallows words. Makes mistakes in writing and talking. Uses wrong words or omits words and syllables.

Confusion in morning. Loses his way in well-known streets. Cretinism. Imbecility of mind and loss of speech after vaccination. Vanishing of thoughts while speaking. Disinclined to talk, worse on awaking mornings.

Sadness. Aversion to life. ***Depression, feels isolated and alone.*** Aversion to company. Feels isolated and different from everyone, that they do not belong. Avoids the sight of people. Mental depression after childbirth (Sep.). Irritable, jealous, quarrelsome towards husband or mother.

Self-contempt. Reproaches himself. ***Thinks she is ugly or unclean.*** Feels unlovable. Emotional sensitivity. Music causes weeping and trembling. When spoken to answers with tears and sobbing.

Anxiety about salvation. Anxiety about health. Anger from contradiction. Overexcited, angry or anxious about trifles. Restlessness with ill-humor. Walks in a circle in room. Talks hastily.

Fear of getting infections, diseases, germs. Despair of recovery. Fear of being incurable, of death. ***Thinks his blood is dirty or poisoned.*** Insane women who will not be touched or approached. Fear of the wind.

Fear of strangers. Nervous, begins to twitch at approach of strangers. Mistrustful, secretive and paranoid. Fear of being discovered, and their secrets will be revealed. Full of hidden plans and secrets. Tells lies to hide real intentions. Manipulates others. Controls herself among strangers and doctors. Fanaticism.

Indifference to opposite sex. ***Fear of getting venereal diseases.*** Religious fanatics. Religious aversion to sex (Puls.). Feels sex is dirty, shameful, sinful. ***Sexual perversions.*** Immoral sexual behavior. Secret and hidden sexual activities. Many sex partners. ***Sexual desires excessive and strange.***

Fixed ideas and delusions, as if a strange person were at his side. Delusions as if soul and body were separated, as if something alive in abdomen (Croc.). Delusions, ***as if body were fragile, made of glass***. Delusion as if being controlled by a stronger power. Imagines himself double or treble. Sudden impulse to kill herself. Time passes too quickly.

Abdomen - Distended. Indurations in abdomen. Intussusception of intestines. ***Flatulence and distention, protruding here and there***. Colic. Gurgling in bowels. Rumbling, flatulence, upper part drawn in. Movements in abdomen, ***as if something alive,*** without pain (Croc.). Soreness of navel. Cutting and squeezing in hypogastrium. Ileus. Cutting, squeezing in hypogastrium, groin. Stinging as from needles. Hernia. Stitches in inguinal glands. Soreness of navel. Yellowish or brownish spots on abdomen. Herpes zoster.

Back - Cramp-like pains. Drawing pain, when sitting, in sacrum, coccyx. Burning in lumbar region. Pulsation in the back. Pressive, bruised sensation in back. Pressing pain over kidney region. Atrophy of long muscles. Spine curved. Spinal curvature after vaccination. Stands bent forward. Boils on back. Blood boils. Steatomous tumors. Cervical glands swollen.

Bladder - Paralysis of sphincter of bladder. Bladder feels paralyzed, must wait for urination. Violent burning pain in fundus of bladder. Burning in urethra. Urethra swollen, inflamed. Cutting pains after urination (Sars.). Pain and burning felt near neck of bladder. Jerking, voluptuous sensation in fossa navicularis. Sensation as if a drop were running down urethra, after urination. ***Urinary stream forked and small.*** Frequent urging to urinate, with profuse flow. Frequent urination at night. Involuntary urination at night. Lithemia. Diabetes mellitus.

Breasts - Aching, pressing pains. Drawing pains, with swelling of both breasts. Sensitiveness and heaviness after the menses. Stinging and itching. Breast cysts, lumps and tumors. Indurations in left breast. Retracted nipples.

Causations - Suppressed sycosis. ***Badly treated or suppressed gonorrhea.*** Syphilis. ***Vaccinations.*** Sulphur, mercury. Sunstroke. ***Sexual excess.*** Tea, coffee, beer, tobacco. Sweets, fat meat, onions.

Chest - Stitches in chest, worse cold drinks. Chest pains take various directions. Pains radiating in various directions. Sensations as if falling drops in chest. Skin of clavicles blue. Brown spots on chest. Brown spots in axilla, like nevi. Skin on clavicles blue. Strong perspiration in axillae.

Constitutions - Suited to hydrogenoid constitutions. Strumous and sycotic pains. Lax muscles, light-haired adults and children. Lymphatic temperament in very fleshy persons, dark complexion, black hair, unhealthy skin.

Coughs - Dry, hacking cough in afternoon, with pain in pit of stomach. Cough only during the day or worse as soon as he eats or drinks anything cold. Constant cough without difficulty in breathing. Cough in morning after rising. Cough evenings after lying down.

Dreams - Anxious dreams. Dreams of teeth breaking off. Dreams of falling, of misfortune. Dreams of dead people, of bodies, of dying.

Ears - Chronic otitis, purulent discharge. Watery, purulent, putrid otorrhea. Chronic otorrhea after vaccination. Ear discharge smells like putrid meat. Polyps. Cracking in ears when empty swallowing. Noise in ear as from boiling water. Inner ear as if swollen with hardness of hearing.

Eyes - Conjunctivitis after vaccination. Blood-red eyes, full of tears, stand open. Styes and tarsal tumors (Staph.). Eyelids agglutinated at night, dry, scaly. Burning and stinging of eyelids. Lids heavy as lead. Jagged iris. Ciliary neuralgia. Iritis. Acute and chronic inflammation of sclera. Chronic scleritis. Chronic keratitis, with excessive photophobia, after vaccination. Small brown spots on cornea. Exophthalmos from tumors behind eyeball. Large, flat phlyctenules, indolent. Constant ache in eye, worse bright light. Feels as if cold air were streaming out of the head through eye, better when warmly covered. Photopsies, beyond visual field. Floating green stripes. Eye symptoms better warmth and covering.

Face - Pale, waxy, shiny, dark under eyes. Greasy skin of face. Light brown, freckles on face. Bloated. Edematous erysipelas of face. Eruptions leaves livid spots. Lips pale, swollen, peeling off. Twitching of lower lip. ***Warts.*** Tumor on cheek. Blood vessels of face and temples distended. Netted with spider-like veins. Boring in malar bones (left), better by touch. Face aches. Burning heat and redness of face. Neuralgia from suppressed gonorrhea or eczema of ear. Cracking of joint of jaw.

Female - Sweaty genitals before menses. Bearing down pain during menses. Menses too early, too short. Scanty, retarded menses. Burning in varicose veins of genitals during menses. ***Leucorrhea,*** profuse, thick, greenish leucorrhea, from one period to the next. ***Vaginitis.*** Vaginal itching. ***Vagina very sensitive,*** prevents sex (Staph., Plat.). ***Venereal warts.*** Fistula of rectum and vagina. Whitish ulcers on labium majorum. Warty growths on vulva and perineum. ***Uterine polyps***, fleshy excrescences. Cauliflower excrescences, bleeding easily. ***Ovarian cysts.*** Severe pain in left ovary and left inguinal region. Chronic ovaritis after gonorrhea. Ovaritis, worse left side, at every menstrual period (Lach.). Erosion of cervix. Fetus moves violently, awakes her. Prolapsed uterus. Miscarriage in the third month. Labor pains weak or ceasing.

Food - Complete loss of appetite. Craving alternating with want of appetite. No appetite, with mental depression. Unable to eat breakfast. Aversion to fresh meat, potatoes, ***onions and garlic.*** Desires chocolate, cold food, drinks and salt. Worse from beer, wine, acids, tobacco, onion, sweets. Bread tastes dry and bitter. Tea-drinking dyspepsia. Thirst increased, at night.

Glands - Adenitis. Tearing pains in glands. Enlarged, swollen glands.

Head - Left-sided headaches. ***Pain as if pierced by a nail*** (Coff., Ign.). Pressing in vertex, as from a nail. Tearing, jerking pain. Headache, worse sexual excess or tea, better bending head backwards. Feeling of numbness in brain. Sensation as if parietal bones were being knocked to pieces. Heaviness of occiput. Boring through the temples. Meningitis. Neuralgia from tea (Sel.). Wants head wrapped up. Honey smelling sweat. White scaly dandruff. Dry hair, splits and falls out. Warts.

Heart - Anxious palpitations, on waking in the morning. Stitches in region of heart. Cramp in heart. Visible palpitations, without anxiety. Excitement and pulsation of arteries before menses. Palpitations during menses. Palpitations from ascending. Violent pulsations in evening. Pulse full and accelerated in evening. Pulse slow and weak in morning. Swelling of veins.

Kidneys - Nephritis with swollen feet. Pains from left kidney to epigastrium, worse motion. Lithemia. Diabetes mellitus. Cutting, squeezing in bladder and urethra. Urethra swollen, inflamed. Forward cutting in urethra on urinating. Desire sudden and urgent, but cannot be controlled. Frequent urination, with profuse flow, with pain in other parts. Urine burns, dribbles, foul, foamy. Sensation of trickling after urinating, as if drop running down urethra. Involuntary urination at night, when coughing.

Limbs - Cracking in joints when stretching them. Muscular twitchings, weakness and trembling. Limbs feel as if made of wood or glass and would break easily. Limbs feels paralyzed. Hip joints give way when walking. Restless knees. Coxalgia with tender soles. Pain in heels and Achilles tendon. Foul, acrid foot sweat. Ingrown toenails. ***Nails brittle, ribbed, soft, distorted, discolored, crumbling.*** Crawling or inflamed finger or toe tips. Trembling of hands and feet. Fingers cold, numb, as if dead, on waking at night.

Lungs - Asthma with red face. ***Asthma in children*** (Ars., Nat-s.), especially vaccinated children, worse at night. Dyspnea from mucus in trachea. Short difficult breathing, worse from deep breathing and talking. Hemoptysis. Expectoration, easy when lying down, green. Expectoration tastes like old cheese. Loose expectoration and easy when he turns from left to right side.

Male - Balanitis. Burning between glans and prepuce. Itching in glans and prepuce. Inflammation, swelling of prepuce and glans, pain in penis. Moisture on glans. Glans very sensitive. Excrescences of prepuce and glans. ***Condylomata,*** fig warts. ***Venereal warts.*** Eczema on genitals. Whitish chancres with hard edges. Pain as from splinters in chancres. Herpes. ***Gonorrhea,*** scalding pain when urinating. ***Impotency*** after suppressed gonorrhea. Painful spermatic cords from suppressed gonorrhea. Rheumatism from suppressed gonorrhea. Prostatic enlargement and weakness (Sabal., Ferr-pic., Iod., Thiosin.). ***Offensive smelling genitals,*** sweetish smelling sweat on scrotum. Testes feel bruised, left drawn up. Chronic induration of testicles. Testes as if contused, worse walking. Chordee, worse at night. Jerking in penis. Masturbation habit. ***Sexual desire increased*** or decreased. ***Sexual excesses.*** Nightly painful erections causes sleeplessness. Nocturnal emissions followed by heaviness and ill-humor. Offensive semen.

Modalities - Better on left side, drawing up limbs, crossing limbs. Better motion. Better pressure, rubbing, scratching. Better wrapping, warmth, air, wind. Better free secretions, sneezing. ***Worse from cold and dampness***. Worse sun, bright light. Worse at night, closing eyes, from heat of bed, left side. Worse from increasing moon, moonlight. Worse at 3 a.m. and 3 p.m. Worse periodically, yearly. Worse touch, stretching. Worse after breakfast, after eating, chewing. Worse during menses. Worse urinating, sex. ***Worse after gonorrhea, after vaccinations, after suppressed warts.***

Mouth - Aphthae, ulcers in the mouth (Bor.). Varicose veins on tongue and mouth. Mouth becomes dry while chewing food. Mouth as if filled with blisters. Mouth as if it has been burnt. Sweetish taste with gonorrhea. Taste as of rotten eggs, in morning. Teeth decay at the edge of gums, crumble, turn yellow. Gnawing pain in teeth, worse cold, tea and blowing nose. Gums, very sensitive and retract. Pyorrhea alveolaris. Drinks fall audibly into stomach.

Nose - Warts on nose. Nose red and hot. Sinusitis. ***Chronic sinus infections***. Chronic catarrh after measles, scarlatina, variola. ***Chronic catarrh, thick, yellow-green mucus,*** blood and pus. Coryza fluent outdoors, dry in room. Violent, sudden coryza. Dryness of nasal cavities. Painful pressure at root of nose. Pain in teeth on blowing nose. Soreness and ulceration of nostrils, worse pressure. Ulceration within the nostrils. Painful scabs in nostrils. Bloody scabs or briny odor in nose. Nosebleed, worse after being over-heated. Smell in nose as of fish-brine or sour beer.

Perspiration - Profuse, sour. Sweetish and strong, smelling like honey. Sweat is foul, oily, pungent, sweetish, sometimes garlicky. Staining brownish, yellow. Profuse sweats at night, staining clothes yellow. Profuse sweat on genitals, gushing, worse company. ***Sweats only on uncovered parts*** or all over except head, when sleeping. Cadaverous exhalation of skin. Profuse, oily sweats, after asthmatic attacks.

Rectum - Constipation with violent rectal pain, causing stool to recede (Sil., Sanic.). Chronic diarrhea, worse after breakfast. ***Diarrhea after vaccination.*** Diarrhea periodically returning at same hour. Noiseless emission of flatus. Moisture oozing from anus, moist perineum. ***Anal fissure,*** painful to touch. ***Anal warts.*** Condylomata at anus. ***Venereal warts.*** Red blotches at anus like fig warts. Swollen hemorrhoids, pain worse sitting with stitching. Hemorrhoids sensitive to touch. Burning pains at the anus. Burning in perineum. Perineal fistula. Perineum moist.

Sensations - As if a strange person were at her side. As if under the influence of a superior power. As if soul and body were separated. As if whole body were very thin and delicate, as if its continuity would be dissolved, as if frail and easily broken, as if made of glass. As if a nail were pressing into vertex, as if a nail were driven from within outward in vertex. As if abdominal muscles were being pushed out by arm of a child. As if a living a animal were in abdomen. Legs as if made of wood when walking. As if lower limbs were elongated. As from flea bites.

Skin - Skin very sensitive to touch. Skin as if pricked with needles. One side cold. Dirty, hairy, dry skin with ***brown spots on hands and arms.*** Freckles and blotches. Eruptions itch or burn violently, worse cold bathing. ***Eruptions only on covered parts,*** worse after scratching. Herpetic eruptions. Herpes zoster. ***Polyps.*** Ringworm. Violent itching on different parts, as from fleabites. Pemphigus. Smallpox, useful during suppurative stage. Chickenpox. ***Warts.*** Warts in ano-genital region. Warts, large, seedy, pedunculated, oozing moisture and bleeding easily. ***Impetigo, with itching.*** Epithelioma. Sarcoma. Nevi, ***Birthmarks.*** Carbuncles and ulcers, in anal-genital region. Ulcers flat with bluish bottom. Foul pustules with sunken apices. Luxuriant growth of hair on parts otherwise not covered by hair. ***Nails crippled,*** brittle and soft.

Sleep - Persistent insomnia. Sleepless when lying on left side. Nocturnal sleeplessness with agitation and coldness of body. Sleeplessness after menses. Nightmare after menses. Dreams of death, of corpses or dead people. Dreams of falling from a height. Lascivious dreams without emission of semen with painful erections on waking. Awakens from too violent movements of fetus. Heavy sleep, can't get awake in morning.

Stomach - Cutting pain in epigastrium. Indurations in stomach. Sinking sensation in epigastrium before food, thirst. Flatulence, pain after food. Noisy swallowing, loud belchings. Gulping up of large quantities of acids. Eructations rancid or acrid. Eructations afford instant relief. Rancid belchings after fat food. Pressing in stomach, with retching, during menses. Vomiting of mucus, or of greasy substances.

Stools - Stools gurgle or pop out, hard, oily, black, lumps. Painless, grass green stools, mixed with gushing water. Stools hurried, explosive, gassy, spraying. Tenesmus of stool with rigidity of penis. Hard stool followed by soft stool. Hard balls. Large, hard stool coated with blood.

Teeth - Very sensitive teeth. Gnawing, in teeth, worse cold. Toothache before and after menses. Toothache on blowing nose. Teeth crumble, turn yellow. Teeth decay next to gums. Gums retracted. Gums swollen, inflamed, dark red. Pyorrhea alveolaris.

Temperature - Chilly from least change of weather. Shaking chill with yawning, worse urinating, not better by heat. Chill, beginning in thighs. Chill without thirst. Coldness of one side. General coldness during menses. Shivering from slightest uncovering in warm air. Heat rises into chest with icy told hands, nosebleed or cough. Orgasm of blood in the evening with throbbing in the blood vessels. Intermittent fever with chronic gonorrheal contamination.

Throat - Throat dry and rough. Polyps of vocal cords. Papilloma of larynx. Chronic laryngitis. Much mucus in throat, hawked up with difficulty. Painful swallowing. Sensations as if constricted when swallowing. Sensations as if a skin in larynx. Much mucus in throat hawked up with difficulty. Mucus tubercles in fauces.

Tongue - Tip of tongue very painful. Tongue as if it has been burnt. ***White blisters on side close to root, painfully sore***. Ranula, varicose veins on tongue and mouth. Frequently bites tongue, from swelling of tongue. Tongue swollen, worse right side. Ranula. Varicose veins on tongue and mouth.

Urine - Foamy urine. Split, small stream. ***Urinary stream forked and small.*** Discharge of glutinous moisture from urethra. ***Weak stream.*** Urine becomes cloudy after standing. Urine yellowish or wine-colored. Urine dark red in morning. Urine deposits a brown mucus. Urine with dark, cloudy sediment, in rheumatism. Urine highly colored and of strong smell. Urine profuse, light-yellow. Urine burns, dribbles, foul, foamy.

Vertigo - Vertigo as from motion of a swing. Vertigo everything seems to jump. Vertigo on closing eyes. Vertigo looking upwards or sideways. Reeling, as after turning in a circle. When rising from sitting; on stooping.

Vision - Shortsighted. Diplopia. Amblyopia with blurring, better rubbing. Misty or obscured, with dilated pupils. Dim vision as from mist or veil, in open air, with confusion of head. Flickering vision. Sees flames of light like fire-flies. Sees clouds and streaks. Muscae volitantes. Streaks of light or sparks passing downward. Objects appear smaller.

COMMENTS - Millspaugh noted that the American Arbor Vitae is a "spiry evergreen attaining a height of from 20 to 50 feet, though generally not above 40 and a diameter of about 10 to 20 feet through the greatest breadth of foliage. It assumes a conical form with such true lines as to appear 'clipped,' thus forming one of our most valued high-hedge trees.

"It abounds in the northern zones of North America from Pennsylvania northwards. There it "often forms what are commonly known as cedar-swamps. It grows upon the rocky banks of rivers and in low, swampy spots, blossoming from May until June and maturing its fruit in autumn."

Teste remarked that in the period when the doctrine of signatures prevailed, the "Resinous callosities of the stems and leaves of Thuja might have seemed an indication that the plant was the specific for sycosis and warts." Teste dismissed this idea, but he did ask whether resinous substances that have the power of modifying vegetable juices in a peculiar way may not affect the animal fluids in the same manner.

He included Castoreum canadense in his Thuj. group and followed by giving an instance in which it acted on fig-warts.

Castoreum canadense is the product of an animal that subsists on the bark of resinous trees.

Hering described Thuj.'s action on fluids as "dissolution of fluids of the body, which become acrid, probably caused by Thuja perverting lymphatic secretions, disturbs digestion and sanguification."

He went on to discuss Thuja's action in the vegetative sphere: "A surplus of producing life, nearly unlimited proliferation of pathological vegetations, condylomata, warty sycotic excrescences, spongy tumors and spongy pock exudates which organize hastily. All morbid manifestations are excessive, but appear quietly, so that the beginning of the diseased state is scarcely know."

Boenninghausen found Thuja both preventive and curative during an epidemic of smallpox. It aborted the disease process and prevented pitting. In veterinary practice, Thuja has proved curative in farcy and in "grease."

These clinical uses point to Thuj.'s affinity to vaccinations. No one has written more forcibly or lucidly on this than Burnett did in his book, Vaccinosis and its Cure by Thuja. "Arbor Vitae: nomen omen," said Burnett on his title page. In his hands, Thuj. proved to be a tree of life to numberless sufferers from the vaccination miasm.

By "vaccinosis" Burnett meant the disease known as vaccinia, the result of vaccination, in addition to "that profound and often long-lasting morbid constitutional state engendered by the vaccine virus." Thuj. is homeopathic to this state, and therefore curative and preventive of it.

Burnett made the observation, which Clarke confirmed, that the vaccination does not need to take in order to produce the vaccination miasm. Many people date their ill health from a so-called unsuccessful vaccination, so vaccinosis may exist apart from vaccinia. The anti-vaccinosis action of Thuj. is part of its anti-sycotic action, therefore vaccinosis is a sycotic disease.

Burnett noted the case of an infant, ten weeks old, whom he was called to see as it was supposed to be dying. He found it ghastly white and in collapse. There was nothing to account for this except that the baby had its wet-nurse changed two or three days before.

The wet-nurse was questioned and declared herself quite well and looked it, but "her arm was a little painful." She had been revaccinated in the Marylebone Workhouse the day before she took charge of the patient.

Burnett found the vaccine eruption just turning into the pustular stage. He concluded that the infant was sucking in the vaccine poison with its nurse's milk.

He gave Thuj. 6c to both infant and nurse. The baby gradually improved the same day and the next morning, though still pale, was practically well and the vaccine vesicles on the nurse's arm had withered.

Burnett quoted a case of vaccine rash in an infant following the vaccination of its mother, who was nursing it.

The effects of chronic vaccinosis are protean. Prominent among them are asthma, neuralgias, skin disorders, indigestion and constipation, warts and new growths of many kinds. Emaciation, brain damage, epilepsy and blindness. Hyperactivity, attention deficit disorder and autism.

In these effects, a favorite method of Burnett's was to give a course of twenty-four numbered powders, only three or four of them medicated with Thuj. 30c, one to be taken at bedtime.

With the same prescription, he cured many cases of paralysis; his indications included paralysis of left side of body, very chilly, worse in morning, in wet weather and in cold. Burnett also found enlargements of the spleen to dissolve with these indications.

The first case Clarke treated homeopathically was one involving new growths. There was a cluster of small warts on the forehead of a boy that had lasted eighteen months, following a cat's scratch. Thuj. in small doses and tincture painted on permanently cured in three weeks.

A gentleman, about 50, consulted Clarke about a wart on the right side of his head. He was then bald and the wart developed in the same locality soon after and has since remained. The patient had been twice vaccinated.

Clarke gave him Thuj. 30c, twenty-eight powders, one in seven medicated, one at bedtime. In one month there was much reduction, Thuj. was repeated and in little over two months the wart was gone.

Burnett suggested Thuj. for fatty tumors, which he regards as sycotic in nature. Thuja not only produces symptoms of the secondary stage of gonorrheal and vaccine affections, it also produces urethritis and a variolous eruption.

Dudgeon reported acute urethritis with yellow discharge lasting altogether a fortnight as the result of chewing a Thuja cone.

Goullon cured a lady who had a headache for a year. On waking, she felt as if a tight hoop enclosed her forehead, not passing away until noon. Eyelids heavy as lead. Thuj. 10x, one dose at bedtime, permanently cured.

Robert Farley related the case of two children, age 5, who had what he graphically termed "urinary tantrums." Two hours after being put to bed they would wake kicking, crying and refusing to answer a question. This lasted an hour or more. Asked if they wanted to urinate they would refuse to answer, strike at attendant, or even say "No."

Finally it was found that if they were taken up and put on the closet they would urinate and then go to sleep readily. One of the children developed signs of incipient inflammation of the left hip joint. The totality led to the selection of Thuj., which was given in the 200c.

After the first night there were no more "tantrums," and in two months the child was perfectly well. This child's father had gonorrhea, treated by injection, some years before the patient was born. But the other child's father had not had gonorrhea. In the latter case, which was exactly like the former, the cure was immediate, in the former case relief occurred on the second night.

C. W. Roberts found Thuj. in five to seven drop doses at bedtime, to control nocturnal seminal emissions better than any other remedy. "Nocturnal seminal emission" is an emphasized symptom.

Percy Wilde recorded the case of a young married woman who had a large epulis on her lower jaw, rapidly increasing in size, ulcerating on the surface, very painful and filling the mouth with an ill-smelling secretion. The entire tumor was removed by operation and also the subjoined bone.

Three weeks later the tumor was as large as before and increased daily. Thuj. 1x was then given. The growth stopped immediately, ulceration ceased, and the pain disappeared. In three weeks the gum was healthy and remained so permanently.

Villers related a case of scalp tumor in a youth of seventeen. The tumor had existed for two years and had somewhat the appearance of a bean. It was situated about the posterior edge of the parietal bone, was devoid of sensation and the hair had disappeared from it, making it very conspicuous.

Thuj. 30c was given, a dose every twenty days. In four months the youth was almost cured, entirely so in five months, and the hair grew again completely covering the spot.

George Royal related a case of persistent cough cured with Thuj. Miss X., 19, fair, had for three months a painless, dry cough. The irritation was only in the throat. There were six small growths at the back of her throat and one near the vocal cord. She had never had a cough before. She also had green, excoriating leucorrhea and menses that were a little too early. Thuj. 30c cured the growths and the cough in about three weeks.

R. B. Johnstone offered some indications for Thuj. in hernia. He found it particularly useful for women with a sycotic history who have a tendency to left-side inguinal hernia after labor. When babies cry a lot, the umbilicus protrudes, growing red and sore, especially when the father has a sycotic history. Left inguinal hernia in infants, child cries all the time and is only quiet when the left inguinal region is relieved from pressure or the thigh is flexed on the abdomen.

Burnett recorded a case of lichen urticatus in a boy of 14, which came into his hands after a long course of treatment, external, internal and dietetic, at the hands of allopathic specialists without result.

The rash came periodically in warm weather; the patient literally tore himself because of the irritation. The rash was worse on the left (vaccinated) side. Thuj. 30c was given in infrequent doses. The spots continued to appear for a week and then disappeared. The skin remained clear in spite of the patient indulging in all kinds of previously forbidden foods.

Birthmarks and stains (Sep., Carc.). Birthmarks and moles in children with a sycotic history. The skin is mottled and discolored, brown or red mottled spots, discoloration of the backs of the hands and feet. Tendency toward acne and greasy skin. Blood blisters. Spider hemangiomas. Benign tumor growths. Polyp formation, particularly on anus, rectum, or cervix.

Severe left ovarian pains, sometimes burning, extend down thigh. Pains worse from any attempt at exercise, especially walking. Pains occur with every menstrual period and are generally worse before and during the flow. The pain compels the patient to lie down, but lying on the left side aggravates.

Gonorrhea with yellow-green discharge. Vaginitis and cervicitis with yellow-green discharge (Puls.). Chronic sinusitis, yellow-green or green mucus. White sinus discharge, with warts and a history of gonorrhea. Sweet smelling perspiration, sickly sweet.

Ailments due to vaccinations (Sil.), especially smallpox. Ailments from gonorrhea or suppressed gonorrhea. Sycotic gonorrhea miasm. AIDS.

Belief that they are somehow separate, that they are different (Nat-m.). Tendency to conceal themselves, cautious as a form of protecting themselves. Difficulty trusting or relying on other people. Self doubt, poor confidence. Don't trust themselves.

Elusive, changeable personality, often distorted. Evasive. Possessive, manipulative (Ars.). Calculating. Males tend to be more reserved, distant, aloof, and manipulative; while females are manipulative, but spacey and soft, with poor confidence.

Distorted sexual desires, often with high sex drive. Tendency to hide their sexual past or desires. Can have a history of sexual, physical (Anac., Staph.) or verbal abuse (Lyc., Nat-m.). Secret obsessions. Can be secret drinkers or drug users. Fixed, distorted ideas. Distorted perceptions (Med.).

Fear of going crazy, or losing control. Fear or sensation of leaving their bodies (Cann., Med.), fear they will not be able to get back into their bodies (Anac.). Can be fearful of demons, spirits or people who can control them or possess them. Idea that there is something bad or dirty in them. Afraid of own thoughts (Arg-n.), that if they think something negative, it will come true.

RELATIONS - ***Antidoted by:*** Cham. (nightly toothache): Cocc. (fever), Camph., Merc., Puls., Sulph. Teste: Colch. the best antidote in his experience. ***Antidote to:*** Merc., Sulph., Iod., Nux-v. ***Compare:*** (1) Med., Nat-s., Calc., Nit-ac., Sil., Psor., Sabin., Puls. (2) Cupre-aust. - sharp, prickling pain, general feeling of warmth, rheumatism and gonorrhea. (3) Cupre-l. - acts like Thuj., terrible pains in the stomach. (4) Sphingurus - falling out of hair from beard, pain in jaw-joint and zygoma. Sil. (5) Med. - suppressed gonorrhea. (6) Merc., Cinnb., Ter., Juni-c., Canth., Cann-i., Ant-t. (7) Bad effect of vaccination, Sil., Maland., Apis, Ant-t., Vac., Var. (8) gonorrheal rheumatism, orchitis, prostatitis, Puls. (the discharge of Puls. is thicker than that of Thuj.). (9) Condylomata, balanorrhea, greenish leucorrhea, Nit-ac. (10) Iritis, green discharges, rheumatism, sweating, Merc. (11) Condylomata, Sabin. (itch and burn, especially in women). (12) Sycotic eruptions, Sars. Ciliary neuralgia, Spig. (Spig. pains radiate downward, Thuj., upward and backward). (13) Nails grow brittle, soft, Sil., Fl-ac. ***Complementary:*** Med., Sabin., Sil., Nat-s. in sycosis. ***Compatible:*** Nit-ac., Sabin. ***Follows well:*** Med., Merc., Nit-ac. ***Followed well by:*** Merc., Sulph. also Calc., Ign., Lyc., Kali-c., Puls., Sil., Vac.

REFERENCES - Boericke. Clarke. Murphy. Phatak.

THYMOLUM

(Thyme Camphor)

PHARMACY - Thymol. Thymolum. Thyme camphor. A phenol from the essences of many Labiatae, Lamiaceae or some Umbelliferae. ***Historical dose:*** Tincture and all potencies.

CLINICAL - Adenoma. Colitis. Diarrhea. Dyspnea. Enterocolitis. Fainting tendency. ***Hookworms.*** Laryngitis. Leucorrhea. Migraines. Neurasthenia. Sexual weakness. Whooping cough.

HERBAL - Thymol exists in the essences of certain plants belonging to the Labiatae family or to the Umbellifers. It is a phenol made up of para-isopropyl-metacresol. Thymol can be extracted from them by combining with alkaline lye (soda or potash). It is used therapeutically as an intestinal anti-septic and as vermifuge against tapeworm.

HOMEOPATHIC - The proving was conducted by Griggs, on eight provers, six males and two females, as well as one control using a placebo, in 1940-41. The experiment began by using 3x for two weeks, 2x for the next two weeks and 1x for about ten days.

The provings show an action limited to the sexual organs, producing a typical sexual neurasthenia. Thymol's general action is on the stomach, genital organs and to a small extent, on the central nervous system.

Genito-urinary diseases. Pathological emissions, priapism and prostatorrhea. Nightly seminal discharge. Blood-streaked leucorrhea. Glairy or membranous diarrhea. ***Hookworm disease*** (Chen-a.).

General weakness with headaches. Constricting headache. Skin blue, cold. Spasmodic laryngeal cough. Excessive salivation with nausea. Frequent urination with compelling urging. Pains in the dorsal and lumbar region, spreading to the buttocks.

MIND - Irritable, arbitrary, must have his own way. Uneasy feeling and agitation. Nervous agitation, loquacity, mental confusion. Bewildered state. Craves company. Morose, sad, uneasy. Energy gone.

Abdomen - Enterocolitis.

Back - Tired, aching throughout lumbar region. Worse mental and physical labor. Back pain during the headaches. Pain in the lumbar and sacral regions, spreading to the buttocks.

Ears - Noises in the ears. Buzzing in the ears. Sound like bells. Temporary deafness.

Female - Brown, blood-streaked, evil-smelling, watery leucorrhea. Menses thick, scanty, drawn-out. Pains before and during menses in the ovaries and uterus. Pain from hypogastric heaviness. Metritis of the cervix. Cancer of the uterus or cervix.

Head - Headache with sadness. Constricting pain in the temples, in women, ameliorated when lying down or from external heat. Bilateral temporal headache and at the occiput. Menstrual migraines.

Kidneys - Pains in the kidneys, spreading to the buttocks. Retention of urine. Frequent urination with urging. Increased urination at night. Urinary burning and subsequent dribbling of urine. Urine copious, proteinuria, hematuria. Urates increased; phosphates decreased.

Limbs - Cyanosed limbs. Numbness at the limbs. Chronic lumbar rheumatism.

Lungs - Dyspnea. Irritating laryngeal and tracheal cough. Whooping cough.

Male - Increased sexual desire. Priapism. Seminal discharge when going to stool. Nightly seminal discharge. Profuse, nightly, seminal emissions with lascivious dreams of a perverted character. Ejaculation with erotic dreams. Prostatitis. Adenoma of the prostate gland. Cancer of the prostate.

Modalities - Better from eating. Worse mental and physical labor. Worse from tobacco.

Mouth - Salivation reduced when eating. Watery salivation with nausea. Ptyalism. Nauseating belchings.

Pulse - Pulse weak, slow or rapid.

Rectum - Hookworms. Diarrhea after constipation. Glairy or membranous diarrhea. Anal pain following diarrhea. Mucous, membranous stools, gray in color.

Skin - Skin blue and cold. Scarlet fever-like or pustulous exanthema.

Sleep - Awakes tired and unrefreshed. Lascivious and fantastic dreams. Erotic dreams.

Stomach - Acrid dyspepsia. Glairy belching with sensation of burning in the stomach, nausea and gastric heaviness. Nausea, ameliorated by eating. Vomiting.

Throat - Spasmodic laryngitis. Irritation of the larynx and trachea.

RELATIONS - ***Compare:*** (1) Carb-tcl. (2) Canth. - Irritation and inflammation of the digestive, urinary and cutaneous mucus membranes. Intense burning in the digestive passages with frequent, compelling need to urinate. (3) Merc-c. - Burning pains in the pharynx, painful, frequent urination, urine comes drop by drop, diarrhea with tenesmus. (4) Ter. - Irritation of the digestive and urinary mucus membranes with tendency to hemorrhage.

REFERENCES - Julian.

THYMUS SERPYLLUM

(Wild Thyme)

PHARMACY - thymu. Thymus serpyllum. Wild thyme. N. O. Labiatae. Tincture of the whole plant. ***Historical dose:*** Tincture and all potencies.

CLINICAL - Asthma. Respiratory, infections. Whooping cough.

HERBAL - Thymus serpyllum belongs to the mint family; all the members have a marked action on the urinary organs and especially on the elimination of uric acid. It contains a volatile oil thymol, tannin, a gum and woody fiber. Thymol is a very powerful germicide, killing the germs of typhoid fever in thirty minutes.

HOMEOPATHIC - Respiratory infections of children, dry nervous asthma, whooping cough, severe spasms but little sputum. Ringing in ears with feeling of pressure in head. Burning in pharynx, sore throat worse empty swallowing, blood vessels distended, dark.

COMMENTS - Small doses of Thymu. act as a sedative and contra-stimulant, the depressive action being preceded by a period of excitation. Large doses dull the nerves and produce motor incoordination and sleep.

Animals poisoned by Thymu. sleep standing and are insensible to the prick of a pin. They have muscular contraction and tremors, vertigo and turning movements.

Increase of diarrhea, vomiting appears, prostration is extreme, the skin becomes cold and death sets in with all the symptoms of a depressant position and with complete anesthesia. These final symptoms are due to the thymic acid, which is a camphor.

REFERENCES - Anshutz. Boericke.

THYROIDINUM

(Thyroid Gland Extract)

PHARMACY - thyr. Thyroidinum. Thyroid gland extract. Thyreoidinum. Thyroidea. Glandula thyreoidea. Thyroidin. A sarcode. Trituration of the fresh or dried thyroid gland of sheep or calf. Potencies of a liquid extract of the gland. ***Historical dose:*** All potencies.

CLINICAL - Abscesses. Acromegaly. Albuminuria. Amblyopia. Amenorrhea. Anemia, pernicious. Angina pectoris. Backache. ***Bedwetting. Breast, tumors.*** Chilblains. Constipation. Convulsions, puerperal. ***Cretinism. Cysts.*** Diabetes. Diarrhea. Diuresis. Dropsy. Dysmenorrhea. Ear, disorders. ***Eczema.*** Edema. Epilepsy. Fainting. Fibroma. Fractures. ***Goiter, exophthalmic.*** Hair, loss. Heart, disorders. Hysteria. Ichthyosis. Idiocy. Leprosy. ***Malnutrition.*** Mania. Milk, deficiency. ***Myxedema.*** Neurasthenia. ***Obesity.*** Optic neuritis. Paralysis, hands and arms. Paraplegia. Pityriasis rubra. ***Psoriasis.*** Puerperal fever. Rupia. Scleroderma. Syphilis. Tetanus. ***Tachycardia. Thyroid, disorders.*** Tuberculosis. ***Uterine, fibroids. Vomiting.***

HOMEOPATHIC - Thyroidinum, also known as Thyroidea, is an organopathic. The sarcode is prepared from the dried thyroid gland taken from a sheep, ox or calf. The thyroid is closely connected with the heart and it exercises a general regulating influence on growth and development.

The homeopathic proving was established by M. Panos, R. Rogers, and J. Stephenson in 1963-64, using a double-blind method. The potencies 12x, 30x, 200c and 1000c were used. The symptomatology completes the work of Ghosh of Calcutta, which dates from 1963. Thyr. symptoms are made up of the toxicological and clinical sources as well as the proving symptoms.

Thyr. affects the central nervous system, skin and left side. Metabolic disorders. ***Goiter. Myxedema*** with hair loss and cretinism. Diuretic action in myxedema and various types of edema.

Anemia, emaciation. Infantile wasting. Rickets. Arrested development of children. Acromegaly, delayed union of fractures. A state of puffiness and obesity. Excessive obesity. Great weakness and hunger, yet loses flesh. Craving for large quantities of sugar.

Rheumatoid arthritis. Nervous tremor of face and limbs. Tingling sensations. Paralysis. Hystero-epilepsy. ***Tetany,*** worse cold. Muscular weakness. Sensation of faintness after acute diseases, weakness. Easy fatigue, weak pulse with a tendency to fainting, palpitations.

Increased heart rate. Dilates arterioles. ***Tachycardia***. Low blood pressure. Cold hands and feet, chilliness and sensitive to cold. As of a cold wind blowing on the body. Sweating, headache. Exophthalmus and dilatation of pupils. Amblyopia. Weak memory. ***Cretinism***. Psoriasis. ***Nocturnal bedwetting***.

Breast tumors. Cystic tumors of the breast (2x trituration). ***Lack of breast milk***. ***Vomiting of pregnancy***. ***Uterine fibroids***. Said to be effective in ***undescended testicles*** in boys when given in half-grain doses twice a day over a considerable period.

Feels tired and sick, easy fatigue, wants to lie down. Fainting fits, tremors, nervous of face and limbs. Stabbing, splitting, clutching sensation. Choking. Convulsion in the nursing children, related to a febrile cutting of teeth.

MIND - Stupor, alternating with restless melancholy. Marked irritability of temper. Irritable, worse least opposition, goes into a rage over trifles. Grumbling, all the time. Irritable before menses.

Difficult concentration. Absent-minded. Nervous and apprehensive. Depression on waking. Depressed, inclined to cry. Weeps when undressing. Morose and sulky, wants to be left alone.

Euphoria. Laughing in a way peculiar to herself. Argues with family. Suspicious. Paranoia that they are being pursued or persecuted. Psychosis from anguish. Homicidal tendency. Insanity, puerperal insanity with fever. Nightmares.

Abdomen - Bearing and aching down through pelvis into anterior thigh. Acute cramping pains with cold sweating. Pain after eating. Pain midway between umbilicus and either anterior superior iliac spine. Sharp, cutting, colicky pains with fullness, worse on pressure and walking, better bending forward and after passage of flatus. Large quantities of flatus passed from bowels often smelling of hydrogen sulphate. Rolling flatulence with gurgling, then loose, gassy stool.

Back - Backache.

Breasts - Breasts tumors and cysts. Deficient in breast milk.

Chest - Angina pectoris. Anxiety about chest. ***Chest feels as if constricted***.

Constitutions - Suited to the phosphoric or carbonic types, generally hyperthyroids. Nervous temperament. Psoric, tubercular and sycotic range of dispositions.

Ears - Sclerosis of ossicles. Difficult hearing. Pain on the right side. Pain in the left ear lobe.

Eyes - Progressive loss of sight with central scotoma (Carbn-s.). Conjunctivitis and chemosis, itching with weeping. Stinging pain in the right eye. Eyeballs prominent. Exophthalmic goiter. Irritation of the eyelids.

Face - Flushed. Dry, red lips, burn with free desquamation. Eruption of acne, worse on the right cheek. Sensation of something heavy, which falls from the cheeks.

Female - Amenorrhea in young girls. Pelvic congestion ameliorated by menses. Amelioration of premenstrual discomforts by the menses. Menses often too early. Metrorrhagia. Endometriosis. Gnawing in the uterus. ***Uterine fibroids.*** Vomiting of pregnancy. Puerperal, convulsions insanity. Tendency to miscarriage or premature birth. Puerperal psychosis. Uterine atony after giving birth. Sterility.

Food - Insatiable appetite, always wants something more interesting to eat. Desire for sweets and thirst for cold water. Aversion to greasy foods.

Head - Feeling of lightness in brain. Fullness and heat. Persistent frontal headache, heaviness over eyes. Headaches ameliorated after menses. Heavy throbbing headache worse in the frontal region, worse from concentrating the mind, better out of doors, worse using the eyes. Fullness in the head with throbbing of the temporal arteries, worse morning and afternoon, from motion, physical or mental, from heat or indoors, better in cool fresh air, often better from external pressure. Falling of hair.

Heart - Ready excitability of heart. Heart's action weak with numbness of fingers. ***Tachycardia*** (Naja.). Palpitations, worse least exertion, hammering, beats felt in ear. Heart pains radiate into axilla. Clutching, constricting pains, worse lying down, causing short breath. Severe heart pains. Angina pectoris. Hypertrophy after hard labor. As if blood were rushing downwards, through the body. Jumping sensation at heart. Large veins on arms and hands. Valvular diseases of heart (Naja). Weak, frequent pulse with inability to lie down.

Kidneys - Pressing urge to urinate. Frequent urination during the day. Burning along urethra, increase of uric acid. Increased flow of urine, polyuria, some albumen and sugar. Urine smells of violets. ***Bedwetting in weakly children*** who are nervous and irritable. Diabetes mellitus.

Limbs - Rheumatic arthritis with tendency to obesity, coldness and cramps of limbs. Aching pains. Trembling of limbs and entire body. Edema of legs. Numbness, left fingers then right leg. Itching without eruption, worse night. Peeling of skin of lower limbs. Cold limbs. Cold, clammy hands. Left hand icy cold. Abnormal growth of limbs due to excessive exertion.

Liver - Cutting pain in liver, worse deep breathing. Jaundice with itching, in the newborn child, accompanied by vomiting.

Lungs - Breathlessness better lying in recumbent position. Dry, painful cough with scanty, difficult expectoration and burning in pharynx. Cough on entering a warm room from cool air. Asthma. Allergies.

Modalities - Better after or during menses. Better evening, rest, lying on abdomen or reclining position. Worse in women, before and during menses. Worse least exertion, stooping. Worse cold. Heart worse lying down.

Mouth - Dryness of mouth. Bad taste, metallic, bitter and sour. Tongue, metallic taste at tip. Tongue coated grayish white in center with red edges or tip. Papillae enlarged and prominent. Tongue thickly coated. Swelling of the upper lip.

Nose - Dry mucus membrane indoors, fluent coryza, profuse, watery and bland outdoors. Dryness and sticking pain in posterior nares, worse on swallowing. Rhinitis with sneezing and edema of the nasal mucus membranes. Pain in the sinuses. Tickling sensation with headaches and dry throat.

Perspiration - Drenching sweats. Oily, musty sweat.

Rectum - Stools dark, fragmented with cadaverous or sulphurous smell. Stools soft, watery.

Skin - ***Eczema***. ***Psoriasis*** associated with obesity. Very dry skin. Itching without eruption, worse night. ***Brown swellings***. Swelling of glands of stony hardness. Symmetrical serpiginous eruptions. Jaundice with itching, in the newborn child, accompanied by vomiting. Urticaria. Ichthyosis. Lupus. Peeling skin of lower limbs. Scleroderma.

Sleep - Insomnia. Difficulty in falling asleep. Nightmares. Wakes for no reason.

Stomach - Increased appetite. Thirst for cold water. Pains, tenderness, aggravated by eating, ameliorated in the evening. Dyspepsia before menses. Flatulence, much flatus in abdomen. Nausea, worse riding in a car, better in cool air. Vomiting of pregnancy.

Temperature - Hot flushes, then chills or drenching sweats.

Throat - Dry larynx, congested, raw, burning, worse on left side. As of a splinter stuck across the throat. Pharynx congested, red and dry, with rawness and burning.

Vertigo - Vertigo, in the morning on rising, on leaning forwards.

COMMENTS - Thyr. has a profound action on the heart. Fatal syncope occurred in a number of cases under "thyroid feeding." Cyanosis was produced in many cases. Burnett gave a patient 3x, producing severe angina pectoris. The connection between the heart and the thyroid gland is very close, as seen in cases of exophthalmic goiter, of which many cases have been cured.

In a case of valvular heart disease following rheumatism in a man, 24, Thyr. 3x, thrice daily, quickly relieved a squeezing pain at the heart with inability to lie down, and hastened the patient's recovery.

Dr. F. C. Skinner cured a case of dysmenorrhea in a goiter subject with Thyr. 1,000c.

In myxedema, cachexia, cretinism and similar conditions, the thyroid gland is absent or defective and the idea is to supply a physiological want. As such, a state of puffiness and obesity may be regarded as a keynote indication for Thyr.

Clarke gave Thyr. 3x to a living skeleton of a child, 5, who looked not older than 2. He had been kept in a box in a cellar all his life until brought into the hospital, when he weighted only 14.25 pounds. Under Bac. 200c and careful feeding he gained .25 pounds per week. When Clarke commenced Thyr. he put on weekly .75 pound and gained the use of his legs, being able to stand by holding on to a chair.

In a case of universal and very aggravated psoriasis in a schoolboy, fair, very chilly, cold, clammy hands and feet, Thyr. 3x and later 30c completely cured after a prolonged course.

An obese lady, age 60, developed diabetes. Clarke cured her completely with Thyr. 3x and 30c. She then could take any kind of food.

H. O. Nicholson related a case of toxemia of pregnancy in a woman, 32, during her third pregnancy. She had a fit on October 3. Thyroid feeding was begun the next day. Marked improvement followed. Edema of face and body diminished. On October 23, the patient was about her usual duties. On November 6, she was delivered of a healthy boy without any untoward symptoms.

Pityriasis rubra, intense redness and scales of legs, and also with intense itching. Ichthyosis, syphilitic eruptions and scleroderma. Acromegaly. Myxedema with hair loss.

Increases the flow of milk in nursing women when the flow has been deficient. Insanity, puerperal insanity with fever. Paranoia that they are being pursued or persecuted. Nightmares.

Optic neuritis and accommodative asthenopia. Exophthalmic goiter, with bulging eyes. Weak heart, valvular problems, shortness of breath. Tachycardia. Operative and idiopathic tetany, worse from spasms by cold. Stitching, aching or heavy pains. Tingling sensations.

Thyr. has poor nutritional development in children. Low thyroid function, with skin problems. It can stimulate function of thyroid gland, or decrease the need for thyroid medications. Thyroid treatment nearly always raises the body heat.

RELATIONS - ***Compare:*** (1) Spong., Calc., Fuc., Lycps. (2) Thyri. (3) Thym-gl. extract - arthritis deformans, metabolic osteoarthritis, 5 grain tablets 3 times daily. High potencies very effective cases of exophthalmic goiter.

REFERENCES - Boericke. Clarke. Murphy. Phatak.

THYROIODINUM

(Iodothyrinum)

PHARMACY - thyri. Thyroiodinum. Iodothyrinum. The iodine exists in organic combination and Thyr. contains 0.003 parts of iodine to every gram. Trituration. ***Historical dose:*** All potencies.

CLINICAL - Emaciation. Dyspnea. Glycosuria. Goiter. Hoarseness. Obesity. Thyroid, disorders. Thyroid, nodules. Urine, increased. Weight, loss.

HOMEOPATHIC - Thyroiodine is now more generally named Iodothyrine, but Clarke retained the former as more convenient.

Hoenigschmied said of it that it is present in only small quantities in the thyroid of sheep. It is completely free from albuminous substances, stable and directly assimilated. The general effects of the drug are increased secretion of urine and corresponding loss of flesh.

Thyri. is the active principle isolated form thyroid gland, a substance rich in Iodine and nitrogen, affects metabolism, reducing weight, may produce glycosuria. It should be used cautiously in obesity, for a fatty heart may not be able to maintain the accelerated metabolic rhythm. Milk contains the internal secretion of the thyroid.

COMMENTS - Hoenigschmied gave some cases, including that of a laborer, 42, for several years had enlargement and induration of all lobes of thyroid, the enlargement caused compression of the structures of the neck, dyspnea, whistling respiration, hoarseness, short, dry cough, vertigo.

Thyri. was given, 5-grain tablets, one every evening, at the end of a week twice daily. After using twenty-five tablets, the gland was smaller and softer, the previously hard and resistant nodules were elastic after two more weeks only remnants of the goiter remained.

Another case, that of a man, 60, thyroid enlarged in all its lobes with a glandular cystic swelling in the right one, dyspnea, loud whistling breathing. Two, three and at last four tablets were given daily for two months, by which time the goiter had vanished, but the cyst was not changed.

A man, 45, medium height, sedentary, suffered from obesity, vertigo, dyspnea, weariness. Pulse feeble, 76, functions normal, appetite and sleep good, weight 230 pounds.

With increasing doses of Thyri., up to ten tablets daily the weight steadily went down to 160 pounds, activity increasing in proportion. When the dose had reached four tablets daily the urine became very abundant, but was free from albumen. The daily dose was increased one tablet every four days.

REFERENCES - Clarke.

TILIA EUROPEA

(Common Lime)

PHARMACY - til. Tilia europea. Common Lime. Linden. Tilia cordata. Tilia sylvestris. N. O. Tiliacae. Tincture of fresh blossoms. ***Historical dose:*** Tincture and all potencies.

CLINICAL - Bedwetting. Dentition. Hemorrhages. Leucorrhea. Lichen. ***Neuralgias.*** Nosebleeds. Peritonitis. Puerperal, metritis. Rheumatism. Toothache. Urticaria. Uterus, prolapsed.

HERBAL - The sap of the linden contains sugar, and the flowers an abundance of honey, which makes the tree particularly attractive to bees.

HOMEOPATHIC - A tincture of the fresh blossoms was proved by the Austrian Society. The most striking characteristic is "an intense sore feeling about the abdomen and profuse warm sweat which gives no relief." This led to its successful use in cases of peritonitis.

In addition to this are marked bearing-down symptoms in the whole genito-urinary and rectal regions, especially in the uterus and these combined with the others have indicated Til. in puerperal metritis and other disorders of the female generative sphere.

Til. is of value in muscular weakness of the eye. Hemorrhages of thin, pale blood. Puerperal metritis. Disease of the antrum (Hydr., Chel.). Intense soreness of the abdomen, uterus. Bearing or dragging down pains in genito-urinary and rectal region. Bed feels too hard. Edema. Neuralgia. Rheumatism. ***The more he sweats the greater the pain***.

MIND - Love-sick. Dread of society. Melancholy, disposed to weep. Irritable. Disinclined to work.

Abdomen - Bloated abdomen, pains as from incarcerated flatulence, repeated noisy discharges of it, which aggravates. Peritonitis. Soreness with warm sweat which gives no relief.

Back - Tearing from nape to top of shoulder. Stitching, drawing, and heat in right back between liver and kidneys. Heaviness in sacral and dorsal region.

Chest - Oppression. Whole chest weak, acute pressure and pinching under sternum. Throbs as from a dull stitch from thorax to back. Bruised pain and swelling. Tearing from left pectoralis major to axilla.

Ears - Stinging in ears.

Eyes - Binocular vision imperfect. Sensation as of gauze or a veil before eyes (Calc., Caust., Nat-m.). As if a piece of cold iron pressed through right eye causing burning.

Face - Face pale, or flushed, frequent alternations. Cutting pains. Sensation of something alive under skin of face. Quivering of lips. Sprained pain in left jaw-point.

Female - ***Intense sore feeling about uterus.*** Bearing-down pains with hot sweat, but without relief. Soreness and redness of external genitals (Thuj., Sulph.). Pelvic inflammation, tympanites, abdominal tenderness and hot sweat which does not relieve. Much slimy leucorrhea when walking (Bov., Carb-an., Graph.). Puerperal metritis.

Head - ***Neuralgias***, first right, then left side, ***with veil before eyes***. Confusion with dimness of vision. Much sneezing with fluent coryza. Bleeding from nose.

Kidneys - Heavy dragging pain in urethra. Constant painful pressure on bladder and urethra. Frequent, copious urination. Scanty urine.

Limbs - Trembling, weariness, bruised feeling in limbs. Paralytic heaviness of arms, especially upper arm. Heaviness and painful lameness in left shoulder. Drawing in small spot left hip while sitting. Cramp in left sole. Ulcerative pain in ball of left great toe.

Lungs - Cough from tickling in throat. Tickling, scraping, irritating, provoking slight cough, especially in left side of larynx. Fine stitches in larynx, worse talking. Hoarseness. Frequent sighing.

Modalities - Better in cool room. Better from motion, walking about in open air. Better closing eyes. Better from coffee. Worse talking, walking, stooping, sneezing. Worse in afternoon and evening. Worse cold water, drafts. ***Worse from sweating,*** warm room, heat of bed, after sleep. Skin symptoms worse heat of bed.

Mouth - Much mucus in mouth, causing fuzzy feeling, affecting speech. Taste bitter, bitter-slimy, pasty. Stinging pain in all the teeth, worse by cold water. Drawing pains in gums.

Nose - Tickling of nose. Much sneezing with fluent coryza. Nosebleeds, blood thin and pale, but coagulates quickly.

Perspiration - ***Sweat warm and profuse*** soon after falling asleep. Sweat increases as rheumatic pains increase.

Sensations - As if a piece of cold iron pierced through right eye, causing burning. Burning as if a piece of ice were drawn over ear and face. As if something living were under skin of face. Tearing in anterior muscles of thigh, as if they were too short.

Skin - Urticaria. Eruption of small, red itching pimples. Violent itching and burning like fire after scratching.

Sleep - Yawning, sleepy, exhausted, worse during pain. Sleeplessness with restlessness, Bed seems too hard. Vivid frightful dreams, bathed in perspiration. Sudden wakings.

Temperature - Profuse warm sweat, soon after falling asleep without relief.

Throat - Burning in throat. Sensation of swelling of the palate, with desire to swallow, and hoarse voice. Tickling in palate causing cough.

Vertigo - Vertigo, with staggering, and like gauze before the eyes. Intoxication.

COMMENTS - An intense facial neuralgia was developed in the proving and also a very aggravated condition of skin irritation with pimples of the lichen order. Pains above the root of the nose, nosebleed of thin, pale blood which coagulated quickly. The left side was most affected. Great sensitiveness to draft of air was induced.

RELATIONS - ***Compare:*** (1) Lil-t., Bell. (2) Puerperal metritis, Bell. (3) Uterine bearing down, Lil-t. (4) Sweat without improvement, Merc.

REFERENCES - Boericke. Clarke. Phatak.

TILLANDSIA USNEOIDES
(Spanish Moss)

PHARMACY - till-u. Tillandsia usneoides. Spanish moss. Tree hair. Old mans beard. Florida moss. N. O. Bromeliaceae (Bromeliad or Pineapple family). ***Historical dose:*** Tincture and all potencies potencies.

CLINICAL - Blood, sugar. Breast, milk. Childbirth. Diabetes. Epilepsy. Hemorrhages. Rheumatism.

HERBAL - Tillandsia is usually an epiphytic plant with reduced to absent stems. Found mostly in tropical to temperate Americas. Hangs in the trees and swamps of the southeast coastal plains.

Many Native American tribes used the moss while cooking to absorb unwanted liquids, for bedding, for tanning hides, and to rub on newborn babies heads for curly hair. It is also used as fodder for animals.

Colonial pickers harvested moss with long poles during the winter. The harvest hung for several months to cure in a moss yard. Curing loosened the outer gray scales making it ready for commercial ginning.

Medicinal use of Spanish moss has a long history. Extracts from it have been used in the treatment of diabetes and it has been used to help control blood sugar levels. Spanish moss was taken, while green, and brewed into tea for expectant mothers, supposedly to aid the flow of breast milk and make the delivery easier. Tea from the plant was also used as a folk remedy for rheumatism.

In Mexico, it has been used to treat infantile epilepsy. In the early 1950s, it was used as an estrogen substitute and scientists have found the plant exhibits anti-bacterial properties. In the West Indies it has been used to make a styptic ointment for the purpose of stopping bleeding.

COMMENTS - Dr. C. W Mayo reported that, in the Feb. 9, 1944 "Staff Meetings of the Mayo Clinic," the absorptive qualities of Spanish Moss for use in surgical dressings had been investigated with interesting results.

"The dried moss will retain its absorptive power better than a substance like cotton, as the liquid taken up is stored chiefly inside the leaves and cells, instead of merely being held between adjoining strands. Spanish moss will take up from six to ten times its dry weight of water."

REFERENCES - Buttimer. Murphy.

TINOSPORA CORDIFOLIA
(Gulancha)

PHARMACY - tinos. Tinospora cordifolia. Gulancha. N. O. Menispermaceae. ***Historical dose:*** Tincture and all potencies.

CLINICAL - Bilious. Cough. Dysuria. Elephantiasis. Fever. Flatulence. Gonorrhea. Hemorrhoids. Impetigo. ***Intermittent, fever.*** Jaundice. Malaria. Palpitations. Rheumatism. Skin, disorders. Syphilis. Urticaria. Vomiting. Worms.

HERBAL - The stem and root are used medicinally; they possess a bitter taste. The root and stem contain starchy extract, bitter principle and a trace of berbornic. Fresh stem is more efficacious than the dry one and is a good substitute for Calumbu.

The Ayurvedic physicians used it as a febrifuge and named it "Indian quinine." They have found it to be bitter tonic and strength giving. It destroys wind, bile and phlegm. It is good for thirst, burning sensation, gonorrhea, cough.

Useful in enlarged spleen. Secondary syphilis, rheumatism, leprosy, skin diseases such as impetigo. Jaundice, torpidity of the liver, splenic affections. Leprosy, rheumatism. Acute and chronic fevers. Worms, vomiting, hemorrhoids, dysuria, flatulence and palpitations of the heart.

As a diuretic and demulcent it is given in dysuria, in scanty, high-colored urine due to catarrh of the bladder. It is stomachic, bitter, tonic, alternative, aphrodisiac, anti-periodic, and demulcent. It is given in dyspepsia and in debility caused by repeated attacks of fever.

HOMEOPATHIC - No proving of Tinos. has been made, but many Indian homeopaths have been using it clinically with excellent results.

Debility. Rheumatism. Skin diseases, leprosy, secondary syphilis. Jaundice, torpidity of the liver. Splenic affections. Acidity of urine, urinary diseases such as gonorrhea and dysuria.

Intermittent fevers. Acute and chronic malarial fevers, the temperature generally rises in the afternoon with chilliness or shaking chill. Fevers with bilious vomiting associated with thirst and headache.

Chronic slow fevers, especially where there is a history of gonorrhea and weakness due to seminal emissions. Fever due to an excessive use or maladministration of quinine. Fever with burning sensation is felt in face, hands and feet, and enlargement of the liver and spleen, jaundice with yellow color of the eyes, no desire for food, and headache.

Vomiting, specially bilious vomiting. Decreased quantity of urine, passes it frequently, burning while urinating. The urine is mixed with pus-like discharges. Gonorrhea. Rheumatism, leprosy and skin diseases. Secondary syphilis.

Tonic, widely used as a stimulant remedy where the patient has become extremely weak owing to repeated attacks of fever and also to exhausting seminal emissions.

COMMENTS - R. N. Khory noted, in the Materia Medica of India, vol. II., that the juice of the Tinospora stem combined with Pakanbhed and honey is given in gonorrhea. The starchy extract is nutritious, largely used in native practice in cold fevers and seminal weakness, also in urinary affections.

W. Dymock, in the Pharmacographia Indica, vol. 1. noted that it is favorably spoken of by those who have tried it as a tonic, anti-periodic and diuretic. Charaka recommended it in chronic fevers, jaundice, bilious vomiting and some other diseases. He found it useful to purify the breast-milk after delivery.

Baghbhata spoke highly of it as an excellent tonic, and noted that it is generally used in chronic fevers and jaundice. Chakradatta reported that Tinospora is an excellent remedy in urticaria, fevers, leprosy, and elephantiasis.

Bangasena recommended it in vomiting and flatulence associated with extreme palpitations of the heart. "It is useful in general and seminal debility, fever, jaundice, torpidity of the liver, skin diseases, secondary syphilis, rheumatism, acidity of urine and urinary diseases, some forms of dyspepsia, splenic affections, chronic gonorrhea, leucorrhea, etc."

Nadkarni wrote "In malaria Tinospora is sometimes more efficacious than quinine." R. N. Chopra, in the Indigenous Drugs of India, wrote "An infusion is prepared from the stem and root which is a valuable tonic in debilitating diseases, intermittent fever and dyspepsia."

RELATIONS - ***Compare:*** Chin., Chin-ars.

REFERENCES - Ghose.

TITANIUM METALLICUM

(Titanium Metal)

PHARMACY - titan. Titanium metallicum. Titanium metal. Trituration of the copper-red crystals obtained from the slag at the bottom of a blast iron furnace. Consisting of Titan. cyanide and Titan. nitride. Titanium is found in the bones and muscles. Apples contain 0.11 percent of Titan. ***Historical dose:*** All potencies.

CLINICAL - Bright's disease. Eczema. ***Hemiopia.*** Lupus. Nasal, catarrh. Premature, ejaculation. Rhinitis. Sexual, weakness.

HOMEOPATHIC - Titanium stands midway between silicon and tin in some of its relations and in other respects it is closely related to iron, chromium and aluminium.

The crystals were proved by Sharp who took 2 grains of the first trituration, daily for a week. It was believed to be the pure metal, but was proved later to be the cyanonitrid.

Titan. has been used in lupus and tuberculosis processes externally, also in skin diseases, nasal catarrh, etc. Giddiness with ***vertical hemiopia***. Bright's disease. Eczema, lupus and rhinitis.

"Imperfect vision, the peculiarity being that ***half an object only could be seen***." Another symptom, which Burnett has turned to good account in cases of sexual weakness is "Too early ejaculation of semen during sex."

RELATIONS - *Compare:* (1) Half-sight, Nat-c., Lyc., Aur., Lith.

REFERENCES - Boericke. Clarke.

TONGO

(Coumarouna Seeds)

PHARMACY - tong. Tongo. Coumarouna seeds. Dipterix odorata. Tonca. Tonka. Tonquin bean. N. O. Leguminosae. Papilionoideae. A tree in Guiana. Tincture of the dried beans. ***Historical dose:*** Tincture and all potencies.

CLINICAL - Hip, pain. Migraines. Neuralgias, face. Toothache. Whooping cough.

HERBAL - The fragrant seeds of Tongo is used by perfumers. Dipteryx odorata, which yields it, is a native of Cayenne. The fruit is something like that of the almond tree.

HOMEOPATHIC - Tong. was proved by Nenning. In the proving Tong. produced "Risings with taste of bitter almonds." The chief uses have been in migraine and neuralgic disorders. Whooping cough.

Eyes - Trembling in right upper lid.

Head - Tearing pain in supra-orbital nerve with heat and throbbing pain in head.

Limbs - Tearing pains in hip joints, femur and knee, especially left side.

Modalities - Better by movement, pressure. Worse by rest, when seated.

Nose - Coryza, nose stopped, must breathe through mouth.

Vertigo - Confused, especially in the occiput with somnolence and a sort of intoxication.

RELATIONS - ***Antidoted by:*** Vinegar. Meli. ***Compare:*** (1) Hay fever, Trif-p., Napht., Sabad. (2) Antho., Asper. and Tong. contain Coumarin, the active principle.

REFERENCES - Boericke. Clarke.

TOPAZ

(Gemstone)

PHARMACY - top. Topaz. Gemstone. Al2SiO4(F,OH)2 + Cr. Hydroxy-fluoro-aluminum silicate. ***Historical dose:*** All potencies.

CLINICAL - Anxiety. Asthma. Blood, sugar. Depression. Diabetes. Exhaustion. Hemorrhages. Indigestion. Insomnia. Liver, disorders. Nightmares. Restlessness. Sexual, dysfunction. Sleepwalking. Tumors.

HOMEOPATHIC - Topaz has been said to cure insomnia, asthma, and hemorrhages. Depression, exhaustion, said to increase stamina. Mood swings, worries, fears, anxiety, stress. It was thought to cure cowardice. Insomnia, sleepwalking, nightmares. Restlessness.

Stomach, liver and pancreas disorders. Disturbed blood sugar. Indigestion. Diabetes. Tumors. Weak eyesight. Strengthens weak tissue and backbone. Said to be a powerful aphrodisiac and was often used to treat sexual dysfunction.

COMMENTS - Topaz occurs not only in the transparent yellow, yellow brown, orangey brown, and pinky brown colors most popularly associated with it, but also in a very light to medium red. In the past, almost any yellow stone was called topaz.

Yellow topaz is used for protective purposes, specifically against envy, jealousy, intrigue, disease, death, negativity and lunacy. Mounting in gold is said to enhance these properties; rings, wrist bracelets and necklaces with the stone next to the heart are thought to be the most projective.

Topaz was also said to change color in the presence of poisoned food or drink. Its curative powers waxed and waned with the phases of the moon. Supposedly helped to break up stagnation of energy within the body, and elimination of toxins.

Powdered and mixed with rosewater, topaz prevented bleeding. Nosebleeds could be stopped by pressing a stone against the side of the nose. It was believed that madness could be cured by a dose of topaz and wine.

REFERENCES - Murphy.

TORULA CEREVISIAE

(Yeast Plant)

PHARMACY - torul. Torula cerevisiae. Yeast plant. Torula sacharomyces. ***Historical dose:*** Tincture and all potencies.

CLINICAL - Boils. ***Constipation***. Eczema. Flatulence. Headaches. Indigestion. Nausea. Sneezing. Sycosis. Tinea versicolor. Wheezing.

HERBAL - Yeast poultices were much used in skin diseases by the ancient Egyptian physicians, for eczema, boils and swelling.

HOMEOPATHIC - Tor. was introduced into homeopathy by Drs. Lehman and Yingling. It has not been proved, but there are many verified clinical symptoms.

A sycotic remedy. Abdominal soreness. Rumbling, flatulence. Sour, yeasty, moldy odor from discharges. Headache. Pains shift around. Tinea versicolor. According to Yingling, useful for anaphylactic states produced by proteins and enzymes.

MIND - Irritable and nervous.

Back - Backache, tired and weak from elbows and knees down.

Head - Aching back of head and neck. Headache and sharp pains all over, worse from constipation.

Limbs - Hands cold like ice and go to sleep easily.

Nose - Sneezing and wheezing. Catarrhal discharge from posterior sinuses.

Rectum - ***Constipation***.

Skin - Boils, recurrent. Itching eczema around ankles. Tinea versicolor.

Sleep - Disturbed with much restlessness.

Stomach - Bad taste. Sense of fullness. Poor digestion. Belching of gas in stomach and abdomen. Nausea.

REFERENCES - Boericke.

TOXICOPHIS PUGNAX

(Moccasin Snake)

PHARMACY - toxi. Toxicophis pugnax. Moccasin snake. N. O. Ophidia. Trituration. ***Historical dose:*** All potencies.

CLINICAL - Edema. Fever. Periodic neuralgia. Skin, dry. Snake, bites.

HOMEOPATHIC - Some effects of bites with this snake have been recorded. A peculiar feature of the cases was that the symptoms of pain and fever recurred annually at exactly the same period for many years with decreasing intensity each year.

In one case, the pains spread to other parts after some years. The right leg became painful and swollen rapidly. For several years the pain was confined to the knee of the bitten limb, in a few years it left the knee and seized the hip and finally attacked the shoulder. Skin rather dry.

Pain and fever recur annually after a bite from this snake (Cedr., Lach.), but without swelling, decreasing in intensity each year. Pains will sometimes change location with disappearance of first symptoms. Unusual dryness of the skin. Edematous swellings and periodical neuralgia.

REFERENCES - Boericke. Clarke.

TRACHINUS DRACO

(Sting-fish)

PHARMACY - trach. Trachinus draco. Sting-fish. Trachinus radiatus. Trachinus vipera. Sting-bull. Great and Lesser Weever. Trituration of the poisonous fins. ***Historical dose:*** All potencies.

CLINICAL - Asthma. Blisters. Blood-poisoning. Delirium. Fever. Gangrene. Headache. Hydrophobia. Insomnia. Nausea. Neuralgia. Palpitations. Rabies. Suffocation. Ulcers. Vomiting.

HOMEOPATHIC - Some very serious effects have been recorded from wounds inflicted with the fins of the sting-fish. Trach. should be indicated in cases of acute blood-poisoning with intense pains.

Swelling of whole body, of wounded arm, then of head and chest. Acute blood poisoning and gangrene. Fever, delirium and the symptoms of hydrophobia.

Intolerable pains. Stinging, burning, throbbing pain increasing to unendurable intensity lasting an hour and then decreasing. Violent burning pain extending from wound to chest.

MIND - Anxiety, raving. Fear of death. Hydrophobia.

Head - Violent headache.

Heart - Palpitations.

Lungs - Paroxysms of suffocation.

Skin - Skin of whole body became yellowish green. Gangrenous blisters on arms.

Sleep - Sleeplessness.

Stomach - Violent thirst. Nausea. Green, bilious vomiting.

Temperature - Constant fever with irregular pulse. Cold, clammy sweat.

Vertigo - Dizzy.

REFERENCES - Boericke. Clarke.

TRADESCANTIA DIURETICA

PHARMACY - trad. Tradescantia diuretica. N. O. Commelynaceae. Tincture of fresh leaves. ***Historical dose:*** Tincture and all potencies.

CLINICAL - Gonorrhea. Hemorrhage. Orchitis. Vertigo.

HOMEOPATHIC - Mure proved Trad., which belongs to a genus of lily-like plants. Disorder of the genito-urinary organs, urethral discharge and inflammation of the scrotum. Embarrassed breathing. Hemorrhage from ear and upper air passages, painful urination, urethral discharge, scrotum inflamed.

Chest - Pain in left side of chest.

Kidneys - Whitish discharge from urethra. Pain when urinating. Stream thin. Urine is acid smelling, yellowish, copious, ash-colored sediment.

Lungs - Breathing is very painful, embarrassed, difficult. Sighing, as from want of air.

Male - Scrotum inflamed, painful and red.

REFERENCES - Boericke. Clarke.

TRIBULUS TERRESTRIS

(Ikshugandha)

PHARMACY - trib. Tribulus terrestris. Ikshugandha. Hygrophila spinosa. N. O. Acanthaceae. India. Tincture of root leaves and seeds. ***Historical dose:*** Tincture and all potencies.

CLINICAL - Apathy. Dropsy. Dysuria. Gonorrhea. Impotency. Incontinence. Insomnia. Kidney, stone. Leucorrhea. Malaria. Masturbation. Pimples. Prostatitis. Rheumatism. Sexual, weakness. Spermatorrhea. Strangury. Urticaria.

HERBAL - Ikshugandha is an East Indian remedy useful in urinary affections, especially dysuria, and in debilitated states of the sexual organs, as expressed in seminal weakness, early emissions and infertile semen.

The root is demulcent, diuretic, and given in dropsy, gonorrhea, hepatic obstruction, and in urinary affections. A paste of the seeds is applied to rheumatic joints. The seeds are used as an aphrodisiac.

HOMEOPATHIC – The Tribulus plant is full of thorns, which cause intolerable burning, swelling and redness. It produces small red pimples and eruptions which look like meals and eruptions due to prickly heat.

Malarial attacks associated with urticaria. Fevers appear in the morning, no chill or thirst, urticaria-like eruptions come on along with the rise of temperature, intense itching which is relieved by cold applications.

Sexual neurasthenia. Impotency. Ailments from masturbation, prostate emissions and spermatorrhea. Impotence caused by overindulgence of advancing age or when accompanied by urinary symptoms incontinence, painful urination, etc. Prostatitis. Leucorrhea. Gonorrhea.

Dropsy. Urinary affections. Urinary calculus. Kidney stones. Hepatic obstruction. Skin diseases, worse from heat and better from cold. Ulcers due to impurities of blood. Rheumatism. Insomnia.

COMMENTS - Charaka found it useful in stone, gravel and calculus in the bladder, and strangury. Sushruta recommended it as a great sexual tonic. Bagbhata recommended it for all skin diseases due to impurities of blood. Chakradatta thought that it could be effectively used in dropsy.

Bangasena acknowledged its efficacy in effecting safe delivery. Harita recommended it for sleeplessness. He also said that it can produce sound sleep if the root is placed on the head.

REFERENCES - Boericke. Clarke. Ghose.

TRICHOSANTHES DIOICA

(Wild Snakegourd)

PHARMACY - trich-d. Trichosanthes dioica. Wild snakegourd. N. O. Cucurbitaceae. Roots and leaves. ***Historical dose:*** All potencies.

CLINICAL - Anasarca. Bilious. Catarrh. Chickenpox. Cholera. Diarrhea. Dropsy. Dysentery. Fever. Headache. Hemoptysis. Jaundice. Kala-azar. Nausea. Rheumatism. Smallpox. Synovitis. Vomiting. Water brash.

HERBAL - The leaves of Trichosanthes dioica are tonic, febrifuge. Fruits of the bitter variety are used in scorpion stings. The fruit is described by Sanskrit writers as febrifuge, laxative and anti-bilious.

Ayurvedic physicians of India found this drug to be of great use in multifarious complaints. Charaka found it to be a sovereign remedy in cases of dropsy, anasarca, bilious and catarrhal fevers, slow chronic fevers associated with hemoptysis and also in synovitis.

Chakradatta recommended it in bilious and catarrhal fevers and rheumatism. Sushruta found it efficacious in hemoptysis and bilious fevers.

Bhavaprakasha recommended its use in smallpox with predominance of bilious symptoms. In the opinion of some Ayurvedic physicians, it is an excellent remedy in smallpox and chickenpox.

HOMEOPATHIC - The root-bark of Trichosanthes dioica possesses highly purgative properties. It causes purging to such a great extent that a little overdose may cause death.

At first the stool appears to be loose, gradually the patient passes bilious and mucous stools, and finally bloody stools and vomiting of blood appear producing the stage of collapse.

Useful for diarrhea, dysentery, cholera and cholerine. Copious loose stools, of green or yellow color, may be mixed with bile and mucus. Prolapsed rectum. Burning in anus. Smarting after stool. Passage of involuntary and bloody stool.

Bloody stools appear without cessation and cause profound prostration and exhaustion. The stools may be mixed with particles of mucus. Frothy stool, during its passage no pain or uneasiness is felt, after stool, urging and straining continue for a long time.

Cholera where there are copious stools and vomiting associated with restlessness, thirst, burning, sweat, extreme weakness, coldness of extremities, pulselessness and other symptoms.

Pain and gurgling in stomach. Gurgling with copious yellow stools. Nausea before vomiting, water brash and rumbling in abdomen. Nausea after drinking water. Constant water brash. Vomiting, copious stringy mucus which may be streaked with blood. Vomiting of bile.

Jaundice. Yellow eyes, with dropsy. Chronic fevers, with enlargement of the liver and spleen. Fevers with bilious symptoms, with headache, water brash, nausea, and especially bilious diarrhea.

Acute, chronic and malarial fevers and also in kala-azar. The fever comes on at 11 a.m. or 12 noon with chilliness, and thirst and headache exist. After this stage headache continues, but it increases with the rise of temperature. The fever may be of short duration one day and of longer duration the next day. Fever with vomiting (Ip.).

Trichosanthes bears a close resemblance to Podo. and it may be safely used in those cases where Podo. is indicated or where Podo. fails to do any good.

RELATIONS - ***Compare:*** Trich-d. may be a grand substitute for Ip. and Podo. or it may be employed where these two medicines fail to do any good.

REFERENCES - Ghose.

TRIFOLIUM PRATENSE

(Red Clover)

PHARMACY - trif-p. Trifolium pratense. Red clover. N. O. Papilionoideae. Tincture of flower heads. ***Historical dose:*** Tincture and all potencies.

CLINICAL - Bladder, catarrh. ***Blood, disorders. Cancer. Cough. Crusta, lactea***. Diabetes.

Dysentery. Fainting. Fibroids, bleeding. Hemorrhages. ***Hoarseness***. Menopause. Menorrhagia. Metrorrhagia. Tumors. ***Whooping cough***. Writer's cramp.

HERBAL - Red clover is an herbal blood tonic and purifier. It has a reputation among herbalists in whooping cough and the coughs of measles and tuberculosis. Felter gave red clover to persons disposed to cancer. He found it retarded the progress of cancerous tumors and improves the general condition of the patient.

HOMEOPATHIC - T. C. Duncan and others proved it and elicited some very decided respiratory symptoms, dry, tickling cough, oppressed breathing with fever. One peculiar symptom was a cough followed by hiccough.

Marked salivation. Feeling of fullness with congestion of salivary glands, followed by increased flow of saliva. ***Crusta lactea,*** dry, scaly crusts. Stiff neck. Feeling as if mumps were coming on. Preventive for mumps and cancer. Retards progress of cancerous tumors before ulceration has taken place. ***Cancerous diathesis***.

MIND - Mental breakdown. Confusion of ideas, morning. Loss of memory.

Abdomen - Griping pains in abdomen and headache. Colicky pains all day.

Back - Neck stiff, cramp in sterno-cleido muscles, relieved by heat and irritation.

Constitutions - Cancer diathesis.

Head - Confusion and headaches on awaking. Dullness in anterior brain.

Limbs - Hands and feet cold. Tingling in palms. Tibial ulcers.

Lungs - Sensation in lungs as if breathing hot air. Air feels as if full of impurities.

Mouth - ***Increased flow of saliva*** (Merc., Syph.).

Lungs - Hay fever. Coryza like that which precedes hay fever, thin mucus with much irritation. ***Hoarse and choking, chills with cough at night***. Cough on coming into the open air. Spasmodic cough. ***Whooping cough***, paroxysms, worse at night.

Throat - Sore throat with hoarseness.

COMMENTS - Trif-p. has many symptoms of congestion. Dull, stupid feeling generally. The head and lungs feel full of blood. Sensation in lungs as if breathing hot air, as if air full of impurities. Persistent headache on waking. Unrefreshing sleep. Weak and intermittent pulse, later full and bounding.

Irritation of the pharynx and trachea. "Sharp pain through uvula causing tears to start." Dryness of trachea causing him to clear throat of some foreign substance. Secretion of urine increased.

Farrington noted "Hoarseness and choking spells at night with cough, the neck is stiff, cramps in sternomastoid muscle better by heat and friction."

Cooper said of Trif-p. that it causes salivation in horses and diarrhea if they eat much of it and that it cures mumps and disorders of the pancreas and salivary glands. Hale said it causes "heaves" in horses.

Felter noted "scaly and ulcerated conditions of the tibial region of the old." The symptoms are worse in close room, better in open air. "When I became very warm with the fever my breathing stopped, lungs felt as if breathing hot air." Worse after sleep.

RELATIONS - *Compare:* (1) Trif-r. ***Complementary:*** Calc-p. - menstrual and hemorrhagic affections.

REFERENCES - Boericke. Clarke.

TRIFOLIUM REPENS

(White Clover)

PHARMACY - trif-r. Trifolium repens. White clover. N. O. Leguminosae. Papilionoideae. Trituration or tincture of flower heads. ***Historical dose:*** Tincture and all potencies.

CLINICAL - Mumps. Salivation.

HOMEOPATHIC - The proving of Trif-r. produced a specific action on the salivary glands. Hale said it produced marked salivation in horses. Feeling of fullness or congestion of all the salivary glands. Discomfort and even pain in glands followed by copious flow of saliva.

Feeling of congestion in salivary glands, pain and hardening, especially submaxillary, worse lying down. Mouth filled with watery saliva, ***worse lying down.*** Taste of blood in mouth and throat.

One prover felt just as if she had mumps coming on. Prophylactic against mumps. Sensation as if heart would stop with great fear, better sitting up or moving about, worse when alone with cold sweat on face.

RELATIONS - ***Compare:*** (1) Jab., Pilo.

REFERENCES - Boericke. Clarke.

TRIGONELLA FOENUM GRAECUM

(Fenugreek)

PHARMACY - trig-f-g. Trigonella foenum graecum. Fenugreek. Foenumgraecum officinale. North Africa, India. N. O. Fabaceae. ***Historical dose:*** Tincture and all potencies.

CLINICAL - Abscesses. Baldness. Beriberi. Boils. Bronchitis. Burns. Cancer. Carbuncles. Cataracts. Cellulitis. Colic. Constipation. Convalescence. Cough. Cysts. Dermatitis. Diabetes. Diarrhea. Eczema. Gout. Hernia. High blood pressure. Hives. Hyperthyroidism. Hypoglycemia. Impotence. Indigestion. Infections. Leg, edema. Leukemia. Lice. Liver disease. Lymphadenitis. Menopausal symptoms. Muscle aches. Peptic ulcer. Rickets. Sores. Spleen, enlargement. Tuberculosis. Ulcers. Vaginal, dryness. Wounds.

HERBAL - Fenugreek is native to southern Europe, the Mediterranean region, and Western Asia. The words foenum - graecum mean Greek hay and arise because of the appearance of the plant which has long slender stems. Fenugreek seeds contain a high percentage of mucilage, a natural gummy substance present in the coatings of many seeds. Although it does not dissolve in water, mucilage forms a thick, gooey mass when exposed to fluids.

The resulting soft mass is not absorbed by the body, but instead passes through the intestines and also triggers intestinal muscle contractions. Both actions promote the emptying of intestinal contents. Therefore, fenugreek is a mild but effective laxative.

In addition, fenugreek seeds contain chemicals that slow down the time that food takes to go through the intestinal tract. As one result, sugars are absorbed from foods more slowly and blood sugar levels may not rise as high or fluctuate as much as usual. Fenugreek may further affect blood sugar levels by decreasing the activity of an enzyme that is involved in releasing stored sugar from the liver into the blood.

Some evidence suggests that fenugreek may also have other medical uses. Fenugreek lowers cholesterol levels as well as blood sugar levels. It may reduce the amounts of calcium oxalate in the kidneys. Calcium oxalate often contributes to kidney stones.

Fenugreek also appeared to lessen the chance of developing colon cancer. It may have some ability to protect the liver against damage from alcohol and other chemicals. Fenugreek is a skin softener and is often an ingredient of soothing facial masks.

Fenugreek is also used for hair care as it prevents hair fall, cures dandruff, and promotes hair growth. A paste of fenugreek seeds is usually applied to the scalp at least 40 minutes before washing hair to help get rid of dandruff, and act as a remedy for hair loss.

The use of shampoo to wash hair can be skipped if fenugreek seed paste is applied on the scalp as the paste helps to remove oil and dirt from the hair and also makes the hair soft. The paste of fresh fenugreek leaves is also used to get rid of dandruff, increase the length of hair, soften the hair, and help preserve its natural color.

Paste of the fresh leaves of fenugreek, applied on the face every night before going to bed and washed with warm water, prevents pimples, blackheads, dryness of the face, and early appearance of wrinkles. It improves complexion and leads to younger looking skin. Fenugreek paste made by grinding fenugreek seeds when used as a mask has a granular texture that helps remove blackheads.

The topical application of the gelatinous texture of fenugreek seed may also have some benefit for soothing skin that is irritated by eczema or other conditions. Fenugreek helps to remove excess oil from the skin. It has also been applied as a warm poultice to relieve muscle aches and gout pain.

A poultice of the leaves can be used for boils, cysts, burns, ulcers, hives, eczema, abscesses, carbuncles, etc. It is also used to treat cuts' and sores. Excessive topical use of fenugreek on the same areas may cause itching, redness, rash, or other reactions. Individuals who have allergies to peanuts or soybeans may also be allergic to fenugreek.

RELATIONS - ***Compare:*** Alf., Avena.

REFERENCES - Murphy.

TRILLIUM PENDULUM

(Lamb's Quarter)

PHARMACY - tril. Trillium pendulum. Lamb's quarter. White bethroot. Trillium erectum. Purple trillium. Bethroot. Birthroot. Rattlesnake root. Wake Robin. Three-leaved nightshade. N. O. Smilaceae or Trilliaceae of the Liliaceae. Tincture of the fresh root. ***Historical dose:*** Tincture and all potencies.

CLINICAL - Bladder, catarrh. Menopause. Diabetes. Dysentery. ***Fainting.*** Fibroids, bleeding. Headache. ***Hemorrhages.*** Menorrhagia. Metrorrhagia. ***Nosebleeds***. Writer's cramp.

HERBAL - The chief uses of Trillium pendulum come to us from herbalists, who learned some of them from the Native Americans. The popular name Birth-root sufficiently indicates one part of its reputation.

HOMEOPATHIC - Tril. is a great hemorrhagic medicine. ***Hemorrhage with great faintness and dizziness***. ***Hemorrhages*** of all kinds with pregnancy. Hemorrhages after childbirth, menopause, from fibroid tumors, gushing, bright red. Uterine hemorrhage.

Threatened miscarriage. Cramp-like pains. Relaxation of pelvic region. Chronic diarrhea of bloody mucus. Tuberculosis with purulent and copious expectoration and spitting of blood.

MIND - Irritable. Anguish, agitation and tossing about, impossible to keep still. Repugnance to conversation. Melancholy with sadness.

Abdomen - Swelling of abdomen as in ascites. Much flatulence and grumbling.

Constitutions - Suited to women who bleed after every labor pain, flabby subjects.

Eyes - Feel too large and as if would fall out from their sockets. Vision blurred, everything looks bluish.

Female - Leucorrhea is copious, yellow, and stringy (Hydr., Kali-bi., Sabin.). Menses every two weeks. Uterine hemorrhages with ***sensation as though hips and back were falling to pieces,*** better tight bandages. Gushing of bright blood on least movement. Hemorrhage from fibroids (Calc., Thal., Spig., Phos., Ust.). Prolapsed uterus with great bearing-down. Metrorrhagia at menopausal. ***Lochia suddenly becomes bloody***. Profuse long-lasting bloody lochia. Varicose veins of pregnancy. Dribbling of urine after labor.

Head - Dull pain, worse noise, walking, coughing, better bending forward. Pain in forehead, worse noise. Headache worse by least noise, walking, coughing. Confused, eyeballs feel too large.

Heart - Palpitations with great anxiety.

Limbs - Cramping pains in muscles of arms and calves.

Lungs - Suffocative attack of irregular breathing with sneezing. Shooting pains through chest. Aching at end of sternum. Cough with spitting of blood. Copious and purulent expectoration. Hemoptysis.

Modalities - Better by exercise in open air. Better from a tight bandage, bending forward. Worse from motion, sitting erect. Worse menopause. Worse after eating. Motion aggravates the hemorrhages. Standing or walking causes bearing down in pelvis.

Mouth - Very offensive taste, especially on rising in morning. Greasy feeling on tongue and gums. Bleeding from gums. ***Bleeding after tooth extraction.***

Nose - ***Profuse nosebleed*** (Mill., Meli.).

Rectum - Chronic diarrhea with bloody discharge. Dysentery with passing of almost pure blood. Diarrhea thin, watery, tinged with blood, painless. Constipation succeeded by thin, watery, very offensive diarrhea.

Sensations - As if eyes too large. As if a crumb were in larynx. As if the chest was tightly bound and could not be expanded. As if hips and small of back were falling to pieces. As if sacroiliac joint were falling apart, wants to be bound tightly.

As if bones were broken. Left side most affected.

Skin - Skin hot and dry, with itching and burning, worse by scratching.

Stomach - Sickness, excessive pain, cramp of stomach. Faintness and sinking at stomach, with heat. Heat and burning stomach rising up in esophagus. Hematemesis.

Temperature - Feverish during pain in abdomen, on the subsidence of which a profuse perspiration broke out.

Vertigo - Vertigo on rising in morning.

COMMENTS - Millspaugh considered Tril. erectum as the proper source of the homeopathic tincture. According to Millspaugh, Tril. pendulum is the white variety of Tril. erectum. The Treasury of Botany gave the names as synonymous. The symptoms of H. Minton, the original prover, were given in Allen under Tril. cernuum.

Minton's proving of Tril. cernuum brought out the hemorrhagic property in the blood tinged diarrhea.

Copious hemorrhages, either active or passive, usually bright red and profuse. Hemorrhage, ante-partum and menopausal, fibroid tumors. Hemorrhage, with faintness and sinking at the stomach, also cold limbs and rapid, feeble pulse. "Flooding with fainting."

Hemorrhages with restlessness and exhaustion. Blue vision, craving for ice water. Tendency to putrescence of fluids. Tril. has been used as a local hemostatic in nosebleed and for bleeding after tooth extraction.

Minton's proving brought out "Sensation of emptiness in abdomen." He also noted extreme debility, palpitation and anxiety. Restless tossing agitation, fear of being sick, and great anguish were experienced by Minton.

RELATIONS - *Compare:* (1) Tril-c. - eye symptoms, everything looks bluish, greasy feeling in mouth. (2) Fic. - hemorrhages, menorrhagia, hematuria, nosebleed, hematemesis, bleeding hemorrhoids. (3) Hir., Leech - hemorrhages, bleeding from anus. (4) Ip., Sabin., Lach., Ham. *Complementary:* Calc-p. (menstrual and hemorrhagic affections).

REFERENCES - Boericke. Clarke.

TRINITROTOLUENUM

(T.N.T.)

PHARMACY - trinit. Trinitrotoluenum. T.N.T. Trotyl. ***Historical dose:*** All potencies.

CLINICAL - Anemia. Cramps. Cyanosis. Depression. Dermatitis. Dyspnea. Faintness. Fatigue. Heart, disorders. ***Hemorrhages***. Insomnia. Jaundice. Palpitations. Vertigo. Vesicles.

HOMEOPATHIC - TNT is a high explosive, obtained by nitrating toluene, a product of coal tar distillation. When the skin or hair is exposed to TNT by contact a characteristic yellow or tawny-orange stain is produced, which lasts for some weeks. Indicated in graver forms of anemia (pernicious) and jaundice. Produces fatal toxic jaundice.

Symptoms were noted in ammunition workers handling TNT who inhale and ingest it, and also absorb some through the skin. They were compiled by Dr. C. Wesselhoeft and published in the December, 1926 issue of the Journal of the American Institute of Homeopathy.

The destructive action of Trinit. on the red blood corpuscles is responsible for the anemia and the jaundice with their secondary symptoms. The hemoglobin is changed so it cannot act satisfactorily as an oxygen carrier and as a result there is breathlessness, dizziness. Headaches, faintness, and palpitations. Undue fatigue, muscle cramps and cyanosis, also drowsiness, depression and insomnia.

Later stages of the poisoning produce toxic jaundice and aplastic anemia. The jaundice is the result of cellular destruction in contrast to obstructive jaundice. Faintness, dizziness, mental sluggishness, delirium, convulsion, coma. Face very dark.

MIND - Depression. Apathetic and cries easily. Aversion to company. Mental sluggishness, delirium.

Food - ***Aversion to tea***. Alcohol aggravates.

Head - Frontal headache and depression.

Heart - Palpitations, tachycardia and bradycardia. Intermittent pulse.

Kidneys - Sudden desire, incontinence and

retention. High colored urine, burning on urination.

Lungs - Nose dry with stuffed sensation. Burning of trachea, choking weight on chest, dry, convulsive cough, raising mucus plugs.

Modalities - Worse alcohol, falls after one or two drinks of whisky.

Nose - Sneezing, coryza.

Skin - ***Tendency to hemorrhage*** under the skin and from the nose. Hands stained yellow. Dermatitis, nodular erythema, vesicles, itching and burning, puffiness. ***Tired pain in back of knees***.

Stomach - Bitter taste, much thirst, sour regurgitation, dull burning behind the ensiform, nausea, vomiting, constipation followed by diarrhea with cramps.

RELATIONS - ***Compare:*** (1) Zinc., Phos., Cina, Ars., Plum.

REFERENCES - Boericke. Clarke.

TRIOSTEUM PERFOLIATUM

(Fever-wort)

PHARMACY - trio. Triosteum perfoliatum. Fever-wort. Fever root. Wild coffee. Horse-gentian. N. O. Caprifliaceae, Tribe, Lonicereae. Tincture of fresh root. ***Historical dose:*** Tincture and all potencies.

CLINICAL - Adenoma. Angina pectoris. Arteritis. Asthma. Backaches. Biliousness. Blepharitis. Breast pain. Conjunctivitis. Coughs. Cystitis. Dyspepsia. Encephalitis. Erysipelas. Erythema. Fevers. Headache, bilious. Herpes zoster. Infections. ***Influenza.*** Joints, stiff. Measles. Menorrhagia. ***Numbness***. Otitis. ***Ozaena.*** Pyelonephritis. Rheumatism. Scarlet, fever. Typhoid, fever. Typhus, fever. ***Urticaria.*** Vomiting.

HERBAL - The name "fever-wort" tells its traditional reputation. Hale said it is one of the ingredients of the "fever powder" of the herbalists.

HOMEOPATHIC - Trio. is an energetically acting drug and has been proved by Williamson, Neidhard, Gatchell and other experienced provers. The symptoms were established by Raeside on fifteen provers (eight men and seven women) in 1959-60. Raeside used the 8c potency, at the rate of one dose every morning until the symptoms appeared.

Trio. is traditionally prescribed as a febrifuge. Above all, it causes vomiting, gastric pains, generalized pains, fever with agitation and insomnia. Talmadge, one of the provers, found it of great value in typhoid and gastric fevers. It produced acute rheumatic symptoms and an intense urticaria.

Biliousness. Gallbladder colic. Diarrhea attended with colicky pains and nausea. ***Numbness of lower limbs after stool***. Increased flow of urine.

Dryness of the mucus membranes of the lips, mouth and throat. Dry cough. ***Influenza with aching pains*** all over with heat in the limbs. Acute encephalitis in infancy, especially after diphtheria, measles, whooping cough.

Sudden weariness around 2 a.m. and 4 p.m. Sensation of sleeping standing up. Sensation of needles all over the body when hot. Generalized pain in the upper and lower limbs. Nervous symptoms (Coff., Hyos.).

Generalized itching, especially on the scalp and limbs of the upper and lower limbs. Erythema, eruption of flat, hard nodules, brown or purple in color, on the joints in the limbs.

MIND - Irritated by noise and in the evening. Irritability, difficulty in controlling himself. In the evening, feels in a rage, difficult to control himself. Tends to quarrel bitterly, argumentative.

Nervous and sleepy, cannot concentrate. Mental exhaustion. All mental activity requires a great effort. Euphoria, followed by a state of depression. Feels isolated, better when alone.

Abdomen - Distended and full of gas. Pain in the coccyx. Sharp pain in the left side of the groin. Epigastric pain spreading to the thorax and throat. Enterocolitis. Colic, especially in the right iliac fossa and the hypogastrium. Flatulence, after drinking milk.

Back - Painful stiffness of the back.

Chest - Angina pectoris. Pressing pain in the precordial region when lying on the left side. Dull ache all over the thorax, predominately in the retro-sternal region with thoracic constriction. Swollen glands in right axilla.

Ears - Otitis. Constant earache in the left ear and discharge. Itching around the ears. Buzzing noises, worse when lying down.

Eyes - Conjunctivitis. Smarting and hot, painful, especially when closed. Left eye swollen, red and hot. Eyes water, difficult to focus. Blepharitis. Eyelids irritated, especially the right side. Twitching of right eyelid in the evening.

Female - Irregular cycle, either late or early menses. Menses long and late. Menses painful, scanty. Menorrhagia.

Food - Loathing of food. Painful hungry feeling, aggravated around 11 a.m. and in the evening. Worse after drinking milk.

Head - Occipital pain with nausea on rising, followed by vomiting. Frontal headache. Dull pain, pulsating or pressing, located at the forehead, occiput or temples. Pressing headache at the left temple and occiput and on the right side of the forehead. Stinging, needle-like pain in the left orbital region. Painful tenderness of the scalp and hair when touched.

Heart - Angina pectoris. Arteritis of the coronary arteries. Pulse slow and weak.

Kidneys - Pyelonephritis. Cystitis. Frequent urination. Smell of ammonia in the urine. Adenoma of the prostate gland.

Limbs - Generalized pains in the upper and lower limbs. Stiffness of all joints, calves numbs, aching in the bones. Rheumatic pain in back. Pains in limbs. Numbness of the lower limbs after going to stool. Burning, pulsating pains in the right axilla, where the glands are swollen. Cramping pain in the left shoulder and arm in the two lower limbs and in the fingers of the right hand.

Lungs - Sensation of choking, has to grope for breath. Asthma. Bronchitis. Dry cough, caused by irritation of the larynx after eating. Cough, especially in the evening, aggravated in a warm room.

Modalities - Better from rest, solitude. Better fresh air, cold drinks. Worse early morning, 3 a.m. to 7 a.m. Worse in the evening, at night, lying, turning in bed, after sleep, rising from bed, waking. Worse sitting up, movement. Worse from heat, drinking cold water.

Mouth - Dry mouth and lips. Mouth like parchment, hot with paresthesia of the lips. Fissure on the lower lip, painful ulcerated areas on the mouth, palate and lips. Sensation of a bitter taste, upper teeth painful. Tongue white and seems swollen.

Nose - Spots on the nose. Dryness of the nose and ears. Dull, continual aching behind the root of the nose. Painful right-sided sinusitis and hyperesthesia of the left side of the face. Rhinitis. ***Ozaena.*** Sinusitis, spasmodic coryza. Coryza with running nose, thick, green discharge with sneezing. Nosebleed and smell of blood in the nose.

Rectum - Proctitis. Constipated, great effort to pass stools, which produces small, hard stools. Stools followed by diarrhea and nauseating wind. Stools watery, frothy. Rectal pains, stabbing, aggravated by pushing to evacuate, worse after passing stools. Rectal burning with anal itching, especially at night. Hemorrhoids.

Skin - Erysipelas. Eczema. Itching welts. ***Urticaria*** from gastric derangement. Itching of the whole body. Itching, especially of the feet, scalp, palms of hands, where there is a dry eruption. Erythematous eruption on the calves, back, scrotum and on the inside of the thighs. Soles of feet itchy in the evening and in bed. Itching eruption on the shoulders and between the scapulae. Patches of brown on the skin. Peeling of the skin on the abdomen. Hyperesthesia of the skin, profuse perspiration, worse at night and from exercise.

Stomach - Acrid dyspepsia. Loathing of food, nausea on rising, followed by vomiting and cramps. Nausea, worse after meals, thirsty for cold drinks, which soothe.

Throat - Painful, irritated, especially at night and on waking. Pharynx red, causing a sensation of constriction. Tickling feeling causes coughing, the left tonsil is painful. Better by drinking cold drinks, even though swallowing is painful. Hoarseness, aggravated when speaking and in fresh air.

Tickling feeling at the back of the throat with constriction, stifling feeling, causing a dry cough.

COMMENTS - Talmadge said of the effect on himself, "Trios. acted promptly and emphatically, causing aching pains in nearly every part of the body, especially of lower limbs and head."

The right side of the head was more affected than the left. The stomach was very much disordered. Severe vomiting and pain in the stomach. Itching at the anus, exudation of mucus.

A peculiar concomitant of the evacuations was numbness of the lower limbs after stool. Many symptoms came on in the early morning hours. One prover, though sleepy, could not sleep after midnight.

RELATIONS - ***Compare:*** (1) Bapt. - Gastric fever. Digestive complaints, putrid excreta, exhaustion, muscle pain. (2) Rheumatism, Bry., Rhus-t. (3) Load at epigastrium, Abies-n. (4) Sleepy but cannot sleep, Bell. Bell. - Fever, heat, restlessness, thirst. (5) Acon. - Skin dry, anxiety, extreme restlessness. (6) Ars. - Anxiety, restlessness, burning pains ameliorated by the heat. (7) Coff. - Palpitations insomnia, restlessness. (8) Lach. - Congestive rush of blood, pharyngeal constriction, worse on waking. (9) Lat-m. - Pre-sternal pains resembling angina. (10) Lyc. - Distention aggravated after 4 p.m. (11) Sulph. - Itching and heat on the feet, alternating with coldness.

REFERENCES - Boericke. Clarke.

TRITICUM REPENS

(Couch Grass)

PHARMACY - tritic. Triticum repens. Couch grass. Agropyrum repens. Cooch-grass. Cutch-grass. Quitch grass. N. O. Gramineae. Tincture of fresh plant. ***Historical dose:*** Tincture and all potencies.

CLINICAL - Bladder, disorders. Cystitis. ***Dysuria.*** Gonorrhea. Incontinence. Prostate, enlarged. Pyelitis. Strangury.

HERBAL - Burnett told how he learned from an herbalist the use of Tritic.; the herbalist cured a patient of Burnett's with it, the man suffered from dysuria. Burnett found it no less valuable for women than for men.

"Frequently in dysuria from an inflamed state of the urethra, Tritic., ten drops in a little water, frequently repeated of prompt effect often giving complete relief in a few hours and if the ailment is primarily in the urethra the relief is an abiding cure, if from a tugging of the heavy womb, it is only relief."

HOMEOPATHIC - Excessive, chronic irritability of the bladder. Dysuria, cystitis and gonorrhea. Strangury, pyelitis. Enlarged prostate. Incontinence, constant desire.

Dysuria, frequent, difficult and painful urination (Pop.). Catarrhal and purulent discharges (Pareir.). Urine is filled with gravel and sediment which causes irritation of the mucus surfaces. Always blowing nose.

COMMENTS - Burnett gave the case of a widow who was suffering from a complete procidentia uterus and very bad hemorrhoidal bleeding. She wrote that she was driven almost mad with painful urination, the burning and straining were truly awful.

Tritic., as above, was ordered and brought a most grateful letter from the patient. She kept a supply always at hand.

RELATIONS - ***Compare:*** (1) Chim., Senec., Pop., Buchu, Uva., Trad. (2) Polytr. - Ground Moss - Painful urination of old people, dropsy, urinary obstruction and suppression).

REFERENCES - Boericke. Clarke.

TROMBIDIUM MUSCAE DOMESTICAE

(Acarus)

PHARMACY - trom. Trombidium muscae domesticae. Acarus. Red acarus of the fly. N. O. Acarudea, class, Arachnida. Tincture of the animals. ***Historical dose:*** All potencies.

CLINICAL - Anus, prolapsed. Diarrhea. ***Dysentery.*** Hip joint, pain. Liver, pain. Nose, catarrh. Sciatica. Tibia, pain. Toothache.

HOMEOPATHIC - Trom. is a parasite found singly or in groups upon the common house-fly of a bright red color, nearly circular in shape. The alcoholic tincture, a brilliant orange in color was prepared from specimens, about 115 in number, collected in Frankfort, Philadelphia in 1864.

The provings, under the supervision of Hering, were made with the 3x, 6x, 9c, 18c. and 30c potencies. Trom. has cured dysentery with brown, thin, bloody stools and tenesmus. Dysentery, ***worse by food and drink.*** Brown, thin, bloody stools, much pain before and after stools. Stools only after eating.

Mucus discharge from nose while eating dinner. Weakness. Felt better in evening, better in open air. Rising up causes fainting. Reading aloud causes toothache. Rheumatic pains in left shoulder, arm, knee, and region of heart. Inability to keep quiet.

MIND - Talkative during day. Disposed to be contrary. Constant disposition to gape. Inability to collect ideas. Absence of ideas. Loss of memory.

Abdomen - Congestion of the liver. Griping in hypochondrium in morning. Much pain in abdomen before and after stool.

Chest - Cutting to right of lower part of sternum. Sharp pain in lower part of chest. Throbbing all over chest from 9 to 11 a.m.

Ears - Shooting in ears in afternoon, worse swallowing or blowing nose. Itching in ears after rising. Burning in ears in evening.

Eyes - Redness of internal part of conjunctiva, similar to a pterygium. Lachrymation in open air. Itching at right inner canthus.

Food - Appetite lost.

Head - Oppressive headache. Dullness of head in forenoon. Head heavy, sometimes sharp pains in temples.

Lungs - Hoarseness. Hacking cough from irritation in throat.

Modalities - Warm drink improves toothache. Open air improves coryza. ***Worse from any food or drink***, after stool. Worse by touch, pressure. Worse shaking head, moving. Cold air aggravates toothache. Cold bath aggravates pain in abdomen.

Mouth - Tongue coated white.

Nose - Nose obstructed on rising. Fluent coryza in open air and on eating. Mucus discharge from nose, worse during dinner. Dryness of nose in evening, with scabs. Nosebleed in morning, afternoon.

Rectum - Burning in anus. Sharp pain in left side, shooting downward during stool. Urgent, loose, stools on rising. Stool only after eating. Brown, thin, bloody stools with tenesmus.

Sensations - As if there were no weight in ear, lightness. As from incarcerated flatus in abdomen. As if excoriated after tenesmus. As if everything were coming out of anus. As if hot air blowing over lower abdomen and thigh. As if abdomen needed support. As if three toes on left foot would be twisted off. As if her breath were leaving her.

Skin - Pimples on nape in evening. Itching in spots on chin and among whiskers, in evening, and about neck.

Sleep - Constant inclination to gape through day, in afternoon. Sleepiness. Restless sleep. Lewd dreams. Wakefulness after 4 a.m., with restlessness.

Stomach - Griping in pit of stomach, worse after dinner. Belching after meals, tasting of ingesta. Vomiting after breakfast, thought it was from drinking coffee.

Teeth - Toothache, better warm drinks. Aching in left decayed tooth, worse lying down, eating, talking, and cold air.

Temperature - Chilliness at night, worse morning on waking. Fever in afternoon, with pulsation in arteries of head and aching on occiput and small of back.

Throat - Throat sore on right side.

Vertigo - Lightness of head. Dizziness, on every attempt to rise from bed, with faintness.

COMMENTS - The grand keynote of Trom. is "worse by eating or drinking," in the nose, teeth or tonsils. On this indication, Clarke cured some of the worst cases of diarrhea and intestinal pains coming on when the patient eat or drinks.

"Much pain before and after stool, stool only after eating." Congested liver with urgent, loose stools on rising from bed. During stool, sharp pain in left side, shooting downward.

Skin symptoms, especially itching of scalp and in whiskers. Restlessness, inability to keep quiet. Fainting on rising up.

RELATIONS - ***Antidoted by:*** Staph. (toothache), Merc-c. (diarrhea), ***Compare:*** (1) Rheumatism, Led. (2) Diarrhea, Sulph. (3) Worse blowing nose. Culx., Thuj. (4) Stitches up anus, Ign., Nit-ac., Sul-ac. with prolapse, Podo.

REFERENCES - Boericke. Clarke.

TROPAEOLUM MAJUS

(Indian Cress)

PHARMACY - trop. Tropaeolum majus. Indian cress. Garden Nasturtium. N. O. Tropaeolaceae. Tincture of fresh plant. ***Historical dose:*** Tincture and all potencies.

HERBAL - Tropaeolum is a native of Peru. The taste of the leaves were considered like the taste of cress, and they have been used like cress in salads. The seeds make pickles and are used as a substitute for capers.

A patient to whom Cooper gave Trop. noted that it made the urine extremely fetid in smell. On this keynote, Cooper relieved several cases of urinary difficulty, giving single doses of the tincture.

REFERENCES - Clarke.

TUBERCULINUM AVIAIRE

(Chicken Tuberculosis)

PHARMACY - tub-a. Tuberculinum aviaire. Chicken tuberculosis. Tuberculinum avis. Nosodes. A preparation of chicken tuberculosis. ***Historical dose:*** All potencies.

CLINICAL - ***Bronchitis. Broncho-pneumonia. Chronic fatigue.*** Colds. ***Coughs.*** Debility. Emaciation. ***Influenza.*** Lung, disorders. Measles. Pneumonia. Prostration. Tuberculosis. Weakness.

HOMEOPATHIC - Tub-a. is prepared from the infected liver of chickens. Dr. Cartier gave an account of this nosode in his paper read at the International Homeopathic Congress, 1896. The bacillus of avian tuberculosis has been identified with that of human tuberculosis. But the clinical properties of the two nosodes are not identical.

Tub-a. acts most prominently on the apices of the lungs and it corresponds most closely to the ***bronchitis of influenza***, which simulates tuberculosis, having cured several hopeless-looking cases. It has also done excellently in some cases of bronchitis following measles. H. D. Baker noted "Tub. aviare has served me better than any remedy in the ***long lasting prostration after the influenza.***"

Dr. Francois Cartier of France found it useful in ***broncho-pneumonia of children*** and persistent cough after influenza and measles.

Symptoms similar to tuberculosis, relieves the debility, diminishes the cough, improves the appetite and braces up the whole organism. Acute broncho-pulmonary diseases of children. Itching of palms and ears. ***Coughs are irritating,*** incessant and tickling, loss of strength and appetite. Emaciation (Hydr. to fatten patients after tuberculosis).

Acts on the mind, spinal nerves and branches, muscles, joints, bronchi and mucus membranes. ***Influenza and its sequelae. Chronic fatigue.*** Muscular or nerve pains are better by motion, but the patient tires easily. Pains and mental symptoms are better in the open air.

Relaxed, degraded conditions of tissues and secretion. Dingy, unhealthy, doughy or aged appearance and feeling of the skin and soft tissues and an old catarrhal aspect of mucus excretions. In acute conditions the rapidity of the emaciation is notable.

MIND - Depressed. Easily frightened. Mentally changeable in feeling and purpose. Desires change. Dissatisfied with present conditions and surroundings. Desperate, wicked feelings. Lack of moral sense. Restlessness, the desire for change is physical as well as mental.

COMMENTS - Anshutz related a case of a woman who entered the hospital suffering from influenza and who, a few days after a slight amelioration of her symptoms, was attacked with a pulmonary congestion, clearly localized in the top of the left lung and accompanied by all the clinical symptoms of tuberculosis.

Rales and moist crepitation, dullness, exaggeration of the thoracic vibration, expectoration, fever, perspiration, spitting of blood. Examination of the sputa showed distinctly the presence of Koch's bacilli.

Anshutz gave her Tub-a. and in three weeks all the symptoms had left. That woman left the hospital completely cured and a year later her health was still perfect. Anshutz noted ten cases of influenzal bronchitis with incessant coughs, fever and expectoration, rapidly cured by Tub-a.

It seems that Tub-a. does not act in diminishing the cough like an anodyne, but braces up the whole organism. The relief of debility and the return of appetite are the phenomena which was observed in conjunction with the diminution of the cough.

In contrast with Bac., Tub-a. has considerable cough and little dyspnea. It has an acute, irritating cough, such as one meets with in acute diseases or sub-acute disorders in young people. A cough which fatigues and which leads to enfeeblement and loss of appetite, a suspicious cough.

Dr. R.E.S. Hayes made the following statement: "My experience has led me to select the Tub. Bovinum for patients presenting more pronounced localizations in the meninges, abdomen, skin, glands or joints. But the Tub. Aviare for patients who were affected by a more evident depreciation of quality in the entire person at the same time, such as occurs after influenza or similar crises. This observation is purely clinical.

"Recurrent influenza with long continued cough. Long continued, annoying, teasing cough remaining after the active symptoms of bronchitis or influenza, in a good many instances Tuberculinum aviare put an immediate end to this cough any related discomforts. Aviare has the usual characteristics of Tuberculinum plus its affinity to influenza and to nerve elements, both sympathetic and cerebro-spinal."

RELATIONS - *Compare:* (1) Bac., Bac-ts., Tub., Ars-i.

REFERENCES - Anshutz. Boericke. Clarke

TUBERCULINUM BOVINUM

(Tuberculosis Nosode)

PHARMACY - tub. Tuberculinum bovinum. Tuberculosis nosode. Tuberculinum bovinum of Kent. Tuberculinum of Koch. Nosode is prepared either from tubercular abscess or from a glycerine extract of pure cultivation of human tubercular bacillus. Dilutions. ***Historical dose:*** Tincture and all potencies.

CLINICAL - Acne. Albuminuria. Allergies. Appendicitis. ***Asthma. Bedwetting.*** Bones, decay. ***Breast, tumors***. Bronchitis. ***Broncho-pneumonia***. Catarrh. Chilblains. Chilly. ***Colds.*** Cornea, opacity, ulceration. ***Coughs.*** Dentition. ***Diarrhea. Dysmenorrhea***. Dyspnea. Ear, infections. Edema. Emaciation. Epilepsy. Erysipelas. Erythema. Glands swollen. Hematuria. Hemoptysis. Headache. Heart, disorders. Hyperactivity. Influenza. Leprosy. Leucorrhea. ***Lungs, disorders.*** Lupus. Mania. Menses, early. Nephritis. Neurasthenia. ***Night sweats.*** Night, terrors. Paralysis. Pleurisy. ***Pneumonia. Throat, sore.*** Tonsillitis. ***Tuberculosis***.

HOMEOPATHIC - Clarke found no appreciable difference between the action of Tub. and that of Bac. His own impression was that they are practically identical and that one will answer to the indications of the other. The first provers were tuberculosis patients and only pathogenetic symptoms are recorded. Tub. 30c was used.

Tub. affects the mind, lungs, head, occiput, glands and larynx. When symptoms are constantly changing and well-selected remedies fail to improve. Relapsing states. Patient always tired, motion causes intense fatigue, aversion to work, wants constant changes.

Tubercular miasm. In ***tuberculosis*** where the symptoms are constantly changing and begin suddenly, ceasing suddenly or of obscure nature. Early stage tuberculosis.

Always tired, motion causes intense fatigue. Increasing exhaustion and lowered vitality. Weakness, emaciation with good appetite. Rapid breakdown of health. General exhaustion. Nervous weakness.

Neurasthenia. Fainting. Trembling, quivering. Epilepsy. Nervous children. Mentally deficient children.

Tendency to ***catch cold easily,*** on slightest exposure, which ends in diarrhea. ***Diarrhea in children*** running for weeks, extreme wasting, bluish pallor, exhaustion. Chronic, enlargement of the glands, adenoids. Enlarged tonsils. Kidney disorders, chronic cystitis.

Bruised pain throughout the body. Bones painful. Formication. Skin affections, acute rheumatism. Arthritis. Clothes feel very damp. Very susceptible to changes of weather. Very sensitive mentally and physically. Sensitive to music.

MIND - Changing moods. Dissatisfied and restless, always wants a change. ***Desire to travel,*** does not want to remain in one place long. ***Deep feeling of being unfulfilled.*** Romantic longing to find inner contentment. Wants to do something different or even to find a new doctor.

Restlessness. Needs stimulating experiences. Constant fight against boredom. Compulsiveness. Desire to break things. ***Impulse to run***. Reckless. Every trifle irritates, worse when waking. Anxious. Anxiety during fever. Children awake screaming with restlessness. Whimpers when spoken to. Whines and complaints with very little ailment. Precocious children.

Contradictory behavior, changing moods. Insomnia and sopor. ***Depressed***, melancholy. Hopeless. Weary of life. ***Sensitive to music.*** Fear something will happen. ***Fear of animals***, particularly averse to dogs and cats. Aversion to mental work. Confusion, everything in the room seems strange. Ritualistic. Superstitious.

Mania and melancholia. ***Maliciousness*** behavior and destructiveness. Abusive. Fits of violent temper, wants to fight, throws anything at anyone even without a cause. Destructive fantasies. Desire to use foul language, curse and swear.

Abdomen - Inguinal glands indurated and visible. Drum belly. Spleen region bulging out, stitching pain in sides after running. Stitching pain in sides after running. Tympanites. Tabes mesenterica.

Back - Tension in nape of neck and down spine. Chilliness between shoulders or up the back. Pain in the back with palpitations. Sensation as if damp clothes on back.

Breasts - Severe pain in breast at the beginning of menses. ***Breast tumors***, benign. Retraction of nipples.

Causations - Tuberculosis.

Chest - Heat in chest. Sore spot, pressure in chest. Sticking pain on both sides of chest in back.

Constitutions - Tubercular constitutions. Lax fiber, low recuperative powers, very susceptible to changes in the weather. Mentally deficient children. Adapted to light complexioned, narrow-chested people.

Coughs - Hard, dry cough during sleep. Hard, hacking cough with profuse sweating and loss of weight, rales all over chest. Cough with chill and red face, worse evening.

Ears - Persistent offensive otorrhea. ***Perforation in eardrum*** with ragged edges. Sticking pain from pharynx to ears. Great aching in ears and teeth. Tinnitus. Rushing in ears with heavy head.

Eyes - Sore, bruised eyeballs, worse turning them. Eczema of margins of eyelids. Meningitis with squint.

Face - Old looking, edematous, pale. Black blisters on lips. Slight swelling and itching of lips. Aching in malar bones.

Female - Burning in genitals. Amenorrhea. Menses too early, too profuse, long-lasting. Menses soon after childbirth. ***Dysmenorrhea, pains increase with the flow.*** Severe pain in breast at beginning of menses. Benign breast tumors. Retraction of nipples.

Food - Loss of appetite, especially in morning. Aversion to all food, particularly meat. Ravenous hunger at night, driving out of bed. Craves alcohol, delicacies, sweets, ***cold milk. Strong craving for smoked meats and fats,*** bacon, ham, pork. Extreme thirst, day and night.

Head - Meningitis. Periodical headaches. Intense pain, as of an iron band around head. Deep violent head pains, tears hair or beats head with fist. Dashes against the wall or floor, worse motion. Shooting from over eyes (right) through the head to back of ear (left) or from right frontal protuberance to right occipital region. Headaches students, worse study or even slight mental exertion. Brain feels loose. Sensitive scalp. Plica polonica (Vinc.).

Heart - Heaviness and pressure over the heart. Palpitations on taking a deep breath after evening meal.

Kidneys - Must strain at stool to pass urine. Sticky urinary sediment. ***Bedwetting.***

Limbs - Acute articular rheumatism. Hands and arms feel lame, unable to write or raise a cup or a glass. Fingertips brown. Sensation of fatigue in limbs. Cold feet in bed. Limbs feel weak or as if paralyzed worse dinner. Rheumatism. Pains in ulnar nerve. Wandering pain in limbs and joints.

Lungs - Shortness of breath. ***Sensation of suffocation,*** even with plenty of fresh air. Longs for cold air. Asthma. ***Pneumonia*** after influenza. ***Tuberculosis.*** Deposits begin in apex of lung. ***Broncho-pneumonia*** in children. Profuse bronchorrhea. Hard, hacking cough, profuse sweating and loss of weight, rales all over chest. Dry, hard cough, more during sleep, worse dyspnea with chill and red face, worse evenings, worse raising arms. Thick, easy, profuse expectoration. Thick yellow or yellow-green sputum. Mucus rattle in chest without expectoration.

Modalities - Better open air, cool wind. ***Better dry mountain air, pine forests***. Better dry, warm weather. ***Worse from close room. Worse change of weather,*** before a storm, ***cold, damp,*** drafts. Worse motion, slightest exertion, standing. Worse noise and music. Worse periodically. Worse after dinner, evening, night, when beginning to sleep. ***Worse on waking***, early morning, after sleep, from 10 a.m. to 3 p.m. Worse in the mornings, much purulent expectoration, sickness and nausea, loss of appetite, thirst, fatigue. Worse or better at seashore.

Mouth - Dryness, stickiness. Black blisters on lips. Grinding of teeth in sleep. Teeth sensitive to cold air. Sensation as if the teeth were all jammed together and there were too many teeth. Delayed dentition.

Nose - Nose and lips somewhat swollen. Sweat on nose. Crops of small boils, intensely painful, successively appear in the nose, ***green, fetid pus.*** Watery pimples, which, suppurating, form scabs. Dryness of posterior nares. Soreness inside of nose. Colds ending in diarrhea.

Perspiration - Clammy sweats. Sweat stains yellow. Offensive, of chest, axillae, palms, nose and feet. Profuse ***night sweats.*** Sweats from coughing, from slightest exertion. Sweats on hands, on upper parts.

Rectum - Constipation, stools large and hard, then diarrhea. Chronic diarrhea with excessive sweat. Early-morning, sudden diarrhea (Sulph.). Brown, foul, watery stools, discharged with much force. Diarrhea of children running for weeks with wasting, exhaustion and bluish pallor. Tearing pain in rectum on coughing. Tearing in rectum on coughing.

Sensations - As if the brain were squeezed with an iron ring. As if the teeth were jammed together and were too many for the mouth. Mucus in the throat of a tumor in the throat. Pressure in stomach going to throat as if the clothes were too tight. As if the clothes on the back were wet (Bac.).

Skin - Skin easily tanned. Dry, harsh, sensitive. ***Acne*** in tuberculous children. Ringworm. Measles. Psoriasis (Thyr.). Bran-like scales. Chronic eczema. Intense itching, changes places on rubbing, worse at night. Itching in cool air, better heat of stove. Itching worse undressing, bathing.

Sleep - Insomnia and sopor. Overpowering sleepiness in daytime. Shuddering sensation on falling to sleep. ***Grinding of teeth*** during sleep. Night, terrors. Nocturnal hallucinations, wakes frightened. Screaming in sleep. ***Nightmares.*** Child wakes screaming. Awakes in horror. ***Night sweats.*** Poor sleep, restless, wakes early. Overpowering sleepiness in daytime. Distressing, vivid dreams. Dreams of shame. Dreams frightful.

Stomach - All gone hungry sensation (Sulph.), which drives one to eat. Cramping pain in stomach. Belchings and sensation of fullness over stomach. Flatulent dyspepsia. Nausea with pains in umbilical region with diarrhea. Nausea before breakfast, with sudden diarrhea. Vomiting.

Temperature - Remittent fever. Loquacious during fever. ***Profuse sweat***, easy, cold, clammy. Sweat on upper parts, on hands, worse coughing, stains yellow. General chilliness. Chilliness between shoulders or up back. Chilly, at beginning of sleep. Chilly, yet wants fresh air. Shuddering like a chill seems to go from brain down spine. Heat on cheek of affected side in spots. Burning in genitals. Flushes of heat, worse eating. Wants covers on in all stages of fever.

Throat - Hoarseness, better talking. ***Enlarged tonsils***. Hawks mucus after eating. Adenoids. Dryness of the posterior sinuses.

Vertigo - Vertigo with obscuration of eyes, is obliged to lean on something. Vertigo with palpitations, nausea. Vertigo with headache, in morning, after dinner.

COMMENTS - Generally a history of tuberculosis in the family. Suppressed acute infections. Tendency for sore throats, colds, and upper respiratory infections or bronchitis. Swollen glands and big tonsils. Sore throats, swollen glands, start losing weight. Recurring tonsillitis in children. Similar to Bac., but more chronic and more severe.

Colds that go into the chest (Phos.). Asthma, associated with frequent colds. Intercurrent for severe, chronic lung disease. Lingering coughs, pneumonias. Coughs where well-indicated remedies don't work.

Rapid emaciation with a good appetite (Iod., Cina.). Emaciation associated with lung diseases. Rickets. Fatigue, faintness, and profuse debility. Great weakness in the limbs, after dinner. Paralysis.

Disturbed circulation, chills and flushes alternating. Extreme exhaustion with sweat. Night sweats and weight loss (Med.). Night terrors. Insomnia from overexcited state and overactive mind. Children grind their teeth during sleep. "Shivering when beginning to sleep." "Cold feet in bed." Low vital heat.

Fontanelles that fail to close. Hydrocephalus. Meningitis. Characteristic desire to hit their head against the wall. Pressure in the head. Insanity. Hair growth in unusual and new places (Syph., Thuj.). Ringworm, particularly in children (Bac.).

Voracious craving for ice-cold milk. Desires sweets, chocolate, fats, smoked meat, pork, bacon, exotic foods and spicy foods. Craves variety in food. Diarrhea.

Better in the mountains, in pine forests. Desire for open air, particularly with respiratory conditions. Better motion, activity, exercise (Rhus-t.). Worse cold, damp with cold hands and feet.

Hyperactive children. Children seem to have two personalities, one very sweet, nice and apologetic, the other destructive, obstinate, and argumentative. Tantrums, behavioral problems. Can be snappy, irritable, peevish, over-reactive (Cham., when due to pain). Very intelligent, but learning disabilities. Too much energy, can't slow down to learn anything (Med., because they can't focus).

Easily bored. Very excitable. Active and very restless. Always needs something new. Strong desire to travel. Sense that there is something missing (Calc-p.), but they don't know what it is. Discontent. Passionate, driven and dissatisfied. Deep feeling of unfulfillment, emptiness. Very romantic, yearning and longing, pining. Falls in love easily and deeply, can be easily grieved (Nat-m.).

Easily upset. Hard to please, capricious. Malicious, conscious intent to do harm or to disrupt their environment (Med. is unconscious, more confused). Characteristic desire to break things. Can bite or mutilate themselves. Insanity. Fear of wasting their life, their time, of not accomplishing something significant before they die. Fear of dying or despair over their recovery. Dislike of dogs and cats, severe allergies to cats.

Nebel used Tub. in exactly the same way as Burnett; others have used Bac., on the indications Burnett laid down and with

Burnett's results.

In 1892, Arnuphy began giving Tub. 6x and 8x trituration in acute and chronic tuberculosis cases, with encouraging success, but with undesired aggravations at times. These were avoided with 12x and 30x.

In one case, originating in influenza, both apices were affected, the right one breaking down and abundant pleuritic effusion on the left side. Six weeks' treatment with Tub. brought about recovery. When seen a year later, the patient was quite well except for retraction of the left side.

Arnuphy frequently used Tub. for bronchitis, catarrhal pneumonia, lobular pneumonia, tubercular pleurisy, parenchymatous nephritis and influenza. He gave two cases of acute lobular pneumonia with characteristic symptoms and high temperatures quickly resolved by Tub.

One case concerned a boy, 3, who received the 12x; the other was a man, 78, who suffered from chronic bronchial catarrh. The latter was taken with influenza, pneumonia developed and he was in a very serious state. Tub. 30x made an almost immediate change for the better and recovery followed.

Arnuphy related that, in this case, an abundant perspiration took place (the skin had been dry) during the night and he observed this in all cases of pneumonia when Tub. acted favorably.

Clarke found Tub. 30c, 100c, 200c and 1000c the best general antidote to the chronic effects of influenza poisoning.

A curious use of Tub. was made by Jauregg of Vienna in a case of insanity. He had observed that cases of insanity are always benefited by an attack of an acute infectious disease, especially if it is accompanied with high fever. The idea then occurred to him to utilize the fever produced by Koch's Tuberculinic injections.

He tried it on some patients and though the favorable symptoms soon disappeared after the fever subsided, there remained a steady clearing of the confused sensorium. Insanity is very frequently a manifestation of the tuberculosis miasm and there is something more than a pyrexial power in Tub.

RELATIONS - Vaccinosis may block the way of action of Tub. until Thuj. has been given. When Tub. fails Syph. often follows, producing a positive reaction. ***Compare:*** (1) Bac., Phos., Sil. (2) Tub-a., Form-ac. Stann., (3) Psor., Lach. (4) Teucr-s. - tuberculosis, garlicky odor of all secretions and breath. ***Complementary:*** Bac., Phos., Calc., Chin., Bry.

REFERENCES - Boericke. Clarke. Murphy. Phatak.

TURQUOISE

(Gemstone)

PHARMACY - turq. Turquoise. Gemstone. Hydrous copper aluminum phosphate. CuAl6(PO4)4(OH)8, 5H2O. ***Historical dose:*** All potencies.

CLINICAL - Asthma. Backache. Cramps. Coryza. Cough. Diarrhea. Faintness. Fractures. Headache. Heat, flushes. Influenza. Injuries. Leucorrhea. Vertigo

HOMEOPATHIC - Injuries after falling from a height. Injuries to bones, fractures. Sharp pains. Internal or external squeezing pain. Sharp pains. Internal trembling. Accelerated pulse. Tension. Faintness on rising. Weakness, lassitude. Emaciation. Influenza.

Worse in the morning, afternoon, 1 to 4 p.m., after midnight, 3 a.m. Worse from waking. Coldness in the morning, in bed. Heat flushes, at noon. Heat aggravates. Better from the moon.

MIND - Fastidious. Industrious. Creative. Memory, active. Dullness, slowness of mind. Difficult concentration. Aversion to mental work. Forgetfulness. Discouraged.

Cheerfulness. Excitement, exhilaration. Laughing, quickly followed by weeping. Alternating moods. Horrible news, sad stories, affect profoundly. Sadness. Grief. Homesickness. Weeping. Despair.

Impatience. Irritability, waking aggravates. Irritability before menses. Confrontational. Censorious. Hatred. Angry, toward husband. Averse to husband. Aversion to company. Anxiety, during cough.

Vivacious. Confidence increased. Amorous disposition. Clairvoyance. Foreboding.

Tranquility. Relaxed feeling. Persistent thoughts. Delusion that she is betrayed. Delusion of being old. As if in a dream. Time passes too slowly, appears longer. Detached. Sensitive to noise, light. Starting during sleep. Restlessness.

Abdomen - Distension. Abdominal pain, better from diarrhea or vomiting. Cutting, squeezing, cramping pain, during diarrhea.

Back - Backache, worse draft of air, bending forward. Back pain, cervical, dorsal, under scapula, lumbar. Dorsal contraction. Lumbar, dorsal tension. Aching pain, cervical, extending to occiput. Cervical stiffness. As if neck gripped by a hand. Pain, swelling in the cervical glands. Pimples. Eruptions, acne.

Breasts - Itching in nipples.

Chest - Compressed sensation. Constriction. Eruptions, acne. Itching, evening. Pain in the ribs. Tingling. Tingling, side.

Ears - Clear discharge. Noises, especially in the left.

Eyes - Dryness, irritation. Heaviness, tired sensation. Swelling. Scratching sensation. Pain, as if from sand.

Face - Discoloration, red flushes. Greasy. Wrinkled skin. Dry lips, posterior nares. Peeling, rough lips. Herpetic eruptions, painful, suppurating. Eruption on lower lip, around mouth. Acne, on forehead. Pimples.

Female - Profuse clotted menses, frequent, too early, too soon, too short. Cramping pain in uterus, during menses. Leucorrhea, lumpy. Itching vagina. Pain, burning vagina. Sexual desire increased, decreased.

Foods - Aversion to meat, sweets. Desires alcohol, cold drinks, cold food, salt, pickles at night. Wine aggravates.

Heads - Sudden headaches. Headaches in the afternoon, evening, on waking. Headaches, worse motion. Forehead pain, behind the eyes, extending to vertex. Temple pain, extending to vertex, forehead. Occiput pain, at night. Vertex pain. Dull pain. Piercing, penetrating pain. Squeezed pain in occiput. Expanded sensation. Sensation of swelling. Sensation of wet towel inside head. Itching scalp.

Kidneys - Urging to urinate. Pain before urination. Frequent urination. Feeble stream, slow, weak.

Limbs - Sharp pain in hip, thigh. Cramps in legs, hips, ankles, feet. Leg cramps at night. Leg weakness, descending stairs with trembling. Burning foot. Blotches, red eruptions. Dry eruptions. Echymoses, in lower limbs. Eruptions in legs, calf, knee, itching. Itching eruption in the forearm, shoulder, hands, palms. Numb finger, second finger. Electrical current sensation in arms. Stiff, tense shoulder.

Lungs - Asthma. Difficult breathing. Dry cough. Night cough.

Mouth - Metallic taste. Numb tongue. Pain, biting in the tongue. Roughness inside lip. Swelling gums.

Nose - Obstruction at night, wakes him. Obstruction, morning. Coryza in the morning, with fluent discharge. Clear discharge. Sneezing in the morning. Acute sense of smell.

Perspiration - Scanty sweat.

Rectum - Constipation, ineffectual urging. Diarrhea. Frequent hard or soft stool. Bloody stool. Flaky stool.

Skin - Abscess. Echymoses. Eruption, pimples, worse warmth. Painful eruptions, red, sudden itching.

Sleep - Yawning, vehement, violent. Falling asleep difficult. Restless. Unrefreshing sleep. Sudden waking, after midnight, 1 a.m., 2 a.m., 3 a.m. Difficult waking. Deep sleep. Vivid dreams. Dreams of cats, insects. Dreams of food, of water, of urinating. Dreams of houses falling apart, of falling, of injuries. Dreams of making purchases, of money, of servants. Dreams of being small, of being very tall, of growing large. Dreams of a man who looks like a woman.

Stomach - Appetite diminished, easy satiety. Appetite increased. Thirst. Tension. Noises, gurgling. Eructations at night. Nausea, with chill, headache. Vomiting.

Throat - Pain. Itching. Thick sensation. Voice rough.

Vertigo - Vertigo with headache, during sleep.

Vision - Acute or blurred vision.

COMMENTS - One of the first gemstones to be mined, turquoise has long been prized for its intense color, which varies from sky blue to green, depending on the quantities of iron and copper within it.

Turquoise symbolizes laughter, humor, confidence, and purpose. Turquoise is said to strengthen eyesight and even cure blindness. Strengthens and calms the mind and body. Stimulates tissue regeneration. Revitalizes blood, nervous system.

It is said to be beneficial for circulation, bowel cramps and the chest area including lungs and respiratory system. Throat, lungs, asthma. Tones and strengthens entire body. Good for internal cleansing. Infections. Headache. High blood pressure. Anorexia. Teeth, jaw ailments. Hearing disorders.

Like amethyst, it protects and detoxifies from alcohol, poison, pollution, x-ray/sun radiation. Induces enthusiasm. Encourages family bonding. Promotes trust, love, kindness and innocence. Empowers artistic traits. Provides discipline, attention and understanding. For fear, depression.

RELATIONS - ***Compare:*** Amethyst. Amber. Ruby.

REFERENCES - Murphy. Rowe.

TUSSILAGO FARFARA

(Coltsfoot)

PHARMACY - tus-fa. Tussilago farfara. Coltsfoot. British herb. Farfara. Tobacco waste. N. O. Compositae. Waste, sandy, clay banks. Tincture of fresh plant. ***Historical dose:*** Tincture and all potencies.

CLINICAL - ***Coughs.*** Gonorrhea. Scrofula. Tuberculosis.

HERBAL - Cooper noted that Tussilago farfara is used in the form of a confection for coughs. The leaves are mucilaginous and were much used in scrofulous disorders. Smoking the dried leaves relieves coughs.

HOMEOPATHIC - Tus-fa. has been used as an intercurrent medicine in tuberculosis of the lungs (Tub.). ***Coughs.*** A popular reputation in gonorrhea.

REFERENCES - Clarke. Cooper.

TUSSILAGO FRAGRANS

PHARMACY - tus-f. Tussilago fragrans. Petasites fragrans. Italian tussilage. Fragrant Tussilage. N. O. Compositae. Tincture of whole plant. ***Historical dose:*** Tincture and all potencies.

CLINICAL - Obesity. Plethora.

HOMEOPATHIC - Demesnes proved Tus-f., taking three drops of the tincture on the tongue. After first causing a disagreeable, spiteful mood, it set up in a few days an opposite condition, which lasted some time. A journey taken on the ninth day of the proving, which usually caused loss of weight, did not do so.

Tus-f. has a peculiar sensation induced was as if a morsel of food lay at the bottom of the cardia and would not pass. Stoutness increased and plethora was added, later on the abdominal protuberance permanently disappeared.

REFERENCES - Clarke.

TUSSILAGO PETASITES

(Bitter-burr)

PHARMACY - tus-p. Tussilago petasites. Bitter-burr. Petasites officinalis. Petasites vulgaris. N. O. Compositae. Grows on sandy meadows on the banks of streams. Tincture of whole fresh plant. ***Historical dose:*** Tincture and all potencies.

CLINICAL - ***Coughs.*** Gallbladder, colic. Gonorrhea. Headache. Kidney colic. Lumbago. Night-sweats. Orchitis. Prostatitis. Pylorus disorders. Sinusitis. Spasmodic cough. Throat, sore. Tibia, pain. Uvula, burning.

HERBAL - Tussilago petasites grows in Central and Northern Europe. Tussilago means "cough-wort." According to Green's Herbal, it is "a genus of Compositae established for three or four species of Tussilago, which have the flower-heads partially dioeceous in racemes, sometimes branching into panicles.

"The essential characters which separate them from the common Coltsfoot (Tussilago farfara) are very slight and the foliage is the same" (Treasury of Botany). Tussilago petasites grows on river-banks that are little trodden on. The roots are an admirable medicine in the worst kind of fevers with boils or buboes."

A medicinal plant, it was used as a diaphoretic in the middle ages. Its pharmacological action is sudorific, diuretic, emmenagogue and anti-asthmatic. It has been used for uterine cramps, coughs, hoarseness and urinary disorders.

HOMEOPATHIC - In 1847 it was the object of a fragmented homeopathic proving by Kuchenmeister and in 1960 of a pharmacological study by Karl Haas. A recent pharmacological study of the root extract revealed a product with antispasmodic action.

Tus-p. has some action on the urinary organs and was found useful in gonorrhea. Affections of pylorus. Irritation of the urethra. Crawling in urethra. Gonorrhea, yellowish, thick discharge. Erections with crawling in the urethra. Inflammation and pain of the spermatic cord. Lumbar pain. Pains in the frontal sinuses.

Modalities - Pains in pylorus worse by pressure. Lumbago worse standing. Drinking causes belchings. Worse from walking.

COMMENTS - Kuchenmeister and five others took substantial doses. Most noticeable among the symptoms were a lumbago of very great severity. Tightness of the chest. Headache shifting from one part of the head to another during two days. Pain about the pylorus. Urethritis with yellow discharge.

Hansen gave the indication "Acute or chronic gonorrhea, yellow or white, thick discharge." Crawling in urethra, jerking in spermatic cord and drawing in right testicle are additional symptoms of the proving.

Rosenberg gave some experiences. The first concerned an extremely violent gonorrhea, penis swollen, painful, emission of urine extremely painful, mixed with blood, patient feverish and restless.

Tus-p. was given in water. There was a great aggravation of all symptoms in thirty-six hours. The remedy was discontinued and marked amelioration followed. Resumed again, much diluted, rapid cure followed. The remedy was used externally as well in this case.

A second case was a chronic ophthalmia, the result of gonorrhea "cured" with turpentine. Tus-p. restored the discharge and then cured.

Rosenberg referred to a writer who said of the plant that if it is macerated in water, the water will not spoil even if kept for years.

RELATIONS - ***Compare:*** (1) Tus-fa. or Tus-f. - pylorus pain, plethora and corpulency. (2) Pain in pylorus - Tus-f. is as if a morsel had lodged at bottom of cardia. (3) Lumbago, Ant-t. (4) gonorrhea, Thuj.

REFERENCES - Boericke. Clarke.

TYPHA LATIFOLIA

(Cat-tail Flag)

PHARMACY - typh. Typha latifolia. Cat-tail flag. Tincture. N. O. Typhaceae. ***Historical dose:*** Tincture and all potencies.

HOMEOPATHIC - Diarrhea, dysentery. Summer diarrhea complaint of children.

RELATIONS - ***Compare:*** Cupr., Chin.

REFERENCES - Boericke.

U

ULMUS FULVA

(Slippery Elm Bark)

PHARMACY - ulm. Ulmus fulva. Slippery elm bark. Ulmus campestris. Red elm. Moose elm. N. O. Ulmaceae of the Urticaceae. Grows in the mountains of Canada and Pennsylvania. Pounded dried inner bark. Decoction of dried bark. Tincture of fresh bark. ***Historical dose:*** Tincture and all potencies.

CLINICAL - Boils. Burns. Chilblains. Constipation. Deafness. Hemorrhoids. Herpes. Inflammations. ***Malnutrition.*** Ophthalmia. Pain. Sore throats. Syphilis. Ulcers. Wounds.

HERBAL - Slippery elm is an herbal diuretic, emollient, and demulcent. A decoction of the viscous inner bark is used as a poultice for painful inflammations. It may be used as such in all cases of weakness, inflammation of the stomach, bronchitis, etc.

The coarse powder forms the finest poultice to be obtained for all inflamed surfaces, ulcers, wounds, burns, boils, skin diseases, purulent ophthalmia, chilblains etc. It soothes the part, disperses the inflammation, draws out impurities, and heals speedily. The finely powdered bark makes an excellent gruel or food, and in addition possesses as much nutrition as oatmeal.

COMMENTS - In a case in which the mucus membrane of the rectum was dry and extremely painful, Burnett relieved the sufferings with 20 drop doses of the tincture.

Cooper mentioned that the triturated bark gives much relief as a snuff in old vascular deafness with tubal obstruction. He could not speak too highly of this remedy, and are confident there is nothing to equal it in the world for its mentioned uses.

Inflammation in the bowels of infants and adults has been cured, when all other remedies have failed, by an injection into the bowels of an infusion of 1 oz of powdered bark to 1 pt of boiling water, used while warm. Slippery elm is also used in lozenges to relieve irritation of the pharynx.

The food or gruel should be made as follows: Take a teaspoonful of the powder, mix well with the same quantity of powdered sugar and add 1 pt of boiling water slowly, mixing as it is poured on. This may be flavored with cinnamon or nutmeg to suit the taste, and makes a very wholesome and sustaining food for infants.

REFERENCES - Clarke. Cooper. Murphy. Potter's Cyclopedia.

UNCARIA TOMENTOSA

(Cat's Claw)

PHARMACY - uncar. Uncaria tomentosa. Cat's claw. Una de Gato. N. O. Rubiaceae. Tincture from the inner bark. ***Historical dose:*** Tincture and all potencies.

CLINICAL - AIDS. Arthritis. Asthma. Brain tumors. Cancer. Chronic fatigue syndrome. Circulation poor. Colitis. Crohn's disease. Exhaustion. Fibromyalgia. ***Immune, weakness.*** Prostate enlarged. Radiation poisoning. Ulcers. Virus effects. Weakness.

HERBAL - Uncaria tomentosa, or cat's claw, has been used by the Ashaninka Indians of the Peruvian Amazon. The inner bark and the root contain similar properties, but the inner bark is preferred over the root, because stripping the bark does not kill the plant.

It is reputed to ***enhance immune functions***, increase energy and stamina. An ideal tonic for those who are mentally, emotionally and physically exhausted from overwork or excessive stress. Helps against viruses, radiation, chemical toxins and chemotherapy effects.

COMMENTS - Hank, age 53, suffered from partial urinary blockage due to an enlarged prostate for over two years. After drinking three cups of cat's claw tea daily, using one teaspoon full of the powdered herb per cup. He reported that his symptoms dramatically diminished after three days.

REFERENCES - Murphy.

UPAS ANTIARIS

PHARMACY - upa-a. Upas antiaris. N. O. Loganiaceae. Resinous exudation of Antiarus toxiearia. ***Historical dose:*** All potencies.

HOMEOPATHIC - Merrel noted that Upa-a. is used in Java as an arrow poison. It is a deadly poison to the muscular system. It suspends both voluntary muscular action and that of the heart without causing convulsions. It produces ***clonic spasms,*** violent vomiting, diarrhea, great prostration.

REFERENCES - Boericke.

UPAS TIEUTE

(Upas Tree)

PHARMACY - upa. Upas tieute. Upas tree. Strychnos tieute. N. O. Loganiaceae. Tincture of the inspissated juice obtained from the root and bark. ***Historical dose:*** The tincture and all potencies, third to higher potencies.

CLINICAL - Asphyxia. Backache. Conjunctivitis. ***Eye, pains.*** Hangnails. Headaches. Palpitations. Sexual, excess. Styes. Tetanus. Vision, disorders.

HOMEOPATHIC - Upa. is obtained from a Strychnos and must not be confounded with Antiaris toxicaria, the concocted juice of which forms the *"Upas antiar"* poison of the Javanese. S. tieute is a climbing shrub. Pitet made a courageous proving of it, carrying it to the length of producing tetanic symptoms.

Upa. produces ***tonic spasms, tetanus and asphyxia.*** A large proportion of the symptoms occurred in the head and eyes. A remarkable headache, "superficial drawing pain traverses left temple from before backward and ceases at outer angle of orbit, the part is hot and painful to touch."

Pressure in the eyes, feeling of a foreign body under the eyelids. Severe pains in orbits inflammation of the conjunctiva of the lids. Distorted vision. "Every morning weakness of the eyes with lachrymation, the lids being so heavy that they close involuntarily as if from drowsiness."

Drowsiness. Pressive and lancinating pains. Pain in the left side of the throat as from a splinter on swallowing. Pain in left sciatic nerve in left iliac fossa. Chiefly affects the left-side.

MIND - Irritable. Disinclined for mental work.

Back - ***Dull backache,*** as after excessive sex.

Causations - Sexual excess.

Chest - Sharp pain throughout right lung toward the liver, stopping breathing.

Eyes - Dull, sunken eyes. ***Pain in eyes and orbits with conjunctivitis***. Styes.

Head - Dull headache deep in brain.

Heart - Violent palpitations, sensation of heaviness in stomach.

Limbs - Hangnails inflamed, itching and redness of nail roots. Numb hands, feet.

Male - Desire increased with loss of power.

Modalities - Better after rising. Better evenings, after dinner. Headache better in open air. Pain in left iliac fossa worse by touch. Throat worse pressure. Worse by motion, walking. Worse morning, afternoon and evening.

Mouth - Herpes on lips. Burning on the tongue. Pain in mouth, as from a splinter (Nit-ac.).

Sensations - As if the brain were rudely shaken. As if a foreign body in eye, as if sand in eyes. As if a splinter in throat on swallowing. As if a foreign body in esophagus preventing swallowing. As if an iron hoop around waist preventing breathing. As after sexual excess.

COMMENTS - Keynote sensitiveness. Irritability, crossness, moroseness increased sensitiveness to cold, the least irritation brought on spasms, pressing in throat causing feeling of suffocation.

Vertigo, ending in pressing headache. Twitching in brain and orbits. Pulsative headache with throbbing all over body. Great exhaustion after convulsive seizures. Itching in patella. Sexual function depressed. Distressing symptoms after sex, as occur after sexual excess.

Left half of face red and hot, right half pale and cold. The tongue is coated white so thickly that it can be scraped off. Aversion to meat and eggs, the very thought of them causes nausea. Smell of manure in nose. Sallow complexion. Severe symptoms in the liver and from the right lung to the liver (cutting as with knives).

RELATIONS - ***Antidote:*** Cur. ***Compare:*** (1) Upas-a., Ox-ac. (2) Upas when Bry. fails (typhoid).

REFERENCES - Boericke. Clarke.

URANIUM MURIATICUM

(Uranium Chloride)

PHARMACY - uran-m. Uranium muriaticum. Uranium chloride. ***Historical dose:*** All potencies.

CLINICAL - Diabetes. Glycosuria. Malassimilation. Pancreas, disorders.

HOMEOPATHIC - Tongue reddish at edges. Malassimilation. Dyspepsia. Prout noted it for diabetes mellitus and insipidus, especially when the diabetes originates in assimilating derangements.

Many cases of diabetes have been cured or much improved by either of these preparations, usually administered in the 1x or 2x trituration or dilution, several times a day for weeks.

REFERENCES - Raue.

URANIUM NITRICUM

(Uranium Nitrate)

PHARMACY - uran-n. Uranium nitricum. Uranium nitrate. Uranyl nitrate. Solution in distilled water. Trituration. ***Historical dose:*** All potencies.

CLINICAL - Albuminuria. Anal, itching. ***Ascites.*** Backache. Bedwetting, nocturnal. Bronchitis. Constipation. ***Debility. Diabetes mellitus. Diabetes insipidus. Dropsy***. Duodenum, ulcer. Dyspepsia. Edema. ***Emaciation.*** Enteritis. Gastric, ulcer. Glycosuria. Impotency. Insomnia. Malassimilation. Milk, secretion. Nephritis. Nephrotic, syndrome. Neuralgia. Ophthalmia. Peritonitis. Phosphaturia. Seminal discharges. Stomach, ulcers. Stomatitis. Styes. Ulcers. Urine, incontinence. Vertigo.

HOMEOPATHIC - Uran-n. belongs to the chromium group of elements. Uran-n. was proved by E. T. Blake, his monograph forms part of Hahnemann's Materia Medica.

Blake's proving was suggested by the observation of an old-school experimenter, Leconte, who found sugar in the urine of dogs slowly poisoned with Uran-n. Blake was not very successful in producing sugar, but his proving is not any less valuable on that account and clinical use has filled out the picture.

Uran-n. causes glycosuria and increased urine. Produces nephritis, diabetes mellitus and insipidus, degeneration of the liver, high blood pressure and dropsy. Its therapeutic keynote is ***great emaciation, debility and tendency to ascites and general dropsy***. Excessive thirst, nausea, vomiting, excessive appetite. Dry mucus membranes and skin.

High blood pressure. Burning in the stomach, gastric ulcer. Incontinence of urine. Burning in urethra while passing urine. Impotency with nightly emissions. Backache and delayed menses. Menses suppressed during diabetes. The left side was more affected than the right.

MIND - Ill-humor, not feeling well all day. Depression.

Abdomen - ***Abdomen bloated.*** Borborygmi. Flatus. Sharp colic with tenesmus and raw feeling in rectum. ***Enteritis and peritonitis with meteorism and great prostration.***

Back - Pain at lower angle of left scapula, worse deep inspiration. Tenderness of spine near and extending to kidneys.

Breasts - Excessive secretion of milk.

Chest - Intermittent pain, radiating from left side to ensiform cartilage, worse fasting.

Cough - Cough with purulent discharge from left nostril. Cough with loss of appetite and great prostration.

Eyes - ***Styes*** in left upper lid. Edema of lower lids, worse than usual. Lids inflamed, agglutinated. Shooting from right orbit to occipital protuberance in evening. Pain over left eye.

Female - Pale, anemic. Menses suppressed during diabetes. Flushing of upper body during menses, with giddiness and faintness. Excessive flow of milk.

Food - Malassimilation. Ravenous appetite.

Eating followed by flatulence. Excessive thirst with intermittent vomiting or with emaciation (diabetes). ***Loss of appetite during menses.*** Craves raw ham, tea, sweets. Intense thirst from sensation of dryness in mouth and fauces. Excessive thirst at night.

Head - Head heavy on waking. Heaviness of head with general languor. Dull, heavy pain. Heavy, burning, in right side of vertex. Shooting from right orbit extending to occipital protuberance, in evening. Frontal headache. Dull aching in right temple. Pain in forehead, over left eye. Pain in left temple, with feeling as if he had taken cold. Severe pain, at posterior edge of right and left temporal bones. Aching at occipital protuberance. Fullness of head. Sensation of blood flowing to head, before eating. Neuralgia on posterior edge of left temporal bone.

Kidneys - Contracted, gouty kidneys, with gastric disturbances. Sore pain in bladder region in evening. Acute nephritis. Diabetes insipidus and mellitus. Incontinence of urine at night. ***Nocturnal bedwetting.*** Burning in urethra, with very acid urine. ***Sugar in the urine.*** Copious urination in cold weather. Diuresis. Unable to retain urine without pain. Urine often excoriating. Urine greenish and smelling fishy. Urine pale, milky, with ammoniacal odour. Profuse, painful urination.

Limbs - Stiffness in loins. White vesicles on arms and legs with red areolae, burn and itch.

Lungs - ***Bronchitis with copious mucus expectoration and much emaciation.*** Chronic colds. Hydrothorax and congestion of lungs. Lung infiltrated with gray tubercle.

Male - Complete impotence with nocturnal emissions. Organs cold, relaxed, sweaty.

Modalities - Better from deep breathing. Worse at night. Headache worse walking.

Mouth - Painless ulcer with one elevated side in mouth, opposite left anterior upper molar, worse evening. Acid saliva. Ulcers in mouth, with copious salivation.

Nose - Itching in nose. Left nostril stuffed. Dry coryza. Nostrils sore with purulent acrid discharge. Chronic scabbing of inner nostril.

Rectum - Borborygmi. Constipation. Urging in rectum and bladder. Soft stool, twice in one day. Anal itching.

Sensations - As if blood were flowing to head. As if he had taken cold with headache.

Skin - White vesicles on hands and legs, with red areola. Burning and itching. Ecchymosis. Epithelioma. Lupus exedens.

Sleep - Restless, with shivering and heat. Extreme languor, on rising from bed. Feeling as if he had taken cold. Great drowsiness and prostration during menses. Restless at night during menses. Sleeplessness.

Stomach - Constant faintness at stomach, even after a hearty meal. Indigestion in afternoon. Dyspepsia, flatus after food, acidity, pain. Tasteless, putrid belchings. ***Sinking at pit***, with acid eructations, flatulence and copious urination. ***Boring pain in pyloric region.*** Burning pain. Gastric and duodenal ulcers. Recurring hematemesis. Nausea and ***vomiting.***

Temperature - Shivering, alternating with heat, at night, with great restlessness. Shivering during day.

Throat - Hawking of tenacious mucus. Contracted feeling in throat.

Vertigo - Vertigo, faint, flushing of upper part of body during menses. Vertigo, worse in evening. Vertigo with heaviness of head. Vertigo with debility and cold feeling.

COMMENTS - Many cases of diabetes have been relieved or cured by Uran-n., usually in the lower potencies. Diabetes with excessive thirst, polyuria and dry tongue. Glycosuria is by no means an essential part of the indications for Uran-n.

Diabetes concomitant with indigestion, belching, burping, and heartburn. Urine with bile and sugar in it, can smell fishy. Kidney disease with protein in the urine, nephrotic syndrome. Stomach ulcers. Very weak (Ph-ac.), debilitated, tendencies toward dizziness.

One case, involving a married woman, was

cured with 5 grain doses of Uran-n. 2x.

She was weak and emaciated, vomited mucus mixed with blood and coffee-ground matter and passed dark, tarry stools, sensitive and tender over region of pylorus.

Dr. Choudhury noted a case of diabetes in a middle-aged man. The patient had progressive weight loss, weakness, and great weariness in the legs with edema. His tongue was coated white, severely dry mouth. Pale, looked haggard with dark circles. Neither Chin. or Phos-ac. helped. Uran-n 30c cured. The patient needed no insulin after treatment.

RELATIONS - ***Compare:*** (1) Elemental relatives, gastro-duodenal affections, Chrom. and Kali-bi. (2) Diabetes, Phos., Ph-ac., Syzyg., Thyr., Lac-def., Lac-ac. (3) Sinking immediately after meals, Ars., Cina, Lyc., Sil., Staph. (4) Craves tea, Sel.

REFERENCES - Boericke. Clarke. Murphy.

UREA PURA
(Carbamide)

PHARMACY - urea. Urea pura. Carbamide. Urea nitrica. The chief solid constituent of the urine of mammals. White crystals. Trituration. Also tincture or solution of the nitrate, Urea nitrica. ***Historical dose:*** Tincture and all potencies.

CLINICAL - Albuminuria. Cirrhosis. Coma. Convulsions. Diabetes. Dropsy. Eczema, gouty. Gout. Kidney stones. Liver, cirrhosis. Pleurisy. ***Skin, disorders.*** Tuberculosis. Uremia.

HOMEOPATHIC - On general indications, Urea. has been used in medicine by both schools. Merck mentioned that it is diuretic and is used in cirrhosis of liver, pleurisy, kidney calculus.

The failure of the kidneys to eliminate urea from the blood leads to uremic intoxication, delirium, convulsions and coma. Tuberculosis. Lumps. Enlarged glands. Kidney dropsy with symptoms of general intoxication. Albuminuria, diabetes, uremia. Urine thin and of low specific gravity. Constant urging, much sediment in urine. Intolerable sensation in abdomen, with burning skin.

Gouty eczema. General uneasiness, felt ill, poisoned.

Urea acted as a nervous tonic in tuberculosis patients. Urea is a hydrogogue diuretic in the treatment of dropsies. 10 grains every 6 hours.

Abdomen - In right hypochondrium, a steady, dull sensation. Intolerable sensation in abdomen and burning of the skin.

Eyes - Itching and profuse watering of eyes.

Head - Head very dull, as if filled with a very heavy lump.

Kidneys - Constant urging to urinate, beginning at root of penis. Profuse diuresis with rapid diminution of dropsy. Albuminuria, bloody urine, general dropsy.

COMMENTS - Burnett used both Urea 6c and Ur-ac. 6c in gouty eczema, "where the gouty eczema has been the cutaneous outlet for the constitution."

Burnett gave Urea in gouty cases where the urine was thin and of low specific gravity, "it thickens the urine and gives great relief to the patient."

Allen cited from Mauthner two cases of kidney dropsy with symptoms of general intoxication in which Urea, 2 grains., divided into three doses and given two hours apart, cured brilliantly.

Arthur Buch related cases of tuberculosis cured, on the plan originated by Harper of Nottingham, with Urea in 20 to 30 grain doses three times a day. Under the treatment, lupoid nodules disappeared, tuberculous glands disappeared, tuberculous joints improved. No ill-effects of the treatment were noticed, "on the contrary, the action has evidently been in many cases that of a nervous tonic."

Villers examined the urine of an intensely neurasthenic woman, suffering from severe asthma and found 4.5 percent of urea instead of the usual 2.5. In order to find out the effect of Urea. on the healthy, he took for five days Urea. 15x., five drops thrice daily.

He was then compelled to stop by the severity of the symptoms. He gave the same dose to a patient, a woman. She begged after a short time to be allowed to discontinue the medicine, as it affected her so painfully, causing constant urging to urinate, much sediment in the urine intolerable sensation in abdomen and burning of the skin.

RELATIONS - ***Compare:*** (1) Ur-ac. - gout, gouty eczema, rheumatism, lipoma. (2) Urt-u., Tub., Thyr. (3) Urin., Ur-ac., Thiosin., Urt-u. (4) Diuresis, Thyr. (5) Tuberculosis, Tub., Bac.

REFERENCES - Allen. Boericke. Clarke.

URICUM ACIDUM

(Uric Acid)

PHARMACY - ur-ac. Uricum acidum. Uric acid. Lithic acid. Trituration. ***Historical dose:*** All potencies.

CLINICAL - Eczema. Gout. Lipoma. Rheumatism. Sebaceous cysts. Tumors. Wens.

HOMEOPATHIC - Ur-ac. has been used on inferential grounds in gouty conditions. Burnett gave it in the 5th and 6th potencies. It is most useful in cases where deposits persist, it stirs them up and helps to eliminate them.

Gouty eczema where the eczema has been the skin outlet for the constitution. Gout. Lipoma. Rheumatism. Headaches with pain as if the head will burst, worse when talking.

COMMENTS - Mersch cured a case of lipoma situated on the left side between abdomen and breast, "as large as a man's head, only lengthened." Relief was almost immediate, the tumor disappeared in a month.

RELATIONS - ***Compare:*** (1) Urea., Urin., Urin-f., Urt-u.

REFERENCES - Clarke.

URINUM FERMENTA

(Fermented Human Urine)

PHARMACY - urin-f. Urinum fermenta. Fermented human urine. Old human urine is fermented naturally in a glass jar for a few years, then made into potencies. ***Historical dose:*** Tincture and all potencies.

CLINICAL - Acne. Bites. ***Blood, disorders.*** Boils. ***Burns.*** Cancer. Dropsy. Dysentery. Eczema. Fungus. Gout. Hair, loss. ***Infections.*** Plague. Psoriasis. Rashes. Ringworm. ***Skin, disorders.*** Scars. Scurvy. Snakebites. Tuberculosis. Ulcers. Uremia. Varicose, ulcers. Warts. ***Wounds.***

HOMEOPATHIC - Old urine has a higher ammonia content that is more effective on skin disorders as eczema and psoriasis. To store urine for later use, one should pour it into a glass bottle and close it tightly. Keep the bottle in a cool, dark place for long periods of time.

Side effects can include headache, ***diarrhea***, itching and rashes, pain, fatigue, soreness of the shoulder, and fever. An increase in symptoms of the specific illness may also occur.

COMMENTS - S. Mills Folwer mentioned the use of urine as a remedy for scurvy in the Civil War. In Andersonville prison the starving prisoners were dying by hundreds of scurvy and Mr. T. (who told the story) was one of the sufferers.

His legs were flexed upon the thighs and the thighs upon the body in such violent contraction that it was impossible to extend them an inch and any attempt to do so was attended with shocks of pain as from an electric battery. He could only move on his elbows and rump.

Within the stockade were growing two large turpentine trees. Of the pitch from these trees the patients would take enough to make their urine "clear and white as crystal." The urine voided was allowed to stand until it began to sour, which took twelve to twenty-four hours.

The patients then took a "good swallow" four or five times a day. They felt the good effect of every dose. The treatment cured Mr. T. and all his companions in misfortune who adopted it.

RELATIONS - ***Compare:*** Urea., Urin., Ur-ac.

REFERENCES - Murphy.

URINUM HUMANUM

(Human Urine)

PHARMACY - urin. Urinum humanum. Human urine. Dilutions. ***Historical dose:*** Tincture and all potencies.

CLINICAL - Acne. AIDS. Albuminuria. Anemia. Ascites. Baldness. ***Blood, disorders.*** Boils. ***Burns.*** Cancer. Chronic fatigue. Cirrhosis. Diabetes. Dropsy. Dysentery. Eczema. Fungus. Gout. Hair, loss. ***Hepatitis.*** Immune, weakness. ***Infections.*** Infertility. Leprosy. Liver, disorders. Multiple sclerosis. Ophthalmia. Plague. Premenstrual syndrome. Psoriasis. Ringworm. ***Skin, disorders.*** Scars. Scurvy. Tuberculosis. Uremia. ***Wounds.***

HOMEOPATHIC - Urine is one of the most ancient remedies and can be used topically, internally and in homeopathic potencies. An important component of urine is urea, a commonly recognized antibacterial, antifungal, and antiviral agent.

The Chinese treated wounds by sprinkling urine on them and the custom is widespread in the Far East. It is a major therapy in Ayurvedic medicine and was commonly used in ancient India.

It is a custom in Yorkshire to wipe the baby's tongue with its own napkin in cases of thrush. For pimples and blotches the natives of Barbados drink their urine and apply it locally. Soldiers in Germany would urinate in their boots so they wouldn't get sores and blisters on their feet from long hikes. In Switzerland, for cases of ophthalmia in children, it is the custom to bathe the eyes in the children's own urine.

Taken internally urine is believed to stimulate the circulation and is valued as an active oxytocic. Anasarca, generally more marked in upper than in lower parts of body. Heaviness, heavy for work, having neither his usual life nor warmth in him. Loses her breath if she walks quickly, is obliged to stop.

Used for multiple sclerosis, colitis, lupus, rheumatoid arthritis. Cancer, hepatitis, pancreatic insufficiency, psoriasis, eczema. Diabetes, herpes, mononucleosis, adrenal failure. Allergies. Premenstrual syndrome, easy labor, mastitis. Cancer.

Abdomen - Ascites. Fluid in abdomen and in parietes of chest and belly.

Face - The face is very much swollen. Countenance pale, expression heavy and vague.

Head - Heaviness of head, worse on stooping.

Kidneys - Urine scanty, thick, deep brown and very offensive.

Rectum - Diarrhea.

Skin - Acne. Boils. Burns and skin rashes. Eczema. Scar tissues. Psoriasis. Wounds.

Stomach - Little thirst.

COMMENTS - In the Brit. Med. Jour. of 1900 a number of instances of Western urine therapy were given. Cooper made some additions to these.

Cooper had a case of a youth with crops of boils which nothing could remedy. He was recommended to drink a cupful of his own urine every morning for three mornings. Then after an intermission of three days to resume and so on until cured. He was cured on the ninth day.

Cooper mentioned the case of a man who suffered very much from weak and inflamed eyes until he began to bathe his eyes in his own urine, which after a time cured him. A case of blackheads was cured in exactly the same way. This patient drank the urine when fresh.

A case of chronic bronchitis was much relieved. This patient was deaf and misunderstood the doctor's direction to bring some of his urine. He thought the doctor said "drink," and acted accordingly. Urine also cured ague and urticaria.

Allen under Urea, gave some symptoms observed on a man who, for a skin affection, drank the morning the urine he had passed the night before. The symptoms were severe, consisting of general dropsy, scanty urine and excessive weakness.

Cooper also mentioned that a celebrated breeder of cattle and horses succeeded in getting his animals' skin into an astonishing condition of fineness by giving them about a tablespoonful of old human urine with every meal. Kraft mentioned that urine has been used as a remedy for croup.

These cures are to some extent analogous with nosode cures, as the patients drank their own urine, but Urin., Urea., and Ur-ac. are also medicines on their own account and rank with the sarcodes. The symptoms of uremia may be taken as a pathogenesis of Urin. for the use of the potencies.

Urea cured kidney dropsy and Urin. produced it. The skin action of Urin. is remarkable in connection with its use in the dressing of leather, no substitute having been found for it in this.

RELATIONS - ***Compare:*** (1) Urea. - probably urine owes its chief effect to urea. (2) Ur-ac., Urt-u.

REFERENCES - Clarke. Murphy.

UROLOPHUS HALLERI

(Round Sting Ray)

PHARMACY - uro-h. Urolophus halleri. Round sting ray. N. O. Urolophidae. ***Historical dose:*** All potencies.

CLINICAL - Acne. Backache. Catarrh. Chilly. Cramping, pain. Cough. Delusion. Diarrhea. ***Fainting.*** Fibromyalgia. Flatulence. Hay fever. Herpes. Hot flushes. Itching. Nausea. Nightmares. Nosebleed. Osteomyelitis. Palpitations. Tinnitus. Trembling. Vertigo.

HOMEOPATHIC - Sting ray venom is a protein which is water soluble. Low concentrations cause heart changes associated with bradycardia, mild hypotension and vasoconstriction. Some degree of respiratory depression is noted and convulsions may also occur.

The pain is immediate and severe. Pain is constant, pulsating or lancinating. The area is quite swollen and pale with a bluish rim, spreading around the wound. Local necrosis, ulceration and secondary infection are common. Bleeding may be profuse.

Symptoms may persist for weeks to months after an injury including a dull ache and swelling which is better on elevation. Osteomyelitis can occur and amputation has been known to be necessary.

The venom is associated with anorexia, nausea, vomiting, diarrhea, frequent urination and salivation. Muscular cramps, tremors, paralysis of the affected limb. Fainting, palpitations, hypotension. Heart rate irregularities. Difficulty breathing, cough, pain on inspiration. Fever at night with copious sweating. Nervousness, confusion or delirium are also known to occur.

Similar to Sep. Chilly, but can't stand stuffy rooms, gets faint in a stuffy room. Very sensitive to weather changes. Needs a lot of sleep. Apt to get headaches. Worse in morning, better in evening. Worse from light or jar. Worse tobacco smoking. Less sensitive than Sep.

Low backache (Sep.), better moving about, does not come back once he moves about. Likes a cushion in the back. Menopausal hot flushes. Palpitations, felt as if heart is pushing out. Fibromyalgia. Hay fever. Chronic nightmares. Dreams of being chased by spirits, of being lost in a house. Tired, self pitying patients.

MIND - Difficult concentration. Dullness of mind, worse mornings. Confusion on waking. Forgetful. Memory weakness, for proper names. Indifference. Want of confidence. Sadness on waking. Indolence. Aversion to company. Disagreeable thoughts. Censorious.

Anxiety, paroxysms. Attacks of anxiety. Fear of animals, snakes. Fear that something bad will happen. Restlessness. Hurried, impatient. Irritability. Shrieking during sleep. Suspiciousness. Talks to himself. Daydreaming. Clairvoyance. Delusion floating in air. Delusion being persecuted. As if in a dream.

Abdomen - Distension, evening. Noises, rumbling. Cramping pain. Flatulence.

Back - Back pain, extending into lower limbs, lying ameliorates. Backache, worse before menses. Aching pains in dorsal region. Lumbar pains.

Breasts - Pain in breasts, worse motion.

Cough - Night aggravates cough. Morning cough. Violent barking, dry cough. Hoarse cough.

Ears - Pain in right ear. Stopped sensation. General noises, synchronous with pulse. Tinnitus. Ringing noises.

Eyes - Discoloration, redness, morning. Itching. Pain, burning, lids.

Face - Eruptions forehead. Acne. Herpes on lips.

Female - Profuse menses. Menopausal hot flushes. Sexual desire decreased or increased.

Food - Appetite diminished. Extreme thirst. Thirst at night. Desires fruit, vegetables, meat, sweets, cinnamon. Aversion to meat.

Head - Fullness. Head pain, in the morning, on waking, in the afternoon, evening, at night. Headache, worse in the afternoon, at night. Dull pain in the forehead. Pulsating pains.

Heart - Palpitations.

Limbs - Eruptions on the hands. Itching of hand, ankles. Cutting pain in foot. Soreness of foot. Swelling of ankles, foot. Tension in shoulders. Twitching, upper arm. Trembling, worse mornings.

Male - Sexual desire increased.

Modalities - Better in evening. Worse change of weather, stuffy room. Worse periodically. ***Worse in morning,*** after midnight, at 3 a.m., at 9 a.m. Worse afternoons. Worse from light, noise or jar. Worse tobacco smoking.

Mouth - Aphthae.

Nose - Catarrh. Sneezing in the morning. Nosebleed, worse in the morning.

Perspiration - Night sweats. Profuse sweats.

Rectum - Diarrhea, in the morning. Painless diarrhea. Flatus after dinner, during diarrhea.

Sensation - Bubbling sensation. Lassitude tendency. Weariness, worse mornings.

Sleep - Restless sleep. Sleeplessness from worries (Ambr.). Waking too early. Waking after midnight, 2 a.m. to 4 a.m. Amorous dream. Chronic nightmares. Dreams of animals, of water. Dreams of being chased by spirits, of being lost in a house, of murder

Stomach - Stomach cramps. Noises, rumbling. Pulsation. As if something alive in stomach. Nausea during cough.

Temperature - Chilly, lack of vital heat. Sensation of heat. Menopausal hot flushes.

Throat - Pain, in the morning, on the right, better warm drinks. Sore or sharp pains. Scratching in throat. Sensation of swelling. Choking, constriction in throat. Lump sensation, worse on swallowing. Swelling of cervical glands.

Urine - Strong odor.

Vertigo - Dizziness. Faintness tendency, worse in the morning. Vertigo on rising, on turning or moving the head.

Vision - Blurred vision.

COMMENTS - Margery Blackie wrote about using Sting Ray in her book Classical Homeopathy. She described patients who needed Sting Ray as "sallow, usually dark who have rather heavy rings around their eyes. They look tired, are chilly yet at the same time cannot stand a stuffy room. They are sensitive to all weather changes, but as a rule can stand real heat. They tell you of their need to sleep, how many hours they need, how they must have it or else they are no good at all.

"They get a slight headache as with Medusa, and like a Sepia headache, but even duller. It usually starts in the morning, strangely enough is usually better in the evening, and is made worse by noise or jarring, rather like Sepia although to a much lesser degree.

"In women, you think the patient must be Sepia. They come in looking pale and drugged and very tired, with rather dark rings. You think they are going to be Sepia, but their chief complaint is of lower backache and gradually they tell you (and Sepia of course also tells you) that it always improves if they walk about. A Sepia backache goes away if the patient walks about. The only difference is that with Sting Ray it does not come back, but in Sepia it always comes back when they sit.

"This type of patient also gets quite a lot of palpitations, the men as well as the women. If the men have a tendency to faint, they think their palpitations has something to do with it.

"The woman gets palpitations quite a lot but forgets it again if she is walking. The history is typically that if she gets bad palpitations, and has to go out because she has a very busy morning, by the time she comes back from shopping it is gone, which surprises her very much but which is a good symptom.

"They are rather tired-out patients, but in no way so despairing or such martyrs as Sepia. Sepia can be real martyrs if they go on getting tired out and have a lot to worry them, especially if they have to look after various members of the family and will not accept any help that is offered to them. Sting Ray patients are much less like this, but they do get rather hopeless.

"One of these patients, the best case I had seen, was a dark, tall, rather tired looking man who used to faint if he had to stand for long. He found it humiliating when he had fainted at two cocktail parties where he had to stand for a long time. He asked if I would give him something to stop him doing that. He had a headache and said that when it came, it lasted more or less all day, but was always better in the evening. These patients also tend to be a bit sensitive to tobacco smoke and I think that this is why he had fainted.

"In one year, just after using Sting Ray the first time, I had two soldiers who fainted continually, especially if they had to stand for an injection. Both of them had fainted half a dozen times each within the last so many weeks. They had had a lot of injections and had had to stand for rather long.

"One of them had taken part in the Queen's birthday parade and had fainted. He had been held up between two other soldiers who had held him on his feet until he came round again, but he felt frightful. Both these men did well on Sting Ray and neither of them ever fainted again."

RELATIONS - ***Compare:*** Sep., Lach., Medus., Murx.

REFERENCES - Blackie.

URTICA URENS

(Stinging Nettle)

PHARMACY - urt-u. Urtica urens. Stinging nettle. Urtica dioica. The Common Nettle has similar if not identical properties. N. O. Urticaceae. Tincture of the fresh plant in flower. ***Historical dose:*** Tincture and all potencies, tincture and lower potencies.

CLINICAL - Agalactia. Ague. ***Allergic, reactions.*** Anemia. Arthritis. Bee, stings. Breastfeeding, disorders. ***Burns.*** Deltoid, rheumatism. Diarrhea. Dysentery. Edema. Erysipelas. Erythema. ***Gout.*** Gravel. Hemorrhages. Hemoptysis. ***Hives.*** Intermittents. Itching. Leucorrhea. Malaria. Menorrhagia. Phlegmasia dolens. ***Kidney, colic. Kidney, stones. Neuritis.*** Rheumatism. Shellfish, allergy. Spleen, disorders. Throat, sore. Uremia. Uric acid, diathesis. ***Urticaria***, nodosa. Vertigo. Whooping cough. Worms.

HERBAL - In Sweden, nettles are regarded as a remedy for anemia. Fresh nettles are cooked and eaten like spinach for the purpose, or a nettle-tea is prepared from dry nettles. The juice of nettles with sugar is popular for hemorrhages of all kinds. Used in gravel and urinary disorders.

Gerarde noted several other uses, including how nettle juice inserted into the nostrils stops nosebleed. He added that it is "good against inflammation of the uvula." Useful in pleurisy, pneumonia, and whooping cough.

"Being eaten," as Dioscorides said, "boiled with periwinkles, it make the body soluble, doing it by a kind of cleansing faculty, it also provoke urine and expels stones out of the kidneys, being boiled with barley cream it is thought to bring up tough humors that stick in the chest."

Gerarde noted that "The leaves or seeds of any kind of nettle do work the like effect, but not with that good speed and so assured as the Roman nettle [U. Pilulifera]." Cooper reported that "A bundle of nettles applied to a rheumatic joint or part, has long been a favorite country remedy.

A leaf of the nettle placed on the tongue and pressed to the roof of the mouth stops bleeding from the nose."

Gerarde mentioned its antidotal action for snakebites. It's also useful for bee stings. An application of the tincture, even on the most sensitive parts of the face or eyelid, gives instant relief. In cases of stings about the eyes, the application may have to be repeated every five minutes and a compress must be kept on all night.

HOMEOPATHIC - Commonly known as stinging nettle, Urt-u. produces stinging or stinging, burning pains. ***First degree burns,*** used locally and given internally. ***Bee stings*** (Apis). Urticaria, associated or alternating with rheumatism. ***Antidotes ill effects of eating shellfish***.

Rheumatic and gouty pains and fever were all evoked. ***Gout and rheumatism*** associated with ***urticaria-like eruptions.*** Among the rheumatic pains a pain in the ***right deltoid muscle*** is very striking. ***Neuritis.*** The right side very much affected, but also the left hypochondrium (spleen).

Uric acid diathesis. Bedwetting and urticaria. ***Kidney stones***. Gout and uric acid diathesis. Spleen disorders. Urine-like odor of the body. Favors elimination.

Dysentery. Burning and itching of anus. Hemorrhages. Angio-neurotic edema. Profuse discharge from mucus surfaces. Very periodic. Ague. Headache with spleen pain, rush of blood to head, sore abdomen.

Affects the ***breast glands,*** genitourinary organs, liver and spleen. Increases milk flow. In the case given in Allen, it caused swelling of the breasts and profuse flow of milk in a woman years after the birth of her last child.

Abdomen - Chronic disease of large intestine characterized by large secretion of mucus. Sore abdomen, when lying. Burnett noted it for liver tumors.

Breasts - Swelling of the breast with stinging, burning pains. ***Diminished secretion of milk*** after childbirth. Arrests the flow of milk after weaning.

Causations - Ill effects of burns, bee-stings, eating shellfish, suppressed milk, urticaria.

Chest - Sore feeling as from a blow to left side of chest. Intermittent soreness in right chest during day. Hemoptysis from least exertion of lungs.

Constitutions - Gouty constitutions. Uric acid diathesis.

Eyes - Eyes feel weak and sore. Pain in eyeballs as from a blow. Feeling as if sand were in eyes.

Female - Uterine hemorrhage. Acid and excoriating leucorrhea. ***Pruritus vulvae with stinging,*** itching and edema.

Head - Headaches, worse over eyes. Headache with stitches in spleen. Dull aching in occiput and over eyes. Stinging pain in right parietal bone. Urticaria of scalp suddenly appearing.

Kidneys - Hemorrhage from bladder. Urine suppressed. Strangury, gravel, disease of bladder and kidneys. Uric acid toxemia. Acrid urine causing itching.

Limbs - Rheumatic pain in arms and ankles, worse right arm. Continuous pain in deltoid. worse rotating arm inwards, difficulty dressing. ***Acute and chronic gout.*** Gout pain in ankles, wrists. Raised, red, itching blisters on skin of hands and fingers. Stiff soreness on inside of left knee.

Lungs - Hemoptysis after violent exertion. Whooping cough. Scanty expectoration, frothy.

Male - Itching and stinging of scrotum, keeps him awake. Swollen scrotum.

Modalities - Better from lying down. Worse water, cool bathing. Worse cool, moist air, snow-air. Worse by touch, lying on arm. Worse yearly. Hemoptysis worse from violent exertion. Burning in skin is worse after sleep.

Rectum - Diarrhea. Frequent urging. Small, painful stool. Stool scanty, a greenish-brown slime, with urging and tenesmus. Mucus mixed with white matter like boiled white of eggs. Ascarides with great rectal irritation. Intense itching of anus from pinworms. Hemorrhoids with raw burning in anus during and after stool.

Sensations - Burning, stinging, itching and soreness are the principal pains. As from a blow in the eyeballs. As of sand in eyes. Muscles of right arm as if bruised.

Skin - ***Burns and scalds. Sunburn*** with intense burning, itching. Vesicles. Burn confined to skin. ***Hives*** with rheumatism, after shellfish, with pinworms. ***Itching, raised, red blotches.*** Nettle rash, worse every year in the same season, suppressed nettle rash. Rheumatism alternates with nettle-rash. ***Chickenpox*** (Dulc.). Urticaria nodosa (Bov.). ***Urticaria***, burning heat with formication, violent itching. Erythema with burning and stinging. Prickly heat. Angio-neurotic edema. Herpes labialis with sensation of heat and itching.

Sleep - Drowsiness when reading.

Stomach - Nausea with burning in throat. Vomiting from suppression of nettle rash.

Temperature - General heat in bed with soreness over abdomen. Fever of gout. Tropical fever. Sweatiness, at night with vertigo, with throbbing all over the body.

Throat - Burning in throat. Frequent hawking of frothy mucus causing cough, expectoration scanty, frothy.

Vertigo - Headache with spleen pains.

COMMENTS - Severe allergic reactions (Apis., worse heat), particularly food allergies (Lyc., Bry.). Urticaria, weals, welts, and hives (Apis., Puls., Nat-m., Sulph.). Allergic reactions to bites or stings (Apis., Led., Hyper.). Dermographia, red and itchy skin, easily marked. Bright red shiny rashes that itch and sting. Vesicles (Canth.).

Burns (Canth.). Old burns that refuse to heal. Shiny sunburns with a stinging, burning pain (Calen.). Palliative for herpes, canker sores. Fever blisters with stinging (Nat-m., Rhus-t.). Burning and itching of the anus and vulva. Allergic vaginitis, vaginal lips are swollen, red and inflamed, especially if due to some dietary reaction. Regulates milk production.

For reactions to the fresh stinging nettle plant. Intermittent fevers, malaria (Ars., Nat-m., Chin.). Enlarged spleen, painful, often associated with viral infections (Nat-m., Cean.). Gout, used in tincture. Arthritis or gout, in packs on the joints.

A woman who had no children for three and a half years and had nursed none of her children took a pint of hot infusion of the herb. Her breasts swelled, then discharged serum, followed by copious milk.

Burnett may be said to have rediscovered Urt-u. as a remedy. The history of how he came to use it is one of the most fascinating passages of his works. Burnett's tincture is made of the small nettle, Urt-u., which is the variety used in homeopathy.

Burnett noted that the nettle springs up everywhere near human habitations. He noticed it flourishing more by the side of ditches that carry off fluid sewage, thus possibly living to some extent on uric acid.

Burnett's discovery of its fever action occurred when a female patient was cured of ague (which he had not succeeded in helping) by drinking nettle-tea on the advice of her herbalist. Urt-u. was useful to him in cases of the fevers of the East India, Burma and Siam. It also has a marked anti-gout action.

Urt-u. causes fever as well as cures it, and one of Burnett's patients was obliged to stop taking it: "It sets all my pulses beating, makes me terribly giddy, makes me feel as if I was going to topple (forwards) on my head and then a bad headache comes on and when I take it at night, it makes me very feverish." When she took the dose in the morning she did not have the fever, and Burnett said, "The fever of gout generally comes on at night."

With Urt-u., Burnett cured severe cases of uremia, vertigo. Burnett used Urt-u. a good deal in spleen disorders and found patients under its use often passed large quantities of gravel.

Burnett gave Urt-u. to a middle-aged, unmarried woman who had enlarged spleen and "who smelled so strongly of nettles that it almost nauseated me whenever it was my duty to examine her."

While taking it, she passed large quantities of gravel, but this did not attract much notice, as the woman was in the habit of passing considerable quantities of gravel with her motions. She had localized abdominal pain preceding such an occasion by a number of days. The painful spot, just under her spleen, she called her "gravel-pit."

Putting this and other points together, including the fever action of Urt-u., Burnett concluded that Urt-u. was a remedy for acute gout, which would cut short the attack "in a safe manner, namely, by ridding the economy of the essence of the disease product, its actual suffering producing material."

He usually ordered five drops of the tincture in a wineglass full of warm water every two or three hours. Under its action the urine became more plentiful, dark and loaded with uric acid.

J. L. Nottingham noted two cases cured with Urt-r. The first concerned Mrs. W., 38, tall, slender, with auburn hair, who had eczema vulvae with violent itching and burning. She had swelling and thickening of her labia. Smooth, pale, dry appearance of the mucus surface. A dry, scaly, fissured appearance of labia majora and skin.

Thirteen years before, she had a sinus from the right ovary emptying into the uterus. The husband had sycotic warts on the glans penis. Urt-u. 1x relieved all the symptoms and removed sexual excitement induced by the itching and uncontrollable desire to rub.

The second case concerned Mr. N., 21, who had swelling, stinging, and burning of his face, hands and feet with redness. Rubbing with a fingertip would leave a white line for some time.

When out in the cold, damp, snowy air, his hands, feet and face became purple-red, puffed and stinging cold. Going into a warm room he had increased swelling, stinging, itching all over him, especially of hands and face. Urt-u. relieved in twenty-four hours. In four days he returned home better than he had been for years.

RELATIONS - ***Antidoted by:*** Dock leaves (Rumex obtus.) rubbed on the stung part lessen the pain, also the nettle's own juice and the juice from the common snail. ***Antidote to:*** Apis (bee-stings). Antidotal to hemlock, mushrooms, quicksilver, henbane, serpents, and scorpions. ***Compare:*** (1) Apis, Medus., Nat-m., Lac-c. (2) Ric. - diminished breast secretion. (3) Bomb-pr., Rhus-t., Chlol., Astac. (4) Puls. - urticaria. (5) Bol-lu. and Anac. - urticaria tuberosa. (6) Lyc. and Hedeo. - uric acid conditions, Form.

REFERENCES - Boericke. Clarke. Murphy. Phatak.

USNEA BARBATA

(Tree Moss)

PHARMACY - usn. Usnea barbata. Tree moss. Old Man's Beard. Tree-hair. N. O. Lichenes. Tincture. The fresh lichen is macerated in five times its weight of alcohol. ***Historical dose:*** Tincture and all potencies.

CLINICAL - Cystitis. Headaches, congestive.

HOMEOPATHIC - Usn. is for some forms of congestive headache, sunstroke. Keynote bursting feeling, ***as if temples would burst or the eyes burst out of the sockets***. Throbbing carotids. Head began to ache, soon could feel the blood press into the brain with domestic attentions he got to sleep and woke next morning uncommonly well. Pain over entire head or front head with feeling as if temples would burst or eyes burst out of sockets.

COMMENTS - Anshutz wrote, "This article appeared in No. 284 of the U. S. Medical Investigator signed 'M.D.' In March 1878, I was cutting wood. I cut down a soft maple, the top was well loaded with moss. It attracted my attention, I viewed it closely.

"I ate a little, about the size of a hickory nut, as I trimmed up my tree. My head began to ache. I cut off one log and had to go to the house. I could feel the blood press to the brain. My wife worked over me and I got to sleep.

"Next morning felt well, never felt better. I did not think of the moss I had eaten. I went on a visit and was gone five days. On my return I went to my tree. The first sight of it reminded me of my headache. I gathered some of the moss and made a tincture. I soon had a case of headache to try my remedy on, it stopped at once.

" In the fall, about September, a load of young folks came to pick cranberries. Two of the young ladies had headache from riding in the hot sun. Both took the lounge. Now for my remedy. I put one drop of tincture in a goblet of water, gave a teaspoonful ordered another in fifteen minutes. The second dose stopped the pain.

"A young married lady came on a visit to a relative - was having pains in her head. I was sent for, found her wild with pain. She said she had been subject to headache for five years, had got tired of doctoring. Gave her one drop in a cup of water, teaspoonful in twenty minutes, no more pain.

"I put ten drops in a two-drachm vial of alcohol, directed her to take one drop when she felt her headache coming on. One year after she wrote her friend it had cured headache, sent thanks to me.

"I could give many more cases where the pain is over the entire head or front head with a feeling as if the temples would burst or the eyes would burst out of their sockets. I have always used the tincture. I have not noticed any other effect from it, would like to see a proving."

RELATIONS - ***Compare:*** (1) Lyc., Glon., Bell. Bry. (2) Tillandsia us. Spanish moss.

REFERENCES - Anshutz. Boericke. Clarke.

USTILAGO MAYDIS

(Corn Smut)

PHARMACY - ust. Ustilago maydis. Corn smut. N. O. Fungi. Fungus on Zea maydis. Trituration. Tincture of the spores. ***Historical dose:*** Trituration and all potencies, tincture to third potency.

CLINICAL - Agalactia. Alopecia. Cancer. Crusta, lactea. Colic. Constipated. Dysmenorrhea. Eczema. ***Fibroids.*** Galactorrhea. Headaches, menstrual. ***Hemorrhages.*** Masturbation. Menopause. Menorrhagia. Menstruation, disorders. ***Miscarriages.*** Nails, disorders. Nosebleeds. Orchitis. Ovary, pain. Psoriasis. Rhinitis. Scald-head. Sexual, organs. Tonsillitis. Tumors. Uterine, hemorrhage.

HOMEOPATHIC - Burt, who proved Ust. on himself and others, introduced the remedy to homeopathy. It had been observed that pregnant animals feeding on maize affected with smut were very liable to abort. Roullin noted that shedding of the hair and sometimes of the teeth, occurred in animals and men, that mules that fed on it cast their hoofs, and that fowls laid eggs without shells.

Ust. affects the female sexual organs, skin, hair and nails. The provings brought out a specific affinity for the reproductive sphere of both sexes, especially for the left ovary and uterus.

Ust. congests the uterus and produces hemorrhages, generally passive or in clots, dark and watery blood. ***Flabby condition of uterus. Uterine hemorrhage,*** menstrual, post-partum and menopausal. ***Bleeding fibroids.*** Bearing down, as if everything would come from her. As of a knot in uterus, bowels, throat etc.

Suppressed menses without cause. Vicarious menstruation, bleeding from the lungs and bowels, and bleeding between the periods with left infra-breast pain. Crusta lactea (Viol-t.). Prostration from sexual abuse.

Warm room causes oppression and faintness. Excessively tired feeling. Loss of hair and nails. Tumors have been seen to disappear after its use.

MIND - Great depression of spirits. Weeps frequently. Irritability, worse being asked a question or to repeat anything. Could not bear to see or talk with anyone. The day seemed like a dream. Restless sleep.

Abdomen - Pain as if intestines were tied in a knot. Colic pains, better by hard stools or constipation. Cutting in umbilical and hypogastric regions. Pain in right lobe of liver.

Back - Pain in back extending to extreme end of spine. Pain in region of right kidney. Dull pain in lumbar region with great despondency and mental irritability. Bearing down in sacral region as in dysmenorrhea. Sensation of boiling water flowing along the back.

Breasts - Pain under left breast, at margin of ribs, between periods, constant.

Constitutions - Adapted to tall, thin women, at menopause.

Chest - Aching, burning distress in sternum. Heat and pressure. Constriction with pain. Oppression along the sternum.

Eyes - Weakness of eyes. Hot feeling on closing lids. Lachrymation in open air. Lids agglutinated in morning. Spots in vision.

Face - Sudden pallor in face, when sitting, in evening. Burning of face and scalp from congestion.

Female - Menses, half liquid, half clotted, bright red, discharge of blood from slightest provocation. Profuse menses after miscarriage. Foul, yellow or brown leucorrhea. Vicarious menstruation from lungs and bowels. Menorrhagia at menopause (Calc., Lach.). Oozing of dark blood, clotted, forming long black strings. ***Uterine fibroids, bleeding.*** Hypertrophy of uterus, sub-involution. ***Cervix spongy, easily bleeding.*** Post-partum hemorrhage. Profuse lochia. Ovaries burn, painful, swollen. Acute ovarian pain, worse left. Pains shoot down thighs. Uterus feels drawn into a knot. Bearing down pains when child nurses.

Food - Poor appetite. Thirst at night.

Head - Sticky secretion matting hair. Milk crusts. Vertigo with white spots before the eyes, at menopause, with profuse menses. Nervous headaches from menstrual irregularities.

Heart - Palpitations. Sudden flying pains from the heart to stomach, arresting breathing.

Kidneys - Tenesmus of bladder and incontinence of urine. Urging. Light-colored, high-colored, red, acid, scanty or increased urine. No desire, but uneasiness.

Limbs - ***Sensation of boiling water along the back.*** Muscular debility. Clonic and tetanic movements. Muscular contractions, especially of lower limbs. Cutting in bones of right hand and foot. Rheumatic symptoms in arms, fingers and legs. Feet swollen in morning.

Male - Irresistible desire to masturbation. Emissions, every night and when talking to a woman. Spermatorrhea with erotic fancies and amorous dreams.

Modalities - Colicky pains better by constipated stool. Ovaries worse from pressure. Menorrhagia worse rising and motion. Abdomen and eyes worse by touch. Riding in carriage aggravates backache. Walking aggravates frontal headache, pain in left groin, pain in loins. Swelling aggravates pains in tonsils. Open air causes lachrymation. Worse from menopause. Worse motion.

Mouth - Bitter, thin salivation. Coppery taste in morning. Tongue coated in morning. Prickling in tongue with feeling as if something were pressing the roots upward with dryness of nostrils.

Nose - Boil in right nostril. Dryness of nostrils in forenoon with dry feeling in skin. Rhinitis, bitter taste offensive odor noticeable to patient himself. Bright nosebleed, better pressure.

Rectum - Loose, soft, dry, lumpy, black stool with pain and rumbling in abdomen. Light-colored diarrhea. Constipated.

Sensations - As if head were being lifted off. As if forehead would burst open. As if something were under root of tongue pressing upward. As of a lump behind larynx. As if intestines were being tied in knots.

Skin - Dry, hot skin. Congested feeling in skin. Tendency to boils. Psoriasis. Eczema, copper-colored spots. Pruritus, sunburn. Painful, destructive disease of nails. Alopecia.

Sleep - Restless night with fever, troubled dreams. Difficult falling asleep, then unpleasant dreams. Sexual dreams without emission.

Stomach - Cutting in stomach. Burning in esophagus at the cardiac orifice. Belchings, of sour fluid, of sour food. Vomiting of blood, passive, venous, accompanied by nausea, better by vomiting.

Teeth - Looseness of teeth. Aching all day in decayed upper first and second molars.

Temperature - Abundant sweat. Pulse at first accelerated then enfeebled. Chills running up and down back. Heat at night. Internal heat with vertigo.

Throat - Dryness of fauces with burning dryness in stomach. Feeling as if there were a lump behind the larynx, which produces constant inclination to swallow. Left tonsil enlarged.

Vertigo - Full feeling. Nervous headache from menstrual irregularities. Aching in eyeballs with much lachrymation.

COMMENTS - Bleeding fibroids (Sec.). Tendency toward miscarriage and passing of dark blood (Sec.). Heavy, dark menstrual flow, debilitating. Alopecia after childbirth.

Hurndall related the case of a small female dog that brought out many features of Ust.'s action. About a fortnight before he saw the dog, she had aborted five fetuses at about the fifth week of gestation. Since then, there had been passive hemorrhage of dark clots.

Moreover, the dog was a perfect specimen of alopecia, not having a hair of any sort on her body and only a little about the head. The cervix os of the uterus was soft, spongy. Great tenderness about the posterior parts when manipulating the hindquarters.

Ust. 3x was prescribed, five drops three times a day. In two days the hemorrhage was completely arrested, tenderness reduced, spirits revived and general health improved. At the end of three months there was a nice coat of hair growing, which in due course became perfectly normal.

RELATIONS - ***Compare:*** (1) Sec., Sabin. Sep. (2) Thlaspi, Zea-i.

REFERENCES - Boericke. Clarke. Murphy.

UVA URSI

(Bearberry)

PHARMACY - uva. Uva ursi. Bearberry. Mountain box. Red berry. Bear's grape. Arctostaphylos. Arbutus uva ursi. N. O. Ericaceae. Tincture or trituration of dried leaves and fruit. Tincture of fresh leaves gathered in autumn. ***Historical dose:*** Tincture and all potencies.

CLINICAL - ***Bladder, disorders.*** Cyanosis. ***Cystitis.*** Dyspnea. Dysuria. Gonorrhea. Hematuria. Kidney, disorders. Kidney, stones. Nausea. ***Pyelitis***. Urinary affections. Urticaria. Uterine, hemorrhage. Vomiting.

HERBAL - Uva ursi is a good kidney tonic (Equis.), it helps prevent the formation of kidney stones and tendencies toward bladder infections. A few experiments have been made with Uva ursi that have seemed to confirm its traditional reputation as an "astringent used to check excessive secretion of mucus, as in urinary and bronchial disorders and even in kidney stones."

The leaves are principally astringent, with which they combine mild tonic and soothing properties. It increase the flow of urine and particularly show their influence upon the uro-genital tissues. In chronic and sub-acute mucus discharges-such as catarrh of the bladder, leucorrhea, gonorrhea, and gleet it lessens the discharge gradually and giving tone to the parts.

The tincture of the leaves may be used in chronic diarrhea and dysentery. Especially suited to an ulcerated condition of the bowels. Uva ursi has been used as a tonic and astringent in a bleeding stomach, bowels and kidneys. It is more soothing to the stomach than nearly any other astringent.

HOMEOPATHIC - Diabetes, gravel and strangury. ***Pyelitis***. Kidney stones. Aching of the kidneys and bladder, congestion and ulceration of the bladder and prostate gland, involuntary seminal emissions, and incontinence of urine. Characteristic shooting pain from hip to hip.

Chronic bladder irritation with pain, tenesmus and catarrhal discharges. ***Cystitis*** with bloody urine. ***Burning after the discharge of slimy urine***. Slime passes with blood. Bladder symptoms are better lying on the back.

Painful dysuria, with frequent but difficult discharge of thick, ropy urine of strong, pungent odor. Constant urging to urinate and straining, with discharge of blood and slime. Straining without any discharge at all, or only a few drops of urine. Cutting and burning pain in urethra, which is followed by discharge of blood.

Dyspnea, nausea, vomiting, pulse small and irregular. Uterine hemorrhage. Cyanosis. Urticaria without itching.

Bladder - ***Cystitis.*** Involuntary urination, green urine. Painful dysuria.

Chest - Uneasy tightness with a sensation of weight at the chest.

Face - Flushing.

Head - Slight vertigo and headache.

Kidneys - *Pyelitis*. Kidney stones. Frequent urging with severe spasms of bladder, burning and tearing pain. Urine contains blood, pus and much tenacious mucus with clots in large masses.

Nose - Fluent coryza with rawness.

Stomach - Weak, sick at stomach, sore all over as if bruised.

Throat - Hoarseness with pain in bowels, stopped up in throat, no appetite. Throat tickles, feels like coughing all the time, sore and bruised all over. Cough, nose raw and burning, cutting and burning on urinating.

COMMENTS - Uva. should be remembered when there is a spasm of the bladder with straining and a discharge of pus, tenacious and clots of blood. It is recommended for hematuria, painful burning urine. Slimy or purulent urine. Calculi of the bladder.

Dropsy, depending on disease of the heart or liver. Leucorrhea and lingering gonorrhea in females. In one cured case there were pains shooting through from hip to hip.

RELATIONS - *Compare:* (1) Sec., Cann-s. (2) Arbin. - a crystallized glucoside of Uva, found also in Kalm., Gaul. and other genera of the family of Eriacee, given in doses of 3 to 8 grains with sugar three times a day. Used as a urinary anti-septic and diuretic. (3) Arctosphylos manzanita - acts on kidney and reproductive organs. Gonorrhea, bladder catarrh, diabetes, menorrhagia. Tincture of leaves. (4) Vacc-m., Huckleberries - dysentery, typhoid, keeps intestines aseptic and prevents absorption and re-infection.

REFERENCES - Boericke. Clarke. Murphy.

V

VACCININUM

(Cowpox Vaccine)

PHARMACY - vac. Vaccininum. Cowpox vaccine. Vaccinia. Vaccinotoxinum. Lymph from cowpox vaccination pustule. Nosode. Trituration of vaccine matter. ***Historical dose:*** Tincture and all potencies.

CLINICAL - Albuminuria. Chickenpox. Conjunctivitis. Eczema. Keloids. Keratitis. Headaches. Hematuria. Herpes. Iritis. Leprosy. Malaise. Menorrhagia. Neuralgias. Nephritis. Nevus. Scars. ***Smallpox.*** Sycosis. Tumors. ***Vaccinosis.*** Whooping cough.

HOMEOPATHIC - Vaccinosis, smallpox and cowpox are inter-related diseases and the nosodes of each are available for the treatment or the prevention of manifestations of all three. The vaccine poison is capable of setting up a morbid state of extreme chronicity, named "vaccinosis" by Burnett. It may do this without causing the primary symptoms, when the vaccination apparently does not "take."

The symptoms of vaccinosis are protean and are, for the most part, identical with the symptoms of the sycosis of Hahnemann; ***vaccinosis*** is a sycotic disease. Leading features of the vaccinosis miasm include neuralgias, inveterate skin eruptions, chilliness, and indigestion with great flatulent distention.

Vac. has skin eruptions, ***new growths,*** sycotic conditions. Restlessness. General malaise. Languor, lassitude. Tired all over with stretching, gaping feeling, unnatural fatigue. Child wants to be carried. Many persons faint when being vaccinated.

Vaccinosis is related to whooping cough. An old-school observer vaccinated a child while they were suffering from whooping cough, and the whooping cough vanished.

Burnett repeated the experiment in other cases with such success that he wrote to the journals to recommend it as a routine practice in the case of unvaccinated children. On the other hand, homeopaths have observed whooping cough immediately after a vaccination and have cured it with Thuj. 30c.

MIND - Capriciousness. Confusion, she does not remember things at the time she wants them. Desired to be carried. Restlessness. Ill-humor, with restless sleep. Irritable, impatient, nervous. Crying. Disposition to be troubled by things. ***Morbid fear of getting smallpox.***

Abdomen - Stitches felt in liver and spleen. Abdomen is bloated up with flatulence.

Arms - Severe pains in left upper arm at vaccination mark. Rheumatic pains in wrists and hands. Keloids on re-vaccination marks.

Back - Backache. Aching pain in back, worse in lumbar region, extending around waist. Chill running down back. Twisting pain in lower back. Weakness in small of back coming on suddenly, ameliorated by lying down.

Chest - Stitch in left side of chest, anteriorly, under short ribs. Stitches in right side under short ribs, in front from right to left, then at corresponding place in left side, but from left to right, lasting five minutes.

Eyes - Keratitis after vaccination. Tinea tarsi and conjunctivitis. Conjunctivae painfully sensitive. Weak eyes. Inflamed and red eyelids. Redness of eyes and face with small pimples on face and hands. Gauzy sensation before eyes in morning, cannot see well.

Face - Redness and distention of face.

Female - Menses rather profuse and too frequent.

Food - Appetite gone. Disgust to taste, smell and appearance of food. Coffee tastes sour.

Head - Eruption like crusta lactea. Frontal headache. Forehead and eyes feel as if split. Forehead felt as if it would split in two in median line from root of nose to top of head. Stitches in right temple. Prickling in left temple, as if going to sleep.

Heart - Febrile action of heart, arteries.

Kidneys - Nephritis with albuminuria, hematuria and dropsy, developed after vaccination.

Limbs - Tearing in left thigh downward.

Soreness of lower limbs, as if heated or over-exerted. Legs ached immoderately, hardly able to get about. Break-bone sensation and a feeling as if bones were undergoing process of comminution (Eupper.). Twisting pains in both knees.

Liver - A stitch in hepatic region, at margin of last lower rib, axillary line.

Lungs - Short breath with aching in pit of stomach and pressure in region of heart. Whooping cough.

Mouth - Dry mouth and tongue. Tongue coated, dry yellow with papillae showing through coat.

Neck - Swelling of neck under right ear (parotid gland), with sensation like being cut.

Nose - Full feeling of head with running at nose. Bleeding at nose preceded by a feeling of contraction above and between eyebrows, soon after eating meat.

Sensations - As if forehead were split. As if head or over-exerted in lower limbs. As if bones of leg were broken and undergoing process of comminution.

Skin - Hot and dry. ***Eruption like variola.*** Small pimples develop at point of vaccination with fourth dilution. Red pimples or blotches in various parts, most evident when warm. Eruption of pustules with a dark-red base and a round or oblong elevation, filled with pus of a greenish-yellow color, resembling varioloid, some as large as a pea, some less without depression in the center, coming with a round, hard feel in the skin (like a shot), very itchy.

Sleep - Waked in middle of night by pain in forehead and eyes as if split and stinging in temples.

Stomach - Aching in pit of stomach with shortness of breath.

Temperature - Fever with heat, thirst tossing about, crying, aversion to food. Chill with shaking.

COMMENTS - Tingling, burning in skin over whole body, most intense in forehead skin and in lower and anterior portion of hairy scalp, which are tinged with a scarlet blush or efflorescence, similar to the immediate precursor of variola-like eruption.

Garrison was consulted by a woman, 50 of a tubercular family. She had consolidation of both apices, had been losing flesh for three months, with severe night sweats. Almost constant, hacking cough with considerable expectoration at times. She was given one dose of Vac. 200c.

In a week she reported that she had not had a severe coughing spell since the dose and for the last three days hardly any cough at all. She received one dose of Vac. a week, and at the end of six weeks returned to business.

Vaccinating on a nevus in a child can destroy the growth by its inflammation and subsequent scarring.

Frolich related the case of a child, age 6, who had well-developed nephritis seven days after vaccination with calf vaccine. The first symptom was puffed eyelids, then pain and swelling of the scrotum. On the fourteenth day, the urine contained blood, the inguinal glands were enlarged and tender, with slight edema of the legs. The urine contained blood and alumen for another month, when he recovered. Other similar cases have been observed.

Burnett said the worse time of Vac. is the early morning. "Waked in middle of night by pain in forehead and eyes as if split and stinging in temples."

Vaccininum 6c in water, for one day with strict diet, repeated after eight days, acted as a preventive in six hundred cases. It treated many cases of variola and varioloid.

Vaccininum 200c quickly relieved the severe symptoms of variola occurring in a child, aged six months. Two days before appearance of eruption the child had been re-vaccinated (after an interval of eight days) on a nevus near right nipple. Swallowing difficult through implication of tongue and fauces. Pustules, many of large size, scattered over scalp, face, body and limbs.

RELATIONS - ***Antidoted by:*** Thuj., Vario., Apis, Sulph., Ant-t., Sil., Maland. ***Compare:*** (1) In smallpox - Vario., Maland., Thuj., Ant-t. Sarr. (2) Nephritis - Apis, Merc-c. (3) Tuberculosis - Bac., Tub. (4) Whooping cough - Dros., Thuj., Meph., Coc-c., Cor-r.

REFERENCES - Boericke. Clarke. Murphy.

VACCINIUM MYRTILLUS
(Bilberry)

PHARMACY - vacc-m. Vaccinium myrtillus. Bilberry. Whortleberry. Black whortles. Whinberry. Trackleberry. Huckleberry. Bleaberry. Hurtleberry. Vaccinium frondosum. N. O. Ericaceae, Vacciniaceae. It is a native of swampy, mountainous regions. Tincture of fresh berries. ***Historical dose:*** Tincture and all potencies.

CLINICAL - Arthritis. Cataracts. Diabetes. Diarrhea. Dropsy. Dysentery. ***Eye, disorders. Eyestrain.*** Glaucoma. Gout. Hemorrhoids. Indigestion. Macular, degeneration. Malaria. Myopia. Nausea. ***Night-blindness.*** Retinitis. Scurvy. Ulcers. Vaccinosis. ***Vision, disorders.*** Wounds.

HERBAL - The name Bilberry (by some old writers "Bulberry") is derived from the Danish "bollebar," meaning dark berry. Bilberry is a close relative of cranberry and the natural order is allied to the Ericaceae. Bilberries are used in making jams, preserves, liqueurs, and wines.

The leaves can be used in the same way as those of Uva ursi. A decoction of the leaves or bark of the root may be used as a local application to ulcers, and in ulceration of the mouth and throat. A tea made of the leaves is also a remedy for diabetes if taken for a prolonged period.

The fruits are astringent, and are especially valuable in diarrhea and dysentery, in the form of syrup. They are also used for discharges, and as antigalactagogues. It is helpful in scurvy and urinary complaints, and when bruised with the roots and steeped in gin has diuretic properties valuable in dropsy and gravel.

Bilberry contains nutrients needed to protect eyes from eyestrain or fatigue, and can improve circulation to the eyes. It works by improving the microcirculation and regeneration of the retina. British Royal Air Force pilots during World War II, ate bilberry preserves before night missions as an aid to night vision.

Clinical experience confirms that, when given orally, it improves visual accuracy in healthy people, and can help those with eye diseases such as pigmentosa, retinitis, glaucoma, and myopia. Cataracts and macular degeneration. ***Poor vision and night blindness.***

The dried fruit and tea has been used as a treatment for diarrhea and as a relief for nausea and indigestion. For mild inflammation of the mucus membranes of the mouth and throat. Stomach problems and irritated digestive tract.

HOMEOPATHIC - Vacc-m. is applicable to vaccinosis, malarial and dysenteric cases. Eye disorders. Diarrhea. Dysentery. Diabetes.

Dr. A. H. Croucher, in an article published in the Homeopathic Review, gave cases of inveterate diarrhea cured by it. His experience has been repeatedly confirmed.

Clarke always used it in the herbal tincture, generally giving 5 drop doses every four hours.

RELATIONS - ***Compare:*** (1) Sima., Chin., Rheum., Merc.

REFERENCES - Clarke. Murphy.

VALERIANA OFFICINALIS
(Valerian)

PHARMACY - valer. Valeriana officinalis. Valerian. N. O. Valerianaceae. Tincture of the fresh root. ***Historical dose:*** Tincture and all potencies.

CLINICAL - Asthma, spasmodic, nervous. Bedsores. Clairvoyance. Coxalgia. Headaches. Heart, palpitations. Heels, pain. Hypochondriasis. Hysteria. ***Insomnia.*** Levitation, sensation. Menopause. ***Nervousness.*** Neuralgia. Sensitive. Sciatica. ***Sleeplessness.*** Toothache.

HERBAL - Valeriana officinalis is usually found in moist hedgerows or on the banks of ditches and streams. The peculiar fetid odor of Valerians is probably due to the presence of Valerianic acid. It is especially agreeable to cats, who become intoxicated with it.

The Treasury of Botany noted that "Volatile oil of Valerian seems not to exist naturally in the plant, but to be developed by the agency of water."

Valerian root is largely relaxant and moderately stimulant. It is a mild stimulant to the circulatory and nervous system. It is an antispasmodic, laxative, diaphoretic and anthelmintic.

A nervine and antispasmodic in cases of irritability, restlessness, hysteria, and nearly all forms of acute nervousness, ***insomnia, calming the brain, inducing quietude and sleep.*** The most valuable uses to which it can be put, are cases of nervousness, restlessness, and hysteria.

If large doses are employed, nausea, vomiting, diarrhea and hiccough, with frequent urination, result. If it is long continued, as state of low, melancholy and hysterical depression results. The heart's action is increased, the temperature raised and formication of the hands and feet is complained of.

HOMEOPATHIC - Valer. first appeared in homeopathic medicine in Stapf's Additions, the article on it was written by Franz, and Hahnemann and Stapf were among the provers.

Valerian produces ***over-sensitiveness of the nerves***, spinal, genitourinary. Affects the mind, muscles, calf, heels, and Achilles tendon. Hysteria, over-sensitiveness, nervous affections. Lack of reaction, when apparently well-chosen remedies fail.

Alternating symptoms. ***Mental and physical dispositions change suddenly*** and go to extreme. Red parts turn white. Constant heat and uneasiness. ***Insomnia.*** Profuse sweat at night. Pains are darting, tearing, move outwards, are felt here and there or come and go, jump from one place to another.

Epileptic fits. Paralysis and contraction of limbs, hysterical. Agitation of all nerves, jerks, twitches, trembling. Restlessness, impulse to move, cannot keep still. Weak, single parts, eyes, arms, wrists, popliteal etc.

Globus hystericus. Illusions of vision, hearing, smell or taste. Slight injury causes spasms. Straightening out limb aggravates sciatica. ***Hysterical flatulence.*** Bedsores form soon in typhoid. Sensation of a thread hanging down from esophagus.

MIND - Mental disturbances passing from one extreme of emotions to another, from the highest joy to deepest grief, from mildness to grumbling. ***Changeable disposition and moods.*** Impatience, passes quickly from one subject to another. Tremulous. Over-sensitiveness (Staph.). ***Irritable***. Anger. Mad, raving, swearing.

Hysterical spasms and disorders generally. Wriggles or squirms about. Inclined to faint. Hysteria, dreads being alone and especially in the dark. Hallucinations at night. Erroneous ideas, thinks she is someone else, as if all around were strange and disagreeable. Delusions of animals, men. Feels light, as if floating in air.

Abdomen - Abdomen inflated and hard. Hysterical cramps. Spasms, cramps in bowels after food and at night in bed. Flatulence. Draws abdomen in involuntarily.

Back - Lancinations in left lumbar region above hip, worse when standing and especially when sitting, than when walking. Rheumatic pains in the shoulder blades.

Causations - Injuries, slightest injury causes spasms.

Chest - Sudden stitches in chest and liver from within out. Eruption of small, hard nodosities on chest.

Constitutions - Hysterical women who have taken too much chamomile tea. Nervous, irritable, and hysterical subjects in whom the intellectual faculties predominate and who suffer from hysteria and neuralgia.

Ears - Otalgia with spasmodic drawings. Jerkings in the ears. Hyperesthesia. ***Earache from exposure to drafts and cold***. Nervous noises. Tinkling and ringing in the ears. Illusions of hearing, imagined he heard the bell tinkle.

Eyes - Swelling and painful sensibility of eyelids. Myopia. Brightness and light before eyes in a dark room, vision sharp. Sparks before eyes. Objects seem too near eyes. Wild look.

Face - Pain appears suddenly and jerks. Muscles twitch. Cheeks red and hot in open air.

Female - Menses late and scanty (Puls.). Neurasthenia of sexual organs.

Food - Voracious hunger with nausea, as if from navel.

Head - Headache, which appears suddenly or in jerks. Fullness as from rush of blood to head. Pressive headache. Headaches, better moving about, worse sunshine. Moving eyes aggravates headache. Sensation of great coldness. Pressure in forehead. Bending head back aggravates pain in occiput.

Heart - Stitching in heart with quick, small and weak pulse.

Kidneys - Much straining and prolapsed rectum during urination. Urine increased and more frequent in nervous women. Urine contains a white, red or turbid sediment.

Limbs - Rheumatic pains in limbs. Heaviness. ***Sciatica, pain worse standing and resting on floor*** (Bell.), stretching limbs, better walking. Pain in heels when sitting. Crampy pain, electric-like shocks in humerus (left), wakes from sleep. ***Constant jerking.*** Tensive pain in the calves, worse crossing legs. Cramps in biceps (right) while writing. Cramps of hands and feet prevent sleep. Pain from calf to heel. Legs feel light after walking.

Lungs - Choking in throat on falling asleep. Wakes as if suffocating. Spasmodic asthma, convulsive movements of the diaphragm. Obstructed respiration and anguish in chest.

Male - Creeping and drawing in of penis, as if it had gone to sleep.

Modalities - Better after a meal, after breakfast. Better after sleep. Better changing position, walking about, motion. Rubbing helps cramp in calf. ***Worse from rest, standing***, sitting, stooping, touch. Worse excitement. Worse fasting. Worse from open air, draft. Worse noon, evening, darkness, before midnight.

Mouth - Rancid, greasy taste. Bitter taste on tip of tongue. Tongue thickly coated. Nausea felt in throat. White blisters on tongue and upper lip, painful when touched. Toothache with shooting pain.

Nose - Violent sneezing.

Rectum - Ascarides. Hemorrhoid pain from worms. Painful borings in rectum. Bubbling pressure above anus in region of coccyx. Loose evacuations, greenish, papescent, and bloody stool. Thin, watery diarrhea with ***lumps of coagulated milk, with violent screaming in children***. Discharge of blood from anus.

Sensations - Pressure of hand or covering with hat causes icy coldness on vertex. As if flying in air. As if eyes would be pierced from within outward. As if smoke in eyes. ***As if a thread were hanging down throat.*** Like lead in limbs. Lightness in leg. As if strained in right ankle. As if bruised in outer malleolus of right foot.

Skin - Skin too dry and warm. Painful eruptions. Eruption of small nodosities, at first red and confluent, then white and hard.

Sleep - Sleeplessness with nightly itching and muscular spasms from excitement, worse on waking. Cannot sleep before midnight. ***Insomnia,*** during pregnancy and menopause. Disturbed sleep with tossing and anxious, confused dreams.

Stomach - Weak stomach and digestion. Sense of something warm rising from stomach and causing suffocation Cramps in stomach. Foul belchings, like bad eggs. Heartburn with gulping of rancid fluid. Nausea with faintness. ***Child vomits curdled milk*** in large lumps after nursing after mother's anger.

Temperature - Chilliness, generally begins in neck and runs down back. Body ice cold with nausea and vomiting. Sensation of icy coldness (Helo., Camp., Abies-c.). ***Heat predominates***. Fever composed of disagreeable heat only. Long lasting heat, often with sweat on face. Sudden gushes of sweat, mostly on forehead.

Throat - Choking in throat-pit on falling asleep, wakes as if suffocating. Pharynx feels constricted. ***Sensation as if a thread were hanging down throat*** with salivation and vomiting. Nausea felt in throat.

Vertigo - Vertigo on stooping, feels light, as if floating. Head confused, as after intoxication. Intoxication and dizziness with absence of ideas. Whirling in head when stooping forwards.

COMMENTS - Franz wrote that it was the custom among women in Germany to take

Valerian almost as frequently as coffee. He attributed much of the nervous suffering, then prevalent, to this practice. "There is scarcely a remedy," he said, "which communicates its primary as well as secondary action to the organism with more intensity than Valer."

He referenced his own eye symptoms, which were both severe and remarkable, though he had no tendency to anything of the kind before. His symptoms were excited at intervals for four months afterwards, the cause was frequently unknown, showing the deep action on the organism.

Franz recorded burning, smarting and pressure in the margins of the eyelids, which seemed sore and swollen. There were also hallucinations of hearing and of sense.

"Imagines she is some one else and moves to the edge of the bed to make room." "Anxious, hypochondriac feeling, as if the objects around him had been taken from him, the room appears to him desolate, he does not feel at home in the room, he is compelled to leave it." "As if in a dream."

"The many inveterate spasms of the stomach and abdomen. The incurable cases of hysteria and hypochondriasis. Moral disturbances, passing from one extreme of emotion to another. From the highest joy to the deepest grief from leniency. Kindness and mildness to grumbling impatience, obstinacy and quarrelsomeness from a sinking of the vital forces. A painful craving for stimulants to the greatest liveliness and extravagance and vice versa."

In Franz's opinion, tedious convalescence after nervous fevers, and paralysis and contractions of the limbs, were owed less to the original intensity of the disease than to the Valer. with which the patients had been dosed. They were only saved from worse effects because Valer. was frequently given in combination with one or more of its antidotes.

Franz noted that the first and most rapid effect of Valer., which precedes any after symptoms, is an acceleration of the pulse and congestion of the head. Symptoms of the upper and lower limbs alternate frequently. Principally produces symptoms at noon and early afternoon, and the hours before midnight. The abdominal symptoms are particularly felt in the evening.

Disturbed digestion. Fetid tallow taste before dinner. Flat, slimy taste early in the morning, on waking. Nausea begins in umbilical region, rising into pharynx.

Darting, tearing pains that come and go. Pains appear suddenly. Tearings, cramps, better morning. Constant heat and uneasiness. Restlessness. Nervous irritation, cannot keep still. Tissot recommended Valer. for epilepsy.

Nash cured a severe case of sciatica in a pregnant woman based on the symptoms, "pain worse standing and letting the foot rest on the floor." She could stand with the foot resting on a chair or lie down in comfort.

Hering said it met "Nervous disorders occurring in excitable temperaments. In hypochondriasis it calms the nervousness, abates the excitement of the circulation.

"It removes the wakefulness, promotes sleep and induces sensation of quietude and comfort. Sadness is removed in globus hystericus in all asthmatic and hysterical coughs. Nervous palpitations, profuse flow of limpid urine. Red parts become white."

RELATIONS - ***Antidoted by:*** Bell., Camph., Cina, Coff., Puls. ***Antidote to:*** Merc., abuse of Chamomile tea. ***Compare:*** (1) Asaf., Ign., Croc., Castor. (2) Am-val., Zinc-val. - in neuralgia, gastric disturbance and great nervous agitation. Insomnia. Feeble, hysterical nervous patients.

REFERENCES - Boericke. Clarke. Murphy.

VALIUM

(Diazepam)

PHARMACY - diaz. Valium. Diazepam. It belongs to a class of drugs known as benzodiazepines. Trituration. ***Historical dose:*** All potencies.

CLINICAL - Anxiety. Athetosis. Bradycardia. Coma. Constipation. Convulsions. Coughing. Cramps. Delirium tremens. Depression. Diplopia. Dysarthria. Dyspnea. Dysuria. Fainting. Fatigue. Hallucinations.

Headaches. Hyperventilation. Hypotension. Incoordination. Nausea. Nystagmus. Photophobia. Rash. Salivation. Sleep, disorders. Tremors. Ulcers. Venous, thrombosis. Vertigo. Vomiting.

HOMEOPATHIC - Valium is used in the treatment of anxiety disorders and for short-term relief of the symptoms of anxiety and panic. It is also used to relieve the symptoms of acute alcohol withdrawal.

To relax muscles, to relieve the uncontrolled muscle movements caused by cerebral palsy and paralysis of the lower body and limbs. Used to control involuntary movement of the hands (athetosis), to relax tight, aching muscles, and to treat convulsive disorders such as epilepsy.

Loss of muscle coordination. Uncontrolled movements of body, including the eyes. Tremors, vertigo, dizziness. Increased sensitivity to touch and pain.

Confusion. Depression. Anxiety. Overstimulation, rage, seizures. Drowsiness, fatigue, light-headedness. Unusual tiredness or weakness. Slow heartbeat. Low blood pressure. Headache. Blurred vision, double vision. Hallucinations.

Yellowing of eyes and skin. Skin rash, sleep disturbances. Changes in salivation. Slurred speech and other speech problems. Nausea. Difficulty urinating, or inability to hold urine. Constipation. Changes in sex drive.

MIND - Mental confusion. Dullness of mind. Memory loss. Disorientation. Slurred speech and other speech problems. Depression. Anxiety. Delirium tremens.

Agitation. Overstimulation and rage. Paradoxical reactions such as acute hyper-excited states. Unusual excitement, nervousness or irritability. Feelings of suspicion or distrust. False sense of well-being.

Abnormal thinking. Behavior changes, including aggressive behavior, bizarre behavior, decreased inhibition, or outbursts of anger. Hallucinations. Delusions, holding false beliefs that cannot be changed by facts. Loss of sense of reality.

Abdomen - Abdominal cramps.

Ears - Increased sense of hearing.

Eyes - Blurred vision. Diplopia. Nystagmus. Yellow eyes. Sensitivity of eyes to light.

Female - Changes in libido.

Head - Headache.

Heart - Fast, pounding, or irregular heartbeat. Bradycardia. Cardiovascular collapse. Hypotension.

Limbs - Muscle spasms, weakness. Ataxia. Staggering. Dysarthria. Tremors. Tingling, burning, or prickly sensations. Trembling or shaking. Venous thrombosis and phlebitis at the site of injection.

Lungs - Increased bronchial secretions. Coughing. Depressed respiration. Dyspnea. Hyperventilation.

Kidneys - Incontinence. Urinary retention.

Male - Changes in libido.

Mouth - Changes in salivation. Watering of mouth. Dryness of mouth. Slurred speech. Ulcers or sores in mouth.

Perspiration - Increased sweating.

Rectum - Constipation.

Skin - Skin rash, itching. Urticaria. Jaundice. Unusual bleeding or bruising.

Sleep - Sleep disturbances and stimulation. Insomnia.

Stomach - Increased thirst. Hiccoughs. Nausea and vomiting.

Temperature - Fever and chills.

Throat - Sore throat. Laryngospasm and pain in throat or chest. Ulcers or sores in throat.

Vertigo - Fainting and dizziness.

COMMENTS - Withdrawal symptoms, similar in character to those noted with barbiturates and alcohol have occurred following abrupt discontinuance of valium. Convulsions, tremors, abdominal and muscle cramps, vomiting and sweating.

REFERENCES - Murphy.

VANADIUM METALLICUM

(Vanadium Metal)

PHARMACY - vanad. Vanadium metallicum. Vanadium metal. (At. Wt. 51.2). Burnett used the soluble ammonium salt. Trituration. ***Historical dose:*** All potencies.

CLINICAL - Addison's disease. AIDS. ***Anemia. Anorexia.*** Arteriosclerosis. Atheroma.

Blindness. Brain, softening. Bronchitis. Bulimia. ***Cachexia.*** Cancer. Colds. Constipation. ***Debility.*** Diabetes. Diarrhea. Emaciation. Eye, disorders. Fatty, heart. Growth, retarded. Hysteria. Immune, weakness. ***Indigestion.*** Liver, disorders. ***Malnutrition.*** Metabolism, disorders. Osteoporosis. Paralysis. Pneumonia. Raynaud's syndrome. Retinitis. Rheumatism. Sciatica. Thyroid, disorders. Tonsillitis. Tuberculosis. Vertigo. Warts. ***Weakness.***

HOMEOPATHIC - Vanad. has never been subjected to the test of a homeopathic proving but something of its effects upon the human body are known from its accidental absorption by workers. It is an ingredient in some black pigments and of a black, permanent ink.

Workers become debilitated. They contract a dry, hard, almost convulsive cough, with hemorrhage. The temperature becomes elevated with a diurnal maximum. Diarrhea sets in soon, and flesh and weight is lost rapidly. They are very apt to go from this state into genuine tuberculosis and die.

These symptoms suggest it as a remedy in the early stages of tuberculosis. It agrees with the general characters of that disease, namely the cough, prostration, fever with daily rise, emaciation, hemorrhage and diarrhea. Vanad. also affects the liver with a degenerative process.

Its action is that of an oxygen carrier and a catalyzer, hence its use in wasting diseases. Increases amount of hemoglobin, also combines its oxygen with toxins and destroys their virulence. It also increases and stimulates phagocytes.

It is a remedy in degenerative conditions of the liver and arteries. Anorexia and symptoms of gastro-intestinal irritation. Tremors, vertigo, neuro-retinitis and blindness. Anemia, emaciation. Cough dry, irritating and paroxysmal, sometimes with hemorrhages. Irritation of nose, eyes and throat.

Acts as ***a tonic to digestive functions*** and in early tuberculosis. Degenerative states with brain softening. Tuberculosis, chronic rheumatism, diabetes. Cold hands and feet. Raynaud's syndrome.

Degenerative conditions of liver and arteries. Fatty degeneration of the heart and liver. Arteriosclerosis, sensation as if heart was compressed, as if blood had no room in the aorta. Deeply pigmented patches on forehead in liver disorders. ***Profound weakness.*** Emaciation and weakness.

MIND - Restlessness. Gloomy. Yielding, easily influenced. Crying easily over trifles. Fears of failure, criticism, being opposed. Anticipation. Fears of being late. Hysteria and melancholia. Mood alternating. Manic depression. Psychosis. ***Anorexia*** alternating with bulimia.

Blood - Anemia and nutritional problems.

Chest - Anxious pressure on whole chest. Sore chest.

Dreams - Dreams of being late, of futile efforts. Dreams of paralysis.

Eyes - Neuro-retinitis and blindness. Opacity. Arcus senilis. Paralysis of optic nerves. Amaurosis.

Female - Premenstrual symptoms. Menses scanty or absent. Pain in ovaries. Worse at ovulation. Lactation problems.

Food - Loss of appetite. ***Anorexia.*** Bulimia. Disturbed fat and glucose metabolism. Retarded growth. Desires licorice, sweets. Weak digestion.

Head - Headaches. Brain softening.

Heart - Fatty degeneration of the heart. Arteriosclerosis. Hypertension. Sensation as if heart was compressed, as if blood had no room in the aorta. Bursting pain. Constriction sensation.

Kidneys - Addison's disease. Albumen, casts and blood in urine.

Limbs - Chronic rheumatism. Sciatica. Restless and itching legs. Paralysis. Osteoporosis.

Liver - Fatty degeneration of the liver.

Lungs - Dyspnea, tiredness, weakness. Pneumonia and bronchitis. Cough dry, irritating. Colds with sneezing. Tuberculosis.

Mouth - Teeth problems. Tongue green.

Rectum - Constipation. Diarrhea.

Skin - Pigmented patches. Warts.

Throat - Tonsillitis and sore throats, coughing up small, greenish-yellow, bitter mucus. Thyroid problems.

COMMENTS - Burnett told how he came to use Vanad. through reading the result of some experiments on animals in which the Salts of Vanadium produced "true cell destruction, the pigment escaping, the liver being hit hardest."

Burnett had at the time a case of "fatty liver, atheroma of the arteries, much pain corresponding to the course of the basilar artery, large, deeply pigmented patches on forehead, profound adynamia." Vanad. restored the patient, who was seventy and at eighty he was "hale and hearty."

Marc Jousset told of experiments with salts of Vanad., chiefly the meta-vanadate of sodium, by Lyonnet and others. Animals poisoned by intravenous injections rapidly develop Cheyne-Stokes respiration with little or no action on circulation or blood.

Cachexia. These clinical observers gave Vanadates to two hundred patients, suffering from neurasthenia, tuberculosis, chlorosis, chronic rheumatism, etc. It produced in nearly all cases increased appetite, strength and weight. The amount of urea was also increased. They regard Vanad. as "an energetic stimulant of nutrition," and probably an oxidant stimulating organic combustion.

RELATIONS - ***Compare:*** (1) Ars., Phos. Am-c. (2) Vanad. - fatty degeneration of liver. (3) fatty degeneration, Phos., Ars. (4) Addison's disease, Adren. (5) Tuberculosis, Tub., Bac.

REFERENCES - Boericke. Clarke.

VANILLA AROMATICA

(Vanilla Beans)

PHARMACY - vanil. Vanilla aromatica. Vanilla beans. Vanilla planifolia. N. O. Orchidaceae. Vanilla beans, tincture of the fruit. (Do not use the synthetic vanilla extract). ***Historical dose:*** All potencies.

CLINICAL - Menses, prolonged. Poison-oak. Skin, disorders.

HERBAL - Vanilla aromatica is an emmagogue and aphrodisiac. Vanilla is supposed to stimulate the brain and sexual propensities.

HOMEOPATHIC - Various disorders of the nervous system and circulation are produced in workers with vanilla. Menses prolonged. It has been found effective in curing skin disorders. Marked skin irritation resembling poison-oak is sometimes produced by handling the beans, also by local use of vanilla essence in a hair wash.

REFERENCES - Boericke.

VARIOLINUM

(Smallpox Nosode)

PHARMACY - vario. Variolinum. Smallpox nosode. Trituration of matter from smallpox vesicle. ***Historical dose:*** All potencies.

CLINICAL - Asthma. ***Backaches.*** Chill. Eczema. Fevers. Headache, occipital. ***Herpes zoster.*** Nausea. Neuralgias. Pustules. ***Shingles. Smallpox.*** Testicle, swelling. Ulcers. Vaccinations, ill effects.

HOMEOPATHIC - The Vario. nosode is prepared from lymph from a smallpox pustule. It has proved as an efficient preventive against smallpox and vaccinial infection. Vario. is used for ***bad effects of vaccinations.*** Seems to be efficacious in protecting against, modifying and aiding in the cure of smallpox.

Vario. was Burnett's chief remedy in ***shingles***, it generally, as he expressed it, wiped out the disease, eruption and pain as well. It will also cure neuralgia left by herpes. Vario. has aborted many cases of smallpox and has proved an efficient preventive against smallpox contagion and vaccinosis infection.

The keynote symptoms of Vario. are the defining symptoms of smallpox. Severe cold, chill, chilly creepings as if cold water were trickling down the back, violent fever with extremely hot skin, with or without high pulse. Violent headache.

General aching in the muscles worse in back, occiput and legs. Nausea. Pain in epigastrium. Pain in limbs as if in bones. ***Severe backache.*** There may be rash or there may not. Calcareous deposits in the blood vessels, spinal cord. etc.

MIND - Delirium with fever. Morbid fear of smallpox. Fear of death. Wild excitement and begging to know if he was to die.

Abdomen - Tympanites, pouting upwards, looks pregnant.

Back - ***Excruciating backache.*** Pain as if back were broken, worse by motion. Terrible pains in back on right side of spine. Pains from back, shift to abdomen.

Ears - Deafness.

Eyes - Inflamed eyelids. Green vision, on rising.

Head - Crazy feeling in the brain. Headache with icy coldness of feet and hands. Pain in occiput.

Limbs - ***Aching in legs.*** Muscular rheumatism, worse on motion. Tired all over with restlessness. Wrist pain.

Lungs - Oppressed breathing. Asthma. Troublesome cough, with serous and sometimes bloody sputa. Cough with thick viscid, slimy, bloody mucus, smelling bad. Feeling of a lump in right side of throat.

Male - Enlargement of testicle. Hard swelling of left testicle from a contusion.

Modalities - Worse from motion. Worse after vaccinations.

Mouth - Tongue protrudes during sleep. Foul, metallic taste. Breath horribly offensive.

Sensations - As if a band tightly encircled head. Crazy feeling through brain. As if throat were closed. As of a lump in right side of throat. Like streams of ice-water running down back.

Skin - Hot, dry. Eczema of palms. Herpes zoster. ***Shingles*** and pains that follow. Eruption of foul pustules. Ulcers look scooped out. Profuse, bad-smelling sweat. As of bugs crawling under the skin.

Stomach - Odor nauseates. Wants to regurgitate food. Vomiting of milk immediately after drinking it.

Temperature - As of cold water trickling down the back. Violent chill. Hot fever with intense, burning, radiating heat.

Throat - Throat very sore, painful swallowing. Deep purplish crimson pharynx and fauces, with gangrenous appearance. Sensation as if throat were closed. Sensation of a lump in right side of throat. Diphtheria with horrible fetor oris.

COMMENTS - Nonspecific shingles (Rhus-t.). Neuralgic pains without defining characteristics. Tendency to herpes, or acutely for herpes zoster or simplex. Acne, with yellow pus, leaving scars and large pock marks (Calc-s.).

G. M. H. recorded the experience he had concerning Vario. 6c given to the mother and children of a family, one of whose members was taken with smallpox and removed to an isolation hospital with his mother to nurse him.

The patient (who did not receive Vario.) was dangerously ill for a month. Neither the mother who nursed him nor any of the other children caught smallpox.

Vaccines were sent by the government, and all the family were vaccinated, but it did not take with any of those who had taken Vario., although the vaccination was repeated.

Moreover, G. M. H. himself, who had taken a dose of Vario., submitted to vaccination, but "although four thorough inoculations were given, they healed up immediately and did not even itch or smart."

A school of two hundred children were "internally variolated" with Vario. (100,000c, Swan) on the evening of February 18th and the morning of February 19th. Of two school mistresses, one was not at all affected, the other was ill for two days in bed.

On February 21st many of the children were ill, by the 23rd, all except forty were. The symptoms were the usual preliminary symptoms of smallpox, and later, Swan found pustules on many.

After the varioloid had passed off, but before the patients had recovered their vitality, twenty-three children were vaccinated without Swan's knowledge. All but one took and had terrible ulcers on the arms and had to be remedied by Vac. (100,000c, Swan).

RELATIONS - ***Antidoted by:*** Maland., Thuj., Ant-t., Vac., Sarr. ***Compare:*** (1) Herpes, Mez., Rhus-t., Ars., Vac. the same action. (2) Maland. - the morbid product of the grease of the horse, a prophylactic of smallpox and a remedy for the ill-effects of vaccination, chronic eczema following vaccination.

REFERENCES - Boericke. Clarke. Murphy.

VENUS MERCENARIA

(American Scallop)

PHARMACY - ven-m. Venus mercenaria. American scallop. American clam. Pelecypoda class, living along the Atlantic Coast of America, France and Southern England. Tincture of the mollusc, plus an equal part of a trituration at 1/100 of the shell. ***Historical dose:*** All potencies.

CLINICAL - Allergies. Amenorrhea. Arthritis. Flatulence. Headaches. ***Indigestion.*** Mania. ***Migraines.*** Schizophrenia. Weakness.

HOMEOPATHIC - Ven-m., the American scallop, is a bi-valvular mollusk. The proving, after a suggestion by D.M. Foubister, was conducted by Raeside in 1961-62 on nineteen provers, plus seven controls during three terms, one dose morning and evening for fourteen days, using the 30c in first term, 12c in second term, and 6c in third term. The third term produced most of the symptoms.

Ven-m. is above all a remedy with cephalic action. For migraine headaches, accompanied by a host of digestive and urinary manifestations. ***Migraines of digestive origin***. Increased frequency of urination.

Frontal and occipital headache, predominantly on the right side, pains of a heavy sort, worse early in the morning and especially in the afternoon. Headache accompanied by vertigo, nausea, vomiting. Furred tongue, flatulence, diarrhea.

Frequency of urination, especially during the day. Scalp and skin of the face and limbs itchy. Predominantly right sided. Sometimes there is a pseudo influenza, weakness at 10 a.m., extreme chilliness from 3 p.m. to 5 p.m. Sensation of contusion when pressure is applied.

MIND - Lack of co-ordination of thoughts. Dull mood, state of indifference and lack of concentration. Sensation of boredom with fear of crying for no reason. Exaggerated irritability from noise and people. Mania. Schizophrenia. Feels cut off from the world. Drunk feeling in the morning.

Abdomen - Abdominal pains around 9 p.m. like menstrual pains. Muco-membranous enterocolitis. Flatulence and rumbling in the morning.

Back - Arthralgia and muscle pain with stiffness in the back and nape of the neck on waking.

Chest - Tender around the sternum.

Constitutions - Allergic, psoric and sycotic types, tending towards a cancerous state following severe self-intoxication.

Female - Amenorrhea. Menses painful, especially at onset, for 2-3 hours. Menstrual pain ameliorated by heat and lying down. Depressed on first day of menstruation.

Food - Desire for cold food, thirsty for cold water, ameliorated in the evening. Food tastes metallic.

Head - Frontal, dull headache, behind the eye to the right with nausea, especially in the afternoon. Occipital headache on the right side, also in the afternoon. ***Migraines of digestive origin***. Frontal and occipital hemicrania of the right or left side with nausea and feeling as if the head were being held tightly. Headache, aggravated in the afternoon, by exercise, ameliorated by sitting quietly in the dark and in the late evening.

Heart - Short stabbing pain in the heart.

Kidneys - Persistent pain in the right kidney on waking up. Fleeting pain in the left kidney. Frequency of urination by day. Urine turbid, frothy with a fetid odor. Frequent need to urinate.

Limbs - Pain and paresthesia of the limbs. Cramps, heaviness, itching of the arms and legs. These pains are ameliorated by movement. Pains in the hip, knee and ankle joints. Right knee swollen, hot and painful. Muscle pain. Arthritis. Arthrosis.

Modalities - Better from movement. Worse on waking, in morning, in afternoon. Worse from noise.

Mouth - Soreness of the left lower lip and corner of lips. Blister on the lips. Tongue coated, furred. Cold feeling in the mouth and throat. Teeth sensitive to hot and cold, especially on the upper left jaw.

Nerves - Incoordination of the mind and body when writing.

Rectum - Slight diarrhea or stubborn constipation with no desire to go to stool.

Skin - Itching eczema. Prurigo simplex.

Itching of the limbs, ears, back and face. Urticaria on the left hand. Boils and eruptions on the face.

Sleep - Sleep disturbed, waking at 2 a.m. Dreams of spiders. Dreams of violence, ending in death. Dreams of death and disease.

Stomach - Dyspepsia. Stomach ulcer. Nausea after eating with headache and vomiting. Flatulence all day long. Pressing stomachache with nausea, ameliorated after eating. Heaviness in the epigastrium, feeling of a stone in the stomach, aggravated by menses and at night.

Throat - Pain on right side, spreading to the ear, aggravated by swallowing with dryness, chill and swollen glands. Constriction in the pharynx and larynx. Boil on the neck.

Vertigo - Vertigo on rising after sitting for a long time, worse when ever tired, ameliorated by pressure.

COMMENTS - Ven-m. in one single dose of 30c or repeated once is a remedy both for attacks of migraine and for complaints based on migraine headaches.

RELATIONS - ***Compare:*** (1) Calc. - digestive complaints with acrid-smelling stools, nausea and headache, chilliness. (2) Iris. - headache around the right eye with gastric complaints, burning and heartburn. (3) Lyc. - meteorism, constipation, depression, aggravated from 4 p.m. to 8 p.m. ***Complementary:*** Carc. is complementary.

REFERENCES - Julian.

VERATRINUM

PHARMACY - verin. Veratrinum. Veratria. Veratroidia. Viridia. Melanthiaceae. An alkaloid obtained chiefly from seeds of Sabadilla and roots of Veratrum album. Trituration. ***Historical dose:*** All potencies.

CLINICAL - Colic. Diarrhea. Dysentery. Dysuria. Esophagus, stricture. Intestines, catarrh. Jaw, snapping. Neuralgias. Pain. Paralysis. Spasms. Spine, neuralgia. Tetanus. Twitchings. Vomiting.

HOMEOPATHIC - Verin. is both a paralyzer and a great pain producer. It causes a sensation like electric streams in nerves, shooting pains like electric-shocks in veins, muscles and joints.

Verin. causes tetanus, which Farrington distinguishes from the convulsive action of Nux-v. in that Verin. causes purgation and vomiting with the spasms and that general paralysis does not take place from exhaustion as with Nux-v., but from devitalization of the muscles.

In large doses, it causes violent sneezing and great gastro-intestinal irritation, vomiting, purging and symptoms of collapse. The pulse is rapid, small and irregular and often involuntary muscular tremors come on. A peculiar creeping and prickling sensation in skin generally accompanies these symptoms.

Externally applied to the unbroken skin it has no marked action. If rubbed on with some fat, it passes through the epidermis and causes first irritation and then paralysis of the ends of the sensory nerves and producing a prickly and creepy sensation, succeeded by numbness.

This effect is produced whether applied locally or taken internally. Brunton noted this irritating action in the sensory nerves is also observed if it is inhaled through the nose, where it causes violent sneezing, which also occurs after absorption through the stomach.

COMMENTS - Subsultus tendinum, fibrillary twitchings are marked. Startings and tremors occur in limbs previously affection by paralysis or pain. The pains are tingling, sparkling, prickling, burning. Twitching of facial muscles. Snapping, closure of lower jaw. Drawing pain along the spine. Shocks in head.

Sensations of oppression in head, suffocation of boiling water running over the back. As if a stream of warm air or drops of hot water issued from various parts. As if a frozen atmosphere around feet to knees or cold water poured on them.

"Dull pain afterwards burning in lower part of spinal column, followed by pain in bowels and prepuce, accompanied with jerking in lower limb."

RELATIONS - ***Antidoted by:*** Coffee mixed with a little lemon-juice. ***Compare:*** (1) Sabad.,

Acon., Con.

REFERENCES - Clarke.

VERATRUM ALBUM

(White Hellebore)

PHARMACY - verat. Veratrum album. White hellebore. White-flowered veratrum. N. O. Melanthacae of the Liliaceae. Alps and Pyrenees. Tincture of the rootstocks collected early in June before flowering. ***Historical dose:*** All potencies, first to thirtieth potency.

CLINICAL - Amenorrhea. Anemia. Anguish. Anasarca. Angina pectoris. Asthma. Bronchitis. ***Cholera.*** Colic. ***Collapse. Coma.*** Constipation. Convulsions. Coprophagia. Coughs. Cramps. Deafness. Debility. ***Dehydration.*** Despair. Diarrhea. Dysmenorrhea. Eclampsia. Emphysema. Epilepsy. Esophagus, stricture. ***Fainting.*** Fevers. Gastric, catarrh. ***Head injury.*** Headaches. ***Heatstroke.*** Hernia. ***Hydrocephalus.*** Hydrophobia. Hysteria. Influenza. ***Insanity, religious.*** Intermittent fever. Intussusception. Labor, constipation. Lips, cracked. Liver, hyperemia. Lockjaw. Lungs, edema. ***Mania.*** Measles. Melancholy. ***Meningitis.*** Menstruation. Neuralgias. Nyctalopia. Paralysis. Peritonitis. Pernicious fevers. Pneumonia. Pregnancy, imaginary. Ptosis. Rheumatism. Salivation. Scarlatina. ***Shock.*** Sleep, whining. Spleen, swollen. Strokes. ***Sunstroke.*** Throat, sore. Toothache. Typhoid fever. Vertigo. Water brash. Whooping cough. Yellow fever.

HERBAL - In his Helleborism of the Ancients, Hahnemann showed that Verat. was the principal agent used at Anticyra and other places in Greece to produce the evacuations which were regarded as an essential of the "cure." Spring was deemed the most favorable season and autumn the next.

The herbal treatment was employed in diseases including "mental derangements, epilepsy, spasms of the facial muscles, hydrophobia, ptyalism of the pancreas, diseases of the spleens, goiter, hidden cancer," etc.

HOMEOPATHIC - Verat. profoundly affects the mind, ***nerves,*** abdominal, heart, blood, blood vessels, respiration, vertex and digestive system. ***Fainting***, from emotions, least exertion, slight injury with hemorrhage after stools, vomiting.

Progressive weakness and emaciation in acute diseases, whooping cough, ague, etc. Sudden sinking of strength. Paralysis after debilitating losses.

Profound prostration, collapse with extreme coldness, blueness and weakness. Post-operative shock with cold sweat on forehead, pale face, rapid, feeble pulse. ***Cold perspiration on the forehead*** with nearly all complaints. ***Vomiting, purging and cramps in limbs. Profuse***, violent retching and vomiting. Breath, tongue, cold as ice.

Effects are violent and sudden. Copious evacuations, vomiting, purging, salivation, sweat, or urine. Excessive dryness of all mucus surfaces. Burnings. Blood seems to run cold, blood sepsis, pyemia. Carphology.

Tonic spasms or cramps in chest, bowels, hands, fingers toes, soles of feet with diarrhea. Convulsions caused by religious mania or excitement, also of children.

MIND - Melancholy with stupor and mania. Head hangs down, sits brooding in silence, wants to be alone. Sits in a stupid manner, notices nothing. ***Sullen indifference***. Amativeness. Haughtiness.

Remorse. Busy restlessness. Deceitful, never speaks the truth. Despair about position in society, feels very unlucky. ***Delusions of impending misfortunes***. Malingering. Anguish, fear of death.

Imaginary diseases. Thinks herself pregnant. Nymphomania, embraces everybody even objects. Kisses everybody, before menses. Puerperal mania.

Religious mania. Despairs of her salvation. Imagines the world on fire. Prays, curses, shrieks in turn. Frenzy of excitement, shrieks, curses. Cursing, howling all night. Insanity. Violent mania alternates with silence and refusal to talk.

Sings, whistles, laughs. Runs from place to place. Delirium with violence, driving to madness, loquacity or lewdness during pain. Mania with desire to cut and tear things (Tarent.). Aimless wandering from home. Talks about the faults of others or scolds.

Swallows his own excrement.

Abdomen - Sinking and empty feeling. ***Cold feeling*** in abdomen. Epigastrium painful. Pain in abdomen preceding stool. Painful retraction of abdomen during vomiting. Abdomen sensitive to pressure, swollen with terrible colic. Cutting colic as if bowels were twisted in knots with cramps in limbs and rapid prostration. Peritonitis. Intussusception. Reversed peristaltic action. Sensation as if hernia would protrude (Nux-v.). As if hot coals in abdomen.

Back - Neck so weak, child can scarcely keep it erect, worse whooping cough. Pain crampy between scapulae better motion. Bruised feeling in sacral region.

Causations - Post-operative shock. Shock of injury. Ill effects of fright, disappointed love, injured pride or honor. Suppressed rashes. Opium, tobacco, alcohol.

Chest - Spasmodic contraction of muscles of chest. Oppressed chest, with pain in side during an inspiration. Sensation of fullness in chest, which induces frequent belchings.

Constitutions - Suited to the extremes of age, children and old people. For lean, choleric or melancholy persons. Young people and women of a sanguine or nervo-sanguine temperament. People who are habitually cold and deficient in vital reaction. Persons of gay disposition, of fitful mood. Anemic persons.

Ears - Shootings in ears. Pressure and constrictive sensations in ears. Alternate sensation of coldness and heat in ears. Deafness, as from obstruction in ears. Humming with sensitiveness to noise. Roaring in ears, especially when rising from a seat.

Eyes - Surrounded by dark rings. Eyes dull, clouded, yellowish. Staring eyes, turned upwards without luster. The eyeballs are turned upwards. Pain, as if the eyeballs were bruised. Lachrymation with redness. Dry, heavy lids.

Face - ***Face very pale, blue, collapsed, cold.*** Features sunken. Deathly pale, on rising, bluish, pinched or distorted, frowning cold, terrified look. Cheek red (left), as if burnt. Tearing in cheeks, temples and eyes. Jaws cramp on chewing. Lockjaw. Lips blue, hang down.

Female - Menses too early, too profuse, suppressed. ***Dysmenorrhea with coldness***, purging, ***cold sweat. Faints from least exertion***. Menorrhagia with nausea, vomiting, diarrhea. Nymphomania, before menses, from disappointed love, unsatisfied passion in lying-in women. Eclampsia. Puerperal mania.

Food - ***Thirst for cold water, but is vomited as soon as swallowed.*** Craves ice water, wants everything cold or sour, drinks, juicy fruits and salt. ***Voracious appetite***, gnawing hunger in spite of nausea and vomiting. Averse to warm food. All fruits disagree, causing painful distention. Potatoes and green vegetables disagree. Better eating meat and drinking milk.

Head - ***Cold sweat on forehead*** in all complaints. ***Sensation of a lump of ice on vertex***. Violent pain driving to despair, better cold. Headaches with nausea, vomiting, pale face, diarrhea, diuresis. Vertex itches during headache. Rubs forehead. Contracted features. Neck too weak to hold head up. As if cold wind blowing through head. Hair bristle, painful.

Heart - Palpitations with anxiety and rapid audible respiration. Visible palpitations with chorea. Weak, cutting at heart. Intermittent, feeble, slow, thready pulse. Intermittent action of heart in feeble persons with some hepatic obstruction. Tobacco heart from chewing. Blood runs like cold water through veins.

Kidneys - Scanty, red brown urine. Thick, greenish, suppressed, involuntary during cough.

Limbs - Brachial neuralgia, paralytic and bruising pain in arms. Fine burning in arms, right to left. Arms feel full and swollen. Tingling in hands and fingers. Feet icy cold. ***Cramps in calves*** during stools. Sciatica, pains like electric flashes in legs, must sit up and let legs hang down out of bed. Soreness and tenderness of joints. Difficulty in walking, like paralysis from debility. Pains in feet or knees as if heavy stones were tied to parts, must move about.

Lungs - Air seems too hot. Asthma, worse in damp, cold weather, better bending head back. Tickling down throat into lungs. Rattling in chest. Much mucus in bronchial tubes that cannot be coughed up. Coarse rales. Chronic bronchitis in the aged (Hippoz.). Continuous violent cough with retching, worse cold drinks. Neglected whooping cough with complication. Barking cough with belchings, worse warm room. Involuntary urination with cough. Cough on entering warm room from cold air (Bry.). Hollow cough, tickling low down with blue face. Urine escapes when coughing.

Modalities - Children feel better when carried about quickly. Better from warmth, covering, hot drinks. Better lying, walking. Better eating meat, milk. ***Worse from drinking,*** cold drinks. Worse wet, cold weather, change of weather. Worse at night. ***Worse exertion,*** touch, pressure. Worse before and during menses. Worse before, during or after stools. Worse fright, during pain. Worse injured pride or honor. Worse opium, tobacco chewing.

Mouth - Dry in center not relieved by water. Salty saliva. Water tastes bitter, like peppermint. Toothache, teeth feel heavy as if filled with lead. Grinding of the teeth. Tongue, cold, pale, cool sensation as from peppermint. Speech lisping, stammering or as if tongue too heavy.

Nose - ***Icy coldness of tip of nose and face.*** Nose grows more pointed. Smell before nose. Nosebleed from right nostril, only at night in sleep.

Rectum - Diarrhea from drinking cold water on hot days. Constipation from inactivity of rectum with heat and headache. Constipation of babies and when produced by very cold weather. ***Large stools with much straining until copious and forcibly evacuated***, followed by great prostration. Evacuations of cholera morbus and true cholera when vomiting accompanies the purging. Cholera morbus. Cholera infantum. Stools, thin like ribbon, flat. Watery, green, odorless or colorless (rice water) stools, or in large masses with straining, until exhausted with cold sweat.

Sensations - As if he had a bad conscience or had committed a crime. As if she would have to fly away. As if in a dream. As if head would burst. As if heat and cold at same time on scalp. Hair as if electrified. Distress over heart and epigastrium. As if something alive running from stomach into throat. As from ravenous hunger, pain in stomach. As of knives cutting bowels. As of hot coals in abdomen. Sinking, empty feeling in abdomen. As if pregnant or in throes of childbirth. As of knives cutting bowels. Electric pains occur in various parts.

Skin - Blue, cold, clammy, ***cold as death***. Skin flabby and without elasticity. Wrinkling of skin of hands and feet. Cold sweat. Skin feels scorched. Dry tetters. Measles, tardy and pale. Nettle rash. Scarlatina in hot weather.

Sleep - Wakes at night trembling. Starts as if frightened. Yawning. Nocturnal sleeplessness with great anguish. Sleep, long, uninterrupted, heavy, too profound. Sleeps with the arms passed over the head. Dreams with frightened waking and a fixed idea that the dream is true, of quarrels. Dreams are anxious, of being bitten by a dog and cannot escape, of being hunted of robbers.

Stomach - Painful, burning at pit of stomach. Hiccough after hot drinks. Cold water brash. ***Copious vomiting with nausea, aggravated by drinking and least motion***. Vomits or belches froth. Violent retching. Nausea while eating, cannot get food down without retching. ***Cold feeling*** in stomach. Gastric irritability with ***chronic vomiting*** of food. Vomiting, worse drinking and least motion. Great weakness after vomiting.

Temperature - Chill with ***extreme coldness*** and thirst. ***General coldness,*** icy, on vertex, nose tongue, mouth, limbs, sweat. Internal heat with cold surface, when drinking. Fevers showing external coldness only.

Throat - Hoarse, weak voice. Loss of voice. Dry, scraping or roughness. When drinking water, it seems to run outside, not going down the esophagus.

Vertigo - Vertigo, especially when walking. Vertigo with cold sweats on forehead with loss of vision, sudden fainting. Vertigo from opium, abuse of tobacco and alcohol.

COMMENTS - Copious discharges, stools, vomiting, urine, salivation and sweat. Discharges drain the tissues. Exhausting discharges, causing vertigo, blackness before the sight, fainting and collapse. "Rapid sinking of forces, complete prostration, cold sweat and cold breath." Useful for collapse with icy cold sweat (Carb-v.).

Fainting from emotions, from the least exertion, from retching, or from stool. Sinking feeling during hemorrhage. "Skin blue, purple, cold, wrinkled, remaining in folds when pinched." "Face hippocratic, nose pointed."

"Hands icy cold." "Face and legs icy cold." "Coldness of the whole body." "Coldness running over whole body soon after taking it." "Continued rigor in back and over arms." "Cold feeling in abdomen."

Coldness predominates in fever, but there is also "heat and redness of face and hands." "Feeling of internal chill ran through him from head to toes of both feet at once." Cold sweats, especially on the forehead.

Cardiac debility, following acute diseases. Thread-like pulse. Low blood pressure. Blood loss, hypovolemic shock. Faints in morning, face red when lying down or sitting up, deadly pale, hands cold, clammy. J. S. Mitchell considered it one of the best heart stimulants in homeopathic doses.

Dryness and burning felt in the nose, mouth, palate, and throat. Pneumonia. Tickling deep in trachea and bronchials. "Tickling in chest, as if it would provoke cough in middle of sternum."

Severe dehydration (Chin.), often associated with heatstroke or sunstroke. Sun headaches or sunstroke. Extreme hunger, craving for cold food and refreshing things. Craves unripe fruit, ice cold drinks, ice cream (Phos.). Great thirst for ice-cold water, during both the chill and heat of fever.

Copious stools. Cholera (Camph. and Cupr.). Rice-water stools. Watery diarrhea in infants. Green vomit, stool, or urine. Characteristic diarrhea, frequent, greenish, gushing, mixed with flakes.

Cutting colic with cramps commencing in hands and feet and spreading all over. Prostrating after fright, worse least movement with vomiting, cold sweat on forehead during stool followed by prostration. "Violent vomiting with profuse diarrhea."

Characteristic constipation without desire. Large, hard stools, in round black balls from inactive rectum. Frequent desire felt in epigastrium. Painful constipation in infants, children, and women after confinement.

Cramps, convulsions, can be tetanic with lockjaw or epileptic. The eyes are particularly convulsed or the lids paralyzed. There may be vanishing of sight, sparks before the sight, or night-blindness. Neuralgic pains, dysmenorrhea, or migraines, accompanied by diarrhea, vomiting, cold sweat, fainting or prostration.

Delirium and prolonged sleep during fever. Violence in delirium. "Fury: tears his clothing, bites her shoes to pieces and swallows the fragments, cursing, stamping, wants to run away, makes a great noise."

Mental alienation. Insanity. Delusions of personal identity. Exalted, religious or sexual mania. Puerperal mania. Nymphomania, mania for kissing everybody. Delusion that she is pregnant, and she gets physical symptoms from it (pseudocyesis). Destructive mania. Despair and hopelessness, "bowed down with great grief."

Hahnemann said that it has the power "to promote a cure of almost one-third of the insane in lunatic asylums (at all events as a homeopathic intermediate remedy)."

One of the symptoms taken by Hahnemann from Grading is "He swallows his own excrement." Goullon verified this in a case of his in which a child had a craze for eating its own feces or dung lying in the street. Verat. 2c. three times daily, cured in a month.

E. F. Watts had the case of Mrs. C., who had severe nervous headaches for years. Any over-exertion, like riding or working on hot days, would excite them. They frequently began in occiput, settling sometimes in one eye, sometimes in the other. Spig. and Sil. gave no relief.

One day, Watts noticed that the brow contracted and the eyelids nearly closed with the intensity of the pain. Verat. was given and relieved at once.

Gee cured, with one dose of Verat. 200c, the case of Mrs. L., a widow, 43. She had sciatica for four years. Pain sharp, transient, darted upwards and downwards and from both sides to center. Heat, worse "the cooler the better."

Cold sweat with the attacks. Headache from both temples to base of brain, worse by heat. Vertex itched during attacks. Pain compelled her to move about, but no better from motion.

RELATIONS - ***Antidoted by:*** (Poisonous doses) Strong coffee, Camph. (pressive pain in head with coldness of body and unconsciousness after), Acon. (anxious, distracted state with coldness of body or burning in brain.), Chin. (other chronic disorders from abuse of Verat. e.g., daily forenoon fever.), Staph. (most cases. Teste). ***Antidote to:*** Ars., Chin., Cupr. (colic), Op., Tab., removes the bad effects of opium and tobacco. ***Compare:*** (1) Chin., Verin. - alkaloid from seed of Sabad. - electric pains, electric shocks in muscles, fibrillary twitchings. (2) Cho. - cramps in calves. (3) Camph., Cupr., Ars., Cupr-ar. - intermittent, cold, clammy sweat. (4) Narc-po. - gastro-enteritis with much griping and cutting pain in bowels. Fainting, trembling, cold limbs, small and irregular pulse. (5) Trychosanthes - diarrhea, pain in liver, dizziness after every stool. (6) Agar-em. Agar-ph. ***Follows well:*** Ars., Arn., Chin., Cupr., Ip., Camph. (cholera), Am-c., Carb-v. Bov. (in dysmenorrhea with vomiting and purging). Lyc. and Nux-v. in painful constipation of infants. ***Followed well by:*** Puls., Acon., Bell., Cham., Rhus-t., Sep., Sulph.

REFERENCES - Boericke. Clarke. Murphy.

VERATRUM NIGRUM

(Dark-flowered Veratrum)

PHARMACY - verat-n. Veratrum nigrum. Dark-flowered veratrum. N. O. Melanthacae. Austria and Siberia. Tincture of fresh leaves and succulent flower-stalks. ***Historical dose:*** All potencies.

HOMEOPATHIC - Cooper gave a few observations for Verat-n. The plant, he said, has much the same botanical characters as Verat, but the flowers are dark-colored. It is native to Austria and Siberia. Verat-n. has headaches, protracted menstruation. Tinnitus aurium.

Ears - Constant buzzing of left ear for two weeks with tenderness of meatus and intense sensitiveness of the head to the motion of an omnibus with beclouding of the brain and pain in nape of neck.

Female - Period continually returning, sometimes light-colored and slight in quantity and sometimes profuse with weak feeling in back.

Head - Constant headache when attempting to move or exert the brain. Fierce headache threatening acute mania.

REFERENCES - Clarke.

VERATRUM VIRIDE

(American Hellebore)

PHARMACY - verat-v. Veratrum viride. American hellebore. Veratrum helonias viridis. Indian Poke. N. O. Melanthacae of the Liliaceae. Tincture of fresh root gathered in autumn. ***Historical dose:*** All potencies.

CLINICAL - Amaurosis. Amenorrhea. Asthma. Bunions. Carphology. Cecum. Chilblains. Chorea. Colds. Convulsions. Delirium. Diplopia. Diaphragmitis. Dysmenorrhea. Eclampsia. ***Esophagitis***. Esophagus, spasms. Erysipelas. Headaches. ***Heart, disorders. Hiccoughs.*** Hyperpyrexia. Influenza. Malarial fever. Measles. Meningitis. Menses, suppressed. Muscle, pains. Orchitis. ***Pneumonia.*** Proctalgia. Puerperal, convulsions. Puerperal mania. ***Pupils, dilated***. Sleep, dream filled. Spinal, congestion. Spleen, congested. Strokes. Sunstroke. Typhoid fever. Uremia. Uterus, congestion.

HERBAL - Growing side by side, Verat. and Verat-v. are scarcely distinguishable when not in flower. Millspaugh, however, said that though much like Verat. in its minor points, Verat-v. is strikingly different in general appearance.

Verat-v. having a much more pointed leaf, panicles looser and more compound, the racemes of Verat. being more compact and as a whole cylindrical, those of Verat-v. scattered, compound and craggy. Verat. flourishes in mountain meadows, Verat-v. grows in swamps and wet meadows and along mountain creeks from Canada to the Carolinas.

Through this confusion, an accidental proving of the latter has been included in the pathogenesis of Verat-v. The plants belong to different orders, though it must be admitted there is a close resemblance in their effects.

The root of Verat-v. contains Veratrine and the other alkaloids found in the root of Verat., but in different proportions.

HOMEOPATHIC - Burt proved Squibb's liquid extract of Verat-v, and said he found no other preparation satisfactory.

Hinsdale noted that it is known clinically that such diseases as Tiegel's contracture, Thompson's disease, athetosis and muscular paralysis present a symptomatology quite like that produced by Verat-v. upon muscular tissue.

Verat-v. produces ***violent congestive*** conditions, base of brain, ***medulla,*** lungs with nausea and vomiting and weakness. Stomach, heart and capillaries are also affected. Congestions, especially to lungs, base of brain with nausea and vomiting. Congestive stage and early manifestations of hepatization in pneumonia.

Twitchings and convulsions, here and there during sleep, jerking and trembling, threatened with convulsions. Chorea, twitching, contortions, unaffected by sleep, froth about the lips. Lies with head low.

Continuous jerking of the head, sexual excitement. Spasms with violent shrieks, opisthotonos, before and after menses. Children tremble as if frightened and on verge of spasm. Furious delirium.

Muscular prostration, pseudo-hypertrophic muscular paralysis. Great prostration. ***Sudden effects***. Sudden fainting, prostration, nausea. Fainting, nausea. Erratic motion, staggering. Lowers blood-pressure.

Numbness. Uneasy sensation in the whole body. Effects of sunstroke. Burning in different places tongue, pharynx, gullet of skin which is cold with prickling. Zigzag of temperature. As if damp clothing on arms and legs or clothes would not fit him, seemed as if they were scratching him somewhere.

Especially adapted to full-blooded and plethoric persons. ***Bloated, livid face.*** Rheumatism of heart. Paroxysms of auricular fibrillation. Induces fall of both systolic and diastolic blood pressure. General pulsations. Eclampsia.

Verat-v. has a pronounced action on the esophagus, it causes a sort of ruminating action or reversed peristalsis. The least food causes vomiting. ***Red streak down the center of the tongue***. Farrington noted it for ***esophagitis***. Uremia.

MIND - Loquacity with exaltation of ideas. Suspicious nature. Fear of seeing her physician, of being poisoned. Quarrelsome. Delirium, furious, screams, howls, strikes incessant muttering. Mania, puerperal. Carphology.

Abdomen - Pain above pelvis with soreness. Cutting at navel to groin. Pain in bowels runs into scrotum. Enteritis with high fever.

Back - Aching pain in back of neck and shoulders. Cannot hold the head up. Opisthotonos.

Causations - Sunstroke. Suppressed menses, lochia.

Chest - Burning in chest.

Constitutions - Suited to full-blooded plethoric persons.

Ears - Deafness from moving quickly with faintness. Cold and pale.

Eyes - Wild, staring during delirium. Blood shot. ***Pupils dilated***. Vision of red spots, purple, on closing eyes, unsteady. Double vision.

Face - ***Face flushed, livid turgid, but becomes faint*** on sitting up. Convulsive twitching of facial muscles (Agar.). Tension across malar bones. Chewing motions of the jaw.

Female - Menstrual colic before the appearance of the discharge with strangury. Suppressed menstruation with congestion to head (Bell.). Rigid os (Bell., Gels.). Puerperal fever, convulsions with mania or mania continues after convulsions have ceased.

Food - Very thirsty, drinks little, which ameliorates for a short time.

Head - Head retracted. ***Pain from nape of neck***, cannot hold head up. Congestion intense, almost apoplectic. Hot head, bloodshot eyes. Bloated, livid face. Hippocratic face. Sunstroke, head full, throbbing arteries (Bell., Glon., Usn.). Aching on vertex and between eyes. Strokes. Pain up occiput with dim vision and dilated pupils. Constant jerking or nodding of the head (chorea), throbs on raising up. Meningitis, basilar.

Heart - Constant, dull, burning pain in region of heart. Valvular disease. ***Beating of pulses throughout body,*** especially in right thigh. Pulse ***slow, soft, weak***, irregular intermittent. Rapid pulse, low tension (Tab., Dig.).

Kidneys - Cystitis with fever. Urine scanty with cloudy sediment.

Limbs - ***Acute rheumatism.*** Severe pain in joints and muscles. Violent electric-like shocks in limbs. Cramps in legs, feet, soles, fingers toes. Convulsive twitching. Pain about the condyles. Pulsation felt in thighs. Restless hands during delirium. Vesicles on hands.

Lungs - Dyspnea. Difficult breathing. Slow and heavy breathing, as of a load on chest. Congestion of lungs. Pneumonia, with faint feeling in stomach and violent congestion. ***Croup***. Violent cough from very start.

Modalities - Better from rubbing, lying with head low. Better eating. Pain in head better by pressure. Closing eyes and resting head helps vertigo. ***Worse from raising up***, lying on back. Worse cold, sunstroke, going from warm to cold. Worse morning, on waking, evening. Worse after confinement. Motion aggravates, sudden motion causes faintness and blindness. Walking causes blindness. Lying down aggravates headache, breathing.

Mouth - Taste like musty odor. Odor from mouth like chloroform or ether. Foul. Increased saliva. Mouth feels as if scalded. Drawn at one corner.

Nose - Pinched and blue. Rapid and continued sneezing with warm biting feeling in mouth.

Rectum - Tenesmus and burning in rectum, better during and after stools.

Sensations - Confused feeling in head as if head would burst. Tongue as if scalded. As if a ball rising into esophagus. As if stomach tightly drawn against spine. As of a load on chest. As of galvanic shocks in limbs. As if damp clothing on arms and legs. As if boiling water poured over parts. As if ankles distorted.

Skin - ***Hot sweating***. Tingling and prickling in skin. Cold, clammy, bluish. Erysipelas with brain symptoms. Erythema. Itching in different parts better rubbing.

Sleep - Sleeplessness. Dreams of drowning of being on water. Coma.

Stomach - Gastritis. Burning in stomach and esophagus. Stomach seems to press against the spine. Constrictive pain increased by warm drinks. ***Hiccoughs***, excessive and painful with ***spasms of esophagus***. Nausea and vomiting. Vomiting, violent without nausea. Smallest quantity of food or drink immediately rejected.

Temperature - Hyperpyrexia or rapidly oscillating temperature with sweat. Cold clammy or hot sweat. Cerebrospinal, suppurative, acute rheumatic, fever. Fever high in the evening, below normal in the morning. Suppurative fevers with great variation of temperature.

Throat - Burning in gullet, esophagitis. As if as ball rising in.

Tongue - Tongue, white as if bleached. ***Tongue dry with red streak down center.***

Vertigo - Vertigo with nausea and sudden prostration, better closing eyes and resting head.

COMMENTS - Hale was instrumental in introducing Verat-v. to homeopathy, using it in fevers and particularly in pneumonia.

Burt made a heroic proving of the liquid extract and his infant daughter (twenty-one months) very nearly died from taking a few drops of the tincture from a phial.

In two minutes she began vomiting. Coffee and camphor were given as antidotes. In five minutes her jaws were rigid, pupils widely dilated, face blue, hands and feet cold, no pulse at wrist.

Her abdomen and back were rubbed with camphor, when she went into spasms with violent shrieks. These spasms were frequently repeated, a hot path being most effective in relaxing the muscles.

Vomiting ropy mucus kept up for three hours. Pulseless, hands and feet shriveled. After three and a half hours she slept quietly and soundly and next morning was well but a little weak.

The congestive symptoms and also of nausea and vomiting, form one of the leading indications of Verat-v. in a great variety of cases. Sensations of fullness. "Head feels full and heavy, rush of blood to the head, face flushed, buzzing in the ears, chest constricted or oppressed as from a heavy load," point to the congestive tendency.

Congestion at the base of brain, chest, spine, stomach. Slowing of the heart's action is a leading effect of the provings (from its action on the heart muscle and cardiac ganglia Dig. on the pneumogastric). Violent pains attending inflammation. Head full, throbbing of arteries, sensitive to sound, double or partial vision.

Chorea, "twitchings during sleep." "Constant jerking or nodding of the head, jerking and trembling. Threatened with convulsions," are other leading symptoms. Puerperal convulsions, Verat-v. has only succeeded when nauseating doses have been given.

Used locally and internally in muscular and joint rheumatism, and in chorea an application to the spine of the tincture, diluted with spirit, has proved a serviceable adjunct.

Verat-v. has been used to "knock down" fever in the same way as Acon. Nash pointed out that there is some risk in this. When Verat-v. was first introduced he used it largely and successfully in a number of cases, but in one case which appeared to be going on favorably, the patient died suddenly. This he attributed to the Verat-v.

D. McLellan was sent for in the middle of the night to see an old woman whom he found sitting up in bed gasping for breath and blue. Rapid congestion of the lungs had occurred. The attack had come on suddenly. Verat-v. quickly rescued the patient from a condition of imminent peril.

Clarke with the 30c, cured a man, 56 of dim sight as if scales over it, numbness, pain in head as if a tight band were around it, rush of blood to head, sleeplessness. Dreaming about water is a characteristic which he has confirmed.

RELATIONS - ***Antidoted by:*** Hot coffee. ***Antidote to:*** Strychnine, use fluid extract, 20-40 drops. ***Compare:*** (1) Puerperal convulsions, Gels. has dull, drowsy state of mind. (2) Verat-v., apoplectic condition between the fits, face red, eyes congested, violent convulsive twitches. (3) Congestions, Ferr-p., Bell. (4) Plethora, Acon. (5) Chorea, Hyos. (6) Pneumonia with engorgement, Sang. (Verat-v. more marked arterial tension). (7) Scalded tongue, Sang. (8) Tetanus, Nux-v., Hyper. (9) Rheumatic fever, Bry., Sal-ac. (10) Sunstroke, double or partial vision, Glon., Gels.

REFERENCES - Boericke. Clarke.

VERBASCUM THAPSUS

(Mullein Oil)

PHARMACY - verb. Verbascum thapsus. Mullein oil. Verbascum thapsiforme. Oleum mullein. Great Mullein. N. O. Scrophulariaceae. Tincture of fresh plant at the commencement of flowering. To prepare mullein oil, fill a bottle with the blossoms from the Verbascum thapsus, cork it tight and hang in the sun for four or five weeks. By that time there will be an oily liquid distilled. Mix with ten percent of alcohol. Tincture of the whole plant beginning to flower. ***Historical dose:*** Tincture and all potencies.

CLINICAL - Anus, itching. ***Bedwetting.*** Colic. Constipation. Cough. ***Deafness. Ear, pain.*** Hemorrhoids. ***Hoarseness.*** Neuralgia. Prosopalgia. Tumors. Urinary, incontinence.

HERBAL - The Treasury of Botany said, "The thick woolly leaves of Verbascum thapsus, the Great Mullein, have a mucilaginous, bitter taste and a decoction of them is employed in domestic practice in catarrhs and diarrhea.

"The leaves are also used as emollient

applications to hard tumors and in pulmonary complaints in cattle hence one of its popular names is Bullock's Lung-wort. It is also called Adam's flannel from its flannel-like leaves."

Among its traditional uses Gerarde mentioned it as a remedy for hemorrhoids and as applications for itching hemorrhoids or anal itching. An ointment is made of the tincture. Gerarde said that the oil of the yellow flowers is also curative in hemorrhoids.

The flowers contain, according to Millspaugh, "A yellow volatile oil and fatty acid, free malic and phosphoric acids and their ate salts of lime, a yellow resinous coloring matter and the general plant constituents including an uncrystallisable sugar." An oil prepared from the flowers has been found useful locally in cases of ***deafness or earache***.

HOMEOPATHIC - Verb. has a pronounced action on the inferior maxillary branch of the fifth pair of the cranial nerves, on the ear and respiratory tract and bladder.

Catarrhs and colds with ***periodical prosopalgia***, spasmodic effects, neuralgias. Nervous and bronchial coughs. Urinary irritation. Tearing, stitching, cramping squeezing, crushing, paralyzing pains. Intermittent pains.

Abdomen - As of a lump or twisting around navel. Incessant gurgling and rumbling beneath left ribs. Inflation of the abdomen, violent and painful pressure on navel. Pinchings and gripings in abdomen.

Back - Lancinations in the back and shoulder blades. Sharp intermittent stitches in left scapula. Backache worse from pressure.

Chest - Shooting in chest, sometimes with oppression and obstructed respiration. Stitches in the chest. Red nodosity near xiphoid cartilage, painful when pressed upon.

Ears - ***Earache.*** Numbness in left ear. Otalgia with a sense of obstruction. Deafness from getting water in, as in swimming or as if stopped by a valve. Dry, scaly condition of meatus (locally).

Eyes - Pains in eyes, as from contraction of the sockets with burning in eyes. Sight confused, as if directed through a veil.

Face - Neuralgia affecting zygoma, temporo-maxillary joint and ear (Meny.), particularly of left side with lachrymation, coryza and sensation ***as if parts were crushed with tongs***. Talking, sneezing and change of temperature aggravate the pains, also, pressing teeth together. Pains seem to come in flashes, excited by least movement, occurring periodically at same hour in morning and afternoon each day.

Food - Mawkish taste with fetid breath. Hunger without relish for food. Insatiable thirst.

Kidneys - Increased urine with pressure in bladder. Burning urination. Constant dribbling. ***Bedwetting***, at night, worse coughing.

Limbs - Stitching in the limbs. Stiffness and ***soreness of joints of lower limbs.*** Lower limbs feel heavy. Cramp-like pain in soles, right foot and knee. Neuralgic pain in left ankle. Thumb feels numb.

Lungs - Asthma. Catarrh with hoarseness and stuffed chest. Frequent attacks of deep, hollow cough with sound like a trumpet, better deep breathing. Soreness in pharynx, cough during sleep. Dry, hoarse cough worse at night. Cough, nervous without waking.

Male - Pollutions without lewd dreams.

Modalities - Better from taking deep inspirations. Worse touch, pressure. Worse cold, drafts, change of temperature. Worse from stooping, walking, talking. Worse sneezing, biting hard (inferior dental nerve). Worse 9 a.m. to 4 p.m., twice a day, at same hour.

Mouth - Copious accumulation of ***salty saliva*** in the mouth. Root of tongue brown. Tongue of a brownish yellow color, loaded with viscid mucus in morning and after dinner.

Nose - Profuse coryza from frontal sinuses with hot, burning, profuse lachrymation. Sensation of stoppage of larynx and ears.

Rectum - Many bowel movements a day with twisting about navel. Feces hard like sheep-dung and expelled with effort. Fearful diarrhea. Hemorrhoids, obstructing stools, itching and inflamed. Inflamed and painful hemorrhoids. Pain extends deep down, causing contraction of anal sphincter.

Sensations - As if everything would press out at forehead. As if temples were pinched and crushed. As if ears were stopped up. As if something had fallen before ear. As if left ramus of jaw were pressed against upper jaw. As if nose and larynx were stopped up. As if intestines were adherent to wall of abdomen and were being torn away. As of a twist around navel. As if cold water were poured over side of body from shoulder to thigh.

Sleep - Strong disposition to sleep after a meal. Disturbed sleep, at night with tossing. Short sleep at night, lasting only until 4 a.m. with anxious, frightful dreams of wars and dead bodies.

Stomach - Aching of stomach. Sensation of emptiness at pit of stomach, which disappears with a rumbling below left ribs. Frequent hiccough. Regurgitation of insipid serum. Empty or else bitter risings with nausea.

Temperature - Internal coldness of whole body of hands and feet, perceptible also externally. Shuddering, especially on one side of body, as if it were bathed in cold water.

Throat - Very severe pain in throat on swallowing. ***Hoarseness,*** voice deep, harsh, sounds like a trumpet, ***"basso profundo."*** Sensation of obstruction in the larynx.

Vertigo - Vertigo when pressing one cheek while supporting the head. Vertigo sudden, as from pressure on whole head.

COMMENTS - Mullein oil is used, locally, for earache and dry, scaly condition of meatus. Also for teasing cough at night or lying down. Bedwetting, five-drop doses night and morning

Cushing introduced this now rather well-known remedy to the medical profession in 1884. He wrote "My father's house was the home for all poor tramps, as well as ministers, etc. He fell into the river, got water in his ears and was quite deaf for months.

"A blind man had called, heard loud conversation, asked the cause, etc., then said for kindness received he would tell us how to make something that would surely cure him and it was worth a thousand dollars in New York City.

"We made the oil, put it in his ears at night and he was well in the morning. For years we kept a bottle of it and it traveled all around the towns and did wonders. That was when I was a youngster."

Hering, in "Hearing and Ears," noticed "In Germany flowers of Verbascum thapsus put in a dark-colored bottle, hung up in the sunlight, give in two or three weeks an oily fluid which has cured many old people and children."

Hahnemann proved Verb. and his proving confirmed many of the old uses. It produced neuralgic pains of very great intensity, pressing and sharp and especially in the facial bones, navel and limbs and a peculiar cough.

Chronic dermatitis of the external meatus and drumhead or exfoliation after furuncle. Catarrhal inflammation of the tympanum Suppurative disease of the tympanum. Accumulations of debris in the case of perforation, scarred eardrum. Chronic inflammation of the eyes. Chilblains. Burns.

Nash described a "Cough, deep, hollow, hoarse in sound like a trumpet." He cured many cases and always used it low. It is more especially a night cough. It occurs in children during their sleep.

Mullein was used as a popular specific for tuberculosis, the leaves being boiled in milk, which was then strained and given warm.

W. B. McCoy gave several illustrations. According to him Verb. (i.e., the "oil") has a "soothing effect on the entire nervous system in many cases acting as a soporific."

In summer diarrhea he gave one to four drops in two ounces of warm water, a teaspoonful every hour. In bedwetting or dribbling of urine one-drop doses in warm water three or four times a day.

Among his cases were those of two boys who had become deaf from getting water in their ears when swimming. They were cured by having three drops of the oil instilled "in each ear alternately night and morning."

O. S. Laws cured a youth of 16 of bedwetting with fifteen drops of the oils three times a day.

The oil plainly acts on the indications of the proving and may be regarded as an alternative preparation to the official tincture. It might be called Verbasci oleum.

Mr. Kemmis spent a large amount of money treating with various physicians for what they pronounced a rose cancer and without any relief. An Indian woman told him to use mullein oil. He distilled it (by sun exposure) and for a short time bathed the cancer with the oil.

The growth of cancer was permanently checked, but it was not healed. Mr. K. lived, perhaps, forty years after the treatment was used and the cancer never again bothered him.

RELATIONS - ***Compare:*** (1) Rhus-a., Caust., Plat., Sphing. - pain in zygoma. (2) in neuralgia, Plat. - pressure, Stann. - gradually increasing and decreasing. (3) Deep cough, Cor-r., Dros., Spong., Sulph. (4) Sheep-dung stools, Mag-m. (5) Cough from tickling in chest, Verat.

REFERENCES - Anshutz. Boericke. Clarke. Murphy.

VERBENA HASTATA
(Blue Vervain)

PHARMACY - verbe-h. Verbena hastata. Blue Vervain. Ironweed. Vervain. Tincture of entire fresh plant. N. O. Verbenaceae. ***Historical dose:*** Tincture and all potencies.

CLINICAL - Depression. ***Epilepsy.*** Insomnia. Intermittent, fever. Mental, exhaustion. Poison oak.

HERBAL - Verbena, in the form of a tea as a diuretic drink, is used by Vannier to aid elimination in tuberculosis cases. In epilepsy it must be continued for a long time.

HOMEOPATHIC - Verbe-h. affects the skin and ***nervous system***. Nervous depression, weakness and irritation and spasms. Promotes the absorption of blood and allays pain in bruises. Passive congestion.

Epilepsy, insomnia, mental exhaustion. In epilepsy, ***it brightens up the patient's mental powers*** and helps the constipation. Intermittent fever. Poison-oak. Vesicular erysipelas.

COMMENTS - Anshutz reported "A[illegible]tract from a paper by Dr. J. N. White, Queen City, Texas, detailing at length the case of a five-year old boy, who after six weeks of whooping cough, developed epileptic symptoms, having as high as twelve spasms in twenty-four hours.

"After two months of treatment with such remedies as Sol-c., Sulfonal, Hyos., Cann-i., Calomel, Zinc., etc. with no results, the cases was given Verbena.

"Another doctor was in consultation and we quote: I told my friend (the Doctor) that when he became satisfied with the zinc treatment, I wanted to try another eclectic remedy. (The Doctor was an allopath). He was perfectly willing and I put him on Verbena hastata tincture, twelve drops, every four hours, skipping the dose at midnight.

"After we both took the case we decided, as there were no curative properties in the sulfonal, we would drop it and not use anything to control the paroxysms. Consequently the boy seemed to get worse to the parents, as now he would have several falling spells a day.

"From the first dose of the Verbena hastata the boy began to improve. He would have contractions of the muscles of the arms and legs and look wild for a minute or more for the first week, but after that he never had another symptom. We kept him on the medicine, as above, for six weeks and now he takes twelve drops three times a day.

"He has not had any symptom in over two months and all that wild vacant look is gone and he plays, eats, sleeps, etc., as if he had never been troubled with epilepsy."

REFERENCES - Anshutz. Boericke.

VERONAL

PHARMACY - veronal. Veronal. A dangerous drug made by the action of alcohol upon urea and contains the same radical that alcohol does. ***Historical dose:*** All potencies.

HOMEOPATHIC - Confluent, reddish spots, dermatitis. Itching of glans and prepuce. Circumscribed dermatitis patch on first metacarpal phalangeal joint. Dr. Varney noted staggering, cannot stand up. Veronal makes a man just as drunk as pure alcohol.

RELATIONS - *Compare:* (1) Chlol.

REFERENCES - Boericke.

VERONICA OFFICINALIS

(Common Speedwell)

PHARMACY - vero-o. Veronica officinalis. Common speedwell. N.O. Scrophulariaceae. *Historical dose:* All potencies.

HOMEOPATHIC - Perspiration at night. Perspiration followed by chills and cold sweats after uncovering. Sleepless at night and desire for naps during the day. Desire to sleep on the right side. Worse right side. Sense of fatigue and lethargy. Weakness, worse missing a meal.

Skin eruptions, red and itching violently. Worse evening, exposure to dampness. Tingling sensation throughout body. Sensation of heat. Dramatic increase in energy, increased clarity of thinking.

Dryness. Sensation of cotton in mouth. Numb sensation in gums, as if having received anesthesia. Burning pain in stomach as from heartburn. Worse beginning to eat. Increased or lost appetite. Increased thirst. Better eructations.

MIND - ***Great mental anxiety.*** Mental confusion and a sense of being overwhelmed, alternates with clarity of thinking. Irritability, particularly with alternating moods. Desire for husband. Homesickness. Detached feeling. Delusion that people are distant, that the body is vibrating. Delusion of having smoked marijuana.

Abdomen - Abdomen pain, better rubbing.

Back - ***Stiffness in lumbar region,*** worse standing. Pain in cervical region, worse cold.

Cough - ***Persistent bronchial cough*** with little or no mucus production.

Ears - Hears popping noises, ringing.

Eyes - Heaviness of eyelids. Pain in right eye, worse touch.

Female - Dark brown, mucus-like discharge during ovulation. Sexual desire decreased or increased.

Food - Desires sweets.

Limbs - ***Sharp pain in hips.*** Perspiration of palms of hands.

Modalities - Worse afternoon, 4 p.m. to 7 p.m.

Nose - Tingling in sinuses.

Rectum - ***Urging followed by loose stool.*** Stool, odor of rotten eggs or sulphur.

Sleep - Dreams of smoking cigarettes. Dreams of riding horses, of snakes.

Throat - Sensation of pinpricks, extending to whole throat. ***Sore throat.*** Skin in external throat around thyroid sensitive to pressure. Fleeting prickling sensation in trachea.

REFERENCES - Riley.

VERVAIN

(Bach-Flower Essence)

PHARMACY - verv-b. Vervain. Verbena officinalis. Bach Flower Essence. The flowering branches are put in a bowl of sunlit water and left to the sun's action for several hours. Subsequently, the water is strained and used as medicine. ***Historical dose:*** Take two drops from the stock bottle into a one ounce dropper bottle (add brandy or alcohol, if this bottle will be used for days or weeks). This is the dosage bottle, take a few drops straight into the mouth or as needed in a little water or juice.

HOMEOPATHIC - Verv-b. belongs to Bach's group of ***Over-Care for Other's Welfare,*** along with Rck-w-b., Beech-b., Vine-b. and Chic-b. Verv-b treats states of over-enthusiasm which lead to exaggerated attempts to convert others to one's own views. Escalating tension and excessive drive of willpower. Gradual depletion of reserves. Manic and catatonic states (Cher-p-b., Imp-b.). Hyperthyroidism.

MIND - Enthusiastic, fixed ideas. Fervency and fanaticism. Excitability, impressionability and quickly aroused motivation and fondness for others. Excessive joy, exaggerated, unbalanced emotions of love and friendship. Extreme disgust and rejection. Hysterical mood swings. Political fanaticism and outbursts of violence. Self-righteous.

Manic states within mental illness. Bipolar disorders and problems with impulse control

(Cher-p-b., Holly, Imp-b.). Obsessive-compulsive disorders. Delusions and psychoses with excessive fervency, ecstasy (Clem-b.) and mania.

REFERENCES - Bach.

VESICARIA COMMUNIS

PHARMACY - vesi. Vesicaria communis. N. O. Cruciferae. Alyssineae. Tincture of whole fresh plant. ***Historical dose:*** Tincture and all potencies.

CLINICAL - Albuminuria. Bladder, pain. ***Cystitis.*** Dropsy. Gleet. Gonorrhea. Gravel. Hematuria. ***Kidney, pain.*** Prostatitis.

HERBAL - According to the Treasury of Botany, Vesicaria is a genus of Cruciferae, natives of the Northern Hemisphere, distinguished by the globose or oboid inflated pouch with hemispherical valves and numerous seeds (generally four to six) in each cell. They are herbs, sometimes shrubby at the base with oblong or linear entire or ripened leaves and terminal racemes of yellow flowers.

The Vesicaria communis tincture is prepared from the whole plant collected fresh. It has been an old home remedy in various parts of Germany for various forms of urinary troubles attendant on gonorrhea, gravel, cystitis, nephralgia, prostatitis etc.

HOMEOPATHIC - George R. Shafter found nephralgia, acute cystitis, irritable bladder, following acute cystitis, and chronic cystitis. particularly amenable to Vesi. Its main indication is a great burning and smarting in urethra with a frequent desire to pass urine. Marked strangury (Thlaspi., Berb., Sars., Chim. and Canth.).

COMMENTS - Shafter recorded many cases, including that of T. S., age 67, who suffered from kidney pain, for which he had received morphine injections in former attacks. Vesi. in 15 drop doses every fifteen minutes, gave marked relief in two hours, which in six hours was complete.

S. B., age 57, had cystitis from cold, high fever, eating, burning pain on voiding urine, which was drop by drop. Vesi. tincture in 10 drop doses. cured in two days.

A woman, age 39, had pain in her back, brick-dust sediment in urine, hands and feet swelling so she could hardly close her hands or walk. Vesi. tincture cured.

Man, age 65, with an irritable bladder, had to rise twenty to thirty times in the night. Vesi. tincture in 20-drop doses, relieved quickly and cured in six weeks.

C. M., 89, chronic cystitis, passing large quantities of mucus, pus. The bladder was at first washed out with boric acid solution, then Vesi. tincture 20 drops every two hours, were given. Improvement followed and in two hours the boric acid washing was stopped and Vesic. given every four hours. This finally cured.

Gonorrhea with smarting and burning on urination and thick creamy discharge. Vesi. tincture a drachm every four hours, soon cured. Gonorrhea, female after being treated for two weeks with injections, was cured in seven days with Vesi. tincture in drachm doses.

Cowperthwaite succeeded in causing albumen to disappear from the urine even in cases of actual Bright's disease. He added that "it is necessary to use only the imported [i.e., European] tincture, 15 drops every four hours" (There are several Vesicarias native to North America).

A. L. Davison treated Mrs. P. for general dropsy of a year's standing, was in uremic spasms when first seen, the kidneys having ceased to secrete urine. Vesi. tincture was prescribed, 15 drops in a teaspoonful of water every hour until urine was freely secreted, then three times a day. The second day the kidneys were pouring out urine and watery stools were passed. In a week all dropsy had disappeared.

Bancroft treated Mrs. T. for irritable kidneys and bladder with polyuria. After a time the urine became bloody with occasional thin clots. Previously there had been for some months a thick, yellow sediment. Vesi. tincture, 6 drops four times a day and later 15 drops three times a day, taken persistently, effected a cure.

Halbert reported the case of Mr. H., a young man whose occupation involved much outdoor exercise and who contracted a chill and had lumbago in consequence.

Under an "orificial" surgeon his rectum was operated on and the sphincter stretched.

Thereafter he had fever, rigors and acute prostatitis. Urination was painful and difficult and soon hematuria ensued. The pain and nervous exhaustion were so extreme that he was put into hospital and for a time only relieved by injections of morphine. The urine contained albumen, blood-clots, much pus. Urine was only passed by means of the catheter and defecation was extremely painful.

Vesi. 1x was given hourly and great relief followed. The painful tenesmus was alleviated and he was soon able to pass urine without the catheter. In three weeks he was able to go home.

Shafer gave Cact. and Thlaspi. in a case of dropsy from heart disease in a woman, age 48. These gave little relief. He then gave Vesi. in combination with the others. There was marked relief in twenty-four hours and in ten days the dropsy had disappeared.

RELATIONS - ***Compare:*** (1) Thlaspi, Berb., Sars., Chim. and Canth. (2) In Gravel, Coc-c., Urt-u., Thlaspi. (3) Hematuria, Chin-s., Fic., Phos. (4) Prostatic affections, Hydrang., Solid., Sabal. (5) Cystitis, Chim. ***Compatible:*** Cact., Thlaspi.

REFERENCES - Clarke.

VESPA CRABRO

(Wasp)

PHARMACY - vesp. Vespa crabro. Wasp. Vespa maculata. Vespa vulgaris. European hornet. Giant hornet. Yellow-jacket. American hornet. N. O. Hymenoptera, Sub-order Vespidae. Tincture of the insects. ***Historical dose:*** All potencies.

CLINICAL - Abscesses, multiple. Alopecia. Bee stings. Bedwetting. ***Boils.*** Cervix, ulcerated. ***Chemosis.*** Edema. ***Erythema.*** Fainting. Flushing. Glottis, spasm. Indigestion. Ophthalmia. Ovary, pain. Quinsy. Tongue, swelling. Uterus, ulcerated. Vertigo.

HOMEOPATHIC - The symptoms are mostly the results of stings although Berridge proved Vesp. 30c on three persons. The symptoms included low spirits, pain in right ear, nausea with faint feeling and trembling, pain in left side of the neck on waking.

Stinging, burning pains, as if pierced with red hot needles. Stinging piercing deeply, as if a hook were pulled out. Sudden stinging and burning in cheek. Burning of the part, then swelling, red with burning pain. Sudden tearing. Indurated feeling.

Cutting like electric shocks through all joints. Arm, head and face swollen. Eyes red and twitching. Red lines along absorbents. Itching over whole body. Insensibility. Vasomotor symptoms of skin and mucus membranes.

Nerve and muscular excitement. Trembling, quaking with chattering of teeth. Convulsions, loss of consciousness, does not answer when spoken to, looks into space, has no recollection of the attack.

Dizzy, better lying on back. Faintness, all day with trembling and nausea. Numbness and blindness. Pulse slow, heart's action scarcely perceptible. Feeling as if dying at night. Heat especially overpowers him. Feet were cold except in summer, when they burned uncomfortably. Perspiration on parts laid on with itching. Axillary glands swollen with soreness of upper arms.

Nausea and vomiting, followed by creeping chills from feet upward. Cramping pain in bowels. Frequent urination. Weakness with bedwetting. Pain in sacrum extending up back. Disorders of left ovary with tenderness.

MIND - Terrible anxiety. Low-spirited. Insensibility. Unconsciousness with inability to move.

Abdomen - Uneasiness in abdomen.

Back - Pain in left side of neck, waking her at night, preventing her from turning it to left side, felt least when lying on back, best on right side. Pain in scapula with soreness.

Ears - Sticking deep in right ear. Purulent catarrh of middle ears.

Eyes - Injection of right conjunctiva. ***Chemosis of conjunctiva***. Inflammation of right eye with baggy swelling of conjunctiva. Itching of right lid in evening with swelling afterwards pain in lid and ball. Erysipelatous inflammation of lid, whole side of face painful and swollen.

Face - Pain in cheek as if pierced with red-hot needles, suddenly awakening him from sleep and recurring periodically. Painful and swollen. Erysipelatous inflammation of lids. Swelling of mouth and throat with violent burning pains. Face livid. Face smooth, dark red, bloated. Anxious look.

Female - Menstruation, preceded by pain, pressure, depression and constipation. Menses intermittent, sometimes brown, accompanied by pain and flatulence, preceded by mental depression, pain, pressure and constipation. ***Left ovary markedly affected with frequent burning, urination***, sacral pains extending up back. ***Erosion around external os.*** Pain in left ovarian region. An irritable ulcer surrounded os tincae. Irritation, worse in groin, passing into pudenda.

Head - Fainting and loss of consciousness. A violent heat came over him, felt sick, then turned giddy and spun around and around like a top until he fell, staggered to the house, got into a chair in a moment, fell out of it, almost fainting, dashed water into his face, at length was able to lie down on his bed. Headache. Face and head swollen and inflamed. Alopecia.

Heart - Aching in heart. Slow beating of heart, almost imperceptible. Pulse rapid and small, feeble, with violent beating of carotids.

Kidneys - Marked tenderness to deep pressure in kidney region. Remittent dysuria with backache. ***Burning pain*** with urination, also itching. Burning urination in women. Hematuria. Incessant bedwetting.

Limbs - Pain in shoulder, axillary glands swollen. Sprained pain in left shoulder joint on moving it, worse lifting arm or twisting it. Aching in hand and arm.

Lungs - Dyspnea. Respiration hurried. Hoarseness. Voice lost. Spasm of glottis (after application of diluted ammonia to tongue), face pale, drops of sweat on forehead, arms thrown out to gasp for air, he got out of bed, sank back on bed, face livid, breath and pulse stopped.

Male - Swelling of scrotum and penis.

Modalities - Better from cold washing of hands. Cold water first relieves then aggravates. Skin better by bathing with vinegar. Worse from hot stove, in a closed room. Worse after sleep, after eating. Worse by motion. Open air aggravates lachrymation.

Mouth - Tongue swollen and tense, swelling below chin, between that and hyoid bone, pain in a point in middle line of tongue, swollen, red, rounded, filled the mouth, immovable, could not speak, only mumbled, swallowing was painful and difficult. Swelling of palate with inflammation. Peculiar taste, as when a nest of wasps is disturbed, worse heat.

Sensations - As if a harpoon were sticking deep in and were drawn on. As if pierced with red-hot needles. As if a cutting instrument were piercing all joints like an electric shock. Cold, chilly sensation around sting. As if left shoulder joint were sprained. As if about to suffocate. As if dying.

Skin - ***Erythema intense itching***, burning. ***Boils***, stinging and soreness, ***relieved by bathing with vinegar.*** Wheals, macules and swellings with burning, stinging and soreness. Erythema multiforme.

Sleep - Night restless. Sleepless all night.

Stomach - Cold feeling in stomach. Heat in stomach. Indigestion with flushing. Belchings. Nausea in evening after coming indoors with weight in stomach with faint feeling and trembling. Vomiting with swelling of head.

Throat - Swelling of throat, soreness, heat of throat. Hypertrophied tonsils which secreted a cheesy matter. Pharyngeal varicosis.

Vertigo - Fainting, loss of consciousness.

COMMENTS - W. Rowbotham was stung on the right cheek. The next day, about 4 a.m., he was suddenly awakened by burning, stinging pain in cheek, "as if pierced with red-hot needles" and soreness and smarting along the lymphatics. After bathing the face he got to sleep and was again suddenly awakened by the pain two hours later, which recurred periodically in paroxysm, throughout the day.

Burnett observed a case of a sting on the tongue in a woman. The tongue entirely filled the buccal cavity. The patient's appearance was exactly like one suffering from severe synanche. The swelling was diffuse and deep-seated. There was not much redness.

Berridge demonstrated that the poison of the hornet and the wasp may answer to each other's indications. He cured with Vesp. 100,000c. (Fincke) a symptom produced by Vespa vulgaris, namely, chemosis of the right eye.

Mr. X. age 66, had his right eye inflamed for six days. When seen there was redness of right lower lid, baggy swelling of conjunctiva partly covering the cornea when pressed upward, lachrymation of right eye worse in open air, right lids adhere in morning. Vesp. three times daily cured in a few days.

E. T. Blake cured with Vesp. face swollen and puffy, skin transparent and blanched, scalding urine followed by itching, itching of right arm.

Blake also related the case of Miss C. J., who at the age of thirty-one was stung on the left thumb, through some calico and was never well after, dying at the age of thirty-eight. She was prone to constipation all her life and at twenty-three had "congestion of the left lung." Most of the abdominal, urinary, ovarian and uterine symptoms were hers. Among the latter was an irritable ulcer.

RELATIONS - ***Antidote:*** Semp., locally. ***Antidoted by:*** Apis, Led., Camph., salt water, vinegar. ***Compare:*** (1) Scorp. - salivation, strabismus, tetanus, Apis. (2) pains as if pierced with red-hot needles, Ars., Apis. (3) Ulcers around os uterus, Mitch., Eup-pur., Apis., Hydrc. ***Incompatible:*** Arg-n.

REFERENCES - Boericke. Clarke.

VIAGRA

(Sildenafil Citrate)

PHARMACY - viag. Viagra. Sildenafil citrate. An allopathic drug. ***Historical dose:*** All potencies.

CLINICAL - Allergic, reactions. Angina pectoris. Arthritis. Asthma. ***Blindness.*** Cataracts. Chest, pain. Chills. Circulation, disorders. Coughs. Depression. Diarrhea. Diplopia. Edema. ***Erectile, dysfunction. Eye, disorders. Facial, flushing.*** Fainting. ***Genital, problems.*** Gout. Headaches. Hemorrhages. ***Heart, disorders.*** Hypertension. Hypotension. ***Impotency.*** Indigestion. Insomnia. Migraines. Numbness. Photophobia. ***Retina, bleeding.*** Seizures. Sexual, disorders. Sinusitis. Strokes. Thrombosis. Tremors. Ulcers. ***Vision, disorders.*** Vertigo.

HOMEOPATHIC - Viagra, used for male impotence, works by dilating blood vessels in the penis, allowing the inflow of blood needed for an erection. Viagra causes erections only during sexual excitement. It does not work in the absence of arousal.

Heart attack, stroke, heart irregularities, dangerous surges in blood pressure, and sudden death have all been reported after use of Viagra, usually in men with existing cardiac risk factors, and typically during or shortly after sex.

Allergic reactions. Chills. Dizziness. Drowsiness. Fainting, falling. Muscle ache. Joint disease. Bone pain. Numbness. Coordination problems. Slow reflexes. Tremors. Seizures. Strokes. Flushing. Thrombosis. Insomnia. Gout. Diabetes. Sinus and throat inflammation.

MIND - Emotional and mental disturbances. Anxiety. Depression. Abnormal dreams.

Abdomen - Abdominal pain. Colitis. Intestinal inflammation. Gastroenteritis.

Bladder - Cystitis. Urinary tract infection. Loss of bladder control. Urinary incontinence. Increased night-time urination.

Chest - Angina pectoris. Breast enlargement.

Ears - Tinnitus. Ringing in the ears. Deafness. Ear pain.

Eyes - Dry eyes. Bloodshot eyes. Increased pressure in the eyes. Eye inflammation and pain. ***Retinal bleeding.*** Cataracts. Dilated pupils. Photophobia. Sensitivity to light. ***Floaters.***

Face - ***Facial flushing.*** Edema.

Female - Vaginal dryness. Anorgasmia.

Head - ***Headaches.*** Migraine headaches.

Cerebral thrombosis.

Heart - Angina pectoris. ***Heart problems.*** Cardiomyopathy. Heart failure. Hypotension. Low blood pressure. Rapid or throbbing heartbeats. Tachycardia, palpitation. Myocardial ischemia.

Lungs - Dyspnea. Breathing difficulty. Asthma. Coughs. Lung inflammation. Bronchitis, sputum increased.

Male - Genital problems. ***Erectile dysfunction.*** Painful erection. ***Prolonged erections.*** Abnormal ejaculation. Anorgasmia. ***Impotency.***

Mouth - Dry mouth. Difficulty swallowing. Gum inflammation. Stomatitis.

Nerves - Ataxia. Hypertonia. Neuralgias. Paresthesia. Tremors, reflexes increased. Hypesthesia.

Nose - ***Nasal congestion.*** Sinusitis. Nosebleeds.

Rectum - Diarrhea. Rectal bleeding.

Skin - Raised skin patches. Itchy skin. Contact dermatitis. Rashes. Ulcers. Urticaria. Herpes simplex. Sweating.

Sleep - Insomnia. Abnormal dreams. Somnolence.

Stomach - Thirst. Stomach inflammation. Dyspepsia. Acid indigestion. Nausea, vomiting.

Throat - Laryngitis, pharyngitis.

Vertigo - Dizziness and fainting.

Vision - Abnormal vision. Double vision. ***Blue color tinge in vision.*** Blurred vision. Color perception changes. Light perception changes. Light sensitivity. ***Blindness.***

REFERENCES - Murphy.

VIBURNUM OPULUS

(Cramp Bark)

PHARMACY - vib. Viburnum opulus. Cramp bark. High cranberry. Bush cramp. Bark water elder. N. O. Caprifliaceae. Great Britain. The Gueldres Rose or Snowball-tree is the cultivated and sterile variety. Tincture of the fresh bark. ***Historical dose:*** Tincture and all potencies.

CLINICAL - After-pains. Cough, pregnancy. ***Cramps. Dysmenorrhea.*** Ears, painful. Epididymitis. Headaches. Hysteria. Labor, false. Labor, pains. Lumbago. Menstruation, painful. ***Miscarriages.*** Ovaries, pain. Paralysis. ***Uterus, pain.***

HOMEOPATHIC - Viburnum opulus, a native of Great Britain, is widely distributed over the northern parts of the continent and America. According to Hale, in America the wild species is called "Cramp bark" and the knowledge of its curative virtues in painful spasmodic diseases, like dysmenorrhea, is derived from the Native Americans. The tincture has a strong odor of Valerianic acid (as also has that of Vib. tinus).

Hale derived his knowledge from herbal sources. In spasmodic dysmenorrhea he gave a few drops of tincture to 3x thrice daily for a week before the period, every hour when the pains set in or every fifteen minutes if the pains are severe.

Cramps in abdomen and legs of pregnant women. To prevent miscarriage when the pains are spasmodic or threatening. False pains preceding labor. After-pains, a dose after each pain.

HOMEOPATHIC - Vib. is a remedy for general cramps. Colicky pains in pelvic organs. Conscious of internal sexual organs. ***Prevents miscarriage.*** False labor-pains. Spasmodic and congestive affections, dependent upon ovarian or uterine origin.

Paralytic conditions after convulsions. Violent, spasmodic, nervous effects, especially in females, dependent upon the ovarian or uterine origin. Pains make her so nervous, she cannot keep still. Sick feeling all over in pelvic complaints. Hemorrhages. ***Left sided symptoms.***

MIND - Very nervous and irritable.

Abdomen - Excruciating crampy colicky pain. Heavy aching, hypogastrium, better menses. ***Sudden cramps and colic pains.*** Tender, worse pressure about umbilicus.

Back - Bruised feeling in back as after severe exertion. Tired backache, better pressure. Lumbago, better walking with a cane pressed, arms across the back. Pains in the back end in a cramp in uterus or go down the thighs.

Chest - Feeling of oppression over whole chest. Sensation as if muscles of chest failed to act, causing dyspnea. Shooting over left sixth rib near sternum.

Constitutions - Suited to tall, slender, dark or fair haired hysterical subjects.

Ears - Stabbing in ears. Pains in bone waking at night. External ear sore as if bruised.

Eyes - Sclerotica streaked with blood. Sensation of sand in eyes. Pain in right eye with congestion. Burning and lachrymation. Sore feeling in eyeballs. Sore feeling on closing lids. Heaviness of eyes.

Face - Flushed and hot. Face swollen and congested. Swelling about right eye with induration. Face and lips pale, dark circles under eyes. Lips dry.

Female - Heavy aching feeling or excruciating cramps in pelvis, better from menses. Bearing-down pains before menses. ***Menses too late, scanty, lasting a few hours,*** offensive in odor with crampy pains, cramps extend down thighs (Bell.). ***Spasmodic and membranous dysmenorrhea*** (Bor.). Leucorrhea, thick, white, blood streaked worse during stools. Leucorrhea, excoriating. Smarting and itching of genitals. Consciousness of internal sexual organs. Pelvic organs turning upside down. Aching in sacrum and pubes with pain in anterior muscles of thighs (Xanth.). Pains from back to loins and womb worse early morning. Uterine pains extend around the pelvis often extending down the thighs. Ovarian region feels heavy and congested. Uterine hemorrhage. ***Frequent and very early miscarriage***, causing seeming infertility. ***False labor pains.*** Violent persistent after-pains. Faint on attempting to sit up.

Food - No appetite. No desire to eat, stomach feels full. Indigestion, food lies heavy.

Head - Head dull and sluggish. Throbbing in head. Terrible crushing pain worse left parietal region with a sensation as if head opening and shutting. Severe pain in temporal region. Head hurt by every cough.

Kidneys - Frequent urging. Frequent, profuse urination during headache, menses, hemorrhages etc. Dysuria, spasmodic. Copious, pale, light-colored urine. Cannot hold water on coughing or walking.

Limbs - Stiff, sore feeling in nape of neck. Feels as if back would break. Sacral backache. Lower limbs weak and heavy. Cramps in calves, before menses.

Lungs - Suffocative spells at night, worse cold, damp. Infantile asthma. Cough during pregnancy.

Modalities - Better by pressure, resting. Better in open air. Worse from motion, sudden jar, lying on left side, lying on affected side. Worse evening and night. Worse in close room, warm room. Worse cold, snow, air. Worse from fright. Worse before menses. Straining at stool aggravates headache. Stooping causes dizziness. Rising causes fainting, nausea and dizziness.

Rectum - Stools large and hard with cutting in rectum and soreness of anus.

Sensations - As if she could not tell where she was or what to do on awaking. As if she could not live, sick feeling at stomach. Emptiness, as if stomach hollow. As if body from waist to lower pelvis would collapse. As if urine continued to flow after urinating. As if menses coming on. As if pelvic organs were turning upside down. As if parts would be forced through vulva and she must support the part. Left side as if strained or bruised by over-lifting.

Skin - Tettery spots on cheeks, arms etc.

Sleep - Very restless sleep, felt sick all over. When asleep, sensation of falling and awakened frequently with a start.

Stomach - Constant nausea, relieved by eating.

Vertigo - Vertigo, feels as if falling forward, worse descending stairs. Feels faint on sitting up.

COMMENTS - The first Vib. provings were by H. C. Allen, assisted by eleven provers, male and female with the tincture and first and 30c dilutions. Dr. Susan Fenton of Oakland, proved Vib. on six provers.

One of the six took the tincture up to drachm doses without obtaining a single symptom. One prover was cured of a number of symptoms, but developed no new ones. All took potencies at first without eliciting any symptoms.

Taking the tincture all had these symptoms with variations: severe backache going through to the front or around the abdomen to uterus. Cramping pelvic pain. Temporal headache. Three had nausea with pains. All had "sick feeling all over." One had omission of a period, two had menses early.

One case was cured; Miss F., 25, a housekeeper, medium height, rather slender, blonde, sanguine, was strong until she had severe pelvic congestion and was fifteen months under treatment and most of the time in bed.

In June, 1892, a double oophorectomy was performed with great relief, but attacks of pelvic congestion with severe pain still persisted, at first every two to four weeks, later less frequently, causing impairment of general health and strength.

Symptoms included excruciating pains through lower abdomen with bearing-down sensation and a feeling as if the body from the waist to lower part of pelvis would collapse, an indescribable sick feeling all over with severe aching in rectum, great depression of spirits, symptoms better when lying down.

Vib. tincture was taken in three-drop doses thrice daily. After taking it for three days she lost all her symptoms and felt "perfectly well for the first time in over four years." It is evident that "sick feeling all over" in connection with pelvic complaints and "worse from movement, better by rest" are keynotes of Vib.

RELATIONS - ***Antidoted by:*** Acon. (epididymitis), Verat. (Diarrhea). ***Compare:*** (1) Vib-p. Cimic., Caul., Sabin., Sep., Thlaspi., Xanth.

REFERENCES - Clarke. Hale.

VIBURNUM PRUNIFOLIUM

(Black Haw)

PHARMACY - Vib-p. Viburnum prunifolium. Black haw. An American species. N. O. Caprifliaceae. Tincture of fresh bark gathered in October and November from trees grown in open situations. Phares. ***Historical dose:*** Tincture and all potencies.

CLINICAL - ***After-pains.*** Dysmenorrhea. Infertility. Menorrhagia. Menstrual disorders. Miscarriage. Morning sickness. Tetanus. Tongue, cancer. Uterine, disorders.

HERBAL - Hale quoted his experiences showing a close resemblance between Vib-p. and Vib. with some additional uses of Vib-p.

Viburnum prunifolium is a ***uterine tonic***. Useful for habitual miscarriage. ***After-pains.*** Menstrual irregularities of infertile females with uterine displacements. Morning sickness. Cancer of the tongue, obstinate hiccough.

Phares said of it, "Vib-p. is particularly valuable in preventing abortion and miscarriage, whether habitual or otherwise, whether threatened from accidental causes or criminal drugging."

COMMENTS - Phares noted the case of Mrs. W. had never gone to full term, had several children at eight months, all of them dying one month after birth. Frequent pregnancies and hemorrhages had seriously impaired her health.

When next pregnant Vib-p. was ordered and at the eighth month when pains set in vigorously with copious bloody discharge, Vib-p. was given freely and she went to term, giving birth to a healthy boy, who survived.

He also recorded the case of Mrs. L., married eighteen months, had miscarried and suffered long and much in consequence. Being again pregnant, Phares gave her Vib-p. tincture, a teaspoonful thrice daily. At the third month, she was severely injured by a fall from her carriage.

Strong uterine contractions ensued, but were arrested by Vib-p., which had to be given freely for several days, the dose being gradually diminished. For nearly a week, miscarriage was threatened whenever Vib-p. was too long suspended. The patient went to term and gave birth to a large boy.

Hale used the tincture in threatened miscarriage, dysmenorrhea and spasmodic uterine pains. It entirely antidotes the effect of Goss., which is much used for procuring abortion in some of the States, one pint of a strong decoction of the cotton-root being sufficient. Vib-p. when taken regularly completely neutralizes this.

E. P. Fowler cured two cases of cancer of the tongue with the decoction of Vib-p. bark, used topically. Phares thinks it perhaps "the best remedy in the world for tetanus."

RELATIONS - ***Antidote to:*** Goss.

REFERENCES - Clarke. Hale.

VIBURNUM TINUS

PHARMACY - vib-t. Viburnum tinus. Laurustinus. N. O. Caprifliaceae. Tincture of fresh leaves. ***Historical dose:*** Tincture and all potencies.

CLINICAL - Deafness. Diaphragm, cramp. Dysmenorrhea Hypochondriasis. Ovary, pain.

HERBAL - Viburnum tinus is the evergreen shrub known in gardens as Laurustinus. Cooper investigated it, giving always single doses of the herbal tincture in cases analogous to those for which Vib. op. is given.

COMMENTS - Using Vib-t., Cooper cured pain in ovary with depression. He considered hypochondriasis an indication for Vib-t. Deafness with sufferings in lower segment of abdomen and dysmenorrhea, erosions about the os uterus. Cramp in diaphragm.

Horrible headache all over head, worse on right side with right-sided deafness, coming on at 7 a.m. and 11 a.m. and 4 a.m. and 7 p.m. with great sinking in pit of chest. Waking at 4 a.m. with horrid depression of spirits that lasts until noon with a weight on chest and back, has to hold herself up to breathe.

REFERENCES - Clarke.

VICHY AQUA

(Vichy Mineral Springs)

PHARMACY - vichy-g. Vichy aqua. Vichy mineral springs. Grande grille. Springs at Vichy, France. Vichy springs containing carbonicum acidum, muriaticum acidum, sulphuricum acidum, silica, phosphoric acidum, arsenicum acidum, ferrum oxidatum, natrum, kalium, calcium and magnesium. Arsenicums. Oxygenums. Silicas. Dilutions. ***Historical dose:*** Tincture and all potencies.

CLINICAL - Bladder, catarrh. Constipation. Diabetes. Gallstones. Gout. Gravel. Heartburn. Indigestion. Intermittent, fevers. Liver, disorders. Neck, stiff. Rheumatism. Salivation. Skin, disorders. Uterus, disorders.

HOMEOPATHIC - The springs of Vichy are alkaline, both hot and cold. Croserio proved Vichy, taking the water and triturations of the salt and dilutions.

Constantin James noted that the springs are used in a large number of maladies, especially diseases of the digestive tract, diseases of the liver with or without stones. Abdominal engorgements consequent on paludal fevers, chronic engorgements of the uterus, catarrh of the bladder, gravel, gout and rheumatism, diabetes mellitus, skin diseases.

Among the most prominent symptoms were stitches below mastoid in chest in right loin and in heart. Across the chest there was a sensation as of a bar impeding breathing. Sinking sensation and sensation as if about to be sick. Burning flatulence. In the nose there were illusions of smell, corpse-like odor, odor of cucumbers. After sex there was excessive weakness as if from hunger.

Modalities - Worse from cold, drafts of air. Worse when seated. Worse after sex. Worse after eating, when eating. Uneasiness is better by dinner.

RELATIONS - ***Compare:*** (1) Nat-m. (2) Stitching pains, Kali-c. (3) Bar sensation, Haematox., Ars., Ox-ac. (4) Worse from sex, Kali-c., Kali-bi., Staph. (5) Illusory smells, Anac.

REFERENCES - Clarke.

VINCA MINOR

(Lesser Periwinkle)

PHARMACY - vinc. Vinca minor. Lesser periwinkle. N. O. Apocynaceae. Grows in woods and shady places. Tincture of whole fresh plant. ***Historical dose:*** All potencies, first to third potency.

CLINICAL - Acne. Alopecia. Diphtheria. Crusta lactea. Eczema. Favus. Hemorrhages. Neck, stiff. Nose, redness. Plica polonica. Seborrhea. Throat, sore. Toothache. Uterus, bleeding.

HOMEOPATHIC - Vinca was proved by Rosenburg on four healthy persons, who took the tincture in 20 to 60 drop doses. It produced a deep impression on the organism and tissues.

Weakness and prostration. "Weakness as if he would die." Inclination to stretch. Trembling and tendency to start, especially on exciting the mind. Trembling in all the blood vessels. Uterine hemorrhages, followed by great debility.

"Toothache better from warmth of bed." Diphtheria. Empty, all gone sensation in the stomach and chest. Distention of abdomen after stool. Stool caused exhaustion. Skin affections, eczema. Plica polonica. Marked affects on the tissues. The left side was most affected.

Abdomen - Abdomen full, tense but painless. Griping. Rumbling and gurgling with passage of much offensive flatus. Distention after a stool.

Back - Painful tension and stiffness of cervical muscles with an illusive sensation as if a weight were lying on them.

Causations - Anger. Mental exertion.

Chest - Pains in chest with sticking and dyspnea. Stitching in sternum. Pressure on sternum with feeling of emptiness in chest.

Ears - Ringing and whistling in ears with feeling of cold wind, especially the 1eft.

Eyes - Itching and burning of lids, which become red. Eye dry, on getting snuff into it there was so little secretion he was obliged to wash it out. Foggy vision while reading, at times also while walking.

Face - Bloated face with pimples. Dry lips. Swelling of upper lip and corner of mouth. Tearing in malar bones.

Female - Menses, profuse, flowing like a stream without interruption with great weakness, at menopause. ***Passive uterine hemorrhages*** (Ust., Trill., Sec.). Menorrhagia, continuous flow, at menopausal (Lach.). Bleeding fibroids.

Food - Hunger alternating with loss of appetite before the hunger has been satisfied. Scarcely any thirst.

Head - Tearing pain in vertex, ringing and whistling in ears. Corrosive itching of scalp. Irresistible desire to scratch. ***Spots on scalp, oozing moisture, matting hair together, plica polonica***. Bald spots covered with short woolly hair. Hair falls out and is replaced by gray hair.

Kidneys - Diminished secretion of urine. Urine pale yellow.

Limbs - Inclination to stretch limbs. Tearing pains in limbs. Arthritic tearing in bones. Swelling and stiffness of first joints of fingers with burning pain in the nails. Cramp-like drawing in feet and toes.

Lungs - Hoarseness. Tenacious mucus in trachea. Spasmodic cough with little tickling in larynx. Rapid respiration.

Modalities - Worse after swallowing, walking, stooping, moving. Worse anger. Worse reading. Worse in open air. Drinking aggravates, liquids (especially beer) causes belchings, coffee causes nausea.

Mouth - Increased secretion of saliva. Insipid taste in mouth to all food. Aphthae. Tearing in teeth better by warmth of bed.

Nose - Becomes red on becoming the least angry. Tip gets red easily. Moist eruption on septum. Seborrhea upper lip and base of nose. Stoppage of one nostril. ***Sores in nose.*** Frequent nose bleeding.

Rectum - Urging to stool. Stool first hard, then soft. Stool exhausting with burning in anus.

Sensations - As if he would die from weakness. As if a hammer were beating from within outwards in vertex. cold wind in ears. As if something sticking low down in esophagus. As if a weight lying on cervical muscles.

Skin - Eczema of head and face. Corrosive itching. ***Great sensitiveness of skin with redness and soreness*** from slight rubbing. Pustules, itching, burning and offensive odor. Hair matted together. Weeping eczema intermingled with foul, thick, crusts. Corrosive itching.

Sleep - Frequent yawning. Sleeplessness and restlessness at night. Lascivious dreams.

Stomach - Emptiness in stomach. Gastric disturbance. Empty belchings after drinking beer and generally worse from taking liquid. Nausea after coffee. Violent, bitter, copious vomiting of yellowish-green liquid.

Throat - Cutting in lower esophagus, which provokes swallowing. ***Diphthe-***

ria. Ulcers. Frequent hawking. Difficult swallowing.

Vertigo - Whirling vertigo with flickering before eyes.

COMMENTS - Vinc. has a wide range in passive uterine hemorrhages. This case is related in Ind. H. R. (ix. 113): uterine hemorrhage, blood dark red, flow copious, uninterrupted with extreme debility. Chin. and Helon. failed to relieved, Vinc. 1x effected a rapid and permanent cure.

Frequent nosebleed. The nose "becomes red from the slightest cause, when the least bit angry." Scabby eruptions about the nose and on the septum, which are part of the general skin effect of the remedy.

Corrosive itching of the skin provoking scratching, moist spots and burning in ulcers. The most characteristic effect is on the scalp, where it produces a condition having many features of crusta lactea, favus and plica polonica.

Clarke cured with Vinc. "sore spots on the scalp" in a young woman. A number of symptoms were produced in the throat and esophagus.

C. M. Boger recorded the case of a women, 31, who had a cutting sensation in lower part of esophagus while swallowing food and continuing after. Empty faintness in stomach better by eating. Stomach sore to touch or pressure of clothing. Constipation from induration of feces. Hemorrhoids constantly sore, smarting after stool. Vinc. 41,000c (Fincke) cured.

RELATIONS - ***Compare:*** (1) Olnd., Staph. (2) peevishness with repentance, Croc. Crusta lactea, Med., Melit., Mez., Jug-r., Olnd. (3) Viol-t. - with strong-smelling urine. (4) Lappa - glands swollen, axillary glands even suppurate. (5) Staph. - sickly children, pale face, dark rings around eyes. (6) Ust. - filthy eruptions, part of hair comes out, part matted. (7) Alopecia, Bac., Phos.

REFERENCES - Boericke. Clarke.

VINE

(Bach Flower Essence)

PHARMACY - vine-b. Vine. Vitis vinifera. Vinum. The flowering clusters, shortly after the stamens have grown out, are put in a sunlit bowl of water and left to the sun's action for several hours. Subsequently, the water is strained and used as medicine. Only the wild vine is used. ***Historical dose:*** Take two drops from the stock bottle into a one ounce dropper bottle (add brandy or alcohol, if this bottle will be used for days or weeks). This is the dosage bottle, take a few drops straight into the mouth or as needed in a little water or juice.

HOMEOPATHIC - Vine-b. belongs to Bach's group of ***Over-Care for Others' Welfare,*** with Rck-w-b., Beech-b., Verv-b. and Chic-b. Vine-b treats the tendency to engage in dominant behavior.

Over-ambitiousness accompanied by envy, frustration and worry, leading to the formation of gastric and duodenal ulcers, or coronary heart disease.

MIND - Assumes control over others. Dominance, preceded by overt attempts to fight back. Disregards peoples' opinions and wishes. Condescending.

Manipulations, schemes and tricks or flattery. Exploitive. Abusive behavior and stubbornness. Passive aggressive personalities. Resistant to change. Very goal-oriented. Tendency to forget one's needs.

Ruthless and violent. Haughty, ego-centered and self-aggrandizing. Anger, impatient and exasperated. Calculating. Reserved. Frustration, a sense of injustice, self-pity, rebelliousness and stubbornness.

REFERENCES - Bach.

VIOLA ODORATA

(Sweet-scented Violet)

PHARMACY - viol-o. Viola odorata. Sweet-scented violet. Violet. N. O. Violaceae, an order most members of which contain emetin, allied to Cinchonaceae. Tincture of fresh plant in flower. ***Historical dose:*** Tincture and all potencies.

CLINICAL - Cancer. Choroiditis. Cough, spasmodic. Deafness. ***Dyspnea. Headaches***. Hoarseness. Hysteria. Neuralgias, supra-orbital. Otorrhea, suppressed. Palpitations. Rheumatism. Seminal emissions. Styes. Whooping cough. ***Worms.*** Wrists, rheumatism.

HOMEOPATHIC - Viol-o. has a specific action on the ear. Affects especially dark-haired patients, supra-orbital and orbital regions, rheumatism in upper parts of the body when on the right side.

Locally, for pain due to uterine fibroids. Marked ***affinity for the wrists***, especially the right. Affects ears, eyes, and skin. Combined eye, ear and kidney symptoms. ***Worm disorders*** in children (Teucr.). For snakebites, bee-stings.

Produces great nervous debility. Nervous activity, then sudden exhaustion. ***Tension***. "Tension of the occiput and forehead," "Tension of the scalp of occiput even when not moving, though worse bending head forward and backward, painful, compelling him to wrinkle forehead, lasting several days." Tension extends to upper half of face and ears.

MIND - Inclined to weep without knowing why. Childish behavior, despondent, refuses eating, talks in low soft voice. Aversion to music, especially the violin.

Abdomen - Distention of abdomen.

Back - Tension in muscles of the neck. Jerking drawing in cervical muscles, near nape, extending down, worse lying on opposite side.

Causations - Suppressed discharges.

Chest - Oppression of chest, as of weight on chest.

Constitutions - Cooper considered it suited to "dark-complexioned people of the Ferr. pic. type." Teste used Viol-o. frequently, described the type as "a lymphatico-nervous temperament, a mild disposition, dry and cool skin." Many patients cured by him were tall and slender. Suited to tall, thin, nervous girls.

Ears - Affections with pain in eyeballs. Otorrhea, recurrent from birth. Deafness. Shooting in ears. Roaring and tickling. Deep stitches beneath ears. Aversion to music.

Eyes - Cramp in eyes. Choroiditis. Pain from eyes (left) to vertex worse cough. Eyeball feels compressed. Lids tend to close without physical sleepiness. Heaviness of lids. Flames before eyes. Myopia. Illusions of vision, fiery, serpentine circles.

Female - Dyspnea during pregnancy.

Food - Craves meat.

Head - Heaviness of head with sensation of weakness in muscles of nape of neck. ***Scalp tense, must knit the brows. Headache across the forehead,*** above the eyebrows. ***Tendency to pain immediately above eyebrows. Burning in the forehead***. Throbbing under eye and temple. Acts upon frontal sinuses. Hysterical attacks in tuberculous patients.

Kidneys - ***Urine milky*** with strong smell. Bedwetting in nervous children.

Limbs - Trembling of limbs. Rheumatism of deltoid muscles and wrists (right) especially in females. Shoulders cold. Pressing pain in bones of fingers. ***Pressing pain in right carpal and metacarpal joints*** (Ulm.).

Lungs - Difficult breathing, anxiety and palpitations. ***Dyspnea during pregnancy.*** Dry, short, spasmodic cough and dyspnea, worse in daytime. Long spells of cough during day time only with dyspnea. Whooping cough with hoarseness.

Modalities - Bone pains, better after rising in morning. Worse from cloudy weather, cold air. Worse music. Worse puberty, suppressed discharges. Worse bending head backward and forward. Cough worse by day. Hoarseness worse in a cold room. Vision worse from dull, wet days.

Nose - Tip numb, as from a blow. Torpor in the end of nose, as from a blow.

Rectum - Itching at anus. ***Worms.***

Sensations - As if everything in head whirled around. As if eyeballs were compressed. As if nose had been beaten and blood were pressing out. As if hard palate were dried up. As if a stone were lying on chest. Burning like a small, transient flame in spots here and there.

Skin - Dry with moist palms.

Sleep - Yawning and stretching without sleepiness.

Vertigo - Vertigo, everything in head seems to whirl around.

COMMENTS - Viol-o. was introduced by Gross and proved by Hahnemann, Gross and Stapf. Gross said of his symptoms that they recurred equally in all positions, were mild, yet more definitely than from other drugs.

Hahnemann had bruised pain in all the bones in the morning in bed after waking, better after rising. Stapf had relaxation of all the muscles.

The mind was greatly excited and disturbed and Viol-o. found its first uses in hysterical cases. Aversion to music, especially the violin is one of the peculiar symptoms.

Increased activity and rush of ideas, generally confused, "Can only grasp half an idea, puts it in its proper place but cannot hold it." Gross experienced the former and Stapf the latter of these.

Gross also noted, "Tension which at times extends to upper half of face, especially of nose, thence to forehead and temples, as far as ears, alternating with a similar sensation in occiput and cervical muscles."

The cure of Lady Margaret Marsha, age 67 of an affection of the throat pronounced to be malignant (apparently epithelia of tonsil) with an infusion of violet leaves is on record. Boiling water was poured on the fresh leaves and allowed to stand twelve hours.

Compresses moistened with this were applied externally to the throat and covered with oil-silk. Relief of pain, dysphagia and suffocative symptoms was immediate. The external swelling disappeared in a week, the growth on the tonsil in a fortnight.

Viol-o. has cured a number of cases of rheumatism, chiefly right-sided. It has a marked affinity for the wrists, especially the right. Ear disorders with pain about the eye orbits indicate Viol-o.

RELATIONS - ***Antidoted by:*** Camph. ***Compatible:*** in whooping cough, Cor-r. in worms, Cina. ***Compare:*** (1) Ulm. - formication in feet, numb, creeping pain in legs and feet, rheumatic pains above wrists, numbness, tingling and full soreness where the gastrocnemius gives off its tendon. (2) Chen-a. (3) Aur., Puls., Sep., Ign., Cina. (4) Caul. - in rheumatism of small joints.

REFERENCES - Boericke. Clarke.

VIOLA TRICOLOR

(Pansy)

PHARMACY - viol-t. Viola tricolor. Pansy. Jacea. Hearts-ease. N. O. Violaceae. Tincture of fresh plant in flower. ***Historical dose:*** Tincture and all potencies.

CLINICAL - Bedwetting. Crusta lactea. Dyspnea. Eczema. Flatulence. Gonorrhea. Gout. ***Impetigo***. Leucorrhea. Ophthalmia. Orchitis. Plica polonica. Rheumatism. Ringworm. Seminal, emissions. Syphilis. Throat, ulceration. Vaginitis.

HERBAL - It had an ancient reputation in asthma and epilepsy and especially in obstinate skin diseases. In Russia a decoction of pansy is a popular remedy for scrofula, swollen glands. Schlegel, of Moscow, used it with good effect in syphilitic affections, especially venereal ulcers.

HOMEOPATHIC - The pansy was proved by Hahnemann and his provers. Skin, scalp and urinary organs are the chief centers of action of Viol-t. The principal uses of this remedy are for eczema in childhood and nocturnal emission accompanied by very vivid dreams. Combined urinary symptoms and skin affection. Nervous paroxysms after suppressed crusta lactea, eczema.

Eczema with urinary disturbances, too copious urination or sudden arrest of secretion. Tinea capitis with frequent involuntary urination. ***Urine smelling like cat's urine***. The male sexual organs were much excited. Emissions with vivid dreams occurred, swelling, itching and pains in prepuce and glans with erections.

Hot face and sweating after eating. Dyspnea after eating. Hands twitch and are clenched in sleep. Nervous paroxysms followed suppressed milk-crust. The axillae and clavicular regions were noticeably affected and stitches and burning stitches were prevailing pains. Lying causes anxiety about heart.

Abdomen - Stitches and cutting pain in abdomen with urging to stool, followed by discharge of lumps of mucus and flatulence. Pressing, stinging in the diaphragm.

Back - Swelling of glands of neck. Spasmodic pain and contraction with pinching between shoulder blades (with cutting, tingling and crawling in the skin).

Causations - Suppressed milk-crust (nervous paroxysms).

Chest - Syphilitic ulcers on clavicles. Shooting in chest. Stitches in the chest, on the ribs, sternum and intercostal muscles.

Eyes - Pain in eyes, as if a hard body were between upper eyelid and eyeball. Smarting and incisive and itching shootings in eye. Contraction and closing of eyelids. Myopia.

Face - Hot and sweating after eating. Thickness and hardness of skin of face. Scabs on face with burning itching,

Female - Stitch in region of mons veneris, right side. Painful pustules on labia. Leucorrhea with stitching pain in children in syphilis. Chancroid ulcers about breasts.

Head - Cracked, gummy crusts on scalp, exuding profuse tenacious yellow fluid, matting the hair together with swelling of cervical glands. Eczema of scalp with swollen glands. Milk crusts. Heavy, pressing-outward pain.

Kidneys - Copious, disagreeable odor. ***Urine offensive, smelling like cat's urine***. Bedwetting.

Limbs - Joint rheumatism. Itching like eruptions around the joints.

Lungs - Stitches in left side of chest, worse during inspiration and expiration.

Male - Seminal emissions with vivid dreams. Involuntary, seminal emissions at stool. Swelling of prepuce, burning in glans. Itching.

Modalities - Open air helps headache, but causes chilliness. Aversion to open air. Worse in winter, when walking in cold air. Worse 11 a.m. Worse by pressure on side opposite to painful side, lying on non-painful side. Walking causes vertigo, stitches through chest and abdomen. Sitting causes stitches in abdomen and groin, standing relieves.

Mouth - Accumulation of saliva in the mouth with sensation of dryness. Tongue loaded with whitish mucus of a bitter taste.

Rectum - Chopped soft stools. Stool with mucus and much flatus.

Skin - Eczema of childhood. Large boils all over the body in scrofulous children. ***Impetigo***. Intolerable itching. Eruptions, particularly over face and head with burning, itching, worse at night. Thick scabs, which crack and exude a tenacious yellow pus. Sycosis.

Sleep - Inclination to sleep in afternoon. Disturbed sleep with frequent waking. Awakens frequently without cause. Sleep retarded by a concourse of ideas with difficulty in waking in morning. Vivid and amorous dreams.

Temperature - Chill or chilliness in forenoon and in open air. Dry, anxious heat at night in bed with red face. General heat, especially in face with anxiety, dyspnea immediately after eating. Night-sweats.

Throat - Sore throat in evening. Swallowing difficult and very painful. Syphilis. Swelling of cervical glands. Much phlegm, causing hawking, worse in the air. Chancroid ulcers.

Vertigo - Vertigo and dizziness when walking. Head bewildered and perplexed.

COMMENTS - Teste put Viol-t. in two groups, whose types are Lyc. and Cham. Homeopathy has brought out some characteristics of Viol-t. which single out its cases.

Teste quoted from old observers the following as cured by Viol-t.: Milk-crust in children at the breast, or recently weaned. Milk-crust with violent cough and excessive oppression.

Impetigo of hairy scalp and face in children and adult females. Favus and serpiginous crusts in children and adults with swelling and induration of cervical glands. Large boils all over body in a scrofulous child. Pustules and ichorous exanthema of feet. Squamous spots on skin.

Rheumatism and gout, joint rheumatism with itch-like eruption around the joints. Impetigo-like exanthema on forehead. Ichorous ulcers with violent itching.

RELATIONS - ***Antidoted by:*** Camph., Merc., Puls., Rhus-t. ***Compare:*** (1) Tension of tissues of face and forehead, Viol-o. (2) Crusta lactea, Vinc. (Viol-t. has urinary concomitants). (3) Eruptions, ulcers, Cham., Graph., Hep., Merc., Olnd., Petr., Staph. (4) Stitches, Kali-c. (5) Viol-o. (6) Lyc. Rhus-t., Calc., Sep. ***Compatible:*** Puls., Rhus-t., Sep., Staph.

REFERENCES - Boericke. Clarke.

VIPERA ASPIS

(Aspis adder)

PHARMACY - vip-a. Vipera aspis. Aspis adder. N. O. Viperidae. ***Historical dose:*** All potencies.

HOMEOPATHIC - Proved in 1970 by Boffa and Dupin on 14 subjects, 7 men, and 7 women. The heart, blood and blood vessels were chiefly affected. Sleepiness during daytime. Chilly. ***Worse left side.***

Nerves. Throbbing pains. Throbbing headache. Heavy sensation in eyes. Dazzling when raising eyes. Dryness of mouth, with pasty tongue, on waking in morning. Dry mouth before menses. Menses with small, very dark clots or with big red clots.

MIND - Pessimism. Nervousness. Irritability. Disposition to contradict. Impatience. Anxiety. Dreams of death.

Food - Intense thirst for cold drinks.

Heart - Palpitations of heart at night, worse lying on left side.

Limbs - Spontaneous ecchymoses on arms. Painful heaviness in legs, worse walking, better raising legs. Veins of thighs distended. Marbled, mottled appearance of thighs.

Modalities - Better during menses. Better gentle motion. Worse warm, damp weather, warm room, heat. ***Worse left side,*** pressure. Worse evening. Worse before menses.

RELATIONS - ***Compare:*** Vip., Lach., Naja., Aran-ix., Buth-aust.

REFERENCES - Julian.

VIPERA BERUS

(German Viper)

PHARMACY - vip. Vipera berus. German viper. Vipera torva. Pelias berus. Adder. Vipera communis. Common Viper. European Viper with other varieties, especially the Red Italian Viper. N. O. Ophidia, family, Viperidae. Dilutions of the venom. ***Historical dose:*** All potencies.

CLINICAL - Bites. Goiter. Hemorrhages. Jaundice. Liver, enlargement. Menopause. Multiple neuritis. Nosebleeds. Paralysis. Paraplegia. Phlebitis. Poliomyelitis. Senility, premature. Tongue, swelling. Varicose veins.

HOMEOPATHIC - The effects of bites by the common viper and related species have been collected and have furnished the data for homeopathic prescribing. The venom of common German Vipera torva affects the blood and blood vessels, leading to hemorrhage and inflammation of the vessels.

Allen related the case of a gold beater who found the veins of his right arm become exceedingly swollen and painful, so that he could no longer work or let his hand hang down. Vip. cured immediately.

A case quoted from Med. Adv. of varicose veins of the popliteal space with the sensation as though the leg would burst and a nervous, fidgety condition of the feet which kept them in constant motion, was cured with Vip. 30c. The bursting feeling appears to be at the root of this characteristic.

A keynote for Vip. in cases of phlebitis and varicose veins is "Worse on letting the limb affected hang down," as if it would burst with fullness. The region of the vessel affected is inflamed and sensitive.

Swan said Vip. was a remedy for all forms of nosebleed.

Vip. affects ***veins,*** causing inflammation and a ***hemorrhagic tendency.*** Inflammation of veins with great swelling. Cardiac dropsy. ***Bursting sensation. enlargement of liver.*** Special action on kidneys and induces hematuria. Edema of glottis. Goiter. Ailments of menopause.

Paralysis, ascending, paraplegia of foot. Multiple neuritis. Poliomyelitis. Temporary increase in reflexes, paresis supervenes, a paraplegia of the lower limbs extending upwards. Resembles acute ascending paralysis of Landry. Vip. has a chronic and periodic action, the symptoms return annually for years.

Abdomen - Excruciating pain in the epigastrium, worse pressure. Violent pain in enlarged liver extends to shoulder and hip, jaundice with fever.

Back - Sticking in kidneys. Pain in loins.

Chest - Oppression with anxiety with violent efforts to breathe and swallow. Veins of chest and abdomen thick and hard. Swelling of chest as far as umbilicus after bite on face.

Eyes - Eyes are dark yellow, red, inflamed and watery, staring, sunken. Pupils are dilated or left dilated, right contracted. Paralysis of lids, dropped over eyes. Vision is dim, dim in left eye, lost in right.

Face - Excessively swollen. Lips and the tongue swollen, livid, protruding. Tongue dry, brown, black. Speech difficult.

Food - Appetite lost. Thirst with moist tongue, for cold drinks.

Female - Menopausal hemorrhage, flow red with dark clots, not profuse but continuous with prostration and faintness from nursing the child.

Kidneys - Strangury. Involuntary urination. Urine is increased, suppressed, dark yellow, as in jaundice. Hematuria. Ineffectual desire.

Limbs - Patient is obliged to keep the limbs elevated. ***When limbs are allowed to hang down, it seems as if they would burst and the pain is unbearable***. Shuffling gait caused by paralysis of foot. ***Varicose veins*** and acute phlebitis. Veins swollen, sensitive, bursting pain. Blue lower limbs. Severe cramps in lower limbs.

Liver - Violent pain in enlarged liver with jaundice and fever, extends to shoulder and hip.

Modalities - ***Worse from letting limbs hang down.*** Worse by pressure. Worse change of weather, from cold touch. Worse yearly.

Mouth - Scorbutic line on gums. Tongue swollen, brownish-black, protruding. Lips, blue, swollen. Speech difficult.

Nose - Nosebleed with vertigo, while nursing the child.

Skin - Livid. Boils, carbuncles with ***bursting*** sensation, relieved by elevating parts. Ulcers. Gangrene. Skin peels in large plates. Lymphangioma.

Stomach - Digestion slow. Pain in epigastrium, worse pressure. Nausea with shuddering with attack of faintness. Retching with suffocative sensation. Vomiting after milk of all food and drink.

Sleep - Disposed to yawn. Sleepiness and heaviness with inability to sleep and also almost constant necessity to change the position. Sleeplessness from pain. Restless at night.

Temperature - Temperature is diminished, resists cold badly. Chilliness with cold sweat, with rigidity and clammy sweat, then fever. Fever of irregular type intermittent fever. Sweat after vomiting.

Throat - Swelling like goiter. Edema of glottis. Closure of throat so that she could swallow only water and milk.

COMMENTS - Vip. patients resist the cold badly. The parts may be paralyzed and ulcers and gangrene follow. Worse from letting limb or part hang down. Sensation as if something ran up the thigh occurred in the bitten limb in one case. In one case there was sweat over the whole body except the bitten limb.

Leonard gave Vip. to a woman suffering from menopausal hemorrhage, flow red with dark clots, excessive to prostration and faintness. She had a small uterine fibroid. A few doses relieved and the excessive hemorrhage did not return.

He also noted the case of a woman nursing a child a year old who was much prostrated by hemorrhage lasting several weeks, not profuse, but continuous: Nosebleed nearly every day, weaning brought no relief. Chin. 200c did no good. Vip. 100,000c cured in three doses.

RELATIONS - ***Compare:*** (1) Hemorrhage of fluid blood, Sanguis. (2) Worse hanging down limbs, Calc., Alumn., Am-c., Sabin., Thuj. (3) Pelius berus, Adder. - Prostration and fainting, faltering pulse, skin yellow, pain about navel. Swelling of arm, tongue, right eye with giddiness, nervousness, faintness, and sickness. Compression of chest, could not breathe properly or take a deep breath, aching and stiffness of limbs, joints stiff, collapsed feeling, great thirst. (4) Ser-ang. - heart and kidney diseases. Failure of compensation and impending asystole.

REFERENCES - Boericke. Clarke.

VISCUM ALBUM

(Mistletoe)

PHARMACY - visc. Viscum album. Mistletoe. N. O. Loranthaceae. Viscaceae. Tincture of ripe berries. Tincture of bruised leaves. Tincture of whole plant. ***Historical dose:*** Tincture and all potencies.

CLINICAL - Ankylosing spondylitis. Arteriosclerosis. ***Asthma***. Aura epileptica. ***Cancer. Chorea.*** Deafness. Dupuytren's disease. Dysphagia. Endometritis. ***Epilepsy.*** Hypertension. Labor pains, slow. Lumbago. Menorrhagia. Metrorrhagia. Migraine. Neuritis. Orchitis. Osteoporosis. Otorrhea. Ovaritis. Raynaud's syndrome. Retained placenta. Sciatica. Spasmodic paralysis. Spleen pain. Throat, sore. Whooping cough.

HERBAL - Viscum Album's active principle is viscotoxin, a mixture of acetylcholine and choline. Viscum is a chlorophyllous plant, which grown on various trees (apple, poplar) and forms large bunches. It is gathered in August and September, before the fruit ripens. The leaves are then blanched and dried quickly in hot air and stabilized.

In the middle ages, it was used as an anti-epileptic. Hypo-tensor and diuretic. Anti-tumors, by external use, as for papilloma, due to the necrotizing properties of the viscotoxin.

Viscine is most abundant in the mistletoe of the apple-tree, Visco-resin in that of the oak and acacia, excites the sexual appetite. The mistletoe of the hawthorn possesses like all the rest, but in a higher degree, the contractile properties of Sec. on the uterus in uterine inertia. That of the oak has a remarkable anti-epileptic power on horses.

According to Laville, all mistletoes are useful in epilepsy and rabies. A breeder had a very fine stock which became epileptic at four or five years old. He cured them with a tincture of the fresh leaves bruised in a mortar.

HOMEOPATHIC - The first homeopathic symptomatology was established by Proll, Stager, Schier and Black during the second half of the 19th century, using the mother tincture and low potencies. Proell made a proving of the tincture and the symptoms developed resembling an epileptic aura and petit mal, which had the additional epileptic feature of recurrence they recurred frequently for two years.

Visc. affects the nerves and female sexual organs. Lowered blood pressure. Dilated blood vessels but does not act on the centers in the medulla. Pulse is slow due to central irritation of the vagus. The symptoms point to rheumatic and gouty complaints, neuralgia, especially sciatica.

Epilepsy, feels a glow that rises up from feet to head. ***Chorea*** and metrorrhagia. Chorea from fright. Symptoms like epileptic aura and petit mal. General tremor as if all muscles are in fibrillary contraction. Neuralgia. Paresthesia.

Rheumatism, ***tearing pains.*** Rheumatoid condition ameliorated in fresh air and by the movement. Gouty. Sciatica with otorrhea. Spinal pains from uterine causes.

Feeling of lightness as if floating on air. The brain is swaying around the inside the skull. Congestion in the head with headaches and vertigo. Blood would not clot and wounds would not heal. Bleeding of bright red blood from the uterus. Valvular disease with disturbances in sexual sphere.

Rheumatic deafness. ***Asthma***. Hypertensive albuminuria. Nausea at the sight of the bottle containing the medicine to be taken. Pruritus. Burning cold under the right shoulder.

MIND - Apathy, sadness. Lack of optimism liveliness. Irritable, sad, morose. Restless, nervous, thoughtless, shakes with impatience. Unable to carry out intellectual activities. Thoughts keep turning to past events, for hours on end. Obsessive persistence of thoughts.

Sensation of strength, optimism, gaiety, desire to undertake anything, full of ideas for the future. Hallucinatory psychosis.

Extremely sensitive to noise. Fear of telephones.

Abdomen - Feels as if someone were dragging her down from the waist. Sore about waist. Violent rumbling and painful distention of the supra-umbilical region, ameliorated by expelling wind and leaning backwards. Colitis. Chronic pancreatitis.

Back - Lumbago from a chill, wants someone to press against the back. Stiffness and muscular pains in the nape of the neck, thoracic cage and back. Torticollis. Sensation of a ***burning coal*** under the right shoulder.

Causations - Chill, wetting. Fright. Suppression of menses.

Chest - Angina pectoris. Nervous dyspnea with feeling of constriction in the chest.

Ears - Deafness from cold. Buzzing and stopped-up feeling in ear. Hypersensitive to noise. Whistling, buzzing. Hears heartbeat. Sclerosis of the ears.

Eyes - Blue rings around eyes. Ocular neuralgia. Conjunctivitis. Mydriasis, ocular neuralgia, conjunctival irritation. Double vision. Bad focusing, eyes weep through fatigue.

Face - Facial muscles in constant agitation. Countenance suffused. Lips livid. Face hot and flushed.

Female - Menses too early, copious with bright red blood and very painful. Menorrhagia. Chronic endometritis. Metrorrhagia. Atonic, post-partum hemorrhage. Hemorrhage with pain. Blood partly clots and bright red. Menopausal complaints (Lach., Sulph.). Pain from sacrum into pelvis with tearing, shooting pains from above downwards. Ovarian pain, especially left. Retained placenta (Sec.).

Food - Felt starving at supper-time. Appetite ravenous.

Head - Feeling as if whole vault of skull were lifted up. Sudden throbbing in vertex. Headache, especially at the forehead, temples and parietal bone, can spread to the whole heat. Dull, heavy aching, numbing and congestive, beating or hammering.

Heart - Hypertrophy with valvular insufficiency, pulse small and weak, unable to rest in a reclining positions. Low blood pressure. Failing compensation, dyspnea worse lying on left side. Weight and oppression of heart, as if a hand were squeezing it, ticking sensation about heart. Inflammation of the coronary arteries. Feeling of tightness of heaviness. As if the heart is being squeezed by a hand. Heartbeat irregular. Agitation and fibrillation. Pulse accelerated or slow with fear of death. Palpitations in the chest, throat and upper part of the abdomen. Palpitations during sex.

Kidneys - Urinary tenesmus and copious urine. Bladder paralyzed. Involuntary passing of urine as a result of an irritating cough. Urine is turbid and evil-smelling. Urine milky after standing. Bedwetting.

Limbs - Chorea-like movements of the arms and legs. A ***glow*** rises from the feet to the head, seems to be on fire. General tremor, as if all muscles were in state of fibrillary contraction. Dropsy of limbs. ***Sciatica.*** Drawing, tearing pains in the arm. Pains alternate in the knee and ankle with shoulder and elbow. Periodic pains from sacrum into pelvis, ***worse in bed*** with pains into thighs and upper limbs. ***Tearing***, shooting pains in both thighs and upper limbs. Cannot keep legs still. Sensation of a spider crawling over back of hand and foot. Itching all over. Compressing pain in feet. Raynaud's syndrome. Walking, bending is painful. Burning sensation in the feet.

Lungs - Dyspnea, ***feeling of suffocating when lying on left side***. Stertorous breathing. Asthma, if connected with gout or rheumatism. Bronchial asthma, connected with gout or rheumatism. Glottal spasms and rattles in the bronchi. Painful, frequent cough, scanty, gray or yellow sputum. Spasmodic cough.

Male - Libido increased or diminished. Disturbed libido. Violent, painful erection. Atonic discharge of seminal fluid. Cramping pain in the prostate. Prostatitis.

Modalities - Better by counter-pressure, resting quietly, walking in the fresh air. Worse by slightest movement. Worse winter, cold, stormy weather, becoming chilled while hot, heat. Worse in bed, lying on left side. Worse suppression of menses. Worse mental effort. Worse tobacco.

Mouth - Lips cracked. Dryness of the mouth. Mouth suddenly fills with saliva. Unpleasant taste on waking tongue coated to tip with ochre-yellow fur. Tongue sore. Buccal mucus membrane is as if tanned. Teeth chattered.

Nose - Catarrh in the nose and pharynx. Catarrhal congestion of the mucus membranes with discharge of a watery or purulent liquid. Purulent rhinitis. Polyps. Nosebleed.

Rectum - Feeling of constriction of the anus with empty urging. Feeling of not having emptied the intestine completely after stool. Stools soft, watery or thick, frothy, stinking, explosive, bulky with nightly urging, forcing him to get out of bed. Stools hard and dry. Pruritus and burning of the anus with splinter-line pain. Bleeding hemorrhoids.

Skin - General itching and tingling with no apparent cause, ameliorated in the evening and by perspiration. Formication along the arms. Pruritus, senile and vulvae.

Sleep - Falls asleep late, wakes early. Sleeps, despite exhaustion and after drinking coffee. Troubled dreams of war, bombardment.

Stomach - Gastritis. Heavy sensation, feeling of a stone in the stomach. Squeamish before breakfast and dinner. Heartburn, cutting pain in the stomach, ameliorated by eating and belching. Nausea ameliorated by vomiting.

Temperature - General shivering followed by sudden hot flush towards the head and feeling of anguish.

Throat - Throat dry, burning with sticky discharge. Sensation of constriction around the neck. The feeling of a lump in the throat disappeared in one female prover.

Vertigo - Vertigo, persistent after epileptic attack. Sensation of lightness, as if floating on air. Severe attacks of vertigo totters and has to hold on to the furniture. Vertigo occurs on rising from movement, by moving the head quickly, tends to fall backwards. Vertigo never occurs when lying down. Vertigo when looking out of a window.

COMMENTS - Two women took Visc. to procure abortion. Every muscle save those of the eyes became paralyzed, as did also the intestinal tract. They could not swallow and died of starvation in consequence, the bowels being obstinately constipated. The muscles of speech were also paralyzed.

A boy, 14, ate some berries, soon after began to feel giddy and then became insensible. He was found with suffused countenance, lips livid, conjunctiva injected, pupils slightly dilated and fixed, pulse slow and full, bounding, breathing slow, stertorous.

On pricking the soles the feet were quickly drawn up. Then, cold applications aroused him, when he began to talk incoherently, had spectral illusions and was inclined to be violent.

In a pamphlet on "Viscum Album" Dr. George Black of Torquay put together most of the facts relating to this plant including four new provings, by himself and three female provers.

Black removed with Visc. 3c lumbago from chill, tearing pain, wants something to press against it. Lumbago, right, extending to right buttock, worse by slightest movement. Pain in sacral region, unable to turn either side, worse slightest movement, "pain of a terrible clutching nature, as if her vitals were affected."

Cooper gave great relief with Visc. in "old spinal irritation pains." He also named "spinal symptoms due to uterine causes" as indicating it. Rheumatism, "the weight of my body on the joint causes it to be very sore," excessive perspiration.

Sciatica associated with otorrhea. Burning pain from center of left buttock to inner ankle, heel as if red-hot coal applied, leg feels heavy as lead. In addition a number of cases of catarrhal deafness with noises in the ears were cured or greatly improved.

Belcher gave to a girl, 17, suffering from chorea, 5 drop doses of a tincture of leaves and berries. On the second day he was called to see her and found her suffering as if under the influence of an opiate.

Black also quoted William Huber's experiences with Visc., the first case was of retained placenta with constitutional symptoms after miscarriage at sixth month. Expulsion rapidly effected by Visc. 3c.

A man, 22, robust, fair took a chill from traveling in ice-cold wind. Got a drawing, tearing pain in left lower jaw, lasting some hours. Succeeded by loud buzzing and stopped-up feeling, ending in complete deafness of that ear. Visc. 3c cured.

Metrorrhagia following suppression from working in water. Sciatica left side, cured with Visc. 3c. Rheumatism from wading ill-shod through great tracts of snow, cured with Visc. 3c. Hydrothorax (right) from chill with shooting in spleen, cured with Visc. 4c and 3c.

John Wilde made a tincture of the bruised leaves and gave 5 drop doses to a boy, 14, who had chorea affecting face and limbs. There was improvement in two days and in a few weeks a complete cure.

A boy, nine, strumous with tendency to skin disease, was affected with chorea after a fright. He was completely changed in expression, speech quite inarticulate, look idiotic.

The movements continued at night and the boy was worn out for want of sleep. Visc., 1 to 2 drop doses, did no good. The dose was then increased to 15 drops. Improvement set in at once and a perfect cure was effected, the doses being diminished after a time because soreness of the tongue and redness of the conjunctiva were set up.

C. M. Boger related a case in which persistent vertigo after epileptic seizures, lasting a month at a time, was cured with Visc. 100,000c.

Huber used the 3x and 6x. He considered it applicable to all kinds of rheumatism, acute and chronic, especially when characterized by tearing pains in cases occurring in winter, the result of exposure to sharp winds and in cases of rheumatic deafness.

RELATIONS - ***Antidoted by:*** Camph., Chin. ***Compare:*** (1) Sec., Conv., Bry., Puls., Rhod. (2) Guipsine - active principle - exalts the hypotensive properties of Viscum. (3) Hed. - Intercranial pressure. (4) Bry. - Vertigo in the morning on rising, prickling pains, aggravated by movement, great thirst, dry constipation, menses copious with brown blood. (5) Bell. - Neuro-vascular congestion, fear of imaginary things, hypersensitivity and hyper-exicitability of the senses, pulse strong, irregular, menses too early with bright red, hot blood. (6) Aran-ix. ***Follows well:*** Acon. (rheumatism).

REFERENCES - Boericke. Clarke. Julian.

VITEX TRIFOLIA

(Indian Arnica)

PHARMACY - vit. Vitex trifolia. Indian arnica. Verbenaceae. ***Historical dose:*** Tincture and all potencies.

CLINICAL - Headaches. Injuries. Sprains.

HOMEOPATHIC - Vit. is a remedy used for many traumatic conditions such as injuries and sprains, etc. Pains in joints, abdomen, testicles. Headache in temples,

REFERENCES - Boericke.

VOESLAU AQUA

(Voeslau Mineral Springs)

PHARMACY - voes. Voeslau aqua. Mineral Spring at Voeslau in Austria, contains calcarea, calcarea sulphurica, calcarea muriatica, magnesia carbonica, magnesia sulphurica, magnesia muriatica, natrum sulphuricum, natrum muriaticum, alumina, silica, ferrum citricum. Dilutions. ***Historical dose:*** Tincture and all potencies.

CLINICAL - Menstruation, disorders. Seminal, emissions. Urticaria. Vertigo.

HOMEOPATHIC - Voes. is the mineral spring at Voeslau in Austria. Rosenberg observed the effects of Voeslau aqua on the healthy.

The waters produced orgasm of blood, pressure and tension. The throat was sensitive to swallowing warm food and drink. Nettle rash with desquamation. In males there was sexual excitement and emissions, and in females increased secretion of mucus in genitals and many troubles connected with menses.

REFERENCES - Clarke.

W

WALNUT

(Bach Flower Essence)

PHARMACY - waln-b. Walnut. Juglans regia. Female flowers are collected and boiled for half an hour. The female flower resembles a green bud with two fuzzy stigmas growing out of the top. After boiling, the water is strained and used as medicine. ***Historical dose:*** Take two drops from the stock bottle into a one ounce dropper bottle (add brandy or alcohol, if this bottle will be used for days or weeks). This is the dosage bottle, take a few drops straight into the mouth or as needed in a little water or juice.

HOMEOPATHIC - Waln-b. belongs to Bach's group of ***Over sensitivity to Influences and Ideas*** with Agri-b., Cent-b. and Holly-b. Waln-b. gives protection from heightened impressionability and sensitivity. Lack of physical stability. Heightened impressionability, may create over-ambitiousness, envy and frustration. Gastric and duodenal ulcers (Vine-b.). Allergies.

MIND - Overly influenced by impressions. Emotional disturbances from impressions. Heightened sensitivity. Exaggerated attraction to sexual matters, even though it may just be mental preoccupation. Delusions when one feels obsessed or influenced by forces beyond one's control (Asp-b.).

REFERENCES - Bach.

WASABIA JAPONICA

(Wasabi)

PHARMACY - wasa. Wasabia japonica. Wasabi. Japanese horseradish. Wasabi pungens. Cochlearia wasabi. The whole plant is used, leaves, stems and rhizomes. N. O. Brassicaceae. ***Historical dose:*** Tincture and all potencies.

CLINICAL - Blood, clots. Cancer. Cerebral, thrombosis. ***Colds.*** Coughs. Diarrhea. Food, poisoning. ***Sinusitis.***

HERBAL - The wasabi plant is native to Japan, and is traditionally found growing in or by cold mountain streams. The earliest cultivation of wasabi in Japan dates back to the 10th century.

The grated rhizome, or above-ground root-like stem, has a fiery hot flavor that quickly dissipates in the mouth, leaving a lingering sweet taste, with no burning sensation. The roots have a strong penetrating odor, which can clear the head and bring tears to the eyes, when inhaled or ingested.

Wasabi is valuable medicinally for its antibacterial properties, and anti-inflammatory action. It has been used for coughs, colds, sinusitis and diarrhea. It is a powerful digestive stimulant, and removes toxins from the body.

As a member of the cruciferous family, wasabi contains the same cancer-fighting isothiocynates as its cabbage relations. Researchers believe that the substances in cruciferous vegetables help prevent cancer by helping the body eliminate excess hormones such as estrogen, thus reducing the risk of hormone-related cancers such as breast and prostate cancer.

Scientists have recently found that a component of the plant inhibits the formation of blood clots and cerebral thrombosis. The plant has exhibited strong antioxidant properties. Research also found that wasabi contains substances that suppress the growth of stomach cancer cells. It has also been used as an antidote to fish poisoning.

RELATIONS - ***Compare:*** Ars.

REFERENCES - Murphy.

WATER VIOLET

(Bach Flower Essence)

PHARMACY - wat-v-b. Water violet. Hottonia palustris. Several flowers are picked by the stalk and left floating in a bowl of sunlit water for several hours. The water is then strained and prepared as medicine. ***Historical dose:*** Take two drops from the stock bottle into a one ounce dropper bottle (add brandy or alcohol, if this bottle will be used for days or weeks). This is the dosage bottle, take a few drops straight into the mouth or as needed in a little water or juice.

HOMEOPATHIC - Wat-v-b. belongs to Bach's group of ***Loneliness,*** with Imp-b and Heath-b. Wat-v-b. treats states of aloofness and haughtiness. Lack of spontaneity and lively involvement. Internal retreating or raising above others may be reflected in a posture of haughtiness and aloofness. Physical stiffness and rigidity.

MIND - Haughty. Feels special, eccentric. Grandiose delusions, narcissistic personality disorder. Reserved dignity. Desire for attention and admiration. Alienates others.

Active engagement with others is avoided or even considered disturbing to inner peace. Disinterest, lack of spontaneity, or even apathy. Tendency to retreat and isolate oneself. Vulnerable and lonely. Insecure. Ailments after severe offense or humiliation.

REFERENCES - Bach.

WHITE CHESTNUT

(Bach Flower Essence)

PHARMACY - wh-ch-b. White chestnut. Aesculus hippocastanum. Individual flowers are picked and placed in a bowl of water which is left to the sun's action for several hours. The water is strained and used as medicine. ***Historical dose:*** Take two drops from the stock bottle into a one ounce dropper bottle (add brandy or alcohol, if this bottle will be used for days or weeks). This is the dosage bottle, take a few drops straight into the mouth or as needed in a little water or juice.

HOMEOPATHIC - Wh-ch-b. belongs to Bach's group of ***Lack of Interest in Present Circumstances,*** with Clem-b., Honey-b., Wld-r-b., Oliv-b., Must-b. and Ch-bd-b.

States of preoccupation and intense worry. Mental preoccupation's and worries. Obsessive-compulsive dwelling on an emotional experience. Insomnia from worry, mental preoccupation. Restlessness from worry. Eyesight failure. Irritable colon, gastrointestinal symptoms. Hyper motility, pylorospasm and ulcers.

MIND - Preoccupied with worrisome, returning thoughts. Anxiety, despair. Obsessions, fixations and persistent thought patterns. Delusions and chronic introspection. Automatic responses and compulsive thinking (Cher-p-b., Crb-a-b., Pine-b.). Worried in a state of regret or self-reproach. Disappointment and annoyance. Frustration and exhaustion. Diverted attention.

REFERENCES - Bach.

WIESBADEN AQUA

PHARMACY - wies. Wiesbaden aqua. The Spring at Wiesbaden in Prussia. Contains in 16 ounces are Carbonic acid 6.416 cubic inches, Nitrogen 0.103 cubic inches of the following solids in grains, Nat-m. 52.49, Kali-m. 1.119 Lith-m. 0.00138, Am-m. 0.128, Calc-m. 3.617, Mag-m. 1.566, Mag-br. 0.027, Calc-s. 0.692, Calc-p. 0.0029, Calc-ar. 0.0015, Calc. 3.210, Mag-c. 0.079, Ferr-c. 0.043, Mang-coll. 0.004, Silicic acid 0.46, Alum-sil. 0.603, traces of Mag-i., Stront-c., Cupr-c. Dilutions. ***Historical dose:*** Tincture and all potencies.

CLINICAL - Amenorrhea. Angina pectoris. Body, odor of offensive. Constipation. Corns. Diarrhea. Earwax, excessive. Glaucoma. Gout. Hair, rapid growth, loss, grows darker. Hemorrhage. Hemorrhoids. Hernia inguinal, femoral. Indigestion. Miscarriages. Nosebleed. Rheumatism. Infertility. Vertigo. Whitlow.

HOMEOPATHIC - The hot, chlorinated saline springs of Wiesbaden contain 8.176 grams of solids to each liter, and of these Nat-m. makes up more than seven grams. The baths, which constitute the chief part of the treatment, are extremely stimulating.

The baths, combined with drinking the water, generally determine at the begining of the cure certain phenomena of saturation which disappear on temporary suspension of the treatment. The most common of these is a saburral state of the stomach and a feeling of fullness and tension in the whole abdomen.

Passive or atonic gout, these cases usually pass through a period of aggravation before improvement sets in. Torpid and rheumatisms, the douche being employed as well as the bath. Paralysis, muscular and tendinous contractions. Sprains in complete anchyloses. Stiffness from old fractures. Gunshot wounds which are slow to heal.

Modalities - Better by nosebleed, by hemorrhoid flux. Worse during menses. Frequent urination worse from coffee. Vertigo worse lying in bed.

COMMENTS - Constantin James noted, "Abdominal plethora and portal obstruction are relieved." By the artificial congestion which they set up in the venous plexus of the rectum they have for a constant effect the disengorgement of the viscera under the diaphragm and the prevention of stasis in their parenchyma.

Pelt observed the effects of drinking the water and excessive bathing.

Magdeburg observed the effects on eight very healthy persons. The stimulating, congestive and evacuant effects mentioned by James appeared in the provings. Blood rushes to the face. Vertigo when lying in bed and vertigo which causes falling. Hemorrhages occur from anus and nose which relieve other symptoms.

Fermentation occurs in the abdomen and there is great exhaustion after diarrhea. Hemorrhoid flow occurs with better of abdominal plethora. In one case nosebleed occurred persistently for six weeks, at the end of which a weakness of vision bordering on blindness was cured. During the menses there is great weakness, also constipation.

A number of remarkable symptoms appeared in reference to the skin and nails. The hair grew rapidly and became darker. Nails also grew rapidly. Corns and callosities dropped off.

Berridge cured with Wies. 200c a Miss B., 21 of a soft corn between the fourth and fifth toes of right foot. There was burning and shooting pain. Itching with the sweat. The sweat on the diseased parts made a brown stain. The urine stiffened linen.

RELATIONS - ***Compare:*** (1) Nat-m. Corns, Ferr-pic. (2) Callosities, Ant-c. (3) Hair turns darker, Jab., Piloc., Wild.

REFERENCES - Clarke.

WILD OAT

(Bach Flower Essence)

PHARMACY - wld-o-b. Wild oat. Bromus ramosus. The flowering ends are picked and placed in a bowl of water which is left standing in bright sunlight for several hours. The water is strained and used as medicine. ***Historical dose:*** Take two drops from the stock bottle into a one ounce dropper bottle (add brandy or alcohol, if this bottle will be used for days or weeks). This is the dosage bottle, take a few drops straight into the mouth or as needed in a little water or juice.

HOMEOPATHIC - Wld-o-b. belongs to Bach's group of ***Uncertainty,*** with Cer-b., Scler-b., Gent-b., Gors-b. and Horn-b. Wld-o-b. deals with lack of motivation and incentive. A depressive mood may permeate the mind and body. Lethargy, a lack of appetite and mental dullness.

Organic mental disorders and mental retardation after head injuries (Horn-b., Must-b., Scler-b.). Obesity. Peptic ulcer. Non-insulin dependent diabetes. Drug abuse.

MIND - Aimless, dissatisfied. Unmotivated. Absent-minded. Lack of motivation and incentive. Lack of concentration. Boredom, lethargy and dissatisfaction.

COMMENTS - Emotions of frustration, joylessness, aversion, dissatisfaction, meaninglessness, boredom and futility. Feelings of being not fully awakened or activated in one's potential. In some forms of mental illness with organic dysfunction and retardation, this remedy will give incentive within the physical limitations of the disease (Horn-b., Must-b.).

RELATIONS - Cer-b., Scler-b., Gent-b., Gors-b. and Horn-b.

REFERENCES - Bach.

WILD ROSE

(Bach Flower Essence)

PHARMACY - wld-r-b. Wild rose. Rosa canina. Sprigs with leaves and flower heads are boiled for half an hour. Subsequently, the water is strained and prepared as medicine. ***Historical dose:*** Take two drops from the stock bottle into a one ounce dropper bottle (add brandy or alcohol, if this bottle will be used for days or weeks). This is the dosage bottle, take a few drops straight into the mouth or as needed in a little water or juice.

HOMEOPATHIC - Wld-r-b. is part of Bach's group of ***Lack of Interest in Present Circumstances,*** with Clem-b., Honey-b., Oliv-b., Wh-ch-b., Must-b. and Ch-b-d.

States of apathy and resignation. Lethargy, listlessness, lack of energy. Passivity. In sickness, when the fighting spirit is gone and recuperation is not proceeding, or even when death is threatened due to resignation.

Schizophrenic states, developmental disorders, psychosis, schizoid personality disorders. Reduced social contact, low emotional involvement.

MIND - Apathy and resignation. Helplessness and powerlessness. Anger or frustration. Disinterest in fighting for health when sick. Retreat from involvement in unfavorable circumstances. Stifled capacity for joy, disinterest in amusement and play, lack of hopes, wishes and dreams.

REFERENCES - Bach.

WILDBAD AQUA

PHARMACY - wild. Wildbad aqua. The Springs at Wildbad in Wurtemburg. The water contains in 16 ounces, Carbonic ac. grains 0.972, Nat-m. 1.808, Nat-c. 0.837, Nat-s. 0.291, Kali-s. 0.018, Calc. 0.738, Silicic acid 0.480, Mag-c. 0.079, Ferr-c. 0.002, Alum. 0.004 and traces of Mang. Dilutions. ***Historical dose:*** Tincture and all potencies.

CLINICAL - Bones, pains. Catarrh. Gout. Hair, disorders. Indigestion. Knees, creaking. Nails, soft. Paralysis, spinal. Paraplegia. Rheumatism. Shoulder, rheumatism.

HOMEOPATHIC - In spite of its very slight mineralization, said Constantin James, the water produces very distinct effects in a graduated series.

The first impression of the bath is delicious, this is succeeded by sensations more clear and distinct: a slight degree of excitement, at times luminous sparks before the sight, a finer blood seems to flow to the brain(Puls.). "One would like to remain in the bath, but something unusual and strange warns you that it is time to get out."

Wildbad is chiefly for ***disorders of the spinal cord,*** more then half the patients being paraplegic. Sensation as if the brain were over-filled. Gnawing, sinking, empty sensation. Pain as if sprained.

Sensation of looseness in the joints, ankles loose, knees loose, the bones seem as if they did not fit. Teeth seem too long. In one prover the hair, which had been greasy, became dry and the beard became of a darker color. Desire to stretch.

Modalities - Worse on waking, at night. Throbbing and heat in occiput worse lying down. Pain in sciatic nerve, looseness of knees worse walking.

RELATIONS - ***Compare:*** (1) Uric acid in urine. (2) pain in right shoulder, Urt-u. Sang.

REFERENCES - Clarke.

WILLOW

(Bach Flower Essence)

PHARMACY - will-b. Willow. Salix vitellina. Twigs with male or female catkins are boiled for half an hour. Subsequently, the water is strained and used as medicine. ***Historical dose:*** Take two drops from the stock bottle into a one ounce dropper bottle (add brandy or alcohol, if this bottle will be used for days or weeks). This is the dosage bottle, take a few drops straight into the mouth or as needed in a little water or juice.

HOMEOPATHIC - Will. belongs to Bach's group of ***Despondency and Despair,*** with Crb-a-b., Oak-b., Star-b-b., Sw-ch-b., Elm-b., Pine-b. and Lar-b. Will-b. deals with states of resentment and bitterness with one's fate. Physical rigidity and worn features may speak of internal bitterness and resentment. Bitterness, disillusionment and depression.

Chronically engaged in repression of aggressive impulses, affecting the heart and intestinal region. Suppressed anger, causing colicky pains, tension headaches, depression. Tachycardia, irregularities in heart activity, hypertension. Hyperventilation. Chronic coughs and constipation (Chic-b., Must-b.) Skin lesions and intermittent insomnia.

MIND - Burdened by an unfavorable and undeserved fate. Blames others for misfortunes. Unfounded resentment, blame. Dissatisfaction and self-pity. Bitterness and dormant despair. Sadness and disappointment. Anger at being mistreated. Outrage and sense of injustice. Self-righteousness, denial of reality, envy and lack of sympathy and compassion.

Malingering (Chic-b.), passive aggressive personality, antisocial and in disruptive behaviors (Holly-b.). Fixed ideas, delusions. Paranoia, as one feels persecuted and thwarted in one's destiny due to the fault of others (Beech-b.).

REFERENCES - Bach.

WITHANIA SOMNIFERA

(Ashwagandha)

PHARMACY - with-s. Withania somnifera. Ashwagandha. Physalis somnifera. Indian winter cherry. Indian ginseng. Winter cherry. N. O. Solanaceae. ***Historical dose:*** Tincture to first potency.

CLINICAL - Alcoholism. AIDS. Alzheimer's disease. Anemia. Arthritis. Asthma. Brain, fatigue. Breathing, difficulty. Bronchitis. Cancer. Carbuncles. ***Convalescence.*** Coughs. Emaciation. Emphysema. ***Exhaustion.*** Hyperglycemia. Immune, disorders. ***Impotency.*** Infertility. Insomnia. Lumbago. Memory, loss. Nerve, weakness. Paralysis. Rheumatism. ***Sexual, debility.*** Spermatorrhea. Skin, disorders. Swollen, glands. Tuberculosis. Tumors. Ulcers. Weakness.

HERBAL - Withania somnifera is an important herb used in Ayurveda, the traditional Indian medicine. A native of India, Pakistan and Sri Lanka, the name comes from the peculiar odor of this herb, smell akin to that of a sweaty horse.

It is an erect branched shrub with a greenish or lurid yellow flowers. In India, it is akin to ginseng in other parts of the orient, both are touted for their longevity enhancing and sexually stimulating properties.

The shoots and seeds are also used as food and to thicken milk in India. It is said to work mainly on the reproductive and nervous systems coupled with rejuvenating qualities. Tumors, inflammation (including arthritis), and a wide range of infectious diseases.

Regulates blood sugar, which aids in suppressing sugar cravings. It is commonly used to increase vitality, recover from chronic illnesses and pain management for arthritic conditions.

HOMEOPATHIC - According to B. Gangooly, M.D., from Calcutta, India, in the Homoeopathic Recorder, vol. 37, 1922, With-s. has been employed successfully in all cases of ***debility***. Nervousness. Brain fatigue. Loss of memory. Spermatorrhea. Problems resulting from masturbation. Speedy emissions, nocturnal emissions.

MIND - Confused. Cannot collect his thoughts. Loss of memory. Brain fatigue. Indifferent. Sadness, low spirits.

Back - Pain in back.

Ears - Whizzing noises.

Limbs - Great debility.

Eyes - Blue margins around eyes. Painful in the morning. Weak sight.

Face - Pale, flushes of heat.

Female - Infertility. Low sex drive.

Food - Desires sweets, sugar.

Head - Dull headache with buzzing in the head.

Heart - Palpitations.

Lungs - Respiratory disorders. Emphysema. Asthma. Bronchitis and coughs,

Male - Impotency. Low sex drive. Masturbation. Spermatorrhea. Emissions at night and at stool.

Sleep - Lascivious dreams with emissions.

Stomach - Pressure as from as load, with drowsiness, nausea, vomiting.

Urine - Frequent desire to urinate. Burning urination.

Vertigo - Vertigo on standing or walking.

COMMENTS - With-s. is specific for a wide range of conditions including arthritic inflammation. Respiratory disorders including emphysema, asthma bronchitis and coughs. gynecological disorders, especially functional female and male infertility and impotence. Low sexual libido.

Chronic neurological diseases especially anxiety, nervousness, depression and insomnia. Weak digestion, fluid retention caused by lowered body metabolism.

Immuno-compromised diseases including tuberculosis and AIDS, chronic upper respiratory diseases, degenerative symptoms attendant to aging, juvenile mal-development and growth.

RELATIONS - ***Compare:*** Phos.

REFERENCES - Gangooly. Murphy.

WYETHIA HELENOIDES

(Poison Weed)

PHARMACY - wye. Wyethia helenoides. Poison weed. Alarconia helenioides. Melarhiza inuloides. N. O. Compositae. Tincture of the root. ***Historical dose:*** Tincture and all potencies, first to sixth potency.

CLINICAL - ***Allergies.*** Asthma. Amenorrhea. Asthma. Bronchitis. Constipation. Coryza. Coughs. Depression. Diarrhea. Dysmenorrhea. Epiglottis disorders. Fatigue. Fevers. ***Hay fever.*** Headache. Hemorrhoids. Hiccoughs. Indigestion. Influenza. ***Itching.*** Leucorrhea. Nervousness, Ovaries, pain. ***Pharyngitis.*** Post-nasal catarrh. Salivation. Sneezing. Throat, sore. Uvula disorders. Weakness.

HOMEOPATHIC - Wye. was introduced and proved with the fresh root or the tincture, on seven men and two women, by Selfridge. The first proving gave Wye. a definite and important place in throat disorders. Those symptoms make up the first pathogenesis.

Wye. has marked effects on the throat and has proven an excellent remedy in ***pharyngitis***, especially the follicular form. Irritable throats of singers and public speakers. Throat feels swollen, epiglottis dry and burning. Constant desire to swallow saliva to relieve the dryness yet affording no comfort. Swallows with difficulty.

Hay fever symptoms, ***itching in posterior sinuses.*** Prickling, dry sensation in posterior sinuses, sensation as if something were in nasal passages, an effort to clear them through the throat affords no relief. Burning sensation in bronchial tubes. Dry, hacking cough, caused by tickling in epiglottis. Useful also in hemorrhoids.

MIND - Nervous, uneasy, apprehensive of calamity. Depressed. Incapacitated for mental work. Averse to company. Impatient and quarrelsome.

Abdomen - Pain and bearing down in abdomen, right side. Pain below ribs of right side.

Back - Swollen and sore glands on right side of neck.

Chest - Deep-seated sharp pain just below right ribs, followed by soreness.

Ears - Itching in right ear. Pain in left ear.

Eyes - Itching in left inner canthus.

Female - Menses commenced with intense burning pain. Leucorrhea. Pain in left ovary, shooting down to knee. Pain in uterus, can outline its contour.

Head - Rush of blood to head. Sharp pain in forehead. Severe headache.

Limbs - Pain in back, extends to end of spine. Pain right arm, stiffness of wrist and hand. Aching pains all over.

Lungs - Dry asthma. ***Dry, hacking cough*** caused by tickling of the epiglottis. Burning sensation in bronchial tubes.

Modalities - Worse afternoon, after eating. Worse motion. Worse exercise, it causes perspiration.

Mouth - Feels as if scalded, sensation of heat down esophagus. Itching of the palate.

Nose - Hay fever symptoms. Sensation as if something in nasal passages.

Rectum - Loose, dark, at night. Constipation with ***hemorrhoids***, not bleeding. Great constriction of rectum. Itching of anus and rectum.

Sensations - Mouth as if scalded. Uvula as if elongated. Epiglottis feels dry and burning. Weight in stomach as if something indigestible had been eaten. Uterus feels as if it enlarged in order to contain all the pain.

Sleep - Wakes frequently and too early.

Stomach - Belching of gas, alternating with hiccough. Nausea and vomiting. Sense of weight in stomach, as if something indigestible had been eaten.

Temperature - Chill at 11 a.m. Thirst for ice water during chill. No thirst with heat. Profuse sweat all night. Terrific headache during sweat.

Throat - Hot, dry throat. Constant clearing and hemming. ***Dry***, posterior sinuses, no relief from clearing. ***Throat feels swollen***, epiglottis dry and burning. Difficult swallowing. Constant desire to swallow saliva. Uvula feels elongated. Tendency to get hoarse talking or singing.

Vertigo - Dizzy.

COMMENTS - Nonspecific hay fever, characteristic itching of the upper palate. Hay asthma, allergic asthma. A history of hay fever going to the lungs, or asthma caused by hay fever treatments or decongestants. Kent used this as a prophylactic hay fever remedy.

Tough, ropy saliva. Belching alternating with hiccough. Pain over left ovary, shooting down to knee. In one case, menses, which had been in abeyance since confinement a year before, returned with much pain.

Hale noted several cases from Selfridge. The first concerned dry asthma in a woman who had several attacks promptly relieved with Wye. The second case noted the effectiveness of Wye. in chronic follicular pharyngitis with dryness of pharynx and burning in epiglottis. In the third case, Hale found Wye. to be successful in a case of severe epidemic influenza.

Clarke had a case reported to him in which a boy had been kept awake many nights by a persistent, dry, hacking, nervous cough. Wye. 30c cured in one dose.

RELATIONS - ***Compare:*** (1) Arum, Sang., Lach. (2) In throat affections, Arum-d., Caust., Hep., Stict., Rumx., Pen., Phos., Sulph. (3) Tough, ropy saliva and headache, Epip. (4) Sensation as if something indigestible eaten, Abies-n. (5) Scalded mouth, Ran-s.

REFERENCES - Boericke. Clarke. Murphy.

X

X-RAY

PHARMACY - x-ray. X-ray. Dilutions made from absolute alcohol irritated with x-rays through a glass bottle. ***Historical dose:*** All potencies.

CLINICAL - ***Anemia.*** Anorexia. Burns. Cancer. ***Chronic fatigue.*** Debility. Dermatitis. Emaciation. Heart, problems. Hemaphila. Hemorrhages. Infertility. ***Leukemia.*** Mastectomy, pains. Memory, weak. Ovaries, atrophy. Psoriasis. Purpura. Radiation, dermatitis. Skin tumors. Sterility. Sun, exposure. Testes, atrophy. ***Vitality, low. Warty growths. Weakness.*** X-ray, poisoning.

HOMEOPATHIC - Roentgen noted that repeated exposure to X-rays produced skin lesions often followed by cancer. Changes take place in the blood lymphatics and bone marrow. Its homeopathic action is centrifugal towards the periphery of the body. The stock comes from the potency 1c of this irradiated alcohol.

The proving on X-ray was conducted by Fincke in 1897, on ten provers, using 6x. This was repeated by W. B. Griggs on two male and one female provers, and published in the Homeopathic Recorder in 1952 using the 30c and 200c potencies.

X-rays have the property of stimulating cellular metabolism. ***Arouses the vitality, mentally and physically.*** Useful for syndromes of deficiency of certain elements present in the blood. ***Leukemia.***

General debility. ***Chronic fatigue and a sick feeling.*** Unexplained weakness. ***Low vitality and anemia.*** Discharges, gray, white with jelly-like lumps. Psoriasis. Corresponds to burns, that refuse to heal. Distressing pain. Sexual glands are particularly affected. Atrophy of ovaries and testicles. Infertility.

X-rays brings to the surface suppressed symptoms, especially the psoric and sycotic due to mixed infections. For cancer patients submitted to treatment by radiation, X-rays, cobalt. For patients submitted for therapy by immuno-suppressors and all anti-tumor chemotherapy.

MIND - Sadness. Aversion to company. Memory, weak. Sleepy. Irritable, desire to kill, especially before and during menses.

Abdomen - Heaviness and fullness in lower abdomen, distended. Flatulence with ineffectual desire for stool.

Back - Lame and stiff in back. Aching whole length of spine. Cramping pains in the back and lumbar region in the morning, on walking. Soreness in small of back.

Blood - Decreased leucocytes and platelets. ***Leukemia.*** Hypochromic anemia. Hemorrhagic syndromes. Hematoma, tendency to hemorrhage, purpura.

Breasts - Nerve pains after mastectomy.

Chest - Thorax painful, palpitations. Contraction of chest at night relieved by belching. Sensation of drops of water trickling down on inside of chest.

Ears - Sensation of fullness, noises in the ear, buzzing. Sore pain in cartilage of left ear when pressing it, later in right ear. Pressing outward in ears. Buzzing in right ear with pressure extending to temples. Intermittent noise as of deep steam-whistle in left ear.

Eyes - Painful to the touch. Eyeballs sore. Sensation in right eye as if bulging. Bearing down of eyelids. Eyelids heavy and sleepy.

Face - Red, smooth eruption on right side of face. Dull pain in right upper jaw. Paralytic feeling in right cheek. Stinging pains in different parts of head and face.

Female - Menses profuse or lacking. Menses dark green one day. Pain darting upward in region of left ovary. Flushes of heat, better afternoons and evenings.

Food - Anorexia, aversion to food. Can eat plenty but does not enjoy it. Desire for sweets.

Head - Sticking pains in different parts of head and face. Ringing in head. Sensation of fullness in the head. Pain in the forehead, occiput, temples, extending to the neck. Better by hot compresses on the forehead.

Heart - Extra systole on coughing or crying. Pain in the precordial region. Noises from the heart prevent him from sleeping on the left side.

Kidneys - Oliguria, tenesmus of the bladder. Retained urine. Kidney colic with vomiting. Clutching pain from left kidney to bladder.

Limbs - Rheumatic pains. Trembling of the limbs. Generalized pains in the limbs, sciatic neuralgia. Sensation of electric current at the limbs.

Lungs - Cough caused by palpitation, in evening. Cough in the morning with green sputum. Grayish expectoration.

Male - Lewd dreams. Sexual desire lost. Sterility. Re-establishes suppressed gonorrhea.

Modalities - Better from hot applications. Worse from cold, open air. Worse movement. Worse afternoon, evening and night, when in bed.

Mouth - Bad taste in the mouth. Tongue dry, rough, sore. Teeth discolored, gray-green color.

Neck - Painful stiffness of the neck, on lifting the head from the pillow. Sudden "cricks" attack first one side of neck, then the other, worse on getting cold. Aching pains in left side of neck.

Nose - Nasal congestion, odor of sulphur vapor.

Rectum - Diarrhea, constipation and anal itching. Green stools.

Skin - Skin is discolored, pale, sclerous, cold. Skin dry, wrinkled. Hyperkeratosis of the skin. ***Warty growths.*** Radiation dermatitis. Chronic itching eruptions. Papular, vesicular, itching eruptions. Dry, itching eczema. Psoriasis. Palms rough and scaly. Erythema around roots of nails. Painful cracks. Nails thicken. Ingrown nails.

Sleep - Sleepy with headache. Sleepy all the time with chronic fatigue. Sleepy, but unable to sleep for some hours after retiring.

Stomach - Nausea with a sick feeling. Nausea and vomiting with profuse sweat after immense stool. Sick feeling in stomach.

Temperature - Chills as soon as beginning to sleep, running up back, preventing sleep. Chilly while undressing in warm room. Chilliness on moving or from draft. Perspires easily. Profuse perspiration on getting into bed, keeping him awake. Night sweats. Spells of fever, perspiration and weakness.

Throat - Throat painful on swallowing. The pharynx has gray-green mucus, discomfort and cramping pain on swallowing. Sensation of narrowness in the throat.

COMMENTS - Dr. John B. Campbell, one of Fincke's original provers, discovered the great value of this remedy in rousing the reactive vitality of the system, both mentally and physically. In doing so, it brings suppressed symptoms to the surface in persons laboring under a combination of Hahnemann's miasms. This is particularly helpful in deep-seated constitutional ailments, sycotic in character, which often terminate in malignant disease, especially cancer.

Useful for conditions lacking presenting symptoms. When well selected anti-psoric remedies (Calc., Med., Psor., Sep., Sulph., Syph., or Tub.) fail to relieve completely. When well-indicated remedies fail with a history of exposure to radiation. Tends to bring out old suppressed eruptions or discharges (Sulph.).

Non-specific chronic fatigue and weakness. Sores that fail to heal. Neuralgias after mastectomy. Extreme thirst and dryness of the mouth.

X-ray burns, whether of the bone or skin. History of exposure to x-rays. Radiation sickness. Weakness after radiation treatments (Sol.).

Dr. King developed an x-ray burn on his left hand. Eighteen months later, seedy warts appeared. Caust. finally helped, so he believed that Caust. may potentially be another antidote for x-rays.

RELATIONS - ***Antidotes:*** Nux-v., Sulph. and the dynamic potencies of the remedy. ***Compare:*** (1) Cadm-s., Carc. - Cancer patients, weak immune system. (2) Electr. - Sugar of milk saturated with the current. Anxiety, nervous tremors, restlessness, palpitation, headaches. Dreads approach of thunder-storms, heaviness of limbs. (3) Magn-ambo. Magn-arct. Magn-aust. (4) Merc. - Desire to hurt, even those dear to him, agitated, confused. Tongue covered with a yellowish coating and retaining the teeth imprints. (5) Phos. - Bleeding of bright red blood, frightened, hypersensitive, afraid of the dark an of storms. (6) Sec. - The limbs are cold with paresthesia, hemorrhaging of black blood, aggravated by the heat, ameliorated by the cold.

REFERENCES - Boericke. Clarke. Murphy.

XANTHIUM SPINOSUM

(Spiny Cocklebur)

PHARMACY - xanth. Xanthium spinosum. Spiny cocklebur. N. O. Compositae. ***Historical dose:*** Tincture and all potencies.

CLINICAL - ***Cystitis.*** Hydrophobia. Rabies.

HOMEOPATHIC - Xanth. is a wildflower that occurs throughout North America. Boericke stated that cockle is known to be a specific for hydrophobia and is recommended for chronic cystitis in women.

Chronic cystitis, that responds to several remedies in the acute phase but keeps recurring. For chronic or interstitial cystitis with a history of sexual abuse at a young age, especially those that include violence and repeated torment. Strong fear of being attacked, especially at night.

RELATIONS - ***Compare:*** Staph., Lyss., Hyos., Lach., Stram., Carc.

REFERENCES - Boericke. Klein.

XANTHORRHIZA APIFOLIA

(Shrub Yellow Root)

PHARMACY - xanrhi. Xanthorrhiza apifolia. Shrub yellow root. Contains Berberine. N. O. Compositae. ***Historical dose:*** Tincture and all potencies.

HOMEOPATHIC - Xanrhi. has dilatation of stomach and intestines, atony, enlarged spleen.

REFERENCES - Boericke.

XANTHORRHEA ARBOREA

PHARMACY - xanrhoe. Xanthorrhea arborea. ***Historical dose:*** Tincture and all potencies.

HOMEOPATHIC - Xanrhoe. has a reputation of being a good kidney tonic. It has severe pain in kidneys, cystitis and gravel. Pain from ureter to bladder and testicles, pain in small of back returns from least chill or damp.

REFERENCES - Clarke.

XANTHOXYLUM FRAXINEUM

(Prickly Ash)

PHARMACY - xan. Xanthoxylum fraxineum. Prickly ash. Xanthoxylum americanum. Toothache tree. N. O. Rutaceae. Tincture of fresh bark. ***Historical dose:*** Tincture and all potencies.

CLINICAL - After-pains. Amenorrhea. Aphonia. Asthma. Cholera. Coccyx, pain. Colic. Dyspepsia. Dysentery. ***Dysmenorrhea.*** Earache. Fibroids. Flatulence. Headaches. ***Hemiplegia.*** Hoarseness. Hysteria. Injuries. Insomnia. Jaw joint, pain. Levitation. Menstruation, painful. Nausea. Nerves, injured. Nervousness. ***Neuralgia.*** Neurasthenia. Ophthalmia. ***Rheumatism.*** Sciatica. Toothache. Ulcers.

HERBAL - Xan. belongs to the Rutaceae and has a vulnerary action (Ruta.). Xan. contains Piperin.

Rafinesque was the first to investigate Xan., which was known to him as "a great article in the Materia Medica of the Indians," who use the root bark in decoction for "colics, gonorrhea, syphilis inward pains toothache, ulcers, etc. It is a great topical stimulant," he continues, "changing the nature of malignant ulcers."

T. C. Duncan, recounting reminiscences of his boyhood, said, "There was another remedy that set my youthful mouth and stomach on fire and that was Prickly Ash. You wanted to open the mouth to let the cool air get in."

This warmth is felt as a warm glow through the entire system with a sensation in the nerves as if gentle shocks of electricity were passing through the body.

HOMEOPATHIC - Xan. exerts its influence on nerves, female sexual organs, respiration and left side. Its action is on the nervous system and mucus membranes.

Injury to nerves. Neurasthenia. Pricking sensation, shocks as from electricity. Numbness of left side. Paralysis, of single parts. ***Hemiplegia***. Insomnia. Occipital headache. ***Neuralgic and rheumatic*** disorders, especially in patients of spare habit and nervous, delicate organization.

Increases mucus secretion of mouth and stimulates the secretion from all glands with ducts opening in the mouth. Poor assimilation, emaciation. Indigestion from over-eating or from too much fluid.

Painful hemorrhages, after-pains, ***dysmenorrhea***. Sluggish capillary circulation. Mucus membranes smart as from pepper. As if floor were soft like wool, on walking. Injury to nerves.

Grinding, shooting, radiating, sudden pains, neuralgia. Many pains are radiating, some are sudden, arouse from sleep and cause the patient to catch her breath. Pains are excruciating, unbearable and are accompanied with red, hot face, but the heart pains causes pallor.

MIND - Nervous, frightened feeling. Mental depression. Did not care if she lived or died.

Abdomen - Some pain in right side below ribs. Griping pain on waking in morning. Colic pain in right iliac region. Rumbling with soreness on pressure. Flatulence.

Back - Very severe pain in cervical and upper sacral region. Back of neck numb. Dull pain from nape to right scapula.

Causations - Injury to nerves. Wetting (getting feet wet). Suppression of menses.

Chest - Oppression of chest.

Constitutions - Suited to women of spare habit, nervous temperament and delicate nerves. Neurasthenic patients who are thin, emaciated, poor assimilation with insomnia and occipital headache.

Ears - Ringing in ears. Loud noise in right ear, as of a valve constantly opening and shutting. Dull pain in right ear. Darting pain under and back or right ear.

Eyes - Watering of eyes and nose. Lachrymation, pain in lid of right eye. Eyes bloodshot with red margins and feel as if full of sand. Dull, heavy, grinding pain in left eye. Ophthalmia. Eyes twitched, pupils dilated. Vision blurred, as if looking through blue lace. Objects seem a long way off.

Face - Hot flushes over face and head. Face much flushed. Pallor even to lips with heart pains. Neuralgia of lower jaw. Pain in right jaw-socket.

Female - Menses too early and painful. Menses thick, almost black. Leucorrhea at time of menses. Leucorrhea with amenorrhea. ***Neuralgic dysmenorrhea*** with neuralgic headaches, pain in ***back and down legs***. Ovarian neuralgia with pain in loins and lower abdomen, ***worse left side,*** extending down the thigh, along genito-crural nerves. ***After pains*** (Arn., Cupr., Cham.).

Food - Very thirsty, drank much at a time. Unusually hungry. No appetite. Anorexia.

Head - Feels full. Weight and pain on vertex. Pain over eyes, throbbing pressure over nose, pressure in forehead, head seems divided, ringing in ears. Occipital headache. Sick headache with dizziness and flatulence. Throbbing headache, pain as if top of head would fly off. As if head is divided into two parts. As of a tight band around.

Kidneys - Urine at night and next morning scanty and high-colored. Profuse, light-colored urine, nervous women.

Limbs - Numbness of left side, impairment of motion. Paralysis of left side following spinal disorders. Hemiplegia. Left arm numb. Neuralgic shooting pain, as from electricity, all over limbs. Anterior neuralgia (Staph.). Sciatica, worse hot weather. Pain in nape, extending down back.

Lungs - Shortness of breath. Constant desire to take a long breath, oppression of chest. Dry cough, day and night. Cough, slight hacking in spells, only in open air.

Modalities - Better from drinking ice-water, vomiting. Better lying down. Headache is better by cold water and in open air. Neck pain is better by pressure and by throwing head back. Worse from sleeping, in morning, 4 a.m. Worse dampness, getting feet wet. Worse suppressed menses. Worse by moving head suddenly.

Mouth - Peppery taste in mouth, fauces and throat. Burning and dry feeling in mouth and tongue. Ptyalism, tongue coated yellow. Tongue seemed to alternately expand and contract. Dryness of mouth and fauces. Pharyngitis (Wye.).

Nose - Fluent coryza. Right nostril seems filled up, discharge of dry and bloody scales of mucus. Discharge of mucus from nose with congested feeling, as if it were about to bleed. Slight nose-bleed. Dryness of both nostrils. Numbness throughout left side of body, division felt in nose.

Rectum - Constipation in morning. Griping and diarrhea. Dysentery with ***tympanites***, tenesmus, inodorous discharges. Epidemic dysentery. Cholera collapse stage.

Sensations - As if top of head would be taken off by flashes of throb-like pain. As if bewildered with pain in back of head. Feeling of looseness of brain. Eyes as if full of sand. As if walking on wool. As if sunk deep in bed. As if body expanded.

Skin - Measles, dullness, bewilderment, drowsiness and want of sufficient development of the eruption. Old, indolent ulcers.

Sleep - Continued gaping, drowsiness. Hard and unrefreshing, dreams of flying. Sleeplessness in neurasthenics. A dream of suffocation woke her.

Stomach - Dyspepsia from excessive eating and drinking. Feeling of fullness of pressure in epigastrium, fluttering. Intense burning and stinging in esophagus with slight nausea. Empty belchings with slight taste of ingesta. Nausea with headache, with sense of oppression at stomach.

Temperature - Slight chill accompanied by death-like nausea. Frequent chills with pains in limbs, nausea. Typhoid fever in stage of collapse. Sense of heat all over veins, flashes of heat from the head to foot.

Throat - Aphonia. Hoarseness with husky feeling in throat, obliged to clear throat frequently. Throat dry, very difficult to talk. Peppery taste in mouth and throat. Feels hollow. Pain and soreness in right side of throat. Throat felt as if in a vice.

COMMENTS - Xan. belongs to the Rutaceae and like Ruta, has a vulnerary action, as Clarke discovered in the case of Miss X., 28, who injured her right ulnar nerve at the elbow by repeatedly striking it against the edge of a bath while washing some articles.

For two months she had to keep the arm in a sling. A few weeks after that the arm was swollen. Some eight months after the injury Clarke saw her. The pain centered in the ulnar nerve where it crosses the inner condyle of the humerus, though there was pain above and below as well.

Clarke gave Ruta 30c, which gave some relief to the pain and relieved a frontal headache to which the patient was subject. The arm becoming less well, Clarke gave Xan. 12c four times a day. This made a distinct improvement in the arm and also relieved a dysmenorrhea to which Miss X. was subject. After treatment with various potencies of Xan. the nerve lost its sensitiveness and the patient could use her arm freely.

In one of Cullis' provers, Miss D. (there were six provers, three of them women, all took the tincture), the entire left half of the body became numb, the left half of the head being sharply divided in sensation from the other half. These symptoms with the many head pains and fullness in the head, give the correspondence in hemiplegia in which Xan. has been given with success.

Two additional provings on women appear in C. D. P. In these provings 20 to 100 drop doses of the tincture were taken and symptoms of great severity were produced. Both provers had severe dysmenorrhea pains with increased and anticipating flow.

The symptoms in each case roused the prover from sleep with pain and suffocation, the pain being confined to head, heart, throat and pelvis. Many of the pains were radiating from above right eye over head from right ovary down thigh and in other directions. Left-sided numbness was present in one, who also had symptoms of levitation and disordered sensation.

Cullis, who had success in cases of dysmenorrhea and amenorrhea, related several cases, including that of Miss A., 25, brunette, who had menstrual irregularity since commencement, would go three, four or five months and then her sufferings were excruciating. When she came under treatment had no menses for two months. Xan. 1c was give, 5 drops thrice daily. Menses appeared in three days and were painless.

Miss B., fair, nervous, had menses suppressed by getting feet wet, being then a week over time. Xan. 1x, 5 drops every three hours, brought on menses the next day.

P. C. Majumdar cured a case of uterine fibroid with Xan. 3x. An emaciated, feeble, wrinkled woman, 56, widow, had been advised by allopaths to have an operation for tumor. Menstruation had ceased fifteen years before. It had been profuse and painful and preceded and followed by leucorrhea.

She had neuralgic pain in right ovarian region, a hard nodular tumor size of a small orange, painful on deep pressure. Fetid, yellowish white discharge from vagina. Nervous, depressed, lazy and sleepy even in daytime. Appetite poor, disgust for food.

Xan. 3x was given night and morning. In a week the pain was better and discharge less. In four weeks Majumdar found the patient a changed person. The tumor was much softer and reduced by half. In six months the tumor had gone and the patient was quite well, Xan. having been taken intermittently all the time.

RELATIONS - ***Compare:*** (1) Gnaph., Cimic., Staph., Mez., Pisc.

REFERENCES - Boericke. Clarke.

XEROPHYLLUM TENAX

(Basket Grass Flower)

PHARMACY - xero. Xerophyllum tenax. Basket grass flower. Tamalpais lily. N. O. Melanthiaceae. ***Historical dose:*** Tincture and all potencies.

CLINICAL - Backache. Constipation. Dermatitis. Dyslexia. Eczema. Flatulence. Leucorrhea. Poison oak. Typhoid.

HOMEOPATHIC - Xero. should prove curative in eczema conditions, poison oak and early typhoid states, etc.

MIND - Dull, cannot concentrate. Forgets names. Dyslexia. ***Writes last letters of words first***. Misspells common words. Bewildered. Loss of consciousness.

Abdomen - Intestinal flatulence. In morning, rumbling with desire for stool.

Back - Feels hot from sacrum to scapulae. Heat deep in spine. Backache, extending down legs. Pain over kidneys.

Eyes - Painful, as if sand, smarting, Hard to focus for close work. Eyes sore, burn.

Face - Bloated, morning. Puffy eyes.

Female - Bearing-down sensation. Vulva inflamed with furious itching. Increased sexual desire with ovarian and uterine pains and leucorrhea.

Head - Feels full, stuffed up, pain across forehead and above eyes. Great pressure at root of nose. Pulsating headache.

Kidneys - Difficulty retaining urine, dribbling when walking. Frequent urination.

Limbs - Limbs feel stiff (Rhus-t.). Muscular lameness, trembling. Inguinal glands and behind knees swollen. Pain in knees.

Lungs - Posterior sinuses raw, discharge thick, yellow mucus. Sneezing. Trachea sore, lumps feel constricted.

Modalities - Better application of hot water. Better in morning. Better moving affected part. Worse application of cold water. Worse in afternoon and evening.

Nose - Stuffed, tightness at bridge of nose, acute nasal catarrh.

Rectum - Constipation, stools hard, small lumps. Difficult, soft stools with much straining. Much flatus. Bearing-down pain in rectum.

Skin - Skin rough and cracked, feels like leather. Dermatitis, especially around knees. Inflammation resembling poison oak. Erythema with vesication and intense itching, stinging and burning. Blisters, little lumps.

Stomach - Feels full and heavy. Belchings sour offensive, an hour after luncheons and dinner. Vomiting at 2 p.m.

Throat - Stitching pain upon swallowing.

RELATIONS - ***Compare:*** Rhus-t., Anac.

REFERENCES - Boericke. Clarke.

Y

YERSIN SERUM

(Anti-plague Serum)

PHARMACY - yersin. Yersin serum. The yersin serum is derived from the anti-plague serum, supplied by Institute Pasteur. ***Historical dose:*** All potencies.

CLINICAL - Abscess. Adenitis. Buboes. Colitis. Crohn's disease. Encephalitis. Erythema. Gastroenteritis. Influenza. Ileitis. Meningitis. Parkinson's disease. Plague. Septicemia.

HOMEOPATHIC - According to Fortier-Bernoville, it is Barishac who proposed Yersin for the treatment of grave or a typical forms of influenza. Severe form of influenza of pulmonary type with hyperthemia, respiratory troubles, soft thick, rosy expectorations, presence of sub-crepitant rales in the base of lungs.

Mesenteric adenitis. Acute entero-colitis, gastro-enteritis with lesion of ilium. Acute enteritis of young children. Crohn's regional ileitis. Influenza of gastro-intestinal form. Pseudo-typho meningitis of milkmen. Meningitis syndromes of influenzal origin. Encephalitis lethargica. Parkinson's disease.

Severe toxic, infectious states, either cutaneous (bubo) or pulmonary. Septicemias accompanied with icterus and hepatic abscess. Acute toxicosis of babies. Lymphoid terminal ileitis of Arnulf and Buffart. Nodulous erythema.

RELATIONS - ***Compare:*** (1) Tub-a., Bapt., Pyrog. (2) Mimosa Pudica - thoracic pain, dry cough, irritation of naso-pharyngeal and laryngeal mucus, frequent irritating stools with colic, better by not bath. (3) Amorphophallus Rivieri - general ill feeling with great weakness, gastro-intestinal troubles with weakening diarrhea, fetid stools.

REFERENCES - Clarke. Julian.

YOHIMBINUM CORYANTHE

(Yohimbe Bark)

PHARMACY - yohim. Yohimbinum coryanthe. Yohimbe bark. N. O. Rubiaceae. A crystalline alkaloid obtained from the bark of the Yohimbeha or Yumbehoa tree of the Cameroons. Trituration. ***Historical dose:*** Tincture and all potencies.

CLINICAL - Aphrodisiac. Diuresis. Hyperemia. Impotence. Menorrhagia. Neurasthenia. Palpitations. Priapism. Urethritis. Sexual, neurasthenia.

HERBAL - The natives of West Africa discovered a potent aphrodisiac in the bark of the Yohimbeha tree, and from this an active principle. It is a powerful stimulant of the genital function in males.

Excites the sexual organs and acts on the central nervous system and respiratory center. An aphrodisiac, used in physiological doses, but contraindicated in all acute and chronic inflammations of abdominal organs.

HOMEOPATHIC - Useful for priapism and congestive states of the sexual organs. Menorrhagia. Hyperemia of the milk glands, stimulates breast-feeding. In animals Yohim. causes increased liveliness and cheerfulness, hyperemia of the conjunctiva, heat and redness of the ears and of the nose also in dogs.

MIND - Intense agitation with trembling.

Abdomen - Flying heat sensations in abdomen.

Back - Flying heat sensations in back.

Face - Sensations of heat, heightening the color.

Food - Appetite almost completely disappeared.

Head - Agitation with flying sensations of heat in face.

Heart - Heart beats more intense and more frequent, pulse, normally 80, became 108. Flying sensation of heat in heart.

Kidneys - Urine clean abundant, foamy, no trace of albumen, had to rise three times in the night. Urethritis.

Limbs - Hands trembled, could scarcely write, writing was illegible.

Male - Sexual neurasthenia with impotence. Priapism. ***Strong and lasting erections*** in the morning without increase of desire. Enlargement of testicles and epididymis.

Mouth - Disagreeable, metallic taste. Copious salivation. Tongue covered with a yellow coat.

Rectum - Intestinal hemorrhage. Bleeding hemorrhoids. Stools frequent, liquid, black and bilious.

Sleep - No sleep all night. ***Sleeplessness***. Thoughts of events of whole past life keep him awake.

Stomach - Nausea and eructation.

Temperature - Rigor intense heat, waves of heat and chilliness, tendency to sweat.

COMMENTS - Lambreghts related the case of a young man, 28, "thin, anemic, nervous and partially impotent," who took a 5 mg. tablet one morning, another in the evening and a third the following morning. The symptoms were so severe that he discontinued the herb in spite of a certain amelioration of the sexual neurasthenia.

Yohim. set up symptoms of fever, disordered the digestion, caused agitation and tremors and increased the action of the heart. Eulenburg used Yohim. in 10 drop doses of a 1 percent solution and "in cases of neurasthenic impotence with excellent result."

RELATIONS - ***Compare:*** (1) Erections - Canth., Pic-ac., Phos., Graph., Canth.

REFERENCES - Boericke. Clarke.

YTTRIUM METALLICUM

PHARMACY - yttr. Yttrium metallicum. ***Historical dose:*** All potencies.

CLINICAL - Aphonia. Cancer. Colds. Eye problems. Headache. Hoarseness. Lung, problems. Voice, problems.

HOMEOPATHIC - Headache in forehead, temples and vertex. Neck problems, stiffness. Eye inflammations, visual disturbances. Colds with watery coryza. Hoarseness. Voice problems. Loss of voice. Stammering. Lung problems. Irritation of lungs. Cancer. Pain in arms. Problems with genitalia, testes and ovaries. Menses profuse.

Bruised pains. Itching. Weakness. Sleepy. ***Nervous trembling***. Worse left side. Worse cold weather, cold feet, ***cold, damp.*** Better being outside.

MIND - Irritability. Humiliation. Mood uncertain, crying. Anticipation. Fear of giving performance, speeches. Fear of heights, ladders. Fear of narrow spaces. Dreams of heights, falling, ladders. Dreams of mountains, volcano, water.

REFERENCES - Scholten.

YUCCA FILAMENTOSA

(Bear Grass)

PHARMACY - yuc. Yucca filamentosa. Bear grass. Agavaceae. N. O. Melanthacae, Liliaceae. Tincture of root and leaves when not in flower. Tincture of flowers. ***Historical dose:*** Tincture and all potencies.

CLINICAL - Biliousness. Coryza. Diarrhea. Flatulence. Headache, temporal. Post-nasal catarrh. Throat, granular.

HOMEOPATHIC - Yuc. was proved by Rowell and four others in the 30c. Farrington gave these Yuc. indications: biliousness with pain going through upper part of liver to back. Diarrhea which contains an excess of bile. Much flatus passed by rectum. Frequent passage of flatus and of watery, yellowish-brown stools. Dull ache in center of liver. Abdomen sensitive.

As with many liver disorders, there is chilliness, cannot bear to be away from the fire. Face sallow. Bilious symptoms with headache. Frontal or temporal headache with frequent flushing of face. Bad taste in mouth. Tongue coated yellow and taking imprint of teeth. The tongue is usually a bluish white.

MIND - Despondent and irritable. Irresolute. Disinclined to study. Mind wanders, uses wrong words. Unable to remember anything read. When others talking to him, hears but doesn't seem to understand.

Abdomen - Deep pain in right side over liver, going through back. Abdomen bloated after dinner and feels sore. Rumbling. Colic. Crampy pains in abdomen after breakfast. Throbbing, painless, right side about twelfth rib. Much flatus emitted, odorless.

Back - Constriction of neck muscles, seems to draw head backward. Tight feeling around neck, evening, had to take off collar. Severe pain in left scapula, at 9 p.m. Backache.

Chest - Constriction in whole chest and in heart. Pain in upper intercostal muscles.

Ears - Pain behind right ear, 6:30 p.m. Very sensitive to least noise.

Eyes - Dark rings under eyes. Eyes feel hot and inflamed. Itching and smarting left eye, left inner canthus. Dull pain over left eye.

Face - Pale, flushed, burning, yellow. Momentary aching in zygoma, recurring several times. Pain in jaw joints.

Food - Appetite increased, food relished, lost.

Head - Headaches frontal, heavy, pressing, throbbing. Headaches as if top of head would fly off. Temporal arteries throb. Sensation of cold air blowing on left side of scalp.

Heart - Constriction in heart. Momentary aching in heart region. Visible throbbing in arteries of hand. Pulse full and heavy, a little irregular.

Kidneys - Circumscribed edematous red swelling, raw sensation around meatus. Irritable bladder, frequent urination. Burning when urinating. Urine increased, high specific gravity.

Limbs - Crampy pains in knees. Sore, crampy pains in muscle of back of left leg, just above ankle, as if sprained.

Lungs - Hard, rattling cough.

Male - Burning and swelling of the prepuce with redness of meatus. Gonorrhea (Cann-s.). Erections, all night long but no emissions, cannot study, mind runs on sexual subjects.

Modalities - Griping pain is better bending forward. Worse by noise. Worse motion, pressure.

Mouth - Bad odor from mouth. Taste as of rotten eggs (Arn.). Back of mouth dry. Yellow tongue yellow, coated, taking imprint of teeth (Merc., Podo., Rhus-t.).

Nose - Nose red. In evening, right side of nose constantly running, left dry. Profuse, bloody, watery discharge. Coryza. Sensation as if something hung down from posterior sinuses, cannot get it up or down.

Rectum - Constant desire for stool. Sudden, violent tenesmus, followed by discharge of wind, which relieves the pain. Diarrhea following pains in abdomen. Stools are watery, copious, thin, yellowish brown with smarting at anus. Stool yellowish brown with bile. Tenesmus after stool.

Sensations - As of something hanging down from back of sinuses. As if cold air blowing on left side of scalp.

Skin - Erythematous redness.

Sleep - Very sleepy in the evening. Restless night. Lewd dreams.

Stomach - Aching and sharp pains in stomach. Region of stomach sore and sensitive.

Temperature - Coldness of scalp, left side, as if cold air blowing on it. Coldness, cannot bear to be away from fire. Restless and feverish. Hot, feverish. Face sweats, evening.

Throat - Tonsils dark red, not sore. Pharynx seems covered with granules is dark red. Stringy, greasy-looking mucus back of throat. Sensation as if something hanging down from posterior sinuses.

RELATIONS - ***Antidoted by:*** Cocc. ***Compare:*** (1) Constriction in heart, Lil-t. (2) Biliousness, Bry. (3) Tongue imprinted with teeth, Merc., Podo. (4) Blue tongue, Gymn.

REFERENCES - Boericke. Clarke.

Z

ZEA ITALICA

(Corn-silk)

PHARMACY - zea-i. Zea italica. Corn-silk. Gramineae. ***Historical dose:*** Tincture and all potencies, tincture in ten to fifty drop doses in water.

HOMEOPATHIC - Zea-i. has curative properties in skin diseases, particularly in psoriasis and eczema rubrum. Appetite increased, voracious, alternating with disgust for food. Heartburn, nausea, vomiting, better from drinking wine.

MIND - Easily angered. Mania for bathing. Impulse to suicide, particularly by drowning.

RELATIONS - ***Antidoted by:*** Cocc. ***Compare:*** (1) Stigm.

REFERENCES - Boericke.

ZINCUM ACETICUM

(Zinc Acetate)

PHARMACY - zinc-acet. Zincum aceticum. Zinc acetate. Trituration of the metal. ***Historical dose:*** All potencies.

CLINICAL - Diarrhea. Erysipelas. Gastritis. Night watching, effects. Toothache.

HOMEOPATHIC - Zinc-acet. was proved by Hahnemann and others. The only clinical uses of Zinc-acet. are from Burnett. He used Rademacher's solution of zinc in acetic acid and gave 5 drop doses three times a day in water to nurses and others who were compelled to work on an insufficient amount of sleep. Clarke verified the great value of this. Burnett also used it for erysipelas of elderly people.

The most peculiar Zinc-acet. symptoms were "Brain feels sore and as if sprinkled with salt." "Throat seems too tight and tongue too short." Empty, hungry sensation. Shaking chill during and after vomiting. Pain and paralytic condition of arms. In the provers it produced a pustular eruption on forehead and knee and the latter was attended with voluptuous itching.

Modalities - Toothache is worse by touch. Worse in evening. Worse by motion, walking in open air.

REFERENCES - Clarke.

ZINCUM ARSENICOSUM

PHARMACY - zinc-ar. Zincum arsenicosum. ***Historical dose:*** All potencies.

CLINICAL - Anemia. Backaches. Chorea. Nervous, disorders. Night watching. Numbness. Prostration. Weakness.

HOMEOPATHIC - Zinc-ar. affects the lumbar region and lower limbs. Chorea. Numbness, right arm then left, better when writing. Lumbar pain, worse from exertion, sitting, jarring or standing. Occipital pain. Blue vision. Burning in bladder.

Anemia. Neurasthenia. Weakness, enervation, exhaustion, prostration, infirmity. Profound exhaustion on slight exertion. Slight exertion aggravates. Soles ache when tired, better pressure.

Worse exertion, ascending stairs. Weakness, in acute diseases. Weakness and infirmity from nursing the sick. Ailments from night watching. Desires to walk. Worse from 10 a.m. and 3 p.m.

REFERENCES - Clarke.

ZINCUM BROMATUM

(Zinc Bromide)

PHARMACY - zinc-br. Zincum bromatum. Zinc bromide. Solution. ***Historical dose:*** All potencies.

CLINICAL - Chorea. Cramps. Dentition. Hydrocephalus.

HOMEOPATHIC - Hale used Zinc-br. on its double indications for teething children who suffer intensely from pain in nerves of head and face. Pains which throw the children into a state of stupor alternating with wakefulness. Hale used the 3c and 6c potencies.

REFERENCES - Clarke.

ZINCUM CHROMATUM

(Zinc Chromate)

PHARMACY - zinc-chr. Zincum chromatum. Zinc chromate. Chrome. Trituration. ***Historical dose:*** All potencies.

HOMEOPATHIC - Zinc-chr. acts upon the ears, nose, throat and left side. Aching, gnawing, grinding, pain or wandering in shocks. Catching stitches that impede motion.

MIND - Aversion to work.

Abdomen - Cannot tolerate her hands on abdomen.

Back - Gnawing and grinding below and above left scapula.

Ears - Throbbing behind the ears.

Eyes - Vision wavering.

Female - Dryness of vagina with sense of a coming sickness, 10 to 12 a.m.

Food - Indefinite craving, knows not for what. Aversion to even thinking of food.

Head - Inward pressure in spot on bregma. Throbbing temples.

Heart - Cutting at apex, at night.

Limbs - Feet sore. Cramps of gnawing, grinding pain in toes, at night.

Lungs - Cough from tickling in throat-pit. Expectoration, sweet, loose, but had to be swallowed or tough with constant spitting spells.

Modalities - ***Worse from motion***. Worse lying on the back. Worse washing the head.

Mouth - Metallic taste in mouth.

Nose - Bad odor within nose. Blowing of pus and blood and scabs.

Throat - Shooting pain from larynx (left side) up through tonsils into ear.

REFERENCES - Clarke.

ZINCUM CYANATUM

(Zinc Cyanide)

PHARMACY - zinc-cy. Zincum cyanatum. Zinc cyanide. Trituration. ***Historical dose:*** All potencies.

CLINICAL - Agitation. Chorea. Congestive Headaches. Constipation. Convulsions. Epilepsy. Hysteria. Meningitis. Parkinson's disease. Petit mal. Trembling.

HOMEOPATHIC - Kopp's proving showed it produces the nervous and mental symptoms of Zinc met. with great intensity. Useful for convulsions and paralytic conditions. Great physical agitation. General trembling. Parkinson's disease. Petit mal.

MIND - Great excitement. Great sensitiveness. Bad temper.

Face - Face suddenly changes color.

Head - Congestion to head.

Rectum - Constipation.

REFERENCES - Clarke.

ZINCUM IODATUM

(Zinc Iodide)

PHARMACY - zinc-i. Zincum iodatum. Zinc iodide. Solution in syrup. Trituration. ***Historical dose:*** All potencies.

CLINICAL - Constipation. Coughs. Throat, pain. Tuberculosis.

HOMEOPATHIC - Zinc-i. has been proved by American provers, producing some well-defined symptoms, including splinter-like pain in throat. A cough from tickling in the throat and the more he coughed the worse the tickling became.

A peculiar tingling in right side of face to vertex with tension in skin of the part. Undulating pain at border of right free ribs, extending to third rib on same side. Coldness in stomach and bowels with tendency to perspire.

RELATIONS - ***Compare:*** (1) Splinter pain in throat, Hep., Arg-n. (2) The more he coughs the worse it tickles, Ign.

REFERENCES - Clarke.

ZINCUM METALLICUM

(Zinc Metal)

PHARMACY - zinc. Zincum metallicum. Zinc metal. An Element, (Zn, At. Wt. 64.9). Trituration of the metal. ***Historical dose:*** All potencies.

CLINICAL - ***Alcoholism.*** Amblyopia. Asthma. Bedwetting. ***Brain-fag.*** Brain, paralysis. Breasts, disorders. Breast-milk, disorders. Cataract. Chilblains. Chin, eruptions. Chlorosis. ***Cholera. Cholera, infantum***. Chorea. Constipation. ***Convulsions***. Cracks. Dentition. Diarrhea. Diphtheria. Dysentery. Dysuria. Earaches. Ear, discharges. Eczema. Emaciation. ***Epilepsy***. ***Eruptions, suppressed.*** Esophagus, spasms. Eyes, affections. Eyelids granular. Fatigue.

Foot sweat, suppressed. Gastralgia. ***Headaches. Head, injury.*** Heels, pains. Hernia, inguinal. Hiccoughs. Hydrocephalus. Hypochondriasis. Hysteria. Joints, cracking. Lips, disorders. Lochia, suppressed. Masturbation. Melancholy. Memory, weakness. ***Meningitis.*** Mental, weakness. Neuralgias. ***Nerve, weakness.*** Nipples, sore. Nymphomania. ***Paralysis.*** Paresis. Photopsia. Prostate, discharge. Ptosis. ***Restless, legs.*** Rheumatism. Sleepiness. Sleepwalking. Spermatorrhea. ***Spinal irritation.*** Spine disorders. Spleen, pain. Strabismus. ***Suppressions.*** Tarsal tumors. Throat, sore. Tibia, burning. Tympanitis. Typhoid, fever. Ulcers. Urinary, retention. Varicose veins. Whooping cough. Worms.

HOMEOPATHIC - Zincum metallicum belongs to the magnesium group of metals, comprising also cadmium and calcium. It has long been known in the arts, especially in its combination with copper (Cupr.) in the manufacture of brass. Zinc was proved by Hahnemann and his associates, and it appears among the remedies in his book Chronic Diseases.

Weyner related the poisoning of cows pasturing near a cadmium mine, near which zinc-smelting was carried on. Effects included general emaciation, skin clinging tightly to the body, eyes pale bluish, drawn back into the orbits, horns and ears unequally warm, mouth hot and shiny and hanging down, at times dry, appetite undisturbed, rumination slower, dung grass-green, thin-flowing and fetid, at times a cough.

As the disease progressed, emaciation increased, the horns became rough, milk dried up and diarrhea increased until the animals could no longer rise and died of total prostration.

Zinc corresponds to the poisoning of nerves and the brain. ***Brain and nerves are fatigued.*** Poisoning from ***suppressed eruptions or discharges.*** Tissues are worn out faster than they are repaired. Decreased number and destruction of red blood corpuscles. Defective vitality. Marked anemia with profound prostration, increasing weariness, worse eating, with restlessness.

Difficulty developing discharges or exanthemata. Great relief from discharges. Bloody discharges. Suppressed eruptions. Chorea from fright or suppressed eruption. Neuralgia after shingles, better touch.

Chronic diseases with brain and spinal symptoms, trembling, convulsive twitching and ***fidgety feet. Convulsions with pale face and no heat.*** Spinal disorders. Twitchings. Convulsive twitching or jerking, worse at night during sleep. Spasms from spinal injuries. Descending paralysis. Impending brain paralysis.

Isolated effects, formication. One part numb another sensitive, one part hot, other part cold. Transverse pain, shooting pains. Pain in spots, between skin and flesh. Disabling bone pains.

Internal trembling. Fidgety feet and other automatic motions of mouth, arms and hands. Feels numb, all over, on lying down. Chilblains, blueness of the surface. ***Intolerance of wine. Wine aggravates all symptoms.***

MIND - Muddled mind. ***Brain-fag.*** Weak memory. Forgets what has been accomplished during day. ***Lethargic, stupid, forgetful.*** Stupefaction after nosebleed. Averse to work, to talk. Excitement over trifles. Excitement after hearing horrible things.

Ill effects of fright, grief, anger. Fretful, peevish, cries if vexed or moved during sleep (children). ***Child repeats everything said to it.*** Chorea from fright. Fear of robbers. Anxiety about thieves. Anxiety from horrible apparition. Desire for company from apprehension and boredom.

Starting in fright. Stares as if frightened on waking and rolls head from side to side. Fears being arrested on account of an imagined crime. ***Confusion, dullness after wine.*** Great fear, as if persecuted by men or the devil on account of crimes which he has never done. Fears of becoming imprisoned or poisoned, or shot, or buried alive.

Changeable moods. Alternately fretful, irritable, quarrelsome, despondent, depressed. ***Irritability in evening.*** Impetuous. Weeps when angry. Hypochondriacal mood with gastric symptoms.

Melancholy. Cerebral depression. Paresis. Sadness when alone. ***Periods of depression with disease.*** Answers very slow and speaks as if in a bad temper. Thinks of death calmly. ***Religious affections.*** Hears voices speaking from within him in abusive and filthy language.

Easily startled, excited or intoxicated. ***Very sensitive to noise.*** Sensitive to others, talking and noise. Easily offended. Weeping from vexation. Screams with pain. ***Torments everyone with his complaints.*** Loquacity. Hysteria better during menses. Kisses everyone before menses. Starting from sleep during menses. Nymphomania during pregnancy. Causeless weeping before menses.

Abdomen - Griping in upper abdomen after soup. Violent cutting pain in abdomen after milk. Sensation as if a lump in liver region or at navel. Neuralgia of spleen. Jerking from groins to penis. Pain after a light meal with tympanitis. Gurgling and griping, distended. Flatulence and rumbling, worse alcohol. Hypogastric flatulence. Hot, putrid flatus. Flatulent colic with retraction of abdomen (Plb.). Reflex symptoms from floating kidney.

Back - Pain in small of back. Backache better seminal emission. Spinal irritation. Spine sensitive, cannot bear it touched (Agar., Ther.). ***Burning along whole spine,*** worse sitting. Aching in spine, small of the back worse turning in bed, sitting and stooping. ***Dull aching about the last dorsal or first lumbar vertebrae, worse sitting.*** Cracking in lumbar region while walking. Lumbar region as if screwed in, on rising from seat. Weakness in lumbar region worse standing. Tension and stinging between shoulders. Tearing pain, burning in shoulder blades, between shoulder blades, better belchings. Small pimples like boils on and between scapulae.

Bladder - Bladder symptoms better urination. Cramp in bladder, preceded by colic. Bladder neuralgia. Pressure upon bladder, but not to urinate. Constant pressure downward in urethra if call to urinate is delayed. Frequent urging at night with scanty discharge. Involuntary urination when walking, coughing or sneezing. Burning urination during menses. Burning in urethra before, during and after urination. Cutting pain in orifice of urethra, in evening while sitting. Bleeding after urination. Vicarious bleeding from suppressed menses.

Breasts - Breasts and genitals painful with suppressed menses (Kali-c.). Breasts swollen and sore to touch. Left breast as if swollen. Violent pressing in right breast. Itching about nipples. Nipples sore. Pressing, sore, about right nipple. Stitching pain, beneath breast.

Causations - Ill effects of fright, grief, anger, surgery, night watching, excessive study. Ill effects from brain concussion, frostbite, suppressions of eruptions, otorrhea, menses, lochia, milk. Chorea from fright or from suppressed eruptions, worse during sleep, the feet especially affected.

Chest - Acute stitches in left clavicle. Dull stitches in right side of chest. Burning pressure beneath sternum. Constriction and cutting in chest. Tightness in chest on walking in open air. Chest as if constricted by a band transversely across it. Pressure in chest as from incarcerated flatus. Pressure under short ribs after eating. Left-sided intercostal neuralgia. Chest as if hollow and cold, after expectoration of tenacious mucus. Weak and burning feeling in sternum. Empty sensation behind sternum. Burning in left axilla. Pain in chest as if beaten. Violent stitches in chest when walking in open air.

Constitutions - Nervous constitutions.

Coughs - Cough, must sit up, with asthmatic breathing. Cough after wine. Debilitating, spasmodic cough, worse eating sweets. Dry cough, before and during menses. Short cough from tickling beneath sternum. Cough much relieved as soon as he brings up something. Child grasps genitals during cough.

Ears - Earache with frequent acute sharp pains in children. Itching, better boring into it. Tearing, stitches and external swelling. Discharge of fetid pus. Offensive moisture from left ear. Neuralgia of middle ear. Cartilage of ear extremely sensitive.

Ringing, whizzing in ear. Impaired, from increase of earwax.

Eyes - Intense burning after eye operation. Pterygium, smarting, lachrymation, itching. Smarting as from salt in eye. Eyes as if pressed inward. Pressure as if pressed into head. Itching and soreness of lids and ***inner canthi.*** Conjunctivitis. Red and inflamed conjunctiva, ***worse inner canthus.*** Pupils contracted during headache. Pupils dilated alternating with contracted. Blurring of one-half of vision, worse stimulants. with severe headache. Photophobia during headache. Dread of sunlight, with dim, watery eyes. Amaurosis Ptosis. Upper lids heavy, as if paralyzed. ***Rolling of eyes.*** Eyes feel drawn together. ***Squinting***.

Face - Face pale and cold, alternating with heat and redness of cheeks. Bluish, miserable. Paleness of face during convulsions. Waxy, white or yellow face. Lips, sticky, dry, cracked. ***Pale lips*** and cracked corners of mouth. Redness and itching eruptions on chin. Tearing pain in facial bones. Bones of face as if bruised. Swelling and itching of left cheek. Spasmodic twitching.

Female - Female symptoms are associated with ***restlessness, depression, coldness, spinal tenderness and restless feet***. Downward pressure on uterus, bladder and rectum, compelling her to sit cross-legged. Stinging pain in pudendum when walking. Bloody leucorrhea, with burning an itching of pudenda, after menses. Menses too early, painful, with bloating of abdomen. Profuse lumpy menses when walking. Menses too late, suppressed, lochia suppressed (Puls.). Menses flow more at night (Bov.). Complaints all ***better during menstrual flow*** (Eupi., Lach.). Ovarian pain, better excessive flow. Ovarian pain, ***especially left, can't keep still*** (Vib.). Sexual desire increased. Nymphomania of lying-in women. Desire for masturbation. Complete loss of sexual desire. Profuse falling of hair from genitals. Varicose veins of external genitals, with fidgety feet.

Food - Loss of appetite, with clean tongue. ***Ravenous hunger*** about 11 a.m. (Sulph.). Great greediness when eating, cannot eat fast enough. Extreme thirst. Thirst, with heat in palms. Desire for beer. Aversion to meat, especially veal, during pregnancy. Aversion to sweets, cooked or warm food. ***Wine aggravates,*** cannot stand smallest quantity of wine.

Head - Brain-fag, headaches of overtaxed school children. ***Forehead cool, base of brain hot***. Roaring in head. Dullness of head after meals. ***Headaches from drinking small quantity of wine.*** Headache with dim vision worse heat. Pressive pain on vertex, at the root of the nose, extending to eyes with weak vision worse warmth, better hard pressure, open air. Heavy aching pain in temples, worse biting. Meningitis. Hydrocephalus after infantile cholera or diarrhea. Rolls head, bores in pillows and grinds teeth. ***Occipital*** pain with weight on vertex. Crashing in head, on falling to sleep. Feels as if he would fall to left side. Hair falls from vertex. Vertex bald with soreness of scalp. Hair brittle, bristle, sensitive. Brain paralysis. Automatic motion of head and hands.

Heart - Pressure, spasmodic tension and heaviness in heart. Sensations if a cap over the heart. Hard heartbeat, taking breath away. Irregular, spasmodic action of the heart, occasionally one violent tnump. Tension and stitches in precordial region. Stitch at every beat of heart, with palpitations. Violent pulsations in blood vessels during fever. Pulse increased by wine.

Kidneys - Floating kidney. Reflex symptoms from floating kidneys. Pressive cutting about kidneys. Pressure in region of left kidney. Can only pass urine if sitting bent backwards. Hysterical retention of urine. Unable to retain the urine unless the feet are in constant motion. Stitches in kidneys. Sticking and bruised pain in left kidney while standing and walking. Left kidney sensitive to touch.

Limbs - ***Restless feet in continued motion, cannot keep them still.*** Lameness, ***weakness, trembling and twitching*** of various muscles. Stumbling, spastic gait totters while walking especially in the dark and with closed eyes. Lightning-like pain of locomotor ataxia, sweaty feet with sore toes. Pains in limbs on becoming heated. Chilblains (Agar.). ***Large varicose veins on legs***. Burning in tibia. ***Soles of feet sensitive.*** Steps with entire sole of foot on floor. Toes, feel swollen, sore, tips ache. Bones of the feet feel broken. Paralysis of feet. Ulcerative pain in heel worse walking. Formication of feet and legs as of insects crawling over the skin, prevents sleep, better rubbing and pressure. ***Transverse pains***, especially in upper extremity. Hysterical contradictions, drawing the fingers out of shape. Weakness and trembling of the hands, when writing during menses. Eczema on hands. Sweaty. Pain in deltoid worse raising arm.

Liver - Liver enlarged, indurated, hard and sore. Squeezing, pressure and shootings in the hepatic region. Sharp stitches in hepatic region after supper.

Lungs - Dyspnea from flatulence after eating. ***Dyspnea, better as soon as expectoration appears,*** worse flatulence. Oppressed and difficult breathing. Very heavy and deep breathing. Breathing, impeded, with apprehension and oppression. Asthmatic bronchitis with constriction of chest. Easy expectoration, at night when lying down, with cough. Copious, expectoration of frothy mucus. Yellow, purulent expectoration. Blood-streaked expectoration. Tenacious, sweetish, putrid expectoration. Metallic tasting expectoration. Large amount of mucus of milky color.

Male - Drawing pain in testicles, spermatic cords. Penis painfully sensitive. Long-lasting and violent erections. Easy sexual excitement, emission too rapid or difficult during embrace. Emissions with hypochondriasis. Sadness after emission. Discharge of prostatic fluid without any cause. Atrophy of testes. Neuralgia of testes worse walking. Testicles swollen, drawn up. Shriveling of scrotum. Falling off of pubic hair. Grasps genitals with cough.

Modalities - Better while eating. ***Better free discharges*** and appearance of eruptions, menses. Better rubbing, scratching. Better motion, hard pressure. Better warm, open air. ***Worse from exhaustion,*** mental or physical. Worse after eating, ***after wine***. Worse sweet things, milk. Worse from noise. ***Worse suppressed eruptions or discharges, menses.*** Worse between 5 p.m. to 7 p.m. Worse being heated, touching anything cold, being touched. Worse approach of storms which causes chills.

Mouth - Bitter or bloody taste. Copious secretion of saliva. Sour, bitter water in mouth. Fetid breath. Inflammation of palate. Ulcers on inner surface of cheek and in throat. Herpes in mouth from sea bathing. Grinds teeth. Gnashing of teeth. Teeth loose. Difficult dentition, child weak, cold and restless feet. Bleeding gums. Echoes speech.

Neck - Pinching feeling on both sides of neck. ***Nape of neck feels weary and tired*** from writing or any mental exertion. Neck feels lame, followed by stupor. Pain in cervical muscles at night.

Nose - Sore feeling high up, pressure upon root. Stoppage of nose. Obstruction of nose. Fluent coryza with hoarseness and burning sensation in chest. Coryza with hoarseness and burning in chest. Frequent sneezing. Sneezing after meals. Frequent blowing of blood from nose. Nosebleed followed by stupefaction. Swollen. Pain as from excoriation in interior of nose. Redness of nose, remaining after freezing, tip of nose easily frosted. Bores finger into nose or picks at dry lips.

Perspiration - Offensive, sour-smelling sweat. Can't tolerate any covering during sweat. Profuse sweat all night, wants to uncover. Easy perspiration, during day, from exercise. Sour sweat with itching over whole body. Sweats on head and hands. Sweats while walking in open air. Sweats at night, especially on lower limbs. Sweaty feet.

Rectum - Desire for stool after eating. Nervous diarrhea. Affections of brain from sudden stoppage of diarrhea. Cholera-like diarrhea in infants. ***Cholera infantum*** with tenesmus. Constipation of newborn infants. Ulceration of hemorrhoids. Hemorrhoids prolapsed, better heat, worse walking. Crawling as from worms in anus. Soreness, drawing pain in rectum. Burning, sticking pain, itching in anus, during and after stool. Itching in anus with oozing of corrosive moisture.

Sensations - Uneasy, as if he had committed a crime. As if he would have a stroke. As if hair bristled. As if scalp were drawn together. As if she had a large goiter which she could not see over. Pains as if between the skin and the flesh. Nauseating weakness as after smoking too strong tobacco. As if kidney would be twisted off. Wrist and foot as if sprained. As if soles swollen. As if tendons of right sole too short. As if ball of great toe frozen.

Skin - Eczema. Eczema of the hands, in the anemic and neurotic. Sudden itching here and there. Itching of thighs. ***Itching in the hollow of knees.*** Formication of feet and legs as from a bug crawling over the skin, preventing sleep. Urticaria-like eruption after scratching. ***Retrocession of eruptions.*** Ulcers. Slight injury of skin bleeds very profusely. ***Varicose veins***, especially of lower limbs (Puls.). Varicose veins of genital organs.

Sleep - Constant yawning. Overpowering sleepiness. Nervous insomnia with intolerable itching of skin at night. Broken, unrefreshing sleep. Sleep disturbed by violent headaches and painful cramps in calves. Jerks and starts on falling asleep. Cries out while sleeping, body jerks, wakes frightened, startled. Nervous motion of feet when asleep (Kali-p.). Loud screaming in sleep without being aware of it. Somnambulism (Kali-p.), after suppressed emotions. Awakens at night from coldness of feet.

Stomach - Atonic dyspepsia, feeling as if stomach were collapsed. Empty feeling at stomach soon after eating. Burning in stomach. Heartburn from sweet things. Hiccough after breakfast. Bitter eructations after eating, followed by vomiting. Sour eructations, after milk. Sweetish rising into throat with sweet taste. Globus hystericus rising from pit of stomach. Sensation as if a worm crawling up to the throat from the pit of stomach, causing coughing. Nausea, vomiting of bitter mucus. Nausea and vomiting, worse wine. Nausea from taking even a small sip of wine. Nausea from sight of meat or anything fatty. Vomiting of almost all food or liquid immediately after swallowing it.

Stools - Hard, small, constipated stool. Stools, large, dry, difficult, followed by involuntary urination. Offensive, diarrheic stools alternating with constipation. Stool at first solid, then liquid. Very soft stool immediately after dinner, with and followed by vertigo and roaring in head. Green mucus discharges.

Teeth - Drawing, tearing, jerking pains. Throbbing in a hollow tooth. Grinding of teeth. Sensations as if teeth would be pulled out. Teeth as if long and loose, with swelling of submaxillary glands. Teeth as if sore. Teeth feel on edge. Difficult dentition. Bleeding gums on slightest touch. Retraction of gums. Gums painful while eating. Gums white, ulcerated.

Temperature - Chills begin after dinner. Chilliness in the back, as if fever would appear. Cold limbs, especially hands and legs. Chills from touching anything cold. Chills on approach of a storm. Frequent, febrile shiverings down back, with flushes of heat, trembling of limbs, short breathing and pulsation throughout whole body. Chills followed by cold sweat. Chill alternating with heat. Fever at night, often with sweat. Febrile flushes, with sudden crying out to be fanned, and thirst.

Throat - Hoarseness with burning in trachea. Dry, constant inclination to hawk up tenacious mucus. Frequent acute tickling in region of larynx. Rawness and dryness in throat and larynx, better eating. Pain in muscles of throat externally while swallowing. Pain in fauces when yawning. Bitter taste in throat. Accumulation of mucus in larynx and posterior nares.

Tongue - Tongue coated at root and dry, in brain affections. Tongue white, as from cheese, without taste. Tongue swollen on left side, hindering talking. Blisters on tongue. Tongue covered with vesicles or with white mucus. Stitches in tip of tongue with salivation.

Urine - Urine turbid, loam-colored in morning. Urine very yellow, deposits white flakes on standing a long time. Emission of urine very slow and in a thin stream. Dribbling urine in evening.

Vertigo - Vertigo in occiput. Violent vertigo with stupor. Vertigo deeply seated in brain. Vertigo as if he would have a stroke. Vertigo, as if the seat were undulating when sitting up in bed in morning. Vertigo while sitting up in bed, as if bed were constantly swaying back and forth. Vertigo as if looking through mist, after eating. Vertigo while smoking.

Vision - Blurring of one-half of vision. Dim and misty vision in morning after waking. Dim vision during severe headache. Dim vision watery eyes in brain affections. Dim vision with itching and stitching pain in inner canthi. Impaired vision, as if a thick fog lay before eyes, during headache. Luminous bodies after eye operation. Objects appear elongated. Yellow, blue and green rings. Diplopia. Flickering vision. Fiery flakes floating in large circles, when looking at sky. Vanishing vision with lachrymation and burning.

COMMENTS - Severe fatigue, nerve or brain-fatigue, muscle-fatigue. Brain-fatigue from over-study or from night watching (Cocc.). Restores suppressed eruptions. Can cure the consequences of suppressions and set free the reactive power in conditions of undeveloped disease.

Symptoms worse from suppressed discharges, particularly foot sweat. "Too weak to develop exanthemata or menstrual function to expectorate or urinate to understand to remember."

"Relief to all suffering as soon as menses begin to flow" or discharge is restored. Nash noted that in asthma "the patient cannot expectorate, but as soon as he can he is relieved."

Sexual excitement in both genders. Seminal losses and prostatorrhea of the male. Nymphomania and masturbation in the female, can be associated with varicose veins or itching of the external genitals. Tendency to press on the pubes or apply the hand to the genitals. Severe boring pain in the left ovary.

Backache with emission, temporarily better by the emission. Backache and spinal irritation in female sexual disorders as well. Dull aching in spine, worse when sitting. Burning pains all along the spine. Burning pains, tension and constriction.

Facial neuralgias, trigeminal neuralgias. Facial twitches and tics (Agar., Spig.). Neuralgia in malar bones with pressive pains. Pressure at root of nose as if it would be pressed in. Grinds teeth, especially in children with worms. "Teeth fail to develop."

Constriction in the chest, connected with both respiration and the heart. "Sudden, spasmodic, bursting sensation about heart, it appears to be beating regularly, when it suddenly seems as if it would burst through the chest." Varicose veins of the thighs and labia, with fidgety feet.

Insatiable hunger and emptiness, notably at 11 a.m. Great thirst. Hasty eating and drinking. Averse to meat, especially veal, sweets, cooked or warm food. Pain is worse from eating or drinking wine. Tearing headache in side of head, worse from wine, after dinner. Intolerance of wine, wine aggravates all symptoms. Drunk easily. Vascular headaches aggravated by the least sip of wine or alcohol. Vertigo from the least alcohol.

Numbness, tingling, formication and fainting spells. "Incessant and violent fidgety feeling in feet or lower limbs, must move them constantly, cannot keep them quiet." These movements may continue during sleep. Insomnia with restless legs.

Great restlessness in the legs and feet. Great urge to stretch the legs. Hyper reflex alternating with low reflex response. Hyperactivity with restlessness. Tendency toward spasms, leg cramps (Cupr.). Jerking and twitchings of the limbs, convulsions, epilepsy. Convulsions in children, with a history of cradle cap (Cupr.). Crawling, numbness, tingling sensation. Legs go to sleep easily, painful. Painful formication of the legs.

Neuralgic shingles. Parkinson's disease where the key trembling is of the legs and feet, as opposed to the arms, with pacing and restlessness. Multiple sclerosis.

Spinal atrophy and deterioration of the spinal cord. Paralysis, but the legs shake or are restless and move. Paralysis after diphtheria (Lac-c.).

Meningitis with sharp pains in the head, worse from the least stimulant. Encephalitis, with brain cry (*cri cephalic*) (Apis.). Hearing loss after meningitis (Hell.). Children with brain disorders have a characteristic "crossness in the evening." On waking there is delirium as if frightened, knows no one, screaming. "Child repeats everything said to it."

Tendency to chilblains, which are swollen and painful and easily made worse by rubbing. Sensitiveness to frostbite, the tip of the nose is easily frostbitten and the nose remains red long after it has been frostbitten. The hands and feet are affected with inflammation, painful eruptions, cracks. There is also a "frost-bitten feeling" in the toes.

Gerstel called attention to Zinc's action in fevers with inflammation of the brain. In these cases the seat of the inflammation was the meninges.

He referred to a case of a child suffering from scarlatina who was "Entirely motionless, limbs icy cold, body cold, skin all over body bluish red, except the parts about the eyes, forehead and chin, which were white." Zinc was then given and the child gradually recovered.

In a case of typhoid in a man in whom mental symptoms had set in, there was a "Muddled feeling in the head, an incapacity to relate anything and a sort of half-smiling loquacity."

Later on he had a "Staring look, almost hippocratic appearance, pale as wax, carphologia, subsultus tendinum, constant trembling of the hands." Zinc 2c saved the patient.

General twitchings and trembling, according to Nash, are equally characteristic of Zinc. He recorded the case of Miss Smith., 20, who had been ill for a week with headache, loss of appetite and especially prostration. Over-study was the cause.

Under Gels., and later Bry., she was improving, when she threw off the bedclothes while sleeping and perspiring and took a chill. The bowels became enormously distended, profuse hemorrhage occurred (finally controlled by Alumn.), a low form of delirium came on and prostration increased in spite of the cessation of hemorrhage.

Her head was retracted, with complete unconsciousness. Staring eyes rolled upward. Lying on back and sliding down in bed, twitching or rather "intense, violent trembling all over so that she shook the bed." Her hands had to be held constantly night and day by nurses. Hippocratic face, limbs deathly cold to knees and elbows. The pulse was intermittent, uncountable, all signs in short of impending paralysis of the brain.

Two drops of Zinc 200c were mixed in two teaspoonfuls of water. One teaspoonful was worked, a little at a time, between the set teeth and the rest half an hour later. About an hour after the latter dose the patient turned down her eyes and said "Milk." Through a bent tube she swallowed half a glass of milk, the first nourishment she had taken for twenty-four hours.

From that time she improved steadily and received no more medicine for four days. Afterwards she had a dose of Nux-v. Recovery was perfect.

F. W. Payne reported a case of cataract in which the right eye was partially affected and the left was practically useless. There was a bruised, sore, smarting, burning, itching and stinging sensation. At intervals, a sudden sensation as if pepper had been thrown into the eye, causing scalding lachrymation and spasm of the lids.

These spells were worse in the evening. Burning dryness as if a stick was under lid scratching eyeball. Flickering before left eye, blue and green rings, green halo around gas-jet at times.

Slight irritation of conjunctiva and tendency of lids to adhere. Worse by warmth, on warm days, by artificial light. Patient nervous, tremulous, impatient, worse by mental emotion. Chorea jerking of individual muscles.

Zinc 200c, given occasionally, steadily improved the case. In six months, the right eye was quite clear and the left steadily gaining. Eleven years later, vision was practically perfect, though some small streaks could still be found in the left lens.

RELATIONS - ***Antidoted by:*** Hep., Ign., Camph. (Lob., Teste). ***Antidote to:*** Bar-c. ***Compare:*** (1) Agar., Ign., Plb., Arg-n., Puls., Hell., Tub. (2) Erratic temperature in fevers, Puls. (3) Colic, Puls., Lyc. (4) Abdominal symptoms, Plb., Podo. (5) Tremors, Arg-n. (6) Spinal pain, Cob., Sep. (7) Asthma with great constriction of chest, Cadm-s., Kali-c, Cact. (8) Boring fingers in nose, Cina, Verat., Arum-t. (9) Scarlatina, Bell. (Zinc follows well when rash fails to come out and child screams whenever moved). (10) Hydrocephalus, Calc-p. (11) Pain in back worse sitting than walking, Sep., Cob., Arg-n. ***Complementary:*** In hydrocephalus, Calc-p. ***Followed well by:*** Sep., Sulph., Puls., Ign. ***Follows well:*** Apis, Bell. ***Incompatible:*** Cham., Nux-v.-v. ***Inimical:*** Nux-v., Cham.

REFERENCES - Boericke. Clarke. Murphy. Phatak.

ZINCUM MURIATICUM

(Zinc Chloride)

PHARMACY - zinc-m. Zinc muriaticum. Zinc chloride. Solutions in water or alcohol. ***Historical dose:*** All potencies.

CLINICAL - Bright's, disease. Chorea. Constipation. Convulsions. Cramps. Diphtheria. Dysentery. Emaciation. Hematemesis. Hiccoughs. Hydrocephalus. Smell, perverted. Taste, perverted. Typhoid fever. Wounds.

HOMEOPATHIC - The bulk of the symptoms of Zinc-m. are derived from poisoning cases. Zinc chloride is an active poison and a powerful disinfectant and, being readily accessible in the form of "Sir Wm. Burnett's Disinfectant Fluid," has occasioned many poisonings, both accidental and suicidal.

Most of the Zinc-m. symptoms are the usual effects of a corrosive poison, but some characteristic symptoms appear. One of them was the perversion of the senses of smell and taste. Things had a putrid smell and taste which were not putrid and feces had no odor at all. Quinine had no bitter taste and acids and alkalis had no acid or alkaline taste. Insipid things were most relished.

Other Zinc-m. symptoms were "No natural appetite, but a morbid craving for something to allay the irritation at the stomach." "Vomiting of all food except boiled milk." "Occasional attacks of tetanic spasms of right forearm and hand."

"Emaciation, skin looked as if stretched tightly over bones of face and hands." "Bluish and blue-mottled skin." "Sleeps on right side with legs drawn up, grinds teeth." Spasmodic twitchings of face and hands, sprains and convulsions were prominent features.

De Noe Walker used a dilution of Zinc-m. as an application to fresh wounds and found it very effectual in securing rapid healing.

REFERENCES - Clarke.

ZINCUM OXYDATUM

(Zinc Oxide)

PHARMACY - zinc-o. Zincum oxydatum. Zinc oxide. Flowers of Zinc. Trituration. ***Historical dose:*** All potencies.

CLINICAL - Anorexia. Coryza. Debility. Deltoid, pain. Diaphragm, neuralgia. Elbow, pain. Hiccough. Hypochondriasis. Laughter, involuntary. Sleeplessness.

HOMEOPATHIC - An extensive proving of Zinc-o. was made by Wernek, Buchner and Michaelis. These symptoms have been included by Allen in the pathogenesis of Zinc. and some of them will be found in the schema of Zinc.

Jahr kept a separate record of Zinc-o. and Clarke added to his account. The contracting, shriveling-up effect of Zinc-o. was marked in these provings.

Among the more peculiar symptoms were an undulating movement in some muscles. Contraction of the risible muscles and constant impulse to laugh. Teeth blunted incisors feel soft and glued together. Hiccoughs, that are better after regurgitation of bile. Liquid stools which better all symptoms.

In the Zinc-o. provings, the left lung was very markedly affected. Coryza, worse after a meal with difficulty to respiration and nasal secretion. Stoppage of the nose. Anorexia better after a meal.

COMMENTS - Farrington said that Zinc-o. is very like Con. in hypochondriasis and melancholy from masturbation, the difference being that Zinc-o. is irritating as well as weakening and depressing.

REFERENCES - Clarke.

ZINCUM PHOSPHORICUM

(Zinc Phosphide)

PHARMACY - zinc-p. Zincum phosphoricum. Zinc phosphide. Trituration. ***Historical dose:*** All potencies.

CLINICAL - Asthma. ***Anemia.*** Brain-fag. Bronchitis. Chorea. Coma. Delirium tremens. Dementia. Epilepsy. Fainting. Headaches. Hemorrhages. Herpes zoster. Hydrocephalus. Hyperventilation. Impotence. Insomnia. Kidneys, irritable. Meningitis. ***Migraine.*** Multiple sclerosis. Nausea. Nerve, disorders. Neuralgia. Paralysis. Parkinson's disease. ***Restlessness.*** Sleeplessness. Tics. Tremors, mercurial. Tuberculosis. Twitchings. Vertigo. Vomiting.

HOMEOPATHIC - According to Hale, Zinc-p. removes the mental depression and paralysis following cerebral congestion and strokes. Hale used it on a combination of the indications of the elements and especially in brain fatigue of business men.

Brain fag, nervousness, and vertigo. Nervous vertigo, better lying. Formication all over body. ***Restless, repetitive movements***, head rolling, head banging, nail biting, tapping, thumb sucking, movements of the mouth, worse talking. Restless legs, worse getting to sleep, grabs the bedclothes. Tics and twitchings. Chorea.

Hands cold, feet perspire. Paralysis. Epilepsy. Burning pains. Hemorrhages of bright red blood. Cerebral hemorrhages. Petechia. ***Anemia.*** Neurological complaints. Meningitis. Hydrocephalus. Multiple sclerosis. Parkinson's disease. Vertigo and fainting. Abuse of bromides.

MIND - Moody. Changeable mood. Happy, open, enthusiastic, then gloomy, discontented, hurried. Complaining. Sentimental. Laughing, hysterical, screaming. Grumbling. Irritability, worse being woken, worse music. Mental depression. Loathing of life.

Mental exhaustion. Fatigue. Brain fatigue of businessmen. Slow mind. Forgetful. ***Loss of memory.*** Indolent. Aversion to talking. Worse talking. Nervousness. ***Restlessness.*** Apprehension, worse afternoon and night.

Anticipation and anxiety. Fear of failure, criticism. Fear of falling, heights. Fear of being alone. Fear of being pursued, thieves. Fear of being observed, touched. Fear of stroke, death. Fear of being buried, the dark. Fear of horror, ghosts. Fear of disease and death of family or friends. Fear of future. Fear of thunder. Superstitious.

Strong sexual, desire. Nymphomania, kisses everyone. Sexual excitement and sleeplessness. Delirious, chaotic, confused. Dementia. Idiotic. Mad, manic. Tourette's. Childish, very active, makes mistakes. Ailments from humiliation, insults, fright, sadness, homesickness. Coma.

Abdomen - Abdominal pains.

Back - Backache, worse carrying heavy loads, worse when sitting.

Bladder - Retention of urine, better when sitting back.

Chest - Neuralgic pains and skin symptoms like those of herpes zoster.

Eyes - Eye infections. Foggy vision. Strabismus.

Face - Sickly and haggard expression.

Female - Menses profuse. Generally better during menses.

Food - Desires sweets, licorice, beer, meat, fruit, starch, cold, fish, anchovies. Aversion to fish, milk, warm foods, sprouts, mushrooms, cloves, salt, oysters. Worse red wine, sweets, coffee.

Head - ***Migraine.*** Pressing pain in forehead, caused by schoolwork. Headache, especially in sides of head. Nervous headache. Neuralgia of head and face.

Heart - Palpitations.

Kidneys - Irritable kidneys with loss of brain power even when calculus is present. Urine becomes cloudy on standing.

Limbs - Bone problems. Growing pains. Rickets. Osteoporosis. ***Restlessness.*** Tingling fingertips. Lightning-like pains in locomotor ataxia.

Lungs - Asthma. Hyperventilation. Gasping for breath. Sighing. Tuberculosis. Bronchitis. Lung problems.

Male - Enlarged prostate. Erections with unusual voluptuousness and desire. Emissions with voluptuous dreams and intense nervous thrill.

Modalities - Better open air, perspiration, discharges. ***Better sitting back,*** lying on left side. Better noise. Better movement. Worse touch, rubbing. ***Worse from suppressed discharges, vaccination.*** Worse noise, music, light. Worse walking. Worse cats, smells, wool. Worse 5 a.m. and 9 p.m. Worse right side. Worse cold weather, thunderstorms. Very sensitive to both wind and wine.

Nose - Hay fever.

Rectum - Constipation. Diarrhea, worse wine.

Sleep - Sleeplessness aggravates. Sleepless after 3 a.m., wakes at three and feels as if under the influence of pleasant and quick music. ***Sexual excitement and sleeplessness.*** Nightmares, caused by lack of sleep. Somnambulism. Sleeps on right side. Better after short sleep. Erotic dreams. Dream of futile efforts. Dream of paralysis, exams. Dream of thieves, fleeing, of being pursued, abduction, ghosts, monsters. Dream of falling, heights. Dream of accidents, murder, quarrels.

Skin - Eczema. Herpes zoster. White spots on nails. Hair loss.

Stomach - Diabetes, worse during pregnancy. Stomach complaints. Empty sensation in stomach. Nausea and vomiting. Vomiting, worse drinking.

Teeth - Late teething. Worse during dentition.

Vertigo - Fainting. Vertigo, better lying down.

COMMENTS - Ashburton Thompson gave pills, each containing 2/3 grains of Zinc-p. to two patients and both experienced a severe frontal headache with frequent stabs of pain backward, deep in the head to occiput.

Hammond cured with it nervousness and vertigo better lying down. In some patients the Zinc-p. 3c potency caused sexual excitement and sleeplessness after 3 a.m.

J. E. Baldwin reported the case of a woman in perfect health prepared a long report and read it to a large audience without undue excitement. The next day, she had some pressure in occiput to cervical spine, lasting four days. Feeling of fatigue with disinclination to any mental exertion. Zinc-p. 2x cured in a few doses.

Zinc-p. 6x has also cured an irritable kidney with loss of memory in an old man.

RELATIONS - ***Compare:*** Phos., Zinc., Staph., Thuj., Viol-o., Viol-t.

REFERENCES - Clarke.

ZINCUM PICRICUM

(Zinc Picrate)

PHARMACY - zinc-pic. Zincum picricum. Zinc picrate. Trituration. ***Historical dose:*** All potencies.

CLINICAL - Brain, fatigue. Bright's disease. Exhaustion. Facial, paralysis. Headaches. Memory, weak. Neurasthenia. Nymphomania. Parkinson's disease. Priapism. Satyriasis. Seminal, emissions. Sexual, mania. Spinal, weakness.

HOMEOPATHIC - Hale gave this indication of Zinc-pic., "Cerebrospinal troubles of the weakness of character." Hugh Pitcairn noted brain-fag and nervous exhaustion from overworked brain or sexual excesses. Chronic occipital headaches, periodic.

Headache occurring in Bright's disease. Threatened cerebral paralysis, especially in children. Profound neurasthenia., when nervous exhaustion has passed beyond stage of weakness. Seminal emissions. Sexual mania.

COMMENTS - Halbert reported the case of recent facial paralysis from cold cured by Zinc-pic. 3x and a case of Parkinson's disease in a woman, 45, very greatly improved by the same.

Hale gave the case of Mr. M., 36, a merchant. Above ordinary intelligence. Single, correct in his habits, but subject to seminal emissions since early manhood, occurring about 3 a.m. every third night, leaving him very weak and debilitated, worse every change of weather, especially in hot weather and before and during thunderstorms. Never masturbated.

Complained of loss of memory and energy, dull, heavy feeling in head, sticky, pasty mouth, dry throat, poor appetite. Belches torrents of tasteless flatus after eating, followed by relief and diarrhea. At other times inclined to constipation. Languid, heavy feeling throughout body. Dull aching pain in back.

Zinc-pic. 2x trituration. caused steady improvement, the emissions being reduced in frequency to one in six weeks.

RELATIONS - ***Compare:*** (1) Fatigue - Pic-ac., Ferr-pic. and picrates generally.

REFERENCES - Clarke.

ZINCUM SULPHURICUM

(Zinc Sulphate)

PHARMACY - zinc-s. Zincum sulphuricum. Zinc sulphate. White Vitriol. Solution. Trituration. ***Historical dose:*** All potencies.

CLINICAL - Anemia. Convulsions. Cornea, opacity. Delirium. Dysentery. Esophagus, stricture. Granular, lids. Headache. Heartburn. Keratitis. Laughter, involuntary. Metrorrhagia. Prostration. Prurigo. Tongue, paralysis. Tremors.

HOMEOPATHIC - A large number of poisonings with Zinc-s. are on record and these have furnished the symptoms of the schema.

The use of Zinc-s. in solution as an eye lotion is founded on a specific relationship, and in homeopathic potencies it has cured corneal opacities. Obstinate keratitis in right eye goes away from a 3x lotion.

Zinc-s. has anemia, tremors and convulsions. Trembling and convulsions. Titillation all over body with irresistible inclination to laugh. Prostration. Heaviness. Feeling as though her blood could scarcely struggle through her being.

MIND - Delirium. Great nervous anxiety and depression. Frightful visions during headache, saw her child with its head shattered (cured with the headache).

Abdomen - Inflammation of abdomen with retraction of umbilicus and terrible colic. Sharp, continuous colic. Pain in abdomen and especially in bladder region in groin.

Chest - Violent burning pains beneath chest. Sense of choking and constriction around chest. Pains in chest with vomiting.

Ears - Roaring in ears.

Eyes - Obstinate keratitis. Bluish rings around eyes. Eyes are heavy and dull, staring, fixed with peculiar bright luster, spasms with upper limbs. Pupils dilated. Lachrymation. Opacity of cornea. Diffuse opacity of each cornea goes away on using a lotion around both orbits externally.

Face - Pale, sunken with cold limbs and convulsed pulse, leaden tint, contracted features.

Female - Metrorrhagia.

Head - Violent headache with thirst. Burning, acute pain in head. Immediately felt as if a painful electric shock had gone through his head, he expected his brains would have burst through his skull.

Heart - Pulse fluttering indistinguishable, dicrotic, almost lost, as in cholera.

Limbs - Trembling and cramps. Convulsive movements of upper limbs and eyeballs.

Lungs - Violent cough with bloody and purulent expectoration. Breathing weak, slow, difficult.

Mouth - Very sour taste. Tongue moist, a little blanched, partially paralyzed. Tongue, mouth and lips greatly swollen. Gums swollen and red on outer edge. Irritation of whole buccal membrane.

Rectum - Rectal tenesmus. Constant desire for stool. Purging and vomiting. Bilious diarrhea. Stools infrequent. After three months stools became bloody with sticking and cutting pains in both sides of abdomen and along colon. Obstinate dysentery with emaciation, pale, bloody stools, painful tenesmus and desire for food that failed to nourish.

Skin - Skin pale yellow. Deadly pallor, skin milky white. Herpes zoster. Blisters on neck discharge first bloody water, later thin, green, ill-smelling pus. Frightful prurigo of children affecting the back.

Sleep - Sleepy and stupid, wanted to sleep and die in peace.

Stomach - Thirst, intolerable and dry mouth. Burning heat in stomach with acute pain in epigastrium. Heartburn. Vomiting and purging with cramps, severe pain and burning in stomach and extreme prostration.

Temperature - Coldness. Shivering violently, slight quivering of lips. Skin and limbs cold and clammy. Hands covered with cold, clammy sweat, but to herself they felt hot and she tried to get hold of anything to cool them. Profuse sweat. Fever followed by profuse sweat. Constant heat, preventing sleep. Burning heat of limbs.

Throat - Inflammation, threatening suffocation. Tenderness in throat. Burning and constriction in fauces. Esophagus is so contracted he fears choking.

Vertigo - Dizziness.

COMMENTS - Severe gastric and dysenteric symptoms. Dysentery, Farrington said it is chiefly in sub-acute cases that it is indicated, when the pains are confined to the sides of the abdomen, probably to the colon. Abdomen contracted.

Burning, acute pain in head. Immediately sensation as if a strong electric shock passed through head, he expected his brains would have burst through his skull. Titillation all over with an irresistible desire to laugh. Sensation as if the blood could scarcely struggle through the veins. A "milk-like pallor of the surface looks like a characteristic."

REFERENCES - Clarke.

ZINCUM VALERIANICUM

(Zinc Valerinate)

PHARMACY - zinc-val. Zincum valerianicum. Zinc valerinate. Zinc Isovalerate. Trituration. ***Historical dose:*** All potencies.

CLINICAL - Angina pectoris. Asthma. Brain, fatigue. Colitis. Deltoids, pain. Diarrhea. Dysmenorrhea. Emaciation. Epilepsy. ***Facial, neuralgia***. ***Headaches***. Hemorrhoids. ***Hiccoughs***. Hypochondriasis. Hystero-epilepsy. ***Insomnia. Neuralgias. Ovarian, disorders.*** Priapism. Sciatica. Seminal, emissions. Stiff-neck.

HOMEOPATHIC - Zinc-val. is a favorite anti-hysteric medicine in old-school practice. One proving, done with substantial doses by C. B. Finney, brought out a strong action on the genital sphere, the usual starting-point of hysteria.

Finney noted the brain-fatigue symptoms of Zinc. and the gastro-intestinal disturbance. The abdominal pains woke him from sleep and he had to rise at 6:30 a.m. for stool, which was partly fecal and partly fluid. Later he was constipated and had tenesmus.

Zinc-val. affects the nerves, ovaries and spine. A remedy for ***neuralgias***, hysteria, angina pectoris and other painful affections, notably in ***ovarian disorders. Facial neuralgia***, violent in left temple and inferior maxillary.

Painful nervous effects. Oversensitive, nervous and sleepless. ***Uncontrollable sleeplessness*** from pain in head with melancholy. Sleeplessness in children. Hysteria. Fidgety feet. Hypochondriasis, groundless fear. Hysterical heart-pain. Epilepsy without an aura. Obstinate ***hiccoughs***.

Finney had distinct heart pains and Hale mentioned angina pectoris as having been cured by Zinc-val. Other conditions named by him are prosopalgia, spinal neuralgia, sciatica, ovarian neuralgia, cerebrospinal meningitis and tubercular meningitis.

MIND - Dullness of mind and headache with erections. Great fullness of head with difficult thinking. Distressed mentally, mind all mixed up. Excitable. Groundless fear.

Abdomen - Mucus colitis. Crampy pains from flatulence in hypogastrium.

Back - Aching up.

Eyes - Tickling over left ear.

Face - Prosopalgia.

Female - Dysmenorrhea, pains down the thighs. ***Ovarian pain that shoots down limbs***, even to foot during and after menses.

Head - Violent, neuralgic ***intermittent headaches***. Becomes almost insane with pain, which is piercing and stabbing.

Limbs - Severe pain in neck and spine. Cannot sit still, must keep legs in constant motion. Sciatic neuralgia.

Modalities - Better from rubbing.

Mouth - Sour taste in morning. Smothers on attempting to eat.

Temperature - Chills after mental excitement or exertion. Cold parts burn as they warm up.

COMMENTS - Hansen gave "epilepsy without aura." Finney had "Sensation as if a very heavy weight on chest," and dull headache and stiffness of muscles of neck.

Hale quoted C. Dradwick as saying that a considerable number of patients who had hemorrhoids, who were taking Zinc-val. for other troubles, had their hemorrhoids relieved by the remedy.

REFERENCES - Boericke. Clarke.

ZINGIBER OFFICINALE

(Ginger Root)

PHARMACY - zing. Zingiber officinale. Ginger root. N. O. Zingiberaceae. Tincture of dried root. ***Historical dose:*** Tincture and all potencies.

CLINICAL - Albuminuria. Asthma. Backaches. Breath, offensive. Colic. Constipation. Deltoid, rheumatism. ***Diarrhea.*** Dropsy. Dyspepsia. ***Dysentery.*** Flatulence. ***Food, poisoning.*** Heartburn. ***Hepatitis. Indigestion.*** Menstrual, cramps. Motion sickness. Morning, sickness. Nausea. Nervous. Ozaena. Post-nasal catarrh. Seminal, emissions. Spleen, pains. Urine, suppressed. Vomiting. ***Water, poisoning.*** Worms.

HERBAL - Ginger tea is a folk remedy for diarrhea from ***food poisoning.*** The herbal tincture (10 to 15 drops in 2 oz. water three times a day) is a preventive remedy for ***traveler's diarrhea*** and food poisoning. Hot ginger tea has also been used for acute colds and respiratory infections.

HOMEOPATHIC - Zing. strongly affects the digestive, genito-urinary and respiratory systems. Like most spices, ginger has a specific action on the liver and digestive organs.

Zing. was proved by Franz and others and their symptoms make a full remedy pathogenesis. Particularly useful for states of debility in the digestive tract, sexual system and respiratory troubles.

Diarrhea or constipation and helps with irritation of the colon. Flatulence. Pressure in the stomach as from a stone. Worse from eating bread and especially from eating melons. Prolonged retention of urine or complete cessation of the function of the kidneys.

MIND - Forgetful, weak memory. Cheerful, good-humored, a pleasing sensation in her system. Increased activity of brain. Nervous and fidgety. Irritable and chilly in evening and during menses. Feet very uncomfortable and did not know what to do.

Abdomen - Colic, diarrhea, extremely loose bowels. Chronic intestinal catarrh.

Back - Stiffness of back of neck with headache and nausea. Back lame. Backache as from weakness, feels stiff.

Chest - Stitches in chest, pleuritic pains.

Causations - Food poisoning. ***Bad food or water.*** Complaints from eating melons. Worms, parasites.

Eyes - Smarting and burning in eyes. Feeling as of sand in eyes. Sensitive to light with stinging pain in them. Pressure on eyes, worse on left. Weakness of sight, dimness of cornea.

Face - Hot, red face. Exhausted look, blue under eyes, before menses. Dry lips and mouth.

Female - Painful menses, cramps. Menstruation too early and too profuse, blood dark, clotted. Irritable with menses.

Food - Much thirst, dry mouth. Taste of food remains long, especially of bread and toast. ***Food or water poisoning.*** Complaints from eating melons.

Head - Headache and pressure in stomach after eating bread. Feels confused and empty in his head. Head feels too large. Frontal headaches. Pain over eyebrows. Pain encircling head. Hemicrania, sudden glimmering before eyes. Congestion of blood to head, especially temples. Itching on scalp, head and cheeks.

Heart - Violent stinging, pressing pain in left side of chest in region of heart.

Kidneys - Dull aching in both kidneys with frequent desire to urinate. Increased secretion of urine. Stinging, burning in orifice. Urine thick, turbid, dark brown of strong smell. Yellow discharge from urethra. After urinating, continues to ooze in drops. Retention of urine after typhus. Complete suppression after typhoid.

Limbs - Joints feel weak, stiff, lame. Dull, heavy feeling in limbs with numbness. Cramps in soles and palms. Rheumatic drawing pains. Painful swelling of feet. Soreness of heels after standing a long time.

Liver - Hepatitis (Chin., Phos.). Liver pains, with weakness. ***Weak digestion.***

Lungs - Painful respiration. ***Asthma*** without anxiety, worse toward morning. Humid asthma. Scratching sensation in throat, stitches in chest. Cough dry and hacking, with copious morning sputa.

Male - Itching of prepuce. Sexual desire excited, painful erections. Emissions.

Modalities - Better sitting, standing. Better uncovering. Worse by touch, motion. Worse evening and night, lying, rising. Worse in cold air, damp air. Worse from bread, melons. Laughing or talking aggravates headache.

Mouth - Slimy, bad taste in mouth in morning. Mouth smells foul to herself, as from disordered stomach. Painful sensibility of teeth with pressive, drawing pain in their roots.

Nose - Feels obstructed and dry. Insupportable itching, tingling in nostrils. Intolerable itching, red pimples. Coryza, watery, sneezing, more in open air. Dryness and obstruction in posterior sinuses with discharge of thick mucus. Ozaena.

Rectum - ***Diarrhea from drinking bad water.*** Diarrhea with much flatulence, cutting pain and relaxation of the anal sphincter (Aloe.). Constipation. Hot, sore, painful anus during pregnancy. Hemorrhoids hot, painful and sore (Aloe.).

Sensations - As if head too large. Confused and empty in head. As if there were an obstacle in throat to swallow over. Pain as from over-work in left deltoid. As of a stone in stomach. Empty feeling in stomach. A shock-like moving downward as from a dropping fluid in left loin. Pain as from weakness in sacral region. As from over-strung muscles in bend of knee. As if going to faint.

Sleep - Sleepy and exhausted, coma. Sleepless, wakes at 3 a.m., falls asleep again late in morning.

Stomach - Weak digestion. ***Acidity*** of stomach (Calc., Rob.). Stomach feels heavy like from a stone (Nux-v.). Heaviness in stomach on waking with gas and rumbling, great thirst and emptiness. Pain from pit to under sternum, worse after eating. Belching and diarrhea. Nausea, vomiting of mucus in alcoholics.

Temperature - Chilliness beginning in lower limbs, going upwards. Chilliness and sensibility in open air. Chilly in evening. Hot and chilly at same time.

Throat - Hoarseness. ***Smarting below larynx,*** breathing difficult. Dryness of throat and difficulty of swallowing, as from an obstruction with dryness of posterior sinuses. Increased mucus secretion, no fever.

Vertigo - Vertigo, limbs heavy. Motion sickness with nausea.

COMMENTS - Motion sickness and morning sickness. Deltoid rheumatism, frozen shoulders (Sang., Ferr.). Farrington said ginger may aggravate kidney affections or Bright's disease.

In asthma, Farrington gave the indication: "Asthma of gastric origin, attacks come in the night towards morning. Patient must sit up to breathe, but despite the severity of the paroxysm, there is no anxiety. The nasal mucus membrane is affected as markedly as that of the lungs. Ozaena and post-nasal catarrh."

RELATIONS - ***Antidoted by:*** Nux-v. ***Compare:*** (1) Ars., Calad., Chin. (2) Abies-n. Weight in stomach. (3) Prepuce cold - Sulph. (4) Wakes at 3 a.m., Nux-v.

REFERENCES - Boericke. Clarke. Murphy.

ZIZIA AUREA

(Meadow Parsnip)

PHARMACY - ziz. Zizia aurea. Meadow parsnip. Thaspium aureum. Carum aureum. N. O. Umbelliferae. Tincture of root. ***Historical dose:*** Tincture and all potencies.

CLINICAL - Asthma. Brain, disorders. Catarrh. Chorea. Convulsions. Depression. Dropsy. Epilepsy. Headaches. Hypochondriasis. Hysteria. Influenza. Leucorrhea. Menses, suppression. Migraine. Ovarian, neuralgia. Pleurisy. Styes.

HOMEOPATHIC - The meadow parsnip is a common plant indigenous to the United States on the moist banks of streams and in open wet woods, where it flowers in June and July. Millspaugh noted that Rafinesque spoke of it as vulnerary, anti-syphilitic and sudorific.

Marcy proved Ziz. on himself and some others, and symptoms of poisoning have been added. Marcy considered Ziz. especially suitable in brain affections, catarrhal, asthmatic and pleuritic diseases, and in ovarian neuralgia.

Exhilaration with increased physical strength, but a slight amount of exercise caused fatigue. The spasms and convulsions of the Umbelliferae were elicited. The generative organs in both sexes were excited.

Ziz. has spasmodic movements of the muscles of face and limbs. Chorea, twitching during sleep. Convulsions, epilepsy. Spasms of face and limbs. Spasms, swooning convulsions and fainting fits, ending in death in three hours. Surface of body sensitive to touch.

Whole body white and puffy. Edema of face and ankles. Aspect of grave and chronic illness. Hypochondriasis, desire to commit suicide. Increased strength with inclination for exertion.

MIND - Exhilaration like intoxication, followed by strong desire to sleep. Laughing and weeping alternately. Depression followed by exhilaration. Nervous irritability and a state of depression. Paroxysms of self-dissatisfaction with weeping. Low-spirited indifferent. Indolence with contentment. Behavior quiet with much apparent suffering and sadness.

Back - Pain in posterior margin of scapula. Aching, smarting, stinging with aching in small of back when at their worst. Smarting burning in small of back. Dull pains in loins, worse by movement.

Chest - Severe pains in pleurae. Pleuritic stitches worse by coughing or deep breath. Bruised feeling in muscles of chest. Pressure causes pain in intercostal muscles. Pain and tenderness on and around xiphoid cartilage. Dull, aching pain under right scapula. Severe shooting from front of thorax to scapula. Sharp pains from sides and chest to both scapula. Severe stitching pains accompanied by feverish symptoms.

Eyes - Redness of both eyes. Pain affects right eye most. Shooting pains through orbits. Sharp pain through right orbit, worse moving eyeballs, stooping or stepping. Eyelids agglutinated on rising by yellowish muco-purulent secretion. Styes, right lid. Styes middle of upper lid, very painful. Sensitive to light (Nat-m.).

Face - Pale and puffy. One cheek red, other pale. Boring pains in cheekbones. Dull pains in jaws. Painful tenderness in lower jawbone, an inch below root of ear.

Female - Increased vascular and nervous excitement. Sudden suppression of menses. Menses appeared in due time but ceased after twelve hours. Profuse menses one day, followed by acrid leucorrhea. Leucorrhea acrid at first, later copious and bland.

Food - Appetite is diminished or lost. Thirst. Craving for acids and stimulants.

Head - Rush of blood to head and face with feeling of fullness (Bell.). Sensation of tightness around head. Intensely painful, sharp headache over right eye (Sang.). Fully developed headache on seventh day, must lie still in dark room, worse evening. Headache associated with backache, worse by coughing. Severe pain in right temple with nausea. Pressure on top of brain. Dull pain in occipital region, extending down neck muscles.

Limbs - Lameness in muscles of both arms

from shoulder to elbow. Pricking sensation in right arm with steadily diminished sensibility of the part. Dragging sensation in both hips. Unusually tired feeling in legs after slightest exertion.

Lungs - Trachea sensitive to touch. Roughness in upper part of larynx when inspiring or coughing. Larynx raw from coughing. Dry cough with shooting pains in chest. Tight cough from deep breath from dryness of larynx. Short, dry cough with severe stitching in right side and sense of suffocation. Breathing oppressed, cannot keep lying down. Asthma.

Male - Excitement. Involuntary emissions at night. Lassitude and prostration after se.

Modalities - Pains fixed, worse by movement. Worse noise, light, evening. Worse contact, touch, motion. Worse lying, stooping, coughing. Pressure causes pain in intercostal muscles. Pressure on stomach causes nausea and faintness.

Mouth - Bitter, bilious taste. Dry mouth. Tongue red and unusually sensitive to cold and warm drinks. Tongue covered with whitish fur, yellow fur. Tongue is broad, furred in middle, red at tip and sides. Oppressed respiration.

Nose - Nasal catarrh with sneezing and coughing from first inhalation. Nasal discharge of thick mucus. Right nostril congested, sore with injection of pharynx and conjunctiva.

Skin - Itching pimples on forehead, wrists and legs.

Sleep - Drowsiness with sense of fatigue. Sleep prevented by pains. During sleep spasmodic twitches, talking, unpleasant dreams.

Stomach - Stomach sensitive to touch, pressure causes nausea and faintness. Nausea. Acid, bilious vomiting, immoderately.

Temperature - Chilliness and heat alternating with faintness, nausea, pain in right temple, redness of eyeballs, dry and red tongue and thirst for cold water. Chilliness accompanied by spasmodic twitchings of muscles of face and upper limbs, followed by fever. Fever with headache, pain in back, thirst. Fever with stitching pain in chest. Some sense of heat and fullness in both cheeks. Redness and heat of cheeks. Hot flushes in face and head followed by perspiration.

Throat - Mucus increased. Slight redness of tonsils and palate with soreness. Inflamed pharynx.

Vertigo - Giddiness, swimming, lightheadedness.

COMMENTS - Ziz. is indicated in uterine disorders characterized by increased nervous and vascular excitement. The menses are profuse and followed by acrid leucorrhea. Uterine congestion with migraine, particularly affecting the region of the right eye.

Rush of blood to the head. Flushed cheeks, hot head. One cheek red. Visible pulsations of carotid and temporal arteries (Bell.). Coldness of hands and feet, drowsiness and irritability. Surface of body paler than natural, white, puffy appearance of whole body. Laughs and weeps alternately. Craves acids and stimulants.

Burning, smarting backache. Spasmodic movements of face and limbs. Mind first exhilarated, then depressed, finally indifferent. Restlessness, running into chorea, the movements continue or are even worse during sleep.

RELATIONS - ***Antidoted by:*** Puls. - migraine, Carb-an., Staph. - styes. ***Compare:*** (1) One cheek red, Cham. (2) Uterine congestion, backache indifference, Sep. (3) Chorea in sleep, Tarent. (4) As if in a dream, Ambr., Anac., Calc., Cann-i., Con., Cupr., Med., Rheum., Valer., Verat. (5) Laughing alternately with weeping, Calc., Ign., Merc., Nux-m., Puls., Stram.

REFERENCES - Clarke.

A

ABANDONED, ailments, from being - **ARS.,** ***aur., calc.,*** carc., ign., ***lac-h.,*** lyc., **NAT-M.,** ***psor.,*** phos., **PULS.,** rhus-t., sac-alb., sep., sil., sulph., ***thuj.***

ABSCESS, acute - acon., ***anan.,*** anthr., apis, ***arn., ars., bell.,*** calc-hp., ***calc-s.,*** calen., canth., ***carb-ac.,*** chin., chin-s., crot-h., fl-ac., **HEP.,** hippoz., ***kreos., lach.,*** lap-a., lob., lyc., **MERC.,** ***merc-s., myris., nit-ac.,*** ph-ac., phos., ***pyrog., rhus-t.,*** **SIL.,** sil-mar., ***sulph., sul-ac.,*** syph., ***tarent-c.,*** vesp.

ABDOMEN, cancer - ***calc-ar., hydr.,*** lob-e., ***orni.***

ABUSE, ailments from - ***acon.,*** alum., ambr., am-m., **ANAC.,** ***arg-n.,*** arn., ars., ***aur., aur-m.,*** bell., ***bry.,*** calc., calc-p., calc-s., **CARC.,** caust., ***cham.,*** **COLOC.,** con., foll., form., gels., grat., hyos., **IGN.,** lac-c., ***lach.,*** **LYC.,** ***lyss.,*** med., merc., **NAT-M.,** ***nux-v., op.,*** **PALL.,** petr., **PH-AC.,** plat., ***puls.,*** rhus-t., ***seneg.,*** sep., sil., **STAPH.,** stram., ***sulph.,*** **THUJ.,** verat., zinc.

ACETONEMIA, blood - ***acet-ac.,*** am-c., ars., carb-ac., caust., op., phenob., sul-ac., ter.

ACETONURIA, urine - acetan., act-sp., ***agar.,*** ars., aur-m., calc., ***calc-m.,*** carb-ac., ***carb-an., caust., cham.,*** cic., ***coc-c.,*** colch., crot-h., cupr-ar., ***euon.,*** **EUP-PER.,** **GRAPH.,** ***insulin, mag-c.,*** **MERC.,** myric., nat-sal., ***nicc., nit-ac.,*** **NUX-V.,** phenob., phos., ***senn., sep.,*** sul-ac., **SULPH.,** ***uran-n., verat.***

ACHILLES TENDON - ***arg.,*** aur-m-n., bry., ***calc., calen.,*** cimic., led., ***merc.,*** mill., rat., rhod., ***rhus-t., ruta,*** thuj., ***zinc.*.**

ACHING, pains, (see Sore, pains)

ACIDOSIS, ailments from excess blood acidity - ***aloe,*** am-c., ***ant-c.,*** arg-n., ars., bar-c., bell., bor., bov., calc., canth., ***carb-v.,*** carc., caust., chin., cimic., dros., ferr., gaert., graph., hep., ***lac-ac., lach., kali-c., kali-n.,*** merc., mur-ac., rheum, rhus-t., nat-c., nat-m., **NAT-P.,** ***nux-v.,*** ph-ac., phos., ran-b., rhus-t., sars., ***sil., staph.,*** sul-ac., sulph., syc-co., zinc.

ACNE, rosacea - agar., ***ars., ars-br.,*** ars-i., aur., ***aur-m.,*** bell., ***calc-p.,*** **CALC-SIL.,** canth., ***caps.,*** carb-ac., ***carb-an.,*** **CARB-V.,** carbn-s., **CAUST.,** chel., chrysar., ***cic.,*** clem., eug., ***hydr-ac., hydrc.,*** iris, kali-br., kali-i., ***kreos.,*** **LACH.,** led., mag-p., ***mez.,*** nux-v., ov., ***petr., plb.,*** **PSOR.,** ***rad.,*** rhus-r., **RHUS-T.,** ***ruta, sep., sil., sul-i., sulo-ac., sulph.,*** sul-ac., syc-co., ***tub., verat.,*** viol-o., ***viol-t.***

ACNE, vulgaris - ***ant-c., ars., ars-i.,*** **AUR.,** bar-c., bell., ***calc.,*** **CALC-SIL.,** ***calc-s.,*** **CARB-AN., CARB-V., CARBN-S., CAUST.,** chel., ***con., cop., crot-h., eug.,*** graph., **HEP.,** iod., **KALI-BR.,** ***kreos., lach.,*** led., med., ***nat-m., nit-ac.,*** **NUX-V.,** ***ph-ac., psor., puls.,*** sabin., sanic., sel., **SEP., SIL.,** ***sulph.,*** sul-i., ***thuj., tub.,*** uran.

ACONITE, ailments from - acet-ac., ***acon.,*** alco., bry., coff., ***sulph.***

ACROMEGALY - ***bar-c.,*** carc., ***pitu-p.,*** thyr.

ACTINOMYCOSIS - hecla., hippoz., kali-i., ***nit-ac.,*** pyrog., thymol.

ADENOCARCINOMA, (see Glands, cancer)

ADDICTIVE, personality - ars., aven., ***carc.,*** lach., ***med., nux-v.,*** op., thuj.

ADDISON'S, disease - ***adren.,*** ant-c., apom., ***arg-n., ars., ars-i.,*** bac., ***bell.,*** **CALC.,** calc-ar., calc-i., calc-p., carb-v., caust., chin., cupr., ***ferr., ferr-i.,*** hydr-ac., **IOD.,** kali-ar., ***kali-c.,*** kreos., lyc., mang., med., **NAT-M.,** nat-s., ***nit-ac.,*** ol-j., petr., **PHOS.,** pic-ac., psor., sec., ***sep.,*** **SIL.,** ***spig., sulph.,*** supren-cort., thal., ther., thuj., ***tub.,*** vanad.

ADENITIS, glands, infection - ***acon.,*** acon-l., ***aln., alumn., anan.,*** apis, arn., ***ars.,*** ars-br., ***ars-i.,*** arum-d., astac., ***aur., aur-m., bad.,*** **BAR-C.,** ***bar-i.,*** **BAR-M., BELL.,** ***bry., brom.,*** bufo, **CALC.,** ***calc-f., calc-i.,*** calc-p., calen., ***camph.,*** canth., caps., ***carb-an.,*** carb-v., **CARC.,** ***cham., cist.,*** clem., ***con.,*** cory., crot-h., **DULC.,** ***echi.,*** ferr-ar., ferr-i., fil., graph., ***hep.,*** hippoz., ***iod.,*** kali-ar., ***kali-c., kali-i.,*** kali-m., kali-p., lac-c., lach., ***lap-a.,*** laur., ***lyc.,*** med., **MERC.,** merc-cy., merc-i-f., ***merc-i-r.,*** nat-s., ***nit-ac., nux-v.,*** petr., ph-ac., **PHOS., PHYT.,** plan., plb., ***psor., puls.,*** **PYROG.,** ***rhus-t., rumx.,*** samb., sars., scirr., **SCROPH-N.,** ***sil.,*** sil-mar., spig., ***spong.,*** squil., staph., sul-ac., **SULPH.,** ***tarent-c.,*** tax., thiosin., thuj., tub., verat., zinc.

ADENOIDS, problems with - ***agra.,*** alum., am-c., apoc., arg., ars., arund., ***asc-t., aur.,*** aur-m., ***bar-c., bar-m.,*** brom., bry., **CALC.,** ***calc-f., calc-i., calc-p.,*** calc-s., carb-an., **CARC.,** chr-ac., ***con.,*** cupr., elaps, fl-ac., gonotox., hep., hip-ac., ***iod.,*** kali-bi., kali-i., kali-m., kali-s., lap-a., lem-m., lob-s., **LYC.,** ***med., merc.,*** mez., mucor, nat-m., nit-ac., **NUX-V.,** osm., phos., phyt., psor., puls., sabad., **SAMB.,** ***sanguin-n.,*** sars., sel., sep., sil., sul-i., sulph., ***syc-co.,*** syph., teucr., ***thuj., tub.,*** vib.

AETHER, ailments from - acet-ac., aether, phos.

AFRICAN, fever - ars., crot-h., **TER.**

AGARICUS, mushroom, ailments from - ***absin., agar.,*** camph., coff.

AGRANULOCYTOSIS, blood - cortico., lach., sulfa., x-ray.

AGORAPHOBIA, fear of open places - ***acon.,*** arg., ***arg-n., arn.,*** ars., bar-c., ***calc., carc.,*** crot-h., ferr., ***gels.,*** glon., hydr-ac., kali-c., ***kali-ar.,*** lac-c., levo., lyc., **LYSS.,** merc., morg., nux-v., ***phos.,*** prot., puls., nux-v., ***sep.,*** sil., stram., succ-ac., tab., visc.

A.I.D.S., acquired immune deficiency syndrome - acon., **ARS.,** ars-i., ***aur.,*** bapt., **CARC.,** ***chin.,*** cortico., crot-h., ***echi., ferr., ferr-p., gels.,*** lach., lyc., **MED.,** **MERC.,** nux-v., op., ph-ac., ***phos.,*** puls., **PYROG.,** sil., stram., sulfa., sulph., ***syph.,*** **THUJ.,** ***tub.,*** urea, urin., vanad., x-ray.

AIR POLLUTION, ailments, from - acet-ac., acon., ***am-c.,*** ant-t., **ARS.,** bell., bov., ***bry.,*** calc., camph., caust., ***carb-diox.,*** **CARB-V.,** carbn-h., carbn-s., cortico., cortiso., ***crot-h.,*** dros., ***euph.,*** ign., just., ***kali-s.,*** lach., lob., ***merc.,*** nat-ar., nat-m., nat-s., nux-v., olnd., op., **PULS.,** rumx., ***sep.,*** sil., **SPIG.,** **SUL-AC.,** sulph.

AIRPLANES, flying in, ailments from - ***acon., arg-n.,*** arn., ***ars.,*** bell., bor., cham., ***coca, cocc.,*** gels., ***kali-m.,*** petr., phos., psor.

ALCOHOLISM, dipsomania, (see Alcohol) - ***absin.,*** acon., adon., **AGAR.,** agav-t., alum., am-m., anac., ange., anis., ***ant-c., ant-t., apoc., apom.,*** arg., arg-n., arn., ars., ars-s-f., ***asaf., asar.,*** **AUR.,** ***aven.,*** bar-c., ***bell.,*** bism., bor., bov., bry., bufo, cadm-s., ***calc.,*** calc-ar., camph., cann-i., ***caps.,*** carb-ac., carb-an., ***carb-v., carbn-s., carc.,*** card-m., caust., cham., ***chel.,*** chim., **CHIN.,** chin-m., cic., ***cimic.,*** coc-c., ***cocc., coff.,*** con., croc., **CROT-H.,** ***cupr-ar.,*** dig., ***eup-per., ferr.,*** fl-ac., ***gels.,*** glon., ***graph., hell.,*** hep., hydr., ***hyos.,*** ichth., ***ign.,*** ip., ***kali-bi.,*** kali-br., kali-c., kali-i., kola, ***lac-c.,*** **LACH.,** ***laur., led.,*** lob., lup., ***lyc.,*** mag-c., meph., merc., mez., mosch., ***nat-c.,*** nat-n., nat-s., ***nux-m.,*** **NUX-V.,** op., passi., petr., ph-ac., ***phos.,*** plat., plb., psor., puls., ***quas., querc.,*** **RAN-B.,** raph., ***rhod., rhus-t.,*** rumx., ruta, sang., sars., sec., **SEL.,** ***sep., sil.,*** staph., ***stram.,*** stront-c., ***stroph.,*** **SUL-AC., SULPH.,** syph., tarax., tub., valer., **VERAT.,** ***zinc.***

ALLERGIES, allergic reactions, (see Hay Fever) - **ALL-C.,** ambro., **APIS, ARS., ARS-I.,** berb-a., ***carb-ac., carb-v., carc.,*** chin-ar., chloram., cortiso., des-ac., dys-co., ergot., ***euphr.,*** flav., foll., form-ac., frag., galph., ***hist.,*** **IOD.,** kali-i., lach., led., levo., ***lyc.,*** mand., **MERC.,** merc-c., morg-g., **NAT-M.,** ***nat-s.,*** nit-ac., ***nux-v., ox-ac.,*** palo., paraph., penic., phenob., phos., pitu-a., pneu., prot., ***psor.,*** puls., **RHUS-T.,** sabad., sal-ac., saroth., ***sin-n.,*** sil., sulfa., ***sul-ac., sulph.,*** syc-co., ***thuj.,*** **URT-U.,** vesp., wye.

ALLERGY, shots, ailments from - carc., sil., ***thuj.***

ALLOXAN, drug, ailments from - allox., lyc., ph-ac., phos.

ALOE, ailments from - aloe., chin., lyc., mur-ac., sulph.

ALTITUDE, sickness, (see Mountain, sickness) - ***acon., arn., ars.,*** aur., bell., **CALC., CARB-V.,** caust., **COCA.,** con., conv., cupr., gels., kola, ***lach.,*** lyc., nat-m., olnd., ***op.,*** puls., **SIL.,** spig., verat.

ALUMINIUM, ailments from - ***alum.,*** alumn., bar-c., ***bry.,*** cadm., cadm-s., calc., camph., cham., con., ferr., ip., nat-m., nux-v., ***plb.,*** puls., sil., sulph., zinc.

ALZHEIMER'S, disease - ***alum., agn.,*** ail., ambr., ***anac.,*** ant-c., arg., ***arg-n., ars.,*** aur., ***aur-i.,*** aza., bapt., bar-acet., ***bar-c.,*** bar-m., bell., bry., calc-p., cann-i., ***con., crot-h.,*** fl-ac., ***helo.,*** **HYOS.,** ign., iod., lach., lil-t., ***lyc., kali-br.,*** kali-p., nat-i., nat-m., nux-m., nux-v., op., ***ov., phos.,*** pic-ac., plb., puls., sec., sep., staph., sulph., thiosin., zinc.

AMAUROSIS, optic nerve, paralysis - acon., agar., alum., am-c., am-m., ambr., anac., anan., ang., ant-c., ant-s., ant-t., apis, ***arg.,*** arg-n., arn., ***ars.,*** ars-s-f., asaf., aur., aur-ar., ***aur-m., aur-m-n., aur-s.,*** bar-c., bar-s., **BELL.,** benz-n., bor., both-l., ***bov.,*** bry., bufo, ***calc., calc-sil.,*** camph., cann-i., cann-s., canth., caps., carb-an., carb-v., carbn-o., card-b., ***caust.,*** cench., cham., ***chel., chin.,*** chin-s., cic., cocc., colch., **CON.,** croc., cycl., daph., dig., dros., dubin., dulc., ***elaps,*** euphr., ***ferr.,*** ferr-ar., ferr-ma., fl-ac., **GELS.,** graph., guai., hep., ***hyos.,*** ign., iod., kali-ar., kali-c., **KALI-I.,** kali-p., ***kali-s.,*** kali-sil., kalm., kreos., laur., led., ***lyc.,*** mag-c., manc., mang., ***meny., merc.,*** merc-c., mez., mom-b., naphtin., nat-ar., nat-c., **NAT-M.,** nat-p., nat-sil., nit-ac., nux-m., ***nux-v.,*** olnd., ***op.,*** oxyt., par., petr., ***ph-ac.,*** **PHOS.,** ***plb., plb-acet., psor.,*** **PULS.,** ***rhus-t., ruta,*** sabad., sabin., sant., sars., **SEC.,** seneg., ***sep.,*** **SIL.,** sol-n., sol-t., spig., staph., **STRAM.,** stront-c., stry., **SULPH.,** syph., tab., thal., ***thuj.,*** upa., vanad., verat., verat-v., verb., vib., ***zinc., zinc-p.***

AMBLYOPIA, dim vision - ***ammc.,*** anag., ant-t., atro., benz-d., caps., carbn-s., **CHIN.,** chin-s., cich., con., crot-h., daph., ***dros.,*** euph., **GELS.,** hyos., ign., ***merc., nat-m.,*** nux-v., ***op.,*** **PHOS.,** ***ph-ac.,*** puls., raph., ***ruta,*** sac-l., ***sant.,*** seneg., sil., ***stram.,*** ter., thyr., zinc.

AMENORRHEA, menses, absent - ***acon.,*** aesc., agar., agn., alet., all-c., aln., ***am-c.,*** am-m., ammc., ***anac., ant-c., apis, apoc.,*** arg-n., ***arist-cl., ars., ars-i.,*** asar., **AUR.,** aur-i., aven., ***bar-c., bell.,*** bell-p., benz-ac., berb., ***bor.,*** brom., ***bry., calc.,*** calc-i., calc-p., calc-s., calc-sil., cann-s., canth., carb-v., **CARBN-S.,** card-m., ***caul., caust., cham.,*** chel., ***chin.,*** chin-ar., chlorpr., cic., ***cimic.,*** cina, ***coca, cocc., coch.,*** colch., ***coll., coloc.,*** **CON.,** cortiso., cortico., croc., croto-t., ***cupr., cycl., cypr.,*** dam., dig., ***dros.,*** **DULC.,** euph., eupi., **FERR.,** ***ferr-ar.,*** **FERR-I.,** ***ferr-m., ferr-p.,*** gast., gels., ***glon., goss.,*** **GRAPH.,** ***guai., ham.,*** hedeo, ***hell., helon.,*** hyper., ***hyos.,*** ictod., **IGN.,** indg., ***iod., kali-ar.,*** **KALI-C.,** kali-i., ***kali-ma., kali-n., kali-p.,*** kali-s., kreos., lac-d., ***lach.,*** lil-t., linu-c., lob., **LYC.,** ***mag-c., mag-m.,*** mag-s., mand., mang., ***merc., merl.,*** mill., ***mit.,*** nat-c., ***nat-m.,*** nat-p., nat-sil., nat-s., nep., ***nux-m., nux-v.,*** ol-an., ***ol-j.,*** op., ovi-g-p., parth., ph-ac., ***phos., phyt.,*** pin-l., pituin., ***plat.,*** plb., podo., ***polyg.,*** **PULS.,** ***rhus-t., sabad.,*** sabin., sang., sanic., sec., **SENEC., SEP.,** sieg., **SIL.,** ***sin-n.,*** spong., ***staph.,*** stram., **SULPH.,** sul-i., symph., tanac., tep., thiop.,

thuj., thyr., **TUB.,** urt-u., ust., ***valer.,*** verat., verat-v., ***vib.,*** wies., wye., x-ray, xan., ***zinc.,*** zinc-p.

AMMONIA, ailments from - ***am-c., am-m.,*** aml-n., ant-t., arn., ***ars.,*** aur., camph., carb-v., glon., hep., lach., merc., mur-ac., phos.

AMPHETAMINES, ailments from - agar., cham., coca, cocc., ***coff.,*** ign., kola, ***nux-v.,*** paull., tarent., zinc.

AMPUTATION, pain, phantom pains - ***acon., all-c.,*** am-m., anh., arg., ***arn., asaf.,*** bell., **CALEN., COFF.,** cupr., haem., hell., **HYPER.,** ign., kalm., ***ph-ac.,*** **PHOS.,** rauw., spig., ***staph.,*** symph., verat.

AMYOTROPHIC, lateral sclerosis - ***arg-n., ars.,*** cupr., hyper., kali-p., ***lach., lath.,*** merc., ***phos.,*** **PLB.,** sec., sep., sulph.

ANASARCA - acet-ac., alco., ars., cham., dig., plb., urea.

ANCHYLOSIS, limbs - acon., ant-s., arn., ars., ba-sv., bell., bor., bry., crot-h., fl-ac., kali-c., merc., rhus-t., ruta, sil., sulph.

ANEMIA, general - abel., abies-c., abrot., absin., ***acet-ac.,*** acetan., acon., agar., agn., ***alet.,*** aloe, alst-s., alum., alum-p., alum-sil., alumn., am-c., ambr., anil., ant-c., ***ant-t., apis,*** apoc., aq-mar., ***arg., arg-n., arg-o., arn.,*** **ARS.,** ars-h., ***ars-i.,*** **ARS-S-F.,** aur-ar., bac., bar-c., ***bell.,*** benz-d., benz-n., berb., beryl., bism., bol., **BOR.,** bov., ***bry.,*** cadm., **CALC.,** calc-ar., calc-i., calc-l., **CALC-P.,** calc-sil., calen., calo., camph-br., cann-i., carb-an., ***carb-v., carbn-s.,*** carc., casc., ***caust.,*** cean., cedr., cham., **CHIN.,** chin-ar., ***chin-s.,*** chlol., chlor., chloram., chlorpr., cic., cina, cob-n., ***cocc.,*** coch., coff., colch., coloc., ***con.,*** cortico., cortiso., crat., ***crot-h., cupr.,*** cupr-ar., cupr-s., ***cycl.,*** dig., eucal., **FERR.,** ferr-acet., **FERR-AR.,** ferr-br., ferr-c., ferr-cit., ***ferr-i., ferr-m.,*** **FERR-P.,** ferr-pic., ferr-prox., ***galeo.,*** ferr-s., franz., galeg., goss., **GRAPH.,** ***ham.,*** **HELL.,** ***helon.,*** hep., ***hydr., ign.,*** iod., ip., ***irid.,*** **KALI-AR.,** ***kali-bi., kali-br., kali-c.,*** kali-chl., kali-fcy., kali-hp., kali-m., kali-ma., kali-n., **KALI-P.,** kali-s., kalm., kres., lac-ac., lac-c., lac-d., ***lach.,*** lec., lyc., lyss., mag-c., mag-m., **MANG., MED., MERC.,** ***merc-c.,*** mez., mill., ***mosch.,*** nat-ar., nat-br., ***nat-c.,*** nat-cac., nat-hchls., **NAT-M.,** nat-n., ***nat-p., nat-s.,*** nat-taur., **NIT-AC.,** nux-m., ***nux-v.,*** ol-j., ***olnd.,*** ost., oxyg., paull-p., peti., petr., ***ph-ac.,*** **PHOS.,** ***phyt., pic-ac.,*** pitu-a., **PLAT., PLB.,** ***plb-acet.,*** psor., **PULS.,** puls-n, rad-br., rhod., ***rhus-t.,*** ric., rob., rub-t., ruta, sabin., sac-alb., sac-l., sal-ac., sarr., ***sec., senec., sep.,*** sil., sin-n., sol-n., spig., **SQUIL.,** ***stann.,*** **STAPH.,** stroph., stry-f-c., **SUL-AC.,** sulfa., sulfonam., **SULPH.,** syc-co., tab., ther., thuj., ***thyr.,*** trif-r., trinit., tub., tub-sp., urt-u., ust., valer., vanad., verat., ***x-ray,*** xan., zinc., zinc-ar., zinc-m., zinc-p., zinc-s.

iron, deficiency, anemia - abies-c., ***abrot., absin., acet-ac.,*** acetan., ***alet., alum.,*** alum-p., alumn., ***am-c., ambr., ant-c., ant-t.,*** aq-mar., ***arg.,*** arg-n., **ARS.,** ars-i., ars-s-f., aur-ar., bar-c., **BELL.,** bry., cadm., **CALC.,** calc-ar., **CALC-P.,** carb-an., ***carb-v.,*** **CARBN-S.,** caust., ***chin., chin-ar.,*** chlor., cina, cob-n., **COCC.,** coch., ***con., cupr., cycl.,*** dig., **FERR., FERR-AR.,** ***ferr-i.,*** **FERR-M., FERR-P.,** ***ferr-s.,*** franz., **GRAPH.,** ***hell., helon., hep.,*** ign., ***ip., kali-ar.,*** kali-bi., ***kali-c., kali-fcy.,*** kali-ma., ***kali-p.,*** kali-s., lac-c., lach., lec., **LYC.,** ***lyss.,*** **MANG.,** ***med.,*** merc., ***mill., nat-c.,*** nat-hchls., **NAT-M.,** nat-p., **NIT-AC.,** ***nux-v.,*** olnd., ***paull-p.,*** peti., ***petr.,*** ph-ac., **PHOS.,** phyt., pic-ac., **PLAT.,** ***plb.,*** **PULS.,** rub-t., sabin., sac-alb., sac-l., **SENEC., SEP.,** ***sin-n., spig.,*** staph., ***stry-f-c.,*** sul-ac., **SULPH.,** thuj., ust., valer., vanad., ***xan.,*** zinc., zinc-m.

ANESTHESIA, poisoning, ailments, from - ***acet-ac.,*** am-c., am-caust., aml-n., ***carb-v., chlf.,*** hep., hyper., ph-ac., **PHOS.**

ANEURISM, general, of large arteries - acet-ac., ***acon.,*** ambr., arn., ars., ars-i., aspar., ***aur.,*** ba-sv., **BAR-C.,** ***bar-m., bell.,*** bry., **CACT., CALC.,** calc-f., calc-p., calc-s., ***calen.,*** cann-s., carb-an., ***carb-v.,*** caust., con., **CUPR.,** ***dig.,*** ferr., ***ferr-p.,*** fl-ac., gall-ac., glon., graph., guai., iod., kali-c., ***kali-i.,*** kalm., ***lach.,*** lith-c., ***lyc.,*** lycps., morph., ***nat-i.,*** nat-m., nux-v., phos., plb., puls., ran-s., rhus-t., ruta, sec., sil., **SPIG.,** ***spong., sulph.,*** thuj., tub., ***verat-v.,*** zinc.

abdomen - bar-m., sec.

aorta, of - acon., ars-i., ***bar-c., bar-m.,*** cact., ***calc.,*** calc-f., calc-p., calen., glon., iod., ***kali-i.,*** kalm., lach., lith-c., ***lyc.,*** morph., ***nat-i.,*** plumbg., puls., ***ran-s.,*** spig., spong., ***verat-v.***

brain - acet-ac., ***acon.,*** alum., ambr., arn., ars., ars-i., aspar., ***aur.,*** ba-sv., **BAR-C.,** ***bar-m., bell.,*** bry., **CACT., CALC.,** calc-f., calc-p., calc-s., ***calen.,*** cann-s., carb-an., ***carb-v.,*** caust., con., **CUPR.,** ***dig.,*** ferr., ***ferr-p.,*** fl-ac., gall-ac., glon., graph., guai., iod., kali-c., ***kali-i.,*** kalm., ***lach.,*** lith-c., ***lyc.,*** lycps., morph., ***nat-i.,*** nat-m., nux-v., phos., plb., puls., ran-s., rhus-t., ruta, sec., sil., **SPIG.,** ***spong., sulph.,*** thuj. tub., ***verat-v.,*** zinc.

heart, of - **CACT.,** ***carb-v.,*** lycps.

ANGER, ailments, from - **ACON.,** agar., alum., alum-sil., am-c., am-m., **ANAC.,** ***androc., ant-t., apis,*** arg., arg-n., arn., ***ars.,*** ars-s-f., ***aur.,*** aur-ar., ***aur-m.,*** aur-m-n., bar-c., ***bell., bry.,*** cadm-s., calc., calc-ar., ***calc-p.,*** calc-s., calc-sil., camph., **CARC.,** ***caust.,*** **CHAM.,** chin., cimic., cina, cist., **COCC.,** ***coch., coff.,*** colch., **COLOC.,** croc., cupr., ferr., ferr-p., ***gels.,*** gink., graph., grat., hecla., hep., hyos., **IGN.,** ilx-a., iod., **IP.,** kali-br., ***kali-p., lach.,*** lachn., **LYC.,** lyss., mag-c., mag-m., mag-p., manc., merc., mez., mur-ac., nat-ar., nat-c., **NAT-M.,** nat-p., nat-s., ***nit-ac.***, nux-m., **NUX-V.,** ol-an., olnd., **OP.,** petr., ***ph-ac., phos.,*** **PLAT.,** ***puls., ran-b.,*** rhus-t., sac-alb., samb., scroph-n., sec., sel., ***sep.,*** sil., stann., **STAPH.,** stram., stront-c., sulph., ***tarent.,*** verat., vinc., zinc., zinc-p.

ANGINA, pectoris, chest, heart pain - acet-ac., **ACON.,** aconin., adren., agar., **AM-C.,** ***aml-n.***, anac., ang., **APIS**, apoc., arg-cy., **ARG-N.**, **ARN.**, **ARS.**, ars-i., ***asim.***, **AUR.**, **AUR-M.**, bism., bry., **CACT.**, calc-f., calc-hp., camph., carb-an., ***carb-v.***, caust., cere-b., ***chel.***, chim-m., **CHIN-AR.**, ***chin-s.***, chlol., chlor., chr-ac., chr-o., ***cimic.***, coca, ***cocain***, coff., conv., **CRAT.,** crot-h., ***cupr.***, ***cupr-acet.***, ***cupr-ar.***, ***dig.***, ***dios.***, foll., glon., ***haem.***, ***hep.***, ***hydr-ac.***, hydro-c., ip., ***jug-c.***, ***kali-c.***, kali-i., kali-p., ***kalm.***, ***lach.***, lact., **LAT-M.**, ***laur.***, lil-t., lith-c., lob., ***lyc.***, ***mag-p.***, magn-gr., mand., mez., morg., morph., ***mosch.***, **NAJA**, ***nat-i.***, nat-n., nat-ns., ***nux-v.***, olnd., **OX-AC.**, petr., **PHOS.**, phyt., pip-n., plb., prot., prun., **RHUS-T.**, sac-l., ***samb.***, samb-c., saroth., scol., **SEC.**, sep., **SPIG.**, **SPONG.**, ***squil.***, staph., stict., ***stram.***, stront-c., stront-i., stry., sulph., ***tab.***, ***tarent.***, thea., ***ther.***, thyr., ***verat.***, verat-v., wies., zinc., zinc-val.

ANGIOMA, hemangioma - abrot., ant-t., **ARS.,** bell., ***calc.,*** **CARB-AN.,** ***carb-v.,*** clem., ***kreos.,*** **LACH.,** ***lyc.,*** manc., ***merc., nat-m., nit-ac.,*** nux-v., **PHOS.,** ***puls., rhus-t.,*** sep., **SIL.,** staph., ***sulph.,*** **THUJ.**

ANKLES, general - arg., **ARN.,** bell-p, **BRY.,** ***calc.,*** calc-f., calc-p., con., hyper., ***led.,*** mill., ***nat-c.,*** nat-m., plb., **RHUS-T., RUTA,** ***stront-c., symph.***

- **injuries,** ankles - anac., ang., **ARN.,** ***bell-p.,*** **BRY.,** ***calc.,*** calc-f., ***calc-p., calen.,*** caust., ***hyper.,*** lach., ***led.,*** nat-c., **RHUS-T., RUTA,** sil., ***stront-c., symph.,*** valer.
- **sprained,** ankles - agar., **ANAC.,** ang., **ARN.,** asc-t., ***bell-p.,*** **BRY.,** ***calc.,*** caust., eup-per., fl-ac., gran., graph., **LED.,** kali-bi., nat-c., nat-s., nit-ac., plb., **RHUS-T., RUTA,** ***sil., stront-c., valer.,*** verat., zinc.

ANKLOSING, spondylitis - **AESC.,** agar., ***arg.,*** caust., cimic., ***con.,*** kali-c., **KALM.,** ***nat-m., rhus-t.,*** tell.

ANOREXIA, nervosa - alf., arg-n., **ARS.,** calc., ***carc.,*** caust., **CHIN.,** hyos., ***ign.,*** kali-p., lach., levo., merc., ***nat-m.,*** perh., ph-ac., phos., puls., rhus-t., ***sac-alb.,*** sep., ***staph.,*** **SULPH.,** syc., tarent., tetox., thuj., vanad., verat.

ANTHRAX, poisoning or infection - **ANTHR.,** apis, **ARS.,** ***camph.,*** carb-ac., ***carb-v.,*** echi., ***kreos.,*** hyos., **LACH.,** ***lyc.,*** rhus-t., sal-ac., sang., ***sec.,*** **SIL.,** stram., ***tarent.,*** ther.

ANTIBIOTICS, poisoning, ailments, from - apis., ***ars.,*** bor., calad., ***chin.,*** chin-ar., ***chin-s.,*** fl-ac., gels., lyc., ***pen.,*** podo., merc., nat-p., ***nit-ac., nux-v., sul-ac., sulfa.,*** thuj.

- **ampicillin**, from - ars., nit-ac., pen.
- **cipro**, from - calc-f., fl-ac.
- **neomycin**, from - ars.
- **nystatin**, from - ars., chin.
- **penicillin**, from - ars., ***calad.,*** chin., chin-s., ***nit-ac.,*** pen.
- **stelazine**, from - nit-ac., pen.
- **streptomycin**, from - ars., chin., ***chin-s.***
- **tetracycline**, from - ars., bell., calad., calc-f., chin., gels., hecla, lyc., nat-p., nit-ac., nux-v., pen., sulph.

ANTICIPATION, ailments, from - **ACON.,** aesc., aeth., agn., alum., am-c., ambr., ***anac.,*** androc., apis, **ARG-N.,** arist-cl., **ARS.,** ***bar-c.,*** bell., bor., ***bry.,*** calad., **CALC.,** calc-s., ***camph.,*** cann-i., canth., ***carb-v.,*** **CARC., CAUST.,** cench., ***chin.,*** chin-s., chlorpr., ***cic.,*** cina, ***cocc., coff.,*** crot-c., crot-h., cypr., dig., dys-co., ***elaps,*** epip., ferr-p., ***fl-ac.,*** **GELS., GRAPH.,** hydrog., **HYOS.,** ***iod.,*** **IGN.,** kali-br., kali-c., kali-i., ***kali-p., lac-c.,*** lach., lec., levo., **LYC.,** ***lyss.,*** **MED.,** ***merc.,*** **MEZ.,** mosch., mur-ac., naja, ***nat-c.,*** **NAT-M.,** nat-p., nat-s., nux-v., ox-ac., oxyg., ***petr., ph-ac.,*** **PHOS.,** pic-ac., plat., **PLB., PSOR., PULS.,** rhus-t., ***sec.,*** sep., **SIL.,** spig., spong., staph., ***still.,*** stram., stroph., ***stront-c.,*** sul-ac., sulph., syc-co., syph., ***thuj., verat.,*** visc., zinc.

ANTI-SPASMODIC, drugs, ailments from - calc., lob., kali-br., mag-p., nux-v., phenob.

ANXIETY, general - ***abrot.,*** **ACON.,** acon-c., ***acon-f., acet-ac.,*** act-sp., ***aeth.,*** aether, agar., agar-ph., agn., ail., alco., ***all-c.,*** all-s., allox., aloe, ***alum., alum-sil.,*** alumn., ***ambr., am-c.,*** am-m., ***aml-n.,*** amyg-am., ***anac., androc.,*** ang., anh., ant-ar., ***ant-c., ant-t.,*** apis, aran., aran-s., ***arg.,*** **ARG-N.,** arge., ***arn.,*** **ARS.,** ***ars-h.,*** **ARS-I., ARS-S-F.,** arum-m., arund., asaf., ***asar., aspar.,*** aster., atro., **AUR.,** aur-m-n., **AUR-S.,** bar-acet., ***bar-c.,*** bar-i., ***bar-m.,*** **BELL.,** benz-ac., berb., **BISM.,** bond., ***bor., bov.,*** brom., **BRY.,** bufo, buni-o., but-ac., buth-aust., **CACT.,** cadm-s., cahin., calad., **CALC.,** calc-acet., **CALC-AR.,** calc-br., ***calc-f.,*** **CALC-P., CALC-S.,** calen., calth., **CAMPH., CANN-I.,** cann-s., ***canth.,*** caps., ***carb-an.,*** **CARB-V.,** ***carbn-o.,*** **CARBN-S., CARC.,** ***carl., casc., cast.,*** **CAUST.,** cedr., ***cench.,*** cent., ***cham., chel.,*** **CHIN.,** ***chin-ar., chin-s., chlol., chlor., cic.,*** cic-m., ***cimx.,*** cimic., cina, cinnam., clem., cob-n., coc-c., coca, **COCC.,** coch., cod., ***coff.,*** coff-t., colch., ***coloc.,*** **CON.,** ***convo-s.,*** corn., cortico., cot., croc., ***crot-c., crot-h.,*** croto-t., cub., culx., ***cupr., cupr-ar.,*** cupr-s., cur., cycl., cypr., cyt-l., der., **DIG.,** ***dros.,*** dulc., elaps, ergot., ***euph.,*** euph-c., eup-per., euon., ***ferr., ferr-ar., ferr-m.,*** ferr-p., ***ferr-i.,*** fil., ***fl-ac.,*** gamb., ***gels.,*** gins., glon., goss., gran., ***graph.,*** grat., grin., guare., haem., hed., ***hell.,*** hell-f., ***hep.,*** hip-ac., hist., hura, ***hydr-ac.,*** hydrog., hydro-c., ***hyos., hyper.,*** hypoth., ***ictod.,***

ign., indg., inul., **IOD.**, ip., ***jal.***, ***jatr.***, kali-ar., **KALI-AR.**, kali-bi., kali-br., **KALI-C.**, kali-chl., ***kali-i.***, ***kali-n.***, **KALI-P.**, **KALI-S.**, ***kalm.***, kiss., kreos., kres., lac-c., lac-e., lac-h., lac-lup., ***lach.***, lact., lat-m., ***laur.***, ***led.***, lip., lipp., ***lil-t.***, ***lith-c.***, lob., **LYC.**, **LYSS.**, ***m-arct.***, ***mag-c.***, mag-f., ***mag-m.***, ***mag-s.***, ***mand.***, manc., mang., med., medus., meny., ***merc.***, **MERC-C.**, merc-n., merc-s-cy., **MEZ.**, mill., morph., mosch., ***mur-ac.***, murx., mygal., naja, **NAT-AR.**, **NAT-C.**, ***nat-p.***, ***nat-m.***, ***nat-s.***, nicc., **NIT-AC.**, nit-s-d., nitro-o., ***nux-m.***, ***nux-v.***, oci-s., oena., ol-an., ol-j., olnd., ***op.***, ***orig.***, osm., ***ox-ac.***, paeon., pall., par., ***petr.***, phel., ***ph-ac.***, **PHOS.**, piloc., pin-s., pituin., plan., ***plat.***, ***plb.***, podo., **PSOR.**, ptel., **PULS.**, puls-n, ***pyrog.***, ran-a., ran-b., ran-s., raph., rat., ***rauw.***, reser., rheum, rhod., rosm., **RHUS-T.**, ***ruta***, ***sabad.***, ***sabin.***, sac-alb., sal-ac., ***samb.***, sang., sars., **SEC.**, sel., ***seneg.***, ***sep.***, ***sil.***, sin-n., ***spig.***, ***spong.***, squil., ***stann.***, staph., still., ***stram.***, stront-c., stroph-s., stry., sul-i., sulo-ac., **SULPH.**, sul-ac., ***sumb.***, ***tab.***, tanac., tarax., ***tarent.***, tax., tep., ter., thea., ***ther.***, thiop., ***thuj.***, thyreotr., tong., trach., tub., valer., **VERAT.**, ***verat-v.***, verb., verin., vesp., viol-o., viol-t., vip., visc., wies., wild., xan., ***zinc.***

AORTA, general, ailments of - acon., adon., ***adren.***, ***ant-ar.***, apis, ***ars-i.***, aur., aur-ar., ***cact.***, chin-s., crat., cupr., glon., kali-i., lyc., spig., stroph., tub.

rupture, of - ***acon.***, apis, ***arn.***, aster., bar-c., ***bell.***, cact., camph., caust., chen-a., chin., croc., crot-h., cupr., form., ***glon.***, hydr-ac., hyos., juni., kali-br., kali-i., ***lach.***, ***laur.***, ***nux-v.***, ***op.***, ***phos.***, sep., stram., sulph., verat., ***verat-v.***

APATHY, indifferance - agn., ***anac-oc.***, ant-t., ***arg-n.***, ars-h., arum-t., berb., bism., bufo, ***calc.***, camph., chlf., **CINCH.**, ***cocc.***, ***con.***, crot-h., cupr-s., **GELS.**, **HELL.**, ign., jatr., ***kali-br.***, lach., **PHOS.**, **PH-AC.**, sec., sil., ***staph.***

APHASIA, lost of speech - agar., alum., ***anac.***, ant-chl., ant-m., ant-t., arag., ***arg-n.***, arn., ***ars.***, arum-m., aur-m., bar-acet., ***bar-c.***, ***both-l.***, ***calc.***, calc-p., cann-i., ***caust.***, cench., cham., ***chen-a.***, chin., chin-ar., cimic., ***colch.***, con., crot-h., cupr., dios., dulc., elaps, ***glon.***, hydr., hyos., ***kali-br.***, ***kali-chl.***, kali-cy., ***kali-m.***, kali-p., lac-c., ***lach.***, ***laur.***, lil-t., ***lyc.***, ***mag-c.***, ***merc.***, mez., naja, **NIT-AC.**, ***nux-m.***, ***nux-v.***, oci., oena., olnd., onos., op., ph-ac., phos., ***plb.***, puls., stram., sulfon., sumb., syph., tab., xero, ***zinc.***

APHONIA, voice, lost of - acal., ***acon.***, ail., ***alum.***, alum-p., **ALUMN.**, am-c., **AM-CAUST.**, am-m., ambr., amyg-am., anan., **ANT-C.**, ***ant-t.***, **ARG.**, **ARG-N.**, arn., ***ars.***, ars-i., ars-s-f., arum-d., **ARUM-T.**, arund., bac., ***bapt.***, ***bar-c.***, bar-i., bar-s., ***bell.***, both-l., bov., **BROM.**, bry., cahin., calad., calc., calc-ar., camph., cann-i., canth., caps., ***carb-ac.***, carb-an., **CARB-V.**, ***carbn-s.***, **CAUST.**, cedr., cham., chin., chin-s., ***chlor.***, choc., cic., ***cina***, coca, cocain, cocc., coch., colch., con., ***crot-c.***, crot-h., croto-t., ***cupr.***, dig., ***dros.***, ***dulc.***, elaps, ery-a., ***euphr.***, ***ferr.***, ferr-ar., ferr-i., ***ferr-p.***, ferr-pic., ***gels.***, glon., graph., haem., ***hep.***, hydr-ac., ***hyos.***, ***ign.***, iod., iodof., ip., ***kali-ar.***, ***kali-bi.***, kali-br., ***kali-c.***, kali-chl., kali-chls., ***kali-i.***, kali-n., ***kali-p.***, kali-s., ***lac-ac.***, lac-c., ***lach.***, lap-c-b., ***laur.***, lyc., mang., meny., ***merc.***, ***merc-c.***, ***merc-i-f.***, mur-ac., ***naja***, nat-ar., nat-c., ***nat-m.***, nat-p., nicc., ***nit-ac.***, ***nux-m.***, ***nux-v.***, ol-an., olnd., ***op.***, ox-ac., oxyg., ozone, paeon., par., petr., **PHOS.**, ***phyt.***, ***plat.***, plb., pop., pop-c., ptel., ***puls.***, pyrus, rhus-g., **RHUS-T.**, ***rumx.***, ruta, sabad., samb., ***sang.***, sec., ***sel.***, ***seneg.***, sep., sil., ***spong.***, ***stann.***, staph., still., **STRAM.**, stry., sul-ac., sul-i., ***sulph.***, syph., tarent., ter., ***verat.***, verb., vesp., vip., xan., zinc., zinc-m.

APHTHOUS, ulcers, (see Ulcers) - acet-ac., ***aeth.***, agar., agav-a., all-s., allox., alum., alum-sil., anan., anis., ***ant-c.***, ant-t., apis, aral., aran-ix., arg., arg-n., **ARS.**, ***ars-i.***, ars-s-f., arum-d., ***arum-t.***, asim., aur., aur-ar., aur-i., aur-m., aur-s., **BAPT.**, ***berb.***, **BOR.**, brom., bry., ***calc.***, calc-i., calc-sil., camph., canth., caps., ***carb-ac.***, ***carb-an.***, ***carb-v.***, carbn-s., carc., casc., caul., cean., cham., chin., chin-ar., ***chin-b.***, chin-s., chlor., chlorpr., cic., cinch., cinnb., clem., coc-c., cocc., colch., corn., cortiso., cub., ***dig.***, dulc., echi., eucal., eup-a., ***ferr.***, ferr-s., ferul., gali., gamb., graph., ham., ***hell.***, ***hep.***, hippoz., hydr., ***hydr-m.***, illec., ***iod.***, ip., ***jug-c.***, ***kali-ar.***, ***kali-bi.***, ***kali-br.***, ***kali-c.***, **KALI-CHL.**, kali-i., kali-p., kali-s., kali-sil., ***kreos.***, ***lac-ac.***, lac-c., lac-d., ***lach.***, ***lyc.***, ***mag-c.***, maland., ***mand.***, med., **MERC.**, **MERC-C.**, merc-cy., merc-d., ***merc-i-r.***, **MUR-AC.**, ***myric.***, ***nat-ar.***, nat-c., nat-h., ***nat-m.***, ***nit-ac.***, nux-m., **NUX-V.**, oci-s., ox-ac., ozone, petr., ***phos.***, phyt., plan., ***plb.***, psil., psor., ran-b., ran-s., rhus-g., rhus-t., ric., sac-alb., sal-ac., sanic., ***sars.***, sec., **SEMP.**, sep., sil., ***staph.***, **SUL-AC.**, sul-i., **SULPH.**, tarent., tarent-c., ter., thal., thuj., tub., vero-b., vib-p., vinc., viol-t.

APPENDICITIS - acon., alf., ammc., **APIS**, arn., ***ars.***, asar., bapt., **BELL.**, bell-p., **BRY.**, but-ac., cadm-s., ***calad.***, calc., ***calc-s.***, canth., carb-v., ***card-m.***, chel., ***chin.***, ***cocc.***, ***colch.***, ***coloc.***, con., cop., ***crot-c.***, ***crot-h.***, ***dios.***, dulc., ***echi.***, ferr-p., gins., graph., ***hep.***, **IGN.**, **IRIS-T.**, kali-c., kali-m., kali-p., lac-d., ***lach.***, ***lyc.***, **MERC.**, **MERC-C.**, merc-d., mur-ac., ***nat-s.***, ***nit-ac.***, ***nux-v.***, **OP.**, ph-ac., **PHOS.**, ***plb.***, puls., pyrog., rham-cath., **RHUS-T.**, rhus-v., sabal., ***samb.***, scroph-n., ***sep.***, **SIL.**, ***stram.***, sul-i., sulph., syc-co., ter., **THUJ.**, tub., tub-k., verat., verat-v., zinc-val.

APOPLEXY, (see Stroke)

ARSENIC, ailments from - ant-t., **ARS.**, ***ars-i.,*** ars-s-f., ars-s-r., bell., camph., ***carb-v.***, chin., chin-ar., chin-s., dig., euph., ***ferr.***, graph., **HEP.**, iod., kali-ar., kali-i., ***ip.***, lach., ***merc.***, nat-c., nux-m., nux-v., op., ***phos.***, plb., samb., sulph., tab., thuj., ***verat.***

ARTERIES, general - acon., aml-n., bell., crat., coff., ferr., ferr-p., gels., glon., lach., ol-an., sec., seneg.

ARTERIOSCLEROSIS, general - adren., alum., ***am***-i, am-van., aml-n., ant-ar., arg-n., ***arn.***, ars., ***ars-i.***, ***aur.***, aur-br., ***aur-i.***, aur-m-n., ***bar-c.***, bar-i., bar-m., bell-p., benz-ac., cact., ***calc.***, calc-ar., calc-f., calcul-r., card-m., chin-s., chlol., con., crat., ***cupr.***, ergot., fl-ac., form., form-ac., fuc., gink., ***glon.***, hed., hyper., iod., ***kali-i.***, kali-sal., kres., lach., lith-c., mag-f., mand., naja, ***nat-i.***, nit-ac., phos., ***plb.***, ***plb-i.***, ***polyg-a.***, rad-br., rauw., saroth., ***sec.***, sil., solid., stront-c., ***stront-i.***, stroph., sumb., ***tab.***, thiosin., thlaspi, thyr., ***vanad.***, ***visc.***, zinc-p.

ARTERITIS - acon., ***ant-t.,*** apis, **ARN.**, **ARS.**, ars-i., **BAR-C.**, ***calc.***, cham., chin., ***cupr.,*** echi., ***ham.,*** hist., ***kali-c.***, ***kali-i.,*** kreos., ***lach.***, lyc., ***nat-i.***, **PULS.**, ***spig.,*** ***puls.***, sec., sil., sulfa., **SULPH.**, thuj., vip., zinc.

ARTHRITIC, nodosities - abrot., acet-ac., acon., aesc., agn., alum., am-be., am-c., am-m., ***am-p.***, ***ant-c.***, ant-t., **APIS**, arg., arn., ars., asaf., ***aur.***, aur-s., benz., **BENZ-AC.**, berb., brom., ***bry.***, bufo, **CALC.**, **CALC-F.**, ***calc-p.***, ***calc-s.***, calc-sil., calcul-r., caps., carb-an., carb-v., carbn-s., **CAUL.**, ***caust.***, ***cic.***, cimic., ***clem.***, cocc., ***colch.***, con., croc., crot-h., ***dig.***, ***elap***s, elat., eucal., eup-per., fago., ***form.***, **GRAPH.**, ***guai.***, ***hecla.***, hed., hep., ign., iod., kali-ar., kali-c., ***kali-i.***, kali-m., kali-s., kali-sil., lach., **LED.**, **LITH-C.**, **LYC.**, mag-c., mag-m., mang., med., ***meny.***, ***merc.***, morg., mur-ac., mut., nat-c., nat-l., nat-m., nat-s., nat-uric., nit-ac., nux-v., ox-ac., paraf., petr., phos., phyt., pipe., plb., ***puls.***, ran-b., ran-s., ***rhod.***, ***rhus-t.***, ruta, ***sabin.***, sars., sep., ***sil.***, ***staph.***, stel., still., sul-ac., sul-i., sulph., syc-co., thuj., tub-r., urea, ***urt-u.***, zinc.

ARTHRITIS, joints - **ACON.**, act-sp., ***ang.***, **APIS**, ***arn.***, ***aur.***, **BELL.**, **BRY.**, ***calc.***, ***caust.***, ***ferr-p.***, ***guai.***, hyper., ***iod.***, **KALI-C.**, ***kali-i.***, ***kalm.***, ***kreos.***, ***lac-ac.***, lach., **LED.**, lith-c., ***lyc.***, ***mang.***, meny., ***merc.***, ***nat-m.***, ***nat-s.***, ***phyt.***, ***psor.***, ***puls.***, ***rhod.***, **RHUS-T.**, ***ruta***, sabin., ***sars.***, ***sep.***, **SIL.**, ***sulph.***, verat-v.

ASBESTOS, ailments from - asbes., cob., con., radon, ***sil.***

ASCITES, dropsy - ***acet-ac.,*** achy-a., acon., ***adon.***, ***agn.***, alco., alf., all-c., ***ambr.***, ampe-qu, anan., ant-c., **APIS**, <u>**APOC.**</u>, apoc-a., aral-h., ***arg-n.***, **ARS.**, ars-s-f., asaf., asc-c., ***aur.***, ***aur-m.***, aur-m-n., aur-s., baros., bell., ***blatta-a.***, ***bry.***, cahin., ***calc.***, calc-sil., camph., cann-s., ***canth.***, carbn-s., <u>**CARD-M.**</u>, caust., **CHEL.**, ***chim.***, **CHIN.**, ***chin-ar.***, cinnam., coc-c., coca, ***colch.***, coll., coloc., cop., crot-h., cur., ***dig.***, ***digin.***, ***dulc.***, equis., eup-per., euph., fel., ferr., ferr-ar., ***fl-ac.***, ***graph.***, ***hell.***, helon., **HYDR.**, hep., iber., iod., iris, juni-c., kali-ar., kali-br., ***kali-c.***, ***kali-chl.***, kali-p., kali-s., kalm., lact., lappa, ***led.***, lept., **LYC.**, mag-m., med., ***merc.***, mill., mur-ac., nat-ch., nat-m., nux-v., oena., op., oxyd., ***phos.***, plb., ***prun.***, ptel., puls., rhus-t., sabin., sac-alb., samb., sars., ***senec.***, seneg., sep., sil., sol-t-ae., spong., squil., stigm., stront-c., ***sulph.***, sumb., tarax., tarent., **TER.**, thuj., tril-c., uran-n., urea.

ASPARTAME, artificial sweetner, ailments from - alum., arg-n., ars., ***aspart.,*** ***carc.,*** fl-ac., gels., kali-br., lyc., merc., ***phos.,*** sulph.

ASPHYXIA, breathing stopped - ***acet-ac.***, acon., am-c., **ANT-T.**, arn., ars., bell., ***camph.,*** **CARB-V.**, ***carbn-s.***, chin., ***chlor.,*** cimic., ***coch.,*** ***coff.***, coloc., crot-h., cupr., ***hydr-ac.,*** hyos., lat-m., laur., merc., nit-ac., nux-v., **OP.**, ph-ac., phos., ***rhus-t.***, sec., ***sin-n.***, stram., sul-ac., sul-h., tab., upa., vip.

ASPIRIN, ailments from - arn., ars., carb-v., ***chin-s.,*** lach., mag-p., nat-m., ***sal-ac.***

ASTHENOPIA, (see Eyestrain) - agar., ***arn.,*** asar., ***cinnb.,*** ***con.,*** ***croc.,*** ***hydr.,*** **KALM.**, ***lach.,*** merl., nicc., **PHOS.**, **RUTA**, **SULPH.**, ***tab.***

ASTHMA, general - acetan., ***acon.***, acon-f., act-sp., adon., adren., aesc., aeth., ***agar.***, ail., all-c., all-s., aloe, alum., alum-p., alum-sil., alumn., ***am-c.***, am-i, am-m., **AMBR.**, ambro., aml-n., ammc., amyg-am., anac., ang., anis., ant-ar., ant-c., ant-i., ***ant-t.***, ***apis***, aral., arg-cy., **ARG-N.**, arist-cl., arn., <u>**ARS.**</u>, **ARS-I.**, ars-s-f., arum-d., arum-dru., arum-m., arum-t., ***asaf.***, asar., asc-i., asc-t., aster., atro., ***aur.***, aur-ar., aur-i., aur-s., ***ba-tn.***, bac., bad., bapt., ***bar-c.***, bar-i., bar-m., bar-s., ***bell.***, benz-ac., **BLATTA,** blatta-a., bomb-pr., bor., ***bov.***, ***brom.***, ***bry.***, ***cact.***, ***calad.***, ***calc.***, calc-ar., calc-hp., calc-i., calc-l., calc-s., ***calc-sil.***, camph., cann-i., ***cann-s.***, ***caps.***, carb-an., ***carb-v.***, carbn-s., **CARC.**, card-m., cast-eq., caust., cedr., cham., chel., chen-a., ***chin.***, ***chin-ar.***, chin-s., ***chlol.***, chlor., ***cic.***, cimic., cina, cist., coc-c., ***coca***, cocain, cocc., coch., ***coff.***, coffin., ***colch.***, coll., coloc., ***con.***, conv., croc., ***crot-h.***, croto-t., **CUPR.**, ***cupr-acet.***, cupr-ar., cycl., cyt-l., daph., der., ***dig.***, digin., ***dros.***, ***dulc.***, erio., eucal., eup-per., ***euph.***, euph-pi., euphr., fel., ***ferr.***, ferr-acet., ***ferr-ar.***, ferr-i., ferr-p., form., form-ac., gad., gall-ac., galv., ***gels.***, glon., glyc-g., ***graph.***, grat., grin., guai., guare., hed., hedeo, ***hep.***, ***hippoz.***, hydr., hydr-ac., hydrc., hyos., hyper., iber., ictod., ***ign.***, ***iod.***, iodof., **IP.**, jatr-u., junc., just., **KALI-AR.**, ***kali-bi.***, ***kali-br.***, <u>**KALI-C.**</u>, ***kali-chl.***, kali-chls., kali-cy., kali-fcy., ***kali-i.***, kali-m., **KALI-N.**, ***kali-p.***, ***kali-s.***, kali-s-chr., kali-sil., kalm., ***kola,*** kreos., lac-c., lac-d., ***lach.***, lact., ***laur.***, ***led.***, lem-m., levo., lil-t., linu-u, lipp., <u>**LOB.**</u>, lob-p., lob-s., ***lyc.***, lycpr., lycps., mag-p., magn-gl., magn-gr., manc., mang., ***med.***, menthol, meny., ***meph.***, merc., merc-i-r., merc-pr-r., mez., mill., moni., morg., morg-g., morph., ***mosch.***, mut., ***naja***, napht., ***naphtin.***, nat-ar., nat-c., ***nat-m.***, nat-n., nat-p., **NAT-S.**, nat-sil., ***nit-ac.***, nuph., nux-m., ***nux-v.***, oci-s., oeno., ol-an., ol-j., onis., ***op.***, osm., ox-ac., pall., par., passi., **PECT.**, petr., ph-ac., phel., phenob., phle., ***phos.***, phos-pchl., ***phyt.***, pitu-a., plat., plb., plb-i., podo., pop-c., ***psor.***, ptel., pulm-v., **PULS.**, queb., ran-s., raph., rat., rhod., rhus-g., rhus-t., rumx., ***ruta***, sabad., sabal., sabin., **SAMB.**, samb-c., ***sang.***, sanguin-n., sanic., sars., scroph-n., sec., sel., ***seneg.***, ***sep.***, **SIL.**, silphu., sin-n., solid., spig., **SPONG.**, squil., ***stann.***, ***staph.***, stict., ***still.***, **STRAM.**, stront-c., stroph., stry., succ., ***sul-ac.***, sul-h., ***sul-i.***, **SULPH.**, sumb., ***syc-co.***, syph., tab., tela, ter., tet., teucr., ***thuj.***, thymu., thyreotr., trach., trif-p., trio., ***tub.***, tub-a., valer., vario., ***verat.***, verat-v., verb., vib., viol-o., viol-t., ***visc.***, wye., xan., zinc., zinc-p., zinc-val., ***zing.***, ziz.

ASTHMA, children - ***acon.***, ambr., **ANT-T.**, **ARS.**, ***carc.***, **CHAM.**, **IP.**, kali-ar., kali-br., kali-c., kali-i., **KALI-N.**, **KALI-S.**, lob., **MED.**, ***mosch.***, **NAT-S.**, nux-v., psor., **PHOS.**, **PULS.**, **SAMB.**, sanic., ***sil.***, stram., sulph., ***thuj.***, **TUB.**, vib.

ASTIGMATISM, eyes - androc., anh., atro., dubin., esin., ***gels.***, helo., ***lil-t.***, onos., ***phys.***, pic-ac., ruta, ***sep.***, ***tub.***

ATAXIA, general - aesc., aesc-g., ***agar.***, ail., **ALUM.**, alum-p., alum-sil., ***alumn.***, am-m., ang., apis, arag., ***arg-n.***, ars., ars-br., ars-i., asar., astra-e., ***atro.***, ***aur.***, aur-m-n., bar-c., bar-m., ***bell.***, berb., brom., bufo, ***calc.***, cann-i., carb-ac., carb-v., carbn-s., ***caust.***, ***cocc.***, ***con.***, crot-c., cund., cupr-ar., cur., dig., dubin., equis., ferr-p., ***ferr-pic.***, ***fl-ac.***, ***gels.***, ***graph.***, guai., ***hell.***, ***helo.***, hyos., ***ign.***, ingluv., ***kali-br.***, ***kali-i.***, kalm., kres., ***lach.***, **LATH.**, ***lil-t.***, lol., lyc., mag-m., mag-p., mang., med., ***merc.***, merc-c., myric., naja, nat-c., nat-n., nit-ac., nux-m., ***nux-v.***, ***onos.***, ***ox-ac.***, oxyt., ped., ***phos.***, ***phys.***, pic-ac., picro., piloc., pip-m., ***plb.***, plb-i., ptel., rhus-t., ruta, sabad., sant., ***sec.***, sieg., ***sil.***, sol-n., ***stram.***, stront-c., ***stry.***, sulfon., ***sulph.***, tarent., thal., thiosin., ***zinc.***, ***zinc-p.***, zinc-s.

ATELECTASIS, lungs, collapsed - **ANT-T.**, ***hyos.***, med., stry-p., sulph.

ATHEROMA, steatoma - adren., agar., ***am-i.***, am-van., ant-ar., ant-c., anthr., arn., ars., ***ars-i.***, aur., ***aur-i.***, aur-m., aur-m-n., ***bar-c.***, bar-m., ***bell.***, benz-ac., brom., cact., ***calc.***, ***calc-f.***, caps., caust., chin-s., clem., ***con.***, crat., ergot., ***glon.***, ***graph.***, ***guare.***, ***hep.***, hydr., iod., kali-br., ***kali-c.***, ***kali-i.***, kali-sal., ***lach.***, ***lac-ac.***, lith-c., ***lob.***, lyc., m-arct., mez., nat-c., ***nat-i.***, ***nit-ac.***, ***ph-ac.***, phos., ***plb.***, ***plb-i.***, ***polyg-a.***, rhus-t., ***sabin.***, sec., ***sil.***, spong., staph., stront-c., ***stront-i.***, stroph., ***sulph.***, sumb., thuj., thyr., ***vanad.***

ATHLETE'S FOOT, fungus - **BAR-C.**, carb-v., **GRAPH.**, ***nit-ac.***, ***sanic.***, sep., **THUJ.**, **SIL.**, zinc.

ATHETOSIS, hammond's disease - lath., stry., verat-v.

ATROPHY, tissues - anan., arg., ars., aur., bar-c., calc-sil., carb-an., **CAUST.**, cham., chim., chin., con., cupr., hep., ***iod.***, kali-ar., kali-c., kali-i., kali-p., kreos., lac-d., ***nat-m.***, nit-ac., nux-m., nux-v., ph-ac., phos., phys., **PLB.**, plb-i., sabal., sars., sec., sil., stann., staph., sul-i., verat.

ATROPINE, ailments from - ***atro.***, ***bell.***, hyos., op., phys., stram.

ATTENTION DEFICIT DISORDER, (see Hyperactivity, Learning disabilities) - agar., amphet., ***anac.***, ***androc.***, aran-ix., ***ars.***, ***aspart.***, ***calc-p.***, caps., **CARC.**, cham., ***cina***, coff., hyos., iod., lyc., lyss., **MED.**, merc., nat-m., ***nux-v.***, plan., ***rital.***, **STRAM.**, ***tarent.***, thuj., tub., verat., ***zinc.***

AUTISTIC, children - aeth., agra., anac., bar-c., bufo, ***carc.***, cann-i., hell., hyos., kali-br., lyc., med., merc., ***nat-m.***, op., stram., syph., thuj., ***tub.***

AUTO-IMMUNE, diseases - ant-c., ***ars.***, ars-i., calen., ***carc.***, cortiso., echi., graph., kali-ar., ***lac-c.***, ***lil-t.***, lach., med., merc., nat-m., nit-ac., psor., rhus-t., syph., thuj.

AVIATOR'S, disease - ars., bell., bor., carc., ***coca***, ***cocc.***, psor.

AXILLA, cancer - ars., **ASTER.**, ***brom.***, ***carb-an.***, chim., ***con.***, ***phyt.***, scroph-m., scroph-n.

AXILLARY, glands - acon-l., **ASTER.**, ***bar-c.***, bufo, cadm-s., bell., calc., calc-s., carb-an., **CON.**, ***crot-h.***, elaps, graph., hep., jug-r., kali-c., ***lac-ac.***, lac-c., **MERC.**, ***merc-i-r.***, nat-m., nat-s., **NIT-AC.**, petr., ph-ac., phos., **PHYT.**, raph., rhus-t., sep., ***sil.***, sulph., thuj.

B

BACK, general - **AESC.**, ***aesc-g.***, ***agar.***, alum., alum-sil., alumn., anan., arg-n., ***arn.***, bar-c., bell-p., berb., ***brach.***, **BRY.**, but-ac., **CALC.**, **CALC-F.**, **CALC-P.**, calc-s., caust., ***cic.***, cimic., ***cocc.***, coloc., ***con.***, cupr-ar., cur., ***eup-per.***, gins., glyc., ***graph.***, guai., hecla, ***helon.***, hydr., **HYPER.**, irid., jac., **KALI-C.**, kali-cy., kali-p., ***lach.***, ***lath.***, ***lyc.***, merc., nat-m., **NAT-S.**, nit-ac., **NUX-V.**, ox-ac., pall., petr., ph-ac., ***phos.***, phys., ***pic-ac.***, ***plb.***, **RHUS-T.**, **RUTA**, ***sel.***, **SEP.**, **SIL.**, staph., stront-c., ***stry.***, **SULPH.**, sul-ac., **SYMPH.**, tell., thuj., **ZINC.**

BACK, injuries - ailments, after - aesc., ***apis***, **ARN.**, ***bell-p.***, bor., **BRY.**, ***calc.***, calc-f., calc-p., carb-an., caust., cic., ***coloc.***, ***con.***, dam., graph., **HYPER.**, kali-bi., ***kali-c.***, ***led.***, ***lyc.***, mez., **NAT-S.**, ***nit-ac.***, nux-v., ph-ac., phos., **RHUS-T.**, **RUTA**, sang., sep., ***sil.***, stront-c., symph., tell., ***thuj.***, zinc.

disks, slipped, herniated, or ruptured - **AESC.**, arn., **AGAR.**, ***berb.***, **BRY.**, ***coloc.***, **HYPER.**, kali-c., mag-p., ruta, tarent., ***tell.***, zinc.

dislocations, vertebrae - **ARN.,** bell-p., **BRY., CALC.,** calc-f., caust., ***coloc.,*** hyper., lyc., nux-v., phos., **RHUS-T.,** ***ruta,*** stront-c., sulph., zinc.

lifting, from - **ARN.,** ***bell-p.,*** bor., **BRY., CALC., GRAPH., HYPER.,** ***lyc., nux-v.,*** ph-ac., **RHUS-T., RUTA,** sang., ***sep.***

pain, after - **ARN.,** bell-p., **BRY.,** calc., ***con.,*** **HYPER.,** ***kali-c., nat-s.,*** **RHUS-T.,** ***ruta, thuj.***

spasms, after - acon., arn., ***ars.,*** bell., bry., calc., ***calc-p.,*** cham., cic., ***cimic., coloc., crot-c.,*** hyper., ***lach.,*** kali-c., **MAG-P.,** ***mygal., nat-m., nat-s., nux-v.,*** oena., ***phys.,*** rhus-t., ruta, sep., stram., syph., tab.

straining, easy - bell-p., bor., bry., **CALC.,** calc-f., ***calc-p.,*** con., **GRAPH.,** ham., kali-c., **LYC.,** mill., ***nux-v.,*** ph-ac., **RHUS-T., RUTA,** sang., ***sep.,*** sil.

BACTERIAL, infections - ant-c., ***ars.,*** **BAPT.,** carb-an., ***echi.,*** hep., merc., nit-ac., ph-ac., phos., puls., **PYROG.,** sil., sulph., ***thuj.***

BAD NEWS, ailments from - acon., aln., alum., alumn., ambr., ***apis, arn.,*** ars., art-v., ***aur.,*** aur-m., bapt., ***bry.,*** **CALC.,** ***calc-p.,*** calc-s., **CARC.,** ***caust., cham.,*** chin., ***cic.,*** cinnb., cocc., colch., ***coloc.,*** cupr., dig., dros., form., **GELS.,** grat., hist., hyos., **IGN.,** kali-c., kali-p., lac-v., lach., ***lyc., lyss.,*** manc., ***med.,*** mez., nat-c., **NAT-M.,** nat-p., ***nit-ac., nux-v.,*** paeon., ***pall.,*** ph-ac., phos., podo., puls., sabin., sep., ***sil., staph.,*** stram., ***sulph.,*** tarent., teucr., zinc.

BALDNESS, (See Hair, loss) - ***anac., apis,*** **BAR-C.,** ***fl-ac., graph.,*** hep., jab., lyc., med., morg., **PH-AC.,** ***phos.,*** piloc., pix., sel., ***sep.,*** **SIL., STANN.,** syc-co., ***zinc.***

BALANITIS, penis, glans - ***acon.,*** alum., ***alumn.,*** antipyrin., ***apis, arg-n.,*** arn., ars., ***aur.,*** aur-ar., aur-s., bry., ***calad., calc., calen.,*** cann-s., canth., carbn-s., caust., chin., **CINNB.,** ***cop., cor-r., cub.,*** cupr., ***dig., gels.,*** graph., ham., iris, ***jac-c.,*** **KALI-CHL.,** kali-p., ***kali-s.,*** lach., led., ***lyc.,*** lyss., ***merc., merc-c.,*** mez., nat-ar., ***nat-c., nat-m.,*** nat-sil., ***nit-ac.,*** nux-v., ozone, petr., ph-ac., ***psor., rhod.,*** rhus-t., sabin., sars., sep., sil., staph., ***sulph., thuj.***

BARBER'S, itch, ringworm of beard - ant-t., anthr., ars., aur-m., ***bac., calc.,*** calc-s., chrysar., ***cic.,*** cinnb., cocc., cypr., ***graph., kali-bi.,*** kali-m., lith-c., ***lyc.,*** mag-p., med., merc-pr-r., nat-s., ***nit-ac.,*** petr., phyt., plan., ***plat.,*** rhus-t., sabad., sep., sil., ***staph.,*** stront-c., sul-i., ***sulph.,*** tell., **THUJ.**

BARIUM, ailments from - ant-t., ***bar-c.,*** bar-m., bell., camph., dulc., mag-s., merc., plb., zinc.

BARTHOLINITIS, genitalia - hep., lach., merc., morg., nit-ac., sep., ***sil.,*** tarent-c., thuj.

BASAL CELL, cancer, (see Epithelioma, Melanoma, Squamos) - ars., **AUR-M.,** ***carc.,*** cinnb., cund., gali., ***hydr.,*** kali-ar., ***kali-bi.,*** petr., rad-br., scroph-n., ***sol,*** thuj.

BAZIN'S, disease - bac., sec., tub.

BEDSORES, decubitus - ***agar.,*** ambr., am-c., am-m., ant-c., ***arg-n.,*** **ARN.,** ars., bapt., bar-c., bell., bov., ***calc.,*** calc-p., canth., carb-an., ***carb-v.,*** caust., cham., **CHIN.,** coff., colch., crot-h., dros., euph., ***fl-ac.,*** **GRAPH.,** ***ham., hep.,*** hippoz., ***hydr.,*** **HYPER.,** ***ign.,*** kali-ar., kali-c., kreos., **LACH., LED.,** ***lyc.,*** mag-m., mang., ***merc.,*** mez., ***nat-c.,*** nat-m., nit-ac., nux-v., olnd., op., paeon., **PETR.,** ph-ac., phos., ***plb., puls.,*** rhus-t., ruta, sel., **SEP., SIL.,** spig., squil., ***sulph., sul-ac.,*** ter., zinc.

BEDWETTING, enuresis - acon., ***aeth.,*** alum., ***am-c.,*** anac., anan., **APIS,** ***apoc., arg.,*** **ARG-N., ARN., ARS.,** ***aur.,*** aur-m., aur-s., bar-c., bar-m., **BELL., BENZ-AC.,** bry., cact., ***calc.,*** canth., ***carb-v., carbn-s.,*** **CAUST.,** ***cham.,*** chin., ***chlol.,*** cimx., ***cina,*** coca, con., ***crot-c.,*** cub., cupr., dulc., **EQUIS.,** ***eup-pur.,*** **FERR.,** ***ferr-acet.,*** ferr-i., ferr-p., ***fl-ac.,*** **GRAPH.,** ***hep.,*** hyos., ign., kali-br., kali-c., ***kali-p.,*** **KREOS., LAC-C.,** lac-d., **LYC.,** m-aust., mag-c., ***mag-m.,*** **MAG-P.,** mag-s., ***med., merc.,*** mur-ac., ***nat-ar., nat-c.,*** **NAT-M.,** ***nat-p.,*** **NIT-AC.,** nux-v., ***op.,*** ox-ac., ***petr.,*** ph-ac., ***phos.,*** physal., ***plan., podo., psor.,*** **PULS.,** quas., rhus-a., **RHUS-T.,** ***ruta,*** sabal., ***sanic.,*** sant., ***sars.,*** sec., sel., ***seneg.,*** **SEP., SIL.,** spig., squil., staph., ***stram.,*** **SULPH.,** ***syc-co.,*** tab., ter., ***thuj.,*** **THYR.,** ***tub., uran., urt-u.,*** uva., verat., ***verb., viol-t.,*** zinc.

BELL'S PALSY, (see Paralysis) - ***acon., agar.,*** all-c., alum., ***am-p.,*** anac., anh., apis, ***arn.,*** ars., bac., bapt., ***bar-c.,*** **BELL.,** ***cadm-s.,*** carb-v., carc., **CAUST.,** ***cocc.,*** colch., con., crot-h., ***cupr., cur., dulc.,*** form., ***gels., graph.,*** hell., hep., hyos., hyper., ***ign.,*** iod., ***kali-chl., kali-i.,*** kali-m., kali-p., lach., lyc., merc., merc-i-f., mur-ac., naja, nat-m., nux-m., ***nux-v.,*** ol-an., op., oxyu-s., peti., petr., phos., phys., physal., phyt., plat., plb., puls., ran-b., rhus-t., ruta, sec., seneg., sep., sil., solid., spig., stram., stry., sulph., syph., zinc., zinc-p., zinc-pic.

BELLADONNA, ailments from - acon., ***atro., bell.,*** camph., coff., hyos., op., phys., stram

BERI-BERI - ars., ***elat.,*** lath., rhus-t.

BERYLLIUM, ailments from - alum., ***beryl.,*** fl-ac., mang., sil., zinc.

BESNIER-BOECK, morbus, sarcoidosis - aq-mar., aran-ix., asar., beryl., hip-ac., hist., kres., lepro., lyc., mand., nat-ar., parathyr., pin-s., puls., thiop., tub., tub-m., v-a-b.

BILE-DUCTS, ailments of - am-m., berb., card-m., ***chel., chin., chion., chol.,*** dios., gels., hippoz., ***hydr.,*** lyc., kali-m., merc-d., nat-p., rheum

BILIOUS, fever - ***acon.***, alum., ant-c., ant-t., arn., ***ars.***, asaf., asar., asc-t., aur., **BAPT.**, ***bell.***, ***bol.***, ***bry.***, calc., card-m., ***cham.***, chin., chol., cocc., ***coff.***, ***coloc.***, corn., croc., **CROT-H.**, cupr., ***dig.***, echi., elat., euon., euon-a., ***eup-per.***, gels., ***graph.***, ham., hydr., hyos., ***ign.***, ip., iris, ***lach.***, lept., ***lyc.***, mag-c., mag-m., malar., ***merc.***, merc-c., merc-d., mez., ***mur-ac.***, nat-c., nat-m., ***nat-s.***, nux-m., ***nux-v.***, nyct., oci-s., ***op.***, petr., ph-ac., ***phos.***, ***plat.***, podo., polyp-p., ***puls.***, **PYROG.**, ran-b., rhus-t., samb., sec., sel., seneg., sep., sil., spong., stann., ***staph.***, stram., stront-c., sulph., tarax., trio., verat., verb., zinc.

BILIOUS, headaches - am-pic., anac., ***arg-n.***, bapt., ***bry.***, card-m., cham., **CHEL.**, ***chion.***, cycl., eup-per., ***ip.***, iris, lob., merc-s., **NUX-V.**, podo., ***puls.***, rob., **SANG.**, stry., tarax.

BIPOLAR, disorder, manic depression - agar., alco., arg., ***anac.***, ***aur.***, bell., cann-i., **CARC.**, cimic., cocc., coff., ***con.***, croc., cyt-l., ***hyos.***, iod., ***kali-br.***, kres., **LACH.**, lil-t., **LITH-C.**, **MED.**, merc., ***nat-s.***, nux-v., op., phos., plat., plb., proz., psor., **STAPH.**, stram., sulfa., syph., tarent., ***verat.***

BIRTHMARKS, nevi - **ACET-AC.**, arn., ars., ***calc.***, calc-f., carb-an., ***carb-v.***, **CARC.**, cund., **FL-AC.**, lach., ***lyc.***, med., nux-v., **PHOS.**, plat., rad., ***sep.***, sol, ***sulph.***, **THUJ.**, ust., vac.

BITES, general, animals and insects, from - acet-ac., all-s., androc., ***apis***, ***arn.***, ***ars.***, aur., ***bell.***, calad., calen., ***cedr.***, ***echi.***, grin., **HYPER.**, ***lach.***, **LED.**, lyss., ***plan.***, ***pyrog.***, seneg., stram., ***sul-ac.***, tarent., ***thuj.***

- **animals,** of poisonous or enraged - ***am-c.***, androc., anthr., ***apis***, arn., ***ars.***, aur., **BELL.**, calad., ***caust.***, ***cedr.***, cist., ***echi.***, hyper., ***lach.***, **LED.**, ***lob-p.***, **LYSS.**, mosch., nat-m., ***plan.***, puls., pyrog., ***seneg.***, ***stram.***, sul-ac., vip.
- **cats,** of - acet-ac., **HYPER.**, ***lach.***, **LED.**
- **dogs,** of (see Rabies) - acet-ac., am-c., am-caust., anthr., ***apis***, arn., ***ars.***, **BELL.**, calad., camph., ***cedr.***, crot-h., ***echi.***, ***grin.***, gua., gymne., hydr-ac., ***hyper.***, kali-ma., ***lach.***, ***led.***, **LYSS.**, ***nat-m.***, mosch., pyrog., sisy., spirae., ***ter.***
- **fleas** - bapt., calad., calc., grin., hyper., ***led.***, pulx., staph.
- **flies,** itch and burn - calad.
- **leeches** - alumn., lach., sec.
- **mosquitoes** - calad., led., staph.
- **rats** - hyper., led.
- **scorpions** - androc., hyper., led.
- **snakes,** venomous - acet-ac., am-c., am-caust., anag., anthr., ***apis***, arist-cl., arn., ***ars.***, aur., **BELL.**, calad., ***camph.***, ***cedr.***, ***crot-h.***, ***echi.***, ***grin.***, gymne., hydr-ac., ***hyper.***, kali-ma., **LACH.**, **LED.**, lob-p., lycps., mosch., ***plan.***, pyrog., seneg., sisy., spirae., stram., sul-ac., ***thuj.***, ***vip.***
- **spiders,** bites - apis., ***hyper.***, lat-m., ***led.***, lycps., tarent.

BLACK WATER, fever - ***ars.***, chin-s., crot-h., lyc., pyrog.

BLADDER, cancer - acet-ac., anil., ars., calc., carb-an., ***carc.***, ***con.***, ***crot-h.***, scirr., sec., stann., tarax., **TER.**, ***thuj.***, visc.

BLADDER, remedies - **ACON.**, am-c., **APIS**, ***arg-n.***, ***arn.***, ***ars.***, aspar., ***bar-m.***, **BELL.**, bell-p., benz-ac., **BERB.**, cact., ***calad.***, calen., ***calc.***, camph., ***cann-i.***, ***cann-s.***, **CANTH.**, ***caps.***, carb-an., **CAUST.**, ***chim.***, ***chin-s.***, coloc., ***con.***, ***cop.***, ***cub.***, ***cupr.***, ***dig.***, ***dulc.***, elat., **EQUIS.**, ***ery-a.***, eucal., ***eup-pur.***, ferr-acet., ferr-p., ***gels.***, ***hep.***, ***hydr.***, ***hyos.***, kali-ar., kali-bi., kali-c., kali-chl., **LACH.**, lil-t., lith-c., **LYC.**, **MED.**, ***merc.***, ***merc-c.***, ***nit-ac.***, ***nux-v.***, ***ol-sant.***, pareir., petr., petros., ph-ac., pip-m., polyg., pop., prun., **PULS.**, ***rhus-t.***, sabal., **SARS.**, ***sabin.***, senec., seneg., **SEP.**, solid., squil., **STAPH.**, ***stigm.***, stram., ***sulph.***, tarent., **TER.**, **THLASPI**, thuj., tub., uva., verat-v.

BLADDER, stones, calculi - acon., ***ambr.***, ant-c., ant-t., arg-n., arn., ars., baros., ***bell.***, **BENZ-AC.**, **BERB.**, cact., **CALC.**, **CALCUL-R.**, calen., cann-s., **CANTH.**, card-m., cham., chim., ***chin.***, chin-s., ***coc-c.***, colch., coloc., con., cupr., dulc., elem., epig., equis., erig., ery-a., ***eup-pur.***, fab., gall-ac., hedeo, hep., hydrang., ***ipom.***, ***lach.***, lipp., ***lith-c.***, **LYC.**, m-aust., ***meny.***, mez., ***mill.***, morg-g., naja, nat-m., nat-s., ***nit-ac.***, ***nux-m.***, ***nux-v.***, oci., oci-s., onon., op., oxyd., ***pareir.***, ***petr.***, ***phos.***, pipe., ***puls.***, ***raph.***, ***ruta***, **SARS.**, **SEP.**, ***sil.***, sol-x., solid., staph., stigm., sulph., ***tab.***, tarent., thlaspi, thuj., ***urt-u.***, ***uva.***, vario., verat., zinc.

BLEEDING, general, (see Blood) - abies-n., acet-ac., ***acon.***, ***adren.***, ***agar.***, aloe, ***alum.***, alumn., ambr., am-c., am-caust., am-m., ***ammc.***, anac., ***ant-c.***, ant-t., anthr., ***apis***, ***aran.***, arg., ***arg-n.***, **ARN.**, ***ars.***, ars-i., arum-t., asar., aur., aur-m., bapt., ***bar-c.***, bar-m., **BELL.**, bell-p., bism., bor., ***bov.***, **BOTH-L.**, brom., bufo, ***bry.***, ***cact.***, **CALC.**, calc-f., **CALC-S.**, cann-s., **CANTH.**, ***caps.***, carb-an., **CARB-V.**, ***carbn-s.***, casc., caust., cina, ***cham.***, **CHIN.**, chin-ar., clem., cinnb., ***cinnam.***, cocc., coc-c., ***coff.***, coff-t., colch., coll., ***coloc.***, con., ***croc.***, crot-c., **CROT-H.**, ***cupr.***, dig., ***dros.***, ***dulc.***, ***elaps***, equis., **ERIG.**, euphr., **FERR.**, ***ferr-ar.***, ***ferr-i.***, ***ferr-m.***, ***ferr-p.***, ***ger.***, glon., ***graph.***, **HAM.**, **HELL.**, hep., hydr., ***hyos.***, ign., ***iod.***, **IP.**, kali-c., ***kali-chl.***, kali-i., kali-n., ***kali-p.***, kreos., **LACH.**, lat-m., ***led.***, ***lyc.***, ***lycps.***, m-arct., m-aust., mag-m., **MELI.**, **MERC.**, **MERC-C.**, ***mez.***, **MILL.**, mosch., mur-ac., **MURX.**, nat-c., **NAT-M.**, ***nat-s.***, nux-m., **NUX-V.**, op., petr., ***ph-ac.***, **PHOS.**, ***plat.***, plb., ***psor.***, **PULS.**, pyrog., rhod., ***rhus-t.***, ruta, sabad., **SABIN.**, sal-ac., sang., sars., **SEC.**, ***senec.***, **SEP.**, sel., ***sil.***, squil., stann., staph., ***stram.***, ***stront-c.***, sulfa., **SULPH.**, **SUL-AC.**, syph., tarax.,

ter., thlaspi, thuj., til., ***tril.,*** urt-u., ust., valer., verat., vib., vinc., vip., wies., x-ray, xan., zinc.

BLENORRHEA, penis, glans - alum., alumn., calad., caust., ***cinnb.,*** cor-r., dig., ***jac-c.,*** lach., ***lyc., merc.,*** mez., nat-c., ***nat-m., nit-ac., nux-v.,*** petr., psor., ***sep., sulph., thuj.***

BLEPHARITIS, eyelids, inflammation - ***acon.,*** act-sp., aeth., aethi-a., alum., am-c., anac., androc., **ANT-C., APIS, ARG., ARG-N.,** ***ars.,*** ars-s-f., arund., aur-m., bac., bar-c., bar-s., bell., berb., bor., bov., bry., ***calc.,*** calc-i., **CALC-S.,** cann-s., canth., ***carb-an.,*** carb-v., **CARBN-S.,** caust., cham., chrys-ac., ***cinnb.,*** clem., ***cocc.,*** com., con., croto-t., ***dig.,*** dulc., euph., euphr., gels., **GRAPH.,** ***hep.,*** hip-ac., ***hydr.,*** hyos., ign., ***iris,*** jug-r., kali-ar., kali-bi., ***kali-c.,*** kali-s., kali-sil., kreos., lach., lap-gr-m., lil-t., **LYC.,** m-aust., m-ambo., mag-c., mag-m., **MED.,** meph., **MERC.,** merc-c., merc-i-f., ***merc-pr-r.,*** ***mez.,*** morbill., morg., morg-g., nat-ar., ***nat-c., nat-m.,*** nat-s., nat-sil., ***nit-ac.,*** nux-v., ozone, **PETR.,** phos., podo., polyg., ***psor.,*** puls., **RHUS-T.,** sabad., ***sang., sanic.,*** sarr., sars., ***seneg., sep., sil., spig.,*** spong., ***squil.,*** stann., **STAPH.,** stram., **SULPH., TELL.,** ***ter., thuj.,*** tub., upa., ***uran-n.,*** vac., vario., verat., zinc., zinc-p.

BLINDNESS, loss of vision, (see Amaurosis) - **ACON.,** aconin., act-sp., ***agar.,*** all-c., alum., am-c., ambr., amyg-am., anac., ant-c., ant-t., apis, apoc., arg., arg-m., arg-n., arn., ars., asaf., asar., aster., ***aur.,*** aur-ar., ***aur-m.,*** aur-s., bar-c., ***bell.,*** benz-d., berb., bor., ***both-l., bov.,*** brom., bry., bufo, cact., cadm-s., ***calc.,*** calc-ar., camph., cann-i., cann-s., canth., caps., carb-an., carb-v., carbn-o., ***carbn-s.,*** cast., ***caust.,*** cedr., cham., chel., chen-a., ***chin., chin-s.,*** chlf., chlol., cic., cimic., cina, clem., coca, cocc., coff., colch., coloc., com., ***con.,*** croc., crot-c., crot-h., croto-t., cupr., cupr-acet., cycl., dict., ***dig.,*** dor., dros., dulc., elaps, eug., euon., eup-per., euph., ***euphr.,*** eupi., ferr., ferr-ar., ferr-p., fil., ***gels.,*** gins., glon., gran., ***graph.,*** grat., guajol., gymn., haem., hedeo, hell., helon., hep., hura, hura-c., hydr-ac., **HYOS.,** ign., indg., iod., iodof., ip., iris, jab., jug-c., kali-ar., kali-bi., kali-br., kali-c., kali-chl., kali-cy., ***kali-i.,*** kali-n., kali-sil., kalm., kreos., lac-ac., lac-d., lac-v., lach., lachn., lact., lam., laur., led., lil-t., ***lith-c., lyc., lyss.,*** mag-c., mag-m., manc., mang., med., meny., meph., **MERC.,** merl., mez., mom-b., morph., mosch., mur-ac., naja, naphtin., nat-c., ***nat-m.,*** nat-p., nat-s., nit-ac., nux-m., ***nux-v.,*** oena., ol-j., olnd., onos., ***op.,*** ox-ac., par., petr., petros., ph-ac., phel., ***phos.,*** phys., phyt., piloc., pitu-p., plat., ***plb.,*** plb-acet., psil., psor., **PULS.,** ran-b., ran-s., raph., rhus-t., rhus-v., rumx., russ., ***ruta,*** sabad., sabin., sang., sant., sars., ***sec.,*** seneg., ***sep.,*** **SIL.,** sol-n., ***spig.,*** squil., stann., staph., **STRAM.,** stront-c., stroph., stry., ***sulph.,*** syph., ***tab.,*** tarax., tep., ter., thea., ***ther.,*** thuj., thyr., til., titan., tub., upa., valer., vanad., verat., ***verat-v.,*** vinc., viol-t., vip., zinc., zinc-m.

BLISTERS, skin - ail., alum., alum-sil., am-c., am-m., ambr., ***anac.,*** **ANT-C.,** anthro., **APIS,** ***ars.,*** ars-s-f., aur., aur-ar., aur-s., bell., bomb-chr., bor., bry., ***bufo,*** **CANTH.,** carb-an., carbn-s., **CAUST.,** ***cham., clem.,*** com., cosm., crot-h., ***dulc.,*** elaps, ***graph.,*** hep., ***kali-ar.,*** kali-bi., ***kali-c.,*** kali-s., kali-sil., lach., lyc., m-ambo., ***mag-c.,*** manc., ***merc.,*** naja, nat-ar., ***nat-c.,*** nat-m., nat-p., nat-s., nit-ac., ***petr.,*** phos., prim-o., ***ran-b., ran-s.,*** **RHUS-T.,** rhus-v., sec., ***sep., sil., sulph.,*** syph., urt-u., verat., verat-v., vip., zinc.

BLOOD, remedies, (see Anemia, Bleeding) - ***acet-ac.,*** agn., am-c., ambr., apoc., aq-mar., **ARS.,** ***ars-i.,*** ars-s-f., aur-ar., cadm-m., cadm-s., calc., calc-ar., ***calc-p.,*** calen., carb-an., **CARB-V.,** ***carbn-s.,*** **CHIN.,** ***chin-ar., chin-s.,*** **CRAT., CROT-H.,** cupr., cupr-ar., cupr-s., dig., **ECHI., ECHI-P., FERR.,** ferr-acet., **FERR-AR.,** ferr-c., ferr-cit., ***ferr-i., ferr-m.,*** ferr-o-r., **FERR-P.,** ferr-pic., ***ferr-o-r.,*** goss., ***ham.,*** ip., kali-ar., kali-br., kali-c., kali-fcy., kali-n., lac-ac., **LACH.,** lyc., nat-ar., nat-n., ***nat-p.,*** nat-s., nit-ac., ***nux-v.,*** ozone, ***ph-ac.,*** **PHOS.,** ***pic-ac.,*** plb., plb-acet., psor., **PULS.,** pyrog., sabin., ***sec., sep.,*** sil., spig., stroph., sul-ac., **SULPH.,** ***thyr.,*** verat., ***x-ray, zinc.,*** zinc-ar., zinc-s.

loss, of blood, ailments from - abrot., ant-c., ***arg-o.,*** arn., ***ars., bac., calc.,*** calc-p., ***cann-i.,*** carb-an., ***carb-v.,*** **CHIN.,** chin-ar., crat., crot-h., ***cycl.,*** **FERR.,** ferr-acet., ferr-p., ferr-pic., goss., ***graph.,*** ham., ***helon., hydr.,*** ign., ip., kali-c., lac-ac., ***lach.,*** mang., nat-br., ***nat-m., nux-v., phos., ph-ac.,*** pic-ac., ***puls.,*** sabin., senec., sep., staph., ***sulph.,*** trif-r., xan.

polycythemia, blood - carc., ferr., phos.

transfusion, blood, ailments from - carc., chin.

BLOOD, vessels, remedies, (see Veins) - abies-c., acon., am-c., aml-n., ant-t., apis, ***arn.,*** ars., aur., ***bell.,*** bell-p., bor., bry., calc., calc-ar., calc-hp., camph., carb-an., **CARB-V.,** caust., chin., chin-s., clem., cocc., coff., croc., crot-h., cupr., cycl., ferr., ferr-p., ***fl-ac.,*** form., gels., glon., graph., **HAM.,** hydr., hydr-ac., ***hyos.,*** iod., kreos., **LACH.,** lyc., med., merc., mill., nat-m., nat-p., nit-ac., nux-v., ol-an., op., petr., ph-ac., phel., **PHOS.,** pip-n., plat., plb., **PULS.,** pyrog., rhus-t., sang., ***sec.,*** seneg., sep., sil., staph., stront-c., sul-ac., sulph., syph., tab., ***thuj.,*** tril., vario., verat., vip., visc., zinc.

injuries, to blood vessels - arn., ham., hyper., led., ***mill.,*** phos.

BOILS, general - abrot., acon., aeth., agar., aloe, alum., alum-p., alum-sil., alumn., am-c., am-m., ambro., ***anac.,*** anan., ***ant-c.,*** ant-t., ***anthr., apis,*** **ARN.,** ***ars., ars-i.,*** ars-s-f., ars-s-r., aur., aur-ar., aur-s., ***bar-c.,*** **BELL.,** ***bell-p.,*** **BERB.,** brom., bry., bufo, cadm-s., ***calc.,*** calc-chln., calc-hp., calc-i., **CALC-M.**, calc-p., ***calc-pic.***, **CALC-S.**, calc-sil., carb-an., carb-v., carbn-s., carc., chin., chin-ar., cist., coc-c., cocc., colch., ***con.***, ***crot-h.***, cupr-ar., dulc., echi., elaps, elat., ***euph.***, ***ferr-i.***, ferr-ma., fl-ac., gaert., gels., ***graph.***, gunp., **HEP.**, hippoz., ho., hydr., ***hyos.***, ***ichth.***, ign., insulin, ***iod.***, iris, jug-r., kali-bi., kali-br., ***kali-i.***, kali-n., kreos., **LACH.**, lappa, laur., ***led.***, lob-p., **LYC.**, m-ambo., mag-c., mag-m., mag-s., maland., ***med.***, **MERC.**, mez., micr., mur-ac., nat-ar., nat-c., ***nat-m.***, nat-p., nat-s., nat-sal., nat-sil., ***nit-ac.***, nux-m., ***nux-v.***, ol-j., ol-myr., op., oper., ozone, **PETR.**, ***ph-ac.***, ***phos.***, ***phyt.***, pic-ac., prot., **PSOR.**, puls., pyrog., **RHUS-T.**, rhus-v., sabin., sanic., sapo., saroth., sars., ***sec.***, senec., ***sep.***, sieg., **SIL.**, sol-a., spong., stann., staph., staphycoc., stram., ***sul-ac.***, ***sul-i.***, **SULPH.**, syph., tarent., ***thuj.***, torul., tub., urine, viol-t., vip., zinc., zinc-o., zinc-p.

BONE, cancer - arg-n., ars., ***aur.***, aur-i., aur-m., **CADM.**, ***calc.***, calc-f., ***carc.***, ***con.***, euph., graph., **HECLA.**, hippoz., merc., methyl., ***phos.***, plut-n., ruta, **SCIRR.**, **SYMPH.**, syph., thuj.

BONES, remedies, (see Periosteum) - acon., agar., am-c., ang., aran., arg., ***arg-n.***, arn., ars., **ASAF.**, ***aur.***, bar-c., bell., berb., both-l., bry., bufo, **CALC.**, **CALC-F.**, ***calc-i.***, **CALC-P.**, ***calc-s.***, carb-an., carb-v., carc., cast-eq., chel., chin., cist., cocc., con., croto-t., cupr., cycl., dulc., eup-per., euph., ferr., ferr-acet., ferr-p., **FL-AC.**, gad., get., graph., ***guai.***, guare., **HECLA.**, hep., iod., kali-bi., kali-c., kali-i., lac-ac., lach., lith-c., lyc., mag-m., mang., med., **MERC.**, ***merc-c.***, ***mez.***, naja, nat-s., ***nit-ac.***, ol-an., ol-j., op., par., parathyr., petr., **PH-AC.**, ***phos.***, ***phyt.***, pip-n., **PLB.**, **PULS.**, pyrog., rad-br., rhod., rhus-t., ***ruta***, sabin., sang., sars., sep., **SIL.**, staph., ***still.***, stront-c., ***sulph.***, **SYMPH.**, syph., tep., ther., thuj., verat.

- **brittle,** bones - asaf., bar-c., bufo, ***calc.***, calc-f., **CALC-P.**, carc., cupr., fl-ac., ***hecla***, ***lac-ac.***, lach., lyc., ***merc.***, par., ph-ac., pip-n., ruta, **SIL.**, sulph., ***symph.***, thuj.
- **curvature**, curving of bones - am-c., **ASAF.**, bar-c., ***bell.***, bufo, ***calc.***, **CALC-F.**, ***calc-p.***, cann-s., caust., cic., ***ferr.***, graph., **HECLA**, hep., iod., ip., kali-c., lyc., ***merc.***, mez., ***nit-ac.***, petr., ***ph-ac.***, ***phos.***, plb., ***puls.***, rhod., ruta, ***sep.***, ***sil.***, staph., ***sulph.***, syph., ther., thuj., tub.
- **decalcification,** (see Osteoporosis) - ***calc.***, ***calc-f.***, **CALC-P.**, cor-r., hecla, sil., symph.
- **tumors,** osteoma - ***arg.***, aur., aur-m., calc., calc-f., crot-c., ***dulc.***, ***fl-ac.***, hecla, ***kali-i.***, lap-a., maland., ***merc-c.***, ***mez.***, ***nit-ac.***, phos., ***puls.***, rhus-t., ***ruta***, sil., sulph., symph.
- **weak,** bones - ang., **ASAF.**, **CALC.**, **CALC-F.**, ***calc-i.***, **CALC-P.**, cic., con., ferr., ***ferr-i.***, ferr-m., ***ferr-p.***, fl-ac., guai., ***hecla.***, ***hep.***, iod., ip., ***kali-i.***, ***lac-c.***, ***lyc.***, **MERC.**, merc-c., mez., ***nit-ac.***, nux-m., ***ol-j.***, parathyr., petr., ph-ac., **PHOS.**, plb., ***psor.***, ***puls.***, rhod., ruta, ***sep.***, **SIL.**, staph., ***sulph.***, **SYMPH.**, syph., ther., thuj.

BONES, injuries, broken, bruised, blows - acon., ang., anthr., **ARN.**, ars., asaf., bell-p., **BRY.**, ***calc.***, ***calc-f.***, **CALC-P.**, ***calen.***, **CARB-AC.**, con., cortico., cortiso., croc., crot-h., des-ac., ***eup-per.***, ferr., fl-ac., hecla., hep., ***hyper.***, iod., kali-i., ***lach.***, lyc., mag-m., mang., merc., mez., nit-ac., ***petr.***, ***ph-ac.***, phos., ***puls.***, rhus-t., **RUTA**, sep., ***sil.***, staph., ***stront-c.***, ***sul-ac.***, sulph., **SYMPH.**, ***thyr.***, valer.

- **ailments,** from - calc., ***calc-p.***, ***hecla.***, ruta, symph.
- **brittle,** bones, fractured often - calc., **CALC-P.**, ***merc.***, ***sil.***
- **callous**, to favor production of - **CALC-P.**, ***symph.***
- **compound,** fracture - ang., ***anthr.***, **ARN.**, bry., ***calc.***, calc-p., ***calen.***, con., crot-h., hep., hyper., iod., ***lach.***, ***petr.***, ph-ac., phos., puls., rhus-t., **RUTA**, sil., staph., symph.
- **fractures**, union of, to promote - arn., asaf., **CALC-P.**, calen., lyc., nit-ac., ruta, sil., sulph., **SYMPH.**
- **infected** and suppurating - **ARN.**, sil.
- **periosteum**, injuries - arn., asaf., bell-p., calc., kali-i., merc., ph-ac., **RUTA**, sil., ***symph.***
- **slow,** healing of broken bones - asaf., **CALC.**, calc-f., **CALC-P.**, calen., des-ac., ***ferr.***, fl-ac., iod., lyc., mang., merc., ***mez.***, nit-ac., ***ph-ac.***, phos., puls., **RUTA**, sep., ***sil.***, staph., sulph., **SYMPH.**, ***thyr.***

BONE SPURS, (see Exostoses, Tumors) - ***arg.***, **AUR.**, **AUR-M.**, calc., **CALC-F.**, crot-c., ***dulc.***, ***fl-ac.***, **HECLA.**, ***kali-i.***, lap-a., maland., ***merc-c.***, ***mez.***, ***nit-ac.***, **PHOS.**, ***puls.***, rhus-t., ***ruta***, **SIL.**, sulph.

BORIC ACID, ailments from - agar., ***bor-ac.***, carb-ac., merc., nat-m.

BRACHIAL, neuralgia - acon., all-c., bell-p., **BRY.**, calc-f., ***caust.***, cham., **HYPER.**, ***kalm.***, merc., nux-v., ***rhus-t.***, ruta, sulph., verat.

BRAIN, remedies - acon., aeth., ***agar.***, **ALUM.**, ***anac.***, apis, ***arg.***, **ARG-N.**, ars., aur., **AVEN.**, **BAR-C.**, bapt., ***bell.***, bov., bry., ***bufo***, calc., calc-f., calc-p., cann-i., cann-s., ***carc.***, caust., ***cic.***, cimic., **CON.**, cob., ***croc.***, ***cupr.***, cycl., dulc., ***gels.***, glon., **HELL.**, helo., hydr-ac., **HYOS.**, ***kali-br.***, **KALI-P.**, laur., lach., laur., merc., naja, nat-s., nux-m., **NUX-V.**, **OP.**, **PHOS.**, phys., ***pic-ac.***, pip-m., ***plb.***, ***plb-i.***, rat., sil., ***stram.***, sulph., ***syph.***, thuj., tub., verat-v., zinc., ziz.

BRAIN, tumors, encephaloma - acet-ac., **AETH.**, apom., arg-n., arn., ***ars.***, ***ars-i.***, art-v., **BAR-C.**, **BAR-I.**, bell., **BUFO**, ***calc.***, ***calc-f.***, carb-ac., ***carb-an.***, ***carc.***, caust., ***cic.***, **CON.**, ***croc.***, crot-h., gali., gels., ***glon.***, graph., hydr., hyper., ***kali-br.***, ***kali-i.***, kali-cy., ***kreos.***, ***lach.***, med., ***merc.***, merc-c., merc-i-r., nit-ac., nux-v., ***op.***, **PHOS.**, pic-ac., **PLB.**, **PLB-I.**, sep., **SIL.**, stram., sulph., ***thuj.***, ***tub.***, ***zinc-s.***

BREAST-FEEDING, nursing, lactation - acon., agn., ***ars.***, ***bell.***, **BOR.**, ***bry.***, **CALC.**, **CALC-P.**, ***calen.***, carb-an., carb-v., ***cham.***, chel., ***chin.***, ***cina***, con., croto-t., ***dulc.***, ferr., graph., ***ign.***, iod., ***ip.***, kali-c., lac-c., lac-d., lach., lyc., ***mag-c.***, merc., nat-c., nat-m., **NAT-P.**, ***nux-v.***, phel., ***ph-ac.***, phos., phyt., **PULS.**, rheum, ***rhus-t.***, samb., sec., sel., **SEP.**, **SIL.**, spig., ***squil.***, stann., ***staph.***, stram., ***sulph.***, zinc.

BREAST-MILK, general

absent - ***acon.***, ***agn.***, alf., apis, ***asaf.***, ***bell.***, bor., **BRY.**, **CALC.**, carb-an., card-m., ***caust.***, cham., ***chel.***, ***coff.***, **DULC.**, ***form.***, frag., ***ign.***, **LAC-C.**, ***lac-d.***, lach., **LACT.**, ***lec.***, merc., ***mill.***, nux-v., ***ph-ac.***, phos., phyt., piloc., **PULS.**, rheum, rhus-t., ***ric.***, samb., ***sec.***, ***sil.***, stict., sulph., ***thyr.***, **URT-U.**, ust., x-ray, **ZINC.**

bad, milk - acet-ac., aeth., ***bor.***, bufo, **CALC.**, **CALC-P.**, carb-an., **CHAM.**, cina, croto-t., lach., lec., ***merc.***, ***nat-p.***, nux-v., op., puls., sil., stann.

increased, too profuse - ***acon.***, anan., arund., asaf., **BELL.**, ***bor.***, **BRY.**, **CALC.**, cham., chim., chin., ***con.***, erig., iod., lac-c., lact., ***medus.***, nux-v., parth., phos., phyt., pip-m., pitu-a., **PULS.**, rheum, ***rhus-t.***, ric., sabal., ***sabin.***, ***salv.***, ***sec.***, ***sol-o.***, spira., stram., ust., yohim.

mother's, milk, agg. - acet-ac., ant-c., ***bor.***, calc., **CALC-P.**, ***cham.***, ***cina***, lach., ***merc.***, ***nat-c.***, ***ph-ac.***, ***sanic.***, **SIL.**, stann., ***valer.***

non-nursing, women, in - ars., ***asaf.***, bell., bor., ***cycl.***, lyc., ***merc.***, phos., **PULS.**, rhus-t., stram., thlaspi., ***tub.***, ***urt-u.***

scanty - acon., apis, ***asaf.***, ***bell.***, ***bry.***, ***calc.***, carb-an., card-m., ***caust.***, **CHAM.**, ***chel.***, ***chin.***, ***coff.***, dulc., ***form.***, ***ign.***, jab., ***lac-d.***, lach., merc., ***mill.***, nux-v., puls., rheum, rhus-t., samb., sec., stict., sulph., **URT-U.**, ust., **ZINC.**

suppression, of breast-milk, ailments from - ***acon.***, agar., ***agn.***, aur., aur-i., aur-s., bell., **BRY.**, calc., calc-sil., camph-br., ***carb-v.***, **CAUST.**, ***cham.***, ***chim.***, cimic., cycl., dulc., frag., ***hyos.***, ign., ***iod.***, lac-d., ***lach.***, ***merc.***, mill., phyt., **PULS.**, ***rhus-t.***, ***sec.***, senec., ***sil.***, sul-i., ***sulph.***, ***urt-u.***, verat., zinc.

BREASTS, cancer - alum., alumn., anag., ***apis***, ***arg-n.***, arn., ***ars.***, ***ars-i.***, ars-s-f., **ASTER.**, ***aur-ar.***, ***aur-m-n.***, ***bad.***, bapt., bar-i., ***bell.***, ***bell-p.***, ***brom.***, bry., **BUFO**, cadm-i., cadm-m., calc., ***calc-f.***, calc-i., calc-ox., calc-p., calc-sil., ***calen.***, ***carb-ac.***, **CARB-AN.**, carb-v., carbn-s., **CARC.**, caust., cham., ***chim.***, cic., cist., ***clem.***, coloc., **CON.**, cory., **CUND.**, dulc., **EUPH.**, ferr-i., form-ac., fuli., ***gali.***, **GRAPH.**, ***hep.***, ***hippoz.***, ho., ***hydr.***, iod., kali-chl., kali-c., ***kali-i.***, kali-m., kreos., ***lac-c.***, ***lach.***, lap-a., ***lob-e.***, ***lyc.***, ***maland.***, med., **MERC.**, ***merc-i-f.***, nat-cac., nat-m., ***nit-ac.***, nux-v., ol-an., ***ox-ac.***, ph-ac., **PHOS.**, **PHYT.**, pic-ac., plb-i., ***psor.***, **PULS.**, rhus-t., ruta, sabin., ***sang.***, sars., **SCIRR.**, **SCROPH-N.**, semp., **SEP.**, **SIL.**, staph., sul-i., ***sulph.***, syc-co., tarent-c., ***thuj.***, tub.

epithelioma - ***arg-n.***, ***ars.***, ***ars-i.***, brom., **BUFO**, calc., calc-p., ***clem.***, **CON.**, ***hydr.***, ***kreos.***, ***lach.***, merc., ***merc-i-f.***, ***phos.***, ***phyt.***, ***sep.***, ***sil.***, sulph., thuj.

fibroadenoma - calc-f.

mastectomy, after - ***calen.***, carc., graph., sil., x-ray.

nipples - aster, chim., phos., ***phyt.***, ***sars.***, sil.

scirrhus - apis, ***arg-n.***, ars., ***ars-i.***, ***aster.***, aur-m-n., ***bar-i.***, bell., ***brom.***, bry., **BUFO**, ***calc-f.***, ***carb-an.***, cham., chim., cist., clem., **CON**, cund., graph., hydr., kreos., lap-a., phyt., puls., rhus-t., sabin., ***sars.***, ***scirr.***, sep., ***sil.***, sulph., tarent-c.

ulceration - **BUFO**, ***calc.***, ***carb-an.***, cund., ***hep.***, ***hippoz.***, ***hydr.***, ***phos.***, **PHYT.**, **SIL.**, sulph.

BREASTS, general - ***acon.***, anan., ***apis***, arn., ars., asc-t., aur-s., **ASTER.**, **BELL.**, **BELL-P.**, bor., **BRY.**, bufo, ***calc.***, ***calc-p.***, carb-an., carb-v., carbn-s., **CARC.**, ***cast-eq.***, ***cham.***, ***cimic.***, ***cist.***, clem., com., **CON.**, croto-t., cycl., ***graph.***, hall, helon., **HEP.**, hyper., ***iod.***, **KALI-C.**, kali-chl., kali-i., kali-m., **LAC-C.**, lac-d., **LAC-H.**, ***lach.***, lepi., ***lyc.***, ***merc.***, nat-s., ol-an., onos., orig., paraf., ***phel.***, ***phos.***, **PHYT.**, plan., plb., ***puls.***, pyrog., rat., rhus-t., rumx., sabal., **SARS.**, sep., **SIL.**, **SULPH.**, ust., verat-v., zinc.

abscess, breasts - acet-ac., apis, ***ars.***, ***bell.***, ***bry.***, bufo, ***calen.***, ***camph.***, ***carb-an.***, cast-eq., cham., ***cist.***, con., crot-c., ***crot-h.***, croto-t., ***graph.***, **HEP.**, kreos., ***lach.***, **MERC.**, **PHOS.**, **PHYT.**, plb., sars., **SIL.**, **SULPH.**, tarent-c.

atrophy, breasts - anac., anan., ars., ars-i., bac., bar-c., cench., cham., ***chim.***, **COFF.**, **CON.**, dulc., fago., ferr., **IOD.**, **KALI-I.**, ***kreos.***, lac-c., ***lac-d.***, ***lach.***, **NAT-M.**, ***nit-ac.***, ***nux-m.***, ***onos.***, ***plb.***, **SABAL.**, sac-alb., sars., ***sec.***, sil.

hypertrophy, breasts - bac., ***calc.***, chim., ***con.***, hydrog., iod., nat-m., nit-ac., nux-v., ***phyt.***, sang., sep., sil., sulph.

induration, breasts - acon., agar., agn., alumn., ambr., anan., apis, arist-cl., arn., ***aster.***, ***aur.***, aur-s., bar-c., ***bar-i.***, ***bell.***, bell-p., ***bry.***, bufo, ***calc.***, ***calc-f.***, calc-i., calc-p., **CARB-AN.**, ***carb-v.***, ***carbn-s.***, carc., **CHAM.**, chim., ***cist.***, ***clem.***, coloc., **CON.**, ***crot-h.***, ***croto-t.***, ***cupr.***, cycl., dulc., fago., ***graph.***, hep., ***hydr.***, ***iod.***, kali-c., ***kali-chl.***, ***kreos.***, ***lac-c.***, ***lap-a.***, ***lyc.***,

merc., nat-m., nit-ac., ***phos.***, ***phyt.***, plb., ***plb-i.***, puls., ***rhus-t.***, ruta, sang., scroph-n., ***sep.***, **SIL.**, spong., ***sul-i.***, ***sulph.***, ***thuj.***, tub., ust., vip.

inflammation, breasts - acet-ac., ***acon.***, acon-l., anan., ant-t., ***apis***, ***arn.***, ars., **BELL.**, **BRY.**, bufo, ***cact.***, cadm-s., calc., cann-s., ***carb-an.***, ***carb-v.***, ***carbn-s.***, carc., ***card-m.***, ***cham.***, ***cist.***, clem., ***con.***, crot-h., ***croto-t.***, cur., dulc., eup-a., ferr., ferr-p., fl-ac., foll., galeg., graph., helon., **HEP.**, kali-m., **LAC-C.**, ***lach.***, laur., ***lyc.***, med., ***merc.***, merc-i-f., petr., ***phel.***, ***phos.***, **PHYT.**, pic-ac., plan., plb., ***puls.***, rhus-t., sabad., sabal., **SIL.**, **SULPH.**, ust., verat-v., verb., x-ray.

lumps, breasts - ***ars-i.,*** bell-p., calc-f., chim., ***con.,*** lyc., **PHYT.,** puls., sep., ***sil.***

nodules, breasts - ars-i., arum-t., ***aster.***, aur., bar-c., ***bell.***, **BELL-P.**, berb-a., ***brom.***, ***bry.***, ***bufo***, calc., ***calc-f.,*** ***calc-i.***, calc-p., calen., **CARB-AN.**, ***carb-v.***, carc., cham., ***chim.***, chin., clem., ***coloc.***, **CON.**, croto-t., cund., cupr., dulc., ferr-i., fl-ac., foll., gnaph., ***graph.***, hecla., ***hydr.***, ***iod.***, kali-m., kreos., ***lac-c.***, lach., lap-a., ***lyc.***, mang., ***merc-i-f.***, murx., ***nit-ac.***, ***phos.***, **PHYT.**, pitu-a., plb-i., psor., ***puls.***, ruta, sabin., sanguin., scirr., scroph-n., sep., **SIL.**, squil., ***sulph.***, thuj., ***thyr.***, tub.

swelling, breasts - acet-ac., acon., aeth., all-s., anan., ***apis,*** arg-n., arn., ars-i., ***asaf.,*** ***aster.***, aur-s., bamb-a., ***bell.***, bell-p., brom., ***bry.***, bufo, cadm-s., **CALC.,** canth., ***carb-an.***, carc., cast., cast-eq., cedr., ***cham.***, cist., ***clem.***, **CON.,** cortiso., ***croto-t.***, cund., ***cupr.***, cur., cycl., ***dulc.***, eupi., fl-ac., foll., graph., ***helon.***, ***hep.***, hydrog., **KALI-C.,** kali-i., kali-m., kali-s., **LAC-C.,** ***lach.***, lap-gr-m., lil-t., lyc., lyss., mag-c., med., ***merc.***, merc-c., merl., murx., naja, nat-c., nat-m., nux-v., oci., onos., orig., ped., ***phos.***, **PHYT.,** pip-n., pitu-a., plb., psor., **PULS.**, rat., ***rhus-t.***, ruta, sabad., sabal., sabin., sac-alb., samb., sang., saroth., **SIL.,** sol-a., sol-o., spig., staph., ***sulph.***, tarent., thuj., tub., urt-u., vip., ***zinc.***

tumors, (see Breasts, cancer) - ***ars-i.,*** ***aster.,*** ***bell.,*** bell-p., berb-a., ***brom.,*** bry., calc., ***calc-f.,*** calen., ***carb-an.,*** cham., ***chim.,*** clem., con., ***cund.,*** ferr-i., gnaph., ***graph.,*** hecla., ***hydr.,*** ***iod.,*** ***kali-i.,*** kali-m., ***lach.,*** lap-a., lyc., ***merc-i-f.,*** murx., nit-ac., ***phos.,*** phyt., ***plb-i.,*** psor., ***puls.,*** sabin., sang., ***scirr.,*** ***scroph-n.,*** sec., sil., skook., thuj., ***thyr.,*** tub.

BREASTS, injuries, to - acon., ***arn.,*** ***bell-p.,*** ***calen.,*** **CON.,** hyper., led., phyt., scirr.

contusion, from - ***bell-p.,*** **CON.**

cut, surgery, from - **CALEN.**

puncture, biopsy, from - ***hyper.,*** **LED.**

BREASTS, nipples, complaints of - ***arn.***, asc-t., **CALEN.,** **CAST-EQ.,** cham., ***con.***, croto-t., cycl., ***graph.,*** lach., lyc., nat-s., phel., puls., ***phyt.***, pyrog., puls., rat., rumx., **SARS.,** sil., ***sulph.***

bleeding, nipples, from - bufo, ***ham.,*** ***lyc.,*** med., ***merc.,*** ***merc-c.,*** ***sep.,*** sil., ***sulph.***

cracks, nipples - aesc., anan., ***arn.,*** ars., aur., ***aur-s.,*** calc., calc-ox., ***calen.,*** carb-an., carb-v., ***cast.,*** **CAST-EQ.,** **CAUST.,** cham., ***con.,*** ***croto-t.,*** ***cund.,*** cur., ***eup-a.,*** ***fl-ac.,*** gali., ger., **GRAPH.,** ham., hep., hipp., ***hydr.,*** ***lyc.,*** merc., ***merc-c.,*** ***mill.,*** nit-ac., ***paeon.,*** **PETR.,** ***phel.,*** phos., **PHYT.,** **RAT.,** **SARS.,** ***sep.,*** **SIL.,** ***sulph.***

inflammation, nipples - acon., arn., ***bry.***, ***cadm-s.***, calc., cann-s., ***cham.***, croto-t., eup-a., helon., med., petr., ***phos.***, ***phyt.***, pic-ac., puls., ***sil.***, sulph.

inverted, nipples - apis, ***con.***, graph., nat-s., phyt., ***sars.***

retraction, nipples - ***ars-i.***, ***aster.***, carb-an., carc., ***chim.***, con., croto-t., cund., graph., hydr., lach., lap-a., lob-e., nat-s., ***nux-m.***, phyt., **BREASTS,** tumors, growths, (see Breast, cancer) - arn., ars-i., **ASTER.,** ***bell.***, **BELL-P.,** berb-a., ***brom.***, bry., calc., ***calc-f.***, calc-i., ***calc-p.***, calen., ***carb-an.***, carb-v., cham., ***chim.***, cist., clem., **CON.**, ***cund.***, ferr-i., fl-ac., gnaph., goss., ***graph.***, hecla., hep., ***hydr.***, ***iod.***, kali-i., ***kali-m.***, ***lach.***, **LAP-A.**, lyc., merc., ***merc-i-f.***, murx., nit-ac., phase., ***phos.***, **PHYT.**, ***plb-i.***, psor., ***puls.***, sabin., sang., ***scirr.***, ***scroph-n.***, sec., ***sil.***, skook., sulph., tep., **THUJ.,** ***thyr.***, tub.

tumors, nipples - carb-an., con.

BREATHING, general, (See Wheezing)

imperceptible, breathing - acon., amyg-am., ***ars.***, bac., benz-ac., carb-ac., ***carb-v.,*** caust., chlor., cic., ***cocc.***, gels., hydr-ac., merc., ***morph.,*** naja, nux-v., ***op.,*** petr., stram., verat.

irregular, breathing - acon., ***acon-f.,*** am-c., ang., antipyrin., atro., bell., ***camph.,*** cann-i., ***carb-v.,*** chlol., coca, cocain., crot-h., ***cupr.,*** cupr-ar., ***dig.,*** ***grin.,*** ***hydr-ac.,*** ***ign.,*** iod., ip., kali-cy., lach., ***laur.,*** led., lob., nux-v., olnd., ***op.,*** ***morph.,*** parth., ***saroth.,*** spong., sul-ac., sulph., vanad., verat.

loud, breathing - acon., agar., alum., am-c., ambr., ant-s., ant-t., aral., ***arn.***, ars., asar., bell., bov., ***brom.***, bry., bufo, calad., **CALC.**, camph., cann-s., ***caps.***, ***carb-v.***, carbn-s., **CHAM.**, **CHIN.**, chin-s., ***chlor.***, ***cina***, cocc., ***colch.***, coloc., con., ***cor-r.***, cub., cupr., dros., dulc., ferr., ferr-m., gamb., graph., guare., hell., ***hep.***, hydr-ac., ***hyos.***, ***ign.***, iod., **KALI-BI.**, ***kali-c.***, ***kalm.***, **LACH.**, laur., lob-s., lyc., mag-m., mag-s., meph., merc., morph., mur-ac., nat-m., ***nat-s.***, nit-ac., nux-v., ***op.***, petr., **PHOS.**, plb.,

puls., rheum, ***rhus-t.***, sabad., sabin., **SAMB.**, ***seneg.***, sep., sil., **SPONG.**, squil., stann., ***stram.***, sul-ac., **SULPH.**, thuj., **VERAT.**

stridulous, breathing - am-caust., ant-t., ars., **BELL.**, calc., ***chlor.***, **GELS.**, **IGN.**, ***lach.***, laur., ***meph.***, merc-i-f., merc-i-r., **MOSCH.**, nit-ac., ***nux-v.***, ***op.***, phos., plb., ***samb.***, ***sang.***, sarr., spong., stram., ulm., verat.

BRIGHT'S disease, (see Nephritis) - adon., alumn., am-be., am-br., ant-t., ***apis***, apoc., arg-n., arge., ***ars.***, ars-br., ars-h., ars-i., atro., **AUR-M.**, ***aur-m-n.***, bell., berb., ***brach.***, bry., ***calc.***, ***calc-ar.***, ***calc-p.***, ***calc-s.***, ***cann-s.***, ***canth.***, ***carb-ac.***, carb-v., caul., ***chel.***, chim., ***chin.***, ***cocc.***, ***colch.***, coloc., con., ***cop.***, ***crot-h.***, ***cupr.***, ***dig.***, dulc., euonin., eup-pur., ***ferr.***, ***ferr-p.***, **GLON.**, glyc-g., hell., ***helon.***, ***hep.***, jab., ***kali-bi.***, ***kali-c.***, ***kali-chl.***, kali-cit., ***kali-i.***, ***kali-p.***, ***kalm.***, kreos., ***lach.***, lith-c., **LYC.**, ***lycps.***, **MERC-C.**, ***merc-cy.***, ***merc-i-r.***, mez., myric., **NAT-C.**, ***nat-m.***, ***nit-ac.***, nux-v., ***ol-j.***, op., **PH-AC.**, ***phos.***, ***phyt.***, **PLB.**, **RHUS-T.**, sars., ***sec.***, seneg., sep., sil., solid., ***sulph.***, **TER.**, uran-n., vesi.

BROMIDES, ailments from - am-c., ***brom.***, camph., cham., helon., ***kali-br.***, lach., mag-c., nat-m., nux-v., op., phenob., phos., zinc., zinc-p.

BRONCHITIS, infection - ***acet-ac.***, ***acon.***, **AESC.**, ***all-c.***, ***alum.***, ***alumn.***, am-c., am-i, ***am-m.***, am-p., ant-ar., ***ant-c.***, **ANT-T.**, ***apis***, ***arn.***, **ARS.**, ars-i., ***asc-t.***, ***aur-m.***, bar-c., **BAR-M.**, ***bell.***, ***benz-ac.***, blatta, ***brom.***, **BRY.**, ***cact.***, ***calc.***, calc-f., ***camph.***, ***cann-s.***, ***carb-v.***, ***carbn-s.***, card-m., ***caust.***, ***cham.***, ***chel.***, chin., chlol., chlor., ***cina***, ***cist.***, ***coc-c.***, colch., cop., dig., **DROS.**, ***dulc.***, eup-per., euphr., ***ferr-i.***, **FERR-P.**, ***gels.***, grin., ***guai.***, **HEP.**, ***hippoz.***, ***hyos.***, ***iod.***, **IP.**, kali-ar., ***kali-bi.***, ***kali-c.***, ***kali-chl.***, kali-p., ***kreos.***, ***lach.***, ***lob.***, **LYC.**, mang., ***merc.***, merc-s., morg., ***naja***, nat-ar., ***nat-m.***, **NAT-S.**, ***nit-ac.***, ***nux-v.***, ***ph-ac.***, **PHOS.**, piloc., pix., ***plb.***, ***psor.***, **PULS.**, ***rhus-t.***, **RUMX.**, **SANG.**, ***sanguin-n.***, **SENEC.**, ***seneg.***, ***sep.***, **SIL.**, solid., **SPONG.**, ***squil.***, **STANN.**, ***stict.***, sul-ac., ***sulph.***, ***ter.***, thuj., **TUB.**, uran., ***verat.***, verat-v., verb., zinc.

BRONCHIECTASIS, chonic dilatation - acet-ac., all-c., all-s., alumn., am-c., **ANT-T.**, ***ars.***, ***bac.***, ***bals-p.***, benz-ac., ***calc.***, cop., crot-h., eucal., ferr-i., grin., ***hep.***, ichth., **KALI-BI.**, ***kali-c.***, kreos., ***lyc.***, med., myos., myrt-c., phel., ***phos.***, ***puls.***, sang., sil., ***stann.***, sulph., tub.

BRUISES, (see Ecchymosis) - absin., acon., aeth., agn., ant-c., anthr., ***arg.***, arg-n., **ARN.**, ars., ***bad.***, bar-c., bar-m., **BELL-P.**, both-l., ***bry.***, calc., ***carb-v.***, caust., cham., chin., chlol., ***cic.***, coca, ***con.***, croc., ***crot-h.***, ***dros.***, dulc., euph., euphr., ***ferr.***, ***form.***, ***glon.***, **HAM.**, ***hep.***, ***hyper.***, ***iod.***, kali-c., kreos., ***lach.***, laur., **LED.**, ***lith-c.***, teucr., mez., mosch., mill., ***olnd.***, ***nux-v.***, par., pareir., petr., **PH-AC.**, **PHOS.**, plan., plat., plb., polyg., ***puls.***, rhod., rhus-t., **RUTA**, **SEC.**, sep., ***sulph.***, **SUL-AC.**, ***symph.***, ***tarent.***, ***ter.***, trinit., uran-n., verat., verb.

BRUXISM, (See Grinding, teeth)

BUBOES, glands - acal., acon., all-c., alum., alumn., anan., ang., ant-t., anthr., apis, ars., ars-i., ars-met., aur., aur-ar., aur-m., aur-m-n., aur-s., bad., bapt., bar-m., bell., blum-o., **BUFO**, calc-s., calen., canth., ***carb-an.***, carb-v., caust., chel., **CINNB.**, clem., ***crot-h.***, dulc., ferr-p., ***graph.***, **HEP.**, hydr., ign., iod., ***iodof.***, ***iris***, jac-c., kali-chl., ***kali-i.***, kali-m., lac-c., lach., ***lith-c.***, lyc., lyss., ***mang.***, med., ***merc.***, merc-c., ***merc-i-f.***, merc-i-r., merc-pr-r., ***merc-s.***, myric., naja, ***nit-ac.***, oci., oper., pest., ph-ac., phyt., puls., **PYROG.**, rhus-t., rob., sep., ***sil.***, sol-x., staph., stram., sul-i., sulph., ***syph.***, ***tarent.***, tarent-c., thuj., tus-p., yersin, zinc.

BUBONIC PLAGUE - alum., ***ars.***, ars-i., aur., aur-m., aur-m-n., bad., ***bapt.***, bar-m., bell., **BUFO**, calc-o-t., ***carb-an.***, ***carc.***, chel., chin., chin-ar., **CINNB.**, clem., crot-h., **HEP.**, ***hippoz.***, ign., iod., kali-chl., ***kali-i.***, lac-c., ***lach.***, lyc., ***merc.***, naja, ***nit-ac.***, phyt., phos., psor., ***pyrog.***, rhus-t., sec., ***sil.***, sulph., sul-ac., tarent-c., verat., zinc.

BULIMIA - abies-c., abies-n., adam., agar., alf., anac., ang., ant-c., ***aq-mar.***, arg-n., ***calc.***, calen., **CARC.**, caust., **CHIN.**, **CINA**, ferr., fl-ac., graph., hell., ign., iod., kali-c., **LYC.**, med., **MERC.**, mur-ac., naja, nat-c., nat-m., nux-m., nux-v., op., petr., ***phos.***, pitu-a., plat., puls., raph., sabad., ***sac-alb.***, **SEP.**, **STAPH.**, sulph., thuj., **VERAT.**, zinc.

BUNIONS, feet - am-c., **ANT-C.**, hyper., ***kali-chl.***, ph-ac., ***phos.***, plb., **SIL.**, zinc.

BURNING, pain - abies-c., acet-ac., achy., **ACON.**, acon-f., aesc., ***agar.***, agro., aloe, ***alum.***, alumn., ***am-br.***, am-c., ***am-m.***, ambr., amor-r., ang., ant-c., ant-t., **ANTHR.**, ***apis***, arg., ***arg-n.***, ***arn.***, **ARS.**, ars-i., **ARS-S-F.**, **ARUM-T.**, ***asaf.***, asar., ***aur.***, aur-i., ***bapt.***, ***bar-c.***, bar-m., **BELL.**, **BERB.**, ***bism.***, bor., bov., brom., **BRY.**, ***bufo***, calad., ***calc.***, ***calc-p.***, calc-sil., ***calen.***, camph., **CANN-I.**, cann-s., **CANTH.**, caps., carb-ac., carb-an., ***carb-v.***, **CARBN-S.**, **CAUST.**, cedr., cham., ***chel.***, ***chin.***, choc., ***cic.***, cina, ***clem.***, cocc., coff., ***colch.***, ***coloc.***, ***com.***, ***con.***, croto-t., cund., ***cupr.***, dig., ***dios.***, dol., ***dros.***, ***dulc.***, equis., eucal., eup-pur., ***euph.***, euphr., ferr., ***fl-ac.***, form., ***gamb.***, **GRAPH.**, hecla., hell., hep., hist., hydr., ***hydrog.***, hyos., ign., iod., ip., ***iris***, kali-ar., **KALI-BI.**, kali-c., ***kali-i.***, kali-n., kali-s., kalm., ***kreos.***, lac-ac., ***lach.***, ***laur.***, led., ***lil-t.***, ***lith-c.***, ***lob.***, ***lyc.***, m-arct., m-aust., mag-c., mag-m., mang., **MERC.**, **MERC-C.**, ***merc-i-f.***, **MEZ.**, mosch., mur-ac., ***nat-ar.***, ***nat-c.***, ***nat-m.***, nat-sil., **NIT-AC.**, nux-m., **NUX-V.**, oena., ol-j., ***op.***, ***osm.***, ***ox-ac.***, par., ***petr.***, ***ph-ac.***, pic-ac., **PHOS.**, phyt., plat., plb., **PRUN.**, ***psor.***, **PULS.**, pyrog., ***ran-b.***, ran-s., rat., ***rhod.***, rhus-r., **RHUS-T.**, rob., ***rumx.***, ruta, **SABAD.**, ***sabin.***, **SANG.**, sanguin-n., ***sars.***,

SEC., *seneg.*, **SEP.**, *sil.*, sin-n., **SPIG.**, **SPONG.**, *stann.*, staph., still., stram., stront-c., sul-ac., **SULPH.**, symph., tab., tarax., **TARENT**., tarent-c., *tell.*, *ter.*, *thuj.*, uran-n., *urt-u.*, ust., uva., *verat.*, verat-v., viol-o., viol-t., wye., **ZINC.**, **ZINC-P.**

BURNS, general, fire, chemicals, ailments, from - acet-ac., *acon.*, agar., aloe, alum., alumn., anac., ant-c., *apis.*, arist-cl., arn., **ARS.**, *bar-c.*, *bell.*, both-l., *bry.*, calc., calc-f., calc-p., calc-s., **CALEN.**, camph., **CANTH.**, carb-ac., *carb-v.*, *carbn-s.*, *caust.*, chin., cic., cosm., crot-h., cycl., des-ac., echi., eucal., euph., ferr., gaul., grin., *ham.*, hed., *hep.*, hoit., hyos., *hyper.*, *ign.*, jab., *kali-bi.*, kali-c., kali-chl., *kreos.*, lach., mag-c., *mag-m.*, *merc.*, mom-b., *nat-c.*, *nux-v.*, op., par., paraf., passi., petr., phos., *pic-ac.*, *plan.*, plat., plb., *puls.*, rad-br., ran-b., *rhus-t.*, ruta, sabad., *sec.*, semp., sep., sieg., *sil.*, **SOL**, spira., *stram.*, *sul-ac.*, *ter.*, thuj., **URT-U.**, verat., x-ray

chemicals, from - canth., carb-ac., *caust.*, pic-ac.

radiation, from - calc-f., calen., fl-ac., phos., rad-br., *sol,* x-ray

scalds - calen., **CANTH.**, *carb-ac.*, *carbn-s.*, **CAUST.**, *crot-h.*, petr., *stram.*

scars - ars., calen., *carb-an.*, *graph.*, lach.

sunburn - acon., *agar.*, *ant-c.*, *apis.*, **BELL.**, bry., bufo, *calen.*, *camph.*, **CANTH.**, clem., cortiso., euphr., *hyos.*, lach., lyc., *mur-ac.*, *nat-c.*, op., **PULS.**, rob., sel., **SOL**, sulph., **URT-U.**, *valer.*, verat.

ulcers, from burns - calen., kali-bi.

vapors, from hot - apis, canth., caust., kali-bi., urt-u.

BURSAE, general - acon., am-c., ant-c., ant-t., apis, **ARN.**, ars-i., aur., bell., *bell-p.*, *benz-ac.*, berb., **BOV.**, bry., calc-f., calc-p., cann-s., canth., caust., chel., cist., ferr., graph., hell., hep., iod., kali-br., kali-c., kali-chl., kali-i., kali-m., *lycpr.*, mag-p., merc., **NAT-M.**, ph-ac., phos., phyt., puls., rhus-t., *ruta*, seneg., **SIL.**, slag, stann., **STICT.**, sul-i., sulph., syc-co., *syph.*, thuj., tub., zinc.

BURSITIS, shoulders - ant-c., **APIS.**, ars., bell., *bell-p.*, *bry.*, graph., hep., iod., *lycpr.*, puls., rhus-t., **RUTA**, **SIL.**, *stict.*, *sulph.*

C

CACHEXIA, cancer, with - acon., **ALF.**, alum., alumn., anan., anil., **ARS.**, ars-i., aster., aur., aur-ar., aur-m., bapt., bar-c., bar-i., brom., bry., bufo, *cadm-i.*, **CADM-S.**, calc., calc-i., calc-ox., calth., carb-an., **CARC.**, caust., chel., cic., cinnam., cist., cit-l., clem., *con.*, crot-h., *cund.*, cur., dubin., elaps., epip., euph-he., ferr-i., gali., graph., ham., hedeo., hippoz., **HYDR.**, hydr-m., *iod.*, kali-ar., kali-cy., *kali-i.*, kreos., kres., lap-a., lob-e., lyc., matth., methyl-bl., mill., myric., *nit-ac.*, ol-an., op., **ORNI.**, oxyg., ph-ac., phos., phyt., pic-ac., *plb.*, psor., rad-br., sang., *sars.*, **SCIRR.**, **SCROPH-N.**, sec., *sed-a.*, sep., **SIL.**, silpho., sol., sulph., sul-ac., thuj., trif-p., viol-o.

CACHEXIA, general, (see Emaciation) - acet-ac., arg., arg-n., arn., **ARS.**, ars-i., bad., bond., calc., caps., carb-ac., chim., chin., clem., *coc-c.*, cund., fl-ac., *form.*, **HYDR.**, *iod.*, *kali-bi.*, kreos., mang., merc., merc-n., morph., mur-ac., nat-m., **NIT-AC.**, nux-v., ol-j., op., phos., phyt., pic-ac., plb., sec., seneg., thal., thuj., vip., x-ray.

appetite, with loss of - **ALF.**, *ars.*, *cadm-i.*, *carc.*, *chin.*, **HYDR.**, sed-a., sil.

chemotherapy, from - alf., ars., **CADM-S.**, chin., hydr., *ip.*, nux-v., phos., sil.

radiation, therapy, from - alf., ars., **CADM-S.**, calc-f., chin., fl-ac., hydr., *ip.*, nux-v., phos., rad-br., sil., **SOL.**, x-ray.

CADMIUM, ailments from - alum., ars., bry., *cadm.*, cadm-f., cadm-i., *cadm-s.*, camph., coff., hydr., ip., op., plb., verat., zinc.

CAFFEINE, poisoning, ailments from, (see Coffee) - acon., aven., *cham.*, *coff.*, cypr., *kola*, nux-v., *paull.*, thea.

CALLOUSES, skin - am-c., **ANT-C.**, bor., calc-f., *dulc.*, elae., *ferr-pic.*, **GRAPH.**, hydr., lach., led., lyc., *nit-ac.*, petr., *ran-b.*, *rhus-t.*, sal-ac., sars., **SEP.**, *sil.*, sulph., *thuj.*

CAMPHOR, ailments from - am-c., *camph.*, camph-br., canth., coff., cupr., dulc., kali-n., lyc., nit-s-d., op., phos., squil., verat.

CANCER, general, (see Tumors) - abr., *acet-ac.*, acon., agar., ail., alum., alumn., *ambr.*, am-c., anac., anan., anil., ant-c., *ant-chl.*, *ant-m.*, ant-t., anthr., *apis*, *ambr.*, apoc., arbu., arg., arg-n., arn., **ARS.**, ars-br., *ars-i.*, ars-s-f., asaf., **ASTER.**, *aur.*, aur-ar., aur-i., *aur-m.*, aur-m-n., aur-s., *bapt.*, bar-c., bar-i., bell., bell-p., bism., **BROM.**, *bry.*, **BUFO**, buni-o., *cadm.*, *cadm-i.*, **CADM-S.**, *calc.*, calc-acet., calc-ar., calc-f., *calc-i.*, calc-o-t., calc-ox., calc-p., *calc-s.*, calc-sil., *calen.*, calth., *carb-ac.*, **CARB-AN.**, *carb-v.*, *carbn-s.*, **CARC.**, card-m., caust., cedr., chel., chim., chol., cholin., chr-ac., cit-l., *cic.*, cinnam., *cist.*, *cit-ac.*, clem., coloc., cory., cot., croc., crot-h., **CON.**, **CUND.**, cupr., cupr-acet., cupr-s., cur., dulc., echi., elaps, elat., eos., epip., eucal., eup-per., euph., ferr-i., ferr-pic., ferr-p., form., formal., form-ac., fuli., gaert., *gali.*, gels., gent-l., *graph.*, gua., *ham.*, hecla., hep., *hippoz.*, *ho.*, **HYDR.**, hydr-ac., hydrc., hydr-m., *iod.*, iodof., *kali-ar.*, *kali-bi.*, kali-c., kali-chl., *kali-cy.*, *kali-i.*, kali-ma., *kali-p.*, *kali-s.*, kres., *kreos.*, *lach.*, lact., **LAP-A.**, laur., lob-c., lob-d., lob-e., lup., lupin., **LYC.**, mag-m., mag-p., mag-s., maland., matth., med., *merc.*, merc-c., *merc-i-f.*, methyl-chl., mez., *mill.*, morg-g., *morph.*, mur-ac., nat-cac., nat-m., nectrin., **NIT-AC.**, nux-v., nym.,

ol-an., op., **ORNI.,** ozone, parat., perh., petr., ph-ac., **PHOS., PHYT.,** pic-ac., ***plb.,*** prot., psor., puls., rad-br., raja-s., ran-b., ran-s., rhod., rhus-t., rumx-a., ruta, sac-alb., ***sang.,*** sarcol-ac., **SCIRR., SCROPH-N.,** ***sec.,*** sed-r., ***semp.,*** senec-j., sep., ***sieg.,*** **SIL.,** silphu., squil., ***sol.,*** spig., spong., staph., sul-ac., sul-i., ***sulph.,*** syc., symph., syph., tarent., tarent-c., tarax., tax., ***ter.,*** thala., ***thuj.,*** toxo., **TRIF-P.,** uran-n., verb., vib-p., viol-o., ***visc., x-ray,*** zinc.

biopsies, cancer from getting - calen., graph., hyper., kreos., led., sil., staph., thuj.

ganglia, cancer - ars-br., ***aur-m.,*** buni-o., **CARB-AN., CON.,** ho., sieg., sul-i., syph.

injury, cancer from - arn., bar-i., ***bell-p.,*** calc-f., calend., **CON.,** phyt., staph., symph.

mediastinum, cancer - carc., iod., ***scirr.,*** **SCROPH-N.,** ***spong., thuj.***

noma, cancrum oris - alum., alumn., anthr., ***ars.,*** bapt., calc., carb-v., ***con.,*** elat., guare., hydr., kali-chl., ***kali-p.,*** kreos., lach., merc., merc-d., mur-ac., sec., sil., sul-ac., sulph., tarent., tarent-c.

pains, cancer - acon., anthr., ***apis*, ARS., *ars-i.,*** **ASTER.,** aur., brom., bry., bufo, calc., ***calc-acet., calc-ar.,*** calc-o-t., calc-ox., ***calen.,*** cadm-i., **CADM-S.,** carb-an., **CARC.,** cedr., cinnam., ***cit-ac.***, cit-l., ***cit-ac., coloc., con.***, cund., echi., **EUPH.,** euph-he., **HYDR.,** hydrc., iodof., kali-bi., kali-c., kali-cy., ***lact.***, lob-d., lup., lupin., lyc., mag-p., merc., morph., op., **OX-AC.,** ph-ac., phyt., psoral., rhus-t., semp., **SCIRR.,** sil., sol., staph., ***syph.,*** tarent., ***x-ray.***

vaccinations, cancer after - crot-h., diph., lach., maland., naja, pyrog., ***sil., thuj.***

weakness, with cancer - **ALF., ARS.,** aur., aur-m-n., **CADM-S., CARC.,** chin., cimic., cocc., **CON.,** gels., **HYDR.,** kreos., nit-ac., nux-v., phos., ph-ac., ***phyt., plb., plb-i.,*** psor., **SCIRR.,** sil., zinc.

wounds, cancer from - calen., con., graph., led., kreos., sil., staph., thuj.

CANDIDA, albicans, infection - ars., calc., calc-p., ***cand-a., cand-p.,*** chin., helon., kreos., lyc., med., moni., nat-p., **NIT-AC.**, nux-v., pen., ***puls.,*** sars., sep., ***thuj.***

CANNABIS, marijuana, ailments from - anh., aven., camph., ***cann-i., cann-s.,*** cit-l., med., merc., nux-v., op., phos., sulph., thuj.

CANTHARIS, ailments from - acon., apis, camph., ***canth.,*** caps., kali-n., merc., ***merc-c.***

CAPILLARIES, blood vessels - bell., caust., ***cupr., fl-ac.,*** hyper., kali-br., lach., phos., sul-ac.

CAPSICUM, ailments from - calad., camph., canth., ***caps.,*** chin., cina, sul-ac.

CARBOLIC ACID, ailments from - acet-ac., am-c., ***apis,*** ars., camph., canth., ***carb-ac.,*** caust., nit-ac., sul-ac.

CARBON DIOXIDE, ailments from - acet-ac., acon., ant-t., bell., bry., bov., camph., carb-an., ***carb-diox., carb-v.,*** carbn-h., ***carbn-s.,*** op.

CARBON GAS, ailments from - acet-ac., acon., am-c., ***apis,*** ant-t., ars., bell., bov., bry., camph., canth., ***carb-ac.,*** carb-an., ***carb-diox.,*** **CARB-V.,** carbn-h., ***carbn-s.,*** caust., lach., laur., nit-ac., op., phos., pic-ac., sul-ac.

CARBON MONOXIDE, ailments from - acet-ac., acon., ant-t., ars., bell., bry., bov., camph., carb-an., ***carb-diox.,*** **CARB-V.,** carbn-h., ***carbn-s.,*** gels., op.

CARBON TETRACHLORIDE, ailments from - carb-tcl., camph.

CARBUNCLES, skin - abrom-aug., achy-a., acon., agar., alco., ant-t., **ANTHR.,** ***apis*, *arn.***, **ARS.**, ars-i., ars-s-f., asim., aza., **BELL.**, bor-ac., both-l., bov., bry., ***bufo***, zirc., calc-chln., calc-f., calc-p., **CALC-S.,** calen., ***canth.***, caps., ***carb-ac.***, carb-an., carb-v., ***cephd.***, ***chin.***, chlor., col-a., coloc., ***crot-c.***, ***crot-h.***, cupr-ar., cyn-d., ***echi.***, echi-p., electr., euph., ferr-p., fl-ac., glyc., gunp., gymne., ham., ***hep.***, ***hippoz.***, ho., ***hyos.***, insulin, iod., ip., jug-r., kali-c., kali-i., kali-m., kali-p., kreos., ***lach.***, lappa, ***led.***, lob., luf-b., **LYC.**, med., merc., mur-ac., myris., nit-ac., op., ***ph-ac.***, phos., phyt., pic-ac., ***pyrog.***, ***rhus-t.***, ***sang.***, ***scol.***, ***sec.***, **SIL.**, staphycoc., stram., sul-ac., ***sulph.***, ***tarent.***, **TARENT-C.,** thuj., torul., tub., vip.

CARPAL TUNNEL SYNDROME - arn., bell-p., brach., calc., ***calc-f., calc-p., caust.,*** guai., ***hyper.,*** plb., rhus-t., **RUTA,** viol-o.

CARTILAGES, complaints of - **ARG.**, asaf., aur., ***calc-f.,*** carb-v., cimic., fl-ac., guai., hep., kali-bi., kali-i., lach., led., merc., merc-c., mez., nat-m., nit-ac., olnd., ph-ac., phos., phyt., plb., ruta, sars., sil., staph., still., sulph.

CASTOR OIL, ailments from - bry., chin., coloc., ***nux-v., ric.***

CATALEPSY, general - abies-c., ***acon.***, acon-c., aether, ***agar.***, aran., ***art-v.***, asaf., bell., bry., camph-br., ***cann-i.***, canth., caust., cham., chin., chlol., ***cic.***, ***cocc.***, ***coff.***, ***con.***, cortico., ***crot-c.***, crot-h., ***cupr.***, ***cur.***, ***ferr.***, ***gels.***, **GRAPH.**, grat., hydr-ac., hyos., ign., indg., iod., ***ip.***, lach., laur., mag-m., merc., ***morph.***, ***mosch.***, ***nat-m.***, ***nux-m.***, nux-v., ol-an., ***op.***, ***petr.***, ***ph-ac.***, pip-m., ***plat.***, plb., raph., rauw., reser., sabad., scut., spong., staph., stram., stry., sulph., tab., tanac., thuj., ***valer.***, verat., ***zinc.***

CATARACT, opacity of lens - acon., agar., alumn., ***am-c.***, ***am-m.***, anac., anag., ang., ant-t., ***apis***, arg-i., arn., ars., aur., ***bar-c.***, bar-s., bell., bov., bry., **CALC., CALC-F.,** ***calc-p.***, calc-s., ***calc-sil.***, calen., ***cann-s.***, caps., ***carb-an.***, **CAUST.,** ***chel.***, chim., chin., cholin., cina, ***cine.***, cocc., coch., ***colch.***, coloc., ***con.***, croc., dig., digin., dulc., ***euph.***, euphr., graph., hed., hep., hyos., ign., iod., ***jab.***, ***kali-c.***, kali-m., kali-s., kali-sil., kreos., lac-c., led., ***lyc.***, **MAG-C.**, mang., merc., naphtin., nat-c., nat-m., nat-s., ***nit-ac.***, op., parathyr., ***phos.***, platan., plb., podo., psor., ***puls.***, quas., rhus-t., ruta, sac-alb., sant., sarr., sars., ***sec.***, seneg., ***sep.***, **SIL.**, spig., stann., staph., stram., sulfa., **SULPH.**, tarax., tell., ***thiosin.***, thuj., verat., ***x-ray***, ***zinc.***, zinc-p.

CATARRH, general - agra., all-c., all-s., aln., alum., ***alumn.***, anis., ***ant-c.***, ant-s., ***ant-t.***, apoc., arg-i., ars., ***ars-i.***, arum-m., arund., asar., asc-t., ***aur.***, bad., bals-p., baros., bell., **CALC.**, calc-f., carb-v., cench., cetr., cham., chin., chlor., cinnb., **CON.**, cop., cor-r., cupr., dros., dulc., erio., eug., euphr., ferr-i., gels., ***graph.***, hepat., hippoz., **HYDR.**, ictod., ign., ip., junc., **KALI-BI.**, kali-c., kali-s., lob-s., mag-c., **MED.**, ***merc.***, merc-d., merc-i-f., merc-k-i., myric., ***nat-m.***, nux-v., ovi-g-p., phel., phos., pulm-v., puls., rumx., sabad., sabal., ***sang.***, sanguin-n., sec., ***sil.***, silphu., sin-n., skook., sol-o., stict., sulph., **THUJ.**, wild., ziz.

CATATONIA, general - cic., cortico., cur., kali-br., puls., rauw.

CATHARTICS, ailments from - ars., carb-v., ***chin.***, ***coloc.***, ***hep.***, ***lyc.***, nit-ac., **NUX-V.**

CATHETER, ailments from - ***acon.***, arn., **CALEN.**, ***camph.***, camph-ac., ***canth.***, kali-c., mag-p., nux-v., petr., **STAPH.**

CAUTERY, ailments, from - arg-n., ***nat-m.***

CELIAC DISEASE - carc., chin., ***lyc.***, phos.

CELIAC PLEXUS, neuralgia - camph., phos.

CELLULITIS, general - ***apis***, ***arn.***, ars., bapt., bell., bry., crot-h., gad., ***hep.***, ***lach.***, mang., merc., ***merc-i-r.***, myris., ***rhus-t.***, ***sil.***, sul-i., tarent-c., vesp.

CEPHALAHEMATOMA, head - arn., ***calc.***, ***calc-f.***, chin., ***merc.***, rhus-t., **SIL.**

CEREBELLAR, disease - hell., helo., plb., sulfon

CEREBRAL HEMORRHAGE, (see Strokes) - **ACON.**, agar., alco., aloe, anthr., apis, **ARN.**, ***aur.***, ***bar-c.***, **BELL.**, **BOTH-L.**, bufo, cadm-br., cadm-s., **CALC.**, calc-f., ***camph.***, carb-ac., carb-v., ***caust.***, chen-a., ***chin.***, **COCC.**, coff., con., ***crot-h.***, ***cupr.***, cur., ***ferr.***, ferr-p., ferr-py., form., **GELS.**, glon., hell., hydr-ac., ***hyos.***, **IP.**, **LACH.**, laur., ***lyc.***, merc., ***mill.***, morg., ***nat-m.***, nit-ac., ***nux-m.***, ***nux-v.***, **OP.**, ***phos.***, pitu-gl., plb., plb-i., ***puls.***, rob., sec., sep., ***sil.***, stram., syph., verat-v., vip., ***zinc.***, zinc-p.

CEREBRAL PALSY - arn., caust., con., gels., hell., ign., lath., op.

CEREBRO-SPINAL, axis, ailments - agar., arg-n., chin., cocc., ***gels.***, ign., ***nux-v.***, phos.

CEREBRO-SPINAL, fever - acon., aeth., agar., am-c., ant-t., **APIS**, ***arg-n.***, arn., ars., bapt., **BELL.**, bry., cact., camph., canth., ***cic.***, ***cimic.***, cocc., crot-h., cupr., dig., **GELS.**, glon., ***hell.***, hydr-ac., hyos., ***ign.***, lyc., ***nat-m.***, **NAT-S.**, ***nux-v.***, **OP.**, ***phos.***, plb., ***rhus-t.***, sol-n., tarent., verat., **VERAT-V.**, ***zinc.***

CERVICITIS, uterine cervix - alum., ant-t., arg-n., ***ars.***, ***bell.***, calen., hydr., kali-bi., kreos., lyc., med., merc., ***merc-c.***, ***nit-ac.***, sep., ***thuj.***

CERVIX, uterine, ailments of - aur-m-n., ***con.***, med., murx., nit-ac., scirr., ***thuj.***

- **erosion**, of - aln., alumn., arg-n., ars., bell-p., bor., bufo, ***calen.***, carb-ac., carb-v., ***caul.***, ***graph.***, ***helon.***, ***hydr.***, hydro-c., ign., kreos., lac-c., ***lach.***, lyc., ***lyss.***, med., merc., ***merc-c.***, merc-i-r., murx., nat-m., nit-ac., ***phyt.***, rhus-t., rob., ***sep.***, sul-ac., ***thuj.***, tril., ***vesp.***

CERVIX, uterine, cancer of - aur., **AUR-M-N.**, calth., ***carb-an.***, carc., **CON.**, hydr., hyper., iod., kreos., nux-v., plat., podo., ***scirr.***, thuj., ust.

- **os** of cervix - ***aur.***, ***aur-m-n.***, ***carb-an.***, hydr., nux-v., plat., podo., ust.

CHAMOMILLA, ailments, from - acon., camph., ***cham.***, chin., cocc., ***coff.***, coloc., ign., nux-v., puls., valer.

CHARCOAL, fumes, ailments from - acet-ac., am-c., ant-t., arn., bell., bor., bov., camph., ***carb-v.***, ***carbn-s.***, coff., op., phos.

CHEMICAL, poisoning, ailments from - acet-ac., acon., agar., ***alum.***, ***alumn.***, **AM-C.**, am-caust., alumn., ang., ant-t., apis., ***asaf.***, arg., arg-n., **ARS.**, ars-i., atro., beryl., brom., cadm-s., calc-f., ***camph.***, carb-ac., carb-v., carbn-s., carc., **CAUST.**, chin., chin-ar., chin-s., chlor., cic., cocc., ***coff.***, cob., con., ***cupr.***, dig., ferr., ***fl-ac.***, formal., ***gels.***, ***glon.***, graph., ***hell.***, ign., iod., ip., kali-bi., kali-br., kali-cy., kali-i., keroso., ***lyc.***, lycps., mang., med., merc-c., **MERC.**, merc-i-f., merc-i-r., ***nat-ar.***, nat-c., nat-m., ***nit-ac.***, nux-v., op., petr., ***ph-ac.***, **PHOS.**, plat., plat-m., **PLB.**, podo., psor., sel., sep., spong., stram., stront-c., sul-ac., sulph., valer., verat., zinc.

CHEMOSIS, edema, conjunctiva - ***acon.***, am-caust., **APIS**, **ARG-N.**, ars., bell., bry., cadm-s., ***con.***, crot-h., dulc., ***euphr.***, ***guare.***, ***hep.***, ***ip.***, ***kali-bi.***, **KALI-I.**, ***lach.***, lyc., merc., merc-i-r., mez., ***nat-m.***, nux-v., phyt., **RHUS-T.**, sil., sul-ac., sulph., syph., ter., thuj., ***vesp.***

CHEMOTHERAPY, treatments, ailments from - ***alf.***, alum., ***ars.***, **BISM.**, ***cadm.***, **CADM-S.**, ***carc.***, ***chel.***, chin., chin-ar., chin-s., ferr., hydr., **IP.**, mercury, nit-ac., ***nux-v.***, phos., plb., sil.

- **nausea**, from - ***ars.***, ***cadm-s.***, ***ip.***, nux-v.
- **vomiting**, from - ars., ***cadm-s.***, ***ip.***, ***nux-v.***
- **weight** loss, from - **ALF.**, ***ars.***, ***cadm-s.***, ***hydr.***, ip., nux-v.

CHEYNE-STOKES, irregular breathing - acon., ***acon-f.***, am-c., ang., antipyrin., atro., bell., ***camph.***, cann-i., ***carb-v.***, chlol., coca, cocain., crot-h., ***cupr.***, cupr-ar., ***dig.***, ***grin.***, ***hydr-ac.***, ***ign.***, iod., ip., kali-cy., lach., ***laur.***, led., lob., nux-v., olnd., ***op.***, ***morph.***, parth., ***saroth.***, spong., sul-ac., sulph., vanad., verat.

CHICKENPOX, infection - acon., **ANT-C.**, ***ant-t.***, apis, ars., asaf., ***bell.***, bry., calc., canth., ***carb-v.***, caust., clem., coff., con., cycl., dulc., gels., graph., hep., hyos., ip., kali-m., ***led.***, ***merc.***, merc-c., nat-c., nat-m., psor., **PULS.**, **RHUS-T.**, sec., ***sep.***, sil., **SULPH.**, ***thuj.***, urt-u., vario.

CHILBLAINS, general - ***abrot.***, acon., **AGAR.**, all-c., aln., aloe, ***alum.***, alum-p., ***alumn.***, am-c., ambr., anac., ant-c., apis, arist-cl., ***arn.***, ***ars.***, asar., aur., aur-ar., bac., ***bad.***, ***bell.***, berb., bor., bry., bufo, cadm-s., calc., calc-l., calc-m., calc-s., calen., camph., ***canth.***, ***carb-an.***, ***carb-v.***, ***cham.***, chin., cocc., ***colch.***, ***cop.***, cortico., ***croc.***, crot-h., croto-t., ***cycl.***, ferr-p., frag., gaert., ham., hep., hydrog., hyos., ign., iod., kali-ar., kali-c., kali-chl., ***kali-m.***, kali-n., kali-p., kalm., lach., led., ***lyc.***, mag-c., merc., morg., ***mur-ac.***, naja, **NIT-AC.**, nux-m., ***nux-v.***, op., **PETR.**, ph-ac., ***phos.***, plan., **PULS.**, ran-b., rheum, rhod., rhus-t., rhus-v., ruta, sal-ac., sec., ***sep.***, ***sil.***, stann., staph., sul-ac., ***sulph.***, syc-co., tam., ***thuj.***, thyr., verat-v., ***zinc.***, zinc-p.

CHILDBIRTH, general, (see Pregnancy, Labor) - ***acon.***, arist-cl., ***arn.***, ***aur.***, ***bell.***, bor., calc., calc-f., ***calen.***, carb-v., **CAUL.**, **CAUST.**, **CHAM.**, ***chin.***, chlf., chlol., ***cic.***, **CIMIC.**, cocc., ***coff.***, ***coff-t.***, ***coll.***, cupr., ferr., ***gels.***, goss., graph., hyos., hyper., ign., ip., **KALI-C.**, kali-p., ***lyc.***, mag-m., mill., mosch., mur-ac., nat-c., nat-m., ***nux-m.***, ***nux-v.***, ***op.***, phos., pitu-gl., plat., **PULS.**, ***pyrog.***, ***rhod.***, rhus-t., ruta, sabin., sars., **SEC.**, **SEP.**, stann., stram., sulph., verat., vib., visc.

after-pains, childbirth - acon., aml-n., arist-cl., **ARN.**, asaf., ***atro.***, aur., **BELL.**, **BELL-P.**, bor., ***bry.***, ***calc.***, calc-f., **CALEN.**, carb-an., carb-v., ***caul.***, **CHAM.**, chin., cic., ***cimic.***, cina, cinnam., cinnb., cocc., ***coff.***, ***coloc.***, ***con.***, croc., crot-h., **CUPR.**, cupr-acet., cupr-ar., cycl., **DIOS.**, ***ferr.***, ***gels.***, goss., ***graph.***, hyos., **HYPER.**, ***ign.***, iod., ip., **KALI-C.**, kreos., ***lac-c.***, lach., lil-t., lyc., ***mill.***, nat-c., nat-m., nux-m., nux-v., ***op.***, **PAR.**, ***phos.***, plat., ***podo.***, **PULS.**, pyrog., **RHUS-T.**, ***ruta***, **SABIN.**, **SEC.**, ***sep.***, sil., sul-ac., ***sulph.***, ter., ust., ***vib.***, ***vib-p.***, vinc., visc., wye., ***xan.***, zinc.

confinement, puerperal - acon., agn., ant-c., ant-t., **ARN.**, asaf., asar., aur., **BELL.**, **BELL-P.**, bor., bov., ***bry.***, ***calc.***, **CALEN.**, camph., canth., ***carb-an.***, carb-v., **CAUL.**, caust., **CHAM.**, chin., cina, cocc., ***coff.***, colch., coloc., con., ***croc.***, cupr., cycl., dros., dulc., equis., ***ferr.***, ***gels.***, glon., graph., helon., rhod., **SEP.**

fever, after - ***acon.***, ail., ant-c., anthr., ***apis***, ***arg-n.***, **ARN.**, ars., ***bapt.***, bell., ***bry.***, calc., cann-i., canth., carb-ac., carb-an., **CARBN-S.**, card-m., **CHAM.**, chin., chin-ar., ***chin-s.***, cimic., cocc., coff., **COLOC.**, con., croc., crot-h., cypr., **ECHI.**, ***ferr.***, gels., helon., ***hydr-ac.***, ***hyos.***, ign., ip., kali-br., kali-c., kali-m., ***kali-p.***, kreos., **LACH.**, **LYC.**, med., merc., merc-c., mill., ***mur-ac.***, **NUX-V.**, op., phos., phyt., plat., **PULS.**, puls-n, **PYROG.**, **RHUS-T.**, sabal., sabin., sal-ac., sec., ***sep.***, sil., stram., **SULPH.**, ter., til., verat., ***verat-v.***, zinc.

CHILDREN, general - abrot., acet-ac., **ACON.**, **AETH.**, agar., ***all-c.***, alum., ***ambr.***, anac., ***ang.***, ***ant-c.***, **ANT-T.**, apis, arg-n., arn., **ARS.**, asaf., **AUR.**, bac., **BAR-C.**, **BELL.**, brom., **BOR.**, ***bry.***, **CALC.**, ***calc-f.***, **CALC-P.**, calc-s., camph., canth., **CAPS.**, **CARC.**, caust., **CHAM.**, chel., chlol., ***cic.***, **CINA**, chin., clem., cocci-s., ***cocc.***, ***coff.***, ***croc.***, con., ***cupr-m.***, ***cypr.***, dig., dros., euph., ferr., **FERR-P.**, ***gels.***, graph., hell., hep., **HYOS.**, **IGN.**, ***iod.***, **IP.**, kali-br., kali-c., ***kali-m.***, ***kali-p.***, kreos., ***lach.***, laur., **LYC.**, mag-c., ***mag-p.***, **MED.**, **MERC.**, mill., ***mosch.***, mur-ac., nat-c., **NAT-M.**, ***nux-m.***, ***nux-v.***, **OP.**, **PHOS.**, plb., ***podo.***, ***psor.***, **PULS.**, **RHEUM**, rhus-t., ruta, sabad., sabin., ***samb.***, ***sanic.***, sec., seneg., senn., sep., **SIL.**, spig., **SPONG.**, squil., stann., **STAPH.**, stram., sul-ac., **SULPH.**, ter., **TEUCR.**, thuj., **THUJ.**, thyr., **TUB.**, ***verat.***, viol-o., viol-t., zinc.

abused, ailments from being - ***acon.***, alum., am-m., **ANAC.**, androc., ***arg-n.***, ars., ***aur.***, ***aur-m.***, bell., ***bry.***, calc., calc-s., **CARC.**, caust., ***cham.***, **COLOC.**, con., form., gels., grat., **IGN.**, ***lach.***, **LYC.**, ***lyss.***, med., merc., **NAT-M.**, ***nux-v.***, ***op.***, **PALL.**, petr., **PH-AC.**, plat., ***puls.***, rhus-t., ***seneg.***, sep., sil., **STAPH.**, stram., ***sulph.***, thuj., verat., zinc.

delicate, puny, sickly - brom., ***calc-p.***, ***caust.***, irid., ***lyc.***, mag-c., phos., psor., **SIL.**

depressed, children - abrot., ***ars.***, **AUR.**, ***calc.***, carc., caust., ***lach.***, lyc., kali-br., **NAT-M.**, rhus-t., sulph.

destructive, behavior - anac., ***bell.***, cham., ***cina***, hep., ***hyos.***, lach., med., ***nux-v.***, ***staph.***, **STRAM.**, tarent., **TUB.**, ***verat.***

development, delayed or arrested - aeth., ***agar.***, ***bac.***, **BAR-C.**, bor., bufo, **CALC.**, **CALC-P.**, **CARC.**, caust., chin., cic., cupr., des-ac., iod., kali-c., kreos., lac-d., med., ***nat-m.***, nat-a., nep., ph-ac., ***phos.***, pin-s., ***sil.***, sulfa., sulph., thyr., vip.

dwarfish, children - ambr., aster., bac., **BAR-C.**, bar-i., ***bar-m.***, bor., bufo, ***calc.***, **CALC-P.**, ***carbn-s.***, ***carc.***, ***con.***, iod., ***lap-a.***, lyc., mag-m., **MED.**, merc., merc-pr-a., nat-m., nep., ***ol-j.***, op., ph-ac., pitu-gl., sec., **SIL.**, sulfa., **SULPH.**, **SYPH.**, ***thyr.***, ***tub.***, zinc.

growth, disorders - **BAR-C.**, **CALC.**, **CALC-P.**, ferr., ferr-acet., iod., irid., kreos., ***ph-ac.***, ***phos.***, ***sil.***, ***syph.***

infants, general - arg-n., aur., ***bar-c.,*** **CALC.,** calc-f., **CALC-P.,** calc-s., cupr., ferr., ***lyc.,*** merc., **PHOS.,** plb., **PULS., SIL.,** stann., ***sulph.***

retarded, mentally - absin., ***aeth.,*** agar., anac., anan., ant-c., ***arg-n.,*** aur., **BAR-C.,** ***bar-m.,*** bell., ***bufo, calc., calc-p.,*** caps., ***carbn-s.,*** **CARC.,** cent., cham., chlol., ***hell.,*** hyos., iod., lyc., ***med.,*** merc., nat-m., nux-m., ***phos., plb.,*** sars., sil., stram., ***sulph.,*** tab., ***tub.,*** zinc.

slowness, mental, children - alum., ***anac.,*** **BAR-C., CALC.,** carc., caust., con., cortiso., gels., ***graph.,*** **HELL.,** hyos., kali-bi., kali-br., lyc., merc., nat-m., ***op.,*** **PH-AC., PHOS.,** puls., ***sil.,*** thuj., ***verat.,*** zinc.

CHILLS, general - abies-c., acon., ***aesc.,*** aeth., ***agar.,*** agn., ail., alst-c., ***alum.,*** alum-p., am-c., am-m., ***ambr., anac.,*** ang., ***ant-c.,*** **ANT-T.,** ***anthr.;*** **APIS, ARAN.,** arg., arg-n., **ARN., ARS.,** ars-i., arum-t., asaf., asar., astac., atha., aur., aur-m., bac., ***bad.,*** bapt., bar-c., bar-m., ***bell.,*** bell-p., berb., ***bism.,*** bol., bor., ***bor-ac.,*** both-l., bov., brom., ***bry.,*** bufo, cact., cadm-s., calad., ***calc., calc-ar.,*** **CALC-F.,** calc-i., ***calc-p.,*** calc-s., **CALC-SIL.,** calen., ***camph.,*** camph-br., cann-i., **CANTH.,** ***caps., carb-an.,*** **CARB-V.,** carbn-o., **CARBN-S.,** cast., caust., **CEDR.,** ***cham.,*** **CHEL., CHIN.,** chin-ar., **CHIN-S.,** ***chlol., cic.,*** cimic., ***cimx.,*** cina, cinnb., ***cist.,*** clem., coca, cocain, cocc., coff., ***colch.,*** coloc., con., cop., corn., corn-f., crat., croc., crot-h., croto-t., cupr., cupr-ar., ***cycl.,*** daph., ***dig.,*** dios., dros., dulc., ***echi., elaps,*** elat., euon., **EUP-PER.,** ***eup-pur.,*** **EUPH.,** ***euphr.,*** eupi., ***ferr.,*** ferr-ar., fl-ac., gamb., **GELS.,** ***graph.,*** grat., guai., hell., **HELO.,** ***hep., hyos.,*** **HYPER., IGN.,** ***iod.,*** **IP.,** ***jatr.,*** **KALI-AR.,** kali-bi., ***kali-c.,*** kali-fcy., ***kali-i., kali-n.,*** **KALI-P.,** kreos., lac-c., lac-d., ***lach., lachn.,*** laur., **LED.,** lil-t., lith-c., lob., luf-op., **LYC.,** lyss., ***mag-c.,*** mag-m., ***mag-p.,*** mag-s., mang., ***med.,*** **MENY.,** merc., merc-c., **MEZ.,** morph., mosch., ***mur-ac.,*** naja, ***nat-ar.,*** nat-c., **NAT-M.,** nat-p., nicc., **NIT-AC., NUX-M., NUX-V.,** ***olnd., op.,*** par., ***petr., ph-ac.,*** phel., ***phos.,*** phyt., pimp., plan., plat., plb., ***podo., psor.,*** **PULS.,** pyrog., rad-br., ran-b., ran-s., rheum, ***rhod.,*** **RHUS-T.,** ***rob.,*** **RUMX.,** ***ruta,*** **SABAD.,** sabin., ***samb.,*** sang., sarr., sars., **SEC.,** sel., senec., seneg., **SEP.,** ***sil.,*** spig., spong., squil., stann., **STAPH.,** ***stram., stront-c., sul-ac.,*** sulph., ***sumb.,*** symph., tab., ***tarax., tarent., tela,*** teucr., ther., **THUJ.,** thyr., ***tub.,*** valer., **VERAT., VERAT-V.,** verb., viol-o., viol-t., vip., ***zinc.***

CHINA BARK, poisoning, ailments from, (see Quinine) - ant-t., aran., arn., **ARS.,** ***bell., calc., carb-v.,*** cham., **CHIN.,** ***chin-ar., chin-s.,*** coff., eup-per., ***ferr., hell.,*** **HEP.,** iod., ***ip.,*** lach., led., meny., merc., nat-c., ***nat-m., nux-v.,*** ph-ac., ***puls.,*** rhus-t., salv., ***sel.,*** sep., ***sulph.,*** thea., ***verat.***

CHLAMYDIAL - med., puls., sulph., thuj.

CHLOASMA, skin - acet-ac., ant-c., ***ars.,*** cadm-s., card-m., caul., coch., ***con.,*** halo., ***lyc.,*** merc-i-r., mez., nat-ar., nux-v., paull., ***plb.,*** pyrar., rob., **SEP.,** ***sol,*** sul-ac., sulph.

chloasma, pregnancy - cadm-s., card-m., caul., ***lyc.,*** nux-v., rob., ***sep., sol.***

CHLORALUM, choral hydrate, ailments from - acet-ac., am-c., anh., atro., cann-i., ***chlf.,*** chlol., dig., mosch., op.

CHLORINE, ailments from - am-c., ant-t., ars., brom., ***chlor.,*** cupr., iod., merc., meph., mur-ac., nat-m., op.

CHLOROFORM, ailments from - acet-ac., am-caust., atro., carbn-h., ***chlf.,*** chlol., hyos., hyper., keroso., op., **PHOS.**

CHLOROSIS, (see Hemolytic, anemia)

CHOKES, easily - ***acon.,*** anac., **ARG., BELL.,** calc., cann-s., cocc., gels., **HYOS.,** ign., kali-c., kali-n., **LACH.,** meph., nat-m., nux-m., op., plat., ***rhus-t.,*** sil., sul-ac., verat.

choking, swallowing, on - acon., ars., ***bar-c.,*** bell., bry., ***cic., cupr.,*** gent-c., ***graph., hyos.,*** kali-c., ***laur.,*** **LYC.,** mag-p., manc., meph., ***merc.,*** mur-ac., ***nat-m.,*** onos., par., ***plb.,*** **PULS.,** rhus-t., stry., tarent., verat., zinc.

CHOLECYSTITIS, inflammation, gallbladder - aran-ix., bell., ***berb.,*** beryl., bold., bry., bufo, but-ac., calc., card-m., ***chel., chin.,*** chion., ***chol.,*** coli., coll., coloc., eberth., flor-p., guat., hed., hoit., ***hydr.,*** ipom., jug-c., ***lach.,*** lept., ***lyc.,*** mag-m., mag-s., malar., morg., morg-g., myric., ***nat-s., nux-v.,*** parat., ***phos.,*** pitu-p., podo., prot., ptel., pyrog., tarax., tell., tere-ch., tub-r.

CHOLERA, infection - acon., ***aeth.,*** agar-ph., am-c., ampe-qu, anil., ant-c., ***ant-t.,*** apis, arg-n., arn., ***ars.,*** ars-i., asar., aven., bac., bell., benz-ac., bism., bov., bry., cadm-s., calc, calc-acet., calc-ar., calc-i., ***calc-p.,*** **CAMPH.,** camph-br., ***canth.,*** carb-ac., ***carb-v.,*** caul., cedr., cham., chin., chin-s., chlol., chlor., cic., coff-t., colch., coloc., colos., corn., crot-h., croto-t., cuph., **CUPR.,** ***cupr-acet., cupr-ar.,*** dig., dios., dulc., elat., epil., epil-a., euon., euon-a., euonin., euph-c., euph-l., ***ferr.,*** ferr-p., gad., ***gamb.,*** gent-q., gnaph., ***graph., grat.,*** gua., ***guai.,*** hell., hell-f., ***hydr-ac.,*** hyos., ign., indol., ***iodof., ip., iris,*** jatr., kali-bi., kali-br., kali-p., kreos., lach., ***laur.,*** lept., lim., mag-c., mag-p., manc., med., merc., merc-c., mom-ch., mur-ac., naja, nat-m., nat-s., nuph., nux-m., nux-v., oeno., ***op.,*** oper., ox-ac., passi., paull-p., ph-ac., ***phos.,*** phyt., plan., plect., ***podo.,*** polyg., polyp-p., prot., ***psor.,*** puls., quas., raph., res., rhus-t., ric., rob., sars., ***sec.,*** sep., ***sil., stram.,*** sul-ac., sulph., ***tab.,*** ter., thuj., tub., **VERAT.,** verat-v., xan., zinc., zinc-m.

cholera, infantum - acon., **AETH.,** ant-c., ant-t., ***apis,*** arg-n., arn., ***ars., ars-i., bac., bell., bism.,*** bry., cadm-s., ***calc.,*** calc-acet., calc-i., ***calc-p.,***

camph., camph-br., canth., ***carb-ac.,*** carb-v., cham., ***chin.,*** colch., coloc., colos., corn., ***croto-t.,*** cuph., ***cupr.,*** cupr-acet., ***cupr-ar., dios., dulc.,*** elat., ***euph-c., ferr.,*** ferr-p., gad., ***gamb., gnaph.,*** graph., grat., **GUAI.,** hydr-ac., ***hyos., ign.,*** indol., ***iodof., ip., iris,*** jatr., kali-bi., kali-br., ***kreos., laur., mag-c., med.,*** merc., nat-m., ***op.,*** ox-ac., passi., ***ph-ac., phos.,*** phyt., ***podo., psor., puls.,*** raph., res., ric., **ROB.,** ***rhus-t.,*** sars., ***sec.,*** sep., ***sil., stram.,*** sulph., ***tab.,*** thuj., ***verat., verat-v., zinc.***

cholera, morbus - ***acon.,*** ant-c., ant-t., arg-n., **ARS.,** asar., bism., camph., camph-br., caul., ***cedr.,*** chlor., ***colch.,*** coloc., crot-h., ***croto-t., cupr., cupr-ar.,*** dios., elat., euph-c., ***ferr., grat.,*** gad., **GUAI.,** hydr-ac., ***ip., iris, jatr.,*** kali-bi., mag-p., op., oper., ph-ac., ***phos.,*** **PODO.,** polyp-p., ***psor.,*** raph., ***ric., sec., tab.,*** thuj., **VERAT.,** ***verat-v.***

CHOLESTEROL, increased - calc., chlf., ***chol.,*** cortiso., dulc., insulin, lyc., mag-f., perh., sulph., thyreotr.

CHONDRITIS, perichondritis - **ARG.,** asaf., ***bell.,*** cham., ***cimic.,*** led., lob-s., merc., ***nat-m.,*** olnd., ***plb., ruta,*** sil., syph.

CHOREA, general - ***abrot.,*** absin., acon., **AGAR.,** agar-ph., agarin., ***ambr., aml-n., ant-t.,*** apis, ***arg-n., ars.,*** ars-i., ars-s-f., **ART-V.,** ***asaf.,*** aster., ***atro.,*** aven., ***bell., bufo, cact.,*** **CALC.,** calc-i., ***calc-p., colch., cast.,*** caul., **CAUST.,** ***cham.,*** cedr., ***chel.,*** **CHIN.,** chlol., **CIC., CIMIC., CINA,** cocain., ***cocc.,*** coch., ***cod.,*** coff., con., ***croc., crot-c.,*** crot-h., **CUPR.,** ***cupr-acet., cupr-ar.,*** cypr., ***dios.,*** dulc., eup-a., ***ferr.,*** ferr-ar., ferr-cit., ferr-cy., ***ferr-i., ferr-r., ferr-s.,*** form., ***gels., guare., hipp., hyos.,*** **IGN.,** ***iod.,*** ip., kali-ar., ***kali-br.,*** kali-c., kali-i., kali-p., ***kali-s.,*** **LACH.,** lat-k., lat-m., laur., levo., ***lil-t.,*** lyss., ***mag-p., mang.,*** merc., mez., ***mill., morph.,*** mur-ac., **MYGAL.,** ***nat-m., nit-ac., nux-m., nux-v.,*** ol-an., ***op.,*** passi., ph-ac., ***phos.,*** phys., phyt., picro., plat., plb., psor., ***puls.,*** rhod., ***rhus-t.,*** russ., sabin., ***sant., scut., sec., sep., sil., sin-n.,*** sol-n., ***spig.,*** stann., ***staph.,*** stict., **STRAM.,** ***stry.,*** stry-p., sul-ter., sulfon., ***sulph., samb., sumb.,*** tanac., **TARENT.,** ***ter.,*** thal., thiop., thuj., ***tub.,*** valer., verat-v., visc., ***zinc.,*** zinc-ar., ***zinc-br.,*** zinc-cy., zinc-p., zinc-val., ziz.

CHRONIC FATIGUE, syndrome, (see Weakness) - **ALUM.,** ***ambr.,*** **AM-C.,** apoc., ***ars., ars-i., aur.,*** bar-c., ***bapt.,*** **CALAD., CALC.,** cann-s., ***carb-v.,*** **CARC.,** ***caust., chel.,*** **CHIN.,** ***chin-s., cocc.,*** **CON.,** ***dig.,*** **FERR.,** ferr-ar., ferr-p., **GELS., GRAPH.,** helon., hyos., ***kali-c.,*** kali-n., ***kali-p.,*** **LACH.,** ***laur., lyc.,*** mag-m., ***mang., merc.,*** mur-ac., nat-ar., ***nat-c., nat-m.,*** nit-ac., ***nux-m.,*** **NUX-V.,** ***op.,*** **PH-AC.,** ***phos.,*** **PIC-AC.,** ***psor.,*** puls., sel., ***seneg., sep.,*** **SIL.,** ***stann.,*** staph., ***stram.,*** stront-c., ***sulph.,*** **SUL-AC.,** ***thuj., valer.,*** verat.

CIRRHOSIS, liver - abies-c., apoc., ***arg-n.,*** arn., ars., ***ars-i.,*** aur., bell., boerh., brom., bry., calc., ***calc-ar.,*** carc., **CARD-M.,** casc., ***chel., chim., chin.,*** chin-ar., chin-s., chol., **CROT-H.,** ***cupr.,*** cur., dig., dulc., fel., fl-ac., graph., hed., ***hep.,*** **HYDR.,** iod., kali-bi., kali-c., kali-i., kali-s., ***lach.,*** lact., lept., levo., luf-b., ***lyc.,*** lyss., mag-c., ***mag-m.,*** menis., merc., merc-d., mez., ***mur-ac., nast.,*** nat-c., nat-hchls., nat-p., nit-ac., nit-m-ac., nux-m., nux-v., **PHOS.,** plb., podo., puls., quas., rauw., sel., senec., sep., sil., **SUL-AC.,** stann., sulph., tarax., urea, urt-u., verat.

CLAUSTROPHOBIA, fear of closed places - **ACON.,** ambr., aran., **ARG-N.,** ***calc.,*** chin-ar., cocc., ***ign.,*** kali-ar., ***lac-d.,*** **LYC.,** med., **NAT-M.,** nit-ac., nux-v., plb., psor., **PULS.,** ruta, staph., **STRAM.,** succ., sulph., tab., valer..

CLOTS, tendency to formation of blood - alum., androc., anthr., ars., bell., **BOTH-L.,** cact., ***crot-h.,*** elaps, ham., ***lach.,*** merc-cy., phos., sabin., sec., stront-c., sul-ac., thlaspi, tril., ust., zinc.

COAL FUMES, ailments from - acet-ac., am-c., ant-t., arn., bell., bor., bov., ***carb-diox., carb-v., carbn-s.,*** coff., ip., lach., ***op.,*** phos., sec.

COBALT, ailments from - bar-c., cadm-s., calc-f., ***cob.,*** cob-n., err., merc., radon, uran-n.

COCAINE, ailments from - aven., camph., carb-v., cham., coff., ***coca., cocain., gels.,*** rital., nux-v.

COCCYX, tailbone, injuries - aesc., ***arn.,*** bell-p., ***carb-an.,*** **HYPER.,** led., ***mez.,*** **SIL.,** tell.

COD LIVER OIL, ailments of - chin., chol., hep.

CODEINE, ailments from - alum., bry., ***cod,*** coff., hyos., morph., nux-v., op.

COFFEE, ailments from, (see Caffeine) - ***aeth.,*** agar., alet., all-c., anac., ars., arum-t., aster., aur-m., bell., bov., bry., ***cact.,*** calc., ***calc-p.,*** cann-i., **CANTH.,** ***caps.,*** carb-v., caul., **CAUST., CHAM.,** chin., cist., clem., ***cocc., coff.,*** colch., coloc., cycl., fl-ac., form., glon., grat., ***hep.,*** **IGN.,** ***ip.,*** kali-bi., kali-c., kali-n., kola, lyc., mag-c., mang., ***merc.,*** nat-m., ***nat-s.,*** nit-ac., **NUX-V.,** ox-ac., ***paull., ph-ac.,*** plat., psor., ***puls.,*** rhus-t., sep., stram., sulph., sul-ac., tab., ***thuj.,*** vinc., xan.

COLCHICINE, ailments from - ars., benz-ac., camph., chin., ***colch.,*** led., urea.

COLDS, tendency to catch - **ACON.,** aesc., agar., ***all-c.,*** **ALUM.,** alum-p., alum-sil., alumn., am-c., am-m., anac., ***ant-c.,*** ant-t., aral., aran., ***arg-n.,*** arn., ***ars., ars-i.,*** ars-s-f., **BAC., BAR-C.,** bar-i., bar-m., bar-s., ***bell.,*** benz-ac., bor., **BRY.,** calad., **CALC.,** calc-i., **CALC-P.,** ***calc-s.,*** calc-sil., ***calen.,*** camph., caps., carb-an., ***carb-v., carbn-s.,*** carc., caust., **CHAM.,** chin., chin-ar., cimic., cinnb., cist., clem., cocc., coc-c., coff., colch., coloc., ***con.,*** croc., cupr., cycl., dig., dros., **DULC.,** dys-co., elaps, eup-per., euphr., ***ferr.,*** ferr-ar., ferr-i., ferr-p., ***form.,*** gast., ***gels.,*** goss., ***graph.,*** ham., hed., **HEP.,** hyos., hyper., ign., iod., ip., kali-ar., ***kali-bi.,*** **KALI-C., KALI-I., KALI-P.,** kali-s., kali-sil., ***lac-d.,*** lach., led., **LYC.,** m-arct., m-aust., mag-c., mag-m., **MED., MERC.,** mez., naja, **NAT-AR.,** ***nat-c.,*** **NAT-M.,** nat-p., nat-sil., **NIT-AC.,** ***nux-m.,*** **NUX-V.,** ol-j., op., osm., ***petr., ph-ac.,*** **PHOS.,** plat., **PSOR.,** ***puls.,*** rhod., ***rhus-t.,*** **RUMX.,** ruta, sabad., sabin., samb., sang., sars., sel., senec., **SEP., SIL.,** solid., spig., stann., staph., sul-i., ***sulph., sul-ac.,*** syph., **THUJ., TUB.,** valer., verat., verb., zinc.

COLIC, infants - aeth., bell., ***calc-p., carb-ac.,*** carb-v., **CHAM.,** chin., ***cina, coloc.,*** dios., ign., kali-br., lyc., ***mag-c.,*** **MAG-P., NUX-V.,** staph.

COLIC, pain - am-m., alum., ***ars.,*** aur., ***bapt.,*** **BELL., BERB.,** ***bry.,*** **CALC., CARD-M.,** ***cham., chel.,*** **CHIN.,** ***chion., chlf.,*** **CHOL., COLOC.,** cupr., dig., **DIOS.,** euon., fel., ferr-s., gels., ***hep., hydr., ip., iris,*** jug-c., kali-ar., ***kali-bi., kali-c., lach.,*** laur., ***lept., lith-c.,*** **LYC., MAG-P.,** mang., merc., merc-d., **MORG.,** myric., **NAT-S.,** ***nux-v.,*** op., osm., ***phos.,*** podo., ptel., puls., rhus-t., sang., ***sep.,*** sulph., tab., tarax., ***ter.,*** thuj., **VERAT.**

COLITIS, enterocolitis - **ACET-AC., ACON.,** alco., aloe, **ANT-T., APIS,** ***ars.,*** **BELL., BRY.,** ***cact.,*** canth., ***cham.,*** chin., ***chin-ar., colch.,*** cop., crot-h., cupr-acet., cupr-s., euph-c., gamb., grat., jal., jug-c., kali-i., kali-s., kali-t., ***lach.,*** lol., lycps., ***merc.,*** mez., ***nit-ac., nuph., ox-ac.,*** phos., plb., rhus-t., sabin., sulph., **TER.,** verat-v.

COLLAPSE, general, (see Fainting) - acet-ac., acetan., acon., aconin., adren., aeth., **AM-C.,** am-caust., ampe-qu, amyg-am., ant-c., ***ant-t.,*** apis, aran-ix., arn., **ARS.,** ***ars-h.,*** bamb-a., bar-c., calc., **CAMPH.,** cann-i., canth., ***carb-ac.,*** carb-an., **CARB-V., CARBN-S.,** carc., cench., **CHIN.,** cina, cit-l., cocc., colch., colchin., con., crat., croc., ***crot-h.,*** croto-t., ***cupr.,*** cupr-acet., cupr-ar., cupr-s., cyt-l., ***dig.,*** diph., dor., euon., eupi., graph., hell., home., hydr., ***hydr-ac.,*** hydrog., ***hyos.,*** hyosin., iod., ip., jab., kali-br., kali-chl., kali-chr., kali-cy., kali-n., kali-p., ***lach.,*** lat-m., ***laur.,*** lob., lob-p., lol., lyc., ***med.,*** merc., merc-c., merc-cy., merc-n., merc-pr-a., mez., morph., ***mosch.,*** mur-ac., naja, nicot., nit-s-d., nux-v., olnd., op., ox-ac., oxyu-s., ozone, petr., ph-ac., ***phos.,*** phys., plb., podo., pyrog., ric., sabad., sant., scam., ***sec., seneg.,*** sep., stann., stram., sul-ac., ***sulph.,*** tab., tarent., tarent-c., tax., ther., ***verat.,*** verat-v., vib., vip., ***zinc.***

COLON, cancer - ***alum.,*** **ALOE,** ***ars., cadm-i., cadm-s.,*** carb-an., carb-v., ***carc.,*** cund., ***graph.,*** **HYDR.,** ***kali-c., lap-a.,*** **LYC.,** mur-ac., ***nit-ac.,*** ORNI., petr., ruta, ***scirr.,*** scroph-n., sed-r., semp., sep., sil., spig., ***thuj.***

COMA, general, unconsciousness - absin., acet-ac., **ACON.,** act-sp., adel., aesc., aesc-g., aeth., aether, agar., agar-cit., agar-pa., agar-ph., agar-pr., agar-se., agar-st., agav-t., agn., agro., ***ail.,*** alco., alet., ***alum.,*** am-caust., ambr., am-c., am-m., ***aml-n.,*** amyg-am., ***anac.,*** ang., anil., ant-m., anthr., ant-c., ant-t., ***apis,*** apoc., apom., aq-mar., arg., ***arg-n., arn., ars.,*** ars-h., art-v., ***arum-t.,*** asar., astac., ***aster.,*** atro., ***bapt.,*** **BAR-C.,** ***bar-m.,*** bar-s., **BELL.,** benz-n., benz-ac., bism., both-l., bov., brom., ***bry.,*** bufo, ***cact., calad.,*** cadm-s., calc., calc-m., calc-s., calc-sil., ***camph.,*** **CANN-I.,** cann-s., ***canth.,*** caps., carb-ac., carb-an., ***carb-v., carbn-h., carbn-o., carbn-s., caust., cedr.,*** cench., ***cham., chel.,*** chen-a., ***chin.,*** chin-s., chlf., ***chlol., chlor., cic.,*** cic-m., cimic., ***cina,*** cit-l., clem., **COCC.,** ***coff.,*** coff-t., ***colch.,*** coloc., ***con.,*** cor-r., cori-r., cortico., croc., ***crot-c., crot-h., cupr., cupr-acet.,*** cupr-s., ***cycl.,*** cyt-l., dat-m., dat-s., der., ***dig.,*** dirc., dor., dubin., dulc., elaps, euph., euphr., ferr., ferr-ar., ferr-m., ferr-p., fil., fl-ac., gaul., ***gels., glon.,*** graph., grat., guai., ham., **HELL.,** ***helon., hep.,*** home., **HYDR-AC., HYOS., IGN.,** iod., ip., jasm., jatr., jatr-u., juni-v., kali-bi., ***kali-br., kali-c.,*** kali-chl., kali-cy., kali-i., kali-m., kali-n., keroso., kreos., ***lac-d.,*** **LACH.,** lact., ***laur., led., lil-t., lyc.,*** lyss., mag-c., mag-m., manc., meli., merc., ***merc-c.,*** merc-n., merc-pr-r., merl., meth-ae-ae., mez., **MOSCH.,** ***mur-ac.,*** naja, nat-c., nat-f., ***nat-m.,*** nat-p., nit-ac., ***nit-s-d.,*** **NUX-M.,** ***nux-v.,*** oena., oeno., ***ol-an., olnd.,*** **OP.,** ox-ac., ***par.,*** past., ***petr.,*** **PH-AC.,** ***phos.,*** phyt., piloc., ***plat., plb.,*** psor., **PULS.,** ran-b., rheum, rhod., ***rhus-t.,*** rumx-a., russ., ruta, sabad., sabin., sang., sapin., sars., ***sec.,*** sel., ***seneg.,*** sep., ***sil., sol-n.,*** sphing., spig., squil., stann., staph., ***stram.,*** sul-ac., sul-h., ***sulph.,*** tab., tanac., tarax., ***tarent.,*** tax., ***ter.,*** tere-ch., tub., uran-n., valer., verb., ***verat.,*** verat-v., verin., vesp., viol-o., vip., vip-a., visc., wies., xero, ***zinc.,*** zinc-p.

CONCUSSION, brain - ***acon.,*** alum., **ARN.,** bar-c., bell., bell-p., bry., calen., carc., chin., **CIC.,** ***cocc.,*** con., gels., glon., ham., **HELL.,** hep., hydr-ac., ***hyos.,*** **HYPER.,** kali-i., ***kali-p., led., lob.,*** mang., merc., ***nat-m.,*** **NAT-S., OP.,** ph-ac., ***rhus-t.,*** sep., sil., stram., sul-ac., sulph., ***teucr.,*** verat-v., zinc.

CONDYLOMATA, skin, (see Excrescences, Warts) - acet-ac., alumn., anac., ant-t., ***apis, arg-n., aur., aur-m.,*** aur-m-n., aur-s., bell., benz-ac., ***calc.,*** carc., caust., cham., **CINNB.,** cub., eucal., euph., euphr., ***euphr., fl-ac.,*** **HEP.,** ***kali-chl., kali-i.,*** kali-m., kreos., lac-c., ***lyc.,*** **MED.,** ***merc.,*** merc-acet., merc-aur., merc-br., **MERC-C.,** ***merc-d.,*** merc-i-f., merc-i-r., merc-s., ***mill.,*** nat-m., **NAT-S., NIT-AC.,** nux-v., **PH-AC.,** ***phos.,*** phyt., plat., psor., sabad., ***sabin.,*** sanic., ***sars.,*** sec., ***sep.,*** sil., ***staph., sulph.,*** syph., ***teucr.,*** **THUJ.**

CONGESTIVE, headaches - ***acon.,*** aml-n., arg-n., **BELL.,** ***bry., cact.,*** chin-s., ***ferr-p., gels.,*** **GLON.,** glyc., joan., **LACH., MELI.,** nat-m., nux-v., op., phase., ***sang.,*** sil., sol-n., sulph., usn., ***verat-v.***

CONGESTIVE, heart disease - **ACON.**, am-c., ***aml-ns.***, **APOC.**, ***asaf.***, asar., carb-v., ***carc.***, cham., **CRAT.**, cycl., cyt-l., dig., ***ferr.***, ***ferr-i.***, **GLON.**, hyper., ign., lach., laur., ***lil-t.***, lyc., merc-c., nit-ac., ***nux-m.***, nux-v., phos., ***puls.***, sep., sil., stront-c., sulph.

CONJUNCTIVITIS, infection - abr., acet-ac., **ACON.**, act-sp., aeth., agar., ail., ***all-c.***, **ALUM.**, alum-p., am-c., ant-c., ant-t., **APIS**, arg., **ARG-N.**, arn., **ARS.**, ars-i., ars-s-f., asaf., asar., asc-t., aur., aur-i., aur-m., bamb-a., bar-c., bar-i., bar-s., **BELL.**, beryl., brom., bry., cadm-s., **CALC.**, ***calc-f.***, calc-hp., calc-i., ***calc-p.***, calc-pic., **CALC-S.**, calen., camph., cann-i., cann-s., ***canth.***, **CARBN-S.**, caust., cedr., ***cham.***, chin., ***chlol.***, chlor., ***cinnb.***, ***clem.***, coc-c., con., cor-r., cortiso., crot-h., ***croto-t.***, ***dig.***, dubin., dulc., dys-co., ery-a., euph., **EUPHR.**, ferr-i., ***ferr-p.***, gels., ***graph.***, grin., guai., guare., ***ham.***, ***hep.***, hist., ***hydr.***, hydro-c., ign., ***iod.***, ***ip.***, jatr-u., jeqol., ***kali-bi.***, kali-chl., kali-i., kali-m., kali-p., kali-s., kali-sil., lach., led., lil-t., linu-u, ***lyc.***, mand., med., meph., ***merc.***, merc-c., merc-cy., merc-d., merc-i-f., merc-n., merc-p., merl., mez., mim-h., morg., myric., ***nat-ar.***, nat-c., nat-m., nat-p., ***nat-s.***, nicc., nit-ac., ***nux-v.***, op., osm., peti., ***petr.***, phys., phyt., pic-ac., psor., **PULS.**, **RHUS-T.**, rhus-v., sanic., sec., ***seneg.***, sep., sil., spig., squil., ***staph.***, staphycoc., stict., sul-ac., sul-i., sulfa., **SULPH.**, sumb., ***syc-co.***, symph., syph., tarent., tela, tell., tep., ter., thal., ***thuj.***, thyr., tub., upa., verat-v., vesp., ***zinc.***, zinc-s.

CONSTIPATION, general - abies-c., abies-n., ***abrot.***, **AESC.**, ***aeth.***, ***agar.***, ***agn.***, alet., ***aloe***, **ALUM.**, **ALUMN.**, ***ambr.***, ***am-c.***, ***am-m.***, ammc., ***anac.***, anan., ***ang.***, ant-c., **APIS**, ***arg.***, ***arg-n.***, arn., **ARS.**, ***ars-i.***, arund., asaf., asc-c., asc-t., aster., ***aur.***, aur-m., bad., ***bar-c.***, ***bar-m.***, bell., ***berb.***, bol., bor., bov., brach., **BRY.**, ***cact.***, calad., **CALC.**, ***calc-p.***, ***calc-s.***, camph., cann-s., caps., ***carb-ac.***, ***carb-an.***, ***carb-v.***, **CARBN-S.**, ***card-m.***, casc., caul., **CAUST.**, ***chel.***, ***chim.***, ***chin.***, chin-ar., chin-s., chr-ac., cimx., cina, **CLEM.**, ***coca***, **COCC.**, **COFF.**, colch., **COLL.**, ***coloc.***, **CON.**, ***cop.***, cor-r., ***croc.***, ***crot-c.***, ***crot-h.***, croto-t., cub., cupr., cycl., ***daph.***, ***dig.***, ***dios.***, ***dulc.***, ***elaps***, ery-a., euon., euph., ***ferr.***, ***ferr-ar.***, ***ferr-i.***, ferr-p., ***fl-ac.***, ***form.***, ***gamb.***, **GRAPH.**, ***guai.***, ***hell.***, hep., hippoz., ***hydr.***, ***hydrc.***, ***hydrog.***, hyos., ***hyper.***, ***ign.***, ***iod.***, ***iris***, jab., jac-c., ***jatr.***, ***kali-ar.***, ***kali-bi.***, ***kali-br.***, ***kali-c.***, ***kali-chl.***, ***kali-i.***, kali-n., kali-p., ***kali-s.***, ***kreos.***, **LACH.**, **LAC-D.**, ***lac-ac.***, ***laur.***, led., ***lept.***, ***lil-t.***, **LYC.**, lycps., ***mag-c.***, **MAG-M.**, mag-s., ***manc.***, mang., med., meli., ***meny.***, ***merc.***, merc-c., ***merc-d.***, ***merc-i-f.***, **MEZ.**, ***mosch.***, murx., ***mur-ac.***, myric., naja, ***nat-acet.***, ***nat-c.***, **NAT-M.**, nat-p., nat-s., nicc., **NIT-AC.**, ***nux-m.***, **NUX-V.**, **OENA.**, olnd., **OP.**, osm., ***ox-ac.***, paeon., pall., petr., ph-ac., **PHOS.**, ***phyt.***, **PLAT.**, **PLB.**, ***podo.***, ***psor.***, ***ptel.***, ***puls.***, ***pyrog.***, ***raph.***, ***rat.***, rhus-t., rob., **RUTA**, ***sabad.***, ***sabin.***, sang., **SANIC.**, ***sars.***, ***sec.***, ***sel.***, ***seneg.***, **SEP.**, **SIL.**, spig., ***spong.***, squil., ***stann.***, **STAPH.**, **STRAM.**, **STRY.**, **SULPH.**, ***sul-ac.***, sumb., ***tab.***, ***tarent.***, tell., ***ter.***, ***ther.***, **THUJ.**, tril., ***tub.***, urt-u., ust., vario., ***verb.***, **VERAT.**, ***vib.***, viol-o., vesp., **ZINC.**

alternating, with diarrhea - ***abrot.***, acet-ac., agar., ail., aloe, am-m., **ANT-C.**, ant-t., ***arg-n.***, ***ars.***, ars-i., ***aur.***, aur-m-n., berb., ***bry.***, calc., ***carb-ac.***, carbn-s., ***card-m.***, ***casc.***, **CHEL.**, choc., ***cimic.***, cina, ***cob.***, coff., ***coll.***, ***con.***, cop., cor-r., crot-h., ***cupr.***, ***dig.***, dios., ferr., ***ferr-i.***, gamb., gnaph., grat., ***hep.***, ho., ***hydr.***, ***ign.***, ***iod.***, kali-ar., kali-bi., ***kali-c.***, kali-s., ***lach.***, ***lac-d.***, ***lact.***, ***lec.***, lil-t., ***lyc.***, mag-s., ***manc.***, ***mang.***, merc., mez., nat-acet., nat-c., ***nat-m.***, nat-p., ***nat-s.***, **NIT-AC.**, ***nux-m.***, **NUX-V.**, **OP.**, ***phos.***, ***plb.***, **PODO.**, polyg., ***ptel.***, ***puls.***, rad., rhus-t., ***ruta***, sang., sars., sep., stram., ***sulph.***, sumb., ***tab.***, ***tub.***, verat., zinc.

CONVALESCENCE, ailments, during or since - ail., ***alet.***, **ALF.**, am-c., apoc., aur., aven., bac., **BELL-P.**, cadm-m., cadm-s., **CALC.**, calc-p., caps., carb-v., **CARC.**, ***cast.***, **CHIN.**, ***chin-ar.***, coca, **COCC.**, cupr., ***cur.***, cypr., echi., ***ferr.***, ferr-acet., foll., form-ac., **GELS.**, graph., guare., hydr., kali-c., kali-chl., kali-m., ***kali-p.***, lach., laur., lob., lyc., mang., med., nat-sal., nat-p., okou., op., paull-p., ***ph-ac.***, phos., pneu., prot., psor., ***scut.***, ***sel.***, **SIL.**, sul-ac., sul-i., sulfonam., ***sulph.***, syph., tarax., thuj., **TUB.**, tub-a., vario., zinc.

CONVULSIONS, (see Epilepsy)

COPPER, poisoning, cuprum, ailments from - bell., camph., ***cupr.***, hep., ***ip.***, lyc., ***merc.***, nux-v., op., puls., sil., zinc.

CORNS, feet - ***acet-ac.***, aesc., ***agar.***, alum., alum-p., ***am-c.***, ambr., anac., anac-oc., **ANT-C.**, aquil., arg., ***arn.***, ars., arum-t., asc-t., aster., ***bar-c.***, bar-s., ***bor.***, bov., ***bry.***, bufo, calad., ***calc.***, zirc., calc-f., ***calc-s.***, calc-sil., camph., carb-ac., ***carb-an.***, carb-v., ***caust.***, cench., chin., chin-b., cist., cocc., coloc., con., ***cur.***, dios., elae., ***ferr-pic.***, fl-ac., ***graph.***, ***hep.***, hydr., hyper., ***ign.***, iod., kali-ar., kali-c., kali-n., kiss., lach., lith-c., **LYC.**, lyss., m-arct., m-ambo., mag-m., med., meph., nat-c., ***nat-m.***, nat-p., nat-sil., nicc., nit-ac., ***nux-v.***, ozone, ***petr.***, **PH-AC.**, **PHOS.**, pimp., plb., **PSOR.**, ptel., puls., puls-n, rad-br., ran-b., ***ran-s.***, rhod., ***rhus-t.***, rumx., ruta, sang., sars., sel., semp., **SEP.**, **SIL.**, spig., staph., sul-ac., sul-i., ***sulph.***, symph., ter., thuj., verat., wies.

CORTISONE, ailments from - apis., ars., ***cortico.***, ***cortiso.***, merc., nat-m., ***sep.***, sulph.

COUGHING, general - **ACON.**, aeth., ***agar.***, ***ambr.***, ***anan.***, ang., ***ant-c.***, **ANT-T.**, anth., ***arg-n.***, ***arn.***, ***ars.***, arum-t., **BAC.**, ***bad.***, **BELL.**, brom., **BRY.**, calad., ***calc.***, **CARB-V.**, ***carbn-h.***, ***carbn-s.***,

CAUST., *cham.*, *chel.*, **CINA**, cocc., **COC-C.**, *con.*, **COR-R.**, croc., *crot-c.*, **CUPR.**, dig., **DROS.**, elaps, ferr-p., **HEP.**, hydr-ac., **HYOS.**, ign., indg., iod., **IP.**, jatr., *kali-c.*, kali-bi., *kali-br.*, *kali-c.*, *kali-chl.*, kali-n., *kali-p.*, kali-s., *kreos.*, *lach.*, lact., laur., lob., lyc., *mag-c.*, mag-p., mang., **MEPH.**, **MERC.**, merc-c., merc-i-r., nat-m., nicc., nit-ac., **NUX-V.**, op., **PHOS.**, phyt., plb., *psor.*, **PULS.**, **RUMX.**, sabad., *sang.*, sarr., *seneg.*, **SEP.**, sil., **SPONG.**, **SQUIL.**, **STANN.**, staph., *sulph.*, *sul-ac.*, **TARENT.**, thuj., **TUB.**, **VERAT.**, zinc.

croupy, coughs - *acet-ac.*, **ACON.**, all-c., alum-sil., anac., ant-t., apis, *ars.*, *ars-i.*, arum-d., *bell.*, *brom.*, *calc-s.*, *carb-ac.*, cham., *chin.*, *chlor.*, *cina*, cinnb., coff., cor-r., cub., cupr-acet., cupr-s., diph., dros., euph., euphr., ferr-p., *gels.*, **HEP.**, *ign.*, **IOD.**, *ip.*, **KALI-BI.**, kali-i., *kali-m.*, kali-s., kreos., *lac-c.*, **LACH.**, lob., merc-cy., *mosch.*, nit-ac., oci-s., **PHOS.**, *phyt.*, *rumx.*, *ruta*, sal-ac., **SAMB.**, *sang.*, sanguin., sarcol-ac., solid., **SPONG.**, staph., stict., **STRAM.**, syc-co.

violent, cough - acal., **AGAR.**, ail., alum., alum-p., alum-sil., am-br., am-c., am-m., ambr., anac., anan., ang., ant-o., ant-t., apis, arg-n., ars., arum-d., asc-t., atro., aur-m-n., bad., **BELL.**, *bor.*, brom., bry., bufo, *calc.*, calc-i., camph., carb-an., **CARB-V.**, carbn-s., **CAUST.**, *cham.*, *chel.*, chin., *cimx.*, *cina*, clem., **COC-C.**, cocc., coll., **CON.**, cop., cor-r., croc., **CUPR.**, *cycl.*, **DROS.**, *dulc.*, elaps, *eup-per.*, *euphr.*, *form.*, gamb., gels., graph., guare., gymn., **HEP.**, hydr-ac., **HYOS.**, **IGN.**, indg., iod., **IP.**, kali-bi., kali-br., **KALI-C.**, kali-chl., kali-sil., *kreos.*, **LACH.**, lact., led., lil-t., lith-c., *lob.*, *lyc.*, lycps., *mag-c.*, mag-p., manc., *meph.*, *merc.*, **MEZ.**, mur-ac., *nat-ar.*, *nat-c.*, nat-p., nicc., nit-ac., *nux-v.*, ol-j., olnd., *op.*, ozone, par., petr., **PH-AC.**, **PHOS.**, phyt., plat., **PULS.**, rhod., *rhus-t.*, rumx., ruta, sabad., *samb.*, sang., seneg., **SEP.**, *sil.*, spig., **SPONG.**, **SQUIL.**, **STANN.**, staph., stict., stront-c., sulph., ther., verat., verb., viol-o., *zinc.*, zinc-p.

COWPOX, vaccinia - *acon.*, ant-t., apis, *bell.*, merc., phos., *sil.*, sulph., *thuj.*, vac., vario.

CRAMPING, pain - acon., agar., alum., am-c., am-m., *ambr.*, **ANAC.**, anan., **ANG.**, arg., *arn.*, *ars.*, *asaf.*, asar., atro., aur., bar-c., **BELL.**, bism., bor., bov., bry., bufo, cact., **CALC.**, calc-s., **CAMPH.**, *cann-s.*, caps., carb-an., carb-v., carbn-o., carbn-s., *cast.*, *caust.*, cedr., *cham.*, chin., cic., **CIMIC.**, **CINA**, clem., *cocc.*, colch., **COLOC.**, *con.*, conin., croc., *crot-c.*, crot-h., **CUPR.**, **CUPR-ACET.**, cyt-l., dig., *dios.*, *dulc.*, euph., euphr., eup-per., ferr., *gels.*, *graph.*, *hell.*, hist., *hyos.*, *ign.*, iod., ip., *iris*, jatr., kali-bi., **KALI-BR.**, *kali-c.*, kali-n., kali-p., kali-s., kreos., lach., lat-m., **LYC.**, mag-m., **MAG-P.**, mang., meny., **MERC.**, merc-c., merc-s., mez., mosch., *mur-ac.*, nat-f., nat-m., *nit-ac.*, **NUX-V.**, olnd., *op.*, ox-ac., *petr.*, ph-ac., phos., *phyt.*, **PLAT.**, *plb.*, plb-acet., puls., ran-b., rheum, rhod., *rhus-t.*, *rob.*, ruta, sabad., samb., sang., sarcol-ac., scopo., *sec.*, sel., **SEP.**, *sil.*, *spig.*, *spong.*, squil., *stann.*, staph., stront-c., **SULPH.**, syph., *tab.*, tarent., *thuj.*, tub., *valer.*, **VERAT.**, verb., vib., viol-o., viol-t., *zinc.*, zinc-s.

CRETINISM - absin., *aeth.*, *anac.*, arn., bac., bar-c., *bufo*, calc-p., carc., hell., ign., iod., *lap-a.*, lol., nat-c., oxyt., ph-ac., plb., sulph., thuj., *thyr.*, tub.

CROHN'S, disease - am-caust., *aloe*, ars., but-ac., carc., chin., hoit., merc-c., *nit-ac.*, phos., prot., raja-s.

CROUP, general, (see Coughing) - **ACON.**, *acet-ac.*, all-c., alumn., anac., *ant-t.*, apis, *ars.*, *ars-i.*, arum-t., asaf., *bell.*, **BROM.**, bry., *calc.*, *calc-f.*, *calc-i.*, **CALC-S.**, *canth.*, *carb-ac.*, *carb-v.*, caust., *cham.*, *chin.*, *chlor.*, *cina*, cinnb., cor-r., cub., *cupr.*, cupr-s., dros., euph., *gels.*, **HEP.**, ictod., ign., **IOD.**, ip., **KALI-BI.**, kali-br., *kali-chl.*, *kali-m.*, *kali-n.*, *kali-p.*, kali-s., kaol., lac-ac., *lac-c.*, **LACH.**, *lob.*, lyc., meph., merc-i-f., mosch., naja, *nat-m.*, *nit-ac.*, petr., **PHOS.**, *phyt.*, *rumx.*, ruta, **SAMB.**, *sang.*, **SPONG.**, staph., stict., *still.*, **STRAM.**, *verat-v.*

CURARE, ailments from - brom., cocc., con., *cur.*, gels., hell., iod., lach., stry.

CUSHING'S, disease - chlorpr.

CUTTING, pain - abies-n., acon., aesc., aeth., agar., agn., ang., all-c., alum., alum-sil., ambr., am-c., am-m., anac., androc., **ANG.**, ant-c., ant-t., arg., arg-n., *arn.*, ars., asaf., asar., aur., bar-c., bar-m., **BELL.**, *berb.*, bism., bor., bov., bry., *calad.*, **CALC.**, calc-i., calc-p., calc-sil., **CALEN.**, camph., cann-i., cann-s., **CANTH.**, caps., carb-an., carb-v., caust., cham., *chel.*, *chin.*, cic., cina, clem., cocc., coc-c., coff., colch., *coll.*, **COLOC.**, **CON.**, conv., croc., crot-h., croto-t., cub., cupr., cycl., dig., **DIOS.**, dros., *dulc.*, *elat.*, *equis.*, ferr., **GAMB.**, gels., graph., guai., hell., hep., hydr., **HYDROG.**, **HYOS.**, ign., iod., *ip.*, iris, **KALI-C.**, kali-chl., *kali-n.*, *kali-s.*, lach., laur., led., **LYC.**, m-arct., m-aust., mag-c., mag-m., mang., meny., **MERC.**, merc-c., mez., mosch., *mur-ac.*, nat-c., **NAT-M.**, nit-ac., nux-m., **NUX-V.**, *op.*, ox-ac., *par.*, *petr.*, ph-ac., *phos.*, plan., plat., plb., polyg., **PULS.**, ran-b., ran-s., rat., *rheum*, rhod., rhus-t., ruta, sabad., sabin., samb., sars., sec., sel., seneg., *sep.*, **SIL.**, *spig.*, spong., squil., *stann.*, **STAPH.**, *stront-c.*, sul-ac., sul-i., **SULPH.**, tell., teucr., thuj., valer., **VERAT.**, verb., *vib.*, viol-t., **ZINC.**, zinc-p., zing.

CUTS, general, (see Punctures, Stabs, Wounds) - androc., anthr., apis., *arn.*, ars., **CALEN.**, *carb-v.*, *cic.*, con., dig., *ham.*, hep., *hyper.*, kali-m., *lach.*, *led.*, merc., nat-c., *nit-ac.*, ph-ac., *phos.*, plan., plb., puls., pyrog., *sil.*, **STAPH.**, sulph., *sul-ac.*

CYANOSIS, breathing - absin., acetan., acon., agar., alum., ***am-c.,*** amyg-am., ang., anil., ant-c., ***ant-ar., ant-t., arg-n.,*** arn., ***ars.,*** asaf., asar., aur., bar-c., ***bell.,*** bism., both-l., benz-n., ***bor.,*** bry., calc., calc-p., **CAMPH.,** canth., carb-an., **CARB-V.,** carbn-o., caust., cedr., cham., chel., chin., chin-ar., cic., cina, cocc., cod., ***con., crot-h.,*** **CUPR.,** cupr-ar., **DIG.,** dros., ferr., glon., hep., ***hydr-ac.,*** hyos., ign., iod., ***ip., kali-chl.,*** kali-n., **LACH., LAUR.,** led., lyc., lycps., mang., merc., merc-c., merc-cy., meth-ae-ae., mez., mosch., mur-ac., ***naja,*** nat-m., nat-n., nit-ac., nux-m., nux-v., **OP.,** ox-ac., petr., ph-ac., phenac., phos., phyt., piloc., plb., puls., psor., ran-b., ***rhus-t.,*** ruta, sabad., ***samb.,*** sant., sars., ***sec.,*** seneg., sil., spong., staph., stram., stry., sulfon., sulph., sul-ac., tab., thuj., **VERAT., VERAT-V.,** vip., xan., zinc., zinc-m.

infants, in - arn., ars., ***bor., cact., camph., carb-v.,*** chin., **DIG., LACH., LAUR.,** ***naja,*** op., ***phos.,*** psor., rhus-t., sec., sulph.

CYSTITIS, bladder, inflammation - **ACON.**, all-c., alth., alum., am-c., anan., ant-c., ***ant-t.***, **APIS**, aq-mar., ***arg-n.***, arist-cl., ***arn.***, ***ars.***, ars-s-f., aspar., bac., bals-p., bamb-a., ***bar-m.***, baros., **BELL.**, benz-ac., ***berb.***, bism., ***bor-ac.***, cact., ***calad.***, ***calc.***, calc-p., calc-s., camph., camph-ac., cand-a., ***cann-i.***, cann-s., **CANTH.**, ***caps.***, carb-an., carb-v., ***caust.***, cham., ***chim.***, ***chin-s.***, cinnb., clem., coc-c., colch., coloc., ***con.***, ***cop.***, ***cub.***, ***dig.***, ***dulc.***, elat., epig., **EQUIS.**, erech., erig., ***ery-a.***, eucal., ***eup-pur.***, fab., ferr-acet., ferr-p., foll., gali., ***gels.***, graph., grin., guai., guare., hedeo, ***hell.***, ***hep.***, ***hydr.*** hydrang., ***hyos.***, ign., iod., ***juni-v.***, kali-ar., kali-bi., kali-c., kali-chl., kali-m., **LACH.**, lil-t., lith-c., **LYC.**, **MED.**, ***merc.***, **MERC-C.,** merc-i-r., methyl., mez., mill., ***morg.***, morg-g., musa, mut., myrt-c., nat-c., ***nit-ac.***, ***nux-v.***, ***ol-sant.***, op., pareir., petr., petros., ph-ac., phos., pip-m., plb., polyg., pop., prot., prun., **PULS.**, rheum, rhus-a., ***rhus-t.***, ruta, sabal., ***sabin.***, sant., **SARS.**, ***saur.***, senec., seneg., **SEP.**, silphu., solid., squil., **STAPH.**, ***stigm.***, stram., sul-ac., ***sulph.***, syc-co., tarent., tax., **TER.**, thal., **THLASPI**, thuj., tritic., tub., uva., verat., verat-v., vesi., xanth., zea-i.

CYSTIC, tumors - agar., ***apis***, apoc., ars., ***aur.***, bar-c., bell-p., benz-ac., bov., ***brom.***, calc., calc-f., calc-p., ***calc-s.***, caust., ***con.***, cory., form-ac., graph., ***hep.***, hydr., ***iod.***, ***kali-br.***, kali-c., kali-m., ***lyc.***, ***med.***, merc-d., nit-ac., phos., platan., ***sabin.***, sil., spong., staph., sulph., thuj.

CYSTOCELE, bladder - calen., staph.

D

DATURA, ailments from - bell., dat-a., dat-m., hyos., ***stram.***

DEAD, appearance of affected parts - ars., carb-v., graph., mez., ***plb.***, ***sec.***, sel., thuj.

DEAFNESS, loss of hearing - acon., ***agar.***, agra., all-s., alum., am-c., ***ambr.***, ***anac.***, ant-c., ant-t., ***arg-n.***, arn., ars., ***ars-i.***, asaf., ***asar.***, aur., aur-ar., ***aur-m.***, ***aur-s.***, bac., bar-c., ***bar-m.***, **BELL.**, bor., bry., caj., calad., ***calc.***, calen., cann-s., caps., ***carb-v.***, ***carbn-s.***, carl., **CAUST.**, cham., cheir., chel., chen-a., chin., chin-s., chin-sal., chlor., ***cic.***, cob-n., coca, cocc., colch., con., cortico., croc., crot-c., croto-t., cupr., dig., dros., dulc., ***elaps***, ferr-pic., gels., ***glon.***, ***graph.***, gua., **HEP.**, hydr-ac., ***hyos.***, ip., jatr., kali-ar., kali-bi., kali-c., kali-cy., ***kali-m.***, ***kali-n.***, kali-p., kali-s., kreos., lach., lachn., lap-c-b., laur., led., lob., lob-e., **LYC.**, ***lyss.***, m-arct., mag-c., mag-m., mang., med., meny., merc., merc-c., merc-d., mez., mosch., mur-ac., nat-c., nat-m., nat-p., nat-s., nicc., nit-ac., oena., ol-an., olnd., peti., petr., ph-ac., phos., piloc., ***plat.***, plb., psor., ***puls.***, puls-n, raph., rheum, rhod., rhus-t., sabad., salin., sang., sanguin-n., scroph-n., ***sec.***, sep., sil., solid., sphing., **SPIG.**, spong., stann., ***stram.***, **SULPH.**, ***syc-co.***, syph., tell., ther., ***thiosin.***, thymol., ulm., vario., verat., **VERB.**, vib-t., vip., visc., zinc.

DEATH, agony, before - **ACON.**, alum., ant-t., **ARS.**, ***carb-v.***, ***carc***, cocc., cupr., gels., **LAT-M.**, plat., puls., ***rhus-t.***, **TARENT.**, ***tarent-c.***, ***verat.***

DEATH, apparent, (see Asphyxia, Dying) - ***acet-ac.***, acon., **ANT-T.**, arn., ars., bell., ***camph.***, **CARB-V.**, ***carbn-s.***, chin., ***chlor.***, ***coch.***, ***coff.***, coloc., crot-h., hydr-ac., laur., merc., nit-ac., **OP.**, ph-ac., phos., ***rhus-t.***, ***sin-n.***, stram., sul-ac., tab.

new-born, infant - acon., **ANT-T.**, ***arn.***, bell., **CAMPH.**, **CARB-V.**, chin., **CUPR.**, **LAUR.**, ***op.***, upa.

DEBAUCHERY, ailments from - agar., ***anan.***, ant-c., arg-n., arn., caj., calad., carb-v., chin., clem., conin., dig., fl-ac., kreos., lach., lact., ***lyc.***, ***med.***, nit-ac., **NUX-V.**, op., ox-ac., pic-ac., sel., sep., spig., stram., sul-ac.

DECALCIFICATION, bones, (see Osteoporosis) - ***calc.***, ***calc-f.***, **CALC-P.**, cor-r., hecla, sil., symph.

DECUBITUS, (see Bedsores)

DEHYDRATION, loss of vital fluids, ailments from - ***ars.***, ars-i., ***calad.***, **CALC.**, **CALC-P.**, ***carb-an.***, **CARB-V.**, caust., **CHIN.**, ***chin-ar.***, **CHIN-S.**, ***con.***, ***crot-h.***, dig., ***ferr.***, **GRAPH.**, ***iod.***, ip., ***kali-c.***, ***kali-p.***, led., lyc., mag-m., ***merc.***, mez., nat-c., nat-m., ***nat-p.***, nit-ac., ***nux-m.***, ***nux-v.***, **PH-AC.**, **PHOS.**, plb., **PULS.**, sec., **SEL.**, **SEP.**, ***sil.***, stann., **STAPH.**, ***sulph.***, thuj., valer., **VERAT.**, zinc.

DELIRIUM, general - absin., acet-ac., ***acon.***, ***act-sp.***, aesc., ***aeth.***, aether, **AGAR.**, agar-cps., agar-pa., agar-ph., agn., ail., **ALCO.**, alum., am-c., amyg-am., ***anac.***, anag., anh., anthr., ant-c., ant-t., anan., apis, arg., arg-n., arn., **ARS.**, **ARUM-T.**, astac., atro., ***aur.***, aur-m., ***bapt.***, bar-c., **BELL.**, bism., bol-lu., bomb-pr., brom., **BRY.**, bufo, calad., cact., ***calc.***, calen., ***camph.,*** **CANN-I.,** cann-s., ***canth.,*** caps., carb-ac., carb-v., ***carbn-s.,*** carc., ***carl.,*** caul., ***cham.,*** **CHEL.,** chin., chin-ar., chin-s., chlf., chol., chloram., chr-ac., **CIC.,** cic-m., cimic., **CINA,** clem., coff., ***colch.,*** coloc., ***con.,*** convo-s., cop., cor-r., croc., **CROT-C.,** ***crot-h., cupr., cupr-acet.,*** cupr-ar., cyt-l., dat-f., dat-m., ***dig.,*** diph., dor., dubin., dubin., ***dulc.,*** euph., fagu., ferr-p., gall-ac., ***gels.,*** glon., graph., guare., ham., hell., hep., hipp., hippoz., hydr., **<u>HYOS.</u>,** hyosin., hyper., ign., iod., iodof., ***ip.,*** iris, iris-fl., iris-foe., jatr., juni-v., kali-ar., kali-bi., **KALI-BR.,** kali-c., ***kali-i., kali-m.,*** kali-n., kali-p., kalm., lac-c., **<u>LACH.</u>,** lachn., lact., lat-k., lept., lil-t., lob., lol., lup., **LYC.,** lyss., manc., mand., ***meli.,*** meny., ***merc., merc-c.,*** merc-cy., merc-i-r., merc-n., merc-s., merl., mez., ***mill.,*** morph., mosch., mur-ac., mygal., naja, nat-m., nat-s., **NIT-AC.,** nit-s-d., nitro-o., ***nux-m., nux-v., oena.,*** **<u>OP.</u>,** oper., ox-ac., paeon., par., ***petr.,*** ph-ac., **PHOS.,** plat., **PLB.,** podo., psor., ***puls.,*** phyt., **<u>PYROG.</u>,** ran-b., ran-s., rheum, rhod., **RHUS-T.,** sabad., sabin., sal-ac., samb., sang., sant., sapin., sarr., **SEC.,** sel., sil., sin-n., sol-n., spig., stigm., **<u>STRAM.</u>,** stry., **SULPH.,** sul-ac., sul-h., sulfa., ***syph.,*** tab., tang., tarax., tarent., tarent-c., tax., ***ter.,*** thea., trinit., tub., valer., vario., **VERAT. VERAT-V.,** verin., vesp., vip., vip-a., xan., zinc., zinc-acet., zinc-s.

<u>DELIRIUM</u>, tremens, mania-a-potu, (see Alcoholism) - acon., aether, **<u>AGAR.</u>,** agar-pr., alco., anac., ant-c., ***ant-t., apoc.,*** apom., ***arn.,*** **ARS.,** ars-s-f., asar., atro., aur., **AVEN.,** ***bell.,*** bism., bry., bufo, ***calc.,*** calc-ar., calc-s., camph-br., ***cann-i.,*** cann-s., ***caps.,*** carb-v., chin., chin-m., chin-s., chim., chlf., chlol., ***chlor., cimic.,*** cocc., ***coff.,*** cori-r., ***crot-h., cupr-ar.,*** cypr., dig., dor., ferr-p., fl-ac., gels., ***glon.,*** grat., hell., hydr., **HYOS.,** ***hyosin.,*** ichth., ign., ***kali-br.,*** kali-i., kali-p., kola, **LACH.,** led., lob., lol., lup., lyc., ***merc.,*** nat-c., **NAT-M., NUX-M., <u>NUX-V.</u>,** oena., **OP.,** passi., ***past., phos.,*** plb., psor., puls., ***querc.,*** **RAN-B.,** raph., rhod., rhus-t., scut., sel., sep., sil., spig., **STRAM.,** stroph., **STRY.,** stry-n., ***sulph., sul-ac.,*** sumb., ***syph.,*** teucr., thea., thuj., tub., tus-p., verat., ***zinc.,*** zinc-acet.

<u>DEMENTIA</u>, madness, (see Delirium, Insanity, Mania, Schizophrenia) - acon., aesc-g., aeth., ***agar.,*** agn., alco., ***alum.,*** **ANAC.,** ant-c., anth., arg., arg-n., ***ars.,*** aur., aur-i., aza., **BAR-C.,** ***bell.,*** calc., calc-p., cann-i., carbn-s., ***carc.,*** cimic., coca, ***con.,*** croc., crot-h., cupr., ferr-i., fl-ac., glyc., hell., **HYOS.,** ign., kali-i., **LACH.,** laur., lith-c., ***lil-t., merc.,*** nat-i., nat-m., ***nat-sal.,*** nit-ac., ***nux-v.,*** oena., op., orch., ov., ***ph-ac., phos., pic-ac., plat.,*** plb., puls., sec., sep., sil., **STRAM.,** sulph., sumb., tarent., thiosin., **VERAT.,** verat-v., vip., zinc., zinc-p.

<u>DENGUE</u>, fever - ***acon.,*** apis, aran., ars., arum-t., bapt., bell., ***bry.,*** canth., chin., coloc., **EUP-PER.,** ferr., gels., ham., ip., merc., nux-v., podo., ***rhus-t.,*** rhus-v., sanic., sec., sul-ac.

<u>DENTITION</u>, difficult, teething - **ACON.,** ***aeth.,*** am-c., ***ant-c., ant-t., apis, arn.,*** **ARS.,** arund., **BELL.,** ***bism.,*** **BOR.,** ***bry.,*** **CALC.,** calc-f., **CALC-P.,** ***canth., caust.,*** **CHAM.,** cheir., chlor., cic., cimic., ***cina, coff., colch., coloc.,*** cupr., cypr., ***dol., dulc., ferr., ferr-p., gels., graph., hecla., hell.,*** hep., hyos., ***ign., ip., kali-br., kreos., lyc., mag-c.,*** **MERC.,** ***merc-c.,*** mill., nat-m., nit-ac., op., passi., ***phyt.,*** plat., ***podo.,*** puls., ***rheum,*** scut., sec., sep., **SIL.,** sol-n., stann., **STAPH., SULPH.,** syph., ***ter.,*** tub., tub-k., zinc., zinc-br.

DEPRESSION, sadness, (see Despair) - ***abies-n.,*** abrot., acal., acet-ac., achy., **ACON.,** acon-f., act-sp., adlu., adon., ***aesc.,*** aeth., aether, agar., agav-t., ***agn.,*** ail., alco., alf., all-c., all-s., allox., aloe, ***alum.,*** alumn., am-br., ***ambr., am-c., am-m., aml-n.,*** ammc., ***anac.,*** anan., ***androc.,*** ang., anh., ***ant-c.,*** anthr., apis, apoc., arag., aran., ***arg., arg-n., arist-cl., arn.,*** **ARS., ARS-I.,** ars-met., ars-s-r., arum-d., arum-m., arum-t., ***asaf.,*** asar., asc-t., astac., aster., astra-e., atro., **<u>AUR.</u>,** aur-i., **AUR-M.,** ***aur-m-n., aur-s.,*** aza., bapt., bar-acet., ***bar-c.,*** bar-i., ***bar-m., bell.,*** benz-ac., berb., bol., bor., bov., ***brom., bry., bufo,*** bufo-s., buni-o., but-ac., ***cact.,*** cadm., caj., calad., **CALC.,** calc-acet., **CALC-AR.,** ***calc-f., calc-p.,*** **CALC-S.,** ***camph.,*** camph-br., cann-i., ***cann-s., canth., caps.,*** carb-ac., **CARB-AN.,** ***carb-v.,*** carbn-o., **CARBN-S., CARC.,** card-m., carl., cass., cast., **CAUST.,** cecr., cedr., cench., **CHAM.,** ***chel.,*** chim., **CHIN.,** ***chin-ar.,*** chin-b., ***chin-s., chlol.,*** chlor., chlorpr., choc., chr-ac., ***cic.,*** **<u>CIMIC.</u>,** ***cina,*** cinnb., ***clem.,*** cob., cob-n., coc-c., coca, ***cocc.,*** coch., ***coff., colch., coloc., con.,*** convo-d., convo-s., cop., ***corn.,*** cortico., cortiso., cot., ***croc.,*** **CROT-C.,** ***crot-h.,*** croto-t., cund., ***cupr., cupr-acet.,*** cupr-ar., ***cur., cycl.,*** cypr., cyt-l., der., ***dig.,*** dirc., ***dros., dulc.,*** echi., elae., elaps, elat., ergot., erig., esp-g., eug., euon., eup-per., eup-pur., euph., euphr., fago., fagu., **FERR.,** ***ferr-ar.,*** **FERR-I.,** ferr-m., ***ferr-p.,*** ferul., fic., fl-ac., flav., flor-p., form., frax., gad., gamb., **GELS.,** glon., goss., gran., **GRAPH.,** ***grat.,*** guai., guat., haem., halo., ham., **HELL.,** ***helon., hep.,*** hera., **HIPP.,** hir., hist., ***hura, hydr.,*** hydr-ac., hydrc., ***hydrog.,*** hydro-c., **HYOS.,** hyper., hypoth., iber., **IGN.,** ind., ***indg.,*** indol., **IOD.,** ***ip.,*** iris, jac-c., jug-c., kali-ar., ***kali-ar.,*** kali-bi., **<u>KALI-BR.</u>,** ***kali-c.,*** kali-fcy., kali-i., kali-n., **KALI-P.,** kali-s., kalm., kreos., kres., ***kola,*** **LAC-C.,** ***lac-d.,*** lac-h., lac-leo., lac-mat., **<u>LACH.</u>,** lachn., lact., lam., lapa., lat-m., lath., ***laur., lec.,*** led., lepi., **LEPT.,** lil-s., **<u>LIL-T.</u>,** lipp., lith-c., lob., ***lob-s.,*** luf-op., lup., **LYC.,** lycps., lyss., m-arct., m-aust., macrin., mag-c., mag-f., mag-m., mag-p., mag-s., ***manc., mand., mang.,*** med., meli., menis., meny., meph., **MERC.,** ***merc-aur., merc-c., merc-i-f., merc-i-r.,*** merl., methys., **MEZ.,** ***mill.,*** mit., moly., morph., mosch., ***mur-ac.,***

MURX., ***mygal.,*** myric., nabal., ***naja,*** **NAT-AR.,** nat-br., **NAT-C.,** nat-f., nat-hchls., **NAT-M.,** nat-n., ***nat-p.,*** **NAT-S.,** nat-sal., nep., nicc., **NIT-AC.,** nux-m., ***nux-v.,*** oena., ***ol-an.,*** olnd., onop., **OP.,** orig., oxyt., palo., parat., paull-p., ped., pen., penic., perh., peti., ***petr.,*** phel., phenob., ***ph-ac.,*** ***phos., phyt.,*** pic-ac., picro., pin-s., plan., **PLAT.,** plect., ***plb.,*** plb-acet., plumbg., pneu., podo., polyg., polyp-p., prot., prun., psil., **PSOR.,** ptel., **PULS.,** pyrog., pyrus., rad., ran-b., ran-s., raph., rauw., reser., rham-f., rheum, rhod., **RHUS-T.,** ***rhus-v.,*** rib-ac., rob., rumx., ***ruta,*** sabad., ***sabin.,*** sac-alb., sal-ac., sang., sanic., sant., sapin., sarcol-ac., saroth., sarr., sars., scut., sec., ***sel.,*** senec., seneg., **SEP.,** sieg., ***sil.,*** sol-c., sol-o., ***spig.,*** spira., ***spong.,*** squil., **STANN.,** stann-i., ***staph., still., stram.,*** stront-c., **STRY.,** ***sul-ac., sul-i.,*** sulfa., sulfonam., **SULPH.,** sumb., ***syph., tab.,*** tarax., tarent., tell., ***ter.,*** thal., thea, thiop., **THUJ.,** thymol., til., tong., tril., trinit., trio., tub., upa., ***uran-n.,*** ust., valer., **VERAT.,** ***verat-v.,*** verb., vesp., ***vib.,*** vip-a., ***vinc.,*** viol-o., viol-t., ***visc.,*** wild., wye., xan., x-ray., yuc., **ZINC., ZINC-P.,** zing., ziz.

DERMAL, trophic lesions - thal.

DERMATITIS, venenata - ***acon.,*** agn., alum., ***anac.,*** ant-c., ***apis, arn., ars., asaf., aur.,*** bad., bar-c., ***bar-m.,*** bell., bor., bry., cadm-s., ***calc.,*** camph., cann-s., canth., carc., caust., **CHAM.,** chlol., cina, cocc., colch., com., con., croc., crot-h., ***dulc.,*** euph., galph., ***gels.,*** graph., **HEP.,** hyos., ***kali-s.,*** kreos., lach., lyc., mang., **MERC.,** mez., nat-c., nat-m., ***nit-ac.,*** petr., phos., ***plb.,*** **PULS.,** rad-br., ran-b., **RHUS-T.,** ruta, sep., **SIL.,** ***staph., sulph.,*** tarent-c., verat., x-ray., zinc.

neurodermatitis - carc., galph.

radiation, dermatitis - cadm-s., rad-br., x-ray.

DERMOID, skin - calc., nat-c., nat-m., nit-ac., sil.

DESPAIR, feelings, (see Depression) - acal., ***acon.,*** act-sp., adam., aesc., agar., agath-a., ***agn.,*** all-c., aloe, ***alum.,*** alum-sil., am-c., am-m., **AMBR.,** ***anac., androc.,*** anh., ant-c., ***ant-t., arg-n.,*** arn., **ARS.,** ars-h., ***ars-i.,*** ars-s-f., aster., **AUR.,** ***aur-ar., aur-m., aur-m-n.,*** bad., bamb-a., bar-c., bell., benz., benz., bov., brom., bry., bufo, cact., cadm., **CALC.,** calc-i., calc-s., ***calc-sil.,*** calen., camph., ***cann-i.,*** canth., carb-an., ***carb-v.,*** carbn-s., **CARC.,** ***caust.,*** cham., chel., ***chin.,*** chin-ar., chin-s., choc., clem., cloth., ***cocc.,*** **COFF.,** colch., ***con.,*** crat., crot-h., ***croto-t.,*** cupr., ***cupr-acet.,*** cur., der., dig., eup-per., ***gad.,*** gamb., gels., ***graph.,*** **HELL.,** helon., hep., hura, hydr-ac., hydrog., hyos., **IGN.,** iod., kali-ar., kali-br., kali-c., kali-i., kali-n., ***kali-p.,*** kola, kreos., lac-c., ***lach.,*** laur., ***lept.,*** **LIL-T.,** lith-c., **LYC.,** med., ***merc., mez.,*** moni., morph., naja, ***nat-ar., nat-c.,*** **NAT-M.,** nat-s., nat-sil., neon, ***nit-ac.,*** nitro-o., ***nux-v., op.,*** orig., ozone, petr., ***ph-ac.,*** phos., pic-ac., plat., plb., plut-n., podo., **PSOR.,** ***puls., rhus-t.,*** ruta, sec., sel., ***sep.,*** sil., spig., stann., ***staph., stram.,*** sul-ac., sul-i., **SULPH.,** sumb., **SYPH.,** tab., ther., thuj., thymol., thyr., tub., valer., **VERAT.,** verb., vip., zinc., zinc-val.

DIABETES, insipidus - acet-ac., acon., ***alf.,*** all-c., am-acet., apis, apoc., ***arg.,*** arg-m., ars., ars-br., ***aur., bell.,*** bry., cahin., ***cann-i.,*** carc., caust., chin-s., chion., cina, ***cod.,*** conv., dulc., **EQUIS.,** ***eup-pur., ferr., ferr-m.,*** **gad.,** ***gels., glon.,*** glyc., gnaph., gua., ***hell., helon., ign.,*** indol., kali-br., ***kali-c.,*** kali-i., ***kali-n., kreos.,*** lac-ac., lac-c., led., ***lil-t., lith-c.,*** lyc., mag-p., merc-c., mosch., ***murx., nat-m.,*** nicc-s., ***nit-ac.,*** nux-v., ***ol-an., oxyt., ph-ac.,*** phos., physal., pic-ac., plat-m-n., puls., quas., ***rhus-a., samb.,*** sang., sant., saroth., sars., ***sin-n., squil.,*** staph., ***stroph., sulph.,*** tarax., ter., thymol., thyr., tril., ***uran-n.,*** verat-v., verb.

DIABETES, mellitus - ***acet-ac., adren.,*** alf., all-s., **ALLOX.,** aln., alumn., am-acet., am-c., aml-n., ant-t., anthro., apoc., ***arg.,*** arg-n., arist-m., arn., ***ars., ars-br.,*** ars-i., aspar., ***aur.,*** aur-m., bar-c., bell., ***benz-ac., bor-ac.,*** **BOV.,** ***bry.,*** cac., cahin., ***calc., calc-p.,*** camph., cann-i., caps., ***carb-ac., carb-v.,*** **CARC.,** carl., caust., cean., ***cham., chel., chim., chin.,*** chin-ar., chin-s., ***chion.,*** chlorpr., cina, ***coca, cod.,*** coff., ***colch.,*** coloc., con., conv., cortiso., crat., ***crot-h.,*** cupr., cupr-ar., ***cur.,*** dulc., ***elaps,*** equis., eup-pur., fel., ferr., ferr-i., ***ferr-m.,*** ferr-p., fl-ac., gad., gels., glon., glyc., gnaph., grin., gua., ***hell.,*** **HELON.,** ***hep.,*** hydrang., ign., indol., inul., ***insulin.,*** iod., ***iris,*** jab., kali-acet., kali-br., kali-c., ***kali-chl.,*** kali-i., kali-n., ***kali-p.,*** kiss., ***kreos., lac-ac., lac-c.,*** lac-d., lac-v., ***lach., lec.,*** led., lith-c., lil-t., **LYC.,** lycpr., ***lycps.,*** lyss., mag-p., mag-s., ***med.,*** meny., merc-c., mosch., morph., mur-ac., murx., nat-ch., nat-l., nat-m., ***nat-p., nat-s.,*** nicc-s., ***nit-ac.,*** nux-v., ol-an., op., oxyg., oxyt., pancreat., petr., **PH-AC.,** phase., phlor., **PHOS.,** physal., ***pic-ac.,*** plan., plat-m-n., **PLB.,** ***podo.,*** puls., quas., ran-b., ***rat., rhus-a.,*** sac-alb., sac-l., sal-ac., samb., sang., sant., saroth., sars., sec., senec., sep., ***sil.,*** sin-n., squil., staph., stict., stigm., stroph., ***sulph., sul-ac.,*** **SYZYG.,** tarax., **TARENT.,** ther., **TER.,** ***thuj.,*** thymol., thyr., tril., tub., **URAN-N.,** urea, vanad., verat-v., verb., vichy-g., vince., zinc., ziz.

DIAPER, rash, buttocks - ***bapt., bor.,*** bry., calen., ***kali-chl., merc., merc-c., mur-ac., nit-ac., sulph.,*** **SUL-AC.**

DIAPHRAGM, ailments of - bry., cact., cimic., cuph., ign., spong., stann., stry.

DIARRHEA, general - ***acet-ac., acon., aesc.,*** aeth., **AGAR.,** alet., all-s., **ALOE,** ***alum.,*** am-m., ammc., anan., ang., anthr., ant-ar., **ANT-C., ANT-T., APIS,** apoc., ***aran.,*** arg., **ARG-N.,** ***arn.,*** **ARS.,** ars-i., arum-m., asaf., ***asar.,*** asc-t., astac., aster., aur., aur-m., **BAPT., BAR-C.,** bar-m., ***bell., benz-ac.,*** berb., bism., ***bor., bov.,*** brach., ***brom.,*** **BRY.,** bufo, cact., **CALC.,** ***calc-ar., calc-p.,*** calc-s., **CANTH.,** ***caps.,*** carb-ac., **CARB-V.,** ***carbn-s., casc.,*** cast., ***caust.,*** cean., **CHAM.,** chel., chim., **CHIN.,** ***chin-ar.,*** chin-s., choc., cic., ***cina,*** cinnam., ***cist.,*** clem., cob., ***cocc., coff., colch., coll., coloc., con., cop.,*** **CORN.,** ***crot-h.,*** **CROTO-T.,** cub., ***cupr.,*** cupr-ar., cycl., ***dig.,*** dios., dros., **DULC.,** ***echi.,*** euph., **FERR., FERR-AR., FERR-I.,** ***ferr-p., ferr-s.,*** **FL-AC., GAMB.,** gels., ***gran., graph., grat.,*** guai., ham., **HELL., HEP.,** ***hydr., hydrog., hyos., ign.,*** ille., ind., **IOD., IP., IRIS,** jab., ***jatr.,*** jug-c., ***kali-ar.,*** **KALI-BI.,** ***kali-c.,*** kali-chl., ***kali-i.,*** kali-n., kali-p., ***kali-s.,*** kreos., ***lach.,*** lac-ac., ***lac-c., lac-d.,*** laur., lec., led., ***lept., lil-t.,*** lith-c., **LYC.,** lyss., ***mag-c., mag-m., mag-p.,*** maland., manc., med., meli., **MERC., MERC-C.,** merc-s., mez., morph., mur-ac., naja, ***nat-acet., nat-c.,*** **NAT-M.,** ***nat-p.,*** **NAT-S.,** nicc., **NIT-AC.,** ***nuph., nux-m., nux-v.,*** ol-an., ***olnd., ol-j.,*** op., ox-ac., par., ***petr.,*** phel., **PH-AC., PHOS.,** phyt., pic-ac., plan., ***plb.,*** **PODO.,** prun., ***psor., ptel., puls.,*** raph., rat., **RHEUM,** rhod., rhus-t., rumx., sabad., samb., ***sang., sanic.,*** sars., **SEC.,** sel., seneg., ***sep.,*** **SIL.,** spong., squil., ***stann.,*** staph., stram., stry., **SULPH.,** ***sul-ac.,*** sumb., tab., tarax., ***tarent., ter.,*** **THUJ.,** trom., ***valer.,*** **VERAT.,** xan., ***zinc., zing.***

<u>DIGITALIS</u>, ailments from - adon., apoc., aur., cact., camph., chin., conv., ***crat., dig.,*** digin., digox., kalm., nit-ac., spig.

<u>DIPHTHERIA</u>, infection - ***acet-ac.,*** ail., alum., alum-sil., ***am-c.,*** am-caust., ant-t., **APIS** arg-n., **ARS.,** ars-i., ***arum-t., bapt.,*** bar-c., bar-i., bar-s., ***bell.,*** bor., **BROM.,** bry., calc-f., calc-p., ***canth., caps., carb-ac.,*** caust., cean-tr., chin., chin-ar., ***chr-ac.,*** cinnb., ***con., crot-c., crot-h.,*** cupr-acet., cupr-ar., ***diph., echi., elaps,*** euph., ferr-p., guai., gymn., hep., hip-ac., hydrog., ign., iod., **KALI-BI.,** kali-br., **KALI-CHL.,** kali-i., ***kali-m.,*** kali-ma., kali-p., ***kreos.,*** **LAC-C., LACH.,** ***lachn.,*** led., lob., **LYC.,** mag-p., manc., ***merc.,*** merc-br., ***merc-c., merc-cy., merc-i-f., merc-i-r.,*** mosch., ***mur-ac.,*** myric., naja, ***nat-ar., nat-m.,*** nat-p., ***nit-ac.,*** nux-m., ***nux-v.,*** ox-ac., ozone, petr., **PHOS., PHYT.,** plb-i., pyrog., **RHUS-T.,** sabad., sal-ac., ***sang.,*** sanic., ***sec.,*** sep., spong., stram., ***sul-ac.,*** sul-i., ***sulph.,*** tarent., ***thuj.,*** tub., vinc., xan., zinc., zinc-m.

<u>DIPLOPIA</u>, double vision - aeth., ***agar., alumn.,*** am-c., anag., anh., ant-t., apis, arag., aran., ***arg-n.,*** arn., art-v., atro., **AUR.,** aur-i., ***aur-s.,*** bamb-a., bar-c., bar-i., ***bell.,*** botul., bry., calc., calc-s., camph., cann-i., cann-s., carb-an., ***carbn-s., caust.,*** cham., ***chel.,*** chlf., chlol., ***cic.,*** cimic., cina, clem., cob-n., coca, ***con.,*** crot-h., croto-t., cupr., ***cycl., daph., dig.,*** dros., eug., euph., **GELS.,** ger., gins., ***graph.,*** hoit., **HYOS.,** ***iod.,*** iodof., kali-bi., kali-c., kali-chl., ***kali-cy.,*** kali-i., lach., led., lith-c., ***lyc., lyss.,*** m-aust., mag-p., med., merc., ***merc-c., morph.,*** **NAT-M.,** ***nicc.,*** **NIT-AC.,** nux-m., ***nux-v., olnd.,*** onos., op., oxyu-s., par., petr., phos., phys., phyt., pitu-a., ***plb.,*** psor., ***puls.,*** raph., rhus-t., sanic., sec., ***seneg.,*** sep., ***spong.,*** stann., ***stram.,*** stroph., sul-i., sulfon., ***sulph.,*** syph., tab., ter., thea., ther., ***thuj.,*** ust., ***verat., verat-v.,*** visc., zinc.

<u>DISAPPOINTMENTS</u>, ailments from - acon., alum., apis, ars., **AUR.,** ***bry.,*** caps., carb-v., carc., caust., ***cham., cocc.,*** colch., ***coloc.,*** dig., ***gels.,*** grat., hyos., **<u>IGN</u>.,** ***lach.,*** **LYC.,** ***merc.,*** **NAT-M.,** ***nux-v., op.,*** **PH-AC.,** phos., plat., **PULS.,** sep., **STAPH.,** verat.

<u>DISLOCATIONS</u>, joints, of - ***agn.,*** ambr., ***am-c.,*** ang., ***arn.,*** bar-c., ***bell.,*** bov., ***bry.,*** **CALC.,** cann-i., ***carb-an.,*** carb-v., caust., con., ***form.,*** graph., hep., ***ign.,*** kreos., **LYC.,** ***merc.,*** mez., mosch., **NAT-C., NAT-M.,** ***kali-n., nit-ac., nux-v.,*** **PETR., PHOS.,** ***puls.,*** rhod., **RHUS-T.,** ***ruta,*** sabin., sep., spig., stann., staph., ***stront-c., sulph.,*** zinc.

<u>DIVERTICULITIS</u>, general - aloe, ars., hydr., chin., chin-ar., nit-ac.

<u>DIVERTICULOSIS</u>, general - aloe, ars., hydr., chin.

<u>DIZZINESS</u>, (see Vertigo)

<u>DROPSY</u>, (see Edema, Swelling)

<u>DOWN'S</u>, syndrome - **BAR-C.,** calc., carc., pitu-gl., thyr.

<u>DROWNED</u>, persons, asphyxia of - ***ant-t.,*** carb-v., lach.

<u>DRUNKEN</u>, state, (see Alcoholism) - absin., agath-a., **AIL.,** ***alco.,*** **BAPT.,** cann-s., gels., hell., ***hyos.,*** **LACH., OP., NUX-V.,** ***stram.,*** sul-ac.

<u>DUPUYTREN'S</u>, contracture - anac., bism., calc., ***caust.,*** cimx., coloc., lyc., mag-p., ***plb.,*** sil., thiosin., zinc.

<u>DYING</u>, agony, while, (see Death, Euthanasia) - **ACON.,** alum., ***ant-t.,*** **ARS.,** cocc., cupr., **LAT-M.,** puls., ***rhus-t., op.,*** **TARENT.,** ***verat.***

<u>DYSENTERY</u>, infection - ***acon., aeth.,*** **<u>ALOE</u>,** alst-c., alumn., ambro., ant-t., ***apis, arg-n., arn.,*** **<u>ARS</u>.,** ars-i., asc-t., ***bapt.,*** bar-m., ***bell., bry.,*** **BUFO, CANTH., CAPS.,** ***carb-ac.,*** **CARB-V., CARBN-S.,** caust., ***cham.,*** chapter, **<u>CHIN</u>.,** chin-ar., ***cinnb.,*** cist., clem., **COLCH., COLL., COLOC.,** ***con.,*** cop., ***corn., crot-c., crot-h.,*** croto-t., cub., cuph., cupr., ***cupr-ar., dirc., dulc.,*** elat., ***erig., eucal.,*** ferr-p., gamb., **GELS., HAM.,** ***hep., ign., iod.,*** **IP.,** ***iris, kali-bi., kali-chl.,*** kali-m., kali-p., ***lach.,*** lept., ***lil-t., lyc.,*** **LYSS., MAG-C.,** mag-m., ***mag-p.,*** manc., **MERC., MERC-C.,** ***merc-cy., merc-d.,*** merc-s., ***mill.,*** mur-ac., ***nit-ac., nux-m.,*** **NUX-V.,** ***op., ox-ac., petr.,*** **PHOS.,** ***phyt.,*** plb., ***psor., puls.,*** raph., rheum, rhod., **RHUS-T.,** sec., ***silphu.,*** staph., **SULPH.,** ***sul-ac., tanac., ter.,*** tril., ***trom.,*** vac., verat., xan., xanth., zinc., zinc-s., ***zing.***

DYSLEXIA, general, (see Learning disabilities) - **AGAR.,** agn., ***anac., ars.,*** **BAR-C.,** bor., **CALC.,** ***calc-p.,*** caps., **CARC.,** caste., caust., cham., con., ign., kali-p., kali-sil., **LYC.,** mag-p., ***med.,*** **MERC.,** ***nat-m.,*** olnd., okou., ph-ac., ***phos.,*** rib-ac., sep., ***sil., thuj.,*** tub., verat.

DYSMENORRHEA, painful menses - abrot., acetan., ***acon.***, aesc., agar., agn., alet., alum., alum-p., alum-sil., alumn., am-acet., am-br., **AM-C.**, am-m., ambr., ammc., amor-r., ***anac.***, anan., ant-c., ***ant-t.***, ap-g., ***apiol.***, apis, apoc-a., aquil., aral., aran., arg-n., arist-cl., arn., ***ars.***, ars-i., ***ars-met.***, asar., asc-c., atro., aur., aven., ba-tn., bac., bamb-a., bar-c., bar-i., bar-m., **BELL.**, bell-p., ***berb.***, ***bor.***, bov., brom., ***bry.***, bufo, buni-o., buth-aust., **CACT.**, caj., ***calc.***, calc-acet., calc-i., **CALC-P.**, calc-s., calc-sil., ***calen.,*** cann-i., cann-s., canth., carb-an., carb-v., carbn-s., carc., cast., ***caul.***, ***caust.***, cer-ox., **CHAM.**, chel., chin., chin-ar., chin-s., chlol., ***chol.***, cic., **CIMIC.**, cinnb., ***cit-v.***, **COCC.**, ***coff.***, coll., **COLOC.**, ***con.***, cortiso., ***croc.***, crot-c., crot-h., ***cupr.***, cur., **CYCL.**, der., dict., ***dios.***, ***dulc.***, dys-co., epip., ergot., **ERIG.**, eug., eup-per., eup-pur., euphr., fago., ferr., ferr-ar., ferr-i., ***ferr-m.***, ***ferr-p.***, foll., frax., ***gels.***, glon., glyc-g., ***gnaph.***, goss., ***graph.***, grat., ***guai.***, ***ham.***, hedeo, ***helon.***, hep., hir., ***hoit.***, ***hydr.***, hydrog., hyos., hyper., **IGN.,** indg., inul., iod., iodof., ***ip.,*** jug-r., juni-c., ***kali-ar.***, kali-bi., **KALI-C.**, kali-chl., kali-fcy., kali-hp., ***kali-i.***, ***kali-ma.***, kali-n., ***kali-p.***, ***kali-s.***, kali-sil., kalm., kreos., ***lac-c.***, lac-v-f., ***lach.***, lam., ***lap-a.***, lap-c-b., lap-gr-m., laur., led., ***lil-t.***, lith-c., lob., ***lyc.***, ***macrin.***, ***mag-c.***, mag-m., **MAG-P.**, mag-s., mang., ***med.***, ***meli.***, meph., ***merc.***, ***merl.***, **MILL.**, ***mit.***, mom-b., morg-g., morph., mosch., mur-ac., murx., ***nat-c.***, nat-m., nat-p., nat-s., nicc., nit-ac., nux-m., **NUX-V.,** ol-an., ***ol-j.***, onop., op., ozone, pall., palo., passi., petr., ph-ac., ***phos.***, phys., phyt., pic-ac., ***pitu-p.***, ***plat.***, plb., podo., **PSOR.**, **PULS.**, puls-n, rauw., rham-cath., ***rhod.***, ***rhus-t.***, ruta, **SABIN.**, ***sac-alb.***, sang., sant., sars., ***sec.***, sel., ***senec.***, **SEP.**, sil., sin-n., spong., stann., ***staph.***, stram., sul-ac., sul-i., **SULPH.**, syc-co., ***syph.***, ***tanac.***, tarax., ***tarent.***, tell., ther., thuj., thyr., thyreotr., trio., ***tub.***, **UST.**, uza., ven-m., ***verat.***, **VERAT-V.**, vesp., **VIB.**, vib-od., vib-p., wye., **XAN.**, xanth., ***zinc.***, ***zinc-val.***

E

EARS, general - ***apis, bar-c.,*** **BELL.,** ***bor.,*** **CALC.,** calc-f., calc-s., **CAPS., CAUST., CHAM.**, ***chin.,*** **CHIN-S.,** ***cur., dulc., ferr-p.,*** gels., **HEP.**, hydr., kali-bi., kali-c., **KALI-M., LYC., MERC., MERC-D., PULS.**, rhus-t., **SIL.,** sulph., ***tell., thiosin., thuj.,*** tub., zinc.

EBOLA, infection - ars., bapt., cadm-s., canth., carb-v., chin., cinnb., ***crot-h.,*** lach., merc-c., mill., phos., sul-ac.

ECCHYMOSIS, general, (see Bruises) - aeth., anthr., arg-n., **ARN.**, ***ars.***, bad., bar-c., bar-m., bell., bell-p., benz-n., bor., both-l., ***bry.***, calc., ***carb-v.***, carc., cham., chin., chlf., chlol., cic., coca, coll., ***con.***, cop., cosm., ***crot-h.***, cub., dulc., erig., euphr., ***ferr.***, foll., ***ham.***, ***hep.***, ***hyper.***, iod., iodof., kali-chl., ***kreos.***, ***lach.***, laur., **LED.**, meli., merc., mill., morg., mur-ac., ***nux-v.***, par., ***petr.***, **PH-AC.**, **PHOS.**, plb., ***puls.***, ***pyrog.***, rhus-t., ruta, **SEC.**, **SUL-AC.**, ***sulph.***, supren., tab., ***tarent.***, ***ter.***, thal., ***thlaspi***, uran-n., verbe-h.

ECLAMPSIA, toxemia - **APIS,** apoc., ***ars.,*** ars-i., ***aur-m.,*** benz-ac., berb., bry., cact., ***calc-acet., canth., chin.,*** cinnb., ***colch., crot-h., cupr-ar.,*** dig., dulc., ferr., ***gels.,*** glon., hell., ***helon.,*** ind., ***kali-ar.,*** kali-br., ***kali-c., kali-chl.,*** kalm., ***lach.,*** led., ***lyc., merc.,*** **MERC-C.,** ***nat-m., ph-ac., phos.,*** rhus-t., sabin., senec., ***sep.,*** sulph., ***ter.,*** thlaspi, thyr., uran., ***verat-v.***

ECZEMA, skin - acon., aethi-a., ***aethi-m.***, aln., alum., alum-p., alum-sil., am-c., am-m., ammc., anac., ant-c., anthro., aq-mar., arbu., arg-n., arist-cl., **ARS.**, **ARS-I.**, **ARS-S-F.**, astac., aur., aur-ar., ***aur-m.***, aur-s., bac., bar-c., **BAR-M.**, bell., ***berb.***, berb-a., bor., ***bov.***, brom., bry., ***calad.***, **CALC.**, calc-f., calc-i., calc-p., **CALC-S.**, ***calc-sil.***, cand-a., ***canth.***, caps., carb-ac., carb-an., ***carb-v.***, carbn-s., carc., cast-eq., ***caust.***, cere-b., chin-s., chlol., chrysar., **CIC.**, cist., clem., com., con., cop., corn., corn-a., cosm., **CROTO-T.**, cupr., cur., cycl., **DULC.**, euph., fago., ferr-ar., fl-ac., foll., form-ac., formal., frax., fuli., **GRAPH.**, guai., hell., **HEP.**, hippoz., ho., hydr., hydrc., insulin, ***iris***, **JUG-C.**, **JUG-R.**, ***kali-ar.***, kali-bi., kali-br., kali-c., ***kali-chl.***, kali-m., ***kali-s.***, kali-sil., kreos., lac-ac., lach., **LAPPA**, led., ***lith-c.***, ***lyc.***, maland., ***mang.***, ***merc.***, merc-c., merc-d., merc-pr-r., **MEZ.**, morg., mur-ac., mut., nat-ar., nat-c., nat-m., nat-p., ***nat-s.***, nit-ac., nux-v., **OLND.**, osm., pers., **PETR.**, ph-ac., phos., ***phyt.***, pic-ac., piloc., ***plb.***, podo., polyg-pe., prim-o., prim-v., **PSOR.**, ***ran-b.***, **RHUS-T.**, rhus-v., rumx., ruta, sabin., sanic., ***sars.***, sec., sel., ***sep.***, ***sil.***, skook., squil., ***staph.***, stry., stry-ar., stry-p., sul-ac., **SUL-I.**, **SULPH.**, tarax., tarent., tarent-c., tell., tere-ch., ***thuj.***, thyr., titan., tub., ur-ac., urea, ust., ***vinc.***, ***viol-t.***, x-ray, xero, zinc., zinc-p.

EDEMA, general, (see Swelling), external - acet-ac., agar., **ANT-C.,** ***ant-t.,*** **APIS, APOC., ARS.,** ars-i., ***asc-c.,*** aur., ***aur-m., bell., bism., bry., cact.,*** calad., ***calc., calc-ar.,*** camph., ***canth., carbn-s., card-m.,*** cedr., chel., **CHIN.,** ***chin-ar.,*** cinnb., coca, **COLCH.,** ***coll.,*** coloc., ***con.,*** conv., cop., ***crot-h.,*** **DIG.,** ***dulc.,*** equis., eup-pur., euph., ***ferr.,*** ferr-ar., ***ferr-i.,*** ferr-p., **GRAPH.,** guai., **HELL.,** hyos., **IOD.,** kali-ar., ***kali-c., kali-i.,*** kali-n., kali-p., kali-s., ***lac-d., lach., led., liatr., lyc.,*** **MED.,** ***merc.,*** mez., mur-ac., nat-ar., nat-c., ***nit-ac., nux-m.,***

OLND., OP., phos., pic-ac., plat., ***plb., puls.,*** rhod., rhus-t., ***ruta, sabin., samb.,*** sars., sec., ***seneg., sep.,*** sil., **SQUIL.,** stram., ***sulph.,*** **TER.,** ***teucr., verat., verb.,*** zinc.

ELBOWS, injuries, to - ***arn.,*** aur., bell-p., **BRY.,** ***hyper., rhus-t.,*** **RUTA.**

ELECTROMAGNETIC, fields, ailments from - agar., apom., arg-n., coff., elect., lyss., m-aust., merc., morph., ***phos.,*** rad-br., ***rhod.,*** sol., ***stront-c.,*** x-ray.

ELECTROSHOCK, ailments, from - arn., ***apom.,*** hell., morph., nat-c., morph., nux-v., op., ***phos.***

ELEPHANTIASIS - abrot., ***anac.,*** ***ars.,*** ars-i., bix., blatta, both-l., caesal., calo., canth., card-m., chin-s., colch., crot-h., cupr., ***elae.,*** graph., ham., hell., hippoz., ***hydrc.,*** iod., kali-bi., lach., led., lyc., malar., ***merc.,*** muru., ***myris.,*** ***nat-c.,*** ***petr.,*** psor., pyrar., raja-s., rauw., sep., ***sil.,*** still., tere-ch., term-c., tinos., verat., vip.

EMACIATION, general, (See Cachexia) - **ABROT.,** ***acet-ac.,*** adren., ***agar.,*** alco., **ALF.,** ***alum.,*** alumn., ***ambr.,*** am-c., am-m., anac., androc., ant-c., ant-t., ***apis,*** aq-mar., ***arg., arg-n.,*** arn., **ARS., ARS-I.,** asc-t., ***aur.,*** aur-m., ba-sv., **BAC.,** bar-acet., **BAR-C.,** ***bar-m.,*** bor., ***bry., bufo, cact.,*** **CALC., CALC-I.,** ***calc-p., camph., canth., carb-v., carbn-s.,*** carc., **CAUST.,** ***cench.,*** cere-b., ***cham., chel.,*** **CHIN.,** chin-ar., ***chlor., chion.,*** cina, ***clem., cocc., colch., coloc.,*** con., cor-r., ***crot-c.,*** croto-t., ***cupr.,*** dig., digin., dros., dulc., **FERR.,** ***ferr-ar., ferr-i., ferr-m., fl-ac.,*** **GRAPH.,** ***guai.,*** hecla., **HELL.,** ***helon., hep., hippoz.,*** hura, **HYDR.,** ***hydrog., ign.,*** **IOD.,** iodof., ***ip.,*** kali-ar., kali-bi., ***kali-br., kali-c., kali-i., kali-p.,*** kali-s., ***kreos., lac-ac.,*** lac-c., ***lac-d., lach.,*** lec., ***lith-c.,*** **LYC.,** mag-c., mag-m., med., ***merc.,*** mez., morph., morg., mur-ac., mygal., ***myos.,*** naja, ***nat-ar., nat-c.,*** **NAT-H., NAT-M.,** ***nat-p., nat-s.,*** **NIT-AC.,** nux-m., **NUX-V.,** ***ol-j., op., orni.,*** ox-ac., ozone, parathyr., ***petr., ph-ac.,*** phel., **PHOS., PLB.,** ***plb-acet.,*** plb-i., ***psor., puls.,*** pyrog., raph., ***rheum,*** rhus-g., ***rhus-t.,*** rhus-v., ric., ruta, sac-alb., sac-l., samb., saroth., ***sars., sec.,*** **SEL.,** sep., **SIL.,** spig., spong., **STANN.,** staph., ***stram., stront-c., sul-ac.,*** sulfa., **SULPH.,** sumb., ***syph.,*** tab., ***tarent., thuj.,*** tthyr., **TUB.,** tub-m., tub-r., ***uran-n.,*** vanad., ***verat., verat-v.,*** vesp., vip., voes., x-ray, xan., zinc.,

EMBOLISM, blood - kali-br., kali-m.

EMOTIONS, ailments, from - acetan., acon., arg-n., ***arn.,*** aster., ***aur., calc.,*** **CAPS., CARC.,** caust., cocc., **COFF.,** ***gels.,*** hyos., **IGN.,** kali-c., kreos., lyc., lyss., med., nat-c., **NAT-M., PH-AC.,** ***phos.,*** plat., psor., ***sep.,*** **STAPH.,** zinc.

EMPHYSEMA, lungs - absin., acet-ac., agar., agarin., agav-t., alco., all-s., alumn., **AM-C.,** aml-n., **ANT-AR.,** ant-s., **ANT-T.,** apom., arg-n., ***ars.,*** ars-i., astra-e., aur., ***bac., bals-p.,*** bar-c., ***bell.,*** benz-ac., benz-n., beryl., blatta-a., ***brom.,*** bry., ***calc.,*** calc-f., ***calc-p.,*** calc-s., ***camph., carb-v.,*** carbn-o., carbn-s., chin., chin-ar., ***chlol., chlor.,*** chlorpr., ***coca,*** con., ***conv.,*** cop., cortico., crot-h., cupr., cupr-ar., cur., ***dig.,*** dros., dulc., eucal., ferr-i., glon., grin., hall, hed., **HEP.,** hist., ichth., iod., ***ip.,*** kali-bi., kali-c., kali-i., kreos., kres., lac-d., **LACH.,** led., leon., lepro., **LOB.,** ***lyc.,*** med., ***merc.,*** morg., myos., myrt-c., myrt-ch., naphtin., ***nat-m.,*** nit-ac., nux-v., op., per., ***phel., phos.,*** plb., pneu., psor., puls., queb., sang., saroth., sars., ***sec.,*** seneg., sep., **SIL.,** silphu., spong., stann., ***stry.,*** sulo-ac., sulph., tell., ter., thal., tub., tub-r., ***verat.***

EMPROSTHOTONOS, back - bell., ***canth.,*** coloc., hyos., ign., ***ip.,*** lach., nux-m., stann.

EMPYEMA, lungs - apis, arn., **ARS.,** ***ars-i.,*** bell., ***calc.,*** **CALC-S.,** carb-an., ***carb-v., carbn-s., chin., chin-ar.,*** dig., echi., ferr., ***hep.,*** iod., ip., ***kali-c.,*** **KALI-S.,** ***lach.,*** lyc., **MERC.,** ***nat-ar.,*** nat-s., ***nit-ac., phos.,*** pyrog., ***sep.,*** **SIL.,** staphycoc., **SULPH.,** tub.

EMPYOCELE, genitalia - ***ars-i., calc.,*** **CALC-SIL., KALI-S.,** ***psor., puls., sep.,*** **SIL., SULPH.**

ENCEPHALITIS, infection, (see Meningitis) - ***acon.,*** aeth., apis, apoc., arn., ars., bapt., **BELL.,** ***bry.,*** cadm-s., calc., calc-p., ***camph.,*** canth., carb-ac., cham., chin., chin-s., chr-ac., chr-o., cic., cina, ***con.,*** crot-h., ***cupr., cupr-ar.,*** dig., **GELS.,** glon., ***hell.,*** hydr-ac., ***hyos.,*** hyper., iod., iodof., kali-i., kreos., lach., ***merc.,*** merc-c., merc-d., mosch., nux-v., ***op.,*** ox-ac., par., ***phos.,*** phys., plb., puls., rhus-t., ***sil.,*** sol-n., stram., sulph., ***tub.,*** verat-v., vip., zinc.

ENCEPHALOMA, brain tumor - acet-ac., **AETH.,** apom., arg-n., arn., ***ars., ars-i.,*** art-v., ***bar-c.,*** bell., **BUFO,** ***calc., calc-f.,*** carb-ac., ***carb-an.,*** caust., cic., **CON.,** ***croc.,*** crot-h., gali., gels., ***glon.,*** graph., hydr., hyper., ***kali-br., kali-i.,*** kali-cy., ***kreos., lach., merc.,*** merc-c., merc-i-r., nit-ac., nux-v., ***op.,*** **PHOS.,** pic-ac., **PLB.,** plb-i., sep., **SIL.,** stram., sulph., ***thuj., tub.***

ENDOCARDITIS, heart, inflammation - ***abrot., acet-ac.,*** **ACON.,** ***adon.,*** agar., **ARS.,** ars-i., **AUR.,** aur-i., ***aur-m.,*** aven., bell., benz-ac., bism., ***bry., cact., calc.,*** chel., chin-s., ***cimic.,*** coc-c., cocc., ***colch.,*** colchin., conv., crot-h., cupr-acet., cupr-ar., dig., diph., ferr., ***ferr-p.,*** hir., hyos., ***iod.,*** kali-ar., ***kali-c., kali-i.,*** kali-n., **KALM.,** ***lach.,*** led., ***lept.,*** lith-c., magn-gr., med., merc-cy., ***naja,*** nat-i., nat-m., ox-ac., pareir., ***phos.,*** phyt., plat., plb., rhus-t., sang., ***sep.,*** **SPIG.,** ***spong., squil.,*** staphycoc., strept., sumb., tab., tarent., verat., ***verat-v.,*** vip., visc., zinc., zinc-i.

ENDOMETRIOSIS, acute - ***acon.,*** ant-i., aphis., ***apis,*** arn., ***ars., bell., bry.,*** calc-f., canth., ***carc.,*** cham., ***cimic.,*** chin., con., flav., ***gels.,*** hep., hyos., ***iod.,*** kali-c., kali-i., lach., lil-t., mag-p., **MED.,** ***mel-c-s., merc-c.,*** nux-v., op., ph-ac., plat., ***puls.,***

rauw., rhus-t., ***sabin., sec., sep., sil.,*** stram., sulph., ter., ***thuj.,*** thyr., til., ***ust.,*** verat-v.

chronic - alet., aloe, ***ars., aur-m., aur-m-n.,*** bell., bor., ***calc., carb-ac.,*** **CARC.,** caul., chin-ar., ***cimic., con.,*** graph., ***helon., hydr.,*** hydrc., inul., ***iod., kali-ar.,*** kali-c., kali-s., kreos., lac-c., ***lach.,*** lyc., ***mag-m., med., mel-c-s., merc.,*** nat-m., nit-ac., ***nux-v., ph-ac.,*** phos., plb., ***puls.,*** rhus-t., ***sabin., sec., sep.,*** sil., stram., ***sulph., thuj., ust.***

ENEMAS, colonics, ailments from - ***chin.,*** lyc., nux-v., op.

ENTEROCOLITIS, (see Colitis) - aloe, ars., chin., nit-ac., ***nuph., ter.***

ENTEROPTOSIS - ars., ***ba-sv.,*** cupr., cupr-ar., lil-t., opun-v., sep., ***stann.,*** syc-co.

EOSINOPHILIA, blood - saroth.

EPIDIDYMITIS, testes - ***acon.,*** apis, arg-n., ars., ***aur., bell.,*** berb., cann-s., ***chin., clem., gels., ham.,*** kali-n., ***med., merc.,*** nit-ac., phyt., **PULS., RHOD.,** sabal., **SPONG.,** sulph., teucr-s., thuj., vib.

EPILEPSY, general - ***absin.,*** acet-ac., acon., ***aeth., agar.,*** alco., all-c., ***alum.,*** alum-p., alum-sil., alumn., ***am-br.,*** am-c., ***ambr.,*** ambro., ***aml-n.,*** amyg-am., ***anac., anag.,*** ang., anil., anis., ant-c., ant-t., antipyrin., apis, **ARG., ARG-N.,** arn., ***ars., art-v.,*** asaf., ***aster., atro.,*** aur., aven., ***bar-c.,*** **BAR-M.,** bar-s., **BELL.,** benz-n., bism., bor., bry., **BUFO,** caj., **CALC., CALC-AR.,** ***calc-p., calc-s.,*** camph., cann-i., ***canth., carb-an.,*** carb-v., carbn-s., ***cast., cast-eq.,*** caste., caul., **CAUST.,** ***cedr., cham.,*** chen-a., ***chin.,*** chin-ar., chin-s., ***chlol.,*** chlorpr., ***cic.,*** cic-m., ***cimic., cina,*** cinnam., ***cocc.,*** coloc., ***con.,*** convo-s., cori-r., ***crot-c., crot-h.,*** **CUPR.,** ***cupr-acet., cupr-ar., cur., cypr.,*** dat-m., des-ac., dig., dros., dulc., fago., ferr., ***ferr-cy.,*** ferr-p., ***form., gels., glon.,*** graph., ***hell.,*** hep., hydr-ac., **HYOS.,** ***hyper., ictod., ign., indg.,*** iod., ***ip.,*** irid., kali-ar., kali-bi., **KALI-BR.,** kali-c., ***kali-chl., kali-cy.,*** kali-m., ***kali-p.,*** kali-s., kres., ***lach., laur.,*** led., levo., lith-br., lol., ***lyc., lyss., mag-c., mag-p.,*** mand., ***med.,*** meli., merc., methyl-chl., mill., mosch., mur-ac., naja, ***nat-m., nat-s.,*** nicot., nit-ac., nitro-o., nux-m., ***nux-v.,*** **OENA.,** oest., onis., onon., ***op.,*** passi., perh., petr., ***ph-ac., phos.,*** phys., ***picro., plat.,*** **PLB.,** polyg-pe., ***psor., puls.,*** ran-b., ran-s., rauw., rhus-t., rib-ac., ruta, ***salam.,*** sant., ***sec.,*** sep., **SIL.,** sin-n., ***sol-c.,*** sol-n., spirae., ***stann.,*** staph., ***stram., stry.,*** sulfon., **SULPH.,** sumb., ***syph.,*** tab., tanac., tarax., ***tarent., ter.,*** thea., thiop., thuj., tub., valer., verat-v., verb., verbe-h., **VISC.,** verat., vip., ***zinc.,*** zinc-o., zinc-p., ***zinc-val., ziz.***

EPITHELIOMA - abr., acet-ac., alum., alumn., arg., arg-n., ***ars.,*** **ARS-I.,** ars-s-f., aur., aur-ar., ***bell.,*** brom., calc., calc-p., calc-sil., carb-ac., carb-an., ***carc.,*** chr-ac., cic., clem., **CON.,** ***cund.,*** euph., fuli., gali., ho., ***hydr., hydrc.,*** kali-ar., kali-chl., kali-m., kali-p., ***kali-s., kreos., lach., lap-a.,*** lob-e., **LYC.,** mag-m., mag-s., merc., merc-c., methyl-chl., nat-cac., nat-m., nectrin., nit-ac., phos., ***phyt.,*** puls., rad-br., raja-s., ***ran-b.,*** ran-s., scroph-n., sep., ***sil., sol.,*** sulph., ***thuj.,*** uran-n.

EPULIS - ***agn.,*** anan., ars., bell., calc., calc-f., canth., ***carb-an., carb-v.,*** chel., clem., cur., graph., hecla., hep., lac-c., lach., ***nat-m.,*** nit-ac., phos., plb., plb-acet., sep., ***sil.,*** staph., sulph., ***thuj.***

ERGOTINE, ailments from - agar., chin., lach., nux-v., ***sec.,*** sol-n.

ERYSIPELAS, general - **ACON.,** ***am-c.,*** am-m., ***anac.,*** anac-oc., anan., ant-c., ***anthr.,*** **APIS, ARIST-CL.,** ***arn., ars., ars-i.,*** ars-s-f., arund., astac., atro., ***aur.,*** aur-ar., aur-s., bar-c., bar-m., **BELL.,** ***bor.,*** both-l., ***bry.,*** bufo, cadm-s., ***calc.,*** calc-i., calc-sil., calen., ***camph., canth.,*** carb-ac., ***carb-an.,*** carb-v., ***carbn-s.,*** caust., ***cham.,*** chel., ***chin., clem.,*** colch., com., cop., **CROT-C.,** ***crot-h.,*** croto-t., cupr., cupr-acet., dor., dulc., ***echi.,*** elat., **EUPH.,** euph-l., ferr., ferr-p., frag., ***gels.,*** **GRAPH.,** gymn., ***hep.,*** hippoz., hydr., hydro-v., hyos., ***iod., ip., jug-c.,*** jug-r., kali-ar., ***kali-c., kali-chl.,*** kali-i., ***kali-p.,*** kali-s., kali-sil., lac-c., **LACH.,** lappa, led., ***lyc.,*** mag-c., mag-s., mang., **MERC.,** mez., mur-ac., nat-ar., nat-c., nat-m., nat-p., nat-s., ***nit-ac.,*** passi., petr., ***ph-ac., phos.,*** plan., plb., podo., polyg., prim-o., psor., ptel., ***puls.,*** pyrog., ran-b., ran-s., rhod., **RHUS-T.,** ***rhus-v., ruta,*** sabad., sabin., samb., sars., sec., semp., sep., ***sil.,*** sol-n., spong., stann., staph., stram., sul-i., ***sulph.,*** syph., ***tarent-c.,*** tax., ***ter., thuj.,*** tub., urt-u., verat., verat-v., verbe-h., verbe-u., vesp., vip., ***xero,*** zinc., zinc-acet.

ERYTHEMA, exsudativum multiforme - antipyrin., bor-ac., cop., vesp.

ERYTHEMA, nodosum - acon., ant-c., ***apis, arn.,*** ars., chin., chin-ar., ***chin-s.,*** ferr., led., morg., nat-c., ptel., ***rhus-t., rhus-v.,*** saroth., ***thal.,*** tub.

ERYTHEMA, simplex - ***acon.,*** antipyrin., apis, ***arn.,*** ars-i., ***bell.,*** bufo, ***canth.,*** chlor., echi., gaul., grin., kali-c., lac-ac., ***merc.,*** mez., narc-ps., nux-v., rhus-t., rob., ter., urt-u., ust., verat-v., xero.

ESOPHAGITIS - acon., alum., arn., **ARS.,** asaf., bell., bufo, ***carb-v.,*** **CAUST.,** cocc., euph., ***gels., iod.,*** laur., merc., merc-c., mez., naja, ***nit-ac.,*** oena., ***phos.,*** **RHUS-T.,** sabad., sec., sul-ac., verat., ***verat-v.,*** vesp.

ESOPHAGUS, cancer - ***arg-n., ars., carc.,*** **CAUST.,** ***con.,*** cund., ***hydr.,*** orni., phos., scirr., ***sil., thuj.***

ESOPHAGUS, injury to - ***cic.***

EUTHANASIA, for relief of death pains, (see Death, Dying) - **ACON.,** aml-n., ant-t., **ARS.,** aur., carb-v., ***crot-h.,*** lach., lachn., med., phos., **TARENT.,** tarent-c.

EXANTEMATIC, fevers - **ACON.**, ***am-c.***, ***ant-c.***, **APIS**, ***arn.***, ***ars.***, ***bell.***, **BRY.**, camph., ***carb-v.***, ***carbn-s.***, cham., ***chel.***, chin., ***chlor.***, ***coff.***, ***cop.***, ***crot-h.***, ***dros.***, **EUPHR.**, ***ferr-p.***, ***gels.***, hyos., ign., ***ip.***, ***kali-bi.***, kali-m., kali-s., mag-c., **MORBILL.**, nux-v., ***phos.***, phyt., **PULS.**, ***rhus-t.***, ***squil.***, stict., ***stram.***, **SULPH.**, verat., zinc.

EXCITEMENT, ailments, from - acet-ac., **ACON.**, agar., aloe, alum., am-m., ***ambr.***, **AML-N.**, anac., ant-t., **ARG-N.**, ***arn.***, ***ars.***, asaf., asar., aster., **AUR.**, bar-c., **BELL.**, **BRY.**, ***calc.***, calc-ar., calc-p., camph., **CAPS.**, carb-an., **CARC.**, **CAUST.**, **CHAM.**, chin., cic., cimic., ***cist.***, cob., **COCC.**, coch., cod., **COFF.**, coff-t., colch., **COLL.**, **COLOC.**, con., croc., convo-s., ***cupr.***, ***cycl.***, cypr., dys-co., epip., ferr., **GELS.**, ***glon.***, goss., graph., hep., **HYOS.**, **IGN.**, ip., kali-ar., ***kali-br.***, ***kali-c.***, kali-n., kreos., **LACH.**, laur., lyc., mag-c., mag-m., ***merc.***, morg-g., mosch., nat-c., ***nat-m.***, ***nit-ac.***, **NUX-M.**, **NUX-V.**, ***olnd.***, **OP.**, ***pall.***, petr., **PH-AC.**, ***phos.***, phys., **PLAT.**, ***podo.***, **PSOR.**, **PULS.**, ran-b., ***rhus-t.***, sac-alb., ***samb.***, sars., scut., sec., sel., ***sep.***, **SIL.**, spong., stann., **STAPH.**, ***stram.***, stront-c., ***sulph.***, ***tarent.***, teucr., **TUB.**, tub-k., **VALER.**, **VERAT.**, verb., ***zinc.***

EXCRESCENCES, growths, (see Condylomata, Warts) - acet-ac., alum., alumn., anac., ***ant-c.***, ant-t., apis, ***arg-n.***, ars., ars-i., ***aur.***, ***aur-m.***, aur-m-n., aur-s., bell., benz-ac., beryl., bry., **CALC.**, calc-sil., ***carb-an.***, ***carb-v.***, ***carbn-s.***, carc., **CAUST.**, cham., ***cinnb.***, clem., cocc., con., ***dulc.***, euph., ***euphr.***, ***fl-ac.***, **GRAPH.**, ***hep.***, iod., kali-bi., ***kali-chl.***, ***kali-i.***, kali-m., kreos., lac-c., **LACH.**, **LYC.**, manc., **MED.**, ***merc.***, **MERC-C.**, merc-d., merc-n., mez., nat-c., nat-m., **NAT-S.**, **NIT-AC.**, nux-v., petr., **PH-AC.**, ***phos.***, phyt., pic-ac., plat-m., plb., psor., puls., ran-b., rhus-t., sabad., ***sabin.***, sang., sanic., ***sars.***, sec., sel., ***sep.***, ***sil.***, **STAPH.**, sul-i., ***sulph.***, syph., teucr., **THUJ.**

EXOSTOSES, general, (see Bone spurs, Tumors).

EXTRAVASATIONS, from injuries - **ARN.**, ***bad.***, bry., cham., chin., cic., ***con.***, dulc., euphr., ferr., ham., ***hep.***, iod., ***lach.***, laur., ***led.***, nux-v., par., plb., ***puls.***, rhus-t., ***ruta***, sec., ***sulph.***, **SUL-AC.**

EYELIDS, cancer - apis, clem., con., cund., hydr., lach., phyt., ran-b., sep., staph., thuj.

EYES, cancer - apis, ars., aur-m-n., aur., ***bell.***, **CALC.**, carb-an., ***carc.***, clem., con., cund., hep., hydr., ***lach.***, **LAUR.**, ***lyc.***, **PHOS.**, phyt., ran-b., sel., ***sep***, ***sil.***, syph., thuj.

EYES, remedies - **ACON.**, ***agar.***, all-c., am-c., anh., **APIS**, arg., ***arg-n.***, **ARN.**, **ARS.**, ars-i., ***aur.***, aur-m., **BELL.**, ***bor.***, calc., calc-p., calc-s., ***calen.***, cann-s., carbn-s., ***caust.***, ***con.***, cop., dig., **EUPHR.**, **GELS.**, ***graph.***, hyos., jab., kali-p., lach., ***lyss.***, mag-m., nat-c., **NAT-M.**, ***nat-s.***, onos., op., ***petr.***, ph-ac., ***phos.***, **PHYS.**, **PULS.**, rhus-t., **RUTA**, sang., sep., sil., ***spig.***, staph., ***stram.***, sulph., verat., ***zinc.***

injuries, eyes - **ACON.**, apis, **ARN.**, ars., asar., bell., bell-p., bry., calad., ***calc.***, calc-s., **CALEN.**, canth., cic., coc-c., coch., con., croc., ***euphr.***, ***ham.***, hep., **HYPER.**, ign., lach., ***led.***, merc., mez., nit-ac., nux-v., petr., phos., phys., ***puls.***, ***rhus-t.***, ruta, seneg., **SIL.**, ***staph.***, sul-ac., sulph., **SYMPH.**, ***zinc.***

EYES, pupils, general

alternately, contracted and dilated in the same light - acet-ac., ***acon.***, aesc., agar., am-c., anac., anh., arn., ars., ***bar-c.***, cann-s., ***carb-ac.***, cham., chin., cic., cocc., con., cycl., dig., dros., dulc., ***hell.***, hyos., ign., ***lach.***, oena., op., ***phys.***, sol-n., stann., staph., stroph., zinc.

contracted - ***acon.***, aesc., agar., amyg-am., ***anac.***, ang., ant-t., ***apis***, arg., arg-n., ***arn.***, ***ars.***, ***aur.***, aur-ar., aur-s., bar-c., ***bell.***, cadm-s., ***calc.***, calc-sil., ***camph.***, canth., caps., carb-ac., carbn-s., cham., ***chel.***, chin., ***chin-s.***, cic., cina, cocc., colch., con., croc., croto-t., cub., ***daph.***, ***dig.***, dros., esin., ***euphr.***, ferr., fl-ac., gamb., gels., ***gins.***, guat., haem., ***hell.***, ***hyos.***, ign., iodof., ip., jab., kali-bi., kali-i., laur., led., lon-c., lycpr., lyss., m-arct., mang., meny., ***merc.***, ***merc-c.***, ***mez.***, ***morph.***, mosch., ***mur-ac.***, naja, nat-c., ***nat-m.***, nat-p., ***nux-m.***, nux-v., ol-an., olnd., onos., **OP.**, oxyt., ph-ac., phos., ***phys.***, phyt., piloc., ***plb.***, podo., ***puls.***, rheum, rhod., ***rhus-t.***, ruta, sabad., samb., sec., seneg., ***sep.***, sil., sol-n., squil., ***stann.***, staph., stram., sul-ac., sulph., tab., tarax., tarent., **THUJ.**, tub., vario., ***verat.***, verat-v., viol-o., viol-t., vip., visc., ***zinc.***, zinc-p.

dilated - acet-ac., acetan., ***acon.***, acon-c., acon-f., adon., aesc., ***aeth.***, ***agar.***, ***agn.***, ***ail.***, alumn., amyg-am., ***anac.***, androc., ang., anh., ***apis***, apom., **ARG-N.**, ***arn.***, ars., ars-i., arund., asaf., asar., astac., atro., aur., bapt., bar-c., bar-i., ***bar-m.***, **BELL.**, bell-p., benz., benz-n., brom., bry., bufo, cadm-s., cahin., **CALC.**, ***calc-i.***, ***camph.***, cann-s., canth., caps., carb-ac., ***carb-an.***, carbn-s., caust., ***cedr.***, cham., ***chel.***, **CHIN.**, ***chin-s.***, ***cic.***, cic-m., cimic., ***cina***, coca, ***cocain.***, ***cocc.***, ***coff.***, ***colch.***, ***coloc.***, ***con.***, ***cor-r.***, ***croc.***, crot-c., crot-h., croto-t., cupr., ***cycl.***, cyt-l., ***dig.***, dor., dros., ***dubin.***, dulc., euph., **GELS.**, ***glon.***, gran., grin., ***guai.***, guare., ***hell.***, hep., hydr-ac., **HYOS.**, ***hyper.***, ign., indol., ***iod.***, ***iodof.***, ip., ipom., kali-bi., ***kali-br.***, kali-cy., ***kali-i.***, kali-n., kreos., lac-ac., lach., lachn., lact., ***laur.***, ***led.***, lyc., lyss., m-arct., m-aust., m-ambo., mand., **MANG.**, meny., ***merc.***, ***merl.***, mez., ***mosch.***, mur-ac., naja, nat-ar., ***nat-c.***, nat-f., ***nat-p.***, ***nit-ac.***, nux-m., ***nux-v.***, oena., olnd., ***op.***, oxyu-s., par., parth., petr., ***ph-ac.***, phase., ***phos.***, phys., phyt., pic-ac., pitu-p., plb., plb-chr., psil., ***puls.***, ran-b., raph., rheum, rhod., rhus-t., samb., ***sang.***, sanguin-t., sant., sars., **SEC.**, sil., sol-n., ***spig.***, squil., stann., staph., **STRAM.**, ***stry.***, sul-i., sulph., tarax., tarent., tax., teucr., thea., thuj., tub., urt-u., valer., ***verat.***, verat-v., verb., vib., vip., xan., zinc., zinc-p.

fixed - acon., ***bar-c.***, ***bell.***, cham., chin., cic., ***cupr.***, dig., ferr., hell., hydr-ac., ***hyos.***, kali-i., lach., ***laur.***, ***nit-ac.***, **OP.**, plb., ran-b., seneg., spig., ***stram.***

insensible, to light - acon., aconin., aeth., agar., amyg-am., arg-n., **ARN.**, ars., aur-m., ***bar-c.***, ***bar-m.***, **BELL.**, benz., benz-n., bufo, cahin., ***camph.***, carb-ac., carb-an., carb-v., carbn-h., cedr., cham., ***chel.***, chin., ***cic.***, ***colch.***, **CUPR.**, ***dig.***, dubin., euph., ferr., gels., ***hell.***, hep., hydr., hydr-ac., **HYOS.**, jab., kali-bi., ***kali-br.***, ***kali-i.***, lach., laur., lyc., ***merc.***, ***merc-c.***, naja, nit-ac., nux-m., **OP.**, ox-ac., oxyt., par., phase., phos., piloc., ***plat.***, puls., ran-b., rhus-t., seneg., sol-n., spig., ***stram.***, sul-ac., sulph., tab., ter., ***tub.***, ***zinc.***

irregular - acon., aur., bar-c., chlor., cinnb., dig., dubin., hyos., **MERC.**, merc-c., nit-ac., **OP.**, plb., sec., sil., sulph., tab.

sluggish - bell., carbn-s., cham., croc., cupr., dig., ***hell.***, ip., jatr., merc., naja, nit-ac., phos., rumx., sec., seneg., sul-ac., tab., tax.

unequal - absin., acon., ***arg.***, ***arg-n.***, aur., bell., cadm-s., cann-i., chlor., colch., cyt-l., dig., hell., hyos., lyss., mang., merc-c., morph., nat-ar., nat-p., onos., **OP.**, ***ph-ac.***, plb., rhod., sil., sulph., ***tarent.***, urt-u., verat-v., zinc.

EYESTRAIN, overexertion, agg., (see Asthenopia) - agar., alum., alum-p., alum-sil., ***am-c.***, am-m., anac., ***apis***, arg., **ARG-N.**, ***arn.***, art-v., ***asaf.***, asar., ***aur.***, bar-c., bar-m., bell., bor., bry., **CALC.**, calc-sil., cann-i., canth., ***carb-v.***, carbn-s., ***caust.***, chlol., ***cic.***, **CINA**, cocc., coff., con., **CROC.**, cupr., dros., dulc., ferr., ***graph.***, hep., ign., ***jab.***, **KALI-C.**, kali-p., kali-s., ***kali-sil.***, kreos., led., lith-c., **LYC.**, mag-c., mag-m., mang., merc., mez., mur-ac., ***naja***, nat-ar., ***nat-c.***, **NAT-M.**, ***nat-p.***, nat-sil., nicc., nicc-s., nicot., nit-ac., nux-m., ***nux-v.***, olnd., **ONOS.**, par., petr., ***ph-ac.***, ***phos.***, phys., ***phyt.***, puls., ran-b., **RHOD.**, ***rhus-t.***, **RUTA**, sabad., sant., ***sars.***, sel., **SENEG.**, ***sep.***, **SIL.**, ***spig.***, ***spong.***, staph., stram., stront-c., sul-ac., sulph., ther., thuj., tril-c., valer., verb., viol-o., zinc., zinc-p.

F

FAINTING, general, (see Vertigo) - abies-c., acet-ac., acetan., **ACON.**, ***aesc.***, aeth., aether, agar., agar-em., alco., alet., ***alf.***, all-c., aloe, ***alum.***, alum-p., alum-sil., alumn., am-br., ***ambr.***, **AM-C.**, am-m., ***aml-n.***, amyg-am., anac., ant-c., ant-m., ***ant-t.***, apis, ***apoc.***, apom., ***arg-n.***, ***arn.***, ***ars.***, ars-h., ***ars-i.***, ars-s-f., ars-s-r., asar., atro., bapt., bar-c., bar-i., ***bar-m.***, ***bar-s.***, bell., benz-n., benz-ac., berb., beryl., bism., bol., bol-s., bor., bov., brom., **BRY.**, bufo, cact., **CADM-S.**, calad., calc., calc-ar., calc-i., calc-m., calc-p., calc-sil., calo., ***camph.***, cann-i., ***cann-s.***, ***canth.***, carb-ac., ***carb-v.***, ***carbn-o.***, ***carbn-s.***, carl., cass., cast., cast-eq., **CAUST.**, cedr., cench., cere-s., **CHAM.**, ***chel.***, chim., **CHIN.**, ***chin-ar.***, chin-s., chlol., ***chlor.***, cic., ***cimic.***, cina, cinnam., cit-v., **COCC.**, ***coch.***, ***coff.***, colch., ***coll.***, ***coloc.***, ***con.***, conin., conv., convo-d., cot., croc., ***crot-c.***, **CROT-H.**, croto-t., ***culx.***, cupr., cupr-acet., ***cupr-ar.***, cupr-s., cur., cycl., **DIG.**, digin., digox., dios., dros., dubo-h., dubin., dulc., elaps, ery-a., eucal., eup-pur., ***euph.***, euph-c., ***ferr.***, ***ferr-ar.***, ***ferr-i.***, ferr-p., ***form.***, gamb., gels., gent-c., **GLON.**, gran., ***graph.***, grin., hedeo, hell., hell-f., **HEP.**, hippoz., hura, ***hydr.***, hydr-ac., ***hydrog.***, ***hyos.***, **IGN.**, ind., **IOD.**, iodof., **IP.**, iris, piloc., jal., jasm., jug-c., kali-ar., kali-bi., kali-br., kali-c., kali-cy., kali-n., kali-ox., kali-p., kali-sil., kalm., ***kreos.***, **LAC-C.**, ***lac-d.***, **LACH.**, lac-ac., lat-k., ***laur.***, ***led.***, lept., ***lil-t.***, ***lina.***, lob., luf-act., lup., ***lyc.***, lycps., lyss., m-arct., mag-c., ***mag-m.***, magn-gr., manc., mang., merc., ***merc-c.***, merc-cy., merc-d., merc-n., merc-pr-r., mez., **MOSCH.**, mur-ac., ***naja***, narc-po., narc-ps., ***nat-h.***, ***nat-m.***, nat-ns., nat-p., nit-ac., nitro-o., **NUX-M.**, **NUX-V.**, oena., ol-an., olnd., ***op.***, ox-ac., ozone, paeon., pana., parth., ped., ***petr.***, ***ph-ac.***, phase., ***phos.***, phys., ***phyt.***, picro., pip-m., plan., plat., **PLB.**, **PODO.**, ***psor.***, ptel., **PULS.**, puls-n, ran-b., ran-s., rhus-t., rob., ruta, sabad., sal-ac., ***sang.***, sapin., ***sars.***, sec., senec., ***seneg.***, **SEP.**, sieg., ***sil.***, sin-n., sol-t., sol-t-ae., ***spig.***, spong., stann., staph., **STRAM.**, stroph., stry., sul-i., **SULPH.**, sul-ac., **SUMB.**, ***tab.***, tarent., tax., ***ter.***, ther., thuj., ***thyr.***, til., ***tril.***, tub., uran-n., ust., valer., **VERAT.**, ***verat-v.***, verin., vesp., ***vib.***, viol-o., vip., zinc., zinc-m., zinc-p., zing., ziz.

FALLS, general, (see Blows, Injuries) - ***acon.***, **ARN.**, aur., ***aur-m.***, ***bad.***, **BELL-P.**, ***bry.***, **CALEN.**, ***cic.***, ***con.***, euph., glon., ***ham.***, ***hep.***, **HYPER.**, ***lach.***, ***led.***, lith-c., **NAT-S.**, puls., pyrog., ***rhus-t.***, **RUTA**, ***sil.***, ***staph.***, stront-c., ***sul-ac.***, ***symph.***

FAT, people, (see Obesity)

FATIGUE, (see Chronic fatigue, Weakness) - **ALUM.**, ***ambr.***, **AM-C.**, apoc., ***ars.***, ***ars-i.***, ***aur.***, bar-c., ***bapt.***, **CALAD.**, **CALC.**, cann-s., ***carb-v.***, **CARC.**, ***caust.***, ***chel.***, **CHIN.**, ***chin-s.***, ***cocc.***, **CON.**, ***dig.***, **FERR.**, ferr-ar., ferr-p., **GELS.**, **GRAPH.**, helon., hyos., ***kali-c.***, kali-n., ***kali-p.***, **LACH.**, ***laur.***, ***lyc.***, mag-m., ***mang.***, ***merc.***, mur-ac., nat-ar., ***nat-c.***, ***nat-m.***, nit-ac., ***nux-m.***, **NUX-V.**, ***op.***, **PH-AC.**, ***phos.***, **PIC-AC.**, ***psor.***, puls., sel., ***seneg.***, ***sep.***, **SIL.**, ***stann.***, staph., ***stram.***, stront-c., ***sulph.***, **SUL-AC.**, ***thuj.***, ***valer.***, verat., zinc., x-ray.

FATTY, degeneration, organs - acon., ***ars.***, **AUR.**, bor., calc., ***calc-ar.***, caust., chin., ***cupr.***, ferr., kali-c., kali-s., ***lac-d.***, ***lyc.***, merc., nux-v., **PHOS.**, puls., sulph., vanad.

blood-vessels - acon., ars., aur., bor., calc., caust., chin., ferr., nux-v., ***phos.***, puls., sulph.

heart - adon., **ARN.**, **ARS.**, ***ars-i.***, **AUR.**, **AUR-M.**, ***bar-c.***, **CACT.**, ***calc.***, caps., cimic., crat., crot-h., cupr., cupr-acet., ***ferr.***, fuc., ***iod.***, **KALI-C.**, kali-fcy., kali-p., ***kalm.***, ***naja,*** ph-ac., **PHOS.**, phys., ***phyt.***, stroph., stry-p., vanad.

liver - alco., am-van., ant-c., ant-t., arg-n., ars., aur., bism., cadm-s., ***calc.***, calc-f., carb-ac., carb-v., carbn-chl., ***card-m.***, ***chel.***, chlf., fl-ac., hippoz., iodof., kali-bi., kali-c., kali-chl., kali-s., lac-d., ***lyc.***, lyss., mag-m., mang., ***merc.***, nat-m., nux-v., phlor., **PHOS.**, ***pic-ac.***, sul-ac., sulph., thal., vanad.

FEARS, phobias, general - abrot., absin., acet-ac., **ACON.**, act-sp., aeth., aether, agar., agn., ***all-c.***, aloe, ***alum.***, alum-sil., am-br., am-c., am-m., ambr., aml-n., anac., **ANDROC.**, ang., ant-c., ant-s., ant-t., apis, aral., arg., **ARG-N.**, arist-cl., ***arn.***, **ARS.**, ars-h., ars-i., ars-s-f., art-v., arum-m., asaf., aspar., astac., aster., atro., **AUR.**, aur-ar., bapt., ***bar-c.***, bar-m., **BELL.**, berb., bism., **BOR.**, brom., ***bry.***, bufo, but-ac., ***cact.***, calad., **CALC.**, calc-f., **CALC-P.**, ***calc-s.***, calc-sil., camph., cann-i., cann-s., canth., ***caps.***, carb-an., ***carb-v.***, **CARBN-S.**, **CARC.**, cast., caul., ***caust.***, cham., chel., chin., chin-ar., chlol., chlor., **CIC.**, cimic., cina, cist., clem., cob-n., ***coca,*** ***cocc.***, coc-c., coff., ***coff-t.***, colch., coloc., ***con.***, cortico., croc., ***crot-h.***, ***cupr.***, cupr-acet., cupr-ar., cycl., cyt-l., daph., **DIG.**, dros., dulc., echi., elaps, euph., euphr., ferr., ferr-ar., ferr-p., fl-ac., ***form.***, **GELS.**, gent-c., gins., glon., **GRAPH.**, grat., hed., hell., ***hep.***, hoit., hydr-ac., ***hyos.***, hyper., iber., **IGN.**, ***iod.***, ip., iris, jatr., **KALI-AR.**, ***kali-br.***, ***kali-c.***, kali-i., kali-n., kali-p., kali-s., kreos., kres., lac-c., lac-del., lach., lact., lat-m., laur., led., ***lil-t.***, lipp., lob., lol., **LYC.**, **LYSS.**, macrin., m-arct., mag-c., ***mag-m.***, mag-s., manc., mang., med., ***meli.***, meny., ***merc.***, merc-c., merc-i-r., mez., ***mosch.***, murx., mur-ac., ***nat-ar.***, **NAT-C.**, ***nat-m.***, ***nat-p.***, nat-s., nicc., nit-ac., ***nux-v.***, ***onos.***, **OP.**, orig., ox-ac., ***petr.***, ph-ac., **PHOS.**, ***phyt.***, pip-m., **PLAT.**, plb., podo., **PSOR.**, ***puls.***, pyrog., rad., ran-b., ran-s., raph., rheum, rhod., ***rhus-t.***, rhus-v., ruta, sabad., sabin., samb., sang., sars., sec., sel., seneg., **SEP.**, sil., ***spig.***, ***spong.***, squil., ***stann.***, staph., **STRAM.**, ***stront-c.***, stroph-s., stry., succ., ***sulph.***, ***sul-ac.***, ***syph.***, ***tab.***, tarax., tarent., tell., ***ther.***, tere-ch., thuj., til., ***tub.***, valer., ***verat.***, visc., wye., xan., ***zinc.***, zinc-m., **ZINC-P.**

FEBRICULA - ***acon.***, arn., ***ars.***, ***bapt.***, bell., bry., camph., ***ferr-p.***, gels., ip., merc., nux-v., puls., ***rhus-t.***

FEVER, general - abies-n., acet-ac., **ACON.**, aesc., aeth., agar., agn., agro., ail., ***all-c.***, all-s., alst-s., alum., am-c., am-m., ***ambr.***, anac., androc., ***ang.***, ant-c., **ANT-T.**, anthr., **APIS**, aran., arg., **ARG-N.**, arist-cl., **ARN.**, **ARS.**, ars-h., **ARS-I.**, ***arum-t.***, asaf., asar., asc-t., atro., aur., **AUR-I.**, aur-m., aur-s., bad., bals-p., ***bapt.***, ***bar-c.***, **BELL.**, bell-p., benz-ac., bism., bol., bor., both-l., bov., brom., **BRY.**, **CACT.**, cadm-s., cahin., calad., ***calc.***, calo., camph., canch., cann-s., ***canth.***, ***caps.***, carb-an., carb-v., ***carbn-chl.***, ***carbn-s.***, carc., card-m., casc., caul., caust., cedr., cham., ***chel.***, chim., ***chin.***, chin-ar., **CHIN-S.**, cic., cimic., cimx., ***cina***, clem., ***coc-c.***, ***cocc.***, ***coff.***, ***colch.***, coloc., colos., **CON.**, cop., corn., corn-f., croc., crot-c., crot-h., cupr., ***cur.***, ***cycl.***, cyt-l., ***dig.***, dor., dros., ***dulc.***, echi., ***elaps***, elat., eucal., ***eup-per.***, eup-pur., euph., euphr., eys., fago., ***ferr.***, ferr-ar., ferr-i., ferr-ma., **FERR-P.**, ***fl-ac.***, **GELS.**, ***glon.***, ***graph.***, guai., guare., gymn., ***hell.***, ***hep.***, hydr., **HYDROG.**, ***hyos.***, iber., ***ign.***, ***iod.***, **IP.**, iris, kali-bi., ***kali-br.***, kali-c., kali-chl., **KALI-I.**, kali-n., ***kali-s.***, ***kreos.***, ***lac-c.***, lach., lachn., lap-gr-m., ***laur.***, ***led.***, lith-c., lob., **LYC.**, m-arct., ***m-aust.***, ***mag-c.***, mag-m., mag-s., mang., ***med.***, meny., ***merc.***, ***merc-c.***, ***merc-cy.***, ***merl.***, **MEZ.**, mill., morph., mosch., ***mur-ac.***, myric., nat-c., **NAT-M.**, nat-p., nat-s., ***nit-ac.***, ***nux-m.***, **NUX-V.**, ol-j., olnd., ***op.***, par., parth., petr., ***ph-ac.***, **PHOS.**, phyt., pic-ac., plan., plat., plb., ***podo.***, pop., ***psor.***, ptel., **PULS.**, puls-n, pulx., **PYROG.**, ran-b., ***ran-s.***, ***rheum***, rhod., **RHUS-T.**, ***rhus-v.***, ruta, sabad., ***sabin.***, ***samb.***, ***sang.***, sarr., sars., **SEC.**, sel., seneg., ***sep.***, **SIL.**, sol-n., spig., spira., spirae., **SPONG.**, **SQUIL.**, ***stann.***, ***staph.***, still., **STRAM.**, stront-c., ***sul-ac.***, ***sul-i.***, ***sulph.***, ***sumb.***, ***tab.***, **TARAX.**, ***tarent.***, ter., teucr., thuj., trio., urt-u., ***valer.***, **VERAT.**, ***verat-v.***, verb., viol-o., ***viol-t.***, zinc., ziz.

high, fever - abrot., **ACON.**, ant-t., ***apis,*** **ARN.**, **ARS.**, ***arum-t.***, ***aur.***, **BAPT.**, **BELL.**, ***bry.***, cact., canth., caps., **CARC.**, chel., chin., ***chin-s.***, cina, coff., ***colch.***, **CON.**, croc., crot-h., cupr., dig., dulc., ferr-ar., **GELS.**, hep., hyos., ***kali-ar.***, kali-i., ***lach.***, ***lyc.***, mag-c., meny., merc-c., **MEZ.**, **NAT-M.**, nat-s., nit-ac., nux-m., ***nux-v.***, ***op.***, ph-ac., ***phos.***, **PULS.**, **PYROG.**, **RHUS-T.**, samb., sang., **SEC.**, ***sil.***, staph., ***stram.***, thuj., ***tub.***

low, fever - ***ail.***, ***arn.***, **ARS.**, **BAPT.**, ***cact.***, camph., carb-ac., carb-v., chim., coca, cocc., ***crot-h.***, eucal., eup-a., **GELS.**, ***lach.***, ***mur-ac.***, nit-s-d., ***ph-ac.***, phos., pyrog., rhus-t., sabin., ter., ***urt-u.***

FIBROMA, tumors - arbu., bell., bry., ***calc.***, calc-f., ***calc-i.***, ***calc-s.***, chol., chr-s., ***con.***, fl-ac., frax., graph., hydr., ***hydr-m.***, ***kali-br.***, ***kali-i.***, ***lap-a.***, led., lil-t., lyc., phos., phyt., ***sec.***, ***sil.***, tarent., ter., teucr., thiosin., thlaspi, thyr., tril., ust., xan.

FIBROIDS, ovaries - apis, calc., coloc., fl-ac., hep., iod., kali-br., lach., merc., plat., ***podo.***, ***sep.***, staph., ***thuj.***, xan.

FIBROIDS, uterine - aesc., agn., ***am-m.***, ***apis***, ars., ***aur.***, ***aur-i.***, **AUR-M-N.**, ***bell.***, brom., bufo, **CALC.**, **CALC-F.**, ***calc-i.***, ***calc-p.***, ***calc-s.***, calc-st-sula., ***calen.***, ***carb-an.***, carc., chin., ***con.***, ***crot-h.***, cub., erod., ferr., foll., **FRAX.**, goss., graph., ham., ***hep.***, hydr., ***hydrc.***, hydrin-m., ***iod.***, ip., kali-br., ***kali-c.***, ***kali-i.***, ***lach.***, lap-a., ***led.***, ***lil-t.***, ***lyc.***, ***lyss.***, med., meph., merc., ***merc-c.***, ***merc-i-r.***, morg., ***nat-c.***, ***nit-ac.***, nux-v., ***pall.***, **PHOS.**, ***phyt.***, plat., plb., podo., puls., sabal., sabin., sang., sanic., sarr., sec., **SEP.**, ***sil.***, solid., staph., sul-ac., sulph., ***tarent.***, ***ter.***, teucr., thiosin., ***thlaspi***, ***thuj.***, **THYR.**, tril., tub., **UST.**, vinc., viol-o., x-ray

FIBROMYALGIA, general, (see Chronic fatigue, Fibrositis) - abrot., anac., ***arn.***, ***ars.***, ***aur.***, ba-sv., ba-tn., ***bell-p.,***, **BRY.**, ***calc.***, calc-f., calc-p., **CARC.**, caust., ***chin.***, chin-ar., cimic., ***cocc.***, ***colch.***, cupr., dys-co., ferr., fl-ac., **GELS.**, ***helon.***, ***irid.***, ***kali-p.***, ***kalm.***, **LAC-AC.**, lach., lob., ***lyc.***, mag-c., mag-m., mang., ***med.***, ***merc.***, ***morg.***, nat-sal., ***nux-v.***, **PH-AC.**, ***phos.***, pic-ac., prot., psor., ***ran-b.***, **RHUS-T.**, **RUTA**, ***sil.***, ***staph.***, ***syc-co.***, ***syph.***, thuj., verat., zinc.

FIBROSITIS, (see Fibromyalgia) - ***ba-sv.***, bell-p., dys-co., gaert., ***morg.***, prot., rhus-t., ***syc-co.***

FINANCIAL, shock, loss of wealth, property - arn., **ARS.**, **AUR.**, calc., ***calc-p.***, caust., ***con.***, ***ign.***, kali-br., lyc., ***psor.***

FISTULA, general - agar., alum., ang., ant-c., ars., asaf., aur., aur-ar., aur-m., aur-s., bac., bar-c., bar-m., bell., ***berb.***, bry., bufo, cact., **CALC.**, ***calc-f.***, calc-hp., calc-m., ***calc-p.***, calc-s., calc-sil., ***calen.***, carb-ac., carb-v., carbn-s., ***caust.***, chel., cinnb., cist., clem., con., cop., cund., eucal., ***fl-ac.***, graph., ***hep.***, hippoz., hydr., iris, kali-c., kali-i., kreos., lach., led., **LYC.**, maland., merc., mez., mill., myris., nat-c., nat-m., nat-p., ***nat-s.***, ***nit-ac.***, ol-j., petr., ph-ac., ***phos.***, phyt., puls., pyrog., querc., rhus-t., ruta, sabin., sel., sep., **SIL.**, stann., staph., stram., stront-c., **SULPH.**, syph., ter., thuj., ***tub.***, tub-k.

FLATUS, flatuence, intestinal - aesc., aeth., ***agar.***, agn., all-c., **ALOE**, alum., alumn., ambr., am-c., **AM-M.**, ammc., ***ant-c.***, ant-t., ***apis***, apoc., **ARG-N.**, arn., **ARS.**, ***ars-i.***, asaf., asar., ***aur.***, bapt., bar-c., bar-i., bar-m., bell., bor., bov., brom., bufo, cahin., **CALC.**, calc-f., ***calc-p.***, **CALC-S.**, ***caps.***, ***carb-ac.***, **CARB-AN.**, **CARB-V.**, **CARBN-S.**, ***caust.***, **CHAM.**, ***chel.***, **CHIN.**, ***chin-ar.***, ***chin-s.***, cic., cinnb., clem., ***coca***, ***cocc.***, coff., **COLCH.**, coll., ***coloc.***, ***con.***, ***cop.***, ***crot-c.***, ***croto-t.***, cycl., dig., ***dios.***, dirc., ***elaps***, eup-per., euph., fago., ferr., ferr-ar., ferr-i., ferr-p., ***fl-ac.***, ***form.***, ***gels.***, gins., glon., **GRAPH.**, gran., ***guai.***, ham., hell., helon., hep., **HYDR.**, hyper., ***ign.***, ***iod.***, indg., ***iod.***, iodof., ip., jug-r., kali-bi., **KALI-C.**, kali-chl., kali-i., ***kali-n.***, kali-p., kali-s., kalm., kreos., ***lac-c.***, ***lac-d.***, ***lach.***, lil-t., **LYC.**, m-arct., m-aust., **MAG-C.**, mag-m., ***mag-p.***, mang., meny., meph., ***merc.***, mez., morg., morg-g., mosch., ***mur-ac.***, myric., ***nat-ar.***, **NAT-C.**, ***nat-m.***, nat-p., **NAT-S.**, nat-sil., **NIT-AC.**, naja, **NUX-M.**, ***nux-v.***, ol-an., **OLND.**, **OP.**, orni., ox-ac., ozone, pall., petr., phel., ***ph-ac.***, ***phos.***, **PIC-AC.**, pitu-a., ***plat.***, plb., ***podo.***, prot., prun., ***psor.***, ***puls.***, puls-n, rad-br., ran-b., ran-s., ***raph.***, rheum, rhod., rhus-t., rumx., sabad., sang., sars., sec., ***sel.***, ***seneg.***, **SENN.**, ***sep.***, **SIL.**, slag, squil., stann., staph., stront-c., stry., sul-ac., sul-i., **SULPH.**, syc-co., ***syph.***, tab., tarax., **TARENT.**, teucr., thea., ther., ***thuj.***, thyr., til., tub., uran-n., valer., **VERAT.**, verat-v., vesp., vinc., xan., ***zinc.***, zinc-p., ***zing.***

FLOURIDE, ailments from - brom., calc-f., ***fl-ac.***, iod., sil.

FONTANELLES, open - ***apis***, ***apoc.***, bac., **CALC.**, calc-f., **CALC-P.**, carb-ac., ***ip.***, mag-c., ***merc.***, ph-ac., ***phos.***, ***puls.***, ***sep.***, **SIL.**, ***sulph.***, ***syph.***, tub., zinc.

FOOD ALLERGIES, hypersensitive, to foods - apis., aloe, ***ant-c.***, arg-n., **ARS.**, cham., chel., ***chin.***, ***chin-ar.***, chin-s., ***coff.***, coloc., ip., kali-c., **LYC.**, med., **MERC.**, **NAT-C.**, ***nat-p.***, ***nit-ac.***, **NUX-V.**, ***phos.***, ***podo.***, psor., sac-alb., sul-ac., sulph., ***urt-u.***, ***zing.***

FOOD POISONING - aeth., ***aloe***, alum., ***ant-c.***, arg-n., **ARS.**, ***bapt.***, bism., bry., carb-an., **CARB-V.**, cham., chel., **CHIN.**, **CHIN-AR.**, chin-s., **COLOC.**, crot-h., hydr., **IP.**, kali-c., lach., lyc., mag-p., nat-c., **NAT-P.**, **NUX-V.**, ph-ac., phos., ***podo.***, psor., ***puls.***, ***pyrog.***, sac-alb., sul-ac., ***urt-u.***, ***zing.***

FOREIGN, bodies, objects, ailments, from - ***acon.***, anag., bell., calc., calc-f., calen., ***cic.***, cocain., ***hep.***, laur., led., ***lob.***, ***myris.***, sep., **SIL.**, spong., sulph.

FORMALDEHYDE, ailments from - ***am-c.***, ***carb-an.***, cupr., ***formal.***, kreos., pyrog., sulph.

FRIGHT, acute - **ACON.**, ***arg-n.***, ***arn.***, ars., ***bell.***, calc., ***caust.***, cham., ***coff.***, **GELS.**, ***hyos.***, **IGN.**, lyc., **OP.**, ***ph-ac.***, ***phos.***, puls., sil.

FRIGHT, ailments from, (see Fears, phobias) - **ACON.**, act-sp., agar., anac., androc., ***apis***, arg., **ARG-N.**, arn., ars., ***art-v.***, ***aur.***, aur-m., ***bell.***, bry., ***bufo***, **CALC.**, calc-sil., camph., canth., carb-v., carbn-s., **CARC.**, **CAUST.**, cham., cic., cimic., cina, cocc., ***coff.***, coloc., crot-h., ***cupr.***, **GELS.**, ***glon.***, ***graph.***, hep., ***hyos.***, hyosin., ***hyper.***, **IGN.**, iod., ***kali-br.***, kali-c., ***kali-p.***, ***lach.***, laur., **LYC.**, lyss., mag-c., merc., morph., nat-c., **NAT-M.**, nicc., nit-ac., nux-m., ***nux-v.***, **OP.**, ***petr.***, **PH-AC.**, **PHOS.**, ***plat.***, psor., **PULS.**, ran-b., ***rhus-t.***, sabad., samb., sec., ***sep.***, **SIL.**, spong., stann., staph., ***stram.***, sulph., tarent., **VERAT.**, verb., vib., visc., zinc., zinc-p.

FROSTBITE, ailments from being frozen - abrot., **AGAR.,** alum., anthr., apis, arist-cl., ars., bell., bor., bry., calc., calen., camph., canth., carb-an., carb-v., coff., colch., croto-t., cycl., ferr-p., frag., ham., hep., kali-c., lach., led., m-aust., merc., mur-ac., nat-c., nit-ac., nux-v., paeon., ***petr.***, ph-ac., ***phos.***, plan., ***puls.***, rhus-t., sec., sep., ***sil.***, staph., sul-ac., sulph., ***tam.***, ***ter.***, thyr., verat-v., **ZINC.**

FROZEN, shoulder - bry., calc., calc-f., caust., ***ferr.***, **RHUS-T.,** ruta, ***sang.***, ***thiosin.*** **SEP.,** ***sil.***, ***sulph.***, syph.

FUMES, gases, poisoning, toxic, ailments, from - acet-ac., ***am-c.***, ant-t., ars., arn., bell., bor., bov., ***bry.***, calc., camph., ***carb-ac.***, ***carbn-s.***, **CARB-V.,** caust., ***chlf.***, chlor., coff., ***crot-h.***, ***euph.***, ip., lach., lyc., ***merc.***, nat-m., nux-v., olnd., ***op.***, ***lob.***, phos., ***puls.***, sec., ***sep.***, sulph., **SPIG.,**

FUNGUS, growths, spongy, (see Tinea) - alum., ant-c., ant-t., ***apis***, ***ars.***, aur., bac., bell., berb., calc., calc-i., ***calc-p.***, **CARB-AN.,** carb-v., caust., cham., ***clem.***, con., graph., hep., iod., kreos., **LACH.,** lyc., merc., mez., **NIT-AC.,** nux-v., petr., ph-ac., ***phos.***, rhus-t., sabin., sang., ***sep.***, ***sil.***, ***staph.***, ***sulph.***, **THUJ.**

FURUNCULOSIS - ***arn.***, bell-p., calen., squil., ter.

G

GALLBLADDER, remedies, (see Cholecystitis) - ars., ars-h., aur., ***bapt.***, bell., **BERB.,** ***bry.***, ***calc.***, **CARD-M.,** ***cham.***, ***chel.***, **CHIN.,** ***chion.***, ***chlf.***, **CHOL.,** **COLOC.,** cupr., dig., ***dios.***, euon., fel., ferr-s., gels., ***hydr.***, ***ip.***, ***iris***, jug-c., kali-ar., ***kali-bi.***, ***kali-c.***, ***lach.***, laur., ***lept.***, ***lith-c.***, **LYC.,** mag-p., mang., merc., merc-d., morg., myric., **NAT-S.,** ***nux-v.***, op., ***phos.***, podo., ptel., puls., rhus-t., sang., ***sep.***, sulph., tab., tarax., ter., **VERAT.**

GALLSTONE, pain, colic from - aml-n., alum., am-m., arge., ***ars.***, atro., aur., bamb-a., ***bapt.***, **BELL.,** **BERB.,** bold., ***bry.***, **CALC.,** calc-f., **CARD-M.,** ***cham.***, ***chel.***, **CHIN.,** ***chion.***, ***chlf.***, ***chlol.***, **CHOL.,** **COLOC.,** cupr., dig., **DIOS.,** erig., euon., fab., fel., ferr-s., gels., ***hep.***, ***hydr.***, ***ip.***, ***iris***, jug-c., kali-ar., ***kali-bi.***, ***kali-c.***, kreos., ***lach.***, laur., ***lept.***, lith-be., ***lith-c.***, lob., **LYC.,** mag-c., ***mag-m.***, mag-p., mag-s., mang., menth., merc., ***merc-d.***, **MORG.,** morph., myric., **NAT-S.,** ***nux-v.***, op., osm., ozone, phos., podo., ptel., puls., rhus-t., ric., sang., ***sep.***, sil., ***sulph.***, tab., tarax., ter., trio., **VERAT.**

GALLSTONES, general - aml-n., alum., am-m., arge., ***ars.***, atro., aur., bamb-a., ***bapt.***, **BELL.,** **BERB.,** bold., ***bry.***, **CALC.,** calc-f., **CARD-M.,** ***cham.***, ***chel.***, **CHIN.,** ***chion.***, ***chlf.***, ***chlol.***, **CHOL.,** **COLOC.,** cupr., dig., **DIOS.,** erig., euon., fab., fel., ferr-s., gels., ***hep.***, ***hydr.***, ***ip.***, ***iris***, jug-c., kali-ar., ***kali-bi.***, ***kali-c.***, kreos., ***lach.***, laur., ***lept.***, lith-be., ***lith-c.***, lob., **LYC.,** mag-c., ***mag-m.***, mag-p., mag-s., mang., menth., merc., ***merc-d.***, **MORG.,** morph., myric., **NAT-S.,** ***nux-v.***, op., osm., ozone, phos., podo., ptel., puls., rhus-t., ric., sang., ***sep.***, sil., ***sulph.***, tab., tarax., ter., trio., **VERAT.**

GANGRENE, general - acon., ***agar.***, ail., all-c., alum., am-c., ant-c., ant-t., **ANTHR.,** ***apis***, arn., **ARS.,** ***ars-s-f.***, ***asaf.***, aur., ***bell.***, both-l., brass., brom., calc., calc-p., calen., **CANTH.,** carb-ac., ***carb-an.***, ***carb-v.***, **CAUST.,** ***chin.***, chlor., chr-o., cist., con., crot-c., ***crot-h.***, cupr., cupr-ar., cycl., ***echi.***, ***euph.***, ferr-p., hell., helo., hep., ***hippoz.***, hyos., ***iod.***, ***iodof.***, kali-chl., kali-n., ***kali-p.***, **KREOS.,** **LACH.,** mag-c., med., merc., ***merc-c.***, mur-ac., **NIT-AC.,** ph-ac., ***phos.***, ***plb.***, ***polyg-pe.***, ran-a., ran-b., ran-fl., ***rhus-t.***, ruta, ***sabin.***, sal-ac., **SEC.,** sieg., **SIL.,** sol-n., solid., ***squil.***, ***stram.***, ***sul-ac.***, sulph., **TARENT.,** tarent-c., ter., ust., verat., vip., zinc.

GANGLION - acon., am-c., ant-c., apis, arn., ars., ars-i., aur-m., ba-sv., bar-c., bell., benz-ac., bov., bufo-s., calc., ***calc-f.***, calc-p., ***carb-v.***, carc., ***caust.***, con., ferr-m., gua., hep., iod., kali-c., kali-chl., kali-m., lach., mag-m., mag-p., merc., ozone, ped., ph-ac., ***phos.***, plb., rhod., rhus-t., **RUTA,** seneg., sil., stict., sul-i., sulph., thuj., zinc.

hands, back of - am-c., caust., ***ph-ac.***, plb., **RUTA,** ***sil.***, zinc.

wrists - am-c., aur-m., ***calc.***, ***calc-f.***, caust., carb-v., **RUTA,** ***sil.***, sulph.

GASOLINE, poisoning - formal., merc., petr., ***ter.***

GASTRITIS, infection - abies-c., abies-n., acon., ***aeth.***, agar-em., all-c., alum., alumn., anis., ***ant-c.***, **ANT-T.,** ***apis***, apoc., ***arg-n.***, arn., **ARS.,** ars-i., asaf., asar., asc-i., aur., aur-m., aur-m-n., bals-p., bapt., bar-c., bar-i., ***bar-m.***, baros., **BELL.,** bell-p., ***benz-ac.***, ***bism.***, brom., **BRY.,** ***cact.***, cadm-s., calc., calc-chln., ***camph.***, cann-s., ***canth.***, caps., carb-ac., carb-an., carb-v., carc., cham., chel., chin., cic., cina, cob-n., coca, ***cocc.***, colch., coll., coloc., cop., cory., crot-h., cund., cupr., cupr-acet., ***dig.***, dulc., **EUPH.,** ferr-p., gaul., gels., ger., ***graph.***, grat., hedeo, hell., ***hydr.***, hydr-ac., **HYOS.,** indg., iod., ***ip.***, iris, kali-ar., kali-bi., kali-br., kali-c., kali-chl., kali-i., kali-m., kali-n., kali-s., lac-ac., ***lac-d.***, lach., laur., lob., **LYC.,** lycps., mag-s., merc., merc-c., mez., nit-ac., **NUX-V.,** op., ox-ac., petr., **PHOS.,** phyt., ***plb.***, podo., ptel., puls., ran-b., ran-s., rheum, rhus-t., rumx., sabad., sabin., ***sang.***, sant., ***sec.***, sep., sil., sin-a., sol-n., spig., squil., stram., sul-ac., sulph., ***ter.***, **VERAT.,** ***verat-v.***, zinc.

GASTROENTERITIS. infection - acon., aloe, ant-c., ant-t., **ARS.,** bapt., bism., ***bry.***, ***cact.***, camph., caul., cedr., **CHIN.,** chlor., ***colch.***, coloc., crot-h., ***croto-t.***, ***cupr.***, ***cupr-ar.***, dios., elat., ***ferr.***, ***grat.***, **GUAI.,** hydr-ac., ***ip.***, ***iris***, ***jatr.***, kali-bi., merc., merc-c., ***nux-v.***, op., oper., ph-ac., ***phos.***, phyt., **PODO.,** ***psor.***, raph., ***rhus-t.***, sant., ***sec.***, ***tab.***, thuj., **VERAT.,** zinc.

GINGIVITIS, inflammation, gums - acon., ***alumn.***, am-c., arg-n., ars., ars-i., aur-m., bell., bor., bufo, ***calc-f.***, calc-s., ***caps.***, ***cham.***, chin-s., ***hecla.***, hep., kali-n., **KREOS.**, lach., lyss., mag-c., **MERC.**, ***merc-c.***, ***mur-ac.***, **NAT-M.**, naja, ***nux-v.***, **PHOS.**, ***phyt.***, plb., rhus-t., **SIL.**, sulph., thuj., tub.

GLANDS, cancer, adenocarcinoma - anthr., ars., ars-br., ***ars-i.***, **ASTER.**, ***aur-m.***, bac., bar-c., ***bar-i.***, ***brom.***, bufo, buni-o., cadm-i., calc-ar., ***calc-f.***, ***calc-i.***, calc-s., **CARB-AN.**, **CARC.**, ***cist.***, **CON.**, ***cory.***, ***cund.***, ferr-i., ferr-pic., ***iod.***, ***lap-a.***, nit-ac., ***phos.***, **PHYT.**, polyp-v., scroph-m., **SCROPH-N.**, sieg., sil., spong., sul-i., syph.

GLANDS, remedies - ars., ars-br., ***ars-i.***, astac., ***aster.***, aur-i., ***bac.***, bad., **BAR-C.**, bar-i., **BAR-M.**, **BELL.**, **BROM.**, bufo, ***calc.***, calc-f., ***calc-i.***, ***calc-p.***, calc-sil., ***carb-an.***, carb-v., **CARC.**, clem., ***cist.***, **CON.**, **DULC.**, echi., ferr-i., gels., ***hep.***, hydr., **IOD.**, iodof., jab., kali-i., lach., ***lap-a.***, ***lyc.***, **MERC.**, ***merc-c.***, merc-d., ***merc-i-f.***, merc-i-r., ***nit-ac.***, nat-m., ***ol-j.***, ph-ac., ***phos.***, **PHYT.**, piloc., plb., ***puls.***, ***pyrog.***, rhus-t., scirr., **SCROPH-N.**, **SIL.**, spong., sul-ac., ***sulph.***, sul-i., syph., thuj., ***thyr.***, tub.

- **injuries,** glands - ***arn.***, aster., cann-s., **BELL-P.**, cic., ***cist.***, **CON.**, ***dulc.***, glon., ***hep.***, ***iod.***, kali-c., kalm., ***iod.***, merc., ***petr.***, ***phos.***, phyt., puls., rhus-t., ***sil.***, ***sul-ac.***, ***sulph.***

GLANDULAR, fever, (see Mononucleosis) - ars., bapt., carc., gels.

GLAUCOMA, eyes - abel., acon., adren., aegle., allox., arec., arg-n., asar., atra-r., atro., aur., bell., berb., bry., camph., caust., ***cedr.***, cob-n., cocain., ***cocc.***, ***colch.***, coloc., **COM.**, cortico., croc., crot-h., dttab., esin., euphr., eys., gels., grin., hed., jab., ***kali-i.***, ***lac-c.***, lach., lyc., mag-c., mag-p., mez., ***nit-ac.***, nux-v., op., ***osm.***, **PHOS.**, ***phys.***, pipe., plb., pot-a., prun., puls., rhod., rhus-t., sapo., saroth., seneg., sil., ***spig.***, sulo-ac., sulph., supren., wies.

GIARDIA, parasites - ars., ***chin.***, cina., nat-p.

GINGIVITIS, inflammation, gums - acon., ***alumn.***, am-c., arg-n., ars., ars-i., aur-m., bell., bor., bufo, ***calc-f.***, calc-s., ***caps.***, ***cham.***, chin-s., ***hecla.***, hep., kali-n., **KREOS.**, lach., lyss., mag-c., **MERC.**, ***merc-c.***, ***mur-ac.***, **NAT-M.**, naja, ***nux-v.***, **PHOS.**, ***phyt.***, plb., rhus-t., **SIL.**, sulph., thuj., tub.

GLANDERS, horse disease - acon., ***ars.***, calc., chin-s., ***crot-h.***, hep., hippoz., ***kali-bi.***, ***lach.***, ***merc.***, ph-ac., phos., sep., sil., sulph., thuj.

GLAUCOMA, eyes - abel., acon., adren., aegle., allox., arec., arg-n., asar., atra-r., atro., aur., bell., berb., bry., camph., caust., ***cedr.***, cob-n., cocain., ***cocc.***, ***colch.***, coloc., **COM.**, cortico., croc., crot-h., dttab., esin., euphr., eys., gels., grin., hed., jab., ***kali-i.***, ***lac-c.***, lach., lyc., mag-c., mag-p., mez., ***nit-ac.***, nux-v., op., ***osm.***, **PHOS.**, ***phys.***, pipe., plb., pot-a., prun., puls., rhod., rhus-t., sapo., saroth., seneg., sil., ***spig.***, sulo-ac., sulph., supren., wies.

GLOSSITIS, infection, tongue - ***acon.***, am-c., anan., ang., **APIS**, apoc., ***arg-n.***, ***arn.***, ***ars.***, ars-s-f., ars-s-r., arum-t., aur-m., bell., ***benz-ac.***, brom., calc., ***calc-s.***, ***canth.***, carb-v., caust., cham., cocc., con., **CROT-C.**, **CROT-H.**, ***cupr.***, ferr-p., gels., hep., kali-ar., kali-chl., **LACH.**, lyc., m-arct., mang., ***merc.***, ***merc-c.***, mez., ***mur-ac.***, nat-ar., nat-c., ***nat-m.***, ***nit-ac.***, nux-v., ox-ac., petr., ph-ac., ***phyt.***, ***plb.***, podo., prun., ptel., ran-b., ran-s., sep., ***sil.***, ***staph.***, ***sul-ac.***, ***sulph.***, thal., ***vip.***

GOITRE, thyroid - adren., aeth., ***ail.***, aln., aloe, am-c., am-m., ***ambr.***, aml-n., anh., antipyrin., ***apis***, aq-mar., aran-ix., ars., ars-i., arum-t., atra-r., ***aur.***, ***aur-i.***, aur-s., bac., ***bad.***, bar-c., bar-i., ***bell.***, berb., brass-o., ***brom.***, bry., bufo, cact., **CALC.**, ***calc-f.***, **CALC-I.**, ***calc-s.***, calc-sil., cann-i., ***carb-an.***, ***carbn-s.***, carc., card-m., ***caust.***, chel., chin., chin-ar., chlol., chr-s., cimic., ***cist.***, cob., colch., con., ***crot-c.***, crot-h., cupr., cyt-l., dig., dros., dubin., dys-co., echi., elaps, ephe., ferr., ***ferr-i.***, ferr-p., ferr-s., ***fl-ac.***, ***flor-p.***, form., ***fuc.***, glon., ***graph.***, ham., hed., ***hep.***, ***hydr.***, hydr-ac., ***ign.***, **IOD.**, ***iris***, jab., kali-c., ***kali-i.***, kali-s., ***lach.***, lam., ***lap-a.***, lap-mar-c., ***lyc.***, ***lycps.***, mag-c., mag-f., mag-m., mag-p., mang., meph., merc., ***merc-i-f.***, ***merc-i-r.***, morg., nat-ar., ***nat-c.***, **NAT-M.**, ***nat-p.***, ***nat-s.***, nat-sil., nit-ac., nux-v., op., petr., ***phos.***, phyt., piloc., plat., podo., puls., rauw., salx-m., saroth., scut., sec., sel., ***sep.***, ***sil.***, spig., **SPONG.**, staph., stram., stroph., sul-i., sulph., syc-co., tab., ***tarent.***, thal., thala., thuj., ***thyr.***, thyreotr., ***tub.***, urt-u., verat., verat-v., vip., zinc-i.

GOLD, aurum, ailments from - arg., aur., aur-m., aur-m-n., bell., chin., cocc., coff., cupr., merc., sol-n., spig.

GONORRHEA, infection - acon., ***agn.***, aloe, ***alum.***, ***alumn.***, am-m., ***anag.***, ***ant-c.***, apis, ***arg-n.***, ars., ars-s-f., aur-m., ***bar-m.***, ***bism.***, ***bor.***, ***calad.***, ***calc.***, **CALC-S.**, cann-i., **CANN-S.**, **CANTH.**, caps., ***caul.***, ***cedr.***, ***cham.***, ***chel.***, chim., ***cinnb.***, ***clem.***, **COCH.**, ***cob.***, ***cub.***, cupr-ar., **DIG.**, dor., erig., ery-a., eucal., ***ferr-i.***, **FERR-P.**, fl-ac., gels., gunp., ***hydr.***, **KALI-CHL.**, ***kali-i.***, ***kali-s.***, lac-c., lachn., led., **MED.**, **MERC.**, ***merc-c.***, ***mez.***, mill., ***nat-m.***, **NAT-S.**, **NIT-AC.**, ***pareir.***, ***petr.***, **PETROS.**, ph-ac., ***phos.***, ***phyt.***, ***plb.***, ***psor.***, **PULS.**, rhod., sabad., sabin., sars., senec., **SEP.**, ***sil.***, still., ***sulph.***, ***tarent.***, **TER.**, **THUJ.**

GOUT, general - acon., anag., ***ant-c.***, ***ant-t.***, anthro., ***apis***, **ARN.**, ***ars.***, aspar., ***bapt.***, ***bell.***, **BENZ-AC.**, **BRY.**, **BUFO**, **CALC.**, calc-p., calc-s., caps., ***carbn-s.***, ***caust.***, cedr., chin., chlol., clem., cocc., coch., **COLCH.**, ***coloc.***, eup-per., ferr-m., ***form.***, ***guai.***, ***hep.***, hyper., ***iod.***, kali-ar., ***kali-c.***, ***kali-i.***, ***kali-m.***, lac-c., **LYC.**, **MAG-C.**, ***mang.***, ***nat-s.***, **NUX-V.**, ol-j., ph-ac., phos., plb., ***puls.***, ***rhod.***, ***sabin.***, sal-ac., ***sars.***, ***sil.***, ***sulph.***, ter., ***urt-u.***, viol-t.

GRIEF, ailments, from - acet-ac., acon., aeth., alum., alum-p., am-m., **AMBR.,** aml-n., anac., ant-c., ***apis***, ***arn.***, ars., art-v., **AUR.**, aur-ar., aur-m., ***aur-m-n.,*** aur-s., bar-s., ***bell., bry., cact.,*** cadm-s., cael., ***calc., calc-p.***, caps., **CARC.**, **CAUST.**, cham., chin., clem., **COCC.**, coff., colch., ***coloc.***, ***con.***, ***crat.***, crot-c., crot-h., cycl., cypr., dig., ***dros., gels., graph.***, ***hura***, ***hyos.***, **IGN.**, ip., ***kali-br.***, kali-c., kali-fcy., kali-p., **LACH.**, lact., laur., lob-c., lob-s., lyc., mag-c., merc., naja, nat-c., **NAT-M.**, nat-p., nat-s., nit-ac., nux-m., ***nux-v.***, ***op.,*** paull., petr., **PH-AC.**, **PHOS.,** phys., pic-ac., ***plat.***, psor., **PULS.,** pyrus, rhus-t., ***samb.***, ***sep.***, seq-s., ***sol-o.***, spig., **STAPH.**, stram., sulph., tarent., tub., ***uran-n.***, verat., ***zinc.***

GRINDING, teeth, bruxism - absin., ***acon.***, agar., agar-ph., agn., alco., anan., ant-c., **APIS**, arg-n., ***arn.***, ***ars.***, ***art-v.***, asaf., atro., aur., aur-ar., aur-s., bac., bar-c., **BELL.**, bond., bor., bov., bruc., ***bry.***, bufo, ***calc.***, camph., cann-i., cann-s., ***canth.***, ***carb-ac.***, carbn-s., carc., carl., cass., ***caust.***, ***cham.***, ***cic.***, **CINA**, cocc., coff., colch., con., conv., ***crot-h.***, ***cupr.***, cupr-s., cur., cycl., cyn-d., emb., ferr., gran., ***grat.***, ***hell.***, **HYOS.**, ign., kali-br., kali-c., kali-p., kara., lac-d., lach., ***laur.***, ***lyc.***, lyss., med., ***merc.***, merc-d., morph., ***mygal.***, nat-p., nux-m., nux-v., oena., op., phos., ***phys.***, phyt., plan., ***plb.***, ***podo.***, psor., rumx-a., ***sant.***, sec., ***sep.***, sol, spig., ***stram.***, sul-ac., ***sulph.***, syph., tab., tarent., thuj., **TUB.,** ***verat.***, vern-a., vip., ***zinc.***

GROWING, pains - acon., agar., bell., calc., **CALC-P.,** ***ferr-acet., guai.,*** mang., ol-an., **PH-AC.,** phos., sil.

GUILLAIN-BARRE syndrome - carc., con., lath., thuj.

GUNSHOT, wounds - apis, **ARN., CALEN.,** chin., ***euph., gunp.,*** **HYPER.**, lach., **LED.,** ***nit-ac., plat., plb.,*** puls., ruta, ***staph., sul-ac.,*** sulph., symph.

H

HAIR, loss, falling out of, (See Baldness) - ail., ***alum., ambr.,*** am-c., ***am-m.,*** anan., ***ant-c.,*** ant-t., apis, ***ars.,*** ars-i., ***arund.,*** asc-t., **AUR.**, ***aur-m.,*** aur-m-n., aur-s., bac., ***bar-c.,*** bell., bov., bry., bufo, ***calc.,*** calc-i., ***calc-p.,*** calc-s., ***canth., carb-an.,*** **CARB-V., CARBN-S.,** carl., caust., ***chel.,*** chlol., chin., colch., ***con.,*** cop., ***elaps, ferr.,*** ferr-ar., ferr-m., ferr-p., **FL-AC.,** ***form.,*** glon., **GRAPH.**, hell., ***hep.,*** hyper., ign., iod., kali-ar., ***kali-bi.,*** **KALI-C.,** kali-i., kali-n., kali-p., **KALI-S.**, kreos., **LACH., LYC.,** ***mag-c.,*** manc., ***merc., merc-c., mez.,*** morg., naja, nat-c., **NAT-M.,** nat-p., **NIT-AC.,** nuph., oena., op., osm., ped., ***petr., ph-ac.,*** **PHOS.**, piloc., plb., psor., puls., rhus-t., rhus-v., sanic., sars., sec., ***sel.,*** **SEP., SIL.,** ***skook., staph.,*** **SULPH.**, sul-ac., ***syph.,*** tab., tep., ***thal.,*** **THUJ.**, thyr., tub., ust., vesp., ***zinc.***

HAIRY, skin - bac., carc., cortico., cortiso., med., nat-m., rauw., ***sep.,*** thuj., thymu.

HAMMOND'S disease, (see Athetosis)

HANGED, strangled persons, asphyxia, of - arn., ars., op.

HANGOVER, from a night of reveling - agar., ambr., ***ant-c., ars.,*** bry., ***carb-v.,*** chel., chin., coff., colch., **IP.,** lac-d., ***laur.,*** led., nat-c., **NUX-V.,** ***puls.,*** ran-b., rhus-t., sabin., staph., sulph.

HAY FEVER, (see Allergies, Coryza) - agar., ail., **ALL-C., AMBRO.,** ***aral.,*** **ARS., ARS-I.,** ***arum-t.,*** **ARUND.,** aspar., bad., benz-ac., ***brom.,*** calc., camph., ***carb-v.,*** chin-ar., chrom-k-s., ***cocain, con., cupr-acet.,*** cycl., ***dulc.,*** euph-pi., ***euphr., gels.,*** graph., grin., hep., iod., ***just.,*** kali-bi., kali-c., ***kali-i.,*** kali-m., ***kali-p.,*** kali-s., lach., linu-u., lyc., mag-m., **MED.,** meph., merc., merc-i-f., ***naja,*** napht., **NAT-M., NAT-S.,** nux-v., phel., phos., **PSOR.,** ***puls., ran-b.,*** ros-d., rhus-t., **SABAD.,** ***sang.,*** sanguin-n., senec., sep., sin-a., **SIN-N.,** ***sil.,*** skook., ***stict.,*** sul-ac., sul-i., sulph., syc-co., teucr., tong., trif-p., **TUB.,** ***wye.***

HEAD, injuries, blows, etc., (see Concussion) - acet-ac., acon., am-c., ***anac.,*** **ARN.**, aur., **BAD.,** ***bell.,*** bell-p., both-l., bry., ***calc., calc-p.,*** calc-s., calen., camph., cann-s., ***carc.,*** caust., chin., ***cic.,*** cina, ***cocc., con.,*** cupr., echi., euphr., ***glon., ham.,*** **HELL.,** ***hyos.,*** **HYPER.,** ***iod., kali-p.,*** kreos., lac-c., lac-d., ***lach.,*** laur., ***led., lob.***, lyc., m-arct., mag-m., ***mang.,*** meli., merc., mez., nat-m., **NAT-S.,** nux-m., ***nux-v.,*** op., ph-ac., ***puls., rhus-t., ruta,*** seneg., ***sep., sil., spig.,*** staph., stram., stry., sul-ac., sulph., ***symph., teucr.,*** valer., ***verat.,*** verb., viol-t., zinc.

epilepsy, after - ***arn., cic.,*** hell., hyper., ***nat-s.,*** zinc.

vertigo, after -bell-p., cic., ***con.,*** **NAT-S.**

HEADACHES, general, head pain, (see Dull, pain) - abrot., absin., acet-ac., acon., act-sp., aesc., aeth., agar., ail., all-c., aloe, ***alum., alumn.,*** ambr., ***am-c.,*** am-m., ammc., anac., ang., **ANTHR.,** ***ant-c.,*** ant-t., **APIS,** ap-g., apoc., **ARG.,** ***arg-n., arn.,*** **ARS.,** ars-i., arum-t., asaf., asar., ***aur.,*** bad., ***bapt.,*** bar-c., bar-m., **BELL.,** berb., benz-ac., berb., bism., ***bor.,*** bov., brom., **BRY.,** bufo, ***cact.,*** calad., **CALC.,** calc-p., **CALC-S.,** camph., cann-i., cann-s., canth., carb-an., ***carb-v.,*** carbn-s., **CARC.,** cast., caul., ***caust.,*** **CEDR.,** ***cham.,*** chel., **CHIN.,** chin-ar., **CHIN-S.,** ***cimic.,*** cina, ***cinnb.,*** clem., cob., coca, **COCC.,** coc-c., ***coff.,*** colch., ***coloc.,*** com., con., conv., corn., croc., **CROT-C.,** ***crot-h., croto-t.,*** cund., ***cupr.,*** cupr-ar., cur., cycl., daph., ***dig., dios., dros., dulc.,*** elaps, elat., eug., eup-per., euph., euphr., eupi., ***ferr., ferr-ar., ferr-i., ferr-p.,*** fl-ac., gamb., **GELS.,** gent-c., gins., **GLON.,** gran., ***graph.,*** grat., guai., gymn., ham., ***hell., hep.,*** hipp., hura, hydr., hydr-ac., **HYDROG.,** ***hyos.,*** hyper., ictod., ***ign.,*** indg., ind., ***iod.,*** ip., **IRIS,** jal., jatr., jug-r., ***kali-ar.,*** **KALI-BI.,** ***kali-c.,*** kali-chl., **KALI-I.,** ***kali-n., kali-p., kali-s., kalm., kreos.,*** **LAC-C.,** ***lac-d.,*** **LACH.,** lachn., lac-ac., lact., laur., ***lec., led.,*** lil-t., lob., ***lyc.,*** lyss., mag-c., ***mag-m.,*** **MAG-P.,** mag-s., ***manc.,*** mang., ***med., meli.,*** meph., **MERC.,** merc-c., merc-i-f., merl., ***mez.,*** mill., morph., mosch., murx., mur-ac., naja, ***nat-ar., nat-c.,*** **NAT-M.,** nat-p., ***nat-s.,*** nicc., **NIT-AC.,** ***nux-m.,*** **NUX-V.,** oena., ol-j., osm., ox-ac., pall., ***par., petr.,*** phel., ***ph-ac.,*** **PHOS.,** phys., phyt., pic-ac., plan., plat., ***plb., podo.,*** prun., **PSOR.,** ptel., **PULS.,** ran-b., ran-s., raph., rheum, rhod., ***rhus-t.,*** rhus-v., rumx., sabad., **SANG.,** sec., sel., seneg., **SEP., SIL.,** sol-n., ***spig.,*** spong., stann., ***staph.,*** stram., stry., **SULPH.,** sul-ac., tab., tanac., tarax., tarent., tax., tell., ***ter.,*** thea., ***ther.,*** **THUJ.,** til., tril., trom., urt-u., ust., valer., verat., viol-o., viol-t., vip., xan., ***zinc.,*** zinc-s., zing., ziz.

left, sided headaches - aloe, alum., ***ambr., ant-c.,*** apis, ***ars., ars-i., asaf., asar., bell.,*** bism., ***bov.,*** **BROM.,** bry., calad., ***calc.,*** calc-p., cann-s., canth., carb-v., carbn-s., caust., ***cham., chin.,*** chin-ar., chin-s., cimic., cina, ***coloc.,*** con., conv., ***croc.,*** crot-h., cupr., ***cycl.,*** eup-pur., ***euph., ferr., ferr-i.,*** fl-ac., ***graph., guai.,*** gymn., ham., hydr., ***hydrog.,*** ign., ***iod., kali-c.,*** lac-c., ***lach.,*** lac-ac., lil-t., lith-c., ***lob.,*** lyc., ***mag-c.,*** med., ***merc.,*** merc-i-f., merc-i-r., murx., nat-m., ***nit-ac., nux-m., olnd.,*** pall., ***par.,*** phel., ***phos.,*** plan., ***plat.,*** plb., ptel., ran-b., ran-s., ***rhod., rhus-t.,*** sabad., ***samb.,*** sec., ***sel.,*** **SEP., SPIG.,** ***sulph.,*** tab., ***tarax., thuj.,*** trom., verat-v., viol-o., viol-t., xan., ***zinc.,*** zing., ziz.

right, sided - ***alum.,*** arg., ars., asaf., **BELL.,** ***bism.,*** bov., ***bry.,*** bufo, ***cact.,*** **CALC.,** carb-an., **CARB-V.,** ***caust.,*** cham., ***chel.,*** cimic., ***cina,*** cist., coca, coc-c., coff., ***con.,*** croc., ***crot-c.,*** crot-h., cycl., euph., ferr-ar., gels., gins., gran., graph., grat., guai., ***hep.,*** **IGN.,** iod., **IRIS,** jac., ***kali-c.,*** lach., **LYC.,** mag-c., meny., merc., merc-i-r., ***mez.,*** mill., ***mosch., nat-m.,*** nit-ac., nux-m., ol-an., plat., ***plb., ran-b., rat.,*** rheum, rhod., ***rhus-t., ruta,*** **SABAD., SANG., SEP.,** sil., spong., sulph., tarax., tarent., thuj., urt-u., verat., zinc.

<u>**HEART ATTACK**</u>, (see Angina pectoris) - **ACON.,** apis, arg-n., **ARN.,** ars., aur., <u>**CACT.**</u>, carb-v., ***dig., glon.,*** iod., ***kalm.,*** **LACH.,** <u>**LAT-M.**</u>, ***laur., naja,*** nux-v., phos., rhus-t., ***spig.,*** verat., ***tarent.***

<u>**HEART**</u>, remedies - **ACON.,** ***adon.,*** agar., alum., ***am-c.,*** am-caust., am-m., ambr., ***aml-n.,*** anac., ang., ant-t., apis, **APOC.,** arg-n., arn., ***ars., ars-i.,*** asaf., asar., **AUR.,** aur-ar., aur-i., **AUR-M.,** ***bad., bar-c.,*** bell., benz-ac., bism., bor., bov., ***brom.,*** bry., bufo, <u>**CACT.**</u>, ***calc., calc-ar.,*** calc-f., camph., cann-s., canth., carb-an., carb-v., ***caust., cench.,*** cham., chin., chin-ar., ***cimic.,*** clem., coca, cocc., colch., ***coll.,*** coloc., con., conch., ***conv.,*** <u>**CRAT.**</u>, ***crot-h., cupr.,*** cycl., **DIG.,** ***digin.,*** dulc., ferr., ***ferr-p.,*** gels., ***glon.,*** graph., grin., hell., hep., ***hydr., hydr-ac.,*** hyos., hyosin., ***iber.,*** ign., ***iod.,*** ip., jab., kali-bi., ***kali-c.,*** kali-chl., kali-n., ***kalm.,*** **LACH., LAT-M.,** ***laur.,*** led., lepi., ***lil-t.,*** **LITH-C., LOB.,** lyc., ***lycps.,*** mag-c., mag-m., mang., med., meny., merc., merc-i-f., mez., ***mosch.,*** mur-ac., myric., **NAJA**, nat-c., nat-i., ***nat-m.,*** nit-ac., nux-m., nux-v., olnd., op., ox-ac., par., petr., ph-ac., ***phase.,*** **PHOS.,** plan., plat., plb., podo., prot., prun., ***psor.,*** **PULS.,** ran-s., rhod., rhus-t., rumx., ruta, sabin., sang., ***saroth.,*** sec., seneg., ***sep.,*** sil., **SPIG., SPONG.,** squil., stront-c., stroph., ***stry.,*** sul-ac., ***sulph.,*** sumb., tab., tarent., ther., thuj., thyr., valer., ***verat.,*** verat-v., verb., viol-o., viol-t., visc., ***zinc.,*** zinc-i.

<u>**HEARTBURN**</u>, general, (see Belching) - acet-ac., acon., adon., ***aesc.,*** agar., ail., all-s., allox., ***alum.,*** alum-p., alum-sil., alumn., **AM-C.,** am-m., **AMBR.,** ***anac.,*** ant-c., ***ant-t.,*** ap-g., ***apis,*** apom., arg., ***arg-n.,*** arn., **ARS.,** ***ars-i.,*** ars-s-f., asaf., asar., aster., ***atro.,*** aur., bamb-a., bar-c., bar-i., bar-m., bar-s., bell., benz-ac., ***berb.,*** **BISM.,** bor., bov., ***bry.,*** cact., cadm-s., caj., **CALC.,** calc-ar., calc-i., calc-p., ***calc-s., calc-sil.,*** calen., camph., canch., cand-a., cann-s., ***canth., caps.,*** carb-ac., ***carb-an.,*** **CARB-V.,** carbn-s., carc., card-m., carl., caul., ***caust.,*** cham., ***chel., chin.,*** chin-ar., ***chin-s.,*** chlor., choc., **CIC.,** coc-c., cocc., coff., coffin., colch., coloc., **CON.,** corn., corn-f., cosm., **CROC.,** crot-h., croto-t., cupr., cycl., daph., dat-a., dig., ***dios.,*** dulc., dys-co., echi., elaps, euph., fago., ferr., ferr-ar., ferr-i., **FERR-P.,** ***fl-ac., gaert.,*** gall-ac., gels., ***graph.,*** grat., grin., guai., gymn., ham., hell., ***hep.,*** hydr., hyos., iber., ign., ***iod.,*** ip., ***iris,*** kali-ar., kali-bi., ***kali-c.,*** kali-chl., ***kali-i.,*** kali-n., kali-p., kali-s., kali-sil., lac-ac., ***lach.,*** lap-mar-c., lath., lith-c., ***lob.,*** lob-s., luna, **LYC., MAG-C.,** mag-m., mag-s., manc., mang., ***merc.,*** merc-c., merc-i-r., merl., ***morg.,*** mosch., mur-ac., myric., naja, nat-ar., ***nat-c., nat-m.,*** nat-p., ***nat-s.,*** nat-sil., nit-ac., nux-m., **NUX-V.,** op., ox-ac., ozone, par., petr., ph-ac., **PHOS.,** phyt., plat., plb., ***podo., prot.,*** prun-c., prun-v., psor., ptel., **PULS.,** puls-n, quas., ran-b., ran-s., rauw., rheum, rhus-t., ***rob.,*** ruta, ***sabad., sabin.,*** sang., sant., sars., sec., ***sep., sil.,*** sin-a., ***sin-n.,*** sol-n., spig., squil., ***stann.,*** staph., still., stram., ***sul-ac.,*** sul-i., sulo-ac., ***sulph.,*** sumb., syc-co., ***syph.,*** tab., tanac., tarax., tarent., tell., ter., thea., thuj., thymol., tub-r., ust., ***valer., verat., verat-v.,*** visc., ***zinc.,*** zing.

<u>**HEMATOCELE**</u>, pelvic - acon., apis, ***arn.,*** ars., bell., canth., chin., coloc., con., dig., ***ferr., ham.,*** ip., ***kali-i.,*** lach., ***merc.,*** mill., nit-ac., ***phos.,*** ruta, sabin., ***sec., sulph.,*** ter., thlaspi

<u>**HEMATOMA**</u> - **ARN.,** calc-f., ham., led., merc., mill., ***nat-s.,*** sil., symph.

<u>**HEMOGLOBINURIA**</u> - ***ars-h.,*** carb-ac., chin-ar., chin-s., ferr-p., kali-bi., ***kali-chl.,*** nat-n., ***phos.,*** pic-ac., sant.

HEMOLYTIC, anemia, chlorosis - abies-c., ***abrot., absin., acet-ac., alet., alum.,*** alum-p., alumn., ***am-c., ambr., ant-c., ant-t.,*** aq-mar., ***arg.,*** arg-n., **ARS.,** ars-i., ars-s-f., aur-ar., bar-c., **BELL.,** bry., cadm-m., **CALC.,** calc-ar., **CALC-P.,** carb-an., ***carb-v.,*** **CARBN-S.,** caust., ***chin., chin-ar.,*** chlor., cob-n., cina, **COCC.,** coch., ***con., cupr., cycl.,*** dig., **FERR., FERR-AR.,** ***ferr-i.,*** **FERR-M.,** ferr-p., ***ferr-s.,*** franz., **GRAPH.,** ***guare., hell., helon., hep.,*** ign., ***ip., kali-ar.,*** kali-bi., ***kali-c., kali-fcy.,*** kali-ma., ***kali-p.,*** kali-s., lac-c., lach., **LYC.,** ***lyss.,*** **MANG., MED.,** merc., ***mill., nat-c.,*** nat-hchls., **NAT-M.,** nat-p., **NIT-AC.,** ***nux-v.,*** olnd., ***petr.,*** ph-ac., **PHOS.,** phyt., pic-ac., **PLAT.,** ***plb.,*** **PULS.,** sabin., sac-l., **SENEC., SEP.,** ***sin-n., spig.,*** staph., **SULPH.,** sul-ac., thuj., ust., valer., vanad., ***xan.,*** zinc.

HEMOPHILIA, blood does not coagulate - ***adren.,*** ail., alum., alumn., am-c., anthr., ***apis,*** aran., ***arn.,*** ars., ars-h., bell., **BOTH-L.,** ***bov., cact.,*** calc., calc-l., calc-p., canth., carb-an., ***carb-v.,*** chin., chin-s., chlol., chloram., ***cinnam.,*** cortico., croc., **CROT-C.,** ***crot-h.,*** dig., dor., ***elaps,*** erech., ergot., ***erig.,*** **FERR.,** ferr-m., ***ferr-p.,*** fic., gall-ac., ***ger., ham.,*** **HIR.,** ***hydrin-m., ip.,*** kali-c., ***kali-p.,*** kreos., **LACH., LAT-M.,** led., meli., merc., merc-cy., mill., mur-ac., nat-m., nat-n., ***nat-s., nat-sil.,*** **NIT-AC.,** op., ph-ac., **PHOS.,** puls., rad-br., ***sabin.,*** sanguis., ***sec.,*** sil., stront-c., ***sul-ac.,*** sulph., ***ter.,*** thlaspi, til., ***tril.,*** ust., verat., vip., visc., x-ray, xanth.

HEMORRHOIDS, general - abrot., acet-ac., acon., **AESC.,** ***aesc-g.,*** aeth., **AGAR.,** agn., ail., all-c., all-s., **ALOE,** alum., alum-p., alum-sil., alumn., am-br., ***am-c.,*** am-m., ambr., anac., anan., androc., ang., ***ant-c.,*** ant-t., ***apis,*** apoc., arg-n., arist-cl., arn., **ARS.,** ***ars-i.,*** ars-s-f., arum-t., arund., asc-t., aster., aur., aur-ar., aur-i., aur-m., aur-m-n., aur-s., ba-sv., ***bac.,*** bad., bapt., ***bar-c.,*** bar-i., bar-m., bar-s., ***bell.,*** berb., bor., bov., ***brom.,*** bry., ***bufo, cact.,*** cadm., ***calc., calc-f.,*** calc-i., ***calc-p., calc-s.,*** calc-sil., cand-a., cann-s., canth., ***caps.,*** carb-ac., **CARB-AN., CARB-V., CARBN-S.,** ***card-m.,*** carl., casc., **CAUST.,** cench., cham., ***chel.,*** chim., chin., chin-ar., chin-s., chr-ac., cic., cimic., ***cimx.,*** cina, cinnb., clem., ***coca,*** cocc., ***coff.,*** colch., **COLL.,** ***coloc.,*** con., cop., croc., crot-h., cub., cupr., cupr-acet., cupr-ar., cur., cycl., cyt-l., dig., ***dios.,*** dol., dulc., elaps, ***erig.,*** ery-a., ***eug.,*** euon., euphr., ***ferr., ferr-ar.,*** ferr-i., ferr-m., ferr-p., ferul., ***fl-ac.,*** gall-ac., gels., glon., gran., **GRAPH.,** grat., gua., **HAM.,** ***hell.,*** helo., ***hep., hydr.,*** hydro-c., ***hyos., hyper., ign., iod., ip.,*** joan., **KALI-AR.,** ***kali-bi.,*** **KALI-C.,** kali-chl., ***kali-m.,*** kali-n., kali-p., **KALI-S.,** kali-sil., kreos., **LACH.,** lact., lam., laps., ***lept.,*** lil-t., lob., **LYC.,** lycps., lyss., m-aust., m-ambo., mag-c., ***mag-m.,*** mag-p., manc., med., meny., ***merc.,*** merc-cy., **MERC-I-R.,** mez., mill., morg., morg-g., mosch., ***muc-u.,*** **MUR-AC.,** nat-c., ***nat-m., nat-s.,*** neg., **NIT-AC.,** nux-m., **NUX-V.,** op., ozone, **PAEON.,** paraf., ***petr.,*** petros., ph-ac., **PHOS.,** phys., ***phyt.,*** pin-s., pitu-a., plan., plat., plb., ***podo., polyg.,*** polyp-p., prot., ***psor.,*** **PULS.,** rad-br., ran-s., ***rat.,*** rhodi., rhodi-o-n., rhus-g., ***rhus-t.,*** rhus-v., rumx., ***ruta, sabin., sang.,*** sars., scroph-n., sec., sed-ac., ***semp.,*** **SEP.,** ***sil.,*** slag, spig., stann., ***staph.,*** stram., stront-c., ***sul-ac.,*** sul-i., **SULPH.,** sumb., symph., syph., ***ter.,*** ther., ***thuj., tub.,*** urt-u., vac., verat., verat-v., verb., ***wye.,*** yohim, zinc., zinc-p., ***zing.***

HEPATITIS, infection, liver - **ACON.,** ***act-sp.,*** adlu., aesc., alco., aloe, alum., am-c., ambr., anag., anan., ant-c., ***ant-t.,*** apis, ***arn.,*** **ARS.,** ars-i., asaf., astac., ***aur.,*** aur-m., bapt., **BELL.,** bol., ***bry.,*** cael., ***calc.,*** calc-f., ***camph.,*** cann-s., canth., ***caps.,*** **CARC., CARD-M.,** ***cham.,*** **CHEL.,** chelo., chim., ***chin.,*** cic., cocc., coloc., ***corn., crot-h.,*** cub., cupr., cupr-acet., ***dig.,*** dol., eup-per., euph-c., fl-ac., ***flor-p.,*** graph., grin., guat., ***hep., hippoz., hydr.,*** ign., iod., kali-ar., kali-bi., ***kali-c.,*** kali-chl., kali-i., kali-n., kali-p., ***lach., laur.,*** lept., **LYC.,** mag-c., ***mag-m.,*** mand., mang., mang-m., mang-s., med., menis., ***merc.,*** merc-c., merc-d., morg-g., nat-ar., nat-c., ***nat-m.,*** **NAT-S.,** ***nit-ac.,*** nit-m-ac., nux-m., **NUX-V.,** ost., petr., ***ph-ac.,*** **PHOS.,** phyt., plb., ***podo., psor., ptel.,*** puls., ran-b., ran-s., rob., sang., sarr., **SCIRR.,** sec., sel., sep., sil., solin., ***stann.,*** staph., stel., sulfa., ***sulph.,*** tab., tell., verat-v., vip., vip-a., wies.

HERNIA, general - acon., aesc., ***all-c., alum.,*** alumn., am-c., am-m., ***apis, asar., aur.,*** bell., berb., ***calc.,*** calc-ar., caps., ***carb-an., carb-v.,*** cham., ***cocc., coff.,*** coloc., ***dig.,*** guai., lach., **LYC.,** ***mag-c.,*** mag-m., mill., ***mur-ac., nit-ac.,*** **NUX-V.,** ***op.,*** petr., phos., plb., prun., psor., puls., ***rhus-t.,*** sars., sep., ***sil., spig.,*** staph., ***sulph., sul-ac.,*** ter., thuj., ***verat., zinc.***

- **inguinal** - aesc., ***all-c., alum.,*** am-c., ***apis, asar., aur.,*** berb., ***calc.,*** calc-ar., caps., ***carb-an., carb-v., cocc., coff.,*** coloc., ***dig.,*** lach., **LYC.,** ***mag-c.,*** mill., ***mur-ac., nit-ac.,*** **NUX-V.,** ***op.,*** petr., phos., prun., psor., ***rhus-t.,*** sars., ***sil., spig.,*** staph., ***sulph., sul-ac.,*** ter., thuj., ***verat., zinc.***
- **scrotal,** congenital - mag-m.
- **strangulated** - acon., ***all-c.,*** alum., alumn., ars., aur., **BELL.,** calc., caps., ***carb-v.,*** cham., ***cocc., coff.,*** coloc., ***dig.,*** lach., lyc., mill., nit-ac., **NUX-V., OP.,** ***plb.,*** rhus-t., sil., ***sulph., sul-ac., tab.,*** verat.
- **umbilical** - ***calc.,*** cocc., ***lach.,*** lyc., ***nux-m.,*** **NUX-V..** ***op.,*** **PLB.,** tub.

HERNIATED, disk syndrome, slipped or ruptured vertebrae - **AESC.,** arn., **AGAR.,** ***berb.,*** **BRY.,** ***coloc.,*** **HYPER.,** kali-c., mag-p., ruta, tarent., ***tell.,*** zinc.

HEROIN, ailments from - agar., apom., ars., aur., **AVEN.**, bell., calc., cann-i., ***cham.,*** cic., cimic., cod., coff., ***herin.,*** hyos., **IP.,** kali-ma., ***lach.,*** lob., ***macrin.,*** merc., ***morph.,*** mur-ac., ***narcot.,*** nat-p., **NUX-V., OP.,** ox-ac., ***passi.,*** phos., plat., puls., stram., valer., zinc.

cravings, for - apom., **AVEN.,** lob., ***ip.,*** nat-p., ***nux-v., op.,*** ox-ac., passi., upa.

HERPES SIMPLEX - acet-ac., acon., aegle-f., aethi-a., agar., aln., ***alum.***, alum-p., alum-sil., am-c., ambr., anac., anag., ***anan.***, ant-c., ant-t., ***anthro.***, ***apis***, arg-n., arn., **ARS.**, ars-br., ***ars-i.***, ars-s-f., aster., aur., aur-ar., aur-i., aur-m., ***aur-s.***, ba-tn., bac., ***bar-c.***, ***bar-m.***, bar-s., bell., berb., bor., **BOV.**, ***bry.***, bufo, cact., cadm-s., calad., **CALC.**, calc-acet., calc-f., calc-i., **CALC-S.**, calc-sil., ***canth.***, caps., ***carb-ac.***, ***carb-an.***, ***carb-v.***, carbn-o., **CARBN-S.**, carc., ***caust.***, cedr., cham., chel., chin., chrys-ac., chrysar., ***cic.***, ***cist.***, **CLEM.**, cocc., com., **CON.**, cop., cortico., cosm., crot-h., ***croto-t.***, cupr., cycl., dip., dol., **DULC.**, dys-co., equis., eucal., eup-per., euph., fl-ac., form-ac., **GRAPH.**, grat., grin., guare., hell., ***hep.***, hydrc., hydrog., hyos., hyper., iod., iris, jug-c., jug-r., ***kali-ar.***, ***kali-bi.***, ***kali-c.***, ***kali-chl.***, ***kali-i.***, kali-n., kali-p., ***kali-s.***, kali-sil., kalm., ***kreos.***, ***lac-c.***, lac-d., ***lach.***, ***led.***, lith-c., **LYC.**, m-arct., mag-c., ***mag-m.***, mag-s., manc., mand., mang., med., menis., menth., **MERC.**, mez., morg., morg-g., morph., mosch., mucor, mur-ac., ***nat-ar.***, ***nat-c.***, **NAT-M.**, nat-p., ***nat-s.***, nat-sil., nit-ac., nux-v., oci-s., ol-j., ***olnd.***, par., ***petr.***, ph-ac., ***phos.***, phyt., pip-m., plb., prot., prun., ***psor.***, puls., **RAN-B.**, ran-s., rhod., **RHUS-T.**, rob., rumx., ruta, sabad., sac-alb., sal-ac., sanic., ***sars.***, sel., semp., **SEP.**, sieg., **SIL.**, sol-n., sphing., spig., spong., squil., stann., ***staph.***, stram., stry-ar., sul-ac., sul-i., **SULPH.**, syc-co., tarax., tax., **TELL.**, ter., teucr., thal., thuj., torul., tub., valer., vario., verat., viol-t., xero, zinc., zinc-p., zinc-val.

HERPES ZOSTER, shingles - acon., agar., apis, arg-n., arn., ***ars.***, aster., ***ba-tn.***, bell., bry., bufo, canth., carbn-o., carbn-s., caust., cedr., cham., cist., **CLEM.,** com., cosm., crot-h., croto-t., dip., dol., dulc., euph., form-ac., ***graph.***, grin., ***hep.***, hyper., iod., **IRIS**, kali-ar., ***kali-bi.***, ***kali-chl.***, kali-i., ***kalm.***, lac-c., ***lach.***, mand., menth., **MERC.**, **MEZ.**, morg-g., morph., nat-c., **NAT-M.,** ***petr.***, phos., pip-m., prun., puls., **RAN-B.**, ran-s., **RHUS-T.**, sal-ac., sel., semp., ***sep.***, sieg., ***sil.***, sphing., staph., stry-ar., ***sulph.***, ***thal.***, ***thuj.***, tub., ***vario.***, zinc., zinc-p., zinc-val.

HICCOUGHS, hiccups - acet-ac., acon., aeth., aether, ***agar.***, agn., all-c., ***alum.***, alum-p., alum-sil., am-c., **AM-M.**, ambr., aml-n., amyg-am., anac., anan., ang., ant-c., ant-t., apoc., arg., arg-m., arg-n., ***arn.***, **ARS.**, ars-h., **ARS-I.**, ars-s-f., arund., asaf., asar., aur., aur-ar., aur-i., **AUR-S.**, ***bar-c.***, ***bar-i.***, bar-m., bar-s., ***bell.***, benz-ac., berb., bism., bor., bov., brom., ***bry.***, bufo, caj., calad., ***calc.***, calc-f., calc-i., calc-sil., calen., cann-s., canth., caps., carb-ac., carb-an., carb-v., carbn-s., carl., cast., caust., ***cham.***, chel., ***chin.***, chin-ar., ***chin-s.***, ***chlf.***, **CIC.**, cimx., cina, cinnam., cob., coca, cocain., ***cocc.***, ***coff.***, colch., coloc., con., cop., crot-h., croto-t., cupr., cupr-ar., cupr-s., cur., **CYCL.**, dig., ***dios.***, ***dros.***, dulc., eug., eup-a., eup-per., ***euph.***, euphr., ferr-p., fil., gamb., ***gels.***, ***gins.***, gnaph., graph., grat., ham., hell., hep., hura, hydr., hydr-ac., **HYOS.**, **IGN.**, indg., **IOD.**, ***ip.***, ipom., jab., ***jatr.***, jug-r., kali-ar., kali-bi., ***kali-br.***, kali-c., kali-chl., kali-i., kali-n., kali-s., kali-sil., ***kreos.***, ***lach.***, lachn., ***laur.***, led., lob., **LYC.**, lyss., mag-c., ***mag-m.***, **MAG-P.**, mand., ***med.***, meny., **MERC.**, merc-c., merc-cy., mez., mill., ***morph.***, ***mosch.***, mur-ac., **NAT-AR.**, **NAT-C.**, **NAT-M.**, nat-s., nat-sil., **NICC.**, nicot., nit-ac., **NUX-M.**, **NUX-V.**, oci-s., ol-suc., ***op.***, ox-ac., ozone, ***par.***, petr., ph-ac., ***phos.***, phys., phyt., piloc., plat., plb., ***psor.***, ***puls.***, ***ran-b.***, ran-s., **RAT.**, rhus-t., rob., ***ruta***, sabad., sabin., samb., sang., ***sars.***, scut., **SEC.**, sel., sep., sil., sin-n., ***spong.***, ***stann.***, staph., **STRAM.**, ***stront-c.***, stroph., succ., ***sul-ac.***, sul-i., sulph., sumb., tab., tarax., tarent., **TEUCR.**, thuj., til., trif-p., ***verat.***, ***verat-v.***, ***verb.***, vib-p., wye., zinc., zinc-o., zinc-p., ***zinc-val.***

HIGH BLOOD, pressure, (see Hypertension)

HIVES, skin - ***acon.,*** agar., all-c., alum., am-c., am-m., ***ant-c.,*** **APIS**, arn., **ARS.**, ***ars-i.***, **ARS-S-F.**, arum-d., **ASTAC.**, aur., bar-c., bell., bell-p., benz-ac., ***bov.,*** ***calad.,*** calc., calc-s., canth., caps., **CARB-AC.,** chlor., croto-t., dulc., dys-co., fago., gaert., gall-ac., ***galph.***, ***graph.,*** hep., **HIST.,** hom., ***ichth.***, ign., iod., ip., **LED.**, ***lyc.,*** med., medus., merc., ***mez.,*** morg-g., mur-ac., nat-c., **NAT-M.**, ***nat-p.,*** nit-ac., ***nux-v.***, ***ox-ac.,*** pic-ac., pin-s., pip-n., ***psor.,*** ***puls.,*** **RHUS-T.**, rhus-v., ***sal-ac.,*** saroth., sulfa., **SULPH.**, ***sul-ac.,*** ter., tet., thuj., ***til.***, ***trio.***, tub., ust., **URT-U.,** valer., vario., vesp., voes., zinc.

HODGKIN'S DISEASE - ***acon.,*** acon-l., ***ars.,*** ***ars-i.,*** **AUR.,** ***aur-i.,*** ***bar-i.,*** buni-o., ***calc-f.,*** ***carc.,*** cist., con., ***cund.,*** ferr-pic., **IOD.,** ***kali-m.,*** lap-a., ***nat-m.,*** ph-ac., ***phos.,*** **PHYT.,** saroth., ***scirr.,*** **SCROPH-N., SPONG.,** syph., ***thuj.,*** ***tub.***

HOMESICKNESS, nostalgia, general - acon., ant-c., **AUR.,** bar-c., ***bell.,*** **BRY.,** ***calc.,*** calc-p., **CAPS.,** **CARB-AN.,** ***carc.,*** carl., ***caust.,*** cent., chlor., cimic., ***clem.,*** ***cocc.,*** ***coff.,*** ***crat.,*** dros., elaps, elat., eup-per., eup-pur., ***hell.,*** hipp., hyos., **IGN.,** iris-t., kali-m., ***kali-p.,*** kreos., lach., lipp., mag-c., **MAG-M.,** manc., meli., ***meny.,*** **MERC., NAT-M.,** ***nit-ac.,*** op., petr., **PH-AC.,** ***phos.,*** plan., plb., puls., puls-n, sac-l., sac-alb., senec., sep., ***sil.,*** ***staph.,*** valer., verat., ***zinc.***

HORMONES, ailments from hormone replacement therapy - adren., agn., apis, arg., arg-n., ars., aur-m-n., bar-c., bell-p., calc., ***carc., caul.,*** cimic., cocc., ***con.,*** cortico., cortiso., croc., cupr., dam., ***estrog.,*** ferr., **FOLL.,** gins., ***helon.,*** ign., insul., iod., kali-c., kali-s., ***lac-c., lac-h.,*** **LACH.,** lap-a., lil-t., luna, lyc., med., ***melat.,*** merc., murx., nat-m., ***orch., ov.,*** pall., phos., phyt., plat., plb., **PULS.,** sabin., sec., **SEP.,** staph., sulph., ***testos.,*** thuj., ***thyr.,*** ust., valer.

birth conrol pills - caul., estrog., foll., ov., ***puls., sep.***

estrogen - agn., carc., caul., cimic., cortico., cortiso., estrog., foll., helon., lac-c., lach., ov., puls., ***sep.,*** thyr.

premarin - estrog., foll., ov., ***sep.***

progestrogen - caul., cimic., estrog., foll., ov., puls., ***sep.***

testosterone - agn., cortico., cortiso., gins., orch., testos., thuj., thyr.

thyroid - calc., calc-i., iris, lyc., sep., thyr.

HOT FLASHES, flushes, (see Menopause) - acet-ac., acon., aesc., agn., ail., alum., ***alumn.,*** ambr., am-c., am-m., aml-n., androc., ang., ant-t., apis, ***arn.,*** ars., ***ars-i.,*** arum-t., asar., aur., bapt., bar-c., bell., berb., bism., bor., bov., brom., bry., bufo, ***cact.,*** **CALC.,** ***calc-s.,*** carb-an., ***carb-v., carbn-s.,*** **CAUST.,** cham., chel., ***chin.,*** chin-s., cimx., **COCC.,** coff., ***colch.,*** coloc., corn., croc., crot-h., croto-t., cupr., dig., dros., ***elaps,*** eup-per., ***ferr.,*** ferr-ar., ferr-i., ferr-p., gamb., **GLON.,** ***graph.,*** hep., helon., hura, ***hydrog.,*** hyos., ***ign., iod., kali-s., kreos.,*** lac-ac., **LACH.,** lob., **LYC.,** lyss., mag-m., **MANG.,** ***meny., merc.,*** nat-ar., nat-c., nat-m., nat-p., **NAT-S.**, **NIT-AC.,** ***nux-v.,*** olnd., op., ***ox-ac., petr.,*** ph-ac., **PHOS.,** plat., podo., **PSOR.**, **PULS.**, raph., rumx., ***rhus-t.,*** ruta, sabad., sabin., ***sang.,*** seneg., **SEP.,** ***sil.,*** spig., ***spong.,*** stann., **SULPH.,** **SUL-AC.**, **SUMB.,** teucr., **THUJ.**, **TUB.,** valer., ***xan.,*** zinc.

HOUSEMAID'S, knee, bursae - **ARN.,** calc-p., cann-s., caust., ***graph.,*** iod., kali-br., kali-m., ***ruta,*** **NAT-M.**, **SIL.,** stann., **STICT.,** ***sulph.***

HUMILIATION, ailments, from, (See Abuse) - ***acon.,*** agath-a., all-c., aloe, alum., am-m., ambr., **ANAC.,** ***apoc., arg-n., ars., aur., aur-m., aur-m-n.,*** bell., ***bry.,*** calc., calc-s., camph., carb-an., carb-v., **CARC.,** ***caust.,*** **CHAM.**, **COLOC.,** ***chin.,*** chin-b., ***cocc.,*** con., cur., form., gels., grat., ham., **IGN.,** ip., lac-c., ***lach.,*** **LYC.,** ***lyss.,*** merc., ***mur-ac.,*** **NAT-M.,** nit-ac., ***nux-v., op.,*** **PALL.,** petr., **PH-AC.,** phel., phos., ***plat., puls.,*** ran-b., rham-p., rhus-g., rhus-t., ***seneg., sep., sil.,*** **STAPH.,** stram., ***sulph.,*** verat., zinc.

HYDROCELE, scrotum - ***abrot.,*** am-c., ambr., ammc., ampe-qu, ant-c., **APIS**, ***arn., ars.,*** ars-i., ***aur.,*** aur-i., aur-s., bell., berb., bry., calad., ***calc.,*** calc-f., ***calc-p., calc-s.,*** calc-sil., canth., carb-v., ***carbn-s.,*** caust., chel., chin., ***clem., con.,*** cor-r., croto-t., cupr-ar., ***dig.,*** dios., dulc., euph., fago., ***fl-ac.,*** gaert., **GRAPH.**, ham., ***hell., hep.,*** **IOD.**, kali-c., ***kali-chl., kali-i., lyc., lyss.,*** med., merc., ***merl.,*** mur-ac., ***nat-m.,*** nat-s., nit-ac., ***nux-v.,*** petr., ph-ac., phos., plb., ***psor.,*** **PULS.**, ran-b., **RHOD.**, rhus-t., samb., sars., ***sel.,*** sep., **SIL.,** ***spong.,*** squil., staph., sul-ac., sul-i., ***sulph.,*** teucr., thuj., tub., uran-n., urt-u., verat-v.

HYDROCEPHALUS - abrot., acon., alco., am-c., amyg-am., **APIS**, apoc., arg-n., ***arn., ars.,*** ars-i., ***art-v., aur.,*** aur-ar., aur-s., bac., bar-c., bell., ***bry.,*** **CALC.,** ***calc-f.,*** calc-hp., calc-i., ***calc-p., calc-sil., camph.,*** canth., carb-ac., caust., ***chin.,*** chin-s., ***cina, colch., con.,*** crot-h., cupr., cupr-acet., ***cupr-m.,*** cur., ***cypr.,*** cyt-l., ***dig., ferr.,*** ferr-i., gels., hed., ***hell., hyos.,*** ign., indg., ***iod.,*** iodof., ***ip., kali-br.,*** kali-hp., ***kali-i.,*** kali-p., lach., **LYC.**, lyss., mag-m., ***merc., nat-m.,*** nux-v., oeno., ***op.,*** petr., ph-ac., ***phos.,*** plat., ***podo., puls.,*** rhus-t., samb., sant., **SIL.,** sol-n., spig., squil., ***stram.,*** sulfon., ***sulph.,*** thuj., **TUB.,** verat., viol-t., vip., zinc., zinc-br., zinc-m.

HYDROPHOBIA, fear of water, (see Rabies) - acet-ac., acon., aconin., agav-a., agn., am-c., anag., anan., ant-c., anthr., apis, aran., arg-n., ars., ***aspar.,*** **BELL.,** brom., calc., camph., camph-br., cann-i., ***canth.,*** carc., cedr., chlol., cocci-s., crot-h., cupr., ***cur.,*** fagu., gels., gent-c., grin., gua., ho., **HYDR-AC.**, **HYOS.,** hyper., iod., jatr., kali-br., ***lach.,*** laur., lith-br., **LYSS.**, mand., merc., naja, nat-m., nux-v., phel., phos., phys., plb., ran-s., ruta, sabad., scut., spirae., **STRAM.**, stry., sulph., tanac., tann-ac., tarent., ter., trach., verat., xanth.

HYPERGLYCEMIA, high blood sugar, (see Diabetes) - **ARG-N.**, ***chin., cina, insulin.,*** iod., **LYC.,** olnd., **PHOS.,** ***sac-alb.,*** stann., verat., ***zinc.***

HYPERSENSITIVE, increased susceptibility - apis., ***ars., coff.,*** med., ***merc.,*** nat-c., ***nit-ac.,*** nux-v., ***phos.,*** psor., sul-ac., sulph.

HYPERTENSION, high blood pressure - acon., adon., ***adren.,*** agar., all-s., **AML-N.**, anh., ant-ar., aran., aran-ix., arg-n., arn., ars., asar., aster., **AUR.,** aur-br., aur-i., aur-m., aur-m-n., ***bar-c.,*** bar-m., bell., ***calc.,*** calc-f., calc-p., calcul-r., caust., chin-s., chloram., chlorpr., choc., coff., con., convo-s., cortico., cortiso., **CRAT.,** cupr., cupr-acet., cupr-ar., cyna., cyt-l., dig., ergot., esp-g., fl-ac., gels., **GLON.,** ***grat.,*** hyosin., ign., iod., ipom., iris, kali-c., ***kali-chl.,*** kali-p., kali-sal., kres., **LACH.,** lat-m., lyc., lycps., mag-c., mand., methys., morg., naja, **NAT-M.**, nit-ac., **NUX-V.**, onop., ph-ac., phos., pic-ac., pitu-p., ***plb.,*** plb-i., psor., puls., rad-br., ***rauw.,*** reser., rhus-t., sang., saroth., ***sec.,*** sep., ser-ang., sil., squil., ***stront-c., stront-i.,*** stroph., sulph., ***sumb.,*** tab., thal., thlaspi, thuj., valer., vanad., **VERAT.**, verat-v., ***visc.***

HYPOSTASIS - am-c., ***carb-v.,*** rhus-t., ***sep.***

HYPOTENSION, low blood pressure - acon., adlu., agar., ***am-c.***, aran., bar-m., ***calc.,*** cact., **CARB-V.,** chlorpr., cortico., cur., ferr., gels., glon., halo., hist., lach., lat-m., levo., lyc., meph., naja, nat-f., ***nat-m.,*** ***phos.***, rad-br., ***rauw.,*** reser., rhus-t., rib-ac., **SEP.**, staph., sulfa., ther., thiop., thymol., ***thyr.,*** v-a-b., verat., visc.

HYPOGLYCEMIA, low blood sugar, agg. - ***alum.,*** arg-n., ***aur., cact.,*** canth., ***caust.,*** chin., ***cina., croto-t.,*** ferr., **GRAPH.,** hell., **IOD., KALI-C., LYC.,** olnd., nux-v., **PHOS.,** plat., ***psor.,*** rhus-t., **SIL.,** ***spig.,*** stann., **SULPH.,** valer., verat., ***zinc.***

HYPOTHERMIA, general - acetan., arg-n., ***ars.,*** ars-h., atra-r., cact., ***carb-v.,*** chin-s., chlor., chlorpr., coli., cupr-acet., diph., eucal., kali-br., kali-p., lycps., nat-sal., pyrog., reser., sapo.

HYSTERICAL, behavior - abies-n., abrot., absin., ***acet-ac., acon.,*** aether, agn., ***agar., aloe, alum.,*** alum-sil., am-val., ***ambr.,*** am-c., aml-n., ***anac.,*** anag., apis, aquil., ***arg-n.,*** arn., ***ars.,*** ars-s-f., ***art-v.,*** arund., **ASAF.,** asar., asc-t., aster., **AUR.,** aur-ar., aur-i., aur-s., bapt., ***bar-c.,*** bar-i., bell., benz-ac., bor., brom., bry., bufo, ***cact., caj.,*** calad., ***calc., calc-s.,*** calc-sil., ***camph.,*** camph-br., cann-i., ***canth.,*** cann-s., ***carbn-s.,*** **CARC.,** ***cast., caul.,*** **CAUST.,** cedr., ***cham., chen-a.,*** chim., chin., chin-s., ***chlf.,*** chlor., cic., ***cimic., chlol., cinnam.,*** cob., ***coca,*** **COCC.,** ***coff., coff-t.,*** **CON.,** convo-s., cop., cor-r., cot., crot-h., croto-t., ***croc.,*** cupr., cypr., ***elaps,*** electr., ***eup-a.,*** eup-pur., ***ferr.,*** ferr-ar., ferr-i., ferr-p., **GELS.,** ***graph., grat.,*** hell., hura, ***hydr-ac., hyos., ictod.,*** **IGN.,** ***indg.,*** iod., ip., kali-ar., ***kali-c.,*** **KALI-P.,** kali-s., kali-sil., ***lac-ac.,*** lac-c., **LACH.,** lact., ***lil-t.,*** lob., ***lyc., mag-c.,*** **MAG-M., MAND.,** mang., **MERC.,** mez., ***mill.,*** morph., **MOSCH.,** mygal., nat-ar., ***nat-c.,*** nat-hchls., **NAT-M.,** nat-p., nat-s., nat-sil., **NIT-AC.,** nitro-o., **NUX-M., NUX-V.,** ol-an., op., orig., ***pall.,*** par., ***ph-ac., phos.,*** phys., **PLAT.,** ***plb.,*** polyg., ictod., **PULS.,** pyrus, ***raph., rhus-t.,*** sabin., sac-alb., sang., scut., ***sec.,*** **SEP.,** senec., **SIL.,** spira., stann., staph., ***stict.,*** stram., stry-p., succ., sul-ac., sul-i., ***sulph., sumb.,*** **TARENT.,** thal., ***ther.,*** thuj., thyr., ust., **VALER., VERAT.,** vib., ***viol-o.,*** visc., xan., zinc., zinc-c., ***zinc-val., ziz.***

I

ICHTHYOSIS, skin - agar., ***am-m.,*** anac., anag., ant-c., **ARS.,** ***ars-i., aur., bar-m., bell.,*** bor., bufo, cact., cadm-s., ***calad., calc.,*** calc-s., canth., chin., cic., **CLEM.,** coloc., com., cupr., cycl., dulc., ***fl-ac., graph.,*** hep., ***hydrc.,*** hyos., ichth., iod., kali-ar., ***kali-bi.,*** kali-c., kali-i., ***kali-s.,*** lac-c., ***led.,*** lyc., ***mag-c.,*** med., ***merc.,*** mez., ***nat-ar.,*** nat-c., ***nat-m., nit-ac.,*** nuph., oena., ol-j., ***olnd.,*** petr., **PHOS., PHYT.,** pip-m., platan., ***plb., psor.,*** rad-br., ***rhus-t.,*** sang., sarr., ***sars.,*** **SEP.,** ***sil.,*** staph., ***sulph.,*** syph., tell., teucr., thuj., ***thyr.***, tub.

ICTERUS, jaundice, newborn - card-m., ***chel.,*** chion., coll., merc., nux-v.

ILEUS, obstruction of intestines - acon., aesc., **ALUM.,** ammc., ***anac.***, ant-t., apoc., arg-n., arn., ars., asaf., atro., bell., bry., calad., cand-a., cann-s., ***caps., carb-an.***, carb-v., cast., ***caust.***, cham., chin., cocc., ***colch.***, coloc., cupr., gels., ***graph.***, kali-bi., ***kali-c.***, karw-h., kreos., lac-d., ***lach.***, lob., lyc., merc., merc-c., nat-m., nit-ac., nux-v., **OP.,** phos., pitu-p., plat., **PLB.,** pyrog., rhus-t., ric., ruta, samb., ***sars.***, sec., ***sep.***, sil., sol-t-ae., staph., stront-c., sulph., tab., tann-ac., tarent., thuj., verat., visc., zinc.

IMPACTION, of bowels, (see Intussusception) - ***alum.,*** **BELL.,** ***caust.,*** coloc., gels., lac-d., ***lach.,*** **OP., PLB.**

paralysis - **OP.,** ***phos.,*** **PLB.,** ***sec.***

IMPETIGO, skin - aln., alum., am-c., **ANT-C.,** ant-s., ant-t., ***ars.,*** ars-i., ***arum-t.***, bac., bar-c., calc., calc-m., ***calen.,*** carb-ac., carb-v., carbn-s., caust., cic., clem., con., croto-t., dys-co., ***dulc.,*** **ECHI.,** euph., ferr-ar., ferr-i., graph., ***hep., iris, jug-c.,*** jug-r., ***kali-bi.,*** kali-n., kreos., lact., lappa, lyc., maland., merc., ***mez.,*** nat-c., nat-m., ***nit-ac.,*** olnd., ***ph-ac.,*** phos., ***rhus-t.,*** rhus-v., sars., sep., ***sil.,*** staph., staphycoc., sulph., ***syc-co.***, thuj., tub., viol-t.

IMPOTENCY, male - ***agar.***, **AGN.,** alco., ***alum.***, alum-p., am-c., ambr., ***anac.***, anil., ***ant-c.***, ant-o., aq-mar., arg., ***arg-n.***, ***arn.***, ars., ars-i., arum-d., aur., aur-i., aur-s., aven., ba-sv., **BAR-C.**, bar-i., bar-s., bart., bell-p., benz-d., berb., bor., ***bufo***, buth-aust., **CALAD., CALC.**, calc-i., **CALC-S.**, ***camph.***, cann-i., cann-s., caps., carb-ac., carb-an., carb-v., carbn-s., carc., card-m., ***caust.***, cere-s., **CHIN.**, chin-s., chlol., chlor., cinnam., clem., ***cob.***, ***coc-c.***, coch., cod., ***coff.***, coloc., **CON.**, corn., cortico., cot., crot-h., croto-t., cub., dam., dig., dios., dol., dulc., elaps, ery-a., ery-m., eug., eup-pur., euph., fab., ***ferr.***, ferr-i., ferr-m., ferr-p., ***fl-ac.***, gast., ***gels.***, gins., glyc., ***graph.***, halo., ***ham.***, ***hell.***, helon., ***hep.***, hydr., hydrc., hyos., ***hyper.***, ign., ***iod.***, kali-bi., ***kali-br.***, kali-c., kali-i., ***kali-p.***, kali-s., kreos., ***lach.***, lact., lappa, lath., ***lec.***, levo., **LYC.**, lyss., m-aust., ***mag-c.***, **MED.**, meny., ***merc.***, merc-n., morph., ***mosch.***, mur-ac., nat-c., ***nat-m.***, ***nat-p.***, ***nit-ac.***, ***nuph.***, ***nux-m.***, **NUX-V.**, oci-s., onis., ***onos.***, ***op.***, orch., ox-ac., oxyt., pall., perh., petr., ***ph-ac.***, phase., **PHOS.**, ***phyt.***, ***pic-ac.***, plan., ***plb.***, polyg., ***psor.***, ***puls.***, rhod., rhodi., rhodi-o-n., ruta, ***sabad.***, ***sabal.***, sabin., ***salx-n.***, saroth., scut., sec., **SEL.**, **SEP.**, sil., sin-a., sin-n., spong., ***stann.***, ***staph.***, stram., ***stry.***, sul-ac., sul-i., **SULPH.**, sumb., syc-co., ***syph.***, tab., teucr., thal., thala., ther., **THUJ.**, trib., tus-p., ***uran-n.***, ust., ***yohim***, zinc., zinc-p.

INCOORDINATION, general - absin., ***agar.***, **ALUM.**, ***arag.***, **ARG-N.**, bar-c., bell., bufo, ***calc.***, carbn-s., caust., chlol., coca, cocc., **CON.**, crot-c., ***cupr.***, ***gels.***, hyos., med., **MERC.**, nux-m., ***onos.***, ***ph-ac.***, ***phos.***, pic-ac., ***plb.***, psil., sec., sil., ***stram.***, stry., ***sulph.***, tab., ***zinc.***

INFANTILISMUS, genitalis - ***bar-c.***, calc-hp., calc-p., chim., con., ferr., helon., iod., ***ov.***, phos., senec., thyr.

INFERTILITY, female, (see Sterility) - **AGN.**, ***alet.***, alum., ***am-c.***, anag., anan., apis, **AUR.**, ***aur-i.***, aur-m., aur-m-n., bar-c., ***bar-m.***, **BOR.**, brom., ***calc.***, calc-i., cann-i., cann-s., ***canth.***, caps., carbn-s., ***caul.***, caust., cic., cocc., ***coff.***, **CON.**, croc., dam., dulc., ***eup-pur.***, ***ferr.***, ***ferr-p.***, ***fil.***, ***foll.***, form., ***goss.***, ***graph.***, helon., ***hyos.***, ***iod.***, ***kali-br.***, kali-c., ***kreos.***, ***lach.***, lappa, lec., lil-t., mand., ***med.***, ***merc.***, mill., mit., **NAT-C.**, **NAT-M.**, nat-p., ***nux-m.***, nux-v., ***orig.***, ***ov.***, ***phos.***, phyt., pituin., ***plat.***, plb., ***puls.***, ruta, ***sabal.***, ***sabin.***, sec., ***senec.***, **SEP.**, ***sil.***, sulph., ***sul-ac.***, ***syph.***, ther., ***thuj.***, vib., wies., x-ray, ***zinc.***

INJECTIONS, ailments, from - androc., ***crot-h.***, **HYPER.**, ***led.***, ***plat.***

INFLUENZA, infection - ***acon.***, aesc., all-c., ant-ar., ant-i., ant-t., ***arn.***, **ARS.**, ***ars-i.***, ars-s-r., asc-t., bac., bad., bamb-a., **BAPT.**, ***bell.***, ***brom.***, **BRY.**, calc., camph., canch., capp., ***carb-ac.***, ***carc.***, card-m., ***caust.***, ***chel.***, ***chin.***, ***chin-s.***, cimic., cupr-ar., cycl., dros., ***dulc.***, ery-a., ***eucal.***, **EUP-PER.**, euph., euphr., ferr-p., **GELS.**, glon., glyc., gymn., indol., ***influ.***, iod., ip., kali-bi., kali-c., kali-i., kali-s., lach., lob-c., ***lob-p.***, lyc., lycps., med., ***merc.***, ***merc-i-r.***, naja, ***nat-sal.***, ***nux-v.***, **OSCILLO.**, ozone, ph-ac., **PHOS.**, phyt., podo., psor., puls., ***pyrog.***, ran-g., **RHUS-T.**, rumx., ***sabad.***, sal-ac., sang., ***sanguin-n.***, sarcol-ac., sars., seneg., sil., silphu., spig., spong., squil., stann., still., ***stict.***, ***sulph.***, trio., verat., verat-v.

INJURIES, general, (see Blows, Bruises and Falls) - abrot., absin., ***acon.***, agar., ***am-c.***, androc., apis, ***arg.***, **ARN.**, aster., ***aur-m.***, ***bad.***, bell., **BELL-P.**, berb., bor., **BRY.**, calc., calc-f., ***calc-p.***, calc-s., **CALEN.**, **CAMPH.**, ***cann-s.***, ***caust.***, cham., ***cic.***, coloc., ***con.***, cortico., cortiso., echi., ferr-p., glon., graph., guai., ***ham.***, hecla., ***hep.***, **HYPER.**, ign., lac-c., lac-d., ***lach.***, laur., ***led.***, mag-p., m-arct., m-aust., ***mill.***, **NAT-S.**, op., ***phos.***, phyt., ***plan.***, puls., pyrog., rad-br., ***rhod.***, **RHUS-T.**, **RUTA**, sec., ***sil.***, ***staph.***, stram., stront-c., ***sul-ac.***, **SYMPH.**, zinc.

- **blows,** from - ***acon.***, **ARN.**, ***aur-m.***, ***bad.***, **BELL-P.**, ***bry.***, **CALEN.**, ***cic.***, ***con.***, glon., ***ham.***, ***hep.***, **HYPER.**, ***lach.***, ***led.***, **NAT-S.**, puls., pyrog., ***rhus-t.***, **RUTA**, ***sil.***, ***staph.***, stront-c., sul-ac., ***symph.***
- **contusions** - **ARN.**, ***bell-p.***, con., ***ham.***, hyper., led., rhus-t., ruta, sul-ac., symph., ter.
- **hematoma** - ***arn.***, calc-f., ham., merc., mill., ***nat-s.***, sil., symph.
- **limping,** from injury - abrot., acon., ant-c., apis, bell., ***bell-p.***, ***bry.***, calc., calc-f., ***caust.***, coloc., dros., dulc., hep., hydrog., kali-bi., kali-c., lyc., merc., nit-ac., phos., ***rhus-t.***, **RUTA**, sabin., sep., spig., sulph., tab., zinc.
- **mental,** symptoms from - ***acon.***, ***arn.***, bell., camph., ***carc.***, cic., ***glon.***, **HELL.**, hyos., ***hyper.***, mag-c., **NAT-S.**, ***op.***, rhus-t., ruta, ***stram.***, sul-ac., verat.
- **nerves** - all-c., bell-p., bry., **CALEN.**, ***coff.***, ***cur.***, glon., **HYPER.**, led., ***mag-p.***, meny., nit-ac., ***phos.***, plan., plat., tarent., ter., ther., xan.
- **pains,** unbearable - **ACON.**, ***arn.***, ***ars.***, **AUR.**, **BRY.**, **CHAM.**, **COFF.**, ***coloc.***, **HEP.**, ***hyper.***, ***nux-v.***, ***phyt.***, ***pip-m.***, ***syph.***
- **soreness,** from injuries - **ARN.**, ***bell-p.***, bry., calc., lac-ac., ***rhus-t.***, ***ruta.***

INSANITY, madness - absin., acon., aeth., aether, ***agar.***, agn., ail., alco., all-c., ***alum.***, alum-p., alum-sil., ***am-c.***, ambr., **ANAC.**, anag., anan., ant-c., ant-t., ***apis***, ***arg.***, arg-n., ***arn.***, **ARS.**, ars-i., ars-s-f., arum-t., aster., atro., **AUR.**, aur-ar., aur-i., aur-s., bac., bar-c., ***bar-m.***, **BELL.**, berb., bor., bov., brom., ***bufo***, cact., calad., ***calc.***, calc-ar., calc-i., calc-s., calc-sil., ***camph.***, cann-i., cann-s., ***canth.***, carb-an., carbn-s., **CARC.**, ***caust.***, cench., cer-b., ***chel.***, chin-s., chlol., ***cic.***, ***cimic.***, ***cocc.***, coff., colch., coloc., ***con.***, cortiso., ***croc.***, ***crot-c.***, crot-h., **CUPR.**, cur., ***cycl.***, dig., dat-a., ***dulc.***, euph., ferr-p., ferul., fl-ac., gels., gins., ***glon.***, ***hell.***, ***hep.***, **HYOS.**, hyper., ***ign.***, indg., iod., ip., kali-ar., kali-bi., ***kali-br.***, kali-c., ***kali-chl.***, kali-i., ***kali-m.***, kali-ox., ***kali-p.***, **LACH.**, led., ***lil-t.***, ***lol.***, **LYC.**, mand., ***manc.***, med., meli., **MERC.**, merc-c., mez., mosch., murx., naja, nat-c., ***nat-m.***, nat-s., ***nux-m.***, **NUX-V.**, oena., olnd., ol-j., ***op.***, opun-v., ***ox-ac.***, par., passi., penic., ph-ac., ***phos.***, phys., **PLAT.**, plb., ***psor.***, ***puls.***, raph., rhod., ***rhus-t.***, rob., sabad., sec., seneg., sep., sil., sol-n., squil., stann., **STRAM.**, ***sulph.***, **SYPH.**, **TARENT.**, ter., ther., thuj., thyr., ***tub.***, **VERAT.**, verat-v., vip., zinc., zinc-p. , zinc-val.

INSOMNIA, sleeplessness - abrot., absin., ***acon.***, acon-c., acon-f., adon., aeth., aether, ***agar.***, agav-t., agn., agra., alco., alet., alf., allox., ***aloe***, alum., alumn., am-caust., ambr., am-br., am-c., am-m., ***ammc.***, anac., ang., anh., anil., ant-c., ant-o., ant-t., anthr., ant-c., aphis., ***apis***, apoc., apoc-a., apom., aquil., aran., arg-c., arg., **ARG-N.**, ***arn.***, **ARS.**, ars-h., ***ars-i.***, **ARS-S-F.**, ***arum-t.***, arund., asaf., asar., asc-t., asim., ***aster.***, ***atro.***, ***aur.***, aur-m., aur-s., ***aven.***, aza., ***bapt.***, bar-c., bar-m., **BELL.**, bell-p., benz., ***benz-ac.***, bism., ***bor.***, brach., **BRY.**, bufo-s., but-ac., **CACT.**, cadm-s., cahin., calad., **CALC.**, calc-ar., calc-caust., calc-i., ***calc-p.***, calc-s., calo., ***camph.***, ***camph-br.***, canch., cann-i., cann-s., ***canth.***, caps., **CARC.**, ***carl.***, carb-an., ***carb-v.***, ***carbn-s.***, cast., caul., ***caust.***, cean., cedr., cer-b., **CHAM.**, chel., **CHIN.**, ***chin-ar.***, ***chin-s.***, chlf., chlol., chrysan., ***cic.***, cimic., ***cina***, cinnb., **CIT-V.**, clem., cob., coca, cocain., ***cocc.***, coc-c., ***cocci-s.***, coch., **COFF.**, coff-t., coffin., colch., ***coloc.***, ***con.***, cop., corn., cot., croc., crot-c., ***crot-h.***, croto-t., ***cupr.***, cupr-acet., **CYCL.**, **CYPR.**, cyt-l., daph., ***dig.***, dios., dip., dirc., ***dros.***, ***dulc.***, elaps, ery-a., eucal., eug., eup-per., eup-pur., euph., euph-pe., euphr., fago., ***ferr.***, ***ferr-ar.***, ferr-i., ferr-p., fil., ***fl-ac.***, form., gad., gamb., ***gels.***, get., ***glon.***, gran., ***graph.***, grin., ***guai.***, guare., haem., ***hell.***, helon., **HEP.**, hipp., hippoz., hura, hydr., hydr-ac., **HYDROG.**, **HYOS.**, ***hyosin.***, iber., ***ign.***, inul., ***iod.***, iodof., ***ip.***, iris, piloc., jac-c., ***jal.***, jatr., jug-c., jug-r., **KALI-AR.**, ***kali-bi.***, ***kali-br.***, **KALI-C.**, kali-cy., ***kali-i.***, kali-n., kali-p., ***kali-s.***, kalm., ***kreos.***, lac-ac., ***lac-c.***, ***lac-d.***, **LACH.**, ***lachn.***, lact., lat-m., laur., lec., ***led.***, lept., lil-t., ***lup.***, lupin., ***lyc.***, ***lycps.***, lyss., ***mag-c.***, ***mag-m.***, mag-p., ***mag-s.***, manc., mang., **MED.**, meph., **MERC.**, **MERC-C.**, merc-cy., merc-i-f., merc-i-r., merl., mez., morph., mosch., mur-ac., myris., naja, nat-ar., ***nat-c.***, ***nat-m.***, ***nat-p.***, ***nat-s.***, nicc., ***nit-ac.***, ***nux-m.***, **NUX-V.**, olnd., **OP.**, ox-ac., passi., petr., ***ph-ac.***, phel., **PHOS.**, phys., phyt., pic-ac., plan., ***plat.***, **PLB.**, ***podo.***, prun., psor., ptel., **PULS.**, ran-b., ran-s., raph., rheum, rhod., **RHUS-T.**, rhus-v., ***rumx.***, ruta, sabad., sabin., samb., sang., sarcol-ac., saroth., sarr., sars., ***scut.***, ***sec.***, ***sel.***, ***senec.***, **SEP.**, **SIL.**, sin-n., sol-t-ae., spig., spong., squil., **STANN.**, **STAPH.**, stict., stram., stront-c., stry., sul-ac., sulfon., ***sulph.***, sul-ac., sumb., **SYPH.**, ***tab.***, tarax., ***tarent.***, tax., tela, tell., teucr., thal., **THUJ.**, thea., til., ***tub.***, ***ust.***, ***valer.***, verat., verb., vesp., vinc., viol-o., ***viol-t.***, vip., x-ray, xan., yohim, zinc., zinc-o., zinc-p., zinc-val., zing.

INSULIN, ailments, from - insul., lyc., phos.

INTERMITTENT FEVER, ague, (See Malaria)

INTERTRIGO, skin, (see Dermatitis) - acon., ***aeth.***, agn., ***am-c.***, ***ambr.***, arist-cl., arn., ars., ***bar-c.***, bell., ***bor.***, calc., ***calc-s.***, calc-sil., ***carb-v.***, **CAUST.**, ***cham.***, ***chin.***, fago., **GRAPH.**, ***hep.***, ***hydr.***, ***ign.***, jug-r., kali-ar., kali-br., ***kali-c.***, kali-chl., kali-s., ***kali-sil.***, **KREOS.**, ***lyc.***, ***mang.***, ***merc.***, mez., morg., ***nat-m.***, nat-s., ***nit-ac.***, nux-v., ol-an., olnd., ox-ac., ***petr.***, ph-ac., phos., ***phyt.***, plb., psor., puls., rhus-t., ruta, sabin., ***sep.***, ***sil.***, squil., ***sul-ac.***, **SULPH.**, syc-co., syph., tub.

INTOXICATION, ailments, from - abies-c., absin., acet-ac., acon., aether, **AGAR.**, agav-a., agn., ***alco.***, ***am-m.***, aml-n., amyg-am., anh., apom., arg., ars., atro., ***aven.***, bart., bell., berb., bov., ***bry.***, camph., cann-i., cann-s., ***caps.***, carb-an., ***carb-v.***, chel., chin., chin-s., cic., ***coca***, ***cocc.***, ***coff.***, coff-t., con., conin., cop., cori-r., dat-m., eucal., euph., fagu., ferr., **GELS.**, grat., **HYOS.**, ign., indol., **IP.**, kali-bi., kali-c., kali-i., kali-n., kiss., kreos., ***lach.***, lact., ***laur.***, led., lol., merc., mez., mill., ***morph.***, nabal., naja, narcot., nat-m., nux-m., **NUX-V.**, **OKOU.**, **OP.**, ph-ac., phenob., phel., pip-m., ***puls.***, pyrog., ran-b., rheum, rhod., sabad., samb., sec., skat., ***spong.***, squil., ***stram.***, tab., tax., ter., teucr., thea., til., tus-f., urea, valer., ***verat.***, vip., zinc.

INTUSSUSCEPTION, intestines - ***acon.***, ***arn.***, **ARS.**, ***bell.***, ***bry.***, ***colch.***, **COLOC.**, ***cupr.***, ***kali-bi.***, kreos., ***lach.***, ***lob.***, ***lyc.***, ***merc.***, ***nux-v.***, **OP.**, ***phos.***, **PLB.**, ***rhus-t.***, ***samb.***, sulph., tab., tarent., thuj., **VERAT.**

IODINE, ailments from - ant-c., ant-t., ***ars.***, bell., brom., ***calc-i.***, camph., chin., chin-s., coff., ***conv.***, ***hep.***, hydr., ***iod.***, kali-i., lycps., merc., ***op.***, ***phos.***, sang., ***sec.***, spong., sulph.

IRITIS, inflammation, iris - ***acon.***, ant-s., ***apis***, ***arg-n.***, **ARN.**, ***ars.***, ars-i., ars-s-f., ***asaf.***, ***aur.***, aur-ar., aur-i., aur-m., aur-s., bar-i., ***bell.***, bry., calc., ***cedr.***, ***chin.***, ***cinnb.***, ***clem.***, ***colch.***, ***coloc.***, ***com.***, con., crot-h., ***croto-t.***, dubin., ***dulc.***, ***euphr.***, ferr-p., form., gels., grin., ham., ***hep.***, iod., ***kali-bi.***, ***kali-i.***, kali-m., kalm., led., ***merc.***, **MERC-C.**, merc-cy., merc-i-f., merc-pr-r., mez., morg., ***nat-m.***, ***nit-ac.***, nux-v., petr., plb., ***puls.***, **RHUS-T.**, sabal., ***seneg.***, sep., ***sil.***, spig., ***staph.***, sul-i., ***sulph.***, ***syph.***, tell., ***ter.***, thal., thuj., tub., zinc.

IRON, ailments from - alum., ars., calc-p., ***chin.***, chin-ar., cupr., ferr-acet., **FERR.**, ferr-i., **FERR-P.**, ***hep.***, iod., ip., merc., nat-m., phos., ***puls.***, ***sulph.***, thea., verat., ***zinc.***

J

JAUNDICE, general, icterus - acal., **ACON.**, aesc., agar., agn., ***aloe***, alum., alum-p., alum-sil., alumn., am-be., am-c., ***am-m.***, ***ambr.***, ant-c., ant-n-l., ***ant-t.***, apis, arg-n., arn., ***ars.***, ars-i., asaf., astac., ***aur.***, aur-ar., aur-m-n., ***bell.***, ***berb.***, blatta-a., bol., both-l., bov., brom., ***bry.***, bufo, cadm., ***calc.***, calc-i., ***calc-p.***, calc-s., calc-sil., cann-s., ***canth.***, ***carb-v.***, carbn-s., **CARD-M.**, casc., ***caust.***, ***cean.***, cedr., ***cham.***, **CHEL.**, chelo., chen-a., **CHIN.**, ***chin-ar.***, chin-s., **CHION.**, chlorpr., chol., cina, coca, cocc., coll., coloc., **CON.**, ***corn.***, corn-f., croc., crot-c., **CROT-H.**, cupr., cur., ***dig.***, ***dol.***, dulc., elaps, elat., eup-per., euph., fel., ***ferr.***, ferr-ar., ***ferr-i.***, gels., graph., hell., ***hep.***, hip-ac., hippoz., ***hydr.***, hydrc., iber., ***ign.***, **IOD.**, ip., iris, jug-c., just., kali-ar., kali-bi., kali-c., kali-chl., kali-i., kali-p., kali-pic., kali-s., kali-sil., **LACH.**, lap-gr-m., laur., ***lept.***, lina., lob., lup., **LYC.**, mag-m., mang., med., **MERC.**, ***merc-c.***, merc-d., ***morg.***, myric., nat-ar., nat-c., ***nat-m.***, nat-p., **NAT-S.**, **NIT-AC.**, **NUX-V.**, olnd., ***op.***, ost., petr., ph-ac., **PHOS.**, pic-ac., **PLB.**, ***podo.***, pop., psor., ***ptel.***, ***puls.***, ran-b., rheum, rhus-t., ric., rumx., ruta, sabad., ***sang.***, ***sec.***, **SEL.**, **SEP.**, ***sil.***, ***spig.***, stann., still., sul-ac., sul-i., ***sulph.***, tab., tarax., tarent., thuj., thyr., trinit., tub., verat., vip., ***yuc.***, zinc.

JAWS, cancer - ***ant-c.,*** arg-n., ***ars.,*** aur., brom., calc., ***calc-f.,*** carc., fl-ac., graph., **HECLA.,** merc., phos., rhus-t., ***scirr.,*** sil., **SYMPH.**

JET LAG - alum., arg-n., ***arn., cocc.,*** con., ***gels., melat.***

JOINTS, remedies - ***abrot.,*** act-sp., aesc., agar., anac., ***ang.,*** apis, ***arg., arn.,*** **BELL., BENZ-AC., BRY., CALC., CALC-F.,** ***calc-p.,*** calen., ***caul.,*** caust., ***cimic.,*** **COLCH.,** graph., ***guai.,*** hyper., kali-bi., **KALI-C.,** kali-i., **KALM.,** ***lac-ac., lac-c.,*** lach., led., lith-c., ***mang., med.,*** meny., phyt., ***puls., sabin., sal-ac.,*** rhod., **RHUS-T., RUTA,** sars., **SIL.,** sulph., thuj., verat-v.

K

KALA AZAR, disease - androg-p., boerh., ***ferr-ar.,*** nat-m., swer-ch., trich-d.

KELOIDS, skin, (see Scars) - alumn., ars., ***bad.,*** bell-p., calc., ***calen.,*** carb-v., **CARC.,** ***caust.,*** crot-h., ***fl-ac.,*** **GRAPH.,** hyper., ***iod.,*** junc., kali-bi., lach., merc., nit-ac., nux-v., phos., phyt., psor., ***rad-br.,*** rhus-t., sabin., **SIL.,** sul-ac., sulph., **THIOSIN.,** tub., vip.

KIDNEYS, remedies - ***adren.,*** **APIS,** apoc., ***ars.,*** bell., ***benz-ac.,*** **BERB.,** ***calc.,*** calc-ar., ***cann-i.,*** **CANTH.,** carc., caust., ***chel., chim.,*** chin., coc-c., coloc., cupr., dig., **EQUIS.,** helon., ***hep.,*** hyosin., kali-c., ***lac-ac.,*** **LYC.,** ***merc., merc-c.,*** **NAT-M.,** ***nit-ac.,*** nux-v., oci., pareir., **PHOS.,** ***polyg., puls.,*** rhus-t., samb., **SARS.,** ***sec.,*** scopo., ***solid.,*** squil., stront-c., **TER.,** uran-n., ***urt-u.,*** uva, viol-o., zinc.

kidney, failure, inactive - acon., **APIS.,** ***coch.,*** **SER-ANG.,** ***stram., ter., zing.***

KIDNEY STONES - act-sp., ant-c., apoc., arn., bell., **BENZ-AC., BERB., CALC.,** ***calcul-r., canth.,*** chin-s., coc-c., ***coloc.,*** equis., eup-pur., hydrang., ***ipom.,*** lach., **LITH-C., LYC.,** med., mill., morg-g., nat-m., nat-s., ***nit-ac., nux-v.,*** oci., **PAREIR.,** ***petr., phos.,*** **SARS., SEP.,** ***sil., tab.,*** ter., **URT-U.,** uva.

KLEPTOMANIA - ***absin.,*** ars., ***art-v.,*** **BELL.,** bry., calc., carb-v., carc., caust., cic., ***cur., herin.,*** hyos., kali-br., kali-c., lach., lyc., mag-m., mand., med., ***morph.,*** nat-m., ***nux-v.,*** **OP.,** oxyt., plat., ***puls.,*** sep., sil., staph., stram., ***sulph.,*** syph., tarent., ***thuj.***

KREOSOTE, ailments from - ars., bapt., carb-an., chin., con., ferr., ***kreos.,*** merc-c., plb.

KRYPTORCHISM, testes - aur., bar-c., calc., canth., con., cory., cupr., lyc., nat-m., psor., sulph., syph., tub., zinc.

L

LABOR PAINS - acon., aeth., alet., aloe, ambr., aml-n., ant-c., apoc-a., arn., ars., asaf., asar-c., aur., bell., bor., bry., cact., calc., camph., cann-i., cann-s., carb-an., carb-v., carbn-s., **CAUL.,** caust., **CHAM.,** chin., chin-s., chlol., cic., ***cimic.,*** cinnam., cinnb., cocc., ***coff.,*** coff-t., con., conv., cupr., cupr-acet., dios., eup-pur., ferr., **GELS.,** goss., graph., guare., hedeo, hyos., hyper., **IGN.,** iod., ip., jab., **KALI-C.,** kali-p., kreos., lach., lob., lyc., mag-c., mag-m., mag-p., merc., mit., morph., mosch., nat-c., nat-m., nux-m., ***nux-v.,*** op., phos., phyt., pitu-p., plat., **PULS.,** rhus-t., ruta, sabad., sabin., ***sec.,*** **SEP.,** stann., stram., stront-c., sul-ac., sulph., thuj., ust., verat., vib., vib-p., visc., zinc., ziz.

false, labor - acon., alet., apoc-a., arn., **BELL.,** bor., ***bry.,*** **CALC., CAUL.,** caust., ***cham., cimic., cinnam., cinnb.,*** coff., ***con.,*** cupr., ***dios., gels.,*** hedeo, hyos., ign., **IP.,** ***kali-c.,*** kali-p., mit., ***nux-m., nux-v., op.,*** **PULS.,** sec., ***sep.,*** stann., vib., ***vib-p.***

painful, too - acon., ant-c., arn., ***aur.,*** **BELL., CHAM.,** ***chin.,*** cimic., ***cocc.,*** **COFF.,** ***con.,*** cupr., hyos., ***lyc.,*** **KALI-C.,** mag-c., nat-c., **NUX-V.,** ***phos.,*** puls., sec., **SEP.,** sulph.

weak, too feeble - aeth., arn., asaf., ***bell.,*** bor., bry., calc., ***camph.,*** cann-i., cann-s., carb-an., ***carb-v., carbn-s.,*** **CAUL.,** ***caust., cham.,*** chin., **CIMIC.,** cinnam., cocc., coff., **GELS.,** goss., ***graph.,*** guare., hyos., ign., **KALI-C.,** kali-p., kreos., lyc., mag-c., mag-m., merc., mit., mosch., ***nat-c.,*** **NAT-M.,** ***nux-m., nux-v.,*** **OP.,** phos., plat., **PULS.,** rhus-t., ***ruta,*** sabad., **SEC.,** sep., stann., sul-ac., sulph., ***thuj.,*** ust., zinc.

LACERATIONS, injuries, (see Wounds) - arist-cl., arn., **CALEN., CARB-AC.,** echi., ***ham.,*** **HYPER.,** led., ***plan., staph.,*** sul-ac., symph.

LACTIC ACID, poisoning, ailments from, (see Acidosis) - arn., colch., ***lac-ac.,*** lith-c., nat-p.

LABRYINTHITIS, (see Otitis, interna)

LARYNGISMUS, stridor - acet-ac., ***acon., agar.,*** alum., am-caust., ***ant-c., ars.,*** ars-i., arum-d., arum-t., arund., ***asaf.,*** **BELL.,** ***brom.,*** calc., calc-f., calc-i., calc-p., carb-v., cham., ***chel.,*** chin., chlf., chlol., ***chlor.,*** cic., ***coff., cor-r.,*** crot-h., ***cupr., cupr-acet.,*** dig., dros., ferr., ***formal.,*** **GELS.,** gran., guai., guare., hep., hydr-ac., hyos., ictod., **IGN.,** ***iod., ip.,*** kali-br., lac-ac., ***lach.,*** laur., lob., ***mag-p., mang.,*** med., meny., ***meph.,*** merc., merc-c., **MOSCH.,** naja, ol-an., ***op., phos.,*** phyt., plat., plb., puls., ***samb.,*** sang., sars., ***sil., spong.,*** stram., ***stry.,*** sul-i., sulph., syc-co., ***tab., tarent.,*** ter., thuj., ***verat.,*** vesp., visc., zinc.

LARYNGITIS - **ACON.,** ***aesc.,*** **ALL-C.,** am-br., am-caust., am-i, am-m., ampe-qu, ***ant-c.,*** ant-s., ant-t., ***apis, arg.,*** **ARG-N.,** arn., ***ars.,*** ars-i., arum-d., arum-t., atro., aur., aur-m., bals-p., bar-c., bar-m., **BELL.,** beryl., ***brom.,*** bry., ***bufo,*** calad., ***calc.,*** calc-i., calc-s., cann-s., canth., caps., carb-ac., carb-an., ***carb-v.,*** carbn-s., ***caust.,*** cedr., ***cham., chel., chin., chlor.,*** cina, cinnb., cist., coc-c., coca, con., cot., ***crot-c., crot-h.,*** cub., cupr., ***dros., dulc.,*** eup-per., euphr., ferr., ferr-p., fl-ac., **GELS.,** ***guai.,***

HEP., hydr-ac., hyos., ign., ***iod.***, ***ip.***, irid., **KALI-BI.**, kali-br., kali-c., kali-chl., kali-i., ***kali-n.***, kreos., ***lach.***, lachn., ***led.***, lyc., mag-c., ***mang.***, menth-pu., menthol, ***merc.***, merc-c., merc-i-f., merc-i-r., mez., morg., mosch., ***naja***, nat-c., ***nat-m.***, nat-sel., ***nit-ac.***, ***nux-v.***, ol-j., osm., par., petr., ph-ac., **PHOS.**, phyt., ***puls.***, ***rhus-t.***, **RUMX.**, sabad., ***samb.***, ***sang.***, sanguin-n., sel., seneg., sep., sil., silphu., spig., ***spong.***, squil., ***stann.***, staph., stict., ***still.***, stram., sul-i., ***sulph.***, tab., thuj., verat., verb., viol-o., zinc.

LARYNX, vocal cords, cancer - arg-cy., ***arg-n.***, ***ars.***, ars-i., bell., carb-an., ***carc.***, clem., ***con.***, hydr., iod., kreos., kres., ***lach.***, lap-a., kali-bi., morph., nit-ac., ***phos.***, ***phyt.***, sang., scirr., **THUJ.**

LEAD, poisoning, ailments from - **ALUM.**, alum-sil., ***alumn.***, ant-c., ars., ***bell.***, cadm., ***cadm-s.***, carbn-s., **CAUST.**, chin., cocc., ***coloc.***, croto-t., cupr., gels., hep., iod., kali-br., ***kali-i.***, kreos., lyc., mang., merc., ***nat-s.***, nux-v., op., petr., ***plat.***, **PLB.**, ***plb—.***, ***sul-ac.***, ***sulph.***, ***ter.***, **TUB.**, uran., ***verat.***, zinc.

LEARNING DISABILITIES, studying, reading, (see Dyslexia) - **AGAR.**, agn., ***anac.***, ***ars.***, **BAR-C.**, bor., **CALC.**, ***calc-p.***, caps., **CARC.**, caste., caust., cham., con., ***kali-p.***, kali-sil., **LYC.**, mag-p., ***med.***, **MERC.**, ***nat-m.***, olnd., okou., ph-ac., ***phos.***, rib-ac., sep., ***sil.***, ***thuj.***, tub., verat.

LEPROSY, general - alum., anac., ant-t., ***ars.***, ars-i., bac., ***bad.***, bar-c., bix., ***calc.***, calo., ***carb-ac.***, ***carb-an.***, ***carb-v.***, ***carbn-s.***, ***caust.***, ***chaul.***, com., con., crot-h., cupr., cupr-acet., cur., daph., ***dip.***, elae., form., ***graph.***, guano, haem., hell., ***ho.***, hura, ***hydrc.***, iod., ***iris***, jatr., kali-c., ***kali-i.***, kam., ***lach.***, mag-c., mang., ***meph.***, merc., ***nat-c.***, nat-m., nit-ac., ***nuph.***, oena., petr., ***phos.***, ***pip-m.***, ***psor.***, **SEC.**, ***sep.***, ***sil.***, still., **SULPH.**, syph., thyr., ***tub.***, zinc.

LEUCOCYTHEMIA - ars., bell., cean., con., iod., lyc., merc., ***nat-ar.***, nit-ac., phos., rhus-t., sulph.

LEUCOCYTOSIS, blood - bar-m., bcg, ter., tub.

LEUKEMIA, blood - acet-ac., acon., apis., ***aran.***, **ARS.**, ***ars-i.***, bar-i., bar-m., benz., benzin., bry., ***calc.***, calc-ar., ***calc-p.***, carb-v., ***carbn-s.***, **CARC.**, **CEAN.**, ***chin.***, chin-s., cit-l., coca, con., cortiso., ***crot-h.***, ergot., ferr-p., ***ferr-pic.***, **HECLA.**, hell., ip., kali-hp., ***kali-p.***, kali-s., kreos., lepro., med., merc., mur-ac., **NAT-AR.**, ***nat-m.***, ***nat-p.***, **NAT-S.**, nit-ac., nux-v., op., phos., ***phyt.***, ***pic-ac.***, querc., rad-br., rhus-t., rib-ac., saroth., ***scirr.***, ***sep.***, sil., ***stront-c.***, succ., sul-ac., sulfa., sulph., ***symph.***, syph., thuj., tub., ***x-ray.***

- **lymphoid** - **ARS.**, ***ars-i.***, carb-v., carbn-s., **CEAN.**, kali-s., mur-ac., nat-ar., nat-m., **PHYT.**, pic-ac., thuj.
- **spleen,** involvement - ***ars.***, **CEAN.**, ***hecla***, ***nat-ar.***, nat-m., nat-s., querc., succ.

LICE, general - am-c., apis, ars., bac., bell-p., ***carb-ac.***, cocc., ferr-ma., lach., led., lob., ***lyc.***, m-ambo., ***merc.***, ***nat-m.***, nit-ac., olnd., ***psor.***, ***sabad.***, **STAPH.**, ***sulph.***, tub., vinc.

LICHEN, planus - agar., anac., ***ant-c.***, apis, arn., ***ars.***, ***ars-i.***, calc., chin., chin-ar., dulc., iod., ***jug-c.***, ***kali-bi.***, kali-i., led., lyc., merc., nux-v., ph-ac., phos., puls., sars., sep., staph., ***sul-i.***, sulph., thal.

LICHEN, simplex - alum., am-m., ***anan.***, ant-c., apis, ***ars.***, ***bell.***, bov., bry., ***calad.***, cast-v., dulc., ***jug-c.***, kali-ar., ***kreos.***, lach., ***led.***, ***lyc.***, merc., nabal., nat-c., ***phyt.***, ***plan.***, ***rumx.***, sep., sul-i., ***sulph.***, thuj., til.

LIFTING, straining of muscles and tendons, from - ***agn.***, alum., ambr., **ARN.**, bar-c., ***bell-p.***, ***bov.***, **BRY.**, **CALC.**, calc-f., calc-p., ***calc-s.***, calc-sil., **CARB-AN.**, calen., ***carb-v.***, ***caust.***, chin., ***cocc.***, coloc., ***con.***, croc., dulc., ***ferr.***, ferr-p., ***form.***, **GRAPH.**, ***hyper.***, iod., ***kali-c.***, ***kalm.***, lach., ***lyc.***, merc., ***mill.***, mur-ac., ***nat-c.***, nat-m., nit-ac., ***nux-v.***, olnd., phos., ***ph-ac.***, plat., podo., rhod., **RHUS-T.**, **RUTA,** sep., **SIL.**, spig., stann., staph., stront-c., sulph., sul-ac., thuj., valer.

LIGHTNING STRIKE, ailments from - arn., apom., crot-h., hell., lach., morph., ***nux-v.***, op., ***phos.***

LIMPING, from injury - abrot., acon., ant-c., apis, bell., ***bell-p.***, ***bry.***, calc., calc-f., ***caust.***, coloc., dros., dulc., hep., hydrog., kali-bi., kali-c., lyc., merc., nit-ac., phos., ***rhus-t.***, **RUTA,** sabin., sep., spig., sulph., tab., zinc.

LIPS, cancer - acet-ac., ant-c., ant-m., ***ars.***, ars-i., aur., ***aur-m.***, ***bell.***, calc., camph., ***carb-an.***, caust., ***cic.***, ***cist.***, clem., com., **CON.**, **CUND.**, hedeo., hydr., kali-chl., kali-s., ***kreos.***, ***lach.***, ***lyc.***, ph-ac., phos., phyt., sabad., ***scirr.***, ***sep.***, ***sil.***, stront-c., sulph., tab., thuj.

- **epithelioma** - acet-ac., ant-c., ant-m., ***ars-i.***, ars-s-f., ars., aur-ar., aur-s., aur., ***cic.***, clem., ***con.***, cund., ***hydr.***, kali-chl., lap-a., med., merc-i-f., merc., morg-g., nat-m., nit-ac., phos., ***sep.***, sil.

LITHIUM, ailments from - aur., benz-ac., lac-ac., ***lith-c.***, lith-m.

LIVER, cancer - **ARS.**, bell., bor., cadm-m., ***calc-ar.***, carb-an., ***carc.***, ***card-m.***, **CHEL.**, chion., ***chlol.***, ***chlor.***, **CHOL.**, cholin., con., cund., echi., euph., ferr-pic., **HYDR.**, ***insul.***, kali-bi., kreos., lach., lept., **LYC.**, mag-m., myric., ***nat-s.***, nit-ac., nux-v., phos., plb., **SCIRR.**, senec., sep., sil., sulph., tarent., ther., uran-n., vanad.

LIVER, remedies - abies-c., abrot., **ACON.**, ***aesc.***, aesc-g., ***agar.***, all-c., ***aloe***, ***alum.***, am-c., ***am-m.***, ant-c., ant-t., ***apoc.***, aq-mar., ***arg-n.***, ***arn.***, **ARS.**, ars-i., asaf., asar., ***astac.***, ***aur.***, aur-ar., aur-i., aur-m., ***aur-m-n.***, ***bapt.***, bar-c., **BELL.**, benz-ac., **BERB.**, berb-a., beryl., bol., bor., brass., **BRY.**, **BUFO**, cadm-s., **CALC.**, ***calc-f.***, **CALC-P.**, calc-sil., camph., ***carb-v.***, **CARBN-S.**, **CARC.**, **CARD-M.**, carl., ***cean.***, ***cham.***, chapter, **CHEL.**, chelo., chen-a., chen-v., **CHIM.**, **CHIN.**, ***chion.***, chol., ***cimx.***, cinnb., clem., cob., ***cocc.***, ***colch.***, ***coll.***, ***coloc.***, ***con.***, **CORN.**, ***croc.***, ***crot-c.***, **CROT-H.**, ***cupr.***, cyna., daph., dig., digin., dios., dol., dros., dulc., echi., ***euon.***, euon-a., euonin., ***eup-per.***, fab., ferr., ferr-ar., ferr-p., ***ferr-pic.***, ***fl-ac.***, frag., gels., gent-l., ***graph.***, grin., ***hep.***, **HYDR.**, iber., ign., **IOD.**, iodof., ip., ***iris***, ***jug-c.***, kalam., ***kali-bi.***, **KALI-C.**, kali-i., kali-m., kali-s., kalm., lac-d., **LACH.**, ***laur.***, **LEPT.**, **LYC.**, mag-c., **MAG-M.**, mang., mang-s., marr., **MERC.**, merc-c., merc-d., merc-i-r., morg., mur-ac., myric., nat-ar., nat-c., ***nat-m.***, nat-p., **NAT-S.**, **NIT-AC.**, nit-m-ac., **NUX-M.**, **NUX-V.**, nyct., ol-j., ost., petr., ***ph-ac.***, **PHOS.**, phyt., plat., ***plb.***, **PODO.**, ***prun.***, ***psor.***, ***ptel.***, ***puls.***, querc., ran-b., ran-s., raph., rheum, rhus-t., ruta, sabad., ***sang.***, sanic., ***scirr.***, sec., sel., senn., **SEP.**, sil., spig., staph., stel., sul-ac., sul-i., **SULPH.**, tab., ***tarax.***, ther., thlaspi, thuj., ***trio.***, upa., uran-n., vanad., verat., veronal, visc., yuc., ***zinc.***

LIVER, spots - am-c., ***ant-c.***, ant-t., ***arg-n.***, arn., ***ars.***, ars-i., ***aur.***, bad., bor., bry., cadm-s., calc, calc-p., calc-s., canth., ***carb-v.***, ***carbn-s.***, ***carc.***, caust., ***con.***, cop., cor-r., crot-h., **CUR.**, dros., ***dulc.***, ferr., ferr-i., graph., ***hyos.***, ***iod.***, kali-ar., kali-bi., kali-c., kali-p., **LACH.**, ***laur.***, **LYC.**, **MERC.**, merc-i-r., ***mez.***, nat-ar., ***nat-c.***, nat-p., **NIT-AC.**, ***nux-v.***, petr., ***phos.***, ***plb.***, puls., ruta, sabad., **SEP.**, sil., stann., **SULPH.**, sul-ac., tarent., **THUJ.**, ***tub.***

LOVE, disappointed, ailments, from, (see Grief) - ***acon.***, am-c., androc., ant-c., ars., **AUR.**, ***aur-m-n.***, ***aur-s.***, ***bell.***, ***bufo***, cact., ***calc-p.***, ***carc.***, ***caust.***, ***cimic.***, cocc., ***coff.***, com., ***con.***, dig., ham., ***hell.***, **HYOS.**, **IGN.**, iod., kali-c., ***kali-p.***, lac-h., ***lach.***, lyc., **NAT-M.**, nat-sil., nat-s., nux-m., nux-v., orig., oxyg., **PH-AC.**, phos., pitu-a., psor., **PULS.**, rhus-g., ***sac-alb.***, sep., seq-s., **STAPH.**, stram., sulph., tarent., til., tub., verat.

LUNGS, cancer - ***asbes.***, ***acal.***, ang., aran., arg., ***arg-n.***, **ARS.**, ars-i., calad., ***carc.***, ***cob.***, cob-m., **CON.**, cordy., crot-h., hydr., ***kali-bi.***, kali-fcy., ***lach.***, ***lap-a.***, **LYC.**, methyl., nicc-s., nit-ac., ***phos.***, plut-n., ***rado.***, ***scirr.***, ***sil.***, ther., ***tub.***, visc.

LUNGS, remedies - ***acon.***, all-c., ambr., ***am-c.***, ant-ar., ant-c., **ANT-T.**, apis, aral., **ARS.**, **ARS-I.**, arum-t., ***bac.***, bar-m., ***bell.***, **BLATTA**, bov., bry., ***cact.***, ***calad.***, ***calc.***, camph., ***carb-v.***, carc., caust., cist., ***coca***, cocain., coc-c., ***cupr.***, cupr-acet., cupr-ar., daph., ***dig.***, ***dros.***, eup-per., ferr-p., grat., ***grin.***, hep., ***ign.***, **IP.**, **KALI-AR.**, ***kali-bi.***, kali-br., **KALI-C.**, ***kali-m.***, ***kali-p.***, ***kali-s.***, lac-d., ***lach.***, ***laur.***, **LOB.**, ***lyc.***, ***med.***, ***meph.***, **MERC.**, merc-i-r., ***naja***, nat-ar., **NAT-S.**, ***nux-v.***, petr., phel., **PHOS.**, ***psor.***, **PULS.**, **RUMX.**, sabad., **SAMB.**, ***sang.***, ***seneg.***, ***sep.***, **SIL.**, sin-n., **SPONG.**, squil., ***stann.***, sulph., ***sul-ac.***, syph., syc-co., ter., ***thuj.***, **TUB.**, ***verat.***, verat-v., zinc.

LUPUS, erythematosum - abr., achy., agar., alum., alum-sil., alumn., ant-c., apis, aran., aran-ix., arg-n., **ARS.**, ars-i., asaf., aur., aur-ar., aur-i., aur-m., bac., ***bar-c.***, bell., cadm., calc., calc-f., calc-i., calc-s., calc-sil., ***carb-ac.***, ***carb-v.***, ***carc.***, ***caust.***, cic., ***cist.***, con., cortiso., cund., ferr-pic., form-ac., graph., guare., hep., hydr., ***hydrc.***, ***iod.***, irid., jug-c., kali-ar., iod., ***kali-bi.***, kali-c., ***kali-chl.***, kali-i., ***kali-s.***, kali-sil., kres., ***kreos.***, ***lac-c.***, lac-lup., lach., ***lil-t.***, **LYC.**, m-arct., mag-c., med., merc-i-r., nat-c., ***nat-m.***, nat-sil-f., **NIT-AC.**, ol-j., paull-p., ***phos.***, ***phyt.***, ***psor.***, pyrar., ran-b., ***rhod.***, **RHUS-T.**, sabin., sec., sep., ***sil.***, spong., staph., sulfa., sulph., thiosin., **THUJ.**, ***thyr.***, titan., ***tub.***, ***tub-a.***, urea, ***x-ray.***

LUPUS, vulgaris - abr., apis, ***ars.***, ***ars-i.***, ***aur.***, aur-ar., aur-i., calc., calc-i., calc-s., ***cist.***, cund., ferr-pic., form-ac., graph., ***hep.***, ***hydr.***, ***hydrc.***, irid., ***kali-bi.***, ***kali-i.***, lyc., nat-sil-f., nit-ac., phyt., staph., ***sulph.***, thiosin., thuj., titan., ***tub.***, urea, x-ray.

LYME, disease - ars., merc., tarent., thuj.

lymphangioma - vip.

LYMPHOMA, lymphatic glands, cancer - am-m., ***ars.***, ***ars-i.***, aur-m., ***bar-i.***, bufo, buni-o., cadm-i., ***calc-f.***, ***calc-i.***, **CARB-AN.**, ***carc.***, cean., cist., ***con.***, cordy., cund., elaps, ferr-pic., iod., lepro., ph-ac., ***phos.***, ***phyt.***, saroth., sec., **SCROPH-N.**, sil., syph., thuj., tub.

LYMPHOID, tumors - lap-a., rad-br., sec.

M

MALABSORPTION - ***alf.***, ***ars.***, calc-p., chin., gaert., ***lyc.***, ***morg.***, nat-p., nux-v., ***sil.***, sulph.

MALARIA, infection, ague - abies-n., acon., agar., alst-c., alst-s., **ALUM.**, am-c., am-m., ***am-pic.***, anac., ang., ant-c., ant-o., ant-t., ***apis***, aran., ***arg-n.***, arist-cl., **ARN.**, **ARS.**, ars-br., ***ars-i.***, ars-s-f., arum-t., asaf., asar., aur., aza., baj., bapt., bar-c., **BELL.**, benz-ac., ***bol.***, bol-lu., bov., ***bry.***, bufo, buth-aust., cact., calad., **CALC.**, calc-ar., ***calc-p.***, calc-s., calli., camph., camph-br., canch., cann-s., canth., ***caps.***, ***carb-ac.***, carb-an., ***carb-v.***, caust., cean., **CEDR.**, cent., ceph., cham., chel., chelo., **CHIN.**, ***chin-ar.***, chin-b., ***chin-m.***, ***chin-s.***, chion., cic., cimx., ***cina***, cist., clem., coc-c., cocc., coff., colch., coloc., corn., ***corn-f.***, croc., crot-h., cupr., cycl., dros., ***echi.***, elat., ***eucal.***, euon-a., eup-per., ***eup-pur.***, euphr., **FERR.**, ferr-ar., ***ferr-i.***, ferr-p., fl-ac., gels., gent-l., gent-q., graph., guare., ***helia.***, hell., ***hep.***, hydr., hyos., ***ign.***, ilx-a., ***iod.***, ***ip.***, ***iris***, kali-ar., kali-bi., kali-c., kali-i., kali-m., kali-n., kali-p., **KALI-S.**, lac-d., ***lach.***, laur., led., lept., lil-t., lob., **LYC.**, lyss., mag-c., mag-m., mag-p., maland., malar., meny., merc., methyl., mosch., mur-ac., naja, nat-c., **NAT-M.**, nat-p., **NAT-S.**, nicc., **NIT-AC.**, nux-m., ***nux-v.***, ol-j., op., ost., par., ***petr.***, ph-ac., phel., ***phos.***, phyt., plan., plb., podo., polyg-a., polyp-p., ***pop.***, prun-c., **PSOR.**, ptel., puls., **PYROG.**, querc., ran-b., ran-s., rheum, rhod., ***rhus-t.***, ***sabad.***, sabin., samb., sang., sec., sed-ac., sel., senec., **SEP.**, ***sil.***, ***spig.***, spong., stann., ***staph.***, stram., sul-ac., **SULPH.**, tarax., **TARENT.**, ***tela***, tell., **TER.**, teucr., ther., ***thuj.***, **TUB.**, urt-u., valer., verat., verat-v., verb., verbe-h., vip., zinc.

MALNUTRITION, (see Marasmus)

MALFORMATIONS - carc., fl-ac., syph.

MAGNESIUM, ailments from - cham., mag-c., mag-m., mag-s., nux-v., rheum.

MANGANESE, ailments from - mang., merc.

MANIA, general, (see Bipolar) - absin., ***acon.***, acon-l., aeth., agar., ail., alco., ***alum.***, **ANAC.**, anag., anan., anh., ant-c., ant-t., ***apis***, ***arn.***, ***arg.***, **ARS.**, ars-s-f., ***arum-t.***, atro., ***aur.***, aur-ar., aur-i., aur-s., bapt., bar-c., ***bar-m.***, **BELL.**, ***brom.***, bry., bufo, cact., ***calad.***, ***calc.***, calc-i., ***camph.***, ***cann-i.***, ***cann-s.***, ***canth.***, carbn-s., **CARC.**, caust., cham., chel., ***chin.***, chin-s., ***chlol.***, cic., ***cimic.***, coca, **COCC.**, coff., colch., ***con.***, cori-r., cortico., croc., ***crot-c.***, crot-h., ***cupr.***, cupr-acet., ***cycl.***, dat-f., dat-m., der., dig., dros., dulc., ferr-p., gels., glon., grat., ***hell.***, ***hep.***, **HYOS.**, hyosin., ***ign.***, indg., ***iod.***, iodof., iris-t., kali-bi., **KALI-BR.**, kali-c., **KALI-CHL.**, kali-i., ***kali-m.***, ***kali-p.***, kres., **LACH.**, laur., led., lil-t., **LITH-C.**, **LYC.**, lyss., mand., ***manc.***, med., **MERC.**, merc-c., murx., nat-m., nit-ac., ***nux-m.***, **NUX-V.**, oena., ***op.***, orig., ***ox-ac.***, par., passi., petr., ph-ac., ***phos.***, pic-ac., pisc., ***plat.***, plb., ***psor.***, puls., raph., rhod., rhus-t., ruta, sabad., sec., senec., seneg., ***sep.***, sil., ***sol-n.***, spig-m., spong., staph., **STRAM.**, sul-h., ***sulph.***, ***tarent.***, ter., thea., thyr., tub-k., ust., **VERAT.**, verat-v., vip., zinc.

MANIC, depression, (see Bipolar)

MARASMUS, general, (see Emaciation) - ***abrot.***, ***acet-ac.***, **AETH.**, alf., ***ant-c.***, ***apis***, arg-n., ***ars.***, bac., ***bar-c.***, ***bell.***, **CALC.**, ***calc-p.***, caps., ***cham.***, ***chin.***, coca, ***con.***, ferr-m., ***hydr.***, ***iod.***, kreos., lac-d., ***lyc.***, ***mag-c.***, med., nat-c., **NAT-M.**, ***nux-m.***, ***nux-v.***, ***ol-j.***, ***op.***, petr., pin-s., ***podo.***, ***sars.***, **SIL.**, ***sulph.***, thyr., tub.

MARIJUANA, (see Cannabis)

MARSH FEVER - abies-n., ***ang.***, arn., **ARS.**, ***asc-t.***, camph., carb-v., ***cedr.***, **CHIN.**, cina, aran., ferr., helo., **IP.**, **NAT-M.**, ***rhus-t.***, ***sang.***, sin-n., verat.

MASTITIS, breast infection - acet-ac., ***acon.***, acon-l., anan., ant-t., ***apis***, ***arn.***, ars., **BELL.**, **BRY.**, bufo, ***cact.***, cadm-s., calc., cann-s., ***carb-an.***, ***carb-v.***, ***carbn-s.***, carc., ***card-m.***, ***cham.***, ***cist.***, clem., ***con.***, crot-h., ***croto-t.***, cur., dulc., eup-a., ferr., ferr-p., fl-ac., foll., galeg., graph., helon., **HEP.**, kali-m., **LAC-C.**, ***lach.***, laur., ***lyc.***, med., ***merc.***, merc-i-f., petr., ***phel.***, ***phos.***, **PHYT.**, pic-ac., plan., plb., ***puls.***, rhus-t., sabad., sabal., **SIL.**, **SULPH.**, ust., verat-v., verb., x-ray.

MASTOIDITIS, infection - ***am-pic.***, asaf., ***aur.***, ***bell.***, benz-ac., calc-p., canth., **CAPS.**, carb-an., ferr-p., ***fl-ac.***, hep., kali-m., ***lach.***, mag-p., menthol, ***merc.***, morg-g., ***nit-ac.***, onis., ***onos.***, ***phos.***, **SIL.**, tell.

MASTURBATION, disposition - agn., ambr., ***anac.***, anan., ***apis***, aster., aur-ar., bamb-a., bell-p., **BUFO**, ***calad.***, calc., ***calc-p.***, carc., caust., ***chin.***, cina, cocc., coff., dys-co., ***gels.***, ***grat.***, hyos., ***kali-br.***, kali-p., ***lach.***, lil-t., **MED.**, ***nat-m.***, ***nux-v.***, op., **ORIG.**, orig-v., ***ph-ac.***, ***phos.***, pic-ac., ***plat.***, puls., raph., salx-n., sec., sep., stann., **STAPH.**, ***sulph.***, tarent., thuj., ***tub.***, ust., ***zinc.***

MEASLES, infection - **ACON.**, aeth., ail., ***am-c.***, ***ant-c.***, **APIS**, aral., ***arn.***, ***ars.***, arum-t., bapt., ***bell.***, **BRY.**, camph., carb-ac., ***carb-v.***, ***carbn-s.***, cham., ***chel.***, chin., ***chlor.***, ***coff.***, ***cop.***, ***crot-h.***, cupr-acet., ***dros.***, ***euph.***, **EUPHR.**, ***ferr-p.***, ***gels.***, hyos., ign., ***ip.***, ***kali-bi.***, kali-c., kali-m., kali-s., ***lach.***, lob., mag-c., merc., merc-c., merc-i-r., **MORBILL.**, mur-ac., nux-v., ***phos.***, phyt., **PULS.**, puls-n, ***rhus-t.***, sang., ***squil.***, ***stict.***, ***stram.***, **SULPH.**, tub., verat., viol-o., zinc.

MEDITERRANEAN, fever - bapt., bry., ***colch.***, merc., rhus-t.

MELANOMA - acet-ac., alum., arg., ***arg-n.***, **ARS.**, **ARS-I.**, ***calc-ar.***, carb-ac., **CARC.**, card-m., ***caust.***, chel., cund., hecla, iod., kreos., ***lach.***, merc., nit-ac., petr., ph-ac., scirr., sil., **SOL.**, squil., sulph., visc., x-ray.

MELANOSIS, eyes - ***aur.***

MEMORY, weakness, of - abrot., absin., acet-ac., ***acon.***, acon-c., act-sp., aesc., aeth., agar., ***agn.***, ail., alco., all-s., allox., **ALUM.**, alum-sil., alumn., **AMBR.**, am-c., am-m., **ANAC.**, ***anac-oc.***, anan., ***androc.***, anh., ***apis***, ***arg.***, **ARG-N.**, ***arn.***, **ARS.**, ars-h., art-v., arum-t., asaf., asc-t., ***atro.***, ***aur.***, aur-ar., aur-m., aur-s., aza., bapt., bar-acet., **BAR-C.**, bar-i., bar-s., **BELL.**, berb., ***bol.***, bor., ***bov.***, brom., ***bry.***, **BUFO**, **BUFO-S.**, cadm., calad., **CALC.**, calc-ar., ***calc-p.***, calc-s., calc-sil., camph., **CANN-I.**, cann-s., caps., carb-ac., ***carb-an.***, ***carb-v.***, carbn-o., **CARBN-S.**, carc., card-m., carl., **CAUST.**, cench., cham., chel., ***chin.***, ***chin-ar.***, chlf., ***chlol.***, chlor., chlorpr., ***cic.***, cimic., ***clem.***, cob-n., coca, **COCC.**, coff., **COLCH.**, coloc., **CON.**, convo-s., cop., cori-r., ***corn.***, cortico., cortiso., cot., croc., crot-c., ***crot-h.***, croto-t., cub., culx., ***cupr.***, cupr-acet., ***cycl.***, der., ***dig.***, dulc., elaps, erio., ***euphr.***, eupi., ferr., ***ferr-p.***, ***fl-ac.***, ***form.***, ***gels.***, **GINK.**, gins., **GLON.**, glyc., ***graph.***, ***guai.***, guare., guat., gymn., haem., ham., **HELL.**, ***helo.***, ***helon.***, **HEP.**, hipp., hist., ***hydr.***, hydrog., **HYOS.**, hyper., ***iber.***, ichth., ***ign.***, iod., ip., iris, jug-c., juni-v., kali-ar., kali-bi., ***kali-br.***, kali-c., kali-cy., ***kali-i.***, kali-n., **KALI-P.**, kali-s., kali-sil., kalm., kreos., ***lac-ac.***, ***lac-c.***, lac-d., lac-e., **LACH.**, ***laur.***, lec., led., lil-t., linu-c., lipp., **LYC.**, lyss., m-arct., mag-c., mand., manc., mang., **MED.**, meli., **MERC.**, ***merc-c., mez.,*** mill., mit., morph., mosch., murx., naja, ***nat-ar., nat-c., nat-m., nat-p.,*** nat-sal., nat-sil., nid., **NIT-AC.,** nitro-o., **NUX-M.,** ***nux-v., oena.,*** okou., ***olnd.,*** onos., ***op.,*** pall., peti., ***petr.,*** **PH-AC.,** phenob., **PHOS.,** phys., **PIC-AC.,** pip-m., plan., **PLAT., PLB.,** pneu., psil., psor., ptel., ***puls.,*** rad., ran-s., raph., rhod., rhus-g., ***rhus-t.,*** ruta, sabad., sabin., sanic., sapin., sarr., sec., ***sel.,*** seneg., **SEP.,** serp., ***sil., spig.,*** spong., ***stann., staph., stram.,*** stront-c., stry., ***sulph.,*** sul-ac., ***syph.,*** tab., tarax., ***tarent.,*** tell., ***thuj.,*** thyr., trif-p., ***tub.,*** valer., **VERAT.,** verat-v., verb., ***viol-o.,*** viol-t., visc., yuc., ***zinc., zinc-m., zinc-p.,*** zinc-pic., zing.

MENIERE'S disease - alum., arg., ***arg-n.,*** arn., ars., asar., bar-m., bell., benz-ac., bry., calc., ***camph.,*** carb-v., carbn-s., ***caust.,*** chen-a., chin., **CHIN-S.,** ***chin-sal., cic., cocc.,*** colch., com., con., crot-h., croto-t., ***dig.,*** eucal., ferr-p., gels., ***glon.,*** gran., hell., hydrobr-ac., jab., kali-c., kali-i., kali-m., kali-p., kalm., laur., mag-c., morg., myric., nat-ar., nat-c., nat-m., nat-p., nat-s., ***nat-sal.,*** nux-v., onos., op., petr., ph-ac., **PHOS.,** pic-ac., psor., puls., rad-br., ***sal-ac., sang.,*** seneg., sep., ***sil.,*** stann., tab., ***ther.,*** thyr., zinc.

MENINGITIS, infection - ***acon.,*** aeth., ***agar.,*** ail., **APIS,** apoc., arg-n., ***arn.,*** ars., atro., ***bapt.,*** **BELL.,** ***bry., calc.,*** calc-br., ***calc-p.,*** camph., canth., carb-ac., chin., chin-s., chr-ac., chr-o., ***cic.,*** cimic., ***cina, cocc.,*** crot-c., crot-h., ***cupr., cupr-acet., cupr-m.,*** dig., echi., **GELS.,** ***glon.,*** **HELL.,** ***hippoz., hydr-ac., hyos.,*** hyper., iod., iodof., ip., ***kali-br.,*** kali-i., kreos., ***lach.,*** med., ***merc.,*** merc-c., merc-d., mosch., ***nat-m., nat-s., op.,*** oreo., ox-ac., ***phos.,*** phys., ***plb., rhus-t., sil.,*** sol-n., **STRAM.,** ***sulph., tub.,*** verat-v., vip., **ZINC.,** ***zinc-c., zinc-m.***

MENOPAUSE, period, ailments, from - absin., acon., aesc., ***agar***., alet., aloe, alum., **AML-N.**, anan., ***apis***, apoc., aquil., arg., ***arg-n***., arist-cl., aur., aur-m., ***bar-c., bell***., ***bell-p***., ***berb***., bor-ac., bov., ***bry., cact***., **CALC.**, ***calc-ar***., camph., caps., carb-ac., carb-an., carb-v., carc., card-m., ***caul***., chen-a., ***chin***., **CIMIC.**, ***cocc***., coff., ***con***., cot., ***croc***., **CROT-C**., ***crot-h***., ***cycl***., cyt-l., dig., ***eucal***., ferr., ferr-i., ferr-p., foll., ***gels***., ***glon***., **GRAPH**., ***helon***., hir., ***hydr***., hydr-ac., ***ign***., ***jab***., ***kali-bi***., kali-br., ***kali-c***., ***kali-s***., ***kreos***., **LACH**., laur., led., lil-t., lyc., m-ambo., mag-c., magn-gl., ***manc***., mand., **MANG**., med., meli., merc., merc-s., mosch., **MURX**., nat-m., nicc-s., nit-ac., ***nux-m***., ***nux-v***., ol-an., onos., orch., ***ov***., ***ph-ac***., ***phos***., phys., piloc., ***plat***., plb., polyg., prun., **PSOR**., **PULS**., rhus-t., **SABIN**., sal-ac., ***sang***., sanguis., sarr., sars., ***sec***., ***sel***., semp., senec., **SEP**., ***stront-c***., stront-n., ***sul-ac***., **SULPH**., sumb., ***tab***., tarent., tell., ***ter***., ***ther***., thlaspi, thuj., trif-r., tril., ***ust***., ***valer***., ***verat***., vinc., vip., visc., x-ray, xan., zinc., ***zinc-val***.

MERCURY, ailments from - acon., agn., alumn., anan., ang., ***ant-c., arg.,*** arn., ars., ***asaf.,*** **AUR.,** aur-m., aur-s., ***bell., bor.,*** bry., calad., ***calc.,*** calo., camph., carb-an., **CARB-V.,** caust., ***chel., chin.,*** cic., cina, ***clem.,*** cocc., coff., ***colch.,*** con., ***cupr.,*** dig., dulc., ***euph.,*** euphr., ferr., fl-ac., graph., ***guai.,*** **HEP.,** ***hydr., iod.,*** iris, kali-bi., ***kali-chl.,*** **KALI-I., LACH.,** laur., ***led., lyc.,*** lycps., merc-c., **MERC.,** merc-i-f., merc-i-r., ***mez., mur-ac., nat-m.,*** **NAT-S., NIT-AC.,** nux-v., op., ***ph-ac.,*** **PHYT.,** plat., plat-m., podo., ***puls.,*** rheum, rhod., rhus-g., rhus-t., sabad., ***sars.,*** sel., sep., ***sil.,*** spong., **STAPH.,** still., stram., stront-c., sul-i., **SULPH.,** thuj., valer., verat., viol-t., zinc.

MICROWAVES, ailments from - cadm-s., rad-br., sol, x-ray.

MIGRAINE, headaches - acon., **AGAR.,** ***anac.,*** **ANT-C.,** apis, ***arg.,*** arn., ***ars.,*** **ASAF.,** ***asar.,*** aster., aur., ***bell.,*** **BRY.,** ***cact.,*** calad., ***calc., calc-p.,*** caust., cedr., ***cham.,*** chel., **CHIN.,** cic., cimic., cina, cocc., **COFF.,** coloc., **CYCL.,** ***eup-per.,*** ferr-p., **GELS.,** glon., graph., **IGN., IP., IRIS, KALI-BI.,** ***kali-p.,*** **LAC-C.,** lac-d., lach., lyc., **NAT-M.,** ***nat-s.,*** **NUX-V.,** op., ***petr.,*** **PHOS., PULS., SANG.,** scut., ***sep.,*** **SIL.,** spig., ***stram., sulph., tab.,*** tarent., ***ther.,*** **THUJ.,** ***valer.,*** **ZINC.**

- **injury**, head after - **ARN.,** ***bell.,*** bry., calc., calc-s., ***cic.,*** cocc., con., dulc., ferr-p., ***glon., hep., hell., hyper.,*** lac-c., lach., merc., ***nat-m.,*** **NAT-S.,** nit-ac., petr., ***phos.,*** puls., ***rhus-t., staph.,*** sulph., sul-ac.

MILK FEVER - **ACON.**, arn., ars., ***bell.***, bor., ***bry.***, ***calc.***, carb-v., ***cham.***, chin., ***coff.***, con., dulc., ign., kali-c., ***lac-c.***, ***lach.***, merc., nux-v., op., ***ph-ac.***, phos., ***phyt.***, ***puls.***, pyrog., rhus-t., ***sep.***, ***sil.***, squil., staph., sulph., zinc.

MINING, ailments, from - ant-t., ars., calc., carbn-s., card-m., mang., nat-ar., plb., ***sil.,*** sulph.

MISCARRIAGE, spontaneous abortion - abrot., absin., ***acon.,*** agar-se., alco., ***alet.***, aloe, ambr., ant-c., **APIS**, apoc-a., arg-n., arist-cl., ***arn.***, ars., art-v., asaf., ***asar.***, asar-c., asc-c., aur., aur-m., aur-m-n., bac., bapt., **BELL.**, bor., ***bry.***, bufo, buni-o., ***calc.***, calc-f., calc-s., camph., cann-i., cann-s., ***canth.***, caps., carb-an., carb-v., carbn-s., **CAUL.**, caust., cedr., **CHAM.**, chim., ***chin.***, chin-s., ***cimic.***, cina, cinnam., ***cocc.***, coff., coll., coloc., con., **CROC.**, crot-h., croto-t., cupr., cycl., dig., dulc., ergot., **ERIG.**, ***eup-pur.***, ***ferr.***, ferr-acet., ***ferr-i.***, ferr-m., ferr-p., fil., **GELS.**, glyc-g., goss., ham., hedeo, ***helon.***, ***hep.***, hippoz., ***hyos.***, ***ign.***, indg., iod., **IP.**, ***iris***, kali-br., ***kali-c.***, kali-chl., kali-i., kali-ma., kali-n., kali-p., kali-s., kou., kreos., lac-c., lach., lil-t., lip., ***lyc.***, ***merc.***, merc-c., ***mill.***, morph., murx., nat-c., nat-m., nit-ac., **NUX-M.**, ***nux-v.***, ***op.***, parth., ***phos.***, phyt., ***pin-l.***, pin-s., ***plat.***, ***plb.***, podo., **PULS.**, pyrog., ***rat.***, rheum, rhod., ***rhus-t.***, rosm., rumx., ruta, sabad., **SABIN.**, sang., sars., **SEC.**, senec., **<u>SEP.</u>**, sieg., ***sil.***, spong., staph., ***stram.***, succ., sul-ac., sul-i., ***sulph.***, ***syph.***, tanac., tarent., ***ter.***, ther., thlaspi, thuj., ***tril.***, ***ust.***, uza., verat., verat-v., ***vib.***, vib-p., visc., wies., xan., zinc.

miscarriage, abortion, ailments, from - alet., asar-c., aur., bapt., calen., carc., **CAUL.**, chin., **CIMIC.**, hedeo, ***helon.***, **IGN.**, ***kali-c.***, ***kali-s.***, ***lac-c.***, lil-t., ***merc.***, murx., ***nat-m.***, ***plat.***, ***podo.***, pyrog., rheum, ruta, ***sabin.***, sec., senec., **SEP.**, **STAPH.**, stram., ***sulph.***, tanac., ***thlaspi.***, tril., ust.

<u>MOLES</u>, skin - ***calc.***, carb-v., ***carc.***, graph., med., nit-ac., petr., ph-ac., **PULS.**, **SEP.**, sil., sol., ***sulph.***, sul-ac., tarent., **THUJ.**

<u>MOLES</u>, uterus - acon., ars., bell., calc., canth., chin., ferr., graph., hyos., ***kali-c.***, lyc., merc., ***nat-c.***, ***puls.***, sabin., sec., sep., ***sil.***, sulph., thuj.

<u>MOLD</u>, ailments from - ars., dulc., nat-s., thuj.

<u>MOLES</u>, hydatids, to promote expulsion, pregnancy - ***ars.***, ***bell.***, ***calc.***, cinch., ***ferr.***, ***lyc.***, merc., ***nat-c.***, ***puls.***, ***sabin.***, sec., ***sil.***, sulph.

<u>MOLLUSCUM</u>, contagiosum - ***brom.***, bry., calc., ***calc-ar.***, kali-i., lyc., merc., merc-s., ***nat-m.***, ***sil.***, sulfa., sulph., teucr., ***thuj.***

<u>MOLLUSCUM</u>, fibrosum - sil.

<u>MOLLUSCUM</u>, granulosum - sulfa.

<u>MONGOLISM</u>, (see Down's Sydrome) - ***bar-c.***, carc., morg., syc-co.

<u>MONOMANIA</u> - ***absin.***, acon., anac., anan., aur., bell., camph., carb-v., ***carc.***, cham., chin., cic., cocc., con., croc., cupr., dros., hell., **HYOS.**, ***ign.***, iod., lach., mag-c., nux-m., oxyt., plat., puls., rhus-t., ***sil.***, stram., sulph., tarent., thuj., ***verat.***

<u>MONONUCLEOSIS</u>, infection - acon., ail., alumn., anan., ***apis***, ars-i., ***ars.***, bapt., bar-c., bar-i., ***bar-m.***, ***bell.***, ***bism.***, **CALC.**, **CARC.**, ***cist.***, clem., ***dulc.***, **GELS.**, graph., ***hep.***, iod., ***iodof.***, ***kali-i.***, **MERC.**, ***merc-i-r.***, ***phos.***, ph-ac., ***phyt.***, rhus-t., sil., ***sil-mar.***, sulph.

<u>MOON</u>, moonlight, agg. - **ALUM.**, ***anac.***, ***apis.***, arg., **ARG-N.**, **ARS.**, bar-c., bell., bov., brom., bry., **CALC.**, calc-p., ***caust.***, ***cina***, ***croc.***, cupr., cycl., fl-ac., gels., ***graph.***, ***hep.***, ign., kali-bi., kali-n., ***lach.***, led., **LUNA**, ***lyc.***, ***merc.***, nat-c., nat-m., nit-ac., nux-v., ph-ac., ***phos.***, psor., **PULS.**, ***rhus-t.***, sabad., sang., ***sep.***, **SIL.**, sol-m., sol-t-ae., spong., sul-i., ***sulph.***, teucr., thuj., verat-v.

full, moon, agg. - ***alum.***, ***anac.***, ***apis.***, **ARG-N.**, **ARS.**, bar-c., bell., bov., brom., bry., **CALC.**, calc-p., ***caust.***, ***cina.***, ***croc.***, cupr., cycl., fl-ac., gels., ***graph.***, ***hep.***, ign., kali-bi., kali-n., ***lach.***, led., **LUNA**, **LYC.**, ***merc.***, nat-c., nat-m., nit-ac., nux-v., ph-ac., **PHOS.**, psor., **PULS.**, ***rhus-t.***, sabad., sang., ***sep.***, **SIL.**, sol-m., sol-t-ae., spong., sul-i., ***sulph.***, teucr., thuj., verat-v.

new, moon, agg. - ***agar.***, alum., am-c., ***apis.***, ***arg-n.***, arn., **ARS.**, ars-i., bell., ***bry.***, bufo, ***calc.***, calc-p., canth., ***caust.***, chin., ***cina.***, clem., croc., ***cupr.***, daph., graph., hep., kali-bi., kali-br., ***lach.***, ***luna***, lyc., merc., merc-c., merc-i-f., nat-m., **NUX-V.**, **PHOS.**, phyt., **PULS.**, **RHUS-T.**, sabad., ***sep.***, ***sil.***, **SULPH.**, thuj.

<u>MORBUS</u>, sudatorius - acon., ars., carb-v., jab., merc.

<u>MORNING</u>, sickness, pregnancy - acet-ac., acon., alet., ***amyg-am.***, **AMYG-P.**, anac., ***ant-c.***, ant-t., ***apom.***, ***ars.***, ***asar.***, bar-c., bism., bry., ***cadm-s.***, calc., carb-ac., carc., cast., chel., cic., cimic., cinnam., ***colch.***, ***con.***, ferr., ferr-p., **GOSS.**, ***graph.***, helon., ***ign.***, ingluv., **IP.**, ***iris***, ***jatr.***, kali-ar., ***kali-br.***, kali-c., ***kreos.***, **LAC-AC.**, lac-c., ***lac-d.***, lac-v-c., lach., ***lil-t.***, ***lob.***, mag-c., mag-m., **MERC.**, ***merc-i-f.***, ***nat-m.***, ***nux-m.***, nat-s., **NUX-V.**, petr., ***phos.***, plat., plb., ***podo.***, psor., ***puls.***, sabin., senec., **SEP.**, sil., sulph., **SYM-R.**, **TAB.**, tarent., ther., thyr., verat.

<u>MORPHINE</u>, ailments from - agar., apom., ars., aur., **AVEN.**, bell., buth-aust., calc., carc., cann-i., ***cham.***, cic., cimic., coff., ***herin.***, hyos., **IP.**, kali-ma., ***lach.***, lob., ***macrin.***, merc., mur-ac., nat-p., ***nux-v.***, **OP.**, ox-ac., ***passi.***, phos., plat., puls., stram., tab., zinc.

craving for - apom., **AVEN.**, lob., ***ip.***, nat-p., ***nux-v.***, ***op.***, ox-ac., passi., upa.

<u>MORVAN'S</u>, disease - aur., bar-m., lach., ***sec.***, sil., thuj.

<u>MOTION SICKNESS</u>, riding in a car, bus or train, while - bor., ***calc.***, ***calc-p.***, **<u>COCC.</u>**, ***cycl.***, ***hep.***, ***iris***, ***lyc.***, ***mag-c.***, naja, ***nux-m.***, ***nux-v.***, **PETR.**, sel., **SEP.**, sulph., **TAB.**, ***ther.***, zinc.

<u>MOUNTAIN SICKNESS</u>, (see Altitude, sickness) - ***acon.***, ***arn.***, ***ars.***, aur., bell., **CALC.**, **CARB-V.**, caust., **<u>COCA.</u>**, con., conv., cupr., gels., kola, ***lach.***, lyc., nat-m., olnd., ***op.***, puls., **SIL.**, spig., verat.

<u>MOUTH</u>, cancer - alumn., apis, ars., aur-m-n., **AUR-M.**, aur., bell., benz-ac., calc., carb-ac., carb-an., ***carc.***, caust., chr-ac., cit-ac., cit-l., ***con.***, crot-h., cund., gali., glyc., hep., ho., **HYDR.**, kali-chl., ***kali-cy.***, kali-i., lach., ***merc.***, mur-ac., nit-ac., phos., phyt., scirr., ***semp.***, sep., sil., silphu., staph., sulph., thuj., vib-p.

<u>MULTIPLE PERSONALITES</u>, disorders, (see Insanity, Schizophrenia) - agar., alum., **ANAC.**, anh., ant-c., arg-n., bapt., ***cann-i.***, cann-s., carc., cic., cycl., ***gels.***, glon., hyos., lac-c., ***lach.***, lil-t., lyc., mosch., ***naja***, nat-m., ***nux-m.***, op., ***petr.***, phos., **PLAT.**, plb., psor., puls., pyrog., pyrus, sec., sil., stram., ther., thuj., ***tril.***, valer., **VERAT.**, xan.

<u>MULTIPLE SCLEROSIS</u> - ***alum.***, arg., ***arg-n.***, ***atro.***, ***aur.***, aur-m., bar-c., bar-m., bell., calc., cann-i., carbn-s., **CAUST.**, ***con.***, ***crot-h.***, des-ac., **GELS.**, halo., irid., ***lath.***, ***lyc.***, mand., merc., **NAT-M.**, nux-v., ox-ac., **PHOS.**, ***phys.***, ***pic-ac.***, ***plb.***, psil., sil., ***stry.***, sulph., tarent., thal., thuj., syph., wild., xan., zinc.

__**MUMPS,**__ infection - abies-c., abrot., ***acon.,*** agar., ail., am-br., ***am-c.,*** ant-t., anthr., apis, arg., ***ars., arum-t., aur.,*** aur-m., bapt., bar-br., **BAR-C.,** bar-i., ***bar-m.,*** **BELL.,** ***brom.,*** bry., ***calc.,*** calc-br., ***carb-an.,*** **CARB-V.,** carc., ***cham.,*** **CIST.,** cocc., ***con., crot-h.,*** dor., dpt, dulc., euphr., ***ferr-p.,*** gink., ***hep.,*** hippoz., hydrog., hyos., iod., **JAB.,** kali-ar., ***kali-bi.,*** kali-br., ***kali-c.,*** kali-m., kali-p., ***lach., lyc.,*** lyss., mag-p., med., **MERC.,** merc-c., merc-i-f., merc-i-r., mmr, ***nat-m.,*** nux-v., pancreat., ***parot.,*** petr., ***phos.,*** phyt., piloc., plb., plut-n., **PULS.,** raja-s., ***rhus-t.,*** sabal., sars., sep., ***sil.,*** staph., sul-ac., sul-i., sulph., thuj., trif-p., trif-r., tub., verb..

__**MUSCLES,**__ remedies, (see Tendons) - alum., **ARN.,** calc., calc-p., calen., caul., **CAUST.,** cimx., coloc., con., dulc., ***gels.,*** **LAC-AC.,** lath., **MAG-P.,** ***plb.,*** rauw., ***rhus-t., ruta,*** sarcol-ac., ***stry.,*** zinc.

__**MUSHROOMS,**__ ailments from - ***absin.,*** agar., ***ars.,*** atro., ***bell.,*** camph., pyrog.

__**MUSTARD GAS,**__ ailments from - antr., ars., carb-ac., petr.

__**MYASTHENIA,**__ gravis - alum., con., gels.

__**MYATROPHY**__, progressive spinal - ars., carb-s., hyper., kali-hp., lath., **PHOS.,** phys., ***plb.,*** sec.

__**MYOCARDITIS**__, heart, inflammation - achy., ***acon., adon.***, ant-ar., apis, ars., ars-i., asar., aur., beryl., bry., ***cact., carb-v.***, caust., chin-ar., chlorpr., ***crat.,*** **DIG.,** diph., eberth., gala., gels., glon., hed., hoit., ***iber.***, iod., kali-bi., kres., ***lach.***, mand., morg., naja, paro-i., ***phos.***, pineal., psor., raja-s., saroth., **SPIG.,** stroph., sulo-ac., sulph., sumb., toxo., verat-v., ***vip.***

__**MYCOSIS**__ - calc., calc-sil., graph., **SIL.,** syc-co.

__**MYOSITIS,**__ muscles - ***arn.,*** bell., bry., calc., ham., hep., kali-i., merc., mez., ***rhus-t., ruta.***

__**MYXEDEMA,**__ thyroid - ***ars.,*** cortico., dor., pen., prim-o., sep., sulfa., ***thyr.***

N

__**NAILS,**__ inflammation, (felon, onychia, paronychia) - all-c., alum., **AM-C.,** ***am-m., anac.,*** ant-c., **ANTHR., APIS,** arn., ***ars.,*** asaf., aur., ba-sv., ba-tn., bar-c., bell., bell-p., benz-ac., berb., bor., bov., bry., ***bufo, calc.,*** calc-f., calc-p., calc-s., calc-sil., canth., carb-ac., ***caust.,*** chin., ***cist.,*** coc-c., con., crot-h., croto-t., cur., **DIOS.,** eug., euph., ferr., **FL-AC.,** gins., gran., graph., **HEP.,** ***hyper., iod., iris,*** kali-c., kali-i., kali-sil., kalm., ***lach.,*** lap-a., ***led.,*** lith-c., ***lyc., m-arct.,*** m-aust., maland., merc., merc-c., mez., mur-ac., ***myris.,*** nat-c., nat-h., ***nat-m., nat-s.,*** **NIT-AC.,** nux-v., ol-myr., op., ozone, par., petr., ph-ac., phos., phyt., plan., plat., plb., psor., ***puls.,*** pyrog., ran-b., ***rhus-t.,*** ruta, sabad., ***sang.***, sec., ***sep.,*** **SIL.,** sin-n., squil., stram., sul-ac., sul-i., ***sulph.,*** syc-co., syph., **TARENT-C.,** teucr., thuj., thyr., ust.

crushed, and lacerated fingernails - arist-cl., ***carb-ac.,*** __**HYPER.**__, ***led., ruta.***

hangnail - ***calc.,*** lyc., ***merc.,*** **NAT-M.,** ***rhus-t.,*** sabad., sep., ***sil., stann.,*** **SULPH.,** ***thuj.***

ingrowing, nails - alum., ***caust.,*** colch., **GRAPH.,** kali-c., kali-chl., lach., __**M-AUST.**__, ***nat-m., nit-ac., ph-ac.,*** plb., **SIL.,** sang., ***sulph.,*** **TEUCR.,** ***thuj.,*** tub.

injuries, toenails - all-c., **ARN.,** calen., __**HYPER.**__, ***led.,*** rhus-t., sep.

splinter, of glass, from - calen., hyper., ***sil.***

__**NARCOLEPSY**__ - aeth., agar., alco., all-c., alum., ***ant-c.,*** **ANT-T.,** ***ars.,*** arum-m., ***aur.,*** bar-acet., bar-c., calc., camph., cann-s., canth., carb-v., carbn-s., ***caust., chin., cimx.,*** cina, cocc., coff., coloc., conin., ***cor-r., crot-h.,*** croto-t., cycl., euph., euphr., ferr., ***gels.,*** grat., ***haem., hydr-ac.,*** hyos., kali-c., ***kali-n., lach.,*** lact., laur., lina., lyc., mag-s., ***merc., mez.,*** naja, nat-c., nat-m., nat-n., nit-ac., **NUX-M.,** ***nux-v.,*** **OP.,** petr., phos., ***phys.,*** pimp., pip-m., plb., ***puls.,*** rhod., ***rhus-t., sabad.,*** scroph-n., sel., ***sep., sil.,*** sol-t-ae., spig., stann., sulph., tab., ***tarax.,*** tarent., verb., ***zinc.***

__**NARCOTICS,**__ ailments from - acet-ac., acon., agar., am-c., apom., ars., aur., **AVEN., BELL.,** bry., calc., ***camph.***, cann-i., canth., carb-v., caust., **CHAM.,** chin., cic., cimic., cod., **COFF.,** colch., coloc., croc., cupr., ***dig.***, dulc., euph., ***ferr.***, ***graph.***, hep., ***hyos.***, ign., **IP.,** kali-ma., **LACH.,** lob., ***lyc.***, macrin., mag-s., merc., morph., mosch., mur-ac., ***narcot.,*** nat-c., nat-m., nat-p., nit-ac., nux-m., **NUX-V., OP.,** ox-ac., ozone., ***passi.,*** ph-ac., phenob., phos., plat., plb., ***puls.***, rhus-t., seneg., ***sep.***, staph., sulph., thuj., ***valer.***, verat., zinc.

__**NAUSEA,**__ general - absin., acet-ac., ***acon.***, act-sp., adon., ***aesc.***, aesc-g., ***aeth.***, ***agar.***, agn., ail., alet., all-c., ***all-s.***, allox., aloe, ***alum.***, alum-p., alum-sil., alumn., am-c., ***am-m.***, ambr., aml-n., amyg-am., ***anac.***, anan., androc., ang., **ANT-C., ANT-T.,** anth., apis, apoc., apoc-a., apom., aq-mar., arag., ***aran.***, aran-s., ***arg.***, **ARG-N.,** arist-cl., arn., **ARS.,** ars-h., ars-i., ars-met., ars-s-f., arund., asaf., ***asar.***, asc-c., asc-i., asc-t., aspar., aster., atro., aur., aur-ar., aur-i., aur-m., aur-m-n., aur-s., ba-tn., bac., bals-p., bamb-a., ***bapt.***, ***bar-c.***, bar-i., bar-m., bar-s., **BELL.,** benz-ac., ***berb.***, berb-a., beryl., ***bism.***, ***bol.***, bor., bor-ac., both-l., ***bov.***, brach., brom., ***bry.***, bufo, cact., cadm., ***cadm-s.***, cahin., caj., calad., ***calc.***, calc-ar., calc-f., calc-i., ***calc-p.***, ***calc-s.***, calc-sil., ***camph.***, cand-a., cann-i., cann-s., ***canth.***, ***caps.***, ***carb-ac.***, ***carb-an.***, ***carb-v.***, **CARBN-S.,** carc., ***card-m.***, carl., casc., cast., caul., ***caust.***, cedr., cench., cer-ox., **CHAM.,** ***chel.***, chim-m., **CHIN.,** chin-ar., ***chin-s.***, ***chion.***, chlf., chlol., choc., ***chr-ac.***, cic., ***cimic.***, cimx., ***cina***, cinnam., cinnb., ***cist.***, cit-v., clem., cob., cob-n., coc-c., coca, cocain, __**COCC.**__, ***cod.***, coff., coff-t., __**COLCH.**__, ***coll.***, ***coloc.***, com., ***con.***, conv., cop., cor-r., ***corn.***, corn-f., corp-l., cortico., cortiso., croc., ***crot-c.***, ***crot-h.***, ***croto-t.***, ***cub.***, cuc-p., cund., **CUPR.,** cupr-acet., ***cupr-ar.***,

cupr-s., cur., ***cycl.***, cyt-l., daph., dict., **DIG.**, digox., dios., dros., **DULC.**, ***echi.***, elaps, ***elat.***, epip., erech., erig., ery-a., eucal., eug., euon., euon-a., ***eup-per.***, eup-pur.,. ***euph.***, euph-c., euphr., eupi., fago., ***ferr.***, ***ferr-ar.***, ferr-i., ferr-m., ***ferr-p.***, fil., ***fl-ac.***, foll., ***form.***, gall-ac., ***gamb.***, ***gels.***, gent-c., gent-l., glon., gnaph., goss., ***gran.***, ***graph.***, grat., ***guai.***, guare., guat., gymn., haem., ham., hed., hedeo, **HELL.**, hell-f., **HEP.**, hip-ac., hipp., hist., hura, ***hydr.***, hydr-ac., hydrc., hydro-c., ***hydrog.***, hyos., hyper., iber., ichth., ***ign.***, ind., indg., indol., inul., ***iod.***, **IP.**, ipom., **IRIS**, **IRIS-FL.**, jab., jac-c., jal., jatr., jug-c., jug-r., **KALI-AR.**, ***kali-bi.***, kali-br., **KALI-C.**, kali-chl., kali-chls., kali-cy., kali-i., kali-m., kali-n., kali-p., ***kali-s.***, kali-sal., kali-sil., kalm., kreos., ***lac-ac.***, ***lac-c.***, lac-d., lac-v., lac-v-c., ***lach.***, lachn., lact., lap-c-b., lap-gr-m., lat-m., ***laur.***, lec., led., lept., lil-t., lith-c., **LOB.**, lob-c., lob-p., ***lyc.***, lycps., lyss., m-aust., mag-c., ***mag-m.***, ***mag-p.***, mag-s., maland., manc., mand., mang., med., meli., menis., menthol, meny., meph., ***merc.***, merc-c., merc-cy., merc-d., ***merc-i-f.***, merc-i-r., merc-s., merl., ***mez.***, mill., mit., morg., ***morph.***, ***mosch.***, ***mur-ac.***, mygal., myric., ***naja***, narc-po., narc-ps., ***nat-ar.***, ***nat-c.***, nat-h., **NAT-M.**, ***nat-p.***, nat-s., nat-sil., nicc., nicot., ***nit-ac.***, nux-m., **NUX-V.**, oena., ***ol-an.***, ol-j., olnd., onos., op., opun-v., osm., ost., ov., ***ox-ac.***, oxyu-s., ozone, paeon., pall., par., parathyr., pareir., paull-p., ped., **PETR.**, ***ph-ac.***, phel., ***phos.***, phys., ***phyt.***, ***pic-ac.***, picro., piloc., pitu-a., plac., plan., ***plat.***, ***plb.***, ***podo.***, polyg., polyp-p., pop., ***prun.***, psil., ***psor.***, ptel., **PULS.**, puls-n, pyrog., rad-br., ***ran-b.***, ***ran-s.***, ***raph.***, rat., ***rheum***, ***rhod.***, rhodi., **RHUS-T.**, ***rhus-v.***, rob., rumx., ruta, ***sabad.***, sabin., sac-l., sal-ac., ***samb.***, **SANG.**, sanic., sant., sarcol-ac., ***sars.***, scol., ***sec.***, sel., senec., ***seneg.***, **SEP.**, **SIL.**, sin-a., sin-n., sol-n., sphing., spig., spong., ***squil.***, ***stann.***, staph., stict., still., stram., stront-c., ***stroph.***, stroph-s., stry., ***sul-ac.***, sul-i., **SULPH.**, sumb., syc-co., **SYM-R.**, syph., **TAB.**, tanac., ***tarax.***, tarent., tax., tell., tep., ***ter.***, teucr., thal., thea., ***ther.***, thlaspi, ***thuj.***, thymol., thyr., torul., tril-c., trinit., trio., tub., upa., uran-n., urt-u., ust., **VALER.**, vario., **VERAT.**, ***verat-v.***, verb., vesp., vib., vib-p., vinc., viol-t., vip., visc., wies., wye., x-ray, xan., yohim, **ZINC.**, **ZINC-P.**, zing., ziz.

NECK, cancer - brom., cadm-i., cist., ***con.***, hydr., ***lach.***, merc., phyt., ***scirr.***, scroph-m., ***scroph-n.***

NECK, injuries - androc., ***arn.***, ***bell-p.***, **BRY.**, ***calc.***, calc-f., caust., cic., **HYPER.**, ***mag-p.***, mez., ***nat-s.***, **RHUS-T.**, ***ruta***, ***symph.***

whiplash - arn., **BRY.**, ***bell-p.***, ***calc.***, caust., cic., **HYPER.**, **RHUS-T.**, ***ruta.***

NECROMANIA, obsessed with death - **AGAR.**, ars., calc-sil.

NEPHRITIS, infection, kidneys - ***acon.***, ***all-c.***, alum., am-c., **APIS**, ***arg-n.***, **ARN.**, ars., arund., ***asc-c.***, ***aur.***, **BELL.**, **BENZ-AC.**, **BERB.**, ***bry.***, cact., calad., calc-s., camph., cann-i., ***cann-s.***, **CANTH.**, ***caps.***, ***carb-ac.***, caust., ***chel.***, ***chim.***, coc-c., ***colch.***, coll., cop., crot-c., crot-h., cub., dig., ***ery-a.***, ***eup-pur.***, ferr., ***gels.***, ***hell.***, ***helon.***, ***hep.***, indg., ***kali-ar.***, ***kali-c.***, **KALI-CHL.**, ***kali-i.***, kali-p., kali-s., lil-t., lith-c., **LYC.**, ***lycps.***, med., ***merc.***, ***merc-c.***, merc-cy., nat-s., nit-ac., ***nux-v.***, **OCI.**, pareir., ph-ac., ***phos.***, ***phyt.***, pic-ac., plb., ***polyg.***, prun., ***puls.***, ***rhus-t.***, ***sabin.***, samb., ***sars.***, sec., ***senec.***, sep., solid., ***stront-c.***, stroph., **SULPH.**, sul-ac., tarent., **TER.**, ***thuj.***, tub., uran., zinc.

NEPHROTIC, syndrome - ars., ***apis.***

NEURALGIC, pains - **ACON.**, acon-f., act-sp., **AGAR.**, ail., all-c., am-val., aml-n., anac., apis, aran., aran-ix., arg-n., arn., **ARS.**, ars-br., arum-d., asaf., atro., aur., bac., bar-c., **BELL.**, ***bry.***, cact., camph., carb-v., carbn-s., ***caust.***, cedr., ***cham.***, chel., chin., chin-ar., chin-s., chlol., cimic., cina, clem., coff., coffin., **COLOC.**, con., crot-h., cupr., cypr., dios., dip., dol., dulc., elat., ergot., ferr., gaul., gels., graph., grat., hed., hep., hyos., **HYPER.**, **IGN.**, iodof., ip., ***iris***, ***kali-bi.***, kali-c., kali-chl., kali-cy., kali-fcy., ***kalm.***, kreos., lach., lim., lob-s., lol., ***lyc.***, lycpr., ***mag-c.***, **MAG-P.**, mand., mang., ***med.***, ***merc.***, methyl., mez., morph., nat-ar., nat-m., nicc-s., nit-ac., ***nux-v.***, oena., ol-j., olnd., onos., op., pall., passi., paull-p., petr., ph-ac., phos., phys., phyt., pime., plan., plat., prun., ***psor.***, puls., ran-b., rauw., rhodi., rhus-r., ***rhus-t.***, rumx., sabad., ***sang.***, sec., sep., sil., sphing., **SPIG.**, stann., staph., still., stry., sul-ac., ***sulph.***, syph., tanac., tarax., tarent., tax., ter., teucr., ***thal.***, thlaspi, thuj., tong., vac., valer., vario., ***verat.***, verb., verin., visc., xan., zinc., zinc-val.

NEURITIS - **ACON.**, ***alum-sil.***, ***ant-c.***, ***ars.***, **BELL.**, ***cact.***, caust., ***cic.***, ***coca***, **COFF.**, ***gels.***, ***hep.***, **HYPER.**, iod., ***ip.***, kali-i., ***kalm.***, lac-c., ***lec.***, ***led.***, ***merc.***, ***nat-m.***, ***nux-v.***, **PHOS.**, ***puls.***, ***rhus-t.***, ***sil.***, stram., sulph., zinc.

NEUROFIBROMATOSIS - calc-f., graph., hyper., lepro.

NEUROSIS, cordis - ***acon.***, adren., agarin., ars., cact., calad., ***calc.***, cham., chin., cimic., ***coff.***, coll., conv., dig., ferr., ***gels.***, ***iber.***, ***ign.***, kalm., lach., ***lil-t.***, lyc., lycps., ***mosch.***, ***nux-v.***, phos., prun., saroth., scut., sep., ***spig.***, staph., stroph., ***tab.***, verat., zinc.

NIGHT-WATCHING, ailments from, (see Nursing, others) - **CARC.**, caust., **COCC.**, cupr., melat., ***nit-ac.***, nux-v., sel., zinc.

NODULES, skin, (see Tubercles) - ***agar.***, am-c., ant-c., arg-n., ars., ***ars-i.***, aur., ***bar-c.***, bor., bufo, calc., ***carb-an.***, caul., caust., ***chel.***, chin., cic., cinnb., ***clem.***, con., ***dulc.***, ***graph.***, guai., ***iod.***, ***kali-c.***, kali-s., lach., ***led.***, lyc., mag-c., mag-m., ***mang.***, ***merc.***, mez., ***mur-ac.***, par., phos., ***puls.***, ***ran-b.***, rhod., **RHUS-T.**, ruta, sars., **SEP.**, **SIL.**, squil., ***staph.***, **SULPH.**, ther., ***thuj.***, tub., verat.

NOSE, cancer - alumn., ***ars.,*** ars-i., **AUR.,** ***aur-m., calc.,*** carb-ac., ***carb-an.,*** con., cund., euphr., hydr., iod., kali-s., ***kreos.,*** med., merc., merc-c., merc-s., nit-ac., ***phyt., sep.,*** sil., sulph., tarent.

NOSEBLEED, epistaxis - abrot., acet-ac., **ACON.,** ***agar.,*** agn., ail., ***all-c.,*** aloe, alum., alum-p., alum-sil., ***alumn.,*** **AM-C.,** am-caust., am-m., **AMBR.,** ambro., aml-n., anac., anag., anan., ang., **ANT-C.,** ant-s., ant-t., apis, aran., ***arg.,*** arg., arg-n., **ARN.,** ***ars., ars-i.,*** ars-s-f., arum-t., asaf., asar., asc-t., astac., aster., aur., aur-ar., aur-i., aur-m., aur-s., bamb-a., ***bapt., bar-c.,*** bar-i., ***bar-m.,*** bar-s., **BELL.,** bell-p., benz-ac., ***berb.,*** beryl., bism., bor., both-a., **BOTH-L., BOV.,** ***brom., bry., bufo,*** **CACT.,** cadm-s., calad., **CALC.,** calc-hp., calc-i., **CALC-P., CALC-S.,** calc-sil., camph., cann-i., ***cann-s.,*** canth., ***caps.,*** carb-ac., ***carb-an.,*** **CARB-V., CARBN-S.,** carc., card-m., **CAUST.,** ***cham.,*** chel., **CHIN.,** chin-ar., ***chin-s.,*** choc., cic., ***cina,*** cinnam., ***cinnb.,*** clem., cob-n., coca, cocc., coff., colch., coloc., ***con.,*** conv., ***cop.,*** cor-r., corn., **CROC.,** crot-c., **CROT-H.,** ***cupr.,*** cyt-l., ***dig.,*** dios., ***dros., dulc.,*** echi., ***elaps,*** erech., ***erig.,*** eup-per., euphr., eupi., ***ferr.,*** ferr-acet., ***ferr-ar.,*** ferr-i., ferr-m., ***ferr-p.,*** **FERR-PIC.,** fic., gall-ac., gamb., gels., ***glon.,*** gran., ***graph.,*** **HAM.,** ***hecla.,*** hedeo, ***hep.,*** hipp., hir., hura, ***hydr.,*** **HYOS.,** ign., ind., indg., ***iod.,*** **IP.,** jug-c., jug-r., kali-ar., ***kali-bi., kali-c.,*** kali-chl., kali-cy., kali-hp., **KALI-I.,** ***kali-n.,*** kali-p., kali-s., kali-sil., ***kreos.,*** lac-ac., lac-c., **LACH.,** lachn., lapa., laur., ***led.,*** lil-t., lob., ***lyc.,*** lycps., ***lyss.,*** m-arct., ***mag-c.,*** mag-m., mag-s., **MED., MELI.,** meny., meph., **MERC.,** ***merc-c.,*** merc-cy., merl., ***mez.,*** **MILL.,** mit., morg., morg-g., ***mosch.,*** mur-ac., naja, nat-ar., ***nat-c.,*** nat-h., ***nat-m., nat-n., nat-p.,*** nat-s., nat-sal., nat-sil., **NIT-AC.,** ***nux-m., nux-v.,*** oena., ol-j., onis., onon., op., orig-v., osm., ox-ac., oxyu-s., ozone, par., paull-p., ***petr., ph-ac.,*** <u>**PHOS.**</u>, phyt., pic-ac., pitu-a., plat., plb., prun., psil., **PULS.,** pyrog., ran-b., ***rat.,*** rauw., ***rhod.,*** rhus-g., **RHUS-T.,** ***rumx.,*** ruta, sabad., sabal., **SABIN.,** samb., ***sang.,*** sanic., sarr., ***sars.,*** scroph-n., **SEC.,** sel., senec., seneg., ***sep., sil.,*** sin-n., spig., ***spong.,*** squil., ***stann.,*** staph., stict., stram., stront-c., ***sul-ac.,*** **SULPH.,** syc-co., syph., tab., tarax., ***tarent., ter.,*** terebe., teucr., thea., ***thlaspi, thuj.,*** thyr., til., trif-p., ***tril.,*** trom., **TUB.,** ***ust.,*** vac., valer., ***verat.,*** verat-v., vib., vinc., viol-o., vip., visc., xan., zinc., zinc-p.

NURSING, of others, ailments, from - abrot., acon., agn., ant-t., ars., ***bell., bor.,*** **BRY., CALC.,** ***calc-p.,*** carb-an., carb-v., <u>**CARC.**</u>, cast-eq., ***caust., cham.,*** chel., ***chin.,*** chin-ar., cina, <u>**COCC.**</u>, con., crot-h., croto-t., ***dulc.,*** ferr., frag., ign., iod., ip., ***kali-c.,*** lac-c., lach., lyc., ***merc.,*** mill., nat-c., nat-m., ***nit-ac.,*** nux-v., olnd., **PH-AC.,** phel., ***phos.,*** **PHYT., PULS.,** rheum, ***rhus-t.,*** samb., sel., **SEP., SIL.,** spig., squil., stann., ***staph.,*** stram., ***sulph.,*** zinc.

O

OBESITY, general - ***acon.,*** adon., agar., ail., alco., all-s., alum., ***am-br., am-c., am-m.,*** ambr., ***ang., ant-c.,*** ant-t., ***apis,*** aq-mar., aran-ix., arist-cl., arn., ***ars., asaf., aur.,*** bac., bad., bar-c., ***bell.,*** blatta, bor., brom., bry., bufo, calad., **CALC.,** calc-acet., ***calc-ar.,*** zirc., ***calo.,*** camph., canth., **CAPS.,** carb-v., carc., carl., caust., cham., chin., chlorpr., cic., cimic., cina, clem., ***coc-c.,*** coca, cocc., coloc., con., cortiso., ***croc., cupr.,*** cyna., dig., ***elaps,*** euph., euphr., **FERR.,** ferr-i., fl-ac., foll., ***fuc.,*** **GRAPH.,** guai., hell., ***hura, hyos.,*** ign., iod., ip., ***kali-bi.,*** kali-br., ***kali-c., lac-d.,*** lach., lap-a., laur., lith-c., lob., ***lyc.,*** lycpr., lycps., mag-c., mag-p., mang., med., merc., merc-d., mur-ac., nat-ar., nat-c., ***nat-m.,*** nux-m., nux-v., olnd., op., ozone, phase., ***phos.,*** **PHYT.,** ***pitu-a.,*** plat., plb., ***puls.,*** rauw., rheum, rhus-t., rumx., sabad., sabal., sac-alb., sars., sec., sel., seneg., sep., sil., spig., spong., stram., stront-c., stroph., ***sulph.,*** syc-co., thuj., ***thyr.,*** thyreotr., tus-f., valer., verat., viol-o.

OBSESSIVE, compulsive disorder - ***anac.,*** anh., ***arg-n.,*** **ARS.,** aur., ***calc.,*** <u>**CARC.**</u>, caust., con., cupr., foll., **HYOS.,** ***ign.,*** iod., kali-c., lyss., manc., **MED.,** merc., ***nat-m., nat-s.,*** **NUX-V.,** pin-s., ***plat.,*** psor., **PULS.,** rat., rhus-t., ***sil., staph.,*** stram., sulph., syph., thuj., tub., ***verat.***

OLD AGE, premature - ***agn.,*** alco., alum., ***ambr.,*** arg., arg-n., ***bar-c.,*** berb., bufo, carb-v., chin-s., coca, ***con.,*** cortico., ***cupr., fl-ac., kali-c.,*** **LYC.,** nux-v., op., ***ph-ac.,*** psor., sars., **SEL.,** sep., staph., stram., sulph., ***vip.,*** zinc.

OOPHORITIS, inflammation, ovaries - abrot., achy., **ACON.,** aesc., am-br., ambr., amor-r., ***ant-c.,*** **APIS,** arg., arg-n., arn., ars., ars-i., aur., aur-ar., ***aur-i.,*** aur-m., aur-m-n., bac., **BELL.,** brom., ***bry., cact., canth.,*** caps., chel., ***chin.,*** chin-s., cimic., cod., coli., coll., coloc., con., crot-h., cub., dulc., euph., eupi., ferr-p., gels., graph., ***guai.,*** ham., hep., hydro-c., ign., ***iod., lac-c., lach., lil-t.,*** **LYC.,** mag-p., ***med.,*** **MERC.,** ***merc-c.,*** nit-ac., ***nux-v., pall., ph-ac.,*** **PHOS.,** ***phyt., plat.,*** **PODO.,** ***puls.,*** pyrog., ran-b., rhus-t., sabad., sabal., **SABIN.,** sep., sil., staph., syc-co., ***syph., thuj.,*** tub-r., ust., ***verat-v.,*** vesp., visc., zinc., zinc-p.

OPIUM, ailments from - agar., ***apom.,*** ars., atro., aur., **AVEN.,** bell., calc., camph., cann-i., ***cham.,*** cic., cimic., coff., cod., hyos., ***ip.,*** kali-ma., ***lach.,*** lob., ***macrin.,*** merc., morph., mur-ac., ***narcot.,*** nat-p., ***nux-v.,*** **OP.,** ox-ac., ***passi.,*** phos., plat., puls., stram., valer., zinc.

craving for - apom., **AVEN.,** lob., ***ip.,*** nat-p., ***nux-v., op.,*** ox-ac., passi., upa.

ORCHITIS, infection, testes - abrot., **ACON.,** agn., am-c., anan., ant-t., apis, arg., ***arg-n.,*** arist-cl., **ARN.,** ***ars., aur.,*** aur-ar., aur-s., **BAPT.,** bar-c., bar-m., ***bell., berb.,*** brom., bufo, calc-i., calen., cann-s., canth., cham., chel., ***chin.***, chin-s., **CLEM.**, **CON.**, cub., der., ***euph.***, gels., ***ham.***, hep., hippoz., hyper., iod., jab., kali-ar., kali-c., kali-chl., ***kali-i.***, kali-n., kali-s., ***lyc.***, med., ***merc.***, merc-i-r., mez., mill., nat-ar., nat-c., ***nat-m.***, ***nit-ac.***, ***nux-v.***, oci., **PAROT.**, phos., ***phyt.***, ***plb.***, podo., polyg., **PULS.**, **RHOD.**, **RHUS-T.**, ruta, sabal., sel., sil., **SPONG.**, ***staph.***, sul-ac., sulph., tarax., teucr-s., thuj., ust., verat-v., verb., vib., zinc.

ORGANS, injury, to - arn., **BELL-P.**, ***mill.***

ORIFICES, ailments of - ***aesc.,*** aloe, ***bell., calen., caust.,*** graph., ign., kali-c., lach., lyc., ***merc.,*** mur-ac., nat-m., **NIT-AC.**, **NUX-V.**, phos., podo., pyrog., rat., ***sep., sil.,*** **STAPH.**, **SULPH.**, syph.

OSGOOD-SCHLATTER'S, disease - ***calc-p., sil.***

OSTEITIS, deformans - calc-p., sil.

OSTEOGENSIS, imperfecta - calc-f., ***calc-p.,*** sil.

OSTEOMALACIA, bones, softening of - am-c., **ASAF.**, ***bell.,*** **CALC.**, calc-f., ***calc-i., calc-p.,*** cic., con., ferr., ***ferr-i.,*** ferr-m., ***ferr-p.,*** fl-ac., guai., hecla., ***hep.,*** iod., ip., ***kali-i., lac-c., lyc.,*** **MERC.**, merc-c., mez., ***nit-ac.,*** nux-m., ***ol-j.,*** parathyr., petr., ph-ac., ***phos.,*** plb., ***psor., puls.,*** rhod., ruta, ***sep.,*** **SIL.**, staph., ***sulph., symph.,*** syph., ther., thuj.

OSTEOMYELITIS, bones - achy., acon., arg., **AUR.**, bell., ***calc.,*** **CALC-P.**, carc., chin-s., conch., des-ac., ***fl-ac.,*** gunp., ***mez., nit-ac., ph-ac.,*** phos., puls., ***pyrog.***, ***ruta, sil., staph., still.,*** symph.

OSTEOPOROSIS, brittle bones - bufo, ***calc.,*** calc-f., **CALC-P.**, calc-sil., carc., hecla, sil., ***symph.***

OTITIS INTERNA, inner ear - ***acon.***, ango., ars., arund., atro., aur., ***bar-c.***, ***bar-m.***, **BELL.**, bor., bov., bry., ***cact.***, **CALC.**, **CALC-S.**, canth., ***caps.***, carb-v., carbn-s., ***caust.***, **CHAM.**, chin., ***con.***, cortico., cur., ferr-p., **GRAPH.**, **HEP.**, ***kali-bi.***, ***kali-c.***, ***kali-chl.***, ***kali-i.***, ***kali-m.,*** kali-n., kino, kreos., ***lach.***, led., **LYC.**, ***mag-c.***, mag-m., **MERC.**, ***merc-c.***, merc-d., merc-i-r., mez., ***nat-s.***, ***nit-ac.***, **NUX-V.**, ***petr.***, ***ph-ac.***, phos., ***pic-ac.***, ***psor.***, ***puls.***, ***rhus-t.***, ***sang.***, sep., ***sil.***, spig., spong., **SULPH.**, ter., ther., ***thuj.***, verat-v., verb., zinc.

OTITIS MEDIA, infection, middle ear - acon., all-c., alum., ***apis***, arist-cl., ***arn.***, ***ars.***, ***asaf.***, asar., ***aur.***, bapt., ***bar-c.***, **BELL.**, ***bor.,*** bry., **CALC.**, calc-f., **CALC-S.**, cand-a., ***caps.***, ***carb-v.***, carbn-s., ***caust.***, **CHAM.**, chin., cocc., colch., con., ***cur., dulc.***, ***ferr-p.***, gels., **HEP.**, ***hydr.,*** **KALI-BI.**, ***kali-c.***, ***kali-chl.***, ***kali-i.***, **KALI-M.**, kali-s., kali-sil., kreos., lac-c., lac-h., lac-v., ***lach.,*** lap-a., **LYC.**, meningoc., **MERC.**, **MERC-D.**, methyl., mill., mur-ac., ***myris.***, ***nat-c.***, ***nat-m.***, ***nux-m.***, nux-v., ***ph-ac.***, phos., pneu., ***psor.***, **PULS.**, rhus-t., sep., **SIL.**, skook., stann., stram., **SULPH.**, ***tell.***, ***ter.***, ***thuj.***, tub., tub-a., tub-m., zinc.

OTOSCLEROSIS, ears - asar., calc., ***calc-f.,*** carb-v., cic., cortico., ferr-pic., graph., iod., iris, kres., mand., petr., syph., ***thiosin.,*** thyr., visc.

OVARIES, cancer - alumn., ***apis,*** ars., **AUR-M-N.**, carb-ac., carb-an., ***carc.,*** **CON.**, graph., kali-br., kreos., ***lach.,*** lap-a., ***lil-t.,*** lyc., med., ***pall.,*** plat., psor., ***sep., scirr., thuj.,*** **VIP.**, visc.

OVARIES, cysts - apis, apoc., arn., ars., aur., ***aur-i.,*** aur-m-n., bell., ***bov.,*** bry., ***bufo,*** canth., carb-an., chin., ***colch., coloc.,*** con., ferr-i., form., graph., ***iod.,*** ***kali-br.,*** kali-fcy., ***lach.,*** lil-t., ***lyc.,*** med., merc., murx., ***ov.,*** pall., ***plat.,*** prun., rhod., ***rhus-t.,*** sabin., sep., syc-co., syph., ter., thuj., zinc.

OVARIES, remedies, (See Oophoritis) - abrot., achy., **ACON.**, aesc., am-br., ambr., amor-r., ***ant-c.***, **APIS**, arg., arg-n., arn., ars., ars-i., aur., aur-ar., ***aur-i.***, aur-m., aur-m-n., bac., **BELL.**, brom., ***bry.***, ***cact.***, ***canth.***, caps., chel., ***chin.***, chin-s., cimic., cod., coli., coll., ***coloc., con.,*** crot-h., cub., dulc., euph., eupi., ferr-p., gels., graph., ***guai.***, ham., hep., hydro-c., ign., ***iod.***, ***lac-c.***, ***lach.***, ***lil-t.***, **LYC.**, mag-p., ***med.***, **MERC.**, ***merc-c.***, nit-ac., ***nux-v.***, **PALL.**, ***ph-ac.***, **PHOS.**, ***phyt.***, ***plat.***, **PODO.**, ***puls.***, pyrog., ran-b., rhus-t., sabad., sabal., **SABIN.**, **SEP.**, sil., staph., syc-co., ***syph.***, **THUJ.**, tub-r., ust., ***verat-v.***, vesp., visc., zinc., zinc-p.

OVARIES, tumors - apis., apoc., ars., ars-i., aur-m-n., bar-m., bov., calc., coloc., con., ferr-i., fl-ac., graph., hep., iod., kali-br., lach., lyc., med., ov., pall., plat., podo., sec., staph., stram., syph., thuj., zinc.

OVARIOTOMY, complaints after - ars., ***bell.***, ***bry.***, chin., coff., ***coloc.***, foll., hyper., ip., lach., lyc., naja, nux-v., orch., ***ov.***, ***staph.***

OVEREXERTION, ailments from - **ARN.**, ***ars.,*** **BELL-P.**, calc., ***ham., mill.,*** kali-p., nux-v., ***rhus-t., ruta.***

OVULATION, ailments during - ***foll.,*** lap-gr-m., sep.

OXALIC ACID, ailments from - ox-ac., urt-u.

OZONE, ailments from - am-c., ars., carb-v., lob., ***ozone., sul-ac.***

P

PAINLESSNESS, of complaints, usually painful - ant-c., ant-t., **ARN.**, asaf., con., ***hell.***, kali-bi., ***laur.***, mosch., **OP.**, ph-ac., psil., sac-alb., sec., **STRAM.**

PAINS, general - ***abrot.***, ***acon.***, act-sp., adon., ***aesc.***, aeth., **AGAR.**, alet., all-c., all-s., allox., ***alum.***, alum-p., alum-sil., alumn., am-be., am-c., am-caust., am-m., am-p., ambr., anac., anag., androc., ang., anh., ant-c., ant-o., ant-t., anthr., anthro., ***apis***, apoc., apoc-a., aq-mar., aran., arbu., arg., arg-n., arge., arist-cl., **ARN.**, **ARS.**, ars-h., ars-i., ars-s-f., asaf., asc-t., aspar., aster., atro., ***aur.***, aur-ar., aur-i., aur-m., aur-m-n., aur-s., aven., aza., bac., bad., ***bapt.***, bar-acet., bar-c., **BELL.**, ***bell-p.,*** benz-ac., **BERB.**, ***bol.***, bor., both-l., bov., brom., **BRY.**, cact., ***calc.***, calc-f., calc-hp., calc-i., ***calc-p.,*** calc-s., calc-sil., ***calen.,*** camph., cann-i., cann-s., **CANTH.**, caps., carb-ac., carb-an., carb-v., carbn-h., carbn-o., carbn-s., **CARC.**, card-m., ***carl.***, casc., cast., ***caul.***, **CAUST.**, cedr., **CHAM.**, **CHEL.**, ***chin.***, chin-ar., chin-s., chlor., cimic., cimx., ***cina***, cinnb., clem., cob-n., coca, cocc., **COFF.**, **COLCH.**, colchin., **COLOC.**, con., cop., corn., croc., crot-c., crot-h., croto-t., ***cupr.***, cur., cycl., daph., dicha., dig., dios., ***dros.***, ***dulc.***, dys-co., ***echi.***, elaps, elat., eucal., euon., **EUP-PER.**, eup-pur., euph., euph-a., euphr., fago., ***ferr.***, ferr-ar., ferr-i., ferr-p., ferr-pic., fl-ac., form., form-ac., franc., gaul., ***gels.***, get., gins., glon., glyc., glyc-g., gnaph., ***graph.***, grat., gua., ***guai.***, haem., ham., ***hecla.***, hed., hedeo, ***hell.***, helo., **HEP.**, hera., hydr., hydrc., hydro-c., hymosa, hyos., **HYPER.**, ign., ind., indg., iod., iodof., ***ip.***, iris, jac., jatr., jug-c., jug-r., **KALI-AR.**, ***kali-bi.***, kali-br., ***kali-c.***, ***kali-i.***, kali-m., kali-n., kali-p., **KALI-S.**, kali-sil., **KALM.**, ***kreos.***, lac-ac., ***lac-c.***, lac-d., lach., lact., lappa, lat-k., lat-m., led., lil-t., lith-c., **LYC.**, lycpr., lycps., ***lyss.***, macrin., mag-c., mag-m., **MAG-P.**, mag-s., magn-gr., mand., mang., **MED.**, meph., **MERC.**, ***merc-c.***, merc-i-f., merc-i-r., merc-s., merl., methyl., methyl-sal., mez., mill., morg., mosch., ***mur-ac.***, myric., naja, ***nat-ar.***, ***nat-c.***, nat-l., nat-m., ***nat-p.***, nat-s., nat-sal., ***nit-ac.***, nit-m-ac., nux-m., **NUX-V.**, nyct., ol-an., ol-j., op., osm., ox-ac., ozone, pall., paull-p., ped., petr., petros., ***ph-ac.***, ***phos.***, phys., **PHYT.**, plan., plat., **PLB.**, plb-acet., podo., prop., prun., psil., psor., ptel., **PULS.**, pyrog., quas., ***rad-br.***, ran-b., ran-s., raph., rat., rauw., rham-cal., rham-cath., **RHOD.**, **RHUS-T.**, rumx., ***ruta***, sabad., sabin., sal-ac., ***sang.***, ***sars.***, scol., ***sec.***, sel., senec., seneg., ***sep.***, sil., skook., sol-n., spig., spirae., spong., squil., stann., staph., ***stel.***, stict., still., stram., strept., stront-c., stroph-s., ***stry.***, stry-p., sul-ac., sul-i., sul-ter., sulfa., **SULPH.**, sumb., syc-co., symph., **SYPH.**, tab., tarax., **TARENT.**, tax., tell., ter., teucr., thal., thuj., thymu., thyr., til., tub., urt-c., urt-u., ***valer.***, **VERAT.**, verat-v., viol-o., viol-t., vip., visc., wye., xan., zinc., zinc-p.

PAINT FUMES, ailments from - ars., carb-ac., form., merc., plb.

PANCREAS, cancer - ars., ***bar-i.***, ***cadm-s.***, ***calc-ar.***, ***carc.***, carb-v., **CEAN.**, ***chel.***, **CON.**, **HYDR.**, nat-s., phos., ***scirr.***

PANCREAS, remedies - acet-ac., achy., adren., agar., ***allox.***, ammc., ant-c., aran-x., ***arg.***, ***arg-n.***, ars., ars-br., ars-i., aspar., ***atro.***, aur., bar-c., bar-m., ***bell.***, bol., bov., but-ac., ***calc.***, calc-ar., calc-f., calc-p., carb-an., carb-v., carc., chel., chim., chion., coloc., ***con.***, cortiso., ferr., ferr-i., fl-ac., glyc., hed., helon., hoit., hydr., ***insulin.***, ***iod.***, **IRIS**, jab., kali-br., kali-c., ***kali-i.***, kali-p., ***lac-ac.***, lac-c., lac-d., lac-v., lach., lept., **LYC.**, mag-f., mand., ***merc.***, merc-i-r., mom-b., nat-p., nat-s., nux-v., ol-j., ***pancreat.***, parathyr., pep., ph-ac., **PHOS.**, piloc., plb., puls., rauw., rhus-t., sac-alb., sac-l., sep., ***spong.***, sulph., ***syzyg.***, tarent., ter., thuj., thyr., ***trif-p.***, uran-n., urea,

PANCREATITIS, infection - achy., agar., allox., aran-x., ars., bar-m., **BELL.**, bol., but-ac., calc-ar., carb-an., ***coloc.***, kali-i., lept., merc., mom-b., parathyr., pep., ***phos.***, plb., puls., rauw., rhus-t., **SPONG.**

PANIC ATTACKS, (se Anxiety, Fear) - **ACON.**, aloe, alum., ang., **ARG-N.**, ***ars.***, ars-i., bar-c., bell., calc., calc-i., ***cann-i.***, ***carb-v.***, **CARC.**, caust., ***cham.***, chel., ***cocc.***, ***cupr.***, ***cupr-ar.***, ferr., **GELS.**, ***hyos.***, ictod., ign., **KALI-AR.**, kali-br., kali-c., **LUNA**, **LYC.**, ***med.***, merc., nat-c., nat-m., nat-s., nit-ac., op., **PHOS.**, plat., ruta, sep., spong., ***sulph.***, ***tab.***, thuj.

PANNUS, cornea - alum., ***apis***, **ARG-N.**, ***aur.***, ***bar-c.***, ***calc.***, cann-s., ***caust.***, ***euphr.***, ***graph.***, ***hep.***, kali-bi., kali-c., merc., ***merc-i-f.***, ***merc-i-r.***, merl., ***nit-ac.***, petr., rhus-t., ***sep.***, sil., syph., ***sulph.***

PARALYSIS, agitans, (see Parkinson's disease)

PARALYSIS, general - absin., ***acon.***, agar., ang., arag., arg-i., ***arg-n.***, ***arn.***, ars-i., asaf., astra-e., aur., ***aur-m.***, ***bar-acet.***, ***bar-c.***, ***bar-m.***, ***bell.***, calc-caust., ***calen.***, carbn-o., carbn-s., **CAUST.**, chen-a., chin-s., cic., **COCC.**, colch., **CON.**, ***cupr.***, ***dulc.***, elaps, **GELS.**, graph., grin., ***gua.***, helo., hydr-ac., hyos., ***hyper.***, ign., iris-fl., kali-br., ***kali-c.***, kali-i., kali-p., **LACH.**, ***lath.***, lol., merc-c., nat-m., ***nux-v.***, ***olnd.***, ***op.***, ***ox-ac.***, oxyt., **PHOS.**, ***phys.***, ***phys.***, pic-ac., plat., **PLB.**, ***plb-acet.***, ***plb-i.***, plect., ***rhus-t.***, sec., stann., staph., stry-f-c., sulph., tab., ***thal.***, verat., xan., zinc., zinc-p.

hemiplegia - acon., ***alum.***, ***anac.***, ***apis***, arg-n., ***ars.***, bapt., bar-m., ***both-l.***, ***cadm-s.***, **CAUST.**, ***cocc.***, coc-c., cop., elaps, ***graph.***, hyos., ***kali-c.***, ***kali-i.***, kali-p., ***lach.***, ***mur-ac.***, nat-c., ***ph-ac.***, ***phos.***, plb., **RHUS-T.**, ***sars.***, ***stann.***, staph., stront-c., ***sul-ac.***, tab., thuj.

paraplegia - agar., anh., ***arg-n.***, ***ars.***, bapt., caul., caust., con., gels., kali-t., kalm., ***lath.***, mang., nat-m., **NUX-V.**, phys., pic-ac., pip-m., plb., rhus-t., rhus-v., ruta, sec., stry., sulph., thal., thyr., vip., wild.

PARANOID, (see Schizophrenia) - **ANAC.**, anh., ars., bell., ***cann-i.***, carc., choc., cupr., hydrog., ***hyos.***, **LACH.**, kali-br., med., ***meli.***, merc., plat., plb., rauw., **STRAM.**, verat.

PARASITES, ailments from, (see Worms) - carc., ***chin.***, ***cina.***

PARKINSON'S, disease - ***agar.***, ant-t., aran., aran-ix., arg., ***arg-n.***, ars., aur., ***aur-s.***, aven., bar-c., bufo, ***camph-br.***, cann-i., chlorpr., cimic., cocain., cocc., ***con.***, dubin., ***dubo-m.***, ***gels.***, halo., ***helo.***, ***hyos.***, ***hyosin.***, ***kali-br.***, kres., lath., levo., lil-t., ***lol.***, lyc., ***mag-p.***, mang., **MERC.**, merc-s., nicot., nux-v., perh., ***phos.***, ***phys.***, ***plb.***, prun., psil., ***puls.***, rauw., reser., **RHUS-t.**, scut., stram., syph., tab., ***tarent.***, thiop., ***thuj.***, **ZINC.**, ***zinc-pic.***

PAROTID, glands, remedies - ***acon.,*** ail., ***am-c.,*** ant-t., anthr., ***ars., arum-t., aur.,*** aur-m., **BAR-C.,** ***bar-m.,*** **BELL.,*****brom., calc., carb-an.,*** **CARB-V.,** ***cham.,*** **CIST.,** cocc., ***con., crot-h.,*** dor., dulc., euphr., ***ferr-p., hep.,*** hippoz., **JAB.,** kali-ar., ***kali-bi., kali-c.,*** kali-m., kali-p., ***lach., lyc.,*** mag-p., **MERC.,** merc-i-f., merc-i-r., ***nat-m.,*** petr., ***phos.,*** phyt., **PILOC., PULS.,** ***rhus-t.,*** sars., ***sil.,*** sul-i., sulph., trif-p., trif-r.

PAROTID, glands, cancer - merc., ***phyt., scirr.***

PELLAGRA, general - ***ars.***, ars-s-r., bov., chin., gels., graph., hep., ign., ped., phos., plb-i., psor., puls., ***sec.***, ***sedi.***, sep., sulph.

PELVIC INFLAMMATORY DISEASE, uterus - ***acon., agn.,*** alum., **APIS,*****arn.,*** **ARS.,*****aur., aur-m.,*** **BELL.,*****bry.,*** bufo, ***cact.,*** calc., **CANTH.,*****carb-an.,*** carbn-s., caul., ***cham.,*** chin., cocc., ***coff.,*** coloc., con., croc., ferr., ferr-ar., graph., ***ham., hep.,*** hydr., ***hyos.,*** hyper., ign., ***iod.,*** ip., iris, kali-c., kali-p., kreos., **LAC-C., LACH., LYC.,** ***lyss.,*** mag-m., **MED.,** ***merc., nux-v.,*** op., ph-ac., ***phos.,*** **PULS.,** ***rhus-t., sabad.,*** **SABIN., SEC.,** ***sep., sil., stram., sulph.,*** **TER.,** thuj., ***verat., verat-v.,*** vib., visc.

PELVIC ORGANS, injuries - ***apis***, arn., ***bell-p.,*** bry., ***calen.***, carb-v., ***ham.***, hyper., lach., ***mill.***, nat-s., rhus-t., ruta. symph.

PEMPHIGUS - acon., am-m., ***anac.***, antipyrin., apis, ***ars.***, arum-t., bell., bufo, calc., calth., canth., carbn-o., caust., chin., chlorpr., ***crot-h.***, ***dulc.***, gamb., hep., hippoz., hydrc., iodof., jug-c., kali-p., lac-c., **LACH.**, lipp., ***lyc.***, ***manc.***, ***merc.***, ***merc-c.***, merc-pr-r., ***nat-m.***, ***nat-s.***, nat-sal., ***nit-ac.***, ph-ac., phos., ***psor.***, ran-b., ran-s., raph., rheum, ***rhus-t.***, rhus-v., ***sars.***, scroph-n., ***sep.***, ***sil.***, sul-ac., sulfonam., ***sulph.***, syph., ter., thuj.

PENIS, cancer - arg-n., ***ars.,*** bell., carbo-an., carbn-s., con., phos., phyt., sil., spong., thuj.

PERICARDITIS, heart, inflammation - achy., **ACON.**, adon., agar., anac., ant-ar., ant-c., ***ant-t.***, ***apis***, apoc., **ARS.**, ***ars-i.***, ars-s-f., ***asc-t.***, aur., aur-i., bell., ***bry.***, ***cact.***, calc-f., calc-s., cann-s., ***canth.***, cham., ***chlol.***, chlor., ***cimic.***, cob-n., coc-c., ***colch.***, colchin., crat., ***dig.***, eberth., ferr-p., fil., franc., glon., hep., hist., hoit., hydr., iber., ***iod.***, kali-ar., ***kali-c.***, kali-chl., ***kali-i.***, kali-m., ***kalm.***, ***lach.***, lycps., magn-gr., ***merc.***, merc-c., naja, nat-m., nat-n., ox-ac., paro-i., phase., plat., **PSOR.**, puls., raja-s., rhus-t., saroth., **SPIG.**, ***spong.***, squil., staphycoc., stroph., **SULPH.**, tere-ch., ***verat.***, ***verat-v.***, x-ray

PERIOSTEUM, cancer - con., ruta, phos., scirr., symph.

PERIOSTEUM, remedies - ***acon.,*** agar., ***apis,*** arg., arn., ***ars., asaf., aur.,*** **AUR-M.,** bell., ***bell-p.,*** **CALC-F.**, calc-p., chin., colch., ***ferr-i., ferr-p.,*** **FL-AC.**, kali-c., ***kali-i.,*** led., ***mang., merc., merc-c.,*** **MEZ.**, ***nit-ac.,*** **PH-AC.,** ***phos.,*** phyt., ***psor.,*** puls., rhus-t., **RUTA,** ***sil., staph.,*** **SYMPH.**

PERIOSTITIS, inflammation, periosteum - ***acon.***, ant-c., ***apis***, aran., ***ars.***, ***asaf.***, aur., aur-ar., ***aur-m.***, ***bell.***, bry., calc., calc-f., calc-p., calc-sil., chin., clem., colch., con., conch., eup-per., ***ferr-i.***, ***ferr-p.***, **FL-AC.**, form-ac., graph., ***guai.***, ***hecla.***, hep., ***iod.***, ***kali-bi.***, ***kali-i.***, lach., led., lyc., ***mang.***, ***merc.***, ***merc-c.***, **MEZ.**, myris., nat-sal., ***nit-ac.***, **PH-AC.**, phos., ***phyt.***, plat., ***psor.***, puls., rhod., rhus-t., **RUTA**, **SABIN.**, sars., sep., ***sil.***, ***staph.***, ***still.***, sulph., ***symph.***, tell., visc.

PERITONITIS, inflammation, enteritis - abrot., ***acet-ac.***, **ACON.**, act-sp., adlu., aethi-a., agar., agn., ail., all-s., aloe, alum., alumn., am-c., am-caust., ambr., ammc., anag., anan., ant-c., **ANT-T.**, **APIS**, aran., aran-ix., arg., arg-n., arist-cl., ***arn.***, **ARS.**, ars-i., asaf., asar., asc-t., astac., atro., aur., aur-m., bac., ***bapt.***, bar-c., bar-m., **BELL.**, bell-p., berb., beryl., bism., bol., bold., **BRY.**, but-ac., ***cact.***, cael., calad., calc-i., calc-s., calc-sil., camph., cann-i., cann-s., ***canth.***, caps., carb-an., ***carb-v.***, carc., ***cham.***, chel., chelo., chion., chloram., chlorpr., cic., cimic., cit-l., clem., cob-n., cocc., coch., coff., **COLCH.**, coli., ***coll.***, **COLOC.,** con., cop., corn., ***crot-c.***, ***crot-h.***, cub., cupr., cupr-acet., cupr-ar., cupr-s., cur., cyn-d., cyt-l., dig., dios., diosm., dol., dros., dulc., eberth., ***echi.***, eucal., eup-per., euph-c., ***ferr.***, ferr-ar., ferr-m., ferr-p., fl-ac., flor-p., gamb., ***gels.***, gins., graph., grat., grin., guat., ham., hed., hep., hip-ac., hippoz., hist., hoit., hydr., hydro-c., **HYOS.**, ign., iod., ***ip.***, ipom., jal., jug-c., junc., kali-ar., kali-bi., ***kali-c.***, ***kali-chl.***, kali-i., kali-m., ***kali-n.***, kali-p., lac-d., **LACH.**, **LAUR.**, **LYC.**, lycps., mag-c., mag-s., malar., mand., mang., mang-m., mang-s., ***med.,*** menis., ***merc.***, ***merc-c.***, merc-d., merc-i-f., merc-i-r., merc-s., ***mez.***, mim-p., morph., mosch., mur-ac., myric., nat-ar., nat-c., nat-m., nat-s., nit-ac., nit-m-ac., ***nuph.***, nux-m., ***nux-v.***, nym., oci., ***op.***, osm., ost., ***ox-ac.***, pall., parat., petr., ph-ac., **PHOS.**, phys., phyt., pin-s., pitu-a., pitu-p., plb., plb-i., polym., psor., ptel., ***puls.***, **PYROG.**, rad-br., raja-s., ran-b., ran-s., rauw., **RHUS-T.**, rhus-v., rob., sabal., sabin., samb., sang., sanguin-n., sant., saroth., sarr., scroph-n., ***sec.***, sel., senec., sep., ***sil.***, ***sin-n.***, sol-n., solin., spig., spong., squil., stann., staph., stel., ***stram.***, stroph-s., succ., sul-ac., sul-i., ***sulph.***, tab., tarax., tell., **TER.**, tere-ch., thlaspi, thuj., thymol., til., trio., tub-k., tub-r., urt-u., ven-m., ***verat.***, ***verat-v.***, vip., vip-a., wies., ***wye.***, xero, zinc-s., zinc-val.

PERSPIRATION, general - ***acet-ac.***, ***acon.***, aesc., aeth., ***agar.***, ail., all-c., alst-c., alst-s., alum., am-acet., am-c., am-m., ambr., aml-n., anac., ang., ***ant-c.***, **ANT-T.**, anthr., anthro., apis, apoc., apoc-a., aq-mar., arg., arg-n., arn., ***ars.***, ars-i., arum-t., arund., asaf., aur., bapt., ***bar-c.***, ***bell.***, benz-ac., berb., bol., bov., brom., ***bry.***, bufo, cact., cahin., calad., **CALC.**, calc-i., calc-s., camph., canch., cann-i., canth., ***caps.***, carb-ac., ***carb-an.***, ***carb-v.***, card-m., caust., ***cedr.***, cham., chel., **CHIN.**, ***chin-s.***, cic., cimic., cimx., cina, cinnb., cist., clem., ***cocc.***, coff., colch., coloc., con., corn., corn-f., crot-c., crot-h., croto-t., cupr., cupr-ar., cur., cycl., daph., ***dig.***, dios., dros., ***dulc.***, ***elaps***, ***elat.***, eup-per., eup-pur., euphr., eupi., **FERR.**, ferr-ar., fl-ac., gamb., ***gels.***, glon., glyc-g., ***graph.***, grat., ***guai.***, guare., hell., **HEP.**, hydr-ac., ***hyos.***, ign., ***iod.***, ***ip.***, iris, jab., jatr., kali-ar., kali-bi., kali-c., kali-i., kali-n., kali-s., kalm., kreos., lac-ac., lach., lachn., lappa, laur., led., lil-t., lob., **LYC.**, ***mag-c.***, mag-s., mang., med., meny., **MERC.**, merc-c., merc-cy., merl., ***mez.***, morph., mosch., mur-ac., myric., naja, ***nat-ar.***, nat-c., **NAT-M.**, nicc., nit-ac., nux-m., **NUX-V.**, ol-j., **OP.**, ***ox-ac.***, oxyg., par., ***petr.***, ***ph-ac.***, **PHOS.**, phys., piloc., plan., plat., plb., ***podo.***, **PSOR.**, ptel., puls., ***ran-s.***, rheum, rhod., ***rhus-t.***, rob., sabad., sabin., sal-ac., **SAMB.**, sang., sarr., ***sec.***, sel., senec., **SEP.**, **SIL.**, sol-n., spig., spong., stann., staph., stram., stry., sul-ac., ***sulph.***, sumb., tab., tarax., tarent., tax., teucr., ther., thuj., trio., tub., ***valer.***, **VERAT.**, ***verat-v.***, vip., wye., zinc., ***zing.***, ziz.

agg., after - ars., bell., bry., ***calc.***, carb-v., **CHIN.,** con., ign., iod., kali-c., lyc., **MERC.,** nat-c., nat-m., nux-v., petr., **PH-AC.,** ***phos.,*** ***puls.,*** sel., **SEP.,** sil., spig., squil., ***staph.,*** ***sulph.***

amel., after - ***acon.,*** aesc., ambr., am-m., ant-t., ***ars.,*** bar-c., bell., bov., ***bry.,*** ***calad.,*** ***canth.,*** **CHAM.,** chel., clem., cocc., coloc., **GELS.,** ***graph.,*** hell., ***hep.,*** hyos., ip., kali-n., led., lyc., mag-m., **NAT-M.,** nit-ac., nux-v., ***olnd.,*** op., **PSOR.,** puls., rhod., **RHUS-T.,** sabad., sabin., samb., sel., spong., stram., ***stront-c.,*** ***sulph.,*** sul-ac., tarax., ***thuj.,*** valer., ***verat.***

PESTICIDES, poisoning, ailments, from - am-c., arg-n., **ARS.,** ***ars-i.,*** cadm., cadm-s., ***carb-ac.,*** carc., gels., ***merc.,*** nit-ac., nux., ozone., ***phos.,*** sep., sil., sulph., thuj.

DDT, poisoning - ars.

dioxin, poisoning - ars., cadm-s., carc., merc., phos., sep., sil., sulph., thuj.

malathion, poisoning - ars., merc., phos.

organophosphates, poisoning - agar., alum., ars., con., gels., kali-br., merc., nit-ac., phos., ***phys.***

paraquat, poisoning - am-c., ars., fl-ac., kali-br., merc., nit-ac.

PETROLEUM, ailments from - graph., ***petr.,*** phos., sil., sulph.

PHARYNX, cancer - cist.

PHARYNGITIS, inflammation of pharynx - bar-m., bell., ***calc.,*** ***fl-ac.,*** kali-i., ***lac-c.,*** lach., merc., naja, ***nat-m.,*** ***petr.,*** ***phyt.,*** ***sep.,*** **SIL.,** sulph.

PHENOBARITAL, ailments from - gels., nux-v., op., ***phenob.***

PHIMOSIS, penis - acon., ***arn.***, ars., bell., bry., calad., ***calc.***, ***cann-s.***, ***canth.***, caps., ***cinnb.***, coloc., cycl., ***dig.***, euph., ***ham.***, ***hep.***, jac., jac-c., kali-i., lach., ***lyc.***, **MERC.**, merc-c., merc-i-r., narz., nat-m., **NIT-AC.**, ***rhus-t.***, rumx., sabin., sep., ***sulph.***, sumb., thuj.

PHLEBITIS, blood - **ACON.**, agar., ***all-c.***, ant-c., ***ant-t.***, apis, arist-cl., ***arn.***, ***ars.***, ***bell.***, both-l., **BRY.**, ***bufo***, **CALC.**, calc-ar., ***calc-f.***, carb-v., carbn-s., ***cham.***, ***chin.***, chlorpr., **CLEM.**, con., crot-h., ferr-p., graph., **HAM.**, hecla., hep., hir., ***iod.***, ***kali-c.***, kali-m., kreos., **LACH.**, ***led.***, ***lyc.***, ***lycps.***, mag-c., mag-f., merc., merc-cy., merc-i-r., mill., morg., mur-ac., ***nat-s.***, nux-v., phos., prot., ***puls.***, rhod., **RHUS-T.**, ruta, ***sep.***, ***sil.***, spig., stront-br., stront-c., sulfa., ***sulph.***, thiop., thuj., verat., ***vip.***, vip-a., zinc.

PHLEGMASIA, alba dolens, (see Phlebitis)

PHOSPHORUS, ailments from - cupr-s., kali-ma., lach., nux-v., ph-ac., ***phos.***, ter.

PITYRIASIS, skin - agar., anac., aran-ix., arg., ***ars.***, ars-i., bac., ***berb-a.***, ***calc.***, carb-ac., caul., clem., ***colch.***, eryth., ***fl-ac.***, graph., kali-ar., kali-br., ***mang.***, ***merc.***, merc-pr-r., ***mez.***, nat-ar., ***nat-m.***, olnd., ***phos.***, phyt., pip-m., psor., ***sep.***, ***sil.***, staph., ***sul-ac.***, sul-i., sulo-ac., sulph., tell., ter., ***thuj.***, thyr., toxo.

PLACENTA, general - ***agn.***, all-s., ***arn.***, ***ars.***, art-v., ***bell.***, **CANTH**., carb-v., ***caul.***, cham., chin., cimic., cocc., con., croc., cupr., ***erig.***, ergot., ferr., gels., ***goss.***, ***hydr.***, hyos., ***ign.***, ***ip.***, ***kali-c.***, mag-p., ***nux-v.***, phos., ***plac.***, plat., ***puls.***, pyrog., rhus-t., ***sabin.***, ***sec.***, **SEP**., stram., sulph., verat., ***verat-v.***, visc.

placenta, praevia - ***erig.***, ***ip.***, ***nux-v.***, phos., ***sabin.***, sec., ***sep.***, verat., ***verat-v.***

retained, placenta - ***agn.***, all-s., ***arn.***, ***ars.***, ***art-v.***, ***bell.***, **CANTH.**, carb-v., **CAUL.**, ***cham.***, chin., cimic., cocc., con., croc., cupr., ergot., ferr., gels., ***goss.***, ***hydr.***, hyos., ***ign.***, ip., ***kali-c.***, mag-p., ***nux-v.***, phos., plat., ***puls.***, pyrog., rhus-t., ***sabin.***, ***sec.***, **SEP.**, stram., sulph., verat-v., visc.

PLAGUE, (see Bubonic) - ars., calc-o-t., crot-h., ign., lach., naja, phos., pyrog., tarent-c.

PLEURA-pneumonia - **ANT-T.,** ***asaf.,*** **BRY.,** ***calc.,*** ***camph.,*** ***caps.,*** ***chin.,*** ***dulc.,*** ***ferr.,*** ***hep.,*** ***iod.,*** ***kali-i.,*** ***lach.,*** **PHOS.,** ***rhus-t.,*** ***seneg.,*** ***sulph.***

PLEURISY, general - abrot., **ACON.,** ant-ar., ant-t., ***apis,*** ***arn.,*** ***arg-n.,*** ***ars.,*** ars-i., arum-t., asc-t., bad., ***bell.,*** ***bor.,*** **BRY.,** ***cact.,*** ***calc.,*** ***cann-s.,*** ***canth.,*** **CARB-AN.,** ***carb-v.,*** ***carbn-s.,*** card-m., ***chel.,*** chin., ***colch.,*** ***dig.,*** ***dulc.,*** erio., ferr-m., ***ferr-p.,*** form., ***guai.,*** ***hep.,*** ***iod.,*** ***kali-ar.,*** **KALI-C.,** ***kali-chl.,*** ***kali-i.,*** kali-p., ***kali-s.,*** ***laur.,*** led., lob-c., ***merc.,*** merc-d., ***mur-ac.,*** nat-m., nat-s., ***nit-ac.,*** op., ***phos.,*** ***ran-b.,*** rhus-t., sabad., ***sang.,*** **SENEG.,** sep., sil., spig., ***squil.,*** ***stann.,*** **SULPH.,** sul-ac., tub., verat-v.

PLEUROSTHOTONOS - acon., bell., bry., hyos., phos., stann., stram.

PNEUMONIA, infection, lungs - **ACON.**, aesc., ***agar.***, ***all-c.***, am-c., am-i, ant-ar., ***ant-c.***, ant-i., ant-s., **ANT-T.**, ***apis***, apom., ***arg-n.***, ***arn.***, **ARS.**, **ARS-I.**, ars-s-f., arum-t., asaf., asc-t., aur., aur-m., ba-tn., bac., ***bad.***, bar-c., bar-i., ***bell.***, ***benz-ac.***, beryl., both-l., ***brom.***, **BRY.**, ***cact.***, cadm., ***calc.***, calc-s., calc-sil., camph., ***cann-s.***, canth., caps., carb-ac., ***carb-an.***, **CARB-V.**, ***carbn-s.***, carc., cham., **CHEL.**, ***chin.***, ***chlor.***, cina, coff., coffin., ***con.***, cop., corn., crot-h., ***cupr.***, ***dig.***, dros., dulc., ***elaps***, eup-per., ***ferr.***, ***ferr-ar.***, ***ferr-i.***, **FERR-P.**, ***gels.***, glyc., graph., **HEP.**, ***hippoz.***, ***hyos.***, hyper., ign., ***iod.***, ***ip.***, kali-ar., ***kali-bi.***, ***kali-br.***, **KALI-C.**, ***kali-chl.***, kali-hp., ***kali-i.***, kali-m., ***kali-n.***, ***kali-p.***, ***kali-s.***, ***kreos.***, ***lach.***, ***lachn.***, ***laur.***, led., **LOB.**, **LYC.**, lycps., **MERC.**, merc-cy., ***mill.***, mur-ac., myos., myrt-c., nat-ar., ***nat-m.***, ***nat-s.***, ***nit-ac.***, nux-v., op., ox-ac., ***ph-ac.***, **PHOS.**, phys., plb., pneu., podo., ***psor.***, **PULS.**, pyrog., ran-b., **RHUS-T.**, rumx., ***sabad.***, samb., ***sang.***, sec., senec., **SENEG.**, **SEP.**, ***sil.***, solin., spig., spong., ***squil.***, stann., stann-i., ***stram.***, stroph., stry., sul-ac., sul-i., **SULPH.**, syc-co., ***ter.***, tub., tub-a., ***tub-k.***, urt-u., ***verat.***, **VERAT-V.**, x-ray

POISON OAK or ivy, (see Rhus poisoning) - agar., am-c., **ANAC.**, arn., ***bry.***, **CLEM.**, **CROTO-T.**, cupr., ***graph.***, ***grin.***, kali-s., led., lob., ***nuph.***, plan., ***rhus-r.***, **RHUS-T.**, ***sang.***, ***sep.***, sulph.

POLIOMYELITIS, infection - ***acon.***, aeth., alum., arg-n., arn., ars., bell., ***bung-f.***, ***calc.***, carb-ac., ***caust.***, chin-ar., chr-s., cur., dulc., ferr-i., ferr-p., **GELS.**, hydr-ac., hydro-c., hyos., kali-i., kali-p., karw-h., kres., lach., **LATH.**, merc., nux-v., phos., phys., ***plb.***, plb-i., ***rhus-t.***, sec., stry-p., sulph., verat., verat-v.

POLYCYTHEMIA, blood - carc., ferr., phos.

POLYPS, general - agra., ***all-c.***, alum., alumn., ambr., ant-c., ***apis***, arn., ***aur.***, bell., berb., bry., cadm-s., **CALC.**, calc-i., **CALC-P.**, ***calc-s.***, ***carb-an.***, carc., ***caust.***, coc-c., **CON.**, dulc., ***form.***, form-ac., graph., hecla., ***hep.***, hydr., ***kali-bi.***, kali-i., kali-m., ***kali-n.***, kali-s., led., ***lem-m.***, ***lyc.***, ***med.***, ***merc.***, merc-c., merc-i-r., ***mez.***, nat-m., nat-s., nit-ac., petr., ph-ac., **PHOS.**, ***psor.***, puls., **SANG.**, ***sanguin-n.***, sep., ***sil.***, **STAPH.**, sul-ac., sulph., syc-co., **TEUCR.**, ***thuj.***, wye., zinc-chr.

POTASSIUM, ailments, from - camph., helon., hydr., ***kali-br.***, kali-c., kali-cy., kail-m., kali-p., kali-s., nux-v., phys., sul-ac., ter., zinc.

PREGNANCY, general, (see Childbirth) - **ACON.**, aesc., ***agar.***, **ALET.**, alum., am-c., am-m., ambr., ang., ***ant-c.***, **ANT-T.**, ***apis***, ***arg.***, arg-n., arist-cl., arn., ars., asaf., ***asar.***, ***bar-c.***, **BELL.**, bell-p., ***benz-ac.***, berb., ***bism.***, ***bor.***, bry., **CALC.**, calc-p., **CAMPH.**, ***canth.***, ***caps.***, **CARB-AC.**, ***carb-v.***, carc., caul., **CAUST.**, **CHAM.**, ***chel.***, ***chin.***, cic., **CIMIC.**, cina, cinnb., **COCC.**, coff., **COLL.**, coloc., con., **CROC.**, cupr., cycl., dig., ***dros.***, dulc., equis., ***ferr.***, ***ferr-p.***, ***gels.***, glon., ***goss.***, graph., ham., **HELL.**, helon., hep., hydr., ***hyos.***, ign., iod., **IP.**, jab., kali-bi., kali-br., kali-c., kali-chl., ***kali-fcy.***, kali-i., kalm., kreos., ***lac-ac.***, ***lach.***, ***lam.***, ***laur.***, lyc., ***lyss.***, mag-c., mag-m., mang., ***merc.***, ***mosch.***, mur-ac., ***murx.***, nat-c., nat-m., nit-ac., ***nux-m.***, **NUX-V.**, op., ***petr.***, ph-ac., phos., ***plat.***, plb., podo., pop., ***psor.***, **PULS.**, pyrog., rat., rhus-t., ***sabad.***, ***sabin.***, ***sec.***, sel., **SEP.**, sil., spig., ***stann.***, staph., ***stram.***, sul-ac., ***sulph.***, tab., ***tarent.***, thuj., valer., **VERAT.**, vib., viol-o., zinc.

PRE-MENSTRUAL, syndrome, (P.M.S.) - alum., ***am-c.***, am-m., arg-n., asaf., asar., ***bar-c.***, bar-m., bell., bor., **BOV.**, bry., **CALC.**, **CALC-P.**, canth., carb-an., ***carb-v.***, carbn-s., caust., cham., chin., cimic., cina, cocc., coff., ***con.***, croc., **CUPR.**, cycl., dulc., ***ferr.***, ferr-i., **FOLL.**, gels., graph., hep., ***hyos.***, ign., iod., ip., ***kali-c.***, kali-n., ***kreos.***, **LAC-C.**, **LACH.**, **LYC.**, mag-c., mag-m., ***mang.***, ***merc.***, mez., mosch., mur-ac., nat-c., **NAT-M.**, ***nat-p.***, nux-m., nux-v., petr., ***ph-ac.***, ***phos.***, ***plat.***, **PULS.**, rhus-t., ruta, sabad., sars., **SEP.**, sil., spig., spong., stann., staph., **SULPH.**, sul-ac., valer., **VERAT.**, ***vib.***, **ZINC.**

PRIAPISM, penis, painful erections - cann-s., canth., lyss.

PROCTITIS, inflammation, rectum and anus - ***aesc.***, aloe, alum., ambr., ***ant-c.***, colch., coll., ferr-p., ***hep.***, hydr., ip., kali-bi., kali-i., ***merc.***, merc-c., ***nit-ac.***, ***op.***, paeon., ***phos.***, podo., ric., sabal., ***sulph.***, zing.

PROLAPSED, uterus - abies-c., acon., ***aesc.***, agar., agn., ***alet.***, ***aloe***, ***alum.***, alum-p., alum-sil., ***alumn.***, am-m., anan., ant-c., ***apis***, **ARG.**, **ARG-N.**, ***arn.***, ***ars.***, ars-i., art-v., asper., aster., **AUR.**, aur-ar., aur-i., aur-m., ***aur-m-n.***, **AUR-S.**, ***bell.***, ***benz-ac.***, berb., **BOR.**, ***bry.***, bufo, **CALC.**, calc-ar., calc-f., ***calc-p.***, calc-s., calc-sil., calen., canth., ***carb-an.***, carb-v., caul., ***cham.***, chel., chim., ***chin.***, chin-ar., ***cimic.***, ***cina***, cocc., coll., ***coloc.***, ***con.***, croc., crot-h., croto-t., dirc., ***dulc.***, erig., eupi., ***ferr.***, ferr-ar., ferr-br., ***ferr-i.***, ferr-p., fl-ac., ***frax.***, gels., ***graph.***, hedeo, ***helon.***, hydr., hydrc., ***ign.***, inul., iod., ***ip.***, kali-ar., ***kali-bi.***, kali-br., ***kali-c.***, kali-cy., kali-p., kali-s., kali-sil., kreos., lac-c., ***lach.***, lappa, led., **LIL-T.**, lyc., ***lyss.***, ***mag-c.***, mag-m., mang., ***mel-c-s.***, merc., mill., ***mur-ac.***, ***murx.***, nat-c., nat-ch., **NAT-H.**, ***nat-m.***, **NAT-P.**, ***nit-ac.***, ***nux-m.***, ***nux-v.***, onos., op., **PALL.**, ***petr.***, ***ph-ac.***, phel., phos., phyt., **PLAT.**, ***podo.***, psor., **PULS.**, pyrog., rheum, ***rhus-t.***, ruta, ***sabin.***, samb., sang., ***sec.***, sel., senec., **SEP.**, ***sil.***, spig., ***squil.***, ***stann.***, ***staph.***, stram., sul-ac., sul-i., ***sulph.***, teucr., ***thuj.***, ***til.***, tril., ***tub.***, ***ust.***, verat., vib., zinc., zinc-p., zinc-val.

PROSTATE, cancer - ars., aur-m., bar-i., cadm-f., cadm-i., ***carc.***, chim., **CON.**, ***crot-h.***, ***cop.***, euph.,

iod., kali-cy., **LYC.**, med., op., pall., phyt., plb., ***psor.***, **SABAL.**, sars., **SCIRR.**, ***sel.***, senec., ***sil.***, ***sulph.***, **THUJ.**, thymol.

PROSTATE, gland, remedies - aesc., ***agn.***, all-s., aloe, alum., ***apis***, aspar., aur., ***bar-c.***, bar-i., baros., bell., ***berb.***, ***calc.***, calc-f., calc-i., cann-i., cann-s., canth., caust., **CHIM.**, clem., **CON.**, crot-h., ***cop.***, cub., **DAM.**, **DIG.**, epig., fab., ***ferr-pic.***, graph., hep., ***hydrang.***, ***iod.***, ***kali-i.***, lach., lith-c., ***lyc.***, ***med.***, ***mela.***, merc., nat-s., ***nit-ac.***, ol-sant., pareir., ***ph-ac.***, phos., phyt., pic-ac., podo., polyg., pop., **PULS.**, **SABAL.**, sars., **SEL.**, ***sep.***, ***sil.***, ***solid.***, **STAPH.**, sul-i., sulph., terebe., **THUJ.**, uva., visc., zinc.

PROSTATITIS, infection - acon., aesc., agn., aloe, alum., alum-sil., anac., **APIS**, arg., arist-cl., arn., aur., bar-c., bell., bov., brach., bry., cact., calad., calc., cann-i., cann-s., canth., ***caps.***, carbn-s., ***caust.***, **CHIM.**, cic., clem., colch., ***con.***, ***cop.***, ***cub.***, cupr., cycl., ***dig.***, ***dulc.***, euphr., ***fab.***, ferr-p., ferr-pic., ***gels.***, graph., ***hep.***, hipp., hydrang., hydrc., iod., ***kali-bi.***, kali-br., kali-c., kali-i., lach., lil-t., lith-c., ***lyc.***, mag-i., **MED.**, ***merc.***, merc-c., merc-d., ***nit-ac.***, ***nux-v.***, ol-sant., pareir., ***petr.***, ph-ac., phyt., pic-ac., pitu-gl., polytr., pop-c., **PULS.**, pyrog., rhus-t., **SABAD.**, ***sabal.***, salx-n., sec., ***sel.***, senec., ***sep.***, ***sil.***, solid., spong., ***staph.***, sul-ac., ***sulph.***, **THUJ.**, trib., tritic., ***verat-v.***, vesi., zinc.

PROZAC, ailments from - ***aur.***, carc., proz., staph.

PRURIGO, nodularis, skin - acon., aln., ***ambr.***, anthro., ***ars.***, ***ars-i.***, ars-s-f., carb-ac., ***chlol.***, ***dol.***, kali-bi., ***lyc.***, ***merc.***, ***mez.***, ***nit-ac.***, ***olnd.***, ov., ped., ***rhus-t.***, ***rhus-v.***, ***rumx.***, sil., ***sulph.***, ter.

PSORIASIS, skin - alum., am-c., ambr., ant-t., aran-ix., ***ars.***, **ARS-I.**, ars-s-f., ars-s-r., asaf., aster., aur., aur-ar., aur-m-n., berb-a., bor., bry., bufo, ***calc.***, ***calc-s.***, ***canth.***, carb-ac., carc., cast-eq., ***chin.***, ***chrysar.***, cic., ***clem.***, cor-r., cortiso., cupr., cupr-acet., des-ac., dulc., dys-co., elae., emetin., ferr., ferr-ar., fl-ac., form., form-ac., **GRAPH.**, hep., hydrc., ichth., iod., ***iris***, ***kali-ar.***, kali-bi., ***kali-br.***, ***kali-c.***, kali-p., ***kali-s.***, lac-c., led., ***lob.***, **LYC.**, mag-c., ***mang.***, med., ***merc.***, merc-aur., merc-c., merc-i-r., ***mez.***, **MORG-G.**, mur-ac., naphtin., nat-ar., **NAT-M.**, ***nit-ac.***, nit-m-ac., nuph., olnd., ***petr.***, ph-ac., ***phos.***, **PHYT.**, plat., ***psor.***, ***puls.***, rad-br., ran-b., ***rhus-t.***, rumx., saroth., ***sarr.***, ***sars.***, **SEP.**, ***sil.***, **STAPH.**, stel., stry-ar., stry-p., sul-i., ***sulph.***, tell., ter., teucr., thuj., **THYR.**, tub., ust., x-ray

PTOMAINE, gas, ailments from - ***absin.***, acet-ac., all-c., ***ars.***, camph., carb-an., carb-v., colch., crot-h., ***cupr-ar.***, gunp., kreos., lach., puls., ***pyrog.***, urt-u., ***verat.***

PUBERTY, ailments from - ***acon.***, agar., ***ant-c.***, apoc., aur., bell., ***calc.***, ***calc-p.***, caust., cimic., croc., cupr., ferr., ***ferr-p.***, **GELS.**, ***graph.***, guai., hell., helon., **IGN.**, iod., ***jug-r.***, kali-br., ***kali-c.***, kali-p., ***lach.***, mag-p., mill., **NAT-M.**, ***ph-ac.***, **PHOS.**, plat., **PULS.**, ***senec.***, **SEP.**, sil., stram., ther., verat., viol-o.

PUERPERAL, fever, (see Childbirth) - ***acon.***, ail., ant-c., anthr., ***apis***, ***arg-n.***, **ARN.**, ars., ***bapt.***, bell., ***bry.***, calc., cann-i., canth., carb-ac., carb-an., **CARBN-S.**, card-m., **CHAM.**, chin., chin-ar., ***chin-s.***, cimic., cocc., coff., **COLOC.**, con., croc., crot-h., cypr., **ECHI.**, ***ferr.***, gels., helon., ***hydr-ac.***, ***hyos.***, ign., ip., kali-br., kali-c., kali-m., ***kali-p.***, kreos., **LACH.**, **LYC.**, med., merc., merc-c., mill., ***mur-ac.***, **NUX-V.**, op., phos., phyt., plat., **PULS.**, puls-n, **PYROG.**, **RHUS-T.**, sabal., sabin., sal-ac., sec., ***sep.***, sil., stram., **SULPH.**, ter., til., verat., ***verat-v.***, zinc.

PULMONARY, edema - acet-ac., ***am-c.***, am-i, ant-ar., **ANT-T.**, **APIS**, **APOC.**, **ARS.**, ars-i., ***asaf.***, ***aspar.***, ***aur-i.***, ***aur-m.***, beryl., **BRY.**, cadm-s., calc., cann-s., ***canth.***, ***carb-v.***, ***carbn-s.***, chel., chin., chin-ar., coch., **COLCH.**, cortico., ***crot-h.***, croto-t., ***dig.***, ***dulc.***, ferr-m., ***fl-ac.***, **HELL.**, ***hyos.***, ***iod.***, ***ip.***, jab., ***kali-ar.***, **KALI-C.**, ***kali-i.***, ***kali-p.***, kres., **LACH.**, ***lact.***, lat-m., **LYC.**, ***merc.***, **MERC-S.**, mez., mur-ac., ***nat-m.***, op., ***phos.***, piloc., plb., ***psor.***, pulm-v., puls., ***ran-b.***, rat., ***sang.***, senec., ***seneg.***, ***sil.***, ***spig.***, ***squil.***, stann., stront-c., stroph., ***sulph.***, ***ter.***, thal., tub., uran., verat., ***zinc.***

PULSE, abnormal - **ACON.**, agar., agn., ambr., am-c., am-m., ant-c., ***ant-t.***, arg., ***arg-n.***, ***arn.***, **ARS.**, **ARS-I.**, asaf., asar., aur., bar-c., **BELL.**, bism., bor., bov., ***bry.***, calad., calc., ***camph.***, cann-s., canth., caps., carb-an., ***carb-v.***, ***carbn-s.***, caust., cham., chel., ***chin.***, cic., cina, cocc., colch., coloc., ***con.***, croc., **CUPR.**, **DIG.**, dulc., ferr., ***gels.***, ***glon.***, graph., guai., hell., ***hep.***, **HYOS.**, ign., **IOD.**, ip., ***kali-c.***, kali-n., **KREOS.**, **LACH.**, ***laur.***, led., lyc., mang., meny., ***merc.***, mez., mosch., mur-ac., nat-m., nit-ac., nux-m., nux-v., olnd., **OP.**, par., petr., **PH-AC.**, **PHOS.**, plat., plb., puls., ran-b., ran-s., rheum, rhod., **RHUS-T.**, sabad., sabin., samb., ***sec.***, seneg., ***sep.***, **SIL.**, spig., spong., squil., stann., staph., **STRAM.**, stront-c., ***sulph.***, sul-ac., thuj., valer., **VERAT.**, viol-o., viol-t., zinc

PUNCTURE, wounds, (see Wounds, general) - **APIS**, aran., arn., **CALEN.**, ***carb-v.***, cic., hep., **HYPER.**, lach., **LED.**, **NIT-AC.**, phase., ***plan.***, plb., sil., sul-ac., sulph.

PURGATIVES, ailments from - ***aloe***, alum., carb-v., chin., chin-s., hydr., ***lyc.***, **NUX-V.**, op., sulph.

PURPURA HEMORRHAGICA - acon., alet., aln., am-m., ***arn.***, ***ars.***, ars-i., ars-s-f., bapt., bell., berb., both-l., bov., bry., ***carb-v.***, carc., chin., chin-s., chlol., chlor., cor-r., croc., ***crot-h.***, ***cupr.***, erig., ferr., ferr-pic., ***ham.***, hyos., iod., ip., jug-r., ***kali-i.***, **LACH.**, **LED.**, meli., merc., merc-c., mill., mur-ac., naja, nat-n., nit-ac., nux-v., ***ph-ac.***, **PHOS.**, ptel., pyrog., ***rhus-t.***, rhus-v., ruta, sabin., sal-ac., **SEC.**, sil., stram., **SUL-AC.**, sulph., sulfon., **TER.**, thlaspi, tub., ust., verat-v.

PYEMIA, blood, (see Septicemia) - **ANTHR.,** ***ars., bapt., calc., crot-h.,*** echi., ***hippoz.,*** **LACH.,** ph-ac., phos., **PYROG.,** verat.

PYLORIC, stenosis - abrot., ***aeth.,*** am-c., carc., ***dys-co., orni.***

PYOMETRA, retained pus in uterus - lach., merc., ***puls., pyrog., sep.***

Q

QUARTAN, fever - acon., anac., ant-c., aran., arn., ***ars.,*** bell., bry., **BUFO,** carb-v., ***chin-s.,*** **CIMX.,** cina, chin., clem., ***coff.,*** cor-r., elat., ***eup-per.,*** hell., ***hyos., ign.,*** iod., ***ip.,*** lach., lap-gr-m., lyc., meny., mill., ***nat-m.,*** **NUX-V.,** oci-s., ***phel.,*** plan., podo., ***puls.,*** rhus-t., ***sabad., sin-n.,*** verat.

QUININE, ailments from - am-c., ant-i., ***ant-t., apis,*** **ARN.,** ***ars.,*** ars-s-f., asaf., aza., ***bell.,*** bry., **CALC.,** calc-ar., caps., carb-an., **CARB-V.,** cham., chelo., **CHIN.,** chin-ar., ***chin-s., cina,*** coloc., corn-f., cupr., cycl., dig., eucal., **FERR.,** ferr-ar., gels., hell., ***hep.,*** **IP.,** kali-ar., lac-d., ***lach.,*** mang., meny., merc., **NAT-M.,** nat-p., nat-s., nux-m., **NUX-V.,** parth., ***ph-ac.,*** phos., plb., **PULS.,** ran-s., samb., sel., ***sep.,*** stann., sul-ac., ***sulph., verat.***

QUINSY, general, (see Tonsillitis) - acon., ***bar-c., bar-m.,*** ferr-m., hep., lach., lyc., merc-i-r.,phos., psor., ran-s., sang., sanguin-n., sep., tarent., vesp.

QUOTIDIAN, fever - acon., aesc., anac., ant-c., ant-t., apis, **ARS.,** bapt., bar-c., bell., bry., cact., calc., calc-s., ***caps.,*** carb-v., ***cedr.,*** cham., ***chin-s.,*** cic., cina, cur., ***aran.,*** elaps, elat., eucal., ***eup-per., eup-pur.,*** gamb., gels., graph., ***hep.,*** hydr., ***ign., ip., kali-br.,*** kali-c., lach., lap-gr-m., ***lob.,*** lyc., mag-c., ***nat-m.,*** nit-ac., nux-v., ***petros.,*** phos., plan., podo., polyp-p, ptel., ***puls., rhus-t.,*** sabad., ***samb., sep.,*** spig., stann., staph., ***stram.,*** sulph., ***tarax., verat.***

R

RABIES, hydrophobia - acet-ac., aconin., agar., agav-a., anag., anan., ant-c., arg-n., ars., ***aspar.,*** **BELL.,** calc., cann-i., ***canth.,*** cedr., chlol., chlor., cocci-s., crot-h., cupr., ***cur.,*** fagu., gua., ho., ***hydr-ac.,*** **HYOS.,** iod., jatr., ***lach.,*** laur., **LYSS.,** merc., nux-v., perh., ***phel., phos.,*** plb., ran-s., ruta, sabad., sant., scut., spirae., **STRAM.,** sulph., tanac., tarent., ter., trach., verat., visc., xan.

RADIATION, sickness, poisoning, ailments, from, (see X-ray) - alf., ars., **BISM.,** ***cadm-i.,*** **CADM-S.,** calc-f., calen., chin., cob., ***fl-ac.,*** hydr., ***ip.,*** nux-v., ***phos.,*** rad-br., sil., **SOL.,** ***stront-c.,*** uran-n., x-ray.

radiation, burns, from - calc-f., canth., caust., fl-ac., phos., rad-br., ***sol.,*** x-ray.

ulcers, from - ***fl-ac.,*** rad-br., x-ray.

RADON, poisoning, ailments from gas - asbes., cob., radon., uran-n.

RANULA - **AMBR., CALC.,** ***canth.,*** cham., chr-ac., eucal., ferr-p., fl-ac., hippoz., lac-c., lacer., ***lach.,*** lyss., ***merc., mez., nat-m., nit-ac., plb.,*** psor., sac-alb., ***staph.,*** syph., ***thuj.,*** verat.

RAPE, victims of - **ACON.,** anac., androc., **ARN., CARC., IGN.,** lyc., ***med.,*** **NAT-M.,** nux-v., **OP.,** ***plat., sep.,*** **STAPH.,** thuj.

RASH, skin - **ACON.,** ***agar.,*** agav-a., ***ail.,*** alum., alum-p., **AM-C.,** am-m., anac., ***anan., ant-c., ant-t., apis,*** aq-mar., ***arn.,*** **ARS.,** ars-i., ars-s-f., arum-t., arund., asaf., atro., bar-c., bar-m., bar-s., **BELL.,** bov., **BRY.,** bufo, ***calad., calc.,*** calc-i., ***calc-s.,*** calc-sil., camph., ***canth., carb-v.,*** carbn-s., **CAUST., CHAM.,** chel., chin-s., ***chlol., clem.,*** cocc., ***coff., com.,*** con., cop., corn., croto-t., cupr., cupr-acet., dig., dros., ***dulc.,*** elaps, euph., euphr., gels., ***graph.,*** hell., ***hep., hyos.,*** iod., iodof., ***ip., jug-c., kali-ar., kali-bi., kali-br., kali-s.,*** kreos., ***lach., led.,*** lyc., **MERC., MEZ.,** mur-ac., ***nat-m.,*** nit-ac., nux-v., op., par., petr., **PH-AC.,** phos., phyt., ***psor.,*** **PULS.,** rheum, **RHUS-T.,** rhus-v., sanic., sars., ***sec., sel., sep., sil.,*** sol-n., spong., ***staph.,*** **STRAM.,** sul-i., **SULPH.,** syph., tab., teucr., tub., urt-u., valer., verat., verat-v., vesp., viol-t., zinc., zinc-p.

RAYNAUD'S, disease - ail., **AGAR.,** ars., astra-e., bac., cact., calc., carb-v., cortico., cupr., cyt-l., ferr-p., foll., halo., hed., **HEP.,** kali-c., kres., lac-c., ***lac-d., merc.,*** nux-v., perh., prot., pull-g., ***pyrog.,*** **RHUS-T.,** sec., **SEP., SIL.,** sulfonam., thala., thiop., thuj., visc., zinc.

RECTUM, cancer - agn., **ALOE,** ***alum.,*** alumn., ***ars.,*** cadm-f., carb-v., ***card-m.,*** cund., ***graph.,*** **HYDR.,** ***kali-c.,*** kali-cy., ***kali-i.,*** kreos., laur., ***lach.,*** lyc., med., mur-ac., ***nat-s.,*** **NIT-AC.,** paro-i., ***phyt., plb.,*** podo., ***ruta,*** sang., ***scirr., sep.,*** spig., sulph., syph., ***thuj.,*** tub., visc.

anus, cancer - cund., hydr., **NIT-AC.,** ruta., ***scirr.***

RECTUM, fissure - acon., aesc., ***agn., all-c.,*** aloe, alum., am-c., anac., androc., ant-c., arg., arn., ***ars.,*** ars-s-f., arum-t., bcg, berb., calc., calc-f., ***calc-p.,*** carb-ac., carb-an., carc., ***caust.,*** **CHAM.,** ***cund.,*** cur., ***fl-ac.,*** **GRAPH.,** grat., hep., ***hydr., ign.,*** kali-c., kali-i., lac-d., ***lach., led.,*** med., ***merc.,*** merc-i-r., mez., morg., morg-g., morph., mur-ac., ***nat-m.,*** **NIT-AC.,** ***nux-v., paeon., petr., phos., phyt.,*** pip-n., plat., ***plb.,*** **RAT.,** rhus-t., sars., ***sed-ac.,*** **SEP.,** ***sil., sulph.,*** syph., tab., **THUJ.,** tub., zing.

RECTUM, fistula - ***aloe, alum.,*** alum-p., am-c., ant-c., ant-t., aur., **AUR-M.,** aur-s., bar-m., bell., **BERB.,** bry., cact., **CALC., CALC-P.,** calc-s., calc-sil., **CARB-V.,** carbn-s., **CARC., CAUST.,** cur., ***fl-ac., graph., hep., hydr.,*** ign., **KALI-C.,** kali-sil., ***kreos., lach., lyc., merc.,*** myris., **NIT-AC.,** nux-v., paeon., ***petr., phos.,*** puls., pyrog., querc., rat., sarr., ***sep.,*** **SIL.,** ***staph., sulph., syph., thuj.***

RECTUM, prolapsed - ***aesc.***, ***aesc-g.***, ail., all-c., **ALOE**, alum., alumn., ang., ant-c., **APIS**, apoc., aral., arg-n., arist-cl., arn., ***ars.***, ars-s-f., arund., ***asar.***, aur., aur-ar., aur-s., ***bell.***, **BELL-P.**, bry., bufo, cadm-i., **CALC.**, calc-acet., calc-p., ***calc-s.***, canth., carb-v., ***carbn-s.***, carc., caust., cench., chel., chin-s., cic., cinnb., cocc., ***colch.***, ***coll.***, ***crot-c.***, croto-t., ***dig.***, dios., ***dulc.***, elaps, ery-a., euph., euph-a., euphr., ***ferr.***, ferr-ar., ***ferr-i.***, ferr-p., fl-ac., ***gamb.***, ***gels.***, gran., ***graph.***, ham., ***hep.***, ***hydr.***, **IGN.**, indg., ***iris***, ***kali-bi.***, kali-c., kali-n., kali-p., ***lach.***, ***lyc.***, m-ambo., ***mag-m.***, mag-p., ***mang.***, med., **MERC.**, ***merc-c.***, mez., morg-g., **MUR-AC.**, nat-c., ***nat-m.***, ***nat-s.***, ***nit-ac.***, nux-m., **NUX-V.**, ph-ac., ***phos.***, phyt., pip-m., plan., plat., ***plb.***, **PODO.**, polyp-p., psor., puls., rad-br., rhus-t., ***ruta***, sec., senn., **SEP.**, **SIL.**, sol-t-ae., stann., ***sulph.***, sumb., syc-co., syph., tab., ther., thuj., trom., tub., valer., zinc., zinc-p.

RECTUM, tumors - cub., cur., kali-br., plb., ruta, sol-t-ae., thuj.

REFLEXES, general

- **diminished** - ***alum.***, arg-n., cur., kali-br., oena., op., oxyt., phys., plb., ***sec.***
- **increased** - anh., bar-c., cann-i., cic., cocc., lath., mang., morph., nux-v., stry.
- **lost** - alum., cur., morph., nat-br., op., sulfon.

REGURGITATION, of food, (see Belching, Vomiting) - ***aesc.***, aeth., ***alum.***, am-m., ***ant-c.***, ***arg-n.***, ars., ***arum-t.***, asaf., ***bell.***, ***bry.***, bufo, ***calc.***, ***calc-s.***, camph., ***cham.***, canth., carb-an., **CARB-V.**, carbn-s., ***caust.***, **CHIN.**, chin-ar., coff., ***con.***, ***cop.***, cycl., ***dig.***, echi., **FERR.**, ferr-i., **FERR-P.**, glon., graph., ***hep.***, ign., ***ip.***, iris, kali-ar., ***kali-bi.***, kali-c., kali-p., kali-s., kalm., ***lach.***, lob., ***lyc.***, mag-m., ***mag-p.***, mang., ***merc.***, ***mez.***, ***mur-ac.***, ***nat-m.***, nat-p., nit-ac., ***nux-v.***, **PHOS.**, **PH-AC.**, pic-ac., plat., plb., ***podo.***, **PULS.**, quas., ran-b., rob., ***rhus-t.***, sars., senec., spig., ***sulph.***, sul-ac., tab., tell., teucr., thuj., ust., valer., verat.

REITER, syndrome - jac., med.

REMITTENT, fever - **ACON.**, ant-c., ***ant-t.***, apis, arn., **ARS.**, ars-s-f., bapt., **BELL.**, bol., **BRY.**, calc., carb-ac., **CHAM.**, chin., ***chin-s.***, ***cina***, ***cocc.***, coff., colch., coloc., crot-h., dor., eucal., eup-per., ferr., ferr-p., ***gels.***, hyos., ign., ***ip.***, ***lach.***, lap-gr-m., lept., ***lyc.***, mag-c., mag-s., **MERC.**, merc-d., mur-ac., ***nat-s.***, nit-ac., ***nux-v.***, nyct., ph-ac., phos., ***podo.***, ***polyp-p.***, psor., ptel., puls., rhus-t., sant., sec., sep., stram., ***sulph.***, tarax., ter., tub., verat., verat-v.

RETINITIS, inflammation, retina - acon., apis, ***ars.***, asaf., aur., bell., benz-d., bry., ***calc.***, con., crot-h., croto-t., dubin., ***gels.***, glon., iod., kali-i., kali-p., ***kalm.***, ***lach.***, ***merc.***, ***merc-c.***, merc-i-r., napht., naphtin., nat-s., nat-sal., nux-v., ***phos.***, pic-ac., ***plb.***, ***prun.***, puls., rhus-t., sal-ac., sant., sec., sil., ***sulph.***, thuj., toxo.

RHEUMATIC, fever - abrot., ***acon.***, act-sp., agn., all-c., ***ant-t.***, apoc., arg., ***arn.***, ars., ars-i., ***ars-s-f.***, asc-t., **AUR.**, **BELL.**, ***benz-ac.***, berb., **BRY.**, ***cact.***, ***calc.***, **CALC-P.**, ***calc-s.***, cann-s., carc., caul., **CAUST.**, cedr., ***cham.***, ***chel.***, ***chim.***, ***chin-s.***, chlf., ***cimic.***, clem., ***cocc.***, **COLCH.**, ***coloc.***, cortiso., ***dulc.***, ***ferr.***, ferr-i., **FERR-P.**, **FORM.**, gels., ***guai.***, ham., ***hep.***, ign., indg., **IOD.**, **KALI-BI.**, kali-c., ***kali-chl.***, ***kali-i.***, ***kali-s.***, **KALM.**, kreos., ***lac-ac.***, ***lac-c.***, ***lach.***, ***led.***, **LYC.**, ***mang.***, ***merc.***, ***nat-m.***, nat-p., ***nat-s.***, ***nux-v.***, ol-j., ox-ac., ***phos.***, ***phyt.***, pic-ac., ***puls.***, ran-b., rheum, ***rhod.***, **RHUS-T.**, ***ruta***, sabin., ***sal-ac.***, ***sang.***, sec., senec., sep., **SPIG.**, spong., ***staph.***, stict., stront-c., ***sulph.***, ***ter.***, teucr., thuj., ***verat-v.***, viol-t.

RHEUMATIC, pain - ***abrot.***, ***acon.***, act-sp., ***aesc.***, ***agar.***, alumn., am-m., ***ant-t.***, ***apis***, ***arg.***, **ARN.**, **ARS.**, ***ars-i.***, ***aur.***, **AUR-M-N.**, **BAD.**, bapt., ***bell.***, **BENZ-AC.**, **BRY.**, ***cact.***, ***calc.***, ***calc-p.***, ***calc-s.***, ***camph.***, cann-s., ***caps.***, ***carb-ac.***, ***carb-v.***, ***carbn-s.***, card-m., ***caul.***, **CAUST.**, cedr., **CHAM.**, **CHEL.**, ***chin.***, ***chin-ar.***, ***cimic.***, clem., **COLCH.**, ***coloc.***, ***corn.***, ***crot-c.***, ***crot-h.***, ***croto-t.***, cupr., ***dig.***, ***dulc.***, elaps, euph., eup-per., ***ferr.***, ***ferr-ar.***, ferr-p., **FORM.**, ***gels.***, grat., ***guai.***, ***ham.***, hell., ***hep.***, hydrc., ***ign.***, ***kali-ar.***, ***kali-bi.***, ***kali-c.***, kali-chl., **KALI-I.**, kali-p., ***kali-s.***, **KALM.**, ***lac-ac.***, ***lac-c.***, ***lach.***, led., **LYC.**, ***mag-c.***, mag-p., mag-s., **MED.**, meph., ***merc.***, merc-i-f., merc-i-r., merc-s., ***mez.***, mill., mur-ac., **NAT-AR.**, ***nit-ac.***, nux-m., ***nux-v.***, ol-an., pall., ***petr.***, ***ph-ac.***, ***phos.***, **PHYT.**, plat., ***psor.***, **PULS.**, ***ran-b.***, **RHOD.**, **RHUS-T.**, ***ruta***, ***sal-ac.***, **SANG.**, **SARS.**, sec., ***sep.***, ***sil.***, spig., squil., stann., ***stel.***, stict., **SULPH.**, ***syph.***, ***tarent.***, ter., thuj., teucr., ***valer.***, ***verat.***, viol-t., zinc.

RHEUMATISM, general - ***abrot.***, ***acon.***, act-sp., ***aesc.***, ***agar.***, alumn., am-m., ***ant-t.***, ***apis***, ***arg.***, **ARN.**, **ARS.**, ***ars-i.***, ***aur.***, **AUR-M-N.**, **BAD.**, bapt., ***bell.***, **BENZ-AC.**, **BRY.**, ***cact.***, ***calc.***, ***calc-p.***, ***calc-s.***, ***camph.***, cann-s., ***caps.***, ***carb-ac.***, ***carb-v.***, ***carbn-s.***, card-m., ***caul.***, **CAUST.**, cedr., **CHAM.**, **CHEL.**, ***chin.***, ***chin-ar.***, ***cimic.***, clem., **COLCH.**, ***coloc.***, ***corn.***, ***crot-c.***, ***crot-h.***, ***croto-t.***, cupr., ***dig.***, ***dulc.***, elaps, euph., eup-per., ***ferr.***, ***ferr-ar.***, ferr-p., **FORM.**, ***gels.***, grat., ***guai.***, ***ham.***, hell., ***hep.***, hydrc., ***ign.***, ***kali-ar.***, ***kali-bi.***, ***kali-c.***, kali-chl., **KALI-I.**, kali-p., ***kali-s.***, **KALM.**, ***lac-ac.***, ***lac-c.***, ***lach.***, led., **LYC.**, ***mag-c.***, mag-p., mag-s., **MED.**, meph., ***merc.***, merc-i-f., merc-i-r., merc-s., ***mez.***, mill., mur-ac., **NAT-AR.**, ***nit-ac.***, nux-m., ***nux-v.***, ol-an., pall., ***petr.***, ***ph-ac.***, ***phos.***, **PHYT.**, plat., ***psor.***, **PULS.**, ***ran-b.***, **RHOD.**, **RHUS-T.**, ***ruta***, ***sal-ac.***, **SANG.**, **SARS.**, sec., ***sep.***, ***sil.***, spig., squil., stann., ***stel.***, stict., **SULPH.**, ***syph.***, ***tarent.***, ter., thuj., teucr., ***valer.***, ***verat.***, viol-t., zinc.

RHUS POISONING, (see Poison oak), ailments from - agar., am-c., **ANAC.**, anac-oc., apis, arn., astac., ***bry.,*** cimic., **CLEM.**, **CROTO-T.**, cupr., cypr., echi., erech., euph-l., ***graph.***, ***grin.***, hedeo, hydro-c., kali-s., ***led.***, lob., mez., ***nuph.***, plan., prim-o., rhus-d., ***rhus-r.***, **RHUS-T.**, ***sang.***, ***sep.***, sulph., tanac., urt-u., vanil., verb., verbe-h., ***xero.***

RICKETS, general, rachitis - am-c., arg., ***ars.***, ars-i., **ASAF.**, bac., bar-c., ***bell.***, bry., bufo, **CALC.**, calc-acet., calc-f., ***calc-hp.***, **CALC-P.**, calc-sil., caust., cic., con., ***ferr.***, ***ferr-i.***, ferr-m., ***ferr-p.***, fl-ac., ***guai.***, hecla, hed., ***hep.***, iod., ***ip.***, iris, ***kali-i.***, ***lac-c.***, ***lyc.***, mag-m., mag-p., med., **MERC.**, mez., ***nit-ac.***, nux-m., nux-v., ***ol-j.***, op., petr., ***ph-ac.***, **PHOS.**, pin-s., plb., ***psor.***, ***puls.***, rhod., ***rhus-t.***, ruta, sac-alb., sac-alb., sanic., ***sep.***, **SIL.**, ***staph.***, ***sulph.***, supren-cort., symph., tarent., ther., thuj., thyr., ***tub.***, verat.

RINGWORM, (see Tinea)

RITALIN, ailments from - amphet., aven., carc., coca., cocc., ***coff.***, hyos., melat., merc., ***rital.***, stram., valer.

ROSEOLA, general - **ACON.**, ail., bad., ***bell.***, **BRY.**, carb-v., ***coff.***, cub., ***hyos.***, iod., ip., kali-i., ***merc.***, merc-c., merc-i-r., nit-ac., nux-v., phos., phyt., **PULS.**, rhus-t., sars., sulph.

RUBELLA - ***acon.***, ***bell.***, ***bry.***, carb-v., ***coff.***, ip., merc., phos., ***puls.***, rhus-t., sulph.

S

SACRO-ILIAC, syndrome - **AESC.**, ***ant-t.***, apis, ***arg-n.***, ***arn.***, bell-p., ***bry.***, ***calc-p.***, ***cimic.***, ***coloc.***, dios., ferr., gels., hep., hyper., jug-c., kali-c., lyc., m-ambo, nat-p., ol-j., plb., rhus-t., rumx., ruta, sabad., spong., sulph., symph., tell., ther., thuj.

SACRUM, injuries - ***aesc.***, arn., bell-p., calc-p., hyper., ruta, symph.

SALPINGITIS, inflammation, fallopian tubes - achy., acon., amor-r., apis, arg., ***ars.***, bry., canth., chin-s., coli., coll., ***coloc.***, eupi., foll., hep., hydro-c., lach., med., merc., ***merc-c.***, ***puls.***, sabal., ***sep.***, sil., staph., syc-co., tub-r.

SARCOCELE, genitalia - **AUR.**, bell., calc., con., hippoz., iod., kali-i., merc., ***merc-i-r.***, psor., ***puls.***, rhod., spong., tarent.

SARCOIDOSIS, besnier-boeck, morbus - aq-mar., aran-ix., asar., beryl., hip-ac., hist., kres., lepro., lyc., mand., nat-ar., parathyr., pin-s., puls., thiop., tub., tub-m., v-a-b.

SARCOMA, cutis - ars., ars-i., asaf., aur., ***bar-c.***, cadm-m., cadm-s., calc., calc-f., calc-p., carb-ac., carb-an., carc., con., ***crot-h.***, ***cund.***, cupr-s., graph., hecla., ***kali-m.***, lach., ***lap-a.***, mez., nit-ac., phos., ***rad-br.***, sil., staph., symph., thiosin., thuj., visc.

SCABIES, general - agn., aloe, alum., ambr., ***ant-c.***, ant-t., anthro., apis, **ARS.**, ***aster.***, ***bar-m.***, bell., bry., ***calc.***, canth., carb-ac., carb-an., **CARB-V.**, **CARBN-S.**, **CAUST.**, chin., ***clem.***, coloc., con., cop., croto-t., ***cupr.***, ***dulc.***, elaps, ferr-ma., ***graph.***, guai., ***hep.***, iod., **KALI-S.**, ***kreos.***, ***lach.***, led., ***lyc.***, m-ambo., ***mang.***, ***merc.***, merc-i-f., mez., ***nat-c.***, nat-m., nat-s., nit-ac., nux-v., olnd., petr., ***ph-ac.***, **PSOR.**, puls., rhus-t., rhus-v., rumx., sabad., sarr., sars., **SEL.**, **SEP.**, ***sil.***, squil., staph., ***sul-ac.***, **SULPH.**, tarax., thuj., valer., ***verat.***, ***zinc.***

SCARLET FEVER, scarlatina - ***acon.***, aeth., **AIL.**, **AM-C.**, am-m., **APIS**, ***arg-n.***, arn., ***ars.***, ars-i., ***arum-t.***, ***asim.***, aur., bapt., bar-c., **BELL.**, ***bry.***, ***calc.***, camph., canth., ***carb-ac.***, ***carb-v.***, caust., ***cham.***, chim., chim-m., chin., ***chin-ar.***, cina, coff., com., con., croc., ***crot-c.***, ***crot-h.***, ***cupr.***, cupr-acet., dubin., dulc., **ECHI.**, eucal., euph., ***gels.***, hep., hoit., hydr-ac., hyos., iod., ip., kali-ar., kali-chl., kali-m., kali-p., kali-s., lac-c., **LACH.**, **LYC.**, **MERC.**, merc-cy., merc-i-r., ***mur-ac.***, **NIT-AC.**, nux-m., nux-v., op., ***ph-ac.***, ***phos.***, phyt., **RHUS-T.**, sang., sec., sil., sol-n., spig., ***stram.***, ***sulph.***, tab., **TER.**, thuj., verat-v., xan., ***zinc.***

SCARS, skin, cicatrices, (see Keloids) - all-c., alum., alumn., ant-c., ant-t., ars., asaf., aster., ***bad.***, bamb-a., ***bell-p.***, bor., both-a., both-l., calc., ***calc-f.***, calc-p., ***calc-sil.***, **CALEN.**, carb-an., carb-v., ***carc.***, caust., cench., chin., con., croc., crot-h., cupre-l., dros., eug., ferr., **FL-AC.**, gast., glon., **GRAPH.**, hep., hyper., ***iod.***, junc., kali-bi., kali-c., kali-i., kali-m., kali-sil., lach., led., lyss., m-ambo., mag-c., mag-m., merc., ***mez.***, naja, nat-c., nat-m., **NIT-AC.**, nux-v., ozone, petr., ***phos.***, phyt., prot., ***psor.***, puls., rad-br., rhus-t., sabin., sars., sep., **SIL.**, ***staph.***, stram., stront-c., sul-ac., sul-i., sulph., syph., tell., **THIOSIN.**, thuj., thyr., tub., vac., vip.

SACRO-ILIAC, syndrome - **AESC.**, ***ant-t.***, apis, ***arg-n.***, ***bry.***, ***calc-p.***, ***cimic.***, ***coloc.***, dios., ferr., gels., hep., hyper., jug-c., m-ambo, nat-p., ol-j., plb., rhus-t., rumx., sabad., spong., sulph., tell., thuj.

S.A.R.S., severe acute respiratory syndrome - acon., ant-t., ars., bac., bapt., bell., bry., camph., carb-v., carbn-s., dulc., eup-per., gels., influ., ip., kali-c., lach., laur., lyc., merc., op., oscillo., phos., pneu., pyrog., samb., sang., seneg., spong., tub., tub-a., verat., verat-v.

SCARS, cancer in old - graph., sil., thiosin.

SCARS, general, cicatrices, (see Keloids) - all-c., alum., alumn., ant-c., ant-t., ars., asaf., aster., ***bad.***, bamb-a., ***bell-p.***, bor., both-a., both-l., calc., ***calc-f.***, calc-p., ***calc-sil.***, **CALEN.**, carb-an., carb-v., ***carc.***, caust., cench., chin., con., croc., crot-h., cupre-l., dros., eug., ferr., **FL-AC.**, gast., glon., **GRAPH.**, hep., hyper., ***iod.***, junc., kali-bi., kali-c., kali-i., kali-m., kali-sil., lach., led., lyss., m-ambo., mag-c., mag-m., merc., ***mez.***, naja, nat-c., nat-m., **NIT-AC.**, nux-v., ozone, petr., ***phos.***, phyt., prot., ***psor.***, puls., rad-br., rhus-t., sabin., sars., sep., **SIL.**, ***staph.***, stram., stront-c., sul-ac., sul-i., sulph., syph., tell., **THIOSIN.**, thuj., thyr., tub., vac., vip.

SCIATICA, pain - acon., agar., ***am-m.,*** anan., ang., ***arg-n., arn., ars.,*** asar., bar-c., ***bell.,*** berb., **BRY., BUFO,** ***calc., calc-p.,*** caps., ***carbn-s.,*** card-m., ***caust., cham.,*** chel., chim., chin-s., ***cimic.,*** cist., cocc., coc-c., ***coff.,*** **COLOC.,** cur., ***dios.,*** dros., ***elaps, elat.,*** euph., eup-pur., ***ferr., ferr-ar.,*** ferr-p., fl-ac., ***gels.,*** **GNAPH.,** ***graph., guai.,*** hep., hyper., ***ign., indg.,*** **IRIS,** ***kali-ar., kali-bi.,*** kali-c., **KALI-I.,** ***kali-p.,*** lac-ac., ***lac-c.,*** lac-d., ***lach.,*** lachn., ***led., lyc.,*** lyss., **MAG-P.,** ***meny.,*** merc., mez., nat-ar., ***nat-m., nat-s.,*** nit-ac., ***nux-m.,*** **NUX-V.,** ***ol-j.,*** pall., ***petr.,*** ph-ac., ***phos., phyt.,*** plan., ***plb., podo.,*** psor., ***puls., ran-b.,*** **RHUS-T.,** ***ruta,*** sal-ac., ***sep.,*** sil., ***staph., still.,*** stram., ***sulph.,*** **TELL.,** ter., ***valer., verat.,*** xan., ***zinc.***

SCIRRHUS, cancer - acet-ac., alum., alumn., ***anac.,*** arg., arg-n., arn., ***ars.,*** ars-i., ars-s-f., ***aster.,*** bell-p., brom., ***calc-s.,*** calen., carb-ac., **CARB-AN.,** ***carb-v., carbn-s.,*** carc., cist., clem., **CON.,** ***cund.,*** gali., ***graph., hydr., lap-a.,*** med., mur-ac., nit-ac., nux-v., ***petr., phos., phyt.,*** **SCIRR.,** sep., **SIL.,** squil., staph., ***sulph.,*** symph.

SCLERODERMA, skin - alum., ***ant-c.,*** arg-n., ars., berb-a., ***bry., calc.,*** calc-f., caust., ***croto-t.,*** echi., ***elae., graph., hydrc.,*** kali-c., kalm., kres., lac-c., lyc., parathyr., petr., phos., ***plb.,*** pyrar., rad-br., ran-b., rhus-r., rhus-t., rhus-v., sarcol-ac., sars., sep., sil., still., sulph., syc-co., thiosin., ***thyr.***

SCRATCHES, general, ailments from - acet-ac., calc-s., ***calen.,*** echi., hep., ***hyper., led., plan.,*** pyrog.

SCROFULA - aln., ampe-qu, bac., bad., bar-i., bell., ***calc.,*** calc-hp., camph., cist., ferr-i., hep., hippoz., kali-m., ol-j., phyt., prun-c., scroph-n., sil., ***sulph.***

SCROFULODERMA - calc-i., calc-s., petr., phos., scroph-n., still., ther.

SCROTUM, cancer - ars., carb-an., fuli., ph-ac., thuj.

SCURVY, scorbutus - acet-ac., ***agav-a.,*** agn., all-s., aln., alum., alumn., ***am-c.,*** am-m., ambr., ant-c., aran., arg., ***ars.,*** ars-i., arum-m., aur., bell., bor., bov., brass., bry., ***calc.,*** canth., caps., carb-ac., ***carb-an.,*** **CARB-V.,** cary., caust., cetr., chin., chin-s., cic., ***cist.,*** cit-ac., cit-l., cit-v., coca, coch., con., ***dulc.,*** elat., ***ferr-p.,*** gali., graph., ***ham., hep., iod.,*** jug-c., jug-r., ***kali-c.,*** kali-chl., kali-n., kali-p., kreos., lach., lyc., mag-m., **MERC., MUR-AC.,** nat-hchls., ***nat-m., nit-ac.,*** nit-m-ac., nux-m., **NUX-V.,** petr., ph-ac., phos., plb., psor., rat., rhus-g., rhus-t., rumx., ruta, sabin., sac-alb., sanic., sed-ac., sep., ***sil.,*** sin-n., sol-t-ae., stann., **STAPH.,** sul-ac., ***sulph.,*** tart-ac., tep., urine, zinc.

SCHIZOPHRENIA, (see Dementia, Insanity, Mania, Multiple personalites) - abrot., absin., alco., am-m., **ANAC.,** anh., ars., **AUR.,** bell., calc., carbn-s., carc., ***chin.,*** chlorpr., cic., ***cocain.,*** con., convo-s., cortico., ***crot-h.,*** cupr., cycl., ***dros.,*** halo., hell., **HYOS.,** ign., ***kali-br.,*** kres., **LACH.,** lepi., levo., lyc., med., ***meli.,*** merc., mosch., nat-c., nat-m., nux-v., op., plat., plb., psil., puls., rauw., reser., ***rhus-t.,*** sil., spong., staph., **STRAM.,** stry., sulfa., syph., thala., thiop., thuj-l., thyr., tub., ven-m., verat., zinc.

SEASICKNESS, (see Motion Sickness) - ***carb-ac.,*** **COCC.,** colch., **CON., EUPH-C.,** ***glon.,*** hyos., ***kali-bi., kreos.,*** lac-ac., nat-m., **NUX-V., PETR.,** sanic., ***sep., staph.,*** **TAB.,** ther.

SEASONAL AFFECTIVE, disorder - ***aur.,*** carc., melat., phos., pineal, sol., stram., ***syph.***

SEBACEOUS, cysts, wens - ***agar.,*** am-c., anac., ant-c., **BAR-C.,** ***benz-ac.,*** brom., **CALC.,** calc-sil., caust., coloc., ***con.,*** daph., **GRAPH.,** ***hep.,*** kali-br., kali-c., ***kali-i.,*** mez., ***nit-ac.,*** ph-ac., phyt., rhus-t., ***sabin.,*** **SIL.,** spong., sulph., thuj.

SEBORRHEA, head - ***am-m., ars.,*** bry., bufo, calc., chin., graph., hera., ***iod.,*** kali-br., kali-c., kali-s., lob., lyc., merc., mez., nat-m., olnd., petr., phos., ***plb.,*** psor., raph., rhus-t., sars., sel., sep., sil., staph., sulph., thuj., ***vinc.***

SEPTIC FEVER - acet-ac., ail., ***am-c.,*** **ANTHR.,** ***apis,*** arg-n., **ARN., ARS., BAPT.,** ***bell.,*** berb., **BRY.,** bufo, ***cadm-s.,*** carb-ac., ***carb-v.,*** **CARBN-S.,** chin-ar., **CROT-C., CROT-H.,** ***cur.,*** **ECHI.,** elaps, ferr., ferr-p., kali-bi., **KALI-P.,** kreos., **LACH., LYC.,** ***merc.,*** merc-cy., **MUR-AC.,** naja, nit-ac., op., ***ph-ac.,*** **PHOS.,** plan., ***puls.,*** **PYROG.,** ***rhus-t., rhus-v.,*** sul-ac., **SULPH.,** tarent., **TARENT-C.,** verat., verat-v., vip.

SEPTICEMIA, blood infection, (see Pyemia) - ***achy., acon.,*** agar., ***ail.,*** am-c., ant-t., ***anthr., apis,*** apisin., arg., arg-n., arist-cl., ***arn.,*** **ARS.,** ars-i., arum-t., asaf., atro., aur., ***bapt.,*** bar-c., bell., bor-ac., both-l., ***bry.,*** bufo, ***calc.,*** calc-ar., calen., ***carb-ac.,*** **CARB-V.,** ***cench.,*** cham., ***chin., chin-ar., chin-s.,*** chlorpr., colch., con., conch., crot-c., **CROT-H.,** dor., **ECHI.,** elaps, eucal., ***ferr.,*** ferr-p., gels., graph., gunp., hell., hep., ***hippoz.,*** hydro-c., hyos., iod., ***ip.,*** irid., kali-bi., kali-br., ***kali-c.,*** kali-chl., kali-ma., ***kali-p.,*** kreos., **LACH.,** lat-k., laur., led., lob-p., ***lyc.,*** mag-c., mang., ***merc.,*** merc-cy., methyl., mur-ac., naja, ***nat-m.,*** nat-s-c., ***nit-ac.,*** nux-v., op., paro-i., ph-ac., ***phos.,*** phyt., ***puls.,*** **PYROG.,** rad-br., raja-s., ***rhus-t.,*** ruta, ***sal-ac., sec.,*** sep., septi., sieg., sil., staph., staphycoc., stram., strept., sul-ac., sulfonam., ***sulph.,*** tarax., tarent., tarent-c., ***ter.,*** trach., vario., ***verat., verat-v., vip.,*** zinc.

SEWER-GAS, poisoning - anthr., ars., ***bapt.,*** kreos., phyt., ***pyrog., tub.***

SHARP, pains, stitching - abrot., absin., ***acon.,*** aconin., aesc., aeth., ***agar.,*** agn., ail., all-c., aloe, alum., alum-p., ***alum-sil., alumn.,*** am-c., ***am-m.,*** ambr., ammc., amyg-am., amyg-p., anac., ang., ant-c., ant-s., ant-t., apis, arg., arg-n., arist-cl., arist-m., ***arn.,*** ars., ars-i., ***ars-s-f.,*** **ASAF.,** asar., ***asc-t.,*** aspar., astac., atro., aur., aur-ar., aur-i., aur-m., aur-s., bad., bamb-a., bar-c., bar-i., bar-m., bar-s., bart., **BELL.**, benz-ac., **BERB.**, bism., bor., ***bov.***, **BRY.**, bufo, buni-o., cac., cact., calad., **CALC.**, calc-f., calc-i., calc-p., ***calc-sil.***, ***calen.***, camph., cann-i., cann-s., **CANTH.**, caps., carb-ac., carb-an., carb-v., carbn-s., card-m., carl., ***caust.***, cedr., cham., ***chel.***, **CHIN.**, chin-ar., chin-s., cic., ***cimic.***, cina, cinnb., cist., clem., coc-c., ***cocc.***, coff., ***colch.***, coll., **COLOC.**, **CON.**, croc., crot-h., croto-t., culx., cupr., ***cycl.***, daph., dig., dios., dol., ***dros.***, dulc., eucal., euonin., euph., euphr., eupi., ferr., ferr-ar., ferr-ma., ferr-p., ferul., fl-ac., form., ***gamb.***, gast., gels., glon., ***graph.***, grat., guai., ham., ***hell.***, hep., hist., hura, hydr., hydro-c., hydrog., hyos., **HYPER.**, **IGN.**, indg., inul., iod., iodof., ip., iris, jac-c., kali-ar., kali-bi., **KALI-C.**, kali-chl., ***kali-i.***, kali-n., kali-p., **KALI-S.**, kali-sil., kalm., ***kreos.***, lac-ac., lac-c., lach., lact., lat-m., ***laur.***, led., lepi., lith-c., lob., lyc., m-arct., m-aust., m-ambo., ***mag-c.***, ***mag-m.***, **MAG-P.**, ***manc.***, mang., med., ***meny.***, **MERC.**, merc-c., merc-i-f., merc-i-r., merc-n., mez., mosch., ***mur-ac.***, murx., naja, nat-ar., ***nat-c.***, nat-h., ***nat-m.***, nat-p., nat-s., ***nat-sil.***, nicc., **NIT-AC.**, nit-s-d., nux-m., nux-v., ol-an., olnd., ***op.***, ***ox-ac.***, paeon., pall., ***par.***, petr., ***ph-ac.***, phel., **PHOS.**, phyt., pitu-a., plan., plat., ***plb.***, plb-i., plect., pneu., prun., psil., psor., **PULS.**, pulx., ran-b., ***ran-s.***, raph., rat., rauw., rheum, rhod., **RHUS-T.**, rumx., ruta, ***sabad.***, **SABIN.**, samb., sang., ***sars.***, scut., sec., sel., seneg., **SEP.**, sil., sin-n., sol-t-ae., sphing., **SPIG.**, ***spong.***, squil., ***stann.***, **STAPH.**, stict., still., stram., stront-c., stroph., stroph-s., stry., sul-ac., sul-i., **SULPH.**, sumb., symph., syph., tab., ***tarax.***, tarent., tax., **TELL.**, teucr., thal., ther., **THUJ.**, tub., urt-c., urt-u., ust., valer., verat., **VERB.**, verin., vesp., viol-o., viol-t., vip., vip-r., zinc., zinc-chr., **ZINC-P.**, ziz.

<u>SHIPBOARD</u>, fever, on - bapt., pyrog.

<u>SHOCK</u>, traumatic - ***acet-ac.***, **<u>ACON</u>.**, ***am-c.***, **<u>ARN</u>.**, ***ars.***, bell., ***calc.***, ***calen.***, **CAMPH.**, ***caps.***, **CARB-V.**, ***cham.***, ***chin.***, ***chlf.***, ***cic.***, cocc., ***coff.***, ***cupr.***, cupr-ar., **DIG.**, ***gels.***, hell., hep., ***hydr-ac.***, hyos., **HYPER.**, ***ip.***, **LACH.**, ***laur.***, lyc., merc., ***nat-m.***, nit-ac., ***nux-m.***, nux-v., **OP.**, ***phos.***, psor., ***ran-b.***, sec., sep., ***staph.***, stront-c., stry-p., sulph., ***tab.***, **VERAT.**

<u>SHOOTING</u>, pains - ***acon.***, ***aesc.***, aeth., **AGAR.**, agn., ail., alum., alumn., am-c., am-m., ambr., amyg-p., anac., ant-c., apis, arg., ***arg-n.***, ars., ars-i., arum-d., asc-t., aster., aur., aur-m., bar-c., bell., **<u>BERB</u>.**, brach., bry., bufo, ***calc.***, calc-p., calc-s., camph., cann-i., cann-s., caps., carb-an., carb-v., carbn-o., carbn-s., caust., cedr., chel., choc., cic., cimic., cinnb., cocc., coff., colch., **COLOC.**, ***con.***, crot-h., croto-t., cupr., cupr-ar., daph., dig., dios., dulc., elat., eup-per., eup-pur., ferr., ferr-p., form., ***gels.***, graph., guai., ham., ***hep.***, hydrog., **<u>HYPER</u>.**, ind., iod., iodof., iris, ***kali-bi.***, kali-c., kali-i., **KALM.**, lac-ac., lach., lec., led., lept., ***lil-t.***, lith-c., lob-s., lyc., lyss., **MAG-P.**, mag-s., magn-gr., manc., med., meph., ***merc.***, merc-c., merc-s., mez., myric., naja, nat-ar., nat-c., nat-f., nat-m., nat-p., nat-s., nicc-s., ***nit-ac.***, ***nux-v.***, osm., ox-ac., ozone, pall., petr., ***phos.***, ***phys.***, phyt., pic-ac., pip-m., ***plan.***, plat., plb., podo., polyg., ptel., puls., rad-br., ran-b., rhod., ***rhus-t.***, rumx., ruta, sabad., sabin., sal-ac., sang., sars., scut., sep., sil., sol-n., **SPIG.**, stann., stict., still., stram., stroph-s., **SULPH.**, sumb., tanac., tarent., tax., **TELL.**, tep., teucr., thal., thuj., trom., urt-u., valer., verat., vib., visc., xan., ***zinc.***

<u>SHOULDER</u>, injuries - ***arn.***, ***bry.***, calc., ***calen.***, ferr., ***ferr-m.***, **RHUS-T.**, **RUTA**, sang., zinc.

<u>SILICOSIS</u>, silica ailments from - agav-t., ars., brom., **CALC.**, calc-sil., camph., **FL-AC.**, hell., hep., ictod., ip., ***lyc.***, mag-m., merc., nat-c., nat-ar., nit-ac., pen., ph-ac., ***puls.***, **SIL.**, sulph.

<u>SILVER</u>, argentum, ailments from - am-caust., arg., arg-n., ars., merc., ***nat-m.***, pall., plat., zinc.

<u>SINUS</u>, headaches, from catarrhal - acon., aesc., ***all-c.***, ***alum.***, ambr., am-m., ***ars.***, ***ars-i.***, ***aur.***, bell., ***bry.***, ***calc.***, **CALC-S.**, camph., ***carb-v.***, carbn-s., caul., cham., chin., chin-ar., ***chlor.***, cic., cimic., cina, **DULC.**, **EUPHR.**, ***ferr.***, ***ferr-ar.***, ferr-p., ***gels.***, **GRAPH.**, gymn., hell., **HEP.**, **HYDR.**, ign., ***iod.***, ***kali-ar.***, **<u>KALI-BI</u>.**, ***kali-c.***, **KALI-I.**, ***kali-s.***, kalm., ***lach.***, laur., ***lyc.***, ***mang.***, **MED.**, **MERC.**, merc-i-f., mez., nat-ar., ***nat-m.***, **NUX-V.**, ***phos.***, ***puls.***, ran-b., rumx., sabad., samb., sang., sil., staph., ***stict.***, still., ***sulph.***, teucr., **THUJ.**

<u>SINUSITIS</u>, infection, nose - ***ars.***, berb., bry., ***calc.***, cinnb., ***cupr.***, ferr., **HYDR.**, **<u>KALI-BI</u>.**, ***kali-chl.***, ***kali-i.***, kali-s., lach., **LYC.**, ***med.***, **MERC.**, merc-i-f., nat-s., ***nux-v.***, phos., **PULS.**, ***sang.***, **SIL.**, stict., syph., **<u>THUJ</u>.**, verb.

post-nasal, catarrh - acon., aesc., ***alum.***, alumn., ant-s., ***arg-n.***, ***aur.***, aur-m., bar-c., bry., ***calc.***, ***calc-s.***, ***canth.***, caust., cinnb., ***cor-r.***, euphr., ***ferr.***, **FERR-P.**, **HEP.**, **HYDR.**, ***iod.***, **KALI-BI.**, ***kali-c.***, ***kali-chl.***, ***kali-i.***, kreos., lith-c., ***lyc.***, mag-s., ***manc.***, ***mang.***, **MED.**, ***merc-i-f.***, ***merc-i-r.***, ***merl.***, ***mez.***, nat-ar., **NAT-C.**, **NAT-M.**, ***nat-s.***, ***nit-ac.***, petr., ***phyt.***, phos., ***plb.***, **PSOR.**, ***rhus-t.***, sang., ***sel.***, **SEP.**, ***sil.***, spig., staph., ***ther.***, **THUJ.**, zinc.

<u>SKIN</u>, cancer, (see Basal, Epithelioma, Melanoma, Squamos) - abr., acet-ac., alum., alumn., arg., arg-n., ***ars.***, **ARS-BR.**, **ARS-I.**, ars-s-f., aur., aur-ar., ***bell.***, brom., calc., calc-p., calc-sil., carb-ac., carb-an., ***carc.***, chr-ac., cic., cinnb., clem., **CON.**, ***cund.***, ***euph.***, fuli., gali., ***hydr.***, ***hydrc.***, kali-ar., kali-chl., kali-m., kali-p., ***kali-s.***, ***kreos.***, ***lach.***, ***lap-a.***, lob-e., **LYC.**, mag-m., mag-s., merc., merc-c., methyl-chl., nat-cac., nat-m., nectrin., nit-ac., petr., phos., ***phyt.***, puls., rad-br., raja-s., ***ran-b.***, ran-s., scirr., scroph-n., sep., ***sil.***, **SOL**, ***sulph.***, ***thuj.***, uran-n.

SLEEPING SICKNESS - arg., ars., gels., ***nat-ar.***, nux-m., op.

SLEEPLESSNESS, (see Insomnia)

SLEEP-TALKING, during sleep - acon., ***ail.,*** alum., alum-p., alum-sil., ambr., am-c., ant-t., apis, ***arn.,*** arg-n., ars., aur., ***bar-acet.,*** bar-c., bar-m., bar-s., **BELL.,** brach., bry., bufo, ***cact., calc.,*** camph., ***cann-i., carb-an.,*** carb-v., carbn-s., cast., caste., caust., ***cham., cina,*** cinnb., dig., ***gels.,*** graph., ***hell.,*** hyos., hyper., coff., com., con., cortico., cupr., graph., ***hyos.,*** ign., indg., kali-c., kali-m., kali-sil., kalm., kali-ar., kali-bi., **KALI-C.,** kali-p., kali-s., ***lac-c.,*** **LACH.,** ***led.,*** lyc., m-aust., mag-c., mag-m., merc., ***mur-ac.,*** nat-c., ***nat-m.,*** nit-ac., ***nux-v., op.,*** ph-ac., phos., plb., podo., psor., ***puls.,*** raph., rheum, ***rhus-t.,*** sabin., sel., ***sep., sil.,*** spig., spong., ***stann., stram., sulph.,*** thuj., tub., zinc., zinc-p.

SLEEP-WALKING, somnambulism - **ACON.,** agar., alum., alum-sil., ***anac.,*** ant-c., arg., ***art-v.,*** bell., ***bry.,*** calc., ***cann-i.,*** caste., cham., cic., croc., crot-h., cur., cycl., des-ac., dict., hyos., ign., ***kali-br.,*** kali-c., kali-p., kali-s., kalm., lach., **LUNA,** lyc., lyss., m-arct., meph., mosch., **NAT-M., OP.,** paeon., petr., **PHOS.,** plat., rheum, rumx., sep., ***sil.,*** spig., ***spong.,*** stann., ***stram., sulph., tarent.,*** teucr., verat., ***zinc.***

SMALLPOX, infection, variola - acon., agar., ail., am-c., am-m., anac., anthr., ***ant-c.,*** **ANT-T.,** ***apis,*** arn., ***ars., bapt., bell., bry.,*** bufo, calc-s., camph., cann-s., canth., ***carb-ac.,*** carb-v., caust., cham., chin., chin-s., cimic., clem., cocc., coff., crot-h., croto-t., cund., cupr-acet., gels., ***hep.,*** hippoz., hydr., hyos., ***kali-bi.,*** kali-br., kreos., lac-c., lach., lepro., **MALAND.,** med., **MERC.,** merc-i-r., mill., mur-ac., ***nat-m.,*** nat-s., nit-ac., op., petr., ph-ac., phos., ***puls.,*** psor., pyrog., **RHUS-T.,** sanic., **SARR.,** sec., sep., sil., sin-n., spig., stram., ***sulph.,*** syph., thea., **THUJ.,** tub., ***vac.,*** **VARIO.,** verat., verat-v., visc., zinc.

SMELL, loss, of - ail., ***alum., alum-p.,*** alum-sil., ***am-m.,*** amyg-p., ***anac., ant-c.,*** ant-s., ***ant-t.,*** apoc-a., arg-n., arist-cl., arn., ***ars., ars-i.,*** ars-s-f., arund., aspar., ***aur.,*** aur-ar., aur-i., aur-s., **BELL.,** ***bry.,*** bufo, **CALC.,** calc-i., **CALC-S.,** calc-sil., camph., ***caps.,*** carb-an., ***carbn-s.,*** card-m., ***caust., cham.,*** chel., chlor., cina, cocc., cod., con., ***cupr.,*** cycl., ***elaps, graph.,*** hell., **HEP.,** ***hyos., ign., iod., ip.,*** joan., just., ***kali-bi., kali-c., kali-i.,*** kali-n., kali-p., ***kali-s.,*** kali-sil., lach., laur., lem-m., ***lyc., mag-m.,*** mag-p., mang., med., **MERC.,** ***mez.,*** morg., ***nat-ar., nat-c.,*** **NAT-M.,** nit-ac., ***nux-m.,*** nux-v., olnd., ***op.,*** phel., **PHOS., PLB.,** ***psor.,*** **PULS.,** rhod., ***rhus-t.,*** ruta, sabad., ***sang., sarr.,*** sec., sel., **SEP., SIL.,** spig., squil., staph., stict., stram., ***sul-ac.,*** sul-i., ***sulph.,*** syc-co., tarent-c., ***teucr.,*** verat., **ZINC.,** zinc-m.

SMOKE, inhalation, (see Fumes, Tobacco), agg. - am-c., ***ars.,*** bell., brom., ***bry.,*** calad., calc., **CARB-V.,** caust., chel., chin., dor., **DROS.,** ***euphr., euph.,*** hep., **IGN.,** just., kali-bi., lob., lyc., naja, nat-ar., nat-m., nux-v., olnd., ph-ac., phos., puls., rumx., ***sep.,*** sil., **SPIG.,** sulph.

SMOKING, cancer from tobacco - ars., calad., cob., ***con.,*** kali-bi., lach., phos.

SNEEZING, general - ***acon., aesc.,*** aeth., ***agar.,*** ail., **ALL-C.,** aloe, alum., alumn., ambr., ***am-m.,*** ammc., ***anac.,*** anag., ***ant-t.,*** aphis., apis, ***arg., arg-n.,*** arn., **ARS.,** ***ars-i.,*** ars-s-r., arum-d., arum-t., ***arund.,*** asar., aspar., ***aur., bad.,*** bapt., ***bar-c.,*** bar-m., ***bell.,*** benz-ac., berb., bor., brach., ***brom.,*** **BRY.,** bufo, ***calc., calc-ar., calc-p., calc-s., camph., caps., carb-an.,*** carb-ac., **CARB-V., CARBN-S.,** cast., ***caust.,*** chel., ***chin., chin-ar., chin-s.,*** chlor., choc., ***cic.,*** cimic., **CINA,** ***cist.,*** clem., cob., cocc., **COC-C.,** coch., colch., ***con.,*** cop., croto-t., crot-h., cupr., ***cycl.,*** dig., ***dros., dulc.,*** euph., ***euphr.,*** **EUP-PER.,** eup-pur., ferr., ***ferr-ar.,*** ferr-i., ***ferr-p.,*** form., ***gamb.,*** gels., glon., ***graph.,*** grat., ham., hell., hep., hydr., **HYDROG.,** hyper., ille., ***indg., ind., iod., ip.,*** ipom., iris, jac-c., ***kali-ar., kali-bi.,*** kali-c., kali-chl., ***kali-i.,*** kali-n., kali-p., kali-s., ***kalm., kreos., lac-c., lach.,*** lac-ac., lil-t., ***lyc.,*** lyss., mag-m., meph., **MERC.,** merc-i-f., merc-s., mez., mur-ac., ***nat-acet., nat-c.,*** **NAT-M.,** ***nat-p., nat-s.,*** nicc., ***nit-ac., nux-m.,*** **NUX-V.,** olnd., ol-j., ox-ac., ***osm., petr., ph-ac., phos.,*** phys., ***plan.,*** prun., psor., ptel., **PULS.,** ran-s., rat., ***rhus-r.,*** **RHUS-T.,** ***rumx.,*** **SABAD.,** ***sal-ac.,*** sac-alb., **SANG.,** sanic., sars., sec., ***senec., seneg., sep., sil., spong., squil., staph.,*** stict., **SULPH.,** ***tarax.,*** tarent., ***teucr.,*** ther., thuj., verat., zinc., zing.

SOLAR PLEXUS, complaints of - bol., eran., grat., hell., ***kali-ar.***

SORE, pains - abrot., ***acon.,*** adon., ***aesc.,*** agar., agn., aloe, ***alum., alum-p.,*** alum-sil., alumn., ***am-c.,*** am-m., ambr., ammc., ampe-qu, anac., androc., ***ang.,*** ant-c., ant-t., apis, apoc., **ARG.,** arg-n., **ARN.,** ***ars.,*** ars-h., ars-i., ars-s-f., arum-t., asaf., ***asar., aur.,*** aur-ar., aur-i., ***bad., bapt.,*** bar-acet., bar-c., bar-i., bar-m., ***bell.,*** **BELL-P.,** benz-ac., berb., bism., bor., bov., brach., ***brom., bry.,*** bufo, calad., calc., calc-p., calc-sil., calen., ***camph.,*** canch., cann-i., cann-s., ***canth.,*** caps., carb-ac., carb-an., carb-v., carbn-o., ***carbn-s., caust.,*** cedr., cent., cerv., cham., chel., **CHIN.,** chion., chlf., chlor., **CIC., CIMIC., CINA,** cinnb., clem., cob., cob-n., **COCC.,** coff., colch., coloc., con., conch., cor-r., cot., ***croc.,*** crot-h., croto-t., culx., cund., cupr., cupr-acet., cycl., cyt-l., ***daph.,*** dig., **DROS.,** dulc., echi., elaps, eucal., eug., **EUP-PER.,** euph., euphr., eupi., fago., **FERR.,** ferr-ar., ferr-i., ferr-p., fl-ac., form., franc., gamb., **GELS.,** glon., goss., gran., graph., grat., guai., guare., **HAM.,** hedeo, hell., helo., helon., hep., hip-ac., hipp., hist., ***hydrc.,***

hydrog., hyos., hyper., iber., ign., ind., iod., iodof., ip., jab., jac., juni-c., kali-bi., kali-c., kali-chl., kali-i., kali-n., kalm., kreos., **LAC-AC.**, lac-d., lach., lap-a., lappa, laur., ***lec.***, ***led.***, lil-t., ***lith-c.***, lyc., lycpr., lyss., m-arct., m-aust., m-ambo., ***mag-c.***, mag-m., mag-p., mag-s., magn-gr., ***mang.***, ***med.***, meny., meph., merc., merc-c., ***merc-i-f.***, merc-i-r., mez., mill., mit., morph., mosch., mur-ac., ***myric.***, narcin., ***nat-ar.***, nat-c., nat-m., nat-n., nat-p., nat-s., nat-sil., nicc., ***nit-ac.***, ***nux-m.***, **NUX-V.**, oci-s., ol-an., ***olnd.***, onos., op., ox-ac., ozone, pall., par., paull-p., petr., ***ph-ac.***, ***phos.***, phys., ***phyt.***, pic-ac., piloc., pitu-a., plan., **PLAT.**, plb., plect., podo., polyp-p., prun., psil., psor., ptel., ***puls.***, puls-n, **PYROG.**, pyrus, ***rad-br.***, ran-a., ***ran-b.***, ran-s., raph., rat., rheum, ***rhod.***, **RHUS-T.**, rhus-v., rumx., **RUTA**, sabad., sabin., samb., sang., sanic., **SARCOL-AC.**, sarr., sars., sec., sel., seneg., sep., **SIL.**, sin-n., sol-n., sol-t-ae., spig., spong., squil., ***stann.***, staph., stel., stict., still., stram., stront-c., stry., ***sul-ac.***, sul-i., **SULPH.**, syph., tab., tarax., tarent., tart-ac., tell., ter., teucr., ther., ***thuj.***, til., ***tub.***, uva., ***valer.***, verat., verb., vib., viol-o., viol-t., wies., wye., x-ray, zinc., zinc-p.

SORENESS, from injuries or overuse - **ARN.**, **BELL-P.,** bry., calc., lac-ac., ***rhus-t.***, ***ruta.***

SPERM, low count of, infertility - agn., carc., rad-br., sulfa., x-ray.

- **aspermatism** - ***agn.***, calc., lyc., nat-m., nux-v., ph-ac., plb., sec., sep., sil., sulph., thuj., x-ray.

SPERMATIC CORD, general - all-c., alum., am-c., arg., bell., ***berb.***, dios., caps., chel., chin-s., ***clem.***, ham., lycps., m-ambo., mag-m., mang., nux-m., nux-v., ***puls.***, rhod., ***sars.***, senec., sil., spong., staph., stront-c.

SPHINCTERS, ailments of - calen., laur., sil., ***staph.***

SPINAL BIFIDA - arn., ars., asaf., bac., bar-c., bell., bry., ***calc.***, calc-f., ***calc-p.***, ***calc-s.***, calen., cann-s., carb-v., dulc., eup-per., graph., hep., iod., lach., lyc., merc., mez., nit-ac., phos., ***psor.***, ruta, **SIL.**, staph., sulph., tub.

SPINAL CORD, complaints - acon., agar., alum., alum-sil., arg-n., ars., aur., bar-m., bell., bry., calc., carb-v., carbn-s., caust., chin., ***cocc.***, con., crot-h., cupr., dig., ***dulc.***, ***hyper.***, ign., kali-m., **KALI-P.**, lach., ***lath.***, mag-p., ***mang.***, med., naja, nat-c., nat-m., ***nux-v.***, ox-ac., ph-ac., ***phos.***, phys., pic-ac., ***plb.***, plb-i., puls., rhus-t., sec., ***staph.***, ***sulph.***, verat., zinc.

SPINAL CURVATURE - acon., aesc., agar., am-c., ant-c., **ASAF.**, aur., ***bac.***, bar-c., ***bar-m.***, ***bell.***, bry., bufo, **CALC.**, **CALC-F.**, calc-hp., calc-i., **CALC-P.**, **CALC-S.**, ***carb-v.***, carbn-s., caust., choc., cic., clem., coloc., ***con.***, dros., dulc., ***ferr.***, ferr-i., get., graph., **HECLA**, ***hep.***, iod., ip., lach., ***lyc.***, mang., ***merc.***, **MERC-C.**, mez., nat-m., ***nit-ac.***, op., petr., **PH-AC.**, **PHOS.**, plb., psor., **PULS.**, rhod., **RHUS-T.**, ruta, sabin., ***sep.***, **SIL.**, staph., **SULPH.**, syph., tarent., ther., thuj., tub.

SPINAL TAP, pain after puncture - arn., led., **HYPER.**

SPINE, injuries, to - aesc., agar., ***apis***, **ARN.**, bell-p., **BRY.**, ***calc.***, ***calen.***, ***cic.***, ***con.***, dam., **HYPER.**, kali-c., ***led.***, **NAT-S.**, ***nit-ac.***, ***rhus-t.***, ***ruta***, ***sil.***, symph., tell., ***thuj.***, zinc.

- **concussion**, from - ***arn.***, bell-p., cic., con., **HYPER.**, **NAT-S.**, phys.
- **lifting**, from - ***arn.***, bell-p., bor., **CALC.**, **GRAPH.**, **LYC.**, ***nux-v.***, ph-ac., **RHUS-T.**, ***ruta***, sang., ***sep.***

SPLEEN, cancer - ars., bor., cadm-m., ***cean.***

SPLEEN, remedies - abies-c., abrot., ***agar.***, alum., ***am-c.***, am-m., anac., anthr., arn., **ARS.**, ***ars-i.***, **ASAF.**, **BELL-P.**, ***bor.***, ***bry.***, cadm-s., calc-p., camph., ***cann-s.***, ***canth.***, caps., carb-an., carb-v., card-m., caust., **CEAN.**, cedr., cham., chel., **CHIN.**, chin-s., cob., coc-c., colch., con., ***dios.***, ***dulc.***, ***ferr.***, ***ferr-m.***, fl-ac., gran., grin., helia., hell-f., **IGN.**, ***iod.***, iris, jug-r., kali-bi., kali-c., kali-n., ***laur.***, mag-c., mag-m., malar., mang., merc., mez., ***mur-ac.***, naja, ***nat-ar.***, ***nat-c.***, ***nat-m.***, ***nat-s.***, nit-ac., ***nux-v.***, parth., ph-ac., phos., ***plat.***, **PLB.**, psor., **RAN-B.**, rhod., rhus-t., rub-t., ***ruta***, sars., sil., squil., ***stann.***, succ., **SUL-AC.**, sulph., ther., thuj., ***urt-u.***, valer., verat., verb., ***zinc.***

SPLEEN, injuries - ***apis***, arn., ***bell-p.***, bry., ***calen.***, carb-v., **CEAN.**, chin., ***ham.***, hyper., lach., ***mill.***, nat-s., rhus-t., ruta

SPLENITIS, infection - acon., ***agn.***, ***apis***, aran., ***arn.***, **ARS.**, ars-i., asaf., bell., ***bry.***, bufo, ***caps.***, carb-v., **CEAN.**, **CHIN.**, chin-s., chlorpr., ***cit-l.***, con., cupr., diosm., dros., ferr., ferr-m., ferr-p., grin., ign., iod., lach., mang., mang-m., mang-s., nat-ar., nat-c., ***nat-m.***, ***nit-ac.***, ***nux-v.***, ***plb.***, plb-i., ***polym.***, rob., sang., sil., ***stann.***, succ., sul-i., sulph., verat-v.

SPLINTERS, wounds, from (see Punctures) - acon., ***anag.***, ***apis***, **ARN.**, ***bar-c.***, calen., ***carb-v.***, **CIC.**, colch., ***hep.***, **HYPER.**, iod., lach., **LED.**, lob., **MYRIS.**, ***nit-ac.***, petr., plat., ran-b., **SIL.**, ***staph.***, sulph.

SPONDYLITIS, back - carc., ph-ac.

SPOTTED FEVER - **CIMIC.**, ***dig.***, ***eup-per.***, ***sil.***, verat-v.

SPRAINS, injuries, distorsions - ***agn.***, ***am-c.***, **ARN.**, ***asaf.***, bell., ***bell-p.***, **BRY.**, **CALC.**, calen., carb-an., carb-v., ***hyper.***, ign., ***led.***, lyc., ***m-aust.***, **MILL.**, **NAT-C.**, nat-m., nit-ac., nux-v., petr., phos., polyg., puls., **RHUS-T.**, rhus-v., **RUTA**, sep., stront-c., sulph., ***symph.***

SQUAMOUS CELL, cancer, (see Skin, cancer) - ars., **AUR-M.**, ***carc.***, cinnb., cund., gali., ***hydr.***, kali-ar., ***kali-bi.***, petr., rad-br., scirr., scroph-n., ***sol***, thuj.

STAB, wounds, (see Punctures) - acet-ac., ***all-c.,*** androc., **APIS,** arn., **CALEN.,** ***carb-v.,*** cic., con., eug., hep., **HYPER.,** lach., **LED.,** nat-m., nit-ac., phase., ***phos.,*** plan., plb., puls., ***rhus-t.,*** sep., sil., ***staph.,*** sul-ac., sulph.

STAGE-FRIGHT, (see Anticipation) - **ACON.,** anac., **ARG-N.,** ***ars.***, bor., calad., calc-p., ***carb-v., carc.,*** cina, coff., crot-c., crot-h., ***cypr.***, **GELS.,** hyos., ign., ***kali-br.***, kali-p., lach., **LYC.,** lyss., ***med., merc.***, nat-m., nat-p., nat-s., ox-ac., petr., ***ph-ac., pic-ac.***, plb., psor., puls., sep., ***sil., stroph.***, sulph., syph., ***thuj.***, tub., ***zinc.***

STAPHYLOCOCCUS, infection - **ANT-C.,** ***ars.,*** ars-i., **BAPT.,** calc., carb-ac., carb-v., caust., cic., clem., con., croto-t., ***dulc.,*** **ECHI.,** graph., ***hep., iris, kali-bi.,*** kreos., lyc., merc., nat-m., ***nit-ac., ph-ac.,*** phos., **PYROG.,** ***rhus-t.,*** sars., sep., ***sil.,*** staph., sul-ac., sulph., viol-t.

STARVATION, general - alf., ars., hydr., ign., psor.

STERILITY, (see Infertility) - agn., ***alet.***, alum., ***am-c***., anag., anan., apis, arist-cl., **AUR.,** ***aur-i.***, aur-m., bar-c., ***bar-m.,*** **BOR.,** brom., ***calc.***, calc-i., cann-i., cann-s., ***canth.***, caps., carbn-s., ***caul.***, caust., cic., cimic., cocc., ***coff., con., croc.***, dam., dulc., ***eup-pur., ferr., ferr-p., fil.***, foll., form., ***goss., graph.***, helon., ***hyos., iod., kali-br.***, kali-c., ***kreos., lach.***, lappa, lec., lil-t., med., ***merc.***, mill., mit., morph., **NAT-C., NAT-M.,** nat-p., nux-m., nux-v., ***orig.***, orig-v., ***ov., phos.***, physala-p., phyt., ***pitu-a.***, pitu-p., ***plat.***, plb., ***puls.***, ruta, ***sabal., sabin.***, sec., ***senec.***, **SEP.,** ***sil., sul-ac.***, sulph., ***syph.***, ther., vib., vib-p., wies., x-ray, ***zinc.***

STERNUM, cancer - ars-s-r., sulph.

STEROIDS, ailments from - apis., ars., ***cortico., cortiso.,*** merc., nat-m., ***sep.,*** sulph.

STIFFNESS, joints - abrot., aesc., ***agar.,*** ant-s., apis, **ARS.,** ***aur., bamb-a.,*** bapt., ***bell.,*** cact., **CALC.,** canth., ***caps., carb-an., carbn-s.,*** **CAUST.,** ***chin-s.,*** cimic., clem., ***cocc.,*** **COLCH.,** ***coloc.,*** ferr-ar., ***form.,*** get., graph., kali-ar., ***kali-bi.,*** **KALI-C.,** ***kali-i.,*** kali-s., lac-ac., ***lac-c.,*** lach., **LED., LYC.,** ***nat-ar., nat-m.,*** nat-p., ***nux-v.,*** **PETR.,** ***phos.,*** psor., ***puls., rhus-r.,*** **RHUS-T.,** ruta, **SEP., SIL.,** ***staph., stict.,*** **SULPH.,** ***zinc.***

STIMULANTS, drugs, ailments, from - agar., am-c., ant-c., chin., chion., ***coca, cocc.,*** **COFF.,** cypr., dig., fl-ac., gels., gins., ***glon., ign.,*** iod., lach., led., lyc., merc., naja, ***nat-c.,*** **NUX-V.,** op., passi., ***paull., phos., rital.,*** thuj., valer., ***zinc.***

- **desires** - alco., aloe, ant-t., ars-s-f., aster., aur., aur-s., calc-i., caps., caust., ***chin., coca, coff.,*** crot-h., ***fl-ac.,*** gins., hep., iber., iod., kali-i., mur-ac., naja, nat-p., **NUX-V.,** ***ph-ac., puls.,*** sol-t-ae., staph., sul-i., ***sulph.,*** sumb., tab., ziz.

STINGING, pains - acon., agar., ***alum-sil.***, ant-c., **APIS**, arn., ***ars.***, bell., berb., bry., caust., cina, con., dulc., ***gels.***, glon., ign., iris, kali-c., ***led.,*** lyc., merc., mez., nit-ac., nux-v., ph-ac., ***phos.***, plat., puls., rhus-t., ruta, ***sep.***, **SIL.**, sul-ac., ***sulph.***, tarent., ther., thuj., **URT-U.,** zinc.

STINGS, insects, jellyfish, etc. - acet-ac., acon., am-c., am-caust., ***am-m., androc.,*** ant-c., ***anthr.***, **APIS,** ***arn.***, ars., bamb-a., ***bell.***, bry., bufo, ***calad.***, camph., ***carb-ac.***, caust., ***cedr.***, coloc., ***crot-h., echi.***, graph., ***grin.***, gua., gymne., hippoz., hydr-ac., **HYPER.,** ip., kali-ma., kreos., ***lach.***, lat-m., **LED.,** merc., mosch., ***nat-m.***, pulx., pyrog., samb., seneg., sep., sil., sisy., spirae., staph., sul-ac., sulph., tab., tarent., **URT-U.**

- **bee stings,** to face, with swelling - **APIS.,** arn., ***carb-ac.,*** **HYPER.,** ***lach.,*** **LED.,** ***nat-m.,*** **URT-U.**
- **jellyfish** - ***apis,*** hyper., ***urt-u.***
- **scorpions** - androc., led., hyper., plan., scorp., urt-u.
- **wasps** - ***acet-ac.,*** apis, carb-ac., hyper., ***led.,*** urt-u., vesp.
- **yellow,** jacket, of - ***apis,*** hyper., ***led.***, urt-u.

STOMACH, cancer - ***acet-ac.,*** act-sp., am-m., ant-c., ***arg-n.,*** **ARS.,** ***ars-i.,*** art-v., asim., aur., bar-c., bell., **BISM., CADM-S.,** ***calc.,*** calc-f., ***caps.,*** **CARB-AC., CARB-AN.,** ***carb-v., carc.,*** caust., chin., coloc., **CON.,** ***crot-h.,*** **CUND.,** dulc., eucal., form-ac., gaert., ger., graph., **HYDR.,** iod., ***ip., iris,*** **KALI-BI.,** kali-br., kali-c., kali-s., ***kreos., lach.,*** lap-a., **LYC.,** mag-p., mang-p., matth., ***merc-c.,*** merl., ***mez.,*** nep., nit-s-d., nux-v., **ORNI.,** pep., **PHOS.,** plat., plat-m., plat-m-n., plb., psor., puls., reser., rob., sal-ac., ***scirr., sec., sep., sil., staph., sulph., verat.***

- **pylorus** - acet-ac., coloc., graph., ***hydr.,*** iris, lap-a., **ORNI.,** sulph.

STOMACH, remedies - abies-n., ***abrot., acet-ac., acon., aesc., aeth.,*** agar., all-c., aloe, alum., alumn., ambr., am-c., aml-n., anac., anan., **ANT-C.,** ***ant-t.,*** apis, ***arg.,*** **ARG-N.,** ***arn.,*** **ARS.,** ars-h., ars-i., arund., ***asaf.,*** asar., aur., bapt., ***bar-c., bar-i., bar-m., bell.,*** benz-ac., **BISM.,** bol., bor., ***brom.,*** **BRY.,** ***cact.,*** **CADM-S.,** calad., ***calc., calc-p., calc-s., camph.,*** cann-s., canth., ***caps., carb-ac., carb-an.,*** **CARB-V., CARBN-S., CARD-M.,** caul., **CAUST.,** ***cham., chel.,*** **CHIN.,** chin-ar., ***chin-s., cina,*** cob., **COCC.,** coc-c., coff., **COLCH., COLOC.,** ***con.,*** cop., croc., ***crot-c., crot-h.,*** croto-t., **CUPR.,** ***cupr-ar.,*** cur., cycl., ***dig., dios.,*** dulc., ***ferr.,*** ferr-ar., ferr-i., ferr-p., ***gels., gran.,*** **GRAPH.,** glon., ***grat.,*** ham., hell., hep., **HYDR.,** ***hydr-ac., hyos., ign., iod.,*** **IP.,** ***iris, kali-ar., kali-bi., kali-c.,*** kali-chl., kali-i., ***kali-n.,*** kali-p., ***kreos., lach., laur.,*** led., ***lept., lob.,*** **LYC.,** ***mag-c., mag-m., mag-p.,*** mag-s., mang., ***med., merc.,*** mez., mosch., mur-ac., naja, ***nat-ar.***, **NAT-C.**, ***nat-m.***, ***nat-p.***, ***nat-s.***, nicc., ***nit-ac.***, ***nux-m.***, **NUX-V.**, ol-an., olnd., ***op.***, ***orni.***, ox-ac., ***petr.***, **PHOS.**, phys., ***phyt.***, plan., **PLB.**, podo., ***ptel.***, prun., **PULS.**, ran-b., ran-s., rhod., rhus-t., rob., ***sang.***, ***sec.***, senec., seneg., ***sep.***, **SIL.**, sol-t-ae., ***spig.***, squil., **STANN.**, ***staph.***, ***stram.***, stront-c., ***stry.***, **SULPH.**, ***sul-ac.***, sumb., **TAB.**, ***tarent.***, ***ter.***, teucr., thuj., ***uran-n.***, ust., valer., **VERAT.**, ***verat-v.***, ***zinc.***, zing.

STOMATITIS, ulcerative - agav-a., aln., ***alum.***, ***arg-n.***, ***ars.***, arum-t., ***arund.***, ***asar.***, **ASTAC.**, aur., ***bapt.***, bor., ***calc.***, ***canth.***, ***caps.***, carb-ac., ***carb-v.***, chin., ***chlol.***, ***cinnb.***, cory., ***crot-h.***, dig., ***dulc.***, ***ferr.***, hell., hep., hydr., ***hydr-m.***, hyos., iod., ***kali-bi.***, ***kali-chl.***, kali-cy., **KALI-I.**, kali-p., ***kreos.***, lac-ac., ***lach.***, mag-c., med., menthol, ***merc.***, ***merc-c.***, mill., mur-ac., myric., ***nat-m.***, nit-ac., nit-m-ac., ***nux-v.***, oxyg., ph-ac., phos., ***podo.***, ***rhus-g.***, ***sal-ac.***, sec., ***sep.***, ***sil.***, staph., ***sul-ac.***, sulo-ac., **SULPH.**, tarax., tril., vero-b.

STONE-CUTTERS, ailments in - asbes., **CALC.**, ip., ***lyc.***, nat-c., nit-ac., ph-ac., ***puls.***, **SIL.**, sulph.

STRABISMUS, eyes - acon., aeth., agar., ***alum.***, alumn., androc., ant-t., **APIS**, apoc., ***arg-n.***, arn., ars., art-v., bac., **BELL.**, benz-d., bufo, buth-aust., ***calc.***, calc-p., camph., cann-i., ***canth.***, caust., ***chel.***, chin., ***chin-s.***, **CIC.**, ***cina***, coloc., ***con.***, cupr., cupr-acet., **CYCL.**, dig., diphtox., ***gels.***, glon., graph., ***hell.***, ***hyos.***, jab., ***kali-br.***, ***kali-i.***, kali-p., lil-t., ***lyc.***, lyss., ***mag-p.***, meny., ***merc.***, ***merc-c.***, merc-i-f., morph., nat-ar., ***nat-m.***, nat-p., nat-sal., nux-m., ***nux-v.***, olnd., op., oxyu-s., phos., phys., plb., podo., psor., puls., rhod., rhus-t., ruta, sant., sec., seneg., sil., ***spig.***, spig-m., ***stram.***, sulph., syph., ***tab.***, tarent., thuj., tub., verat., ***zinc.***

STRAINS, ailments from overexertion, (see Lifting) - **arn.**, ***ars.***, **CALC.**, calc-f., carb-an., carb-v., cocc., ***con.***, ***ham.***, lyc., ***mill.***, nat-c., ovi-g-p., **RHUS-T.**, **RUTA,** sanic., sil., ter.

STRAMONIUM, poisoning, datura, ailments from - acet-ac., ***bell.***, ***hyos.***, ***stram.***, nux-v., tab.

STRANGLED, victims of being - arn., ars., op.

STREPTOCOCCUS, infection - ail., arn., ***ars.***, ***bell.***, strept., sul-ac., x-ray.

STROKE, apoplexy - **ACON.**, agar., ail., ***alco.***, am-c., **ANAC.**, ant-c., ant-t., apis, ***arg-n.***, **ARN.**, ***ars.***, ars-met., ars-s-f., asar., ***aster.***, ***aur.***, bapt., **BAR-C.**, **BELL.**, both-l., brom., **BRY.**, bufo, cact., cadm-br., cadm-s., caj., calc., calc-f., ***camph.***, camph-br., carb-v., carbn-h., carbn-s., **CAUST.**, chen-a., ***chin.***, chin-ar., chin-s., chlol., cinnam., **COCC.**, ***coff.***, con., croc., ***crot-h.***, ***cupr.***, cupr-acet., cupr-m., cur., dig., erig., ***ferr.***, fl-ac., ***form.***, form-ac., gast., **GELS.**, **GLON.**, gua., guare., hell., hep., **HYDR-AC.**, ***hyos.***, hyper., ign., iod., **IP.**, juni-c., juni-v., kali-br., kali-chl., kali-cy., kali-i., kali-n., kreos., **LACH.**, ***laur.***, lim., lith-br., lol., ***lyc.***, ***merc.***, methyl., ***mill.***, morph., nat-m., nat-n., nat-ns., nit-ac., ***nux-m.***, **NUX-V.**, ***oena.***, olnd., **OP.**, ox-ac., ph-ac., ***phos.***, **PLB.**, prim-v., ***puls.***, ran-g., rhus-t., sabad., samb., sang., sars., sec., sep., ***sil.***, sin-n., sol-a., sol-n., ***stram.***, stront-c., sulph., tab., tanac., ter., thuj., verat., ***verat-v.***, viol-o., vip., zinc., zinc-p.

STROPHULUS, volaticus in children - kam.

STRYCHNINE, ailments from - cham., cur., ***eucal.***, ign., kali-br., ***nux-v.***, oxyg., phys., ***stry.***

STYES, eyelids - agar., allox., alum., alum-p., alum-sil., am-c., ambr., ant-t., ***apis***, ars., ***aur.***, aur-ar., aur-m-n., aur-s., bar-c., bell., bry., cahin., calc., calc-f., calc-pic., **CARBN-S.**, carc., caust., ***chel.***, colch., **CON.**, cortiso., cypr., ***dig.***, dys-co., elaps, euphr., ferr., ferr-p., gaert., **GRAPH.**, hep., hip-ac., hydr., hydro-c., hyper., ***jug-c.***, kali-c., kali-p., kreos., lac-f., lach., lappa, **LYC.**, m-aust., mag-m., mand., med., meny., ***merc.***, morg., morg-g., mygal., nat-m., ozone, petr., ***ph-ac.***, phos., pic-ac., ***psor.***, **PULS.**, pyrog., ***rhus-t.***, sabad., seneg., **SEP.**, ***sil.***, skook., stann., **STAPH.**, sulfa., **SULPH.**, ***thuj.***, tub., upa., uran-n., valer., zinc.

SUBMAXILLARY, glands, cancer - ***anthr.***, calc-s., carb-an., ferr-i.

SUBSULTUS, tendinum - ***agar.***, ambr., am-c., ***ars.***, ***asaf.***, bell., ***calc.***, ***camph.***, ***canth.***, ***chel.***, ***chlor.***, **HYOS.**, **IOD.**, ***kali-i.***, ***lyc.***, ***mez.***, ***mur-ac.***, ***ph-ac.***, ***phos.***, rhus-t., ***sec.***, ***stry.***, sul-ac., **ZINC.**

SUICIDAL, depression - acon., ***accu.***, aeth., agn., alco., ***alum.***, alum-p., alum-sil., am-c., ambr., ***anac.***, anan., anh., ***ant-c.***, ***ant-t.***, aq-mar., arg-n., ***ars.***, asaf., **AUR.**, aur-ar., **AUR-M.**, aur-m-n., aur-s., ***bell.***, berb., bov., bry., buni-o., but-ac., ***calc.***, calc-sil., camph., ***caps.***, carb-v., carbn-s., ***carc.***, caust., chel., ***chin.***, chin-ar., cic., ***cimic.***, clem., con., crot-c., crot-h., cur., der., dros., fuli., gamb., gels., glon., graph., grat., hell., ***hep.***, hipp., hydr-ac., hydrog., ***hyos.***, ***ign.***, iod., ***iodof.***, iris, kali-ar., ***kali-br.***, kali-chl., kreos., ***lac-d.***, ***lach.***, laur., led., lil-t., lyc., lyss., med., meli., ***merc.***, ***merc-aur.***, mez., morg., morg-p., morph., ***naja,*** nat-c., ***nat-m.***, **NAT-S.**, nit-ac., ***nux-m.***, ***nux-v.***, op., orig., orni., oxyg., ped., phos., plat., ***plb.***, plut-n., prot., ***proz.***, **PSOR.**, ***puls.***, rauw., reser., rhus-t., rumx., ruta, sarr., scirr., scut., sec., sel., ***sep.***, sil., ***spig.***, spong., stann., **STAPH.**, ***stram.***, sul-ac., sulph., symph., tab., tarent., ter., thal., thea., thlaspi, thuj., thuj-l., tub., ust., valer., verat., x-ray, xan., ***zinc.***, zinc-p., ziz.

SULPHUR, ailments from - acon., ars., ***calc.***, camph., cham., chin., iod., ***merc.***, nit-ac., nux-v., **PULS.**, rhus-t., sel., sep., ***sulph.***, thuj.

SULPHURATED, hydrogen, fumes, ailments from - ***acet-ac.***, ant-t., carb-v., ***carbn-h.***, carbn-s., chlor., sul-ac., sulph.

SUN, sunlight, ailments from - ***acon.***, adlu., aeth., ***agar.***, aloe, aml-n., anh., **ANT-C.**, apis, ***arg.***, arn., ***ars.***, bac., ***bar-c.***, **BELL.**, bov., brom., ***bry.***, bufo, cact., cadm-s., calc., calc-f., ***camph.***, canth., ***carb-v.***, cina, cit-l., clem., cob-n., cocc., cortiso., crot-h., cyt-l., euph-pi., ***euphr.***, fago., ***gels.***, **GLON.**, gran., graph., hell., hist., hydr-ac., hyos., ign., iod., ip., kali-c., ***kalm.***, **LACH.**, lappa, lyc., ***lyss.***, mag-m., med., merc-c., mur-ac., murx., **NAT-C.**, **NAT-M.**, nat-n., ***nux-v.***, ***op.***, pop-c., prot., prun., psil., ***psor.***, **PULS.**, rhus-t., rob., ***sang.***, ***sel.***, **SOL.**, spig., stann., stram., sul-i., sulph., symph., syph., ther., thuj., usn., ***uva.***, ***valer.***, **VERAT.**, verat-v., x-ray, zinc.

SUNBURN, ailments from - acon., ***agar.***, ***ant-c.***, ***apis.***, **BELL.**, bov., bry., bufo, ***calen.***, ***camph.***, **CANTH.**, clem., cortiso., cyt-l., euphr., hist., ***hyos.***, kali-c., lach., ***lyc.***, ***mur-ac.***, ***nat-c.***, op., **PULS.**, rob., sel., **SOL,** ***sulph.***, **URT-U.**, ***valer.***, verat.

SUNSTROKE, ailments from - ***acon.***, agar., **AML-N.**, ***ant-c.***, apis, arg., ***arn.***, ***ars.***, **BELL.**, bry., ***cact.***, ***cadm.***, ***camph.***, ***carb-v.***, crot-h., cyt-l., euph-pi., ***gels.***, **GLON.**, ***gran.***, ***hell.***, hydr-ac., hyos., kalm., **LACH.**, lyc., lyss., **NAT-C.**, nat-m., nux-v., ***op.***, pop-c., rhus-t., **SOL.**, stram., syph., ***ther.***, thuj., usn., valer., **VERAT.**, ***verat-v.***

SURGERY, ailments, from - acet-ac., ***acon.***, all-c., ***anthr.***, apis., **ARN.**, ars., ars-i., ***bell.***, **BELL-P.**, berb., bry., calc-f., calc-p., calc-s., **CALEN.**, camph., ***carb-v.***, ***chin.***, ***chlf.***, croc., echi., ferr-p., graph., gunp., ham., ***hyper.***, iod., kali-s., led., merc., merc-c., merc-i-r., mill., myrt-c., naja, nit-ac., nux-v., ***op.***, ph-ac., ***phos.***, ***piloc.***, pop., ***pyrog.***, rad-br., raph., rhus-t., ruta, ***sil.***, **STAPH.**, ***stront-c.***, sul-ac., ***thiosin.***, verat., zinc.

SWELLING, general, (see Edema) - ***acon.***, agar., agn., alum., ambr., am-c., am-m., anac., ant-c., **APIS**, **APOC.**, arg., ***arn.***, **ARS.**, ars-i., asaf., aur., ***bar-c.***, **BELL.**, bism., bor., bov., **BRY.**, bufo, calad., ***calc.***, camph., cann-s., ***canth.***, caps., carb-an., carb-v., ***carbn-s.***, caust., ***cham.***, chel., ***chin.***, cic., clem., cocc., coff., colch., coloc., com., con., cop., croc., crot-h., cupr., cycl., dig., dros., ***dulc.***, euph., euphr., ***ferr.***, graph., guai., hell., ***hep.***, hyos., ign., iod., ***kali-ar.***, **KALI-BI.**, ***kali-c.***, kali-n., kreos., lach., laur., led., ***lyc.***, mag-c., mag-m., mang., **MERC.**, mez., mosch., mur-ac., naja, ***nat-c.***, nat-m., ***nit-ac.***, nux-m., **NUX-V.**, olnd., op., par., petr., ***ph-ac.***, ***phos.***, ***plb.***, **PULS.**, ran-b., rhod., **RHUS-T.**, ruta, sabad., sabin., samb., sars., sec., seneg., ***sep.***, ***sil.***, ***spig.***, spong., squil., stann., staph., ***stram.***, stront-c., ***sulph.***, sul-ac., ***thuj.***, valer., verat., ***vip.***, zinc.

SYNOVITIS, joints - **APIS**, bell., **BRY.**, calc., ***caust.***, ferr-p., iod., ***kali-c.***, kali-i., led., lyc., merc., **PHYT.**, puls., **RHUS-T.**, sep., sil., sulph., verat-v.

SYSTOLE, extra - dys-co.

T

TAR, ailments from local applications - bov., cupr., petr., zinc.

TEETH, decayed, rotten, hollowed - abrot., acon., aloe, alum., alumn., ***am-c.***, ***ambr.***, anac., anan., ang., **ANT-C.**, ars., asar., aur., aur-ar., aur-s., bac., ***bar-c.***, **BELL.**, **BOR.**, ***bov.***, bry., cadm-s., ***calc.***, **CALC-F.**, **CALC-P.**, ***calc-s.***, calc-sil., carb-an., ***carb-v.***, carbn-s., carc., caust., ***cham.***, ***chin.***, clem., coca, cocc., coff., con., euph., **FL-AC.**, ***glon.***, graph., ***hecla.***, ***hep.***, ***hyos.***, ip., ***kali-bi.***, ***kali-c.***, ***kali-i.***, kali-n., kali-p., **KREOS.**, ***lach.***, lob-s., ***lyc.***, ***mag-c.***, mag-m., mang., med., meph., **MERC.**, **MEZ.**, naja, **NAT-C.**, nat-m., nat-p., nat-s., ***nit-ac.***, ***nux-v.***, ox-ac., par., ***parathyr.***, petr., ***ph-ac.***, ***phos.***, ***plan.***, plat., **PLB.**, ***puls.***, rheum, ***rhod.***, ***rhus-t.***, ruta, sabad., sabin., sang., sel., **SEP.**, ***sil.***, spig., **STAPH.**, sul-ac., ***sulph.***, syph., tab., ***tarax.***, thuj., **TUB.**, verat., zinc.

TEETH, deformed, distorted - ***calc-f.***, calc-p., kreos., staph., syph.

TEETH, enamel, deficient - **CALC-F.**, fl-ac., ***sil.***

TEETH, extraction, complaints after tooth - **ARN.**, calen., ferr-p., hecla, **HYPER.**, ***phos.***, ruta, staph., symph.

TEETHING, dentition, difficult - **ACON.**, ***aeth.***, am-c., ***ant-c.***, ***ant-t.***, ***apis***, ***arn.***, **ARS.**, arund., **BELL.**, ***bism.***, **BOR.**, ***bry.***, **CALC.**, calc-f., **CALC-P.**, ***canth.***, ***caust.***, **CHAM.**, cheir., chlor., cic., cimic., ***cina***, ***coff.***, ***colch.***, ***coloc.***, cupr., cypr., ***dol.***, ***dulc.***, ***ferr.***, ***ferr-p.***, ***gels.***, ***graph.***, ***hecla.***, ***hell.***, hep., hyos., ***ign.***, ***ip.***, ***kali-br.***, ***kreos.***, ***lyc.***, ***mag-c.***, **MERC.**, ***merc-c.***, mill., nat-m., nit-ac., op., passi., ***phyt.***, plat., ***podo.***, puls., ***rheum***, scut., sec., sep., **SIL.**, sol-n., stann., **STAPH.**, **SULPH.**, syph., ***ter.***, tub., tub-k., zinc., zinc-br.

TEMPOROMANDIBULAR, T.M.J., jaws, pain in joints - agar., acet-ac., alum., alumn., ***arum-t.***, asaf., asar., brom., calc., **CAUST.**, cimic., cist., cor-r., dros., fl-ac., glon., hyper., ***ign.***, laur., mang., mez., nicc., op., **RHUS-T.**, spig., spong., staph., ***stry.***, sul-ac., vesp.

TENDONS, general - agar., anac., ant-c., ***arg.***, arn., ***bry.***, calc-p., calen., caust., form-ac., get., iod., phyt., ***rhod.***, **RHUS-T.**, **RUTA.**, sabin., thuj.

injuries - arn., ***anac.***, ***arg.***, calen., **RHUS-T.**, **RUTA.**

TENDONITIS - anac., ant-c., ***arg.***, bell-p., calen., mag-p., ***rhod.***, ***rhus-t.***, ***ruta.***

TENNIS, elbow - arn., aur., bell-p., ***bry.***, calc-f., hyper., ***rhus-t.***, ***ruta.***

TERTIAN, fever - aesc., ***alum.***, anac., **ANT-C.**, ***ant-t.***, ***apis***, aran., arn., ***ars.***, bar-c., ***bar-m.***, ***bell.***, ***bry.***, calc., calc-s., canch., ***canth.***, ***caps.***, carb-v., ***cedr.***, ***cham.***, cic., cina, ***chin.***, ***chin-s.***, ***cimx.***, ***chin.***, cor-r., ***aran.***, ***dig.***, dros., dulc., elat., eucal., **EUP-PER.**, ferr., gamb., gels., graph., hell., ***hep.***, hyos., ***ign.,*** iod., ***ip.,*** ***lach.,*** lap-gr-m., lyc., meny., merc., mez., mill., ***nat-m.,*** nux-m., **NUX-V.,** oci-s., ol-j., petr., ptel., plan., podo., polyp-p, ***puls.,*** ran-b., ***rhus-t.,*** ***sabad.,*** sep., sil., staph., stram., ***sulph.,*** ***thuj.,*** verat., zinc.

TESTES, cancer - arg., ars., ***aur.,*** bell., ***carb-an.,*** ***carc.,*** clem., **CON.,** fuli., hippoz., ox-ac., phos., ***phyt.,*** puls., ***sil.,*** ***spong.,*** sulph., thuj.

TESTES, general - acet-ac., **AGN.,** aloe, am-c., ant-t., arn., astac., ***aur.,*** bell., cahin., **CALAD.,** ***calc.,*** calc-p., camph., caps., carb-ac., carb-an., carb-v., carbn-s., chin., chin-s., **CLEM.,** cocc., ***coff.,*** con., crot-h., croto-t., ***dios.,*** ***ferr.,*** ferr-i., ***gels.,*** get., ***hell.,*** hep., hydr., hydrc., ign., iod., iris, lach., ***lec.,*** **LYC.,** mag-c., ***mag-m.,*** mag-p., merc., merc-c., ***nat-m.,*** nit-ac., ***nuph.,*** nux-m., ol-an., op., ***ph-ac.,*** phos., phyt., pic-ac., ***psor.,*** **PULS.,** pyrog., ***rhus-t.,*** sanic., sep., ***sil.,*** **STAPH.,** sul-ac., sul-i., **SULPH.,** sumb., **TAB.,** tarent., ***tub.,*** ***uran-n.,*** ust.

TESTES, tumors - clem., con., sil., tarent., thuj.

TETANUS, lockjaw - absin., acet-ac., ***acon.,*** act-sp., aeth., agar., alum., alumn., ambro., aml-n., amyg-am., anan., ***ang.,*** anthr., ant-t., ***arg-n.,*** arn., ars., art-v., aster., aur., aur-m-n., bapt., **BELL.,** bry., bufo, calc., ***calen.,*** ***camph.,*** cann-i., ***canth.,*** carbn-s., cast-eq., ***caust.,*** ***cedr.,*** cham., chin., chin-s., chlf., chlol., **CIC.,** cimic., cina, cob., ***cocc.,*** coffin., colch., con., ***crot-c.,*** crot-h., ***cupr.,*** ***cupr-acet.,*** cur., dig., dios., dulc., ***gels.,*** ***glon.,*** grat., ***guare.,*** ***hep.,*** hydr-ac., ***hyos.,*** **HYPER.,** ***ign.,*** iod., ***ip.,*** kali-br., kali-cy., kreos., lach., lat-m., ***laur.,*** **LED.,** ***lyc.,*** lyss., mag-c., mag-p., mang., ***merc.,*** merc-c., merc-i-f., morph., ***mosch.,*** naja, ***nux-m.,*** **NUX-V.,** ***oena.,*** **OP.,** ox-ac., ***passi.,*** **PETR.,** ph-ac., phos., phys., ***plan.,*** phyt., **PLAT.,** ***plb.,*** podo., puls., rhus-t., ***sec.,*** seneg., **SEP.,** sil., sol-n., spong., stann., staph., ***stram.,*** **STRY.,** sulph., tab., tarent., ter., ***tetox.,*** ther., ***upa.,*** ***verat.,*** verat-v., vip., zinc-m.

THALLASEMIA, blood - carc.

THROAT, cancer - cadm-i., ***carb-an.,*** ***hydr.,*** led., mur-ac., silphu., tarent., thuj.

THROBBING, pains - **ACON.,** ***agar.,*** **ALUM.,** ***am-m.,*** **ANT-T.,** ***arg.,*** ***arg-n.,*** ars-met., ***asaf.,*** **BELL.,** berb., ***bor.,*** ***bry.,*** **CALC.,** ***cann-i.,*** ***caps.,*** ***caust.,*** ***cham.,*** **COCC.,** **GLON.,** **HEP.,** ***ign.,*** ***iod.,*** **KALI-C.,** ***kreos.,*** ***laur.,*** **LED.,** ***lyc.,*** ***meli.,*** ***merc.,*** ***nat-c.,*** ***nat-m.,*** ***nit-ac.,*** **OLND.,** **PHOS.,** ***plat.,*** ***plb.,*** **PULS.,** ***rhod.,*** ***rhus-t.,*** ***ruta,*** **SABAD.,** **SEP.,** **SIL.,** ***spig.,*** ***spong.,*** **SULPH.,** ***tarax.,*** ***thuj.,*** zinc.

THROMBOSIS, blood - acetan., am-c., am-caust., antipyrin., ***apis,*** arn., ***ars.,*** **BOTH-L.,** bufo, calc-ar., carb-v., card-m., cortico., fl-ac., ham., hir., ***kali-chl.,*** ***kali-m.,*** kres., ***lach.,*** mag-f., ***nat-s.,*** prot., sec., ***vip.***

THYROID, cancer - cadm-i., calc-i., ***carc.,*** ***iod.,*** kali-i., ***lach.,*** lap-a., ***scirr.,*** sil., ***spong.,*** **THUJ.**

THYROID, gland, remedies - aloe, am-c., am-m., **AMBR.,** apis, ars., ars-i., aur., ***bad.,*** bar-c., bell., **BROM.,** bufo, **CALC.,** calc-f., **CALC-I.,** calc-p., calc-s., caust., cist., crot-c., ***con.,*** dig., ferr-i., fl-ac., form., graph., ham., ***hep.,*** **IOD.,** ***iris,*** kali-c., **KALI-I.,** ***lach.,*** lap-a., lycps., **LYC.,** mag-c., ***merc.,*** ***merc-i-f.,*** ***merc-i-r.,*** nat-ar., **NAT-C.,** **NAT-M.,** nat-p., nat-s., nit-ac., petr., phos., **SEP.,** sil., **SPONG.,** staph., sul-i., sulph., thuj., **THYR.**

enlargement, of thyroid - ail., ***calc-i.,*** ferr-i., iod., kali-i., mag-c., nat-c., ***spong.***

hyperthyroid - adren., aml-n., ars-i., aur-i., bad., ***bell.,*** brom., ***cact.,*** ***calc.,*** calc-i., ***ferr-i.,*** ***fl-ac.,*** ***glon.,*** **IOD.,** ***kali-i.,*** lycps., ***nat-m.,*** nux-v., ***phos.,*** ***piloc.,*** sel., ***spong.,*** stram., ***thyr.,*** verat.

hypertrophy - ***brom.,*** calc-i., cist., ferr-i., ***iod.,*** kali-i., spong.

hypothyroid - aq-mar., bad., ***brom.,*** bufo, **CALC.,** calc-f., **CALC-I.,** calc-p., cist., con., ferr-i., fl-ac., form., fuc., **GRAPH.,** iod., kali-c., **KALI-I.,** ***lach.,*** lycps., ***lyc.,*** nat-c., **NAT-M.,** phos., pineal, **SEP.,** sil., **SPONG.,** thuj., **THYR.**

parathyroid, gland - calc., calc-f., ***calc-p.***

THRUSH, mouth - arum-t., **BOR.,** cand-a., iod., lac-c., ***kali-chl.,*** **MERC.,** merc-cy., mur-ac., **NAT-M.,** nit-ac., sang., sulph., **SUL-AC.,** syph., thuj.

TINEA, ringworm, general - ***ail.,*** anac., anag., arg-n., ars-s-f., **BAC.,** ***bar-c.,*** **CALC.,** calc-acet., ***carb-an.,*** ***carb-v.,*** ***carbn-s.,*** chin., chrysar., cina, clem., cupr., cupr-acet., cur., dulc., dys-co., equis., ***eup-per.,*** ***fil.,*** ***form.,*** frag., ***gran.,*** ***graph.,*** grat., hell., hep., iod., kali-c., kali-i., ***lith-c.,*** mag-c., mag-m., med., merc., ***nat-c.,*** **NAT-M.,** nat-s., ***nit-ac.,*** nux-v., petr., phos., **PHYT.,** ***plat.,*** ***puls.,*** ***sabad.,*** ***sanic.,*** sant., **SEP.,** ***sil.,*** sol, spong., ***stann.,*** sulph., syc-co., **TELL.,** ter., **THUJ.,** torul., **TUB.,** valer.

TINEA, capitis, favosa - aethi-a., agar., ars., ars-i., ***brom.,*** calc., calc-i., ***calc-m.,*** calc-s., ***dulc.,*** ferr-i., graph., ***hep.,*** jug-r., ***kali-c.,*** kali-s., lappa, ***lyc.,*** med., ***mez.,*** nit-ac., olnd., phos., ***sep.,*** ***sil.,*** sul-ac., sulph., ust., vinc., ***viol-t.***

TINEA, circinate, ringworm - aesc., ant-c., ***bac.,*** calc., dulc., graph., hep., lyc., merc., mez., psor., rhus-t., ***sep.,*** sulph., ***thuj.***

TINEA, tonsurans - ant-c., ant-t., ***ars.,*** ***bac.,*** calc., calc-i., ***chrysar.,*** graph., hep., jug-c., jug-r., kali-s., lyc., mez., nat-m., petr., psor., puls., rhus-t., semp., ***sep.,*** sulph., ***tell.,*** thuj., tub., viol-t.

TINEA, versicolor - ars., ars-i., bac., calc., carb-an., carb-v., chrysar., kali-s., mez., ***nat-ar.,*** nit-ac., phos., phyt., psor., ***sep.,*** sil., sulph., tell., **THUJ.**

TINNITUS, hearing, (see Noises in ears, ringing) - anac., ***bell.,*** bism., ***caust.,*** cedr., all-c., chin-ar., ***chin.,*** **CHIN-S.,** ***coc-c.,*** ***iod.,*** kali-br., lac-c., merc., ***nat-s.,*** ***phos.,*** plat., ***plb.,*** ***puls.,*** ***sal-ac.,*** ***sil.,*** **THIOSIN.**

<u>**TOBACCO**</u>, smoke, agg. - ***abies-n.***, acon., act-sp., agar., ***alum.***, ***alumn.***, ambr., anac., ang., arg., arg-n., **ARS.**, ars-i., asc-t., aur-m-n., bell., bor., brom., ***bry.***, cact., ***calad.***, calc., calc-caust., calc-p., ***camph.***, cann-i., carb-an., carbn-s., caust., cham., chel., chin., chin-ar., chin-m., cic., ***clem.***, coca, coc-c., ***cocc.***, ***coff.***, coloc., con., conv., cupr., ***cycl.***, dig., dor., ***euphr.***, ferr., ***gels.***, ***hell.***, hep., hydr., <u>**IGN.**</u>, iod., ***ip.***, kali-bi., kali-br., kalm., lac-ac., ***lach.***, lob., ***lyc.***, ***mag-c.***, mag-m., mand., ***meny.***, merc., mur-ac., naja, nat-c., ***nat-m.***, nicot., **NUX-V.**, okou., olnd., osm., ***par.***, petr., ***phos.***, **PLAN.**, plb., psil., **PULS.**, rad-br., ran-b., rhus-t., ***ruta***, sabad., sabin., sars., scut., sec., ***sel.***, sep., sil., sol-m., **SPIG.**, **SPONG.**, **STAPH.**, stel., stroph., sulph., tab., ***tarax.***, ***thuj.***, verat.

desire, for smoking - ***ars.***, ***asar.***, ***aven.***, bell., **CALAD.**, ***calc-p.***, ***camph.***, carb-ac., carb-an., carb-v., card-m., cast-eq., ***chin.***, chlor., ***coca***, coff., con., daph., eug., ***glon.***, ham., hydrog., kreos., lap-gr-m., led., **LOB.**, lyc., m-arct., m-aust., manc., med., narz., nat-c., nicot., nicot-r., nux-v., ox-ac., ***phos.***, plan., plat., plb., rhus-t., ***spig.***, ***staph.***, **TAB.**, ther., ***thuj.***

<u>**TONGUE**</u>, cancer - ***alumn.***, ***apis***, arg-cy., ***ars.***, ***aur.***, **AUR-M.**, aur-m-n., bell., benz-ac., calc., carb-ac., ***carb-an.***, ***carc.***, caust., chr-ac., cit-ac., cit-l., ***con.***, crot-h., cund., gali., glyc., hep., ho., ***hydr.***, kali-chl., **KALI-CY.**, ***kali-i.***, ***lach.***, merc., ***mur-ac.***, ***nit-ac.***, ***phos.***, ***phyt.***, rad-br., ***scirr.***, ***semp.***, sep., ***sil.***, staph., sulph., ***thuj.***, vib-p.

<u>**TONSILLECTOMY**</u>, ailments after - arn., calc., calen., carc., strept., sulph.

<u>**TONSILLITIS**</u>, infection - ***acon.***, aesc., ***ail.***, **ALUMN.**, aml-n., anan., ant-t., anthr., ***apis***, ***ars.***, bad., ***bapt.***, **BAR-C.**, ***bar-m.***, <u>**BELL.**</u>, benz-ac., berb., bufo, ***canth.***, ***caps.***, cedr., ***cham.***, chel., ***chen-a.***, ***colch.***, ***crot-h.***, ***cupr.***, cur., ***dulc.***, <u>**FERR-P.**</u>, ***fl-ac.***, ***gels.***, **GUAI.**, ham., **HEP.**, ***ign.***, ***iod.***, ***kali-bi.***, ***kali-chl.***, kali-p., **LAC-C.**, **LACH.**, ***lyc.***, <u>**MERC.**</u>, ***merc-cy.***, **MERC-D.**, ***merc-i-f.***, ***merc-i-r.***, naja, ***nat-s.***, **NIT-AC.**, ***phyt.***, ***plb.***, ***psor.***, puls., ***sabad.***, ***sang.***, sep., **SIL.**, ***staph.***, still., ***sulph.***, tarent., ust., verat., vesp., zinc.

<u>**TONSILS**</u>, cancer - ***carb-an.***, ***hydr.***, led., mur-ac., silphu., tarent.

<u>**TONSILS**</u>, remedies - ***acon.***, aesc., agra., ail., ***alumn.***, am-c., anan., anthr., ars-i., ars-s-f., aur., ***bac.***, bad., ***bapt.***, **BAR-C.**, bar-i., **BAR-M.**, **BELL.**, benz-ac., berb., brom., bufo, ***calc.***, **CALC-F.**, **CALC-I.**, **CALC-P.**, ***calc-s.***, ***canth.***, caps., ***carc.***, ***cedr.***, ***cham.***, chel., ***chen-a.***, chin., cist., ***colch.***, con., ***crot-h.***, ***cupr.***, cur., euph., fago., ***ferr.***, ferr-p., ***gels.***, goss., **GUAI.**, guare., ham., **HEP.**, iber., ign., iod., ***kali-bi.***, ***kali-c.***, ***kali-i.***, kali-m., kali-p., **LAC-C.**, **LACH.**, lob., luf-op., **LYC.**, mag-f., mag-i., med., **MERC.**, **MERC-D.**, merc-i-f., merc-i-r., mit., nat-ar., ***nat-m.***, ***nit-ac.***, petr., phos., ***phyt.***, plb., plb-i., ***psor.***, puls., sabad., ***sang.***, sanguin-n., ***sep.***, **SIL.**, sol-n., spig., spong., ***staph.***, still., sul-i., ***sulph.***, syc-co., ***syph.***, tarent., thuj., **TUB.**, ust., vesp., zinc.

<u>**TOOTHACHES**</u> - ***acet-ac.***, **ACON.**, ***agar.***, ***ail.***, all-c., alum., ***ambr.***, am-c., am-m., anac., anag., ang., ***ant-c.***, ant-t., apis, ***aran.***, arg., ***arg-n.***, arn., ***ars.***, ars-h., ***ars-i.***, asar., asc-t., ***aspar.***, aur., aur-m., ***bar-c.***, bar-m., **BELL.**, berb., ***benz-ac.***, bism., ***bor.***, bov., **BRY.**, ***bufo***, calad., ***calc.***, calc-f., calc-p., canth., ***carb-ac.***, carb-an., ***carb-v.***, ***carbn-s.***, ***caust.***, **CHAM.**, ***chel.***, chen-a., **CHIN.**, chin-ar., clem., cocc., coch., **COFF.**, colch., coloc., con., cor-r., croc., cycl., dios., dros., dulc., ***echi.***, ***euph.***, ***ferr.***, ferr-i., ferr-p., ***fl-ac.***, **GLON.**, ***graph.***, grat., guai., guare., ***hell.***, **HEP.**, **HYDROG.**, ***hyos.***, hyper., ign., ***iod.***, ip., ***kali-c.***, ***kali-i.***, kali-n., ***kali-p.***, kali-s., ***kalm.***, ***kreos.***, **LACH.**, laur., led., lob., ***lyc.***, ***mag-c.***, ***mag-m.***, mag-p., ***mag-s.***, m-arct., m-aust., mang., **MERC.**, ***merc-c.***, merl., ***mez.***, mur-ac., ***nat-ar.***, **NAT-C.**, ***nat-m.***, ***nat-p.***, ***nat-s.***, nicc., ***nit-ac.***, ***nux-m.***, ***nux-v.***, olnd., par., ***petr.***, ph-ac., ***phos.***, ***phyt.***, plat., ***plan.***, plb., prun., ***puls.***, ran-s., raph., rat., rheum, **RHOD.**, ***rhus-t.***, ruta, sabad., ***sars.***, sel., seneg., **SEP.**, sil., spig., spong., squil., **STAPH.**, stront-c., stry., ***sulph.***, sul-ac., tab., tarax., ***tarent.***, teucr., ther., thuj., ***valer.***, verat., verb., vinc., **ZINC.**

<u>**TORTICOLLIS**</u>, neck - ***acon.***, alum., ant-c., ***apis***, ars., asar., **BELL.**, ***calc.***, camph., cann-i., caul., **CAUST.**, cedr., ***cham.***, chel., chin., **CIC.**, **CIMIC.**, ***cina***, ***colch.***, ***cupr.***, con., dulc., eup-per., eup-pur., ***gels.***, ***glon.***, ***graph.***, guai., ***hell.***, ***hep.***, hura, ***hyos.***, hyper., ***ign.***, ***ip.***, kreos., lac-ac., lac-c., lach., <u>**LACHN.**</u>, **LYC.**, mag-c., merc., ***mez.***, mur-ac., ***nat-m.***, ***nat-s.***, ***nux-v.***, **OP.**, ***phel.***, **PHOS.**, ***ran-b.***, **RHUS-T.**, samb., stram., sulph., syc-co., ***tab.***, verat-v., ***zinc.***

<u>**TRACHEA**</u>, cancer - arg-cy., arg-n., ars-i., ***ars.***, bell., carb-an., clem., ***con.***, hydr., iod., kreos., kres., lach., lap-a., morph., nit-ac., phos., ***phyt.***, sang., thuj.

<u>**TRANSFUSIONS**</u>, blood, ailments of - carc., ***chin.***

<u>**TRICHINOSIS**</u> - ars., bapt., cina.

<u>**TRICHOPHYTOSIS**</u>, (see Ringworm) - abr., ant-c., ant-t., ***ars.***, ***bac.***, calc., calc-i., ***chrysar.***, ***graph.***, hep., jug-c., jug-r., kali-s., lyc., mez., psor., ran-b., rhus-t., semp., ***sep.***, sulph., ***tell.***, ter., tub., viol-t.

<u>**TUBERCLES**</u>, general, (see Nodules) - agar., alum., am-c., ***am-m.***, anac., ang., ***ant-c.***, apis, aran., arn., ***ars.***, ars-i., aur., bac., ***bar-c.***, bar-m., bar-s., bell., berb., bov., ***bry.***, **CALC.**, calc-p., calc-s., canth., ***carb-an.***, ***carb-v.***, carbn-s., **CAUST.**, cham., ***cic.***, cocc., ***con.***, crot-h., dig., ***dulc.***, ***fl-ac.***, ***graph.***, hell., ***hep.***, hydrc., ign., kali-ar., ***kali-bi.***, ***kali-br.***, kali-c., kali-chl., ***kali-i.***, kali-n., kali-s., **LACH.**, **LED.**, ***lyc.***, mag-c., mag-m., mag-s., mang., ***merc.***, merc-c., merc-i-r., ***mez.***, ***mur-ac.***, nat-ar., ***nat-c.***, ***nat-m.***,

nicc., ***nit-ac.***, nux-v., ***olnd.***, op., ***petr.***, ph-ac., ***phos.***, phyt., puls., ***rhus-t.***, rhus-v., sang., sec., sel., sep., ***sil.***, spig., squil., stann., ***staph.***, still., stram., stront-c., sul-ac., ***sulph.***, syph., tarax., ***thuj.***, tub., valer., verat., zinc.

TUBERCULOSIS, infection - abr., ***acal., acet-ac.***, acon., aesc., aethi-a., **AGAR.**, agarin., ***all-s.***, alum., alum-sil., alumn., am-acet., am-c., am-m., ant-ar., ant-c., ant-i., ant-t., ***aq-mar.***, arg., arg-n., arist-cl., arn., ***ars.***, ***ars-i.***, ars-s-f., arum-t., asaf., atro., aur., aur-ar., aur-m., aur-m-n., **BAC.**, bals-p., ***bapt.***, bar-c., ***bar-m.***, bell., berb., beta., betin., blatta, ***brom.***, ***bry.***, ***bufo***, cact., calag., **CALC.**, calc-ar., calc-f., calc-hp., ***calc-i.***, **CALC-P.**, ***calc-s.***, ***calc-sil.***, calo., cann-s., ***carb-an.***, ***carb-v.***, ***carbn-s.***, carc., card-m., caust., cetr., cham., ***chin.***, ***chin-ar.***, chin-s., chlor., ***cimic.***, coc-c., cod., ***con.***, ***crot-h.***, ***cupr.***, cupr-ar., dig., ***dros.***, ***dulc.***, ***elaps***, erig., erio., eucal., euon., eupi., **FERR.**, ferr-acet., ***ferr-ar.***, ***ferr-i.***, ferr-m., ***ferr-p.***, fil., fl-ac., form., form-ac., gall-ac., gamb., ***graph.***, ***guai.***, guare., ***ham.***, helx., **HEP.**, hippoz., hydr., hydrc., hyos., hyosin., ichth., **IOD.**, ***iodof.***, ***ip.***, jug-c., just., kali-acet., kali-ar., ***kali-bi.***, **KALI-C.**, kali-chl., kali-i., kali-m., ***kali-n.***, ***kali-p.***, **KALI-S.**, kali-sil., ***kreos.***, lac-c., ***lac-d.***, ***lach.***, lachn., laur., lec., led., lipp., lob., **LYC.**, lycps., mag-c., malar., mang., ***med.***, ***merc.***, merc-c., merc-i-r., mill., ***myos-a.***, myris., ***myrt-c.***, naphtin., nat-ar., nat-c., ***nat-cac.***, ***nat-m.***, nat-p., ***nat-s.***, ***nat-sel.***, ***nit-ac.***, nux-m., nux-v., ***ol-j.***, ox-ac., petr., ***ph-ac.***, phel., **PHOS.**, phyt., piloc., pineal., ***plb.***, polyg., polyg-a., prun-c., **PSOR.**, ptel., **PULS.**, pyrog., rhus-t., ***rumx.***, ruta, ***salv.***, samb., ***sang.***, sec., **SENEC.**, ***seneg.***, ***sep.***, **SIL.**, silpho., **SPONG.**, **STANN.**, stann-i., staph., stict., still., succ., sul-ac., sul-i., **SULPH.**, tarent., tarent-c., teucr., teucr-s., thea., **THER.**, thiosin., thuj., ***tril.***, **TUB.**, tub-a., ***tub-k.***, tub-r., tus-fa., uran-n., urea, vac., vanad., verat., verb., x-ray, **ZINC.**, zinc-p.

last, stage - am-c., ars., bac., bry., **CALC.**, calc-hp., **CARB-V.**, ***chin.***, ***dros.***, ***euon.***, kali-n., **LACH.**, led., lob., **LYC.**, ***phel.***, ***phos.***, ***psor.***, **PULS.**, ***pyrog.***, **SANG.**, senec., ***seneg.***, **STANN.**, stann-i., **TARENT.**

TUMORS, general, (see Cancer) - abr., abrot., acet-ac., acon., agar., all-c., aloe, alum., alumn., am-c., am-m., anan., ***ant-c.***, ant-t., anthr., apis, apoc., arbu., arg-n., arn., ars., ars-i., art-v., ***aster.***, aur., aur-m., **AUR-M-N.**, ba-tn., bad., bapt., ***bar.***, **BAR-C.**, bar-i., bar-m., bell., bell-p., benz-ac., beryl., bov., brom., bry., cact., ***calc.***, calc-ar., ***calc-f.***, calc-i., calc-p., calc-s., calen., carb-ac., carb-an., carb-v., ***carc.***, caust., chin., chol., chr-s., cic., ***cist.***, clem., coloc., **CON.**, conch., croc., crot-h., cund., cupre-l., cypr., daph., dios., elat., eucal., euph., ***ferr-i.***, ferr-ma., ferr-pic., fl-ac., foll., form-ac., frax., fuli., gali., gast., ***graph.***, guare., ***hecla.***, hep., ho., **HYDR.**, hydr-m., hyper., iod., junc., kali-ar., kali-bi., ***kali-br.***, kali-c., kali-chl., kali-i., kali-m., kali-p., kali-s., kreos., lac-ac., lach., **LAP-A.**, led., lil-t., lob., ***lob-e.***, lyc., m-arct., maland., manc., med., merc., merc-c., merc-d., merc-i-r., merc-p., mez., mur-ac., **ORNI.**, nat-c., nat-cac., nat-m., nat-sil., ***nit-ac.***, nux-v., ph-ac., ***phos.***, **PHYT.**, platan., ***plb.***, ***plb-i.***, psor., puls., rad-br., ran-b., rhus-t., ruta, sabin., scroph-n., sec., ***sem-t.***, sep., **SIL.**, sol-t-ae., spong., ***staph.***, stram., sul-ac., sulph., syph., tarent., tarent-c., ter., teucr., thiosin., thlaspi, **THUJ.**, ***thyr.***, tril., tub., ***ur-ac.***, urea, ust., vac., vanad., verb., vip., xan., zinc.

injuries, tumors, after - arn., bell-p., con.

neuroma - acon., all-c., arn., bell., bry., calc., calc-f., calen., chin., con., lyc., merc., rhus-t., ***ruta,*** sil., staph., sulph., thuj.

papillomata - ant-c., ***calc.***, nit-ac., staph., ***thuj.***

steatoma, suppurating - ***calc.***, ***carb-v.***

TURPENTINE, ailments from - benz-ac., colch., ***ter.***, nux-m.

TWITCHING, pain - acon., **AGAR.**, all-c., am-c., am-m., ammc., amyg-p., anag., ang., arn., ars., ars-h., arund., asaf., bell., berb., bry., calc., calc-p., carb-an., carbn-s., cast., cast-eq., caust., cedr., chin., **CIC.**, cimic., cinnb., coch., ***coloc.***, dig., dulc., eupi., hyos., ***ign.***, junc., kali-c., kali-n., lact., led., lith-c., lyc., ***m-aust.***, mag-c., mag-m., ***mag-p.***, mang., meny., meph., mez., morph., nat-c., nat-s., nux-v., op., pall., petr., ph-ac., phos., plat., prun., puls., rhod., sil., spig., squil., stann., sul-ac., sulph., tarax., tet., thuj., verat., verin., visc., **ZINC.**

TYPHLITIS - **APIS**, ***ars.***, **BELL.**, **BRY.**, ***calad.***, ***card-m.***, ***chin.***, ***colch.***, ***crot-h.***, gins., **LACH.**, ***lyc.***, **MERC.**, ***nat-s.***, **OP.**, ***phos.***, ***plb.***, **RHUS-T.**, ***samb.***, ***sep.***, ***sil.***, ***stram.***, sulph., **THUJ.**

TYPHOID, fever, salmonella - acet-ac., achy., acon., aeth., agar., ail., alum., alumn., am-c., ant-c., ant-t., anthr., apis, arg., arg-n., arn., **ARS.**, ars-s-f., **ARUM-T.**, asar., atro., **BAPT.**, bell., bor., **BRY.**, cadm-s., calad., calc., ***camph.***, cann-i., ***canth.***, ***caps.***, carb-ac., ***carb-an.***, **CARB-V.**, caust., cham., chel., **CHIN.**, ***chin-ar.***, ***chin-s.***, **CHLOR.**, cic., cimic., cina, ***cocc.***, **COLCH.**, con., **CROT-H.**, cupr., cupr-ar., cyt-l., dig., dor., dulc., **ECHI.**, elaps, ***eucal.***, eup-a., ***eup-per.***, euphr., ferr., ferr-m., ferr-p., **GELS.**, glon., graph., gymn., haem., ham., ***hell.***, hep., hydr., hydr-ac., hydrin-s., **HYOS.**, ign., iod., ip., iris, kali-bi., kali-c., kali-m., kali-n., ***kali-p.***, kreos., **LACH.**, lachn., laur., lept., ***lyc.***, lycps., maland., mang., **MERC.**, merc-c., merc-cy., merc-i-r., methyl., mez., mill., ***mosch.***, **MUR-AC.**, nat-m., nat-s., ***nit-ac.***, nux-m., ***nux-v.***, oci-s., ***op.***, par., petr., ***ph-ac.***, **PHOS.**, plan., plb., ***psor.***, puls., ***pyrog.***, rheum, rhus-g., **RHUS-T.**, ***rhus-v.***, sang., sars., ***sec.***, sel., seneg., sep., ***sil.***, spig., stann., staph., **STRAM.**, stry., ***sul-ac.***, **SULPH.**, sumb., tarax., tarent., ***ter.***, thuj., trio., tub., ***urt-u.***, vac., valer., verat., verat-v., xan., xero, zinc.

TYPHO-MALARIAL, fever - lycps.

TYPHUS, fever, rickettsia - agar., ail., alum., apis, ***ars.***, asar., ***bapt.***, calad., carb-v., cast., chin., chin-s., chlf., chlor., echni., hell., hydr., hyos., hyosin., lach., mang., merc., merc-i-r., mur-ac., pest., ph-ac., phos., plb., ***pyrog.***, rhus-t., stram.

U

ULCERS, cancerous - ***ambr.***, ***anthr.***, ant-c., apis, **ARN.**, **ARS.**, ***ars-i.***, **ARS-S-F.**, ***aster.***, aur., aur-ar., aur-i., **AUR-S.**, ***bell.***, **BUFO**, calc., ***calc-s.***, ***carb-ac.***, ***carb-an.***, ***carb-v.***, ***carbn-s.***, caust., chel., chim., chin-s., clem., **CON.**, ***crot-c.***, **CUND.**, dor., dulc., ***ferr.***, fl-ac., fuli., ***gali.***, ***graph.***, **HEP.**, ***hippoz.***, ***hydr.***, kali-ar., kali-bi., kali-c., ***kali-i.***, ***kreos.***, ***lach.***, **LYC.**, ***lyss.***, mang., ***merc.***, merc-i-f., ***mill.***, mur-ac., ***nit-ac.***, ***petr.***, ***ph-ac.***, ***phos.***, ***phyt.***, ***rhus-t.***, rumx., sars., ***scirr.***, ***sep.***, **SIL.**, spong., squil., ***staph.***, **SULPH.**, sul-ac., sul-i., syph., tarent-c., ***thuj.***, x-ray., ***zinc.***

ULCERS, general, (see Aphthous, ulcers) - abrot., acet-ac., ***acon.***, aesc., agar., agn., ail., all-c., ***alum.***, alum-p., alum-sil., alumn., ***am-c.***, am-m., ambr., ampe-qu, anac., anac-oc., anag., ***anan.***, ang., ant-c., ant-t., ***anthr.***, ap-g., apis, aq-sil., arg., ***arg-n.***, arist-cl., arn., **ARS.**, **ARS-I.**, ars-s-f., **ASAF.**, aster., ***aur.***, aur-ar., aur-i., aur-m., aur-m-n., ***aur-s.***, bals-p., bapt., bar-c., bar-i., ***bar-m.***, ***bell.***, benz-ac., berb., beryl., bism., bor., both-l., bov., ***brom.***, ***bry.***, bufo, calc., calc-f., calc-i., calc-m., calc-p., ***calc-s.***, ***calc-sil.***, calen., camph., canth., caps., carb-ac., carb-an., **CARB-V.**, **CARBN-S.**, card-m., ***caust.***, cench., ***cham.***, chel., chim., chin., chin-ar., chin-s., chlor., cic., cina, ***cinnb.***, cist., clem., cocc., coff., colch., coloc., com., ***con.***, cor-r., croc., crot-c., crot-h., croto-t., cund., ***cupr.***, cupr-ar., cycl., dig., dor., dros., dulc., ***echi.***, eucal., euph., ferr., ferr-ar., ferr-i., ferr-ma., ferr-p., ***fl-ac.***, fuli., gali., gast., gels., ***ger.***, ***graph.***, grat., grin., guai., ham., hecla., hell., hell-v., **HEP.**, hippoz., ho., hydr., hydrc., hyos., hyper., ign., insulin, ***iod.***, ip., jac., jug-r., ***kali-ar.***, **KALI-BI.**, ***kali-c.***, **KALI-CHL.**, kali-i., kali-n., kali-p., **KALI-S.**, kali-sil., kalm., ***kreos.***, lac-c., **LACH.**, lap-a., laur., led., liatr., **LYC.**, lyss., m-ambo., mag-c., mag-i., mag-m., mang., med., **MERC.**, merc-acet., merc-c., merc-cy., merc-d., merc-i-f., merc-i-r., merc-pr-r., merc-s., ***mez.***, mill., morg., mosch., mur-ac., naja, ***nat-ar.***, ***nat-c.***, nat-i., ***nat-m.***, nat-p., nat-s., **NIT-AC.**, nux-m., nux-v., olnd., op., ***paeon.***, par., ***petr.***, ***ph-ac.***, ***phos.***, **PHYT.**, plat., plb., plb-i., polyg., prun-c., ***psor.***, **PULS.**, ***pyrog.***, rad-br., ran-a., ran-b., ran-s., rat., rhus-r., ***rhus-t.***, rumx., ruta, sabad., sabin., samb., sang., ***sars.***, scroph-n., ***sec.***, sel., seneg., ***sep.***, **SIL.**, sol-n., spig., spong., squil., stann., ***staph.***, still., stram., stront-c., sul-ac., sul-i., **SULPH.**, syph., syzyg., tarax., tarent., tarent-c., tell., ter., thlaspi, ***thuj.***, valer., vario., verat., vinc., viol-t., vip., xan., ***zinc.***, zinc-i., zinc-p., zinc-s.

UNCONSCIOUSNESS, (see Coma)

UREMIA, blood - ***ail.***, aloe, am-be., ***am-c.***, ***apis***, apoc., ars., asc-c., aur-m., bapt., ***bell.***, benz-ac., berb., botul., calc., cann-i., ***canth.***, ***carb-ac.***, chlf., cic., ***cupr.***, cupr-acet., cupr-ar., dig., eup-pur., gels., **COLCH.**, ***glon.***, glyc-g., graph., ***hell.***, hydr-ac., ***hyos.***, iod., jab., kali-br., ***kali-s.***, lach., lyc., merc-n., methyl., ***morph.***, mosch., ***op.***, ***phos.***, ***pic-ac.***, piloc., ***plb.***, queb., senec., seneg., ser-ang., ***stram.***, sulfa., ***ter.***, thlaspi., tub., urea, urine, **URT-U.**, ***verat-v.***

URETHRA, stricture - acon., agar., alumn., ant-t., ***apis***, ***arg-n.***, arn., baros., bell., ***berb.***, bry., ***calc.***, calc-i., calc-sil., camph., ***cann-s.***, **CANTH.**, carb-v., ***chim.***, chin., cic., cinnb., **CLEM.**, coc-c., ***con.***, cop., ***dig.***, dios., ***dulc.***, ery-a., eucal., gels., ***graph.***, hep., hydrang., ***indg.***, ***iod.***, ***kali-i.***, lob., lyc., mag-m., ***merc.***, nast., ***nat-m.***, nat-s., **NIT-AC.**, nux-v., op., **PETR.**, ***petros.***, ph-ac., phos., plb., prun., **PULS.**, rhus-t., sabal., sec., sep., ***sil.***, spong., stram., ***sul-i.***, ***sulph.***, tarent., ***thiosin.***, thuj.

URETHRITIS, inflammation, urethra - ***acon.***, alum., anemps., ant-t., apis, arg., **ARG-N.**, **ARIST-CL.**, ***ars.***, ***aur.***, aur-ar., bell., bov., ***cact.***, calc., calc-p., camph., cann-i., **CANN-S.**, **CANTH.**, caps., caust., ***chim.***, ***clem.***, coch., ***cop.***, croto-t., ***cub.***, cypr., dig., ***dor.***, dulc., erig., eup-pur., fab., ferr-p., ***gels.***, gran., ham., hedy., ***hep.***, jac-c., kali-bi., ***kali-i.***, led., lyc., manz., mati., med., ***merc.***, **MERC-C.**, merc-n., mez., nat-m., nit-ac., ***nux-v.***, oci-s., ol-sant., pareir., ***petr.***, ***petros.***, ph-ac., puls., rhus-t., sabal., ***sabin.***, salx-n., sars., sel., sep., sil., ***sulph.***, syc-co., tab., **TER.**, teucr., thlaspi, **THUJ.**, tritic., tub., tus-p., yohim, yuc.

URIC ACID, diathesis - adren., agn., alco., ant-c., ***apis***, aran., arg-n., arn., aspar., ***bar-m.***, bell., **BENZ-AC.**, berb., bry., calc., calc-m., ***calc-p.***, ***canth.***, ***caps.***, ***carbn-s.***, caust., ***cham.***, chel., chim., chin., chin-s., chlf., cimic., coc-c., coff-t., **COLCH.**, coloc., cortico., cortiso., ***crot-h.***, dig., dulc., ***epig.***, fab., form., gins., guai., hedeo, kali-c., kali-i., kali-m., kalm., led., lith-be., lith-c., lob., ***lyc.***, ***mag-c.***, med., ***meny.***, mez., mit., nat-m., nat-s., nit-ac., nux-v., ***oci.***, oxyg., **PAREIR.**, phase., phos., phyt., pic-ac., pipe., plb., **PULS.**, rhod., rhus-t., sabin., sang., sars., sep., skook., solid., sulph., ter., thlaspi, thuj., thymol., thyr., **UR-AC.**, ***urea***, **URT-U.**

URINATION, painful, dysuria, (See Cystitis) - **ACON.**, aesc., aeth., ***agar.***, ***all-c.***, all-s., aloe, ***alum.***, ang., ant-c., ant-t., ***apis***, ***apoc.***, **ARG-N.**, arn., ***ars.***, ars-s-f., asim., atro., aur., aur-ar., aur-m., bar-c., bar-m., bar-s., **BELL.**, ***benz-ac.***, ***berb.***, bor., cact., calc., ***calc-p.***, ***camph.***, ***cann-i.***, **CANN-S.**, **CANTH.**, caps., carb-v., carbn-s., casc., caul., caust., cedr., ***cham.***, chel., ***chim.***, cic., cina, ***clem.***, ***coc-c.***, cocc., coff., colch., ***coloc.***, ***con.***, **COP.**, corn., crot-h., cub., cuc-c., ***cupr.***, ***dig.***, ***dor.***, dros., dulc., epig., equis., erig., ery-a., ***eup-pur.***, euph., fab., ferr., ferr-p., gali., gamb., ***gels.***, graph., ham., hell., ***hep.***, ***hydr.***, hydrang., ***hyos.***, hyper., ign., ind., jatr., junc., juni-c., ***kali-ar.***, ***kali-c.***, kali-chl., kali-n., kali-p., kali-s., ***kreos.***, ***lac-c.***, lach., lappa, laur., **LIL-T.**, ***lith-c.***, ***lyc.***, lycps., m-aust., mag-m., med., meph., merc., **MERC-C.**, mit., morph., mur-ac., nat-ar., nat-c., ***nat-m.***, nat-p., ***nit-ac.***, nux-m., **NUX-V.**, oci., ***ol-sant.***, **OP.**, **PAREIR.**, petr., **PETROS.**, ph-ac., phos., plat., ***plb.***, podo., ***polyg.***, pop., prun., psor., **PULS.**, rad-br., ran-b., ***rheum***, ***rhus-a.***, ***rhus-t.***, ruta, ***sabal.***, ***sabin.***, sang., sanic., ***sant.***, sars., saur., sec., sel., ***senec.***, ***sep.***, sil., solid., spig., stann., staph., stigm., stram., **SULPH.**, sumb., tab., tanac., tarax., ***tarent.***, tax., **TER.**, thlaspi, ***thuj.***, ***tritic.***, urotrop., urt-u., ***uva.***, ***verat.***, verat-v., verb., vesp., vib., vib-od., zinc., zinc-p., zing.

URINE, retention of - abr., **ACON.**, aesc., agar., all-c., alum., alum-p., alum-sil., **AM-C.**, ant-t., ap-g., **APIS**, ***apoc.***, arg., arg-n., **ARN.**, **ARS.**, ***ars-i.***, ars-s-f., art-v., aspar., atro., aur., aur-ar., aur-i., aur-s., ***bar-c.***, bar-i., bar-m., bar-s., **BELL.**, benz-ac., berb., bism., ***bor.***, bry., bufo, ***cact.***, ***calc.***, calc-i., calc-p., calc-s., calc-sil., ***camph.***, ***cann-i.***, ***cann-s.***, **CANTH.**, ***caps.***, carb-v., carbn-s., card-m., **CAUST.**, cham., chel., ***chim.***, chin., chin-ar., ***cic.***, cimic., cina, cinnb., ***clem.***, coc-c., cocc., coch., ***colch.***, ***coloc.***, **CON.**, cop., ***crot-h.***, **CUPR.**, cycl., ***dig.***, dios., dor., ***dulc.***, elaps, equis., erig., ery-a., eup-pur., ***euph.***, ferr., ferr-p., **GELS.**, graph., ham., ***hell.***, helon., ***hep.***, ***hyos.***, hyper., ign., ***iod.***, ***ip.***, iris, kali-ar., kali-bi., ***kali-chl.***, kali-cy., kali-i., kreos., lach., ***laur.***, led., **LYC.**, lyss., ***mag-p.***, mag-s., **MENY.**, merc., ***merc-c.***, merc-cy., merc-d., mez., morph., mur-ac., nat-m., ***nit-ac.***, nux-m., **NUX-V.**, **OP.**, ox-ac., **PAREIR.**, petr., ph-ac., phos., ***phyt.***, **PLB.**, podo., ***polyg.***, ***prun.***, psor., ***puls.***, ran-s., ***rhus-t.***, ***ruta***, ***sabin.***, ***sars.***, ***sec.***, **SEL.**, **SEP.**, sil., solid., stann., ***staph.***, ***stigm.***, ***stram.***, stry., sul-ac., sul-i., ***sulph.***, **TARENT.**, **TER.**, thlaspi, ***thuj.***, trinit., tub., urt-u., ***verat.***, ***zinc.***, zinc-p.

URTICARIA, (See Hives)

UTERUS, bleeding, uterus, metrorrhagia - abrot., acal., ***acet-ac.***, ***acon.***, adren., agar., ***agn.***, alet., aloe, alum., alum-acet., alumn., am-br., am-c., am-m., **AMBR.**, aml-n., amor-r., anac., ant-c., ***apis***, ***apoc.***, aran., arg., ***arg-n.***, arg-o., ***arn.***, ***ars.***, ***ars-i.***, art-v., asaf., asar., asc-t., aur., aur-m-k., aur-m-n., aza., ba-sv., bad., bapt., **BELL.**, bell-p., bor., **BOTH-L.**, ***bov.***, brom., ***bry.***, bufo, buni-o., ***cact.***, **CALC.**, calc-acet., calc-ar., calc-f., calc-i., calc-p., calc-s., calc-sil., calc-st-sula., calen., camph., cann-i., cann-s., ***canth.***, caps., ***carb-an.***, ***carb-v.***, ***carbn-s.***, carc., ***card-m.***, ***caul.***, caust., ***cean.***, ***cham.***, chel., **CHIN.**, chin-ar., ***chin-s.***, ***cimic.***, cina, ***cinnam.***, cit-v., cob-n., ***coc-c.***, ***cocc.***, coch., ***coff.***, coff-t., ***colch.***, coll., ***coloc.***, con., cop., **CROC.**, crot-c., **CROT-H.**, cupr., cycl., dict., dig., ***elaps***, epip., erech., ergot., ***erig.***, erod., eupi., **FERR.**, ***ferr-acet.***, ferr-ar., ***ferr-i.***, ***ferr-m.***, ***ferr-p.***, ***ferr-s.***, fic., fl-ac., flav., foll., fuli., gall-ac., gels., ger., glon., goss., graph., guare., **HAM.**, hed., hell., ***helon.***, ***hep.***, hydr., hydrin-m., hydrin-s., ***hyos.***, ***ign.***, ind., ***iod.***, **IP.**, iris, joan., jug-r., juni-c., juni-v., kali-ar., kali-bi., ***kali-br.***, ***kali-c.***, ***kali-chl.***, **KALI-FCY.**, kali-i., ***kali-n.***, kali-p., kali-s., kali-sil., kalm., ***kreos.***, ***lac-c.***, **LACH.**, lap-a., laur., ***led.***, lil-t., lob., lup., ***lyc.***, lycps., lyss., m-aust., mag-c., mag-m., mag-s., mamm., mang., mang-m., mangi., ***med.***, ***meli.***, ***merc.***, **MILL.**, mit., ***morg.***, mosch., mur-ac., **MURX.**, nat-ar., ***nat-c.***, ***nat-hchls.***, nat-m., nat-s., **NIT-AC.**, ***nux-m.***, **NUX-V.**, ***oci-s.***, op., ozone, paro-i., petr., ph-ac., **PHOS.**, ***phyt.***, pitu-a., **PLAT.**, plb., podo., ***polyg.***, polyg-pe., prun., **PSOR.**, **PULS.**, pyrog., **RAT.**, ***rhus-a.***, ***rhus-t.***, rob., rosm., ruta, sabal., **SABIN.**, samb., ***sang.***, sanguis., **SEC.**, sed-ac., sed-t., ***senec.***, ***sep.***, ***sil.***, spong., squil., stann., staph., ***stram.***, sul-ac., sul-i., ***sulph.***, syc-co., sym-r., ***tarent.***, tep., ter., ther., thiop., ***thlaspi***, thuj., trif-r., **TRIL.**, ***tub.***, urt-u., **UST.**, verat., verat-v., **VIB.**, vib-p., ***vinc.***, ***visc.***, x-ray, ***xan.***, yohim, zinc., zinc-s., zinc-val.

UTERUS, cancer - alum., alumn., amor-r., anan., apis, ***arg.***, ***arg-n.***, **ARS.**, **ARS-I.**, asaf., aug., aur-ar., **AUR-M-N.**, aur-s., aur., bell., bov., brom., bry., ***bufo***, buni-o., calc-ar., calc-o-t., calc-s., ***calc.***, calen., calth., cand-a., canth., carb-ac., ***carb-an.***, ***carb-v.***, carbn-s., ***carc.***, caust., cham., chin., cic., ***cinnam.***, cist., clem., cocc., **CON.**, ***crot-h.***, cund., elaps, equis., fuli., **GRAPH.**, hep., hir., hist., hoit., **HYDR.**, ***iod.***, irid., kali-ar., kali-bi., kali-c., kali-i., kali-p., kali-s., kaol., **KREOS.**, **LACH.**, ***lap-a.***, laur., ***lil-t.***, **LYC.**, mag-m., mag-p., med., ***merc-i-f.***, merc., **MURX.**, ***nat-c.***, nat-cac., ***nat-m.***, nat-sil., ***nit-ac.***, nux-v., nym., ov., paro-i., **PHOS.**, ***phyt.***, plat., psor., psoral., rheum, rhus-t., rob., ruta, sabin., sang., sars., ***scirr.***, ***sec.***, **SEP.**, **SIL.**, ***staph.***, sul-ac., sul-i., sulph., tarent-c., tarent., thlaspi, **THUJ.**, thymol., tril., ust., **VIP.**, ***zinc.***

- **cervix** - anan., **AUR-M-N.**, calth., carb-an., ***carc.***, **CON.**, hir., hist., hydr., iod., kali-i., kreos., ***lil-t.***, nat-sil., **PULS.**, ***scirr.***, sec., ***sep.***, tarent., ***thuj.***
- **scirrhus** - alum., ***alumn.***, anan., ***arg.***, ***ars.***, aug., ***aur-m-n.***, aur., bell., carb-an., chin., cit-l., **CON.**, graph., kreos., lyc., mag-m., phos., ***phyt.***, rhus-t., rob., sep., staph., tarent., thlaspi.

UTERUS, tumors - **AUR-M-N.**, bell-p., ***calc.***, carc., con., ***crot-h.***, lyc., nat-m., pall., sep., sil., ter., ***thuj.***

V

VACCINATIONS, reactions, ailments, from - ***acon.***, all-c., am-c., ***ant-t.***, anthr., **APIS**, arg-n., arn., ***ars.***, ars-i., bac., bad., ***bapt.***, bar-c., ***bell.***, ***brom.***, bufo, ***calc.***, calc-p., calen., ***carb-v.***, carb-ac., **CARC.**, caust., chin., ***cic.***, con., ***crot-c.***, ***crot-h.***, **DIPH.**, ***echi.***, ferr-p., **GELS.**, graph., gunp., **HEP.**, ***hist.***, hyos., **HYPER.**, ign., **INFLU.**, kali-chl., ***kali-m.***, kali-p., lac-v., ***lac-c.***, **LACH.**, ***lachn.***, laur., **LED.**, lob., lyc., **MALAND.**, ***med.***, ***merc.***, merc-i-r., merc-s., **MEZ.**, **MORBILL.**, ***naja***, ***nat-m.***, ***nit-ac.***, op., ***ped.***, ***per.***, **PERT.**, phos., ***phyt.***, **PLAN.**, plb., podo., ***psor.***, puls., ***pyrog.***, rhus-t., sabin., sal-ac., sarr., **SARS.**, sep., **SIL.**, skook., staph., stram., **SULPH.**, syc-co., tetox., **THUJ.**, ***tub.***, **VAC.**, valer., **VARIO.**, vinc., zinc., zinc-m.

- **asthma**, after vaccination - ambro., **ALL-C.**, **ANT-T.**, **ARS.**, ***ars-i.***, ***bad.***, ***carb-v.***, carc., chin-ar., ***dulc.***, ***euphr.***, **IOD.**, kali-i., lach., linu-u, lob., ***naja***, nat-c., ***nat-s.***, ***nux-v.***, op., ***sabad.***, sang., ***sin-n.***, ***sil.***, stict., sulph., **THUJ.**
- **autism,** children, after vaccination - agra., anac., bar-c., bufo, **CARC.**, cann-i., hyos., kali-br., lyc., med., ***merc.***, ***nat-m.***, op., stram., syph., ***thuj.***, tub.
- **cancer**, after - crot-h., diph., lach., maland., naja, pyrog., ***sil.***, ***thuj.***
- **developement,** arrested - agar., ***bac.***, **BAR-C.**, bor., bufo, ***calc.***, **CALC-P.**, **CARC.**, caust., chin., cupr., des-ac., kali-c., kreos., lac-d., med., nat-m., nep., ph-ac., ***phos.***, pin-s., ***sil.***, sulfa., sulph., thyr., vip.
- **diptheria,** pertussis, tetnus, **(D.P.T.)**, vaccination, ailments from - ant-t., **APIS**, arg-n., **ARS.**, ***bapt.***, bar-c., ***bell.***, **BROM.**, bry., calc-p., ***canth.***, ***caps.***, ***carb-ac.***, **CARC.**, ***con.***, ***crot-c.***, ***crot-h.***, **DIPH.**, **DROS.**, ***echi.***, hep., **HYPER.**, ign., iod., ***kali-c.***, kali-p., **LAC-C.**, **LACH.**, ***lachn.***, **LED.**, lob., **LYC.**, ***merc.***, ***merc-cy.***, ***mur-ac.***, naja, ***nat-m.***, ***nit-ac.***, **PERT.**, ***phos.***, ***phyt.***, ***rhus-t.***, sal-ac., ***sulph.***, ***sul-ac.***, tetox., **THUJ**, vinc., zinc-m.
- **hyperactive,** children, from - anac., ***ars.***, ars-i., calc-p., ***carc.***, ***cina***, coff., **HYOS.**, ***iod.***, ***med.***, merc., nux-v., **STRAM.**, ***tarent.***, thuj., ***tub.***, ***verat.***
- **influenza,** vaccination, after - abrot., bapt., ***carc.***, con., chin., cypr., ***gels.***, ***influ.***, kali-p., merc., ***ph-ac.***, rhus-t., scut., thuj., x-ray.
- **measles,** mumps, rubella, **(M.M.R.)** vaccination, ailments from - ***acon.***, ***ant-c.***, ant-t., anthr., **APIS**, ***ars.***, ***aur.***, **BAR-C.**, ***bar-m.***, **BELL.**, ***brom.***, **BRY.**, ***calc.***, ***carb-v.***, **CARC.**, cham., chin., ***chlor.***, **CIST.**, cocc., ***coff.***, ***con.***, ***crot-h.***, ***dros.***, dulc., **EUPHR.**, ***ferr-p.***, ***gels.***, ***hep.***, hyper., hyos., ign., ***ip.***, **JAB.**, kali-ar., ***kali-bi.***, ***kali-c.***, kali-m., kali-p., kali-s., ***lach.***, led., ***lyc.***, mag-c., mag-p., **MERC.**, **MORBILL.**, ***nat-m.***, nux-v., ***parot.***, petr., ***phos.***, phyt., piloc., **PULS.**, ***rhus-t.***, sars., ***sil.***, ***squil.***, stict., ***stram.***, sul-i., **SULPH.**, **THUJ.**, trif-p., trif-r., verat., zinc.
- **preventive,** prophylactic for side effects - arn., **HYPER.**, **LED.**, phys., plan., ***sil.***, sulph., tetox., ***thuj.***, vario.
- **rabies,** vaccination, ailments from - agar., agav-a., anag., **BELL.**, calc., ***canth.***, cupr., ***cur.***, **HYOS.**, iod., ***lach.***, laur., **LYSS.**, scut., **STRAM.**, verat.
- **smallpox,** vaccination, ailments from - agar., ***ant-c.***, **ANT-T.**, ***apis***, ***ars.***, bapt., ***bell.***, ***bry.***, clem., hyos., **MALAND.**, ***merc.***, nit-ac., phos., ***puls.***, ***rhus-t.***, sarr., sil., stram., ***sulph.***, **THUJ.**, **VAC.**, **VARIO.**, ***zinc.***
- **tetanus,** vaccination, ailments from - all-c., arn., cic., **HYPER.**, **LED.**, mill., phys., ***plan.***, sil., ***tetox.***, ***thuj.***

VACCINIA, general, (see Cowpox) - ***acon.***, ant-t., apis, ***bell.***, merc., phos., ***sil.***, sulph., ***thuj.***, vac.

VAGINA, cancer - ars., camph., ***con.***, cund., ***ferr-i.***, hep., hydr., **KREOS.**, ***scirr.***, sil., thuj.

VAGINA, remedies - achy., ***acon.***, alum., amor-r., apis, arg., arn., ars., aur-m., ***bell.***, bor., cact., ***calad.***, calc., ***cann-s.***, canth., caul., cimic., ***coc-c.***, con., croto-t., ***cur.***, fab., ferr., ferr-p., gels., ***graph.***, grin., ***ham.***, helon., hep., ***hydr.***, hyper., ign., iod., iodof., kali-bi., kali-c., kali-m., kali-n., kreos., **MED.**, ***merc.***, merc-c., ***morg.***, ***nat-acet.***, nat-p., nit-ac., petros., plat., prot., **PULS.**, rhus-t., sabal., sep., sil., sulph., syc-co., **THUJ.**

- **vagina**, cysts - foll., ***lyc.***, ***puls.***, ***rhod.***, sil., teucr., thuj.

VAGINISMUS, vagina - ***acon.***, aln., alumn., apis, aq-mar., arg-n., atro., aur., ***bell.***, ***berb.***, bor., cac., **CACT.**, calc., calc-p., ***canth.***, carb-v., ***caul.***, caust., ***cimic.***, coc-c., cocc., ***coff.***, con., **CUPR.**, cupr-acet., ferr., ferr-i., ferr-m., ferr-ma., ***ferr-p.***, gels., ***ham.***, hep., hydr., **IGN.**, kali-bi., kali-br., kali-c., kreos., lac-c., lach., ***lyc.***, lyss., mag-p., med., merc., mur-ac., ***murx.***, ***nat-m.***, nit-ac., nux-m., nux-v., orig., **PLAT.**, **PLB.**, plumbg., pop., ***puls.***, rhus-t., sabin., sep., ***sil.***, **STAPH.**, sulph., syph., tarent., ***thuj.***

VAGINITIS, infection - achy., ***acon.***, alum., amor-r., apis, arg., arn., ars., aur-m., ***bell.***, bor., cact., ***calad.***, calc., ***cann-s.***, canth., caul., cimic., ***coc-c.***, con., croto-t., ***cur.***, fab., ferr., ferr-p., gels., ***graph.***, grin., ***ham.***, helon., hep., ***hydr.***, hyper., ign., iod., iodof., kali-bi., kali-c., kali-m., kali-n., kreos., **MED.**, ***merc.***, merc-c., ***morg.***, ***nat-acet.***, nat-p., nit-ac., petros., plat., prot., **PULS.**, rhus-t., sabal., sep., sil., sulph., syc-co., **THUJ.**

VARICELLA, (see Chickenpox)

VARICOSE, ulcers - aesc., am-m., anac., ant-t., arn., ***ars.***, ***calc.***, calc-f., calen., ***carb-v.***, ***card-m.***, **CAUST.**, chin., cinnb., clem., crot-h., cund., eucal., **FL-AC.**, graph., grin., ***ham.***, hydr., insulin, kreos., ***lach.***, **LYC.**, merc., merc-c., mez., morg., phyt., psor., **PULS.**, pyrog., ***rhus-t.***, sars., sec., ***sil.***, sul-ac., ***sulph.***, thuj., verat., ***zinc.***

VARICOSE, veins - acet-ac., aesc., alum., alum-sil., ***alumn.***, ***am-c.***, ***ambr.***, ang., ***ant-t.***, apis, arist-cl., **ARN.**, ***arg-n.***, ***ars.***, ars-s-f., asaf., ***bar-c.***, ***bell.***, bell-p., ***berb.***, brom., ***bry.***, **CALC.**, **CALC-F.**, ***calc-i.***, calc-p., calc-s., calen., camph., ***carb-an.***, **CARB-V.**, carbn-s., carc., card-b., ***card-m.***, ***caust.***, chel., ***chin.***, chin-s., cic., clem., coll., coloc., con., ***croc.***, ***crot-h.***, cycl., ***ferr.***, ferr-ar., ferr-p., **FL-AC.**, form., form-ac., ***graph.***, **HAM.**, hecla., ***hep.***, hyos., kali-ar., kali-n., ***kreos.***, lac-c., lach., ***lyc.***, **LYCPS.**, m-aust., mag-c., mag-f., mand., mangi., meli., meny., merc-cy., mez., mill., morg., mosch., mur-ac., ***nat-m.***, ***nux-v.***, olnd., op., ***paeon.***, petr., ph-ac., ***phos.***, ***plb.***, polyg., **PULS.**, pyrog., ***ran-s.***, rhod., ***rhus-t.***, ruta, sabin., sars., scirr., sec., **SEP.**, sil., sol-n., ***spig.***, spong., ***staph.***, stront-br., stront-c., sul-ac., ***sulph.***, thuj., ***vip.***, ***zinc.***

VARIOCELE, spermatic, cord - acon., aesc., arn., ars., ***aur.***, bell., ***calc.***, carb-v., colch., ***coll.***, crot-h., ferr-p., fl-ac., graph., ***ham.***, ***lach.***, ***lyc.***, ***merc-i-r.***, ***nux-v.***, osm., ***ph-ac.***, plb., ***podo.***, ***puls.***, ruta, sep., ***sil.***, ***sulph.***, tab.

VARIOLA, (see Smallpox)

VEINS, general, (see Blood, vessels) - acet-ac., aesc., alum., alum-sil., ***alumn.***, ***am-c.***, ***ambr.***, ang., ***ant-t.***, apis, arist-cl., **ARN.**, ***arg-n.***, ***ars.***, ars-s-f., asaf., ***bar-c.***, ***bell.***, bell-p., ***berb.***, brom., ***bry.***, **CALC.**, ***calc-f.***, ***calc-i.***, calc-p., calc-s., calen., camph., ***carb-an.***, **CARB-V.**, carbn-s., carc., card-b., ***card-m.***, ***caust.***, chel., ***chin.***, chin-s., cic., clem., coll., coloc., con., ***croc.***, ***crot-h.***, cycl., ***ferr.***, ferr-ar., ferr-p., **FL-AC.**, form., form-ac., ***graph.***, **HAM.**, hecla., ***hep.***, hyos., kali-ar., kali-n., ***kreos.***, lac-c., lach., ***lyc.***, **LYCPS.**, m-aust., mag-c., mag-f., mand., mangi., meli., meny., merc-cy., mez., mill., morg., mosch., mur-ac., ***nat-m.***, ***nux-v.***, olnd., op., ***paeon.***, petr., ph-ac., ***phos.***, ***plb.***, polyg., **PULS.**, pyrog., ***ran-s.***, rhod., ***rhus-t.***, ruta, sabin., sars., scirr., sec., **SEP.**, sil., sol-n., ***spig.***, spong., ***staph.***, stront-br., stront-c., sul-ac., ***sulph.***, thuj., ***vip.***, ***zinc.***

VENESECTION, ailments from - echi., chin., ferr., ferr-p., ham., **HYPER.**, ign., lach., **LED.**, ***plan.***, plat., pyrog., senec., sil., squil., thuj.

VERATRUM, ailments from - camph., coff., verat.

VERTIGO, general - abies-c., abies-n., absin., acet-ac., **ACON.**, act-sp., ***aesc.***, ***aeth.***, **AGAR.**, agn., **AIL.**, alet., all-c., ***aloe***, alumn., ***alum.***, ***ambr.***, ***am-c.***, am-m., aml-n., anac., anan., ***ant-c.***, ant-t., **APIS**, apoc., **ARG.**, ***arg-n.***, ***arn.***, ***ars.***, ***ars-h.***, ars-i., arum-t., arund., asaf., asar., asc-c., asc-t., aspar., ***aster.***, ***aur.***, ***aur-m.***, bad., **BAPT.**, ***bar-c.***, bar-m., **BELL.**, benz-ac., ***berb.***, bism., bor., both-l., bov., brach., brom., **BRY.**, bufo, ***cact.***, cahin., calad., **CALC.**, calc-ar., calc-f., ***calc-p.***, **CALC-S.**, ***camph.***, **CANN-I.**, ***cann-s.***, ***canth.***, caps., carb-ac., ***carb-an.***, ***carb-v.***, carbn-h., carbn-o., **CARBN-S.**, carl., cast-eq., caul., ***caust.***, ***cedr.***, ***cham.***, **CHEL.**, chen-a., chim., ***chin.***, chin-ar., **CHIN-S.**, chlol., chlf., chlor., ***cic.***, ***cimic.***, cina, cinnb., cist., clem., cob., coca, **COCC.**, coc-c., ***coff.***, colch., ***coloc.***, com., **CON.**, ***cop.***, corn., croc., ***crot-c.***, crot-h., croto-t., ***cupr.***, cupr-ar., **CYCL.**, daph., **DIG.**, dios., dirc., dros., **DULC.**, echi., ***elaps***, equis., euon., eup-per., eup-pur., euph., euphr., eupi., fago., ***ferr.***, ***ferr-ar.***, ferr-i., ***ferr-p.***, ferr-ma., fl-ac., form., gamb., **GELS.**, ***glon.***, goss., gran., ***graph.***, grat., ***guare.***, ham., hell., helon., ***hep.***, hura, hydr-ac., ***hydrc.***, **HYDROG.**, ***hyos.***, hyper., ign., ille., indg., ***iod.***, ip., iris, jab., jatr., jug-c., jug-r., kali-ar., ***kali-bi.***, ***kali-br.***, ***kali-c.***, ***kali-i.***, ***kali-n.***, kali-p., ***kali-s.***, ***kalm.***, kreos., lac-c., ***lac-d.***, ***lach.***, lachn., lact., laur., ***led.***, lept., lil-t., lob., **LYC.**, lycps., lyss., mag-c., mag-m., mag-s., maland., ***manc.***, mang., med., meny., ***merc.***, ***merc-c.***, merc-i-f., merc-i-r., ***mez.***, mill., ***mosch.***, ***mur-ac.***, murx., ***mygal.***, naja, ***nat-ar.***, ***nat-c.***, ***nat-h.***, **NAT-M.**, ***nat-p.***, ***nat-s.***, nicc., ***nit-ac.***, par., **PETR.**, phel., ***ph-ac.***, **PHOS.**, ***phyt.***, pic-ac., plan., ***plat.***, plb., ***podo.***, ***psor.***, ptel., **PULS.**, ***ran-b.***, ran-s., raph., rheum, ***rhod.***, **RHUS-T.**, ***rhus-v.***, rumx., ruta, sabad., ***sabin.***, samb., **SANG.**, sanic., sars., **SEC.**, sel., senec., ***seneg.***, ***sep.***, **SIL.**, ***spig.***, ***spong.***, squil., ***stann.***, staph., ***stram.***, ***stront-c.***, ***stry.***, **SULPH.**, sul-ac., sumb., ***syph.***, **TAB.**, tarent., tarax., tell., ***ter.***, teucr., ther., ***thuj.***, uran., ***urt-u.***, ust., ***valer.***, ***verat.***, ***verat-v.***, ***vesp.***, vib., ***zinc.***, zing.

VIOLENCE, ailments from - acon., ***anac.***, **ARN.**, ***aur.***, ***bry.***, **CARC.**, ***caust.***, coff., lyc., nat-m., ***op.***, **STAPH.**

VIOLENT, behavior - abrot., absin., acon., aesc., ***agar.***, agav-t., **ALCO.**, aloe, alum., am-c., am-m., ambr., **ANAC.**, ***androc.***, ang., ***ant-t.***, apis, arn., ars., **AUR.**, aur-ar., aur-s., bar-c., **BELL.**, bor., ***bry.***, calc., calc-p., camph., canth., ***carb-v.***, ***carbn-s.***, caste., carc., **CAUST.**, ***cham.***, chin., **CIC.**, cocc., coff., coloc., con., corn., croc., cupr., cyna., dros., dulc., ferr., gall-ac., gamb., graph., grat., **HEP.**, **HYOS.**, ictod., ign., **IOD.**, iodof., kali-ar., kali-bi., kali-c., ***kali-i.***, ***kali-p.***, **LACH.**, ***led.***, lil-t., ***lyc.***, ***m-arct.***, mag-s., mang., med., merc., merc-c., merl., mez., mill., mosch., nat-c., ***nat-m.***, nat-s., nit-ac., **NUX-V.**, oena., olnd., ox-ac., ***petr.***, ph-ac., ***phos.***, plat., plb., prot., ran-b., sabad., sac-alb., seneg., ***sep.***, sil., spig., stann., ***staph.***, **STRAM.**, stront-c., ***sulph.***, syph., ***tarent.***, teucr., thuj., **TUB.**, tub-k., ***verat.***, verat-v., ***visc.***, zinc.

VIOLENT, illnesses - **ACON.**, alum., anac., ***ars.***, ***bapt.***, **BELL.**, bry., canth., carb-v., **CARC.**, **CHAM.**, **CIC.**, cupr., ***glon.***, hep., ***hyos.***, ign., iod., ***lach.***, merc., **NUX-V.**, **PYROG.**, **STRAM.**, sulph., ***tarent.***, ***verat.***

VIRAL, infection, fever with - acon., ars., ***bapt.***, bell., bry., ***carc.***, **GELS.**, influ., merc., nat-m., ph-ac., rhus-t.

VITILIGO, leucoderma, general - ***alum.***, am-c., ant-t., **ARS.**, ***ars-s-f.***, ***aur.***, ***berb.***, ***calc.***, calc-f., ***calc-sil.***, carb-ac., carb-an., carc., cob-n., coca, graph., kali-i., kres., lyc., med., ***merc.***, mica, ***nat-c.***, nat-m., nit-ac., ozone, ***phos.***, pip-m., ***pitu-a.***, pitu-p., prot., pyrar., sel., **SEP.**, **SIL.**, ***sulph.***, sumb., syph., ***thuj.***, zinc., zinc-p.

VOMITING, general - absin., acet-ac., **ACON.**, ***aesc.***, **AETH.**, ***agar.***, alet., all-c., alumn., ambr., am-c., ***am-m.***, anac., ***anthr.***, **ANT-C.**, **ANT-T.**, **APIS**, ***apoc.***, **APOM.**, aran., arg-c., **ARG-N.**, ***arn.***, **ARS.**, ars-h., ars-i., arum-m., ***asar.***, asc-t., aur., aur-m., bapt., ***bar-c.***, bar-i., ***bar-m.***, ***bell.***, ***bism.***, ***bor.***, ***both-l.***, **BRY.**, bufo, ***cact.***, **CADM-S.**, cahin., ***calc.***, ***calc-p.***, ***calc-s.***, ***camph.***, cann-i., cann-s., ***canth.***, carb-ac., carbn-s., **CARC.**, caust., **CHAM.**, ***chel.***, **CHIN.**, chin-ar., ***chin-s.***, chlol., cic., ***cimic.***, ***cina***, ***cocc.***, ***coc-c.***, coff., **COLCH.**, coll., coloc., ***con.***, cop., ***crot-c.***, crot-h., croto-t., ***cub.***, **CUPR.**, ***cupr-ar.***, ***cupr-s.***, cycl., ***dig.***, ***dor.***, ***dros.***, ***dulc.***, elaps, ***eup-per.***, ***euph.***, **FERR.**, ***ferr-ar.***, ***ferr-i.***, ferr-p., ***form.***, **GAMB.**, gels., glon., ***gran.***, ***graph.***, ***grat.***, ***hell.***, ***hep.***, hydr., ***hyos.***, ***ign.***, indg., ***iod.***, **IP.**, **IRIS**, kali-ar., ***kali-bi.***, ***kali-br.***, kali-c., ***kali-i.***, kali-p., kali-s., kalm., **KREOS.**, ***lac-d.***, ***lach.***, ***laur.***, **LOB.**, ***lyc.***, ***mang.***, ***merc.***, ***merc-c.***, ***merc-d.***, ***mez.***, mosch., mur-ac., naja, ***nat-m.***, nat-p., ***nit-ac.***, ***nux-m.***, **NUX-V.**, olnd., op., ***ox-ac.***, paeon., ***petr.***, ph-ac., **PHOS.**, phyt., **PLB.**, podo., ***psor.***, ptel., **PULS.**, rat., rhod., rhus-t., ruta, sabin., sal-ac., ***samb.***, ***sang.***, ***sec.***, seneg., sel., ***sep.***, **SIL.**, squil., sol-n., ***stry.***, **SULPH.**, sul-ac., **TAB.**, ***tarent.***, tep., ***ter.***, ***ther.***, thuj., ***tub.***, uran., ***valer.***, **VERAT.**, **VERAT-V.**, wye., ***zinc.***, **ZINC-P.**, zinc-s., zing., ziz.

W

WARTS, skin, (see Condylomata or Excrescences) - acet-ac., alum., am-c., ambr., anac., anac-oc., anag., anan., ***ant-c.***, ant-t., arg-n., ***ars.***, ars-br., ars-i., ***aur.***, aur-ar., aur-m., aur-m-n., aur-s., ba-tn., **BAR-C.**, **BAR-S.**, **BELL.**, ***benz-ac.***, berb., bor., ***bov.***, bufo, **CALC.**, calc-cal., calc-o-t., **CALC-S.**, calc-sil., camph., caps., carb-an., carb-v., carc., cast., cast-eq., **CAUST.**, cham., chel., chin., chr-o., cinnb., clem., cocc., colch., con., croc., cund., cupr., **DULC.**, dys-co., euph., euphr., ferr., ferr-ar., ferr-ma., ferr-p., ferr-pic., ***fl-ac.***, graph., hecla., hell., ***hep.***, hyos., iod., kali-ar., kali-br., kali-c., ***kali-chl.***, kali-i., kali-m., kali-ma., kali-n., kali-s., kali-sil., ***lac-c.***, lac-h., ***lach.***, lyc., mag-m., ***mag-s.***, ***med.***, meny., merc., **MERC-C.**, merc-i-f., mill., ***nat-c.***, ***nat-m.***, nat-p., **NAT-S.**, **NIT-AC.**, nit-s-d., ***ox-ac.***, petr., ***ph-ac.***, phase., phos., phyt., pic-ac., pitu-a., ***psor.***, rad-br., ran-b., rheum, rhod., ***rhus-t.***, ruta, sabad., sabin., sars., sec., semp., seneg., ***sep.***, sil., spig., spong., staph., sul-ac., **SULPH.**, syc-co., syph., **THUJ.**, verat., x-ray

- **cancerous** - aur-m., ferr-pic., nit-ac., thuj.
- **genitalia** - ***calc.***, euphr., ***lyc.***, ***med.***, ***merc.***, **NAT-S.**, **NIT-AC.**, ***sabin.***, ***sars.***, sep., ***staph.***, **THUJ.**
- **bleeding** - ambr., calc., **CAUST.**, cinnb., ferr., ferr-ma., hep., iod., kali-c., lyc., merc., nat-c., ***nit-ac.***, ph-ac., ***rhus-t.***, staph., syc-co., **THUJ.**
- **flat** - acet-ac., ant-c., ba-tn., berb., calc., ***caust.***, **DULC.**, dys-co., fl-ac., lach., merc-i-f., nat-m., ruta, ***sep.***, ***thuj.***

WATER-BRASH, (see Belching) - ***abies-n.***, acet-ac., acon., aesc., aeth., alum., alum-p., alum-sil., ***alumn.***, ***am-c.***, ***am-m.***, ambr., anac., ant-c., ***ant-t.***, ***apis***, arg., arg-n., arn., **ARS.**, ars-i., asar., **BAR-C.**, ***bar-i.***, bar-m., **BAR-S.**, bell., ***bism.***, bov., **BRY.**, **CALC.**, calc-ar., calc-i., ***calc-p.***, ***calc-s.***, ***calc-sil.***, cann-s., canth., ***caps.***, ***carb-an.***, **CARB-V.**, carbn-s., ***caust.***, chel., ***chin.***, chin-ar., ***cic.***, ***cina***, clem., cob., ***cocc.***, colch., coloc., con., croc., cupr., cupr-o., cur., cycl., ***daph.***, dig., dios., ***dros.***, dulc., euph., fago., ferr., ferr-ar., ferr-i., ferr-p., genist., ***graph.***, grat., hell., ***hep.***, hip-ac., hydr., hydr-ac., ***ign.***, iod., ***ip.***, kali-ar., ***kali-bi.***, ***kali-c.***, kali-chl., kali-i., kali-p., kali-s., kali-sil., kreos., ***lac-ac.***, lac-d., lach., laur., ***led.***, lil-t., ***lob.***, lob-s., lol., **LYC.**, mag-c., ***mag-m.***, manc., mang., meny., ***merc.***, merl., **MEZ.**, ***morg.***, mosch., mur-ac., ***nat-ar.***, ***nat-c.***, ***nat-m.***, nat-p., ***nat-s.***, nat-sil., ***nit-ac.***, nux-m., **NUX-V.**, ol-an., olnd., ox-ac., **PAR.**, **PETR.**, ph-ac., ***phos.***, phys., pic-ac., pitu-a., plat., plb., podo., psil., psor., **PULS.**, pyrar., ***ran-b.***, ran-s., rat., ***rhod.***, ***rhus-t.***, rob., **SABAD.**, sabin., **SANG.**, ***sars.***, sec., seneg., ***sep.***, **SIL.**, spig., spong., squil., stann., **STAPH.**, still., **STRAM.**, ***sul-ac.***, sul-i., **SULPH.**, sumb., sym-r., tab., tarax., tarent., ter., thea., thuj., tub-r., valer., **VERAT.**, verb., zinc., zinc-p.

WEAKNESS, sensation, (see Fatigue) - acon., aesc., agar., **ALF.**, **ALUM.**, ambr., ***am-c.***, ***anac.***, **ANDROC.**, ***ant-c.***, ***ant-t.***, arg., ***arg-n.***, ***arn.***, **ARS.**, ***ars-i.***, asaf., asar., aur., aur-m., ***bapt.***, bar-c., bar-m., bell., **BENZ-AC.**, berb., bism., bov., ***bry.***, calc., **CALC-P.**, camph., **CANN-S.**, canth., caps., ***carb-ac.***, carb-an., ***carb-v.***, **CARBN-S.**, **CARC.**, caust., cham., **CHEL.**, **CHIN.**, cic., cimic., cimx., cina, clem., cocc., ***coc-c.***, coff., colch., coloc., ***con.***, **CROC.**, ***crot-c.***, ***cupr.***, cycl., dig., dros., dulc., euph., euphr., **FERR.**, ferr-p., **GELS.**, **GRAPH.**, ***ham.***, hell., helon., ***hep.***, **HYDROG.**, ***hyos.***, ign., ***ip.***, kali-c., kali-n., **KALI-P.**, kali-s., ***kreos.***, **LACH.**, lac-ac., ***laur.***, led., **LYC.**, ***mag-c.***, mag-m., mang., meny., **MERC.**, mez., mosch., **MUR-AC.**, ***nat-c.***, **NAT-M.**, ***nat-s.***, nit-ac., ***nux-m.***, **NUX-V.**, olnd., op., ***par., petr.,*** **PH-AC., PHOS., PIC-AC.,** ***plat., plb., psor.,*** **PULS.,** ran-b., ***rheum, rhod., rhus-t.,*** **RUTA,** sabad., sabin., samb., sars., sec., senec., seneg., **SEP., SIL.,** spig., spong., squil., ***stann.,*** **STAPH.,** ***stram.,*** stront-c., **SULPH.,** sumb., ***sul-ac., tab.,*** teucr., thuj., **TUB.,** valer., ***verat.,*** verb., viol-o., **X-RAY., ZINC.**

WEIGHT, loss, (see Cachexia, Emaciation)

WENS, (see Sebaceous cysts)

WHEEZING, breathing, (see Asthma) - acon., agar., ail., aloe, ***alum.***, alum-p., alum-sil., ***am-c.***, ***ambr.***, anac., ang., ***ant-t.***, ***apoc.***, aral., arg., arg-n., arn., **ARS.**, ***ars-i.***, ars-s-f., ***asaf.***, ***aur.***, ***bac.***, **BELL.**, bov., ***brom.***, bry., calad., calc., calc-s., camph., ***cann-s.***, ***caps.***, carb-an., **CARB-V.**, carbn-s., card-m., caust., ***cham.***, ***chin.***, ***chin-ar.***, chlol., ***cic.***, ***cina***, ***cocc.***, coloc., con., croc., croto-t., ***cupr.***, ***dig.***, dol., ***dros.***, dulc., erio., euphr., ferr., ferr-i., ***fl-ac.***, form., graph., ***grin.***, hell., hep., hydr-ac., hydrog., ***hyos.***, ign., ***iod.***, iodof., **IP.**, just., ***kali-ar.***, ***kali-bi.***, **KALI-C.**, ***kali-i.***, kali-m., kali-n., ***kali-s.***, ***lach.***, lap-c-b., laur., ***led.***, **LOB.**, ***lyc.***, ***lycps.***, mag-m., manc., merc., mez., mosch., mur-ac., murx., naja, nat-c., ***nat-m.***, ***nat-n.***, ***nat-s.***, ***nit-ac.***, ***nux-m.***, nux-v., op., ox-ac., par., ph-ac., phos., plb., prun., ***puls.***, pyrog., ran-b., ran-s., ***rhod.***, rhus-t., ruta, sabad., ***samb.***, sang., sanic., sars., **SENEG.**, sep., ***sil.***, spong., squil., stann., staph., stram., sul-ac., sul-i., sulph., syc-co., ***syph.***, teucr., ***thuj.***, ***verat.***, ***visc.***, ***zinc.***

WHOOPING COUGH, pertussis - acon., agar., all-c., alum., alumn., ***am-br.***, am-c., am-m., am-pic., ***ambr.***, ambro., ***anac.***, ***anan.***, ang., ant-c., **ANT-T.**, ***arg-n.***, ***arn.***, ***ars.***, ars-i., ars-s-f., arum-t., asaf., asar., bad., ***bar-c.***, bar-m., bar-s., **BELL.**, ***brom.***, ***bry.***, ***calc.***, ***calc-p.***, caps., ***carb-ac.***, ***carb-an.***, **CARB-V.**, carbn-h., ***carbn-s.***, carc., cast., ***cast-v.***, ***caust.***, cer-ox., ***cham.***, ***chel.***, ***chin.***, chlol., chlor., **CINA**, ***coc-c.***, cocain, con., ***cor-r.***, ***crot-h.***, **CUPR.**, ***cupr-acet.***, cupr-ar., dig., dios., **DIRC.**, **DROS.**, ***dulc.***, dys-co., erio., eucal., euph., ***euphr.***, ***ferr.***, ferr-ar., ***ferr-p.***, ***formal.***, glyc-g., ***graph.***, grin., guare., ***hep.***, ***hippoz.***, hydr-ac., ***hyos.***, hyper., ictod., ign., ind., indg., iod., ***ip.***, ***just.***, ***kali-bi.***, kali-br., ***kali-c.***, kali-chl., kali-i., ***kali-m.***, ***kali-p.***, **KALI-S.**, kali-sil., ***kreos.***, lach., ***lact.***, laur., ***led.***, ***lob.***, ***lyc.***, ***mag-m.***, mag-p., **MEPH.**, merc., ***mez.***, mosch., mur-ac., naphtin., narc-ps., nat-c., ***nat-m.***, nicc., ***nit-ac.***, **NUX-V.**, oeno., ol-j., op., osm., oxyg., par., passi., **PER.**, ph-ac., phel., **PHOS.**, podo., ***puls.***, rhus-t., ***rumx.***, ruta, ***samb.***, **SANG.**, sanguin-n., sec., senec., ***seneg.***, ***sep.***, ***sil.***, spig., ***spong.***, ***squil.***, stann., stict., ***stram.***, sul-ac., ***sulph.***, syph., ***tab.***, tere-ch., thymu., tong., ***trif-p.***, tub., urt-u., vac., ***verat.***, verat-v., viol-o., ***visc.***, zinc., zinc-p.

WILSON'S, disease - cupr., mang.

WISDOM TEETH, ailments from - ***calc.***, calc-p., **CHAM.**, ***fl-ac.***, hecla, m-aust., ***mag-c.***, ***sil.***

WORMS, parasites - acon., aesc., all-c., all-s., ***ambro.***, apoc., apoc-a., arg-n., ***ars.***, art-v., bapt., bell., calad., **CALC.**, ***calc-p.***, carb-v., ***carc.***, ***chelo.***, **CHIN.**, ***cic.***, **CINA**, cupr-acet., cupr-o., dol., ***ferr.***, ***ferr-m.***, ferr-s., fil., ***gaert.***, ***gran.***, graph., helm., ign., indg., ip., kali-m., luna, lyc., med., merc., merc-c., morg., ***naphtin.***, **NAT-M.**, **NAT-P.**, ***nux-m.***, nux-v., passi., petr., podo., puls., quas., ***rat.***, ***ruta***, ***sabad.***, ***sant.***, sec., ***sil.***, ***sin-n.***, **SPIG.**, spong., squil., ***stann.***, **SULPH.**, sumb., ***ter.***, ***teucr.***, tub., ***valer.***, verat., ***viol-o.***, ***viol-t.***

ancylostomiasis - carb-tcl., chen-a., ***thymol.***

ascarides - abrot., acet-ac., acon., aesc., agn., ant-c., ant-t., ***ars.***, asar., asc-t., **BAR-C.**, bar-m., ***calc.***, carb-v., carbn-s., ***chelo.***, chin., **CINA**, croto-t., cupr., dig., dol., ***ferr.***, ferr-m., gran., graph., grat., hyos., ***ign.***, indg., ip., kali-chl., lyc., mag-c., ***mag-s.***, merc., merc-d., naphtin., **NAT-M.**, ***nat-p.***, nux-v., petr., phos., pin-s., plat., ***ptel.***, ***rat.***, **SABAD.**, ***sant.***, ***scirr.***, ***sep.***, sil., ***sin-n.***, ***spig.***, ***spong.***, squil., stann., ***sulph.***, tell., **TER.**, ***teucr.***, thuj., urt-u., ***valer.***, viol-o.

hookworm - ***carb-tcl.***, card-m., chen-a., cina, cupr., thymol.

lumbricoides - acon., all-s., anac., ***ars.***, asar., art-v., bar-c., bell., calc., carbn-s., cic., cham., ***chel.***, **CINA**, ***ferr-s.***, ***gran.***, graph., hyos., kali-c., lyc., mag-c., merc., nat-m., nux-v., rhus-t., ruta, ***sabad.***, sec., ***sil.***, **SPIG.**, stann., **SULPH.**, ter.

oxyuris, vermicularis - ars., bapt., ***chelo.***, ***cina***, ign., indg., lyc., ***merc-d.***, ***merc-s.***, nat-p., rat., ***sant.***, sil., sin-n., spig., teucr., valer.

schistosomiasis - ant-t., ars., chin., ip.

teniae - ***ail.***, arg-n., **CALC.**, ***carb-an.***, ***carb-v.***, carbn-s., chin., cina, cupr., cupr-acet., cur., ***fil.***, ***form.***, frag., ***gran.***, ***graph.***, grat., kali-c., kali-i., mag-m., merc., ***nat-c.***, nat-s., nux-v., petr., phos., ***plat.***, ***puls.***, ***sabad.***, sant., ***sep.***, ***sil.***, ***stann.***, sulph., ter., thuj., valer.

trichinae, trichinosis - ars., bapt., cina.

WOUNDS, general, (see Cuts, Lacerations, Punctures, Stab) - anag., androc., ***anthr.***, ***apis***, arist-cl., ***arn.***, ***ars.***, bell-p., bor., bor-ac., bov., bry., bufo, calc-p., **CALEN.**, carb-ac., carb-v., cham., cic., cist., con., croc., ***crot-h.***, ***echi.***, erig., ery-a., eup-per., ferr-p., ham., helia., hell., hep., hydrog., **HYPER.**, iod., kali-p., kreos., ***lach.***, ***lappa***, **LED.**, merc., mez., mill., nat-c., nat-m., nit-ac., ph-ac., ***phos.***, phys., ***plan.***, plb., ***puls.***, **PYROG.**, rhus-t., ruta, sec., senec., seneg., sil., ***staph.***, stront-c., sulph., ***sul-ac.***, symph., ***ter.***, zinc.

bleeding, freely - ***acon.***, am-c., ant-t., aran., ***arn.***, ars., asaf., bell-p., bor., both-l., **CALEN.**, ***carb-v.***, caust., cench., ***chin.***, clem., con., ***cop.***, croc., ***crot-h.***, ***dor.***, eug., ***euphr.***, ferr., ***ferr-p.***, ham., ***hydr.***, ***kreos.***, **LACH.**, **LAT-M.**, led., merc., mez., **MILL.**, ***nat-c.***, nat-m., **NIT-AC.**, ***nux-m.***, ***nux-v.***, ***ph-ac.***, **PHOS.**, plb., puls., rhus-t., ruta, sec., sep., sil., ***staph.***, sul-ac., ***sulph.***, vip., ***zinc.***

gangrenous - acon., am-c., ***anthr.***, **ARS.**, ***bell.***, ***brom.***, calen., ***carb-v.***, ***chin.***, ***eucal.***, euph., **LACH.**, sal-ac., ***sec.***, ***sil.***, sul-ac., trach., vip., vip-a.

painful - ***all-c.***, am-c., ***anthr.***, ***apis***, arist-cl., ***arn.***, bell., calc., calc-f., **CALEN.**, cham., con., croc., crot-h., eug., ***hep.***, **HYPER.**, led., nat-c., ***nat-m.***, ***nit-ac.***, nux-v., ***ph-ac.***, plan., **STAPH.**, sulph.

slow, to heal - ***all-c.***, alum., alum-p., alum-sil., am-c., ars., ***bar-c.***, ***bor.***, both-l., ***calc.***, calc-s., **CALEN.**, ***carb-v.***, **CARC.**, caust., ***cham.***, chel., clem., con., cortiso., croc., crot-h., echi., ***graph.***, ***gunp.***, hell., **HEP.**, hydrog., hyper., kali-c., kreos., **LACH.**, lyc., lyss., mag-c., mang., ***merc.***, ***merc-c.***, mur-ac., nat-c., **NIT-AC.**, nux-v., **PETR.**, ph-ac., phos., plb., puls., psor., ***rhus-t.***, sars., sep., **SIL.**, squil., ***staph.***, **SULPH.**, ***tub.***, x-ray.

suppurating - arn., asaf., ***bell.***, bor., ***bufo***, ***calc.***, calc-f., **CALC-S.**, ***calen.***, caust., ***cham.***, ***chin.***, ***croc.***, echi., **HEP.**, hydrog., ign., lach., led., ***merc.***, ***nat-m.***, plb., ***puls.***, ***pyrog.***, **SIL.**, ***sulph.***, syph., vip-a.

WRIST, weak - aloe, amyg-p., arn., ars., bell-p., bov., brach., bry., calad., ***calc.***, ***calc-f.***, ***carb-v.***, **CAUST.**, choc., ***cur.***, dig., dor., **GUAI.**, ***glon.***, hura, kali-bi., kali-br., kali-c., kali-n., kalm., lil-t., lyc., manc., ***merc.***, mez., nat-m., nat-p., phos., phys., **PLB.**, ***plb-acet.***, podo., rhod., ***rhus-t.***, **RUTA**, sarcol-ac., sep., ***sil.***, spong., sul-ac., sulph., tub., valer., ***viol-o.***, zinc.

WRITER'S CRAMP - brach., calc., calc-f., cupr., cycl., **MAG-P.**, **STANN.**, ruta, tril.

X

X-RAYS, ailments from, (see Radiation, poisoning) - ***cadm-s.***, cob., m-aust., phos., rad-br., sol, sulph., uran-n., x-ray.

Y

YELLOW FEVER - **ACON.**, ***all-c.***, am-c., ***ant-t.***, ***apis***, arg., ***arg-n.***, ***ant-t.***, ***arn.***, **ARS.**, ***ars-h.***, **BELL.**, ***bry.***, **CADM-S.**, calc., **CAMPH.**, **CANTH.**, caps., carb-ac., **CARB-V.**, cham., cean., ***chin.***, chin-s., coff., coloc., crot-c., **CROT-H.**, cupr., daph., dig., eup-per., ***gels.***, ***glon.***, gua., hell., hep., ***hyos.***, ip., kali-p., **LACH.**, lept., ***lob.***, **MERC.**, mur-ac., ***nat-s.***, nit-ac., **NUX-V.**, op., ***phos.***, plat., plb., ***psor.***, puls., ***rhus-t.***, sabad., sabin., ***sep.***, ***sul-ac.***, sulph., ***ter.***, ***verat.***, ***verat-v.***

Z

ZINC, poisoning, ailments from - agar., nux-v., zinc.

ZYMOTIC FEVER - acet-ac., ail., alum., alumn., am-c., anthr., apis, arg-n., **ARN.**, **ARS.**, ars-s-f., arum-t., **BAPT.**, ***bell.***, berb., **BRY.**, ***cadm-s.***, canth., carb-v., **CARBN-S.**, ***chin.***, **CROT-H.**, ***cur.***, dig., **ECHI.**, ham., **HYOS.**, ip., kali-bi., **KALI-P.**, kreos., **LACH.**, **LYC.**, **MERC.**, merc-c., **MUR-AC.**, nit-ac., nux-m., **NUX-V.**, op., ph-ac., ***phos.***, pic-ac., psor., ***puls.***, **PYROG.**, **RHUS-T.**, rhus-v., sal-ac., staph., sul-ac., **SULPH.**, tarent., ter.

Index

A

Index

Index

B

Index

C

Index

D

E

F

G

I

J

K

L

M

Index

S

T

U

References

A

Agrawal, M.L. Mat. Med. of Human Mind. 1989.

Ahmad, S., Homeopathy and Adverse Reactions of Allopathic Drugs.

Allen, Henry Clay. Keynotes and Characteristics.

Allen, Henry Clay. Mat. Med. of Nosodes. 1910.

Allen, Henry Clay. Therapeutics of Fevers. 1902.

Allen, Henry Clay. Therapeutics of Intermittent Fever. 1879.

Allen, John Henry. Diseases and Therapeutics of the Skin. 1902.

Allen, John Henry. The Chronic Miasms. 1902.

Allen, Timothy F. Encyclopedia of Pure Mat. Med.. 1874-79.

Allen, Timothy F. Handbook of Mat. Med.. 1889.

Allen, Timothy F. Symptom-Register. Index of the Encyclopedia of Pure Mat. Med.. 1874-79.

Anshutz, Edward P. New, Old and Forgotten Remedies. 2nd edition. 1917.

Anshutz, Edward P. Therapeutic By-Ways.

Armstrong, W.P. A Handbook of the Diseases of the Heart. 1882.

Assilem, M. Folliculinum. 1990.

Assilem, M. The Mad Hatter's Tea Party. 1994.

Assilem, M. Women Ripening through the Menopause.

B

Barthel, Horst/Klunker, Wil. Synthetic Repertory Vol. I-III. 3rd edition. 1987.

Bhattacharya, A. K. Gem Therapy, Septenate Mixures..

Berridge, Edward W. Repertory to the Mat. Med., Diseases of the Eye. 1873.

Bidwell, Glen I. How to use the Repertory. 1915.

Blackwood, Alex. A Manual of Mat. Med., Therapeutics and Pharmacology, with Index.

Blackwood, Alex. Diseases of the Heart. 1901.

Boericke, Garth., Compendium of Homeopathy..

Boericke, Wm. and Oscar E., Manual of Hom. Mat. Med. and Repertory.

Boericke, Wm. and Dewey, W. A., Twelve Tissue Remedies of Schussler.

Boger, Cyrus. Additions to Kent's Repertory..

Boger, Cyrus Boenninghausen's Characteristics and Repertory. 1905.

Boger, Cyrus Synoptic Key of Mat. Med.. 1915.

Boger, Cyrus Times and Moon phases. 1910.

Bonninghausen, Clemens von. A Systematic Alphabetic Repertory of Homeopathic Remedies, ed. Cyrus M Boger. 1900.

Bonninghausen, Clemens von. Therapeutic Pocketbook, ed. T F Allen. 1891.

Borland, Douglas M. Homeopathic Practice.

Borland, Douglas M. Childrens Types. 1939.

Borland, Douglas M. Homoeopathy for Mother and Infant. 1950.

Burnett, James Compton. Delicate, Backward, Puny and Stunted Children. 1895.

Burnett, James Compton. Diseases of the Liver and Spleen.

Burnett, James Compton. Enlarged tonsils cured by medicine. 1901.

Burnett, James Compton. Fifty Reasons for being a Homeopath.

Burnett, James Compton. Organ Diseases of Women.

Burnett, James Compton. Organ Remedies.

Burnett, James Compton. Vaccinosis.

Burt, William H. Characteristic Mat. Med.. 2nd edition. 1873.

Burt, William H. Physiological Mat. Med.. 3rd edition. 1883.

C

Carey, George W. Biochemic System of Medicine. 1894.

Case, Erastus E. Some Clinical Experiences of Erastus E. Case MD. 1916.

Carleton, Edmund. Homeopathy in Medicine and Surgery.

Castro, David. Encyclopaedia of Repertories. 1989.

Castro, David. Logic of Repertories. 1992.

Chitkara, H.L., Update Additions to Repertory of Mind.

Choudhuri, N.M. A Study on Mat. Med. and Repertory. 2nd edition 1929.

Clarke, John Henry. The Prescriber.

Clarke, John Henry. A Dictionary of Practical Mat. Med.. 1900-02.

Clarke, John Henry. Clinical Repertory of Mat. Med.. 1904.

Clarke, John Henry. Therapeutics of the Serpent Poisons.

Cooper, Robert T. Cancer and Cancer Symptoms. 2nd edition. 1900.

References

Coulter, C. and Ramakrishnan, A.U., A Homeopathic Approach to Cancer.

Cowperthwaite, Allen Corson. A Textbook of Gynaecology. 1888.

Cowperthwaite, Allen Corson. An Elementary Textbook of Mat. Med. and Therapeutics. 1909.

D

Das, Bishamber. Select Your Remedy. 1988.

Das, Eswara, Synopsis and Homeopathic Aetiology, A Complete Work on Causation.

Dewey, W. A. Practical Homeo. Therapeutics,

Dewey, Willis A. 12 Tissue Remedies.

Dewey, Willis A. Essentials of Homoepathic Mat. Med.. 1908.

Dockx, R. & Kokelenberg, G., Kent's Comparative Repertory of Homeopathic Mat. Med.. 1988.

Douglass, Melford E. Repertory of Tongue. 1896.

Dunham, Caroll. Lectures on Mat. Med.. 1879.

Dunham, Caroll. Science of Therapeutics. 1877.

E

Eizayaga, Francisco. El moderno Repertorio de Kent. 1979.

Eizayaga, Francisco. Treatise on Homeopathic Medicine,

Eizayaga, Francisco. Lectures and Practice. 1991.

F

Farrington, Ernest A. Clinical Mat. Med., 1887.

Farrington, Ernest A. Comparative Mat. Med.

Fincke, Bernhardt. Imponderables, provings and comments, Sol.

Foubister, Donald M. A Clinical Study of Carcinosin as a Constitutional remedy. 1953.

Foubister, Donald M. Carcinosin Drug Picture. 1958.

Foubister, Donald M. Clinical impressions of Carcinosin. 1954.

Foubister, Donald M. Tutorials on Homoeopathy. 1989.

G

Gallavardin, J., Repertory of Psychic Medicines and Mat. Med..

Gallavardin, Jean Pierre. Repertory of psychic medicines with Mat. Med.. 1986.

Gentry, W. D. Concordance Repertory. 1890-92.

Ghosh, B.K., Food, Desires and Aversions.

Gibson, D. M. Studies of Homeopathic Remedies.

Gilchrist, James G. Homeopathic Treatment of Surgical Diseases. 1873.

Gladwin, Fredericka E. A Study and Revision of Kent's Repertory. 1928.

Grimmer, Arthur H. Applications of Remedies to Cancer cases. 1930.

Grimmer, Arthur H. Differentiating symptoms of some of the cadmium salts. 1930.

Gross, R.H. Comparative Mat. Med.. 1867.

Guernsey, Henry N.l. Keynotes to Mat. Med., Obstetrics.

Guernsey, Henry Newell. Obstetrics. 1883.

Guernsey, William Jefferson. Desires and Aversions.

Gupta, B. P., Encyclopedia of Homeopathy.

H

Hahnemann, Samuel. Mat. Med. Pura.

Hahnemann, Samuel. Organon of Medicine.

Hahnemann, Samuel. The Chronic Diseases.

Hale, Edwin M. Diseases of the Heart.

Hale, Edwin M. Mat. Med. of New Remedies, Therapeutics. 1875.

Hamilton, Edward. Flora homoeopathica.

Hansen, Oscar. A Text-book of Mat. Med. and Therapeutics of Rare Homeo. Remedies, 1899.

Hardy, Mary. The Alchemist Handbook to Homeopathy.

Hartmann, Franz. Diseases of Children, Transl. Hempel C.J. 1853.

Herrick, Nancy. Sacred Plants, Human Voices.

Hering, Constantine. Analytical Repertory of Symptoms of the Mind. 1881.

Hering, Constantine. Condensed Mat. Med.. 1884.

Hering, Constantine. Guiding Symptoms of our Mat. Med.. 1879-1891.

Hoyne, Temple S. Clinical therapeutics. 1993.

Hughes, Richard. Cyclopaedia of drug pathogenesy. 1886-91.

Hughes, Richard. Repertory to the Cyclopaedia Drug Pathogenesis. 1897-1900.

I

Imhauser, H., Homeopathy in Pediatric Practice.

J

Jahr, George Heinrich G. A New Manual of Homeopathic Practice.

Jahr, George Heinrich G. Hulls "Jahr", Transl. Hempel, 6 th american Edition. 1874.

Jahr, George Heinrich G. Mental Diseases, 1857.

Jahr, George Heinrich G., 40 years Practice.

Jones, Eli. Definite Medication. also Cancer.

Julian, O. A., Dictionary of Homeo. Mat. Med.

Julian, O. A., Mat. Med. of New Homeo. Remedies.

Julian, O. A., Mat. Med. of Nosodes.

K

Kent, James Tyler. Lectures on Homoepathic Mat. Med.. 1911.

Kent, James Tyler. Lesser Writings, New Remedies, Clinical Cases. 1985.

Kent, James Tyler. Repertory. 6th edition. 1957.

Kent, James Tyler. The Development and Formation of the Repertory. 1914.

Kichlu and Bose, A Textbook of Descriptive Medicine.

King, John C. Headaches/Repertory. 1891.

Kishore, J., Integrated Homeopathic Repertory.

Knerr, Calvin B. Repertory of Herings Guiding Symptoms of our Mat. Med.

Knerr, Calvin B. Drug Relationships. 1936.

Krishnamoorty, V., Homeopathy in Accidents and Injuries with a Short Repertory on Emergencies.

Kunzli, Jost. Kent's Repertorium Generale. 1987.

L

Lathoud, J. A., Homeopathic Mat. Med..

Lee, Edmund Jennings. Repertory of Characteric Symptoms of Hom. Mat. Medica. 1889.

Lee, Edmund Jennings. Repertory of Mind and Head. 1889.

Leeser, Otto. Homeopathic Mat. Med.. 1935.

Lillienthal, Samuel. Homoeopathic Therapeutics. 1890.

Lippe, Adolph. Text-Book of Mat. Med.. 1866.

Lippe, Adolph. Keynotes and Red line symptoms of the Mat. Med.. 1854.

Lippe, Constantine. Repertory to the More Characterics of the Mat. Med.. 1879.

M

Mills, E. J., Public Health & Homeopathy for HIV in India.

Minton, Henry. Uterine Therapeutics. 1906.

Mukherji, R.K., O.A. Julians's Intestinal Nosodes of Bach-Paterson.

Murphy, Robin. Homeopathic Clinical Repertory. 3rd ed., 2005.

Murphy, Robin. Homeopathic Remedy Guide, 2nd ed., 2005

Murphy, Robin. Homeopathy and Cancer, 1979

Murphy, Robin. Keynotes of Mat. Med., Lectures 1995.

Murphy, Robin. Lectures on Homeopathic Philosophy & Practice, (Audio Lecture Series).

Murphy, Robin. Lotus Mat. Med., 1st ed., 1995.

N

Nash, E.. Leaders in Homoeopathic Therapeutics, 6th edition.

Nash, E. Regional Leaders.

Nash, E. Testimony of the Clinic.

P

Panos, M. Homeopathic Medicine at Home.

Patel, Ramanlal P. Analysis and Evaluation of Symptoms. 1974.

Patel, Ramanlal P. Repertory of the Homoeopathic Mat. Med. by J.T. Kent, 6th edition. 1990.

Patel, Ramanlal P. Word-index with rubrics of Dr. Kent's Repertory, 3rd edition. 1977.

Paterson, John. The Bowel Nosodes. 1950.

Perko, Sandra Homeopathy for Pregnant Women and Her Infant.

Perko, Sandra The Homeopathic Treatment of Influenza.

Phatak, S.R. Phatak's Concise Repertory of Homoeopathic Medicines, 2nd, edition.1977.

Phatak, S.R. Phatak's Mat. Med. of Homoeopathic Medicines.1988.

Pulford, A. Key to the Homeo. Mat. Med.. 1947.

R

Rachemacher, J. G. Rachemacher.s Universal and Organ Remedies.

Ramakrishnan, A.U. and Coulter, C., A Homeopathic Approach to Cancer.

Rastogi, D.P., Overview of Repertories.

Rastogi, Corrections to Boger's Repertory.1990.

Raue, C. Diseases of Children.

Roberts, Herbert A. Sensations As If. 1937.

Roberts, Herbert. Homeopathy: Principles and Practice.

Roberts, Herbert A. Study of Remedies by Comparison. 1941.

Roy, S.P. Word index to Boger-Boenninghausen's Repertory. 1990.

Royal, George. Textbook of Homeopathic Mat. Med..1920.

Ruddock, E. Harris. Diseases of Infants and Children. 1886.

Ruddock, E. Harris. Lady's Homoeopathic Manual. London. 1865.

S

Sankaran, P. Some Cross References to Kent's Repertory. 1966.

Schroyens, Frederik. Synthesis Repertory, ed. 8.1.

Scholten, Jan Homeopathy and Minerals.

Schussler, W.H. The Biochemic System, The Twelve Tissue Remedies.

Schussler, W.H. Biochemical Treatment of Disease. 1931.

Schuster, Bernd. Bamboo (Bambusa) Proving.

Sethi, B., Repertory, Likes and Dislikes.

Sheppard, Dorthy. Epidemic Diseases,

Sheppard, Dorthy. Magic of the Minimum Dose.

Sheppard, Dorthy. Physician's Posey.

Sherr, Jeremy. The Homoeopathic Proving of Hydrogen. 1992.

Sherr, Jeremy. The Homoeopathic Proving of Chocolate. 1993.

Sherr, Jeremy. The Homoeopathic Proving of Scorpion. 2nd edition. 1992.

Sinha, Y., Unique Repertory.

Sirker, C., A Keynote Repertory of Mat. Med..

Sirker, K.K., A Handbook of Repertory.

Sivaraman, P. Corrections and Additions to Kent's Repertory.

Sivaraman, P. Kent's Repertory of the Homeopathic Mat. Med. Expanded. 1995.

Sivaraman, P., A Concise Repertory of Aggravations and Ameliorations.

Smits. Tinus. Practical Materia Medica.

Squire, B., Repertory of Homeopathic, Nosodes and Sarcodes.

Stephenson, James. A Mat. Med. and Repertory.

Stephenson, James. Hahnemanns Provings 1924-1959. 1963.

Swan, Samuel. Nosodes. 1888.

T

Talcott, Selden H. Mental Diseases and their Modern Treatment. 1901.

Templeton, W. Lees. Provings of Carcinosin. 1954.

Tiwari, S. K., Essentials of Repertorization.

Tiwari, S. K., Homeopathy and Childcare.

Tyler, Margaret L. A Study of Kent's Repertory. 1914.

Tyler, Margaret L. Homoeopathic Drug Pictures.

Tyler, Margaret L. Pointers to the Common Remedies.

U

Underwood B. F., The Diseases of Childhood and Their Homeopathic Treatment.

Underwood B. F., Headaches and Its Mat. Med..

V

Vakil, P. Leprosy Proving.

Vannier, Homeopathy Human Medicine.

Vermeulen, F. Concorant Materia Medica.

Vermeulen, F. Synoptic Materia Medica.

Von Lippe, A., Keynotes and Redline Symptoms of the Mat. Med..

W

Ward, James William. Unabridged Dictionary of the Sensations As If. 1939.

Warkentin, David. MacRepertory, Computer Software. Kent Homeopathic Associates.

Warkentin, David. MacRepertory, Reference Works Homeopathic Software. Kent Homeopathic Associates.

Watson, Ian. A Guide to the Methodologies of Homeopathy.

Wood, James C. Clinical Gynecology. 2nd edition. 1898.

Worcester, S. H., Repertory to the Modalities.

Wright-Hubbard, Elizabeth. Homoeopathy as Art and Science. 1990.

Wright-Hubbard, Elizabeth. Index to Remedies in Kent's Mat. Med.. 1928.

Y

Yasgur, Jay. A Dictionary of Homeopathic Medical Terminology. 3rd edition. 1994.

Yingling, William A. Accoucheur's Emergency Manual. 1895.

Homeopathic-Herbal Glossary

Abscess - A localized collection in a cavity or lump formed by the process of suppuration and disintegration of tissue.

Absinthism - The pathological state resulting from the excessive and habitual use of absinth, characterized by neuritis, hyperesthesia, hallucinations, convulsions, acute mania and general paralysis.

Accoucheur - To assist in childbirth, from old French meaning to lay down. A midwife, obstetrician, one who helps deliver babies.

Acne rosacea - Acne of cheeks and nose associated with congestion and formation of telangiectases (stretching and dilation of small vessels).

Acne vulgaris - Acne simplex or common acne. It is considered an abnormal response to normal levels of the male hormone testosterone. Acne lesions are commonly referred to as pimples, spots or zits.

Acromegaly - Acromegaly (from Greek akros "high" and megas "large" extremities enlargement) is a hormonal disorder that results when the pituitary gland produces excess human growth hormone (HGH). Most commonly from a benign HGH producing tumor called pituitary adenoma.

Actinomycosis - An infectious disease caused by a parasite. The jaw is most commonly affected being the site of slow growing suppurating tumors. (Lumpy jaw, clyers, wooden tongue).

Acute remedies - These are the type of homeopathic remedies prescribed for acute infections and fevers. Examples: Aconite, Arsenicum album, Baptisia, Belladonna, Bryonia, Chamomille, Gelsemium, Ferrum phos., Pulsatilla, Pyrogen.

Adaptogen - The word adaptogen, coined by Russian Dr. Nicolai Lazarev in 1947, refers to any natural herbal remedy that increases the body's resistance to stresses such as trauma, anxiety, aging and bodily fatigue.

Addison's disease - A disease caused by partial or total failure of adrenocortical functions. This is characterized by a bronze-like pigmentation of the skin and mucous membranes, anemia, weakness, and low blood pressure.

Adenitis - Inflammation of the lymph nodes or glands.

Adenoma - A glandular tumor.

Aggravated, (Agg.) - A term used to denote when a symptom or state is becoming worse from some kind of action. Example: Aggravated by motion, heat, pressure, etc.

Aggravation - In homeopathy, an aggravation is an intensification of symptoms experienced after the remedy is taken. A healing aggravation, in which current symptoms temporarily intensify or old symptoms temporarily reappear is often a positive sign that the curative process has begun. This phenomenon is also known as a 'healing crisis'.

Agoraphobia - Fear of being in open spaces or crossing open spaces.

Ague - A chill. Recurrent chill. An intermittent fever with alternating fits of hot and cold. Oftens refers to malaria and periodic fevers.

AIDS - Acquired Immune Deficiency Syndrome (AIDS or Aids) is a collection of symptoms and infections in humans resulting from the specific weakness of the immune system caused by the human immunodeficiency virus (HIV). The late stage of the condition leaves individuals prone to opportunistic infections and tumors.

Alexia - An inability to read, word blindness.

Allopathy - Remedies or treatments that are in opposition to the immune response are antipathic or allopathic. Conventional western medicine. Chemical/drug medicine. The term was coined by Samuel Hahnemann to differentiate homeopathic practices from conventional medicine, based on the types of treatments used. Hahnemann used this term to distinguish medicine as practiced in his time from his use of infinitesimally small doses of substances to treat the vital causes of illness. As used by homeopaths, the term "allopathy" has always referred to a principle of curing disease by administering substances that produce the opposite effect of the disease when given to a healthy human. The term "allopath" comes from the Greek roots meaning "opposite" and "disease." the form "allopathy."

Alterative - Any herbal remedy which causes a favorable change or alteration in the processes of nutrition and repair, probably through some unknown way improving metabolism.

Alzheimer's disease - Senile dementia with cerebral atrophy, memory failure, disorientation. It is the most common type of dementia. The most striking early symptom is loss of short term memory (amnesia).

Amblyopia - Dimness of vision without any apparent defect of eye. Blurred or weak vision.

Ameliorated, (Amel.) - A term used to denote when a symptom or state is becoming better from some kind of action. Example: Ameliorated by motion, heat, pressure, etc.

Amenorrhea - The absence of menstruation means no menstrual flow. Absent menstruation may be primary (no menstruation before age 16) or secondary (menstruation begins at the appropriate age, but later stops for more than 3 cycles or 6 months).

Homeopathic-Herbal Glossary

Analgesic - Same as Anodyne. An agent that relieves pain.

Anaphrodisiac - An agent that lessens sexual desire or depresses sexual power.

Anasarca - (Hyposarca). A generalized systemic edema.

Anesthetic (Anaesthetic) - An agent which temporarily abolishes sensation, producing insensibility to contact and pain. There are local and general anesthetics, the latter being administered by inhalation.

Aneurysm - An abnormal dilatation of an artery, generally producing a sac as a result of arterial wall stretching. The sac is thin, weak and prone to rupture.

Anodyne - An agent that relieves pain, but does not necessarily produce unconsciousness.

Anorexia - Absence or loss of appetite.

Anorexia nervosa - An abnormal or hysterical aversion to food. Anorexia nervosa is a psychiatric diagnosis that describes an eating disorder characterized by low body weight and body image distortion. Individuals with anorexia often control body weight by voluntary starvation, purging, vomiting, excessive exercise, or other weight control measures, such as diet pills or diuretic drugs.

Antacid - An agent that will correct acidity by neutralization, chiefly acidity of the stomach.

Anthelmintic - A remedy against intestinal worms.

Antidote - A agent to counteract poisons. It is (a) chemical, neutralizes the poison, (b) mechanical, preventing absorption, (c) physiological, opposing the effect upon the system after absorption of the poison.

Antidotes - An antidote is anything that counteracts the effect of a homeopathic remedy, which may prevent the remedy from working. In relation to homeopathic remedies, some remedies act to neutralize or antidote other remedies.

Antiperiodic - An agent that diminishes or arrests the periodicity of malarial attacks. In general, an antimalarial agent.

Antipyretic - An agent which reduces the temperature of fevers.

Antiscorbutic - A remedy that prevents or corrects scurvy.

Antiseptic - An agent that opposes or prevents sepsis. An agent which prevents the growth of microbes and cripples their activity while in contact with them.

Antisudorific - An agent to prevent or relieve excessive sweating.

Antitoxin - Any defensive protein acting as a neutralizer of poison. Most therapeutic antitoxins are derived from the blood-serum of animals in which a specific disease has been purposely developed. *Examples*: Anti-diphtheric and Anti-tetanic serums.

Antitussive - A remedy to relieve or prevent cough.

Aperient - A gentle and nonirritating purgative causing but little increase of peristalsis and producing soft feces.

Aphasia - The loss of power of speech, the inability to talk.

Aphonia - Loss of voice, as in clergyman's sore throat.

Aphrodisiac - An agent which increases sexual desire, or increases sexual power.

Aphthous ulcer - A small sensitive painful ulcer crater in the lining of the mouth. Commonly called a type of canker sore. Aphthous ulcers are one of the most common problems that occur in the mouth. Aphthous ulcers typically last for 10-14 days and they heal without leaving a scar.

Apoplexy - The word "apoplexy" comes from the Greek "apoplexia" meaning a seizure, in the sense of being struck down. In Greek "plexe" is "a stroke." The ancients believed that someone suffering a stroke (or any sudden incapacity) had been struck down by the gods. Apoplexy is a venerable term for a stroke, a cerebrovascular accident (CVA), often associated with loss of consciousness and paralysis of various parts of the body.

Ascarides - Roundworms. Intestinal worms.

Ascites - It is an accumulation of fluid in the peritoneal cavity. Ascites is also known as hydroperitoneum or more archaically as abdominal dropsy. Although most commonly due to cirrhosis and severe liver disease, its presence can portend other significant medical problems.

Astigmatism - Ophthalmic astigmatism is a refraction error of the eye in which there is a difference in degree of refraction in different meridians. Astigmatism causes difficulties in seeing fine detail. In some cases vertical lines and objects such as walls may appear to the patient to be leaning over.

Astringent - An agent which, by acting upon the tissues, causes condensation and contraction, and restrains discharges.

Homeopathic-Herbal Glossary

Ataxia - Incoordination and unsteadiness due to the brain's failure to regulate the body's posture and regulate the strength and direction of limb movements. Wobbliness. Ataxia is usually a consequence of disease in the brain, specifically in the cerebellum which lies beneath the back part of the cerebrum.

Atelectasis - Collapsed lung. Incomplete expansion of lobules (clusters of alveoli) or lung segments may result in partial or complete lung collapse. Atelectasis can be present at birth (incomplete expansion of the lungs), or during adulthood (from a collapsed lung).

Autism - A mental condition, present from early childhood, characterized by great difficulty in communicating and forming relationships with other people and in using language and abstract concepts. Some now speculate that autism is not a single condition but a group of several distinct conditions that manifest in similar ways.

Auto-nosodes - The auto-nosodes are homeopathic remedies made from the patient's own diseased blood, urine, pus, discharges or tissues.

Autopathy - A little-known method of healing which has developed out of the tradition of homeopathy. In essence it consists of using homeopathically highly diluted secretions from the body of the person who is being treated. (Autopathic remedies: Blood, Saliva, Urine, etc).

Auto-sarcodes - The auto-sarcodes are homeopathic remedies made from the patient's own heaalthy blood, urine, pus, discharges or tissues.

Avogadro's number - The number of molecules in a mole of a substance, approximately 6.023 x 1023. A mole is the number of grams of a substance equal to its molecular weight.

Bach Flower Essences - A group of herbal essences derived from various flowers by the British physician and homeopath Edward Bach in the early 20th century. In 1929 he left London in search for simple herbal treatments for illness. He eventually developed the "Bach Flower Essences." The Flower Essences may be given single or combined. There are 38 original flower remedies that heal disorders of the emotions and mind: Agrimony, Aspen, Beech, Centaury, Cerato, Cherry Plum, Chestnut, Chicory, Clematis, Crab Apple, Elm, Gentitian, Gorse, Heather, Holly, Honeysuckle, Hornbeam, Impatiens, Larch, Mimulus, Mustard, Oak, Olive, Pine, Red Chestnut, Rock Rose, Rock Water, Scleranthus, Star of Bethlehem, Sweet Chestnut, Vervain, Vine, Walnut, Water Violet, White Chestnut, Wild Oat, Wild Rose, Willow.

Balanitis - Inflammation of the glans of the penis. Inflammation of the foreskin is called posthitis. In the uncircumcised male, balanitis and posthitis generally occur together as balanoposthitis: inflammation of both the glans and foreskin.

Barber's itch - Ringworm of the beard. Pustular folliculitis affecting facial hair.

Basedow's disease - see Graves's disease.

Bazin's disease - Bazin-tuberculosis indurativa cutanea et subcutanea. Also known as Bazin's malady. Chronic skin disease characterized by hard cutaneous nodules that break down to form indolent necrotic ulcers leaving atrophic, pigmented scars. Initially, it was considered a form of skin tuberculosis, and most frequently seen in adolescent girls and menopausal women with tuberculosis or positive tuberculin test. However, cases that appear to be unrelated to tuberculosis have been observed. Etiology is still uncertain.

Bell's palsy - Facial paralysis. Peripheral paralysis of the facial nerve.

Beri-beri - Polyneuritis, the muscles are stiff and atrophied with accompanying nerve pains.

Besotted - A muddled or stupified expression. Often relating to malaise and fever states.

Bilious - Relating to bile. Marked by or suffering from liver-gallbladder dysfunction and especially excessive secretion of bile. Appearing as if affected by a bilious disorder.

Bilious fever - Fever with digestive disturbances, and relating to bilious conditions.

Bilious humor - See Choleric. A person described as "bilious" is mean-spirited, suspicious, and angry.

Biochemic remedies - See Tissue salts.

Bitter - An agent which increases the tone and activity of the gastric mucosa, thereby improving the appetite.

Blackwater fever - Hemolytic malaria, a contagious and fatal malarial disease of the tropics.

Blennorrhea - Copious mucous discharge from the vagina or urethra.

Borborygmi - Intestinal rumblings caused by gas in the intestines.

Bowel nosodes - These remedies were developed by Edward Bach and Dr. John Paterson followed up the research. The bowel nosodes were derived from stool cultures and they were prescribed on the percentages of bacteria found in the stools of patients. These nosodes are potentized from a culture of the intestinal bacterial flora. Bach observed a sympathy between certain disease states and which bacteria was associated with them. The following is a list of the bowel nosodes:

Bacillus number seven, Bacillus number ten, Dysentery bacillus, Gaertner bacillus, Morgan bacillus, Mutabile bacillus, Proteus bacillus, Sycotic bacillus.

Brain fag - Term for brain fatigue. Exhaustion of the mental faculties through intellectual overwork.

Bright's disease - Bright's disease is a historical classification of kidney diseases that would be described in modern medicine as acute or chronic nephritis. The term is no longer used, as diseases are now classified according to their more fully-understood etiologies. It is typically denoted by the presence of albumin in the urine, and frequently accompanied by edema.

Bronchiectasis - Dilatation of bronchi due to inflammation.

Bruxism - Clenching and/or grinding of the teeth. Bruxism is caused by the activation of reflex chewing activity.

Bubo - The ancient word "bubo" comes from the Greek "boubon" meaning groin or swollen groin. Bubo is an enlarged lymph node that is tender and painful, particularly in the groin and armpit (the axilla). A feature of a number of infectious diseases including gonorrhea, syphilis, tuberculosis, and the plague. Hence, the term bubonic plague.

Bulimia - An eating disorder in which a large quantity of food is consumed in a short period of time, often followed by feelings of guilt or shame. Also called binge-eating syndrome.

Bursa - A fluid filled cavity between joints.

Cachexia - Physical wasting with loss of weight and muscle mass caused by disease. Cachexia is a wasting syndrome that causes weakness and a loss of weight, fat, and muscle. Patients with advanced cancer, AIDS, and some other major chronic progressive diseases may appear cachectic. Anorexia (loss of apppetite) and cachexia often occur together. Cachexia can occur in people who are eating enough, but who cannot absorb the nutrients. Cachexia is not the same as starvation. A healthy person's body can adjust to starvation by slowing down its use of nutrients, but in cachectic patients, the body does not make this adjustment.

Calculi - Stones, as in kidney or gallbladder stones.

Cancer miasm - This is several miasms combined. Tendency toward inflammatory illness, whooping cough or high fevers of unknown origin, pneumonia, or *severe acute diseases.* History of diabetes, pernicious anemia, or cancer. Periodic high fevers, immune diseases. *Cancer* miasm can be result of abuse, emotional suppressions, prolong stress and fear. Insomnia and sleep loss.

Carbuncle - A severe abscess or multiple boils in the skin, typically infected with staphylococcus bacteria.

Cardiac - An agent which stimulates and tones the heart, also a cordial or restorative.

Caries - Decay of the bone. Bones become fragile, thin, breaks down with the formation of pus.

Carminative - An herbal agent that prevents or relieves flatulence and thereby allays pain.

Caruncle - A fleshy outgrowth at the meatus of female urethra.

Catalepsy - A condition characterized most often by rigidity of the extremities and by decreased sensitivity to pain.

Catarrh - A discharge or mucus blockage caused by the swelling of the mucous membranes. The symptom is usually associated with the common cold, but can also be found in patients with middle ear infections, tonsillitis, sinusitis or an adenoid infection. Some blockages may be chronic.

Catatonia - Catatonic patients will sometimes hold rigid poses for hours and will ignore any external stimuli. Catatonia is not a mental disorder is thought of as a syndrome accompanying other mental disorders. There is a sub-type of schizophrenia called "catatonic schizophrenia" in which the patient experiences an extreme loss of motor ability or constant hyperactive motor activity.

Cathartic - An agent that hastens and increases evacuation of the bowels. (See Purgative).

Causative remedies - The etiology or initial cause of a disorder is very important in determining the most similar remedy for any emergency, acute or chronic case. Etiologies can be described as shocks, traumas, injuries, excesses, mental and emotional stress and vital energy or fluid leaks. These causative factors can be looked up as rubrics in the Clinical Repertory and the major remedies can then be studied in the Materia Medica. The following group gives some of the major causes of diseases and suffering: Abuse, Accidents, Alcohol, Allergies, Anger, Anticipation, Bad news, Blows, Burns, Depletions, Cuts, Diet, Disappointed Love, Drugs, side effects, Emotional shocks, mental traumas, Environmental influences, Excesses, Forsaken, Fright, Genetic weakness, Greed, Grief, Humiliation, Infections, Injuries, Meat-eating, Medical, side effects, Miasms, Physical traumas, Poor hygiene, Poisons, Sexual excesses, Sleep, deprivations. Surgical, side effects, Work, Worry, Tobacco, Toxins, Vaccinations.

Caustic - An agent having an escharotic or corrosive action on living tissue. Used interchangeably with Cauterant.

Homeopathic-Herbal Glossary

Cell salts - See Tissue salts.

Cellulitis - Inflammation of cellular or connective tissue.

Centesimal potency - A homeopathic remedy that is produced by a series of dilution of one part substance to 99 parts water or alcohol. Also known as a 'c potency.' The designation "c," (centismal) which is the Roman numeral for 100, represents the dilutions that are manufactured by mixing one part of the starting material with 99 parts of the diluting solution. Each subsequent dilution repeats the process of 1:100 dilution.

Cerates - These are waxy herbal pastes intermediate in consistency between the ointment and plaster. They are sufficiently soft to be easily spread upon muslin with a spatula. When applied to the skin they adhere, but do not become soft enough to liquefy at the body temperature. The most abundant constituent is wax, hence their name. They are (1) *simple* and (2) *medicated*. Examples: Calendula Cerate and Graphites Cerate.

Chalazion - Stye, tumor cyst or lump on the border of the eyelid due to inflammation of the Meibomian gland.

Chemosis - A swelling of the eye surface membranes because of accumulation of fluid. This symptom is often related to an allergic response.

Cheyne-Stokes - Irregular intermittent breathing. Heavy breathing followed by very shallow breathing.

Chloasma - Deposit of pigment in the skin, occurring in patches of various sizes. A blotchy discoloration of a woman's face that is associated with pregnancy or with the use of oral contraceptives.

Chlorosis - Green sickness. A form of anemia seen in young women marked by a greenish pale color of the skin and menstrual disorders.

Cholagogue - A medicine which stimulates and increases the flow of bile.

Cholecystitis - Inflammation of the gall bladder. It is commonly due to impaction (sticking) of a gallstone within the neck of the gall bladder, leading to inspissation of bile, bile stasis, and infection by gut organisms.

Cholera infantum - Acute intestinal poisoning of bacterial origin in infants and young children.

Choleric - In ancient medicine choleric was one of the four bodily humors, believed to be associated with a sensitive, irritable, or peevish ill-natured temperament. Choleric corresponds to the fluid of yellow bile, the season of summer (dry and hot), and the element of fire. Bad-tempered or irritable, easily angered. Choleric also refers to cholera. Choleric refers to the condition of the bile. The disease cholera gained its name from choler (bile).

Chondroma - A benign bone tumor located within the marrow cavity.

Chordee - A painful downward curved erection of penis usually caused by gonorrhea inflammation.

Chronic remedies - These are homeopathic remedies for chronic degenerative diseases and weaknesses. Therefore the goals and method of approaching the case is different than in acute or emergency prescribing. Low potencies repeated daily are very effective for these long term conditions.

Chyle - A milk white emulsion of fat globules in lymph formed in intestines.

Cicatrice - Scars. Fibrous tissue that replaces the normal tissues destroyed by injury or disease.

Clap - Gonorrhea.

Classical homeopathy - Historical homeopathic traditions and practices. Use of a single homeopathic remedy prescribed according to the individual's presentation and history.

Clergyman's sore throat - loss of voice due to inflammation of the mucous membrane and underlying parts of pharynx.

Clinkers - Clumps of nasal mucus.

Coma vigil - State of delirium in which the person is lethargic and partly conscious, yet never actually sleeping or comatose.

Combination remedies - Preparations made by combining two or more homeopathic remedies.

Complex homeopathy - More than one remedy is used concurrently.

Complex remedies - See Combination remedies.

Concomitant - Occurring simultaneously. A symptom or other phenomenon that occurs at the same time as another symptom or phenomenon.

Condylomata - Condylomata acuminata. Genital warts. Human papilloma virus (HPV). Venereal wart. A viral skin disease characterized by a soft wart-like growth on the genitals. In adults, the disorder is considered a sexually-transmitted disease, but in children the virus appears to be transmitted with or without sexual contact.

Constitution - The constitution is the genetic makeup of the vitality, body and tissues. It is also the temperament, emotional disposition and personality of a person. This state involves the inherited strengths and weaknesses with which a person is born. These traits are very individual and reflect the health of the parents at the time of conception, the mother's health during pregnancy and the circumstances of the birth.

Homeopathic-Herbal Glossary

Constitutional remedies - The proper constitutional remedy will enhance and help maintain the general health. These are homeopathic remedies are prescribed for the genetic vitality of the person. Constitutional remedies are often given to children while they are developing and to the weak and elderly. Constitutional remedies help fortify people through times of stress or help one to recover from debilitating diseases. When the vitality is weakened, then one's susceptibility is increased to certain diseases. Some important constitutional remedies are: Bar-c., Calc., Calc-p., Sil., Phos., Graph., Sulphur and Lyc.

Consumption - A generic term for wasting away or atrophy usually referring to tuberculosis.

Corrosive - An agent destructive to tissue.

Coryza - A cold in the head. The word "coryza" came from the Greek "koryza" which is thought to have been compounded from "kara", head + "zeein", to boil. The "boiling over from the head" refers to the runny nose, an all-too-familiar feature of a head cold.

Counterirritant - An agent which, by inducing local irritation or hyperaemia, acts as a derivative to relieve irritation, inflammation or pain in some part remote from that to which it is applied.

Cretinism - A condition of severely stunted physical and mental growth due to untreated congenital deficiency of thyroid hormones (hypothyroidism). The term cretin refers to a person so affected.

Cri encephalique - Brain cry due to swelling and inflammation of the brain. Encephalitic cry. Brain cry, the characteristic crying sound made by infants and children suffering from encephalitis or meningitis, or other intracranial pathology of some severity.

Cushing's disease - A complex hormonal condition that involves many areas of the body. The symptoms and signs caused by an excess of cortisol hormone. Common symptoms are thinning of the skin, weakness, weight gain, bruising, hypertension, diabetes, thin weak bones (osteoporosis), facial puffiness and, in women, cessation of menstrual periods

Cyanosis - Refers to the bluish coloration of the skin due to the presence of deoxygenated hemoglobin in blood vessels near the skin surface.

Cystocele - Prolapse of bladder into the vagina. Hernia of the bladder.

Dacryagogue - An agent which causes a flow of tears.

Debauchery - Extreme indulgence, intemperance. Overindulging in alcohol, intoxicants, food, sex, etc.

Decimal potency - A homeopathic remedy that is produced by a series of dilution of one part substance to 9 parts water or alcohol. Also known as a 'X' or 'D' potency. The designation "X," which is the Roman numeral for 10, represents dilutions that are manufactured by mixing 1 part of the starting material with 9 parts of the diluting solution. Each subsequent dilution repeats the process of 1:10 dilution.

Decoctions - Freshly prepared aqueous solutions of the soluble parts of herbs, but, unlike infusions, are prepared by *boiling* the herb in water. One part of herb to twenty parts of water, unless otherwise specified. Decoctions are usually boiled for fifteen minutes and then allowed to cool. After it has been cooled and strained, the preparation can be made to measure up to the original quantity of menstruum by the addition of cold water passed through the mass in the strainer. The process is the opposite to that for preparing infusions. In the latter, hot or cold water is employed, and if hot, the product is allowed to *cool*; in the decoction, cold or warm water is employed and the preparation is *boiled*.

Decubitus - A decubitus ulcer is a pressure sore or what is commonly called a "bed sore."

Delirium tremens - (the DT's) A delirious state marked by delusions, illusions, hallucinations, insomnia, exhaustion and constant tremor. Often associated with alcohol poisoning and alcohol withdrawal.

Demulcent - (See Emollient.) A bland and soothing oily or mucilaginous application or medicine to relieve irritation of inflamed or abraded surfaces, usually intended for use upon the mucosa.

Dentition - Teething, cutting of teeth.

Deodorant - An agent that masks, removes, or destroys odor.

Depilatory - A substance that removes or destroys hair.

Depressant - An agent that will depress function and vital energies by causing relaxation of muscular tissues and sweating; a medicine that depresses any function.

Diabetes insipidus - Passage of large quantities of urine, intense thirst and dehydration due to inadequate of pituitary antidiuretic hormone (ADH).

Diabetes mellitus - Sugar diabetes, inability to metabolize sugars normally. Hypergycemia.

Diaphoretic - An agent that will stimulate and cause increased perspiration: a sedative diaphoretic is one that acts by dilation of the vessels of the skin, as when induced by heart sedatives or emetics.

Homeopathic-Herbal Glossary

Diathesis - A constitutional, hereditary or predisposition to a disease. A state or disposition of the body, most often present from birth. Diathesis means to be susceptible to certain types of diseases, stresses.

Digestant - An agent, which digests, or assists the digestion of food.

Diplopia - Double vision.

Dipsomania - Uncontrollable craving for alcohol. Term for alcoholism.

Disinfectant - An agent that prevents, or frees from infection, acting chiefly by destroying pathogenic germs or rendering organic ferments inactive.

Diuretic - An agent which causes and increases secretion and flow of urine.

Doctrine of Signatures - An ancient belief, which says that external characteristics of a plant, including color, serve to indicate possible theraputic effects. For centuries this has been used in herbal medicine to draw a correspondence between a particular plant and its medicinal use.

Down's syndrome - Down's syndrome or trisomy 21 (British Down's syndrome) is a genetic condition resulting from the presence of all or part of an extra 21st chromosome. A birth defect often associated with moderate mental retardation and various phyical malformations.

Dromomania - Intense desire to wander about from place to place.

Dropsy - Edema, an abnormal accumulation of fluids in tissues or a body cavity.

Drug - Original meaning for the term drug was a dry herb. Modern meaning of drug, refers to the chemical or synthetic medicines used by allopathic doctors.

Dupuytren's contraction - A contracted state of palm and fingers causing a permanent flexion of one or more fingers.

Dynamization - reducing the volume and increasing the effectiveness of a medicinal substance by repeated dilution with succussion.

Dyslexia - The word "dyslexia" comes from the Greek words dys- ("difficulty with") and lexis ("words" or "lexicon"). A general term for disorders that involve difficulty in learning to read or interpret words, letters, and other symbols, but that do not affect general intelligence. Mistakes in writing and understanding. Dyslexia is not limited to reversing the order of letters in reading or writing. Other difficulties have been reported including deficits in processing spoken language as well as non-language difficulties.

Dysmenorrhea - It is defined as painful menses. Menstrual cramps.

Ecbolic - An agent which excites and accelerates parturition, (childbirth).

Ecchymosis - Bruises. Skin discoloration caused by the escape of blood into the tissues from ruptured blood vessels. Ecchymoses can similarly occur in mucous membranes as, for example, in the mouth.

Eclampsia - Toxemia of pregnancy. Convulsions occurring with pregnancy associated high blood pressure, proteinuria and having no other cause.

Eclectic Medicine - The term was coined by Constantine Rafinesque (1784-1841), a doctor living among the Native Americans, and observing their use of medicinal plants. He coined the word "eclectic" to refer to those physicians who adopted in practice whatever was found to be beneficial to their patients. Eclectic medicine is still practiced today, mainly by medical herbalists rather than physicians.

Effervescent salts - Mixtures in the form of a fine or granulated powder of soluble chemical compounds with citric or tartaric acid, or both, and sodium bicarbonate. When added to water they form an effervescent draught which should be swallowed while it is foaming.

Elephantiasis - A chronic, often extreme enlargement and hardening of the cutaneous and subcutaneous tissue, especially of the legs and scrotum. Elephantiasis generally results from obstructions of the lymphatic vessels.

Elixirs - These herbal elixirs are sweetened, aromatic and alcoholic solutions, designed as vehicles for small amounts of active medicines. Example: Elixir Glycyrrhizae.

Emergency remedies - Homeopathic remedies prescribed for injuries, bites, burns, shocks and traumas in any form. The important things to know are the causative factors and different remedies for each condition. The 30c and 200c are effective potencies for first aid problems. Emergency and acute dosage. One dose equals a few of the pellets, tablets or two to four drops of the liquid remedies. Take one dose of a 30c, 3 times daily for a few days, or as needed or take a dose of 200c, a few times daily for a few days, again repeat as needed. In severe cases, one may need to repeat the remedy more often if needed.

Emetic - An agent that causes vomiting (emesis).

Emmenagogue - An agent that stimulates menstruation.

Emollient - A medicine or agent which softens or soothes the skin, or soothes the mucosa, when irritated. (see Demulcent.)

Emulsions - Aqueous fluid preparations holding in suspension oils or resinous substances by means of a mucilaginous or viscid media. Examples: Emulsum Asafœtidae (milk of asafetida).

Enchondroma - Benign cartilaginous growth occurring in parts where cartilage does not normally exist.

Endometriosis - A condition in which the tissue that normally lines the uterus (endometrium) grows in other areas of the body, causing pain, irregular bleeding, and possible infertility. The tissue growth (implant) typically occurs in the pelvic area, outside of the uterus, on the ovaries, bowel, rectum, bladder, and the delicate lining of the pelvis. However, the implants can occur in other areas of the body, too

Enemas - Enemas or Cylsters are fluids designed for injection into the rectum. They may be (1) *simple* or (2) *medicated,* or (3) *nutritional*. Examples: water, herbal, or nutritional retention enemas, to feed a patient rectally.

Energetic remedies - See Imponderables.

Enteritis - Inflammation of the intestines.

Entero-colitis - Inflammation of the intestines and colon.

Enuresis - Bedwetting. Involuntary urination, incontinence.

Epidemic remedies - These are homeopathic remedies prescribed for epidemic dieases. These remedies are found by using the frequent appearing symptoms and the strong symptoms of the epidemic disease. The epidemic remedy can be given preventively to those who have been exposed to infected individuals. The epidemic remedy is given in repeated doses for a short period of time, a few days or longer if needed.

Epulis - This is a benign, localised swelling of the gingiva, (gums).

Erysipelas - Erysipelas in Greek means red skin. It is an acute streptococcus bacterial skin infection, resulting in skin inflammation and often extending into underlying fat tissue.

Escharotic - A caustic or corrosive agent capable of producing an eschar or slough.

Etiology - The study of the cause of diseases. One of the aspects of a complete symptom.

Excitant - A medicine which causes excitation of the vital functions, as of the nervous (nervous excitant), muscular (motor excitant), circulatory (vaso-motor and cardiac excitants) systems.

Exostosis - Bone spurs.

Expectorant - An agent which promotes expectoration. Stimulant expectorants excite in atony while sedative expectorants allay irritation, both facilitating the expulsion of mucus from the lungs.

Expectoration - The ejection, by spitting of mucus, fluids secreted by the bronchials-lung tissue.

Extracts - These are prepared by evaporating the solutions, alcoholic or otherwise, of vegetable medicines at a low heat. They are either solid or semisolid in consistence. They are (1) *simple* or (2) *compound*. Dry extracts are fine dry powders. Examples: Powdered Extract of Cascara Sagrada.

Fag - Fatigue, exhaustion, weariness.

Febricula - A simple continued fever. A mild fever of short duration. Fever of indefinite origin, and without any distinctive pathology.

Febrifuge - An agent that will reduce temperature in fevers.

Felon - An abscess or inflammation of the finger tip, especially around the nail.

Fig wart - See Condylomata.

Fistula - An abnormal passage or communication, usually between two internal organs or leading from an internal organ to the surface of the body.

Flower essence - A general term for a liquid prepared by immersing a flower in water and then exposing it to sunlight or heat.

Fluid extracts - Fluid extracts are fluid alcoholic preparations of herbal products. Fluid extracts are concentrated tinctures. Alcohol constitutes the bulk of the solution, though water and glycerin, are often used with it. Prepared by percolation and subsequent concentration of a portion of the percolate by evaporation. Fluid extracts are so constructed as to represent one grain of the crude drug in each minim of fluid extract. They may be (1) *simple* or (2) *compound*. Examples: Fluid Extract of Lobelia or Sarsaparilla.

Fundamental remedies - The fundamental remedies give the personality types of the medicine. In some cases, the fundamental will be the same remedy as it is for the pathological layer. That is the first stage of development of a fixed pathology from a mutable one. The following list contains the major fundamental remedies: Arg-n., Ars., Aur., Bar-c., Calc., Calc-p., Carc., Caust., Cham., Graph., Ign., Kali-c., Lach., Lyc., Med., Merc., Nat-c., Nat-m., Nat-s., Nit-ac., Nux-v., Ph-ac., Phos., Plat., Psor., Puls., Rhus-t., Sep., Sil., Staph., Sulph., Tub.

Fungus hematode - A spongoid or soft cancer. A soft bleeding malignant tumor.

Homeopathic-Herbal Glossary

Furunculosis - Furunculosis crops of boils that occur over a period of time. The boils can develop continuously, or occur from time to time.

Galactagogue - An agent that stimulates the secretion or promotes the flow of milk.

Galactophyge - An agent that diminishes or arrests the flow of milk.

Galactorrhea - An excessive flow of milk.

Genus epidemicus - The group of symptoms which characterizes an epidemic. This 'symptom complex' is then used to select a particular homeopathic remedy which can be used both curatively and prophylactically during the epidemic.

Germicide - An agent destructive to germs or micro-organisms.

Glairy - Resembling the white of an egg, as in 'glairy mucus.'

Glandular fever - Infectious mononucleosis. An infectious disease with fever, swollen cervical lymph nodes and enlargement of liver or spleen.

Glossitis - Tongue inflammation, infection. It is an abnormality of the tongue that results from inflammation.

Glycerites - These are mixtures or solutions of medicines in glycerin. They are intended for both external, (chiefly) and internal exhibition. Example: Glyceritum Hydrastis.

Graves disease - Hyperthyroidism. It is a medical condition in which an overactive thyroid gland secretes an excess amount of thyroid hormone. As a result, there maybe an enlarged thyroid gland, palpitations, fast pulse, profuse sweating, high blood pressure, irritability, and a number of symptoms related to the eyes.

Hahnemann, Samuel - (April, 10, 1755-1843) The German physician who founded and brought to prominence Homeopathic Medicine.

Healing crisis - A temporary intensification of symptoms that occurs as part of the healing process - It occurs as the body detoxifies and rebalances.

Helminthiasis - The condition having intestinal worms.

Hematic (haematic) - An agent which improves the quality of the blood.

Hepatic - Refers to the liver. A remedy that stimulates the function of the liver.

Herbal tinctures - These are tinctures are alcoholic solutions of plant materials. Herbal tinctures are given as tonics to heal and regulate the organs and systems of the body. They are prepared by maceration. The plants are picked at the most harmonious time and chopped up and put into a glass bottle to which pure alcohol is added. Tinctures are almost identical in nature with fluid extracts. Tinctures made from fresh bruised or crushed herbs, by maceration, were known as Tincture Herbarum Recentium or Tinctures of Fresh Herbs. Tinctures are also (1) *simple* and (2) *compound*. Example: Alfalfa Tincture or Hoxsey formula.

Hering's Law of Cure - Three observations made by Constantine Hering, M.D. (1800-1880), who is considered "the father of American homeopathy": 1. The human body seeks to externalize disease, to dislodge it from more serious internal levels to more superficial external levels. Thus, someone with asthma may develop an external skin rash as part of the curative process. 2. Healing progresses from the top of the body to the bottom. Thus, someone with arthritis in many joints will generally notice relief in the upper part of the body before the lower part. 3. Healing proceeds in the reverse order of the symptoms. Thus, the most recent symptoms will generally be the first to be healed, and in the process of cure a person may re-experience previous symptoms.

Heroic Medicine - The practice of "conventional" medicine in both Europe and America during the 19th century is sometimes referred to as the age of 'heroic medicine' (because of the 'heroic' measures such as bleeding and purging).

Homeopathic Pharmacopeia of the United States (HPUS) - A compilation of standards for source, composition, and preparation of homeopathic drugs. It contains more than 1,300 "monographs" of ingredients used in homeopathic products. It is recognized as an official compendium under Section 201(j) of the Federal Food, Drug, and Cosmetic Act. The Homeopathic Pharmacopeia provides no information about the alleged uses of these substances. It merely states how plants, minerals, or other substances are processed into "medicinal" form.

Homeopathic remedies - Homeopathic remedies are energy medicines prescribed on the principle of similarity. Homeopathic remedies work by the principles of harmonic resonance. Their function is to neutralized disorders and to arouse the Vix Medicatrix Naturae, (the healing power of nature). Sympathy reflects the principle of likes cures likes. Remedies or treatments that are in opposition to the immune response are antipathic or allopathic.

Homeopathy - The treatment of disease by minute doses of natural substances that in a healthy person would produce similar symptoms. Homeopathy is a system of natural medicine developed by Samuel Hahnemann. The selection of the remedies is based on the Law of Similars (Like cures Like). Often contrasted with allopathy.

Homeopathic-Herbal Glossary

Homotoxicology - A system developed by German homeopath Hans Heinrich Reckeweg, who claimed that symptoms are the result of the body's attempt to use "homotoxins" to detoxify the body. Reckeweg developed many homeopathic mixtures said to enhance "homotoxin" production. He also claimed that his remedies can neutralize and excrete homotoxins.

Honeys - These are preparations related to the syrups, but differing in the substitution of clarified honey for syrup. Example: Mel Rosae. In ancient Egypt honey was a general remedy for many complaints such as burns, wounds, rashes, ulcers, sores, bites, etc.

Housemaid's knee - Synovitis, an inflammation and swelling of the bursa, just behind the knee-cap.

Hydragogue - An agent that causes watery discharge; especially a purge which produces watery catharsis.

Hydrocele - It is a collection of watery fluid around the testicle.

Hydrocephalus - An abnormal accumulation of fluid in the cerebral ventricles of the skull and compression of the brain. Also known as 'water on the brain'.

Hydrogenoid - An excess of water in the tissues and blood. Corresponds with the sycotic miasm.

Hypnotic - A medicine which induces sleep simulating that of normal slumber. Some pain relievers are also hypnotic, but true hypnotics only cause sleep.

Hypochondria - The section of the abdomen lying below the ribs.

Hypochondriac - Someone who is obsessive or anxious about health. Low spirits, fear, anxiety, especially about health.

Hysteria - Abnormal extreme emotional excitability, mania, overdramatic or attention-seeking behavior. The term was formerly regarded as a disease specific to women, from the Greek hustera, 'womb'.

Ichthyosis - Its literal translation is "fish skin." People with ichthyosis have scaly skin which can vaguely resemble the scales of a fish. The conditions are caused by genetic abnormalities. The term ichthyosis is sometimes used to mean the specific condition ichthyosis vulgaris. Ichthyosis was formerly referred to as "pseudo-leprosy," as it can produce an appearance superficially similar to that of leprosy.

Icterus - It is a synonym of jaundice. It is usually reserved for the discoloration of the conjunctiva which makes the sclera (whites of the eyes) appear yellow.

Ileus - Ileus, refers to limited or absent intestinal passage. Blocked intestines.

Impetigo - A contagious skin infection that usually produces blisters or sores on the face and hands. It is one of the most common skin infections among kids.

Imponderables - Homeopathic remedies made from energy sources are called the imponderables. Some examples are: Sol, (sunlight) and Luna, (moonlight), the Magnetic poles, Radiation, X-rays, Electricity, etc.

Indolent - Inactive, sluggish, painless, as in an indolent ulcer.

Infusions - Infusions are teas of the soluble herbs prepared usually by pouring upon the dried plant, hot water and allowing the product to macerate and cool. If the properties of the herb are impaired by hot water, cold water is employed. They are often prepared in the strength of one part of the plant to sixteen of parts of water. Unless otherwise specified they should be prepared of 1 part of herb to 15 to 20 parts of water for ordinary infusions. Infusions differ from decoctions in not being prepared by boiling.

Intussusception - It occurs when one portion of the bowel slides into the next, much like the pieces of a telescope. When this occurs, it creates an obstruction in the bowel, with the walls of the intestines pressing against one another. This, in turn, leads to swelling, inflammation, and decreased blood flow to the intestines involved.

Irritant - An agent which, when applied locally, excites hyperaemia or inflammation.

Isopathic remedies - These remedies are made from discharges, toxins, allergens and nosodes. Isopathic remedies help eliminate toxic chemicals and heavy metals.

Isopathy - Isopathy means giving a substance that is the same as the disease, which is slightly different from the principle of similars. A system which undertakes to cure a disease by means of the agent which causes the disease. While in certain aspects similar to homeopathy and often using homeopathically prepared substances, Isopathy bases the selection of remedies on the 'Law of Similars'.

Kala-azar - A chronic, often fatal disease occurring chiefly in Asia, caused by the protozoan parasite (Leishmania donovani) and characterized by irregular fever, enlargement of the spleen and liver, and emaciation.

Keloids - A special type of scar which results in an overgrowth of tissue at the site of a healed skin injury. Keloids are firm, rubbery lesions or shiny, fibrous nodules and can vary from pink to flesh-colored or red to dark brown in color.

Keynotes - A unique feature or fundamental aspect of a remedy. A keynote symptom is one which has been shown over time to appear in many different individuals who need the same certain remedy. Such a symptom then becomes associated with that remedy. When it appears strongly in an individual case, that remedy would be more strongly considered.

Koplik's spots - Small red spots on the mucous membrane of the mouth occurring early in measles.

Kwashiorkor - A malnutrition syndrome most commonly seen in children between the ages of 6 months to four years, and most prevalent in developing nations.

Laconic - Using very few words, terse.

Laryngismus - Laryngeal spasm caused by the sudden contraction of laryngeal muscles.

Lascivious - Excessive sexual desire and behavior. Lustful.

Law of Similars - See Similia.

Laxative - A medicine causing a mild and painless evacuation of the bowels.

Lead colic - Chronic intestinal pains and constipation caused by lead poisoning.

Lenitive - A medicine which has the soothing action of a demulcent on the internal membranes.

Leucoderma - see Vitiligo.

Leucoplakia - Irregular white patches on tongue.

Leucorrhea - A thick, whitish discharge from the vagina or cervical canal.

Life Force - See "Vital Force"

Liniments - These are fluid, or semifluid preparations, usually oleaginous, though alcohol or even water may be employed as the base, intended for external use, and to be applied with friction. Cotton seed or olive oil is usually preferred as a base. Some liniments are perfect solutions, while others are mixtures of soft solids, which liquefy at the temperature of the body, are also denominated liniments. Most liniments are designed to be rubbed into the skin.

LM potencies - The second potency scale developed by Hahnemann, introduced in the sixth edition of the Organon. Also called 50 millesimal or Q potencies. Start with a 3c triturate of a remedy. One part is placed into 500 drops liquid (4 parts water, 1 part pure alcohol 95%). One drop is placed into 2 ml pure alcohol. This is succussed by hand 100 times. One drop of this mixture is used to medicate 500 #10 pellets. This is the Lm 1 potency (sometimes written 0/1). The Lm 2 is made by taking 1 of these medicated pellet and placing it into 2 ml alcohol 95%. This mixture is succussed 100 times by hand."

Lochia - Discharge from the vagina of mucous, and tissue debris following childbirth.

Loquacious - Abnormally talkative.

Lotions - Lotions are solutions of medicinal bodies in water or other menstruum, designed chiefly to be applied to localized regions for their topical influence. They are (1) *simple* or (2) *compound.*

Lozenges - These are solid, candy-like masses, usually flattened and discoid or round or cylindrical in shape, composed of powdered drugs combined with sugar and mucilage and sometimes flavored. Lozenges are designed to influence the mouth or throat.

Lumbago - A term used to describe general lower back pain. The exact cause of the lumbago/back pain is maybe unknown. The back pain can come on after lifting things, or overuse or it may come on without previous exercise or training.

Lumbricoides - A parasitic round worm found in the human intestine.

Mania-a-potu - See Delirium tremens.

Marasmus - A form of severe protein malnutrition characterised by calorie deficiency and weakness. Some other conditions are emaciation, kwashiorkor and cachexia.

Materia Medica - In homeopathy the material medica refers to the written descriptions of the effects of homeopathic medicines. Literally meaning "medical material", it comprises hundreds of volumes of remedy descriptions. A reference book that lists the curative indications and therapeutic actions of homeopathic medicines. This information is derived from provings and clinical experience.

Meatus - An opening, passage or canal.

Melancholic - In ancient medicine melancholic was one of the four bodily humors, believed to be associated with a serious, sad, or depressed temperament. Melancholic is the temperment of an individual characterized by black bile; hence (Greek melas, "black", + kholé, "bile"). It also indicates the season of autumn (dry and cold) and the element of earth. A person who was a thoughtful ponderer had a melancholic disposition. Also can become overly obsessed on the tragedy and cruelty in the world, thus becoming depressed. A melancholic is also often a perfectionist, being very particular about what they want and how they want it in some cases.

Melancholy - A mental state characterized by a deep, pensive, and long-lasting sadness. A serious, sad, gloomy and depressive mood.

Menarche - The commencing of the menstrual cycle in a young girl.

Meniere's disease - A disorder of the inner ear that can affect hearing and balance. It is characterized by episodes of dizziness and tinnitus and progressive hearing loss, usually in one ear. It is caused by an increase in volume and pressure of the endolymph of the inner ear.

Miasms - These are the tendencies and predispositions to certain diseases, like allergies, infections or diseases. The term is used in homeopathy to describe an underlying pattern of weakness and susceptibility. As defined by Hahneman, miasms are the susceptibility principle, or diathesis, which, when taken into the organism that may set up a tendency towards specific diseases. Miasms may be inherited, aquired, or acute. Miasms can be dormant or active. Miasms may occur as the result of some suppressive theraphy like drugs or vaccinations. Hahnemann originally described them as inherited tendencies passed down from generation to generation. There are five major miasms: Psora, Cancer, Sycosis, Syphilis and the Tuberculosis miasm.

Milk fever - An elevation of temperature following childbirth, possibly due to the establishment of the secretion of milk.

Milk leg - A painful swelling of the leg occurring in women after childbirth as a result of clotting and inflammation of the femoral veins.

Minimum dose - The smallest dose or lowest potency of a similimum that will result in the most efficient healing with least aggravation.

Miotic (myotic) - A medicine which causes the pupil to contract (miosis).

Modality - A condition that makes a person or their symptom better or worse. (see Aggravation, Amelioration). For example, better in a hot bath, abdominal pain better while bending over, worse in rainy weather, etc. Modalities are one of the parts of a complete symptom in homeopathy.

Mongolism - see Down's Syndrome.

Monomania - In psychiatry, monomania (from Greek monos, one, and mania, mania) is a type of paranoia in which the patient has only one idea or type of ideas. Emotional monomania is that in which the patient is obsessed with only one emotion or several related to it. Intellectual monomania is that which is related to only one kind of delirious idea or ideas

Mother tincture - The starting alcoholic liquid from which homeopathic potencies are made. A solution of a substance in alcohol, that is not succussed but is used as the starting source for all homeopathic prepared liquid remedies.

Mucilages - More or less viscid, thick, and adhesive fluids. These are prepared by taking the mucilaginous constituents out with water or aqueous solutions of gums or of starch, as these bodies swell with water. Some are prepared with heat, while others are not. Mucilage of slippery elm, and some others, are best prepared with ice-cold water.

Mydriatic - An agent which dilates the pupil (mydriasis).

Myotic - See Miotic.

Myxedema - A skin and tissue disorder usually due to severe prolonged hypothyroidism. Hypothyroidism can be caused by Hashimoto's thyroiditis, surgical removal of the thyroid, and rarer conditions. Partial forms of myxedema, especially of the lower legs (called pre-tibial myxedema], occasionally occur in adults with Graves' disease or Hashimoto's thyroiditis without severe hypothyroidism

Narcotic - A drug that will induce stuporous sleep, at the same time relieving pain and abolishing consciousness.

Naturopathy - A medical approach to natural healing that uses many different modalities. Naturopaths may use homeopathic remedies in addition to other methods. The initials N.D. stand for Doctor of Naturopathy.

Night terrors - A type of severe nightmare often seen in children.

Night-watching - Staying up at night to care for the sick or for an ailing loved one. An inability to sleep, wherein a person is alert and restless at night. Insomnia due to keeping late nights, nursing of sick ones, nursing of others, night work, etc.

Noli-me-tangere - A form of malignant epithelial ulcer found in many tissues and bones most commonly on the face.

Nosode - The word "Nosode" comes from a Greek root word for disease. In the ancient days "Nosocomium" was the name for a hospital. Homeopathic remedies made from pathological organs or tissues; causative agents such as bacteria, fungi, ova, parasites, virus particles and yeast; disease products; or excretions. Some nosode remedies: Anthracinum, Bacill., Carcinosin, Diptherinum, Hippozenin., Lyssin, Malandrin., Medorr., Ocillococcinum, Pestinum, Psorinum, Pyrogen, Secale, Staphylococcinum, Streptococcinum, Syphilinum, Tuber. aviaire, Tuberculinum, Ustilago maidis, Vaccininum, Variolinum.

Nostrums - It is a medicine whose efficacy maybe questionable and whose ingredients are usually kept secret. In ancient times, patent medicines were called nostrum remedium, "our remedy" in Latin, hence the name "nostrum."

Nymphomania - An abnormal, uncontrollable or excessive sexual desire in a woman. (see Satyriasis).

Occipital - Pertaing to the back of the head.

Oils - Solids, semi-solids, and fluid, greasy and water insoluble preparations obtained by expression. Some oils were extracted by the methods of maceration and distillation. Oils were a part of Egyptian Medicine, the two important ones were Castor Oil and Olive Oil. Edgar Cayce recommended Castor oil to be rubbed in arthritic or sore joints and muscles.

Ointments - Some contain either one or more of the following: glycerin, wax, paraffin, expressed oil of almond, according to the use to be made of them. When applied to the skin they are softened and rendered fluid by the heat of the body. They may be medicated or unmedicated. Ointments are applied generally by to irritated areas of the skin. Chapped skin, burns, sores, etc. Example: Calendula ointment.

Onychia - Inflammation of the nail bed with loss of nail.

Oophoritis - An inflammation of the ovaries.

Opisthotonos - The back muscles, the head and lower limbs are bent backward and the trunk is arched forward caused by a tetanic spasm.

Orchititis - A very painful condition of the testicles involving inflammation, swelling and frequently infection.

Organ remedies - Herbal tonics for the organs. Some herbal remedies have strong affinities for certain organs, such as Chelidonium for the liver, Crataegus for the heart, Avena for the brain, Lobelia for the lungs, Echinacea for the blood, Ceanothus for the spleen, Equisteum for the kidneys. These organ remedies should be given in drop doses of the tincture, five to twenty five drops per dose.

Organon - The Organon of Medicine is the title of Samuel Hahnemann's book outlining the principles of homeopathy. Hahneman was the "re-discoverer" of modern homeopathy and his book was written in six editions over a thirty two year period. The final addition was finished in 1842. This book describes the principles and practice of homeopathy. Hahnemann wrote six editions of the Organon from 1810-1842. The sixth edition, though finished in 1842, was not published until 1921.

Osgood-schlatter's disease - An inflammation of the growth plate at the tibial tuberosity. It is one of a group of conditions called Osteochondritis. The disease is most common in boys aged 10-14.

Osteitis deformans - See Paget's disease.

Osteomalacia - See Rickets.

Osteoporosis - Osteoporosis is a disease of bone in which the bone mineral density (BMD) is reduced. Osteoporotic bones are more susceptible to fracture. Due to its hormonal component, more women, particularly after menopause, suffer from osteoporosis than men. In addition it may be caused by various hormonal conditions, smoking and medications (specifically glucocorticoids).

Otosclerosis - A hardening of the tissues in the inner ear.

Oxytocic - A drug which accelerates or hastens the process of delivery in childbirth.

Paget's disease - Otherwise known as osteitis deformans, is a chronic disorder that typically results in enlarged and deformed bones. It is named after Sir James Paget, the British surgeon who first described this disease. The excessive breakdown and formation of bone tissue that occurs with Paget's disease can cause bone to weaken, resulting in bone pain, arthritis, deformities, and fractures.

Paget's disease, breast - Disease of the breast areola preceding cancer of the breast. Paget's disease of the breast, also known as Paget's disease of the nipple, is a condition that outwardly may have the appearance of eczema with skin changes involving the nipple of the breast. Because of its seemingly innocuous and surface appearance, it often presents late.

Painter's colic - Colic, spasms and pain of the stomach due to lead poisoning.

Palliation - Palliation (from Latin palliare, to cloak) is any form of medical care or treatment that concentrates on reducing the severity of the symptoms of a disease, or slow the disease's progress, rather than provide a cure. However, it may occasionally be used in conjunction with curative therapy, providing that the curative therapy will not cause additional morbidity. It aims at improving quality of life, by reducing or eliminating pain and other physical symptoms, enabling the patient to ease or resolve psychological and spiritual problems, and supporting the partner and family.

Pannus - A medical term for a hanging flap of skin. It is usually found in the abdomen of people who have recently lost a significant amount of weight. Pannus is commonly referred to as "fat folds" or "rolls."

Papilloma – A benign, circumscribed skin tumor projecting from the surrounding surface.

Paralyzant - A drug that causes temporary functional paralysis of some part of the body.

Parturifacient - A medicine that induces or facilitates childbirth.

Parturuition - Childbirth, giving birth.

Partus praeparator - An agent that strengthens preparatory to labor.

Patent medicines - (See Nostrums). Patent medicine is the term given to various medical compounds sold under a variety of names and labels, though they were for the most part actually trademarked medicines, not patented.

Pathological remedies - These remedies are given for their similarity to the disease, as opposed to the fundamental and constitutional remedies which are aimed at the person in general. Pathological states are not limited to physical diseases alone. Mental and emotional diseases can form pathological layers and diseases. Examples are depression, mania, personality disorders, senility, violence behavior, insanity, etc.

Pellagra - A vitamin deficiency disease caused by dietary lack of niacin (vitamin B3) and protein, especially proteins containing the essential amino acid tryptophan.

Pertussis - see Whooping cough.

Phimosis - A medical condition in which the foreskin of the penis of an uncircumcised male cannot be fully retracted.

Phlebitis - An inflammation of a vein, usually in the legs.

Phlegmasia alba dolens - See Milk leg.

Phlegm - The thick viscous substance secreted by the mucous membranes of the respiratory passages, esp. when produced in excessive or abnormal quantities, e.g., when someone is suffering from a cold.

Phlegmatic - In ancient medicine phlegmatic was one of the four bodily humors, believed to be associated with a calm, stolid, or apathetic temperament. Phlegmatic means pertaining to phlegm, corresponds to the season of winter (wet and cold), and connotes the element of water. Having a slow, sluggish, apathetic temperment, unemotional. A phlegmatic person is calm and unemotional.

Pityriasis - Shedding of the skin in fine flaky scales.

Placenta praevia - A placeta which has superimposed itself upon and around the internal opening f the vagina causing bleeding during labor.

Plant juices - A succus is fresh plant juice preserved in alcohol. Example: Calendula Succus, and Cineria Maritima.

Plasters - These are tenacious substances usually spread upon some kind of pliable skin or fabric, and intended to be applied to the exterior of the body either for purposes of counter irritation or as simple adhesives. They require heat to spread them. When applied to the body they adhere but do not become soft. They are composed chiefly of some resinous body and may be simple or medicated. Commercial plasters have largely supplanted those prepared by the ordinary pharmacist. Examples: Emplastrum Capsicum or Mustard.

Plica polonica - A matted condition of the hair caused by filth and neglect.

Plussing - A method, of which there are several variations, to slightly increase the potency or quantity of a remedy administered in water. Plussing means one takes a few drops and then dilutes and shakes the remedy each time before he takes it again.

Polycrest remedies - This is the group of often used remedies, they are the polycrests. "Poly" means "many" and "crest" means "time." The polycrests are the most often prescribed remedies for: acute, chronic, emergency, fundamental, pathological and constitutional remedies. It is good to learn the polycrest remedies first when studying homeopathic medicine.

Potions - A liquid with healing, magical, or poisonous properties. Example: *a love potion.*

Potency - The power, vitality, or strength which a homeopathic possesses. Determined by how many times the remedy has been succussed and diluted during preparation. A number and a letter are associated with the remedy name to indicate which potency scale has been used. An example of the decimal scale would be Arnica 6x. An example of the centesimal scale would be Arnica 6c. An example of the 50 millesimal scale (Lm) would be Arnica Lm 6. These are the three major potency scales currently in use.

Potentization - Usually refers to a substance prepared according to homeopathic pharmaceutical standards. This means that it has gone through a series dilutions and succussions.

Pott's disease - Tuberculosis spondlylitis. Weakness and collapse of spinal vertebrae due to tuberculosis.

Poultices - A poultice is formed of such substances as, when wet, will be more or less tenacious, and will accommodate themselves to parts to which they are applied. They are employed to soften and relax the tissues, and at the same time exclude the air, to stimulate, induce hyperemia, or to apply counterirritants. A poultice should be prepared from flax seed, oats, elm, bread, bran or meal, as desired, by gradually adding them to hot water in a hot vessel, and spreading them in convenient thickness upon a hot fabric with a hot knife or spatula. Examples: Oat meal, Linseed, Flaxseed Poultice.

Prana - This term refers to the breath, vital force, qi or vital energy.

Prana remedies - Homeopathic and herbal remedies are pure prana remedies. These remedies contain prana or qi, (chi), they also affect the seven pranas of the body. When prana is suspended in a fluid or dry medium it can be potentized through a series of dilutions and succusions. The higher the potency means the prana of the remedy has become purer and more exalted in its healing energy, therefore these remedies work deeper and last alot longer in their action. Prana remedies have gentle power to restore or to heal. Prana remedies facilitate the self-restoration and healing processes.

Priapism - A persistant abnormal and painful erection of the penis due to disease and not provked by sexual desire.

Proctitis - Inflammation of rectum.

Prophylactic remedies - These are remedies that are given to prevent diseases. Prophylactic remedies are given to prevent acute and epidemic diseases. Prophylactic treatment can also be given to prevent any disease from returning.

Proving - A homeopathic proving is an experiment undertaken by a group of healthy individuals in order to test the medicinal effects of a particular substance. After taking one or more doses of the remedy, the symptoms produced are recorded, collated and organized into a comprehensive description of the action of the remedy. Provings can also happen during the therapeutic process if the patient is very sensitive, or by repeating an incorrect remedy too often. Proving symptoms usually disappear of their own accord after a little time has passed.

Prurigo - A term used to describe skin eruptions.

Psoric miasm - According to Hahnemann, Psora is the original miasm or inherited disposition that is shared by most of humanity. It is represented by intense itching and is often correlated with scabies. *Psora is the tendency to get sick is due to poor living habits* that are perpetuated from generation to generation. It has a tendency towards nutritional, allergic, digestive and skin disorders. Poor hygiene leads to psoric diseases and conditions.

Ptosis - Drooping of upper eyelid; prolapse or falling down of an organ part.

Puerperal fever - Also called childbed fever, is caused by infection of the genital tract shortly after giving birth. Any fever within two weeks of childbirth is dangerous since it can cause infertility or septicemia. Puerperal fever is now rare due to improved hygiene during delivery, and deaths have been reduced.

Purgative - A cathartic. An agent that will cause evacuation of the contents of the bowels.

Pustulant - An agent that attacks isolated areas of the skin, as the sudoriferous glands, causing pustules (pustulation).

Q potencies - (see LM potencies).

Quartan - Occurring every fourth day (especially the fever and weakness of malaria)

Quinsy - Peritonsillar abscess, quinsy also called PTA a recognised complication of tonsillitis and consists of a collection of pus beside the tonsil (peritonsillar space).

Quotidian - Recurring daily. Term used relating to attacks of malaria.

Rachitis - Inflammation of spine, rickets.

Raynaud's disease - A condition that affects blood flow to the extremities which include the fingers, toes, nose and ears when exposed to temperature changes or stress. It was named after Maurice Raynaud.

Refrigerant - An agent which imparts a cooling sensation to the mucosa and allays thirst; externally it cools by evaporation.

Reiter syndrome - Reiter's syndrome is a disorder that causes three seemingly unrelated symptoms: arthritis, redness of the eyes, and urinary tract signs.

Remedy - A medicine, application, or treatment that relieves or cures a disease. A homeopathic or herbal medicine. Something that corrects or counteracts.

Repertory - An index of the homeopathic materia medica by symptom or clinical topic. A list of remedies is indicated for each symptom. It is an exhaustive list of symptoms, each of which is followed by a list of remedies that have either produced the symptom during a proving or cured it clinically.

Rescue Remedy - A combination of Bach Flower Remedies used for emergencies and shocks. Bach discovered a unique combination of five remedies which aim at restoring balance and calm to a person in acute emergency situations. Rescue remedy is of great value immediately after accidents or similar moments of shock and panic when there is faintness, trembling, or other failing of normal physical functioning. Rescue Remedy cream is very effective as a topic applications for stings, bites, chapped skin, sores, etc. Rescue Remedy contains the following flower remedies: Star of Bethlehem, Rock Rose, Cherry Plum, Impatiens, and Clematis.

Restorative - An herbal agent that restores to consciousness, or one that aids in restoring tone, function, vigor, or health.

Reyes syndrome - A potentially fatal disease that causes numerous detrimental effects to many organs, especially the brain and liver. All body organs are affected, research has established a link between Reye's syndrome and the use of aspirin and other salicylate containing medications.

Rickets - Osteomalacia, also known as rickets, is among the most frequent childhood diseases in developing countries. The predominant cause is a vitamin D deficiency, but lack of adequate calcium in the diet may also lead to rickets. Although it can occur in adults, the majority of cases occur in children suffering from severe malnutrition, usually resulting from famine or starvation during the early stages of childhood.

Rigors - Coldness experienced will shivering.

Ringworm - see Tinea.

Rosacea - Vascular dilation involving the skin on nose and cheeks.

Roseola - Roseola is a benign disease of children, generally under two years old. It symptoms are usually limited to a transient rash ("exanthum") that occurs following a fever of about three day's duration. Exanthem subitum (meaning sudden rash), also referred to as roseola infantum (or rose rash of infants), sixth disease and (confusingly) baby measles.

Rubefacient - An agent which, when locally applied, reddens the skin.

Rubric - A rubric is a listing in the homeopathic repertory. Under this symptom may be listed any number of remedies which have produced and/or cured this symptoms. An example would be "Vertigo, eating after."

Salpingitis - The inflammation of the fallopian tubes.

Sanguine - In ancient medicine sanguine was one of the four bodily humors, believed to be associated with a optimistic, cheerful, confident, rational, popular, and fun-loving temperament. Cheerfully optimistic, or having the constitution associated with the predominance of blood among the bodily humors. Sanguine indicates the personality of an individual with the temperament of blood, the season of spring (wet and hot), and the element of air.

Sarcodes - A tissue or glandular extract made into a homeopathic remedy. The term "sarcodes" is useful for designating the remedies prepared from healthy tissues and organs. This is in contrast to a nosode, taken from diseased tissue. They are often used as "organ" remedies, to help stimulate or regulate the organs or glands. The auto-sarcodes are also in this group. The blood, urine, mucus and discharges are also part of the materia medica.

Sarcoidosis - Involves inflammation that produces tiny lumps of cells in various organs in your body. The lumps are called granulomas because they look like grains of sugar or sand. They are very small and can be seen only with a microscope.

Sarcoma - A general class of uncommon cancers in which the cancer cells arise from or resemble normal cells in the body known as "connective tissues"

Satyriasis - An excessive, uncontrollable sexual desire in men.

Scabies - A common skin infection that causes small itchy bumps and blisters due to tiny mites that burrow into the top layer of human skin to lay their eggs.

Scirrhus - Scirrhus hard tumor.

Scleroderma - A rare, chronic disease characterized by excessive deposits of collagen. Progressive systemic scleroderma or systemic sclerosis, the generalised type of the disease, can be fatal. The localised type of the disease tends not to be fatal. The term "localised, generalised scleroderma" can be used to describe cases where the disease covers a large area of the body, typically more than 40%.

Scrofula - (Scrophula or Struma). Refers to a variety of skin diseases, in particular, a form of tuberculosis, affecting the lymph nodes of the neck. In adults it is caused by Mycobacterium tuberculosis and in children by nontuberculous mycobacteria. The word comes from the Latin scrofulae, meaning brood sow.

Seborrhea - Seborrhea dermatitis is a skin disorder affecting the scalp, face and trunk causing scaly, flaky, itchy, red skin. It particularly affects the sebum-gland rich areas of skin.

Sedative - A drug that allays or calms excitement.

Sensation - the experience of a symptom, what it feels like. One of the parts of a complete symptom.

Septicemia - The presence of bacteria in the blood (bacteremia) and is often associated with severe fever and disease.

Similia similibus curentur - These words were first coined by Paracelsus, a medical alchemist of the 16th century. The similarity principle that "like cures like", upon which Homeopathic treatment is based. Law of Similars is the principle tenet of homeopathy stating that a substance which is capable of inducing a symptom or set of symptoms in a healthy individual has the curative power to eliminate similar symptoms when they manifest in an individual as part of a disease state.

Simillimum - The most similar remedy corresponding to a case. As such, the remedy most likely to cure. A remedy that most closely matches the symptom picture of the patient. Simila similibus curentur (Let like be cured with like). The concept of the simillimum refers to a homeopathic remedy that perfectly matches the state of an individual for whom it is prescribed.

Somnambulism - Sleepwalking.

Somnifacient - An agent which induces sleep. A hypnotic herb or drug.

Spagyric - This word was coined by Paracelsus, a medical alchemist of the 16th century. Spagyria is from two Greek words, 'spao', to draw out, to extract, to divide and 'ageiro' to bind, join, combine, gather. The spagyric art translates as plant alchemy, the art of separating, exalting and recombining medicinal herbs and roots. Traditionally, these remedies prepared in strict accordance with ancient alchemical principles. Each of these formulated tinctures contains the purified salts, oil, and natural alcohol of the herbs.

Specific - An agent supposed to have a selective curative action in a special disease, or in some phases of disease.

Sternutatory - An agent that excites sneezing.

Stimulant - An agent that excites functional activity. Stimulants are diffusible when they excite the circulation and general functions of the body; nervous, when they act chiefly upon the nerve centers; hepatic, when they arouse the functions of the liver; cardiac, when they increase the heart's action; gastric, when they quicken digestion; respiratory, when they increase respiratory movements; etc. Also applied to medicines in which the action of the contained ethyl alcohol is desired,

Stomatitis - Stomatitis, or viral stomatitis, is a common infection in kids, usually between ages one to two years or so. The child will typically run a fair amount of fever, drool quite a bit, and will be very uncomfortable.

Strabismus - Also known as "heterotropia", "squint", "crossed eye", "cockeyed', "wandering eye", or "wall eyed." It is a condition in which the eyes are not properly aligned with each other. It typically involves a lack of coordination between the extraocular muscles which prevents bringing the gaze of each eye to the same point in space, preventing proper binocular vision, which may adversely affect depth perception.

Strange, Rare and Peculiar - A homeopathic term referring to symptoms that are unique to the individual. They refer to symptoms that sound odd or out of context. An example might be if someone describes their headache "as if my head were made of glass and could shatter at any second." Most people would not say this.

Styptic - A local agent that, through a strongly astringent action, will arrest bleeding.

Succussion - This is one way of making a homeopathic remedy. It involves striking the bottle of homeopathic medicine firmly against an object such as a thick book. Proponents claim that this "releases energy" that "potentizes" the mixture for each dilution and that the process and outcome differ from that of ordinary serial dilution. The c potency is succussed 100 times per dilution. In the 3c potency, the original substance is diluted 1part to 100, and then shaken 100 times. This process is repeated 3 times.

Sudorific - An agent that will cause active or droplet perspiration, a more intense action than that of the ordinary diaphoretic.

Suppression - The driving inward of a disease, so that a person experiences more serious symptoms than originally, causing a deterioration of health.

Susceptibility - Vunerability, sensitivity to catching a disease. Tendency to catch certain diseases.

Sycotic miasm - Syscosis. A sycosis miasm is a weakness related to the history of gonorrhea in the family or person. The skin is stimulated in an unnatural way to produce growth of all sizes and shapes. These growths are usually benign, but they can be cancerous later; i.e., all types of warts, moles, discoloration of the skin, especially brown spots, birth marks, liver spots, polyps, lymphomas, cysts, nodules, skin tags, etc. Also excess discharges from the mucous membranes. The suppression of moles, warts, and their removal, including cysts, leads to problems. These growths occur where they do because these areas are weak; surgery to remove them insults and traumatizes a weak area. The sycosis type patient is less healthy, their minds are more foggy and spacey, and then these growths appear.

Symptom - Any change in the body's functioning on a mental, emotional , or physical level. Usually associated with a particular disease or a specific stress.

Synthetic remedies - These remedies are prescribed when the symptoms of two different mineral remedies appear in the same case. For example, when a case looks like Calc-carb., and Phos., one should consider giving Calc-phos., which is the synthetic form of the other two remedies. Calc-phos. in some cases will do more healing than either the Calc-carb. or the Phos., could do separately. Many mineral remedies exist naturally combined as salts. Natrum mur. is a synthetic or combined form of sodium and chloride. The general energy of the sodium and chloride portions of salt are combined in Natrum mur.

Syphilis miasm - The main idea of syphilis is destructiveness. It's a destructive and usually attacks the nervous system, the brain, the bones, also the mental and emotional state. Syphilis has *severe* phobias, neurotic behavior, anxieties, and the indicated remedies aren't working. *Worse from sunset to sunrise*. The neuralgias, bone pains, depression, insomnia are worse at night. Alcoholism, depression, insanity.

Syrups - These are concentrated aqueous solutions of sugar or thick solutions of sugar in aqueous medicated or flavoring solutions. They are (1) *simple,* (2) *medicated*, or (3) *flavored*. Examples: Syrupus Pruni Virginianæ, Syrupus Aurantii.

Tabes dorsalis - see Locomotor Ataxia.

Tabes mesenterica - Tuberculosis of the abdominal mesenteric glands.

Taeniacide (Taenicide) - An agent that will kill and expel the tapeworm.

Taenifuge (Taeniafuge) - An agent that will expel the tapeworm.

Tautopathy - This term applies to a method of homeopathic prescribing. Tautopathic means using the 'same' substance potentised as a remedy (rather than a 'similar' substance). These are mainly remedies made from allopathic drugs or toxic chemicals. Tautopathics are made from cortisone, morphine, penicillin, histamine, etc. If there is a strong history that a certain drug caused a person's condition then one should consider giving a tautopathic remedy.

Tenesmus - Ineffective straining at stool or while urinating.

Tertian fever - A fever caused by malaria parasites with a periodicity of 48 hours.

Thrombosis - The formation of a clot or thrombus inside a blood vessel, obstructing the flow of blood through the circulatory system.

Thrush - A disorder caused by infection of the mouth with the fungus (yeast) Candida albicans.

Tic douloureux - A twitching facial neuralgia.

Tincture - An alcoholic extract (e.g. of an herb) or solution of a nonvolatile substance. Solutions of volatile substances were called spirits, although that name was also given to several other materials obtained by distillation, even when they did not include alcohol.

Tinea - A skin infection with a dermatophyte (ringworm) fungus.

Tinnitus - The perception of sound in the absence of a corresponding external sound. It can be perceived in one or both ears or in the head. Tinnitus is the Latin word for "ringing", and usually it is described as a ringing noise, but in some patients it takes the form of a buzzing, hissing, humming, or whistling sound, ticking, clicking, roaring, "crickets," tunes, songs, or beeping. It has also been described as a "whooshing" sound, as of wind or waves.

Tissue salts - A set of 12 mineral salts created by a German homeopath, W. H. Schuessler, in the late 19th century. These are the Schussler's Tissue Salts that are used for treating organ, blood and biochemical disorders. Cell or tissue salts are some of the major minerals found in the body. Biochemic remedies are usually given in a low potency, such as 6x or 12x, three times a day, over a long period of time, i.e. months. These cell salts restore organ functions because of their ability to balance the biochemistry of the blood. The twelve biochemic remedies are mineral tonics to the blood, organs and tissues: Calc-fl., Calc-p., Calc-s., Ferr-p., Kali-m., Kali-p., Kali-s., Mag-p., Nat-m., Nat-p., Nat-s., Sil.

Tonic - A medicinal substance taken to give a feeling of vigor or well-being. An agent which tends to produce or restore normal tone to the functions and tissues of the body. Something with an invigorating effect.

Torticollis - Commonly known as "wry neck." It is a deformity of the neck in which the head tilts toward one shoulder and is simultanously the chin rotates toward the opposite shoulder.

Totality of Symptoms - The complete set of mental, emotional, and physical manifestations of an individual's illness. The totality of symptoms is a somewhat scientific and somewhat artistic method of determining which symptoms represent the entire state of the vital disturbance of the patient. It does not simply mean taking all the symptoms and adding them together. It means taking all the important symptoms without including too much or too little.

Tourette's syndrome - Tourette's is an inherited neurological disorder, characterized by the presence of multiple physical (motor) tics and at least one vocal (phonic) tic. These tics characteristically wax and wane. Involuntary repetition of a word, or of vulgar words.

Toxicology - The study of toxins, poisons and the poisonous effects of plants or drugs. It includes their description, detection, symptoms, antidotes, antagonists, and treatment.

Trituration - This is a method for preparing a homeopathic remedy. The crude substance is mixed with milk sugar and ground together in a mortar and pestle for 20 minutes. Triturations containing one part in ten are named the first decimal triturations, the 1x potency. One part of the 1x with nine parts of milk sugar, becomes the second decimal, the 2x potency, etc. Triturations containing one part in a hundred are named the first centismal triturations, the 1c potency. One part of the foregoing with ninety nine parts of milk sugar, becomes the second centismal, 2c potency, etc.

Tuberculosis miasm - A weakness in the lungs and respiratory tract. That means there's a *tendency to respiratory infections*. Colds, sore throats, swollen glands, and bronchitis, asthma, pneumonia, and emphysema. Weight loss, night sweats. People who sweat a lot, especially with fevers. Tendency to catch colds, and influenzas.

Tympanites - Bloating of the belly caused by excess gas.

Undulant fever - Undulating degrees of temperature with enlargement of the spleen, profuse sweating and painful joints.

Uremia - A toxic condition resulting from renal failure, when kidney function is compromised and urea, a waste product normally excreted in the urine, is retained in the blood. Uremia can lead to disturbances in the platelets and hypersomnia, among other effects.

Urticaria - Edematous hives or rashes. often due to an allergic reaction.

Vaccinia - Vaccinia virus is a large, complex enveloped virus belonging to the poxvirus family of viruses. Vaccinia virus is well-known for its role as a vaccine that eradicated the smallpox disease from our world, making it the first human disease to be successfully eradicated by mankind.

Vaccinosis - Ill effects of vaccines on healthy persons. A state of being never well since recieving vaccinations.

Vaginismus - A condition which affects a woman's ability to have sexual intercourse, insert tampons and undergo gynecological examinations. This is the result of a conditioned muscle reflex of the pubococcygeus muscle in which they clamp shut, making penetration either extremely painful or impossible. The severity of vaginismus varies from woman to woman.

Vapor medicines - These are usually employed as *inhalations*, or as *steaming vapors*. Medicated steam produced by means of atomization, with a spray-apparatus, nebulizer or any other means. Lobelia was a famous vapor remedy, the herb was put into boiling water, while the patient put a towel over their head as they inhaled the lobelia vapors. This was effective for asthma, coughs, colds, bronchitis, pneumonia, lung disorders, etc. Also, the homeopathic and bach flower remedies can be inhaled into the nose as vapor medicines. Ancient Egyptians used a bowl with a straw holed lid to swallow the vaporous herbal remedies.

Varicella - Chickenpox. An acute contagious disease, usually occurring in children, caused by the varicella-zoster virus, a member of the family Herpesviridae, and marked by a sparse eruption of papules, which become vesicles and then pustules, like that of smallpox although less severe and varying in stages, usually with mild constitutional symptoms. Incubation period is about 14 to 17 days.

Variocele - Varicose veins of the testes. Varicosities of the scrotal veins forming a soft, elastic swelling which feels like a collection of worms, causing a painful and weighty sensation.

Venesection - Opening a vein to let blood out. Bloodletting.

Vermicide - A medicine that will kill intestinal worms.

Vermifuge - A medicine that will cause the expulsion of intestinal worms.

Verruca - A common wart. Verruca vulgaris

Vesicant - A drug which causes blistering (vesication).

Vinegars - Acetums are vinegars that are filtered solutions of the active constituents of botanicals in diluted acetic acid. Certain remedies, such as Lobelia and Sanguinaria are excellent Acetum medicines. Vinegar was formerly and to some extent is still is used in many excellent products. Examples: Acetum Lobelia, Acetum Sanguinaria.

Vital Force - The concept of the Vital force is central to homeopathic philosophy. The Vital Force is the life energy that keeps us alive and breathing. It is the energy that helps us grow and evolve. In homeopathy, we become sick when the Vital Force become "mistuned" or misdirected. The correct homeopathic remedy will "retune" us.

Vitiligo - Vitiligo or leukoderma is a chronic skin condition that causes loss of pigment, resulting in irregular pale patches of skin. The precise etiology of vitiligo is not fully understood. There is some evidence suggesting it is caused by a combination of auto-immune, genetic and environmental factors.

Waterbrash - Heartburn, rising of water from the stomach into the mouth.

Waters - Medicated Waters are solutions of volatile substances, usually of oils or camphors, in water. Aromatic Waters are solutions prepared by several methods, as by direct solution in hot or cold water or by filtering water through some inert powder or cotton impregnated with the volatile body. These waters are employed chiefly as vehicles for other medicines. Example: Aqua Menthæ Piperitæ.

Whitlow - An inflammation around the nail which may be deep seated, effecting the bone.

Whooping cough - An acute infectious disease marked by recurrent attacks of spasmodic coughing continued until the breath is exhausted, then ending with a deep, noisy inspiration.

Wines - Medicated Wines are fluid preparations, in which the soluble medicinal principles are dissolved in or extracted with wine.

Wry neck - See Torticollis.

Xanthopsia - Yellow vision. Sometimes occurs with jaundice.

Xerostomia - Dry mouth due to lack of saliva.

Yellow saddle - A yellowish discoloration of the skin over the bridge of the nose. A well known symptom of the remedy Sepia.

Zona - See Herpes zoster.

Zymosis - Fermentation. An infection due to a fungus. Prostration and septicemia.

Zymotic fever - Zymotic diseases (for the Greek term zumoun for "ferment"), an obsolete term in medicine, formerly applied to the class of acute infectious maladies, presumed to be due to some virus or organism which acts in the system like a ferment. The term, however, came to be restricted in medical nomenclature to the chief fevers and contagious diseases (e.g. typhus and typhoid fevers, smallpox, scarlet fever, measles, erysipelas, cholera, whooping-cough, diphtheria.

1-800-Homeopathy, US - PO Box 8080. Richford, VT, USA 05476. (800)Homeopathy. (877)999-0090 (fax). info@1800homeopathy.com. www.1-800homeopathy.com.

A. Nelson & Co. Ltd, UK - 5 Endeavour Way, London SW19 9UH, tel: 0208 946 8527.

Abha Light Foundation, Kenya - PO Box 471-00606. Nairobi, Kenya. telephone: (+254 20) 4450181. cell phones (+254) 733-895466/0723-869133. www.abhalight.org. www.abhalight.org/college.

Academy of Classical Homeopathy, UK - 11 Steyning Close, Crawley, Sussex RH10 8HR, tel 01293 547185, mail@achom.co.uk

Academy of Veterinary Homeopathy, US - PO Box 9280. Wilmington, DE, USA 19809. (866)652-1590. (866)652-1590 (fax). office@theavh.org. www.theavh.org.

Ainsworths Homeopathic Pharmacy, UK - 36 Cavendish Street, London W1M 7LH, tel 0207 935 5330, fax 0207 486 4313; enquiries@ainsworths.com.

Allen Academy, US - 2321 Fells Ln., Wilmington DE, USA 19808. 302-994-6838. rbann@delanet.com.

Allen College of Homeopathy, UK - 382 Baddow Road, Great Baddow. Chelmsford, Essex, UK, CM2 9RA. 44 (0) 1245 505858. Fax: 44 (0) 1245 505859. allencollege@btinternet.com.

Alliance of Registered Homeopaths, UK - Millbrook, Millbrook Hill, Nutley, East Sussex, UK TN22 3PJ. tel/fax: 08700 736339 (Remedy). info@a-r-h.org

Alternative Medicine College of Canada, Canada - 1120 East, Belanger Street, Montreal, Quebec, H2S 1H4. Tel.: 1 (514) 990-5229. Toll Free Telephone (Canada Only): 1-800-663-8380. Fax: (514) 278-2637. www.alternativemedicinecollege.com.

Alternativa Publishing Ltd., Czech Republic - Elišky Přemyslovny 380, 156 00 Prague 16, Czech Republic, fax: +420 257 921631, e-mail: info@alternativa.cz, http://www.autopathy.info.

American Association of Homeopathic Pharmacists, US - 5112 Wilshire Dr. Santa Rosa, CA, USA 95404. (800)478-0421. (800)478-0421 (fax). info@homeopathyresource.org. www.homeopathyresource.org.

American Botanical Council, US - 6200 Manor Rd, Austin, TX 78723. Phone: 512-926-4900 | Fax: 512-926-2345. Website: www.herbalgram.org. Email: abc@herbalgram.org

American Herbal Pharmacopoeia, US - PO Box 66809 Scotts Valley, CA. 95067. Telephone: 831-461-6318. Fax: 831-475-6219. Email: admin@herbal-ahp.org

American Herbal Products Association, US - 8484 Georgia Ave., Suite 370. Silver Spring, MD 20910. Phone: (301) 588-1171. Fax: (301) 588-1174. Email: ahpa@ahpa.org.

American Herbalists Guild, 141 Nob Hill Road, Cheshire, CT 06410. Phone: 203.272.6731. Fax: 203.272.8550. Email: ahgoffice@earthlink.net.

American Institute of Homeopathy, US - 801 N Fairfax St Ste 306. Alexandria, VA, USA 22314-1757. (888)445-9988. (888)445-9988 (fax). aih@homeopathyusa.org. www.homeopathyusa.org.

American Medical College of Homeopathy, US - 2001 W. Camelback Rd. Suite 150, Phoenix, AZ 85015.

American University of Complementary Medicine, US - 11543 Olympic Blvd. Los Angeles, CA, USA 90064. (310)914-4116. (310)479-3376 (fax). marketing@aucm.org. www.aucm.org.

Apothecary Homeopathic Pharmacy, UK - Morthen Road, Wickersley, Rotherham, South Yorkshire S66 OBU. tel 01709 531177, 01709 530302; andy@healthc.demon.co.uk

Archibel, Belgium - Rue Fontaine St. Pierre 1E. Zoning Industriel de la Fagne. 5330 Assesse. Tel: +32 83 66 05 00. Fax: +32 83 65 62 82. info@archibel.com. www.archibel.com

Arrowroot Standard Direct Ltd., US - 83 East Lancaster Ave., Paoli, PA, USA 19301, tel (800) 234-8879, customerservice@arrowroot.com

Auckland College of Classical Homeopathy, New Zealand - PO Box 56 655, Dominion R, Mt Eden, Auckland 1446, New Zealand.

Australasian College of Hahnemannian Homeopathy, Australia - P.O. Box 155. Daylesford Victoria, Australia. 3460. Phone/Fax: (03) 5348 3667. i_golden@netconnect.com.au.

Australian Federation of Homeopaths, Australia - 6 Mugara Street, Chermside, Australia, 4032. 61-7-3350-2960

B. Jain Publishers, India - 1921/10 Chuna Mandi Pahargani. Post Box 5775, New Delhi, India, 100-055. 91-11-2358-0800, 5169-8991.

Bastyr University, US - 4500 Juanita Dr. NE. Kenmore, WA, 98028-4966. (425) 823-1300 Fax (425) 823-6222. admiss@bastyr.edu.

Bay of Plenty College of Homeopathy, New Zealand - PO Box 784. Tauranga, New Zealand, 3001. 64-7-578-1331. bopcoh@wave.co.nz. www.homeopathycollege.com.

Bengal Allen Medical Institute, India - 'Similimum', 46 Creek Row, Calcutta - 700 01. tel (91-33)246 8438 / 9255. fax (91-33)246 5178. hahnemann@vsnl.com

Boericke & Tafel, US - A division of Nature's Way Products Inc. 1375 N Mountain Springs Pky. Springville, UT, USA 84663. (800)962-8873. (801)489-1700 (fax). www.naturesway.com.

Boericke and Tafel, US - 2381 Circadian Way, Santa Rosa, CA, USA 95407, tel (707) 571-8202, fax (707) 571-8237

Boiron-Bornemann, US - 6 Campus Blvd. Newtown Square, PA, USA 19073. (800)BLU-TUBE (258-8823) orders. (610)325-7480 (fax). info@boironusa.com. www.boiron.com.

Brighter Day Nautral Foods, US - 1102 Bull St. Savannah, GA 31401. (912) 236-4703. (912) 236-9026 (fax). www.brighterdayfoods.com.

British Homeopathic Association, UK - 15 Clerkenwell Close, London EC1R 0AA. tel 020 7566 7800. fax 020 7566 7815. info@trusthomeopathy.org

British Homeopathic Dental Association, UK - 2B Franklin Road, Watford, Herts WD1 1QD. tel 01923 233 336.

British Homeopathic Library, UK - Glasgow Homeopathic Hospital, 1053 Great Western Road, Glasgow, UK G12 0XQ. tel: 0141 211 1617. Fax:0141 211 1610. Email: hom-inform@dial.pipex.com

British Institute of Homeopathy, UK - Cygnet House, Market Square, Staines TW18 4RH, tel 01784 44067 or 01784 466251, fax 01784 449887. britinsthom@compuserve.com

British School of Homeopathy, UK - Juniper House, Bath Road, Leonard Stanley, Glos. GL10 3LU. bshadmin@btconnect.com.

Caduceus Institute of Classical Homeopathy, US - 3070 Prather Lane. Santa Cruz, CA, USA 95065. (800)396-9778. (831)726-3192 (fax). willa@homeopathyhome.net. www.homeopathytraining.org.

California Homeopathic Medical Society, US. - 169 E El Roblar Dr. Ojai, CA, USA 93023. (805)646-1495. (805)646-8159 (fax). rhiltner@sbcglobal.net. www.homeopathywest.org.

Canadian Academy of Homeopathy, Canada - 1173 Blvd du Mont Royal. Montreal, PQ, Canada H2V 2H6. (514)279-6629. (514)279-0111 (fax). cah@videotron.ca. www.homeopathy.ca.

Canadian College of Naturopathic Medicine, Canada - 1255 Sheppard Avenue East. Toronto, Ontario, M2K 1E2. 416-498-1255. Fax: 416-498-1576. info@ccnm.edu.

Castle Remedies, US - 2345 South Huron Parkway, Ann Arbor, MI USA 48104. 734-973-8990

Centre for Homeopathy Education, UK - Regents College, Inner Circle, Regents Park, London NW1. Administrator, - 1st Floor, 243 Upper Street, Islington, London N1 1RU, tel. 020 7359 7424; homeopathy@london.com. www.homeopathycollege.org.

Central Council for Research in Homeopathy, India - 61- 65, Institutional Area, D Block, Janakpuri, New Delhi, 110058

Chiropractic Academy of Homeopathy, US - 6536 Stadium Drive. Zephyrhills, Florida, USA 33540. tel (813) 782-2690. fax (813) 782-3275. DANdc1@aol.com.

College of Classical Homeopathy, UK - Othergates Clinic, 45 Barrington Street. Tiverton, Devon, EX16 6QP.

College of Practical Homeopathy (London) UK - 760 High Road, North Finchley. London N12 9QH. (44) 0 20 8445 6123. admin@collegeofpracticalhomeopathy.com. www.college-of-practical-homeopathy.com.

College of Practical Homeopathy (Midlands), UK - 186 Wolverhampton Street, Dudley, West Midlands, DY1 3AD, tel 01384-233664; admin@Homeopathytraining.co.uk

Combined Colleges of Homœopathy, UK - Hahnemann House. 32 Welbeck Street, London W1G 8EU, tel 0207 487 4322, fax 0207 487 4299; admissions@homoeopathic-education.com

Contemporary College of Homeopathy Ltd., UK - 71 Hartland Road. Queens Park, London NW6 6BH. 0845 6032878. info@conhom.com.

Dave's Health and Nutrition, US - 1108 E. 3300 South, Salt Lake City, UT, USA 84106. 801-483-9024

Desert Institute School of Classical Homeopathy, US - 2001 W Camelback Rd #150. Phoenix, AZ, USA 85015. (602)347-7950. (602)864-2949 (fax). disch@igc.org. www.weteachhomeopathy.com.

Dolisos America, US - 3014 Rigel Avenue, Las Vegas, NV, USA 89102, tel 1-800-DOLISOS, ie. (800) 365-4767

Dr. Nielsen's Homoeopathic Medical Education and Research Centre, Canada - 185 Henderson Highway. Winnipeg, Canada, MB R2P 0N8. (204) 982 0780 - Clinic & Institution. (204) 982 0787 - Fax. drnielsen@shaw.ca.

Dynamis School for Advanced Homoeopathic Studies, UK - P.O. Box 652, Worcester, WR5 3WN. Telephone +44 (0) 1905 828272 Fax +44 (0) 1905 828264. dynamis@dynamis.edu. www.dynamis.edu.

Edinburgh College of Classical Homeopathy, UK - 39A York Place, Edinburgh, EH1 3HP, tel 031 558 3118

Elixirs.com, US - 422 N Earl Rd. Moses Lake, WA, USA 98837. (800)390-9970 orders/questions. (206)350-1556 (fax). consult@elixirs.com. www.elixirs.com.

Emryss Publishers, The Netherlands - Duinoordstraat 78, 2023 WE Haarlem, The Netherlands. 31 (0)23 527 50 60

Farrington Homeopathy School, US - 20 Cedar Blvd. Suite 303. Pittsburgh, PA, 15228. 800 430-9328. Director: Edward C. Kondrot, MD, CCH. www.farringtonschool.com.

Five Elements School of Classical Homeopathy, US - PO Box 537. Boonton NJ, 07005. 973 402-8510. remedy@gti.net.

Florida Academy of Classical Homeopathy, US - 320 W Minnesota Ave. Deland, FL, USA 32720-3350. (386)736-8685. (386)736-8685 (fax). info@floridahomeopathy.org. www.floridahomeopathy.org.

Homeopathic-Herbal Directory

Florida Homeopathic Medical Society, US - 1539 Hunters Stand Run. Oviedo, FL, 32765. (407)766-3710. wrcolwell@earthlink.net.

Foundation for Homeopathic Education, US - 356 Middle St. Amherst, MA, USA 01002. (413)256-5949. (413)256-6223 (fax). fhe@nesh.com. www.nesh.com.

Freemans Homoeopathic Pharmacy, UK - 20 Main Street, Busby, Glasgow G76 8DU, tel +44 (0)141-644-1165, fax +44 (0)141-644-5735, info@freechem.co.uk

Frontline Homeopathy, UK - Frontline, Bush Master House, 204 Uxbridge Road, London, W12 7JD. tel/fax +44 208 749 0093. frontlinehom@btinternet.com

Frontier Cooperative Herbs, US - 800-669-3275; 3021 78th St.; PO Box 299; Norway IA 52318 USA. A well-stocked and high-quality wholesale source for herbs; mostly Western herbs, but some Chinese herbs are available, as well as miscellaneous health products including essential oils, incense, vegetable oils, and homeopathic preparations.

Galen Homoeopathic Pharmacy, UK - Lewell Mill, West Stafford, Dorchester, Dorset DT2 8AN, tel 01305 263996.

Galway College of Homeopathy, UK - Clare Sheehan. Ballinderreen, Kilcolgan. Co Galway, Ireland. 00353 91 776886. admin@galwayhomeopathy.com.

Hahnemann Academy of North America, US - 1315 S. Main St. #148, Blacksburg, VA USA 24060. www.lotushealthinstitute.com

Hahnemann College for Homeopathy and Heilkunst, Canada - 2411 River Road. Manotick ON, K4M 1B4. Phone: 613 830-2556. Fax: 613 830-2056. in Canada: 1-800-579-HEAL. registrar@homeopathy.com.

Hahnemann College of Homeopathy, US - 80 Nicholl Avenue. Pt. Richmond CA, USA 94801. 510-232-2079 Fax 510-412-9044. hahnemann@igc.apc.org.

Hahnemann Laboratories, US - 1940 4th St. San Rafael, CA, USA 94901. (888)427-6422 toll free. (415)451-6981 (fax). info@hahnemannlabs.com. www.hahnemannlabs.com.

HealthCo Northwest, US - 170 W. Ellendale, Dallas, OR, USA 97338, tel 503-831-0871, Toll Free: 888-715-6398, fax 503-831-0873

Heel Inc., US - 11600 Cochiti S.E., Albuquerque, NM, USA 87123, tel 1-800-621-7644, fax 505-275-1672

Helios Homoeopathic Pharmacy, UK - 97 Camden Road, Tunbridge Wells, Kent TN1 2QR, UK. Telephone (01892) 536393 (24hr) / (01892) 537254 (9:45am-5:30pm) Fax (01892) 546850. pharmacy@helios.co.uk, www.helios.co.uk.

Herb Research Foundation, US - 4140 15th St. Boulder, CO 80304. (303) 449-2265 (Office). (303) 449-7849 (FAX).

Herbalist and Alchemist, US - 51 S. Wandling Ave. Washington, NJ 07882. 800-611-8235. 908-689-9071 fax. herbalist@nac.net. www.herbalist-alchemist.com.

Hogan Pharmacy, Canada - Bayside Mall, 150 Christina St. Sarnia, Ontario, N7T7W5. Bus:1-800-799-8198. Bus:1-519-344-6111

Hickey Chemist, US - 888 2nd Ave., New York, NY, USA 10017, tel 212-223-6333

Homeopathic Academy of Southern California, US - 2236 Rutherford Rd Ste 115. Carlsbad, CA, USA 92008. (877)800-4197. info@homeopathic-academy.com. www.homeopathic-academy.com.

Homeopathic College of Canada - 280 Eglinton Ave E. Toronto, Ontario, M4P 1L4. (416) 481-8816 Fax:(416) 481-4444. 888-374-6636. info@homeopathy.edu.

Homeopathic College of East Anglia, UK - Complementary Health Care Centre, 34 Exchange Street, Norwich, Norfolk NR2 1AX, tel 01603 665173, fax 01603 455656; enquiries@homeopathic-college.com

Homeopathic Educational Services, US - 2124 Kittredge St #N. Berkeley, CA, USA 94704. (800)359-9051 orders only. (510)649-1955 (fax). mail@homeopathic.com. www.homeopathic.com.

Homeopathic Education Society, India - Irla, R.G. Gadkari Road, Irla Naka, Vile Parle (west), Mumbai 400056. tel 91-22-6201135, fax 91-22-6243841. helpline@homeopathyinstitute.com

Homeopathy India Foundation, India - 203-A, Trimurty Arcade, LBS Road, Next to Sarvodaya Hosp., Ghatkopar(w), Mumbai 400086. tel 91-22-5119080, fax 91-22-3434818. hif@classicalhomoeopathy.com

Homeopathic Medical Association, UK - 7 Darnley Road, Gravesend, Kent, UK, DA11 0RU. Email: info@the-hma.org. Tel: 01474 560336

Homeopathic Medical Society of the State of New York, US - 6250 Route 9. Rhinebeck, NY, USA 12572. (845)876-6323. (845)876-2627 (fax). homeopathicmd@earthlink.net. www.hmssny.org.

Homeopathic Nurses Association, US - 8403 Tahona Dr. Silver Spring, MD, USA 20903. (866)240-0495. hnanurses@lycos.com. www.nursehomeopaths.org.

Homeopathic Pharmacopœia Convention of the United States, US - PO Box 2221. Southeastern, PA, USA 19399-2221. (610)783-0987. (610)783-5180 (fax). hpus@aol.com. www.hpcus.com.

Homeopathic Publishing Ltd., Japan - Homeopathy Japan Tokyo HQ bldg. 3-49-13 Nishihara. Shibuya-ku, Tokyo, Japan 151-0066. (03) 5790 8705

Homeopathic Resources & Services, US - Library Homœopathia (Historical Research). PO Box 131. Old Chatham, NY, USA 12136. (518)794-8653. wkirtsos@taconic.net.

Homeopathic-Herbal Directory

Homeopathic Symposium, US - 7904 SE Main St. Portland, OR, USA 97215. (800)600-1024. info@homeopathicsymposium.com. www.homeopathicsymposium.com.

Homeopathy College, UK - 454 Hagley Road West. Quinton, Birmingham, B68 0DL. 0121 423 1913. admin@Homeopathytraining.co.uk.

Homeopathy Japan, Japan - HQ bldg. 3-49-13 Nishihara. Shibuya-ku, Tokyo, Japan 151-0066. (03) 5790 8705

Homeopathy Overnight, US - 929 Shelburne Ave. Absecon, NJ, USA 08201. (800)276-4223. (609)646-0347 (fax). remedy@homeopathyovernight.com. www.homeopathyovernight.com.

Homeopathy School of Colorado, US - P.O. Box 20340. Boulder, Colorado, USA 80308-3340. Tel 303.440.3717. Fax: 303.440.6525. info@homeopathyschool.org.

Homeopathy Works, US - 124 Fairfax St., Berkeley Springs, WV, USA 25411, tel 304-258-2541

Homeopathywest, US - 1442A Walnut St #138. Berkeley, CA, USA 94709. (877)850-5078. (877)850-5078 (fax). seminars@homeopathywest.com. www.homeopathywest.com.

Homeopathic Supply Co, UK - The Street, Bodham, Holt, Norfolk NR25. 6AD, tel 01263 588788, fax 01263 588875. orders@homeopathicsupply.com.

Hompath, Computer Software, India - P. N. Exports [Hompath], 8, New Hari Niwas, Dattatray Road, Santacruz (W), Mumbai - 400 054, India. Tele: 022 - 2661 4532 / 2661 6561. Fax : 022 - 2605 2505. hompath@vsnl.com. www.hompath.com.

Illinois Homeopathic Medical Association, US - 400 E 22nd St Ste F. Lombard, IL, USA 60148. (630)792-9311. (630)792-9316 (fax). www.homeopathyillinois.org.

Indian Books & Periodicals Syndicate, India - B-5/62, Dev Nagar, P.L.Road, Karol Bagh, New Delhi-110005. tel 0091-11-5725444. fax 2576 66 99. ibps@del3.vsnl.net.in.

Institute of Classical Homœopathy, US - 2325 Third St Ste 426. San Francisco, CA, USA 94107. (415)551-1020. (415)551-1021 (fax). ich@classicalHomeopathy.org. www.classicalHomeopathy.org.

Institute of Natural Health Sciences, US - 20270 Middlebelt Rd Ste 4. Livonia, MI, USA 48152. (248)473-8522. (248)473-8141 (fax). instituteofmich@aol.com. www.naturalhealthsciences.org.

Integrative College, UK - 24 Primrose Street. Lancaster, LA1 3BN. tel: 01524 67009. mail@theintegrativecollege.co.uk.

International Academy of Classical Homeopathy, Greece - vithoulkas@n-skiathos.gr. www.vithoulkas.com.

Irish College of Homoeopathic Medicine, Ireland - Training courses, Homeopathy and Alternative Therapies. Ray Nolan. info@ichm.ie.

Irish School of Homeopathy, Ireland - Contact Administrator Angie Murphy. Irish School of Homeopathy. 47 Ratoath Estate. Cabra, Dublin 7. Phone/Fax 00-353-1-8682581. info@Homeopathy.ie.

Kent Homeopathic Associates, US - 710 mission Avenue, San Rafael, CA, 94901, 415-457-0678

King Bio Homeopathics, US - 3 Westside Dr. Asheville, NC, USA 28806. (828)255-0201. (828)255-0940 (fax). jake@kingbio.com. www.kingbio.com.

Lakeland College, UK - Postal Building, Ash Street. Bowness on Windermere. Cumbria, LA23 3EB, England. Tel +44 (0)15394 47666. Fax +44 (0)15394 47676. mail@thelakelandcollege.co.uk.

Leicester Pharmacy, US - 1060 Main St., Leicester, MA, USA 01524, tel:(508) 892-8166, fax:(508) 892-1896

London College of Classical Homeopathy, UK - Hahnemann House, 32 Welbeck Street. London W1M 7PG. 0171 487 4322 Fax 0171 487 4299. lcch@msn.com.

London International College of Homeopathy, UK - Bush Master House. 204 Uxbridge Road, London W12 7JD. tel/fax +44 181 749 0093. lich@btinternet.com.

London School of Classical Homeopathy, UK - 159 Ladysmith Road , Enfield , London UK EN1 3AH. Telephone/Fax:+44(0)2083608757. info@homeopathy-lsch.co.uk.

Longevity Pure Medicines, US. 9595 Wilshire Blvd.#706, Beverly Hills, CA, USA 90212

Los Angeles School of Homeopathy, US - 13323 W Washington Blvd Ste 202. Los Angeles, CA, USA 90066. (310)772-8235. avghi@homeopathycourses.com. www.lahomeopathicschool.com.

Lotus Health Institute - 125 N. Main St. #500-350, Blacksburg, VA USA 24060. www.lotushealthinstitute.com

Luminos Homeopathic Courses Ltd, US - F-31. Bowen Island, B.C., Canada V0N 1G0. (604)947-0757. (604)947-0764 (fax). info@homeopathycourses.com. www.homeopathycourses.com.

Luyties Pharmacal Co., US - 4200 Laclede St., St. Louis, MO, USA 63108, tel 1-800-HOMEOPATHY, 1-800-466-3672, fax 314-535-9600, info@1800homeopathy.com

Manitoba College of Homeopathic Medicine, US - 601 Corydon Ave. Winnipeg, Canada MB R3L 0P3. Tel: 204 475-5461. Clinic: 204 475-7127.

Mediral International, US - 10550 E 54th Ave Unit E. Denver, CO, USA 80239-2131. (877)633-4725 toll free. (303)355-4155 (fax). homeopathy@mediral.com. www.mediral.com.

Miccant Ltd, UK - 14 Mulberry Close, West Bridgford, Nottingham, UK, NG2 7SS. Tel + 44 (0) 870 141 7053. miccant@miccant.com. www.miccant.com.

Minerva Homeopathic Books, UK - 17 Harpurs, Tadworth Park, Tadworth, Surrey, UK, KT20 5UD. Tel: 01737 370 009. minervabks@aol.com. www.minervabooks.co.uk

Minimum Price Homeopathic Books, US - P.O. Box 2187. 250 "H" St. Blaine, WA, USA 98230. (800)663-8272 orders only. (604)597-8304 (fax). orders@minimum.com. www.minimum.com.

Montreal Institute of Classical Homeopathy, Canada - 2356 Regent Avenue. Montreal, Quebec, H4A 2R1. Tel: 514 486-2716. info@m-i-c-h.com.

Narayana Verlag, Germany - Blumenplatz 2, D-79400 Kandern, Germany. 49-7626-970 145

National Center for Homeopathy, US - 801 North Fairfax Street, Suite 306. Alexandria, VA, USA 22314. (703) 548-7790. nchinfo@igc.apc.org.

National College of Naturopathic Medicine, US - 049 SW Porter St. Portland, OR, USA 97201. admissions@ncnm.edu. (503) 499-4343 Fax: (503) 499-0027.

National Vaccine Information Center, US - 421-E Church Street, Vienna, VA 22180. Phone: (703) 938-DPT3. Fax (703) 938-5768. www.909shot.com

Natural Health Supply, US - 6410 Avenida Christina, Santa Fe, NM, USA 87507, tel 505 474 9175 and 888 689 1608, fax (505) 473–0336, nhs@a2zhomeopathy.com

Natural Path, US - PO Box 70, Lewis, Colorado, USA 81327. cheyannewest@frontier.net. www.cheyannewest.com.

Nelson's Pharmacy, UK - 73 Duke Street, Mayfair, London, UK W1K 5BY. Tele: 020 7629 3118. pharmacy@nelsons.net. www.nelsonspharmacy.com.

New England Homeopathic Academy, US - 24 Minot Ave. Acton, MA, USA 01720. (978)635-0605. (978)263-6646 (fax). bwood@igc.org. www.newenglandhomeopathy.org.

New England School of Homeopathy, US - 356 Middle St. Amherst, MA, USA 01002. (413)256-5949. (413)256-6223 (fax). nesh@nesh.com. www.nesh.com.

New Mexico School of Classical Homeopathy, US - 202 Morningside SE. Albuquerque, NM, USA 87108. (505) 268-6870 ext 115.

New York Luminos School of Homeopathy, US - 158 Franklin St. #3. New York, NY, USA 10013. (212)925-4623 phone/fax. faculty@nyhomeopathy.com. www.nyhomeopathy.com.

North American Society of Homeopaths, US - PO Box 450039. Sunrise, FL, USA 33345-0039. (206)720-7000. (208)248-1942 (fax). nashinfo@aol.com. www.homeopathy.org.

North West College of Homœopathy, UK - 23 Wilbraham Road, Fallowfield, Manchester, M14 6FR, tel & fax 0161 257 2445. info@nwch.co.uk

Northern College of Homoeopathic Medicine, UK - Swinburne House, Swinburne Street. Gateshead, NE8 1AX. tel/fax 0191 4900276. n.c.h.m@tynebridge8.freeserve.co.uk.

Northwestern Academy of Homeopathy, US - 5201 Eden Ave Ste 245. Minneapolis, MN, USA 55436. (612)794-6445. info@homeopathicschool.org. www.homeopathicschool.org.

Ontario College of Homeopathic Medicine, US - 332 Dupont Street. Toronto, Ontario, Canada M5R 1V9. 416 535-5995. fax: 416 535-2964. info@ochm.ca.

Optimum Health Centre, Hong Kong - Alexander Yuan, ND. 2/F, Prosperous Commercial Building. 54 - 58 Jardine's **Bazaar, Causeway Bay**, Hong Kong . Tel : 2577-3798.

Pacific Academy of Homeopathy, US - 1199 Sanchez St. San Francisco, CA, USA 94114. (415)695-2710. (415)695-8220 (fax). health@homeopathy-academy.org. www.homeopathy-academy.org.

Purton House School of Homeopathy, UK - Penley Grange, Marlow Road, Stokenchurch, Bucks HP14 3UW, tel 01494 485 952, fax 01494 484 668. info@purtonhouse.com

Remedy Professional Software, UK - 5 Foxhill Road, Burton Joyce, Nottingham, UK NG14 5DB United Kingdom. Tel: 0044 115 9 31 42 64.

Renaissance Institute of Classical Homeopathy, US - 5A Lancaster St. Cambridge, MA, USA 02140. drluc@cybermesa.com.

Resonance School of Homeopathy, US - 3621 Big Bend. Reno, NV, USA 89509. (775)827-0222. (775)827-0222 (fax). robertfieldhomeopath@hotmail.com. www.resonanceschoolofhomeopathy.com.

Royal Academy of Homeopathy, Japan - Homeopathy Japan Co. Tokyo headquarters blgd., 3-49-13 Nishihara, Shibuya-Ku, Tokyo 151 0066, Japan. Tel: (03)5790 8705. Fax: (03)5790 8706. office@Homeopathy.co.jp. www.rah.Homeopathy.co.jp.

Samurai International Ltd, UK - 5 Foxhill Road, Burton Joyce, Nottingham, UK NG14 5DB United Kingdom. Tel: 0044 115 9 31 42 64.

San Diego Center for Homeopathic Education and Training, US - 1268 Birch Avenue, Escondido, CA, 92027, (760)741-7875. (E-Mail: mannkind@adnc.com)

Santa Monica Homeopathic Pharmacy, US - 629 Broadway (at 7th Street), Santa Monica, CA, USA 90401, tel (310) 395-1131, fax (310) 395-7861

Homeopathic-Herbal Directory

School of Homeopathy, UK - Yondercott House, Uffculme, Devon EX15 3DR, tel UK only 0800 0439 349, +44 (0)845 257 8887, fax +44 (0)845 257 8885. info@homeopathyschool.com

Scottish College of Homeopathy, UK - 17 Edinburgh Road, Biggar S., Lanarkshire ML12 6AX, tel 01899 2220931

Sheffield School of Homeopathy, UK - 46 Long Meadow Road, Alfreton, Derbyshire DE5 7PD, tel 01773 831291; ian@sheffhom.demon.uk

Similasan Corporation, US - 1745 Shea Center Dr Ste 380. Highlands Ranch, CO, USA 80129. (800)426-1644. (303)539-4061 (fax). getinfo@healthyrelief.com. www.healthyrelief.com.

Society of Homeopaths, UK - 11 Brookfield, Duncan Close, Moulton Park, Northampton NN3 6WL. Tel 0845 450 6611 Fax 0845 450 6622.

Soluna School of Homeopathy, UK - College Business Centre. Uttoxeter New Road Derby, UK DE22 3WZ. 01332 383355. adam@solunahomeopathy.co.uk.

South Downs School of Homeopathy, UK - 35 Victoria Road, Shoreham-by-Sea, Sussex BN43 5LA, tel/fax: 01273 454310; littlemiracle@freeuk.com

South East College of Homeopathy, UK - 41 Terminus Road, Eastbourne, East Sussex BN21 3QL, tel (01323) 430025, fax (01323) 648452; sjosling@aol.com

Southwest College of Botanical Medicine, US - P.O. Box 4565, Bisbee, Arizona 85603

Southwest College of Naturopathic Medicine, US - 2140 E Broadway Rd. Tempe, AZ, USA 85282. (480)858-9100. (480)858-9116 (fax). admissions@scnm.edu. www.scnm.edu.

Standard Homeopathic Company, US - 210 W 131st St. PO Box 61067. Los Angeles, CA, USA 90061. (800)624-9659. (310)516-8579 (fax). shcinfo@hylands.com. www.hylands.com.

Teleosis Institute, US - 1521 5th St Ste B. Berkeley, CA, USA 94710. (510)558-7285. (510)527-1682 (fax). info@teleosis.org. www.teleosis.org.

Teleosis School of Homeopathy, US - 5A Lancaster St. Cambridge, MA, 02140. (617)547-8500. (617)812-0282 (fax). teleosis@verizon.net. www.teleosisschool.org.

Texas Institute for Homeopathy, US - 1406 Brookstone. San Antonio, TX, USA 78248-1425. (210)492-3162. (210)492-9152 (fax). texashomeopathy@aol.com. www.texashomeopathy.com.

Texas Society of Homeopathy, US - 4200 Westheimer Ste 100. Houston, TX, USA 77027. (713)621-3184. (713)877-8035 (fax). info@txsoho.com. www.txsoho.com.

Toronto School of Homeopathic Medicine, US - Director: Raymond Edge, RSHom(NA), CCH. 1881 Yonge Street, Suite 500. Toronto, Ontario, Canada M4S 3C4. 416 966-2350. 800 572-6001. fax: 416 966-1724. info@homeopathycanada.com.

University of Bridgeport: College of Naturopathic Medicine, US - 60 Lafayette Street. Bridgeport, CT, USA 06601. 203 576-4109. natmed@bridgeport.edu.

Van Hoy Publishing, US - PO Box 636, Greenville, PA 16125. E-mail: jay@yasgur.net. www.yasgur.net.

Vancouver Homeopathic Academy, US - PO Box 34095, Station D. Vancouver, BC, Canada, V6J 4M1. Phone: 604-708-9387. Fax: 604-708-1547. Email: info@HomeopathyVancouver.com.

Victorian College of Classical Homeopathy, Australia - 3A/574 Whitehorse Rd. Mitcham, Victoria.,3132. Phone: (03) 9873 0567. Fax - (03) 9787 5145. admin@vcch.org.

Washington Homeopathic Products, US - 33 Fairfax St. Berkeley Springs, WV, USA 25411. (800)336-1695 orders only. (877)286-0601 (fax). joelillard@homeopathyworks.com. www.homeopathyworks.com.

Weise Pharmacy, Homeopathic and Natural Medicines, US - 4343 Colonial Ave. Jacksonville, FL, USA 32210. (800)554-6670. (904)384-0569 (fax). gillthepill@aol.com. www.naturallyweise.com.

Weleda, Ltd, US - PO Box 675. Palisades, NY, USA 10964. (800)241-1030. (800)280-4899 (fax). rx@weleda.com. www.usa.weleda.com.

Welsh School of Homeopathy, UK - 27 Holtsfield, Murton. Swansea, SA3 3AQ. 01792 234059. demurph54@tiscali.co.uk. tele: 01792 234059.

Whole Health Now, Books, US - 1685 H St #311. Blaine, WA, USA 98230. (866) 599-5950. (604)599-5911 (fax). books@whnow.com. www.wholehealthnow.com/books.

Yorkshire School of Homeopathy (Leeds), UK - Lansdown, 24 Rosebank, Burley-in-Wharfedale, Ilkley, West Yorkshire, LS29 7PQ, tel/fax 01943 862549; yorkshireHomeopathy@btopenworld.com

Homeopathic Medical Repertory

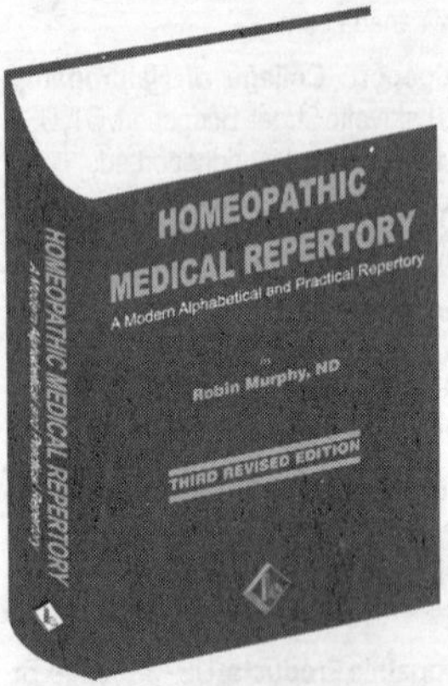

New Third Edition! Now Available!
*2,432 pages

*** Alphabetical Chapters and Rubrics**

*** New Remedies from Modern Provings**

*** 20,000 New Clinical Rubrics**

*** 100,000 New Additions and Updates**

*** Contains 74 chapters**

ISBN : 978-81-319-0858-7 | Price : Rs. 999.00 | Page : 2432pp | HB

* The Homeopathic Medical Repertory was designed to be a modern, practical and easy to use reference guide to the homeopathic materia medica. This alphabetical repertory contains thousands of new clinical rubrics, especially in the areas of mental disorders, emergencies, infections, pathologies and organs. Also, consistent alphabetical formatting, (chapters, rubrics and sub-rubrics) with updated medical terminology and modern disorders. The Homeopathic Medical Repertory includes all of the original Kent's Repertory and additions from Allen, Hering, Boericke, Knerr, Kunzli, Phatak Repertories etc., plus thousands of clinical updates from Dr Murphy's years of homeopathic and herbal research.

* **New Remedies and Updates - New Remedies added from modern provings.** Also additions from Allen, Boericke, Boenninghausen, Burnett, Clarke, Grimmer, Hahnemann, Hering, Julian, Kent, Knerr, Kunzli, Nash, Phatak and many more.

* **New Chapters** - Homeopathic Medical Repertory-3rd edition chapters: Abdomen, Ankles, Arms, Back, Bladder, Bones, Brain, Breasts, Breathing, **Cancer,** Chest, Children, Chills, **Clinical**, Constitutions, Coughing, Dreams, Ears, Elbows, Eyes, Face, **Fainting**, Feet, Female, Fevers, Food, **Gallbladder**, Generals, Glands, Hands, Head, Headaches, Hearing, Heart, Hips, Intestines, Joints, Kidneys, Knees, Larynx, Legs, Limbs, Liver, Lungs, Male, Mind, Mouth, Muscles, Neck, Nose, Pelvis, Perspiration, Pregnancy, Pulse, Rectum, Shoulders, Skin, Sleep, **Speech, Spleen,** Stomach, Stool, **Taste,** Teeth, Throat, **Time,** Tongue, Toxicity, Urine, **Vaccinations,** Vertigo, Vision, **Weakness,** Wrists.

* **New Clinical Rubrics** - Addictions, A.I.D.S., Allergies, Anxiety attacks, Asphyxia, Appendicitis Auto-immune disorders, Bi-Polar, Blood poisoning, Burns, Bubonic Plague, Cancers, Chemotherapy Chronic Fatigue, Compulsive-Obessive Disorder, Chemical Poisoning, Coma, Dehydration, Diabetes Drug overdose, Ebola, Endometriosis, Food Poisoning, Gastroenteritis, Hepatitis, Herpes, Infections Infertility, Infl uenza, Malaria, Mononucleosis, Motion sickness, Multiple Sclerosis, Parkinson' disease, Radiation Sickness, Retinitis, SARS, Seasonal Affective Disorder, Sea sickness, Surgery Tetanus, Tourette's syndrome, Typhoid fever, Vaccinations, Vaginitis, etc.